Pharmacotherapy
Principles & Practice

NOTICE

Medicine is an ever-changing science. As new research and clinical experience broaden our knowledge, changes in treatment and drug therapy are required. The authors and the publisher of this work have checked with sources believed to be reliable in their efforts to provide information that is complete and generally in accord with the standards accepted at the time of publication. However, in view of the possibility of human error or changes in medical sciences, neither the authors nor the publisher nor any other party who has been involved in the preparation or publication of this work warrants that the information contained herein is in every respect accurate or complete, and they disclaim all responsibility for any errors or omissions or for the results obtained from use of the information contained in this work. Readers are encouraged to confirm the information contained herein with other sources. For example, and in particular, readers are advised to check the product information sheet included in the package of each drug they plan to administer to be certain that the information contained in this work is accurate and that changes have not been made in the recommended dose or in the contraindications for administration. This recommendation is of particular importance in connection with new or infrequently used drugs.

Pharmacotherapy Principles & Practice

SECOND EDITION

Editors

Marie A. Chisholm-Burns, PharmD, MPH, FCCP, FASHP

Professor and Head
Department of Pharmacy Practice and Science
The University of Arizona College of Pharmacy
Tucson, Arizona

Terry L. Schwinghammer, PharmD, FCCP, FASHP, BCPS

Professor and Chair
Department of Clinical Pharmacy
West Virginia University
School of Pharmacy
Morgantown, West Virginia

Barbara G. Wells, PharmD, FASHP, FCCP, BCPP

Professor and Dean
Executive Director, Research Institute
   of Pharmaceutical Sciences
School of Pharmacy
The University of Mississippi
Oxford, Mississippi

Patrick M. Malone, PharmD, FASHP

Professor and Associate Dean, Internal Affairs
College of Pharmacy
The University of Findlay
Findlay, Ohio

Jill M. Kolesar, PharmD, BCPS, FCCP

Professor
University of Wisconsin School of Pharmacy
Director, 3P
Analytical Instrumentation Laboratory
University of Wisconsin Paul P. Carbone Comprehensive
   Cancer Center
Madison, Wisconsin

Joseph T. DiPiro, PharmD, FCCP

Professor and Executive Dean
South Carolina College of Pharmacy
University of South Carolina, Columbia
Medical University of South Carolina
Charleston, South Carolina

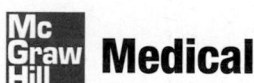

New York   Chicago   San Francisco   Lisbon   London   Madrid   Mexico City
Milan   New Delhi   San Juan   Seoul   Singapore   Sydney   Toronto

The McGraw·Hill Companies

Pharmacotherapy Principles & Practice, Second Edition

Copyright © 2010, 2008 by The McGraw-Hill Companies, Inc. All rights reserved. Printed in the United States of America. Except as permitted under the United States Copyright Act of 1976, no part of this publication may be reproduced or distributed in any form or by any means, or stored in a database or retrieval system, without the prior written permission of the publisher.

3 4 5 6 7 8 9 0   DOW/DOW   14 13 12 11

ISBN 978-0-07-162180-9
MHID 0-07-162180-6

This book was set in Minion by Newgen North America.
The editors were Michael Weitz and Peter J. Boyle.
The production supervisor was Phil Galea.
Project management was provided by Newgen North America.
The interior designer was Alan Barnett; the cover designer was Pehrsson Design.
Cover image, left to right: 1. Anatomical Travelogue/Photo Researchers, Inc. 2. Image Source.
3. Jim Dowdalls/Photo Researchers, Inc. 4. ER productions Ltd. 5. John Bavosi/Photo Researchers, Inc.
Art management was by Armen Ovsepyan.
RR Donnelley was printer and binder.

This book was printed on acid-free paper.

Library of Congress Cataloging-in-Publication Data

Pharmacotherapy principles & practice / editors, Marie A. Chisholm-Burns ... [et al.]. — 2nd ed.
   p. ; cm.
  Other title: Pharmacotherapy principles and practice
  Includes bibliographical references and index.
  ISBN 978-0-07-162180-9 (hardback : alk. paper) 1. Chemotherapy–Textbooks. I. Chisholm-Burns,
Marie A. II. Title: Pharmacotherapy principles and practice.
  [DNLM: 1. Drug Therapy. WB 330 P53592 2010]
RM262.P475   2010
615.5′8—dc22   2010004385

McGraw-Hill books are available at special quantity discounts to use as premiums and sales promotions, or for use in corporate training programs. To contact a representative please e-mail us at bulksales@mcgraw-hill.com.

CONTENTS

About the Editors ix

Contributors xi

Reviewers xxv

Preface xxxiii

PART I BASIC CONCEPTS OF PHARMACOTHERAPY PRINCIPLES AND PRACTICE

1. Introduction 3
   Jack E. Fincham

2. Geriatrics 7
   Jeannie K. Lee, Damian M. Mendoza, M. Jane Mohler, and Susan J. Morris

3. Pediatrics 23
   Hanna Phan, Vinita B. Pai, Milap C. Nahata

4. Palliative Care 35
   Marc A. Sweeney and Phyllis A. Grauer

PART II DISORDERS OF ORGAN SYSTEMS

SECTION 1 Cardiovascular Disorders 51

5. Hypertension 51
   Robert J. Straka, David Parra, and Kade T. Birkeland

6. Heart Failure 79
   Orly Vardeny and Tien M.H. Ng

7. Ischemic Heart Disease 109
   Larisa H. Cavallari and Robert J. DiDomenico

8. Acute Coronary Syndromes 131
   Sarah A. Spinler and Simon de Denus

9. Arrhythmias 157
   James E. Tisdale

10. Venous Thromboembolism 185
    Edith A. Nutescu and Stuart T. Haines

11. Stroke 215
    Susan R. Winkler

12. Dyslipidemias 229
    Matthew K. Ito

13. Hypovolemic Shock 251
    Bradley A. Boucher and G. Christopher Wood

SECTION 2 Respiratory Disorders 265

14. Asthma 265
    W. Greg Leader

15. Chronic Obstructive Pulmonary Disease 289
    Tara R. Whetsel and Nicole D. Verkleeren

16. Cystic Fibrosis 303
    Kimberly J. Novak

SECTION 3 Gastrointestinal Disorders 315

17. Gastroesophageal Reflux Disease 315
    Dianne B. Williams and Marie A. Chisholm-Burns

18. Peptic Ulcer Disease 327
    John W. Devlin

19. Inflammatory Bowel Disease 341
    Brian A. Hemstreet

20. Nausea and Vomiting 357
    Sheila Wilhelm

21. Constipation, Diarrhea, and Irritable Bowel Syndrome 371
    Beverly C. Mims and Clarence E. Curry Jr.

22. Portal Hypertension and Cirrhosis 387
    Laurajo Ryan

23. Pancreatitis 403
    Joseph J. Kishel

24. Viral Hepatitis 413
    Juliana Chan

SECTION 4 Renal Disorders 431

25. Acute Kidney Injury 431
    Mary K. Stamatakis

26. Chronic and End-Stage Kidney Disease 445
    Kristine S. Schonder

27. Fluids and Electrolytes 479
    Mark A. Malesker and Lee E. Morrow

28. Acid–Base Disturbances 495
    Lee E. Morrow and Mark A. Malesker

SECTION 5 Neurologic Disorders 507

29. Multiple Sclerosis 507
    Melody Ryan

30. Epilepsy   521
Timothy E. Welty and Edward Faught

31. Status Epilepticus   541
Gretchen M. Brophy and Eljim P. Tesoro

32. Parkinson's Disease   553
Mary L. Wagner

33. Pain Management   567
Christine K. O'Neil

34. Headache   583
Leigh Ann Ross and Brendan S. Ross

SECTION 6 Psychiatric Disorders   595

35. Alzheimer's Disease   595
Megan J. Ehret, Gary M. Levin, and
Toya M. Bowles

36. Substance-Related Disorders   607
Sally K. Guthrie and Theadia L. Carey

37. Schizophrenia   631
Deanna L. Kelly, Elaine Weiner, and
Heidi J. Wehring

38. Major Depressive Disorder   653
Cherry W. Jackson, Marshall E. Cates, and
Jacqueline M. Feldman

39. Bipolar Disorder   669
Brian L. Crabtree and Martha J. Faulkner

40. Generalized Anxiety Disorder, Panic Disorder,
and Social Anxiety Disorder   691
Sheila Botts, Anna Lockwood, and
Timothy Allen

41. Sleep Disorders   709
John M. Dopp and Bradley G. Phillips

42. Attention-Deficit Hyperactivity Disorder   723
John Erramouspe and Kevin W. Cleveland

SECTION 7 Endocrinologic Disorders   735

43. Diabetes Mellitus   735
John T. Johnson, Susan Cornell, and
William E. Wade

44. Thyroid Disorders   763
Michael D. Katz

45. Adrenal Gland Disorders   783
Devra K. Dang, Judy T. Chen, Frank Pucino Jr.,
and Karim Anton Calis

46. Pituitary Gland Disorders   801
Judy T. Chen, Devra K. Dang, Frank Pucino Jr.,
and Karim Anton Calis

SECTION 8 Gynecologic and
Obstetric Disorders   821

47. Pregnancy and Lactation: Therapeutic
Considerations   821
Ema Ferreira, Évelyne Rey, and Caroline Morin

48. Contraception   841
Julia M. Koehler and Kathleen B. Haynes

49. Menstruation-Related Disorders   855
Elena M. Umland, Lara C. Weinstein, and
Edward Buchanan

50. Hormone Therapy in Menopause   869
Nicole S. Culhane and Kelly R. Ragucci

SECTION 9 Urologic Disorders   883

51. Erectile Dysfunction   883
Cara Liday and Catherine Heyneman

52. Benign Prostatic Hyperplasia   895
Mary Lee and Roohollah Sharifi

53. Urinary Incontinence and Pediatric Enuresis   909
David R.P. Guay

SECTION 10 Immunologic Disorders   927

54. Allergic and Pseudoallergic Drug Reactions   927
J. Russell May and Philip H. Smith

55. Solid Organ Transplantation   939
Steven Gabardi and Ali J. Olyaei

SECTION 11 Bone and Joint Disorders   965

56. Osteoporosis   965
Beth Bryles Phillips

57. Rheumatoid Arthritis   981
Susan P. Bruce

58. Osteoarthritis   997
Steven M. Smith, Benjamin J. Epstein, and
John G. Gums

59. Gout and Hyperuricemia   1011
Geoffrey C. Wall

60. Musculoskeletal Disorders   1019
Jill S. Burkiewicz

SECTION 12 Disorders of the Eyes, Ears, Nose, and Throat   1031

61. Glaucoma   1031
Mikael D. Jones

62. Allergic Rhinitis   1047
David A. Apgar

63. Ophthalmic Disorders   1063
Kendra J. Grande

SECTION 13 Dermatologic Disorders   1079

64. Psoriasis   1079
Rebecca M.T. Law

65. Common Skin Disorders   1093
Angie L. Goeser

SECTION 14 Hematologic Disorders   1109

66. Anemia   1109
Edward C. Li and James M. Hoffman

67. Coagulation and Platelet Disorders   1121
Anastasia Rivkin

68. Sickle Cell Anemia   1139
Tracy M. Hagemann and Teresa V. Lewis

SECTION 15 Diseases of Infectious Origin   1155

69. Antimicrobial Regimen Selection   1155
Catherine M. Oliphant and Karl Madaras-Kelly

70. Central Nervous System Infections   1169
P. Brandon Bookstaver and April D. Miller

71. Lower Respiratory Tract Infections   1189
Diane M. Cappelletty

72. Upper Respiratory Tract Infections   1203
Heather VandenBussche

73. Skin and Soft Tissue Infections   1221
Christie Nelson, Jaime R. Hornecker, and Randy Wesnitzer

74. Infective Endocarditis   1235
Ronda L. Akins

75. Tuberculosis   1253
Charles A. Peloquin and Rocsanna Namdar

76. Gastrointestinal Infections   1267
Elizabeth D. Hermsen and Ziba Jalali

77. Intra-Abdominal Infections   1281
Joseph T. DiPiro and Thomas R. Howdieshell

78. Parasitic Diseases   1293
J.V. Anandan

79. Urinary Tract Infections   1307
Kathryn R. Matthias and Brian A. Potoski

80. Sexually Transmitted Infections   1317
Marlon S. Honeywell and Michael D. Thompson

81. Osteomyelitis   1337
Melinda M. Neuhauser and Susan L. Pendland

82. Sepsis and Septic Shock   1347
S. Scott Sutton

83. Superficial Fungal Infections   1361
Lauren S. Schlesselman

84. Invasive Fungal Infections   1375
Russell E. Lewis and P. David Rogers

85. Antimicrobial Prophylaxis in Surgery   1395
Mary A. Ullman, Jeremy A. Schafer, and John C. Rotschafer

86. Vaccines and Toxoids   1405
Marianne Billeter

87. Human Immunodeficiency Virus Infection   1419
Amanda Corbett, Rosa Yeh, Julie Dumond, and Angela D.M. Kashuba

SECTION 16 Oncologic Disorders   1445

88. Cancer Chemotherapy and Treatment   1445
Dianne Brundage

89. Breast Cancer   1475
Gerald Higa

90. Lung Cancer   1499
Val Adams and Justin Balko

91. Colorectal Cancer   1517
Patrick J. Medina

92. Prostate Cancer   1535
Trevor McKibbin and Jill M. Kolesar

93. Malignant Lymphomas   1551
Christopher Fausel and Patrick J. Kiel

94. Ovarian Cancer   1565
Judith A. Smith

95. Acute Leukemia   1579
Nancy Heideman

96. Chronic Leukemias and Multiple Myeloma   1597
Amy M. Pick

97. Skin Cancer   1611
Trinh Pham and Jennifer Nam Choi

98. Hematopoietic Stem Cell Transplantation   1629
Amber P. Lawson

99. Supportive Care in Oncology   1649
Sarah L. Scarpace

SECTION 17 Nutrition and Nutritional
Disorders   1681

100. Parenteral Nutrition   1681
Michael D. Kraft and Imad F. Btaiche

101. Enteral Nutrition   1701
Sarah J. Miller

102. Overweight and Obesity   1719
Maqual R. Graham and Cameron C. Lindsey

Appendix A: Conversion Factors and Anthropometrics   1731

Appendix B: Common Laboratory Tests   1735

Appendix C: Common Medical Abbreviations   1743

Appendix D: Glossary   1751

Index   1777

Marie A. Chisholm-Burns, BPharm, PharmD, MPH, FCCP, FASHP, is professor and head of the Department of Pharmacy Practice and Science at The University of Arizona College of Pharmacy. She received her BS and PharmD degrees from The University of Georgia and completed a residency at Mercer University Southern School of Pharmacy and at Piedmont Hospital in Atlanta, Georgia. She is the founder and executive director of the Medication Access Program. She has also served in elected positions in numerous professional organizations. She has authored more than 200 publications and has received more than $6.3 million in external funding as principal investigator. She has also received numerous awards and honors including the Robert K. Chalmers Distinguished Pharmacy Educator Award from the American Association of Colleges of Pharmacy, the Clinical Pharmacy Education Award from the American College of Clinical Pharmacy, the Daniel B. Smith Practice Excellence Award from the American Pharmacists Association, and the Rufus A. Lyman Award for most outstanding publication in the American Journal of Pharmaceutical Education (in 1996 and 2007). She lives in Tucson, is married, and has one child, John Fitzgerald Burns, Jr. She enjoys writing, playing chess, and cycling.

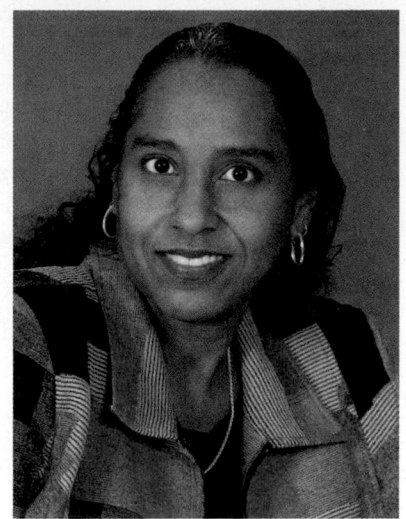

Terry L. Schwinghammer, BPharm, PharmD, BCPS, FCCP, FASHP, is professor and chair of the Department of Clinical Pharmacy at the West Virginia University School of Pharmacy. He received his BS and PharmD degrees from Purdue University and completed a pharmacy residency at Indiana University Hospitals. He has practiced in adult inpatient and ambulatory care settings. He is a past recipient of the APhA-APPM Distinguished Achievement Award in Clinical/Pharmacotherapeutic Practice and is a Distinguished Practitioner in the National Academies of Practice. His teaching focuses on pharmacotherapy of rheumatic diseases and physical assessment. In addition to authoring more than 60 publications, he is co-editor of the *Pharmacotherapy Casebook* and *Pharmacotherapy Handbook* and is editor-in-chief of AccessPharmacy (www.AccessPharmacy.com). He has been elected to membership in the Rho Chi Pharmaceutical Honor Society and the Phi Lambda Sigma Pharmacy Leadership Society. He was named a Distinguished Alumnus of Purdue University in 2004. His hobby is collecting apothecary antiques, and he enjoys boating and water skiing with his family.

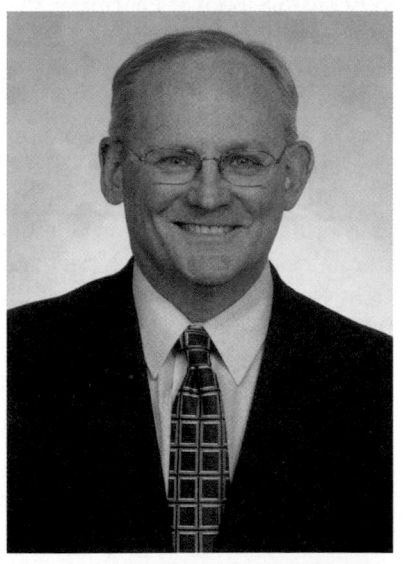

Barbara G. Wells, BPharm, PharmD, BCPP, FCCP, FASHP, is dean and professor at the University of Mississippi School of Pharmacy and Executive Director of the Research Institute of Pharmaceutical Sciences. She completed a residency in psychiatric pharmacy practice at the University of Tennessee. She is a past president and chair of the board of the American Association of Colleges of Pharmacy (AACP) and the American College of Clinical Pharmacy (ACCP). She is a past member of the NIH Advisory Committee on Research on Women's Health and of the FDA Psychopharmacologic Drugs Advisory Committee. Her primary instructional interests are in psychiatric therapeutics, and she has received six teaching awards, including the Robert K. Chalmers Distinguished Pharmacy Educator Award from AACP. Other books that she co-edits are *Pharmacotherapy: A Pathophysiologic Approach* and the *Pharmacotherapy Handbook*. She enjoys a leisurely or working weekend on her houseboat named Euphoria on Pickwick Lake.

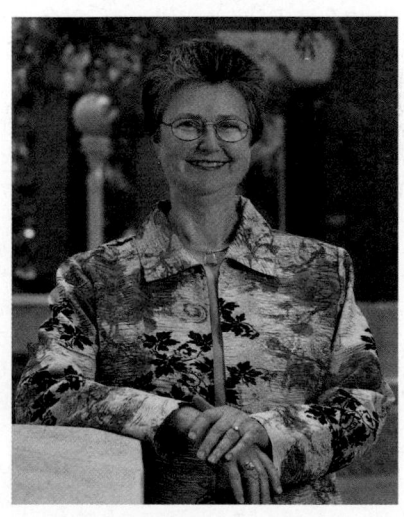

Patrick M. Malone, BPharm, PharmD, FASHP, is professor and associate dean of Internal Affairs at The University of Findlay College of Pharmacy. He received his BS in Pharmacy from Albany College of Pharmacy and PharmD from the University of Michigan. He completed a clinical pharmacy residency at the Buffalo General Hospital, Drug Information Fellowship at the University of Nebraska Medical Center, and U.S. West Fellowship in Academic Development and Technology at Creighton University. His practice and teaching have centered on drug information, and he is the first author for all three editions of *Drug Information—A Guide for Pharmacists*. He was also the drug information pharmacist at the XIII Winter Olympics. He has approximately 100 publications, numerous presentations and has held various offices in national organizations. He was the director of the Web-Based Pharmacy Pathway at Creighton University Medical Center, from its initial establishment until after graduation of the first class. His hobby is building and flying radio-controlled aircraft.

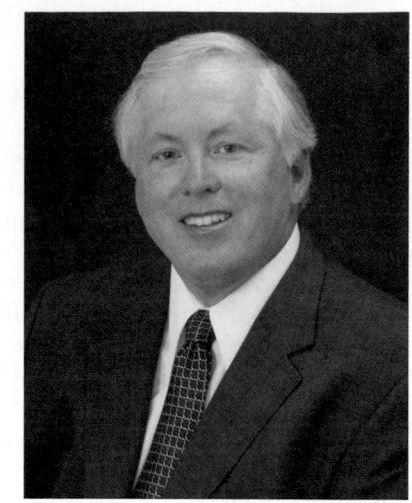

Jill M. Kolesar, BPharm, PharmD, BCPS, FCCP, is a professor at the University of Wisconsin School of Pharmacy, the Director of the 3P Laboratory at the University of Wisconsin Paul P. Carbone Comprehensive Cancer Center, and a clinical specialist in the Hematology Clinic at the William S. Middleton VA Hospital. She received a BS in Pharmacy from the University of Wisconsin and a PharmD from the University of Texas. She also completed an oncology residency and fellowship at the University of Texas Health Science Center in San Antonio. She has authored more than 100 publications and has received more than $1.2 million in external funding as a principal investigator. She holds two U.S. and international patents for novel technologies invented in her laboratory and founded Helix Diagnostics based on this technology. She is a member of the National Cancer Institute Central IRB and has received the Innovations in Teaching Award from AACP. Other books she co-edits are *Pharmacogenomics: Applications to Patient Care* and *The Pharmacogenomics Handbook*, both in their second edition. She loves to read, run, ski, and travel with her husband and five children. They plan to visit all of our National Parks.

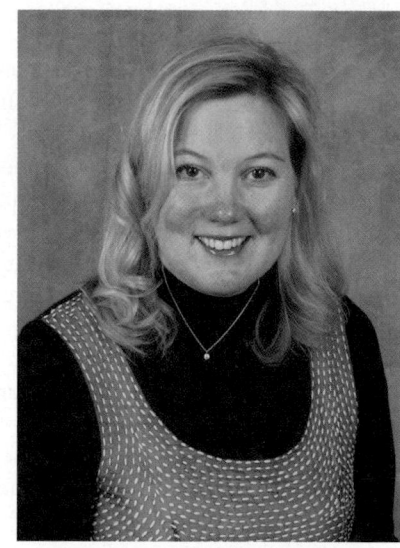

Joseph T. DiPiro, BPharm, PharmD, FCCP, is executive dean of the South Carolina College of Pharmacy, which is an integrated program of the Colleges of Pharmacy at the University of South Carolina and the Medical University of South Carolina. He received his BS in Pharmacy from the University of Connecticut and PharmD from the University of Kentucky. He served a residency at the University of Kentucky Medical Center and a fellowship in Clinical Immunology at Johns Hopkins University. He is the editor of the *American Journal of Pharmaceutical Education*. He has published more than 120 refereed papers in academic and professional journals. He is also an editor for *Pharmacotherapy: A Pathophysiologic Approach* and an author of *Concepts in Clinical Pharmacokinetics*. He was a president of the American College of Clinical Pharmacy and has served on the Research Institute Board of Trustees. In 2002, the American Association of Colleges of Pharmacy selected Dr. DiPiro for the Robert K. Chalmers Distinguished Educator Award. He has also received the Russell R. Miller Literature Award and the Education Award from the American College of Clinical Pharmacy and the Award for Sustained Contributions to the Literature from the American Society of Health-System Pharmacists. He is an avid runner and has completed 15 marathons.

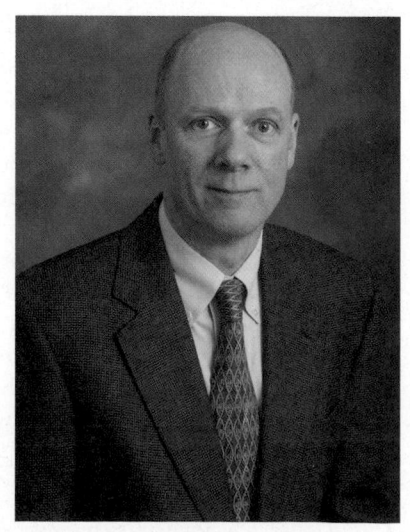

CONTRIBUTORS

Val R. Adams, PharmD, FCCP, BCOP
Associate Professor
University of Kentucky
Oncology Clinical Specialist
Markey Cancer Center
Lexington, Kentucky
Chapter 90: Lung Cancer

Ronda L. Akins, PharmD
Associate Professor
Infectious Diseases
University of Louisiana Monroe
College of Pharmacy
Monroe, Louisiana
Chapter 74: Infective Endocarditis

Timothy Allen, MD
Assistant Professor
Department of Psychiatry
College of Medicine
University of Kentucky
Director of Forensic Services
Kentucky Correctional Psychiatric Center
Lexington, Kentucky
*Chapter 40: Generalized Anxiety Disorder, Panic Disorder,
    and Social Anxiety Disorder*

J.V. Anandan, PharmD
Adjunct Associate Professor
Eugene Appelbaum College of Pharmacy and Health
    Sciences
Wayne State University
Detroit, Michigan
Chapter 78: Parasitic Diseases

David A. Apgar, PharmD
Clinical Assistant Professor
Department of Pharmacy Practice and Science
The University of Arizona College of Pharmacy
Tucson, Arizona
Chapter 62: Allergic Rhinitis

Justin Balko, PharmD, PhD
Postdoctoral Fellow
Vanderbilt-Ingram Cancer Center
Vanderbilt University
Nashville, Tennessee
Chapter 90: Lung Cancer

Marianne Billeter, PharmD, BCPS
Manager
Clinical and Ambulatory Pharmacy Services
Ochsner Clinic Foundation
New Orleans, Louisiana
Chapter 86: Vaccines and Toxoids

Kade T. Birkeland, PharmD
PGY2 Cardiology Practice Resident
Veterans Affairs Medical Center
West Palm Beach, Florida
Chapter 5: Hypertension

P. Brandon Bookstaver, PharmD, BCPS, AAHIVE
Clinical Assistant Professor
South Carolina College of Pharmacy, USC Campus
Clinical Specialist, Infectious Diseases
Palmetto Health Richland
Columbia, South Carolina
Chapter 70: Central Nervous System Infections

Sheila Botts, PharmD, BCPP
Assistant Professor
Pharmacy Practice and Science College of Pharmacy
University of Kentucky
Clinical Pharmacy Specialist
Psychiatry
Lexington Veterans Affairs Medical Center
Lexington, Kentucky
*Chapter 40: Generalized Anxiety Disorder, Panic Disorder,
    and Social Anxiety Disorder*

Bradley A. Boucher, PharmD, FCCP, FCCM, BCPS
Professor of Clinical Pharmacy
University of Tennessee Health Science Center
Critical Care Pharmacist
Regional Medical Center at Memphis
Memphis, Tennessee
Chapter 13: Hypovolemic Shock

Toya M. Bowles, PharmD, BCPP
Medical Science Liaison
Schering Plough Corporation
Bradenton, Florida
Chapter 35: Alzheimer's Disease

Gretchen M. Brophy, PharmD, BCPS, FCCP, FCCM
Associate Professor of Pharmacy and Neurosurgery
Virginia Commonwealth University
Medical College of Virginia Campus
Richmond, Virginia
Chapter 31: Status Epilepticus

Susan P. Bruce, PharmD, BCPS
Chair and Associate Professor
Department of Pharmacy Practice
Northeastern Ohio Universities College of Pharmacy
Rootstown, Ohio
Chapter 57: Rheumatoid Arthritis

Dianne Brundage, PharmD, FCCP, BCPS, BCOP
Oncology Clinical Pharmacy Specialist
Park Nicollet Health Services/Methodist Hospital
Minneapolis, Minnesota
Chapter 88: Cancer Chemotherapy and Treatment

Imad F. Btaiche, BS, PharmD, BCNSP
Clinical Associate Professor
Department of Clinical, Social and Administrative Sciences
University of Michigan College of Pharmacy
Clinical Pharmacist
Department of Pharmacy Services
University of Michigan Hospitals and Health Centers
Ann Arbor, Michigan
Chapter 100: Parenteral Nutrition

Edward Buchanan, MD
Professor
Department of Family and Community Medicine
Thomas Jefferson University Hospital
Philadelphia, Pennsylvania
Chapter 49: Menstruation-Related Disorders

Jill S. Burkiewicz, PharmD, BCPS
Professor
Pharmacy Practice
Chicago College of Pharmacy
Midwestern University
Clinical Pharmacist
Mercy Family Health Center
Downers Grove, Illinois
Chapter 60: Musculoskeletal Disorders

Karim Anton Calis, PharmD, MPH, FASHP, FCCP
Clinical Investigator
Eunice Kennedy Shriver National Institute of Child Health and Human Development and National Institute of Diabetes and Digestive and Kidney Diseases
National Institutes of Health
Bethesda, Maryland
Professor
Virginia Commonwealth University
Richmond, Virginia
Clinical Professor
University of Maryland
Baltimore, Maryland
Chapter 45: Adrenal Gland Disorders
Chapter 46: Pituitary Gland Disorders

Diane M. Cappelletty, PharmD
Associate Professor
University of Toledo College of Pharmacy
Toledo, Ohio
Chapter 71: Lower Respiratory Tract Infections

Theadia L. Carey, MD
Clinical Assistant Professor
University of Michigan Medical School
Ann Arbor, Michigan
Chapter 36: Substance-Related Disorders

Marshall E. Cates, PharmD, BCPP, FASHP
Assistant Dean for Student Affairs and Professor of Pharmacy Practice
Samford University McWhorter School of Pharmacy
Clinical Professor of Psychiatry
University of Alabama at Birmingham School of Medicine
Birmingham, Alabama
Chapter 38: Major Depressive Disorder

Larisa H. Cavallari, BS, PharmD, BCPS
Associate Professor
Department of Pharmacy Practice
University of Illinois at Chicago College of Pharmacy
Chicago, Illinois
Chapter 7: Ischemic Heart Disease

Juliana Chan, PharmD
Associate Director of Pharmacy Clinical Services
Clinical Assistant Professor
Department of Pharmacy Practice
College of Pharmacy and Department of Medicine
   Sections of Digestive Diseases & Nutrition and Section of Hepatology
University of Illinois at Chicago
Chicago, Illinois
Chapter 24: Viral Hepatitis

Judy T. Chen, PharmD, BCPS, CDE
Clinical Assistant Professor of Pharmacy Practice
Purdue University School of Pharmacy and Pharmaceutical Sciences
Indianapolis, Indiana
Chapter 45: Adrenal Gland Disorders
Chapter 46: Pituitary Gland Disorders

Marie A. Chisholm-Burns, PharmD, MPH, FCCP, FASHP
Professor and Head
Department of Pharmacy Practice and Science
The University of Arizona College of Pharmacy
Tucson, Arizona
Chapter 17: Gastroesophageal Reflux Disease

Jennifer Nam Choi, MD
Assistant Professor of Dermatology
Yale University School of Medicine
Department of Dermatology
New Haven, Connecticut
Chapter 97: Skin Cancer

Kevin W. Cleveland, PharmD
Assistant Professor
Idaho State University College of Pharmacy
Director of Idaho Drug Information Service
Pocatello, Idaho
Chapter 42: Attention-Deficit Hyperactivity Disorder

Amanda H. Corbett, PharmD, BCPS
Clinical Assistant Professor
University of North Carolina
Eshelman School of Pharmacy
Clinical Specialist
UNC Infectious Diseases Clinic
Chapel Hill, North Carolina
Chapter 87: Human Immunodeficiency Virus Infection

Susan Cornell, PharmD, CDE, FAPhA, FAADE
Assistant Director of Experimental Education
Assistant Professor of Pharmacy Practice
Pharmacy Practice
Midwestern University Chicago College of Pharmacy
Clinical Pharmacist, Certified Diabetes Educator
DuPage Community Clinic
Wheaton, Illinois
Chapter 43: Diabetes Mellitus

Brian L. Crabtree, PharmD, BCPP
Associate Professor of Pharmacy Practice
Clinical Associate Professor of Psychiatry
University of Mississippi School of Pharmacy
University of Mississippi Medical Center
Psychopharmacologist
Mississippi State Hospital
Whitfield, Mississippi
Chapter 39: Bipolar Disorder

Nicole S. Culhane, PharmD, BCPS
Director of Experiential Education and Associate Professor
    of Clinical and Administrative Sciences
College of Notre Dame of Maryland School of Pharmacy
Baltimore, Maryland
Chapter 50: Hormone Therapy in Menopause

Clarence E. Curry Jr., PharmD
Interim Associate Dean and Associate Professor
Howard University School of Pharmacy
Washington, DC
*Chapter 21: Constipation, Diarrhea, and Irritable Bowel
    Syndrome*

Devra K. Dang, PharmD, BCPS, CDE
Associate Clinical Professor
University of Connecticut School of Pharmacy
Storrs, Connecticut
Chapter 45: Adrenal Gland Disorders
Chapter 46: Pituitary Gland Disorders

Simon de Denus, BPharm, PhD, MSc
Assistant Professor
Faculty of Pharmacy
Universite de Montreal
Montreal, Quebec, Canada
Chapter 8: Acute Coronary Syndromes

John W. Devlin, PharmD, BCPS, FCCM, FCCP
Associate Professor
Department of Pharmacy Practice
Northeastern University School of Pharmacy
Adjunct Associate Professor
Tufts University School of Medicine
Boston, Massachusetts
Chapter 18: Peptic Ulcer Disease

Robert J. DiDomenico, PharmD
Clinical Associate Professor
University of Illinois at Chicago
Cardiovascular Clinical Pharmacist
University of Illinois Medical Center at Chicago
Chicago, Illinois
Chapter 7: Ischemic Heart Disease

Joseph T. DiPiro, PharmD
Professor and Executive Dean
South Carolina College of Pharmacy
University of South Carolina, Columbia
Medical University of South Carolina
Charleston, South Carolina
Chapter 77: Intra-Abdominal Infections

John M. Dopp, PharmD
Assistant Professor
University of Wisconsin School of Pharmacy
Clinical Pharmacist
Wisconsin Sleep Center
Madison, Wisconsin
Chapter 41: Sleep Disorders

Julie B. Dumond, PharmD
Research Assistant Professor
University of North Carolina at Chapel Hill Eshelman School
    of Pharmacy
Chapel Hill, North Carolina
Chapter 87: Human Immunodeficiency Virus Infection

Megan J. Ehret, PharmD, BCPP
Assistant Professor
University of Connecticut
Clinical Pharmacist
Institute of Living
Storrs, Connecticut
Chapter 35: Alzheimer's Disease

Benjamin J. Epstein, PharmD, BCPS
Assistant Professor of Pharmacy and Medicine
Department of Pharmacotherapy and Traslational Research
    and Medicine
Director, Internal Medicine Pharmacotherapy Clinic
University of Florida
Gainesville, Florida
Chapter 58: Osteoarthritis

John Erramouspe, PharmD, MS
Professor of Pharmacy Practice
Idaho State University
Pocatello, Idaho
Chapter 42: Attention-Deficit Hyperactivity Disorder

Edward Faught Jr., MD
Professor of Neurology
University of Alabama at Birmingham
Birmingham, Alabama
Chapter 30: Epilepsy

Martha J. Faulkner, PhDc, CNP, LISW
Staff
Department of Psychiatry
Nurse Practitioner
University of New Mexico
Albuquerque, New Mexico
Chapter 39: Bipolar Disorder

Christopher A. Fausel, PharmD, BCPS, BCOP
Clinical Associate Professor of Medicine
Indiana University School of Medicine
Clinical Director
Oncology Pharmacy Services
Simon Indiana University Cancer Center
Indianapolis, Indiana
Chapter 93: Malignant Lymphomas

Jacqueline M. Feldman, MD
Patrick H. Linton Professor
Director Division of Public Psychiatry
University of Alabama at Birmingham
Birmingham, Alabama
Chapter 38: Major Depressive Disorder

Ema Ferreira, BPharm, MSc, PharmD, FCSHP
Clinical Associate Professor
Universite de Montreal
Pharmacist
Obstetrics and Gynecology
Centre Hospitalier Ste-Justine
Montreal
Quebec, Canada
Chapter 47: Pregnancy and Lactation: Therapeutic Considerations

Jack E. Fincham, BS, PhD
Professor of Pharmacy Practice and Administrative Sciences
University of Missouri Kansas City School of Pharmacy
Kansas City, Missouri
Chapter 1: Introduction

Steven Gabardi, PharmD, BCPS
Abdominal Organ Transplant Clinical Specialist
Brigham and Women's Hospital
Assistant Professor of Medicine
Harvard Medical School
Boston, Massachusetts
Chapter 55: Solid Organ Transplantation

Angie L. Goeser, PharmD
Assistant Professor of Pharmacy Practice
Creighton University School of Pharmacy and Health Professions
Omaha, Nebraska
Chapter 65: Common Skin Disorders

Maqual R. Graham, PharmD
Associate Professor of Pharmacy Practice
University of Missouri-Kansas City
Clinical Pharmacy Specialist
Veterans Affairs Medical Center
Kansas City, Missouri
Chapter 102: Overweight and Obesity

Kendra J. Grande, RPh
Consultant Pharmacist
Abelian Consulting
Parker, Colorado
Chapter 63: Ophthalmic Disorders

Phyllis A. Grauer, PharmD, CGP
Assistant Clinical Professor
Ohio State University College of Pharmacy
Vice President Clinical Services
HospiScript Services
Dublin, Ohio
Chapter 4: Palliative Care

David R.P. Guay, PharmD
Professor
Department of Experimental and Clinical Pharmacology
University of Minnesota College of Pharmacy
Division of Geriatrics
HealthPartners Inc.
Minneapolis, Minnesota
Chapter 53: Urinary Incontinence and Pediatric Enuresis

John G. Gums, PharmD, FCCP
Associate Chair
Department of Pharmacotherapy and Translational Research
Professor of Pharmacy and Medicine
Departments of Pharmacotherapy and Translational Research and Community Health and Family Medicine
University of Florida
Gainesville, Florida
Chapter 58: Osteoarthritis

Sally K. Guthrie, PharmD, FCCP, BCPP
Associate Professor of Pharmacy
University of Michigan
College of Pharmacy
Ann Arbor, Michigan
Chapter 36: Substance-Related Disorders

Tracy M. Hagemann, PharmD, FCCP, FASHP, FAPhA, BCPS
Associate Professor
University of Oklahoma College of Pharmacy
Clinical Pediatric Specialist
Oklahoma City, Oklahoma
Chapter 68: Sickle Cell Anemia

Stuart T. Haines, PharmD, FCCP, FASHP, FAPhA, BCPS
Professor
Department of Pharmacy Practice and Science
University of Maryland School of Pharmacy
Clinical Pharmacy Specialist
West Palm Beach Veteran's Administration Medical Center
West Palm Beach, Florida
Chapter 10: Venous Thromboembolism

Kathleen B. Haynes, PharmD, BCPS
Disease Management Pharmacist
Visionary Enterprises, Inc.
Community Health Network
Indianapolis, Indiana
Chapter 48: Contraception

Nancy Heideman, PharmD, BCPS
Clinical Pharmacy Specialist—Pediatrics
University of New Mexico Hospital
Albuquerque, New Mexico
Chapter 95: Acute Leukemia

Brian A. Hemstreet, PharmD, BCPS
Associate Professor
University of Colorado Denver School of Pharmacy
Aurora, Colorado
Chapter 19: Inflammatory Bowel Disease

Elizabeth D. Hermsen, PharmD, MBA, BCPS-ID
Adjunct Assistant Professor
University of Nebraska Medical Center
College of Medicine and Pharmacy
Antimicrobial Stewardship Program Coordinator
Nebraska Medical Center
Omaha, Nebraska
Chapter 76: Gastrointestinal Infections

Catherine Heyneman, PharmD, MS, ANP, FASCP
Associate Professor of Pharmacy Practice and Administrative Sciences
Idaho State University College of Pharmacy
Pharmacist-in-Charge
Advanced Isotopes of Idaho
Pocatello, Idaho
Chapter 51: Erectile Dysfunction

Gerald Higa, PharmD
Associate Professor
West Virginia University Schools of Pharmacy and Medicine
Mary Babb Randolph Cancer Center
Morgantown, West Virginia
Chapter 89: Breast Cancer

James M. Hoffman, PharmD, MS, BCPS
Assistant Professor
College of Pharmacy
University of Tennessee Health Science Center
Medication Outcomes and Safety Officer
St. Jude Children's Research Hospital
Memphis, Tennessee
Chapter 66: Anemia

Marlon S. Honeywell, PharmD
Associate Professor of Pharmacy Practice
Florida A&M University
Clinical Pharmacist
Bond Community Health Center
Tallahassee, Florida
Chapter 80: Sexually Transmitted Infections

Jamie R. Hornecker, PharmD, BCPS
Clinical Assistant Professor
University of Wyoming School of Pharmacy
University of Wyoming Family Medicine Residency Program/ Community Health Center of Central Wyoming
Casper, Wyoming
Chapter 73: Skin and Soft Tissue Infections

Thomas R. Howdieshell, MD, FACS, FCCP
Professor of Surgery
University of New Mexico Health Science Center
Department of Surgery
Division of Trauma/Surgical Critical Care
Albuquerque, New Mexico
Chapter 77: Intra-Abdominal Infections

Matthew K. Ito, PharmD, FCCP, FNLA, CLS
Professor
Oregon State University/Oregon Health and Science University College of Pharmacy
Portland, Oregon
Chapter 12: Dyslipidemias

Cherry W. Jackson, BS, BS Pharm, PharmD
Professor of Pharmacy and Medicine
Auburn University School of Pharmacy
School of Medicine
Clinical Specialist
University of Alabama
Birmingham, Alabama
Chapter 38: Major Depressive Disorder

Ziba Jalali
Assistant Professor
College of Medicine
University of Nebraska Medical Center
Omaha, Nebraska
Chapter 76: Gastrointestinal Infections

John T. Johnson, PharmD, CDE, BC-ADM, FAADE
Chair, Professor of Pharmacy Practice
Presbyterian College School of Pharmacy
Clinton, South Carolina
Chapter 43: Diabetes Mellitus

Mikael D. Jones, PharmD, BCPS
Clinical Assistant Professor
University of Kentucky College of Pharmacy
College of Nursing
Lexington, Kentucky
Chapter 61: Glaucoma

Angela D.M. Kashuba, PharmD, DABCP
Associate Professor
Eshelman School of Pharmacy
University of North Carolina
Chapel Hill, North Carolina
Chapter 87: Human Immunodeficiency Virus Infection

Michael D. Katz, PharmD
Clinical Associate Professor
Department of Pharmacy Practice and Science
The University of Arizona College of Pharmacy
Tucson, Arizona
Chapter 44: Thyroid Disorders

Deanna L. Kelly, PharmD, BCPP
Associate Professor of Psychiatry
University of Maryland School of Medicine
Acting Director of the Treatment Research Program
Maryland Psychiatric Research Center
Baltimore, Maryland
Chapter 37: Schizophrenia

Patrick J. Kiel, PharmD, BCPS
Clinical Pharmacy Specialist
Hematology/Stem Cell Transplant
IU Simon Cancer Center-Clarian Health
Indianapolis, Indiana
Chapter 93: Malignant Lymphomas

Joseph J. Kishel, PharmD, BCPS (AQ-ID)
Clinical Scientific Director
Penn State College of Medicine
Cubist Pharmaceuticals, Inc.
Lexington, Massachusetts
Chapter 23: Pancreatitis

Julia M. Koehler, PharmD
Associate Professor and Chair of Pharmacy Practice
Butler University College of Pharmacy and Health Sciences
Clinical Pharmacist in Family Medicine
Clarian Health Partners
Department of Pharmacy and the Indiana University-
    Methodist Residency Program/Department of Family
    Medicine
Indianapolis, Indiana
Chapter 48: Contraception

Jill M. Kolesar, PharmD, BCPS, FCCP
Professor
University of Wisconsin School of Pharmacy
Director
3P Analytical Instrumentation Laboratory
University of Wisconsin Comprehensive Cancer Center
Madison, Wisconsin
Chapter 92: Prostate Cancer

Michael D. Kraft, PharmD, BCNSP
Clinical Associate Professor
University of Michigan
College of Pharmacy
Clinical Coordinator and Clinical Pharmacist
Department of Pharmacy Services
University of Michigan Health System
Ann Arbor, Michigan
Chapter 100: Parenteral Nutrition

Rebecca M.T. Law, PharmD
Associate Professor
School of Pharmacy
Memorial University of Newfoundland
St. John's
Newfoundland and Labrador, Canada
Chapter 64: Psoriasis

Amber P. Lawson, PharmD, BCOP
Clinical Pharmacy Specialist
University of Kentucky HealthCare
Lexington, Kentucky
Chapter 98: Hematopoietic Stem Cell Transplantation

W. Greg Leader, PharmD
Interim Dean
Professor of Clinical Pharmacy
University of Louisiana at Monroe College of Pharmacy
Monroe, Louisiana
Chapter 14: Asthma

Jeannie K. Lee, PharmD, BCPS
Clinical Assistant Professor
The University of Arizona
College of Pharmacy
Clinical Pharmacist in Geriatrics
Southern Arizona VA Health Care System
Tucson, Arizona
Chapter 2: Geriatrics

Mary Lee, PharmD, BCPS, FCCP
Vice President and Chief Academic Officer
Midwestern University
Professor of Pharmacy Practice
Chicago College of Pharmacy
Downers Grove, Illinois
Chapter 52: Benign Prostatic Hyperplasia

Gary M. Levin, PharmD, BCPP, FCCP
Dean and Professor
LECOM School of Pharmacy
Bradenton, Florida
Chapter 35: Alzheimer's Disease

Russell E. Lewis, PharmD, FCCP, BCPS
Associate Professor
University of Houston College of Pharmacy
Clinical Pharmacy Specialist
Infections Diseases
University of Texas M.D. Anderson Cancer Center
Houston, Texas
Chapter 84: Invasive Fungal Infections

Teresa V. Lewis, PharmD, BCPS
Clinical Assistant Professor
University of Oklahoma College of Pharmacy
Clinical Pediatric Specialist
Oklahoma City, Oklahoma
Chapter 68: Sickle Cell Anemia

Edward C. Li, PharmD, BCOP
Oncology Scientist–Compendium
National Comprehensive Cancer Network (NCCN)
Fort Washington, Pennsylvania
Chapter 66: Anemia

Cara Liday, PharmD, BCPS, CDE
Associate Professor
College of Pharmacy
Idaho State University
Intermountain Medical Clinic
Pocatello, Idaho
Chapter 51: Erectile Dysfunction

Cameron C. Lindsey, PharmD, BC-ADM
Associate Professor of Pharmacy Practice
University of Missouri-Kansas City
Clinical Pharmacy Specialist
Veterans Affairs Medical Center
Kansas City, Missouri
Chapter 102: Overweight and Obesity

Anna Lockwood, PharmD
Pharmacy Practice and Science College of Pharmacy
University of Kentucky
Clinical Pharmacy Specialist
Psychiatry
Lexington VA Medical Center
Lexington, Kentucky
Chapter 40: Generalized Anxiety Disorder, Panic Disorder, and Social Anxiety Disorder

Karl Madaras-Kelly, PharmD, MPH
Associate Professor
Department of Pharmacy Practice
College of Pharmacy
Idaho State University
Clinical Pharmacy Specialist
Veterans Affairs Medical Center
Boise, Idaho
Chapter 69: Antimicrobial Regimen Selection

Mark A. Malesker, PharmD, FCCP, BCPS
Professor of Pharmacy Practice and Medicine
Creighton University
Clinical Pharmacy Specialist
Creighton University Medical Center
Omaha, Nebraska
Chapter 27: Fluids and Electrolytes
Chapter 28: Acid–Base Disturbances

Kathryn R. Matthias, PharmD
Clinical Assistant Professor
The University of Arizona
University Medical Center
Tucson, Arizona
Chapter 79: Urinary Tract Infections

J. Russell May, PharmD, FASHP
Clinical Professor
The University of Georgia College of Pharmacy
Clinical Pharmacist
Medical College of Georgia Health System
Augusta, Georgia
Chapter 54: Allergic and Pseudoallergic Drug Reactions

Trevor McKibbin, PharmD, MS, BCPS
Assistant Professor
University of Tennessee College of Pharmacy
Memphis, Tennessee
Chapter 92: Prostate Cancer

Patrick J. Medina, PharmD, BCOP
Associate Professor
University of Oklahoma College of Pharmacy
OU Cancer Institute
Oklahoma City, Oklahoma
Chapter 91: Colorectal Cancer

Damian M. Mendoza, PharmD, CGP
Clinical Instructor in Pharmacy Practice and Science
University of Arizona College of Pharmacy
Clinical Pharmacy Specialist
Southern Arizona VA Health Care System
Tucson, Arizona
Chapter 2: Geriatrics

April D. Miller, PharmD
Clinical Assistant Professor
South Carolina College of Pharmacy
University of South Carolina Campus
Clinical Pharmacy Specialist
Critical Care
Palmetto Health Richland
Columbia, South Carolina
Chapter 70: Central Nervous System Infections

Sarah J. Miller, PharmD, MS, BCNSP
Professor
University of Montana Skaggs School of Pharmacy
Clinical Coordinator
Saint Patrick Hospital
Missoula, Montana
Chapter 101: Enteral Nutrition

Beverly C. Mims, PharmD
Associate Professor of Pharmacy Practice
Howard University College of Pharmacy
Nursing and Allied Health Sciences
Clinical Pharmacist
Howard University Hospital
Washington DC
Chapter 21: Constipation, Diarrhea, and Irritable Bowel Syndrome

M. Jane Mohler, RN, MPH, PhD
Associate Research Professor
Colleges of Medicine, Pharmacy, and Public Health
Associate Director of Research
Arizona Center on Aging
University of Arizona
Tucson, Arizona
Chapter 2: Geriatrics

Caroline Morin, BPharm, MSc
Associated Clinician
Universite de Montreal
Pharmacist
Obstetrics and Gynecology
CHU Ste-Justine
Montreal, Quebec, Canada
Chapter 47: Pregnancy and Lactation: Therapeutic Considerations

Susan J. Morris, MD
Assistant Professor of Geriartrics
Section of Geriatrics
Texas Tech University Health Sciences Center
El Paso, Texas
Chapter 2: Geriatrics

Lee E. Morrow, MD, MSc
Associate Professor of Medicine and Pharmacy Practice
Creighton University Medical Center
Pulmonary and Critical Care Fellowship Program Director
Creighton University Medical Center
Omaha, Nebraska
Chapter 27: Fluids and Electrolytes
Chapter 28: Acid–Base Disturbances

Milap C. Nahata, PharmD, MS
Professor of Pharmacy, Pediatrics and Internal Medicine
Chair, Division of Pharmacy Practice and Administration
College of Pharmacy
The Ohio State University
Associate Director
Department of Pharmacy
Ohio State University Medical Center
Columbus, Ohio
Chapter 3: Pediatrics

Rocsanna Namdar, PharmD
Assistant Professor
University of Colorado
Aurora, Colorado
Chapter 75: Tuberculosis

Christie Nelson, PharmD
Clinical Assistant Professor
University of Wyoming School of Pharmacy
Wyoming Medical Center
Casper, Wyoming
Chapter 73: Skin and Soft Tissue Infections

Melinda M. Neuhauser, PharmD, MPH
Clinical Pharmacy Specialist
Infectious Diseases
VA Pharmacy Benefits Management Services
Hines, Illinois
Chapter 81: Osteomyelitis

Tien M.H. Ng, PharmD, BCPS
Associate Professor of Clinical Pharmacy
University of Southern California School of Pharmacy
Los Angeles, California
Chapter 6: Heart Failure

Kimberly J. Novak, PharmD, BCPS
Clinical Assistant Professor
Ohio State University College of Pharmacy
Clinical Pharmacy Specialist
Pediatric Pulmonary Medicine
Nationwide Children's Hospital
Columbus, Ohio
Chapter 16: Cystic Fibrosis

Edith A. Nutescu, PharmD, FCCP
Clinical Professor
University of Illinois at Chicago
College of Pharmacy
Department of Pharmacy Practice and Center for
    Pharmacoeconomic Research
Clinical Manager
Antithrombosis Center
University of Illinois Medical Center
Chicago, Illinois
Chapter 10: Venous Thromboembolism

Catherine M. Oliphant, PharmD
Associate Professor of Pharmacy Practice
Idaho State University
Clinical Pharmacist
St. Luke's Internal Medicine/St. Luke's Regional Medical
    Center
Boise, Idaho
Chapter 69: Antimicrobial Regimen Selection

Ali J. Olyaei, PharmD, BCPS
Associate Professor of Medicine
Nephrology and Hypertension
Oregon Health and Sciences University
Portland, Oregon
Chapter 55: Solid Organ Transplantation

Christine K. O'Neil, PharmD, BCPS, FCCP, CGP
Professor
Mylan School of Pharmacy
Duquesne University
Director
Center for Pharmacy Care
Pittsburgh, Pennsylvania
Chapter 33: Pain Management

Vinita B. Pai, PharmD, MS
Assistant Professor of Clinical Pharmacy
The Ohio State University
College of Pharmacy
Clinical Pharmacy Specialist
Pediatric Blood and Transplantation Program
Nationwide Children's Hospital
Columbus, Ohio
Chapter 3: Pediatrics

David Parra, PharmD, FCCP, BCPS
Clinical Assistant Professor
Department of Experimental and Clinical Pharmacology
College of Pharmacy
University of Minnesota
Clinical Pharmacy Specialist in Cardiology
Veterans Affairs Medical Center
West Palm Beach, Florida
Chapter 5: Hypertension

Charles A. Peloquin, PharmD
Professor
University of Florida
Gainesville, Florida
Chapter 75: Tuberculosis

Susan L. Pendland, MS, PharmD
Adjunct Associate Professor
University of Illinois at Chicago
Clinical Staff Pharmacist
Saint Joseph Berea Hospital
Berea, Kentucky
Chapter 81: Osteomyelitis

Trinh Pham, PharmD, BCOP
Assistant Clinical Professor
University of Connecticut
School of Pharmacy
Assistant Clinical Professor
Yale New Haven Hospital
New Haven, Connecticut
Chapter 97: Skin Cancer

Hanna Phan, PharmD, BCPS
Clinical Assistant Professor
The University of Arizona
College of Pharmacy
Clinical Pharmacy Specialist
Pediatric Pulmonary Medicine
University Medical Center
Tucson, Arizona
Chapter 3: Pediatrics

Beth Bryles Phillips, PharmD, FCCP, BCPS
Clinical Associate Professor
The University of Georgia
Clinical Pharmacy Specialist
Charlie Norwood VA Medical Center
Athens, Georgia
Chapter 56: Osteoporosis

Bradley G. Phillips, PharmD, FCCP, BCPS
Millikan-Reeve Professor and Head
University of Georgia College of Pharmacy
Department of Clinical and Administrative Pharmacy
Athens, Georgia
Chapter 41: Sleep Disorders

Amy M. Pick, PharmD, BCOP
Assistant Professor Pharmacy Practice
Creighton University School of Pharmacy and Health
   Professions
Omaha, Nebraska
Chapter 96: Chronic Leukemias and Multiple Myeloma

Brian A. Potoski, PharmD, BCPS (AQ-ID)
Assistant Professor
Department of Pharmacy and Therapeutics
University of Pittsburgh School of Pharmacy
Associate Director
Antibiotic Management Program
University of Pittsburgh Medical Center
Presbyterian University Hospital
Pittsburgh, Pennsylvania
Chapter 79: Urinary Tract Infections

Frank Pucino Jr., PharmD, MPH, BCPS, FASHP, FCCP,
   FDPGEC
Clinical Investigator
National Institute of Arthritis and Muculoskeletal and Skins
   Disease
National Institute of Diabetes abd Digestive and Kidney Diseases
National Institute of Health
Bethesda, Maryland
Chapter 45: Adrenal Gland Disorders
Chapter 46: Pituitary Gland Disorders

Kelly R. Ragucci, PharmD, FCCP, BCPS, CDE
Associate Professor
Clinical Pharmacy and Outcome Sciences/Family Medicine
South Carolina College of Pharmacy
MUSC Campus
Charleston, South Carolina
Chapter 50: Hormone Therapy in Menopause

Évelyne Rey, MD, MSc, FRCPC
Professor and Head
Division of Obstetrics Medicine
Department of Obstetrics and Gynecology
CHU Sainte-Justine
Montreal, Quebec, Canada
Chapter 47: Pregnancy and Lactation: Therapeutic
   Considerations

Anastasia Rivkin, BS, PharmD, BCPS
Associate Professor and Division Director of Pharmacy
   Practice
Arnold and Marie Schwartz College of Pharmacy and Health
   Sciences
Long Island University
Brooklyn, New York
Critical Care Pharmacist
St. Luke's Roosevelt Hospital Center
New York
Chapter 67: Coagulation and Platelet Disorders

P. David Rogers, PhD, FCCP
First Tennessee Chair of Excellence in Clinical Pharmacy
Professor and Associate Dean for Transitional Research
Department of Clinical Pharmacy
University of Tennessee College of Pharmacy
Memphis, Tennessee
Chapter 84: Invasive Fungal Infections

Brendan S. Ross, MD
Clinical Associate Professor
Department of Pharmacy Practice
University of Mississippi School of Pharmacy
Staff Physician
G.V. (Sonny) Montgomery Veterans Affairs
   Medical Center
Jackson, Mississippi
Chapter 34: Headache

Leigh Ann Ross, PharmD
Associate Professor and Chair
Department of Pharmacy Practice
University of Mississippi School of Pharmacy
Associate Dean for Clinical Affairs
University of Mississippi School of Pharmacy
Jackson, Mississippi
Chapter 34: Headache

John C. Rotschafer, PharmD
Professor
University of Minnesota
College of Pharmacy
Minneapolis, Minnesota
Chapter 85: Antimicrobial Prophylaxis in Surgery

Laurajo Ryan, PharmD, MSc, BCPS, CDE
Clinical Assistant Professor
University of Texas at Austin College of Pharmacy
University of Texas Health Science Center San Antonio
Pharmacotherapy Education and Research Center
San Antonio, Texas
Chapter 22: Portal Hypertension and Cirrhosis

Melody Ryan, PharmD, MPH
Associate Professor
Departments of Pharmacy Practice and Science and
    Neurology
University of Kentucky
Clinical Pharmacy Specialist
Lexington Veterans Affairs Medical Center
Lexington, Kentucky
Chapter 29: Multiple Sclerosis

Sarah L. Scarpace, PharmD, BCOP
Assistant Professor
Pharmacy Practice
Albany College of Pharmacy
Clinical Oncology Pharmacist
Stratton Veterans Affairs Medical Center
Albany, New York
Chapter 99: Supportive Care in Oncology

Jeremy A. Schafer, PharmD
Manager of Formulary Development
Prime Therapeutics
Eagan, Minnesota
Chapter 85: Antimicrobial Prophylaxis in Surgery

Lauren S. Schlesselman, PharmD
Assistant Clinical Professor and Director of Assessment and
    Accreditation
University of Connecticut School of Pharmacy
Storrs, Connecticut
Chapter 83: Superficial Fungal Infections

Kristine S. Schonder, PharmD
Assistant Professor
University of Pittsburg School of Pharmacy
Clinical Specialist
Thomas E. Starzl Transplantation Institute
Pittsburgh, Pennsylvania
Chapter 26: Chronic and End-Stage Kidney Disease

Roohollah Sharifi, MD, FACS
Professor of Surgery/Urology
University of Illinois
Department of Urology
College of Medicine
Chicago, Illinois
Chapter 52: Benign Prostatic Hyperplasia

Judith A. Smith, PharmD, FCCP, BCOP, FISOPP
Associate Professor
University of Texas
M.D. Anderson Cancer Center
Houston, Texas
Chapter 94: Ovarian Cancer

Philip H. Smith, MD
Assistant Professor of Medicine
Allergy and Immunology
Medical College of Georgia
Augusta, Georgia
Chapter 54: Allergic and Pseudoallergic Drug Reactions

Steven M. Smith, PharmD
Postdoctoral Fellow in Family Medicine
Departments of Pharmacotherapy and Translational Research
    and Community Health and Family Medicine
University of Florida
Gainesville, Florida
Chapter 58: Osteoarthritis

Sarah A. Spinler, PharmD, FCCP, BCPS (AQ Cardiology)
Professor of Clinical Pharmacy
Philadelphia College of Pharmacy
University of the Sciences in Philadelphia
Philadelphia, Pennsylvania
Chapter 8: Acute Coronary Syndromes

Mary K. Stamatakis, BS, PharmD
Associate Dean and Associate Professor
West Virginia University School of Pharmacy
Morgantown, West Virginia
Chapter 25: Acute Kidney Injury

Robert J. Straka, PharmD, FCCP
Professor
Department of Experimental and Clinical Pharmacology
University of Minnesota
Minneapolis, Minnesota
Chapter 5: Hypertension

S. Scott Sutton, PharmD, BCPS AQ ID
Associate Clinical Professor
South Carolina College of Pharmacy
University of South Carolina
Clinical Pharmacist
Medicine and Infectious Diseases
Dorn Veterans Affairs Medical Center
Columbia, South Carolina
Chapter 82: Sepsis and Septic Shock

Marc A. Sweeney PharmD, MDiv
Dean and Professor of Pharmacy Practice
Cedarville University School of Pharmacy
Cedarville, Ohio
Chapter 4: Palliative Care

Eljim P. Tesoro, PharmD
Clinical Assistant Professor
University of Illinois at Chicago
Clinical Pharmacist
University of Illinois Medical Center at Chicago
Chicago, Illinois
Chapter 31: Status Epilepticus

Michael D. Thompson, PharmD, BCNSP
Assistant Dean for Clinical Affairs and Professor
Florida A&M University
Training Partner
Florida Caribbean AIDS Education and Training Center
Tallahassee, Florida
Chapter 80: Sexually Transmitted Infections

James E. Tisdale, PharmD
Professor
School of Pharmacy and Pharmaceutical Sciences
Purdue University
Indianapolis, Indiana
Chapter 9: Arrhythmias

Mary A. Ullman, PharmD
Infectious Diseases Research Fellow
University of Minnesota
Minneapolis, Minnesota
Chapter 85: Antimicrobial Prophylaxis in Surgery

Elena M. Umland, BS, PharmD
Associate Dean for Academic Affairs
Associate Professor of Clinical Pharmacy
Jefferson School of Pharmacy
Thomas Jefferson University
Philadelphia, Pennsylvania
Chapter 49: Menstruation-Related Disorders

Heather VandenBussche, PharmD
Professor
Department of Pharmacy Practice
Ferris State University College of Pharmacy
Kalamazoo, Michigan
Chapter 72: Upper Respiratory Tract Infections

Orly Vardeny, PharmD
Assistant Professor
University of Wisconsin School of Pharmacy
Madison, Wisconsin
Chapter 6: Heart Failure

Nicole D. Verkleeren, PharmD, BCPS
Clinical Pharmacist
Western Pennsylvania Hospital–Forbes Regional Campus
Monroeville, Pennsylvania
Chapter 15: Chronic Obstructive Pulmonary Disease

William E. Wade, PharmD
College of Pharmacy
The University of Georgia
St. Mary's Health Care System
Athens, Georgia
Chapter 43: Diabetes Mellitus

Mary L. Wagner, PharmD, MS
Associate Professor
Rutgers State University of New Jersey
Ernest Mario School of Pharmacy
Clinical Pharmacist of Ambulatory Care Neurology
Robert Wood Johnson University Hospital
Piscataway, New Jersey
Chapter 32: Parkinson's Disease

Geoffrey C. Wall, PharmD, BCPS, CGP, FCCP
Associate Professor of Pharmacy Practice
Drake University College of Pharmacy and Health Sciences
Internal Medicine Clinical Pharmacist
Iowa Methodist Medical Center
Des Moines, Iowa
Chapter 59: Gout and Hyperuricemia

Heidi J. Wehring, PharmD, BCPP
Academic Fellow
Maryland Psychiatric Research Center
University of Maryland School of Medicine
Catonsville, Maryland
Chapter 37: Schizophrenia

Elaine Weiner, MD
Assistant Professor
University of Maryland School of Medicine
Medical Director
Maryland Psychiatric Research Center
Outpatient Research Program
Catonsville, Maryland
Chapter 37: Schizophrenia

Lara C. Weinstein, MD
Assistant Professor
Department of Family and Community Medicine
Thomas Jefferson University Hospital
Philadelphia, Pennsylvania
Chapter 49: Menstruation-Related Disorders

Timothy E. Welty, BS Pharm, PharmD, MA, FCCP, BCPS
Professor and Chair
School of Pharmacy
Department of Neurology
Department of Pharmacy Practice
University of Kansas
Kansas City, Kansas
Chapter 30: Epilepsy

Randy C. Wesnitzer, PharmD
Consultant Pharmacist
Casper, New York
Chapter 73: Skin and Soft Tissue Infections

Tara R. Whetsel, PharmD
Clinical Assistant Professor
West Virginia University School of Pharmacy
Morgantown, West Virginia
Chapter 15: Chronic Obstructive Pulmonary Disease

Sheila Wilhelm, PharmD, BCPS
Assistant Professor
Wayne State University
Clinical Pharmacy Specialist
Harper University Hospital
Detroit, Michigan
Chapter 20: Nausea and Vomiting

Dianne B. Williams, PharmD, BCPS
Clinical Associate Professor
University of Georgia College of Pharmacy
Clinical Pharmacist
Medical College of Georgia Health, Inc.
Augusta, Georgia
Chapter 17: Gastroesophageal Reflux Disease

Susan R. Winkler, PharmD, BCPS
Assistant Dean
Professor and Interim Chair
Pharmacy Practice
Chicago College of Pharmacy
Midwestern University
Downers Grove, Illinois
Chapter 11: Stroke

G. Christopher Wood, PharmD, FCCP, BCPS
Associate Professor of Clinical Pharmacy
University of Tennessee Health Science Center
Critical Care Clinical Pharmacist
Regional Medical Center at Memphis
Memphis, Tennessee
Chapter 13: Hypovolemic Shock

Rosa Yeh, PharmD, BCPS, AAHIVE
Assistant Professor
University of Houston
Houston, Texas
Chapter 87: Human Immunodeficiency Virus Infection

REVIEWERS

Dona Alberti, BSN, RN
Programs Administrator
Phase I and GU Programs
Assistant Director, Translational Research and International
  Collaborations
Carbone Cancer Center
University of Wisconsin
Madison, Wisconsin

Rita R. Alloway, PharmD, BCPS, FCCP
Research Professor of Medicine
Director of Transplant Clinical Research
University of Cincinnati
Cincinnati, Ohio

L.E. Ashworth, PharmD
Professor of Pharmacy Practice
Director of Drug Information
Vicechair
Department of Pharmacy Practice
Mercer University College of Pharmacy and Health Sciences
Atlanta, Georgia

Sara Grimsley Augustin, PharmD, BCPP
Clinical Pharmacist
DeKalb Regional Crisis Center
Decatur, Georgia

Jodie Linn Bakus, PharmD, BCPS
Clinical Assistant Professor
Department of Clinical,
Social, and Administrative Sciences
University of Michigan College of Pharmacy
Ann Arbor, Michigan

Marialice S. Bennett, BS, RPh, FAPhA
Professor of Clinical Pharmacy
Ohio State University
Pharmacy Director
University Health Connection
Columbus, Ohio

Sarah E. Bland, RPh
Clinical Instructor
University of Wisconsin School of Pharmacy
Senior Clinical Pharmacist
University of Wisconsin Hospital and Clinics
Madison, Wisconsin

Ebrahim A. Blbisi, PharmD
Associate Clinical Professor
St. John's University
Queens, New York
Clinical Coordinator Ambulatory Medicine
Queens Hospital Center
Jamaica, New York

Patty Bluml, MSN, ARNP, OCN
ARNP for Blood and Marrow Transplant Program
CNS-Oncology
Via Christi Regional Medical Center
Wichita, Kansas

Scott Bolesta, PharmD
Clinical Pharmacist
Critical Care/Internal Medicine
Mercy Hospital
Scranton, Pennsylvania
Assistant Professor
Nesbitt College of Pharmacy and Nursing
Wilkes University
Wilkes-Barre, Pennsylvania

P. Branden Bookstaver, PharmD, BCPS, AAHIVE
Clinical Assistant Professor
South Carolina College of Pharmacy, USC Campus
Clinical Specialist, Infectious Diseases
Palmetto Health Richland
Columbia, South Carolina

Margaret T. Bowers, MSM
Assistant Clinical Professor
Duke University School of Nursing
Family Nursing Practitioner
Duke Heart Failure Disease Management Program
Durham, North Carolina

Daniel Patrick Boyle, RPh, BCOP
Adjunct Assistant Professor of Pharmacy Practice
University of Connecticut School of Pharmacy
Oncology Pharmacist
Maine General Medical Center
Augusta, Maine

Jeffrey Paul Bratberg, PharmD, BCPS
Clinical Associate Professor of Pharmacy Practice
University of Rhode Island College of Pharmacy
Infectious Diseases Specialist
Roger Williams Medical Center
Kingston, Rhode Island

Kelsey Briggs, PharmD
Pediatric Clinical Specialist
West Virginia University Hospitals
Morgantown, West Virginia

Denise Buonocore, MSN, ACNP-BC, CCRN
Acute Care Nurse Practitioner
Yale New Haven Hospital
New Haven, Connecticut

Bethaney Campbell, RN, MN, RN, AOCNS
Oncology/Hematology
Stem Cell Transplant Clinical Nurse Specialist
University of Wisconsin Hospital & Clinics and the Paul P.
    Carbone Comprehensive Cancer Center
Madison, Wisconsin

Katie E. Cardone, PharmD
Assistant Professor of Pharmacy Practice
Albany College of Pharmacy and Health Sciences
Pharmacist
Hortense and Louis
Rubin Dialysis Center
Albany, New York

Cynthia Carnes, PharmD, PhD
Associate Professor of Pharmacy
Ohio State University
Specialty Practice Pharmacist
Ohio State University Medical Center
Columbus, Ohio

Barry L. Carter, PharmD
Professor
Colleges of Pharmacy and Medicine
University of Iowa
Iowa City, Iowa

Elias B. Chahine, PharmD, BCPS
Assistant Professor of Pharmacy Practice
Palm Beach Atlantic University
Clinical Pharmacist
JFK Medical Center
West Palm Beach, Florida

Alexandre Chan, PharmD, BCPS, BCOP
Assistant Professor
National University of Singapore
Faculty of Science
Department of Pharmacy
Clinical Pharmacist National Cancer Centre
Singapore

Nina Han Cheigh, PharmD
Clinical Associate Professor
University of Illinois College of Pharmacy
Chicago, Illinois

Deborah A. Chyun, PhD, RN, FAHA, FAAN
Associate Professor and Director
Florence S. Downs PhD Program in Nursing Research and
    Theory Development
College of Nursing
New York University
New York, New York

John D. Cleary, PharmD, FCCP
Professor
University of Mississippi Medical Center
Jackson, Mississippi

Kelli L. Coover, PharmD, CGP
Assistant Professor of Pharmacy Practice
Creighton University School of Pharmacy and Health
    Professions
Omaha, Nebraska

Jessica Shank Coviello, MSN, APRN
Assistant Professor
Yale University School of Nursing
Adult Nurse Practitioner
The Connecticut Heart Group
New Haven, Connecticut

Joseph E. Crea, DO, MHA
Assistant Professor
University of Findlay College of Pharmacy
Findlay, Ohio

Bonnie Dadig, EdD, PA-C
Associate Professor and Chair of the Physician Assistant
    Department
Physician Assistant Certified
Medical College of Georgia
Augusta, Georgia

Lawrence Davidow, PhD, RPh
Clinical Assistant Professor
University of Kansas School of Pharmacy
Lawrence Kansas

Christopher J. Destache, PharmD
Professor of Pharmacy Practice
Creighton University School of Pharmacy & Health
    Professions
Infectious Diseases Clinical Pharmacist
Creighton University Medical Center
Omaha, Nebraska

Thomas C. Dowling, PharmD, PhD
Associate Professor and Vice Chair
School of Pharmacy
University of Maryland
Baltimore, Maryland

Jingyang Fan, PharmD, BCPS
Clinical Associate Professor
Southern Illinois University Edwardsville
Clinical Pharmacist in Cardiology
St. John's Mercy Medical Center
Edwardsville, Illinois

Roberta M. Farrah, PharmD, BCPS
Assistant Professor
Department of Pharmacy and Therapeutics
University of Pittsburgh School of Pharmacy
Director of Outpatient Pharmacotherapy Education
UPMC St. Margaret Family Medicine Residency Program,
    Pittsburgh, Pennsylvania

Pamela A. Foral, PharmD, BCPS
Associate Professor of Pharmacy Practice
Creighton University School of Pharmacy and Health
  Professions
Omaha, Nebraska

Maisha Kelly Freeman, PharmD, BCPS
Associate Professor
Samford University
Director
Samford University Global Drug Information Service
Birmingham, Alabama

Cynthia L. Gaston, PharmD
Clinical Associate Professor
University of Wisconsin School of Pharmacy
Senior Clinical Pharmacist
University of Wisconsin Hospital and Clinics
Madison, Wisconsin

Nancy S. Goldstein, CRNP, MSN, RNC
Instructor
Johns Hopkins University School of Nursing
Nurse Practitioner
Sidney Kimmel Cancer Center at the Johns Hopkins Medical
  Institute
Baltimore, Maryland

Marjorie J. Good, RN, BSN, MPH, OCN
Manager
Wichita Community Clinical Oncology Program
Wichita, Kansas

Justine Schuller Gortney, PharmD, BCPS
Clinical Assistant Professor
Mercer University College of Pharmacy and Health Sciences
Internal Medicine
DeKalb Medical Center
Atlanta, Georgia

Erich Jason Grant, MMS, PA-C
Instructor
Wake Forest University School of Medicine
Department of PA Studies
Wake Forest University Health Sciences
Winston-Salem, North Carolina

Myke R. Green, BS, PharmD, BCOP
Oncology Clinical Pharmacy Specialist
University Medical Center
Arizona Cancer Center
Tucson, Arizona

Hillary Wall Grillo, PharmD
Adjunct Assistant Professor
Bernard J. Dunn School of Pharmacy
Shenandoah University
Winchester, Virginia

Robert Hadley, PhD, PA-C
Associate Professor
Jefferson College of Health Sciences
Roanoke, Virginia

Deborah Anne Hass, PharmD, BCOP
Hematology/Oncology Clinical Pharmacist
Stanford Hospital and Clinics
Stanford, California

David Hawkins, PharmD
Professor and Dean
California Northstate College of Pharmacy
Rancho Cordova, California

Keith A. Hecht, PharmD, BCOP
Clinical Associate Professor of Pharmacy Practice
Southern Illinois University Edwardsville
School of Pharmacy
Clinical Pharmacy Specialist
Hematology/Oncology
St. John's Mercy Medical Center
Edwardsville, Illinois

Mark A. Heisler, PharmD, BCPS
Manager
Pharmacy Clinical Decision Support
Banner Health
Phoenix, Arizona

Shirley Hogan, PharmD
Clinical Assistant Professor
University of Mississippi School of Pharmacy
Department of Pharmacy Practice
Pediatric Oncology Clinical Pharmacy Specialist
University of Mississippi Medical Center–Blair E. Batson
  Children's Hospital
Jackson, Mississippi

Wendy M. Horton, PharmD, BCPS
Clinical Instructor
University of Wisconsin School of Pharmacy
Senior Clinical Pharmacist
University of Wisconsin Hospital and Clinics
Madison, Wisconsin

Hiroaki Ikesue, PhD
Clinical Pharmacist
Kyushu University Hospital
Fukuoka, Japan

Arthur I. Jacknowitz, PharmD
Professor and Distinguished Chair in Clinical Pharmacy
West Virginia University School of Pharmacy
Morgantown, West Virginia

Michael K. Jensen, RPh, MS
Clinical Associate Professor of Pharmacy Practice
University of Utah College of Pharmacy
University Hospital
Clinical Pharmacist
Ophthalmic Specialist
John A. Moran Eye Center
University of Utah Hospital
Salt Lake City, Utah

Jill T. Johnson, PharmD, BCPS
Associate Professor
University of Arkansas for Medical Sciences College of
    Pharmacy
The University Hospital
Little Rock, Arkansas

Charles M. Karnack, PharmD, BCNSP
Assistant Professor of Clinical Pharmacy
Duquesne University Mylan School of Pharmacy
Clinical Pharmacy Specialist
University of Pittsburgh Medical Center–Mercy Hospital
Pittsburgh, Pennsylvania

Nikki Katalanos, PhD, PA-C
Assistant Professor
University of New Mexico
Director
UNM Physician Assistant Program
Department of Family and Community Medicine
Albuquerque, New Mexico

Julie C. Kissack, PharmD, BCPP
Professor and Chair of Pharmacy Practice
Harding University College of Pharmacy
Searcy, Arkansas

Shawna L. Kraft, PharmD
Adjunct Clinical Assistant Professor
University of Michigan College of Pharmacy
Clinical Pharmacist
Hematology/Oncology
University of Michigan Health System
Ann Arbor, Michigan

Sin Hung (Masha) Lam, BS, PharmD
Oncology Pharmacist
Hematology/Oncology Outpatient Infusion Clinic
Kaiser Permanente
Antioch Medical Center
Antioch, California

Rebecca M.T. Law, PharmD
Associate Professor
School of Pharmacy
Memorial University of Newfoundland
St. John's
Newfoundland and Labrador, Canada
Chapter 64: Psoriasis

Thomas L. Lenz, PharmD, MA
Associate Professor of Pharmacy Practice
Creighton University
Clinical Director
Creighton Cardiovascular Risk Reduction Program
Creighton University
Omaha, Nebraska

Chin Yeh Liu, MS, PharmD, BCOP
Adjunct Assistant Professor
Wayne State University
Manager
Clinical Pharmacy Services
Karmanos Cancer Center
Detroit, Michigan

Sam J. Lubner, MD
Medical Oncology Fellow
University of Wisconsin
Madison, Wisconsin

Carolyn Ma, PharmD, BCOP
Associate Professor and Chair
University of Hawaii at Hilo College of Pharmacy
Hilo, Hawaii

Carrie M. Maffeo, PharmD, BCPS, CDE
Assistant Professor of Pharmacy Practice
Butler University College Pharmacy and Health Sciences
Director
Health Education Center
Indianapolis, Indiana

Michael A. Mancano, PharmD
Clinical Associate Professor of Pharmacy
Associate Chair
Department of Pharmacy Practice
Temple University School of Pharmacy
Clinical Consultant
Northeastern Hospital
Philadelphia, Pennsylvania

Joel C. Marrs, PharmD, BCPS, CLS
Clinical Assistant Professor
Oregon State University/Oregon Health & Science
    University
Clinical Pharmacy Specialist
Oregon Health & Science University Hospital
Portland, Oregon

Trevor McKibbin, PharmD, MS, BCPS
Assistant Professor
University of Tennessee College of Pharmacy
Memphis, Tennessee

Mary Grace Mihalyo, BS, PharmD
Assistant Professor Pharmacy Practice
Duquesne University Mylan School of Pharmacy
President and Clinical Pharmacy Specialist
Palliative Therapeutics, LLC
Pittsburgh, Pennsylvania

Donald R. Miller, PharmD, FASHP
Professor and Chair
Department of Pharmacy Practice
North Dakota State University
Fargo, North Dakota

Candis M. Morello, PharmD, CDE, FCSHP
Associate Professor of Clinical Pharmacy
University of California, San Diego
Skaggs School of Pharmacy and Pharmaceutical Sciences
Ambulatory Care Pharmacist Specialist
Veterans Affairs San Diego Healthcare System
La Jolla, California

Jadwiga Najib, BS, PharmD
Professor of Pharmacy Practice
Arnold and Marie Schwartz College of Pharmacy
Long Island University
Clinical Psychiatric Pharmacist
St. Luke's/Roosevelt Hospital Center
New York, New York

Robert Nelson, PharmD, BCPS (AQ-ID)
Assistant Professor
North Dakota State University College of Pharmacy
Nursing & Allied Sciences
Clinical Pharmacy Manager
MeritCare Health System
Fargo, North Dakota

Jacob A. Ninan, MD
Hematology/Oncology Fellow
University of Wisconsin Hospitals and Clinics
Madison, Wisconsin

Jacqueline L. Olin, MS, PharmD, BCPS
Associate Professor of Pharmacy
Wingate University School of Pharmacy
Wingate, North Carolina

Keith M. Olsen, PharmD, FCCP, FCCM
Professor and Chair
Department of Pharmacy Practice
College of Pharmacy
University of Nebraska Medical Center
Critical Care Specialist
The Nebraska Medical Center
Omaha, Nebraska

Victor A. Padron, RPe, PhD
Associate Professor of Pharmacy Sciences
Creighton University School of Pharmacy and Health Professions
Creighton University Medical Center
Omaha, Nebraska

Emily Farthing Papineau, PharmD, BCPS
Assistant Professor of Pharmacy Practice
Butler University College Pharmacy and Health Sciences
Clinical Pharmacy Specialist
Community Family Medical Center
Indianapolis, Indiana

Todd Pillen, PA-C/SA, MPAS
Master of Physician Assistant Sciences
Children's Healthcare of Atlanta
Liver Transplant Department
Atlanta, Georgia

Charles D. Ponte, PharmD, BC-ADM, BCPS, CDE, FAPhA, FASHP, FCCP
Professor of Clinical Pharmacy and Family Medicine
West Virginia University Robert C. Byrd Health Sciences Center
Schools of Pharmacy and Medicine
Morgantown, West Virginia

Kalen B. Porter, PharmD, BCPS, AE-C
Clinical Assistant Professor
University of Georgia College of Pharmacy
Clinical Pharmacy Specialist
Pediatrics
Medical College of Georgia Health Inc.
Augusta, Georgia

Michael D. Reed, PharmD, FCCP, FCP
Professor and Associate Chair
Department of Pediatrics
Northeastern Ohio Universities Colleges of Medicine and Pharmacy
Director
Division of Clinical Pharmacology/Toxicology and The Clinical Research Center
Children's Hospital Medical Center of Akron
Akron, Ohio

Kathleen Reeve, DrPH, MSN, ANP-BC, AOCN
Associate Professor
University of Texas Health Science Center at Houston
Adult Nurse Practitioner
University of Houston Downtown
Houston, Texas

Randolph E. Regal, BS, PharmD
Clinical Assistant Professor
University of Michigan College of Pharmacy
Clinical Pharmacist
Adult Internal Medicine
University of Michigan Hospitals and Health Centers
Ann Arbor, Michigan

James Roch, MPAS, PA-C
Assistant Professor
Midwestern University Physician Assistant Professor
    Program
Physician Assistant
Nextcare Urgent Care
Glendale, Arizona

Carol J. Rollins, MS, RD, PharmD, BCNSP
Clinical Associate Professor
The University of Arizona College of Pharmacy
Coordinator, Nutrition Support Team
University Medical Center
Tucson, Arizona

Warren E. Rose, PharmD
Assistant Professor of Pharmacy
University of Wisconsin School of Pharmacy
Pharmacy Practice Division
Madison, Wisconsin

Polly Royal, DNP
Clinical Assistant Professor
Purdue University
West Lafayette, Indiana

Celeste Nicole Rudisill, PharmD
Clinical Assistant Professor
South Carolina College of Pharmacy–USC Campus
Clinical Specialist, Infectious Diseases
Palmetto Health Richland
Columbia, South Carolina

Maha Saad, PharmD, CGP, BCPS
Assistant Clinical Professor
St. John's University
College of Pharmacy and Allied Health Professions
Clinical Coordinator
Long Island Jewish Medical Center
New Hyde Park, New York

JoAnne M. Saxe, RN, ANP, MS
Health Sciences Clinical Professor
University of California San Francisco School of Nursing
Department of Community Health Systems
Adult Nurse Practitioner
Glide health Services
San Francisco, California

Denise M. Schentrup, DNP, ARNP-BC
Clinical Assistant Professor
University of Florida
College of Nursing
Gainesville, Florida

Laura S. Schlesselman, PharmD
Assistant Clinical Professor and Director of Assesment and
    Accreditation
University of Connecticut School of Pharmacy
Storrs, Connecticut

Bradley W. Shinn, PharmD
Associate Professor of Pharmacy Practice
University of Findlay College of Pharmacy
Findlay, Ohio

Catherine Neal Shull, PA-C, MPAS
Instructor
Department of Physicians Assistant Studies
Wake Forest University School of Medicine
Physician Assistant
Wake Forest University Family Physicians
Wake Forest University Health Sciences
Winston-Salem, North Carolina

Douglas Slain, PharmD, BCPS, FCCP
Associate Professor
West Virginia University School of Pharmacy
Anti-infective Specialist
West Virginia University Hospitals
Morgantown, West Virginia

Candace Smith, PharmD
Associate Clinical Professor
Chair
Clinical Pharmacy Practice Department
St. John's University College of Pharmacy and Allied Health
    Professions
Coordinator of Pharmacokinetics
ICU Specialist
Neurology Specialist
Long Island Jewish Medical Center
Queens, New York

Jacqueline Jordan Spiegel, MS, PA-C
Assistant Professor
Physician Assistant
Midwestern University
Glendale, Arizona

Darcie D. Streetman, PharmD
Adjunct Clinical Assistant Professor
University of Michigan College of Pharmacy
Clinical Pediatric Pharmacist
University of Michigan Hospitals
Ann Arbor, Michigan

Shawn Scott Sutton, PharmD, BCPS
Associate Clinical Professor
South Carolina College of Pharmacy
University of South Carolina
Clinical Pharmacist
Medicine and Infectious Diseases
Dorn Veterans Affairs Medical Center
Columbia, South Carolina

Joseph M. Swanson, PharmD, BCPS
Assistant Professor of Clinical Pharmacy
University of Tennessee College of Pharmacy
Memphis, Tennessee

Marc A. Sweeney, PharmD, MDiv
Dean and Professor of Pharmacy Practice
Cedarville University School of Pharmacy
Cedarville, Ohio

Javad Tafreshi, PharmD, BCPS, AQ Cardiology
Professor
Loma Linda University School of Pharmacy
Loma Linda University Medical Center
Loma Linda, California

Damary C. Torres, BS, PharmD
Associate Clinical Professor
St. John's University
Clinical Pharmacy Specialist
Winthrop University Hospital
Queens, New York

Tanya Vadala, PharmD
Instructor
Albany College of Pharmacy and Health Sciences
Clinical Pharmacist
Hannaford Bros. Co.
Albany, New York

Lee Vermeulen, RPh, MS, FCCP
Clinical Professor
University of Wisconsin School of Pharmacy
Madison, Wisconsin

Catherine A. Voge, RN, MS, AOCN
Clinical Assistant Professor
University of Wisconsin School of Nursing
Madison, Wisconsin

Christine Marie Walko, PharmD, BCOP
Assistant Professor
Hematology and Oncology
University of North Carolina School of Pharmacy
Institute of Pharmacogenomics and Personalized Therapy
Lineberger Comprehensive Cancer Center
Chapel Hill, North Carolina

Terri M. Wensel, PharmD, BCPS
Assistant Professor
Samford University McWhorter School of Pharmacy
Drug Information Specialist
Samford University Global Drug Information Service
Birmingham, Alabama

Christine Werner, PA-C, PhD, RD
Associate Professor
St. Louis University Physician Assistant Education
Physician Assistant
Registered Dietitian
St. Louis, Missouri

Amy Whitaker, PharmD
Assistant Professor
Virginia Commonwealth University
Richmond, Virginia

Thomas G. White, JD, PA-C
Lecturer
University of New Mexico School of Medicine
Physician Assistant
University of New Mexico
Albuquerque, New Mexico

Mihkaila Maurine Wickline, MN, RN, AOCN
Clinical Faculty
University of Washington School of Nursing
Hematopoietic Stem Cell Transplant Clinical Nurse
    Specialist
Seattle Cancer Care Alliance
Seattle, Washington

Eric A. Wright, PharmD, BCPS
Associate Professor
Wilkes University
Wilkes-Barre, Pennsylvania

Monty Yoder, PharmD, BCPS
Clinical Coordinator
Wake Forest University Baptist Medical Center
Winston-Salem, North Carolina

PREFACE

The first edition of *Pharmacotherapy Principles & Practice* received the Medical Book Award, Healthcare Professionals Category, from the American Medical Writers Association. We credit this award to our outstanding team of authors, reviewers, and assistants who worked tirelessly to deliver a quality pharmacotherapy textbook.

The second edition, with fully updated clinical content, additional chapters, and enhanced features, is designed to prepare the next generation of pharmacists, nurse practitioners, and physician assistants. Now more than ever, health care practitioners who design, implement, monitor, and evaluate medication therapy bear an important responsibility to their patients and society. Development of these practice abilities requires an integration of knowledge, skills, attitudes, beliefs, and values that can be acquired only through a structured learning process that includes classroom work, independent study, mentorship, and, ultimately, direct involvement in the care of patients.

Pharmacotherapy Principles & Practice is designed to meet the classroom and independent study needs of today's learners in the health care professions. The first edition was accepted enthusiastically by pharmacy, nursing, and physician assistant schools. Chapters are written by content experts and reviewed critically by pharmacists, nurse practitioners, physician assistants, and physicians who are authorities in their fields. The book is written in a concise style that facilitates in-depth understanding of essential concepts. The disease states and treatments discussed focus on those disorders most often seen in practice.

The second edition of *Pharmacotherapy Principles & Practice* contains 102 chapters. The Introduction chapter is followed by three new chapters on pediatrics, geriatrics, and palliative care. The remainder of the book consists of 98 disease-based chapters that review disease etiology, epidemiology, pathophysiology, and clinical presentation, followed by clear therapeutic recommendations for drug selection, dosing, and patient monitoring. The following features in *Pharmacotherapy Principles & Practice* were designed in collaboration with educational design specialists to enhance learning and retention:

- *Structured learning objectives* are included at the beginning of each chapter, with information in the text that corresponds to each learning objective identified by a vertical rule with a circle in the margin, allowing the reader to find content related to each objective quickly.

- *Key concepts related to patient assessment and treatment* are listed at the beginning of each chapter to help focus learning. Numbered icons are used throughout the chapter to identify content that develops these concepts.

- *Patient encounters* are distributed throughout each chapter to facilitate critical thinking skills and lend clinical relevance to the scientific foundation provided. This feature has been expanded in the second edition.

- *Patient care and monitoring guidelines* are placed near the end of each chapter to assist students in their general approach to assessing, treating, and monitoring patients for therapeutic response and adverse events.

- *Up-to-date literature citations* for each chapter are provided to support treatment recommendations.

- *Key references and readings* provide a mechanism to acquire a deeper understanding of the subject matter.

- *Tables, figures, text boxes, and algorithms are used liberally* to enhance understanding of pathophysiology, clinical presentation, drug selection, pharmacokinetics, and patient monitoring.

- *Medical abbreviations and their meanings* are placed at the end of each chapter to facilitate learning the accepted shorthand used in real-world medical practice.

- *A glossary of medical terms* is included as an appendix to the book; the first use of each glossary term in a chapter appears in bold font.

- *Self-assessment questions and answers for each chapter* are located in the Online Learning Center to evaluate student learning.

- *Laboratory values are expressed as both conventional units and Systemè International (SI) units* to facilitate learning by those in countries where these units of measure are used.

- *Appendices* contain: (1) conversion factors and anthropometrics; (2) common laboratory tests and their reference ranges; and (3) common medical abbreviations.

Enhancements found in the second edition include:

- *Additional drug dosing guidelines for renal failure and hepatic failure.*

- *More drug dosing information for special populations (e.g., pediatric and geriatric patients).*

- *Issues related to cultural competency in patient encounters.*

- *Incorporation of pharmacogenomic information as appropriate.*

The Online Learning Center at www.ChisholmPharmaco therapy.com provides complete reference lists, self-assessment questions, a testing center that has the ability to grade and provide immediate feedback on the self-assessment questions as well as reporting capabilities, and other features designed to support learning.

We would like to acknowledge the commitment and dedication of the more than 170 contributing authors and more than 110 reviewers of the chapters contained in this text. We also would like to thank the many educators who have adopted this text in their courses. We also extend our thanks to McGraw-Hill Medical, especially Michael Weitz, Peter Boyle, and Laura Libretti, as well as the support teams at our individual universities including Christina Spivey, Tricia Pierre, and Barb Beinborn for their dedication to this project. Finally, we thank those students, practitioners, and educators who provided feedback on the first edition to help us make the second edition even better.

The Editors
March 2010

Part I

Basic Concepts of Pharmacotherapy Principles and Practice

1 Introduction

Jack E. Fincham

INTRODUCTION

Many roles are assigned to health professionals; the daily fulfillment of these roles in an exemplary fashion is the hallmark of health professional practice and delivery of health care to patients in the United States. Patients are thus well served, and fellow health professionals share knowledge and expertise specific to their profession. Despite this, many problems remain in the U.S. health care system; there are 46 million uninsured individuals in the United States, representing between 16% and 17% of the population. Many more in our midst are underinsured. They may have coverage after a fashion, but the deductibles, co-pays, and monthly payments for insurance create an economic dilemma for individuals each time they seek care or pay premiums. According to the U.S. Centers for Medicare and Medicaid Services, National Health Expenditure data, well over $2.2 trillion was spent on health care in the United States during 2007 amounting to $7,400 per person, some of it no doubt unnecessarily so.[1]

The use of medications in the health care system provides enormous help to many; lives are saved or enhanced, and lifespans are lengthened. Many other uses of medications lead to significant side effects, worsening states of health, and premature deaths. So, how to separate these disparate pictures of drug use outcomes? You, within your practices and within your networks in the health workplace, can help to promote the former and diminish the latter. The authors of the chapters in this book have written sterling chapters that can empower you to positively influence medication use.

DRUG USE IN THE HEALTH CARE SYSTEM

Spending on drugs, as a percentage of what was spent on health care in total, increased from 5.8% to 8.5% from 2005 to 2006.[2] This amounts to a percentage increase of 47% in 1 year. Drivers for this significant increase include increasing available technologies, increasing numbers of patients and prescriptions per patient, and an increasing number of seniors taking advantage of the Medicare Part D Drug Benefit.[2] Generic drug use accounts for over 50% of prescriptions filled in the United States, but, as a percentage of expenditures on drugs in total, remains less than 30%. Brand-name drug purchases fuel the increase in spending on drugs as evidenced by the 2006 data.[2]

There are significant numbers of medications used daily in the United States. Over one decade (from 1997 to 2007) prescriptions purchased zoomed from 2.2 billion to 3.8 billion.[3] The average number of prescriptions per capita in the United States rose from 8.9 in 1997 to 12.6 in 2007.[3] Problems occurring with the use of drugs can include:

- Medication errors
- Suboptimal drug, dose, regimen, dosage form, and duration of use
- Unnecessary drug therapy
- Therapeutic duplication
- Drug–drug, drug–disease, drug–food, or drug–nutrient interactions
- Drug allergies
- Adverse drug effects, some of which are preventable

Clinicians are often called upon to identify, resolve, and prevent problems that occur due to undertreatment, overtreatment, or inappropriate treatment. Individuals can purchase medications through numerous outlets. Over-the-counter (OTC) medications can be purchased in pharmacies, supermarkets, convenience stores, via the Internet, and through any number of additional outlets. OTCs are widely used by all age groups. Prescription medications can be purchased through traditional channels (community chain and independent pharmacies), from mail-order pharmacies, through the Internet, from physicians, from health care institutions, and elsewhere. Herbal remedies are marketed and sold in numerous outlets. The monitoring of the positive and negative outcomes of the use of these drugs, both prescription and OTC, can be disjointed and incomplete. Clinicians and health professions students need to take ownership of these problems and improve patient outcomes resulting from drug use.

It is important to realize that, although clinicians are the gatekeepers for patients to obtain prescription drugs, patients can obtain prescription medications from numerous sources. Patients may also borrow from friends, relatives, or even casual acquaintances. In addition, patients obtain OTC medications from physicians through prescriptions, on advice from pharmacists and other health professionals, through self-selection, or through the recommendations of friends or acquaintances. Through all of this, it must be recognized that there are both formal (structural) and informal (word-of-mouth) components at play. Health professionals may or may not be consulted regarding the use of medications, and in some cases are unaware of the drugs patients are taking. In addition, herbal remedies or health supplements may be taken without the knowledge or input of a health professional.

External variables may greatly influence patients and their drug-taking behaviors. Coverage for prescribed drugs allows those with coverage to obtain medications with varying cost sharing requirements. However, many do not have insurance coverage for drugs or other health-related needs. With the advent of Medicare Part D coverage for outpatient prescription medications, we have seen more of the elderly with access to needed therapy—more than ever before.[4]

Self-Medication

Self-medication can be broadly defined as a decision made by a patient to consume a drug with or without the approval or direction of a health professional. The self-medication activities of patients have increased dramatically in the late 20th and early 21st centuries. Many factors affecting patients have continued to fuel this increase in self-medication. There are ever increasing ways to purchase OTC medications. There have been many prescription items switched to OTC classification in the last 50 years, which is dramatically and significantly fueling the rapid expansion of OTC drug usage. In addition, patients are increasingly becoming comfortable with self-diagnosing and self-selection of OTC remedies. In many studies,[5] self-medication with nonprescribed therapies exceeds the use of prescription medications in the patient groups assessed.

Patients' use of self-selected products has the potential to provide enormous benefits.[6] Through the rational use of drugs, patients may avoid more costly therapies or expenditures for other professional services. Self-limiting conditions, and even some chronic health conditions (e.g., allergies and dermatologic conditions), if appropriately treated through patient self-medication, allow the patient to have a degree of autonomy in health care decisions.

Compliance Issues

Patient noncompliance with prescription regimens is one of the most understated problems in the health care system. The effects of noncompliance have enormous ramifications for patients, caregivers, and health professionals. Noncompliance is a multifaceted problem with a need for interprofessional, multidisciplinary solutions. Interventions that are organizational (how clinics are structured), educational (patient counseling, supportive approach), and behavioral (impacting health beliefs and expectations) are necessary. Noncompliance leads to lack of control of hypertension and a high discrepancy in how patients respond to therapies.[7] Helping to identify psychosocial interventions, which engage patients to self-manage their therapies, has proven efficacy.[7] Acknowledging the barriers that people perceive in complying helps to identify how to assist patients to overcome these distracters.[7] Compliant behavior can be enhanced through your actions with the patients for whom you provide care. Many times what is necessary is referral to specific clinicians for individualized treatment and monitoring to enhance compliance. The case histories provided in this text will allow you to follow what others have done in similar situations to optimally help patients succeed in improving compliance rates and subsequent positive health outcomes.

Drug Use by the Elderly

Various components of drug use in the elderly are worth noting. Problems with health literacy (i.e., the understanding of medical terminology and directions from providers) are more common among the elderly.[8] The burgeoning population of the elderly, coupled with their lack of health literacy, means that this issue will become even more problematic in the future.[9]

Over the next decade, seniors will spend $1.8 trillion on prescription medications. Medicare proposals to provide a drug benefit for seniors have been suggested to cost $400 billion over a 10-year period. Thus, the most elaborate of the current drug programs will pay only 22% of seniors' drug costs. Enhanced use of pharmacoeconomic tenets to select appropriate therapy, while considering cost and therapeutic benefits for seniors and others, will become even more crucial for clinicians in the future.

Unnecessary drug therapy and over medication are problems with drug use in the elderly. A joint effort by health professionals working together is the best approach to aiding seniors in achieving optimal drug therapy. Evaluation of all medications taken by seniors at each patient visit can help prevent polypharmacy from occurring.[10]

IMPACTING THE PROBLEMS OF DRUG USE
Medication Errors

There is more glaring issue in medication use and monitoring than the need to reduce medication errors. Untold morbidity and mortality occur due to the many errors occurring in medication use. Studies have shown that reconciling the medications that patients take, with coordination by various caregivers providing care, can help reduce medication errors in patient populations.[11] Current changes in how drugs are prescribed, such as electronic prescribing, barcode identification of patients, and electronic medication records, can all help reduce medication errors.[12,13] As these technologies are increasingly used, the benefits will expand.

The incorporation of three key interventions (computerized physician order entry [CPOE], additional staffing, and bar coding) have been shown in an institutional setting to help reduce medication errors.[13] Being able to track drug ordering, dispensing, and administration electronically has been shown to be cost effective in the long run.[14] Nurses and office staff have been proven as a valuable resource for reporting prescribing errors, especially with ongoing reminders to scrutinize orders.[15]

The Epidemic of Prescribed Drug Abuse

According to data from the U.S. National Institute on Drug Abuse, in 2006, "approximately 7 million persons were current users of psychotherapeutic drugs taken nonmedically (2.8% of the U.S. population)."[16] The main classes of drugs abused that were obtained via legitimate channels through prescribers and pharmacies include:

- Pain relievers—5.2 million
- Tranquilizers—1.8 million
- Stimulants—1.2 million
- Sedatives—0.4 million[15]

The main source for these drugs is the family medicine cabinet. The abuse of prescription medications by adolescents is an ascending problem that all health professionals must address and work together to try to lessen in intensity.

SUMMARY

Health professionals are at a crucial juncture as we face an uncertain, yet promising future. Technological advances, including electronic prescribing, may stem the tide of medication errors and inappropriate prescribing. These technological enhancements for physician order entry (via personal data assistants or through web access to pharmacies) have been implemented to reduce drug errors. The skills and knowledge that enable effective pharmacotherapy practice have never been more daunting among the numerous health professions. Sophisticated computer technology can further empower health professionals to play an ever increasing and effective role in helping patients and fellow health professionals to practice safe and effective medicine.

This book provides a thorough analysis of common disease states, discussion of therapies to treat these conditions, and specific advice to provide to patients to help them self-medicate when appropriate and safe to do so. The use of material in this text, which incorporates materials written by some of the finest minds in pharmacy practice and education, can enable the reader to play a crucial role in improving the drug use process for patients, providers, payers, and society. The purpose of this book is to help hone your skills, so you can make a real improvement in the therapies you provide to your patients. Current and future clinicians can rely on the information laid out here to enhance your knowledge and allow you to assist your patients with the sound advice that they expect you to provide. Use the text, case histories, and numerous examples detailed here to expand your therapeutic skills, and to help positively impact your patients in the years to come.

You can help to reverse medication related problems, improve outcomes of care both clinically and economically, and enable drug use to meet stated goals and objectives. This text provides a thorough analysis and summary of treatment options for commonly occurring diseases and the medications or alternative therapies used to successfully treat these conditions.

Abbreviations Introduced in This Chapter

CPOE   Computerized physician order entry
OTC   Over-the-counter

REFERENCES

1. U.S. Centers for Medicare and Medicaid Services, National Health Expenditures. Washington, DC, January 9, 2009. *http://www.cms.hhs.gov/NationalHealthExpendData/*
2. Catlin A, Cowan C, Hartman M, Heffler S. National health spending in 2006: A year of change for prescription drugs. Health Aff 2008;27(1): 14–29.
3. Kaiser Family Foundation Washington, DC, September, 2008. Prescription Drug Trends, Fact Sheet (#3057-07), *http://kff.org/rxdrugs/upload/3057_07.pdf.*
4. Fincham JE. Pharmacy curricula and bellwether changes in payment for pharmacy practice services. Am J Pharm Educ 2005;69(3):392–393.
5. Johnson G, Helman C. Remedy or cure? Lay beliefs about over-the-counter medicines for coughs and colds. Br J Gen Pract. 2004;54(499): 98–102.
6. Hughes CM, McElnay JC, Fleming GF. Benefits and risks of self medication. Drug Safety 2001;24(14):1027–1037.
7. Vrijens B, Vincze G, Kristanto P, Urquhart J, Burnier M. Adherence to prescribed antihypertensive drug treatments: Longitudinal study of electronically compiled dosing histories. BMJ 2008;336(7653):1114–1117.
8. Williams A, Manias E, Walker R. Interventions to improve medication adherence in people with multiple chronic conditions: A systematic review. J Adv Nurs 2008;63(2):132–143.
9. Parker RM, Ratzan SC, Lurie N. Health literacy: A policy challenge for advancing high-quality health care. Health Aff 2003;22(4):147–153.
10. Hajjar ER, Cafiero AC, Hanlon JT. Polypharmacy in elderly patients. Am J Geriatr Pharmacother 2007;5:345–351.
11. Delate T, Chester EA, Stubbings TW, Barnes CA. Clinical outcomes of a home-based medication reconciliation program after discharge from a skilled nursing facility. Pharmacotherapy 2008;28:444–452.
12. Fincham JE. e-prescribing: The electronic transformation of medicine. Sudbury MA: Jones and Bartlett Publishers, Inc. 2009.
13. Franklin BD, O'Grady K, Donyai P, Jacklin A, Barber N. The impact of a closed-loop electronic prescribing and administration system on prescribing errors, administration errors and staff time: A before-and-after study. Qual Saf Health Care 2007; 16:279–284.
14. Karnon J, McIntosh A, Dean J, et al. Modelling the expected net benefits of interventions to reduce the burden of medication errors. J Health Serv Res Policy 2008;13:85–91.
15. Kennedy AG, Littenberg B, Senders JW. Using nurses and office staff to report prescribing errors in primary care. Int J Qual Health Care 2008;20:238–245.
16. U.S. National Institute on Drug Abuse, Topics in Brief, Prescription Drug Abuse March 2008. *http://www.nida.nih.gov/pdf/tib/prescription.pdf.*

2 Geriatrics

Jeannie K. Lee, Damian M. Mendoza,
M. Jane Mohler, and Susan J. Morris

LEARNING OBJECTIVES

● **Upon completion of the chapter, the reader will be able to:**

1. Explain the growth pattern of the elderly population.
2. Discuss age-related pharmacokinetic and pharmacodynamic changes.
3. Identify drug-related problems and associated morbidities commonly experienced by elderly.
4. Describe major components of geriatric assessment.
5. Recognize multidisciplinary patient care functions in various geriatric practice settings.

KEY CONCEPTS

❶ Population aging is an incontrovertible trend.

❷ Older Americans use considerably more health care services than younger Americans, and their health care needs are often complex.

❸ All four components of pharmacokinetics—absorption, distribution, metabolism, and excretion—are affected by aging, the most clinically important and consistent being the reduction of renal elimination of drugs.

❹ In general, the pharmacodynamic changes that occur in the elderly tend to increase their sensitivity to drug effects.

❺ Comorbidities and polypharmacy complicate elderly health status, particularly when polypharmacy includes inappropriate medications that lead to drug-related problems.

❻ Elderly patients are at greater risk for medication nonadherence due to high prevalence of multiple comorbidities and polypharmacy use leading to complex regimens.

❼ The clinical approach to assessing older adults frequently goes beyond a traditional "history and physical" used in general internal medicine practice.

❽ Considering geriatric patients' vision, hearing, swallowing, cognitive impairment, motor impairment, and education and literacy levels during the education sessions can lead to successful drug regimen adherence.

❾ Long-term care geriatric practices emphasize the interdisciplinary team approach.

The continual growth of the aging population requires that health care professionals gain knowledge specific to meeting the needs of this patient group. Despite the availability and benefit of the numerous pharmacotherapies to treat their diseases, elderly patients often experience various drug-related problems resulting in additional morbidities. Therefore, it is essential for clinicians serving older adults in diverse health care settings to understand epidemiology of aging, age-related physiologic changes, drug-related problems prevalent in elderly, comprehensive geriatric assessment, and multidisciplinary approaches to geriatric care.

EPIDEMIOLOGY AND ETIOLOGY

As humans age, they are at increasingly elevated risk of disease, disability, and death primarily for three reasons: (a) genetic predisposition, (b) reduced immunological surveillance, and (c) the accumulated effects of physical, social, environmental, and behavioral exposures over the life course. Human relationships, social conditions, and networks interact with these accumulating exposures, and differences in time and place influence health outcomes by age cohort. Combined, these factors result in considerable variation in health states and health care requirements, by age. All elders experience increasing vulnerability and homeostenosis. Although resilient elders are able to successfully maintain high levels of physical and cognitive functioning, avoid chronic conditions, and remain socially engaged, others suffer functional decline, frailty, disability, or death. There is an urgent need for all clinicians to better understand the epidemiology of aging in order that health care needs of the elderly can be comprehensively addressed, and so that safe, quality services can be provided efficiently to optimize functioning and health-related quality of life for the aged.[1]

Sociodemographics

▶ Population

❶ *Population aging is an incontrovertible trend.* In 2006, 37 million U.S. residents were aged 65 and above years (more than 12.4% of the total population), nearly 5.3 million people were aged more than or equal to 85 years (the "oldest-old"), and over 73,000 were centenarians.[2] When the Baby Boomers (those born between 1946 and 1964) begin turning 65 years in 2011, the number of elders will double to 71.5 million in 2030, representing nearly 20% of the total U.S. population.[2] In 2006, there were a total of 21.6 million women and 15.7 million men (a ratio of 138:100, respectively) aged more than or equal to 65 years; this ratio widens as elders age. The oldest-old are projected to increase from 5.3 million in 2006 to nearly 21 million in 2050.[2] In addition, minority elder populations are projected to increase to 8.1 million in 2010 (20.1%), and up to 12.9 million in 2020 (23.6%), including disproportionate increases in Hispanics (254%); Asians and Pacific Islanders (208%); African Americans (147%); and Native Americans, Eskimos, and Aleuts (143%).[2] Surviving Baby Boomers will be proportionally more women, more racially diverse, better educated, and have more financial resources than were elders in previous generations.

▶ Economics

More elders are enjoying higher economic prosperity than ever before, with net worth increasing by nearly 80% for older Americans over the past 20 years. Still, major inequalities persist, with older blacks and those without high school diplomas reporting smaller economic gains, and fewer financial resources.[3] Considerable disparities exist; the 2005 median net worth of households headed by Caucasians greater than or equal to 65 years was $226,900 compared to black elder household net worth of $37,800 (a sixfold difference).[3]

▶ Education and Health Literacy

By 2007, more than 75% of U.S. elders had graduated from high school, and nearly 20% had a bachelor's degree or higher. Still, substantial educational differences exist among racial and ethnic minorities. While over 80% of non-Hispanic white elders had high school degrees in 2007, only 72% of Asians, 58% of blacks, and 42% of Hispanic elders were graduates. Nearly 40% of people aged more than or equal to 75 years have low health literacy, more than any other age group.[3] Despite these limitations, the Pew Trust reports that over 8 million Americans (22%) aged more than or equal to 65 years increasingly use the Internet,[4] and large health care plans such as the Veterans Administration are increasingly offering online health information to support this need. These advances in literacy are important because communication between health care providers and elders is vitally important in providing quality care, supporting self-care, and in negotiating the health care system.

Health Status

▶ Life Expectancy

Though Americans are living longer than ever before, an estimated average of 78.14 years overall in 2008, U.S. life expectancy lags behind that of many other industrialized nations.[5] There is nearly a 6-year gap between 2008 estimated life expectancy in males (75.29 years) and females (81.13 years).[6] Disparities in mortality persist, with estimated 2008 life expectancy in the white population nearly 5 years higher than that of the black population.[6] More than one-third of U.S. deaths in 2000 were attributed to three risk behaviors: smoking, poor diet, and physical inactivity, accounting for nearly 35% of deaths in 2000 (Table 2–1). Currently, only 9% of Americans over 65 years smoke; however, nearly 54% of men and 21% of women are former smokers.[7] Overweight elders aged 65 to 74 years increased from 57% to 73% in 2004 largely due to inactivity and a diet high in refined foods, saturated fats, and sugared beverages, and deficient in whole grains, fruits, vegetables, nuts, and seeds.[3] Despite the proven health benefits of regular physical activity, more than half of the older population is sedentary; 47% of those aged 65 to 74 years, and 61% over 75 years report no physical activity.[8]

The 2007 National Health Interview Survey indicated that 39% of non-Hispanic, white elders reported "very good" or "excellent" health, compared with 29% of Hispanics, and 24% of blacks.[9] Chronic diseases disproportionately affect older adults and are associated with disability, diminished quality of life, and increased costs for health care and long-term care. About 80% of older adults have at least one chronic condition, and 50% have at least two. The prevalence of certain chronic conditions differs by sex, with women reporting higher levels of arthritis (54% versus 43%), and men reporting higher levels of heart disease (37% versus 26%) and cancer (24% versus 19%).[4] Though many older Americans report multiple chronic health conditions, the rate of functional limitations among elderly has actually declined between 1992 and 2005 from 49% to 42%.[4] Among the 15 leading causes of death, age-adjusted death rates decreased significantly from 2004 to 2005 for the top three leading causes—heart disease (33%), cancer (22%), and stroke (8%),

Table 2–1

Top Five Actual Causes of Death Among Persons of All Ages in the United States, 2000

Actual Cause	Percentage
Tobacco use	18.1
Poor diet and physical inactivity	15.2
Alcohol consumption	3.5
Microbial agents (e.g., influenza, pneumonia)	3.1
Toxic agents (e.g., particulate air pollution, environmental tobacco smoke, radon)	2.3

Adapted from Ref. 5.

though chronic lower respiratory diseases, unintentional injuries, Alzheimer's disease, influenza and pneumonia, hypertension, and Parkinson's disease increased.[5] Figure 2–1 specifies the most common chronic conditions of elders, by sex. Frailty is a common biological syndrome in the elderly. Once frail, elders may rapidly progress toward failure to thrive and death. Only 3% to 7% of elders between the ages of 65 and 75 years are frail, increasing to more than 32% in those aged more than 90 years.[10]

▶ Health Care Utilization and Cost

❷ *Older Americans use considerably more health care services than younger Americans, and their health care needs are often complex.* Although in 2005, hospital stays for those 65 years or older were one-half of what they had been in 1970 (5.5 versus 12.6 days), they accounted for over 65% of hospitalizations overall, with longer lengths of stay corresponding to increasing age.[11] Nine persons per 1,000 aged 65 to 74 years lived in nursing homes in 2004, compared with 36 of 1,000 aged 75 to 84 years, and 139 of 1,000 aged 85 years or older;[11] as the aged live longer, more will require institutional care. After adjusting for inflation, health care costs increased significantly among older Americans from $8,644 in 1992 to $13,052 in 2004, three to five times greater than the cost for someone younger than 65 years. Medicare spending has grown nearly ninefold in the past 25 years, to over $507 billion in 2008, and Medicare roles are expected to increase to $78 million by 2030.[4]

By knowing and applying the epidemiology of aging, clinicians can better understand the multiple points of potential pharmaceutical intervention to postpone disease, disability, and mortality, to avoid error, and to promote health, functioning, and health-related quality of life.

Patient Encounter 1

JM is a 69-year-old Hispanic male who understands English, speaks English fairly well, but does not read. He came into the Geriatric Primary Care Clinic for a cholesterol screening because he "has been eating bad food" for over 10 years and not exercising. He smokes one pack of cigarettes and drinks two to three beers a day. He takes a "baby aspirin" daily ever since he suffered a "mini-stroke" 2 years ago. His other medical conditions include hypertension, arthritis, chronic obstructive pulmonary disease, allergies, and Parkinson's disease. He was hospitalized for pneumonia 2 months ago. He takes nine chronic medications including his inhalers.

What information is consistent with epidemiology of aging?

Which of JM's medical conditions are commonly found in older adults?

What additional information do you need before recommending drug therapy for JM?

AGE-RELATED CHANGES

In basic terms, pharmacokinetics is what the body does to the drug, whereas pharmacodynamics is what the drug does to the body. **❸** *All four components of pharmacokinetics—absorption, distribution, metabolism, and excretion—are affected by aging, the most clinically important and consistent being the reduction of renal elimination of drugs.*[12] As people age, they become frailer and are more likely to experience altered and variable drug pharmacokinetics and pharmacodynamics than younger patients. Even though this alteration is influenced more by a patient's clinical state

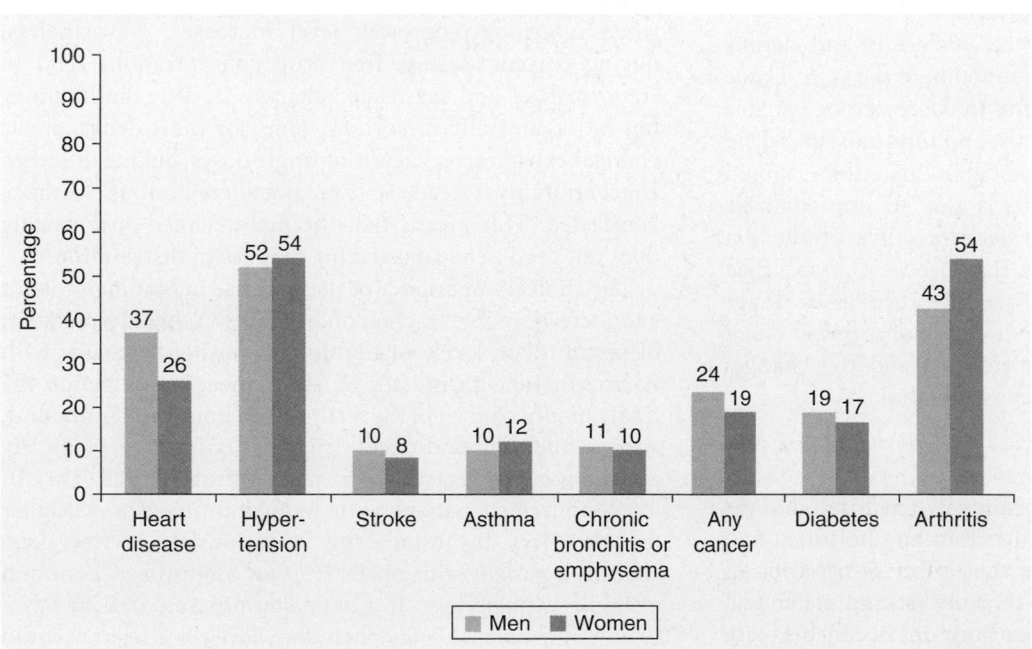

FIGURE 2–1 Percentage of people aged 65 years and over who reported having selected chronic conditions, by sex, 2005 to 2006. Note: Data are based on 2-year average from 2005 to 2006. Reference population: These data refer to the civilian noninstitutionalized population. (From Centers for Disease Control and Prevention, National Center for Health Statistics, National Health Interview Survey.)

than their chronological age, the older patient is more likely to be malnourished and suffering from diseases that affect pharmacokinetics and pharmacodynamics.[13] An example is the greater impact chronic, uncontrolled diabetes has on reducing renal function than the age-related decline. Clinicians have the responsibility to use pharmacokinetic and pharmacodynamic principles to improve the care of elderly patients and avoid harmful side effects of the drugs used.

Pharmacokinetic Changes

▶ Absorption

Multiple changes occur throughout the GI tract with aging, but there is little evidence that drug absorption is significantly altered. The changes include decreases in overall surface of the intestinal epithelium, gastric acid secretion, and splanchnic blood flow.[12] Peristalsis is weaker and also gastric emptying is delayed. These changes slow absorption in the stomach, especially for enteric-coated and delayed-release preparations. Despite the decreased rate, the extent of absorption is not significantly altered. Similarly, reduced gastric acid with aging has not been shown to affect drug absorption. Relative achlorhydria and reduction in intrinsic factor production are caused by atrophy of gastric cells in the stomach. These changes can decrease the absorption of nutrients such as vitamin B_{12}, calcium, and iron.[13]

The majority of medications are absorbed by passive diffusion in the GI tract. Drugs that require passive diffusion have a slower absorption in the elderly due to decreased jejunal surface area and reduced splanchnic blood flow. Delayed absorption may lead to a longer time required to achieve peak drug effects, but it does not significantly alter the amount of drug absorbed.[12,13] Thus, despite the well-reported changes in gastric motility and blood flow with aging, the efficiency of drug movement from the GI tract into circulation is not meaningfully altered.

Aging facilitates atrophy of the epidermis and dermis along with a reduction in barrier function of the skin. Tissue blood perfusion is reduced leading to decreased or variable rates of transdermal, subcutaneous, and intramuscular drug absorption. Therefore, intramuscular injections should generally be avoided in the elderly due to unpredictable drug absorption.[12] Additionally, because saliva production decreases with age, medications that need to be absorbed rapidly by the buccal mucosa are absorbed at a slower rate.[13] However, for the majority of drugs, absorption is not significantly changed in elderly patients and the changes described above are clinically inconsequential.[14]

▶ Distribution

Elderly patients can undergo significant structural changes in the body that alter drug distribution, half-life, and duration of action. Main factors that affect distribution of drugs in the body are changes in body fat and water and changes in protein binding. Lean body mass can decrease by as much as 12% to 19% through loss of skeletal muscle in the elderly. Thus, blood levels of drugs primarily distributed in muscle increase, an example being digoxin. Low body weight, in addition to advanced age, represents a risk factor for overmedication.[13] A concern with frail elderly, having low muscle mass, is the risk of adverse effects when they receive higher doses per unit of body weight. While lean muscle mass decreases, adipose tissue can increase by 14% to 35% in the elderly (18% to 36% in men and 33% to 45% in women). Fat-soluble drugs have an increased volume of distribution (V_d), leading to higher tissue concentrations and prolonged duration of action. Higher V_d leads to an increased half-life and an increase in time required to reach a steady-state serum concentration with regular use. Examples of lipophilic drugs with increased V_d are diazepam (lipophilic benzodiazepine), amiodarone, and verapamil.[12,13]

Total body water decreases by about 10% to 15% by the age of 80 years. This lowers the volume of distribution of hydrophilic drugs leading to higher plasma drug concentrations than in younger adults when equal doses are used.[12,13] Toxic drug effects may be enhanced when dehydration occurs and when the extracellular space is reduced by diuretic use. Examples of commonly used hydrophilic drugs are aspirin, lithium, and ethanol. Elderly also experience a decline in gastric alcohol dehydrogenase, further increasing the peak effect of ethanol. Likewise, plasma albumin concentration decreases by 10% to 20%, though disease and malnutrition contribute more to this decrease than age alone.[12] In patients with an acute illness or malnutrition, rapid decreases in serum albumin can increase drug effects. Examples of highly protein-bound drugs include warfarin, phenytoin, nonsteroidal anti-inflammatory drugs (NSAIDs), furosemide, diazepam, and sulfonylureas.[13] While plasma albumin, which primarily binds acidic drugs, decreases, α_1-acid glycoprotein, which primarily binds alkaline drugs, increases, although this increase is attributed more to inflammatory disease, cancer, or trauma than to aging. Serum concentration of basic drugs such as propranolol and imipramine can be reduced when α_1-acid glycoprotein level increases. Nevertheless, during chronic dosing, free drug concentrations tend to "renormalize" and age-related changes in drug binding may not be as clinically important. Thus for most drugs, above changes can alter peak levels of single doses, but mean serum concentrations at steady state are not altered unless clearance is affected. This means that the maintenance dose usually does not need to be adjusted for changes in distribution.[13]

The clinical importance of the decrease in binding proteins and increase in free fraction of drugs lies in the interpretation of serum drug levels of highly protein-bound drugs with narrow therapeutic indices. Most labs measure and report the total amount of drug in the serum, both bound and unbound. As it is the unbound (free) drug that is pharmacologically active, this concentration is more clinically relevant. In a malnourished patient with hypoalbuminemia, a higher percentage of the total drug level consists of free drug than in a patient with normal serum albumin. A common example is phenytoin. If a hypoalbuminemic patient has a low or low-normal total phenytoin level, a clinician could increase the phenytoin dose for greater effect. This may actually cause the free phenytoin concentration to increase to a toxic level.[14]

▶ *Metabolism*

Drug metabolism is affected by age, acute and chronic diseases, and drug–drug interactions. The liver is the primary site of drug metabolism, which undergoes changes with age. The effect of age on hepatic drug metabolism is somewhat controversial, and there is not a consistent decline in the capacity of the liver to metabolize all drugs, but older patients have decreased metabolism of many drugs.[12,14] There is also a decline with age in the liver's ability to recover from injury. Liver mass is reduced by 20% to 30% with advancing age, and hepatic blood flow is decreased by as much as 40%. These changes can drastically reduce the amount of drug delivered to the liver per unit of time, reduce its metabolism, and increase the elimination half-life.[13] Metabolic clearance of some drugs is decreased by 20% to 40% (e.g., amiodarone, amitriptyline, warfarin, and verapamil), but for others it is unchanged. This is partially due to whether the drug has a high or low extraction by the liver. Drugs that have high **extraction ratios** also have significant first-pass metabolism resulting in a higher bioavailability in older adults. For example, the effect of morphine is increased due to a decrease in clearance by around 33%. Similar increases in bioavailability associated with reduced clearance can be seen with propranolol, levodopa, and hydroxymethylglutaryl coenzyme-A (HMG-CoA) reductase inhibitors (statins). Elderly patients may experience a similar clinical response to that of younger patients, but at lower doses.[13] Drugs with a low hepatic extraction are usually not affected by hepatic hemoperfusion.[13]

The effect of aging on liver enzymes (cytochrome P450 system, known as the CYP450 system) may lead to a decreased elimination rate of drugs that undergo oxidative phase-I metabolism, but this is controversial.[13] Originally, it was thought that the CYP450 system was impaired in the elderly, leading to a decrease in drug clearance and increase in serum half-life. Studies have not consistently confirmed this and although there is an age-related increase in half-life of some drugs, it may be attributed to other factors like changes in volume of distribution. Thus, variations in the CYP450 activity may not be due to aging, but due to lifestyle (e.g., smoking), illness, and drug interactions.[13,14] A patient's nutritional status plays a role in drug metabolism as well. Frail elderly have a more diminished drug metabolism than those with healthy body weight.[12] Age does not have an effect on phase-II hepatic metabolism, known as conjugation or glucuronidation, but conjugation is reduced with frailty. Temazepam and lorazepam are examples of drugs that undergo phase-II metabolism.[13]

▶ *Elimination*

The most clinically important pharmacokinetic change in the elderly is the decrease in renal drug elimination.[12] As people age, renal blood flow, renal mass, glomerular filtration rate, filtration fraction, and tubular secretion decrease. After age 40, there is a decrease in the number of functional glomeruli, and renal blood flow declines by approximately 1% yearly. From age 25 to 85 years, average renal clearance declines by as much as 50% and is independent of the effects of disease.[12–14] The effect of age on renal function can be variable and is not always a linear decline.[14] Longitudinal studies have suggested that a percentage (up to 33%) of elderly patients do not experience this age-related decline in renal function. Clinically significant effects of decreased renal clearance include prolonged drug half-life, increased serum drug level, and increased potential for **adverse drug reaction** (ADR).[12] Special attention should be given to renally eliminated drugs with a narrow therapeutic index (e.g., digoxin, aminoglycosides). Monitoring serum concentration and making appropriate dose adjustment for these agents can prevent serious ADR that may result from drug accumulation.[13] It is important to note that despite a dramatic decrease in renal function (creatinine clearance) with aging, serum creatinine may remain fairly unchanged and within normal limits. This is because elderly patients, especially the frail elderly, have decreased muscle mass resulting in less creatinine production for input into circulation.[12,13] Because chronic kidney disease can be overlooked if a clinician focuses only on the serum creatinine value, drugs can be dosed inappropriately.

For reasons stated above, creatinine clearance should always be calculated when starting or adjusting drugs in the elderly. Clearance measure using 24-hour urine collection is impractical, costly, and often done inaccurately. The Cockcroft-Gault equation is the most widely used formula for estimating renal function and adjusting drug doses. It incorporates serum creatinine, age, gender, and weight. See Chapter 25 (Table 25–1) in this book for more details.

$$\text{Creatinine clearance} = \frac{(140 - \text{Age}) \times \text{Weight (kg)}}{\text{Serum creatinine} \times 72} \times (0.85 \text{ if female})$$

This equation is also used by drug manufacturers to determine dosing guidelines. The Cockcroft-Gault equation provided the best balance between predictive ability and bias in a study that compared it to the Modification of Diet in Renal Disease (MDRD) and Jeliffe "bedside" clearance equations.[13] A limitation of the MDRD equation is that it was not validated for patients older than 70 years.[14] Understand that the predictive formulas can significantly overestimate actual renal function, especially in the chronically ill, debilitated elderly.

Pharmacodynamic Changes

Pharmacodynamics refers to the actions of a drug at its target site and the body's response to that drug. Pharmacodynamic changes associated with aging are not as well known as that of pharmacokinetics, but a better understanding of these effects can enhance the quality of medication prescribing. ❹ *In general, the pharmacodynamic changes that occur in the elderly tend to increase their sensitivity to drug effects.* Most pharmacodynamic changes in the elderly are associated with a progressive reduction in homeostatic mechanisms

Patient Encounter 2

KS is a 79-year-old white female who has a long history of seizure disorder. She has been taking phenytoin 100 mg three times a day, but states that her doctor thought she may need to double her dose. She was recently hospitalized for dehydration and is recovering from "low kidney function."

PE:

VS: BP 122/70, P 72, RR 14, T 38.6°C (101.5°F), ht: 5'2" (1.57 m), wt: 55 kg

Labs: Na 140 mEq/L (140 mmol/L), K 4.7 mEq/L (4.7 mmol/L), Cl 99 mEq/L (99 mmol/L), CO_2 25 mEq/L (25 mmol/L), BUN 60 mg/dL (21.4 mmol/L), creatinine 1.8 mg/dL (1.59 micromoles/L), albumin 2.5 g/dL (25 g/L)

What is KS's estimated creatinine clearance?

How does phenytoin serum concentration react to KS's albumin level?

What other factors need to be considered before making phenytoin dosage adjustment in this patient?

and changes in receptor properties. Although the end result of these changes is an increased sensitivity to the effects of many drugs, a decrease in response can also occur.[15] The changes in the receptor site include alterations in binding affinity of the drug, number or density of active receptors at the target organ, structural features, and postreceptor effects (biochemical processes/signal transmission). These include receptors in the adrenergic, cholinergic, and dopaminergic systems, as well as *gamma aminobutyric acid* (GABA) and opioid receptors.[12,13]

▶ Cardiovascular System

Decreased homeostatic mechanisms in elderly patients increase their susceptibility to orthostatic hypotension when taking drugs that affect the cardiovascular system and lower the arterial blood pressure. This is explained by a decrease in arterial compliance and a decreased baroreceptor reflex response, which limits their ability to quickly compensate for postural changes in blood pressure. It has been estimated that as many as 5% to 33% of the elderly experience drug-induced orthostasis. Examples of drugs, other than typical antihypertensives, that have a higher likelihood of causing orthostatic hypotension in geriatric patients are tricyclic antidepressants, antipsychotics, loop diuretics, direct vasodilators, and opioids.[12,13,15] Although older patients have a decreased β-adrenergic receptor function and are less sensitive to β-agonists and β-adrenergic antagonists effects in the cardiovascular system and possibly in the lungs, their response to α-agonists and antagonists is unchanged.[13,15] Increased hypotensive and heart rate response (to lesser degree) to calcium channel blockers (e.g., verapamil) are reported. Increased risk of developing drug-induced QT prolongation and torsades de pointes is also present.[15]

Therefore, clinicians must start medications at low doses and titrate slowly, closely monitoring the patient for any adverse response.

▶ Central Nervous System

Overall, geriatric patients exhibit a greater sensitivity to the effects of drugs that gain access to the CNS. In most cases, lower doses are required for adequate response and patients have a higher incidence of adverse effects. The blood–brain barrier becomes more permeable as people age; thus, more medications can cross the barrier. Examples of problematic medications include benzodiazepines, antidepressants, neuroleptics, and antihistamines. There is a decrease in the number of cholinergic neurons as well as nicotinic and muscarinic receptors, decreased choline uptake from the periphery, and increased acetylcholinesterase.[13,15] The elderly have a decreased ability to compensate for these imbalances in the neurotransmitters, which can lead to movement and memory disorders. Older patients have increased number of dopamine type 2 receptors, which makes them more susceptible to delirium from anticholinergic and dopaminergic drugs. On the other hand, they have reduced number of dopamine and dopaminergic neurons in the *substantia nigra* of the brain resulting in higher incidence of extrapyramidal symptoms from antidopaminergic medications (e.g., antipsychotics).[12,15] Lower doses of opioids provide sufficient pain relief for older patients, whereas conventional doses can cause oversedation and respiratory depression due to increased response to the drug.[12,13,15]

▶ Fluids and Electrolytes

Fluid and electrolyte homeostatic mechanism is decreased in the geriatric population. The elderly experience more severe dehydration with equal amounts of fluid loss compared to younger patients. The multitude of factors involved include decreased thirst and cardiovascular reflexes, decreased fluid intake, decreased ability of the kidneys to concentrate urine, increased atrial natriuretic peptide, decreased aldosterone response to hyperkalemia, and decreased response to antidiuretic hormone. The result is an increased incidence of hyponatremia, hyperkalemia, and prerenal azotemia, especially when the patient is taking a thiazide or loop diuretic (e.g., hydrochlorothiazide, furosemide). Angiotensin-converting enzyme inhibitors also have an increased potential to cause hyperkalemia and acute renal failure, thus the need to start low, titrate slowly, and monitor frequently.[12,15]

▶ Glucose Metabolism

An inverse relationship between glucose tolerance and age has been reported. This is likely due to a reduction in insulin secretion and sensitivity (greater insulin resistance). Consequently, there is an increased incidence of hypoglycemia when using sulfonylureas (e.g., glyburide, glipizide).[12] Due to an impaired autonomic nervous system, elderly patients may have a decreased response to, or awareness of, hypoglycemia (may not experience the sweating, palpitations, or tremors, but instead will experience the neurologic symptoms of syncope, ataxia, confusion, or seizures).

▶ *Anticoagulants*

The geriatric population is more sensitive to anticoagulant effects of warfarin compared to younger people. When similar plasma concentrations of warfarin are attained, there is greater inhibition of vitamin K–dependent clotting factors in older patients than in young. Overall the risk of bleeding is increased in the elderly, and when overanticoagulated, the likelihood of morbidity and mortality is higher. This is further complicated by presence of concomitant herbals/supplements, multiple drug–drug interactions, nonadherence, confusion, and acute illness. Close monitoring of international normalized ratio (INR) and screening for appropriate use is paramount. In contrast, there is no association between age and response to heparin.[12]

DRUG-RELATED PROBLEMS

❺ *Comorbidities and polypharmacy complicate elderly health status, particularly when polypharmacy includes inappropriate medications that lead to drug-related problems.* It is reported that 28% of hospitalizations in older adults are due to medication-related problems including nonadherence and ADRs. Studies using the Beers' criteria indicate that 14% to 40% of the frail elderly are prescribed at least one inappropriate drug, and unnecessary medication use was detected in 44% of older veterans at the time of hospital discharge.[16] Drug-related problems, including ADRs and therapeutic failure, lead to morbidity and mortality in nursing facilities and accrue health care cost of nearly $4 billion yearly.[17] Collaboration among multidisciplinary providers and older patients can minimize adverse drug events, maximize medication adherence, and ensure appropriate therapy.

Polypharmacy

Polypharmacy is defined as taking multiple medications concurrently (some report at least four and others at least five). Polypharmacy is prevalent in older adults who comprise 14% of the U.S. population, but receive 36.5% of all prescription drugs.[16] According to the Centers for Disease Control and Prevention, polypharmacy is the primary cause of drug-related adverse events in older adults. Medication use rises with age, resulting in over 90% of elders in the United States taking at least one medication a week. An estimated 50% of the community-dwelling elderly take five or more medications and 12% of them take 10 or more.[18] Also, common use of dietary supplements and herbal products in this population adds to the polypharmacy. In nursing home settings, patients receiving nine or more chronic medications increased from 17% in 1997 to 27% in 2000.[16] Among various reasons for polypharmacy, an apparent one is a patient receiving multiple medications from different providers who treat the patient's comorbidities. Thus, medication

reconciliation will become increasingly important as aging population continues to grow.

A recent review that analyzed studies aimed at reducing polypharmacy in elderly emphasized complete evaluation of all medications by health care providers at each patient visit to prevent polypharmacy.[19] Efforts should be made to reduce polypharmacy by discontinuation of any medication without an indication. However, clinicians should also understand that appropriate polypharmacy is indicated for patients who have multiple diseases, and support should be provided for optimal adherence. Drug-related problems associated with polypharmacy can be identified by performing a comprehensive medication review during each patient encounter (see Patient Care and Monitoring box).

Inappropriate Prescribing

Inappropriate prescribing is defined as prescribing medications that cause a significant risk of an adverse event when there is an effective and safer alternative. It also includes prescribing a medication outside the bounds of accepted medical standards. The incidence of prescribing potentially inappropriate drugs to elderly patients has been reported to be as high as 12% in those living in the community and 40% in nursing home residents.[20,21] At times, medications are continued long after the initial indication has resolved. The clinician prescribing for older adults must understand the rate of adverse reactions and drug–drug interactions, the evidence available for using a specific medication, and patient use of over-the-counter (OTC) medications and herbal supplements.[20,22]

Screening tools have been developed to help the clinician identify potentially inappropriate drugs. The most utilized and well known is the Beers' criteria, which was first developed in 1991. It was revised in 2003 to include community-dwelling individuals, lists of specific medications to avoid, and warnings regarding disease/medication combinations. It identifies 48 medications and 20 disease/medication combinations that are deemed inappropriate in elderly patients.

Some of the more common medications referred to in the Beers' criteria[23] include the following:

- Amitriptyline (strong anticholinergic and sedative properties)
- Propoxyphene and combination products (side effects of narcotics with similar analgesic benefits to acetaminophen)
- Indomethacin (most CNS side effects of all the NSAIDs)
- Long-acting benzodiazepines like diazepam (increased sedation; risk of falls and fractures)
- Antihistamines like diphenhydramine (confusion and sedation with a prolonged effect)
- Long-term use of full-dose NSAIDs (increased potential to cause GI bleeding, renal failure, hypertension, and heart failure)
- Fluoxetine (long-acting selective serotonin-reuptake inhibitor [SSRI] that causes sleep disturbance, increased agitation and excessive CNS stimulation)

Examples of drug/disease combinations reported as potentially inappropriate are as follows:

- NSAIDs and aspirin 325 mg or higher daily in patients with gastric/duodenal ulcers
- Anticholinergic antihistamines and patients with bladder outlet obstruction or benign prostatic hyperplasia
- Metoclopramide and typical antipsychotics and patients with Parkinson's disease
- Barbiturates, anticholinergics, antispasmodics, and muscle relaxants with cognitive impairment
- Bupropion and seizure disorders (lowers seizure threshold)

As noted above, the consequences of inappropriate prescribing are widespread and vary in severity. It is important to note that these medications are "potentially" inappropriate and alternatives should be used or focused monitoring for adverse effects should be provided. Practical strategies for appropriate medication prescribing include establishing a partnership with patients and caregivers to enable them to understand and self-monitor their medication regimen. Providers should perform drug–drug and drug–disease interaction screening, and use time-limited trials to evaluate the benefits and risks of new regimens.[22]

Undertreatment

Much has been written about the consequences of overmedication and polypharmacy in the elderly. However, underutilization of medications is harmful in the elderly as well, resulting in reduced functioning and quality of life, and increased morbidity and mortality. There are instances when an indicated drug is truly contraindicated appropriately preventing its use, when a lower dose is indicated, or when prognoses dictate withholding of aggressive therapy. Outside of these scenarios, many elders do not receive the therapeutic interventions that would clearly provide benefit. This occurs for many reasons including the belief that treatment of the patient's primary problem is enough intervention, cost, concerns of nonadherence, fear of adverse effects and associated liability, starting low and slow and failing to increase to an appropriate dose, skepticism regarding secondary prevention for elders, or frank ageism. A study found evidence of underprescribing in 64% of older patients, and those on more than eight medications at the highest risk. Interestingly, the lack of proven beneficial therapy was not dependent on age, race, sex, comorbidity, cognitive status, and dependence in activities of daily living.[24] Common categories of geriatric undertreatment are listed in Table 2–2.

A reasoned clinical assessment strategy to weigh the potential benefit versus harm of the older patient's complete medication regimen is required. Once frank contraindications have been dismissed, the patient's (a) goals and preferences, (b) remaining life expectancy, and (c) time until therapeutic benefit will be achieved should be taken into consideration to determine whether the therapy can meet treatment goals. Underprescribing can best be avoided

Table 2–2	
Common Categories of Geriatric Undertreatment	
Therapy	**Concern**
Anticoagulation in patients with atrial fibrillation	Providers may be overly concerned with general risk of bleeding, or the risk of falls if anticoagulated
Malignant and nonmalignant pain complaints or uncontrolled pain	Providers are often hesitant to prescribe opioids due to possible cognitive and bowel side effects, or concerns about addiction, and patients may often be hesitant to take opioids
Antihypertensive therapy	Providers may underestimate the benefit on stroke and cardiovascular events, and/or fail to add the second or third medication needed to attain control
β-Blocker treatment in heart failure	Providers are concerned about complications in high-risk patients despite the substantial evidence of mortality reduction
Statin treatment for hyperlipidemia	Providers may underestimate benefit, or have high concern for adverse events
Treatment of osteopenia/ osteoporosis in men and women at risk of fractures	Providers often fail to screen for bone mineral density and are therefore unprepared to offer treatment

by using careful clinical assessment strategies, improving adherence support, and increasing financial coverage of expensive drugs.

Adverse Drug Reaction

ADR is defined by the World Health Organization as a reaction that is noxious and unintended, which occurs at dosages normally used in humans for prophylaxis, diagnosis, or therapy, increases with polypharmacy. (See the glossary for the American Society of Health-System Pharmacists' definition of an ADR.[25]) Older adults commonly experience ADRs. In fact, ADR is the most frequently occurring drug-related problem among elderly nursing home residents, and the yearly occurrence in outpatient elderly is noted to be 5% to 33%.[26]

Seven predictors of ADRs in older patients have been identified[26]: (a) taking more than four medications; (b) longer than 14-day hospital stay; (c) having more than four active medical problems; (d) general medical unit admission versus geriatric ward; (e) alcohol use history; (f) lower Mini-Mental State Exam score (confusion, dementia); and (g) two to four new medications added during a hospitalization. Similarly, there are four predictors for severe ADRs experienced by the elderly[27]: (a) use of certain medications including diuretics, NSAIDs, antiplatelets, and digoxin; (b) number of drugs taken; (c) age; and (d) comorbidities. Suggested strategies to preventing ADRs in older adults are described in Table 2–3.[27] Particular care must be taken when prescribing drugs that can alter cognition of the elderly, including antiarrhythmics,

Table 2–3
Strategies to Preventing ADRs in Older Adults
• Evaluating comorbidities, frailty, and cognitive function
• Identifying caregivers to take responsibility for medication management
• Evaluating renal function and adjusting doses appropriately
• Monitoring drug effects
• Recognizing that clinical signs or symptoms can be an ADR
• Minimizing number of medications prescribed
• Adapting treatment to patient's life expectancy
• Realizing that self-medication and nonadherence are common and can induce ADRs

From Ref. 27.

Table 2–4	
Factors Influencing Medication Nonadherence	
Three or more chronic medical conditions	Living alone in the community
Five or more chronic medications	Recent hospital discharge
Three times or more per day dosing or 12 or more medication doses per day	Caregiver reliance
Four or more medication changes in past 12 months	Low literacy
Three or more prescribers	Medication cost
Significant cognitive or physical impairments	History of medication nonadherence

From Ref. 31.

antidepressants, antiemetics, antihistamines, anti-Parkinson's, antipsychotics, benzodiazepines, digoxin, histamine-2 receptor antagonists, NSAIDs, opioids, and skeletal muscle relaxants.[21]

One of the most damaging ADRs occurring in older adults is medication-related falls. Falls are associated with poor prognosis ranging from premature institutionalization to early mortality. Extrinsic factors for falling include taking certain medications or polypharmacy. A recent systematic review concluded that psychotropic medications including benzodiazepines, antidepressants, and antipsychotics have strong association to increased risk for falls, where antiepileptics and antihypertensives have weak association.[28] Multifactorial interventions to preventing falls should always involve medication simplification and modification in order to prevent and resolve ADRs.

Nonadherence

"America's other drug problem" is the term given to medication nonadherence by the National Council on Patient Information and Education.[29] Nonadherence to chronic pharmacotherapies is prevalent and escalates health care costs associated with worsening disease and increased hospitalization.[29] Medication adherence is a term describing a patient's medication-taking behavior, generally defined as the extent to which a patient adheres to an agreed regimen derived from collaboration between the patient and their health care provider. The word "adherence" is often preferred over "compliance" because medication compliance implies the patient passively complying to provider's medication orders with no attempts made at collaboration.[30]

❻ *Elderly patients are at greater risk for medication nonadherence due to high prevalence of multiple comorbidities and polypharmacy use leading to complex regimens.* Numerous barriers to optimal medication adherence exist and include patient's lack of understanding, provider's failure to educate, polypharmacy leading to complex regimen and inconvenience, treatment of asymptomatic conditions (such as hypertension and hyperlipidemia), and cost of medications.[30] Factors influencing medication nonadherence are listed in Table 2–4.

Following is a list of six questions that can be asked when assessing medication adherence[32]:

1. How do you take your medications?
2. How do you organize your medications to help you remember to take them?
3. How do you schedule your meal and medication times?
4. How do you pay for your medications?
5. How do you think the medications are working for your condition?
6. How many times in the last week/month have you missed a dose?

Although no one intervention has found to consistently improve adherence, patient-centered, multicomponent interventions such as combining education, convenience aid, and serial follow-up have resulted in positive impact on medication adherence and associated health outcomes.[33] Additionally, there is a need for adherence studies evaluating belief-related variables, including personal and cultural beliefs, in larger and more ethnically diverse samples of older populations.

GERIATRIC ASSESSMENT

The term geriatric assessment is used to describe the interdisciplinary team evaluation of the frail, complex elderly patient. Such a team may include but is not limited to a geriatrician, nurse, pharmacist, case manager/social worker, physical therapist, occupational therapist, speech therapist, psychologist, nutritionist, dentist, optometrist, and audiologist. Assessment may be performed in a centralized geriatric clinic, or by a series of evaluations performed in separate settings. The team may conduct an interdisciplinary case conference to discuss the patient's assessment and plan. For a healthy, active elderly patient, the assessment might require only two to three members of this team, with coordination of care provided by the patient's geriatrician.

Patient Interview

❼ *The clinical approach to assessing older adults frequently goes beyond a traditional "history and physical" used in*

Patient Encounter 3

PW is an 83-year-old African American male who has been living in a long-term care facility for 4 years after his wife passed away. He has been eating one to two meals a day with complaints of trouble swallowing, constipation, depressed mood, and fatigue. He has lost 2 kg in last 6 months and has developed a new coccyx ulcer.

PMH: Hypertension, diabetes, hyperlipidemia, hypothyroidism, Parkinson's disease, osteoarthritis, constipation, allergic rhinitis

FH: Father died of stroke at age 82; mother died of breast cancer at age 67

SH: 40-year smoking history but quit 9 years ago; no alcohol drinking

Allergies: NKDA

Meds: (1) Aspirin 81 mg daily, (2) hydrochlorothiazide 25 mg daily, (3) lisinopril 10 mg twice daily, (4) glipizide 5 mg twice daily, (5) metformin 500 mg twice daily, (6) levothyroxine 25 mcg daily, (7) carbidopa/levodopa 25 mg/100 mg three times daily, (8) ibuprofen 600 mg three times daily, (9) docusate sodium 100 mg twice daily, (10) lorazepam 2 mg twice daily, (11) diphenhydramine 25 mg at bedtime, (12) amitriptyline 10 mg at bedtime

PE: Ht: 5'8″, wt: 65 kg, BMI: 21.8 kg/m²

VS: BP 122/62, P 60, RR 14, T 36.8°C (98.3°F), pain 3/10 (on scale of 0–10)

Labs: Complete metabolic panel is within normal limits; CBC pending

What potential drug-related problems does PW have?

What quality indicators can you identify in this nursing home resident?

What recommendations can be made about his medication regimen?

Table 2–5

ADL and IADL

ADL

Transfers	Dressing	Mobility	Eating
Bathing	Toileting	Grooming	

IADL

Using transportation	If still driving, assess driving ability (including cognitive function, medications that can inhibit ability to drive, vision, neuromuscular conditions that may interfere with reaction time, ability to turn head) at the time of license renewal
Using the telephone	Check for emergency phone numbers located near the telephone
Management of finances	Assess the ability to balance checkbook and pay bills on time
Cooking	Check for safe operation of appliances and cooking tools as well as ability to prepare balanced meals
Housekeeping	Check for decline in cleanliness or neatness
Medication administration	Assess organization skills and adherence

ADL, activities of daily living; IADL, instrumental activities of daily living.

Three item recall
1. Ask the patient if you may test his or her memory.
2. Give the patient 3 words (e.g., apple, table, penny) to repeat and remember.
3. Have the patient repeat the 3 words from memory later (e.g., after the clock drawing test).

Clock drawing test
1. Have the patient draw the face of a clock, including numbers.
2. Instruct the patient to place the hands at a specific time, such as 11:10.

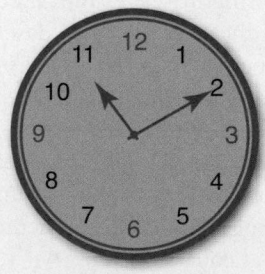
Correct

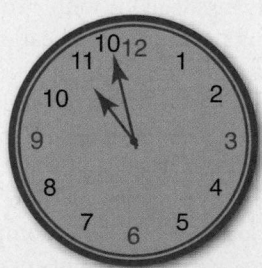
Incorrect hands and inserted number

A positive dementia screen
1. Failure to remember all 3 words.
2. Failure to remember 1-2 words plus an abnormal clock drawing.

FIGURE 2–2 The mini-cog mental status exam. (Adapted from Ref. 35.)

general internal medicine practice.[31] Functional status must be determined, which includes the patient's activities of daily living (ADLs) and instrumental activities of daily living (IADLs). Refer to Table 2–5 for descriptions of ADLs and IADLs. Evidence of declining function in specific organ systems is sought. Of particular importance is cognitive assessment, which may require history gathering from family, friends, or other caregivers, and is important in determination of the patient's competence to consent to medical treatment.[34] The mini-cog mental status exam,[35] shown in Figure 2–2, is a quick tool to assess patient's cognitive impairment. Commonly there is decreased visual acuity, hearing loss, dysphagia, and manual dexterity. Decreased skin integrity, if present, greatly increases risk for pressure ulcers. Sexual function is a sensitive but important area, which should be specifically inquired

Table 2–6
The *Is* of Geriatrics: Common Problems in Older Adults

Immobility	Instability
Isolation	Intellectual impairment
Incontinence	Impotence
Infection	Immunodeficiency
Inanition (malnutrition)	Insomnia
Impaction	Iatrogenesis
Impaired senses	

Reprinted with permission from DiPiro JT, Talbert RL, Yee GC, et al.: Pharmacotherapy: A Pathophysiologic Approach, 7th ed. New York: McGraw-Hill, 2008.

about. Cardiac, renal, hepatic, and digestive insufficiencies can have significant implications for pharmacotherapy. Inadequate nutritional status may lead to weight loss, and impaired functioning at the cellular or organ level as discussed previously. See Table 2–6 for common problems experienced by older adults.

It is important to identify "geriatric syndromes" which may be present in the patient. Frailty, instability and falls, osteoporosis, insomnia, and incontinence impact quality of life and must be recognized. Common diseases such as thyroid dysfunction and depression often present in an atypical manner in the geriatric population as many common conditions may present as delirium. It is also important to assess for caregiver stress and be aware of the support systems the older patient relies on. These may include family, friends, religious and social networks, as well as home health aides, homemakers, or sitters. Without such networks, the older adult may not be able to continue to live independently. Assessment of safety in the home is often necessary for the frail elderly. In addition, look for signs and symptoms of elder abuse, neglect, or exploitation. Health professionals are required to report suspicion of elder mistreatment to Adult Protective Services.[36]

Drug Therapy Monitoring

Geriatric patients often are frail, and have multiple drugs, medical comorbidities, and prescribers. It is essential that there be a single individual, a pharmacist, nurse, or primary care physician, who oversees the patient's drug therapy. The providers need to be aware of the patient's Medicare Part C or D plan, and what type of coverage these plans afford. What is the copayment for generic, preferred, and nonpreferred drugs? Is the patient responsible for all drug costs during the Medicare "donut hole" period? (The first $2,250 of medication is partially subsidized, but the patient pays 100% of the next $2,850.[37]) Many Medicare patients, especially the socioeconomically challenged, have limited understanding of the complex Medicare drug benefit. This problem is compounded when the prescriber also does not understand the patient's insurance program.[38] Providers can

assist patients by prescribing generic medication that are offered through retail pharmacy discount plans ($4 retail pharmacy programs do not bill insurance, so the cost of those medications are not counted toward the $2,250 benefit), and help patients apply for the medication assistance programs offered by drug manufacturers. Particularly challenging in the geriatric population is identifying the cause(s) of nonadherence to medical regimens. Providers assessing elderly patients' medication regimens should keep the following questions in mind:

- Are medications skipped or reduced due to cost?
- Can the patient benefit from sample drugs? Starting a patient on a free drug sample may increase patient costs in the long term, since samples typically are newer, expensive drugs.[38]
- Is there an educational barrier such as low health literacy?
- Does the patient speak English, but only read in another language?
- Can the patient see labels and written instructions?
- Does the patient have hearing problems? Patients with deficits might not admit they cannot hear or understand questions or instructions.
- Can the patient manipulate pill bottles, syringes, inhalers, eye/ear drops?
- Has the patient's cognitive functioning worsened over time such that they can no longer follow the medication regimen?

Homeostenosis and comorbidities require more frequent monitoring for adverse effects: symptoms, abnormal laboratory results, drug interactions, and drug levels—see Table 2–7.

Documentation

Clear, current, and correct medication lists must be available to patients and all individuals involved with their care. It is especially important for geriatric patients to bring their list, or preferably their medication containers, to each visit with medical providers. Medications taken may require verification with the pharmacist, caregivers, or family. Transitions in patient care, such as hospital to subacute nursing facility or home, are points of vulnerability to medication errors because medications may have been deleted or added.[39] It is now standard of care to conduct medication reconciliation upon hospital admission and discharge to facilitate appropriate medication use and documentation.

Patient Education

Poor adherence in the geriatric age group could be related to inadequate patient education. "Ask me 3" cues the patient to ask three important questions of their providers to improve health literacy:

1. What is my main problem?
2. What do I need to do?
3. Why is it important for me to do this?

Table 2–7	
Centers for Medicare and Medicaid Services Guidelines for Monitoring Medication Use	
Drug	**Monitoring**
Acetaminophen (greater than 4 g/day)	Hepatic function tests
Aminoglycosides	Serum creatinine, drug levels
Hypoglycemic agents	Blood sugar levels
Antiepileptic agents (older)	Drug levels
Angiotensin-converting enzyme inhibitors	Potassium levels
Antipsychotic agents	Extrapyramidal adverse effects
Appetite stimulants	Weight, appetite
Digoxin	Serum creatinine, drug levels
Diuretic	Potassium levels
Erythropoiesis stimulants	Blood pressure, iron and ferritin levels, complete blood count
Fibrates	Hepatic function test, complete blood count
Iron	Iron and ferritin levels, complete blood count
Lithium	Drug levels
Niacin	Blood sugar levels, hepatic function tests
Statins	Hepatic function tests
Theophylline	Drug levels
Thyroid replacement	Thyroid function tests
Warfarin	Prothrombin time/international normalized ratio

Reprinted with permission from DiPiro JT, Talbert RL, Yee GC, et al.: Pharmacotherapy: A Pathophysiologic Approach, 7th ed. New York: McGraw-Hill, 2008.

The provider can assess patient grasp of medication instructions by asking the patient to repeat instructions initially and again in 3 minutes.[40]

8 *Considering geriatric patients' vision, hearing, swallowing, cognitive impairment, motor impairment, and education and literacy levels during the education sessions can lead to successful drug regimen adherence.* Specific routes of drug administration, such as metered dose inhalers, ophthalmic/otic drops, and subcutaneous injections, may be difficult for older patients. More time needs to be spent in advising the patient and/or caregivers of potential ADRs and when to notify the provider about ADRs. (See Patient Care and Monitoring box for detailed information regarding patient education.)

GERIATRIC PRACTICE SITES

Ambulatory Geriatric Clinic

Ambulatory geriatric clinics are established to provide a multitude of primary care needs specifically tailored to the elderly population. Patients are usually referred by their primary care physicians due to the desire for increased access to services (patients-to-physician ratio), the complexity of the patient's chronic conditions and medications, and the need for specialized knowledge in geriatric treatment. It is common for the appearance of cognitive impairment to be the catalyst for a referral to such clinic. These clinics take advantage of the enhanced knowledge base gained from utilizing multiple members of the health care team. Interdisciplinary geriatrics primary care teams can consist of one or more of the following: geriatrician, clinical pharmacist, nurses (registered nurse [RN], licensed practical nurse [LPN]), social worker, physical/occupational therapist, and nutritionist. Regular interdisciplinary meetings to discuss patients and combine input on their care plans from each specialty area are conducted. The geriatrician assumes the overall care of the patient. They have specialized training in treating the older population encompassing patient's physical, medical, emotional, and social needs. The clinical pharmacist assists in optimizing medication regimen by conducting comprehensive medication review, screening and resolving potential drug-related problems, and educating patients and caregivers about medications and monitoring parameters. Clinical pharmacists' effectiveness can be enhanced with the specialty certification in geriatrics. Nurses provide medical triage and day-to-day patient care activities such as obtaining vitals and providing wound care. Social workers are involved in various aspects from assessing mood and cognitive status of patients to obtaining placement in higher levels of care. Physical/occupational therapists are often involved in assessing the patient's functional status and the need for further therapy, and help maintain a safe home environment. They provide adaptive equipments such as grab bars, raised toilet seat and shower bench for the bathroom, and cane or walker for ambulation. Nutritionists evaluate the patient's nutritional status and educate on proper diet and weight management. From these successful clinical strategies, specialty geriatric clinics have developed including multidisciplinary geriatric oncology clinic[41] and community-based memory clinic.[42]

Long-Term Care

Long-term care provides support for people who are dependent to varying degrees in ADLs and IADLs, numbering about 9 million people over age 65 years as of 2008.[43] Care is provided in the patient's home, in community settings such as adult care homes or assisted living facilities, as well as in nursing homes. Long-term care is expensive, typically several thousand dollars per month. Most care is provided at home by unpaid family members or friends. Medicare covers all or part of the cost of skilled nursing care for a limited period posthospitalization.[43,44] Medicare does not cover long-term care. Financing of long-term care comes from patients' and family savings and/or private long-term care insurance. When a patient's assets have been depleted, Medicaid provides basic nursing home care.[44] However, this care is heavily discounted, often resulting in economizing such as lower caregiver-to-patient ratios and higher number of patients per room. Nursing homes are highly regulated by state and federal government through the Center for Medicare and Medicaid Services.[43,45] Initial and continuing certification of the facility depends upon periodic state and federal review of the facility. Auditors' ratings are available to consumers in an online Nursing Home Report Card.[46,47] **Quality indicators** are used by facility administrators and government overseers to identify problem areas, including[48]:

- Use of nine or more medications in single patient
- Prevalence of indwelling catheters
- Prevalence of antipsychotic, anxiolytic, and hypnotic use
- Use of physical restraints
- Prevalence of depression in patients without antidepressant therapy

- Clinical quality measures such as decubitus ulcers
- Moderate daily pain or any excruciating pain in residents

❾ *Long-term care geriatric practices emphasize the interdisciplinary team approach.* The medical director leads regular meetings with all disciplines delivering care. These may include director of nursing, rehabilitation services (physical, occupation, and speech therapy), pharmacist, social worker, nutritionist, case manager, and psychologist. The pharmacist conducts a monthly drug regimen review of each patient's medication list.[39] The physician is alerted to medication concerns and must approve the patient's orders every 60 days. Such a team approach is vital to coordinate care for the typical frail, complex long-term care patient.

Patient Care and Monitoring

1. Drug-related problems in the elderly patient can be identified by performing a comprehensive medication review.
2. Have the patient bring all of their medication bottles to the medication review including:
   - Prescription medications
   - OTC drugs
   - Vitamin supplements
   - Herbal products
3. Review the indication for all medications taken by the patient.
4. Review the doses taken to identify any underdose or overdose of medications.
5. Screen for any drug–drug, drug–disease, drug–vitamin/herbal, drug–food interactions.
6. Ensure that patient is not taking any medications to which he/she has allergies or intolerances.
7. Assess medication adherence by single or combination methods (use combination methods whenever possible):
   - Self-report
   - Refill history
   - Tablet count
8. Inquire about any adverse drug reactions experienced by the patient.
9. Identify any untreated indication or suboptimal treatment, including preventative therapy such as aspirin, calcium + vitamin D, etc.
10. Assess vitals signs including pain.
11. Evaluate laboratory findings to assess the following:
    - Renal function
    - Hepatic function

- Therapeutic drug monitoring (e.g., digoxin, warfarin, phenytoin)
- Therapeutic goals for chronic disease (e.g., HgbA1c, LDL-C)
12. Perform medication regimen tailoring when indicated:
    - Discontinue unnecessary drugs
    - Simplify dosing times to minimize complex regimen
    - Tailor regimen to patient's daily routine to improve adherence
13. Recognize any physical or functional barriers that can be overcome, such as providing nonchild-resistant caps and tablet cutters.
14. Provide medication education and adherence aid:
    - Verbal and written information about medications and/or disease states
    - Special product counseling for inhalers, insulins, ophthalmic/otic drops, etc.
    - List of medications to include generic and brand names, indications, doses, directions for use, timing of doses, etc.
    - Information on medication storage
    - Pill box or patient-specific blister packs
    - List of future appointments
15. Promote self-monitoring and lifestyle modification:
    - Use of blood pressure device and glucometer
    - Diet and exercise
    - Smoking cessation
    - Immunizations

Abbreviations Introduced in This Chapter

ADL	Activities of daily living
ADR	Adverse drug reaction
GABA	Gamma aminobutyric acid
Hgb_{A1c}	$Hemoglobin_{A1c}$
IADL	Instrumental activities of daily living
INR	International Normalized Ratio
LDL-C	Low density lipoprotein-cholesterol
MDRD	Modification of Diet in Renal Disease
NSAID	Nonsteroidal anti-inflammatory drug
OTC	Over-the-counter
SSRI	Selective serotonin reuptake inhibitor
V_d	Volume of distribution

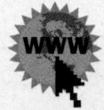 Self-assessment questions and answers are available at *http://www.mhpharmacotherapy. com/pp.html.*

REFERENCES

1. IOM: Retooling for an Aging America: Building the Health Care Workforce. Washington, DC: Institute of Medicine. 2008, *http://www. iom.edu/.*
2. U.S. Census Bureau, Population Division: Population Estimates. Washington, DC: U.S. Census Bureau, 2008, *http://www.census.gov/ popest/.*
3. Federal Interagency Forum on Aging-Related Statistics. Older Americans 2008: Key Indicators of Well-Being. Federal Interagency Forum on Aging-Related Statistics. Washington, DC: U.S. Government Printing Office, March 2008.
4. Centers for Disease Control and Prevention and the Merck Company Foundation. The State of Aging and Health in America 2007. Whitehouse Station, NJ: The Merck Company Foundation, 2007.
5. Mokdad AH, Marks JS, Stroup DF, Gerberding JL. Actual causes of death in the United States, 2000 [published correction appears in JAMA 2005;293(3):293–294]. JAMA 2004;291(10):1240.
6. Kung HC, Hoyert DL, Xu JQ, Murphy SL. Deaths: Final Data for 2005. National Vital Statistics Reports; vol 56 no 10. Hyattsville, MD: National Center for Health Statistics, 2008.
7. Office of the Surgeon General. Health Consequences of Smoking: A Report of the Surgeon General. Washington, DC: U.S. Department of Health and Human Services, 2004, *http://www.surgeongeneral.gov/ library/Smokingconsequences/.*
8. National Committee for Quality Assurance (NCQA). HEDIS 2008: Healthcare Effectiveness Data & Information Set. Vol. 2, Technical Specifications. Washington, DC: National Committee for Quality Assurance (NCQA); 2007 Jul.
9. U.S. Vital and Health Statistics. Summary Health Statistics for U.S. Adults: National Health Interview Survey, 2007 Series 10: Data from the National Health Interview Survey No. 240
10. Ahmed N, Mandel R, Fain MJ. Frailty: An emerging geriatric syndrome. Am J Med 2007;120(9):748–753.
11. DeFrances CJ, Hall MJ. 2005 National Hospital Discharge Survey. Advance Data from Vital and Health Statistics; no 385. Hyattsville, MD: National Center for Health Statistics. 2007.
12. Turnmeim K. Drug therapy in the elderly. Exp Gerontol 2004;39:1731–1738.
13. Elliott DP. Pharmacokinetics and Pharmacodynamics in the Elderly. Pharmacotherapy Self-Assessment Program. 5th ed. 2004:115–130.
14. Huilmer SN, McLachlan AJ, Le Couteur DG. Clinical pharmacology in the geriatric patient. Fundam Clin Pharmacol 2007;21:217–230.
15. Hutchison LC, O'Brien CE. Changes in pharmacokinetics and pharmacodynamics in the elderly patient. J Pharm Prac 2007;20.1:4–12.
16. Chutka DS, Takahashi PY, Hoel RW. Inappropriate medications for elderly patients. Mayo Clin Proc 2004;79:122–139.
17. Bootman JL, Harrison DL, Cox E. The health care cost of drug-related morbidity and mortality in nursing facilities. Arch Intern Med 1997;157:2089–2096.
18. Cannon KT, Choi MM, Zuniga MA. Potentially inappropriate medication use in elderly patients receiving home health care: A retrospective data analysis. Am J Geriatr Pharmacother 2006;4(2):134–143.
19. Hajjar ER, Cafiero AC, Hanlon JT. Polypharmacy in elderly patients. Am J Geriatr Pharmacother 2007;5:345–351.
20. Gallagher P, Barry P, O'Mahony D. Inappropriate prescribing in the elderly. J Clin Pharm Ther 2007;32:113–121.
21. Starner CI, Gray SL, Guay DR, et al. Geriatrics. In: DiPiro JT, Talbert RL, Yee GC, et al., eds. Pharmacotherapy: A Pathophysiologic Approach. 7th ed. New York City: McGraw-Hill; 2008:57–66.
22. Petrone K, Katz P. Approaches to appropriate drug prescribing for the older adult. Prim Care Clin Office Pract 2005;32:755–775.
23. Fick DM, Cooper JW, Wade WE, et al. Updating the Beers criteria for potentially inappropriate medication use in older adults. Arch Intern Med 2003;163:2716–2723.
24. American Geriatrics Society Clinical Practice Committee. The use of oral anticoagulants (warfarin) in older people. J Am Geriatr Soc 2002;50:1439.
25. American Society of Health-System Pharmacists. ASHP guidelines on adverse drug reaction monitoring and reporting. Am J Health-Syst Pharm 1995;52:417–419.
26. Gurwitz JH, Field TS, Harrold LR, et al. Incidence and preventability of adverse drug events among older persons in the ambulatory setting. JAMA 2003;289:1107–1116.
27. Merle L, Laroche ML, Dantoine T, et al. Predicting and preventing adverse drug reactions in the very old. Drugs Aging 2005;22(5):375–392.
28. Hartikainen S, Lonnroos E, Louhivuori K. Medication as a risk factor for falls: Critical systematic review. J Gerontol Med Sci 2007;62A(10):1172–1181.
29. Sokol MC, McGuigan KA, Verbrugge RR, Epstein RS. Impact of medication adherence on hospitalization risk and healthcare cost. Med Care 2005;43:521–530.
30. Osterberg L, Blaschke T. Adherence to medication. N Engl J Med 2005;353:487–497.
31. Miller KE, Zylstra RG, Standridge JB. The geriatric patient: A systematic approach to maintaining health. Am Fam Physician 2000;61:1089–1104.
32. MacLaughlin EJ, Raehl CL, Treadway AK, et al. Assessing medication adherence in the elderly: Which tools to use in clinical practice? Drugs Aging 2005;22(3):231–255.
33. Lee JK, Grace KA, Taylor, AJ. Effect of a pharmacy care program on medication adherence and persistence, blood pressure, and low-density lipoprotein cholesterol: A randomized controlled trial. JAMA 2006;296:2563–2571.
34. Appelbaum PS. Clinical practice. Assessment of patients' competence to consent to treatment. N Engl J Med 2007;357(18):1834–1840.
35. Borson S, Scanlan J, Brush M, Vitaliano P, Dokmak A. The mini-cog: A cognitive "vital signs" measure for dementia screening in multi-lingual elderly. Int J Geriatr Psychiat 2000;15(11):1021–1027.
36. Armstrong J, Mitchell E. Comprehensive nursing assessment in the care of older people. Nurs Older People 2008;20(1):36–40.
37. CMS: Prescription Drug Coverage: Basic Information. Washington, DC: Centers for Medicare & Medicaid Services. 2008, *http://www. medicare.gov/pdp-basic-information.asp*
38. Piette JD, Heisler M. The relationship between older adults' knowledge of their drug coverage and medication cost problems. J Am Geriatr Soc 2006;54:91–96.
39. Levenson SA, Saffel DA. The consultant pharmacist and the physician in the nursing home: Roles, relationships, and a recipe for success. J Am Med Dir Assoc 2007;8:55–64.

40. NPSF: Ask Me 3. BOSTON (MA): National Patient Safety Foundation. 2007–2009, *http://www.npsf.org/askme3/*.

41. Lynch MP, Marcone D, Kagan SH. Developing a multidisciplinary geriatric oncology program in a community cancer center. Clin J Onc Nursing 2004;11:929–933.

42. Grizzell M, Fairhurst A, Lyle S, Jolley D, Willmott S, Bawn S. Creating a community-based memory clinic for older people. Nurs Times 2006;102:32–34.

43. CMS: Long Term Care. Washington, DC: Centers for Medicare & Medicaid Services. 2007–2008, *http://www.medicare.gov/LongTermCare/Static/Home.asp*.

44. Gozalo PL, Miller SC, Intrator O, et al. Hospice effect on government expenditures among nursing home residents. Health Serv Res 2008;43(1):134–153.

45. Harrington C, Swan JH, Carillo H. Nursing staffing levels and Medicaid reimbursement rates in nursing facilities. Health Serv Res 2007;42(3):1105–1129.

46. Mukamel DV, Spector WD, Zinn JS, et al. Nursing homes' response to the Nursing Home Compare Report Card. J Gerontol B Psychol Sci Soc Sci 2007;62(4):S218–S225.

47. CMS: Nursing Home Compare. Washington, DC: Centers for Medicare & Medicaid Services. 2008, *http://www.medicare.gov/NHCompare/*.

48. Hawes C, Mor V, Phillips CD, et al. The OBRA-87 nursing home regulations and implementation of the resident assessment instrument: Effects on process quality. J Am Geriatr Soc 1997;45:977–985.

3 Pediatrics

Hanna Phan, Vinita B. Pai, and Milap C. Nahata

LEARNING OBJECTIVES

Upon completion of the chapter, the reader will be able to:

1. Define different age groups within the pediatric population.
2. Explain general pharmacokinetic and pharmacodynamic differences in pediatric versus adult patients.
3. Identify factors that affect selection of safe and effective drug therapy in pediatric patients.
4. Identify strategies for appropriate medication administration to infants and young children.
5. Apply pediatric pharmacotherapy concepts to make drug therapy recommendations, assess outcomes, and effectively communicate with patients and caregivers.

KEY CONCEPTS

❶ Pediatric patients are not just "smaller adult patients," where doses are scaled only for their smaller size; there are multiple factors to consider when selecting and providing drug therapy for patients in this specific population.

❷ Due to multiple differences including age-dependent development of organ function in pediatric patients, pharmacokinetics, efficacy, and safety of drugs within the pediatric population often differs from adults; thus, pediatric dosing should not be calculated based on a single factor of difference.

❸ Medication errors among pediatric patients are possible due to differences in dose calculation and preparation; it is important to identify potential errors through careful review of calculations, dispensing and administration of drug therapy to infants and children.

❹ Safety and efficacy data of drugs in pediatric patients may be limited to small studies and case reports, leading to frequent off-label use of drugs in this population.

❺ Caregiver education is essential, as they are often responsible for administration and monitoring of drug therapy in infants and young children.

INTRODUCTION

Pediatric clinical practice involves the care of infants, children, and adolescents with the goal of optimizing their health, growth, and development toward adulthood. Clinicians serve as advocates for this unique and vulnerable patient population to maximize their well-being.

There is a continued need for pediatric health care resources, evidenced by the annual increase in the number of infants born in the United States.[1] Ambulatory care settings, such as the pediatrician office and emergency department as well as hospitals, require the expertise of knowledgeable clinicians with pediatric experience. In fact, national data have noted the lack of appropriate services and supplies for pediatric patients at many institutions.[2] Pediatric care accounts for a considerable amount of total patient care annually. For example, patients less than 15 years of age accounted for 16.7% of physician office visits in the United States during 1995 to 2005, with 60% of the drugs used during the 2005 visits being new drug therapies.[3] The overall inpatient hospitalization rate of patients less than 20 years of age was 10.8%, with an average length of stay between 3.8 and 4.5 days, similar to the overall U.S. national average length of stay of 4.8 days for all pediatric and adult patients.[4]

Despite the common misconception of pediatric patients as "smaller adults," they significantly differ within their age groups and from adults regarding drug administration, psychosocial development, and organ function development, which affect efficacy and safety of pharmacotherapy.

FUNDAMENTALS OF PEDIATRIC PATIENTS

Classification of Pediatric Patients

Pediatric patients are those less than 18 years of age. Unlike an adult patient, whose age is commonly measured in years, a pediatric patient's age can be expressed in days, weeks, months, and years. Patients are classified based on age and may be further described based on other factors, including birth weight and prematurity status (Table 3–1).[5]

Growth and Development

Children are monitored for physical, motor, cognitive, and psychosocial development through clinical recognition of timely milestones during routine well-child visits. As a newborn continues to progress to infant, child, and adolescent stages, different variables are monitored to assess growth compared to the general population of similar age and size. The Centers for Disease Control and Prevention (CDC) Growth Charts (Fig. 3–1) are used to plot head circumference, weight, length or stature, and body mass index for a graphical representation of a child's growth compared to the general pediatric population.[6] These tools assess whether a child is meeting the appropriate physical growth milestones, thereby allowing identification of nutritional issues such as poor weight and height gain (e.g., failure to thrive).

Differences in Vital Signs

Normal values for heart rate and respiratory rate vary based on their age. Normal values for blood pressure vary based on gender and age for all pediatric patients, and also height percentile for patients greater than 1 year of age. Normal values for blood pressure in pediatric patients can be found in various national guidelines and other pediatric diagnostic references.[7] Heart rates are highest in neonates and infants, ranging from 95 to 180 beats per minute (bpm) and decrease with age, reaching adult rates (60–100 bpm) around 10 years of age.[8] Respiratory rates are also higher in neonates and infants (24–38 breaths/min), decreasing with age to adult rates around 15 years of age (12–20 breaths/min).[9] Another vital sign commonly monitored in children by their caregivers is body temperature, especially when they seem "warm to the touch." The American Academy of Pediatrics (AAP) recommends rectal temperature measurement in children 4 years of age or younger, using a digital thermometer. For children 4 years of age or older, axillary or oral temperature measurement is appropriate as the child is more able to cooperate when asked. Axillary thermometers can be used in children as young as 3 months, but may be less accurate.[10] Tympanic (otic) temperature readings are also safe for all ages; however, these temperatures may be less accurate and can be affected by cerumen accumulation. Generally, rectal temperature is greater than oral temperature by 0.6°C (1°F), and oral temperature is 0.6°C (1°F) higher than axillary temperatures. Also known as the fifth vital sign, pain assessment is more challenging to assess in neonate, infants, and young children due to inability to communicate symptoms. Indicators of possible pain include physiologic changes such as increased heart rate, respiratory rate, and blood pressure, decreased oxygen saturation, as well as behavior changes such as prolonged, higher pitch crying and facial expressions. Laboratory values also vary depending on age. Normal ranges are often noted by the laboratory facility on reported results.

Table 3–1

Pediatric Age Groups, Age Terminology, and Weight Classification

Age Group	Age
Neonate	28 days (4 weeks) of life or less
Infant	29 days to less than 12 months
Child	1–12 years
Adolescent	13–17 years

Age Terminology	Definition
GA	Age from date of mother's first day of last menstrual period to date of birth
Full term	Describes infants born at 38-weeks gestation or less
Premature	Describes infants born before 37-week gestation
Small for GA	Neonates with birth weight below the 10th percentile among neonates of the same GA
Large for GA	Neonates with birth weight above the 90th percentile among neonates of the same GA
Chronological or postnatal age	Age from birth to present, measured in days, weeks, months, or years
Corrected or adjusted age	May be used to describe the age of a premature child up to 3 years of age: Corrected age = Chronological age in months – [(40 – GA at birth in weeks) ÷ 4 weeks] For example, if a former 29-week GA child is now 10 months old chronologically, his corrected age is approximately 7 months: 10 months – [(40–29 weeks) ÷ 4 weeks] = 7.25 months

Weight Classification	Definition
LBW infant	Premature infant with birth weight between 1,500 and 2,500 g
VLBW infant	Premature infant with birth weight 1,000 g to less than 1,500 g
Extreme LBW	Premature infant with birth weight less than 1,000 g

GA, gestational age; LBW, low birth weight; VLBW, very low birth weight.

Compiled from data in Ref. 5.

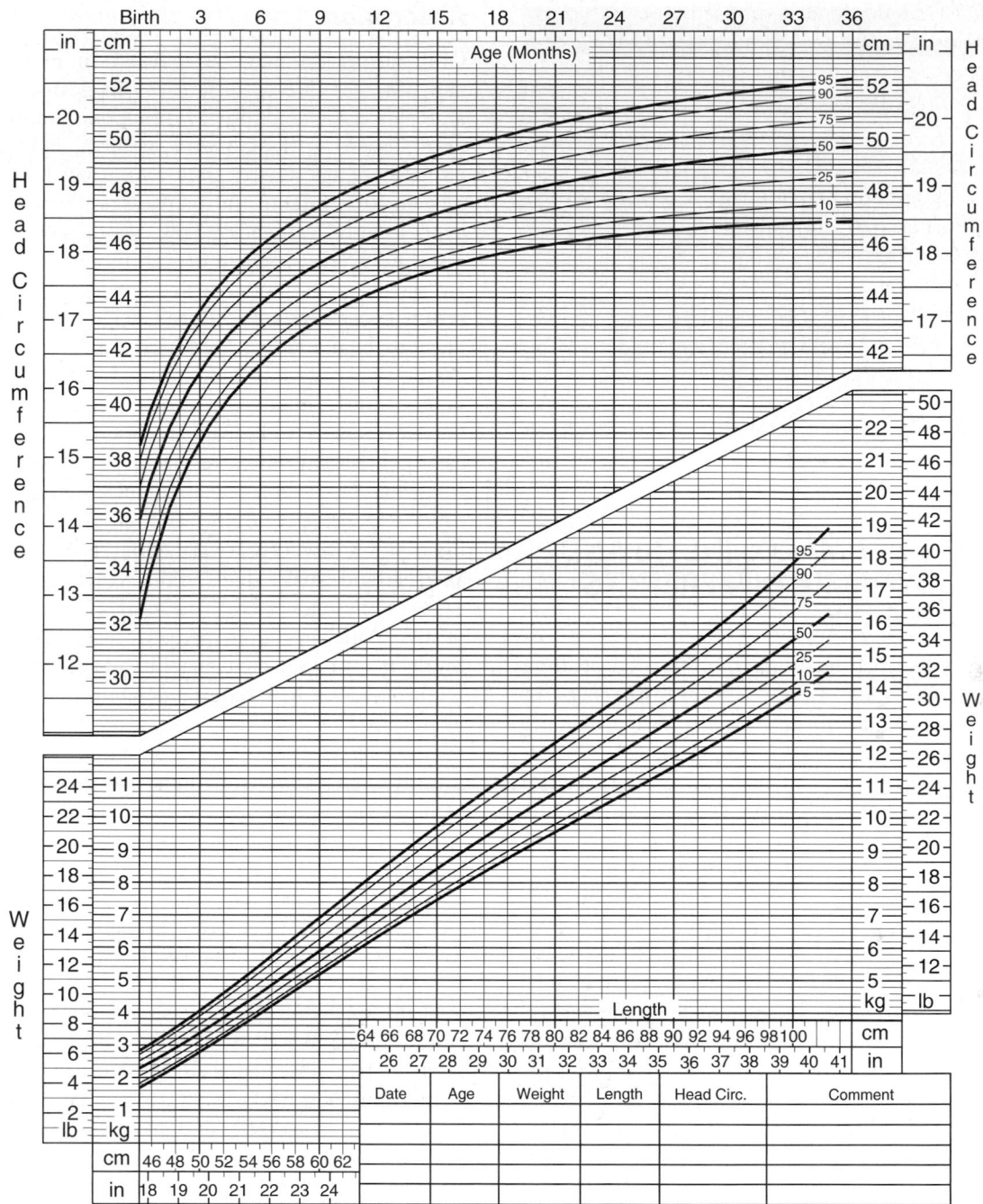

FIGURE 3–1 Example of CDC growth chart of boys, birth to 36 months: Head circumference-for-age and weight-for-length percentile, 2000. (From Ref. 6.)

Fluid Requirements

Fluid requirement and balance are important to monitor in pediatric patients, especially in premature neonates and infants. Maintenance fluid requirement can be calculated based on body surface area for patients greater than 10 kg with a range of 1,500 to 2,000 mL/m²/day. However, a weight-based method of determining normal maintenance fluid for children is often used (Table 3–2).

Table 3–2	
Maintenance Fluid Calculations by Body Weight	
Patient Body Weight	**Maintenance Fluid Requirement**
Less than 10 kg	100 mL/kg/day
11–20 kg	1,000 mL + 50 mL/kg over 10 kg
Greater than 20 kg	1,500 mL + 20 mL/kg over 20 kg

Patient Encounter, Part 1

BB, a 27-week gestational age (GA) premature baby boy weighing 1,000 g, length 48.5 cm, was born to a 19-year-old female this morning. He is admitted to the neonatal intensive care unit, was found to have blood oxygen saturation of 84%, and was placed under an oxygen hood with FiO_2 of 40%. His chest x-ray exhibited ground glass appearance of lung fields and right lower lobe atelectasis. He was intubated and requires maintenance IV fluids until his total parenteral nutrition can be started.

Calculate corrected age for BB 4 months from today.

How much maintenance fluid would you recommend for BB?

EFFECTS OF PHARMACOKINETIC AND PHARMACODYNAMIC DIFFERENCES ON DRUG THERAPY

● Drug selection strategy may be similar or different depending on age and disease state, as a result of differences in pathophysiology of certain diseases, and pharmacokinetic and pharmacodynamic parameters among pediatric and adult patients. It is noteworthy that pediatric patients may require the use of different medications from those used in adults affected by certain diseases. For example, phenobarbital is commonly used for treatment of neonatal seizures, but not often used for treatment of seizures in adults, due to differences in seizure etiology and availability of extensive data regarding its use in neonates compared to newer antiepileptic medications. There also exist commonalties between pediatric and adult patients, such as therapeutic serum drug concentrations required to treat certain diseases. For example, gentamicin peak and trough serum concentrations needed to treat Gram-negative pneumonia are the same in children as in adults. **❶** *The appropriate selection and dosing of drug therapy for a pediatric patient depends on specific factors such as age, weight, height, disease being treated, comorbidities, organ function, and available drug dosage forms.* Often, pediatric drug doses are calculated as mg/kg/day or mg/kg/dose based on body weight compared to mg/day or mg/dose for adult patients. Thus, accurate weight should be available while writing or dispensing medications for this patient population. Pediatric doses may exceed adult doses for certain medications due to differences in pharmacokinetics and pharmacodynamics; hence, the use of pediatric drug dosing guides is recommended.

❷ *Equations proposed to calculate pediatric doses based on adjusted age or weight such as Clark's, Fried's, or Young's Rule should not be routinely used to calculate pediatric doses, as they account for only one factor of difference, age or weight, and lack integration of the effect of growth and development on drug pharmacokinetics and pharmacodynamics in this population.*

Absorption

Oral absorption may be reduced in premature infants and neonates due to differences in gastric acid secretion and pancreatic and biliary function. Full-term neonates have a gastric pH of 6 to 8 at birth and pH 1 to 3 by 48 hours of age. Gastric acid output per kilogram is lower in premature infants and increases with age to adult levels by 6 months of age.[11,12] Low gastric acid secretion can result in increased serum concentrations of weak bases and acid-labile medications, such as penicillin, and decreased serum concentrations of weak acid medications, such as phenobarbital, due to increased ionization. Additionally, gastric emptying time and intestinal transit time are delayed in premature infants, increasing drug contact time with the GI mucosa and drug absorption.[13] Diseases such as gastroesophageal reflux, respiratory distress syndrome, and congenital heart disease may further delay gastric emptying time. Pancreatic exocrine and biliary function are also reduced in newborns, with about 50% less secretion of amylase and lipase than adults, reaching adult values as early as the end of the first year and as late as 5 years of age. Deficiency in pancreatic secretions and bile salts results in decreased bioavailability of prodrug esters, such as erythromycin, which requires solubilization or intraluminal hydrolysis.[12] Due to limited data on oral bioavailability of medications in infants and children for newer agents, some drug dosing recommendations may be extrapolated from adult safety and efficacy studies and case reports.

Topical or percutaneous absorption in neonates and infants is increased due to a thinner stratum corneum, increased cutaneous perfusion, and greater body surface-to-weight ratio. Hence, application of topical medications should be limited to the smallest amount possible. Increased percutaneous absorption can lead to high serum concentrations of topically applied drugs such as corticosteroids, lidocaine, or chlorhexidine, as well as inactive additives such as propylene glycol, potentially causing adverse effects.

Intramuscular absorption in premature and full-term infants can be erratic due to variable perfusion, poor muscle contraction, and decreased muscle mass compared to older patients.[14] Intramuscular administration may be appropriate for some medications; however, use of this route of administration can be painful and is usually reserved when others (e.g., IV) are not accessible, such as initial doses of ampicillin and gentamicin for neonatal sepsis.

Rectal absorption can also be erratic and is not a commonly recommended route of administration if there are other routes available (e.g., oral). This route is useful in cases of severe nausea and vomiting or status epilepticus. For medications that undergo extensive first-pass metabolism, bioavailability increases as the blood supply bypasses the liver from the lower rectum directly to the inferior vena cava. Availability of rectal dosage forms varies, with acetaminophen suppositories and diazepam gel as examples of medications used by the rectal route in pediatric patients. Rectal use of oral medications or other dosage forms is based on limited studies and case reports.

Volume of Distribution

In pediatric patients, apparent volume of distribution (V_d) is normalized based on body weight and expressed as L/kg. Extracellular fluid and total body water per kilogram of body weight are increased in neonates and infants, resulting in higher V_d for water-soluble drugs such as aminoglycosides and decreases with age. Therefore, neonates and infants often require higher individualized doses by weight (mg/kg) than older children and adolescents to achieve the same therapeutic serum concentrations.[14–17] Neonates and infants have a lower normal range for serum albumin (2–4 g/dL, 20–40 g/L), reaching adult levels after 1 year of age. This affects highly protein-bound drugs such as phenytoin, resulting in lower total serum concentrations needed to achieve therapeutic, unbound serum concentrations.[14]

As premature neonates have lower body adipose composition compared to older children and adults, they have a decreased V_d for lipid-soluble drugs such as midazolam and require lower doses by body weight. Lipid-soluble drugs may also reach higher concentrations in the CNS due to an immature blood–brain barrier.[18]

Metabolism

Drug metabolism is slower at birth in full-term infants compared to adolescents and adults, with further delay in premature neonates. Phase I reactions and enzymes, such as oxidation and alcohol dehydrogenase, are impaired in premature neonates and infants and do not fully develop until later childhood or adolescence. Accordingly, the use of products containing ethanol or propylene glycol can result in increased toxicities, including respiratory depression, hyperosmolarity, metabolic acidosis, and seizures, and should be avoided in neonates and infants. Cytochrome P450 isoenzymes (e.g., CYP2C9, CYP1A2) develop at various ages, ranging from a few months to 3 years of age, with delayed development in premature infants.[15]

Among phase II reactions, sulfate conjugation by sulfotransferases is well developed at birth in term infants. Glucuronidation by the uridine diphosphate glucuronosyl transferases, on the other hand, is immature in neonates and infants, requiring at least several months to develop to adult values at approximately 4 years of age. In neonates this deficiency results in adverse effects including cyanosis, ash gray color of the skin, limp body tone, and hypotension, also known as "gray baby syndrome" with use of chloramphenicol.[19] Products containing benzyl alcohol or benzoic acid should be avoided in neonates due to immature glycine conjugation, resulting in accumulation of benzoic acid. This accumulation can lead to "gasping syndrome," which includes respiratory depression, metabolic acidosis, hypotension, seizures or convulsions, and gasping respirations.[20] Acetylation via *N*-acetyltransferase reaches adult maturation at around 1 year of life, but its impact is not well understood regarding neonatal drug therapy.[12] Thus, reduced dosing of medications undergoing hepatic metabolism may be required for full-term and premature neonates. Conversely, hepatic enzyme activity increases to nearly twice as much as adults at 6 months of age and may continue to be high through puberty, around 9 to 12 years of age.[14] These children may require higher doses per kilogram of body weight for hepatically metabolized medications. Common examples include antiepileptic medications such as phenytoin, carbamazepine, and valproic acid. This increase in metabolism slows to adult levels as the child goes through puberty into adulthood.[14]

Elimination

Renal drug clearance is reduced in infants and slowest in premature neonates, due to immature renal function, resulting in the need for longer dosing intervals for renally cleared medications, such as vancomycin, to prevent accumulation. Glomerular filtration rate (GFR) is lowest in premature neonates, increasing with age and peaking at 3 to 12 years of age, after which there is a gradual decline to approximate adult value. For example, vancomycin is often given every 18 to 24 hours in a low birth weight (LBW) premature neonate, every 6 hours in children with normal renal function, and every 8 to 12 hours in adult patients with normal renal function. Children with cystic fibrosis also present with greater renal clearance of drugs such as aminoglycosides, compared to children without the disease, requiring higher doses by weight and more frequent dosing intervals.[21]

Pediatric creatinine clearance (CrCl), an indicator of GFR, is normalized due to variable body size (mL/min/1.73 m²). The use of the Cockroft-Gault or Jelliffe equations for estimating CrCl in adults is not recommended for patients less than 18 years of age.[22,23] Schwartz's equation is a common method of estimating pediatric CrCl for LBW infants up to 21 years of age (Fig. 3–2). This equation utilizes patient length (cm), serum creatinine (mg/dL), and a constant, k,

$$CrCl = \frac{k \times L}{SCr}$$

Age	r
Low birth weight ≤1 year of age	0.33
Full term ≤1 year of age	0.45
2–12 years (male or female) **or** 13–21 years (female)	0.55
13–21 years (male)	0.70

k = Proportionality constant

L = Length in cm

SCr = Serum creatinine in mg/dL

CrCl = Creatinine clearance in mL/min/1.73 m²

FIGURE 3–2 Estimation of creatinine clearance (CrCl) in pediatric patients up to 21 years of age. (Redrawn from Ref. 24.)

Patient Encounter, Part 2

BB is now 3 days old and presents with body temperature fluctuations and hypotension. A workup to rule out sepsis was initiated with collection of blood cultures. He was empirically started on ampicillin 50 mg (50 mg/kg/dose) IV every 8 hours and gentamicin 4 mg (4 mg/kg/dose) IV daily.

BB's Laboratory Values	Normal Ranges
WBC 10.2 × 10³/μL	9–35 × 10³/mm³
(10.2 × 10⁹/L)	(9–35 × 10⁹/L)
Bands 0%	10–18%
Segs 41%	32–62%
Lymphs 49%	19–29%
Monocytes 6%	5–7%
SCr 0.4 mg/dL (35.4 μmol/L)	Less than or equal to 0.6 mg/dL (53 μmol/L)

Using the most appropriate method, calculate a creatinine clearance for BB.

The mg/kg dose of gentamicin administered to BB is high compared to a child or an adolescent; however, the dosing frequency is less often. How would you explain this difference?

which is dependent on age for all patients and also gender for those greater than 2 years of age.[24] Urine output is also a parameter used to assess renal function in pediatric patients, with a urine output of greater than 1 to 2 mL/kg/h considered normal.

COMMON PEDIATRIC ILLNESSES

There may be similarities and differences in illnesses such as infections, asthma, allergic rhinitis, attention deficient hyperactivity disorder, diabetes, and seizure disorders between children and adults. These have been discussed throughout the textbook. The incidence of previously common childhood illness such as measles, mumps, and rubella has significantly decreased as a result of en masse vaccination of infants and children. The Advisory Committee on Immunization Practices (ACIP) within the CDC release and update child and adolescent immunization schedules every year. Patients' immunization records should be reviewed routinely for needed immunizations based on these schedules.[25,26] Most of the common illnesses in children leading to missed school and/or need for clinician consultation are ambulatory in nature; however, some complications may require hospitalization.

Presentation of common childhood illnesses may vary depending on age and development. Older children and adolescents are able to communicate symptoms verbally, making assessment and treatment easier, unlike infants and younger children who are less able to do so. In such cases, changes in vital signs, such as respiratory rate, heart rate, body temperature, and changes in oral intake, feeding pattern, and urine output are used as indicators of potential illness. Parents may also note subjective items such as changes in mood (e.g., increased irritability or "fussiness").

SPECIFIC CONSIDERATIONS IN DRUG THERAPY

In addition to differences in pharmacokinetics and pharmacodynamic parameters, other factors including dosage formulations, medication administration techniques, and parent/caregiver education should be considered when selecting drug therapy.

Routes of Administration and Drug Formulations

Depending on age, disease, and disease severity, different routes of administration may be considered. Use of rectal route of administration is reserved in cases where oral administration is not possible and IV route is not necessary. Topical administration is often used for treatment of dermatologic ailments. Transdermal routes are often not recommended, unless it is an approved indication such as the methylphenidate transdermal patch for treatment of attention deficit hyperactivity disorder. The injectable route of administration is used in patients with severe illnesses or when other routes of administration are not possible. As done with adult patients, IV compatibility and access should be evaluated when giving parenteral medications. However, dilution of parenteral medications may be necessary to measure smaller doses for neonates. On the other hand, higher concentration of parenteral medications may be necessary for patients with fluid restrictions such as premature infants, and patients with cardiac anomalies and/or renal disease. Appropriate stability and diluent selection data should be obtained from the literature.

When oral drug therapy is needed, one must also consider the type of dosage form available. Children less than 6 years of age are often not able to swallow oral tablets or capsules and may require oral liquid formulations. The child's ability to swallow a solid dosage form should be determined before selecting a drug product. Not all oral medications, especially those unapproved for use in infants and children, have a commercially available liquid dosage form. Use of a liquid formulation compounded from a solid oral dosage form is an option, when data are available. Factors such as stability, suspendability, dose uniformity, and palatability should be considered when compounding a liquid formulation.[27] Commonly used suspending agents include methylcellulose and carboxymethylcellulose (e.g., Ora-Plus). Palatability of a liquid formulation can be enhanced by using simple syrup or OraSweet. If no dietary contraindications or interactions exist, doses can be mixed with food items such as pudding, chocolate syrup, or applesauce immediately before administration of individual doses. Honey, although capable of masking unpleasant taste of medication, may contain spores of *Clostridium botulinum* and should not be given to infants less than 1 year of age due to increased risk for developing illness. Most hospitals caring for pediatric patients compound formulations in their inpatient pharmacy. Limited accessibility to compounded oral liquids in community pharmacies poses a greater challenge. A list of community pharmacies with compounding capabilities should be maintained and provided to the parents and caregivers before discharge from the hospital.

Common Errors in Pediatric Drug Therapy

Prevention of errors in pediatric drug therapy begins with identification of possible sources. Reports have shown that nearly 50% of medication errors in the United States in neonatal and pediatric critical care units are attributable to prescribing and transcribing errors.[28] Up to 69.5% of overall calculation errors affect pediatric patients.[29] ❸ *As pediatric drug therapy is based on weight, body surface area, and age, it is crucial to verify accurate weight, height, and age for dosing calculations and dispensing of prescriptions.* Consistent units of measurements in reporting patient weight (kg), height (cm), and age (weeks and years) should be used. Dosing units such as mg/kg, mcg/kg, mEq/kg, or units/kg should also be used accurately. Given the age-related differences in metabolism of additives such as propylene glycol and benzyl alcohol, careful consideration should be given to the active and inactive ingredients when selecting a formulation.

Decimal errors, including trailing zeroes (e.g., 1.0 mg misread as 10 mg) and missing leading zeroes (e.g., .5 mg misread as 5 mg) in drug dosing or body weight documentation are possible, resulting in several fold overdosing. Strength or concentration of drug should also be clearly communicated by the clinician in prescription orders. Similarly, labels that look alike may lead to drug therapy errors, e.g., mistaking a vial of heparin for insulin, when compounding parenteral solutions. Dosing errors of combination drug products can be prevented by using the right component for dose calculation (e.g., dose of sulfamethoxazole/trimethoprim is calculated based on the trimethoprim component).

The use of the "rule of six" was previously used to calculate infusions of medication such as inotropes for critically ill patients in hospitals.[30] However, the Institute for Safe Medication Practice (ISMP) has found a relationship between medication errors and use of nonstandard injectable concentrations, such as those resulting from use of the "rule of six." The Joint Commission on Accreditation of Healthcare Organizations determined that "the rule of six" did not meet its goals of standardizing and limiting the number of drug concentrations. Use of standardized concentrations and programmable infusion pumps, such as smart pumps with built-in libraries, is encouraged to minimize errors with parenteral medications. Some hospitals have also adopted the use of enhanced photoemission spectroscopy to scan small samples of compounded IV solution in verification of high-risk IV solutions.[31] Introduction of technological advances such as computer physician order entry (CPOE) systems

with ability for dose range checks by weight for pediatric medication orders and the use of bar code technology for dispensing of medications have decreased medication errors.[32,33]

Prevention of medication errors is a joint effort between health care professionals and parents/caregivers. Obtaining a complete medication history including over-the-counter (OTC) and complementary and alternative medicines (CAMs), simplification of medication regimen, clinician awareness for potential errors, and appropriate patient/parent/caregiver education on measurement and administration of medications are essential in preventing medication errors.

CAM and OTC Medication Use

An estimated 31% to 84% of children with cancer, 74% with autism spectrum disorder, 71% with asthma, and 15% seen in the emergency department utilize CAM or other OTC products.[34-37] Over 50% of parents/caregivers do not disclose this use to the physicians.[35] CAM can include mind-body therapy (e.g., imagery, hypnosis), energy field therapies (e.g., acupuncture, acupressure), massage, antioxidants (e.g., vitamins C and E), herbs (e.g., St. John's wort, kava, ginger, valerian), prayer, immune modulators (e.g., echinacea), or other folk/home remedies.

It is critical to realize that there are limited data establishing efficacy of various CAM therapies in children. For example, colic is a condition of unclear etiology in which an infant cries inconsolably for over a few hours in a 24-hour period, usually during the same time of day. Symptoms of excessive crying usually improve by the third month of life and often resolve by 9 months of age. No medication has been approved by the FDA for this condition. This condition is self-limiting and infants will outgrow it as they age. Some parents are advised by family and friends to use alternative treatments, such as gripe water, to treat colic. Gripe water is an oral solution containing a combination of ingredients such as chamomile, peppermint, fennel, ginger, aloe, sodium bicarbonate, and lemon balm. Combinations of ingredients vary among manufacturers as there is no defined formulation. These options have not been proven safe or effective in the treatment of colic in infants and are not regulated by the FDA. Further, some of these therapies (e.g., St. John's wort) can interact with prescription drugs and produce toxicities. St. John's wort can increase adverse effects of selective serotonin receptor antagonists and 5-HT1 serotonin receptor agonists due to serotonergic syndrome and decrease effectiveness of anticonvulsants, warfarin, cyclosporine, digoxin, and protease inhibitors due to their increased metabolism and reduced serum concentration.[38]

It is important to assess OTC product use in pediatric patients. For example, treatment of the common cold in children is similar to adults, including symptom control with adequate fluid intake, rest, use of saline nasal spray, and acetaminophen (15 mg/kg/dose every 6–8 hours) or ibuprofen (4–10 mg/kg/dose every 8 hours) for relief of discomfort and fever. Unlike adults, symptomatic relief through the use of pharmacologic agents, such as OTC combination cold remedies, is not recommended for pediatric patients younger than 4 years of age. Currently, the FDA does not recommend the use of OTC cough and cold medications (e.g., diphenhydramine and dextromethorphan) in children less than 2 years of age; however, the Consumer Healthcare Products Association, with the support of the FDA, has voluntarily changed product labeling of OTC cough and cold medications to state "do not use in children under 4 years of age." This is due to increased risk for adverse effects (e.g., excessive sedation, respiratory depression) and no docu-mented benefit in relieving symptoms. It has also been noted that these medications may also be less effective in children under 6 years of age compared with older children and adults.[39,40] Also noteworthy is the potential for medication error with use of OTC products in older children, such as cold medications containing diphenhydramine and acetaminophen. A parent/caregiver may inadvertently overdose a child on one active ingredient, such as acetaminophen, by administering acetaminophen suspension for fever and an acetaminophen-containing combination product for cold symptoms. The use of aspirin in patients less than 18 years of age with viral infections is not recommended due to risk of Reye's syndrome. While making an appropriate recommendation for an OTC product for a pediatric patient, the parent/caregiver should always be referred to their pediatrician for further advice and evaluation, especially in the care of a neonate.

Clinicians should respect parents'/caregivers' beliefs in use of CAM and OTC products and encourage a discussion with the intention of providing information regarding their risks and benefits to achieve desired health outcomes as well as optimize medication safety.

Off-Label Medication Use

Pharmacotherapy in pediatric patients often includes use of approved and unapproved (off-label) drugs. Off-label use of medication is the use of a drug outside of its approved labeled indication. This includes the use of a medication in the treatment of illnesses not listed on the manufacturer's package insert, use outside the licensed age range, dosing outside those recommended, or use of a different route of administration.[41] Such off-label use in infants and children is frequently based on limited data.

Currently, there is a lack of pediatric dosing, safety, and efficacy information for over 75% of drugs approved in adults. Off-label use occurs in both outpatient and inpatient settings. About 80% of hospitalized pediatric patients receive at least one off-label medication.[42] **4** *It is appropriate to use a drug off-label when no alternatives are available; however, clinicians should refer to published studies and case reports for available safety, efficacy, and dosing information.* FDA regulatory changes, such as patent exclusivity, provide incentives for a pharmaceutical manufacturer to market drugs for pediatric patients.

Medication Administration to Pediatric Patients and Caregiver Education

Considering the challenges in cooperation from infants and younger children, medication administration can become a difficult task for any parent or caregiver. Clinicians should consider ease of measurement and administration when selecting and dosing pediatric drug therapy. Clinicians should check concentrations of available products and round doses to a measurable amount. For example, if a patient were to receive an oral formulation, such as amoxicillin 400 mg/5 mL suspension, and the dose was calculated to be 4.9 mL, the dose should be rounded to 5 mL for ease of administration. Rounding the dose by 10% to the closest easily measureable amount is commonly practiced for most medications; however, drugs with narrow therapeutic indices are exceptions to this guideline.

The means or devices for measuring and administering medications by the caregivers should also be closely considered. Special measuring devices as well as clear and complete education about their use are essential. Oral syringes are accurate and offered at most community pharmacies for measurement of oral liquid medications. Oral droppers that are included specifically with a medication may be appropriate for use in infants and young children. Medicine cups are not recommended for measuring doses for infants and young children due to possible inaccuracy of measuring smaller doses. Household dining or measuring spoons are not accurate or consistent and should not be used for administration of oral liquids.

5 *Comprehensive and clear parent/caregiver education improves medication adherences, safety, and therapeutic outcomes.* Information about the drug including appropriate and safe storage from children, possible drug interactions, duration of therapy and importance of adherence, adverse effects, and expected therapeutic outcomes should be provided. Parent/caregiver education is important in both inpatient and outpatient care settings and should be reviewed at each point of care.

As parents/caregivers are often sole providers of home care for ill children, it is important to demonstrate appropriate dose preparation and administration techniques

---

Patient Encounter, Part 3

BB is now older (6 months corrected age) and his mother calls the clinic and tells you that her son is "just miserable" with a runny nose, cough, and a fever (axillary temperature) of 38.3°C (101°F). She wanted to know if she could use baby aspirin instead of the acetaminophen, which doesn't seem to help. She also wanted to know which cough and cold preparation would be most appropriate for BB.

What additional information would you need to help BB and his mom?

What is your recommendation regarding use of aspirin for BB?

What cough and cold preparation would you recommend for BB?

to the caregivers before medication dispensing. First, a child should be calm for successful dose administration. Yet, calming a child is often a challenge during many methods of administration (e.g., otic, ophthalmic, rectal). Parents/caregivers should explain the process in a simple and understandable form to the child as this may decrease child's potential anxiety. In addition, it is also recommended to distract younger children using a favorite item such as toy, or reward cooperative or "good" behavior during medication administration. Administration of ophthalmic drops or ointment is best when the child is calm and laying in a supine position, with similar instructions of washing hands before administration, avoiding contact of the applicator tip to the eye or other surfaces as noted in adult administration. Otic drop administration should begin with the child lying in a prone position with head tilted to expose the treated ear followed by gentle pulling of the outer ear outward, followed by pulling downward and upward for patients less than and greater than 3 years of age, respectively, due to the change in angle of the eustachian tube with age. Another challenging route of administration for caregivers is use of nasal drops, which should be administered when the child is in a supine position with the head slightly tilted back, remaining in position for a few minutes for appropriate distribution of medication. Rectal administration, also a difficult route to achieve patient cooperation, is similar to adults regarding preparation of dose; however, for patients under 3 years of age, a smaller finger (e.g., pinky finger) should be used to insert the suppository, whereas the index finger can be used in older children for administration.[43]

Accidental Ingestion in Pediatric Patients

Over 1.2 million accidental ingestions occurred in children less than 6 years of age in 2001; these often occur in the home.[44] Ingested substances can vary, from household cleaning solutions to prescription and nonprescription medications. Management of accidental ingestions varies depending on the ingested substance, the amount, and the age and size of the child. Clinicians receiving calls regarding management of accidental ingestions should direct them to the local or regional poison control center for specific recommendations, which can be located through the American Association of Poison Control Centers (*www.aapcc.org*).

Inducing emesis is not recommended for suspected ingestions of acidic or alkaline substances. The American Academy of Clinical Toxicology and the AAP do not recommend the use of ipecac syrup as it can decrease effectiveness of activated charcoal treatment administered in the emergency department and compromise patient outcomes.[45] Activated charcoal use is preferred for treatment of ingestion in the emergency department at a dose of 1 g/kg for infants less than 1 year of age, 1 to 2 g/kg orally for children greater than 1 year of age and adults, as a single dose.[46] Monitor symptoms of toxicities from the substance ingested

---

Patient Encounter, Part 4

BB is now 23 months old, brought by his father to the pediatrician. He has a 4-day history of left ear pain, excessive crying, decreased appetite, and difficulty sleeping over the past 2 days. The child's temperature last night was 39°C (102.2°F) by electronic axial thermometer. The father gave the child several doses of acetaminophen drops (80 mg/0.8 mL), but the pain or temperature did not improve and none was given this morning. His immunizations are up to date. He was last treated for acute otitis media 4 months ago using oral amoxicillin 40 mg/kg/day divided every 12 hours. He has no known drug allergies.

Medications prior to admission: Acetaminophen drops as needed for pain and fever.

PE:
General: Crying, tugging on his left ear
VS: T 39°C (102.2°F), BP 104/58 mm Hg (90th percentile), HR 133 bpm, RR 36 bpm, wt 14 kg (30.8 lb) (75th percentile), ht 89 cm (75th percentile)
HEENT: Tympanic membranes erythematosus (L>R); left ear is bulging and nonmobile. Throat erythematous; nares patent.
Diagnosis: Acute otitis media, left ear

You and the pediatrician decide to start BB on high-dose oral amoxicillin (90 mg/kg/day divided every 12 hours, using a 400 mg/5 mL suspension) for a total of 10 days and continue acetaminophen drops (10 mg/kg/dose every 6 hours as needed for fever or pain).

Based on the information available, create a care plan for BB. The plan should include:

(a) *Statement of the drug-related needs and/or problems,*

(b) *Patient-specific detailed therapeutic plan with specific dosing, and*

(c) *Parent/caregiver education points.*

---

during hospitalization. Parents/caregivers should continue monitoring at home following discharge.

Abbreviations Introduced in This Chapter

AAP	American Academy of Pediatrics
ACIP	Advisory Committee on Immunization Practices
bpm	Beats per minute
CAM	Complementary and alternative medicine
CDC	Centers for Disease Control and Prevention
CPOE	Computer physician order entry
CrCl	Creatinine clearance
GA	Gestational age
GFR	Glomerular filtration rate

Patient Care and Monitoring

For all pediatric patients, review and consider the following when selecting and monitoring drug therapy:

- Gestational age, postnatal age, and corrected age if the patient is a neonate
- Patient's demographic information including age, weight (and birth weight if a neonate), and gender
- Disease or illness for which treatment is needed
- Past medical history, including comorbidities
- Medication history current and past (including OTC and complementary and alternative products)
- History of medication adherence
- Other concurrent medications
- Previous therapy failures
- Available routes of administration
  - Can the patient take medications orally?
  - If IV medication is needed what types of IV accesses are available? For example, does the patient have a central or peripheral line?
  - Is intramuscular administration needed?
- Fluid status—Is the patient dehydrated, balanced, or edematous?
- Available data regarding safe and effective dosing of selected drug
- Verification of accurate dose calculation
  - Verify weight and dosing units (e.g., mg/kg/day, mg/kg/dose)
  - Is the dosing interval appropriate?

- Is the dose an easily measurable amount for the caregiver?
- Will the drug be administered at home and/or a daycare facility or school?
  - Does the parent/caregiver need additional documentation for medication administration at other locations?
  - Are additional supplies for medication administration at other locations needed?
- Educate parent/caregiver/patient, regarding selected drug therapy
- Regular assessment of weight
  - Premature neonates and infants can change frequently, check weight daily
  - Depending on illness in older children, daily weight check may be necessary
- Organ function
  - For drugs that undergo extensive hepatic metabolism and clearance, assess liver function at baseline and periodically (depending on severity of illness)
  - For drugs that undergo extensive renal elimination
    - Note changes in serum creatinine and urine output
    - Calculate serum creatinine clearance using Schwartz's or Traub–Johnson's equations
- Measure drug serum concentrations when appropriate
- Monitor clinical outcomes of pharmacotherapy
- Monitor, manage, and prevent adverse drug events
- Monitor for drug–drug or drug–food interactions

ISMP	Institute for Safe Medication Practices
LBW	Low birth weight
OTC	Over-the-counter
V_d	Volume of distribution (apparent)
VLBW	Very low birth weight

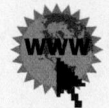 Self-assessment questions and answers are available at *http://www.mhpharmacotherapy.com/pp.html.*

REFERENCES

1. Hamilton BE, Martin JA, Ventura SJ. Births: Preliminary data for 2006. National vital statistics reports; vol 56 no 7. Hyattsville, MD: National Center for Health Statistics. 2007.
2. Committee on the Future of Emergency Care in the United States Health System. Emergency Care for Children, Growing Pains. Executive Summary. The Institute of Medicine, 2007, *http://books.nap.edu/catalog/11655.html.*
3. Cherry DK, Woodwell DA, Rechtsteiner EA. National Ambulatory Medical Care Survey: 2005 Summary. Advance data from vital and health statistics; no. 387. Hyattsville, MD: National Center for Health Statistics. 2007.
4. Kozak LJ, DeFrances CJ, Hall MJ. National Hospital Discharge Survey: 2004 annual summary with detailed diagnosis and procedure data. National Center for Health Statistics. Vital Health Stat 13(162). 2006.
5. American Academy of Pediatrics, Committee on Fetus and Newborn. Age terminology during the perinatal period. Pediatrics 2004;114: 1362–1364.
6. Center for Disease Control Growth Charts, 2000. Developed by the National Center for Health Statistics in collaboration with the National Center for Chronic Disease Prevention and Health Promotion. *http://www.cdc.gov/growthcharts.*
7. National High Blood Pressure Education Program Working Group on High Blood Pressure in Children and Adolescents. The Fourth Report on the Diagnosis, Evaluation, and Treatment of High Blood Pressure in Children and Adolescents. NIH Publication No. 05-5268. Bethesda, MD: National Heart, Lung, and Blood Institute. Pediatrics 2004;114:555–576.
8. Gajewski KK. Cardiology. In: Robertson J, Shilkofski N, eds. The Harriet Lane Handbook: A Manual for Pediatric House Officers, 17th ed. Philadelphia: Mosby, 2005.
9. Loughlin CE. Pulmonology. In: Robertson J, Shilkofski N, eds. The Harriet Lane Handbook: A Manual for Pediatric House Officers, 17th ed. Philadelphia: Mosby, 2005.

10. American Academy of Pediatrics. Fever and Your Child. 2007.
11. Boyle JT. Acid secretion from birth to adulthood. J Pediatr Gastroenterol Nutr 2003;37:S12–S16.
12. Alcorn J, Nakamura PJ. Pharmacokinetics in the newborn. Adv Drug Deliv Rev 2003;55:667–686.
13. Ramirez A, Wong WW, Shulman RJ. Factors regulating gastric emptying in preterm infants. J Pediatr 2006;149:475–479.
14. Soldin OP, Soldin SJ. Therapeutic drug monitoring in pediatric patients. Ther Drug Monit 2002;24:1–8.
15. Strolin Benedetti M, Baltes EL. Drug metabolism and disposition in children. Fundam Clin Pharmacol 2003;17:281–299.
16. Semchuk W, Shevchuk YM, Sankaran K, Wallace SM. Prospective, randomized, controlled evaluation of a gentamicin loading dose in neonates. Biol Neonate 1995;67(1):13–20.
17. Shevchuk YM, Taylor DM. Aminoglycoside volume of distribution in pediatric patients. DICP Ann Pharmacother 1990 Mar;24(3):273–276.
18. Blumer JL. Clinical pharmacology of midazolam in infants and children. Clin Pharmacokinet 1998;35(1):37–47.
19. Mulhall A, de Louvois J, Hurley R. Chloramphenicol toxicity in neonates: Its incidence and prevention. Br Med J (Clin Res Ed) 1983 Nov 12;287(6403):1424–1427.
20. Menon PA, Thach BT, Smith CH, et al. Benzyl alcohol toxicity in a neonatal intensive care unit. Incidence, symptomatology, and mortality. Am J Perinatol 1984;1(4):288–292.
21. Rey E, Tréluyer JM, Pons G. Drug disposition in cystic fibrosis. Clin Pharmacokinet 1998 Oct;35(4):313–329.
22. Cockroft DW, Gault MH. Prediction of creatinine clearance from serum creatinine. Nephron 1976;16:31–41.
23. Jelliffe RW. Creatinine clearance: Bedside estimate. Ann Intern Med 1973;79:604–605.
24. Schwartz GJ, Brion LP, Spitzer A. The use of plasma creatinine concentration for estimating glomerular filtration rate in infants, children, and adolescents. Pediatr Clin N Am 1987;34:571–590.
25. General Recommendations on Immunization: Recommendations of the Advisory Committee on Immunization Practices (ACIP). Advisory Committee on Immunization Practices (ACIP), Centers for Disease Control and Prevention. MMWR 2006:55(RR15); 1–48.
26. Department of Health and Human Services, Center for Disease Control and Prevention. Recommended immunization schedules for persons aged 0–18 years, United States, 2008.
27. Nahata MC, Hipple TF, Pai VB. Pediatric Drug Formulations, 5th ed. Cincinnati, OH: Harvey Whitney Books Co., 2003:1–293.
28. Swanson A. Nix the six: Raise the bar on medication delivery. Newborn Infant Nursing Rev 2006;6:230–236.
29. Lesar TS. Errors in the use of medication dosage equations. Arch Pediatr Adolesc Med 1998;152(4):340–344.
30. McLeroy PA. The rule of six: Calculating intravenous infusions in a pediatric crisis situation. Hosp Pharm 1994;29:939–940, 943.
31. Kaakeh Y, Phan H, DeSmet BD, et al. Enhanced photoemission spectroscopy for verification of high-risk i.v. medications. Am J Health Syst Pharm 2008;65:49–54.
32. Cordero L, Kuehn L, Kumar RR, Mekhjian HS. Impact of computerized physician order entry on clinical practice in a newborn intensive care unit. J Perinatol 2004;24(2):88–93.
33. Potts AL, Barr FE, Gregory DF, et al. Computerized physician order entry and medication errors in a pediatric critical care unit. Pediatrics 2004;113(1 Pt 1):59–63.
34. Sencer SF, Kelly KM. Complementary and alternative therapies in pediatric oncology. Pediatr Clin N Am 2007;54:1043–1060.
35. Hanson E, Kalish LA, Bunce E, et al. Use of complementary and alternative medicine among children diagnosed with autism spectrum disorder. J Autism Dev Disord 2007;37:627–636.
36. Sidora-Arcoleo K, Yoos HL, Kitzman H, McMullen A, Anson E. Don't ask, don't tell: Parental nondisclosure of complementary and alternative medicine and over-the-counter medication use in children's asthma management. J Pediatr Health Care 2008;22:221–229.
37. Sawni A, Ragothaman R, Thomas RL, Mahajan P. The Use of complementary/alternative therapies among children attending an urban pediatric emergency department. Clin Pediatr 2007;46:36–41.
38. Rey JM, Walter G, Soh N. Complementary and alternative medicine (CAM) treatments and pediatric psychopharmacology. J Am Acad Child Adoles Psych 2008;47:4:364–368.
39. US Food and Drug Administration. Public Health Advisory: Nonprescription Cough and Cold Medicine Use in Children. January 17, 2008, *http://www.fda.gov/Cder/drug/advisory/cough_cold_2008.htm.*
40. MedWatch Safety Summary, October 8, 2008. FDA Statement Following CHPA's Announcement on Nonprescription Over-the-Counter Cough and Cold Medicines in Children, *http://www.fda.gov/bbs/topics/NEWS/2008/NEW01899.html.*
41. Conroy S. Unlicensed and off-label drug use: Issues and recommendations. Pediatr Drugs 2002;4:363–369.
42. Shah SS, Hall M, Goodman DM, et al. Off-label drug use in hospitalized children. Arch Pediatr Adolesc Med 2007;161:282–290.
43. Pediatric Medication Administration. In: Taketomo CK, Hodding JH, Kraus DM, eds. Pediatric Dosage Handbook, 14th ed, Hudson, OH: Lexi-Comp, Inc., 2007: Miscellaneous Appendix.
44. American Academy of Pediatrics Committee on Injury, Violence, and Poison Prevention. Poison treatment in the home. Pediatrics 2006;112:1182–1185.
45. Manoguerra AS, Cobaugh DJ. Guideline on the use of ipecac syrup in the out-of-hospital management of ingested poisons. Clin Toxicol (Phila) 2005;43(1):1–10.
46. Burns MM. Activated charcoal as the sole intervention for treatment after childhood poisoning. Curr Opin Pediatr 2000;12:166–171.

4 Palliative Care

Marc A. Sweeney and Phyllis A. Grauer

LEARNING OBJECTIVES

● **Upon completion of the chapter, the reader will be able to:**

1. Describe the philosophy of palliative care and its impact on drug therapy.

2. Discuss the therapeutic management of palliative care patients and how it differs and is similar to traditional patient care.

3. List the most common symptoms experienced by the terminally ill patient.

4. Explain the pathophysiology of the common symptoms experienced in the terminally ill patient.

5. Assess the etiology of symptoms in the terminally ill patient.

6. Describe the pharmacologic rationale of drug therapy used for symptom management in the terminally ill patient.

7. Recommend nonpharmacologic and pharmacologic management for symptoms in a terminally ill patient.

8. Develop a patient monitoring plan for palliative care management.

9. Educate patients and caregivers regarding palliative care management plan, including rationale of treatment, assessment of success and importance of adherence.

KEY CONCEPTS

❶ According to the World Health Organization (WHO), "Palliative care is defined as the active total care of patients whose disease is not responsive to curative treatment. The goal of palliative care is to achieve the best quality of life for patients and their families."

❷ The goals of palliative care include enhancing quality of life while maintaining or improving functionality.

❸ Palliative care is appropriate for all incurable diseases including cancer; chronic obstructive pulmonary disease; dementia, including Alzheimer's disease; Parkinson's disease; chronic cardiac disease; stroke, renal failure; hepatic failure; multiorgan failure; diabetes mellitus; etc.

❹ Following a complete assessment of the patient, developing a comprehensive therapeutic plan that utilizes the fewest number of medications to achieve the highest quality of life is essential.

❺ Palliative care is more than just pain management. It includes the treatment of symptoms resulting in the discomfort for the patient, which may include nausea, agitation, anxiety, depression, dyspnea, cachexia, constipation, diarrhea, pressure ulcers, edema, etc.

❻ Involving the patient and caregivers into the development of the therapeutic plan demonstrates responsible palliative medicine.

❼ Assessing positive therapeutic outcomes includes resolution of symptoms while minimizing adverse drug events.

❽ Patient and caregiver education is vital to ensuring positive outcomes.

INTRODUCTION

❶ *According to the World Health Organization (WHO), "Palliative care is defined as the active total care of patients whose disease is not responsive to curative treatment. The goal of palliative care is to achieve the best quality of life for patients and their families."*[1] Since the word, "palliate," literally means "to cloak," the WHO goal of achieving high quality of life is consistent with managing disease-related symptoms.[2] Palliative care is an approach to care focusing on patients and their families and the challenges they face associated with life-threatening illness.[3] The goal of care is to prevent and relieve suffering by means of early identification, assessment and treatment of pain and other physical symptoms, including associated psychosocial, emotional, and spiritual concerns.[1] The WHO goes on to state that the most effective palliative care is provided by a team of health care professionals. Palliative medicine is rapidly becoming a well-recognized medical specialty throughout the world.[4] This expanding specialty in medicine is much needed due to the increased number of patients with chronic, slowly debilitating diseases.[2]

The term palliative care is frequently used synonymously with hospice, and although hospice programs provide palliative care, palliative care has a much broader application. The goals for both types of care are similar; however, differences exist. In the United States, hospice is defined by Medicare and other third-party payers as a medical benefit available to individuals who have 6 months or less life expectancy if the disease runs its typical course.[5] Hospice care guidelines and regulations are typically defined by federal regulations. Palliative care, on the other hand, may be provided at any point during the disease process and is not limited to the last 6 months of life as is the case with hospice care. Patients and families may receive some aspects of palliative care beginning at the time of diagnosis of a life-limiting illness. Palliative care, whether it is through a hospice program or a palliative care service may be delivered to patients in all care settings including the hospital, outpatient clinic, extended care facility, or at home.[6]

Palliative care is not only a philosophy of patient care, but also a highly organized system to deliver care.[7] The foundation for providing quality palliative care centers around the active participation of an interdisciplinary group or team of professionals who work closely together to meet the goals of the patient and family. Palliative care team members include representatives from medicine, nursing, social work, pharmacy, chaplaincy, nutrition, rehabilitation, and other professional disciplines. The involvement of multiple disciplines provides a holistic approach to the patient's care. Figure 4–1 provides a diagrammatic view of how a palliative care team may work together in caring for the patient.

❷ *The goals of palliative care include enhancing quality of life while maintaining or improving functionality.*[8] Given this goal of patient care, palliative care should most logically be delivered to patients from the onset of any chronic, life-altering disease. Palliative care is not a new concept, in fact, it is one of the oldest approaches to patient care. Before many of our modern medical and therapeutic advancements were developed, curative treatments were not normally available.[9] Provision of comfort and addressing quality of life during illness was considered the mainstay for patient care. During the 20th century, advances in medical care, nutrition, public health, and trauma care resulted in fewer patient deaths

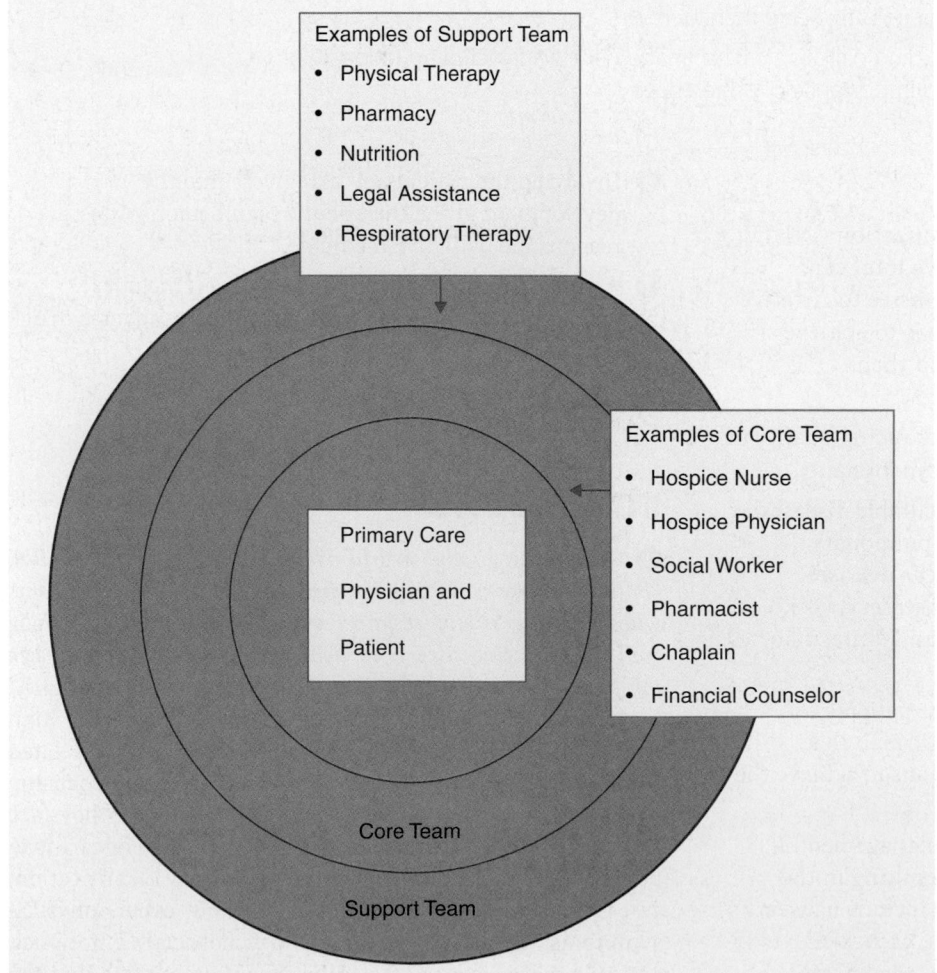

FIGURE 4–1. An illustrative view of how a palliative care team works together.

Examples of Support Team
- Physical Therapy
- Pharmacy
- Nutrition
- Legal Assistance
- Respiratory Therapy

Examples of Core Team
- Hospice Nurse
- Hospice Physician
- Social Worker
- Pharmacist
- Chaplain
- Financial Counselor

Primary Care Physician and Patient

Core Team

Support Team

attributed to acute illness or injury. Medical management shifted focus from comfort to a death-denying approach with prolonging life as the primary goal. With this shift in focus, palliative care became less of an emphasis until 1967, when the first modern hospice was established in London, England. Today the palliative care philosophy attempts to combine enhanced quality of life, compassionate care, and patient and family support with modern medical advances.

EPIDEMIOLOGY AND ETIOLOGY

Although the modern hospice model of care originated in England in 1967, the first hospice in the United States was founded in 1974. Since that time, hospice acceptance and utilization has increased in the United States. The number of Medicare beneficiaries enrolled in hospice increased by 100% between 2000 and 2005.[10] Medicare spending for hospice care tripled during that same time period, reflecting a greater number of patients receiving the benefits of this type of care. The Medicare Hospice Benefit is now the fastest growing benefit in the Medicare program, representing 3% of Medicare costs.[11] The growth between the early 1990s and 2005 was significant.

When the hospice Medicare benefit was introduced in 1982, most patients had a terminal diagnosis of cancer, representing over 90% of beneficiaries.[12] In 2005, less than 50% of patients receiving the Medicare Hospice Benefit have a cancer diagnosis, with the majority of hospice patients having other chronic or life-limiting diseases. Unfortunately, the average length of time a patient receives hospice care also decreased over time. Initially, the mean length of stay was 70 days per patient, but in 2005, the mean length of stay fell to approximately 20 days, resulting in less time for patients and families to benefit from the many services offered through hospice care.

Because palliative care and hospice have not typically been part of the traditional medical mindset, ongoing education has been directed toward physicians and other health care professionals to encourage them to introduce palliative care before a life-limiting disease has progressed to advanced stages. The goal is to offer hospice to patients when they have several months of life expectancy rather than waiting until the last days or weeks of life. In order to accomplish that, physicians are encouraged to discuss advanced care planning with individuals at the time of diagnosis of any chronic, life-limiting disease. As the health care community and the public recognize that psychosocial, spiritual, and emotional support of the patient, family, and caregiving system provides the foundation for coping with changes as patients decline, health care professionals are beginning to incorporate aspects of palliative care in the treatment plan sooner.

As health care providers recognize the benefit of palliative care for patients with any life-limiting illness, the approach to patient care has expanded beyond the cancer model of care. Understanding differences and similarities in pathophysiology of various disease states and their respective symptoms equips palliative care providers to develop appropriate individualized plans of care for their patients.

PATHOPHYSIOLOGY

● In many respects, understanding the pathophysiology of multiple end-stage disease states is daunting, yet, in palliative care, the emphasis is not so much on the disease as it is on the associated physical, psychological, social, and spiritual symptoms. Palliative care focuses on symptom management for patients with progressive, life-limiting illnesses from diagnosis through death where the pathophysiological impact of disease on a patient's symptoms may vary greatly depending on the stage of a patient's illness. ❸ *Palliative care is appropriate for all incurable diseases including cancer; chronic obstructive pulmonary disease; dementia, including Alzheimer's disease; Parkinson's disease; chronic cardiac disease; stroke; renal failure; hepatic failure; multiorgan failure; diabetes mellitus; etc.*

For the purpose of this chapter, pathophysiology will not be a primary focus. Rather, the philosophy of managing physical, psychological, social, and spiritual symptoms in order to maintain quality of life and prevent suffering is discussed within the context of progressively incurable illnesses. This philosophy frequently deviates from principles and concerns related to the management of patients where prolonging life is the goal.

CLINICAL PRESENTATION AND DIAGNOSIS

Cancer

Palliative care is most commonly associated with patients who have cancer. Regardless of whether or not the cancer is curable, most patients have various degrees of physical, psychological, social, and spiritual symptoms which arise once a diagnosis is confirmed. The primary site of solid tumor and hematologic cancers associated with limited life include, but are not limited to, lung, bronchus, breast, colon, rectum, pancreas, prostate, ovaries, uterus, brain, esophagus, liver, kidneys, bladder, lymph system, bone marrow, and skin. The spread of cancer cells (metastases) to distant areas are associated with poorer prognosis. Once a cancer patient has failed curative and life-prolonging therapy, prognosis and disease trajectory is easier to determine than in patients with other life-limiting diseases. The change in focus from cure to symptom control becomes apparent and, therefore, more acceptable. Symptoms associated with cancer are dependent on both the primary tumor site and the location of metastatic spread. Symptoms may also result from the effects of cancer treatments such as chemotherapy and radiation. (See Chaps. 88–99 for specific cancers and their treatments.)

End-Stage Heart Failure

Heart disease is the leading cause of death by disease. Many forms of heart disease result in sudden death; however, the disease progression of heart failure is protracted yet unpredictable. Advanced heart failure (class III–IV or stage C or D) is characterized by persistent symptoms that

Patient Encounter 1

TS is a 78-year-old white female admitted to a hospice program for palliative care. The patient has a primary diagnosis of breast cancer with metastases to the lung and bone. TS has a past medical history that includes chronic heart failure (CHF), hypothyroidism, osteoporosis, and gastroesophageal reflux disease (GERD). She has no known drug allergies. The patient's chief complaint upon admission is pain that is rated 5 on the pain scale (0–10), nausea and vomiting, depression, and constipation. She describes her pain as an aching pain in the areas of her bone metastases. The pain increases with movement. She also has a constant deep pain in her left chest area but it is not as severe. TS is currently bedbound.

VS: BP 120/82, RR 40, P 100, wt 44.5 kg (98 lb), ht 5'4"

Meds: Albuterol two inhalations every 2 hours; digoxin 0.25 mg by mouth daily; omeprazole 40 mg by mouth daily; furosemide 40 mg by mouth twice daily; oxycodone/acetaminophen 10/325; 1–2 tablets by mouth every 4 hours as needed; fentanyl patch 50 mcg/h; apply one patch every 72 hours; levothyroxine 25 mcg by mouth daily; alendronate 70 mg by mouth weekly; celecoxib 100 mg by mouth daily; multivitamin 1 tablet by mouth daily

What are potential etiologies of the nausea and vomiting TS is experiencing?

What type of the pain is TS experiencing?

What questions would you ask TS during your assessment?

What potential drug–drug interactions may exist and how would you monitor the patient for them?

Outline three interventions that the practitioner should make to improve the care of TS.

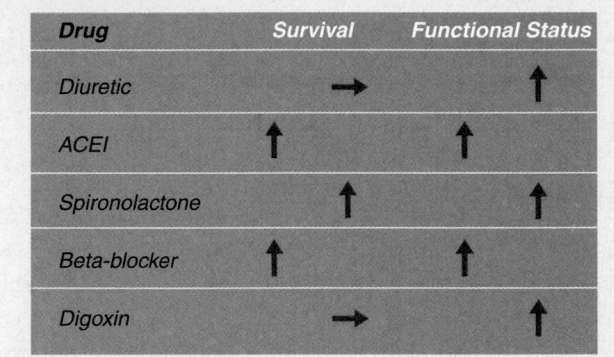

FIGURE 4–2. Drugs, their use in Class III–IV heart failure, and their effects on survival, hospital admissions, and functional status. →, survival does not increase or decrease, but stays the same; ↑, survival increases. (Data from Ref. 8, p. 172.)

limit activities of daily living despite optimal drug therapy. Common symptoms include fatigue, breathlessness, anxiety, fluid retention, and pain. In heart failure, standard medication management is intended to reduce the progression of cardiac remodeling and is considered disease modifying (Fig. 4–2). However, with the exception of cholesterol-lowering agents, these same cardiac medications are also palliative and should not be discontinued prematurely without cause. Exacerbations of heart failure symptoms should be aggressively treated as long as the patient is responsive to therapy and wishes to receive treatment. In hospice, this can often be accomplished through medication manipulation in the patient's home without the need for hospitalization (see Chap. 6).

Chronic Obstructive Pulmonary Disease

Chronic obstructive pulmonary disease (COPD) has a prolonged and variable course. Patients with COPD have a high number of physician visits and hospital admissions. Palliative care treatment is directed at reducing symptoms, reducing the rate of decline in lung function, preventing and treating exacerbations, and maintaining quality of life. In end-stage COPD, bronchodilators and anti-inflammatory agents become less effective. Symptoms of late-stage disease include wheezing, chronic sputum production, cough, frequent respiratory infections, dyspnea with exertion progressing to dyspnea at rest, fatigue, pain, hypoxia, and weight loss. Pulmonary hypertension frequently occurs and can lead to cor pulmonale or right-sided heart failure (see Chap. 15).

End-Stage Renal Disease

Chronic kidney disease is progressive and leads to renal failure. In end-stage renal disease (ESRD) the only life-sustaining treatments are dialysis or renal transplant. Without treatment, kidney failure causes uremia, oliguria, hyperkalemia and other electrolyte disorders, fluid overload and hypertension unresponsive to treatment, anemia, hepatorenal syndrome, and uremic pericarditis. Symptoms associated with chronic kidney disease (stage 5) include fatigue, pruritus, nausea, vomiting, constipation, dysgeusia, muscle pain, and bleeding abnormalities. Palliative care in these patients includes the minimization of listed symptoms; however, because many options for drug therapy will be cleared through the kidneys, agents should be chosen cautiously to avoid other complications (see Chap. 26).

End-Stage Liver Disease

Like kidney disease, the only treatment to prolong life in advanced liver disease is transplant. Patients with end-stage liver disease typically present with ascites, jaundice, pruritus, or encephalopathy and frequently with all four symptoms. Additionally, bleeding disorders are common and associated esophageal or gastric varices bleeds are the cause of death in about one-third of those who die from liver disease. Palliative care in these patients focuses on the symptom management of end-stage liver disease complications.

HIV/AIDS

Pharmacologic advances have changed the prognosis and progression of HIV/AIDS. Today, palliative care is predominately directed toward patients who have not had access to drug therapy in the early stages of their disease. Patients with progressed HIV/AIDS are susceptible to acquire opportunistic infections and cancer which may hasten their death. Common symptoms observed in individuals with HIV/AIDS at the end of their life include fatigue, profound weight loss, breathlessness, nausea, GI disturbances, and pain. The goal of palliative care in these patients is to minimize common AIDS-related symptoms (see Chap. 87).

Stroke/Cerebral Vascular Accident

Stroke can be a result of hemorrhage or ischemia. The prognosis of patients who have had a cerebral vascular accident (CVA) is unpredictable and may be extended, resulting in caregiver fatigue. Approximately one-third of patients who have a stroke will die within 2 years. Patients with stroke deal with loss of physical and cognitive function, poststroke pain and frequent depression. Incontinence, aphasia and dysphagia and seizures are also common. Patients who have dysphagia have a high incidence of aspiration pneumonia, which often is the cause of death (see Chap. 11).

Parkinson's Disease

Parkinson's disease is a degenerative neurologic disease with a long chronic, progressive course evidenced by akinesia, rigidity, and tremor. The goal of therapy is to reduce symptoms and maintain or improve quality of life. Palliative care provides support to both the patient and caregiving system as patients become more disabled and as neuropsychiatric problems arise. Symptoms that frequently occur are skin infections and breakdown, constipation, pain, depression, hallucinations, and confusion. Individuals with Parkinson's disease often die from bronchial pneumonia due to dysphagia and complication from falls (see Chap. 32).

Amyotrophic Lateral Sclerosis (Lou Gehrig's Disease)

Amyotrophic lateral sclerosis (ALS) is a chronic neurodegenerative disorder that is characterized by progressive loss of motor neurons. The median survival is approximately 3 years from the onset of symptoms with less than 15% of patients surviving 10 years. Initially symptoms of ALS present as limb weakness, with other symptoms developing in no particular order including cramps, spasticity, pain, dysarthria, sialorrhea, fatigue, insomnia, depression, fear and anxiety, involuntary emotional expression disorder,

constipation, aspiration, and laryngospasm. Many patients do not have cognitive impairment; however, one-fourth to one-half of patients with ALS may have associated frontal lobe dementia. Disease progression eventually involves all systems except sphincter control and eye movement. Unless the individual has long-term mechanical ventilation, the cause of death is typically respiratory failure.

Alzheimer's and Other Dementia

Dementia is a progressive, nonreversible deterioration in cognitive function with associated behavioral dysfunction. Alzheimer's disease accounts for the majority of dementia cases while vascular, Parkinson's disease, dementia with Lewy body, and frontotemporal dementias are less prevalent. Drug therapy is targeted at slowing the progression of the cognitive symptoms and preserving the patient function. As patients progress toward end-stage dementia, in addition to memory loss and personality and behavioral changes, they require assistance in basic activities of daily living such as feeding, dressing, and toileting. At this point they may not respond to their surroundings, may not communicate, or have impaired movements and dysphagia. Depression, agitation, delusions, compulsions, confusion, hallucinations, incontinence, and disruption of sleep/wake cycles are all common symptoms in end-stage dementias. Assessment of symptoms is challenging due to the cognitive impairment and frequent aphasia. Palliative care is not only directed toward the patient but also emotional support is needed for those close to them (see Chap. 35).

TREATMENT

❹ *Following a complete assessment of the patient, developing a comprehensive therapeutic plan that utilizes the fewest number of medications to achieve the highest quality of life is essential.* Many times, one drug may provide relief for multiple symptoms, resulting in better patient care, lower costs, and fewer medications for the patient to take. Cost-effective drug recommendations are essential for hospice agencies to control costs, given that Medicare and most other third-party payors reimburse hospice at a fixed per-diem rate. Avoiding polypharmacy will reduce the incidence of adverse drug events related to drug interactions, excessive side effects, and duplications of therapy. The following list of symptoms addressed by palliative care includes common symptoms observed in end of life; however, it is not comprehensive. ❺ *Palliative care is more than just pain management. It includes the treatment of symptoms resulting in the discomfort for the patient, which may include nausea, agitation, anxiety, depression, dyspnea, cachexia, constipation, diarrhea, pressure ulcers, edema, etc.*

It should be noted that many drugs used for the treatment of symptoms in end-of-life care are often prescribed for unapproved uses, administered by unapproved routes or in dosages higher than that recommended by the package insert. This "off-label" use of medication is not unique to palliative care.

Anxiety

A comprehensive review of anxiety disorders may be found in Chapter 40.

▶ Palliative Care Considerations

- Anxiety is "a state of fearfulness, apprehension, worry, emotional discomfort, or uneasiness that results from an unknown internal stimulus, is excessive, or is otherwise inappropriate to a given situation."[13]

- Anxiety is closely related to fear, but fear has an identified cause or source of worry (e.g., fear of death). Fear may be more responsive to counseling than an anxiety state that the patient cannot attribute to a particular fearful stimulus. Anxiety disorders are the most prevalent class of mental disorders overall, so it is not surprising that anxiety is a common cause of distress at life's end.[14]

- In addition to anxiety disorders, a variety of conditions can cause, mimic, or exacerbate anxiety[15,16]:
  - Delirium, particularly in its early stages, can easily be confused with anxiety.
  - Physical complications of illness, especially dyspnea and undertreated pain, are common precipitants.
  - Significant anxiety is present in the majority of patients with advanced lung disease and is closely related to periods of oxygen desaturation.
  - Medication side effects, especially akathisia from older antipsychotics and antiemetics (including and especially metoclopramide), can present as anxiety.
  - Interpersonal, spiritual, or existential concerns can mimic anxiety.
  - Patients with an anxious or dependent coping style are at high risk of anxiety as a complication of advanced illness.
  - Short of making a diagnosis of a formal anxiety disorder, differentiating normal worry and apprehension from pathologic anxiety requires clinical judgment.

- Behaviors indicative of pathological anxiety include:
  - Intense worry or dread
  - Physical distress (e.g., tension, jitteriness, or restlessness)
  - Maladaptive behaviors (e.g., treatment nonadherence, social withdrawal, or avoidance)
  - Diminished coping and inability to relax
  - Pathologic anxiety may be complicated by insomnia, depression, fatigue, GI upset, dyspnea, or dysphagia. Anxiety can also worsen these conditions if they are already present.
  - Untreated anxiety may lead to numerous complications, including withdrawal from social support, poor coping, limited participation in palliative care treatment goals, and family distress.

- Reassess the patient for anxiety with any change in behavior or any change in the underlying medical condition.
  - Search for probable etiologies
  - Assess for formal anxiety disorders
  - Assess for other contributing factors

- Appropriate assessment of anxiety is key to its management.

▶ Nonpharmacologic Treatment in Palliative Care

Regardless of what treatment approach is chosen, the following principles apply:

- Offer emotional support and reassurance when appropriate.
- Err on the side of treatment—be willing to palliate anxiety.
- Assess treatment response and side effects frequently.
- Aim to provide maximum resolution of anxiety.
- Educate patients and families about anxiety and its treatments.
- Psychotherapies can help in the management of anxiety, though the availability of trained therapists willing to make home visits, and limited stamina and attention span of seriously ill patients, typically make such therapies impractical in the hospice setting.
- Cognitive and behavioral therapies can be beneficial, including simple relaxation exercises or distraction strategies (i.e., focusing on something pleasurable or at least emotionally neutral).
- Encourage chaplain visits, especially if spiritual and existential concerns predominate.
- When an underlying cause of anxiety can be identified, treatment is initially aimed at the precipitating problem, with monitoring to see if anxiety improves or resolves as the underlying cause is addressed.

▶ Pharmacotherapy in Palliative Care

- In most cases, management of pathological anxiety in the hospice setting involves pharmacologic therapies. Benzodiazepines are the gold standard for treatment; however, selective serotonin reuptake inhibitors (SSRIs), typical and atypical antipsychotics, and tricyclic antidepressants may also be appropriate.[17]
- The primary goal of therapy for anxiety in hospice is patient comfort. Aim to prevent anxiety, not just treat it with as needed medications when it flares. Think of pain management as an analogy.
- Start at the lower end of the dose range of a given anxiolytic agent to prevent unnecessary sedation, but recognize that standard or higher doses may be required.
- Avoid use of bupropion and psychostimulants for anxiety. While effective for depression, they are ineffective for anxiety and may make anxiety worse.

- Lorazepam, alprazolam, and diazepam are commonly crushed and placed under the tongue with a few drops of water for patients who have difficulty swallowing.
- Low dose haloperidol is also used to treat anxiety in palliative care particularly if delirium is present.
- Chapter 40 provides more detailed information on appropriate use of anxiolytic agents.

Delirium

▶ *Palliative Care Considerations*

- Delirium is a very common disorder in hospice, occurring in more than 80% of terminally ill patients, most often in the last few days of life.[13]
- Potential causes of delirium in the hospice setting include, but are not limited to, medical illness, dehydration, hypoxia, metabolic disturbances, sepsis, side effects of drugs, urinary retention, constipation or impaction, uncontrolled pain, or alcohol or drug withdrawal.[18,19]
- A classic symptom of delirium is clouding of consciousness. This can be manifested by an inability to either maintain or shift attention. Patients also have impaired cognitive functioning, which may or may not include memory disturbances.
- "Sundowning" is very common phenomenon in end of life and especially in the presence of delirium. It presents as daytime sleepiness and nighttime agitation and restlessness.
- Another common characteristic is fluctuation in severity of delirium symptoms during the course of the day. This can even occur within the course of a single hour or also from day to day.
- Patients who exhibit agitation from their delirium are easy to identify, but those who present as withdrawn and with diminished responsiveness ("quiet" delirium) are more difficult to diagnose. It is not uncommon for patients to exhibit both quiet and agitated delirium. Treatment is the same for both types of delirium.
- Delirium is difficult to distinguish from dementia. Delirium more commonly presents as a sudden onset (e.g., hours to days), with an altered level of consciousness and a clouded sensorium. However, dementia more commonly presents gradually and with an unimpaired level of consciousness.

▶ *Nonpharmacologic Treatment in Palliative Care*

- Establishing a safe, soothing environment where there are familiar objects such as photographs and familiar music can be helpful to calm the patient.
- Minimizing risk of injury is important when the patient is agitated.
- Providing education to families and caregivers about the causes of delirium, signs and symptoms, and how to best manage it will help to reduce their anxiety and distress when it occurs.

▶ *Pharmacotherapy in Palliative Care*

- The most important initial step is to determine the goal of care. If possible, reverse the underlying cause of delirium in order to restore the patient to a meaningful cognitive status.[18]
- If the precipitating factors cannot be reversed, initiate therapy to treat the symptoms. Patients who are not agitated may not require any treatment other than comfort measures. If the patient is irreversibly delirious and agitated, drug therapy is generally indicated.
- Neuroleptic drugs (conventional or atypical antipsychotics) are the drugs most commonly used to treat confusion and agitation associated with delirium. However, treatment of delirium with these drugs is an "off-label" indication.
- Atypical antipsychotics such as risperidone, olanzapine, quetiapine, ziprasidone, paliperidone, and aripiprazole account for a major portion of increasing medication costs in the geriatric population.[20]
- Haloperidol, when given in doses less than 2 mg/day is well-tolerated and nonsedating and is within the recommended dosing parameters for long-term care facilities.
- When sedation is beneficial for terminal aggressive, agitated delirium, chlorpromazine is useful to provide patient comfort as they approach death. When patients are bedbound and in the final stages of life, orthostatic hypotension common with chlorpromazine is not a concern.
- Haloperidol and chlorpromazine are commonly given sublingually or rectally if swallowing becomes difficult, although these are not approved routes of administration. Haloperidol, but not chlorpromazine, can be given subcutaneously.[21,22]
- Administering benzodiazepines alone in a patient with delirium can actually make the delirium and confusion worse, although it is sometimes helpful to add benzodiazepines along with antipsychotics if sedation is desired. Phenobarbital may also be used for this purpose

Dyspnea

▶ *Palliative Care Considerations*

- Dyspnea is described as an uncomfortable awareness of breathing. It is a subjective sensation, and patient self-report is the only reliable indicator. Respiratory rate or Po_2 often does not correlate with the feeling of breathlessness.[23,24]
- Respiratory effort and dyspnea are not the same. Patients may report substantial relief of dyspnea from opioids with no change in respiratory rate.
- The prevalence of dyspnea varies from 12% to 74% and tends to worsen in the last week of life in terminally ill cancer patients to between 50% and 70%.

Patient Encounter 2

JK is an 80-year-old white male admitted to hospice with a primary diagnosis of CHF. Other comorbidities include renal failure, diabetes mellitus, coronary artery disease, hyperlipidemia, anemia, arthritis and hypothyroidism. The patient also has a percutaneous endoscopic gastrostomy (PEG) tube, peripherally inserted central catheter (PICC) and Foley catheter. The patient has no known drug allergies. JK's chief complaint is lower leg edema and shortness of breath.

Meds: Sliding scale insulin (e.g., regular insulin administered with fasting blood glucose greater than 250 mg/dL); potassium chloride 20 mEq daily via PEG; furosemide 20 mg twice daily via PEG; levothyroxine 88 mcg crushed daily via PEG; loperamide liquid 4 mg twice daily via PEG; famotidine liquid 20 mg daily via PEG; simvastatin 20 mg daily via PEG; ibuprofen liquid 400 mg every 6 hours via PEG

What potential interventions could the practitioner make to improve JK's care?

What medications could be discontinued?

How does the presence of a percutaneous endoscopic gastrostomy tube impact the drug therapy decisions?

Would the use of a positive inotropic agent in this patient provide benefit? What would be the risks and benefits?

What potential drug–drug interactions may exist? How would you monitor the patient for them?

- A thorough history and physical examination should be taken and possible reversible causes of dyspnea should be identified and treated, if present.

▶ *Nonpharmacologic Treatment in Palliative Care*

- Provide information and anticipate and proactively prepare the patient and family for worsening symptoms.
- Identify triggers that cause dyspnea attacks and minimize as much as possible.
- Educate patient and family regarding treatment of dyspnea, including the use of opioids.
- Prevent isolation and address spiritual issues that can worsen symptom.
- Encourage relaxation and minimize the need for exertion.
- Reposition to comfort, usually to a more upright position or with the compromised lung down.
- Avoid strong odors, perfumes, and smoking in the patient's presence or in close proximity.
- Improve air circulation/quality.
  - Provide a draft, use fans, or open windows.
  - Adjust temperature/humidity with air conditioner or humidifier.

▶ *Pharmacotherapy in Palliative Care*

- If no treatable causes can be identified or when treatments do not completely alleviate distressing symptoms, opioids are first-line agents for treating dyspnea.[25,26]
- Opioids suppress respiratory awareness, decrease response to hypoxia and hypercapnia, vasodilate, and have sedative properties.
- Low-dose opioids (e.g., starting oral dose of morphine approximately 5 mg) have been shown to be safe and effective in the treatment of dyspnea. Doses should be titrated judiciously.

- As anxiety can exacerbate dyspnea, benzodiazepines and antidepressants that have anxiolytic properties can be beneficial.[27]
- Once an effective dose of an opioid has been established, converting to an extended-release preparation may simplify dosing.
- When using opioids, anticipate side effects and prevent constipation by initiating a stimulant laxative/stool softener combination.
- Nebulized opioids for treatment of dyspnea are controversial. Study results have been inconsistent.[28–30]
  - Nonrandomized studies, case reports, and chart reviews describe anecdotal improvement in dyspnea using nebulized opioids; however, several controlled studies using nebulized opioids have provided inconclusive or negative results.
  - Nebulized opioids may be advantageous in patients that are not able to or willing to take an oral agent or cannot tolerate adverse effects of systemic administration.
  - Fentanyl appears to be the safest nebulized opioid.
- Nebulized furosemide appears effective for dyspnea refractory to other conventional therapies.[31–33]
  - Hypothesized mechanism of action of nebulized furosemide is its ability to enhance pulmonary stretch receptor activity, inhibition of chloride movement through the membrane of the epithelial cell, and its ability to increase the synthesis of bronchodilating prostaglandins.
- Oxygen therapy may be useful to patients with dyspnea and can reverse hypoxemia.
- For known etiologies of dyspnea, consider the following:[23,25,27]
  - **Bronchospasm or COPD exacerbation**: Albuterol, ipratropium, and/or oral steroids should be used for

symptoms management. Nebulizing bronchodilators are more effective than using handheld inhalers in patients who are weak and have difficulty controlling their breathing.

- **Thick secretions**: If cough reflex is strong, loosen secretions with guaifenesin or nebulized saline. If the cough is weak, hyoscyamine, glycopyrrolate, or scopolamine patch can effectively dry secretions.
- **Anxiety associated with dyspnea**: Consider benzodiazepines (e.g., diazepam, lorazepam).
- **Effusions**: Thoracentesis will be necessary.
- **Low hemoglobin**: Red blood cell transfusion (controversial) or erythropoietin (rarely used in hospice, but might have a larger role in palliative care patients).
- **Infections:** Antibiotic therapy as appropriate.
- **Pulmonary emboli**: Anticoagulants for prevention and treatment or vena cava filter placement (rarely used in hospice, but might have a larger role in palliative care patients).
- **Rales due to volume overload**: Reduction of fluid intake or diuretic therapy as appropriate.

Nausea and Vomiting

A comprehensive review of nausea and vomiting may be found in Chapter 20.

▶ Palliative Care Considerations

- Up to 71% of palliative care patients will develop nausea and vomiting with approximately 40% experiencing these symptoms in the last 6 weeks of life. Chronic nausea can be defined as lasting longer than a week and without a well-identified or self-limiting cause, such as chemotherapy, radiation, or infection.[34-37]
- Four major mechanisms are correlated with the stimulation of the vomiting center (Fig. 4–3). Potentially reversible causes of nausea and vomiting should not be overlooked.
- Causes of chronic nausea in end-of-life patients may include: autonomic dysfunction, constipation, antibiotics, nonsteroidal anti-inflammatory drugs (NSAIDs), other drugs, infection, bowel obstruction, metabolic abnormalities (e.g., renal or hepatic failure, hypercalcemia), increased intracranial pressure, anxiety, radiation therapy, chemotherapy, or untreated pain.

▶ Nonpharmacologic Treatment in Palliative Care

- Relaxation techniques may prove beneficial in some patients.
- Strong foods or odors should be avoided.
- If possible, eliminate offending medications.

▶ Pharmacotherapy in Palliative Care

- The clinical features of nausea and vomiting should guide the choice of antiemetics used (for a more comprehensive review, refer to Chap. 20). The following are examples of managing nausea and vomiting as it correlates with the etiology:
- **Chemoreceptor trigger zone** (CTZ)-induced nausea and vomiting are caused by chemotherapeutic agents, bacterial toxins, metabolic products (e.g., uremia), and opioids. Dopamine (D_2), serotonin (5-HT), and neurokinin-1 are the primary neurotransmitters involved in this process. Therapy is based on blocking D_2 with D_2-antagonists including butyrophenones (e.g., haloperidol), phenothiazines, and metoclopramide. Serotonin (5-HT$_3$) antagonists (e.g., ondansetron) are mainly used for chemotherapy and radiotherapy-induced nausea.[38,39]
- **Cerebral cortex**-induced nausea and vomiting can be caused by anxiety, taste, and smell, as well as by increased intracranial pressure. Corticosteroids are

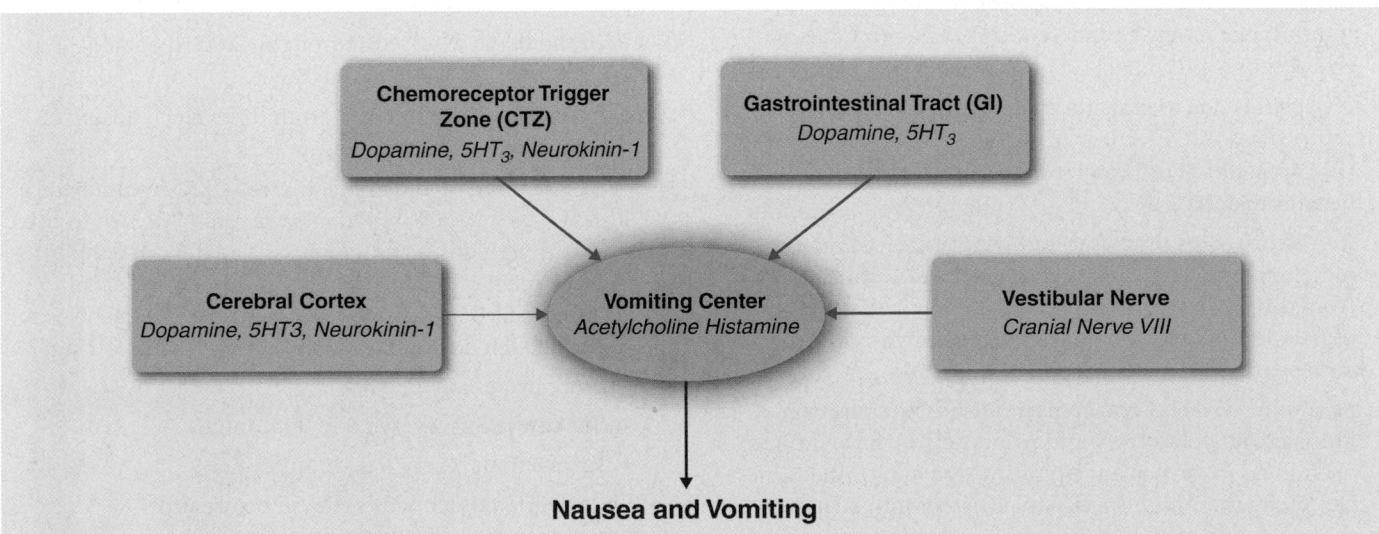

FIGURE 4–3. Mechanisms and associated neurotransmitters involved in nausea and vomiting.

administered to decrease intracranial pressure while anxiolytics such as benzodiazepines are used to treat the "anticipatory," gustatory, and olfactory stimulation.

- **Vestibular** nausea and vomiting is triggered by motion. Opioids can sensitize the vestibular center resulting in movement-induced nausea. Ambulatory patients are more susceptible to vestibular nausea and vomiting then bedbound patients. Because histamine and acetylcholine are the predominant neurotransmitters here, antihistamines and anticholinergics are the drugs of choice in movement-induced nausea and vomiting.

- **GI tract** stimulation occurs through vagal and sympathetic pathways. These pathways can be triggered by stimulation of either mechanoreceptors or chemoreceptors located in the gut. Gastric stasis, GI obstruction, drugs, metastatic disease, bacterial toxins, chemotherapeutic agents, and irradiation can lead to nausea and vomiting. Glossopharyngeal or vagus nerve stimulation in the pharynx by sputum, mucosal lesions, or infection (e.g., *Candida*) can also evoke nausea. The major neurotransmitters in the upper GI tract are D_2, acetylcholine, and 5-HT. Metoclopramide blocks $5-HT_4$ and increases gastric motility above the jejunum, whereas anticholinergics will decrease GI spasticity and motility in nausea induced by gut hyperactivity. In high doses, metoclopramide will also act as a $5-HT_3$ antagonist.

- **Autonomic failure** causes gastroparesis resulting in anorexia, nausea, early satiety, and constipation. Delayed gastric emptying is frequently observed in patients with diabetes mellitus, chronic renal failure, and neurologic disorders. Malnutrition, cachexia, lung and pancreatic cancers, HIV, radiotherapy, and drugs such as opioids, anticholinergics, antidepressants, and vasodilators have been associated with autonomic failure and resulting chronic nausea, poor performance, tachycardia, and malnutrition.

- In addition to their usefulness in reducing intracranial pressure, corticosteriods have been found to be effective in nonspecific nausea and vomiting. The mechanism of this action is unknown.

- If nausea is due to gastritis, hiatal hernia, gastroesophageal reflux disease (GERD), or peptic ulcer disease, histamine$_2$ (H_2) antagonists or proton pump inhibitors (PPIs) should be administered.

- Refractory cases of nausea and vomiting often require judiciously selected combinations of medications from different classes (e.g., various combinations of haloperidol, metoclopramide, diphenhydramine, lorazepam, dexamethasone).

- Serotonin$_3$ (5-HT$_3$) antagonists, such as ondansetron, granisetron, dolasetron, and palonosetron, have limited usefulness in nausea and vomiting due to terminal illness caused by their high specificity for serotonin$_3$. They are typically indicated with emetogenic chemotherapy and up to 10 to 14 days post-treatment.

- Aprepitant is a neurokinin-1 antagonist that is indicated for the treatment of nausea due to highly emetogenic chemotherapy and in combination with a 5-HT$_3$ antagonist and corticosteroid. Aprepitrant should not be used as a sole agent.

Pain

A comprehensive review of pain management may be found in Chapter 33.

▶ *Palliative Care Considerations*

- According to the SUPPORT study, 74% to 95% of very ill or dying patients still experience uncontrolled pain.[3] Although existing drug therapy affords the opportunity to manage over 90% of pain, many patients needlessly suffer.[40]

- As with any pain management, patient assessment is key to choosing appropriate therapeutic interventions. Because pain is subjective, both physical and humanistic factors must be considered.

- Patients in an end-of-life setting must also be evaluated for anxiety, depression, delirium, and other neurologic influences that may heighten a patient's awareness or response to pain.

▶ *Nonpharmacologic Treatment in Palliative Care*

- Nonpharmacologic treatment is essential in chronic pain management.

- Physical, complementary, and cognitive behavioral interventions reduce the perception of pain and decrease the dose requirements of medications. Examples of such strategies may include education and information about medical treatments (e.g., misconceptions about pain medications), massage, ice, heat, physical therapy, music therapy, imagery, pet therapy, psychotherapy, etc.

▶ *Pharmacotherapy in Palliative Care*

- The WHO's approach to pain management is still appropriate for most nociceptive pain (see Chap. 33).

- Pain should be assessed thoroughly and frequently, especially at the onset of treatment.

- For chronic, constant pain, around the clock dosing of analgesics are usually necessary.[41,42]

- When titrating opioid doses, increase daily maintenance doses by 25% to 50% if patients are requiring two to three breakthrough doses per 24 hours. The dose of opioids for the treatment of breakthrough pain should be equal to 5% to 15% of the daily maintenance dose. Frequencies for breakthrough dosing should not exceed the following:

  - **Oral**: every 1 to 2 hours
  - **Subcutaneous**: every 20 to 30 minutes
  - **Intravenous**: every 6 to 20 minutes

- Only short acting opioids should be used for breakthrough pain (e.g., immediate-release morphine, oxycodone, and hydromorphone are common examples).

- Monitor for and appropriately treat common side effects of opioids. Common side effects of opioids include constipation, nausea and vomiting, itching, and transient sedation.
  - Because constipation occurs with all chronic opioid therapy, prevention is imperative. Stimulant laxatives (senna or bisacodyl) with or without a stool softener (docusate) are the drugs of choice for opioid-induced constipation.
- Myoclonus, delirium, hallucinations, and hyperalgesia are possible signs of opioid neurotoxicity and require a change in opioid therapy or dose reduction.
- Respiratory depression is very uncommon with appropriate opioid dose titration. However, if it does occur, small doses (0.1 mg) of the mu receptor antagonist, naloxone, are appropriate and can be repeated if necessary. The goal is to increase respirations to a safe level while preventing the patient from experiencing a loss of pain control.
- Fentanyl transdermal patches may be appropriate in some patients however many end-of-life patients experience muscle wasting and dehydration resulting in reduced and variable absorption. Fentanyl transdermal patches have a slow onset of action contributing to difficulty in dose titration.
- Drugs that should not be used for treatment of pain during end-of-life care are listed in Table 4–1.

Table 4–1

Drugs NOT Recommended for Treatment in End-of-Life Care

Drug	Rationale
Meperidine	Meperidine has a short duration of analgesia (e.g., 2–3 hours) and its metabolite, normeperidine, may accumulate with repeated dosing, especially in geriatric patients, resulting in neurotoxicity
Propoxyphene	Propoxyphene's metabolite, norpropoxyphene, may accumulate with repeated dosing, especially in geriatric patients, resulting in cardiotoxicity
Opioid agonist-antagonists (e.g., pentazocine, butorphanol, nalbuphine)	The risk of precipitating withdrawal symptoms in opioid-dependent patients in addition to their ceiling dose and possible induction of psychomimetic effects (e.g., dysphoria, delusions, hallucinations) make this group of analgesics inappropriate for use
Anxiolytics (e.g., alprazolam, diazepam, lorazepam) and other sedative-hypnotic drugs (e.g., barbiturates)	These agents have not shown benefit in patients with nociceptive pain. The added sedative properties of these agents compromise neurologic assessment in patients receiving opioids

- Different types of pain may require other analgesics or adjuvant medications. For example:
  - Visceral pain (nociceptive pain that is caused by stretching or spasms of visceral organs such as the GI tract, liver, and pancreas) should be treated with the standard WHO step approach to pain, with the addition of anticholinergic agents or, if inflammation is associated with the pain, corticosteroids.
  - Bone pain (a common metastatic site of various cancers) is best treated with NSAIDs or corticosteroids in addition to standard opioid therapy.
  - Neuropathic pain (pain caused by damage to the afferent nociceptive fibers) can be managed with tricyclic antidepressants, antiepileptic drugs, tramadol, or N-methyl-D-aspartate antagonists such as ketamine. Methadone is an opioid mu agonist that has a role in neuropathic pain given its added N-methyl-D-aspartate antagonist activity.

Terminal Secretions

▶ Palliative Care Considerations

- Terminal secretions, or death rattle, is the noise produced by the oscillatory movements of secretions in the upper airways in association with the inspiratory and expiratory phases of respiration.[43,44]
- As patients lose their ability to swallow and clear oral secretions, accumulation of mucus results in a rattling or gurgling sound produced by air passing through mucus in the lungs and air passages.
- The sound does not represent any discomfort for the patient. However, the sound is sometimes so distressing to the family that it should be treated.
- Terminal secretions are typically seen only in patients who are obtunded or are too weak to expectorate.
- Drugs that decrease secretions are best initiated at the first sign of death rattle, as they do not affect existing respiratory secretions.
- These agents have limited or no impact when the secretions are secondary to pneumonia or pulmonary edema.

▶ Nonpharmacologic Treatment in Palliative Care

- Position the patient on his/her side or in a semiprone position to help facilitate drainage of secretions.
- If necessary, place the patient in the Trendelenburg position (lowering the head of the bed); this allows fluids to move into the oropharnyx, facilitating an easy removal. Do not maintain this position for long, as there is a risk of aspiration.
- Oropharyngeal suctioning is another option, but may be disturbing to both the patient and visitors.
- Fluid intake can also be decreased, as appropriate.

▶ *Pharmacotherapy in Palliative Care*

- Anticholinergic drugs remain the standard of therapy for prevention and treatment of terminal secretions due to their ability to effectively dry secretions.[45–47]

- Drugs used for this indication are similar pharmacologically, and one can be selected by anticholinergic potency, onset of action, route of administration, alertness of patient, and cost.

- The most commonly used anticholinergic agents are atropine, hyoscyamine, scopolamine, and glycopyrrolate.

- Anticholinergic side effects are common and include blurred vision, constipation, urinary retention, confusion, delirium, restlessness, hallucinations, dry mouth, and heart palpitations.

- Unlike the other anticholinergics, glycopyrrolate does not cross the blood–brain barrier and is associated with fewer central nervous system side effects. Glycopyrrolate is a potent drying agent when compared to others agents and has the potential to cause excessive dryness.[48]

Advanced Heart Failure

▶ *Palliative Care Considerations*

- Heart failure symptoms at the end of life may include hypotension, volume overload, edema, and fatigue. Patients should be assessed to confirm symptoms are related to heart failure rather than other disease states to ensure appropriate treatment strategies.[49,50]

- The goals for advanced heart failure treatment will differ from traditional heart failure management. Drug therapy will be focused on symptom management rather than improving mortality. Prevention of cardiovascular disease through cholesterol reduction is no longer necessary at this point.

▶ *Nonpharmacologic Treatment in Palliative Care*

- Patients should be maintained in a comfortable position with feet elevated to minimize lower leg fluid accumulation.

- Patients should minimize high-salt foods to reduce fluid accumulation associated with a failing heart.

- The patient should not over exert during physical activity. At this stage in heart failure, comfort becomes the primary initiative.

▶ *Pharmacotherapy in Palliative Care*

- If patient becomes symptomatic of hypotension, reduce dose of angiotensin-converting enzyme (ACE) inhibitor, angiotensin receptor blocker (ARB), and/or β-adrenergic blocker. For β-adrenergic blockers, in particular, this should be done gradually to avoid significant clinical deterioration.

- If volume overload occurs or persists, consider tapering off β-adrenergic blocker therapy.

- If the patient is fatigued while taking a β-adrenergic blocking agent *and* their heart rate does not increase with exertion, consider tapering down the dose of β-adrenergic blocker.

- If patient's renal function deteriorates (e.g., cardiorenal syndrome), consider discontinuing the ACE inhibitor (or the ARB).

- If the patient restricts sodium and water intake, consider reducing the dose of diuretic or potentially discontinuing therapy.

- Digoxin toxicity is common; therefore, patients should be carefully monitored, and therapy adjusted or discontinued as appropriate. Monitoring should include complaints of anorexia, nausea and vomiting, visual disturbances, disorientation, confusion, or cardiac arrhythmias.

- Hydroxymethylglutaryl coenzyme-A (HMG-CoA) reductase inhibitors (and other cholesterol lowering medications) 2 are likely to have a long-term effect rather than a palliative effect; consider discontinuing therapy.

- Figure 4–2 provides a list of agents that improve functional status in advanced heart failure patients.

OUTCOME EVALUATION

6 *Involving the patient and caregivers in the development of the therapeutic plan demonstrates responsible palliative medicine.* Before the implementation of drug therapy, the patient and caregiver should be involved with the decision-making process. The practitioner should ensure that his or her understanding of the patient's goals are being addressed. **7** *Assessing positive therapeutic outcomes includes resolution of symptoms while minimizing adverse drug events.* Resolution of symptoms is very important to patients and their caregivers. The hallmark of palliative medicine is specializing in symptom management while preventing adverse drug events. Cultural diversity is an extremely important consideration when establishing goals. Various cultures may perceive some symptoms as more or less important and the practitioner should be aware of those differences.

Nearly all physical symptoms are exacerbated by humanistic suffering. Patients with life-limiting diseases have emotional and spiritual issues that deserve attention by trained professionals. Addressing these concerns and providing support and coping skills can dramatically reduce the medication requirements for symptom control. Psychosocial and spiritual support is not only directed toward the patient in palliative care, but also supports the family during the time of the illness and after the death of their loved one. This bereavement support of the family is mandated under the Medicare Hospice Benefit and is unique to hospice care.

8 *Patient and caregiver education is vital to ensuring positive outcomes.* If the patient and caregiver are unaware of the purposes of the strategies used in palliative medicine, adherence to regimens will be hindered and outcomes will be compromised. Practitioners who are challenged in the area of palliative medicine are greatly rewarded through achieving positive outcomes and observing immediate results of good decision making.

Patient Encounter 3

TT, a 76-year-old white female, presents to the outpatient clinic with a complaint of nausea and occasional vomiting. Her nausea started approximately 2 weeks ago and has progressively worsened. The patient also has a recent complaint of constipation (the past few weeks). The patient has a past medical history of non-small cell lung cancer (completed last chemotherapy regimen 3 weeks ago), osteoarthris, and hypertension. The patient has smoked one pack per day for the past 20 years and drinks occasional alcohol. The patient's family history is unknown. The patient reports an allergy to morphine.

Meds: Naproxen 500 mg every 6 hours as needed for osteoarthritis pain (started 4 weeks ago); enalapril 10 mg twice daily; celecoxib 100 mg twice daily; acetaminophen 500 mg every 6 hours as needed for pain; hydrocodone/acetaminophen 5/500 mg two tablets every 6 hours as needed for cancer pain; ginseng (the patient takes as needed for energy)

What potential drug–drug interactions exist in this patient?

What medications could be discontinued and/or changed?

How does the patient's allergy to morphine impact potential treatment options?

How could this patient's pain regimen be improved? Should the different types of pain the patient is experiencing be managed differently?

Patient Care and Monitoring

Other symptoms that are commonly observed in palliative care that the practitioner should monitor:

- **Depression**: Patients may need to experience quicker symptom relief than typical antidepressants may provide. In some cases, methylphenidate may be an appropriate, short-term option for treatment.

- **Insomnia**: Many times, patients experience insomnia due to a lack of appropriate symptom management. Treatment should begin with uncontrolled symptoms. Sleep disruption should be minimized and good patient assessment is necessary to effectively manage insomnia.

- **Constipation**: Most patients experience constipation as a result of opioid use, which requires management with a stimulant laxative; other drugs, poor hydration, dietary supplements, and immobility may contribute to constipation as well. Careful assessment of etiology is important before implementing treatment.

- **Diarrhea**: Patients experiencing fluid loss through excessive diarrhea need to be monitored for dehydration and electrolyte imbalance. Fluid replacement is typically the first line of therapy in addition to drug therapy to minimize the symptom. Overflow diarrhea from constipation or a bowel obstruction is often misdiagnosed and treated inappropriately, worsening the problem.

- **Dysphagia**: Difficulty swallowing is common in end-of-life patients and may necessitate that medications be given through alternative routes of administration. Knowledge of drug absorption and disposition when administered rectally, sublingually, and topically is key in good clinical decision making.

Abbreviations Introduced in This Chapter

5-HT	5-Hydroxytriptophan (serotonin)
ACE	Angiotensin-converting enzyme
ALS	Amyotrophic lateral sclerosis
ARB	Angiotensin receptor blocker
CHF	Chronic heart failure
COPD	Chronic obstructive pulmonary disease
CTZ	Chemoreceptor trigger zone
CVA	Cerebrovascular accident
ESRD	End-stage renal disease
GERD	Gastroesophogeal reflux disease
HMG-CoA	Hydroxymethylglutaryl coenzyme-A
NSAID	Nonsteroidal anti-inflammatory drug
PEG	Percutaneous endoscopic gastrostomy
PICC	Peripherally inserted central catheter
PPI	Proton pump inhibitors
SSRI	Selective serotonin reuptake inhibitor
WHO	World Health Organization

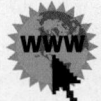 Self-assessment questions and answers are available at *http://www.mhpharmacotherapy.com/pp.html.*

REFERENCES

1. World Health Organization. National Cancer Control Programmes: Policies and Managerial Guidelines, 2nd ed; 2002. *www.who.int/cancer/media/en/408.pdf.*
2. Higginson I, Astin P, Dolan S. Where do cancer patients die? Ten year trends in place of death of cancer patients in England. Palliat Med 1998;12:353–363.
3. The SUPPORT Principles Investigators. A controlled trial to improve care for seriously ill hospitalized patients: The Study to

Understand Prognoses and Preferences for Outcomes and Risks of Treatments (SUPPORT). JAMA 1995;274:1591–1598. [Erratum, JAMA, 1996;275:1232.]

4. Billings JA. What is palliative care. J Palliat Med 1998;1:73–81.

5. Higginson I, Astin P, Dolan S. Where do cancer patients die? Ten year trends in place of death of cancer patients in England. Palliat Med 1998;12:353–363.

6. Hill RR. Clinical pharmacy services in a home-based palliative care program. Am J Health Syst Pharm 2007;64:806–810.

7. Lipman AG. Evidence-based palliative care. In: Lipman AG, Jackson KC, Tyler LS, eds. Evidence-Based Symptom Control in Palliative Care: Systemic Reviews and Validated Clinical Practice Guidelines. Binghamton, NY: Hawthorn Press, 2000.

8. Grauer P, Shuster J, Protus BM. Palliative Care Consultant, 3rd ed. Dubuque, IA: Kendall/Hunt Publishing, 2008.

9. Goldstein NE, Fischberg D. Update in palliative medicine. Ann Intern Med 2008;148:135–140.

10. Strickland JM, Huskey AG. Palliative Care. Pharmacotherapy Self-Assessment Program, 5th ed. 2004:191–218.

11. Hospice Care. Health Letter. Harvard Health Publications. July, 2008.

12. Connor SR. Development of hospice and palliative care in the United States. Omega (Westport) 2007–08;56(1):89–99.

13. American Psychiatric Association. Diagnostic and Statistics Manual of Mental Disorders, 4th ed. Washington DC: American Psychiatric Press, 1994.

14. Portenoy RK, Thaler HT, Kornblith AB, et al. The Memorial Symptom Assessment Scale: An instrument for the evaluation of symptom prevalence, characteristics and distress. Eur J Cancer 1994;30A:1326–1336.

15. Hocking LB, Koenig HG. Anxiety in medically ill older patients: A review and update. Int J Psychiatry Med 1995;25:221–238.

16. Stoudemire A. Epidemiology and psychopharmacology of anxiety in medical patients. J Clin Psychiatry 1996;57(Suppl 7):64–72, 73–75.

17. Rubey RN, Lydiard RB. Pharmacological treatment of anxiety in the medically ill patient. Semin Clin Neuropsychiatry 1999;4:133–147.

18. Grauer PA, Shuster J, Protus BM. Palliative Care Consultant, 3rd ed. Dubuque, IA: Kendall-Hunt, 2008:29–31, 40–47, 78–85.

19. Shuster JL. Confusion, agitation, and delirium at the end-of-life. J Palliat Med 1998;1:177–186.

20. Katz IR. Optimizing atypical antipsychotic treatment strategies in the elderly. J Am Geriatr Soc 2004;52:272–277.

21. Breitbart W, Marotta R, Platt MM, et al. A double-blind trial of haloperidol, chlorpromazine, and lorazepam in the treatment of delirium in hospitalized AIDS patients. Am J Psychiatry 1996;153:231–237.

22. Fainsinger R, MacEachern T, Hanson J, et al. Symptom control during the last week of life on a palliative care unit. J Palliat Care 1991;7:5–11.

23. Tyler LS, Lipman AG. Dyspnea. In: Evidence Based Symptom Control in Palliative Care. Systematic Review and Validated Clinical Practice Guidelines for 15 Common Problems in Patients with Life Limiting Disease, 1st ed. New York: Pharmaceutical Products Press, 2000:109–124.

24. Storey P, Knight CF. UNIPAC Four: Management of Selected Non-Pain Symptoms in the Terminally Ill, 2nd ed. New York: Mary Ann Liebert, 2003;29–35.

25. Thomas JR, vonGunten CF. Management of dyspnea. J Support Oncol 2003;1:23–24.

26. LeGrand SB, Khawam EA, Walsh D, Rivera NI. Opioids, respiratory function, and dyspnea. Am J Hosp Palliat Care 2003;1:57–61.

27. Weissman DE. Fast Facts and Concepts 27: Terminal Dyspnea. November, 2000. End-of-Life Physician Education Resource Center. www.eperc.mcw.edu.

28. Zepetella G. Nebulized morphine in the palliation of dyspnea. Palliat Med 1997;11(4):267–275.

29. Ferraresi V. Inhaled opioids for the treatment of dyspnea. Am J Health Syst Pharm 2005;62:319–320.

30. Emanuel LL, von Gunten CF, Ferris FD, HauserJM, eds. The Education for Physicians on End-of-life Care (EPEC) Curriculum. Module 10: Common Physical Symptoms, 2003:5–10.

31. Kohara H, Ueoka H, Aoe K, et al. Effect of nebulized furosemide in terminally ill cancer patients with dyspnea. J Pain Symptom Manage 2003;26:962–967.

32. Shimoyama N, Shimoyama M. Nebulized furosemide as a novel treatment for dyspnea in terminal cancer patients. J Pain Symptom Manage 2002;23:73–76.

33. Stone P, Kurowska A. Re: Nebulized furosemide for dyspnea in terminal cancer patients. J Pain Symptom Manage 2002;24:274–275.

34. Bruera E, Sweeney C. In: Principles & Practices of Palliative Care & Supportive Oncology, 2nd ed. Philadelphia: Lippincott Williams & Wilkins, 2002:Ch 14.

35. Ferris FD, von Gunten CF, Emanuel LL. Ensuring competency in end-of-life care: Controlling symptoms. BMC Palliat Care 2002;1:5.

36. Gralla RJ, Osoba D, Kris MG, et al. Recommendations for the use of antiemetics: Evidence-based, clinical practice guidelines. American Society of Clinical Oncology. J Clin Oncol 1999;17:2971–2994.

37. Tyler LS. Nausea and vomiting in palliative care. In: Evidence Based Symptom Control in Palliative Care. Binghamton, NY: The Haworth Press, 2000:163–181.

38. Vella-Brincat J, Macleod AD. Haloperidol in palliative care. Palliat Med 2004;18:195–201.

39. Study to understand prognoses and preferences for outcomes and risks of treatment (SUPPORT). JAMA 1995;274:1591–1598.

40. American Pain Society. Principles of Analgesic Use in the Treatment of Acute Pain and Cancer pain, 5th ed. Glenview, IL: American Pain Society, 2003.

41. Berger AM, Portenoy RK, Weissman DE. Principles and Practice of Palliative Care and Supportive Oncology, 2nd ed. Philadelphia: Lippincott Williams & Wilkins, 2002.

42. McCaffery M, Pasero C. Pain: Clinical Manual, 2nd ed. St. Louis: Elsevier Mosby, 1999.

43. Wildiers H, Menten J. Death rattle: Prevalence, prevention and treatment. J Pain Symptom Manage 2002;34:310–317.

44. Morita T, Tsunoda J, Inone S, Chihara S. Risk factors for death rattle in terminally ill cancer patients: A prospective exploratory study. Palliat Med 2000;14:19–23.

45. Bennett M, Lucas V, Brennan M, Hughes A, O'Donnell V, Wee B. Using anti-muscarinic drugs in the management of death rattle: Evidence-Based guidelines for palliative care. Palliat Med 2002;16:369–374.

46. Varkey B. Palliative care for end-stage lung disease patients. Clin Pulm Med 2003;10(5):269–277.

47. Hyson HC, Johnson AM, Jog MS. Sublingual atropine for sialorrhea secondary to parkinsonism: A pilot study. Mov Disorder 2002;17(6):1318–1320.

48. Back IN, Jenkins K, Blower A, Beckhelling J. A study comparing hyoscine hydrobromide and glycopyrrolate in the treatment of death rattle. Palliat Med 2001 July 1;15(4):329–336.

49. Hauptman PJ, Havranek EP. Integrating palliative care into heart failure care. Arch Intern Med 2005;165:374–378.

50. McPherson ML. Palliative Care and Appropriate Medication Use in End-Stage Heart Failure. Medscape Nurses. 2007, www.medscape.com.

Part II

Disorders of Organ Systems

5 Hypertension

Robert J. Straka, David Parra, and
Kade T. Birkeland

LEARNING OBJECTIVES

● **Upon completion of the chapter, the reader will be able to:**

1. Classify blood pressure (BP) levels and treatment goals.
2. Recognize the underlying causes and contributing factors in the development of hypertension.
3. Describe the appropriate measurement of BP.
4. Recommend appropriate lifestyle modifications and pharmacotherapy for patients with hypertension.
5. Identify populations requiring special consideration when designing a treatment plan.
6. Construct an appropriate monitoring plan to assess hypertension treatment.

KEY CONCEPTS

❶ Hypertension is widely prevalent and accounts for significant morbidity and mortality, as well as billions of dollars in direct and indirect costs.

❷ The cause of hypertension is unknown in the majority of cases (primary hypertension), but for patients with secondary hypertension, specific causes can be identified.

❸ Patients failing to achieve goal BP despite maximum doses of three antihypertensives including a diuretic should be carefully screened for resistant hypertension.

❹ The pathophysiology of primary hypertension is heterogeneous, but ultimately exerts its effects through the two primary determinants of BP: cardiac output (CO) and peripheral resistance (PR).

❺ Appropriate technique in measuring BP is a vital component to the diagnosis and continued management of hypertension in the outpatient setting.

❻ Drug selection for the management of patients with hypertension should be considered as adjunctive to nonpharmacologic approaches for BP lowering, and ultimately the attainment of target BP in many cases may be more important than the antihypertensive agent used.

❼ Implementation of lifestyle modifications successfully lowers BP, often with results similar to those of therapy with a single antihypertensive agent.

❽ An approach to selection of drugs for the treatment of patients with hypertension should be evidence-based. Consideration should be given to the individual's comorbidities, coprescribed medications, and practical patient-specific issues including costs.

❾ Specific antihypertensive therapy is warranted for certain patients with comorbid conditions that may elevate their level of risk for cardiovascular disease (CVD).

❿ The frequency of follow-up visits for patients with hypertension will vary based on individual cases, but will be influenced by severity of hypertension, comorbidities, and choice of agent selected.

INTRODUCTION

Despite efforts to promote awareness, treatment, and the means available to aggressively manage high blood pressure (BP), trends over the past 15 years demonstrate only modest improvements in its treatment and control. National and international organizations continually refine their recommendations of how clinicians should approach the management of patients with high BP, and although approaches vary to some degree, there are clear themes that emerge regardless of which national or international organization's algorithm is followed. The purpose of this chapter is to provide a summary of key issues associated with the management of patients with hypertension. We will discuss the basic approach to treating patients with hypertension and provide a functional summary of the currently prevailing themes of national guidelines, including their grounding in relevant landmark trials. Finally, we will summarize salient pharmacotherapeutic issues essential for clinicians to consider when managing patients with hypertension.

Various algorithms recommending nonpharmacologic and pharmacologic management for typical and atypical patients are proposed, with the underlying theme that achievement of BP targets mitigate end-organ damage, leading to substantial reductions in stroke, myocardial infarction (MI), end-stage renal disease, and heart failure. Although references to other algorithms will be mentioned, this chapter will focus primarily on the *Seventh Report of the Joint National Committee on Prevention, Detection, Evaluation and Treatment of High Blood Pressure,* more commonly referred to as the Joint National Committee Seventh Report (JNC 7) report,[1] with additional reference to recent recommendations from the American Heart Association[2] and European Society of Cardiology.[3] It should be noted that an update of the JNC 7 report (JNC 8), as part of an integrated set of cardiovascular risk reduction guidelines, is expected to be released in 2010.[3]

The JNC 7 report describes four stages of BP classification and provides guidance on nonpharmacologic and pharmacologic approaches to managing patients with hypertension. The four stages of BP classification include normal, prehypertension, stage 1 hypertension, and stage 2 hypertension (Table 5–1). These stages are defined as such to connote a level of risk and thus the need for varying intensities of intervention with drug therapy (Fig. 5–1). With the exception of individuals with "compelling indications," recommendations for drug therapy typically begin with one or two (in the case of stage 2) antihypertensive drugs as an initial step. Specific drug selection is guided by the presence of compelling indications—specific comorbid conditions. These compelling indications, such as heart failure, diabetes, and chronic kidney disease (CKD), represent specific conditions for which explicit evidence in the literature exists to document the utility of a particular agent or class of agents. Selection of drug therapy consequently involves an iterative process of considering multiple antihypertensive drugs as needed to achieve target BPs of less than 140/90 mm Hg for all patients, with more aggressive targets of less than 130/80 mm Hg for patients with diabetes or chronic (greater than 3 months) kidney disease (estimated glomerular filtration rate [GFR] less than 60 mL/min/1.73 m^2 or the presence of albuminuria [300mg/day or 200 mg/g creatinine]).[1] In addition, the AHA scientific statement expands those in whom a lower BP target of less than 130/80 mm Hg should be pursued to include patients with known coronary artery disease or coronary artery disease risk equivalents (carotid artery disease, peripheral arterial disease, abdominal aortic aneurysm), or a 10-year Framingham risk score of greater than 10%. See Dyslipidemias chapter. In patients with left ventricular dysfunction, additional BP lowering to a target of less than 120/80 mm Hg may also be considered.[2]

EPIDEMIOLOGY

① *Hypertension is widely prevalent and accounts for significant morbidity and mortality, as well as billions of dollars in direct and indirect costs.* Worldwide prevalence of hypertension is estimated to include 1 billion individuals. There are an estimated 7 million deaths per year that may be related to the diagnosis of hypertension.[4] The prevalence of hypertension in the United States is among the highest in the world and is estimated to include 73 million individuals (1 in 3 adults) with an estimated 69.4 billion dollars spent annually in direct and indirect costs.[5] Furthermore, it is estimated that 37.4% of the U.S. population older than 20 years of age has prehypertension.

The prevalence of hypertension differs based on age, sex, and ethnicity. As individuals become older, their risk of systolic hypertension increases. Individuals 55 years of age who do not have hypertension are estimated to have a lifetime risk of 90% of eventually developing hypertension. In the United States, hypertension is slightly more prevalent

---

Table 5–1

Classification of BP in Children, Adolescents, and Adults[a]

BP Classification	Adult SBP (mm Hg)	Adult DBP (mm Hg)	Children/Adolescents SBP or DBP Percentile[b]
Normal	Less than 120	and less than 80	Less than 90th
Prehypertension	120–139	or 80–89	90–95th or 120/80 mm Hg
Stage 1 hypertension	140–159	or 90–99	95–99th + 5 mm Hg[c]
Stage 2 hypertension	Greater than or equal to 160	Greater than or equal to 100	Greater than 99th + 5 mm Hg[d]

BP, blood pressure; DBP, diastolic blood pressure; SBP, systolic blood pressure.

[a]Defined as 18 years old or more.

[b]Tables contain the 50th, 90th, and 99th percentiles of SBP and DBP standards based on percentile height by age and sex, which is used to compare the child's measured BP on three separate occasions. The difference in BP of the 95th and 99th percentiles are 7 to 10 mm Hg, which requires an adjustment of 5 mm Hg to accurately categorize stage 1 or 2 hypertension. If the systolic and diastolic percentile categories are different, then classify hypertension by the higher BP value.

[c]Children and adolescents' stage 1 hypertension is classified by BP levels that range from the 95th percentile to 5 mm Hg above the 99th percentile.

[d]Children and adolescents' stage 2 hypertension is classified by BP levels that are greater than 5 mm Hg above the 99th percentile.

From Ref. 1.

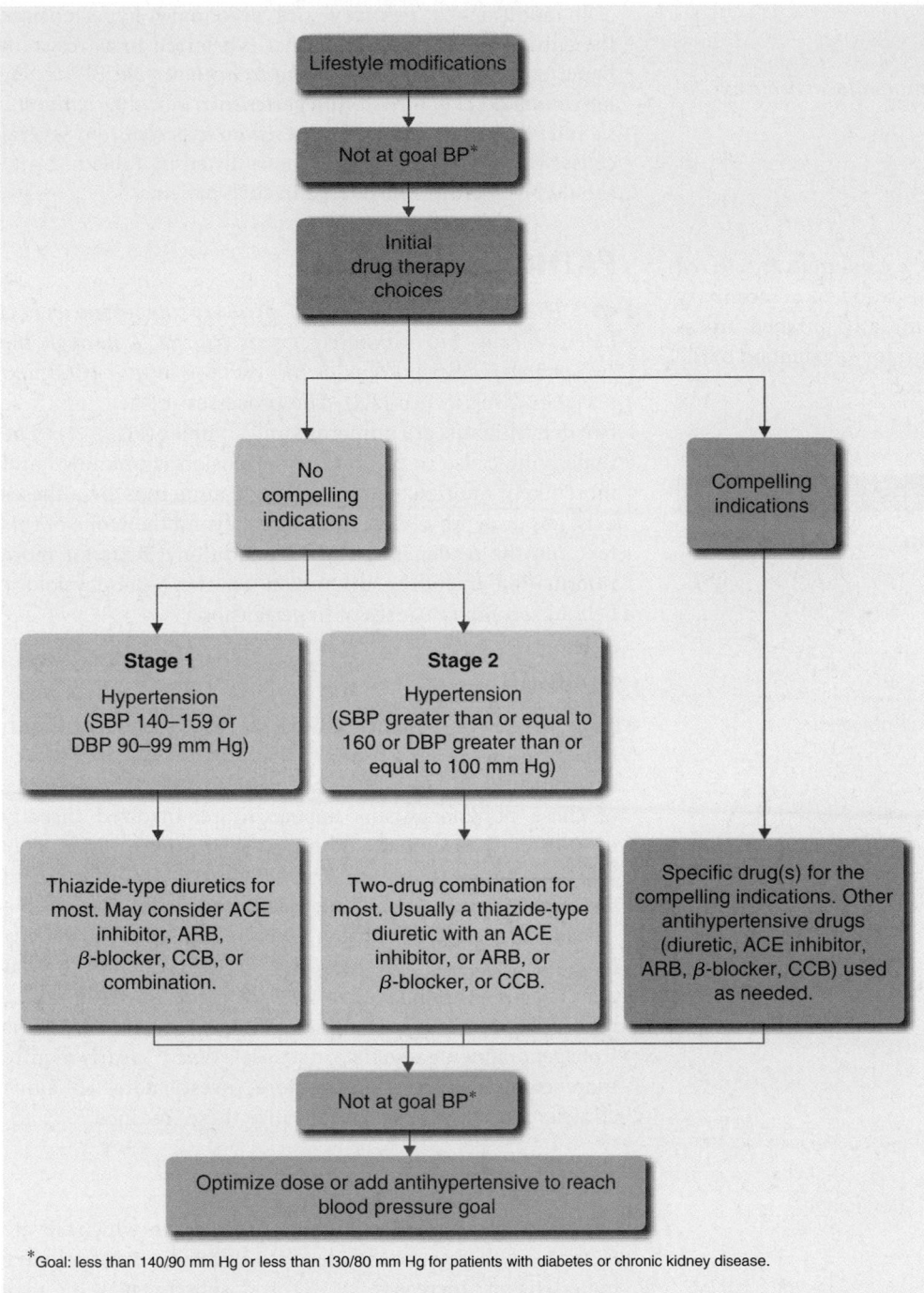

FIGURE 5–1. Algorithm for treatment of hypertension when patients are not at their goal BP. Compelling indications refer to specific indications where the selection of a particular antihypertensive drug class for a defined high-risk population is highly recommended. These recommendations are usually based on results from landmark randomized placebo-controlled outcome trials or consensus statements from clinical guidelines and are usually based on findings documenting superior outcomes in terms of morbidity and mortality. (ACE, angiotensin-converting enzyme; ARB, angiotensin receptor blocker; BP, blood pressure; CCB, calcium channel blocker; DBP, diastolic blood pressure; SBP, systolic blood pressure.) (From Ref. 1.)

Within figure:

Lifestyle modifications

Not at goal BP*

Initial drug therapy choices

No compelling indications

Compelling indications

Stage 1
Hypertension (SBP 140–159 or DBP 90–99 mm Hg)

Stage 2
Hypertension (SBP greater than or equal to 160 or DBP greater than or equal to 100 mm Hg)

Thiazide-type diuretics for most. May consider ACE inhibitor, ARB, β-blocker, CCB, or combination.

Two-drug combination for most. Usually a thiazide-type diuretic with an ACE inhibitor, or ARB, or β-blocker, or CCB.

Specific drug(s) for the compelling indications. Other antihypertensive drugs (diuretic, ACE inhibitor, ARB, β-blocker, CCB) used as needed.

Not at goal BP*

Optimize dose or add antihypertensive to reach blood pressure goal

*Goal: less than 140/90 mm Hg or less than 130/80 mm Hg for patients with diabetes or chronic kidney disease.

in women (33.6%) than men (33.2%).[5] In addition, age-adjusted prevalence of hypertension is highest in non-Hispanic blacks or African Americans (41%) when compared to non-Hispanic whites (28.1%) and Mexican Americans (22%). However, Mexican Americans have lower rates of treatment and control.[6]

Hypertension is strongly associated with type 2 diabetes.[7] The added comorbidity of hypertension in diabetes leads to a higher risk of cardiovascular disease (CVD), stroke, renal disease, and diabetic retinopathy leading to greater health care costs.[8]

ETIOLOGY

❷ *In the majority of patients (greater than 90%), the cause of hypertension is unknown and is referred to as essential, or more appropriately, as primary hypertension.[9] However, in some patients there is an identifiable cause of which the most common are:[2]*

- *CKD*
- *Coarctation of the aorta*
- *Cushing's syndrome and other glucocorticoid excess states*

- *Drug induced/related* (*Table 5–2*)
- *Pheochromocytoma*
- *Primary aldosteronism and other mineralocorticoid excess states*
- *Renovascular hypertension*
- *Sleep apnea*
- *Thyroid or parathyroid disease*

Hypertension caused by any of these conditions is referred to as secondary hypertension. Identification of a secondary cause of hypertension is often not initially pursued unless suggested by routine clinical and laboratory evaluation of the patient, or failure to achieve BP control.

Table 5–2

Causes of Resistant Hypertension

Apparent Resistance
Improper BP measurement
Failure to receive or take antihypertensive medication
Inadequate doses (subtherapeutic)
Improper antihypertensive selection or combination
White coat effect

True Resistance
Secondary hypertension
Medication effects and interactions
  Nonsteroidal anti-inflammatory medications
  Sympathomimetics (decongestants, anorectics, and stimulants)
  Cocaine, amphetamines, and other illict drugs
  Recent caffeine or nicotine intake
  Oral contraceptive hormones
  Adrenal steroid hormones
  Erythropoietin
  Natural licorice (including some chewing tobacco)
  Cyclosporine and tacrolimus
  Herbal products (ma huang, guarana, bitter orange)
  Volume overload
  Excess sodium intake
  Inadequate diuretic therapy
  Fluid retention from kidney disease or potent vasodilators (e.g., minoxidil)
Comorbidities
  Obesity
  Excess alcohol intake
  Chronic pain syndromes
  Intense vasoconstriction (arteritis)
  Anxiety-induced hyperventilation/panic attacks
Genetic variation
  Genetic differences in drug efficacy or metabolism

From Ref. 1 and Kaplan NM, Sica DA. Resistant Hypertension in Izzo JL Jr, Black HR eds. Hypertension Primer. The Essentials of High Blood Pressure. 4th ed. Philadelphia: Lippincott Williams & Wilkins; 2008: 348–350.

In addition to primary and secondary hypertension, the clinician may encounter what is referred to as resistant hypertension. ❸ *Patients failing to achieve goal BP despite maximum doses of three antihypertensives including a diuretic should be carefully screened for resistant hypertension.* Several causes of resistant hypertension are listed in Table 5–2 and should be carefully considered in such patients.

PATHOPHYSIOLOGY

❹ *The pathophysiology of primary hypertension is heterogeneous, but ultimately exerts its effects through the two primary determinants of BP: cardiac output (CO) and peripheral resistance (PR).* The processes influencing these two determinants are numerous and complex (Fig. 5–2).[9] The underlying cause of primary hypertension is unknown and most likely multifactorial. Although numerous hypotheses exist, an in-depth review of these is beyond the scope of this text and the reader is referred to additional texts for more information including discussion on the pathophysiology behind secondary causes of hypertension.[10]

Genetics

Multiple genetic polymorphisms have been associated with hypertension. It is estimated that up to 30% to 50% of variability in BP may have a genetic basis.[11] The majority of these polymorphisms appear to be involved directly or indirectly in renal sodium reabsorption, which may represent future therapeutic drug targets.[12] In addition to the identification of genetic factors contributing to the development of hypertension, explorations into the genetic basis of variability in response to drug therapy are at early stages. Although advances are made on both fronts, replication of early findings identifying genetic variations from genome-wide association scans (GWAS)[13] clearly require more comprehensive study before investigators, let alone clinicians, are in a position to utilize these findings.[14]

Cardiac Output

CO is an important determinant of BP. Factors which elevate CO may, in theory, contribute to the development of primary hypertension. Increases in CO and subsequently BP may arise from factors that increase preload (fluid volume) or myocardial contractility. Nonetheless, even if increased CO may be involved in the development of primary hypertension, these increases do not appear to persist over time. As a consequence, elevated CO is not considered a hemodynamic hallmark of established primary hypertension.

Sodium Regulation

The contribution of sodium to the development of primary hypertension is related to excess sodium intake and/or abnormal sodium excretion by the kidneys. Proposed mechanisms supporting either of these are numerous and complex. However, it is generally accepted that dietary salt is associated with increases in BP that can be lowered with

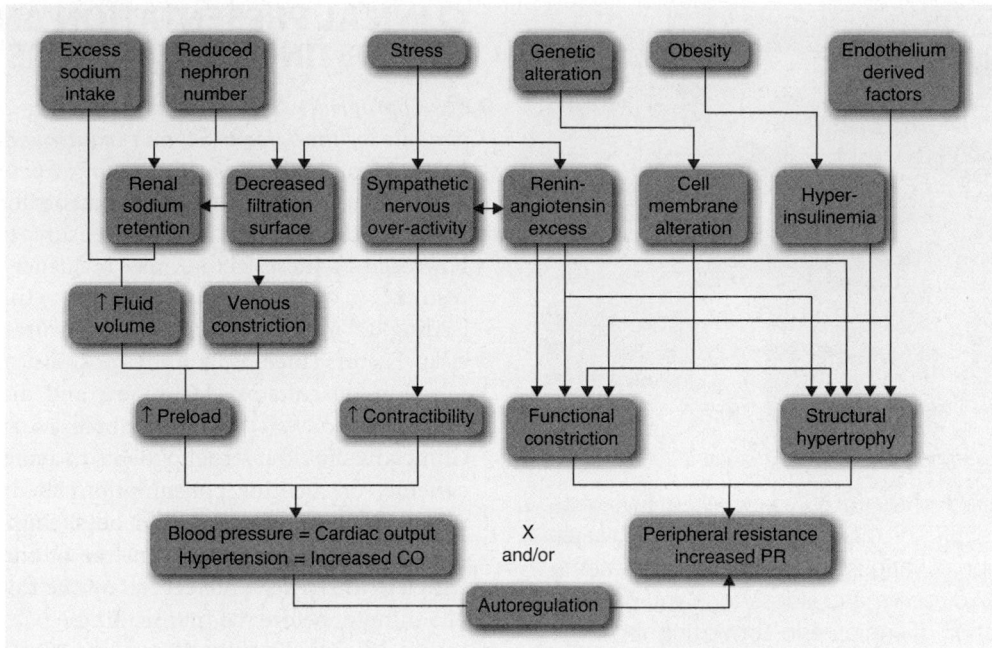

FIGURE 5–2. Factors involved in the pathogenesis of hypertension are summarized. Some of the factors involved in the control of BP affect the basic equation: BP = CO × PR. The figure depicts the complex nature of various factors that may play a role in the development of hypertension. Each of these factors may individually or collectively modulate BP through its actions on various physiologic systems at the cellular, organ, and organ system level. (BP, blood pressure; CO, cardiac output; PR, peripheral resistance.) *(From Kaplan NM. Primary hypertension: Pathogenesis. In: Kaplan's Clinical Hypertension. 9th ed. Philadelphia: Lippincott Williams & Wilkins; 2006: 63, with permission.)*

reduction of sodium intake.[1,15] There appears to be a threshold effect of sodium intake in the range of 50 to 100 mmol/day (1.2–2.4 g of sodium per day, which is equivalent to 3–6 g of sodium chloride per day [50–100 mmol/day]) and its impact on BP. The mean sodium intake per day is 175 mmol (4.1 g) for men and 120 mmol (2.7 g) for women in the United States, with the majority derived from processed foods.[1] Adherence to sodium restriction is important as up to 50% of all individuals appear to be sodium-sensitive and thus susceptible to a high dietary sodium intake.[9]

Renin-Angiotensin-Aldosterone System

Since the discovery of renin over 100 years ago, the renin-angiotensin-aldosterone system (RAAS) has been extensively studied as a prime target or site of action for many effective antihypertensives.[16] Renin is produced and stored in the juxtaglomerular cells of the kidney, and its release is stimulated by impaired renal perfusion, salt depletion, and β_1-adrenergic stimulation. The release of renin is the rate-limiting step in the eventual formation of angiotensin II, which is primarily responsible for the pressor effects mediated by the RAAS (Fig. 5–3). Evidence indicates that renin's pressor effects occur at the cellular level (autocrine), the local environment (paracrine), and throughout the systemic circulation (endocrine).[17] The role of the RAAS in primary hypertension is supported by the presence of high levels of renin, suggesting that the system is inappropriately

activated. Proposed mechanisms behind this inappropriate activation include increased sympathetic drive, defective regulation of the RAAS (nonmodulation), and the existence of a subpopulation of ischemic nephrons that release excess renin.[9] However, there are also patients with primary hypertension and low levels of renin. This observation suggests that alternate mechanisms for hypertension unrelated to renin levels or activity may be in play.[18] Ongoing studies utilizing the oral direct renin inhibitor (DRI) known as aliskiren may advance our understanding of the role this DRI may play when combined with other agents affecting the RAAS.[19]

Sympathetic Overactivity

Overactivation of the sympathetic nervous system (SNS) may also play a role in the development and maintenance of primary hypertension for some individuals. Among other effects, direct activation of the SNS may lead to enhanced sodium retention, insulin resistance, and baroreceptor dysfunction.[9] Regardless of which mechanism(s) underlies the role the SNS may play in the development of primary hypertension, the SNS remains a target of many antihypertensive agents.

Peripheral Resistance

Elevated peripheral arterial resistance is the hemodynamic hallmark of primary hypertension. The increase in PR

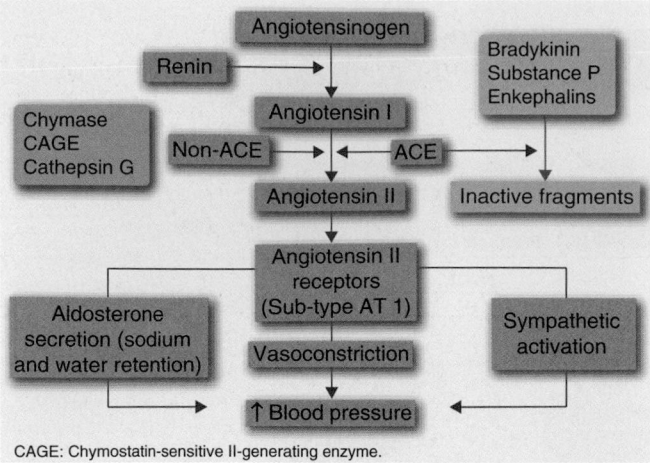

CAGE: Chymostatin-sensitive II-generating enzyme.

FIGURE 5–3. Diagram of the RAAS, a key system involved in the modulation of BP. The diagram depicts the pathways involved in the action of various antihypertensives including ACE inhibitors, ARBs, diuretics, and aldosterone antagonists. By inhibiting the action of angiotensin-converting enzymes, ACE inhibitors reduce both the formation of the vasoconstrictor angiotensin II, and the degradation of vasodilating substances including bradykinin. ARBs primarily act through inhibition of the action of angiotensin II on the angiotensin-1 receptors that modulate vasoconstriction. Aldosterone antagonists directly inhibit the actions of aldosterone, while diuretics affect sodium and water retention at a renal level. (ACE, angiotensin-converting enzyme; ARB, angiotensin receptor blockers; AT1, angiotensin-1; BP, blood pressure; RAAS, renin-anglotensin aldosterone system.)

typically observed may be due to a reduction in the arterial lumen size as a result of vascular remodeling. This remodeling, or change in vascular tone, may be modulated by various endothelium-derived vasoactive substances, growth factors, and cytokines. This increase in arterial stiffness or reduced compliance results in the observed increase in systolic BP.[9]

Other Contributing Processes and Factors

Many other processes are proposed to contribute to the development of hypertension, including obesity, physical inactivity, insulin resistance, potassium and magnesium depletion, chronic moderate alcohol consumption, and transient effects of cigarette smoking and caffeine intake.[9] The assessment of global cardiovascular risk in all hypertensive patients should be part of the management plan while also pursuing target BPs through nonpharmacologic and pharmacologic means. Regardless of the initiating process or processes leading to the development of hypertension, the ultimate goal is to reduce the risk of cardiovascular events and minimize target organ damage. This clearly requires the early identification of risk factors and treatment of patients with hypertension.

CLINICAL PRESENTATION AND CO-EXISTING RISK FACTORS

⑤ *Appropriate technique in measuring BP is a vital component to the diagnosis and continued management of hypertension in the outpatient setting.* Accurate measurement of a patient's BP identifies and controls for factors that may influence the variability in the measure. Failure to consider how each of these factors may influence BP measurement results in significant variation in measurements, leading to misclassification or inaccurate assessments of risk. Factors including body position, cuff size, device selection, auscultatory technique, and dietary intake prior to the clinic visit may contribute to such inaccuracies. Clinicians should instruct patients to avoid exercise, alcohol, caffeine, or nicotine consumption 30 minutes before BP measurement. Patients should be sitting comfortably with their back supported and arm free of constrictive clothing with legs uncrossed and feet flat on the floor for a minimum of 5 minutes before the first reading.

Systolic and diastolic BP tend to increase when the cuff size is too small. Ideally, the cuff bladder should encircle at least 80% of the arm's circumference to ensure a more accurate measurement of BP.

Mercury sphygmomanometers are recommended for routine office measurements, but concerns of patient exposure and environmental contamination of mercury has fostered the development of other devices to measure BP. However, there is no general consensus among health care providers as to an acceptable replacement for mercury sphygmomanometers.

To reduce deviations in BP measurement in the clinic, the patient and clinician should not talk during BP readings. The measurement arm is supported and positioned at heart level. If a mercury or aneroid device is used, then the palpatory method must be used first to estimate the systolic BP.[20] If an automated device is used, this is not necessary. After the patient's cuff is inflated above the systolic pressure, the mercury column should drop at a rate of 2 to 3 mm Hg/s. A stethoscope placed over the brachial artery in the antecubital fossa identifies the first and last audible Korotkoff sounds, which should be taken as systolic and diastolic pressure, respectively. A minimum of two readings at least 1 minute apart are then averaged. If measurements vary by more than 5 mm Hg between the two readings, then one or two additional BP measurements are collected and the multiple readings averaged. BP classification is based on the average of two or more properly measured, seated BP readings on each of two or more office visits. Details and further recommendations for accurate measurement of BP in special populations can be reviewed in the American College of Cardiology/American Heart Association (ACC/AHA) BP Measurement in Humans Statement for health care professionals.[20]

Finally, the measurement of clinic or office BPs is poorly correlated with assessments of BP in other settings. Consequently, under select circumstances, clinicians are increasingly using 24-hour ambulatory BP monitoring devices and home BP monitors. These tools are useful in

Clinical Presentation and Diagnosis of Primary Hypertension

General

Age: Prevalence of hypertension is likely to be highest with middle-aged or older patients

Sex: In the United States, hypertension is slightly more prevalent in women (33.6%) than men (33.2%)

Symptoms

The patient with primary hypertension may be asymptomatic yet still have major CVD risk factors

Signs

Adult patients have an average of two or more BP readings (SBP and DBP) on two seperate occassions indicating either:

	SBP (mm Hg)	DBP (mm Hg)
Normal	Less than 120	Less than 80
Prehypertension	120–139	or 80–89
Stage 1 hypertension	140–159	or 90–99
Stage 2 hypertension	Greater than or equal to 160	Greater than or equal to 100

Laboratory Tests (not necessarily indicative of hypertension, but should be measured in patients with hypertension)

Fasting lipid panel:

- Low-density lipoprotein greater than 160 mg/dL (4.14 mmol/L)
- Total cholesterol greater than 240 mg/dL (6.22 mmol/L)
- HDL less than 40 mg/dL (1.04 mmol/L)
- Triglycerides greater than 200 mg/dL (2.26 mmol/L)

Fasting plasma glucose or hemoglobin A1c (does not need to be fasting):

- Impaired fasting glucose is a glucose of 100–125 mg/dL (5.55–6.94 mmol/L)
- Diagnosis of diabetes with fasting glucose greater than or equal to 126 mg/dL (6.99 mmol/L) or a hemoglobin A1c greater than or equal to 6.5% on two separate occasions,

or a random plasma glucose reading of greater than or equal to 200 mg/L (11.1 mmol/L) with symptoms of diabetes

The following abnormal tests may indicate hypertension related damage

- Serum creatinine elevated (greater than 1.2 mg/dL [106 μmol/L])
- **Microalbuminuria,** which is diagnosed either from a 24-hour urine collection (20–200 μg/min) or from elevated concentrations (30–300 mg/L) on at least two occassions. Use of the albumin-to-creatinine ratio (ACR) in a spot urine sample is becoming more common and microalbuminuria is defined by this measure as 30–300 mg/g creatinine

Common Comorbidities and Factors Contributing to CV Risk

Diabetes mellitus

Metabolic syndrome

Insulin resistance

Dyslipidemia

Microalbuminuria

Family history

Central obesity

Physical inactivity

Tobacco use

Target Organ Damage

Heart (left ventricular hypertrophy, angina, prior myocardial infarction, prior coronary revascularization, heart failure)

Brain (stroke or transient ischemic attack, dementia)

Chronic kidney disease

Peripheral arterial disease

Retinopathy

identifying patients with white coat hypertension or with elevations of BP during nighttime. They may also aid in the management of refractory hypertensives with minor target organ damage, those with suspected autonomic neuropathy, those with hypotensive symptoms, and patients with large differences between home and clinic BP measurements. Benefits derived from alternative BP monitoring may be of greater prognostic significance than traditional office based measurements.[20]

TREATMENT

Desired Outcomes

Hypertension management by nonpharmacologic and pharmacologic therapies has proven useful in reducing the risk of heart attack, heart failure, stroke, and kidney disease morbidity and mortality. For every 20 mm Hg systolic or 10 mm Hg diastolic increase in BP, there is a doubling of mortality for both ischemic heart disease and stroke.[21] The

Patient Encounter 1

A 62-year-old Caucasian man comes to your clinic with results from a health fair he attended earlier this month. He was concerned as his BP at that time was 170/86 mm Hg, and when repeated 184/96 mm Hg. Upon examination, seated BP in the left arm is 144/82 mm Hg and 148/80 mm Hg in the right arm. Repeat measurements 5 minutes later are 142/84 mm Hg in the left arm and 144/76 mm Hg in the right. Much relieved, he declines any further evaluation or intervention, but promises to return in 1 week. BP at this 1 week follow-up is 146/84 as averaged from two readings in his right arm. The physical exam and past medical history are unremarkable, and all laboratory measurements are within normal limits with the exception of a high-density lipoprotein cholesterol of 45 mg/dL (1.17 mmol/L), triglyceride level of 155 mg/dL (1.75 mmol/L), total cholesterol of 180 mg/dL (4.66 mmol/L) and calculated LDL cholesterol of 104 mg/dL (2.69 mmol/L). Of note, he does not smoke.

Based on above information should this patient be classified as having hypertension?

What is this patient's BP target using recommendations from JNC 7?

Does the BP target differ using recommendations from the 2007 American Heart Association Statement on the treatment of hypertension in the prevention and management of ischemic heart disease?

What factors may have contributed to the discrepancy between the health fair and office based BP readings?

goal of BP management is to reduce the risk of CVD and target organ damage. Targeting a specific BP is actually a surrogate goal that has been associated with reductions in CVD and target organ damage.

General Approach to Treatment

❻ *As is the case with dyslipidemia and other cardiovascular conditions, drug selection for the management of patients with hypertension should be considered as adjunctive to nonpharmacologic approaches for BP lowering. Previous clinical research has established the relative value of using individual antihypertensive drugs versus placebo to achieve reduction in morbidity and mortality by lowering BP. However, as newer antihypertensive agents are developed, it is difficult to justify the comparison of newer agents to placebo on ethical grounds. Consequently, contemporary large outcome-based, multicenter trials have been designed to compare one specific agent-based therapy (along with options to add others) versus another agent-based therapy (along with options to add others of a different class). These attempts at "head-to-head" comparisons and meta-analyses of multidrug regimen*

trials have, in general, provided evidence supporting the position that the main benefits of pharmacologic therapy are related to the achievement of BP lowering and are generally largely independent of the selection of an individual drug regimen. Inherent in this position is the realization that nonpharmacologic approaches alone are rarely successful in attaining target BPs, and multidrug therapy (sometimes as many as three or more agents) is necessary for most patients with hypertension.[22] While JNC 7 focuses on utilizing BP levels in determining the threshold and target for treatment, the European Society of Cardiology also incorporates total cardiovascular risk in determining thresholds for treatment. This approach results in a "flexible" definition of hypertension which is dependent on an individual's total cardiovascular risk.[3] While acknowledging that there are several approaches currently employed to manage patients with hypertension, this chapter will use as its basis the JNC 7 guidelines while recognizing important changes outlined within the American Heart Association Guidelines.

Nonpharmacologic Treatment: Lifestyle Modifications

● Therapeutic lifestyle modifications consisting of nonpharmacologic approaches to BP reduction should be an active part of all treatment plans for patients with hypertension. The most widely studied interventions demonstrating effectiveness include:

- Weight reduction in overweight or obese individuals
- Adoption of a diet rich in potassium and calcium
- Dietary sodium restriction
- Physical activity
- Moderation of alcohol consumption

❼ *Implementation of these lifestyle modifications successfully lowers BP (Table 5–3), often with results similar to those of therapy with a single antihypertensive agent.[23]* Combinations of two or more lifestyle modifications can have even greater effects with BP lowering. BP lowering in overweight patients may be seen by a weight loss of as few as 4.5 kg (10 lb). The Dietary Approaches to Stop Hypertension (DASH) trial demonstrated that a diet high in fruits, vegetables, and low-fat dairy products, along with a reduced intake of total and saturated fat, significantly reduced BP in as little as 8 weeks.[23] Sodium restriction in moderate amounts lowers BP, is generally well-accepted, and is free of adverse effects. Restriction of sodium intake to 2.4 g (100 mmol) of elemental sodium (6 g of sodium chloride [100 mmol] or 1 teaspoon of table salt) should be easily achievable in most patients simply by avoidance of highly salted processed foods.[24] Simple dietary advice and instructions on reading packaging labels should be introduced to the patient initially and assessed and reinforced at subsequent office visits. As is the case with weight loss, changes in physical activity do not need to be profound in order to have a significant effect on BP. It is generally accepted that 30 minutes of moderately intense aerobic activity (e.g., brisk walking) most days of the week will lower BP.[25] While many

Table 5–3

Lifestyle Modifications to Manage Hypertension[a]

Modification	Recommendation	Approximate Systolic BP Reduction (Range)
Weight reduction	Maintain normal body weight (body mass index 18.5–24.9 kg/m²)	5–20 mm Hg/10 kg
Adopt DASH eating plan	Consume a diet rich in fruits, vegetables, and low-fat dairy products with a reduced content of saturated and total fat	8–14 mm Hg
Dietary sodium restriction	Reduce dietary sodium intake to no more than 100 mmol/day (2.4 g sodium or 6 g sodium chloride)	2–8 mm Hg
Physical activity	Engage in regular aerobic physical activity such as brisk walking (at least 30 min/day, most days of the week)	4–9 mm Hg
Moderation of alcohol consumption	Limit consumption to no more than 2 drinks (e.g., 24 oz [710 mL] beer, 10 oz [296 mL] wine, or 3 oz [89 mL] 80-proof whiskey) per day in most men and to no more than 1 drink per day in women and lighter weight persons	2–4 mm Hg

BP, blood pressure; DASH, Dietary Approaches to Stop Hypertension.

[a]For overall cardiovascular risk reduction, stop smoking. The effects of implementing these modifications are dose- and time-dependent and could be greater for some individuals.

From Ref. 1.

patients can safely engage in moderately intense aerobic activity, individuals with known CVD, multiple risk factors with symptoms, or selected diabetic patients should undergo medical examination, possibly including exercise testing, prior to participation.[26,27] The effects of alcohol on BP are variable. Initially, acute ingestion leads to a fall in BP followed by a rise several hours later,[28] and binge drinking is associated with a higher risk of stroke. Furthermore, abstinence from alcohol in heavy drinkers leads to a reduction in BP.[29] Alcohol also attenuates the effects of antihypertensive therapy, which is mostly reversible within 1 to 2 weeks with moderation of intake.

In addition to their beneficial effects on lowering BP, lifestyle modifications also have a favorable effect on other risk factors such as dyslipidemia and insulin resistance, which are commonly encountered in the hypertensive population, and lifestyle modifications should be encouraged for this reason as well. Smoking cessation should also be encouraged for overall cardiovascular health despite its lack of chronic effects on BP.[30,31] Although lifestyle modifications have never been documented to reduce cardiovascular morbidity and mortality in patients with hypertension, they do effectively lower BP to some extent in most hypertensive patients. This may obviate the need for drug therapy in those with mild elevations in BP or minimize the doses or number of antihypertensive agents required in those with greater elevations in BP.

Pharmacologic Treatment

❽ *An approach to selection of drugs for the treatment of patients with hypertension should be evidence-based with considerations regarding the individual's coexisting disease states, coprescribed medications, and practical patient-specific issues including cost. The JNC 7 report and statements from other global organizations recommend drug therapy that is largely grounded in the best available evidence for superiority in outcomes—specifically morbidity and mortality.[1] The approach is often tempered with practical considerations related to competing options for specific comorbidities and issues regarding a patient's experience or tolerance for side effects, and in some cases, the cost of medications.*

Although landmark trials, such as the Antihypertensive and Lipid-Lowering Treatment to Prevent Heart Attack Trial (ALLHAT), have provided some objective basis for comparisons between initiating antihypertensive drug therapy with one class of antihypertensives versus another, there is room for criticism of these studies.[22,32,33] Consequently, practical interpretations of their conclusions must always leave room for individualization based on clinical judgment. Overall current clinical guidelines provide a reasonable basis for guiding the selection of drug classes for individuals based on their stage of hypertension, comorbidities, and special circumstances. The following section will summarize key features of specific drug classes and guideline recommendations for patients with hypertension. Finally, an overview of the specific oral antihypertensive drug classes in common use is summarized in Table 5–4.

Diuretics

Many authorities recognize the value of diuretics as first-line agents for the majority of patients with hypertension. Among others, the basis for endorsement of diuretics as choice initial drug therapy for a variety of patient types includes their practical attributes (acquisition cost and availability as combination agents), extent of experience and favorable outcomes in placebo-controlled trials.[1,2] These virtues are further supported by results of studies such as ALLHAT.[22]

Table 5–4

Commonly Used Oral Antihypertensive Drugs by Pharmacologic Class

Class	Drug Name and Usual Oral Dosage Range (mg/day)	Compelling Indications	Clinical Trials	Select Adverse Events	Comments[a]
Diuretic					
Thiazides	Chlorthalidone (Hygroton) 6.25–25	Heart failure stage A [chlorthalidone]	ALLHAT[34] PROGRESS[35]	Hypokalemia and other electrolyte imbalances	Chlorthalidone is about twice as potent as hydrochlorothiazide
	Indapamide (Lozol) 1.25–5	High coronary disease risk [chlorthalidone]	HYVET[36]	Negative effect on glucose and lipids	Thiazide diuretics are generally more effective antihypertensive agents than loop diuretics
	Hydrochlorothiazide 12.5–50	Diabetes [chlorthalidone]			Not first-line agents in pregnancy, but probably safe per JNC 7
	Metolazone (Zaroxolyn) 2.5–5	Stroke [perindopril + indapamide]			Monitor electrolytes (i.e., decreased serum potassium) and metabolic abnormalities (i.e., dyslipidemia, hyperglycemia)
					Use caution in patients with gout
					Contraindications include hypersensitivity, anuria, renal decompensation
Loops	Bumetanide (Bumex) 1–4		RALES[37] EPHESUS[38]	Potassium-sparing diuretics may enhance hyperkalemic effects of drug therapies (i.e., ACE inhibitor, aldosterone antagonist)	Monitor electrolytes (i.e., decreased potassium) and metabolic abnormalities (i.e., dyslipidemia, hyperglycemia)
	Furosemide (Lasix) 40–160				Use with caution in patients with gout
	Torsemide (Demadex) 2.5–10			Hyperkalemia	Contraindications include hypersensitivity, anuria, acute renal insufficiency, hyperkalemia
Potassium-sparing aldosterone antagonists	Amiloride (Midamor) 5–20 Triamterene (Dyrenium) 50–200	Heart failure [spironolactone]			Monitor electrolytes (i.e., decreased potassium) and metabolic abnormalities (i.e., dyslipidemias, hyperglycemia)
		Heart failure post-MI [eplerenone]			Use with caution in patients with gout
	Spironolactone (Aldactone) 25–100			Gynecomastia [spironolactone]	Contraindications include hypersensitivity, anuria, acute renal insufficiency, hyperkalemia
	Eplerenone (Inspra) 50–200				Eplerenone contraindicated as an antihypertensive in patients with estimated creatinine clearance less than 50 mL/min or serum creatinine greater than 1.8 mg/dL (159 μmol/L) for women or 2 mg/dL (177 μmol/L) in men as well as type 2 diabetes mellitus with microalbuminuria. Also contraindicated in patients concomitantly receiving strong CYP3A4 inhibitors or a serum potassium greater than 5.5 mEq/L (5.5 mmol/L) at initiation

Class	Drug (range)	Compelling indication [drug]	Trial	Side effects	Comments
β-Blocker					
Cardioselective	Atenolol (Tenormin) 25–100 Bisoprolol (Zebeta) 2.5–10 Metoprolol tartrate (Lopressor) 100–200 Metoprolol succinate (Toprol XL) 50–100	Heart failure [metoprolol XL, carvedilol, bisoprolol] Heart failure post-MI [carvedilol] Post-MI [propranolol, β₁-antagonists] High coronary disease risk	MERIT-HF[39] COPERNICUS[40] CAPRICORN[41] BHAT[42] CIBIS-II[43]	Bradycardia Heart block Heart failure Hypotension/syncope Dyspnea, bronchospasm Fatigue, dizziness, lethargy, depression Hyper/hypoglycemia, hyperkalemia, hyperlipidemia	Caution with heart rate less than 60 and respiratory disease Selectivity of β_1 agents is diminished at higher doses Abrupt discontinuation may cause rebound hypertension May mask signs/symptoms of hypoglycemia in diabetic patients Contraindicated in hypersensitivity, sinus node dysfunction or severe sinus bradycardia (in the absence of a pacemaker), heart block (greater than first-degree), cardiogenic shock, acute decompensated heart failure
Nonselective	Nadolol (Corgard) 40–120 Nebivolol (Bystolic) 2.5–40 Propranolol (Inderal) 40–160 Propranolol long-acting (Inderal LA, Innopran XL) 60–180 Timolol (Blocadren) 20–40				
Mixed α- and β-blocker	Carvedilol (Coreg) 25–100 Carvedilol CR (Coreg CR) 20–80 Labetalol (Trandate) 200–800				
CCBA					
Nondihydropyridines	Diltiazem long-acting (Cardizem SR, Cardizem CD, others) 180–420 Verapamil sustained-release (Calan SR, Isoptin SR, Verelan) 120–360	High coronary disease risk [verapamil-tandolapril] Diabetes	INVEST[44] VALUE[33] ASCOT[32]	Bradycardia, heart block [nondihydropyridines] Constipation [nondihydropyridines] Hypotension Peripheral edema, headache, flushing Gingival hyperplasia [dihydropyridines] Reflex tachycardia [dihydroyridine]	Caution with heart rate less than 60 [verapamil, diltiazem] Use caution in concomitant use with β-blocker, may potentiate heart block Extended release formulations are preferred for once or twice daily medication administration Contraindicated in hypersensitivity, sinus node dysfunction, or severe sinus bradycardia (in the absence of a pacemaker) [nondihydropyridines], heart block (greater than first-degree) in the absence of a pacemaker [nondihydropyridines], atrial fibrillation/flutter associated with accessory bypass tract [nondihydropyridines], severe hypotension (systolic less than 90 mm Hg) [nondihydropyridines], severe left ventricular dysfunction [nondihydropyridines]
Dihydropyridines	Amlodipine (Norvasc) 2.5–10 Felodipine (Plendil) 5–20 Isradipine SR (DynaCirc SR) 2.5–10 Nicardipine SR (Cardene SR) 60–120 Nifedipine long-acting (Adalat CC, Procardia XL) 30–60 Nisoldipine (Sular) 10–40				

Table 5–4

Commonly Used Oral Antihypertensive Drugs by Pharmacologic Class (Continued)

Class	Drug Name and Usual Oral Dosage Range (mg/day)	Compelling Indications	Clinical Trials	Select Adverse Events	Comments[a]
ACE Inhibitor	Benazepril (Lotensin) 20–80 Captopril (Capoten) 25–100 Enalapril (Vasotec) 2.5–40 Fosinopril (Monopril) 10–40 Lisinopril (Prinivil, Zestril) 10–40 Moexipril (Univasc) 7.5–30 Perindopril (Aceon) 4–8 Quinapril (Accupril) 10–40 Ramipril (Altace) 2.5–20 Trandolapril (Mavik) 1–4	Heart failure [enalapril] Heart failure post-MI [ramipril, trandolapril] Post-MI [captopril] High coronary disease risk [ramipril, perindopril] Diabetes [captopril] Chronic kidney disease [captopril, ramipril] Stroke [perindopril + indapamide]	SOLVD[45] AIRE[46] TRACE[47] SAVE[48] HOPE[49] EUROPA[50] Captopril Trial[49] PROGRESS[35]	Cough Hyperkalemia Renal function deterioration Angioedema Hypotension/syncope	Monitor electrolytes (i.e., increased serum potassium) Monitor renal function with serum creatinine and blood urea nitrogen Initial dose may be reduced in renal impairment; the elderly, patients who are volume depleted or maintained on diuretic therapy Contraindicated in pregnancy and hypersensitivity; bilateral renal artery stenosis or unilateral renal artery stenosis in a solitary functional kidney, serum potassium greater than 5.5 mEq/L (5.5 mmol/L) that cannot be reduced
ARB	Candesartan (Atacand) 8–32 Eprosartan (Tevetan) 400–800 Irbesartan (Avapro) 150–300 Losartan (Cozar) 25–100 Olmesartan (Benicar) 20–40 Telmisartan (Micardis) 20–80 Valsartan (Diovan) 80–320	Heart failure [valsartan, candesartan] High coronary disease risk [losartan] Diabetes CKD [irbesartan, losartan]	CHARM[51] LIFE[52] RENAAL[53] IDNT[54] IRMA-2[55] ValHeFT[56]	Hyperkalemia Renal function deterioration Angioedema Hypotension/syncope	Monitor electrolytes (i.e., increased serum potassium) Monitor renal function with serum creatinine and blood urea nitrogen Contraindicated in pregnancy and hypersensitivity
Central α-2 Agonists	Methyldopa 250–1,000 Clonidine (Catapres) 0.1–0.8 Clonidine patch (Catapres TTS) 0.1–0.3 Guanabenz 4–32 Guanfacine 0.5–2	No recommendations at this time		Transient sedation initially Hepatotoxicity, hemolytic anemia, peripheral edema (methyldopa) Orthostatic hypotension (methyldopa, clonidine) Dry mouth, muscle weakness (clonidine)	First-line agent in pregnancy [methyldopa] Tolerance may occur 2–3 months after initiation of methyldopa; increase dose or add diuretic Contraindications include hypersensitivity, concurrent use of MAO inhibitor [methyldopa], hepatic disease [methyldopa]

Class	Drug (dose, mg/day)	Compelling indications	Trial	Adverse effects	Cautions/Contraindications
α-1 Blockers	Doxazosin (Cardura) 1–16 Prazosin (Minipress) 2–20 Terazosin (Hytrin) 1–20	Benign prostatic hyperplasia		Syncope Dizziness Palpitations	Contraindicated in hypersensitivity
Direct Vasodilators	Isosorbide dinitrate 20 mg and hydralazine 37.5 (BiDil) 1–2 tablets three times a day Hydralazine (Apresoline) 25–100 Minoxidil (Loniten) 2.5–80	Heart failure [isosorbide dinitrate + hydralazine in African Americans]	A-HeFT[57]	Edema [minoxidil] Tachycardia Lupus-like syndrome [hydralzine]	Give minoxidil with diuretic and β-blocker Contraindicated in hypersensitivity, pheochromocytoma (minoxidil), acute closure glaucoma, head trauma or cerebral hemorrhage (isosorbide dinitrate + hyralazine)
Direct Renin Inhibitors	Aliskiren (Tekturna) 150–300	No recommendations at this time		Hyperkalemia Hypotension	Use caution in patients with severe renal impairment and in patients with deteriorating renal function or renal artery stenosis, both bi- and unilateral
Peripheral Sympathetic Inhibitors	Reserpine 0.05–0.25 Guanethidine 10–50 Guanadrel 10–75	No recommendations at this time		Mental depression Orthostatic hypotension Peripheral vascular disease Nasal congestion, fluid retention, peripheral edema Diarrhea, increased gastric secretion	Contraindications include hypersensitivity, peptic ulcer disease or ulcerative colitis [reserpine], history of mental depression or electroconvulsive therapy [reserpine], pheochromocytoma [guanethidine, guanadrel], concurrent use (within 1 week) of MAO inhibitor [guanethidine, guanadrel], heart failure exacerbation [guanethidine, guanadrel]

A-HeFT, African American Heart Failure Trial; ACE, angiotensin–converting enzyme; AIRE, Acute Infarction Ramipril Efficacy study; ALLHAT, Antihypertensive and Lipid-Lowering Treatment to Prevent Heart Attack Trial; ARB, angiotensin receptor blocker; ASCOT, Anglo-Scandinavian Cardiac Output Trial; BHAT, Beta-Blocker Heart Attack Trial; bpm, beats per minute; CAPRICORN, Carvedilol Post-Infarct Survival Control in Left Ventricular Dysfunction Trial; Captopril Trial, Collaborative Study Captopril Trial ("The Effect of Angiotensin-Converting Enzyme Inhibition on Diabetic Nephropathy"); CCBA, calcium channel blocker agent; CHARM, Candesartan in Heart Failure Assessment of Reduction in Morbidity and Mortality Trial; CIBIS-II, The Cardiac Insufficiency Bisoprolol Study II; COPERNICUS, Carvedilol Prospective Randomized Cumulative Survival Trial; EPHESUS, Eplerenone Post-Acute Myocardial Infarction Heart Failure Efficacy and Survival Study; EUROPA, European Trial on Reduction of Cardiac Events with Perindopril in Stable Coronary Artery Disease Trial; HOPE, Heart Outcomes Prevention Evaluation Study; HYVET, Hypertension in the Very Elderly Trial; IDNT, Irbesartan Diabetic Nephropathy Trial; INVEST, International Verapamil-Trandolapril Study; IRMA-II, Irbesartan in Patients with Type 2 Diabetes and Microalbuminuria study; ISA, intrinsic sympathomimetic activity; LIFE, Losartan Intervention For Endpoint reduction in hypertension study; MAO, monoamine oxidase; MERIT-HF, Metoprolol CR/XL Randomised Intervention Trial in Congestive Heart Failure; MI, myocardial infarction; PROGRESS, Perindopril Protection Against Recurrent Stroke Study; RALES, Randomized Aldactone Evaluation Study; RENAAL, Reduction of Endpoints in NIDDM with the Angiotensin II Antagonist Losartan study; SAVE, Survival and Ventricular Enlargement trial; SOLVD, Studies of Left Ventricular Dysfunction; TRACE, Trandolapril Cardiac Evaluation; VALUE, Valsartan Antihypertensive Long-term Use Evaluation; ValHeFT, Veterans Affairs Cooperative I study.

*Comments listed are not intended to be inclusive of all adverse effects, monitoring parameters, cautions or contraindications and may vary by source.

This landmark double-blind study tested the hypothesis that newer antihypertensive agents would outperform thiazide-type diuretics when selected as initial drug therapy. After 4.9 years of follow-up in over 42,000 patients, the primary endpoint of fatal coronary heart disease and nonfatal MI was indistinguishable between chlorthalidone versus either amlodipine or lisinopril. A fourth arm examining doxazosin was terminated early based on a higher risk of heart failure for doxazosin compared with chlorthalidone.[58] In spite of these findings for the primary endpoint, differences in outcomes for select secondary endpoints demonstrated superiority of chlorthalidone over either of the two remaining comparison groups. These observations, along with perceived cost-effectiveness (which was not specifically evaluated in this study), led the authors of JNC 7 to endorse diuretics as initial drug therapy for most patients with hypertension. Nonetheless, substantial criticism of this trial has undermined the enthusiasm for diuretics as first-line therapy in the minds of some clinicians' as well as members of international guideline committees.[3] Criticism of the differential BPs achieved in the various treatment groups, the artificial construct guiding the use of add-on drugs to base therapy, and the over-representation of African Americans exhibiting select endpoints have weakened the interpretability of the authors' conclusions. Furthermore, other contemporary studies[32,59] have also challenged the status of diuretics as ideal baseline choices for initial antihypertensive drug therapy for all patients. Specifically, the Australian-New Zealand Blood Pressure-2 (ANBP2) Study[59] seemingly demonstrated (in particular for the male cohort) a superior outcome for angiotensin-converting enzyme (ACE) inhibitor-based therapy versus diuretic-based therapy in over 6,000 relatively older patients treated for over 4 years. Similarly, the Anglo-Scandinavian Cardiac Outcomes Trial-Blood Pressure Lowering Arm (ASCOT-BPLA)[32] study demonstrated outcomes which seemingly favored the calcium channel blocker agent (CCBA)/ACE inhibitor-based approach versus a β-blocker/diuretic-based approach in over 19,000 patients treated for approximately 5 years. Needless to say, all three of these major trials are subject to significant criticism including heterogeneity of achievement in BP targets between treatment arms for both the ALLHAT and ASCOT-BPLA studies.[60] In addition, the recently completed Avoiding Cardiovascular Events in Combination Therapy in Patients Living with Systolic Hypertension (ACCOMPLISH) trial failed to demonstrate superiority of a low-dose diuretic-ACE inhibitor combination versus a calcium channel blocker-ACE inhibitor combination in hypertensive patients. This has refueled the debate over whether the means by which BP is lowered (drug selection) is more or less important than the extent and or time taken to lower BP.[61] Furthermore, controversy has ignited as to whether the choice and dose of diuretic (chlorthalidone, ALLHAT) versus hydrochlorothiazide (ANBP2, ACCOMPLISH) was partly responsible for the difference in study results, and raised the question whether chlorthalidone should be the preferred thiazide type diuretic.[62,63] Nonetheless, diuretics remain supported by most as baseline initial therapy for

the majority of hypertensive patients without compelling indications.[60]

Key features of diuretics that must be kept in mind, along with evidence from outcome-based studies, include the diversity between the subtypes of diuretics and their corresponding diversity of pharmacologic actions. The four subtypes include thiazides, loop diuretics, potassium-sparing agents, and aldosterone antagonists. The latter will be discussed as a separate entity. Each subtype has clinically based properties which distinguish their roles in select patient populations. Thiazide diuretics are by far the most commonly prescribed subtype with the greatest number of outcome-based studies supporting their use. In the United States, hydrochlorothiazide and chlorthalidone represent the most commonly prescribed thiazide-type diuretics and have been the subject of the majority of large outcome-based studies. Although subtle differences in pharmacokinetics between these agents exist, practical differences are limited to their relative diuretic potency. Chlorthalidone is considered approximately 1.5 to 2 times more potent than hydrochlorothiazide for BP reduction.[64] Since the relationship between antihypertensive efficacy and metabolic/electrolyte-related side effects of thiazide diuretics is considered to be dose-related, attention to this differential in potency may be important. Specifically, select metabolic effects (hyperlipidemic and hyperglycemic) and electrolyte-related effects (hypokalemic, hypomagnesemic, hyperuricemic, and hypercalcemic) seem to increase with higher doses. This has led to national guidelines[1] recommending doses not exceed 6.25 to 25 mg/day for chlorthalidone or 12.5 to 50 mg/day for hydrochlorothiazide. These metabolic effects may clearly complicate the management of higher-risk patients with common comorbidities such as dyslipidemia or diabetes, or even those likely to be sensitive to the potassium- or magnesium-wasting effects of diuretics (patients with dysrhythmias or those taking digoxin). While rates of diabetes are higher following administration of thiazides, there is evidence that this can be greatly minimized by keeping potassium in the high normal range (i.e., above 4.0 mEq/L [4 mmol/L]).[65] Furthermore, whether the development of new-onset diabetes in association with thiazide diuretic is of clinical significance is in question as the large ALLHAT and the Systolic Hypertension in the Elderly Program [SHEP]) trials showed no significant adverse CV events from new diuretic-associated diabetes whereas a smaller trial did.[66] Nonetheless, clinicians should rarely approach the upper limits of these dosage ranges without careful assessment of their metabolic effects or potential to induce electrolyte disturbances. In this way, optimization of BP lowering potential may be achieved while minimizing potential adverse outcomes.

Another key feature of the thiazide-type diuretics is their limited efficacy in patients whose renal function is reduced simply by age. Estimated by a calculated GFR, as renal function declines with age to less than 30 mL/min, loop type diuretics such as furosemide emerge as superior to thiazide type diuretics for lowering BP. Clinicians often fail to reevaluate the use of thiazide diuretics prescribed to individuals whose renal function has been declining with age.

The loop diuretics, such as furosemide, bumetanide, torsemide, and ethacrynic acid, have a common site of action in the thick ascending limb of the loop of Henle.[67] Responsible for reabsorption of over 65% of the filtered sodium, their diuretic efficacy is clearly superior to that of the thiazides, potassium-sparing diuretics, and mineralocorticoids. Practically speaking, furosemide is the most common agent used as an alternative to thiazide type agents for patients whose renal function has been compromised. With the exception of torsemide, which has a longer half-life, the loop diuretics should be administered twice daily versus once when utilized primarily for their antihypertensive (versus diuretic) effect. The most significant adverse effects related to loop diuretic use concerns their potential for excessive diuresis leading to hyponatremia or hypotension. Additionally, hypokalemia, hypomagnesemia, and hypocalcemia may develop over time and contribute to the potential for cardiac arrhythmias. Overall relevance of drug-drug interactions and potential for aggravating select conditions (hyperglycemia, dyslipidemias, and hyperuricemia) should be routinely considered in the monitoring plan for those taking loop diuretics for extended periods of time.

Potassium-sparing diuretics that do not act through mineralocorticoid receptors include triamterene and amiloride. These agents are often prescribed with potassium-wasting diuretics in an attempt to mitigate the loss of potassium. When administered as a single entity or as one component of a combination product, these agents result in moderate diuresis. Potassium-sparing diuretics act on the late distal tubule and collecting duct, and thereby have limited ability to affect sodium reabsorption, which translates into modest diuresis. The most important adverse effects associated with these agents are their potential to contribute to hyperkalemia. This is especially relevant in the context of those patients receiving other agents with potassium-sparing properties, such as ACE inhibitors, angiotensin receptor blockers (ARBs), and potassium supplements, as well nonsteroidal anti-inflammatory drugs (NSAIDs). It is also relevant in those with more than mild renal impairment.

Aldosterone Antagonists

Aldosterone antagonists such as spironolactone, and eplerenone (Fig. 5–3) modulate vascular tone through a variety of mechanisms besides diuresis. Their potassium-sparing effects mediated through aldosterone antagonism, complement the potassium-wasting effects of more potent diuretics such as thiazide or loop diuretics. Patients with resistant hypertension (with or without primary aldosteronism) experience significant BP reductions with the addition of low-dose spironolactone (12.5–50 mg/day) to diuretics, ACE inhibitors, and ARBs.[68] Although functional in this circumstance, it is important to recognize their potential to enhance the risk for hyperkalemia when used in conjunction with ACE inhibitors, ARBs, and now potentially DRIs. This is particularly relevant for individuals with comorbidities associated with reduced renal function or those receiving either potassium supplements or NSAIDs. The most commonly used potassium-sparing diuretic is spironolactone; however, eplerenone has been used with increasing frequency in patients with heart failure following acute myocardial infarction (AMI).[38] Although spironolactone is commonly associated with gynecomastia, eplerenone rarely causes this complication.[69] The risk of hyperkalemia is also more commonly reported with patients on spironolactone.[70]

β-Blockers

Controversy surrounds the JNC 7 recommended role of β-blockers as first-line antihypertensive agents. For example, a meta-analysis by Lindholm et al.[71] demonstrated a higher risk of stroke in patients treated for primary hypertension with β-blockers compared to other antihypertensives. Moreover, Messerli et al.[72] showed that β-blockers were ineffective in preventing coronary heart disease, cardiovascular mortality, and all-cause mortality compared to diuretics for elderly patients (60 years of age or older) treated for primary hypertension. Consequently, current evidence suggests patients with uncomplicated hypertension may not benefit as much, if at all, from β-blocker therapy relative to other antihypertensives.[2] This may be in part due to their tendency to reduce central aortic pressure and cardiac afterload to a lesser degree relative to other agents.[73] It must be noted that all of these analyses were conducted with a limited number of β-blockers such as atenolol and metoprolol tartrate. Whether newer formulations such as metoprolol succinate, or agents with unique properties such as carvedilol would be more efficacious in reducing morbidity and mortality is unknown. The drug with the most prominent difference in the increased risk of stroke between the three β-blocker subgroups was atenolol. The concern regarding β-blocker use in hypertensive patients without compelling indications is reflected in American Heart Association's recommendations and the European Society of Cardiology's abandonment of β-blockers as first-line antihypertensive agents. On the other hand, the role of β-blockers in patients with specific select comorbidities is well established (Table 5–5). Specific outcome-based studies conducted in patients with comorbidities such as heart failure and recent MI have clearly demonstrated a benefit from β-blocker use.[74] Their hemodynamic effects and antiarrhythmic properties make them desirable agents for hypertensive patients who suffer from ischemic conditions including AMI.[67] When used judiciously in hypertensive patients with heart failure, β-blocker inhibition of neurohormonal mediated cardiac remodeling reduces morbidity and mortality relative to standard heart failure therapies. The mechanisms through which β-blockers affect BP are complex, but most certainly include their modulation of renin (Fig. 5–3) which appears to result in a reduction in CO and/or reduction in PR along with their negative inotropic/chronotropic actions.

The specific pharmacologic properties of β-blockers are varied and diverse. An understanding of these properties

Table 5–5

Compelling Indications for Individual Drug Classes

Compelling Indication	Recommended Drug Class						
	Diuretic	Ald Ant	BB	CCBA	ACE-I	ARB	Dir Vaso
Heart failure	X	X	X		X	X	X
Postmyocardial infarction		X	X		X		
High coronary disease risk	X		X	X	X		
Diabetes	X		X	X	X	X	
Chronic kidney disease					X	X	
Recurrent stroke prevention	X				X		

ACE-I, angiotensin-converting enzyme inhibitor; Ald Ant, aldosterone antagonist; ARB, angiotensin receptor blocker; BB, β-blocker; CCBA, calcium channel blocking agent; Dir Vaso, direct vasodilator.

From Ref. 1.

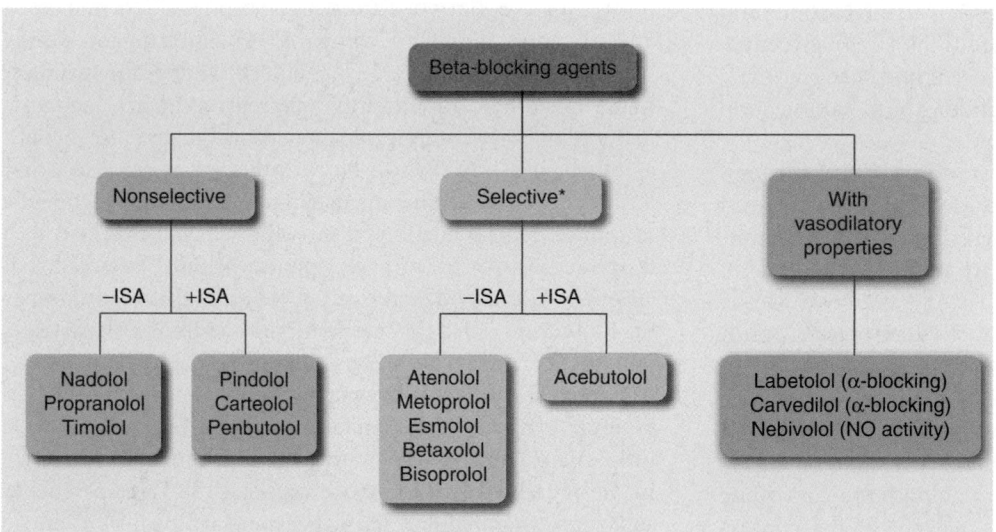

FIGURE 5–4. Flowchart listing various β-blocking agents separated by β-receptor activity and intrinsic sympathomimetic activity. *β-1 Cardioselective. (ISA, intrinsic sympathomimetic activity; NO, nitrous oxide.)

may assist in the selection of one agent over others given a patient's specific condition(s). One of these properties is cardioselectivity—the property of some β-blockers that preferentially block β_1- versus β_2-receptors. Another property exhibited by some β-blockers is membrane stabilization activity, which relates to the propensity of the β-blocker to possess some capacity for antiarrhythmic properties, in addition to β-receptor blocking properties. Some β-blockers (Fig. 5–4) possess properties referred to as intrinsic sympathomimetic activity (ISA). β-Blockers possessing this property effectively block the β-receptor at higher circulating catecholamine levels, such as during exercise, while having modest β-blocking activity at times of lower catecholamine levels, such as at rest.[75]

When selecting a β-blocker, some of these properties may be of practical value while others, such as membrane stabilization activity and ISA, are of theoretical interest only. Because neither membrane stablization activity nor ISA has been directly proven value in the clinical setting, they will not

be discussed further other than to point out that β-blockers with ISA are not recommended for use in the post-MI patient.[76] With regards to cardioselectivity, consider a patient with mild asthma, chronic obstructive pulmonary disease, or peripheral vascular disease (intermittent claudication). A β-blocker with relative cardioselectivity to block β_1-receptors may be more desirable in such a patient, while a nonselective β-blocker (Fig. 5–4) may be potentially disadvantageous. In such a patient, low doses of cardioselective β-blockers may achieve adequate blockade of β_1-receptors in the heart and kidneys while minimizing the undesirable effects of β_2-receptor blockade on the smooth muscle lining the bronchioles. In doing so, hypertension may be managed while avoiding complications of the coexisting reactive airway disease, which is mediated by β_2-receptor stimulation. Similarly, either because of a reduction in the β_2-mediated vascular blood flow or by enhanced unopposed α-agonist–mediated vasoconstriction, a patient with peripheral vascular disease (intermittent claudication) may experience a worsening of symptoms with use of a nonselective β-blocker (Fig. 5–4). It is important to remember that cardioselectivity is dependent upon dose, with diminished selectivity exhibited with higher doses.

A limited number of β-blockers also possess vasodilatory properties that are either mediated through α_1-receptor blockade (carvedilol, labetalol) or via L-arginine/nitric oxide-induced release from endothelial cells with subsequent increased nitric oxide bioavailability in the endothelium (nebivolol; Fig. 5–4). Reductions in PR through α_1-receptor mediated blockade or via L-arginine/nitric oxide-induced release, in addition to β-blockade, may benefit patients with hypertension. Such combinations should theoretically contribute to enhanced reductions in vascular tone. Nonetheless, there has been no proven evidence of superior outcomes from the use of β-blockers with vasodilatory properties through either means compared to those with only β-blocking activity.

The adverse effects of β-blockers logically follow their pharmacology. Initiating β-blockers to treat patients with hypertension may have the potential to precipitate bradycardia, various degrees of heart block, or signs and symptoms of heart failure. The latter is usually limited to those with a subclinical diagnosis and should be considered in the elderly or those with documented reductions in left ventricular function. Conversely, abrupt discontinuation of β-blockers has been cited as a precipitating factor in the development of ischemic syndromes—especially for those patients in whom β-blockers were used for extended periods of time, at higher doses, or who had underlying ischemic heart disease. In such cases, the dose of these agents should be reduced (tapered) over a period of several days to perhaps 1 or even 2 weeks depending on patient-related factors.

Calcium Channel Blocking Agents

Exhibiting considerable interclass diversity, CCBAs are recognized as effective antihypertensives, particularly in the elderly. Patients with isolated systolic hypertension who were taking CCBAs experienced reduced CVD endpoints during several clinical trials. Several trials comparing a CCBA-based approach versus non-CCBA-based approach have been published. Specifically, the Valsartan Antihypertensive Long-term Use Evaluation (VALUE) trial compared valsartan-based therapy to amlodipine-based therapy in over 15,000 patients who were at high-risk for cardiac events. In spite of an attempt to achieve identical BP reductions, differences were noted early and sustained throughout the 4.2-year length of the study.[32] Overall the primary endpoint (composite cardiac mortality and morbidity) was not statistically significantly different between the groups, but cause-specific outcomes did favor the regimen affording the achievement of lower BPs—namely the amlodipine-based therapy. This theme of unequal reductions in BP accounting for differences in cause-specific outcomes was shared by the findings of the ASCOT-BPLA study, which compared amlodipine-based therapy versus atenolol-based therapy in over 19,000 hypertensives for 5.5 years. Again although no

statistically significant reduction in the primary endpoint was observed, the study was stopped prematurely. The basis for this early termination was grounded in the association of a higher mortality rate and worse outcome for those allocated to the atenolol-based regimen compared to those receiving the amlodipine-based regimen. These observations support the argument that regardless of the agents used, the evidence appears to indicate that the amount of BP lowering achieved has more to do with event reduction than with the agents or combinations of agents used to achieve them. Primary endpoints aside, certain secondary endpoints demonstrated differences between regimens. Protection from the development of new-onset diabetes over the duration of the study was noted for the amlodipine-based therapy in the ASCOT-BPLA study and favored the ARB-based regimen over the CCBA-based regimen in the VALUE study.

The diversity of pharmacologic properties among the subclasses of CCBAs is significant. A clinician's familiarity with these differences among subclasses helps categorize their expected effects on the cardiovascular system and potential risk of toxicities. Dihydropyridine CCBAs such as amlodipine are commonly associated with edema, especially when used at higher doses. Phenylalkylamine-verapamil and benzothiazepine-diltiazem are more commonly recognized for their electrophysiological effects, negative chronotropic and negative inotropic effects. Many of these pharmacologic properties are exploited for their specific clinical utility. Given that verapamil and diltiazem (both are nondihydropyridine CCBAs) effectively block cardiac conduction through the atrioventricular node, their value in the management of patients with atrial fibrillation in addition to hypertension is obvious. In contrast, the dihydropyridine subclass of agents has no utility in managing atrial dysrhythmias. Similarly, all three subclasses of CCBAs possess some coronary vasodilating properties and hence may be used in select patients for the management of patients with angina, in addition to their antihypertensive benefits.

ACE Inhibitors

ACE inhibitors are widely used for the treatment of hypertension in a variety of patients with or without comorbidities and/or cardiovascular risk factors. Supported by the findings of numerous outcome trials, they have been extensively studied. This broad utility extends to the list of compelling indications (Table 5–5) for patients as described in JNC 7. These compelling indications include their qualified role in managing patients with hypertension who have type 1 diabetes,[33] heart failure,[77] post-MI,[76] type 2 diabetes,[78] CKD,[79,80] or recurrent stroke prevention.[35] Comparative trials between ACE inhibitors and various other agents as initial drug therapy have also demonstrated some differences in outcomes for this class. In ALLHAT,[22] ACE inhibitors appeared to perform less well than diuretics in terms of incidence of combined CVD and heart failure. On the other hand, the ANBP2 trial[59] seemed to suggest that ACE inhibitors may be equivalent to diuretics in terms of overall outcomes. Because there are legitimate criticisms of both these trials (including the smaller number of overall events and choice of hydrochlorothiazide as the diuretic in ANBP2), it may only be safe to conclude that both diuretics and ACE inhibitors represent formidable agents as either first- or second-line hypertensive therapies that effectively achieve a target BP goal for most patients with or without comorbidities.

Although generally well-tolerated, classic side effects associated with ACE inhibitors include their potential to cause hyperkalemia and a persistent dry cough. Modest elevations in serum potassium should be anticipated, particularly in patients with compromised renal function, those receiving concurrent NSAIDs, or those taking potassium supplementation or using a potassium containing salt substitute. The elevations in potassium should be anticipated, if not prospectively considered, when starting or increasing the dose of an ACE inhibitor. Hyperkalemia is rarely a reason for discontinuation of therapy. Nonetheless, periodic monitoring of serum potassium is prudent for patients receiving ACE inhibitors. The dry cough associated with ACE inhibitors is thought to be caused by accumulation of bradykinin resulting from a direct effect of inhibiting ACE. Although mild forms are tolerable, should cough jeopardize compliance with the agent, ARBs should be considered as possible alternative agents since there is less incidence of cough.

In general, the effects of ACE inhibitors on diminished renal function and potassium can be predicted given an understanding of their pharmacologic actions (Fig. 5–3). Inhibition of the generation of angiotensin II through ACE inhibition (or direct blockage of the angiotensin II receptor by angiotensin II receptor blockers) naturally would reduce the efferent renal artery tone thereby changing the intraglomerular pressure. Although changes in the afferent renal artery tone also occur, the overall effects usually translate into a reduction in GFR[80] with resulting elevations of up to 30% in serum creatinine values. It is important to recognize that such elevations in serum creatinine are not usually indications to discontinue use of the ACE inhibitor. Rather, possible dose reduction and continued monitoring for further increases in serum creatinine remains prudent. Alternatively, should elevations in serum creatinine exceed 30%, discontinuation is prudent until further evaluation can be made.

More rare forms of adverse effects of ACE inhibitors include blood dyscrasias, angioedema, and more serious effects of ACE inhibitors on renal function. The latter include acute renal failure in those with pre-existing kidney dysfunction, bilateral renal artery stenosis, or unilateral renal artery stenosis in a patient with one functioning kidney.

Angiotensin Receptor Blockers

ARBs are another key class of agents whose role in managing patients with hypertension has been further defined by recently completed studies. ARBs are inhibitors of the angiotensin-1 (AT1) receptors (Fig. 5–3). AT1 receptor stimulation evokes a pressor response via a host of accompanying effects on catecholamines, aldosterone, and thirst.[67] Consequently, inhibition of AT1 receptors directly prevents this pressor response and results in up-regulation of the RAAS. Up-regulation of the RAAS results in elevated levels of angiotensin II, which have the added effect of stimulating the angiotensin-2 (AT2) receptors. AT2-receptor stimulation is generally associated with antihypertensive activity; however, long-term effects of AT2-receptor stimulation that involve cellular growth and repair are relatively unknown. What is clear is that ARBs differ from ACE inhibitors in that the former causes up-regulation of the RAAS while the latter blocks the breakdown of bradykinin. The therapeutic relevance resulting from these pharmacologic differences has yet to be fully evaluated through long-term clinical comparative trials in hypertensive patients. However, data from other patient populations (heart failure, high-risk coronary artery disease patients) suggest that the clinical benefits of ARBs are less robust than those of ACE inhibitors.[81,82]

At this point, ARBs have emerged as an effective class of antihypertensives whose low incidence of side effects and demonstrated clinical role in patients with specific comorbidities have afforded them an attractive position in the antihypertensive armamentarium. Like ACE inhibitors, the antihypertensive effectiveness of ARBs is greatly enhanced by combining them with diuretics. Furthermore, they have proven their value as well-tolerated alternatives to ACE inhibitors for patients with CKD, diabetes mellitus, and post-AMI (Table 5–5). As of late, the addition of ARBs to standard therapy for patients with heart failure (HF), including ACE inhibitors, have demonstrated additional incremental benefits for patients with systolic dysfunction[83] or diastolic dysfunction[84] or as alternatives to ACE inhibitors when ACE inhibitors are not tolerated.[85] Comparative studies with alternate (non-ACE inhibitors) antihypertensive regimens in patients with type 2 diabetes[84] and left ventricular hypertrophy[52] have demonstrated their usefulness as effective antihypertensives in these special populations. Studies (the Irbesartan Diabetic Nephropathy Trial [IDNT] and Reduction of Endpoints in NIDDM with the Angiotensin II Antagonist Losartan [RENAAL; NIDDM refers to noninsulin-dependent diabetes mellitus]) have demonstrated superiority of delaying progression toward renal dysfunction for ARBs relative to alternative antihypertensives in type 2 diabetics.[84] Although better tolerated than ACE inhibitors, ARBs have not been shown to demonstrate superiority of outcomes relative to ACE inhibitors. This key observation, in addition to their relatively higher acquisition cost, has mitigated the growth of ARB use relative to ACE inhibitors.

Renin Inhibitors

Aliskiren is the first agent in the newest class of antihypertensive agents. While similar to ACE inhibitors and ARBs in that it acts within the RAAS, it is unique in that it directly blocks renin thereby reducing plasma renin activity (PRA), and subsequently angiotensin I and angiotensin II, with a resultant reduction in BP. This disruption of the negative feedback loop results in a compensatory increase in renin levels—the significance of which is not yet known. Aliskiren has been shown to be well tolerated and effective in reducing BP when used as monotherapy and in combination with hydrochlorothiazide or valsartan for patients with mild to moderate HTN. However, long-term clinical trials evaluating efficacy and safety have yet to be completed, and thus the effects of aliskiren on morbidity and mortality are as of yet unknown. Because of aliskiren's role in the RAAS, recommendations and precautions for monitoring serum potassium and kidney function should be similar to those of ACE inhibitors and ARBs.

α-Blockers

Generally, α_1-blockers are considered as inferior agents and should not be used as monotherapy. The ALLHAT trial had an α_1-blocker arm that was discontinued early as terazosin was associated with an increase in cardiovascular events. α_1-Blockers may be considered as add-on therapy to other agents (i.e., 3rd or 4th line) when hypertension is not adequately controlled. In addition, they may have a specific role in the antihypertensive regimen for elderly males with prostatism; however, their use is often curtailed by complaints of syncope, dizziness, or palpitations following the first dose

Patient Encounter 2

A 55-year-old African American woman comes to your clinic with a recent diagnosis of hypertension. She is 5′5″ (165 cm) tall and weighs 73 kg (160 lb; body mass index 26.6 kg/m²). She reports that she does not use tobacco or drink alcohol, and exercises about once a week. Physical exam was unremarkable, but an ECG revealed left ventricular hypertrophy. Baseline laboratory tests were significant for fasting blood glucose of 124 mg/dL (6.88 mmol/L), serum creatinine of 1.5 mg/dL (133 μmol/L), potassium of 4.8 mEq/L (4.8 mmol/L), total cholesterol of 200 mg/dL (5.18 mmol/L), high-density lipoprotein cholesterol of 40 mg/dL (1.04 mmol/L), triglycerides of 200 mg/dL (2.26 mmol/L), and low-density lipoprotein cholesterol of 120 mg/dL (3.11 mmol/L). She has a history of an elevated serum creatinine ranging from 1.3 to 1.5 mg/dL (115–133 μmol/L) over the past 6 months. Urinalysis was positive for microalbuminuria. BP today was 165/86 mm Hg with a pulse of 55 bpm.

What signs of target-organ damage does this patient exhibit?

Is more extensive testing for identifiable causes of hypertension indicated at this time?

Based on the information presented, create a care plan for this patient's hypertension. This should include (a) goals of therapy, (b) a patient-specific therapeutic plan, and (c) a plan for appropriate monitoring to achieve goals and avoid adverse effects.

and orthostatic hypotension with chronic use. The roles of doxazosin, terazosin, and prazosin in the management of patients with hypertension are limited due to the paucity of outcome data and the absence of a unique role for special populations or compelling indications from JNC 7.

Central α₂-Agonists

Limited by their tendency to cause orthostasis, sedation, dry mouth, and vision disturbances, clonidine, methyldopa, guanfacine, and guanabenz represent rare choices in contemporary treatment of patients with hypertension. Their central α_2-adrenergic stimulation is thought to reduce sympathetic outflow and enhance parasympathetic activity thereby reducing heart rate, CO, and total PR. Occasionally used for cases of resistant hypertension, these agents may have a role when other more conventional therapies appear ineffective. The availability of a transdermal clonidine patch that is applied once weekly may offer an alternative to hypertensive patients with adherence problems. Of particular importance is the issue of severe rebound hypertension when clonidine is abruptly discontinued. The dose of this agent should be tapered when discontinuation is considered. If the patient is also receiving concomitant β-blocker therapy, the β-blocker should be tapered to discontinuation ideally several days before discontinuation of clonidine is initiated.

Other Agents

Direct vasodilators such as hydralazine and minoxidil represent additional alternative agents used for patients with resistant hypertension. Primarily acting to relax smooth muscles in arterioles and activate baroreceptors, their use in the absence of concurrently administered β-blockers and diuretics is uncommon. This is due to the need to offset their tendency to cause reflex tachycardia and fluid retention. Other, more rare adverse effects include hydralazine-induced lupus-like syndrome and hypertrichosis from minoxidil. Finally, reserpine, although slow to act, represents another rarely used alternative agent for those who are recalcitrant to more standard therapy. This agent is a long-acting depleter of the catecholamine norepinephrine from sympathetic nerve endings and via blockade of norepinephrine transport into its storage granules which causes reduced sympathetic tone leading to reductions in PR. Reserpine's association with numerous side effects including gastric ulceration, depression, and sexual side effects has limited its perception as a useful agent, but in low doses it can be well tolerated. In fact, the SHEP trial[86] demonstrated the BP lowering effectiveness of low-dose reserpine (0.05 mg/day) when combined with a diuretic, with similar cardiopulmonary and psychosocial side effects between the treatment and placebo groups. In addition, low-dose reserpine was also used as add-on therapy in the ALLHAT trial. Two additional agents, guanethidine and guanadrel, act as postganglionic sympathetic inhibitors inhibiting the release of norepinephrine as well as depleting norepinephrine from these nerve terminals. However, these agents have little role in the management of hypertension because of significant adverse effects.

SPECIAL PATIENT POPULATIONS

Compelling Indications and Special Considerations

❾ *Specific antihypertensive therapy is warranted for certain patients with comorbid conditions that may elevate their level of risk for CVD.* Clinical conditions for which there is compelling evidence supporting one or more classes of drug therapy include:[1]

- Ischemic heart disease
- Heart failure
- Diabetes
- CKD
- Cerebrovascular disease

Compelling indications for specific drug therapies are summarized in Table 5–5.[1,87] In patients with hypertension and angina, β-blockers and long-acting CCBAs are indicated due to their antihypertensive and antianginal effects.[1,26] In addition, patients may benefit from the potential atherosclerotic plaque stabilizing effects of amlodipine.[2] In patients at high-risk of ischemic heart disease, such as diabetic patients with additional cardiovascular risk factors or chronic coronary artery or vascular disease, ACE inhibitors are particularly useful in reducing the risk of cardiovascular events regardless of whether the patient carries a concurrent diagnosis of hypertension.[1,50,88] In patients intolerant to an ACE inhibitor, an ARB may be substituted given the findings of the recently completed ONgoing Telmisartan Alone and in combination with Ramipril Global Endpoint Trial (ONTARGET).[89]

β-Blockers and ACE inhibitors are indicated for post-MI patients due to their proven reduction of cardiovascular morbidity and mortality in this population. Aldosterone antagonists are also indicated for the post-MI patient with reduced left ventricular systolic function and diabetes or signs and symptoms of heart failure.[1,76]

Patients with asymptomatic left ventricular systolic dysfunction and hypertension should be treated with β-blockers and ACE inhibitors. Those with heart failure secondary to left ventricular dysfunction and hypertension should be treated with drugs proven to also reduce the morbidity and mortality of heart failure, including β-blockers, ACE inhibitors, ARBs, aldosterone antagonists, and diuretics for symptom control as well as antihypertensive effect. In African Americans with heart failure and left ventricular systolic dysfunction, combination therapy with nitrates and hydralazine not only affords a morbidity and mortality benefit, but may also be useful as antihypertensive therapy if needed.[57] The dihydropyridine CCBAs amlodipine or felodipine may also be used in patients with heart failure and left ventricular systolic dysfunction for uncontrolled BP, although they have no effect on heart failure morbidity and mortality in these patients.[77] For patients with heart failure

and preserved ejection fraction, antihypertensive therapies that should be considered include diuretics, β-blockers, ACE inhibitors, ARBs, CCBAs (including nondihydropyridine agents), and others as needed to control BP.[1,77]

Patients with diabetes and hypertension should initially be treated with either ACE inhibitors, ARBs, β-blockers, diuretics, or CCBAs. There is a general consensus that therapy focused on RAAS inhibition by ACE inhibitors or ARBs may be optimal if the patient has additional cardiovascular risk factors such as left ventricular hypertrophy or CKD.[1,78,79,52]

In patients with CKD and hypertension, ACE inhibitors and ARBs are preferred, usually in combination with a diuretic.[79] ACE inhibitors in combination with a thiazide diuretic are also preferred in patients with a history of prior stroke or transient ischemic attack. This therapy reduces the risk of recurrent stroke, making it particularly attractive in these patients for BP control.[83]

There are several situations in the management of hypertension requiring special considerations including, but not limited to:

- Hypertensive crisis
- Elderly populations
- Isolated systolic hypertension
- Minority populations
- Pregnancy
- Pediatrics

Hypertensive crisis can be divided into hypertensive emergencies and hypertensive urgencies. A hypertensive emergency occurs when severe elevations in BP are accompanied by acute or life-threatening target organ damage such as AMI, unstable angina, encephalopathy, intracerebral hemorrhage, acute left ventricular failure with pulmonary edema, dissecting aortic aneurysm, rapidly progressive renal failure, accelerated malignant hypertension with papilledema, and eclampsia, among others. BP is generally greater than 220/140 mm Hg, although a hypertensive emergency can occur at lower levels, particularly in individuals without previous hypertension. The goal in a hypertensive emergency is to reduce mean arterial pressure by up to 25% to the range of 160/100 to 110 mm Hg in minutes to hours.[1,90] IV therapy is generally required and may consist of the agents listed in Table 5–6.[87] A hypertensive urgency is manifested as a severe elevation in BP without evidence of acute or life-threatening target organ damage. In these individuals, BP can usually be managed with orally administered short-acting medications (i.e., captopril, clonidine, or labetalol) and observation in the emergency department over several hours, with subsequent discharge on oral medications and follow-up in the outpatient setting within 24 hours.[1,87]

The treatment of elderly patients with hypertension, as well as those with isolated systolic hypertension, should follow the same approach as with other populations with the exception that lower starting doses may be warranted to avoid symptoms. Special attention should be paid to postural hypotension. This should include a careful assessment of orthostatic symptoms, measurement of BP in the upright position, and caution to

Table 5–6

Parenteral Antihypertensive Agents for Hypertensive Emergency[a]

Drug	Dose Range	Onset of Action	Duration of Action	Adverse Effects[b]	Special Indications
Vasodilators					
Sodium nitroprusside	0.25–10 mcg/kg/min as IV infusion[c]	Immediate	1–2 minutes	Nausea, vomiting, muscle twitching, sweating, thiocyanate and cyanide intoxication	Most hypertensive emergencies; use with caution with high intracranial pressure or azotemia
Nicardipine hydrochloride	5–15 mg/h IV	5–10 minutes	15–30 minutes, may exceed 4 hours	Tachycardia, headache, flushing, local phlebitis	Most hypertensive emergencies except acute heart failure; use with caution with coronary ischemia
Fenoldopam mesylate	0.1–0.3 mcg/kg/min as IV infusion[c]	Less than 5 minutes	30 minutes	Tachycardia, headache, nausea, flushing	Most hypertensive emergencies; use with caution with glaucoma
Nitroglycerin	5–100 mcg/kg/min as IV infusion	2–5 minutes	5–10 minutes	Headache, vomiting, methemoglobinemia, tolerance with prolonged use	Coronary ischemia
Enalaprilat	1.25–5 mg every 6 hours IV	15–30 minutes	6–12 hours	Precipitous fall in pressure in high-renin states; variable response	Acute left ventricular failure; avoid in acute myocardial infarction
Hydralazine hydrochloride	10–20 mg IV / 10–40 mg IM	10–20 minutes / 20–30 minutes	1–4 hours IV / 4–6 hours IM	Tachycardia, flushing, headache, vomiting, aggravation of angina	Eclampsia
Clevidipine	1–21 mg/h IV	2–4 minutes	5–15 minutes	Atrial fibrillation, fever, insomnia, nausea, headache, vomiting, postprocedural hemorrhage, acute renal failure, respiratory failure	Contraindicated in severe aortic stenosis, defective lipid metabolism
Diazoxide	1–3 mg/kg or 50–100 mg every 5-15 minutes	2 minutes	3–12 hours	Hyperglycemia, sodium and water retention	Preeclampsia, eclampsia, impaired renal function
Furosemide	10–40 mg/h IV, maximum 80–160 mg/h IV	5 minutes	2 hours	Hypotension, electrolyte abnormalities, hearing impairment	Heart failure, fluid overload, adjunct therapy to vasodilators
Adrenergic Inhibitors					
Labetalol hydrochloride	20–80 mg IV bolus every 10 minutes	5–10 minutes	3–6 hours	Vomiting, scalp tingling, dizziness, bronchoconstriction, nausea, heart block, orthostatic hypotension	Most hypertensive emergencies except acute heart failure
Esmolol hydrochloride	250–500 mcg/kg/min IV bolus, then 50–100 mcg/kg/min by infusion; may repeat bolus after 5 minutes or increase infusion to 300 mcg/min	1–2 minutes	10–30 minutes	Hypotension, nausea, asthma, first-degree heart block, heart failure	Aortic dissection, perioperative
Phentolamine	5–15 mg IV bolus	1–2 minutes	10–30 minutes	Tachycardia flushing, headache	Catecholamine excess

IM, intramuscular.

[a]These doses may vary from those in the *Physicians' Desk Reference* (63rd ed.).

[b]Hypotension may occur with all agents.

[c]Requires special delivery system.

Adapted from Saseen JJ, Maclaughlin EJ. Hypertension. In: DiPiro JT, Talbert RL, Yee GC, et al. (eds.) Pharmacotherapy: A Pathophysiologic Approach. 7th ed. New York: McGraw-Hill; 2008: 165, with permission.

avoid volume depletion and rapid titration of antihypertensive therapy.[1] In individuals with isolated systolic hypertension, the optimal level of diastolic pressure is not known, and although treated patients who achieve diastolic pressures less than 60 to 70 mm Hg had poorer outcomes in a landmark trial, their cardiovascular event rate was still lower than those receiving placebo.[90] In addition, a recently completed trial (HYVET) documented the benefits of antihypertensive therapy in patients over the age of 80 as they experienced a significant reduction in all-cause mortality, fatal stroke and heart failure when treated with a diuretic (indapamide) with or without an ACE inhibitor (Perindopril).[36]

While the treatment approach of hypertension in minority populations is similar, special consideration should be paid to socioeconomic and lifestyle factors that may be important barriers to BP control. In addition, in patients of African origin, diminished BP responses have been seen with ACE inhibitors and ARBs compared to diuretics or calcium channel blockers.[1] Hypertension in pregnancy is a major cause of maternal, fetal, and neonatal morbidity and mortality. There are many categories of hypertension in pregnancy; however, pre-existing hypertension and pre-eclampsia are treated differently. The therapeutic selection of an oral antihypertensive agent (Table 5–7) in a pregnant patient with chronic hypertension is determined with regard to fetal safety. Therapeutic options for acute severe hypertension in pre-eclampsia may be reviewed in JNC 7.[1]

Similar to the JNC 7 criteria (which has four stages for BP classification in adults), the measurement of three or more BPs in children and adolescents are compared to tables listing the 90th-, 95th-, and 99th-percentile BPs based on age, height, and gender that classify BP as normal, prehypertension, and stage 1 and stage 2 hypertension (Table 5–1).[91] The prevalence of hypertension in adolescent populations is increasing and is associated with obesity, sedentary lifestyle, or a positive family history, which increases the risk of CVD. The clinician should be aware that secondary causes are common in adolescent hypertensives, and the identification and aggressive modification of risk factors with nonpharmacologic and pharmacologic interventions is paramount for

---

Patient Encounter 3

A 78-year-old Caucasian man presents to the emergency department with complaints of a headache persisting over the last 3 days. Repeated BP measurements average 200/110 mm Hg. He reports no other symptoms; physical examination and laboratory tests are unremarkable as is his past medical history with exception of hypertension diagnosed in his early 60s. He reports he is struggling on a fixed retirement income with no prescription coverage and takes "what I can afford." BP medications are metoprolol succinate (Toprol XL) 200mg once daily, amlodipine 10mg (Norvasc) once daily, torsemide (Demadex) 10 mg once daily, and valsartan (Diovan) 320 mg once daily.

What type of hypertensive crisis is this patient experiencing?

What are likely causes of this patient's loss of BP control?

Create a care plan for this patient's hypertensive crisis. This should include (a) acute goals of therapy, (b) a patient-specific therapeutic plan to achieve this, and (c) a plan for appropriate outpatient follow-up.

Table 5–7

Treatment of Chronic Hypertension in Pregnancy

Agent	Comments
Methyldopa	Preferred first-line therapy on the basis of long-term follow-up studies supporting safety after exposure in utero. Surveillance data do not support an association between drug and congenital defects when the mother took the drug early in the first trimester
Labetalol	Increasingly preferred to methyldopa because of reduced side effects. The agent does not seem to pose a risk to the fetus, except possibly in the first trimester
β-Blockers	Generally acceptable on the basis of limited data. Reports of intrauterine growth restriction with atenolol in the first and second trimesters
Clonidine	Limited data; no association between drug and congenital defects when the mother took the drug early in the first trimester, but number of exposures is small
Calcium channel antagonists	Limited data; nifedipine in the first trimester was not associated with increased rates of major birth defects, but animal data were associated with fetal hypoxemia and acidosis. This agent should probably be limited to mothers with severe hypertension
Diuretics	Not first-line agents; probably safe; available data suggest that throughout gestation a diuretic is not associated with an increased risk of major fetal anomalies or adverse fetal-neonatal events
Angiotensin-converting enzyme inhibitors and angiotensin II receptor antagonists	Contraindicated; reported fetal toxicity and death

From Ref. 1.

risk reduction of target organ damage. The 2004 National High Blood Pressure Education Program (NHBPEP) Working Group Report on Hypertension in Children and Adolescents provides specific recommendations to modify and treat risk factors in this population of patients. In addition, the American Heart Association has recently released a source guiding the role of ambulatory BP measurements in children and adolescents.[91,92] The *Nelson Textbook of Pediatrics* is also recommended for a comprehensive review of treatment of congenital and pediatric hypertension.[93]

PATIENT CARE AND MONITORING

⑩ *The frequency of follow-up visits for patients with hypertension will vary based on individual cases, but will be influenced by severity of hypertension, comorbidities, and choice of agent selected.* A recent analysis of the VALUE trial found that achieving BP control within 6 months reduced CV events compared to a longer time to achieve goal. In addition, another recent analysis of the INSIGHT trial found that the more times a patient is below goal, the lower the risk.[94,95] These studies suggest that there is an urgency to achieve and maintain BP control, and this may necessitate frequent assessment and adjustments (i.e., 2 weeks). At a minimum, assessment of response to medications should be done at 1-month intervals.[1] In patients with stage 2 hypertension or those with comorbidities (e.g., diabetes, vascular disease, CHF, or CKD), shorter time frames of 2 weeks or less are more appropriate.[79] Once BP is controlled, annual or semiannual monitoring for changes in serum biochemistries such as serum creatinine or potassium are recommended.[1] However, for patients with CHF, CKD, or diabetes, more frequent monitoring will be necessary to adequately control comorbid conditions. Another aspect to monitoring relates to the importance of medication adherence. Confirmation of continued use of antihypertensive medications should be considered in the routine monitoring of patients on numerous medications for hypertension. Evaluation of side effects, lab abnormalities, and/or progression to target organ damage should also be considered at appropriate intervals. Given the generally asymptomatic nature of hypertension, patient motivation to adhere to prescribed medications becomes a key tool in controlling hypertension.[2]

Given the chronic nature of hypertension, parsimony of medication regimens is a virtue of a good therapeutic plan. Minimizing the number of medications a patient is required to take has the potential to enhance adherence and mitigate cost. Often, control of BP is achieved by use of two or even three or more BP lowering medications.[34,96] Many combination products contain a diuretic as one of their active components. However, combination therapy may limit the ability of the clinician to titrate the dose of a specific agent. As such, the number of medications ("pill count") may often be reduced through use of combination products. This inherently simplifies the number of medications and copays a patient may have to endure to achieve effective BP control. These practicalities, although obvious, go a long way to optimize adherence, another challenge to maximizing therapy effectiveness.

Patient Care and Monitoring

1. Measure patient BP twice, at least 1 minute apart in a sitting position, and then average the readings to determine if BP is adequately controlled.

2. Conduct a medical history. Does the patient have any compelling indications? Is the patient pregnant?

3. Conduct a medication history (prescription, over-the-counter, and dietary supplements) to determine conditions or causes of hypertension. Does the patient take any medications, supplements, herbal products, or foods that may elevate SBP or DBP? Does the patient have drug allergies?

4. Review available laboratory tests to examine electrolyte balance and renal function.

5. Discuss lifestyle modifications that may reduce BP with the patient. Determine what nonpharmacologic approaches might be or have been helpful to the patient.

6. Evaluate the patient if pharmacologic treatment has reached the target BP goal. If the patient is at the goal, skip to step 9.

7. If patient is not at goal BP, assess efficacy, safety, and compliance of the antihypertensive regimen to determine if a dose increase or additional antihypertensive agent (step 8) is needed to achieve goal BP.

8. Select an agent to minimize adverse drug reactions and interactions when additional drug therapy is needed. Does the patient have prescription coverage or is the recommended agent in the formulary?

9. Open a dialogue to address patient concerns about hypertension and management of the condition.

10. Provide a plan to assess effectiveness and safety of therapy. Follow-up at monthly intervals or less until BP is achieved, otherwise semiannual or annual clinic visits to assess electrolyte balance and renal function once BP target is achieved. Presence of comorbidities (i.e., CKD) may require more frequent follow-up.

OUTCOME EVALUATION

- Short-term goals are to safely achieve reduction in BP through the iterative process of employing drug therapy, along with nondrug therapy or lifestyle changes.

- Lifestyle changes should address other risk factors for CVD including obesity, physical inactivity, insulin resistance, dyslipidemia, smoking cessation, and others.

- Monitoring for efficacy, adverse events, and adherence to therapy is key to achieving the long-term goals of reducing the risk of morbidity and mortality associated with CVD.

Abbreviations Introduced in This Chapter

ACC/AHA	American College of Cardiology/ American Heart Association
ACCOMPLISH	Avoiding Cardiovascular Events in Combination Therapy in Patients Living with Systolic Hypertension
ACE	Angiotensin-converting enzyme
ACE-I	Angiotensin-converting enzyme inhibitor
A-HeFT	African American Heart Failure trial
AIRE	Acute Infarction Ramipril Efficacy Study
ALLHAT	Antihypertensive and Lipid-Lowering Treatment to Prevent Heart Attack Trial
AMI	Acute myocardial infarction
ANBP2	Australian-New Zealand Blood Pressure-2 study
ARB	Angiotensin-receptor blocker
ASCOT-BPLA	Anglo-Scandinavian Cardiac Outcomes Trial-Blood Pressure Lowering Arm study
AT1	Angiotensin-1
AT2	Angiotensin-2
BHAT	β-Blocker Heart Attack Trial
BUN	Blood urea nitrogen
CAGE	Chymostatin-sensitive II-generating enzyme
CAPRICORN	Carvedilol Post-Infarct Survival Control in Left Ventricular Dysfunction Trial
Captopril Trial	Collaborative Study Captopril Trial ("The Effect of Angiotensin-Converting Enzyme Inhibition on Diabetic Nephropathy")
CCBA	Calcium channel blocker agent
CHARM	Candesartan in Heart Failure Assessment of Reduction in Morbidity and Mortality Trial
CIBIS-II	The Cardiac Insufficiency Bisoprolol Study II
CKD	Chronic kidney disease
CO	Cardiac output
COPERNICUS	Carvedilol Prospective Randomized Cumulative Survival Trial
CVD	Cardiovascular disease
DASH	Dietary Approaches to Stop Hypertension
DBP	Diastolic blood pressure
DRI	Direct renin inhibitor
EPHESUS	Eplerenone Post-Acute Myocardial Infarction Heart Failure Efficacy and Survival Study
EUROPA	European Trial on Reduction of Cardiac Events with Perindopril in Stable Coronary Artery Disease Trial
GFR	Glomerular filtration rate
GWAS	Genome-wide association scans
HF	Heart failure
HOPE	Heart Outcomes Prevention Evaluation Study
HYVET	Hypertension in the Very Elderly Trial
IDNT	Irbesartan Diabetic Nephropathy Trial
INVEST	International Verapamil-Trandolapril Study
IRMA-II	Irbesartan in Patients with Type 2 Diabetes and Microalbuminuria study
ISA	Intrinsic sympathomimetic activity
JNC 7	Joint National Committee Seventh Report
LIFE	Losartan Intervention For Endpoint reduction in hypertension study
MAO	Monoamine oxidase
MERIT-HF	Metoprolol CR/XL Randomised Intervention Trial in Congestive Heart Failure
MI	Myocardial infarction
NHBPEP	National High Blood Pressure Education Program
NIDDM	Noninsulin-dependent diabetes mellitus
NO	Nitric or nitrous oxide
NSAID	Nonsteroidal anti-inflammatory drug
ONTARGET	Ongoing Telmisartan Alone and in combination with Ramipril Global Endpoint Trial
PR	Peripheral resistance
PRA	Plasma rennin activity
PROGRESS	Perindopril Protection Against Recurrent Stroke Study
RAAS	Renin-angiotensin-aldosterone system
RALES	Randomized Aldactone Evaluation Study
RENAAL	Reduction of Endpoints in NIDDM with the Angiotensin II Antagonist Losartan study
SAVE	Survival and Ventricular Enlargement Trial
SBP	Systolic blood pressure
SHEP	Systolic Hypertension in the Elderly Program
SNS	Sympathetic nervous system
SOLVD	Studies of Left Ventricular Dysfunction
TRACE	Trandolapril Cardiac Evaluation
VALUE	Valsartan Antihypertensive Long-term Use Evaluation
ValHeFT	Veterans Affairs Cooperative I study

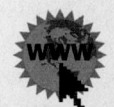 Self-assessment questions and answers are available at *http://www.mhpharmacotherapy. com/pp.html.*

REFERENCES

1. Chobanian AV, Bakris GL, Black HR, et al. Seventh report of the Joint National Committee on Prevention, Detection, Evaluation, and Treatment of High Blood Pressure. Hypertension 2003;42(6):1206–1252.

2. Rosendorff C, Black HR, Cannon CP, et al. Treatment of hypertension in the prevention and management of ischemic heart disease: A scientific statement from the American Heart Association Council for High Blood Pressure Research and the Councils on Clinical Cardiology and Epidemiology and Prevention. Circulation 2007 29;115(21):2761–2788.

3. Mancia G, De Backer G, Dominiczak A, et al. 2007 Guidelines for the management of arterial hypertension: The Task Force for the Management of Arterial Hypertension of the European Society of Hypertension (ESH) and of the European Society of Cardiology (ESC). Eur Heart J 28 2007;(12):1462–1536.

4. WHO. The world health report 2002-reducing risks, promoting healthy life.. Available at: *http://www.who.int/whr/2002/en/whr02_en.pdf*

5. Rosamond W, Flegal K, Furie K, et al. Heart disease and stroke statistics—2008 update: A report from the American Heart Association Statistics Committee and Stroke Statistics Subcommittee. Circulation 29 2008;117(4):e25–e146.

6. Ostchega Y, Hughes JP, Wright JD, McDowell MA, Louis T. Are demographic characteristics, health care access and utilization, and comorbid conditions associated with hypertension among US adults? Am J Hypertens 2008;(2):159–165.

7. Sowers JR, Haffner S. Treatment of cardiovascular and renal risk factors in the diabetic hypertensive. Hypertension Dec 2002;40(6):781–788.

8. Arauz-Pacheco C, Parrott MA, Raskin P. Hypertension management in adults with diabetes. Diabetes Care 2004;27(Suppl 1):S65–S67.

9. Kaplan NM, Flynn JT. Kaplan's Clinical Hypertension, 9th ed. Philadelphia, PA: Lippincott Williams & Wilkins, 2006.

10. Izzo JL, Sica DA, Black HR. Council for High Blood Pressure Research (American Heart Association). Hypertension Primer, 4th ed. Philadelphia, PA: Lippincott Williams & Wilkins, 2008.

11. Dominiczak AF, Negrin DC, Clark JS, Brosnan MJ, McBride MW, Alexander MY. Genes and hypertension: From gene mapping in experimental models to vascular gene transfer strategies. Hypertension 2000;35(1 Pt 2):164–172.

12. Meneton PG, Warnock D. Involvement of renal apical Na transport systems in the control of blood pressure. Am J Kidney Dis 2001;37 (1 Suppl 2):S39–S47.

13. Genome-wide association study of 14,000 cases of seven common diseases and 3,000 shared controls. Nature 2007;447(7145): 661–678.

14. Ehret GB, Morrison AC, O'Connor AA, et al. Replication of the Wellcome Trust genome-wide association study of essential hypertension: The Family Blood Pressure Program. Eur J Hum Genet 2008;16:1507–1511.

15. Chobanian AV, Hill M. National Heart, Lung, and Blood Institute Workshop on Sodium and Blood Pressure: A critical review of current scientific evidence. Hypertension 2000;35(4):858–863.

16. Phillips MI, Schmidt-Ott KM. The Discovery of Renin 100 Years Ago. News Physiol Sci 1999;14:271–274.

17. Lavoie JL, Sigmund CD. Minireview: Overview of the renin-angiotensin system—An endocrine and paracrine system. Endocrinology 2003; 144(6):2179–2183.

18. Laragh J. Laragh's lessons in pathophysiology and clinical pearls for treating hypertension. Am J Hypertens 2001;14(1):84–89.

19. Brown MJ. Aliskiren. Circulation 2008;118(7):773–784.

20. Pickering TG, Hall JE, Appel LJ, et al. Recommendations for blood pressure measurement in humans and experimental animals: Part 1: Blood pressure measurement in humans: A statement for professionals from the subcommittee of professional and public education of the American heart association council on high blood pressure research. Circulation 2005;111(5):697–716.

21. Lewington S, Clarke R, Qizilbash N, Peto R, Collins R. Age-specific relevance of usual blood pressure to vascular mortality: A meta-analysis of individual data for one million adults in 61 prospective studies. Lancet 2002;360(9349):1903–1913.

22. Major outcomes in high-risk hypertensive patients randomized to angiotensin-converting enzyme inhibitor or calcium channel blocker vs diuretic: The Antihypertensive and Lipid-Lowering Treatment to Prevent Heart Attack Trial (ALLHAT). JAMA 2002;288(23): 2981–2997.

23. Sacks FM, Svetkey LP, Vollmer WM, et al. Effects on blood pressure of reduced dietary sodium and the Dietary Approaches to Stop Hypertension (DASH) diet. DASH-Sodium Collaborative Research Group. N Engl J Med 2001;344(1):3–10.

24. Beard TC. The bread of the 21st century. Aust J Nutr Diet 1997;54: 198–203.

25. Whelton SP, Chin A, Xin X, He J. Effect of aerobic exercise on blood pressure: A meta-analysis of randomized, controlled trials. Ann Intern Med 2002;136(7):493–503.

26. Gibbons RJ, Abrams J, Chatterjee K, et al. ACC/AHA 2002 guideline update for the management of patients with chronic stable angina—summary article: A report of the American College of Cardiology/American Heart Association Task Force on practice guidelines (Committee on the Management of Patients With Chronic Stable Angina). J Am Coll Cardiol 2003;41(1):159–168.

27. Simmons-Morton DG. Exercise Therapy. In: Izzo JL, Jr, Black HR, eds. *Hypertension Primer: The Essentials of High Blood Pressure*, 3rd ed. Philadelphia: Lippincott Williams & Wilkins, 2003:388–389.

28. Rosito GA, Fuchs FD, Duncan BB. Dose-dependent biphasic effect of ethanol on 24-h blood pressure in normotensive subjects. Am J Hypertens 1999;12(2 Pt 1):236–240.

29. Xin X, He J, Frontini MG, Ogden LG, Motsamai OI, Whelton PK. Effects of alcohol reduction on blood pressure: A meta-analysis of randomized controlled trials. Hypertension 2001;38(5):1112–1117.

30. Omvik P. How smoking affects blood pressure. Blood Press 1996;5(2): 71–77.

31. Primatesta P, Falaschetti E, Gupta S, Marmot MG, Poulter NR. Association between smoking and blood pressure: Evidence from the health survey for England. Hypertension 2001;37(2):187–193.

32. Dahlof B, Sever PS, Poulter NR, et al. Prevention of cardiovascular events with an antihypertensive regimen of amlodipine adding perindopril as required versus atenolol adding bendroflumethiazide as required, in the Anglo-Scandinavian Cardiac Outcomes Trial-Blood Pressure Lowering Arm (ASCOT-BPLA): A multicentre randomised controlled trial. Lancet 2005;366(9489):895–906.

33. Julius S, Kjeldsen SE, Weber M, et al. Outcomes in hypertensive patients at high cardiovascular risk treated with regimens based on valsartan or amlodipine: The VALUE randomised trial. Lancet 2004;363(9426):2022–2031.

34. ALLHAT Collaborative Research Group. Major cardiovascular events in hypertensive patients randomized to doxazosin vs chlorthalidone: The antihypertensive and lipid-lowering treatment to prevent heart attack trial (ALLHAT). JAMA 2000;283(15):1967–1975.

35. Randomised trial of a perindopril-based blood-pressure-lowering regimen among 6,105 individuals with previous stroke or transient ischaemic attack. Lancet 2001;358(9287):1033–1041.

36. Beckett NS, Peters R, Fletcher AE, et al. Treatment of hypertension in patients 80 years of age or older. N Engl J Med 2008;358(18):1887–1898.

37. Pitt B, Zannad F, Remme WJ, et al. The effect of spironolactone on morbidity and mortality in patients with severe heart failure. Randomized Aldactone Evaluation Study Investigators. N Engl J Med 1999;341(10):709–717.

38. Pitt B, Remme W, Zannad F, et al. Eplerenone, a selective aldosterone blocker, in patients with left ventricular dysfunction after myocardial infarction. N Engl J Med 2003;348(14):1309–1321. Epub 2003 Mar 1331.

39. Effect of metoprolol CR/XL in chronic heart failure: Metoprolol CR/XL Randomised Intervention Trial in Congestive Heart Failure (MERIT-HF). Lancet 1999;353(9169):2001–2007.

40. Krum H, Roecker EB, Mohacsi P, et al. Effects of initiating carvedilol in patients with severe chronic heart failure: Results from the COPERNICUS Study. JAMA 2003;289(6):712–718.

41. Dargie HJ. Effect of carvedilol on outcome after myocardial infarction in patients with left-ventricular dysfunction: The CAPRICORN randomised trial. Lancet 2001;357(9266):1385–1390.

42. Lampert R, Ickovics JR, Viscoli CJ, Horwitz RI, Lee FA. Effects of propranolol on recovery of heart rate variability following acute

myocardial infarction and relation to outcome in the Beta-Blocker Heart Attack Trial. Am J Cardiol 2003;91(2):137–142.

43. The Cardiac Insufficiency Bisoprolol Study II (CIBIS-II): A randomised trial. Lancet 1999;353(9146):9–13.

44. Pepine CJ, Handberg EM, Cooper-DeHoff RM, et al. A calcium antagonist vs a non-calcium antagonist hypertension treatment strategy for patients with coronary artery disease. The International Verapamil-Trandolapril Study (INVEST): A randomized controlled trial. JAMA 2003;290(21):2805–2816.

45. Effect of enalapril on mortality and the development of heart failure in asymptomatic patients with reduced left ventricular ejection fractions. The SOLVD Investigattors. N Engl J Med 1992;327(10):685–691.

46. Effect of ramipril on mortality and morbidity of survivors of acute myocardial infarction with clinical evidence of heart failure. The Acute Infarction Ramipril Efficacy (AIRE) Study Investigators. Lancet 1993;342(8875):821–828.

47. Kober L, Torp-Pedersen C, Carlsen JE, et al. A clinical trial of the angiotensin-converting-enzyme inhibitor trandolapril in patients with left ventricular dysfunction after myocardial infarction. Trandolapril Cardiac Evaluation (TRACE) Study Group. N Engl J Med 1995;333(25):1670–1676.

48. Pfeffer MA, Braunwald E, Moye LA, et al. Effect of captopril on mortality and morbidity in patients with left ventricular dysfunction after myocardial infarction. Results of the survival and ventricular enlargement trial. The SAVE Investigators. N Engl J Med 1992;327(10):669–677.

49. Lewis EJ, Hunsicker LG, Bain RP, Rohde RD. The effect of angiotensin-converting-enzyme inhibition on diabetic nephropathy. The Collaborative Study Group. N Engl J Med 1993;329(20):1456–1462.

50. Fox KM. Efficacy of perindopril in reduction of cardiovascular events among patients with stable coronary artery disease: Randomised, double-blind, placebo-controlled, multicentre trial (the EUROPA study). Lancet 2003;362(9386):782–788.

51. Pfeffer MA, Swedberg K, Granger CB, et al. Effects of candesartan on mortality and morbidity in patients with chronic heart failure: The CHARM-Overall programme. Lancet 2003;362(9386):759–766.

52. Dahlof B, Devereux RB, Kjeldsen SE, et al. Cardiovascular morbidity and mortality in the Losartan Intervention For Endpoint reduction in hypertension study (LIFE): A randomised trial against atenolol. Lancet 2002;359(9311):995–1003.

53. Brenner BM, Cooper ME, de Zeeuw D, et al. Effects of losartan on renal and cardiovascular outcomes in patients with type 2 diabetes and nephropathy. N Engl J Med 2001;345(12):861–869.

54. Lewis EJ, Hunsicker LG, Clarke WR, et al. Renoprotective effect of the angiotensin-receptor antagonist irbesartan in patients with nephropathy due to type 2 diabetes. N Engl J Med 2001;345(12): 851–860.

55. Parving HH, Lehnert H, Brochner-Mortensen J, Gomis R, Andersen S, Arner P. The effect of irbesartan on the development of diabetic nephropathy in patients with type 2 diabetes. N Engl J Med 2001;345(12):870–878.

56. Cohn JN, Tognoni G. A randomized trial of the angiotensin-receptor blocker valsartan in chronic heart failure. N Engl J Med 2001;345(23):1667–1675.

57. Taylor AL, Ziesche S, Yancy C, et al. Combination of isosorbide dinitrate and hydralazine in blacks with heart failure. N Engl J Med 2004;351(20):2049–2057.

58. Diuretic versus alpha-blocker as first-step antihypertensive therapy: Final results from the Antihypertensive and Lipid-Lowering Treatment to Prevent Heart Attack Trial (ALLHAT). Hypertension 2003;42(3): 239–246.

59. Wing LM, Reid CM, Ryan P, et al. A comparison of outcomes with angiotensin-converting—enzyme inhibitors and diuretics for hypertension in the elderly. N Engl J Med 2003;348(7):583–592.

60. Psaty BM, Lumley T, Furberg CD, et al. Health outcomes associated with various antihypertensive therapies used as first-line agents: A network meta-analysis. JAMA 2003;289(19):2534–2544.

61. Jamerson K, Weber MA, Bakris GL, et al. Benazepril plus amlodipine or hydrochlorothiazide for hypertension in high-risk patients. N Engl J Med 2008;359:2417–2428.

62. Ernst ME, Carter BL, Goerdt CJ, et al. Comparative antihypertensive effects of hydrochlorothiazide and chlorthalidone on ambulatory and office blood pressure. Hypertension 2006;47(3):352–358.

63. Sica DA. Chlorthalidone: Has it always been the best thiazide-type diuretic? Hypertension 2006;47(3):321–322.

64. Carter BL, Ernst ME, Cohen JD. Hydrochlorothiazide versus chlorthalidone: Evidence supporting their interchangeability. Hypertension 2004;43(1):4–9.

65. Zillich AJ, Garg J, Basu S, Bakris GL, Carter BL. Thiazide diuretics, potassium, and the development of diabetes: A quantitative review. Hypertension 2006;48(2):219–224.

66. Carter BL, Einhorn PT, Brands M, et al. Thiazide-induced dysglycemia: Call for research from a working group from the national heart, lung, and blood institute. Hypertension 2008;52(1):30–36.

67. Goodman LS, Hardman JG, Limbird LE, Gilman AG. Goodman & Gilman's the pharmacological Basis of Therapeutics, 10th ed. New York: McGraw-Hill, 2001.

68. Nishizaka MK, Zaman MA, Calhoun DA. Efficacy of low-dose spironolactone in subjects with resistant hypertension. Am J Hypertens 2003;16(11 Pt 1):925–930.

69. Menard J. The 45-year story of the development of an anti-aldosterone more specific than spironolactone. Mol Cell Endocrinol 2004;217(1–2): 45–52.

70. Sica DA. Pharmacokinetics and pharmacodynamics of mineralocorticoid blocking agents and their effects on potassium homeostasis. Heart Fail Rev 2005;10(1):23–29.

71. Lindholm LH, Carlberg B, Samuelsson O. Should beta blockers remain first choice in the treatment of primary hypertension? A meta-analysis. Lancet 2005;366(9496):1545–1553.

72. Messerli FH, Grossman E, Goldbourt U. Are beta-blockers efficacious as first-line therapy for hypertension in the elderly? A systematic review. JAMA 1998;279(23):1903–1907.

73. Williams B, Lacy PS, Thom SM, et al. Differential impact of blood pressure-lowering drugs on central aortic pressure and clinical outcomes: Principal results of the Conduit Artery Function Evaluation (CAFE) study. Circulation 2006;113(9):1213–1225.

74. Bangalore S, Messerli FH, Kostis JB, Pepine CJ. Cardiovascular protection using beta-blockers: A critical review of the evidence. J Am Coll Cardiol 2007;50(7):563–572.

75. Weber MA. The role of the new beta-blockers in treating cardiovascular disease. Am J Hypertens 2005;18(12 Pt 2):169S–176S.

76. Antman EM, Anbe DT, Armstrong PW, et al. ACC/AHA guidelines for the management of patients with ST-elevation myocardial infarction-executive summary: A report of the American College of Cardiology/American Heart Association Task Force on Practice Guidelines (Writing Committee to Revise the 1999 Guidelines for the Management of Patients With Acute Myocardial Infarction). Circulation 2004; 110(5):588–636.

77. Hunt SA, Abraham WT, Chin MH, et al. ACC/AHA 2005 Guideline Update for the Diagnosis and Management of Chronic Heart Failure in the Adult—Summary Article: A Report of the American College of Cardiology/American Heart Association Task Force on Practice Guidelines (Writing Committee to Update the 2001 Guidelines for the Evaluation and Management of Heart Failure): Developed in Collaboration With the American College of Chest Physicians and the International Society for Heart and Lung Transplantation: Endorsed by the Heart Rhythm Society. Circulation Sep 20, 2005;112(12):1825–1852.

78. Standards of medical care in diabetes. Diabetes Care 2005;28(Suppl 1): S4–S36.

79. K/DOQI clinical practice guidelines on hypertension and antihypertensive agents in chronic kidney disease. Am J Kidney Dis 2004;43(5 Suppl 1):S1–S290.

80. Bakris GL, Williams M, Dworkin L, et al. Preserving renal function in adults with hypertension and diabetes: A consensus approach. National Kidney Foundation Hypertension and Diabetes Executive Committees Working Group. Am J Kidney Dis 2000;36(3):646–661.

81. The Telmisartan Randomised AssesmeNt Study in ACE iNtolerant subject with cardiovascular Disease (TRANSCEND) investigator. Effects of the angiotensin-receptor blocker telmisartan on

cardiovascular events in high-risk patients intolerant to angiotensin-converting enzyme inhibitors: a randomised controlled trial. Lancet 2008; published online Aug 31. DOI: 10.1016/S0140-6736(08)61242-8.

82. Ripley TL, Harrison D. The power to TRANSCEND. Lancet 2008.

83. McMurray JJ, Ostergren J, Swedberg K, et al. Effects of candesartan in patients with chronic heart failure and reduced left-ventricular systolic function taking angiotensin-converting-enzyme inhibitors: The CHARM-Added trial. Lancet 2003;362(9386):767–771.

84. Yusuf S, Pfeffer MA, Swedberg K, et al. Effects of candesartan in patients with chronic heart failure and preserved left-ventricular ejection fraction: the CHARM-Preserved Trial. Lancet 2003;362(9386):777–781.

85. Granger CB, McMurray JJ, Yusuf S, et al. Effects of candesartan in patients with chronic heart failure and reduced left-ventricular systolic function intolerant to angiotensin-converting-enzyme inhibitors: The CHARM-Alternative trial. Lancet 2003;362(9386):772–776.

86. Prevention of stroke by antihypertensive drug treatment in older persons with isolated systolic hypertension. Final results of the Systolic Hypertension in the Elderly Program (SHEP). SHEP Cooperative Research Group. JAMA 1991;265(24):3255–3264.

87. DiPiro JT. Pharmacotherapy: A pathophysiologic Approach, 7th ed. New York: McGraw-Hill Medical, 2008.

88. Yusuf S, Sleight P, Pogue J, Bosch J, Davies R, Dagenais G. Effects of an angiotensin-converting-enzyme inhibitor, ramipril, on cardiovascular events in high-risk patients. The Heart Outcomes Prevention Evaluation Study Investigators. N Engl J Med 2000;342(3):145–153.

89. Yusuf S, Teo KK, Pogue J, et al. Telmisartan, ramipril, or both in patients at high risk for vascular events. N Engl J Med 2008;358(15):1547–1559.

90. Somes GW, Pahor M, Shorr RI, Cushman WC, Applegate WB. The role of diastolic blood pressure when treating isolated systolic hypertension. Arch Intern Med 1999;159(17):2004–2009.

91. The fourth report on the diagnosis, evaluation, and treatment of high blood pressure in children and adolescents. Pediatrics 2004;114(2 Suppl 4th Report):555–576.

92. Urbina E, Alpert B, Flynn J, et al. Ambulatory blood pressure monitoring in children and adolescents: Recommendations for standard assessment: A scientific statement from the American Heart Association Atherosclerosis, Hypertension, and Obesity in Youth Committee of the Council on Cardiovascular Disease in the Young and the Council for High Blood Pressure Research. Hypertension 2008;52(3):433–451.

93. Kliegman R, Nelson WE. Nelson Textbook of Pediatrics, 18th ed. Philadelphia: Saunders, 2007.

94. Mancia G, Messerli F, Bakris G, Zhou Q, Champion A, Pepine CJ. Blood pressure control and improved cardiovascular outcomes in the International Verapamil SR-Trandolapril Study. Hypertension 2007;50(2):299–305.

95. Weber MA, Julius S, Kjeldsen SE, et al. Blood pressure dependent and independent effects of antihypertensive treatment on clinical events in the VALUE Trial. Lancet 2004;363(9426):2049–2051.

96. Hansson L, Zanchetti A, Carruthers SG, et al. Effects of intensive blood-pressure lowering and low-dose aspirin in patients with hypertension: Principal results of the Hypertension Optimal Treatment (HOT) randomised trial. HOT Study Group. Lancet 1998;351(9118):1755–1762.

6

Heart Failure

Orly Vardeny and Tien M.H. Ng

LEARNING OBJECTIVES

● **Upon completion of the chapter, the reader will be able to:**

1. Differentiate between the common underlying etiologies of heart failure, including ischemic, nonischemic, and idiopathic causes.

2. Describe the pathophysiology of heart failure as it relates to neurohormonal activation of the renin-angiotensin-aldosterone system and the sympathetic nervous system (SNS).

3. Identify signs and symptoms of heart failure and classify a given patient by the New York Heart Association (NYHA) Functional Classification (FC) system and American College of Cardiology/American Heart Association (ACC/AHA) Heart Failure Staging.

4. Describe the goals of therapy for a patient with acute or chronic heart failure.

5. Develop a nonpharmacologic treatment plan which includes patient education for managing heart failure.

6. Develop a specific evidence-based pharmacologic treatment plan for a patient with acute or chronic heart failure based on disease severity and symptoms.

7. Formulate a monitoring plan for the nonpharmacologic and pharmacologic treatment of a patient with heart failure.

KEY CONCEPTS

❶ The most common causes of heart failure are coronary artery disease (CAD), hypertension, and dilated cardiomyopathy.

❷ Development and progression of heart failure involve activation of neurohormonal pathways, including the sympathetic nervous system (SNS) and the renin-angiotensin-aldosterone system (RAAS).

❸ The clinician must identify potential reversible causes of heart failure exacerbations including prescription and nonprescription drug therapies, dietary indiscretions, and medication nonadherence.

❹ Symptoms of left-sided heart failure include dyspnea, orthopnea, and paroxysmal nocturnal dyspnea (PND), whereas symptoms of right-sided heart failure include fluid retention, GI bloating, and fatigue.

❺ Therapeutic goals focus on alleviating symptoms, slowing or preventing disease progression, maintaining quality of life, and improving patient survival.

❻ Nonpharmacologic treatment involves dietary modifications such as sodium and fluid restriction, risk factor reduction including smoking cessation, timely immunizations, and supervised regular physical activity.

❼ Diuretics are used for relief of acute symptoms of congestion and maintenance of euvolemia.

❽ Agents with proven benefits in improving symptoms, slowing disease progression, and improving survival in chronic heart failure target neurohormonal blockade; these include angiotensin-converting enzyme (ACE) inhibitors or angiotensin receptor blockers (ARBs), β-adrenergic blockers, and aldosterone antagonists.

❾ Combination therapy with hydralazine and isosorbide dinitrate is an appropriate substitute for angiotensin II antagonism in those unable to tolerate an ACE inhibitor or ARB, or as add-on therapy in African Americans.

❿ Treatment of acute heart failure (AHF) targets relief of congestion and optimization of cardiac output utilizing oral or IV diuretics, IV vasodilators, and, when appropriate, inotropes.

INTRODUCTION

Heart failure (HF) is defined as the inadequate ability of the heart to pump enough blood to meet the blood flow and metabolic demands of the body.[1] High-output HF is characterized by an inordinate increase in the body's metabolic demands, which outpaces an increase in cardiac output (CO) of a generally normally functioning heart. More commonly, low-output HF is a result of low CO secondary to impaired cardiac function. In this chapter, HF will refer to low-output HF.

HF is a clinical syndrome characterized by a history of specific signs and symptoms related to congestion and hypoperfusion. As HF can occur in the presence or absence of fluid overload, the term "heart failure" is preferred over the former term "congestive heart failure." HF results from any structural or functional cardiac disorder that impairs the ability of the ventricle to fill with or eject blood.[1] Many disorders such as those of the pericardium, epicardium, endocardium, or great vessels may lead to HF, but most patients develop symptoms due to impairment in left ventricular (LV) myocardial function.

The phrase "acute heart failure" (AHF) is used to signify either an acute decompensation of a patient with a history of chronic HF or a patient presenting with new-onset HF symptoms. Terms commonly associated with HF, such as cardiomyopathy and LV dysfunction, are not equivalent to HF but describe possible structural or functional reasons for the development of HF.

EPIDEMIOLOGY AND ETIOLOGY

Epidemiology

HF is a major public health concern affecting approximately 5 million people in the United States. An additional 550,000 new cases are diagnosed each year. HF manifests most commonly in adults over the age of 60.[2] The growing prevalence of HF corresponds to: (a) better treatment of patients with acute myocardial infarctions (MIs) who will survive to develop HF later in life, and (b) the increasing proportion of older adults due to the aging "Baby Boomer" population. The relative incidence of HF is lower in women compared to men, but there is a greater prevalence in women overall due to their longer life expectancy. AHF accounts for 12 to 15 million office visits per year and 6.5 million hospitalizations annually.[2] According to national registries, patients presenting with AHF are older (mean age 75 years) and have numerous comorbidities such as coronary artery disease (CAD), renal insufficiency, and diabetes.[2]

Total estimated direct and indirect costs for managing both chronic and acute HF in the United States for 2008 was approximately $34.8 billion. Medications account for approximately 10% of that cost.[3] HF is the most common hospital discharge diagnosis for Medicare patients and is the most costly diagnosis in this population.

The prognosis for patients hospitalized for AHF remains poor. Average hospital length of stay is estimated to be between 4 and 6 days, a number which has remained constant over the past decade.[3] The in-hospital mortality rate has been estimated at approximately 4%, but ranges from 2% to 20% depending on the report.[4] In-hospital mortality

increases to an average of 10.6% in patients requiring an intensive care unit admission. Readmissions are also high, with up to 30% to 60% of patients readmitted within 6 months of their initial discharge date.[4] The 5-year mortality rate for chronic HF remains approximately 50%. Survival strongly correlates with severity of symptoms and functional capacity. Sudden cardiac death is the most common cause of death, occurring in approximately 40% of patients with HF.[2] Although therapies targeting the upregulated neurohormonal response contributing to the pathophysiology of HF have clearly impacted morbidity and mortality, long-term survival remains low.

Etiology

HF is the eventual outcome of numerous cardiac diseases or disorders (Table 6–1).[5] HF can be classified by the primary underlying etiology as ischemic or nonischemic, with 70% of HF related to ischemia. ❶ *The most common causes of HF are CAD, hypertension, and dilated cardiomyopathy.* CAD resulting in an acute MI and reduced ventricular function is a common presenting history. Nonischemic etiologies include hypertension, viral illness, thyroid disease, excessive alcohol use, illicit drug use, pregnancy-related heart disease, familial congenital disease, and valvular disorders such as mitral or tricuspid valve regurgitation or stenosis.

HF can also be classified based on the main component of the cardiac cycle leading to impaired ventricular function. A normal cardiac cycle is dependent on two components: systole and diastole. Expulsion of blood occurs during systole or contraction of the ventricles, while diastole relates

Table 6–1
Causes of Heart Failure

Systolic Dysfunction (Decreased Contractility)
- Reduction in muscle mass (e.g., MI)
- Dilated cardiomyopathies
- Ventricular hypertrophy
  - Pressure overload (e.g., systemic or pulmonary hypertension, aortic or pulmonic valve stenosis)
  - Volume overload (e.g., valvular regurgitation, shunts, high-output states)

Diastolic Dysfunction (Restriction in Ventricular Filling)
- Increased ventricular stiffness
- Ventricular hypertrophy (e.g., hypertrophic cardiomyopathy, other examples above)
- Infiltrative myocardial diseases (e.g., amyloidosis, sarcoidosis, endomyocardial fibrosis)
- Myocardial ischemia and infarction
- Mitral or tricuspid valve stenosis
- Pericardial disease (e.g., pericarditis, pericardial tamponade)

MI, myocardial infarction.

From Parker RB, Rodgers JE, Cavallari LH. Heart failure. In: DiPiro JT, Talbert RL, Yee GC, et al. (eds.) Pharmacotherapy: A Pathophysiologic Approach, 7th ed. New York: McGraw-Hill, 2008:174.

to filling of the ventricles. Ejection fraction (EF) is the fraction of the volume present at the end of diastole that is pushed into the aorta during systole. Abnormal ventricular filling (diastolic dysfunction) and/or ventricular contraction (systolic dysfunction) can result in a similar decrease in CO and cause HF symptoms. Most HF is associated with evidence of LV systolic dysfunction (evidenced by a reduced EF) with or without a component of diastolic dysfunction, which coexists in up to two-thirds of patients. Isolated diastolic dysfunction, occurring in approximately one-third of HF patients, is diagnosed when a patient exhibits impaired ventricular filling with or without accompanying HF symptoms but normal systolic function. Long-standing hypertension is the leading cause of diastolic dysfunction. Ventricular dysfunction can also involve either the left or right chamber of the heart or both. This has implications for symptomatology, as right-sided failure manifests as systemic congestion, whereas left-sided failure results in pulmonary symptoms.

PATHOPHYSIOLOGY

A basic grasp of normal cardiac function sets the stage for understanding the pathophysiologic processes leading to HF and selecting appropriate therapy for HF. CO is defined as the volume of blood ejected per unit of time (liters per minute) and is a major determinant of tissue perfusion. CO is the product of heart rate (HR) and stroke volume (SV): CO = HR × SV. The following describes how each parameter relates to CO.

HR is controlled by the autonomic nervous system, where sympathetic stimulation of β-adrenergic receptors results in an increase in HR and CO. SV is the volume of blood ejected with each systole. SV is determined by factors regulating preload, afterload, and contractility. Preload is a measure of ventricular filling pressure, or the volume of blood in the left ventricle (also known as LV end-diastolic volume). Preload is determined by venous return as well as atrial contraction. An increase in venous return to the left ventricle results in the stretch of cardiomyocyte sarcomeres (or contractile units) and a subsequent increase in the number of cross-bridges formed between actin and myosin myofilaments. This results in an increase in the force of contraction based on the Frank-Starling mechanism.[6] Afterload is the resistance to ventricular ejection and is regulated by ejection impedence, wall tension, and regional wall geometry. Thus, elevated aortic and systemic pressures result in an increase in afterload and reduced SV. Contractility, also known as the inotropic state of the heart, is an intrinsic property of cardiac muscle incorporating fiber shortening and tension development. Contractility is influenced to a large degree by adrenergic nerve activity and circulating catecholamines such as epinephrine and norepinephrine.

Compensatory Mechanisms

In the setting of a sustained loss of myocardium, a number of mechanisms aid the heart when faced with an increased hemodynamic burden and reduced CO. They include the Frank-Starling mechanism, tachycardia and increased afterload, and cardiac hypertrophy and remodeling (Table 6–2).[5,7]

Table 6–2

Beneficial and Detrimental Effects of the Compensatory Responses in Heart Failure

Compensatory Response	Beneficial Effects of Compensation	Detrimental Effects of Compensation
Increased preload (through sodium and water retention)	Optimized SV via Frank–Starling mechanism	Pulmonary and systemic congestion and edema formation Increased MVO_2
Vasoconstriction	Maintained BP and perfusion in the face of reduced CO	Increased MVO_2 Increased afterload decreases SV and further activates the compensatory responses
Tachycardia and increased contractility (due to SNS activation)	Increased CO	Increased MVO_2 Shortened diastolic filling time β_1-Receptor downregulation, decreased receptor sensitivity Precipitation of ventricular arrhythmias Increased risk of myocardial cell death
Ventricular hypertrophy and remodeling	Maintained CO Reduced myocardial wall stress	Diastolic dysfunction Systolic dysfunction Increased risk of myocardial cell death Increased risk of myocardial ischemia Increased arrhythmia risk

BP, blood pressure; CO, cardiac output; MVO_2, myocardial oxygen consumption; SNS, sympathetic nervous system; SV, stroke volume.

▶ *Preload and the Frank-Starling Mechanism*

In the setting of a sudden decrease in CO, the natural response of the body is to decrease blood flow to the periphery in order to maintain perfusion to the vital organs such as the heart and brain. Therefore, renal perfusion is compromised due to both the decreased CO, as well as shunting of blood away from peripheral tissues. This results in activation of the renin-angiotensin-aldosterone system (RAAS). The decrease in renal perfusion is sensed by the juxtaglomerular cells of the kidneys leading to the release of renin and initiation of the cascade for production of angiotensin II (AT_2). AT_2 stimulates the synthesis and release of aldosterone. Aldosterone in turn stimulates sodium and water retention in an attempt to increase intravascular volume, and hence preload. In a healthy heart, a large increase in CO is usually accomplished with just a small change in preload. However, in a failing heart, alterations in the contractile filaments reduce the ability of cardiomyocytes to adapt to increases in preload. Thus, an increase in preload actually impairs contractile function in the failing heart and results in a further decrease in CO.

▶ *Tachycardia and Increased Afterload*

Another mechanism to maintain CO when contractility is low is to increase HR. This is achieved through sympathetic nervous system (SNS) activation and the agonist effect of norepinephrine on β-adrenergic receptors in the heart. Sympathetic activation also enhances contractility by increasing cytosolic calcium concentrations. SV is relatively fixed in HF, thus HR becomes the major determinant of CO. Although this mechanism increases CO acutely, the chronotropic and inotropic responses to sympathetic activation increase myocardial oxygen demand, worsen underlying ischemia, contribute to proarrhythmia, and further impair both systolic and diastolic function.

Activation of both the RAAS and the SNS also contribute to vasoconstriction in an attempt to redistribute blood flow from peripheral organs such as the kidneys to coronary and cerebral circulation.[7] However, arterial vasoconstriction leads to impaired forward ejection of blood from the heart due to an increase in afterload. This results in a decrease in CO and continued stimulation of compensatory responses, creating a vicious cycle of neurohormonal activation.

▶ *Cardiac Hypertrophy and Remodeling*

Ventricular hypertrophy, an adaptive increase in ventricular muscle mass due to growth of existing myocytes, occurs in response to an increased hemodynamic burden such as volume or pressure overload.[5] Hypertrophy can be concentric or eccentric. Concentric hypertrophy occurs in response to pressure overload such as in long-standing hypertension or pulmonary hypertension, whereas eccentric hypertrophy occurs after an acute MI. Eccentric hypertrophy involves an increase in myocyte size in a segmental fashion, as opposed to the global hypertrophy occurring in concentric hypertrophy. Although hypertrophy helps to reduce cardiac wall stress in the short term, continued hypertrophy accelerates myocyte cell death through an overall increase in myocardial oxygen demand.

Cardiac remodeling occurs as a compensatory adaptation to a change in wall stress and is largely regulated by neurohormonal activation, with AT_2 and aldosterone being key stimuli.[7] The process entails changes in myocardial and extracellular matrix composition and function, which results in both structural and functional alterations to the heart. In HF, the changes in cardiac size, shape, and composition are pathologic and detrimental to heart function. In addition to myocyte size and extracellular matrix changes, heart geometry shifts from an elliptical to a less efficient spherical shape. Even after remodeling occurs, the heart can maintain CO for many years. However, heart function will continue to deteriorate until progression to clinical HF. The timeline for remodeling varies depending on the cardiac insult. For example, in the setting of an acute MI, remodeling starts within a few days.[5] Chronic remodeling, however, is what progressively worsens HF and therefore is a major target of drug therapy.

Models of HF

Earlier models of HF focused on the hemodynamic consequences of volume overload from excess sodium and water retention, decreased CO secondary to impaired ventricular function, and vasoconstriction.[8] Congestion was a result of fluid backup due to inadequate pump function. Therefore, drug therapy was focused on relieving excess volume using diuretics, improving pump function with inotropic agents, and alleviating vasoconstriction with vasodilators. Although these agents improved HF symptoms, they did little to slow the progressive decline in cardiac function or to improve survival.

▶ *Neurohormonal Model*

❷ *Development and progression of HF involves activation of neurohormonal pathways including the SNS and the RAAS.* This model begins with an initial precipitating event or myocardial injury resulting in a decline in CO, followed by the compensatory mechanisms previously discussed. This includes activation of neurohormonal pathways with pathologic consequences including the RAAS, SNS, endothelin and vasopressin, and those with counterregulatory properties such as the natriuretic peptides and nitric oxide. This model currently guides our therapy for chronic HF in terms of preventing disease progression and mortality.

Angiotensin II AT_2 is a key neurohormone in the pathophysiology of HF. The vasoconstrictive effects of AT_2 lead to an increase in systemic vascular resistance (SVR) and blood pressure (BP). The resulting increase in afterload contributes to an increase in myocardial oxygen demand and opposes the desired increase in SV. In the kidneys, AT_2 enhances renal function acutely by raising intraglomerular pressure through constriction of the efferent arterioles.[6] However, the increase in glomerular filtration pressure may be offset by a reduction in renal perfusion secondary to AT_2's influence over the release of other vasoactive neurohormones such as vasopressin and endothelin-1 (ET-1). AT_2 also potentiates the release of aldosterone from the adrenal glands and norepinephrine from adrenergic nerve terminals. Additionally, AT_2 induces vascular hypertrophy and remodeling in both cardiac and renal cells. Clinical studies show that blocking the effects of the RAAS in HF is associated with improved cardiac function and prolonged survival. Thus, angiotensin-converting enzyme (ACE) inhibitors and angiotensin receptor blockers (ARBs) are the cornerstone of HF treatment.

Aldosterone Aldosterone's contribution to HF pathophysiology is also multifaceted. Renally, aldosterone causes sodium and water retention in an attempt to enhance intravascular volume and CO. This adaptive mechanism has deleterious consequences because excessive sodium and water retention worsen the already-elevated ventricular filling pressures. Aldosterone also contributes to electrolyte abnormalities seen in HF patients. Hypokalemia and hypomagnesemia contribute to the increased risk of arrhythmias. In addition, evidence supports the role of aldosterone as an etiologic factor for myocardial fibrosis and cardiac remodeling by causing increased extracellular matrix collagen deposition and cardiac fibrosis.[6] Aldosterone potentially contributes to disease progression via sympathetic potentiation and ventricular remodeling. In addition, the combination of these multiple effects is likely responsible for the increased risk of sudden cardiac death attributed to aldosterone. As elevated aldosterone concentrations have been associated with a poorer prognosis in HF, its blockade has become an important therapeutic target for improvement of long-term prognosis.

Norepinephrine Norepinephrine is a classic marker for SNS activation. It plays an adaptive role in the failing heart by stimulating HR and myocardial contractility to augment CO and by producing vasoconstriction to maintain organ perfusion. However, excess levels are directly cardiotoxic. In addition, sympathetic activation increases the risk for arrhythmias, ischemia, and myocyte cell death through increased myocardial workload and accelerated apoptosis (i.e., programmed cell death). Ventricular hypertrophy and remodeling are also influenced by norepinephrine.[8]

Plasma norepinephrine concentrations are elevated proportionally to HF severity, with the highest levels correlating to the poorest prognosis. Several mechanisms relate to diminished responsiveness to catecholamines (e.g., norepinephrine) as cardiac function declines.[6] Adrenergic receptor desensitization and downregulation (decreased postreceptor responses and signaling and decreased receptor number) occur under sustained sympathetic stimulation. The desensitization contributes to further release of norepinephrine.[5] β-Adrenergic blocking agents, although intrinsically negatively inotropic, have become an essential therapy for chronic HF. β-Adrenergic blockers negate deleterious effects of norepinephrine, and therefore decrease HF disease progression.

Endothelin ET-1, one of the most potent physiologic vasoconstrictors, is an important contributor to HF pathophysiology.[9] ET-1 binds to two G-protein–coupled receptors, endothelin-A (ET-A) and endothelin-B (ET-B). ET-A receptors mediate vasoconstriction and are prevalent in vascular smooth muscle and cardiac cells. ET-B receptors are expressed on the endothelium and in vascular smooth muscle, and receptor stimulation mediates vasodilation. Levels of ET-1 correlate with HF functional class and mortality.

Arginine Vasopressin Higher vasopressin concentrations are linked to dilutional hyponatremia and a poor prognosis in HF. Vasopressin exerts its effects through vasopressin type 1a (V_{1a}) and vasopressin type 2 (V_2) receptors.[5,7] V_{1a} stimulation leads to vasoconstriction, while actions on the V_2 receptor cause free water retention through aquaporin channels in the collecting duct. Vasopressin increases preload, afterload, and myocardial oxygen demand in the failing heart.

Counterregulatory Hormones (Natriuretic Peptides, Bradykinin, and Nitric Oxide) Atrial natriuretic peptide (ANP) and B-type (formerly brain) natriuretic peptide (BNP) are endogenous neurohormones that regulate sodium and water balance. Natriuretic peptides decrease sodium reabsorption in the collecting duct of the kidney.[10] Natriuretic peptides also cause vasodilation through the cyclic guanosine monophosphate (cGMP) pathway. ANP is synthesized and stored in the atria, while BNP is produced mainly in the ventricles. Release of ANP and BNP is stimulated by increased cardiac chamber wall stretch, usually indicative of volume load. Higher concentrations of natriuretic peptides correlate with a more severe HF functional class and prognosis. BNP is sensitive to volume status; thus, the plasma concentration can be used as a diagnostic marker in HF.[10]

Bradykinin is part of the kallikrein-kinin system, which shares a link to the RAAS through ACE. Bradykinin is a vasodilatory peptide that is released in response to a variety of stimuli, including neurohormonal and inflammatory mediators known to be activated in HF.[9] As a consequence, bradykinin levels are elevated in HF patients and thought to partially antagonize the vasoconstrictive peptides.

Nitric oxide, a vasodilatory hormone released by the endothelium, is found in higher concentrations in HF patients and provides two main benefits in HF: vasodilation and neurohormonal antagonism of ET.[9] Nitric oxide production is affected by the enzyme inducible nitric oxide synthetase (iNOS), which is upregulated in the setting of HF, likely due to increased levels of AT_2, norepinephrine, and multiple cytokines. In HF, the physiologic response to nitric oxide appears to be blunted, which contributes to the imbalance between vasoconstriction and vasodilation.

▶ Cardiorenal Model

There is growing evidence of a link between renal disease and HF.[8] Renal insufficiency is present in one-third of HF patients and is associated with a worse prognosis. In hospitalized HF patients, the presence of renal insufficiency is associated with longer lengths of stay, increased in-hospital morbidity and mortality, and detrimental neurohormonal alterations. Conversely, renal dysfunction is a common complication of HF or results from its treatment. Renal failure is also a common cause for HF decompensation.

▶ Proinflammatory Cytokines

Inflammatory cytokines have been implicated in the pathophysiology of HF.[9] Several proinflammatory (e.g., tumor necrosis factor-α [TNF-α], interleukin-1, interleukin-6, and interferon-γ) and anti-inflammatory cytokines (e.g., interleukin-10) are overexpressed in the failing heart. The most is known about TNF-α, a pleiotrophic cytokine that acts as a negative inotrope, stimulates cardiac cell apoptosis, uncouples β-adrenergic receptors from adenylyl cyclase, and is related to cardiac cachexia. The exact role of cytokines and inflammation in HF pathophysiology continues to be studied.

Precipitating and Exacerbating Factors in HF

HF patients exist in one of two clinical states. When a patient's volume status and symptoms are stable, their HF condition is said to be "compensated." In situations of volume overload or other worsening symptoms, the patient is considered "decompensated." Acute decompensation can be precipitated by numerous etiologies that can be grouped into cardiac, metabolic, or patient-related causes (Table 6–3).[5]

❸ *The clinician must identify potential pharmacologic and dietary reversible causes of HF exacerbations including prescription and nonprescription drug therapies, dietary indiscretions, and medication nonadherence. Nonadherence with dietary restrictions or chronic HF medications deserves special attention, as it is the most common cause of acute decompensation and can be prevented. As such, an accurate history regarding diet, food choices, and the patient's knowledge regarding sodium and fluid intake (including alcohol) is valuable in assessing dietary indiscretion.* Nonadherence

Table 6–3		
Exacerbating or Precipitating Factors in HF		
Cardiac	**Metabolic**	**Patient Related**
Acute ischemia	Anemia	Dietary/fluid
Arrhythmia	Hyperthyroidism/	nonadherence
Endocarditis	thyrotoxicosis	HF therapy nonadherence
Myocarditis	Infection	Use of cardiotoxins
Pulmonary	Pregnancy	(cocaine, chronic
embolus	Worsening renal	alcohol, amphetamines,
Uncontrolled	function	sympathomimetics)
hypertension		Offending medications
Valvular		(NSAIDs, COX-2 inhibitors,
disorders		steroids, lithium,
		β-blockers, calcium
		channel blockers,
		antiarrhythmics, alcohol,
		thiazolidinediones)

COX-2, cyclooxygenase-2; HF, heart failure; NSAID, nonsteroidal anti-inflammatory drug.

Patient Encounter, Part 1

BE is a 62-year-old female with a history of known CAD and type 2 diabetes mellitus who presents for a belated follow-up clinic visit (her last visit was 2 years ago). She states that she used to be able to walk over one-half mile (0.8 km) and two flights of stairs before experiencing chest pain and becoming short of breath. Since her last visit, she has had increasing symptoms and has now progressed to shortness of breath (SOB) with walking only half a block and doing chores around the house. She also notes her ankles are always swollen and her shoes no longer fit, therefore she only wears slippers. Additionally, her appetite is decreased, and she often feels bloated. She also feels full after eating only a few bites of each meal.

What information is suggestive of a diagnosis of HF?

What additional information do you need to know before creating a treatment plan for BE?

with medical recommendations such as laboratory and other follow-up appointments can also be indicative of nonadherence with diet or medications.

CLINICAL PRESENTATION AND DIAGNOSIS OF CHRONIC HF

In low-output HF, symptoms are generally related to either congestion behind the failing ventricle(s), hypoperfusion (decreased tissue blood supply), or both. Congestion is the most common symptom in HF, followed by symptoms related to decreased perfusion to peripheral tissues including decreased renal output, mental confusion, and cold extremities. Activation of the compensatory mechanisms occurs in an effort to increase CO and preserve blood flow to vital organs. However, the increase in preload and afterload in the setting of a failing ventricle leads to elevated filling pressures and further impairment of cardiac function, which manifests as systemic and/or pulmonary congestion. It is important to remember that congestion develops behind the failing ventricle, caused by the inability of that ventricle to eject the blood that it receives from the atria and venous return. As such, signs and symptoms may be classified as left sided or right sided. ❹ *Symptoms of left-sided HF include dyspnea, orthopnea, and paroxysmal nocturnal dyspnea (PND), whereas symptoms of right-sided HF include fluid retention, GI bloating, and fatigue. Although most patients initially have left ventricular failure (LVF; pulmonary congestion), the ventricles share a septal wall, and because LVF increases the workload of the right ventricle, both ventricles eventually fail and contribute to the HF syndrome. Because of the complex nature of this syndrome, it has become exceedingly more difficult to attribute a specific sign or symptom as caused by either right ventricular failure (RVF; systemic congestion) or LVF. Therefore, the numerous signs and symptoms associated*

Clinical Presentation and Diagnosis of Chronic HF

General

Patient presentation may range from asymptomatic to cardiogenic shock.

Symptoms

- Dyspnea, particularly on exertion
- **Orthopnea**
- SOB
- PND
- Exercise intolerance
- Tachypnea
- Cough
- Fatigue
- **Nocturia** and/or **polyuria**
- Hemoptysis
- Abdominal pain
- Anorexia
- Nausea
- Bloating
- Ascites
- Mental status changes
- Weakness
- Lethargy

Signs

- Pulmonary rales
- Pulmonary edema
- S$_3$ gallop
- Pleural effusion

- Cheyne-Stokes respiration
- Tachycardia
- Cardiomegaly
- Peripheral edema (e.g., pedal edema, which is swelling of feet and ankles)
- Jugular venous distention (JVD)
- Hepatojugular reflux (HJR)
- Hepatomegaly
- Cyanosis of the digits
- Pallor or cool extremities

Laboratory Tests

- BNP greater than 100 pg/mL (greater than 100 ng/L or 28.9 pmol/L) or N-terminal proBNP (NT-proBNP) greater than 300 pg/mL (greater than 300 ng/L or greater than 35.4 pmol/L)
- ECG: May be normal or could show numerous abnormalities including acute ST-T wave changes from myocardial ischemia, atrial fibrillation, bradycardia, and LV hypertrophy
- Serum creatinine: May be increased owing to hypoperfusion; pre-existing renal dysfunction can contribute to volume overload
- CBC: Useful to determine if HF is due to reduced oxygen-carrying capacity
- CXR: Useful for detection of cardiac enlargement, pulmonary edema, and pleural effusions
- Echocardiogram: Used to assess LV size, valve function, pericardial effusion, wall motion abnormalities, and EF

BNP, B-type natriuretic peptide; CBC, complete blood cell count; CXR, chest x-ray; EF, ejection fraction; LV, left ventricular.

with this disorder are collectively attributed to HF rather than to dysfunction of a specific ventricle.

General Signs and Symptoms

Hypoperfusion of skeletal muscles leads to fatigue, weakness, and exercise intolerance. Decreased perfusion of the CNS is related to confusion, hallucinations, insomnia, and lethargy. Peripheral vasoconstriction due to SNS activity causes pallor, cool extremities, and cyanosis of the digits. Tachycardia is also common in these patients and may reflect increased SNS activity. Patients will often exhibit polyuria and nocturia. Polyuria is a result of increased release of natriuretic peptides caused by volume overload. Nocturia occurs due to increased renal perfusion as a consequence of reduced SNS renal vasoconstrictive effects at night. In chronic severe HF, unintentional weight loss can occur which leads to a syndrome of cardiac cachexia. Cardiac cachexia can be

defined as a nonedematous weight loss greater than 6% of the previous normal weight over a period of at least 6 months. HF prognosis worsens considerably once cardiac cachexia has been diagnosed, regardless of HF severity. This results from several factors including loss of appetite, malabsorption due to GI edema, elevated metabolic rate, and elevated levels of norepinephrine and pro-inflammatory cytokines. Absorption of fats is especially affected, leading to deficiencies of fat soluble vitamins.

Patients can experience a variety of symptoms related to buildup of fluid in the lungs. Dyspnea, or shortness of breath (SOB), can result from pulmonary congestion or systemic hypoperfusion due to LVF. Exertional dyspnea occurs when patients describe breathlessness induced by physical activity or a lower level of activity than previously known to cause breathlessness. Patients often state that activities such as stair climbing, carrying groceries, or walking a particular distance cause SOB. Severity of HF is inversely proportional to the amount of activity required to produce dyspnea. In severe HF, dyspnea will be present even at rest.

Orthopnea is dyspnea that is positional. Orthopnea is present if a patient is unable to breathe while lying flat on a bed (i.e., in the recumbent position). It manifests within minutes of a patient lying down and is relieved immediately when the patient sits upright. Patients can relieve orthopnea by elevating their head and shoulders with pillows. The practitioner should inquire as to the number of pillows needed to prevent dyspnea as a marker of worsening HF. PND occurs when patients awaken suddenly with a feeling of breathlessness and suffocation. PND is caused by increased venous return and mobilization of interstitial fluid from the extremities leading to alveolar edema, and usually occurs within 1 to 4 hours of sleep. In contrast to orthopnea, PND is not relieved immediately by sitting upright and often takes up to 30 minutes for symptoms to subside.

Pulmonary congestion may also cause a nonproductive cough that occurs at night or with exertion. Cheyne-Stokes respiration, or periodic breathing, is also common in advanced HF. It is usually associated with low-output states and may be perceived by the patient as either severe dyspnea or transient cessation of breathing. In cases of pulmonary edema, the most severe form of pulmonary congestion, patients may produce a pink, frothy sputum and experience extreme breathlessness and anxiety due to feelings of suffocation and drowning. If not treated aggressively, patients can become cyanotic and acidotic. Severe pulmonary edema can progress to respiratory failure, necessitating mechanical ventilation.

Systemic venous congestion results mainly from RVF. A clinically validated assessment of the jugular venous pressure (JVP) is performed by examining the right internal jugular vein for distention or elevation of the pulsation while reclining at a 45-degree angle. A JVP of more than 4 cm above the sternal angle is indicative of elevated right atrial pressure. JVP may be normal at rest, but if application of pressure to the abdomen can elicit a sustained elevation of JVP, this is defined as hepatojugular reflux (HJR). A positive finding of HJR indicates hepatic congestion and results from displacement of volume from the abdomen into the jugular vein because the right atrium is unable to accept this additional blood. Hepatic congestion can cause abnormalities in liver function, which can be evident in liver function tests and/or clotting times. Development of hepatomegaly occurs infrequently and is caused by long-term systemic venous congestion. Intestinal or abdominal congestion can also be present, but usually doesn't lead to characteristic signs unless overt ascites is evident. In advanced RVF, evidence of pulmonary hypertension may be present (e.g., right ventricular heave).

The most recognized finding of systemic congestion is peripheral edema. It usually occurs in dependent areas of the body, such as the ankles (pedal edema) for ambulatory patients, or the sacral region for bedridden patients. Weight gain often precedes signs of overt peripheral edema. Therefore, it is crucial for patients to weigh themselves daily even in the absence of symptoms to assess fluid status.

Patients may complain of swelling of their feet and ankles, which can extend up to their calves or thighs. Abdominal congestion may cause a bloated feeling, abdominal pain, early satiety, nausea, anorexia, and constipation. Often patients may have difficulty fitting into their shoes or pants due to edema.

▶ *Patient History*

A thorough history is crucial to identify cardiac and noncardiac disorders or behaviors that may lead to or accelerate the development of HF. Past medical history, family history, and social history are important for identifying comorbid illnesses that are risk factors for the development of HF or underlying etiologic factors. A complete medication history (including prescription and nonprescription drugs, herbal therapy, and vitamin supplements) should be obtained each time a patient is seen to evaluate adherence, to assess appropriateness of therapy, to eliminate drugs that may be harmful in HF (Table 6–4), and to determine additional monitoring requirements. For newly diagnosed HF, previous use of chemotherapeutic agents as well as current or past use of alcohol and illicit drugs should be assessed. In addition, for patients with a known history of HF, questions related to symptomatology and exercise tolerance are essential for assessing any changes in clinical status that may warrant further evaluation or adjustment of the medication regimen.

HF Classification

There are two common systems for categorizing patients with HF. The New York Heart Association (NYHA) Functional

---

Table 6–4
Drugs That May Precipitate or Exacerbate HF

Agents Causing Negative Inotropic Effect
Antiarrhythmics (e.g., disopyramide, flecainide, and others)
β-Blockers (e.g., propranolol, metoprolol, atenolol, and others)
Calcium channel blockers (e.g., verapamil and diltiazem)
Itraconazole
Terbinafine

Cardiotoxic Agents
Doxorubicin
Daunomycin
Cyclophosphamide

Agents Causing Sodium and Water Retention
NSAIDs
COX-2 inhibitors
Glucocorticoids
Androgens
Estrogens
Salicylates (high dose)
Sodium-containing drugs (e.g., carbenicillin disodium, ticarcillin disodium)
Thiazolidinediones (e.g., rosiglitazone, pioglitazone)

COX-2, cyclooxygenase-2; NSAIDs, nonsteroidal anti-inflammatory drugs.

From Parker RB, Rodgers JE, Cavallari JH. Heart failure. In: DiPiro JT, Talbert RL, Yee GC, et al. (eds.) Pharmacotherapy: A Pathophysiologic Approach, 7th ed. New York: McGraw-Hill, 2008:180.

Table 6–5

NYHA Functional Classification and ACC/AHA Staging

NYHA FC	ACC/AHA Stage	Description
N/A	A	Patients at high risk for HF but without structural heart disease or symptoms of HF
I	B	Patients with cardiac disease but without limitations of physical activity. Ordinary physical activity does not cause undue fatigue, dyspnea, or palpitation
II	C	Patients with cardiac disease that results in slight limitations of physical activity. Ordinary physical activity results in fatigue, palpitations, dyspnea, or angina
III	C	Patients with cardiac disease that results in marked limitation of physical activity. Although patients are comfortable at rest, less than ordinary activity will lead to symptoms
IV	C, D	Patients with cardiac disease that results in an inability to carry on physical activity without discomfort. Symptoms of HF are present at rest. With any physical activity, increased discomfort is experienced. Stage D refers to end-stage HF patients

ACC/AHA, American College of Cardiology/American Heart Association; FC, functional class; HF, heart failure; NYHA FC, New York Heart Association Functional Class.

Classification (FC) system is based on the patient's activity level and exercise tolerance. It divides patients into one of four classes, with FC I patients exhibiting no symptoms or limitations of daily activities, and FC IV patients who are symptomatic at rest (Table 6–5). The NYHA FC system reflects a subjective assessment by a health care provider and can change frequently over short periods of time. FC correlates poorly with EF; however, EF is one of the strongest predictors of prognosis. In general, anticipated survival declines in conjunction with a decline in functional ability.

The American College of Cardiology/American Heart Association (ACC/AHA) has proposed another system based on the development and progression of the disease. Instead of classifications, patients are placed into stages A through D (Table 6–5).[11] Because the staging system is related to development and progression of HF, it also proposes management strategies for each stage including risk factor modification. The staging system is meant to complement the NYHA FC system; however, patients can move between NYHA FCs as symptoms improve with treatment, whereas HF staging does not allow for patients to move to a lower stage (e.g., patients cannot be categorized as stage C and move to stage B after treatment). Currently, patients are categorized based on both systems. NYHA FC and ACC/AHA staging are useful from a clinician's perspective,

Patient Encounter, Part 2

BE's medical history, physical exam, and diagnostic test results.

PMH: Type 2 diabetes mellitus for 15 years; coronary artery disease for 10 years (MIs in 1999 and 2002); tobacco use; history of back surgery in 2001

Allergies: NKDA

Meds: Diltiazem CD 240 mg once daily; nitroglycerin 0.4 mg sublingual (SL) as needed (last use yesterday after showering); glipizide 10 mg twice daily for diabetes; ibuprofen 600 mg twice daily for arthritis pain; vitamin B_{12} once daily; multivitamin daily; aspirin 325 mg once daily

FH: Significant for early heart disease in father (MI at age 53)

SH: Disabled from a previous accident; married, has six children, and runs her own business; she does not drink alcohol and smokes one to two packs of cigarettes per day

PE:

BP 126/70 mm Hg, P 60 bpm and regular, RR 16/min, ht 5'8" (173 cm), wt 114 kg (251 lb), BMI 38.2 kg/m²

Lungs: Clear to auscultation with a prolonged expiratory phase; rales are present bilaterally

CV: RRR with normal S_1 and S_2; there is an S_3 and a soft S_4 present; there is a 2/6 systolic ejection murmur heard best at the left lower sternal border; point of maximal impulse is within normal limits at the midclavicular line; there is no JVD

Abd: Soft, nontender, and bowel sounds are present; 2+ pitting edema of extremities extending to below the knees is observed

CXR: Bilateral pleural effusions and cardiomegaly

Echo: EF 35%

Laboratory Values

Hct: 41.1%

WBC: $5.3 \times 10^3/mm^3$ ($5.3 \times 10^9/L$)

Sodium: 132 mEq/L (132 mmol/L)

Potassium: 3.2 mEq/L (3.2 mmol/L)

Bicarb: 30 mEq/L (30 mmol/L)

Chloride: 90 mEq/L (90 mmol/L)

Magnesium: 1.5 mEq/L (0.8 mmol/L)

Fasting blood sugar: 120 mg/dL (6.7 mmol/L)

Uric acid: 8 mg/dL (476 μmol/L)

Blood urea nitrogen (BUN): 40 mg/dL (14 mmol/L)

SCr: 0.8 mg/dL (71 μmol/L)

Alk phos: 120 IU/L (2 μKat/L)

Aspartate aminotransferase: 100 IU/L (1.7 μKat/L)

(Continued)

Patient Encounter, Part 2 (Continued)

What other laboratory or other diagnostic tests are required for assessment of BE's condition?

How would you classify BE's NYHA FC and ACC/AHA HF stage?

Identify exacerbating or precipitating factors that may worsen BE's HF.

What are your treatment goals for BE?

allowing for a longitudinal assessment of a patient's risk and progress, requirements for nonpharmacologic interventions, response to medications, and overall prognosis.

TREATMENT OF CHRONIC HF

Desired Therapeutic Outcomes

There is no cure for HF. ❺ *The general management goals for chronic HF include preventing the onset of clinical symptoms or reducing symptoms, preventing or reducing hospitalizations, slowing progression of the disease, improving quality of life, and prolonging survival.* The ACC/AHA staging system described earlier provides a guide for application of these goals based on the clinical progression of HF for a given patient. The goals are additive as one moves from stage A to stage D.[1,11] For stage A, risk factor management is the primary goal. Stage B includes the addition of pharmacologic therapies known to slow the progression of the disease in an attempt to prevent the onset of clinical symptoms. Stage C involves the use of additional therapies aimed at controlling symptoms and decreasing morbidity. Finally, in stage D, the goals shift toward quality of life related issues. Only with aggressive management throughout all the stages of the disease will the ultimate goal of improving survival be realized. The attainment of these goals is based on designing a therapeutic approach that encompasses strategies aimed at control and treatment of contributing disorders, nonpharmacologic interventions, and optimal use of pharmacologic therapies.[12,13]

Control and Treatment of Contributing Disorders

All causes of HF must be investigated to determine the etiology of cardiac dysfunction in a given patient. Because the most common etiology of HF in the United States is ischemic heart disease, assessment for cardiac ischemia, which may include stress testing, echocardiography, and/or coronary angiography is warranted in the majority of patients with a history suggestive of underlying CAD. Revascularization of those with significant CAD may help restore some cardiac function in patients with reversible ischemic defects. Aggressive control of hypertension, diabetes, and obesity is also essential because each of these conditions can cause

further cardiac damage. Surgical repair of valvular disease or congenital malformations may be warranted if detected. Because clinical HF is partly dependent on metabolic processes, correction of imbalances such as thyroid disease, anemia, and nutritional deficiencies is required. Other more rare causes such as autoimmune disorders or acquired illnesses may have specific treatments. Identifying and discontinuing medications that can exacerbate HF is also an important intervention, as is eliminating alcohol for those with alcohol-related cardiomyopathy.

Nonpharmacologic Interventions

It is imperative that patients recognize the role of self-management in HF. ❻ *Nonpharmacologic treatment involves dietary modifications such as sodium and fluid restriction, risk factor reduction including smoking cessation, timely immunizations, and supervised regular physical activity. Patient education regarding monitoring symptoms, dietary and medication adherence, exercise and physical fitness, risk factor reduction, and immunizations are important for prevention of AHF exacerbations.*

Patients should be encouraged to become involved in their own care through several avenues, the first of which is self-monitoring. Home monitoring should include daily assessment of weight and exercise tolerance. Daily weights should be done first thing in the morning upon arising and before any food intake to maintain consistency. Patients should record their weight daily in a journal and bring this log to each clinic or office visit. Changes in weight can indicate fluid retention and congestion prior to onset of peripheral or pulmonary symptoms. Individuals who have an increase of 0.9 to 1.4 kg (2–3 lb) in a single day or 2.3 kg (5 lb) over 5 days should alert their HF care provider. Some patients may be educated about self-adjusting diuretic doses based on daily weights. In addition to weight changes, a marked decline in exercise tolerance should also be reported to the HF care provider.

Nonadherence is an important issue as it relates to acute exacerbations of HF. Ensuring an understanding of the importance of each medication used to treat HF, proper administration, and potential adverse effects may improve adherence. Stressing the rationale for each medication is important, especially for NYHA FC I or ACC/AHA stage B patients who are asymptomatic, yet started on drugs that may worsen symptoms initially. A clinician's involvement in emphasizing medication adherence, offering adherence suggestions such as optimal timing of medications or use of weekly pill containers, and providing intensive follow-up care has been shown to reduce AHF hospitalizations.

Dietary modifications in HF consist of initiation of an AHA step II diet as part of cardiac risk factor reduction, sodium restriction, and sometimes fluid restriction. As sodium and water retention is a compensatory mechanism that contributes to volume overload in HF, salt and fluid restriction is often necessary to help avoid or minimize congestion. The normal American diet includes 3 to 6 g of sodium per day. Most patients with HF should limit salt intake to a maximum of 2 g/day. Patients should be educated to avoid cooking with salt and to limit intake of foods with high salt content, such as fried or processed food (lunchmeats, soups, cheeses, salted snack foods, canned food, and some ethnic food). Salt restriction can be challenging for many patients. The clinician should counsel to restrict salt slowly over time. Drastic dietary changes may lead to nonadherence due to an unpalatable diet. Substituting spices to flavor food is a useful recommendation. Salt substitutes should be used judiciously, as many contain significant amounts of potassium, which can increase the risk of hyperkalemia. Fluid restriction may not be necessary in many patients. When applicable, fluid intake is generally limited from all sources to less than 2 L/day.

Exercise, while discouraged when the patient is acutely decompensated to ease cardiac workload, is recommended when patients are stable. The heart is a muscle that requires activity to prevent atrophy. In addition, exercise improves peripheral muscle conditioning and efficiency, which may contribute to better exercise tolerance despite the low CO state. Regular, low-intensity aerobic exercise that includes walking, swimming, or riding a bike is encouraged, while heavy weight training is discouraged. The prescribed exercise regimen needs to be tailored to the individual's functional ability, and thus it is suggested that patients participate in cardiac rehabilitation programs, at least initially. It is important that patients not overexert themselves to fatigue or exertional dyspnea.

Modification of classic risk factors, such as tobacco and alcohol consumption, is important to minimize the potential for further aggravation of heart function. Data from observational studies suggest that patients with HF who smoke have a mortality rate 40% higher than those who do not consume tobacco products.[1] All HF patients who smoke should be counseled on the importance of tobacco cessation and offered a referral to a cessation program. Patients with an alcoholic cardiomyopathy should abstain from alcohol. Whether all patients with other forms of HF should abstain from any alcohol intake remains controversial. Proponents of moderation of alcohol base their rationale on the potential cardio-protective effects. However, opponents to any alcohol intake point out that alcohol is cardiotoxic and should be avoided.

In general, it is suggested that patients remain up to date on standard immunizations. Patients with HF should be counseled to receive yearly influenza vaccinations. Additionally, a pneumococcal vaccine is recommended.

Pharmacologic Treatment

In addition to determining therapeutic goals, the ACC/AHA staging system delineates specific therapy options based on disease progression.[1,11] For patients in stage A, every effort is made to minimize the impact of diseases that can injure the heart. Antihypertensive and lipid-lowering therapies should be utilized when appropriate to decrease the risk for stroke, MI, and HF. ACE inhibitors should be considered in high-risk vascular disease patients. For stage B patients, the goal is to prevent or slow disease progression by interfering with neurohormonal pathways that lead to cardiac damage and mediate pathologic remodeling. The goal is to prevent the onset of HF symptoms. The backbone of therapy in these patients includes ACE inhibitors or ARBs and β-blockers. In stage C patients with symptomatic LV systolic dysfunction (EF less than 40%), the goals focus on alleviating fluid retention, minimizing disability, slowing disease progression, and reducing long-term risk for hospitalizations and death. Treatment entails a strategy that combines diuretics to control intravascular fluid balance with neurohormonal antagonists to minimize the effects of the RAAS and SNS. Additional neurohormonal blockade with aldosterone antagonists or other therapies such as digoxin are often added as cardiac function continues to decline. Patients with advanced stage D disease are offered more modest goals, such as improvement in quality of life. Enhancing quality of life is often achieved at the expense of expected survival. Treatment options include mechanical support, transplantation, and continuous use of IV vasoactive therapies, in addition to maintaining an optimal regimen of chronic oral medications (Fig. 6–1).

▶ *Diuretics*

Diuretics have been the mainstay for HF symptom management for many years. **❼** *Diuretics are used for relief of acute symptoms of congestion and maintenance of euvolemia.* These agents interfere with sodium retention by increasing urinary sodium and free water excretion. No prospective data exist on the effects of diuretics on patient outcomes.[14] Therefore, the primary rationale for the use of diuretic therapy is to maintain euvolemia in symptomatic or stages C and D HF. Diuretic therapy is recommended for all patients with clinical evidence of fluid overload retention.[15,16] In more mild HF, diuretics may be used on an as-needed basis. However, once the development of edema is persistent, regularly scheduled doses will be required.

Two types of diuretics are used for volume management in HF: thiazides and loop diuretics. Thiazide diuretics such as hydrochlorothiazide, chlorthalidone, and metolazone block sodium and chloride reabsorption in the distal convoluted tubule. Thiazides are weaker than loop diuretics in terms of effecting an increase in urine output and therefore are not utilized frequently as monotherapy in HF. They are optimally suited for patients with hypertension who have mild congestion. Additionally, the action of thiazides is limited in patients with renal insufficiency (creatinine clearance [CrCl] less than 30 mL/min) due to reduced secretion into their site of action. An exception is metolazone, which retains its potent action in patients with renal dysfunction. Metolazone is often used in combination with loop diuretics when patients exhibit diuretic resistance, defined as edema unresponsive to loop diuretics alone.

Loop diuretics are the most widely used diuretics in HF. These agents, including furosemide, bumetanide, and torsemide, exert their action at the thick ascending loop of Henle. Loop diuretics are not filtered through the glomerulus, but instead undergo active transport into the

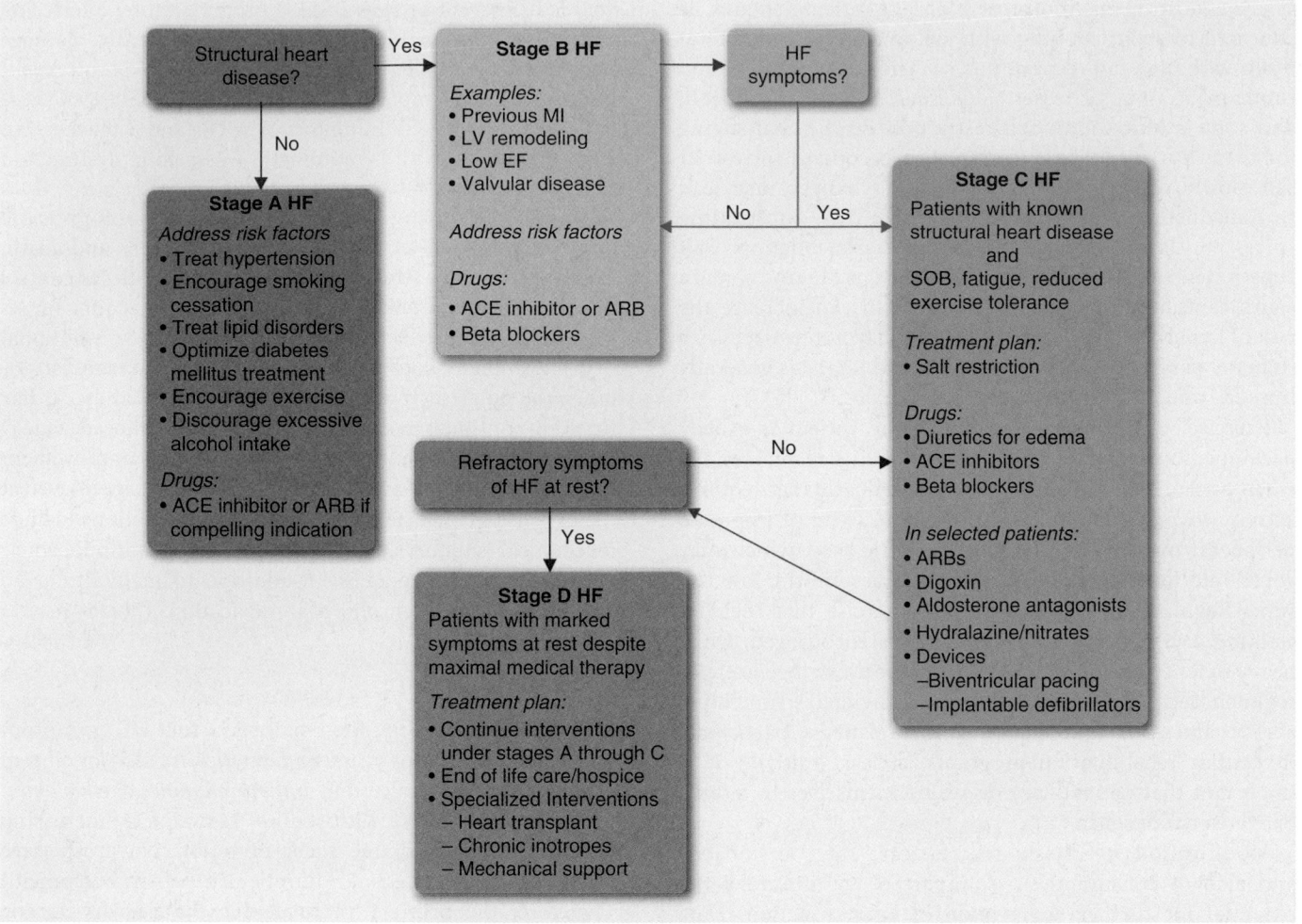

FIGURE 6–1. Treatment algorithm for chronic HF. Table 6–5 describes staging of heart failure. (ACE, angiotensin-converting enzyme; ARB, angiotensin receptor blocker; EF, ejection fraction; HF, heart failure; LV, left ventricular; MI, myocardial infarction; SOB, shortness of breath.)

tubular lumen via the organic acid pathway. As a result, drugs that compete for this active transport (e.g., probenecid and organic byproducts of uremia) can lower efficacy of loop diuretics. Loop diuretics increase sodium and water excretion, and induce a prostaglandin-mediated increase in renal blood flow which contributes to their natriuretic effect. Unlike thiazides, they retain their diuretic ability in patients with poor renal function. The various loop diuretics are equally effective when used at equipotent doses, although there are intrinsic differences in pharmacokinetics and pharmacodynamics (Table 6–6).[5] The choice of which loop diuretic to use and the route of administration depends on clinical factors, such as presence of intestinal edema and rapidity of desired effect. Oral diuretic efficacy may vary based on differing bioavailability, which is almost complete for torsemide and bumetanide, but averages only 50% for furosemide. Therefore, oral torsemide can be considered an alternative to the IV route of administration for patients who do not respond to oral furosemide in the setting of profound edema. The onset of effect is slightly delayed after oral administration but occurs within a few minutes with IV

Table 6–6

Loop Diuretics Used in HF

	Furosemide	Bumetanide	Torsemide
Usual daily dose (oral)	20–160 mg	0.5–4 mg	10–80 mg
Ceiling dose:			
Normal renal function	80–160 mg	1–2 mg	20–40 mg
CrCl 20–50 mL/min	160 mg	2 mg	40 mg
CrCl less than 20 mL/min	400 mg	8–10 mg	100 mg
Bioavailability	10–100% (average 50%)	80–90%	80–100%
Affected by food	Yes	Yes	No
Half-life	0.3–3.4 hours	0.3–1.5 hours	3–4 hours

CrCl, creatinine clearance; HF, heart failure.

From Parker RB, Rodgers JE, Cavallari JH. Heart failure. In: DiPiro JT, Talbert RL, Yee GC, et al. (eds.) Pharmacotherapy: A Pathophysiologic Approach, 7th ed. New York: McGraw-Hill, 2008:187.

dosing. Consequently, bioequivalent doses of IV furosemide are half the oral dose, whereas bumetanide and torsemide IV doses are generally equivalent to the oral doses.

In patients with evidence of mild to moderate volume overload, diuretics should be initiated at a low dose and titrated to achieve a weight loss of up to 0.91 kg/day (2 lb/day). Patients with severe volume overload should be managed in an inpatient setting. Once diuretic therapy is initiated, dosage adjustments are based on symptomatic improvement and daily body weight. As body weight changes are a sensitive marker of fluid retention or loss, patients should continue to weigh themselves daily. Once a patient reaches a euvolemic state, diuretics may be cautiously tapered and then withdrawn in appropriate patients. In stable, educated, and adherent patients, another option is self-adjusted diuretic dosing. Based on daily body weight, patients may temporarily increase their diuretic regimen in order to reduce the incidence of overt edema. This also avoids overuse of diuretics and possible complications of overdiuresis such as hypotension, fatigue, and renal impairment.

The maximal response to diuretics is reduced in HF, creating a "ceiling dose" above which there is limited added benefit. This diuretic resistance is due to a compensatory increase in sodium reabsorption in the distal tubules, which decreases the effect of blocking sodium reabsorption in the loop of Henle.[17] In addition, there is a simultaneous increase in the reabsorption of sodium from the proximal tubule, allowing less to reach the site of action for loop diuretics. Apart from increasing diuretic doses, strategies to improve diuretic efficacy include increasing the frequency of dosing to two or three times daily, utilizing a continuous infusion of a loop diuretic, and/or combining a loop diuretic with a thiazide diuretic.[17,18] The latter strategy theoretically prevents sodium and water reabsorption at both the loop of Henle and the compensating distal convoluted tubule. Metolazone is used most often for this purpose, as it retains its activity in settings of a low CrCl. Metolazone can be dosed daily or as little as once weekly. This combination is usually maintained until the patient reaches his or her baseline weight. The clinician must use metolazone cautiously, as its potent activity predisposes a patient to metabolic abnormalities as outlined below.

Diuretics cause numerous adverse effects and metabolic abnormalities, with severity linked to diuretic potency. A particularly worrisome adverse effect in the setting of HF is hypokalemia. Low serum potassium can predispose patients to arrhythmias and sudden death. Hypomagnesemia often occurs concomitantly with diuretic-induced hypokalemia, and therefore both should be assessed and replaced in patients needing correction of hypokalemia. Magnesium is an essential cofactor for movement of potassium intracellularly to restore body stores. Patients taking diuretics are also at risk for renal insufficiency due to overdiuresis and reflex activation of the renin-angiotensin system. The potential reduction in renal blood flow and glomerular pressure is amplified by concomitant use of ACE inhibitors or ARBs.

▶ *Neurohormonal Blocking Agents*

❽ *Agents with proven benefits in improving symptoms, slowing disease progression, and improving survival in chronic HF target neurohormonal blockade. These include ACE inhibitors, ARBs, β-adrenergic blockers, and aldosterone antagonists.*

ACE Inhibitors ACE inhibitors are the cornerstone of treatment for HF. ACE inhibitors decrease neurohormonal activation by blocking the conversion of angiotensin I (AT_1) to AT_2, a potent mediator of vasoconstriction and cardiac remodeling. The breakdown of bradykinin is also reduced. Bradykinin enhances the release of vasodilatory prostaglandins and histamines. These effects result in arterial and venous dilatation, and a decrease in myocardial workload through reduction of both preload and afterload. ACE inhibitors demonstrate favorable effects on cardiac hemodynamics, such as long-term increases in cardiac index (CI), stroke work index, and SV index, as well as significant reductions in LV filling pressure, SVR, mean arterial pressure, and HR.

There is extensive clinical experience with ACE inhibitors in systolic HF. Numerous clinical studies show ACE inhibitor therapy is associated with improvements in clinical symptoms, exercise tolerance, NYHA functional class, LV size and function, and quality of life as compared with placebo.[18–21] ACE inhibitors significantly reduce hospitalization rates and mortality regardless of underlying disease severity or etiology. ACE inhibitors are also effective in preventing HF development in high-risk patients. Studies in acute MI patients show a reduction in new-onset HF and death with ACE inhibitors whether they are initiated early (within 36 hours) or started later. In addition, ACE inhibition decreases the risk of HF hospitalization and death in patients with asymptomatic LV dysfunction. The exact mechanisms for decreased HF progression and mortality are postulated to involve both the hemodynamic improvement and the inhibition of AT_2's growth promoting and remodeling effects. All patients with documented LV systolic dysfunction, regardless of existing HF symptoms, should receive ACE inhibitors unless a contraindication or intolerance is present.

There is no evidence to suggest that one ACE inhibitor is preferred over another. ACE inhibitors should be initiated using low doses and titrated up to target doses over several weeks depending on tolerability (adverse effects and BP). The ACC/AHA 2005 guidelines advocate using the doses that were proven to decrease mortality in clinical trials as the target doses (Table 6–7).[1] If the target dose cannot be attained in a given patient, the highest tolerated dose should be used chronically. Although there is incremental benefit with higher doses of ACE inhibitors, it is accepted that lower doses provide substantial if not the majority of the effect.[22] Because ACE inhibitors are only one component of a mortality-reducing treatment plan in HF, targeting a high ACE inhibitor dose should not interfere with starting a β-blocker or aldosterone antagonist by accentuating the hypotensive effects. Higher ACE inhibitor dosing may also limit tolerability of a regimen that also includes β-blockers and aldosterone antagonists.

Table 6–7

Dosing and Monitoring for Neurohormonal Blocking Agents

Drug	Initial Daily Dose	Target or Maximum Daily Dose	Monitoring
ACE Inhibitors[a]			
Captopril	6.25 mg three times	50 mg three times	BP
Enalapril	2.5 mg twice	10–20 mg twice	Electrolytes (K$^+$, BUN, SCr) at baseline,
Fosinopril	5–10 mg once	40 mg once	2 weeks, and after dose titration, CBC
Lisinopril	2.5–5 mg once	20–40 mg once	periodically
Perindopril	2 mg once	8–16 mg once	Adverse effects: cough, angioedema
Quinopril	5 mg once	20 mg twice	
Ramipril	1.25–2.5 mg once	10 mg once	
Trandolapril	1 mg once	4 mg once	
ARBs[a]			
Candesartan	4–8 mg once	32 mg once	BP
Losartan	25–50 mg once	50–100 mg once	Electrolytes (K$^+$, BUN, SCr) at baseline,
Valsartan	20–40 mg once	160 mg twice	2 weeks, and after dose titration; CBC
			periodically
			Adverse effects: cough, angioedema
Aldosterone Antagonists			
Spironolactone	12.5–25 mg once	25 mg once or twice	BP
Eplerenone	25 mg once	50 mg once	Electrolytes (K$^+$) at baseline and within 1 week of initiation and dose titration
			Adverse effects: gynecomastia or breast tenderness, menstrual changes, hirsutism
β-Blockers			
Bisoprolol	1.25 mg once	10 mg once	BP, HR baseline and after each dose titration, ECG
Carvedilol	3.125 mg twice	25 mg twice (50 mg twice for patients greater than 85 kg or 187 lb)	Adverse effects: worsening HF symptoms (edema, SOB, fatigue), depression, sexual dysfunction
Metoprolol succinate	12.5–25 mg once	200 mg once	

ACE, angiotensin-converting enzyme; ARB, angiotensin receptor blocker; BP, blood pressure; BUN, blood urea nitrogen; CBC, complete blood cell count; HF, heart failure; HR, heart rate; K$^+$, potassium; SCr, serum creatinine; SOB, shortness of breath.

[a]Use lower dose listed in patients with renal failure.

Despite their clear benefits, ACE inhibitors are still underutilized in HF. One reason is undue concern or confusion regarding absolute versus relative contraindications for their use. Absolute contraindications include a history of angioedema, bilateral renal artery stenosis, and pregnancy. Relative contraindications include unilateral renal artery stenosis, renal insufficiency, hypotension, hyperkalemia, and cough. Relative contraindications provide a warning that close monitoring is required, but they do not necessarily preclude their use.

Clinicians are especially concerned about the use of ACE inhibitors in patients with renal insufficiency. It is important to recognize that ACE inhibitors can potentially contribute to preservation or decline in renal function depending on the clinical scenario. Through preferential efferent arteriole vasodilation, ACE inhibitors can reduce intraglomerular pressure. Reduced glomerular pressures are renoprotective chronically; however, in situations of reduced or fixed renal blood flow, this leads to a reduction in filtration. In general,

ACE inhibitors can be used in patients with serum creatinine less than 2.5 to 3 mg/dL (221–265 μmol/L). In HF, their addition can result in improved renal function through an increase in CO and renal perfusion. Although a small increase in serum creatinine (less than 0.5 mg/dL [44 μmol/L]) is possible with the addition of an ACE inhibitor, it is usually transient or becomes the patient's new serum creatinine baseline level. However, ACE inhibition can also worsen renal function as glomerular filtration is maintained in the setting of reduced CO through AT$_2$'s constriction of the efferent arteriole. Patients most dependent on AT$_2$ for maintenance of glomerular filtration pressure, and hence most susceptible to ACE inhibitor worsening of renal function, include those with hyponatremia, severely depressed LV function, or dehydration. The most common reason for creatinine elevation in a patient without a history of renal dysfunction is overdiuresis. Therefore, clinicians should consider decreasing or holding diuretic doses if an elevation in serum creatinine occurs concomitantly with a rise in blood urea nitrogen.

Hypotension occurs commonly at the initiation of therapy or with dosage increases but may happen any time during therapy. Hypotension can manifest as dizziness, lightheadedness, presyncope, or syncope. The risk of hypotension due to possible volume depletion increases when ACE inhibitors are initiated or used concomitantly in patients on high diuretic doses. Therefore, in euvolemic patients, diuretic doses may often be decreased or withheld during ACE inhibitor dose titration. Initiating at a low dose and titrating slowly can also minimize hypotension. It may be advisable to initiate therapy with a short-acting ACE inhibitor, such as captopril, and subsequently switch to a longer-acting agent, such as lisinopril or enalapril, once the patient is stabilized.

Hyperkalemia results from reduced AT_2-stimulated aldosterone release. The risk of hyperkalemia with ACE inhibitors is also increased in HF due to a propensity for impaired renal function and additive effects with aldosterone antagonists. The ACE inhibitor dose may need to be decreased or held if serum potassium increases above 5 mEq/L (5 mmol/L). Persistent hyperkalemia in the setting of renal insufficiency may preclude the use of an ACE inhibitor.

Cough is commonly seen with ACE inhibitors (5–15%) and may be related to accumulation of tissue bradykinins.[5] It can be challenging to distinguish an ACE inhibitor-induced cough from cough caused by pulmonary congestion. A productive or wet cough usually signifies congestion, whereas a dry, hacking cough is more indicative of a drug-related etiology. If a cough is determined to be ACE inhibitor-induced, its severity should be evaluated before deciding on a course of action. If the cough is truly bothersome, a trial with a different ACE inhibitor or switching to an ARB is warranted.

ARBs ARBs selectively antagonize the effects of AT_2 directly at the AT_1-receptor. AT_1-receptor stimulation is associated with vasoconstriction, release of aldosterone, and cellular growth promoting effects, while AT_2 stimulation causes vasodilation. By selectively blocking AT_1 but leaving AT_2 unaffected, ARBs block the detrimental AT_1 effects on cardiac function while allowing AT_2-mediated vasodilation and inhibition of ventricular remodeling. ARBs are considered an equally effective replacement for ACE inhibitors in patients who are intolerant or have a contraindication to an ACE inhibitor.

It was hoped that the more complete blockade of AT_2's AT_1 effects would confer greater long-term efficacy with ARBs compared to ACE inhibitors. However, prospective, randomized trials suggest that the clinical efficacy of ARBs is similar to that of ACE inhibitors for reduction of hospitalizations for HF, sudden cardiac death, and all-cause mortality.[23-25] Despite poorer suppression of AT_2, comparable efficacy of ACE inhibitors may be due to the additional effects on the kallikrein-kinin system. Although ARBs produce hemodynamic and neurohormonal effects similar to those of ACE inhibitors, they are considered second-line therapy due to the overwhelming clinical trial experience with ACE inhibitors.

Because the mechanism for long-term benefit appears different for ACE inhibitors and ARBs, the combination has been studied for additive benefits. One study evaluated the addition of the ARB candesartan versus placebo in HF patients with systolic dysfunction intolerant to an ACE inhibitor, systolic dysfunction currently on ACE inhibitor therapy, or patients with preserved systolic function.[25] Candesartan reduced the combined incidence of cardiovascular death and hospitalization for HF in all three groups; the greatest benefit was noted in those not on an ACE inhibitor. Candesartan significantly decreased mortality compared to placebo when all three groups were combined. Based on this study, the addition of an ARB to ACE inhibitor therapy can be considered in patients with evidence of disease progression despite optimal ACE inhibitor therapy.[1] This study also demonstrates the importance of having some form of AT_2 antagonism as part of a treatment regimen.

ARBs show similar tolerability to ACE inhibitors with regard to hypotension and hyperkalemia, but they have markedly less incidence of cough as ARBs do not cause an accumulation of bradykinin. ARBs can be considered in patients with ACE inhibitor-induced angioedema, but they should be initiated cautiously, as cross-reactivity has been reported. Many of the other considerations for the use of ARBs are similar to those of ACE inhibitors, including the need for monitoring renal function, BP, and potassium. Contraindications are similar to those of ACE inhibitors. In patients truly intolerant or contraindicated to ACE inhibitors or ARBs, the combination of hydralazine and isosorbide dinitrate should be considered.

Hydralazine and Isosorbide Dinitrate Complementary hemodynamic actions originally led to the combination of nitrates with hydralazine. Nitrates reduce preload by causing primarily venous vasodilation through activating guanylate cyclase and a subsequent increase in cGMP in vascular smooth muscle. Hydralazine reduces afterload through direct arterial smooth muscle relaxation via an unknown mechanism. More recently, nitric oxide has been implicated in modulating numerous pathophysiologic processes in the failing heart, including inflammation, cardiac remodeling, and oxidative damage. Supplementation of nitric oxide via administration of nitrates has also been proposed as a mechanism for benefit from this combination therapy. The beneficial effect of an external nitric oxide source may be more apparent in the African American population, which appears to be predisposed to having an imbalance in nitric oxide production. In addition, hydralazine may reduce the development of nitrate tolerance when nitrates are given chronically.

The combination of hydralazine and isosorbide dinitrate was the first therapy shown to improve long-term survival in patients with systolic HF, but has largely been supplanted by AT_2 antagonist therapy (ACE inhibitors and ARBs).[26,27] Therefore, until recently, this combination therapy was reserved for patients intolerant to ACE inhibitors or ARBs secondary to renal impairment, angioedema, or hyperkalemia. New insight into the pathophysiologic role of nitric oxide has reinvigorated research into this combination therapy.

The nitrate-hydralazine combination was first shown to improve survival compared to placebo.[26] Subsequently, the combination of isosorbide dinitrate 40 mg and hydralazine 75 mg, both given four times daily, was compared to the ACE inhibitor enalapril.[27] Enalapril produced a 28% greater decrease in mortality. Therefore, the combination is considered a third-line vasodilatory option for patients truly intolerant of ACE inhibitors and ARBs.

More recently, the value of adding the combination of isosorbide dinitrate 40 mg and hydralazine 75 mg three times daily to therapy including ACE inhibitors, β-blockers, digoxin, and diuretics was shown in a prospective, randomized trial in African American patients.[28] ❾ *Combination therapy with hydralazine and isosorbide dinitrate is an appropriate substitute for AT$_2$ antagonism in those unable to tolerate an ACE inhibitor or ARB or as add-on therapy in African Americans. The ACC/AHA HF guidelines now recommend considering the addition of isosorbide dinitrate and hydralazine in African Americans already on ACE inhibitors or ARBs.*[1] Combination therapy with isosorbide dinitrate and hydralazine should be initiated and titrated as are other neurohormonal agents such as ACE inhibitors and β-blockers. Low doses are used to initiate therapy with subsequent titration of the dose toward target doses based on tolerability. Adverse effects such as hypotension and headache cause frequent discontinuations in patients taking this combination, and full doses often cannot be tolerated. Patients should be monitored for headache, hypotension, and tachycardia. Hydralazine is also associated with a dose-dependent risk for lupus.

The frequent dosing of isosorbide dinitrate (e.g., three of four times daily) is not conducive to patient adherence; therefore, a once-daily isosorbide mononitrate is commonly substituted for isosorbide dinitrate to simplify the dosing regimen. A nitrate-free interval is still required when using nitrates for HF.

β-Adrenergic Antagonists β-Adrenergic antagonists, or β-blockers, competitively block the influence of the SNS at β-adrenergic receptors. As recently as 15 years ago, β-adrenergic blockers were thought to be detrimental in HF due to their negative inotropic actions, which could potentially worsen symptoms and cause acute decompensations. Since then, the benefits of inhibiting the SNS have been recognized as far outweighing the acute negative inotropic effects. Chronic β-blockade reduces ventricular mass, improves ventricular shape, and reduces LV end-systolic and diastolic volumes.[6,8] β-Blockers also exhibit antiarrhythmic effects, slow or reverse catecholamine-induced ventricular remodeling, decrease myocyte death from catecholamine-induced necrosis or apoptosis, and prevent myocardial fetal gene expression. Consequently, β-blockers improve EF, reduce all-cause and HF-related hospitalizations, and decrease all-cause mortality in patients with systolic HF.[29–33]

The ACC/AHA recommends that β-blockers be initiated in all patients with NYHA FC I to IV or ACC/AHA stages B through D HF if clinically stable.[1] To date, only three β-blockers have been shown to reduce mortality in systolic HF, including the selective β$_1$-antagonists bisoprolol and metoprolol succinate, and the nonselective β$_1$-, β$_2$-, and α$_1$-antagonist carvedilol.[29–33] The positive findings of β-blockers are not a class effect, as bucindolol did not exhibit a beneficial effect on mortality when studied for HF, and there is limited information with propranolol and atenolol.

Although metoprolol and carvedilol are the most commonly used β-antagonists in HF, it is unknown whether one agent should be considered first-line. To compare their relative effects on patient outcomes, one study compared immediate-release metoprolol tartrate to carvedilol in 3,000 patients with mild to severe HF.[33] Carvedilol lowered all-cause mortality significantly more than metoprolol tartrate. However, there are questions about the validity of using immediate-release metoprolol tartrate as the comparison agent, and the low average dose of metoprolol tartrate achieved in the study.

The key to utilizing β-blockers in systolic HF is initiation with low doses and slow titration to target doses over weeks to months. It is important that the β-blocker be initiated when a patient is clinically stable and euvolemic. Volume overload at the time of β-blocker initiation increases the risk for worsening symptoms. β-Blockade should begin with the lowest possible dose (Table 6–7), after which the dose may be doubled every 2 to 4 weeks depending on patient tolerability. β-Blockers may cause an acute decrease in left ventricular ejection fraction (LVEF) and short-term worsening of HF symptoms upon initiation and at each dosage titration. After each dose titration, if the patient experiences symptomatic hypotension, bradycardia, orthostasis, or worsening symptoms, further increases in dose should be withheld until the patient stabilizes. After stabilization, attempts to increase the dose should be reinstituted. If mild congestion ensues as a result of the β-blocker, an increase in diuretic dose may be warranted. If moderate or severe symptoms of congestion occur, a reduction in β-blocker dose should be considered along with an increase in diuretic dose. Dose titration should continue until target clinical trial doses are achieved (Table 6–7) or until limited by repeated hemodynamic or symptomatic intolerance. Patient education regarding the possibility of acutely worsening symptoms but improved long-term function and survival is essential to ensure adherence.

Apart from possible clinical differences between the β-blockers approved for HF, selection of a β-blocker may also be affected by pharmacologic differences. Carvedilol exhibits a more pronounced BP lowering effect and thus causes more frequent dizziness and hypotension as a consequence of its β$_1$- and α$_1$-receptor blocking activities. Therefore, in patients predisposed to symptomatic hypotension, such as those with advanced LV dysfunction (LVEF less than 20%) who normally exhibit low systolic BPs, metoprolol succinate may be the more desirable first-line β-blocker. In patients with uncontrolled hypertension, carvedilol may provide additional antihypertensive efficacy.

β-Blockers may be used by those with reactive airway disease or peripheral vascular disease, but should be used with considerable caution or avoided if patients display active respiratory symptoms. Care must also be used in interpreting SOB in these patients, as the etiology could be either cardiac or pulmonary. A selective β_1-blocker such as metoprolol is a reasonable option for patients with reactive airway disease. The risk versus benefit of using any β-blocker in peripheral vascular disease must be weighed based on the severity of the peripheral disease.

Both metoprolol and carvedilol are metabolized by the liver through cytochrome P-450 (CYP450) 2D6 and undergo extensive first-pass metabolism. β-Blockers should not be used in patients with severe hepatic failure. Bisoprolol is not as commonly used since it is not FDA-approved for this use.

Aldosterone Antagonists Currently, the aldosterone antagonists available are spironolactone and eplerenone. Both agents are inhibitors of aldosterone that produce weak diuretic effects while sparing potassium concentrations. Eplerenone is selective for the mineralocorticoid receptor and hence does not exhibit the endocrine adverse-effect profile commonly seen with spironolactone. The initial rationale for specifically targeting aldosterone for treatment of HF was based on the knowledge that ACE inhibitors do not suppress the chronic production and release of aldosterone. Aldosterone is a key pathologic neurohormone that exerts multiple detrimental effects in HF. Similar to norepinephrine and AT_2, aldosterone levels are increased in HF and have been shown to correlate with disease severity and patient outcomes.

Each agent (spironolactone and eplerenone) has been studied in a defined population of patients with HF. One study established efficacy with low-dose spironolactone in NYHA FC III and IV HF patients in reducing HF hospitalizations, improving functional class, reducing sudden cardiac death, and improving all-cause mortality.[34] Another study investigated the use of eplerenone in patients within 14 days of MI and LVEF less than 40%.[35] Eplerenone was found to decrease mortality as well as cardiovascular death and related hospitalization, mainly due to reducing occurrence of sudden cardiac death. Based on these two studies, the ACC/AHA guidelines recommend that the addition of spironolactone be considered in NYHA FC III and IV (ACC/AHA stages C and D) patients, and eplerenone in directly post-MI patients with evidence of LV dysfunction.[1]

The major risk related to aldosterone antagonists is hyperkalemia. Therefore, the decision for use of these agents should balance the benefit of decreasing death and hospitalization from HF and the potential risks of life-threatening hyperkalemia. Before and within 1 week of initiating therapy, two parameters must be assessed: serum potassium and CrCl (or serum creatinine). Aldosterone antagonists should not be initiated in patients with potassium concentrations greater than 5.5 mEq/L (5.5 mmol/L). Likewise, these agents should not be given when CrCl is less than 30 mL/min or serum creatinine is greater than 2.5 mg/dL (221 µmol/L).

In patients without contraindications, spironolactone is initiated at a dose of 12.5 to 25 mg daily, or occasionally on alternate days for patients with baseline renal insufficiency. Eplerenone is used at a dose of 25 mg daily, with the option to titrate up to 50 mg daily. Doses should be halved or switched to alternate-day dosing if CrCl falls below 50 mL/min. Potassium supplementation is often decreased or stopped after aldosterone antagonists are initiated, and patients should be counseled to avoid high-potassium foods. At any time after initiation of therapy, if potassium concentrations exceed 5.5 mEq/L (5.5 mmol/L), the dose of the aldosterone antagonist should be reduced or discontinued. In addition, worsening renal function dictates consideration for stopping the aldosterone antagonist. Other adverse effects observed mainly with spironolactone include gynecomastia for men and breast tenderness and menstrual irregularities for women. Gynecomastia leads to discontinuation in up to 10% of patients on spironolactone. Eplerenone is a CYP3A4 substrate and should not be used concomitantly with strong inhibitors of 3A4.

▶ *Digoxin*

Digoxin has been used for several decades in the treatment of HF. Traditionally, it was considered useful for its positive inotropic effects, but more recently its benefits are thought to be related to neurohormonal modulation. Digoxin exerts positive inotropic effects through binding to sodium- and potassium-activated adenosine triphosphate (ATP) pumps, leading to increased intracellular sodium concentrations and subsequently more available intracellular calcium during systole. The mechanism of digoxin's neurohormonal blocking effect is less well understood, but may be related to restoration of baroreceptor sensitivity and reduced central sympathetic outflow.[5]

The exact role of digoxin in therapy remains controversial largely due to disagreement on the risk versus benefit of routinely using this drug in patients with systolic HF. Digoxin was shown to decrease HF-related hospitalizations but did not decrease HF progression or improve survival.[36] Moreover, digoxin was associated with an increased risk for concentration related toxicity and numerous adverse effects. Post hoc study analyses demonstrated a clear relationship between digoxin plasma concentration and outcomes. Concentrations below 1.2 ng/mL (1.5 nmol/L) were associated with no apparent adverse effect on survival, whereas higher concentrations increased the relative risk of mortality.[37,38]

Current recommendations are for the addition of digoxin for patients who remain symptomatic despite an optimal HF regimen consisting of an ACE inhibitor or ARB, β-blocker, and diuretic. In patients with concomitant atrial fibrillation, digoxin may be added to slow ventricular rate regardless of HF symptomology.

Digoxin is initiated at a dose of 0.125 to 0.25 mg daily depending on age, renal function, weight, and risk for toxicity. The lower dose should be used if the patient satisfies any of the following criteria: over 65 years of age, CrCl less than 60 mL/min, or ideal body weight less than 70 kg (154 lb). The 0.125 mg daily dose is adequate in the majority of patients. Doses are halved or switched to alternate-day dosing in patients with moderate to severe renal failure. The desired concentration range for digoxin is 0.5 to 1.2 ng/mL (0.64–1.5 nmol/L), preferably with concentrations at or less than 0.8 ng/mL (1 nmol/L). Routine monitoring of serum drug concentrations is not required but recommended in those with changes in renal function, suspected toxicity, or after addition or subtraction of an interacting drug.

Digoxin toxicity may manifest as nonspecific findings such as fatigue or weakness, and other CNS effects such as confusion, delirium, and psychosis. GI manifestations include nausea, vomiting, or anorexia, and visual disturbances may occur such as halos, photophobia, and color perception problems (red–green or yellow–green vision). Cardiac findings include numerous types of arrhythmias related to enhanced automaticity, slowed or accelerated conduction, or delayed after depolarizations. These include ventricular tachycardia and fibrillation, atrioventricular nodal block, and sinus bradycardia. Risk of digoxin toxicity, in particular the cardiac manifestations, are increased with electrolyte disturbances such as hypokalemia, hypercalcemia, and hypomagnesemia. To reduce the proarrhythmic risk of digoxin, serum potassium and magnesium should be monitored closely and supplemented when appropriate to ensure adequate concentrations (potassium greater than 4.0 mEq/L [4.0 mmol/L] and magnesium greater than 2.0 mEq/L [1 mmol/L]). In patients with life-threatening toxicity due to cardiac or other findings, administration of digoxin-specific Fab antibody fragments usually reverses adverse effects within an hour in most cases.

▶ Calcium Channel Blockers

Treatment with nondihydropyridine calcium channel blockers (diltiazem and verapamil) may worsen HF and increase the risk of death in patients with advanced LV systolic dysfunction due to their negative inotropic effects. Conversely, dihydropyridine calcium channel blockers, although negative inotropes in vitro, do not appear to decrease contractility in vivo. Amlodipine and felodipine are the two most extensively studied dihydropyridine calcium channel blockers for systolic HF.[39,40] These two agents have not been shown to affect patient survival, either positively or negatively. As such, they are not routinely recommended as part of a standard HF regimen; however, amlodipine and felodipine can safely be used in HF patients to treat uncontrolled hypertension or angina once all other appropriate drugs are maximized.

▶ Antiplatelets and Anticoagulation

Patients with HF are at an increased risk of thromboembolic events secondary to a combination of hypercoagulability, relative stasis of blood, and endothelial dysfunction. However, the role of antiplatelets and anticoagulants remains debatable due to a lack of prospective clinical trials.

Aspirin is generally used in HF patients with an underlying ischemic etiology, a history of ischemic heart disease, or other compelling indications such as history of embolic stroke. Routine use in nonischemic cardiomyopathy patients is currently discouraged because of a lack of data supporting any long-term benefit, as well as the potential negative drug–drug interaction with ACE inhibitors and ARBs. If aspirin is indicated, the preference is to use a low dose (81 mg daily).[41]

Current consensus recommendations support the use of warfarin in patients with reduced LV systolic dysfunction and a compelling indication such as atrial fibrillation or prosthetic heart valves.[42] In addition, warfarin is empirically used in patients with echocardiographic evidence of a mural thrombus or severely depressed (LVEF less than 20%) LV function.[43] However, there are limited data supporting the use of empiric warfarin based on echocardiographic findings. Patients with HF often have difficulty maintaining a therapeutic International Normalized Ratio (INR) due to fluctuating volume status and varying drug absorption. Therefore, the benefit of using warfarin should be evaluated in the context of the risk for bleeding.

▶ Complementary and Alternative Medicine

Complementary and alternative medicines (CAM) are treatment strategies not commonly used in Western medicine. Natural health products (NHP) are one component of CAM and are considered nutrition supplements by the FDA. Some patients with HF use NHP for heart problems, weight loss, anxiety, and arthritis. Fish oils, n-3 polyunsaturated fatty acids, or omega-3 fatty acids were recently studied for HF and found to mildly decrease cardiovascular admissions and mortality without significant adverse effects. Fish oils are more commonly used for treatment of hypertriglyceridemia. Their mechanism in HF is incompletely understood, but postulated to involve decreased membrane excitability (thus reducing arrhythmias), decreased inflammation and platelet aggregation, and favorable changes in autonomic tone. Hawthorn is another NHP studied in HF, shown to increase exercise capacity and reduce HF symptoms. Its benefits are thought to be due to flavonoids, which increase force of contraction and CO. The ACC/AHA guidelines do not currently advocate the use of fish oils and hawthorn for HF. It is important to counsel patients to remain on their other HF medications if they decide to initiate a NHP, and to let their health care providers know when starting a new supplement.

HF With Preserved LVEF

It is now recognized that a significant number of patients exhibiting HF symptoms have normal systolic function or preserved LVEF (40–60%). It is believed that the primary defect in these patients is impaired ventricular relaxation and filling, commonly referred to as diastolic dysfunction or diastolic HF. HF with preserved EF is more prevalent in older women and is closely associated with hypertension or diabetes, and to a lesser extent, CAD and atrial fibrillation.[44] Morbidity in HF patients with preserved EF is comparable to those with depressed EF, as both are characterized by frequent, repeated hospitalizations.[44] However, HF with preserved EF is associated with better survival. The diagnosis is based on findings of typical signs and symptoms of HF, in

Patient Encounter, Part 3

Based on the information presented and your problem-based assessment, create a care plan for BE's HF. Your plan should include:

Nonpharmacologic treatment options.

Acute and chronic treatment plans to address BE's symptoms and prevent disease deterioration.

Monitoring plan for acute and chronic treatments.

conjunction with echocardiographic evidence of normal LV systolic function and no valvular disease.

Unlike systolic HF, few prospective trials have evaluated the safety and efficacy of various cardiac medications in patients with diastolic HF or preserved EF. The Candesartan in Heart Failure Assessment of Reduction in Mortality and Morbidity (CHARM) study demonstrated that angiotensin receptor blockade with candesartan resulted in beneficial effects on HF morbidity in patients with preserved LVEF similar to those seen in depressed LV function.[25]

In the absence of more landmark clinical studies, the current treatment approach for diastolic dysfunction or preserved LVEF is: (a) correction or control of underlying etiologies (including optimal treatment of hypertension and CAD and maintenance of normal sinus rhythm); (b) reduction of cardiac filling pressures at rest and during exertion; and (c) increased diastolic filling time. Diuretics are frequently used to control congestion. Recent studies failed to show significant reductions in mortality or hospitalizations with use of ARBs. β-Blockers and calcium channel blockers can theoretically improve ventricular relaxation through negative inotropic and chronotropic effects. Unlike in systolic HF, nondihydropyridine calcium channel blockers (diltiazem and verapamil) may be especially useful in improving diastolic function by limiting the availability of calcium that mediates contractility. A recent study did not find favorable effects with digoxin in patients with mild to moderate diastolic HF. Therefore, the role of digoxin for symptom management and HR control in these patients is not well established.

Special Populations and Patients With Concomitant Disorders

▶ Ethnic and Genetic Considerations

HF is more prevalent and associated with a worse prognosis in African Americans compared to the general population.[1] Unfortunately, deficiencies in disease prevention, detection, and access to treatment are well documented in minority populations. African Americans and other races are underrepresented in clinical trials, compromising the extrapolation of results from these studies to ethnic subpopulations. The influence of race on efficacy and safety of medications used in HF treatment has received additional attention with the

advent of pharmacogenomics (the influence of genetics on drug response). The application of race and genetics to pharmacotherapeutic decision making for HF is in the early stages. However, these concepts are being applied to the use of hydralazine and isosorbide dinitrate in African American patients.[28] It is anticipated that further investigation will lead to better insight relating to the clinical applicability of genetic variations to drug responses.

▶ Peripartum Cardiomyopathy and Pregnancy

Peripartum cardiomyopathy (PPCM) is currently defined as clinical and echocardiographic evidence for new-onset HF occurring during pregnancy and up to 6 months after delivery, with other etiologies excluded. Although PPCM is not well understood, it manifests in pregnant women of all ages, but the risk is elevated in women older than 30 years of age.[45] The true incidence of idiopathic PPCM is debatable, with reported rates for peripartum HF at 1 case per 100 to 4,000 deliveries.[46] The leading hypothesis for PPCM pathogenesis is myocarditis caused by a viral infection or an abnormal immune response to pregnancy. HF may persist after delivery but can be reversible (with partial or full recovery of cardiac function) in many cases.[45]

The clinical presentation of peripartum HF is indistinguishable from that of other types of HF. Initial treatment is also similar, with the exception of ACE inhibitors and ARBs being contraindicated during the antepartum period. Treatment includes reducing preload by sodium restriction and diuretics, afterload reduction with vasodilators, and sometimes inotropic support with digoxin. Hydralazine is utilized frequently in pregnancy and is classified as FDA pregnancy category C. Labetalol is used for acute parenteral control of BP, but long-term β-blocker use corresponds with low birth-weight infants. Management of the cardiomyopathy after delivery includes use of ACE inhibitors and β-blockers, although these treatment guidelines have been extrapolated from studies in patients with idiopathic dilated cardiomyopathy rather than specific trials in PPCM. Patients with PPCM also have a high rate of thromboembolism. Treatment options during pregnancy are limited to unfractionated heparin and low-molecular-weight heparin as warfarin is contraindicated. After delivery, anticoagulation is recommended in patients with LVEF less than 20%.[46]

OUTCOME EVALUATION OF CHRONIC HF

- The evaluation of therapy is influenced by the ability of treatment to successfully reduce symptoms, improve quality of life, decrease frequency of hospitalizations for AHF, reduce disease progression, and prolong survival (Fig. 6–1).

- The major outcome parameters focus on: (a) volume status; (b) exercise tolerance; (c) overall symptoms/quality of life; (d) adverse drug reactions; and (e) disease progression and cardiac function. Assess quality of life by evaluating patients' ability to continue their activities of daily living.

- Assess symptoms of HF such as dyspnea on exertion, orthopnea, weight gain, and edema, and abdominal manifestations such as nausea, bloating, and loss of appetite.
- If diuretic therapy is warranted, monitor for therapeutic response by assessing weight loss and improvement of fluid retention, as well as exercise tolerance and presence of fatigue.
- Once therapy for preventing disease progression is initiated, monitoring for symptomatic improvement continues.
- It is important to keep in mind that patients' symptoms of HF can worsen with β-blockers, and it may take weeks or months before patients notice improvement.
- Monitor BP to evaluate for hypotension caused by drug therapy.
- To assess for prevention of disease progression, practitioners may utilize serial echocardiograms every 6 months to assess cardiac function and evaluate the effects of drug therapy.
- Occasional exercise testing is conducted in order to ascertain disease prognosis or suitability for heart transplant. Even though these tests can demonstrate improvement in heart function and therefore slowed disease progression, patient symptoms may not improve.

ACUTE AND ADVANCED HF

Clinical Presentation and Diagnosis of AHF

Patients with AHF present with symptoms of worsening fluid retention or decreasing exercise tolerance and fatigue (typically worsening of symptoms presented in the chronic HF clinical presentation text box). These symptoms reflect congestion behind the failing ventricle and/or hypoperfusion. Patients can be categorized into hemodynamic subsets based on assessment of physical signs and symptoms of congestion and/or hypoperfusion.[47] Patients can be described as "wet" or "dry" depending on volume status, as well as "warm" or "cool" based on adequacy of tissue perfusion. "Wet" refers to patients with volume/fluid overload (e.g., edema and jugular venous distention [JVD]), whereas "dry" refers to euvolemic patients. "Warm" refers to patients with adequate CO to perfuse peripheral tissues (and hence the skin will be warm to touch), whereas "cool" refers to patients with evidence of hypoperfusion (skin cool to touch with diminished pulses). Additionally, invasive hemodynamic monitoring can be used to provide objective data for assessing volume status (pulmonary capillary wedge pressure [PCWP]) and perfusion (CO). A CI below 2.2 L/min/m² is consistent with hypoperfusion and reduced contractility, and a PCWP above 18 mm Hg correlates with congestion and an elevated preload. The four possible hemodynamic subsets a patient may fall into are "warm and dry," "warm and wet," "cool and dry," or "cool and wet."

Clinical Presentation and Diagnosis of AHF

Subset I (Warm and Dry)

- CI greater than 2.2 L/min/m², pulmonary capillary wedge pressure (PCWP) less than 18 mm Hg
- Patients considered well compensated and perfused, without evidence of congestion
- No immediate interventions necessary except optimizing oral medications and monitoring

Subset II (Warm and Wet)

- CI greater than 2.2 L/min/m², PCWP greater than 18 mm Hg
- Patients adequately perfused and display signs and symptoms of congestion
- Main goal is to reduce preload (PCWP) carefully with loop diuretics and vasodilators

Subset III (Cool and Dry)

- CI less than 2.2 L/min/m², PCWP less than 18 mm Hg
- Patients are inadequately perfused and not congested
- Hypoperfusion leads to increased mortality, elevating death rates fourfold compared to those who are adequately perfused
- Treatment focuses on increasing CO with positive inotropic agents and/or replacing intravascular fluids
- Fluid replacement must be performed cautiously, as patients can rapidly become congested

Subset IV (Cool and Wet)

- CI less than 2.2 L/min/m², PCWP greater than 18 mm Hg
- Patients are inadequately perfused and congested
- Classified as the most complicated clinical presentation of AHF with the worst prognosis
- Most challenging to treat; therapy targets alleviating signs and symptoms of congestion by increasing CI as well as reducing PCWP, while maintaining adequate mean arterial pressure
- Treatment involves a delicate balance among diuretics, vasodilators, and inotropic agents
- Use of vasopressors is sometimes necessary to maintain BP

Clinical Assessment and Diagnosis

▶ Precipitating Factors

❸ *It is important for the clinician to identify the cause(s) of AHF in order to maximize treatment efficacy and reduce future disease exacerbations. Cardiovascular, metabolic, and lifestyle factors can all precipitate AHF. The most common* precipitating factors for acute decompensation and how they contribute pathophysiologically are listed in Table 6–3.

▶ Laboratory Assessment

Routine laboratory testing of patients with AHF includes electrolytes and blood glucose, as well as serum creatinine and blood urea nitrogen to assess renal function. CBC count is measured to determine if anemia or infection is present. Creatine kinase and/or troponin concentrations are used to diagnose ischemia, and hepatic transaminases are measured to assess hepatic congestion. Thyroid function tests are measured to assess hyperthyroidism or hypothyroidism as causes of AHF. A urinalysis is obtained in patients with an unknown history of renal disease to rule out nephrotic syndrome. Lastly, a toxicology screen is obtained in patients in whom use of illicit drugs is suspected.

Assays measuring BNP and its degradation product NT-proBNP are being used with greater frequency in clinical practice.[10] BNP is synthesized, stored, and released from the ventricles in response to increased ventricular filling pressures. Hence, plasma levels of BNP can be used as a marker for volume overload. The most widely accepted indication for BNP measurement is as an adjunctive aid for diagnosing a cardiac etiology for dyspnea.[10]

The current values for ruling out a cardiac etiology for dyspnea are a BNP less than 100 pg/mL (100 ng/L or 28.9 pmol/L) or an NT-proBNP less than 300 pg/mL (300 ng/L or 35.4 pmol/L). BNP measurements require cautious interpretation, as numerous conditions can also elevate BNP concentrations. These include older age, renal dysfunction, pulmonary embolism, and chronic pulmonary disease. Nesiritide, a recombinant BNP drug, has an identical structure to native BNP and will interfere with the commercial BNP assay, resulting in a falsely elevated level. Therefore, blood for BNP determination should be obtained 2 hours after the end of a nesiritide infusion, or alternatively the NT-proBNP assay should be utilized.

Other diagnostic tests should also be obtained in order to help determine precipitating factors (chest radiograph) and to evaluate cardiac function (ECG).

Invasive hemodynamic monitoring in patients with HF entails placement of a right heart or pulmonary artery catheter (PAC). The catheter is inserted percutaneously through a central vein and advanced through the right side of the heart to the pulmonary artery. Inflation of a balloon proximal to the end port allows the catheter to "wedge," yielding the PCWP, which estimates pressures in the left ventricle during diastole. Additionally, CO can be estimated and SVR calculated (Table 6–8).

There are no universally accepted guidelines dictating when invasive monitoring in HF is required. The use of a PAC remains an essential component of management and monitoring of patients in cardiogenic shock; however, the use of inotropic agents does not mandate invasive monitoring. Invasive hemodynamic monitoring is most commonly used to aid in the assessment of hemodynamics when there is disagreement between signs and symptoms and clinical

Table 6–8

Hemodynamic Monitoring: Normal Values

Hemodynamic Variable	Normal Value
Central venous (right atrial) pressure, mean	Less than 5 mm Hg
Right ventricular pressure	25/0 mm Hg
Pulmonary artery pressure	25/10 mm Hg
Pulmonary artery pressure, mean	Less than 18 mm Hg
Pulmonary artery occlusion pressure, mean	Less than 12 mm Hg
Systemic arterial pressure	120/80 mm Hg
Mean arterial pressure	90–120 mm Hg
CI	2.8–4.2 L/min/m^2
SV index	30–65 mL/beat/m^2
SVR	900–1,400 dyn·s·m^{-5}
Pulmonary vascular resistance	150–250 dyn·s·m^{-5}
Arterial oxygen content	20 mL/dL
Mixed venous oxygen content	15 mL/dL
Arteriovenous oxygen content difference	3–5 mL/dL

CI, cardiac index; SV, stroke volume; SVR, systemic vascular resistance.

From Parker RB, Rodgers JE, Cavallari JH. Heart failure. In: DiPiro JT, Talbert RL, Yee GC, et al. (eds.) Pharmacotherapy: A Pathophysiologic Approach, 7th ed. New York: McGraw-Hill, 2008:203.

response. In addition, invasive monitoring is helpful in guiding ongoing therapy for AHF. Invasive monitoring offers the advantage of immediate hemodynamic assessment of an intervention, allowing for prompt adjustments. Risks with PACs include infection, bleeding, thrombosis, catheter malfunction, and ventricular ectopy.

Treatment of AHF

Desired Therapeutic Outcomes

The goals of therapy for AHF are to: (a) correct the underlying precipitating factor(s); (b) relieve the patient's symptoms; (c) improve hemodynamics; (d) optimize a chronic oral medication regimen; and (e) educate the patient, reinforcing adherence to lifestyle modifications and the drug regimen. The ultimate goal for a patient hospitalized for AHF is the return to a compensated HF state and discharge to the outpatient setting on oral medications. Only through aggressive management to achieve all of these goals will a patient's prognosis be improved and future hospitalizations for acute decompensations prevented.

Removal or control of precipitating factors is essential for an optimal response to pharmacologic therapy. Relief of symptoms should occur rapidly to minimize length of hospitalization. Although a rapid discharge from the hospital is desirable, a patient should not be discharged before ensuring that he or she is in a euvolemic, or nearly euvolemic, state with a body weight and functional capacity similar to before the acute decompensation. Oral agents such as β-blockers,

ACE inhibitors or ARBs, and aldosterone antagonists should be initiated as soon as possible during the hospitalization. These chronic oral medications not only improve mortality and prevent readmissions, acutely they also contribute to improvement in hemodynamics. Patient education prior to discharge from the hospital is recommended to assist in minimizing adverse effects and nonadherence. Dissemination of written information, in addition to verbal information, is helpful for patient comprehension and retention. This can include therapy goals, lifestyle modifications, drug regimen, dosage information, and relevant adverse effects, as well as symptom and diary cards.

Pharmacologic Approaches to Treatment

❿ *Treatment of AHF targets relief of congestion and optimization of CO utilizing oral or IV diuretics, IV vasodilators, and when appropriate inotropes based on presenting hemodynamics. Current treatment strategies in AHF target improving hemodynamics while preserving organ function.* A specific treatment approach is formulated depending on the patient's symptoms (congestion versus hypoperfusion) and hemodynamic indices (CI and PCWP).[48,49] If the patient primarily exhibits signs and symptoms of congestion, treatment entails use of diuretics as first-line agents to decrease PCWP. Additionally, IV vasodilators are added to provide rapid relief of congestion and additional reductions in PCWP. By reducing congestion in the heart, cardiac contractile function may improve, which results in an increase in SV and CO, and hence perfusion to vital organs. For patients primarily displaying symptoms of hypoperfusion, treatment relies on use of agents that increase cardiac contractility, known as positive inotropes. Some patients display both symptoms of congestion as well as hypoperfusion, and thus require use of combination therapies. One of the current challenges to the treatment of AHF is achieving hemodynamic improvement without adversely affecting organ function. In the case of inotropes, the increased contractility occurs at the expense of an increase in cardiac workload and proarrhythmia. In addition, high-dose diuretic therapy is associated with worsened renal function and possibly neurohormonal activation.

▶ Diuretics

Loop diuretics, including furosemide, bumetanide, and torsemide, are the diuretics of choice in the management of AHF. Furosemide is the most commonly used agent. Diuretics decrease preload by functional venodilation within 5 to 15 minutes of administration and subsequently by an increase in sodium and water excretion. This provides rapid improvement in symptoms of pulmonary congestion. Diuretics reduce PCWP but do not increase CI as do positive inotropes and arterial vasodilators. Patients who have significant volume overload often have impaired absorption of oral loop diuretics because of intestinal edema or altered transit time. Therefore, doses are usually administered via IV boluses or continuous IV infusions, given either at the same dose as the home oral dose for those taking diuretics regularly or at lower doses for diuretic-naïve patients (Table 6–9). Higher doses may be required for patients with renal insufficiency due to decreased drug delivery to the site of action in the loop of Henle.

There is a paucity of clinical trial evidence comparing the benefit of diuretics to other therapies for symptom relief or long-term outcomes. Additionally, excessive preload reduction can lead to a decrease in CO resulting in reflex increase in sympathetic activation, renin release, and the expected consequences of vasoconstriction, tachycardia, and increased myocardial oxygen demand. Careful use of diuretics is recommended to avoid overdiuresis. Monitoring of serum electrolytes such as potassium, sodium, and magnesium is done frequently to identify and correct imbalances. Monitor serum creatinine and blood urea nitrogen daily at a minimum to assess volume depletion and renal function.

Occasionally, patients with HF do not respond to a diuretic, defined as failure to achieve a weight reduction of at least 0.5 kg (1.1 lb; or negative net fluid balance of at least 500 mL) after several increasing bolus doses.[17]

Several strategies are employed to overcome diuretic resistance. These include using larger oral doses, converting to IV dosing, or increasing the frequency of administration. Small studies using low-dose continuous infusions of furosemide and torsemide have shown an increase in urine output compared to intermittent bolus dosing.[50] Continuous infusions may provide a theoretical advantage of continuous presence of high drug levels within the tubular lumen, causing a sustained natriuresis. Most regimens include a bolus dose followed by a maintenance infusion (Table 6–9).[51] Another useful strategy is to combine two diuretics with different sites of action within the nephron. The most common combination is the use of a loop diuretic with a

Table 6–9					
IV Diuretics Used to Treat HF-Related Fluid Retention					
	Onset of Action (minutes)	Duration of Action (hours)	Relative Potency	Intermittent Bolus Dosing (mg)	Continuous Infusion Dosing (Bolus/Infusion)
Furosemide	2–5	6	40	20–200+	20–40/2.5–10
Torsemide	Less than 10	6–12	20	10–100	20/2–5
Bumetanide	2–3	4–6	0.5	1–10	1–4/0.5–1
Ethacrynic acid	5–15	2–7		0.5–1 mg/kg/dose up to 100 mg/dose	

thiazide diuretic such as metolazone. Combining diuretics should be used with caution due to an increased risk for cardiovascular collapse due to rapid intravascular volume depletion. Strict monitoring of electrolytes, vital signs, and fluid balance is warranted.

Finally, poor CO may contribute to diuretic resistance. In these patients, it may become necessary to add vasodilators or inotropes to enhance perfusion to the kidneys. Care must be taken, as vasodilators can decrease renal blood flow despite increasing CO through dilation of central and peripheral vascular beds.

▶ Vasodilators

IV vasodilators cause a rapid decrease in arterial tone, resulting in a decrease in SVR and a subsequent increase in SV and CO. Additionally, vasodilators reduce ventricular filling pressures (PCWP) within 24 to 48 hours, reduce myocardial oxygen consumption, and decrease ventricular workload. Vasodilators are commonly used in patients presenting with AHF accompanied by moderate to severe congestion. This class includes nitroglycerin, nitroprusside, and nesiritide. Hemodynamic effects and dosages for these agents are included in Tables 6–10 and 6–11, respectively. Although vasodilators are generally safe and effective, identification of the proper patient for use is important to minimize the risk of significant hypotension. In addition, vasodilators are contraindicated in patients whose cardiac filling (and hence CO) depends on venous return or intravascular volume, as well as patients who present with shock.

Nitroglycerin Nitroglycerin acts as a source of nitric oxide, which induces smooth muscle relaxation in venous and arterial vascular beds. Nitroglycerin is primarily a venous vasodilator at lower doses, but exerts potent arterial vasodilatory effects at higher doses. Thus, at lower doses, nitroglycerin causes decreases in preload (or filling pressures) and improved coronary blood flow. At higher doses (greater than 100 mcg/min), additional reduction in preload is achieved, along with a decrease in afterload and subsequent increase in SV and CO. IV nitroglycerin is primarily used as a preload reducer for patients exhibiting pulmonary

Table 6–11
Usual Doses and Monitoring of Commonly Used Hemodynamic Medications

Drug	Dose	Monitoring Variables[a]
Dopamine	0.5–10 mcg/kg/min	BP, HR, urinary output and kidney function, ECG, extremity perfusion (higher doses only)
Dobutamine	2.5–20 mcg/kg/min	BP, HR urinary output and function, ECG
Milrinone	0.375–0.75 mcg/kg/min	BP, HR, urinary output and function, ECG, changes in ischemic symptoms (e.g., chest pain), electrolytes
Nitroprusside	0.1–3 mcg/kg/min	BP, HR, liver and kidney function, blood cyanide and/or thiocyanate concentrations if toxicity suspected (nausea, vomiting, altered mental function)
Nitroglycerin	5–200+ mcg/kg/min	BP, HR, ECG, changes in ischemic symptoms
Nesiritide	Bolus: 2 mcg/kg; Infusion: 0.01 mcg/kg/min	BP, HR, urinary output and kidney function, blood BNP concentrations

BNP, B-type natriuretic peptide; BP, blood pressure; HR, heart rate.

[a]In addition to pulmonary capillary wedge pressure and cardiac output.

congestion or in combination with inotropes for congested patients with severely reduced CO.[52]

Continuous infusions of nitroglycerin should be initiated at a dose of 5 to 10 mcg/min and increased every 5 to 10 minutes until symptomatic or hemodynamic improvement. Effective doses range from 35 to 200 mcg/min. The most common adverse events reported are headache, dose-related hypotension, and tachycardia. A limitation to nitroglycerin's use is the development of tachyphylaxis, or tolerance to its effects, which can be evident within 12 hours after initiation of continuous infusion and necessitate additional titrations to higher doses.

Nitroprusside Nitroprusside, like nitroglycerin, causes the formation of nitric oxide and vascular smooth muscle relaxation. In contrast to nitroglycerin, nitroprusside is both a venous and arterial vasodilator regardless of dosage. Nitroprusside causes a pronounced decrease in PCWP, SVR, and BP, with a modest increase in CO. Nitroprusside has been studied to a limited extent in AHF and no studies have evaluated its effects on mortality.[48] Nitroprusside is initiated at 0.1 to 0.25 mcg/kg/min, followed by dose adjustments in 0.1 to 0.2 mcg/kg/min increments if necessary to achieve desired effect. Because of its rapid onset of action and metabolism, nitroprusside is administered as a continuous infusion that is easy to titrate and provides predictable hemodynamic effects. Nitroprusside requires strict

Table 6–10
Usual Hemodynamic Effects of Commonly Used IV Agents for Treatment of Acute or Severe HF

Drug	CO	PCWP	SVR	BP	HR
Diuretics	↑/↓/0	↓		↓	0
Nitroglycerin	↑	↓↓	↓	↓↓	↑/0
Nitroprusside	↑	↓↓↓	↓↓↓	↓↓↓	↑
Nesiritide	↑	↓↓	↓↓	↓↓	0
Dobutamine	↑↑	↓/0	↓/0	↓/0	↑↑
Milrinone	↑↑	↓↓	↓	↓	↑

BP, blood pressure; CO, cardiac output; HR, heart rate; PCWP, pulmonary capillary wedge pressure; SVR, systemic vascular resistance; ↑, increase; ↓, decrease; 0, no or little change.

monitoring of BP and HR. Nitroprusside's use is limited in AHF due to recommended hemodynamic monitoring with an arterial line and mandatory intensive care unit admission at many institutions. Abrupt withdrawal of therapy should be avoided, as rebound neurohormonal activation may occur. Therefore, the dose should be tapered slowly. Nitroprusside has the potential to cause cyanide and thiocyanate toxicity, especially in patients with hepatic and renal insufficiency, respectively. Toxicity is most common with use longer than 3 days and with higher doses. Nitroprusside should be avoided in patients with active ischemia, because its powerful afterload-reducing effects within the myocardium can "steal" coronary blood flow from myocardial segments that are supplied by epicardial vessels with high-grade lesions.

Nesiritide BNP is an endogenous neurohormone that is synthesized and released from the ventricles in response to chamber wall stretch or increased filling pressures. Recombinant BNP, or nesiritide, is the newest compound developed for AHF. Nesiritide binds to guanylate cyclase receptors in vascular smooth muscle and endothelial cells, causing an increase in cGMP concentrations leading to vasodilation (venous and arterial) and natriuresis. Nesiritide also antagonizes the effects of the RAAS and ET. Nesiritide reduces PCWP, right atrial pressure, and SVR. Consequently, it also increases SV and CO without affecting HR. Continuous infusions result in sustained effects for 24 hours without tachyphylaxis, although experience with its use beyond 72 hours is limited.

Nesiritide has been shown to improve symptoms of dyspnea and fatigue. In a randomized clinical trial,[53] nesiritide was found to significantly decrease PCWP more than nitroglycerin and placebo over 3 hours. Nesiritide improved patients' self-reported dyspnea scores compared to placebo at 3 hours, but there was no difference compared to nitroglycerin. There are no prospective mortality studies with nesiritide in AHF.

Currently, nesiritide is indicated for patients with AHF exhibiting dyspnea at rest or with minimal activity. The recommended dose regimen is a bolus of 2 mcg/kg, followed by a continuous infusion for up to 24 hours of 0.01 mcg/kg/min. Because nesiritide's effects are predictable and sustained at the recommended dosage, titration of the infusion rate (maximum of 0.03 mcg/kg/min) is not commonly required nor is invasive hemodynamic monitoring. Nesiritide should be avoided in patients with systolic BP less than 90 mm Hg. Although nesiritide's place in AHF therapy is not firmly defined, it is used as one of the first-line agents (in combination with diuretics) for many patients presenting in moderate to severe decompensation, mainly due to its proven benefits and unique mechanism of action. One potential disadvantage compared to other vasodilators is its longer half-life. If hypotension occurs, the effect can be prolonged (2 hours). There are also concerns relating to elevations in serum creatinine observed with nesiritide; however, whether this effect is clinically relevant remains unanswered.

▶ Inotropic Agents

Currently available positive inotropic agents act via increasing intracellular cyclic adenosine monophosphate (cAMP) concentrations through different mechanisms. β-Agonists activate adenylate cyclase through stimulation of β-adrenergic receptors, which subsequently catalyzes the conversion of ATP to cAMP. In contrast, phosphodiesterase inhibitors reduce degradation of cAMP. The resulting elevation in cAMP levels leads to enhanced phospholipase activity, which then increases the rate and extent of calcium influx during systole, thereby enhancing contractility. Additionally, during diastole, cAMP promotes uptake of calcium by the sarcoplasmic reticulum which improves cardiac relaxation. The inotropes approved for use in AHF are discussed in the following sections. Inotropes have been associated with increased risk for arrhythmias and higher mortality rates, and therefore require careful monitoring.

Dobutamine Dobutamine has historically been the inotrope of choice for AHF. As a synthetic catecholamine, it acts as an agonist mainly on β_1- and β_2-receptors and minimally on α_1-receptors. The resulting hemodynamic effects are due to both receptor- and reflex-mediated activities. These effects include increased contractility and HR through β_1- (and β_2-) receptors and vasodilation through a relatively greater effect on β_2- than α_1-receptors. Dobutamine can increase, decrease, or cause little change in mean arterial pressure depending on whether the resulting increase in CO is enough to offset the modest vasodilation. Although dobutamine displays a half-life of approximately 2 minutes, its positive hemodynamic effects can be observed for several days to months after administration. The use of dobutamine is supported by several small studies documenting improved hemodynamics, but large-scale clinical trials in AHF are lacking.[54]

Dobutamine is initiated at a dose of 2.5 to 5 mcg/kg/min, which can be gradually titrated to 20 mcg/kg/min based on clinical response. There are several practical considerations to dobutamine therapy in AHF. First, owing to its vasodilatory potential, monotherapy with dobutamine is reserved for patients with systolic BPs greater than 90 mm Hg. However, it is commonly used in combination with vasopressors in patients with lower systolic BPs. Second, due to downregulation of β_1-receptors or uncoupling of β_2-receptors from adenylate cyclase with prolonged exposure to dobutamine, attenuation of hemodynamic effects has been reported to occur as early as 48 hours after initiation of a continuous infusion, although tachyphylaxis is more evident with use spanning longer than 72 hours. Full sensitivity to dobutamine's effects can be restored 7 to 10 days after the drug is withdrawn. Third, many patients with AHF will be taking β-blockers on a chronic basis. Because of β-blockers' high affinity for β-receptors, the effectiveness of β-agonists such as dobutamine will be reduced. In patients on β-blocker therapy, it is recommended that consideration be given to the use of phosphodiesterase inhibitors such as milrinone, which are not dependent on β-receptors for effect.[55,56] Although commonly practiced, use of high doses of dobutamine to overcome the β-blockade should be discouraged, as this negates any of the protective benefits of the β-blocker.

Dopamine Dopamine is most commonly reserved for patients with low systolic BPs and those approaching cardiogenic shock. It may also be used in low doses (less than 3 mcg/kg/min) to improve renal function in a patient with inadequate urine output despite high filling pressures and volume overload, although this indication is controversial.

Dopamine exerts its effects through direct stimulation of adrenergic receptors, as well as release of norepinephrine from adrenergic nerve terminals. Dopamine produces hemodynamic effects that differ based on dosing. At lower doses, dopamine stimulates dopamine type 1 (D1) receptors and thus increases renal perfusion. Positive inotropic effects are more pronounced at doses of 3 to 10 mcg/kg/min. CI is increased due to increased SV and HR. At doses higher than 10 mcg/kg/min, chronotropic and α_1-mediated vasoconstriction effects are evident. This causes an increase in mean arterial pressure due to higher CI and SVR. The ultimate effect on cardiac hemodynamics will depend largely on the dosage prescribed and must be individually tailored to the patient's clinical status. Dopamine is generally associated with an increase in CO and BP, with a concomitant increase in PCWP. Dopamine increases myocardial oxygen demand and may decrease coronary blood flow through vasoconstriction and increased wall tension. As with other inotropes, dopamine is associated with a risk for arrhythmias.

Phosphodiesterase Inhibitors Milrinone and inamrinone work by inhibiting phosphodiesterase III, the enzyme responsible for the breakdown of cAMP. The increase in cAMP levels leads to increased intracellular calcium concentrations and enhanced contractile force generation. Milrinone has replaced inamrinone as the phosphodiesterase inhibitor of choice due to the higher frequency of thrombocytopenia seen with inamrinone.

Milrinone has both positive inotropic and vasodilating properties and as such is referred to as an "inodilator." Its vasodilating activities are especially prominent on venous capacitance vessels and pulmonary vascular beds, although a reduction in arterial tone is also noted. IV administration results in an increase in SV and CO, and usually only minor changes in HR. Milrinone also lowers PCWP through venodilation. Routine use of milrinone during acute decompensations in NYHA FC II to IV HF is not recommended, and milrinone use remains limited to patients who require inotropic support.[57]

Dosing recommendations for milrinone include a loading dose of 50 mcg/kg, followed by an infusion beginning at 0.5 mcg/kg/min (range 0.23 mcg/kg/min for patients with renal failure up to 0.75 mcg/kg/min). A loading dose is not necessary if immediate hemodynamic effects are not required or if patients have low systolic BPs (less than 90 mm Hg). Decreases in BP during an infusion may necessitate dose reductions as well. Lower doses are also used in patients with renal insufficiency.

Milrinone is a good option for patients requiring an inotrope who are also chronically receiving β-blockers, as the inotropic effects are achieved independent of β-adrenergic receptors. However, milrinone exhibits a long distribution and elimination half-life compared to β-agonists, thus requiring a loading dose when an immediate response is desired. Potential adverse effects include hypotension, arrhythmias, and less commonly, thrombocytopenia. Milrinone should not be used in patients in whom vasodilation is contraindicated.

Mechanical, Surgical, and Device Therapies

▶ Implantable Cardioverter Defibrillators

Implantable cardioverter defibrillators (ICDs) are the most effective modality for primary and secondary prevention of sudden cardiac death in patients with LV dysfunction. Studies universally demonstrate greater efficacy compared to antiarrhythmic therapy and a significant reduction in mortality compared to placebo.[58-60] Recent studies have expanded the eligible patient populations beyond classic indications, such as prior MI and nonsustained ventricular tachycardia or nonsuppressible ventricular tachycardia during an electrophysiologic study. A clear advantage of implanting ICDs in all symptomatic patients with LVEF less than 35% regardless of etiology or other cardiac parameters has been demonstrated.[60] Because ICD implantation and follow-up is associated with a significant economic burden, the cost effectiveness of widespread ICD use continues to be debated. Defining subgroups that would derive the greatest benefit and determining the optimal ICD configuration will aid in improving the potential costs compared to benefits.

▶ Cardiac Resynchronization Therapy

Dyssynchronous contraction, as a reflection of intra- and interventricular conduction delays between chambers of the heart, is common in advanced HF patients. Dyssynchrony contributes to diminished cardiac function and unfavorable myocardial energetics through altered filling times, valvular dysfunction, and wall motion defects. Cardiac resynchronization therapy (CRT) with biventricular pacing devices improves cardiac function, quality of life, and mortality in patients with NYHA FC III or IV HF, evidence of intraventricular conduction delay (QRS greater than 120 msec), depressed LV function (LVEF less than 35%), and on an optimal pharmacologic regimen. A recent study also showed that the addition of an ICD to CRT with biventricular pacing further reduced hospitalizations and mortality.[61]

▶ Intra-aortic Balloon Counterpulsation

Intra-aortic balloon counterpulsation (IABC) or intra-aortic balloon pumps (IABPs) are one of the most widely used mechanical circulatory assistance devices for patients with cardiac failure who do not respond to standard therapies. An IABP is placed percutaneously into the femoral artery and advanced to the high descending thoracic aorta. Once in

Patient Encounter, Part 4

After 6 months, BE returns to clinic complaining of extreme SOB with any activity, including dressing and showering, as well as at rest. She sleeps sitting up due to severe orthopnea, is unable to eat without nausea, and states she has gained 10 kg (22 lb) from her baseline weight. She also states that she does not feel her furosemide therapy is working. She is admitted to the cardiology unit.

SH: BE admits to resuming smoking after quitting for 2 months; additionally, she has been eating out in restaurants more often in the past 2 weeks.

Meds: Lisinopril 10 mg once daily; furosemide 80 mg twice daily; glipizide 10 mg twice daily for diabetes; metformin 1,000 mg twice daily for diabetes; nitroglycerin 0.4 mg sublingual (SL) as needed; multivitamin daily; Aspirin 325 mg daily

VS: BP 146/94 mm Hg, pulse 102 bpm and regular, RR 22/min, temperature 37°C (98.6°F), Wt 123 kg (271 lb), BMI 41.2

Lungs: There are rales present bilaterally

CV: RRR with normal S_1 and S_2; there is an S_3 and an S_4; a 4/6 systolic ejection murmur is present and heard best at the left lower sternal border; point of maximal impulse is displaced laterally; jugular veins are distended, JVP is 11 cm above sternal angle; a positive HJR is observed

Abd: Hard, tender, and bowel sounds are absent; 3+ pitting edema of extremities is observed

CXR: Bilateral pleural effusions and cardiomegaly

Echo: EF 20%

Labs: BNP 740 pg/mL (740 ng/L or 214 pmol/L), K 4.2 mEq/L (4.2 mmol/L), BUN 64 mg/dL (23 mmol/L), SCr 2.4 mg/dL (212 mmol/L), Mg 1.8 mEq/L (0.9 mmol/L)

A pulmonary catheter is placed, revealing the following: PCWP 37 mm Hg; CI 2.2 L/min/m²

What NYHA FC, ACC/AHA stage, and hemodynamic subset is BE currently in?

What are your initial treatment goals?

What pharmacologic agents are appropriate to use at this time?

Identify a monitoring plan to assess for efficacy and toxicity of the recommended drug therapy.

Once BE's symptoms are improved, how would you optimize her oral medication therapy for HF?

(afterload). As such, IABC increases myocardial oxygen supply and decreases oxygen demand. This device has many indications including cardiogenic shock, high-risk unstable angina in conjunction with percutaneous interventions, preoperative stabilization of high-risk patients prior to surgery, and patients who cannot be weaned from cardiopulmonary bypass. Possible complications include infection, bleeding, thrombosis, limb ischemia, and device malfunction. The device is typically useful for short-term therapy due to the invasiveness of the device, the need for limb immobilization, and the requirement for anticoagulation.

▶ *Ventricular Assist Device*

The ventricular assist device (VAD) is a surgically implanted pump that reduces or replaces the work of the right, left, or both ventricles. VADs are currently indicated for short-term support in patients refractory to pharmacologic therapies, as long-term bridge therapy (a temporary transition treatment) in patients awaiting cardiac transplant, or in some instances, as the destination therapy (treatment for patients in lieu of cardiac transplant for those who are not appropriate candidates for transplantation).[1] The most common complications are infection and thromboembolism. Other adverse effects include bleeding, air embolism, device failure, and multiorgan failure.

▶ *Surgical Therapy*

Heart transplantation represents the final option for refractory, end-stage HF patients who have exhausted medical and device therapies. Heart transplantation is not a cure, but should be considered a trade between a life-threatening syndrome and the risks associated with the operation and long-term immunosuppression. Assessment of appropriate candidates includes comorbid illnesses, psychosocial behavior, available financial and social support, and patient willingness to adhere to lifelong therapy and close medical follow-up.[1] Overall, the transplant recipient's quality of life may be improved, but not all patients receive this benefit. Post-transplant survival continues to improve due to advances in immunosuppression, treatment and prevention of infection, and optimal management of patient comorbidities.

Investigational Therapies

Clinical trials are currently investigating new agents for the treatment of AHF. These compounds offer unique mechanisms of action by targeting different neurohormonal receptors (vasopressin, ET, ANP, and adenosine) or through completely novel pharmacologic profiles (myosin ATPase agonists). Some agents or drug classes being studied include tolvaptan, a V_2-selective vasopressin antagonist; various ET-A selective and nonselective antagonists; and an adenosine-1 receptor agonist.

OUTCOME EVALUATION OF AHF

- Focus on: (a) acute improvement of symptoms and hemodynamics due to IV therapies; (b) criteria for a safe

position, the balloon is programmed to inflate during diastole and deflate during systole. Two main beneficial mechanisms are: (a) inflation during diastole increases aortic pressure and perfusion of the coronary arteries, and (b) deflation just prior to the aortic valve opening reduces arterial impedence

Patient Care and Monitoring

1. Assess the severity and duration of the patient's symptoms including limitations in activity. Rule out potential exacerbating factors.

2. Obtain a thorough history of prescription, nonprescription, and herbal medication use. Is the patient taking any medications that can exacerbate HF?

3. Review available diagnostic information from the chest radiograph, ECG, and echocardiogram.

4. Review the patient's lifestyle habits including salt and alcohol intake, tobacco product use, and exercise routine.

5. If unknown, investigate the patient's underlying etiology of HF. Verify that comorbidities that lead to or worsen HF are optimally managed with appropriate drug therapy.

6. Educate the patient on lifestyle modifications such as salt restriction (maximum 2 g/day), fluid restriction if appropriate, limitation of alcohol, tobacco cessation, participation in a cardiac rehabilitation and exercise program, and proper immunizations such as the pneumococcal vaccine and yearly influenza vaccine.

7. Develop a treatment plan to alleviate symptoms and maintain euvolemia with diuretics. Daily weights to assess fluid retention are recommended.

8. Develop a medication regimen to slow the progression of HF with the use of neurohormonal blockers such as vasodilators (ACE inhibitors, ARBs, or hydralazine/isosorbide dinitrate), β-blockers, and aldosterone antagonists. Utilize digoxin if the patient remains symptomatic despite optimization of the above therapies.

   - Is the patient at goal or maximally tolerated doses of vasodilator and β-blocker therapy?

   - Are aldosterone antagonists utilized in appropriate patients with proper electrolyte and renal function monitoring?

9. Stress the importance of adherence to the therapeutic regimen and lifestyle changes for maintenance of a compensated state and slowing of disease progression.

10. Evaluate the patient for presence of adverse drug reactions, drug allergies, and drug interactions.

11. Provide patient education with regard to disease state and drug therapy, and reinforce self-monitoring for symptoms of HF that necessitate follow-up with a health care practitioner.

---

discharge from the hospital; and (c) optimization of oral therapy.

- Initially, monitor patients for rapid relief of symptoms related to the chief complaint on admission. This includes improvement of dyspnea, oxygenation, fatigue, JVD, and other markers of congestion or distress.

- Monitor for adequate perfusion of vital organs through assessment of mental status, CrCl, liver function tests, and a stable HR between 50 and 100 bpm. Additionally, adequate skin and muscle blood perfusion and normal pH is desirable.

- Monitor changes in hemodynamic variables if available. CI should increase, with a goal to maintain it above 2.2 L/min/m². PCWP should decrease in volume overloaded patients to a goal of less than 18 mm Hg.

- Closely monitor BPs and renal function while decreasing preload with diuretics and vasodilators.

- Ensure patients are euvolemic or nearly euvolemic prior to discharge.

- Because oral therapies can both improve symptoms and prolong survival, optimizing outpatient HF management is a priority when preparing a patient for hospital discharge. Ensure that the patient's regimen includes a vasodilator, β-blocker, a diuretic at an adequate dose to maintain euvolemia, and digoxin or aldosterone antagonist if indicated.

Abbreviations Introduced in This Chapter

ACC/AHA	American College of Cardiology/American Heart Association
ACE	Angiotensin-converting enzyme
AHF	Acute heart failure
ANP	Atrial natriuretic peptide
ARB	Angiotensin receptor blocker
AT_1	Angiotensin type 1
AT_2	Angiotensin type 2
ATP	Adenosine triphosphate
BMI	Body mass index
BNP	B-type natriuretic peptide
bpm	Beats per minute
BUN	Blood urea nitrogen
CAD	Coronary artery disease
CAM	Complementary and alternative medicine
cAMP	Cyclic adenosine monophosphate
CBC	Complete blood cell count
cGMP	Cyclic guanosine monophosphate
CHARM	Candesartan in Heart Failure Assessment of Reduction in Mortality and Morbidity
CI	Cardiac index
CO	Cardiac output
COX-2	Cyclooxygenase-2
CrCl	Creatinine clearance
CRT	Cardiac resynchronization therapy

CYP450	Cytochrome P-450 isoenzyme
D1	Dopamine receptor type 1
EF	Ejection fraction
ET-1	Endothelin-1
ET-A	Endothelin-A
ET-B	Endothelin-B
HF	Heart failure
HJR	Hepatojugular reflux
HR	Heart rate
IABC	Intra-aortic balloon counterpulsation
IABP	Intra-aortic balloon pump
ICD	Implantable cardioverter defibrillator
iNOS	Inducible nitric oxide synthetase
INR	International Normalized Ratio
JVD	Jugular venous distention
JVP	Jugular venous pressure
LV	Left ventricular
LVEF	Left ventricular ejection fraction
LVF	Left ventricular failure
MI	Myocardial infarction
MVO_2	Myocardial oxygen consumption
NHP	Natural health products
NSAID	Nonsteroidal anti-inflammatory drug
NT-proBNP	N-terminal proBNP
NYHA FC	New York Heart Association Functional Class
PAC	Pulmonary artery catheter
PCWP	Pulmonary capillary wedge pressure
PE	Physical exam
PND	Paroxysmal nocturnal dyspnea
PPCM	Peripartum cardiomyopathy
RAAS	Renin-angiotensin-aldosterone system
RVF	Right ventricular failure
SCr	Serum creatinine
SL	Sublingual
SNS	Sympathetic nervous system
SOB	Shortness of breath
SV	Stroke volume
SVR	Systemic vascular resistance
TNF-α	Tumor necrosis factor-α
V_{1a}	Vasopressin type 1a
V_2	Vasopressin type 2
VAD	Ventricular assist device

 Self-assessment questions and answers are available at *http://www.mhpharmacotherapy.com/pp.html.*

REFERENCES

1. Hunt SA, Abraham WT, Chin MH, et al., for the Committee to Revise the 2001 Guidelines for the Evaluation and Management of Heart Failure. ACC/AHA guideline update for the diagnosis and management of chronic heart failure in the adult—Summary article. A report of the American College of Cardiology/American Heart Association Task Force on Practice Guidelines (Committee to revise the 2001 Guidelines for the Evaluation and Management of Heart Failure). J Am Coll Cardiol 2005;46:1116–1143.
2. Centers for Disease Control and Prevention. Heart Failure Fact Sheet. September 2006, http://www.cdc.gov/DHDSP/library/pdfs/fs_heart_failure.pdf.
3. Nieminen MS, Harjola VP. Definition and epidemiology of acute heart failure syndromes. Am J Cardiol 2005;96(Suppl):5–10.
4. Bonow RO, Bennett S, Casey DE Jr, et al., for the Writing Committee to Develop Heart Failure Clinical Performance Measures. ACC/AHA clinical performance measures for adults with chronic heart failure: A report of the American College of Cardiology/American Heart Association Task Force on Performance Measures (Writing Committee to Develop Heart Failure Clinical Performance Measures) endorsed by the Heart Failure Society of America. J Am Coll Cardiol 2005(Sept 20);46(6):1144–1178.
5. Johnson JA, Parker RB, Patterson JH. Heart failure. In: Dipiro JT, Talbert RL, Yee GC, et al., eds. Pharmacotherapy: A Pathophysiologic Approach, 5th ed. New York: McGraw-Hill, 2002:185–218.
6. Jessup M, Brozena S. Heart failure. N Engl J Med 2003;348:2007–2018.
7. Schrier RW, Abraham WT. Hormones and hemodynamics in heart failure. N Engl J Med 1999;341(8):577–585.
8. Mann DL. Mechanisms and models in heart failure—A combinatorial approach. Circulation 1999;100:999–1008.
9. Mann DL. Inflammatory mediators and the failing heart—Past, present, and the foreseeable future. Circ Res 2002;91:988–998.
10. Silver MA, Maisel A, Yancy CW, et al. BNP Consensus Panel 2004: A clinical approach for the diagnostic, prognostic, screening, treatment monitoring, and therapeutic roles of natriuretic peptides in cardiovascular diseases. Congest Heart Fail 2004(Sept-Oct);10(5 Suppl 3):1–30.
11. Hunt SA, Baker DW, Chin MH, et al., for the Committee to Revise the 1995 Guidelines for the Evaluation and Management of Heart Failure. ACC/AHA guidelines for the evaluation and management of chronic heart failure in the adult: Executive summary. A report of the American College of Cardiology/American Heart Association Task Force on Practice Guidelines. (Committee to revise the 1995 Guidelines for the Evaluation and Management of Heart Failure). J Am Coll Cardiol 2001;38:2101–2113.
12. Consensus recommendations for the management of chronic heart failure. On behalf of the membership of the advisory council to improve outcomes nationwide in heart failure. Am J Cardiol 1999;83(2A):1A–38A.
13. Heart Failure Society of America. Heart failure in patients with left ventricular systolic dysfunction. J Card Fail 2006;12(1):e38–e57.
14. Ng TMH, Carter O, Guillory GS, et al. High-impact articles related to the pharmacotherapeutic management of systolic heart failure. Pharmacotherapy 2004;24(11):1594–1633.
15. Brater DC. Diuretic therapy. N Engl J Med 1998(Aug 6);339(6):387–395.
16. Brater DC. Diuretic therapy in congestive heart failure. Congest Heart Fail 2000(May);6(4):197–201.
17. De Bruyne LK. Mechanisms and management of diuretic resistance in congestive heart failure. Postgrad Med J 2003;79:268–271.
18. The CONSENSUS Trial Study Group. Effects of enalapril on mortality in severe congestive heart failure. N Engl J Med 1987;316:1429–1435.
19. The SOLVD Investigators. Effect of enalapril on survival in patients with reduced left ventricular ejection fractions and congestive heart failure. N Engl J Med 1991;325:293–302.
20. The SOLVD Investigators. Effect of enalapril on mortality and the development of heart failure in asymptomatic patients with reduced left ventricular ejection fractions. N Engl J Med 1992;327:685–691.
21. Pfeffer MA, Braunwald E, Move LA, et al. Effect of captopril on mortality and morbidity in patients with left ventricular dysfunction after myocardial infarction. Results of the survival and ventricular enlargement trial. N Engl J Med 1992;327:669–677.
22. Packer M, Wilson-Poole PA, Armstrong PW, et al. Comparative effects of low- and high doses of the angiotensin-converting enzyme inhibitor, lisinopril, or morbidity and mortality in chronic heart failure. Circulation 1999;100:2312–2318.
23. Pitt B, Poole-Wilson PA, Segal R, et al., for the ELITE II Investigators. Effect of losartan compared with captopril on mortality in patients

with symptomatic heart failure: Randomised trial—The Losartan Heart Failure Survival Study ELITE II. Lancet 2000;355:1582–1587.

24. Cohn JN, Tognoni G, for the Valsartan Heart Failure Trial Investigators. A randomized trial of the angiotensin-receptor blocker valsartan in chronic heart failure. N Engl J Med 2001;345:1667–1675.

25. Pfeffer MA, Swedberg K, Granger CB, et al., for the CHARM Investigators and Committees. Effects of candesartan on mortality and morbidity in patients with chronic heart failure: The CHARM-Overall programme. Lancet 2003;362:759–766.

26. Cohn JN, Archibald DG, Ziesche S, et al. Effect of vasodilator therapy on mortality in chronic congestive heart failure. N Engl J Med 1986;314:1547–1552.

27. Cohn JN, Johnson G, Ziesche S, et al. A comparison of enalapril with hydralazine-isosorbide dinitrate in the treatment of chronic congestive heart failure. N Engl J Med 1991;325:303–310.

28. Taylor AL, Ziesche S, Yancy C, et al. Combination of isosorbide dinitrate and hydralazine in blacks with heart failure. N Engl J Med 2004;351(20):2049–2057.

29. Packer M, Bristow MR, Cohn JN, et al., for the U.S. Carvedilol Heart Failure Study Group. The effect of carvedilol on morbidity and mortality in patients with chronic heart failure. N Engl J Med 1996;334:1349–1355.

30. CIBIS-II Investigators and Committees. The cardiac insufficiency bisoprolol study II (CIBIS-II): A randomized trial. Lancet. 1999;353:9–13.

31. MERIT-HF Study Group. Effect of metoprolol CR/XL in chronic heart failure: Metoprolol CR/XL randomized intervention trial in congestive heart failure (MERIT-HF). Lancet 1999;353:2001–2007.

32. Packer M, Coats AJ, Fowler MB, et al., for the Carvedilol Prospective Randomized Cumulative Survival Study Group. N Engl J Med 2001;344(22):1651–1658.

33. Poole-Wilson PA, Swedberg K, Cleland JG, et al., for the COMET Investigators. Comparison of carvedilol and metoprolol on clinical outcomes in patients with chronic heart failure in the Carvedilol or Metoprolol European Trial (COMET): Randomized controlled trial. Lancet 2003;362:7–13.

34. Pitt B, Zannad F, Remme WJ, et al. The effect of spironolactone on morbidity and mortality in patients with severe heart failure. N Engl J Med 1999;341(10):709–717.

35. Pitt B, Williams G, Remme W, et al. Eplerenone, a selective aldosterone antagonist, in patients with left ventricular dysfunction after myocardial infarction (EPHESUS). N Engl J Med 2003;348(14):1309–1321.

36. The Digitalis Investigation Group. The effect of digoxin on mortality and morbidity in patients with heart failure. The Digitalis Investigation Group. N Engl J Med 1997;336:525–533.

37. Adams KF, Gheorghiade M, Uretsky BF, et al. Clinical benefits of low serum digoxin concentrations in heart failure. J Am Coll Cardiol 2002;39:946–953.

38. Rathore SS, Curtis JP, Wang Yongfei, et al. Association of serum digoxin concentration and outcomes in patients with heart failure. JAMA 2003;289:871–878.

39. Packer M, O'Connor CH, Ghali JK, et al. Effect of amlodipine on morbidity and mortality in severe chronic heart failure. N Engl J Med 1996;335:1107–1114.

40. Cohn JN, Ziesche S, Smith R, et al. Effect of the calcium antagonist felodipine as supplementary vasodilator therapy in patients with chronic heart failure treated with enalapril. Circulation 1997;96:856–863.

41. Lip GY, Gibbs CR. Antiplatelet agents versus control or anticoagulation for heart failure in sinus rhythm: A Cochrane systematic review. Q J Med 2002;95:461–468.

42. Fuster V, Ryde'n LE, Asinger RW, et al., for the Committee to Develop Guidelines for the Management of Patients with Atrial Fibrillation. ACC/AHA/ESC guidelines for the management of patients with atrial fibrillation: A report of the American College of Cardiology/American Heart Association Task Force on Practice Guidelines and the European Society of Cardiology Committee for Practice Guidelines and Policy Conferences. (Committee to Develop Guidelines for the Management of Patients With Atrial Fibrillation). J Am Coll Cardiol 2001;38:1231–1266.

43. Lip GY, Gibbs CR. Anticoagulation for heart failure in sinus rhythm: A Cochrane systematic review. Q J Med 2002;95:451–459.

44. Aurigenuna GP, Gaasch WH. Diastolic heart failure. N Engl J Med 2004;351(11):1097–1105.

45. Pearson GD, Veille JC, Rahimtoola S, et al. Peripartum cardiomyopathy: National Heart, Lung, and Blood Institute and Office of Rare Diseases (National Institutes of Health) workshop recommendations and review. JAMA 2000;283(9):1183–1188.

46. Tidswell M. Peripartum cardiomyopathy. Crit Care Clin 2004;20:777–788.

47. Stevenson LW. Tailored therapy to hemodynamic goals for advanced heart failure. Eur J Heart Fail 1999(Aug);1(3):251–257.

48. DiDomenico RJ, Park HY, Southworth MR, et al. Guidelines for acute decompensated heart failure treatment. Ann Pharmacother 2004(Apr);38(4):649–660.

49. Nohria A, Lewis E, Stevenson LW. Medical management of advanced heart failure. JAMA 2002;287:628–640.

50. Howard PA, Dunn MI. Severe heart failure in the elderly: Potential benefits of high-dose and continuous infusion diuretics. Drugs Aging 2002;19:249–256.

51. Licata G, Pasquale PD, Parrinello G, et al. Effects of high-dose furosemide and small-volume hypertonic saline infusion in comparison with a high dose of furosemide as bolus in refractory congestive heart failure: Long term effects. A Heart J 2003;145:459–466.

52. Jain P, Massie BM, Gattis WA, et al. Current medical treatment for the exacerbation of chronic heart failure resulting in hospitalization. Am Heart J 2003;145:S3–S17.

53. VMAC Investigators. Intravenous nesiritide versus nitroglycerin for treatment of decompensated congestive heart failure. JAMA 2002;287:1531–1540.

54. Felker GM, O'Connor CM. Inotropic therapy for heart failure: An evidence-based approach. Am Heart J 2001;142:393–401.

55. Stevenson LW. Clinical use of inotropic therapy for heart failure: Looking backward or forward? Part I: Inotropic infusions during hospitalizations. Circulation 2003;109:367–372.

56. Stevenson LW. Clinical use of inotropic therapy for heart failure: Looking backward or forward? Part II: Chronic inotropic therapy. Circulation 2003;108:492–497.

57. Cuffe MS, Califf RM, Adams KF, et al., for the OPTIME-CHF Investigators. Short-term intravenous milrinone for acute exacerbation of chronic heart failure. JAMA 2002;287:1541–1547.

58. Rose EA, Gelijns AC, Moskowitz AJ, et al.; Heitjan DF, Stevenson LW, Dembitsky W, et al., for the Randomized Evaluation of Mechanical Assistance for the Treatment of Congestive Heart Failure (REMATCH) Study Group. Long-term mechanical left ventricular assistance for end-stage heart failure. N Engl J Med 2001;345(20):1435–1443.

59. Abraham WT, Fisher WG, Smith AL, et al., for the MIRACLE Study Group. Cardiac resynchronization in chronic heart failure. N Engl J Med 2002;346(24):1845–1853.

60. Bardy GH, Lee KL, Mark DB, et al. Amiodarone or an implantable cardioverter-defibrillator for congestive heart failure. N Engl J Med 2005;352:225–237.

61. Abraham WT, Fisher WG, Smith AL, et al. Cardiac resynchronization in chronic heart failure. N Engl J Med 2002;346(24):1845–1853.

7 Ischemic Heart Disease

Larisa H. Cavallari and Robert J. DiDomenico

LEARNING OBJECTIVES

● **Upon completion of the chapter, the reader will be able to:**

1. Identify risk factors for the development of ischemic heart disease (IHD).

2. Differentiate between the pathophysiology of chronic stable angina and acute coronary syndromes (ACSs).

3. Recognize the symptoms and diagnostic criteria of IHD in a specific patient.

4. Identify the treatment goals of IHD and appropriate lifestyle modifications and pharmacologic therapy to address each goal.

5. Design an appropriate therapeutic regimen for the management of IHD based on patient-specific information.

6. Formulate a monitoring plan to assess effectiveness and adverse effects of an IHD drug regimen.

KEY CONCEPTS

❶ Ischemic heart disease (IHD) results from an imbalance between myocardial oxygen demand and oxygen supply that is most often due to coronary atherosclerosis. Common clinical manifestations of IHD include chronic stable angina and the acute coronary syndromes (ACSs) of unstable angina, non-ST-segment elevation myocardial infarction (MI), and ST-segment elevation MI.

❷ Early detection and aggressive modification of risk factors is one of the primary strategies for delaying IHD progression and preventing IHD-related events including death.

❸ Patients with chest pressure or heaviness that is provoked by activity and relieved with rest should be assessed for IHD. Sharp pain is not a typical symptom of IHD. Some patients may experience discomfort in the neck, jaw, shoulder, or arm rather than, or in addition to, the chest. Pain may be accompanied by nausea, vomiting, or diaphoresis.

❹ The major goals for the treatment of IHD are to prevent ACSs and death, alleviate acute symptoms of myocardial ischemia, prevent recurrent symptoms of myocardial ischemia, and avoid or minimize adverse treatment effects.

❺ Both 3-hydroxy-3-methylglutaryl coenzyme A reductase inhibitors (statins) and angiotensin-converting enzyme (ACE) inhibitors are believed to provide vasculoprotective effects, and in addition to antiplatelet agents, have been shown to reduce the risk of acute coronary events and death in patients with IHD. Angiotensin receptor blockers (ARBs) may be used in patients who cannot tolerate ACE inhibitors because of side effects (e.g., chronic cough). β-Blockers have been shown to decrease morbidity and improve survival in patients who have suffered a MI.

❻ Antiplatelet therapy with aspirin should be considered for all patients without contraindications, particularly in patients with a history of MI. Clopidogrel may be considered in patients with allergies or intolerance to aspirin. In some patients, combination antiplatelet therapy with aspirin and clopidogrel may be used.

❼ To control risk factors and prevent major adverse cardiac events, statin therapy should be considered in all patients with IHD, particularly in those with elevated low-density lipoprotein cholesterol. In the absence of contraindications, ACE inhibitors should be considered in IHD patients who also have diabetes mellitus, left ventricular dysfunction, history of MI, or any combination of these. Angiotensin receptor blockers may be used in patients who cannot tolerate ACE inhibitors because of side effects.

❽ All patients with a history of angina should have sublingual nitroglycerin tablets or spray to relieve acute ischemic symptoms. Patients should be instructed to use one dose (tablet or spray) every 5 minutes until pain is relieved and to call 911 if pain is unimproved or worsens 5 minutes after the first dose.

❾ β-Blockers are first-line therapy for preventing ischemic symptoms, particularly in patients with a history of MI. Long-acting calcium channel blockers and long-acting nitrates may be added for refractory symptoms or substituted if a β-blocker is not tolerated.

❿ Patients should be monitored to assess for drug effectiveness, adverse drug reactions, and potential drug–drug interactions. Patients should be assessed for adherence to their pharmacotherapeutic regimens and lifestyle modifications.

INTRODUCTION

Ischemic heart disease (IHD) is also called coronary heart disease (CHD) or coronary artery disease. The term "ischemic" refers to a decreased supply of oxygenated blood, in this case to the heart muscle. IHD is caused by the narrowing of one or more of the major coronary arteries that supply blood to the heart, most commonly by atherosclerotic plaques. Atherosclerotic plaques may impede coronary blood flow to the extent that cardiac tissue distal to the site of the coronary artery narrowing is deprived of sufficient oxygen in the face of increased oxygen demand. **❶** *IHD results from an imbalance between myocardial oxygen supply and oxygen demand (Fig. 7–1). Common clinical manifestations of IHD include chronic stable angina and the acute coronary syndromes (ACSs) of unstable angina, non-ST-segment elevation myocardial infarction (MI), and ST-segment elevation MI.*

Angina pectoris, or simply angina, is the most common symptom of IHD. Angina is discomfort in the chest that occurs when the blood supply to the myocardium is compromised. Chronic stable angina is defined as a chronic and predictable occurrence of chest discomfort due to transient myocardial ischemia with physical exertion or other conditions that increase oxygen demand. The primary focus of this chapter is on the management of chronic stable angina. However, some information is also provided related to ACS, given the overlap between the two disease states. The American College of Cardiology and the American Heart Association have jointly published practice guidelines for the management of patients with chronic stable angina, and the reader is referred to these guidelines for further information.[1,2]

EPIDEMIOLOGY AND ETIOLOGY

IHD affects over 16 million Americans and is the leading cause of death for both men and women in the United States.[3] The incidence of IHD is higher in middle-aged men compared to women. However, the rate of IHD increases two- to threefold in women after menopause. Chronic stable angina is the initial manifestation of IHD in about 50% of patients, whereas unstable angina or MI is the first sign of IHD in other patients. Chronic stable angina is associated with considerable patient morbidity, with many affected patients eventually requiring hospitalization for ACS. In addition, chronic stable angina has a major negative impact

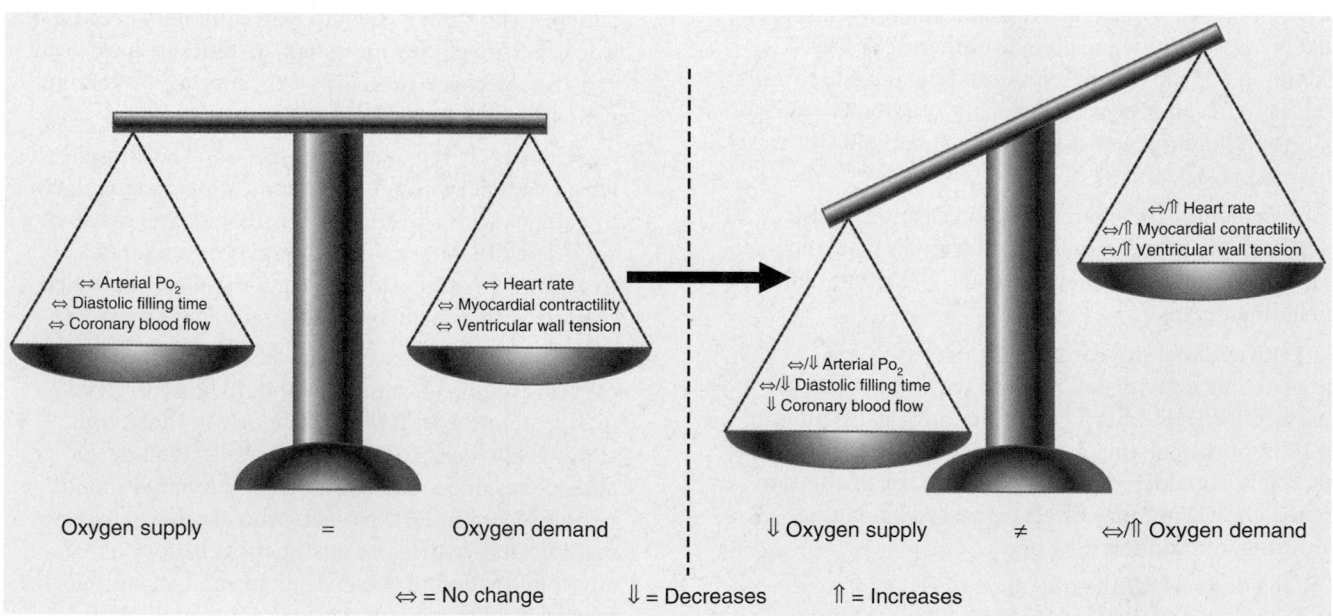

FIGURE 7–1. This illustration depicts the balance between myocardial oxygen supply and demand and the various factors that affect each. It should be noted that diastolic filling time is not an independent predictor of myocardial oxygen supply per se, but rather a determinant of coronary blood flow. On the left is myocardial oxygen supply and demand under normal circumstances. On the right is the mismatch between oxygen supply and demand in patients with IHD. In patients without IHD, coronary blood flow increases in response to increases in myocardial oxygen demand. However, in patients with IHD, coronary blood flow cannot sufficiently increase (and may decrease) in response to increased oxygen demand resulting in angina. (IHD, ischemic heart disease; Po_2, partial pressure of oxygen.)

on health-related quality of life. Thus, in patients with chronic stable angina, it is important to optimize pharmacotherapy to reduce symptoms, improve quality of life, slow disease progression, and prevent ACS.

Conditions Associated With Angina

Figure 7–2 shows the anatomy of the coronary arteries. The major epicardial coronary arteries are the left main, left anterior descending, left circumflex, and right coronary arteries. Atherosclerosis involving one or more of the major coronary arteries or their principal branches is the major cause of angina. Vasospasm at the site of an atherosclerotic plaque may contribute to angina by further restricting blood supply to the distal myocardium. Less commonly, vasospasm in coronary arteries with no or minimal atherosclerotic disease can produce angina and even precipitate ACS. This type of vasospasm is referred to as variant or Prinzmetal angina. Other nonatherosclerotic conditions that can cause angina-like symptoms are listed in Table 7–1. It is important to differentiate the etiology of chest discomfort since treatment varies depending on the underlying disease process.

Risk Factors

Factors that predispose an individual to IHD are listed in Table 7–2. Hypertension, diabetes, dyslipidemia, and cigarette smoking are associated with endothelial dysfunction and potentiate atherosclerosis of the coronary arteries. The risk for IHD increases twofold for every 20 mm Hg increment in systolic blood pressure and up to eightfold in

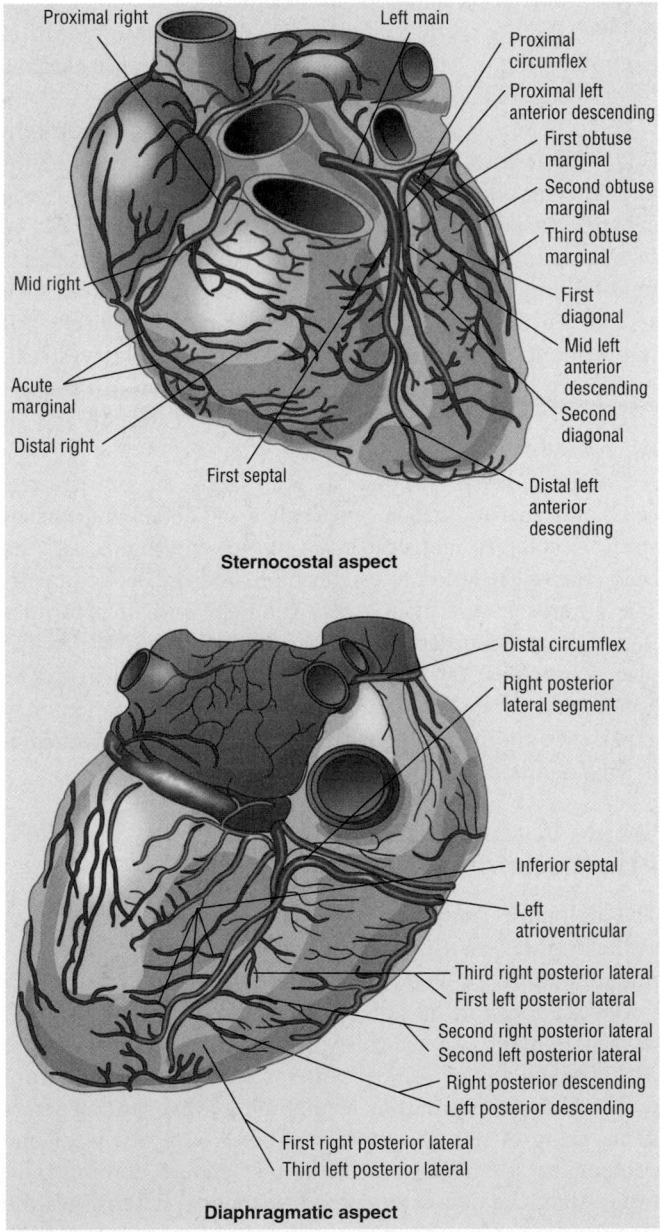

FIGURE 7–2. Coronary artery anatomy with sternocostal and diaphragmatic views. (Reproduced from Talbert RL. Ischemic heart disease. In: DiPiro JT, Talbert RL, Yee GC, et al. (eds.) Pharmacotherapy: A Pathophysiologic Approach. 6th ed. New York: McGraw-Hill; 2005: 263, with permission.)

Table 7–1

Nonatherosclerotic Conditions That Can Cause Angina-Like Symptoms

Organ System	Condition
Cardiac	Aortic dissection, coronary artery vasospasm, pericarditis, valvular heart disease, severe uncontrolled hypertension
Noncardiac	Anemia, anxiety disorders, carbon monoxide poisoning, cocaine use, esophageal reflux, peptic ulcer, pleuritis, pneumonia, pneumothorax, pulmonary embolus, pulmonary hypertension, thyrotoxicosis

---

Table 7–2

Major Risk Factors for Ischemic Heart Disease

Modifiable	Nonmodifiable
Cigarette smoking	Age 45 years or greater for males, age 55 years or greater for females
Dyslipidemia	
• Elevated LDL or total cholesterol	Gender (men and post menopausal women)
• Reduced HDL cholesterol	Family history of premature cardiovascular disease, defined as cardiovascular disease in a male first-degree relative (i.e., father or brother) younger than 55 years old or a female first-degree relative (i.e., mother or sister) younger than 65 years
Diabetes mellitus	
Hypertension	
Physical inactivity	
Obesity (body mass index greater than or equal to 30 kg/m²)	

HDL, high-density lipoprotein; LDL, low-density lipoprotein.

the presence of diabetes.[4,5] Physical inactivity and obesity independently increase the risk for IHD, in addition to predisposing individuals to other cardiovascular risk factors, namely hypertension, dyslipidemia, and diabetes.

Patients with multiple risk factors, particularly those with diabetes, are at the greatest risk for IHD. While there are alternative definitions for metabolic syndrome, it is generally considered as a constellation of cardiovascular risk factors related to hypertension, abdominal obesity, dyslipidemia, and insulin resistance. Metabolic syndrome increases the risk of developing IHD and related complications by twofold.[6] According to the American Heart Association, patients must meet at least three of the following criteria for the diagnosis of metabolic syndrome[7]:

- Increased waist circumference (more than or equal to 40 inches or 102 centimeters in males and more than or equal to 35 inches or 89 centimeters in females).
- Triglycerides of 150 mg/dL (1.70 mmol/L) or greater or active treatment to lower triglycerides.
- Low high-density lipoprotein (HDL) cholesterol (less than 40 mg/dL or 1.04 mmol/L in males and less than 50 mg/dL or 1.3 mmol/L in females) or active treatment to raise HDL cholesterol.
- Systolic blood pressure of 130 mm Hg or greater, diastolic blood pressure of 85 mm Hg or greater, or active treatment with antihypertensive therapy.
- Fasting blood glucose of 100 mg/dL (5.55 mmol/L) or greater or active treatment for diabetes.

❷ *Early detection and aggressive modification of risk factors are among the primary strategies for delaying IHD progression and preventing IHD-related events including death.*

PATHOPHYSIOLOGY

The determinants of oxygen supply and demand are shown in Figure 7–1. Increases in heart rate, cardiac contractility, and left ventricular wall tension increase the rate of myocardial oxygen consumption (MVO$_2$). Ventricular wall tension is a function of blood pressure, left ventricular end-diastolic volume, and ventricular wall thickness. Physical exertion increases MVO$_2$ and commonly precipitates symptoms of angina in patients with significant coronary atherosclerosis. Medications that reduce heart rate, cardiac contractility, and/or ventricular wall tension are commonly prescribed to prevent ischemic symptoms in chronic stable angina.

Reductions in coronary blood flow (secondary to atherosclerotic plaques, vasospasm, or thrombus formation) and arterial oxygen content (secondary to hypoxia) decrease myocardial oxygen supply. Because the coronary arteries fill during diastole, decreases in diastolic filling time (e.g., tachycardia) can also reduce coronary perfusion and myocardial oxygen supply. In chronic stable angina, atherosclerotic plaques are the most common cause of coronary artery narrowing and reductions in coronary blood flow. In contrast, in ACS, disruption of an atherosclerotic plaque with subsequent thrombus (blood clot) formation causes abrupt reductions in coronary blood flow and oxygen supply. Anemia, carbon monoxide poisoning, and cyanotic congenital heart disease are examples of conditions that reduce the oxygen-carrying capacity of the blood, potentially causing ischemia in the face of adequate coronary perfusion. Interventional procedures to compress, cut away, or bypass atherosclerotic plaques are effective methods of improving myocardial oxygen supply in patients with IHD.

Coronary Atherosclerosis

The normal arterial wall is illustrated in Figure 7–3A. The intima consists of a layer of endothelial cells that line the lumen of the artery and form a selective barrier between the vessel wall and blood contents. Vascular smooth muscle cells are found in the media. The vascular adventitia comprises the artery's outer layer. Atherosclerotic lesions form in the subendothelial space in the intimal layer.

Endothelial dysfunction allows low-density lipoprotein (LDL) cholesterol and inflammatory cells (e.g., monocytes and T lymphocytes) to migrate from the plasma to the subendothelial space, as illustrated in Figure 12–5 in the Dyslipidemias chapter. Monocyte-derived macrophages ingest lipoproteins to form foam cells. Macrophages also secrete growth factors that promote smooth muscle cell migration from the media to the intima. A fatty streak consisting of lipid-laden macrophages and smooth muscle cells is formed. The fatty streak is the earliest type of atherosclerotic lesion.

The fatty streak enlarges as foam cells, smooth muscle cells, and necrotic debris accumulate in the subendothelial space. A collagen matrix forms a fibrous cap that covers the lipid core of the lesion to establish an atherosclerotic plaque. The atherosclerotic plaque may progress until it protrudes into the artery lumen and impedes blood flow. When the plaque occludes 70% or more of a major coronary artery or 50% or more of the left main coronary artery, the patient may experience angina during activities that increase myocardial oxygen demand.

Stable Versus Unstable Atherosclerotic Plaques

The hallmark feature in the pathophysiology of chronic stable angina is an established atherosclerotic plaque that impedes coronary blood flow to the extent that myocardial oxygen supply can no longer meet increases in myocardial oxygen demand. In contrast, the hallmark feature in the pathophysiology of ACS is atherosclerotic plaque rupture with subsequent thrombus formation. Plaque rupture refers to fissuring of the fibrous cap and exposure of the plaque contents to elements in the blood. Plaque composition, rather than the degree of coronary stenosis, determines the stability of the plaque and the likelihood of rupture and ACS. As depicted in Figure 7–3B, a stable lesion characteristic of chronic stable angina consists of a small lipid core that is surrounded by a thick fibrous cap that protects the lesion from the shear stress of blood flow. In contrast, an unstable plaque consists of a thin, weak cap in combination with

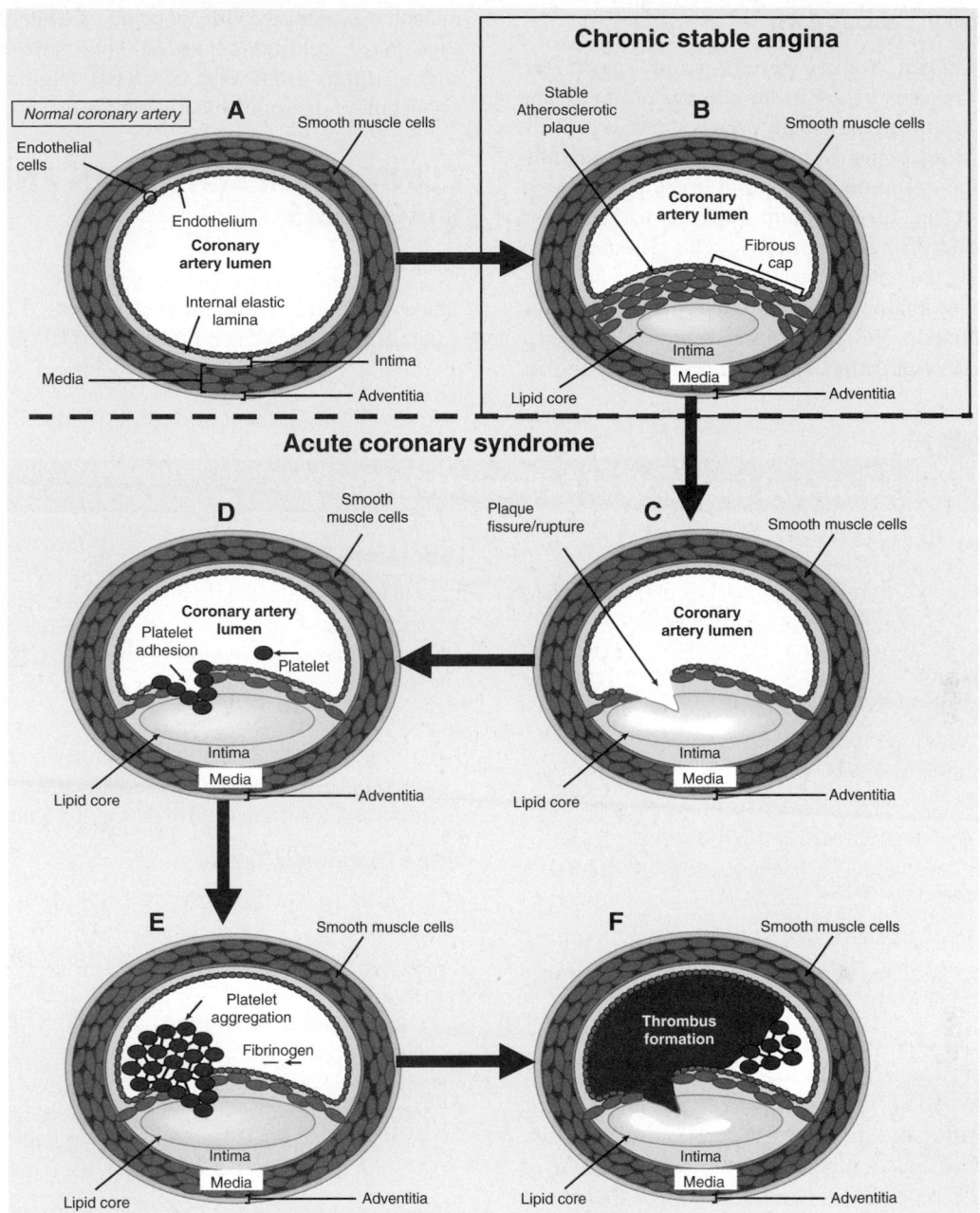

FIGURE 7–3. Pathophysiology of chronic stable angina versus acute coronary syndromes. **A** depicts the cross section of a normal coronary artery. **B** depicts the cross section of a coronary artery with a stable atherosclerotic plaque. Note that the lipid core is relatively small in size and the fibrous cap is made up of several layers of smooth muscle cells. **C** depicts an unstable atherosclerotic plaque with a larger lipid core, and a thin fibrous cap comprised of a single layer of smooth muscle cells with a fissure or rupture. **D** depicts platelet adhesion in response to the fissured plaque. Platelet activation may ensue leading to platelet aggregation as fibrinogen binds platelets to one another to form a meshlike occlusion in the coronary lumen (**E**). At this stage, patients may experience symptoms of acute coronary syndrome. If endogenous anticoagulant proteins fail to halt this process, platelet aggregation continues and fibrinogen is converted to fibrin, resulting in an occlusive thrombus (**F**).

a large, rich lipid core that renders the plaque vulnerable to rupture (Fig. 7–3C). The transformation of a stable plaque into an unstable plaque involves the degradation of the fibrous cap by substances released from macrophages and other inflammatory cells. Following plaque rupture, platelets adhere to the site of rupture, aggregate, and generate thrombin and a fibrin clot (Fig. 7–3D–F). Coronary thrombi extend into the vessel lumen, where they either partially or

completely occlude blood flow, resulting in unstable angina or MI.

An unstable plaque often produces minimal occlusion of the coronary vessel, and the patient remains asymptomatic until the plaque ruptures. In fact, the majority of MIs arise from vulnerable plaques that occlude less than 50% of the coronary lumen.[8] As a result, unstable angina or MI is the initial manifestation of IHD in about one-half of affected patients.

Coronary Artery Vasospasm

Prinzmetal or variant angina results from spasm (or contraction) of a coronary artery in the absence of significant atherosclerosis. Variant angina usually occurs at rest, especially in the early morning hours. While vasospasm is generally transient, in some instances vasospasm may persist long enough to infarct the myocardium. Patients with variant angina are typically younger than those with chronic stable angina and often do not possess the classic risk factors for IHD. The cause of variant angina is unclear but appears to involve endothelial dysfunction and paradoxical response to agents that normally cause vasodilation. Precipitants of variant angina include cigarette smoking, cocaine use, hyperventilation, and exposure to cold temperatures. The management of variant angina differs from that of classic angina, and thus it is important to distinguish between the two.

CLINICAL PRESENTATION AND DIAGNOSIS

History

The evaluation of a patient with suspected IHD begins with a detailed history of symptoms. ❸ *The classic presentation of angina is described in the Clinical Presentation and*

---

❸ Clinical Presentation and Diagnosis of Ischemic Heart Disease

General

- Patients with chronic stable angina will generally be in no acute distress. In patients presenting in acute distress, the clinician should be suspicious of ACS.

Symptoms of Angina Pectoris

- The five components commonly used to characterize chest pain are quality, location, and duration of pain; factors that provoke pain; and factors that relieve pain.
- Patients typically describe pain as a sensation of pressure, heaviness, or squeezing in the anterior chest area. Sharp pain is not a typical symptom of IHD.
- Pain may radiate to the neck, jaw, shoulder, back, or arm.
- Pain may be accompanied by dyspnea, nausea, vomiting, or diaphoresis.
- Symptoms are often provoked by exertion (e.g., walking, climbing stairs, and doing yard- or housework) or emotional stress and relieved within minutes by rest or sublingual nitroglycerin. Other precipitating factors include exposure to cold temperatures and heavy meals. Pain that occurs at rest (without provocation) or that is prolonged and unrelieved by sublingual nitroglycerin is indicative of an ACS.
- Some patients, most commonly women and patients with diabetes, may present with atypical symptoms including indigestion, gastric fullness, and shortness of breath. Patients with diabetes may experience associated symptoms, such as dyspnea and diaphoresis, without having any of the classic chest pain symptoms
- In some cases, ischemia may not produce any symptoms and is termed "silent ischemia."

Signs

- Findings on the physical exam are often normal in patients with chronic stable angina. However, during episodes of ischemia, patients may present with abnormal heart sounds, such as paradoxical splitting of the second heart sound, a third heart sound, or a loud fourth heart sound.

Laboratory Tests

- Cardiac enzymes (creatine kinase [CK], CK-MB fraction, troponin I and troponin T) are elevated in MI (ST-segment elevation MI and non-ST-segment elevation MI), but normal in chronic stable angina and unstable angina.
- Hemoglobin, fasting glucose, and fasting lipid profile should be determined for assessing cardiovascular risk factors and establishing the differential diagnosis.

Other Diagnostic Tests

- A 12-lead ECG recorded during rest is often normal in patients with chronic stable angina in the absence of active ischemia. Significant Q waves indicate prior MI. ST-segment or T-wave changes in two or more contiguous leads during symptoms of angina support the diagnosis of IHD. ST-segment depression or T-wave inversion is typically observed in chronic stable angina, unstable angina, and non-ST-segment elevation MI, whereas ST-segment elevation occurs with ST-segment elevation MI and Prinzmetal (variant) angina.
- Treadmill or bicycle exercise ECG, commonly referred to as a "stress test," is considered positive for IHD if the ECG shows at least a 1 mm deviation of the ST-segment (depression or elevation).
- Wall motion abnormalities or left ventricular dilation with stress echocardiography are indicative of IHD.
- Stress myocardial perfusion imaging with the radionuclides technetium-99m sestamibi or thallium-201 allows for the identification of multivessel disease and assessment of myocardial viability.
- Coronary angiography detects the location and degree of coronary atherosclerosis and is used to evaluate the potential benefit from revascularization procedures. Stenosis of at least 70% of the diameter of at least one of the major epicardial arteries on coronary angiography is indicative of significant IHD.

Diagnosis box. Chronic stable angina should be distinguished from unstable angina since the latter is associated with a greater risk for MI and death and requires more aggressive treatment. Because the pathophysiology of chronic stable angina is due primarily to increases in oxygen demand, rather than acute changes in oxygen supply, symptoms are typically reproducible. Specifically, a patient with angina secondary to significant coronary atherosclerosis will generally experience a similar pattern of discomfort (i.e., same quality, location, and accompanying symptoms) with a similar level of exertion with each angina attack. The exception may be a patient with coronary artery vasospasm, in whom symptoms may be more variable and unpredictable. In contrast to chronic stable angina, ACS is due to an acute decrease in coronary blood flow leading to insufficient oxygen supply. Consequently, ACS is marked by prolonged symptoms, symptoms that occur at rest, or an escalation in the frequency or severity of angina over a short period of time. The presentation of unstable angina is described in Table 7–3.[9]

The Canadian Cardiovascular Society Classification System

The Canadian Cardiovascular Society Classification System (Table 7–4) is commonly used to assess the degree of disability resulting from IHD.[10] Patients are categorized into one of four classes depending on the extent of activity that produces angina. Grouping patients according to this or a similar method is commonly used to assess changes in IHD severity over time and the effectiveness of pharmacologic therapy.

Physical Findings and Laboratory Analysis

A thorough medical history, physical exam, and laboratory analysis are necessary to ascertain cardiovascular risk factors and to exclude nonischemic and noncardiac conditions that could cause angina-like symptoms. Laboratory analyses should assess for glycemic control (i.e., fasting glucose, glycosylated hemoglobin), fasting lipids, hemoglobin, and organ function (i.e., blood urea nitrogen, creatinine, liver function tests, thyroid function tests). Additionally, serial measurements of cardiac enzymes (usually three measurements within 24 hours) are used to exclude the

---

Table 7–3

Presentations of Acute Coronary Syndromes

- Angina at rest that is prolonged in duration, usually lasting over 20 minutes
- Angina of recent onset (within 2 months) that markedly limits usual activity
- Angina that increases in severity (i.e., by Canadian Cardiovascular Society Classification System of one level or more), frequency, or duration, or that occurs with less provocation over a short time period (i.e., within 2 months)

From Ref. 9.

Table 7–4

The Canadian Cardiovascular Society Classification System of Angina

Class	Description
I	Able to perform ordinary physical activity (e.g., walking and climbing stairs) without symptoms. Strenuous, rapid, or prolonged exertion causes symptoms
II	Symptoms slightly limit ordinary physical activity. Walking rapidly or for more than two blocks, climbing stairs rapidly or climbing more than one flight of stairs causes symptoms
III	Symptoms markedly limit ordinary physical activity. Walking less than two blocks or climbing one flight of stairs causes symptoms
IV	Angina may occur at rest. Any physical activity causes symptoms

From Ref. 10.

Patient Encounter, Part 1

RJ is a 47-year-old man with a history of hypertension who presents to your clinic complaining of chest pain that occurred several times over the past few weeks. RJ describes his chest pain as "a heaviness." He states that it first occurred while he was mowing the grass. He later felt the same heavy sensation while raking leaves and again while carrying some boxes. The pain was located in the substernal area and radiated to his neck. The pain resolved after about 5 minutes of rest.

What information is suggestive of angina?

What tests would be beneficial in establishing a diagnosis?

What additional information do you need to create a treatment plan for this patient?

---

diagnosis of MI. Cardiac findings on the physical exam are often normal in patients with chronic stable angina. However, findings such as **carotid bruits** or abnormal peripheral pulses would indicate atherosclerosis in other vessel systems and raise the suspicion for IHD.

Diagnostic Tests

A resting ECG is indicated in all patients with angina-like symptoms. A 12-lead ECG should be done within 10 minutes of presentation to the emergency department in patients with symptoms of ischemia. Patients with ST-segment elevation are at the highest risk of death and need interventions to restore blood flow to the myocardium as quickly as possible. In patients without ST-segment elevation, biochemical markers are used to distinguish between unstable angina and non-ST-segment elevation MI.

"Stress" testing with either exercise or pharmacologic stressors increases myocardial oxygen demand and is commonly used to evaluate the patient with suspected IHD. Approximately 50% of patients with IHD who have a normal ECG at rest will develop ECG changes with exercise on a treadmill (most commonly) or bicycle ergometer. Dobutamine is a pharmacologic stressor used in patients who are unable to exercise. Dobutamine increases oxygen demand by stimulating the β_1-receptor, leading to increases in heart rate and contractility. Dobutamine is commonly used with echocardiography (referred to as dobutamine stress echocardiography) to identify stress-induced wall motion abnormalities indicative of coronary disease.

Adenosine and dipyridamole are coronary vasodilators commonly combined with radionuclide myocardial perfusion imaging (nuclear imaging studies). These agents increase coronary blood flow in vessels free of disease, but not in diseased vessels. An IV radioactive tracer is used to detect areas of the heart that receive less blood after adenosine or dipyridamole infusion, indicating a myocardial perfusion defect and coronary disease.

Coronary artery calcium scoring via CT, also known as electron beam CT (EBCT) or "ultra-fast CT," may be performed as a noninvasive means to assess for IHD. Calcium deposits within the coronary arteries which are indicative of IHD are detected on CT. A calcium score is calculated, and the risk for IHD-related events is estimated.

Coronary angiography (also referred to as a cardiac catheterization or "cardiac cath") is considered the gold standard for the diagnosis of IHD. Coronary angiography is indicated when stress testing results are abnormal or symptoms of angina are poorly controlled. Angiography involves catheter insertion, usually into the femoral artery, and advancement into the aorta and into the coronary arteries. Contrast medium is injected through the catheter into the coronary arteries allowing visualization of the coronary anatomy by fluoroscopy. Contrast medium must be used cautiously with adequate hydration in patients with pre-existing renal disease (especially in those with diabetes) to avoid contrast-induced nephropathy.

TREATMENT

Desired Outcomes

Once the diagnosis of IHD is established in a patient, the clinician should provide counseling on lifestyle modifications, institute appropriate pharmacologic therapy, and evaluate the need for surgical revascularization. ❹ *The major goals for the treatment of IHD are to:*

- *Prevent ACSs and death*
- *Alleviate acute symptoms of myocardial ischemia*
- *Prevent recurrent symptoms of myocardial ischemia*
- *Avoid or minimize adverse treatment effects*

The treatment approach to address these goals is illustrated in Figure 7–4.

Patient Encounter, Part 2: Medical History, Physical Exam, and Diagnostic Tests

PMH: Hypertension, diagnosed 7 years ago

FH: Father with coronary artery disease, had a myocardial infarction at age 50 years; mother alive and well

SH: Smokes half a pack to a pack per day; denies alcohol and illicit drug use; no regular exercise program

Allergies: NKDA

Meds: Hydrochlorothiazide 25 mg orally once daily; nifedipine XL 60 mg orally once daily

PE:

VS: BP 154/90 mm Hg, HR 84 bpm, RR 16 per minute, T 37°C (98.6°F), Ht 5'10" (178 cm), wt 105 kg (230 lb)

CV: RRR, normal S_1 and S_2, no S_3 or S_4; no murmurs, rubs, gallops

Lungs: Clear to auscultation and percussion

Abd: Nontender, nondistended, + bowel sounds

Labs: Fasting lipid profile: total cholesterol 233 mg/dL (6.03 mmol/L), HDL cholesterol 30 mg/dL (0.78 mmol/L), LDL cholesterol 165 mg/dL (4.27 mmol/L), triglycerides 188 mg/dL (2.12 mmol/L); other labs within normal limits

Exercise treadmill test: Positive for ischemia

Identify RJ's risk factors for ischemic heart disease.

How might RJ's current drug regimen adversely affect his ischemic heart disease?

What therapeutic alternatives are available to manage RJ's IHD?

General Approach to Treatment

The primary strategies for preventing ACS and death are to:

- Modify cardiovascular risk factors
- Slow the progression of coronary atherosclerosis
- Stabilize existing atherosclerotic plaques

The treatment algorithm in Figure 7–5 summarizes the appropriate management of IHD. Risk factor modification is accomplished through lifestyle changes and pharmacologic therapy. ❺ *Both 3-hydroxy-3-methylglutaryl coenzyme A reductase inhibitors (HMG-CoA reductase inhibitors or statins) and angiotensin-converting enzyme (ACE) inhibitors are believed to provide vasculoprotective effects (properties that are generally protective of the vasculature, which may include anti-inflammatory effects, antiplatelet effects, improvement in endothelial function, and improvement in arterial compliance and tone), and in addition to aspirin, have been shown to reduce the risk of acute coronary events as well as mortality in patients with IHD. Angiotensin receptor blockers (ARBs) may*

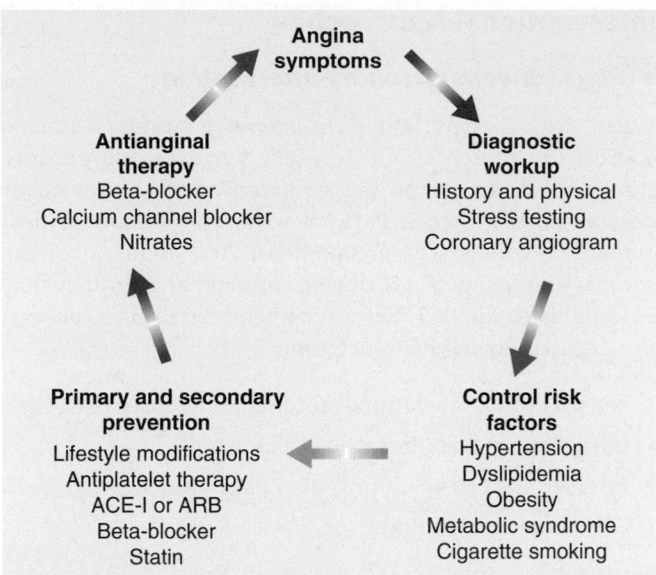

FIGURE 7–4. General treatment strategies for angina follow in clockwise fashion from the top center. (ACE-I, angiotensin-converting enzyme inhibitor; ARB, angiotensin receptor blocker.)

be used in patients who cannot tolerate ACE inhibitors because of side effects (e.g., chronic cough). β-Blockers have been shown to decrease morbidity and improve survival in patients who have suffered an MI.

Therapies to alleviate and prevent angina are aimed at improving the balance between myocardial oxygen demand and supply. Since angina usually results from increased myocardial oxygen demand in the face of a relatively fixed reduction in oxygen supply, drug treatment is primarily aimed at reducing oxygen demand. Short-acting nitrates are indicated to acutely relieve angina. β-Blockers, calcium channel blockers (CCBs), and long-acting nitrates are traditionally used to reduce the frequency of angina and improve exercise tolerance. In most patients with IHD, the most effective treatments to improve myocardial oxygen supply are invasive mechanical interventions, percutaneous coronary intervention (PCI), and coronary artery bypass graft (CABG) surgery, which are described later in the chapter in the section on interventional approaches.

Adverse treatment effects can largely be averted by avoiding drug interactions and the use of drugs that may have unfavorable effects on comorbid diseases. For example, β-blockers may exacerbate pre-existing bronchospasm. β-Blockers are not absolutely contraindicated in broncho-spastic disease, but should be avoided in patients with poorly controlled symptoms. While patients often require combination antianginal therapy, there is a potential pharmacodynamic drug interaction with the concurrent use of β-blockers and nondihydropyridine CCBs. Since both drug classes slow electrical conduction through the atrioventricular (AV) node, serious bradycardia or heart block may result with their concomitant use. Appropriate drug dosing and monitoring also reduces the risk for adverse

treatment effects. Drugs should be initiated in low doses, with careful up-titration as necessary to control symptoms of angina and cardiovascular risk factors.

Lifestyle Modifications

Lifestyle modifications, including smoking cessation, avoidance of second-hand smoke, dietary modifications, increased physical activity, and weight loss, reduce cardiovascular risk factors, slow the progression of IHD, and decrease the risk for IHD-related complications. Cigarette smoking is the single most preventable cause of IHD and IHD-related death. Smoking may also attenuate the antianginal effects of drug therapy. The clinician should ascertain smoking status for the patient and family members on the patient's initial clinic visit. For patients and/or family members who smoke, clinicians should provide counseling on the importance of smoking cessation at each subsequent visit and referral to special smoking cessation programs. There are several pharmacologic aids for smoking cessation. Transdermal nicotine replacement therapy and bupropion have been studied in patients with IHD and appear safe.[8,11]

Weight loss, through caloric restriction and increased physical activity, should be encouraged in patients who have a body mass index greater than 25 kg/m^2. Dietary modification is important for risk factor management, and dietary counseling should be provided to all patients with newly diagnosed angina regardless of weight. The American Heart Association recommends a diet that includes a variety of fruits, vegetables, grains, low-fat or nonfat dairy products, fish, legumes, poultry, and lean meats.[12] Fatty fish, such as salmon and herring, are high in omega-3 fatty acids, which have been shown to reduce triglyceride concentrations and slow atherosclerotic plaque progression.[12] Specific dietary recommendations for patients with IHD should include the following[2,12]:

- Limit fat intake to less than 30% of total caloric consumption.
- Limit cholesterol intake to less than 200 mg/day.
- Limit consumption of saturated fat and *trans* unsaturated fat found in fatty meats, full-fat dairy products, and hydrogenated vegetable oils to less than 7% of total calories.
- Consume at least two servings of fish per week. Alternatively patients may take omega-3 fatty acid supplements (1 g/day).
- Consume at least six servings of grains, five servings of fruits and vegetables, and two servings of nonfat or low-fat dairy products per day.
- Consider adding plant stanol/sterols (2 g/day) and/or viscous fiber (over 10 g/day) to lower LDL cholesterol. It is recommended that patients with diabetes consume 14 g of fiber for every 1,000 kcal consumed.
- Limit daily sodium intake to 2.4 g (6 g of salt) for blood pressure control.

Exercise facilitates both weight loss and blood pressure reduction. In addition, regular exercise improves functional

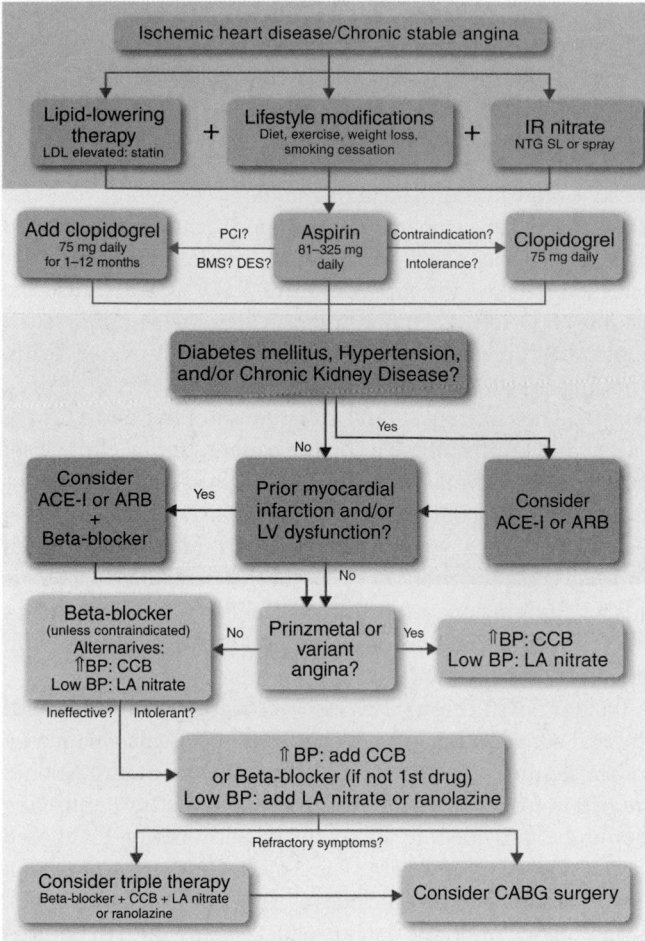

FIGURE 7–5. The treatment algorithm for ischemic heart disease. It begins at the top (blue section), which suggests risk factor modifications as the first treatment modality. Moving down to the green section, appropriate antiplatelet therapy is selected. The purple section identifies patients at high risk for major adverse cardiac events and suggests appropriate drug therapy to decrease cardiovascular risk. The yellow section at the bottom recommends appropriate antianginal therapy. The minimum duration of clopidogrel therapy following intracoronary stent placement is as follows: at least 1 month for bare metal stents and at least 12 months for drug-eluting stents. (ACE-I, angiotensin-converting enzyme inhibitor; ARB, angiotensin receptor blocker; BMS, bare metal stent; BP, blood pressure; CABG, coronary artery bypass graft; CCB, calcium channel blocker; DES, drug-eluting stent; IR, immediate-release; LA, long-acting; LDL, low-density lipoprotein; LV, left ventricular; NTG, nitroglycerin; PCI, percutaneous coronary intervention; SL, sublingual.)

capacity and symptoms in chronic stable angina.[1] Recent guidelines recommend moderate intensity aerobic activity, such as brisk walking, ideally for 30 to 60 minutes every day.[2] Medically supervised cardiac rehabilitation programs are recommended for high-risk patients.

Interventional Approaches

▶ Percutaneous Coronary Intervention

When drug therapy fails or if extensive coronary atherosclerosis is present, PCI is often performed to restore coronary blood flow, relieve symptoms, and prevent major adverse cardiac events. Patients with one or more critical coronary stenoses (i.e., greater than 70% occlusion of the coronary lumen) detected during coronary angiography may be candidates for PCI. Several catheter-based interventions may be used during PCI, including:

- Percutaneous transluminal coronary angioplasty (PTCA)
- Intracoronary bare metal stent placement
- Intracoronary drug-eluting stent placement
- Rotational atherectomy

During PCI, a catheter is advanced into the blocked coronary artery, as described for cardiac catheterization. If PTCA (i.e., balloon angioplasty) is performed, a balloon at the end of the catheter is inflated inside the artery at the site of the critical stenosis. When inflated, this balloon catheter displaces the atherosclerotic plaque out of the lumen of the artery, restoring normal myocardial blood flow. Most PCI procedures involve the placement of a small wire stent (similar in size and shape to the spring at the tip of a ball point pen) at the site of angioplasty. Coronary stenting involves use of a special balloon catheter containing the stent. When the balloon is inflated, the stent is deployed in the wall of the coronary artery, forming a sort of bridge or scaffold to maintain normal coronary blood flow. Either a bare metal stent or a drug-eluting stent may be used. Drug-eluting stents are impregnated with low concentrations of an antiproliferative drug (either paclitaxel or sirolimus), which is released locally over a period of weeks to inhibit restenosis or renarrowing of the coronary artery after PCI. A recent observational study demonstrated a significant reduction in all-cause mortality over a 4.5-year interval among patients who received a drug-eluting stent compared to those with a bare metal stent.[13] Stents themselves are thrombogenic, especially until they become endothelialized (covered in endothelial cells like a normal coronary artery). As such, dual antiplatelet therapy (discussed later) is required until the stent becomes endothelialized and perhaps indefinitely following stent placement to reduce the risk for stent thrombosis, MI, or death. Lastly, rotational atherectomy may be performed wherein a special catheter is used to essentially cut away the atherosclerotic plaque, restoring coronary blood flow.

▶ Coronary Artery Bypass Graft Surgery

As an alternative to PCI, CABG surgery, or open-heart surgery, may be performed if the patient is found to have extensive coronary atherosclerosis (generally greater than 70% occlusion of three or more coronary arteries) or is refractory to medical treatment. In the former case, CABG surgery has been shown to reduce mortality from IHD.

During CABG surgery, veins from the leg (i.e., saphenous veins) or arteries from the arm (i.e., radial artery) or chest wall (i.e., internal mammary arteries) are surgically removed. In the case of venous or radial artery conduits, one end of the removed blood vessel is attached to the aorta, and the other end is attached to the coronary artery distal to the atherosclerotic plaque. However, when internal mammary arteries are used, the distal end of the artery is detached from the chest wall and anastomosed to the coronary artery distal to the plaque. A median sternotomy, in which an incision the length of the sternum is made, is commonly required to gain access to the thoracic cavity and expose the heart. As the "new" blood vessels are being engrafted, the patient is typically placed on cardiopulmonary bypass (i.e., heart-lung machine) to maintain appropriate myocardial and systemic perfusion. Alternative surgical approaches for advanced IHD may be used in some settings including "off-pump" CABG (cardiopulmonary bypass is not required) and minimally invasive CABG (i.e., thorascopic surgery), although these techniques are not the norm. Because of the extremely invasive nature of this surgery, CABG surgery is generally reserved for patients with extensive coronary disease or as a treatment of last resort in patients with symptoms refractory to medical therapy.

Pharmacologic Therapy

▶ *Pharmacotherapy to Prevent ACSs and Death*

Control of Risk Factors A major component of any IHD treatment plan is control of modifiable risk factors, including dyslipidemia, hypertension, and diabetes. In addition, although not discussed in detail in this chapter, mental depression is common among patients with IHD and increases the risk for cardiac events and death. Thus, patients with IHD should be assessed for depression, and if present, appropriate management of depression should ensue.

Treatment strategies for dyslipidemia and hypertension in the patient with IHD are summarized in the following paragraphs. Visit chapters in this textbook on the management of hypertension and dyslipidemia for further information.

Because lipoprotein metabolism and the pathophysiology of atherosclerosis are closely linked, treatment of dyslipidemias is critical for both primary and secondary prevention of IHD-related cardiac events. In 2001, the Adult Treatment Panel III of the National Cholesterol Education Program issued guidelines for the management of dyslipidemia and recommended an LDL cholesterol goal of less than 100 mg/dL (2.59 mmol/L) for patients with documented IHD or IHD-risk equivalents such as diabetes or other vascular disease.[14] Since the publication of these guidelines, new evidence from several primary and secondary prevention trials suggests that there are additional clinical benefits from further reduction in LDL cholesterol.[15] In response to this evidence, more aggressive cholesterol-lowering goals were established for patients at *high risk* for developing IHD-related events, including those with diabetes or known cardiovascular disease. The following modifications were made to national treatment guidelines[15,16]:

- Statin or other LDL-lowering therapy is indicated along with lifestyle modifications in patients with cardiovascular disease or diabetes and multiple cardiovascular risk factors, regardless of baseline LDL cholesterol.
- Intensity of LDL-lowering therapy should be sufficient to decrease LDL cholesterol by 30% to 40%.
- Goal LDL cholesterol in patients with known clinical cardiovascular disease or diabetes plus one or more cardiovascular risk factors is less than 70 mg/dL (1.81 mmol/L).

Like dyslipidemia, hypertension is a major, modifiable risk factor for the development of IHD and related complications. Unfortunately, awareness, treatment, and control of blood pressure are suboptimal.[17] Aggressive identification and control of hypertension is warranted in patients with IHD to minimize the risk of major adverse cardiac events. Goal blood pressure in patients with IHD is less than 130/80 mm Hg with consideration of reducing blood pressure to less than 120/80 mm Hg in patients with left ventricular dysfunction or heart failure.[18] Because of their cardioprotective benefits, β-blockers and ACE inhibitors (or ARBs in ACE-inhibitor-intolerant patients), either alone or in combination, are appropriate for most patients with both hypertension and IHD.

Antiplatelet Agents Platelets play a major role in the pathophysiology of ACS. Specifically, platelets adhere to the site of atherosclerotic plaque rupture where they become activated, aggregate, and stimulate thrombus formation and ACS. Thromboxane is a potent platelet activator. Aspirin inhibits cyclooxygenase, an enzyme responsible for the production of thromboxane, thereby inhibiting platelet activation and aggregation. ❺ *In patients with stable or unstable angina, aspirin has been consistently shown to reduce the risk of major adverse cardiac events, particularly MI.*[19] ❻ *Antiplatelet therapy with aspirin should be considered for all patients without contraindications, particularly in patients with a history of MI.* Aspirin doses of 75 to 162 mg daily are recommended in patients with or at risk for IHD.[2,20] If aspirin is contraindicated (e.g., aspirin allergy) or is not tolerated by the patient, other antiplatelet agents such as clopidogrel should be considered.

Dual antiplatelet therapy with aspirin and a thienopyridine is recommended following PCI with stent placement to prevent stent thrombosis prior to stent endothelialization. Historically, ticlopidine was the thienopyridine agent used in combination with aspirin. However, clopidogrel has essentially replaced ticlopidine due to hematologic toxicity (leukopenia) of ticlopidine and the growing body of evidence supporting the use of clopidogrel. Antiproliferative drugs in drug eluting stents delay endothelialization, and thus a longer period of combination antiplatelet therapy is recommended for drug-eluting stents compared to bare metal stents to prevent thrombosis. Recent guidelines advocate combination antiplatelet therapy for at least 1 month after a bare metal stent and at least 12 months after a drug-eluting stent, although there are some data to support indefinite use of combination antiplatelet therapy after stent placement.[21] Because of the risk for stent thrombosis with premature discontinuation of dual antiplatelet therapy, it is imperative for clinicians to educate patients on this risk and the need for continuation of combination antiplatelet therapy for the recommended duration.

There are also data to support use of dual antiplatelet therapy in patients with ACS regardless of whether PCI with stent implantation is performed. In this population, the combination of aspirin and clopidogrel was more effective than aspirin alone in decreasing the risk of death, MI, and stroke.[22,23] For more information regarding the use of dual antiplatelet therapy in the setting of ACS, the reader is referred to the Acute Coronary Syndromes Chapter.

Statins Statins are the preferred drugs to achieve LDL cholesterol goals based on their potency in lowering LDL cholesterol and efficacy in preventing cardiac events. Specifically, over the last decade, several studies in tens of thousands of patients have revealed that lowering cholesterol with statins is effective for both primary and secondary prevention of IHD-related events.[15] Statins shown to decrease morbidity and mortality associated with IHD include lovastatin, simvastatin, pravastatin, and atorvastatin. A recent meta-analysis showed that the risk of major adverse cardiac events is reduced by 21% with the use of statins in patients at high risk for IHD-related events.[24]

Several studies have investigated whether statins possess pharmacologic properties in addition to their LDL cholesterol-lowering effect that may confer additional benefits in IHD.[25] These studies were prompted by evidence that patients with "normal" LDL cholesterol derived benefit from statins. Statins have been shown to modulate the following characteristics thought to stabilize atherosclerotic plaques and contribute to the cardiovascular risk reduction seen with these drugs:

- Shift LDL cholesterol particle size from predominantly small, dense, highly atherogenic particles to larger, less atherogenic particles.

- Improve endothelial function leading to more effective vasoactive response of the coronary arteries.

- Prevent or inhibit inflammation by lowering C-reactive protein and other inflammatory mediators thought to be involved in atherosclerosis.

- Possibly improving atherosclerotic plaque stability.

❼ *In summary, to control risk factors and prevent major adverse cardiac events, statin therapy should be considered in all patients with IHD, particularly in those with elevated low-density lipoprotein cholesterol or diabetes. Statins are potent lipid-lowering agents, possess non–lipid-lowering effects that may provide additional benefit to patients with IHD, and have been shown to reduce morbidity and mortality in patients with IHD. Based on these benefits, statins are generally considered the drugs of choice in patients with dyslipidemias. Moreover, based on evidence that statins improve outcomes in patients with IHD and "normal" LDL cholesterol concentration, statins should be considered in all patients with IHD at high risk of major adverse cardiac events, regardless of baseline LDL cholesterol.*

ACE-Is and ARBs Angiotensin II is a neurohormone produced primarily in the kidney. It is a potent vasoconstrictor and stimulates the production of aldosterone. Together, angiotensin II and aldosterone increase blood pressure and sodium and water retention (increasing ventricular wall tension), cause endothelial dysfunction, promote blood clot formation, and cause myocardial fibrosis.

ACE inhibitors decrease angiotensin II production and have consistently been shown to decrease morbidity and mortality in patients with heart failure or a history of MI.[26,27] A meta-analysis of 22 clinical trials with ACE inhibitors in post-MI patients found that ACE inhibitors reduced 1-year mortality by 16% to 32%, and the mortality-reducing effects were sustained for up to 4 years.[27] In addition, there is evidence that ACE inhibitors reduce the risk of vascular events in patients with chronic stable angina or risk factors for IHD.[28,29] Specifically, in nearly 10,000 patients with vascular disease (including IHD) or risk factors for vascular disease, such as diabetes, ramipril reduced the risk of death, acute MI, and stroke by 22% compared to placebo after an average of 5 years of treatment.[28] Similar results have been demonstrated with perindopril in patients with IHD.[29]

❼ *In the absence of contraindications, ACE inhibitors should be considered in all patients with IHD, particularly those who also have hypertension, diabetes mellitus, chronic kidney disease, left ventricular dysfunction, history of MI, or any combination of these.[2] Additionally, ACE inhibitors should also be considered in patients at high risk for developing IHD based on findings from the studies summarized above. ARBs may be used in patients with indications for ACE inhibitors but who cannot tolerate them due to side effects (e.g., chronic cough).* ARBs also antagonize the effects of angiotensin II. In one large trial, valsartan was as effective as captopril at reducing morbidity and mortality in post-MI patients.[26] However, there are far more data supporting the use of ACE inhibitors in IHD. Therefore, ACE inhibitors should remain first-line in patients with a history of MI, diabetes, chronic kidney disease, or left ventricular dysfunction. The ACE inhibitors and ARBs with indications for patients with or at risk for IHD or IHD-related complications are listed in Table 7–5.

Side effects with ACE inhibitors and ARBs include hyperkalemia, deterioration in renal function, and rarely, angioedema. Serum potassium increases are secondary to aldosterone inhibition and are more likely in the presence of pre-existing renal impairment, diabetes, or concomitant therapy with nonsteroidal anti-inflammatory drugs (NSAIDs), potassium supplements, or potassium-sparing diuretics. Reductions in glomerular filtration may occur during ACE inhibitor or ARB initiation or up-titration due to inhibition of angiotensin II-mediated vasoconstriction of the efferent arteriole. This type of renal impairment is usually temporary and is more common in patients with

Table 7–5

Doses of ACE Inhibitors and ARBs Indicated in IHD

Drug	Indications	Usual Dosage in IHD[a]
ACE Inhibitors		
Captopril	HTN, HF, post-MI, diabetic nephropathy	6.25–50 mg 3 × daily
Enalapril	HTN, HF	2.5–40 mg daily in 1–2 divided doses
Fosinopril	HTN, HF	10–80 mg daily in 1–2 divided doses
Lisinopril	HTN, HF, post-MI	2.5–40 mg daily
Perindopril	HTN, IHD	4–8 mg daily
Quinapril	HTN, HF, post-MI	5–20 mg twice daily
Ramipril	HTN, high-risk for IHD, HF, post-MI	2.5–10 mg daily in 1–2 divided doses
Trandolapril	HTN, HF, post-MI	1–4 mg daily
ARBs		
Candesartan	HTN, HF	4–32 mg daily
Valsartan	HTN, HF, post-MI	80–320 mg daily in 1–2 divided doses

ACE, angiotensin-converting enzyme; ARB, angiotensin-receptor blockers; HF, heart failure; HTN, hypertension; IHD, ischemic heart disease; MI, myocardial infarction.

[a]Reduce initial dose and gradually titrate upward as tolerated in renal impairment.

pre-existing renal dysfunction or unilateral renal artery stenosis. Bilateral renal artery stenosis is a contraindication for ACE inhibitors and ARBs because of the risk for overt renal failure. Angioedema is a potentially life-threatening adverse effect that occurs in less than 1% of ACE inhibitor-treated patients and may also occur with ARBs. Substitution of an ARB for an ACE inhibitor is appropriate for patients who develop a persistent cough with ACE inhibitor therapy, as this cough is believed to be due to accumulation of bradykinin secondary to ACE inhibition. Both ACE inhibitors and ARBs can cause fetal injury and death and are contraindicated in pregnancy.

▶ Nitroglycerin to Relieve Acute Symptoms

Short-acting nitrates are first-line treatment to terminate acute episodes of angina. ❽ *All patients with a history of angina should have sublingual nitroglycerin tablets or spray to relieve acute ischemic symptoms.* Nitrates undergo biotransformation to nitric oxide. Nitric oxide activates soluble guanylate cyclase and leads to increased intracellular concentrations of cyclic guanosine monophosphate, and ultimately, to smooth muscle relaxation. Nitrates primarily cause venodilation, leading to reductions in preload. The resultant decrease in ventricular volume and wall tension leads to a reduction in myocardial oxygen demand. In higher doses, nitrates may also cause arterial dilation and reduce afterload. In addition to reducing oxygen demand, nitrates increase myocardial oxygen supply by dilating the epicardial coronary arteries and collateral vessels, as well as relieving vasospasm.

Short-acting nitrates are available in tablet and spray formulations for sublingual administration. Sublingual nitroglycerin tablets are most commonly used to alleviate angina and are less expensive than the spray. However, the spray is preferred for patients who have difficulty opening the tablet container or produce insufficient saliva for rapid dissolution of sublingual tablets. ❽ *At the onset of an angina attack, a 0.3 to 0.4 mg dose of nitroglycerin (tablet or spray) should be administered sublingually, and repeated every 5 minutes until symptoms resolve. Sitting or standing enhances venous pooling and the effectiveness of nitroglycerin. Sublingual nitroglycerin can also be used to prevent effort-induced angina (i.e., angina that occurs with exertion). In this case, the patient should use sublingual nitroglycerin 2 to 5 minutes prior to an activity known to cause angina, with the effects persisting for approximately 30 minutes.* Isosorbide dinitrate, also available in a sublingual form, has a longer half-life with antianginal effects lasting up to 2 hours. The use of short-acting nitrates alone, without concomitant long-acting antianginal therapy, may be acceptable for patients who experience angina symptoms once every few days. However, for patients with more frequent attacks, long-acting antianginal therapy with β-blockers, CCBs, or long-acting nitrates is recommended.

The use of nitrates with phosphodiesterase type 5 inhibitors (e.g., sildenafil, vardenafil, and tadalafil), commonly prescribed for erectile dysfunction, is contraindicated. Phosphodiesterase degrades cyclic guanosine monophosphate (GMP), which is responsible for the vasodilatory effects of nitrates. Concomitant use of nitrates and phosphodiesterase type 5 inhibitors enhances cyclic GMP-mediated vasodilation and can result in serious hypotension and even death. All patients with IHD should receive a prescription for sublingual nitrates and education regarding their use. Points to emphasize when counseling a patient on nitroglycerin use include:

- The seated position is generally preferred when using nitroglycerin because the drug may cause dizziness.
- Call 911 if symptoms are unimproved or worsen 5 minutes after the first dose.
- Keep nitroglycerin tablets in the original glass container and close the cap tightly after use.
- Nitroglycerin should not be stored in the same container as other medications since this may reduce nitroglycerin's effectiveness.
- Repeated use of nitroglycerin is not harmful or addictive and does not result in any long-term side effects. Patients should not hesitate to use nitroglycerin whenever needed.
- Nitroglycerin should not be used within 24 hours of taking sildenafil or vardenafil or within 48 hours of taking tadalafil because of the potential for life-threatening hypotension.

▶ Pharmacotherapy to Prevent Recurrent Ischemic Symptoms

The overall goal of antianginal therapy is to allow patients with IHD to resume normal activities without symptoms of angina and to experience minimal to no adverse drug effects. The drugs traditionally used to prevent ischemic symptoms are β-blockers, CCBs, and nitrates. These drugs exert their antianginal effects by improving the balance between myocardial oxygen supply and demand, with specific effects listed in Table 7–6. β-Blockers, CCBs, and nitrates decrease the frequency of angina and delay the onset of angina during exercise. However, there is no evidence that any of these agents prevent ACS or improve survival in patients with chronic stable angina. Ranolazine is a newer molecular entity indicated for the treatment of chronic stable angina in patients unresponsive to traditional antianginal medications. Combination therapy with two or three antianginal drugs is often needed.

β-Blockers Stimulation of the β_1- and β_2-adrenergic receptors in the heart increases heart rate and cardiac contractility. β-Blockers antagonize these effects and decrease myocardial oxygen demand. β-Blockers may also reduce oxygen demand by lowering blood pressure and ventricular wall tension through blockade of plasma renin release. However, with marked reductions in heart rate, β-blockers may actually increase ventricular wall tension. This is because slower heart rates allow the ventricle more time to fill during diastole, leading to increased left ventricular volume, end-diastolic pressure, and wall tension. However, the net effect of β-blockade is usually a reduction in myocardial oxygen demand. β-Blockers do not improve myocardial oxygen supply.

The properties and recommended doses of various β-blockers are summarized in Table 7–7. β-Blockers with intrinsic sympathomimetic activity have partial β-agonist effects and cause lesser reductions in heart rate at rest. As a result, β-blockers with intrinsic sympathomimetic activity may produce lesser reductions in myocardial oxygen demand and should be avoided in patients with IHD. Other β-blockers appear equally effective at controlling symptoms of angina. The frequency of dosing and drug cost should be taken into consideration when choosing a particular drug. Agents that can be dosed once or twice daily are preferred. Most β-blockers are available in inexpensive generic versions. β-Blockers should be initiated in doses at the lower end of the usual dosing range, with titration according to symptom and hemodynamic response. The β-blocker dose is commonly titrated to achieve the following:

- Resting heart rate between 50 and 60 beats per minute (bpm).
- Maximum heart rate with exercise of 100 bpm or less or 20 bpm above the resting heart rate.

❾ *β-Blockers are first-line therapy for preventing ischemic symptoms, particularly in patients with a history of MI. In*

Table 7–6

Effects of Antianginal Medications on Myocardial Oxygen Demand and Supply

Antianginal Agent	Oxygen Demand			Oxygen Supply
	Heart Rate	Wall Tension	Cardiac Contractility	
β-Blockers	↓	↔ or ↑	↓	↔
Calcium channel blockers				
Verapamil, diltiazem	↓	↓	↓	↑
Dihydropyridines	↔ or ↑	↓	↓	↑
Nitrates	↑	↓	↔	↑

↓, decreases; ↔, no change; ↑, increases.

Table 7–7

Properties and Dosing of β-Blockers in Ischemic Heart Disease

Drug	Receptor Affinity	Intrinsic Sympathomimetic Activity	Usual Dose Range
Acebutolol	β_1-Selective	Yes	100–400 mg twice daily[a,b]
Atenolol	β_1-Selective	No	25–100 mg once daily[b]
Betaxolol	β_1-Selective	No	5–20 mg once daily[b]
Bisoprolol	β_1-Selective	No	2.5–10 mg once daily[a,b]
Carvedilol	α_1, β_1, and β_2	No	6.25–25 mg twice daily[c]
Labetalol	α_1, β_1, and β_2	Yes, at β_2-receptors	100–400 mg twice daily[a]
Metoprolol	β_1-Selective	No	50–100 mg twice daily (once daily for extended-release)[a]
Nadolol	β_1 and β_2	No	40–120 mg once daily[b]
Penbutolol	β_1 and β_2	Yes	10–40 mg once daily[a]
Pindolol	β_1 and β_2	Yes	10–40 mg twice daily[a]
Propranolol	β_1 and β_2	No	20–80 mg twice daily (60–180 mg once daily for long-acting formulation)[a]
Timolol	β_1 and β_2	No	10–20 mg twice daily[a,b]

[a]Dose adjust in hepatic impairment.

[b]Dose adjust in renal impairment

[c]Avoid in patients with hepatic impairment.

the absence of contraindications, β-blockers are preferred because of their potential cardioprotective effects. Specifically, β-blockers may prevent cardiac arrhythmias by decreasing the rate of spontaneous depolarization of ectopic pacemakers. Second, while the long-term effects of β-blockers on morbidity and mortality in patients with chronic stable angina are largely unknown, certain β-blockers have been shown to decrease the risk for reinfarction and improve survival in patients who have suffered an MI.[30] Specific β-blockers associated with mortality reductions in clinical trials include metoprolol, propranolol, and carvedilol.[30,31] In a meta-analysis of 82 clinical trials investigating the use of β-blockers in patients following MI, the relative risk of death was reduced by 23% in patients treated with β-blockers compared to control subjects.[30] Long-term therapy (for at least 6 months) was associated with greater mortality benefit compared to short-term β-blockade (6 weeks or less).

β-Blockers are contraindicated in patients with severe bradycardia (heart rate less than 50 bpm) or AV conduction defects in the absence of a pacemaker. β-Blockers should be used with particular caution in combination with other agents that depress AV conduction (e.g., digoxin, verapamil, and diltiazem) because of increased risk for bradycardia and heart block. Relative contraindications include asthma, bronchospastic disease, and severe depression. β_1-Selective blockers are preferred in patients with asthma or chronic obstructive pulmonary disease. However, selectivity is dose dependent, and β_1-selective agents may induce bronchospasm in higher doses.

There are several precautions to consider with the use of β-blockers in patients with diabetes or heart failure. All β-blockers may mask the tachycardia and tremor (but not sweating) that commonly accompany episodes of hypoglycemia in diabetes. In addition, nonselective β-blockers may alter glucose metabolism and slow recovery from hypoglycemia in insulin-dependent diabetes. β_1-Selective agents are preferred because they are less likely to prolong recovery from hypoglycemia. Importantly, β-blockers should not be avoided in patients with IHD and diabetes, particularly in patients with a history of MI who are at a high risk for recurrent cardiovascular events. β-Blockers are negative inotropes (i.e., they decrease cardiac contractility). Cardiac contractility is impaired in patients with left ventricular systolic dysfunction. Therefore, β-blockers may worsen symptoms of heart failure in patients with left ventricular systolic dysfunction (i.e., ejection fraction less than 40%). While certain β-blockers are indicated in patients with heart failure because they have been shown to reduce morbidity and mortality in this population, they must be used cautiously. In particular, when used for management of IHD in a patient with heart failure, β-blockers should be initiated in very low doses with slow up-titration to avoid worsening heart failure symptoms. The initiation of a β-blocker in a patient with acute cardiac decompensation should be delayed until the patient has stabilized.

Other potential adverse effects from β-blockers include fatigue, sleep disturbances, malaise, depression, and sexual dysfunction. Abrupt β-blocker withdrawal may increase the frequency and severity of angina, possibly because of increased receptor sensitivity to catecholamines after long-term β-blockade. If the decision is made to stop β-blocker therapy, the dose should be tapered over several days to weeks to avoid exacerbating angina.

Calcium Channel Blockers CCBs inhibit calcium entry into vascular smooth muscle and cardiac cells, resulting in the inhibition of the calcium-dependent process leading to muscle contraction. Inhibition of calcium entry into the vascular smooth muscle cells leads to systemic vasodilation and reductions in afterload. Inhibition of calcium entry into the cardiac cells leads to reductions in cardiac contractility. Thus, CCBs reduce myocardial oxygen demand by lowering both wall tension (through reductions in afterload) and cardiac contractility. In addition, the nondihydropyridine CCBs, verapamil and diltiazem, further decrease myocardial oxygen demand by slowing cardiac conduction through the AV node and lowering heart rate. In contrast, dihydropyridine CCBs, nifedipine in particular, are potent vasodilators that can cause baroreflex-mediated increases in sympathetic tone and heart rate. Because of their negative **chronotropic** effects, verapamil and diltiazem are generally more effective antianginal agents than the dihydropyridine CCBs. In addition to decreasing myocardial oxygen demand, all CCBs increase myocardial oxygen supply by dilating coronary arteries, thus increasing coronary blood flow and relieving vasospasm.

In randomized, controlled, clinical trials, CCBs were as effective as β-blockers at preventing ischemic symptoms. ❾ *CCBs are recommended as initial treatment in IHD when β-blockers are contraindicated or not tolerated. In addition, CCBs may be used in combination with β-blockers when initial treatment is unsuccessful.* However, the combination of a β-blocker with either verapamil or diltiazem should be used with extreme caution since all of these drugs decrease AV nodal conduction, increasing the risk for severe bradycardia or AV block when used together. If combination therapy is warranted, a long-acting dihydropyridine CCB is preferred. β-Blockers will prevent reflex increases in sympathetic tone and heart rate with the use of CCBs with potent vasodilatory effects. For patients with variable and unpredictable occurrences of angina, indicating possible coronary vasospasm, CCBs may be more effective than β-blockers in preventing angina episodes. The dosing of CCBs in IHD is described in Table 7–8.

Verapamil and diltiazem are contraindicated in patients with bradycardia and pre-existing conduction disease in the absence of a pacemaker. As noted above, verapamil and diltiazem should be used with particular caution in combination with other drugs that depress AV nodal conduction (e.g., β-blockers and digoxin). Because of their negative **inotropic** effects, CCBs may cause or exacerbate heart failure in patients with pre-existing left ventricular systolic dysfunction and should be avoided in this population. The exceptions are amlodipine and felodipine, which have less negative inotropic effects compared to other CCBs and appear to be safe in patients with left ventricular

Table 7–8	
Dosing of CCBs in Ischemic Heart Disease	
Drug	Usual Dose Range
Diltiazem, extended-release	120–360 mg once daily; consider dose adjustment in hepatic dysfunction
Verapamil, extended-release	180–480 mg once daily; use initial dose of 120 mg in hepatic dysfunction
Dihydropyridines	
Amlodipine	5–10 mg once daily
Felodipine	5–10 mg once daily; use initial dose of 2.5 mg once daily in hepatic dysfunction
Nifedipine, extended release	30–90 mg once daily; dose adjust and monitor closely in hepatic dysfunction
Nicardipine	20–40 mg 3 × daily; dose twice daily in hepatic dysfunction and up-titrate slowly in both hepatic and renal dysfunction

CCB, calcium channel blockers.

Table 7–9	
Nitrate Formulations and Dosing for Chronic Use	
Formulation	Dose
Oral	
Nitroglycerin extended-release capsules	2.5 mg 3 × daily initially, with up-titration according to symptoms and tolerance; allow a 10–12-hour nitrate-free interval
Isosorbide dinitrate tablets	5–20 mg 2–3 × daily, with a daily nitrate-free interval of at least 14 hours (e.g., dose at 7 AM, noon, and 5 PM)
Isosorbide dinitrate slow-release capsules	40 mg 1–2 × daily, with a daily nitrate-free interval of at least 18 hours (e.g., dose at 8 AM and 2 PM)
Isosorbide mononitrate tablets	5–20 mg 2 × daily initially, with up-titration according to symptoms and tolerance; doses should be taken 7 hours apart (e.g., 8 AM and 3 PM)
Isosorbide mononitrate extended-release tablets	30–120 mg once daily
Transdermal	
Nitroglycerin extended-release film	0.2–0.8 mg/h, on for 12–14 hours, off for 10–12 hours

systolic dysfunction.[32,33] Finally, there is some evidence that short-acting CCBs (particularly short-acting nifedipine and nicardipine) may increase the risk of cardiovascular events.[34] Therefore, short-acting agents should be avoided in the management of IHD.

Long-Acting Nitrates Nitrate products are available in both oral and transdermal formulations for chronic use. Commonly used products are listed in Table 7–9. All nitrate products are equally effective at preventing the recurrence of angina when used appropriately.

The major limitation of nitrate therapy is the development of tolerance with continuous use. The loss of antianginal effects may occur within the first 24 hours of continuous nitrate therapy. While the cause of tolerance is unclear, several mechanisms have been proposed, including the generation of free radicals that degrade nitric oxide. The most effective method to avoid tolerance and maintain the antianginal efficacy of nitrates is to allow a daily nitrate-free interval of at least 8 to 12 hours. Nitrates do not provide protection from ischemia during the nitrate-free period. Therefore, the nitrate-free interval should occur when the patient is least likely to experience angina. Generally, angina is less common during the nighttime hours when the patient is sleeping and myocardial oxygen demand is reduced. Thus, it is common to dose long-acting nitrates so that the nitrate-free interval begins in the evening. For example, isosorbide dinitrate is typically dosed on awakening and again 7 hours later.

Monotherapy with nitrates for the prevention of ischemia should generally be avoided for a couple of reasons. First, reflex increases in sympathetic activity and heart rate, with resultant increases in myocardial oxygen demand, may occur secondary to nitrate-induced venodilation. Second, patients are unprotected from ischemia during the nitrate-free interval. β-Blockers and CCBs are dosed to provide 24-hour protection from ischemia. ❾ *Treatment with long-acting nitrates should be added to baseline therapy with either a β-blocker or CCB or a combination of the two.* β-Blockers attenuate the increase in sympathetic tone and heart rate that occurs during nitrate therapy. In turn, nitrates attenuate the increase in wall tension during β-blocker therapy. As a result, the combination of β-blockers and nitrates is particularly effective at preventing angina and provides greater protection from ischemia than therapy with either agent alone. Monotherapy with nitrates may be appropriate in patients who have low blood pressure at baseline or who experience symptomatic hypotension with low doses of β-blockers or CCBs.

Common adverse effects of nitrates include postural hypotension, flushing, and headache secondary to venodilation. Headache often resolves with continued therapy and may be treated with acetaminophen. Hypotension is generally of no serious consequence. However, in patients with hypertrophic obstructive cardiomyopathy or severe aortic valve stenosis, nitroglycerin may cause serious hypotension and syncope. Therefore, long-acting nitrates are relatively contraindicated in these conditions. Because life-threatening hypotension may occur with concomitant use of nitrates and phosphodiesterase type 5 inhibitors, nitrates should not be used within 24 hours of taking sildenafil or vardenafil or within 48 hours of taking tadalafil. Skin erythema and inflammation may occur with transdermal nitroglycerin administration and may be minimized by rotating the application site.

Ranolazine Ranolazine is an anti-ischemic agent that exerts its effects by inhibiting the late inward sodium current during the plateau phase of the cardiac action potential. Under ischemic conditions, excess sodium may enter the myocardial cell during systole. The resultant intracellular sodium overload leads to intracellular calcium accumulation (calcium overload) though a sodium/calcium exchange mechanism. Calcium overload results in increases in left ventricular wall tension and myocardial oxygen consumption. By reducing intracellular sodium concentrations, ranolazine decreases calcium overload, left ventricular wall tension, and myocardial oxygen consumption.

In clinical trials, ranolazine at a dose of 750 to 1,000 mg twice daily improved angina and increased exercise capacity when added to other antianginal therapy.[35,36] Ranolazine has minimal effects on heart rate or blood pressure; however, it has the potential to prolong the QT interval and increase the risk for the life-threatening arrhythmia, torsades de pointes. Therefore, ranolazine should be reserved for patients with angina that is refractory to traditional antianginal medications. Contraindications to ranolazine are shown in Table 7–10. Common adverse effects with ranolazine include dizziness, headache, constipation, and nausea. Syncope may occur infrequently. Ranolazine is a substrate for CYP3A4 and both an inhibitor and substrate of p-glycoprotein. Concomitant use of ranolazine with moderate to potent CYP3A4 inhibitors, including verapamil and diltiazem, is contraindicated. Ranolazine should be used cautiously with p-glycoprotein inhibitors (e.g., cyclosporine) and substrates (e.g., digoxin).

▶ *Pharmacotherapy With No Benefit or Potentially Harmful Effects*

Hormone Replacement Therapy Hormone replacement therapy (HRT) has favorable effects on lipoprotein cholesterol concentrations. Data from several observational studies suggested that HRT might reduce the risk of cardiovascular events in women with IHD. However, subsequent randomized, controlled, clinical trials failed to demonstrate a reduction in the risk for IHD or cardiovascular events with HRT in postmenopausal women.[37,38] In fact, HRT appeared to be harmful in this patient population, increasing the risk of thromboembolic events and breast cancer. Current guidelines recommend against the use of HRT to reduce cardiovascular risk.[1] Furthermore, the clinician should consider discontinuing HRT therapy in women who suffer an acute coronary event while receiving such therapy.

Antioxidants Oxidization of LDL-cholesterol is believed to play a significant role in the atherosclerotic process. The antioxidant vitamins, vitamin E, vitamin C, and β-carotene, protect LDL cholesterol from oxidation. Evidence from observational and animal studies suggested that increased intake of antioxidant vitamins might inhibit the formation of atherosclerotic lesions and decrease the risk for cardiovascular events.[39] However, a meta-analysis of several large, randomized, prospective studies found no beneficial effect of vitamin E or β-carotene on cardiovascular

Table 7–10	
Contraindications and Precautions With Ranolazine	
Contraindications	**Precautions**
Pre-existing QT prolongation	Treatment with CYP3A4 inducers, including rifampin, phenobarbital, phenytoin, and carbamezpine, may significantly decrease the efficacy of ranolazine (by 95% with rifampil)
History of torsades de pointes	
Uncorrected hypokalemia	
Hepatic impairment	Treatment with a p-glycoprotein inhibitor may increase ranolazine absorption
Treatment with other QT-prolonging drugs	
Treatment with moderate to potent CYP3A4 inhibitors, including ketaconazole, verapamil, diltiazem, and St. John's wort	Ranolazine may increase bioavailability of p-glycoprotein substrates (increases digoxin plasma concentrations by 1.5-fold)
	Ranolazine may cause syncope; use caution when driving or operating machinery
	Ranolazine may cause reduced metabolism of CYP2D6 substrates

outcomes in patients with IHD or IHD risk factors.[40,41] Similarly disappointing results were demonstrated with vitamin C supplementation.[42] Based on this evidence, current guidelines do not recommend supplementation with vitamin E or other antioxidants for the sole purpose of preventing cardiovascular events.

Folic Acid Elevated homocysteine concentrations have been associated with an increased risk for cardiovascular disease in both epidemiologic and clinical studies.[43] Several studies have evaluated the benefit of lowering homocysteine levels with folic acid, vitamin B_6 and/or vitamin B_{12} supplementation. Despite lowering homocysteine levels, neither folic acid nor other vitamin B supplementation has been shown to reduce cardiovascular events in randomized controlled clinical trials.[44,45] Based on available evidence, the use of folate or vitamin B supplementation for the purpose of preventing cardiovascular events in patients with pre-existing IHD or at risk for IHD is not recommended.

Herbal Supplements Herbal products are widely used for their purported cardiovascular benefits; examples of such products include danshen, dong quai, feverfew, garlic, hawthorn, and hellebore. However, strong evidence supporting their benefits in cardiovascular disease is generally lacking. While small randomized controlled trials have shown benefits with some herbal supplements, the potential for drug interactions and the lack of product standardization limits the products' usefulness in clinical practice. Safety with herbal supplements in patients with IHD is a major concern. Unlike prescription and OTC medicines, the FDA does not require manufacturers of herbal products to submit proof of safety prior to product marketing. Numerous case reports of adverse cardiovascular events, including stroke, MI, and lethal cardiac arrhythmias with ephedra-based products (e.g.,

Ma huang) led the FDA to ban ephedra-containing products in 2004. However, other herbal supplements with potentially serious adverse cardiovascular effects remain easily accessible to the consumer (e.g., bitter orange). Some herbal supplements may interact with antiplatelet and antithrombotic therapy and increase bleeding risk (e.g., ginkgo biloba). Others may reduce the effectiveness of antianginal medications. Thus, it is important to assess the use of herbal products in patients with IHD and to counsel patients about the potential for drug interactions and adverse events with herbal therapies.

Cyclooxygenase-2 (COX-2) Inhibitors and NSAIDs Data suggest that COX-2 inhibitors and nonselective NSAIDs may increase the risk for MI and stroke.[46,47] The cardiovascular risk with COX-2 inhibitors and NSAIDs may be greatest in patients with a history of, or with risk factors for, cardiovascular disease. The COX-2 inhibitors rofecoxib and valdecoxib were withdrawn from the market in recent years because of safety concerns. The FDA requested the manufacturers of other COX-2 and nonselective NSAIDs (prescription and OTC) to include information about the potential adverse cardiovascular effects of these drugs in their product labeling. The American Heart Association recommends that the use of COX-2 inhibitors be limited to low-dose, short-term therapy in patients for whom there is no appropriate alternative.[46] Patients with cardiovascular disease should consult a clinician before using OTC NSAIDs.

SPECIAL POPULATIONS

Variant Angina

Vasospasm as the sole etiology of angina (Prinzmetal or variant angina) is relatively uncommon. As a result, treatment options are not well studied. Nevertheless, based on the pharmacology of available drugs, several recommendations can be made. First, β-blockers should be avoided in patients with variant angina because of their potential to worsen vasospasm due to unopposed α-adrenergic receptor stimulation. In contrast, both CCBs and nitrates are effective in relieving vasospasm and are preferred in the management of variant angina. Nitrates have several limitations outlined above, most notably the need for an 8- to 12-hour nitrate-free interval. Therefore, the role of monotherapy with long-acting nitrates as prophylaxis for anginal attacks due to vasospasm is limited. However, immediate-release nitroglycerin is effective at terminating acute anginal attacks due to vasospasm. Therefore, all patients diagnosed with variant angina should be prescribed immediate-release nitroglycerin. CCBs are effective for monotherapy of variant angina. Since short-acting CCBs have been associated with increased risk of adverse cardiac events, they should be avoided.[34] Long-acting nitrates may be added to CCB therapy if needed.

Elderly Patients With IHD

Elderly patients are more likely than younger patients to have other comorbidities that may influence drug selection for

Patient Encounter, Part 3: Creating a Care Plan

Based on the information presented, create a specific plan for the management of RJ's ischemic heart disease. Your plan should include:

(1) the goals of therapy;
(2) specific nonpharmacologic and pharmacologic interventions to address these goals; and
(3) a plan for follow-up to assess drug tolerance and whether the therapeutic goals have been achieved.

the treatment of angina. As a result, polypharmacy is more common in elderly patients, increasing the risk of drug–drug interactions, and perhaps decreasing medication adherence. Additionally, elderly patients are often more susceptible to adverse effects of antianginal therapies, particularly the negative chronotropic and inotropic effects of β-blockers and CCBs. Therefore, drugs should be initiated in low doses with close monitoring of elderly patients with IHD.

Acute Coronary Syndrome

The management of ACS is discussed in further detail in the chapter on acute coronary syndromes. It is important to educate patients with IHD on the signs of ACS and what to do if they appear. Importantly, patients should be instructed to seek emergent care if symptoms of angina last longer than 20 to 30 minutes, do not improve after 5 minutes of using sublingual nitroglycerin, or worsen after 5 minutes of using sublingual nitroglycerin. In patients with a history of ACS, it is crucial to select appropriate pharmacotherapy to prevent recurrent ACS and death. Appropriate pharmacotherapy for patients with a history of ACS includes aspirin (perhaps in combination with clopidogrel), ACE inhibitors or ARBs, β-blockers, and statins. In addition, determining appropriate goals and instituting appropriate therapy to meet the goals for cardiovascular risk factors (e.g., dyslipidemia, hypertension, and diabetes) is critical.

OUTCOME EVALUATION

Assessing for Drug Effectiveness and Safety

- ⑩ *Monitor symptoms of angina at baseline and at each clinic visit for patients with IHD to assess the effectiveness of antianginal therapy. In particular, assess the frequency and intensity of anginal symptoms.* Determining the frequency of sublingual nitroglycerin use is helpful in making this assessment. If angina is occurring with increasing frequency or intensity, adjust antianginal therapy and refer the patient for additional diagnostic testing (e.g., coronary angiography) and possibly for coronary interventions (e.g., PCI or CABG surgery).

- Assess the patient for IHD-related complications, such as heart failure. The presence of new comorbidities may indicate worsening IHD requiring additional workup or pharmacologic therapy.

- ⓾ *Routinely monitor hemodynamic parameters to assess drug tolerance. Assess blood pressure at baseline, after drug initiation and dose titration, then periodically thereafter in patients treated with β-blockers, CCBs, nitrates, ACE inhibitors, and/or ARBs.*

- Blood pressure reduction may be particularly pronounced after initiation and dose titration of β-blockers that also possess α-blocking effects (e.g., labetalol and carvedilol).

- Because of the potential for postural hypotension, warn patients that dizziness, presyncope, and even syncope may result from abrupt changes in body position during initiation or up-titration of drugs with α-blocking effects.

- ⓾ *Closely monitor heart rate in patients treated with drugs that have negative chronotropic effects (e.g., β-blockers, verapamil, or diltiazem) or drugs that may cause reflex tachycardia (e.g., nitrates or dihydropyridine CCBs).*

- Treatment with β-blockers, verapamil, or diltiazem can usually be continued in patients with asymptomatic bradycardia. However, reduce or discontinue treatment with these agents in patients who develop symptomatic bradycardia or serious conduction abnormalities.

- Regularly assess control of existing risk factors and the presence of new risk factors for IHD. Routine screening for the presence of metabolic syndrome will help in assessing the control of known major risk factors and identifying new risk factors. If new risk factors are identified and/or the presence of metabolic syndrome is detected, modify the pharmacotherapy regimen, as discussed previously, to control these risk factors and lower the risk of IHD and IHD-related adverse events.

- ⓾ *In patients treated with ACE inhibitors and/or ARBs, routinely monitor renal function and potassium levels at baseline, after drug initiation and dose titration, then periodically thereafter. This is particularly important when using these therapies in patients with pre-existing renal impairment or diabetes as they may be more susceptible to these adverse events.*

Duration of Therapy

- Drugs that modify platelet activity, lipoprotein concentrations, and neurohormonal systems reduce the risk for coronary events and death. However, these therapies do not cure IHD.

- Treatment with antiplatelet (aspirin or clopidogrel), lipid-lowering, and neurohormonal-modifying therapy for IHD is generally lifelong. Similarly, antianginal therapy with a β-blocker, CCB, and/or nitrate is usually long term.

- A patient with severe symptoms managed with combination antianginal drugs who undergoes successful coronary revascularization may be able to reduce antianginal therapy. However, treatment with at least one agent that improves the balance between myocardial oxygen demand and supply is usually warranted.

Patient Care and Monitoring

1. Assess the patient's symptoms to determine whether the patient should be evaluated by a physician.
   - Determine the quality, location, and duration of pain.
   - Determine factors that provoke and relieve pain.
   - Are symptoms characteristic of angina?
2. Identify risk factors for IHD.
   - Are there any modifiable risk factors?
3. Obtain a thorough history of prescription drug, nonprescription drug, and herbal product use.
   - Is the patient taking any medications/supplements that may exacerbate angina or interact with antianginal drug therapy?
4. Educate the patient on lifestyle modifications to control risk factors for IHD.
5. Is the patient taking appropriate drug therapy to prevent ACS and death? If not, why?
6. Is the patient taking appropriate antianginal therapy? If not, why?
7. Develop a plan to assess effectiveness of anti-ischemic therapy after 1 to 2 weeks.
8. Evaluate the patient to assess for adverse drug reactions, drug intolerance, and drug interactions.
9. Stress the importance of adherence with the therapeutic regimen, including lifestyle modifications.
10. Provide patient education regarding disease state, lifestyle modifications, and drug therapy:
    - What are the consequences of untreated IHD?
    - What lifestyle modifications should the patient follow?
    - When should the patient take his or her medications?
    - What potential adverse drug effects may occur?
    - Teach the patient how to monitor heart rate and blood pressure to assess tolerance to antianginal therapy.
    - Which drugs may interact with therapy or worsen IHD?
    - What should the patient do when chest pain or its equivalent occurs?
    - When should the patient seek emergent care?

Abbreviations Introduced in This Chapter

ACE	Angiotensin-converting enzyme
ACE-I	Angiotensin-converting enzyme inhibitor
ACS	Acute coronary syndrome
ARB	Angiotensin receptor blocker

AV	Atrioventricular
BMS	Bare metal stent
BPM	Beats per minute
CABG	Coronary artery bypass graft
CCB	Calcium channel blocker
CHD	Coronary heart disease
CK	Creatinine kinase
CK-MB	Creatinine kinase, MB fraction
COX-2	Cyclooxygenase-2
DES	Drug-eluting stent
EBCT	Electron beam computed tomography
GMP	Guanosine monophosphate
HDL	High-density lipoprotein
HF	Heart failure
HMG-CoA	3-Hydroxy-3-methylglutaryl coenzyme A reductase inhibitor
HRT	Hormone replacement therapy
IHD	Ischemic heart disease
IR	Immediate-release
LA	Long-acting
LDL	Low-density lipoprotein
LV	Left ventricular
MI	Myocardial infarction
MVO_2	Myocardial oxygen consumption
NSAID	Nonsteroidal anti-inflammatory drug
PCI	Percutaneous coronary intervention
Po_2	Partial pressure of oxygen
PTCA	Percutaneous transluminal coronary angioplasty
SL	Sublingual

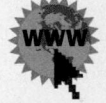 Self-assessment questions and answers are available at *http://www.mhpharmacotherapy.com/pp.html.*

REFERENCES

1. Gibbons RJ, Abrams J, Chatterjee K, et al. ACC/AHA 2002 guideline update for the management of patients with chronic stable angina—Summary article: A report of the American College of Cardiology/American Heart Association Task Force on practice guidelines (Committee on the Management of Patients With Chronic Stable Angina). J Am Coll Cardiol 2003;41:159–168.

2. Fraker TD Jr., Fihn SD, Gibbons RJ, et al. Chronic angina focused update of the ACC/AHA 2002 guidelines for the management of patients with chronic stable angina: A report of the American College of Cardiology/American Heart Association Task Force on Practice Guidelines Writing Group to develop the focused update of the 2002 guidelines for the management of patients with chronic stable angina. J Am Coll Cardiol 2007;50:2264–2274.

3. Rosamond W, Flegal K, Furie K, et al. Heart disease and stroke statistics—2008 update: A report from the American Heart Association Statistics Committee and Stroke Statistics Subcommittee. Circulation 2008;117:e25–e146.

4. Lewington S, Clarke R, Qizilbash N, Peto R, Collins R. Age-specific relevance of usual blood pressure to vascular mortality: A meta-analysis of individual data for one million adults in 61 prospective studies. Lancet 2002;360:1903–1913.

5. Grundy SM, Howard B, Smith S Jr, et al. Prevention Conference VI: Diabetes and Cardiovascular Disease: Executive summary: Conference proceeding for healthcare professionals from a special writing group of the American Heart Association. Circulation 2002;105:2231–2239.

6. Ninomiya JK, L'Italien G, Criqui MH, et al. Association of the metabolic syndrome with history of myocardial infarction and stroke in the Third National Health and Nutrition Examination Survey. Circulation 2004;109:42–46.

7. Grundy SM, Cleeman JI, Daniels SR, et al. Diagnosis and management of the metabolic syndrome: An American Heart Association/National Heart, Lung, and Blood Institute Scientific Statement. Circulation 2005;112:2735–2752.

8. Tzivoni D, Keren A, Meyler S, et al. Cardiovascular safety of transdermal nicotine patches in patients with coronary artery disease who try to quit smoking. Cardiovasc Drugs Ther 1998;12:239–244.

9. Braunwald E, Jones RH, Mark DB, et al. Diagnosing and managing unstable angina. Agency for Health Care Policy and Research. Circulation 1994;90:613–622.

10. Sangareddi V, Chockalingam A, Gnanavelu G, et al. Canadian Cardiovascular Society classification of effort angina: An angiographic correlation. Coron Artery Dis 2004;15:1111–1114.

11. Tonstad S, Farsang C, Klaene G, et al. Bupropion SR for smoking cessation in smokers with cardiovascular disease: A multicentre, randomised study. Eur Heart J 2003;24:946–955.

12. Krauss RM, Eckel RH, Howard B, et al. AHA Dietary Guidelines: Revision 2000: A statement for healthcare professionals from the Nutrition Committee of the American Heart Association. *Stroke* 2000;31:2751–2766.

13. Shishehbor MH, Goel SS, Kapadia SR, et al. Long-term impact of drug-eluting stents versus bare-metal stents on all-cause mortality. J Am Coll Cardiol 2008;52:1041–1048.

14. Executive Summary of The Third Report of The National Cholesterol Education Program (NCEP) expert panel on detection, evaluation, and treatment of high blood Cholesterol in adults (adult treatment panel III). JAMA 2001;285:2486–2497.

15. Grundy SM, Cleeman JI, Merz CN, et al. Implications of recent clinical trials for the National Cholesterol Education Program Adult Treatment Panel III guidelines. Circulation 2004;110:227–239.

16. Brunzell JD, Davidson M, Furberg CD, et al. Lipoprotein management in patients with cardiometabolic risk: Consensus conference report from the American Diabetes Association and the American College of Cardiology Foundation. J Am Coll Cardiol 2008;51:1512–1524.

17. Chobanian AV, Bakris GL, Black HR, et al. Seventh report of the Joint National Committee on prevention, detection, evaluation, and treatment of high blood pressure. Hypertension 2003;42:1206–1252.

18. Rosendorff C, Black HR, Cannon CP, et al. Treatment of hypertension in the prevention and management of ischemic heart disease: A scientific statement from the American Heart Association Council for High Blood Pressure Research and the Councils on Clinical Cardiology and Epidemiology and Prevention. Circulation 2007;115:2761–2788.

19. Tran H, Anand SS. Oral antiplatelet therapy in cerebrovascular disease, coronary artery disease, and peripheral arterial disease. JAMA 2004;292:1867–1874.

20. Patrono C, Baigent C, Hirsh J, Roth G. Antiplatelet drugs: American College of Chest Physicians Evidence-Based Clinical Practice Guidelines (8th Edition). Chest 2008;133:199S–233S.

21. Grines CL, Bonow RO, Casey DE Jr, et al. Prevention of premature discontinuation of dual antiplatelet therapy in patients with coronary artery stents: A science advisory from the American Heart Association, American College of Cardiology, Society for Cardiovascular Angiography and Interventions, American College of Surgeons, and American Dental Association, with representation from the American College of Physicians. Circulation 2007;115:813–818.

22. Yusuf S, Zhao F, Mehta SR, et al. Effects of clopidogrel in addition to aspirin in patients with acute coronary syndromes without ST-segment elevation. N Engl J Med 2001;345:494–502.

23. Chen ZM, Jiang LX, Chen YP, et al. Addition of clopidogrel to aspirin in 45,852 patients with acute myocardial infarction: Randomised placebo-controlled trial. Lancet 2005;366:1607–1621.

24. Baigent C, Keech A, Kearney PM, et al. Efficacy and safety of cholesterol-lowering treatment: Prospective meta-analysis of data from 90,056 participants in 14 randomised trials of statins. Lancet 2005;366:1267–1278.

25. Liao JK. Effects of statins on 3-hydroxy-3-methylglutaryl coenzyme A reductase inhibition beyond low-density lipoprotein cholesterol. Am J Cardiol 2005;96:24F–33F.

26. Pfeffer MA, McMurray JJ, Velazquez EJ, et al. Valsartan, captopril, or both in myocardial infarction complicated by heart failure, left ventricular dysfunction, or both. N Engl J Med 2003;349:1893–1906.

27. Rodrigues EJ, Eisenberg MJ, Pilote L. Effects of early and late administration of angiotensin-converting enzyme inhibitors on mortality after myocardial infarction. Am J Med 2003;115:473–479.

28. Yusuf S, Sleight P, Pogue J, et al. Effects of an angiotensin-converting-enzyme inhibitor, ramipril, on cardiovascular events in high-risk patients. The Heart Outcomes Prevention Evaluation Study Investigators. N Engl J Med 2000;342:145–153.

29. Fox KM. Efficacy of perindopril in reduction of cardiovascular events among patients with stable coronary artery disease: Randomised, double-blind, placebo-controlled, multicentre trial (the EUROPA study). Lancet 2003;362:782–788.

30. Freemantle N, Cleland J, Young P, Mason J, Harrison J. Beta Blockade after myocardial infarction: Systematic review and meta regression analysis. BMJ 1999;318:1730–1737.

31. Dargie HJ. Effect of carvedilol on outcome after myocardial infarction in patients with left-ventricular dysfunction: the CAPRICORN randomised trial. Lancet 2001;357:1385–1390.

32. Packer M, O'Connor CM, Ghali JK, et al. Effect of amlodipine on morbidity and mortality in severe chronic heart failure. Prospective Randomized Amlodipine Survival Evaluation Study Group. N Engl J Med 1996;335:1107–1114.

33. Cohn JN, Ziesche S, Smith R, et al. Effect of the calcium antagonist felodipine as supplementary vasodilator therapy in patients with chronic heart failure treated with enalapril: V-HeFT III. Vasodilator-Heart Failure Trial (V-HeFT) Study Group. Circulation 1997;96:856–863.

34. Psaty BM, Smith NL, Siscovick DS, et al. Health outcomes associated with antihypertensive therapies used as first-line agents. A systematic review and meta-analysis. JAMA 1997;277:739–745.

35. Morrow DA, Scirica BM, Karwatowska-Prokopczuk E, et al. Effects of ranolazine on recurrent cardiovascular events in patients with non-ST-elevation acute coronary syndromes: The MERLIN-TIMI 36 randomized trial. JAMA 2007;297:1775–1783.

36. Chaitman BR, Pepine CJ, Parker JO, et al. Effects of ranolazine with atenolol, amlodipine, or diltiazem on exercise tolerance and angina frequency in patients with severe chronic angina: A randomized controlled trial. JAMA 2004;291:309–316.

37. Hulley S, Grady D, Bush T, et al. Randomized trial of estrogen plus progestin for secondary prevention of coronary heart disease in postmenopausal women. Heart and Estrogen/progestin Replacement Study (HERS) Research Group. JAMA 1998;280:605–613.

38. Heiss G, Wallace R, Anderson GL, et al. Health risks and benefits 3 years after stopping randomized treatment with estrogen and progestin. JAMA 2008;299:1036–1045.

39. Willcox BJ, Curb JD, Rodriguez BL. Antioxidants in cardiovascular health and disease: key lessons from epidemiologic studies. Am J Cardiol 2008;101:75D–86D.

40. Bleys J, Miller ER, 3rd, Pastor-Barriuso R, Appel LJ, Guallar E. Vitamin-mineral supplementation and the progression of atherosclerosis: A meta-analysis of randomized controlled trials. Am J Clin Nutr 2006;84:880–887; quiz 954–955.

41. Vivekananthan DP, Penn MS, Sapp SK, Hsu A, Topol EJ. Use of antioxidant vitamins for the prevention of cardiovascular disease: Meta-analysis of randomised trials. Lancet 2003;361:2017–2023.

42. Cook NR, Albert CM, Gaziano JM, et al. A randomized factorial trial of vitamins C and E and beta carotene in the secondary prevention of cardiovascular events in women: Results from the Women's Antioxidant Cardiovascular Study. Arch Intern Med 2007;167:1610–1618.

43. Malinow MR, Bostom AG, Krauss RM. Homocyst(e)ine, diet, and cardiovascular diseases: A statement for healthcare professionals from the Nutrition Committee, American Heart Association. Circulation 1999;99:178–182.

44. Bazzano LA, Reynolds K, Holder KN, He J. Effect of folic acid supplementation on risk of cardiovascular diseases: A meta-analysis of randomized controlled trials. JAMA 2006;296:2720–2726.

45. Albert CM, Cook NR, Gaziano JM, et al. Effect of folic acid and B vitamins on risk of cardiovascular events and total mortality among women at high risk for cardiovascular disease: A randomized trial. JAMA 2008;299:2027–2036.

46. Bennett JS, Daugherty A, Herrington D, et al. The use of nonsteroidal antiinflammatory drugs (NSAIDs): A science advisory from the American Heart Association. Circulation 2005;111:1713–1716.

47. Gislason GH, Jacobsen S, Rasmussen JN, et al. Risk of death or reinfarction associated with the use of selective cyclooxygenase-2 inhibitors and nonselective nonsteroidal antiinflammatory drugs after acute myocardial infarction. Circulation 2006;113:2906–2913.

8 Acute Coronary Syndromes

Sarah A. Spinler and Simon de Denus

LEARNING OBJECTIVES

● **Upon completion of the chapter, the reader will be able to:**

1. Define the role of atherosclerotic plaque, platelets, and the coagulation system in an acute coronary syndrome (ACS).

2. List key ECG and clinical features identifying a patient with non-ST-segment elevation (NSTE) ACS who is at high risk of myocardial infarction (MI) or death.

3. Devise a pharmacotherapy treatment plan for a patient undergoing primary percutaneous coronary intervention (PCI) in ST-segment elevation (STE) MI given patient-specific data.

4. Devise a pharmacotherapy treatment plan for a patient with STE MI given patient-specific data.

5. List the quality performance measures of care for MI.

6. Formulate a monitoring plan for a patient with STE ACS receiving fibrinolytics, aspirin (ASA), clopidogrel, an anticoagulant, IV nitroglycerin, IV β-blockers followed by oral β-blockers, an angiotensin-converting enzyme (ACE) inhibitor, and a statin.

7. Devise a pharmacotherapy treatment and monitoring plan for a patient with NSTE ACS given patient-specific data.

8. Formulate a monitoring plan for a patient with NSTE ACS receiving ASA, clopidogrel, β-blocker, anticoagulant, and glycoprotein IIb/IIIa receptor inhibitor.

9. Devise a pharmacotherapy and risk-factor modification treatment plan for secondary prevention of coronary heart disease events in a patient following MI.

KEY CONCEPTS

❶ The cause of an acute coronary syndrome (ACS) is the rupture of an atherosclerotic plaque with subsequent platelet adherence, activation, and aggregation, and the activation of the clotting cascade. Ultimately, a clot forms composed of fibrin and platelets.

❷ The American Heart Association (AHA) and the American College of Cardiology (ACC) recommend strategies, or guidelines, for ACS patient care for ST-segment elevation(STE) and non-ST-segment elevation (NSTE) ACS.

❸ Patients with ischemic chest discomfort and suspected ACS are risk-stratified based upon a 12-lead electrocardiogram, past medical history, and results of the creatine kinase (CK) myocardial band (MB) and troponin tests. The diagnosis of myocardial infarction (MI) is confirmed based on the results of the CK MB and troponin tests.

❹ Early reperfusion therapy with primary percutaneous coronary intervention (PCI) within 90 minutes from time of hospital presentation is the reperfusion treatment of choice for patients presenting with STE ACS.

❺ The most recent NSTE ACC/AHA clinical practice guidelines recommend coronary angiography with either PCI or coronary artery bypass graft surgery revascularization as an early treatment (early invasive strategy) for high-risk and moderate-risk NSTE ACS patients.

❻ According to the ACC/AHA Association STE ACS practice guidelines, in addition to reperfusion therapy, early pharmacotherapy of STE should include intranasal oxygen (if oxygen saturation is less than 90%), sublingual (SL) nitroglycerin (NTG) followed by IV NTG in selected patients, ASA, clopidogrel, selective use of β-blockers, an anticoagulant, and fibrinolysis in eligible candidates.

❼ According to the ACC/AHA NSTE ACS practice guidelines, in the absence of contraindications, early pharmacotherapy of NSTE ACS should include intranasal oxygen (if oxygen saturation is low), SL NTG followed by IV NTG in selected patients, ASA, clopidogrel, β-blocker, and anticoagulant. High-risk patients should undergo early coronary angiography and revascularization with PCI or coronary artery bypass graft surgery. Administration of a glycoprotein IIb/IIIa receptor inhibitor may be considered in high-risk patients.

❽ Guidelines from the ACC/AHA suggest that, in the absence of contraindications, following MI from either STE or NSTE ACS, patients should receive indefinite treatment with ASA, a β-blocker, and an angiotensin-converting enzyme (ACE) inhibitor. For NSTE ACS, most patients should receive clopidogrel, in addition to ASA, for up to 12 months. For STE ACS, clopidogrel is administered during hospitalization and for at least 14 days (unless they undergo PCI where the duration of clopidogrel therapy depends on stent type), and up to 1 year. Most patients will receive a statin to reduce low-density lipoprotein cholesterol to less than 100 mg/dL (2.59 mmol/L).

❾ Secondary prevention of death, reinfarction, and stroke is more cost effective than primary prevention of coronary heart disease events.

INTRODUCTION

Cardiovascular disease (CVD) is the leading cause of death in the United States and one of the major causes of death worldwide. Acute coronary syndromes (ACSs), including unstable angina (UA) and myocardial infarction (MI), are a form of coronary heart disease (CHD) that comprises the most common cause of CVD death.[1] **❶** *The cause of an ACS is primarily the rupture of an atherosclerotic plaque with subsequent platelet adherence, activation, and aggregation, and the activation of the clotting cascade. Ultimately, a clot forms composed of fibrin and platelets.* **❷** *The American Heart Association (AHA) and the American College of Cardiology (ACC) recommend strategies, or guidelines, for ACS patient care for ST-segment elevation (STE) and non-ST-segment elevation (NSTE) ACS.* These joint practice guidelines are based upon a review of available clinical evidence, have graded recommendations based upon evidence, and are updated periodically. These guidelines form the cornerstone for quality care of the ACS patient.[2–4]

EPIDEMIOLOGY

Each year, more than one million Americans will experience an ACS and 150,000 will die of an MI.[1] In the United States, more than 8 million living persons have survived an MI.[1] Chest discomfort is a frequent reason for patient presentation to emergency departments, with up to 6 million, or approximately 5%, of all emergency department visits linked to chest discomfort and possible ACS. Coronary heart disease is the leading cause of premature, chronic disability in the United States. The risks of CHD events, such as death, recurrent MI, and stroke, are higher for patients with established CHD and a history of MI than for patients with no known CHD. The cost of CHD is high, with estimated direct and indirect costs of more than 156 billion dollars.[1] The median length of hospital stay for MI in 2005 was approximately 3.3 days.

In patients with STE ACS, in-hospital death rates are approximately 3% in patients receiving primary percutaneous coronary intervention (PCI), 7% for patients who are treated with fibrinolytics and 16% for patients who do not receive reperfusion therapy. In patients with NSTE MI, in-hospital mortality is less than 5%. In-hospital and 1-year mortality rates are higher for women and elderly patients.[1] At 1 year, rates of mortality and reinfarction are similar between STE and NSTE MI.

Because reinfarction and death are major outcomes following ACS, therapeutic strategies to reduce morbidity and mortality, particularly utilization of coronary angiography, revascularization, and pharmacotherapy, will have a significant impact on the social and economic burden of CHD in the United States.

ETIOLOGY

Endothelial dysfunction, inflammation, and the formation of fatty streaks contribute to the formation of atherosclerotic coronary artery plaques, the underlying cause of coronary artery disease (CAD). **❶** *The predominant cause of ACS in more than 90% of patients is atheromatous plaque rupture, fissuring, or erosion of an unstable atherosclerotic plaque that occludes less than 50% of the coronary lumen prior to the event, rather than a more stable 70% to 90% stenosis of the coronary artery.*[3] Stable stenoses are characteristic of stable angina.

PATHOPHYSIOLOGY

Spectrum of ACSs

ACSs include all clinical syndromes compatible with acute MI resulting from an imbalance between myocardial oxygen demand and supply.[3] In contrast to stable angina, an ACS results primarily from diminished myocardial blood flow secondary to an occlusive or partially occlusive coronary artery thrombus. ACSs are classified according to electrocardiogram (ECG) changes into STE ACS (STE MI) or NSTE ACS (NSTE MI and UA) (Fig. 8–1). An STE MI, formerly known as Q-wave or transmural MI, typically results in an injury that transects the thickness of the myocardial wall. Following an STE MI, pathologic Q waves are frequently seen on the ECG, indicating transmural MI, while such an ECG manifestation is seen less commonly in patients with NSTE MI.[5] NSTE MI, formerly known as non-Q-wave or nontransmural MI, is limited to the subendocardial myocardium. Patients in this case do not

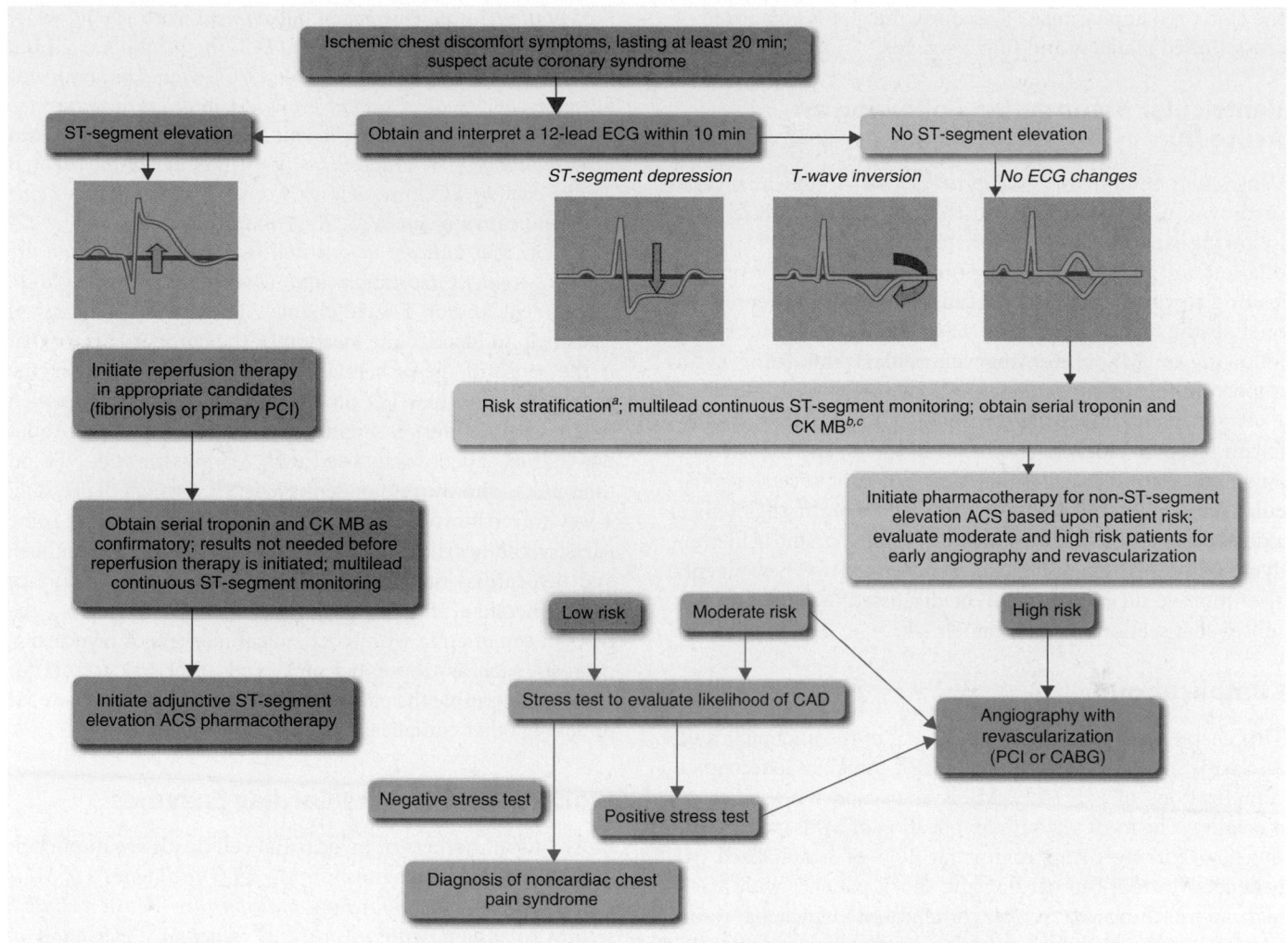

FIGURE 8–1. Evaluation of the ACS patient. [a]As described in Table 8–1. [b]Positive = above the myocardial infarction decision limit. [c]Negative = below the myocardial infarction decision limit. (ACSs, acute coronary syndromes; CABG, coronary artery bypass graft; CAD, coronary artery disease; CKMB, creatine kinase myocardial band; ECG, electrocardiogram; min, minute; PCI, percutaneous coronary intervention.) Refer to Figure 9–2 for further details regarding ECG interpretation. (From Spinler SA, de Denus S. Acute Coronary Syndromes. In DiPiro JT, Talbert RL, Yee GC, et al., (eds.) Pharmacotherapy: A Pathophysiologic Approach. 7th ed. New York: McGraw-Hill; 2008: 251, with permission.)

usually develop a pathologic Q wave on the ECG. Moreover, an NSTE MI is smaller and not as extensive as an STE MI. Approximately two-thirds of all MIs are NSTE MI, whereas one-third of patients with MI present with STE. NSTE MI differs from UA in that ischemia is severe enough to produce myocardial necrosis resulting in the release of a detectable amount of biomarkers, mainly **troponins T** or **I**, but also **creatine kinase** (CK) **myocardial band** (MB), from the necrotic myocytes in the bloodstream.[3] The clinical significance of serum markers will be discussed in greater detail in later sections of this chapter.

Plaque Rupture and Clot Formation

Following plaque rupture, a clot (a partially occlusive or completely occlusive thrombus), forms on top of the ruptured plaque. The thrombogenic contents of the plaque are exposed

to blood elements. Exposure of collagen and tissue factor induce platelet adhesion and activation, which promote the release of platelet-derived vasoactive substances including adenosine diphosphate (ADP) and thromboxane A_2 (TXA_2).[6] These produce vasoconstriction and potentiate platelet activation. Furthermore, during platelet activation, a change in the conformation in the glycoprotein IIb/IIIa surface receptors of platelets occurs which cross-links platelets to each other through fibrinogen bridges. This is considered the final common pathway of platelet aggregation. Inclusion of platelets gives the clot a white appearance. Simultaneously, the extrinsic coagulation cascade pathway is activated as a result of exposure of blood components to the thrombogenic lipid core and endothelium, which are rich in tissue factor. This leads to the production of thrombin (factor IIa), which converts fibrinogen to fibrin through enzymatic activity.[6] Fibrin stabilizes the clot and traps red blood cells, which gives the clot a red appearance. Therefore, the clot is composed of cross-linked platelets and fibrin strands.[6]

Ventricular Remodeling Following an Acute MI

Ventricular remodeling is a process that occurs in several cardiovascular conditions including heart failure and following an MI. It is characterized by left ventricular dilation and reduced pumping function of the left ventricle, leading to cardiac failure.[7] Because heart failure represents one of the principal causes of mortality and morbidity following an MI, preventing ventricular remodeling is an important therapeutic goal.[7]

Angiotensin-converting enzyme (ACE) inhibitors, angiotensin receptor blockers (ARBs), β-blockers, and aldosterone antagonists are all agents that slow down or reverse ventricular remodeling through inhibition of the renin-angiotensin aldosterone system and/or through improvement in hemodynamics (decreasing preload or afterload).[7] These agents also improve survival and will be discussed in more detail in subsequent sections of this chapter.

Complications

This chapter will focus on management of the uncomplicated ACS patient. However, it is important for clinicians to recognize complications of MI, since MI is associated with increased mortality. The most serious complication of MI is cardiogenic shock, occurring in approximately 10% of hospitalized MI patients. Mortality in cardiogenic shock patients with MI is high, approaching 60%.[8] Other complications which may result from MI are heart failure, valvular dysfunction, bradycardia, heart block, pericarditis, stroke secondary to left ventricular thrombus embolization, venous thromboembolism, left ventricular free wall rupture, and ventricular and atrial tachyarrhythmias.[9] In fact, more than one-quarter of MI patients die, presumably from ventricular fibrillation, prior to reaching the hospital.[1]

Symptoms and Physical Examination Findings

● The classic symptom of an ACS is midline anterior anginal chest discomfort, most often occurring when an individual is at rest, as a severe new onset, or as an increasing angina that is at least 20 minutes in duration. The chest discomfort may radiate to the shoulder, down the left arm, and to the back or to the jaw. Associated symptoms which may accompany the chest discomfort include nausea, vomiting, diaphoresis, or shortness of breath. While similar to stable angina, the duration may be longer and the intensity greater. On physical examination, no specific features are indicative of ACS.

12-Lead ECG

❸ *There are key features of a 12-lead ECG that identify and risk-stratify a patient with an ACS. Within 10 minutes of* *presentation to an emergency department with symptoms of ischemic chest discomfort, a 12-lead ECG should be obtained and interpreted. When possible, a 12-lead ECG should be performed by emergency medical system providers in order to reduce the delay until myocardial reperfusion. If available, a prior 12-lead ECG should be reviewed to identify whether or not the findings on the current ECG are new or old, with new findings being more indicative of an ACS. Key findings on review of a 12-lead ECG that indicate myocardial ischemia or infarction are STE, ST-segment depression, and T-wave inversion (Fig. 8–1).* ST-segment and/or T-wave changes in certain groupings of leads help to identify the location of the coronary artery that is the cause of the ischemia or infarction. In addition, the appearance of a new left bundle-branch block accompanied by chest discomfort is highly specific for acute MI. About one-half of patients diagnosed with MI present with STE on their ECG, with the remainder having ST-segment depression, T-wave inversion, or in some instances, no ECG changes. Some parts of the heart are more "electrically silent" than others, and myocardial ischemia may not be detected on a surface ECG. Therefore, it is important to review findings from the ECG in conjunction with biochemical markers of myocardial necrosis, such as troponin I or T, and other risk factors for CHD to determine the patient's risk for experiencing a new MI or having other complications.

Biochemical Markers/Cardiac Enzymes

Biochemical markers of myocardial cell death are important for confirming the diagnosis of MI. ❸ *The diagnosis of MI is confirmed when the following conditions are met in a clinical setting consistent with myocardial ischemia: "Detection of a rise and/or fall of cardiac biomarkers (troponin preferred) with at least one value above the 99th percentile of the upper reference limit together with evidence of myocardial ischemia as recognized by at least one of the following: (a) symptoms of ischemia; (b) ECG changes of new ischemia or development of pathological Q waves; or (c) imaging evidence of new loss of viable myocardium or new regional wall motion abnormality."*[10] Typically, a blood sample is obtained once in the emergency department, then 6 to 9 hours later, and in patients at a high suspicion of MI but in whom previous measurements did not reveal elevations in biomarkers, 12 to 24 hours after. A single measurement of a biochemical marker is not adequate to exclude a diagnosis of MI, as up to 15% of values which were initially below the level of detection (a "negative" test) rise to the level of detection (a "positive" test) in subsequent hours. While troponins and CK-MB appear in the blood within 6 hours of infarction, troponins stay elevated for up to 10 days while CK-MB returns to normal values within 48 hours. Hence, traditionally, CK-MB was used to detect reinfarction. However, more recent data have suggested that troponins provide similar information to CK-MB in such a situation which has lead to the use of troponins in this setting as well. Current guidelines suggest that, in patients in whom a recurrent MI is suspected, a cardiac biomarker should be immediately measured, followed by a second measurement three to six hours later. A recurrent

Clinical Presentation and Diagnosis of ACSs

General

- The patient is typically in acute distress and may develop or present with heart failure or cardiogenic shock.

Symptoms

- The classic symptom of ACS is midline anterior chest discomfort. Accompanying symptoms may include arm, back, or jaw pain; nausea; vomiting; or shortness of breath.
- Patients less likely to present with classic symptoms include elderly patients, diabetic patients, and women.

Signs

- No signs are classic for ACS.
- However, patients with ACS may present with signs of acute heart failure including jugular venous distention and an S_3 sound on auscultation.
- Patients may also present with arrhythmias and therefore may have tachycardia, bradycardia, or heart block.

Laboratory Tests

- Troponin I or T (and creatine kinase myocardial band [CK-MB]) are measured.
- Blood chemistry tests are performed with particular attention given to potassium and magnesium, which may affect heart rhythm.

- The SCr is measured to identify patients who may need dosing adjustments for some medications, as well as those who are at high risk of morbidity and mortality.
- Baseline CBC and coagulation tests (activated partial thromboplastin time and International Normalized Ratio [INR]) should be obtained, as most patients will receive antithrombotic therapy which increases the risk for bleeding.
- Fasting lipid panel.

Other Diagnostic Tests

- The 12-lead ECG is the first step in management. Patients are risk-stratified into two groups: ST-segment elevation ACS and suspected non-ST-segment elevation ACS.
- During hospitalization, a measurement of left ventricular function, such as an echocardiogram, is performed to identify patients with low EFs (less than 40%) who are at high risk of death following hospital discharge.
- Selected low-risk patients may undergo early stress testing.

Adapted from Spinler SA, de Denus S. Acute Coronary Syndromes. In: DiPiro JT, Talbert RL, Yee GC, et al., (eds.) Pharmacotherapy: A Pathophysiologic Approach. 7th ed. New York: McGraw-Hill; 2008: 252, with permission.

MI is diagnosed when there is an increase of at least 20% in the second measurement of the biomarker, if this value exceeds the 99th percentile of the upper reference limit.[10]

Risk Stratification

Patient symptoms, past medical history, ECG, and biomarkers, particularly troponins, are utilized to stratify patients into low, medium, or high risk of death, MI, or likelihood of failing pharmacotherapy and needing urgent coronary angiography and percutaneous coronary intervention (PCI). ❸ ❹ *Initial treatment according to risk stratification is depicted in Figure 8–1. Patients with STE are at the highest risk of death.* Initial treatment of STE ACS should proceed without evaluation of the troponins, as these patients have a greater than 97% chance of having an MI subsequently diagnosed with biochemical markers. The ACC/AHA define a target time to initiate reperfusion treatment as within 30 minutes of hospital presentation for fibrinolytics (e.g., streptokinase, alteplase, reteplase, and tenecteplase) and within 90 minutes or less from presentation for primary PCI.[3] The sooner the infarct-related coronary artery is opened for these patients, the lower their mortality and the greater the amount of myocardium that is preserved.[11,12] While all

patients should be evaluated for reperfusion therapy, not all patients may be eligible. Indications and contraindications for fibrinolytic therapy are described in the treatment section of this chapter. Less than 25% of hospitals in the United States are equipped to perform primary PCI. If patients are not eligible for reperfusion therapy, additional pharmacotherapy for STE patients should be initiated in the emergency department and the patient transferred to a coronary intensive care unit. The typical length of stay for a patient with uncomplicated STE MI is less than 4 days.

Risk-stratification of the patient with NSTE ACS is more complex, as in-hospital outcomes for this group of patients varies with reported rates of death of 0% to 12%, reinfarction rates of 0% to 3%, and recurrent severe ischemia rates of 5% to 20%.[12] Not all patients presenting with suspected NSTE ACS will even have CAD. Some will eventually be diagnosed with nonischemic chest discomfort. ❸ *In general, among NSTE patients, those with ST-segment depression (Fig. 8–1) and/or elevated biomarkers are at higher risk of death or recurrent infarction.*

TREATMENT

Desired Outcomes

Short-term desired outcomes in a patient with ACS are: (a) early restoration of blood flow to the infarct-related

Patient Encounter 1, Part 1

SD is a 55-year-old, 85 kg (187 lb) male who developed chest tightness while skiing at 20:30 hours. He became short of breath and diaphoretic. Local paramedics were summoned and he was given three 0.4-mg sublingual nitroglycerin tablets by mouth, 325 mg ASA by mouth, and morphine 2-mg IV push without relief of chest discomfort. SD presented to the hospital at 21:15 hours. The hospital does not have a cardiac catheterization laboratory and transport time to the nearest hospital with interventional facilities is more than 1.5 hours away via air transport.

PMH: HTN for 10 years; dyslipidemia for 6 months; two-vessel CAD (60% right coronary artery [RCA] and 80% left anterior descending artery [LAD] occlusion) after intracoronary sirolimus-eluting stent placement to the mid-LAD artery lesion 10 months ago

FH: Father with myocardial infarction at age 65; mother alive and well; one sibling with HTN

SH: Smoked one pack per day for 30 years, quit 10 weeks ago

Allergies: NKDA

Meds: Metoprolol 25 mg by mouth twice daily; ASA 325 mg by mouth once daily; lovastatin 20 mg by mouth once daily at bedtime; enalapril 5 mg by mouth once daily

ROS: 7/10 chest pain/squeezing, diaphoretic

PE:

HEENT: Normocephalic atraumatic

CR: Regular rate and rhythm S_1, S_2, $+S_3$, $+S_4$, no murmurs or rubs

VS: BP 110/70 mm Hg; HR 98 bpm; T 37°C (98.6°F)

Lungs: Rales bilaterally ¼ way up

Abd: Nontender, nondistended

GI: Normal bowel sounds

GU: Stool guaiac negative

Exts: No bruits, pulses 2+, femoral pulse present, good range of motion

Neuro: Alert and oriented × 3, cranial nerves intact

Labs: Sodium 138 mEq/L (138 mmol/L), potassium 4.2 mEq/L (4.2 mmol/L), chloride 105 mEq/L (105 mmol/L), bicarbonate 24 mEq/L (24 mmol/L), SCr 1.0 mg/dL (88 μmol/L), glucose 95 mg/dL (5.27 mmol/L), WBC 9.9 × 10³/mm³(9.9 × 10⁹/L), hemoglobin 15.7 g/dL (157 g/L or 9.7 mmol/L), hematocrit 47%, platelets 220 × 10³/mm³ (220 × 10⁹/L), brain natriuretic peptide 3,238 pg/mL (3,238 ng/L), troponin I 16 ng/mL (16 mcg/L), oxygen saturation 99% on room air

ECG: Normal sinus rhythm, PR 0.16 seconds, QRS 0.08 seconds, QT$_c$ 0.38 seconds, occasional polymorphic premature ventricular contractions, 3 mm ST-segment elevation anterior leads

CXR: Congestive heart failure, borderline upper normal heart size

Echo: Hypocontractile left ventricle, akinesis of anterior apical wall, EF 20%

What information is suggestive of acute MI?

What complications of MI are present?

---

artery to prevent infarct expansion (in the case of MI) or prevent complete occlusion and MI (in UA); (b) prevention of death and other complications; (c) resolve ECG changes; (d) prevention of coronary artery reocclusion; and (e) relief of ischemic chest discomfort.

Long-term desired outcomes are control of risk factors, prevention of additional cardiovascular events, including reinfarction, stroke and heart failure, and improvement in quality of life.

General Approach to Treatment

General treatment measures for all STE ACS and high- and intermediate-risk NSTE patients include admission to hospital, oxygen administration (if oxygen saturation is low, less than 90%), continuous multi-lead ST-segment monitoring for arrhythmias and ischemia, frequent measurement of vital signs, bed rest for 12 hours in hemodynamically stable patients, avoidance of the Valsalva maneuver (prescribe stool softeners routinely), and pain relief (Figs. 8–2 and 8–3).

Because risk varies and resources are limited, it is important to triage and treat patients according to their risk category. Initial approaches to treatment of STE and NSTE ACS patients are outlined in Figure 8–1. Patients with STE are at high risk of death, and efforts to reestablish coronary perfusion, as well as adjunctive pharmacotherapy, should be initiated immediately.

❸ *Features identifying low-, moderate-, and high-risk NSTE ACS patients are described using the thrombolysis in myocardial infarction (TIMI) risk score in Table 8–1.*[2]

Nonpharmacologic Therapy

▶ Primary PCI for STE ACSs

❹ *Early reperfusion therapy with primary PCI within 90 minutes from time of hospital presentation is the reperfusion treatment of choice for patients presenting with STE ACS.*[3,4] (Fig. 8–2) For primary PCI, the patient is taken from the emergency department to the cardiac catheterization laboratory and undergoes coronary angiography with either

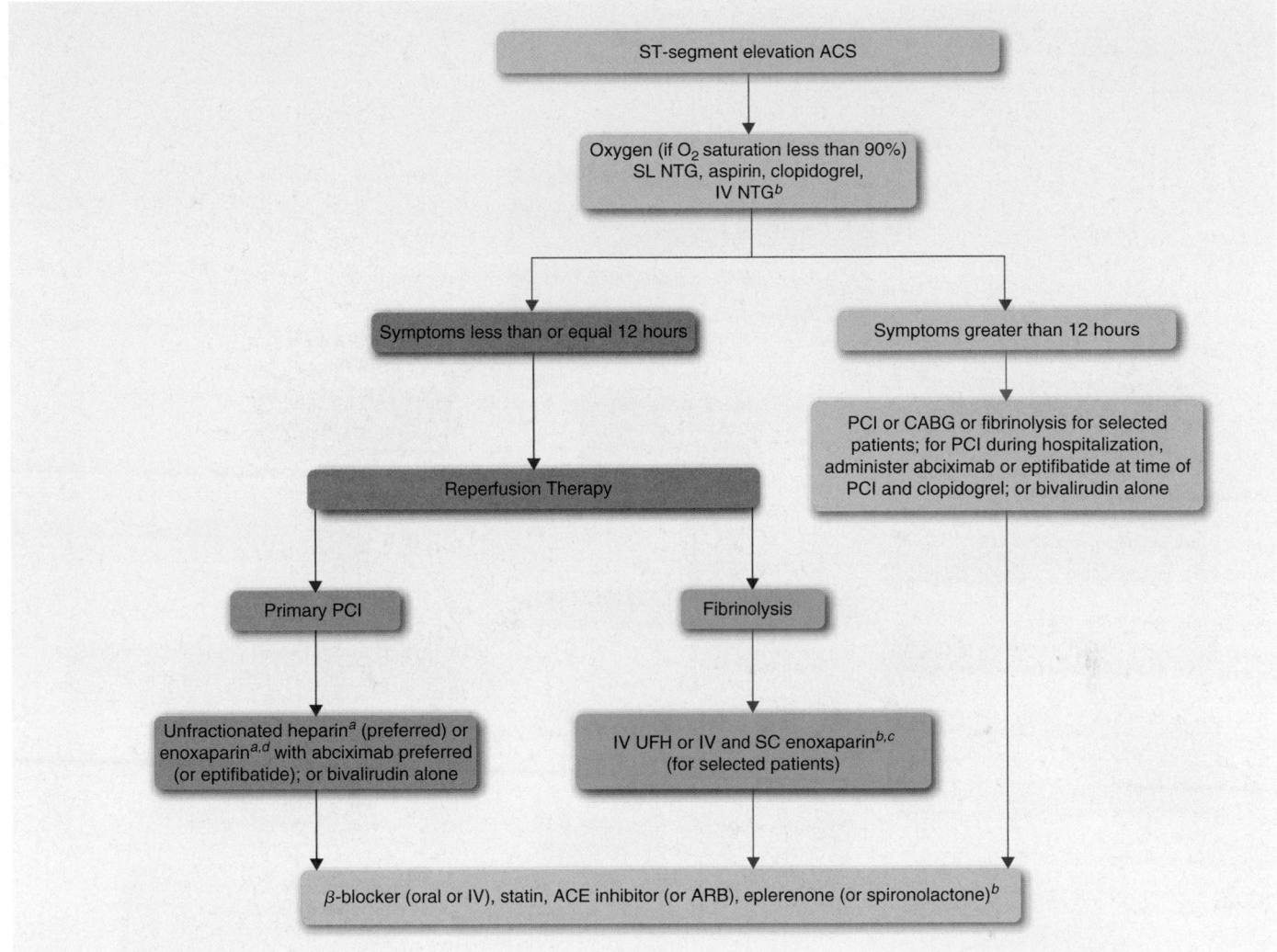

FIGURE 8–2. Initial pharmacotherapy for ST-segment elevation MI. [a]For at least 48 hours. [b]For selected patients, see Table 8–2. [c]For the duration of hospitalization, up to 8 days. [d]Exact dose not known. (ACSs, acute coronary syndromes; CABG, coronary artery bypass graft surgery; hrs, hours; IV, intravenous; NTG, nitroglycerin; PCI, percutaneous coronary intervention; SC, subcutaneous; SL, sublingual; UFH, unfractionated heparin.) (Adapted from Spinler SA, de Denus S. Acute Coronary Syndromes. In DiPiro JT, Talbert RL, Yee GC, et al., eds. Pharmacotherapy: A Pathophysiologic Approach. 7th ed. New York: McGraw-Hill; 2008: 256, with permission.) From Refs. 3, 9.

balloon angioplasty or placement of a bare metal or drug-eluting intracoronary stent. About 62% of patients with STE ACS are treated with primary PCI and 18% are treated with fibrinolytics. Results from a meta-analysis of trials comparing fibrinolysis to primary PCI indicate a lower mortality rate with primary PCI.[13] One reason for the superiority of primary PCI compared to fibrinolysis is that more than 90% of occluded infarct-related coronary arteries are opened with primary PCI compared to fewer than 60% of coronary arteries opened with currently available fibrinolytics.[9] In addition, intracranial hemorrhage and major bleeding risks from primary PCI are lower than the risks of severe bleeding events following fibrinolysis. An invasive strategy of primary PCI is generally preferred in patients presenting to institutions with skilled interventional cardiologists and a catheterization laboratory immediately

available, in patients in cardiogenic shock, those with contraindications to fibrinolytics, and those presenting with symptom onset greater than 3 hours ago.[3] A quality performance measure (quality performance measures are measures of quality health care developed from practice guidelines and intended to permit the quality of patient care to be assessed, compared between institutions and over time, and ultimately, improved) in the care of MI patients with STE is the time from hospital presentation to the time that the occluded artery is opened with PCI. This "door-to-primary PCI" time should be equal to or less than 90 minutes.[3,14] Currently, the median time for primary PCI is 87 minutes with only 54% of patients being treated within 90 minutes. Hospitals should have policies in place describing triage and catheterization laboratory personnel mobilization for implementing primary PCI for the patient with STE MI.

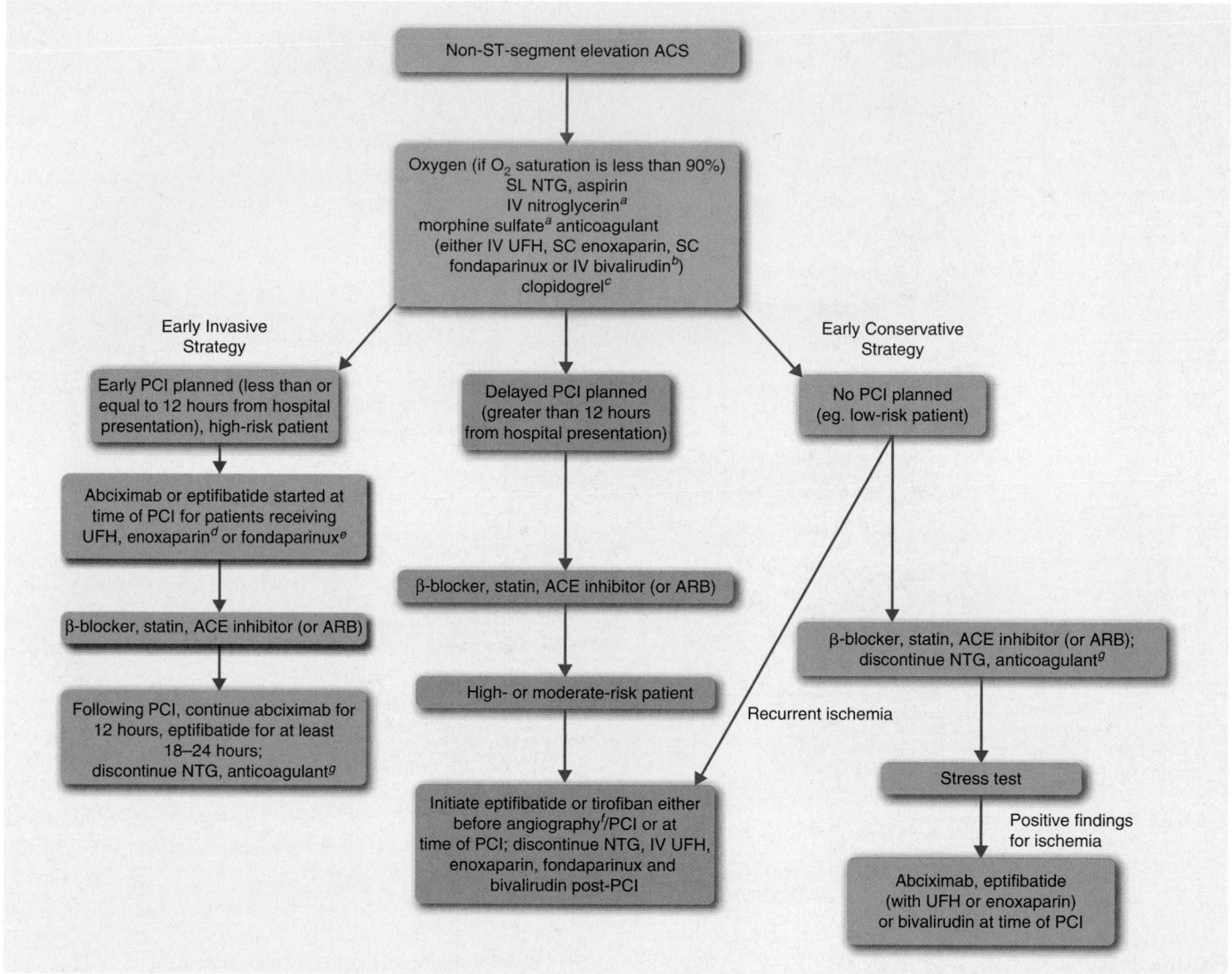

FIGURE 8–3. Initial pharmacotherapy for non-ST-segment elevation ACS. [a]For selected patients, see Table 8–2. [b]Enoxaparin, UFH, fondaparinux plus UFH, or bivalirudin for early invasive strategy; enoxaparin or fondaprinux if no angiography/PCI planned. [c]In patients unlikely to undergo coronary artery bypass graft surgery. [d]May require an IV supplemental dose of enoxaparin, see Table 8–2. [e]May require an IV supplemental dose of UFH, see Table 8–2. [f]For signs and symptoms of recurrent ischemia. [g]SC enoxaparin or UFH can be continued at a lower dose for venous thromboembolism prophylaxis. (ACE, angiotensin-converting enzyme; ACSs, acute coronary syndromes; ARB, angiotensin receptor blocker; hrs, hours; IV, intravenous; NTG, nitroglycerin; PCI, percutaneous coronary intervention; SC, subcutaneous; SL, sublingual; UFH, unfractionated heparin.) (Adapted from Spinler SA, de Denus S. Acute Coronary Syndromes. In DiPiro JT, Talbert RL, Yee GC, et al., (eds.) Pharmacotherapy: A Pathophysiologic Approach. 7th ed. New York: McGraw-Hill; 2008: 264, with permission.)

Patient Encounter 1, Part 2

Identify your acute treatment goals for SD.

Is reperfusion therapy with fibrinolysis indicated at this time?

What adjunctive pharmacotherapy should be administered to SD in the emergency department?

What additional pharmacotherapy should be initiated on the first day of SD's hospitalization following successful reperfusion?

PCI during hospitalization for STE MI may also be appropriate in other patients following STE MI, such as those in whom fibrinolysis is not successful, those presenting later in cardiogenic shock, those with life-threatening ventricular arrhythmias, and those with persistent rest ischemia or signs of ischemia on stress testing following MI.[3,4]

▶ *PCI in NSTE ACSs*

⑤ *The most recent NSTE ACC/AHA clinical practice guidelines recommend coronary angiography with either PCI or coronary artery bypass graft (CABG) surgery revascularization as*

Table 8–1

TIMI Risk Score for NSTE ACSs

Past Medical History	Clinical Presentation

• Age 65 years or older
• Three or more risk factors for CAD:
  Hypercholesterolemia
  HTN
  DM
  Smoking
  Family history of premature CHD
• Known CAD (50% or greater stenosis of a coronary artery)
• Use of ASA within the past 7 days
	• ST-segment depression (0.5 mm or greater)
	• Two or more episodes of chest discomfort within the past 24 hours
	• Positive biochemical marker for infarction[a]

Using the TIMI Risk Score

One point is assigned for each of the seven medical history and clinical presentation findings. The point total is calculated and the patient is assigned a risk for experiencing the composite endpoint of death, MI, or urgent need for revascularization as follows:

High risk	Medium risk	Low risk
TIMI risk score 5–7 points	TIMI risk score 3–4 points	TIMI risk score 0–2 points

Other Ways to Identify High-Risk Patients

Other findings that alone or in combination may identify a high-risk patient:
• ST-segment depression
• Positive biochemical marker for infarction
• Deep symmetric T-wave inversions (2 mm or greater)
• Acute heart failure
• DM
• Chronic kidney disease
• Refractory chest discomfort despite maximal pharmacotherapy for ACS
• Recent MI within the past 2 weeks

ACSs, acute coronary syndromes; CAD, coronary artery disease; CHD, coronary heart disease; DM, diabetes mellitus; HTN, hypertension; MI, myocardial infarction; NSTE, non-ST-segment elevation; TIMI, thrombolysis in myocardial infarction.

[a]A positive biochemical marker for infarction is a value of troponin I, troponin T, or creatine kinase myocardial band of greater than the MI detection limit.

From Spinler SA, de Denus S. Acute Coronary Syndromes. In DiPiro JT, Talbert RL, Yee GC, et al., (eds.) Pharmacotherapy: A Pathophysiologic Approach. 7th ed. New York: McGraw-Hill; 2008: 254, with permission.

an early treatment (early invasive strategy) for high-risk and moderate-risk NSTE ACS patients[2] (Fig. 8–3). Several clinical trials support an "invasive" interventional strategy with early angiography and PCI or CABG versus a "conservative medical management" strategy, whereby coronary angiography with revascularization is reserved for patients with symptoms refractory to pharmacotherapy and patients with signs of ischemia on stress testing.[2] An "invasive" approach results in fewer MIs, less need for additional revascularization procedures over the next year following hospitalization, and less cost than

the conservative "medical stabilization" approach in patients at moderate to high risk in most trials.[2,15] All patients undergoing PCI should receive aspirin (ASA) therapy indefinitely. Clopidogrel is administered (concomitantly with ASA) for at least 30 days following PCI for a patient receiving a bare metal stent and for at least 1 month and ideally up to 12 months following PCI for a patient receiving a drug eluting stent (DES) who is not at high risk for bleeding (Table 8–2).[4] Drug-eluting stents reduce the rate of smooth muscle cell growth causing stent restenosis. However, there is a delay in endothelial cell regrowth at the site of the stent which places the patient at higher risk of thrombotic events following PCI. Therefore, dual antiplatelet therapy is indicated for a longer period of time following PCI with a drug-eluting stent.[4] Regardless of whether or not a patient with NSTE receives a stent, the preferred duration of clopidogrel therapy is at least a year.[2]

Additional Testing and Risk Stratification

At some point during hospitalization but prior to discharge, patients with MI should have their left ventricular function (LVF) evaluated for risk stratification.[2,3] The most common way LVF is measured is using an echocardiogram to calculate the patient's left ventricular ejection fraction (LVEF). Left ventricular function is the single best predictor of mortality following MI. Patients with LVEFs less than 40% are at highest risk of death. Patients with ventricular fibrillation or sustained ventricular tachycardia occurring more than 2 days following MI and those with LVEF less than 30% (measured at least 1 month after STE MI and 3 months after coronary artery revascularization with either PCI or CABG) benefit from placement of an implantable cardioverter defibrillator (ICD).[3,16]

Predischarge from the hospital, stress testing (Fig. 8–3) may be indicated in: (a) moderate- or low-risk patients in order to determine who would benefit from coronary angiography to establish the diagnosis of CAD, and (b) patients following MI to predict intermediate- and long-term risk of recurrent MI and death.[2] In most cases, patients with a positive stress test indicating coronary ischemia will then undergo coronary angiography and subsequent revascularization of significantly occluded coronary arteries. If a patient has a negative exercise stress test for ischemia, the patient is at lower risk for subsequent CHD events.

Early Pharmacologic Therapy for STE ACSs

Pharmacotherapy for early treatment of ACS is outlined in Figure 8–2. ❻ *According to the ACC/AHA STE ACS practice guidelines, in addition to reperfusion therapy, early pharmacotherapy of STE should include intranasal oxygen (if oxygen saturation is less than 90%), sublingual (SL) nitroglycerin (NTG) followed by IV NTG in selected patients, ASA, clopidogrel, an anticoagulant, a β-blocker in selected patients, and fibrinolysis in eligible candidates (not undergoing primary PCI). Recent results from two clinical trials in patients with STE ACS indicate that clopidogrel should be administered along with ASA to patients receiving fibrinolytics to reduce mortality and reinfarction as well as to improve the patency of the infarcted artery.*[17,18] Morphine is administered to patients

Table 8-2

Evidence-Based Pharmacotherapy for STE and NSTE ACSs

Drug	Clinical Condition and ACC/AHA Guideline Recommendation[a]	Contraindications[b]	Dose and Duration of Therapy
Aspirin	STE MI, class I recommendation for all patients NSTE ACS, class I recommendation for all patients	Hypersensitivity, active bleeding, severe bleeding risk	160–325 mg orally once on hospital day 1. 75–162 mg once daily orally starting hospital day 2 and continued indefinitely in patients not receiving an intracoronary stent. 162–325 mg once daily orally for a minimum of 30 days in patients undergoing PCI receiving a bare metal stent, 3 months with a sirolimus-eluting stent, and 6 months with a paclitaxel-eluting, followed by 75–162 mg once daily orally thereafter. Continue indefinitely.
Clopidogrel	STE MI, class I recommendation in patients allergic to aspirin; class I recommendation to add to aspirin. NSTE ACS, class I recommendation for all hospitalized In PCI in STE and NSTE ACS, class I recommendation	Hypersensitivity, active bleeding, severe bleeding risk	300 mg (class I recommendation) to 600 mg (class IIa recommendation) loading dose on hospital day 1 followed by a maintenance dose of 75 mg po once daily starting on hospital day 2 in patients with NSTE ACS or STEMI undergoing PCI. 300 mg loading dose followed by 75 mg po daily in patients receiving a fibrinolytic or that do not receive reperfusion therapy in patients with a STE MI (avoid loading dose in patients aged 75 years or more). Administer indefinitely in patients with aspirin allergy (class I recommendation). Administer at least 9 months in patients with NSTE ACS who are managed medically (class I recommendation). For post-PCI stented patients with DES, administer at least 12 months (AHA Science Advisory). For bare-metal stents, administer for at least 1 month, ideally for 12 months. In patients receiving a fibrinolytic or that do not receive reperfusion therapy in patients with a STE MI, administer for at least 14 days (Class I) and up to 1 year (Class IIa).
Unfractionated heparin	STE MI, class I recommendation in patients undergoing PCI, and for those patients treated with fibrinolytics, class IIa recommendation for patients not treated with fibrinolytic therapy NSTE ACS, class I recommendation in combination with antiplatelet therapy for conservative or invasive approach PCI, class I recommendation (NSTE ACS and STE MI)	Active bleeding, heparin-induced thrombocytopenia, severe bleeding risk, recent stroke	For STE MI with fibrinolytics, administer 60 Units/kg IV bolus (maximum 4,000 Units) followed by a constant IV infusion at 12 units/kg/h (maximum 1,000 Units/h). For STE MI primary PCI administer 60–70 units/kg followed by a constant infusion of 12–15 units/kg/h. For NSTE ACS, administer 60 Units/kg IV bolus (maximum 400 Units) followed by a constant IV infusion at 12 Units/kg/h (maximum 1,000 Units/h). Titrated to maintain an aPTT of 1.5–2.0 × control (approximately 50–70 seconds) for STE MI and for NSTE ACS. The first aPTT should be measured at 4–6 hours for NSTE ACS and STE ACS in patients not treated with fibrinolytics. The first aPTT should be measured at 3 hours in patients with STE ACS who are treated with fibrinolytics. Continue for 48 hours or until the end of PCI.
Enoxaparin	STE MI class I recommendation in patients receiving fibrinolytics and class IIa for patients not undergoing reperfusion therapy NSTE ACS, class I recommendation in combination with aspirin for conservative or invasive approach For PCI, class IIa recommendation as an alternative to UFH in patients with NSTE ACS For primary PCI in STE MI, class IIb recommendation as an alternative to UFH	Active bleeding, history of heparin-induced thrombocytopenia, severe bleeding risk, recent stroke, avoid enoxaparin if CrCl less than 15 mL/min, avoid if CABG surgery	Enoxaparin 1 mg/kg SC every 12 hours for patients with NSTE ACS (CrCl greater than or equal to 30 mL/min). Enoxaparin 1 mg/kg SC every 24 hours (CrCl 15–29 mL/min) for NSTE or STE MI. For patients undergoing PCI following initiation of SC enoxaparin for NSTE ACS, a supplemental 0.3 mg/kg IV dose of enoxaparin should be administered at the time of PCI if the last dose of SC enoxaparin was given 8–12 hours prior to PCI. For patients with STE MI receiving fibrinolytics: Age less than 75 yrs: administer enoxaparin 30 mg IV bolus followed immediately by 1 mg/kg SC every 12 hours (first 2 doses administer maximum of 100 mg for patients weighing more than 100 kg). Age greater than or equal to 75 yrs: administer enoxaparin 0.75 mg/kg SC every 12 hours (first 2 doses administer maximum of 75 mg for patients weighing more than 75 kg). Continue throughout hospitalization or up to 8 days for STE MI. Continue for 24–48 hours for NSTE ACS or until the end of PCI.

Drug	Recommendation	Contraindications/Precautions	Dosing
Bivalirudin	NSTE ACS class I recommendation for invasive strategy PCI in STE MI (no recommendation; clinical trial data)	Active bleeding, severe bleeding risk	For NSTE ACS, administer 0.1 mg/kg IV bolus followed by 0.25 mg/kg/h infusion. For PCI in NSTE ACS, administer a second bolus of 0.5 mg/kg IV and increase infusion rate to 1.75 mg/kg/h. Alternatively for PCI (in either NSTE ACS or STE MI), administer a 0.75 mg/kg IV bolus followed by a 1.75 mg/kg/h IV infusion Discontinue at end of PCI or continue for up to 4 hours.
Fondaparinux	Class I recommendation for STE MI receiving thrombolytics and IIa for patients not undergoing reperfusion therapy. Class I for NSTE ACS for invasive or conservative approach.	Active bleeding, severe bleeding risk, SCr greater than or equal to 3.0 mg/dL (265 µmol/L) or CrCl less than 30 mL/min	For STE MI, 2.5 mg IV bolus followed by 2.5 mg SC once daily starting on hospital day 2. For NSTE ACS, 2.5 mg SC once daily. For PCI, give 50–60 units/kg IV bolus of UFH (regimen not rigorously studied). Continue until hospital discharge or up to 8 days.
Fibrinolytic therapy	STE MI, class I recommendation for patients presenting within 12 hours following the onset of symptoms, class IIa in patients presenting between 12 and 24 hours, following the onset of symptoms with continuing signs of ischemia NSTE ACS, class III recommendation	Any prior intracranial hemorrhage, known structural cerebrovascular lesions, such as an arterial venous malformation, known intracranial malignant neoplasm, ischemic stroke within 3 months, active bleeding (excluding menses), significant closed head or facial trauma within 3 months	Streptokinase: 1.5 MU IV over 60 minutes. Alteplase: 15 mg IV bolus followed by 0.75 mg/kg IV over 30 min (max 50 mg) followed by 0.5 mg/kg (max 35 mg) over 60 min (maximum dose = 100 mg). Reteplase: 10 Units IV × 2, 30 minutes apart. Tenecteplase: less than 60 kg = 30 mg IV bolus 60–69.9 kg = 35 mg IV bolus 70–79.9 kg = 40 mg IV bolus
Glycoprotein IIb/IIIa receptor blockers	NSTE ACS, class IIa recommendation for either tirofiban or eptifibatide for patients with either continuing ischemia, elevated troponin, or other high-risk features, class I recommendation for patients undergoing PCI, class IIb recommendation for patients without high-risk features who are not undergoing PCI STE MI, class IIa for abciximab for primary PCI and class IIb for either tirofiban or eptifibatide for primary PCI	Active bleeding, thrombocytopenia, prior stroke	

Drug	Dose for PCI	Dose for NSTE ACS with/without PCI	Dose adjustment for renal insufficiency
Abciximab	0.25 mg/kg IV bolus followed by 0.125 mcg/kg/min (maximum 10 mcg/min) for 12 hours	Not recommended	None
Eptifibatide	180 µg/kg IV bolus × 2, 10 minutes apart with an infusion of 2 mcg/kg/min for 18–24 hours after PCI	180 µg/kg IV bolus followed by an infusion of 2 mcg/kg/min for 12–72 hours	Reduce maintenance infusion to 1 µg/kg/min for patients with CrCl less than 50 mL/min; not studied in patients with serum creatinine greater than 4.0 mg/dL (354 µmol/L); Patients weighing 121 kg or more should receive a maximum infusion rate of 22.6 mg per bolus and a maximum infusion rate of 15 mg/h
Tirofiban	Not FDA approved	0.4 mg/kg IV bolus administered over 30 minutes followed by an infusion of 0.1 mcg/kg/min for 18–72 hours	Reduce maintenance infusion to 0.05 mcg/kg/min for patients with CrCl less than 30 mL/min

(Continued)

Table 8–2

Evidence-Based Pharmacotherapy for STE and NSTE ACSs (Continued)

Drug	Clinical Condition and ACC/AHA Guideline Recommendation[a]	Contraindications[b]	Dose and Duration of Therapy
Nitroglycerin	STE MI and NSTE ACS, class I indication in patients with ongoing ischemic discomfort, control of hypertension or management of pulmonary congestion	Hypotension, sildenafil or vardenafil within 24 hours or tadalafil within 48 hours	0.4 mg SL, repeated every 5 minutes × 3 doses 5–10 mcg/min IV infusion titrated up to 75–100 mcg/min until relief of symptoms or limiting side-effects (headache) with a systolic blood pressure less than 90 mmHg or more than 30 percent below starting mean arterial pressure levels if significant hypertension is present. Topical patches or oral nitrates and acceptable alternatives for patients without ongoing or refractory symptoms
β-blockers[c]	STE MI and NSTE ACS, class I recommendation for oral β-blockers in all patients without contraindications in the first 24 hours, class IIa for IV β-blockers in hypertensive patients	PR ECG segment greater than 0.24 seconds, 2nd degree or 3rd degree atrioventricular heart block, heart rate less than 60 beats/min, systolic blood pressure less than 90 mm Hg, shock, left ventricular failure with congestive heart failure, severe reactive airway disease	Continue IV infusion for 24–48 hours. Target resting heart rate of 50–60 beats/min. Metoprolol 5 mg slow IV push (over 1–2 min), repeated every 5 minutes for a total of 15 mg followed in 1–2 hours by 25–50 mg by mouth every 6 hours; if a very conservative regimen is desired, initial doses can be reduced to 1–2 mg. Propranolol 0.5–1 mg IV dose followed in 1–2 hours by 40–80 mg by mouth every 6–8 hours. Atenolol 5 mg IV dose followed in 5 minutes by a second 5 mg IV dose for a total of 10 mg followed in 1–2 hours by 50–100 mg by mouth once daily. Alternatively, initial intravenous therapy can be omitted. Continue oral β-blocker indefinitely ▼
Calcium channel blockers	STE MI class IIa recommendation and NSTE ACS class I recommendation for patients with ongoing ischemia who are already taking adequate doses of nitrates and β-blockers or in patients with contraindications to or intolerance to β-blockers (diltiazem or verapamil preferred during initial presentation) NSTE ACS, class IIb recommendation for diltiazem for patients with AMI	Pulmonary edema, evidence of left ventricular dysfunction, systolic blood pressure less than 100 mm Hg, PR ECG segment greater than 0.24 seconds for verapamil and diltiazem, 2nd or 3rd degree atrioventricular heart block for verapamil or diltiazem, heart rate less than 60 beats/min for diltiazem or verapamil	Diltiazem 120–360 mg sustained release orally once daily. Verapamil 180–480 mg sustained release orally once daily. Nifedipine 30–90 mg sustained release orally once daily. Amlodipine 5–10 mg orally once daily. Continue indefinitely if contraindication to oral β-blocker persists.

Drug	Clinical Condition and ACC/AHA Guideline Recommendation[a]	Contraindications[b]			
ACE Inhibitors	NSTE ACS or STE MI, class I recommendation for patients with heart failure, left ventricular dysfunction and EF less than or equal to 40%, type 2 diabetes mellitus or chronic kidney disease	Systolic blood pressure less than 100 mm Hg, history of intolerance to an ACE inhibitor bilateral renal artery stenosis serum potassium greater than 5.5 mEq/L (greater than 5.5 mmol/L) acute renal failure, pregnancy	**Drug** Captopril Enalapril Lisinopril Ramipril Trandolapril	**Initial Dose** 6.25–12.5 mg 2.5–5.0 mg 2.5–5.0 mg 1.25–2.5 mg 1.0 mg	**Target Dose** 50 mg twice daily orally to 50 three times daily 10 mg twice daily orally 10–20 mg once daily orally 5 mg twice daily or 10 mg once daily orally 4 mg once daily orally

Drug category	Indications[a]	Contraindications/cautions[b]	Drug	Initial Dose	Target Dose
	Consider in all patients with CAD (class I recommendation, class IIa in low risk patients)				
	Indicated indefinitely for all patients with EF less than 40% (class I recommendation)				
Angiotensin receptor blockers	NSTE MI or STE MI, class I recommendation in patients with clinical signs of heart failure or left ventricular EF less than 40% and intolerant of an ACE inhibitor, class IIa recommendation in patients with clinical signs of heart failure or EF less than 40% and no documentation of ACE inhibitor intolerance. Class I in other intolerant patients with hypertension.	Systolic blood pressure less than 100 mm Hg, bilateral renal artery stenosis, serum potassium greater than 5.5 mg/dL (greater than 5.5 mmol/L), acute renal failure, pregnancy	Candesartan Valsartan Continue indefinitely.	4–8 mg 40 mg	32 mg once daily orally 160 mg twice daily orally

Drug category	Indications[a]	Contraindications/cautions[b]	Drug	Initial Dose	Maximum Dose
Aldosterone antagonists	STE ACS, class I recommendation for patients with MI and EF less than or equal to 40% and either diabetes mellitus or heart failure symptoms who are already receiving an ACE inhibitor	Hypotension hyperkalemia, serum potassium greater than 5.0 mEq/L (greater than 5.5 mmol/L), SCr greater than 2.5 mg/dL (greater than 221 µmol/L)	Eplerenone Spironolactone Continue indefinitely.	25 mg 12.5 mg	50 mg once daily orally 25–50 mg once daily orally
Morphine sulfate	STE and NSTE ACS, class I recommendation for patients whose symptoms are not relieved after three serial SL nitroglycerin tablets or whose symptoms recur with adequate anti-ischemic therapy	Hypotension, respiratory depression, confusion obtundation	2–4 mg IV bolus dose May be repeated every 5–15 minutes as needed to relieve symptoms and maintain patient comfort.		

[a]Class I recommendations are conditions for which there is evidence and/or general agreement that a given procedure or treatment is useful and effective.

Class II recommendations are those conditions for which there is conflicting evidence and/or divergence of opinion about the usefulness/efficacy of a procedure or treatment. For Class IIa recommendations, the weight of the evidence/opinion is in favor of usefulness/efficacy. Class IIb recommendations are those for which usefulness/efficacy is less well established by evidence/opinion. Class III recommendations are those where the procedure or treatment is not useful and may be harmful.

[b]Allergy or prior intolerance contraindication for all categories of drugs listed in this chart.

[c]Choice of the specific agent is not as important as ensuring that appropriate candidates receive this therapy. If there are concerns about patient intolerance due to existing pulmonary disease, especially asthma, selection should favor a short-acting agent, such as propranolol or metoprolol or the ultra short-acting agent, esmolol. Mild wheezing or a history of chronic obstructive pulmonary disease should prompt a trial of a short-acting agent at a reduced dose (e.g., 2.5 mg intravenous metoprolol, 12.5 mg oral metoprolol, or 25 mcg/kg/min esmolol as initial doses) rather than complete avoidance of β-blocker therapy.

ACC, American College of Cardiology; ACE, angiotensin converting enzyme inhibitor; AHA, American Heart Association; ACS, acute coronary syndrome; aPTT, activated partial thromboplastin time; CABG, coronary artery bypass graft; CAD, coronary artery disease; CrCl, Creatinine clearance; DES, drug eluting stent; ECG, electrocardiogram; EF, ejection fraction; FDA, Food and Drug Administration; IV, intravenous; MI, myocardial infarction; NSTE, non-ST-segment elevation; PCI, percutaneous coronary intervention; SC, subcutaneous; SCr, serum creatinine; SL, sublingual; STE, ST-segment elevation; UFH, unfractionated heparin.

From Refs. 2, 3, 4, 9, 22, 32, 50.

with refractory angina as an analgesic and a venodilator that lowers preload. These agents should be administered early, while the patient is still in the emergency department. Dosing and contraindications for SL and IV NTG, ASA, clopidogrel, β-blockers, anticoagulants, and fibrinolytics are listed in Table 8–2.[2-4]

▶ *Fibrinolytic Therapy*

Administration of a fibrinolytic agent is indicated in patients with STE ACS who present to the hospital within 24 hours of the onset of chest discomfort, have at least a 1 mm STE in two or more contiguous ECG leads, and are not able to undergo primary PCI within 90 minutes of hospital presentation.[3] The mortality benefit of fibrinolysis is highest with early administration and diminishes after 12 hours. The use of fibrinolytics between 12 and 24 hours after symptom onset should be limited to patients with ongoing ischemia. Fibrinolytic therapy is preferred over primary PCI where there is no cardiac catheterization laboratory or there would be a delay in "door-to-primary PCI" of more than 90 minutes. Indications and contraindications for fibrinolysis are listed in Table 8–3.[9] It is not necessary to obtain the results of biochemical markers before initiating fibrinolytic therapy. Because administration of fibrinolytics result in clot lysis, patients who are at high risk of major bleeding (including intracranial hemorrhage) presenting with an absolute contraindication will likely not receive fibrinolytic therapy, as primary PCI is preferred. In patients who have a contraindication to fibrinolytics and PCI, or who don't have access to a facility that can perform PCIs, treatment with an anticoagulant (other than unfractionated heparin [UFH]) for up to 8 days can be administered.

In patients with symptoms lasting less than 6 hours, a more fibrin-specific agent such as alteplase, reteplase, or tenecteplase is preferred over a non-fibrin-specific agent such as streptokinase.[9,19] Fibrin-specific fibrinolytics open a greater percentage of infarcted arteries. In a large clinical trial, administration of alteplase reduced mortality by 1% (absolute reduction) and cost about $30,000 per year of life saved compared to streptokinase.[20] Two other trials compared alteplase to reteplase and alteplase to tenecteplase and found similar mortality between agents.[21,22] Therefore, either alteplase, reteplase, or tenecteplase are acceptable as first-line agents. Intracranial hemorrhage and major bleeding are the most serious side effects of fibrinolytic agents. The risk of intracranial hemorrhage is higher with fibrin-specific agents than with streptokinase. However, the risk of systemic bleeding other than intracranial hemorrhage is higher with streptokinase than with other more fibrin-specific agents and was higher with alteplase versus tenecteplase in one study.[19,20,22]

As mentioned previously, less than 20% of patients with STE ACS receive fibrinolysis compared with more than 60% receiving primary PCI. However, 17% of eligible patients receive neither primary PCI nor fibrinolysis despite being eligible. The primary reason for lack of reperfusion therapy is that most patients present more than 12 hours after the

Table 8–3
Indications and Contraindications to Fibrinolytic Therapy per ACC/AHA Guidelines for Management of Patients With STE MI

Indications

1. Ischemic chest discomfort at least 20 minutes in duration but 12 hours or less since symptom onset
   and
   STE of at least 1 mm in height in two or more contiguous leads, or new or presumed new left bundle-branch block
2. Ongoing ischemic chest discomfort at least 20 minutes in duration 12–24 hours since symptom onset
   and
   STE of at least 1 mm in height in two or more contiguous leads

Absolute Contraindications

- Active internal bleeding (not including menses)
- Previous intracranial hemorrhage at any time; ischemic stroke within 3 months
- Known intracranial neoplasm
- Known structural vascular lesion (e.g., arteriovenous malformation)
- Suspected aortic dissection
- Significant closed head or facial trauma within 3 months

ACC, American College of Cardiology; AHA, American Heart Association.

From Ref. 3.

time of symptom onset. The percentage of eligible patients who receive reperfusion therapy is a quality performance measure of care in patients with MI.[3,14] The "door-to-needle time," the time from hospital presentation to start of fibrinolytic therapy, is another quality performance measure.[3,14] The ACC/AHA guidelines recommend a "door-to-needle time" of less than 30 minutes from the time of hospital presentation until start of fibrinolytic therapy. The median national average is decreasing and is currently 30 minutes. All hospitals should have protocols addressing fibrinolysis eligibility, dosing and monitoring.

▶ *Aspirin*

ASA has become the preferred antiplatelet agent in the treatment of all ACS.[2,3] ASA administration to all patients who do not have contraindications to ASA therapy within 24 hours before or after hospital arrival is a quality performance measure for MI.[3,14] The antiplatelet effects of ASA are mediated by inhibiting the synthesis of TXA_2 through an irreversible inhibition of platelet cyclooxygenase-1. In patients undergoing PCI, ASA prevents acute thrombotic occlusion during the procedure. In patients receiving fibrinolytics, ASA reduces mortality, and its effects are additive to fibrinolysis alone.[23]

Although an initial dose of 160 to 325 mg is required to achieve rapid platelet inhibition, long-term therapy with doses of 75 to 150 mg daily are as effective as higher doses. In addition, doses of less than 325 mg daily are associated with a lower rate of bleeding.[24,25] The major bleeding rate associated with chronic ASA administration in doses less than 100 mg per day is 1.6%, whereas the rate with doses more than 100 mg per day is 2.3%.[25] Therefore, a daily maintenance dose of 75 to 162 mg is recommended.[2] Although evidence-based data are sparse, a dose of 162 to 325 mg daily is recommended for at least 1 month following intracoronary placement of a bare metal stent, 3 months after a sirolimus stent and 6 months after a paclitaxel stent.[3,4]

Nonsteroidal anti-inflammatory drugs other than ASA should not be used because they increase the risk of mortality, reinfarction, hypertension (HTN), heart failure and myocardial rupture.[3] In response to shear stress, endothelial cells produce cyclooxygenase-2 (COX-2). COX-2 inhibition may be associated with a reduction in prostacyclin synthesis, sodium and water retention and increased blood pressure (BP). During MI, the balance between thrombosis and inhibition of thrombosis may be shifted to a prothrombotic state, increasing infarct size. Other GI disturbances, including dyspepsia and nausea, are infrequent when low-dose ASA is used. ASA therapy should be continued indefinitely.

▶ Thienopyridines

Administration of clopidogrel, in addition to ASA, is recommended for all patients with STE ACS (Table 8–2).[3] Clopidogrel blocks adenosine diphosphate receptors on platelets, preventing the expression of glycoprotein IIb/IIIa receptors and thus platelet activation and aggregation.

Clopidogrel reduces death, MI, or stroke in patients with NSTE ACS when combined with ASA.[26] Early therapy with clopidogrel 75 mg once daily administered during hospitalization and up to 28 days (mean 14 days) in patients with STE ACS reduced mortality and reinfarction in patients treated with fibrinolytics without increasing the risk of major bleeding.[17,18] Therefore, the combination of clopidogrel and ASA is indicated for all patients with ACS. For PCI, clopidogrel is administered as a 300 to 600 mg loading dose followed by a 75 mg per day maintenance dose, in combination with ASA, to prevent subacute stent thrombosis and long-term events, such as the composite endpoint of death, MI, or need to undergo repeat PCI.[3,4] Clopidogrel should be continued for at least 14 days (and up to one year) for patients with STE ACS who do not undergo PCI and a minimum of 4 weeks up to 12 months for patients undergoing primary PCI with a bare metal stent.[3,4] In patients receiving a DES, clopidogrel should be administered for at least 12 months.[4] For patients not undergoing PCI or early revascularization with CABG surgery, clopidogrel should be administered for 14 days.[2,3] If CABG is planned, clopidogrel should be withheld preferably for 5 days, to reduce the risk of postoperative bleeding, unless the need for revascularization outweighs the bleeding risk. The most frequent side effect of clopidogrel is rash or GI events (nausea, vomiting, or diarrhea). Rarely, thrombotic thrombocytopenic purpura has been reported with clopidogrel.

▶ Glycoprotein IIb/IIIa Receptor Inhibitors

Abciximab is a first-line glycoprotein IIb/IIIa receptor inhibitor for patients undergoing primary PCI[3,16] who have not received fibrinolytics. It should not be administered for medical management of the STE ACS patient who will not be undergoing PCI. Abciximab, in combination with ASA, a thienopyridine, and UFH (administered as an infusion for the duration of the procedure), is given a higher recommendation in the ACC/AHA guidelines over eptifibatide and tirofiban in this setting because abciximab is the most common glycoprotein IIb/IIIa receptor inhibitor studied in primary PCI trials, and a meta-analysis of trials demonstrated a reduction in short- and long-term mortality.[3,19,27]

Dosing and contraindications for abciximab are described in Table 8–2. Glycoprotein IIb/IIIa receptor inhibitors block the final common pathway of platelet aggregation; namely, cross-linking of platelets by fibrinogen bridges between the glycoprotein IIb and IIIa receptors on the platelet surface. Administration of a glycoprotein IIb/IIIa receptor inhibitor increases the risk of bleeding, especially if it is given in the setting of recent (less than 4 hours) administration of fibrinolytic therapy.[27] It is important to note that failure to decrease the dose of eptifibatide and tirofiban in patients with renal dysfunction increases bleeding risk. Glycoprotein IIb/IIIa inhibitors are given in addition to ASA, clopidogrel and an anticoagulant, usually UFH or enoxaparin and not bivalirudin. An immune-mediated thrombocytopenia occurs in approximately 5% of patients receiving abciximab.[28]

▶ Anticoagulants

UFH, administered as a continuous infusion, is a first-line anticoagulant for treatment of patients with STE ACS for patients undergoing PCI.[2–4,19,29] In those patients, UFH is initiated in the emergency department and continued until the end of the PCI procedure. For patients undergoing reperfusion with fibrinolytics, newer guidelines have favored the use of enoxaparin.[3,19] Anticoagulant therapy should be initiated in the emergency department and continued for at least 48 hours, and up to eight days when fibrinolytics are administered.[3] UFH and enoxaparin dosing for STE ACS are described in Table 8–2. The dose of the UFH infusion is adjusted frequently to a target activated partial thromboplastin time (aPTT) (Table 8–2). When coadministered with a fibrinolytic, aPTTs above the target range are associated with an increased rate of bleeding, while aPTTs below the target range are associated with increased mortality and reinfarction.[30]

A meta-analysis of small randomized studies from the 1970s and 1980s suggests that UFH reduces mortality by approximately 17% compared to no anticoagulant therapy.[9] In studies of patients receiving fibrinolytics, both fondaparinux and reviparin have shown mortality reductions compared to placebo (no anticoagulant therapy).[31,32] Other beneficial effects of anticoagulation are prevention of cardioembolic stroke, as well as venous thromboembolism in MI patients.[3] Besides bleeding, the most frequent adverse effect of UFH is an immune-mediated clotting disorder, heparin-induced thrombocytopenia, which occurs in up to 5% of patients treated with UFH. Heparin-induced thrombocytopenia is less common in patients receiving low–molecular weight heparins (LMWHs), such as enoxaparin or dalteparin.

Low-molecular-weight heparins have not been studied in the setting of primary PCI. Low-molecular-weight heparins, like UFH, bind to antithrombin and inhibit both factor Xa and IIa. However, because their composition contains mostly short saccharide chain lengths, they preferentially inhibit factor Xa over factor IIa, which requires larger chain lengths for binding and inhibition. A large trial comparing enoxaparin administered for up to 8 days or until hospital discharge versus UFH administered for 48 hours in patients who received fibrinolytics found that enoxaparin reduced the rate of death or MI by 17% but also increased the risk of major bleeding (2.1% versus 1.4%).[33] Fondaparinux, an indirect-acting specific inhibitor of factor Xa, has also been compared to UFH in conjunction with fibrinolytics in the setting of STE MI. The rate of death or MI was similar between fondaparinux (administered as a low-dose for 8 days) and UFH. There was no significant difference in bleeding rates between fondaparinux and UFH.[34] Current guidelines by both the AHA/ACC and the American College of Chest Physicians (ACCP) recommend that patients undergoing reperfusion with fibrinolytics receive an anticoagulation treatment with enoxaparin for up to eight days, over a 48-hour regimen of UFH.[3,19] Nonetheless, these organizations have provided conflicting recommendations regarding the use of fondaparinux in such patients, illustrating well the more modest results of this agent compared to UFH.[3,19]

Bivalirudin, an IV direct thrombin inhibitor, may also be a choice of an anticoagulant for patients undergoing primary PCI. Potential advantages of direct thrombin inhibitors over UFH are that they bind to and inhibit clot-bound thrombin in addition to circulating thrombin and have no significant binding to plasma proteins. Thereby, they have a more predictable anticoagulant response. In addition, because thrombin is a potent stimulus for platelet aggregation, direct thrombin inhibitors have antiplatelet as well as anticoagulant activity. Like lepirudin, bivalirudin exhibits bivalent binding to thrombin, that is, it binds to both the active site and exosite-1, while argatroban binds only to the active site. Unlike lepirudin, both argatroban and bivalirudin exhibit reversible binding to thrombin, whereas lepirudin binds irreversibly. After bivalirudin binds to thrombin, thrombin cleaves a bivalirudin Arg3-Pro4 bond, re-exposing the thrombin catalytic site. Thus, bivalirudin provides consistent anticoagulation when administered as an IV bolus and infusion, but its activity is short-lived when discontinued. These potential advantages suggest that bivalirudin may have similar or superior efficacy and fewer bleeding complications compared to traditional anticoagulants. Recently, the results of a clinical trial demonstrated lower mortality at 30 days (34% reduction) and 1 year (31% reduction), with a 40% reduction in bleeding and similar rates of reinfarction with bivalirudin (administered during primary PCI) compared to UFH plus a glycoprotein IIb/IIIa inhibitor (administered during and for 12–18 hours following primary PCI).[35]

▶ *Nitrates*

One SL NTG tablet should be administered every 5 minutes for up to three doses in order to relieve myocardial ischemia. If patients have been previously prescribed SL NTG and ischemic chest discomfort persists for more than 5 minutes after the first dose, the patient should be instructed to contact emergency medical services before self-administering subsequent doses in order to activate emergency care sooner. IV NTG should then be initiated in all patients with an ACS who have persistent ischemia, heart failure, or uncontrolled high BP, in the absence of contraindications.[9] IV NTG should be continued for approximately 24 hours after ischemia is relieved (Table 8–2). Nitrates promote the release of nitric oxide from the endothelium, which results in venous and arterial vasodilation. Venodilation lowers preload and myocardial oxygen demand. Arterial vasodilation may lower BP, thus reducing myocardial oxygen demand. Arterial vasodilation also relieves coronary artery vasospasm, dilating coronary arteries to improve myocardial blood flow and oxygenation. Although used to treat ACS, nitrates have been suggested to play a limited role in the treatment of ACS patients, as two large, randomized clinical trials failed to show a mortality benefit for IV nitrate therapy followed by oral nitrate therapy in acute MI.[36,37] The most significant adverse effects of nitrates are tachycardia, flushing, headache, and hypotension. Nitrate administration is contraindicated in patients who have received oral phosphodiesterase 5 inhibitors, such as sildenafil and vardenafil, within the past 24 hours, and tadalafil within the past 48 hours.[9]

▶ *β-Blockers*

A β-blocker should be administered early in the care of a patient with STE ACS and continued indefinitely. Early administration of a β-blocker to patients lacking a contraindication within the first 24 hours of hospital arrival as well as prescription at hospital discharge for patients with MI is a quality performance measure.[14] In ACS, the benefit of β-blockers mainly results from the competitive blockade of β_1-adrenergic receptors located on the myocardium. β_1-Blockade produces a reduction in heart rate (HR), myocardial contractility, and BP, decreasing myocardial oxygen demand. As a result of these effects, β-blockers reduce the risk for recurrent ischemia, infarct size and risk of reinfarction, and occurrence of ventricular arrhythmias in the hours and days following MI.[38]

Landmark clinical trials have established the role of early β-blocker therapy in reducing MI mortality, reinfarction, and arrhythmias. Most of these trials were performed in the 1970s and 1980s before routine use of early reperfusion therapy.[39,40] However, data regarding the acute benefit of β-blockers in MI in the reperfusion era is derived mainly from a recently reported large clinical trial, which suggests that there may be an early risk of cardiogenic shock when initiating IV β-blockers followed by oral β-blockers early in the course of STE MI, especially in patients presenting with pulmonary congestion.[41] Therefore, a low-dose of an oral β-blocker should be initiated, followed by careful assessment for signs of hypotension and heart failure prior to any dose titration in patients with STE MI. IV β-blockers are reserved for patients presenting with HTN.[3]

The most serious side effects of β-blocker administration early in ACS are hypotension, bradycardia, and heart block. While initial acute administration of β-blockers is not appropriate for patients who present with decompensated heart failure, initiation of β-blockers may be attempted before hospital discharge in the majority of patients following treatment of acute heart failure.

▶ Calcium Channel Blockers

Calcium channel blockers in the setting of STE ACS are used for relief of ischemic symptoms in patients who have certain contraindications to β-blockers. Current data suggest little benefit on clinical outcomes beyond symptom relief for calcium channel blockers in the setting of ACS.[42] Therefore, calcium channel blockers should be avoided in the acute management of MI unless there is a clear symptomatic need or a contraindication to β-blockers. Agent selection is based on HR and left ventricular dysfunction (diltiazem and verapamil are contraindicated in patients with bradycardia, heart block, or systolic heart failure). Dosing and contraindications are described in Table 8–2.

Early Pharmacotherapy for NSTE ACSs

In general, early pharmacotherapy of NSTE ACS (Fig. 8–3) is similar to that of STE ACS with three exceptions: (a) fibrinolytic therapy is not administered; (b) glycoprotein IIb/IIIa receptor inhibitors are administered to high-risk patients for medical therapy as well as to PCI patients; and (c) at this time, there are no standard quality performance measures for patients with NSTE ACS who are not diagnosed with MI.

❼ *According to the ACC/AHA NSTE ACS practice guidelines, in the absence of contraindications, early pharmacotherapy of NSTE ACS should include intranasal oxygen (if oxygen saturation is low), SL NTG followed by IV NTG in selected patients, ASA, clopidogrel, β-blocker, and anticoagulant. High-risk patients should undergo early coronary angiography and revascularization with PCI or CABG. Administration of a glycoprotein IIb/IIIa receptor inhibitor may be considered in high-risk patients.* Morphine is also administered to patients with refractory angina as described previously. These agents should be administered early, while the patient is still in the emergency department. Dosing and contraindications for SL and IV NTG (for selected patients), ASA, clopidogrel, β-blockers, and the anticoagulants UFH, LMWHs, bivalirudin, and fondaparinux are listed in Table 8–2.[2,4]

▶ Fibrinolytic Therapy

Fibrinolytic therapy is not indicated in any patient with NSTE ACS, as increased mortality has been reported with fibrinolytics compared to controls in clinical trials in which fibrinolytics have been administered to patients with NSTE ACS (patients with normal or ST-segment depression ECGs).

▶ Aspirin

ASA reduces the risk of death or developing MI by about 50% (compared to no antiplatelet therapy) in patients with NSTE ACS.[24] Therefore, ASA remains the cornerstone of early treatment for all ACS.[43] Dosing of ASA for NSTE ACS is the same as that for STE ACS (Table 8–2). ASA is continued indefinitely.

▶ Thienopyridines

For patients with NSTE ACS, clopidogrel added to ASA and started on the first day of hospitalization as a 300 to 600 mg loading dose and followed the next day by 75 mg orally per day is recommended for most patients.[2] Clopidogrel, administered as a 300 mg loading dose followed by 75 mg once daily for at least 1 month and up to 12 months is recommended in patients who do not undergo a coronary stent placement, because its use reduces the combined risk of death from cardiovascular causes, nonfatal MI, or stroke by 20%.[2,26] In patients who undergo a coronary stent placement, it should be used in a similar fashion as described for STEMI.[2,4] Because of the potential for increased risk of bleeding, clopidogrel should be discontinued for at least 5 days before elective CABG surgery.[2]

▶ Glycoprotein IIb/IIIa Receptor Inhibitors

In patients with NSTE ACS scheduled for early PCI, administration of either abciximab or eptifibatide (double bolus) at the time of PCI is recommended. The use of tirofiban in these patients is not recommended, because it has been shown to be inferior to abciximab.[2] Medical therapy with either eptifibatide or tirofiban in patients without a planned PCI or as therapy started before PCI is reserved for higher-risk patients, such as those with positive troponin or ST-segment depression, and patients who have continued or recurrent ischemia despite other antithrombotic therapy.[2] Abciximab started as medical therapy prior to proceeding to PCI should not be used because it has not been shown to be beneficial in that setting.[2]

Doses and contraindications to glycoprotein IIb/IIIa receptor inhibitors are described in Table 8–2. Major bleeding and rates of transfusion are increased with administration of a glycoprotein IIb/IIIa receptor inhibitor in combination with ASA and an anticoagulant,[25] but there is no increased risk of intracranial hemorrhage in the absence of concomitant fibrinolytic treatment. The risk of thrombocytopenia with tirofiban and eptifibatide is lower than that with abciximab. Bleeding risks appear similar between agents.

▶ Anticoagulants

The choice of anticoagulant for a patient with NSTE ACS is guided by risk stratification, treatment strategy, and the results of recent clinical trials.[2,44-46] For patients undergoing an early invasive strategy with early coronary angiography and PCI, either UFH, LMWH, low-dose fondaparinux or bivalirudin should be administered. If fondaparinux is chosen for a patient who undergoes PCI, it should be administered in

Patient Encounter 2, Part 1

RR is a 66-year-old, 90-kg (198-lb) male who presents to the emergency department by ambulance complaining of 4 hours of continuous chest pressure that started while mowing the lawn. RR developed substernal chest pressure about 30 minutes after starting to mow his lawn. He stopped and rested but the chest pressure did not resolve. Local paramedics were summoned and he was given three 0.4 mg sublingual nitroglycerin tablets by mouth, 325 mg ASA by mouth, and morphine 2 mg IV push without relief of chest discomfort.

PMH: HTN for 5 years; type 2 DM for 5 years

FH: Father with myocardial infarction at age 75; mother and sister alive with type 2 DM

SH: Nonsmoker

Allergies: NKDA

Meds: Metformin 1,000 mg by mouth twice daily; ASA 325 mg by mouth once daily; lisinopril 20 mg by mouth once daily

ROS: 10/10 chest pain/squeezing

PE:

HEENT: Normocephalic atraumatic

CV: Regular rate and rhythm S_1, S_2, $-S_3$, $-S_4$, no murmurs or rubs

VS: BP 140/88; HR 88 bpm; T 37°C (98.6°F)

Lungs: Clear to auscultation and percussion

Abd: Nontender, nondistended

GI: Normal bowel sounds

GU: Stool guaiac negative

Exts: No bruits, pulses 2+, femoral pulse present, good range of motion

Neuro: Alert and oriented × 3, cranial nerves intact

Labs: Sodium 136 mEq/L (136 mmol/L), potassium 4.0 mEq/L (4.0 mmol/L), chloride 105 mEq/L (105 mmol/L), bicarbonate 22 mEq/L (24 mmol/L), SCr 1.0 mg/dL (88 μmol/L), glucose 160 mg/dL (8.9 mmol/L), WBC $6.9 \times 10^3/mm^3$ ($6.9 \times 10^9/L$), hemoglobin 14.7 g/dL (147 g/L or 9.1 mmol/L), hematocrit 42%, platelets $320 \times 10^3/mm^3$ ($320 \times 10^9/L$), troponin I 10 ng/mL (10 mcg/L), oxygen saturation 99% on room air

ECG: Normal sinus rhythm, PR 0.16 seconds, QRS 0.08 seconds, QT_c 0.38 seconds, occasional polymorphic premature ventricular contractions, 2 mm ST-segment depression inferior leads

CXR: Normal

What type of ACS is this?

What information is suggestive of acute MI?

---

combination with UFH as the dose of fondaparinux studied appears too low to prevent thrombotic events during PCI. UFH is the preferred anticoagulant following angiography in patients subsequently undergoing CABG during the same hospitalization.[2]

In patients in whom an initial conservative strategy is planned (i.e., are not anticipated to receive angiography and revascularization), either enoxaparin, UFH or low-dose fondaparinux is recommended.[2] Bivalirudin has not been studied in this setting. Because there are more data supporting the use of enoxaparin,[2] it is the preferred LMWH for ACS.

In comparative trials, the rate of bleeding with enoxaparin has been higher than other anticoagulants.[2] For patients presenting with NSTE ACS in whom cardiologists suspect a high risk for bleeding while receiving an anticoagulant, fondaparinux (for conservatively managed patients) and bivalirudin (for interventionally managed patients) are the preferred anticoagulants recommended by the ACC/AHA NSTE ACS guidelines.[2] Neither fondaparinux or bivalirudin are FDA approved for NSTE ACS despite being recommended by the ACC/AHA NSTE ACS guidelines.

Guideline recommended dosing and contraindications are described in Table 8–2. Because LMWHs are eliminated renally and patients with renal insufficiency generally have been excluded from clinical trials, some practice protocols recommend UFH for patients with creatinine clearance (CrCl) rates of less than 30 mL/min. (CrCl is calculated based on total patient body weight using the Cockroft-Gault equation.[2,3]) However, while recommendations for dosing adjustment of enoxaparin in patients with CrCl between 10 and 30 mL/min are listed in the product manufacturer's label, the safety and efficacy of LMWH in this patient population remain vastly understudied. Administration of LMWHs should be avoided in dialysis patients with ACS. It is unclear whether or not bivalirudin requires dose adjustment for patients with significant renal dysfunction. While bivalirudin is eliminated renally, the duration of infusion in recent trials has been short (several hours only), and therefore the actual need for dosing adjustment is unlikely. Patients with serum creatinine (SCr) greater than 3.0 mg/dL (265 μmol/L) were excluded from ACS trials with fondaparinux and the product label states that fondaparinux is contraindicated in patients with CrCl less than 30 mL/min and in patients weighing less than 50 kg (110 lb).

UFH is monitored and the dose adjusted to a target aPTT, whereas LMWHs are administered by a fixed, actual body weight-based dose without routine monitoring of antifactor Xa levels. Some experts recommend antifactor Xa monitoring for LMWHs in patients with renal impairment

Patient Encounter 2, Part 2

Is reperfusion therapy with fibrinolysis indicated at this time for patient RR?

What adjunctive pharmacotherapy should be administered to RR in the emergency department?

What additional pharmacotherapy should be initiated on the first day of RR's hospitalization following successful reperfusion?

during prolonged courses of administration of more than several days. No monitoring of coagulation is recommended for bivalirudin and fondaparinux.

▶ *Nitrates*

SL NTG followed by IV NTG should be administered to patients with NSTE ACS and ongoing ischemia (Table 8–2). The mechanism of action, dosing, contraindications, and adverse effects are the same as those described in the section on early pharmacologic therapy for STE ACS. IV NTG is typically continued for approximately 24 hours following ischemia relief.

▶ *β-Blockers*

The use of β-blockers in NSTE ACS is similar to STE ACS in that oral β-blockers should be initiated within 24 hours of hospital admission to all patients in the absence of contraindications. Benefits of β-blockers in this patient group are assumed to be similar to those seen in patients with STE ACS. β-Blockers are continued indefinitely. The prescription of a β-blocker at hospital discharge used to be reported as a quality measure.

▶ *Calcium Channel Blockers*

As described in the previous section, calcium channel blockers should not be administered to most patients with ACS. Their role is a second-line treatment for patients with certain contraindications to β-blockers and those with continued ischemia despite β-blocker and nitrate therapy. Administration of either amlodipine, diltiazem, or verapamil is preferred.[2]

Secondary Prevention Following MI

The long-term goals following MI are to: (a) control modifiable CHD risk-factors; (b) prevent the development of heart failure; (c) prevent recurrent MI and stroke; and (d) prevent death, including sudden cardiac death. Pharmacotherapy, which has been proven to decrease mortality, heart failure, reinfarction, or stroke, should be initiated prior to hospital discharge for secondary prevention. ❽ *Guidelines from the ACC/AHA suggest that in the absence of contraindications, following MI from either STE ACS or NSTE ACS, patients should receive indefinite treatment with ASA, a β-blocker, and an ACE inhibitor.[2,3,47] For NSTE ACS, clopidogrel should be added to ASA for at least 1 month and ideally for up to 12 months[2] and for STE ACS for at least 2 weeks (unless they undergo PCI where the duration of clopidogrel therapy depends on stent type), and up to 1 year.[3] Most patients will receive a statin to reduce low-density lipoprotein cholesterol to less than 100 mg/dL (2.59 mmol/L), and ideally less than 70 mg/dL (1.81 mmol/L). Newer therapies include eplerenone, an aldosterone antagonist. For all ACS patients, treatment and control of modifiable risk factors such as HTN, dyslipidemia, and diabetes mellitus (DM) is essential.* Benefits and adverse effects of long-term treatment with these medications are discussed in more detail below.

❾ *Because the costs for chronic preventative pharmacotherapy are the same for primary and secondary prevention, while the risk of events is higher with secondary prevention, secondary prevention is more cost effective than primary prevention of CHD.* Pharmacotherapy demonstrating cost effectiveness to prevent death in the ACS and post-MI patient includes fibrinolytics ($2,000 to $33,000 cost per year of life saved), ASA, glycoprotein IIb/IIIa receptor inhibitors ($13,700 to $16,500 per year of life added), β-blockers (less than $5,000 to $15,000 cost per year of life saved), ACE inhibitors ($3,000 to $5,000 cost per year of life saved), eplerenone ($15,300 to $32,400 per year of life gained), statins ($4,500 to $9,500 per year of life saved) and gemfibrozil ($17,000 per year of life saved).[46–55] Because cost-effectiveness ratios of less than $50,000 per added life-year are considered economically attractive from a societal perspective,[48] pharmacotherapy described above for ACS and secondary prevention are standards of care because of their efficacy and cost attractiveness to payors.

▶ *Aspirin*

ASA decreases the risk of death, recurrent infarction, and stroke following MI. ASA prescription at hospital discharge is a quality care performance measure in MI patients.[9,14] All patients should receive ASA indefinitely; those patients with a contraindication to ASA should receive clopidogrel.[2,3] The risk of major bleeding from chronic ASA therapy is approximately 2% and is dose-related. ASA doses higher than 75 to 81 mg are no less effective than doses of 160 to 325 mg, but do have lower rates of bleeding. Therefore, chronic doses of ASA should not exceed 81 mg.[46] For patients receiving intracoronary stents, the dose of ASA recommended by the ACC/AHA PCI guidelines in combination with clopidogrel is 162–325 mg for the duration specified by type of stent followed by low-dose ASA (see Table 8–2) but this is based upon consensus recommendations and not on randomized trials of ASA dosing.[4] In contrast, the American College of Chest Physician guidelines recommend low-dose ASA in combination with clopidogrel for all patients, including those with stents.[19,29,47]

▶ *Clopidogrel*

For patients with either STE or NSTE ACS, clopidogrel decreases the risk of cardiovascular events.[17,18,26] The ACC/

AHA guidelines suggest a minimum therapy duration of 1 month in patients following NSTE ACS who are managed conservatively, and ideally up to 12 months.[2] In patients receiving clopidogrel for STE MI who do not undergo PCI, clopidogrel should be administered for at least 14 to 28 days.[26] Patients who have undergone a PCI with a bare metal stent should receive clopidogrel for at least 1 month, ideally up to 1 year, and for patients receiving a drug-eluting stent for at least 12 months.[4]

β-Blockers, Nitrates, and Calcium Channel Blockers

Current treatment guidelines recommend that following an ACS, patients should receive a β-blocker indefinitely[2,3] whether they have residual symptoms of angina or not.[59] Overwhelming data support the use of β-blockers in patients with a previous MI. Currently, there are no data to support the superiority of one β-blocker over another.

Although β-blockers should be avoided in patients with decompensated heart failure from left ventricular systolic dysfunction complicating an MI, clinical trial data suggest that it is safe to initiate β-blockers prior to hospital discharge in these patients once heart failure symptoms have resolved.[49] These patients may actually benefit more than those without left ventricular dysfunction.[50] In patients who cannot tolerate or have a contraindication to a β-blocker, a calcium channel blocker can be used to prevent anginal symptoms, but should not be used routinely in the absence of such symptoms.[2,3,51]

Finally, all patients should be prescribed short-acting, SL NTG or lingual NTG spray to relieve any anginal symptoms when necessary and instructed on its use.[2,3] Chronic long-acting nitrate therapy has not been shown to reduce CHD events following MI. Therefore, IV NTG is not routinely followed by chronic, long-acting oral nitrate therapy in ACS patients who have undergone revascularization, unless the patient has chronic stable angina or significant coronary stenoses that were not revascularized.[51]

ACE Inhibitors and ARBs

ACE inhibitors should be initiated in all patients following MI to reduce mortality, decrease reinfarction, and prevent the development of heart failure.[2,3,9] Dosing and contraindications are described in Table 8–2. The benefit of ACE inhibitors in patients with MI most likely comes from their ability to prevent cardiac remodeling. The largest reduction in mortality is observed in patients with left ventricular dysfunction (low LVEF) or heart failure symptoms. Early initiation (within 24 hours) of an *oral* ACE inhibitor appears to be crucial during an acute MI, as 40% of the 30-day survival benefit is observed during the first day, 45% from days 2 to 7, and approximately 15% from days 8 to 30.[52] However, current data do not support the early administration of *IV* ACE inhibitors in patients experiencing an MI, as mortality may be increased.[53] Administration of ACE inhibitors should be continued indefinitely. Hypotension should be avoided, as coronary artery filling may be compromised. Additional

trials suggest that most patients with CAD, not just ACS or heart failure patients, benefit from ACE inhibitors. Therefore, ACE inhibitors should be considered in all patients following an ACS in the absence of a contraindication.

Many patients cannot tolerate chronic ACE inhibitor therapy secondary to adverse effects outlined below. The ARBs, candesartan and valsartan, have been documented in trials to improve clinical outcomes in patients with heart failure.[54,55] Therefore, either an ACE inhibitor or candesartan or valsartan are acceptable choices for chronic therapy for patients who have a low LVEF and heart failure following MI. Since more than five different ACE inhibitors have proven benefits in MI while only two ARBs have been studied, the benefits of ACE inhibitors are generally considered a class effect while the benefits of ARBs are still under study. More recently, telmisartan has been shown to be equivalent to ramipril for prevention of CVD events or hospitalization for heart failure in patients with CAD or at high risk of CVD events.[56] Nevertheless, a subsequent trial in ACE inhibitor intolerant patients produced more modest results.[57] ACE inhibitor prescription (or alternatively an ARB) at hospital discharge following MI, in the absence of contraindications, to patients with depressed LVF (EF less than 40%) is currently a quality performance measure for MI.[3,14]

Besides hypotension, the most frequent adverse reaction to an ACE inhibitor is cough, which may occur in up to 30% of patients. Patients with an ACE inhibitor cough and either clinical signs of heart failure or LVEF less than 40% may be prescribed an ARB.[3] Other, less common but more serious adverse effects to ACE inhibitors and ARBs include acute renal failure, hyperkalemia, and angioedema.

Aldosterone Antagonists

To reduce mortality, administration of an aldosterone antagonist, either eplerenone or spironolactone, should be considered within the first 2 weeks following MI in all patients who are already receiving an ACE inhibitor (or ARB) and have an LVEF of equal to or less than 40% and either heart failure symptoms or diagnosis of DM.[3] Aldosterone plays an important role in heart failure and in MI because it promotes vascular and myocardial fibrosis, endothelial dysfunction, HTN, left ventricular hypertrophy, sodium retention, potassium and magnesium loss, and arrhythmias. Aldosterone antagonists have been shown in experimental and human studies to attenuate these adverse effects.[58] Spironolactone decreases all-cause mortality in patients with stable, severe heart failure.[59]

Eplerenone, like spironolactone, is an aldosterone antagonist that blocks the mineralocorticoid receptor. In contrast to spironolactone, eplerenone has no effect on the progesterone or androgen receptor, thereby minimizing the risk of gynecomastia, sexual dysfunction, and menstrual irregularities. In a large clinical trial,[60] eplerenone significantly reduced mortality, as well as hospitalization for heart failure in post-MI patients with an EF less than 40% and symptoms of heart failure at any time during hospitalization. The risk of hyperkalemia, however, was increased. Therefore, patients with a SCr greater than 2.5 mg/dL (221 μmol/L) or CrCl less than 50 mL/min or serum potassium concentration of greater than 5.0 mmol/L (5.0 mEq/L) should not receive eplerenone (in addition to either an ACE inhibitor or ARB). Currently, there are no data to support that the more selective, more expensive eplerenone is superior to, or should be preferred to, the less expensive generic spironolactone unless a patient has experienced gynecomastia, breast pain, or impotence while receiving spironolactone. Finally, it should be noted that hyperkalemia is just as likely to appear with both of these agents, and is more common in patients receiving concomitant ACE inhibitors.

▶ Lipid-Lowering Agents

There are now overwhelming data supporting the benefits of statins in patients with CAD in prevention of total mortality, cardiovascular mortality, and stroke. According to the National Cholesterol Education Program (NCEP) Adult Treatment Panel recommendations, all patients with CAD should receive dietary counseling and pharmacologic therapy in order to reach a low-density lipoprotein (LDL) cholesterol of less than 100 mg/dL (2.59 mmol/L), with statins being the preferred agents to lower LDL cholesterol.[61] Results from landmark clinical trials have unequivocally demonstrated the value of statins in secondary prevention following MI in patients with moderate to high cholesterol.[62,63] Although the primary effect of statins is to decrease LDL cholesterol, statins are believed to produce many non-lipid-lowering or "pleiotropic" effects such as anti-inflammatory and antithrombotic properties. Newer recommendations from the NCEP give an optional LDL cholesterol goal of less than 70 mg/dL (1.81 mmol/L).[63,64] In patients with an ACS, statin therapy initiation should not be delayed and statins should be prescribed at or prior to discharge in most patients.[65] Statin prescription at hospital discharge is currently a quality performance measure for MI.[14]

A fibrate derivative or niacin should be considered in select patients with a low high-density lipoprotein (HDL) cholesterol less than 40 mg/dL (1.04 mmol/L) and/or a high triglyceride level greater than 200 mg/dL (2.26 mmol/L). In a large randomized trial of men with established CAD and low levels of HDL cholesterol, the use of gemfibrozil (600 mg twice daily) significantly decreased the risk of nonfatal MI or death from coronary causes.[66] Studies with fenofibrate have produced less definitive results.

▶ Other Modifiable Risk Factors

Smoking cessation, managing HTN, weight loss, and tight glucose control for patients with DM, in addition to treatment of dyslipidemia, are important treatments for secondary prevention of CHD events.[3] Smoking cessation counseling at the time of discharge following MI is a quality care performance measure.[3] The use of nicotine patches or gum, or of bupropion alone or in combination with nicotine patches, should be considered in appropriate patients.[3] HTN should be strictly controlled according to published guidelines.[67] Patients who are overweight should be educated on the importance of regular exercise, healthy eating habits, and reaching and maintaining an ideal weight.[68] Finally, because diabetics have up to a four-fold increased risk of mortality compared to nondiabetics, the importance of tight glucose control, as well as other CHD risk factor modifications, cannot be overstated.[69]

OUTCOME EVALUATION

- To determine the efficacy of nonpharmacologic and pharmacotherapy for both STE and NSTE ACS, monitor patients for: (a) relief of ischemic discomfort; (b) return of ECG changes to baseline; and (c) absence or resolution of heart failure signs.

- Monitoring parameters for recognition and prevention of adverse effects from ACS pharmacotherapy are described in Table 8–4. In general, the most common adverse reactions from ACS therapies are hypotension and bleeding. To treat for bleeding and hypotension, discontinue the offending agent(s) until symptoms resolve. Severe bleeding resulting in hypotension secondary to hypovolemia may require blood transfusion.

Patient Encounter 1, Part 3

Identify the long-term treatment goals for SD.

What additional pharmacotherapy should be initiated prior to hospital discharge?

Create a care plan for SD for hospital discharge which includes pharmacotherapy, desired treatment outcomes, and monitoring for efficacy and adverse effects.

Patient Encounter 2, Part 3

Patient RR undergoes coronary angiography and PCI with a drug-eluting stent placed for a 90% stenosis in his right coronary artery on hospital day 1.

Identify the long-term treatment goals for RR.

What additional pharmacotherapy should be initiated prior to hospital discharge?

Create a care plan for RR for hospital discharge that includes pharmacotherapy, desired treatment outcomes, and monitoring for efficacy and adverse effects.

Table 8–4

Therapeutic Drug Monitoring for Adverse Effects of Pharmacotherapy for ACSs

Drug	Adverse Effects	Monitoring
ASA	Dyspepsia, bleeding, gastritis	Clinical signs of bleeding,[a] GI upset; baseline CBC and platelet count; CBC and platelet count every 6 months
Clopidogrel	Bleeding, TTP (rare), diarrhea, rash	Clinical signs of bleeding[a]; baseline CBC and platelet count; CBC and platelet count every 6 months following hospital discharge
UFH	Bleeding, heparin-induced thrombocytopenia	Clinical signs of bleeding[a]; baseline CBC, platelet count, aPTT and INR; aPTT every 6 hours until target then every 24 hours; daily CBC; platelet count every 2–3 days from day 4 to 14 until heparin is stopped (minimum, preferably every day)
Enoxaparin	Bleeding, heparin-induced thrombocytopenia	Clinical signs of bleeding[a]; baseline CBC and platelet count, SCr, aPTT and INR; daily CBC, No routine platelet count monitoring unless recent UFH (less than 100 days) then baseline and within 24 hours; SCr daily
Fondaparinux	Bleeding	Clinical signs of bleeding[a]; baseline CBC and platelet count, SCr, aPTT and INR; daily CBC and SCr
Bivalirudin	Bleeding	Clinical signs of bleeding[a]; baseline CBC and platelet count, SCr, aPTT and INR; daily CBC and SCr
Fibrinolytics	Bleeding, especially intracranial hemorrhage	Clinical signs of bleeding[a]; baseline CBC, platelet count, INR and aPTT; mental status every 2 hours for signs of intracranial hemorrhage; daily CBC
Glycoprotein IIb/IIIa receptor inhibitors	Bleeding, acute profound thrombocytopenia	Clinical signs of bleeding[a]; baseline CBC, platelet count; SCr; daily CBC; platelet count at 2–4 hours after initiation then daily
Intravenous nitrates	Hypotension, flushing, headache, tachycardia	BP and HR every 2 hours
β-Blockers	Hypotension, bradycardia, heart block, bronchospasm, heart failure, fatigue, depression, sexual dysfunction, nightmares, masking hypoglycemia symptoms in diabetics	BP, RR, HR, 12-lead ECG and clinical signs of heart failure every 5 minutes during bolus intravenous dosing; BP, RR, HR, and clinical signs of heart failure every shift during oral administration during hospitalization, then BP and HR every 6 months following hospital discharge
Diltiazem and verapamil	Hypotension, bradycardia, heart block, heart failure, gingival hyperplasia	BP and HR every shift during oral administration during hospitalization then every 6 months following hospital discharge; dental exam and teeth cleaning every 6 months
Amlodipine	Hypotension, dependent peripheral edema, gingival hyperplasia	BP every shift during oral administration during hospitalization, then every 6 months following hospital discharge; dental exam and teeth cleaning every 6 months
ACE inhibitors and ARBs	Hypotension, cough (with ACE inhibitors), hyperkalemia, prerenal azotemia, angioedema (ACE inhibitors more so than ARBs)	BP every 2 hours × 3 for first dose, then every shift during oral administration during hospitalization, then once every 6 months following hospital discharge; baseline SCr and potassium; daily SCr and potassium while hospitalized then every 6 months (or 1–2 weeks after each outpatient dose titration); closer monitoring required in selected patients using spironolactone or eplerenone or if renal insufficiency; counsel patient on throat, tongue, and facial swelling
Aldosterone antagonists	Hypotension, hyperkalemia, increased SCr	BP and HR every shift during oral administration during hospitalization, then once every 6 months; baseline SCr and serum potassium concentration; SCr and potassium at 48 hours, at 7 days, then monthly for 3 months, then every 3 months thereafter following hospital discharge
Morphine	Hypotension, respiratory depression	BP and RR 5 minutes after each bolus dose

ACE, angiotensin-converting enzyme; aPTT, activated partial thromboplastin time; ARB, angiotensin receptor blocker; BP, blood pressure; CBC, complete blood count; ECG, electrocardiogram; HR, heart rate; INR, International Normalized Ratio; RR, respiratory rate; SCr, serum creatinine, TTP, thrombotic thrombocytopenic purpura; UFH, unfractionated heparin.

[a]Clinical signs of bleeding include bloody stools, melena, hematuria, hematemesis, bruising, and oozing from arterial or venous puncture sites.

Adapted from Spinler SA, de Denus S. Acute Coronary Syndromes. In: DiPiro JT, Talbert RL, Yee GC, et al., (eds.) Pharmacotherapy: A Pathophysiologic Approach. 7th ed. New York: McGraw-Hill; 2008: 272, with permission.

Patient Care and Monitoring

For patients in acute distress and ACS is suspected:

- Follow recommendations in Figures 8–1 and 8–2 and Table 8–2. Also incorporate into your plan the recommendations detailed below under "For patients diagnosed with ACS."

For patients diagnosed with ACS:

1. Review patient's medical record to determine indications for each medication.

2. Review patient's medical record to determine contraindications for each medication. For ASA, β-blockers, ACE inhibitors, and ARBs, document contraindications in patient's medical record.

3. Review doses of medications for appropriateness. Titration toward target doses of ACE inhibitors and β-blockers should be in progress. Evaluate if the dose of ASA may be reduced to less than 100 mg if no recent stent.

4. Interview the patient to assess complementary or alternative medication use. Counsel appropriately based on indications and drug interactions.

5. Evaluate the patient's medical record and medication history, and conduct a patient interview to assess for the presence of drug allergies, adverse drug reactions, drug interactions, and medication adherence.

6. Educate the patient and evaluate their success with lifestyle modifications, including smoking cessation, diet, weight loss, and exercise. For patients with DM, tight glucose control should be emphasized.

7. Provide patient education with regard to CAD, MI, indications for medications, and potential adverse effects and drug interactions.
   - What is CAD?
   - How can the progression of CAD and MI be prevented?
   - How does each medication benefit the patient?
   - Why is adherence important?
   - What potential adverse effects may occur?
   - What potential drug interactions may occur?
   - Warning signs to report to the physician or emergency medical services include chest squeezing, burning, or pain; jaw pain; pain radiation down the arm; bleeding; and loss of consciousness.
   - Dial 911 if there is no chest discomfort relief after one SL NTG tablet.
   - Important to train caregiver or relative to administer cardiopulmonary resuscitation (CPR).

8. Document smoking cessation counseling and patient receipt of discharge instructions in the patient's medical record.

Abbreviations Introduced in This Chapter

ACC	American College of Cardiology
ACCP	American College of Chest Physicians
ACE	Angiotensin-converting enzyme
ACS	Acute coronary syndrome
ADP	Adenosine diphosphate
AHA	American Heart Association
AMI	Acute myocardial infarction
aPTT	Activated partial thromboplastin time
ARB	Angiotensin receptor blocker
ASA	Aspirin
BP	Blood pressure
CABG	Coronary artery bypass graft (surgery)
CAD	Coronary artery disease
CHD	Coronary heart disease
CK	Creatine kinase
CK-MB	Creatine kinase myocardial band
COX-2	Cyclooxygenase-2
CPR	Cardiopulmonary resuscitation
CrCl	Creatinine clearance
CVD	Cardiovascular disease
DES	Drug eluting stent
DM	Diabetes mellitus
EF	Ejection fraction
HDL	High-density lipoprotein
HTN	Hypertension
ICD	Implantable cardioverter defibrillator
INR	International Normalized Ratio
LAD	Left anterior descending (artery)
LDL	Low-density lipoprotein
LMWH	Low–molecular weight heparin
LVEF	Left ventricular ejection fraction
LVF	Left ventricular function
MB	Myocardial band
MI	Myocardial infarction
NCEP	National Cholesterol Education Program
NSTE	Non-ST-segment elevation
NTG	Nitroglycerin
PCI	Percutaneous coronary intervention
SCr	Serum creatinine
SL	Sublingual
STE	ST-Segment elevation
TIMI	Thrombolysis in myocardial infarction
TNK-tPA	Tenecteplase
TTP	Thrombotic thrombocytopenic purpura
TXA_2	Thromboxane A_2
UA	Unstable angina
UFH	Unfractionated heparin

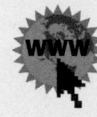 Self-assessment questions and answers are available at *http://www.mhpharmacotherapy.com/pp.html.*

REFERENCES

1. Rosamond W, Flegal K, Furie K, et al. Heart disease and stroke statistics—2008 update: A report from the American Heart Association Statistic s Committee and Stroke Statistics Subcommittee. Circulation 2008;117:e25–e146.

2. Anderson JL, Adams CD, Antman EM, et al. ACC/AHA 2007 guidelines for the management of patients with unstable angina/non ST-elevation myocardial infarction: A report of the American College of Cardiology/American Heart Association Task Force on Practice Guidelines (Writing Committee to Revise the 2002 Guidelines for the Management of Patients With Unstable Angina/Non ST-Elevation Myocardial Infarction): Developed in collaboration with the American College of Emergency Physicians, the Society for Cardiovascular Angiography and Interventions, and the Society of Thoracic Surgeons: Endorsed by the American Association of Cardiovascular and Pulmonary Rehabilitation and the Society for Academic Emergency Medicine. Circulation 2007;116:e148–e304.

3. Antman EM, Hand M, Armstrong PW, et al. 2007 Focused Update of the ACC/AHA 2004 Guidelines for the Management of Patients With ST-Elevation Myocardial Infarction: A report of the American College of Cardiology/American Heart Association Task Force on Practice Guidelines: Developed in collaboration With the Canadian Cardiovascular Society endorsed by the American Academy of Family Physicians: 2007 Writing Group to Review New Evidence and Update the ACC/AHA 2004 Guidelines for the Management of Patients With ST-Elevation Myocardial Infarction, Writing on Behalf of the 2004 Writing Committee. Circulation 2008;117:296–329.

4. King SB 3rd, Smith SC Jr, Hirshfeld JW Jr, et al. 2007 focused update of the ACC/AHA/SCAI 2005 guideline update for percutaneous coronary intervention: A report of the American College of Cardiology/American Heart Association Task Force on Practice guidelines. J Am Coll Cardiol 2008;51:172–209.

5. Libby P. Current concepts of the pathogenesis of the acute coronary syndromes. Circulation 2001;104:365–372.

6. Ruberg FL, Leopold JA, Loscalzo J. Atherothrombosis: Plaque instability and thrombogenesis. Prog Cardiovas Dis 2003;44:381–394.

7. St John Sutton M, Ferrari VA. Prevention of left ventricular remodeling after myocardial infarction 2002;4:97–108.

8. Goldberg RJ, Gore JM, Thompson CA, et al. Recent magnitude of and temporal trends (1994–1997) in the incidence and hospital death rates of cardiogenic shock complicating acute myocardial infarction: The second National Registry of Myocardial Infarction. Am Heart J 2001;141:65–72.

9. Antman EM, Anbe DR, Armstrong PW, et al. ACC/AHA guidelines for the management of patients with ST-elevation myocardial infarction: A report of the American College of Cardiology/American Heart Association Task Force on Practice Guidelines (Committee to Revise the 1999 Guidelines for the Management of Patients with Acute Myocardial Infarction). Circulation 2004;110(9):e82–e292. Erratum in: Circulation 2005;111:2013–2014. Circulation 2007;17:115(15):e411.

10. Thygesen K, Alpert JS, White HD. Universal definition of myocardial infarction. J Am Coll Cardiol 2007;50(22):2173–2195.

11. Fibrinolytic Therapy Trialists' (FTT) Collaborative Group. Indications for fibrinolytic therapy in suspected myocardial infarction: Collaborative overview of early mortality and major morbidity results from all randomized trials of more than 1,000 patients. Lancet 1994;343:311–322.

12. Berger P, Ellis SG, Holmes DR, Jr, et al. Relationship between delay in performing direct coronary angioplasty and early clinical outcome in patients with acute myocardial infarction: Results from the Global Use of Strategies to Open Occluded Arteries in Acute Coronary Syndromes (GUSTO-IIb) trial. Circulation 1999;100:14–20.

13. Boersma E. Does time matter? A pooled analysis of randomized clinical trials comparing primary percutaneous coronary intervention and in-hospital fibrinolysis in acute myocardial infarction patients. Eur Heart J 2006;27:779–788.

14. Krumholz HM, Anderson JL, Bachelder BL, et al. ACC/AHA 2008 performance measures for adults with ST-elevation and non-ST-elevation myocardial infarction: A report of the American College of Cardiology/American Heart Association Task Force on Performance Measures (Writing Committee to Develop Performance Measures for ST-Elevation and Non-ST-Elevation Myocardial Infarction) Developed in Collaboration With the American Academy of Family Physicians and American College of Emergency Physicians Endorsed by the American Association of Cardiovascular and Pulmonary Rehabilitation, Society for Cardiovascular Angiography and Interventions, and Society of Hospital Medicine. J Am Coll Cardiol 2008;52:2046–2099.

15. Fox KAA, Poole-Wilson PA, Henderson RA, et al. Interventional versus conservative treatment for patients with unstable angina or non-ST-elevation myocardial infarction: the British Heart Foundation RITA 3 randomised trial. Lancet 2002;360:743–751.

16. Epstein AE, DiMarco JP, Ellenbogen KA, et al. ACC/AHA/HRS 2008 Guidelines for Device-Based Therapy of Cardiac Rhythm Abnormalities: A report of the American College of Cardiology/American Heart Association Task Force on Practice Guidelines (Writing Committee to Revise the ACC/AHA/NASPE 2002 Guideline Update for Implantation of Cardiac Pacemakers and Antiarrhythmia Devices) developed in collaboration with the American Association for Thoracic Surgery and Society of Thoracic Surgeons. J Am Coll Cardiol 2008;51(21):e1–e62.

17. Sabatine MS, Cannon CP, Gibson CM, et al. Addition of clopidogrel to aspirin and fibrinolytic therapy for myocardial infarction with ST-segment elevation. N Engl J Med 2005;352:1179–1189.

18. COMMIT (Clopidogrel and Metoprolol in Myocardial Infarction Trial [collaborative group]). Addition of clopidogrel to aspirin in 45852 patients with acute myocardial infarction: randomised placebo-controlled trial. Lancet 2005;366:1607–1621.

19. Goodman SG, Menon V, Cannon CP, et al. Acute ST-segment elevation myocardial infarction: American College of Chest Physicians Evidence-Based Clinical Practice Guidelines (8th Edition). Chest. 2008;133(6 Suppl):708S–775S.

20. The GUSTO Investigators. An international randomized trial comparing four thrombolytic strategies for acute myocardial infarction. N Engl J Med 1993;329:673–682.

21. The Global Use of Strategies to Open Occluded Coronary Arteries (GUSTO III) Investigators. A comparison of reteplase with alteplase for acute myocardial infarction. N Engl J Med 1997;337:1118–1123.

22. Assessment of the Safety and Efficacy of a New Thrombolytic (ASSENT-2) Investigators. Single-bolus tenecteplase compared with front-loaded alteplase in acute myocardial infarction: The ASSENT-2 double-blind randomized trial. Lancet 2000;354:716–722.

23. ISIS-2 (Second International Study of Infarct Survival) Collaborative Group. Randomised trial of intravenous streptokinase, oral aspirin, both, or neither among 17,187 cases of suspected acute myocardial infarction: ISIS-2. Lancet 1988;2:349–360.

24. Antiplatelet Trialists' Collaboration. Collaborative meta-analysis of randomised trials of antiplatelet therapy for prevention of death, myocardial infarction, and stroke in high risk patients. BMJ 2002;324: 71–86.

25. Serebruany VL, Malinin AI, Sane DC, et al. The risk of bleeding complications with antiplatelet agents: A meta-analysis of 338,191 patients enrolled in 50 randomized controlled trials. Am J Cardiol 2005;95: 1218–1222.

26. Yusuf S, Zhao F, Mehta SR, et al. Effects of clopidogrel in addition to aspirin in patients with acute coronary syndromes without ST-segment elevation. N Engl J Med 2001;345:494–502. Erratum in: N Engl J Med 2001;345(23):1716. N Engl J Med 2001;345(20):1506.

27. De Luca G, Suryapranata H, Stone GW, et al. Abciximab as adjunctive therapy to reperfusion in acute ST-segment elevation myocardial infarction: A meta-analysis of randomized trials. JAMA 2005;293:1759–1765.

28. Dasgupta H, Blankenship JC, Wood C, et al. Thrombocytopenia complicating treatment with intravenous glycoprotein IIb/IIIa receptor inhibitors: A pooled analysis. Am Heart J 2000;140:206–211.

29. Harrington RA, Becker RC, Cannon CP, et al. Antithrombotic therapy for non-ST-segment elevation acute coronary syndromes: American College of Chest Physicians Evidence-Based Clinical Practice Guidelines (8th Edition). Chest. 2008;133(6 Suppl):670S–707S.

30. Granger CB, Hirsh J, Califf RM, et al. Activated partial thromboplastin time and outcome after thrombolytic therapy for acute myocardial infarction. Circulation 1996;93:870–878.

31. Peters RJ, Joyner C, Bassand JP et al. The role of fondaparinux as an adjunct to thrombolytic therapy in acute myocardial infarction: A subgroup analysis of the OASIS-6 trial. Eur Heart J 2008;29(3):324–331.

32. Yusuf S, Mehta SR, Xie C, et al. Effects of reviparin, a low-molecular-weight heparin, on mortality, reinfarction, and strokes in patients with acute myocardial infarction presenting with ST-segment elevation JAMA 2005;293(4):427–435.

33. Antman EM, Morrow DA, McCabe CH, et al. Enoxaparin versus unfractionated heparin with fibrinolysis for ST-elevation myocardial infarction. N Engl J Med 2006 Apr 6;354(14):1477–1488.

34. Yusuf S, Mehta SR, Chrolavicius S, et al. Effects of fondaparinux on mortality and reinfarction in patients with acute ST-segment elevation myocardial infarction: The OASIS-6 randomized trial. JAMA 2006;295:1519–1530.

35. Stone GE, Witzenbitchler B, Guagliumi G, et al. Bivalirudin during primary PCI in acute myocardial infarction. N Engl J Med 2008;358:2218–2230.

36. Gruppo Italioano per Lo Studio della Sopravvivenza Nell'infarcto Myocardio. GISSI-3: Effects of lisinopril and transdermal glyceryl trinitrate singly and together on 6-week mortality and ventricular function after acute myocardial infarction. Lancet 1994;343:1115–1122.

37. ISIS-4 (Fourth International Study of Infarct Survival [collaborative group]). ISIS-4: A randomised factorial trial assessing early oral captopril, oral mononitrate, and intravenous magnesium sulphate in 58,050 patients with suspected acute myocardial infarction. Lancet 1995;345:669–685.

38. Gheorghiade M, Goldstein S. β-Blockers in the post-myocardial infarction patient. Circulation 2002;106:394–398.

39. First International Study of Infarct Survival Collaborative Group. Randomised trial of intravenous atenolol among 16,027 cases of suspected acute myocardial infarction: ISIS-1. Lancet 1986;2:57–661.

40. Metoprolol in acute myocardial infarction (MIAMI). A randomised placebo-controlled international trial. Eur Heart J 1985;6:199–226.

41. COMMIT (Clopidogrel and Metoprolol in Myocardial Infarction Trial [collaborative group]). Early intravenous then oral metoprolol in 45,852 patients with acute myocardial infarction: Randomised placebo-controlled trial. Lancet 2005;366:1622–1632.

42. Abernethy DR, Schwartz JB. Calcium-antagonist drugs. N Engl J Med 1999;341:1447–1457.

43. Watson RD, Chin BS, Lip GY. Antithrombotic therapy in acute coronary syndromes. BMJ 2002; 325:1348–1351.

44. Yusuf S, Mehta SR, Chrolavicius S, et al. Comparison of fondaparinux and enoxaparin in acute coronary syndromes. N Engl J Med 2006 Apr 6;354(14):1464–1476.

45. The Synergy Trial Investigators. Enoxaparin vs unfractionated heparin in high-risk patients with non-ST-segment elevation acute coronary syndromes managed with an intended early invasive strategy. JAMA 2004;292:45–54.

46. Stone GW, McLaurin BT, Cox DA, et al. Bivalirudin for patients with acute coronary syndromes. N Engl J Med 2006;355:2203–2216.

47. Becker RC, Meade TW, Berger PB, et al. The primary and secondary prevention of coronary artery disease: American College of Chest Physicians Evidence-Based Clinical Practice Guidelines. 8th ed. Chest 2008;133(Suppl 6):776S–814S.

48. Mark DB. Medical economics in cardiovascular medicine. In: Textbook of cardiovascular medicine. Topol EJ, Califf RM, Isner J, et al. Philadelphia: Lippincott Williams & Wilkins, Inc.;2003:957–979.

49. Dargie HJ. Effect of carvedilol on outcome after myocardial infarction in patients with left-ventricular dysfunction: The CAPRICORN randomised trial. Lancet 2001;357:1385–1390.

50. Houghton T, Freemantle N, Cleland JG, et al. Are beta-blockers effective in patients who develop heart failure soon after myocardial infarction? A meta-regression analysis of randomised trials. Eur J Heart Fail 2000;2:333–340.

51. Gibbons RJ, Abrams J, Chatterjee K, et al, for the Committee on the Management of Patients with Chronic Stable Angina. ACC/AHA 2002 guideline update for the management of patients with chronic stable angina—summary article: A report of the American College of Cardiology/American Heart Association Task Force on practice guidelines. J Am Coll Cardiol 2003;41:159–168.

52. ACE Inhibitor Myocardial Infarction Collaborative Group. Indications for ACE inhibitors in the early treatment of acute myocardial infarction: Systematic overview of individual data from 100,000 patients in randomized trials. Circulation 1998;97:2202–2212.

53. Swedberg K, Held P, Kjekshus J, et al. Effects of the early administration of enalapril on mortality in patients with acute myocardial infarction. Results of the Cooperative New Scandinavian Enalapril Survival Study II (CONSENSUS II). N Engl J Med 1992;327:678–684.

54. Pfeffer MA, McMurray JJV, Velazquez EJ, et al. Valsartan, captopril, or both in myocardial infarction complicated by heart failure, left ventricular dysfunction, or both. N Engl J Med 2003;349:1893–1906.

55. Granger CB, McMurray JV, Yusuf S, et al. Effects of candesartan in patients with chronic heart failure and reduced left-ventricular systolic function intolerant to angiotensin-converting-enzyme inhibitors: The CHARM-Alternative trial. Lancet 2004;362:772–776.

56. ONTARGET Investigators. Telmisartan, ramipril, or both in patients at high risk for vascular events. N Engl J Med 2007;358:1547–1559.

57. The Telmisartan Randomised Assessment Study in ACE intolerant subjects with cardiovascular Disease (TRANSCEND) Investigators. Effects of the angiotensin-receptor blocker telmisartan on cardiovascular events in high-risk patients intolerant to angiotensin-converting enzyme inhibitors: A randomised controlled trial. Lancet 2008;372:1174–1183.

58. Makkar KM, Sanoski CA, Spinler SA. The role of angiotensin-converting enzyme inhibitors, angiotensin receptor blockers and aldosterone antagonists in the prevention of atrial and ventricular arrhythmias. Pharmacother 2009;(In Press).

59. Pitt B, Zannad F, Remme WJ, et al, for the Randomized Aldactone Evaluation Study Investigators.. The effect of spironolactone on morbidity and mortality in patients with severe heart failure. N Engl J Med 1999;341:709–717.

60. Pitt B, Remme W, Zannad F, et al. Eplerenone, a selective aldosterone blocker in patients with left ventricular dysfunction after myocardial infarction. N Engl J Med 2003;348:1309–1321.

61. Executive Summary of the Third Report of the National Cholesterol Education Program (NCEP) Expert Panel on Detection, Evaluation, and Treatment of High Blood Cholesterol in Adults (Adult Treatment Panel III). JAMA 2001;285:2486–2497.

62. Studer M, Briel M, Leimenstoll B, et al. Effect of different antilipidemic agents and diets on mortality. Arch Intern Med 2005;165:725–730.

63. Grundy SM, Cleeman JI, Merz CN, et al. Implications of Recent Clinical Trials for the National Cholesterol Education Program Adult Treatment Panel III Guidelines. Circulation 2004;110: 227–239.

64. Cannon CP, Braunwald E, McCabe CH, et al. Intensive versus moderate lipid lowering with statins after acute coronary syndromes. N Engl J Med 2004;350:1495–1504.

65. Muhlestein JB, Horne BD, Bair TL, et al. Usefulness of in-hospital prescription of statin agents after angiographic diagnosis of coronary artery disease in improving continued compliance and reduced mortality. Am J Cardiol 2001;87:257–261.

66. Rubins HB, Robins SJ, Collins D, et al, for the Veterans Affairs High-Density Lipoprotein Cholesterol Intervention Trial Study Group. Gemfibrozil for the secondary prevention of coronary heart disease in men with low levels of high-density lipoprotein cholesterol. N Engl J Med 1999;341:410–418.

67. Chobanian AV, Bakris GL, Black HR, et al. The seventh report of the Joint National Committee on Prevention, Detection, Evaluation, and Treatment of High Blood Pressure: The JNC 7 Report. JAMA 2003;289:2560–2572.

68. Haskell WL, Lee IM, Pate RR, et al. Physical activity and public health: Updated recommendation for adults from the American College of Sports Medicine and the American Heart Association. Circulation 2007;116:1081–1093.

69. American Diabetes Association. Standards of medical care in diabetes—2008. Diabetes Care 2008;31(Suppl 1):S12–S54.

9 Arrhythmias

James E. Tisdale

LEARNING OBJECTIVES

● **Upon completion of the chapter, the reader will be able to:**

1. Describe the phases of the cardiac action potential, compare and contrast the cellular ionic changes corresponding to each phase, and explain the relationship between the cardiac action potential and the ECG.

2. Describe the modified Vaughan Williams classification of antiarrhythmic drugs, and compare and contrast the effects of available antiarrhythmic drugs on ventricular conduction velocity, refractory period, automaticity, and inhibition of ion flux through specific myocardial ion channels.

3. Compare and contrast the risk factors for and the features, mechanisms, etiologies, symptoms, and goals of therapy of: (a) sinus bradycardia; (b) atrioventricular (AV) nodal blockade; (c) atrial fibrillation (AF); (d) paroxysmal supraventricular tachycardia (PSVT); (e) ventricular premature depolarizations (VPDs); (f) ventricular tachycardia (VT, including torsades de pointes); and (g) ventricular fibrillation (VF).

4. Compare and contrast appropriate nonpharmacologic and pharmacologic treatment options for sinus bradycardia and AV nodal blockade.

5. Compare and contrast the mechanisms of action of drugs used for ventricular rate control, conversion to sinus rhythm and maintenance of sinus rhythm in patients with AF, and explain the importance of anticoagulation for patients with AF.

6. Compare and contrast the mechanisms of action of drugs used for acute termination of PSVT.

7. Compare and contrast the role of drug therapy versus nonpharmacologic therapy for long-term prevention of recurrence of PSVT.

8. Describe the role of drug therapy for management of asymptomatic and symptomatic VPDs.

9. Compare and contrast the mechanisms of action of drugs used for the treatment of acute episodes of VT (including torsades de pointes), and describe options and indications for nonpharmacologic treatment of VT and VF.

10. Design individualized drug-therapy treatment plans for patients with: (a) sinus bradycardia; (b) AV nodal blockade; (c) AF; (d) PSVT; (e) VPDs; (f) VT (including torsades de pointes); and (g) VF.

KEY CONCEPTS

❶ Cardiac arrhythmias may be caused by abnormal impulse formation (automaticity), abnormal impulse conduction (re-entry), or both.

❷ Numerous drugs (β-blockers, diltiazem, verapamil, digoxin, dronedarone, and amiodarone) can cause bradyarrhythmias (sinus bradycardia and/or atrioventricular [AV] nodal blockade).

❸ Individualized goals of treatment of atrial fibrillation (AF) include: (a) ventricular rate control with drugs that inhibit AV nodal conduction, (b) restoration of sinus rhythm with direct current cardioversion or antiarrhythmic drugs (commonly referred to as "cardioversion" or "conversion to sinus rhythm"), (c) maintenance of sinus rhythm/reduction in the frequency of episodes using antiarrhythmic drugs, and (d) prevention of stroke.

❹ Antiarrhythmic drug therapy for maintenance of sinus rhythm/reduction in frequency of episodes of AF should be initiated only in patients in whom symptoms persist despite maximal tolerated doses of appropriate drugs for ventricular rate control.

❺ The majority of patients with AF should receive warfarin therapy (titrated to an International Normalized Ratio [INR] of 2–3) for stroke prevention, particularly if they have other risk factors for stroke.

6 Adenosine is the drug of choice for termination of paroxysmal supraventricular tachycardia.

7 Asymptomatic ventricular premature depolarizations (VPDs) should not be treated with antiarrhythmic drug therapy.

8 Implantable cardioverter-defibrillators are more effective than antiarrhythmic drugs for reduction in the risk of sudden cardiac death due to ventricular tachycardia (VT) or ventricular fibrillation (VF).

9 The purpose of drug therapy for VF is facilitation of electrical defibrillation; in the absence of electrical defibrillation, drug therapy alone will not terminate VF.

10 Drugs with the potential to cause QT interval prolongation and torsades de pointes should be avoided or used with extreme caution in patients with other risk factors for torsades de pointes.

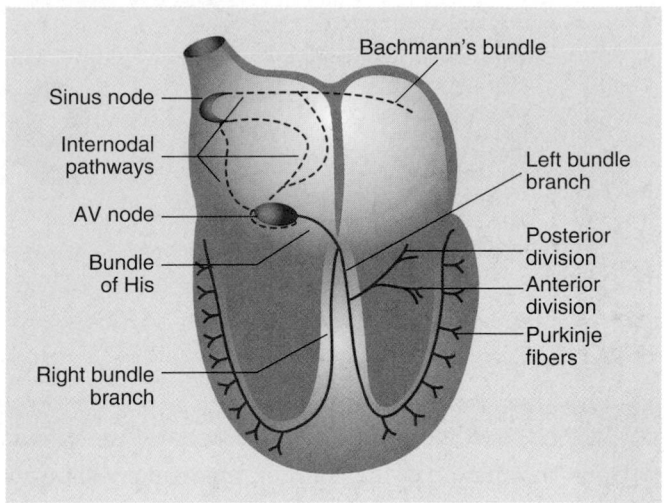

FIGURE 9–1. The cardiac conduction system. (AV, atrioventricular.)

NORMAL AND ABNORMAL CARDIAC CONDUCTION AND ELECTROPHYSIOLOGY

The heart functions via both mechanical and electrical activity. The mechanical activity of the heart refers to atrial and ventricular contraction, the mechanism by which blood is delivered to tissue. When circulated blood returns to the heart via the venous circulation, the blood enters the right atrium. Right atrial contraction and changes in right-ventricular pressure result in delivery of blood to the right ventricle through the tricuspid valve. Right-ventricular contraction pumps blood through the pulmonic valve through the pulmonary arteries to the lungs, where the blood becomes oxygenated. The blood then flows through the pulmonary veins into the left atrium. Left-atrial contraction and changes in left-ventricular (LV) pressure result in delivery of blood through the mitral valve into the left ventricle. Contraction of the left ventricle results in pumping of blood through the aortic valve and to the tissues of the body.

The mechanical activity of the heart (contraction of the atria and ventricles) occurs as a result of the electrical activity of the heart. The heart possesses an intrinsic electrical conduction system (Fig. 9–1).[1] Normal myocardial contraction cannot occur without proper and normal function of the heart's electrical conduction system. Electrical depolarization of the atria results in atrial contraction, and ventricular depolarization is followed by ventricular contraction. Malfunction of the heart's electrical conduction system may result in dysfunctional atrial and/or ventricular contraction and may reduce cardiac output.

The Cardiac Conduction System

Under normal circumstances, the sinoatrial (SA) node (also known as the sinus node), located in the upper portion of the right atrium, serves as the pacemaker of the heart

and generates the electrical impulses that subsequently result in atrial and ventricular depolarization (Fig. 9–1).[1] The SA node serves as the heart's pacemaker because it has the greatest degree of automaticity, which is defined as the ability of a cardiac fiber or tissue to initiate depolarizations spontaneously. In adults at rest, the normal intrinsic depolarization rate of the SA node is 60 to 100 per minute. Other cardiac fibers also possess the property of automaticity, but normally the intrinsic depolarization rates are slower than that of the SA node. For example, the normal intrinsic depolarization rate of the atrioventricular (AV) node is 40 to 60 per minute, while that of the ventricular tissue is 30 to 40 per minute. Therefore, because of greater automaticity, the SA node normally serves as the pacemaker of the heart. However, if the SA node fails to generate depolarizations at a rate faster than that of the AV node, the AV node may take over as the pacemaker. Similarly, if the SA node and AV node fail to generate depolarizations at a rate greater than 30 to 40 per minute, ventricular tissue may take over as the pacemaker.

Following initiation of the electrical impulse from the SA node, the impulse travels through the internodal pathways of the specialized atrial conduction system and Bachmann's bundle (Fig. 9–1).[1] The atrial conducting fibers do not traverse the entire breadth of the left and right atria; as impulse conduction occurs across the internodal pathways, and when the impulse reaches the end of Bachmann's bundle, atrial depolarization spreads as a wave, conceptually similar to that which occurs upon throwing a pebble into water. As the impulse is conducted across the atria, each depolarized cell excites and depolarizes the surrounding connected cells, until both atria have been completely depolarized. Atrial contraction follows normal atrial depolarization.

Following atrial depolarization, impulses are conducted through the AV node, located in the lower right atrium (Fig. 9–1).[1] The impulse then enters the bundle of His, and is conducted through the ventricular conduction system, consisting of the left and right bundle branches. The left ventricle requires a larger conduction system than the right ventricle due to its larger mass; therefore, the left bundle branch bifurcates into the left anterior and posterior divisions (also commonly known as "fascicles"). The bundle branches further divide into the Purkinje fibers, through which impulse conduction results in ventricular depolarization, after which ventricular contraction occurs.

The Ventricular Action Potential

The ventricular **action potential** is depicted in Figure 9–2.[2] Cardiac myocyte resting membrane potential is usually 70 to 90 mV, due to the action of the sodium–potassium adenosine triphosphatase (ATPase) pump, which maintains relatively high extracellular sodium concentrations and relatively low extracellular potassium concentrations. During each action-potential cycle, the potential of the membrane increases to a threshold potential, usually 60 to 80 mV. When the membrane potential reaches this threshold, the fast sodium channels open, allowing sodium ions to rapidly enter the cell. This rapid influx of positive ions creates a vertical upstroke of the action potential, such that the potential reaches 20 to 30 mV. This is phase 0, which represents ventricular depolarization. At this point, the fast sodium channels become inactivated, and ventricular repolarization begins, consisting of phases 1 through 3 of the action potential. Phase 1 repolarization occurs primarily as a result of an efflux of potassium ions (Fig. 9–2).[2] During phase 2, potassium ions continue to exit the cell, but the membrane potential is balanced by an influx of calcium and sodium ions, transported through slow calcium and slow sodium channels, resulting in a plateau. During phase 3, the efflux of potassium ions greatly exceeds calcium and sodium influx, resulting in the major component of ventricular repolarization. During phase 4, sodium ions are actively pumped out of the myocyte via the sodium-potassium ATPase pump, resulting in restoration of ion concentrations to their resting values. An understanding of the ionic fluxes that are responsible for each phase of the action potential facilitates understanding of the effects of specific drugs on the action potential. For example, drugs that primarily inhibit ion flux through sodium channels influence phase 0 (ventricular depolarization), while drugs that primarily inhibit ion flux through potassium channels influence the repolarization phases, particularly phase 3.

The Electrocardiogram

The ECG is a noninvasive means of measuring the electrical activity of the heart. The relationship between the ventricular action potential and the ECG is depicted in Figure 9–2.[2] The P wave on the ECG represents atrial depolarization (atrial depolarization is not depicted in the action potential shown in Figure 9–2, which shows only the ventricular action potential). Phase 0 of the action potential corresponds to the QRS complex; therefore, the QRS complex on the ECG is a noninvasive representation of ventricular depolarization. The T wave on the ECG corresponds to phase 3 ventricular repolarization. The interval from the beginning of the Q wave to the end of the T wave, known as the QT interval, is

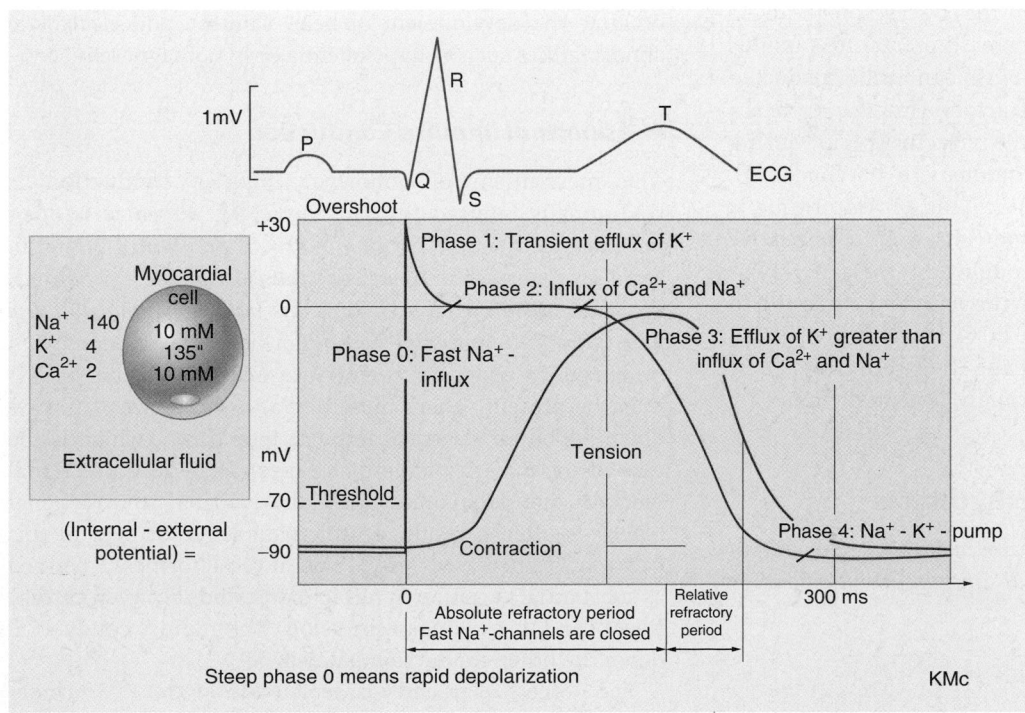

FIGURE 9–2. The ventricular action potential depicting the flow of specific ions responsible for each phase. The specific phases of the action potential that correspond to the absolute and relative refractory periods are portrayed, and the relationship between phases of the action potential and the ECG are shown. (Ca, calcium; K, potassium; Na, sodium.) (From Ref. 2.)

used as a noninvasive marker of ventricular repolarization time. Atrial repolarization is not displayed on the ECG, because it occurs during ventricular depolarization and is obscured by the QRS complex.

Several intervals and durations are routinely measured on the ECG. The PR interval represents the time of conduction of impulses from the atria to the ventricles through the AV node; the normal PR interval in adults is 0.12 to 0.2 seconds. The QRS duration represents the time required for ventricular depolarization, which is normally 0.08 to 0.12 seconds in adults. The QT interval represents the time required for ventricular repolarization. The QT interval varies with heart rate—the faster the heart rate, the shorter the QT interval, and vice versa. Therefore, the QT interval is corrected for heart rate using Bazett's equation,[3] which is:

$$QT_c = \frac{QT}{\sqrt{RR}}$$

where QT_c is the QT interval corrected for heart rate, and RR is the interval from the onset of one QRS complex to the onset of the next QRS complex, measured in seconds (i.e., the heart rate, expressed in different terminology). The normal QT_c interval in adults is 0.36 to 0.44 seconds.

Refractory Periods

After an electrical impulse is initiated and conducted, there is a period of time during which cells and fibers cannot be depolarized again. This period of time is referred to as the absolute refractory period (Fig. 9–2),[2] and corresponds to phases 1, 2, and approximately one-third of phase 3 repolarization on the action potential. The absolute refractory period also corresponds to the period from the Q wave to approximately the first half of the T wave on the ECG (Fig. 9–2). During this period, if there is a premature stimulus for an electrical impulse, this impulse cannot be conducted because the tissue is absolutely refractory. However, there is a period of time following the absolute refractory period during which a premature electrical stimulus can be conducted, and is often conducted abnormally. This period of time is called the relative refractory period (Fig. 9–2).[2] The relative refractory period corresponds roughly to the latter two-thirds of phase 3 repolarization on the action potential and to the latter half of the T wave on the ECG. If a new (premature) electrical stimulus is initiated during the relative refractory period, it can be conducted abnormally, potentially resulting in an arrhythmia.

Mechanisms of Cardiac Arrhythmias

❶ *In general, cardiac arrhythmias are caused by: (a) abnormal impulse formation, (b) abnormal impulse conduction, or (c) both.*

▶ Abnormal Impulse Initiation

Abnormal initiation of electrical impulses occurs as a result of abnormal automaticity. If the automaticity of the

SA node decreases, this results in a decreased rate of impulse generation and a slow heart rate (sinus bradycardia). Conversely, if the automaticity of the SA node increases, this results in an increased rate of generation of impulses and a rapid heart rate (sinus tachycardia). If other cardiac fibers become abnormally automatic, such that the rate of initiation of spontaneous impulses exceeds that of the SA node, or premature impulses are generated, other types of tachyarrhythmias may occur. Many cardiac fibers possess the capability for automaticity including the atrial tissue, the AV node, the Purkinje fibers, and the ventricular tissue. In addition, fibers with the capability of initiating and conducting electrical impulses are present in the pulmonary veins. Abnormal atrial automaticity may result in premature atrial contractions or may precipitate atrial tachycardia or atrial fibrillation (AF); abnormal AV nodal automaticity may result in "junctional tachycardia" (the AV node is also sometimes referred to as the AV junction). Abnormal automaticity in the ventricles may result in ventricular premature depolarizations (VPDs) or may precipitate ventricular tachycardia (VT) or ventricular fibrillation (VF). In addition, abnormal automaticity originating from the pulmonary veins is a precipitant of AF.

Automaticity of cardiac fibers is controlled in part by activity of the sympathetic and parasympathetic nervous systems. Enhanced activity of the sympathetic nervous system may result in increased automaticity of the SA node or other automatic cardiac fibers. Enhanced activity of the parasympathetic nervous system tends to suppress automaticity; conversely, inhibition of activity of the parasympathetic nervous system increases automaticity. Other factors may lead to abnormal increases in automaticity of extra-SA nodal tissues, including hypoxia, atrial or ventricular stretch (as might occur following long-standing hypertension or after the development of heart failure), and electrolyte abnormalities such as hypokalemia or hypomagnesemia.

▶ Abnormal Impulse Conduction

The mechanism of abnormal impulse conduction is traditionally referred to as re-entry. **❶** *Re-entry is often initiated as a result of an abnormal premature electrical impulse (abnormal automaticity); therefore, in these situations, the mechanism of the arrhythmia is both abnormal impulse formation (automaticity) and abnormal impulse conduction (re-entry).* In order for re-entry to occur, three conditions must be present. There must be: (a) at least two pathways down which an electrical impulse may travel (which is the case in the majority of cardiac fibers); (b) a "unidirectional block" in one of the conduction pathways (this "unidirectional block" is often a result of prolonged refractoriness in this pathway, or increased "dispersion of refractoriness," defined as substantial variation in refractory periods between cardiac fibers); and (c) slowing of the velocity of impulse conduction down the other conduction pathway.

The process of re-entry is depicted in Figure 9–3.[4] Under normal circumstances, when a premature impulse is initiated, it cannot be conducted in either direction down either

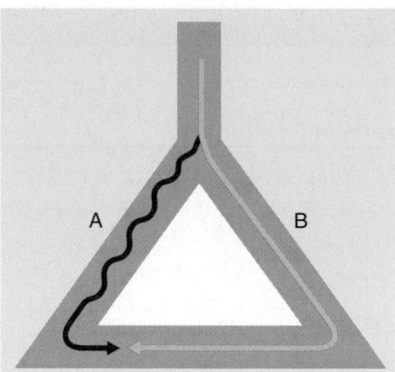

FIGURE 9–3. The process of initiation of re-entry. There are two pathways for impulse conduction, slowed impulse conduction down pathway A, and a longer refractory period in pathway B. A precisely timed premature impulse usually initiates re-entry; the premature impulse cannot be conducted down pathway B, because the tissue is still in the absolute refractory period from the previous, normal impulse. However, because of dispersion of refractoriness (i.e., different refractory periods down the two pathways), the impulse can be conducted down pathway A. Because conduction down pathway A is slowed, by the time the impulse reaches pathway B in a retrograde direction, the impulse can be conducted retrogradely up the pathway, because the pathway is now beyond its refractory period from the previous impulse. This creates re-entry, in which the impulse continuously and repeatedly travels in a circular fashion around the loop.

pathway because the tissue is in its absolute refractory period from the previous impulse. A premature impulse may be conducted down both pathways if it is only slightly premature and arrives after the tissue is no longer refractory. However, when refractoriness is prolonged down one of the pathways, a precisely-timed premature beat may be conducted down one pathway, but cannot be conducted in either direction in the pathway with prolonged refractoriness because the tissue is still in its absolute refractory period (Fig. 9–3).[4] When the third condition for re-entry is present, that is, when the velocity of impulse conduction in one is slowed, the impulse traveling forward down the other pathway still cannot be conducted. However, because the impulse in one is traveling more slowly than normal, by the time it circles around and travels upward along the other pathway, sufficient time has passed so the pathway is no longer in its absolute refractory period, and now the impulse may travel upward in that pathway. In other words, the electrical impulse "re-enters" a previously stimulated pathway in the reverse (retrograde) direction. This results in circular movement of electrical impulses; as the impulse travels in this circular fashion, it excites each cell around it, and if the impulse is traveling at a rate faster than the intrinsic rate of the SA node, a tachycardia occurs in the tissue in question. Re-entry may occur in numerous tissues, including the atria, the AV node, and the ventricles.

Prolonged refractoriness and/or slowed impulse conduction velocity may be present in cardiac tissues for a variety of reasons. Myocardial ischemia may alter ventricular refractory periods or impulse conduction velocity, facilitating ventricular re-entry. In patients with past myocardial infarction, the infarcted myocardium is dead and cannot conduct impulses. However, there is typically a border zone of tissue which is damaged and in which refractory periods and conduction velocity are often deranged, facilitating ventricular re-entry. In patients with left-atrial or LV hypertrophy as a result of long-standing hypertension, refractory periods and conduction velocity are often perturbed. In patients with heart failure due to LV dysfunction, ventricular refractoriness and conduction velocity are often altered due to LV hypertrophy, collagen deposition, and other anatomic and structural changes.

Vaughan Williams Classification of Antiarrhythmic Drugs

The Vaughan Williams classification of antiarrhythmic drugs, first described in 1970[5] and subsequently further expanded,[6,7] is presented in Table 9–1. This classification is based on the effects of specific drugs on ventricular conduction velocity, repolarization/refractoriness, and automaticity. Class I drugs, which are the sodium channel blocking agents, primarily inhibit ventricular automaticity and slow conduction velocity. However, due to differences in the potency of the drugs to slow conduction velocity, the class I drugs are subdivided into class IA, IB, and IC. The class IC drugs have the greatest potency for slowing ventricular conduction, the class IA drugs have intermediate potency, and the class IB drugs have the lowest potency, with minimal effects on conduction velocity at normal heart rates. Class II drugs are the adrenergic β-receptor inhibitors (β-blockers), class III drugs are those that inhibit ventricular repolarization or prolong refractoriness, and class IV drugs are the calcium channel blockers (CCBs) diltiazem and verapamil.

The Vaughan Williams classification of antiarrhythmic drugs has been criticized for a number of reasons. The classification is based on the effects of drugs on normal, rather than diseased, myocardium. In addition, many of the drugs may be placed into more than one class. For example, the class IA drugs prolong repolarization/refractoriness, either via the parent drug[8,9] or an active metabolite,[10] and therefore also may be placed in class III. Sotalol is also a β-blocker, and therefore fits into class II. Amiodarone inhibits sodium and potassium channels, is a noncompetitive inhibitor of β-receptors, and inhibits calcium channels, and therefore may be placed into any of the four classes. For this reason, drugs within each class cannot be considered "interchangeable." Nonetheless, despite attempts to develop mechanism-based classifications that better distinguish the actions of antiarrhythmic drugs,[11] the Vaughan Williams classification continues to be widely used because of its simplicity and the fact that it is relatively easy to remember and understand.

Table 9–1

Vaughan Williams Classification of Antiarrhythmic Agents[a]

Class	Drug	Conduction Velocity[b]	Repolarization/Refractoriness[b]	Automaticity[b]
IA	Quinidine Procainamide Disopyramide	↓	↑	↓
IB	Lidocaine Mexiletine Tocainide	0/↓	↓/0	↓
IC	Flecainide Propafenone	↓↓	0	↓
II	β-blockers[c] Acebutolol Atenolol Betaxolol Bisoprolol Carteolol Carvedilol[d] Esmolol Labetalol[d] Metoprolol Nadolol Nebivolol Penbutolol Pindolol Propranolol Timolol	0	0	0
III	Amiodarone[e] Dofetilide Dronedarone Ibutilide Sotalol	0	↑	0
IV	CCBs[c] Diltiazem Verapamil	0	0	0

CCB, calcium channel blocker; ↑, increase/prolong; ↓, decrease; 0, no effect; 0/↓, does not change or may decrease: ↓/0, decreases or does not change.

[a]Adenosine and digoxin are agents used for the management of arrhythmias that do not fit into the Vaughan Williams classification.

[b]In ventricular tissue only; effects may differ in atria, sinus node or atrioventricular node.

[c]Slows conduction, prolongs refractory period, and reduces automaticity in sinoatrial node and AV node tissue, but not in the ventricles.

[d]Combined α- and β-blocker.

[e]Amiodarone also slows conduction velocity and inhibits automaticity.

CARDIAC ARRHYTHMIAS

In general, cardiac arrhythmias are classified into two broad categories: supraventricular (those occurring above the ventricles) and ventricular (those occurring in the ventricles). The names of specific arrhythmias are generally composed of two words; the first word indicates the location of the electrophysiologic abnormality resulting in the arrhythmia (sinus, AV node, atrial, or ventricular), and the second word describes the arrhythmia in terms of whether it is abnormally slow (bradycardia) or fast (tachycardia), or the type of arrhythmia (block, fibrillation, or flutter).

SUPRAVENTRICULAR ARRHYTHMIAS

Sinus Bradycardia

Sinus bradycardia is an arrhythmia that originates in the SA node, and is defined by a sinus rate less than 60 bpm.[12]

▶ Epidemiology and Etiology

Many individuals, particularly those who partake in regular vigorous exercise, have resting heart rates less than 60 bpm. For those individuals, sinus bradycardia is normal

Clinical Presentation and Diagnosis of Sinus Bradycardia

Symptoms

- Many patients are asymptomatic, particularly those with normal resting heart rates less than 60 bpm as a result of physical fitness due to regular vigorous exercise
- Susceptible patients may develop symptoms, depending on the degree of heart rate lowering
- Symptoms of bradyarrhythmias include dizziness, fatigue, light-headedness, syncope, chest pain (in patients with underlying CAD), and shortness of breath and other symptoms of heart failure (in patients with underlying left ventricular dysfunction)

Diagnosis

- Cannot be made on the basis of symptoms alone, as the symptoms of all bradyarrhythmias are similar

- History of present illness, presenting symptoms, and 12-lead ECG that reveals sinus bradycardia
- Assess possible correctable etiologies, including myocardial ischemia, serum potassium concentration (for hyperkalemia), thyroid function tests (for hypothyroidism)
- Determine whether patient is taking any drugs known to cause sinus bradycardia. If the patient is currently taking digoxin, determine the serum digoxin concentration and ascertain whether it is supratherapeutic (less than 2 ng/mL [2.6 nmol/L])

and healthy, and does not require evaluation or treatment. However, some individuals develop symptomatic sinus-node dysfunction. In the absence of correctable underlying causes, idiopathic sinus-node dysfunction is referred to as sick sinus syndrome,[12] and occurs with greater frequency in association with advancing age. The prevalence of sick sinus syndrome is approximately 1 in 600 individuals over the age of 65 years.[12]

Sick sinus syndrome leading to sinus bradycardia may be caused by degenerative changes in the sinus node that occur with advancing age. ❷ *However, there are other possible etiologies of sinus bradycardia including drugs* (Table 9–2).[13]

▶ *Pathophysiology*

Sick sinus syndrome leading to sinus bradycardia occurs as a result of fibrotic tissue in the SA node, which replaces normal SA node tissue.[12]

▶ *Treatment*

Desired Outcomes The desired outcomes of treatment are to restore normal heart rate and alleviate patient symptoms.

Pharmacologic Therapy Treatment of sinus bradycardia is only necessary in patients who become symptomatic. ❷ *If the patient is taking any medication(s) that may cause sinus bradycardia, the drug(s) should be discontinued whenever possible.* If the patient remains in sinus bradycardia after discontinuation of the drug(s) and after five half-lives of the drug(s) have elapsed, then the drugs(s) can usually be excluded as the etiology of the arrhythmia. In certain circumstances, however, discontinuation of the medication(s) may be undesirable, even if it may be the cause of symptomatic sinus bradycardia. For example, if the patient has a history of myocardial infarction or heart failure, discontinuation of a β-blocker is undesirable, because β-blockers have been shown to reduce mortality and

Table 9–2
Etiologies of Sinus Bradycardia

Idiopathic ("sick sinus syndrome")
Myocardial ischemia
Carotid-sinus hypersensitivity
Neurocardiac syncope
Electrolyte abnormalities: hypokalemia or hyperkalemia
Hypothyroidism
Hypothermia
Amyloidosis
Sarcoidosis
Systemic lupus erythematosus
Scleroderma
Sleep apnea
Drugs:

Adenosine	Fluoxetine
Amiodarone	Halothane
β-Blockers	Isradipine
Cisplatin	Neostigmine
Citalopram	Nicardipine
Clonidine	Nitroglycerin
Cocaine	Paclitaxel
Dexmedetomidine	Propafenone
Digoxin	Propofol
Diltiazem	Sevoflurane
Dipyridamole	Sotalol
Disopyramide	Succinylcholine
Donepezil	Thalidomide
Dronedarone	Verapamil
Flecainide	

From Refs. 12, 13.

prolong life in patients with those diseases, and the benefits of therapy with β-blockers outweigh the risks associated with sinus bradycardia. In these patients, clinicians and patients may elect to implant a permanent pacemaker in order to allow the patient to continue therapy with β-blockers.

Acute treatment of the symptomatic patient consists primarily of administration of the anticholinergic drug atropine, which may be given in doses of 0.5 mg IV every 3 to 5 minutes. The maximum recommended total dose of atropine is 3 mg;[14] however, this total dose should not be administered to patients with sinus bradycardia, but rather should be reserved for patients with cardiac arrest due to asystole, as complete vagal inhibition at this dose can increase myocardial oxygen demand and precipitate ischemia or tachyarrhythmias in patients with underlying coronary artery disease (CAD). Therefore, for management of sinus bradycardia, the maximum atropine dose should be approximately 2 mg. In patients with hemodynamically unstable or severely symptomatic sinus bradycardia that is unresponsive to atropine and in whom temporary or transvenous pacing is not available or is ineffective, epinephrine (2–10 mcg/min, titrate to response) and/or dopamine (2–10 mcg/kg/min) may be administered.[14] Both drugs stimulate adrenergic α- and β-receptors.

In patients with sinus bradycardia due to underlying correctable disorders (such as electrolyte abnormalities or hypothyroidism), management consists of correcting those disorders.

Nonpharmacologic Therapy Long-term management of patients with sick sinus syndrome requires implantation of a permanent pacemaker.[12]

▶ Outcome Evaluation

- Monitor the patient's heart rate and alleviation of symptoms.
- Monitor for adverse effects of medications, such as atropine (dry mouth, mydriasis, urinary retention, and tachycardia).

AV Nodal Blockade

AV nodal blockade occurs when conduction of electrical impulses through the AV node is impaired to varying degrees. AV nodal blockade is classified into three categories. First-degree AV block is defined simply as prolongation of the PR interval to greater than 0.2 seconds. During first-degree AV block, all impulses initiated by the SA node that have resulted in atrial depolarization are conducted through the AV node; the abnormality is simply that the impulses are conducted more slowly than normal, resulting in prolongation of the PR interval.[15] Second-degree AV block is further distinguished into two types: Mobitz type I (also known as Wenckebach) and Mobitz type II. In both types of second-degree AV block, some of the impulses initiated by the SA node are not conducted through the AV node. This often occurs in a regular pattern; for example, every third or fourth impulse generated by the SA node may not be conducted. During third-degree AV block, which is also referred to as "complete heart block," none of the impulses generated by the SA node are conducted through the AV node. This results in "AV dissociation," during which the atria continue to depolarize normally as a result of normal impulses initiated by the SA node; however, the ventricles initiate their own depolarizations, because no SA node–generated impulses are conducted to the ventricles. Therefore, on the ECG, there is no relationship between the P waves and the QRS complexes.

▶ Epidemiology and Etiology

The overall incidence of AV nodal blockade is unknown. AV nodal blockade may be caused by degenerative changes in the AV node. ❷ *In addition, there are many other possible etiologies of AV nodal blockade including drugs* (Table 9–3).[12,13,15]

▶ Pathophysiology

First-degree AV nodal blockade occurs due to inhibition of conduction within the upper portion of the node.[15] Mobitz type I second-degree AV nodal blockade occurs as a result of inhibition of conduction further down within the node.[12,15] Mobitz type II second-degree AV nodal blockade is caused by inhibition of conduction within or below the level of the bundle of His.[12,15] Third-degree AV nodal blockade may be a result of inhibition of conduction either within the AV node or within the bundle of His or the His-Purkinje system.[12,15] AV block may occur as a result of age-related AV node degeneration.

▶ Treatment

Desired Outcomes The desired outcomes of treatment are to restore normal sinus rhythm and alleviate patient symptoms.

Table 9–3

Etiologies of AV Nodal Blockade

Idiopathic degeneration of the AV node
Myocardial ischemia or infarction
Neurocardiac syncope
Carotid-sinus hypersensitivity
Electrolyte abnormalities: hypokalemia or hyperkalemia
Hypothyroidism
Hypothermia
Infectious diseases: Chagas' disease or endocarditis
Amyloidosis
Sarcoidosis
Systemic lupus erythematosus
Scleroderma
Sleep apnea
Drugs:

Adenosine	Hydroxychloroquine
Amiodarone	Paclitaxel
β-Blockers	Phenylpropanolamine
Bupivicaine	Propafenone
Carbamazepine	Propofol
Chloroquine	Sotalol
Digoxin	Thioridazine
Diltiazem	Tricyclic antidepressants
Dronedarone	Verapamil
Flecainide	

AV, atrioventricular.
From Refs. 12, 13, 15.

Clinical Presentation and Diagnosis of AV Nodal Blockade

Symptoms

- First-degree AV nodal blockade is rarely symptomatic, because it rarely results in bradycardia
- Second-degree AV nodal blockade may cause bradycardia, as not all impulses generated by the SA node are conducted through the AV node to the ventricles
- In third-degree AV nodal blockade, or complete heart block, the heart rate is usually 30 to 40 bpm, resulting in symptoms
- Symptoms of bradyarrhythmias such as second- or third-degree AV block consist of dizziness, fatigue, light-headedness, syncope, chest pain (in patients with underlying CAD), and shortness of breath and other symptoms of heart failure (in patients with underlying left ventricular dysfunction)

Diagnosis

- Made on the basis of patient presentation, including history of present illness and presenting symptoms, as well as a 12-lead ECG that reveals AV nodal blockade
- Assess potentially correctable etiologies, including myocardial ischemia, serum potassium concentration (for hyperkalemia), and thyroid function tests (for hypothyroidism)
- Determine whether the patient is taking any drugs known to cause AV block
- If the patient is currently taking digoxin, determine the serum digoxin concentration and ascertain whether it is supratherapeutic (less than 2 ng/mL [2.6 nmol/L])

Pharmacologic Therapy Treatment of first-degree AV nodal blockade is rarely necessary, because symptoms rarely occur. However, the ECGs of patients with first-degree AV nodal blockade should be monitored to assess the possibility of progression of first-degree AV nodal blockade to second- or third-degree block. Second- or third-degree AV nodal blockade requires treatment, because bradycardia usually results in symptoms. If the patient is taking any medication(s) that may cause AV nodal blockade, the drug(s) should be discontinued whenever possible. If the patient's rhythm still exhibits AV nodal blockade after discontinuing the medication(s) and after five half-lives of the drug(s) have elapsed, then the drug(s) can usually be excluded as the etiology of the arrhythmia. However, in certain circumstances, discontinuation of a medication that is inducing AV nodal blockade may be undesirable. For example, if the patient has a history of myocardial infarction or heart failure, discontinuation of a β-blocker is undesirable because β-blockers have been shown to reduce mortality and prolong life in patients with those diseases, and the benefits of therapy with β-blockers outweigh the risks associated with AV nodal blockade. In these patients, clinicians and patients may elect to implant a permanent pacemaker in order to allow the patient to continue therapy with β-blockers.

Acute treatment of patients with second- or third-degree AV nodal blockade consists primarily of administration of atropine, which may be administered in the same doses as recommended for management of sinus bradycardia. In patients with hemodynamically unstable or severely symptomatic AV nodal blockade that is unresponsive to atropine and in whom temporary or transvenous pacing is not available or is ineffective, epinephrine (2–10 mcg/min, titrate to response) and/or dopamine (2–10 mcg/kg/min) may be administered.[14]

In patients with second- or third-degree AV block due to underlying correctable disorders (such as electrolyte abnormalities or hypothyroidism), management consists of correcting those disorders.

Nonpharmacologic Therapy Long-term management of patients with second- or third-degree AV nodal blockade due to idiopathic degeneration of the AV node requires implantation of a permanent pacemaker.[12]

Outcome Evaluation

- Monitor the patient for termination of AV nodal blockade and restoration of normal sinus rhythm, heart rate, and alleviation of symptoms.
- If atropine is administered, monitor the patient for adverse effects including dry mouth, mydriasis, urinary retention, and tachycardia.

Atrial Fibrillation

AF is the most common arrhythmia encountered in clinical practice. It is important for clinicians to understand AF, because it is associated with substantial morbidity and mortality and because many strategies for drug therapy are available. Drugs used to treat AF often have a narrow therapeutic index and a broad adverse-effect profile.

▶ Epidemiology and Etiology

Approximately 2.3 million Americans have AF. The prevalence of AF increases with advancing age; roughly 9% of patients between the ages of 80 and 89 years have AF.[16] Similarly, the incidence of AF increases with age, and it occurs more commonly in men than in women.[16]

Etiologies of AF are presented in Table 9–4. The common feature of the majority of etiologies of AF is the development of left atrial hypertrophy. Hypertension may be the most important risk factor for development of AF. However, AF occurs commonly in patients with CAD. In addition, heart failure is

Clinical Presentation and Diagnosis of AF

Symptoms

- Approximately 20% to 30% of patients with AF remain asymptomatic

- Symptoms typical of tachyarrhythmias such as AF include palpitations, dizziness, light-headedness, shortness of breath, chest pain (if underlying CAD is present), near-syncope, and syncope. Patients commonly complain of palpitations; often the complaint is "I can feel my heart beating fast" or "I can feel my heart fluttering" or "It feels like my heart is going to beat out of my chest."

- Other symptoms are dependent on the degree to which cardiac output is diminished, which is in turn dependent on the ventricular rate and the degree to which stroke volume is reduced by the rapidly beating heart

- In some patients, the first symptom of AF is stroke

Diagnosis

- Because the symptoms of all tachyarrhythmias are dependent on heart rate and are therefore essentially the same, the diagnosis depends on the presence of AF on the ECG

- AF is characterized on ECG by an absence of P waves, an undulating baseline that represents roughly 350 to 600 attempted atrial depolarizations per minute, and an irregularly irregular rhythm, meaning that the intervals between the R waves are irregular and that there is no pattern to the irregularity

Table 9–4

Etiologies of AF

Hypertension
Coronary artery disease
Heart failure
Diabetes
Hyperthyroidism
Rheumatic heart disease
Diseases of the heart valves:
  Mitral stenosis or regurgitation
  Mitral valve prolapse
Chronic obstructive pulmonary disease
Pulmonary embolism
Idiopathic ("lone" AF)
Thoracic surgery:
  Coronary artery bypass graft surgery
  Pulmonary resection
  Thoracoabdominal esophagectomy
Drugs:
  Adenosine
  Albuterol
  Alcohol
  Alendronate
  Dobutamine
  Enoximone
  Ipratropium bromide
  Methylprednisolone
  Milrinone
  Mitoxantrone
  Paclitaxel
  Propafenone
  Theophylline
  Verapamil
  Zoledronic acid

AF, atrial fibrillation.
From Refs. 13, 20, 21.

increasingly recognized as a cause of AF; approximately 25% to 30% of patients with New York Heart Association (NYHA) class III heart failure have AF,[17] and the arrhythmia is present in as many as 50% of patients with NYHA class IV heart failure.[18]

Drug-induced AF is relatively uncommon, but has been reported (Table 9–4).[13] Acute ingestion of large amounts of alcohol may cause AF; this phenomenon has been referred to as the "holiday heart" syndrome.[19] In addition, recent reports have associated use of the bisphosphonate drugs zoledronic acid[20] and alendronate[21] with new-onset serious AF. The potential relationship between bisphosphonate use and new-onset AF requires further study.

▶ Pathophysiology

❶ *AF may be caused by both abnormal impulse formation and abnormal impulse conduction.* Traditionally, AF was believed to be initiated by premature impulses initiated in the atria. However, it is now understood that in many patients AF is triggered by electrical impulses generated within the pulmonary veins.[22] These impulses initiate the process of re-entry within the atria, and AF is believed to be sustained by multiple re-entrant wavelets operating simultaneously within the atria.[23] Some believe that, at least in some patients, the increased automaticity in the pulmonary veins may be the sole mechanism of AF and that the multiple re-entrant wavelet hypothesis may be incorrect. However, the concept of multiple simultaneous re-entrant wavelets remains the predominant hypothesis regarding the mechanism of AF.[23]

AF leads to electrical remodeling of the atria. Episodes of AF that are of longer duration and episodes that occur with increasing frequency result in progressive shortening of atrial refractory periods, further potentiating the re-entrant circuits in the atria.[24] Therefore, it is often said that "atrial fibrillation begets atrial fibrillation," that is, AF causes atrial electrophysiologic alterations that promote further AF.[23,24] AF is associated with 400 to 600 attempted atrial depolarizations per minute and chaotic, disorganized atrial electrical activity.

The AV node is incapable of conducting 400 to 600 impulses per minute; however, it may conduct 100 to 200 impulses per minute, resulting in ventricular rates ranging from 100 to 200 bpm.

AF is classified as **paroxysmal**, persistent, or permanent (Fig. 9–4).[25] Patients with paroxysmal AF have episodes that begin suddenly and spontaneously, last minutes to hours, or rarely as long as 7 days, and terminate suddenly and spontaneously. Some patients with paroxysmal AF have episodes that do not terminate spontaneously but require intervention, and this is known as persistent AF. Approximately 18% to 30% of patients with AF progress to the point of permanent AF; these patients are subsequently never in normal sinus rhythm but rather are always in AF.

AF is associated with substantial morbidity and mortality. This arrhythmia is associated with a risk of ischemic stroke of approximately 5% per year.[25] The risk of stroke is increased two- to sevenfold in patients with AF compared to patients without this arrhythmia.[25] AF is the cause of roughly one of every six strokes. During AF, atrial contraction is absent. Due to the fact that atrial contraction is responsible for

approximately 30% of left ventricular filling, this blood that is not ejected from the left atrium to the left ventricle pools in the atrium, particularly in the left atrial appendage. Blood pooling facilitates the formation of a thrombus, which subsequently may travel through the mitral valve into the left ventricle and may be ejected during ventricular contraction. The thrombus then may travel through a carotid artery into the brain, resulting in an ischemic stroke.

AF may lead to the development of heart failure as a result of tachycardia-induced cardiomyopathy.[26] AF increases the risk of mortality approximately twofold compared to that in patients without AF;[25] the causes of death are likely stroke or heart failure.

▶ Treatment

● **Desired Outcomes** ❸ *The goals of individualized therapy of AF are: (a) ventricular rate control, (b) termination of AF and restoration of sinus rhythm (commonly referred to as "cardioversion" or "conversion to sinus rhythm"), (c) maintenance of sinus rhythm, or reduction in the frequency of episodes of paroxysmal AF, and/or (d) prevention of stroke. These goals of therapy do not necessarily apply to all patients; the specific goal(s) that apply depend on the patient's AF classification* (Table 9–5).

● **Hemodynamically Unstable AF** For patients who present with an episode of AF that is hemodynamically unstable, emergent conversion to sinus rhythm is necessary using **direct current cardioversion** (DCC). Hemodynamic instability may be defined as the presence of any one of the following[14]: (a) patient has altered mental status, (b) hypotension (systolic blood pressure less than 90 mm Hg) or other signs of shock,

Patient Encounter, Part 1

DA is a 58-year-old male who presents to the emergency department (ED) complaining that he can "feel my heart beating fast," which started when he was taking out the garbage. He also complains of feeling light-headed and short of breath. His pulse is irregularly irregular, with a rate of 135 bpm.

His physical exam is completely normal and no focal neurologic deficits were observed.

What information is suggestive of AF?

What additional information do you need in order to develop a treatment plan?

Patient Encounter, Part 2: Medical History, Physical Exam, and Diagnostic Tests

PMH: Hypertension × 15 years; coronary artery disease × 5 years; myocardial infarction 2005; heart failure × 5 years

Meds: Aspirin 81 mg once daily; metoprolol 50 mg twice daily; enalapril 5 mg twice daily; furosemide 40 mg daily

PE:

Ht 5′10″ (178 cm), wt 80 kg (176 lb), BP 110/70 mm Hg, P 135 bpm, RR 20/min; remainder of PE noncontributory

Labs: All within normal limits

CXR: Mild pulmonary edema

Echo: Moderately reduced LV function, LVEF 35%

ECG: Atrial fibrillation

What is your assessment of DA's condition?

What are your treatment goals?

What pharmacologic or nonpharmacologic alternatives are available for each treatment goal?

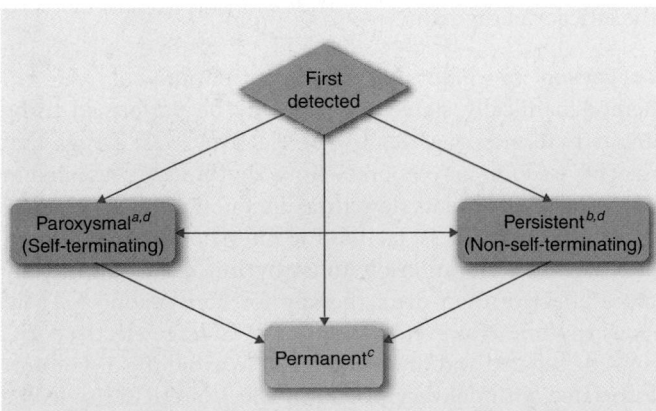

FIGURE 9–4. Classification of atrial fibrillation. [a]Episodes that generally last 7 days or less (most less than 24 hours). [b]Episodes that usually last 7 days. [c]Cardioversion failed or not attempted. [d]Either paroxysmal or persistent atrial fibrillation may be recurrent. AF, atrial fibrillation. (From Ref. 25.)

Table 9–5

Treatment Goals According to AF Classification

First Detected Episode	Paroxysmal AF	Persistent AF	Permanent AF
Ventricular rate control Stroke prevention Conversion to sinus rhythm	Ventricular rate control Stroke prevention Maintenance of sinus rhythm *if ventricular rate control is not* *sufficient to control symptoms*	Ventricular rate control Stroke prevention Conversion to sinus rhythm	Ventricular rate control Stroke prevention

AF, atrial fibrillation.

(c) ventricular rate greater than 150 bpm, and/or (d) patient is experiencing squeezing, crushing chest pain suggestive of myocardial ischemia.

DCC is the process of administering a synchronized electrical shock to the chest. The purpose of DCC is to simultaneously depolarize all of the myocardial cells, resulting in interruption and termination of the multiple re-entrant circuits and restoration of normal sinus rhythm. The initial energy level of the shock is 100 joules (J); if the DCC attempt is unsuccessful, successive cardioversion attempts may be made at 200 J, 300 J, and 360 J.[14] Delivery of the shock is synchronized to the ECG by the cardioverter machine, such that the electrical charge is not delivered during the latter portion of the T wave (i.e., the relative refractory period), to avoid delivering an electrical impulse that may be conducted abnormally, which may result in a life-threatening ventricular arrhythmia.

The remainder of this section will be devoted to management of hemodynamically stable AF. The specific goals of therapy that apply to patients in each AF classification are presented in Table 9–5.

Pharmacologic Therapy

Ventricular Rate Control. Ventricular rate control can be achieved by inhibiting the proportion of electrical impulses conducted from the atria to the ventricles through the AV node. Therefore, drugs that are effective for ventricular rate control are those that inhibit AV nodal impulse conduction: β-blockers, diltiazem, verapamil, digoxin, and amiodarone (Tables 9–6 and 9–7).

In patients who present with their first detected episode of AF, or for those who present with an episode of persistent AF, ventricular rate control is usually initially achieved using IV drugs. A decision algorithm for selecting a specific drug for acute ventricular rate control is presented in Figure 9–5. In general, an IV CCB or β-blocker is preferred for ventricular rate control in patients with normal LV function, as ventricular rate control can often be achieved within several minutes. In patients with heart failure due to LV dysfunction, IV digoxin or amiodarone is preferred, because diltiazem and verapamil are associated with negative inotropic effects and may exacerbate heart failure.[27] Similarly, although oral β-blockers are indicated in patients with heart failure due to LV dysfunction, IV β-blockers are generally avoided due to the potential for acutely exacerbating heart failure.

A decision strategy for long-term rate control in patients with paroxysmal or permanent AF is presented in Figure 9–6. In general, while digoxin is effective for ventricular rate control in patients at rest, digoxin is less effective than CCBs or β-blockers for ventricular rate control in patients undergoing physical activity including activities of daily living. This is likely because activation of the sympathetic nervous system during exercise and activity overwhelms the stimulating effect of digoxin on the parasympathetic nervous system. Therefore, in patients with normal LV function, CCBs or β-blockers are preferred for long-term ventricular rate control. Diltiazem may be preferable to verapamil in older patients due to a lower incidence of constipation. However, in patients with heart failure, oral diltiazem and verapamil are contraindicated as a result of their negative inotropic activity and propensity to exacerbate heart failure. Therefore, the options in this population are β-blockers or digoxin. The majority of patients with heart failure should be receiving therapy with an oral β-blocker with the goal of achieving mortality risk reduction. In patients with heart failure who develop rapid AF while receiving therapy with β-blockers, digoxin should be administered for purposes of ventricular rate control. Fortunately, studies have found the combination of digoxin and β-blockers to be effective for ventricular rate control, likely as a result of β-blocker-induced attenuation of the inhibitory effects of the sympathetic nervous system on the efficacy of digoxin.

Conversion to Sinus Rhythm. Termination of AF in hemodynamically stable patients may be performed using antiarrhythmic drug therapy or elective DCC. Drugs that may be used for conversion to sinus rhythm are presented in Table 9–8; these agents slow atrial conduction velocity and/or prolong refractoriness, facilitating interruption of re-entrant circuits and restoration of sinus rhythm. DCC is generally more effective than drug therapy for conversion of AF to sinus rhythm. However, patients who undergo elective DCC must be sedated and/or anesthetized to avoid the discomfort associated with delivery of 100 to 360 J of electricity to the chest. Therefore, it is important that patients scheduled to undergo elective DCC do not eat within approximately 8 to 12 hours of the procedure to avoid aspiration of stomach contents during the period of sedation/anesthesia. This often factors into the decision as to whether to employ elective DCC or drug therapy for conversion of AF to sinus rhythm. If a

Table 9–6

Drugs for Ventricular Rate Control in AF

Drug	Mechanism of Action	Loading Dose	Daily Dose	Drug Interactions
Amiodarone	β-Blocker CCB	150 mg IV over 10 min	0.5–1 mg/min IV continuous infusion 200 mg everyday orally	Inhibits clearance of digoxin, warfarin, and other drugs
β-Blockers[a]	Inhibit AV nodal conduction by slowing AV nodal conduction and prolonging AV nodal refractoriness	Esmolol 500 mcg/kg IV over 1 minute Propranolol 0.15 mg/kg IV Metoprolol 2.5–5 mg IV × 2–3 doses	Esmolol 50–200 mcg/kg/min continuous IV infusion Propranolol 80–240 mg/day Metoprolol 50–200 mg/day	
Diltiazem	Inhibits AV nodal conduction by slowing AV nodal conduction and prolonging AV nodal refractoriness	0.25 mg/kg IV load over 2 minutes. If necessary, 0.35 mg/kg IV over 2 minutes after first dose	Continuous infusion of 5–15 mg/h 120–360 mg/day orally	Inhibits elimination of cyclosporine
Verapamil	Inhibits AV nodal conduction by slowing AV nodal conduction and prolonging AV nodal refractoriness	0.075–0.15 mg/kg IV over 2 minutes. If necessary, an additional dose of 0.075–0.15 mg/kg IV may be administered 30 minutes later	120–360 mg/day	Inhibits digoxin elimination
Digoxin	Inhibits AV nodal conduction by (a) vagal stimulation, (b) directly slowing AV, nodal conduction and prolonging AV nodal refractoriness	0.25 mg IV every 2 hours up to 1.5 mg	0.125–0.375 mg orally once daily	Amiodarone, verapamil, quinidine inhibit digoxin elimination

AF, atrial fibrillation; AV, atrioventricular; CCB, calcium channel blocker.

[a]While oral β-blockers are important agents for mortality reduction in patients with heart failure, IV β-blockers should be avoided due to the potential for heart failure exacerbation.

Table 9–7

Adverse Effects of Drugs Used to Treat Arrhythmias

Drug	Adverse Effects
Adenosine	Chest pain, flushing, shortness of breath, sinus bradycardia/AV block
Amiodarone	IV: Hypotension, sinus bradycardia Oral: Blue–gray skin discoloration, photosensitivity, corneal microdeposits, pulmonary fibrosis, hepatotoxicity, sinus bradycardia, hypo- or hyperthyroidism, peripheral neuropathy, weakness, AV block
Atropine	Tachycardia, urinary retention, blurred vision, dry mouth, mydriasis
Digoxin	Nausea, vomiting, anorexia, green–yellow halos around objects, ventricular arrhythmias
Diltiazem	Hypotension, sinus bradycardia, heart failure exacerbation, AV block
Dofetilide	Torsades de pointes
Dronedarone	Diarrhea, asthenia, nausea and vomiting, abdominal pain, bradycardia, GI distress
Esmolol	Hypotension, sinus bradycardia, AV block, heart failure exacerbation
Flecainide	Dizziness, blurred vision, heart failure exacerbation
Ibutilide	Torsades de pointes
Lidocaine	Dizziness, confusion, seizures (if dose too high)
Metoprolol	Hypotension, sinus bradycardia, AV block, fatigue, heart failure exacerbation[a]
Mexiletine	Nausea, vomiting, GI distress, tremor, dizziness, fatigue, seizures (if dose too high)
Procainamide	Hypotension, torsades de pointes
Propafenone	Dizziness, blurred vision
Propranolol	Hypotension, bradycardia, AV block, heart failure exacerbation[a]
Sotalol	Sinus bradycardia, AV block, fatigue, torsades de pointes
Verapamil	Hypotension, heart failure exacerbation, bradycardia, AV block, constipation (oral)

AV, atrioventricular.

[a]Associated with IV administration, inappropriately high oral doses at initiation of therapy, or overly aggressive and rapid dose titration.

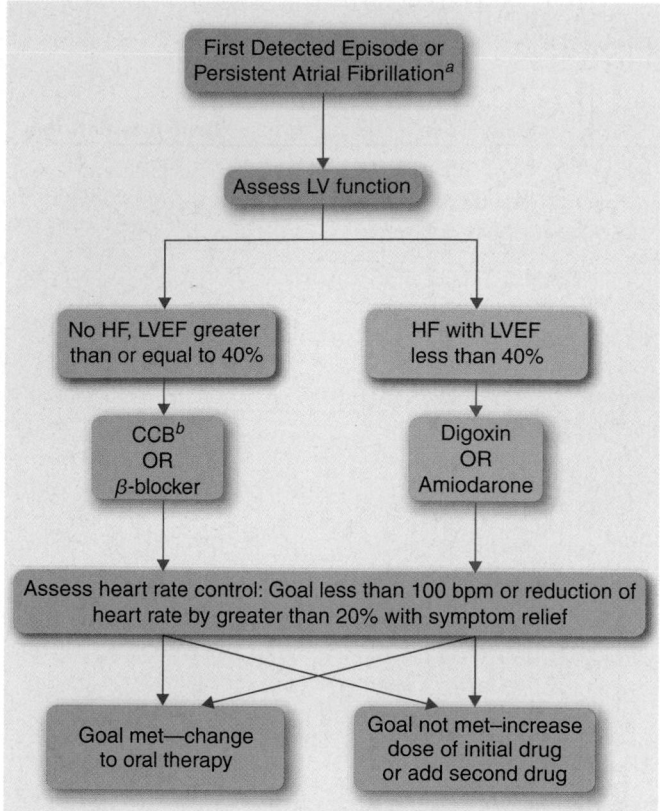

FIGURE 9–5. Decision algorithm for ventricular rate control using IV drug therapy for patients presenting with the first detected episode or an episode of persistent atrial fibrillation that is hemodynamically stable. ^aDrugs administered IV. ^bDiltiazem is generally preferred over verapamil because of a lower risk of severe hypotension. (β-blocker, esmolol, metoprolol, or propranolol; bpm, beats per minute; CCB, calcium channel blocker [diltiazem or verapamil]; HF, heart failure; LV, left ventricular; LVEF, left ventricular ejection fraction.)

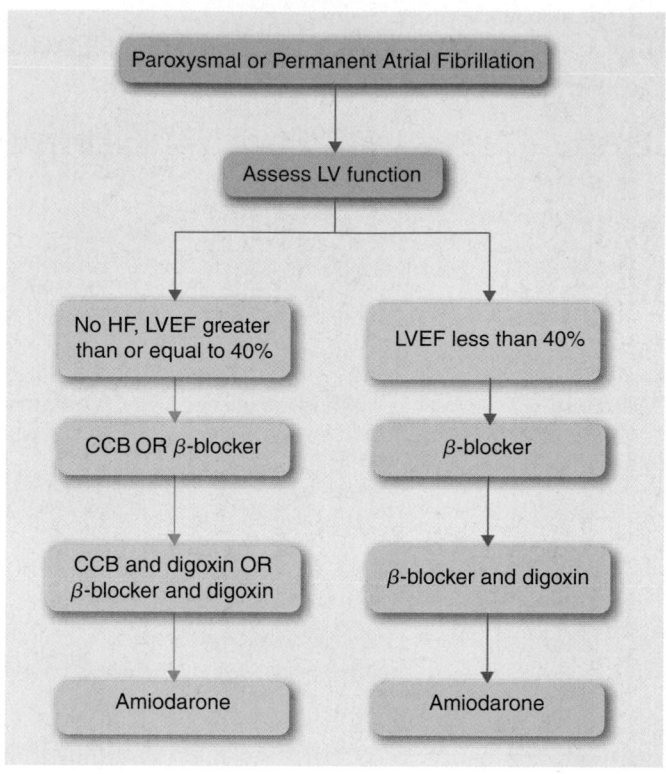

FIGURE 9–6. Decision algorithm for long-term ventricular rate control with oral drug therapy for patients with paroxysmal or permanent atrial fibrillation. With each therapy/dose change, assess heart rate control. Goal less than 100 bpm or reduction of heart rate by more than 20% with symptom relief. If goal is not met, move to next step in algorithm. (bpm, beats per minute; CCB, calcium channel blocker [diltiazem or verapamil]; HF, heart failure; LV, left ventricular function; LVEF, left ventricular ejection fraction.)

Table 9–8

Drugs for Conversion of AF to Normal Sinus Rhythm

Treatment	Loading Dose	Continuous Infusion Rate	Drug Interactions
Amiodarone	5–7 mg/kg IV over 30–60 minutes	1.2–1.8 g/24 h	Inhibits elimination of digoxin and warfarin
Dofetilide	See below^a; patients must be hospitalized for 3 days during initiation of therapy	—	Cimetidine, hydrochlorothiazide, ketoconazole, medroxyprogesterone, promethazine, trimethoprim, verapamil (all inhibit dofetilide elimination)
Ibutilide	1 mg IV over 10 minutes, followed by a second 1 mg IV dose if necessary	—	—
Propafenone	600 mg single oral dose	—	—
Flecainide	200–300 mg single oral dose	—	—

AF, atrial fibrillation.

^aDofetilide dosing:

Calculated Creatinine Clearance	Dofetilide Dose
Greater than 60 mL/min	500 mcg twice daily
40–60 mL/min	250 mcg twice daily
20–40 mL/min	125 mcg twice daily
Less than 20 mL/min	Contraindicated

patient presents with AF requiring nonemergent conversion to sinus rhythm, and the patient has eaten a meal that day, then pharmacologic methods must be used for cardioversion on that day, or DCC must be postponed to the following day to allow for a period of fasting prior to the procedure.

A decision strategy for conversion of AF to sinus rhythm is presented in Figure 9–7. The cardioversion decision strategy depends greatly on the duration of AF. If the AF episode began within 48 hours, conversion to sinus rhythm is safe and may be attempted with elective DCC or specific drug therapy (Fig. 9–7). However, if the duration of the AF episode is longer than 48 hours or if there is uncertainty regarding the duration of the episode, two strategies for conversion may be considered. Data indicate that a thrombus may form in the left atrium during AF episodes of 48 hours or longer; if an atrial thrombus is present, the process of conversion to sinus rhythm, whether with DCC or drugs, can dislodge the atrial thrombus and cause a stroke. Therefore, in patients experiencing an AF episode of 48 hours or longer, conversion to sinus rhythm should be deferred unless it is known that an atrial thrombus is not present. In the past, common practice in patients with AF of greater than 48 hours duration was to anticoagulate with warfarin, maintaining a therapeutic International Normalized Ratio (INR) for 3 weeks, after

which cardioversion may be performed. Patients were subsequently anticoagulated for a minimum of 4 weeks following the restoration of sinus rhythm. Today, rather than se nd patients with ongoing AF home for 3 weeks of anticoagulation, it has become standard practice at many institutions to perform a transesophageal echocardiogram (TEE) to determine whether an atrial thrombus is present; if such a thrombus is not present, DCC or pharmacologic cardioversion may be performed within 24 hours. If this strategy is selected, hospitalized patients should undergo anticoagulation with IV unfractionated heparin, with the dose targeted to a partial thromboplastin time (PTT) of 60 seconds (range 50–70 seconds), or warfarin therapy (target INR 2.5; range 2–3) during the hospitalization period prior to the TEE and cardioversion procedure. If no thrombus is present during TEE and cardioversion is successful, patients should maintain anticoagulation with warfarin (target INR 2.5; range 2–3) for at least 4 weeks. If a thrombus is observed during TEE, then cardioversion should be postponed and anticoagulation should be continued indefinitely. Another TEE should be performed prior to a subsequent cardioversion attempt.[28]

Conversion of AF to sinus rhythm is usually performed in patients with the first detected episode of AF or in patients with an episode of persistent AF. In patients with permanent AF, conversion to sinus rhythm is usually not attempted because cardioversion is unlikely to be successful, and in those rare patients in whom sinus rhythm is restored successfully, AF usually recurs shortly thereafter.

Maintenance of Sinus Rhythm/Reduction in the Frequency of Episodes of Paroxysmal AF. In many patients, permanent maintenance of sinus rhythm following cardioversion is an unrealistic goal. Many, if not most, patients experience recurrence of AF after cardioversion. Therefore, a more realistic goal for many patients is not permanent maintenance of sinus rhythm, but rather reduction in the frequency of episodes of paroxysmal AF.

In recent years, numerous studies have been performed to determine whether drug therapy for maintenance of sinus rhythm is preferred to drug therapy for ventricular rate control.[29–32] In these studies, patients have been assigned randomly to receive therapy either with drugs for rate control or with drugs for rhythm control (Table 9–9).

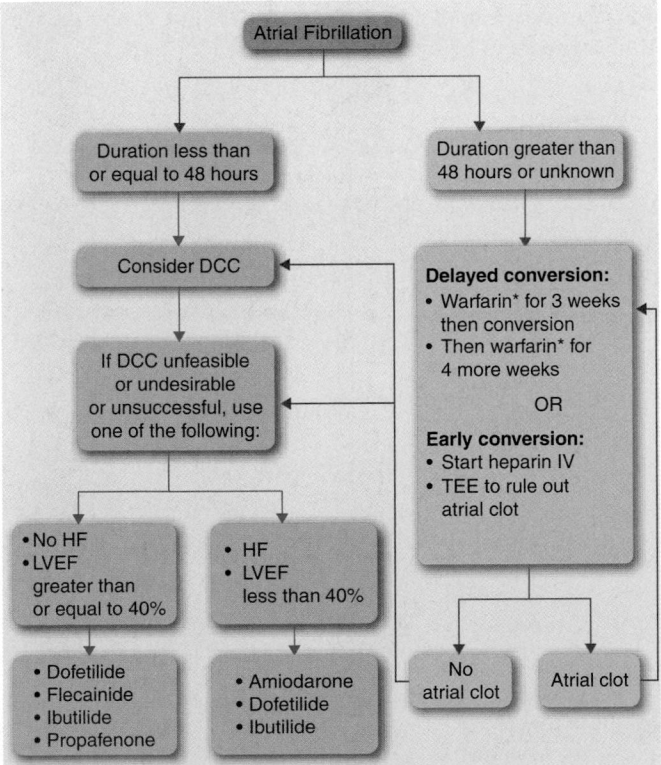

FIGURE 9–7. Decision algorithm for conversion of hemodynamically stable atrial fibrillation to normal sinus rhythm. (DCC, direct current cardioversion; HF, heart failure; LVEF, left ventricular ejection fraction; TEE, transesophageal echocardiogram.) *International Normalized Ratio 2–3.

Table 9–9

Drugs for Maintenance of Sinus Rhythm/Reduction in the Frequency of Episodes of AF

Drug	Dose
Amiodarone	100–400 mg orally once daily
Dofetilide	As described in Table 9–8
Dronedarone	400 mg orally twice daily
Sotalol	80–160 mg orally twice daily
Propafenone	150–300 mg orally thrice daily
Flecainide	100–150 mg orally three times daily

AF, atrial fibrillation.

These studies have found no significant differences in mortality in patients who received rhythm control therapy versus those who received rate control therapy.[29-32] However, patients assigned to the rhythm control strategy were more likely to be hospitalized[29,31,32] and were more likely to experience adverse effects associated with drug therapy.[29,30] ❹ *Therefore, drug therapy for the purpose of maintaining sinus rhythm or reducing the frequency of episodes of AF should be initiated only in those patients with episodes of paroxysmal AF who continue to experience symptoms despite maximum tolerated doses of drugs for ventricular rate control.* A decision strategy for maintenance therapy of sinus rhythm is presented in Figure 9–8. Drug therapy for maintenance of sinus rhythm and/or reduction in the frequency of episodes of paroxysmal AF should not be initiated in patients with underlying correctable causes of AF, such as hyperthyroidism; rather, the underlying cause of the arrhythmia should be corrected.

Stroke Prevention. All patients with paroxysmal, persistent, or permanent AF should receive therapy for stroke prevention unless compelling contraindications exist. A number of decision strategies for assigning patients to receive anticoagulation for stroke prevention in AF have been suggested; two commonly used strategies are presented in Tables 9–10[28] and 9–11.[33] ❺ *In general, most patients require therapy with warfarin; in some patients with no or few additional risk factors for stroke, aspirin may be acceptable.* For some patients, serious consideration of the benefits of warfarin versus the risks of bleeding associated with warfarin therapy is warranted. The potential bleeding risks associated with warfarin may outweigh the benefits in patients with a pretreatment INR of greater than 2, alcoholism, anticipated poor compliance, a history of falls, or current bleeding diathesis. In these situations, patients are at risk of severe bleeding associated with warfarin, including intracerebral hemorrhage, which may be associated with consequences as serious as those associated with a thrombotic stroke, and aspirin therapy may be associated with a more favorable benefit:risk ratio.

Recently, specific genetic tests to guide the initiation of warfarin therapy have been approved by the FDA. These tests assess single nucleotide polymorphisms on the gene that encodes cytochrome P-450 2C19, the primary hepatic enzyme responsible for warfarin metabolism, and the gene *VKORC1*, which encodes vitamin K epoxide reductase, the enzyme that is inhibited by warfarin as its mechanism of anticoagulation. Some advocate that all patients in whom warfarin therapy is being initiated should undergo genetic testing to guide the initiation of therapy; patients with specific polymorphisms of one or both of these genes may require adjustment of the initial warfarin dose to achieve adequate anticoagulation or avoid overanticoagulation and toxicity. Genetic testing to guide the initiation of warfarin therapy has not yet become standard practice, and many have questioned the efficacy and cost effectiveness of incorporation of routine genetic testing into warfarin therapy. The role of genetic testing in selecting initial warfarin doses may continue to evolve, but at the present time, appears to be limited.

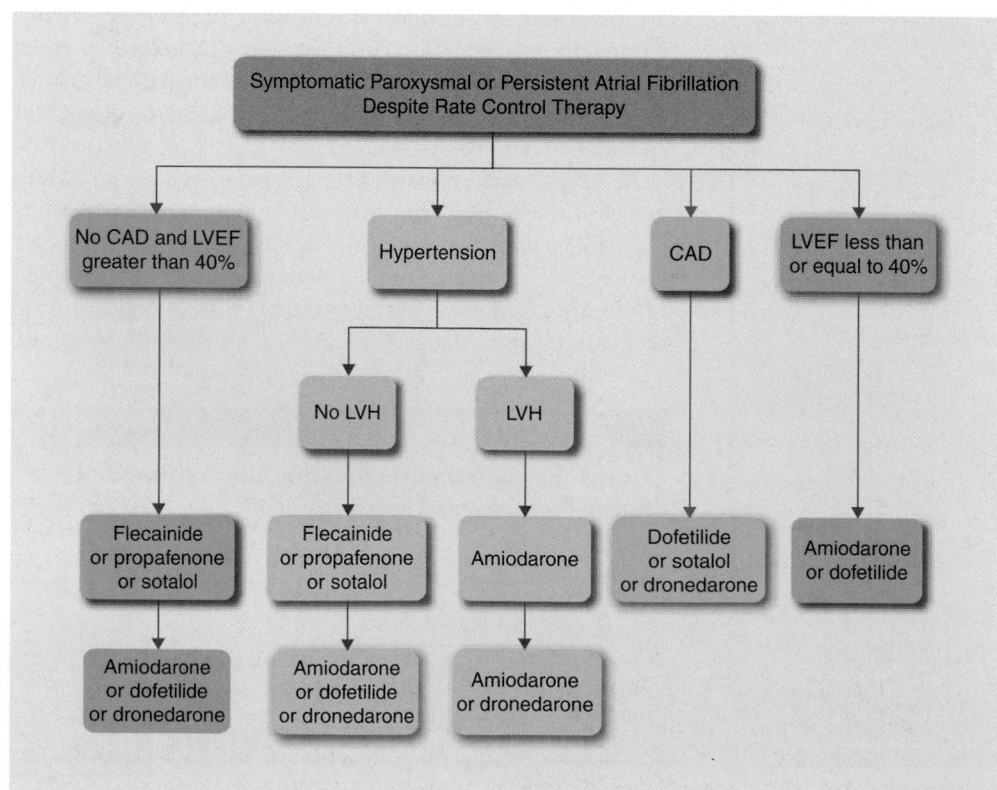

FIGURE 9–8. Decision algorithm for maintenance of sinus rhythm/reduction in the frequency of episodes of atrial fibrillation. (CAD, coronary artery disease; LVEF, left ventricular ejection fraction; LVH, left ventricular hypertrophy.)

Table 9–10

American College of Chest Physicians Recommendations for Stroke Prevention in AF

Patient Category (Risk Factors)	Recommended Drug	Dose/Target
Prior ischemic stroke, TIA, or systemic embolism	Warfarin	INR 2.5 (range 2–3)
Two or more of the following: Age greater than 75 years Hypertension Diabetes mellitus Heart failure	Warfarin	INR 2.5 (range 2–3)
One of the following: Age greater than 75 years Hypertension Diabetes mellitus Heart failure	Warfarin or aspirin; however, guidelines strongly recommend warfarin in this population	INR 2.5 (range 2–3) 75–325 mg orally daily
Less than 75 years of age and no other risk factors for ischemic stroke	Aspirin	75–325 mg orally daily

AF, atrial fibrillation; INR, International Normalized Ratio; TIA, transient ischemic attack.

From Ref. 28.

Table 9–11

Drugs for Stroke Prevention in AF—CHADS$_2$ Risk Stratification

CHADS$_2$ Score	Degree of Risk	Recommended Stroke Prevention Strategy
0	Low	Aspirin 325 mg orally daily
1	Moderate	Aspirin 325 mg orally daily or warfarin (INR 2–3)
Greater than or equal to 2	High	Warfarin (INR 2–3)

CHADS$_2$ score calculated as follows:

Congestive heart failure	1 point
Hypertension	1 point
Age greater than or equal to 75 years	1 point
Diabetes mellitus	1 point
Stroke or TIA history	2 points

AF, atrial fibrillation; INR, International Normalized Ratio; TIA, transient ischemic attack.

From Ref. 33.

▶ Outcome Evaluation

- Monitor the patient to determine whether the goal of ventricular rate control is met: heart rate less than 100 bpm or decrease in heart rate of 20% from the pretreatment value.

Patient Encounter, Part 3: Creating a Care Plan

Based on the information presented, create a care plan for DA's acute AF episode, and for long-term management of his AF.

Your plan should include: (a) a statement of the drug-related needs and/or problems, (b) the goals of therapy, (c) a patient-specific detailed therapeutic plan, and (d) a plan for follow-up to determine whether the goals have been achieved and adverse effects avoided.

- Monitor ECG to assess continued presence of AF and to determine whether conversion to sinus rhythm has occurred.
- Monitor INR approximately monthly to make sure it is therapeutic (target 2.5; range 2–3).
- Monitor patients for adverse effects of specific drug therapy (Table 9–7). Monitor patients receiving warfarin for signs and symptoms of bruising or bleeding.

Paroxysmal Supraventricular Tachycardia

Paroxysmal supraventricular tachycardia (PSVT) is a term that refers to a number of arrhythmias that occur above the ventricles and that require atrial or AV nodal tissue for initiation and maintenance.[34] The most common of these arrhythmias is known as AV re-entrant tachycardia, in which the arrhythmia is caused by a re-entrant circuit that involves the AV node or tissue adjacent to the AV node. Other types of PSVT include the relatively uncommon Wolff-Parkinson-White syndrome, which is caused by re-entry through an accessory extra-AV nodal pathway. For the purposes of this section, the term PSVT will refer to AV nodal re-entrant tachycardia.

▶ Epidemiology and Etiology

While PSVT can occur in patients experiencing myocardial ischemia or infarction, it often occurs in relatively young individuals with no history of cardiac disease. The overall incidence of PSVT is unknown.

▶ Pathophysiology

❶ *Paroxysmal supraventricular tachycardia is caused by re-entry that includes the AV node as a part of the re-entrant circuit.* Typically, electrical impulses travel forward (antegrade) down the AV node and then travel back up the AV node (retrograde) in a repetitive circuit. In some patients, the retrograde conduction pathway of the re-entrant circuit may exist in extra-AV nodal tissue adjacent to the AV node. One of these pathways usually conducts impulses rapidly, while the other usually conducts impulses slowly. Most commonly, during PSVT the impulse conducts antegrade through the slow pathway and retrograde through the faster

Clinical Presentation and Diagnosis of PSVT

- May occur at any age, but most commonly during the fourth and fifth decades of life[34]
- Occurs more commonly in females than in males; approximately two-thirds of patients that experience PSVT are women[34]

Symptoms

- Symptoms typical of tachyarrhythmias such as PSVT include palpitations, dizziness, light-headedness, shortness of breath, chest pain (if underlying CAD is present), near-syncope, and syncope. Patients commonly complain of palpitations; often the complaint is "I can feel my heart beating fast" or "I can feel my heart fluttering" or "It feels like my heart is going to beat out of my chest."

- Other symptoms are dependent on the degree to which cardiac output is diminished, which is in turn dependent on the heart rate and the degree to which stroke volume is reduced by the rapidly beating heart

Diagnosis

- Because the symptoms of all tachyarrhythmias are dependent on heart rate and are therefore essentially the same, diagnosis depends on the presence of PSVT on the ECG, characterized by narrow QRS complexes (usually less than 0.12 seconds). P waves may or may not be visible, depending on the heart rate
- PSVT is a regular rhythm and occurs at rates ranging from 100 to 250 bpm

---

pathway; in approximately 10% of patients, the re-entrant circuit is reversed.[34]

▶ Treatment

Desired Outcomes The desired outcomes for treatment are to terminate the arrhythmia, restore sinus rhythm, and prevent recurrence. Drug therapy is employed to terminate the arrhythmia and restore sinus rhythm; nonpharmacologic measures are employed to prevent recurrence.

Termination of PSVT Hemodynamically unstable PSVT should be treated with immediate synchronized DCC, using an initial energy level of 50 J; if the DCC attempt is unsuccessful, successive cardioversion attempts may be made at 100, 200, 300, and 360 J.[14]

The primary method of termination of hemodynamically stable PSVT is inhibition of impulse conduction and/or prolongation of the refractory period within the AV node. Because PSVT is propagated via a re-entrant circuit involving the AV node, inhibition of conduction within the AV node interrupts and terminates the re-entrant circuit.

Prior to initiation of drug therapy for termination of hemodynamically stable PSVT, some simple nonpharmacologic methods known as vagal maneuvers may be attempted.[35] Vagal maneuvers stimulate the activity of the parasympathetic nervous system, which inhibits AV nodal conduction, facilitating termination of the arrhythmia. Perhaps the simplest vagal maneuver is cough, which stimulates the vagus nerve. Instructing the patient to cough two or three times may successfully terminate the PSVT. Another vagal maneuver that may be attempted is carotid sinus massage; one of the carotid sinuses, located in the neck in the vicinity of the carotid arteries, may be gently massaged, stimulating vagal activity.[35] Carotid sinus massage should not be performed in patients with a history of stroke or transient ischemic attack, or in those in whom carotid bruits may be heard on auscultation. The Valsalva

maneuver, during which patients bear down against a closed glottis, may also be attempted.[35]

If vagal maneuvers are unsuccessful, IV drug therapy should be initiated.[34] Drugs that may be used for termination of hemodynamically stable PSVT are presented in Table 9–12. A decision strategy for pharmacologic termination of hemodynamically stable PSVT is presented in Figure 9–9.[35] ❻ *Adenosine is the drug of choice for pharmacologic termination of PSVT and is successful in 90% to 95% of patients.* Adenosine is associated with adverse effects (Table 9–7) including flushing, sinus bradycardia or AV nodal blockade, and bronchospasm in susceptible patients. In addition, adenosine may cause chest pain that mimics the discomfort of myocardial ischemia, but which is not actually associated with ischemia. The half-life of adenosine is approximately 10 seconds, due to deamination in the blood; therefore, in the vast majority of patients, adverse effects are of short duration.

If adenosine therapy is unsuccessful for termination of PSVT, subsequent choices of therapy depend on whether the patient has heart failure and/or a depressed left ventricular ejection fraction (LVEF).

Nonpharmacologic Therapy: Prevention of Recurrence In the past, prevention of recurrence of PSVT was attempted using long-term oral therapy with drugs such as verapamil or digoxin. Unfortunately, oral therapy with these drugs was associated with relatively limited success. Currently, the treatment of choice for long-term prevention of recurrence of PSVT is radiofrequency catheter ablation. During this procedure, a catheter is introduced transvenously and directed to the right atrium under fluoroscopic guidance. The catheter is advanced to the AV node, and radiofrequency energy is delivered to ablate, or destroy, one of the pathways of the re-entrant circuit. This procedure usually achieves a complete cure of PSVT and is associated with a relatively low risk of complications, and therefore obviates the need for long-term antiarrhythmic drug therapy in this population.

Table 9–12

Drugs for Termination of PSVT

Drug	Mechanism	Dose	Drug Interactions
Adenosine	Direct AV nodal inhibition	6 mg IV rapid bolus. If no response in 1–2 minutes, 12 mg IV rapid bolus. If no response in 1–2 minutes, 12 mg IV rapid bolus	Theophylline inhibits response to adenosine Dipyridamole accentuates response to adenosine
Verapamil	Direct AV nodal inhibition	1. 0.075–0.15 mg/kg IV over 2–3 minutes 2. If necessary, an additional dose of 0.075–0.15 mg/kg may be administered 30 minutes later	Inhibits digoxin elimination
Diltiazem	Direct AV nodal inhibition	1. 0.25 mg/kg IV load over 2 minutes 2. If necessary, 0.35 mg/kg IV over 2 minutes after first dose 3. Maintenance infusion: 5–15 mg/h	Inhibits elimination of cyclosporine
Digoxin	1. Vagal stimulation 2. Direct AV nodal inhibition	0.25 mg IV every 2 hours, up to 1.5 mg	Amiodarone and verapamil (inhibit digoxin elimination)
β-Blockers	Direct AV nodal inhibition	Esmolol 500 mcg/kg IV over 1 minute then 50–200 mcg/kg/min continuous infusion Propranolol 0.15 mg/kg IV Metoprolol 2.5–5 mg IV × 2–3 doses	
Amiodarone	β-blocker Calcium channel blocker	5–7 mg/kg IV over 30–60 minutes then 1.2–1.8 g per 24 hours IV infusion	Inhibits elimination of digoxin and warfarin

AV, atrioventricular; PSVT, paroxysmal supraventricular tachycardia.

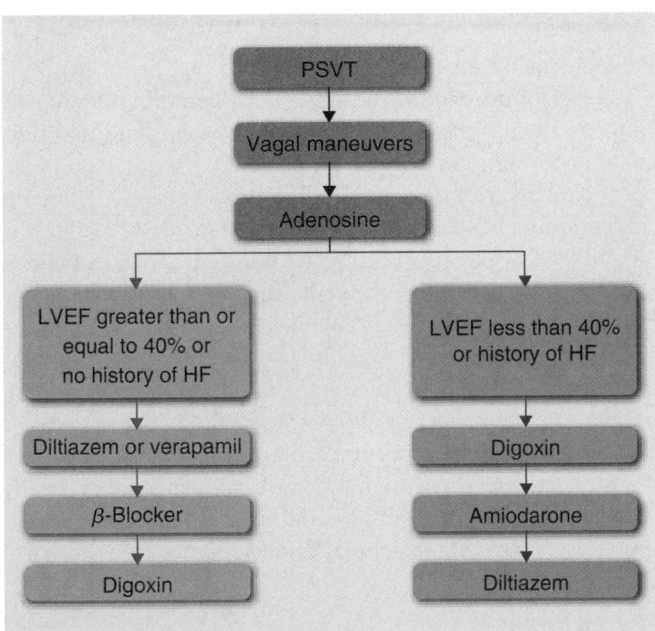

FIGURE 9–9. Decision algorithm for termination of PSVT. (HF, heart failure; LVEF, left ventricular ejection fraction; PSVT, paroxysmal supraventricular tachycardia.)

▶ Outcome Evaluation

- Monitor patients for termination of PSVT and restoration of normal sinus rhythm.
- Monitor patients for adverse effects of adenosine or any other antiarrhythmic agents administered (Table 9–7).

VENTRICULAR ARRHYTHMIAS

Ventricular Premature Depolarizations

VPDs are ectopic electrical impulses originating in ventricular tissue, resulting in wide, misshapen, abnormal QRS complexes. VPDs are also commonly known by other terms, including premature ventricular contractions (PVCs), ventricular premature beats (VPBs), and ventricular premature contractions (VPCs).

▶ Epidemiology, Etiology, and Pathophysiology

VPDs occur with variable frequency, depending on underlying comorbid conditions. The prevalence of complex or frequent VPDs is approximately 33% and 12% in men with and without CAD, respectively[36]; in women, the prevalence of complex or frequent VPDs is 26% and 12% in those with and without CAD, respectively.[37] VPDs occur more commonly in patients with ischemic heart disease, a history of myocardial infarction, and heart failure due to LV dysfunction. They may also occur as a result of hypoxia, anemia, and following cardiac surgery.

❶ *VPDs occur as a result of abnormal ventricular automaticity, due to enhanced activity of the sympathetic nervous system and altered electrophysiologic characteristics of the heart during myocardial ischemia and following myocardial infarction.*

In patients with underlying CAD or a history of myocardial infarction, the presence of complex or frequent VPDs is associated with an increased risk of mortality due to sudden cardiac death.[38]

Clinical Presentation and Diagnosis of VPD

- VPDs are usually categorized as simple or complex: simple VPDs are those that occur as infrequent, isolated single abnormal beats; complex VPDs are those that occur more frequently and/or in specific patterns

- Two consecutive VPDs are referred to as a couplet.[37] The term bigeminy refers to VPDs occurring with every other beat; trigeminy means VPDs occurring with every third beat; quadrigeminy means VPDs occurring every fourth beat.[37] VPDs occurring at a rate of more than 10 per hour or 6 or more per minute are defined as frequent[37]

Symptoms

- The majority of patients who experience simple or complex VPDs are asymptomatic. Occasionally, patients with complex or frequent VPDs may experience symptoms of palpitations, light-headedness, fatigue, near-syncope or syncope

▶ Treatment

Desired Outcomes The desired outcomes for treatment are to alleviate patient symptoms.

Pharmacologic Therapy ❼ *Asymptomatic VPDs should not be treated with antiarrhythmic drug therapy.* Based on the knowledge that complex or frequent VPDs increase the risk of sudden cardiac death in patients with a history of myocardial infarction, the Cardiac Arrhythmia Suppression Trials (CAST I and II)[39,40] tested the hypothesis that suppression of asymptomatic VPDs with the drugs flecainide, encainide, or moricizine in patients with a relatively recent history of myocardial infarction would lead to a reduction in the incidence of sudden cardiac death. However, the results of the trial showed that not only did these antiarrhythmic agents not reduce the risk of sudden cardiac death, there was a significant *increase* in the risk of death in patients who received therapy with encainide or flecainide compared to those that received placebo.[39] During the continuation of the study with moricizine, a trend was found toward an increase in the incidence of death in the patients who received this antiarrhythmic drug as well.[40] A subsequent meta-analysis of studies of other Vaughan Williams class I agents, including quinidine, procainamide, and disopyramide, found that the patients with complex VPDs who received these drugs following myocardial infarction were also at increased risk of death.[41] Therefore, all available evidence shows that patients with complex VPDs following myocardial infarction do not benefit from therapy with antiarrhythmic agents and that many of these drugs increase the risk of death. ❼ *Therefore, asymptomatic VPDs should not be treated.*

Patients with symptomatic VPDs should be treated with β-blockers, as the majority of patients with symptomatic VPDs have underlying CAD. β-Blockers have been shown to reduce mortality in this population and have been shown to be effective for VPD suppression.[42]

▶ Outcome Evaluation

- Monitor patients for relief of symptoms.
- Monitor for adverse effects of β-blockers—heart rate, blood pressure, fatigue, masking of symptoms of hypoglycemia and/or glucose intolerance (in patients with

diabetes), wheezing or shortness of breath (in patients with asthma or chronic obstructive pulmonary disease).

Ventricular Tachycardia

Ventricular tachycardia (VT) is a series of three or more consecutive VPDs at a rate greater than 100 bpm. VT is defined as nonsustained if it lasts less than 30 seconds and terminates spontaneously; sustained VT lasts greater than 30 seconds and does not terminate spontaneously but rather requires therapeutic intervention for termination.

▶ Epidemiology, Etiology, and Pathophysiology

Etiologies of VT are presented in Table 9–13. The incidence of VT is variable, depending on underlying comorbidities. Up to 20% of patients who experience acute myocardial infarction experience ventricular arrhythmias.[43] Approximately 2% to 4% of patients with myocardial infarction develop VT during the period of hospitalization.[42] Nonsustained VT occurs in 34% to 79% of patients with heart failure.[44] Other etiologies of VT include electrolyte abnormalities such as hypokalemia, hypoxia, and some drugs (Table 9–13).

❶ *Ventricular tachycardia is usually initiated by a precisely timed VPD, occurring during the relative refractory period, which provokes re-entry within ventricular tissue.*

Sustained VT requires immediate intervention, because if untreated, the rhythm may cause sudden cardiac death via hemodynamic instability and the absence of a pulse (pulseless VT) or via degeneration of VT into VF.

▶ Treatment

Desired Outcomes The desired outcomes for treatment are to terminate the arrhythmia and restore sinus rhythm, and to prevent sudden cardiac death.

Pharmacologic Therapy Hemodynamically unstable VT should be terminated immediately using synchronized DCC beginning with 100 J and increasing subsequent shocks to 200 J, 300 J, and 360 J.[14] In the event that VT is present but the patient has no pulse (and therefore no blood pressure), asynchronous defibrillation should be performed, starting with 200 J and increasing to 300 and 360 J.[14]

Clinical Presentation and Diagnosis of VT

Symptoms

- As with other tachyarrhythmias, symptoms associated with VT are dependent primarily on heart rate and include palpitations, dizziness, light-headedness, shortness of breath, chest pain (if underlying CAD is present), near-syncope, and syncope

- Patients with nonsustained VT may be asymptomatic if the duration of the arrhythmia is sufficiently short. However, if the rate is sufficiently rapid, patients with nonsustained VT may experience symptoms

- Patients with sustained VT are usually symptomatic, provided that the rate is fast enough to provoke symptoms. Patients with rapid sustained VT may be hemodynamically unstable

- In some patients, sustained VT results in the absence of a pulse or may deteriorate to ventricular fibrillation, resulting in the syndrome of sudden cardiac death

Diagnosis

- Diagnosis of VT requires ECG confirmation of the arrhythmia
- VT is characterized by wide, misshapen QRS complexes, with the rate varying from 140 to 280 bpm
- In the majority of patients with VT, the shape and appearance of the QRS complexes are consistent and similar, and referred to as monomorphic VT. However, some patients experience polymorphic VT, in which the shape and appearance of the QRS complexes vary

---

Table 9–13

Etiologies of VT and VF

Coronary artery disease
Myocardial infarction
Heart failure
Electrolyte abnormalities: hypokalemia and hypomagnesemia
Drugs:

Adenosine	Propafenone
Amiodarone	Sotalol
Chlorpromazine	Terbutaline
Digoxin	Theophylline
Disopyramide	Thioridazine
Flecainide	Trazodone
Ibutilide	Tricyclic antidepressants
Procainamide	Venlafaxine

VF, ventricular fibrillation; VT, ventricular tachycardia.

Drugs used for the termination of hemodynamically stable VT are presented in Table 9–14. IV drug administration is required. A decision algorithm for management of hemodynamically stable VT is presented in Figure 9–10. The initial choice of drug is dependent on whether the patient's VT is occurring in the setting of acute myocardial ischemia or infarction; if this is the case, the initial drug of choice is lidocaine, followed by procainamide and amiodarone.[45] However, if the patient's VT is not associated with myocardial ischemia or infarction, there is evidence that procainamide may be more effective for termination of VT;[46] therefore, procainamide is the drug of choice in this situation.[45]

Nonpharmacologic Therapy: Prevention of Sudden Cardiac Death ❽ *In patients who have experienced VT and are at risk for sudden cardiac death, implantation of an implantable cardioverter-defibrillator (ICD) is the treatment of choice.*[47] An ICD is a device that provides internal electrical cardioversion of VT or defibrillation of VF; the ICD does not prevent the patient from developing the arrhythmia, but it reduces the risk that the patient will die of sudden cardiac death as a result of the arrhythmia. Whereas early versions of ICDs required a thoracotomy for implantation, these devices now may be implanted transvenously, similarly to pacemakers, markedly reducing the incidence of complications.

ICDs have been found to be significantly more effective than antiarrhythmic agents such as amiodarone or sotalol for reducing the risk of sudden cardiac death[48,49]; therefore, ICDs are preferred therapy.[47] However, many patients with ICDs receive concurrent antiarrhythmic drug therapy to reduce the frequency with which patients experience the discomfort of shocks and to prolong battery life of the devices. Combined pharmacotherapy with amiodarone and a β-blocker is more effective than monotherapy with sotalol or β-blockers for reduction in the frequency of ICD shocks.[50]

▶ Outcome Evaluation

- Monitor patients for termination of VT and restoration of normal sinus rhythm.
- Monitor patients for adverse effects of antiarrhythmic drugs administered (Table 9–7).

Ventricular Fibrillation

VF is irregular, disorganized, chaotic electrical activity in the ventricles resulting in absence of ventricular depolarizations, and, consequently, lack of pulse, cardiac output, and blood pressure.

▶ Epidemiology and Etiology

Approximately 400,000 people die of sudden cardiac death annually in the United States. While some of these deaths

Table 9–14		
Drugs for Termination of VT		
Drug	**Loading Dose**	**Maintenance Dose**
Procainamide	12–17 mg/kg IV, no faster than 20 mg/min	1–4 mg/min continuous infusion
Lidocaine	0.5–0.75 mg/kg IV bolus Repeat every 5–10 minutes to a total of 3 mg/kg	1–4 mg/min continuous infusion
Amiodarone	150 mg IV over 10 minutes	1 mg/min continuous infusion for 6 hours, 0.5 mg/min for 18 hours

VT, ventricular tachycardia.

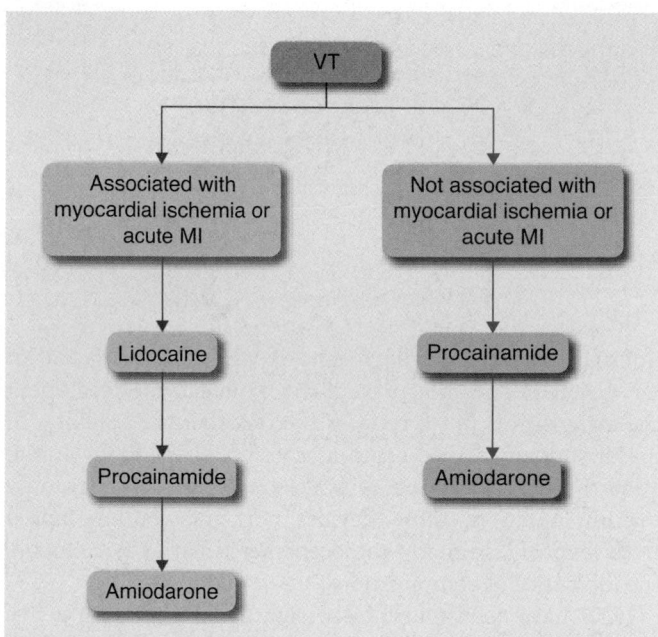

FIGURE 9–10. Decision algorithm for termination of hemodynamically stable ventricular tachycardia. (MI, myocardial infarction; VT, ventricular tachycardia.)

occur as a result of asystole, the majority occur as a result of VT that degenerates into VF or primary VF. Etiologies of VF are presented in Table 9–13 and are similar to those of VT.

► *Treatment*

Desired Outcomes The desired outcomes for treatment are to: (a) terminate VF, (b) achieve return of spontaneous circulation, and (c) achieve patient survival to hospital admission (in those with out-of-hospital cardiac arrest) and to hospital discharge.

Pharmacologic and Nonpharmacologic Therapy VF is by definition hemodynamically unstable, due to the absence of a pulse and blood pressure. Initial management includes provision of basic life support, including calling for help and initiation of cardiopulmonary resuscitation (CPR).[51] Oxygen should be administered as soon as it is available. Most importantly, defibrillation should be performed as soon as possible. It is critically important to understand that the only means of successfully terminating VF and restoring sinus rhythm is electrical defibrillation. Defibrillation should be

Clinical Presentation and Diagnosis of VF

Symptoms
- VF results in immediate loss of pulse and blood pressure. Patients who are in the standing position at the onset of VF suddenly and immediately collapse to the ground

Diagnosis
- The absence of a pulse does not guarantee VF, as the pulse may also be absent in patients with asystole, VT, or pulseless electrical activity
- Confirmation of the diagnosis with an ECG is necessary in order to determine appropriate treatment. ECG reveals no organized, recognizable QRS complexes. If treatment is not initiated within a few minutes, death will occur, or at best, resuscitation of the patient with permanent anoxic brain injury

attempted using 200 J, after which CPR should be resumed immediately while the defibrillator charges; if the first shock was unsuccessful, subsequent defibrillation shocks should be 360 J.[51]

If VF persists following one or two defibrillation shocks, drug therapy may be administered. ❾ *The purpose of drug administration for treatment of VF is to facilitate successful defibrillation. Drug therapy alone will not result in termination of VF.* Drugs that are used for facilitation of defibrillation in patients with VF are listed in Table 9–15. Drug administration should occur during CPR, before or after delivery of a defibrillation shock. The vasopressor agents epinephrine or vasopressin are administered initially because it has been shown that a critical factor in successful defibrillation is maintenance of coronary perfusion pressure, which is achieved via the vasoconstricting effects of these drugs. A decision algorithm for the treatment of VF is presented in Figure 9–11. Epinephrine and vasopressin are equally effective for facilitation of defibrillation leading to survival to hospital admission in patients with out-of-hospital cardiac arrest due to VF. Amiodarone is more effective than lidocaine for facilitation of defibrillation leading to survival to hospital admission in patients with VF,[52] which is the reason that amiodarone administration is recommended earlier than lidocaine administration in the decision algorithm.[51] Note

Table 9–15

Drugs for Facilitation of Defibrillation in Patients with VF

Drug	Dose
Epinephrine	1 mg IV every 3–5 minutes
Vasopressin	40 units IV single dose
Amiodarone	300 mg IV diluted in 20–30 mL D₅W. One subsequent dose of 150 mg IV may be administered
Lidocaine	1–1.5 mg/kg IV bolus. Follow with additional IV boluses of 0.5–0.75 mg/kg up to total of 3 mg/kg

D₅W, 5% dextrose in water; VF, ventricular fibrillation.

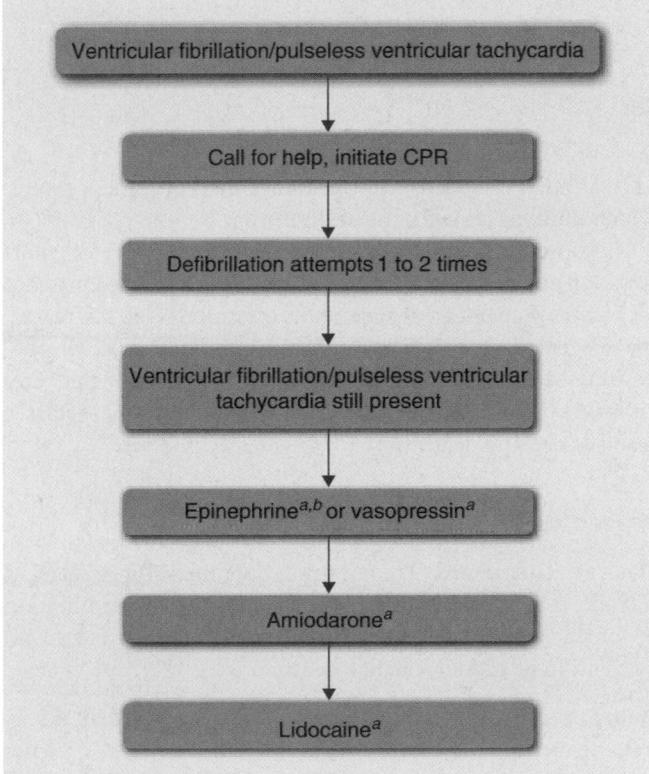

FIGURE 9–11. Decision algorithm for resuscitation of VF or pulseless ventricular tachycardia. (CPR, cardiopulmonary resuscitation.) ᵃDefibrillation attempt should be made after every dose of drug. ᵇEpinephrine should continue to be administered every 3 to 5 minutes throughout the remainder of the resuscitation.

that the amiodarone doses recommended for administration during a resuscitation attempt for VF (Table 9–15) are different than those recommended for administration for termination of VT (Table 9–14).

▶ Outcome Evaluation

- Monitor the patient for return of pulse and blood pressure, and for termination of VF and restoration of normal sinus rhythm.

- After successful resuscitation, monitor the patient for adverse effects of drugs administered (Table 9–7).

Torsades de Pointes

Torsades de pointes is a specific polymorphic VT that is associated with prolongation of the QT interval in the sinus beats that precede the arrhythmia.[13]

▶ Epidemiology and Etiology

The incidence of torsades de pointes in the population at large is unknown. The incidence of torsades de pointes associated with specific drugs ranges from less than 1% to as high as 8% to 10%, depending on dose and plasma concentration of the drug and the presence of other risk factors for the arrhythmia.

Torsades de pointes may be inherited or acquired. Patients with specific genetic mutations may have an inherited long QT syndrome, in which the QT interval is prolonged, and these patients are at risk for torsades de pointes. Acquired torsades de pointes may be caused by numerous drugs (Table 9–16); the list of drugs that are known to cause torsades de pointes continues to expand.

▶ Pathophysiology

Torsades de pointes is caused by circumstances, often drugs, that lead to prolongation in the repolarization phase of the ventricular action potential (Fig. 9–2) manifested on the ECG by prolongation of the QT interval. Prolongation of ventricular repolarization occurs via inhibition of efflux of potassium through potassium channels; therefore, drugs that inhibit conductance through potassium channels may cause QT interval prolongation and torsades de pointes.

Table 9–16

Drugs That Have Been Reported to Cause Torsades de Pointes

Amiodarone	Indapamide
Amitriptyline	Levofloxacin
Arsenic	Levomethadyl
Bepridil	Methadone
Chloroquine	Metoclopramide
Chlorpromazine	Pentamidine
Ciprofloxacin	Pimozide
Clarithromycin	Procainamide
Disopyramide	Propafenone
Dofetilide	Quinidine
Doxepin	Risperidone
Droperidol	Sertraline
Erythromycin	Sotalol
Famotidine	Tacrolimus
Flecainide	Thioridazine
Fluconazole	Trazodone
Fluoxetine	Trimethoprim-sulfamethoxazole
Haloperidol	Voriconazole
Ibutilide	

From Ref. 13.

Clinical Presentation and Diagnosis of Torsades de Pointes

Symptoms

- As with other tachyarrhythmias, symptoms associated with torsades de pointes are dependent primarily on heart rate and arrhythmia duration, and include palpitations, dizziness, light-headedness, shortness of breath, chest pain (if underlying CAD is present), near-syncope, and syncope
- Torsades de pointes may be hemodynamically unstable if the rate is sufficiently rapid
- Like sustained monomorphic VT, torsades de pointes may result in the absence of a pulse, or may rapidly degenerate into VF, resulting in the syndrome of sudden cardiac death

Diagnosis

- Diagnosis of torsades de pointes requires examination of the arrhythmia on ECG

- Torsades de pointes, or "twisting of the points," appears on ECG as apparent twisting of the wide QRS complexes around the isoelectric baseline
- The arrhythmia is associated with heart rates from 140 to 280 bpm
- Characteristic feature: a "long-short" initiating sequence that occurs as a result of a ventricular premature beat followed by a compensatory pause which is followed by the first beat of the torsades de pointes
- Episodes of torsades de pointes may self-terminate, with frequent recurrence

❶ *Prolongation of ventricular repolarization likely promotes the development of early ventricular afterdepolarizations during the relative refractory period, which may provoke re-entry leading to torsades de pointes.*

❿ *Drug-induced torsades de pointes rarely occurs in patients without specific risk factors for the arrhythmia (Table 9–17).* In most cases, administration of a drug known to cause torsades de pointes is unlikely to cause the arrhythmia; however, the likelihood of the arrhythmia increases markedly in patients with concomitant risk factors.

The onset of torsades de pointes associated with oral drug therapy is somewhat variable and in some cases may be delayed; often, a patient can be taking a drug known to cause torsades de pointes for months or longer without problem

until another risk factor for the arrhythmia becomes present, which then may trigger the arrhythmia.

In some patients, torsades de pointes may be of short duration and may terminate spontaneously. However, torsades de pointes may not terminate on its own, and if left untreated, may degenerate into VF and result in sudden cardiac death.[13] Several drugs, including terfenadine, astemizole, and cisapride, have been withdrawn from the U.S. market as a result of causing deaths due to torsades de pointes.

▶ Treatment

Desired Outcomes The desired outcomes for treatment include: (a) prevention of torsades de pointes, (b) termination of torsades de pointes, (c) prevention of recurrence, and (d) prevention of sudden cardiac death.

Pharmacologic and Nonpharmacologic Therapy ❿ *In patients with risk factors for torsades de pointes, drugs with the potential to cause QT interval prolongation and torsades de pointes should be avoided or used with extreme caution, and diligent QT interval monitoring should be performed.*

Management of drug-induced torsades de pointes includes discontinuation of the potentially causative agent. Patients with hemodynamically unstable torsades de pointes should undergo immediate synchronized DCC. In patients with hemodynamically stable torsades de pointes, electrolyte abnormalities such as hypokalemia and hypomagnesemia should be corrected. Hemodynamically stable torsades de pointes is often treated with IV magnesium, irrespective of whether the patient is hypomagnesemic; magnesium has been shown to terminate torsades de pointes in normomagnesemic patients. Magnesium may be administered IV in doses of 1 to 2 g, diluted in 50 to 100 mL 5% dextrose in water (D_5W), administered over 5 to 10 minutes; doses may be repeated to a total of 12 g.

Table 9–17

Risk Factors for Drug-Induced Torsades de Pointes

QTc interval greater than 500 milliseconds
Increase in QTc interval by more than 60 milliseconds compared with the pretreatment value
Female sex
Age greater than 65 years
Heart failure
Electrolyte abnormalities: hypokalemia and hypomagnesemia
Bradycardia
Elevated plasma concentrations of QT interval-prolonging drugs due to drug interactions or absence of dose adjustment for organ dysfunction
Rapid IV infusion of torsades-inducing drugs
Concomitant administration of more than one agent known to cause QT interval prolongation/torsades de pointes
Possible genetic predisposition
Previous history of drug-induced torsades de pointes

QTc, corrected QT interval.

From Ref. 13.

Alternatively, a continuous magnesium infusion may be initiated after the first bolus, at a rate of 0.5 to 1 g/h. Alternative treatments include: transvenous insertion of a temporary pacemaker for overdrive pacing, which shortens the QT interval and may terminate torsades de pointes and reduce the risk of recurrence; IV isoproterenol 2 to 10 mcg/min, to increase the heart rate and shorten the QT interval; IV lidocaine, which may shorten the duration of ventricular repolarization; or IV phenytoin, which may also shorten the duration of ventricular repolarization, administered at a dose of 10 to 15 mg/kg infused at a rate of 25 to 50 mg/min.

▶ *Outcome Evaluation*

- Monitor vital signs (heart rate and blood pressure).
- Monitor the ECG to determine the QTc interval (maintain less than 450 milliseconds) and for the presence of torsades de pointes.
- Monitor serum potassium and magnesium concentrations.
- Monitor for symptoms of tachycardia.

Abbreviations Introduced in This Chapter

AF	Atrial fibrillation
ATPase	Adenosine triphosphatase
AV	Atrioventricular
Ca	Calcium
CAD	Coronary artery disease
CAST	Cardiac Arrhythmia Suppression Trial
CCB	Calcium channel blocker
CPR	Cardiopulmonary resuscitation
DCC	Direct current cardioversion
D_5W	5% Dextrose in water
ED	Emergency department
HF	Heart failure
ICD	Implantable cardioverter-defibrillator
INR	International Normalized Ratio
J	Joules
K	Potassium
LV	Left ventricular
LVEF	Left ventricular ejection fraction
LVH	Left ventricular hypertrophy
MI	Myocardial infarction
Na	Sodium
NYHA	New York Heart Association
PSVT	Paroxysmal supraventricular tachycardia
PTT	Partial thromboplastin time
PVC	Premature ventricular contraction
QTc	Corrected QT interval
RR	RR interval
SA	Sinoatrial
TEE	Transesophageal echocardiogram
TIA	Transient ischemic attack
VPB	Ventricular premature beat
VPC	Ventricular premature contraction
VPD	Ventricular premature depolarization
VF	Ventricular fibrillation
VT	Ventricular tachycardia

Patient Care and Monitoring

1. Perform a thorough medication history to determine whether the patient is receiving any prescription or nonprescription drugs that may cause or contribute to the development of an arrhythmia.

2. Evaluate the patient for the presence of drug-induced diseases, drug allergies, and drug interactions.

3. Determine and monitor the patient's serum electrolyte concentrations to determine the presence or absence of hypokalemia, hyperkalemia, hypomagnesemia, or hypermagnesemia.

4. Consider the patient's heart rate, blood pressure, and symptoms to determine whether he or she is hemodynamically stable or unstable.

5. Monitor the patient's 12-lead ECG or single rhythm strips to determine if an arrhythmia is present and to identify the specific arrhythmia, and evaluate and monitor the patient's symptoms.

6. Develop drug therapy treatment plans for management of the specific arrhythmia that the patient is experiencing: sinus bradycardia, AV nodal blockade, AF, PSVT, VPDs, VT (including torsades de pointes), or VF.

7. Develop specific drug therapy monitoring plans for the treatment plan implemented. Monitoring includes assessment of symptoms, ECG, adverse effects of drugs, and potential drug interactions.

8. In those receiving warfarin for AF, determine whether the patient's INR is therapeutic.

9. Provide information regarding safe and effective warfarin therapy:
   - Notify appropriate clinicians in the event of severe bruising, blood in urine or stool, or frequent nosebleeds.
   - Avoid radical changes in diet.
   - Avoid alcohol.
   - Do not take nonprescription medications or herbal/alternative/complementary medicines without notifying your physician, pharmacist, and/or health care team members.

10. Stress the importance of adherence to the therapeutic regimen.

11. Provide patient education regarding disease state and drug therapy.

Self-assessment questions and answers are available at *http://www.mhpharmacotherapy.com/pp.html.*

REFERENCES

1. Cummins RO, ed. ACLS Provider Manual. Dallas: American Heart Association, 2006.
2. Paulev PE. Textbook in Medical Physiology and Pathophysiology. Essentials and Clinical Problems. Copenhagen: Copenhagen Medical Publishers, 2000, *http://www.mfi.ku.dk/ppaulev/chapter11/Chapter%2011.htm.*
3. Bazett HC. An analysis of time relationships of the electrocardiogram. Heart 1920;7:353–370.
4. Fogoros RN. Electrophysiologic Testing, 4th ed. Malden, MA: Blackwell, 2006:17.
5. Vaughan Williams EM. Classification of anti-arrhythmic drugs. In: Sandoe E, Flensted-Jansen E, Olesen KH, eds. Symposium on Cardiac Arrhythmias. Sodertalje, Sweden: AB Astra, 1970:449–472.
6. Singh BN, Vaughan Williams EM. A third class of anti-arrhythmic action. Effects on atrial and ventricular intracellular potentials, and other pharmacological actions on cardiac muscle, of MJ 1999 and AH 3474. Br J Pharmacol 1970;39:675–687.
7. Singh BN, Vaughan Williams EM. A fourth class of anti-arrhythmic action? Effect of verapamil on ouabain toxicity, on atrial and ventricular intracellular potentials, and on other features of cardiac function. Cardiovasc Res 1972;6:109–119.
8. Snyders J, Knoth KM, Roberds SL, Tamkun MM. Time-, voltage-, and state-dependent block by quinidine of a cloned human cardiac potassium channel. Mol Pharmacol 1992;41:322–330.
9. Coraboeuf E, Deroubaix E, Escande D, Coulombe A. Comparative effects of three class I antiarrhythmic drugs on plateau and pacemaker currents of sheep cardiac Purkinje fibres. Cardiovasc Res 1988;22:375–384.
10. Komeichi K, Tohse N, Nakaya H, et al. Effects of N-acetylprocainamide and sotalol on ion currents in isolated guinea-pig ventricular myocytes. Eur J Pharmacol 1990;187:313–322.
11. Task Force of the Working Group on Arrhythmias of the European Society of Cardiology. The Sicilian gambit. A new approach to the classification of antiarrhythmic drugs based on their actions on arrhythmogenic mechanisms. Circulation 1991;84:1831–1851.
12. Mangrum JM, DiMarco JP. The evaluation and management of bradycardia. N Engl J Med 2000;342: 703–709.
13. Tisdale JE. Arrhythmias. In: Tisdale JE, Miller DM. Drug-Induced Diseases. Prevention, Detection, and Management. Bethesda, MD: American Society of Health-Systems Pharmacists, 2005:289–327.
14. 2005 American Heart Association Guidelines for Cardiopulmonary Resuscitation and Emergency Cardiac Care, Part 7.3. Management of symptomatic bradycardia and tachycardia. Circulation 2005;112:Iv-67–Iv-77.
15. Kaushik V, Leon AR, Forrester JS, Trohman RG. Bradyarrhythmias, temporary and permanent pacing. Crit Care Med 2000;28(Suppl):N121–N128.
16. Kannel WB, Wolf PA, Benjamin EJ, Levy D. Prevalence, incidence, prognosis, and predisposing conditions for atrial fibrillation: Population-based estimates. Am J Cardiol 1998;82:2N–9N.
17. Torp-Pedersen C, Moller M, Bloch-Thomsen PE, et al., for the Danish Investigations of Arrhythmia and Mortality on Dofetilide Study Group. Dofetilide in patients with congestive heart failure and left ventricular dysfunction. Danish Investigations of Arrhythmia and Mortality on Dofetilide Study Group. N Engl J Med 1999;341: 857–865.
18. Maisel WH, Stevenson LW. Atrial fibrillation heart failure: Epidemiology, pathophysiology, and rationale for therapy. Am J Cardiol 2003;91:2D–8D.
19. Rich EC, Siebold C, Campion B. Alcohol-related acute atrial fibrillation. A case-control study and review of 40 patients. Arch Intern Med 1985;145:830–833.
20. Black DM, Delmas PD, Eastell R, et al. Once-yearly zoledronic acid for treatment of postmenopausal osteoporosis. N Engl J Med 2007;356:1809–1822.
21. Heckbert SR, Li G, Cummings SR, et al. Use of alendronate and risk of incident atrial fibrillation in women. Arch Intern Med 2008;168: 826–831.
22. Haissaguerre M, Jais P, Shah DC, et al. Spontaneous initiation of atrial fibrillation by ectopic beats originating in the pulmonary veins. N Engl J Med 1998;339(10): 659–666.
23. Cohen M, Naccarelli GV. Pathophysiology and disease progression of atrial fibrillation: Importance of achieving and maintaining sinus rhythm. J Cardiovasc Electrophysiol 2008;19:885–890.
24. Wijffels MC, Kirchhof CJ, Dorland R, Allessie MA. Atrial fibrillation begets atrial fibrillation. A study in awake chronically instrumented goats. Circulation 1995;92:1954–1968.
25. Fuster V, Rydén LE, Cannom DS, et al. ACC/AHA/ESC 2006 guidelines for the management of patients with atrial fibrillation—Executive summary: A report of the American College of Cardiology/American Heart Association Task Force on Practice Guidelines and the European Society of Cardiology Committee for Practice Guidelines (Writing Committee to Revise the 2001 Guidelines for the Management of Patients With Atrial Fibrillation). Circulation 2006;114:700–752.
26. Krahn AD, Manfreda J, Tate RB, et al. The natural history of atrial fibrillation: Incidence, risk factors, and prognosis in the Manitoba Follow-Up Study. Am J Med 1995;98:476–484.
27. Elkayam U, Shotan A, Mehra A, Ostrzega E. Calcium channel blockers in heart failure. J Am Coll Cardiol 1993;22(4 Suppl A):139A–144A.
28. Singer DE, Albers GW, Dalen JE, et al. Antithrombotic therapy in atrial fibrillation: American College of Chest Physicians Evidence-Based Practice Guidelines (8th ed). Chest 2008;133:546–592.
29. The Atrial Fibrillation Follow-up Investigation of Rhythm Management (AFFIRM) Investigators. A comparison of rate control and rhythm control in patients with atrial fibrillation. N Engl J Med 2002;347: 1825–1833.
30. Van Gelder IC, Hagens VE, Bosker HA, et al., for the Rate Control versus Electrical Cardioversion for Persistent Atrial Fibrillation Study Group. A comparison of rate control and rhythm control in patients with recurrent persistent atrial fibrillation. N Engl J Med 2002;347: 1834–1840.
31. Carlsson J, Miketic S, Windeler J, et al. Randomized trial of rate-control versus rhythm-control in persistent atrial fibrillation: The Strategies of Treatment of Atrial Fibrillation (STAF) study. J Am Coll Cardiol 2003;41:1690–1696.
32. Opolski G, Torbicki A, Kosior D, et al. Rhythm control versus rate control in patients with persistent atrial fibrillation. Results of the HOT CAFE Polish Study. Kardiol Pol 2003;59:1–16.
33. Gage BF, Waterman AD, Shannon W, Boechler M, Rich MW, Radford MJ. Validation of clinical classification schemes for predicting stroke: Results from the National Registry of Atrial Fibrillation. JAMA 2001;285:2864–2870.
34. Ganz LI, Friedman PL. Supraventricular tachycardia. N Engl J Med 1995;332:162–173.
35. Blomstrom-Lundqvist C, Scheinman MM, Aliot EM, et al., for the Writing Committee to Develop Guidelines for the Management of Patients with Supraventricular Arrhythmias. ACC/AHA/ESC guidelines for the management of patients with supraventricular arrhythmias—Executive summary: A report of the American College of Cardiology/American Heart Association Task Force on practice guidelines and the European Society of Cardiology Committee for Practice Guidelines (Writing Committee to Develop Guidelines for the Management of Patients with Supraventricular Arrhythmias). J Am Coll Cardiol 2003;42:1493–1531.
36. Bikkina M, Larson MG, Levy D. Prognostic implications of asymptomatic ventricular arrhythmias: The Framingham Heart Study. Am J Cardiol 1994;74:232–235.

37. Lown B, Wolf M. Approaches to sudden death from coronary heart disease. Circulation 1971;44:130–144.

38. Ruberman W, Weinblatt E, Goldberg JD, et al. Ventricular premature beats and mortality after myocardial infarction. N Engl J Med 1977;297:750–757.

39. Echt DS, Liebson PR, Mitchell LB, et al. Mortality and morbidity in patients receiving encainide, flecainide, or placebo. The Cardiac Arrhythmia Suppression Trial. N Engl J Med 1991;324:781–788.

40. The Cardiac Arrhythmia Suppression Trial II Investigators. Effect of the antiarrhythmic agent moricizine on survival after myocardial infarction. N Engl J Med 1992;327:227–233.

41. Teo KK, Yusuf S, Furberg CD. Effects of prophylactic antiarrhythmic drug therapy in acute myocardial infarction. An overview of results from randomized controlled trials. JAMA 1993;270:1589–1595.

42. Chandraratna PA. Comparison of acebutolol with propranolol, quinidine, and placebo: Results of three multicenter arrhythmia trials. Am Heart J 1985;109: 1198–1204.

43. Al-Khatib SM, Stebbins AL, Califf RM, et al. Sustained ventricular arrhythmias and mortality among patients with acute myocardial infarction: Results from the GUSTO-III trial. Am Heart J 2003;145:515–521.

44. Stevenson WG, Ellison KE, Sweeney MO, et al. Management of arrhythmias in heart failure. Cardiol Rev 2002;10:8–14.

45. Zipes DP, Camm AJ, Borggrefe M, et al. ACC/AHA/ESC 2006 Guidelines for management of patients with ventricular arrhythmias and the prevention of sudden cardiac death: A report of the American College of Cardiology/American Heart Association Task Force and the European Society of Cardiology Committee for Practice Guidelines (Writing Committee to Develop Guidelines for Management of Patients With Ventricular Arrhythmias and the Prevention of Sudden Cardiac Death): Developed in collaboration with the European Heart Rhythm Association and the Heart Rhythm Society. Circulation 2006;114:e385–e484.

46. Gorgels AP, van den Dool A, Hofs A, et al. Comparison of procainamide and lidocaine in terminating sustained monomorphic ventricular tachycardia. Am J Cardiol 1996;78:43–46.

47. Epstein AE, DiMarco JP, Ellenbogen KA, et al. ACC/AHA/HRS 2008 Guidelines for Device-Based Therapy of Cardiac Rhythm Abnormalities: Executive summary: A report of the American College of Cardiology/American Heart Association Task Force on Practice Guidelines (Writing Committee to Revise the ACC/AHA/NASPE 2002 Guideline Update for Implantation of Cardiac Pacemakers and Antiarrhythmia Devices). Circulation 2008;117:2820–2840.

48. The Antiarrhythmics versus Implantable Defibrillators (AVID) Investigators. A comparison of antiarrhythmic-drug therapy with implantable defibrillators in patients resuscitated from near-fatal ventricular arrhythmias. N Engl J Med 1997;337:1576–1583.

49. Connolly SJ, Gent M, Roberts RS, et al. Canadian implantable defibrillator study (CIDS): A randomized trial of the implantable cardioverter defibrillator against amiodarone. Circulation 2000;101:1297–1302.

50. Connolly SJ, Dorian P, Roberts RS, et al. Comparison of β-blockers, amiodarone plus ß-blockers, or sotalol for prevention of shocks from implantable cardioverter-defibrillators. The OPTIC study: A randomized trial. JAMA 2006;295:165–171.

51. 2005 American Heart Association Guidelines for Cardiopulmonary Resuscitation and Emergency Cardiac Care, Part 7.2. Management of cardiac arrest. Circulation 2005;112:IV-57–IV-66.

52. Dorian P, Cass D, Schwartz B, et al. Amiodarone as compared with lidocaine for shock-resistant ventricular fibrillation. N Engl J Med 2002;346:884–890.

10 Venous Thromboembolism

Edith A. Nutescu and Stuart T. Haines

LEARNING OBJECTIVES

● **Upon completion of the chapter, the reader will be able to:**

1. Identify risk factors and signs and symptoms of deep vein thrombosis (DVT) and pulmonary embolism (PE).

2. Describe the processes of hemostasis and thrombosis, including the role of the vascular endothelium, platelets, coagulation cascade, and thrombolytic proteins.

3. Determine a patient's relative risk (low, moderate, or high) of developing venous thrombosis.

4. Formulate an appropriate prevention strategy for a patient at risk for DVT.

5. State at least two potential advantages of the low–molecular weight heparins (LMWHs) and fondaparinux over unfractionated heparin (UFH).

6. Select and interpret laboratory test(s) to monitor antithrombotic drugs.

7. Identify factors that place a patient at high-risk of bleeding while receiving antithrombotic drugs.

8. Identify warfarin drug–drug and drug–food interactions.

9. Manage a patient with an elevated International Normalized Ratio (INR) with or without bleeding.

10. Formulate an appropriate treatment plan for a patient who develops a DVT or PE, and develop a comprehensive education plan for a patient who is receiving an antithrombotic drug.

KEY CONCEPTS

❶ Antithrombotic therapies require meticulous and systematic monitoring, as well as ongoing patient education. Well-organized anticoagulation management services improve the quality of patient care and reduce the overall cost.

❷ The risk of venous thromboembolism (VTE) is related to several identifiable factors including age, prior history of VTE, major surgery (particularly orthopedic procedures of the lower extremities), trauma, malignancy, pregnancy, estrogen use, and hypercoagulable states. These risks are additive.

❸ The diagnosis of VTE must be confirmed by objective testing.

❹ At the time of hospital admission, all patients should be evaluated for their risk of VTE, and strategies to prevent VTE appropriate for each patient's level of risk should be routinely employed. Prophylaxis should be continued throughout the period of risk.

❺ In the absence of contraindications, the treatment of VTE should initially include a rapid-acting anticoagulant (e.g., unfractional heparin [UFH], low-molecular

weight heparin [LMWH], or fondaparinux) overlapped with warfarin for at least 5 days and until the patient's International Normalized Ratio (INR) is greater than 2 and stable. Anticoagulation therapy should be continued for a minimum of 3 months. However, the duration of anticoagulation therapy should be based on the patient's risk of VTE recurrence and major bleeding.

❻ Bleeding is the most common adverse effect associated with antithrombotic drugs. A patient's risk of major hemorrhage is related to the intensity and stability of therapy, age, concurrent drug use, history of gastrointestinal bleeding, risk of falls or trauma, and recent surgery.

❼ Most patients with an uncomplicated deep vein thrombosis (DVT) can be managed safely at home.

❽ Warfarin is prone to numerous clinically important drug–drug and drug–food interactions.

INTRODUCTION

Venous thromboembolism (VTE) is one of the most common cardiovascular disorders in the United States. VTE is manifested as deep vein thrombosis (DVT) and pulmonary embolism (PE) resulting from thrombus formation in the

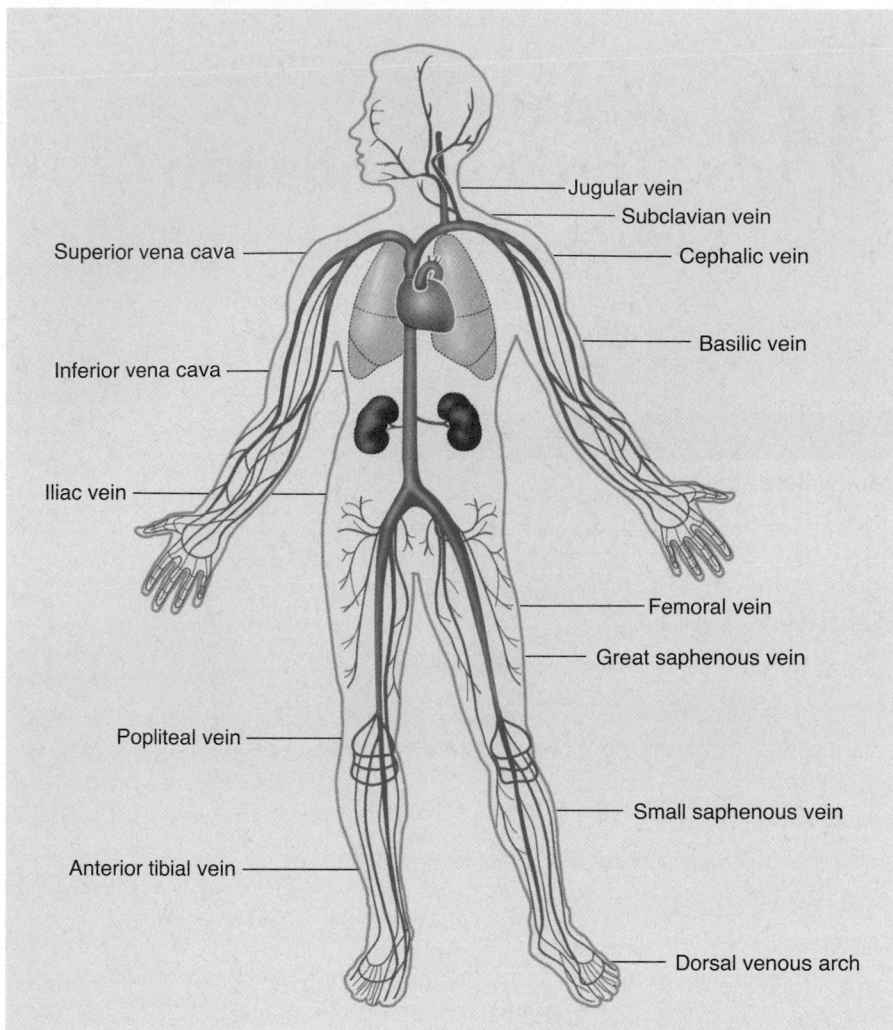

FIGURE 10–1. Venous circulation. (From Haines ST, Witt DM, Nutescu EA. Venous thromboembolism. In: DiPiro JT, Talbert RL, Yee GC, et al., eds. Pharmacotherapy: A Pathophysiologic Approach, 7th ed. New York: McGraw-Hill; 2008:332.)

Labels in figure:
- Jugular vein
- Subclavian vein
- Superior vena cava
- Cephalic vein
- Basilic vein
- Inferior vena cava
- Iliac vein
- Femoral vein
- Great saphenous vein
- Popliteal vein
- Small saphenous vein
- Anterior tibial vein
- Dorsal venous arch

venous circulation (**Fig. 10–1**).[1] It is often provoked by prolonged immobility and vascular injury and is most frequently seen in patients who have been hospitalized for a serious medical illness, trauma, or major surgery. VTE can also occur with little or no provocation in patients who have an underlying hypercoagulable disorder.

While VTE may initially cause few or no symptoms, the first overt manifestation of the disease may be sudden death.[2] Death from PE can occur within minutes, before effective treatment can be given. In addition to the symptoms produced by the acute event, the long-term sequelae of VTE such as the post-thrombotic syndrome (PTS; a complication of VTE occurring due to damage to the vein caused by a blood clot and that leads to development of symptomatic venous insufficiency such as chronic lower extremity swelling, pain, tenderness, skin discoloration, and ulceration) and recurrent thromboembolic events cause long-term pain and suffering.

The treatment of VTE is fraught with substantial risks.[3] ❶ *Antithrombotic drugs require precise dosing and meticulous monitoring, as well as ongoing patient education.[4,5] Well-organized anticoagulation management services improve the quality of patient care and reduce the overall cost.* A systematic approach to drug therapy management substantially reduces these risks, but bleeding remains a common and serious complication.[5] Therefore, preventing VTE is paramount to improving outcomes. When VTE is suspected, a rapid and accurate diagnosis is critical to making appropriate treatment decisions. The optimal use of antithrombotic drugs requires not only an in-depth knowledge of their pharmacology and pharmacokinetic properties, but also a comprehensive approach to patient management.[6]

EPIDEMIOLOGY AND ETIOLOGY

The true incidence of VTE in the general population is unknown because many patients, perhaps more than 50%, have no overt symptoms or go undiagnosed.[7] An estimated 2 million people in the United States develop VTE each year; 600,000 are hospitalized and 60,000 die. The estimated annual direct medical costs of managing the disease are well over $1 billion. The incidence of VTE nearly doubles in each decade of life over the age of 50 and is slightly higher in men. As the population ages, the total number of cases of DVT and PE continues to rise.[2]

❷ *The risk of VTE is related to several factors including age, prior history of VTE, major surgery (particularly orthopedic procedures of the lower extremities), trauma, malignancy, pregnancy, estrogen use, and hypercoagulable states*

Table 10–1

Risk Factors for VTE

Risk Factor	Example
Age	Risk doubles with each decade after age 50
Prior history of VTE	Strongest known risk factor for DVT and PE
Venous stasis	Major medical illness (e.g., congestive heart failure)
	Major surgery (e.g., general anesthesia for greater than 30 minutes)
	Paralysis (e.g., due to stroke or spinal cord injury)
	Polycythemia vera
	Obesity
	Varicose veins
Vascular injury	Major orthopedic surgery (e.g., knee and hip replacement)
	Trauma (especially fractures of the pelvis, hip, or leg)
	Indwelling venous catheters
Hypercoagulable states	Malignancy, diagnosed or occult
	Activated protein C resistance/factor V Leiden
	Prothrombin (20210A) gene mutation
	Protein C deficiency
	Protein S deficiency
	AT deficiency
	Factor VIII excess (greater than 90th percentile)
	Factor XI excess (greater than 90th percentile)
	Antiphospholipid antibodies
	Dysfibrinogenemia
	PAI-I excess
	Pregnancy/postpartum
Drug therapy	Estrogen-containing oral contraceptive pills
	Estrogen replacement therapy
	SERMs
	HIT
	Chemotherapy

AT, antithrombin; DVT, deep vein thrombosis; HIT, heparin-induced thrombocytopenia; PAI-I, plasminogen activator inhibitor; PE, pulmonary embolism; SERMs, selective estrogen receptor modulators.

(Table 10–1).[2] *VTE risk factors can be categorized in one of the three elements of Virchow's triad: stasis in blood flow, vascular endothelial injury, and inherited or acquired changes in blood constituents that cause hypercoagulation states. These risk factors are additive and some can be easily identified in clinical practice.* A prior history of venous thrombosis is perhaps the strongest risk factor for recurrent VTE, presumably because of the destruction of venous valves and obstruction of blood flow caused by the initial event. Rapid blood flow has an inhibitory effect on thrombus formation, but a slow rate of flow reduces the clearance of activated clotting factors in the zone of injury and slows the influx of regulatory substances. Stasis tips the delicate balance of procoagulation and anticoagulation in favor of thrombogenesis. The rate of blood flow in the venous circulation, particularly in the deep veins of the lower extremities, is relatively slow. Valves in the deep veins of the legs, as well as contraction of the

calf and thigh muscles, facilitate the flow of blood back to the heart and lungs. Damage to the venous valves and periods of prolonged immobility result in venous stasis. Vessel obstruction, either from a thrombus or external compression, promotes clot propagation. Numerous medical conditions and surgical procedures are associated with reduced venous blood flow and increase the risk of VTE (Table 10–1). Greater than normal blood viscosity, seen in myeloproliferative disorders like polycythemia vera, for example, may also contribute to slowed blood flow and thrombus formation.

A growing list of hereditary deficiencies, gene mutations, and acquired diseases have been linked to hypercoagulability (Table 10–1).[8] Activated protein C resistance is the most common genetic disorder of hypercoagulability, found in nearly 5% of individuals of northern European descent and in as many as 40% of those who suffer an idiopathic DVT. Although these patients have normal plasma concentrations of protein C, they have a mutation on factor V that renders it resistant to degradation by activated protein C. This mutation is known as factor V Leiden, named after the city of Leiden, Holland, where the defect was initially reported. The prothrombin gene 20210A mutation is also a relatively common defect, occurring in as many as 3% of healthy individuals of southern European descent and 16% of those with an idiopathic DVT. Although less common, inherited deficiencies of the natural anticoagulants protein C, protein S, and antithrombin (AT) place patients at a high lifetime risk for VTE. Conversely, high concentrations of factors VIII, IX, and XI also increase the risk of VTE. Some patients have multiple genetic defects.

Acquired disorders of hypercoagulability include malignancy, antiphospholipid antibodies, estrogen use, and pregnancy.[2] The strong link between cancer and thrombosis has been recognized since the late 1800s.[9] Tumor cells secrete a number of procoagulant substances that activate the clotting cascade. Furthermore, patients with cancer often have suppressed levels of protein C, protein S, and AT. Antiphospholipid antibodies, commonly found in patients with autoimmune disorders such as systemic lupus erythematosus and inflammatory bowel disease, can cause venous and arterial thrombosis.[8] The antiphospholipid antibody syndrome is associated with repeated pregnancy loss. The precise mechanism by which these antibodies provoke thrombosis is unclear, but they activate the coagulation cascade and platelets, as well as inhibit the anticoagulant activity of proteins C and S. Estrogen-containing contraceptives, estrogen replacement therapy, and many of the selective estrogen receptor modulators (SERMs) increase the risk of venous thrombosis.[2,10,11] While the mechanisms are not clearly understood, estrogens increase serum clotting factor concentrations and induce activated protein C resistance. Increased serum estrogen concentrations may explain, in part, the increased risk of VTE during pregnancy and the postpartum period.[11]

PATHOPHYSIOLOGY

Hemostasis, the arrest of bleeding following vascular injury, is essential to life.[12] Within the vascular system, blood remains in a fluid state, transporting oxygen, nutrients, plasma proteins, and waste. When a vessel is injured, a dynamic interplay between thrombogenic (activating) and antithrombotic (inhibiting) forces result in the local formation of a hemostatic plug that seals the vessel wall and prevents further blood loss (Figs. 10–2, 10–3, and 10–4). A disruption of this delicate system of checks and balances may lead to inappropriate clot formation within the blood vessel that can obstruct blood flow or embolize to a distant vascular bed.

Under normal circumstances, the endothelial cells that line the inside of blood vessels maintain blood flow by producing a number of substances that inhibit platelet adherence, prevent the activation of the coagulation cascade, and facilitate fibrinolysis.[12] Vascular injury exposes the subendothelium (Fig. 10–3). Platelets readily adhere to the subendothelium, using glycoprotein (GP) Ib receptors found on their surfaces and facilitated by von Willebrand's factor (vWF). This causes platelets to become activated, releasing a number of procoagulant substances that stimulate circulating platelets to expose GP IIb–IIIa receptors and allow platelets to adhere to one another, resulting in platelet aggregation. The damaged vascular tissue releases tissue factor which activates the extrinsic pathway of the coagulation cascade (Fig. 10–4).

The clotting cascade is a stepwise series of enzymatic reactions that result in the formation of a fibrin mesh.[12] Clotting factors circulate in the blood in inactive forms. Once a precursor is activated by specific stimuli, it activates the next precursor in the sequence. The final steps in the cascade are the conversion of prothrombin to thrombin and fibrinogen to fibrin. Thrombin plays a key role in the coagulation cascade; it is responsible not only for the production of fibrin, but also for the conversion of factors V and VIII, creating a positive feedback loop that greatly accelerates the entire cascade. Thrombin also enhances platelet aggregation. Traditionally, the coagulation cascade has been divided into three distinct parts: the intrinsic, the extrinsic, and the common pathways (Fig. 10–4). This artificial division is misleading because there are numerous interactions between the three pathways.

A number of tempering mechanisms control coagulation (Fig. 10–2).[12] Without effective self-regulation, the coagulation cascade would proceed unabated until all the clotting factors and platelets are consumed. AT and heparin cofactor II (HCII) are circulating proteins that inhibit thrombin and factor Xa. The intact endothelium adjacent to the damaged tissue actively secretes several antithrombotic substances including heparan sulfate and thrombomodulin. Heparan sulfate exponentially accelerates AT and HCII activity. Protein C and its cofactor, protein S, are vitamin K-dependent anticoagulant proteins made in the liver. Activation of the clotting cascade activates protein C that, in turn, inhibits factor Va and VIIIa activity. Tissue factor pathway inhibitor (TFPI) inhibits the extrinsic coagulation pathway. When these self-regulatory mechanisms are intact, the formation of the fibrin clot is limited to the zone of tissue injury. However, disruptions in the system often result in inappropriate clot formation.

The fibrinolytic protein plasmin degrades the fibrin mesh into soluble end products collectively known as fibrin split products or fibrin degradation products.[13] The fibrinolytic system is also under the control of a series of stimulatory and inhibitory substances. Tissue plasminogen activator (t-PA) and urokinase plasminogen activator (u-PA) convert plasminogen to plasmin. Plasminogen activator inhibitor-1 (PAI-1) inhibits the plasminogen activators and α_2-antiplasmin inhibits plasmin activity. Aberrations in the fibrinolytic system have also been linked to hypercoagulability.

CLINICAL PRESENTATION AND DIAGNOSIS

Although a thrombus can form in any part of the venous circulation, the majority begin in the lower extremities. Once formed, a venous thrombus may behave in a combination of ways including: (a) remain asymptomatic, (b) spontaneously lyse, (c) obstruct the venous circulation, (d) propagate into more proximal veins, (e) embolize, and/or (f) slowly incorporate into the endothelial layer of the vessel.[14] The majority of patients with VTE never develop symptoms.[2] However, even those who initially experience no symptoms may suffer long-term consequences, such as

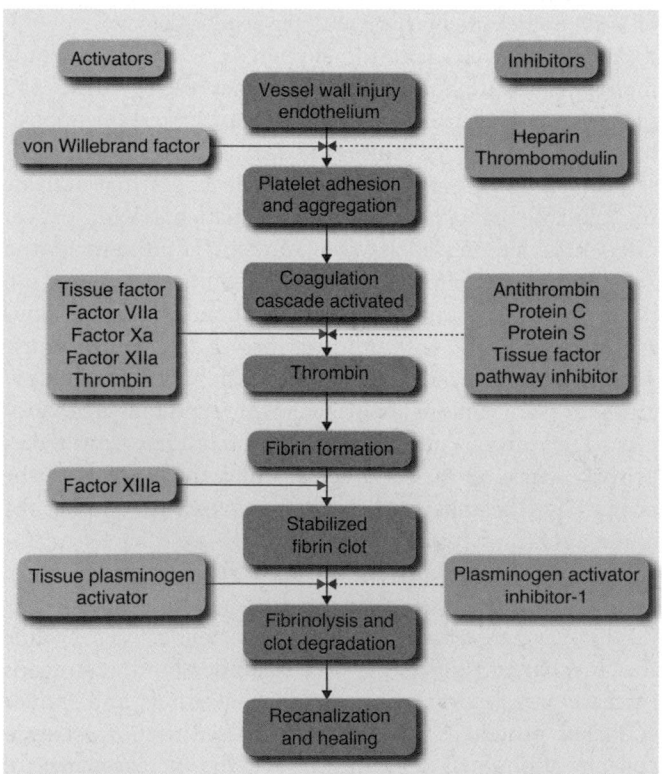

FIGURE 10–2. Hemostasis and thrombosis. (From Haines ST, Witt DM, Nutescu EA. Venous thromboembolism. In: DiPiro JT, Talbert RL, Yee GC, et al., eds. Pharmacotherapy: A Pathophysiologic Approach, 7th ed. New York: McGraw-Hill; 2008:334.)

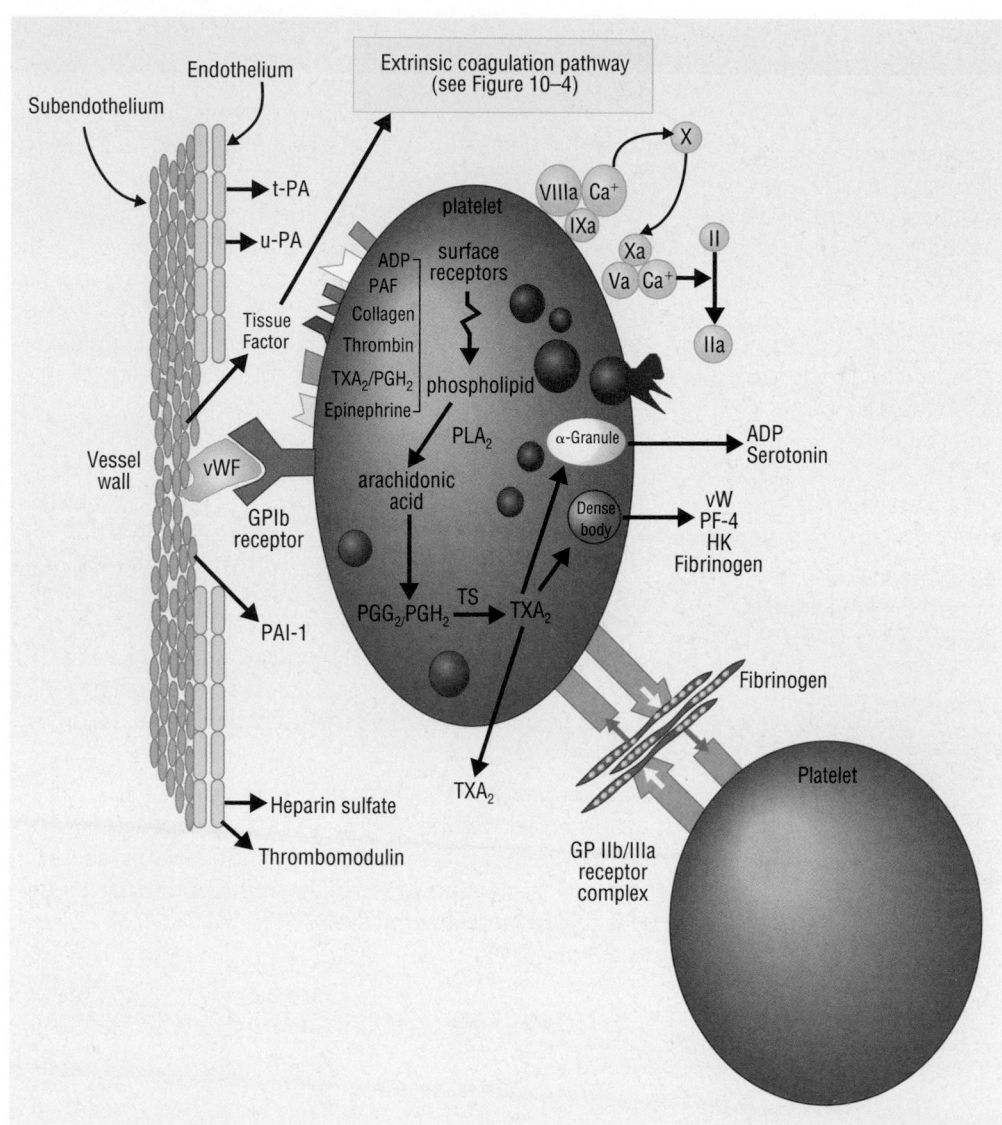

FIGURE 10–3. Vascular injury and thrombosis. (ADP, adenosine diphosphate; GP Ib, glycoprotein Ib; GP IIb/IIa, glycoprotein IIb/IIa; HK, high–molecular weight kininogen; PAF, platelet activating factor-1; PAI-1, plasminogen activator inhibitor; PF-4, platelet factor-4; PGG/PGH, prostaglandins; PLA, phospholipase A; TS, thromboxane synthetase; TXA_2, thromboxane A_2; t-PA, tissue plasminogen activator; u-PA, urokinase plasminogen activator; vWF, von Willebrand's factor.) (From Haines ST, Witt DM, Nutescu EA. Venous thromboembolism. In: DiPiro JT, Talbert RL, Yee GC, et al., eds. Pharmacotherapy: A Pathophysiologic Approach, 7th ed. New York: McGraw-Hill; 2008:335.)

PTS and recurrent VTE. ❸ *The symptoms of DVT or PE are nonspecific, and it is extremely difficult to distinguish VTE from other disorders on clinical signs alone.*[15] *Therefore, objective tests are required to confirm or exclude the diagnosis.* Patients with DVT frequently present with unilateral leg pain and swelling. Similarly, the PTS, a long-term complication of DVT caused by damage to the venous valves, produces chronic lower extremity swelling, pain, and tenderness that lead to skin discoloration and ulceration. The D-dimer test, a quantitative measure of fibrin breakdown in the serum, is a marker of acute thrombotic activity and may help to distinguish between an acute DVT and the PTS. Symptomatic PE usually produces shortness of breath, tachypnea, and tachycardia.[16] Hemoptysis occurs in less than one-third of patients. The physical exam may reveal diminished breath sounds, crackles, wheezes, or a pleural friction rub during auscultation of the lungs. Cardiovascular collapse, characterized by cyanosis, shock, and oliguria, is an ominous sign.

Given that VTE can be debilitating or fatal, it is important to treat it quickly and aggressively.[17] On the other hand, because major bleeding induced by antithrombotic drugs can be equally harmful, it is important to avoid treatment when the diagnosis is not reasonably certain. Assessment of the patient's status should focus on the search for risk factors in the patient's medical history (Table 10–1).[15,16] Venous thrombosis is uncommon in the absence of risk factors, and the effects of these risks are additive. Indeed, if a patient has multiple risk factors, VTE should be strongly suspected even when the symptoms are very subtle.

Because radiographic contrast studies are the most accurate and reliable methods for the diagnosis of VTE, they are considered the gold standards in clinical trials.[18,19] Contrast venography allows visualization of the entire venous system in the lower extremities and abdomen. Pulmonary angiography allows the visualization of the pulmonary arteries. The diagnosis of VTE can be made if there is a persistent intraluminal filling defect observed on multiple x-ray films.

Clinical Presentation and Diagnosis of DVT

General

VTE most commonly develops in patients with identifiable risk factors (Table 10–1) during or following a hospitalization. Many, perhaps the majority of patients, have asymptomatic disease. Patients may die suddenly of PE.

Symptoms

- The patient may complain of leg swelling, pain, warmth, skin discoloration. Symptoms are nonspecific and objective testing must be performed to establish the diagnosis.

Signs

- The patient's superficial veins may be dilated and a "palpable cord" may be felt in the affected leg.

- The patient may experience unilateral leg edema with measurable difference in leg circumference, erythema, increase in warmth, tenderness with palpation of calf muscles.

- The patient may experience pain in back of the knee in the affected leg when the examiner dorsiflexes the foot while the knee is slightly bent (Homan's sign).

NOTE: The physical exam signs can be unreliable. Homan's sign (an increased resistance to foot dorsiflexion without pain or discomfort as criteria for the positive test) can also be unreliable.

Laboratory Tests

- The initial lab evaluation should include CBC with differential, coagulation studies, serum chemistries with renal and liver function, and urinalysis.

- Serum concentrations of D-dimer, a by-product of thrombin generation, will be elevated in an acute event. The patient may have an elevated erythrocyte sedimentation rate (ESR) and WBC.

- The D-dimer test cannot be used alone to prove the presence of a DVT because it can be elevated in many other conditions. A D-dimer level of less than 500 ng/mL (less than 500 mcg/L) with a low clinical probability of DVT is helpful and cost effective in excluding DVT without the need for ultrasound testing.

Diagnostic Tests

- Duplex ultrasonography is the most commonly used test to diagnose DVT. It is a noninvasive test that can measure the rate and direction of blood flow and visualize clot formation in proximal veins of the legs. It cannot reliably detect small blood clots in distal veins. Coupled with a careful clinical assessment, it can rule in or out (include or exclude) the diagnosis in the majority of cases.

- Venography (also known as phlebography) is the gold standard for the diagnosis of DVT. However, it is an invasive test that involves injection of radiopaque contrast dye into a foot vein. It is expensive and can cause anaphylaxis and nephrotoxicity.

Contrast studies are expensive, invasive procedures that are technically difficult to perform and evaluate. Severely ill patients often are unable to tolerate the procedure, and many develop hypotension and cardiac arrhythmias. Furthermore, the contrast medium is irritating to vessel walls and toxic to the kidneys. For these reasons, noninvasive tests, such as ultrasonography, CT scans, MRI, and ventilation/perfusion (V/Q) scans are frequently used in clinical practice for the initial evaluation of patients with suspected VTE. See the Clinical Presentation and Diagnosis of PE, and Clinical Presentation and Diagnosis of DVT textboxes.

PREVENTION

Given that VTE is often clinically silent and potentially fatal, prevention strategies have the greatest potential to improve patient outcomes.[2] To rely on the early diagnosis and treatment of VTE is unacceptable because many patients will die before treatment can be initiated. Furthermore, even clinically silent disease is associated with long-term morbidity from the PTS and predisposes the patient to future thromboembolic events. Despite an immense body of literature that overwhelmingly supports the widespread use of pharmacologic and nonpharmacologic strategies to prevent VTE, prophylaxis is underutilized in most hospitals. Even when prophylaxis is given, many patients receive prophylaxis that is less than optimal. Educational programs and computerized clinical decision support systems have been shown to improve the appropriate use of VTE prevention methods.[2]

The goal of an effective VTE prophylaxis program is to identify all patients at risk, determine each patient's level of risk, and select and implement regimens that provide sufficient protection for the level of risk.[20] ❹ *At the time of hospital admission, all patients should be evaluated for their risk of VTE, and strategies to prevent VTE appropriate for each patient's level of risk should be routinely employed. Prophylaxis should be continued throughout the period of risk.* The risk classification criteria and recommended prophylaxis strategies published by the American College of Chest Physicians (ACCP) Conference on Antithrombotic Therapy are widely used in North America (Table 10–2).[2]

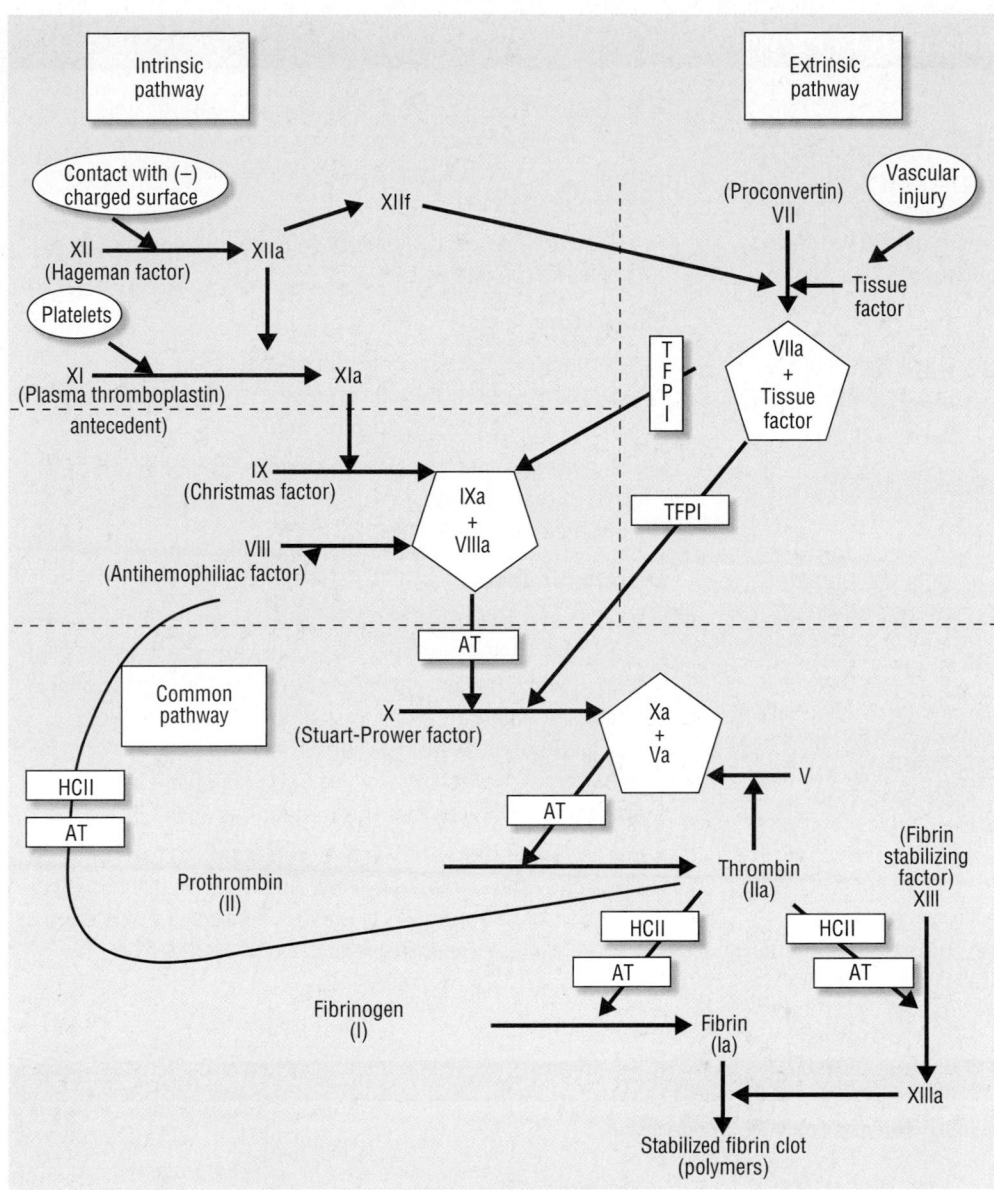

FIGURE 10–4. Coagulation cascade. (AT, antithrombin; HCII, heparin cofactor II; TFPI, tissue factor pathway inhibitor.) (From Haines ST, Witt DM, Nutescu EA. Venous thromboembolism. In: DiPiro JT, Talbert RL, Yee GC, et al., eds. Pharmacotherapy: A Pathophysiologic Approach, 7th ed. New York: McGraw-Hill; 2008:336.)

Several pharmacologic and nonpharmacologic methods are effective for preventing VTE, and these can be used alone or in combination. Nonpharmacologic methods improve venous blood flow by mechanical means, while drug therapy prevents thrombus formation by inhibiting the coagulation cascade.

Nonpharmacologic Therapy

Ambulation as soon as possible following surgery lowers the incidence of VTE in low-risk patients.[2] Walking increases venous blood flow and promotes the flow of natural antithrombotic factors into the lower extremities. Graduated compression stockings (GCS) reduce the incidence of VTE by approximately 60% following general surgery, neurosurgery, and stroke. Compared with anticoagulant drugs, GCS are relatively inexpensive and safe; however, in higher risk patients they are less effective then pharmacologic agents. They are a good choice in low- to moderate-risk patients when pharmacologic interventions are contraindicated. When combined with pharmacologic interventions, GCS have an additive effect. However, some patients are unable to wear compression stockings because of the size or shape of their legs.

Similar to GCS, intermittent pneumatic compression (IPC) devices increase the velocity of blood flow in the lower extremities.[2] These devices sequentially inflate a series of cuffs wrapped around the patient's legs from the ankles to the thighs and then deflate in 1- to 2-minute cycles. IPC has been shown to reduce the risk of VTE by more than 60% following general surgery, neurosurgery, and orthopedic surgery. Although IPC is well tolerated and safe to use in patients who have contraindications to pharmacologic therapies, it does have a few drawbacks: it is more expensive

Clinical Presentation and Diagnosis of PE

General

PE most commonly develops in patients with risk factors for VTE (Table 10–1) during or following a hospitalization. While many patients will have symptoms of DVT prior to developing a PE, many do not. Patients may die suddenly before effective treatment can be initiated.

Symptoms

- The patient may complain of cough, chest pain, chest tightness, shortness of breath, wheezing, or palpitations.
- The patient may present with hemoptysis (spit or cough up blood).
- The patient may complain of dizziness or lightheadedness.
- Symptoms may be confused for a myocardial infarction or pneumonia, and objective testing must be performed to establish the diagnosis.

Signs

- The patient may have tachypnea (increased respiratory rate) and tachycardia (increased heart rate).
- The patient may appear diaphoretic (sweaty).
- The patient's neck veins may be distended reflecting increased jugular venous pressure.
- The examiner may hear diminished breath sounds, crackles, wheezes, or pleural friction rub, right ventricular S_3, or parasternal lift during auscultation of the lungs.

- In massive PE, the patient may appear cyanotic and hypotensive. In such cases, oxygen saturation by pulse oximetry or arterial blood gas will likely indicate that the patient is hypoxic.
- In the worst cases, the patient may go into circulatory shock and die within minutes.

Laboratory Tests

- Serum concentrations of D-dimer, a by-product of thrombin generation, will be elevated. The patient may have an elevated ESR and WBC count.
- The patient may have elevated serum LDH or AST (SGOT) with normal bilirubin. Serum troponin I and troponin T can be elevated in a large PE.

Diagnostic Tests

- A CT scan is the most commonly used test to diagnose PE but some institutions still use a ventilation/perfusion (V/Q) scan. Spiral CT scans can detect emboli in the pulmonary arteries. A V/Q scan measures the distribution of blood and air flow in the lungs. When there is a large mismatch between blood and air flow in one area of the lung, there is a high probability that the patient has a PE.
- Pulmonary angiography is the gold standard for the diagnosis of PE. However, it is an invasive test that involves injection of radiopaque contrast dye into the pulmonary artery. The test is expensive and associated with a significant risk of mortality.

Table 10–2

Risk Classification and Consensus Guidelines for VTE Prevention

Level of Risk	Risk of VTE	Prevention Strategies
Low		
Minor surgery, in mobile patients	Less than 10%	Early and aggressive ambulation
Medical patients who are fully mobile		
Moderate		
Major surgery, and no clinical risk factors	10–40%	UFH 5,000 units SC every 8–12 hours
Acutely ill medical patients (e.g., myocardial infarction, ischemic stroke, heart failure exacerbation) at bed rest		Dalteparin 2,500–5,000 units SC every 24 hours
		Enoxaparin 40 mg SC every 24 hours
		Fondaparinux 2.5 mg SC every 24 hours
		Tinzaparin 3,500 units SC every 24 hours
		IPC[a]; GCS[a]
High		
Major lower extremity orthopedic surgery	40–80%	Dalteparin 5,000 units SC every 24 hours
Hip fracture		Enoxaparin 30 mg SC every 12 hours or 40 mg SC every 24 hours
Major trauma		Fondaparinux 2.5 mg SC every 24 hours
		Tinzaparin 75 units/kg SC every 24 hours
		Warfarin (target INR = 2–3)
		IPC[a]; GCS[a]

GCS, graduated compression stockings; INR, International Normalized Ratio; IPC, intermittent pneumatic compression; SC, subcutaneous; UFH, unfractionated heparin; VTE, venous thromboembolism.

[a]Mechanical methods of prophylaxis are used in patients at high risk of bleeding complications

From Ref. 2.

than the use of GCS, it is a relatively cumbersome technique, and some patients may have difficulty sleeping while using it. To be effective, IPC needs to be used throughout the day. In practice, this has been difficult to achieve and special efforts should be made to ensure that the devices are worn and operational for the majority of the day.

Inferior vena cava (IVC) filters, also known as Greenfield filters, provide short-term protection against PE in very-high-risk patients by preventing the embolization of a thrombus formed in the lower extremities into the pulmonary circulation.[2] Insertion of a filter into the IVC is a minimally invasive procedure. Despite the widespread use of IVC filters, there are very limited data regarding their effectiveness and long-term safety. The evidence suggests that IVC filters, particularly in the absence of effective antithrombotic therapy, increase the long-term risk of recurrent DVT. In the only randomized clinical trial examining the short- and long-term effectiveness of the filters in patients with a documented proximal DVT, treatment with IVC filters reduced the risk of PE by more than 75% during the first 12 days following insertion.[21] However, this benefit was not sustained during 2 years of follow-up and the long-term risk of recurrent DVT was nearly two-fold higher in those who received a filter. Although IVC filters can reduce the short-term risk of PE in patients at highest risk, they should be reserved for patients in whom other prophylactic strategies cannot be used. To further reduce the long-term risk of VTE in association with IVC filters, pharmacologic prophylaxis is necessary and warfarin therapy should begin as soon as the patient is able to tolerate it.[2]

Pharmacologic Therapy

Numerous randomized clinical trials have extensively evaluated pharmacologic strategies for VTE prophylaxis.[2] Appropriately selected drug therapies can dramatically reduce the incidence of VTE following hip replacement, knee replacement, general surgery, myocardial infarction, and ischemic stroke (Table 10–2). The choice of medication and dose to use for VTE prevention must be based on the patient's level of risk for thrombosis and bleeding complications, as well as the cost and availability of an adequate drug therapy monitoring system.

The ACCP Conference on Antithrombotic Therapy recommends against the use of aspirin as the primary method of VTE prophylaxis.[2] Antiplatelet drugs clearly reduce the risk of coronary artery and cerebrovascular events in patients with arterial disease, but aspirin produces a very modest reduction in VTE following orthopedic surgeries of the lower extremities. The relative contribution of venous stasis in the pathogenesis of venous thrombosis compared with that of platelets in arterial thrombosis likely explains the reason for this difference.

The most extensively studied drugs for the prevention of VTE are unfractionated heparin (UFH), the low–molecular weight heparins (LMWHs; dalteparin, enoxaparin, and tinzaparin), fondaparinux, and warfarin.[2] The LMWHs and fondaparinux provide superior protection against VTE when compared to low-dose UFH after hip and knee replacement surgery and in other high-risk populations. Even so, UFH remains an effective, cost-conscious choice for moderate-risk patient populations, provided that it is given in the appropriate dose (Table 10–2). Low-dose UFH (5,000 units every 12 or 8 hours) given subcutaneously (SC) has been shown to significantly reduce the risk of VTE in patients undergoing a wide range of general surgical procedures as well as following a myocardial infarction or stroke. For patients who are hospitalized with an acute medical illness, the available evidence supports the use of UFH (5,000 units every 12 or 8 hours), enoxaparin 40 mg SC daily, dalteparin 5,000 units SC daily, or fondaparinux 2.5 mg SC daily.

For the prevention of VTE following hip and knee replacement surgery, the effectiveness of low-dose UFH is considerably lower. Adjusted-dose UFH therapy provided SC, which requires dose adjustments to maintain the activated partial thromboplastin time (aPTT) at the high end of the normal range, may be used in the highest-risk patient populations. However, adjusted-dose UFH has been studied in only a few, relatively small clinical trials and requires frequent laboratory monitoring. The LMWHs and fondaparinux appear to provide a high degree of protection against VTE in most high-risk populations. The appropriate prophylactic dose for each LMWH product is indication-specific (Table 10–2). There is no evidence that one LMWH is superior to another for the prevention of VTE. Fondaparinux was significantly more effective than enoxaparin in several clinical trials that enrolled patients undergoing high-risk orthopedic procedures, but has not been shown to reduce the incidence of symptomatic PE or mortality, and heightened the risk of bleeding.[22] To provide optimal protection, some experts believe that the LMWHs should be initiated prior to surgery.[2]

Warfarin is another commonly used option for the prevention of VTE following orthopedic surgeries of the lower extremities.[2] Warfarin appears to be as effective as the LMWHs for the prevention of symptomatic VTE events in the highest-risk populations. When used to prevent VTE, the dose of warfarin must be adjusted to maintain an International Normalized Ratio (INR) between 2 and 3. Oral administration and low drug cost give warfarin some advantages over the LMWHs and fondaparinux. However, warfarin does not achieve its full antithrombotic effect for several days and requires frequent monitoring and periodic dosage adjustments, making therapy cumbersome. Warfarin should only be used when a systematic patient monitoring system is available.

The optimal duration for VTE prophylaxis is not well established.[2] Prophylaxis should be given throughout the period of risk. For general surgical procedures and medical conditions, once the patient is able to ambulate regularly and other risk factors are no longer present, prophylaxis can be discontinued. The risk of VTE in the first month following hospital discharge among patients who have undergone total knee replacement, total hip replacement or hip fracture repair is very high. Therefore, extended prophylaxis for 21 to 35 days following hospital discharge with an LMWH, fondaparinux, or warfarin is recommended.

Patient Encounter 1, Part 1

KK is a 69-year-old, obese female who fell on her way to church and fractured her right hip. She is hospitalized and will undergo surgery to repair her fractured right hip.

PMH: Hypertension × 12 years; dyslipidemia × 10 years; obesity × 20 years; degenerative joint disease × 5 years; recurrent urinary tract infections

FH: Nonsignificant

SH: Smoked half a pack per day for 25 years; occasional alcohol use. The patient has Medicare, but due to her fixed income, has difficulty paying for medications, leading to occasional periods of noncompliance

Current Meds: Metoprolol 100 mg by mouth twice daily; hydrochlorothiazide 25 mg by mouth daily; simvastatin 40 mg by mouth daily; salsalate 750 mg by mouth twice daily; trimethoprim-sulfamethoxazole SS tablets by mouth twice daily for 7 days (last treatment was 1 month ago); shark cartilage three tablets by mouth daily; enteric-coated aspirin 81 mg by mouth daily; ginseng two tablets by mouth daily

Allergies: NKDA

PE:

VS: BP 145/90 mm Hg, HR 72, RR 16, T 37.4°C (99.3°F), wt 127 kg (280 lb), BMI 40 kg/m²

Labs: Within normal limits; estimated glomerular filtration rate (GFR) = 74 mL/min

Which risk factor(s) predispose KK to VTE?

What is KK's estimated risk for developing VTE?

Given KK's presentation and history, create an appropriate VTE prophylaxis plan including the pharmacologic agent, dose, route and frequency of administration, duration of therapy, monitoring parameters, and patient education.

TREATMENT

Desired Therapeutic Outcomes

The goal of VTE treatment is to prevent short- and long-term complications of the disease. In the short term (i.e., the first few days to 6 months), the aim of therapy is to prevent propagation or local extension of the clot, embolization, and death. In the long term (i.e., more than 6 months after the first event), the aim of therapy is to prevent complications, such as PTS, pulmonary hypertension, and recurrent VTE.[17,23]

General Treatment Principles

Anticoagulant drugs are considered the mainstay of therapy for patients with VTE, and the therapeutic strategies for

DVT and PE are essentially identical.[17,23] **❺** *In the absence of contraindications, the treatment of VTE should initially include a rapid-acting anticoagulant (e.g., UFH, LMWH, or fondaparinux) overlapped with warfarin for at least 5 days and until the patient's INR is greater than 2. Anticoagulation therapy should be continued for a minimum of 3 months. However, the duration of anticoagulation therapy should be based on the patient's risk of VTE recurrence and major bleeding.* The treatment of VTE can be divided into acute, subacute, and chronic phases (Fig. 10–5).[23,24] The acute treatment phase of VTE is typically accomplished by administering a fast-acting parenteral anticoagulant (Table 10–3). The subacute and chronic phase treatments of VTE are usually accomplished using oral anticoagulant agents, such as warfarin.[17,23] In certain populations, such as patients with cancer and women who are pregnant, the LMWHs are the preferred agents during subacute and chronic treatment phases.[17] In the last decade, several novel anticoagulants, such as direct thrombin inhibitors (DTIs) and factor Xa inhibitors have emerged as potential alternatives for the acute, subacute, and chronic phases of treatment. As data from clinical trials using these new agents in VTE treatment continue to emerge, their role in clinical practice will be better understood.[17,23]

Treatment Options

► *Pharmacologic Therapy*

Thrombolytics The role of thrombolysis in the treatment of VTE is controversial. Thrombolytic agents are proteolytic enzymes that have the ability to dissolve, or lyse, the fibrin clot (Table 10–4). Thrombolytics are administered systemically or directly into the thrombus using a catheter-directed infusion.[17] Compared to anticoagulants, thrombolytics restore venous patency more quickly; however, the bleeding risk associated with their use is significantly higher.[25] In patients with DVT, thrombolytics decrease short-term pain and swelling and prevent destruction of the venous valves. It is not clear if thrombolytics decrease the incidence and severity

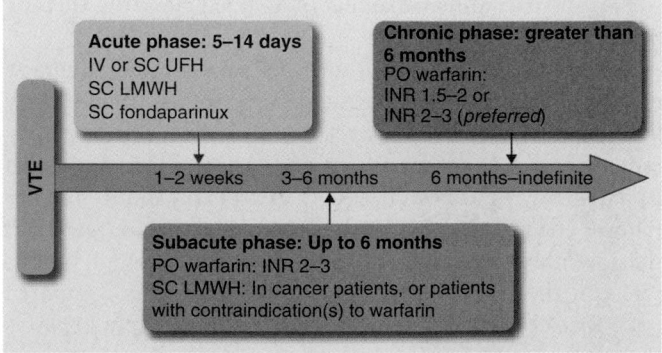

FIGURE 10–5. Treatment approach for patients with VTE. (INR, International Normalized Ratio; IV, intravenous; LMWH, low–molecular weight heparin; PO, oral; SC, subcutaneous; UFH, unfractionated heparin; VTE, venous thromboembolism.) (From Ref. 24.)

Table 10–3

Pharmacologic Options for the Initial Treatment of Acute VTE

UFH

IV administration:[a] use weight-based dosing nomogram (Table 10–5)

or

SC administration: 17,500 units (250 units/kg) given every 12 hours (an initial 5,000 unit IV bolus dose is recommended to obtain rapid anticoagulation)

Adjust subsequent doses to attain a goal aPTT based on the institution-specific therapeutic range

or

SC administration: 333 units/kg followed by 250 units/kg given every 12 hours (fixed-dose unmonitored dosing regimen)

LMWHs

Dalteparin: 200 units/kg SC once daily or 100 units/kg SC twice daily[b]

Enoxaparin: 1.5 mg/kg SC once daily or 1 mg/kg SC twice daily; if CrCl is less than 30 mL/min: 1 mg/kg SC once daily

Tinzaparin: 175 units/kg SC once daily

Factor Xa Inhibitor

Fondaparinux:

For body weight less than 50 kg (110 lb), use 5 mg SC once daily

For body weight 50–100 kg (110–220 lb), use 7.5 mg SC once daily

For body weight greater than 100 kg (220 lb), use 10 mg SC once daily

---

aPTT, activated partial thromboplastin time; CrCl, creatinine clearance; SC, subcutaneous; VTE, venous thromboembolism; UFH, unfractionated heparin; LMWHs, low–molecular weight heparins.

[a]IV administration preferred due to improved dosing precision.

[b]Not FDA-approved for treatment of VTE in noncancer patients.

From Ref. 17.

Table 10–4

Thrombolysis for the Treatment of VTE

- Thrombolytic therapy should be reserved for patients who present with shock, hypotension, right ventricular strain, or massive DVT with limb gangrene
- Diagnosis must be objectively confirmed before initiating thrombolytic therapy
- Thrombolytic therapy is most effective when administered as soon as possible after PE diagnosis, but benefit may extend up to 14 days after symptom onset
- Approved PE thrombolytic regimens:
  - Streptokinase 250,000 units IV over 30 minutes followed by 100,000 units/h for 24 hours[a]
  - Urokinase 4,400 units/kg IV over 10 minutes followed by 4,400 units/kg/h for 12–24 hours[a]
  - Alteplase 100 mg IV over 2 hours
- Factors that increase the risk of bleeding must be evaluated before thrombolytic therapy is initiated (i.e., recent surgery, trauma or internal bleeding, uncontrolled hypertension, recent stroke, or ICH)
- Baseline labs should include CBC and blood typing in case transfusion is needed
- UFH should not be used during thrombolytic therapy. Neither the aPTT nor any other anticoagulation parameter should be monitored during the thrombolytic infusion
- aPTT should be measured following the completion of thrombolytic therapy:
  - If aPTT less than 2.5 times the control value, UFH infusion should be started and adjusted to maintain aPTT in therapeutic range
  - If aPTT greater than 2.5 times the control value, remeasure every 2–4 hours and start UFH infusion when aPTT is less than 2.5
- Avoid phlebotomy, arterial puncture, and other invasive procedures during thrombolytic therapy to minimize the risk of bleeding

---

aPTT, activated partial thromboplastin time; DVT, deep vein thrombosis; PE, pulmonary embolism; UFH, unfractionated heparin; VTE, venous thromboembolism.

[a]Two-hour infusions of streptokinase and urokinase are as effective and safe as alteplase.

---

of PTS. Clinical trials have failed to show any long-term benefits from the routine use of thrombolytics; therefore, their use in the majority of patients is not recommended.[17,25] In a select group of high-risk patients with massive iliofemoral DVT who are at risk of limb gangrene, thrombolysis may be considered.[17]

In patients with acute PE, the use of thrombolytics provides short-term benefits such as restoring pulmonary artery patency and hemodynamic stability.[17,26] A recent meta-analysis of nine small randomized clinical trials showed a slightly lower risk of death or recurrent PE in patients treated with thrombolytics when compared to those treated with heparin alone. However, this small benefit was offset by a higher risk of major bleeding.[27] Streptokinase, urokinase, and tissue plasminogen activator (t-PA) have all been studied and are FDA-approved in the treatment of PE. All three agents have comparable thrombolytic capacity but t-PA has the potential advantage of a shorter infusion time. Reteplase is not currently FDA-approved for the treatment of PE, but it has also been studied. Reteplase is administered as two 10 unit IV boluses given 30 minutes apart.[17,28]

Given the relative lack of data to support their routine use, thrombolytics should be reserved for select high-risk circumstances (Table 10–4). Candidates for thrombolytic therapy are patients with acute massive **embolism** who are hemodynamically unstable (systolic blood pressure [SBP] less than 90 mm Hg) and at low risk for bleeding.[17] The use of thrombolytics in hemodynamically stable patients with right ventricular dysfunction is controversial but some experts support their use.

Unfractionated Heparin UFH has traditionally been the drug of choice for indications requiring a rapid anticoagulation including the acute treatment of VTE. Commercially available UFH preparations are derived from porcine intestinal mucosa or bovine lung. UFH is composed of a heterogeneous mixture of glycosaminoglycans with variable length, molecular weight, and pharmacologic properties. Unlike thrombolytics, UFH and other anticoagulants will not dissolve a formed clot but prevent its propagation and growth.[4,29]

Heparin exerts its anticoagulant effect by augmenting the natural anticoagulant, AT. A specific pentasaccharide sequence on the heparin molecule binds to AT and causes a conformational change that greatly accelerates its activity (Fig. 10–6). This complex inhibits thrombin (factor IIa), as well as factors Xa, IXa, XIa, and XIIa. Thrombin and factor Xa are most sensitive to this inhibition and are inactivated in an equal 1:1 ratio. In order to inactivate thrombin, the UFH molecule needs to form a ternary complex by binding to both AT and thrombin. Only UFH molecules that are at least 18 saccharide units long are able to form this bridge between AT and thrombin. In contrast, inhibition of factor Xa does not require the formation of a ternary complex. UFH molecules as short as five saccharide units can catalyze the inactivation of factor Xa. Due to its nonspecific binding to cellular proteins, UFH has several limitations, including poor bioavailability when given SC and significant intra- and interpatient variability in anticoagulant response.[4,29]

UFH can be administered via the IV or SC route.[4] When rapid anticoagulation is required, UFH should be administered IV and an initial bolus dose should be given. For the treatment of VTE, UFH is generally given as a continuous IV infusion. Intermittent IV bolus dosing is associated with a higher risk of bleeding and is therefore not recommended. When given SC, the bioavailability of UFH ranges from 30% to 70%, depending on the dose given. Therefore, higher doses of UFH must be given if the SC route of administration is used. Onset of anticoagulation is delayed by 1 to 2 hours after the SC injection. Due to the risk of hematomas and erratic absorption, intramuscular (IM) administration is not recommended. The half-life of UFH is dose dependent and ranges from 30 to 90 minutes, but may be significantly longer, up to 150 minutes, with high doses. UFH is eliminated by two mechanisms: (a) enzymatic degradation via a saturable zero-order process, and (b) renally via a first-order process. Lower UFH doses are primarily cleared via enzymatic processes, while higher doses are primarily renally eliminated. Clearance of UFH can be impaired in patients with renal and hepatic dysfunction. Patients with active thrombosis may require higher UFH doses due to a more rapid elimination or variations in the plasma concentrations of heparin-binding proteins. AT deficiency and elevated factor VIII levels are common in pregnant patients. AT deficiency has been linked to higher UFH dose requirements. The requirement of these higher UFH doses is termed "heparin resistance." Factor VIII elevations can result in altered aPTT response to UFH and monitoring with antifactor Xa levels is recommended.[4,29]

The dose of UFH required to achieve a therapeutic anticoagulant response is correlated to the patient's weight.[4] Weight-based dosing regimens should be utilized in order to exceed the therapeutic threshold in the first 24 hours after initiating treatment.[30] Achieving a therapeutic aPTT in the first 24 hours after initiating UFH is critical because this

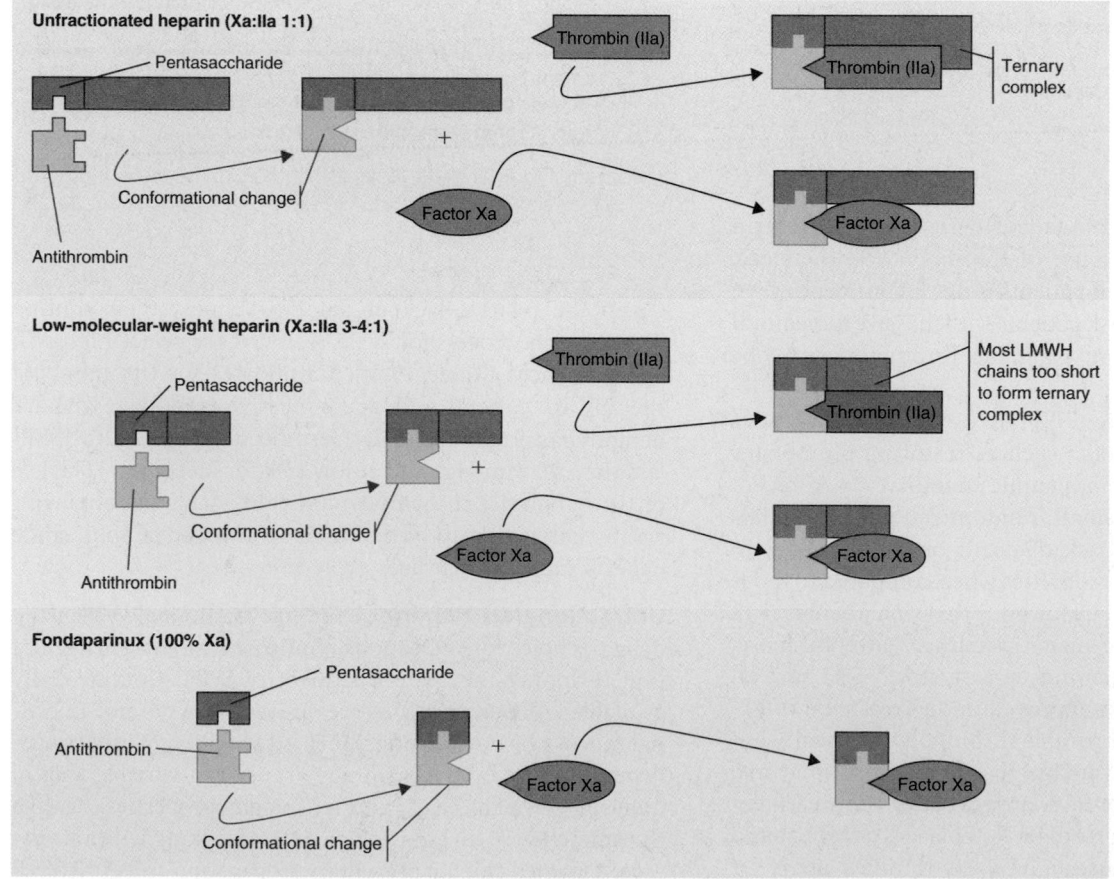

FIGURE 10–6.

Mechanism of action of unfractionated heparin, low–molecular weight heparin (LMWH), and fondaparinux. (From Haines ST, Witt DM, Nutescu EA. Venous thromboembolism. In: DiPiro JT, Talbert RL, Yee GC, et al., eds. Pharmacotherapy: A Pathophysiologic Approach, 7th ed. New York: McGraw-Hill; 2008:338.)

has been shown to lower the risk of recurrent VTE.[4,30] For nonobese patients, the actual body weight should be used to calculate the initial UFH dose (Table 10–5). For obese patients, using the actual body weight to calculate the initial dose is also generally recommended; however, data are more limited in morbidly obese patients; that is, weight greater than 150 kg (330 lb). Some experts recommend using an adjusted body weight (ABW) in these patients instead. The infusion rate is then adjusted based on laboratory monitoring of the patient's response. UFH can also be administered via the SC route; however, IV infusion is preferred by most clinicians because it can be dosed more precisely. If the SC route is selected, an initial 5,000 unit IV bolus should be given followed by 17,500 units given SC every 12 hours. Subsequent doses of SC-UFH need to be adjusted based on the patient's response.[17,23,31] Alternatively, in patients with DVT, a fixed-dose, weight-based dose of unmonitored UFH regimen can also be used with an initial dose of 333 units/kg followed by 250 units/kg given SC every 12 hours.[17,32]

❶ *Due to significant variability in interpatient response and changes in patient response over time, UFH requires close monitoring and periodic dose adjustment.* The response to UFH can be monitored using a variety of laboratory tests including the aPTT, the whole blood clotting time, activated clotting time (ACT), antifactor Xa activity, and the plasma heparin concentration.[4,33] Although it has several limitations, the aPTT is the most widely used test in clinical practice to monitor UFH. Traditionally, therapeutic aPTT range is defined as 1.5 to 2.5 times the control aPTT value. However, due to variations in the reagents and instruments used to measure the aPTT in different laboratories, each institution should establish a therapeutic range for UFH. The institution-specific therapy range should correlate with a plasma heparin concentration of 0.2 to 0.4 units/mL by protamine titration or 0.3 to 0.7 units/mL by an amidolytic antifactor Xa assay.[4,33] An aPTT should be obtained at baseline, 6 hours after initiating the heparin infusion, and 6 hours after each dose change, as this is the time required to reach steady state. The UFH dose is then adjusted based on the aPTT measurement and the institutional-specific therapeutic range (Table 10–5). In patients with "heparin resistance," antifactor Xa concentrations may be a more accurate method of monitoring the patient's response.[4,33]

Side effects associated with UFH include bleeding, thrombocytopenia, hypersensitivity reactions, and with prolonged use, alopecia, hyperkalemia, and osteoporosis.[4,29] ❻ *Bleeding is the most common adverse effect associated with antithrombotic drugs, including UFH therapy. A patient's risk of major hemorrhage is related to the intensity and stability of therapy, age, concurrent drug use, history of GI bleeding, risk of falls or trauma, and recent surgery.* Several risk factors can increase the risk of UFH-induced bleeding (Table 10–6). The risk of bleeding is related to the intensity of anticoagulation. Higher aPTT values are associated with an increased risk of bleeding. The risk of major bleeding is 1% to 5% during the first few days of treatment.[3] In addition to the aPTT, hemoglobin, hematocrit, and blood pressure should also be monitored. Concurrent use of UFH with other antithrombotic agents, such as thrombolytics and antiplatelet agents, also increases the risk of bleeding. Patients receiving UFH therapy should be closely monitored for signs and symptoms of bleeding, including epistaxis, hemoptysis, hematuria, hematochezia, melena, severe

---

Table 10–5

Weight-Based[a] Dosing for UFH Administered by Continuous IV Infusion for VTE

Initial Loading Dose	Initial Infusion Rate
80 units/kg (maximum = 10,000 units)	18 units/kg/h (maximum = 2,300 units/h)

aPTT (seconds)	Maintenance Infusion Rate *Dose Adjustment*
Less than 37 (or less than 12 seconds below institution-specific therapeutic range)	80 units/kg bolus then increase infusion by 4 units/kg/h
37–47 (or 1–12 seconds below institution-specific therapeutic range)	40 units/kg bolus then increase infusion by 2 units/kg/h
48–71 (within institution-specific therapeutic range)	No change
72–93 (or 1–22 seconds above institution-specific therapeutic range)	Decrease infusion by 2 units/kg/h
Greater than 93 (or greater than 22 seconds above institution-specific therapeutic range)	Hold infusion for 1 hour then decrease by 3 units/kg/h

aPTT, activated partial thromboplastin time; IBW, ideal body weight; UFH, unfractionated heparin; VTE, venous thromboembolism.

[a]Use actual body weight for all calculations. Adjusted body weight (ABW) may be used for morbidly obese patients (greater than 130% of IBW).

ABW = IBW + (Actual body weight – IBW) × 0.7.

Table 10–6

Risk Factors for Major Bleeding While Taking Anticoagulation Therapy

Anticoagulation intensity (e.g., INR greater than 5, aPTT greater than 120 seconds)
Initiation of therapy (first few days and weeks)
Unstable anticoagulation response
Age greater than 65 years
Concurrent antiplatelet drug use
Concurrent nonsteroidal anti-inflammatory drug or aspirin use
History of GI bleeding
Recent surgery or trauma
High risk for fall/trauma
Heavy alcohol use
Renal failure
Cerebrovascular disease
Malignancy

aPTT, activated partial thromboplastin time; INR, International Normalized Ratio.

headache, and joint pain. If major bleeding occurs, UFH should be stopped immediately and the source of bleeding treated.[3,4] If necessary, use protamine sulfate to reverse the effects of UFH. The usual dose is 1 mg protamine sulfate per 100 units of UFH, up to a maximum of 50 mg, given as a slow IV infusion over 10 minutes. The effects of UFH are neutralized in 5 minutes, and the effects of protamine persist for 2 hours. If the bleeding is not controlled or the anticoagulant effect rebounds, repeated doses of protamine may be administered.[4]

Heparin-induced thrombocytopenia (HIT) is a very serious adverse effect associated with UFH use. Platelet counts should be monitored every 2 to 3 days during the course of UFH therapy.[4] HIT should be suspected if the platelet count drops by more than 50% from baseline or to below $120 \times 10^3/mm^3$ ($120 \times 10^9/L$). HIT should also be suspected if thrombosis occurs despite UFH use. Immediate discontinuation of all heparin-containing products, including the use of LMWHs is in order. Alternative anticoagulation should be initiated. In patients with contraindications to anticoagulation therapy, UFH should not be administered (Table 10–7).

UFH is an FDA pregnancy category C drug and may be used to treat VTE during pregnancy. UFH should be used with caution in the peripartum period due to the risk of maternal hemorrhage. UFH is not secreted into the breast milk and is safe for use by women who wish to breast-feed.[11] For the treatment of VTE in children, the UFH dose is 50 units/kg bolus followed by an infusion of 20,000 units/m[2] per 24 hours. Alternatively, a loading dose of 75 units/kg followed by an infusion of 28 units/kg/h if less than 12 months old and 20 units/kg/h if greater than 1 year old may be considered.[34]

Low–Molecular Weight Heparins The LMWHs are smaller heparin fragments obtained by chemical or enzymatic depolymerization of UFH. LMWHs are heterogeneous mixtures of glycosaminoglycans, and each product has slightly different molecular weight distributions and pharmacologic properties.[4] Compared with UFH, LMWHs have improved pharmacodynamic and pharmacokinetic properties. They exhibit less binding to plasma and cellular proteins, resulting in a more predictable anticoagulant response. Consequently, routine monitoring of anticoagulation activity and dose adjustments are not required in the majority of patients. LMWHs have longer plasma half-lives, allowing once- or twice-daily administration, improved SC bioavailability, and dose-independent renal clearance. In addition, LMWHs have a more favorable side effect profile than UFH. They are also associated with a lower incidence of HIT and osteopenia. Three LMWHs are currently available in the United States: dalteparin, enoxaparin, and tinzaparin.[4,29]

Like UFH, LMWHs prevent the propagation and growth of formed thrombi. The anticoagulant effect is mediated through a specific pentasaccharide sequence that binds to AT. The primary difference in the pharmacologic activity of UFH and LMWH is their relative inhibition of thrombin (factor IIa) and factor Xa. Smaller heparin fragments cannot bind

---

Table 10–7

Contraindications to Anticoagulation Therapy

General
Active bleeding
Hemophilia or other hemorrhagic tendencies
Severe liver disease with elevated baseline PT
Severe thrombocytopenia (platelet count less than $20 \times 10^3/mm^3$ [$20 \times 10^9/L$])
Malignant hypertension
Inability to meticulously supervise and monitor treatment

Product-Specific Contraindications
UFH
Hypersensitivity to UFH
History of HIT

LMWHs
Hypersensitivity to LMWH, UFH, pork products, methylparaben, or propylparaben
History of HIT or suspected HIT

Fondaparinux
Hypersensitivity to fondaparinux
Severe renal insufficiency (CrCl less than 30 mL/min)
Body weight less than 50 kg (110 lb)
Bacterial endocarditis
Thrombocytopenia with a positive in vitro test for antiplatelet antibodies in the presence of fondaparinux

Lepirudin
Hypersensitivity to hirudins

Argatroban
Hypersensitivity to argatroban

Warfarin
Hypersensitivity to warfarin
Pregnancy
History of warfarin-induced skin necrosis
Inability to obtain follow-up PT/INR measurements
Inappropriate medication use or lifestyle behaviors

CrCl, creatinine clearance; HIT, heparin-induced thrombocytopenia; INR, International Normalized Ratio; LMWHs, low–molecular weight heparins; PT, prothrombin time; UFH, unfractionated heparin.

AT and thrombin simultaneously (Fig. 10–6). Due to their smaller chain length, LMWHs have relatively greater activity against factor Xa and inhibit thrombin to a lesser degree. The antifactor Xa:IIa activity ratio for the LMWHs ranges from 2:1 to 4:1. The SC bioavailability of the LMWHs is greater than 90%. The peak anticoagulant effect of the LMWHs is reached 3 to 5 hours after a SC dose. The elimination half-life is 3 to 6 hours and is agent-specific. In patients with renal impairment, the half-life of LMWHs is prolonged.[4,29]

The dose of LMWHs for the treatment of VTE is determined based on the patient's weight and is administered SC once or twice daily (Table 10–3). Once-daily dosing of enoxaparin appears to be as effective as twice-daily dosing; however, some data suggest that twice-daily dosing may be more effective in patients who are obese or have cancer.[17,23,35] The dose of enoxaparin is expressed in milligrams, whereas the doses of dalteparin and tinzaparin are expressed in units of antifactor Xa activity. Due to their predictable anticoagulant effect, routine monitoring is not necessary in the majority of patients.[4] LMWHs have been evaluated in a large number of randomized trials and have been shown to be at least as safe and effective as UFH for the treatment of VTE.[17,23] Indeed, the rate of mortality was lower in patients treated with a LMWH in clinical trials. This mortality benefit was primarily seen in patients with cancer.[31,36]

Prior to initiating treatment with a LMWH, baseline laboratory tests should include prothrombin time (PT)/INR, aPTT, CBC, and serum creatinine. Monitor the CBC with platelet count every 2 to 3 days during the first 2 weeks of therapy, and every 2 to 4 weeks with extended use.[4] Use LMWHs cautiously in patients with renal impairment due to the potential of drug accumulation and risk of bleeding. Specific dosing recommendations for patients with a creatinine clearance (CrCl) less than 30 mL/min are currently available for enoxaparin but are lacking for other agents of the class (Table 10–3). Higher mortality rate has been reported in elderly patients with renal dysfunction who were treated with the LMWH tinzaparin. Current guidelines recommend the use of UFH over LMWH in patients with severe renal dysfunction (CrCl less than 30 mL/min).[17,37]

❼ *Most patients with an uncomplicated DVT can be managed safely at home.* LMWHs can be easily administered in the outpatient setting, thus enabling the treatment of VTE at home. Several large clinical trials have demonstrated the efficacy and safety of LMWHs for outpatient treatment of DVT.[17,20,31] Acceptance of this treatment approach has increased tremendously over the last several years among clinicians. Patients with DVT with normal vital signs, low-bleeding risk, no other comorbid conditions requiring hospitalization, and who are stable, may have anticoagulant initiated at home. Although the treatment of patients with PE in the outpatient setting is controversial, patients with submassive PE who are hemodynamically stable can be safely treated in the outpatient setting as well.[17,26] Patients considered for outpatient therapy must be reliable or have adequate caregiver support and must be able to strictly adhere to the prescribed treatment regimen and recommended follow-up visits. Close patient follow-up is critical to the success of any outpatient DVT treatment program. Home DVT treatment results in cost savings and improved patient satisfaction and quality of life.[20,37,38]

Laboratory methods of measuring a patient's response to LMWH may be warranted in certain situations.[4,39] Although controversial, measurement of antifactor Xa activity has been the most widely used method in clinical practice and is recommended by the College of American Pathologists.[39] Monitoring of antifactor Xa activity may be considered in adult patients who are morbidly obese (weight greater than 150 kg [330 lb] or BMI greater than 50 kg/m²), weigh less than 50 kg (110 lb), or have significant renal impairment (CrCl less than 30 mL/min). Laboratory monitoring may also be useful in children and pregnant women. When monitoring antifactor Xa activity, the sample should be obtained approximately 4 hours after the SC dose is administered, when peak concentration is anticipated. The therapeutic range for antifactor Xa activity has not been clearly defined, and there is a limited correlation between antifactor Xa

activity and safety or efficacy.[39] For the treatment of VTE, an acceptable antifactor Xa activity range is 0.5 to 1 unit/mL with twice-daily dosing. In patients treated with once-daily LMWH regimens, a target level between 1 and 2 units/mL is recommended by some experts.[4,17,35,39]

Similar to UFH, bleeding is the major complication associated with LMWHs. The frequency of major bleeding appears to be numerically lower with LMWHs than with UFH.[31] The incidence of major bleeding reported in clinical trials is less than 3%.[17] Minor bleeding, especially bruising at the injection site, occurs frequently. Protamine sulfate will partially reverse the anticoagulant effects of the LMWHs and should be administered in the event of major bleeding. Due to its limited binding to LMWH chains, protamine only neutralizes 60% of their antithrombotic activity. If the LMWH was administered within the previous 8 hours, give 1 mg protamine sulfate per 1 mg of enoxaparin or 100 antifactor Xa units of dalteparin or tinzaparin. If the bleeding is not controlled, give 0.5 mg of protamine sulfate for every antifactor Xa 100 units of LMWH. Give smaller protamine doses if more than 8 hours have lapsed since the last LMWH dose.[4]

The incidence of HIT is lower with LMWHs than with UFH. However, LMWHs cross-react with heparin antibodies in vitro and should not be given as an alternative anticoagulant in patients with a diagnosis or history of HIT. Monitor platelet counts every few days during the first 2 weeks and periodically thereafter.[4]

In patients undergoing spinal and epidural anesthesia or spinal puncture, spinal and epidural hematomas have been linked to the use of LMWHs. In patients with in-dwelling epidural catheters, concurrent use of LMWHs and all other agents that impact hemostasis should be avoided. When inserting and removing the in-dwelling epidural catheters, the timing of LMWH administration around catheter manipulation should be carefully coordinated. Catheter manipulation should only occur at minimal or trough anticoagulant levels.[4]

LMWHs are an excellent alternative to UFH for the treatment of VTE in pregnant women.[11] The LMWHs do not cross the placenta, and they are FDA pregnancy category B. Because the pharmacokinetics of LMWHs may change during pregnancy, monitor antifactor Xa activity every 4 to 6 weeks to make dose adjustments.[11,40] LMWHs have also been used to treat VTE in pediatric patients. Children less than 1 year old require higher doses (e.g., enoxaparin 1.5 mg/kg SC every 12 hours). Monitor antifactor Xa activity to guide dosing in children.[34]

Factor Xa Inhibitors Fondaparinux, the first agent in this class, is an indirect inhibitor of factor Xa, and exerts its anticoagulant activity by accelerating AT. Fondaparinux contains the specific five-saccharide sequence found in UFH that is responsible for its pharmacologic activity. Due to its small size, fondaparinux exerts inhibitory activity specifically against factor Xa and has no effect on thrombin (factor IIa; Fig. 10–6).[29,41] Fondaparinux is currently the only agent of the class that is commercially available in the United

States. Idraparinux, rivaroxaban, and apixaban are antifactor Xa inhibitors currently undergoing Phase III clinical trials. Fondaparinux and idraparinux are administered SC; rivaroxaban and apixaban are administered orally. After SC administration, fondaparinux is completely absorbed, and peak plasma concentrations are reached within 2 to 3 hours.[41,42]

As synthetic drugs (unlike UFH and the LMWHs), factor Xa inhibitors cannot transmit animal pathogens, are consistent from batch-to-batch, and are available in an unlimited supply. Other favorable attributes of factor Xa inhibitors include a predictable and linear dose–response relationship, rapid onset of activity, and long half-life.[29,41,42] Factor Xa inhibitors do not require routine coagulation monitoring or dose adjustments. Fondaparinux has a half-life of 17 to 21 hours, permitting once-daily administration, but the anticoagulant effects of fondaparinux will persist for 2 to 4 days after stopping the drug. In patients with renal impairment, the anticoagulant effect persists even longer. Idraparinux has a significantly longer duration of activity and is being developed for once-weekly injection. The oral agents, rivaroxaban and apixaban, have half-lives ranging from 5 to 14 hours allowing once- or twice-daily administration.[41,42] Neither fondaparinux nor idraparinux are metabolized in the liver and therefore have few drug interactions. However, concurrent use with other antithrombotic agents increases the risk of bleeding. Unlike the heparins, factor Xa inhibitors do not affect platelet function and do not react with the heparin platelet factor-4 (PF-4) antibodies seen in patients with HIT. Some centers use fondaparinux in patients with subacute HIT or a history of HIT who require anticoagulation therapy.[4,29,41]

Fondaparinux has been evaluated for the treatment of DVT and PE in two large phase 3 trials and is approved by the FDA for these indications. Fondaparinux is as safe and effective as IV UFH for the treatment of PE and SC LMWH for DVT treatment.[43,44] The recommended dose for fondaparinux in the treatment of VTE is based on the patient's weight (Table 10–3). Fondaparinux is renally eliminated and accumulation can occur in patients with renal dysfunction. Due to the lack of specific dosing guidelines, fondaparinux is contraindicated in patients with severe renal impairment (CrCl less than 30 mL/min). Baseline renal function should be measured and monitored closely during the course of therapy. Based on limited available data at this time, monitoring antifactor Xa activity to guide fondaparinux dosing is not recommended.[4,17,29]

As with other anticoagulants, the major side effect associated with fondaparinux is bleeding. Fondaparinux should be used with caution in elderly patients because their risk of bleeding is higher. Patients receiving fondaparinux should be carefully monitored for signs and symptoms of bleeding. A CBC should be obtained at baseline and monitored periodically to detect the possibility of occult bleeding. In the event of major bleeding, fresh frozen plasma and factor concentrates should be given. In the case of a life-threatening bleed, recombinant factor VIIa may be considered, but this is a very costly option and it can also

increase the risk of thrombosis. Fondaparinux is not reversed by protamine.[4,17,29,41]

Fondaparinux is pregnancy category B, but there are very limited data regarding its use during pregnancy. Use in pediatric patients has not been studied.[4,29,41]

DTIs Given that thrombin is the central mediator of coagulation and amplifies its own production, it is a natural target for pharmacologic intervention. DTIs bind thrombin and prevent interactions with its substrates (Fig. 10–7). Several injectable DTIs are approved for use in the United States including lepirudin, bivalirudin, argatroban, and desirudin. Several oral DTIs are currently in development. These agents differ in terms of their chemical structure, molecular weight, and binding to the thrombin molecule. Potential advantages of DTIs include a targeted specificity for thrombin, the ability to inactivate clot-bound thrombin, and an absence of platelet interactions that can lead to HIT. Unlike heparins, DTIs do not require AT as a cofactor and do not bind to plasma proteins. Therefore they produce a more predictable anticoagulant effect. DTIs are considered the drugs of choice for the treatment of VTE in patients with a diagnosis or history of HIT.[29,41,45]

The prototype of this class is hirudin, which was originally isolated from the salivary glands of the medicinal leech, *Hirudo medicinalis*. Hirudin itself is not commercially available, but recombinant technology has permitted production of hirudin derivatives, namely lepirudin and desirudin.[29,41,45] Lepirudin has a short half-life of approximately 40 minutes after IV administration and

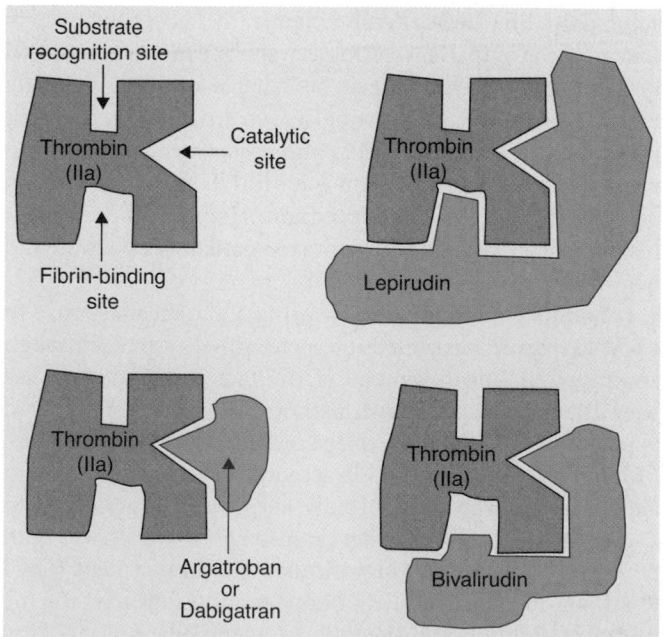

FIGURE 10–7. Mechanism of action of direct thrombin inhibitors. (From Haines ST, Witt DM, Nutescu EA. Venous thromboembolism. In: DiPiro JT, Talbert RL, Yee GC, et al., eds. Pharmacotherapy: A Pathophysiologic Approach, 7th ed. New York: McGraw-Hill; 2008:345.)

120 minutes when given SC. Elimination of lepirudin is primarily renal; therefore, doses must be adjusted based on the patient's renal function. The dose should be monitored and adjusted to achieve an aPTT ratio of 1.5 to 2.5 times the baseline measurement. Lepirudin is currently approved for use in patients with HIT and related thrombosis. Up to 40% of patients treated with lepirudin will develop antibodies to the drug.[29,41,45]

Bivalirudin, a smaller-molecular-weight DTI, is given by IV infusion. Bivalirudin has a shorter elimination half-life (approximately 25 minutes) than lepirudin and is only partially eliminated renally. Unlike lepirudin, bivalirudin is a reversible inhibitor of thrombin and provides transient antithrombotic activity. Patients with moderate or severe renal impairment (CrCl less than 60 mL/min) may require dose adjustment because clearance of bivalirudin is reduced by approximately 20% in these patients. Bivalirudin is approved for use in patients with unstable angina undergoing percutaneous transluminal coronary angioplasty. The ACT is used to monitor the anticoagulant effect of bivalirudin during percutaneous coronary intervention (PCI).[29,41,45]

Desirudin is a SC administered DTI approved for VTE prevention after hip replacement surgery but is not yet commercially available in the United States. Desirudin has an elimination half-life of 2 to 3 hours and is typically dosed every 12 hours. It is primarily eliminated through the kidneys, so dose reduction is needed in patients with renal impairment. The aPTT should be used to measure desirudin's anticoagulant activity.[29,41,45]

Argatroban is a small synthetic molecule that binds reversibly to the active site of thrombin (Fig. 10–7). Argatroban is IV administered and has a 40- to 50-minute elimination half-life. The aPTT must be monitored to assess its anticoagulant activity. Argatroban is hepatically metabolized; therefore, dose reductions and careful monitoring are recommended in patients with hepatic dysfunction. Renal impairment has no influence on the elimination half-life or dosing of argatroban. Argatroban is approved for prevention and treatment of thrombosis in patients with HIT and in patients with HIT undergoing PCI.[29,41,45]

Small-molecule DTIs have been structurally modified for oral administration. Several oral DTIs are in development. Dabigatran is one of the oral DTI agents that is in the most advanced phases of clinical development. Dabigatran is undergoing phase 3 clinical trials for the treatment and prevention of VTE and for stroke prevention in patients with atrial fibrillation. The potential advantages of oral DTIs include the ability to give them in fixed once- or twice-daily doses, and without the need for routine coagulation monitoring. In addition, there appear to be a significantly lower number of drug and food interactions associated with oral DTIs as compared to some of the traditional oral anticoagulants such as warfarin.[41,45]

Contraindications to the use of DTIs and risk factors for bleeding are similar to those of other antithrombotic agents (Tables 10–6 and 10–7). Bleeding is the most common side effect reported with the use of DTIs. Concurrent use of DTIs with thrombolytics significantly increases bleeding complications. Currently, there are no known antidotes to reverse the effects of the DTIs. Fresh frozen plasma, factor concentrates, or recombinant factor VIIa should be given in the event of a major bleed. DTIs can increase the PT/INR and can interfere with the accuracy of monitoring and dosing of warfarin therapy. Data on the use of DTIs in pregnancy and pediatric patients are very limited.[29,41,45]

Warfarin Warfarin has been the primary oral anticoagulant used in the United States for the past 60 years. Warfarin is the anticoagulant of choice when long-term or extended anticoagulation is required. Warfarin is FDA-approved for the prevention and treatment of VTE, as well as the prevention of thromboembolic complications in patients with myocardial infarction, atrial fibrillation, and heart valve replacement. While very effective, warfarin has a narrow therapeutic index, requiring frequent dose adjustments and careful patient monitoring.[5,29]

Warfarin exerts its anticoagulant effect by inhibiting the production of the vitamin K-dependent coagulation factors II (prothrombin), VII, IX, and X, as well as the anticoagulant proteins C and S (Fig. 10–8). Warfarin has no effect on circulating coagulation factors that have been previously formed, and its full antithrombotic activity is delayed for 5 to 7 days, and potentially longer in slower metabolizers. This delay is related to half-lives of the clotting factors: 60 to 100 hours for factor II (prothrombin), 6 to 8 hours for factor VII, 20 to 30 hours for factor IX, and 24 to 40 hours for factor X. Proteins C and S, the natural anticoagulants, are inhibited more rapidly due to their shorter half-lives, 8 to 10 hours and 40 to 60 hours, respectively. Reductions in the concentration of natural anticoagulants before the clotting factors are depleted can lead to a paradoxical hypercoagulable state during the first few days of warfarin therapy. It is for this reason that patients with acute thrombosis should receive a fast-acting anticoagulant (heparin, LMWH, or fondaparinux) while transitioning to warfarin therapy.[5,20,29]

Warfarin is a racemic mixture of two isomers, the S and the R forms. The S-isomer is two to five times more potent than the R-isomer. Both isomers are extensively bound to albumin. The two isomers are metabolized in the liver via several isoenzymes including cytochrome P-450 (CYP) 1A2, 2C9, 2C19, 2C18, and 3A4 (Fig. 10–8). Hepatic metabolism of warfarin varies greatly among patients, leading to very large interpatient differences in dose requirements and genetic variations in these isoenzymes; specifically, polymorphisms in the CYP2C9*2, CYP2C9*3 genotype result in significantly lower warfarin dose requirement to achieve a therapeutic response, and VKORC1 haplotype mutations can result in hereditary warfarin resistance and increased warfarin requirements.[5] Several algorithms that incorporate CYP2C9 genotype and the VKORC1 haplotype with other patient characteristics to predict warfarin maintenance dosing requirements have been developed and are being tested in large populations. Whether pharmacogenomic-based dosing will improve clinical outcomes has yet to be determined and is not recommended at this time, but it does hold promise for a more personalized approach to warfarin dosing.[5,46]

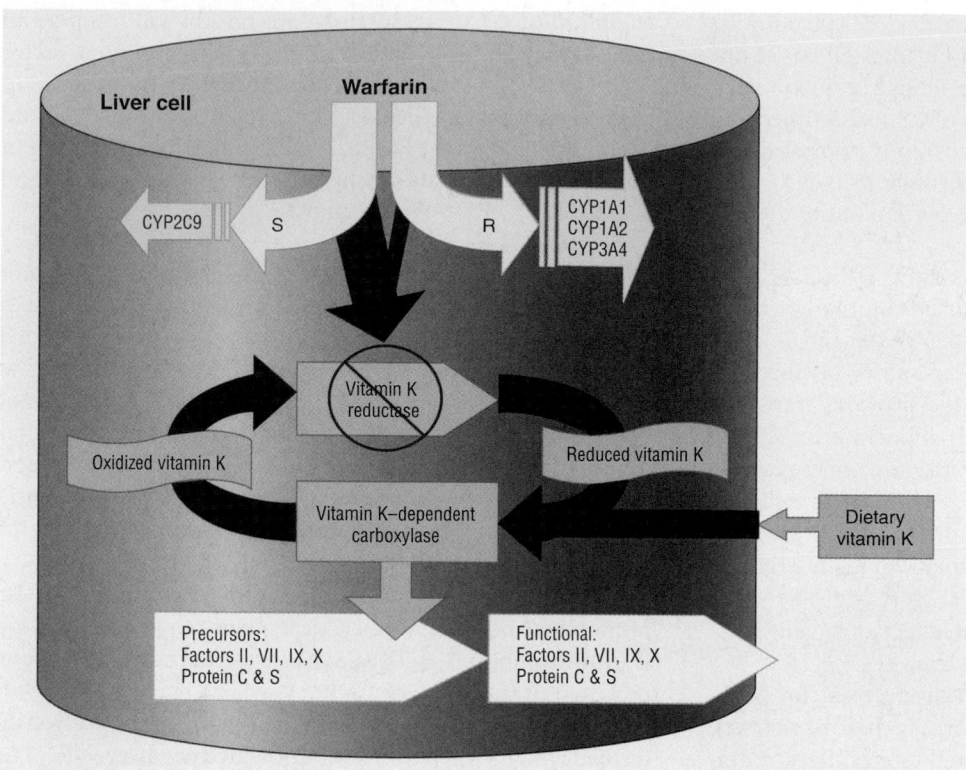

FIGURE 10–8. Pharmacologic activity and metabolism of warfarin. (CYP, cytochrome P-450 isoenzyme.) (From Haines ST, Witt DM, Nutescu EA. Venous thromboembolism. In: DiPiro JT, Talbert RL, Yee GC, et al., eds. Pharmacotherapy: A Pathophysiologic Approach, 7th ed. New York: McGraw-Hill; 2008:347.)

Warfarin does not follow linear kinetics. Small dose adjustments can lead to large changes in anticoagulant response. The dose of warfarin is determined by each patient's individual response to therapy and the desired intensity of anticoagulation. In addition to hepatic metabolism, warfarin dose requirements are influenced by diet, drug–drug interactions, and health status. Therefore, the dose of warfarin must be determined by frequent clinical and laboratory monitoring.[5,20,29] While there are conflicting data regarding the optimal warfarin induction regimen, most patients can start with 5 mg daily, and subsequent doses are determined based on INR response (Fig. 10–9). When initiating therapy, it is difficult to predict the precise warfarin maintenance dose that a patient will require. Patients who are younger (less than 55 years of age) and otherwise healthy can safely use higher warfarin "initiation" doses (e.g., 7.5 or 10 mg). A more conservative "initiation" dose (e.g., 5 mg or less) should be given to elderly patients (greater than 75 years of age), patients with heart failure, liver disease, or poor nutritional status, and patients who are taking interacting medications or are at high risk of bleeding.[5,23] Loading doses of warfarin (e.g., 15 to 20 mg) are not recommended. These large doses can lead to the false impression that a therapeutic INR has been achieved in 2 to 3 days and lead to potential future overdosing.[5] Before initiating therapy, screen the patient for any contraindications to anticoagulation therapy and risk factors for major bleeding (Tables 10–6 and 10–7). In addition, conduct a thorough medication history including the use of prescription and over-the-counter drugs, and any herbal supplements to detect interactions that may affect warfarin dosing requirements. In patients with acute VTE, a rapid-acting anticoagulant (UFH, LMWH, or fondaparinux)

should be overlapped with warfarin for a minimum of 5 days and until the INR is greater than 2 and stable. This is important because the full antithrombotic effect will not be reached until 5 to 7 days or even longer after initiating warfarin therapy.[5,17] The typical maintenance dose of warfarin for most patients will be between 25 and 55 mg per week, although some patients require higher or lower doses. Adjustments in the maintenance warfarin dose should be determined based on the total weekly dose and by reducing or increasing the weekly dose by increments of 5% to 25%. When adjusting the maintenance dose, wait at least 7 days to ensure that a steady state has been attained on the new dose before checking the INR again. Checking the INR too soon can lead to inappropriate dose adjustments and unstable anticoagulation status.[5]

❶ *Warfarin requires frequent laboratory monitoring to ensure optimal outcomes and minimize complications.* The PT is the most frequently used test to monitor warfarin's anticoagulant effect. The PT measures the biological activity of factors II, VII, and X. Due to wide variation in reagent sensitivity, different **thromboplastins** will result in different PT results, potentially leading to inappropriate dosing decisions.[5] In order to standardize result reporting, the World Health Organization (WHO) developed a reference thromboplastin and recommended the INR to monitor warfarin therapy. The INR corrects for the differences in thromboplastin reagents and uses the following formula: $INR = (PT^{Patient}/PT^{Control})^{ISI}$. The International Sensitivity Index (ISI) is a measure of the thromboplastin's responsiveness compared to the WHO reference.[5] The goal or target INR for each patient is based on the indication for warfarin therapy. For the treatment and prevention of VTE, the INR target is

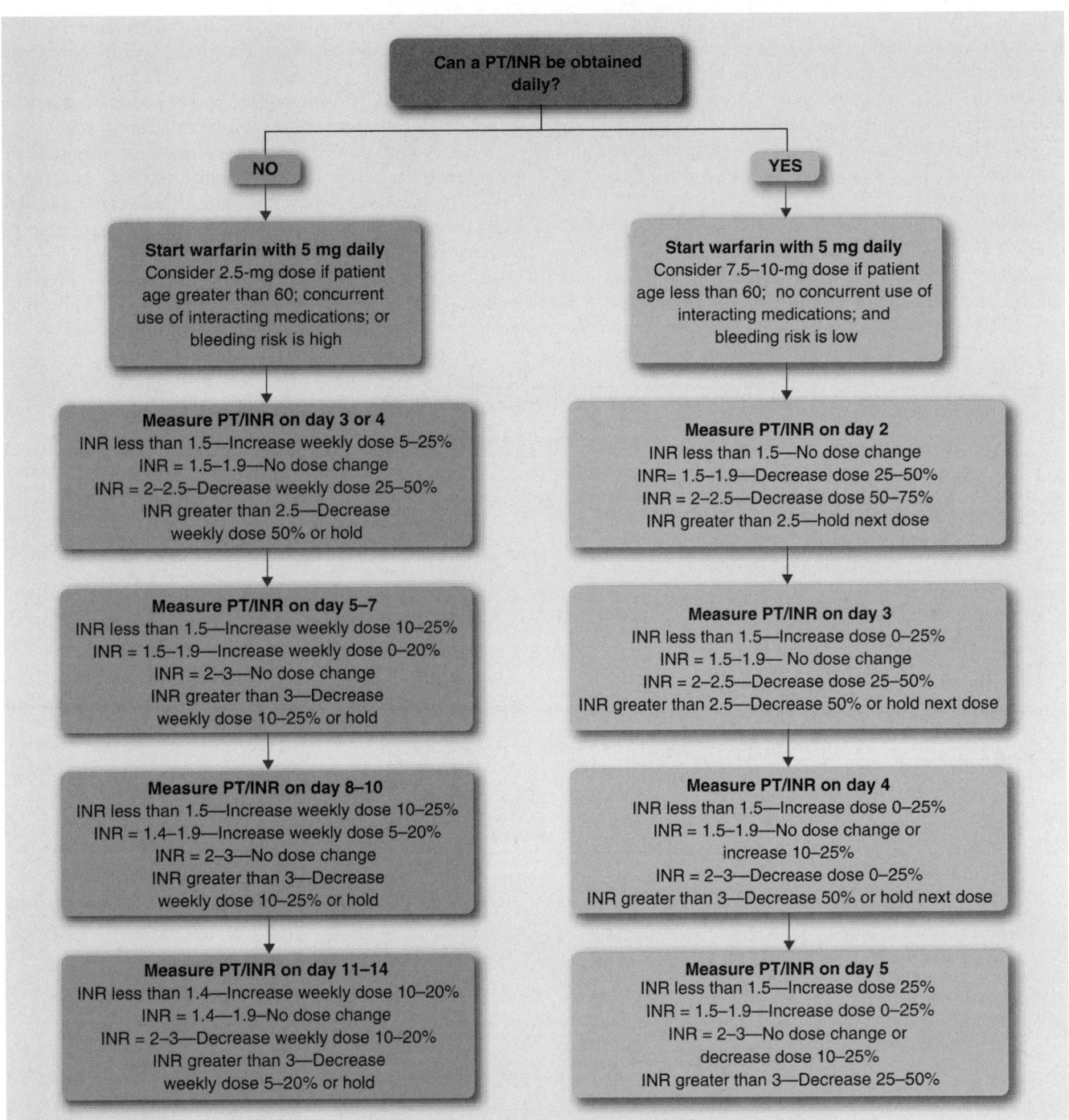

FIGURE 10–9. Initiation of warfarin therapy. (INR, International Normalized Ratio; PT, prothrombin time.) (From Haines ST, Witt DM, Nutescu EA. Venous thromboembolism. In: DiPiro JT, Talbert RL, Yee GC, et al, eds. Pharmacotherapy: A Pathophysiologic Approach, 7th ed. New York: McGraw-Hill; 2008:350.)

2.5 with an acceptable range of 2 to 3. In certain high-risk patients (e.g., certain mechanical heart valves), a higher target INR of 3 with a range of 2.5 to 3.5 is recommended.[5] Before initiating warfarin therapy, a baseline PT/INR and CBC should be obtained. After initiating warfarin therapy, the INR should be monitored at least every 2 to 3 days during the first week of therapy. Once a stable response to therapy is achieved, INR monitoring is performed less frequently, weekly for the first 1 to 2 weeks, then every 2 weeks, and

monthly thereafter.[5,47] At each encounter, the patient should be carefully questioned regarding any factors that may influence the INR result. These factors include adherence to therapy, the use of interacting medications, consumption of vitamin K-rich foods, alcohol use, and general health status. Patients should also be questioned about symptoms related to bleeding and thromboembolic events. Warfarin dose adjustments should take into account not only the INR result, but also patient-related factors that influence the result. Structured anticoagulation therapy management services (anticoagulation clinics) have been demonstrated to improve the efficacy and safety of warfarin therapy when compared to "usual" medical care.[5,47] Some patients engage in self-testing and self-management by using a point of care PT/INR device approved for home use. Highly motivated and well-trained patients are good candidates for self-testing or self-management.[5,47]

❻ *Similar to other anticoagulants, warfarin's primary side effect is bleeding.* Warfarin can "unmask" an existing lesion. The incidence of warfarin-related bleeding appears to be highest during the first few weeks of therapy. The annual incidence of major bleeding ranges from 1% to 10% depending on the quality of warfarin therapy management. Bleeding in the GI tract is most common. Intracranial hemorrhage (ICH) is one of the most serious complications, as it often causes severe disability and death. The intensity of anticoagulation therapy is related to bleeding risk. ● Higher INRs result in higher bleeding risk, and the risk of ICH increases when the INR exceeds 4.[3,5] Instability and wide fluctuations in the INR are also associated with higher bleeding risk. In cases of warfarin overdose or over-anticoagulation, vitamin K may be used to reverse warfarin's effect (Fig. 10–10).[5] Vitamin K can be given by the IV or oral

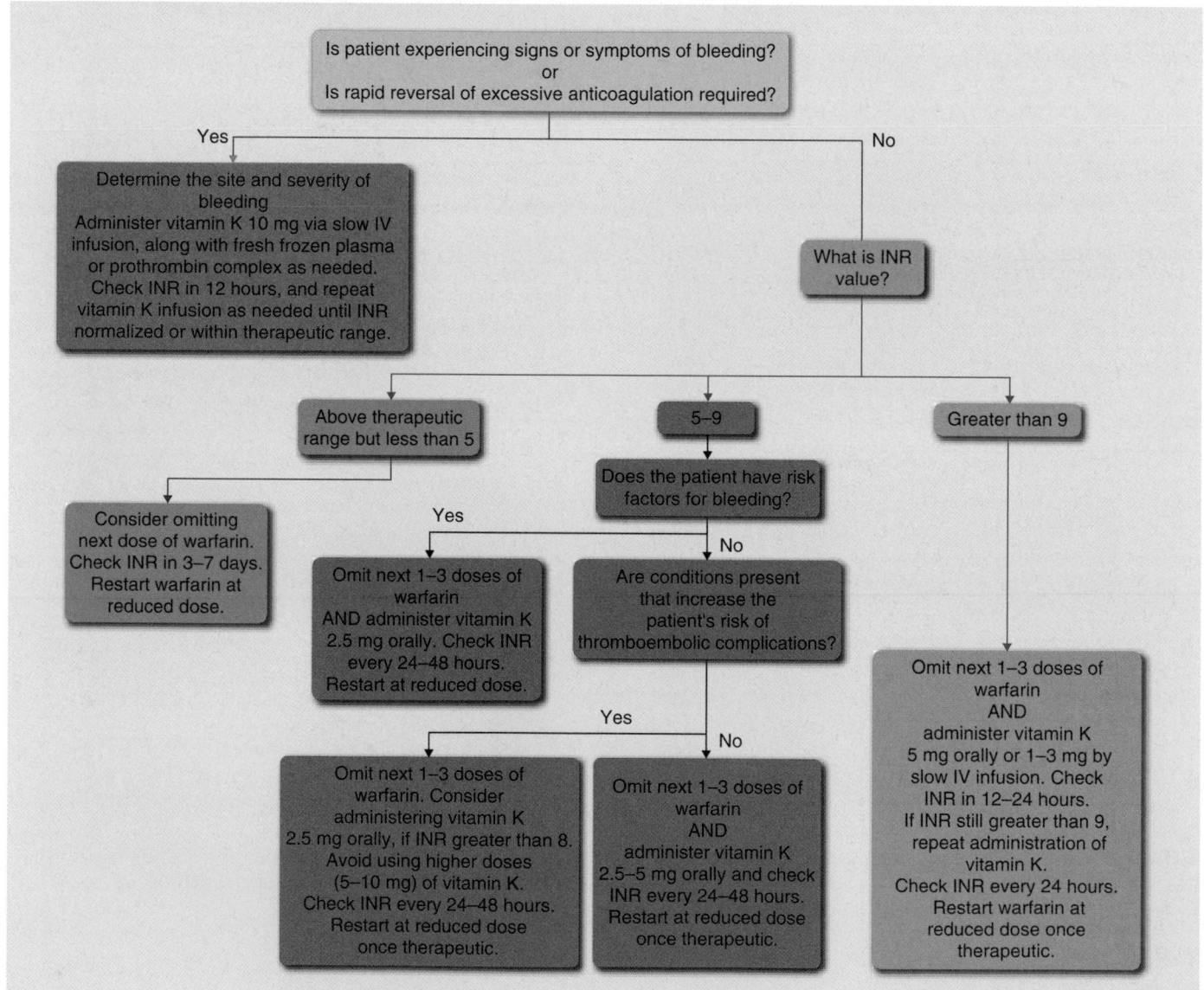

FIGURE 10–10. Management of an elevated INR in patients taking warfarin. Dose reductions should be made by determining the weekly warfarin dose and reducing the weekly dose by 10% to 25% based on the degree of INR elevation. Conditions that increase the risk of thromboembolic complications include history of hypercoagulability disorders (e.g., protein C or S deficiency, presence of antiphospholipid antibodies, antithrombin deficiency, or activated protein C resistance), arterial or venous thrombosis within the previous month, thromboembolism associated with malignancy, mechanical mitral valve in conjunction with atrial fibrillation, previous stroke, poor ventricular function, or coexisting mechanical aortic valve. (INR, International Normalized Ratio.) (From Haines ST, Witt DM, Nutescu EA. Venous thromboembolism. In: DiPiro JT, Talbert RL, Yee GC, et al., eds. Pharmacotherapy: A Pathophysiologic Approach, 7th ed. New York: McGraw-Hill; 2008:353.)

route; the SC route is not recommended. When given SC, vitamin K is erratically absorbed and frequently ineffective. The IV route is reserved for cases of severe warfarin overdose (e.g., INR greater than 20) or major bleeding. Anaphylactoid reactions have been reported with rapid IV administration, therefore slow infusion is recommended. An oral dose of vitamin K will reduce the INR within 24 hours. If the INR is still elevated after 24 hours, another dose of oral vitamin K can be given. The dose of vitamin K should be based on the INR elevation. A dose of 1 to 2.5 mg is sufficient when the INR is between 5 and 9, but 5 mg may be required for INRs greater than 9. Higher doses (e.g., 10 mg) can lead to prolonged warfarin resistance. In cases of life-threatening bleeding, fresh frozen plasma or clotting factor concentrates should be administered, in addition to IV vitamin K. In patients in whom the INR is less than 9 and there is no active bleeding or imminent risk of bleeding, simply withholding warfarin until the INR decreases to within therapeutic range and reducing the weekly dose with more frequent monitoring is appropriate.[5]

Nonhemorrhagic side effects related to warfarin are rare but can be severe when they occur. Warfarin-induced skin necrosis presents as an eggplant-colored skin lesion or a maculopapular rash that can progress to necrotic gangrene. It usually manifests in fatty areas such as the abdomen, buttocks, and breasts. The incidence is less than 0.1%, and it generally appears during the first week of therapy. Patients with protein C or S deficiency or those who receive large loading doses of warfarin are at greatest risk.[5,11] The mechanism is thought to be due to imbalances between procoagulant and anticoagulant proteins early in the course of warfarin therapy. Warfarin-induced purple toe syndrome is another rare side effect; patients present with a purplish discoloration of their toes. If these side effects are suspected, warfarin therapy should be discontinued immediately and an alternative anticoagulant given. There is a theoretical risk that warfarin may cause accelerated bone loss with long-term use, but to date there is no evidence to support this concern. Warfarin is teratogenic and is FDA pregnancy category X. It should be avoided during pregnancy, and women of child-bearing potential should be instructed to use an effective form of contraception. UFH and LMWH are the agents of choice for the treatment of VTE during pregnancy.[5,11]

❽ *Warfarin is prone to numerous clinically significant drug–drug and drug–food interactions* (Tables 10–8, 10–9, and 10–10). Patients on warfarin should be questioned at every encounter to assess for any potential interactions with foods, drugs, herbal products, and nutritional supplements. When an interacting drug is initiated or discontinued, more frequent monitoring should be instituted. In addition, the dose of warfarin can be modified (increased or decreased) in anticipation of the expected impact on the INR.[5,48] Warfarin-related drug interactions can generally be divided into two major categories: pharmacokinetic and pharmacodynamic. Pharmacokinetic interactions are most commonly due to changes in hepatic metabolism or

Table 10–8
Clinically Significant Warfarin Drug Interactions

Increase Anticoagulation Effect (↑ INR)	Decrease Anticoagulation Effect (↓ INR)	Increase Bleeding Risk
Acetaminophen	Amobarbital	Argatroban
Alcohol binge	Butabarbital	Aspirin
Allopurinol	Carbamazepine	Clopidogrel
Amiodarone	Cholestyramine	Danaparoid
Cephalosporins (with MTP side chain)	Dicloxacillin	Dipyridamole
Chloral hydrate	Griseofulvin	LMWHs
Chloramphenicol	Nafcillin	Nonsteroidal anti-inflammatory drugs
Cimetidine	Phenobarbital	Ticlopidine
Ciprofloxacin	Phenytoin	UFH
Clofibrate	Primidone	
Danazol	Rifampin	
Disulfiram	Secobarbital	
Doxycycline	Sucralfate	
Erythromycin	Vitamin K	
Fenofibrate		
Fluconazole		
Fluorouracil		
Fluoxetine		
Fluvoxamine		
Gemfibrozil		
Influenza vaccine		
Isoniazid		
Itraconazole		
Lovastatin		
Metronidazole		
Miconazole		
Moxalactam		
Neomycin		
Norfloxacin		
Ofloxacin		
Omeprazole		
Phenylbutazone		
Piroxicam		
Propafenone		
Propoyxphene		
Quinidine		
Sertraline		
Sulfamethoxazole		
Sulfinpyrazone		
Tamoxifen		
Testosterone		
Vitamin E		
Zafirlukast		

INR, International Normalized Ratio; LMWHs, low–molecular weight heparins; UFH, unfractionated heparin.

binding to plasma proteins. Drugs that affect the CYP2C9, CYP3A4, and CYP1A2 have the greatest impact on warfarin metabolism. Interactions that impact the metabolism of the S-isomer result in greater changes in the INR than interactions affecting the R-isomer. Pharmacodynamic drug interactions enhance or diminish the anticoagulant effect of warfarin, increasing the risk of bleeding or clotting, but may not alter the INR.[5,48] There are increasing reports regarding dietary supplements, nutraceuticals, and

Table 10–9		
Potential Warfarin Interactions With Herbal and Nutritional Products		
Increased Anticoagulation Effect (Increase Bleeding Risk or ↑ INR)		**Decreased Anticoagulation Effect (↓ INR)**
Amica flower	Ginkgo	Coenzyme Q$_{10}$
Angelica root	Horse chestnut	Ginseng
Anise	Licorice root	Green tea
Asafoetida	Lovage root	St. John's wort
Bogbean	Meadowsweet	
Borage seed oil	Onion	
Bromelain	Papain	
Capsicum	Parsley	
Celery	Passionflower herb	
Chamomile	Poplar	
Clove	Quassia	
Danshen	Red clover	
Devil's claw	Rue	
Dong quai	Sweet clover	
Fenugreek	Turmeric	
Feverfew	Vitamin E	
Garlic	Willow bark	
Ginger		

INR, International Normalized Ratio.

Table 10–10			
Vitamin K Content of Select Foods[a]			
Very High (Greater Than 200 mcg)	**High (100–200 mcg)**	**Medium (50–100 mcg)**	**Low (Less Than 50 mcg)**
Brussels sprouts	Basil	Apple, green	Apple, red
Chickpea	Broccoli	Asparagus	Avocado
Collard greens	Canola oil	Cabbage	Beans
Coriander	Chive	Cauliflower	Breads and
Endive	Coleslaw	Mayonnaise	grains
Kale	Cucumber	Pistachios	Carrot
Lettuce, red	(unpeeled)	Squash,	Celery
leaf	Green onion/	summer	Cereal
Parsley	scallion		Coffee
Spinach	Lettuce,		Corn
Swiss chard	butterhead		Cucumber
Tea, black	Mustard greens		(peeled)
Tea, green	Soybean oil		Dairy
Turnip greens			products
Watercress			Eggs
			Fruit (varies)
			Lettuce,
			iceberg
			Meats, fish,
			poultry
			Pasta
			Peanuts
			Peas
			Potato
			Rice
			Tomato

[a]Approximate amount of vitamin K per 100 g (3.5 oz) serving.

vitamins that can interact with warfarin.[49] Patients on warfarin may experience changes in the INR due to fluctuating intake of dietary vitamin K. Patients should be instructed to maintain a consistent diet and avoid large fluctuations in vitamin K intake rather than strictly avoiding vitamin K-rich foods.[49]

▶ Nonpharmacologic

Thrombectomy Most cases of VTE can be successfully treated with anticoagulation. In some cases, removal of the occluding thrombus by surgical intervention may be warranted. Surgical or mechanical thrombectomy can be considered in patients with massive iliofemoral DVT when there is a risk of limb gangrene due to venous occlusion. The procedure can be complicated by recurrence of thrombus formation. In patients who present with massive PE, pulmonary embolectomy can be performed in emergency cases when conservative measures have failed. Patients who are hemodynamically unstable and have a contraindication to thrombolysis are candidates for pulmonary embolectomy. Administer heparin by IV infusion to achieve a therapeutic aPTT during the operation and postoperatively. Thereafter, give warfarin for the usual recommended duration.[17,23]

Vena Cava Interruption IVC interruption is indicated in patients with PE who have a contraindication to anticoagulation therapy and in patients who have recurrent VTE while taking anticoagulation therapy.[17,23] IVC interruption is accomplished by inserting a filter through the internal

Patient Encounter 1, Part 2

KK has been hospitalized for right hip fracture repair. Two weeks after her discharge from the hospital, she presents to the emergency department with complaints of swelling, redness, and pain in her right lower extremity. KK states her symptoms started 3 days ago and have gotten progressively worse. During your interview, the patient states that she was sent home with a prescription for fondaparinux 2.5 mg SC daily. A duplex ultrasound shows a proximal DVT in her right lower extremity. All of her other laboratory values are within normal limits.

Which of KK's symptoms are consistent with an acute DVT?

Design an appropriate treatment plan for KK. Your plan should include acute and chronic therapy—specify the drug(s), dose(s), route, frequency of administration, and duration of each therapy, as well monitoring parameters, patient education, and follow-up plan.

Assuming KK continues to take the prescription and over-the-counter medications listed in her medication history obtained during her hospitalization, should any of these medications be discontinued or changed? If changed, what alternative therapy would you recommend?

Is KK a candidate for outpatient treatment of her DVT?

jugular vein or femoral vein and advancing it into the IVC using ultrasound or fluoroscopic guidance. IVC filters reduce the short-term risk of PE, but this benefit is not sustained in the long term. The incidence of DVT at 1 year after IVC filter insertion is higher when compared to patients without filters. Survival after a PE is no different in patients with filters versus patients without filters.[21] Therefore, anticoagulation therapy should be resumed as soon as possible after filter insertion and continued as long as the filter is in place due to the high risk of DVT.[17] Temporary or removable filters are now increasingly used and are replacing the use of permanent filters.[17]

Compression Stockings PTS occurs in 20% to 50% of patients within 8 years after a DVT. Wearing GCS after a DVT reduces the risk of PTS by as much as 50%. Current guidelines recommend the use of GCS with an ankle pressure of 30 to 40 mm Hg for 2 years after a DVT. To be effective, GCS must fit properly. Traditionally, strict bed rest has been recommended after a DVT, but this approach has now been refuted and patients should be encouraged to ambulate as tolerated.[17,20]

APPROACH TO TREATING PATIENTS WITH VTE

❺ *Once the diagnosis of VTE has been confirmed with an objective test, promptly start anticoagulation therapy in full therapeutic doses. If there is high clinical suspicion of VTE, anticoagulation therapy can be initiated while waiting for the results of diagnostic tests.[17] Initiate therapy with a quick-acting anticoagulant such as UFH (given IV or SC), an LMWH (given SC), or fondaparinux (given SC; Figs. 10–5 and 10–11). In patients with adequate renal function, the LMWHs are preferred over UFH.[17] Recent evidence also supports the use of SC fondaparinux as an alternative option to UFH or LMWH for the initial treatment of VTE.[17] For the long-term treatment phase, warfarin is the preferred approach except for patients with cancer, in whom an LMWH is recommended due to better efficacy in preventing recurrent thromboembolic events. Initiate warfarin on the first day of therapy after the first dose of UFH, LMWH, or fondaparinux is given. Overlap the injectable agent with warfarin therapy for a minimum of 5 days. Warfarin should be dosed to achieve a goal INR range of 2 to 3. Once the INR is stable and above 2, the injectable anticoagulant should be discontinued. Anticoagulation therapy is continued for a minimum of 3 months but should be given longer depending on the underlying etiology of the VTE and the patient's risk factors (Table 10–11).[17,20,23] Use a thrombolytic only if the patient has a massive iliofemoral DVT and is at risk of limb gangrene. In patients with PE, use a thrombolytic if the patient is hemodynamically unstable (i.e., SBP less than 90 mm Hg). If there is a contraindication to anticoagulation therapy or the patient has failed therapy with an anticoagulant, a vena cava filter should be inserted. Encourage early ambulation as tolerated by the patient during the initial treatment phase.[17,20,23]*

Patient Encounter 2, Part 1

BA is a 38-year-old female who presents to the emergency department complaining of chest pain, shortness of breath, and lightheadedness. The patient states that her symptoms started with some mild left calf pain approximately 5 days ago. She started feeling short of breath and experiencing chest pain last evening. She could not sleep and her shortness of breath has gotten progressively worse in the last several hours. BA was hospitalized because she was suspected to have a PE.

PMH: Obesity × 12 years; asthma

FH: Mother died of a stroke; paternal grandmother had clots in her legs

SH: The patient is a school teacher

Current Meds: Albuterol (salbutamol) metered-dose inhaler as needed; ortho-Tri-Cyclen Lo by mouth daily; echinacea one to two tablets by mouth daily as needed; multivitamin one tablet by mouth daily

Allergies: Shellfish, NKDA

PE:

VS: BP 104/64 mm Hg, HR 102, RR 20, T 38°C (100.4°F), wt 96 kg (211 lb), ht 65 in. (165 cm)

Labs: Within normal limits; estimated GFR 101 mL/min

Procedures/Tests

ECG: Normal sinus rhythm

CXR: Slightly enlarged heart

V/Q scan: High probability of PE

What signs and symptoms are consistent with the diagnosis of PE in BA's case? What are the most likely etiologies for PE in this case?

What are appropriate initial and chronic treatment options for BA?

If UFH is chosen as the initial anticoagulation treatment option, what is the goal aPTT?

What is BA's goal INR for warfarin therapy?

How long should BA remain on anticoagulation therapy?

Given the list of medications BA took prior to hospitalization, should any of these medications be discontinued or changed? If changed, what alternative therapy would you recommend?

OUTCOME EVALUATION

• Achieve optimal outcomes by: (a) preventing the occurrence of VTE in patients who are at risk, (b) administering effective treatments in a timely manner to patients who develop VTE, (c) preventing treatment-related complications, and (d) reducing the

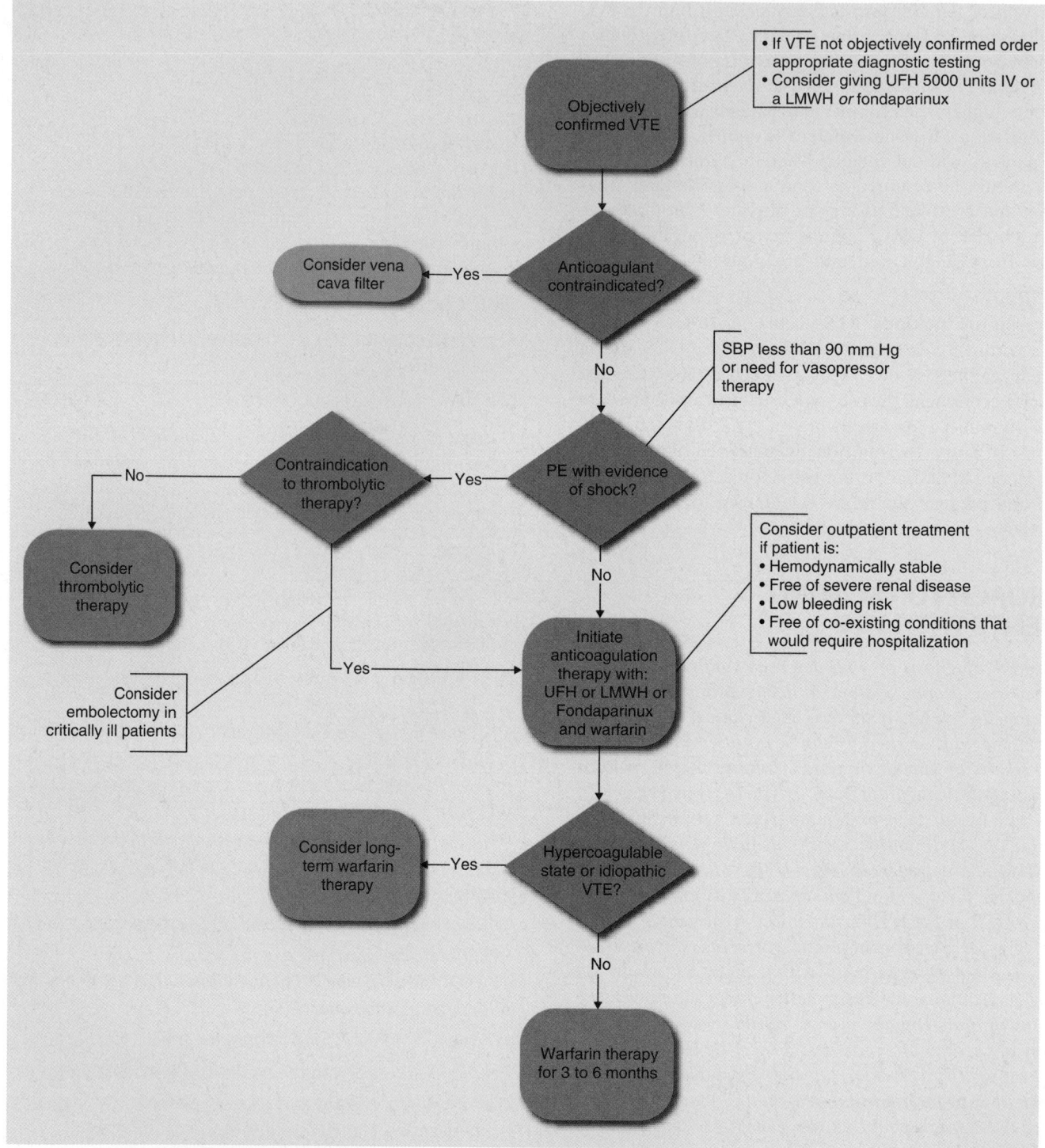

FIGURE 10–11. Treatment of VTE. (LMWH, low–molecular weight heparin; PE, pulmonary embolism; SBP, systolic blood pressure; UFH, unfractionated heparin; VTE, venous thromboembolism.) (From Haines ST, Witt DM, Nutescu EA. Venous thromboembolism. In: DiPiro JT, Talbert RL, Yee GC, et al., eds. Pharmacotherapy: A Pathophysiologic Approach, 7th ed. New York: McGraw-Hill; 2008:357.)

likelihood of long-term complications including recurrent events.

- Given that VTE is often clinically silent and potentially fatal, strategies to increase the widespread use of prophylaxis have the greatest potential to improve patient outcomes. Thus, relying on the early diagnosis and

treatment of VTE is unacceptable because many patients will die before treatment can be initiated.

- Effective VTE prophylaxis programs screen and identify all patients at risk, determine each patient's level of risk, and select and implement regimens that provide sufficient protection for the level of risk.

Table 10–11

Duration of Anticoagulation Therapy for the Treatment of VTE

Patient Characteristics	Drug	Duration of Therapy (Months)	Comments
First episode of VTE secondary to a transient (reversible) risk factor	Warfarin	3	Recommendation applies to both proximal and calf vein thrombosis
First episode, unprovoked VTE	Warfarin	At least 3	After 3 months of therapy, evaluate patient for risk–benefit of long-term therapy
First episode, unprovoked proximal DVT or unprovoked PE		Long term	If risk factors for bleeding are absent and good anticoagulant monitoring is achieved
First episode of VTE and cancer	LMWH	6	LMWH is recommended over warfarin for the initial 6 months Subsequent therapy (beyond the initial 6 months) until cancer is resolved is recommended with warfarin or LMWH
Second episode of unprovoked VTE	Warfarin	Long term	

DVT, deep vein thrombosis; LMWH, low–molecular weight heparins; PE, pulmonary embolism; VTE, venous thromboembolism.

From Ref. 17.

Patient Encounter 2, Part 2

BA is discharged home on warfarin therapy. She was referred to a local area antithrombosis center for monitoring of her oral anticoagulation therapy and has been maintained on warfarin 6 mg daily for the last 3 months. The patient presents today for a routine visit for anticoagulation monitoring and her INR is 8.3. She reports that 6 days ago she was started on metronidazole 500 mg by mouth twice daily, which was prescribed by her primary care physician for a vaginal infection. In addition, the primary care physician told the patient that her thyroid gland was enlarged and ordered some lab tests to determine if she has a thyroid problem. The patient has not heard what the results are. She also reports that her intake of vitamin K-rich foods (spinach, broccoli, and cabbage) has increased significantly over the last month because she is trying to lose weight. BA has no other complaints today and denies any signs or symptoms of bleeding.

What is the most likely explanation for elevated INR in BA's case?

Should BA be given vitamin K? If yes, discuss the dose, route of administration, and an appropriate patient monitoring plan.

How will you manage BA's warfarin therapy? Outline a plan including specific dose changes, timing of monitoring, and patient education.

- Periodically evaluate patients who receive prophylaxis during the course of treatment for signs and symptoms of VTE, such as swelling, pain, warmth, and redness of lower extremities, and for DVT, as well as chest pain, shortness of breath, palpitations, and hemoptysis.

- Providing effective treatment in a timely manner is the primary goal for patients who develop VTE. Treat DVT and PE quickly and aggressively with effective doses of anticoagulant drugs.

- The short-term aim of therapy is to prevent propagation or local extension of the clot, embolization, and death.

- Regularly monitor patients for the development of new symptoms or worsening of existing symptoms.

- Anticoagulant drugs require precise dosing and meticulous monitoring. Closely monitor patients receiving anticoagulant therapy for signs and symptoms of bleeding including epistaxis, hemoptysis, hematuria, bright red blood per rectum, tarry stools, severe headache, and joint pain. If major bleeding occurs, stop therapy immediately and treat the source of bleeding. In addition, closely monitor patients for potential drug–drug and drug–food interactions and adherence with the prescribed regimen.

- The long-term (more than 3 months after the first event) goals of therapy are to prevent complications such as the PTS, pulmonary hypertension, and recurrent VTE.

- Encourage all patients who have had DVT to wear GCS.

- Continue warfarin therapy for an appropriate duration based on the etiology of the initial clot and the presence of ongoing risk factors.

Patient Care and Monitoring

Day 1

1. It is critical to first confirm diagnosis of VTE
   - Clinical assessment: look for risk factors for VTE
   - If DVT symptoms are present, obtain a venous ultrasound
   - If PE is suspected, obtain a V/Q or CT scan
   - D-dimer: this test may be a helpful adjunct to either a venous ultrasound or V/Q scan

2. Obtain baseline laboratory tests. These tests must be obtained prior to initiating anticoagulation therapy:
   - PT and calculated INR
   - aPTT
   - Serum creatinine
   - CBC with platelets

3. Medications:
   - Screen the patient's pharmacy profile for potential drug–drug interactions with anticoagulation therapy
   - Initiate UFH or LMWH or fondaparinux by injection (see Table 10–3 for dosing guidelines)
   - Start warfarin sodium orally every evening (see Fig. 10–9 for dosing guidelines)
   - Start pain medication if necessary (avoid nonsteroidal anti-inflammatory drugs)

4. Patient education:
   - Educate the patient regarding the purpose of therapy and importance of proper monitoring of anticoagulant drugs. Assist the patient to determine an appropriate provider for long-term monitoring of anticoagulation therapy.
   - If LMWH or fondaparinux is selected, teach the patient how to self-administer (if the patient or a family member is unwilling or unable to self-administer, visiting nurse services should be arranged). Initial injection should be administered in the medical office or hospital.
   - Inform patient about the effects of vitamin K-rich foods on warfarin therapy. Moderate intake (less than 500–1,000 mcg) of vitamin K is acceptable. Provide patient with written material regarding vitamin K content of foods.
   - Inform the patient about the potential drug–drug interactions with warfarin, including over-the-counter medications and dietary supplements (Tables 10–8, 10–9, and 10–10). Instruct the patient to call the health care practitioner responsible for monitoring warfarin therapy before starting any new medications or dietary supplements.
   - Instruct the patient regarding nonpharmacologic strategies including elevation of the affected extremity and antiembolic exercises such as flexion/extension of the ankle (for lower extremity VTE) or hand squeezing/relaxation (for upper extremity VTE).

5. Next steps:
   - If the patient is to be treated at home, dispense to the patient a 5- to 7-day supply of prefilled LMWH or fondaparinux syringes in patient-specific dose.
   - If the patient is to be treated with UFH, measure aPTT (or antifactor Xa activity) 6 hours after initiating the IV infusion. Adjust dose if necessary (Table 10–5) and measure aPTT (or antifactor Xa activity) every 6 hours after each dose change until therapeutic. Measure aPTT (or antifactor Xa activity) daily thereafter.
   - Arrange for follow-up and long-term anticoagulation therapy management. Communicate with the patient's primary care physician and/or refer to a local antithrombosis service, if available. If the patient is to be treated primarily in the hospital, these arrangements can be made 1 to 2 days prior to hospital discharge.

6. Document all activities in medical record.

Day 2

1. If the patient is being treated with UFH, remeasure the aPTT, and adjust dose if necessary. If patient is being treated with LMWH or fondaparinux, continue therapy.

2. Interview the patient to determine if there is worsening or new symptoms related to VTE. Ask the patient about overt bruising or bleeding, particularly at the injection site, as well as changes in stool or urine color.

3. Advise the patient to limit physical activity if pain persists and to elevate the extremity; increase activity as tolerated.

4. Document activities in medical record.

Days 3 to 5

1. Measure PT/INR every 1 to 2 days.

2. Interview the patient to determine if there is worsening or new symptoms related to VTE. Inquire about and evaluate patient adherence to therapy. Ask the patient about overt bruising or bleeding, particularly at the injection site, as well as changes in stool or urine color. Advise the patient to limit physical activity if pain persists and to elevate the extremity; increase activity as tolerated. Reinforce previous patient education regarding vitamin K intake and potential drug–drug interactions with warfarin.

3. Hold or adjust warfarin dose as necessary. If the patient is being treated with UFH, measure aPTT daily, and adjust dose if necessary. If the patient is being treated with an LMWH or fondaparinux, continue therapy.

4. Document activities in medical record.

(Continued)

Patient Care and Monitoring *(Continued)*

Days 6 to 8

1. Measure PT/INR every 2 to 3 days. Obtain CBC or platelet count.

2. Interview the patient to determine if there is worsening or new symptoms related to VTE. Inquire about and evaluate patient adherence to therapy. Ask the patient about overt bruising or bleeding, particularly at the injection site, as well as changes in stool or urine color. Advise the patient to limit physical activity if pain persists and to elevate the extremity; increase activity as tolerated. Reinforce previous patient education regarding vitamin K intake and potential drug–drug interactions with warfarin.

3. Hold or adjust warfarin dose as necessary. Discontinue UFH, LMWH, or fondaparinux if INR is greater than 2 on two consecutive occasions. If the patient requires continued treatment with UFH, measure aPTT, and adjust dose if necessary.

4. If the patient is treated with UFH or LMWH and platelet count has dropped by greater than 50% from baseline or is less than $120 \times 10^3/\mu l$, evaluate the patient for HIT.

5. Document activities in medical record.

Days 9 to 14

1. Measure PT/INR every 3 to 5 days.

2. Interview the patient to determine if there is worsening or new symptoms related to VTE. Inquire about and evaluate patient adherence to therapy. Ask the patient about overt bruising or bleeding, particularly at the injection site, as well as changes in stool or urine color. Advise the patient to elevate the extremity and increase activity as tolerated. Reinforce previous patient education regarding vitamin K intake and potential drug–drug interactions with warfarin.

3. Hold or adjust warfarin dose as necessary. Discontinue UFH, LMWH, or fondaparinux if INR is greater than 2 on two consecutive occasions. If the patient requires

continued treatment with UFH, remeasure aPTT, and adjust dose if necessary.

4. Obtain CBC or platelet count. If the patient is treated with UFH or LMWH and platelet count has dropped by more than 50% from baseline or is less than $120 \times 10^3/mm^3$ ($120 \times 10^9/L$), evaluate the patient for HIT.

5. Document activities in medical record.

Days 15 to 90

1. Measure PT/INR every 1 to 4 weeks based on the stability of the INR and patient's health status.

2. Interview the patient to determine if there is worsening or new symptoms related to VTE. Inquire about and evaluate patient adherence to therapy. Ask the patient about overt bruising or bleeding as well as changes in stool or urine color. Encourage the patient to increase activity as tolerated. Reinforce previous patient education regarding vitamin K intake and potential drug–drug interactions with warfarin.

3. Adjust warfarin dose as necessary. Consider restarting LMWH or fondaparinux if INR drops below 1.5.

4. Document activities in medical record.

Three Months and Beyond

1. Measure PT/INR every 1 to 4 weeks based on the stability of the INR and patient's health status.

2. Interview the patient to determine if there is worsening or new symptoms related to VTE. Inquire about and evaluate patient adherence to therapy. Ask the patient about overt bruising or bleeding as well as changes in stool or urine color. Reinforce previous patient education regarding vitamin K intake and potential drug–drug interactions with warfarin.

3. Reevaluate the risks and benefits of continuing warfarin therapy.

4. Document activities in medical record.

Abbreviations Introduced in This Chapter

ABW	Adjusted body weight
ACCP	American College of Chest Physicians
ACT	Activated clotting time
ADP	Adenosine diphosphate
aPTT	Activated partial thromboplastin time
AT	Antithrombin
BMI	Body mass index
CrCl	Creatinine clearance
CYP	Cytochrome P-450 isoenzyme
DTI	Direct thrombin inhibitor
DVT	Deep vein thrombosis
ESR	Erythrocyte sedimentation rate
GCS	Graduated compression stockings
GFR	Glomerular filtration rate
GP	Glycoprotein
HCII	Heparin cofactor II
HIT	Heparin-induced thrombocytopenia
HK	High–molecular weight kininogen
IBW	Ideal body weight
ICH	Intracranial hemorrhage
IM	Intramuscular
INR	International Normalized Ratio
IPC	Intermittent pneumatic compression (device)
ISI	International Sensitivity Index
IVC	Inferior vena cava

LMWH	Low-molecular weight heparin
PAF	Platelet activating factor
PAI-1	Plasminogen activator inhibitor-1
PCI	Percutaneous coronary intervention
PE	Pulmonary embolism
PF-4	Platelet factor-4
PGG/PGH	Prostaglandins
PLA	Phospholipase A
PT	Prothrombin time
PTS	Post-thrombotic syndrome
SBP	Systolic blood pressure
SC	Subcutaneous
SERM	Selective estrogen receptor modulator
TFPI	Tissue factor pathway inhibitor
t-PA	Tissue plasminogen activator
TS	Thromboxane synthetase
TXA	Thromboxane A
UFH	Unfractionated heparin
u-PA	Urokinase plasminogen activator
V/Q	Ventilation/perfusion (scan)
VTE	Venous thromboembolism
vWF	von Willebrand's factor

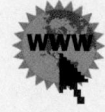 Self-assessment questions and answers are available at *http://www.mhpharmacotherapy.com/pp.html.*

REFERENCES

1. Turpie AGG, Chin BSP, Lip GYH. Venous thromboembolism: Pathophysiology, clinical features, and prevention. BMJ 2002;325:887–890.
2. Geerts WH, Bergqvist D, Pineo GF, et al. Prevention of venous thromboembolism: American College of Chest Physicians Evidence-Based Clinical Practice Guidelines, 8th ed. Chest 2008;133:381S–453S.
3. Schulman S, Beyth RJ, Kearon C, Levine MN; American College of Chest Physicians. Hemorrhagic complications of anticoagulant and thrombolytic treatment: American College of Chest Physicians Evidence-Based Clinical Practice Guidelines, 8th ed. Chest 2008;133:257S–298S.
4. Hirsh J, Bauer KA, Donati MB, et al. Parenteral anticoagulants: American College of Chest Physicians Evidence-Based Clinical Practice Guidelines, 8th ed. Chest 2008;133:141S–159S.
5. Ansell J, Hirsh J, Hylek E, et al. Pharmacology and management of the vitamin K antagonists: American College of Chest Physicians Evidence-Based Clinical Practice Guidelines, 8th ed. Chest 2008;133:160S–198S.
6. Haines ST, Nutescu EA. Current and emerging treatment options for venous thrombosis: A case discussion. Am J Health Syst Pharm 2005;62:593–605.
7. Spencer FA, Emery C, Lessard D, et al. The Worcester venous thromboembolism study: A population-based study of the clinical epidemiology of venous thromboembolism. J General Intern Med 2006;21:722–727.
8. Johnson CM, Mureebe L, Silver D. Hypercoagulable states: A review. Vasc Endovascular Surg 2005;39:123–133.
9. Khorana AA. The NCCN Clinical Practice Guidelines on venous thromboembolic disease: Strategies for improving VTE prophylaxis in hospitalized cancer patients. Oncologist 2007;12:1361–1370.
10. Canonico M, Plu-Bureau G, Lowe GDO, Scarabin P-Y. Hormone replacement therapy and risk of venous thromboembolism in postmenopausal women: Systematic review and meta-analysis. BMJ 2008; 336:1227–1231.
11. Bates SM, Greer IA, Pabinger I, Sofaer S, Hirsh J. American College of Chest Physicians. Venous thromboembolism, thrombophilia, antithrombotic therapy, and pregnancy: American College of Chest Physicians Evidence-Based Clinical Practice Guidelines, 8th ed. Chest 2008;133:844S–886S.
12. Aird WC. Coagulation. Crit Care Med 2005;33:S485–S487.
13. Cesarman-Maus G, Hajjar KA. Molecular mechanisms of fibrinolysis. Br J Haematol 2005;129:307–321.
14. Kearon C. Natural history of venous thromboembolism. Circulation 2003;107:I22–I30.
15. Wells PS, Owen C, Doucette S, Fergusson D, Tran H. Does this patient have deep vein thrombosis? JAMA 2006;295:199–207.
16. Sinert R, Foley M. Clinical assessment of the patient with a suspected pulmonary embolism. Ann Emerg Med 2008;52:76–79.
17. Kearon C, Kahn SR, Agnelli G, et al. Antithrombotic therapy for venous thromboembolic disease: American College of Chest Physicians Evidence-Based Clinical Practice Guidelines, 8th ed. Chest 2008;133:454S–545S.
18. Kanne JP, Lalani TA. Role of computed tomography and magnetic resonance imaging for deep venous thrombosis and pulmonary embolism. Circulation 2004;109:I15–I21.
19. Zierler BK. Ultrasonography and diagnosis of venous thromboembolism. Circulation 2004;109:I9–I14.
20. Bates SM, Ginsberg JS. Clinical practice. Treatment of deep-vein thrombosis. N Engl J Med 2004;351:268–277.
21. Decousus H, Leizorovicz A, Parent F, et al. A clinical trial of vena caval filters in the prevention of pulmonary embolism in patients with proximal deep-vein thrombosis. N Engl J Med 1998;338:409–415.
22. Turpie AG, Bauer KA, Eriksson BI, Lassen MR. Fondaparinux vs enoxaparin for the prevention of venous thromboembolism in major orthopedic surgery: A meta-analysis of 4 randomized double-blind studies. Arch Intern Med 2002;162:1833–1840.
23. Buller HR, Sohne M, Middeldorp S. Treatment of venous thromboembolism. J Thromb Haemost 2005;3:1554–1560.
24. Nutescu EA. Emerging options in the treatment of venous thromboembolism. Am J Health Syst Pharm 2004;61:S12–S17.
25. Watson LI, Armon MP. Thrombolysis for acute deep vein thrombosis. Cochrane Database Syst Rev 2004:CD002783.
26. Tapson VF. Acute pulmonary embolism. N Engl J Med 2008;358:1037–1052.
27. Agnelli G, Becattini C, Kirschstein T. Thrombolysis vs heparin in the treatment of pulmonary embolism: A clinical outcome-based meta-analysis. Arch Intern Med 2002;162:2537–2541.
28. Wood KE. Major pulmonary embolism: Review of a pathophysiologic approach to the golden hour of hemodynamically significant pulmonary embolism. Chest 2002;121:877–905.
29. Nutescu EA, Shapiro NL, Chevalier A, Amin AN. A pharmacologic overview of current and emerging anticoagulants. Cleve Clin J Med 2005;72(Suppl 1):S2–S6.
30. Raschke RA, Reilly BM, Guidry JR, et al. The weight-based heparin dosing nomogram compared with a "standard care" nomogram. Ann Intern Med 1993;119:874–881.
31. Segal JB, Streiff MB, Hofmann LV, et al. Management of venous thromboembolism: A systematic review for a practice guideline. Ann Intern Med 2007;146(3):211–222.
32. Kearon C, Ginsberg JS, Julian JA, et al. Comparison of fixed-dose weight-adjusted unfractionated heparin and low-molecular-weight heparin for acute treatment of venous thromboembolism. JAMA 2006;296(8):935–948.
33. Olson JD, Arkin CF, Brandt JT, et al. College of American Pathologists Conference XXXI on laboratory monitoring of anticoagulation therapy. Laboratory monitoring of unfractionated heparin therapy. Arch Pathol Lab Med 1998;122:782–788.
34. Monagle P, Chalmers E, Chan A, et al. Antithrombotic therapy in neonates and children: American College of Chest Physicians Evidence-Based Clinical Practice Guidelines, 8th ed. Chest 2008;133:887S–968S.

35. Nutescu EA, Wittkowsky AK, Dobesh PP, Hawkins DW, Dager WE. Choosing the appropriate antithrombotic agent for the prevention and treatment of VTE: A case-based approach. Ann Pharmacother 2006;40(9):1558–1571.

36. Akl EA, Rohilla S, Barba M, et al. Anticoagulation for the initial treatment of venous thromboembolism in patients with cancer. Cochrane Database Syst Rev 2008(1):CD006649.

37. Nutescu EA. Assessing, preventing, and treating venous thromboembolism: Evidence-based approaches. Am J Health Syst Pharm 2007;64(11 Suppl 7):S5–S13.

38. Scarvelis D, Wells PS. Diagnosis and treatment of deep-vein thrombosis. CMAJ 2006;175(9):1087–1092.

39. Laposata M, Green D, Van Cott EM, et al. College of American Pathologists Conference XXXI on laboratory monitoring of anticoagulant therapy: The clinical use and laboratory monitoring of low-molecular-weight heparin, danaparoid, hirudin and related compounds, and argatroban. Arch Pathol Lab Med 1998;122:799–807.

40. Duhl AJ, Paidas MJ, Ural SH, et al., Pregnancy and Thrombosis Working Group. Antithrombotic therapy and pregnancy: Consensus report and recommendations for prevention and treatment of venous thromboembolism and adverse pregnancy outcomes. Am J Obstet Gynecol 2007;197(5):457.e1–e21.

41. Weitz J, Hirsh J, Samama MM. New antithrombotic drugs: American College of Chest Physicians Evidence-Based Clinical Practice Guidelines, 8th ed. Chest 2008;133:234S–256S.

42. Gulseth MP, Michaud J, Nutescu EA. Rivaroxaban: An oral direct inhibitor of factor Xa. Am J Health Syst Pharm 2008;65(16)1520–1529.

43. Buller HR, Davidson BL, Decousus H, et al. Subcutaneous fondaparinux versus intravenous unfractionated heparin in the initial treatment of pulmonary embolism. N Engl J Med 2003;349:1695–1702.

44. Buller HR, Davidson BL, Decousus H, et al. Fondaparinux or enoxaparin for the initial treatment of symptomatic deep venous thrombosis: A randomized trial. Ann Intern Med 2004;140:867–873.

45. Nutescu EA, Shapiro NL, Chevalier A. New anticoagulant agents: Direct thrombin inhibitors. Cardiol Clin 2008;26(2):169–187.

46. Lenzini PA, Grice GR, Milligan PE, et al. Laboratory and clinical outcomes of pharmacogenetic vs. clinical protocols for warfarin initiation in orthopedic patients. J Thromb Haemost 2008;6(10):1655–1662.

47. Garcia DA, Witt DM, Hylek E, et al. Delivery of optimized anticoagulant therapy: Consensus statement from the Anticoagulation Forum. Ann Pharmacother 2008;42(7):979–988.

48. Holbrook AMMDPMF, Pereira JAM, Labiris RP, et al. Systematic overview of warfarin and its drug and food interactions. Arch Intern Med 2005;165:1095–1106.

49. Nutescu EA, Shapiro NL, Ibrahim S, West P. Warfarin and its interactions with foods, herbs and other dietary supplements. Expert Opin Drug Saf 2006;5(3):433–451.

11 Stroke

Susan R. Winkler

LEARNING OBJECTIVES

Upon completion of the chapter, the reader will be able to:

1. Understand the types of cerebrovascular disease including transient ischemic attack, cerebral infarction, and cerebral hemorrhage.

2. Understand the pathophysiology of cerebral ischemia and cerebral hemorrhage.

3. Identify the modifiable and nonmodifiable risk factors associated with ischemic stroke and hemorrhagic stroke.

4. Identify risk factors for ischemic stroke in a patient and provide the appropriate patient education.

5. Discuss the various treatment options for acute ischemic stroke and hemorrhagic stroke.

6. Determine whether thrombolytic therapy is indicated in a patient with acute ischemic stroke.

7. Develop an appropriate patient-specific therapeutic plan for acute ischemic stroke.

8. Develop an appropriate therapeutic plan for the outpatient management of a patient with ischemic stroke, including an appropriate agent to prevent stroke recurrence.

KEY CONCEPTS

❶ Strokes can either be ischemic (88%) or hemorrhagic (12%).

❷ Ischemic stroke is the abrupt development of a focal neurologic deficit that occurs due to inadequate blood supply to an area of the brain. Most often, this is due to a thrombotic or embolic arterial occlusion leading to cerebral infarction.

❸ Hemorrhagic stroke is a result of bleeding into the brain and other spaces within the CNS and includes subarachnoid hemorrhage (SAH), intracerebral hemorrhage (ICH), and subdural hematomas.

❹ There are two main classifications of cerebral ischemic events: transient ischemic attacks and cerebral infarction.

❺ A major goal in the long-term treatment of ischemic stroke involves the prevention of a recurrent stroke through the reduction and modification of risk factors.

❻ All patients should have a brain CT scan or MRI scan to differentiate an ischemic stroke from a hemorrhagic stroke, as the treatment will differ accordingly and thrombolytic (fibrinolytic) therapy must be avoided until a hemorrhagic stroke is ruled out.

❼ In carefully selected patients, alteplase is effective in limiting the infarct size and protecting brain tissue from ischemia and cell death by restoring blood flow. Treatment should preferably be given within 3 hours and not more than 4.5 hours after symptom onset. Earlier treatment is preferred due to improved outcomes.

❽ Early aspirin (ASA) therapy with an initial dose of 50 to 325 mg is recommended in most patients with acute ischemic stroke within 48 hours after stroke onset.

❾ Selection of the initial antiplatelet agent for secondary prevention of ischemic stroke should be individualized. Clopidogrel and the combination of extended-release dipyridamole and immediate-release ASA are preferred over ASA monotherapy.

❿ There is no proven treatment for ICH. Management is based on neurointensive care treatment and prevention of complications. Oral nimodipine is recommended in SAH to prevent delayed cerebral ischemia.

EPIDEMIOLOGY

Cerebrovascular disease (CVD), or stroke, is the third leading cause of death in the United States and the second most common cause of death worldwide. Approximately 780,000 strokes occur in the United States each year. New strokes account for 600,000 of this total, while recurrent strokes account for the remaining 180,000 strokes each year. Stroke is the leading cause of long-term disability in adults, with 90% of survivors having residual deficits. Moderate to severe disability is seen in 70% of survivors. The American Heart Association estimates that there are over 4.7 million survivors of stroke in the United States. The societal impact and economic burden is great, with costs exceeding $65 billion per year in the United States. Stroke mortality has declined due to improved recognition and treatment of risk factors; however, risk factor management is still inadequate. Stroke incidence increases with age, especially after age 55, resulting in an increased stroke incidence due to aging of the population.[1]

ETIOLOGY

❶ *Strokes can either be ischemic (88% of all strokes) or hemorrhagic (12% of all strokes).* Figure 11–1 provides a classification of stroke by mechanism. ❷ *Ischemic stroke is the abrupt development of a focal neurologic deficit that occurs due to inadequate blood supply to an area of the brain. Most often, this is due to a thrombotic or embolic arterial occlusion leading to cerebral infarction.* A thrombotic occlusion occurs when a thrombus forms inside an artery in the brain. An embolism refers to a clot originating either inside or outside of the cerebral vessels in which a piece of the clot breaks loose and is carried either further through or into the cerebral vessels until it lodges causing occlusion. An outside source of emboli is often the heart causing cardioembolic stroke.

❸ *Hemorrhagic stroke is a result of bleeding into the brain and other spaces within the CNS and includes subarachnoid hemorrhage (SAH), intracerebral hemorrhage (ICH), and subdural hematomas.* SAH results from sudden bleeding into the space between the inner layer and middle layer of the meninges, most often due to trauma or rupture of a cerebral aneurysm or arteriovenous malformation (AVM). ICH is bleeding directly into the brain parenchyma, often as a result of chronic, uncontrolled hypertension. Subdural hematomas result from bleeding under the dura which covers the brain and most often occur as a result of head trauma.

CLASSIFICATION

Cerebral Ischemic Events

❹ *There are two main classifications of cerebral ischemic events: transient ischemic attack (TIA) and cerebral infarction.* A TIA is a temporary reduction in perfusion to a focal region of the brain causing a short-lived disturbance of function. TIAs have a rapid onset (5 minutes) and short duration (2–15 minutes, up to 24 hours). The symptoms vary depending on the area of the brain affected; however, no deficit remains after the attack. The classic definition of TIA is based on symptom duration of less than 24 hours, while symptoms lasting 24 hours or greater have been categorized as cerebral infarction. Improved brain imaging techniques have revealed that clinical symptoms lasting greater than 1 hour but less than 24 hours are often cerebral infarction. For this reason, it has been proposed that the definition of TIA be changed to include clinical symptoms lasting less than

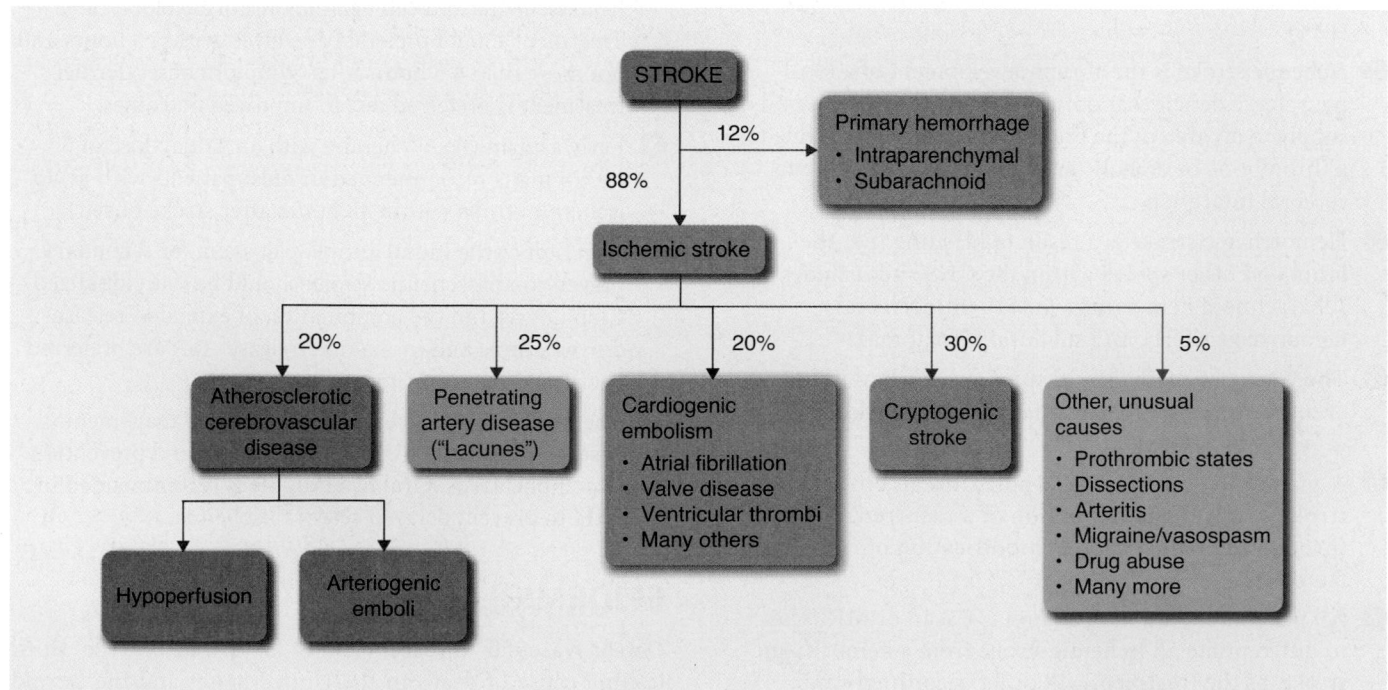

FIGURE 11–1. Classification of stroke. (From Fagan SC, Hess DC. Stroke. In: DiPiro JT, Talbert RL, Yee GC, et al., eds. Pharmacotherapy: A Pathophysiologic Approach. 7th ed. New York: McGraw-Hill; 2008: 374, with permission.)

1 hour with no evidence of cerebral infarction. A TIA may be the only warning of an impending stroke, with the greatest risk occurring in the first week. Cerebral infarction is similar to a TIA; however, symptoms last longer than 24 hours, and in 90% of patients residual deficits remain after the event.

Hemorrhagic Events

A sudden severe headache, nausea and vomiting, and photophobia may be the first signs and symptoms of hemorrhagic stroke. Neck pain and nuchal rigidity may also be experienced at the time of the hemorrhage. Patients may complain that the headache is "the worst headache of my life," especially if the cause is a SAH. It is important to note that a diagnosis of the type of stroke cannot be made solely on signs and symptoms, as overlap occurs between the types of stroke.

Risk Factors

Assessment of risk factors for ischemic stroke as well as for hemorrhagic stroke is an important component of the

Table 11–1
Nonmodifiable and Modifiable Risk Factors for Ischemic Stroke

Nonmodifiable Factors
- Age (greater than 55 years of age)
- Gender (males greater than females)
- Race and ethnicity (African American, Hispanic, or Asian/Pacific Islander)
- Heredity
- Low birth weight

Modifiable Factors
- Hypertension (single most important risk factor)
- Cardiac disease
  - Atrial fibrillation (most important and treatable cardiac cause of stroke)
  - Mitral stenosis
  - Mitral annular calcification
  - Left atrial enlargement
  - Structural abnormalities such as atrial-septal aneurysm
  - MI
- Transient ischemic attacks or prior stroke (major independent risk factor)
- Diabetes (independent risk factor)
- Dyslipidemia
- Lifestyle factors
  - Cigarette smoking
  - Excessive alcohol use
  - Physical inactivity
  - Obesity
  - Diet
  - Cocaine and IV drug use
  - Low socioeconomic status
- Increased hematocrit
- Sickle cell disease
- Elevated homocysteine level (still under study, but may be related to stroke risk)
- Migraine (risk not clear)
- Asymptomatic carotid stenosis
- Oral contraceptive use (with estrogen content greater than 50 mcg)

MI, myocardial infarction.

diagnosis and treatment of patients. ❺ *A major goal in the long-term treatment of ischemic stroke involves the prevention of a recurrent stroke through the reduction and modification of risk factors.* This is also a major focus of primary prevention (prevention of the first stroke). Risk factors for ischemic stroke can be divided into modifiable and nonmodifiable. Table 11–1 provides a list of risk factors for ischemic stroke. Every patient should have risk factors assessed and treated, if possible, as management of risk factors can decrease the occurrence and/or recurrence of stroke.[2]

Nonmodifiable risk factors include age, gender, race/ethnicity, and heredity. Ischemic stroke risk is increased in those greater than 55 years of age, in men, and in African Americans, Hispanics, and Asian Pacific Islanders. It is also increased in those with a family history of stroke. Modifiable risk factors include a number of treatable disease states and lifestyle factors that can greatly influence overall stroke risk. Hypertension is one of the major risk factors for both ischemic and hemorrhagic stroke. For ICH specifically, hypertension has been shown to increase risk by a factor of 3.68.[3] Other risk factors for hemorrhagic stroke include trauma, cigarette smoking, cocaine use, heavy alcohol use, and cerebral aneurysm and AVM rupture.

PATHOPHYSIOLOGY

Ischemic Stroke

In ischemic stroke, there is an interruption of the blood supply to an area of the brain either due to thrombus formation or an embolism. Loss of cerebral blood flow results in tissue hypoperfusion, tissue hypoxia, and cell death. Lipid deposits in the vessel wall cause turbulent blood flow and lead to vessel injury, exposing vessel collagen to blood. This vessel injury initiates the platelet aggregation process due to the exposed subendothelium. Platelets release adenosine diphosphate (ADP), which causes platelet aggregation and consolidation of the platelet plug. Thromboxane A_2 is released, contributing to platelet aggregation and vasoconstriction. The vessel injury also activates the coagulation cascade, which leads to thrombin production. Thrombin converts fibrinogen to fibrin, leading to clot formation as fibrin molecules, platelets, and blood cells aggregate. Refer to Figures 7–3, 10–3, and 10–4 for a depiction of these processes.

After the initial event, secondary events occur at the cellular level that contribute to cell death. Regardless of the initiating event, the cellular processes that follow may be similar. Excitatory amino acids such as glutamate accumulate within the cells, causing intracellular calcium accumulation. Inflammation occurs and oxygen free radicals are formed resulting in the common pathway of cell death.

There is often a core of ischemia containing unsalvageable brain cells. Surrounding this core is an area termed the ischemic penumbra. In this area cells are still salvageable; however, this is a time-sensitive endeavor. Without restoration of adequate perfusion, cell death continues throughout a larger area of the brain ultimately leading to neurologic deficits. No agents have been shown to be effective at providing neuroprotection at this time.

Hemorrhagic Stroke

● The pathophysiology of hemorrhagic stroke is not as well studied as that of ischemic stroke; however, it is more complex than previously thought. Much of the process is related to the presence of blood in the brain tissue and/or surrounding spaces resulting in compression. The hematoma that forms may continue to grow and enlarge after the initial bleed and early growth of the hematoma is associated with a poor outcome. Brain tissue swelling and injury is a result of inflammation caused by thrombin and other blood products. This can lead to increased intracranial pressure (ICP) and herniation.[4,5]

DESIRED TREATMENT OUTCOMES

The short-term treatment goals for acute ischemic stroke include reducing secondary brain damage by re-establishing and maintaining adequate perfusion to marginally ischemic areas of the brain and to protect these areas from the effects of ischemia (i.e., neuroprotection). The long-term treatment goals include prevention of a recurrent stroke through reduction and modification of risk factors and by use of appropriate treatments.

Patient Encounter, Part 1

GR is a 68-year-old, 64 kg African American male who presents to the emergency department with dizziness and loss of speech that began 1 hour ago. His past medical history is significant for hypertension, diabetes mellitus, dyslipidemia, and benign prostatic hypertrophy (BPH). Social history is significant for smoking one pack per day for the last 38 years. Current medications include metoprolol 50 mg twice daily, insulin NPH 20 units twice daily, and simvastatin 20 mg daily.

What signs and symptoms does GR have that are suggestive of stroke?

What nonmodifiable and modifiable risk factors does GR have for acute ischemic stroke?

Clinical Presentation and Diagnosis of Stroke

General

- The patient may not be able to reliably report the history owing to cognitive or language deficits. A reliable history may have to come from a family member or another witness.

Symptoms

- The patient may complain of weakness on one side of the body, inability to speak, loss of vision, vertigo, or falling. Stroke patients may complain of headache; however, with hemorrhagic stroke, the headache can be severe.

Signs

- Patients usually have multiple signs of neurologic dysfunction, and the specific deficits are determined by the area of the brain involved.
- Hemiparesis or monoparesis occur commonly, as does a hemisensory deficit.
- Patients with vertigo and double vision are likely to have posterior circulation involvement.
- Aphasia is seen commonly in patients with anterior circulation strokes.
- Patients may also suffer from dysarthria, visual field defects, and altered levels of consciousness.

Laboratory Tests

- There are no specific laboratory tests for stroke.

- Tests for hypercoagulable states, such as protein C deficiency and antiphospholipid antibody, should be done only when the cause of stroke cannot be determined based on the presence of well-known risk factors for stroke.

Other Diagnostic Tests

- A CT scan of the head will reveal an area of hyperintensity (white) identifying that a hemorrhage has occurred. The CT scan will either be normal or hypointense (dark) in an area where an infarction has occurred. It may take 24 hours (and rarely longer) to reveal the area of infarction on a CT scan.
- MRI of the head will reveal areas of ischemia earlier and with better resolution than a CT scan. Diffusion-weighted imaging can reveal an evolving infarct within minutes.
- Carotid Doppler studies will determine whether the patient has a high degree of stenosis in the carotid arteries supplying blood to the brain (extracranial disease).
- The ECG will determine whether the patient has atrial fibrillation, which is a major risk factor for stroke.
- A transthoracic echocardiogram will identify whether there are heart valve abnormalities or problems with wall motion resulting in emboli to the brain.

Short-term treatment goals for hemorrhagic stroke include rapid neurointensive care treatment to maintain adequate oxygenation, breathing, and circulation. Management of increased ICP and blood pressure (BP) are important in the acute setting. Long-term management includes prevention of complications and prevention of a recurrent bleed and delayed cerebral ischemia.

Prevention of long-term disability and death related to the stroke are important regardless of stroke type.

GENERAL APPROACH TO TREATMENT

❻ *All patients should have a brain CT scan or MRI scan to differentiate an ischemic stroke from a hemorrhagic stroke, as the treatment will differ accordingly and thrombolytic (fibrinolytic) therapy must be avoided until a hemorrhagic stroke is ruled out.* A CT scan is the most important diagnostic test in patients with acute stroke. For those with an ischemic stroke, an evaluation should be done to determine the appropriateness of reperfusion therapy. In hemorrhagic stroke, a surgical evaluation should be completed to assess the need for surgical clipping of an aneurysm or other procedure to control the bleed and prevent rebleeding and other complications. Figure 11–2 provides an algorithm for the initial management of the acute stroke patient.

TREATMENT OF ACUTE ISCHEMIC STROKE

Acute ischemic stroke is a medical emergency. Identification of the time and manner of stroke onset is an important

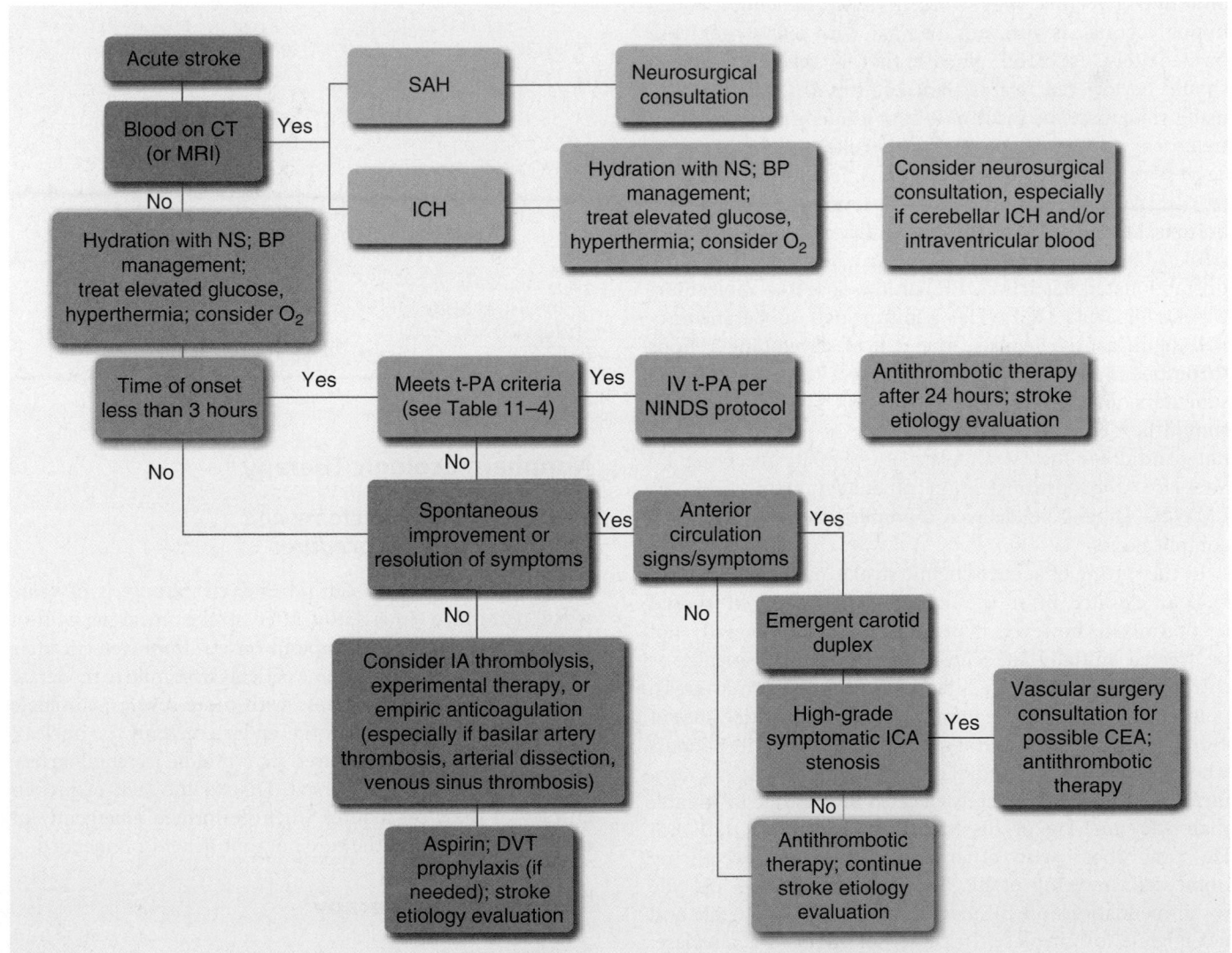

FIGURE 11–2. Acute stroke treatment algorithm. (BP, blood pressure; CEA, carotid endarterectomy; DVT, deep vein thrombosis; IA, intra-arterial; ICA, internal carotid artery; ICH, intracerebral hemorrhage; NINDS, National Institute of Neurological Disorders and Stroke; NS, normal saline; SAH, subarachnoid hemorrhage; t-PA, tissue plasminogen activator.)

determinant in treatment. The time the patient was last without symptoms is used as the time of stroke onset. Because patients typically do not experience pain, determining the onset time can be difficult. It is also important to document risk factors and the previous functional status of the patient to assess current disability due to stroke.

Supportive Measures

Acute complications of ischemic stroke include cerebral edema, increased ICP, seizures, and hemorrhagic conversion. In the acute setting, supportive interventions and treatments to prevent acute complications should be initiated.

Tissue oxygenation should be maintained acutely. Measure the oxygen saturation using pulse oximetry and supplement the patient with oxygen if necessary. The oxygen saturation should be maintained at 92% or greater.[6] Volume status and electrolytes should be corrected. If required, the blood glucose should be corrected, as both hyperglycemia and hypoglycemia may worsen brain ischemia. When hypoglycemia is present, bolus with 50% dextrose immediately. A blood glucose that is severely elevated should be lowered to less than 200 mg/dL (11.1 mmol/L) using subcutaneous insulin. Recent guidelines suggest that treatment of hyperglycemia poststroke should be more aggressive than previously recommended.[7] If the patient is febrile, treat with acetaminophen, as fever is associated with brain ischemia and increased morbidity and mortality after stroke. Alternately, cooling devices can be used.[7,8] Low-dose unfractionated heparin (UFH) or low-dose low–molecular-weight heparins (LMWHs) administered subcutaneously will significantly decrease the risk of developing venous thromboembolism (VTE) poststroke. UFH 5,000 units subcutaneously every 8 to 12 hours or low-dose LMWHs should be given for VTE prophylaxis in patients who are not candidates for IV alteplase. In patients receiving IV alteplase, the administration of subcutaneous UFH or LMWHs should be delayed 24 hours to avoid bleeding complications.

In the setting of acute ischemic stroke, many patients will have an elevated BP in the first 24 to 48 hours.[9] BP should be optimized; however, hypertension should generally not be treated initially in acute ischemic stroke patients, as this may cause decreased blood flow in ischemic areas, potentially increasing the infarction size. The cautious use of antihypertensive medications may be necessary in patients who are otherwise candidates for thrombolytic therapy, including those with severely elevated BP (systolic BP greater than 220 mm Hg or diastolic BP greater than 120 mm Hg), and those with other medical disorders requiring immediate lowering of BP. Tables 11–2 and 11–3 provide recommendations on BP management in those eligible and not eligible for alteplase. In those not eligible for alteplase, when BP is lowered, aim for a 10% to 15% reduction. Avoid using sublingual calcium channel blockers, as these may lower BP too rapidly. BP should be checked three times with each reading taken 5 minutes apart.

Table 11–2

BP Recommendations for Ischemic Stroke (Not Eligible for Alteplase)

Systolic BP less than 220 mm Hg or diastolic BP less than 120 mm Hg	Observe unless other end-organ involvement
Systolic BP greater than 220 mm Hg or diastolic BP 121–140 mm Hg	Labetalol 10–20 mg IV over 1–2 minutes (may repeat every 10–20 minutes; maximum dose 300 mg); nicardipine infusion 5 mg/h titrated to response
Diastolic BP greater than 140 mm Hg	Nitroprusside 0.25–0.3 mcg/kg/min titrated to response

BP, blood pressure.

Table 11–3

BP Recommendations for Ischemic Stroke (Eligible for Alteplase)

Before treatment, if systolic BP is greater than 185 mm Hg or diastolic BP is greater than 110 mm Hg	Labetalol 10–20 mg IV over 1–2 minutes (may repeat after 10 minutes); nicardipine infusion 5 mg/h titrated to response
During and after treatment, if diastolic BP is greater than 140 mm Hg	Nitroprusside 0.25–0.3 mcg/kg/min titrated to response
If systolic BP is greater than 230 mm Hg or diastolic BP is 121–140 mm Hg	Labetalol 10 mg IV over 1–2 minutes (may repeat every 10–20 minutes; maximum dose 300 mg) or nicardipine infusion 5 mg/h titrated to response
If systolic BP is 180–230 mm Hg or diastolic BP is 105–120 mm Hg	Labetalol 10–20 mg IV over 1–2 minutes (may repeat every 10–20 minutes; maximum dose 300 mg)

BP, blood pressure.

Nonpharmacologic Therapy

► Carotid Endarterectomy and Other Surgical Procedures

It is unknown whether carotid endarterectomy is of value when performed emergently after stroke, meaning within the first 24 hours after symptom onset.[7] Improvement after surgery has been shown in some patients with mild to moderate neurologic deficits. In patients with more severe neurologic deficits, the utility of carotid endarterectomy is unclear. Emergency bypass procedures and middle cerebral artery embolectomy are controversial. Due to the lack of proven efficacy of these procedures when performed emergently in acute ischemic stroke, they are not routinely recommended.

Thrombolytic Therapy

► Alteplase

Alteplase (rt-PA; Activase) is an IV thrombolytic (fibrinolytic) that was approved for acute stroke treatment in 1996 based on the results of the National Institute of Neurological

Disorders and Stroke (NINDS) rt-PA Stroke Trial.[10] The American Stroke Association guidelines include alteplase as the only FDA-approved acute treatment for ischemic stroke and strongly encourage early diagnosis and treatment of appropriate patients.[7]

Based on several assessment scales, patients treated with alteplase were 30% more likely to have minimal or no disability at 3 months compared with patients given placebo. Alteplase treatment resulted in an 11% to 13% absolute increase in patients with excellent outcomes at 3 months independent of patient age, stroke subtype, stroke severity, or prior use of ASA.[11] ICH within 36 hours after stroke onset occurred in 6.4% of those given alteplase versus 0.6% in those given placebo. There was no significant difference in mortality between the two groups at 3 months or 1 year.
❼ *In carefully selected patients, alteplase is effective in limiting the infarct size and protecting brain tissue from ischemia and cell death by restoring blood flow. Treatment should preferably be given within 3 hours and not more than 4.5 hours after symptom onset. Earlier treatment is preferred due to improved outcomes.* A dose of 0.9 mg/kg (maximum 90 mg) is recommended; the first 10% is given as an IV bolus and the remainder is infused over 1 hour. Table 11–4 details the inclusion and exclusion criteria for the administration of alteplase in acute ischemic stroke.

Studies following the NINDS trial protocol have supported alteplase use in acute ischemic stroke and have shown similar rates for both response and ICH occurrence. When the clinical trials are pooled, study results show that the sooner alteplase is given after the onset of stroke symptoms, the greater the benefit seen in neurologic outcome.[12] Current guidelines recommend alteplase use within 3 hours after stroke onset in appropriate patients and further recommend that alteplase be started as soon as possible within this window of time.[11] Based upon a pooled analysis of the clinical trials and the ECASS III trial results, alteplase may provide some benefit if administered within 4.5 hours of symptom onset.[11,13]

Antiplatelet agents, anticoagulants, and invasive procedures such as insertion of a central line or placement of a nasogastric tube should be avoided for 24 hours after the infusion of alteplase to prevent bleeding complications. Bladder catheterization should be avoided for 30 minutes postinfusion.

Efficacy is measured by the elimination of existing neurologic deficits and the long-term improvement in neurologic status and functioning based on neurologic examinations and other outcome measures. Neurologic examinations should be completed every 15 minutes during the infusion of alteplase, every 30 minutes for the first 6 hours after the infusion, and then every 4 hours up to 24 hours after alteplase administration. In the NINDS trial, neurologic function was assessed 24 hours after the administration of alteplase using the National Institutes of Health Stroke Scale (NIHSS). This scale quantifies neurologic deficits in patients who have had a stroke and is easily performed. At 3 months, the NIHSS and other neurologic assessments were completed.

The major adverse effects of thrombolytic therapy are bleeding, including ICH and serious systemic bleeding. Mental status changes and a severe headache may indicate ICH. Signs of bleeding include easy bruising, hematemesis, guaiac-positive stools, black, tarry stools, hematoma formation, hematuria, bleeding gums, and nosebleeds. Angioedema is a potential side effect that may cause airway obstruction.

▶ Streptokinase

Streptokinase and other thrombolytics, except alteplase, are not indicated for use in acute ischemic stroke. Three large randomized controlled trials evaluating streptokinase were stopped early due to a high incidence of hemorrhage in the streptokinase-treated patients.[14–16] Other thrombolytic agents, including tenecteplase, reteplase, desmoteplase, and urokinase, are not recommended for treatment unless associated with a clinical trial.[7,17]

Table 11–4

Inclusion and Exclusion Criteria for Alteplase Use in Acute Ischemic Stroke

Inclusion Criteria
- 18 years of age or older
- Clinical diagnosis of ischemic stroke causing a measurable neurologic deficit
- Time of symptom onset well established to be less than 180 minutes before treatment would begin

Exclusion Criteria
- Evidence of intracranial hemorrhage on CT scan of the brain prior to treatment
- Only minor or rapidly improving stroke symptoms
- Clinical presentation suggestive of SAH even with a normal head CT
- Active internal bleeding
- Known bleeding diathesis, including but not limited to (a) platelet count less than $100 \times 10^3/mm^3$ ($100 \times 10^9/L$); (b) heparin within 48 hours with an elevated aPTT; or (c) current oral anticoagulant use (e.g., warfarin) or recent use with an elevated PT (greater than 15 seconds) or INR (greater than 1.7)
- Intracranial surgery, serious head trauma, or previous stroke within 3 months
- Suspected aortic dissection associated with stroke
- Suspected subacute bacterial endocarditis or vasculitis
- History of GI or urinary tract hemorrhage within 21 days
- Major surgery or serious trauma within 14 days
- Recent arterial puncture at a noncompressible site
- Lumbar puncture within 7 days
- History of intracranial hemorrhage
- Known AVM or aneurysm
- Witnessed seizure at the same time as the onset of stroke symptoms occurred
- Recent acute MI
- SBP greater than 185 mm Hg or DBP greater than 110 mm Hg at the time of treatment, or patient requires aggressive treatment to reduce BP to within these limits

aPTT, activated partial thromboplastin time; AVM, arteriovenous malformation; DBP, diastolic blood pressure; INR, International Normalized Ratio; MI, myocardial infarction; PT, prothrombin time; SBP, systolic blood pressure.

▶ Intra-arterial Thrombolytics

Intra-arterial (IA) thrombolytics may improve outcomes in selected patients with acute ischemic stroke due to large-vessel occlusion. Patients in two clinical trials received prourokinase (r-pro UK) plus heparin or heparin alone within 6 hours of symptom onset.[18,19] Results from the first trial were not statistically significant, but favored r-pro UK, while the results of the second trial showed a statistically significant benefit to r-pro UK. No difference in mortality was found, although the incidence of intracranial hemorrhage was greater in the r-pro UK plus heparin group versus heparin alone. Note in particular, r-pro UK is not FDA approved and is not available for clinical use. Interest in IA thrombolysis has continued as an option for patients who have contraindications to IV alteplase. It may be used in patients with middle cerebral artery occlusion within 6 hours of symptom onset. IA thrombolysis should be performed by qualified personnel and should not delay treatment with IV alteplase in eligible patients.[7]

Heparin

Full dose IV UFH has been commonly used in acute stroke therapy; however, no adequately designed trials have been conducted to establish its efficacy and safety. Current acute ischemic stroke treatment guidelines do not recommend routine, urgent, full dose anticoagulation with UFH or LMWHs due to the lack of a proven benefit in improving neurologic function and the risk of intracranial bleeding.[7,11,20] Full dose UFH may prevent early recurrent stroke in patients with large-vessel atherothrombosis or those thought to be at high-risk of recurrent stroke (i.e., cardioembolic stroke); however, more study is required.

The major complications of heparin include evolution of the ischemic stroke into a hemorrhagic stroke, bleeding, and thrombocytopenia. The occurrence of severe headache and mental status changes may indicate ICH. Signs of bleeding mirror those listed for alteplase therapy. The hemoglobin, hematocrit, and platelet count should be obtained at least every 3 days to detect bleeding and thrombocytopenia.

▶ LMWHs and Heparinoids

Full dose LMWHs and heparinoids are not recommended in the treatment of acute ischemic stroke.[7,11,21] Studies with these agents have generally been negative and no convincing evidence exists that these agents improve outcomes after ischemic stroke. An increased risk of bleeding complications and hemorrhagic transformation have been observed.

Aspirin

ASA in acute ischemic stroke has been studied in two large, randomized trials, the International Stroke Trial and the Chinese Acute Stroke Trial.[22,23] Patients who received ASA within 24 to 48 hours of the onset of acute stroke symptoms were less likely to suffer early recurrent stroke, death, and disability. ❽ *Early ASA therapy with an initial dose of 150 to 325 mg is recommended in most patients with acute ischemic stroke within 48 hours after stroke onset.* The ASA dose may then be reduced to 50 to 100 mg daily to reduce bleeding complications.[11]

The administration of anticoagulants and antiplatelet agents should be delayed for 24 hours in those patients receiving alteplase. Clopidogrel either alone or in combination with ASA is not recommended in acute ischemic stroke. Glycoprotein IIb/IIIa receptor inhibitors are not recommended except in the setting of research.[7]

Ancrod

Ancrod is an investigational agent that acts to decrease plasma fibrinogen levels. It may be beneficial in patients with acute ischemic stroke when administered within 3 hours of symptom onset. Based upon available clinical trials, ancrod appears to have a potential benefit; however, studies are ongoing. It is not recommended for clinical use because efficacy and safety have not been definitively established.[7,24]

PREVENTION OF ACUTE ISCHEMIC STROKE

Primary Prevention

▶ Aspirin

The use of ASA in patients with no history of stroke or ischemic heart disease reduced the incidence of nonfatal myocardial infarction (MI) but not of stroke. A meta-analysis of eight trials found that the risk of stroke, especially hemorrhagic stroke, was slightly increased with ASA use. Major bleeding risk was also increased with ASA use.[25] The Women's Health Study evaluated over 38,000 women and found a benefit with ASA use in high-risk women 65 years and older.[26] A recent meta-analysis found a higher risk of hemorrhagic stroke in men and a greater risk of major bleeding in both men and women.[27] Primary prevention guidelines recommend ASA use in older women who are at high-risk for stroke; however, the benefit must be weighed against the risk of major bleeding. No benefit and potentially more risk of hemorrhagic stroke has been found in men, therefore, ASA is not recommended in this group.[28]

▶ Statin Therapy

Dyslipidemia has not previously been identified as an independent risk factor for stroke; however, recent studies have found a relationship between total cholesterol levels and stroke rate.[28] Statin use may reduce the incidence of a first stroke in high-risk patients (e.g., hypertension, coronary heart disease, or diabetes) including patients with normal lipid levels. Stroke risk was decreased by 27% to 32% overall in large clinical trials.[29,30] Patients with a history of MI, coronary artery disease (CAD), elevated lipid levels, diabetes, and other risk factors benefit from treatment with a lipid-lowering agent including patients with normal lipid levels.

▶ BP Management

Lowering BP in patients who are hypertensive has been shown to reduce the relative risk of stroke, both ischemic and hemorrhagic, by 35% to 44%.[31] All patients should have their BP monitored and controlled appropriately based on current guidelines for BP management.[32] Reduction in BP is the main goal as one agent has not been clearly shown to be more beneficial than any other for the primary prevention of stroke.

▶ Smoking Cessation

The relationship between smoking and both ischemic and hemorrhagic stroke is clear. Patients should be assisted and encouraged in smoking cessation as the stroke risk after cessation has been shown to decline over time. Effective treatment options are available including counseling, nicotine replacement products, and oral agents.

▶ Other Treatments

A number of other disease states and lifestyle factors should be addressed as primary prevention of stroke. Atrial fibrillation is an important and well documented risk for stroke. See Chapter 9 for information on stroke prevention in atrial fibrillation. Diabetes, carotid stenosis, cardiac disease, obesity, and physical inactivity are other risks that should be assessed and managed appropriately.

Secondary Prevention

▶ Nonpharmacologic Therapy

Carotid Endarterectomy The benefit of carotid endarterectomy for prevention of recurrent stroke has been studied previously in major trials.[33,34] A recent meta-analysis has been completed that has combined these clinical trials to evaluate 6,092 patients.[35] Carotid endarterectomy has been shown to be beneficial for preventing ipsilateral stroke in patients with symptomatic carotid artery stenosis of 70% or greater and is recommended in these patients. In patients with symptomatic stenosis of 50% to 69%, a moderate reduction in risk is seen in clinical trials. In those patients with stenosis of 50% to 69% and a recent stroke, carotid endarterectomy is appropriate. In other patients, surgical risk factors and surgeon skill should be considered prior to surgery. Carotid endarterectomy is not beneficial for symptomatic carotid stenosis less than 50% and should not be considered in these patients.

Patients with asymptomatic carotid artery stenosis of 60% or more may benefit from carotid endarterectomy if it is performed by a qualified surgeon with low complication rates (less than 3%). There is considerable controversy over how this information can be applied to clinical practice. Currently, recommendations suggest considering carotid endarterectomy in patients with carotid artery stenosis of 60% to 99% who are between 40 and 75 years of age if there is a 5-year life expectancy and the operative risks are low.[36]

Carotid Angioplasty Carotid angioplasty with or without stenting is typically restricted to patients who are refractory to medical therapy and are not surgical candidates. Clinical trials are currently ongoing to further define the role of carotid angioplasty in both symptomatic and asymptomatic patients.

▶ Pharmacologic Therapy

Aspirin In a recent meta-analysis including 144,051 patients with previous MI, acute MI, previous TIA or stroke, and acute stroke, as well as others at high risk, ASA was found to decrease the risk of recurrent stroke by approximately 25%.[37] ASA is an option for initial therapy for secondary prevention of ischemic stroke and decreases the risk of subsequent stroke by approximately 22% in both men and women with previous TIA or stroke.[37] A wide range of doses have been used (30 to 1,500 mg/day); however, the FDA has approved doses of 50 to 325 mg for secondary ischemic stroke prevention. Current guidelines recommend varying ASA doses including ASA 50 to 100 mg daily and 50 to 325 mg daily.[2,11] Lower ASA doses are currently recommended to prevent the bleeding complications associated with higher doses of ASA. Adverse effects of ASA include GI intolerance, GI bleeding, and hypersensitivity reactions.

Warfarin Recent clinical trials have not found oral anticoagulation in those patients without atrial fibrillation or carotid stenosis to be better than antiplatelet therapy. In patients without atrial fibrillation, antiplatelet therapy is recommended over warfarin. Patients with atrial fibrillation and a previous TIA or stroke have the highest risk of recurrent stroke. Long-term anticoagulation with warfarin is recommended and is effective in both the primary and secondary prevention of stroke.[2,11] The goal International Normalized Ratio (INR) for this indication is 2 to 3.

Ticlopidine Ticlopidine is slightly more beneficial in stroke prevention than ASA in men and women.[38,39] The usual recommended dosage is 250 mg orally twice daily. Ticlopidine is costly, and side effects include bone marrow suppression, rash, diarrhea, and an increased cholesterol level. Neutropenia is seen in approximately 2% of patients. Thrombotic thrombocytopenic purpura (TTP) occurs in 1 of every 2,000 to 4,000 patients treated with ticlopidine.

Patient Encounter, Part 2

In the emergency department an IV line is placed, a physical and neurologic exam is completed, and GR is moved to the stroke unit. The CT scan is negative for hemorrhagic stroke.

Identify your treatment goals for GR.

What acute management would be appropriate for GR at this time?

Monitoring of the complete blood count (CBC) is required every 2 weeks for the first 3 months of therapy. Due to the costly laboratory monitoring required and the adverse effect profile, ticlopidine is typically avoided clinically.

Clopidogrel Clopidogrel is slightly more effective than ASA with a relative-risk reduction of 7.3% more than that provided by ASA.[40] The usual dose is 75 mg orally taken once daily. Clopidogrel has a lower incidence of diarrhea and neutropenia than ticlopidine, and laboratory monitoring is not required. There have been eleven case reports of TTP occurring secondary to clopidogrel, with the majority occurring within the first 2 weeks of therapy, therefore, clinicians need to be aware of the potential for the development of TTP with clopidogrel. Clopidogrel should be used as monotherapy for stroke prevention. It is an option for initial therapy and is considered first-line therapy in patients with peripheral arterial disease.

Extended-Release Dipyridamole Plus Immediate-Release Aspirin Combination therapy with extended-release (ER) dipyridamole plus immediate-release (IR) ASA was more effective than either treatment alone in the European Stroke Prevention Study 2.[41] In this study, patients received either placebo, ASA 25 mg twice daily, ER dipyridamole 200 mg twice daily, or a combination of both agents. The individual agents produced risk reductions of 18.1% with ASA and 16.3% with ER dipyridamole, whereas the combination produced a 37% risk reduction. Headache and diarrhea were common adverse effects of dipyridamole, while bleeding was more common in the treatment groups receiving ASA. This is the first study showing that combination antiplatelet therapy has additive effects over each agent alone. The currently available formulation is a combination product containing 25 mg ASA and 200 mg ER dipyridamole. This combination is an option for initial therapy, but is not appropriate for patients who are intolerant to ASA.

Current Clinical Trials Recent trials have been completed to evaluate other combinations of antiplatelet agents and to compare them against one another. In the MATCH trial, low-dose ASA plus clopidogrel combination therapy did not show a significant benefit compared to clopidogrel alone.[42] This trial found that the addition of ASA to clopidogrel increased the risk of major bleeding. The combination of ASA and clopidogrel is not recommended due to these concerns. The ESPRIT trial compared the combination of ASA and dipyridamole to ASA alone.[43] ASA was dosed between 30 and 325 mg daily and dipyridamole was dosed at 200 mg twice daily with 83% of patients using ER dipyridamole. This trial showed that the combination of ASA and dipyridamole was more effective at preventing recurrent stroke than ASA alone. Another trial by the PRoFESS Study Group compared the combination of ASA and ER dipyridamole to clopidogrel. Neither agent was shown to be superior.[44]

▶ *Antiplatelet Therapy*

The current stroke treatment guidelines from the American College of Chest Physicians recommend ASA, clopidogrel, or combination therapy with ER dipyridamole plus IR ASA as initial antiplatelet therapy for the secondary prevention of stroke.[2,11] **9** *Selection of the initial antiplatelet agent for the secondary prevention of ischemic stroke should be individualized. Clopidogrel and the combination of ER dipyridamole and IR ASA are preferred over ASA monotherapy.* Therapy is individualized based on patient factors and cost.

Therapeutic failure in this patient population is challenging as no data are available to guide a treatment decision. When a patient is on therapeutic doses of ASA, yet experiences a recurrent TIA or stroke, switching to either clopidogrel or the combination of ASA and ER dipyridamole is a reasonable option. If failure occurs on either clopidogrel or the combination of ASA and ER dipyridamole, switching to the alternate drug may be appropriate.

BP Management Hypertension is an important risk factor for stroke; however, it had been unclear if lowering BP reduced the incidence of secondary ischemic stroke. In the PROGRESS trial, it was shown that BP reduction using the angiotensin-converting enzyme inhibitor (ACE-I) perindopril alone resulted in a 28% reduction in recurrent stroke compared to placebo. With the addition of the diuretic indapamide to perindopril, a 43% reduction in stroke recurrence was seen.[45] This reduction in stroke incidence occurred even in patients who were not hypertensive. In patients with a previous history of TIA or stroke, the Joint National Committee on the Prevention, Detection, Evaluation, and Treatment of High Blood Pressure (JNC 7) recommends a diuretic and an ACE-I.[32] Table 11–5 provides drug and dosing recommendations for the treatment of ischemic stroke.

TREATMENT OF ACUTE HEMORRHAGIC STROKE

Supportive Measures

Acute hemorrhagic stroke is considered to be an acute medical emergency. Initially, patients experiencing a hemorrhagic stroke should be transported to a neurointensive care unit. **10** *There is no proven treatment for ICH. Management is based on neurointensive care treatment and prevention of complications.* Treatment should be provided to manage the needs of the critically ill patient including management of increased ICP, seizures, infections, and prevention of rebleeding and delayed cerebral ischemia. In those with

---

Patient Encounter, Part 3

GR is ready for discharge after spending 5 days in the hospital.

What would be an appropriate discharge plan for GR at this time?

What specific medications would you recommend upon discharge?

Table 11–5		
Recommendations for Pharmacotherapy of Ischemic Stroke		
	Primary Agents	**Alternatives**
Acute Treatment	Alteplase 0.9 mg/kg IV (maximum 90 mg) over 1 hour in selected patients within 3 hours of onset ASA 150–325 mg started within 48 hours of onset (may reduce dose to 50–100 mg daily)	Alteplase 0.9 mg/kg IV (maximum 90 mg) over 1 hour in selected patients between 3 and 4.5 hours of onset Alteplase (various doses) intra-arterially up to 6 hours after onset in selected patients
Secondary Prevention	ASA 50–325 mg daily Clopidogrel 75 mg daily ASA 25 mg + ER dipyridamole 200 mg twice daily	Ticlopidine 250 mg twice daily
Cardioembolic	Warfarin (INR 2–3)	
All	ACE-I + diuretic or ARB; BP lowering: Perindopril 2–8 mg daily Indapamide 1.25–5 mg daily Statin therapy	

ACE-I, angiotensin-converting enzyme inhibitor; ARB, angiotensin receptor blocker; ASA, aspirin; BP, blood pressure; ER, extended-release; INR, International Normalized Ratio.

severely depressed consciousness, rapid endotracheal intubation and mechanical ventilation may be necessary. BP is often elevated after hemorrhagic stroke and appropriate management is important to prevent rebleeding and expansion of the hematoma.[46] BP can be controlled with IV boluses of labetalol 10 to 80 mg every 10 minutes up to a maximum of 300 mg or with IV infusions of labetalol (0.5–2 mg/min) or nicardipine (5–15 mg/h). Deep vein thrombosis prophylaxis with intermittent compression stockings should be implemented early after admission. In those patients with SAH, once the aneurysm has been treated, heparin may be instituted.[4,5]

Nonpharmacologic Therapy

Patients with hemorrhagic stroke are evaluated for surgical treatment of SAH and ICH. In SAH, either clipping of the aneurysm or coil embolization is recommended within 72 hours after the initial event to prevent rebleeding. Coil embolization, also called coiling, is a minimally invasive procedure in which a platinum coil is threaded into the aneurysm. The flexible coil fills up the space to block blood flow into the aneurysm thereby preventing rebleeding. Surgical removal of the blood in patients with ICH is controversial, as one large randomized trial did not show a benefit to removal compared with those treated conservatively according to the current guidelines.[46,47]

Pharmacologic Therapy

▶ Calcium Antagonists

🔟 *Oral nimodipine is recommended in SAH to prevent delayed cerebral ischemia.* Delayed cerebral ischemia occurs 4 to 14 days after the initial aneurysm rupture and is a common cause of neurologic deficits and death. A meta-analysis of 12 studies was conducted and concluded that oral nimodipine 60 mg every 4 hours for 21 days following aneurysmal SAH reduced the risk of a poor outcome and delayed cerebral ischemia.[48]

▶ Hemostatic Therapy

Recombinant factor VIIa has been shown to have a benefit in the treatment of ICH. The Recombinant Activated Factor VII Intracerebral Hemorrhage Trial compared three different doses and placebo. Doses were 40, 80, or 160 mcg/kg or placebo given as an IV infusion over 1 to 2 minutes within 4 hours after the onset of symptoms. Hematoma growth was decreased at 24 hours, mortality was decreased at 90 days, and overall functioning was increased at 90 days.[49] A recent phase III trial showed that recombinant factor VIIa decreased growth of the hematoma, but did not improve survival or functional outcome.[50] Current treatment guidelines suggest that recombinant factor VIIa infused within the first 3 to 4 hours after onset may be beneficial; however, further study is required before this treatment can be recommended outside of a clinical trial.[46]

OUTCOME EVALUATION

- Stroke outcomes are measured based on the neurologic status and functioning of the patient after the acute event. The NIHSS is a measure of daily functioning and is used to assess patient status following a stroke.

- Early rehabilitation can reduce functional impairment after a stroke. Recent stroke rehabilitation guidelines have been endorsed by the American Heart Association and the American Stroke Association. These guidelines recommend that patients receive care in a multidisciplinary setting or stroke unit, receive early assessment using the NIHSS, and recommend that rehabilitation is started as soon as possible after the

Table 11–6

Monitoring the Stroke Patient

Treatment	Parameter(s)	Monitoring Frequency	Comments
Ischemic Stroke			
Alteplase	BP, neurologic function, bleeding	Every 15 minutes × 1 hour, every 0.5 hour × 6 hours, every 1 hour × 17 hours; then every shift	
ASA	Bleeding	Daily	
Clopidogrel	Bleeding	Daily	
ASA/ER dipyridamole	Headache, bleeding	Daily	
Warfarin	Bleeding, INR, Hb/Hct	INR daily × 3 days; weekly until stable; then monthly	
Hemorrhagic Stroke			
	BP, neurologic function, ICP	Every 2 hours in ICU	May require treatments to lower BP to less than 180 mm Hg systolic
Nimodipine for SAH	BP, neurologic function, fluid status	Every 2 hours in ICU	

ASA, aspirin; BP, blood pressure; ER, extended-release; Hb, hemoglobin; Hct, hematocrit; ICP, intracranial pressure; ICU, intensive care unit; INR, International Normalized Ratio; SAH, subarachnoid hemorrhage.

stroke. Other recommendations include screening for **dysphagia** and aggressive secondary stroke prevention treatments.[51]

- Table 11–6 provides monitoring guidelines for the acute stroke patient.

Patient Care and Monitoring

1. Assess the patient's signs and symptoms including the time of symptom onset and the time of arrival in the emergency department.

2. Perform thorough neurologic and physical examinations evaluating for potential causes of the stroke.

3. Perform a CT scan to rule out a hemorrhagic stroke prior to administering any treatment.

4. Evaluate the inclusion and exclusion criteria for thrombolytic therapy to determine appropriateness for the patient.

5. Transfer the patient to a stroke center if available and develop a plan for the acute management of the patient.

6. Determine the patient's risk factors for stroke.

7. Develop a plan for the long-term management of risk factors in order to prevent a recurrent stroke.

8. Educate the patient on appropriate lifestyle modifications that will reduce stroke risk.

9. Educate the patient on their medication regimen stressing the importance of adherence.

Abbreviations Introduced in This Chapter

ACE-I	Angiotensin-converting enzyme inhibitor
ADP	Adenosine diphosphate
aPTT	Activated partial thromboplastin time
ARB	Angiotensin receptor blocker
ASA	Aspirin
AVM	Arteriovenous malformation
BPH	Benign prostatic hypertrophy
CAD	Coronary artery disease
CBC	Complete blood count
CEA	Carotid endarterectomy
CVD	Cerebrovascular disease
DBP	Diastolic blood pressure
ER	Extended-release
ESPS2	European Stroke Prevention Study 2
Hb	Hemoglobin
Hct	Hematocrit
IA	Intra-arterial
ICA	Internal carotid artery
ICH	Intracerebral hemorrhage
ICP	Intracranial pressure
ICU	Intensive care unit
INR	International Normalized Ratio
IR	Immediate-release
JNC 7	Joint National Committee on the Prevention, Detection, Evaluation, and Treatment of High Blood Pressure
LMWH	Low–molecular-weight heparin
MI	Myocardial infarction
NIHSS	National Institutes of Health Stroke Scale
NINDS	National Institute of Neurological Disorders and Stroke
NS	Normal saline

PROACT II   Prolyse in Acute Cerebral
             Thromboembolism II
PT   Prothrombin time
rt-PA   Alteplase
r-pro UK   Prourokinase
SAH   Subarachnoid hemorrhage
SBP   Systolic blood pressure
TIA   Transient ischemic attack
TTP   Thrombotic thrombocytopenic purpura
VTE   Venous thromboembolism

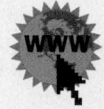 Self-assessment questions and answers are available at *http://www.mhpharmacotherapy.com/pp.html.*

REFERENCES

1. American Heart Association. Heart Disease and Stroke Statistics—2008 Update. A Report from the American Heart Association Statistics Committee and Stroke Statistics Subcommittee. Circulation 2008;117:e25–e146.
2. Sacco RL, Adams R, Albers G, et al. Guidelines for prevention of stroke in patients with ischemic stroke or transient ischemic attack: A statement for healthcare professionals from the American Heart Association/American Stroke Association Council on Stroke: Cosponsored by the Council on Cardiovascular Radiology and Intervention: The American Academy of Neurology affirms the value of the guidelines. Stroke 2006;37(2):577–617.
3. Ariesen MJ, Claus SP, Rinkel GJE, Algra A. Risk factors for intracerebral hemorrhage in the general population: A systematic review. Stroke 2003;34:2060–2065.
4. Suarez JI, Tarr RW, Selman WR. Aneurysmal subarachnoid hemorrhage. N Engl J Med 2006;354:387–396.
5. Mayer SA, Rincon F. Treatment of intracerebral hemorrhage. Lancet Neurol 2005;4:662–672.
6. Treib J, Grauer MT, Woessner R, Morganthaler M. Treatment of stroke on an intensive stroke unit: A novel concept. Intensive Care Med 2000;26:1598–1611.
7. Adams HP, del Zoppo G, Alberts MJ, et al. Guidelines for the early management of adults with ischemic stroke: A guideline from the American Heart Association/ American Stroke Association Stroke Council, Clinical Cardiology Council, Cardiovascular Radiology and Intervention Council, and the Atherosclerotic Peripheral Vascular Disease and Quality of Care Outcomes in Research Interdisciplinary Working Groups: The American Academy of Neurology affirms the value of this guideline as an educational tool for neurologists. Stroke 2007;38:1655–1711.
8. Sulter G, Elting JW, Maurits N, Luyckx GJ, De Keyser J. Acetylsalicylic acid and acetaminophen to combat elevated body temperature in acute ischemic stroke. Cerebrovasc Dis 2004;17:118–122.
9. Morfis L, Schwartz RS, Poulos R, Howes LG. Blood pressure changes in acute cerebral infarction and hemorrhage. Stroke 1997;28:141–145.
10. National Institute of Neurological Disorders and Stroke rt-PA Stroke Study Group. Tissue plasminogen activator for acute ischemic stroke. N Engl J Med 1995;333:1581–1587.
11. Albers GW, Amarenco P, Easton JD, Sacco RL, Teal P. Antithrombotic and thrombolytic therapy for ischemic stroke: American College of Chest Physicians evidence-based clinical practice guidelines. 8th ed. Chest 2008;133:630–669.
12. The ATLANTIS, ECASS, and NINDS rt-PA Study Group Investigators. Association of outcome with early stroke treatment: Pooled analysis of ATLANTIS, ECASS, and NINDS rt-PA stroke trials. Lancet 2004;363:768–774.
13. Hacke W, Kaste M, Bluhmki E, et al. Thrombolysis with alteplase 3 to 4.5 hours after acute ischemic stroke. N Engl J Med 2008;359(13):1317–1329.
14. Donnan GA, Davis SM, Chambers BR, et al. Streptokinase for acute ischemic stroke with relationship to time of administration: Australian Streptokinase (ASK) Trial Study Group. JAMA 1996;276:961–966.
15. Multicenter Acute Stroke Trial—Europe Study Group. Thrombolytic therapy with streptokinase in acute ischemic stroke. N Engl J Med 1996;335:145–150.
16. Multicentre Acute Stroke Trial—Italy (MAST-I) Group. Randomised controlled trial of streptokinase, aspirin, and combination of both in treatment of acute ischaemic stroke. Lancet 1995;346:1509–1514.
17. Blakeley JO, Llinas RH. Thrombolytic therapy for acute ischemic stroke. J Neurol Sci 2007;261:55–62.
18. del Zoppo GJ, Higashida RT, Furlan AJ, et al. PROACT: A phase II randomized trial of recombinant pro-urokinase by direct arterial delivery in acute middle cerebral artery stroke. Stroke 1998;29:4–11.
19. Furlan A, Higashida R, Wechsler L, et al. Intra-arterial prourokinase for acute ischemic stroke. The PROACT II study: A randomized controlled trial. Prolyse in acute cerebral thromboembolism. JAMA 1999;282:2003–2011.
20. Sandercock PA, Counsell C, Kamal AK. Anticoagulants for acute ischaemic stroke. Cochrane Database Syst Rev 2008;8(4):CD000024.
21. Sandercock PA, Counsell C, Tseng MC. Low-molecular-weight heparins or heparinoids versus standard unfractionated heparin for acute ischaemic stroke. Cochrane Database Syst Rev 2008;16(3):CD000119.
22. Chinese Acute Stroke Trial (CAST) Collaborative Group. CAST: A randomized, placebo-controlled trial of early aspirin use in 20,000 patients with acute ischemic stroke. Lancet 1997;349:1641–1649.
23. International Stroke Trial Collaborative Group. The International Stroke Trial (IST): A randomized trial of aspirin, subcutaneous heparin, both, or neither among 19,435 patients with acute ischemic stroke. Lancet 1997;349:1560–1581.
24. Lui M, Counsell C, Zhao XL, Wardlow J. Fibrinogen depleting agents for acute ischaemic stroke. Cochrane Database Syst Rev 2003;(3):CD000091.
25. Straus SE, Majumdar SR, McAlister FA. New evidence for stroke prevention: Scientific review. JAMA 2002;288: 388–395.
26. Ridker PM, Cook NR, Lee IM, et al. A randomized trial of low-dose aspirin in the primary prevention of cardiovascular disease in women. N Engl J Med 2005;352:1293–1304.
27. Berger JS, Roncaglioni MC, Avanzini F, et al. Aspirin for the primary prevention of cardiovascular events in women and men: A sex-specific meta-analysis of randomized controlled trials. JAMA 2006;295:306–313.
28. Goldstein LB, Adam R, Alberts MJ, et al. Primary prevention of ischemic stroke: A guideline from the American Heart Association/ American Stroke Association Stroke Council: Cosponsored by the Atherosclerotic Peripheral Vascular Disease Interdisciplinary Working Group; Cardiovascular Nursing Council; Clinical Cardiology Council; Nutrition, Physical Activity, and Metabolism Council; and the Quality of Care and Outcomes Research Interdisciplinary Working Group: The American Academy of Neurology affirms the value of this guideline. Stroke 2006;37:1583–1633.
29. Sever PS, Dahlof B, Poulter NR, et al. ASCOT Investigators. Prevention of coronary and stroke events with atorvastatin in hypertensive patients who have average or lower-than-average cholesterol concentrations, in the Anglo-Scandinavian Cardiac Outcomes Trial-Lipid Lowering Arm (ASCOT-LLA): A multicentre randomised controlled trial. Lancet 2003;361:1149–1158.
30. Collins R, Armitage J, Parish S, et al. Heart Protection Study Collaborative Group. Effects of cholesterol-lowering with simvastatin on stroke and other major vascular events in 20536 people with cerebrovascular disease or other high-risk conditions. Lancet 2004;363:757–767.
31. Neal B, MacMahon S, Chapman N. Blood Pressure Lowering Treatment Trialists' Collaboration. Effects of ACE inhibitors, calcium antagonists,

and other blood-pressure-lowering drugs: Results of prospectively designed overviews of randomized trials. Blood Pressure Lowering Treatment Trialists' Collaboration. Lancet 2000;356:1955–1964.

32. Chobanian AV, Bakris GL, Black HR, et al. National Heart, Lung, and Blood Institute Joint National Committee on Prevention, Detection, Evaluation, and Treatment of High Blood Pressure; National High Blood Pressure Education Program Coordinating Committee. The Seventh Report of the Joint National Committee on Prevention, Detection, Evaluation, and Treatment of High Blood Pressure: The JNC 7 report. JAMA 2003;289:2560–2572.

33. North American Symptomatic Carotid Endarterectomy Trial Collaborators. Beneficial effect of carotid endarterectomy in symptomatic patients with high-grade carotid stenosis. N Engl J Med 1991;325:445–453.

34. European Carotid Surgery Trialists' Collaborative Group. Randomised trial of endarterectomy for recently symptomatic carotid stenosis: Final results of the MRC European Carotid Surgery Trial (ECST). Lancet 1998;351:1379–1387.

35. Rothwell PM, Eliasziw M, Fox AJ, et al., for the Carotid Endarterectomy Trialists' Collaboration. Analysis of pooled data from the randomised controlled trials of endarterectomy for symptomatic carotid stenosis. Lancet 2003;361:107–116.

36. Chaturvedi A, Bruno A, Feasby T, et al. Carotid endarterectomy—An evidence-based review. Neurology 2005;65:794–801.

37. Collaborative meta-analysis of randomised trials of antiplatelet therapy for prevention of death, myocardial infarction, and stroke in high risk patients. BMJ 2002;324:71–86.

38. Hass WK, Easton JD, Adams HP Jr., et al, for the Ticlopidine Aspirin Stroke Study Group. A randomized trial comparing ticlopidine hydrochloride with aspirin for the prevention of stroke in high-risk patients. Ticlopidine Aspirin Stroke Study Group. N Engl J Med 1989;321:501–507.

39. Gent M, Blakely JA, Easton JD, et al. The Canadian American Ticlopidine Study (CATS) in thromboembolic stroke. Lancet 1989;1:1215–1220.

40. CAPRIE Steering Committee. A randomized, blinded, trial of clopidogrel versus aspirin in patients at risk of ischaemic events. Lancet 1996;348:1329–1339.

41. Diener HC, Cunha L, Forbes C, et al. European Stroke Prevention Study 2. Dipyridamole and acetylsalicylic acid in the secondary prevention of stroke. J Neurol Sci 1996;143:1–13.

42. Deiner HC, Bogousslavsky J, Brass LM, et al, for the MATCH Investigators. Aspirin and clopidogrel compared with clopidogrel alone after recent ischaemic stroke or transient ischaemic attack in high-risk patients (MATCH): Randomised, double-blind, placebo-controlled trial. Lancet 2004;364:331–337.

43. The ESPRIT Study Group. Aspirin plus dipyridamole versus aspirin alone after cerebral ischaemia of arterial origin (ESPRIT): Randomized controlled trial. Lancet 2006;367:1665–1673.

44. Sacco RL, Deiner HC, Yusuf S, et al. Aspirin and extended-release dipyridamole versus clopidogrel for recurrent stroke. N Engl J Med 2008;359:1238-1251.

45. PROGRESS Collaborative Group. Randomized trial of perindopril-based blood-pressure-lowering regimen among 6105 individuals with previous stroke or transient ischaemic attack. Lancet 2001;358:1033–1041.

46. Broderick J, Connolly S, Feldmann E, et al. Guidelines for the management of spontaneous intracerebral hemorrhage in adults: 2007 update: A guideline from the American Heart Association/American Stroke Association Stroke Council, High Blood Pressure Research Council, and the Quality of Care and Outcomes in Research Interdisciplinary Working Group: The American Academy of Neurology affirms the value of this guideline as an educational tool for neurologists. Stroke 2007;38:2001–2023.

47. Mendelow DA, Gregson BA, Fernandes HM, et al, for the STICH Investigators. Early surgery versus initial conservative treatment in patients with spontaneous supratentorial intracerebral haematomas in the International Surgical Trial in Intracerebral Haemorrhage (STICH): A randomised trial. Lancet 2005;365:387–397.

48. Rinkel GJ, Feigin VL, Algra A, van den Bergh WM, Vermeulen M, van Gijn J. Calcium antagonists for aneurysmal subarachnoid haemorrhage. Cochrane Database Syst Rev 2005;1:CD000277.

49. Mayer SA, Brun NC, Begtrup K, et al, for the Recombinant Activated Factor VII Intracerebral Hemorrhage Trial Investigators. Recombinant activated factor VII for acute intracerebral hemorrhage. N Engl J Med 2005;352:777–785.

50. Mayer SA, Brun NC, Begtrup K. et al. Efficacy and safety of recombinant activated factor VII for acute intracerebral hemorrhage. N Engl J Med 2008;358:2127–2137.

51. Bates B, Choi JY, Duncan PW. et al. Veterans Affairs/Department of Defense clinical practice guideline for the management of adult stroke rehabilitation care: Executive summary. Stroke 2005;36:2049–2056.

12 Dyslipidemias

Matthew K. Ito

LEARNING OBJECTIVES

● **Upon completion of the chapter, the reader will be able to:**

1. Identify the major components within each lipoprotein and their role in lipoprotein metabolism and the development of atherosclerosis.

2. Identify the common types of lipid disorders.

3. Determine a patient's coronary heart disease risk and corresponding treatment goals according to the National Cholesterol Education Program Adult Treatment Panel III guidelines.

4. Recommend appropriate therapeutic lifestyle changes (TLC) and pharmacotherapy interventions for patients with dyslipidemia.

5. Identify the diagnostic criteria and treatment strategies for the metabolic syndrome.

6. Describe the components of a monitoring plan to assess effectiveness and adverse effects of pharmacotherapy for dyslipidemias.

7. Educate patients about the disease state, appropriate TLC, and drug therapy required for effective treatment.

KEY CONCEPTS

❶ The risk of atherosclerosis is directly related to increasing levels of serum cholesterol.

❷ The National Cholesterol Education Program Adult Treatment Panel III guidelines have set the "optimal" level for low-density lipoprotein (LDL) cholesterol for all adults as less than 100 mg/dL (2.59 mmol/L).

❸ All adults greater than 20 years of age should be screened at least every 5 years using a fasting blood sample.

❹ The benefits of lowering LDL cholesterol to as low as 70 mg/dL (1.81 mmol/L) have been demonstrated in clinical trials; however, the lowest level at which to treat LDL cholesterol where there are no further benefits in coronary heart disease (CHD) risk has not yet been determined.

❺ An adequate trial of therapeutic lifestyle changes (TLC) should be employed in all patients, but pharmacotherapy should be instituted concurrently in higher-risk patients.

❻ Typically, statins are the medications of choice to treat high LDL cholesterol because of their ability to substantially reduce LDL cholesterol, ability to reduce morbidity and mortality from atherosclerotic disease, convenient once-daily dosing, and low risk of side effects.

❼ Patients with metabolic syndrome have an additional lipid parameter that needs to be assessed, namely non–high-density lipoprotein (non-HDL) cholesterol (total cholesterol minus HDL cholesterol). The target for non-HDL cholesterol is less than the patient's LDL cholesterol target plus 30 mg/dL (0.78 mmol/L).

❽ After assessment and control of LDL cholesterol, patients with serum triglycerides of 200 to 499 mg/dL (2.26–5.64 mmol/L) should be assessed for atherogenic dyslipidemia (low HDL cholesterol and increased small-dense LDL particles) and the metabolic syndrome.

❾ Combination drug therapy is an effective means to achieve greater reductions in LDL cholesterol (statin + ezetimibe or bile acid resin, bile acid resin + ezetimibe, or three-drug combinations) as well as raising HDL cholesterol and lowering serum triglycerides (statin + niacin or fibrate).

❿ Reducing LDL cholesterol while substantially raising HDL cholesterol (statin + niacin) appears to reduce the risk of atherosclerotic disease progression to a greater degree than statin monotherapy.

INTRODUCTION

❶ *The risk of atherosclerosis is directly related to increasing levels of serum cholesterol.* Hypercholesterolemia (elevation in serum cholesterol) and other abnormalities in serum lipids play a major role in plaque formation leading to coronary heart disease (CHD) as well as other forms of atherosclerosis, such as **carotid** and peripheral artery disease (atherosclerosis of the peripheral arteries). This predictive relationship has been demonstrated from large epidemiologic,[1] animal, and genetic studies. CHD is the leading cause of death in both men and women in the United States and most industrialized nations. It is also the chief cause of premature, permanent disability in the U.S. workforce. Annually, approximately 700,000 Americans will suffer a new heart attack and 500,000 will have a recurrent event. The average age of a first heart attack is 66 years for American men and 70 years for women. The direct and indirect cost of CHD to the U.S. economy in 2007 was almost $151.6 billion.[2] Clinical trials have consistently demonstrated that lowering serum cholesterol reduces atherosclerotic progression and mortality from CHD.

The development of CHD is a lifelong process. Except in rare cases of severely elevated serum cholesterol levels, years of poor dietary habits, sedentary lifestyle, and life-habit risk factors (e.g., smoking and obesity) contribute to the development of atherosclerosis.[3] Unfortunately, many individuals at risk for CHD do not receive lipid-lowering therapy or are not optimally treated. This chapter will help identify individuals at risk, assess treatment goals based on the level of CHD risk, and implement optimal treatment strategies and monitoring plans.

PATHOPHYSIOLOGY

Lipid and Lipoprotein Metabolism

Cholesterol is an essential substance manufactured by most cells in the body. Cholesterol is used to maintain cell wall integrity and for the biosynthesis of **bile acids** and steroid hormones. Other major lipids in our body are triglycerides and phospholipids. Since cholesterol is a relatively water-insoluble molecule, it is unable to circulate through the blood alone. Cholesterol along with triglycerides and phospholipids are packaged in a large carrier-protein called a lipoprotein (Fig. 12–1). Lipoproteins are water soluble, which allows transportation of the major lipids in the blood. These lipoproteins are spherical and vary in size (approximately 1,000 to 6 nm) and density (less than 0.94 to 1.21 g/mL) (Table 12–1). The amount of cholesterol and triglycerides vary by lipoprotein size. The major lipoproteins in descending size and ascending density are chylomicrons, very low-density lipoprotein (VLDL), intermediate-density lipoprotein (IDL), low-density lipoprotein (LDL), and high-density lipoprotein (HDL). When clinical laboratories measure and report serum total cholesterol, what they are measuring and reporting are the total cholesterol molecules in all the major lipoproteins. The estimated value of LDL cholesterol is found using the following equation:

LDL cholesterol = total cholesterol − (HDL cholesterol + triglycerides/5) using traditional units of mg/dL; or

LDL cholesterol = total cholesterol − (HDL cholesterol + triglycerides/2.2) using SI units of mmol/L.

If serum triglycerides are greater than 400 mg/dL (4.52 mmol/L), chylomicrons are present, or the patient has type III

hyperlipoproteinemia, this formula becomes inaccurate and LDL cholesterol must be directly measured.[3]

Each lipoprotein has various proteins called apolipo-proteins (Apos) embedded on the surface (Fig. 12–1). These Apos serve four main purposes, they: (a) are required for assembly and secretion of lipoproteins (such as Apos B-48 and B-100); (b) serve as major structural components of lipo-proteins; (c) act as ligands (Apo B-100 and Apo E) for binding to receptors on cell surfaces (LDL receptors); and (d) can be cofactors (such as Apo C-II) for activation of enzymes (such as lipoprotein lipase [LPL]) involved in the breakdown of triglycerides from chylomicrons and VLDL.[4] Apos A-I and A-II are major structural proteins on the surface of HDL. Apo A-I interacts with adenosine triphosphate (ATP) binding cassette A1 and G1 to traffic cholesterol from extrahepatic tissue (such as the arterial wall) to immature or **nascent** HDL.

Cholesterol from the diet as well as from bile enters the small intestine, where it is emulsified by bile salts into **micelles** (Fig. 12–2). These micelles interact with the duodenal and jejunal enterocyte surfaces, and cholesterol is transported from the micelles into these cells by the Niemann-Pick C1 Like 1 (NPC1L1) transporter.[5] Some cholesterol and most plant sterols, which are structurally similar to cholesterol, are exported back from the enterocyte into the intestinal lumen by the ATP-binding cassette (ABC) G5/G8 transporter. Cholesterol within enterocytes is esterified and packaged into chylomicrons along with triglycerides, phospholipids, and Apo B-48 as well as Apos C and E, which are then released into the **lymphatic** circulation. In the circulation, chylomicrons are converted to chylomicron remnants (through loss of

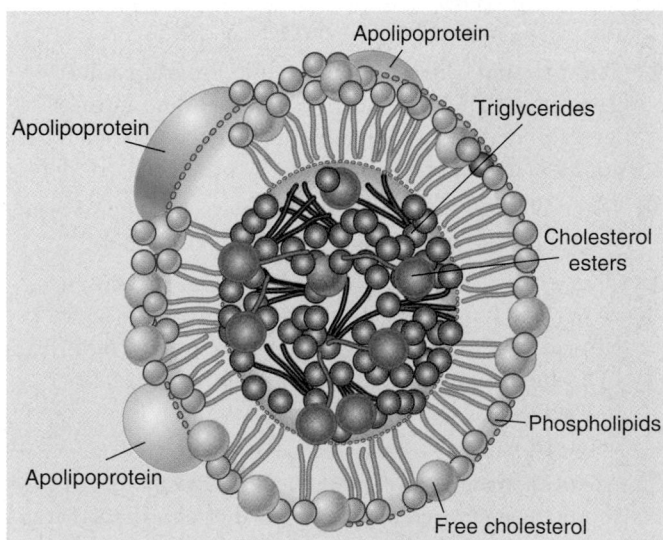

FIGURE 12–1. Lipoprotein structure. Lipoproteins are a diverse group of particles with varying size and density. They contain variable amounts of core cholesterol esters and triglycerides, and have varying numbers and types of surface apolipoproteins. The apolipoproteins function to direct the processing and removal of individual lipoprotein particles. (From LipoScience, Inc. with permission.)

Table 12–1

Physical Characteristics of Lipoproteins

| Lipoprotein | Density Range (g/mL) | Size (nm) | Composition (%) | | Apolipoprotein |
			Cholesterol	Triglycerides	
Chylomicrons	Less than 0.95	100–1,000	3–7	85–95	A-I, A-II, A-IV, B-48, C-I, C-II, E
VLDL	Less than 1.006	40–50	20–30	50–65	B-100, C-I, C-II, C-III, E
IDL	1.006–1.019	25–30	40	20	B-100, E
LDL	1.019–1.063	20–25	51–58	4–8	B-100
HDL	1.063–1.21	6–10	18–25	2–7	A-I, A-II, C-I, C-II, C-III, E

HDL, high-density lipoprotein; IDL, intermediate-density lipoprotein; LDL, low-density lipoprotein; VLDL, very low-density lipoprotein.

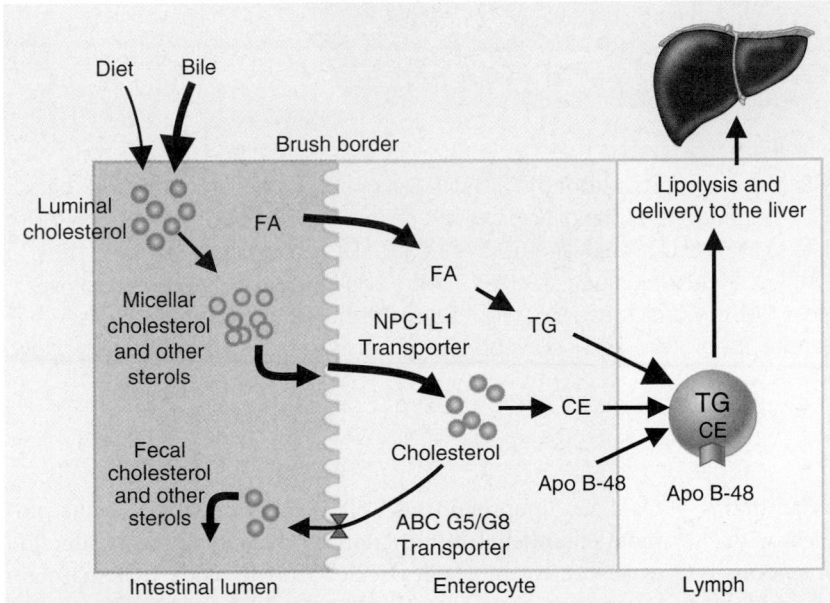

FIGURE 12–2. Intestinal cholesterol absorption and transport. Cholesterol from food and bile enter the gut lumen and are emulsified by bile acids into micelles. Micelles binding to the intestinal enterocytes, and cholesterol and other sterols are transported from the micelles into the enterocytes by a sterol transporter. Triglycerides synthesized by absorbed fatty acids along with cholesterol and apolipoprotein B-48 are incorporated into chylomicrons. Chylomicrons are released into the lymphatic circulation and are converted to chylomicron remnants (through loss of triglyceride), and then taken up by the hepatic LDL receptor-related protein (LRP). (ABC G5/G8, ATP-binding cassette G5/G8; Apo, apolipoprotein; CE, cholesterol ester; FA, fatty acid; NPC1L1, Niemann-Pick C1 Like 1; TG, triglyceride.)

triglycerides by the interaction of Apo C-II and LPL). During this process, chylomicrons also interact with HDL particles (Fig. 12–3) and exchange triglyceride and cholesterol content, and HDL particles acquire Apos A and C. Chylomicron remnant particles are then taken up by LDL-related protein (LRP).

In the liver, cholesterol and triglycerides are incorporated into VLDL along with phospholipids and Apo B-100 (Fig. 12–4). VLDL particles are released into the circulation where they acquire Apo E and Apo C-II from HDL. VLDL loses its triglyceride content through the interaction with LPL to form VLDL remnant and IDL. IDL can be cleared from the circulation by hepatic LDL receptors or further converted to LDL (by further depletion of triglycerides) through the action of hepatic lipases (HL). Approximately 50% of IDL is converted to LDL. LDL particles are cleared from the circulation primarily by hepatic LDL receptors by interaction with Apo B-100. They can also be taken up by extrahepatic tissues or enter the arterial wall, contributing to atherogenesis.[6]

Cholesterol is transported from the arterial wall or other extrahepatic tissues back to the liver by HDL (Fig. 12–3). Apo A-I (derived from the intestine and liver) on nascent HDL interacts with ATP-binding cassette A1 (ABCA1) and G1 transporter on extrahepatic tissue. Cholesterol in nascent HDL is esterified by lecithin-cholesterol acyltransferase (LCAT) resulting in mature HDL. The esterified cholesterol can be transferred as noted above to Apo B-containing particles in exchange for triglycerides. Triglyceride-rich HDL is hydrolyzed by HL, generating fatty acids and nascent HDL particles, or the mature HDL can bind to the scavenger receptors (SR-BI) on hepatocytes and transfer their cholesterol ester content for excretion in the bile.

A variety of genetic mutations occur in the above steps during lipoprotein synthesis and metabolism that cause lipid disorders. The major genetic disorders and their effect on serum lipids are presented in Table 12–2. Disorders that increase serum cholesterol are generally those that affect the number or affinity of LDL receptors (also known as Apo B-E receptors) known as familial hypercholesterolemia, or the

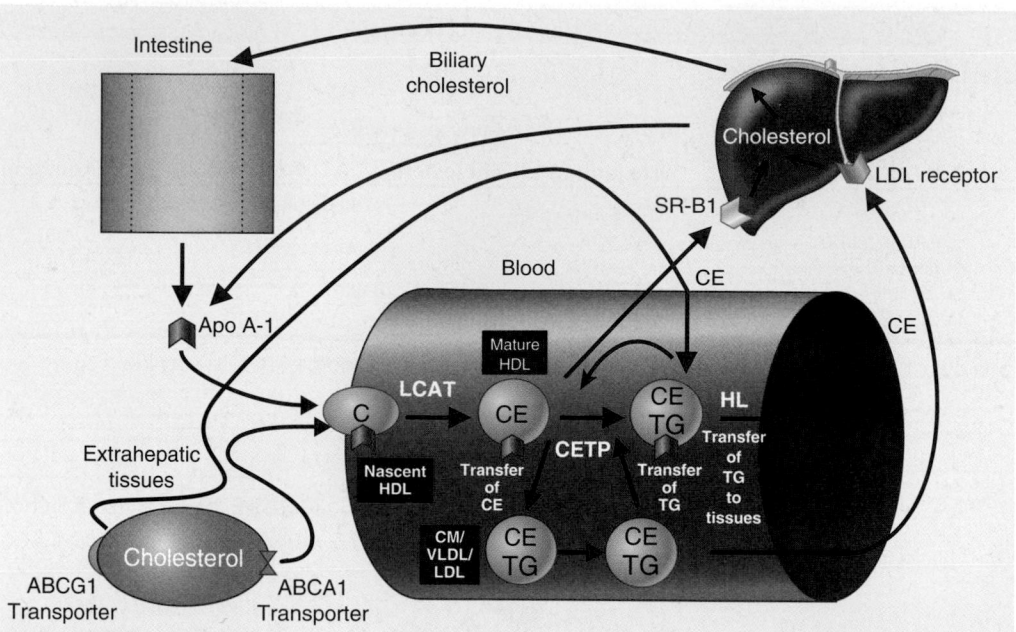

FIGURE 12–3. Reverse cholesterol transport. Cholesterol is transported from the arterial wall or other extrahepatic tissues back to the liver by HDL. Esterified cholesterol from HDL can be transferred to apolipoprotein B-containing particles in exchange for triglycerides. Cholesterol esters transferred from HDL to VLDL and LDL are taken up by hepatic LDL receptors or delivered back to extrahepatic tissue. (ABCA1, ATP-binding cassette A1; ABCG1, ATP-binding cassette G1; Apo, apolipoprotein; C, cholesterol; CE, cholesterol ester; CETP, cholesterol ester transfer protein; CM, chylomicrons; HDL, high-density lipoprotein; HL, hepatic lipase; LCAT, lecithin-cholesterol acyltransferase; LDL, low-density lipoprotein; SR-B1, scavenger receptors; TG, triglyceride; VLDL, very low-density lipoprotein.)

ability of Apo B-100 to bind to the receptor known as familial defective Apo B-100. These patients commonly present with **corneal arcus** of the eye and **xanthomas** of extensor tendons of the hand and Achilles tendon. Elevations in triglycerides are generally associated with overproduction of VLDL, mutations in Apo E, or lack of LPL. Patients with extremely elevated serum triglycerides can develop **pancreatitis** and **tuberoeruptive xanthomas**. Most individuals have mild to moderate elevations in cholesterol caused by a polygenic disorder. Polygenic hypercholesterolemia is not as well understood as the single-gene disorders discussed above. Polygenic hypercholesterolemia is thought to be caused by various, more subtle genetic defects as well as environmental factors such as diet and lack of physical activity.[3]

Pathophysiology of CAD

The most widely accepted theory of the process of atherosclerosis is that it is a low-grade inflammatory response due to injury of the vascular endothelium induced by lipoprotein retention in the arterial wall.[6] The process begins when lipoproteins migrate between the **endothelial cells** into the arterial wall and bind to **proteoglycans** (Fig. 12–5). The initial lesion, known as a fatty streak, appears to form after accumulation of lipoproteins within the **intima**. After entering the intima, lipoproteins are then structurally modified by oxidation.

Oxidized lipoproteins as well as other cytotoxic agents promote endothelial dysfunction by disturbing the production of vasoactive molecules such as nitric oxide that maintain vasomotor tone. Small, denser LDL particles migrate into the arterial wall more readily and are particularly susceptible to oxidation. The oxidized particles cause an increased expression of cell-adhesion molecules on vascular endothelial cells leading to recruitment of **monocytes** into the intima. The monocytes differentiate into **macrophages** and express scavenger receptors allowing enhanced uptake of Apo B-containing lipoproteins. The macrophages continue to accumulate lipoproteins and ultimately develop into lipid-laden **foam cells**. Accumulation of foam cells leads to formation of a lipid-rich core, which marks the transition to a more complicated atherosclerotic plaque. Vascular wall remodeling leading to outward growth of the wall occurs to accommodate this lipid-rich core. Thus, the vascular lumen is relatively well preserved and generally the lesion would not be detected using traditional coronary angiographic techniques. Initially, smooth muscle cells migrate and proliferate from the **media** to the intima forming a protective fibrous cap which separates the potentially thrombogenic lipid core from circulating blood. As the plaque matures, inflammatory cells secrete **matrix metalloproteinases** that degrade collagen and fibrin produced by smooth muscle cells that lead to a weakened fibrous cap. Ischemic events result when the fibrous

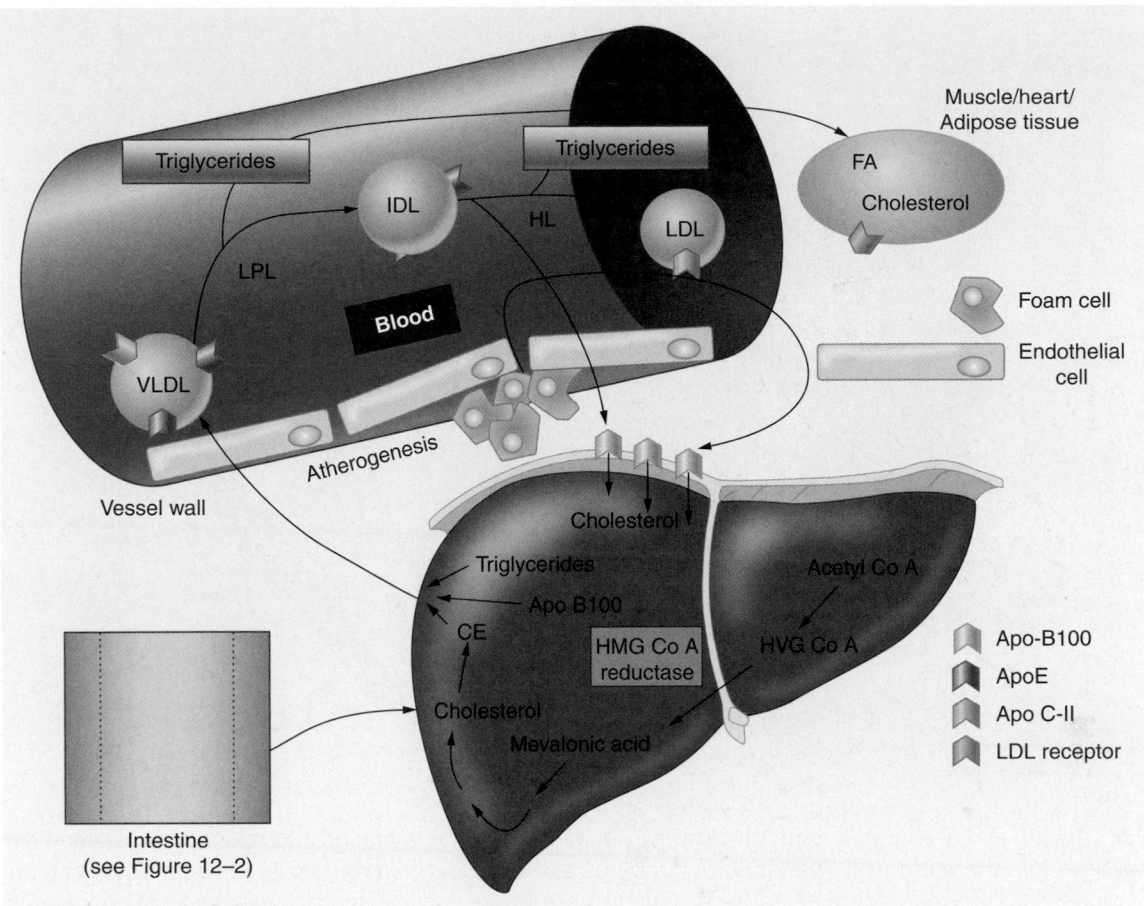

FIGURE 12–4. Endogenous lipoprotein metabolism. In liver cells, cholesterol and triglycerides are packaged into VLDL particles and exported into blood where VLDL is converted to IDL. Intermediate-density lipoprotein can be either cleared by hepatic LDL receptors or further metabolized to LDL. LDL can be cleared by hepatic LDL receptors or can enter the arterial wall, contributing to atherosclerosis. (Acetyl CoA, acetyl coenzyme A; Apo, apolipoprotein; CE, cholesterol ester; FA, fatty acid; HL, hepatic lipase; HMG-CoA, 3-hydroxy-3-methyglutaryl coenzyme A; IDL, intermediate-density lipoprotein; LCAT, lecithin-cholesterol acyltransferase; LDL, low-density lipoprotein; LPL, lipoprotein lipase; VLDL, very low-density lipoprotein.)

Table 12–2

Selected Characteristics of Primary (Genetic) Dyslipidemias

Disorder	Estimated Frequency	Metabolic Defect	Main Lipid Parameter
Familial hypercholesterolemia homozygous	1/1 million	LDL-receptor negative	LDL-C greater than 500 mg/dL (12.95 mmol/L)
Heterozygous	1/500	Reduction in LDL receptors	LDL-C 250–500 mg/dL (6.48–12.95 mmol/L)
Familial defective Apo B-100	1/1,000	Single nucleotide mutation	LDL-C 250–500 mg/L (6.48–12.95 mmol/L)
Polygenic hypercholesterolemia	Common	Metabolic and environmental	LDL-C 160–250 mg/dL (4.14–6.48 mmol/L)
Familial combined dyslipidemia	1/200–300	Overproduction of VLDL and/or LDL	LDL-C 250–350 mg/dL (6.48–9.07 mmol/L) TG 200–800 mg/dL (2.26–9.04 mmol/L)
Familial hyperapobetalipoproteinemia	5%	Increase Apo B production	Apo B greater than 125 mg/dL (0.25 g/L)
Familial dysbetalipoproteinemia	0.5%	Apo E2/2 phenotype	LDL-C 300–600 mg/dL (7.77–15.54 mmol/L) TG 400–800 mg/dL (4.52–9.04 mmol/L)
Familial hypertriglyceridemia			
Type IV	1/300	Unknown	TG 200–500 mg/dL (2.26–5.65 mmol/L)
Type V	1/205,000	Unknown	TG greater than 1,000 mg/dL (11.3 mmol/L)
Hypoalphalipoproteinemia	3–5%	Defect in HDL catabolism	HDL-C less than 35 mg/dL (0.91 mmol/L)

Apo, apolipoprotein; C, cholesterol; HDL, high-density lipoprotein; LDL, low-density lipoprotein; TG, triglyceride; VLDL, very low-density lipoprotein.

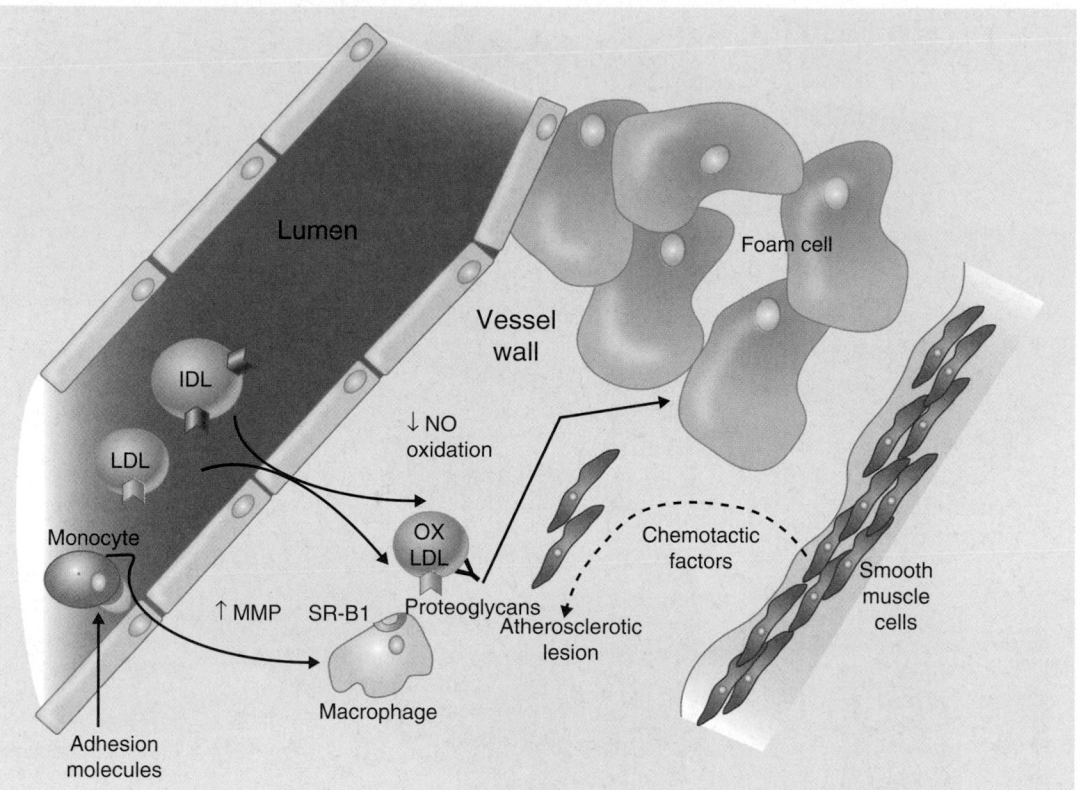

FIGURE 12–5. The process of atherogenesis. Atherosclerosis is initiated by the migration and retention of LDL and remnant lipoprotein particles into the vessel wall. These particles undergo oxidation and are taken up by macrophages in an unregulated fashion. The oxidized particles participate to induce endothelial cell dysfunction leading to a reduced ability of the endothelium to dilate the artery and cause a prothrombotic state. The unregulated uptake of cholesterol by macrophages leads to foam cell formation and the development of a blood clot–favoring fatty lipid core. The enlarging lipid core eventually causes an encroachment of the vessel lumen. Early in the process, smooth muscle cells are activated and recruited from the media to the intima, helping to produce a collagen matrix that covers the growing clot protecting it from circulating blood. Later, macrophages produce and secrete matrix metalloproteinases which degrade the collagen matrix, leading to unstable plaque which may cause a myocardial infarction. (IDL, intermediate-density lipoprotein; LDL, low-density lipoprotein; MMP, matrix metalloproteinases; NO, nitric oxide.)

cap of these unstable plaques rupture and produce an occlusive **thrombus**. In contrast, repeated wound healing secondary to less significant plaque disruption that causes no symptoms might produce a more stable plaque as a consequence of smooth muscle cell, collagen, and fibrin accumulation and a resolution of the lipid core.[6] These more stable plaques usually cause luminal encroachment (detected by traditional coronary angiographic techniques) and may produce **angina pectoris**. Unstable lesions usually outnumber the more stable plaques, thus accounting for a majority of **acute coronary syndromes**. Evidence demonstrates that aggressive lipid-lowering does stabilize these vulnerable lesions and restores endothelial function.[3,6,7]

TREATMENT

In the United States, prevention and treatment of CHD is based primarily on guidelines issued in 2001 by the National Cholesterol Education Program (NCEP) Expert Panel on Detection, Evaluation, and Treatment of High Blood Cholesterol in Adults (Adult Treatment Panel III [ATP III]).[3] The ATP IV guidelines are in development and will be available in 2010.[8] LDL cholesterol is the primary diagnostic and therapeutic target. ❷ *The NCEP ATP III guidelines have set the "optimal" level for LDL cholesterol for all adults as less than 100 mg/dL (2.59 mmol/L).* The NCEP panel issued an update in 2004 to the ATP III guidelines based on more recent clinical trial evidence.[9] The update outlines additional treatment options for certain patient populations, mainly those who are at very high risk of recurrent CHD events. These treatment options emphasize the benefits of diet, exercise, and weight control and the use of 3-hydroxy-3-methylglutaryl coenzyme A (HMG-CoA) reductase inhibitors (or statins) as first-line drugs. If statins or other drugs used to treat hyperlipidemia are prescribed, doses that reduce LDL cholesterol by at least 30% to 40% should be recommended.[9]

Most recently, the American Heart Association and American College of Cardiology issued guidelines for

Clinical Presentation and Diagnosis of Dyslipidemias

Lipid Panel

- Patients presenting with a total cholesterol level exceeding 200 mg/dL (5.18 mmol/L) or LDL cholesterol exceeding 100 mg/dL (2.59 mmol/L) should be evaluated for high cholesterol.
- Patients with serum triglycerides from 150 to 500 mg/dL (1.70–5.65 mmol/L) and serum HDL cholesterol less than 40 mg/dL (1.04 mmol/L) may have metabolic syndrome and need to be evaluated.

Physical Findings

- Patients with genetic disorders that cause a marked increase in serum LDL cholesterol (greater than 250 mg/dL [6.48 mmol/L]) may present with corneal arcus of the eye and xanthomas of extensor tendons of the hand and Achilles tendon.
- Patients with extremely elevated serum triglycerides (greater than 1,000 mg/dL [11.3 mmol/L]) can develop pancreatitis and tuberoeruptive xanthomas.

Indications for Lipid Panel

- All adults greater than 20 years of age should be screened at least every 5 years using a fasting blood sample to obtain a lipid profile (total cholesterol, LDL cholesterol, HDL cholesterol, and triglycerides). A fasting lipid profile is preferred so an accurate assessment of LDL cholesterol can be performed, and fasting will allow the clearance of triglycerides carried by chylomicrons from the circulation, allowing VLDL cholesterol to be determined.
- Children between 2 and 20 years old should be screened for high cholesterol if their parents have premature CHD or if one of their parents has a total cholesterol greater than 240 mg/dL (6.22 mmol/L). Early screening will help to identify children at highest risk of developing CHD in whom early education and dietary intervention is warranted.

Indications for Other Tests

- Conditions that may produce lipid abnormalities (such as those listed in Table 12–3) should be screened for using appropriate tests. If present, these conditions should be properly addressed.

---

secondary prevention in patients with established CHD based on the results of two additional trials published after the 2004 NCEP update.[10] These guidelines suggest it is reasonable to set an LDL cholesterol goal of less than 70 mg/dL (1.81 mmol/L) in all patients with CHD. If it is not possible to attain LDL cholesterol less than 70 mg/dL (1.81 mmol/L) due to a high baseline LDL cholesterol, it is generally possible to achieve an LDL cholesterol reduction of greater than 50% with more intensive LDL-lowering therapy, including combination drug therapy.

Guidelines for Treatment

▶ Step 1: Patient Assessment

Determine lipoprotein profile after fasting for 9 to 12 hours. ❸ *The NCEP guidelines recommend that all adults greater than 20 years of age should be screened at least every 5 years using a fasting blood sample to obtain a lipid profile (total cholesterol, LDL cholesterol, HDL cholesterol, and triglycerides).* A fasting lipid profile is preferred so an accurate assessment of LDL cholesterol can be performed. Fasting permits the clearance of triglycerides carried by chylomicrons from the circulation, thus allowing VLDL cholesterol to be determined. Children between 2 and 20 years old should be screened for high cholesterol if their parents have premature CHD or if one of their parents has a total cholesterol greater than 240 mg/dL (6.22 mmol/L).[3]

Early screening will help to identify children at highest risk of developing CHD, in whom early education and dietary intervention is warranted.

▶ Step 2: Rule Out Secondary Causes of Dyslipidemia

Certain drugs and diseases can cause abnormalities in serum lipids and should be evaluated (Table 12–3). Every effort should be made to correct or control underlying diseases such as hypothyroidism and diabetes. Concurrent medications known to induce lipid abnormalities should be evaluated for discontinuation prior to instituting long-term lipid-lowering therapy.[3]

▶ Step 3: Identify the Presence of Clinical Atherosclerotic Disease or Other Conditions That Confer High Risk for CHD Events

Individuals with established CHD, other clinical atherosclerotic disease (CAD), or diabetes have a greater than 20% risk over a 10-year period of developing CHD events.[3] The ATP III guidelines set the target LDL cholesterol level at less than 100 mg/dL (2.59 mmol/L) for high-risk patients who have a history of one or more of the following:

- Myocardial infarction (MI)
- Unstable angina
- Chronic stable angina

Table 12–3

Secondary Conditions and Drugs That May Cause Hyperlipidemias

	↑ LDL Cholesterol	↑ Triglycerides	↓ HDL Cholesterol
Diabetes		√	√
Hypothyroidism	√	√	
Obstructive liver disease/biliary cirrhosis	√		
Renal disease		√	
Nephrotic syndrome	√	√	
Chronic renal failure		√	
Hemodialysis patients		√	
Obesity		√	√
Drugs:			
Estrogen		√	
Progestins	√		√
Protease inhibitors		√	√
Anabolic steroids	√		√
Corticosteroids	√	√	
Isotretinoin		√	√
Cyclosporine	√		
Atypical antipsychotics		√	√
Thiazide diuretics	√	√	
β-Blockers		√	√

LDL, low-density lipoprotein; HDL, high-density lipoprotein.

- Coronary interventions (coronary bypass, percutaneous transluminal coronary angioplasty, or stents)
- Peripheral arterial disease (claudication or ankle-brachial index less than 0.9)
- Symptomatic carotid artery disease (stroke or transient ischemic attack)
- Diabetes (types 1 and 2)
- Multiple risk factors with a Framingham calculated risk (Fig. 12–6) greater than 20%

❹ *The benefits of lowering LDL cholesterol to as low as 70 mg/dL (1.81 mmol/L) have been demonstrated in clinical trials.* Thus, in patients considered very high risk, an LDL cholesterol goal of less than 70 mg/dL (1.81 mmol/L) is a therapeutic option.[9,10] These individuals have established CAD or present with acute coronary syndromes. *The lowest level of LDL cholesterol where there is no further reduction in CHD risk has not yet been determined.*

▶ Step 4: Determine the Presence of Major Risk Factors

In individuals who do not have established CHD or CHD risk equivalent, the next step is to count major risk factors

for CHD as presented in Table 12–4. These risk factors are considered independent predictors of CHD. HDL cholesterol of greater than or equal to 60 mg/dL (1.55 mmol/L) is considered a negative risk factor and means one risk factor can be subtracted from the total count.[3]

▶ Step 5: If Two or More Risk Factors Are Present Without CHD or CHD Risk Equivalent, Assess 10-Year CHD Risk

● Listed in Table 12–5 are the risk groups that require risk calculations using the Framingham scoring system.[3] Because individuals with two or more risk factors may carry a risk equivalent to individuals with established CHD, and therefore should be treated with the same intensity, a scoring system developed from the Framingham Coronary Heart Disease Study is used to estimate this 10-year risk (Fig. 12–6). This system assigns points to the following risk factors: age, total cholesterol level, smoking status, HDL cholesterol level, and systolic blood pressure. The score is used to determine a patient's risk category and the intensity of treatment to lower their LDL cholesterol. To calculate a Framingham score, visit the following website: *http://www.nhlbi.nih.gov/guidelines/cholesterol/index.htm.*

▶ Step 6: Determine Treatment Goals and Therapy

● Treatment goals for LDL cholesterol and thresholds for the institution of therapeutic lifestyle changes (TLC) and pharmacotherapy is the next step (Table 12–6).

▶ Step 7: Initiate TLC If LDL Is Above Goal

● TLC should be the first approach tried in all patients (Table 12–7).[3] ❺ *An adequate trial of TLC should be employed in all patients, but pharmacotherapy should be instituted concurrently in higher-risk patients (Table 12–6).* This includes dietary restrictions of cholesterol and saturated fats as well as regular exercise and weight reduction. In addition, therapeutic options to enhance LDL cholesterol lowering such as consumption of plant stanols/sterols (which competitively inhibit incorporation of cholesterol into micelles) and dietary fiber should be encouraged. These therapeutic options collectively may reduce LDL cholesterol by 20% to 25%. For a more detailed overview of lifestyle modifications, the reader should refer to the ATP III guidelines[3] and the American Heart Association's diet and lifestyle recommendations.[11]

▶ Step 8: Consider Adding Drug Therapy If LDL Is Above Threshold Level

● Patients unable or unlikely to achieve their LDL cholesterol goals following a reasonable trial of TLC (typically 12 weeks for patients without CHD and sooner for those at high risk or with LDL cholesterol greater than 190 mg/dL [4.92 mmol/L] at baseline) are candidates for drug therapy (Table 12–6). ❻ *Typically, statins are the medications of choice to treat high*

Men Estimate of 10-year risk for men		Women Estimate of 10-year risk for women	

(Framingham point scores)

Age	Points
20–34	−9
35–39	−4
40–44	0
45–49	3
50–54	6
55–59	8
60–64	10
65–69	11
70–74	12
75–79	13

(Framingham point scores)

Age	Points
20–34	−7
35–39	−3
40–44	0
45–49	3
50–54	6
55–59	8
60–64	10
65–69	12
70–74	14
75–79	15

Men — Points

Total cholesterol	Age 20–39	Age 40–49	Age 50–59	Age 60–69	Age 70–79
Less than 160	0	0	0	0	0
160–199	4	3	2	1	0
200–239	7	5	3	1	0
240–279	9	6	4	2	1
Greater than or equal to 280	11	8	5	3	1

Women — Points

Total cholesterol	Age 20–39	Age 40–49	Age 50–59	Age 60–69	Age 70–79
Less than 160	0	0	0	0	0
160–199	4	3	2	1	1
200–239	8	6	4	2	1
240–279	11	8	5	3	2
Greater than or equal to 280	13	10	7	4	2

Men — Points

	Age 20–39	Age 40–49	Age 50–59	Age 60–69	Age 70–79
Nonsmoker	0	0	0	0	0
Smoker	8	5	3	1	1

Women — Points

	Age 20–39	Age 40–49	Age 50–59	Age 60–69	Age 70–79
Nonsmoker	0	0	0	0	0
Smoker	9	7	4	2	1

HDL (mg/dL)	Points
Greater than or equal to 60	−1
50–59	0
40–49	1
Less than 40	2

HDL (mg/dL)	Points
Greater than or equal to 60	−1
50–59	0
40–49	1
Less than 40	2

Systolic BP (mm Hg)	If untreated	If treated
Less than 120	0	0
120–129	0	1
130–139	1	2
140–159	1	2
Greater than or equal to 160	2	3

Systolic BP (mmHg)	If untreated	If treated
Less than 120	0	0
120–129	1	3
130–139	2	4
140–159	3	5
Greater than or equal to 160	4	6

Point total	10-year risk %
Less than 0	Less than 1
0	1
1	1
2	1
3	1
4	1
5	2
6	2
7	3
8	4
9	5
10	6
11	8
12	10
13	12
14	16
15	20
16	25
Greater than or equal to 17	Greater than or equal to 30

10-year risk _____ %

Point total	10-year risk %
Less than 9	Less than 1
9	1
10	1
11	1
12	1
13	2
14	2
15	3
16	4
17	5
18	6
19	8
20	11
21	14
22	17
23	22
24	27
Greater than or equal to 25	Greater than or equal to 30

10-year risk _____ %

FIGURE 12–6. Framingham Point Scale for estimating 10-year CHD risk. The Framingham score is used to determine a patient's CHD risk category when they are found to have two or more CHD risk factors (Table 12–4). This system assigns points to the following risk factors: age, total cholesterol level (in mg/dL), smoking status, HDL cholesterol level, and systolic blood pressure. The point total corresponds to the 10-year risk (%) of a CHD event (nonfatal myocardial infarction and coronary death), which serves as a basis for deciding how intensively to treat hypercholesterolemia and other risk factors. To calculate risk factor using the Framingham Point Scale, go to the following website: *http://www.nhlbi.nih.gov/guidelines/cholesterol/index.htm*. The Système International units for the corresponding conventional units in the Framingham Point Scale illustration include: (1) total cholesterol (160 mg/dL = 4.14 mmol/L; 160–199 mg/dL = 4.14–5.15 mmol/L; 200–239 mg/dL = 5.18–6.19 mmol/L; 240–279 mg/dL = 6.22–7.23 mmol/L; 280 mg/dL = 7.25 mmol/L) and (2) HDL (60 mg/dL = 1.55 mmol/L; 50–59 mg/dL = 1.3–1.53 mmol/L; 40–49 mg/dL = 1.04–1.27 mmol/L; 40 mg/dL = 1.04 mmol/L). (BP, blood pressure; CHD, coronary heart disease; HDL, high-density lipoprotein.) (From *http://www.nhlbi.nih.gov/guidelines/cholesterol/index.htm*.)

Patient Encounter 1, Part 1

MN is a 48-year-old man with a history of hypertension and smoking who presents to the clinic for evaluation of his cholesterol. He denies having chest pain or history of myocardial infarction, stroke, or peripheral artery disease. He has no siblings and both parents are alive with no history of CHD. MN says that he smokes about one pack of cigarettes per day. He does not exercise on a regular basis. He has been fasting for approximately 11 hours.

Can MN be evaluated today for his cholesterol?

Does he have risk factors for CHD?

What additional information do you need to know for the evaluation of MN?

Table 12–4

Risk Factors for CHD

Risk Factor	Definition
Age (years)	Male 45 years or older; female 55 years or older
Family history of premature CHD events	Male first-degree relative at less than 55 years Female first-degree relative at less than 65 years
Hypertension	SBP greater than or equal to 140 mm Hg DBP greater than or equal to 90 mm Hg
HDL cholesterol	Less than 40 mg/dL (1.04 mmol/L)
Cigarette smoking	Within the past month

CHD, coronary heart disease; DBP, diastolic blood pressure; HDL, high-density lipoprotein; SBP, systolic blood pressure.

HDL cholesterol greater than or equal to 60 mg/dL (1.55 mmol/L) is considered a negative risk factor; thus, subtract one risk factor from the total from above.

Table 12–5

CHD Risk Factors and Needed Risk Factors for Framingham Score Calculation

Risk Profile	10-Year Risk for CHD	Need for Framingham Calculation
Less than or equal to 1 risk factor	Less than 10%	No
Greater than or equal to 2 risk factors	0–10%	Yes
	10–20%	Yes
CAD or CAD risk equivalent	Greater than 20%	No
Very high risk	Much greater than 20%	No

CAD, clinical atherosclerotic disease; CHD, coronary heart disease.

LDL cholesterol because of their ability to substantially reduce LDL cholesterol, ability to reduce morbidity and mortality from atherosclerotic disease, convenient once-daily dosing, and low risk of side effects.

▶ Step 9: Identify Patients With the Metabolic Syndrome

Diagnosis of the metabolic syndrome is made when three or more of the following risk factors are present:[3,12]

- Waist circumference greater than or equal to 40 in. (102 cm) in men (35 in. [89 cm] in Asian males), or 35 in. (89 cm) in women (31 in. [79 cm] in Asian females)

- Triglycerides greater than or equal to 150 mg/dL (1.70 mmol/L) or on drug treatment for elevated triglycerides

- HDL cholesterol less than 40 mg/dL (1.04 mmol/L) in men or 50 mg/dL (1.3 mmol/L) in women or on drug treatment for reduced HDL cholesterol

- Blood pressure greater than or equal to 130/85 mm Hg or on drug treatment for hypertension

- Fasting blood glucose greater than or equal to 100 mg/dL (5.55 mmol/L) or on drug treatment for elevated glucose

Patients with the metabolic syndrome are twice as likely to develop type 2 diabetes and four times more likely to develop CHD.[3,13] These individuals are usually insulin resistant, obese, have hypertension, are in a **prothrombotic state**, and have atherogenic dyslipidemia characterized by low HDL cholesterol and elevated triglycerides, and an increased proportion of their LDL particles are small and dense.[3]

NCEP ATP III identified the metabolic syndrome as an important target for further reducing CHD risk. Treatment of the metabolic syndrome starts with increased physical activity, weight reduction (which also enhances LDL cholesterol lowering and insulin sensitivity), and moderation of ethanol use and carbohydrate intake, which effectively reduce many of the associated risk factors. Each of the risk factors should be addressed independently as appropriate, including treatment of hypertension and use of aspirin in CHD patients to reduce the prothrombotic state. **7** *Patients with metabolic syndrome have an additional lipid parameter that needs to be assessed, namely non-HDL cholesterol (total cholesterol minus HDL cholesterol).*[3] *The target for non-HDL cholesterol is less than the patient's LDL cholesterol target plus 30 mg/dL (0.78 mmol/L).* **8** *After assessment and control of LDL cholesterol, patients with serum triglycerides between 200 and 499 mg/dL (2.26 and 5.64 mmol/L) should be assessed for atherogenic dyslipidemia (low HDL cholesterol, increased small-dense LDL particles) and metabolic syndrome.* Non-HDL cholesterol estimates the cholesterol carried by all Apo B-containing lipoprotein particles. Thus, non-HDL cholesterol represents the sum of LDL cholesterol, VLDL cholesterol, and other triglyceride-rich remnant particles. The non-HDL cholesterol goal is 30 mg/dL (0.78 mmol/L) higher than the LDL cholesterol goal. This is based on the premise that a VLDL cholesterol level less than or equal to 30 mg/dL (0.78 mmol/L) is normal.

Table 12–6

National Cholesterol Education Program (NCEP) Expert Panel on Detection, Evaluation, and Treatment of High Blood Cholesterol in Adults (Adult Treatment Panel III [ATP III]) Treatment Goals for LDL Cholesterol and Thresholds for Starting TLC and Pharmacotherapy

Risk Category	LDL cholesterol Goal	Initiate Therapeutic Lifestyle Changes (TLC)	Consider Drug Therapy
High Risk CHD or CHD risk equivalents (10-year risk greater than 20%)	Less than 100 mg/dL (2.59 mmol/L)	Greater than or equal to 100 mg/dL (2.59 mmol/L)	Greater than or equal to 100 mg/dL (2.59 mmol/L)
Very-High Risk	Optional goal of less than 70 mg/dL[a] (1.81 mmol/L)		
Moderately-High Risk Greater than or equal to 2 risk factors (10-year risk 10–20%)	Less than 130 mg/dL (3.37 mmol/L) (Optional goal of less than 100 mg/dL[a] [2.59 mmol/L])	Greater than or equal to 130 mg/dL (3.37 mmol/L)	Greater than or equal to 130 mg/dL (3.37 mmol/L) (consider drug options if LDL cholesterol 100–129 mg/dL [2.59–3.34 mmol/L])
Moderate Risk Greater than or equal to 2 risk factors (10-year risk less than 10%)	Less than 130 mg/dL (3.37 mmol/L)	Greater than or equal to 130 mg/dL (3.37 mmol/L)	Greater than 160 mg/dL (4.14 mmol/L)
Low Risk	Less than 160 mg/dL (4.14 mmol/L)	Greater than or equal to 160 mg/dL (4.14 mmol/L)	Greater than or equal to 190 mg/dL (4.92 mmol/L) (consider drug options if LDL cholesterol 160–189 mg/dL [4.14–4.90 mmol/L])

CHD, coronary heart disease; LDL, low-density lipoprotein; TLC, therapeutic lifestyle changes.

[a]Optional goals indicated in the NCEP ATP III 2004 update of the guidelines.

Table 12–7

Essential Components of TLC

Component	Recommendation
LDL-raising nutrients Saturated fats Dietary cholesterol	Total fat range should be 25–35% for most cases Less than 7% of total calories and reduce intake of trans fatty acids Less than 200 mg/day
Therapeutic options for LDL-lowering plant stanols/sterols	2 g per day
Increased viscous (soluble) fiber	10–25 g per day
Total calories	Adjust caloric intake to maintain desirable body weight and prevent weight gain
Physical activity	Include enough moderate exercise to expend at least 200 kcal (837 kJ) per day

LDL, low-density lipoprotein; TLC, therapeutic lifestyle changes.

For example, the LDL cholesterol goal is less than 100 mg/dL (2.59 mmol/L) and the non-HDL cholesterol goal is less than 130 mg/dL (3.37 mmol/L) for a diabetic patient without a history of CHD. Two treatment approaches can be considered for achieving the non-HDL cholesterol goal: titrating existing LDL-lowering therapy or adding niacin or a fibrate to the LDL-lowering therapy.[3] The reader is referred to the Ischemic Heart Disease and Diabetes Mellitus chapters for further information regarding metabolic syndrome.

▶ *Step 10: Treatment of Elevated Triglycerides*

Patients with serum triglycerides exceeding 500 mg/dL (5.65 mmol/L) are at increased risk of pancreatitis, especially when levels exceed 1,000 mg/dL (11.3 mmol/L).[3] Reducing triglycerides in these individuals becomes the primary target for intervention. Reduction in fats, ethanol, and carbohydrates should be considered, and secondary causes (Table 12–3) should be assessed. When pharmacotherapy is instituted, the intensity of therapy should be to reduce

Patient Encounter 1, Part 2: Medical History, Physical Exam, and Diagnostic Tests

PMH: Hypertension for 9 years; history of gout

FH: Father and mother both alive with no history of CHD or diabetes.

SH: Works as a computer programmer and sits at his desk most of the day; does not exercise on a regular basis; drinks alcohol (2 to 3 beers) mainly on the weekends while watching sports on TV

Meds: Aspirin 80 mg once daily, verapamil SR 180 mg once daily

ROS: No chest pain, shortness of breath, or dizziness

PE:

VS: BP 142/86 mm Hg, p 71 bpm, RR 16 bpm, T 37°C (98.6°F), waist circumference 38 in. (97 cm)

CV: RRR, normal S_1, S_2; no murmurs, rubs, or gallops

Abd: Soft, nontender, nondistended; positive for bowel sounds, no hepatosplenomegaly or abdominal aortic aneurysm

Exts: Ankle-brachial index 1.1

Neck: No carotid and basilar bruits

Labs:

Total cholesterol 256 mg/dL (6.63 mmol/L), triglycerides 235 mg/dL (2.66 mmol/L), HDL cholesterol 27 mg/dL (0.70 mmol/L), glucose 115 mg/dL (6.38 mmol/L), all other labs within normal limits

Given this additional information, what is your assessment of MN's CHD risk?

Identify your treatment goals for MN.

What diagnostic parameters does MN have for the metabolic syndrome?

What nonpharmacologic and pharmacologic alternatives are available for MN?

Develop a care plan for MN.

triglycerides to less than 150 mg/dL (1.70 mmol/L). Once triglycerides are less than 500 mg/dL (5.65 mmol/L) and the risk of pancreatitis is reduced, the primary focus of intervention should once again be on LDL cholesterol. As noted above, individuals with triglycerides between 200 and 499 mg/dL (2.26 and 5.64 mmol/L) identified as having metabolic syndrome have an increase in triglyceride-rich remnant lipoproteins and small-dense LDL particles. Non-HDL cholesterol should be a secondary target in these individuals. Niacin, fibrates, and omega-3-fatty acids (O3FA) are the most effective agents in patients with hypertriglyceridemia.[3]

Emerging and Life-Habit Risk Factors

In addition to the five major risks, the ATP III guidelines recognize other factors that contribute to CHD risk. These are classified as life-habit risk factors and emerging risk factors. Life-habit risk factors, consisting of obesity, physical inactivity, and an atherogenic diet, require direct intervention. For example, emerging risk factors are lipoprotein(a), homocysteine, prothrombotic/proinflammatory factors, lipoprotein-associated phospholipase A2 (Lp-PLA2), and C-reactive protein (CRP). CRP is a marker of low-level inflammation and appears to help in predicting CHD risk beyond LDL cholesterol and major CHD risk factors.[13] In a recent trial, rosuvastatin significantly reduced the incidence of major cardiovascular events in apparently healthy persons without hyperlipidemia (LDL cholesterol less than 130 mg/dL [3.37 mmol/L]) but with elevated high-sensitivity CRP levels.[14] These results will need to be considered by the ATP IV writing committee.[8] In some patients, emerging risk factors may be used to guide the intensity of risk-reduction therapy. Deciding when to consider emerging risk factors requires the use of clinical judgment.

Pharmacotherapy

▶ Statins (HMG-CoA Reductase Inhibitors)

Statins are very effective LDL-lowering medications and are proven to reduce the risk of CHD, stroke, and death. Thus, NCEP ATP III considers statins the preferred LDL-lowering medications. Data concerning the efficacy and safety of the statins now go back nearly 25 years. Statins are effective in reducing MIs, strokes, revascularization procedures, cardiovascular deaths, and in some cases, total mortality. This effectiveness has been demonstrated in both genders, the elderly, patients with diabetes and hypertension, those with and without pre-existing CHD, and following an acute coronary syndrome.[14-25] Statins inhibit conversion of HMG-CoA to L-mevalonic acid and subsequently cholesterol. Statins lower LDL cholesterol levels by approximately 25% to 62% (Table 12–8). A substantial reduction in LDL cholesterol occurs at the usual starting dose and each doubling of the daily dose only produces an additional 6% average reduction (known as the "rule of 6"). This is important when considering dose escalation versus adding on an additional LDL-lowering drug. Statins are moderately effective at reducing triglycerides and modestly raise HDL cholesterol (Table 12–8). By inhibiting the synthesis of L-mevalonic acid, statins in turn inhibit other important by-products in the cholesterol biosynthetic pathway that affect intracellular transport, membrane trafficking, and gene transcription.[26] This may explain some of the cholesterol-independent benefits (so-called "pleiotropic" effects) of statins such as reducing lipoprotein oxidation, enhancing endothelial synthesis of nitric oxide, and inhibiting thrombosis. These pleiotropic effects are thought to contribute to the rapid/earlier benefits of statins on CHD risk while the decrease in serum lipids accounts for the slower late benefit.

Table 12–8

Effects of Lipid-Lowering Drugs on Serum Lipids at FDA-Approved Doses

Lipid-Lowering Drug	LDL Cholesterol	HDL Cholesterol	Triglycerides	Total Cholesterol
Statins				
Atorvastatin	−26% to −60%	+5% to +13%	−17% to −53%	−25% to −45%
Fluvastatin	−22% to −36%	+3% to +11%	−12% to −25%	−16% to −27%
Fluvastatin ER	−33% to −35%	+7% to +11%	−19% to −25%	−25%
Lovastatin	−21% to −42%	+2% to +10%	−6% to −27%	−16% to −34%
Lovastatin ER	−24% to −41%	+9% to +13%	−10% to −25%	−18% to −29%
Pravastatin	−22% to −34%	+2% to +12%	−15% to −24%	−16% to −25%
Rosuvastatin	−45% to −63%	+8% to +14%	−10% to −35%	−33% to −46%
Simvastatin	−26% to −47%	+8% to +16%	−12% to −34%	−19% to −36%
Bile Acid Sequestrants				
Cholestyramine	−15% to −30%	+3% to +5%	May increase in patients with elevated triglycerides	−10% to −25%
Colesevelam	−8% to −15%	+3% to +5%		−70% to −10%
Colestipol	−15% to −30%	+3% to +5%		−10% to 25%
Cholesterol Absorption Inhibitor				
Ezetimibe	−18%	+1% to +2%	−7% to −9%	−12% to −13%
Nicotinic Acid				
Niacin ER	−5% to −17%	+14% to +26%	−11% to −38%	−3% to −12%
Niacin IR	−5% to −25%	+15% to +39%	−20% to −60%	−3% to −25%
Fibric Acid Derivatives				
Fenofibrate	−31% to +45%	+9% to +23%	−23% to −54%	−9% to −22%
Gemfibrozil	−30% to +30%	+10% to +30%	−20% to −60%	−2% to −16%
Combination Products				
Niacin ER and lovastatin	−30% to −42%	+20% to +30%	−32 to −44%	Not stated
Niacin ER and simvastatin[a]	−12% to −14%	+21% to +29%	−27% to −38%	−9% to −11%
Simvastatin and ezetimibe	−46% to −59%	+8% to +12%	−26% to −25%	−34% to −43%
Omega-3-Fatty Acids				
Lovaza	+45%	+9%	−44.9%	−9.7%

ER, extended-release; FDA, Food and Drug Administration; HDL, high-density lipoprotein; IR, immediate-release; LDL, low-density lipoprotein; SR, sustained-release.

[a]Additional percent changes with treatment with niacin ER and simvastatin 1,000 mg/20 mg to 2,000 mg/20 mg after initial treatment with simvastatin 20 mg.

Statins are well tolerated with less than 4% of patients in clinical trials discontinuing therapy due to adverse side effects (Table 12–9). Elevations in liver function tests (LFTs) and myopathy, including rhabdomyolysis, are important adverse effects associated with the statins. Liver toxicity, defined as LFT elevations greater than three times the upper limit of normal, is reported in less than 2% of patients; however, the incidence is higher at higher doses and the progression to liver failure is thought to be exceedingly rare. LFTs should be obtained at baseline and 6 to 12 weeks after starting therapy or any dose escalation. Annual monitoring of LFTs is usually sufficient. Myopathy, defined as muscle symptoms with creatine kinase (CK; or creatine phosphokinase [CPK]) 10 times the upper limit of normal, is reported to range from 0% to less than 0.5% for the currently marketed statins at FDA-approved doses. Rhabdomyolysis, defined as muscle symptoms with marked elevation in CK 10 times the upper limit of normal with creatinine elevation usually associated with myoglobinuria and brown urine, is very rare.[27] The concern of statin-associated myopathy has increased since the voluntary removal of cerivastatin from the world market

in 2001 because the reported rate of fatal rhabdomyolysis was 16 to 80 times higher than the rate for any other statin, and many of these cases were reported in patients treated with concomitant gemfibrozil.[28] The American College of Cardiology/American Heart Association/National Heart, Lung and Blood Institute published a clinical advisory with a focus on myopathy.[27] Listed below are the risks associated with statin-induced myopathy published in this report:

- Small body frame and frailty
- Multisystem disease (e.g., chronic renal insufficiency, especially due to diabetes)
- Multiple medications (see below)
- Perioperative periods
- Specific concomitant medications or consumptions (check specific statin package insert for warnings): fibrates (especially gemfibrozil, but other fibrates too), nicotinic acid (rarely), cyclosporine, azole antifungals such as itraconazole and ketoconazole, macrolide antibiotics such as erythromycin and clarithromycin, protease inhibitors

Table 12-9

Formulation, Dosing, and Common Adverse Effects of Lipid-Lowering Drugs

Lipid-Lowering Drug	Dosage Forms	Usual Adult Maintenance Dose Range	Adverse Effects
Statins			
Atorvastatin	10, 20, 40, 80 mg tablets	10–80 mg once daily (at any time of day). Dose adjustment in patients with renal dysfunction is not necessary	Most frequent side effects are constipation, abdominal pain, diarrhea, dyspepsia, and nausea. Statins should be discontinued promptly if serum transaminase levels (liver function tests) rise to 3 times upper limit of normal, or if patient develops signs or symptoms of myopathy. Approximate equivalent doses of HMG-CoA reductase inhibitors are: atorvastatin 10 mg, fluvastatin 80 mg, lovastatin 40 mg, pravastatin 40 mg, simvastatin 20 mg, and rosuvastatin 5 mg
Fluvastatin	20, 40 mg capsules; 80 mg ER tablets	20–40 mg/day as a single dose (evening) or 40 mg twice daily; 80 mg once daily (evening). Dose adjustments for mild to moderate renal impairment are not necessary	
Lovastatin	10, 20, 40 mg tablets	10–80 mg/day as a single dose (with evening meal) or divided twice daily with food. In patients with severe renal insufficiency (creatinine clearance less than 30 mL/min), dosage increases above 20 mg/day should be carefully considered and, if deemed necessary, implemented cautiously	
Lovastatin ER	20, 30, 60 mg tablets	20–60 mg/day as a single dose. In patients with severe renal insufficiency (creatinine clearance less than 30 mL/min), dosage increases above 20 mg/day should be carefully considered and, if deemed necessary, implemented cautiously	
Pravastatin	10, 20, 40, 80 mg tablets	10–80 mg/day as a single dose at bedtime. In patients with a history of significant renal or hepatic dysfunction, a starting dose of 10 mg daily is recommended.	
Rosuvastatin	5, 10, 20, 40 mg tablets	5–40 mg/day (at any time of day). 40 mg reserved for those who don't achieve LDL cholesterol goal on 20 mg. In patients with a history of significant renal or hepatic dysfunction, a starting dose of 10 mg daily is recommended.	
Simvastatin	5, 10, 20, 40, 80 mg tablets	5–80 mg/day as a single dose in the evening, or divided. In patients with mild to moderate renal insufficiency dosage adjustment is not necessary. However, caution should be exercised in patients with severe renal insufficiency; such patients should be started at 5 mg/day and be closely monitored	

(Continued)

Table 12-9

Formulation, Dosing, and Common Adverse Effects of Lipid-Lowering Drugs (*Continued*)

Lipid-Lowering Drug	Dosage Forms	Usual Adult Maintenance Dose Range	Adverse Effects
Bile Acid Sequestrants			
Cholestyramine	4 g packets	4–24 g/day in two or more divided doses	Main side effects are nausea, constipation, bloating, and flatulence, although these may be less with Colesevelam. Increasing fluid and dietary fiber intake may relieve constipation and bloating. Impair absorption of fat-soluble vitamins
Colesevelam	625 mg tablets	3,750–4,375 mg/day as a single dose or divided twice daily, with meals	
Colestipol	5 g packets	5–30 g/day as a single dose or divided	
	1 g tablets	2–16 g/day as a single dose or divided	
Cholesterol Absorption Inhibitors			
Ezetimibe	10 mg tablet	10 mg once daily. No dosage adjustment is necessary in patients with renal or mild hepatic insufficiency	The overall incidence of adverse events reported with ezetimibe alone was similar to that reported with placebo and generally similar between ezetimibe with a statin and statin alone. The frequency of increased transaminases was slightly higher in patients receiving ezetimibe plus a statin compared with those receiving statin monotherapy (1.3% versus 0.4%)
Nicotinic Acid			
Niacin ER	500, 750, 1,000 mg ER tablets	1,000–2,000 mg once daily at bedtime. Decrease dose by 50% when GFR less than 15 mL/min	Side effects include flushing, itching, gastric distress, headache, hepatotoxicity, hyperglycemia, and hyperuricemia
Niacin	50–750 mg tabs or caps, immediate-release	1–5 g/day in three or more divided doses. Decrease dose by 50% when GFR less than 15 mL/min	
	250–750 mg sustained-release	1–2 g/day (never exceed 2 g/day due to increased risk of hepatotoxicity). Decrease dose by 50% when GFR less than 15 mL/min	
Fibric Acid Derivatives			
Fenofibrate	54, 160 mg tablets	54–160 mg/day; the dosage should be minimized in severe renal impairment	Most common side effects are nausea, diarrhea, abdominal pain, and rash. Increased risk of rhabdomyolysis when given with a statin. Fibric acids are associated with gallstones, myositis, and hepatitis
Gemfibrozil	600 mg tablets	1,200 mg/day in two doses, 30 minutes before meals; should be avoided in hepatic or severe renal impairment	
Combination Products			
Niacin ER and lovastatin	500 mg/20 mg, 750 mg/20 mg, 1,000 mg/20 mg tablets	500 mg/20 mg to 2,000 mg/40 mg daily, at bedtime	See prior entries for each drug (niacin ER and lovastatin)
Niacin ER and simvastatin	500 mg/20 mg, 750 mg/20 mg, 1,000 mg/20 mg tablets	1,000 mg/20 mg to 2,000 mg/40 mg (two 1,000 mg/20 mg tablets), at bedtime	See prior entries for each drug (niacin ER and simvastatin)
Ezetimibe and simvastatin	10 mg/10 mg, 10 mg/20 mg, 10 mg/40 mg, 10 mg/80 mg	The dosage range is 10/10 mg/day through 10/80 mg/day. The recommended usual starting dose is 10/20 mg/day. Initiation of therapy with 10/10 mg/day may be considered for patients requiring less aggressive LDL cholesterol reductions	See prior entries for each drug (ezetimibe and simvastatin)

ER, extended release; GFR, glomerular filtration rate; HMG-CoA, 3-hydroxy-3-methyglutaryl coenzyme A; LDL, low-density lipoprotein; min, minute.

used to treat AIDS, nefazodone (antidepressant), verapamil, amiodarone, large quantities of grapefruit juice (usually more than 1 quart [about 950 mL] per day), and alcohol abuse (independently predisposes to myopathy)

Baseline CK should be obtained in all patients prior to starting statin therapy. Follow-up CK should only be obtained in patients complaining of muscle pain, weakness, tenderness, or brown urine. Routine monitoring of CK is of little value in the absence of clinical signs or symptoms. Patient assessment for symptoms of myopathy should be done 6 to 12 weeks after starting therapy and at each visit. More frequent monitoring should be done in higher-risk individuals such as those identified above.

With the exception of pravastatin which is mainly metabolized by isomerization in the gut to a relatively inactive metabolite, the other statins undergo biotransformation by the cytochrome P-450 system. Therefore, drugs known to inhibit statin metabolism should be used cautiously. The time until maximum effect on lipids for statins is generally 4 to 6 weeks.

► Cholesterol Absorption Inhibitors

Ezetimibe is the first drug in a new class of agents referred to as cholesterol absorption inhibitors. Ezetimibe blocks biliary and dietary cholesterol as well as phytosterol (plant sterol) absorption by interacting with the NPC1L1 transporter located in the brush border membrane of enterocytes (Fig. 12–2).[5] Ezetimibe inhibits 54% of all intestinal cholesterol absorption on average. By reducing the cholesterol content within chylomicrons delivered to the liver, ezetimibe reduces liver cholesterol stores, inducing an upregulation of LDL receptors resulting in a decrease in serum cholesterol. As a result, ezetimibe also induces a compensatory increase in cholesterol biosynthesis. Since statins inhibit cholesterol biosynthesis, the compensatory increase in cholesterol biosynthesis by ezetimibe can be blocked by combining ezetimibe with a statin.

Ezetimibe reduces LDL cholesterol by an average of 18% (Table 12–8). However, larger reductions can be seen in some individuals, presumably due to higher absorption of cholesterol. These individuals appear to have a blunted response to statin therapy. Ezetimibe lowers triglycerides by 7% to 9% and modestly increases HDL cholesterol.

Once absorbed, ezetimibe undergoes extensive glucuronidation in the intestinal wall to the active metabolite (ezetimibe glucuronide). Ezetimibe and the active metabolite are enterohepatically recirculated back to the site of action, which limits systemic exposure and may explain the low incidence of adverse effects (Table 12–9). Ezetimibe alone or with a statin is contraindicated in patients with active liver disease or unexplained persistent elevations in LFTs. Ezetimibe combined with simvastatin and simvastatin monotherapy were not associated with a reduction in carotid intima-media thickness in patients with heterozygous familial hypercholesterolemia.[29] The patients studied in this trial were well managed (80% were receiving statins prior to enrollment) and had "near normal" measurements of carotid intima-media thickness at baseline which may

***

> ### Patient Encounter 2
>
> LC is a 51-year-old female with a history of CHD (stent placement in the left anterior descending coronary artery 3 years prior) and type 2 diabetes who is referred to you for follow-up of her cholesterol. She is taking simvastatin 20 mg once daily in the evening for her cholesterol, metformin 2,000 mg once daily in the evening, and pioglitizone 15 mg once daily for diabetes. Her diabetes is well controlled. Her laboratory test results are within normal limits, except for her fasting lipid profile: total cholesterol 215 mg/dL (5.57 mmol/L), triglycerides 135 mg/dL (1.53 mmol/L), HDL cholesterol 51 mg/dL (1.32 mmol/L), and LDL cholesterol 137 mg/dL (3.55 mmol/L).
>
> *What is your assessment of LC's cholesterol results?*
>
> *Identify treatment goals for LC.*
>
> *Assess LC's risk for statin-induced side effects.*
>
> *Design a treatment plan for LC.*

explain the study findings. However, ezetimibe combined with simvastatin was associated with a reduced incidence of ischemic cardiovascular events in low risk patients with mild to moderate asymptomatic aortic stenosis compared to placebo.[30] Other clinical trials designed to determine ezetimibe's effects on CHD morbidity and mortality have not been completed. The time until maximum effect on lipids for ezetemibe is generally 2 weeks.

► Bile Acid Sequestrants

Cholestyramine, colestipol, and colesevelam are the bile acid-binding resins or sequestrants (BAS) currently available in the United States. Resins are highly charged molecules that bind to bile acids (which are produced from cholesterol) in the gut. The resin-bile acid complex is then excreted in the feces. The loss of bile causes a compensatory conversion of hepatic cholesterol to bile, reducing hepatocellular stores of cholesterol resulting in an upregulation of LDL receptors to replenish hepatocellular stores which then result in a decrease in serum cholesterol. Resins have been shown to reduce CHD events in patients without CHD.[31]

Resins are moderately effective in lowering LDL cholesterol but do not lower triglycerides (Table 12–8). Moreover, in patients with elevated triglycerides, the use of a resin may worsen the condition. This may be due to a compensatory increase in HMG-CoA reductase activity and results in an increase in assembly and secretion of VLDL. The increase in HMG-CoA reductase activity can be blocked with a statin, resulting in enhanced reductions in serum lipids (see section on combination therapy). Resins reduce LDL cholesterol from 15% to 30%, with a modest increase in HDL cholesterol (3%–5%) (Table 12–8). Resins are most often used as adjuncts to statins in patients who require additional lowering of LDL cholesterol. Because these drugs are not absorbed, adverse effects are limited to the GI tract (Table 12–9). About 20% of patients taking cholestyramine or colestipol report constipation and symptoms such as flatulence and bloating. A large number of patients stop therapy because of this. Resins should be started at the lowest dose and escalated slowly over weeks to months as tolerated until the desired response is obtained. Patients should be instructed to prepare the powder formulations in 6 to 8 ounces (approximately 180–240 mL) of noncarbonated fluids, usually juice (enhances palatability) or water. Fluid intake should be increased to minimize constipation. Colesevelam is better tolerated with fewer gastrointestinal side effects, although it is more expensive. All resins have the potential to prevent the absorption of other drugs such as digoxin, warfarin, thyroxine, thiazides, β-blockers, fat-soluble vitamins, and folic acid. Potential drug interactions can be avoided by taking a resin either 1 hour before or 4 hours after these other agents. Colesevelam appears less likely than the older agents to reduce drug absorption, and the manufacturer does state that colesevelam has to be dosed hours apart from other medications that have been tested in in vitro binding or in vivo drug interaction testing or with postmarketing reports to interact. Orally administered drugs that have not been tested for interaction with colesevelam, especially those with a narrow therapeutic index, should be administered at least 4 hours prior to colesevelam.[32] The time until maximum effect on lipids for resins is generally 2 to 4 weeks.

▶ Niacin

Niacin (vitamin B$_3$) has broad applications in the treatment of lipid disorders when used at higher doses than those used as a nutritional supplement. Niacin inhibits fatty acid release from adipose tissue and inhibits fatty acid and triglyceride production in liver cells. This results in an increased intracellular degradation of Apo B, and in turn, a reduction in the number of VLDL particles secreted (Fig. 12–4). The lower VLDL levels and the lower triglyceride content in these particles leads to an overall reduction in LDL cholesterol as well as a decrease in the number of small, dense LDL particles. Niacin also reduces the uptake of HDL-Apo A1 particles and increases uptake of cholesterol esters by the liver, thus improving the efficiency of reverse cholesterol transport between HDL particles and vascular tissue (Fig. 12–4). Niacin is indicated for patients with elevated triglycerides, low HDL cholesterol, and elevated LDL cholesterol.[3]

Several different niacin formulations are available: niacin immediate-release (IR), niacin sustained-release (SR), and niacin extended-release (ER).[33,34] These formulations differ in terms of dissolution and absorption rates, metabolism, efficacy, and side effects. Limitations of niacin IR and SR are flushing and **hepatotoxicity**, respectively. These differences appear related to the dissolution and absorption rates of niacin formulations and its subsequent metabolism. Niacin IR is available by prescription (Niacor) as well as a dietary supplement which is not regulated by the FDA.[33] Currently, there are no FDA-approved niacin SR products; thus, all SR products are available only as dietary supplements.

Niacin IR is usually completely absorbed within 1 to 2 hours; thus, it quickly saturates a high-affinity, low-capacity metabolic pathway, and the majority of the drug is metabolized by a second low-affinity, high-capacity system with metabolites associated with flushing.[35] Conversely, absorption of niacin SR may exceed 12 hours. Because niacin SR is absorbed over 12 or more hours, the high-affinity pathway metabolizes the majority of the drug, resulting in the production of metabolites associated with hepatotoxicity. Niacin ER was developed as a once-daily formulation to be taken at bedtime, with the goal of reducing the incidence of flushing without increasing the risk of hepatotoxicity. Niacin ER (Niaspan) is the only long-acting niacin product approved by the FDA for dyslipidemia. Niacin ER has an absorption rate of 8 to 12 hours, intermediate to niacin IR and SR, and therefore balances metabolism more evenly over the high-affinity, low-capacity pathway and the low-affinity, high-capacity pathway. Furthermore, taking niacin ER at bedtime can minimize the impact of flushing.

Niacin use is limited by cutaneous reactions such as flushing and pruritus of the face and body. The use of aspirin or a nonsteroidal anti-inflammatory drug (NSAID) 30 minutes prior to taking niacin can help alleviate these reactions, as they are mediated by an increase in prostaglandin D2.[3] In addition, taking niacin with food and avoiding hot liquids at the time niacin is taken is helpful in minimizing flushing and pruritus.

In general, niacin reduces LDL cholesterol from 5% to 25%, reduces triglycerides by 20% to 50%, and increases HDL cholesterol by 15% to 35% (Table 12–8). Niacin has been shown to reduce CHD events and total mortality[36] as well as the progression of atherosclerosis when combined with a statin.[37]

Niacin can raise uric acid levels, and in diabetics can raise blood glucose levels. However, several clinical trials have shown that niacin can be used safely and effectively in patients with diabetes.[38] Due to the high cardiovascular risk of patients with diabetes, the benefits of improving the lipid profile appear to outweigh any adjustment in diabetic medication(s) that is needed.[39]

Niacin should be instituted at the lowest dose and gradually titrated to a maximum dose of 2 g daily for ER and SR products and no more than 5 g daily for IR products. FDA-approved niacin products are preferred because of product consistency. Moreover, niacin products labeled as "no flush" don't contain nicotinic acid and therefore have no therapeutic role in the treatment of lipid disorders.[33] The time until maximum effect on lipids for niacins is generally 3 to 5 weeks.

▶ Fibrates

The predominant effects of fibrates are a decrease in triglyceride levels by 20% to 50% and an increase in HDL cholesterol levels by 9% to 30% (Table 12–8). The effect on LDL cholesterol is less predictable. In patients with high triglycerides, however, LDL cholesterol may increase. Fibrates increase the size and reduce the density of LDL particles much like niacin. Fibrates are the most effective triglyceride-lowering drugs and are used primarily in patients with elevated triglycerides and low HDL cholesterol.

Fibrates work by reducing Apos B, C-III (an inhibitor of LPL), and E, and increasing Apos A-I and A-II through activation of peroxisome proliferator-activated receptors-alpha (PPAR-α), a nuclear receptor involved in cellular function. The changes in these Apos result in a reduction in triglyceride-rich lipoproteins (VLDL and IDL) and an increase in HDL.

Clinical trials of fibrate therapy in patients with elevated cholesterol and no history of CHD demonstrated a reduction in CHD incidence, although less than the reduction attained with statin therapy.[40] In addition, a large study of men with CHD, low HDL cholesterol, low LDL cholesterol, and elevated triglycerides demonstrated a 24% reduction in the risk of death from CHD, nonfatal MI, and stroke with gemfibrozil.[41] Fibrates may be appropriate in the prevention of CHD events for patients with established CHD, low HDL cholesterol, and triglycerides below 200 mg/dL (2.26 mmol/L). However, LDL-lowering therapy should be the primary target if LDL cholesterol is elevated. Evidence of a reduction in CHD risk among patients with established CHD has not been demonstrated with fenofibrate.

The fibric acid derivatives are generally well tolerated. The most common adverse effects include dyspepsia, abdominal pain, diarrhea, flatulence, rash, muscle pain, and fatigue (Table 12–9). Myopathy and rhabdomyolysis can occur, and the risk appears to increase with renal insufficiency or concurrent statin therapy. If a fibrate is used with a statin, fenofibrate is preferred because it appears to inhibit the glucuronidation of the statin hydroxy and moiety less than gemfibrozil, allowing greater renal clearance of the statins.[27,42] A CK level should be checked before therapy is started and if symptoms occur. Liver dysfunction has been reported, and LFTs should be monitored. Fibrates increase cholesterol in the bile and have caused gallbladder and bile duct disorders, such as cholelithiasis and cholecystitis. Unlike niacin, these agents do not increase glucose or uric acid levels. Fibrates are contraindicated in patients with gallbladder disease, liver dysfunction, or severe kidney dysfunction. The risk of bleeding is increased in patients taking both a fibrate and warfarin. The time until maximum effect on lipids is generally 2 weeks for fenofibrate and 3 to 4 weeks for gemfibrozil.

▶ Omega-3 Fatty Acids

O3FAs (eicosapentaenoic acid and docosahexaenoic acid), the predominant fatty acids in the oil of cold-water fish, lower triglycerides by as much as 35% when taken in large amounts. Fish oil supplements may be useful for patients with high triglycerides despite diet, alcohol restriction, and fibrate therapy. This effect may be modulated through PPAR-α and a reduction in Apo B-100 secretion. O3FAs reduce platelet aggregation and have antiarrhythmic properties, and therefore their use has been associated with a reduction in MI and sudden cardiac death, respectively.[43]

Prescription grade O3FAs are FDA approved at a dose of 4 g daily for the treatment of elevated triglycerides. Use of high-quality O3FAs free of contaminants such as mercury and organic pollutants should be encouraged when using these agents. Common side effects associated with O3FAs are diarrhea and excess bleeding. Patients taking anticoagulant or antiplatelet agents should be monitored more closely when consuming these products because excessive amounts of O3FAs (e.g., greater than 3 g daily) may lead to bleeding and may increase the risk of hemorrhagic stroke.

Combination Therapy

A large proportion of the U.S. population won't achieve their NCEP cholesterol targets for a variety of reasons.[44] These include inadequate patient adherence, adverse events, inadequate starting doses, lack of dose escalation, and lower treatment targets.[3,45] Moreover, patients with concomitant elevations in triglycerides and/or low levels of HDL cholesterol may need combination drug therapy to normalize their lipid profile. ❾ *Combination drug therapy is an effective means to achieve greater reductions in LDL cholesterol (statin + ezetimibe or bile acid resin, bile acid resin + ezetimibe, or three-drug combinations) as well as raising HDL cholesterol and lowering serum triglycerides (statin + niacin or fibrate).*

▶ Combination Therapy for Elevated LDL Cholesterol

For patients who don't achieve their LDL or non-HDL cholesterol goals with statin monotherapy and lifestyle modifications including those unable to tolerate high doses due to adverse effects, combination therapy may be appropriate. Resins or ezetimibe combine effectively with statins to augment LDL cholesterol reduction. When added to a statin, ezetimibe can reduce LDL cholesterol levels by an additional 18% to 21% or up to 65% total reduction with maximum doses of the more potent statins. Ezetimibe and simvastatin are available as a combination tablet (Vytorin) and indicated as adjunctive therapy to diet for the reduction of elevated total cholesterol, LDL cholesterol, Apo B, triglycerides, and non-HDL cholesterol, and to increase HDL cholesterol. The usual starting dose is 10 mg/20 mg, and the maximum dose is 10 mg/80 mg (Table 12–9). Adverse events are similar to those of each product taken separately; however, the percentage of patients with LFT elevations greater than three times normal is slightly higher than with a statin alone, and there appears to be a slightly higher risk of myopathy and rhabdomyolysis when statins and ezetimibe are combined. The time until maximum effect on lipids for this combination is generally 2 to 6 weeks.

A statin combined with a resin results in similar reductions in LDL cholesterol as those seen with ezetimibe. However, the magnitude of triglyceride reduction is less with a resin compared to ezetimibe, and this should be considered in patients with higher baseline triglyceride levels. In addition, gastrointestinal adverse events and potential drug interactions limit the utility of this combination.

Ezetimibe and a resin can also be combined. A study which assessed the effects of adding ezetimibe to ongoing resin therapy showed an additional 19% reduction in LDL cholesterol and an additional 14% reduction in triglycerides. This combination was well tolerated.[46]

Some patients, in particular those with genetic forms of hypercholesterolemia (Table 12–2), will require three or more drugs to manage their disorder. Regimens using a statin, resin, and niacin were found to reduce LDL cholesterol up to 75%.[47] These early studies were conducted with lovastatin, so larger reductions would be expected with the more potent statins available today.

▶ Combination Therapy for Elevated Cholesterol and Triglyceridemia With or Without Low HDL Cholesterol

Fibrates are the most effective triglyceride-lowering agents and also raise HDL cholesterol levels. Combination therapy with a fibrate, particularly gemfibrozil, and a statin has been found to increase the risk for myopathy. Of the 31 rhabdomyolysis deaths reported with cerivastatin use, 12 involved concomitant gemfibrozil.[28] Therefore, more frequent monitoring, thorough patient education, and consideration of factors that increase the risk as reviewed previously should be considered.

⑩ *Reducing LDL cholesterol while substantially raising HDL cholesterol (statin + niacin) appears to reduce the risk of atherosclerotic disease progression to a greater degree than statin monotherapy.* Combining niacin with a statin augments the LDL cholesterol lowering potential of niacin while enhancing both the HDL cholesterol-raising effects and triglyceride-lowering effects of the statin. A statin combined with niacin appears to offer greater benefits for reducing atherosclerosis progression compared to a statin alone.[37] Formulations combining ER niacin and lovastatin (Advicor) and ER niacin and simvastatin (Simcor) are available, and are indicated for treatment of primary hypercholesterolemia and mixed dyslipidemia in patients treated with lovastatin or simvastatin who require further triglyceride lowering or HDL cholesterol raising and may benefit from having niacin added to their regimen. The combination is also indicated for patients treated with niacin who require further LDL-cholesterol lowering and may benefit from having lovastatin or simvastatin added to their regimen. The time until maximum effect on lipids for this combination is generally 3 to 6 weeks.

Niacin can be combined with a fibrate in patients with high elevations in serum triglycerides. The combination may increase the risk of myopathy compared to either agent alone.

Compared with monotherapy, combination therapy is relatively unstudied in terms of the effects on CHD event reduction and may reduce patient compliance through increased side effects and increased costs. When used appropriately and with proper precautions, however, they are effective in normalizing lipid abnormalities, particularly in patients who cannot tolerate adequate doses of statin therapy for more severe forms of dyslipidemia.

▶ Investigational Agents

There are numerous investigational drugs in development for the treatment of lipid disorders and prevention of atherosclerosis. Many of these will likely be used in combination with currently available lipid-modulating drugs. The most promising is an antisense drug that significantly reduced Apo B-100 and LDL cholesterol.[48] Other agents in development include newer statins; bile acid transport inhibitors; phytostanol analogues; acyl coenzyme A: cholesterol acyltransferase (ACAT) inhibitors; squalene synthase inhibitors; and newer PPAR-α, -γ, and -δ agonists, as well as dual PPAR-α/γ agonists. In addition, weekly infusions of genetically engineered HDL (Apo A1 Milano) in patients with atherosclerosis has been shown to cause significant reduction in atheroma volume compared to placebo after just 5 weeks of therapy.[49]

These novel therapies will provide opportunities for developing different combination strategies to further reduce the risk of CHD even after adequate treatment with existing agents. Well-designed studies using noninvasive imaging technology and long-term follow-up periods are needed to ensure that there is a favorable risk-to-benefit ratio.

OUTCOME EVALUATION

- The successful outcome in cholesterol management is to reduce cholesterol and triglycerides below the NCEP ATP III goals in an effort to alter the natural course of atherosclerosis and decrease future cardiovascular events.

- **⑤** *Employ an adequate trial of TLC in all patients, but institute pharmacotherapy concurrently in higher-risk patients.*

- When indicated, initiate drug therapy at a dose that will reduce LDL cholesterol in the range of 30% to 40%.

- **⑥** *Typically, statins are the medications of choice to treat high LDL cholesterol because of their ability to substantially reduce LDL cholesterol, ability to reduce morbidity and mortality from atherosclerotic disease, convenient once-daily dosing, and low risk of side effects.*

- Employ an individualized patient monitoring plan in an effort to minimize side effects and maintain treatment adherence and lipid goals.

Patient Care and Monitoring

1. Assess the patient for the presence of CHD or other atherosclerosis disorders.

2. Assess major risk factors for CHD.

3. For patients without CHD or CHD risk equivalent, but two or more major CHD risk factors, perform Framingham risk assessment.

4. Obtain fasting cholesterol profile and assess any abnormal lipid levels.

5. Obtain a thorough history of prescription, nonprescription, and natural drug product use. Determine what treatments for cholesterol the patient has used in the past (if any). Assess if the patient is taking any medications that may contribute to his or her abnormal lipid levels.

6. Assess concomitant diseases that may contribute to the patient's abnormal lipid levels.

7. Assess risk factors for metabolic syndrome.

8. Determine the treatment goal for LDL cholesterol based on the patient's CHD risk and non-HDL cholesterol goal if patient meets criteria for metabolic syndrome.

9. Educate all patients on TLC and the importance of regular physical activity.

10. For patients exceeding their LDL cholesterol goal, initiate TLCs. Consider starting concurrent pharmacotherapy in patients in the high-risk or moderately high-risk categories. Pharmacotherapy should be initiated at a dose to reduce LDL cholesterol by 30% to 40% at a minimum.

11. TLC should be continued and intensified (consider adding plant sterols/stanols and increase fiber) after 6 weeks if not below LDL cholesterol target. For those patients above their LDL cholesterol target after adequate trial of TLC (12 to 18 weeks), pharmacotherapy should be strongly considered.

12. Institute appropriate pharmacotherapy based on lipid abnormality. Obtain appropriate baseline labs to monitor for adverse drug effects. Assess potential disease and drug interactions that may affect choice or intensity of pharmacotherapy.

13. Monitor response, safety, and adherence after a minimum of 4 to 6 weeks. Titrate therapy or add a second drug as needed.

14. Once the LDL cholesterol goal is achieved, assess non-HDL cholesterol in those with metabolic syndrome and intensify LDL-lowering therapy further or consider adding niacin or fibrate.

15. Provide patient education regarding CHD, hyperlipidemia, therapeutic lifestyle modifications, drug therapy, and therapy adherence.

Abbreviations Introduced in This Chapter

ABC	ATP-binding cassette
ABCA1	ATP-binding cassette A1
ABCG1	ATP-binding cassette G1
ABCG5/G8	ATP-binding cassette G5/G8
ACAT	Acyl coenzyme A: cholesterol acyltransferase
Acetyl CoA	Acetyl coenzyme A
Apo	Apolipoprotein
ATP	Adenosine triphosphate
ATP III	Adult Treatment Panel III edition
BAS	Bile acid sequestrant
CAD	Coronary artery disease
CE	Cholesterol ester
CETP	Cholesterol ester transfer protein
CHD	Coronary heart disease
CK	Creatine kinase
CM	Chylomicrons
CPK	Creatine phosphokinase
CRP	C-reactive protein
DBP	Diastolic blood pressure
ER	Extended-release
FA	Fatty acid
GFR	Glomerular filtration rate
HDL	High-density lipoprotein
HMG-CoA	3-hydroxy-3-methyglutaryl coenzyme A
HL	Hepatic lipase
IDL	Intermediate-density lipoprotein
IR	Immediate-release
LCAT	Lecithin-cholesterol acyltransferase
LDL	Low-density lipoprotein
LFT	Liver function test
LPL	Lipoprotein lipase
Lp-PLA2	Lipoprotein-associated phospholipase A2
LRP	LDL-related protein
MI	Myocardial infarction
MMP	Matrix metalloproteinase
NCEP	National Cholesterol Education Program
NO	Nitric oxide
NPC1L1	Niemann-Pick C1 Like 1
NSAID	Nonsteroidal anti-inflammatory drug
O3FA	Omega-3-fatty acids
PPAR-α	Peroxisome proliferator-activated receptor-alpha
SBP	Systolic blood pressure
SR	Sustained-release
SR-BI	Scavenger receptors
TG	Triglyceride
TLC	Therapeutic lifestyle changes
VLDL	Very low-density lipoprotein

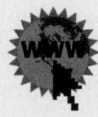 Self-assessment questions and answers are available at *http://www.mhpharmacotherapy.com/pp.html.*

REFERENCES

1. Kronmal RA, Cain KC, Ye Z, Omenn GS. Total serum cholesterol levels and mortality risk as a function of age. A report based on the Framingham data. Arch Intern Med 1993;153:1065–1073.

2. Rosamond W, Flegal K, Friday G, et al. Heart Disease and Stroke Statistics—2007 Update A Report From the American Heart Association Statistics Committee and Stroke Statistics Subcommittee. Circulation. 2007;115:e69–e171.

3. Third Report of the National Cholesterol Education Program (NCEP) Expert Panel on Detection, Evaluation, and Treatment of High Blood Cholesterol in Adults (Adult Treatment Panel III) Final Report. Circulation 2002;106 (25):3143–3421.

4. Genest J. Lipoprotein disorders and cardiovascular risk. J Inherit Metab Dis 2003;26:267–287.

5. Garcia-Calvo M, Lisnock J, Bull HG, et al. The target of ezetimibe is Niemann-Pick C1-Like 1 (NPC1L1). Proc Natl Acad Sci 2005;102(23):8132–8137.

6. Libby P. Molecular basis of the acute coronary syndrome. Circulation 1995;91:2844–2850.

7. Brown BG, Zhao XQ, Chait A, et al. Simvastatin and niacin, antioxidant vitamins, or the combination for the prevention of coronary disease. N Engl J Med 2001;345:1583–1592.

8. Grundy SM, Cleeman JI, Bairey Merz CN, et al. for the Coordinating Committee of the National Cholesterol Education Program endorsed by the National Heart, Lung, and Blood Institute, American College of Cardiology Foundation, and American Heart Association. Update implications of recent clinical trials for the national cholesterol education program adult treatment panel III guidelines. Circulation 2004;110:227–239.

9. National Heart Lung and Blood Institute. Detection, Evaluation, and Treatment of High Blood Cholesterol in Adults (Adult Treatment Panel IV). Available at *http://www.nhlbi.nih.gov/guidelines/cholesterol/atp4/index.htm.*

10. Smith SC Jr., Allen J, Blair SN, et al. AHA/ACC Guidelines for Secondary Prevention for Patients With Coronary and Other Atherosclerotic Vascular Disease: 2006 Update: Endorsed by the National Heart, Lung, and Blood Institute. Circulation 2006;113:2363–2372.

11. Lichtenstein AH, Appel LJ, Brands M, et al. Diet and lifestyle recommendations revision 2006: A scientific statement from the American Heart Association Nutritional Committee. Circulation. 2006;114:82–96.

12. Grundy SM, Cleeman JI, Daniels SR, et al. Diagnosis and management of the metabolic syndrome: An American Heart Association/National Heart, Lung, and Blood Institute scientific statement. Curr Opin Cardiol 2006;21:1–6.

13. Pearson TA, Mensah GA, Alexander RW, et al. Markers of inflammation and cardiovascular disease: Application to clinical and public health practice: A statement for healthcare professionals from the Centers for Disease Control and Prevention and the American Heart Association. Circulation 2003;107(3):499–511.

14. Ridker PM, Danielson E, Fonseca FA, et al. Rosuvastatin to prevent vascular events in men and women with elevated C-reactive protein. N Engl J Med. 2008;359(21): 2195–2207.

15. Shepherd J, Cobbe SM, Ford I, et al. for The West of Scotland Coronary Prevention Study Group. Prevention of coronary heart disease with pravastatin in men with hypercholesterolemia. N Engl J Med 1995;333:1301–1307.

16. Sever PS, Dahlof B, Poulter NR, et al. Prevention of coronary and stroke events with atorvastatin in hypertensive patients who have average or lower-than-average cholesterol concentrations, in the Anglo-Scandinavian Cardiac Outcomes Trial—Lipid-Lowering Arm (ASCOT-LLA): A multicentre randomised controlled trial. Lancet. 2003;361:1149–1158.

17. The ALLHAT Officers and Coordinators for the ALLHAT Collaborative Research Group. Major outcomes in moderately hypercholesterolemia, hypertensive patients randomized to pravastatin vs usual care: The Antihypertensive and Lipid-Lowering Treatment to Prevent Heart Attack Trial (ALLHAT-LLT). JAMA 2002;288:2998–3007.

18. Calhoun HM, Betteridge DJ, Durrington PN, et al. Primary prevention of cardiovascular disease with atorvastatin in type 2 diabetes in the Collaborative Atorvastatin Diabetes Study (CARDS): Multicentre randomised placebo-controlled trial. Lancet 2004;364:685–696.

19. Scandinavian Simvastatin Survival Study Group. Randomised trial of cholesterol lowering in 4444 patients with coronary heart disease: The Scandinavian Simvastatin Survival Study (4S). Lancet 1994;344:1383–1389.

20. Sacks FM, Pfeffer MA, Moye LA, et al. for the Cholesterol and Recurrent Events Trial Investigators. The effect of pravastatin on coronary events after myocardial infarction in patients with average cholesterol levels. Cholesterol and Recurrent Events Trial investigators. N Engl J Med 1996;335:1001–1009.

21. Heart Protection Study Collaborative Group. MRC/BHF Heart Protection Study of cholesterol lowering with simvastatin in 20,536 high-risk individuals: A randomized placebo-controlled trial. Lancet 2002;360(9326):7–22.

22. The Long-Term Intervention with Pravastatin in Ischemic Disease (LIPID) Study Group. Prevention of cardiovascular events and death with pravastatin in patients with coronary heart disease and a broad range of initial cholesterol levels. N Engl J Med 1998;399(19):1349–1357.

23. Cannon CP, Braunwald E, McCabe CH, et al. Intensive versus moderate lipid-lowering with statins after acute coronary syndromes. N Engl J Med 2004;350:1495–1504.

24. LaRosa JC, Grundy SM, Waters DD, et al. Treating to New Targets (TNT) Investigators. Intensive lipid lowering with atorvastatin in patients with stable coronary disease. N Engl J Med 2005;352:1425–1435.

25. Downs JR, Clearfield M, Weis S, et al. for the AFCAPS/TexCAPS Research Group. Primary prevention of acute coronary events with lovastatin in men and women with average cholesterol levels: Results of AFCAPS/TexCAPS. JAMA 1998;270:1615–1622.

26. Liao JK. Clinical implications for statin pleiotropy. Curr Opin Lipidol 2005;16(6):624–629.

27. Pasternak RC, Smith SC Jr, Bairey-Merz CN, et al. ACC/AHA/NHLBI clinical advisory on the use and safety of statins. J Am Coll Cardiol 2002;40:568–573.

28. Staffa JA, Chang J, Green L. Cerivastatin and reports of fatal rhabdomyolysis. New Engl J Med 2002;346(7):539–540.

29. Kastelein JJ, Akdim F, Stroes ES, et al. Simvastatin with or without ezetimibe in familial hypercholesterolemia. N Engl J Med 2008;358(14):1431–1443.

30. Rossebø AB, Pedersen TR, Boman K, et al. Intensive Lipid Lowering with Simvastatin and Ezetimibe in Aortic Stenosis. N Engl J Med 2008;359:1343–1356.

31. The Lipid Research Clinics Coronary Primary Prevention Trial results. II. The relationship of reduction in incidence of coronary heart disease to cholesterol lowering. JAMA 1984;251:365–374.

32. Sankyo Pharma, Inc., Parsippany, New Jersey: Drug Prescribing Information: WelChol (2008). Parsippany, NJ: Author.

33. Meyers CD, Carr MC, Park S, et al. Varing cost and free nicotinic acid content in over-the-counter niacin preparations for dyslipidemia. Ann Intern Med 2003;139:996–1002.

34. McKenney JM, Proctor JD, Harris S, et al. A comparison of the efficacy and toxic effects of sustained- vs immediate-release niacin in hypercholesterolemic patients. JAMA 1994;271:672–677.

35. Pieper JA. Overview of niacin formulations: Differences in pharmacokinetics, efficacy, and safety. Am J Health Syst Pharm 2003;60(13 suppl 2):S9–S14.

36. Canner PL, Berge GK, Wender NK, et al. Fifteen-year mortality in Coronary Drug Project patients: Long-term benefit with niacin. J Am Coll Cardiol 1986;18:1245–1255.

37. Taylor AJ, Sullenberger LE, Lee HJ, et al. Arterial biology for the investigation of the treatment effects of reducing cholesterol (ARBITER) 2. A double-blind, placebo-controlled study of extended-release niacin on atherosclerosis progression in secondary prevention patients treated with statins. Circulation 2004;110:3512–3517.

38. Bays HE, Dujovne CA, McGovern ME, et al. ADvicor versus Other Cholesterol-Modulating Agents Trial Evaluation. Comparison of once-daily, niacin extended-release/lovastatin with standard doses of

atorvastatin and simvastatin (the ADvicor versus Other Cholesterol-Modulating Agents Trial Evaluation [ADVOCATE]). Am J Cardiol 2003;91(6):667–672.

39. Canner PL, Furberg CD, Terrin ML, et al. Benefits of niacin by glycemic status in patients with healed myocardial infarction (from the Coronary Drug Project). Am J Cardiol 2005;95:254–257.

40. Frick MH, Elo O, Haapa K, et al. Helsinki Heart Study: Primary prevention trial with gemfibrozil in middle aged men with dyslipidemia. Safety of treatment, changes in risk factors, and incidence of coronary heart disease. N Engl J Med 1987;317:1237–1245.

41. Robins SJ, Collins D, Wittes JT, et al. for the VA-HIT Study Group. Veterans Affairs High-Density Lipoprotein Intervention Trial. Relation of gemfibrozil treatment and lipid levels with major coronary events: VA-HIT: A randomized controlled trial. JAMA 2001;285(12):1585–1591.

42. Prueksaritanont T, Zhao JJ, Ma B, et al. Mechanistic studies on metabolic interactions between gemfibrozil and statins. J Pharmacol Exp Ther 2002;301(3):1042–1051.

43. Kris-Etherton PM Harris WS, Appel LJ, for the Nutrition Committee: Fish consumption, fish oil, omega-3 fatty acids, and cardiovascular disease. Circulation 2002;106:2747–2757.

44. Pearson TA, Laurora I, Chu H, et al. The lipid treatment assessment project (L-TAP): A multicenter survey to evaluate the percentages of dyslipidemic patients receiving lipid-lowering therapy and achieving low-density lipoprotein cholesterol goals. Arch Intern Med 2000;160:459–467.

45. Ito MK, Lin JC, Morreale AP, et al. Effect of pravastatin-to-simvastatin conversion on reducing low-density lipoprotein cholesterol. Am J Health Syst Pharm 2001;58:1734–1739.

46. Xydakis AM, Guyton JR, Chiou P, et al. Effectiveness and tolerability of ezetimibe add-on therapy to a bile acid resin-based regimen for hypercholesterolemia. Am J Cardiol 2004;94(6):795–797.

47. Leitersdorf E, Muratti EN, Eliav O, et al. Efficacy and safety of triple therapy (fluvastatin-bezafibrate-cholestyramine) for severe familial hypercholesterolemia. Am J Cardiol 1995;76:84A–88A.

48. Ito MK. ISIS 301012 Gene Therapy for Hypercholesterolemia: Sense, Antisense, or Nonsense. Ann Pharmacother 2007;41:1669–1678.

49. Nissen SE, Tsunoda T, Tuzcu EM, et al. Effect of recombinant ApoA-I Milano on coronary atherosclerosis in patients with acute coronary syndromes: A randomized controlled trial. JAMA 2003;290(17):2292–2300.

13 Hypovolemic Shock

Bradley A. Boucher and G. Christopher Wood

LEARNING OBJECTIVES

● **Upon completion of the chapter, the reader will be able to:**

1. List the most common etiologies of decreased intravascular volume in hypovolemic shock patients.

2. Describe the major hemodynamic and metabolic abnormalities that occur in patients with hypovolemic shock.

3. Describe the clinical presentation, including signs, symptoms, and laboratory test measurements, for the typical hypovolemic shock patient.

4. Prepare a treatment plan with clearly defined outcome criteria for a hypovolemic shock patient that includes both fluid management and other pharmacologic therapy.

5. Compare and contrast the relative advantages and disadvantages of crystalloids, colloids, and blood products in the treatment of hypovolemic shock.

6. Formulate a stepwise monitoring strategy for a hypovolemic shock patient.

KEY CONCEPTS

❶ Hypovolemic shock occurs as a consequence of inadequate intravascular volume to meet the oxygen and metabolic needs of the body.

❷ Protracted tissue hypoxia sets in motion a downward spiral of events leading to organ dysfunction and eventual failure if untreated.

❸ The overarching goals in treating hypovolemic shock are to restore effective circulating blood volume, as well as managing its underlying cause, thereby reversing organ dysfunction and returning to homeostasis.

❹ Three major therapeutic options are available to clinicians for restoring circulating blood volume: crystalloids (electrolyte-based solutions), colloids (large-molecular-weight solutions), and blood products.

❺ In the absence of ongoing blood loss, administration of 2,000 to 4,000 mL (about 4 to 8 pints) of isotonic crystalloid will normally re-establish baseline vital signs in adult hypovolemic shock patients.

❻ Colloid solutions administered are primarily confined to the intravascular space, in contrast to isotonic crystalloid solutions that distribute throughout the extracellular fluid space.

❼ Blood products are indicated in adult hypovolemic shock patients who have sustained blood loss from hemorrhage exceeding 1,500 mL (about 3 pints).

❽ Vasopressors may be warranted as a temporary measure in patients with profound hypotension or evidence of organ dysfunction in the early stages of shock.

❾ Major treatment goals in hypovolemic shock following fluid resuscitation are as follows: arterial systolic blood pressure (SBP) greater than 90 mm Hg within 1 hour, organ dysfunction reversal, and normalization of laboratory measurements as rapidly as possible (less than 24 hours).

INTRODUCTION

The principal function of the circulatory system is to supply oxygen and vital metabolic compounds to cells throughout the body, as well as removal of metabolic waste products. Circulatory shock is a life-threatening condition whereby this principal function is compromised. When circulatory shock is caused by a severe loss of blood volume or body water it is called **hypovolemic shock**, which is the focus of this chapter. Regardless of etiology, the most distinctive manifestations of hypovolemic shock are arterial hypotension and **metabolic acidosis.** Metabolic acidosis is a consequence of an accumulation of lactic acid resulting from tissue hypoxia and anaerobic metabolism. If the decrease in arterial blood pressure (BP) is severe and protracted, such hypotension will inevitably lead to severe hypoperfusion and organ dysfunction. Rapid and effective restoration of circulatory homeostasis through the use of fluids, pharmacologic agents, and/or blood products is imperative to prevent complications of untreated shock and ultimately death.

ETIOLOGY AND EPIDEMIOLOGY

Practitioners must have a good understanding of cardiovascular physiology to diagnose, treat, and monitor circulatory problems in critically ill patients. The inter-relationships between the major hemodynamic variables are depicted in Figure 13–1.[1] These variables include: arterial BP, cardiac output (CO), systemic vascular resistance (SVR), heart rate (HR), stroke volume (SV), left ventricular size, afterload, myocardial contractility, and preload. While an oversimplification, Figure 13–1 is beneficial in conceptualizing where the major abnormalities occur in patients with circulatory shock as well as predicting the body's compensatory responses.

Shock can be effectively categorized by etiology into four major types: hypovolemic, obstructive, cardiogenic, and distributive (Table 13–1).[2,3] As noted, all patients with shock have profound decreases in arterial BP. Understanding the primary cause of the circulatory abnormality in these respective shock states is invaluable to their management. Hypovolemic shock is caused by a loss of intravascular volume either by hemorrhage or fluid loss (e.g., dehydration). Obstructive shock is caused by an obstruction that directly compromises inflow or outflow of blood from the heart. Cardiogenic shock is caused by diminished myocardial contractility which results in decreased CO with an increase in SVR. Lastly, distributive shock is caused by a major decrease in SVR with an increase in CO. Differentiating between the underlying abnormality and the associated compensatory response is also essential in terms of treatment and monitoring. Hypovolemic shock is considered to be essentially a profound deficit in preload. Preload is defined as the volume in the left ventricle at the end of diastole. Decreased preload results in subsequent decreases in SV, CO, and eventually, mean arterial pressure (MAP). As such, restoration of preload becomes an over-riding goal in the management of hypovolemic shock.

The prognosis of shock patients depends on several variables including severity, duration, underlying etiology, pre-existing organ dysfunction, and reversibility.[4] Data are not readily available as to the incidence of hypovolemic

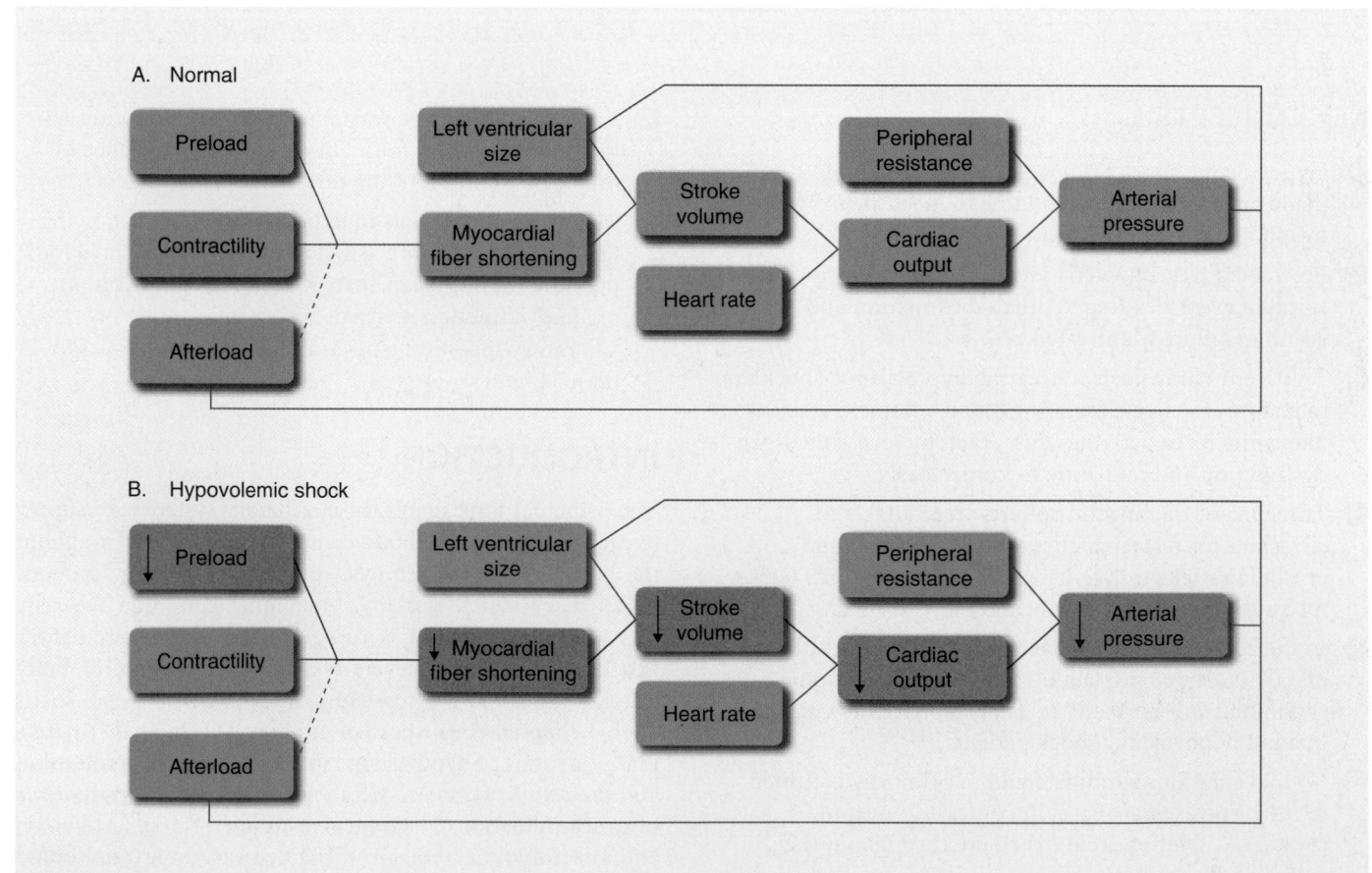

FIGURE 13–1. Hemodynamic relationships among key cardiovascular parameters (A). Solid lines represent a direct relationship; the broken line represents an inverse relationship. In B, the alterations typically observed in hypovolemic shock are highlighted with arrows depicting the likely direction of the alteration. (From Ref. 1.)

Table 13–1
Major Shock Classifications and Etiologies

I. Hypovolemic
Hemorrhagic
 Trauma
 GI
 Abdominal aortic aneurysm
Nonhemorrhagic (dehydration)
 Vomiting
 Diarrhea
 Third spacing

II. Cardiogenic
Myocardial infarction
Septal wall rupture
Acute mitral valve regurgitation
Myocarditis
Arrhythmias

III. Obstructive
Pericardial tamponade
Pulmonary embolism
Amniotic fluid embolism
Tumor embolism

IV. Distributive
Sepsis
Anaphylactic
Spinal cord injury

From Refs. 2, 3.

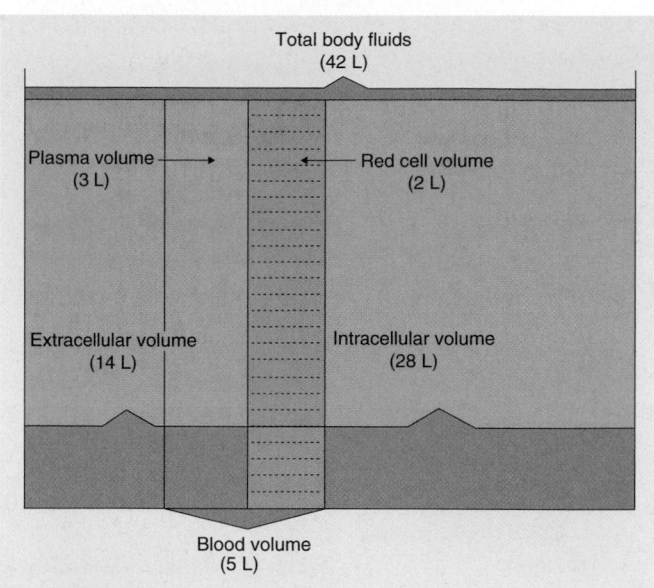

FIGURE 13–2. Distribution of body fluids showing the extracellular fluid volume, intracellular body fluid volume, and total body fluids in a 70 kg (154 lb) adult. Extracellular volume (ECV) comprises 14 L of total body fluid (42 L). Plasma volume makes up approximately 3 L of the 14 L of ECV. Intracellular volume accounts for the remaining 28 L of total body fluids with roughly 2 L being located within the red blood cells. Blood volume (approximately 5 L) is also depicted and is made up of primarily red blood cells and plasma. (From Guyton AC, Hall JE. *Textbook of Medical Physiology*. 8th ed. Philadelphia: Saunders, 1991: 275, with permission.)

shock, although hypovolemia due to hemorrhage is a major factor in 40% to 50% of trauma deaths annually.[5]

PATHOPHYSIOLOGY

The total amount of water in a typical 70 kg (154 lb) adult is approximately 42 L (Fig. 13–2). About 28 of the 42 L are inside the cells of the body (intracellular fluid) while the remaining 14 L are in the extracellular fluid space (fluid outside of cells: interstitial fluid and plasma). Circulating blood volume for a normal adult is roughly 5 L (70 mL/kg) and is comprised of 2 L of red blood cell fluid (intracellular) and 3 L of plasma (extracellular). ❶ *By definition, hypovolemic shock occurs as a consequence of inadequate intravascular volume to meet the oxygen and metabolic needs of the body.* Diminished intravascular volume can result from severe external or internal bleeding, profound fluid losses from GI sources such as diarrhea or vomiting, or urinary losses such as diuretic use, diabetic ketoacidosis, or diabetes insipidus (Table 13–1).[3] Other sources of intravascular fluid loss can occur through damaged skin, as seen with burns, or via "capillary leak" into the interstitial space or peritoneal cavity, as seen with edema or ascites. This latter phenomenon is often referred to as "third spacing" since fluid accumulates in the interstitial space disproportionately to the intracellular and extracellular fluid spaces. Regional ischemia may also develop as blood flow is naturally shunted from organs such as the GI tract or the kidneys to more immediately vital organs such as the heart and brain.

Hypovolemic shock symptoms begin to occur with decreases in intravascular volume in excess of 750 mL or 15% of the circulating blood volume (20 mL/kg in pediatric patients).[6] As previously stated, decreases in preload or left ventricular end-diastolic volumes result in decreases in SV. Initially, CO may be partially maintained by compensatory tachycardia. Similarly, reflex increases in SVR and myocardial contractility may diminish arterial hypotension. This neurohumoral response to hypovolemia is mediated by the sympathetic nervous system in an attempt to preserve perfusion to vital organs such as the heart and brain (Fig. 13–3). Two major endpoints of this response are to conserve water to maximize intravascular volume and to improve tissue perfusion by increasing BP and CO (oxygen delivery). The body attempts to maximize its fluid status by decreasing water and sodium excretion through release of ADH, aldosterone, and cortisol. BP is maintained by peripheral vasoconstriction mediated by catecholamine release and the renin-angiotensin system.[5] CO is augmented by catecholamine release and fluid retention.[3,7] However, when intravascular volume losses exceed 1,500 mL (about 3 pints), the compensatory mechanisms are inadequate, typically resulting in a fall in CO and arterial BP, while acute losses greater than 2,000 mL (about 4 pints) are

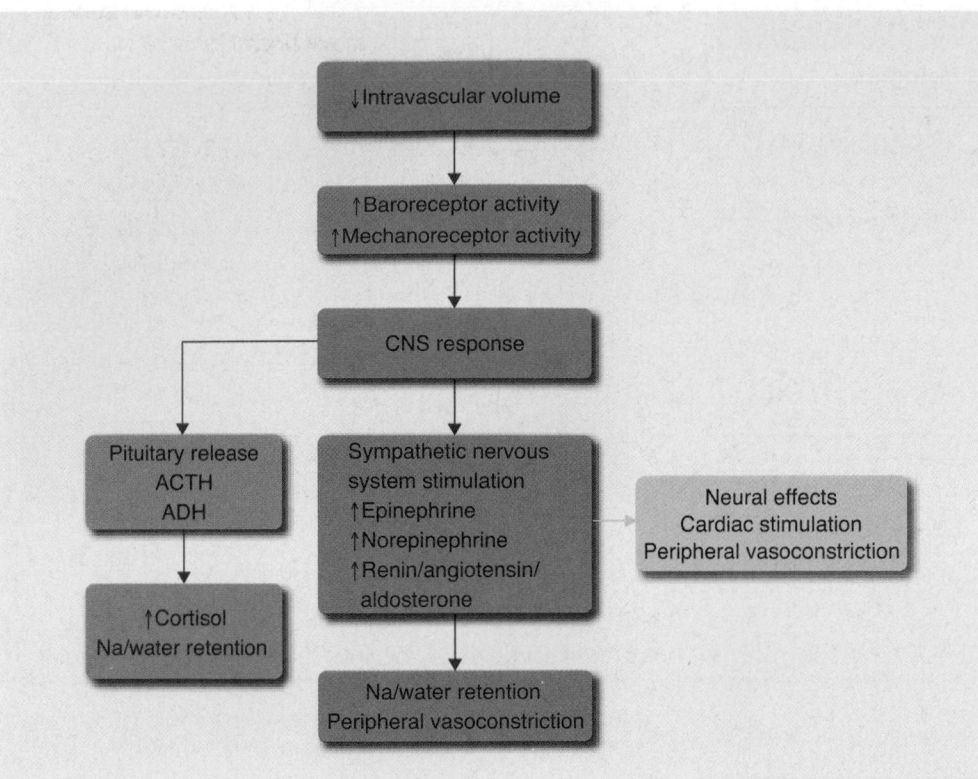

FIGURE 13–3. Expected neurohumoural response to hypovolemia. (ACTH, adrenocorticotropic hormone; ADH, antidiuretic hormone; Na, sodium.) (From Jimenez EJ. Shock. In: Civetta JM, Taylor RW, Kirby RR, eds. Critical Care. New York: Lippincott-Raven; 1997: 369, with permission.)

life-threatening (35 mL/kg in pediatric patients).[7] The decrease in CO results in a diminished delivery of oxygen to tissues within the body and activation of an acute inflammatory response.[5] Oxygen delivery can be further compromised by inadequate blood hemoglobin levels due to hemorrhage and/or diminished hemoglobin saturation due to impaired ventilation. Decreased delivery of oxygen and other vital nutrients results in diminished production of the energy substrate, adenosine triphosphate (ATP). Lactic acid is then produced as a by-product of anaerobic metabolism within tissues throughout the body.[3] Hyperglycemia produced during the stress response from cortisol release is also a contributing factor in the development of lactic acidosis. Lactic acidosis indicates that inadequate tissue perfusion has occurred.[3] ❷ *Protracted tissue hypoxia sets in motion a downward spiral of events leading to organ dysfunction and eventual failure if untreated.*[6] Table 13–2 describes the effects of shock on the body's major organs. Relative failure of more than one organ, regardless of etiology, is referred to as the multiple organ dysfunction syndrome (MODS). Involvement of the heart is particularly devastating considering the central role it plays in oxygen delivery and the potential for myocardial dysfunction to perpetuate the shock state. Pre-existing organ dysfunction and build up of inflammatory mediators can also exacerbate the effects of hypovolemic shock to the point of irreversibility.[5] For example, acute or chronic heart failure can lead to pulmonary edema, further aggravating gas exchange in the lungs and, ultimately, tissue hypoxia. MODS develops in approximately 20% of trauma patients

who require fluid resuscitation. Only about one-third of early-onset MODS is quickly reversible (within 48 hours) with proper fluid resuscitation. Thus, it is imperative that hypovolemic shock be treated quickly to avoid MODS.[8]

Table 13–2
Shock Manifestations on Major Organs

Heart
• Myocardial ischemia
• Dysrhythmias
Brain
• Restlessness, confusion, obtundation
• Global cerebral ischemia
Liver
• Release of liver enzymes
• Biliary stasis
Lungs
• Pulmonary edema
• ARDS
Kidneys
• Oliguria
• Decreased glomerular filtration
• Acute kidney injury
GI tract
• Stress-related mucosal disease
• Bacterial translocation
Hematologic
• Thrombocytopenia
• Coagulopathies

ARDS, acute respiratory distress syndrome; GI, gastrointestinal.

Clinical Presentation and Diagnosis of Hypovolemic Shock

General

Patients will be in acute distress, although symptoms and signs will vary depending on the severity of the hypovolemia and whether the etiology is hemorrhagic versus nonhemorrhagic.

Symptoms

- Thirst
- Weakness
- Lightheadedness

Signs

- Hypotension, arterial systolic BP (SBP) less than 90 mm Hg or fall in SBP greater than 40 mm Hg
- Tachycardia
- Tachypnea
- Hypothermia
- Oliguria

- Dark, yellow-colored urine
- Skin color: pale to ashen; may be cyanotic in severe cases
- Skin temperature: cool to cold
- Mental status: confusion to coma
- Pulmonary artery catheter measurements: decreased CO, decreased SV, increased SVR, low pulmonary artery occlusion pressure (PAOP)

Laboratory Tests

- Hypernatremia
- Elevated serum creatinine
- Elevated blood urea nitrogen
- Decreased hemoglobin/hematocrit (hemorrhagic hypovolemic shock)
- Hyperglycemia
- Increased serum lactate
- Decreased arterial pH

Patient Encounter, Part 1

JT is a 65-year-old male admitted to the emergency department (ED) after a 3-day history of severe vomiting and diarrhea. The patient's wife states that a "stomach virus" causing vomiting and diarrhea has been recently affecting several family members. JT is weak and confused, his breathing is labored, and he is losing consciousness. The initial diagnosis by the ED team is hypovolemic shock. A physical exam is being performed and blood samples are being sent to the laboratory.

What type of hypovolemic shock does JT have and what is the cause?

What signs and symptoms would you expect to see in this patient with hypovolemic shock?

What laboratory abnormalities might be expected in this patient?

What are the first nonpharmacologic steps in treating the patient?

TREATMENT

Desired Outcomes

❸ *The overarching goals in treating hypovolemic shock are to restore effective circulating blood volume, as well as manage its underlying cause.* In achieving this goal, the downward spiral of events that can perpetuate severe or protracted hypovolemic shock is interrupted. This is accomplished through the delivery of adequate oxygen and metabolic substrates such as glucose and electrolytes to the tissues throughout the body that will optimally bring about a restoration of organ function and return to homeostasis. Evidence of the latter is a return to the patient's baseline vital signs, relative normalization of laboratory test results, and alleviation of the other signs and symptoms of hypovolemic shock previously discussed.[9] Concurrent supportive therapies are also warranted to avoid exacerbation of organ dysfunction associated with the hypovolemic shock event.

General Approach to Therapy

Securing an adequate airway and ventilation is imperative in hypovolemic shock patients consistent with the airway, breathing, and circulation (ABCs) of life support. Any compromise in ventilation will only accentuate the tissue hypoxia occurring secondary to inadequate perfusion. Thus, tracheal intubation and mechanical ventilation may be needed (Fig. 13–4). IV access is also essential for administration of IV fluids and medications. IV access can be accomplished through the placement of peripheral IV lines or catheterization with central venous lines if rapid or large volumes of resuscitative fluids are indicated. While primarily facilitating fluid administration, the IV lines provide access for blood samples for obtaining appropriate laboratory tests. Placement of an arterial catheter is advantageous to allow for accurate and continual monitoring of BP, as well as arterial blood gas (ABG) sampling. A bladder catheter should be inserted for ongoing monitoring of urine output.

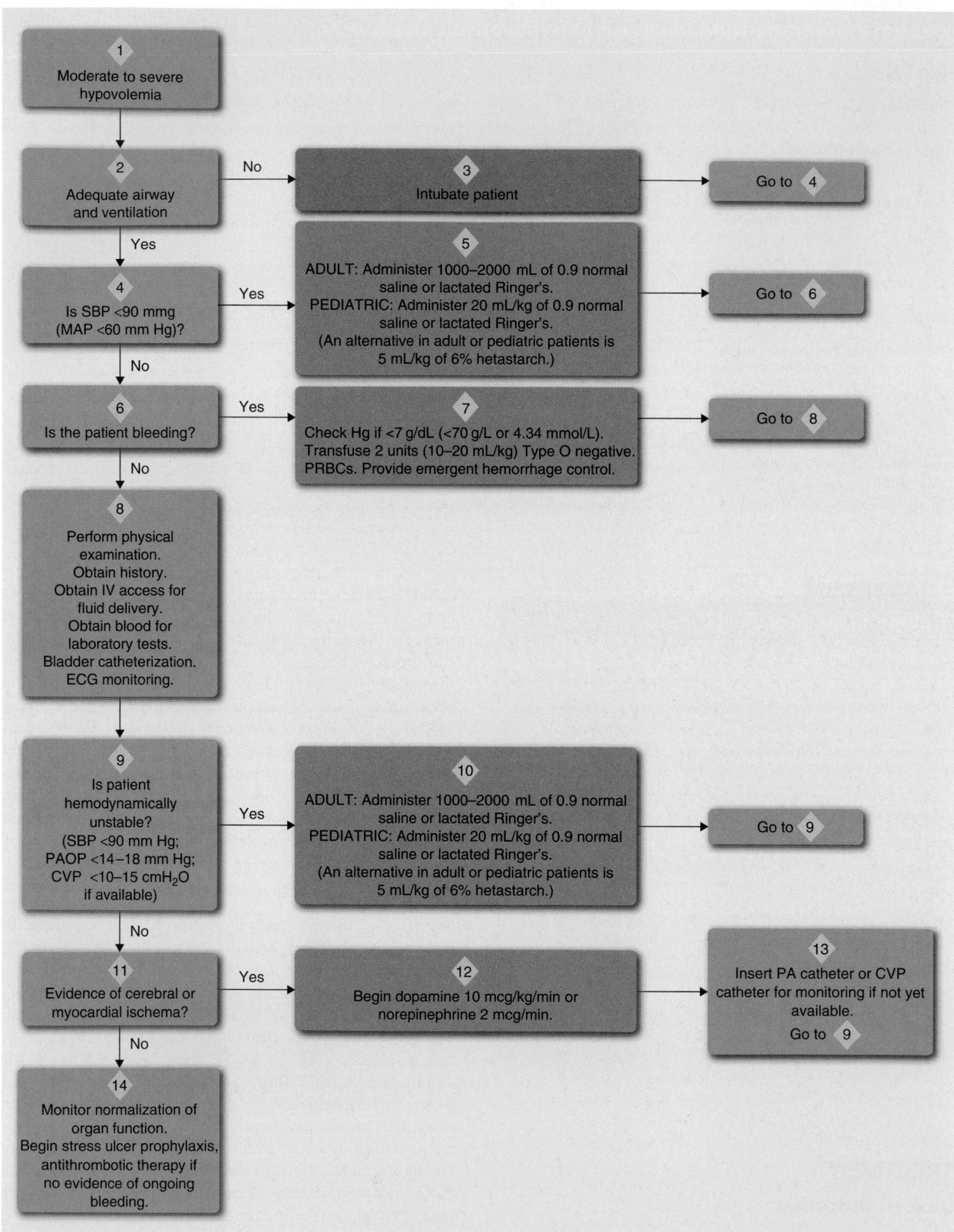

FIGURE 13–4. Treatment algorithm for the management of moderate to severe hypovolemia. (CVP, central venous pressure; MAP, mean arterial pressure; PA, pulmonary artery; PAOP, pulmonary artery occlusion pressure; PRBCs, packed red blood cells; SBP, systolic blood pressure.)

Baseline laboratory tests that should be done immediately include: complete blood cell counts with differentials, serum chemistry profile, liver enzymes, prothrombin and partial thromboplastin times, and serum lactate. A urinalysis and an ABG should also be obtained and ongoing ECG monitoring should be performed. In addition to restoring circulating blood volume, it is necessary to prevent further losses from the vascular space. This is especially true with hemorrhagic hypovolemic shock where identifying the bleeding site and achievement of hemostasis are critical in the successful resuscitation of the patient. This frequently involves surgical treatment of hemorrhages.

Upon stabilization, placement of a pulmonary artery (PA) catheter may be indicated based on the need for more extensive cardiovascular monitoring than is available from noninvasive measurements such as vital signs, cardiac rhythm, and urine output.[9,10] Key measured parameters that can be obtained from a PA catheter are the pulmonary artery occlusion pressure (PAOP), which is a measure of preload, and CO. From these values and simultaneous measurement of HR and BP, one can calculate the left ventricular SV and SVR.[10] Placement of a PA catheter should be reserved for patients at high risk of death due to the severity of shock or pre-existing medical conditions such as heart failure.[11] Use of PA catheters in broad populations of critically ill patients is somewhat controversial because clinical trials have not shown consistent benefits with their use.[12–14] However, critically ill patients with a high severity of illness may have improved outcomes from PA catheter placement. It is not clear why this was seen, but it could be that more severely ill patients have less physiologic reserve and less "room for error" and benefit from the therapeutic decisions that come from detailed PA catheter data.[15] An alternative to the PA catheter is placement of a central venous catheter that typically resides in the superior vena cava to monitor central venous pressure (CVP). While central venous catheters are less expensive and more readily placed, they are not particularly accurate in monitoring effective fluid resuscitation.[10]

▶ Fluid Therapy

④ *Three major therapeutic options are available to clinicians for restoring circulating blood volume: crystalloids (electrolyte-based solutions), colloids (large-molecular-weight solutions), and blood products.* Blood products are used only in instances involving hemorrhage (or severe pre-existing anemia), thus leaving crystalloids and colloids as the mainstay of therapy in all types of hypovolemic shock, along with adjunctive vasopressor support. The aggressiveness of fluid resuscitation (rate and volume) will be dictated by the severity of the hypovolemic shock and the underlying cause. Warming of all fluids to 37°C (98.6°F) prior to administration is an important consideration to prevent hypothermia, arrhythmias, and coagulopathy, as they will have a negative impact on the success of the resuscitation effort.[16]

Crystalloids Conventional, "balanced" crystalloids are fluids with (a) electrolyte composition that approximates plasma, such as lactated Ringer's (LR), or (b) a total calculated osmolality similar to that of plasma (280 to 295 mOsm/kg), such as 0.9% sodium chloride (also known as normal saline [NS] or 0.9% NaCl) (Table 13–3).[17] Thus, conventional crystalloids will distribute in normal proportions throughout the extracellular fluid space upon administration. In other words, expansion of the intravascular space will only increase by roughly 200 to 250 mL for every liter of isotonic crystalloid fluid administered.[5] Hypertonic crystalloid solutions such as 3% NaCl or 7.5% NaCl have osmolalities substantially higher than plasma. The effect observed with these fluids is a relatively larger volume expansion of the intravascular space. By comparison to conventional crystalloids, administration of 250 mL of 7.5% sodium chloride will result in an intravascular space increase of 500 mL.[5] This increase is a result of the fluid administered as well as osmotic drawing of intracellular fluid into the intravascular and interstitial spaces. This occurs because the hypertonic saline increases the osmolality of the intravascular and interstitial fluid compared to the intracellular fluid. Hypertonic saline also has the potential for decreasing the inflammatory response.[18] Despite these theoretical advantages, data are lacking demonstrating superiority of hypertonic crystalloid solutions compared with isotonic solutions.[19] Crystalloids are generally advocated as the initial resuscitation fluid in hypovolemic shock because of their availability, low cost, and equivalent outcomes compared with colloids.[9] A reasonable initial volume of an isotonic crystalloid (0.9% NaCl or LR) in adult patients is 1,000 to 2,000 mL (about 2 to 4 pints) administered over the first hour of therapy. Ongoing external or internal bleeding will require more aggressive fluid resuscitation. **⑤** *In the absence of ongoing blood loss, administration of 2,000 to 4,000 mL (about 4 to 8 pints) of isotonic crystalloid will normally re-establish baseline vital signs in adult hypovolemic shock patients.*[20] Selected populations, such as burn patients, may require more aggressive fluid resuscitation, while other patient subsets such as those with cardiogenic shock or heart failure may warrant less aggressive fluid administration to avoid over-resuscitation.[21] In hemorrhagic shock patients, approximately three to four times the shed blood volume of isotonic crystalloids is needed for effective resuscitation.[20,21]

Side effects from crystalloids primarily involve fluid overload and electrolyte disturbances of sodium, potassium, and chloride.[22] Dilution of coagulation factors can also occur resulting in a dilutional coagulopathy.[5] Two clinically significant reasons LR is different from NS is that LR contains potassium and has a lower sodium content (130 versus 154 mEq/L or mmol/L). Thus, LR has a greater potential than NS to cause hyponatremia and/or hyperkalemia. Alternatively, NS can cause hypernatremia and hypokalemia. Nevertheless, there is no clear cut advantage when comparing NS and LR.

Colloids Understanding the effects of colloid administration on circulating blood volume necessitates a review of those physiologic forces that determine fluid movement between capillaries and the interstitial space throughout the circulation (Fig. 13–5).[5,23] Relative hydrostatic pressure between the capillary lumen and the interstitial space is

Table 13–3

Composition of Common Resuscitation Fluids

Fluid	Na (mEq/L)[a]	Cl (mEq/L)[a]	K (mEq/L)[a]	Mg (mEq/L)[b]	Ca (mEq/L)[b]	Lactate (mEq/L)[a]	Other	pH	Osmolality (mOsm/kg)[c]
0.9% NaCl	154	154						5.0	308
3% NaCl	513	513						5.0	1,027
7.5% NaCl	1,283	1,283						5.0	2,567
Lactated Ringer's	130	109	4		3	28			
Hetastarch (Hextend)	143	124	3	0.9	5	28	Hetastarch 6 g/dL	5.9	307
Hetastarch (Hespan)	154	154					Hetastarch 6 g/dL	5.5	310
Pentastarch	154	154					Pentastarch 10 g/dL	5.0	326
5% Albumin	130–160	130–160					Albumin 5 g/dL (50 g/L)	6.9	
25% Albumin	130–160	130–160					Albumin 25 g/dL (250 g/L)	6.9	
5% PPF	130–160	130–160	0.25				Plasma proteins 5 g/dL (50 g/L) (88% albumin)	7.0	
Dextran 40	154	154					Dextran 10 g/dL (avg. molecular weight 40 kDa)		
Dextran 70	154	154					Dextran 6 gm/dL (avg. molecular weight 70 kDa)	5.5	308
Dextran 75	154	154					Dextran 6 gm/dL (avg. molecular weight 75 kDa)	5.5	308

avg., average; Ca, calcium; Cl, chloride; K, potassium; kDa, kilodalton; Mg, magnesium; Na, sodium; PPF, plasma protein fraction.

[a]For these values, mEq/L = mmol/L; e.g., 154 mEq/L Na = 154 mmol/L.

[b]For these values, mEq/L × 0.5 = mmol/L; e.g., 0.9 mEq/L Mg = 0.45 mmol/L Mg.

[c]For this value, mOsm/kg = mmol/kg; e.g., 308 mOsm/kg = 308 mmol/kg.

From Ref. 17.

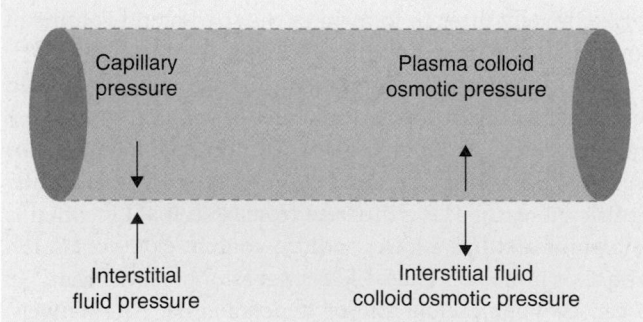

FIGURE 13–5 Operative forces at the capillary membrane tend to move fluid either outward or inward through the capillary membrane. In hypovolemic shock, one therapeutic strategy is the administration of colloids that can sustain and/or draw fluid from the interstitial space by increasing the plasma colloid osmotic pressure. (From Guyton AC, Hall JE. *Textbook of Medical Physiology*. 8th ed. Philadelphia: Saunders; 1991: 174, with permission.)

one of the major determinants of net fluid flow into or out of the circulation. The other major determinant is the relative colloid osmotic pressure between the two spaces. Administration of exogenous colloids results in an increase in the intravascular colloid osmotic pressure. The effects of colloids on intravascular volume are a consequence of their relatively large molecular size (greater than 30 kilodaltons [kDa]), limiting their passage across the capillary membrane in large amounts. Alternatively stated, colloids can be thought of as "sponges" drawing fluid into the intravascular space from the interstitial space. In the case of isosmotic colloids (5% albumin, 6% hetastarch, and dextran products), initial expansion of the intravascular space is essentially 65% to 75% of the volume of colloid administered accounting for some "leakage" of the colloid from the intravascular space.[5] ❻ *Thus, in contrast to isotonic crystalloid solutions that distribute throughout the extracellular fluid space, the volume of isooncotic colloids administered remains relatively confined to the intravascular space.* In the case of hyperoncotic solutions such as 25% albumin, fluid is pulled from the interstitial space into the vasculature resulting in an increase in the intravascular volume that is much greater than the original volume of the 25% albumin that was administered. While theoretically attractive, hyperoncotic solutions should not be used for hypovolemic shock since the expansion of the intravascular space is at the expense of depletion of the interstitial space. Exogenous colloids available in the United States include 5% albumin, 25% albumin, 5% plasma protein fraction (PPF), 6% hetastarch, 10% pentastarch, 10% dextran 40, 6% dextran 70, and 6% dextran 75 (Table 13–3). The first three products are derived from pooled human plasma. Hetastarch and pentastarch are semisynthetic hydroxyethyl starches derived from amylopectin. The dextran products are semisynthetic glucose polymers that vary in terms of the average molecular weight of the polymers. Superiority of one colloid solution over another has not been clearly established.[24]

For years within the critical care literature a controversy known as the "colloid versus crystalloid debate" raged over the relative merits of the two types of resuscitation fluids. At the center of the debate was what the goal of fluid resuscitation in shock should be: immediate expansion of the intravascular space with colloids versus expansion of the entire extracellular fluid space with crystalloids. A randomized controlled study involving 6,997 critically ill patients (Saline versus Albumin Fluid Evaluation [SAFE] study) demonstrated no difference in mortality between patients receiving saline versus albumin.[25] Largely in response to the SAFE trial, the FDA issued a notice to health care providers in May 2005 declaring albumin safe for use in most critically ill patients.[26] Burn, traumatic brain injury, and septic shock patients were excluded from the SAFE trial; however, based on previous data there do not appear to be a clear-cut overall advantage for either crystalloids or colloids in these patient groups.[26] Thus, while the debate is not fully resolved, most clinicians today prefer using crystalloids based on their availability and inexpensive cost compared with colloids.[21,27]

Generally, the major adverse effects associated with colloids are fluid overload, dilutional coagulopathy, and anaphylactoid/anaphylactic reactions.[28,29] Although derived from pooled human plasma, there is no risk of disease transmission from commercially available albumin or PPF products since they are heated and sterilized by ultrafiltration prior to distribution.[28] Because of direct effects on the coagulation system with the hydroxyethyl starch and dextran products, they should be used cautiously in hemorrhagic shock patients. This is another reason why crystalloids may be preferred in hemorrhagic shock. Furthermore, hetastarch can result in an increase in amylase not associated with pancreatitis. As such, the adverse-effect profiles of the various fluid types should also be considered when selecting a resuscitation fluid.

Blood Products ❼ *Blood products are indicated in hypovolemic shock patients who have sustained blood losses from hemorrhage exceeding 1,500 mL.* This, in fact, is the only setting in which freshly procured whole blood is administered. In virtually all other settings, blood products are given as the individual components of whole blood units, such as packed red blood cells (PRBCs), fresh frozen plasma (FFP), platelets, cryoprecipitate, and concentrated coagulation factors.[30] This includes ongoing resuscitation of hemorrhagic shock, when PRBCs can be transfused to increase oxygen-carrying capacity in concert with crystalloid solutions to increase blood volume. In patients with documented coagulopathies, FFP for global replacement of lost or diluted clotting factors, or platelets for patients with severe thrombocytopenia (less than $20 \times 10^3/mm^3$ or $20 \times 10^9/L$) should be administered.[31] Type O negative blood or "universal donor blood" is given in emergent cases of hemorrhagic shock. Thereafter, blood that has been typed and cross-matched with the recipient's blood is given. The traditional threshold for PRBC transfusion in hypovolemic shock has been a serum hemoglobin of less than 10 g/dL (100 g/L or 6.2 mmol/L) and hematocrit less than 30%. However, a more restrictive transfusion threshold of 7 g/dL (70 g/L or 4.34 mmol/L) appears to be safe for critically ill patients after they have received appropriate fluid resuscitation and have no signs of ongoing bleeding.[32] Traditional risks from allogeneic blood product administration include hemolytic and nonhemolytic transfusion reactions and transmission of bloodborne infections in contaminated blood. However, recent large studies have also shown that transfusions are associated with higher mortality, possibly because of adverse immune and inflammatory effects.[30] Based on limitations of homologous blood donations, intraoperative salvage techniques can be employed in patients with massive hemorrhage in an effort to conserve blood.[6,32,33]

Due to blood shortages and associated risks with transfusions, there are ongoing research efforts concerning the development of red blood cell substitutes as a possible therapy alternative. Products that have reached clinical trials include perfluorocarbon emulsions and hemoglobin-based oxygen carriers (HBOCs).[34] These blood products have several advantages over PRBCs including greater availability (because donors aren't needed), increased shelf-life, absence of infectious risks, and no need for cross-matching. As such, red blood cell substitutes have the potential to serve as temporizing measures in hypovolemic shock patients until conventional red blood cell transfusions can be administered or in instances in which availability of donated PRBCs is extremely limited. Nonetheless, lack of adequate efficacy data and additional side effects associated with each of the respective red blood cell substitutes have precluded their approval in the United States at present.[34]

Research also continues into the use of recombinant activated factor VII (rFVIIa) as an adjunctive agent to treat uncontrolled hemorrhage. Initial experiences with rFVIIa show that it can decrease transfusions, though large studies have not been performed.[35] A major unresolved issue surrounding the use of rFVIIa is its safety where the risk of thromboembolic events in patients receiving this agent off-label was recently highlighted.[36] The optimal dose of rFVIIa in nonhemophilic patients is also unknown. This latter issue is particularly important in light of the high acquisition costs for rFVIIa, and ultimately, pharmacoeconomic analyses of rFVIIa will be needed.

► *Pharmacologic Therapy*

Vasopressor Therapy Vasopressor is the term used to describe any pharmacologic agent that can induce arterial vasoconstriction through stimulation of the α_1-adrenergic receptors. ❽ *While replenishment of intravascular volume is undoubtedly the cornerstone of hypovolemic shock therapy, use of vasopressors may be warranted as a temporary measure in patients with profound hypotension or evidence of organ dysfunction in the early stages of shock.*[2,9] Typically, vasopressors are used concurrently with fluid administration. Table 13–4 is a list of those vasopressors used in the management of hypovolemic shock. Dopamine or norepinephrine may be preferred over epinephrine because epinephrine has an increased potential for causing cardiac arrhythmias and impaired abdominal organ (splanchnic) circulation.[37] In cases involving concurrent heart failure, an inotropic agent such as dobutamine may be needed, in addition to the use of a vasopressor.

Vasopressors are almost exclusively administered as continuous infusions because of their very short duration of action and the need for close titration of their dose-related effects. Starting doses should be at the lower end of the dosing range followed by rapid titration upward if needed to maintain adequate BP. Monitoring of end-organ function such as adequate urine output should also be used to monitor therapy. Once BP is restored, vasopressors should be weaned and discontinued as soon as possible to avoid any untoward events. The most significant systemic adverse events associated with vasopressors are excessive vasoconstriction resulting in decreased organ perfusion and potential to induce arrhythmias (Table 13–4). Central venous catheters should be used to minimize the risk of local tissue necrosis that can occur with extravasation of peripheral IV catheters.

Supportive Care Measures

Lactic acidosis, which typically accompanies hypovolemic shock as a consequence of tissue hypoxia, is best treated by reversal of the underlying cause. Administration of alkalizing agents such as sodium bicarbonate has not been demonstrated to have any beneficial effects and may actually worsen intracellular acidosis.[38] Since GI ischemia is a common complication of hypovolemic shock, prevention of

---

Patient Encounter, Part 2: Physical Exam, Diagnostic Tests, and Initial Treatment

PMH: Hypertension, congestive heart failure

Meds: Benazepril 10 mg daily, atenolol 50 mg daily, furosemide 40 mg daily as needed for edema

SH: Occasional alcohol use (per family)

FH: Noncontributory

PE: Ht 5′9″ (175 cm), Wt 65 kg (143 lb)

VS: 80/40 mm Hg, P 130 bpm, RR 22, T 35.0°C (95.0°F), urine output: none since catheterization 10 minutes ago

Neuro: Recent loss of consciousness

Pulmonary: Normal breath sounds, undergoing tracheal intubation for mechanical ventilation

CV: ECG shows sinus tachycardia, otherwise normal

Abd: WNL

Extremities: Noncontributory

Pertinent labs: pH 7.20, $PaCO_2$ 50 mm Hg (6.65 kPa), PaO_2 70 mm Hg (9.31 kPa), Na 153 mEq/L (153 mmol/L), HCO_3 18 mEq/L (18 mmol/L), lactate 7.0 mg/dL (0.78 mmol/L), SCr 1.7 mg/dL (150 μmol/L), Hct 51%

Identify treatment goals for JT in the next hour.

Identify treatment goals for JT in the next 24 hours.

What initial pharmacologic/fluid therapy is required?

Comment on the need for blood products or sodium bicarbonate in JT.

---

stress-related mucosal disease should be instituted as soon as the patient is stabilized. The most common agents used for stress ulcer prophylaxis are the histamine$_2$-receptor antagonists and proton pump inhibitors. Prevention of thromboembolic events is another secondary consideration in hypovolemic shock patients. This can be accomplished with the use of external devices such as sequential compression devices and/or antithrombotic therapy such as the low-molecular-weight heparin products or unfractionated heparin. Patients with adrenal insufficiency due to pre-existing disease, glucocorticoid use, or critical illness

---

Table 13–4

Vasopressor Drugs

Drug	Usual IV Dose	Adrenergic Effects			Potential to Cause Arrhythmias
		α_1	β_1	Dopaminergic	
Dopamine	10–20 mcg/kg/min[a]	+++	++	+++	+++
Norepinephrine	0.5–80 mcg/min	+++	++	0	++
Epinephrine	1–200 mcg/min	++	+++	0	+++
Phenylephrine	0.5–9 mcg/kg/min	+++	0	0	0

[a]Lower dosages of dopamine may not produce desired α_1-adrenergic (vasopressor) effects.

may have refractory hypotension despite resuscitation. Such patients should receive appropriate glucocorticoid replacement therapy (e.g., hydrocortisone).

OUTCOME EVALUATION

❾ *Successful treatment of hypovolemic shock is measured by the restoration of BP to baseline values and reversal of associated organ dysfunction.* The likelihood of a successful fluid resuscitation will be directly related to the expediency of treatment. Therapy goals include:

- Arterial SBP greater than 90 mm Hg (MAP greater than 60 mm Hg) within 1 hour
- Organ dysfunction reversal evident by increased urine output to greater than 0.5 mL/kg/h (1.0 mL/kg/h in pediatrics), return of mental status to baseline, and normalization of skin color and temperature over the first 24 hours
- HR should begin to decrease reciprocally to increases in the intravascular volume within minutes to hours

Patient Encounter, Part 3: Care Plan/Ongoing Therapy

One hour after the initial fluid bolus, JT's vital signs are:

BP 85/50 mm Hg, HR 120 bpm, RR 20, urine output: 15 mL in past hour. Pertinent new labs: lactate 4.8 mg/dL (0.53 mmol/L). JT has regained consciousness but is weak and confused.

What is your assessment of the patient's condition compared to 1 hour ago?

What therapy is required at this time?

How does JT's past medical history affect therapy decisions?

Describe monitoring over the next 24 hours.

Patient Care and Monitoring

1. Does the patient have an adequate airway and ventilation (hemoglobin saturation greater than 92%)? If not, trained emergency personnel should consider performing tracheal intubation with initiation of mechanical ventilation.

2. Is there a detectable BP? If yes, obtain history, perform physical examination, obtain blood for baseline laboratory tests, and monitor ECG. If not, begin isotonic crystalloid fluid resuscitation immediately (see step 4).

3. Monitor the following serial laboratories for comparison to baseline values every 6 hours in the first 24 hours and daily thereafter until normalized: sodium, serum creatinine, blood urea nitrogen, serum lactate, glucose, bilirubin, hemoglobin, hematocrit, platelets, prothrombin time, partial thromboplastin time, ABGs, and pH.

4. Is the systolic BP less than 90 mm Hg (MAP less than 60 mm Hg)? If yes, start aggressive fluid therapy beginning with 1,000 to 2,000 mL lactated Ringer's over 1 hour in adults (20 mL/kg in pediatrics). Monitor BP at least every 15 minutes (or continuously via an arterial catheter).

5. Is the patient bleeding? If yes, transfuse 5 to 10 mL/kg PRBCs. (Note: 1 unit PRBCs will provide approximately 3% increase in hematocrit or 1 g/dL [10 g/L or 0.62 mmol/L] increase in hemoglobin.) Do not allow hemoglobin concentrations to fall below 7 g/dL (70 g/L or 4.34 mmol/L; hematocrit 20%). Conventional goal hemoglobin concentration is 10 g/dL (100 g/L or 6.2 mmol/L; alternatively, hematocrit greater than or equal to 30%). Provide emergent control of ongoing hemorrhaging.

6. Is there evidence of cerebral or myocardial ischemia? If yes, begin vasopressor therapy of dopamine 10 mcg/kg/min or norepineprhine 2 mcg/min. Titrate dosage every 5 minutes as needed. Wean and discontinue vasopressor as soon as the goal arterial BP has been achieved.

7. Has the goal arterial BP been achieved? If not, give additional fluid therapy hourly blending crystalloids and isooncotic colloids based on inadequate BP response.

8. Is the patient hemodynamically stable? If not, admit to the intensive care unit for ongoing treatment and monitoring. A PA catheter (or CVP catheter) should be inserted by trained medical personnel. Monitor PAOP to a goal pressure of 14 to 18 mm Hg and minimum cardiac index of 2.2 L/min/m² (alternatively CVP 8 to 15 cm H$_2$O).

9. Monitor normalization of organ function to baseline state including mental status, urine output to greater than 0.5 mL/kg/h (1 mL/kg/h in pediatric patients), normal skin color and temperature, and normalization of base deficit and/or lactate. Begin supportive care measures including stress ulcer prophylaxis and antithrombotic therapy if there is no evidence of ongoing bleeding.

10. Has the underlying cause of the hypovolemic shock been addressed to prevent its recurrence? If not, treat as necessary.

11. Is there any evidence of adverse events from the resuscitation therapies employed such as fluid overload, electrolyte disturbances, transfusion reactions, and/or alterations in coagulation? If yes, manage the particular adverse event accordingly.

- Normalization of laboratory measurements expected within hours to days following fluid resuscitation. Specifically, normalization of base deficit and serum lactate is recommended within 24 hours to potentially decrease mortality[39] and

- Achievement of PAOP to a goal pressure of 14 to 18 mm Hg occurs (alternatively, CVP 8 to 15 mm Hg)

Abbreviations Introduced in This Chapter

ABCs	Airway, breathing, and circulation
ABG	Arterial blood gas
ACTH	Adrenocorticotropic hormone
ADH	Antidiuretic hormone
ARDS	Acute respiratory distress syndrome
ATP	Adenosine triphosphate
Ca	Calcium
Cl	Chloride
CO	Cardiac output
CVP	Central venous pressure
ECV	Extracellular volume
ED	Emergency department
FFP	Fresh frozen plasma
HBOC	Hemoglobin-based oxygen carrier
HCO_3	Bicarbonate
Hct	Hematocrit
HR	Heart rate
K	Potassium
kDa	Kilodalton
LR	Lactated Ringer's
MAP	Mean arterial pressure
Mg	Magnesium
MODS	Multiple organ dysfunction syndrome
Na	Sodium
NaCl	Sodium chloride
NS	Normal saline
PA	Pulmonary artery
Pao_2	Partial pressure of arterial oxygen
PAOP	Pulmonary artery occlusion pressure
$PaCo_2$	Partial pressure of carbon dioxide
PPF	Plasma protein fraction
PRBCs	Packed red blood cells
rFVIIa	Recombinant activated factor VII
SAFE	Saline versus Albumin Fluid Evaluation
SBP	Systolic blood pressure
SCr	Serum creatinine
SV	Stroke volume
SVR	Systemic vascular resistance

 Self-assessment questions and answers are available at *http://www.mhpharmacotherapy.com/pp.html.*

REFERENCES

1. Braunwald E. Regulation of the circulation. I. N Engl J Med 1974;290:1124–1129.
2. Astiz ME. Pathophysiology and classification of shock states. In: Fink MP, Abraham E, Vincent JL, et al., eds. Textbook of Critical Care. Philadelphia: Elsevier Saunders, 2005:897–904.
3. Jones AE, Kline JA. Shock. In: Marx JA, Hockberger RS, Walls RM. eds. Rosen's Emergency Medicine: Concepts and Clinical Practice. Philadelphia: Mosby Elsevier, 2006:41–56.
4. Vallet B, Wiel E, Lebuffe G. Resuscitation from circulatory shock. In: Fink MP, Abraham E, Vincent JL, et al., eds. Textbook of Critical Care. Philadelphia: Elsevier Saunders, 2005:905–910.
5. Puyana JC. Resuscitation of hypovolemic shock. In: Fink MP, Abraham E, Vincent JL, et al., eds. Textbook of Critical Care. Philadelphia: Elsevier Saunders, 2006:1933–1943.
6. Stern SA, Bobke EMK. Resuscitation: Management of shock. In: Ferrera PC, Colucciello SA, Marx JA, et al., eds. Trauma Management: An Emergency Medicine Approach. St. Louis: Mosby, 2002:75–102.
7. Harbrecht BG, Alarcon LH, Peitzman AB. Management of shock. In: Moore EE, Feliciano DV, Mattox KL, eds. Trauma. New York: McGraw-Hill, 2004:201–226.
8. Ciesla DJ, Moore EE, Johnson JL, et al. Multiple organ dysfunction during resuscitation is not postinjury multiple organ failure. Arch Surg 2004;139:590–594.
9. Moore FA, McKinley BA, Moore EE. The next generation in shock resuscitation. Lancet 2004;36:1988–1996.
10. Rhodes A, Grounds RM, Bennett ED. Hemodynamic monitoring. In: Fink MP, Abraham E, Vincent JL, et al., eds. Textbook of Critical Care. Philadelphia: Elsevier Saunders, 2005:735–739.
11. Practice guidelines for pulmonary artery catheterization: An updated report by the American Society of Anesthesiologists Task Force on Pulmonary Artery Catheterization. Anesthesiology 2003;99: 988–1014.
12. Ivanov R, Allen J, Calvin JE. The incidence of major morbidity in critically ill patients managed with pulmonary artery catheters: A meta-analysis. Crit Care Med 2000;28:615–619.
13. Richard C, Warszawski J, Anguel N, et al. Early use of the pulmonary artery catheter and outcomes in patients with shock and acute respiratory distress syndrome: A randomized controlled trial. JAMA 2003;290: 2713–2720.
14. Sandham JD, Hull RD, Brant RF, et al. A randomized, controlled trial of the use of pulmonary-artery catheters in high-risk surgical patients. N Engl J Med 2003;348:5–14.
15. Chittock DR, Dhingra VK, Ronco JJ, et al. Severity of illness and risk of death associated with pulmonary artery catheter use. Crit Care Med 2004;32:911–915.
16. Hoffman GL. Blood and blood components. In: Marx JA, Hockberger RS, Walls RM. eds. Rosen's Emergency Medicine. Concepts and Clinical Practice. Philadelphia: Mosby Elsevier, 2006:56–61.
17. Zaloga GP, Kirby RR, Bernards WC, et al. Fluids and electrolytes. In: Civetta JM, Taylor RW, Kirby RR, eds. Critical Care. New York: Lippincott-Raven, 1997:413–441.
18. Rhee P, Koustova E, Alam HB. Searching for the optimal resuscitation method: Recommendations for the initial fluid resuscitation of combat casualties. J Trauma 2003;54:S52–S62.
19. Bunn F, Roberts I, Tasker R, et al. Hypertonic versus near isotonic crystalloid for fluid resuscitation in critically ill patients. Cochrane Database Syst Rev 2004:CD002045.
20. Mullins RJ. Management of shock. In: Mattox KL, Feliciano DV, Moore EE, eds. Trauma. New York: McGraw-Hill, 2000:195–232.
21. Shafi S, Kauder DR. Fluid resuscitation and blood replacement in patients with polytrauma. Clin Orthop Relat Res 2004:37–42.
22. Revell M, Greaves I, Porter K. Endpoints for fluid resuscitation in hemorrhagic shock. J Trauma 2003;54:S63–S67.
23. Guyton AC, Hall JE. Textbook of Medical Physiology. 10th ed. Philadelphia: Saunders, 2000.
24. Bunn F, Alderson P, Hawkins V. Colloid solutions for fluid resuscitation. Cochrane Database Syst Rev 2003:CD001319.

25. Finfer S, Bellomo R, Boyce N, et al. A comparison of albumin and saline for fluid resuscitation in the intensive care unit. N Engl J Med 2004;350:2247–2256.

26. Safety of albumin administration in critically ill patients. Rockville, MD: U.S. Food and Drug Administration, 2005.

27. Perel P, Roberts I. Colloids versus crystalloids for fluid resuscitation in critically ill patients. Cochrane Database Syst Rev 2007:CD000567.

28. Boldt J. Volume replacement in the surgical patient—Does the type of solution make a difference? Br J Anaesth 2000;84:783–793.

29. Barron ME, Wilkes MM, Navickis RJ. A systematic review of the comparative safety of colloids. Arch Surg 2004;139:552–563.

30. Boucher BA, Hannon TJ. Blood management: A primer for clinicians. Pharmacotherapy 2007;27:1394–1411.

31. Kelley DM. Hypovolemic shock: An overview. Crit Care Nurs Q 2005;28:2–19.

32. McIntyre LA, Hebert PC. Can we safely restrict transfusion in trauma patients? Curr Opin Crit Care 2006;12:575–583.

33. Fowler RA, Berenson M. Blood conservation in the intensive care unit. Crit Care Med 2003;31:S715–S720.

34. Stollings JL, Oyen LJ. Oxygen therapeutics: Oxygen delivery without blood. Pharmacotherapy 2006;26:1453–1464.

35. Holcomb JB. Use of recombinant activated factor VII to treat the acquired coagulopathy of trauma. J Trauma 2005;58:1298–1303.

36. O'Connell KA, Wood JJ, Wise RP, et al. Thromboembolic adverse events after use of recombinant human coagulation factor VIIa. JAMA 2006;295:293–298.

37. Dellinger RP, Levy MM, Carlet JM, et al. Surviving Sepsis Campaign: International guidelines for management of severe sepsis and septic shock: 2008. Crit Care Med 2008;36:296–327.

38. Boyd JH, Walley KR. Is there a role for sodium bicarbonate in treating lactic acidosis from shock? Curr Opin Crit Care 2008;14:379–383.

39. Tisherman SA, Barie P, Bokhari F, et al. Clinical practice guideline: Endpoints of resuscitation. J Trauma 2004;57:898–912.

14 Asthma

W. Greg Leader

LEARNING OBJECTIVES

● **Upon completion of the chapter, the reader will be able to:**

1. Discuss the economic and health burden caused by asthma.
2. Explain the pathophysiology of asthma.
3. Describe the clinical presentation of acute and chronic asthma.
4. Identify factors that affect asthma severity.
5. Identify the goals of asthma management.
6. Classify asthma severity based on impairment due to asthma and future risk for negative outcomes due to asthma.
7. Recommend environmental control strategies for patients with identified allergies.
8. Educate patients on the use of inhaled drug delivery devices, peak flow meters, and asthma education plans.
9. Develop a therapeutic plan for patients with chronic asthma that maximizes patient response while minimizing adverse drug events and other drug-related problems.
10. Evaluate current asthma control and make therapeutic changes when necessary.
11. Develop a therapeutic plan for treating patients with acute asthma.

KEY CONCEPTS

❶ Asthma is a complex disease that presents in a heterogeneous manner.

❷ Asthma is the most prevalent chronic disease of childhood, and it causes significant morbidity and mortality in both adults and children.

❸ Asthma is characterized by inflammation, airway hyper-responsiveness (AHR), and airway obstruction.

❹ In chronic asthma, initial classification of asthma severity is based on current disease impairment and future risk.

❺ Direct airway administration of asthma medications through inhalation is the most efficient route and minimizes systemic adverse effects.

❻ Short-acting-inhaled β_2-agonists are the most effective agents for reversing acute airway obstruction caused by bronchoconstriction and are the drugs of choice for treating acute severe asthma and symptoms of chronic asthma.

❼ Inhaled corticosteroids (ICS) are the preferred therapy for all forms of persistent asthma in all age groups.

❽ The intensity of pharmacotherapy for chronic asthma is based on disease severity for initial therapy and level of control for subsequent therapies.

❾ In acute severe asthma, early and appropriate intensification of therapy is important to resolve the exacerbation and prevent relapse and severe airflow obstruction in the future.

INTRODUCTION

In 2007, the National Heart, Lung, and Blood Institute's (NHLBI) National Asthma Education and Prevention Program (NAEPP) updated its *Guidelines for the Diagnosis and Management of Asthma.*[1] In this update, the Expert Panel Report-3 (EPR-3) defines asthma as "… a common chronic disorder of the airways that is complex and characterized by variable and recurring symptoms, airflow obstruction, bronchial hyperresponsiveness and underlying inflammation."[1]

❶ *Asthma is a complex disease that presents in a hete-rogeneous manner.* Severity of chronic disease ranges from mild intermittent symptoms to severe and disabling disease if left untreated. Despite variances in the underlying severity of chronic asthma, all asthmatics are at risk of acute severe disease when exposed to the appropriate trigger or if inadequately treated. The NAEPP guidelines[1] emphasize the importance of treating underlying airway inflammation to control asthma and reduce asthma-associated risks.

EPIDEMIOLOGY AND ETIOLOGY

❷ *Asthma is the most prevalent chronic disease of childhood, and it causes significant morbidity and mortality in both adults and children.* Approximately 22.9 million people in the United States carry the diagnosis of asthma, and nearly 6.8 million of these are younger than 18 years of age. The highest prevalence is in children 5 to 17 years of age.[2] Puerto Ricans and non-Hispanic blacks have a higher prevalence than non-Hispanic whites.[2,3]

Approximately 10.1 million workdays and 12.8 million school days are missed every year due to asthma.[2] In 2005, there were 1.77 million emergency department visits and 488,594 hospital discharges related to asthma.[2] Children have the highest rates of emergency department visits and hospitalizations.[2,3] There were approximately 3,816 asthma-related deaths in 2004. The total number of asthma deaths have decreased every year since 1999.[2]

Asthma is also a significant economic burden in the United States, costing $19.7 billion in 2007. Prescription drugs are the single largest direct medical expenditure and account for 42% of direct medical costs.[3] Costs increase with disease severity, and it has been suggested that less than 20% of asthma patients account for over 80% of direct medical expenditures.[4]

Asthma results from a complex interaction of genetic and environmental factors, but the underlying cause is not well understood. The onset of asthma occurs early in life for most patients.[1] There appears to be an inherited component, as the presence of asthma in a parent is a strong risk factor for development of asthma in a child. This risk increases when a family history of atopy is also present.[1] The presence of atopy is a strong prognostic factor for continued asthma as an adult. Furthermore, the severity of early childhood asthma is a predictor of adult asthma severity.[5]

Environmental exposure also appears to be an important factor in the etiology of asthma. Patients with occupational asthma develop the disease late in life upon exposure to specific allergens in the workplace. Exposure to second-hand smoke after birth increases the risk of childhood asthma.[1] Adult-onset asthma may be related to atopy, nasal polyps, aspirin sensitivity, occupational exposure, or a recurrence of childhood asthma.

PATHOPHYSIOLOGY

❸ *Asthma is characterized by inflammation, airway hyper-responsiveness (AHR), and airway obstruction.* Inhaled antigens induce a type 2 T-helper CD4+ (T_H2) response. Antigens are taken up by antigen-presenting cells, and presentation of antigens to T-lymphocytes causes activation of the T_H2 type response. This leads to B-cell production of antigen-specific immunoglobulin E (IgE) as well as proinflammatory cytokines and chemokines that recruit and activate eosinophils, neutrophils, and alveolar macrophages.[6,7] Further exposure to the antigen results in cross-linking of cell-bound IgE in mast cells and basophils, causing the release of preformed inflammatory mediators such as histamine or generation of new inflammatory mediators such as leukotriene C_4 and prostaglandins.[8] Activation and degranulation of mast cells and basophils result in an early-phase response involving acute bronchoconstriction that lasts approximately 1 hour after allergen exposure.[6] This early-phase response can be blocked by pretreatment with inhaled short-acting β_2-agonists (SABA) or cromolyn.

In the late-phase response, activated airway cells release inflammatory cytokines and chemokines, thereby recruiting more inflammatory cells into the lungs. The late-phase response occurs 4 to 6 hours after the initial allergen challenge and results in a less intense bronchoconstriction as well as increased AHR and airway inflammation.[6]

Airway Inflammation and Hyper-responsiveness

Although the symptoms of asthma are intermittent, airway inflammation is chronic.[7] Considerable variations in the pattern of inflammation may exist, resulting in phenotypic differences.[1] T-lymphocytes release cytokines that coordinate eosinophilic infiltration and IgE production by B-lymphocytes.[9] Mast cells, eosinophils, macrophages, neutrophils, fibroblasts, and airway smooth muscle cells are also activated in asthma. Mast cells infiltrate airway smooth muscle and bronchial epithelium and may cause mucous gland hyperplasia. Proinflammatory mediators generated during mast cell degranulation propagate the inflammatory response and contribute to AHR and airway remodeling.[10]

AHR is the exaggerated ability of the airways to narrow in response to a variety of stimuli. AHR is a characteristic feature of asthma and is related to airway inflammation and structural changes in the airways.[1] Treatment of airway inflammation with inhaled corticosteroids (ICS) attenuates AHR in asthma but does not eliminate it.[1] Clinically, AHR manifests as increased variability of airway function. Although not commonly used to diagnose asthma, AHR can be evaluated clinically using a methacholine or histamine bronchoprovocation test.

Airway Obstruction

Symptoms of airway obstruction include chest tightness, cough, and wheezing. Airway obstruction can be caused by multiple factors including airway smooth muscle constriction, airway edema, mucus hypersecretion, and airway remodeling. Airway smooth muscle tone is maintained by an interaction between sympathetic, parasympathetic, and nonadrenergic mechanisms. Acute bronchoconstriction usually results from mediators such as histamine, cysteinyl leukotrienes, prostaglandins, and tryptase released or generated during degranulation of mast cells and basophils.[1] Inflammatory mediators such as histamine, leukotrienes, and bradykinin increase microvascular permeability leading to mucosal edema, which causes the airways to become more rigid and limits airflow.[11] These changes exaggerate the consequences of acute bronchoconstriction. In asthmatics, there is an increased number and volume of mucous glands, with increased mucus secretion.[12] Extensive mucus plugging may be a cause of persistent airway obstruction in acute severe attacks.

Although airway obstruction in asthma is generally reversible, some asthmatics have an irreversible or fixed obstruction. *Airway remodeling* is the term used to describe the process that produces the structural airway changes leading to this fixed obstruction; it is characterized by airway epithelial damage, subepithelial fibrosis, airway smooth muscle hypertrophy, increased mucus production, and increased vascularity of the airways.[1,12] These changes increase airflow obstruction and airway responsiveness and may decrease patient responsiveness to therapy.[1]

CLINICAL PRESENTATION AND DIAGNOSIS

The diagnosis of asthma is based on a detailed medical history, a physical examination of the upper respiratory tract and skin, and spirometry. The clinician should determine that episodic symptoms of airflow obstruction are present, airflow obstruction is at least partially reversible, and alternative diagnoses are excluded.[1] Spirometry is required for diagnosing asthma because the medical history and physical examination are not reliable for characterizing the status of lung impairment or excluding other diagnoses.[1]

Factors Affecting Asthma Severity

Major factors that may contribute to the severity of asthma include allergens, environmental chemical exposures or pollution, and exposure to tobacco smoke. Up to 80% of asthmatics have symptoms of rhinitis, and treatment of rhinitis with intranasal corticosteroids may relieve the symptoms.[13] Gastroesophageal reflux has been associated with increased asthma symptoms, especially nighttime symptoms. Obesity has been associated with asthma persistence and severity.

Nonselective β-blockers, including those in ophthalmic preparations, may cause asthma symptoms, and these agents should be avoided in asthmatics unless the benefits of therapy outweigh the risks.[1] In asthmatic patients requiring β-blocker therapy, a β_1-selective agent should be chosen. Because selectivity is dose related, the lowest effective dose should be used. β-blockers may inhibit β-agonist reversal

---

Clinical Presentation and Diagnosis of Chronic Asthma

General

Asthma severity ranges from normal pulmonary function and symptoms with only acute exacerbations to significantly decreased pulmonary function with continuous symptoms.

Symptoms

- Symptoms may include **dyspnea**, cough, wheezing, and chest tightness that may be continual, episodic, seasonal, or occur in association with known triggers.
- Symptoms may occur more often at night, early in the morning, or with exercise.
- Patients with intermittent asthma may be symptom-free and have normal pulmonary function between exacerbations.

Signs

- Patients may have end-expiratory wheezing and dry cough.

Laboratory Tests

- Increased serum concentrations of IgE or eosinophils may help confirm the diagnosis of asthma but are not diagnostic for asthma.

Other Diagnostic Tests

- Spirometry, an objective measure of pulmonary function, can be used to assist in confirming the diagnosis of asthma.

- Useful pulmonary function tests include the forced expiratory volume in 1 second (FEV_1) and forced vital capacity (FVC). The following values support a diagnosis of asthma:

  - Decreased FEV_1/FVC relative to predicted values demonstrates airway obstruction. The ratio may be normal between exacerbations.

  - 12% or greater (at least 200 mL) improvement in FEV_1 after an inhaled bronchodilator demonstrates a reversible obstruction. A 2- to 3-week course of oral corticosteroids may be necessary to demonstrate reversibility in airway obstruction.

  - A decrease in FEV_1 of 15% or more after an exercise test is diagnostic for exercise-induced asthma.

  - Assessment of diurnal variation in peak expiratory flow (PEF) may be useful in patients who have asthma symptoms and normal spirometry.

  - When spirometry is equivocal, a 20% or greater decrease in FEV_1 after the administration of methacholine is diagnostic for asthma. A negative bronchoprovocation test with methacholine may help rule out asthma.

- A positive allergen test may help guide nonpharmacologic therapy but is not diagnostic for asthma.

Clinical Presentation and Diagnosis of Acute Asthma

General

Acute asthma can present rapidly (within 3 to 6 hours) but more commonly, deterioration occurs over several hours, days, or even weeks. Typically, there is gradual deterioration over several days followed by a more rapid decline over 2 to 3 days. Acute asthma can be a life-threatening event, and severity does not correspond to severity of the chronic disease.

Symptoms

- The patient usually presents with complaints of dyspnea, cough, shortness of breath, and chest tightness.
- Because of their inability to breathe, patients are generally anxious and may be agitated. In acute severe asthma, patients may be unable to communicate in complete sentences.
- Mental status changes may indicate impending respiratory failure.

Signs

- The patient usually has tachypnea and may have tachycardia.
- Wheezing may vary from end-expiratory wheezing in mild exacerbations to wheezing throughout inspiration and expiration in severe exacerbations.
- Bradycardia and absence of wheezing may indicate impending respiratory failure.

- Patients may also present with hyperinflation, use of accessory muscles to breathe, pulsus paradoxus, diaphoresis, and cyanosis.

Laboratory Tests

- Arterial blood gases for evaluating partial arterial pressure of carbon dioxide (Pco_2) should be considered for patients in severe distress, suspected hypoventilation, or when PEF or FEV_1 is 30% or less after initial treatment.
- A CBC with differential should be obtained in patients with fever or purulent sputum.
- Serum electrolytes should be obtained, because frequent β_2-agonist administration may decrease serum potassium, magnesium, and phosphate.

Other Diagnostic Tests

- Patients may present with PEF rates ranging from greater than 80% and oxygen saturation greater than 95% in mild exacerbations to PEF rates less than 50%, oxygen saturations less than 91%, partial arterial oxygen pressures (Pao_2) less than 50 mm Hg (less than 6.65 kPa), and Pco_2 greater than 42 mm Hg (greater than 5.59 kPa) in severe exacerbations.
- A chest x-ray should be performed when pneumonia is suspected.

Patient Encounter, Part 1

RB is a 13-year-old African American female who presents with complaints of shortness of breath when she exercises. She recently joined the cross-country team. She finishes her training runs, but she is having trouble keeping up with the other girls on the team because she gets extremely short of breath 5 or 10 minutes into her run, her chest begins to feel tight, and she coughs. The symptoms usually go away 30 minutes to an hour after she stops running. She also wakes up at night about once a week because she is having trouble catching her breath.

What information is suggestive of asthma?

Based on the information presented, how would you classify this patient's asthma severity?

What additional information do you need to know before creating a treatment plan for this patient?

of bronchospasm, and a larger dose of β-agonist or the use of an anticholinergic agent may be necessary to reverse bronchospasm.

TREATMENT OF ASTHMA

Desired Outcomes

▶ Chronic Asthma

Therapy for chronic asthma is directed at maintaining long-term control of asthma using the least amount of medications and minimizing adverse effects.[1] Treatment goals are to: (a) prevent chronic and troublesome symptoms; (b) require infrequent use (2 or fewer days/week) of SABA for quick relief of symptoms; (c) maintain normal or near-normal pulmonary function; (d) maintain normal activity levels; (e) meet patients' and families' expectations of satisfaction with asthma care; (f) prevent exacerbations of asthma and the need for emergency department visits or hospitalizations; (g) prevent progressive loss of lung function; and (h) provide optimal pharmacotherapy with minimal or no adverse effects.

▶ *Acute Severe Asthma*

Acute or worsening asthma can be a life-threatening situation and requires rapid assessment and appropriate intensification of therapy. Mortality associated with asthma exacerbations is usually related to an inappropriate assessment of the severity of the exacerbation resulting in insufficient treatment or referral for medical care.[14] The goals of therapy are to: (a correct significant **hypoxemia**; (b) reverse airflow obstruction rapidly; and (c) reduce the likelihood of exacerbation relapse or recurrence of severe airflow obstruction in the future.[1]

General Approach to Treatment

▶ *Chronic Asthma*

Chronic asthma is classified as: (a) intermittent asthma or (b) persistent asthma that may be graded as mild, moderate, or severe. ❹ *In chronic asthma, initial classification of asthma severity is based on current disease impairment and future risk.* The term *impairment* refers to the frequency and severity of symptoms, use of SABA for quick relief of symptoms, pulmonary function, and impact on normal activity and quality of life. *Risk* refers to the potential for future severe exacerbations and asthma-related death, progressive loss of lung function (adults) or reduced lung growth (children), and the occurrence of drug-related adverse effects. Initial assessment of severity is made at the time of diagnosis, and initial therapy is based on this assessment. Future therapy decisions are based on ongoing assessments of asthma control.

Treatment of chronic asthma involves avoidance of triggers known to precipitate or worsen asthma and the use of long-term control and quick-relief medications. Long-term control medications include ICS, inhaled long-acting β_2-agonists (LABA), oral theophylline, oral leukotriene modifying agents, and omalizumab (Table 14–1). In patients with severe asthma, systemic corticosteroids may be used as a long-term control medication. Quick-relief medications include SABA, anticholinergics, and systemic corticosteroids. A stepwise approach to therapy is recommended to achieve the treatment goals.[1]

▶ *Acute Severe Asthma*

In acute severe asthma, the severity of an exacerbation is not dependent upon the classification of the patient's chronic asthma because even patients with intermittent asthma can have life-threatening acute exacerbations. Treatment of acute or worsening asthma primarily involves pharmacologic therapy. Early and aggressive treatment is necessary for quick resolution.[1]

Important elements of an early treatment plan include: (a) a written action plan; (b) recognition of early indicators of an acute exacerbation (e.g., asthma symptoms or worsening PEF or FEV$_1$) and taking prompt action; (c) appropriate intensification of pharmacotherapy by increasing inhaled SABA, and in some cases adding a short course of oral corticosteroids; (d) removal of triggers or irritants that may be contributing to the acute exacerbation; and (e) timely communication between patient and clinician about worsening symptoms, declining PEF, and decreased responsiveness to SABA.[1]

Initial treatment of acute severe asthma includes use of oxygen for rapid reversal of hypoxemia, a SABA and perhaps inhaled ipratropium bromide to reverse airway constriction, and a systemic corticosteroid to attenuate the inflammatory response. Close monitoring of objective measures such as FEV$_1$ or PEF is important to quantify the response to therapy. Because recovery from exacerbations is often gradual, intensified therapy should be continued for several days.

Nonpharmacologic Therapy

Patients should play an active role in their therapy, and an active partnership should be developed with the patient and family. Goals for asthma treatment should be shared, and the patient and health care provider should jointly agree on the patient's personal treatment goals.

Nonpharmacologic therapy should be incorporated into each step of therapy, and patient education should occur at all points where health care professionals interact with patients. Patient education should begin at the time of diagnosis and be tailored to meet individual patient needs.[1] Patients should understand: the difference between the asthmatic and normal lung, what happens to the lung during an asthma attack, differences between controller and relief medications, how to take inhaled medications correctly, and environmental control measures. Patients should also learn: self-management of asthma, including assessing level of control, recognizing signs and symptoms of worsening asthma, skills for self-monitoring of pulmonary function, when and how to take rescue actions, and when to seek medical care.

The importance of understanding asthma as a chronic disease and the need for daily treatment with long-term control medications should be stressed. The importance of proper use of medication-delivery devices should be reinforced.[1]

▶ *Risk Factor Avoidance*

Patients who smoke should be strongly encouraged to quit; cigarette smoking decreases the efficacy of ICS and can trigger an acute asthmatic response.[1] All patients should also avoid second-hand smoke. Patients should avoid outdoor activities when air quality is poor and avoid exposure to other irritants such as hairspray, paint, exhaust fumes, and smoke from any fire.

Patients sensitive to specific allergens should be educated on ways to avoid them. Environmental controls to reduce the allergen load in the patient's home may reduce

Table 14–1

Usual Dosages for Quick-Relief Medications in Asthma

Medication	Dosage Form	0–4 Years	5–11 Years	Adults	Comments
Inhaled Short-Acting β₂-Agonists					
Albuterol HFA	*MDI:* 90 mcg/puff, 200 puffs/canister	1–2 puffs 5 minutes before exercise 2 puffs every 4–6 hours as needed	2 puffs 5 minutes before exercise 2 puffs every 4–6 hours as needed	2 puffs 5 minutes before exercise 2 puffs every 4–6 hours as needed	*Applies to both SABAs.* Increasing use or lack of expected effect indicates diminished control of asthma Not recommended for long-term daily treatment. Regular use exceeding 2 days/week for symptom control (not prevention of EIB) indicates the need for additional long-term control therapy May double usual dose for mild exacerbations
Levalbuterol HFA	45 mcg/puff, 200 puffs/canister	N/A	2 puffs every 4–6 hours as needed	2 puffs 5 minutes before exercise 2 puffs every 4–6 hours as needed	Prime the inhaler by releasing 4 actuations prior to use Periodically clean HFA actuator, as drug may plug orifice Nonselective agents (i.e., epinephrine, isoproterenol, metaproterenol) are not recommended due to their potential for excessive cardiac stimulation, especially in high doses
Albuterol	*Nebulizer Solution:* 0.63 mg/3 mL 1.25 mg/3 mL 2.5 mg/3 mL 5 mg/mL (0.5%)	0.63–2.5 mg in 3 mL saline every 4–6 hours as needed	1.25–5 mg in 3 mL saline every 4–8 hours as needed	1.25–5 mg in 3 mL saline every 4–8 hours as needed	May mix with cromolyn solution, budesonide inhalant suspension, or ipratropium solution for nebulization. May double dose for severe exacerbations
Levalbuterol	0.31 mg/3 mL 0.63 mg/3 mL 1.25 mg/0.5 mL 1.25 mg/3 mL	0.31–1.25 mg in 3 mL every 4–6 hours as needed	0.31–0.63 mg every 8 hours as needed	0.63–1.25 mg every 8 hours as needed	Does not have FDA-approved labeling for children less than 6 years of age The product is a sterile-filled preservative-free unit dose vial Compatible with budesonide inhalant suspension
Anticholinergics					
Ipratropium HFA	*MDI:* 17 mcg/puff, 200 puffs/canister	N/A	N/A	2–3 puffs every 6 hours	Evidence is lacking for anticholinergics producing added benefit to β₂-agonists in long-term control asthma therapy.
	Nebulizer Solution: 0.25 mg/mL (0.025%)	N/A	N/A	0.25 mg every 6 hours	
Ipratropium with albuterol	18 mcg/puff ipratropium bromide and 90 mcg/puff albuterol, 200 puffs/canister	N/A	N/A	2–3 puffs every 6 hours	
	Nebulizer Solution: 0.5 mg/3 mL ipratropium and 2.5 mg/3 mL albuterol	N/A	N/A	3 mL every 4–6 hours	Contains EDTA to prevent discoloration of the solution. This additive does not induce bronchospasm
Systemic Corticosteroids					
Methylprednisolone	2, 4, 6, 8, 16, 32 mg oral tablets	Short course-"burst"; 1–2 mg/kg/day po, maximum 60 mg/day po, for 3–10 days	Short course-"burst": 40–60 mg/day po as single or 2 divided doses for 3–10 days	Short course "burst": 40–60 mg/day po as single or 2 divided doses for 3–10 days	*Applies to the first three corticosteroids.* Short courses or "bursts" are effective for establishing control when initiating therapy or during a period of gradual deterioration The burst should be continued until patient achieves 80% PEF personal best or symptoms resolve. This usually requires 3–10 days but may require longer. There is no evidence that tapering the dose following improvement prevents relapse
Prednisolone	5 mg oral tablets; 5 mg/5 mL and 15 mg/5 mL oral liquid				
Prednisone	1, 2.5, 5, 10, 20, 50 mg tablets; 5 mg/mL and 5 mg/5 mL oral liquid				

(Continued)

Table 14–1					
Usual Dosages for Quick-Relief Medications in Asthma (Continued)					
Medication	**Dosage Form**	**0–4 Years**	**5–11 Years**	**Adults**	**Comments**
Methylprednisolone acetate	*Repository Injection:* 40 mg/mL 80 mg/mL	7.5 mg/kg IM once	240 mg IM once	240 mg IM once	May be used in place of a short burst of oral steroids in patients who are vomiting or if adherence is a problem

CFC, chlorofluorocarbon; EDTA, ethylinediamine tetraacetic acid; EIB, exercise-induced bronchospasm; HFA, hydrofluoroalkane; IM, intramuscular; MDI, metered-dose inhaler; N/A, safety and efficacy not established; PEF, peak expiratory flow; SABA, short-acting β_2-agonist.

Dosages are provided for products that have been approved by the U.S. FDA or have sufficient clinical trial safety and efficacy data in the appropriate age ranges to support their use.

From Ref. 1.

asthma symptoms, school absences because of asthma, and unscheduled clinic and emergency visits for asthma.[15] Patients allergic to warm-blooded pets should remove them from home if possible or at least keep them out of the bedroom. Allergies to cockroach antigens and dust mites should be identified and appropriate measures taken to reduce or eliminate them.

The inactivated influenza vaccine should be considered in patients having asthma to decrease their risk of complications from influenza.[1] The pneumococcal vaccine may decrease the risk of invasive pneumococcal disease in asthmatics, but current guidelines do not include routine administration to asthma patients.[1,16]

▶ Drug Delivery Devices

⑤ *Direct airway administration of asthma medications through inhalation is the most efficient route and minimizes systemic adverse effects.* Poor inhaler technique can result in increased oropharyngeal deposition of the drug with decreased efficacy and increased adverse effects. Figure 14–1 provides steps for the appropriate use of inhaled delivery devices. Inhaled asthma medications are available in metered-dose inhalers (MDIs), dry powder inhalers (DPIs), and nebulized solutions. Because inhaler technique deteriorates over time, health care providers should take every opportunity to reinforce appropriate inhaler technique. Although nebulizers have often been used for drug delivery in children, their use is expensive and time consuming.

Patients should be educated to keep track of inhaler use. Some inhalers have a built-in counter or device to notify the patient of how many doses are remaining (e.g., Ventolin, hydrofluoroalkane [HFA], and Twisthaler).

Spacers or holding chambers with valves decrease the need for coordination of actuation of MDI devices with inhalation, decrease oropharyngeal deposition of drug, and increase pulmonary drug delivery.[17,18] Patients using a spacer or holding chamber should be counseled to place only one puff of the drug into the chamber at a time, because

actuating the MDI more than once into the chamber before inhalation decreases drug delivery. However, taking multiple breaths after a single actuation is appropriate and does not decrease drug efficacy.[17] Spacers or holding chambers with valves are equipped with a mouthpiece or a facemask allowing the use of an MDI in children younger than 5 years of age.

▶ Asthma Self-Management

Asthma self-management plans give patients the freedom to adjust therapy based on personal assessment of disease severity and a predetermined action plan. These plans reduce morbidity and the need for medical services.[19] For self-management plans to be effective, patients should be given a written action plan that is part of a global educational program.[1] The plan should include instructions on daily management and how to recognize and handle worsening asthma.[1]

Asthma control is assessed by evaluating signs and symptoms of worsening asthma and/or monitoring PEF. Early signs of deterioration include increasing nocturnal symptoms, increasing use of inhaled SABA, or symptoms that do not respond to increased use of inhaled SABAs. Measurement of PEF should be considered for patients with moderate to severe asthma, a poor perception of worsening asthma or airflow obstruction, and those with an unexplained response to environmental or occupational exposures.[1] If PEF measurements are used to assess control, the patient must be able to use a peak flow meter properly. PEF should be measured daily in the morning on waking, before using a bronchodilator. For PEF-based asthma action plans, the patient's personal best PEF should be established over a 2- to 3-week period using established methods when the patient is receiving optimal treatment.[1] Subsequent PEF measurements are evaluated in relation to their variability from the patient's best.[19] PEF measurements in the range of 80% to 100% of personal best (green zone) indicate that current therapy is acceptable. A PEF in the range of 50% to 79% of personal best

Please demonstrate your inhaler technique at every visit.

1. Remove the cap and hold inhaler upright.
2. Shake the inhaler.
3. Tilt your head back slightly and breathe out slowly.
4. Position the inhaler in one of the following ways (A or B is optimal, but C is acceptable for those who have difficulty with A or B.
   C is required for breath-activated inhalers.):

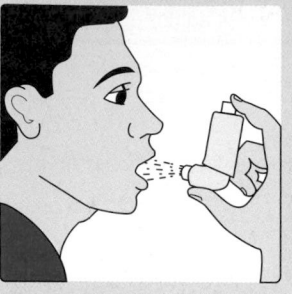 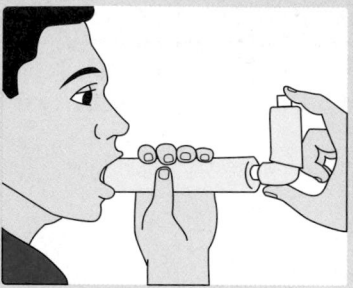 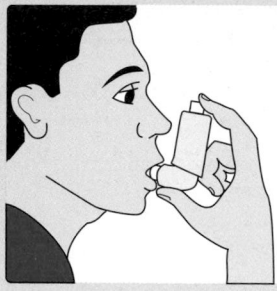 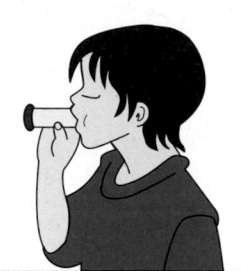

A Open mouth with inhaler 1 to 2 inches away.

B Use spacer/holding chamber (that is recommended especially for young children and for people using corticosteroids).

C In the mouth. Do not use for corticosteroids

D NOTE: Inhaled dry powder capsules require a different inhalation technique. To use a dry powder inhaler, it is important to close the mouth tightly around the mouthpiece of the inhaler and to inhale rapidly.

5. Press down on the inhaler to release medication as you start to breathe in slowly.
6. Breathe in slowly (3 to 5 seconds).
7. Hold your breath for 10 seconds to allow the medicine to reach deeply into your lungs.
8. Repeat puff as directed. Waiting 1 minute between puffs may permit second puff to penetrate your lungs better.
9. Spacers/holding chambers are useful for all patients. They are particularly recommended for young children and older adults and for use with corticosteroids.

Avoid common inhaler mistakes. Follow these inhaler tips:
• Breathe out before pressing your inhaler.
• Inhale slowly.
• Breathe in through your mouth, not your nose.
• Press down on your inhaler at the start of inhalation (or within the first second of inhalation).
• Keep inhaling as you press down on inhaler.
• Press your inhaler only once while you are inhaling (one breath for each puff).
• Make sure you breathe in evenly and deeply.

NOTE: Other inhalers are becoming available in addition to those illustrated above. Different types of inhalers require different techniques.

FIGURE 14–1. Instructions for using an inhaler. (From Ref. 20.)

(yellow zone) may indicate an impending exacerbation, and therapy should be intensified based on the self-management plan. A PEF less than 50% (red zone) signals a medical alert; patients should use their SABA immediately and consult their asthma action plan.

Pharmacologic Therapy

▶ β₂-Adrenergic Agonists

β_2-Agonists relax airway smooth muscle by directly stimulating β_2-adrenergic receptors.[20] They also increase mucociliary clearance and stabilize mast cell membranes. Inhalation dosage forms are most commonly used, but oral and injectable dosage forms are also available. β_2-Agonists have significantly better bronchodilating activity in acute asthma than theophylline or anticholinergic agents.

Adverse effects include tachycardia, tremor, and hypokalemia, which are usually not troublesome with inhaled dosage forms. Oral β_2-agonists have increased adverse effects and should be avoided in patients who are able to use inhaled medications. Oral β_2-agonists should not be used in acute asthma because of a delayed onset of action compared to the inhaled route. Inhaled β_2-agonists are classified as either short- or long-acting based on duration of action.

Short-Acting Inhaled β₂-Agonists ⑥ *Inhaled SABAs are the most effective agents for reversing acute airway obstruction caused by bronchoconstriction and are the drugs of choice for treating acute severe asthma and symptoms of chronic asthma as well as preventing exercise-induced bronchospasm.*[1] Inhaled SABA have an onset of action of less than 5 minutes and a duration of action of 4 to 6 hours. Using an MDI with a spacer is quicker and at least as effective as administration by nebulization.

Albuterol (known as salbutamol outside the United States), the most commonly used inhaled SABA, is a racemic mixture (50:50) of albuterol enantiomers. The R-enantiomer is the active component, whereas the S-enantiomer is inactive and may be associated with unwanted effects. Levalbuterol, the pure R-enantiomer of albuterol (and referred to as R-salbutamol outside the United States), is available as an MDI and solution for nebulization. Levalbuterol and albuterol are similar in efficacy, but the acquisition cost of levalbuterol is substantially higher.[21] Nonselective β_2-agonists (e.g., metaproterenol) are not used commonly due to the potential for increased adverse effects.

Doses used for quick relief in chronic asthma are provided in Table 14–1. Usual rescue doses may be doubled for mild exacerbations. The regular use of inhaled SABAs is not recommended.[1]

Long-Acting Inhaled β$_2$-Agonists Salmeterol and formoterol are LABA that provide up to 12 hours of bronchodilation after a single dose. Both agents are approved for chronic prevention of asthma symptoms. Salmeterol is a partial agonist with an onset of action of approximately 30 minutes. Because of this delayed onset, patients should be cautioned not to use salmeterol as a quick-relief medication. Formoterol is a full agonist that has an onset of action similar to that of albuterol, but it is not currently approved for the treatment of acute bronchospasm.

Inhaled LABA are indicated for add-on therapy for asthma not controlled on low to medium doses of ICS. Adding an LABA is at least as effective in improving symptoms and decreasing asthma exacerbations as doubling the dose of an ICS.[22,23] Adding an LABA to ICS therapy also reduces the amount of ICS necessary for asthma control.[24]

Although both formoterol and salmeterol are effective as add-on therapy for moderate persistent asthma, neither agent should be used as monotherapy for chronic asthma. There may be an increased risk of severe asthma exacerbations and asthma-related deaths when LABA are used alone or added to standard therapy.[25,26] The labeling for all drugs containing LABA contains a "black-box" warning against their use without an ICS. The risk of increased severe asthma exacerbations does not appear to be increased in adults receiving both an LABA and ICS.[27,28]

Salmeterol and formoterol are available in fixed ratio combination products containing fluticasone and budesonide, respectively. Combination products may increase adherence because of the need for fewer inhalers and inhalations. However, they offer less flexibility in dosage adjustment of individual ingredients when that is considered necessary. Doses used for long-term control of chronic asthma are provided in Table 14–2.

▶ Corticosteroids

Corticosteroids are the most potent anti-inflammatory agents available for the treatment of asthma and are available in inhaled, oral, and injectable dosage forms. They decrease airway inflammation, AHR, and mucus production and secretion. Corticosteroids also improve the response to β_2-agonists.[20]

Inhaled Corticosteroids ❼ *ICS are the preferred therapy for all forms of persistent asthma in all age groups.*[1] ICS are more effective than cromolyn, leukotriene modifiers, nedocromil, and theophylline in improving lung function and preventing emergency department visits and

hospitalizations due to asthma exacerbations.[1,22] The primary advantage of using ICS compared to systemic corticosteroids is the targeted drug delivery to the lungs, which decreases the risk of systemic adverse effects. All ICS are equally effective if given in equipotent doses (Table 14–3). Product selection should be based on preference for dosage form, delivery device, and cost.

Although some beneficial effect is seen within 12 hours of administration, 2 weeks of therapy is necessary to see significant clinical effects. Longer treatment may be necessary to realize the full effects on airway inflammation and remodeling.

ICS have a flat dose–response curve; doubling the dose has a limited additional effect on asthma control.[1,29] Considerable variability in response to ICS exists,[30,31] and increasing the doses may be of greater benefit in severe asthma than in mild-to-moderate asthma.[32] The ICS are effective when given twice daily and may be effective when given once daily for mild asthma.

Local adverse effects of ICS include oral candidiasis, cough, hoarse voice, and dysphonia. The incidence of local adverse effects can be reduced by using a spacer or valved holding chamber and by having the patient rinse the mouth with water and expectorate after using the ICS. Decreasing the dose reduces the incidence of hoarseness. For most delivery devices, the majority of the drug is deposited in the mouth and throat and swallowed. Systemic absorption occurs via the pulmonary and oral routes. Although only a fraction of the drug is delivered to the lungs, 100% of the drug reaching the lungs is absorbed systemically.[1]

Systemic adverse effects are dose dependent and rare at low to medium doses. However, high-dose ICS have been associated with adrenal suppression, decreased bone mineral density, skin thinning, cataracts, and easy bruising.[1] Growth suppression in children occurs primarily in the first year of treatment and may be due to delayed growth with the potential of future catch-up growth.[33]

Systemic Corticosteroids Systemic corticosteroids are effective as both long-term control and rescue medications. Because of serious potential adverse effects, systemic corticosteroids should be used for long-term asthma control only in patients who have failed other therapies. If systemic therapy is necessary, once-daily or every-other-day therapy should be used with repeated attempts to decrease the dose or discontinue the drug.

Systemic corticosteroids are the cornerstone of treatment for worsening asthma not responding to bronchodilators and for acute severe asthma. For patients with nonresponsive worsening asthma, a short course or "burst" of systemic corticosteroids is effective for gaining control and preventing progression.[1]

In acute severe asthma, systemic corticosteroids should be given to all patients who have moderate to severe exacerbations or who do not respond to initial bronchodilator therapy. Corticosteroids reduce inflammation, increase the response to β_2-agonists, hasten recovery, decrease hospital admissions, and reduce relapse rates. The onset

Table 14–2

Usual Dosages for Long-Term Control Medications in Asthma

Medication	Dosage Form	0–4 Years	5–11 Years	Adult Dose	Comments
Inhaled Corticosteroids (see Table 14–3, Estimated Comparative Daily Dosages for Inhaled Corticosteroids)					
Systemic (Oral) Corticosteroids:					**Applies to all three corticosteroids.**
Methylprednisolone	2, 4, 8, 16, 32 mg oral tablets	0.25–2 mg/kg daily in single dose or every other day	0.25–2 mg/kg daily in single dose or every other day	7.5–60 mg daily in a single dose or every other day	For long-term treatment of severe persistent asthma, administer a single dose in a.m. either daily or on alternate days (alternate-day therapy may produce less adrenal suppression)
Prednisolone	5 mg oral tablets; 5 mg/5 mL and 15 mg/5 mL oral liquid	Short-course "burst": 1–2 mg/kg/day, maximum 30 mg/day for 3–10 days	Short-course "burst": 1–2 mg/kg/day, maximum 60 mg/day for 3–10 days	Short-course "burst": 40–60 mg/day as single or 2 divided doses for 3–10 days	Short courses or "bursts" are effective for establishing control when initiating therapy or during a period of gradual deterioration. There is no evidence that tapering the dose following improvement in symptom control and pulmonary function prevents relapse
Prednisone	1, 2.5, 5, 10, 20, 50 mg oral tablets; 5 mg/mL, 5 mg/5 mL oral liquid				*For children 0–11 years of age:* Patients receiving the lower dose (1 mg/kg/day) experience fewer behavioral side effects and it appears to be equally effective
Long-Acting β₂-Agonists					**Should not be used for symptom relief or exacerbations. Use only with ICS**
Salmeterol[a]	DPI 50 mcg/blister	N/A	Contents of one blister every 12 hours	Contents of one blister every 12 hours	Decreased duration of protection against EIB may occur with regular use. Most children younger than 4 years of age cannot provide sufficient inspiratory flow for adequate lung delivery. Do not blow into inhaler after dose is activated
Formoterol[a]	PI 12 mcg/capsule	N/A	Contents of one capsule every 12 hours	Contents of one capsule every 12 hours	Most children younger than 4 years of age cannot provide sufficient inspiratory flow for adequate lung delivery. Each capsule is for single use only; additional doses should not be administered for at least 12 hours. Capsules should be used only with the Aerolizer inhaler and should not be taken orally
Combined medication					
Fluticasone/Salmeterol[a]	DPI 100 mcg/50 mcg, 250 mcg/50 mcg, 500 mcg/50 mcg; HFA MDI 45 mcg/21 mcg, 115 mcg/21 mcg, 230 mcg/21 mcg	N/A	One inhalation twice a day	One inhalation twice a day; dose depends on severity of asthma	*For adults:* 100/50 DPI or 45/21 HFA for patients not controlled on low- to medium-dose ICS. 250/50 DPI or 115/21 HFA for patients not controlled on medium- to high-dose ICS. There have been no clinical trials in children less than 4 years of age. Most children younger than 4 years of age cannot provide sufficient inspiratory flow for adequate lung delivery. Do not blow into inhaler after dose is activated
Budesonide/Formoterol[a]	HFA MDI 80 mcg/4.5 mcg, 160 mcg/4.5 mcg	N/A	Two puffs twice a day	Two puffs twice a day; dose depends on severity of asthma	*For adults:* 80/4.5 for patients not controlled on low- to medium-dose ICS. 160/4.5 for patients not controlled on medium- to high-dose ICS. There have been no clinical trials in children younger than 4 years of age. Currently approved for use individuals 12 years of age and older. Dose for children 5–12 years of age based on clinical trials using DPI with slightly different delivery characteristics

(Continued)

Table 14–2

Usual Dosages for Long-Term Control Medications in Asthma (*Continued*)

Medication	Dosage Form	0–4 Years	5–11 Years	Adult Dose	Comments
Cromolyn/Nedocromil:					
Cromolyn	MDI 0.8 mg/puff	N/A	Two puffs 4 times a day	Two puffs 4 times a day	4–6 week trial may be needed to determine maximum benefit
	Nebulizer 20 mg/ampule	one ampule 4 times a day; safety and efficacy not established below age 2 years	One ampule 4 times a day	One ampule 4 times a day	Dose by MDI may be inadequate to affect hyper-responsiveness One dose before exercise or allergen exposure provides effective prophylaxis for 1–2 hours. Not as effective as inhaled β_2-agonists for EIB Once control is achieved, the frequency of dosing may be reduced
Nedocromil	MDI 1.75 mg/puff	N/A	Two puffs 4 times a day	Two puffs 4 times a day	
Leukotriene Modifiers:					
Montelukast	4 mg or 5 mg chewable tablet; 4 mg granule packets 10 mg tablets	4 mg at bedtime (1–5 years of age)	5 mg at bedtime (6–14 years of age)	10 mg at bedtime	Montelukast exhibits a flat dose-response curve. Doses above 10 mg will not produce a greater response in adults No more efficacious than placebo in infants 6–24 months
Zafirlukast	10 or 20 mg tablets	N/A	10 mg twice a day (7–11 years of age)	40 mg daily (20 mg tablet twice a day)	For zafirlukast, administration with meals decreases bioavailability; take at least 1 hour before or 2 hours after meals Monitor for signs and symptoms of hepatic dysfunction
Zileuton	600 mg tablets	N/A	N/A	600 mg 4 times a day	For zileuton, monitor hepatic enzymes (ALT)
Methylxanthines:					
Theophylline	Liquids, sustained-release tablets and capsules	Starting dose 10 mg/kg/day; usual maximum: Less than 1 year old: 0.2 (age in weeks) + 5 = mg/kg/day 1 year of age and older: 16 mg/kg/day	Starting dose 10 mg/kg/day; usual maximum: 16 mg/kg/day	Starting dose 10 mg/kg/day up to 300 mg maximum; usual maximum 800 mg/day	Adjust dosage to achieve serum concentration of 5–15 mcg/mL at steady-state (at least 48 hours on same dosage) Due to wide interpatient variability in theophylline metabolic clearance, routine serum theophylline level monitoring is essential
Immunomodulators:					
Omalizumab	Subcutaneous injection, 150 mg/1.2 mL after reconstitution with 1.4 mL sterile water for injection	N/A	N/A	150–375 mg SC every 2–4 weeks, depending on body weight and pretreatment serum IgE level	Do not administer more than 150 mg per injection site Monitor for anaphylaxis for two hours after at least the first three injections

DPI, dry powder inhaler; EIB exercise-induced bronchospasm; HFA, hydrofluoroalkane (inhaler propellant); ICS, inhaled corticosteroids; IgE; immunoglobulin E; MDI, metered-dose inhaler; N/A, safety and efficacy not established; SABA, short-acting β_2-agonist; SC, subcutaneously.

[a]In December 2008, an FDA Advisory Panel recommended banning use of (Serevent) salmeterol and Foradil (formoterol) for treatment of asthma. Use of the combination products Advair (fluticasone/salmeterol) and Symbicort (budesonide/formoterol) were not included in the recommended ban.

Dosages are provided for products that have been approved by the U.S. Food and Drug Administration or have sufficient clinical trial safety and efficacy data in the appropriate age ranges to support their use.

From Ref. 1.

Table 14–3

Estimated Comparative Daily Dosages for Inhaled Corticosteroids for Asthma

Medication	Low Daily Dose			Medium Daily Dose			High Daily Dose		
	Child 0–4 Years	Child 5–11 Years	Adults	Child 0–4 Years	Child 5–11 Years	Adults	Child 0–4 Years	Child 5–11 Years	Adults
Beclomethasone HFA (MDI) 40 or 80 mcg/puff	N/A	80–160 mcg	80–240 mcg	N/A	Above 160–320 mcg	Above 240–480 mcg	N/A	Above 320 mcg	Above 480 mcg
Budesonide DPI 90, 180, or 200 mcg/inhalation	N/A	180–400 mcg	180–600 mcg	N/A	Above 400–800 mcg	Above 600–1,200 mcg	N/A	Above 800 mcg	Above 1,200 mcg
Budesonide inhalation suspension for nebulization	0.25–0.5 mg	0.5 mg	N/A	Above 0.5–1 mg	1 mg	N/A	Above 1 mg	2 mg	N/A
Flunisolide HFA 80 mcg/puff	N/A	160 mcg	320 mcg	N/A	320 mcg	Above 320–640 mcg	N/A	640 mcg and above	Above 640 mcg
Fluticasone HFA (MDI) 44, 110, or 220 mcg/puff	176 mcg	88–176 mcg	88–264 mcg	Above 176–352 mcg	Above 176–352 mcg	Above 264–440 mcg	Above 352 mcg	Above 352 mcg	Above 440 mcg
Fluticasone DPI 50, 100, or 250 mcg/inhalation	N/A	100–200 mcg	100–300 mcg	N/A	Above 200–400 mcg	Above 300–500 mcg	N/A	Above 400 mcg	Above 500 mcg
Mometasone DPI 200 mcg/inhalation	N/A	N/A	200 mcg	N/A	N/A	400 mcg	N/A	N/A	Above 400 mcg

DPI, dry powder inhaler; HFA, hydrofluoroalkane; MDI, metered-dose inhaler, N/A, safety and efficacy not established.

From Ref. 1.

of action is delayed, and a clinical response may not be seen for 4 to 12 hours.[20] For this reason, systemic corticosteroids should be started early in the course of acute exacerbations or worsening asthma. The oral route is preferred in acute severe asthma; there is no evidence that IV corticosteroid administration is more effective.[1] Recommended doses for acute asthma exacerbations are shown in Table 14–4.

Therapy with systemic corticosteroids should generally be continued until the PEF is 70% or more of the predicted value or personal best. The duration of therapy usually ranges from 3 to 10 days, but longer therapy may be necessary for severe exacerbations. Tapering the corticosteroid dose in patients receiving short bursts (up to 10 days) is not necessary because any adrenal suppression is transient and rapidly reversible.[1,20]

▶ Anticholinergics

Anticholinergic agents (see Tables 14–1 and 14–4) act by inhibiting the effects of acetylcholine on muscarinic receptors in the airways. They only protect against cholinergic-mediated bronchoconstriction and are not as effective as β_2-agonists in asthma.[20] Anticholinergic drugs may cause bothersome adverse effects such as blurred vision, dry mouth, urinary retention, and constipation. However, the inhaled anticholinergic agents are quaternary amines that are not absorbed systemically and have limited adverse effects.

Ipratropium bromide (Atrovent) is available as an MDI and solution for nebulization. It has an onset of action of approximately 30 minutes and a duration of action of 4 to 8 hours. Care should be taken to avoid contact of the spray or nebulized solution with the eyes, as it can cause mydriasis and blurred vision.

The addition of ipratropium bromide to inhaled β_2-agonist therapy in acute severe asthma improves pulmonary function and decreases hospitalization rates in both adult and pediatric patients.[34] The benefit of combining ipratropium and albuterol appears to be greatest in moderate to severe exacerbations, and the combination should be considered first-line therapy in severe exacerbations.

Tiotropium bromide (Spiriva) is a long-acting inhaled anticholinergic available in a DPI; it has an onset of action of approximately 30 minutes and a duration of action longer than 24 hours. There is little evidence supporting the use of tiotropium bromide in asthma.

▶ Leukotriene Modifiers

Leukotriene modifiers (see Table 14–2) either inhibit 5-lipoxygenase (zileuton) or competitively antagonize the effects of leukotriene D_4 (montelukast and zafirlukast). These agents improve FEV_1 and decrease asthma symptoms, rescue

Table 14–4

Dosages of Selected Drugs for Asthma Exacerbations

Medication	Child Dose[a]	Adult Dose	Comments
Inhaled Short-Acting β_2-Agonists			
Albuterol			
Nebulizer solution 0.63 mg/ 3 mL, 1.25 mg/ 3 mL, 2.5 mg/3 mL, 5 mg/mL	0.15 mg/kg (minimum dose 2.5 mg) every 20 minutes for 3 doses then 0.15–0.3 mg/kg up to 10 mg every 1–4 hours as needed; or 0.5 mg/kg/hour by continuous nebulization	2.5–5 mg every 20 minutes for 3 doses, then 2.5–10 mg every 1–4 hours as needed; or 10–15 mg/hour by continuous nebulization	Only selective β_2-agonists are recommended. For optimal delivery, dilute aerosols to minimum of 3 mL at gas flow of 6–8 L/min. Use large volume nebulizers for continuous administration. May mix with ipratropium nebulizer solution
MDI 90 mcg/puff	4–8 puffs every 20 minutes for 3 doses, then every 1–4 hours inhalation maneuver as needed. Use VHC; add mask in children less than 4 years	4–8 puffs every 20 minutes up to 4 hours, then every 1–4 hours as needed	In mild-to-moderate exacerbations, MDI plus VHC is as effective as nebulized therapy with appropriate administration technique and coaching by trained personnel
Levalbuterol			
Nebulizer solution 0.31 mg/ 3 mL, 0.63 mg/3 mL, 1.25 mg/0.5 mL, 1.25 mg/ 3 mL	0.075 mg/kg (minimum dose 1.25 mg) every 20 minutes for 3 doses, then 0.075–0.15 mg/kg up to 5 mg every 1–4 hours as needed	1.25–2.5 mg every 20 minutes for 3 doses, then 1.25–5 mg every 1–4 hours as needed	Levalbuterol administered in one-half the mg dose of albuterol provides comparable efficacy and safety. Has not been evaluated by continuous nebulization
MDI 45 mcg/puff	See albuterol MDI dose	See albuterol MDI dose	
Pirbuterol			
MDI 200 mcg/puff	See albuterol MDI dose; thought to be half as potent as albuterol on a mg basis	See albuterol MDI dose	Has not been studied in severe asthma exacerbations
Systemic (Subcutaneous) β_2-Agonists			
Epinephrine			
1:1,000 (1 mg/mL)	0.01 mg/kg up to 0.3–0.5 mg every 20 minutes for 3 doses SC	0.3–0.5 mg every 20 minutes for 3 doses SC	No proven advantage of systemic therapy over aerosol
Terbutaline			
(1 mg/mL)	0.01 mg/kg every 20 minutes for 3 doses then every 2–6 hours as needed SC	0.25 mg every 20 minutes for 3 doses SC	No proven advantage of systemic therapy over aerosol
Anticholinergics			
Ipratropium bromide			
Nebulizer solution 0.25 mg/mL	0.25–0.5 mg every 20 minutes for 3 doses, then as needed	0.5 mg every 20 minutes for 3 doses then as needed	May mix in same nebulizer with albuterol. Should not be used as first-line therapy; should be added to SABA therapy for severe exacerbations. Addition of ipratropium does not provide further benefit once the patient is hospitalized
MDI 18 mcg/puff	4–8 puffs every 20 minutes as needed up to 3 hours	8 puffs every 20 minutes as needed up to 3 hours	Use with VHC and face mask for children younger than age 4. Studies have examined ipratropium bromide MDI for up to 3 hours
Ipratropium with albuterol			
Nebulizer solution (0.5 mg ipratropium bromide/ 2.5 mg albuterol per 3 mL vial.)	1.5 mL every 20 minutes for 3 doses, then as needed	3 mL every 20 minutes for 3 doses, then as needed	May be used for up to 3 hours in the initial management of severe exacerbations. Addition of ipratropium to albuterol does not provide further benefit once the patient is hospitalized
MDI (18 mcg ipratropium bromide/90 mcg albuterol per puff)	4–8 puffs every 20 minutes as needed up to 3 hours	8 puffs every 20 minutes as needed up to 3 hours	Use with VHC and face mask for children younger than age 4
Systemic (Oral) Corticosteroids			
Prednisone, Methylprednisolone Prednisolone	1 mg/kg po in 2 divided doses (maximum 60 mg/day) until PEF is 70% of predicted or personal best	40–80 mg/day po in 1 or 2 divided doses until PEF reaches 70% of predicted or personal best	For outpatient "burst", use 40–60 mg po in single or 2 divided doses for total of 5–10 days in adults (children: 1–2 mg/kg/day; maximum 60 mg/day for 3–10 days)

ED, emergency department; MDI, metered-dose inhaler; PEF, peak expiratory flow; SC, subcutaneously; VHC, valved holding chamber.

[a]Children 12 years of age and younger.

Notes: There is no known advantage for higher doses of corticosteroids in severe asthma exacerbations, nor is there any advantage of IV administration over oral therapy provided GI transit time or absorption is not impaired.

The total course of systemic corticosteroids for an asthma exacerbation requiring an ED visit of hospitalization may last from 3 to 10 days. For corticosteroid courses of less than 1 week, there is no need to taper the dose. For slightly longer courses (e.g., up to 10 days), there probably is no need to taper, especially if patients are concurrently taking ICS.

ICS can be started at any point in the treatment of an asthma exacerbation.

From Ref. 1.

drug use, and exacerbations due to asthma. Although these agents offer the convenience of oral therapy for asthma, they are significantly less effective than low doses of ICS.[1,35] Combining a leukotriene receptor antagonist with an ICS or LABA is not as effective as an ICS plus an LABA.[1]

The leukotriene receptor antagonists zafirlukast (Accolate) and montelukast (Singulair) are generally well tolerated and dosed twice daily and once daily, respectively. Significant increases in hepatic enzymes have been reported in postmarketing studies for zafirlukast but not montelukast. Zafirlukast also inhibits the CYP2C9 and CYP3A4 isoenzymes and may increase prothrombin time in patients receiving warfarin; the International Normalized Ratio should be monitored if warfarin and zafirlukast are used concomitantly. Montelukast does not appear to inhibit the cytochrome P-450 enzymes.

Zileuton (Zyflo) is not commonly used because of the need for dosing four times daily, potential drug interactions, and potential hepatotoxicity with the resulting need for frequent monitoring of hepatic enzymes.

▶ Cromolyn and Nedocromil

Cromolyn sodium (Intal) and nedocromil sodium (Tilade) are inhaled anti-inflammatory agents that block both the early- and late-phase response possibly by inhibiting release of mediators from mast cells. Both agents are alternatives to ICS for treatment of mild persistent asthma, but they are significantly less effective than low doses of ICS (see Table 14–2).[1] Cromolyn and nedocromil are similar in efficacy to the leukotriene antagonists and theophylline for persistent asthma.[20] Both drugs require dosing four times daily until symptoms stabilize, after which the dosage frequency can be reduced to three times a day for cromolyn and twice daily for nedocromil.[20] Patients may notice improvement in 1 to 2 weeks, but maximal benefit may not be seen for 4 to 6 weeks.

One dose of cromolyn or nedocromil prior to exercise or allergen exposure will provide prophylaxis for 1 to 2 hours. These agents are not as effective as albuterol for prophylaxis of exercise-induced asthma.

Both agents are well tolerated with adverse effects limited to cough and wheezing. Bad taste and headache have also been reported with nedocromil.

▶ Methylxanthines

Theophylline (see Table 14–2) causes bronchodilation by inhibiting phosphodiesterase and antagonizing adenosine. It may also have mild anti-inflammatory and immunomodulatory properties.[36] Its use is limited because of inferior efficacy as a controller medication compared to ICS, a narrow therapeutic index with potentially life-threatening toxicity, and multiple clinically important drug interactions.

Target serum theophylline concentrations are 5 to 15 mg/L (28–83 μmol/L); an increased risk of adverse effects outweighs the increased bronchodilation in most patients above 15 mg/L (83 μmol/L).[37] Headache, nausea, vomiting, and irritability may occur at serum concentrations less than 20 mg/L (110 μmol/L) but are rare when the dose is started low and increased slowly. More serious adverse effects, including cardiac arrhythmias, seizures, toxic encephalopathy, and death can occur at higher concentrations.[20]

Theophylline is primarily metabolized by CYP1A2 and CYP3A4 and is involved in a large number of disease and drug interactions. Theophylline exhibits nonlinear pharmacokinetics in the therapeutic range; therefore, serum concentration changes due to dosage adjustments and drug interactions may not always be predictable.[20] Theophylline also exhibits interpatient variability in hepatic clearance; consequently, serum theophylline concentrations should be monitored.

▶ Omalizumab

Omalizumab (Xolair) is a recombinant humanized monoclonal anti-IgE antibody that inhibits binding of IgE to receptors on mast cells and basophils, resulting in inhibition of mediator release and attenuation of the early- and late-phase allergic response. It is indicated for treatment of moderate to severe persistent asthma in patients 12 years of age or older whose asthma is not controlled by ICS and who have a positive skin test or in vitro reactivity to perennial allergens.[38] Omalizumab significantly decreases ICS use, reduces the number and length of exacerbations, and increases asthma-related quality of life. It is also effective in improving asthma control in severe asthmatics receiving combination therapy with high-dose ICS and LABAs.[1] However, its place in therapy is limited by its high cost.[39]

Omalizumab is given as a subcutaneous injection every 2 to 4 weeks, and the initial dose is based on the patient's weight and initial total IgE serum concentration. The dosage should not be adjusted based on subsequent total serum IgE measurements (see Table 14–2). Drug clearance depends on patient weight, and dosage should be adjusted if there is a significant change in body weight. Doses greater than 150 mg should be administered as separate injections at multiple sites.

The most common adverse effects are injection site reactions and include bruising, redness, pain, stinging, itching, and burning. Anaphylactic reactions are rare but may be delayed 2 hours or more after drug administration.[40] Reports of delayed anaphylactic reactions have led to a "black box" warning in the labeling and a medication guide warning of this risk.

Treatment of Chronic Asthma

8 *The intensity of pharmacotherapy for chronic asthma is based on disease severity for initial therapy and level of control for subsequent therapies.* The least amount of medications necessary to meet the goals of asthma therapy should be used.[1] Current recommendations for stepwise therapy for chronic asthma are shown in Figure 14–2. However, because of varying asthma presentations, the therapeutic plan must be individualized. The EPR-3 separates treatment recommendations into three categories based on patient age: (a) children younger than 5 years of age, (b) children

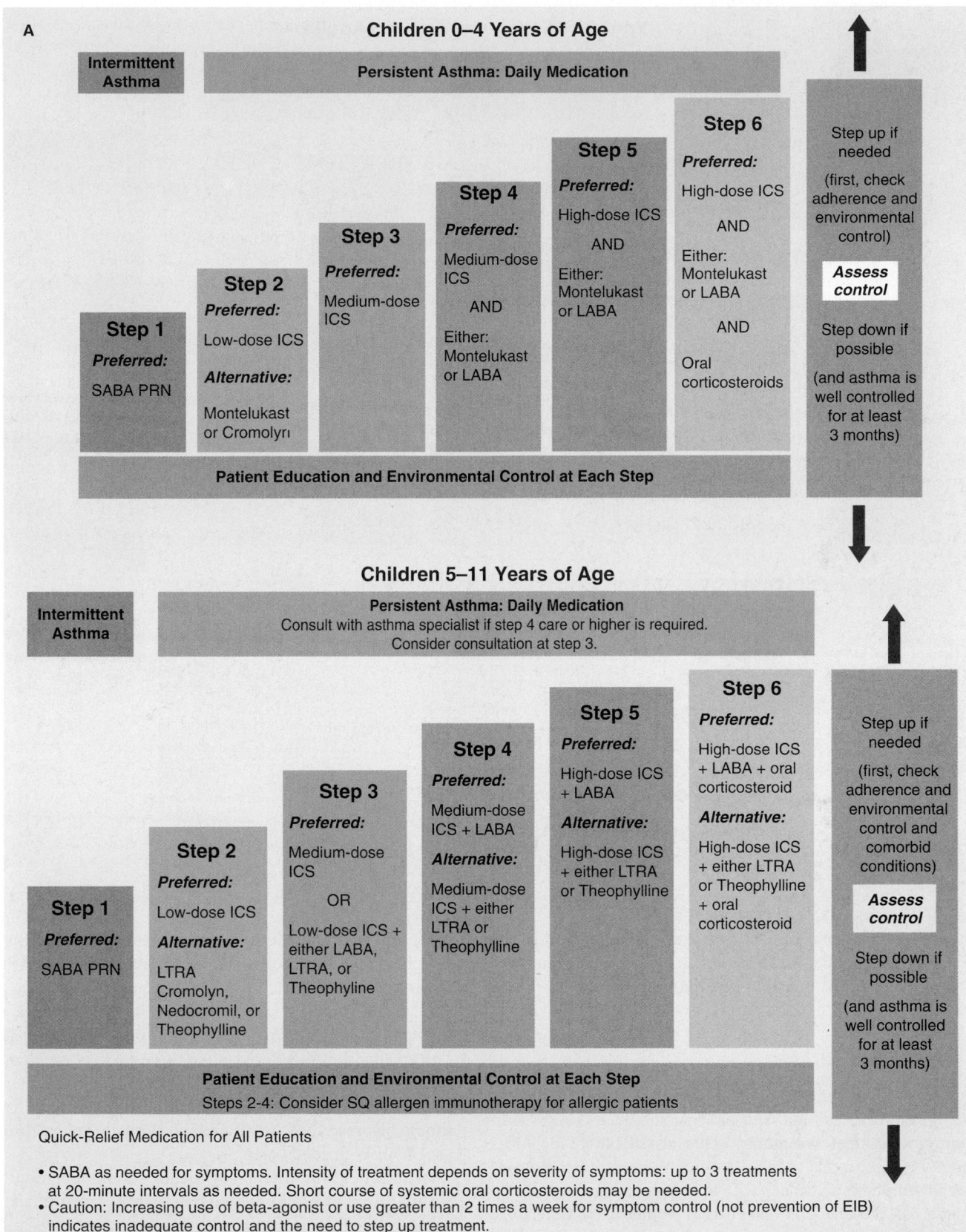

FIGURE 14–2. Stepwise approach for managing asthma in children (A) and adults (B).
(ICS, inhaled corticosteroids; LABA, long-acting β-agonists; LTRA, leukotriene receptor antagonist; PRN, as needed; SABA, short-acting β-agonist.) (From Ref. 20.)

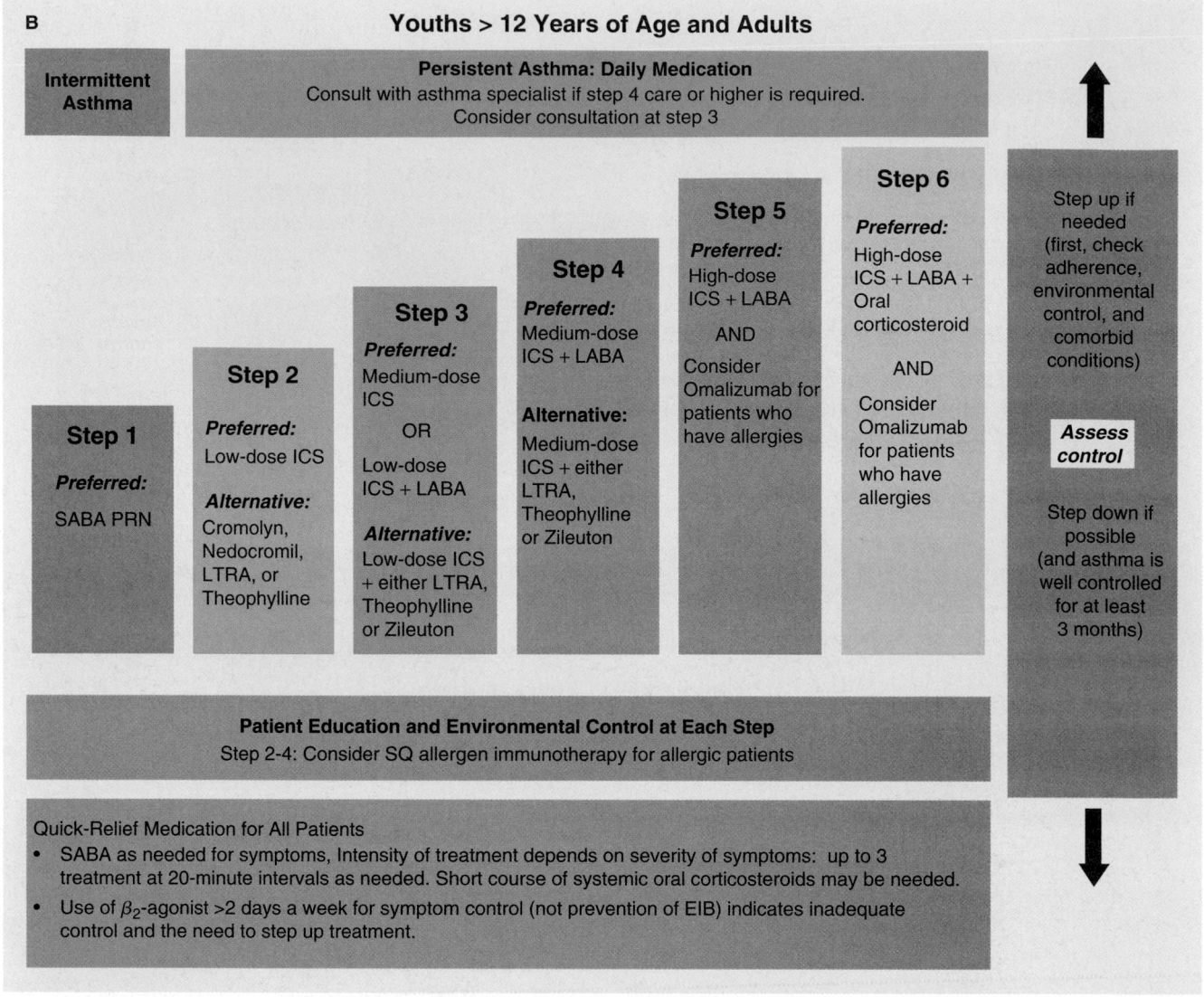

FIGURE 14–2. *(Continued)*

between the ages of 5 and 11 years, and (c) individuals 12 years of age and older. Refer to Ref. 1 for more information on assessing asthma control and adjusting therapy in these three categories.[1]

▶ Intermittent Asthma

Long-term control medications are not necessary in patients with intermittent asthma, and patients should use an SABA to prevent or treat symptoms.[1] This classification includes patients with exercise-induced asthma, seasonal asthma, or asthma symptoms associated with infrequent trigger exposure. Patients can pretreat with two puffs of albuterol, cromolyn, or nedocromil prior to exposure to a known trigger.

▶ Persistent Asthma

Patients who use an SABA more than twice a week for symptom control (not exercise-induced bronchospasm) should be treated as persistent asthma. Patients who experienced two or more exacerbations requiring oral corticosteroids in the past year may also be categorized as having persistent asthma.[1] Patients with persistent asthma require daily long-term control therapy (see Tables 14–2 and 14–3). However, daily therapy limited to a predefined period of risk (e.g., seasonal asthma) may be considered when these periods are identified by history. ICS are the long-term control medication of choice at all levels of severity and in all age groups.[1] SABAs should be prescribed for all patients with chronic asthma for use on an as-needed basis.

After initiating therapy, patients should be monitored within 2 to 6 weeks to ensure that asthma control has been achieved. Before increasing therapy, the patient's inhaler technique and adherence to therapy should be evaluated.[1] Patients with controlled asthma should be monitored at 1- to 6-month intervals to ensure control is maintained. A gradual stepdown in control therapy should be initiated when possible, usually once control has been maintained for at least 3 months.[1]

Patient Encounter, Part 2: The Medical History, Physical Exam, and Diagnostic Tests

HPI: As presented in Part 1. In addition, the patient does not report any daytime symptoms and states that she does not get short of breath walking up the stairs at school.

PMH: Allergic rhinitis for 6 years (allergic to dust mites per skin testing; no other allergies positive on the skin testing panel). Bronchitis 3 times in the last 6 years (all treated with azithromycin and Robitussin DM); last episode 6 months ago. Hospitalized with viral lower respiratory tract infections twice at ages 1 and 2.

FH: Mother had asthma as a child, but "outgrew it" and has had no problems with it since she was 12 or 13 years old; both her mother and father have allergic rhinitis.

SH: Only child who lives at home with her mother and father in a two-bedroom duplex built on a concrete slab. Neither the patient nor her parents smoke or drink alcohol. They have no animals inside or outside the home.

Meds: Cetirizine 10 mg by mouth daily

ROS: Unremarkable except as described above.

PE:

Gen: Small for her age but appears to be well nourished and healthy

VS: BP 112/68 mm Hg, P 78 bpm, RR 18 bpm, T 37.0°C (98.7°F), ht 4'6" (137 cm), wt 28 kg (62 lb)

Chest: CTA bilaterally, no wheezing

CV: RRR; S_1 and S_2 normal; no rubs, gallops, or murmurs

Ext: No clubbing, cyanosis, or edema

Labs: Normal except for WBC differential with 7% eosinophils

Pulmonary Function Tests

FEV_1: 1.5 L (84% predicted)

FVC: 1.75 L (92% predicted)

FEV_1/FVC: 0.857

Postbronchodilator FEV_1: 1.70 L (13.3% increase)

FEV_1 after exercise: 1.23 L (23.1% decrease)

Given this additional information, what is your assessment of the patient's asthma severity?

Identify your treatment goals for this patient.

What nonpharmacologic and pharmacologic alternatives are feasible for this patient?

Outline a treatment plan for this patient that includes nonpharmacologic therapy, pharmacologic therapy, and a monitoring plan. Justify your therapeutic selections.

Children Up to 4 Years of Age (Fig. 14–2) Long-term control medications should be initiated in patients who have had: (a) four or more episodes within the last year that have lasted for a day or longer and affected sleep *and* (b) have one major or two minor risk factors for developing persistent asthma. Major risk factors include a parental history of asthma, diagnosis of atopic dermatitis, and evidence of sensitization to aeroallergens. Minor risk factors include sensitization to food, 4% or more eosinophils in peripheral blood, and wheezing apart from colds. In addition, controller therapy should be considered if the patient requires symptomatic treatment for more than 2 days a week for more than 4 weeks or has two asthma exacerbations requiring systemic corticosteroids within 6 months.[1,33]

Daily ICS are the preferred long-term control therapy in all steps, and nonpreferred alternatives are cromolyn or a leukotriene receptor antagonist. Patients not controlled on low doses of ICS should be increased to medium doses before adding other therapies. Because high-dose ICS may be associated with significant adverse effects, addition of a leukotriene receptor antagonist or LABA to medium-dose therapy is preferred before increasing the ICS dose further. Theophylline is not recommended as an alternative at any step in this age group.[1]

Children 5 to 11 Years of Age (Fig. 14–2) Daily ICS are the preferred long-term control therapy in all steps.

Nonpreferred alternatives are cromolyn, a leukotriene receptor antagonist, nedocromil, or theophylline. For patients not controlled on low-dose ICS, the addition of an LABA, leukotriene receptor antagonist, or theophylline to current therapy or increasing to medium-dose ICS are equivalent options.[1] In patients not controlled on medium-dose ICS or low-dose ICS plus adjunctive therapy, the addition of an LABA to medium-dose ICS is preferred over other adjunctive therapies.[1]

Individuals 12 Years of Age and Older (Fig. 14–2) Daily ICS are the preferred long-term control therapy in all steps. Nonpreferred alternatives include cromolyn, a leukotriene receptor antagonist, nedocromil or sustained-release theophylline. For patients not controlled on low doses of ICS, the addition of a LABA, or increasing to medium-dose ICS are equivalent options.[1] The addition of other add-on therapies (leukotriene receptor antagonist, sustained-release theophylline, or zileuton) are nonpreferred options.[1] Omalizumab may be considered in patients not controlled on high-dose ICS and an LABA.

Treatment of Acute Severe Asthma

The optimal treatment of acute severe asthma depends on the severity of the exacerbation. The patient's condition usually deteriorates over several hours, days, or weeks.

Gradual deterioration may indicate failure of long-term controller therapy. However, rapid deterioration can occur in some patients; these patients usually respond well to bronchodilator therapy.[41] Severity at the time of the evaluation can be estimated by signs and symptoms or presenting PEF or FEV$_1$, but patient response 30 minutes after inhalation of a bronchodilator is the best predictor of outcome.[14]

⑨ *In acute severe asthma, early and appropriate intensification of therapy is important to resolve the exacerbation, prevent relapse, and prevent severe airflow obstruction in the future.* Starting therapy at home allows

for rapid initiation and early assessment of response (see Fig. 14–3). Patients should follow their written action plan as symptoms intensify or lung function deteriorates. Based on the initial response to β_2-agonist therapy, the severity of the exacerbation can be assessed, and treatment can be appropriately intensified.[1]

In patients with a good response to therapy, doubling the dose of ICS is no longer recommended, and a short course of oral corticosteroids should be considered. All patients with an incomplete response or whose response to an inhaled SABA lasts less than 1 hour should receive a short

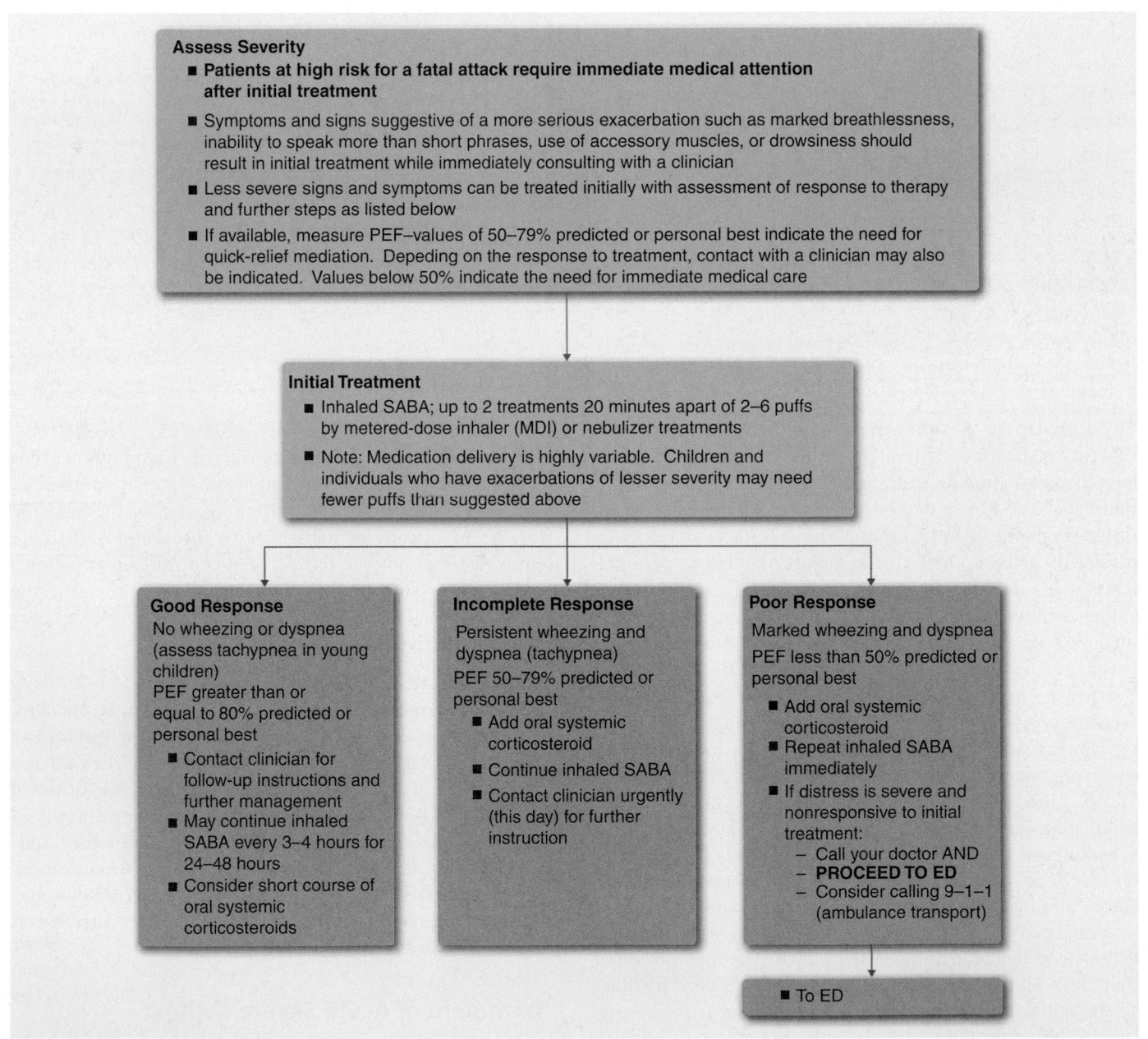

FIGURE 14–3. Management of Asthma Exacerbations: Home Treatment. (ED, emergency department; MDI, metered-dose inhaler; PEF, peak expiratory flow; SABA, short-acting β_2-agonist.) (From Ref. 1.)

Patient Encounter, Part 3

Follow-up: Six months later, RB's mother brings her back for a checkup. The patient has been using her albuterol inhaler 3 to 4 days a week to treat symptoms, and she is waking up about one to two times a month with shortness of breath. She has developed a sore mouth. White patches on the back of her tongue and the inside of her cheek are observed on examination.

Meds: Pulmicort Flexhaler 180 mcg/puff, one puff twice a day; proventil HFA two puffs as needed for symptoms; fluticasone nasal spray one puff in each nostril daily

What further information do you need to assess this patient's asthma control?

How would you counsel this patient to prevent further adverse reactions?

Assuming that the patient is using her medications appropriately, how would you adjust this patient's medication?

course of systemic corticosteorids.[1] Corticosteroid therapy should continue until PEF is at least 70% of predicted or personal best.[1] The SABA therapy can be continued at two to four inhalations every 3 to 4 hours for 24 to 48 hours until symptoms resolve. Continued reliance on an SABA for prolonged periods indicates a need to seek medical care.

Patients with incomplete responses should contact their health care provider immediately for instructions. Those with a poor response should proceed directly to the emergency department.[1] In the emergency department, baseline PEF measurements and oxygen saturation should be monitored. PEF should be monitored before and 15 to 20 minutes after bronchodilator administration. Treatment should be initiated as soon as lung function is assessed (Fig. 14–4). Multiple doses of inhaled ipratropium should be added to SABA therapy in patients with severe airflow obstruction.[1] Dosages for emergency department and hospital use of quick-relief medications are shown in Table 14–4.

Patients with oxygen saturation less than 90% (less than 95% in children, pregnant women, and patients with coexisting heart disease) should receive oxygen with the dose adjusted to keep oxygen saturation above these levels.[14] Administration of low concentrations of oxygen (less than 30% of the fraction of inspired air) by nasal cannula or facemask is usually sufficient to reverse hypoxemia in most patients.

Routine antibiotic use is not warranted because the primary infectious agents associated with asthma exacerbations are viruses.[1] Antibiotics should be reserved for situations when bacterial infection is strongly suspected (e.g., fever and purulent sputum, pneumonia, and suspected sinusitis).

In patients with impending respiratory failure, IV magnesium and heliox, a mixture of helium and oxygen that results in a lower density of inspired air and improved oxygen delivery, should be considered.[1] Theophylline is not recommended for treatment of acute asthma.[1]

Patients responding to therapy in the emergency department with a sustained response to inhaled β_2-agonists (PEF greater than 70%) can be discharged home.[1] Patients should have an inhaled SABA, be restarted on maintenance medications, and receive a 3- to 10-day course of oral corticosteroids. Patients who do not respond adequately to intensive therapy in the emergency department within 3 to 4 hours should be admitted to the hospital.

Special Populations

▶ Pregnancy

Approximately 4% to 8% of pregnant women are affected by asthma with about one-third of them experiencing worsening asthma during pregnancy.[42] Because uncontrolled asthma is a greater risk to the fetus than the risk of asthma medication use, it is safer for pregnant women to have asthma treated with medications than to experience worsening asthma. Consequently, asthma exacerbations should be managed aggressively with pharmacotherapy. The stepwise approach to asthma therapy in pregnancy is similar to that for the general population.

Budesonide has the most safety data in humans and is the preferred ICS; it is the only ICS classified as pregnancy category B. However, there are no data indicating that other ICS contribute to increased risk to the mother or fetus. Albuterol is the drug of choice for the treatment of asthma symptoms and exacerbations in pregnancy.[42]

▶ Exercise-Induced Asthma

Exercise is one of the most common precipitants of asthma symptoms. Shortness of breath, wheezing, or chest tightness usually occur during or shortly after vigorous exercise, peak 5 to 10 minutes after stopping the activity, and resolve within 20 to 30 minutes.

Patients with exercise-induced asthma should warm up prior to vigorous exercise and cover the mouth and nose with a scarf or mask during cold weather. Increased physical conditioning and gradually decreasing the intensity of exercise prior to stopping may also help prevent bronchospasm. Pretreatment with albuterol 5 minutes prior to exercise is the treatment of choice and will protect against bronchospasm for 2 to 3 hours.[1] Pretreatment with cromolyn sodium or nedocromil may also be effective in preventing bronchospasm but is not as effective as albuterol.[20] Pretreatment with a leukotriene modifier and regular treatment with ICS also prevents bronchospasm associated with exercise. Consideration should be given to initiating long-term control therapy in mild intermittent asthmatics using multiple weekly doses of a bronchodilator to prevent asthma symptoms associated with exercise.

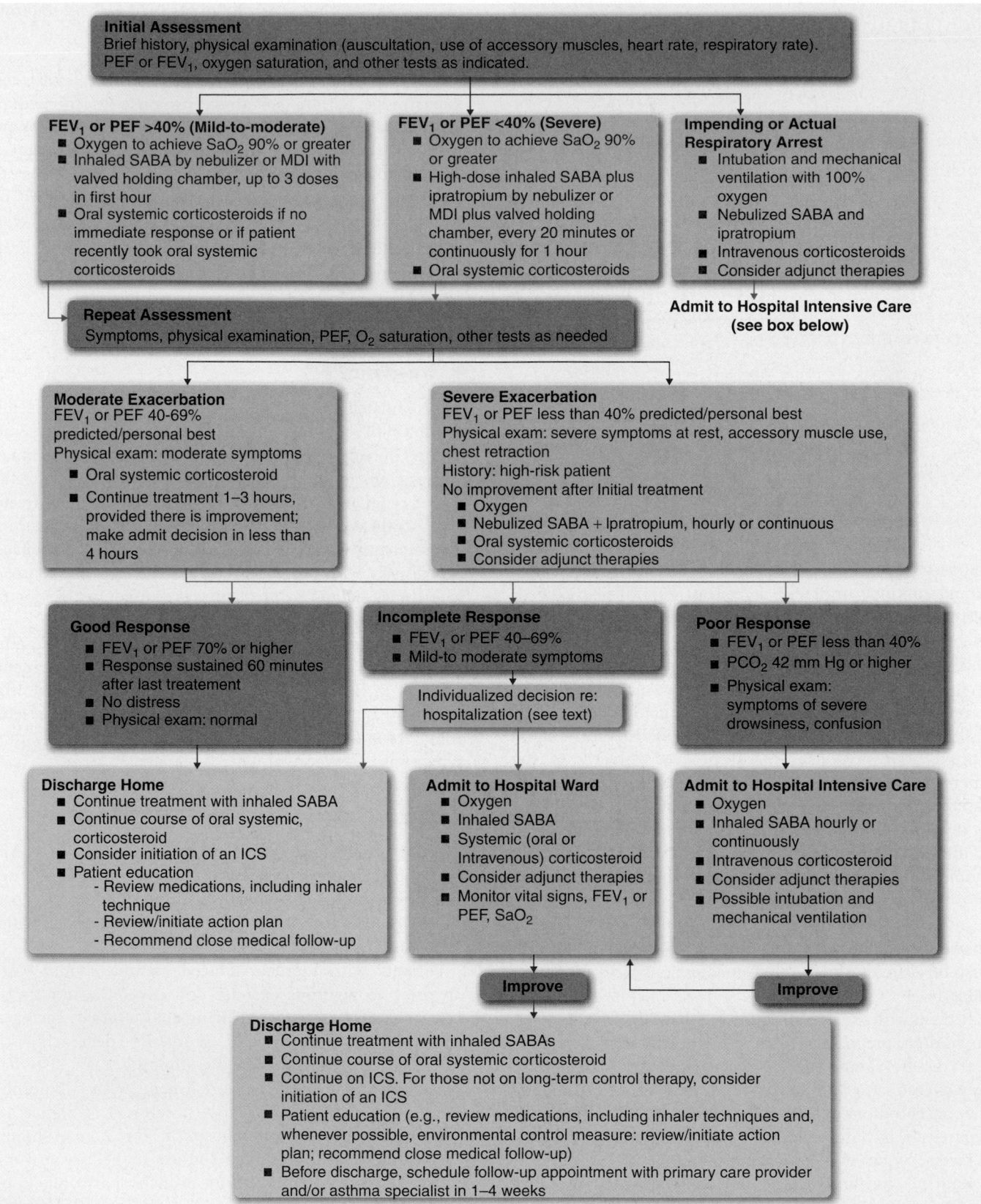

FIGURE 14–4. Management of asthma exacerbations: Emergency department and hospital-based care. (FEV₁, forced expiratory volume in 1 second; ICS, inhaled corticosteroid; MDI, metered-dose inhaler, P_{CO_2}, partial arterial pressure of carbon dioxide; PEF, peak expiratory flow; SABA, short-acting β₂-agonist [(quick-relief inhaler]; SaO₂, oxygen saturation.) (From Ref. 1.)

Patient Encounter, Part 4: Emergency Department Visit

RB is brought to the emergency department short of breath and unable to speak in complete sentences. The symptoms started approximately 1½ hours ago, and she has already used four puffs of albuterol every 20 minutes for three doses. She has never been hospitalized for asthma previously. On exam, she has inspiratory and expiratory wheezes and appears to be in distress. She is leaning forward to breathe, pursing her lips, and has intercostal and supraclavicular retractions. Her heart rate is 120 bpm and her respiratory rate is 26 breaths per minute. A PEF measurement is 35% of predicted value and her O_2 saturation is 87%.

Home Meds: Symbicort 160 mcg/4.5 mcg, one inhalation twice a day; proventil HFA two puffs as needed for symptoms; fluticasone nasal spray one puff in each nostril daily

Based on the information presented above, what initial treatment would you recommend for this patient?

What are the goals of treatment in this patient?

If RB does not respond to therapy, what adjunctive therapies should be considered?

▶ *Aspirin Sensitivity*

Patients with aspirin-sensitive asthma are usually adults and often present with the triad of rhinitis, nasal polyps, and asthma. In these patients, acute asthma may occur within minutes of ingesting aspirin or another nonsteroidal anti-inflammatory drug (NSAID). These patients should be counseled against using NSAIDs.[1] Although acetaminophen is generally safe in this population, doses larger than 1 gram may cause acute asthmatic reactions in some patients.[43] Patients with aspirin-sensitive asthma may tolerate cyclooxygenase-2 inhibitors; however, given the potentially serious adverse events that could occur in aspirin-sensitive asthmatics, the first dose of a cyclooxygenase-2 inhibitor should be given under the observation of a health care provider with rescue drugs available.[44]

OUTCOME EVALUATION

Chronic Asthma

- Assess the patient's inhaler technique frequently and always assess technique before stepping up therapy. Reeducate the patient on appropriate inhaler technique at every visit.

- Monitor symptoms such as wheezing, shortness of breath, chest tightness, cough, and nocturnal awakenings. Daytime symptoms should occur no more than twice a week, and nocturnal symptoms should occur no more than twice a month in adolescents and adults and no more than once a month in children younger than 12 years of age. Patients with more frequent symptoms should have their long-term control medications increased.

- In persons 12 years of age and older, monitor lung function. FEV_1 or PEF should remain above 80% of predicted or personal best. Patients with PEF rates consistently greater than 80% over several months should be evaluated for a stepdown in long-term control therapy. Patients with a PEF less than 80% of personal best should begin to monitor PEF twice daily and consult their asthma action plan. Patients with a PEF less than 50% of personal best should immediately use their SABA and consult their asthma action plan.

- Monitor patient activity levels. Inability of a patient to perform routine physical activities indicates inappropriate therapy, and long-term control medications should be increased.

- In individuals 12 years of age and older, monitor asthma impairment using a validated questionnaire to ensure asthma is well controlled.

- Monitor frequency of patient exacerbations. Frequent exacerbations, unscheduled clinic visits, emergency department visits, and hospitalizations due to asthma may indicate a nonadherent patient or the need to step up long-term control medications.

- Monitor use of long-term control medications to ensure adherence. Reeducate nonadherent patients on the importance of these medications for asthma control.

- Monitor use of inhaled SABAs. Their use more than twice a week in intermittent asthma may indicate the need to initiate long-term control therapy. Use of more than one canister per month indicates the need to step up long-term control therapy.

- Monitor for adverse events from medications, including candidiasis and dysphonia from ICS.

- Monitor the patient's immunization status and provide an annual influenza vaccination if warranted.

Acute Severe Asthma

- Monitor PEF, which should increase to greater than 70% of personal best or predicted after the first three doses of an inhaled SABA.

- Monitor patients for hypoxemia. Oxygen saturation should be greater than 90% in adults and greater than 95% in children, pregnant women, and patients with coexisting cardiovascular disease.

- In patients with severe exacerbations, monitoring of P_{CO_2} should be considered. Patients with acute asthma usually have a respiratory alkalosis, and a normal or increased P_{CO_2} indicates the potential for respiratory failure.

- Monitor serum potassium in patients receiving high-dose or continuous nebulization of SABA. Serum potassium concentrations should be obtained upon hospital admission, and if the patient is hypokalemic,

Patient Care and Monitoring

Chronic Asthma

1. Obtain a thorough medical history focusing on disease states that may worsen asthma severity.

2. Ask the patient about the frequency and severity of symptoms, when symptoms occur, and whether or not symptoms are associated with exposure to known allergens. Ask about previous emergency department visits and hospitalizations due to asthma.

3. Use the patient's level of impairment and risk of future adverse outcomes to classify disease severity.

4. Explain the goals of therapy and ask whether the patient has any personal treatment goals.

5. Develop a patient education plan that fits the patient's needs. Educate about the differences between the asthmatic and normal lung and what happens to the lung during an asthma attack. Counsel the patient on how their medications work and differentiate between long-term control and quick relief medications.

6. Provide a specific allergen avoidance plan and counsel all patients to avoid second-hand tobacco smoke.

7. Demonstrate the appropriate use of drug delivery devices and peak flow meters; then have the patient perform these activities for you. If the task is performed incorrectly, demonstrate the skill again, emphasizing the incorrect step and have the patient redemonstrate the skill.

8. Prepare a patient-specific self-monitoring plan and review it with the patient. Educate the patient on the signs and symptoms of asthma deterioration and when and how to take rescue actions.

9. Assess the patient's adherence to long-term control therapy. Stress the importance of adherence if necessary. Evaluate the complexity of the treatment plan and simplify it if possible.

10. Assess the patient for adverse effects such as candidiasis and dysphonia associated with ICS.

11. Evaluate therapy on a regular basis. Assess the patient's control of asthma by evaluating the patient's impairment due to asthma and their risk for future adverse events due to asthma. Step long-term control therapy up or down based on these parameters. Before stepping up therapy, reassess the patient's inhaler technique to assure appropriate drug delivery.

Acute Severe Asthma

1. Assess the patient's PEF.

2. Assess whether or not the patient can use an MDI with a spacer or holding chamber. If the patient cannot use the device, determine whether someone can assist the patient with the inhaler device, or whether a nebulizer is necessary.

3. Initiate therapy with an SABA and 2 to 6 L/min of oxygen if needed.

4. Perform a brief medical history to determine the time of symptom onset, symptom severity, symptom severity in relation to previous exacerbations, current medications, previous emergency department visits or hospitalizations due to asthma, previous history of respiratory failure, and psychiatric or psychological disorders.

5. Assess the patient's general appearance, use of accessory muscles, respiratory rate, heart rate, lung sounds, presence of pulsus paradoxus, PEF, and oxygen saturation.

6. Reassess pulmonary function every 20 to 30 minutes. If there was not an immediate response to the inhaled SABA, initiate systemic corticosteroid therapy. If the patient is not improving, add ipratropium to the patient's therapy and continue with a high-dose inhaled SABA.

7. Assess the patient for hospitalization or discharge home.

8. If the patient is discharged home, ensure that the patient has an SABA, review the appropriate technique for inhaler use, and ensure that the patient has a prescription for 3 to 10 days of an oral corticosteroid. Consider starting ICS and providing the patient with a 1 to 2 month supply of the medication.

9. Restart the patient on maintenance therapy. Instruct the patient on what to do if asthma worsens and to follow-up with his/her health care provider in 1 to 4 weeks.

every 4 hours (after each 30 to 40 mEq [mmol] of replacement) until the serum potassium is stable. Serum potassium should be monitored every 3 to 6 months after discharge.

Abbreviations Introduced in This Chapter

AHR	Airway hyper-responsiveness
CFC	Chlorofluorocarbon
CYP	Cytochrome P-450 isoenzyme
DPI	Dry powder inhaler
EPR-3	Expert Panel Report-3
FEV_1	Forced expiratory volume in 1 second
FVC	Forced vital capacity
HFA	Hydrofluoroalkane
ICS	Inhaled corticosteroid
IgE	Immunoglobulin E
LABA	Long-acting β_2-agonist
MDI	Metered-dose inhaler
NAEPP	National Asthma Education and Prevention Program

NHLBI   National Heart, Lung, and Blood Institute
NSAID   Nonsteroidal anti-inflammatory drug
Pao$_2$ Partial arterial oxygen pressure
Pco$_2$ Partial arterial pressure of carbon dioxide
PEF   Peak expiratory flow
SABA   Short-acting β_2-agonist
T$_H$2   Type 2 T-helper CD4+ cell

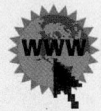 Self-assessment questions and answers are available at *http://www.mhpharmacotherapy. com/pp.html.*

REFERENCES

1. NHLBI National Asthma Education and Prevention Program, Expert Panel Report-3. Guidelines for the Diagnosis and Management of Asthma. NIH Publication No. 07-4051. Bethesda, MD: U.S. Department of Health and Human Services, 2007, *http://www.nhlbi.nih.gov/ guidelines/asthma*
2. American Lung Association. Trends in asthma morbidity and mortality. American Lung Association Epidemiology & Statistics Unit Research and Program Services. November 2007, *http://www.lungusa.org.*
3. Moorman JE, Rudd RA, Johnson CA, et al. National surveillance for asthma—United States, 1980–2004. MMWR Morb Mortal Wkly Rep 2007;56(08):1–14, 18–54.
4. Weiss KB, Sullivan SD. The health economics of asthma and rhinitis. I. Assessing the economic impact. J Allergy Clin Immunol 2001;107:3–8.
5. Reed CE. The natural history of asthma. J Allergy Clin Immunol 2006;110:543–548.
6. Busse WW, Lemanske RF Jr. Advances in immunology: Asthma. N Engl J Med 2001;344:350–362.
7. Larché M, Robinson DS, Kay AB. The role of T lymphocytes in the pathogenesis of asthma. J Allergy Clin Immunol 2003;111:450–463.
8. Robinson DS. The role of mast cells in asthma: Induction of airway hyperresponsiveness by interaction with smooth muscle? J Allergy Clin Immunol 2004;114:58–65.
9. Cohn L, Elias JA, Chupp GL. Asthma: Mechanisms of disease persistence and progression. Annu Rev Immunol 2004;22:789–815.
10. Bradding P, Walls AF, Holgate ST. The role of the mast cell in the pathophysiology of asthma. J Allergy Clin Immunol 2006;117:1277–1284.
11. Lemanske RF Jr, Busse WW. Asthma. J Allergy Clin Immunol 2003;111:S502–S519.
12. Beckett PA, Howarth PH. Pharmacotherapy and airway remodeling in asthma? Thorax 2003;58:163–174.
13. Bousquet J, Khaltaev N, Cruz AA, et al. Allergic rhinitis and its impact on asthma (ARIA) 2008 update (in collaboration with the World Health Organization, GA(2)LEN and AllerGen). Allergy 2008;63(Suppl 86):8–160.
14. Rodrigo GJ, Rodrigo C, Hall JB. Acute asthma in adults: A review. Chest 2004;125:1081–1102.
15. O'Connor GT. Allergen avoidance in asthma: What do we do now? J Allergy Clin Immunol 2005;116:26–30.
16. Talbot TR, Hartert TV, Mitchel E, et al. Asthma as a risk factor for invasive pneumococcal disease. N Engl J Med 2005;352:2082–2090.
17. Newman SP. Spacer devices for metered dose inhalers. Clin Pharmacokinet 2004;43:349–360.
18. de Benedictis FM, Selvaggio D. Use of inhaler devices in pediatric asthma. Paediatr Drugs 2003;5:629–638.
19. Gibson PG, Powell H. Written action plans for asthma: An evidence-based review of the key components. Thorax 2004;59:94–99.
20. Kelly HW, Sorkness CA. Asthma. In: Dipiro JT, Talbert RL, Yee GC, et al., eds. Pharmacotherapy: A Pathophysiologic Approach. 7th ed. New York: McGraw-Hill, 2008:464–493.
21. Nowak RM, Emerman CL, Shaefer K, et al. Levalbuterol compared with racemic albuterol in the treatment of acute asthma: Results of a pilot study. Am J Emerg Med 2004;22:29–36.
22. Sin DD, Man J, Sharpe H, et al. Pharmacological management to reduce exacerbations in adults with asthma: A systematic review and meta-analysis. JAMA 2004;292:367–376.
23. Bateman ED, Boushey HA, Bousquet J, et al. Can guideline-defined asthma control be achieved? The gaining optimal asthma control study. Am J Respir Crit Care Med 2004;170:836–844.
24. Masoli M, Weatherall M, Holt S. Moderate dose inhaled corticosteroids plus salmeterol versus higher doses of inhaled corticosteroids in symptomatic asthma. Thorax 2005;60:730–734.
25. Nelson HS, Weiss ST, Bleeker ER, et al., and the Smart Study Group. The salmeterol multicenter asthma research trial: A comparison of usual pharmacotherapy for asthma or usual pharmacotherapy plus salmeterol. Chest 2006;129:15–26.
26. Kelly HW. Rationale for the major changes in the pharmacotherapy section of the National Asthma Education and Prevention Program Guidelines. J Allergy Clin Immunol 2007;120:989–994.
27. Nelson HS. Is there a problem with inhaled long-acting β-adrenergic agonists? J Allergy Clin Immunol 2006;117:3–16.
28. Bateman E, Neslon H, Bousquet J, et al. Meta-analysis: Effects of adding salmeterol to inhaled corticosteroids on serious asthma-related events. Ann Intern Med 2008;149:33–42.
29. Currie GP, Devereux GS, Lee DKC, et al. Recent developments in asthma management. BMJ 2005;330:585–589.
30. Szefler SJ, Martin RJ, King TS, et al. Significant variability in response to inhaled corticosteroids for persistent asthma. J Allergy Clin Immunol 2002;109:410–418.
31. Martin RJ, Szefler SJ, Chinchilli VM, et al. Systemic effect comparisons of six inhaled corticosteroid preparations. Am J Respir Crit Care Med 2002;165:1377–1383.
32. Masoli M, Weatherall M, Holt S, et al. Clinical dose response relationship of fluticasone propionate in adults with asthma. Thorax 2004;59:16–20.
33. Guilbert TW, Morgan WJ, Zeiger RS, et al. Long-term inhaled corticosteroids in preschool children at high risk for asthma. N Engl J Med 2006;354:1985–1997.
34. Rodrigo GJ, Castro-Rodrigo JA. Anticholinergics in the treatment of children and adults with acute asthma: A systematic review with meta-analysis. Thorax 2005;60:740–746.
35. Sorkness CA, Lemanske RF Jr, Mauger DT, et al. Long-term comparison of 3 controller regiments for mild-moderate persistent childhood asthma: The pediatric asthma controller trial. J Allergy Clin Immunol 2007;119:64–72.
36. Barnes PJ. Theophylline. New perspective on an old drug. Am J Respir Crit Care Med 2003;167:813–818.
37. Barnes PJ. Theophylline: New perspective on an old drug. Am J Resp Crit Care Med 2003;167:813–818.
38. Davis LA. Omalizumab: A novel therapy for allergic asthma. Ann Pharmacother 2004;38:1236–1242.
39. Wu AC, Paltiel D, Kuntz KM, et al. Cost-effectiveness of omaluzimab in adults with severe asthma: Results from the asthma policy model. J Allergy Clin Immunol 2007;120:1146–1152.
40. Limb SL, Starke PR, Lee CE, et al. Delayed onset and protracted progression of anaphylaxis after omalizumab administration in patients with asthma. J Allergy Clin Immunol 2007;120:1378–1381.
41. McFadden ER Jr. Acute severe asthma. Am J Respir Crit Care Med 2003;168:740–759.
42. National Heart Lung and Blood Institute, National Asthma Education and Prevention Program Asthma and Pregnancy Working Group. NAEPP expert panel report. Managing asthma during pregnancy: Recommendations for pharmacologic treatment—2004 update. J Allergy Clin Immunol 2005;115:34–46.
43. Eneli I, Sadri K, Camargo C, et al. Acetaminophen and the risk of asthma: The epidemiologic and pathophysiologic evidence. Chest 2005;127:604–612.
44. West PM, Fernández C. Safety of Cox-2 inhibitors in asthma patients with aspirin hypersensitivity. Ann Pharmacother 2003;37:1497–1501.

15 Chronic Obstructive Pulmonary Disease

Tara R. Whetsel and Nicole D. Verkleeren

LEARNING OBJECTIVES

● **Upon completion of the chapter, the reader will be able to:**

1. Describe the pathophysiology of chronic obstructive pulmonary disease (COPD).

2. Identify signs and symptoms of COPD.

3. List the treatment goals for a patient with COPD.

4. Design an appropriate COPD treatment regimen based on patient-specific data.

5. Develop a monitoring plan to assess effectiveness and adverse effects of pharmacotherapy for COPD.

6. Formulate an appropriate education plan for a patient with COPD.

KEY CONCEPTS

❶ Inflammation plays a key role in the pathophysiology of chronic obstructive pulmonary disease (COPD), but it differs from that seen in asthma; therefore, the use of and response to anti-inflammatory medications are different.

❷ An integrated approach of health maintenance (e.g., smoking cessation), drug therapy, and supplemental therapy (e.g., oxygen and pulmonary rehabilitation) should be used in a stepwise manner.

❸ Smoking cessation slows the rate of decline in pulmonary function in patients with COPD.

❹ Bronchodilators are the mainstay of treatment for symptomatic COPD. They reduce symptoms and improve exercise tolerance and quality of life. In patients with moderate to severe COPD, bronchodilators may reduce the rate of decline in pulmonary function.

❺ In symptomatic patients with severe COPD and frequent exacerbations, regular treatment with inhaled corticosteroids decreases the number of exacerbations per year and improves health status. Corticosteroids may reduce the rate of decline in pulmonary function in patients with moderate to severe COPD.

❻ Antibiotics should be used in patients with COPD exacerbations who: (a) have all three cardinal symptoms (increased dyspnea, increased sputum volume, and increased purulence); (b) have increased sputum purulence along with one other cardinal symptom; or (c) experience a severe exacerbation requiring mechanical ventilation.

INTRODUCTION

Chronic obstructive pulmonary disease (COPD) is a progressive disease characterized by airflow limitation that is not fully reversible. It is caused by exposure to noxious particles or gases, most commonly cigarette smoke. It is a major cause of morbidity and mortality and a leading cause of disability in the United States.

COPD includes chronic bronchitis and emphysema. Chronic bronchitis is defined clinically as a chronic productive cough for at least 3 months in each of two consecutive years in a patient in whom other causes have been excluded.[1] Emphysema is defined pathologically as the presence of permanent enlargement of the airspaces distal to the terminal bronchioles, accompanied by destruction of their walls without obvious fibrosis.[1] The major risk factor for both conditions is cigarette smoking, and many patients share characteristics of each condition. Therefore, new consensus guidelines have moved away from using these subsets and instead focus on chronic airflow limitation.

The Global Initiative for Chronic Obstructive Lung Disease (GOLD) is an expert panel of health professionals who have developed a consensus document with recommendations for the diagnosis and care of patients with COPD.[2] The online document is updated annually and is commonly referred to as the GOLD guidelines. The American Thoracic Society (ATS) and the European Respiratory Society (ERS) have jointly published standards for the diagnosis and treatment of patients with COPD.[1] The ATS–ERS guidelines provide more specific recommendations on oxygen therapy, pulmonary rehabilitation, and other treatment issues than the broader GOLD guidelines.

EPIDEMIOLOGY AND ETIOLOGY

In 2006, 12.1 million U.S. adults 18 years of age and older reported having COPD.[3] The true prevalence is larger; COPD is underdiagnosed because many patients have few or no symptoms in the early stages.

COPD is the fourth leading cause of death in the United States; in 2005, 127,049 adults died from the disease.[3] In 2007, COPD was estimated to cost the United States $42.6 billion, with direct medical costs accounting for $26.7 billion of the total.[3] Morbidity, mortality, and costs are all expected to increase over the next decade; by 2020, it is expected to be the third leading cause of death worldwide.[2]

Exposures and host factors play a role in the development of COPD. Cigarette smoking is the leading cause of COPD and accounts for 80% to 90% of cases in developed countries.[4] Environmental tobacco smoke (i.e., secondhand smoke) may increase the risk of COPD.[2] Occupational exposure to dusts and chemicals (vapors, irritants, and fumes) also plays a role. Environmental air pollution has been implicated as an etiologic factor, but its exact role is unclear. Not all smokers develop clinically significant COPD, which suggests that genetic susceptibility plays a role. The best documented genetic factor is a rare hereditary deficiency of α_1-antitrypsin (AAT). Severe deficiency of this enzyme results in premature and accelerated development of emphysema. Asthma and airway hyper-responsiveness have been identified as risk factors, but how they influence the development of COPD is unknown. Failure to reach maximal lung function, due to recurrent infections or exposure to tobacco smoke during childhood, may also increase the risk of COPD.

PATHOPHYSIOLOGY

COPD is characterized by pathologic changes in the central airways, peripheral airways, lung parenchyma, and pulmonary vasculature. Chronic inflammation in the lung from repeated exposure to noxious particles and gases is primarily responsible for these changes.[2] An imbalance between proteinases and antiproteinases in the lung and oxidative stress are also thought to be important in the pathogenesis of COPD. These processes may be a result of ongoing inflammation or may arise from environmental (e.g., oxidants in cigarette smoke) or genetic (e.g., AAT deficiency) factors (Fig. 15–1).[2] In addition to these destructive processes, chronic inflammation and exposure to noxious particles and gases disrupts or impairs the normal protective and repair mechanisms.

Inflammation is present in the lungs of all smokers. It is unclear why only 15% to 20% of smokers develop COPD, but susceptible individuals appear to have an exaggerated inflammatory response.[5] ❶ *The inflammation of COPD differs from that seen in asthma, so the use of anti-inflammatory medications and the response to those medications are different.* The inflammation of asthma is

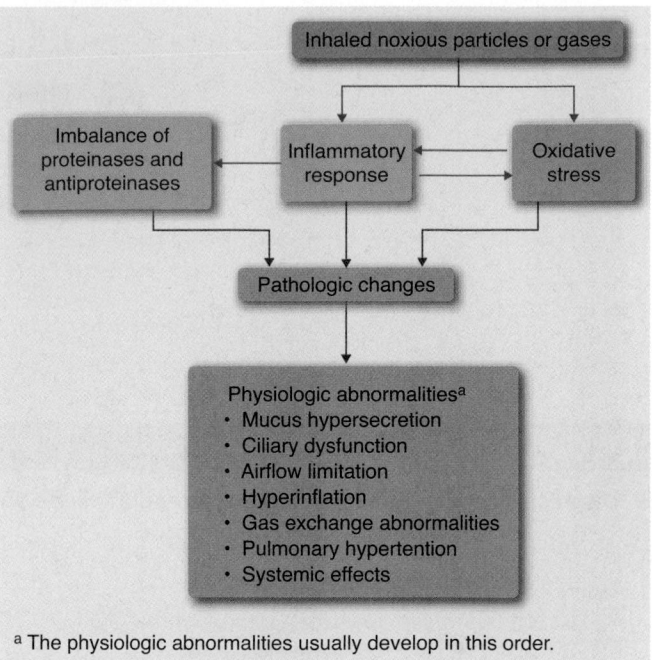

FIGURE 15–1. Pathophysiology of COPD.

mainly mediated through eosinophils and mast cells. In COPD, the primary inflammatory cells include neutrophils, macrophages, and CD8+ T lymphocytes. Eosinophils may be increased in some patients, particularly during exacerbations. Activated inflammatory cells release a variety of mediators, most notably leukotriene B$_4$, interleukin-8, and tumor necrosis factor-α (TNF-α). Various proteinases, such as elastase, cathepsin G, and proteinase-3, are secreted by activated neutrophils. These mediators and proteinases are capable of sustaining inflammation and damaging lung structures.

Proteinases and antiproteinases are part of the normal protective and repair mechanisms in the lungs. The imbalance of proteinase-antiproteinase activity in COPD is a result of either increased production or activity of destructive proteinases or inactivation or reduced production of protective antiproteinases. AAT (an antiproteinase) inhibits trypsin, elastase, and several other proteolytic enzymes. Deficiency of AAT results in unopposed proteinase activity, which promotes destruction of alveolar walls and lung parenchyma, leading to emphysema.

Markers of oxidative stress (e.g., hydrogen peroxide, nitric oxide, and isoprostane F$_2\alpha$-III) have been found in the epithelial fluid, breath, and urine of cigarette smokers and patients with COPD.[2] Increased oxidative stress contributes to COPD in a variety of ways. Oxidants (e.g., reactive oxygen species, superoxide, and nitric oxide) can react with and damage a variety of molecules leading to cell dysfunction and damage to the lung extracellular matrix. Oxidative stress promotes inflammation and contributes to the proteinase–antiproteinase imbalance by reducing antiproteinase activity. In addition, oxidants constrict airway smooth muscle, contributing to reversible airway narrowing.

In the central airways (the trachea, bronchi, and bronchioles greater than 2 to 4 mm in internal diameter), inflammatory cells and mediators stimulate mucus-secreting gland **hyperplasia** and mucus hypersecretion. Mucus hypersecretion and ciliary dysfunction lead to chronic cough and sputum production. The major site of airflow obstruction is the peripheral airways (small bronchi and bronchioles with an internal diameter less than 2 mm). Three mechanisms are postulated to be involved in the narrowing of these small airways.[2] Airways may be blocked by inflammatory exudates and mucus hypersecretion. Loss of elasticity and destruction of alveolar attachments leads to loss of support and closure of small airways during expiration. Infiltration of inflammatory cells, increased smooth muscle tissue, and fibrosis cause thickening of airway walls. Of these mechanisms, the structural changes in the airway walls are the most important cause of fixed airflow obstruction.

As airflow obstruction worsens, the rate of lung emptying is slowed and the interval between inspirations does not allow expiration to the relaxation volume of the lungs. This leads to pulmonary hyperinflation, which initially only occurs during exercise, but later is also seen at rest. Hyperinflation contributes to the discomfort associated with airflow obstruction by flattening the diaphragm and placing it at a mechanical disadvantage.

In advanced COPD, airflow obstruction, damaged bronchioles and alveoli, and pulmonary vascular abnormalities lead to impaired gas exchange. This results in **hypoxemia** and eventually **hypercapnia**. Hypoxemia is initially present only during exercise but occurs at rest as the disease progresses. Inequality in the **ventilation-to-perfusion ratio** (V_A/Q) is the major mechanism behind hypoxemia in COPD. As hypoxemia worsens, the body may compensate by increasing the production of erythrocytes in an attempt to increase oxygen delivery to tissues.

Pulmonary hypertension develops late in the course of COPD, usually after the development of severe hypoxemia. It is the most common cardiovascular complication of COPD and can result in **cor pulmonale**, or right-sided heart failure. Hypoxemia plays the primary role in the development of pulmonary hypertension by causing vasoconstriction of the pulmonary arteries and promoting vessel wall remodeling. Destruction of the pulmonary capillary bed by emphysema further contributes by increasing the pressure required to perfuse the pulmonary vascular bed. Cor pulmonale is associated with venous stasis and thrombosis that may result in pulmonary embolism. Another important systemic effect is the progressive loss of skeletal muscle mass, which contributes to exercise limitations and declining health status. These extrapulmonary effects may contribute to disease severity and should not be overlooked.

CLINICAL PRESENTATION AND DIAGNOSIS

Diagnosis

A suspected diagnosis of COPD should be based on the patient's symptoms and/or history of exposure to risk factors.

Clinical Presentation and Diagnosis of COPD

General

- Patients with COPD are initially asymptomatic. The disease is usually not diagnosed until declining lung function leads to significant symptoms and prompts patients to seek medical care.

Symptoms

- The onset of symptoms is variable but often does not occur until the FEV_1 has fallen to approximately 50% of predicted.[2]

- Initial symptoms include chronic cough (duration greater than 3 months), which may be intermittent at first, chronic sputum production, and dyspnea on exertion.

- As COPD progresses, dyspnea at rest develops and the ability to perform activities of daily living declines.

Signs

- Observation of the patient may reveal use of accessory muscles of respiration (manifested as paradoxical movements of the chest and abdomen, in a "seesaw"-type motion), pursed-lips breathing, and hyperinflation of the chest with increased anterior–posterior diameter ("barrel chest").

- On auscultation of the lungs, patients may have distant breath sounds, wheezing, a prolonged expiratory phase of respiration, and rhonchi.

- In advanced COPD, signs of hypoxemia may include cyanosis and tachycardia.

- Signs of cor pulmonale include increased pulmonic component of the second heart sound, jugular venous distention (JVD), lower extremity edema, and hepatomegaly.

Laboratory Tests

- Hematocrit may be elevated and may exceed 55% (polycythemia).

- Arterial blood gases (ABGs) should be obtained in patients with an FEV_1 less than 40% predicted or signs or symptoms suggestive of cor pulmonale or respiratory failure.[2] COPD patients characteristically exhibit normal or increased arterial carbon dioxide tension ($PaCO_2$) and decreased arterial oxygen tension (PaO_2).

- An AAT level should be obtained in younger patients (less than 45 years old) presenting with COPD signs and symptoms, especially if there is a strong family history of emphysema.

Table 15–1				
GOLD Classification of COPD Severity[a]				
Stage	**Category**	**FEV$_1$/FVC (%)**	**FEV$_1$**	**Symptoms**
I	Mild	Less than 70	Greater than or equal to 80% predicted	With or without chronic cough and sputum production
II	Moderate	Less than 70	50% to 79% predicted	With or without chronic cough and sputum production
III	Severe	Less than 70	30% to 49% predicted	With or without chronic cough and sputum production
IV	Very severe	Less than 70	Less than 30% predicted or less than 50% predicted plus chronic respiratory failure[b]	

FEV$_1$, forced expiratory volume in 1 second; FVC, forced vital capacity; GOLD, Global Initiative for Chronic Obstructive Lung Disease.

[a]Classification based on postbronchodilator FEV$_1$.

[b]Respiratory failure: Arterial partial pressure of oxygen (PaO$_2$) less than 60 mm Hg (7.98 kPa) with or without arterial partial pressure of carbon dioxide (PaCO$_2$) greater than 50 mm Hg (6.65 kPa) while breathing air at sea level.

From Ref. 2.

Spirometry is required to confirm the diagnosis. The presence of a postbronchodilator FEV$_1$/FVC ratio less than 70% (the ratio of forced expiratory volume in 1 second [FEV$_1$] to forced vital capacity [FVC]) confirms the presence of airflow limitation that is not fully reversible.[1,2] Spirometry results can further be used to classify COPD severity (Table 15–1). Full pulmonary function tests (PFTs) with lung volumes and diffusion capacity and arterial blood gases (ABGs) are not necessary to establish the diagnosis or severity of COPD.

It is important to distinguish COPD from asthma because treatment and prognosis differ. Differentiating factors include age of onset, smoking history, triggers, occupational history, and degree of reversibility measured by pre- and postbronchodilator spirometry. In some patients, a clear distinction between asthma and COPD is not possible. Management of these patients should be similar to that of asthma. Bronchiectasis, cystic fibrosis, obliterative bronchiolitis, congestive heart failure, and tuberculosis are other possible differential diagnoses that are usually easier to distinguish from COPD. Chest radiography or high-resolution CT along with patient presentation help rule out these other lung diseases.

TREATMENT

Desired Outcomes

The goals of COPD management include: (a) smoking cessation; (b) reducing symptoms; (c) minimizing the rate of decline in lung function; (d) maintaining or improving the quality of life; (e) preventing and treating exacerbations; and (f) limiting complications.

General Approach to Treatment

❷ *An integrated approach of health maintenance (e.g., smoking cessation), drug therapy, and supplemental therapy (e.g., oxygen and pulmonary rehabilitation) should be used in*

Patient Encounter, Part 1

A 49-year-old man with a medical history of hypertension presents to the clinic complaining of shortness of breath that began about 3 to 4 years ago. His symptoms have gradually gotten worse since then. He is now unable to walk 100 yards without having to stop and rest. He also has a daily cough that is usually productive of yellowish sputum. He smokes about one and a half packs of cigarettes a day and has done so for the last 30 years. He also drinks on average six to seven beers a day. He does not have any significant occupational exposures to dust, gases, or fumes.

What information is suggestive of COPD?

What risk factors does he have for COPD?

What additional information do you need to know before creating a treatment plan for this patient?

a stepwise manner. Table 15–2 provides an overview of the management of stable COPD.

Nonpharmacologic Therapy

▶ Smoking Cessation

❸ *Smoking cessation slows the rate of decline in pulmonary function in patients with COPD.*[6,7] Stopping smoking can also reduce cough and sputum production and decrease airway reactivity. Therefore, it is a critical part of any treatment plan for patients with COPD. Unfortunately, achieving and maintaining cessation is a major challenge. A clinical practice guideline from the U.S. Public Health Service recommends a specific action plan depending on the current smoking status and desire to quit (Fig. 15–2).[8] Brief interventions are effective and can increase cessation rates significantly. The five As and the five Rs can be used to guide brief interventions (Table 15–3).

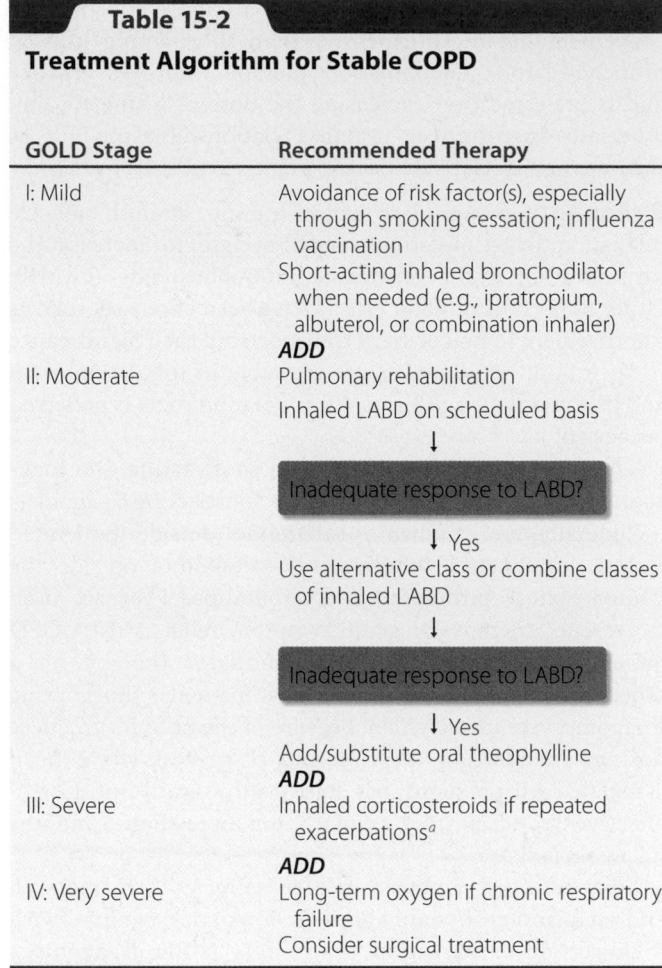

Table 15-2

Treatment Algorithm for Stable COPD

GOLD Stage	Recommended Therapy
I: Mild	Avoidance of risk factor(s), especially through smoking cessation; influenza vaccination
	Short-acting inhaled bronchodilator when needed (e.g., ipratropium, albuterol, or combination inhaler)
	ADD
II: Moderate	Pulmonary rehabilitation
	Inhaled LABD on scheduled basis
	↓
	Inadequate response to LABD?
	↓ Yes
	Use alternative class or combine classes of inhaled LABD
	↓
	Inadequate response to LABD?
	↓ Yes
	Add/substitute oral theophylline
	ADD
III: Severe	Inhaled corticosteroids if repeated exacerbations[a]
	ADD
IV: Very severe	Long-term oxygen if chronic respiratory failure
	Consider surgical treatment

LABD, long-acting bronchodilator (tiotropium[b], salmeterol, or formoterol).

[a]Defined as three exacerbations in the last 3 years by GOLD and as at least one exacerbation requiring a course of oral corticosteroid or antibiotic within the last year by American Thoracic Society/European Respiratory Society. Other authorities define frequent exacerbations as at least two within the past year.

[b]Albuterol should be used as rescue therapy for patients treated with tiotropium.

All tobacco users should be assessed for their readiness to quit and appropriate strategies implemented. Those who are ready to quit should be treated with a combination of counseling on behavioral and cognitive strategies and pharmacotherapy (nicotine replacement therapy, sustained-release bupropion, or varenicline; refer to Smoking Cessation in **Chap. 36**). In COPD patients, the likelihood of sustained abstinence is higher with nicotine replacement therapy than that with sustained-release bupropion.[9]

▶ *Pulmonary Rehabilitation*

Pulmonary rehabilitation results in significant and clinically meaningful improvements in dyspnea, exercise capacity, health status, and health care utilization.[10] It should be considered for patients with COPD who have dyspnea or other respiratory symptoms, reduced exercise capacity, a restriction

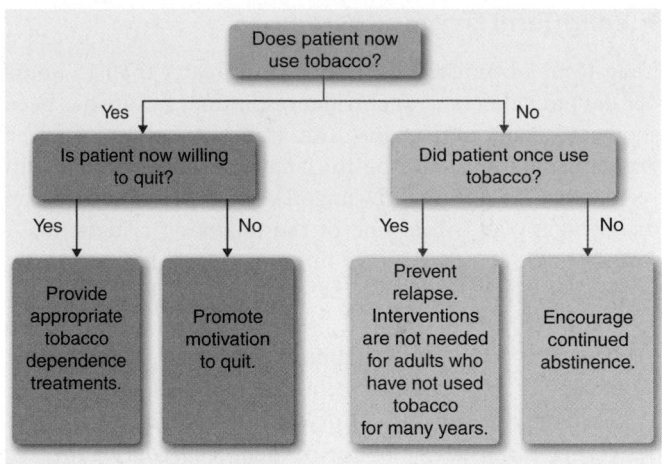

FIGURE 15-2. Algorithm for routine assessment of tobacco use status. (From Ref. 8.)

in activities because of their disease, or impaired health status.[1] A comprehensive pulmonary rehabilitation program should include exercise training, nutrition counseling, and education. It should cover a range of nonpulmonary problems including exercise deconditioning, relative social isolation, altered mood states (especially depression), muscle wasting, and weight loss.

Rehabilitation programs may be conducted in the inpatient, outpatient (most common), or home setting. The minimum length of an effective program is 2 months; the longer the program, the more sustained the results.[10] It is important for patients to continue with a home exercise program to maintain the benefits gained from the pulmonary rehabilitation program.

Table 15-3

Components of Brief Interventions for Tobacco Users

The 5 As for Brief Intervention

Ask: Identify and document tobacco-use status for every patient at every visit

Advise: Urge every tobacco user to quit

Assess: Is the tobacco user willing to make a quit attempt at this time?

Assist: Use counseling and pharmacotherapy to help patients willing to make a quit attempt

Arrange: Schedule follow-up contact, preferably within the first week after the quit date

The 5 Rs to Motivate Smokers Unwilling to Quit at Present

Relevance: Tailor advice and discussion to each smoker

Risks: Help the patient identify potential negative consequences of tobacco use

Rewards: Help the patient identify the potential benefits of quitting

Roadblocks: Help the patient identify barriers to quitting

Repetition: Repeat the motivational message at every visit

▶ *Long-Term Oxygen Therapy*

Long-term administration of oxygen (greater than 15 hours per day) to patients with chronic respiratory failure has been shown to reduce mortality and improve quality of life.[1,2] Oxygen therapy should be initiated in stable patients with very severe COPD (GOLD stage IV) who are optimized on drug therapy and meet one of the following criteria: (a) A resting PaO_2 at or below 55 mm Hg (7.32 kPa) or oxygen saturation (SaO_2) at or below 88%; or (b) PaO_2 between 55 and 60 mm Hg (7.32 and 7.98 kPa) or SaO_2 of 89% and evidence of pulmonary hypertension, peripheral edema suggesting congestive heart failure, or polycythemia.[1,2]

The dual-prong nasal cannula is the standard means of delivering continuous flow of oxygen. The goal of therapy is to increase the baseline oxygen saturation to at least 90% and/or PaO_2 to at least 60 mm Hg (7.98 kPa), allowing adequate oxygenation of vital organs. The flow rate, expressed as liters per minute (L/min), must be increased during exercise and sleep and can be adjusted based on pulse oximetry. Hypoxemia also worsens during air travel; patients requiring oxygen should generally increase their flow rate by 2 L/min during flight.[1]

Oxygen therapy should be continued indefinitely if it was initiated while the patient was in a stable state (rather than during an acute episode). Withdrawal of oxygen because of improved PaO_2 in such a patient may be detrimental.

▶ *Surgery*

Bullectomy, lung volume reduction surgery, and lung transplantation are surgical options for very severe COPD. These procedures may result in improved spirometry, lung volumes, exercise capacity, dyspnea, health-related quality of life, and possibly survival. Patient selection is critical because not all patients benefit. Refer to the ATS/ERS COPD standards for a detailed discussion of appropriate selection of surgical candidates.[1]

Pharmacologic Therapy of Stable COPD

The medications available for COPD are effective for reducing or relieving symptoms, improving exercise tolerance, reducing the number and severity of exacerbations, and improving quality of life. Evidence showing that medications slow the rate of decline in pulmonary function are conflicting, with more recent studies showing a benefit.[11]

▶ *Bronchodilators*

❹ *Bronchodilators are the mainstay of treatment for symptomatic COPD. They reduce symptoms and improve exercise tolerance and quality of life.*[2] They can be used as needed for symptoms or on a scheduled basis to prevent or reduce symptoms. Bronchodilator drugs commonly used in COPD include β_2-agonists, anticholinergics, and theophylline. The choice depends on availability, individual response, and preferences. The inhaled route is preferred, but attention must be paid to proper inhaler technique training.

Long-acting inhaled bronchodilators are more effective and convenient but more expensive than short-acting inhaled bronchodilators. Combination therapy improves efficacy and is preferred over increasing the dose of a single agent, especially since the dose–response relationship using FEV_1 as the outcome is relatively flat for single-agent therapy.

β_2-Agonists β_2-Agonists cause airway smooth muscle relaxation by stimulating adenyl cyclase to increase the formation of cyclic adenosine monophosphate (cAMP). Other nonbronchodilator effects have been observed, such as improvement in mucociliary transport, but their significance is uncertain.[12] β_2-Agonists are available in inhalation, oral, and parenteral dosage forms; the inhalation route is preferred because of fewer adverse effects.

These drugs are also available in short-acting and long-acting formulations (Table 15–4). The short-acting β_2-agonists include albuterol (known as salbutamol outside the United States), levalbuterol (known as R-salbutamol outside the United States), pirbuterol, and terbutaline. They are used as "rescue" therapy for acute symptom relief. Most COPD patients need continuous bronchodilator therapy on a scheduled basis every day. For these patients, short-acting β_2-agonists are inconvenient because of the need for frequent dosing. In addition, short-acting β_2-agonists have been associated with a slight, but statistically significant, loss of effectiveness when used regularly for more than 3 months (tachyphylaxis).[13]

Long-acting β_2-agonists include salmeterol, formoterol, and arformoterol. Salmeterol is a partial agonist with a slower onset of action than short-acting β_2-agonists. Formoterol is a more complete agonist and has an onset of action similar to that of albuterol. Arformoterol is the (R,R)-isomer of formoterol; both are available for nebulization, providing an alternative for patients with poor inhaler technique. Full agonists (formoterol and arformoterol) produce greater response at full receptor capacity than partial agonists (salmeterol). Bronchodilator effects of long-acting β_2-agonists last at least 12 hours, allowing for twice-daily dosing. Long-acting bronchodilators (LABDs) are superior to scheduled short-acting bronchodilators on important clinical outcomes, including frequency of exacerbations, degree of dyspnea, and health-related quality of life.[12] For symptomatic patients, these are preferred over short-acting agents for maintenance therapy. In patients with moderate-to-severe COPD, salmeterol can reduce the rate of decline of FEV_1.[11] Patients should also have a short-acting β_2-agonist such as albuterol available for as-needed use ("rescue" medication).

Adverse effects of both long- and short-acting β_2-agonists are dose-related and include palpitations, tachycardia, hypokalemia, and tremor. Sleep disturbance may also occur and appears to be worse with higher doses of inhaled long-acting β_2-agonists. Increasing doses beyond those clinically recommended is without benefit and could be associated with increased adverse effects.

Anticholinergics Ipratropium and tiotropium are inhaled anticholinergic medications commonly used for COPD.

Table 15–4

Maintenance Medications for COPD

	Medication	Onset	Peak	Duration	Usual Dose
Short-Acting β₂-Agonists	**Albuterol[a]**				
	Nebulization	5–15 minutes	0.5–2 hours	2–6 hours	2.5 mg every 6–8 hours (max: 30 mg/day)
	Inhalation	5–15 minutes	0.5–2 hours	2–6 hours	MDI (90 mcg/puff) 1–2 puffs every 4–6 hours (max: 1,080 mcg/day)
	Oral	7–30 minutes	2–3 hours	4–6 hours ER: 8–12 hours	2–4 mg 3–4 times a day ER: 4–8 mg every 12 hours (max: 32 mg/day)
	Levalbuterol				
	Nebulization	10–20 minutes	1.5 hours	5–8 hours	0.63–1.25 mg 3 times/day, 6–8 hours apart (max: 3.75 mg/day)
	Inhalation	5–10 minutes	1–1.5 hours	3–6 hours	MDI (45 mcg/puff) 1–2 puffs every 4–6 hours (max: 540 mcg/day)
	Pirbuterol				
	Inhalation	5 minutes	0.5–1.5 hours	4–5 hours	MDI (200 mcg/puff) 1–2 puffs every 4–6 hours (max: 2,400 mcg/day)
	Terbutaline				
	Oral	0.5–2 hours	1–3 hours	6–8 hours	2.5–5 mg 3 times/day, 6 hours apart[b] (max: 15 mg/day)
Long-Acting β₂-Agonists	**Formoterol**				
	Inhalation	1–3 minutes	1–3 hours	12 hours	Powder (12 mcg/inhalation) 1 inhalation every 12 hours (max: 24 mcg/day)
	Nebulization	1–3 minutes	1–3 hours	12 hours	20 mcg every 12 hours (max: 40 mcg/day)
	Salmeterol				
	Inhalation	10 minutes to 2 hours	2–5 hours	12 hours	Powder (50 mcg/inhalation) 1 inhalation every 12 hours (max: 100 mcg/day)
	Arformoterol				
	Nebulization	7–20 minutes	1–3 hours	12 hours	15 mcg every 12 hours (max: 30 mcg/day)
Short-Acting Anticholinergic	**Ipratropium**				
	Nebulization	1–30 minutes	1.5–2 hours	4–6 hours	500 mcg every 6–8 hours (max: 2,000 mcg/day)
	Inhalation	1–30 minutes	1.5–2 hours	4–6 hours	MDI (18 mcg/puff) 2 puffs 4 times/day (max: 216 mcg/day)
Long-Acting Anticholinergic	**Tiotropium**				
	Inhalation	30 minutes	1–4 hours	24 hours	Powder (18 mcg/inhalation) 1 inhalation every 24 hours (max: 18 mcg/day)[c]
Methylxanthine	**Theophylline**				
	Oral	0.5–2 hours	Up to 24 hours, depending on formulation	6–24 hours	400–600 mg/day divided every 6–24 hours based on formulation (max: 800 mg/day) Adjust dose to serum concentrations of 5–15 mcg/mL (28–83 µmol/L)
Inhaled Corticosteroids	**Beclomethasone**	1–7 days	1–4 weeks		MDI (40, 80 mcg/puff) 40–160 mcg twice a day (max: 640 mcg/day)
	Budesonide	1–7 days	1–2 weeks		Powder (90, 180 mcg/inhalation) 180–360 mcg twice a day (max: 1,440 mcg/day)
	Ciclesonide	1–7 days	1–4 weeks		MDI (80, 160 mcg/puff) 80–160 mcg 1 or 2 times/day (max: 640 mcg/day)
	Fluticasone	1–7 days	1–2 weeks		MDI (44, 110, 220 mcg/puff) 88–440 mcg twice a day (max: 1,760 mcg/day) Powder (50, 100, 250 mcg/inhalation) 100–250 mcg twice a day (max: 2,000 mcg/day)
	Triamcinolone	1–7 days	1–2 weeks		MDI (75 mcg/puff) 2 puffs 3–4 times/day or 4 puffs twice a day (max: 1,200 mcg/day)
	Mometasone	1–7 days	1–2 weeks		Powder (110, 220 mcg/inhalation) 220–440 mcg once daily (max: 880 mcg/day)

In elderly patients, start with the lowest recommended dose and increase as necessary.

ER, extended-release; MDI, metered-dose inhaler.

[a]Albuterol is known as salbutamol outside the United States.

[b]Not recommended if creatinine clearance (CrCl) less than or equal to 10 mL/min; for CrCl 11 to 50 mL/min, reduce dose by 50%.

[c]Patients with reduced activity in the CYP2D6 pathway (poor metabolizers; PMs) have higher plasma concentrations than those with normal activity (extensive metabolizers, EMs); PMs may require lower doses and should be monitored closely for adverse effects.

They produce bronchodilation by competitively blocking muscarinic receptors in bronchial smooth muscle. They may also decrease mucus secretion, although this effect is variable. Tiotropium dissociates from receptors extremely slowly, resulting in a half-life longer than 36 hours, allowing for once-daily dosing. Ipratropium has an elimination half-life of about 2 hours, necessitating dosing every 6 to 8 hours.

Tiotropium provides the most consistent improvements on the widest range of outcomes among all the bronchodilators. It has been shown to be superior to ipratropium and salmeterol in improving lung function and superior to ipratropium in relieving symptoms, reducing exacerbation frequency, and improving health status.[14,15] Because of its superior efficacy, tiotropium is considered first-line therapy for all COPD patients with persistent symptoms (e.g., dyspnea, need for rescue medication more than twice a week, and night waking). The largest drawback to widespread use of tiotropium is the high cost of therapy. Patients using tiotropium as maintenance therapy should be prescribed albuterol as their rescue therapy. The combination of ipratropium and tiotropium is not recommended because of the risks of excessive anticholinergic effects.

Inhaled anticholinergics are well tolerated with the most common adverse effect being dry mouth. Occasional metallic taste has also been reported with ipratropium. Other anticholinergic adverse effects include constipation, tachycardia, blurred vision, and precipitation of narrow-angle glaucoma symptoms. Urinary retention could be a problem, especially for those with concurrent bladder outlet obstruction. Recent studies suggest that inhaled anticholinergics may increase the risk of myocardial infarction and cardiovascular death in patients with COPD.[16,17] Further study is needed to clarify this risk. When initiating anticholinergic medications in patients with COPD, this potential risk should be weighed against the symptomatic benefits.

Methylxanthines Theophylline is a nonspecific phosphodiesterase inhibitor that increases intracellular cAMP within airway smooth muscle resulting in bronchodilation. It has a modest bronchodilator effect in patients with COPD, and its use is limited due to a narrow therapeutic index, multiple drug interactions, and adverse effects. Theophylline should be reserved for patients who cannot use inhaled medications or who remain symptomatic despite appropriate use of inhaled bronchodilators.

Theophylline's bronchodilatory effects are dependent upon achieving adequate serum concentrations, and therapeutic drug monitoring is needed to optimize therapy because of wide interpatient variability. If theophylline is used, serum concentrations in the range of 5 to 15 mcg/mL (28–83 μmol/L) provide adequate clinical response with a greater margin of safety than the traditionally recommended range of 10 to 20 mcg/mL (55–110 μmol/L). The most common adverse effects include heartburn, restlessness, insomnia, irritability, tachycardia, and tremor. Dose-related adverse effects include nausea and vomiting, seizures, and arrhythmias.

Tobacco smoke contains chemicals that induce the cytochrome P-450 isoenzymes 1A1, 1A2, and 2E1. Theophylline is metabolized by 1A2 and 2E1, and therefore smoking leads to increased clearance and subsequently decreased plasma levels of the drug.[18] Because most patients with COPD are current or past smokers, it is important to assess current tobacco use and adjust the theophylline dose as required based on altered plasma theophylline levels if tobacco use changes.

Combinations of Bronchodilators Patients with COPD often need maintenance treatment with two or three bronchodilators. Combining albuterol plus ipratropium, a long-acting β_2-agonist plus theophylline, or a long-acting β_2-agonist plus tiotropium, produces a greater change in spirometry than either drug alone.[1,2,19,20] Administering a long-acting β_2-agonist plus ipratropium leads to fewer exacerbations than either drug alone.[21] A combination of all three bronchodilator classes (β_2-agonist, anticholinergic, and theophylline) can be used if the response to a two-drug combination is inadequate. However, this approach has not been evaluated adequately in clinical trials.

▶ *Corticosteroids*

⑤ *In symptomatic patients with severe COPD (FEV$_1$ less than 50% predicted) and frequent exacerbations, regular treatment with inhaled corticosteroids decreases the number of exacerbations per year and improves health status.*[2,22–26] Corticosteroids may reduce the rate of decline in pulmonary function in patients with moderate to severe COPD.[11] They do not appear to improve mortality.[27] A combination inhaler device is recommended when using a long-acting β_2-agonist with an inhaled corticosteroid (e.g., Advair [fluticasone/salmeterol] and Symbicort [budesonide/formoterol]).

Patients should be reassessed 6 to 8 weeks after initiating inhaled corticosteroids to determine whether there has been a positive response. A positive response is indicated by an increase in FEV$_1$ of 15% or more, improvement in symptoms, and/or improvement in 6-minute walking distance.[28] Treatment should be discontinued if no substantial clinical or physiologic improvement is seen.[1,28]

Upon discontinuation of inhaled corticosteroids, some patients may experience deterioration in lung function and an increase in dyspnea and mild exacerbations; it is reasonable to reinstitute the medication in these patients.[29]

The most common adverse effects from inhaled corticosteroids include oropharyngeal candidiasis and hoarse voice. These can be minimized by rinsing the mouth after use and by using a spacer device with metered-dose inhalers (MDIs). Increased bruising, decreased bone density, and increased incidence of pneumonia have also been reported; the clinical importance of these effects remains uncertain.[1,2,22,27]

Long-term use of oral corticosteroids should be avoided due to an unfavorable risk-to-benefit ratio. The steroid myopathy that can result from long-term use of oral corticosteroids weakens muscles, further decreasing the respiratory drive in patients with advanced disease.

▶ *Immunizations*

● Serious illness and death in COPD patients can be reduced by about 50% with annual influenza vaccination. The optimal time for vaccination is usually from early October through mid-November. All patients with COPD should also receive a one-time vaccination with the pneumococcal polysaccharide vaccine, even though sufficient data supporting its use in COPD patients are lacking.[1,2] Patients over 65 years of age should be revaccinated if it has been more than 5 years since initial vaccination and they were less than 65 years of age at the time.

▶ *a₁-Antitrypsin Augmentation Therapy*

The ATS and the ERS have published standards for the diagnosis and management of individuals with AAT deficiency.[30] They recommend IV augmentation therapy for individuals with AAT deficiency and moderate airflow obstruction (FEV₁ 35–60% predicted). In these patients, augmentation therapy appears to reduce overall mortality and slow the decline in FEV₁, although large randomized controlled trials have not been conducted.

Augmentation therapy consists of weekly transfusions of pooled human AAT with the goal of maintaining adequate plasma levels of the enzyme. The benefits of augmentation therapy are unclear in patients with severe (FEV₁ less than 35% predicted) or mild (FEV₁ greater than 60% predicted) airflow obstruction. Augmentation therapy is not recommended for individuals with AAT deficiency who do not have lung disease.

▶ *Other Pharmacologic Therapies*

● Leukotriene modifiers (e.g., zafirlukast and montelukast) have not been adequately evaluated in COPD patients and are not recommended for routine use. Small, short-term studies showed improvement in pulmonary function, dyspnea, and quality of life when leukotriene modifiers were added to inhaled bronchodilator therapy.[31,32] Additional long-term studies are needed to clarify their role.

Nedocromil, a mast cell stabilizer, has not been adequately tested in COPD patients and is not included in the GOLD recommendations.

N-acetylcysteine has antioxidant and mucolytic activity, which makes it a promising agent for COPD treatment, but clinical trials have produced conflicting results. One of the largest trials found *N*-acetylcysteine to be ineffective in reducing the decline in lung function and preventing exacerbations.[33] Routine use cannot be recommended at this time.

Prophylactic, continuous use of antibiotics has no effect on the frequency of exacerbations; antibiotics should only be used for treating infectious exacerbations. Antitussives are

---

Patient Encounter, Part 2: The Medical History, Physical Exam, and Diagnostic Tests

PMH: Hypertension for 6 years, currently controlled

SH: Patient works as an accountant; married with two children

FH: Father with emphysema and lung cancer. There is no family history of type 2 diabetes or heart disease

Meds: Lisinopril 40 mg orally once daily; hydrochloro-thiazide 25 mg orally once daily

ROS: (–) skin rash; (–) nasal congestion, drainage; (–) chest pain, paroxysmal nocturnal dyspnea, orthopnea; (+) shortness of breath, cough, intermittent wheezing; (–) hemoptysis; (–) heartburn, reflux symptoms, N/V/D, change in appetite, change in bowel habits; (–) joint pain or swelling; (–) pedal edema

PE:

VS: BP 134/82 mm Hg, P 80 bpm, RR 20/min, T 35.8°C (96.4°F), wt 60 kg (132 lb), ht 64 in. (163 cm), BMI 22.7 kg/m²

HEENT: EOMI; mucosal membranes are moist; no evidence of jugular venous distention; no palpably enlarged cervical lymph nodes

Lungs: Barrel-shaped chest; hyper-resonant on percussion bilaterally; lung sounds are distant, no rhonchi or crackles.

CV: RRR, normal S₁, S₂; no murmur, gallop, or rub
Abd: Soft, nontender, no hepatosplenomegaly
Ext: No cyanosis, edema, or finger clubbing; evidence of onychomycosis on all fingernails

Pulmonary Function Tests

	Prebronchodilator		Postbronchodilator	
	Actual	**% Predicted**	**Actual**	**% Predicted**
FVC (L)	4.4	107%	4.0	97%
FEV₁ (L)	1.68	50%	1.59	47%
FEV₁/FVC (%)			39%	

CXR: Hyperlucency and hyperinflation of the lungs suggestive of emphysematous change

Given this additional information, what is your assessment of the patient's condition?

This patient's COPD can be classified as what stage?

What are the treatment goals for this patient?

What nonpharmacologic and pharmacologic alternatives are feasible for this patient?

Develop a treatment plan for this patient.

contraindicated because cough has an important protective role. Opioids may be effective for dyspnea in advanced disease but may have serious adverse effects; they may be used to manage symptoms in terminal patients.

Therapy of COPD Exacerbations

An exacerbation is a sustained worsening of the patient's symptoms from his or her usual stable state that is beyond normal day-to-day variations. It is acute in onset and sufficient to warrant a change in management. Commonly reported symptoms are worsening of dyspnea, increased sputum production, and change in sputum color. The most common causes of an exacerbation are respiratory infection and air pollution, but the cause cannot be identified in about one-third of severe exacerbations.[2]

Treatment depends on the symptoms and severity of the exacerbation. Mild exacerbations can often be treated at home with an increase in bronchodilator therapy with or without oral corticosteroids (Fig. 15–3). Antibiotics are indicated when there are specific signs of airway infection (e.g., change in color of sputum and/or increased sputum production or dyspnea) or when mechanical ventilation is needed. Moderate to severe exacerbations require management in the emergency department or hospital. Management should consist of controlled oxygen therapy, bronchodilators, oral or IV corticosteroids, antibiotics if indicated, and consideration of mechanical ventilation (noninvasive or invasive).

▶ Bronchodilators

Albuterol is the preferred bronchodilator for treatment of acute exacerbations because of its rapid onset of action. Ipratropium can be added to allow for lower doses of albuterol, thus reducing dose-dependent adverse effects such as tachycardia and tremor. Delivery can be accomplished through MDI and spacer or nebulizer. The nebulizer route is preferred in patients with severe dyspnea and/or cough that would limit delivery of medication through an MDI with spacer. If response is inadequate, theophylline can be considered; however, clinical evidence supporting its use is lacking.

▶ Oral Corticosteroids

Systemic corticosteroids shorten the recovery time, help to restore lung function more quickly, and may reduce the risk of early relapse.[34] The GOLD guidelines recommend that corticosteroids be considered in addition to bronchodilators in all hospitalized patients and in outpatients with baseline FEV_1 less than 50% predicted.[2] Other authorities recommend corticosteroids for all patients experiencing a COPD exacerbation.[1] Oral prednisone 30 to 40 mg/day for 10 to 14 days is recommended. Prolonged treatment does not result in greater efficacy and increases the risk of adverse effects. If inhaled corticosteroids are part of the patient's usual treatment regimen, they should be continued during systemic therapy.

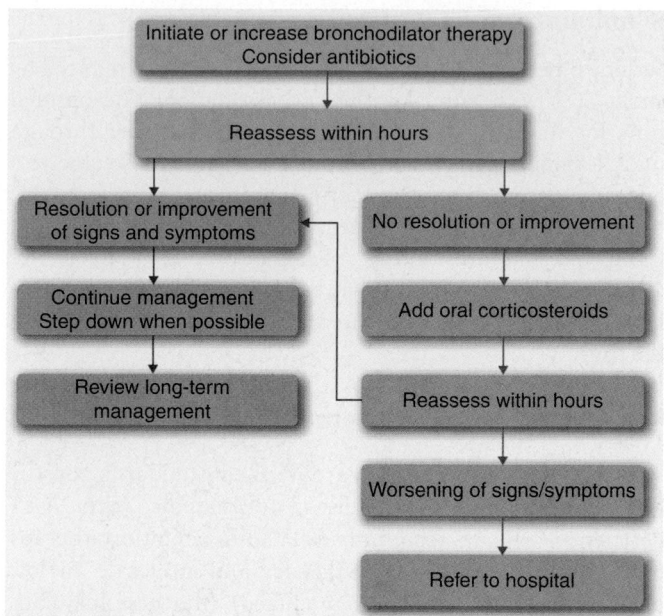

FIGURE 15–3. Algorithm for the management of an exacerbation of COPD at home. (From Ref. 2.)

▶ Antibiotics

The role of antibiotic treatment in treating COPD exacerbation is evolving, and recent evidence suggests that subsets of patients may benefit from antibiotic treatment. ❻ *Antibiotics should be used in patients with COPD exacerbations who: (a) have all three cardinal symptoms (increased dyspnea, increased sputum volume, and increased purulence); (b) have increased sputum purulence along with one other cardinal symptom; or (c) experience a severe exacerbation requiring mechanical ventilation.*[2]

The predominant bacterial organisms in patients with mild exacerbations are *Streptococcus pneumoniae*, *Haemophilus influenzae*, and *Moraxella catarrhalis*. In patients with more severe underlying COPD, other bacteria such as enteric Gram-negative bacilli (*Escherichia coli*, *Klebsiella pneumoniae*, and *Enterobacter cloacae*) and *Pseudomonas aeruginosa* may be more common. Selection of empiric antibiotic therapy should be based on the most likely organism(s) thought to be responsible for the infection and on local resistance patterns. A risk stratification approach has been advocated to help guide antibiotic selection.[1,2,35] This approach is based on risk factors found to be predictive of treatment failure or early relapse. Patients at risk for poor outcome are candidates for more aggressive initial antibiotic treatment. Table 15–5 provides recommended antibiotic treatment based on this risk stratification approach.[2,35] Antibiotic treatment for most patients should be maintained for 3 to 7 days, until the patient has been afebrile for 3 consecutive days. Exacerbations due to certain infecting organisms (*P. aeruginosa*, *E. cloacae*, and methicillin-resistant *Staphylococcus aureus*), while not common, require more lengthy courses of therapy (21–42 days).

If there is worsening clinical status or inadequate clinical response in 48 to 72 hours, reevaluate the patient, consider sputum Gram stain and culture if not already obtained, and adjust antimicrobial therapy. If Gram stain and culture results are available, narrow the antibiotic therapy according to cultured organism(s) and sensitivities. If no cultures have been obtained, or cultures remain negative, consider additional antibiotics and/or change to antibiotics with a broader spectrum of activity.

▶ *Oxygen*

The goal of oxygen therapy is to maintain PaO_2 above 60 mm Hg (7.98 kPa) or SaO_2 above 90% to prevent tissue hypoxia and preserve cellular oxygenation.[1] Increasing the PaO_2 much further confers little added benefit and may increase the risk of CO_2 retention, which may lead to respiratory acidosis. ABGs should be obtained after 1 to 2 hours to assess for hypercapnia.

Table 15–5

Recommended Antibiotic Therapy in Acute Exacerbations of COPD

Patient Characteristics	Likely Pathogens	Recommended Antibiotics[a,b]
Mild Exacerbation Without Risk Factors for Poor Outcome		
Not requiring hospitalization Less than three exacerbations per year No comorbid illness FEV_1 greater than 50% predicted No recent antibiotic therapy	*Streptococcus pneumoniae* *Haemophilus influenzae* *Moraxella catarrhalis* *Chlamydia pneumoniae* Viruses	*Oral First-Line Therapy:* β-Lactam (high-dose amoxicillin)[c] β-Lactam/β-lactamase inhibitor (amoxicillin-clavulanate) Tetracycline Trimethoprim/sulfamethoxazole *Alternative Oral Therapy:* Macrolides (azithromycin, clarithromycin) Second- or third-generation cephalosporins (cefuroxime, cefpodoxime, cefdinir, cefprozil) *IV Therapy:* Not recommended
Moderate Exacerbation With Risk Factors for Poor Outcome		
FEV_1 less than 50% predicted Comorbid diseases Three or more exacerbations per year Antibiotic therapy in the previous 3 months	Above organisms *plus:* Resistant pneumococci (β-lactamase producing, penicillin-resistant), *Escherichia coli, Proteus* spp, *Enterobacter* spp, *Klebsiella pneumoniae*	*Oral First-Line Therapy:* β-Lactam/β-lactamase inhibitor (amoxicillin-clavulanate) *Alternative Oral Therapy:* Fluoroquinolone with enhanced pneumococcal activity (levofloxacin, gemifloxacin, moxifloxacin) *IV Therapy:* β-lactam/β-lactamase inhibitor (ampicillin–sulbactam) Second- or third-generation cephalosporin (cefuroxime, ceftriaxone) Fluoroquinolone with enhanced pneumococcal activity (levofloxacin, moxifloxacin)
Severe Exacerbation With Risk Factors for *Pseudomonas aeruginosa*		
Recent hospitalization Four or more courses of antibiotics in the last year Very severe COPD (GOLD stage IV) Previous isolation of *P. aeruginosa*	Above organisms *plus:* *P. aeruginosa*	*Oral First-Line Therapy:* Antipseudomonal fluoroquinolone (ciprofloxacin, high-dose levofloxacin) *IV Therapy:* Antipseudomonal β-lactamase-resistant penicillin (piperacillin-tazobactam) Third- or fourth-generation cephalosporin with antipseudomonal activity (ceftazidime, cefepime) Antipseudomonal fluoroquinolone (ciprofloxacin, high-dose levofloxacin)

COPD, chronic obstructive pulmonary disease; FEV_1, forced expiratory volume in 1 second.

[a]Antibiotics are indicated for patients with COPD exacerbations who: (a) have all three cardinal symptoms (increased dyspnea, increased sputum volume, and increased purulence); (b) have increased sputum purulence along with one other cardinal symptom; or (c) experience a severe exacerbation requiring mechanical ventilation.

[b]Antibiotic choices should take into consideration local resistance patterns.

[c]High-dose amoxicillin is recommended due to the prevalence of penicillin-resistant *S. pneumoniae*.

In advanced COPD, caution should be used because overly aggressive administration of oxygen to patients with chronic hypercapnia may result in respiratory depression and respiratory failure. In these patients, mild hypoxemia, rather than CO_2 accumulation, triggers their drive to breathe.

▶ Assisted Ventilation

Mechanical ventilation can be administered as follows: (a) invasive (conventional) mechanical ventilation through an endotracheal tube; and (b) noninvasive mechanical ventilation using either negative (e.g., iron lung—not recommended) or positive pressure devices. Noninvasive positive pressure ventilation (NPPV) is preferred whenever possible. It improves signs and symptoms, decreases the length of hospital stay, and most importantly, reduces mortality.[36] Appropriate patients to consider for NPPV include those with the following characteristics: (a) moderate-to-severe dyspnea with use of accessory muscles and paradoxical abdominal motion; (b) moderate-to-severe acidosis (pH between 7.25 and 7.35) and hypercapnia ($PaCO_2$ between 45 and 60 mm Hg [6–8 kPa]); and (c) respiratory rate between 25 and 35 breaths/min.[2] Invasive mechanical ventilation should be used in patients with more severe symptoms and in those failing NPPV.

OUTCOME EVALUATION

- Monitor the patient for improvement in symptoms (dyspnea, cough, sputum production, and fatigue).

- Changes in FEV_1 should not be the main outcome assessed. FEV_1 changes are weakly related to symptoms, exacerbations, and health-related quality of life (outcomes that are important to patients).

- The Medical Research Council dyspnea scale can be used to monitor physical limitation due to breathlessness (Table 15–6). The scale is simple to administer and correlates well with scores of health status.[37]

- The BODE index is a validated predictor of mortality and a better predictor than FEV_1 alone.[38] It is a composite score derived from body mass index or BMI (**B**), FEV_1 or degree of airflow obstruction (**O**), modified Medical Research Council (MMRC) dyspnea scale (**D**), and 6-minute walking distance (**E**, exercise capacity). All of these variables predict important outcomes such as health-related quality of life, the rate of exacerbations, and the risk of death. The composite score is based on a 10-point scale in which higher scores indicate a higher risk of death (Table 15–7). The BODE index can be used clinically to monitor disease progression. Its usefulness in measuring outcomes of drug therapy, pulmonary rehabilitation, and the degree of health care resource utilization needs further study.

- Assess quality of life using the St. George's Respiratory Questionnaire, which has been validated and is specific for COPD patients.[39]

- Monitor theophylline levels with goal serum concentrations in the range of 5 to 15 mcg/mL (28–83 μmol/L). Trough levels should be obtained 1 to 2 weeks after initiation of treatment and after any dosage adjustment. Routine levels are not necessary unless toxicity is suspected or disease has worsened.

Table 15–6

Medical Research Council Dyspnea Scale

Grade	Modified Grade[a]	Statement About Perceived Breathlessness[b]
1	0	"I only get breathless with strenuous activity"
2	1	"I get short of breath when hurrying on the level or up a slight hill"
3	2	"I walk slower than people of the same age on the level because of breathlessness or I have to stop for breath after a mile or so on the level at my own pace"
4	3	"I stop for breath after walking 100 yards or after a few minutes on the level"
5	4	"I am too breathless to leave the house or I get breathless while dressing"

[a]The modified grade is used in the BODE index.
[b]The last statement to which the patient answers "yes" is their grade.

Table 15–7

The BODE Index

Variable	Points on BODE Index[a]			
	0	1	2	3
FEV_1 (% of predicted)	65 or greater	50–64	36–49	35 or less
Distance walked in 6 minutes (m)	350 or greater	250–349	150–249	149 or less
Modified Medical Research Council Dyspnea Scale	0–1	2	3	4
BMI (kg/m²)	Greater than 21	21 or less		

FEV_1, forced expiratory volume in 1 second.
[a]The cutoff values for the assignment of points are shown for each variable.
From Ref. 38.

Patient Care and Monitoring

1. Assess the patient's symptoms and history of exposure to risk factors. For new patients, obtain a detailed medical history including:
   - Medical conditions, especially history of respiratory disorders
   - Immunization status (pneumococcal and influenza)
   - Family history of COPD or other chronic respiratory disease
   - History of exacerbations or previous hospitalizations for respiratory disorders
   - Impact of disease on the patient's life, including limitation of activity, missed work, and feelings of depression or anxiety

2. Obtain spirometry measurements to assess airflow limitation and aid in severity classification and treatment decisions. Measure arterial blood gases if FEV_1 is less than 40% predicted or if the patient has clinical signs suggestive of respiratory failure or right heart failure.

3. Obtain a thorough history of prescription, nonprescription, and dietary supplement use. Assess inhaler technique and adherence to the medication regimen. Ask the patient about effectiveness of medications at controlling symptoms and adverse effects.

4. Ask current tobacco users about daily quantity, past quit attempts, and current readiness to quit.

5. Design a therapeutic plan including lifestyle modifications (e.g., smoking cessation) and optimal drug therapy. Consider need for pulmonary rehabilitation, oxygen therapy, and/or surgery.

6. Provide patient education about the disease state and therapeutic plan:
   - What COPD is, and what its natural course is like
   - Smoking cessation counseling
   - Role of regular exercise and healthy eating
   - How and when to take medications; importance of adherence to the medication plan; adverse effects and how to minimize them
   - Signs and symptoms of an exacerbation and what to do if one occurs
   - Advanced directives and end-of-life issues for patients with more severe disease

7. Determine the follow-up period based on patient status and needs (typically 3–6 months).

8. Follow-up visits should include:
   - Assessment of tobacco use and/or quit attempts
   - Assessment of change in symptoms. Obtain spirometry if there is a substantial increase in symptoms or a complication
   - Review of drug therapy (dosages, adherence, inhaler technique, effectiveness, adverse effects, and drug interactions)
   - Evaluation of exacerbation frequency, severity, and likely causes

9. Perform spirometry at least annually to assess disease progression.

10. Provide annual influenza vaccination.

11. Assess inhaler technique at every visit. Have the patient demonstrate proper use of each device using a placebo inhaler or personal inhaler. Proper use of these devices is critical for therapeutic success.

Abbreviations Introduced in This Chapter

AAT	α_1-Antitrypsin
ABG	Arterial blood gas
ATS	American Thoracic Society
BMI	Body mass index
cAMP	Cyclic adenosine monophosphate
COPD	Chronic obstructive pulmonary disease
EOMI	Extraocular movements intact
ERS	European Respiratory Society
FEV_1	Forced expiratory volume in 1 second
FVC	Forced vital capacity
GOLD	Global Initiative for Chronic Obstructive Lung Disease
JVD	Jugular venous distention
LABD	Long-acting bronchodilator
MDI	Metered-dose inhaler
MMRC	Modified Medical Research Council
NPPV	Noninvasive positive pressure ventilation
$PaCO_2$	Partial pressure of arterial carbon dioxide
PaO_2	Partial pressure of arterial oxygen
PFTs	Pulmonary function tests
SaO_2	Arterial oxygen saturation
TNF-α	Tumor necrosis factor-α
V_A/Q	Ventilation-to-perfusion ratio

Self-assessment questions and answers are available at *http://www.mhpharmacotherapy. com/pp.html*.

REFERENCES

1. American Thoracic Society/European Respiratory Society Task Force. Standards for the diagnosis and management of patients with COPD. Version 1.2. New York: American Thoracic Society; 2004, *www.thoracic.org/go/copd.*

2. GOLD Science Committee. Global strategy for the diagnosis, management, and prevention of chronic obstructive pulmonary disease. *www.goldcopd.com.*

3. American Lung Association. Chronic Obstructive Pulmonary Disease (COPD) Fact Sheet. 2008 (June), *www.lungusa.org.*

4. Altose MD. Approaches to slowing the progression of COPD. Curr Opin Pulm Med 2003;9:125–130.

5. Hogg JC. Pathophysiology of airflow limitation in chronic obstructive pulmonary disease. Lancet 2004;364:709–721.

6. Anthonisen NR, Connett JE, Murray RP. Smoking and lung function of the lung health study participants after 11 years. Am J Respir Crit Care Med 2002;166:675–679.

7. Scanlon PD, Connett JE, Waller LA, et al. Smoking cessation and lung function in mild-to-moderate chronic obstructive pulmonary disease. The Lung Health Study. Am J Respir Crit Care Med 2000;161:381–390.

8. Fiore MC, Jaén CR, Baker TB, et al. Treating tobacco use and dependence, *www.surgeongeneral.gov/tobacco/treating_tobacco_use08.pdf.*

9. Wagena EJ, van der Meer RM, Ostelo RJWG, et al. The efficacy of smoking cessation strategies in people with chronic obstructive pulmonary disease: Results from a systematic review. Respir Med 2004;98:805–815.

10. Troosters T, Casaburi R, Gosselink R, Decramer M. Pulmonary rehabilitation in chronic obstructive pulmonary disease. Am J Respir Crit Care Med 2005;172:19–38.

11. Celli BR, Thomas NE, Anderson JA, et al. Effect of pharmacotherapy on rate of decline of lung function in chronic obstructive pulmonary disease. Results from the TORCH study. Am J Respir Crit Care Med 2008;178:332–338.

12. Tashkin DP, Cooper CB. The role of long-acting bronchodilators in the management of stable COPD. Chest 2004;125:249–259.

13. Rennard SI, Serby CW, Ghafouri M, et al. Extended therapy with ipratropium is associated with improved lung function in patients with COPD. A retrospective analysis of data from seven clinical trials. Chest 1996;110:62–70.

14. Vincken W, van Noord JA, Greefhorst APM, et al. Improved health outcomes in patients with COPD during 1 year's treatment with tiotropium. Eur Respir J 2002;19:209–216.

15. Brusasco V, Hodder R, Miravitlles M, et al. Health outcomes following treatment for six months with once daily tiotropium compared with twice daily salmeterol in patients with COPD. Thorax 2003;58:399–404.

16. Singh S, Loke YK, Furberg CD. Inhaled anticholinergics and risk of major adverse cardiovascular events in patients with chronic obstructive pulmonary disease. JAMA 2008;300:1439–1450.

17. Lee TA, Pickard AS, Au DH, et al. Risk for death associated with medications for recently diagnosed chronic obstructive pulmonary disease. Ann Intern Med 2008;149:380–390.

18. Zevin S, Benowitz NL. Drug interactions with tobacco smoking. An update. Clin Pharmacokinet 1999;36:425–438.

19. ZuWallack RL, Mahler DA, Reilly D, et al. Salmeterol plus theophylline combination therapy in the treatment of COPD. Chest 2001;119:1661–1670.

20. Cazzola M, Noschese P, Salzillo A, et al. Bronchodilator response to formoterol after regular tiotropium or to tiotropium after regular formoterol in COPD patients. Respir Med 2005;99:524–528.

21. van Noord JA, de Munck DRAJ, Bantje TA, et al. Long-term treatment of chronic obstructive pulmonary disease with salmeterol and the additive effect of ipratropium. Eur Respir J 2000;15:878–885.

22. The Lung Health Study Research Group. Effect of inhaled triamcinolone on the decline in pulmonary function in chronic obstructive pulmonary disease: Lung Health Study II. N Engl J Med 2000;343:1902–1909.

23. Burge PS, Calverley PM, Jones PW, et al. Randomised, double blind, placebo controlled study of fluticasone propionate in patients with moderate to severe chronic obstructive pulmonary disease: The ISOLDE trial. BMJ 2000;320:1297–1303.

24. Mahler DA, Wire P, Horstman D, et al. Effectiveness of fluticasone propionate and salmeterol combination delivered via the Diskus device in the treatment of chronic obstructive pulmonary disease. Am J Respir Crit Care Med 2002;166:1084–1091.

25. Jones PW, Willits LR, Burge PS, Calverley PM. Disease severity and the effect of fluticasone propionate on chronic obstructive pulmonary disease exacerbations. Eur Respir J 2003;21:68–73.

26. Calverley P, Pauwels R, Vestbo J, et al. Combined salmeterol and fluticasone in the treatment of chronic obstructive pulmonary disease: A randomised controlled trial. Lancet 2003;361:449–456.

27. Calverley PMA, Anderson JA, Celli B, et al. Salmeterol and fluticasone propionate and survival in chronic obstructive pulmonary disease. N Engl J Med 2007;356:775–789.

28. Institute for Clinical Systems Improvement. Health care guideline: Chronic Obstructive Pulmonary Disease. *www.icsi.org.*

29. Wouters EF, Postma DS, Fokkens B, et al. Withdrawal of fluticasone propionate from combined salmeterol/fluticasone treatment in patients with COPD causes immediate and sustained disease deterioration: A randomised controlled trial. Thorax 2005;60:480–487.

30. Alpha-1 Antitrypsin Deficiency Task Force. American Thoracic Society/European Respiratory Society statement: Standards for the diagnosis and management of individuals with alpha-1 antitrypsin deficiency. Am J Respir Crit Care Med 2003;168:818–900.

31. Celik P, Sakar A, Havlucu Y, et al. Short-term effects of montelukast in stable patients with moderate to severe COPD. Respir Med 2005;99:444–450.

32. Cazzola M, Centanni S, Boveri B, et al. Comparison of the bronchodilating effect of salmeterol and zafirlukast in combination with that of their use as single treatments in asthma and chronic obstructive pulmonary disease. Respiration 2001;68:452–459.

33. Decramer M, Rutten-van Molken M, Dekhuijzen PNR, et al. Effects of N-acetylcysteine on outcomes in chronic obstructive pulmonary disease (Bronchitis Randomized on NAD Cost-Utility Study, BRONCUS): A randomised placebo-controlled trial. Lancet 2005;365:1552–1560.

34. Wood-Baker RR, Gibson PG, Hannay M, et al. Systemic corticosteroids for acute exacerbations of chronic obstructive pulmonary disease. Cochrane Database Syst Rev 2005;CD001288.

35. Sethi S, Murphy TF. Acute exacerbations of chronic bronchitis: New developments concerning microbiology and pathophysiology—impact on approaches to risk stratification and therapy. Infect Dis Clin N Am 2004;18:861–882.

36. American Thoracic Society. International Consensus Conferences in Intensive Care Medicine: noninvasive positive pressure ventilation in acute respiratory failure. Am J Respir Crit Care Med 2001;163:283–291.

37. Bestall JC, Paul EA, Garrod R, et al. Usefulness of the Medical Research Council (MRC) dyspnoea scale as a measure of disability in patients with chronic obstructive pulmonary disease. Thorax 1999;54:581–586.

38. Celli BR, Cote CG, Marin JM, et al. The body-mass index, airflow obstruction, dyspnea, and exercise capacity index in chronic obstructive pulmonary disease. N Engl J Med 2004;350:1005–1012.

39. Jones PW, Quirk FH, Baveystock GM, Littlejohns P. A self-complete measure of health status for chronic airflow limitation. The St. George's Respiratory Questionnaire. Am Rev Respir Dis 1992;145:1321–1327.

16 Cystic Fibrosis

Kimberly J. Novak

LEARNING OBJECTIVES

● **Upon completion of the chapter, the reader will be able to:**

1. Explain the pathophysiology of cystic fibrosis (CF) and its multiorgan system involvement.
2. Describe the common clinical presentation and diagnosis of CF.
3. Consider long-term treatment goals with respect to clinical course and prognosis of CF.
4. Identify nonpharmacologic therapies for CF management.
5. Recommend appropriate pharmacologic therapies for chronic CF management.
6. Design appropriate antibiotic regimens for acute pulmonary exacerbations of CF.
7. Employ pharmacokinetic principles when calculating drug doses in CF patients.
8. Formulate monitoring plans for acute and chronic CF pharmacotherapy.

KEY CONCEPTS

❶ In cystic fibrosis (CF), the CF transmembrane regulator (CFTR) chloride channel is dysfunctional and usually results in decreased chloride secretion and increased sodium absorption, leading to altered viscosity of fluid excreted by the exocrine glands and mucosal obstruction.

❷ Pulmonary disease is characterized by thick mucus secretions, impaired mucus clearance, chronic airway infection and colonization, obstruction, and an exaggerated neutrophil-dominated inflammatory response.

❸ Maximizing nutritional status through pancreatic enzyme replacement and vitamin and nutritional supplements is necessary for normal growth and development and for maintaining long-term lung function.

❹ Airway clearance therapy is a necessary routine for all CF patients to clear secretions and control infection.

❺ Antibiotic therapy is indicated in three distinct situations over the course of CF: (a) early eradication and delay of colonization; (b) suppression of bacterial growth once colonization occurs; and (c) reduction of bacterial load in acute overgrowth.

❻ Antibiotic selection is based on periodic culture and sensitivity data, typically covering all organisms identified during the preceding year. If no culture data are available, empiric antibiotics should cover the most likely organisms for the patient's age group.

❼ Antibiotic regimens in severe CF exacerbations usually include an IV antipseudomonal β-lactam plus an aminoglycoside.

❽ CF patients have larger volumes of distribution for many antibiotics due to an increased ratio of lean body mass to total body mass and lower fat stores. CF patients also have an enhanced total body clearance, although the exact mechanism has not been determined.

❾ Titration of pancreatic enzyme doses is based on control of steatorrhea, stool output, and abdominal symptoms.

❿ Because CF-related diabetes results from insulin insufficiency, exogenous insulin replacement is usually required.

INTRODUCTION

Cystic fibrosis (CF) is an inherited multiorgan system disorder affecting children and an ever-growing adult population. It is the most common life-threatening genetic disease among Caucasians and the major cause of severe chronic lung disease and pancreatic insufficiency in children. The disease generally manifests as mucosal obstruction of exocrine glands caused by defective ion transport within epithelial cells. Due to the array of affected organ systems and complicated medical therapies, appropriate CF treatment necessitates multidisciplinary team collaboration.

EPIDEMIOLOGY AND ETIOLOGY

In the United States, CF most commonly occurs in the Caucasian population, ranging from 1 in 1,900 to 3,700 individuals. CF is less common in Hispanics (1 in 9,000), African Americans (1 in 15,000), and Asian Americans (1 in 32,000).[1] CF is inherited as an autosomal recessive trait, and approximately 1 in 25 Caucasians are heterozygous carriers. Offspring of a carrier couple (each parent being heterozygous) have a 1 in 4 chance of having the disease (homozygous), a 1 in 2 chance of being a carrier (heterozygous), and a 1 in 4 chance of receiving no trait. The gene mutation is found on the long arm of chromosome 7 and encodes for the CF transmembrane regulator (CFTR) protein, which functions as a chloride channel to transport water and electrolytes. Over 1,000 mutations have been described in the CF gene; however, the ΔF508 mutation is the most common and is present in 70% to 90% of CF patients in the United States.[2]

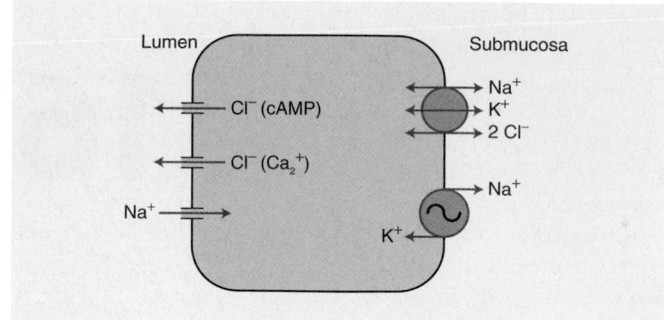

FIGURE 16–1. Electrolyte transport in the airway epithelial cell. (Ca, calcium; cAMP, cyclic-3′, 5′-adenosine monophosphate; Cl, chloride; Na, sodium; K potassium.) (From Milavetz G, Smith JJ. Cystic fibrosis. In: DiPiro JT, Talbert RL, Yee GC, et al. (eds.) Pharmacotherapy: A Pathophysiologic Approach. 7th ed. New York: McGraw-Hill, 2008: 536.)

PATHOPHYSIOLOGY

CF is a disease of exocrine gland epithelial cells where CFTR expression is prevalent. Normally, these cells transport chloride through CFTR chloride channels with sodium and water accompanying this flux across the cell membrane (Fig. 16–1). CFTR is regulated by protein kinases in response to varying levels of the intracellular second messenger cyclic-3′,5′-adenosine monophosphate (cAMP). CFTR also downregulates the epithelial sodium channel, regulates calcium-activated chloride and potassium channels, and may function in exocytosis and formation of plasma membrane molecular complexes and proteins important in inflammatory responses.[2] ❶ *In CF, the CFTR chloride channel is dysfunctional and usually results in decreased chloride secretion and increased sodium absorption, leading to altered viscosity of fluid excreted by the exocrine glands and mucosal obstruction.*

Pulmonary System

Chronic lung disease is a hallmark of CF, leading to death in 90% of patients.[3] ❷ *Pulmonary disease is characterized by thick mucus secretions, impaired mucus clearance, chronic airway infection and colonization, obstruction, and an exaggerated neutrophil-dominated inflammatory response.*[4] Over time, chronic obstruction and inflammations lead to air trapping, atelectasis, mucus plugging, bronchiectasis, cystic lesions, pulmonary hypertension, and eventual respiratory failure. In the U.S.-CF population, pulmonary function declines at an average yearly rate of 2%, as measured by forced expiratory volume in 1 second (FEV_1). The rate in an individual patient may be higher or lower depending on severity of CFTR dysfunction and comorbidities. Patients may show a slow steady decline over time, or they may have stable lung function with intermittent periods of sharp decline.[1] In the upper airways, sinusitis and nasal polyps are also common, and microbial colonization is similar to that of the lungs.

Bacterial pathogens are often acquired in an age-dependent sequence, and prevalence is tracked in the Cystic Fibrosis Foundation Patient Registry. Early infection is most often caused by *Staphylococcus aureus* and nontypeable *Haemophilus influenzae* (and thus is not prevented by childhood *H. influenzae* type b immunization). *Pseudomonas aeruginosa* infection also occurs early in life and is the most significant CF pathogen among all age groups. *P. aeruginosa* expresses extracellular toxins that perpetuate lung inflammation. Mucoid strains of *P. aeruginosa* produce an alginate biofilm layer that interferes with antibiotic penetration. Other organisms identified later in the disease course include *Stenotrophomonas maltophilia*, *Achromobacter (Alcaligenes) xylosoxidans*, *Burkholderia cepacia*, fungi including *Candida* and *Aspergillus* species, and nontuberculous mycobacteria.[1] Other organisms may also present chronically or intermittently. Similarly, cultured organisms may represent an initial infection, chronic colonization, or microbial overgrowth in an acute exacerbation.

Gastrointestinal System

GI involvement may present initially as small bowel obstruction shortly after birth due to abnormally thick meconium that cannot be passed (meconium ileus). Older CF patients may develop distal intestinal obstruction syndrome (DIOS), formerly called meconium ileus equivalent, which occurs due to fecal impaction in the terminal ileum and cecum.

Maldigestion due to pancreatic enzyme insufficiency is present in about 85% to 90% of CF patients.[5] Thick pancreatic secretions and cellular debris obstruct the pancreatic ducts and lead to fibrosis. Volume and concentration of pancreatic enzymes and bicarbonate are reduced, leading to maldigestion of fat and protein and subsequent malabsorption of fat-soluble vitamins (A, D, E, and K). Maldigestion is characterized by abdominal distention, steatorrhea, flatulence, and malnourishment despite voracious intake. Maldigestion is progressive and may develop later in a previously pancreatic sufficient patient. Other complications may include gastroesophageal reflux, dysmotility, salivary dysfunction, intussusception, volvulus, atresia, rectal prolapse, and complications related to corrective surgery for meconium ileus.[6]

Hepatobiliary disease occurs due to bile duct obstruction from abnormal bile composition and flow. Hepatomegaly, splenomegaly, and cholecystitis may be present. Hepatic steatosis may also be present due to effects of malnutrition. The progression from cholestasis (impaired bile flow) to portal fibrosis and to focal and multilobar cirrhosis, esophageal varices, and portal hypertension takes several years. Many patients are compensated and asymptomatic but may be susceptible to acute decompensation in the event of extrinsic hepatic insult from viruses, medications, or other factors.[7]

Endocrine System

CF-related diabetes (CFRD) shares characteristics of both type 1 and type 2 diabetes mellitus, but CFRD is categorized separately. Reduced functional pancreatic islet cells and increased islet amyloid deposition results in insulin deficiency, the primary cause of CFRD. Insulin secretion is delayed in response to glucose challenge, and absolute insulin secretion over time is reduced. Some insulin resistance may also be present in CFRD; however, sensitivity may be increased in CF patients without diabetes.[8]

Postprandial hyperglycemia is common, but because some basal insulin secretion is maintained, fasting hyperglycemia is less severe and ketosis is rare.[5] Diet, acute and chronic infection, and corticosteroid use lead to fluctuations in glucose tolerance over time.[8] CFRD is associated with greater nutritional failure, increased pulmonary disease, and earlier death. The average age of onset is 18 to 21 years; but underdiagnosis is thought to be common.

Reproductive System

CF patients often experience delayed puberty. In females, menarche occurs 18 months later than average, and menstrual irregularity is common. Females also have reduced fertility due to increased viscosity of cervical mucus. Due to increasing life expectancy, pregnancy is becoming more common; however, outcomes depend on prepartum nutritional and pulmonary status. Almost all males with CF are azoospermic due to congenital absence of the vas deferens with resultant obstruction; however, conception still occurs occasionally. Conception can also occur through application of assisted reproductive technologies.[9]

Musculoskeletal System

Several factors contribute to development of bone disease in CF: (a) malabsorption of vitamins D and K and calcium; (b) poor nutrition and decreased body mass; (c) physical inactivity; (d) corticosteroid therapy; and (e) delayed puberty.

Chronic pulmonary infection, through release of inflammatory cytokines, can cause increased bone resorption and decreased formation. Osteopenia, osteoporosis, pathological fractures, and kyphosis can then occur.[10] Episodic or chronic arthritis and hypertrophic pulmonary osteoarthropathy may also occur due to immune complex formation in response to chronic inflammation.[11] Digital clubbing is commonly observed and is a marker for hypoxia.

Hematologic System

Anemia may be present in some patients due to impaired erythropoietin regulation, nutritional factors (vitamin E and iron malabsorption), or chronic inflammation. With chronic pulmonary disease, increased cytokine production can lead to shortened red blood cell survival, reduced erythropoietin response, and impaired mobilization of iron stores. Additionally, with chronic hypoxia, normal hemoglobin and hematocrit values may represent relative anemia.[12] Increased red blood cell production is a physiological response to hypoxia; however, this response may be blunted in CF and may result in symptoms of anemia despite normal lab values.

Abnormal bleeding may also be observed as a result of vitamin K malabsorption or antibiotic-associated depletion of GI flora and vitamin K synthesis.

Integumentary System

Abnormally high concentrations of sodium and chloride are found in sweat due to impaired reabsorption within the sweat duct from loss of CFTR channels. Patients are usually asymptomatic (other than a characteristic salty taste to the skin).[2] In rare instances such as hot weather or excessive sweating during physical activity, patients may become dehydrated and experience symptoms of hyponatremia (nausea, headache, lethargy, and confusion).

CLINICAL PRESENTATION AND DIAGNOSIS

Diagnosis

Diagnosis of CF is based on two separate elevated sweat chloride concentrations of 60 mEq/L (60 mmol/L) or greater obtained through pilocarpine iontophoresis (referred to as the "sweat test"). Genetic testing (CFTR mutation analysis) may be performed to confirm the diagnosis, screen in utero, or detect carrier status. More than 70% of diagnoses are made by 12 months of age and almost all are made by age 12. Many states have added CF to their routine newborn screening panels in an effort to identify patients prior to symptom development. This allows for early intervention with CF therapies and improvement in long-term outcomes. A positive newborn screen for CF is not diagnostic (due to false-positive results among CF carriers), nor does a negative screen universally exclude the diagnosis. All "positive screens" are referred to a CF care center for sweat chloride test and genetic evaluation.

Clinical Presentation of CF

General

- CF is usually diagnosed in neonates (due to meconium ileus at birth or newborn screening programs) or during early childhood. Some patients may present much later in life due to less severe symptoms or misdiagnosis

Symptoms

- Pulmonary: chronic cough, sputum production, decreased exercise tolerance, and recurrent respiratory tract infections (pneumonia and sinusitis). Acute infection may be marked by increased cough, changes in sputum (darker and thicker), dyspnea, and fever
- GI: numerous large, foul-smelling loose stools (steatorrhea), flatulence, and abdominal pain. Intestinal obstruction may present as abdominal pain and distention and/or decreased bowel movements
- Nutritional: poor weight gain, voracious appetite, and hunger. Dry skin, skin rash, and visual disturbances may be noted in vitamin deficiency
- CFRD: weight loss, increased thirst, and more frequent urination

Signs

- Obstructive airway disease: tachypnea, dyspnea, cyanosis, wheezes, crackles, sternal retractions, digital clubbing, and barrel chest
- Failure to thrive: despite apparent adequate caloric intake, children may be below age-based normal in both height and weight, and adults may be near/below ideal body weight or have a low BMI
- Salty taste to the skin
- Hepatobiliary disease: asymptomatic or evidenced by hepatomegaly, splenomegaly, or prolonged bleeding
- Recurrent pancreatitis (usually in pancreatic-sufficient patients): episodic epigastric abdominal pain, persistent vomiting, and fever

Laboratory Tests

- WBC with an associated increase in polymorphonuclear (PMN) leukocytes and bands may occur in acute pulmonary infection; however, infection may occur without these laboratory abnormalities
- Maldigestion: decreased serum levels of fat-soluble vitamins (A, D, E, and K). Decreased vitamin K levels may result in elevated prothrombin time (PT) and international normalized ratio (INR)
- Glucose intolerance: blood glucose between 140 and 199 mg/dL (7.77–11.04 mmol/L) 2 hours after an oral glucose-tolerance test
- CFRD: blood glucose 200 mg/dL (11.1 mmol/L) or higher 2 hours after an oral glucose-tolerance test or fasting hyperglycemia (fasting blood glucose 126 mg/dL (6.99 mmol/L) or more regardless of the postglucose challenge level)
- Hepatobiliary disease: serum aspartate aminotransferase, alanine aminotransferase, alkaline phosphatase, γ-glutamyltransferase, and bilirubin may be elevated

Other Tests

- Microbial cultures (sputum, throat, bronchoalveolar lavage, or sinus): isolation of *P. aeruginosa*, *S. aureus*, *S. maltophilia*, and other CF-related organisms
- PFTs: decreased FEV_1, decreased forced vital capacity (FVC), and increased residual volume. Values are typically lower during acute pulmonary exacerbations
- Chest x-ray or chest CT scan: infiltrates, atelectasis, bronchiectasis, and mucus plugging
- Abdominal x-ray or CT scan: if present, intestinal obstruction may be manifested as meconium ileus, DIOS, or intussusception. Rectal prolapse may be noted on physical exam
- Maldigestion: elevated fecal fat content, reduced fecal pancreatic elastase-1 (less than or equal to 200 mcg/g of feces)

Clinical Course and Prognosis

Life expectancy has greatly increased from a predicted survival of 16 years in 1970 to more than 40 years for patients born in the 1990s.[5] The average age of patients in the Cystic Fibrosis Foundation Registry is now more than 16 years, and almost 45% of CF patients in the 2006 Registry annual report are over 18 years old with the oldest being age 78.[13]

The clinical course varies greatly among patients because of the multiple genetic mutations and heterogeneous profile of the ΔF508 mutation. Some patients develop severe lung disease early in childhood and reach end-stage lung disease by their teens, whereas others maintain near-normal lung function into adulthood. Newly diagnosed adults tend to present with chronic respiratory symptoms but usually have milder lung disease, less frequent *Pseudomonas* infection, and less severe pancreatic insufficiency.[5]

Patient Encounter, Part 1

Jessica is an 18-month-old female who is brought to her pediatrician because of difficulty gaining weight. Her mother states that Jessica has had four to five loose stools daily "ever since I can remember." She was previously diagnosed with reflux and milk allergy. Oral ranitidine and elimination of cow's milk-based dairy products have not helped. Jessica is plotted on the growth chart at less than the third percentile for both height and weight. Mom also reports that she has been treated in the emergency department for pneumonia twice since birth. Mom is concerned because her mother's older sister died from some strange "wasting illness" when she was a young child.

What information is consistent with a diagnosis of CF?

What other information would you like to gather?

How would you pursue making the diagnosis of CF?

TREATMENT

Desired Outcomes

Therapeutic outcomes in CF care relate to both chronic and acute treatment goals. With chronic management, the primary goals are to delay disease progression and optimize quality of life. ❸ *Maximizing nutritional status through pancreatic enzyme replacement and vitamin and nutritional supplements is necessary for normal growth and development and for maintaining long-term lung function.* Reduction of airway inflammation and infection and aggressive preventive therapies minimize acute pulmonary exacerbations and delay pulmonary decline. In pulmonary exacerbations, therapy is directed toward reducing acute airway inflammation and obstruction. This is accomplished through more aggressive airway clearance regimens and antibiotic therapy with a goal of returning lung function to pre-exacerbation levels or greater.

Nonpharmacologic Therapy

▶ Airway Clearance Therapy

❹ *Airway clearance therapy is a necessary routine for all CF patients to clear secretions and control infection, even at diagnosis prior to becoming symptomatic.* Waiting until development of a first pneumonia or until daily symptoms are present delays benefits and may contribute to a faster pulmonary decline. The traditional form of chest physiotherapy (CPT) is known as percussion and postural drainage. Areas of the patient's chest, sides, and back are rapidly "clapped" by hand in different patient positions, followed by cough or forced expiration to mobilize secretions. Patients may also be taught autogenic drainage, which consists of deep breathing exercises followed by forced cough.

Several devices are also available to promote airway clearance. Flutter valve devices employ oscillating positive expiratory pressure (OPEP) to cause vibratory airflow obstruction and an internal percussive effect to mobilize secretions. Intrapulmonary percussive ventilation (IPV) provides continuous oscillating pressures during inhalation and exhalation. Finally, the most commonly used technique is high-frequency chest compression (HFCC) with an inflatable vest that provides external oscillation. Vest therapy is often preferred by patients because they can independently perform the therapy even from an early age.[5,14]

If performed appropriately, airway clearance techniques provide similar clearance results, so choice should be based on patient preference and compliance. Airway clearance therapy is typically performed once or twice daily for maintenance care and is increased to three or four times per day for acute exacerbations. Inhaled medications are usually given with the therapies and will be discussed in a later section.

▶ Nutrition

Most CF patients have an increased caloric need due to increased energy expenditure through increased work of breathing, increased basal metabolism, and maldigestion. Prevention of malnutrition requires early patient-specific nutritional intervention. Caloric requirements to promote age-appropriate weight gain or maintenance are typically 110% to 200% of the recommended daily allowance (RDA) for age, gender, and size and increase as disease progresses.[15]

Nutrition in malnourished patients consists of baseline required calories plus additional calories for weight gain. Even with aggressive diet and oral supplements, the caloric requirement may not be achieved, and placement of a gastrostomy or jejunostomy tube to allow for nighttime supplemental feeds may be necessary.[5] Patients with refractory malabsorption, CFRD, and/or tube feedings are especially challenging due to their unique caloric needs. Collaboration with a dietician specially trained in CF nutrition is essential.

Pharmacologic Therapy

▶ Pulmonary System

Treating Obstruction and Inflammation (Table 16–1) Airway clearance therapy is usually accompanied by bronchodilator treatment (albuterol [also known as salbutamol outside the United States] by nebulizer or metered-dose inhaler) to stimulate mucociliary clearance and prevent bronchospasm associated with other inhaled agents.

A mucolytic agent may be administered subsequently to reduce sputum viscosity and enhance clearance. Dornase alfa (Pulmozyme) is a recombinant human (rh) DNase that selectively cleaves extracellular DNA. This DNA is released during neutrophil degradation and contributes to the high viscosity of CF sputum. Nebulization of dornase alfa 2.5 mg once or twice daily improves daily pulmonary symptoms and function, reduces pulmonary exacerbations, and improves quality of life.[16]

Table 16–1

Common Pulmonary Medications in CF

Medication	Pediatric Dose	Adult Dose
Albuterol (salbutamol)	2.5 mg nebulized with chest physiotherapy 2 to 4 times daily; alternatively, two puffs via metered-dose inhaler may be substituted	2.5 mg nebulized with chest physiotherapy 2 to 4 times daily; alternatively, two puffs via metered-dose inhaler may be substituted
Dornase alfa	2.5 mg nebulized once or twice daily	2.5 mg nebulized once or twice daily
Hypertonic saline 7%, 3.5%, or 3%	4 mL nebulized 1–4 times/day	4 mL nebulized 1–4 times/day
Intranasal corticosteroids[a,b]		
Beclomethasone	1–2 sprays each nostril twice daily	1–2 sprays each nostril twice daily
Budesonide	1–2 sprays each nostril daily	2–4 sprays each nostril daily
Flunisolide	1–2 sprays each nostril twice daily	2–4 sprays each nostril twice daily
Fluticasone	1–2 sprays each nostril daily	2 sprays each nostril daily
Mometasone	1 spray each nostril daily	2 sprays each nostril daily or twice daily
Triamcinolone	1 spray each nostril daily	2 sprays each nostril daily or twice daily
Antihistamines[a]		
Azelastine	1 spray each nostril twice daily	2 sprays each nostril twice daily
Cetirizine	2.5–5 mg daily or divided twice daily	5–10 mg daily or divided twice daily
Desloratadine	1–2.5 mg daily	5 mg daily
Fexofenadine	15–30 mg twice daily	60 mg twice daily or 180 mg daily
Levocetirizine	2.5 mg daily	5 mg daily
Loratadine	5–10 mg daily	10 mg daily
Montelukast[a]	4–5 mg daily	10 mg daily
Azithromycin	Body weight 25–39 kg: 250 mg on Mondays, Wednesdays, and Fridays	Body weight 40 kg or more: 500 mg on Mondays, Wednesdays, and Fridays
Ibuprofen[c]	20–30 mg/kg/dose given twice daily	20–30 mg/kg/dose given twice daily

[a]Consult a pediatric dosing reference and/or package insert for more specific age-related recommendations. Each product has different age ranges and dosing recommendations.

[b]Intranasal corticosteroids may be titrated based on response and occasionally exceed labeled dosages for age.

[c]Adjusted to achieve peak plasma concentrations of 50 to 100 mcg/mL (243–485 μmol/L). Maintain chronic dosing with same dosage form and manufacturer. Note that therapy is not always continued into adulthood.

Hypertonic saline for inhalation (Hyper-Sal) 7% or 3.5% is sometimes used as an add-on mucolytic agent or for sputum induction. It must be preceded by a bronchodilator due to a greater incidence of bronchospasm and may not be tolerated by some patients.[17] N-acetylcysteine is another mucolytic agent, but its unpleasant odor and taste limit patient acceptance.[5]

Many patients with CF also have reactive airways or concurrent asthma and benefit from long-acting β_2-agonists.[5] Patients with recurrent wheezing or dyspnea who have demonstrated improvement with albuterol (known as salbutamol outside the United States) should be considered for maintenance therapy, as should patients with bronchodilator-responsive pulmonary function tests (PFTs). Inhaled corticosteroids may also attenuate reactive airways and reduce airway inflammation in some patients; however, clear benefit in CF has not been established.[1,18] Drug delivery to the site of inflammation is limited by the severity of lung disease, which may limit efficacy. Patients on inhaled corticosteroids and/or long-acting β_2-agonists should administer these medications after airway clearance therapies to optimize drug delivery. Montelukast, antihistamines, and/or intranasal steroids are sometimes used for CF patients with reactive airways or allergic rhinitis symptoms.

Long-term systemic corticosteroids have been shown to reduce airway inflammation and improve lung function. However, beneficial effects diminish upon discontinuation, and concern for long-term adverse effects limits their use as maintenance therapy.[18] In clinical practice, systemic corticosteroids may be added for short courses in acute exacerbations or for treatment of allergic response to *Aspergillus* colonization (allergic bronchopulmonary aspergillosis or ABPA); however, dose and duration of therapy should be minimized.[1,19]

High-dose ibuprofen to achieve peak concentrations of 50 to 100 mcg/mL (243–485 μmol/L) has been shown to slow progression of disease, particularly in children 5 to 13 years of age with mild lung disease (FEV$_1$ greater than 60%). At high doses, ibuprofen inhibits the lipoxygenase pathway, reducing neutrophil migration and function as well as release of lysosomal enzymes. At the lower concentrations achieved with analgesic dosing, neutrophil migration increases, potentially increasing inflammation.[20,21] A dose of 20 to 30 mg/kg given twice daily is usually needed to attain target levels, but interpatient variability necessitates serum concentration monitoring.[20] Due to the need for pharmacokinetic monitoring and concerns regarding long-term safety and tolerability, only a few CF centers currently prescribe high-dose ibuprofen.[1,18]

Azithromycin is a macrolide antibiotic commonly used in CF as an anti-inflammatory agent. The exact mechanism for this activity is unclear, but azithromycin has been shown to improve overall lung function. Proposed mechanisms include interference with *Pseudomonas* alginate biofilm production, bactericidal activity during stationary *Pseudomonas* growth, neutrophil inhibition, interleukin-8 reduction, and reduction in sputum viscosity.[22,23] Due to its long tissue half-life, azithromycin is typically dosed 3 days per week (Monday, Wednesday, and Friday), with a dose of 500 mg for patients weighing at least 40 kg and 250 mg for patients weighing 25 to 39 kg. Alternatively, patients may take 500 mg or 250 mg either every day or only Monday through Friday, based on the same weight parameters. To minimize the risk of selecting for macrolide-resistant nontuberculous mycobacteria (a contraindication to chronic azithromycin therapy), patients should have a screening acid-fast bacillus sputum culture obtained prior to initiation and then every 6 months.[18]

Antibiotic Therapy ❺ *Antibiotic therapy is used in three distinct clinical settings within the course of CF: (a) eradication and delay of colonization in early lung disease; (b) suppression of bacterial growth once colonization is present; and (c) reduction of bacterial load in acute exacerbations in an attempt to return lung function to pre-exacerbation levels or greater.*[1] ❻ *Antibiotic selection is based on periodic culture and sensitivity data, typically covering all organisms identified during the preceding year. If no culture data are available, empiric antibiotics should cover the most likely organisms for the patient's age group.* Due to altered pharmacokinetics and microorganism resistance, care must be taken to ensure that optimal doses are prescribed (Table 16–2).

Severity of pulmonary symptoms also guides selection of antibiotic regimens for treatment of acute exacerbations. For recent-onset or mild symptoms, patients may be treated with outpatient oral and inhaled antibiotics for 14 to 21 days. Oral fluoroquinolones are a mainstay among CF patients infected with *P. aeruginosa*, even in children. Despite concerns regarding cartilage and tendon toxicity in young animals, clinical practice has not shown an increased risk in human children.[24] To prevent development of resistance and promote synergy, inhaled tobramycin or colistin is usually added for double coverage.[1,3] Methicillin-sensitive *S. aureus* (MSSA) may be treated with oral amoxicillin-clavulanic acid, dicloxacillin, first- or second-generation cephalosporins, trimethoprim–sulfamethoxazole, or clindamycin, depending on sensitivity. Likewise, methicillin-resistant *S. aureus* (MRSA) may be treated with oral trimethoprim–sulfamethoxazole, clindamycin, minocycline, or linezolid. *H. influenzae* often produces β-lactamases but can usually be treated with amoxicillin–clavulanic acid, a cephalosporin, or trimethoprim–sulfamethoxazole. Oral trimethoprim–sulfamethoxazole or minocycline may be used to treat *S. maltophilia*.

Table 16–2

Antibiotic Dosing in CF[a]

Antibiotic	Pediatric Dose (mg/kg/day)	Adult Maximum Daily Dose	Interval (hours)
Intravenous			
Tobramycin, gentamicin[b]	10	None	8–24
Amikacin[b]	30	None	8–24
Ceftazidime	150	6 g	8
Cefepime	150	6 g	8
Piperacillin–tazobactam	400	16 g	6
Ticarcillin–clavulanate	400–600	12–18 g	4–6
Meropenem	120	6 g	8
Imipenem–cilastatin	100	2 g	6
Aztreonam	200	8 g	6
Ciprofloxacin	30	1.2 g	8–12
Levofloxacin	10–20	750 mg	12–24
Nafcillin	200	12 g	4–6
Vancomycin[b]	40–60	None	6–12
Linezolid	20–30	1.2 g	8–12
Colistin	5–8	480 mg	8
Chloramphenicol[b]	60–80	4 g	6
Oral			
Amoxicillin ± clavulanic acid	45–90	4 g	12
Dicloxacillin	100	2 g	6
Cephalexin	50–100	4 g	6–8
Cefuroxime	30	1 g	12
Trimethoprim–sulfamethoxazole[c]	10–20	1,280 mg	6–12
Clindamycin	30	1.8 g	6–8
Ciprofloxacin	40	2 g	12
Levofloxacin	10–20	750 mg	12–24
Minocycline[d]	4	200 mg	12
Linezolid	20–30	1.2 g	8–12
Inhaled			
Tobramycin	160–600 mg/day	600 mg	12
Colistin	75–150 mg/day	300 mg	12

[a]All doses assume normal renal and hepatic function. Consult a specialized drug reference for dosage adjustment if function is impaired. Dose and/or interval may require adjustment.

[b]Empiric starting doses only. Adjust dose per therapeutic drug monitoring.

[c]Dose based on trimethoprim component.

[d]Children older than 8 years of age.

For more severe infections or patients failing outpatient therapy, IV antibiotic therapy is prescribed for 2 to 3 weeks as inpatient therapy. However, depending on the availability of home health services, some patients may be discharged to finish their course or even receive their entire course at home. ❼ *Typical regimens for severe infections include an antipseudomonal β-lactam plus an aminoglycoside for added synergy and delay of resistance development.*[1,3] Cephalosporins tend to be better tolerated and offer the benefit of administration every 8 hours. Extended-spectrum penicillins have been associated with a higher incidence of allergy. Aztreonam offers the added benefit of little cross-reactivity in penicillin- or cephalosporin-allergic patients; however, it has no gram-positive coverage. Meropenem should be reserved for organisms resistant to all other antibiotics to minimize development of resistance in the carbapenem drug class, as it is the last line of defense against extended-spectrum β-lactamase (ESBL)-producing organisms.

Tobramycin IV is generally the first-line aminoglycoside. Isolates are usually resistant to gentamicin, and amikacin is reserved for tobramycin-resistant strains. Pharmacokinetic goals are listed in Table 16–3. In general, higher peak serum concentrations are targeted to maximize efficacy, whereas lower serum trough levels are targeted to reduce the risk of toxicity. Some centers use once-daily aminoglycoside dosing (tobramycin 10–15 mg/kg/day or amikacin 35 mg/kg/day) to achieve higher peaks and lower troughs. Because aminoglycosides exhibit concentration-dependent killing, once-daily dosing may optimize this effect. However, time below the minimum inhibitory concentration (MIC) is prolonged with once-daily administration in children, possibly leading to loss of synergy for a substantial portion of the dosing interval. Due to a shorter half-life, once-daily aminoglycoside dosing is not optimal for younger children. However, it may be a reasonable option in adults and older teens, in whom the time below the MIC can be minimized. Long-term studies are needed to examine the efficacy and resistance patterns associated with once-daily aminoglycosides in the CF population.[1,3]

Most other serious gram-negative infections are also treated with combination therapy. S. maltophilia is highly resistant and is most often treated with trimethoprim–sulfamethoxazole or ticarcillin–clavulanate. A. xylosoxidans and B. cepacia are also highly resistant and may have minimal therapeutic options. In some cases, fluoroquinolones may be substituted for aminoglycosides based on sensitivity data or if renal dysfunction and/or ototoxicity are present. Due to excellent bioavailability, oral fluoroquinolones, trimethoprim–sulfamethoxazole, minocycline, and linezolid should be used whenever possible. Due to toxicity risk, colistin and chloramphenicol are reserved for life-threatening, highly resistant infections. Additional combinations of two or three drugs may be used for highly resistant organisms based on synergy studies that test susceptibility of different antibiotic combinations.

Inpatient treatment of MRSA can consist of IV vancomycin or oral agents as described above, depending on the severity of infection and concomitant organisms. Vancomycin IV may also be converted to oral step-down therapy upon discharge.

Chronic maintenance antibiotic therapy may be used in patients with Pseudomonas colonization in an attempt to prevent bacterial overgrowth. However, long-term systemic antibiotics are not recommended due to emergence of resistance.[1] Chronic or rotating inhaled-antibiotic maintenance therapy is used for suppressing P. aeruginosa colonization. Inhaled tobramycin (TOBI) is typically administered to patients 6 years of age and older in alternating 28-day cycles of 300 mg nebulized twice daily, followed by a 28-day washout period to minimize development of resistance. Long-term intermittent administration improves pulmonary function, decreases microbial burden, and reduces the need for hospitalization for IV therapy.[25,26] Due to minimal systemic absorption, pharmacokinetic monitoring is not necessary with normal renal function. Lower doses of nebulized tobramycin solution for injection have been used in younger children, and studies are underway using 300 mg twice daily in children under age 6 years. Nebulized colistin using the IV formulation may be an option in patients with tobramycin-resistant strains or intolerance to inhaled tobramycin, but pretreatment with albuterol is necessary due to increased risk of bronchoconstriction.[1,5] Inhaled antibiotics are typically stopped during an acute exacerbation requiring IV therapy. Drug delivery is reduced with increased sputum production, and concomitant use of IV aminoglycosides may increase risk of toxicity.

Pharmacokinetic Considerations ⑧ *CF patients have larger volumes of distribution for many antibiotics due to an increased ratio of lean body mass to total body mass and lower fat stores. CF patients also have an enhanced total body clearance, although the exact mechanism has not been determined.* Increased renal clearance, increased glomerular filtration rate, decreased protein binding, increased tubular secretion, decreased tubular reabsorption, extrarenal

---

Table 16–3

Pharmacokinetic Goals in Cystic Fibrosis

Antibiotic	Traditional Units of Measurement		SI Units of Measurement	
	Goal Peak[a] (mcg/mL)	Goal Trough[b] (mcg/mL)	Goal Peak[a] (μmol/L)	Goal Trough[b] (μmol/L)
Tobramycin, gentamicin	10–12	Less than 1.5	21.4–25.7	Less than 3.2
Amikacin	30–40	Less than 5.0	51.3–68.4	Less than 8.6
Vancomycin	—[c]	10–20	—[c]	7–13.8

[a]Peaks calculated 30 minutes after end of infusion for aminoglycosides. Higher peaks may be targeted with corresponding lower trough concentrations for aminoglycosides based on cystic fibrosis center practice.

[b]Troughs calculated immediately prior to the time the dose is due.

[c]Not routinely measured.

elimination, and increased metabolism have all been proposed as possible reasons for the increased clearance.

Because of these pharmacokinetic changes, higher doses of aminoglycosides are needed to achieve target serum levels and promote adequate tissue penetration. Higher doses of β-lactam antibiotics are also needed to achieve and sustain levels above the MIC. Trimethoprim–sulfamethoxazole displays enhanced renal clearance and hepatic metabolism in the CF population. Fluoroquinolones and vancomycin have fewer pharmacokinetic deviations in the CF population; however, higher doses are typically needed to attain inhibitory serum and tissue concentrations against CF pathogens.[27]

Although most CF patients have shorter half-lives and larger volumes of distribution than non-CF patients, some patients exhibit decreased renal clearance. Reasons may include concomitant use of nephrotoxic medications, presence of diabetic nephropathy, history of transplantation (immunosuppressant use and/or procedural hypoxic injury), age-related decline in renal function in adult patients, and multiple lifetime exposures to aminoglycosides. Evaluation of previous pharmacokinetic parameters and trends, along with incorporation of new health information, is key to appropriate dosing.

▶ Gastrointestinal System

Pancreatic enzyme replacement is the mainstay of GI therapy. Most enzyme products are formulated as capsules containing enteric-coated microspheres or microtablets to avoid inactivation of enzymes by gastric acid; instead, they dissolve in the more alkaline environment of the duodenum. Capsules may be opened and the microbeads swallowed with food (for infants and young children), as long as they are not chewed or mixed with alkaline or hot foods, as enzymes may be denatured. A powder form is available for patients unable to swallow the capsules or microbeads, but bioavailability is poor. While products may contain similar enzyme ratios, they are not bioequivalent and cannot be substituted. Generic enzyme products generally display poor dissolution and should not be used.[5,28] Table 16–4 lists commonly used enzyme replacement products. Note that enzyme formulations are frequently changing due to a newly mandated FDA approval process. Consult a specialized drug reference for updated product availability.

Pancreatic enzymes are initiated at 500 to 1,000 units/kg/meal of lipase component (because fats are the most difficult food components to digest) with half-doses given for snacks. Enzymes should be taken at the beginning or divided throughout the meal and must be given with any fat-containing snack. Infants are typically started at 1,500 to 2,500 units of lipase per 120 mL of formula or breast milk and may require division of capsule contents via visual estimation to obtain appropriate doses. Pancreatic enzymes cannot be placed in formula bottles due to inability to consistently pass through the nipple slit. Instead, enzyme microbeads are placed on a small dot of infant applesauce (or moistened infant rice cereal) and administered via infant spoon with subsequent nursing or bottle-feeding to facilitate swallowing. The oral mucosa must be examined afterward

Table 16–4
Common Pancreatic Enzyme Replacement Products

Trade Name[a]	Lipase (Units)	Amylase (Units)	Protease (Units)
Enteric-Coated			
Creon 6,000	4,000	30,000	19,000
Creon 12,000	12,000	40,000	38,000
Creon 24,000	24,000	120,000	76,000
Pancrease	4,500	20,000	25,000
Pancrease MT 4	4,000	12,000	12,000
Pancrease MT 10	10,000	30,000	30,000
Pancrease MT 16	16,000	48,000	48,000
Pancrease MT 20	20,000	56,000	44,000
Pancrecarb MS-4	4,000	25,500	25,000
Pancrecarb MS-8	8,000	40,000	45,000
Pancrecarb MS-16	16,000	52,000	52,000
Ultrase	4,500	20,000	25,000
Ultrase MT 12	12,000	39,000	39,000
Ultrase MT 18	18,000	58,500	58,500
Ultrase MT 20	20,000	65,000	65,000
NonEnteric Coated			
Viokase 8 tablet	8,000	30,000	30,000
Viokase 16 tablet	16,000	60,000	60,000
Viokase powder (amount per 0.7 g)	16,800	70,000	70,000

[a]The number after a trade name refers to the number of thousands of units of lipase contained per dosage form.

to ensure that all enzymes are swallowed, because remnant microbeads can cause oral erosions (ulcers).

❾ *Titration of pancreatic enzyme doses is based on control of steatorrhea, stool output, and abdominal symptoms.* Infants should have no more than three to four stools per day, whereas older patients should have no more than two to three (children) or one to two (adolescents/adults) well-formed stools per day. Pancreatic enzymes are titrated at 2- to 3-week intervals in increments of 150 to 250 units of lipase/kg/meal (or the next easily administered capsule or half-capsule). Doses up to 2,500 units/kg/meal may be needed, but higher doses should be used with caution due to the risk of fibrosing colonopathy.[5,6,28] Patients who respond poorly to maximal doses of one product may benefit from changing to another product[6] and/or addition of a histamine H_2-receptor antagonist or proton pump inhibitor. Acid suppression may boost effective enzyme dose if duodenal pH is not alkaline enough to neutralize residual gastric acid and dissolve enteric coating as well as treat concomitant gastroesophageal reflux.[5,6,28]

Fat-soluble vitamin supplementation is usually required in pancreatic insufficiency. Specially-formulated products for CF patients (e.g., ADEKs, AquADEKs, SourceCF, and Vitamax) are usually sufficient to attain normal serum vitamin levels at a dose of one tablet daily for younger children and one tablet twice daily for teenagers and adults. Additional supplementation may be needed in uncontrolled malabsorption or for replacement of severe vitamin deficiency.[5,28] Appetite stimulants such as cyproheptadine may be an option for promoting nutrition and weight gain, but efficacy has not been established.

Patient Encounter, Part 2

Laboratory testing confirms the diagnosis of CF, and Jessica has been referred to her regional CF center for treatment. Additional stool studies indicate the presence of severe fat maldigestion. The pulmonologist indicates that she would like to start Jessica (weight 8.2 kg) on pancreatic enzyme replacement therapy.

What formulation and dose would you recommend?

How would you administer the enzymes?

How would you titrate the dose?

Patient Encounter, Part 3

At Jessica's follow-up appointment 1 month later, her weight is up to 8.8 kg. Her mother reports that she seems to have caught a cold and has been coughing quite a bit of late and has not been eating as well as usual. In clinic, the following vitals are noted: respiratory rate 40/min, temperature 38.3°C (100.9°F), and oxygen saturation 92%. The throat culture from her previous visit was positive for *S. aureus* (sensitive to cefazolin, nafcillin, trimethoprim–sulfamethoxazole, clindamycin, vancomycin, doxycycline, and linezolid; resistant to erythromycin) and *P. aeruginosa* (sensitive to ceftazidime, cefepime, piperacillin, aztreonam, meropenem, ciprofloxacin, tobramycin, and amikacin; resistant to gentamicin). She has no drug allergies.

What antibiotic(s) and dose(s) would you recommend for outpatient therapy?

What antibiotic(s) and dose(s) would you recommend for inpatient therapy?

Develop a monitoring plan to assess antibiotic response.

Ursodiol at 15 to 20 mg/kg/day in two divided doses may slow progression of liver disease. It improves bile flow and may displace toxic bile acids that accumulate in a cholestatic liver, stimulate bicarbonate secretion into the bile, offer a cytoprotective effect, and reduce elevated liver tests.[5,7]

Treatment of DIOS consists of oral or nasogastric administration of polyethylene glycol (PEG) electrolyte solutions. Enemas may also be used to facilitate stool clearance, and severe presentations may require surgical resection. IV fluids are often required to correct dehydration due to vomiting or decreased oral intake. Reevaluation of enzyme compliance and dosing is essential to prevent further episodes, and some patients with recurrent symptoms may require daily PEG administration (Miralax).[5]

▶ Endocrine System

Patients with mild CFRD may be managed with carbohydrate modification if their nutritional status is optimal. However, most patients present with poor nutrition and weight loss and require more aggressive treatment. ⑩ *Because CFRD results from insulin insufficiency, exogenous insulin replacement is usually required.* Many patients can be successfully managed by meal coverage with short- or rapid-acting insulin (regular, lispro, or aspart) dosed per carbohydrate counting. Patients with fasting hyperglycemia or patients receiving nighttime tube feedings typically also require longer-acting basal insulin. Regular home glucose monitoring is essential to appropriate therapy. Little information is available regarding use of oral antidiabetic agents in CFRD, and routine use is not recommended.[5,8]

▶ Musculoskeletal System

CF patients with low bone mineral density and low serum vitamin D levels may improve bone health through supplemental vitamin D analogs beyond those found in standard CF vitamins. For ergocalciferol, a minimum of 400 IU and 800 IU should be taken daily by infants and patients over 1 year of age, respectively.[28] Total weekly doses of 12,000 IU for children less than 5 years of age and 50,000 IU for patients 5 years of age and older may be required to achieve target vitamin D concentrations. Supplemental calcium should be provided if 1,300 to 1,500 mg of elemental calcium intake cannot be achieved through diet.[27]

Antiresorptive agents (oral or IV bisphosphonates) may be used to treat adult CF patients with osteoporosis. Remaining upright each day for 30 minutes after dosing may be difficult for patients needing to perform airway clearance therapy, so products offering less frequent dosing should be considered. Gastroesophageal reflux or cirrhosis-associated esophageal varices may also complicate therapy and increase the risk of erosive esophagitis. Pamidronate 30 mg IV every 3 months has increased bone mineral density in adult CF patients, and studies using IV bisphosphonates in children with CF are underway.[29] Androgen replacement in male CF patients with documented hypogonadism may also benefit bone health but should be decided on an individual basis.[10,29]

Short courses of nonsteroidal anti-inflammatory drugs (NSAIDs) can be used to treat CF-related arthritis and hypertrophic pulmonary osteoarthropathy.[5] The impact on neutrophil recruitment in the lung with long-term NSAID therapy at lower analgesic doses is unknown.

▶ Future Therapeutic Directions

Development of new therapies has extended the CF lifespan over the past several decades. Since the discovery of the CF gene and the CFTR protein defect, research has focused on gene therapy to restore normal CFTR function through DNA transfer. Pharmacologic approaches are being investigated to correct dysfunctional CFTR by suppressing premature stop codons in the CFTR gene and to activate alternative chloride channels, effectively bypassing dysfunctional CFTR. Additional research is being conducted with anti-inflammatory therapies, antipseudomonal vaccines, and development of exogenous cationic antimicrobial peptides to mimic those found naturally in the lung.[1] Development of more effective systemic and inhaled antibiotic agents (such

Patient Care and Monitoring

1. Perform a thorough history of prescription, nonprescription, and alternative medications. Assess adherence to the prescribed regimen, including timing of inhaled medications with respect to airway clearance therapies and timing of enzymes and insulin with regard to meals. Is the patient taking any medications not prescribed by the CF center team?

2. Is the patient on all appropriate maintenance medications? Are medications at the appropriate doses for weight and/or age? If the patient is admitted, are maintenance medications ordered?

3. Evaluate the medication regimen for drug interactions, adverse reactions, and allergies.

4. Assess pulmonary symptoms. Review the incidence and quality of cough, dyspnea, respiratory rate, sputum production, and fever. Are the patient's PFTs decreased? Is there an oxygen requirement?

5. Review culture and sensitivity history over the last 1 to 2 years. What antibiotics were used in the past, and did the patient appear to respond better to a particular regimen? Is the patient currently on antibiotics, and if so, are the symptoms improving? Recommend an appropriate antibiotic regimen based on culture and sensitivity data.

6. Review the pharmacokinetic history. Are there any possible changes in clearance since the last antibiotic course? Will the patient be discharged home on IV antibiotics? Can the IV regimen be simplified or made more convenient for home administration? Recommend appropriate doses based on the patient's clearance and an appropriate but convenient schedule.

7. Perform pharmacokinetic adjustments as necessary. Recommend a monitoring plan for the antibiotic course. Are any other laboratory tests necessary? Are signs of toxicity present?

8. Assess nutritional status. Is the patient gaining or maintaining weight according to age? Are any oral supplements or tube feedings being used?

9. Assess GI symptoms. What is the quantity and quality of bowel movements? Does the patient have bloating, flatulence, or abdominal pain?

10. Assess quality-of-life measures such as physical, psychological, and social well-being.

11. Understand that CF therapy is complicated, and recommend regimens to ease the care burden if possible.

12. Educate the patient and family, stressing the importance of adherence to the regimen.

as tobramycin powder for inhalation, aztreonam lysine, and amikacin) continues to be a major focus as well.

OUTCOME EVALUATION

Pulmonary System

- Monitor for changes in pulmonary symptoms such as cough, sputum production, respiratory rate, and oxygen saturation. Symptoms should improve with antibiotics and aggressive airway clearance therapy. PFTs should be markedly increased after 1 week and trend back to pre-exacerbation levels after 2 weeks of therapy. If improvement lags, 3 weeks of therapy may be needed.

- For IV antimicrobial therapy, obtain serum drug levels for aminoglycosides and/or vancomycin and perform pharmacokinetic analysis. Adjust the dose, if needed, according to the parameters in Table 16–3. Obtain follow-up trough levels at weekly intervals or sooner if renal function is unstable. Follow serum creatinine levels if renal function is unstable. Hearing tests may be scheduled yearly or per patient preference.

Gastrointestinal System

- Monitor short- and long-term nutritional status through evaluation of height, weight, and body mass index (BMI). Ideally, parameters should be near the normals for non-CF patients.

- Evaluate the patient's stool patterns. Steatorrhea indicates suboptimal enzyme replacement or noncompliance. Infants should have two to three well-formed stools daily, whereas older children and adults may have one or two stools daily.

- Monitor efficacy of vitamin supplementation through yearly serum vitamin levels. Obtain levels more frequently if an identified deficiency is being treated.

Endocrine System

- Monitor blood glucose several times daily in patients with CFRD or those taking systemic corticosteroids. Follow glycosylated hemoglobin levels on an outpatient basis to assess long-term glucose control. Levels may be falsely low in CF due to a shorter red blood cell half-life.

Abbreviations Introduced in This Chapter

ABPA	Allergic bronchopulmonary aspergillosis
BMI	Body mass index
cAMP	Cyclic 3′,5′-adenosine monophosphate
CF	Cystic fibrosis
CFRD	Cystic fibrosis-related diabetes
CFTR	Cystic fibrosis transmembrane regulator
CPT	Chest physiotherapy
DIOS	Distal intestinal obstruction syndrome
ESBL	Extended-spectrum β-lactamase

FEV$_1$	Forced expiratory volume in 1 second
FVC	Forced vital capacity
HFCC	High-frequency chest compression
INR	International Normalized Ratio
IPV	Intrapulmonary percussive ventilation
MIC	Minimum inhibitory concentration
MRSA	Methicillin-resistant *Staphylococcus aureus*
MSSA	Methicillin-sensitive *S. aureus*
NSAID	Nonsteroidal anti-inflammatory drug
OPEP	Oscillating positive expiratory pressure
PEG	Polyethylene glycol
PFT	Pulmonary function test
PMN	Polymorphonuclear
PT	Prothrombin time
RDA	Recommended daily allowance

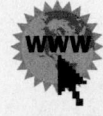 Self-assessment questions and answers are available at http://*www.mhpharmacotherapy. com/pp.html.*

REFERENCES

1. Gibson RL, Burns JL, Ramsey BW. State of the art: Pathophysiology and management of pulmonary infections in cystic fibrosis. Am J Respir Crit Care Med 2003;168:918–951.
2. Rowe SM, Miller SM, Sorscher EJ. Mechanisms of disease: Cystic fibrosis. N Engl J Med 2005;352:1992–2001.
3. Doring G, Conway SP, Heijerman, et al. Antibiotic therapy against pseudomonas aeruginosa in cystic fibrosis: A European consensus. Eur Respir J 2000;16:749–767.
4. Conese M, Copreni E, Di Gioia S, et al. Neutrophil recruitment and airway epithelial cell involvement in chronic cystic fibrosis lung disease. J Cyst Fibros 2003;2:129–135.
5. Yankaskas JR, Marshall BC, Sufian JD, et al. Cystic fibrosis adult care consensus conference report. Chest 2004;125:1S–39S.
6. Littlewood JM, Wolfe SP. Control of malabsorption in cystic fibrosis. Paediatr Drugs 2000;2:205–222.
7. Sokol RJ, Durie PR. Recommendations for management of liver and biliary tract disease in cystic fibrosis. Cystic Fibrosis Foundation Hepatobiliary Disease Consensus Group. J Pediatr Gastroenterol Nutr 1999;28(suppl 1):S1–S13.
8. Moran A, Hardin D, Rodman D, et al. Diagnosis, screening and management of cystic fibrosis related diabetes mellitus: A consensus conference report. Diabetes Res Clin Pract 1999;45:61–73.
9. Phillipson G. Cystic fibrosis and reproduction. Reprod Fertil Dev 1998;10:113–119.
10. Aris RM, Merkel PA, Bachrach LK, et al. Consensus statement: Guide to bone health and disease in cystic fibrosis. J Clin Endocrinol Metab 2005;90:1888–1896.
11. Botton E, Saraux A, Laselve H, et al. Muscular manifestations in cystic fibrosis. Joint Bone Spine 2003; 70:327–335.
12. O'Conner TM, McGrath DS, Short C, et al. Subclinical anaemia of chronic disease in adult patients with cystic fibrosis. J Cyst Fibros 2002;1:31–34.
13. Cystic Fibrosis Foundation. Cystic fibrosis foundation patient registry annual report 2006. Bethesda, MD: Cystic Fibrosis Foundation, 2008.
14. Wagener JS, Headley AA. Cystic fibrosis: Current trends in respiratory care. Respir Care 2003;48:234–245.
15. Stallings VA, Stark LJ, Robinson KA, et al. Evidence-based practice recommendations for nutrition-related management of children and adults with cystic fibrosis and pancreatic insufficiency: Results of a systematic review. J Am Diet Assoc 2008;108:832–839.
16. Fuchs HJ, Borowitz DS, Christiansen DH, et al. Effect of aerosolized recombinant human DNase on exacerbations of respiratory symptoms and on pulmonary function in patients with cystic fibrosis. N Engl J Med 1994;331: 637–642.
17. Elkins MR, Robinson M, Rose BR, et al. A controlled trial of long-term inhaled hypertonic saline in patients with cystic fibrosis. N Engl J Med 2006;354:229–240.
18. Prescott WA, Johnson CE. Antiinflammatory therapies for cystic fibrosis: Past, present, and future. Pharmacotherapy 2005;25(4):555–573.
19. Konstan MW, Davis PB. Pharmacological approaches for the discovery and development of new anti-inflammatory agents for the treatment of cystic fibrosis. Adv Drug Deliv Rev 2002;54:1409–1423.
20. Konstan MW, Byard PJ, Hoppel CL, Davis PB. Effect of high-dose ibuprofen in patients with cystic fibrosis. N Engl J Med 1995;332:848–854.
21. Konstan MW, Krenicky JE, Finney MR, et al. Effect of ibuprofen on neutrophil migration in vivo in cystic fibrosis and healthy subjects. J Pharmacol Exp Ther 2003;306:1086–1091.
22. Equi A Balfour-Lynn IM, Bush A, Rosenthal AB. Long term azithromycin in children with cystic fibrosis: A randomized, placebo-controlled crossover trial. Lancet 2002;360:978–984.
23. Saiman L, Marshall BC, Mayer-Hamblett N, et al. Azithromycin in patients with cystic fibrosis chronically infected with pseudomonas aeruginosa: A randomized controlled trial. JAMA 2003;290:1749–1756.
24. Yee CL, Duffy C, Gerbino PG, et al. Tendon or joint disorders in children after treatment with fluoroquinolones or azithromycin. Pediatr Infect Dis J 2002;21:525–529.
25. Ramsey BW, Pepe MS, Quan JM, et al. Intermittent administration of inhaled tobramycin in patients with cystic fibrosis. N Engl J Med 1999;340:23–30.
26. Moss RB. Long-term benefits of inhaled tobramycin in adolescent patients with cystic fibrosis. Chest 2002;121:55–63.
27. Touw DJ, Vinks AA, Mouton JW, Horrevorts. Pharmacokinetic optimisation of antibacterial treatment in patients with cystic fibrosis: Current practice and suggestions for future directions. Clin Pharmacokinet 1998;35:437–459.
28. Borowitz D, Baker RD, Stallings V. Consensus report on nutrition for pediatric patients with cystic fibrosis. J Pediatr Gastroenterol Nutr 2002;35(3):246–259.
29. Hecker TM, Aris RM. Management of osteoporosis in adults with cystic fibrosis. Drugs 2004;64:133–147.

17 Gastroesophageal Reflux Disease

Dianne B. Williams and Marie A. Chisholm-Burns

LEARNING OBJECTIVES

● **Upon completion of the chapter, the reader will be able to:**

1. Explain the underlying causes of gastroesophageal reflux disease (GERD).

2. Differentiate among typical, atypical, and complicated symptoms of GERD.

3. Determine which diagnostic test should be recommended based on the patient's clinical presentation.

4. Identify the desired therapeutic outcomes for patients with GERD.

5. Recommend appropriate lifestyle modifications and pharmacotherapy interventions for patients with GERD.

6. Discuss other nonpharmacologic interventions that may be appropriate for patients with GERD.

7. Formulate a monitoring plan to assess the effectiveness and safety of pharmacotherapy for GERD.

8. Educate patients on appropriate lifestyle modifications and drug therapy issues, including compliance, adverse effects, and drug interactions.

KEY CONCEPTS

❶ Esophageal gastroesophageal reflux disease (GERD) syndromes can be divided into two distinct categories: (a) symptomatic esophageal syndromes and (b) syndromes associated with esophageal tissue injury.

❷ Patients with GERD may display symptoms described as: (a) typical, (b) atypical, or (c) complicated.

❸ Patients presenting with uncomplicated, typical symptoms of reflux (heartburn and regurgitation) do not usually require invasive esophageal evaluation.

❹ The goals of treatment of GERD are to alleviate symptoms, decrease the frequency of recurrent disease, promote healing of mucosal injury, and prevent complications.

❺ Treatment for GERD involves one or more of the following modalities: (a) patient-specific lifestyle changes and patient-directed therapy; (b) pharmacologic intervention primarily with acid-suppressing agents; (c) antireflux surgery, or (d) endoscopic therapies.

❻ Acid-suppressing therapy is the mainstay of GERD treatment and should be considered for anyone not responding to lifestyle changes and patient-directed therapy after 2 weeks.

❼ Antireflux surgery or endoscopic therapies offer an alternative treatment for refractory GERD or when pharmacologic management is undesirable.

❽ Many patients with GERD experience relapse if medication is withdrawn, and long-term maintenance treatment is required in such patients.

❾ Patient medication profiles should be reviewed for drugs that may aggravate GERD.

INTRODUCTION

Previously, **gastroesophageal reflux disease** (GERD) was defined as symptoms or mucosal damage produced by the abnormal reflux of gastric contents into the esophagus.[1] In late 2008, the American College of Gastroenterology redefined GERD as troublesome symptoms and/or complications caused by refluxing the stomach contents into the esophagus.[2] The key is that these troublesome symptoms adversely affect the well-being of the patient.[2] ❶ *Esophageal GERD syndromes can be divided into two distinct categories: (a) symptomatic (or "symptom-based") esophageal syndromes and (b) syndromes associated with esophageal tissue injury.*[2] Symptomatic esophageal syndrome is associated with severe reflux symptoms with normal endoscopic findings. Erosive **esophagitis**, a syndrome associated with esophageal tissue injury, occurs when the esophagus is repeatedly exposed to refluxed material for prolonged periods (Fig. 17–1). The inflammation that occurs progresses to erosions of the squamous epithelium. Barrett's esophagus is a complication of GERD, characterized by replacement of the normal squamous

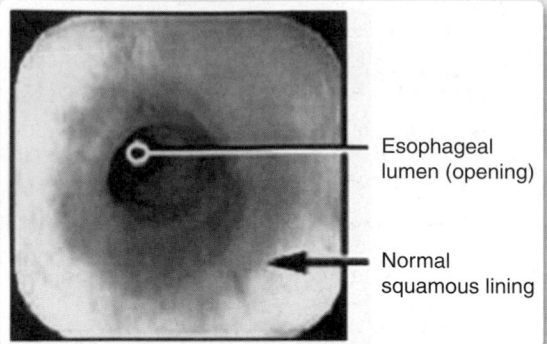
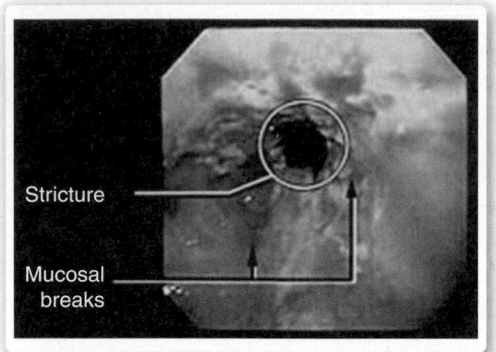

FIGURE 17–1. Endoscopic images of the esophagus. *Left:* Image taken during an endoscopy of the esophagus revealing normal smooth squamous cell lining. *Right:* Narrowed esophageal lumen (stricture) due to chronic GERD with inflammation and scarring. The surrounding esophageal lining has ulcerations and erosions from chronic acid injury. (From Barrett's esophagus website: *http://www.barrettsinfo.com*)

epithelial lining of the esophagus by specialized columnar-type epithelium. Barrett's esophagus is more likely to occur in patients with a long history (years) of symptomatic reflux and may be a risk factor for developing adenocarcinoma of the esophagus.

EPIDEMIOLOGY AND ETIOLOGY

GERD is prevalent in patients of all ages and appears to be increasing in both adults and children. The prevalence of GERD in Western countries is approximately 10% to 20%.[3] Although mortality associated with GERD is rare, symptoms can significantly decrease quality of life. The true prevalence and incidence of GERD are unknown because: (a) many patients do not seek medical treatment, (b) symptoms do not always correlate well with disease severity, and (c) there is no gold standard for diagnosing the disease. The prevalence of erosive esophagitis increases in adults older than 40 years. There does not appear to be a major gender difference in incidence except for its association with pregnancy. Gender is an important factor in the development of Barrett's esophagus that occurs more frequently in males.

PATHOPHYSIOLOGY

The retrograde movement of acid or other noxious substances from the stomach into the esophagus is a major factor in the development of GERD.[4] Commonly, gastroesophageal reflux is associated with defective lower esophageal sphincter (LES) pressure or function. Problems with other normal mucosal defense mechanisms such as anatomic factors, esophageal clearance, mucosal resistance, gastric emptying, epidermal growth factor, and salivary buffering may also contribute to the development of GERD. Other factors that may promote esophageal damage upon reflux into the esophagus include gastric acid, pepsin, bile acids, and pancreatic enzymes. Therapeutic regimens for GERD are designed to maximize normal mucosal defense mechanisms and attenuate these other factors that contribute to the disease.

LES Pressure

The LES is a manometrically defined zone of the distal esophagus with an elevated basal resting pressure. The sphincter is normally in a tonic, contracted state, preventing the reflux of gastric material from the stomach. It relaxes on swallowing to permit the free passage of food into the stomach.

Mechanisms by which defective LES pressure may cause gastroesophageal reflux are threefold. First, and probably most important, reflux may occur after spontaneous transient LES relaxations that are not associated with swallowing.[5] Esophageal distention, vomiting, belching, and retching can cause relaxation of the LES. These transient relaxations may play an important role in intermittent nonerosive reflux.[6] Transient decreases in sphincter pressure are responsible for approximately 65% of the reflux episodes in patients with GERD.

Second, reflux may occur after transient increases in intra-abdominal pressure (stress reflux).[4] An increase in intra-abdominal pressure such as that occurring during straining, bending over, or a Valsalva maneuver may overcome a weak LES, and thus may lead to reflux.

Third, the LES may be atonic, thus permitting free reflux. Although transient relaxations are more likely to occur when there is normal LES pressure, the latter two mechanisms are more likely when the LES pressure is decreased by such factors as fatty foods, gastric distention, or smoking.[4] Certain foods and medications may worsen esophageal reflux by decreasing LES pressure or by irritating the esophageal mucosa (Table 17–1).[7]

Anatomic Factors

Disruption of the normal anatomic barriers by a hiatal hernia was once thought to be a primary etiology of gastroesophageal reflux and esophagitis. Currently, the presence of a hiatal hernia is generally considered to be a separate entity that may or may not be associated with reflux.

Esophageal Clearance

Many patients with GERD produce normal amounts of acid, but the acid produced spends too much time in contact with

Table 17–1

Foods and Medications That May Worsen GERD Symptoms

Decreased LES Pressure

Foods

Fatty meal	Coffee, cola, tea
Carminatives (peppermint, spearmint)	Garlic
	Onions
Chocolate	Chili peppers

Medications

Anticholinergics	Isoproterenol
Barbiturates	Narcotics (meperidine, morphine)
Benzodiazepines (e.g., diazepam)	
Caffeine	Nicotine (smoking)
Dihydropyridine calcium channel blockers	Nitrates
	Phentolamine
Dopamine	Progesterone
Estrogen	Theophylline
Ethanol	

Direct Irritants to the Esophageal Mucosa

Foods

Spicy foods	Tomato juice
Orange juice	Coffee

Medications

Alendronate	NSAIDs
Aspirin	Quinidine
Iron	Potassium chloride

GERD, gastroesophageal reflux disease; LES, lower esophageal sphincter; NSAIDs, nonsteroidal anti-inflammatory drugs.

Adapted from Williams DB, Schade RR. Gastroesophageal reflux disease. In: DiPiro JT, Talbert RL, Yee GC, et al., eds. Pharmacotherapy: A Pathophysiologic Approach, 7th ed. New York: McGraw-Hill, 2008: 556, with permission.

the esophageal mucosa. The contact time is dependent on the rate at which the esophagus clears the noxious material, as well as the frequency of reflux. The esophagus is cleared by primary peristalsis in response to swallowing, or by secondary peristalsis in response to esophageal distention and gravitational effects.

Swallowing contributes to esophageal clearance by increasing salivary flow. Saliva contains bicarbonate that buffers the residual gastric material on the surface of the esophagus. The production of saliva decreases with increasing age, making it more difficult to maintain a neutral intraesophageal pH. Therefore, esophageal damage due to reflux occurs more often in the elderly and patients with Sjögren's syndrome or xerostomia. Swallowing is also decreased during sleep, which contributes to nocturnal GERD in some patients.

Mucosal Resistance

The esophageal mucosa and submucosa consist of mucus-secreting glands that contain bicarbonate. Bicarbonate moving from the blood to the lumen can neutralize acidic refluxate in the esophagus. A decrease in this normal defense mechanism can potentially lead to erosions in the esophagus. When the mucosa is repeatedly exposed to the refluxate in

GERD, or if there is a defect in the normal mucosal defenses, hydrogen ions diffuse into the mucosa, leading to the cellular acidification and necrosis that ultimately cause esophagitis.[4]

Gastric Emptying

Gastric volume is related to the amount of material ingested, rate of gastric secretion, rate of gastric emptying, and amount and frequency of duodenal reflux into the stomach. Delayed gastric emptying can lead to increased gastric volume and can contribute to reflux. Factors that increase gastric volume and/or decrease gastric emptying, such as smoking and high-fat meals, are often associated with gastroesophageal reflux. This partially explains the prevalence of postprandial gastroesophageal reflux.

Composition of Refluxate

The composition, pH, and volume of the refluxate are other factors associated with gastroesophageal reflux. Duodeno-gastric reflux esophagitis or "alkaline esophagitis" refers to esophagitis induced by the reflux of bilious and pancreatic fluid. Although bile acids have both a direct irritant effect on the esophageal mucosa and an indirect effect of increasing hydrogen ion permeability of the mucosa, symptoms are more often related to acid reflux than to bile reflux. The percentage of time that esophageal pH is below 4 is greater for patients with severe disease than for those with mild disease.

The pathophysiology of GERD is a complex process. It is difficult to determine which occurs first: gastroesophageal reflux leading to defective peristalsis with delayed clearing or an incompetent LES pressure leading to gastroesophageal reflux. Understanding factors associated with the development of GERD is essential to providing effective treatment (Fig. 17–2).

CLINICAL PRESENTATION AND DIAGNOSIS

❷ *Patients with GERD may display symptoms described as: (a) typical, (b) atypical, or (c) complicated (see Clinical Presentation box).*[8]

Diagnosis of GERD

The most useful tool in the diagnosis of GERD is the clinical history, including both the presenting symptoms and associated risk factors. ❸ *Patients presenting with uncomplicated, typical symptoms of reflux (heartburn and regurgitation) do not usually require invasive esophageal evaluation.* These patients generally benefit from a trial of patient-specific lifestyle modifications and empiric acid-suppressing therapy.[1] A clinical diagnosis of GERD is assumed in those responding to appropriate therapy.

Endoscopy with biopsy is the preferred diagnostic test for assessing the mucosa for esophagitis and Barrett's esophagus. It should also be performed in patients with troublesome dysphagia, weight loss, or epigastric mass and

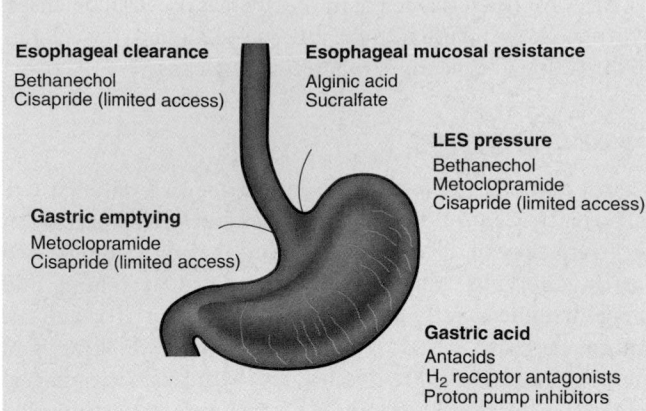

FIGURE 17–2. Therapeutic interventions in the management of gastroesophageal reflux disease. Pharmacologic interventions are targeted at improving defense mechanisms or decreasing aggressive factors. LES, lower esophageal sphincter. (Adapted with permission from Williams DB, Schade RR. Gastroesophageal reflux disease. In: DiPiro JT, Talbert RL, Yee GC, et al., eds. Pharmacotherapy: A Pathophysiologic Approach, 7th ed. New York: McGraw-Hill, 2008: 559.)

Patient Encounter, Part 1

A 42-year-old man with a history of diabetes and hypertension presents complaining of "heartburn." He reports a burning sensation in his upper chest and some regurgitation of sour-tasting material into his throat. The symptoms began about 1 month ago, occur about twice a week, and are associated with heavy meals and lying down after eating. He says that he smokes about one pack of cigarettes per day and drinks coffee and alcohol-containing beverages on most days. His weight is 116 kg (255 lb).

What information is suggestive of GERD?

Does he have any factors contributing to GERD?

What additional information do you need before creating a treatment plan for this patient?

Clinical Presentation of GERD

- Heartburn is the hallmark symptom of GERD and is described as a substernal sensation of warmth or burning rising up from the abdomen that may radiate to the neck. It may be waxing and waning in character.
- Regurgitation is common.
- Symptoms may be worse after a fatty meal, when bending over, or when lying in a recumbent position.[1]
- Hypersalivation and belching.

Atypical Symptoms

- Asthma, chronic cough, hoarseness, pharyngitis, chest pain, and dental erosions.
- It is important to distinguish GERD symptoms from those of other diseases, especially when chest pain or pulmonary symptoms are present.

Complicated Symptoms

- Continual pain, dysphagia (difficulty swallowing), odynophagia (painful swallowing), bleeding, unexplained weight loss, unexplained anemia, and choking.
- These symptoms may be indicative of complications of GERD such as Barrett's esophagus, esophageal strictures (Fig. 17–1), or esophageal cancer.

in patients with esophageal GERD syndrome who have not responded to an empiric trial of twice-daily proton pump inhibitor (PPI) therapy.[2] While controversial, some feel that screening for Barrett's esophagus should be performed in patients more than 50 years of age and those with longstanding heartburn.

Newer technology involves a camera-containing capsule swallowed by the patient, which can perform noninvasive endoscopy but cannot adequately assess for Barrett's esophagus. The procedure can be performed in the practitioner's office in approximately 15 minutes.

Patients with esophageal GERD syndromes who have failed twice-daily PPI therapy and have normal findings on endoscopy may benefit from manometry. Manometry helps to localize the LES for ambulatory pH monitoring, evaluates peristaltic function in patients considering surgery, and identifies possible motor disorders.[2]

Ambulatory pH monitoring objectively proves that symptoms are reflux related in patients with esophageal GERD syndromes not responding to twice-daily PPI therapy. Impedance monitoring allows reflux episodes to be characterized as acid or nonacid.[9] This method may be useful in patients with refractory symptoms. Duodenogastroesophageal reflux monitoring may be useful in identifying nonacid reflux (e.g., bile reflux), especially in patients not responding to twice-daily PPI therapy. It is preferable that PPI therapy be held for 7 days prior to ambulatory impedance pH, catheter pH, or wireless pH monitoring for best results.[2]

TREATMENT

Desired Outcomes

❹ *The goals of treatment of GERD are to alleviate symptoms, decrease the frequency of recurrent disease, promote healing*

Patient Encounter, Part 2: Medical History, Physical Exam, and Diagnostic Tests

PMH: Type-2 diabetes mellitus since age 36, it is often not well controlled because of poor patient compliance; hypertension × 3 years, currently controlled; history of hepatitis B

FH: Father died of MI at the age of 68, mother is still alive with history of colon cancer and diabetes

SH: Works as a laborer in a warehouse, drinks alcohol most days but denies any alcohol-related problems

Meds: Metformin 1,000 mg orally twice daily; hydrochlorothiazide 25 mg orally once daily; nifedipine XL 60 mg orally once daily; regular insulin 4 units subcutaneously 3 times daily with meals; insulin glargine 20 units subcutaneously at bedtime

ROS: (+) Heartburn, regurgitation; (–) chest pain, nausea, vomiting, diarrhea, weight loss, change in appetite, shortness of breath or cough, difficulty or painful swallowing

PE:

VS: BP 134/84 mm Hg, P 82 bpm, RR 16 per minute, T 37°C (98.6°F)

CV: RRR, normal S_1, S_2; no murmurs, rubs, or gallops

Abd: Soft, nontender, nondistended; (+) bowel sounds, (–) hepatosplenomegaly, heme (–) stool

Given this additional information, what findings are consistent with a diagnosis of GERD?

Could any of the medications listed aggravate GERD symptoms in this patient?

Identify your treatment goals for this patient.

What nonpharmacologic and pharmacologic options are feasible for this patient?

of mucosal injury, and prevent complications. Inadequate treatment and consequent long-term acid exposure may lead to complications such as Barrett's esophagus, which may be an independent risk factor for esophageal adenocarcinoma.[10]

General Approach to Treatment

5 *Treatment for GERD involves one or more of the following modalities: (a) lifestyle changes and patient-directed therapy; (b) pharmacologic intervention primarily with acid-suppressing agents; (c) antireflux surgery; or (d) endoscopic therapies.* The first therapeutic option used depends upon the patient's condition (i.e., frequency of symptoms, degree of esophagitis, and presence of complications; Table 17–2).

6 *Acid-suppressing therapy is the mainstay of GERD treatment and should be considered for anyone not responding to patient-specific lifestyle changes and patient-directed therapy after 2 weeks.* The PPIs provide the greatest relief of symptoms and highest rates of healing, especially in patients with erosive disease or moderate to severe symptoms.

Maintenance therapy is generally necessary to control symptoms and prevent complications. GERD that is refractory to adequate acid suppression is rare. In these cases, the diagnosis should be confirmed through further diagnostic tests before long-term, high-dose therapy or antireflux surgery or endoscopic therapies are considered.[1]

Nonpharmacologic Therapy

Nonpharmacologic treatment of GERD includes patient-specific lifestyle modifications, antireflux surgery, or endoscopic therapies.

▶ Lifestyle Modifications

Although most patients do not respond to lifestyle changes alone, the importance of maintaining these lifestyle changes throughout the course of GERD therapy should be stressed to selected patients on a routine basis. The most common lifestyle changes that a patient should be educated about include: (a) losing weight and (b) elevating the head of the bed if symptoms are worse when recumbent. Elevating the head of the bed about 6 to 10 in. (15–25 cm) with an undermattress foam wedge (not just elevating the head with pillows) decreases nocturnal esophageal acid contact time and should be recommended.[4]

Other lifestyle modifications should be considered based on the circumstances of the individual patient. These include: (a) eating smaller meals and avoiding meals 3 hours before sleeping, (b) avoiding foods or medications that exacerbate GERD, (c) smoking cessation, and (d) avoiding alcohol.

Patient medications and food histories should be evaluated to identify potential factors that may exacerbate GERD symptoms (see Table 17–1).[7,11,12] Patients should be monitored closely for symptoms when medications known to worsen GERD are started.

▶ Antireflux Surgery and Endoscopic Therapies

7 *Antireflux surgery or endoscopic therapies offer alternative treatments for refractory GERD or when pharmacologic management is undesirable.*

Antireflux Surgery Surgical intervention is a viable alternative for selected patients with well-documented GERD.[1] The goal of surgery is to re-establish the antireflux barrier, to position the LES within the abdomen where it is under positive (intra-abdominal) pressure, and to close any associated hiatal defect.[13] It should be considered in patients who: (a) fail to respond to pharmacologic treatment; (b) opt for surgery despite successful treatment because of lifestyle considerations including age, time, or expense of medications; (c) have complications of GERD (Barrett's

Table 17–2

Therapeutic Approach to GERD in Adults

Patient Presentation	Recommended Treatment Regimen	Comments

Intermittent, mild heartburn	A. Lifestyle modifications based on patient-specific circumstances
	PLUS
	B. Antacids
	• Magnesium/aluminum hydroxide 30 mL after meals and at bedtime as needed
	• Antacid/alginic acid (Gaviscon) 2 tablets or 15 mL after meals and at bedtime
	AND/OR
	C. Patient-directed therapy
	• Over-the-counter H₂RAs (each taken up to twice daily)
	    Cimetidine 200 mg
	    Famotidine 10 mg
	    Nizatidine 75 mg
	    Ranitidine 75 mg
	OR
	• Over-the-counter PPI (taken once daily)
	    Omeprazole 20 mg
		• If symptoms are unrelieved with lifestyle changes and over-the-counter medications after 2 weeks, begin therapy with a standard dose acid-suppressing agent
		• Aluminum-containing antacids may accumulate in renal failure. May need to decrease dose or avoid
		• Calcium-containing antacids may need to be decreased in patients with CrCl less than 25 mL/min (based on serum calcium level)
		• In general, give 50% of H₂RA dose with CrCl less than 50 mL/min

Symptomatic GERD	A. Lifestyle modifications based on patient-specific circumstances
	PLUS
	B. Standard dose acid-suppressing therapy
	• H₂RAs (taken twice daily) for 6 to 12 weeks
	    Cimetidine 400 mg
	    Famotidine 20 mg
	    Nizatidine 150 mg
	    Ranitidine 150 mg
	
	OR
	• PPIs (taken once daily) for 4 to 8 weeks; increase to twice daily in patients with inadequate symptom response to once daily therapy.
	    Dexlansoprazole 30 mg
	    Esomeprazole 20 mg
	    Lansoprazole 15 to 30 mg
	    Omeprazole 20 mg
	    Pantoprazole 40 mg
	    Rabeprazole 20 mg
		• For typical symptoms, treat empirically with standard doses of acid-suppressing therapy
		• Mild GERD can usually be treated effectively with H₂RAs. Patients with moderate-to-severe symptoms should receive a PPI as initial therapy. If symptoms are relieved, treat recurrences on an as-needed basis
		• If symptoms recur frequently, consider maintenance therapy with the lowest effective dose
		• Most patients require standard doses for maintenance therapy
		• May need to decrease dose of omeprazole, esomeprazole, and lansoprazole with severe liver impairment. No specific recommendations available. No adjustment needed for pantoprazole

Healing of erosive esophagitis or treatment of moderate to severe symptoms or complications	A. Lifestyle modifications
	PLUS
	B. PPIs (taken once or twice daily) for 4 to 16 weeks
	    Dexlansoprazole 60 mg
	    Esomeprazole 20 to 40 mg
	    Lansoprazole 30 mg
	    Omeprazole 20 mg
	    Rabeprazole 20 mg
	    Pantoprazole 40 mg
		• For atypical symptoms, give a trial of a PPI or H₂RA
		• If symptoms are relieved, consider maintenance therapy
		• PPIs are the most effective maintenance therapy in patients with atypical symptoms, complicated symptoms, or erosive disease
		• Patients not responding to acid-suppressing therapy, including those with persistent atypical symptoms, may be candidates for antireflux surgery or endoscopic therapies

GERD, gastroesophageal reflux disease; H₂RA, histamine₂-receptor antagonist; PPI, proton pump inhibitor.

Adapted from Williams DB, Schade RR. Gastroesophageal reflux disease. In: DiPiro JT, Talbert RL, Yee GC, et al., eds. Pharmacotherapy: A Pathophysiologic Approach, 7th ed. New York: McGraw-Hill. 2008: 560, with permission.

esophagus or strictures); or (d) have atypical symptoms and reflux documented on 24-hour ambulatory pH monitoring.[13] In the latter situation, the benefits of surgery must be carefully weighed against the risks including flatulence, inability to belch, and postsurgery bowel symptoms.[2]

Unfortunately, up to 60% of patients still require use of antireflux medications approximately 10 years postsurgery, and surgery is not superior to PPIs in terms of esophagitis grade, complications, or quality of life with long-term follow-up.[14]

● **Endoscopic Therapies** Three endoscopic approaches to the management of GERD are available.[15] They include: (a) application of radiofrequency energy to the LES area (**Stretta procedure**), (b) endoscopic suturing to produce a plication (**Endocinch**), and (c) endoscopic injection of a biopolymer at the gastroesophageal junction.[1] More studies and experience are needed to determine their exact role in the management of GERD. They cannot currently be recommended for routine use in patients with esophageal GERD syndromes.[2]

Pharmacologic Therapy

▶ Antacids and Antacid–Alginic Acid Products

Antacids are an appropriate component of treating mild GERD as they are clearly effective for immediate, symptomatic relief. They are often used concurrently with other acid-suppressing therapies.

An antacid product combined with alginic acid (Gaviscon) is not a potent neutralizing agent but forms a highly viscous solution that floats on the surface of the gastric contents. This viscous solution serves as a protective barrier for the esophagus against reflux of gastric contents. It also reduces the frequency of the reflux episodes.[16]

Dosage recommendations for antacids vary and range from hourly dosing to administration on an as-needed basis. In general, antacids have a short duration of action, which requires frequent administration throughout the day to provide continuous acid neutralization.

Antacids also have clinically significant drug interactions with ferrous sulfate, isoniazid, sulfonylureas, and quinolone antibiotics. Antacid–drug interactions are influenced by antacid composition, dose, dosage schedule, and formulation.

▶ Histamine₂-Receptor Antagonists

The histamine$_2$-receptor antagonists (H$_2$RAs)—cimetidine, famotidine, nizatidine, and ranitidine—decrease acid secretion by inhibiting the histamine$_2$-receptors in gastric parietal cells. When given in divided doses, they are effective for patients with mild to moderate GERD.[1] Standard doses provide symptomatic improvement in about 60% of patients after 12 weeks of therapy.[1] Healing rates per endoscopy tend to be lower (50%).[1] Response to the H$_2$RAs is dependent on: (a) the severity of disease, (b) the dosage regimen used, and (c) the duration of therapy.

For symptomatic relief of mild GERD, low-dose, nonprescription H$_2$RAs may be beneficial. For patients not responding to patient-directed therapy with over-the-counter agents after 2 weeks, standard-dose acid-suppressing therapy is warranted. Although higher doses of H$_2$RAs may provide greater symptomatic and endoscopic healing rates, limited information exists regarding the safety of these regimens and they can be less effective and more costly than once-daily PPIs.

Because all H$_2$RAs have similar efficacy, selection of the specific agent should be based on factors such as differences in dosage regimen, safety profile, and cost. In general, H$_2$RAs are well tolerated. Patients should be monitored for adverse effects and potential drug interactions. Cimetidine may inhibit the metabolism of certain medications such as theophylline, warfarin, or phenytoin. An alternate H$_2$RA should be selected if the patient is taking any of these medications.

▶ Proton Pump Inhibitors

The PPIs—esomeprazole, lansoprazole, omeprazole, pantoprazole, rabeprazole, and dexlansoprazole—block gastric acid secretion by inhibiting gastric H$^+$/K$^+$-adenosine triphosphatase in gastric parietal cells.[17] This produces a profound, long-lasting antisecretory effect capable of maintaining the gastric pH above 4, even during acid surges seen postprandially.[4,6]

The PPIs are superior to H$_2$RAs in patients with moderate-to-severe GERD. This includes not only patients with erosive esophagitis or complicated symptoms (Barrett's esophagus or strictures) but also those with symptomatic esophageal syndromes. Symptomatic relief is seen in approximately 83% of patients, and healing rates at 8 weeks as judged by endoscopy are 78%.[1]

A PPI should be given empirically to patients with troublesome symptoms of GERD. If the standard once-daily course of therapy is not effective in eliminating symptoms, then empiric therapy with twice-daily dosing should be given. Patients not responding to twice-daily PPI therapy should be considered treatment failures and further diagnostic evaluation should be performed.[2]

Whether PPIs can reverse Barrett's esophagus remains a topic for debate. The use of high-dose omeprazole (40 mg twice daily) caused partial regression of Barrett's esophagitis, but no change was noted in patients receiving ranitidine 150 mg twice daily.[17] Others propose that islands of normal squamous cells that appear in patients with Barrett's esophagus after high-dose PPIs may be covering gastric mucosa and may mask the development of cancerous changes in the mucosa.[18] It is unknown whether regression of Barrett's esophagus reduces the risk of adenocarcinoma, but aggressive therapy to suppress acid reflux early in the disease may help prevent Barrett's esophagus.

Comparable daily doses of PPIs are omeprazole 20 mg = esomeprazole 20 mg = lansoprazole 30 mg = dexlansoprazole 30 mg = rabeprazole 20 mg = pantoprazole 40 mg. The PPIs degrade in acidic environments and are therefore formulated in delayed-release capsules or tablets.[19] Lansoprazole, esomeprazole, and omeprazole contain enteric-coated (pH-sensitive) granules in a capsule form. For patients unable to swallow the capsule or in pediatric patients, the contents of the capsule can be mixed in applesauce or placed in orange juice. Lansoprazole is also available in a packet for oral suspension and a delayed-release orally disintegrating tablet. Patients taking pantoprazole or rabeprazole should be instructed not to crush, chew, or split the delayed-release tablets.

Omeprazole is also available in an immediate-release formulation combined with sodium bicarbonate (Zegerid). The proposed benefit of this combination product is fast onset of action and increase in pH by the sodium bicarbonate, which helps prevent degradation of omeprazole in the stomach. Sodium bicarbonate may also stimulate gastrin production, which may activate the proton pumps and optimize the effectiveness of omeprazole.

Pantoprazole and esomeprazole are available in IV formulations that offer an alternative route for patients unable to take oral medications. The IV product is not more effective than the oral forms and is significantly more expensive.

Patients should be instructed to take their PPI in the morning, 15 to 30 minutes before breakfast to maximize efficacy, because these agents inhibit only actively secreting proton pumps.[6,20] While usually given prior to breakfast, patients with night-time symptoms may benefit from taking their PPI prior to the evening meal.[1] If a second dose is needed, it should be administered before the evening meal and not at bedtime.[1] Regardless of the time of day, PPIs should be given prior to a meal to gain the most benefit. The exception to this is the immediate-release omeprazole–sodium bicarbonate combination product, which can be given at bedtime.

The PPIs are generally well tolerated, and the choice of a particular agent is often based on cost and tolerability. The most common side effects are headache, diarrhea, constipation, and abdominal pain. All PPIs can decrease the absorption of drugs (e.g., ketoconazole) that require an acidic environment to be absorbed. All PPIs are metabolized by the cytochrome P-450 system to some extent. Omeprazole and lansoprazole are metabolized by CYP2C19 enzymes. Concerns have been raised in patients taking PPIs concurrently with clopidogrel, a prodrug, that must be converted to its active form by CYP2C19. Inhibition of CYP2C19 by PPIs has been suggested to decrease the effectiveness of clopidogrel and increase the risk of cardiac events. More study is needed to determine this effect. No interactions with lansoprazole, pantoprazole, or rabeprazole have been seen with CYP2C19 substrates such as diazepam, warfarin, or phenytoin.[21] Esomeprazole does not appear to interact with warfarin or phenytoin. Pantoprazole is metabolized by a cytosolic sulfotransferase and is therefore less likely to have significant drug interactions than other PPIs.[20]

While generally not of major concern, omeprazole may inhibit the metabolism of warfarin, diazepam, and phenytoin; lansoprazole may decrease theophylline concentrations. Drug interactions with omeprazole are of particular concern in patients who are considered "slow metabolizers," as are approximately 3% of the Caucasian population. Unfortunately, it is unclear which patients have the polymorphic gene variation that makes them slow metabolizers.[20] Alternatively, patients who are considered rapid metabolizers, which is most common in the Asian population (12–20%), may not respond as well as those who are considered slow metabolizers.[22,23] This genetic variation among patients may alter the effect of PPIs due to the ability of their enzyme system to metabolize the drug.[22] Esomeprazole is metabolized more by CYP3A4 enzymes and may be affected less by the patient's genotype.[24] Patients on potentially interacting drugs should be monitored for development of drug-related problems.

Other potential concerns with PPIs include hypergastrinemia, vitamin B_{12} deficiency, and risk for enteric infections or fractures. Prolonged hypergastrinemia leading to the development of colonic polyps and potentially adenocarcinoma in rats was a concern that has proven to be unfounded with long-term use in humans.[25] The FDA has stated that there is insufficient evidence linking PPI use to atrophic gastritis, intestinal metaplasia, or gastric cancer.[26] PPIs may inhibit the secretion of intrinsic factor by the parietal cells, which may lead to decreased absorption of vitamin B_{12} with subsequent deficiency. Patients receiving long-term PPI therapy should have periodic complete blood counts performed to detect signs of vitamin B_{12} deficiency. More recently, concerns include risk of enteric infections and risk of fractures with long-term use of PPIs. Although the incidence is low, further evaluation is needed to adequately quantify the risk of developing these effects. Routine bone density studies or calcium supplementation is not warranted based on PPI use alone.[2]

▶ Prokinetic Agents

The prokinetic agents include cisapride, metoclopramide, and bethanechol. The inferior efficacy and side-effect profiles of metoclopramide and bethanechol limit their use in the treatment of GERD, and they are not recommended.

▶ Mucosal Protectants

Sucralfate, a nonabsorbable aluminum salt of sucrose octasulfate, has very limited value in the treatment of GERD and is not recommended.

Combination Therapy

Two agents of different therapeutic classes should not be used routinely. Only modest improvements have been shown when a prokinetic agent is combined with a standard dose of an H_2RA. Therefore, patients not responding to standard H_2RA doses should be switched to a PPI instead of adding a prokinetic agent. Monotherapy with a PPI is not only more effective, but it also improves compliance with once-daily dosing and is ultimately more cost effective.

The addition of an H_2RA at bedtime to PPI therapy has been suggested to decrease nocturnal acid breakthrough. While there may be an immediate effect to control symptoms and keep the pH greater than 4, tachyphylaxis may develop within 1 week. If H_2RAs are used at night, it may be preferable to only use them as needed to provide a "drug holiday" that may lessen the occurrence of tachyphylaxis.[27] Immediate-release omeprazole–sodium bicarbonate has been shown to decrease nocturnal acid exposure compared with pantoprazole administered daily with the evening meal and lansoprazole administered at bedtime. Although more studies are needed, immediate-release omeprazole may offer an effective option for controlling nocturnal acid exposure and symptoms.

Maintenance Therapy

❽ *Many patients with GERD experience relapse if medication is withdrawn, and long-term maintenance treatment is required in such patients.*[1] Candidates for maintenance therapy include patients whose symptoms return once therapy is discontinued or decreased, patients with a history of esophagitis healed by PPIs, patients with complications such as Barrett's esophagus or strictures, and perhaps patients with atypical symptoms. In some patients, the dose of acid-suppressing therapy may be titrated to the lowest dose that controls symptoms.[2]

The goal of maintenance therapy is to improve quality of life by controlling symptoms and preventing complications. These goals cannot generally be achieved by decreasing the dose or switching to a less potent acid-suppressing agent. Most patients require standard doses to prevent relapses.[28] Patients should be counseled on the importance of complying with patient-specific lifestyle changes and long-term maintenance therapy to prevent recurrence or worsening of disease.

The H$_2$RAs may be effective maintenance therapy for patients with mild disease.[6] The PPIs are first choice for maintenance treatment of moderate-to-severe GERD.[29] A short course of "on-demand" therapy may be appropriate in patients with symptomatic esophageal syndromes without esophagitis when symptom control is the primary outcome of interest.[2] With on-demand therapy, patients take the medication only when symptoms occur. Antacids have the fastest onset and may be used in combination with an H$_2$RA or PPI for "on-demand" symptom relief. However, patients with a history of esophagitis and/or complications should be maintained on standard daily doses of PPIs for maximum benefit. PPIs significantly decrease the incidence of dysplasia in patients with Barrett's esophagus for over 20 years.[30]

Long-term use of higher PPI doses is not indicated unless the patient has complicated symptoms, has erosive esophagitis per endoscopy, or has had further diagnostic evaluation to determine degree and frequency of acid exposure. Antireflux surgery and endoscopic therapies may be viable alternatives to long-term drug use for maintenance therapy in selected patients.

Special Population Considerations

▶ Patients With Atypical GERD

In patients presenting with extraesophageal GERD syndromes such as laryngitis or asthma, treatment with twice-daily PPI therapy for 2 months is probably warranted when there is a concomitant esophageal GERD syndrome.[2] Patients with suspected reflux chest pain syndrome should receive twice-daily PPI therapy after cardiac causes have been excluded. Manometry and pH or impedance pH monitoring should be considered in patients who do not respond to PPI therapy.[2]

Maintenance therapy is generally indicated in patients with extraesophageal GERD syndromes and concomitant esophageal GERD syndromes but not with reflux chest pain syndrome alone.[2] Stepdown therapy can be attempted based on symptom control.

▶ Pediatric Patients With GERD

Gastroesophageal reflux occurs in approximately 18% of infants. As in adults, transient LES relaxations appear to be the most common cause.[31] This is due to developmental immaturity of the LES.[32] Other causes include impaired luminal clearance of gastric acid, neurologic impairment, and type of infant formula. Most infants with gastroesophageal reflux have physiologic reflux with no clinical consequence.[31]

Uncomplicated GERD usually resolves by 12 to 18 months of life and responds to supportive therapy, including dietary adjustments such as smaller meals, more frequent feedings, or thickened infant formula. Postural management (e.g., positioning the infant in an upright position, especially after meals) may also be helpful.[32] Medical therapy may be indicated if there is no improvement.

The combination of a prokinetic agent and acid-suppressing drug is used commonly in pediatric patients with GERD.[32] Monotherapy with an H$_2$RA is also used frequently; ranitidine 2 to 4 mg/kg/day IV (or 4–6 mg/kg/day orally) is effective in neonates and pediatric patients.

Use of PPIs is becoming more common in pediatrics. Lansoprazole is FDA approved for treating symptomatic and erosive GERD in patients 1 through 11 years of age. Studies in adolescents (12–17 years old) demonstrated pharmacokinetics similar to those seen in adults.[33] The recommended dose is 15 mg once daily for children weighing 30 kg or less and 30 mg once daily for those weighing more than 30 kg. Although omeprazole is not FDA approved for use in children, evidence supports its effectiveness in children with GERD. A common dose for esophagitis is omeprazole 1 mg/kg/day (given once or twice daily).[34] Although no major adverse events have been reported in children receiving PPIs for up to 7 years, the safety of prolonged use in children is unknown.[34]

▶ Elderly Patients With GERD

Older individuals have decreased host defense mechanisms such as slowed gastric emptying and decreased saliva production. These patients often do not seek medical attention because they believe their symptoms are part of the normal aging process. PPIs are the most useful option in this population because they have superior efficacy and are dosed once daily.[35] In addition, there are fewer drug–drug and drug–disease state interactions compared with H$_2$RAs and metoclopramide. Elderly patients may be sensitive to the CNS effects of metoclopramide and H$_2$RAs.

▶ Patients With Refractory GERD

Refractory GERD may be present in patients not responding to 4 to 8 weeks of twice-daily PPI therapy. Compliance should always be assessed prior to deciding that a patient is refractory to acid-suppressing therapy. Endoscopy is indicated to determine if underlying pathology exists. In addition, patients with esophagitis may have a genotype that renders the PPIs less effective.[22] Patients with normal

Patient Encounter, Part 3: Creating a Care Plan

Based on the information presented, create a care plan for this patient's GERD. Your plan should include:

A statement of the drug-related needs and/or problems.

The goals of therapy.

A patient-specific, detailed therapeutic plan.

Cultural biases the practitioner should avoid in order to make the best treatment decisions for the patient.

A plan for follow-up to determine whether the goals have been achieved and adverse effects avoided.

endoscopy should undergo further testing with ambulatory pH monitoring or impedance monitoring to identify acid and nonacid reflux episodes, respectively.[22] Patients not responding to PPI therapy may in fact have nonacid reflux approximately 20% to 30% of the time.[9] Consideration should be made to switch a patient to an alternative PPI due to variability of patient responses. As many as 20% of patients on twice-daily PPI therapy with continued symptoms may have nonacid reflux.[36,37]

OUTCOME EVALUATION

- Monitor for symptom relief and the presence of complicated symptoms, such as difficulty swallowing, painful swallowing, or unexplained weight loss.
- Record the frequency and severity of symptoms by interviewing the patient after 4 to 8 weeks of acid-suppressing therapy. Continued symptoms may indicate the need for long-term maintenance therapy.
- Monitor for adverse drug reactions, drug–drug interactions, and compliance with the therapeutic regimen initially and any time there is a change in symptoms or medications.
- Educate patients about symptoms that suggest the presence of complications requiring immediate medical attention, such as dysphagia or odynophagia.
- Refer patients who present with atypical symptoms such as cough, nonallergic asthma, or chest pain to their physician for further diagnostic evaluation.
- ❾ *Review patient profiles for drugs that may aggravate GERD.*

Patient Care and Monitoring

1. Assess patient symptoms to determine if further diagnostic evaluation is necessary. Does the patient have any GERD-related complications such as difficulty in swallowing or unexplained weight loss?

2. Perform a thorough medication history by evaluating nonprescription, prescription, natural drug products, food, and patient history to determine exacerbating factors.

3. Determine what treatments have been helpful in the past.

4. Instruct the patient to avoid foods that aggravate GERD symptoms.

5. Educate the patient on lifestyle modifications to improve symptoms.

6. Review the results of diagnostic tests such as hemoglobin and hematocrit to rule out unexplained anemia.

7. Recommend appropriate therapy and develop a plan to assess effectiveness. Patients should receive 4 to 8 weeks of empiric acid-suppressing therapy. Patients who fail to respond should be assessed for compliance and proper medication administration. Twice-daily PPI therapy should be considered in patients not responding to once-daily therapy.

8. Evaluate the patient for the presence of adverse drug reactions, drug allergies, and drug interactions.

9. Stress the importance of compliance with the regimen, especially in patients with more severe erosive esophagitis or complicated symptoms.

10. Determine if long-term maintenance treatment is necessary.

11. Assess improvement in quality-of-life measures such as physical, psychological, and social functioning and well-being.

12. Provide patient education on disease, lifestyle modifications, and drug therapy:

    - What causes GERD and what are things to avoid?
    - What are possible complications of GERD?
    - When should medications be taken?
    - What potential adverse effects may occur?
    - Which drugs may interact with their therapy?
    - What warning signs should be reported to the physician?

Abbreviations Introduced in This Chapter

GERD	Gastroesophageal reflux disease
H$_2$RA	Histamine$_2$-receptor antagonist
LES	Lower esophageal sphincter
NSAID	Nonsteroidal anti-inflammatory drug
PPI	Proton pump inhibitor

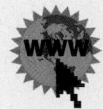 Self-assessment questions and answers are available at *http://www.mhpharmacotherapy.com/pp.html.*

REFERENCES

1. DeVault KR, Castell DO. Updated guidelines for the diagnosis and treatment of gastroesophageal reflux disease. Am J Gastroenterol 2005;100:190–200.
2. AGA Institute Medical Position Panel. American Gastroenterological Association Medical Position Statement on the management of gastroestophageal reflux disease. Gastroenterology 2008;135:1383–1391.
3. Dean BB, Crawley JA, Schmitt CM, et al. The burden of illness of gastro-oesophageal reflux disease: Impact on work productivity. Aliment Pharmacol Ther 2003;17:1309–1317.
4. Fennerty MB, Castell D, Fendrick AM, et al. The diagnosis and treatment of gastroesophageal reflux disease in a managed care environment. Suggested disease management guidelines. Arch Intern Med 1996;156:477–484.
5. Lambert R. Current practices and future perspectives in the management of gastroesophageal reflux disease. Aliment Pharmacol Ther 1997;11:661–662.
6. Johnson DA. Medical therapy of GERD: Current state of the art. Hosp Pract (Off Ed) 1996;31:135–148.
7. Weinberg DS, Caddish SL. The diagnosis and management of gastroesophageal reflux disease. Med Clin North Am 1996;80:411–429.
8. Krueger KJ. Changing clinical perspectives toward gastroesophageal reflux [Editorial]. South Med J 1996;89:548–550.
9. Karamonolis G, Sifrim D. Developments in pathogenesis and diagnosis of gastroesophageal reflux disease. Curr Opin Gastroenterol 2007;23(4):428–433.
10. Lagergren J, Bergstrom R, Lindgren A, et al. Symptomatic gastroesophageal reflux as a risk factor for esophageal adenocarcinoma. N Engl J Med 1999;340:825–831.
11. Kitchin LI, Castell DO. Rationale and efficacy of conservative therapy for gastroesophageal reflux disease. Arch Intern Med 1991;151:448–454.
12 Richter JE, Castell DO. Drugs, foods and other substances in the cause and treatment of reflux esophagitis. Med Clin North Am 1981;65:1223–1234.
13. Anon. Guideline for the surgical treatment of gastroesophageal reflux disease (GERD). Surg Endosc 1998;12:186–188.
14. Spechler SJ, Lee E, Ahnen D, et al. Long-term outcome of medical and surgical therapies for gastroesophageal reflux disease: Follow-up of a randomized controlled trial. JAMA 2001;285:2331–2338.
15. Johnson DA. Endoscopic therapy for GERD—Baking, sewing, or stuffing: An evidence-based perspective. Rev Gastroenterol Disord 2003;3(3):142–149.
16. Washington N, Steele RJ, Jackson SJ, et al. Patterns of food and acid reflux in patients with low-grade oesophagitis—The role of an antireflux agent. Aliment Pharmacol Ther 1998;12:53–58.
17. Peters FT, Ganesh S, Kuipers EJ, et al. Endoscopic regression of Barrett oesophagus during omeprazole treatment: A randomised double blind study. Gut 1999;45:489–494.
18. Sampliner RE, Camargo E. Normalization of esophageal pH with high-dose proton pump inhibitor therapy does not result in regression of Barrett esophagus. Am J Gastroenterol 1997;92:582–585.
19. Horn J. The proton-pump inhibitors: Similarities and differences. Clin Ther 2000;22:266–280.
20. Richardson P, Hawkey CJ, Stack WA. Proton pump inhibitors. Pharmacology and rationale for use in gastrointestinal disorders. Drugs 1998;56:307–335.
21. Welage LS, Berardi RR. Evaluation of omeprazole, lansoprazole, pantoprazole, and rabeprazole in the treatment of acid-related disorders. J Am Pharm Assoc 2000;40:52–62.
22. Richter JE. How to manage refractory gastroesophageal reflux disease. Nat Clin Pract Gastroenterol Hepatol 2007;4(12):658–664.
23. Furuta T, Shirai N, Watanabe F, et al. Effect of the cytochrome P4502C19 genotypic differences on cure rates for gastroesophageal reflux disease by lansoprazole. Clin Pharmacol Ther 2002;72:453–460.
24. Schwab M, et al. Esomeprazole-induced healing of gastroesophageal reflux disease is unrelated to the genotype of CYP2C19: Evidence from clinical and pharmacokinetic data. Clin Pharmacol Ther 2005;78:627–634.
25. Garrett WR. Considerations for long-term use of proton-pump inhibitors. Am J Health Syst Pharm 1998;55:2268–2279.
26. Anonymous. Proton pump inhibitor relabeling for cancer risk not warranted. FD& C Report 1996 (Nov 1);58:T&G 1–2.
27. Fackler WK, Ours T, Vaezi M, Richter J. Long-term effect of H2RA therapy on nocturnal gastric acid breakthrough. Gastroenterology 2002;122:625–632.
28. Robinson M, Lanza F, Avner D, Haber M. Effective maintenance therapy of reflux esophagitis with low dose lansoprazole: A randomized, double blind placebo-controlled trial. Ann Intern Med 1996;124:859–867.
29. Vigneri S, Termini R, Leandro G, et al. A comparison of five maintenance therapies for reflux esophagitis. N Engl J Med 1995;333:1106–1110.
30. El-Serag HB, Aguirre T, Davis S, et al. Proton pump inhibitors reduce incidence of dysplasia in BE. Am J Gastroenterol 2004;99:1877–1883.
31. Vandenplas Y, Belli D, Benhamou P-H, et al. Current concepts and issues in the management of regurgitation in infants: A reappraisal. Management guidelines from a working party. Acta Paediatr 1996;85:531–534.
32. Faubion WA, Zein NN. Gastroesophageal reflux in infants and children. Mayo Clin Proc 1998;73:166–173.
33. Prevacid® (Lansoprazole). Package Insert. Takeda Pharmaceuticals America, Inc. Deerfield, IL. November 2008.
34. Patel AS, Pohl JF, Easley DJ. Proton pump inhibitors in pediatrics. Pediatr Rev 2003;24(1):12–15.
35. Katz PO. Gastroesophageal reflux disease. J Am Geriatr Soc 1998;46:1558–1565.
36. Zerbib F, Roman S, Ropert A, et al. Esophageal pH-impedance monitoring and symptom analysis in GERD: A study in patients on and off therapy. Am J Gastroenterol 2006;101:1956–1963.
37. Mainie I, Tutuian R, Shay S, et al. Acid and non-acid reflux in patients with persistent symptoms despite acid suppressive therapy: A multicenter study using ambulatory impedance-pH monitoring. Gut 2006;55:1398–1402.

18 | Peptic Ulcer Disease

John W. Devlin

LEARNING OBJECTIVES

Upon completion of the chapter, the reader will be able to:

1. Recognize differences between ulcers induced by *Helicobacter pylori* and nonsteroidal anti-inflammatory drugs (NSAIDs) in terms of risk factors, pathogenesis, signs and symptoms, clinical course, and prognosis.

2. Identify desired therapeutic outcomes for patients with *H. pylori*–associated ulcers and NSAID-induced ulcers.

3. Identify factors that guide selection of an *H. pylori* eradication regimen and improve compliance with these regimens.

4. Determine the appropriate management for a patient taking a nonselective NSAID who is at high risk for ulcer-related GI complications or who develops an ulcer.

5. Devise an algorithm for evaluation and treatment of a patient with signs and symptoms suggestive of an *H. pylori*–associated or NSAID-induced ulcer.

6. Given patient-specific information and the prescribed drug treatment regimen, formulate a monitoring plan for a patient who is receiving drug therapy to either eradicate *H. pylori* or to treat an active NSAID-induced ulcer or GI complication.

KEY CONCEPTS

❶ Patients with peptic ulcer disease (PUD) should avoid exposure to factors known to worsen the disease, exacerbate symptoms, or lead to ulcer recurrence (e.g., nonsteroidal anti-inflammatory drug [NSAID] use, alcohol consumption, or cigarette smoking).

❷ Reliance on conventional antiulcer drug therapy as an alternative to *Helicobacter pylori* eradication is inappropriate because it is associated with a higher incidence of ulcer recurrence and ulcer-related complications.

❸ Eradication therapy with a proton pump inhibitor (PPI) based three-drug regimen should be considered for all patients who test positive for *H. pylori* and have an active ulcer or a documented history of either an ulcer or ulcer-related complication. Different antibiotics should be used if a second course of *H. pylori* eradication therapy is required.

❹ In patients at risk for NSAID-induced ulcers, PPIs at standard doses reduce the risk of both gastric and duodenal ulcers (DU) as effectively as misoprostol and are generally better tolerated.

❺ Selective cyclooxygenase-2 (COX-2) inhibitors are no more effective than the combination of a PPI and a nonselective NSAID in reducing the incidence of ulcers and are associated with a greater incidence of cardiovascular (CV) events (e.g., ischemic stroke).

❻ Low-dose maintenance therapy with a PPI or histamine$_2$-receptor antagonist (H$_2$RA) is only indicated for patients who fail *H. pylori* eradication, have *H. pylori*-negative ulcers, are heavy smokers, or develop severe complications related to their ulcer disease.

INTRODUCTION

Peptic ulcer disease (PUD) refers to an ulceration that forms on the muscular mucosa in the wall of the GI tract. The most common types of PUD are duodenal ulcers (DU) and gastric ulcers (GU). GU are usually located in the antrum or lesser curvature of the stomach. PUD is common and may adversely affect quality of life unless properly diagnosed and treated. The high prevalence and relapse rate associated with PUD pose a substantial economic burden. Peptic ulcers are most commonly caused by one of three etiologies: (a) *Helicobacter pylori* infection; (b) use of nonsteroidal anti-inflammatory drugs (NSAIDs); or (c) stress-related mucosal damage (SRMD). A number of pathophysiologic variables can be used to distinguish these three common types of peptic ulcer (Table 18–1). This chapter will focus on strategies to

Table 18–1
Characteristics of Common Causes of PUD

	H. pylori	NSAID	SRMD
Onset	Chronic	Chronic	Acute
Primary location of damage	Duodenum	Stomach	Stomach
Presence of symptoms	Frequent	Rare	Rare
Primary mechanism for ulceration	Infection resulting in inflammatory state	Loss of defense mechanisms	Loss of defense mechanisms
Depth of ulcers	Superficial	Deep	Superficial
Dependence on acid for mucosal damage	Greater	Lesser	Lesser
Characterization of GI bleeding	Minor	Major	Major
Responsive to acid-suppressive therapy	No	Yes	Yes

NSAID, nonsteroidal anti-inflammatory drug; PUD, peptic ulcer disease; SRMD, stress-related mucosal damage.

optimize pharmacotherapy for patients with PUD related to *H. pylori* or NSAID therapy.

SRMD occurs most frequently in critically ill patients and is thought to be caused by factors such as compromised mesenteric perfusion rather than *H. pylori* or NSAIDs. Its onset is usually acute, and in a small proportion of patients may progress to deep ulceration and hemorrhage.

Less common causes of peptic ulceration include Zollinger-Ellison syndrome (ZES), cancer chemotherapy, radiation, and vascular insufficiency. ZES is caused by a gastrin-producing tumor called a gastrinoma and results in gastric acid hypersecretion. High-dose oral proton pump inhibitor (PPI) therapy is the initial treatment of choice for ZES; intermittent IV PPI therapy may be required for any patient in whom oral therapy is contraindicated.[1]

EPIDEMIOLOGY AND ETIOLOGY

Approximately, 25 million Americans are affected by PUD, with the lifetime prevalence estimated to be 12% in men and 10% in women.[2] Annual direct and indirect costs associated with PUD in the United States are estimated to be more than $9 billion. Despite the widespread use of conventional anti-ulcer therapy that effectively reduces gastric acid secretion, ulcers frequently recur, with 1-year recurrence rates (after ulcer initial healing) estimated to range from 60% to 100%.[1]

H. pylori infection and NSAID use account for most cases of PUD. The relatively high incidence of PUD in the elderly may be due to higher NSAID use. Although hospitalizations related to PUD have decreased over the past two decades, the incidence of PUD-related complications such as bleeding and perforation remain unchanged.

In general, ulcers related to *H. pylori* infection more commonly affect the duodenum whereas ulcers related to NSAIDs more frequently affect the stomach (Fig. 18–1). However, ulcers may be found in either location from either cause. GU tend to occur much later in life than DU, with the peak incidence of GU occurring in patients over 60 years of age. Malignancy is more commonly found with GU than DU.

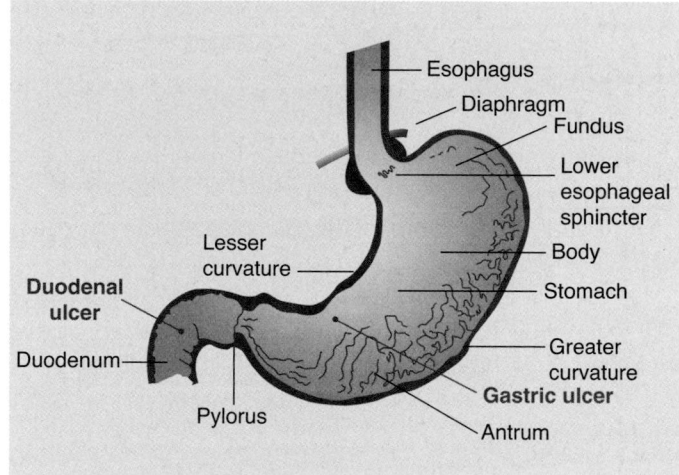

FIGURE 18–1. Anatomic structure of the stomach and duodenum and most common locations of gastric and duodenal ulcers. (From Ref. 37.)

Helicobacter pylori

Since its discovery nearly 25 years ago, the role of *H. pylori* in PUD has been increasingly recognized, and it is now one of the most common causes of PUD.[3] While *H. pylori* causes gastritis in all infected patients, only a small proportion (less than 20%) of patients actually develop symptomatic PUD.

H. pylori normally resides in the human stomach and is transmitted via the fecal–oral route or through ingestion of fecal-contaminated water or food. Infection with *H. pylori* is more common in developing countries because of crowded conditions and the presence of contaminated food and water. *H. pylori* colonization does not necessarily reflect an active infection since the organism can attach itself to the gastric epithelium without invading cells. Cellular invasion by *H. pylori* is necessary for an active infection, which is usually asymptomatic and leads to chronic active gastritis.

Patient Encounter 1, Part 1

PUD Secondary to *Helicobacter pylori*

A 51-year-old woman presents to the emergency department complaining of abdominal pain for the past 3 days and dark tarry stools over the past 2 days. She states that she has never had these symptoms before and that she has been feeling weak and tired for the past 2 weeks. She denies having bright red blood in her stools or vomiting. She does not take any prescription medications and only takes extra-strength acetaminophen for occasional headaches.

PMH: Hypertension × 10 years

FH: Mother died of a stroke at age 81; father died of pneumonia at age 71

SH: Denies alcohol, tobacco, or illicit drug use

Allergies: NKDA

Meds: Acetaminophen extra-strength two tablets every 6 hours as needed for occasional headache

Which signs and symptoms are suggestive of PUD?

What are this patient's risk factors for PUD?

What additional information do you need to know before creating a treatment plan for this patient?

Nonsteroidal Anti-Inflammatory Drugs

NSAIDs are one of the most widely used classes of medications in the United States, particularly in the elderly.[4] More than 20,000 deaths and 100,000 hospitalizations occur in the United States per year as a direct result of adverse events related to NSAID use. Chronic NSAID ingestion leads to symptoms of nausea and dyspepsia in nearly half of the patients. Peptic ulceration occurs in up to 30% of patients who use NSAIDs (including aspirin) chronically, with GI bleeding or perforation occurring in 1.5% of patients who develop an ulcer. NSAID-related peptic ulcers usually occur in the stomach; DU are much less common.

Risk factors for NSAID-induced peptic ulcers and complications are presented in Table 18–2. Several important principles should be considered when estimating the risk for developing PUD in a patient taking an NSAID: (a) risk factors are generally additive; (b) some risk factors (e.g., corticosteroid therapy) are not by themselves a risk factor for ulceration but increase PUD risk substantially when combined with NSAID therapy; and (c) many of the risk factors postulated to increase PUD risk in a patient taking an NSAID (e.g., rheumatoid arthritis, tobacco smoking, and alcohol consumption) remain unproven and thus should not generally be considered independent risk factors for NSAID-induced ulceration.[5] Whether *H. pylori* infection is a risk factor for NSAID-induced ulcers remains controversial. However, *H. pylori* and NSAIDs act independently to

Table 18–2

Established Risk Factors for Ulcers and GI Complications Related to NSAID Use

Age over 60
Concomitant anticoagulant use
Pre-existing coagulopathy (elevated INR or thrombocytopenia)
Concomitant corticosteroid or selective serotonin reuptake inhibitor therapy
Previous PUD or upper GI bleeding
CV disease and other comorbid conditions
Multiple NSAID use (e.g., low-dose aspirin in conjunction with another NSAID)
Duration of NSAID use (greater than 1 month)
High-dose NSAID use
NSAID-related dyspepsia
Cigarette smokers

CV, cardiovascular; INR, International Normalized Ratio; NSAID, nonsteroidal anti-inflammatory drug; PUD, peptic ulcer disease.

increase ulcer risk and ulcer-related bleeding and appear to have additive effects.

Other Causative Factors

Cigarette smoking is associated with a higher prevalence of ulcers and may also impair healing of ulcers that develop.[6] The exact mechanism(s) for the detrimental effects of smoking on the gastric mucosa are unclear but may involve increased pepsin secretion, duodenogastric reflux of bile salts, elevated levels of free radicals, and reduced bicarbonate and prostaglandin (PG) production.[7,8] It is unknown whether nicotine or one of the many other ingredients found in cigarettes is responsible for these deleterious effects.

Until the discovery of *H. pylori*, psychological stress was considered one of the primary causes of PUD. Although psychosocial factors such as life stress, baseline personality patterns, and depression may influence PUD prevalence, a clear causal relationship has not been demonstrated.

Dietary factors such as coffee, tea, cola, beer, and a highly spiced diet may cause dyspepsia, but they have not been shown to independently increase PUD risk. Although caffeine increases gastric acid secretion and alcohol ingestion causes acute gastritis, there is inconclusive evidence to confirm that either of these substances are independent risk factors for peptic ulcers.

PATHOPHYSIOLOGY

Ulcer formation is the net result of a lack of homeostasis between factors within the GI tract responsible for the breakdown of food (e.g., gastric acid and pepsin) and factors that promote mucosal defense and repair (e.g., bicarbonate, mucus secretion, and PGs).

Gastric Acid and Pepsin

Hydrochloric acid and pepsin are the primary substances that cause gastric mucosal damage in PUD. Three different stimuli

Patient Encounter 2, Part 1

PUD Secondary to NSAID Use

A 65-year-old man with a history of osteoarthritis and chronic obstructive pulmonary disease (COPD) comes to your clinic complaining of burning abdominal pain. The pain has worsened over the past 2 weeks; it is worse at night and after meals.

PMH: Osteoarthritis for 5 years, started diclofenac within the past 2 months; COPD for 15 years

FH: Noncontributory

SH: Tobacco one pack per day × 40 years; drinks two beers per day

Meds: Ipratropium metered-dose inhaler (MDI) two puffs every 6 hours; albuterol (known as salbutamol outside the United States) MDI two puffs every 4 hours as needed; prednisone 10 mg orally daily; diclofenac 75 mg orally two times a day; aspirin 81 mg orally daily

Which signs and symptoms are suggestive of PUD?

What are this patient's risk factors for PUD?

What additional information do you need to know before creating a treatment plan for this patient?

(i.e., histamine, acetylcholine, and gastrin) are responsible for acid secretion through their interactions with the histaminic, cholinergic, and gastrin receptors on the surface of parietal cells. Gastric acid output occurs in two stages: (a) basal acid output (BAO), which reflects the baseline output of acid during the fasting state; and (b) maximal acid output (MAO), which occurs in response to meals. Basal acid secretion follows a circadian cycle in which it is highest at night and lowest in the morning and is modulated by the effects of acetylcholine and histamine acting on the parietal cell.

Food can cause maximal gastric acid secretion in two ways. In the cephalic phase of acid secretion, the vagus nerve stimulates acid secretion in response to the sight, smell, or taste of food. In both the gastric and intestinal phases of acid secretion, the physical distention caused by food in the gastric fundus and small intestine induces gastrin secretion resulting in acid production. After stimulation by histamine, acetylcholine, and gastrin, acid is secreted by the H⁺-K⁺-ATPase (proton) pump, located on the luminal side of parietal cells. Acid secretion in PUD is usually normal or slightly elevated. NSAID ingestion usually does not affect acid secretion, whereas *H. pylori* infection usually leads to a slight increase in acid output. This is in contrast to ZES, in which acid secretion is substantially elevated.

Pepsinogen released from chief cells in the body of the stomach during food digestion is converted to pepsin in the presence of an acidic environment and plays a key role in the initiation of protein digestion, proteolysis of collagen, and as a signal for the release of other digestive enzymes such as gastrin and cholecystokinin. The proteolytic activity of pepsin appears to influence ulcer formation.

Mucosal Defense and Repair

Several defense and repair mechanisms are responsible for preventing mucosal damage and subsequent ulcer formation. Mucus gel, through its buffering action, is the primary source of defense for the gastric epithelial surface against gastric acid. It allows an acidic environment to be maintained in the lumen but a near neutral pH to be maintained on the epithelial lining. On the epithelial lining, a number of protective mechanisms are responsible for the repair of damaged cells, production of defense mechanisms, and the promotion of epithelial growth.

PGs inhibit gastric acid secretion and have numerous mucosal protective effects, the most important of which include the stimulation of both mucus and phospholipid production, promotion of bicarbonate secretion, and increased mucosal cell turnover. Damage to the mucosal defense system is the primary method by which *H. pylori* or NSAIDs cause peptic ulcers.

Helicobacter pylori

H. pylori are a gram-negative microaerophilic rod that has a number of adaptive functions allowing it to live within the acidic environment of the stomach. It is an S-shaped bacterium with multiple flagella that initially inhabits the gastric antrum but migrates to the more proximal sections of the stomach over time. The motility provided by the flagella allows it to penetrate the mucous gel barrier, thus permitting a direct interaction with epithelial cells—the site where acute infection occurs. *H. pylori* are able to survive in the acidic conditions of the stomach because of its ability to induce a transient hypochlorhydria via production of urease, an enzyme that hydrolyzes urea into carbon dioxide and ammonia. Ammonia can both protect *H. pylori* and damage tissue.

A number of host and pathogenic factors contribute to the ability of *H. pylori* to cause gastroduodenal mucosal injury including: (a) direct mucosal damage; (b) alterations to host inflammatory responses; and (c) hypergastrinemia leading to a state of elevated acid secretion. Bacterial-surface adhesion components facilitate binding of *H. pylori* to epithelial cells, and vacuolating cytotoxin (vac A) facilitates the binding of *H. pylori* to the cell membrane, thus enabling the *H. pylori* organism better access to nutrients. The cag pathogenicity island (*cag*-PAI) leads to the release of cytokines thus leading to a chronic inflammatory state in *H. pylori*-infected patients.[3] The complex interplay between bacterial virulence factors and an enhanced inflammatory response results in a chronic *H. pylori* infection that elevates acid production and reduces various protective factors.

Nonsteroidal Anti-Inflammatory Drugs

Nonselective NSAIDs (those that inhibit both cyclo-oxygenase-1 and -2 [COX-1 and COX-2]) cause gastric mucosal damage by two primary mechanisms: (a) direct or topical irritation of the gastric epithelium; and (b) systemic inhibition of endogenous mucosal PG synthesis.

Direct irritation of the mucosal lining by NSAIDs occurs because NSAIDs are weak acids. Topical irritation is therefore most pronounced with more acidic NSAIDs such as aspirin. While the direct irritant effects of NSAIDs play a contributory role in the development of NSAID-induced gastritis, this mechanism generally plays a minor role in the evolution of NSAID-induced PUD.

The systemic effects of NSAIDs are the primary cause of PUD. COX is the rate-limiting enzyme in the PG synthesis pathway (Fig. 18–2). Inhibition of PG production is the primary therapeutic effect of NSAIDs. COX is responsible for the conversion of arachidonic acid to PGs such as PGG_2 and PGH_2. There are two forms of the COX enzyme, COX-1 and COX-2. COX-1 is routinely found in body tissues that produce PGs for normal physiological maintenance. In contrast, COX-2 is an inducible enzyme that is expressed during states in which cytokines and inflammatory mediators are elevated (e.g., fever and pain). Inhibition of the COX-1 isoenzyme decreases production of endogenous PGs, particularly PGE_1, PGE_2, and PGI_2. Administration of NSAIDs parenterally (e.g., ketorolac) and rectally (e.g., indomethacin) is associated with an incidence of PUD that is similar to that with oral NSAIDs. Topical NSAIDs (e.g., diclofenac) would be unlikely to cause PUD given the very low serum concentrations that are achieved with this route of administration compared to that observed with oral therapy.

PGs, through their effects on mucous cell secretion, basal bicarbonate secretion, and mucosal growth, are important factors in gastric healing and protection. Inhibition of PG production by NSAIDs compromises these important protective mechanisms. Finally, the antiplatelet effects of NSAIDs may worsen bleeding complications associated with PUD.

Complications

Hemorrhage is the most common complication of PUD and may occur when an ulcer erodes the wall of a gastric or duodenal artery. Bleeding may be occult (hidden) or may present as melena or hematemesis. Bleeding occurs in approximately 15% of PUD patients and is more common in patients more than 60 years of age, particularly those who ingest NSAIDs. Up to 20% of patients who develop a PUD-related hemorrhage do not have prior symptoms. Death occurs primarily in patients who continue to bleed, or in those who rebleed after the initial bleeding has stopped.

Gastric outlet obstruction occurs in approximately 2% of patients with PUD and is usually caused by ulcer-related inflammation or scar formation near the peripyloric region. Signs and symptoms of outlet obstruction include early satiety after meals, nausea, vomiting, abdominal pain, and weight loss. Ulcer healing with conventional acid-suppressive therapy is the primary treatment, but if this is unsuccessful then an endoscopic procedure (e.g., balloon dilation) is required.

CLINICAL PRESENTATION AND DIAGNOSIS

Diagnosis

Diagnostic tests for the presence of *H. pylori* can be either endoscopic or nonendoscopic. Endoscopic diagnosis requires the extraction of gastric tissue samples that are subsequently tested for *H. pylori*.[9] Recent antibiotic use can lead to a false negative biopsy result. Although endoscopy is the gold standard for detecting *H. pylori* infections, it may be associated with rare but severe complications and greater expense than nonendoscopic diagnostic methods. Endoscopy is therefore usually reserved for patients more than 50 years of age who have anemia, GI bleeding, or unexplained weight loss.

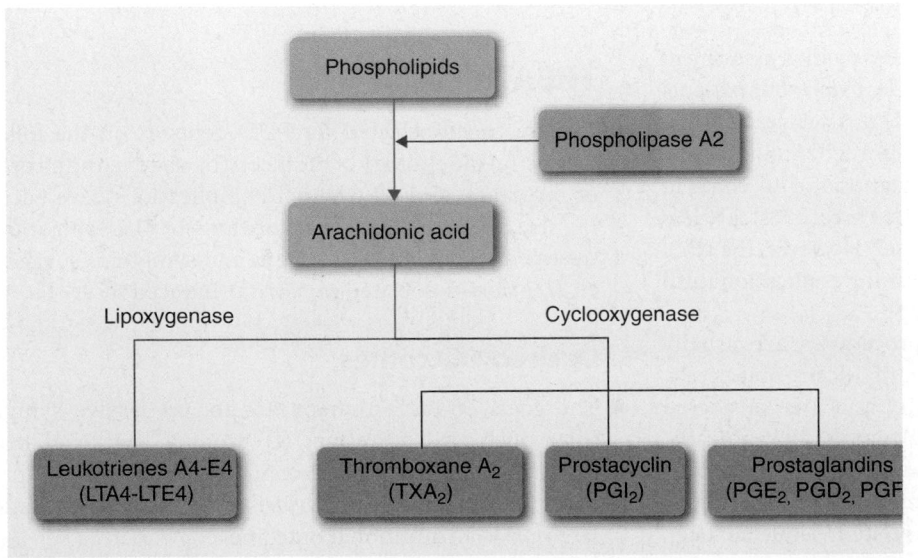

FIGURE 18–2. The arachidonic acid pathway.

Clinical Presentation and Diagnosis of PUD

Symptoms

- Mild epigastric pain that may be described as burning, gnawing, or aching in character.
- Abdominal pain may be described as burning or a feeling of discomfort.
- Some patients report nocturnal pain.
- The severity of pain often fluctuates.
- The intensity of pain can vary widely (e.g., from dull to sharp).
- DU pain occurs 1 to 3 hours after meals and may be relieved by food ingestion.
- GU pain occurs immediately after meals and is often aggravated by food.
- Patients may also complain of heartburn, belching, bloating, nausea, or vomiting.

Signs

- Weight loss may be associated with nausea and vomiting.
- Complications such as bleeding, perforation, or obstruction may occur.
- Alarm signs and symptoms include: bleeding, anemia, tarry stools or "coffee-grounds" emesis, and weight loss.

Patient Encounter 1, Part 2: Physical Examination, Laboratory Tests, and Diagnostic Procedures

PE:

VS: BP 135/90 mm Hg, P 89 bpm, RR 14/min, T 37.5°C (99.5°F)

Gen: NAD

Skin: Normal turgor

HEENT: PERRL

CV: RRR; S_1, S_2 normal; no S_3 or S_4

Lungs: Computed tomographic angiography (CTA) bilaterally

Abd: Soft, nontender, nondistended, (+) bowel sounds × 4 quadrants, 7/10 pain

Neuro: A&O × 3, cranial nerves intact, DTR 2+

Labs: WBC 4.6 × 10³/mm³ (4.6 × 10⁹/L), hemoglobin 8.5 g/dL (85 g/L or 5.3 mmol/L), hematocrit 24.7%, platelets 327 × 10³/mm³ (327 × 10⁹/L), aPTT 32.5 seconds, PT 12.1 seconds, INR 1.02

Fecal occult blood: (+)

EGD: Multiple superficial ulcerations in the duodenum; largest ulcer measures 2 cm in diameter; no active bleeding noted.

Campylobacter-like organism (CLO) test (urease test): (+) for *H. pylori*

Given this information, what is your assessment of the patient's condition?

What are your treatment goals?

What nonpharmacologic and pharmacologic alternatives are available for this patient?

Nonendoscopic testing methods include the urea breath test, serological testing, and the stool antigen assay. Compared to endoscopic procedures, these tests are more comfortable, less expensive, and do not require a special procedure. The urea breath test is usually the first-line test to detect active *H. pylori* infection because it has a sensitivity and specificity greater than 95% and a short turnaround time. The BreathTek urea breath test used with a desktop infrared spectrometer can provide results within a few minutes. Concomitant acid-suppressive or antibiotic therapy may give false-negative results with this test.

Office-based serological testing provides a quick assessment (within 15 minutes) of an exposure to *H. pylori*, but patients can remain seropositive for up to 1 year after eradication, making the clinical utility of this test limited. Stool antigen assays can be useful for the initial diagnosis or to confirm *H. pylori* eradication, and unlike the urea breath test, are less affected by concomitant medication use.[9] However, the stool antigen assay should not be used to test for eradication until 6 to 8 weeks after completion of therapy.

Radiological and/or endoscopic procedures are usually required to document the presence of ulcers objectively. Barium studies have a high sensitivity and are considered first-line tests to document an ulcer radiographically. However, the cost and complexity of all of these tests has led to the promotion of an early empiric treatment strategy for patients at low risk for PUD-related sequelae (e.g.,

malignancy). An empiric treatment strategy is appropriate for patients less than 50 years of age who have mild or intermittent epigastric symptoms and no evidence of PUD-related systemic symptoms or complications.

TREATMENT

The treatment selected for PUD depends on the following factors: (a) the etiology of the ulcer; (b) whether the ulcer is new or recurrent; and (c) whether complications have occurred. Figure 18–3 contains an algorithm for the evaluation and treatment of a patient with signs and symptoms suggestive of an *H. pylori*–associated or NSAID-induced ulcer.

Desired Outcomes

The goals of PUD therapy are to: (a) resolve symptoms; (b) reduce acid secretion; (c) promote epithelial healing; (d) prevent ulcer-related complications; and (e) prevent ulcer recurrence. For *H. pylori*-related PUD, eradication of *H. pylori* is an additional outcome.

Patient Encounter 2, Part 2: Physical Examination, Laboratory Tests, and Diagnostic Procedures

PE:

VS: BP 125/85 mm Hg, P 72 bpm, RR 12/min, T 37.5°C (99.5°F)

Gen: NAD

Skin: Dry, intact

HEENT: PERRL

CV: RRR, S_1, S_2

Lungs: CTA B/L

Abd: Soft, nontender, nondistended, (+) bowel sounds, 5/10 pain on the epigastric region

Neuro: A&O × 3, cranial nerves intact, DTR 2+

Labs: WBC 9.9 × 10³/mm³ (9.9 × 10⁹/L), hemoglobin 12.1 g/dL (121 g/L or 7.5 mmol/L), hematocrit 38.3%, platelets 108 × 10³/mm³ (108 × 10⁹/L), aPTT 27.9 seconds, PT 12.4 seconds, INR 1.09

EGD: One ulcer located on the antrum of the stomach measuring 3 cm in diameter; no bleeding or obstruction noted

Given this information, what is your assessment of the patient's condition?

What are your treatment goals?

What nonpharmacologic and pharmacologic treatment alternatives are available for this patient?

Nonpharmacologic Therapy

❶ *Patients with PUD should avoid exposure to factors known to worsen the disease, exacerbate symptoms, or lead to ulcer recurrence.* Patients should be advised to reduce psychological stress and avoid cigarette smoking, alcohol consumption, foods or beverages that exacerbate ulcer symptoms, and NSAID or aspirin use.[10,11] Patients who require chronic NSAID therapy (e.g., rheumatoid arthritis) may be given prophylaxis with misoprostol or a PPI (see Treatment of NSAID-Induced Ulcers).

The high-success rates of medical therapies have reduced the number of surgical procedures performed and relegated surgery primarily to elective situations. For this reason, surgical interventions are generally reserved for complicated or refractory PUD. Some surgical procedures include: (a) vagotomy and pyloroplasty; (b) highly selective vagotomy; or (c) vagotomy combined with antrectomy. Vagotomy is the central component of most procedures because of its targeted effects on blocking further acid secretion. These procedures have a high success rate. Complications are rare but can include dumping syndrome, bile reflux, diarrhea, malabsorption, and gastric atony.[12]

Pharmacologic Therapy

▶ *Treatment of H. pylori–Associated Ulcers*

The primary goal of *H. pylori* therapy is to completely eradicate the organism using an effective antibiotic-containing regimen. ❷ *Reliance on conventional acid-suppressive drug therapy alone as an alternative to* H. pylori *eradication is inappropriate because it is associated with a higher incidence of ulcer recurrence and ulcer-related complications.* Reinfection rates are generally low after the initial course of therapy as long as the patient has received a regimen with proven efficacy and is compliant with it. The *H. pylori* regimen that is chosen should have a per-protocol cure rate of 90% or more or a cure rate based on intention-to-treat analysis of 80% or more.[9] In addition to proven efficacy, the optimal treatment regimen should cause minimal adverse events, have low risk for the development of bacterial resistance, and be cost effective.[9]

H. pylori treatment regimens are presented in Table 18–3. ❸ *Eradication therapy with a PPI-based three-drug regimen should be considered for all patients who test positive for* H. pylori *and have an active ulcer or a documented history of either an ulcer or ulcer-related complication. Different antibiotics should be used if a second course of* H. pylori *eradication therapy is required.*

The first-line regimen should contain a PPI plus clarithromycin and either amoxicillin or metronidazole. Amoxicillin should not be used in penicillin-allergic patients, and metronidazole should be avoided if alcohol is going to be consumed. The combination of two antimicrobials and a PPI leads to cure rates greater than 80% (by intention-to-treat basis) and reduces the risk of selecting out resistant organisms.[13] A single daily dose of a PPI may be less effective than twice daily dosing when used as part of a triple-drug regimen. Substitution of one PPI for another is acceptable and does not appear to affect eradication rates. Monotherapy with a single antibiotic or antiulcer agent is not recommended due to high failure rates. In the United States, two-drug regimens consisting of a PPI and an antibiotic are also not recommended.

The duration of therapy is controversial and varies by continent. Europeans routinely treat patients for 7 days whereas Americans usually rely on a 14-day regimen. While these seven additional days of therapy improves the absolute cure rate by approximately 9%,[14] longer courses decrease compliance and increase drug cost.

Bismuth-based four-drug regimens have clinical cure rates similar to three-drug, PPI-based regimens. Bismuth-based regimens usually include tetracycline, metronidazole, and an antisecretory agent (e.g., PPI or histamine₂-receptor antagonist [H_2RA]). Bismuth salts promote ulcer healing through antibacterial and mucosal protective effects. While cheaper than most other regimens, drawbacks of bismuth-based regimens include the frequency of administration (four times a day), risk for salicylate toxicity in patients with renal impairment, and propensity for bothersome side effects (e.g., stool and tongue discoloration, constipation, nausea, and vomiting).

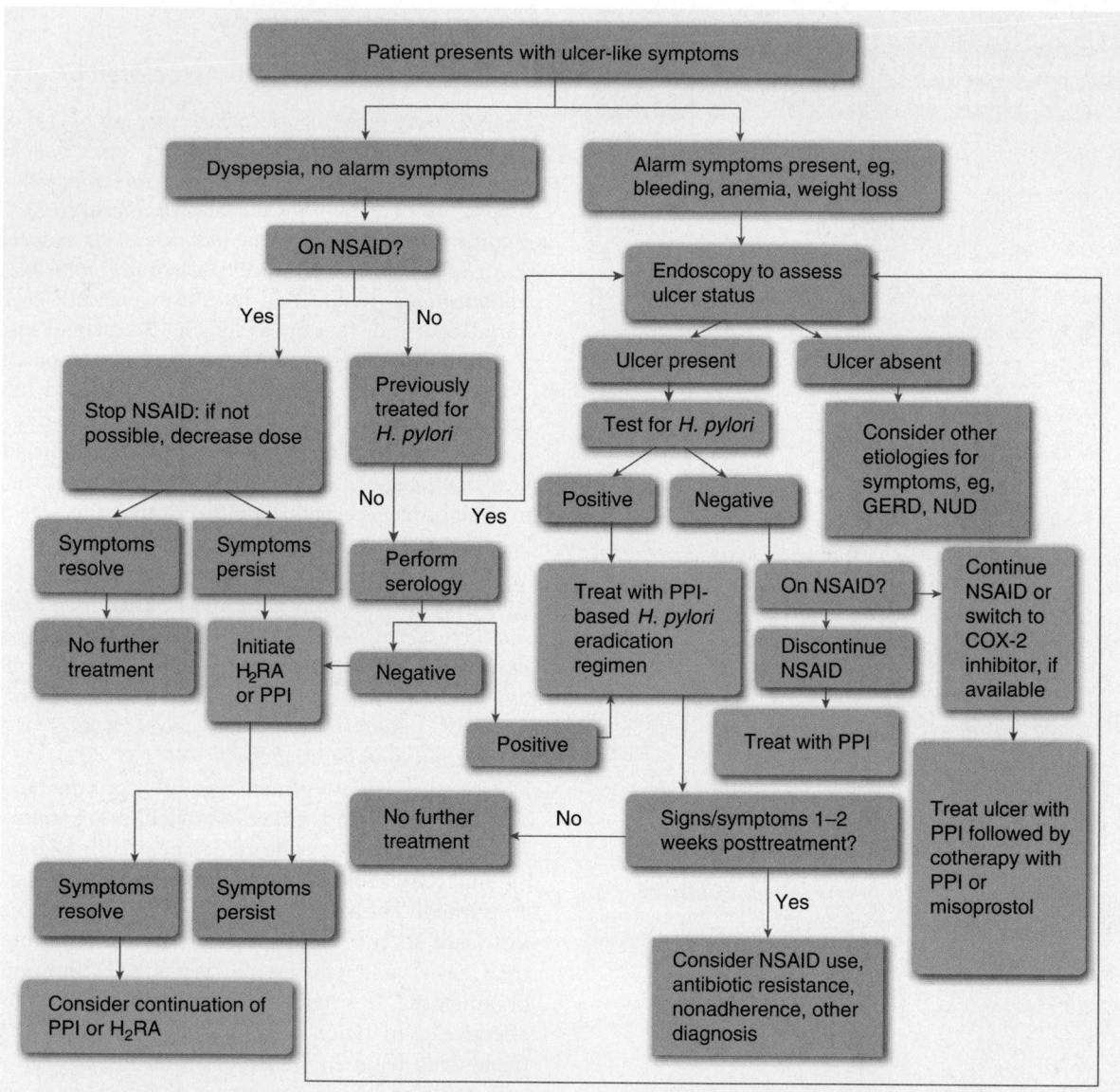

FIGURE 18–3. Approach to the patient presenting with ulcer-like symptoms. (GERD, gastroesophageal reflux disease; HP *Helicobacter pylori*; H₂RA, histamine₂-receptor antagonist; NSAID, nonsteroidal anti-inflammatory drug; NUD, nonulcer dyspepsia; PPI, proton pump inhibitor.) (From Ref. 37.)

The combination product Pylera (bikalcitrate potassium 140 mg, metronidazole 125 mg, and tetracycline 125 mg) when used in combination with omeprazole 20 mg twice daily (before breakfast and dinner) is as effective as omeprazole–amoxicillin–clarithromycin (OAC) in eradicating *H. pylori* in patients with DU. Although not FDA-approved for patients with GU, it would be expected to be effective in eradicating *H. pylori* in patients with GUs. The usual dose of Pylera is three capsules four times daily after meals and at bedtime with 8 oz. water for 10 days. The simultaneous administration of tetracycline and a metal-containing product (e.g., many antacids) may result in complexation and reduced tetracycline absorption. Consequently, the bismuth salt and tetracycline are physically separated in the capsule formulation of Pylera.

Helidac is a package of 14 blister cards with each card containing a single-day supply of bismuth subsalicylate (two 262.4-mg chewable tablets four times daily), metronidazole (250 mg tablet four times daily), and tetracycline (500 mg capsule four times daily). Unlike Pylera, Helidac is not a combination product; all three medications must be taken four times daily for 14 days in combination with an H₂RA rather than a PPI.

The acquisition cost for a 10-day course of Pylera and a 14-day course of Helidac is more than $200, which is substantially more expensive than the cost of prescriptions for generic metronidazole and tetracycline and a bottle of nonprescription bismuth subsalicylate.

Patients may remain infected with *H. pylori* after the initial course of therapy because of reinfection, nonadherence with the initial regimen, or antimicrobial resistance.

Table 18–3

Drug Regimens to Eradicate *Helicobacter pylori*[a]

Treatment Regimen	Cure Rates[b]
Two Drugs	
Amoxicillin 1 g three times a day + omeprazole 20 mg two times a day	Poor
Clarithromycin 500 mg three times a day + omeprazole 40 mg daily	Poor
Clarithromycin 500 mg three times a day + RBC 400 mg two times a day	Fair
Three Drugs	
Clarithromycin 500 mg two times a day + metronidazole 500 mg two times a day + omeprazole 20 mg two times a day	Good–excellent
Clarithromycin 500 mg two times a day + amoxicillin 1 g two times a day + lansoprazole 30 mg two times a day	Good–excellent
Clarithromycin 500 mg two times a day + metronidazole 500 mg two times a day + RBC 400 mg two times a day	Good
Amoxicillin 1 g two times a day + clarithromycin 500 mg two times a day + RBC 400 mg two times a day	Good
Four Drugs	
BSS 525 mg four times a day + metronidazole 250 mg four times a day + tetracycline 500 mg four times a day + H$_2$RA (conventional ulcer-healing dose)[c]	Good–excellent
BSS 525 mg four times a day + metronidazole 250 mg four times a day + amoxicillin 500 mg four times a day + H$_2$RA (conventional ulcer-healing doses)[c]	Good
BSS 525 mg four times a day + metronidazole + amoxicillin + PPI[d]	Good
Pylera (bismuth subcitrate potassium 140 mg + metronidazole 125 mg + tetracycline 125 mg) two times a day and omeprazole 20 mg two times a day	Good–excellent
Rescue Therapy[e]	
BSS 525 mg four times a day + metronidazole 500 mg four times a day + tetracycline 500 mg four times a day + omeprazole 20 mg two times a day[d]	Good–excellent
Furazolidone 200 mg two times a day + amoxicillin 1 g two times a day + omeprazole 20 mg two times a day[e]	Good
Amoxicillin 1 g two times a day + rifabutin 300 mg daily + pantoprazole 40 mg two times a day[f]	Good–excellent

BSS, bismuth subsalicylate; H$_2$RA, H2-receptor antagonist; PPI, proton pump inhibitor; RBC, ranitidine bismuth citrate (not available in the United States).

[a]These regimens based on efficacy for a 14-day treatment duration unless otherwise noted.

[b]Cure rates based on intention-to-treat analysis from references 3, 12, 14, and 35, where: poor = less than 70% eradication, fair = 70% to 80%, good = 80% to 90%, and excellent = greater than 90%.

[c]H$_2$RA therapy should be continued for an additional 2 weeks.

[d]Duration of therapy is 7 to 10 days.

[e]Given for 7 days.

[f]Given for 10 days.

Factors associated with decreased adherence include use of a large number of medications, a need for frequent drug administration or long treatment duration, and the use of drugs that may cause intolerable side effects. Potential adverse drug events include taste disturbances (clarithromycin and metronidazole), nausea, vomiting, abdominal pain, and diarrhea. Superinfections with oral thrush or vaginal candidiasis can occur.

Pre-existing antimicrobial resistance is an increasing cause of treatment failure and is estimated to account for up to 70% of all treatment failures. Geography is the most important factor in *H. pylori* resistance. Metronidazole-resistant strains are more prevalent in Asia (85%) than North America (30%).[15] Primary resistance to amoxicillin and tetracycline remains low in both the United States and Europe. Clarithromycin resistance rates are estimated to be approximately 10% in the United States. Another confounding factor when evaluating potential antibiotic resistance is that culture and sensitivity studies are not routinely performed with *H. pylori* infection.

Initiation of a second *H. pylori* treatment regimen after failure of the initial treatment regimen is usually associated with a lower success rate. Reasons for failure are often the same as those reported with failure of the initial regimen: patient noncompliance and/or antimicrobial resistance. In these situations, quadruple therapy for 14 days is generally required, and metronidazole or clarithromycin should be replaced by another antibiotic if either one of these agents was used in the initial regimen. If both clarithromycin and metronidazole were used as initial therapy, a regimen consisting of furazolidone 100 mg four times a day with tetracycline, bismuth, and a PPI can be used. Another second-line regimen consisting of a PPI, amoxicillin 1 g twice daily, and rifabutin 300 mg once daily for 10 days resulted in eradication rates greater than 80%.[16,17]

▶ Treatment of NSAID-Induced Ulcers

Treatment and dosing recommendations to heal NSAID-induced GU or provide maintenance therapy in patients receiving NSAIDS are shown in Table 18–4. Choice of regimen in a patient with PUD related to NSAID use depends on whether NSAID use is to be continued. NSAIDs should be discontinued if possible and replaced with alternatives (such as acetaminophen) although this may not be desirable or feasible in some patients. For patients discontinuing NSAID

Table 18–4

Oral Drug Regimens to Heal Peptic Ulcers or Maintain Ulcer Healing in the Absence of Antibiotic Therapy

Drug	DU or GU Healing (mg/day)[a]	Maintenance of DU or GU Healing (mg/day)[a]
Mucosal Protectant		
Sucralfate	1 g four times a day	1 g four times a day
	2 g two times a day	1–2 g two times a day
H$_2$-Receptor Antagonists		
Cimetidine	300 mg four times a day	400–800 mg daily
	400 mg two times a day	
	800 mg at bedtime	
Famotidine	20 mg two times a day	20–40 mg daily
	40 mg at bedtime	
Nizatidine	150 mg two times a day	150–300 mg daily
	300 mg at bedtime	
Ranitidine	150 mg two times a day	150–300 mg daily
	300 mg at bedtime	
Proton Pump Inhibitors		
Esomeprazole	20–40 mg daily	20–40 mg daily
Lansoprazole	15–30 mg daily	15–30 mg daily
Omeprazole	20–40 mg daily	20–40 mg daily
Pantoprazole	40 mg daily	40 mg daily
Rabeprazole	20 mg daily	20 mg daily

DU, duodenal ulcer; GU, gastric ulcer.

[a]The lower dose in each dosing range is recommended for DU; the higher dose is recommended for GU.

therapy, PPIs, H$_2$RAs, or sucralfate are all effective for ulcer healing. PPIs are usually preferred because they provide more rapid relief of symptoms and ulcer healing than H$_2$RAs or sucralfate.[16,17] For patients continuing NSAID therapy, PPIs are preferred over H$_2$RAs or sucralfate because potent acid suppression is required to accelerate ulcer healing.[18–21] If the decision is made to continue NSAID therapy, adjunctive strategies may be required to promote ulcer healing and prevent future recurrences.

▶ Prevention of NSAID-Induced Ulcers

Prophylactic regimens against PUD are often required in patients who require long-term NSAID or aspirin therapy for osteoarthritis, rheumatoid arthritis, or cardioprotection. Misoprostol, H$_2$RAs, PPIs, and COX-2 selective inhibitors have been evaluated in controlled trials to reduce the risk of NSAID-induced PUD. ❹ *In patients at risk for NSAID-induced ulcers, PPIs at standard doses reduce the risk of both gastric and DU as effectively as misoprostol and are generally better tolerated.*

Although acute GI bleeding is the most serious adverse outcome of NSAID therapy and is ultimately what clinicians are trying to prevent with prophylactic therapy, few studies have compared PUD prophylaxis strategies using this outcome measure. Acute GI bleeding is not usually evaluated in studies because of the low frequency with which bleeding

occurs in NSAID users, the small size of most prophylaxis studies, and their short duration. Instead, studies usually rely on secondary outcome variables to evaluate efficacy such as the incidence of ulcers during screening endoscopy or the incidence of patient-reported ulcer symptoms. Correlation between these secondary outcomes and PUD-related bleeding events is poor and thus, clinicians must be cautious when extrapolating the results of these studies to patient care.

Misoprostol Misoprostol is a synthetic PG E$_1$ analog that exogenously replaces PG stores. It is indicated for reducing the risk of NSAID-induced GU in patients at high risk of complications from GU (e.g., the elderly and patients with concomitant debilitating disease), as well as patients at high risk of developing gastric ulceration, such as patients with a history of ulcer. The minimum effective dose shown to inhibit acid secretion and promote mucosal defense is 400 mcg/day.[22,23] Misoprostol use is limited by a high frequency of bothersome GI effects such as abdominal pain, flatulence, and diarrhea.[24–26] Misoprostol is contraindicated in pregnancy due to potential abortifacient effects. Arthrotec is a combination product that contains diclofenac (either 50 or 75 mg) and misoprostol 200 mcg in a single tablet.

H$_2$-Receptor Antagonists Refer to Chapter 17, for more information on the H$_2$RAs. Standard doses of H$_2$RAs (e.g., famotidine 40 mg/day) are effective in preventing NSAID-related duodenal ulceration but not gastric ulceration (the most frequent type of ulcer-associated with NSAIDs). Higher doses (e.g., famotidine 40 mg twice daily) may reduce the risk of gastric and duodenal ulceration in NSAID users, but results from clinical trials are variable.

Proton Pump Inhibitors Refer to Chapter 17 for more information on the PPIs. PPI therapy is more effective than H$_2$RAs in reducing the risk of nonselective NSAID-related gastric and duodenal ulceration. PPIs are also as effective as misoprostol but better tolerated. All PPIs are effective when used in standard doses. In patients who experience a PUD-related bleeding event while taking aspirin but who require continued aspirin therapy, the addition of a PPI reduces the incidence of recurrent GI bleeding.[27] Prevacid NapraPAC provides naproxen (either 250, 375, or 500 mg) and lansoprazole 15 mg in individual blister packages.

COX-2 Selective Inhibitors With the availability of NSAIDs with COX-2 selectivity, clinicians postulated that these agents would avoid the need to add an additional prophylactic agent in patients with PUD risk factors. ❺ *However, selective COX-2 inhibitors are no more effective than the combination of a PPI and a nonselective NSAID in reducing the incidence of ulcers and are associated with a greater incidence of CV events (e.g., ischemic stroke).* Celecoxib is the only agent in this class that remains on the market; its postulated improved GI safety when compared to nonselective NSAIDs has not been established.[28,29] In addition, controlled studies demonstrated that celecoxib is no better than the combination of diclofenac and omeprazole.[30]

Longer-term studies evaluating the CV risks associated with the use of COX-2 inhibitors have found a higher incidence of CV mortality with these agents compared to traditional NSAIDs.[31,32] This prompted the withdrawal of both rofecoxib and valdecoxib from the market and the inclusion of a black box warning in the celecoxib package insert.[33] Given the CV risk of the COX-2 inhibitors, a nonselective NSAID and a PPI is recommended instead of celecoxib in patients at high risk for NSAID-related PUD.[5,34]

Sucralfate Sucralfate is a negatively charged, nonabsorbable agent that forms a complex by binding with positively-charged proteins in exudates, forming a viscous, paste-like, adhesive substance. This forms a coating that protects the ulcerated area of the gastric mucosa against gastric acid, pepsin, and bile salts. Limitations of sucralfate include the need for multiple daily dosing, large tablet size, and interaction with a number of other medications (e.g., digoxin and fluoroquinolones).

Adverse effects of sucralfate include constipation, nausea, metallic taste, and the possibility for aluminum toxicity in patients with renal failure. While sucralfate may be used for the treatment of an NSAID-related ulcer when NSAID therapy is being stopped, it is not recommended for use as prophylaxis against NSAID-induced ulcers.

▶ ***Conventional Treatment of Active DU and GU and Long-Term Maintenance of Ulcer Healing***

Conventional therapy prior to the advent of *H. pylori* eradication therapy consisted of standard doses of sucralfate or an H_2RA for 6 to 8 weeks. A PPI provides equivalent efficacy with treatment duration of only 4 weeks. Long-term antiulcer therapy is ineffective for treating *H. pylori* infections.

❻ *Low-dose maintenance therapy with a PPI or H_2RA is only indicated for patients who fail* H. pylori *eradication, have* H. pylori-*negative ulcers, or develop severe complications related to ulcer disease.* Drug regimens and doses are presented in Table 18–4.

▶ ***Treatment of Refractory Ulcers***

The presence of refractory ulcers (ulcers that persist beyond 8 weeks [DU] or 12 weeks [GU]) requires thorough assessment, including evaluation of medication compliance. The patient should be questioned regarding recent NSAID ingestion. Tolerance has been reported with as few as 4 weeks of H_2RA therapy, and thus a change to PPI therapy should be considered in this situation.[35] Other assessments that may be considered include an ulcer biopsy to exclude malignancy, *H. pylori* testing (if not done initially), a serum gastrin measurement to exclude ZES, and gastric acid studies. In one study, increasing the starting dose of PPI therapy healed 90% of refractory ulcers after 8 weeks of therapy.[36]

Patient Care and Monitoring

General Recommendations: *H. pylori*–Associated and NSAID-Induced Ulcers

1. Assess the severity of signs and symptoms. Identify the presence of any alarm signs and symptoms.

2. Educate the patient on monitoring for alarm signs and symptoms.

3. Obtain a history of prescription medication, over-the-counter medication, and dietary supplement use.

4. Encourage lifestyle modifications such as reducing tobacco use and ethanol ingestion and decreasing psychological stress.

5. Determine the appropriate duration for acid-suppressive therapy.

6. Define the current impact of PUD on the patient's quality of life and the improvement in these outcomes sought with drug therapy.

7. Evaluate current drug therapy for potential adverse drug reactions and drug interactions.

H. pylori–Associated Ulcers

1. Recommend an appropriate drug regimen that will eradicate the organism.

2. Identify the patient's drug allergies and avoid drug classes a patient is allergic to.

3. Educate patients on specific adverse drug effects, particularly with metronidazole (avoidance of alcohol), bismuth (change in stool color), and clarithromycin (taste disturbance).

4. Assess the potential for drug interactions, particularly in patients taking regimens containing metronidazole, clarithromycin, and/or cimetidine.

5. Recommend different antibiotics if this treatment regimen is a result of failure of a prior *H. pylori* regimen.

6. Educate the patient on the importance of adherence to eradication therapy.

NSAID-Associated Ulcers

1. Assess for risk factors for NSAID ulcers and recommend an appropriate strategy to reduce ulcer risk.

2. Monitor for signs and symptoms of complications associated with NSAID-related ulceration.

3. Recommend an appropriate treatment regimen to heal the ulcer.

4. Assess and counsel patients on potential adverse drug events and drug interactions.

5. Inform patients who are receiving prophylactic therapy on the importance of its use, potential adverse drug events, and the possible alarm symptoms associated with PUD.

OUTCOME EVALUATION[37]

- Obtain a baseline CBC. Recheck the CBC if the patient exhibits alarm signs or symptoms.
- Obtain a baseline serum creatinine measurement. Calculate the estimated creatinine clearance and adjust the dose of H_2RAs and sucralfate according to package insert recommendations.
- Obtain a history of symptoms from the patient. Monitor for improvements in pain symptoms (e.g., epigastric or abdominal pain) daily.
- Monitor the patient for the development of any alarm signs and symptoms.
- Recommend a follow-up visit if signs and symptoms worsen at any time or do not improve within the defined treatment period.
- Assess for potential drug interactions whenever there is a change in the patient's medications, particularly for patients taking cimetidine, omeprazole, or sucralfate.
- Educate the patient on the importance of adhering to the *H. pylori*-eradication regimen.
- Monitor the patient for complications related to antibiotic therapy (e.g., diarrhea or oral thrush) during and after completion of *H. pylori* eradication therapy.
- Recommend follow-up care if the patient's signs and symptoms do not improve after completion of *H. pylori*-eradication therapy.

Abbreviations Introduced in This Chapter

BAO	Basal acid output
cag-PAI	Cag pathogenicity island
CLO	Campylobacter-like organism
COX	Cyclooxygenase
DU	Duodenal ulcer
EGD	Esophagogastroduodenoscopy
GU	Gastric ulcer
H_2RA	Histamine$_2$-receptor antagonist
MALT	Mucosa-associated lymphoid tissue
MAO	Maximal acid output
NSAID	Nonsteroidal anti-inflammatory drug
PG	Prostaglandin
PPI	Proton pump inhibitor
PUD	Peptic ulcer disease
SRMD	Stress-related mucosal damage
ZES	Zollinger-Ellison syndrome

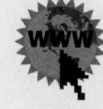

Self-assessment questions and answers are available at *http://www.mhpharmacotherapy. com/pp.html.*

REFERENCES

1. Del Valle J, Chey WD, Scheiman JM. Acid peptic disorders. In: T Yamada, DH Alpers, N Kaplowitz et al., eds. Textbook of Gastroenterology, 4th ed. Vol. 1. New York: Lippincott Williams & Wilkins, 2003:1321–1376.
2. Sonnenberg A. Peptic ulcer. In: J Everhart, ed. Digestive Diseases in the United States: Epidemiology and Impact. Washington, DC: US Department of Health and Human Services, Public Health Service, National Institutes of Health, 1994:359–408. NIH publication no. 94:1447.
3. Suerbaum S, Michetti P. *Helicobacter pylori* infection. N Engl J Med 2002;347:1175–1186.
4. Weaver AL. Review article: Aspirin, non-steroidal anti-inflammatory drugs and cyclo-oxygenase-1 sparing agents. AP&T Symposium Series 2005;1:2–5.
5. Chan FK, Graham DY. Review article: Prevention of non-steroidal anti-inflammatory drug gastrointestinal complications: Review and recommendations based on risk assessment. Aliment Pharmacol Ther 2004;19:1051–1061.
6. Friedman GD, Siegelaub AB, Seltzer CC. Cigarettes, alcohol, coffee and peptic ulcer. N Engl J Med 1974;290:469–473.
7. Wu WK, Cho CH. The pharmacological actions of nicotine on the gastrointestinal tract. J Pharmacol Sci 2004;94:348–358.
8. Quan C, Talley NJ. Management of peptic ulcer disease not related to *Helicobacter pylori* or NSAIDs. Am J Gastroenterol 2002;97:2950–2961.
9. Chey WD, Wong BCY, et al. American College of Gastroenterology guideline in the management of *helicobacter pylori* infection. Am J Gastroenterol 2007;102:1808–1825.
10. Laine L, Bombardier C, Hawkey CJ, et al. Stratifying the risk of NSAID-related upper gastrointestinal clinical events: Results of a double-blind outcomes study in patients with rheumatoid arthritis. Gastroenterology 2002;123:1006–1012.
11. Van Deventer G, Elashoff J, Reedy T, et al. A randomized study of maintenance therapy with ranitidine to prevent the recurrence of duodenal ulcer. N Engl J Med 1989;320:1113–1119.
12. Behrman SW. Management of complicated peptic ulcer disease. Arch Surg 2005;140:201–208.
13. Laheij RJ, Rossum LG, Jansen JB, et al. Evaluation of treatment regimens to cure *Helicobacter pylori* infection: A meta-analysis. Aliment Pharmacol Ther 1999;13:857–864.
14. Calvet X, Garcia N, Lopez T, et al. A meta-analysis of short versus long therapy with a proton pump inhibitor, clarithromycin and either metronidazole or amoxycillin for treating *Helicobacter pylori* infection. Aliment Pharmacol Ther 2000;14:603–609.
15. Meyer JM, Silliman NP, Wang W, et al. Risk factors for *Helicobacter pylori* resistance in the United States: The surveillance of *H. pylori* antimicrobial resistance partnership (SHARP) study, 1993–1999. Ann Intern Med 2002;136:13–24.
16. Jodlowski TZ, Lam S, Ashby CR. Emerging therapies for the treatment of *helicobacter pylori* infections. Ann Pharmacother 2008;42:1621–1639.
17. Qasim A, Sebastian S, Thornton O, et al. Rifabutin- and furazolidone-based *Helicobacter pylori* eradication therapies after failure of standard first- and second-line eradication attempts in dyspepsia patients. Aliment Pharmacol Ther 2005;21:91–96.
18. Agrawal NM, Campbell DR, Safdi MA, et al. Superiority of lansoprazole vs ranitidine in healing nonsteroidal anti-inflammatory drug-associated gastric ulcers: Results of a double-blind, randomized, multicenter study. NSAID-associated gastric ulcer study group. Arch Intern Med 2000;160:1455–1461.
19. Yeomans ND, Tulassay Z, Juhasz L, et al. A comparison of omeprazole with ranitidine for ulcers associated with nonsteroidal antiinflammatory drugs. Acid suppression trial: Ranitidine versus omeprazole for NSAID-associated ulcer treatment (ASTRONAUT) study group. N Engl J Med 1998;338:719–726.
20. Wolfe MM, Lichtenstein DR, Singh G. Gastrointestinal toxicity of nonsteroidal antiinflammatory drugs. N Engl J Med 1999;340:1888–1899.

21. Targownik LE, Metge CJ, Leung S, et al. The relative efficacies of gastroprotective strategies in chronic users of nonsteroidal anti-inflammatory drugs. Gastronenterology 2008;134:937–944.
22. Graham DY, White RH, Moreland LW, et al. Duodenal and gastric ulcer prevention with misoprostol in arthritis patients taking NSAIDs. Misoprostol study group. Ann Intern Med 1993;119:257–262.
23. Raskin JB, White RH, Jaszewski R, et al. Misoprostol and ranitidine in the prevention of NSAID-induced ulcers: A prospective, double-blind, multicenter study. Am J Gastroenterol 1996;91:223–227.
24. Silverstein FE, Graham DY, Senior JR, et al. Misoprostol reduces serious gastrointestinal complications in patients with rheumatoid arthritis receiving nonsteroidal anti-inflammatory drugs: A randomized, double-blind, placebo-controlled trial. Ann Intern Med 1995;123:241–249.
25. Taha AS, Hudson N, Hawkey CJ, et al. Famotidine for the prevention of gastric and duodenal ulcers caused by nonsteroidal antiinflammatory drugs. N Engl J Med 1996;334:1435–1439.
26. Hawkey CJ, Karrasch JA, Szczepanski L, et al. Omeprazole compared with misoprostol for ulcers associated with nonsteroidal antiinflammatory drugs. Omeprazole versus misoprostol for NSAID-induced ulcer management (OMNIUM) study group. N Engl J Med 1998;338:727–734.
27. Chan FK, Ching JY, Hung LC, et al. Clopidogrel versus aspirin and esomeprazole to prevent recurrent ulcer bleeding. N Engl J Med 2005;352:238–244.
28. Silverstein FE, Faich G, Goldstein JL, et al. Gastrointestinal toxicity with celecoxib vs nonsteroidal anti-inflammatory drugs for osteoarthritis and rheumatoid arthritis: The CLASS study: A randomized controlled trial. Celecoxib long-term arthritis safety study. JAMA 2000;284:1247–1255.
29. Hrachovec JB, Mora M, Wright JM, et al. Reporting of 6-Month vs 12-Month data in a clinical trial of celecoxib. JAMA 2001;286:2398–2400.
30. Chan FK, Hung LC, Suen BY, et al. Celecoxib versus diclofenac and omeprazole in reducing the risk of recurrent ulcer bleeding in patients with arthritis. N Engl J Med 2002;347:2104–2110.
31. Nussmeier NA, Whelton AA, Brown MT, et al. Complications of the COX-2 inhibitors parecoxib and valdecoxib after cardiac surgery. N Engl J Med 2005;352:1081–1091.
32. Bresalier RS, Sandler RS, Quan H, et al. Cardiovascular events associated with rofecoxib in a colorectal adenoma chemoprevention trial. N Engl J Med 2005;352:1092–1102.
33. Administration FDA. FDA alert for practitioners celecoxib (marketed as Celebrex) 2005.
34. Chan FK, Abraham NS, Scheiman JM, et al. Management of patients on nonsteroidal anti-inflammatory drugs: A clinical practice recommendation from the first international working party on gastrointestinal and cardiovascular effects of nonsteroidal anti-inflammatory effects and anti-platelet agents. Am J Gastroenterol 2008;103:2908–2918.
35. Prewett EJ, Hudson M, Nwokolo CU, et al. Nocturnal intragastric acidity during and after a period of dosing with either ranitidine or omeprazole. Gastroenterology 1991;100:873–877.
36. Brunner G, Arnold R, Hennig U, Fuchs W. An open trial of long-term therapy with lansoprazole in patients with peptic ulceration resistant to extended high-dose ranitidine treatment. Aliment Pharmacol Ther 1993;7(Suppl 1):51–55, discussion 61–66.
37. Berardi R, Welage L. Peptic ulcer disease. In: DiPiro JT; Talbert RA; Yee GC, et al., eds. Pharmacotherapy: A Pathophysiologic Approach, 7th ed. New York:McGraw-Hill, 2008:576–587.

19 Inflammatory Bowel Disease

Brian A. Hemstreet

LEARNING OBJECTIVES

● **Upon completion of the chapter, the reader will be able to:**

1. Characterize the pathophysiologic mechanisms underlying inflammatory bowel disease (IBD).

2. Recognize the signs and symptoms of IBD, including major differences between ulcerative colitis (UC) and Crohn's disease (CD).

3. Identify appropriate therapeutic outcomes for patients with IBD.

4. Describe pharmacologic treatment options for patients with acute or chronic symptoms of UC and CD.

5. Create a patient-specific drug treatment plan based on symptoms, severity, and location of UC or CD.

6. Recommend appropriate monitoring parameters and patient education for selected drug regimens for treatment of IBD.

KEY CONCEPTS

❶ Inflammatory bowel disease (IBD) includes both ulcerative colitis (UC) and Crohn's disease (CD) and is associated with inflammation of various areas of the GI tract.

❷ Differentiation of UC and CD is based on signs and symptoms as well as characteristic endoscopic findings including the extent, pattern, and depth of inflammation.

❸ Patients may manifest extraintestinal symptoms of IBD, such as arthritis, primary sclerosing cholangitis, erythema nodosum, and pyoderma gangrenosum, among others.

❹ Major treatment goals for patients with IBD include alleviation of signs and symptoms and suppression of inflammation during acute episodes and maintenance of remission thereafter.

❺ When designing a drug regimen for treatment of IBD, several factors should be considered, including the patient's symptoms, medical history, current medication use, drug allergies, and location and severity of disease.

❻ Antidiarrheal medications that reduce GI motility, such as loperamide, diphenoxylate/atropine, and codeine should be avoided in patients with active IBD due to the risk of precipitating acute colonic dilation (toxic megacolon).

❼ Treatment of acute episodes of UC is dictated by the severity and extent of disease, and first-line therapy of mild to moderate disease involves oral or topical aminosalicylate derivatives.

❽ Maintenance of remission of UC may be achieved with oral or topical aminosalicylates. Immunosuppressants such as azathioprine, 6-mercaptopurine (6-MP), or infliximab can be used for unresponsive patients or those who develop corticosteroid dependency.

❾ Treatment of active mild to moderate CD involves use of oral or topical aminosalicylate derivatives, whereas moderate to severe disease may require systemic corticosteroid therapy.

❿ Maintenance of remission of CD may be achieved with oral or topical aminosalicylate derivatives, immunosuppressants (such as azathioprine, 6-MP, and methotrexate), or infliximab, adalimumab, certolizumab, or natalizumab.

INTRODUCTION

❶ *Inflammatory bowel disease (IBD) encompasses both Crohn's disease (CD) and ulcerative colitis (UC). Both disorders are associated with inflammation of various regions within the GI tract.* Differences exist between UC and CD with regard to the regions of the GI tract that may be affected as well as in the distribution and depth of inflammation. Some patients with IBD may also have inflammation involving organs other than the GI tract, known as extraintestinal manifestations. Symptoms of IBD are associated with significant morbidity, reduction in quality of life, and substantial costs to the health care system. For purposes of this chapter, references made to IBD will include both UC and CD. Significant differences between UC and CD will be discussed separately when applicable.

EPIDEMIOLOGY

IBD is most common in Westernized countries such as the United States. UC affects up to 500,000 people and CD affects up to 480,000 people in the United States.[1-5] The age of initial presentation of IBD is bimodal, with patients typically diagnosed between the age ranges of 20 to 40 years or 60 to 80 years.[5] The peak incidence of CD occurs in the second and third decades of life, with a smaller peak in the fifth decade.[2,5] Peak incidence of UC occurs between the ages of 15 and 25 years.[6]

Men and women are approximately equally affected by IBD. In general, whites are affected more often than blacks, and persons of Jewish descent also have higher reported incidences of IBD. One of the greatest risk factors for development of IBD is a positive family history of the disease. The incidence of IBD is 10 to 40 times greater in patients with a first-degree relative who has IBD compared to the general population.[4,5,7] A positive family history may be more of a contributing factor for development of CD than UC.[7-9]

ETIOLOGY

The exact cause of IBD is not fully understood. Processes thought to be involved in its development include genetic predisposition, dysregulation of the inflammatory response within the GI tract, or perhaps environmental or antigenic factors.[3,4] The fact that a positive family history is a strong predictor of IBD supports the theory that genetic predisposition may be responsible in many cases. Many potential candidate genes have been identified. An example is a gene found on chromosome 16 that encodes for nucleotide oligomerization domain 2 (NOD2). NOD2 is a cytoplasmic protein expressed in macrophages, monocytes, and gut epithelial cells thought to be involved in recognition and degradation of bacterial products by the gut wall. Less is known about genetic alterations that may predispose patients to UC, but UC may share common genetic features with CD.

An alteration in the inflammatory response regulated by intestinal epithelial cells may also contribute to development of IBD. This may involve inappropriate processing of antigens presented to the GI epithelial cells.[3,4,10,11] The inflammatory response in IBD may actually be directed at bacteria that normally colonize the GI tract. Products derived from these bacteria may translocate across the mucosal layer of the GI tract and interact with various cells involved in immunologic recognition. The result is T-cell stimulation, excess production of proinflammatory cytokines, and persistent inflammation within the GI tract.

The intestinal mucosa of patients with CD has a preponderance of CD4+ type 1 helper T cells, while patients with UC have more CD4+ lymphocytes with atypical type 2 helper T cells.[10] Likewise, drugs such as nonsteroidal anti-inflammatory drugs (NSAIDs) that disrupt the integrity of the GI mucosa may facilitate mucosal entry of intestinal antigens and lead to disease flares in patients with IBD.[12]

The role of antigens derived from dietary intake in the development of IBD is less well defined. There is some speculation that ingestion of large quantities of refined carbohydrates or margarine leads to higher rates of CD. Use of oral contraceptives has been associated with increased development of IBD in some cohort studies, but a strong causal relationship has not been proven.[8]

Lastly, positive smoking status has been shown to have protective effects in UC, leading to reductions in disease severity. The opposite is true in CD, as smoking may lead to increases in symptoms or worsening of the disease.[10]

PATHOPHYSIOLOGY
Ulcerative Colitis

The inflammatory response in UC is propagated by atypical type 2 helper T cells that produce proinflammatory cytokines such as interleukin-1 (IL-1), IL-6, and tumor necrosis factor (TNF).[8] As discussed previously, a genetic predisposition to UC may partially explain the development of excessive colonic and rectal inflammation. The finding of positive perinuclear antineutrophil cytoplasmic antibodies (pANCA) in association with the human leukocyte antigen (HLA)-DR2 allele in a large percentage of patients with UC supports this theory.[13]

The potential role of environmental factors in development of UC implies that the immune response is directed against an unknown antigen. The findings that development and severity of UC are reduced in patients who smoke, or in those with appendectomies, may support the theory that these factors may somehow modify either the genetic component or phenotypic response to immunologic stimuli.[12,14]

The inflammatory process within the GI tract is limited to the colon and rectum in patients with UC (Fig. 19–1). Most patients with UC have involvement of the rectum (*proctitis*) or both the rectum and the sigmoid colon (proctosigmoiditis). Inflammation involving the majority of the colon is referred to as *pancolitis*. Left-sided disease, defined as inflammation extending from the rectum to the splenic flexure, occurs in 30% to 40% of patients.[12] A small number of cases of UC involve mild inflammation of the terminal ileum, referred to as "backwash ileitis."

The pattern of inflammation in UC is continuous and confluent throughout the affected areas of the GI tract. The inflammation is also superficial and does not typically extend below the submucosal layer of the GI tract (Fig. 19–2). Ulceration or erosion of the GI mucosa may be present and varies with disease severity. The formation of *crypt abscesses* within the mucosal layers of the GI tract is characteristic of UC and may help to distinguish it from CD. Severe inflammation may also result in areas of hypertrophied GI mucosa, which may manifest as *pseudopolyps* within the

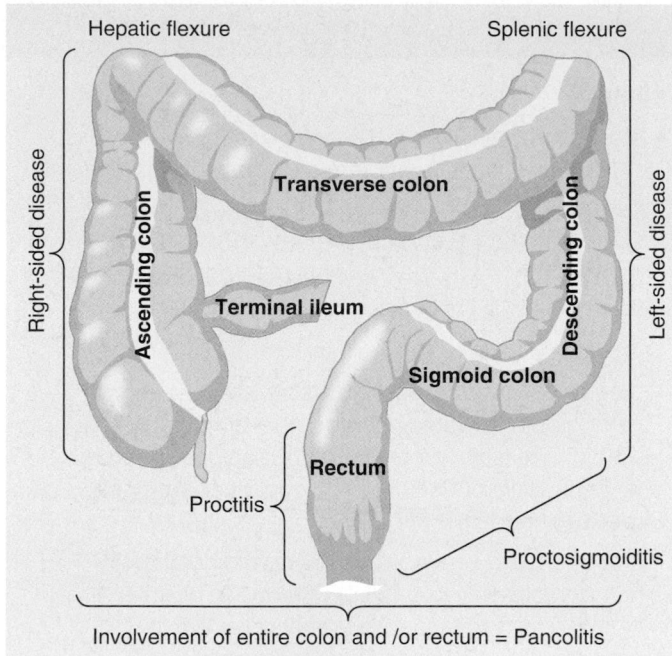

FIGURE 19–1. Major GI landmarks and disease distribution in inflammatory bowel disease.

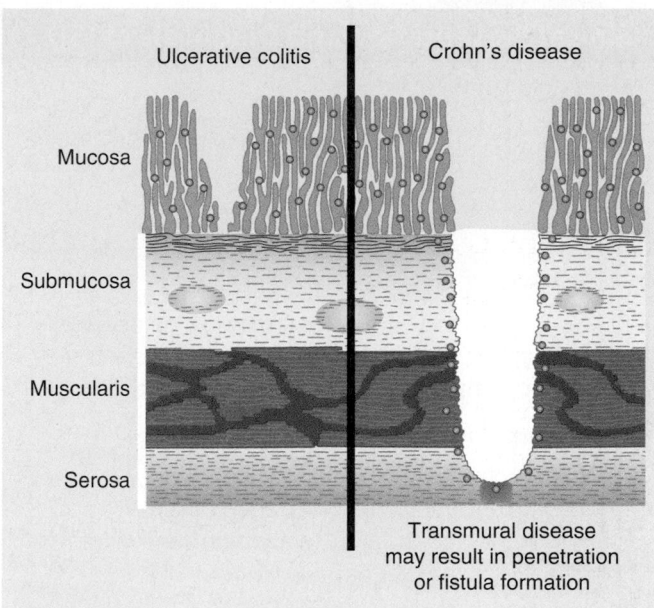

FIGURE 19–2. Depth of disease penetration in ulcerative colitis and Crohn's disease.

colon.[13] The inflammatory response may progress in severity, leading to mucosal friability and significant GI bleeding.

Crohn's Disease

As with UC, the immune activation seen in CD involves the release of many proinflammatory cytokines. Cytokines thought to play major roles in CD are derived from T-helper type 1 cells and include interferon-γ, TNF-α, and IL-1, IL-6, and IL-12. TNF-α is a major contributor to the inflammatory process seen in CD. Its physiologic effects include activation of macrophages, procoagulant effects in the vascular endothelium, and increases in production of matrix metalloproteinases in mucosal cells.[13,15] Excessive production of both interferon-γ and TNF-α may account for the excessive clinical evidence of granulomatous disease in patients with CD.[11] TNF-α is also thought to induce production of nuclear factor $\kappa\beta$, which stimulates further production of TNF-α and other proinflammatory cytokines.[3,16]

The role of an immune response directed against endogenous bacteria as the initiating factor is more evident in CD, as evidenced by the apparent strong T-helper 1 activation against bacteria seen in animal models of this disease. The role of dietary antigens in the development of CD compared to UC is also another potential initiating factor. Excess ingestion of refined sugars or margarine may be higher in patients who develop CD.[8]

The distribution of inflammation in CD differs from that seen in UC, as any part of the entire GI tract may be affected in CD. The small intestine is the site most commonly involved. Within the small intestine, the terminal ileum and cecum are almost always affected. Approximately 20% of patients have isolated colonic involvement, whereas inflammation proximal to the small intestine is almost never seen without the presence of small or large intestinal disease.[13]

In contrast to UC, the pattern of inflammation in CD is described as discontinuous. Areas of inflammation are intermixed with areas of normal GI mucosa, resulting in characteristic "skip lesions." Superficial **aphthous ulcers** may also develop in the GI mucosa. These ulcers may coalesce into larger linear ulcers, resulting in fissure formation as they increase in depth, giving rise to the characteristic "cobblestone" pattern observed upon examination of the mucosa.

Furthermore, the inflammation may be **transmural**, penetrating to the muscularis or serosal layers of the GI tract (Fig. 19–2). The propensity for transmural involvement may lead to serious complications of CD, such as **strictures**, **fistulae**, abscesses, and perforation.[13] While rectal inflammation is typically less common in CD than UC, several types of perianal lesions may be observed in patients with CD. These include skin tags, hemorrhoids, fissures, anal ulcers, abscesses, and fistulae.[15]

CLINICAL PRESENTATION AND DIAGNOSIS

❷ *Differentiation between UC and CD is based on signs and symptoms as well as characteristic endoscopic findings, including the extent, pattern, and depth of inflammation (see Clinical Presentation box).*

Extraintestinal Manifestations and Complications of IBD

❸ *Patients may manifest signs and symptoms of disease in areas outside the GI tract. These extraintestinal manifestations*

Clinical Presentation and Diagnosis of IBD

General

- Patients with CD or UC may present with similar symptoms.
- The onset may be insidious and subacute.
- Some patients present with extraintestinal manifestations before GI symptoms occur.
- In approximately 10% of cases it may not be possible to distinguish between UC and CD. These patients are described as having "indeterminate colitis."

Symptoms

- *Ulcerative colitis*: Diarrhea (bloody, watery, or mucopurulent), rectal bleeding, abdominal pain/ cramping, weight loss and malnutrition, tenesmus, constipation (with proctitis)
- *Crohn's disease*: Diarrhea (less bloody than UC), rectal bleeding (less than UC), abdominal pain/cramping, weight loss and malnutrition (more common than UC), fatigue/malaise

Signs

- *Ulcerative colitis*: Fever, tachycardia (with severe disease), dehydration, arthritis, hemorrhoids, anal fissures, perirectal abscesses
- *Crohn's disease*: Fever, tachycardia (with severe disease), dehydration, arthritis, abdominal mass and tenderness, perianal fissure or fistula

Laboratory Tests

- *Ulcerative colitis*: Leukocytosis, decreased hematocrit/ hemoglobin, elevated erythrocyte sedimentation rate (ESR) or C-reactive protein (CRP), guaiac-positive stool, (+) perinuclear antineutrophil cytoplasmic antibodies (pANCA; up to 70% of patients)
- *Crohn's disease*: Leukocytosis, decreased hematocrit/ hemoglobin, elevated ESR or CRP, guaiac-positive stool, (+) anti–*Saccharomyces cerevisiae* antibodies (up to 50% of patients), hypoalbuminemia with severe disease

may occur in various body regions.[5,13] Painful joint complications associated with IBD include sacroiliitis and ankylosing spondylitis. Ocular involvement with episcleritis, uveitis, or iritis may manifest as blurred vision, eye pain, and photophobia. Associated skin findings include pyoderma gangrenosum (involving papules and vesicles that develop into painful ulcerations) and erythema nodosum (red nodules of varying size typically found on the lower extremities). Nephrolithiasis may also develop at a higher rate in patients with IBD. Oxalate stones are more common in CD, and uric acid–containing stones are more common in UC.[13]

Liver and biliary manifestations of IBD include an increased incidence of gallstone formation in patients with CD and development of sclerosing cholangitis or cholangiocarcinoma in patients with UC. Patients with UC are also at increased risk for development of colorectal cancer. Ongoing inflammation due to active IBD may induce a hypercoagulable state, resulting in higher rates of both arterial and venous thromboembolism. Likewise, inflammation and recurrent blood loss may result in the development of chronic anemia. Patients with IBD also have higher rates of osteopenia, osteoporosis, and fractures, which are most strongly associated with use of corticosteroids.[17]

A serious complication of UC is toxic megacolon, defined as dilation of the transverse colon of greater than 6 cm (2.4 in.). Patients with toxic megacolon typically manifest systemic signs of severe inflammation such as fever, tachycardia, and abdominal distention.[3,13] Surgical intervention, including colonic resection, may be necessary to acutely manage toxic megacolon.

Formation of strictures, abscesses, fistulae, and obstructions in patients with CD is possible. Patients with CD may develop significant weight loss or nutritional deficiencies secondary to malabsorption of nutrients in the small intestine, or as a consequence of multiple small- or large-bowel resections. Common nutritional deficiencies encountered in IBD include vitamin B_{12}, fat-soluble vitamins, zinc, folate, and iron. Malabsorption in children with CD may contribute to significant reductions in growth and development.

Diagnosis

Because patients often present with nonspecific GI symptoms, initial diagnostic evaluation includes methods to characterize the disease and rule out other potential etiologies. This may include stool cultures to examine for infectious causes of diarrhea.

Endoscopic approaches are typically used and may include colonoscopy, proctosigmoidoscopy, or possibly upper GI endoscopy in patients with suspected CD. Endoscopy is useful for determining the disease distribution, pattern and depth of inflammation, and to obtain mucosal biopsy specimens. Supplemental information from imaging procedures, such as CT, abdominal x-ray, abdominal ultrasound, or intestinal barium studies may provide evidence of complications such as obstruction, abscess, perforation, or colonic dilation.[3]

After the diagnosis is made, the information derived from diagnostic testing and the patient's medical history and symptoms are used to gauge disease severity. The severity of active UC is generally classified as mild, moderate, severe, or fulminant.[1] Mild UC typically involves up to four bloody or watery stools per day without systemic signs of toxicity or elevation of erythrocyte sedimentation rate (ESR). Moderate disease is classified as more than four stools per day with evidence of systemic toxicity. Severe disease is considered

Patient Encounter 1, Part 1

A 25-year-old Caucasian woman presents to the university student clinic with complaints of intermittent crampy abdominal pain and four to five loose stools per day. She describes some visible mucus and blood in the stool and states that these symptoms have been present for 6 to 8 weeks. She also has intermittent lower back pain, fatigue, fever, and a 4.5-kg (10-lb) weight loss. The back pain started about the same time as her GI symptoms. She denies any sick contacts and has not eaten any take-out or restaurant food over the last 2 months. She takes nonprescription naproxen as needed for aches and pains. She has been using more naproxen recently because of the back pain. She also takes an oral contraceptive pill once daily. She consumes alcohol socially and currently smokes one-half to one pack of cigarettes per day.

What symptoms are suggestive of IBD in this patient?

Are these symptoms more suggestive of UC or CD?

What factors may be contributing to her IBD symptoms?

What additional information would you acquire prior to recommending drug therapy?

more than six stools per day and evidence of anemia, tachycardia, or an elevated ESR or C-reactive protein (CRP). Lastly, fulminant UC may present as more than 10 stools per day with continuous bleeding, signs of systemic toxicity, abdominal distention or tenderness, colonic dilation, or a requirement for blood transfusion.

A similar classification scheme is used to gauge the severity of active CD.[2] Patients with mild to moderate CD are typically ambulatory and have no evidence of dehydration; systemic toxicity; loss of body weight; or abdominal tenderness, mass, or obstruction. Moderate to severe disease is considered in patients who fail to respond to treatment for mild to moderate disease, or those with fever, weight loss, abdominal pain or tenderness, vomiting, intestinal obstruction, or significant anemia. Severe to fulminant CD is classified as the presence of persistent symptoms or evidence of systemic toxicity despite outpatient corticosteroid treatment, or presence of cachexia, rebound tenderness, intestinal obstruction, or abscess.

TREATMENT

Desired Outcomes

● Pharmacologic interventions for IBD are designed to target the underlying inflammatory response. Treatment goals involve both management of active disease and prevention of disease relapse. ❹ *Major treatment goals include alleviation of signs and symptoms and suppression of inflammation during acute episodes and maintenance of remission thereafter.* Addressing active IBD in a timely and appropriate manner may prevent major complications such as perforation and may reduce the need for hospitalization

or surgical intervention. Once control of active disease is obtained, treatment regimens are designed to achieve the following long-term goals: (a) maintenance of remission and prevention of disease relapse; (b) improvement in the patient's quality of life; (c) prevention of surgical intervention or hospitalization; (d) management of extraintestinal manifestations; (e) prevention of malnutrition; and (f) prevention of treatment-associated adverse effects.

General Approach to Treatment

❺ *When designing a drug regimen for treatment of IBD, several factors should be considered, including the patient's symptoms; medical history; current medication use; drug allergies; and extent, location, and severity of disease.* A thorough patient history may also help to identify a family history of IBD or potential exacerbating factors, such as tobacco or NSAID use.

Nonpharmacologic Therapy

No specific dietary restrictions are recommended for patients with IBD, but avoidance of high-residue foods in patients with strictures may help to prevent obstruction. Avoidance of excess fat in the diet may be preferred as well. Nutritional strategies in patients with long-standing IBD may include use of vitamin and mineral supplementation. Administration of vitamin B_{12}, folic acid, fat-soluble vitamins, and iron may be needed to prevent or treat deficiencies. In severe cases, enteral or parenteral nutrition may be needed to achieve adequate caloric intake.

Patients with IBD, particularly those with CD, are also at risk for bone loss. This may be a function of malabsorption or an effect of repeated courses of corticosteroids.[17] Risk factors for osteoporosis should be determined, and baseline bone density measurement may be considered.[17] Vitamin D and calcium supplementation should be used in all patients receiving long-term corticosteroids. Oral bisphosphonate therapy may also be considered in patients receiving prolonged courses of corticosteroids or in those with osteopenia or osteoporosis.

Surgical intervention is a potential treatment option in patients with complications such as fistulae or abscesses, or in patients with medically refractory disease. UC is curable with performance of a total colectomy. Patients with UC may opt to have a colectomy to reduce the chance of developing colorectal cancer. Patients with CD may have affected areas of intestine resected. Unfortunately, CD may recur following surgical resection. Repeated surgeries may lead to significant malabsorption of nutrients and drugs consistent with development of short-bowel syndrome.

Pharmacologic Therapy

Several pharmacologic classes are available for the acute treatment and maintenance therapy of IBD. Because there may be differences in the underlying disease process, distribution, and severity between CD and UC, response rates to drugs in the same pharmacologic class may differ between these two diseases. Therefore, initial selection of an appropriate agent for patients with active IBD should be designed to deliver maximum efficacy while minimizing toxicity. Response rates to individual classes of medications for both UC and CD will be discussed within the specific treatment section for each disease.

▶ Symptomatic Interventions

Patients with active IBD often have severe abdominal pain and diarrhea. Medications used to manage these types of symptoms may have adverse consequences in patients with active IBD. ❻ *Antidiarrheal medications that reduce GI motility, such as loperamide, diphenoxylate/atropine, and codeine should be avoided in patients with active IBD due to the risk of precipitating acute colonic dilation (toxic megacolon).*[13] Drugs with anticholinergic properties, such as hyoscyamine and dicyclomine, are often used to treat intestinal spasm and pain, but these drugs may also reduce GI motility and should generally be avoided in active IBD.

Patients who have had multiple intestinal resections due to CD may have diarrhea related to the inability to reabsorb bile salts. Cholestyramine has been demonstrated to improve diarrheal symptoms in this population.[15] NSAIDs should be avoided for pain management due to their ability to worsen IBD symptoms. Opioid analgesics should be used with caution, as they may significantly reduce GI motility.

▶ Aminosalicylates

The aminosalicylates are among the most commonly used drugs for inducing and maintaining remission in patients with IBD (Table 19–1). These drugs are designed to deliver 5-aminosalicylate (5-ASA, mesalamine) to areas of inflammation within the GI tract. While the mechanism of mesalamine is not fully understood, it appears to have favorable anti-inflammatory effects. The delivery of mesalamine to the affected sites is accomplished by either linking mesalamine to a carrier molecule or altering the formulation to release drug in response to changes in intestinal pH. Topical suppositories and enemas are designed to deliver mesalamine directly to the distal colon and rectum.[7,18–21]

The prototypical aminosalicylate is sulfasalazine, which is comprised of mesalamine linked by a diazo bond to the carrier molecule sulfapyridine. This linkage prevents premature absorption of mesalamine in the small intestine. Once sulfasalazine is delivered to the colon, bacterial degradation of the diazo bond frees mesalamine from sulfapyridine. Sulfapyridine is then absorbed and excreted renally, while mesalamine acts locally within the GI tract.

Newer mesalamine products utilize nonsulfapyridine methods for drug delivery. Olsalazine uses two mesalamine molecules linked together, while balsalazide uses the inert carrier molecule 4-aminobenzoyl-β-alanine. Both drugs use a diazo bond similar to sulfasalazine. Other mesalamine formulations are pH-dependent formulations that release mesalamine at various points throughout the GI tract. The newest mesalamine products include Lialda, a multimatrix (MMX) formulation with a pH-sensitive coat that releases in the terminal ileum, allowing for once-daily dosing.[18] Enteric-coated mesalamine granules that also use a polymer matrix for extended release (Apriso) are also able to be given in a once-daily fashion.

Sulfasalazine is associated with various adverse effects, most of which are thought to be due to the sulfapyridine component. Common adverse effects that may be dose related include headache, dyspepsia, nausea, vomiting, and fatigue.[19–21] Idiosyncratic effects include bone marrow suppression, reduction in sperm counts in males, hepatitis,

---

Table 19–1

Aminosalicylates for Treatment of IBD

Drug	Trade Names	Formulation	Strengths	Daily Dosage Range (g)	Site of Action
Sulfasalazine	Azulfidine Azulfidine Entabs Sulfazine Sulfazine EC	Immediate-release or enteric-coated tablets	500 mg	2–6	Colon
Mesalamine	Rowasa	Enema	4 g/60 mL	4	Distal left colon and rectum
	Asacol	Delayed-release resin tablet	400 mg	1.6–4.8	Distal ileum and colon
	Canasa	Rectal suppository	1,000 mg	1	Rectum
	Pentasa	Microgranule controlled-release capsule	250 mg 500 mg	2–4 2–4	Small bowel Colon
	Lialda	MMX formulated pH-dependent polymer film coated tablet	1.2 g	1.2–4.8	Terminal ileum and colon
	Apriso	Enteric-coated granules in polymer matrix	375 mg	1.5	Colon
Olsalazine	Dipentum	Delayed-release capsule	250 mg	1–3	Colon
Balsalazide	Colazal	Delayed-release capsule	750 mg	2–6.75	Colon

MMX, multimatrix.

Table 19–2

Corticosteroids for Treatment of IBD

Drug	Trade Names	Daily Dose
Prednisone	Generic	20–60 mg orally
Prednisolone	Generic	20–60 mg orally
Budesonide	Entocort EC	Induction: 9 mg orally Maintenance: 6 mg orally
Methylprednisolone	Medrol (orally) Solu-Medrol (IV)	15–60 mg orally or IV
Hydrocortisone	Solu-Cortef	300 mg IV in three divided doses
	Cortenema	100 mg rectally at bedtime
	Cortifoam	90 mg rectally once or twice daily
	Anucort 25 mg	25–50 mg rectally twice daily
	Proctocort 30 mg	25–50 mg rectally twice daily

Table 19–3

Immunosuppressant and Biologic Agents for Treatment of IBD

Drug	Trade Name(s)	Dose
Azathioprine	Imuran, Azasan	1.5–2.5 mg/kg/day orally
6-Mercaptopurine	Purinethol	1.5–2.5 mg/kg/day orally
Methotrexate	Rheumatrex, Trexall	15–25 mg weekly (IM/SC/ orally)
Cyclosporine	Sandimmune	4 mg/kg/day IV continuous infusion
Infliximab	Remicade	Induction: 5 mg/kg IV at 0, 2, and 6 weeks; 10 mg/kg per dose IV for nonresponders Maintenance: 5 mg/kg IV every 8 weeks
Adalimumab	Humira	Induction: 160 mg SC day 1 (given as four 40-mg injections in one day or as two 40-mg injections per day for two consecutive days), then 80 mg SC 2 weeks later (day 15) Maintenance: 40 mg SC every other week, starting on day 29 of therapy
Certolizumab	Cimzia	Induction: 400 mg SC initially, then 400 mg SC at 2 and 4 weeks Maintenance: 400 mg SC every 4 weeks if initial response
Natalizumab	Tysabri	Induction/maintenance: 300 mg IV every 4 weeks

IM, intramuscular; PEG, polyethylene glycol.

and pulmonitis. Hypersensitivity reactions may occur in patients allergic to sulfonamide-containing medications.

The use of nonsulfapyridine-based aminosalicylates has led to greater tolerability. Although the adverse effects are similar to those of sulfasalazine, they occur at a much lower rate. Olsalazine, in particular, is associated with a higher incidence of secretory diarrhea. These agents can also be used safely in patients with a reported sulfonamide allergy.

▶ Corticosteroids

Corticosteroids have potent anti-inflammatory properties and are used in active IBD to suppress inflammation rapidly. They may be administered systemically or delivered locally to the site of action by altering the drug formulation (Table 19–2). Because these drugs usually improve symptoms and disease severity rapidly, they should be restricted to short-term management of active disease. Long-term use of systemic corticosteroids is associated with significant adverse effects, including cataracts, skin atrophy, hypertension, hyperglycemia, adrenal suppression, osteoporosis, and increased risk of infection, among others.[21–23]

Budesonide is a high-potency glucocorticoid used in CD that has low systemic bioavailability when administered orally.[24] The formulation releases budesonide in the terminal ileum for treatment of disease involving the ileum or ascending colon. Due to its reduced bioavailability, budesonide may prevent some long-term adverse effects in patients who have steroid-dependent IBD.[23,24]

▶ Immunosuppressants

Agents targeting the excessive immune response or cytokines involved in IBD are potential treatment options (Table 19–3). Azathioprine and its active metabolite 6-mercaptopurine (6-MP) are inhibitors of purine biosynthesis and reduce

IBD-associated GI inflammation. They are most useful for maintaining remission of IBD or reducing the need for long-term use of corticosteroids.[23,25] Use in active disease is limited by their slow onset of action, which may be as long as 3 to 12 months. Adverse effects associated with azathioprine and 6-MP include hypersensitivity reactions resulting in pancreatitis, fever, rash, hepatitis, and leukopenia.[22,23,25] Patients should be tested for activity of thiopurine methyltransferase, the major enzyme responsible for metabolism of azathioprine. Deficiency or reduced activity of thiopurine methyltransferase may result in excess toxicity from azathioprine and 6-MP.

Methotrexate is a folate antagonist used primarily for maintaining remission of CD. It may be administered orally, subcutaneously, or IV and may result in a steroid-sparing effect in patients with steroid-dependent disease.[23,26,27] Long-term methotrexate use may result in serious adverse effects, including hepatotoxicity, pulmonary fibrosis, and bone marrow suppression.

Cyclosporine is a cyclic polypeptide immunosuppressant typically used to prevent organ rejection in transplant patients. Its use is restricted to patients with fulminant or refractory symptoms in patients with active IBD. Significant toxicities associated with cyclosporine are nephrotoxicity, risk of infection, seizures, hypertension, and liver function test abnormalities.[1,23]

▶ Biologic Agents

Several biologic agents targeting TNF-α are used for treatment of IBD (Table 19–3). Reduction in TNF-α activity is associated with improvement in the underlying inflammatory process. Infliximab is the prototypical agent and is used in both UC and CD, whereas the other agents are approved for use only in CD. Due to its chimeric structure (i.e., part human, part mouse) antibodies to infliximab may develop, resulting in loss of efficacy over time. Newer biologic agents are humanized and have a lower propensity for antibody development.[28]

Disadvantages of anti-TNF biologic therapy include need for parenteral administration, significant drug cost, and potential for serious adverse effects. Adverse effects may include infusion-related reactions such as fever, chest pain, hypotension, and dyspnea. All of the TNF-α inhibitors have also been associated with reactivation of serious infections, particularly intracellular pathogens such as tuberculosis, as well as hepatitis B.[16,22] These agents should not be used in patients with current infections, and patients should be screened for tuberculosis prior to initiating therapy. Exacerbation of heart failure is also a potential adverse effect, and biologic agents should be avoided in patients with advanced or decompensated heart failure.[16,21,22]

Natalizumab is a humanized monoclonal antibody that antagonizes integrin heterodimers, prevents α_4-mediated leukocyte adhesion to adhesion molecules, and prevents migration across the endothelium.[29] It has been associated with development of progressive multifocal leukoencephalopathy, and its use is restricted to patients with CD who have failed other therapies. Natalizumab should not be used concomitantly with immunosuppressants or TNF-α inhibitors.

▶ Other Agents

Antibiotics have been studied based on the rationale that they may interrupt the inflammatory response directed against endogenous bacterial flora. Metronidazole and ciprofloxacin have been the two most widely studied agents.[30] Metronidazole may benefit some patients with pouchitis (inflammation of surgically created intestinal pouches) and patients with CD who have had ileal resection or have perianal fistulas. Ciprofloxacin has shown some efficacy in refractory active CD. Both drugs may cause diarrhea, and long-term use of metronidazole is associated with the development of peripheral neuropathy.

Patient Encounter 1, Part 2: Medical History and Physical Examination

PMH: Tonsillectomy at age 5, fractured right clavicle (sports related)

FH: Both parents alive; father has history of hypertension, type 2 DM, and dyslipidemia; mother has a history of colon cancer with subtotal colectomy; brother with history of "indeterminate colitis"

SH: College student, social alcohol use and one-half to one pack per day tobacco use for 6 years

Allergies: sulfa drugs (rash)

Meds: Naproxen 220 mg orally as needed, Lo-Ovral orally once daily

ROS: (+) Diarrhea, abdominal pain, fatigue, back pain, fever, weight loss

PE:

VS: BP 118/65 mm Hg, P 92 bpm, RR 13/min, T 37.9°C (100.2°F)

CV: Tachycardia with normal rhythm. No murmurs, rubs, or gallops

HEENT: Dry mucous membranes

Abd: Soft, nondistended, mild diffuse tenderness, (+) bowel sounds, (−) hepatosplenomegaly, (−) masses, heme (+) stool

MS: Point tenderness over sacral area, (−) erythema, reduced lower back ROM

Labs: Sodium 139 mEq/L (139 mmol/L), potassium 3.2 mEq/L (3.2 mmol/L), chloride 100 mEq/L (100 mmol/L), bicarbonate 27 mEq/L (27 mmol/L), blood urea nitrogen 12 mg/dL (4.3 mmol/L urea), serum creatinine 1.0 mg/dL (88.4 µmol/L), albumin 4.2 g/dL (42 g/L), hemoglobin 11 g/dL (110 g/L or 6.82 mmol/L), hematocrit 33%, white blood cell count 11.0 × 10³/mm³ (11 × 10⁹/L), platelets 300 × 10³/mm³ (300 × 10⁹/L), ESR 120 mm/hour, CRP 12 mg/L

Imaging: Abdominal x-ray: (−) obstruction, perforation, or colonic dilation

Colonoscopy: Patchy "cobblestone" inflammation in the terminal ileum and ascending colon with evidence of recent bleeding, (−) polyps or strictures, biopsy taken

Path: Evidence of disease extension to muscularis with noncaseating granulomas

How is this additional information helpful in determining disease type and severity?

What are your treatment goals for this patient?

What factors should you consider in choosing appropriate therapy for this patient?

Because smoking is associated with reduced symptoms of UC, nicotine has been studied as a potential treatment option. Transdermal nicotine may result in some improvement in mild to moderate UC symptoms and may be more effective in patients who are ex- smokers.[1,31] Daily doses between 15 and 25 mg appear to be most effective.

Probiotics, such as *Lactobacillus acidophilus* or *Bifidobacterium*, may offer possible benefit, based on the rationale that modification of the host flora may alter the inflammatory response. Some evidence exists for improvement in disease symptoms, but further well-controlled trials are needed.[26]

Treatment of UC

Drug and dosing guidelines based on disease severity and location are presented in Table 19–4.

▶ Mild to Moderate Active UC

❼ *Treatment of acute episodes of UC is dictated by the severity and extent of disease, and first-line therapy of mild to moderate disease involves oral or topical aminosalicylate derivatives.*

Topical suppositories and enemas are preferred for active distal UC (left-sided disease and proctitis), as they deliver mesalamine directly to the site of inflammation. Topical mesalamine is superior to both topical corticosteroids and oral aminosalicylates for inducing remission in active mild to moderate UC.[1,31–34] Enemas are appropriate for patients with left-sided disease, as the medication will reach the splenic flexure. Suppositories deliver mesalamine up to approximately 20 cm and are most appropriate for treating proctitis.[6,7,31]

Topical mesalamine products provide a more rapid response than oral preparations. Improvement in symptoms may be seen in as little as 2 days, but up to 4 weeks of treatment may be necessary for maximal response. Oral and topical mesalamine preparations may be used together to provide maximal effect. Oral mesalamine may also be used for patients who are unwilling to use topical preparations.[31–34]

Topical corticosteroids are typically reserved for patients who do not respond to topical mesalamine.[1,23] Patients should be properly educated regarding appropriate use of topical products. This includes proper administration and adequate retention of topical mesalamine products in order to maximize efficacy.

Table 19–4

Treatment Recommendations for UC

Disease Severity and Location	Active Disease	Maintenance of Remission
Mild Disease		
Proctitis	Mesalamine suppository 1 g rectally daily	May reduce suppository frequency to 1 g 3 times/week
Left-sided disease	Mesalamine enema 1 g rectally daily, *or* Mesalamine 2.4–4.8 g/day or sulfasalazine 4–6 g/day orally	May reduce enema frequency to 1 g every other day, *or* Taper to mesalamine 1.6–2.4 g/day or sulfasalazine 2–4 g/day orally
Colitis	Mesalamine 2.4–4.8 g/day or sulfasalazine 4–6 g/day orally	Taper to mesalamine 1.6–2.4 g/day or sulfasalazine 2–4 g/day orally
Moderate Disease		
Proctitis	Mesalamine suppository 1 g rectally daily; If no response to mesalamine: • Prednisone 40–60 mg/day orally	May reduce suppository frequency to 1 g 3 times/week; taper prednisone as soon as possible; Consider adding azathioprine or 6-MP 1.5–2.5 mg/kg/day orally
Left-sided disease	Mesalamine enema 1 g rectally at bedtime daily, *or* Mesalamine 2.4–4.8 g/day or sulfasalazine 4–6 g/day orally May combine enema and oral therapies	May reduce enema frequency to 1 g 3 times/week if symptoms permit; May reduce dose of oral agents if symptoms permit; Consider adding azathioprine or 6-MP 1.5–2.5 mg/kg/day orally
Colitis	Mesalamine 2.4–4.8 g/day or sulfasalazine 4–6 g/day orally; If no response to mesalamine or sulfasalazine: • Prednisone 40–60 mg/day orally; *or* • Infliximab 5 mg/kg IV at weeks 0, 2, and 6	Taper mesalamine to 1.6–2.4 g/day or sulfasalazine 2–4 g/day orally; If prednisone or infliximab were required: • Taper prednisone as soon as possible; • Give infliximab 5 mg/kg IV every 8 weeks Consider adding azathioprine or 6-MP 1.5–2.5 mg/kg/day orally
Severe or Fulminant Disease	Hydrocortisone 300 mg IV daily (or equivalent) × 7 days, *or* Infliximab 5 mg/kg IV at weeks 0, 2, and 6 If no response to IV corticosteroids or infliximab: • Cyclosporine 4 mg/kg/day IV	Change to oral corticosteroid and taper as soon as possible; Restart oral mesalamine or sulfasalazine May continue infliximab at maintenance doses of 5 mg/kg every 8 weeks

6-MP, 6-mercaptopurine.

For patients with more extensive disease extending proximal to the splenic flexure, oral sulfasalazine or any of the newer oral mesalamine products is considered first-line therapy.[1] Doses should provide 4 to 6 g of sulfasalazine or 4.8 g of mesalamine. While little differences in efficacy exist between mesalamine products, sulfasalazine and olsalazine have a higher incidence of adverse effects.[18] Use of the once-daily formulations of mesalamine may improve patient adherence.[18,34] Induction of remission may require 4 to 8 weeks of therapy at appropriate treatment doses.

Oral corticosteroids may be used for patients who are unresponsive to sulfasalazine or mesalamine. Prednisone doses of 40 to 60 mg/day (or equivalent) are recommended.[1,23] Azathioprine or 6-MP is used for patients unresponsive to corticosteroids or those who become steroid dependent. Infliximab 5 mg/kg may also be used for patients who are unresponsive to conventional oral therapies and may reduce the need for colectomy after 3 months of treatment. Infliximab may also be used in patients who are refractory to or dependent on corticosteroids.[35,36]

▶ Severe or Fulminant UC

Patients with severe UC symptoms require hospitalization for management of their disease. If the patient is unresponsive to oral or topical mesalamine and oral corticosteroids, then a course of IV corticosteroids should be initiated.[1] Hydrocortisone 300 mg/day given in three divided doses or methylprednisolone 60 mg daily for 7 to 10 days are the preferred therapies.[23]

Infliximab 5 mg/kg is also an option for severe UC. Cyclosporine 2 to 4 mg/kg/day given as a continuous IV infusion should be reserved for patients unresponsive to 7 to 10 days of IV corticosteroid therapy.

Patients with fulminant disease are treated similarly, although infliximab is not indicated for this population. Patients with fulminant UC should be assessed for signs of significant systemic toxicity or colonic dilation, which may require earlier surgical intervention.

▶ Maintenance of Remission

Unfortunately, up to 50% of patients receiving oral therapies and up to 70% of untreated patients relapse within 1 year after achieving remission.[26] For this reason, patients may require maintenance drug therapy indefinitely to preserve remission.

❽ *Maintenance of remission of UC may be achieved with oral or topical aminosalicylates.* In patients with proctitis, mesalamine suppositories 1 g daily may prevent relapse in up to 90% of patients.[1,7,31] Mesalamine enemas are appropriate for left-sided disease and may often be dosed two to three times weekly. Oral mesalamine at lower doses (e.g., 1.2 to 1.6 g/day) may be combined with topical therapies to maintain remission. Topical or oral corticosteroids are not effective for maintaining remission of distal UC and should be avoided.

Oral sulfasalazine or mesalamine is effective in maintaining remission in patients with more extensive disease.[1,26] Lower daily doses (e.g., 2 to 4 g sulfasalazine or 1.6

to 2.4 g mesalamine) may be used for disease maintenance. As with distal UC, oral corticosteroids are not effective for maintaining remission and should be avoided due to the high incidence of adverse effects.

❽ *Immunosuppressants such as azathioprine or 6-MP can be used for unresponsive patients or those who develop corticosteroid dependency.* Remission may be maintained in up to 58% of patients after 5 years of treatment.[1,25] Intermittent infliximab dosing (5 mg/kg IV every 8 weeks) may be used to maintain disease remission and reduce the need for corticosteroids in patients with moderate to severe UC. Colectomy is an option for patients with progressive disease who cannot be maintained on drug therapy alone.

Treatment of CD

Drug and dosing guidelines based on disease severity and location are presented in Table 19–5.

▶ Mild to Moderate Active CD

❾ *Induction of remission of mild to moderate active CD may be accomplished with oral aminosalicylates or budesonide.* Sulfasalazine 4 to 6 g/day is most effective for patients with active colonic or ileocolonic involvement, with response rates of approximately 50%.[2,5,37] Mesalamine products have shown more variable results but may be used for patients with ileal, ileocolonic, or colonic CD.[2,37] These drugs are typically better tolerated than sulfasalazine at full treatment doses. Induction of remission may require up to 16 weeks of treatment at full doses.[37]

Budesonide 9 mg orally once daily for up to 8 weeks may be used for mild to moderate active CD in patients with involvement of the terminal ileum or ascending colon, with success expected in 50% to 69% of patients.[23,24,37] Because the

---

Patient Encounter 2

A 57-year-old African American man presents to the clinic for follow-up management of UC. He has had left-sided disease for 3 years and has been maintained in remission on maximal doses of oral mesalamine and prednisone 35 mg orally once daily. His provider has attempted several times to taper the prednisone dose, but the patient experiences a reappearance of symptoms if the dose is lowered below this level. Medical history is also significant for hypertension and heart failure. He has no known drug allergies.

What are the risks of long-term corticosteroid use in this patient?

What treatment options are available for reducing corticosteroid dependency in this patient?

What other information is needed before recommending a pharmacologic intervention?

Table 19–5		
Treatment Recommendations for CD		
Disease Location and Severity	**Active Disease**	**Maintenance of Remission**
Mild Disease		
Ileal or ileocolonic	Mesalamine 3.2–4.8 g/day or sulfasalazine 4–6 g/day orally	Taper mesalamine 1.6–2.4 g/day or sulfasalazine 2–4 g/day orally
Ileal +/– ascending colon	Budesonide 9 mg daily orally for up to 8 weeks	Taper budesonide to 6 mg daily for up to 3 months
Perianal	Mesalamine 2.4–4.8 g/day or sulfasalazine 4–6 g/day orally; May add metronidazole 10–20 mg/kg/day or ciprofloxacin 1 g daily	Taper mesalamine to 1.6–2.4 g/day or sulfasalazine 2–4 g/day orally
Moderate Disease	Same treatment as for mild disease; If inadequate response to aminosalicylate, consider: • Infliximab *or* adalimumab *or* certolizumab (see Table 19–3 for dosage regimens) or • Prednisone 40–60 mg/day orally, *or* • Budesonide 9 mg/day orally for up to 8 weeks; • Consider natalizumab if no response to prior therapies If fistulizing disease, consider: • Infliximab or adalimumab	Continue aminosalicylate at maintenance dose; May continue infliximab at maintenance doses (see Table 19–3); If loss of response to infliximab, consider adalimumab Taper prednisone as soon as possible; Taper budesonide to 6 mg daily for 3 months; Consider adding azathioprine or 6-MP 1.5–2.5 mg/kg/day orally or methotrexate 12.5–25 mg orally or IM/SC once weekly Consider natalizumab if no response to previous therapies
Severe or Fulminant Disease	Hydrocortisone 300 mg IV daily (or equivalent) × 7 days, *or* Infliximab (severe or fistulizing disease) 5 mg/kg IV at 0, 2, and 6 weeks; • Adalimumab or certolizumab *or* • Consider natalizumab if no response to prior therapies Consider cyclosporine 4 mg/kg/day for refractory disease	Taper corticosteroid as soon as possible; May continue infliximab, adalimumab, certolizumab, or natalizumab (see Table 19–3 for dosage regimens) Consider adding azathioprine or 6-MP 1.5–2.5 mg/kg/day orally or methotrexate 12.5–25 mg orally or IM/SC weekly

6-MP, 6-mercaptopurine; IM, intramuscular; SC, subcutaneous.

formulation releases budesonide in the terminal ileum, it is not effective in reaching sites distal to the ascending colon.[24,37] Conventional oral corticosteroids such as prednisone and methylprednisolone may be used for patients who are unresponsive to aminosalicylates or budesonide.

Metronidazole or ciprofloxacin can be used in patients who do not respond to oral aminosalicylates. Response rates of up to 50% are reported, but data are conflicting, and these agents should generally not be considered first-line therapy.[2,37]

▶ Moderate to Severe Active CD

⑨ *Patients with moderate to severe active CD may be treated with oral corticosteroids, such as prednisone 40 to 60 mg daily.[2]* Budesonide 9 mg orally once daily may be used for moderate active CD involving the terminal ileum or ascending colon.

Infliximab is an effective alternative to corticosteroid therapy for patients with moderate to severe CD, including patients with fistulizing or perianal disease.[14,24,37] The recommended regimen for induction of remission is infliximab 5 mg/kg at weeks 0, 2, and 6; it is effective in inducing remission in approximately 80% of patients at 8 weeks. Complete closure of existing enterocutaneous fistulae occurs in approximately 50% of patients.

Adalimumab is effective in moderate to severe active CD and is used preferably in patients with diminished response to infliximab. The approved adult dose of 160 mg on day 1, 80 mg at 2 weeks, and 40 mg at day 29 resulted in a remission rate of 36% at 4 weeks.[16,38]

Certolizumab is also effective, with a dose of 400 mg subcutaneously initially, and then at 2 and 4 weeks resulting in a clinical response rate of 37% at 6 weeks.[16,38] Natalizumab 300 mg IV every 4 weeks has been reported to induce remission in up to 37% of patients at 10 weeks, which was similar to placebo.[16,38]

For patients with simple perianal fistulae, antibiotics, infliximab, or adalimumab are appropriate treatment options. Complex perianal fistulae are those associated with multiple openings, abscess, stricture, or penetration into the vaginal wall. These types of perianal fistulae may require surgical intervention but may also be amenable to treatment with antibiotics, infliximab, azathioprine, or 6-MP.[2,15,16,23]

▶ Severe to Fulminant Active CD

Most patients with severe to fulminant CD require hospitalization for appropriate treatment. Patients should be assessed for possible surgical intervention if abdominal distention, masses, abscess, or obstruction are present. Daily IV doses of corticosteroids equivalent to prednisone 40 to 60 mg are recommended as initial therapy to rapidly suppress severe inflammation.

If there are no contraindications, infliximab 5 mg/kg followed by 5 mg/kg at weeks 2 and 6 may be used for severe active CD. There is no evidence that infliximab is either safe or effective for fulminant disease. Adalimumab or certolizumab are also options for patients with severe CD, particularly those who have lost response to infliximab or those who are nonresponsive to traditional therapies. Natalizumab can be used for severe CD but is reserved for patients failing other available therapies, including TNF-α inhibitors.

Adjunctive therapy with fluid and electrolyte replacement should be initiated. Nutritional support with enteral or parenteral nutrition may be indicated for patients unable to eat for more than 5 to 7 days.[2] Some evidence suggests that enteral nutrition provides anti-inflammatory effects in patients with active CD.[39,40]

Limited evidence indicates that cyclosporine, or possibly tacrolimus, may be effective as salvage therapy for patients who fail IV corticosteroid therapy.[2,23] Surgical intervention may ultimately be necessary for medically refractory disease.

▶ Maintenance of Remission in CD

Patients with CD are at high risk for disease relapse after induction of remission. Within 2 years, up to 80% of patients suffer a relapse; therefore, most patients should be evaluated for indefinite maintenance therapy. ❿ *Maintenance of remission of CD may be achieved with oral or topical aminosalicylate derivatives, immunosuppressants (such as azathioprine, 6-MP, and methotrexate), or infliximab, adalimumab, certolizumab, or natalizumab.*

In contrast to their use in UC, sulfasalazine and the newer aminosalicylates are marginally effective in preventing CD relapse in patients with medically induced remission, with success rates of only 10% to 20% at 1 year.[26] Nevertheless, aminosalicylates are routinely used to maintain remission of CD. Some evidence does exist that the aminosalicylates may prevent or delay disease recurrence in patients with surgically induced remisson.[2,26]

Several other treatment options exist for maintaining remission that may also reduce the need for corticosteroids. Infliximab has been shown to maintain remission in 46% of patients compared to 23% of those treated with placebo over a 54-week period.[15,23,38] Adalimumab 40 mg subcutaneously given every other week has been shown to maintain remission in up to 36% of patients at 56 weeks of treatment.[15,38] Certolizumab 400 mg IV every 4 weeks has also been effective in maintaining remission in up to 61% of patients at 26 weeks.[15,38] Patients with a baseline CRP of greater than 10 mg/L may have a more favorable response. Natalizumab may also be used for maintenance in patients unresponsive to anti-TNF-α agents. Up to 40% of patients may maintain remission at 15 months.[15,38]

Azathioprine and 6-MP in oral doses up to 2.5 mg/kg/day have been shown to maintain remission in 45% of patients

for up to 5 years.[2,23,25,26] These drugs may be used to prevent disease recurrence after surgically induced remission. Methotrexate in doses ranging from 12.5 to 25 mg/week given orally, intramuscularly, or subcutaneously has resulted in remission rates of up to 52% at 3 years.[26,27]

Corticosteroids, while effective for inducing remission rapidly, are not effective for maintenance therapy and are associated with significant adverse effects with long-term use. Therefore, systemic or topical corticosteroids should not be used for maintaining remission in patients with IBD. Unfortunately up to 50% of patients treated acutely with corticosteroids become dependent on them to prevent symptoms.[2]

In place of conventional corticosteroids, budesonide 6 mg orally once daily may be used for up to 3 months after remission induction for mild to moderate CD.

Treatment of IBD in Special Populations
(Table 19–6)

▶ Elderly Patients

Approximately 8% to 20% of patients with UC and 7% to 26% of patients with CD are elderly at initial diagnosis.[41] In general, IBD presents similarly in elderly patients compared to younger individuals. Elderly patients may have more comorbid diseases, some of which may make the diagnosis of IBD more difficult. Such conditions include ischemic colitis, diverticular disease, and microscopic colitis. Increased age is also associated with a higher incidence of adenomatous polyps, but the onset of IBD at an advanced age does not appear to increase the risk of developing colorectal cancer. Elderly patients may also use more medications, particularly NSAIDs, which may induce or exacerbate colitis.

Treatment of elderly patients with IBD is similar to that for younger patients, but special consideration should be given to some of the medications used. Corticosteroids may worsen diabetes, hypertension, heart failure, or osteoporosis. The TNF-α inhibitors should be used cautiously in patients with heart failure and should be avoided in New York Heart Association Class III or IV disease. Lastly, elderly patients requiring major surgical interventions may be at higher risk for surgical complications or may not meet eligibility criteria for surgery because of comorbid conditions, age-related organ dysfunction, or reduced functional status.

▶ Children and Adolescents

CD occurs in approximately 4.56 per 100,000 pediatric patients, and UC occurs in about 2.14 cases per 100,000.[42] A major issue in children with IBD is the risk of growth failure secondary to inadequate nutritional intake. Failure to thrive may be an initial presentation of IBD in this population. Aggressive nutritional interventions may be required to facilitate adequate caloric intake. Chronic corticosteroid therapy may also be associated with reductions in growth and bone demineralization. Exploration of using lower doses in patients who are corticosteroid dependent may result in fewer problems with altered height velocity.[43]

Table 19–6

Dosing Considerations of IBD Therapies in Special Populations

Therapy	Pediatric Patients	Elderly Patients	Pregnancy[44–46]
Sulfasalazine	Age more than 2 years: 40–60 mg/kg/day in 3–6 divided doses; 30 mg/kg/day in 3–6 divided doses for maintenance	No specific changes	Category B Administer folic acid 2 mg daily during prenatal period and pregnancy
Mesalamine	No specific changes; Balsalazide indicated for age more than 5 years	No specific changes	Category B (Olsalazine Category C) Generally considered safe and effective
Corticosteroids	No specific changes	No specific changes Elderly patients at high risk for osteoporosis	Older agents not rated; Budesonide Category C Generally considered safe and effective
TNF-a inhibitors	Infliximab indicated for pediatric patients: 5 mg/kg at 0, 2, and 6 weeks, then every 8 weeks. Adalimumab has been used at doses of 80 mg SC day 0, then 40 mg SC every other week	Avoid in patients with heart failure Elderly patients at higher risk for infections	Category B Pregnancy registry for adalimumab via manufacturer
Natalizumab	Dose of 3 mg/kg IV at 0, 4, and 8 weeks reported; data are lacking in children	No specific changes	Category C Report pregnancy to manufacturer's pregnancy registry
Azathioprine 6-Mercaptopurine	1.5–2 mg/kg/day to start	No specific changes	Category D Accepted as safe Avoid initiating during pregnancy, but continue if patient is already receiving when pregnant
Methotrexate	17 mg/m² orally/SC/IM	No specific changes	Category X Contraindicated
Cyclosporine	No specific changes	No specific changes	Category C Use only in refractory patients
Metronidazole	30–50 mg/kg/day divided every 6 hours	No specific changes	Category B Use short courses if possible
Ciprofloxacin	Avoid use	Adjust dose for CrCl less than 50 mL/min	Category C Consider other alternatives

CrCl, creatinine clearance; IM, intramuscular; SC, subcutaneously.

The aminosalicylates, azathioprine, 6-MP, and infliximab are all viable options for treatment and maintenance of IBD in pediatric patients. Use of immunosuppressive therapy or infliximab may help reduce overall corticosteroid exposure. Adalimumab is approved for use in patients age 4 years or greater with juvenile rheumatoid arthritis. Limited recent information suggests that adalimumab may be effective in pediatric patients with CD.[44–46] Certolizumab and natalizumab have only recently been approved for use in adult patients with IBD; therefore, data in children are limited.[47]

▶ Pregnant Women

Inducing and maintaining remission of IBD prior to conception is the optimal approach in women planning to become pregnant. Active IBD may result in prematurity and low birth weight. Thus, pregnant women with IBD should be monitored closely, particularly during the third trimester.[48–50]

Patients do not need to discontinue drug therapy for IBD once they become pregnant, but certain adjustments may be required.[48–50] The aminosalicylates are considered safe to use in pregnancy, but sulfasalazine is associated with folate malabsorption. Because pregnancy results in a higher folate requirement, pregnant patients treated with sulfasalazine should be supplemented with folic acid 1 mg orally twice daily.[48]

As with nonpregnant patients, corticosteroids may be used for treatment of active disease but not for maintenance of remission. Generally, corticosteroids confer no additional risk on the mother or fetus and are generally well tolerated. Both azathioprine and 6-MP have been used successfully in pregnant patients and appear to carry minimal risk, despite carrying an FDA pregnancy category D rating.[49] Infliximab, adalimumab, and certolizumab are all FDA category B drugs and appear to carry minimal risk in pregnant patients.[50] Little is known about excretion of these drugs in breast milk, so benefit versus risk should be considered if they are used during nursing. Natalizumab is a pregnancy category C drug and should be used only when other therapies have been exhausted.

Methotrexate is a known abortifacient and carries an FDA category X pregnancy rating. Thus, it is contraindicated during pregnancy. Metronidazole carries a theoretical risk of mutagenicity in humans, but short courses are safe during pregnancy. Prolonged use of metronidazole should be avoided in pregnant patients due to lack of safety data supporting its use.[48] Ciprofloxacin should be avoided in pregnant women. First-trimester use of the antidiarrheal diphenoxylate has been associated with fetal malformations and should be avoided.

OUTCOME EVALUATION

- Monitor for improvement of symptoms in patients with active IBD, such as reduction in the number of daily stools, abdominal pain, fever, and heart rate.

- For patients in remission, assure that proper maintenance doses of medications are used and educate the patient to seek medical attention if symptoms recur or worsen.

- Evaluate patients receiving systemic corticosteroid therapy for improvement in symptoms and opportunities

to taper or discontinue corticosteroid therapy. For patients using more than 5 mg daily of prednisone for more than 2 months or for steroid-dependent patients consider the following:

- Central bone mineral density testing to evaluate the need for preventive or therapeutic bisphosphonate therapy;

- Periodic monitoring of blood glucose, lipids, and blood pressure;

- Evaluation for evidence of cushingoid features or signs or symptoms of infection.

- When considering treatment with azathioprine or 6-MP, obtain baseline CBC, liver function tests, and TPMT activity. These tests should be monitored closely (every 2–4 weeks) at the start of therapy and then approximately every 3 months during maintenance therapy.

- With azathioprine and 6-MP, monitor for hypersensitivity reactions, including severe skin rashes and pancreatitis. Educate the patient regarding signs

---

Patient Care and Monitoring

1. Evaluate the patient's symptoms to determine if they are consistent with UC or CD. Determine whether the patient has evidence of extraintestinal manifestations or GI complications related to IBD. Identify any psychosocial problems related to the presence of IBD.

2. If the patient is presenting with an exacerbation of preexisting IBD, determine if the symptoms are similar in type and severity to the patient's previous episodes.

3. Assess the patient's medical history for pertinent drug allergies, tobacco use, and current prescription and nonprescription drug therapies. Determine if any of the medications could exacerbate IBD. If applicable, inquire about adherence or recent changes to the patient's current IBD drug regimen.

4. Use available diagnostic laboratory, endoscopic, and imaging data to gauge the extent and severity of the patient's disease.

5. Construct a drug treatment plan based on the disease severity and location. Identify potential contraindications or financial barriers to drug therapy. Inquire if the patient has an aversion to or inability to properly use certain drug formulations that you may wish to recommend, such as topical (rectal) products.

6. Assess whether the patient will require maintenance therapy after remission induction. If so, identify the treatment duration. Decide when the patient should receive follow-up care.

7. Outline parameters to evaluate the efficacy and toxicity of the drug regimen you are recommending. Determine whether the patient will need preventive drug therapy or

diagnostic testing to prevent or screen for potential drug-related toxicities.

8. Educate the patient on proper use of drug therapy, including when to expect symptom improvement after initiation of treatment and which signs or symptoms to report that might be related to adverse drug effects.

9. Provide patient education on the proper use of aminosalicylate medications and assess regularly for adherence. Include the following:

   - Proper use of suppositories and enemas

   - The appropriate number of tablets or capsules to take per day. Reinforce that tablets and capsules are delayed-release and should not be crushed, opened, or chewed.

   - Appropriate dose titration, particularly with oral sulfasalazine

   - The time frame the patient can expect improvement based on drug dose and disease severity

   - Signs or symptoms of potential adverse effects

10. Once remission is achieved, evaluate the patient's drug regimen to determine if dose reductions or changes in frequency of administration are required. Reinforce the need for adherence to drug therapy in order to maximize effectiveness.

11. Educate patients about their disease state. Refer patients to available support groups or IBD organizational resources if they are having difficulty in coping with their disease.

and symptoms of pancreatitis (nausea, vomiting, and abdominal pain).

- Prior to initiating methotrexate therapy, obtain complete blood count, serum creatinine, liver function tests, chest x-ray, and pregnancy test (if female). Monitor blood counts weekly for 1 month, then monthly thereafter.

- Prior to initiating infliximab, adalimumab, or certolizumab obtain a tuberculin skin test to rule out latent tuberculosis. Also monitor patients with a prior history of hepatitis B virus infection for signs of liver disease, such as jaundice. Assure that patients do not have a clinically significant systemic infection or New York Heart Association Class III or IV heart failure.

- In patients receiving infliximab, monitor for infusion-related reactions such as hypotension, dyspnea, fever, chills, or chest pain when administering IV doses.

- In patients with fistulae, monitor at every infliximab, adalimumab, or certolizumab dosing interval for evidence of fistula closure and overall reduction in the number of fistulae.

- Obtain a magnetic resonance imaging procedure prior to initiation of natalizumab therapy. Monitor patients for signs of progressive multifocal leukoencephalopathy, such as mental status changes, signs of liver disease (e.g., jaundice), and hypersensitivity reactions following administration.

Abbreviations Introduced in This Chapter

5-ASA	5-Aminosalicylate
6-MP	6-Mercaptopurine
CD	Crohn's disease
CRP	C-reactive protein
ESR	Erythrocyte sedimentation rate
HLA	Human leukocyte antigen
IBD	Inflammatory bowel disease
IL	Interleukin
NOD2	Nucleotide oligomerization domain 2
NSAID	Nonsteroidal anti-inflammatory drug
pANCA	Perinuclear antineutrophil cytoplasmic antibodies
PPAR-γ	Peroxisome proliferator activated receptor-γ
PR	Per rectum
TNF-α	Tumor necrosis factor-α
UC	Ulcerative colitis

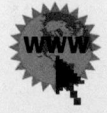
Self-assessment questions and answers are available at http://*www.mhpharmacotherapy.com/pp.html.*

REFERENCES

1. Kornbluth A, Sachar DB. Ulcerative colitis practice guidelines in adults (update): American College of Gastroenterology, Practice Parameters Committee. Am J Gastroenterol 2004;99:1371–1385.

2. Lichtenstein GR, Hanauer SB, Sandborn WJ. The Practice Parameters Committee of the American College of Gastroenterology. Management of Crohn's disease in adults. Am J Gastroenterol 2009;104:465–483.

3. Viscido A, Aratari A, Maccioni F, et al. Inflammatory bowel diseases: Clinical update of practical guidelines. Nucl Med Commun 2005;26:649–655.

4. Lakatos PL, Fischer S, Lakatos L, Gal I, Papp J. Current concept on the pathogenesis of inflammatory bowel disease-crosstalk between genetic and microbial factors: Pathogenic bacteria and altered bacterial sensing or changes in mucosal integrity take "toll." World J Gastroenterol 2006;12(12):1829–1841.

5. Gismera CS, Aladrén BS. Inflammatory bowel diseases: A disease(s) of modern times? Is incidence still increasing? World J Gastroenterol 2008;14(36):5491–5498.

6. Knutson D, Greenberg G, Cronau H. Management of Crohn's disease— A practical approach. Am Fam Physician 2003;68:707–714, 717–718.

7. Regueiro MD. Diagnosis and treatment of ulcerative proctitis. J Clin Gastroenterol 2004;38:733–740.

8. Sandler RS, Eisen GM. Epidemiology of inflammatory bowel disease. In: Kirsner JB, ed. Inflammatory Bowel Diseases. Philadelphia: WB Saunders, 2000:89–112.

9. Achkara JP, Duerr R. The expanding universe of inflammatory bowel disease genetics. Curr Opin Gastroenterol 2008;24:429–434.

10. Podolsky DK. Inflammatory bowel disease. N Engl J Med 2002;347:417–429.

11. MacDonald TT, DiSabatino A, Gordon JN. Immunopathogenesis of Crohn's disease. JPEN 2005;29(4):S118–S125.

12. Cipolla G, Crema F, Sacco S, et al. Nonsteroidal anti-inflammatory drugs and inflammatory bowel disease: Current perspectives. Pharmacol Res 2002;46:1–6.

13. Judge TA, Lichtenstein GR. Inflammatory bowel disease. In: Current Diagnosis & Treatment in Gastroenterology. 2nd ed. *http://online.statref.com/document.aspx? fxid=23&docid=72.*

14. Sands BE. Therapy of inflammatory bowel disease. Gastroenterology 2000;118:S68–S82.

15. American Gastroenterological Association. AGA technical review on perianal Crohn's disease. Gastroenterology 2003;125:1508–1530.

16. Jones J, Panaccione R. Biologic therapy in Crohn's disease: State of the art. Curr Opin Gastroenterol 2008, 24:475–481.

17. American Gastroenterological Association. AGA technical review osteoporosis in gastrointestinal diseases. Gastroenterology 2003;124:795–841.

18. Ng SC, Kamm MA. Review article: New drug formulations, chemical entities and therapeutic approaches for the management of ulcerative colitis. Aliment Pharmacol Ther 2008;28:815–829.

19. Sandborn WJ, Hanauer SB. Systematic review: The pharmacokinetic profiles of oral mesalamine formulations and mesalazine pro-drugs used in the management of ulcerative colitis. Aliment Pharmacol Ther 2003;17:29–42.

20. Sandborn WJ. Rational selection of oral 5-aminosalicylate formulations and prodrugs for the treatment of ulcerative colitis [Editorial]. Am J Gastroenterol 2002;97(12):2939–2941.

21. Navarro F, Hanauer SB. Treatment of inflammatory bowel disease: Safety and tolerability issues. Am J Gastroenterol 2003;98(12 Suppl):S18–S23.

22. Pascal J, Valérie P, Felley C, et al. Drug safety in Crohn's disease therapy. Digestion 2007;76:161–168.

23. American Gastroenterological Association Institute Technical Review on Corticosteroids, Immunomodulators, and Infliximab in Inflammatory Bowel Disease. Gastroenterology 2006;130:940–987.

24. Hofer KN. Oral budesonide in the management of Crohn's disease. Ann Pharmacother 2003;37:1457–1464.

25. Fraser AG, Orchard TR, Jewell DP. The efficacy of azathioprine for the treatment of inflammatory bowel disease: A 30 year review. Gut 2002;50:485–489.

26. Feagan BG. Maintenance therapy for inflammatory bowel disease. Am J Gastroenterol 2003;98(12 Suppl):S6–S17.

27. Vandell AG, DiPiro JT. Low-dosage methotrexate for treatment and maintenance of remission in patients with inflammatory bowel disease. Pharmacotherapy 2002;22:613–620.

28. Tracey D, Klareskog L, Sasso, et al. Tumor necrosis factor antagonist mechanism of action: A comprehensive review. Pharmacol Ther 2008;117:244–279.

29. Stefanelli T, Malesci A, De La Rue SA, Danese S. Anti-adhesion molecule therapies in inflammatory bowel disease: Touch and go. Autoimmun Rev 2008;7: 364–369.

30. Guslandi M. Antibiotics for inflammatory bowel disease: Do they work? Eur J Gastroenterol Hepatol 2005 ;17: 145–147.

31. Regueiro M, Loftus, EV, Steinhart H, Cohen RD. Clinical guidelines for the medical management of left-sided ulcerative colitis and ulcerative proctitis: Summary statement. Inflamm Bowel Dis 2006;12:972–978.

32. Marshall JK, Irvine EJ. Putting rectal 5-aminosalicylic acid in its place: The role in distal ulcerative colitis. Am J Gastroenterol 2000;95:1628–1636.

33. Cohen RD, Woseth DM, Thisted RA, Hanauer SB. A meta-analysis and overview of the literature on treatment options for left-sided ulcerative colitis and ulcerative proctitis. Am J Gastroenterol 2000;95:1263–1276.

34. Brain O, Travis SPL. Therapy of ulcerative colitis: State of the art. Curr Opin Gastroenterol 2008;24:469–474.

35. Willert RP, Lawrance IC. Use of infliximab in the prevention and delay of colectomy in severe steroid dependant and refractory ulcerative colitis. World J Gastroenterol 2008;14(16):2544–2549.

36. Janerot G, Hertervig E, Friid-liby I, et al. Infliximab as rescue therapy in severe to moderately severe ulcerative colitis: A randomized, placebo-controlled study. Gastroenterology 2005;128:1805–1811.

37. Sandborn WJ, Feagan BG, Lichtenstein GR. Medical management of mild to moderate Crohn's disease: Evidence-based treatment algorithms for induction and maintenance of remission. Drugs 2007;67(17):2511–2537.

38. Panes J, Gomollon F, Taxonera C, et al. Crohn's disease: A review of current treatment with a focus on biologics. Drugs 2007;67(17):2511–2537.

39. Griffiths AM. Enteral nutrition in the management of Crohn's disease. JPEN 2005;29(4 Suppl):S108–S117.

40. Sanderson IR, Croft NM. The anti-inflammatory effects of enteral nutrition. JPEN 2005;29(4 Suppl): S134–S140.

41. Robertson DJ, Grimm IS. Inflammatory bowel disease in the elderly. Gastroenterol Clin North Am 2001;30:409–426.

42. Kim SC, Ferry GD. Inflammatory bowel diseases in pediatric and adolescent patients: Clinical, therapeutic, and psychosocial considerations. Gastroenterology 2004;126:1550–1560.

43. Navarro FA, Hanauer SB, Kirschner BS. Effect of long-term low-dose prednisone on height velocity and disease activity in pediatric and adolescent patients with Crohn's disease. J Pediatr Gastroenterol Nutr 2007;45:312–318.

44. Hadziselimovic F. Adalimumab induces and maintains remission in severe, resistant paediatric crohn disease. J Pediatric Gastroenterol Nutr 2008;46:208–211.

45. Noe JD, Pfefferkorn M. Short-term response to adalimumab in childhood inflammatory bowel disease. Inflamm Bowel Dis 2008;14:1683–1687.

46. Wyneski MJ, Green A, Kay M, et al. Safety and efficacy of adalimumab in pediatric patients with Crohn disease. J Pediatr Gastroenterol Nutr 2008;47:19–25.

47. Hyams JS, Wilson DC, Thomas A, et al. Natalizumab therapy for moderate to severe Crohn disease in adolescents. J Pediatr Gastroenterol Nutr 2007;44:185–191.

48. Steinlauf AF, Present DH. Medical management of the pregnant patient with inflammatory bowel disease. Gastroenterol Clin N Am 2004;33:361–385.

49. Ferrero S, Ragni N. Inflammatory bowel disease: Management issues during pregnancy. Arch Gynecol Obstet 2004;270:79–85.

50. Dubinsky M, Abraham B, Mahadevan U. Management of the pregnant IBD patient. Inflamm Bowel Dis 2008;14:1736–1750.

20 Nausea and Vomiting

Sheila Wilhelm

LEARNING OBJECTIVES

Upon completion of the chapter, the reader will be able to:

1. Identify several causes of nausea and vomiting.
2. Describe the pathophysiologic mechanisms of nausea and vomiting.
3. Identify the three stages of nausea and vomiting.
4. Distinguish between simple and complex nausea and vomiting.
5. Create goals for treating nausea and vomiting.
6. Recommend a treatment regimen for a patient with nausea and vomiting associated with cancer chemotherapy, surgery, pregnancy, or motion sickness.
7. Outline a monitoring plan to evaluate the treatment outcomes for nausea and vomiting.

KEY CONCEPTS

❶ Nausea and vomiting are symptoms that can be due to a number of different causes.

❷ To treat nausea and vomiting most effectively, it is important to first identify the underlying cause of the symptoms.

❸ Nonpharmacologic approaches to treating nausea and vomiting include dietary, physical, and psychological changes.

❹ For prevention of acute chemotherapy-induced nausea and vomiting (CINV) for patients receiving moderately or highly emetogenic chemotherapy, a combination of antiemetics with different mechanisms of action is recommended.

❺ Droperidol or a 5-hydroxytryptamine (serotonin) type 3 (5-HT$_3$) receptor antagonist should be administered at the end of surgery to patients at high risk for developing postoperative nausea and vomiting (PONV).

❻ Nausea and vomiting affect the majority of pregnant women; the teratogenic potential of the therapy is the primary consideration in drug selection.

❼ Because the vestibular system is replete with muscarinic type cholinergic and histaminic (H$_1$) receptors, anticholinergics and antihistamines are the most commonly used pharmacologic agents to prevent and treat motion sickness.

INTRODUCTION

Nausea and vomiting are due to complex interactions of the GI system, the vestibular system, and various portions of the brain. Nausea and vomiting have a variety of causes that can be simple or complex. Preventing and treating nausea and vomiting require pharmacologic and nonpharmacologic measures tailored to individual patients and situations.

ETIOLOGY AND EPIDEMIOLOGY

❶ *Nausea and vomiting are symptoms that can be due to a number of different causes.* Various disorders of the GI, cardiac, neurologic, and endocrine systems can lead to nausea and vomiting (Table 20–1).[1-4] Cancer chemotherapy agents are rated according to their emetogenic potential, and antiemetic therapy is prescribed based on these ratings. Due to potentially severe nausea and vomiting, some patients are unable to complete their chemotherapy treatment regimen. Radiation therapy can induce nausea and vomiting, especially when it is used to treat abdominal malignancies.[5]

Oral contraceptives, hormone therapy, oral hypoglycemic agents, anticonvulsants, and opioids are other common therapies that can cause nausea and vomiting.[1,6] Some medications, such as digoxin and theophylline, cause nausea and vomiting in a dose-related fashion. Nausea and vomiting may indicate higher-than-desired drug concentrations. Ethanol and other toxins also cause nausea and vomiting.

Table 20–1					
Causes of Nausea and Vomiting					
GI or Intraperitoneal	**Cardiac**	**Neurologic**	**Other Causes**	**Therapy Induced**	**Endocrine/Metabolic**
Obstructing disorders	Cardiopulmonary	Vestibular disease	Bulimia and	Cancer chemotherapy	Pregnancy (morning
Pyloric obstruction	disease	Motion sickness	anorexia	Antibiotics	sickness and
Small bowel obstruction	Cardiomyopathy	Labyrinthitis	nervosa	Cardiac antiarrhythmics	hyperemesis
Colonic obstruction	Myocardial	Head trauma	Cyclic vomiting	Digoxin	gravidarum)
Achalasia	infarction	Migraine headache	syndrome	Oral hypoglycemics	Renal disease (uremia)
Superior mesenteric artery	Congestive heart	Increased		Oral contraceptives	Diabetes (ketoacidosis)
syndrome	failure	intracranial		Theophylline	Thyroid and parathyroid
Enteric infections		pressure		Opioids	disease
Inflammatory bowel		Intracranial		Anticonvulsants	Adrenal insufficiency
diseases		hemorrhage		Radiation therapy	Electrolyte
Pancreatitis		Meningitis		Ethanol	abnormalities
Appendicitis		Hydrocephalus		Toxins	(hyponatremia,
Cholecystitis		Psychogenic		Operative procedures	hypercalcemia)
Biliary colic		causes			
Gastroparesis		Psychogenic			
Postvagotomy syndrome		vomiting			
Intestinal pseudo-		Depression			
obstruction		Psychiatric illness			
Functional dyspepsia		Self-induced			
Gastroesophageal reflux		Anticipatory			
Peptic ulcer disease		Rumination			
Hepatitis					
Peritonitis					
Gastric malignancy					
Liver failure					

Postoperative nausea and vomiting (PONV) occurs in 30% of surgical patients overall and in up to 70% of high-risk patients.[7–9] This can be due to severing or disturbing the vagus nerve leading to gastric motility abnormalities. Additional risk factors for PONV include female gender, history of motion sickness or PONV, nonsmoking status, and use of opioids in the postoperative period.[9–11] The choice of anesthetic agents and the duration of surgery may also contribute to PONV.[7,9,11]

Pregnancy-associated nausea and vomiting is common, affecting 70% to 85% of pregnant women, especially early in pregnancy.[12] Approximately one-half of pregnant women experience nausea and vomiting of pregnancy (NVP), one-quarter experience nausea alone, and one-quarter are not affected.[12] In 0.5% to 2% of pregnancies, this can lead to **hyperemesis gravidarum**, a potentially life-threatening condition of prolonged nausea, vomiting, and consequently, malnutrition.[12]

PATHOPHYSIOLOGY

Nausea and vomiting consist of three stages: (a) **nausea**; (b) **retching**; and (c) **vomiting**. Nausea is the subjective feeling of a need to vomit.[1,6] It is often accompanied by autonomic symptoms such as pallor, tachycardia, diaphoresis, and salivation. Retching, which follows nausea, consists of diaphragm, abdominal wall, and chest wall contractions and spasmodic breathing against a closed glottis.[1] Retching can occur without vomiting, but this stage produces the pressure gradient needed for vomiting, although no gastric contents are expelled. Vomiting, or emesis, is a reflexive, rapid, and forceful oral expulsion of upper GI contents due to powerful and sustained contractions in the abdominal and thoracic musculature.[1] Vomiting, like nausea, can be accompanied by autonomic symptoms.

Regurgitation, unlike vomiting, is a passive process without involvement of the abdominal wall and diaphragm wherein gastric or esophageal contents move into the mouth.[1] In patients with gastroesophageal reflux disease (GERD), one hallmark symptom is acid regurgitation.

Various areas in the brain and the GI tract are stimulated when the body is exposed to noxious stimuli (e.g., toxins), GI irritants (e.g., infectious agents), or chemotherapy. These areas include the **chemoreceptor trigger zone** (CTZ) in the area postrema of the fourth ventricle of the brain, the vestibular system, visceral afferents from the GI tract, and the cerebral cortex.[2,3,6] These in turn stimulate regions of the reticular areas of the medulla within the brain stem. This area is the central vomiting center, the area of the brain stem that coordinates the impulses sent to the salivation center, respiratory center, and the pharyngeal, GI, and abdominal muscles that lead to vomiting (Fig. 20–1).[13]

The CTZ, located outside the blood–brain barrier, is exposed to cerebrospinal fluid and blood.[2,3] Therefore, it is easily stimulated by uremia, acidosis, and the circulation of toxins such as chemotherapeutic agents. The CTZ has many 5-hydroxytryptamine (serotonin) type 3 (5-HT$_3$), neurokinin-1 (NK_1), and dopamine (D_2) receptors.[2,14] Visceral vagal nerve fibers are rich in $5\text{-}HT_3$ receptors. They respond to GI distention, mucosal irritation, and infection.

Motion sickness is caused by stimulation of the vestibular system.[15] This area contains many histaminic (H_1) and muscarinic cholinergic receptors. The higher brain (i.e., cerebral cortex) is affected by sensory input such as sights, smells, or emotions that can lead to vomiting. This area is involved in anticipatory nausea and vomiting associated with chemotherapy.

Nausea and vomiting can be classified as either simple or complex.[4] Simple nausea and vomiting occurs occasionally and is either self-limiting or relieved by minimal therapy. It does not have detrimental effects on hydration status, electrolyte balance, or weight because it is short-lived. Alternatively, complex nausea and vomiting requires more aggressive therapy because electrolyte imbalances, dehydration, and weight loss may occur. Unlike simple nausea and vomiting, complex nausea and vomiting can be caused by exposure to noxious agents.

CLINICAL PRESENTATION AND DIAGNOSIS

TREATMENT

Desired Outcomes

● The primary goal of treatment is to relieve the symptoms of nausea and vomiting, which should increase the patient's quality of life. Drug therapy for nausea and vomiting should be safe, effective, and economical.

General Approach to Treatment

❷ *To treat nausea and vomiting most effectively, it is important to first identify the underlying cause of the symptoms.* Treating the cause (if possible) will in turn eliminate the nausea and vomiting.

Profuse or prolonged vomiting can lead to complications of dehydration and metabolic abnormalities. Patients must have adequate hydration and electrolyte replacement orally (if tolerated) or IV to prevent and correct these problems. Some pharmacologic treatments work locally in the GI tract (e.g., antacids and prokinetic agents), whereas others work in the CNS (e.g., antihistamines and anticholinergics).[1]

Nonpharmacologic Therapy

A variety of effective pharmacologic treatments exist for nausea and vomiting, but they all have unwanted adverse treatment effects. For this reason, nonpharmacologic treatment options may be considered in selected patients.

Nonpharmacologic options are desirable for treating NVP due to concern for teratogenic effects with drug therapies. When treating PONV, the nonpharmacologic approach is appealing to minimize additive CNS depression with antiemetics and anesthetic agents. ❸ *Nonpharmacologic approaches to treating nausea and vomiting include dietary, physical, and psychological changes.*

Dietary approaches are the cornerstone of treatment for NVP.[16] They are included in treatment guidelines even though there is little evidence to support their effectiveness.[12] Recommendations include eating frequent, small meals; avoiding spicy or fatty foods; eating high-protein snacks; and eating bland or dry foods the first thing

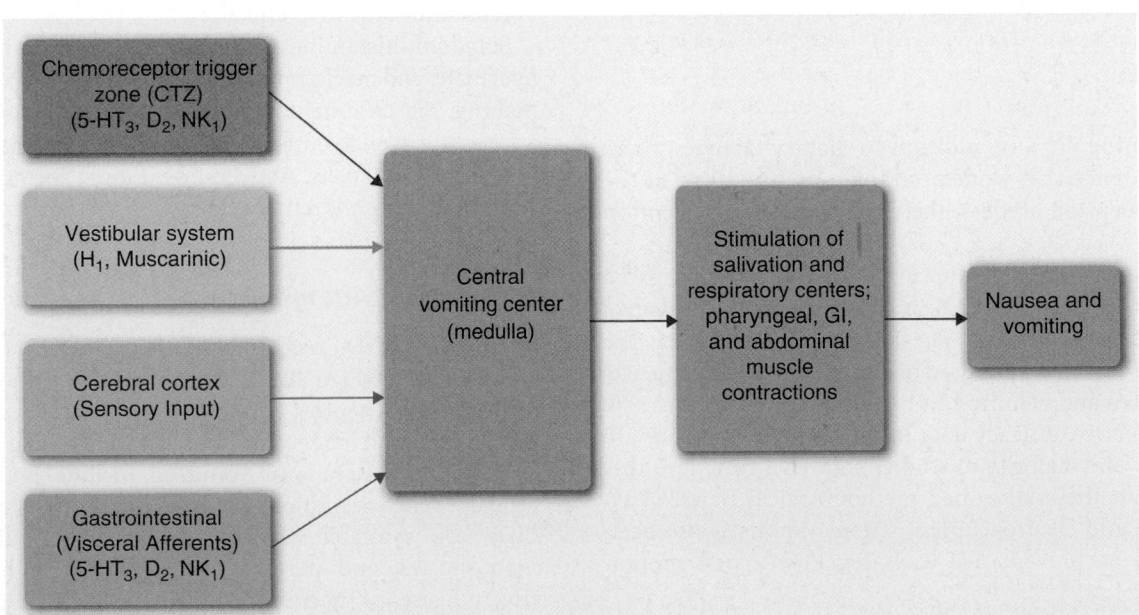

FIGURE 20–1. Physiologic pathways that result in nausea and vomiting. ($5\text{-}HT_3$, serotonin type 3 receptor; D_2, dopamine type 2 receptor; H_1, histamine type 1 receptor, NK_1, neurokinin-1.) (From Ref. 13.)

Clinical Presentation and Diagnosis of Nausea and Vomiting

Symptoms

- Patients with nausea often complain of autonomic symptoms such as diaphoresis, general disinterest in surroundings, pallor, faintness, and salivation.

Signs

- With complex and prolonged nausea and vomiting, patients may show signs of malnourishment, weight loss, and dehydration (dry mucous membranes, skin tenting, tachycardia, and lack of axillary sweat).

Laboratory Tests

- Dehydration, electrolyte imbalances, and acid–base disturbances may be evident in complex and prolonged nausea and vomiting.
- Dehydration is suggested by elevated blood urea nitrogen (BUN) and serum creatinine (SCr) concentrations, especially with a BUN to SCr ratio of 20:1 or greater (using traditional units of measurement).
- Calculated fractional excretion of sodium (FeNa) less than 1% in patients with compromised baseline renal function and less than 0.2% in patients with normal baseline renal function indicates dehydration and reduced renal perfusion.
- Low serum chloride and elevated serum bicarbonate levels indicate metabolic alkalosis.
- Arterial blood gases with a normal or elevated pH indicates metabolic alkalosis that may or may not be compensated.
- Hypokalemia may occur from GI potassium losses and intracellular potassium shifts to compensate for alkalosis.

in the morning.[12,16,17] In addition to dietary changes, there is some evidence that women taking a multivitamin at the time of conception are less likely to seek medical attention for NVP.[12]

Acupressure and acupuncture have been investigated based on the theory that certain points on the body control specific bodily functions.[16] The P6 (Neiguan) point on the inside of the wrist has been used historically by acupuncturists to treat nausea and vomiting. While this approach seems safe and cost effective, efficacy data in the treatment of NVP are conflicting. The majority of studies showed a benefit to this approach, but the studies had methodological flaws.[12,18] P6 acupressure and electroacupoint stimulation have also been investigated as preventative tools for PONV and motion sickness.[19–21]

Hypnosis may be effective for severe NVP.[22] Psychotherapy is another noninvasive treatment approach that is safe during pregnancy or in situations in which adverse treatment effects and drug interactions are a concern. One small study suggested that patients with hyperemesis gravidarum may benefit from the combination of psychotherapy and antiemetics.

Pharmacologic Therapy

Table 20–2 contains the names, usual dosages, and common adverse effects of the pharmacologic treatments for nausea and vomiting.[1,4,5,9]

▶ Anticholinergics (Scopolamine)

The anticholinergic agent scopolamine blocks muscarinic receptors in the vestibular system, thereby halting signaling to the CNS. It is effective for preventing and treating motion sickness and perhaps for preventing PONV as well.[23,24] Scopolamine is available as an adhesive transdermal patch (Transderm Scop) that is effective for up to 72 hours after application. This may be beneficial for patients unable to tolerate oral medications or those requiring continuous prevention of motion sickness (e.g., passengers on cruise ships). Scopolamine is associated with adverse anticholinergic effects such as sedation, visual disturbances, dry mouth, and dizziness.

▶ Antihistamines

Antihistamines are commonly used to prevent and treat nausea and vomiting due to motion sickness, vertigo, or migraine headache.[1,15,25] Their efficacy is presumably due to the high concentration of H_1 and muscarinic cholinergic receptors within the vestibular system. Similarly to scopolamine, antihistamines such as diphenhydramine and meclizine cause undesired effects including drowsiness and blurred vision. Cetirizine and fexofenadine, two second-generation antihistamines without CNS depressant properties, were found to be ineffective for treating motion sickness, perhaps because they lack CNS effects.[25]

Some antihistamines such as diphenhydramine, dimenhydrinate, and meclizine are available without a prescription, making self-treatment convenient for patients. Antihistamines are available in a variety of dosage forms, including oral capsules, tablets, and liquids. Liquid formulations are convenient for children or adults who are unable to swallow solid dosage forms.

▶ Dopamine Antagonists

Stimulation of D_2 receptors in the CTZ leads to nausea and vomiting (Fig. 20–1). Phenothiazine antiemetics act primarily via a central antidopaminergic mechanism in the CTZ.[1] Common phenothiazines that have long been used for treating nausea and vomiting include promethazine, prochlorperazine, chlorpromazine, and thiethylperazine. They are available as oral solids and liquids, rectal suppositories, and parenteral formulations. This permits effective use of phenothiazines in a variety of settings including treatment of severe motion sickness or vertigo, gastritis or gastroenteritis, NVP, PONV, or chemotherapy-induced nausea and vomiting (CINV).[5,7,9,12,26–29]

Table 20–2

Antiemetic Agents: Doses for Adults and Children and Adverse Effects

Drug	Adult Dosing	Pediatric Dosing	Adverse Effects[a]
Anticholinergics			
Scopolamine (Transderm Scop)	TD: 1.5 mg patch applied every 72 hours as needed	N/A	Most common: Dry mouth, drowsiness, impaired eye accommodation Rare: Disorientation, memory disturbances, dizziness, hallucinations
Antihistamines			
Cyclizine (Marezine)	Orally: 50 mg every 4–6 hours as needed	N/A	Most common: Sedation, dry mouth, constipation
Dimenhydrinate (Dramamine)	Orally: 50–100 mg every 4–6 hours as needed	Orally, 2–6 years: 12.5–25 mg every 6–8 hours; Orally, 6–12 years 25–50 mg every 6–8 hours	Less common: Confusion, blurred vision, urinary retention
Diphenhydramine (Benadryl)	Orally: 25–50 mg every 4–6 hours IV/IM: 10–50 mg every 2–4 hours as needed	Orally/IV/IM: 2–6 years: 6.25 mg every 4–6 hours, max 37.5 mg/day; 6–12 years: 12.5–25 mg every 4–6 hours, max 150 mg/day	
Hydoxyzine (Atarax, Vistaril)	Orally/IV/IM: 25–100 mg every 4–6 hours as needed	Orally: 0.6 mg/kg IM: 0.5–1 mg/kg	
Meclizine (Bonine, Antivert)	Orally: 25–50 mg once daily as needed	Orally: 12 years or older: use adult dose	
Phenothiazines			
Chlorpromazine (Thorazine)	Orally: 10–25 mg every 4–6 hours as needed IV/IM: 25–50 mg every 4–6 hours as needed	Orally, 6 months and older: 0.5 mg/kg every 4–6 hours as needed IV/IM: 6 months and older: 0.5–1 mg/kg every 6–8 hours; max dose less than 5 years: 40 mg/day; max for 5–12 years: 75 mg/day	Most common: Sedation, lethargy, skin sensitization Less common: Cardiovascular effects, extrapyramidal effects, cholestatic jaundice, hyperprolactinemia Rare: Neuroleptic malignant syndrome, hematologic abnormalities, respiratory depression
	Supp: 50–100 mg every 6–8 hours as needed	Supp: over 6 months: 1 mg/kg every 6–8 hours as needed	
Prochlorperazine (Compazine)	Orally: 5–10 mg 3–4 times a day as needed	Orally: over 2 years and more than 9 kg: 0.4 mg/kg/day or 10 mg/m² daily in 2–3 divided doses; Max daily dose: 9–13 kg, 7.5 mg; 13.1–17 kg, 10 mg; 17.1–37 kg, 15 mg	
	Supp: 25 mg twice daily as needed IV/IM 2.5–10 mg every 3–4 hours as needed	Supp: See po dosing IM: over 2 years and more than 9 kg: 0.13 mg/kg	
Promethazine (Phenergan)	Orally/IM/IV/Supp: 12.5–25 mg every 4–6 hours as needed	Orally/IM/IV/Supp: 2 years and older: 0.25–0.5 mg/kg or 7.5–15 mg/m² 4–6 times daily; maximum 25 mg/dose	
Thiethylperazine (Torecan)	Orally/IM: 10 mg 3 times a day	N/A	
Butyrophenones			
Droperidol (Inapsine)[b]	IM/IV: 0.625–2.5 mg every 4–6 hours as needed	IM/IV: 2–12 years: 0.05–0.1 mg/kg (max 2.5 mg) every 4–6 hours as needed	Most common: Sedation, hypotension, tachycardia
Haloperidol (Haldol)	Orally, IM/IV: 0.5–5 mg every 12 hours as needed	N/A	Less common: Extrapyramidal effects, dizziness, increase in blood pressure, chills, hallucinations
Benzamides			
Domperidone (Motilium)[c]	Orally: 10–20 mg every 4–8 hours as needed Supp: 30–60 mg every 4–8 hours as needed	Orally: 0.2–0.4 mg/kg every 4–8 hours as needed for CINV prophylaxis Supp: Max daily dose based on weight: 10–15 kg, 30 mg; 15.5–25 kg, 60 mg; 25.5–35 kg, 90 mg; 35.5–45 kg, 120 mg	Most common: Sedation, restlessness, diarrhea (metoclopramide), agitation, CNS depression

(Continued)

Table 20–2

Antiemetic Agents: Doses for Adults and Children and Adverse Effects (Continued)

Drug	Adult Dosing	Pediatric Dosing	Adverse Effects[a]
Metoclopramide (Reglan)[d]	PONV: 10–20 mg po/IV/IM 10 minutes prior to anesthesia CINV Prophylaxis: 1–2 mg/kg po/IV every 2–4 hours	N/A	Less common: Extrapyramidal effects (more frequent with higher doses), hypotension, neuroleptic syndrome, supraventricular tachycardia (with IV administration)
Trimethobenzamide (Tigan)	Orally: 300 mg 3–4 times a day as needed IM: 200 mg 2–4 times a day as needed	Orally: 15–20 mg/kg/day divided into 3–4 doses Not recommended	
Corticosteroids			
Dexamethasone (Decadron)	CINV: 12–20 mg orally/IV day 1, then 8–12 mg po/IV daily PONV: 4–5 mg orally/IV at induction of anesthesia	CINV: 10 mg/m² prior to chemotherapy then 5 mg/m²	Most common: GI upset, anxiety, insomnia
Methylprednisolone (Solu-Medrol)	125–500 mg orally/IV every 6 hours for total of 4 doses	N/A	Less common: Hyperglycemia, facial flushing, euphoria, perineal itching or burning (with dexamethasone, probably secondary to vehicle and rate of injection)
Cannabinoids			
Dronabinol (Marinol)	Orally: 5–15 mg/m² every 2–4 hours as needed	Use adult dose, use with caution and adjust dose based on response	Most common: Drowsiness, euphoria, somnolence, vasodilation, vision difficulties, abnormal thinking, dysphoria
Nabilone (Cesamet)	Orally: 1–2 mg 2–3 times a day as needed	N/A	Less common: Diarrhea, flushing, tremor, myalgia
Benzodiazepines			
Lorazepam (Ativan)	Orally/IV: 0.5–2 mg prior to chemotherapy	Orally/IV: 2–15 years old: 0.05 mg/kg (up to 2 mg) prior to chemotherapy	Most common: Sedation, amnesia
Alprazolam (Xanax)	Orally: 0.5–2 mg 3 times a day prior to chemotherapy	N/A	Rare: Respiratory depression, ataxia, blurred vision, hallucinations, paradoxical reactions (weeping, emotional reactions)
Serotonin Antagonists			
Dolasetron (Anzemet)	CINV: 1.8 mg/kg or 100 mg IV/po before chemotherapy; PONV: 12.5 mg IV 15 minutes before end of anesthesia or at onset of N/V OR 100 mg po within 2 hours before surgery	CINV, 2–16 years: 1.8 mg/kg IV/po (maximum 100 mg) PONV: 0.35 mg/kg IV (maximum 12.5 mg) OR 1.2 mg/kg po (maximum 100 mg) within 2 hours before surgery	Most common: Headache, asymptomatic prolongation of electrocardiographic interval
Granisetron (Kytril)	CINV: 10 mcg/kg IV prior to chemotherapy; or 1 mg orally 1 hour before chemotherapy and 1 mg 12 hours after the first dose, or 2 mg 1 hour before chemotherapy PONV: 1 mg IV before induction of anesthesia OR immediately before reversal of anesthesia, OR at onset of N/V	CINV: 2–16 years: Use adult dosing IV or po regimen PONV: Not recommended for pediatric patients	Less common: Constipation, asthenia, somnolence, diarrhea, fever, tremor or twitching, ataxia, lightheadedness, dizziness, nervousness, thirst, muscle pain, warm or flushing sensation on IV administration
Granisetron (Sancuso)	CINV: 1 patch 24–48 hours before chemotherapy; may be worn for up to 7 days (delivers 3.1 mg granisetron per 24 hours)	N/A	Rare: Transient elevations in hepatic transaminases
Ondansetron (Zofran)[e]	CINV: orally: 24 mg prior to chemotherapy as a single dose, or 8 mg prior to chemotherapy, repeat every 12 hours. IV: 8–12 mg IV 30 minutes prior to chemotherapy, or 0.15 mg/kg 3 times a day beginning prior to chemotherapy	CINV: orally: 4–11 years: 4 mg 30 minutes prior to chemotherapy, repeat at 4 and 8 hours and every 8 hours for 1–2 days after chemotherapy completion IV: over 6 months: 0.15 mg/kg 3 times a day beginning prior to chemotherapy	Granisetron may be degraded by direct sunlight or exposure to sunlamps. Patients should be advised to cover the patch application site (e.g., with clothing) if there is a risk of exposure to sunlight or sunlamps during use and for 10 days after removal

(Continued)

Table 20–2

Antiemetic Agents: Doses for Adults and Children and Adverse Effects (Continued)

Drug	Adult Dosing	Pediatric Dosing	Adverse Effects[a]
	PONV: 4 mg IV/IM before anesthesia induction or at onset of N/V; 16 mg orally once given 1 hour before anesthesia induction	PONV: 1 month–12 years: 4 mg IV/IM before anesthesia induction for over 40 kg and 0.1 mg/kg IV for under 40 kg Oral recommendations not available	
Palonosetron (Aloxi)	CINV: 0.25 mg IV 30 minutes before chemotherapy; 0.5 mg orally 1 hour before chemotherapy PONV: 0.075 mg IV before anesthesia induction	N/A	
Neurokinin-1 Antagonist			
Aprepitant (Emend)	CINV: 115 mg IV (fosaprepitant) 30 minutes before chemotherapy on first day of chemotherapy only, as a substitute for 125 mg orally dose; 125 mg orally on day 1, 1 hour prior to chemotherapy; 80 mg on days 2 and 3 PONV: 40 mg orally 3 hours prior to anesthesia induction	N/A	Most common: Fatigue, hiccups Less common: Dizziness, headache, insomnia Rare: Transient elevations in hepatic transaminases

CINV, chemotherapy-induced nausea and vomiting; IM, intramuscularly; Inj, injectable dosage form for IV or IM use; N/A, not available; PONV, postoperative nausea and vomiting; TD, transdermal; Supp, rectal suppository.

[a]Most common, greater than 10%; less common, 1% to 10%; rare, less than 1%. On the basis of U.S. FDA-approved labeling and generalized to drug class.

[b]See text for warnings.

[c]Not available in the United States.

[d]Reduce dose by half if creatinine clearance is less than 40 mL/min.

[e]Daily dose not to exceed 8 mg in severe hepatic impairment (Child-Pugh score 10 or more).

Phenothiazines may cause sedation, orthostatic hypotension, and extrapyramidal symptoms (EPS) such as dystonia (involuntary muscle contractions), tardive dyskinesia (irreversible and permanent involuntary movements), and akathisia (motor restlessness or anxiety).[1,30,31] Chronic phenothiazine use has been associated with EPS, but single doses have also caused these effects.[32]

Akathisia is disturbing for patients and can be disruptive to patient care. Giving diphenhydramine with prochlorperazine may reduce the incidence of akathisia, but the combination increases the risk of sedation.[33] Slowing the IV infusion rate of prochlorperazine does not decrease akathisia.[31,32]

Droperidol, a butyrophenone derivative, is another centrally acting antidopaminergic agent effective for preventing PONV and treating opioid-induced nausea and vomiting.[1,7] It may also be used for treating CINV for patients who are intolerant to serotonin receptor antagonists and corticosteroids.[26]

Adverse effects of droperidol include sedation, agitation, and restlessness. In addition, droperidol carries a U.S. FDA black box warning regarding the potential for QT interval prolongation and cardiac arrhythmias that may result in torsades de pointes and sudden cardiac death.[34] Droperidol should not be used in patients with a prolonged QT interval or in those who are at risk for developing a prolonged QT interval (e.g., heart failure, electrolyte abnormalities, or concurrently taking other medications that may prolong the QT interval).[34] A 12-lead ECG is recommended prior to treatment with droperidol. Haloperidol is another butyrophenone with some antiemetic effects at low doses (0.5–2 mg).[9] It has been explored as an alternative to droperidol.[35-37]

The substituted benzamides metoclopramide and domperidone (not available in the United States) act as D_2 antagonists both centrally in the CTZ and peripherally in the GI tract.[1,38] They also display cholinergic activity, which increases lower esophageal sphincter tone and promotes gastric motility. Metoclopramide at high doses has antiserotonergic properties as well. Because metoclopramide and domperidone have both antiemetic and prokinetic effects, both are used for a variety of disorders including PONV, CINV, NVP, gastroparesis, GERD, and migraine headaches.[1,7,12,26,39,40] Metoclopramide is available in injectable, oral solid, and oral liquid dosage forms, allowing for its use in both hospitalized and ambulatory patients. Other substituted benzamides include trimethobenzamide and benzquinamide.

Metoclopramide crosses the blood–brain barrier and has centrally mediated adverse effects. Young children and the elderly are especially susceptible to these effects, which include somnolence, reduced mental acuity, anxiety, depression, and EPS (akathisia, dystonia, and tardive dyskinesia).[41] The overall incidence of adverse effects is estimated to be 10% to 20%.[1]

Domperidone minimally crosses the blood–brain barrier; it acts in the CTZ that lies outside of the blood–brain barrier. As such, domperidone is less likely to cause the centrally mediated adverse effects seen with metoclopramide and has an estimated overall incidence of 5% to 10%.[1,41] However, domperidone has been associated with prolonged QT intervals, cardiac arrhythmias, and sudden death.[42] It should not be used for patients with underlying long QT interval or for those on other medications that prolong the QT interval. Both metoclopramide and domperidone can cause hyperprolactinemia, galactorrhea, and gynecomastia.

▶ Corticosteroids

Corticosteroids, especially dexamethasone and methylprednisolone, are used alone or in combination with other antiemetics for preventing and treating PONV, CINV, or radiation-induced nausea and vomiting.[5,9,14,43] They are administered either orally or IV. Their efficacy is thought to be due to release of 5-HT, reduction in the permeability of the blood–brain barrier, and reduction of inflammation.[44] Common adverse effects with short-term use include GI upset, anxiety, insomnia, and hyperglycemia.[5] Because their use is generally of short duration, long-term adverse effects (e.g., reduction in bone mineral density, corticosteroid-related diabetes, and cataracts) are not usually seen.

▶ Cannabinoids

Cannabinoids have antiemetic activity when used alone or in combination with other antiemetics.[45,46] Dronabinol and nabilone are commercially available oral formulations used for preventing and treating refractory CINV.[5,45,46] Cannabinoids are thought to exert their antiemetic effect centrally, although the exact mechanism of action is unknown.[45,46] Sedation, euphoria, hypotension, ataxia, dizziness, and vision difficulties can occur with cannabinoids.

▶ Benzodiazepines

Benzodiazepines, especially lorazepam, are used to prevent and treat CINV.[5,14,43] Lorazepam is thought to prevent input from the cerebral cortex and limbic system from reaching the central vomiting center in the brain stem.[13] Sedation and amnesia are common side effects. Respiratory depression can occur with high doses or when other central depressants such as alcohol are combined with benzodiazepines.

▶ Serotonin Antagonists

Chemotherapeutic agents cause release of 5-HT from enterochromaffin cells in the intestinal mucosa.[44] This increase in 5-HT concentrations leads to stimulation of the visceral vagal nerve fibers and CTZ, thereby triggering nausea and vomiting. Both the CTZ and the vagal visceral nerve fibers are rich in 5-HT$_3$ receptors.[2] Selective 5-HT$_3$ receptor antagonists (ondansetron, granisetron, dolasetron, and palonosetron) are available to prevent and treat nausea and vomiting due to stimulation of these receptors, especially for prevention and treatment of CINV and PONV.[5,7,9,11,14,43,44,47] These agents are well tolerated; the most common adverse effects are headache, somnolence, diarrhea, and constipation.[5]

The 5-HT$_3$ antagonist palonosetron is the first of its class to be approved for prevention of both acute and delayed CINV.[5] Compared to the other 5-HT$_3$ antagonists, palonosetron has a longer serum half-life (40 hours compared to 4–9 hours) and a higher receptor-binding affinity, which may contribute to its efficacy in preventing delayed CINV.[48] Despite these pharmacokinetic properties, palonosetron has not been shown to be superior to other 5-HT$_3$ antagonists. It is recommended as an alternative and equally effective 5-HT$_3$ antagonist in the most recent (2006) American Society of Clinical Oncology (ASCO) guideline.[5]

▶ NK$_1$ Receptor Antagonists

Aprepitant is the first NK$_1$ receptor antagonist antiemetic drug.[49] NK$_1$ receptors are present in the CTZ and GI tract and are involved in the nausea and vomiting response, especially CINV.[5,44] Aprepitant is effective for preventing acute and delayed CINV when used with a 5-HT$_3$ antagonist and a corticosteroid.[5,49,50] It is also effective for the prevention of PONV.[9,51]

Chemotherapy-Induced Nausea and Vomiting

CINV is classified as: (a) acute (occurring within 24 hours after receiving chemotherapy); (b) delayed (occurring more than 24 hours after receiving chemotherapy); or (c) anticipatory (occurring prior to chemotherapy in patients who experienced acute or delayed nausea and vomiting with previous courses).[5,43,47] Risk factors for CINV include poor emetic control with prior chemotherapy, female gender, low chronic alcohol intake, and younger age.[43,52]

Chemotherapeutic agents are classified according to their emetogenic potential (Table 20–3), which aids in predicting CINV.[5,14,53] Risk factors that are useful in predicting anticipatory nausea and vomiting include poor prior control of CINV and a history of motion sickness or NVP.[5,47]

❹ *For prevention of acute CINV for patients receiving moderately or highly emetogenic chemotherapy, a combination of antiemetics with different mechanisms of action is recommended* (Table 20–4).[5,14,43,47] Patients receiving chemotherapeutic agents with low emetogenic potential should receive a corticosteroid as CINV prophylaxis, and those receiving chemotherapy with minimal emetogenic risk do not require prophylaxis. Delayed nausea and vomiting is more difficult to prevent and treat. It occurs most often with cisplatin- and cyclophosphamide-based regimens, especially if delayed nausea and vomiting occurred with previous courses

Table 20–3

Emetogenicity of Chemotherapeutic Agents

Minimal Emetogenic Potential (Less Than 10% Risk)[a]	Moderate Emetogenic Potential (30–90% Risk)
Bevacizumab	Carboplatin
Bleomycin	Cyclophosphamide less than
Busulfan	1,500 mg/m²
Chlorambucil	Cytarabine greater than
2-Chlorodeoxyadenosine	1,000 mg/m²
Cladarabine	Daunorubicin
Erlotinib	Doxorubicin
Fludarabine	Epirubicin
Gefitinib	Idarubicin
Hydroxyurea	Ifosfamide
Rituximab	Irinotecan
Vinblastine	Melphalan
Vincristine	Oxaliplatin
Vinorelbine	Trabectedin
	Temozolomide
	Treosulfan

Low Emetogenic Potential (10–30% Risk)	High Emetogenic Potential (Greater Than 90% Risk)
Asparaginase	Carmustine
Bortezomib	Cisplatin
Cetuximab	Cyclophosphamide 1,500 mg/m²
Cytarabine 1 g/m² or less	or more
Docetaxel	Dactinomycin
Etoposide	Dacarbazine
Fluorouracil	Lomustine
Gemcitabine	Mechlorethamine
Methotrexate	Pentostatin
Mitomycin	Streptozotocin
Mitoxantrone	
Paclitaxel	
Pegasparaginase	
Premetrexed	
Thiotepa	
Topotecan	
Trastuzumab	

[a]"% risk" is the incidence of emesis without the administration of antiemetics.

From Refs. 5, 14, 43, 47.

of chemotherapy.[5,43] Patients at greatest risk are those who previously had poorly controlled acute CINV.[5]

Antiemetics can be administered either IV or orally in this situation, depending on patient characteristics such as ability to take oral medications, dosage form availability, and cost considerations.[5] The IV and oral routes are equally effective. When used at equipotent doses, the 5-HT$_3$ antagonists have similar efficacy in preventing acute CINV, despite pharmacokinetic and receptor-binding affinity differences.[5,14]

Patients undergoing chemotherapy should have antiemetics available to treat breakthrough nausea and vomiting even if prophylactic antiemetics were given.[5,43] A variety of antiemetics may be used, including lorazepam, dexamethasone, methylprednisolone, prochlorperazine,

---

Patient Encounter 1, Part 1

A 28-year-old healthy woman seeks your advice. She is about to leave on a 7-day Caribbean cruise and is concerned about motion sickness. She recently experienced nausea and one episode of vomiting while on a sailboat on Lake Michigan for an afternoon. She is not allergic to any medications. She does not smoke and only occasionally drinks alcohol. She takes an oral contraceptive (ethinyl estradiol and norgestimate) and occasional ibuprofen for headaches.

What nonpharmacologic and pharmacologic options are available for this woman?

How would you instruct her to use the recommended modalities?

What adverse effects would you discuss with her?

---

promethazine, metoclopramide, and dronabinol. If breakthrough CINV occurs, it may be best treated with an antiemetic with a mechanism of action that differs from the medications already administered. The 5-HT$_3$ antagonists are effective for treating breakthrough nausea and vomiting, but they have not been shown to be superior to more traditional and less expensive antiemetics.

The best strategy for preventing anticipatory nausea and vomiting is to prevent acute and delayed CINV by using the most effective antiemetic regimens recommended based on the emetogenic potential of the chemotherapy and patient factors. CINV should be aggressively prevented with the first cycle of therapy rather than waiting to assess patient response to less effective regimens. If anticipatory nausea and vomiting occurs, benzodiazepines and behavioral therapy such as relaxation techniques are the recommended approaches.[5,14]

Postoperative Nausea and Vomiting

PONV is a common complication of surgery and can lead to delayed discharge and unanticipated hospitalization.[7] The overall incidence of PONV for all surgeries and patient populations is 25% to 30%, but PONV can occur in 70% to 80% of high-risk patients.[7,9,11] Risk factors for PONV include patient factors (female gender, nonsmoking status, and history of PONV or motion sickness), anesthetic factors (use of volatile anesthetics, nitrous oxide, or intraoperative or postoperative opioids), and surgical factors (duration and type of surgery).[7,9–11]

The first step in preventing PONV is reducing baseline risk factors when appropriate.[7,9] For example, the incidence of PONV may be less with regional anesthesia than general anesthesia, and nonsteroidal anti-inflammatory drugs may cause less PONV than opioid analgesics.

❺ *Droperidol or a 5-HT$_3$ receptor antagonist should be administered at the end of surgery to patients at high risk for developing PONV.*[1,7,8,11,54] Dexamethasone is also effective when given as a single dose prior to induction of

Table 20–4

Recommended Drug Regimens for Prevention of CINV Based on Emetogenic Risk

Emetogenic Risk		Acute CINV (Day 1)	Delayed CINV (Days 2–4)
Minimal		None	None
Low		Dexamethasone	None
Moderate	Non-AC chemotherapy regimen	5-HT$_3$ antagonist + dexamethasone	5-HT$_3$ antagonist or dexamethasone (days 2 and 3)
	AC chemotherapy regimen	5-HT$_3$ antagonist + dexamethasone + aprepitant	Aprepitant or dexamethasone (days 2 and 3)
High		5-HT$_3$ antagonist + dexamethasone + aprepitant	Aprepitant (days 2 and 3) + dexamethasone (days 2–4)

AC, anthracycline (daunorubicin, doxorubicine, epirubicin, or idarubicin) plus cyclophosphamide; CINV, chemotherapy-induced nausea and vomiting.

From Refs. 5, 14, 43, 47, 52.

Patient Encounter 2

A 57-year-old woman is scheduled for an abdominal hysterectomy due to uterine fibroids. She is very anxious about her surgery.

PMH: Uterine fibroids; hypertension for 6 years; hypercholesterolemia for 6 years

FH: Father died of lung cancer; mother is still alive with a history of hypertension and cerebrovascular accident

SH: Works as a high school teacher; drinks one glass of wine with dinner three times per week; does not use tobacco

Meds: Hydrochlorothiazide 25 mg orally once daily; lisinopril 20 mg orally once daily; simvastatin 40 mg orally once daily at bedtime; aspirin 81 mg orally once daily; acetaminophen as needed for headache or body aches

Labs: Within normal limits

ECG: Normal sinus rhythm

Anesthesia for the surgery will be thiopental 4.5 mg/kg, atracurium 0.5 mg/kg, and fentanyl 0.05 mg followed by tracheal intubation, 70% nitrous oxide, and 0.5% to 2% isoflurane in oxygen.

What risk factors for PONV does this patient have?

Identify your treatment goals for this patient.

What nonpharmacologic and pharmacologic measures can be taken to prevent PONV?

Discuss any contraindications or adverse effects associated with your recommended treatments.

---

anesthesia.[7,54] Anticholinergics and antihistamines are also effective for preventing PONV.[7]

Aprepitant, an NK$_1$ receptor antagonist, prevents PONV; however, it does not appear to be more effective than other available agents and is costly.[9] Conversely, metoclopramide, ginger, and cannabinoids have been shown to be of limited utility for PONV and are not recommended.[9]

Combinations of antiemetics are the recommended method of preventing PONV for high-risk patients.[9] Droperidol plus a 5-HT$_3$ antagonist or dexamethasone plus a 5-HT$_3$ antagonist are effective combinations.[9] Three-drug combinations such as dexamethasone, droperidol, and a 5-HT$_3$ antagonist have not been formally studied but may be a reasonable approach.[54]

If PONV occurs despite appropriate prophylaxis, it should be treated with an antiemetic from a pharmacologic class not already administered.[9,11] If no prophylaxis was used, a low-dose 5-HT$_3$ antagonist should be used.[9,11]

Nausea and Vomiting of Pregnancy

⑥ *Nausea and vomiting affect the majority of pregnant women; the teratogenic potential of the therapy is the primary consideration in drug selection.*[12] Risks and benefits of any therapy must be weighed by the health care professional and the patient.

Nonpharmacologic therapy such as dietary, physical, and behavioral approaches should be considered first.[12,16] Pyridoxine (vitamin B$_6$) 10 to 25 mg three to four times daily alone or in combination with an antihistamine such as doxylamine is often used for NVP.[12,16–18] This combination was previously marketed as Bendectin or Debendox but was withdrawn due to concerns over possible teratogenic effects, although the literature did not support this claim.[17,18] Pyridoxine is well tolerated, but doxylamine and other antihistamines commonly cause drowsiness. For more severe NVP, promethazine, metoclopramide, and trimethobenzamide may be effective and have not been associated with teratogenic effects.[12,16] Ondansetron, which is pregnancy category B, has been used to treat severe NVP. Animal data do not indicate a safety concern in pregnancy, but safety and efficacy data in humans for NVP are sparse.

In rare instances (0.5–2% of pregnancies), NVP progresses to hyperemesis gravidarum.[12] Treatment may require the use of enteral or parenteral nutrition if weight loss is present. A corticosteroid such as methylprednisolone may be considered. Methylprednisolone is associated with oral clefts in the fetus when used during the first trimester. Therefore, corticosteroids should be reserved as a last resort and should be avoided during the first 10 weeks of gestation.[12,16,17]

Motion Sickness and Vestibular Disturbances

Nausea and vomiting can be caused by disturbances of the vestibular system in the inner ear.[15,55] Vestibular disturbances can result from infection, traumatic injury, neoplasm, and motion. Patients may experience dizziness and vertigo in addition to nausea and vomiting. If a patient is susceptible to motion sickness, some general preventive measures include minimizing exposure to movement, restricting visual activity, ensuring adequate ventilation, reducing the magnitude of movement, and taking part in distracting activities.[15]

❼ *Because the vestibular system is replete with muscarinic type cholinergic and histaminic (H₁) receptors, anticholinergics and antihistamines are the most commonly used pharmacologic agents to prevent and treat motion sickness.* Oral medications should be taken prior to motion exposure to allow time for adequate absorption. Once nausea and vomiting due to motion sickness occur, oral medication absorption may be unreliable, making the therapies ineffective. Scopolamine, the anticholinergic medication used for motion sickness, is available as a transdermal patch delivery system, which may be helpful for patients who cannot tolerate oral medications or who require treatment for a prolonged period.[23] Drowsiness and reduced mental acuity are the most bothersome side effects of antihistamines and anticholinergics. Visual disturbances, dry mouth, and urinary retention can also occur.

Patient Encounter 1, Part 2

Four months later, the patient returns to your practice. She is 8 weeks pregnant and complains of nausea and occasional vomiting. She is only taking prenatal vitamins. She does not smoke or drink alcohol. She was told at her last prenatal visit that she was appropriately gaining weight. She asks for your advice about preventing and treating nausea and vomiting.

What general considerations about treating NVP will you discuss with this patient?

What nonpharmacologic and pharmacologic treatment options are available for her?

Patient Care and Monitoring

1. Identify the underlying cause of the nausea and vomiting and eliminate it if possible. Counsel the patient to avoid known triggers.

2. Assess the patient to determine whether the nausea and vomiting is simple or complex and whether patient-directed therapy is appropriate.

3. Obtain a thorough patient history including the prescription, nonprescription, and herbal medications being used. Identify any substances that may be causing or worsening nausea and vomiting. Determine which treatments for nausea and vomiting have been used in the past and their degree of efficacy.

4. Develop a treatment plan with the patient and other health care professionals if appropriate. Choose therapeutic options based on the underlying cause of nausea and vomiting, duration and severity of symptoms, comorbid conditions, medication allergies, presence of contraindications, risk of drug–drug interactions, and treatment adverse-effect profiles.

5. Use the oral route of administration if the patient has mild nausea with minimal or no vomiting. Seek an alternative route (e.g., transdermal, rectal suppository, or parenteral) if the patient is unable to retain oral medications due to vomiting.

6. Educate the patient about nonpharmacologic measures such as stimulus avoidance, dietary changes, acupressure or acupuncture, and psychotherapy.

7. To assess efficacy, ask the patient whether he or she is still experiencing nausea or vomiting while using the therapy. Assess whether treatment failure is due to inappropriate medication use or the need for additional or different treatments and proceed accordingly.

8. Assess adverse effects by asking the patient what he or she has experienced. Also, patient observation or examination is useful for diagnosing adverse effects such as EPS.

9. Provide patient education regarding causes of nausea and vomiting, avoidance of triggers, potential complications, therapeutic options, medication adverse effects, and when to seek medical attention.

OUTCOME EVALUATION

- The symptoms of simple nausea and vomiting are self-limited or can be relieved with minimal treatment. Monitor patients for adequate oral intake and alleviation of nausea and vomiting.

- Patients with complex nausea and vomiting may have malnourishment, dehydration, and electrolyte abnormalities.

- Monitor patients for adequate oral intake. If the patient has weight loss, assess whether enteral or parenteral nutrition is needed.

- Assess for dry mucous membranes, skin tenting, tachycardia, and lack of axillary sweat to determine if dehydration is present.

- Obtain blood urea nitrogen (BUN), serum creatinine (SCr), calculated fractional excretion of sodium (FeNa), serum electrolytes, and arterial blood gases.

- Ask patients to rate the severity of nausea.

- Monitor the number and volume of vomiting episodes.

- Ask patients about adverse effects to the antiemetics used. Use this information to assess efficacy and tailor the patient's antiemetic regimen.

Abbreviations Introduced in This Chapter

ASCO	American Society of Clinical Oncology
BUN	Blood urea nitrogen
CINV	Chemotherapy-induced nausea and vomiting
CTZ	Chemoreceptor trigger zone
D_2	Dopamine type 2 receptor
EPS	Extrapyramidal symptoms
FeNa	Fractional excretion of sodium
GERD	Gastroesophageal reflux disease
H_1	Histamine type 1 receptor
5-HT_3	5-Hydroxytryptamine (serotonin) type 3 receptors
NK_1	Neurokinin type 1 receptors
NVP	Nausea and vomiting of pregnancy
PONV	Postoperative nausea and vomiting
SCr	Serum creatinine

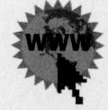 Self-assessment questions and answers are available at *http://www.mhpharmacotherapy.com/pp.html*.

REFERENCES

1. Quigley EM, Hasler WL, Parkman HP. AGA technical review on nausea and vomiting. Gastroenterology 2001;120:263–286.
2. Kearney DJ. Approach to the patient with gastrointestinal disorders. In: Friedman SL, McQuaid KR, Grendell JH, eds. Current Diagnosis and Treatment in Gastroenterology, 2nd ed. New York: McGraw-Hill, 2003:1–33.
3. Proctor DD. Approach to the patient with gastrointestinal disease. In: Goldman L, Ausiello D, Arend W, et al., eds. Cecil Medicine: Expert Consult (Cecil Textbook of Medicine), 23rd ed. Philadelphia: WB Saunders, 2007.
4. DiPiro CV, Taylor AT. Nausea and Vomiting. In: DiPiro JT, Talbert RL, Yee GC, Matzke GR, Wells BG, Posey LM, eds. Pharmacotherapy: A Pathophysiologic Approach, 6th ed. New York: McGraw-Hill, 2005:665–676.
5. Kris MG, Hesketh PJ, Somerfield MR, et al. American Society of Clinical Oncology guideline for antiemetics in oncology: Update 2006. J Clin Oncol 2006;24:2932–2947.
6. Chepyala P, Olden KW. Nausea and vomiting. Curr Treat Options Gastroenterol 2008;11:135–144.
7. Gan TJ, Meyer T, Apfel CC, et al. Consensus guidelines for managing postoperative nausea and vomiting. Anesth Analg 2003;97:62–71.
8. Gan TJ. Postoperative nausea and vomiting—Can it be eliminated? JAMA 2002;287:1233–1236.
9. Gan TJ, Meyer TA, Apfel CC, et al. Society for Ambulatory Anesthesia guidelines for the management of postoperative nausea and vomiting. Anesth Analg 2007;105:1615–1628.
10. Apfel CC, Laara E, Koivuranta M, et al. A simplified risk score for predicting postoperative nausea and vomiting: Conclusions from cross-validations between two centers. Anesthesiology 1999;91:693–700.
11. Wilhelm SM, Dehoorne-Smith ML, Kale-Pradhan PB. Prevention of postoperative nausea and vomiting. Ann Pharmacother 2007;41:68–78.
12. ACOG (American College of Obstetrics and Gynecology) Practice Bulletin: Nausea and vomiting of pregnancy. Obstet Gynecol 2004;103:803–814.
13. ASHP Therapeutic Guidelines on the Pharmacologic Management of Nausea and Vomiting in Adult and Pediatric Patients Receiving Chemotherapy or Radiation Therapy or Undergoing Surgery. Am J Health Syst Pharm 1999;56:729–764.
14. Hesketh PJ. Chemotherapy-induced nausea and vomiting. N Engl J Med 2008;358:2482–2494.
15. Shupak A, Gordon CR. Motion sickness: Advances in pathogenesis, prediction, prevention, and treatment. Aviat Space Environ Med 2006;77:1213–1223.
16. Badell ML, Ramin SM, Smith JA. Treatment options for nausea and vomiting during pregnancy. Pharmacotherapy 2006;26:1273–1287.
17. Lane CA. Nausea and vomiting of pregnancy: A tailored approach to treatment. Clin Obstet Gynecol 2007;50:100–111.
18. Jewell D, Young G. Interventions for nausea and vomiting in early pregnancy. Cochrane Database Syst Rev 2003:CD000145.
19. Miller KE, Muth ER. Efficacy of acupressure and acustimulation bands for the prevention of motion sickness. Aviat Space Environ Med 2004;75:227–234.
20. Lee A, Done ML. Stimulation of the wrist acupuncture point P6 for preventing postoperative nausea and vomiting. Cochrane Database Syst Rev 2004:CD003281.
21. Arnberger M, Stadelmann K, Alischer P, et al. Monitoring of neuromuscular blockade at the P6 acupuncture point reduces the incidence of postoperative nausea and vomiting. Anesthesiology 2007;107:903–908.
22. Mazzotta P, Magee LA. A risk-benefit assessment of pharmacological and nonpharmacological treatments for nausea and vomiting of pregnancy. Drugs 2000;59:781–800.
23. Spinks AB, Wasiak J, Villanueva EV, Bernath V. Scopolamine (hyoscine) for preventing and treating motion sickness. Cochrane Database Syst Rev 2007:CD002851.
24. Kranke P, Morin AM, Roewer N, et al. The efficacy and safety of transdermal scopolamine for the prevention of postoperative nausea and vomiting: A quantitative systematic review. Anesth Analg 2002;95:133–143.
25. Cheung BS, Heskin R, Hofer KD. Failure of cetirizine and fexofenadine to prevent motion sickness. Ann Pharmacother 2003;37:173–177.
26. Gralla RJ, Osoba D, Kris MG, et al. Recommendations for the use of antiemetics: Evidence-based, clinical practice guidelines. American Society of Clinical Oncology. J Clin Oncol 1999;17:2971–2994.
27. Bles W, Bos JE, Kruit H. Motion sickness. Curr Opin Neurol 2000;13:19–25.
28. Ernst AA, Weiss SJ, Park S, et al. Prochlorperazine versus promethazine for uncomplicated nausea and vomiting in the emergency department: A randomized, double-blind clinical trial. Ann Emerg Med 2000;36:89–94.
29. Habib AS, Gan TJ. The effectiveness of rescue antiemetics after failure of prophylaxis with ondansetron or droperidol: A preliminary report. J Clin Anesth 2005;17:62–65.
30. Olsen JC, Keng JA, Clark JA. Frequency of adverse reactions to prochlorperazine in the ED. Am J Emerg Med 2000;18:609–611.
31. Vinson DR, Migala AF, Quesenberry CP, Jr. Slow infusion for the prevention of akathisia induced by prochlorperazine: A randomized controlled trial. J Emerg Med 2001;20:113–119.

32. Collins RW, Jones JB, Walthall JD, et al. Intravenous administration of prochlorperazine by 15-minute infusion versus 2-minute bolus does not affect the incidence of akathisia: A prospective, randomized, controlled trial. Ann Emerg Med 2001;38:491–496.

33. Vinson DR, Drotts DL. Diphenhydramine for the prevention of akathisia induced by prochlorperazine: A randomized, controlled trial. Ann Emerg Med 2001;37:125–131.

34. MedWatch 2001 Safety Information Summaries: Inapsine (Droperidol). *www.fda.gov/Safety/MedWatch/SafetyInformation/SafetyAlerts forHumanMedicalProducts/ucm173778.htm.*

35. Grecu L, Bittner EA, Kher J, et al. Haloperidol plus ondansetron versus ondansetron alone for prophylaxis of postoperative nausea and vomiting. Anesth Analg 2008;106:1410–1413.

36. Rosow CE, Haspel KL, Smith SE, et al. Haloperidol versus ondansetron for prophylaxis of postoperative nausea and vomiting. Anesth Analg 2008;106:1407–1409.

37. Chu CC, Shieh JP, Tzeng JI, et al. The prophylactic effect of haloperidol plus dexamethasone on postoperative nausea and vomiting in patients undergoing laparoscopically assisted vaginal hysterectomy. Anesth Analg 2008;106:1402–1406.

38. Kovac AL. Prevention and treatment of postoperative nausea and vomiting. Drugs 2000;59:213–243.

39. Bsat FA, Hoffman DE, Seubert DE. Comparison of three outpatient regimens in the management of nausea and vomiting in pregnancy. J Perinatol 2003;23:531–535.

40. Colman I, Brown MD, Innes GD, et al. Parenteral metoclopramide for acute migraine: Meta-analysis of randomised controlled trials. BMJ 2004;329:1369–1373.

41. Patterson D, Abell T, Rothstein R, et al. A double-blind multicenter comparison of domperidone and metoclopramide in the treatment of diabetic patients with symptoms of gastroparesis. Am J Gastroenterol 1999;94:1230–1234.

42. Drolet B, Rousseau G, Daleau P, et al. Domperidone should not be considered a no-risk alternative to cisapride in the treatment of gastrointestinal motility disorders. Circulation 2000;102:1883–1885.

43. Lohr L. Chemotherapy-induced nausea and vomiting. Cancer J 2008;14: 85–93.

44. Minami M, Endo T, Hirafuji M, et al. Pharmacological aspects of anticancer drug-induced emesis with emphasis on serotonin release and vagal nerve activity. Pharmacol Ther 2003;99:149–165.

45. Davis M, Maida V, Daeninck P, Pergolizzi J. The emerging role of cannabinoid neuromodulators in symptom management. Support Care Cancer 2007;15:63–71.

46. Davis MP. Oral nabilone capsules in the treatment of chemotherapy-induced nausea and vomiting and pain. Expert Opin Investig Drugs 2008;17:85–95.

47. Jordan K, Sippel C, Schmoll HJ. Guidelines for antiemetic treatment of chemotherapy-induced nausea and vomiting: Past, present, and future recommendations. Oncologist 2007;12:1143–1150.

48. Gralla R, Lichinitser M, Van Der Vegt S, et al. Palonosetron improves prevention of chemotherapy-induced nausea and vomiting following moderately emetogenic chemotherapy: Results of a double-blind randomized phase III trial comparing single doses of palonosetron with ondansetron. Ann Oncol 2003;14:1570–1577.

49. Warr DG, Hesketh PJ, Gralla RJ, et al. Efficacy and tolerability of aprepitant for the prevention of chemotherapy-induced nausea and vomiting in patients with breast cancer after moderately emetogenic chemotherapy. J Clin Oncol 2005;23:2822–2830.

50. Hesketh PJ, Grunberg SM, Gralla RJ, et al. The oral neurokinin-1 antagonist aprepitant for the prevention of chemotherapy-induced nausea and vomiting: A multinational, randomized, double-blind, placebo-controlled trial in patients receiving high-dose cisplatin—The Aprepitant Protocol 052 Study Group. J Clin Oncol 2003;21:4112–4119.

51. Golembiewski J, Tokumaru S. Pharmacological prophylaxis and management of adult postoperative/postdischarge nausea and vomiting. J Perianesth Nurs 2006;21:385–397.

52. Herrstedt J, Dombernowsky P. Anti-emetic therapy in cancer chemotherapy: Current status. Basic Clin Pharmacol Toxicol 2007;101: 143–150.

53. Hesketh PJ, Kris MG, Grunberg SM, et al. Proposal for classifying the acute emetogenicity of cancer chemotherapy. J Clin Oncol 1997;15: 103–109.

54. Tramer MR. Strategies for postoperative nausea and vomiting. Best Pract Res Clin Anaesthesiol 2004;18:693–701.

55. Zajonc TP, Roland PS. Vertigo and motion sickness. Part I: Vestibular anatomy and physiology. Ear Nose Throat J 2005;84:581–584.

21 Constipation, Diarrhea, and Irritable Bowel Syndrome

Beverly C. Mims and Clarence E. Curry Jr.

LEARNING OBJECTIVES

● **Upon completion of the chapter, the reader will be able to:**

1. Identify the causes of constipation.

2. Compare the features of functional constipation with those of irritable bowel syndrome (IBS) with constipation (IBS-C).

3. Recommend general and dietary modifications and therapeutic interventions for the treatment of functional constipation.

4. Distinguish between acute and chronic diarrhea.

5. Compare and contrast diarrhea caused by different infectious agents.

6. Explain how medication use can lead to diarrhea.

7. Discuss nonpharmacologic strategies for treating diarrhea.

8. Identify the signs and symptoms of IBS.

9. Contrast IBS with diarrhea (IBS-D) and IBS with constipation (IBS-C).

10. Discuss the goals of IBS treatment.

11. Evaluate the effectiveness of principal pharmaceutical therapies for IBS.

KEY CONCEPTS

❶ Constipation is defined in many ways, and it is important to know what is meant when the term is used.

❷ Functional constipation exists when criteria are fulfilled for at least 3 months with symptom onset at least 6 months before diagnosis.

❸ General and dietary modifications should be employed prior to the use of laxatives in most instances of constipation.

❹ Oral laxatives are the primary pharmacologic intervention for relief of constipation.

❺ When diarrhea is severe and oral intake is limited, dehydration can occur, particularly in the elderly and infants.

❻ The primary treatment of acute diarrhea includes fluid and electrolyte replacement, dietary modifications, and drug therapy.

❼ Irritable bowel syndrome (IBS) is generally described as a functional disorder rather than a distinct disease entity.

❽ IBS symptoms typically cluster around two main types: IBS with diarrhea and IBS with constipation.

❾ Diagnosis of IBS is made by symptom-based criteria and the exclusion of organic disease.

❿ The principal goal of IBS treatment is to reduce or control symptoms.

CONSTIPATION

❶ *Constipation is defined in many ways, and it is important to know what is meant when the term is used.* Constipation, when not associated with symptoms of irritable bowel syndrome (IBS), can be defined as a heterogeneous disorder characterized by disorganized passage of feces resulting in infrequent stools, difficult passage of stools, or both.[1] It may be described as difficulty in passing stool with too much effort, unproductive urges, too small amount of stool, too hard consistency of stool, painful elimination of stool, or a feeling of incomplete evacuation. The existence of some or all of these symptoms suggests the presence of constipation when the frequency of elimination of feces is limited to less than two times weekly or when more than 3 days have passed without elimination of stool.[1] ❷ *Functional constipation exists when symptoms last for at least 3 months with onset at least 6 months prior to diagnosis.[2]*

EPIDEMIOLOGY AND ETIOLOGY

Constipation is a common complaint of patients seeking medical attention, and about one-third of patients with constipation seek medical treatment. Constipation occurs in approximately 20% of the population.[3] Approximately 2.5 million physician visits and 90,000 hospitalizations per year in the United States are due to constipation.[4,5] Many medications and some disease states are associated with constipation. Constipation is associated with high socioeconomic costs and has considerable quality-of-life ramifications.[6]

Elderly patients, non-Caucasians, women, and those of lower educational and socioeconomic levels are more likely to report being constipated. Constipation in children can occur because of a change in the usual diet or fluid intake, a deviation from usual toileting routines such as during vacations, avoidance of bowel movements because of pain associated with having a stool, or due to the use of medications. Children who are diagnosed with severe constipation at a young age are likely to continue to suffer through puberty.

PATHOPHYSIOLOGY

Constipation can be due to primary and secondary causes (Table 21–1). Primary or idiopathic constipation is typified by normal-transit constipation, slow-transit constipation, and dyssynergic defecation. In the normal-transit type, colonic motility is unchanged and patients tend to experience hard stools despite normal movements. In the slow-transit type, motility is decreased leading to infrequent, harder, drier stools. In dyssynergic defecation (also known as pelvic floor dysfunction), patients have lost the ability to relax the anal sphincter while coordinating muscle contractions of the pelvic floor. Some causes of secondary constipation are listed in Table 21–1.

Constipation affects about 50% of pregnant women. Progesterone levels may be responsible in part for slowing digestion. Reabsorption mechanisms may affect colon water during pregnancy leading to harder stools and more difficult bowel movements. Intake of iron supplements may also contribute to constipation during pregnancy.

CLINICAL PRESENTATION AND DIAGNOSIS

Diagnosis

A complete history should be obtained so that the patient's symptoms can be evaluated and the diagnosis of functional constipation confirmed. The diagnosis of functional

---

Table 21–1

Causes of Constipation

Primary Causes

Normal-transit constipation (includes idiopathic or functional disorders)
Slow-transit constipation (includes motility disorders)
Defecatory or rectal evacuation disorders (e.g., Hirschsprung's disease, pelvic floor dyssynergia)

Secondary Causes (Selected)

Endocrine/metabolic conditions (diabetes mellitus, hypothyroidism, hypercalcemia)
GI conditions (IBS, diverticulitis, hemorrhoids)
Neurogenic conditions (brain trauma, spinal cord injury, cerebrovascular accident, Parkinson's disease)
Psychogenic (postponing the urge to defecate, psychiatric conditions)
Medications (analgesics, anticholinergics, calcium channel blockers, clonidine, diuretics, phenothiazines, tricyclic antidepressants [TCAs], iron supplements, calcium- and aluminum-containing antacids)
Miscellaneous (immobility, poor diet, laxative abuse, hormonal disturbances)

Clinical Presentation of Constipation

Symptoms

- Functional constipation (constipation occurring in the absence of a demonstrated pathologic condition) involves the presence of at least two of the following symptoms: straining, lumpy or hard stools, sensation of incomplete evacuation, sensation of anorectal obstruction or blockage, need for manual maneuvers to facilitate defecation, and/or infrequent bowel movements (fewer than 3 per week).

- Other complaints may include painful or difficult defecation, bloating, and absence of loose stools.

- Alarm (or red flag) symptoms include worsening of constipation, blood in the stools, weight loss, fever, anorexia, nausea, and vomiting.

- The patient should seek medical attention when symptoms are severe, last longer than 3 weeks, are disabling, when alarm symptoms occur, or whenever a significant change in usual bowel habits occurs.

Laboratory Tests (to Identify Secondary Causes)

- Thyroid function tests; abnormal thyroid hormone levels may suggest hypothyroidism, which may be associated with constipation.

- Serum calcium; either increased or decreased serum calcium levels may be associated with constipation.

- Glucose; increased blood glucose may indicate diabetes mellitus, which may be associated with constipation.

- Serum electrolytes; dehydration may be associated with constipation.

- Urinalysis may also indicate dehydration, if present.

- Complete blood count; anemia may be due to cancer or another systemic disorder accompanied by constipation.

constipation is suggested by the presence of two or more of the following criteria: (a) straining, (b) hard or lumpy stools, (c) sensation of incomplete evacuation, (d) sensation of anorectal blockage/obstruction, (e) need for manual maneuvers, or (f) fewer than three defecations per week for at least 25% of defecations. The symptoms must have been present for the last 3 months with onset at least 6 months prior to diagnosis. In addition the criteria for meeting the diagnosis of IBS are not met.[2]

Dietary habits should be evaluated; patients should be encouraged to maintain adequate fiber intake and hydration. Evaluation of psychosocial status is recommended. Constipation may occur in patients who are depressed or in psychosocial distress. A complete family history should be obtained, particularly as it relates to inflammatory bowel disease and colon cancer. A full record of prescription and over-the-counter medications is mandatory to identify drug-related causes of constipation.

In most cases, there is no underlying cause of constipation, and the physical examination and rectal examination are normal. Endoscopic evaluation is required in patients who have weight loss, rectal bleeding, or anemia with constipation. These examinations can be used to exclude the presence of cancer or strictures, especially in patients over the age of 50 years. Endoscopic evaluation is appropriate in patients without alarm symptoms and those younger than 50 years of age. However, all adults older than 50 years of age who present with new-onset constipation should undergo endoscopic evaluation to rule out malignancy.[7]

TREATMENT

Desired Outcomes

In patients with constipation, the principal goals are to: (a) identify and treat secondary causes, (b) relieve symptoms, and (c) restore normal bowel function.

Nonpharmacologic Therapy

❸ *General and dietary modifications should be employed prior to the use of laxatives in most instances of constipation.* Treatment of constipation depends upon the characteristics and severity of symptoms. Intake of dietary fiber increases fecal bulk by promoting movement of water into the feces and bacterial proliferation. Increasing fiber intake to 20 to 35 g/day may help improve symptoms. Foods high in fiber include beans, whole grains, bran cereals, fresh fruits, and vegetables such as asparagus, brussels sprouts, cabbage, and carrots. Persons with constipation should avoid excessively processed low-fiber foods such as luncheon meats, hot dogs, certain cheeses, and ice cream.

Adequate fluid intake is also important; patients should be encouraged to drink when thirsty. The thirst mechanism changes with age; maintenance of a daily intake diary may assist patients who need to be reminded to drink fluids.

Walking and other aerobic exercises help to tone the muscles of the lower abdominal area, which promotes propulsion in the bowel. Constipation is a frequent complaint of sedentary persons.

Each day most persons experience a strong peristaltic wave known as the gastrocolic reflex. A bowel movement usually follows. When the urge to have a bowel movement occurs, it should not be ignored. Some people put off having a stool for various reasons, which may lead to more difficulty in passing stool. Time should be planned daily to attempt having a stool. A busy lifestyle should not be allowed to interfere with normal bowel function.

Pharmacologic Therapy

❹ *Oral laxatives are the primary pharmacologic intervention for relief of constipation* (Table 21–2). There are several different drug classes, as described below.

▶ Bulk Producers

These agents are either naturally derived (psyllium), semisynthetic (polycarbophil), or synthetic (methylcellulose). They act by swelling in intestinal fluid, forming a gel that aids in fecal elimination and promoting peristalsis. They may cause flatulence (which is less common with methylcellulose) and abdominal cramping. Bulk-forming laxatives must be taken with sufficient water (8 oz or 240 mL/dose) to avoid becoming lodged in the esophagus and producing obstruction or worsening constipation. Hypersensitivity reactions may occur and rarely may be manifested as an anaphylactic reaction.

▶ Hyperosmotics

These products cause water to enter the lumen of the colon. Lactulose, sorbitol, and glycerin are osmolar sugars. Polyethylene glycol 3350 with electrolytes is most useful for acute complete bowel evacuation prior to GI examination. Polyethylene glycol 3350 without electrolytes is useful in patients who are experiencing acute constipation or who have had inadequate response to other agents.[8] Lactulose causes acidification of the contents of the colon, increases water content of the gut, and softens the stool. Glycerin causes local irritation and possesses hyperosmotic action. Osmotic agents may cause flatulence, abdominal cramping, and bloating.

Sorbitol and glycerin may be administered rectally for treatment of constipation. Rectal discomfort and irritation may occur when administered rectally. Glucose levels should be monitored in diabetic patients who ingest oral sorbitol.

▶ Lubricants

Lubricant laxatives work by coating the stool, which allows it to be expelled more easily. The oily film covering the stool also keeps the stool from losing its water to intestinal reabsorption processes. Mineral oil (liquid petrolatum) is a nonprescription heavy oil that should be used with caution, if at all, because it can be aspirated into the lungs and cause lipoid pneumonia when ingested orally. This is of particular concern in the young or the elderly. It may also interfere with the absorption of fat-soluble vitamins.

Table 21–2
Dosage Recommendations for Selected Laxatives and Cathartics

Agent	Adults and Children Ages 12 and Over	Children Ages 6–11 Years
Agents That Cause Softening of Feces in 1–3 Days		
Bulk-forming agents		
Methylcellulose	0.45–3 g po per dose up to 6 g/day	0.45–1.5 g po per dose up to 3 g/day
Polycarbophil	1–4 g po daily	On advice of practitioner
Psyllium	2.5–30 g po daily	On advice of practitioner
Emollients		
Docusate sodium	100–300 mg po daily	50–100 mg po daily
Docusate calcium	240 mg po daily	On advice of practitioner
Docusate potassium	100–300 mg po daily	100 mg po daily
Lactulose	15–30 mL (10–20 g) up to 60 mL (40 g) po daily	7.5 mL (5 g) po daily
Sorbitol	30–150 mL (as 70% solution) po daily	2 mL/kg (as 70% solution) po daily
Mineral oil	15–45 mL po daily	5–15 mL po daily
Agents That Result in Soft or Semifluid Stool in 6–12 Hours		
Bisacodyl (oral)	5–15 mg po daily 30 mg po daily for complete bowel evacuation	5–10 mg (0.3 mg/kg) po daily
Senna	12–50 mg po once or twice daily	6–25 mg po once or twice daily
Agents That Cause Watery Evacuation in 1–6 Hours		
Magnesium citrate[a]	120–300 mL po daily	100–150 mL po daily
Magnesium hydroxide[a]	30–60 mL po daily (15–30 mL of concentrate po daily)	2.5–5 mL po up to 4 × daily
Magnesium sulfate[a]	10–30 g po daily	5–10 g po daily
Bisacodyl (suppository)	10 mg rectally	5 mg rectally (1/2 suppository)
Polyethylene glycol 3350	17 g in 8 oz (240 mL) water po once daily; do not use longer than 2 weeks	Safety and efficacy not established

po, orally.

[a]Magnesium can accumulate in renal dysfunction.

Adapted from Spruill WJ, Wade WE. Diarrhea, constipation and irritable bowel syndrome. In: DiPiro JT, Talbert RL, Yee GC, et al. (eds.), Pharmacotherapy: A Pathophysiologic Approach. 7th ed. New York: McGraw-Hill; 2008:617–632, with permission.

▶ Stimulant Laxatives

Diphenylmethane derivatives (e.g., bisacodyl) and anthraquinones (e.g., senna) have a selective action on the nerve plexus of intestinal smooth muscle leading to enhanced motility. Enteric-coated bisacodyl tablets should be swallowed whole to avoid gastric irritation and vomiting. Ingestion should be avoided within 1 to 2 hours of antacids, H_2-receptor antagonists, proton pump inhibitors, and milk. The onset of effect is rapid but the effects can be harsh (cramping), depending on the dose taken. Castor oil is another member of this class that is used less frequently. Castor oil is classified as Pregnancy Category X. It is associated with uterine contractions and rupture. The use of castor oil in breast-feeding is considered as "possibly unsafe."

▶ Emollients

Also known as surfactants and stool softeners, emollients (e.g., salts of docusate) act by increasing the surface-wetting action on the stool leading to a softening effect. They reduce friction and make the stool easier to pass. These agents are not recommended for treating constipation of long duration.

▶ Saline Agents

Salts of sodium, magnesium, and phosphate pull water into the lumen of the intestines resulting in increased enteral pressure. Magnesium and phosphate may accumulate in patients with renal dysfunction. Principal concerns with sodium phosphate derivative use include dehydration, hypernatremia, hyperphosphotemia, acidosis, hypocalcemia, and worsening renal function. Patients with congestive heart failure and renal dysfunction should be advised to avoid these agents. In 2009, nonprescription oral sodium phosphate solutions were voluntarily recalled by the manufacturer because of the risk of acute phosphate nephropathy. Prescription products contain a black-box warning about use in high-risk patients.

▶ Tegaserod Maleate

Tegaserod maleate (Zelnorm) is a partial serotonin (5-HT$_4$) receptor agonist that causes an increase in peristaltic activity and intestinal secretion, and moderation of visceral sensitivity. It increases the frequency of bowel movements and reduces abdominal discomfort, bloating, and straining. The availability of tegaserod maleate is limited to emergency situations in women who are under the age of 55 years and who have a diagnosis of chronic idiopathic constipation who meet specific guidelines. Tegaserod availability was limited because postmarketing safety evaluation found that patients receiving it were at higher risk of suffering cardiac events such as stroke, heart attack, and unstable angina when compared with patients receiving placebo.

▶ Lubiprostone

Lubiprostone (Amitiza), a bicyclic acid oral agent, is approved for treatment of chronic idiopathic constipation in adults. It has not been studied in children. Lubiprostone acts locally on intestinal chloride channels and increases intestinal fluid secretion, resulting in increased intestinal motility and thereby increasing the passage of stool.[9]

Lubiprostone is contraindicated in patients with a history of mechanical GI obstruction and should not be used in patients suspected of having GI obstruction. Safety has not been established in pregnant women; animal studies indicated the potential to cause fetal loss. Women who could become pregnant should have a negative pregnancy test result prior to beginning therapy with lubiprostone.

GI adverse events reported with lubiprostone include nausea, diarrhea, abdominal distention, abdominal pain, flatulence, vomiting, loose stools, and dyspepsia. Nausea is a prominent adverse effect and may be minimized when lubiprostone is taken with food.

The recommended dose of lubiprostone is 24 mcg orally twice daily with food and water. Studies evaluated lubiprostone use for no longer than 4 weeks. Patients should be assessed periodically for the need to continue therapy.

▶ Methylnaltrexone Bromide

Methylnaltrexone bromide (Relistor) is indicated for opioid-induced constipation in patients with advanced illness, receiving palliative care, and who have experienced insufficient response to laxative therapy. It is a selective antagonist of opioid binding at the μ-receptor. It has limited ability to cross to the blood–brain barrier and causes laxation in patients with opioid-induced constipation without reducing the analgesic effects of opioids or inducing opioid withdrawal. Methynaltrexone bromide is administered subcutaneously no more than once daily or every other day at individualized dosages based on patient weight. In patients with renal impairment (creatinine clearance less than 30 mL/min) the dose should be reduced by 50%. The most common side effects are abdominal pain, flatulence, nausea, dizziness, and diarrhea. It is contraindicated in known or suspected GI obstruction.

▶ Treatment Recommendations

Slow-transit constipation can be treated with chronic administration of hyperosmotic laxatives. Senna, bisacodyl, and other stimulants should be used only when the others fail to deliver the desired effect.

Laxatives may provide appropriate relief when constipation occurs during the postpartum period, when not breastfeeding, and in immobile patients. Patients who are not constipated but who need to avoid straining (e.g., patients with hemorrhoids, hernia, or myocardial infarction) may benefit from stool softeners or mild laxatives such as polyethylene glycol 3350.

Laxatives should not be given to children younger than 6 years of age unless prescribed by a physician. Because children may not be able to describe their symptoms well, they should be evaluated by a physician before being given a laxative. Treating secondary causes may resolve the constipation without the use of laxatives. As in adults, children benefit from a healthy balanced diet, adequate fluid, and regular exercise.

Because many elderly persons experience constipation, laxative use is sometimes viewed as a normal part of daily

---

> ## Patient Encounter 1
>
> DB is a 72-year-old woman who complains of small, hard stools for the last 3 weeks. She noted that lately she has to strain to have bowel movements. She states that this difficulty with having bowel movements has occurred off and on for several months. She denies abdominal pain. She has a history of hypertension, osteoarthritis, and Type 2 diabetes mellitus.
>
> *What general approach to this patient should be employed?*
>
> *What are the possible contributing causes of her constipation?*
>
> *What nonpharmacologic and pharmacologic therapies would be appropriate for her condition?*

life. However, oral ingestion of mineral oil can be a special hazard in bedridden elderly persons because it can lead to pneumonia through inhalation of oil droplets into the lungs. Lactulose may be a better choice in this situation. Regular use of any laxative that affects fluid and electrolytes may result in significant unwanted adverse effects.

Bulk producers are commonly used during pregnancy. Stool softeners (Pregnancy Category C) are probably safe to use at any time during a pregnancy because they are poorly absorbed. Lactulose and magnesium products are classified as Pregnancy Category B. Specifically, no human studies are available concerning use of lactulose in pregnant women. Magnesium-based antacids are not classified according to pregnancy categories and are associated with low-risk and minimal absorption in pregnant women. Long-term use of magnesium citrate should be avoided (Pregnancy Category B).

To avoid constipation, pregnant women should be advised to eat regular meals that are balanced among fruits, vegetables, and whole grains; maintain adequate water intake; and get appropriate exercise.

Patients with the following conditions should use laxatives only under the supervision of a health care provider: (a) colostomy, (b) diabetes mellitus (some laxatives contain large amounts of sugars such as dextrose, galactose, and/or sucrose), (c) heart disease (some products contain sodium), (d) kidney disease, and (e) swallowing difficulty (bulk-formers may produce esophageal obstruction).

OUTCOME EVALUATION

- Ask the patient about the absence or improvement in symptoms to determine whether laxative therapy is effective. Patients should have an increase in stool frequency to three or more well-formed stools per week. Patients should report the absence of prolonged defecation time or the absence of the need for excessive straining.

Patient Care and Monitoring for Constipation

1. Assess the patient's symptoms to determine if patient-directed therapy is appropriate or whether the patient should be evaluated by a physician. Determine type and frequency of symptoms.

2. Review available information to determine the most likely cause or type of constipation.

3. Obtain a thorough history of prescription, nonprescription, and dietary supplement use. Determine what treatments have been helpful in the past. Is the patient taking any medications that may contribute to constipation?

4. Remember that no single therapy has proven effective for all patients who present with constipation.

5. Develop a plan to assess the effectiveness of laxative use in cases of functional constipation.

6. Evaluate the patient for the presence of adverse drug reactions, drug allergies, and drug interactions.

7. Provide patient education about constipation, general and dietary modifications, and drug therapy.

• When acute overuse or chronic misuse of saline or stimulant laxatives is suspected, it may be necessary to check for electrolyte disturbances (e.g., hypokalemia, hypernatremia, hyperphosphatemia, or hypocalcemia).

• Some laxatives (e.g., bulk producers) contain significant amounts of sodium or sugar and may be unsuitable for salt-restricted or diabetic patients. Monitoring of fluid retention (edema) and blood pressure changes are indicated in patients on sodium-restricted diets. Glucose monitoring may be required in diabetic patients as needed with chronic use. Use of low-sodium or sugar-free products may be indicated.

• Saline laxatives containing magnesium, potassium, or phosphates should be used cautiously in persons with reduced kidney function. Monitor appropriate serum electrolyte concentrations in patients with unstable renal function evidenced by changing serum creatinine or creatinine clearance.

• All laxatives are contraindicated in patients with abdominal pain, nausea, vomiting, symptoms of appendicitis, or undiagnosed abdominal pain. Patients should consult their physicians if sudden changes in bowel habits persist for more than 14 days or if use of a laxative for 7 days results in no effect.

DIARRHEA

Diarrhea is a symptom of an underlying problem, not a disease. It is characterized by increased stool frequency (usually more than three times daily), stool weight, liquidity, and decreased consistency of stools compared to a patient's usual pattern. Acute diarrhea is defined as diarrhea lasting for 14 days or less. Diarrhea lasting more than 30 days is called chronic diarrhea. Illness of 15 to 30 days is referred to as persistent diarrhea.[10]

EPIDEMIOLOGY AND ETIOLOGY

Most cases of diarrhea in adults are mild and resolve quickly. Infants and children (especially under 3 years of age) are highly susceptible to the dehydrating effect of diarrhea, and its occurrence in this age group should be taken seriously.

Acute Diarrhea

Acute diarrhea has many possible causes, but infection is the most common. Infectious diarrhea occurs because of food and water contamination via the fecal–oral route. Viruses are the cause in a large proportion of cases. Likely viral suspects include Rotavirus, Norwalk, and adenovirus. Patients usually exhibit sudden low-grade fever, vomiting, and watery stools.

Bacterial precipitants in many other cases include *Escherichia coli*, *Salmonella* species, *Shigella* species, *Vibrio cholerae*, and *Clostridium difficile*. The term dysentery describes some of these bacterial infections when associated with serious occurrences of bloody diarrhea. Additionally, acute diarrheal conditions can be prompted by parasites–protozoa such as *Entamoeba histolytica*, *Microsporidium*, *Giardia lamblia*, and *Cryptosporidium parvum*. Most of these infectious agents can cause traveler's diarrhea, a common malady afflicting travelers worldwide. It usually occurs during or just after travel following the ingestion of fecally contaminated food or water. It has an abrupt onset but usually subsides within 2 to 3 days.

Noninfectious causes of acute diarrhea include drugs and toxins (Table 21–3), laxative abuse, food intolerance, IBS, inflammatory bowel disease, ischemic bowel disease, lactase deficiency, Whipple's disease, pernicious anemia, diabetes mellitus, malabsorption, fecal impaction, diverticulosis, and celiac sprue.

Table 21–3

Selected Drugs and Substances That May Cause Acute Diarrhea

Drugs

Antibiotics	Hydralazine	Metformin	Sorbitol
Colchicine	Laxatives	Misoprostol	Theophylline
Digitalis	Mannitol	Quinidine	Thyroid products

Dietary Supplements

St. John's wort	Echinacea	Ginseng	Aloe vera

Poisons

Arsenic	Cadmium	Mercury	Monosodium glutamate

Lactose intolerance is responsible for many cases of acute diarrhea, especially in patients of African descent, Asians, and Native Americans. Possible food-related causes include fat substitutes, dairy products, and products containing nonabsorbable carbohydrates.

The diarrhea of IBS is sudden and perhaps watery but likely loose, usually accompanied by urgency, bloating, and abdominal pain occurring upon arising in the morning or immediately following a meal. Inflammatory bowel disease is typically associated with the sudden onset of bloody diarrhea accompanied by urgency, crampy abdominal pain, and fever. Patients who experience bowel ischemia may develop bloody diarrhea, particularly if they progress to shock.

Chronic Diarrhea

Chronic diarrhea lasts 4 weeks or more. Most cases result from functional or inflammatory bowel disorders, endocrine disorders, malabsorption syndromes, and drugs (including laxative abuse). In chronic diarrhea, daily watery stools may not occur. Diarrhea may be either intermittent or persistent.

PATHOPHYSIOLOGY

During normal processes, approximately 9 L (about 2.4 gallons) of fluid traverse the GI tract daily. Of this amount, 2 L represent gastric juice, 1 L is saliva, 1 L is bile, 2 L are pancreatic juice, 1 L is intestinal secretions, and 2 L are ingested. Of these 9 L of fluid presented to the intestine, only about 150 to 200 mL remain in the stool after reabsorptive processes occur.

Any event that leads to a significant increase in the amount of fluid retained in the stool may result in diarrhea. Large-stool diarrhea often signifies small intestinal involvement, whereas small-stool diarrhea usually originates in the colon. Diarrhea may be classified according to pathophysiologic mechanisms, which include osmotic, secretory, inflammatory, and altered motility.

Osmotic diarrhea results from the intake of unabsorbable but water-soluble solutes in the intestinal lumen leading to water retention. Common causes include lactose intolerance and ingestion of magnesium-containing antacids.

Secretory diarrhea results in an increase in the net movement (secretion) of ions into the intestinal lumen leading to an increase in intraluminal fluid. Medications, hormones, and toxins may be responsible for secretory activity.

Inflammatory (or exudative) diarrhea results from changes to the intestinal mucosa that damage absorption processes and lead to an increase in proteins and other products in the intestinal lumen with fluid retention. The presence of blood or fecal leukocytes in the stool is indicative of an inflammatory process. The diarrhea of inflammatory bowel disease (e.g., ulcerative colitis) is inflammatory in nature.

Increased motility results in decreased contact between ingested food and drink and the intestinal mucosa, leading to reduced reabsorption and increased fluid in the stool. Diarrhea resulting from altered motility is often established after other mechanisms have been excluded. IBS-related diarrhea is due to altered motility.

Although diarrhea can often be attributed to a specific mechanism, some patients develop diarrhea due to overlapping mechanisms. For example, malabsorption syndromes and traveler's diarrhea are associated with both secretory and osmotic diarrhea.

Drug-induced diarrhea can occur by several mechanisms. First, water can be drawn into the intestinal lumen osmotically. Second, the intestinal bacterial ecosystem can be upset leading to the emergence of invasive pathologic organisms triggering secretory and inflammatory processes. Saline laxatives are an example of the first mechanism, and many antibiotics act by the second. A third way is through altered motility as may occur with tegaserod maleate. Other drugs such as procainamide or colchicine produce diarrhea through undetermined mechanisms. Discontinuation of the offending drug may be the only measure needed to ameliorate the diarrhea.

CLINICAL PRESENTATION AND DIAGNOSIS

Diagnosis

Patients with diarrhea should be questioned about the onset of symptoms, recent travel, diet, source of water, and medication use. Other important considerations include duration and severity of the diarrhea along with an accounting of the presence of associated abdominal pain or vomiting, blood in the stool, stool consistency, stool appearance, stool frequency, and weight loss. Although most cases of diarrhea are self-limited, infants, children, elderly persons, and immunocompromised patients are at risk for increased morbidity.

Findings on physical examination can assist in determining hydration status and disease severity. The presence of blood in the stool suggests an invasive organism, an inflammatory process, or perhaps a neoplasm. Large-volume stools suggest a small-intestinal disorder, whereas small-volume stools suggest a colon or rectal disorder. Patients with prolonged or severe symptoms may require colonoscopic evaluation to identify the underlying cause.

TREATMENT

Most healthy adults with diarrhea do not develop significant dehydration or other complications and can be treated symptomatically by self-medication. ❺ *When diarrhea is severe and oral intake is limited, dehydration can occur, particularly in the elderly and infants.* Other complications of diarrhea resulting from fluid loss include electrolyte disturbances, metabolic acidosis, and cardiovascular collapse.

Children are more susceptible to dehydration (particularly when vomiting occurs) and may require medical attention early in their course, especially if younger than 3 years of age. Physician intervention is also necessary for elderly patients who are sensitive to fluid loss and electrolyte changes due to concurrent chronic illness.

Clinical Presentation of Diarrhea

Signs and Symptoms of Acute Diarrhea

- Patients with acute diarrhea have the abrupt onset of loose, watery, or semi-formed stools.
- Abdominal cramps and tenderness, rectal urgency, nausea, bloating, and fever may be present.
- The disorder is generally self-limited, lasting 3 to 4 days even without treatment.
- Patients with acute infectious diarrhea from invasive organisms also have bloody stools and severe abdominal pain.

Laboratory Tests in Acute Diarrhea

- Stool cultures can help identify infectious causes. Cultures are subject to time delay. New methodology using real-time polymerase chain reaction (PCR) shortens the reporting time.
- Stool may also be analyzed for mucus, fat, osmolality, fecal leukocytes, and pH. The presence of mucus suggests colonic involvement. Fat in the stool may be due to a malabsorption disorder. Fecal leukocytes can be found in inflammatory diarrheas including infections and caused by invasive bacteria (e.g., *E. coli,* and *Shigella* and *Campylobacter* species). Stool pH (normally greater than 6) is decreased by bacterial fermentation processes.

- Stool volume and electrolytes can be assessed in large-volume watery stools to determine whether the diarrhea is osmotic or secretory.
- CBC and blood chemistries may be helpful in patients whose symptoms persist. The presence of anemia, leukocytosis, or neutropenia may provide further clues to the underlying cause.

Signs and Symptoms of Chronic Diarrhea

- In patients with chronic diarrhea, symptoms may be severe or mild. Weight loss can be demonstrated, and weakness may be present.
- Dehydration may be manifested by decreased urination, dark-colored urine, dry mucous membranes, increased thirst, and tachycardia.

Laboratory Tests in Chronic Diarrhea

- All of the tests described for acute diarrhea would be used to establish a diagnosis of chronic diarrhea because the differential diagnosis is more complicated. The data obtained can help categorize the diarrhea as watery, inflammatory, or fatty, narrowing the focus on a primary disorder.
- Colonoscopy allows visualization and biopsy of the colon and is preferred if blood has been found in the stool or if the patient has AIDS.

Patients should undergo medical evaluation in the following circumstances: (a) moderate to severe abdominal tenderness, distention, or cramping; (b) bloody stools; (c) evidence of dehydration (e.g., thirst, dry mouth, fatigue, dark-colored urine, infrequent urination, reduced urine, dry skin, lack of skin elasticity, rapid pulse, rapid breathing, muscle cramps, muscle weakness, sunken eyes, or lightheadedness); (d) high fever (greater than or equal to 38°C or 101°F); (e) evidence of weight loss greater than 5% of total body weight; and (f) diarrhea that lasts longer than 48 hours.

Desired Outcomes

The goals of treatment for diarrhea are to relieve symptoms, maintain hydration, treat the underlying cause(s), and maintain nutrition. ❻ *The primary treatment of acute diarrhea includes fluid and electrolyte replacement, dietary modifications, and drug therapy.*

Nonpharmacologic Therapy

▶ *Fluid and Electrolytes*

Fluid replacement is not a treatment to relieve diarrhea but rather an attempt to restore fluid balance. In many parts of the world where diarrheal states are frequent and severe, fluid replacement is accomplished using oral rehydration solution (ORS), a measured mixture of water, salts, and glucose. The WHO-recognized solution consists of 75 mEq/L sodium, 75 mmol/L glucose, 65 mEq/L chloride, 20 mEq/L potassium, and 10 mEq/L citrate, having a total osmolarity of 245 mOsm/L. A simple solution can be prepared from 1 L water mixed with eight teaspoonfuls of sugar and one teaspoonful of table salt. Some commercial products include Pedialyte, Rehydralyte, and Ceralyte.

Consistent intake of water (perhaps by slowly sipping) along with eating as tolerated, should restore lost fluids and salt for typical diarrhea sufferers. Patients may also replace lost fluid by drinking flat soft drinks such as ginger ale, tea, fruit juice, broth, or soup. Caution is advised in using sports drinks for dehydration, as they may not provide an appropriate amount of electrolytes. Severe diarrhea may require the use of parenteral solutions such as lactated Ringer's or normal saline solution to replace large and life-threatening fluid losses.[10]

▶ *Dietary Modifications*

Once an acute diarrheal situation ensues, patients typically eat less as they become focused on the diarrhea. Both children and adults should attempt to maintain nutrition. Food provides nutrients and fluid volume that help replace what is lost. However, food-related fluid may not be enough to compensate for diarrheal losses. Some foods may be inappropriate if they irritate the GI tract or if they are implicated as the cause of the diarrhea. Patients with chronic diarrhea may find that increasing bulk in the diet may help (e.g., rice, bananas, whole wheat, and bran).

Pharmacologic Therapy

The goal of drug therapy is to control symptoms, enabling the patient to continue with as normal a routine as possible while avoiding complications (Table 21–4). Most infectious diarrheas are self-limited or curable with anti-infective agents.

▶ Adsorbents and Bulk Agents

Attapulgite adsorbs excess fluid in the stool with few adverse effects. Calcium polycarbophil is a hydrophilic polyacrylic resin that also works as an adsorbent, binding about 60 times its weight in water and leading to the formation of a gel that enhances stool formation. Neither attapulgite nor polycarbophil is systemically absorbed. Not only are both products effective in reducing fluid in the stool but they can also adsorb nutrients and other medications. Their administration should be separated from other oral medications by 2 to 3 hours. Psyllium and methylcellulose products may also be used to reduce fluid in the stool and relieve chronic diarrhea.

▶ Antiperistaltic (Antimotility) Agents

Antiperistaltic drugs prolong intestinal transit time, thereby reducing the amount of fluid lost in the stool. The two drugs in this category are loperamide HCl (available over-the-counter as Imodium A–D and generically) and diphenoxylate HCl with atropine sulfate (available by prescription as Lomotil and generically). The atropine is included only as an abuse deterrent; when taken in large doses, the unpleasant anticholinergic effects of atropine negate the euphoric effect of diphenoxylate. Both loperamide and diphenoxylate are effective in relieving symptoms of acute noninfectious diarrhea and are safe for most patients experiencing chronic diarrhea. These products should be discontinued in patients whose diarrhea worsens despite therapy.

▶ Antisecretory Agents

Bismuth subsalicylate (BSS) is thought to have antisecretory and antimicrobial effects and is used to treat acute diarrhea. Although it passes largely unchanged through the GI tract, the salicylate portion is absorbed in the stomach and small intestine. For this reason, BSS should not be given to people who are allergic to salicylates, including aspirin. Caution should be exercised with regard to the total dose given to patients taking salicylates for other reasons to avoid salicylism. Patients taking BSS should be informed that their stool will turn black.

Octreotide is an antisecretory agent that has been used for severe secretory diarrhea associated with cancer chemotherapy, HIV, diabetes, gastric resection, and GI tumors. It is administered as a subcutaneous or IV bolus injection in an initial dose of 500 mcg three times daily to assess the patient's tolerance to GI adverse effects. Biweekly serum levels of insulin-like growth factor-1 (IGF-1 or somatomedin C) can be used as a guide to dose titration. Possible adverse effects include nausea, bloating, pain at the injection site, and gallstones (with prolonged therapy).

▶ Probiotics

Probiotics are dietary supplements containing bacteria that may promote health by enhancing the normal microflora of the GI tract while resisting colonization by potential pathogens. Probiotics can stimulate the immune response and suppress the inflammatory response. Yogurt can provide relief from diarrhea due to lactose intolerance. It supports digestion of lactose because the bacteria used to make yogurt

Table 21–4

Pharmacotherapy for Diarrhea

Drug	Usual Oral Dose	Type of Diarrhea
Attapulgite	Adults: 1,200–1,500 mg after each loose stool. Maximum 9,000 mg in 24 hours Children aged 6–12: 750 mg after each loose stool. Maximum 4,500 mg in 24 hours	Acute and chronic
Calcium polycarbophil	Adults: 1,000 mg 4 × daily or after each loose stool, not to exceed 12 tablets per day Children aged 6–12: 500 mg 3 × daily Children aged 3–6: 500 mg twice daily	Chronic
Loperamide	Adults: 4 mg initially, then 2 mg after each subsequent loose stool. Maximum 16 mg in 24 hours Children maximum doses: Age 2–5: 3 mg Age 6–8: 4 mg Age 8–12: 6 mg	Acute and chronic
Diphenoxylate/ atropine	Adults: Two tablets (5 mg) initially, then one tablet every 3–4 hours, not to exceed 20 mg in 24 hours Children aged 2–12 : Oral solution (avoid tablets) 0.3–0.4 mg/kg/day in divided doses. Do not administer to children less than 2 years of age	Acute and chronic
Bismuth subsalicylate	Adults: 30 mL (regular strength) or 2 tablets, repeated every 30–60 minutes as needed. Maximum 8 doses daily Children: Consumers should speak with a physician before giving to children under 12 years of age	Traveler's and

Patient Encounter 2

KW, a 31-year-old day care teacher, complains of nausea, vomiting, abdominal cramps, and frequent watery stools for the past 2 days. She also indicates that her heart has been "beating faster" and her mouth has been dry. Although she looks ill, she does not have a fever. She does not have any current medical problems or drug therapy.

What is the likelihood that her diarrhea is due to an invasive microorganism?

Which of her symptoms suggest the presence of dehydration?

Discuss potential treatment measures for this woman.

produce lactase and digest the lactose before it reaches the colon. The *Lactobacillus acidophilus* in yogurt, cottage cheese, and acidophilus milk improve digestion of lactose and may prevent or relieve diarrhea related to lactose deficiency and milk intake. Although lactase is not a probiotic, lactase tablets may also be used to prevent diarrhea in susceptible patients.

▶ Anti-infectives

Empiric antibiotic therapy is an appropriate approach to traveler's diarrhea. Eradication of the causal microbe depends on the etiologic agent and its antibiotic sensitivity. Most cases of traveler's diarrhea and other community-acquired infections result from enterotoxigenic (ETEC) or enteropathogenic *Escherichia coli* (EPEC). Routine stool cultures do not identify these strains; primary empiric antibiotic choices include fluoroquinolones such as ciprofloxacin or levofloxacin. Azithromycin may be a feasible option when fluoroquinolone resistance is encountered.

Although most cases of infectious diarrhea resolve with therapy, routine antibiotic use may contribute to antimicrobial resistance. Empiric treatment should be considered for other acute infectious diarrhea including those caused by nonhospital-acquired invasive organisms such as Shiga toxin-producing *Escherichia coli* (STEC) O157, *Campylobacter*, *Salmonella*, and *Shigella* organisms producing moderate to severe fever, tenesmus, and bloody stools.[11]

OUTCOME EVALUATION

- Monitor the patient with diarrhea from the point of first contact until symptoms resolve, keeping in mind that most episodes are self-limiting.
- Question the patient to determine whether symptom resolution occurs within 48 to 72 hours in acute diarrhea.
- Monitor for the maintenance of hydration, particularly when symptoms continue for more than 48 hours. Look for increasing thirst, decreased urination, dark-colored urine, dry mucous membranes, and rapid heartbeat as suggestive of dehydration, especially when nausea and vomiting have been present.

Patient Care and Monitoring for Diarrhea

1. Assess the patient's symptoms to determine if patient-directed therapy is appropriate or whether the patient should be evaluated by a physician. Determine the type of symptoms, severity, frequency, and exacerbating factors. Remember to inquire about recent foreign travel.

2. Determine if the patient is dehydrated.

3. Determine whether the patient has a history of disease that might be associated with diarrhea.

4. Obtain a thorough current history of prescription, nonprescription, and dietary supplement use. Remember to review the current therapy as a potential cause of diarrhea.

5. Determine if any diarrhea treatments have been attempted, including home remedies.

6. Medical referral is advised if the patient is pregnant, breast-feeding, younger than 3 or older than 70 years of age, or suffers from multiple medical conditions.

7. If home care is recommended, provide clear instructions about how to proceed if symptoms do not improve or new symptoms emerge.

8. Discuss the importance of maintaining nutrition by modifying the diet to include low-residue meals (low-fiber meals).

9. Educate the patient about: (a) the causes of acute and chronic diarrhea, (b) the possible complications of diarrhea, (c) the goals of treatment for diarrhea, (d) the antidiarrheal medication used to manage acute or chronic diarrhea, and (e) if appropriate, the circumstances when antibiotics are used to treat diarrhea.

- Monitor for symptom control in patients with chronic diarrhea.
- When antibiotics are used, monitor for completion of the course of therapy.

IRRITABLE BOWEL SYNDROME

IBS is a disorder of the GI tract that interferes with the normal functions of the colon. At various points in the past, IBS has been referred to as mucous colitis, spastic colon, irritable colon, or nervous stomach. ❼ *IBS is generally described as a functional disorder rather than a disease per se. A functional disorder involves symptoms that cannot be attributed to a specific injury, infection, or other physical problem.* A functional disorder occurs because of altered physiologic processes rather than structural or biochemical defects and may be subject to nervous system influence.

IBS is associated with frequent fluctuation in symptoms, loss of productivity, and decreased quality of life. Although IBS has been referred to as functional bowel disease, true functional bowel disease may be more indicative of widespread GI involvement including (but not limited to) the colon.

EPIDEMIOLOGY AND ETIOLOGY

IBS is one of the most common disorders seen in primary care and the most common reason for referral to gastroenterologists. Although between 15% and 20% of Americans suffer from IBS, only about one-quarter of those affected seek medical attention. The associated costs to society are significant, and the recurrent nature of IBS contributes to these costs through missed workdays, inattention on the job, and high consumption of health services.[12]

In the United States, IBS affects women about twice as often as men. However, this may reflect a woman's tendency to seek medical care more often than a man's. IBS can occur at any age but is most common between 20 and 50 years; onset beyond age 60 is rare. However, prevalence for older adults is the same as for young persons. Prevalence is similar in Caucasians and African Americans but may be lower in people of Hispanic origin. A genetic link is unproven, but IBS seems more common in certain families.

There is a strong association between emotional distress and IBS. Psychosocial trauma (e.g., a history of abuse, recent death of a close relative or friend, or divorce) is more likely to be found in patients presenting with IBS than in the general population. An increased prevalence of psychiatric disorders such as anxiety, depression, personality disorders, and somatization (psychological distress expressed as physical symptoms) occurs among adult patients with IBS. Alcohol consumption and smoking have not been shown to be risk factors for developing IBS.[13]

Some people show first evidence of IBS after contracting gastroenteritis, which has led to speculation about whether infection heightens GI tract susceptibility. Women with IBS may have symptoms triggered by menstrual periods.

PATHOPHYSIOLOGY

Enteric nerves control intestinal smooth muscle action and are connected to the brain by the autonomic nervous system. IBS is thought to result from dysregulation of this "brain–gut axis." The enteric nervous system is composed of two ganglionated plexuses that control gut innervation: the submucous plexus (Meissner's plexus) and the myenteric plexus (Auerbach's plexus). The enteric nervous system and the CNS are interconnected and interdependent. A number of neurochemicals mediate their function, including serotonin (5-hydroxytryptamine or 5-HT), acetylcholine, substance P, and nitric oxide, among others.

Two 5-HT receptor subtypes, $5-HT_3$ and $5-HT_4$, are involved in gut motility, visceral sensitivity, and gut secretion. The $5-HT_3$ receptors slow colonic transit and increase fluid absorption, whereas $5-HT_4$ receptor stimulation results in accelerated colonic transit.

Although no single pathologic defect has been found to account for the pattern of exacerbations and remissions seen in IBS, CNS abnormalities, dysmotility, visceral hypersensitivity, and a number of other factors have been implicated.[14]

The passage of fluids into and out of the colon is regulated by epithelial cells. In IBS, the colonic lining (epithelium) appears to work properly. However, increased movement of the contents in the colon can overwhelm its absorptive capacity. Disturbed intestinal motility appears to be a central feature of IBS, which leads to altered stool consistency. Studies suggest that the colon of IBS sufferers is abnormally sensitive to normal stimuli.[15] This enhanced visceral sensitivity manifests as pain, especially related to gut distention.

IBS activity may be affected by the immune system. Some IBS patients have been found to have antibodies that may indicate food hypersensitivity that might be involved in symptom production.[16] Specifically, sensitivity has been demonstrated to common foods such as wheat, beef, pork, soy, and eggs.

CLINICAL PRESENTATION AND DIAGNOSIS

Diagnosis

❾ *The diagnosis of IBS is made by symptom-based criteria and the exclusion of organic disease.* IBS is diagnosed by obtaining a careful and thorough history to identify symptoms characteristic of the disorder. It is equally important to distinguish among IBS and conditions having similar symptoms. Patients should be questioned about the character of their stools. This should include questions about frequency, consistency, color, and size. Moreover, because of the functional nature of IBS, a patient may present with symptoms of upper GI problems such as gastroesophageal reflux disease or with excessive flatulence. Patients should also be questioned about diet to determine whether symptoms seem to occur in relationship to meals or specifically after consumption of certain dietary products.

Barium enema, sigmoidoscopy, or colonoscopy may be indicated in the presence of red flag symptoms (fever, weight loss, bleeding, and anemia, which may be accompanied by persistent severe pain), which often point to a potentially serious non-IBS problem. A barium enema may identify polyps, diverticulosis, tumors, or other abnormalities that might be responsible for the symptoms. In addition, exaggerated haustral contractions may be noted with barium enema. Such contractions impede stool movement and contribute to constipation. Flexible sigmoidoscopy can be performed to identify obstruction in the rectum and lower colon, whereas colonoscopy can evaluate the entire colon for organic disease.

Clinical Presentation of IBS

Symptoms

- Patients report a history of abdominal pain or discomfort that is relieved with defecation. Symptom onset is associated with change in frequency or appearance of stool. Some persons experience hard, dry stools whereas others experience loose or watery stools. Some stools may be small and pellet-like in appearance while others may be narrow and pencil-like.

- ❽ *Symptoms can typically be categorized as either IBS with diarrhea (IBS-D) or IBS with constipation (IBS-C). Patients with IBS-D usually report more than three loose or watery stools daily. Those with IBS-C usually have fewer than three bowel movements per week; stools are typically hard and lumpy and accompanied by straining. However, stool frequency may be normal in many cases. The Rome III diagnostic criteria (see Diagnosis) place more emphasis on stool form unlike Rome II, which emphasized frequency.*

- While many patients fit into one of these subtypes, some patients report alternating episodes of diarrhea and constipation (irritable bowel syndrome with constipation and diarrhea [IBS-M], where M represents mixed).

- Other common symptoms include: (a) feelings of incomplete evacuation, (b) abdominal fullness, (c) bloating, (d) flatulence, (e) passage of clear or white mucus with a stool, and (f) occasional fecal incontinence.

- Periods of normal stools and bowel function are punctuated by episodes of sudden symptoms.

- Symptoms are often exacerbated by stress.

- Left lower quadrant abdominal pain is often brought on or made worse by eating. Passage of stool or flatus may provide some relief.

- IBS-C can often be distinguished from functional constipation primarily by the presence of abdominal pain and discomfort. Although pain and discomfort may be present in some patients with functional constipation, it is an expected feature of IBS.

- Patients with IBS may experience comorbidities outside the GI tract such as fibromyalgia, sleep disturbances, headaches, dyspareunia, and temporomandibular joint syndrome.

Signs

- The physical examination is often normal in IBS.

- The patient may appear to be anxious.

- Palpation of the abdomen may reveal left lower quadrant tenderness, which may indicate a tender sigmoid colon.

- Abdominal distention may be present in some cases.

- The following "red flag" or alarm features are *not* associated with IBS and may indicate inflammatory bowel disease, cancer, or other disorders: fever, weight loss, bleeding, and anemia, which may be accompanied by persistent severe pain.

Laboratory Tests

- In most cases, laboratory testing reveals no abnormalities in IBS, but certain tests can be used to identify other causes for the patient's symptoms.

- CBC may identify anemia, which may suggest blood loss and an organic source for GI symptoms.

- Serum electrolytes and chemistries may indicate metabolic causes of symptoms.

- Thyroid-stimulating hormone (TSH) should be ordered when thyroid dysfunction is suspected. Hypothyroidism may be responsible for constipation and related symptoms.

- Stool testing for ova and parasites may identify *C. difficile* and amoebae as possible causes of diarrhea rather than IBS.

- Fecal leukocytes can be found in inflammatory diarrhea, especially when due to invasive microorganisms.

- A positive stool guaiac test indicating blood in the GI tract does not support a diagnosis of IBS.

- An elevated erythrocyte sedimentation rate is consistent with a systemic inflammatory process such as inflammatory bowel disease rather than IBS.

- Testing for lactase deficiency can confirm the presence of lactose intolerance, which may explain the symptoms.

IBS diagnosis has long been symptom based. Manning defined the first widely used practical criteria: (a) abdominal pain relieved by defecation with either (i) looser stools with pain onset, or (ii) frequent stools with pain onset; (b) abdominal distention; (c) mucus in the stool; and (d) sensation of incomplete evacuation.[17,18]

The Rome III criteria are the most current diagnostic criteria and can also be applied clinically.[19] They presume the absence of a structural or biochemical explanation for the symptoms. The Rome III criteria define IBS as occurring when symptoms of recurrent abdominal pain or discomfort exist for at least 3 days/month in the last 3 months associated with two or more of the following: (a) improvement with defecation, (b) onset associated with a change in the frequency of stool, and/ or (c) onset associated with a change in the form (appearance) of stool. These criteria should be fulfilled for the previous 3 months with symptom onset at least 6 months prior to diagnosis. IBS is unlikely if symptom onset occurs in old age, the disorder has a steady but aggressive course, or the patient experiences frequent awakening because of symptoms.

Patient Encounter 3, Part 1

A 38-year-old woman presents complaining of headache, abdominal pain, bloating, occasional nausea, and excessive belching. These symptoms have occurred with increasing frequency over the past 2 to 3 weeks. She has missed 2 days of work recently. The abdominal pain is crampy in character and located in the left lower abdominal area. She has also had alternating episodes of loose stools and hard dry stools and the presence of white thread-like material in her stool during some of the past 3 weeks. She reports no family history of GI problems.

Which of the patient's symptoms are characteristics of IBS?

How well does this woman fit the typical epidemiologic profile of patients with IBS?

TREATMENT

General Approach to Treatment

❿ *The principal goal of IBS treatment is to reduce or control symptoms.* The treatment strategy is based on: (a) the prevailing symptoms and their severity, (b) the degree of functional impairment, and (c) the presence of psychological components. A standard treatment regimen is not possible because of the heterogeneous nature of the IBS patient population. Patients suffering from IBS can benefit from clinician support and reassurance, because specific pathology is unlikely to be found.

Nonpharmacologic Therapy

▶ Diet and Other General Modifications

Dietary modification is a standard therapeutic modality. Food hypersensitivities and adverse effects are thought to occur widely in IBS patients, especially those with IBS with diarrhea subtype. Elimination diets are the most commonly used strategy, usually focusing on milk and dairy products, fructose and sorbitol, wheat, and beef. Flatulence may be controlled by reducing gas-causing foods such as beans, celery, onions, prunes, bananas, carrots, and raisins. Response to elimination diets varies widely, but they may be useful in individual patients. Care must be taken to avoid creating nutritional deficits while attempting to eliminate an offending food.

Probiotics may also be an option for some patients with IBS. *Bifidobacterium infantis* is one product used for its effect in constipation, diarrhea, gaseousness, bloating, and abdominal discomfort. Reportedly, it is not associated with significant untoward effects.[2] The usual dose is one 4-mg capsule daily.

▶ Psychological Treatments

Psychotherapy focused on reducing the influence of the CNS on the gut has been studied. Cognitive behavioral therapy (CBT), dynamic psychotherapy, relaxation therapy, and hypnotherapy have been reported to be effective in some patients. However, CBT and relaxation therapy do not appear to be better than standard approaches.[20] Biofeedback may provide relief in cases of severe constipation, but definitive evidence is lacking.[21,22] Psychotherapy interventions provide relief from pain and diarrhea but not from constipation.[23]

Pharmacologic Therapy

▶ Botanicals

Peppermint oil is widely advocated; it acts as an antispasmodic agent due to its ability to relax GI smooth muscle. However, it also relaxes the lower esophageal sphincter, which could allow reflux of gastric contents into the esophagus. The usual dose is 1 to 2 enteric-coated capsules containing 0.2 mL of peppermint oil two to three times daily.

Matricaria recutita, known as German chamomile, is also purported to have antispasmodic properties. It is taken most often as a tea up to four times a day. Benzodiazepine, alcohol, and warfarin users should be cautioned against taking this product because it can cause drowsiness, and it contains coumarin derivatives.[24]

▶ Antispasmodics

Antispasmodic agents such as dicyclomine or hyoscyamine have been among the most frequently used medications for treating abdominal pain in patients with IBS (Table 21–5). Side effects include blurred vision, constipation, urinary retention, and (rarely) psychosis. Although their effectiveness remains unconfirmed, these drugs may deserve a trial in patients with intermittent postprandial pain.[18]

▶ Antidepressants

Tricyclic antidepressants (TCAs) such as amitriptyline and doxepin have been used with some success in the treatment of IBS-related pain (Table 21–5). They modulate pain principally through their effect on neurotransmitter reuptake, especially norepinephrine and serotonin. Their helpfulness in functional GI disorders seems independent of mood-altering effects normally associated with these agents. Low-dose TCAs (e.g., amitriptyline, desipramine, or doxepin 10–25 mg daily) may help patients with IBS who predominantly experience diarrhea or pain.

The selective serotonin-reuptake inhibitors (SSRIs) paroxetine, fluoxetine, and sertraline are potentially useful due to the significant effect of serotonin in the gut. SSRIs principally act on $5\text{-}HT_1$ or $5\text{-}HT_2$ receptors, but they can also have some effect on gut-predominant $5\text{-}HT_3$ and $5\text{-}HT_4$ receptors, perhaps reducing visceral hypersensitivity. They may be beneficial for patients with IBS-C or when the patient presents with IBS complicated by a mood disorder.[24] SSRIs should be reserved for use when TCAs are not effective because evidence supporting their use solely in IBS is lacking.

Table 21–5

Common Pharmacologic Treatments for IBS

Generic (Brand) Name	Dose
Antispasmodics	
Dicyclomine (Bentyl)	10–20 mg po every 4–6 hours as needed
Hyoscyamine (Levsin)	0.125–0.25 po mg or sublingually every 4 hours as needed
Propantheline bromide (Pro-Banthine)	15 mg po 3 × a day (before meals) and 30 mg at bedtime
Clidinium bromide plus chlordiazepoxide HCl (Librax)	5–10 mg po 3–4 × a day
Hyoscyamine, scopolamine, atropine, phenobarbital (Donnatal)	1–2 tablets po 3–4 × daily
Tricyclic antidepressants (TCAs)	**In IBS With Diarrhea:**
Amitriptyline	50–150 mg po daily
Doxepin	10–150 mg po daily
Selective Serotonin-Reuptake Inhibitors	**In IBS With Constipation:**
Paroxetine (others can be used)	10–40 mg po daily
Bulk-Forming Laxatives	
Psyllium (Metamucil)	2.5–4 g po daily
Methylcellulose (Citrucel)	4–6 g po daily
Antimotility Agents	
Loperamide (Imodium A/D)	4 mg po; then 2 mg po after each loose stool; daily maximum 16 mg
5-HT$_3$ Receptor Antagonist	
Alosetron (Lotronex)[a]	1 mg po daily
5-HT$_4$ Receptor Agonist	
Tegaserod maleate (Zelnorm)[b]	6 mg po twice daily

[a]Withdrawn from general use; available only under special circumstances.

[b]Withdrawn from general use; available only as emergency treatment.

▶ Bulk Producers

Bulk producers may improve stool passage in IBS-C but are unlikely to have a favorable effect on pain or global IBS symptoms.[25] Psyllium may increase flatulence, which may worsen discomfort in some patients. Methylcellulose products are less likely to increase gas production. Although fiber-based supplements are more likely to be useful in IBS-C, these products may be dose-adjusted in diarrhea to increase stool consistency. Other laxative products might be used in IBS-C, but most are less desirable than bulking agents due to the potential for unwanted effects.

▶ Antimotility Agents

Loperamide stimulates enteric nervous system receptors, inhibiting peristalsis and fluid secretion. It improves stool consistency and reduces the number of stools.[25] Consequently, it is most useful in patients who have diarrhea as a prominent symptom. However, it can occasionally aggravate abdominal pain.

▶ Alosetron

Stimulation of 5-HT$_3$ receptors triggers hypersensitivity and hyperactivity of the large intestine. Alosetron (Lotronex) is a selective 5-HT$_3$ antagonist that blocks these receptors and is used to treat women with severe IBS-D. Eligible patients should have frequent and severe abdominal pain, frequent bowel urgency or incontinence, and restricted daily activities. Alosetron has been shown to improve overall symptoms and quality of life. Alosetron can cause constipation in some patients.

Because alosetron has been associated with ischemic colitis, it may be prescribed only under strict guidelines, including signing of a consent form by both patient and physician. Patients selected for therapy should exhibit severe chronic IBS symptoms and should have failed to respond to conventional therapy.

▶ Tegaserod Maleate

Tegaserod maleate (Zelnorm) stimulates 5-HT$_4$ receptors in the GI tract, thereby increasing intestinal secretion, peristalsis, and small bowel transit. It also reduces sensitivity related to abdominal distention. It has been shown to be more effective than placebo in improving global IBS symptoms and altered bowel habits in IBS-C.[25] However, because a higher risk of heart attack, stroke, and unstable angina (heart/chest pain) in patients treated with tegaserod maleate is suspected, the drug has been withdrawn from general use. The FDA can authorize use of tegaserod maleate for emergency situations only. The FDA must also authorize the drug to be shipped.

OUTCOME EVALUATION

- Because symptoms vary in intensity and among patients, a specific drug therapy may not lead to equivalent symptom abatement in different patients.

- Monitor for adequate relief of symptoms. Patients whose pain does not respond to drug therapy may have a psychological comorbid condition and may require psychiatric intervention.

- Specifically, monitor for relief of pain if present initially. Monitor patients with symptoms of constipation or diarrhea for frequency, appearance, and size of stools in relationship to their normal characteristics. As stools normalize, associated symptoms such as bloating and abdominal distention should resolve.

- For IBS-C patients taking bulk producers, monitor for relief of constipation. Hard stools should become softer within 72 hours. IBS-M patients may gain relief with these agents as well.

Patient Encounter 3, Part 2

Upon further questioning, the patient states that she had similar symptoms (often following menses) near the end of graduate school 6 years ago. The symptoms gradually subsided after graduation, so she did not seek medical attention. She is an accountant and recently received a promotion at work. As a result, she has taken on considerably more responsibility.

PMH: Anxiety; muscle contractions; headaches

FH: Mother has migraine headaches

SH: Nonsmoker; drinks a glass of wine occasionally

Meds: Naproxen 220 mg every 12 hours as needed for headaches and menstrual pain; loperamide 2 mg as needed for diarrhea

Allergies: No known drug allergies

PE:

Gen: Alert and oriented; well-developed and well-nourished, anxious black woman

VS: BP 137/88 mm Hg, P 80 bpm, RR 21 per minute, T 37.1°C (98.7°F), Ht 5'7" (170 cm), Wt 74 kg (173 lb)

Integ: Hair and nails unremarkable; scalp dry and flaky; skin otherwise unremarkable

HEENT: PERRLA, EOMI

Chest: Clear to A & P bilaterally

CV: RRR, normal S_1 and S_2; no S_3 or S_4

Abd: (+) BS, mildly tender LLQ

Rectal: No palpable masses; no hemorrhoids; stool negative for occult blood

What information is consistent with a diagnosis of IBS?

Outline an appropriate therapeutic plan for this patient.

- Monitor antidepressant therapy for relief of lower abdominal pain.
- Antispasmodics may provide limited relief of crampy abdominal pain.
- Assess 5-HT$_4$ receptor agonists (tegaserod) for relief of crampy abdominal pain and bloating.
- Evaluate 5-HT$_3$ receptor antagonists (alosetron) for relief of abdominal pain and fecal incontinence.
- Antimotility agents should be expected to reduce stool frequency and control diarrhea.
- Monitor complete blood cell count, serum electrolytes and chemistries, stool guaiac, and erythrocyte sedimentation rate yearly for changes that might signal an overlapping organic problem.
- Refer any patient presenting with red flag signs for medical evaluation.

Patient Care and Monitoring for IBS

1. Assess symptoms to determine if patient-directed therapy is appropriate or whether physician evaluation is needed.
2. Determine the type, severity, and frequency of symptoms and possible exacerbating factors.
3. Listen attentively to the patient's complaints and reassure the patient to allay fears about invasive disease.
4. Obtain a thorough current history of prescription, nonprescription, and dietary supplement use.
5. Determine if any IBS treatments have been attempted and how effective they have been.
6. Determine whether the patient has received educational intervention about IBS, health promotion, and symptom prevention measures.
7. Provide patient education about IBS symptoms, lifestyle modifications, and drug therapy for IBS:
   - Explain how to use medications relative to symptom intensity.
   - If taking alosetron, determine nonadherence with special use requirements.
   - Describe potential adverse effects.
   - List drugs that may interact with the therapy.
   - Discuss what to do if red flag symptoms occur.

Abbreviations Introduced in This Chapter

BSS	Bismuth subsalicylate
CBT	Cognitive behavioral therapy
EPEC	Enteropathogenic *Escherichia coli*
ETEC	Enterotoxigenic *E coli*
FGID	Functional gastrointestinal disorder
IBS	Irritable bowel syndrome
IBS-C	Irritable bowel syndrome with constipation
IBS-D	Irritable bowel syndrome with diarrhea
IBS-M	Irritable bowel syndrome with constipation and diarrhea (mixed)
ORS	Oral rehydration solution
TCA	Tricyclic antidepressant

Self-assessment questions and answers are available at *http://www.mhpharmacotherapy.com/pp.html.*

REFERENCES

1. Brandt L, Schoenfeld P, Prather C, et al. American College of Gastroenterology Functional Gastrointestinal Disorders Task Force.

An evidence based approach to the management of chronic constipation in North America. Am J Gastroenterol 2005;100:S1–S21.

2. Drossman DA. The functional gastrointestinal disorders and the Rome III process. Gastroenterology 2006;130:1377–1390.

3. Locke GR, Pemberton JH, Phillips SF. American Gastroenterological Association medical position statement on constipation. Gastroenterology 2000;119:1766–1778.

4. Irvine EJ, Ferrazzi S, Pare P. Health-related quality of life in functional GI disorders: Focus on constipation and resource utilization. Am J Gastroenterol 1998;97:1986–1993.

5. Sonnenberg A, Koch TR. Physician visits in the United States for constipation: 1958 to 1986. Dig Dis Sci 1989;34:606–611.

6. Drossman DA, Li Z, Andruzzi E, et al. US householder survey of functional gastrointestinal disorders: Prevalence, sociodemography, and health impact. Dig Dis Sci 1993;38:1569–1580.

7. Longstreth GF, Thompson WG, Chey WD. Functional bowel disorders. Gastroenterology 2006;130:1480–1491.

8. Lembo A, Camilleri M. Chronic constipation. N Engl J Med 2003;349:1360–1368.

9. Amitiza package insert. Bethesda, MD: Sucampo Pharmaceuticals, 2006.

10. Guerrant RL, Van Gilder T, Steiner TS, et al. Practice guidelines for the management of infectious diarrhea. Clin Infect Dis 2001;32:331–351.

11. King CK, Glass R, Bresee JS, et al. Managing acute gastroenteritis among children: Oral rehydration, maintenance, and nutritional therapy. Morbid Mortal Wkly Rep 2003;52(RR16):1–16.

12. Gore JI, Surawicz C. Severe acute diarrhea. Gastroenterol Clin North Am 2003;32:1249–1267.

13. Cash B, Sullivan S, Barghout V. Total costs of IBS: Employer and managed care perspective. Am J Manag Care 2005;11(Suppl):S7–S16.

14. Cremonini F, Talley NJ. Irritable bowel syndrome: Epidemiology, natural history, health care seeking, and emerging risk factors. Gastroenterol Clin North Am 2005;34:189–204.

15. Morgan T, Robson KM. Irritable bowel syndrome: Diagnosis is based on clinical criteria. Postgrad Med 2002;112(5):30–40.

16. Schwetz I, Bradesi S, Mayer EA. The pathophysiology of irritable bowel syndrome. Minerva Med 2004;95:418–426.

17. Atkinson W, Sheldon TA, Shaath N, et al. Food elimination based on IgG antibodies in irritable bowel syndrome: A randomised controlled trial. Gut 2004;53:1459–1464.

18. Fass R, Longstreth GF, Pimentel M, et al. Evidence- and consensus-based practice guidelines for the diagnosis of irritable bowel syndrome. Arch Intern Med 2001;161:2081–2088.

19. Talley NJ, Spiller R. Irritable bowel syndrome: A little understood organic bowel disease? Lancet 2002;359:555–564.

20. O'Mahony L, McCarthy J, Kelly P, et al. *Lactobacillus and Bifidobacterium* in irritable bowel syndrome: Symptom responses and relationship to cytokine profiles. Gastroenterology 2005;128:541–551.

21. Boyce PM, Talley NJ, Balaam B, et al. A randomized controlled trial of cognitive behavior therapy, relaxation training, and routine clinical care for the irritable bowel syndrome. Am J Gastroenterol 2003;98:2209–2218.

22. Mertz HR. Drug therapy: Irritable bowel syndrome. N Engl J Med 2003;349:2136–2146.

23. Miller LG. Herbal medicinals: Selected clinical considerations focusing on known or potential drug-herb interactions. Arch Intern Med 1998;158:2200–2211.

24. Schoenfeld P. Efficacy of current drug therapies in irritable bowel syndrome: What works and does not work. Gastroenterol Clin North Am 2005;34:319–335.

25. Jones MP, Dilley JB, Drossman D, Crowell MD. Brain–gut connections in functional GI disorders: Anatomic and physiologic relationships. Neurogastroent Motil 2006;18:91–103.

22 Portal Hypertension and Cirrhosis

Laurajo Ryan

LEARNING OBJECTIVES

Upon completion of the chapter, the reader will be able to:

1. Describe the epidemiology and social impact of portal hypertension and cirrhosis.
2. Explain the pathophysiology of cirrhosis and portal hypertension.
3. Outline the progression of liver damage from excessive alcohol intake.
4. Identify the signs and symptoms of liver disease in a given patient.
5. Describe the consequences associated with decreased hepatic function.
6. List the treatment goals for a patient with portal hypertension and its complications.
7. Evaluate patient history and physical exam findings to determine the etiology of cirrhosis.
8. Recommend a specific treatment regimen that includes lifestyle changes, pharmacologic therapy, and nonpharmacologic therapy.

KEY CONCEPTS

❶ Portal hypertension is the precipitating factor for the complications of cirrhotic liver disease: ascites, spontaneous bacterial peritonitis (SBP), variceal bleeding, and hepatic encephalopathy (HE). Lowering portal pressure can reduce the complications of cirrhosis and decrease morbidity and mortality.

❷ Chronic excessive ingestion of ethanol causes progressive liver damage because both ethanol and its metabolic products are direct hepatotoxins.

❸ Cirrhosis is irreversible; treatments are directed at limiting disease progression and minimizing complications.

❹ Nonselective β-blockers are first-line treatment for preventing variceal bleeding; they vasoconstrict the splanchnic bed through multiple mechanisms.

❺ The goals of treating ascites are to minimize acute discomfort, reequilibrate ascitic fluid, and prevent SBP. Treatment should modify the underlying disease pathology; without directed therapy, fluid will rapidly reaccumulate.

❻ Cirrhosis is a high aldosterone state; spironolactone is a direct aldosterone antagonist and a primary treatment for ascites.

❼ During acute variceal hemorrhage, it is crucial to control bleeding, prevent rebleeding, and avoid acute complications such as SBP.

❽ Long-term antibiotic prophylaxis for SBP decreases mortality in patients with a history of SBP or low-

protein ascites (ascitic fluid albumin less than 1 g/dL [10 g/L]).

❾ Lactulose is the foundation of pharmacologic therapy to prevent and treat HE. It binds ammonia in its ionic form in the gut and facilitates its excretion.

INTRODUCTION

Cirrhosis is the progressive replacement of normal hepatic cells with fibrous scar tissue. This scarring is accompanied by the loss of viable hepatocytes, which are the functional cells of the liver. ❶ *Progressive cirrhosis is irreversible and leads to* **portal hypertension**, *which is in turn responsible for many of the complications of advanced liver disease. These consequences include (but are not limited to)* **spontaneous bacterial peritonitis (SBP)**, **hepatic encephalopathy (HE)**, *and* **variceal bleeding.**[1]

EPIDEMIOLOGY AND ETIOLOGY

Cirrhosis is the result of long-term insult to the liver, so damage is typically not evident clinically until the fourth decade of life. Chronic liver disease and cirrhosis combined were the 12th leading cause of death in the United States in 2002. In patients between the ages of 25 and 64 years, damage from excessive alcohol use accounted for over one-half of the deaths.[2] Alcoholic liver disease and viral hepatitis C are the most common causes of cirrhosis in the United States, whereas hepatitis B accounts for the majority of cases worldwide.[3] Once cirrhosis is diagnosed, the disease progression is relentless, regardless of the initial insult to the liver.

Variations occur, but cirrhosis secondary to alcohol abuse typically develops after 10 or more years of daily ingestion of 80 g of ethyl alcohol; this is an average of 6 to 8 drinks per day (a drink is equivalent to 1 ounce [30 mL] of hard liquor, 4 ounces [120 mL] of wine, or a 12-ounce [360-mL] beer).[4] With equivalent alcohol intake, women usually develop cirrhosis more quickly than men do. Differences in the rate of alcohol metabolism may account for this gender disparity; women metabolize less alcohol in the GI tract; this allows delivery of higher levels of ethanol (which is directly hepatotoxic) to the liver.[5] Genetic factors also play a role in development of alcoholic liver disease; some persons will progress to cirrhosis with much less cumulative alcohol intake than that of a typical cirrhotic patient (either fewer drinks per day, or faster disease development), while others do not develop the disease with even more excessive intake.

Infection with one or more strains of viral hepatitis causes an acute inflammation of the liver, whereas chronic infection with hepatitis B or C can lead to cirrhosis. Hepatitis B and C are common in IV drug users and can also be transmitted through sexual contact, but many cases of hepatitis C are idiopathic.[6,7] See Chapter 24 (Viral Hepatitis) for a complete discussion of infectious hepatitis.

Approximately 30% of patients with cirrhosis experience variceal bleeding at some point during the course of the disease. Variceal bleeding carries a remarkably high mortality rate. Up to 55% of patients with advanced disease die from their first episode. Mortality correlates with disease severity; risk factors include poor liver function, large varices, and red signs (wales) on endoscopic examination.[8] More than two-thirds of patients who survive the first incidence of variceal bleeding experience a repeat episode.

Development of ascites in cirrhotic patients is a particularly ominous marker; 1-year mortality after initial presentation with ascites is approximately 50%.[9] In addition to the high mortality rate, cirrhosis carries an enormous economic and social burden from hospitalizations, lost wages, and decreased productivity, not to mention the emotional strain of the disease on both patients and families.

Determining the specific cause of cirrhosis requires examination of both physical presentation and a thorough past medical history. An accurate social history is particularly important because few factors in the physical and laboratory examination aid in determining disease etiology. Understanding the cause of a patient's cirrhosis is imperative because it can affect therapeutic options and treatment decisions, even though cirrhosis itself cannot be reversed.

PATHOPHYSIOLOGY

Portal Hypertension and Cirrhosis

The portal vein is the primary vessel leading into the liver; it receives the deoxygenated venous blood flow from the splanchnic bed (intestines, stomach, pancreas, and spleen) (Fig. 22–1). Portal flow accounts for approximately 75% of all the blood delivered to the liver. The hepatic artery provides the remaining 25% of the blood supply in the form of oxygenated blood from the abdominal aorta. Normal portal vein pressure is between 5 and 10 mm Hg; this level maintains blood flow to the liver at approximately 1 to 1.5 L/min. Portal hypertension occurs when the hepatic venous pressure gradient (the pressure difference between the portal vein and the inferior vena cava) exceeds 10 to 12 mm Hg.[10,11]

Portal hypertension is a consequence of increased resistance to blood flow through the portal vein. This is usually due to restructuring of intrahepatic tissue (sinusoidal damage) but may also be caused by presinusoidal damage such as portal vein occlusion from trauma, malignancy, or thrombosis. The third (and the least common) cause of portal hypertension is outflow obstruction of the hepatic vein. This latter damage is posthepatic, and normal liver structure is maintained. This chapter will focus on portal hypertension caused by intrahepatic damage from cirrhosis.

Sinusoidal damage from cirrhosis is the most common cause of portal hypertension. The sinusoids are porous vessels within the liver that surround radiating rows of hepatocytes, which are the basic functional cells of the liver (Fig. 22–2). Progressive destruction of hepatocytes and an increase in fibroblasts and connective tissue surrounding the hepatocytes culminate in cirrhosis. Fibrosis and regenerative

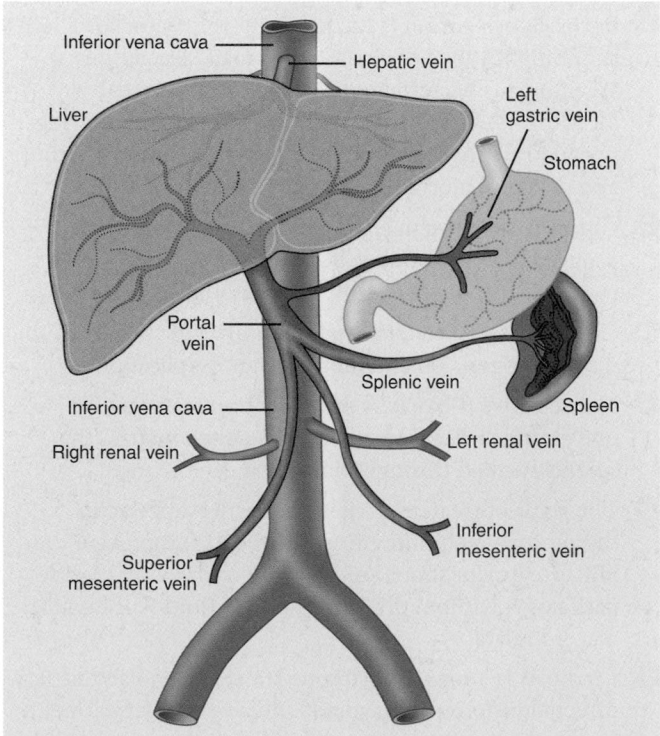

FIGURE 22–1. The portal venous system. (From Sease JM, Timm EJ, Stragand JJ. Portal hypertension and cirrhosis. In: DiPiro JT, Talbert RL, Yee GC, et al., eds. Pharmacotherapy: A Pathophysiologic Approach, 7th ed. New York: McGraw-Hill; 2008: 634, with permission.)

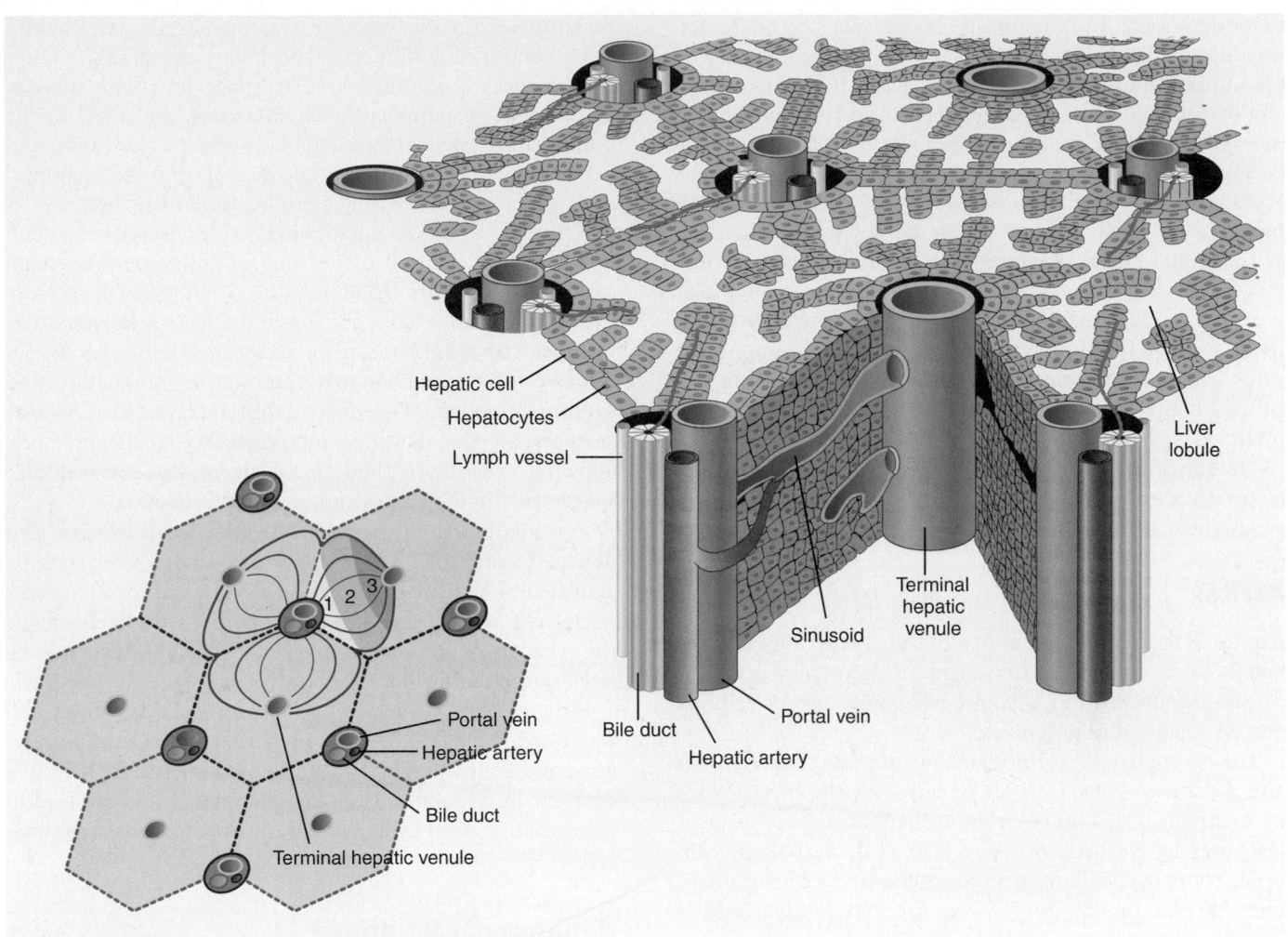

FIGURE 22–2. Relationship of sinusoids to hepatocytes and the venous system. (From Sease JM, Timm EJ, Stragand JJ. Portal hypertension and cirrhosis. In: DiPiro JT, Talbert RL, Yee GC, et al., eds. Pharmacotherapy: A Pathophysiologic Approach, 7th ed. New York: McGraw-Hill; 2008: 634, with permission.)

nodules of scar tissue modify the basic architecture of the liver, disrupting and reducing hepatic blood flow as well as normal liver function. Reduced hepatic blood flow alters the normal metabolic breakdown processes and decreases protein synthesis within the liver.

The sinusoids transport both portal and arterial blood to the hepatocytes. The systemic blood delivered to the liver contains nutrients, drugs, and ingested toxins. The liver processes nutrients (carbohydrates, proteins, lipids, vitamins, and minerals) for either immediate use or for storage, while drugs and toxins are broken down through a variety of metabolic processes. Changes in hepatic blood flow can significantly alter metabolism. Processing of drugs eliminated by first-pass metabolism is reduced, extending the half-life. In the case of prodrugs that are activated by the liver, the time to therapeutic effect is delayed. The liver also processes metabolic waste products for excretion. In cirrhosis, bilirubin (from the enzymatic breakdown of heme) can accumulate; this causes jaundice (yellowing of the skin), scleral icterus (yellowing of the sclera), and tea-colored urine (urinary bilirubin excretion).

Changes in steroid hormone production, as well as changes in the conversion and handling of steroids are also prominent features of cirrhosis. These changes can result in decreased libido, gynecomastia (development of breast tissue in men), testicular atrophy, and features of feminization in male patients. Another deleterious effect of changes in sex hormone metabolism is the development of spider angiomata (nevi). Spider angiomata are vascular lesions found mainly on the trunk. The lesion has a central arteriole (body) surrounded by radiating "legs." When blanched, the lesions fill from the center body outward toward the legs. Spider angiomata are not specific to cirrhosis, but the number and size do correlate with disease severity, and their presence relates to risk of variceal hemorrhage.[12]

Increased intrahepatic resistance to portal flow increases pressure on the entire splanchnic bed; an enlarged spleen (splenomegaly) is a common finding in cirrhotic patients. Splenic sequestration secondary to splenomegaly is one of the causes of thrombocytopenia in cirrhotic patients. Portal hypertension mediates systemic and splanchnic arterial vasodilation through production of nitric oxide and other vasodilators in an attempt to counteract the increased pressure gradient. Nitric oxide causes a fall in systemic arterial pressure; unfortunately, this activates both the renninangiotensin–aldosterone system (RAAS) and the sympathetic nervous system, as well as increasing antidiuretic hormone (vasopressin) production.[13] The activation of these systems is an attempt to maintain arterial blood pressure through increases in renal sodium and water retention. Increased systemic and portal pressure put increased pressure on the vascular system. As a consequence, the umbilical vein, which is usually eradicated in infancy, may become patent and increase blood flow to the abdominal veins. These prominent veins, which are visible on the surface of the abdomen, are called caput medusae because they resemble the head of the mythical Gorgon Medusa.

The aim of pharmacologic treatment in portal hypertension is to decrease portal pressure and reduce the effects of sympathetic activation.

Ascites

Ascites is the accumulation of fluid in the peritoneal space and is often one of the first signs of decompensated liver disease. Ascites is the most common complication of cirrhosis and portends a dire prognosis.[14]

The pathophysiologic mechanisms of portal hypertension and of cirrhosis itself are entwined with the mechanisms of ascites (Fig. 22–3). Cirrhotic changes and subsequent decreases in synthetic function lead to decreased albumin production (hypoalbuminemia). Albumin is the primary intravascular protein responsible for maintaining oncotic

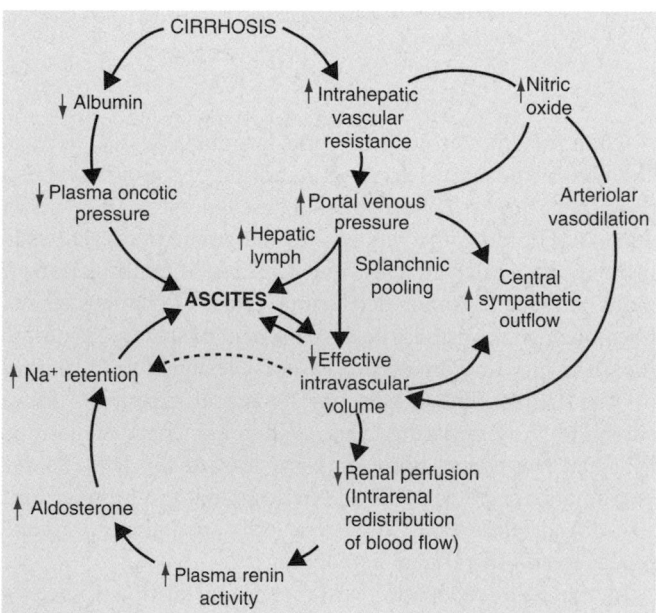

FIGURE 22–3. Factors involved in the development of ascites. (From Chung RT, Podolsky DK. Cirrhosis and its complications. In: Kasper DL, Braunwald E, Fauci AS, et al., eds. Harrison's Principles of Internal Medicine, 17th ed. New York: McGraw-Hill, 2005: 1858–1869, with permission.)

pressure within the vascular system; low serum albumin levels combined with increased capillary permeability allow fluid to leak from the vascular space into body tissues. This results in peripheral edema, ascites, and fluid in the pulmonary system. Obstruction of hepatic sinusoids and hepatic lymph nodes allows fluid to seep into the peritoneal cavity, further contributing to ascitic fluid formation.

As previously discussed, the nitric oxide released in reaction to portal hypertension dilates the systemic arterial system, causing a decrease in blood pressure. There is also a decrease in renal perfusion from the lowered effective intravascular volume. The kidney reacts by activating the RAAS, which increases plasma renin activity, aldosterone production, and sodium retention. This increase in intravascular volume furthers the imbalance of intravascular oncotic pressure, allowing even more fluid to escape to the extravascular spaces, furthering ascites and peripheral edema.

Vasodilation and decreased arterial pressure are also detected centrally. The sympathetic nervous system is activated to increase blood pressure, which in turn increases portal pressure. Unchecked, these combined effects enable the cycle of portal pressure and ascites to continue, creating a self-perpetuating loop of ascites formation.

Most patients with large ascites also retain sodium and water avidly, partially due to activation of antidiuretic hormone. Patients may become hyponatremic if there is a decrease in free water excretion. Untreated, this can lead to a decrease in renal function and the hepatorenal syndrome (HRS).[4,13]

Hepatorenal Syndrome

Type 1 HRS is characterized by rapid deterioration of renal function in the presence of decompensated cirrhosis. HRS is not reversible with volume repletion and is rapidly fatal, with a 50% mortality rate at 14 days if left untreated. Renal artery vasoconstriction (stimulated by activation of the sympathetic nervous system) and decreased mean arterial pressure (mediated by nitric oxide) combine to decrease renal perfusion and precipitate renal failure in patients with cirrhosis. The kidneys attempt to counteract this drop in renal perfusion by activating the RAAS. Production of renin stimulates a cascade that causes fluid retention and peripheral vasoconstriction in an attempt to increase blood flow to the kidneys. Production of prostaglandin E_2 and prostacyclin are increased to stimulate renal vasodilation. HRS develops when these mechanisms are overwhelmed and renal perfusion drops acutely. SBP is often implicated as a trigger for HRS, and nonsteroidal anti-inflammatory drugs (NSAIDs) can precipitate HRS by inhibiting prostaglandins.

Varices

The splanchnic system drains venous blood from the GI tract to the liver. In portal hypertension, there is increased resistance to drainage from the originating organ so collateral vessels (varices) develop in the esophagus, stomach, and rectum to compensate for the increased blood volume. Varices divert blood meant for hepatic circulation back to the systemic circulation; this has the unintended deleterious effect of decreasing clearance of medications and potential toxins through loss of first-pass metabolism. Varices are weak superficial vessels, so any additional increase in pressure can cause these vessels to rupture and bleed.[15]

Spontaneous Bacterial Peritonitis

SBP is an acute bacterial infection of peritoneal (ascitic) fluid in the absence of intra-abdominal infection or intestinal perforation. Estimates of the prevalence of SBP in patients with ascites range from 10% to 30%.[16] The peritoneal cavity is usually a sterile space. One proposed mechanism of bacterial contamination is translocation of intestinal bacteria into the peritoneal cavity, which then seeds the ascitic fluid.[17] Bacterial translocation correlates with the delay in intestinal transit time and increased intestinal wall permeability observed in cirrhotic patients. Another possible mechanism is the hematogenous spread of bacteria into the peritoneal space.[18]

Enteric gram-negative aerobes are the most common bacteria isolated from ascitic fluid, usually *Escherichia coli* or *Klebsiella pneumoniae*. *Streptococcus pneumoniae* is the most common gram-positive pathogen associated with SBP.[19] Once a bacterial pathogen has been identified, the antibiotic spectrum can be narrowed; SBP is rarely polymicrobial.

Hepatic Encephalopathy

Decreased cognition, confusion, and changes in behavior combined with physical signs such as asterixis (characteristic flapping of hands upon extension of arms with wrist flexion) indicate HE. To objectively stage the degree of impairment, the patient should be assessed in five distinct categories:

1. Level of consciousness
2. Cognition (e.g., attention, memory, and disorientation)
3. Behavior (e.g., mood, anger, and paranoia)
4. Motor function (e.g., coordination, reflexes, and asterixis)
5. Response to psychometric tests

Changes in mental status may be acute and therefore possibly reversible. Identifiable triggers can often be detected and reversed in acute HE. Changes may also be of a more chronic, insidious nature. Patients rarely recover from chronic HE.

Numerous factors, many of them poorly understood, are involved in the development of HE. In severe hepatic disease, systemic circulation bypasses the liver, so many of the substances normally metabolized by the liver remain in the systemic circulation and accumulate to toxic levels. In excess, these metabolic byproducts, especially nitrogenous waste, cause alterations in CNS functioning.[20]

Ammonia (NH_3) is just one of the toxins implicated in HE. It is a metabolic byproduct of protein catabolism and is also generated by bacteria in the GI tract. In a normally functioning liver, hepatocytes take up ammonia and degrade it to form urea, which is later renally excreted. In patients with cirrhosis, this conversion to urea is retarded and ammonia accumulates, resulting in encephalopathy. The decrease in urea formation is manifest on laboratory assessment as decreased blood urea nitrogen (BUN), but BUN levels do not correlate with degree of HE. Patients with HE commonly have elevated serum ammonia concentrations, but again, the levels do not correlate well with the degree of CNS impairment.[20]

False neurotransmitters resulting from increased levels of aromatic amino acids, γ-aminobutyric acid and endogenous benzodiazepines have also been implicated in HE. These substances bind to both the γ-aminobutyric acid and benzodiazepine receptors and act as agonists at the active receptor sites.[20]

Patients with previously stable cirrhosis who develop acute encephalopathy often have an identifiable precipitating event that can account for the increased production and/or decreased elimination of these toxins. Infections, variceal hemorrhage, renal insufficiency, electrolyte abnormalities, and increased dietary protein have all been associated with acute development of HE.

Bleeding Diathesis and Synthetic Failure

Coagulopathies signal end-stage liver disease. The liver manufactures coagulation factors essential for blood clotting and maintenance of blood homeostasis. With advanced disease, the liver is unable to synthesize these proteins, resulting in extended clotting times (e.g., prothrombin time) and bleeding irregularities.[21] Thrombocytopenia is another coagulation abnormality seen in advanced liver disease. This is a result of decreased platelet production in the bone marrow (triggered by a lack of thrombopoietin stimulation by the liver) as well as the splenic sequestration of formed platelets. Macrocytic anemia may also occur because of decreased intake, metabolism, and storage of folate and vitamin B_{12}. In individuals who continue to drink, blood abnormalities are also aggravated further because ethanol is toxic to bone marrow.

Alcoholic Liver Disease

The course of alcoholic liver disease moves through several distinct phases from development of fatty liver to the development of alcoholic hepatitis and cirrhosis. Fatty liver and alcoholic hepatitis may be reversible with cessation of alcohol intake, but cirrhosis itself is irreversible. Although the scarring of cirrhosis is permanent, maintaining abstinence from alcohol can still decrease complications and slow progression to end-stage liver disease.[22] Continuing to imbibe ethanol speeds the advancement of liver dysfunction and its complications.

Metabolism of ethanol begins even prior to absorption, as alcohol dehydrogenase (ADH) within the gastric mucosa oxidizes a portion of ingested alcohol to acetaldehyde. The remaining alcohol is rapidly absorbed from the GI tract, and since it is highly lipid soluble, it enters the body tissues quite easily. ❷ *ADH oxidizes ethanol in body tissues, primarily the liver, producing hypoxic damage.*[23] High levels of ethanol saturate the ADH enzyme system; when the ADH system is overwhelmed, the microsomal ethanol oxidizing system must take over the detoxification process. The microsomal ethanol oxidizing system is an inducible cytochrome P-450 (CYP 450) enzyme system; it participates in phase 1 metabolism and also produces acetaldehyde as its end product.[24,25] Acetaldehyde exerts direct toxic effects on the liver by damaging hepatocytes, inducing fibrosis, and by directly coupling to proteins, interfering with their intended actions. Metabolism of large amounts of ethanol shifts hepatic metabolic processes away from oxidation and toward reduction. These changes in metabolism account for the fatty liver, hypertriglyceridemia, and acidemia observed in alcoholic liver disease.

Less Common Causes of Cirrhosis

Genetics and metabolic risk factors mediate other less common causes of cirrhosis. These diseases vary widely in prevalence, disease progression, and treatment options.

Primary biliary cirrhosis is characterized by progressive inflammatory destruction of the bile ducts. This immune-mediated inflammation of the intrahepatic bile ducts results in remodeling and scarring, causing retention of bile within the liver and subsequent hepatocellular damage and cirrhosis. The number of patients affected with primary biliary cirrhosis is difficult to estimate because many people are asymptomatic; it is often diagnosed incidentally during a routine health care visit.

Nonalcoholic fatty liver disease (NAFLD) begins with asymptomatic fatty liver but may progress to cirrhosis. NAFLD is a disease of exclusion; elimination of any possible viral, genetic, or environmental causes must be made prior to making this diagnosis. NAFLD is directly related to numerous metabolic abnormalities. Risk factors include diabetes mellitus, dyslipidemia, obesity, and other conditions associated with increased hepatic fat.[26]

Hereditary hemochromatosis is an autosomal recessive disease of increased intestinal iron absorption and deposition in hepatic, cardiac, and pancreatic tissue. Hepatic iron overload results in the development of fibrosis, hepatic scarring, cirrhosis, and hepatocellular carcinoma. Hemochromatosis can also be caused by repeated blood transfusions, but this mechanism rarely leads to cirrhosis.

Wilson's disease is another autosomal recessive disease that leads to cirrhosis through protein abnormalities. The protein that is responsible for facilitating copper excretion in the bile is faulty, so copper accumulates in hepatic tissue. High copper levels within hepatocytes are toxic, and fibrosis and cirrhosis may develop in untreated patients. Those with Wilson's disease usually present with symptoms of liver and/or neurologic disease while still in their teens.

A third autosomal recessive genetic disease is α_1-antitrypsin deficiency. Abnormalities in the α_1-antitrypsin protein impair its secretion from the liver. α_1-Antitrypsin deficiency causes cirrhosis in children as well as adults; adults usually have concomitant pulmonary disease such as chronic obstructive pulmonary disease.

CLINICAL PRESENTATION AND DIAGNOSIS

Diagnosis of Cirrhosis

In some cases, cirrhosis is diagnosed incidentally before the patient develops symptoms or acute complications. Other patients may have decompensated cirrhosis at initial presentation; they may present with variceal bleeding, ascites, SBP, or HE. At diagnosis, patients may have some, all, or none of the laboratory abnormalities and/or signs and symptoms that are associated with cirrhosis.[28]

Ultrasound examination is used routinely to evaluate cirrhosis; a small, nodular liver with increased echogenicity is consistent with cirrhosis. Liver biopsy is the only way to diagnose cirrhosis definitively, but this is often deferred in lieu of a presumptive diagnosis. Because it is an invasive

---

Clinical Presentation of Cirrhosis and Complications of Portal Hypertension

General

- Most signs and symptoms that bring a patient to the attention of medical personnel are specific to the complication the patient is experiencing at that time. The signs and symptoms vary with severity and suddenness of onset.

Symptoms

- Patients with cirrhosis may exhibit nonspecific symptoms such as fatigue and weakness but may be asymptomatic until acute complications develop.

- Nonspecific symptoms include anorexia, fatigue, and changes in libido and sleep patterns. Patients may also experience easy bruising and may bleed from minor injuries. Pruritus may be present, particularly with biliary involvement.

- Patients with ascites may complain of abdominal pain, nausea, increasing tightness and fullness in the abdomen, shortness of breath and early satiety.

- Hemorrhage from esophageal or gastric varices may be associated with melena, pallor, fatigue, and weakness from blood loss. Patients often present with nausea, vomiting, and hematemesis because blood in the GI tract

Continued

Clinical Presentation of Cirrhosis and Complications of Portal Hypertension (*Continued*)

is nauseating. Bleeding from rectal varices may present as hematochezia.

- In patients with bleeding varices, digestion of swallowed blood represents a high protein load; this causes nausea and can precipitate symptoms of HE.

- In patients with HE, neurologic changes can be overwhelming or so subtle that they are not clinically apparent except during a targeted clinical evaluation.

- Patients with HE may complain of disruption of sleep patterns and day-to-night inversion; patients have delayed to-bed and wake times, which may progress to complete inversion of the normal diurnal cycle.

- If SBP occurs, symptoms of infection may include fever, chills, abdominal pain, and mental status changes.

Signs

- Nonspecific signs on physical exam include jaundice, scleral icterus, tea-colored urine, bruising, hepatomegaly, splenomegaly, spider angiomata, caput medusae, palmar erythema, gynecomastia, and testicular atrophy.

- Ascites can be detected by increased abdominal girth accompanied by shifting dullness and a fluid wave.

- Signs of variceal bleeding depend on the degree of blood loss and abruptness of onset. Rapid and massive blood loss is more likely to result in hemodynamic instability than is slow, steady bleeding. Signs of acute bleeding may include pallor, hypotension, tachycardia, mental status changes, and hematemesis.

- Markers of hepatic encephalopathy (HE) include decreased cognition, confusion, changes in behavior, and asterixis.

- Patients with SBP may present with fever, painful tympanic abdomen, and changes in mental status.

- Decreases in clotting factors may manifest as abnormal bruising and bleeding.

- Dupuytren contracture is a contraction of the palmar fascia that usually affects the fourth and fifth digits.[27] It is not specific to cirrhosis and can also be seen in repetitive use injuries.

Laboratory Abnormalities

- Hepatocellular damage manifests as elevated serum aminotransferases (alanine aminotransferase [ALT] and aspartate aminotransferase [AST]). The degree of transaminase elevation does not correlate with the remaining functional metabolic capacity of the liver. An AST level two-fold higher than ALT is suggestive of alcoholic liver damage.

- Elevated alkaline phosphatase is nonspecific and may correlate with liver or bone disease; it tends to be elevated in biliary tract disease.

- γ-Glutamyl transferase (GGT) is specific to the bile ducts, and in conjunction with an elevated alkaline phosphatase, suggests hepatic disease. Extremely elevated GGT levels further indicate obstructive biliary disease. GGT is also elevated in those who drink three or more alcoholic drinks daily.

- Increased total, direct, and indirect bilirubin concentrations indicate defects in transport, conjugation, or excretion of bilirubin.

- Lactate dehydrogenase (LDH) is a nonspecific marker of hepatocyte damage; disproportionate elevation of LDH indicates ischemic injury.

- Thrombocytopenia may occur because of decreased platelet production and splenic platelet sequestration.

- Anemia (decreased hemoglobin and hematocrit) occurs as a result of variceal bleeding, decreased erythrocyte production, and hypersplenism.

- Elevated prothrombin time (PT) and international normalized ratio (INR) are coagulation derangements that indicate loss of synthetic capacity in the liver and correlate with functional loss of hepatocytes.

- Decreased serum albumin and total protein occur in chronic liver damage due to loss of synthetic capacity within the liver.

- The serum albumin-to-ascites gradient is 1.1 g/dL (11 g/L) or greater caused by portal hypertension.

- Increased blood ammonia concentration is characteristic of HE, but levels do not correlate well with the degree of impairment.

- Increased serum creatinine signaling a decline in renal function may be seen with hepatorenal syndrome.

- Signs and symptoms of SBP in a patient with cirrhosis and ascites should prompt a diagnostic paracentesis (Fig. 22–5). In SBP, there is decreased total serum protein, elevated white blood cell count (with left shift), and the ascitic fluid contains at least $250/mm^3$ (250×10^6/L) neutrophils. Bacterial culture of ascitic fluid may be positive, but lack of growth does not exclude the diagnosis.

procedure, the decision to perform a biopsy is based on the expected clinical utility of the biopsy results. If the results have the potential to change the course of treatment, it may be advisable to perform a biopsy. The modified Child-Pugh and Model for End-Stage Liver Disease (MELD) classifi- cation systems (Table 22–1) are used to classify disease severity and evaluate the need for transplantation.

Patients with ascites or known varices must be assumed to have portal hypertension and are treated as such, even if direct measurements of portal pressure have not been made.[29]

TABLE 22–1

Child-Pugh and MELD Classifications for Determining Severity of Liver Damage

Child-Pugh Classification[a]

Variable	1 Point	2 Points	3 Points
Bilirubin (mg/dL) (μmol/L)	Less than 2 Less than 34	2–3 34–51	Greater than 3 Greater than 51
Albumin (g/dL) (g/L)	Greater than 3.5 Greater than 35	2.8–3.5 28–35	Less than 2.8 Less than 28
Prothrombin time (seconds prolonged) or	1–3	4–6	Greater than 6
INR	Less than 1.8	1.8–2.3	Greater than 2.3
Ascites Encephalopathy	None None	Slight Stages 1–2	Moderate Stages 3–4

MELD Classification

The formula for the MELD score is $3.8 \times \mathrm{Ln}$ (bilirubin [mg/dL]) + $11.2 \times \mathrm{Ln}(\mathrm{INR}) + 9.6 \times \mathrm{Ln}$(creatinine [mg/dL]) + $6.4 \times$ (etiology: 0 if cholestatic or alcoholic, 1 otherwise)

Using SI units, the MELD score is $3.8 \times \mathrm{Ln}$(bilirubin [μmol/L] / 17.1) + $11.2 \times \mathrm{Ln}(\mathrm{INR}) + 9.6 \times \mathrm{Ln}$(creatinine [μmol/L] /88.4) + $6.4 \times$ (etiology: 0 if cholestatic or alcoholic, 1 otherwise)

INR, International Normalized Ratio; MELD, Model for End-Stage Liver Disease; Ln, natural logarithm.

[a]Class A: 1 to 6 total points; B: 7 to 9 points; C: 10 to 15 points.

From Lucey MR, Brown KA, Everson GT, et al. Minimal criteria for placement of adults on the liver transplant waiting list: A report of a national conference organized by the American Society of Transplant Physicians and the American Association for the Study of Liver Diseases. Liver Transpl Surg 1997;3:628–637; and Kamath PS, Wiesner RH, Malinchoc M, et al. A model to predict survival in patients with end-stage liver disease. Hepatology 2001;33:464–470.

Diagnosis of Ascites

In obese patients or those with only small amounts of fluid accumulation, ultrasound evaluation may be necessary to detect ascites with certainty. Analysis of ascitic fluid obtained during paracentesis provides diagnostic clues to the etiology of the ascites. Diagnostic evaluation should include cell count with differential, albumin, total protein, Gram stain, and bacterial cultures. In patients without an established diagnosis of liver disease, the serum ascites–albumin gradient (SAAG) is sensitive in determining if the ascites is caused by portal hypertension.[22] SAAG compares the serum albumin concentration to the ascitic fluid albumin concentration:

$$\mathrm{Alb}_{serum} - \mathrm{Alb}_{ascites} = \mathrm{SAAG}$$

A value of 1.1 g/dL or greater (11 g/L or greater) identifies portal hypertension as the cause of the ascites with 97% accuracy.[22,30] In portal hypertension, the ascitic fluid is low in albumin; this balances the oncotic pressure gradient with the hydrostatic pressure gradient of portal hypertension. The differential diagnoses for SAAG values less than 1.1 g/dL (less than 11 g/L) include peritoneal carcinoma, peritoneal

infection (tuberculosis, fungal, or cytomegalovirus), and nephrotic syndrome. Serum albumin measurements should be made at the same time ascitic fluid is obtained for an accurate comparison.[22]

TREATMENT OF CIRRHOSIS, PORTAL HYPERTENSION, AND COMPLICATIONS

Desired Outcomes

Recognizing and treating the cause of cirrhosis is paramount. ❸ *Cirrhosis is irreversible; treatments are directed at limiting disease progression and minimizing complications.* The immediate treatment goals are to stabilize acute complications such as variceal bleeding and prevent SBP. Once life-threatening conditions have stabilized, the focus shifts to preventing complications and preventing further liver damage. Complication prevention involves both primary and secondary prophylaxis. To determine appropriate prophylactic therapy, a careful analysis of patient characteristics and disease history is mandatory. The sections that follow concentrate on treatment and prevention of cirrhotic complications.

Nonpharmacologic Therapy

Lifestyle modifications can limit disease complications and slow further liver damage. Avoidance of additional hepatic insult is critical for successful cirrhosis treatment. The only proven treatment for alcoholic liver disease is the immediate cessation of alcohol consumption. Patients who have cirrhosis from etiologies other than alcoholic liver disease should also abstain from alcohol consumption to prevent further liver damage.

All patients with ascites require counseling on dietary sodium restriction. Salt intake should be limited to less than 800 mg sodium (2 g sodium chloride) per day. More stringent restriction may cause faster mobilization of ascitic fluid, but adherence to such strict limits is very difficult. Ascites usually responds well to sodium restriction accompanied by diuretic therapy.[14,22,31,32] The goal of therapy is to achieve urinary sodium excretion of at least 78 mEq (78 mmol) per day.[22] While a 24-hour urine collection will provide this information, a spot urine sodium:potassium ratio greater than 1 provides the same information and is much less cumbersome to perform.

Medication use must be monitored carefully for potential hepatotoxicity. Hepatically metabolized medications have the potential to accumulate in patients with liver disease. Little guidance is available on drug dosing in hepatic impairment because these patients have historically been excluded from drug trials. Daily acetaminophen use should not exceed 2 g. Dietary supplements, herbal remedies, and nutraceuticals have not been well studied in hepatic impairment and cannot be recommended.

In patients with variceal bleeding, nasogastric (NG) suction reduces the risk of aspirating stomach contents. Aspiration pneumonia is a major cause of death in patients with variceal bleeding. NG suction is also helpful in decreasing vomiting

Patient Encounter, Part 1

ES is a 44-year-old Hispanic man who presents to the emergency department with complaints of abdominal pain and fatigue.

Chief complaint: "My belly feels tight"

HPI: Increasing feelings of fullness and abdominal tightness that have become noticeable over the past 2 weeks, accompanied by nausea and decreased food intake, but without vomiting

PMH: Hypertension × 15 years, acute pancreatitis × 2 episodes

PSH: No surgeries

SH: Married, currently separated; denies tobacco and illicit drug use; for the past 20 years typically drinks a 12-pack of beer daily and several shots of tequila; use has recently increased due to depression over marital separation

FH: Father with cirrhosis, died at age 45 from coronary disease; mother alive at age 62 with type 2 diabetes mellitus, hypertension, hyperlipidemia, and gastroesophageal reflux disease

Outpatient Meds: Chlorthalidone 25 mg daily

ROS: (+) Anorexia and nausea; denies vomiting, constipation, or diarrhea; patient reports moderate shortness of breath and dyspnea on exertion

PE

VS: BP 125/75 mm Hg, P 84 bpm, T 37.3°C (99.1°F), RR 18/min, oxygen saturation 98% on room air

HEENT: PERRL, EOMI, (+) sclera icterus

CV: RRR, no murmurs, rubs, or gallops

Chest: CTA bilaterally, no crackles or wheezes

Abd: Tense, distended abdomen that is tender to palpation, decreased bowel sounds, (+) hepatosplenomegaly

Ext: 2+ pedal pulses, 2+ pitting edema

What are this patient's risk factors for liver disease?

Identify features of his presentation that are consistent with cirrhosis.

---

during acute episodes of variceal bleeding.[33,34] Blood within the GI tract is very nauseating; removal of the blood can decrease vomiting.

Endoscopic band ligation and sclerotherapy are both means to stop acutely bleeding varices. Endoscopic band ligation is the application of a stricture around the varix, whereas sclerotherapy involves injecting the varix with substances designed to decrease blood flow to the area and prevent rebleeding. Endoscopic band ligation has replaced sclerotherapy as the preferred endoscopic treatment and is effective in stopping acute variceal bleeding in up to 90% of patients.[35] It is the standard of care for secondary prophylaxis of repeat bleeding in patients with a history of either esophageal or gastric variceal bleeding. Endoscopic band ligation is best used in conjunction with pharmacologic treatment.[36–38]

Balloon tamponade involves the application of direct pressure to the area of bleeding with an inflatable balloon attached to an NG tube. It is an option for patients in whom drug therapy and band ligation fail to stop variceal bleeding. Balloon tamponade is used only when other methods have failed. Once the direct pressure of the balloon is removed, rebleeding often occurs, so balloon tamponade is only a temporary measure prior to more definitive treatment such as shunting.[11]

During episodes of acute HE, temporary protein restriction to decrease ammonia production can be a useful adjuvant to pharmacologic therapy. Long-term protein restriction in cirrhotic patients is not recommended. Cirrhotic patients are already in a nutritionally deficient state, and prolonged protein restriction will exacerbate the problem.[20]

Vaccination against hepatitis A and B is recommended in patients with underlying cirrhosis to prevent additional liver damage from an acute viral infection.[39] Pneumococcal and influenza vaccination may also be appropriate and can reduce hospitalizations due to influenza or pneumonia.

Shunts are long-term solutions to decrease elevated portal pressure. Shunts divert blood flow either through or around the diseased liver, depending on the location and type of shunt employed. Transjugular intrahepatic portosystemic shunts (TIPS) create a communication pathway between the intrahepatic portal vein and the hepatic vein. TIPS procedures have an advantage over surgically inserted shunts because they are placed through the vascular system rather than through a more invasive surgical procedure, but they still carry a risk of bleeding and infection. TIPS placement is associated with an improvement in HRS but an increased incidence of HE.[40] HE associated with TIPS placement results from decreased detoxification of nitrogenous waste products because the shunt allows blood to evade metabolic processing.

Pharmacologic Therapy

Drug therapy targeted to reduce portal hypertension and cirrhosis can alleviate symptoms and prevent complications but cannot reverse cirrhosis. Drug therapy is available to treat the complications of ascites, varices, SBP, HE, HRS, and coagulation abnormalities.

▶ Portal Hypertension

4 *Nonselective β-blockers such as propranolol and nadolol are first-line treatments to reduce portal hypertension. They* reduce bleeding and decrease mortality in patients with known varices. Use of β-blockers for primary prevention of variceal formation is controversial.

Only nonselective β-blockers reduce bleeding complications in patients with known varices. Blockade of β_1 receptors reduces cardiac output and splanchnic blood flow. β_2-Adrenergic blockade prevents β_2-receptor–mediated splanchnic vasodilation while allowing unopposed α-adrenergic effects; this enhances vasoconstriction of both the systemic and splanchnic vascular beds. The combination of β_1 and β_2 effects makes the nonselective β-blockers preferable to cardioselective agents in treating portal hypertension.[1,35,41] Cardioselective β-blockers do lose their cardioselectivity at higher doses, but most patients with cirrhosis cannot tolerate the high doses.

Because β-blockers decrease blood pressure and heart rate, they should be started at low doses to increase tolerability. Propranolol is hepatically metabolized, and its half-life and pharmacologic effects are prolonged in portal hypertension. A reasonable starting dose of propranolol is 10 mg two to three times daily.

Doses should be titrated as tolerated with the goal of decreasing heart rate by 25% or to approximately 55 to 60 bpm.[11,35] Heart rate is not an accurate marker for portal pressure reduction, but it is the acknowledged surrogate marker for effectiveness because there are no other acceptable alternatives.

Nitrates have been suggested in patients who do not achieve therapeutic goals (heart rate reduction) with β-blocker therapy alone. Trials to evaluate the effects of nitrates (e.g., isosorbide mononitrate) on portal pressure, both alone and in combination with β-blockers, show enhanced reduction of portal pressure; however, there is an increase in mortality when nitrates are used alone. Adverse effects are significantly higher in patients treated with the combination of nonselective β-blockers and nitrates as opposed to β-blocker monotherapy.[42,43] The current evidence only supports use of the combination to prevent rebleeding, not for primary prophylaxis. Unfortunately, β-blockers either alone or in combination may be intolerable for many patients with cirrhosis.

▶ Ascites

⑤ *The goals of treating ascites are to minimize acute discomfort, reequilibrate ascitic fluid, and prevent SBP. Treatment should modify the underlying disease pathology; without directed therapy, fluid will rapidly reaccumulate.*

In the case of tense ascites, relief of acute discomfort may be accomplished by therapeutic paracentesis. Often the removal of just 1 to 2 L of ascitic fluid provides relief from pain and fullness. When removing 5 L or more of fluid at one time, volume resuscitation with 8 to 10 g of albumin given IV should be provided for each liter of fluid removed. Large-volume paracentesis without albumin administration is a known precipitant of HRS, secondary to decreased perfusion. If less than 5 L of fluid is removed in a hemodynamically stable patient, albumin use is not warranted.[22]

▶ Diuretics

Diuretics are often required in addition to sodium restriction (see Nonpharmacologic Therapy). **⑥** *Spironolactone and*

Patient Encounter, Part 2

In the emergency department, a chest x-ray was normal. The following laboratory test results were obtained:

Sodium 128 mEq/L (mmol/L)	Platelets $118 \times 10^3/mm^3$ ($\times 10^9$/L)
Potassium 3.1 mEq/L (mmol/L)	Albumin 2.7 g/dL (27 g/L)
Chloride 106 mEq/L (mmol/L)	Total bilirubin 2.3 mg/dL (39.3 μmol/L)
Bicarbonate 24 mEq/L (mmol/L)	Alk phos 177 IU/L (2.95 μKat/L)
BUN 10 mg/dL (3.57 mmol/L)	AST 443 IU/L (7.38 μKat/L)
Scr 1.1 mg/dL (97 μmol/L)	ALT 206 IU/L (3.43 μKat/L)
Glucose 145 mg/dL (8.0 mmol/L)	INR 1.6
Hemoglobin 12.5 g/dL (125 g/L or 7.75 mmol/L)	GGT 185 IU/L (3.1 μKat/L)
Hematocrit 38% (0.38)	LDH 203 IU/L (3.38 μKat/L)
WBC $7.4 \times 10^3/mm^3$ ($\times 10^9$/L)	PT 29 seconds

Which of these values are consistent with the diagnosis of cirrhosis?

What (if anything) in the current presentation implies the underlying cause of the disease?

Which of the laboratory results are suggestive of complications related to cirrhosis?

ALT, alanine aminotransferase; AST, aspartate aminotransferase; GGT, γ-glutamyl transferase; INR, International Normalized Ratio; IU, international units; LDH, lactate dehydrogenase; PT, prothrombin time.

furosemide form the basis of pharmacologic therapy for ascites. Spironolactone is an aldosterone antagonist and counteracts the effects of activation of the RAAS. In hepatic disease, not only is aldosterone production increased, but the half-life is prolonged because of decreased hepatic metabolism. Spironolactone also acts to conserve the potassium that would otherwise be excreted because of elevated aldosterone levels.

Spironolactone is usually used in combination with a loop diuretic (e.g., furosemide) for more potent diuresis. A ratio of 40 mg furosemide (the most commonly used loop diuretic) to each 100 mg spironolactone can usually maintain serum potassium concentrations within the normal range. Therapy is commonly initiated with oral spironolactone 100 mg and furosemide 40 mg/day.

Doses should be titrated at intervals no more frequent than every 2 to 3 days. Because spironolactone is used for its antialdosterone effects, much higher doses (up to 400 mg/day) are needed than those used when treating hypertension. If intolerable side effects such as gynecomastia occur with spironolactone, other potassium-sparing diuretics may be used, but clinical trials have not shown equivalent efficacy.[22]

The target in treating ascites is to cause a fluid loss of approximately 0.5 L/day.[22] Because ascites equilibrates with vascular fluid at a much slower rate than does peripheral edema, aggressive diuresis is associated with intravascular volume depletion and should be avoided unless patients have concomitant peripheral edema. Patients with peripheral edema in addition to ascites may require increasing furosemide doses until euvolemia is achieved; IV diuretics are often necessary.[22] Diuretic therapy in cirrhosis is typically lifelong.

▶ Varices

Unfortunately, variceal bleeding is common in cirrhotic patients; it accounts for between 10% and 30% of all cases of upper GI hemorrhage. ❼ *During acute variceal hemorrhage, it is crucial to control bleeding, prevent rebleeding, and avoid acute complications such as SBP; mortality from first bleeding episode is up to 55%, and patients must be treated aggressively.* A treatment algorithm for acute variceal bleeding is depicted in Figure 22–4.

▶ Octreotide

Octreotide is a synthetic analogue of somatostatin; it causes selective vasoconstriction of the splanchnic bed, decreasing portal venous pressure with few serious side effects. Vasopressin has also been used to achieve this effect, but since vasopressin causes nonselective vasoconstriction, it carries the risk of systemic consequences, which limits its usefulness.

The recommended octreotide dose is a 50- to 100-mcg IV loading dose followed by a continuous IV infusion of 25 to 50 mcg/hour. Therapy should continue for at least 24 to 72 hours after bleeding has stopped. Some clinicians continue octreotide for a full 5 days since this is the time frame during which the risk of rebleeding is highest. Octreotide combined with endoscopic therapy results in decreased rebleeding rates and transfusion needs when compared to endoscopic treatment alone.[35]

▶ Spontaneous Bacterial Peritonitis

Initiation of prophylactic antibiotic therapy to prevent SBP is recommended during acute variceal bleeding; this is typically initiated with a fluoroquinolone (e.g., ciprofloxacin 500 mg twice daily for 7 days) or an IV third-generation cephalosporin. Some institutions would not use a fluoroquinolone antibiotic in patients who have been on long-term prophylactic therapy with that class of drugs. Prophylactic antibiotic therapy reduces in-hospital infections and mortality in patients hospitalized for variceal bleeding.[44]

If the presence of SBP is suspected, empiric antibiotic therapy with a broad-spectrum anti-infective agent should be initiated after ascitic fluid collection, pending cultures and susceptibilities (Fig. 22–5).[45,46] In the setting of presumed infection, delaying treatment while awaiting laboratory confirmation is inappropriate and may result in death. The initial antibiotic should be an IV third-generation cephalosporin (e.g., cefotaxime 2 g every 8 hours, ceftriaxone 1 g every 24 hours), an IV extended-spectrum penicillin (e.g., piperacillin–tazobactam 3.375 g every 6 hours or 4.5 g every 8 hours), or a fluoroquinolone (e.g., ciprofloxacin 400 mg IV every 12 hours), because these agents cover the most common gram-negative and gram-positive agents implicated in SBP. Third-generation cephalosporins are usually recommended as first-line therapy. Fluoroquinolones may be used if resistant (extended-spectrum β-lactamase positive) organisms are suspected based on local susceptibility patterns or patient history. Once an infectious agent has been identified, antibiotic coverage can be narrowed to an agent that is highly active against that particular organism.

SBP has been identified as a cause of HRS. The risk of renal failure is lessened with IV albumin therapy, dosed at 1.5 g/kg of body weight initially, followed by 1 g/kg of body weight on day 3 of SBP therapy.[47]

Patient Encounter, Part 3

ES is found to have ascites. Therapeutic paracentesis is ordered to relieve shortness of breath and abdominal pain; 4 L of ascitic fluid is removed.

What are the goals for treating ascites in this patient?

What lifestyle modifications should the patient make that may decrease his risk of hospitalization and death from cirrhosis?

What pharmacologic options are available to treat ascites in this patient?

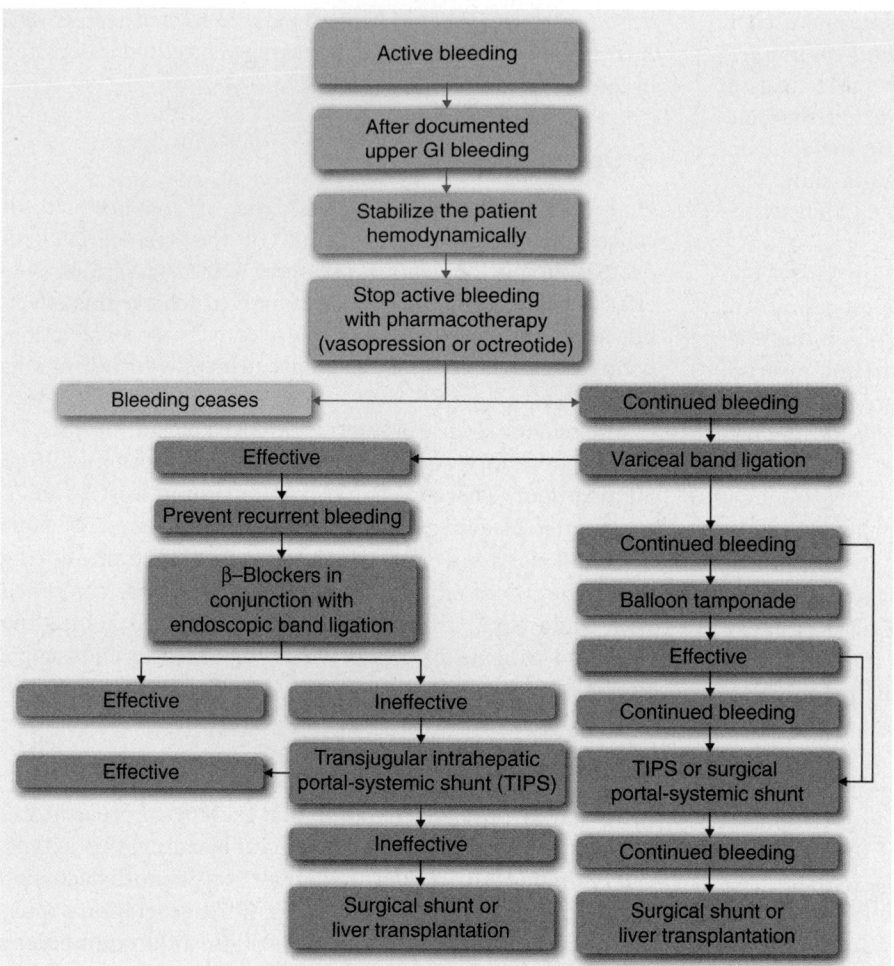

FIGURE 22–4. Treatment algorithm for active GI bleeding resulting from portal hypertension. (Adapted from Schiano TD, Bodenheimer HC. Complications of chronic liver disease. In: Friedman SL, McQuaid KR, Grendell JH, eds. Current Diagnosis and Treatment in Gastroenterology, 2nd ed. New York: McGraw-Hill, 2003, p. 649, with permission).

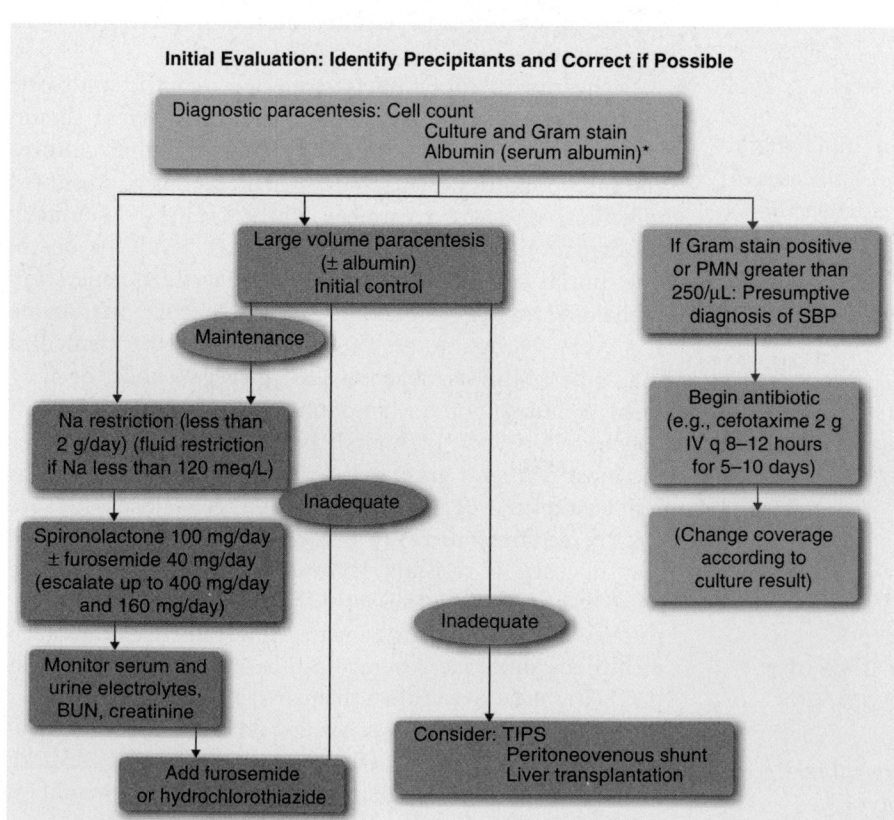

FIGURE 22–5. Approach to the patient with ascites and spontaneous bacterial peritonitis (SBP). (BUN, blood urea nitrogen; Na, sodium; PMN polymorphonuclear leukocyte; TIPS, transjugular intrahepatic portosystemic shunt.) (From Chung RT, Podolsky DK. Cirrhosis and its complications. In: Kasper DL, Braunwald E, Fauci AS, et al., eds. Harrison's Principles of Internal Medicine, 17th ed. New York: McGraw-Hill, 2005: 1858–1869, with permission.)
*If PMN is greater than 250/μL but culture is negative (culture-negative neutrocytic ascites) begin empiric antibiotics and retap after 48 hours. If culture is positive but PMN less than 250/μL, treat as if PMN greater than 250/μL (presumed SBP). If polymicrobial infection exists, exclude SBP.

Patient Encounter, Part 4

ES is brought to the emergency department by ambulance 2 months after the initial presentation.

Chief Complaint: "I've been vomiting black stuff and I'm really tired."

HPI: Hematemesis for the past 2 days, worsening today and accompanied by profound weakness; patient is continuing to drink alcohol at the same rate as he was at his first visit.

Outpatient Meds: Spironolactone 100 mg daily; furosemide 40 mg daily

ROS: (+) Nausea, coffee-ground emesis, and melena; denies constipation or diarrhea; (+) bilateral lower extremity edema

PE:

VS: BP 98/60 mm Hg, P 122 bpm, T 37.1°C (98.8°F), RR 21/min, oxygen saturation 91% on room air

CV: Tachycardia; no murmurs, rubs, or gallops

Chest: CTA bilaterally

Abd: Mildly distended, tender to deep palpation, decreased bowel sounds, (+) hepatosplenomegaly and fecal occult blood test

Ext: Decreased pedal pulses, 3+ pitting edema

What are the immediate treatment goals for ES? How will these goals be achieved?

Does this presentation warrant prophylaxis to prevent further disease complications? If so, what therapy is appropriate for this patient?

❽ *Patients who have previously experienced SBP and those with low-protein ascites (ascitic fluid albumin less than 1 g/dL [less than 10 g/L]) are candidates for long-term prophylactic antibiotic therapy.* Recommended regimens include either a single trimethoprim–sulfamethoxazole double-strength tablet 5 days per week (Monday through Friday) or ciprofloxacin 750 mg once weekly.[19,46]

▶ Encephalopathy

Lactulose **❾** *Lactulose is the foundation of pharmacologic therapy to prevent and treat HE. It is a nondigestible synthetic disaccharide laxative that is hydrolyzed in the gut to an osmotically active compound that draws water into the colon and stimulates defecation. Lactulose lowers colonic pH, which favors the conversion of ammonia (NH_3) to ammonium (NH_4^+).*[48] *Ammonium is ionic and cannot cross back into systemic circulation; it is eliminated in the feces.* Lactulose is usually initiated at 15 to 30 mL two to three times per day

and titrated to a therapeutic goal of two to four soft bowel movements daily.[20,49,50]

Antibiotic Therapy Prior to the introduction of lactulose, neomycin was the only treatment available for HE. Neomycin exerts its antibiotic action in the gut, thereby eliminating urease-producing bacteria. Elimination of these organisms decreases ammonia production. Although neomycin is classified as a nonabsorbable antibiotic, patients with cirrhosis have been shown to have detectable plasma concentrations. This is thought to be due to decreased integrity of the intestinal mucosa and may lead to nephrotoxicity. Neomycin is given orally in doses of 3 to 6 g daily.

Rifaximin is another nonabsorbable antibiotic that is used extensively in Europe as first-line therapy for HE. Rifaximin therapy has been shown to be both efficacious and well tolerated, but the expense in the United States (where it is not licensed for HE) may be prohibitive for long-term use. Rifaximin given at the typical dose of 1,200 mg/day costs approximately tenfold more than lactulose.

Flumazenil Evidence for the false transmitter theory as the cause of encephalopathy is demonstrated by the fact that administration of flumazenil (a benzodiazepine antagonist) has resulted in functional improvement. Unfortunately, long-term benefit has not been shown, and since flumazenil can only be administered parenterally, it is not an appropriate choice for clinical use. Its use is limited to the research setting.

▶ Hepatorenal Syndrome

HRS is a life-threatening complication of cirrhosis. Targeted treatment increases volume within the central venous system. Peripheral vasoconstriction redistributes fluid from the periphery to the venous system, and the fluid is contained thereby increases in oncotic pressure from albumin administration. The ultimate goal is to increase renal perfusion.

A common regimen involves administration of albumin 1 g/kg on day one, followed by 20 to 40 g on subsequent treatment days. This regimen is used in combination with midodrine (an α-agonist) and octreotide. Midodrine is typically initiated at 7.5 mg three times daily, and octreotide is administered subcutaneously (as opposed to IV during variceal bleeding) 100 mcg three times daily. Both of these regimens can be titrated as tolerated to achieve increases in mean arterial pressure of 15 mm Hg or greater.

Terlipressin, a vasopressin analog available in Europe, has been used with success in patients with HRS, but it is not currently available in the United States.

▶ Coagulation Abnormalities

Vitamin K is essential for the production of coagulation factors within the liver. Elevated clotting times from decreased protein synthesis are indistinguishable from those produced by low vitamin K levels resulting from malnutrition or poor

Patient Encounter, Part 5

During the hospital stay, ES had endoscopic band ligation to treat esophageal and gastric varices. Propranolol 20 mg three times a day was initiated; IV furosemide 60 mg twice daily resolved the pedal edema. Prescriptions for spironolactone 200 mg daily and furosemide 40 mg twice daily were provided at discharge. Three weeks later, ES is brought to clinic by his daughter who states that he is confused and "hasn't been himself." She is unsure if he has been taking his medication but says he continues to drink and has been eating poorly. Patient will only speak to staff in Spanish.

What are the presenting signs and symptoms of hepatic encephalopathy (HE)?

What factors could contribute to HE in this patient?

What is the prognosis for this patient who has developed ascites, variceal bleeding, and HE within 3 months?

Patient Care and Monitoring

1. Obtain a complete history of alcohol intake and hepatotoxic drug use, including over-the-counter products and dietary supplements.

2. At each encounter, ask the patient specific questions about adherence to prescribed therapy, dietary restrictions and cessation of alcohol intake.

3. At each visit, evaluate the pharmacotherapy regimen for appropriate drug choice and dose, nonprescription drug use, adverse effects, and use of potentially hepatotoxic medications.

4. Question the patient about adverse effects, since hepatically metabolized medications may accumulate and cause adverse effects.

5. Consider antibiotic prophylaxis for SBP in patients with low-protein ascites or prior SBP.

6. Conduct a review of systems and physical examination at each visit to determine if the patient has had progression of complications.

7. Ask specific questions about bleeding, bruising, and fatigue. There is a direct link between loss of synthetic function and disease progression.

8. Refer the patient to substance abuse counseling for education about alcohol cessation if appropriate.

9. Provide education regarding dietary sodium restriction at each visit; consider referral to a dietician if appropriate.

intestinal absorption. Vitamin K_1 (phytonadione) 10 mg given subcutaneously daily for 3 days can help to establish whether the prolonged bleeding time results from loss of synthetic function in the liver or vitamin K deficiency. It is unusual to completely reverse clotting abnormalities, but most patients experience a decrease in international normalized ratio (INR), conferring a decreased risk of bleeding.

OUTCOME EVALUATION

- Reevaluate the pharmacotherapy regimen at each visit to assess adherence, effectiveness, adverse events, and need for drug titration.

- Determine adherence to lifestyle changes such as cessation of ethanol intake and avoidance of over-the-counter medications (particularly NSAIDs) and herbal remedies that may exacerbate complications of cirrhosis.

- Assess the effectiveness of β-blocker therapy by measuring heart rate. Heart rate reduction of 25% from baseline or to 55 to 60 bpm is desirable. Ask the patient specific, directed questions regarding adverse effects of β-blockers; inquire about symptoms of orthostatic hypotension (e.g., lightheadedness, dizziness, or fainting).

- Evaluate effectiveness of diuretic therapy with regard to ascitic fluid accumulation and development of peripheral edema. Ask the patient directed questions about abdominal girth, fullness, tenderness, and pain. Weigh the patient at each visit, and ask the patient to keep a weight diary. Assess for peripheral edema at each visit.

- Assess dietary sodium intake by patient food recall. Objectively measure dietary sodium adherence using spot urine sodium-to-potassium ratio. Assess for appropriate sodium excretion.

- Obtain complete blood count and prothrombin time (PT)/INR to assess for anemia, thrombocytopenia, or coagulopathy. Ask about increases in bruising, bleeding, or development of hematemesis, hematochezia, or melena to assess for bleeding.

- Review biopsy reports and laboratory data. Transaminases and blood ammonia levels do not correlate well with disease progression, but increased coagulation times are markers of loss of synthetic function.

- Evaluate for signs and symptoms of HE. Mental status changes may be subtle; questioning family members or caregivers about confusion or personality changes may reveal mild HE even if the patient is unaware of the deficits.

- In patients taking lactulose therapy, titrate the dose to achieve two to four soft bowel movements daily.

Abbreviations Introduced in This Chapter

ADH	Alcohol dehydrogenase
ALT	Alanine aminotransferase
AST	Aspartate aminotransferase

BUN	Blood urea nitrogen
CYP450	Cytochrome P-450 isoenzyme
GGT	γ-Glutamyl transpeptidase
HE	Hepatic encephalopathy
HRS	Hepatorenal syndrome
INR	International normalized ratio
LDH	Lactate dehydrogenase
MELD	Model for End-Stage Liver Disease
NAFLD	Nonalcoholic fatty liver disease
NG	Nasogastric
NH_3	Ammonia
NH_4^+	Ammonium
NSAID	Nonsteroidal anti-inflammatory drug
PT	Prothrombin time
RAAS	Renin–angiotensin–aldosterone system
SAAG	Serum–ascites albumin gradient
SBP	Spontaneous bacterial peritonitis
TIPS	Transjugular intrahepatic portosystemic shunt

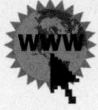 Self-assessment questions and answers are available at *http://www.mhpharmacotherapy.com/pp.html.*

REFERENCES

1. Lubel JS, Angus PW. Modern management of portal hypertension. Int Med J 2005;35:45–49.
2. Anderson RN, Smith BL. Deaths: Leading causes for 2002. Natl Vital Stat Rep 2005;53:17.
3. National Digestive Diseases Information Clearinghouse. Cirrhosis of the liver. NIH Publication No. 04-1134. Bethesda, MD: Author; 2003(December).
4. Lelbach WK. Cirrhosis in the alcoholic and its relation to the volume of alcohol abuse. Ann N Y Acad Sci 1975;252:85–105.
5. Frezza M, DiPadova C, Pozzato G, et al. High blood alcohol levels in women. The role of decreased alcohol dehydrogenase activity and first pass metabolism. N Engl J Med 1990;322:95–99.
6. Alter MJ, Hadler SC, Margolis HS, et al. The changing epidemiology of hepatitis B in the United States. Need for alternative vaccination strategies. JAMA 1990;263:1218–1222.
7. Alter MJ, Gerety RJ, Smallwood LA, et al. Sporadic non-A, non-B hepatitis: Frequency and epidemiology in an urban U.S. population. J Infect Dis 1982;145:886–893.
8. The North Italian Endoscopic Club for the Study and Treatment of Esophageal Varices. Prediction of the first variceal hemorrhage in patients with cirrhosis of the liver and esophageal varices. A prospective multicenter study. N Engl J Med 1988;319:983–989.
9. Krige JEJ, Beckingham IJ. ABC of diseases of liver, pancreas, and biliary system: Portal hypertension 2: Ascites, encephalopathy, and other conditions. BMJ 2001;322:416–418.
10. Krige JEJ, Beckingham IJ. ABC of diseases of liver, pancreas, and biliary system: Portal hypertension 1: Varices. BMJ 2001;322:348–351.
11. DeFranchis R. Updating consensus in portal hypertension: Report of the Baveno III workshop on definitions, methodology and therapeutic strategies in portal hypertension. J Hepatol 2000;33:846–852.
12. Zaman A, Hapke R, Flora K, et al. Factors predicting the presence of esophageal or gastric varices in patient with advanced liver disease. Am J Gastroenterol 1999;94:3292–3296.
13. Martin PY, Gines P, Schrier RW. Nitric oxide as a mediator of hemodynamic abnormalities of sodium and water retention in cirrhosis. N Engl J Med 1998;339:533–541.
14. Gines P, Cardena A, Arroyo V, Rodes J. Management of cirrhosis and ascites. N Engl J Med 2004;350:1646–1654.
15. Sarin SK, Lahoti D, Saxena SP, et al. Prevalence, classification and natural history of gastric varices: A long-term follow-up study in 568 portal hypertension patients. Hepatology 1992;16:1343–1349.
16. Rimola A, Garcia-Tsao G, Navasa M, et al. Diagnosis, treatment and prophylaxis of spontaneous bacterial peritonitis: A consensus document. J Hepatol 2000;32:142–145.
17. Guarner C, Runyon BA. Spontaneous bacterial peritonitis: Pathogenesis, diagnosis, and management. Gastroenterology 1995;3:311–328.
18. Such J, Frances R, Munoz C, et al. Detection and identification of bacterial DNA in patients with cirrhosis and culture-negative, nonneutrocytic ascites. Hepatology 2002;36:135–141.
19. Rimola A, Garcia-Tsao G, Navasa M, et al. Diagnosis, treatment and prophylaxis of spontaneous bacterial peritonitis: A consensus document. J Hepatol 2000;32:142–153.
20. Blei AT, Cordoba J. The Practice Parameters Committee of the American College of Gastroenterology. Hepatic encephalopathy practice guidelines. Am J Gastroenterol 2001;96:1968–1976.
21. Robert A, Chazouilleres O. Prothrombin time in liver failure: Time, ratio, activity percentage, or international normalized ratio. Hepatology 1996;24:1392–1394.
22. Runyon BA. American Association for the Study of Liver Diseases (AASLD) practice guideline: Management of adult patients with ascites due to cirrhosis. Hepatology 2004;39:841–856.
23. Lieber CS. Biochemical and molecular basis of alcohol-induced injury to liver and other tissues. N Engl J Med 1988;319:1639–1650.
24. Tsutsumi M, Lasker JM, Shimuzu M, et al. The intralobular distribution of ethanol inducible P450IIE1 in rat and human liver. Hepatology 1989;10:437–446.
25. Tsutsumi M, Lasker JM, Takahashi T, Lieber CS. In vivo induction of hepatic P4502E1 by ethanol: Role of increased enzyme synthesis. Arch Biochem Biophys 1993;304(1):209–218.
26. Chitturi S, Abeygunasekera S, Farrell GC, et al. NASH and insulin resistance: Insulin hypersecretion and specific association with the insulin resistance syndrome. Hepatology 2002;35:373–379.
27. Attali P, Ink O, Pelletier G, et al. Dupuytren's contracture, alcohol consumption, and chronic liver disease. Arch Intern Med 1987;147:1065–1067.
28. Bravo A, Sheth S, Chopra S. Liver biopsy. N Engl J Med 2001;344:495–500.
29. Garcia-Tsao G, Groszmann RJ, Fisher RL, et al. Portal pressure, presence of gastroesophageal varices and variceal bleeding. Hepatology 1985;5:419–424.
30. Runyon BA, Montano A, Akrivadis E, et al. The serum ascites albumin gradient is superior to the exudate-transudate concept in the differential diagnosis of ascites. Ann Intern Med 1992;117:215–220.
31. Runyon BA. Care of patients with ascites. N Engl J Med 1994;330:337–342.
32. Runyon BA. Management of adult patients with ascites caused by cirrhosis. Hepatology 1998;27:264–272.
33. D'Amico G, Morabito A, Pagliaro L. Six week prognostic indicators in upper gastrointestinal hemorrhage in cirrhotics. Front Gastrointest Res 1986;9:247.
34. Garden OJ, Motyl H, Gilmour WH, et al. Prediction of outcome following acute variceal haemorrhage. Br J Surg 1985;72:91–95.
35. Sharara AI, Rockey DC. Gastroesophageal variceal hemorrhage. N Engl J Med 2001;345:669–681.
36. Grace ND, American College of Gastroenterology Practice Parameters Committee. Diagnosis and treatment of gastrointestinal bleeding secondary to portal hypertension. Am J Gastroenterol 1997;92:1081–1091.
37. Lo GH, Lai KH, Cheng JS, et al. Endoscopic variceal ligation plus nadolol and sucralfate compared with ligation alone for the prevention of variceal rebleeding: A prospective, randomized trial. Hepatology 2000;32:461–465.

38. De La Pena J, Brullet E, Sanchez-Hernandez E, et al. Variceal ligation plus nadolol compared with ligation for prophylaxis of variceal rebleeding: A multicenter trial. Hepatology 2005;41:572–578.

39. Centers for Disease Control and Prevention. Sexually transmitted diseases treatment guidelines 2002. MMWR Recomm Rep; 2002(May 10);51(RR-6):1–78.

40. Boyer TD, Haskal ZJ. American Association for the Study of Liver Diseases (AASLD) practice guideline: The role of transjugular intrahepatic portosystemic shunt in the management of portal hypertension. Hepatology 2005;41:386–401.

41. Pagliaro L, D'Amico G, Sorensen TI, et al. Prevention of first bleeding in cirrhosis. A meta-analysis of randomized trials of nonsurgical treatment. Ann Intern Med 1992;117:59–70.

42. Merkel C, Sacerdoti D, Bolognesi M, et al. Hemodynamic evaluation of the addition of isosorbide-5-mononitrate to nadolol in cirrhotic patients with insufficient response to the beta-blocker alone. Hepatology 1997;26:34–39.

43. Gournay J, Masliah C, Martin T, et al. Isosorbide mononitrate and propranolol compared with propranolol alone for the prevention of variceal rebleeding. Hepatology 2000;6:1239–1245.

44. Soares-Weiser K, Brezis M, Tur-Kaspa R, Leibovici L. Antibiotic prophylaxis for cirrhotic patients with gastrointestinal bleeding. Cochrane Database Syst Rev 2002;(2):CD002907.

45. Such J, Runyon BA. Spontaneous bacterial peritonitis. Clin Infect Dis 1998;27:669–674.

46. Soares-Weiser K, Brezis M, Tur-Kaspa R, et al. Antibiotic prophylaxis of bacterial infections in cirrhotic inpatients: A meta-analysis of randomized controlled trials. Scand J Gastroenterol 2003;38:193–200.

47. Sort P, Navasa M, Arroyo V, et al. Effect of intravenous albumin on renal impairment and mortality in patients with cirrhosis and spontaneous bacterial peritonitis. N Engl J Med 1999;341:403–409.

48. Pasricha PJ. Treatment of disorders of bowel motility and water flux; antiemetics; agents used in biliary and pancreatic disease. In: Brunton LL, LAZO JS, Parker KL, eds. Goodman & Gilman's the Pharmacologic Basis of Therapeutics, 11th ed. New York: McGraw-Hill, 2005:1335–1358.

49. Mortensen PB. The effect of oral-administered lactulose on colonic nitrogen metabolism and excretion. Hepatology 1992;16:1350–1356.

50. Mortensen PB, Holtug K, Bonnen H, Clausen MR. The degradation of amino acids, proteins, and blood to short-chain fatty acids in colon is prevented by lactulose. Gastroenterology 1990;98:353–360.

23 Pancreatitis

Joseph J. Kishel

LEARNING OBJECTIVES

Upon completion of the chapter, the reader will be able to:

1. Describe the pathophysiology of acute and chronic pancreatitis.
2. Differentiate the signs and symptoms of acute from chronic pancreatitis.
3. Discuss the clinical implications of pancreatic fluid collections, pancreatic abscess, and pancreatic necrosis in acute pancreatitis.
4. Formulate care plans for managing acute pancreatitis.
5. Identify pharmacologic and nonpharmacologic means of preventing repeat episodes of chronic pancreatitis.
6. Choose appropriate pancreatic enzyme supplementation for patients with chronic pancreatitis.

KEY CONCEPTS

❶ The most common causes of acute and chronic pancreatitis in adults are ethanol abuse and biliary stones.

❷ Pancreatic necrosis occurs within the first 2 weeks of acute pancreatitis and develops in 10% to 30% of patients with acute pancreatitis.

❸ Therapy of acute pancreatitis is primarily supportive unless a specific etiology is identified. Supportive therapy involves fluid repletion, nutrition support, and analgesia.

❹ Medications aimed at decreasing pancreatic enzyme release (e.g., somatostatin), nasogastric suction, and anticholinergic medications have all failed to show benefit in the treatment of acute pancreatitis.

❺ Long-term sequelae of chronic pancreatitis include dietary malabsorption, impaired glucose tolerance, cholangitis, and potential addiction to opioid analgesics.

❻ Treatment of chronic pancreatitis is aimed at removing the cause (ethanol abuse or biliary stones), providing analgesia, supplementing with pancreatic enzyme preparations, and implementing dietary restrictions.

INTRODUCTION

The pancreas is a gland in the abdomen lying in the curvature of the stomach as it empties into the duodenum. The pancreas functions primarily as an exocrine gland, although it also has endocrine function. The exocrine cells of the pancreas are called acinar cells that produce an alkaline fluid known as pancreatic juice that contains various digestive enzymes. The pancreatic juice is released through the ampulla of Vater into the duodenum to aid in the digestive process as well as buffer acidic fluid released from the stomach (Fig. 23–1).

These enzymes are produced and stored as inactive proenzymes within zymogen granules to prevent autolysis

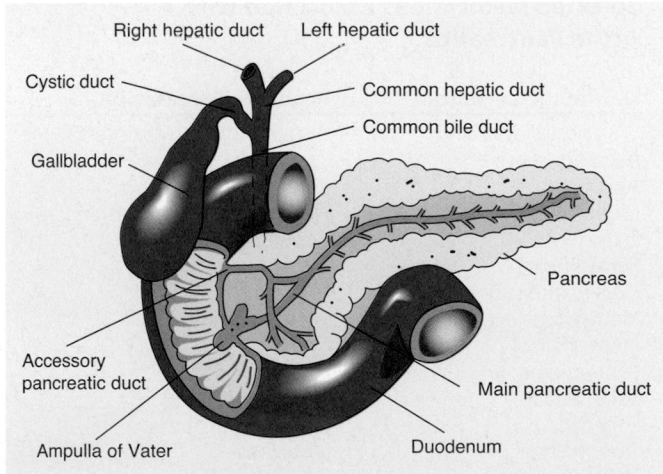

FIGURE 23–1. Anatomic structure of the pancreas and biliary tract. (From Berardi RR, Montgomery PA. Pancreatitis. In: DiPiro JT, Talbert RL, Yee GC, et al., eds. Pharmacotherapy: A Pathophysiologic Approach, 7th ed. New York: McGraw-Hill, 2005:660, with permission.)

and digestion of the pancreas. The zymogen granules are also responsible for enzyme transport to the pancreatic duct. Amylase and lipase are released from the zymogen granules in the active form, whereas the proteolytic enzymes are activated in the duodenum by enterokinase. Enterokinase triggers the conversion of trypsinogen to the active protease, trypsin. Trypsin then activates the other proenzymes to their active enzymes. The pancreas contains a trypsin inhibitor to prevent autolysis.

ACUTE PANCREATITIS

EPIDEMIOLOGY AND ETIOLOGY

1 *In the Western hemisphere, acute pancreatitis is caused mainly by ethanol use/abuse and gallstones (choleli-thiasis).* Other common causes of acute pancreatitis include hypertriglyceridemia, endoscopic retrograde chol-angiopancreatography (ERCP), pregnancy, and autodigestion due to early activation of pancreatic enzymes. Numerous medications have also been implicated as causes of acute pancreatitis (Table 23–1).

PATHOPHYSIOLOGY

Ethanol abuse may cause precipitation of pancreatic enzymes in the ducts of the pancreas, leading to chronic inflammation and fibrosis resulting in loss of exocrine function. Ethanol itself may be directly toxic to the pancreatic cells, compounding this effect. Gallstones may obstruct the ampulla of Vater causing pancreatic enzymes or bile to move in a retrograde

fashion into the pancreas. This retrograde movement may be responsible for pancreatic autolysis.[1]

Autolysis of the pancreas can occur when zymogens are activated in the pancreas before being released into the duodenum. Acute pancreatitis can result from the initial injury to the zymogen-producing cells, which is followed by neutrophil invasion of the pancreas and further activation of enzymes within the pancreas. This cascade of events is destructive to the pancreas and harmful to the patient.

Acute pancreatitis can progress to several distinct consequences. A pancreatic fluid collection (or pancreatic pseudocyst) is a collection of tissue, pancreatic enzymes, and blood that forms weeks after acute pancreatitis. Many pancreatic pseudocysts resolve spontaneously, but some require surgical drainage.[2] Rupture of a pancreatic pseudocyst with associated erosion and hemorrhage of major abdominal blood vessels can have a mortality approaching 60%; thus, continued monitoring of a pseudocyst is prudent.[3]

Pancreatic necrosis is a diffuse inflammation of the pancreas with infectious etiology. **2** *Pancreatic necrosis occurs within the first 2 weeks of acute pancreatitis and develops in 10% to 30% of patients with acute pancreatitis.* The necrotic pancreas can become secondarily infected with enteric gram-negative bacteria (such as *Escherichia coli*), and disseminated infection may result from pancreatic necrosis.[4,5]

Pancreatic abscess is a collection of pus that forms in the pancreas 4 to 6 weeks after acute pancreatitis. Pancreatic abscess is usually less life-threatening than pancreatic necrosis or pancreatic pseudocyst and can be managed with percutaneous drainage.[2] Pancreatic fluid collections and pancreatic abscesses can form during the course of acute pancreatitis. Pancreatic necrosis can occur when pancreatic enzymes damage the pancreatic tissue or when pancreatic abscesses become secondarily infected. This infection is usually due to bacteria that are normally found in the GI tract, including *E. coli*, Enterobacteriaceae, *Staphylococcus aureus*, viridans group streptococci, and anaerobes.

CLINICAL PRESENTATION AND DIAGNOSIS

A patient with acute pancreatitis may develop many severe local and systemic complications. Abdominal pain and distention may be due to local complications such as fluid collection, necrosis, or abscess in the pancreas. Hypotension, tachycardia, and fever may result from systemic complications, which can affect virtually any organ system but tend to target the pulmonary and cardiovascular systems and the kidneys. Multiorgan failure is a poor prognostic indicator. Acute respiratory distress syndrome (ARDS) is a life-threatening syndrome of acute lung injury with resulting hypoxia. ARDS may be due to the systemic release of pancreatic enzymes causing destruction of pulmonary surfactant, which is required for proper lung function.[7] Circulating pancreatic enzymes can cause cardiovascular shock. Acute renal failure may result from hypovolemia.[8]

Patients at greatest risk for mortality from acute pancreatitis are those who have multiorgan failure (e.g.,

---

Table 23–1
Selected Medications Associated With Acute Pancreatitis

Definite Association	Probable Association
5-Aminosalicylic acid	Angiotensin-converting enzyme inhibitors
Asparaginase	Bumetamide
Azathioprine	HMG-CoA reductase inhibitors
Didanosine	Cimetidine
Estrogens	Cisplatin
Furosemide	Clozapine
6-Mercaptopurine	Corticosteroids
Methyldopa	Cytarabine
Metronidazole	Ethacrynic acid
Pentamidine	Ifosfamide
Sulfonamides	Interferon *a*-2b
Sulindac	Losartan
Tigecycline	Procainamide
Thiazide diuretics	Salicylates
Valproic acid/salts	

Adapted from Berardi RR, Montgomery PA. Pancreatitis. In: DiPiro JT, Talbert RL, Yee GC, et al., eds. Pharmacotherapy: A Pathophysiologic Approach, 7th ed. New York: McGraw-Hill, 2008; Table 41–2, p. 661, with permission.

Clinical Presentation and Diagnosis of Acute Pancreatitis

Symptoms

- Abdominal pain radiating to the back is the most common presenting symptom. Pain can be due to intestinal immobility or chemical peritonitis induced by pancreatic enzymes.
- Other common symptoms include nausea, vomiting, and abdominal pain.

Signs

- Tachycardia, hypotension, fever, and abdominal distention may be present.
- There may be a positive Cullen's sign (bluish discoloration of the periumbilical skin indicating blood in the peritoneum).
- After 2 to 3 days of acute hemorrhagic pancreatitis, there may be a positive Turner's sign (local areas of discoloration [bruising] and induration of the skin near the umbilicus due to extravasation of blood).

Laboratory Tests

- The serum **amylase** can be elevated three times the upper limit of normal within the first 12 hours of the onset of acute pancreatitis. The degree of elevation does not predict the severity of disease.
- As acute pancreatitis progresses, serum **lipase** and colipase become elevated.[6]
- Other possible laboratory abnormalities include elevated WBC count, hyperglycemia, hypocalcemia, hyperbilirubinemia, elevated serum lactate dehydrogenase (LDH), and hypertriglyceridemia.

Patient Encounter, Part 1

A 32-year-old woman in her second trimester of pregnancy presents to the emergency department complaining of sharp persistent pain in the RUQ of the abdomen. The pain started 3 days ago and has progressed to become severe. She was nauseated at home and has vomited twice in the emergency department. The patient is at normal weight for this stage in her pregnancy. All prenatal visits were normal. The patient does not smoke or consume ethanol but does have a history of cholelithiasis.

What information about the patient presentation is consistent with acute pancreatitis?

What risk factors does the patient have for acute pancreatitis?

What additional laboratory tests would you recommend?

hypotension, respiratory failure, or renal failure), pancreatic necrosis, obesity, volume depletion, above 70 years of age, and an elevated Acute Physiology, Age, and Chronic Health Evaluation (APACHE) II score.[9,10]

DIAGNOSIS

Diagnosis of acute pancreatitis is based on the patient's history and presenting signs and symptoms. Evaluation of laboratory results, specifically the serum lipase, aids in diagnosis. Serum amylase is elevated early in the disease process but may return to normal within 12 hours.[8] Although an elevated serum amylase had been the diagnostic standard, its utility is limited by lack of specificity. Serum lipase and colipase are now the gold standards for laboratory testing due to greater than 90% specificity for acute pancreatitis. Serum lipase will remain elevated for days after the acute event and may be more useful for diagnosis depending on when the patient presents for evaluation.[8,11] CT is more complicated than abdominal radiography or ultrasound, but it is the most useful tool for diagnosis and staging of acute pancreatitis.[12]

The patient's history will identify risk factors for acute pancreatitis, such as age above 70 years or history of alcohol abuse. Finally, CT scan or ultrasound of the abdomen can help identify pancreatic fluid collections.[12] The APACHE II score is a rating scale of disease severity in critically ill patients. The CT severity index has the highest sensitivity and specificity in the diagnosis of acute pancreatitis.

TREATMENT

Desired Outcomes

The goals of treatment for acute pancreatitis include: (a) resolution of nausea, vomiting, abdominal pain, and fever; (b) ability to tolerate oral intake; (c) normalization of serum amylase, lipase, and WBC count; and (d) resolution of abscess, pseudocyst, or fluid collection as measured by CT scan.

Nonpharmacologic Therapy

Many medications can precipitate an attack of acute pancreatitis. If a medication is determined to be the cause of acute pancreatitis, it should be discontinued and an alternative therapy be considered.[13,14]

❸ *Therapy of acute pancreatitis is primarily supportive unless a specific etiology is identified (Fig. 23–2). Supportive therapy involves fluid repletion, nutrition support, and analgesia.* Patients with acute pancreatitis are administered IV fluids to maintain hydration and blood pressure. Fluids may be given in the form of crystalloids (e.g., 0.9% sodium chloride for infusion) or colloids (e.g., dextran or albumin for infusion).[15] Sodium chloride 0.9% for infusion (normal saline) at a rate of 50 to 100 mL/h is reasonable for patients

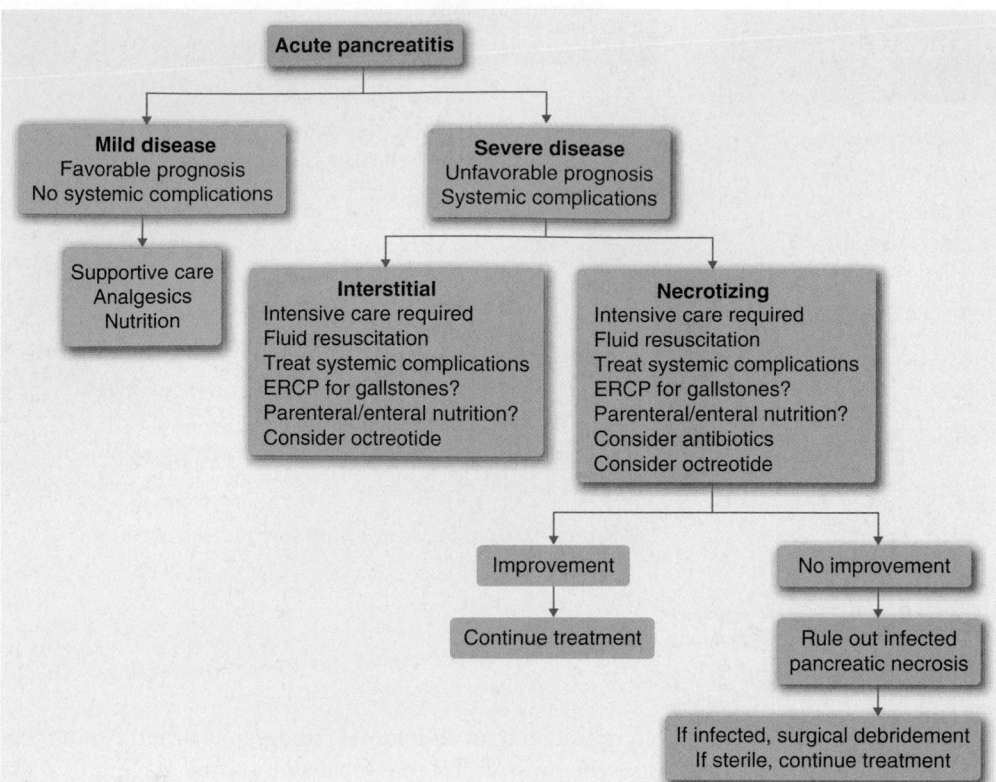

FIGURE 23–2. Algorithm for evaluation and treatment of acute pancreatitis. (ERCP, endoscopic retrograde cholangiopancreatography.) (From Berardi RR, Montgomery PA. Pancreatitis. In: DiPiro JT, Talbert RL, Yee GC, et al., eds. Pharmacotherapy: A Pathophysiologic Approach, 7th ed. New York: McGraw-Hill, 2008:664, with permission.)

with mild to moderate fluid depletion. However, as much as 200 mL/h may be required for patients with severe fluid losses.[16] Electrolytes such as potassium and magnesium may be added to the infusions if necessary. Hyperglycemia can be managed with insulin-containing IV infusions.

It is common practice to discontinue oral feedings during an attack of acute pancreatitis. In theory, discontinuation of oral intake will decrease the secretory functions of the pancreas and minimize further complications from the disease. Some patients can be fed with minimal oral intake, even in severe acute pancreatitis. Tube feeding delivered via a nasojejunal tube will feed the patient beyond the ampulla of Vater, minimizing stimulation of the pancreas.[15,16] If oral intake is discontinued for a protracted period, total parenteral nutrition must be used to maintain adequate nutrition.[17,18]

If pancreatic necrosis has been identified, surgical debridement is necessary because mortality approaches 100% without drainage or surgical intervention. Percutaneous drainage is an option for managing pancreatic necrosis but is best used only in unstable patients as a bridge to surgery. Repeated surgery may be required in patients with a protracted or progressing disease state.[2,19]

Pharmacologic Therapy

▶ Analgesics

Meperidine has historically been the most popular analgesic in acute pancreatitis because it is purported to cause less spasm and resulting pain in the sphincter of Oddi than other opioids. However, the clinical importance of this phenomenon is unclear.[15,20] As a result, patients with acute pancreatitis should be given the most effective analgesic. Hydromorphone and fentanyl are reasonable alternatives to meperidine and may be more desirable due to other adverse effects associated with meperidine. Refer to Chapter 30 on pain management for guidance in selecting an analgesic dose.

▶ Antibiotics

Empiric antibiotics are not necessary if the patient has mild disease or a noninfectious etiology of acute pancreatitis. Antibiotics have not been shown to prevent the formation of pancreatic abscess or necrosis when given early in the course of acute pancreatitis.

Antibiotics may be appropriate for pancreatic necrosis, which can be infected initially or be susceptible to a secondary infection; however, published data yield conflicting results regarding mortality and infection rate in this setting.[16,21,22] As such, the decision to use antibiotics is highly individualized. Selected intravenous antibiotic regimens are shown in Table 23–2. If necrosis is confirmed, antibiotics are insufficient as sole therapy; surgical debridement is necessary for cure.

Broad-spectrum antibiotics with activity against enteric gram-negative bacilli are appropriate. It is often difficult to narrow the spectrum of activity of the antibiotic choice since the infections are usually polymicrobial. As such, patients may receive long courses of broad-spectrum antibiotics such as meropenem and may develop superinfections due to more resistant bacteria or bacteria not susceptible to meropenem. Antifungal agents such as fluconazole may be considered if

Patient Encounter, Part 2: Medical History, Physical Exam, and Diagnostic Tests

PMH: Gravida 2, para 1; cholelithiasis

Allergies: No known allergies

FH: Father and mother alive and well

SH: No ethanol currently, but one to two drinks per night before pregnancy; no tobacco

Meds: No prescription medications; multivitamin one tablet orally once daily; ferrous sulfate 324 mg orally once daily; calcium carbonate 500 mg orally twice daily

ROS: Positive for sharp RUQ abdominal pain radiating to the back, nausea, vomiting, negative for chest pain, or shortness of breath

PE:

VS: wt 80 kg (176 lb), ht 5'5" (165 cm), BP 110/60 mm Hg, p 120 bpm, RR 18 per minute, T 37.9°C (100.2°F)

CV: Regular rate and rhythm, no murmurs

Abd: Pregnant, (+) rebound tenderness, (+) bowel sounds, no hepatosplenomegaly

Labs: Amylase 50 units/L (0.83 μKat/L), lipase 1,000 units/L (16.7 μKat/L)

Abdominal Ultrasound: Results pending

Given this additional information, what is your assessment of the patient's condition?

Why is the amylase low and the lipase high?

Patient Encounter, Part 3: Treatment and Monitoring

The patient acutely decompensates upon leaving the CT scanner and is therefore transferred to the surgical intensive care unit for mechanical ventilation, blood pressure support, and surgical evaluation. A diagnosis of acute pancreatitis with pancreatic necrosis is made.

Formulate a care plan for this patient.

What are some possible causes of respiratory failure and hypotension in this patient? Are these findings poor prognostic indicators?

What is the recommended treatment for pancreatic necrosis?

What empiric antibiotic regimen would be a reasonable choice in this patient? Provide a drug, dose, route, and frequency.

Suppose a surgeon requested clindamycin 600 mg IV every 8 hours for this patient. Would this be a reasonable choice? Why or why not?

Ineffective therapies include: reducing pancreatic secretion by administering somatostatin or atropine, reducing gastric acidity and decreasing pancreatic secretion with histamine$_2$-receptor antagonists, inhibition of pancreatic enzymes using protease inhibitors such as aprotinin, probiotics, and immunomodulation.[11,24–27] Nasogastric suction has only been effective in patients with ileus or persistent vomiting.[28]

OUTCOME EVALUATION

Given the severity of acute pancreatitis, patients are monitored closely in the intensive care setting. Patients with mild disease can be managed more conservatively with observation and supportive care. Critically ill patients may require surgery and aggressive life support measures.[16,29]

CHRONIC PANCREATITIS

EPIDEMIOLOGY AND ETIOLOGY

The incidence of chronic pancreatitis is approximately one in 10,000 people. ❶ *The most common cause of chronic pancreatitis in adults in Western countries is ethanol abuse.* The most common cause in children is cystic fibrosis due to pre-existing pancreatic insufficiency inherent in the disease. Gallstones can occur at the same time as chronic pancreatitis but are not often implicated as the cause. Unlike acute pancreatitis, chronic pancreatitis has an unknown etiology in a significant number of cases (30%).[29,30]

Table 23–2

Selected IV Antimicrobial Regimens for Pancreatic Necrosis

Drug	Usual Dose^a	Notes
Meropenem	1 g every 8 hours	Risk of superinfection
Piperacillin/ tazobactam	3.375 g every 6 hours	Avoid if allergic to penicillin
Cefepime + metronidazole	2 g every 12 hours + 500 mg every 6 hours	Will not cover enterococci
Aztreonam + vancomycin + metronidazole	1 g every 8 hours + 15 mg/kg every 8–12 hours + 500 mg every 6 hours	Option for penicillin-allergic patients

^{a}Doses must be adjusted for the degree of renal impairment.

peritonitis or GI perforation develops due to the presence of fungi such as *Candida albicans* in the GI tract.[23]

▶ *Ineffective Therapies*

❹ *Several pharmacologic therapies have been proven to be ineffective in reducing morbidity or mortality from the disease.*

PATHOPHYSIOLOGY

Chronic pancreatitis is an inflammatory process that occurs over a long period of time. The inflammation damages the enzyme-producing cells in the pancreas and can also disrupt or destroy the endocrine function of the pancreas by causing diffuse scarring and fibrosis.[30,31] Ethanol abuse may cause precipitation of pancreatic enzymes in the ducts of the pancreas leading to chronic inflammation and damage. Ethanol may also be directly toxic to pancreatic cells.[32] Counterintuitively, the amount of ethanol consumed does not correlate with the incidence or progression of chronic pancreatitis.[33] A patient who "binge drinks" by consuming large amounts of ethanol over short periods of time is as likely to develop chronic pancreatitis as someone who chronically consumes socially acceptable amounts of alcohol. Patients who die from the first diagnosed episode of chronic pancreatitis may have had undiagnosed chronic pancreatitis for some time.[34]

⑤ *Long-term sequelae of chronic pancreatitis include dietary malabsorption, impaired glucose tolerance, cholangitis, and potential addiction to opioid analgesics.* As patients lose exocrine function of the pancreas, they have decreased ability to absorb lipids and protein ingested with normal dietary intake. Weight loss from nutritional malabsorption is a common symptom of chronic pancreatitis not often seen in acute pancreatitis. Fatty- or protein-containing stools are also common; carbohydrate absorption is usually unaffected. Even though patients with chronic pancreatitis have decreased ability to absorb lipid from the GI tract, there does not appear to be an increased incidence of fat-soluble vitamin deficiency in these patients.[36]

CLINICAL PRESENTATION AND DIAGNOSIS

Differentiating an episode of acute from chronic pancreatitis may be difficult because the clinical presentations can be similar. The diagnosis of chronic pancreatitis is made by looking for the effects of chronic pancreatic inflammation and scarring on the pancreas and the patient as a whole. CT or ERCP will allow visualization of chronic calcified lesions in the pancreas when present.[39]

TREATMENT

Desired Outcomes

The goals of pharmacotherapy for chronic pancreatitis are: (a) prevention and resolution of chronic abdominal pain and (b) correction of dietary malabsorption with exogenous pancreatic enzymes.

Nonpharmacologic Therapy

Lifestyle modifications are an important part of the therapy for chronic pancreatitis. Patients who completely avoid ethanol after an attack of ethanol-induced pancreatitis are significantly less likely to have a recurrence than patients

---

Clinical Presentation and Diagnosis of Chronic Pancreatitis

General

- The presentation of chronic pancreatitis can be similar to that of acute pancreatitis.

Symptoms

- Pain is the most common chief complaint. Pain can be dull or sharp, and it may be localized to the area around the stomach or can radiate to the back. The pain is not relieved by antacids and can be provoked by ethanol ingestion or a fatty meal.[35]
- Weight loss can result from chronic fat and protein malabsorption.

Signs

- Patients often present with chronic fat-containing diarrhea due to dietary lipid malabsorption.
- GI bleeding can result from erosion of intestinal blood vessels by pancreatic enzymes or as a result of thrombosis.
- Chronic obstruction of the common bile duct by the inflamed pancreas can cause icterus, cholangitis, and biliary cirrhosis.[37]

Laboratory Tests

- Glucose intolerance may occur because of chronic destruction of the endocrine function of the pancreas.[38]
- Serum amylase and lipase levels are not usually elevated in chronic pancreatitis.
- The serum bilirubin or alkaline phosphatase may be elevated due to inflammation near the common bile duct.

---

who ingest even casual amounts of ethanol. ⑥ *Avoidance of ethanol and fatty meals can decrease the pain of chronic pancreatitis.*

Many surgical procedures have been employed to reduce the inflammation or remove the strictures that cause pain in chronic pancreatitis. However, most procedures, including nerve blocks, have not been proven effective in clinical trials and carry a high risk of morbidity and mortality.[40]

Pharmacologic Therapy

▶ Analgesics

⑥ *Pain management is an important component of therapy and is similar to that of acute pancreatitis.* Nonopioid analgesics (e.g., tramadol) are preferred, but the severe and persistent nature of the pain often requires opioid therapy. Patients can require chronic doses of opioid analgesics, with a resulting risk of addiction. Pain can also be managed by removing the stimulus of exacerbation if identified.[32,41]

▶ *Pancreatic Enzymes*

The goal of pancreatic enzyme supplementation is to deliver exogenous enzyme to the duodenum without causing further GI side effects from the medication, risking noncompliance due to the large number of dosage units required, or causing undue medication expense.[42]

❻ *Supplementation with pancreatic enzymes may reduce the pain and fatty diarrhea associated with chronic pancreatitis* (Table 23–3). Best results are achieved in patients who have mild nonalcoholic pancreatic disease. Common pancreatic enzyme supplements contain lipase, amylase, and protease in varying proportions. Thus, the dose can be tailored to the patient's requirement for exogenous enzyme supplementation and response to therapy.

Nonenteric-coated pancreatic enzyme supplements require high doses to compensate for loss of enzyme due to destruction by the low pH of the stomach. This effect can be minimized by administering a histamine$_2$-receptor antagonist or proton pump inhibitor (PPI). Nonenteric-coated pancreatic enzyme supplements may have an advantage in minimizing pain early in the disease state through regulation of proteases in the duodenum.

Nonenteric-coated pancreatic enzyme supplements can be used for initial therapy. The relative dose of amylase, lipase, and protease may be increased until control of pain and fatty diarrhea are achieved or the patient experiences intolerable side effects. If pain and diarrhea control are achieved, the patient can be transitioned to an enteric-coated supplement to maximize compliance. A reasonable example starting regimen is Viokase-8, six tablets with each meal and at bedtime, given with famotidine 20 mg at bedtime.

Table 23–3

Frequently Used Pancreatic Enzyme Preparations

Product	Dosage Form	Enzyme Content (Units)[a] Lipase	Amylase	Protease
Creon-10	ECMS	10,000	33,200	37,500
Creon-20	ECMS	20,000	66,400	75,000
Ku-Zyme HP	C	8,000	30,000	30,000
Lipram-CR10	ECMS	10,000	33,200	37,500
Lipram-PN16	ECMS	16,000	48,000	48,000
Lipram-CR20	ECMS	20,000	66,400	75,000
Lipram-PN20	ECMS	20,000	56,000	44,000
Lipram-UL12	ECMS	12,000	39,000	39,000
Lipram-PN10	ECMS	10,000	30,000	30,000
Lipram-UL18	ECMS	18,000	58,500	58,500
Lipram-UL20	ECMS	20,000	65,000	65,000
Pancrease	ECMS	4,500	20,000	25,000
Pancrease MT-4	ECMT	4,000	12,000	12,000
Pancrease MT-10	ECMT	10,000	30,000	30,000
Pancrease MT-16	ECMT	16,000	48,000	48,000
Pancrease MT-20	ECMT	20,000	56,000	44,000
Ultrase MT 12	ECMT	12,000	39,000	39,000
Ultrase MT 18	ECMT	18,000	58,500	58,500
Ultrase MT 20	ECMT	20,000	65,000	65,000
Viokase[b]	P	16,800	70,000	70,000
Viokase 8	UCT	8,000	30,000	30,000
Viokase 16	UCT	16,000	60,000	60,000

C, powder encased in a cellulose capsule; ECMS, enteric-coated microspheres encased in a cellulose or gelatin capsule; ECMT, enteric-coated microtablets encased in a cellulose capsule; P, powder; UCT, uncoated tablet.

[a]All listed products contain pancrelipase. Pancrelipase contains not less than 24 USP units of lipase activity, not less than 100 USP units of amylase activity, and not less than 100 USP units of protease activity per milligram.

[b]Units of 0.7 g of powder.

From Berardi RR, Montgomery PA. Pancreatitis. In: DiPiro JT, Talbert RL, Yee GC, et al., eds. Pharmacotherapy: A Pathophysiologic Approach, 7th ed. New York: McGraw-Hill, 2008:670, with permission.

Patient Encounter 2

The same patient described in the first encounter is now 34 years old (she delivered a healthy baby boy without complications). She presents to the clinic with RUQ pain radiating to her back. She is also jaundiced and nauseated.

PMH: Gravida 2 para 2, cholelithiasis

SH: Consumes one to two alcoholic beverages per evening; no tobacco

Meds: Multivitamin one tablet daily; pantoprazole 40 mg orally once daily; maalox 15 mL orally four times daily as needed for heartburn/stomach upset; acetaminophen 325 mg orally every 6 hours as needed for pain/headache

ROS: Positive for sharp RUQ abdominal pain radiating to the back, nausea, and recent unintentional weight loss; negative for chest pain or shortness of breath, fatty diarrhea present for months

PE:

VS: BP 130/86 mm Hg, p 80 bpm, RR 16 per minute, T 37.0°C (98.6°F), wt 80 kg (176 lb), ht 5′5″ (165 cm).

CV: Regular rate and rhythm, no murmurs noted

Abd: Distended, (+) rebound tenderness, (+) bowel sounds, marked hepatosplenomegaly

Labs: Amylase 100 units/L (1.67 μKat/L), lipase 100 units/L (1.67 μKat/L)

CT Scan: Diffuse pancreatic scarring and calcifications

Formulate a care plan for this patient.

Why are the serum amylase and lipase normal?

What lifestyle modifications can this patient make to minimize impact from her disease state?

Is this patient taking any medication(s) that could exacerbate pancreatitis? If so, what alternatives can you offer?

What medications may help alleviate the fatty diarrhea the patient is experiencing?

How would you monitor the effectiveness of your recommendations?

Most pancreatic enzyme supplements are enteric coated to release enzymes in the alkaline environment of the intestine; this minimizes enzyme destruction in the stomach. Enteric-coated pancreatic enzyme supplements require fewer daily dosage units, but delivery of the drug to the site of action and effectiveness may be delayed by gastric emptying time.[43]

Pancreatic enzyme supplements should be taken immediately prior to meals to aid in the digestion and absorption of food. Alternately, patients can supplement their diet with medium-chain triglycerides (MCTs) or ingest foods rich in MCTs since they do not require pancreatic enzymes for absorption. An appropriate regimen incorporates the successful doses of each enzyme (amylase, lipase, and protease) from the starting Nonenteric-coated regimen. As with the previous example, a patient stabilized on Viokase-8, six tablets with each meal, can be transitioned to Pancrease MT-16 three tablets with meals. The famotidine can then be discontinued.

OUTCOME EVALUATION

- Monitor for adequate pain control and the need for escalation or de-escalation of analgesia.

Patient Care and Monitoring

1. Determine whether ethanol is a contributing causative factor. If so, reinforce counseling on the need for abstinence and provide appropriate resources to maintain abstinence (e.g., professional counseling, alcoholics anonymous).

2. Obtain a thorough history of prescription, nonprescription, and dietary supplement use to identify products that may exacerbate chronic pancreatitis.

3. Refer the patient for nutritional counseling if there is decreased caloric intake and weight loss. Compare actual body weight to ideal body weight.

4. Make a plan for analgesia, in conjunction with a pain management service if possible, to control and prevent pain. Recommend an analgesic with ease of dosing and minimal side effects, realizing that patients with chronic pancreatitis may require large doses of opioids.

5. Optimize pancreatic enzyme supplementation, starting first with a nonenteric-coated enzyme supplement and a histamine$_2$-receptor antagonist. When pain and diarrhea are stabilized, consider switching to an enteric-coated enzyme supplement for ease of dosing.

6. Develop a plan for reassessing pancreatic enzyme supplementation and analgesia on an outpatient basis.

7. Assess improvement in quality of life measures such as physical, psychological, and social functioning and well-being.

- If pain relief is achieved by avoiding ethanol or fatty meals, encourage continuation of these practices.

- When dietary malabsorption exists, monitor patients for weight gain or loss, activity level, and ability to perform activities of daily living.

- Ask patients to monitor the frequency and consistency of stool output as an indicator of malabsorption.

- Educate patients that compliance with and proper use of dietary pancreatic enzyme supplementation is key to improved outcomes.[32,35,41-43]

Abbreviations Introduced in This Chapter

ARDS	Acute respiratory distress syndrome
ERCP	Endoscopic retrograde Cholangiopancreatography
LDH	Lactate dehydrogenase
MCT	Medium-chain triglycerides
PPIs	Proton pump inhibitors
RUQ	Right upper quadrant

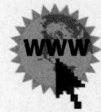

Self-assessment questions and answers are available at *http://www.mhpharmacotherapy.com/pp.html.*

REFERENCES

1. Ros E, Navarro S, Bru C, et al. Occult microlithiasis in "idiopathic" acute pancreatitis: Prevention of relapses by cholecystectomy or ursodeoxycholic acid therapy. Gastroenterology 1991;101:1701–1709.
2. Bradley EL, III. A clinically based classification system for acute pancreatitis. Summary of the International Symposium on Acute Pancreatitis, Atlanta, GA, September 11 through 13, 1992. Arch Surg 1993;128:586–590.
3. Balthazar EJ. Staging of acute pancreatitis. Radiol Clin North Am 2002;40:1199–1209.
4. Perez A, Whang EE, Brooks DC, et al. Is severity of necrotizing pancreatitis increased in extended necrosis and infected necrosis? Pancreas 2002;25:229–233.
5. Lankisch PG, Pflichthofer D, Lehnick D. Acute pancreatitis: Which patient is most at risk? Pancreas 1999;19:321–324.
6. Kazmierczak S. Biochemical indicators of acute pancreatitis. In: Lott J, ed. Clinical Pathology of Pancreatic Disorders. Totowa, NJ: Humana Press, 1997:75.
7. Isenmann R, Rau B, Beger HG. Early severe acute pancreatitis: Characteristics of a new subgroup. Pancreas 2001;22:274–278.
8. Cappell MS. Acute pancreatitis: Etiology, clinical presentation, diagnosis, and therapy. Med Clin North Am 2008;92:889–923.
9. Tenner S, Sica G, Hughes M, et al. Relationship of necrosis to organ failure in severe acute pancreatitis. Gastroenterology 1997;113:899–903.
10. Dervenis C, Johnson CD, Bassi C, et al. Diagnosis, objective assessment of severity, and management of acute pancreatitis. Santorini consensus conference. Int J Pancreatol 1999;25:195–210.
11. Marshall JB. Acute pancreatitis. A review with an emphasis on new developments. Arch Intern Med 1993;153:1185–1198.
12. Gurleyik G, Emir S, Kilicoglu G, et al. Computed tomography severity index, APACHE II score, serum CRP concentration for predicting the severity of acute pancreatitis. JOP 2005;6:562–567.

13. Badalov N, Baradarian R, Iswara K, et al. Drug-induced acute pancreatitis: An evidence-based review. Clin Gastroenterol Hepatol 2007;5:648–661.

14. Pezzilli R, Billi P, Melandri R, et al. Anticonvulsant-induced chronic pancreatitis. A case report. Ital J Gastroenterol 1992;24:245–246.

15. Mayerle J, Simon P, Lerch MM. Medical treatment of acute pancreatitis. Gastroenterol Clin North Am 2004;33:855–869.

16. Banks PA, Freeman ML. Practice guidelines in acute pancreatitis. Am J Gastroenterol 2006;101:2379–2400.

17. Petrov MS, Correia MI, Windsor JA. Nasogastric tube feeding in predicted severe acute pancreatitis. A systematic review of the literature to determine safety and tolerance. JOP 2008;9:440–448.

18. Ioannidis O, Lavrentieva A, Botsios D. Nutrition support in acute pancreatitis. JOP 2008;9:375–390.

19. Bradley EL, III, Allen K. A prospective longitudinal study of observation versus surgical intervention in the management of necrotizing pancreatitis. Am J Surg 1991;161:19–24; discussion 24–25.

20. Thompson DR. Narcotic analgesic effects on the sphincter of Oddi: A review of the data and therapeutic implications in treating pancreatitis. Am J Gastroenterol 2001;96:1266–1272.

21. Yu B, Gao J, Zou D, et al. Prophylactic antibiotics cannot reduce infected pancreatic necrosis and mortality in acute necrotizing pancreatitis: Evidence from a meta-analysis of randomized controlled trials. Am J Gastroenterol 2008;103:104–110.

22. Sainio V, Kemppainen E, Puolakkainen P, et al. Early antibiotic treatment in acute necrotising pancreatitis. Lancet 1995;346:663–667.

23. Bassi C, Larvin M, Villatoro E. Antibiotic therapy for prophylaxis against infection of pancreatic necrosis in acute pancreatitis. Cochrane Database Syst Rev 2003(4):CD002941.

24. Pezzilli R. Gabexate mesilate in acute pancreatitis: Neither a miracle nor a mirage, merely the search of optimal dosage. Digest Liver Dis 2001;33:502.

25. Pederzoli P, Bassi C, Falconi M, et al. Gabexate mesilate in the treatment of acute pancreatitis. Annali Italiani di Chirurgia 1995;66:191–195.

26. Norman JG. New approaches to acute pancreatitis: Role of inflammatory mediators. Digestion 1999;60(Suppl 1):57–60.

27. Besselink MG, van Santvoort HC, Buskens E, et al. Dutch Acute Pancreatitis Study Group. Probiotic prophylaxis in predicted severe acute pancreatitis: A randomised, double-blind, placebo-controlled trial. Lancet 2008;37:651–659.

28. Levant JA, Secrist DM, Resin H, et al. Nasogastric suction in the treatment of alcoholic pancreatitis. A controlled study. JAMA 1974;229:51–52.

29. Nathens AB, Curtis JR, Beale RJ, et al. Management of the critically ill patient with severe acute pancreatitis. Crit Care Med 2004;32:2524–2536.

30. Sarles H, Bernard JP, Johnson C. Pathogenesis and epidemiology of chronic pancreatitis. Annu Rev Med 1989;40:453–468.

31. Sarles H, Adler G, Dani R, et al. The pancreatitis classification of Marseilles-Rome 1988. Scand J Gastroenterol 1989;24:641–642.

32. Steer ML, Waxman I, Freedman S. Chronic pancreatitis. N Engl J Med 1995;332:1482–1490.

33. Pelli H, Lappalainen-Lehto R, Piironen A, et al. Risk factors for recurrent acute alcohol-associated pancreatitis: A prospective analysis. Scand J Gastroenterol 2008;43:614–621.

34. Lowenfels AB, Maisonneuve P, Cavallini G, et al. Prognosis of chronic pancreatitis: An international multicenter study. International Pancreatitis Study Group. Am J Gastroenterol 1994;89:1467–1471.

35. Bornman PC, Marks IN, Girdwood AW, et al. Pathogenesis of pain in chronic pancreatitis: Ongoing enigma. World J Surg 2003;27:1175–1182.

36. Beglinger C. Relevant aspects of physiology in chronic pancreatitis. Digest Dis 1992;10:326–329.

37. Ammann RW, Akovbiantz A, Largiader F, Schueler G. Course and outcome of chronic pancreatitis. Longitudinal study of a mixed medical-surgical series of 245 patients. Gastroenterology 1984;86(5 Pt 1):820–828.

38. Malka D, Hammel P, Sauvanet A, et al. Risk factors for diabetes mellitus in chronic pancreatitis. Gastroenterology 2000;119:1324–1332.

39. Etemad B, Whitcomb DC. Chronic pancreatitis: Diagnosis, classification, and new genetic developments. Gastroenterology 2001;120:682–707.

40. Warshaw AL, Banks PA, Fernandez-Del Castillo C. AGA technical review: Treatment of pain in chronic pancreatitis. Gastroenterology 1998;115:765–776.

41. Ammann RW, Muellhaupt B. The natural history of pain in alcoholic chronic pancreatitis. Gastroenterology 1999;116:1132–1140.

42. Brown A, Hughes M, Tenner S, Banks PA. Does pancreatic enzyme supplementation reduce pain in patients with chronic pancreatitis: A meta-analysis. Am J Gastroenterol 1997;92:2032–2035.

43. Layer P, Keller J. Pancreatic enzymes: Secretion and luminal nutrient digestion in health and disease. J Clin Gastroenterol 1999;28:3–10.

24 Viral Hepatitis

Juliana Chan

LEARNING OBJECTIVES

● Upon completion of the chapter, the reader will be able to:

1. Differentiate the five types of viral hepatitides by their epidemiology, etiology, pathophysiology, clinical presentation, and natural history.

2. Identify modes of transmission and risk factors among the major types of viral hepatitis.

3. Evaluate hepatic serologies to understand how the type of hepatitis is diagnosed.

4. Create treatment goals for a patient with viral hepatitis.

5. Recommend an appropriate pharmacotherapy for prevention of viral hepatitis.

6. Develop a pharmaceutical care plan for treatment of viral hepatitis.

7. Formulate a monitoring plan to assess adverse effects of pharmacotherapy for viral hepatitis.

KEY CONCEPTS

❶ Prevention and treatment of viral hepatitis may prevent progression to chronic hepatitis, cirrhosis, end-stage liver disease, and hepatocellular carcinoma.

❷ Acute viral hepatitis A, B, C, D, and E are primarily managed with supportive care.

❸ Good personal hygiene and proper disposal of sanitary waste are required to prevent fecal–oral transmission of the hepatitis A and E virus.

❹ Individuals may minimize their risk of acquiring both hepatitis B and C infection by avoiding contaminated blood products and not indulging in high-risk behavior such as IV drug use.

❺ Persons at high risk of acquiring the hepatitis B virus (HBV) should be vaccinated with the hepatitis B vaccine at months 0, 1, and 6.

❻ A vaccine that combines both inactivated hepatitis A and recombinant hepatitis B (Twinrix) is approved for immunizing individuals more than 18 years of age with indications for both hepatitis A and B vaccines.

❼ The drug of choice for chronic hepatitis B depends on the patient's past medical history, alanine aminotransferase (ALT) level, HBV DNA level, HBeAg status, severity of liver disease, and history of previous HBV therapy.

❽ Hepatitis D infection is possible only if the patient also has the hepatitis B virus; therefore, hepatitis B vaccination can indirectly prevent hepatitis D infection.

INTRODUCTION

There are five types of viral hepatitis: hepatitis A (HAV), B (HBV), C (HCV), D (HDV), and E (HEV). Acute hepatitis may be associated with all five types of hepatitis and rarely exceeds 6 months in duration. Chronic hepatitis (disease lasting longer than 6 months) is usually associated with hepatitis B, C, and D.

❶ *Chronic viral hepatitis may lead to the development of cirrhosis, which may lead to end-stage liver disease (ESLD) and hepatocellular carcinoma (HCC).* Complications of ESLD include ascites, edema, hepatic encephalopathy, infections (e.g., spontaneous bacterial peritonitis), hepatorenal syndrome, and bleeding esophageal varices. Therefore, prevention and treatment of viral hepatitis may prevent ESLD and HCC.

Viral hepatitis can occur at any age and is the most common cause of liver disease in the world. The true prevalence and incidence may be under-reported because most patients are asymptomatic. The epidemiology, etiology, and pathogenesis vary depending on the type of hepatitis and are considered separately below.

EPIDEMIOLOGY AND ETIOLOGY

Hepatitis A

Hepatitis A affects 1.4 million people yearly worldwide.[1] The prevalence is highest in underdeveloped countries including Africa, parts of South America, the Middle East, and Southeast Asia. Australia, parts of western and northern

Table 24–1

Risk Factors for Acquiring Viral Hepatitis

Hepatitis A
International travelers to endemic areas (e.g., Africa, Asia, and parts of South America)
Sexual contact with infected persons (e.g., men having sex with other men)
Shellfish infected with HAV (e.g., raw oysters)
Day-care centers or household contacts with people infected with HAV
Health care workers
IV drug users using unsterilized needles
Workers involved with nonhuman primates
Food service handlers
Patients with clotting factor disorders
Individuals residing in health care institutions

Hepatitis B and D
Men having sex with other men
Individuals with multiple heterosexual partners
IV drug users using unsterilized needles
Recipients of blood products
Household contacts with acute hepatitis B with open cuts
Health care providers in contact with contaminated needles
Patients undergoing dialysis

Hepatitis C
Recipients of blood products
Health care providers in contact with infected needles
Individuals having multiple sexual partners
Perinatal transmission (less than 5%)
Unprofessional body piercing and tattooing

Hepatitis E
International travelers to endemic areas (e.g., parts of Asia, Africa, and Mexico)
Ingesting foods and drinks contaminated with bodily waste

Europe, Japan, and the United States have a lower prevalence. This is primarily due to vaccination programs, but outbreaks still can happen as evidenced by an outbreak in Pennsylvania in 2003.[2,3] The number of infections and hospitalizations due to HAV infection annually have decreased markedly since the introduction of the hepatitis A vaccine in 1996.[4,5]

HAV is primarily detected in contaminated feces and infects people via the fecal-oral route.[4,6] Outbreaks occur primarily in areas of poor sanitation.[1,4,5] Individuals at greatest risk of acquiring HAV are listed in Table 24–1.[4,7] Approximately 50% of the reported cases have no identifiable risk factors.[4]

To date, there are no documented cases of chronic hepatitis A.[1,4] Death associated with HAV is rare and is mostly associated with fulminant hepatitis, with which approximately 100 people die annually.[4]

Hepatitis B

Hepatitis B is a bloodborne infection affecting more than 2 billion people worldwide.[8] Approximately 400 million people have chronic infection, which may lead to cirrhosis and complications of ESLD.[8] There are 500,000 to 700,000 deaths annually due to hepatitis B.[9] Despite having an effective vaccine against HBV, more than 300,000 newly diagnosed infections emerge each year. Fewer than 1% of individuals in North America and western Europe are chronically infected compared with 8% to 10% in developing areas such as Southeast Asia.[8]

The highest concentration of the HBV is found in blood and serous fluids. Therefore, the primary mode of hepatitis B transmission is either by blood or body fluids through perinatal, sexual, or percutaneous exposure.[10] Infants born of mothers who are infected with HBV that is actively replicating have a 90% risk of developing chronic hepatitis B. If an infant residing in an endemic area is not infected at birth, the risk of acquiring chronic hepatitis B is still 30% to 60% within the first 5 years of life from horizontal transmission.[11,12] Individuals at greatest risk of acquiring HBV are listed in Table 24–1. Approximately 33% of the reported hepatitis B cases have no identifiable risk factors.[10]

Hepatitis C

More than 170 million people are infected with hepatitis C worldwide, and more than 4 million have the disease in the United States.[13] The prevalence is higher among non-Hispanic blacks than non-Hispanic whites, and men are more likely to be infected than women.[14,15] Additionally, genotypes are geographically specific. For example, genotype 1 is commonly found in patients in the United States whereas genotype 4 is common in the Middle East.[14,16] Approximately 75% of those infected with HCV in the United States have genotype 1, and about 14% and 5% have genotypes 2 and 3, respectively.[14,16] Genotype does not dictate disease severity or clinical outcomes but is used to determine the duration of therapy and the likelihood of therapeutic response.[15]

IV drug users utilizing contaminated paraphernalia are responsible for about 60% of HCV transmissions.[13] Because of the routine screening of blood products, the risk of HCV transmission via blood transfusion is very low (0.004–0.0004% per unit transfused).[13,17] Other populations at risk for acquiring HCV are listed in Table 24–1. Approximately 10% of the individuals infected with HCV have no identifiable risk factors.[17]

Hepatitis D

Hepatitis D affects approximately 10 million people worldwide. Eastern Asia has the lowest prevalence of HDV despite having the highest prevalence of HBV infections. Areas with the highest prevalence of HDV include the Middle East, West Africa, Western and Central Asia, parts of South America, and the South Pacific islands.[18,19]

There are three major HDV genotypes that are geographically specific. Genotype 1 primarily affects individuals residing in North America, Europe, Middle East, East Asia, and North Africa.[18] Individuals residing in Japan and Taiwan are mostly diagnosed with genotype 2. Patients in northern parts of South America are mostly infected with genotype 3.[18,20]

The most likely modes of transmitting the HDV are similar to those of HBV, including IV drug users using unsterilized needles and recipients of contaminated blood products. Sexual and perinatal transmission are rare for HDV.[18,19] Individuals at greatest risk of acquiring HDV are listed in Table 24–1.

Hepatitis E

Hepatitis E is found worldwide, but acute cases occur primarily in Central and Southeast Asia, the Middle East, and North Africa.[21,22] The HEV prevalence rate in the United States is 1% to 3%. The virus is primarily transmitted by the fecal–oral route. Transmission of HEV is more prominent in underdeveloped countries where sanitation is poor.

PATHOPHYSIOLOGY

Hepatitis A

Hepatitis A is a nonenveloped single-stranded RNA virus classified as the *Hepatovirus* genus under the Picornaviridae family.[1,4] The only host for the HAV is humans, with hepatic cells as the primary site for viral replication. As part of the viral degradation process, the HAV is released into the biliary system causing elevated concentrations of the virus in the feces.[23]

Hepatitis B

Hepatitis B (also known as the Dane particle) belongs to the Hepadnaviridae family.[24] The HBV is a partially double-stranded DNA virus with a phospholipid layer containing hepatitis B surface antigen (HBsAg) that surrounds the nucleocapsid. The nucleocapsid contains the core protein that produces hepatitis B core antigen (HBcAg), which is undetectable in the serum. Hepatocellular injury from HBV is thought to be due to a cytotoxic immune reaction that occurs when HBcAg is expressed on the surface of the hepatic cells. Fortunately, antibodies against hepatitis B core antigen (anti-HBc) are measurable in the blood, where anti-HBc to immunoglobulin M (IgM) indicates active infection and anti-HBc to IgG relates to either chronic infection or possible immunity against HBV.

Viral replication occurs when hepatitis B envelope antigen (HBeAg) is present and circulating in the blood. The serum HBV DNA concentration is a measure of viral infectivity and quantifies viral replication. Once the hepatitis B infection resolves, antibodies against hepatitis B envelope (anti-HBe) and antibodies against hepatitis B surface antigen (anti-HBs) develop, and HBV DNA levels become undetectable. However, if these antibodies do not develop, then the likelihood of developing chronic hepatitis B increases. This is primarily dependent on the host's immune system at the time the infection was attained. In immunocompetent individuals, the disease resolves spontaneously in most cases with no further sequelae. In immunocompromised persons, the infection is less likely to be eradicated.[24]

▶ *Natural History of Hepatitis B*

The natural history of hepatitis B depends on the age at which infection is acquired. Chronic HBV occurs in less than 5% of those who are older than 5 years of age, whereas the rate is more than 90% in infants born to mothers infected with HBV.[10] Approximately 90% of adults infected with HBV develop anti-HBs, which results in lifelong immunity. About 30% of adults with initial symptoms of HBV present with jaundice or fatigue, and about 0.5% exhibit fulminant hepatitis.[11,25] Cirrhosis and HCC are the two major complications associated with chronic hepatitis B infections. Patients who develop cirrhosis have a higher mortality rate than those without this complication.[11]

Hepatitis C

Hepatitis C, first known as non-A, non-B hepatitis, is a bloodborne infection caused by a single-stranded RNA virus belonging to the Flaviviridae family and the *Hepacivirus* genus.[13,16] It is theorized that structural and nonstructural (NS) peptides may be responsible for RNA viral replication, specifically the NS5 peptide. There are 11 genotypes (numbered 1–11) and more than 90 subtypes (genotypes 1a, 1b, 2a, 3b, etc.) that are unique to hepatitis C.[13]

Antibodies against HCV (anti-HCV) in the blood indicate infection with the HCV. If the infection persists for more than 6 months and viral replication is confirmed by HCV RNA levels, then the person has chronic hepatitis C. Chronic disease may be due to an ineffective host immune system against the HCV. Cytotoxic T lymphocytes are ineffective in eradicating the HCV, thus allowing persistent damage to hepatic cells. Therefore, immunocompromised individuals are less likely to eradicate the HCV.[16]

▶ *Natural History of Hepatitis C*

Only 10% to 15% of patients have acute hepatitis C that resolves without any further sequelae. In more than 70% of cases, hepatitis C develops into a chronic disease that is asymptomatic in about 60% to 80% of patients.[12,13] Approximately 70% of chronic HCV cases progress to mild, moderate, or severe hepatitis. Cirrhosis and its complications occur in 15% to 20% of patients infected with HCV. In 10% to 20% of cases, 20 to 40 years may elapse between the time of exposure and the development of cirrhosis.[12] Once cirrhosis is confirmed, the rate of developing HCC increases by 1% to 4% per year.[12] Approximately 25% of patients infected with the HCV who develop cirrhosis ultimately die from the disease.[13]

Hepatitis D

Hepatitis D (originally called delta hepatitis) belongs to the genus *Deltavirus* of the Deltaviridae family.[18,19] The HDV virion is a defective single-stranded circular RNA virus that requires the presence of HBV for HDV viral replication. This is because the hepatitis D virus antigen (HDVAg) is coated by the HBsAg.

The mechanism of hepatic damage induced by HDV is undetermined, but it is known that replication of HDV cannot occur without HBV being present causing either coinfection (both hepatitis B and D infection occurring simultaneously) or superinfection (acquiring HDV after having longstanding disease with HBV).[18,19]

Hepatitis E

Hepatitis E is a nonenveloped single-stranded messenger RNA virus of unclassified genus.[21] The HEV is similar to HAV in that the virus is found in contaminated feces, thus infecting people via the fecal–oral route. High HEV levels in the bile often prompt viral shedding in the feces. The severity of hepatic damage is dependent on the HEV strain: Mex 14, Sar 55, or the US 2 strain.[22] No cases of chronic hepatitis E have been documented.

CLINICAL PRESENTATION AND DIAGNOSIS

Diagnosis of Viral Hepatitis

Diagnosing viral hepatitis may be difficult because most infected individuals are asymptomatic.[4,10,12,13] Because symptoms cannot identify the specific type of hepatitis, laboratory serologies must be obtained (Table 24–2). In addition, liver function tests may be obtained to assess the extent of cholestatic and hepatocellular injury. However, the definitive test to determine the amount of damage and inflammation of hepatic cells is a liver biopsy.

▶ Hepatitis A

The diagnosis of hepatitis A is made by detecting immunoglobulin antibody to the capsid proteins of the HAV. The presence of IgM anti-HAV in the serum indicates an acute infection. IgM appears approximately 3 weeks after exposure and becomes undetectable within 6 months. In contrast, IgG anti-HAV appears in the serum at approximately the same time IgM anti-HAV develops but indicates protection and lifelong immunity against hepatitis A.[1]

▶ Hepatitis B

Hepatitis B is diagnosed when HBsAg is detectable in the serum. The nucleocapsid of the HBsAg contains the core protein that produces HBcAg, which is undetectable in the serum. The presence of antibodies against anti-HBc to IgM indicates active infection, and anti-HBc to IgG relates to either chronic infection or possible immunity against HBV.[8,10]

Viral replication occurs when HBeAg is present. Measurement of HBV DNA is used to determine viral infectivity and assess and quantify viral replication. Once the hepatitis B infection resolves, anti-HBe and anti-HBs develop, and HBV DNA levels becomes undetectable. Chronic hepatitis B is separated into two types, HBeAg-positive or HBeAg-negative.

▶ Hepatitis C

Hepatitis C is diagnosed by testing for anti-HCV in the serum. The disease is confirmed by the presence of HCV RNA. HCV RNA levels quantify viral replication and are used to determine if antiviral treatment for HCV is effective. Once a hepatitis C infection has been confirmed, further blood work should be obtained to determine the individual's genotype (1–11). HCV genotyping is used to determine the likelihood of response to antiviral therapy.[13]

▶ Hepatitis D

Hepatitis D infection requires the presence of HBV for HDV viral replication. Measuring HDV RNA levels in the serum by polymerase chain reaction (PCR) confirms the presence of HDV and is the most accurate diagnostic test. The presence of IgM antibodies to HDV Ag (IgM anti-HD) indicates active disease, and IgG anti-HD also becomes detectable if the infection does not resolve spontaneously. Unlike the antibodies developed against HAV, HDV antibodies do not confer immunity.

▶ Hepatitis E

The diagnosis of hepatitis E is based on the presence of anti-HEV antibodies; IgM anti-HEV. A test for hepatitis E RNA levels is available for use in clinical trials.[21]

Clinical Presentation and Diagnosis of Viral Hepatitis

Symptoms
- Most patients infected with any type of viral hepatitis have no symptoms.
- Patients with symptoms may experience any of the following: flu-like symptoms, fevers, fatigue/malaise, anorexia, nausea, vomiting, diarrhea, dark urine, pale-appearing stools, pruritus, and abdominal pain.

Signs
- Jaundice may be evident in the whites of the eyes (scleral icterus) or skin.

- An enlarged liver (hepatomegaly) and spleen (splenomegaly) may be present.
- In fulminant hepatitis with hepatic encephalopathy, patients may have asterixis and coma.
- In rare instances, extrahepatic symptoms may develop: arthritis, postcervical lymphadenopathy, palmar erythema, cryoglobulinemia, and vasculitis.

Laboratory Tests
- See Table 24–2.

Table 24–2

Interpretation of Viral Hepatitis Serology Panels

Type	Laboratory Test	Result	Interpretation of Panel
Hepatitis A	IgM anti-HAV IgG anti-HAV	Negative Negative	Susceptible to infection
	IgM anti-HAV	Positive	Acutely infected
	IgG anti-HAV	Positive	Immune due to either natural infection or HAV vaccine
Hepatitis B[a]	HBsAg Anti-HBc Anti-HBs	Negative Negative Negative	Susceptible to infection
	HBsAg Anti-HBc Anti-HBs	Negative Positive Positive	Immune due to natural infection
	HBsAg Anti-HBc Anti-HBs	Negative Negative Positive	Immune due to hepatitis B vaccination
	HBsAg Anti-HBc IgM anti-HBc Anti-HBs	Positive Positive Positive Negative	Acutely infected
	HBsAg Anti-HBc IgM anti-HBc Anti-HBs	Positive Positive Negative Negative	Chronically infected
	HBsAg Anti-HBc Anti-HBs	Negative Positive Negative	Four interpretations possible: (a) Resolved infection (most common); (b) false-positive anti-HBc, thus susceptible; (c) low-level chronic infection; (d) resolving acute infection
Hepatitis C	Anti-HCV	Negative	Susceptible to infection
	Anti-HCV	Positive	Acutely or chronically infected
Hepatitis D[b]	IgM anti-HDV HDVAg HBsAg HBeAg Anti-HBc	Positive Positive Positive Positive Positive	Acute HBV-HDV coinfection
Hepatitis E	IgM anti-HEV IgG anti-HEV	Negative Negative	Susceptible to infection
	IgM anti-HEV	Positive	Acutely infected
	IgG anti-HEV	Positive	Immune due to natural infection

Anti-HAV, hepatitis A antibody; anti-HBc, hepatitis B core antibody; anti-HBs, hepatitis B surface antibody; HBsAg, hepatitis B surface antigen; anti-HCV, hepatitis C antibody; anti-HDV, hepatitis D antibody; anti-HEV, hepatitis E antibody; HAV, hepatitis A virus; HBV, hepatitis B virus; HDV, hepatitis D virus; HDVAg, hepatitis D antigen; IgG, immunoglobulin G; IgM, immunoglobulin M.

[a]Centers for Disease Control and Prevention. Hepatology, *http://www.cdc.gov/hepatitis/HBV/PDFs/SerologicChartv8.pdf*.

[b]Hepatitis D should be suspected in those who have HBsAg positivity. Hepatitis D may present as either coinfection where both HDV and HBV serologies appear simultaneously, whereas for superinfection, HBV has been present for some time and later HDV develops.

PREVENTION AND TREATMENT OF VIRAL HEPATITIS

Desired Outcomes

General desired outcomes for treating hepatitis are to: (a) prevent the spread of the disease; (b) prevent and treat symptoms; (c) suppress viral replication; (d) normalize hepatic aminotransferases; (e) improve histology on liver biopsy; and (f) decrease morbidity and mortality by preventing cirrhosis, HCC, and ESLD.

For hepatitis B, additional treatment goals include: (a) seroconversion or loss of HBsAg; (b) seroconversion or loss of HBeAg; and (c) achieving undetectable HBV DNA levels. Additional goals for chronic hepatitis C include achieving undetectable HCV RNA 6 months post hepatitis C therapy by obtaining a sustained virologic response (SVR).[26]

General Approach

Managing viral hepatitis involves both prevention and treatment. Prevention of hepatitis A and B (and indirectly for hepatitis D) can be achieved with immune globulin or vaccines. ❷ *Acute viral hepatitis A, B, C, D, and E are primarily managed with supportive care.* Individuals with

Patient Encounter, Part 1

A 41-year-old Caucasian man is required by his employer to obtain a physical exam. His only complaint is fatigue for the past year that he attributes to working overtime at the steel mill. He has no significant past medical history. He reports being stressed at times from an impending divorce and from needing to take care of his five young children.

PMH: Patient never had any suicidal ideations in the past or history of depression.

PSH: Appendectomy in 1987 at the age of 27 that required blood transfusions

FH: Mother with osteoporosis and father alive and well

SH: He was in a monogamous relationship. Single now with no significant other. Smoked a pack of cigarettes per day times 15 years but quit 5 years ago; used illicit drugs once in the past; drinks daily for the past 30 years; has one tattoo on the left arm done unprofessionally; employed as a steel mill worker

Meds: None

ROS: Complains only of irritability and mild depression; no nausea, vomiting, diarrhea, abdominal pain, or anorexia; never had an episode of jaundice, pale stools, or tea-colored urine

PE:

VS: BP 128/80 mm Hg, P 80 bpm, RR 20/minute, T 37.0°C (98.6°F), wt 70 kg (154 lb), ht 5'9" (175 cm)

Abd: Soft, nontender, normal liver span; no hepato-splenomegaly, no ascites.

Labs:

- Sodium 141 mEq/L (mmol/L), potassium 4.1 mEq/L (mmol/L), chloride 99 mEq/L (mmol/L), CO_2 21 mEq/L (mmol/L), BUN 20 mg/dL (7.14 mmol/L), serum creatinine 1.2 mg/dL (106 μmol/L), glucose 98 mg/dL (5.4 mmol/L)

- Hemoglobin 16.1 g/dL (161 g/L or 10.0 mmol/L), hematocrit 48.4% (0.484), WBC $5.1 \times 10^3/mm^3$ ($\times 10^9$/L), platelets $135 \times 10^3/mm^3$ ($\times 10^9$/L)

- Aspartate aminotransferase (AST) 69 IU/L (1.15 μKat/L), alanine aminotransferase (ALT) 92 IU/L (1.53 μKat/L)

- Total bilirubin 1.0 mg/dL (17.1 μmol/L), albumin 3.7 g/dL (37 g/L), alkaline phosphatase 164 IU/L (2.73 μKat/L), TSH 1.3 micro IU/mL (mIU/L)

- Anti-HAV IgM (−), anti-HAV IgG (−), anti-HBs (+), HBsAg (−), HBeAg (−), anti-HBc IgG (−), anti-HBc IgM (−), anti-HBe (−), HBV DNA less than 2,000 IU/mL, anti-HCV (+), genotype 2; HCV RNA 91,230 IU/mL

- **Liver biopsy:** Mild inflammation and minimal fibrosis (grade 1, stage 1 disease) consistent with chronic hepatitis C

What information is suggestive of viral hepatitis?

What risk factors does he have for viral hepatitis?

What additional information do you need before creating a treatment plan for this patient?

---

mild to moderate symptoms rarely require hospitalization. Occasionally, hospitalization is required in individuals experiencing significant nausea, vomiting, diarrhea, and encephalopathy. Liver transplantation may be required in rare instances if fulminant hepatitis develops.

Patients with viral hepatitis B, C, and D may develop chronic disease leading to ESLD and HCC. Treatment is available for chronic liver disease associated with HBV, HCV, and HDV.[26]

Hepatitis A Prevention

❸ *Good personal hygiene and proper disposal of sanitary waste are required to prevent fecal–oral transmission of the HAV.*[1,4,6] This includes frequent handwashing with soap and water after using the bathroom and prior to eating meals. Drinking bottled water, avoiding fruits, vegetables, and raw shellfish harvested from sewage-contaminated water in areas where HAV is most endemic will also minimize the risk of becoming infected with hepatitis A.

Individuals at high risk of acquiring hepatitis A (Table 24–1) should receive either serum immune globulin or the hepatitis A vaccine, depending on their personal circumstances, as described below.[4,27]

▶ Immune Globulin

Immune globulin (IG) is a solution containing antibodies from sterilized pooled human plasma that provides passive immunization against various infectious diseases, including hepatitis A.[4] Immune globulin is available for either intravenous (IGIV) or intramuscular (IGIM) administration, but only IGIM is used for prevention of hepatitis A. IGIM does not confer lifelong immunity, but it is effective in providing pre- and postexposure prophylaxis against HAV.[4]

Adverse effects of IGIM are rare. There have been reports of anaphylaxis in individuals who have immunoglobulin A deficiency after receiving repeated IG administration. Therefore, these patients should not receive IGIM. IGIM is not contraindicated in pregnant or lactating women or infants requiring hepatitis A immunization. The thimerosal-free preparation should be used in infants.[4]

IGIM should be injected into a deltoid or gluteal muscle. It does not affect the immune response of inactivated vaccines, oral polio virus, or yellow fever vaccine. The administration of live vaccines (e.g., measles, mumps, rubella [MMR] vaccine) concomitantly with IGIM may decrease the immune response significantly; thus, MMR and varicella vaccines should be delayed for at least 3 and 5 months, respectively, after IGIM has been administered. Additionally, IGIM should not be given within 2 weeks of the MMR administration or within 3 weeks of the varicella vaccine to maximize the efficacy of the immunization.[4]

Pre-exposure Prophylaxis Pre-exposure prophylaxis with IGIM is indicated for individuals at high risk of acquiring the HAV who: (a) are less than 12 months of age; (b) elect not to receive the hepatitis A vaccine; or (c) cannot receive the hepatitis A vaccine (e.g., because of allergy to the components alum or 2-phenoxyethanol). Because active vaccine immunity takes several weeks to develop, travelers who are older adults, immunocompromised, have chronic liver disease or other chronic medical conditions who plan to depart for endemic areas within 2 weeks *and* have not received the hepatitis A vaccine should receive IGIM. If the duration of travel is less than 3 months, these individual should receive a dose of IG 0.02 mL/kg and hepatitis A vaccine at the same time, but administered at different injection sites.[4,27]

If the travel duration is expected to be greater than 2 months, then IG at a dose of 0.06 mL/kg should be administered as the higher dose provides immunity up to 5 months. If protection against HAV is required beyond 5 months, then readministration of IGIM is recommended.[4,27]

Postexposure Prophylaxis Individuals in contact with people infected with acute HAV (including household and sexual partners), staff and children from day care facilities, and food handlers of restaurant establishments may be candidates for postexposure prophylaxis. IG is preferred in individuals who are less than 12 months or more than 40 years of age, immunocompromised, diagnosed with chronic liver disease, or have contraindications to the hepatitis A vaccine.[4,27]

The risk of infection may be decreased by 90% if IGIM 0.02 mL/kg is given within 2 weeks of being exposed to the HAV. IGIM may still be beneficial if it is given more than 2 weeks after exposure to a known case of HAV, as it may decrease the severity of hepatic damage.[4,27]

▶ Hepatitis A Vaccine

Persons at risk of acquiring the HAV should receive the hepatitis A vaccine when appropriate. The vaccine is effective in providing pre- and postexposure prophylaxis against clinical hepatitis A infections.[27,28]

Two inactivated hepatitis A vaccines, HAVRIX and VAQTA, are available in the United States and are effective in providing active immunization and preventing clinical hepatitis A. The two vaccines are considered interchangeable, and doses are dependent on age (Table 24–3).[4]

HAVRIX and VAQTA are effective in providing active pre- or postexposure prophylaxis when given in two injections 6 months apart (referred to as months 0 and 6). Efficacy is defined by measuring antibody response with the modified enzyme immunoassay. For HAVRIX, levels greater than 20 mIU/mL (20 IU/L), and for VAQTA, levels greater than 10 mIU/mL (10 IU/L) are considered protective. After administration of the first dose of vaccine, 94% to 100% of adults and 97% to 100% of children and adolescents develop protective antibody concentrations against the HAV. All recipients over 2 years of age receiving the second dose at month 6 have 100% antibody coverage; therefore, postvaccination measurement of antibody response is not required.[4]

For pre-exposure prophylaxis, the hepatitis A vaccine is recommended for travelers to endemic hepatitis A countries. It should be administered to healthy international travelers aged 40 years of age and younger regardless of the scheduled dates for departure. This recommendation does not apply to adults more than 40 years old, the immunocompromised, or those with chronic medical conditions with or without chronic liver disease. These individual who plan to depart to an endemic country in less than 2 weeks should receive both the hepatitis A vaccine and IG (0.02 mL/kg).[27]

For postexposure prophylaxis, the hepatitis A vaccine is effective in preventing clinical infection in healthy individuals between 12 months and 40 years of age when administered within 14 days after exposure.[27,28] Individuals outside these age ranges or with significant comorbid conditions should receive IG for postexposure prophylaxis rather than the hepatitis A vaccine because this population has not been studied.[27]

	Table 24–3				
Recommended Intramuscular Doses of Hepatitis A Vaccines					
Product	Recipient Age (years)	Dose	Volume (mL)	No. of Doses	Schedule (months)
VAQTA	1–18	25 units	0.5	2	0, 6–18
	19 or more	50 units	1	2	0, 6
HAVRIX	1–18	720 ELISA units	0.5	2	0, 6–12
	19 or more	1,440 ELISA units	1	2	0, 6–12

ELISA, enzyme-linked immunosorbent assay.

From Chan J. Viral hepatitis. Pharmacotherapy Self-Assessment Program. 5th ed. Kansas City: MO, American College of Clinical Pharmacy, 2005:1, 4, with permission.

The hepatitis A vaccine may provide effective immunity for 8 years in adults and children. Kinetic models have theorized that immunity may last longer than 20 years, but this has not been confirmed in clinical trials.[4]

The most common adverse effects in adults include injection site reactions (e.g., tenderness, pain, and warmth), headaches within 5 days after vaccination, and fatigue. Children may have feeding disturbances. Local reactions may be minimized by using an appropriate needle length based on the person's age and size and by administering the injection intramuscularly in the deltoid muscle. Hepatitis A vaccine given during pregnancy has not been evaluated in clinical trials. Since both brands of vaccine are made from inactivated HAV, the risk of developing fetal complications should be minimal.

Hepatitis B Prevention

④ *Individuals may minimize their risk of acquiring the hepatitis B infection by avoiding contaminated blood products or indulging in high-risk behavior such as IV drug use.* In addition, those who are at high risk of acquiring the HBV (Table 24–1) should be vaccinated with the hepatitis B vaccine.[10] Screening pregnant women for hepatitis B and providing universal hepatitis B vaccinations to all newborns is effective in preventing hepatitis B infections.[29] In some cases, postexposure prophylaxis with hepatitis B immune globulin (HBIG) may be recommended to prevent the development of acute infection and complications associated with HBV.

▶ *Hepatitis B Immune Globulin*

Hepatitis B immune globulin (HBIG) is a sterile solution containing antibodies prepared from pooled human plasma that has a high concentration of anti-HBs (antibodies to hepatitis B surface antigen). HBIG provides passive immunization for postexposure prophylaxis against the HBV. A single dose of HBIG of 0.06 mL/kg is effective in preventing chronic hepatitis B infections in adults.[10] Similar to IGIM, HBIG should only be administered intramuscularly.

The most common side effects of HBIG include erythema at the injection site, headaches, myalgia, fatigue, urticaria, nausea, and vomiting. Serious adverse effects are rare and may include liver function test abnormalities, arthralgias, and anaphylactic reactions. HBIG should be used with caution in individuals who have experienced hypersensitivity reactions to immune globulin or those who have immunoglobulin A deficiency. Similar to IGIM, concomitant administration of HBIG and live vaccines should be avoided because the efficacy of the immunization may decrease significantly.

▶ *Hepatitis B Vaccine*

The two hepatitis B vaccines available in the United States are Recombivax HB and Engerix-B. These vaccines are produced with recombinant DNA technology by inserting the gene for HBsAg into the plasmid that is synthesized by *Saccharomyces cerevisiae* cells. ⑤ *Persons at high risk (Table 24–1) of acquiring the hepatitis B virus should be vaccinated with the hepatitis B vaccine at months 0, 1, and 6.* The hepatitis B vaccine dose depends on the person's age (Table 24–4).

In addition to pre-exposure prophylaxis, the hepatitis B vaccine is indicated after exposure to the HBV to prevent chronic hepatitis B disease. Adults acutely exposed to blood containing HBsAg from an accidental needlestick, sexual contacts, or IV drug use should be offered hepatitis B vaccine with or without HBIG, preferably within 24 hours of exposure based on the source of exposure and the vaccination status of the exposed person (Table 24–5). Postexposure prophylaxis for perinatal exposure is dependent on several factors, including

---

Table 24–4

Recommended Intramuscular Dosing Regimens for Hepatitis B Vaccines

Product	Patient Categories	Dose (mcg)	Volume (mL)	No. of Doses	Schedule (months)
Recombivax HB	0–19 years of age	5	0.5	3	0, 1, 6
	11–15 years of age[a]	10	1	2	1, 4–6
	20 years of age or older	10	1	3	0, 1, 6
	Hemodialysis[b] less than 20 years of age	5	0.5	3	0, 1, 6
	Hemodialysis 20 years of age or older	40	1	3	0, 1, 6
Engerix-B	0–19 years of age	10	0.5	3	0, 1, 6
	20 years of age or older	20	1	3	0, 1, 6
	Hemodialysis[b] less than 20 years of age	10	0.5	3	0, 1, 6
	Hemodialysis 20 years of age or older	40[c]	2	4	0, 1, 2, 6

[a]Adolescents 11 through 15 years of age may receive either the 5 mcg, three-dose pediatric formulation or a 10 mcg, two-dose regimen using the adult formulation.

[b]Higher doses might be more immunogenic, but no specific recommendations have been made.

[c]Two 1.0-mL doses administered at one site.

Modified from Chan J. Viral hepatitis. Pharmacotherapy Self-Assessment Program. 5th ed. Kansas City, MO: American College of Clinical Pharmacy, 2005:1, 8, with permission.

Table 24–5

Recommendations for Prophylaxis After Nonoccupational Exposure to the Hepatitis B Virus

	Treatment to Administer if Serology Test of Source Person Is:	
Exposed Person's Vaccination Status	HBsAg-Positive	Unknown HBsAg Status
Unvaccinated	HBIG × 1 and initiate HB vaccine series	Initiate HB vaccine series
Previously vaccinated[a]	Administer HB vaccine booster dose	No treatment

HB, hepatitis B; HBsAg, hepatitis B surface antigen; HBIG, hepatitis B immune globulin.

[a]A person who has written documentation of a complete hepatitis B vaccine series and did not receive postvaccination testing.

Table 24–6

Recommendations for Hepatitis B Prophylaxis to Prevent Perinatal Transmission

	Mother's HBsAg Status		
Treatment	Positive	Negative	Unknown
HBIG[a]	Given within 12 hours of birth	None	Test HBsAg. If positive, give within 7 days; if negative, give none
AND			
Hepatitis B vaccine[b]			
Dose 1	Within 12 hours of birth	Based on infant's weight[c]	Within 12 hours of birth
Dose 2	At month 1–2	At month 1–2	At month 1–2
Dose 3[d]	At month 6	At month 6–18	At month 6

[a]0.5 mL intramuscularly in a different site from vaccine.

[b]See Table 24–4 for appropriate hepatitis B vaccine dose.

[c]Full-term infants who are medically stable and weigh 2,000 g or more born to HBsAg-negative mothers should receive the hepatitis B vaccine before hospital discharge. Preterm infants weighing less than 2,000 g born to HBsAg-negative mothers should receive the first dose of hepatitis B vaccine 1 month after birth or at hospital discharge.

[d]The final dose in the vaccine series should not be administered before age 24 weeks (164 days).

From Centers for Disease Control and Prevention. A Comprehensive Immunization Strategy to Eliminate Transmission of Hepatitis B Virus Infection in the United States. Recommendations of the Advisory Committee on Immunization Practices (ACIP) Part 1: Immunization of Infants, Children, and Adolescents.

maternal HBsAg status and newborns weight.[29] For mothers who are HBsAg-positive, newborns should be immunized within 12 to 24 hours after birth with both the hepatitis B vaccine and HBIG 0.5 mL. If the mother is HBsAg-negative, the newborn should be given only the hepatitis B vaccine (Table 24–6).

For optimal response, the hepatitis B vaccine should only be administered intramuscularly (into the anterolateral thigh region in neonates and infants; the deltoid region in older children and adults) and not intravenously or intradermally. The vaccine should not be given in the gluteal region, as it may result in lower rates of immunity.

The efficacy of the hepatitis B vaccine occurs when antibody concentrations are greater than 10 mIU/mL (10 IU/L). Because most people who complete the vaccination series obtain adequate antibody levels, postvaccination testing is not routinely recommended. The immunogenicity rate is greater than 90% at completion of the three-dose hepatitis B immunization series.[10] This regimen is also 85% to 95% effective in preventing perinatal HBV infections.[29] The hepatitis B vaccine may provide effective immunity for 10 to 15 years in children and adolescents; however, there may be an anamnestic response requiring booster doses.[30,31]

Protective antibody levels may be lower in older adults and immunocompromised patients, so postvaccine testing may be warranted 1 to 6 months after completing the vaccination series in these patients.[10]

The most frequent adverse effects are local reactions at the injection site (pain, tenderness, erythema, swelling, and pruritus), fever, headaches, dizziness, and irritability. Anaphylaxis, a serum sickness–like hypersensitivity syndrome, chronic fatigue syndrome, and neurologic diseases (leukoencephalitis, optic neuritis, and transverse myelitis) have been reported rarely.[10] Hepatitis B vaccine is not contraindicated during pregnancy.[10]

▶ *Hepatitis A and B Combination Vaccine*

6 *A vaccine that combines both inactivated hepatitis A and recombinant hepatitis B (Twinrix) is approved for immunizing individuals more than 18 years of age with indications for* *both hepatitis A and B vaccines.*[10] A 1-mL dose of Twinrix contains the antigenic components of not less than 720 ELISA units of Havrix and 20 mcg of recombinant HBsAg protein of Engerix-B and should be administered at months 0, 1, and 6. Antibody seroconversion for hepatitis A and B was greater than 98% in adult volunteers tested 1 month after a three-dose vaccine series. The side-effect profile of Twinrix is similar to giving each vaccine separately.[32]

Chronic Hepatitis B Treatment

Patients who are immune tolerant or have inactive hepatitis B (defined as having a positive HBsAg, normal ALT, high or low HBV DNA levels, and mild/minimal inflammation and fibrosis) should not receive treatment because hepatitis B antiviral agents rarely result in HBeAg seroconversion, and long-term treatment leads to drug resistance.[33] Patients with elevated ALT (more than two times the upper limit of normal) and positive HBV DNA levels require treatment to delay progression to cirrhosis and prevent the development of ESLD.

Chronic hepatitis B may be separated into two main types: (a) HBeAg-positive (also known as wild type), and (b) HBeAg-negative (known as precore mutant or promoter mutant). The treatment endpoints for HBeAg-positive patients are different from those who are HBeAg-negative because the latter disease does not allow for HBeAg seroconversion.

Patients with HBeAg-positive chronic hepatitis B have elevated HBV DNA concentrations greater than 20,000 IU/mL and detectable HBeAg. In contrast, patients with HBeAg-negative chronic hepatitis B have HBV DNA concentrations greater than 2,000 IU/mL and undetectable serum HBeAg. Thus, an undetectable HBV DNA level, not seroconversion, is considered a treatment endpoint. HBeAg-negative HBV infections are more likely to lead to liver fibrosis and may require lifelong treatment because undetectable HBV DNA levels are difficult to achieve.

❼ *The drug of choice for chronic hepatitis B depends upon the patient's past medical history, ALT, HBV DNA level, HBeAg status, severity of liver disease, and history of previous HBV therapy.* The safety and efficacy profile of the medication and the likelihood of developing drug resistance should also be considered.

Entecavir and tenofovir are recommended as first-line chronic hepatitis B treatments due to profound HBV DNA suppression and minimal resistance.[34] Pegylated interferon α-2a is also considered a first-line agent because it lacks drug resistance. Pegylated interferon has replaced unmodified interferon because the pegylated form may be given subcutaneously once weekly rather than three times weekly.

Adefovir is second-line to tenofovir because adefovir is less potent in suppressing hepatitis B viral replication in treatment-naïve patients. Lamivudine is no longer recommended as first-line therapy due to its high rate of resistance.[34,35] Patients who are being treated with adefovir or lamivudine and currently responding to treatment should continue with the regimen. However, if there is inadequate virologic response or drug resistance develops, then adding

another hepatitis B antiretroviral agent or switching to a more potent drug should be considered. The role of telbivudine in therapy is undetermined due to its intermediate rate of resistance.[35] Each therapeutic agent will be described briefly in the sections that follow.

▶ *Interferon and Peyglated Interferon*

Interferon α-2b and pegylated interferon α-2a are the only interferon therapies approved for treatment of chronic hepatitis B. Unlike other antiretroviral treatments, interferon therapy is effective in suppressing, and in some cases ceasing, viral replication without inducing resistance.

Approximately one-third of HBeAg-positive patients become seronegative after 4 to 6 months of treatment.[36,37] Patients with HBeAg-negative hepatitis B may require 12 to 24 months of therapy to achieve an SVR.[38,39] The durability of response (likelihood of achieving and sustaining HBeAg seroconversion) is greater than 80% after treatment discontinuation.

Pegylated interferon is interferon that is attached to a polyethylene glycol molecule that increases the half-life of the drug allowing once-weekly dosing versus thrice-weekly administration of unmodified interferon. Pegylated interferon is well-tolerated with similar or better efficacy than unmodified interferon for the treatment of chronic hepatitis B.[34,35] However, it should not be used in patients with decompensated liver disease (because it may induce hepatic failure) or in those with significant and unstable medical comorbidities.[33]

The subcutaneous dose of interferon α-2b (Intron-A) is either 5 million units daily (better tolerated) or 10 million units three times weekly. The recommended treatment duration is 16 to 24 *weeks* for HBeAg-positive disease and 12 to 24 *months* for HBeAg-negative disease.[35] The approved dose of pegylated interferon α-2a (Pegasys) for chronic hepatitis B is 180 mcg subcutaneously once weekly for 48 weeks.[37] Interferon doses may need to be adjusted in patients with cytopenias and renal impairment.

Even though the advantages of interferon or pegylated interferon include a finite duration of treatment, lack of resistance, and possible HBsAg loss or seroconversion (development of anti-HBs), there are several significant disadvantages. These include the need for subcutaneous injections and a pronounced adverse-effect profile that may require dosage reductions or treatment discontinuation. The most common adverse effects include injection site reactions and flu-like symptoms (fevers, chills, joint pain, and muscle aches). Systemic adverse effects include fatigue, headache, insomnia, irritability, depression, suicidal ideation, alopecia, and dermatitis. Other rare but significant systemic untoward effects include endocrine abnormalities (thyroid, diabetes), hypertriglyceridemia, GI (diarrhea, anorexia, nausea) and possible ophthalmic changes. Hematologic abnormalities are common including neutropenia, anemia, and thrombocytopenia, which may require either a dose reduction or treatment discontinuation. Refer to the subsequent section on hepatitis C for management of these adverse effects. Approximately 35% of patients develop an ALT flare when treated with interferon. An increase in ALT has been associated with a positive response, but it may lead to hepatic decompensation, which can be fatal. Thus, only patients with compensated liver disease should be considered for treatment with interferon therapy.

▶ Entecavir

Entecavir (Baraclude) is a guanosine nucleoside analogue that is highly potent in inhibiting HBV DNA polymerase. Entecavir is effective against HBeAg-positive, HBeAg-negative, and lamivudine-resistant chronic hepatitis B.[34,40–43] Resistance rates are low (1–2%) in patients treated with entecavir for up to 5 years in lamivudine-naïve individuals. For patients who were previously treated with lamivudine and switched to entecavir, the resistance rate is approximately 50% at 5 years.[34]

The dose of entecavir is 0.5 mg once daily for patients naïve to lamivudine and 1 mg once daily for those with lamivudine resistance. Dosage adjustments are required in patients with renal dysfunction. The side effect profile for entecavir is similar to lamivudine and adefovir dipivoxil. Patients treated with entecavir should be monitored for signs and symptoms of lactic acidosis and severe hepatomegaly with steatosis, because some cases have been fatal.

The package labeling for entecavir contains a "black-box" warning indicating that there is a potential for development of resistance to HIV nucleoside reverse transcriptase inhibitors if entecavir is used to treat chronic hepatitis B in patients with untreated HIV infection. Therefore, entecavir monotherapy should not be initiated in patients coinfected with HIV and HBV because resistance to highly active antiretroviral therapy (HAART) may occur.[44]

▶ Tenofovir Disoproxil Fumarate

Tenofovir disoproxil fumarate (Viread) is an acyclic adenine nucleotide reverse transcriptase inhibitor that is similar in structure to adefovir dipivoxil. Tenofovir inhibits HIV and hepatitis B viral replication and is indicated for HBeAg-positive and HBeAg-negative chronic hepatitis B with compensated liver disease.

Tenofovir is preferred over adefovir for chronic hepatitis B infections because of greater effectiveness in inhibiting viral replication and lack of resistance at week 72.[34,45,46] Patients who developed resistance to lamivudine, entecavir or adefovir may benefit from tenofovir.[47–49]

The dose of tenofovir disoproxil fumarate is 300 mg orally once daily. Dose adjustments are required in patients with renal dysfunction because tenofovir is primarily renally excreted. Tenofovir is well-tolerated with adverse effects similar to adefovir and other hepatitis B oral agents. Several case reports have implicated tenofovir in causing nephrotoxicity and Fanconi's syndrome in patients coinfected with HIV and HBV.[50,51] Patients should be monitored for signs and symptoms of lactic acidosis and severe hepatomegaly with steatosis because some cases have been fatal. Hepatic function should be carefully monitored if treatment is to be discontinued because severe acute exacerbations of hepatitis have been reported with antihepatitis B viral agents.

▶ Adefovir Dipivoxil

Adefovir dipivoxil (Hepsera) is a prodrug of adefovir, an adenosine nucleotide analog that inhibits DNA polymerase. It is effective against HIV and HBV, including HBV resistant to lamivudine, entecavir, tenofovir, and telbivudine. Treatment with adefovir dipivoxil 10 mg daily is comparable to lamivudine in normalizing aminotransferase levels and improving histologic activity.[52–54] Resistance to adefovir dipivoxil is minimal for the first few years of treatment but increases to approximately 30% after 5 years of therapy.[35,55]

The dose of adefovir dipivoxil is 10 mg once daily. The most common side effects include asthenia, abdominal pain, diarrhea, dyspepsia, headaches, nausea, and flatulence. Adefovir dipivoxil is also associated with dose-related nephrotoxicity, which was most commonly seen in HIV patients receiving doses larger than 60 mg. Serum creatinine monitoring is recommended to detect renal tubular injury. The dose must be reduced in patients with renal insufficiency.

▶ Lamivudine

Lamivudine (Epivir-HBV) is an oral synthetic cytosine nucleoside analogue having antiviral effects against HIV and hepatitis B virus. In patients with chronic hepatitis B, lamivudine is effective in suppressing hepatitis B viral replication, normalizing ALT levels, and improving liver histology.[33,56,57] Patients with chronic hepatitis B may have a similar or a superior response in achieving these endpoints when compared to interferon or pegylated interferon.[34]

However, prolonged lamivudine therapy (up to 5 years) may be needed to sustain seroconversion, and lamivudine resistance is as high as 60% to 70% at 5 years.[34,35] Due to the high rate of resistance, lamivudine is no longer recommended as first-line therapy for chronic hepatitis B.[34]

The dose of lamivudine is 100 mg orally once daily for treatment of chronic hepatitis B without HIV coinfections. The dose must be adjusted in patients with renal dysfunction.

Adverse effects are minimal and include fatigue, diarrhea, nausea, vomiting, and headaches. ALT levels should be monitored carefully, as two- to threefold increases may be observed. ALT should also be monitored closely when lamivudine therapy is being discontinued, as increased levels may indicate a flare in disease activity leading to liver failure.

▶ Telbivudine

Telbivudine (Tyzeka) is an L-nucleoside analogue that inhibits HBV replication. It is indicated for HBeAg-positive and HBeAg-negative chronic hepatitis B with compensated liver disease.

Telbivudine offers a slightly more effective reduction in HBV DNA levels and normalization of aminotransferases when compared to lamivudine. However, its benefits in improving histology, HBeAg seroconversion, and HBeAg loss remain to be confirmed.[58] Telbivudine resistance is lower than with lamivudine, but rates are significant with continued treatment.

The dose of telbivudine is 600 mg orally once daily. Dosage adjustments are required in patients with renal dysfunction.

Adverse effects are similar to other HBV oral agents. Patients should be monitored for signs and symptoms of lactic acidosis and severe hepatomegaly with steatosis, because some cases have been fatal. Myopathy characterized by elevated creatine kinase levels and muscle weakness have been associated with telbivudine.[58] ALT and AST levels may become elevated while on treatment at rates similar to lamivudine. Telbivudine lacks HIV activity, and it is not recommended for use in patients coinfected with HIV and HBV because HIV drug resistance may develop with telbivudine monotherapy.

Hepatitis C Prevention

The risk factors for hepatitis C and hepatitis B are quite similar; thus, the risk of acquiring the HCV is minimized by avoiding contaminated blood products and high-risk behaviors such as sharing needles among IV drug users. The risk of HCV transmission through a blood transfusion is 1 in 2 million.[59] No vaccines are available for preventing hepatitis C, but several are under development.[60] High-risk individuals (Table 24–1) should be tested for HCV since most patients will be asymptomatic and unaware they are infected.[17]

Chronic Hepatitis C Treatment

Individuals with confirmed chronic hepatitis C should be evaluated for treatment with pegylated interferon with or without ribavirin. Interferon α-2a (Roferon A), interferon α-2b (Intron-A), and interferon alfacon-1 (Infergen) are approved for chronic hepatitis C but are no longer recommended because only 12% to 16% of patients achieve an SVR.[61,62]

Pegylated interferon α-2a (Pegasys) and pegylated interferon α-2b (PEG-Intron) are the preferred treatments for hepatitis C.[63,64] Pegylated interferons (interferon attached to polyethylene glycol) have an extended half-life, allowing for once-weekly administration. The SVR to pegylated interferon alone (SVR 25–40%) can be increased by adding ribavirin, a synthetic guanosine analog that inhibits viral polymerase (SVR 45–55%). Consequently, pegylated interferon plus ribavirin is the regimen of choice for chronic hepatitis C.[61,62]

The most important predictor of response to pegylated interferon is the patient's genotype. Individuals with genotype 2 or 3 achieve a higher SVR than patients with genotype 1.[63,64] Genotype also determines the duration of therapy. The recommended treatment duration for individuals with genotype 2 and 3 is 24 weeks and 48 weeks for genotype 1.[61,62]

Pegylated interferon is administered subcutaneously and may be given as either a fixed dose or based on body weight. The recommended dose of pegylated interferon α-2a (Pegasys) is 180 mcg once weekly and the adult dose of pegylated interferon α-2b (PEG-Intron) is 1.5 mcg/kg/week.

According to recommended treatment guidelines, the dose of ribavirin is weight based for patients with genotype 1 (less than 75 kg = 1,000 mg daily; 75 kg or more = 1,200 mg daily), whereas genotype 2 and 3 patients receive 800 mg daily regardless of weight.[61,62] The ribavirin dose must be reduced in patients with renal impairment and is contraindicated in patients with creatinine clearance less than 50 mL/min.

Adherence to therapy is an important factor in increasing and maintaining SVR. Patients who were adherent with pegylated interferon and ribavirin therapy (taking more than 80% of doses for more than 80% of the treatment duration) had an SVR of 52% whereas those who were not compliant had an SVR of 44%.[65]

▶ *Management of Adverse Effects From Interferon, Pegylated Interferon, and Ribavirin*

The type and incidence of adverse effects associated with unmodified interferon and pegylated interferon are similar. Approximately 10% to 30% of patients receiving hepatitis C medications require a dose reduction or treatment discontinuation to minimize side effects.

Most patients treated with pegylated interferon experience flu-like symptoms (fevers, chills, rigors, and myalgias). These symptoms may be mild to moderate in severity and usually occur with the first injection and diminish with continued treatment. The flu-like symptoms may be minimized by premedication with acetaminophen or nonsteroidal anti-inflammatory drugs. Patients may also self-administer pegylated interferon prior to bedtime so they can sleep through it.

Psychiatric adverse effects occur frequently and may include irritability, depression, and rarely, suicidal ideation. Individuals with a history of uncontrolled psychiatric disorders must weigh the risk versus benefit of treatment, as pegylated interferon may exacerbate or worsen the psychiatric condition. Patients who develop mild to moderate psychiatric symptoms may require antidepressants or anxiolytics. Those with severe symptoms including suicidal ideation should discontinue treatment immediately.[62]

Several hematologic abnormalities are associated with pegylated interferon plus ribavirin therapy. Up to 35% of patients require either a dosage reduction or drug discontinuation due to thrombocytopenia, neutropenia, or anemia.[66] A decrease in platelet count of 25% to 30% usually occurs within 6 to 8 weeks after initiation of treatment. Decreasing the dose or discontinuing interferon therapy is rarely required because of significant thrombocytopenia (defined as a platelet count less than $50 \times 10^3/mm^3$ [less than $50 \times 10^9/L$]). However, caution is required in patients with cirrhosis because they may already have low platelet counts prior to starting treatment. Approved therapies for thrombocytopenia are not recommended for interferon-induced thrombocytopenia due to significant adverse effects including pulmonary edema and cardiac arrhythmias. Several pharmacologic agents are under investigation for patients with thrombocytopenia due to chronic liver disease and interferon-induced thrombocytopenia.[67] The interferon dose should either be reduced or discontinued if the platelet count declines significantly or symptoms of bruising and bleeding are present.

Neutropenia associated with interferon therapy is defined as an absolute neutrophil count (ANC) of less than $1.0 \times 10^3/mm^3$ ($1.0 \times 10^9/L$). In rare cases, an ANC less than $0.5 \times 10^3/mm^3$ ($0.5 \times 10^9/L$) may be observed. The neutropenia is more common and in some cases more severe with pegylated interferon than with unmodified interferon. Neutropenia usually occurs within the first 2 weeks after initiating either formulation of interferon, with the WBC count stabilizing by week 4 or 6. Neutropenia is reversible upon discontinuing therapy. Granulocyte colony-stimulating factor has been used as an adjunctive therapy for pegylated interferon-induced neutropenia.[68,69]

Ribavirin causes a dose-related hemolytic anemia, which is more common in patients receiving weight-base dosing than in those taking fixed doses.[70] After treatment initiation, the hemoglobin concentration may decrease by 2.5 to 3 g/dL (25–30 g/L or 1.55–1.86 mmol/L) from baseline within 4 weeks. In addition, interferon may slightly suppress bone marrow erythroprogenitor cells. Therefore, a "mixed" anemia (hemolytic anemia and bone marrow suppression occurring simultaneously) develops when both pegylated interferon and ribavirin are used. This is a reversible process with the hemoglobin level returning to baseline within 7 to 8 weeks after either drug has been discontinued. Patients treated taking pegylated interferon and ribavirin may require dosage reductions when hemoglobin levels decrease to less than 10.5 g/dL (105 g/L or 6.51 mmol/L) or they develop intolerable symptoms such as shortness of breath or severe fatigue. Discontinuing ribavirin and blood transfusions may be needed in rare cases when the hemoglobin level falls below 8.5 g/dL (85 g/L or 5.27 mmol/L). If warranted, erythropoietin or darbepoetin-α may be used as adjunctive therapy for ribavirin-induced hemolytic anemia.[68,70]

All women of childbearing age and men who are able to father a child should use two forms of contraception during ribavirin therapy and 6 months after treatment because ribavirin has been documented to cause teratogenic and embryocidal effects.

Hepatitis D Prevention and Treatment

8 *Hepatitis D infection is possible only if the patient also has the hepatitis B virus present; therefore, hepatitis B vaccination can indirectly prevent hepatitis D infection.* Although there are no FDA-approved treatments for hepatitis D, interferon and pegylated interferon have been shown to be effective in normalizing aminotransferase levels and sustaining virologic response.[71] Various interferon doses have been evaluated, with the most effective treatment being 9 million units three times weekly.[72] Seventy-one percent of patients who were treated with

this regimen for 48 weeks had normalized ALT levels.[72] Several small trials have evaluated pegylated interferon for HDV with conflicting results.[71] Adverse effects and monitoring parameters for interferon and pegylated interferon are similar to treatment for hepatitis C. In some situations, patients infected with hepatitis D who develop hepatic decompensation and ESLD may need to undergo liver transplantation.

Hepatitis E Prevention and Treatment

Hepatitis E is similar to hepatitis A in that the mode of transmission is via the fecal–oral route. Therefore, the most effective ways to prevent acquiring the virus are good personal hygiene and proper disposal of sanitary waste. Frequent handwashing and avoiding contaminated foods and vegetables decrease the risk of infection.

At present, only acute cases of hepatitis E have been documented.[21,22] Currently there are no commercially approved vaccines available to prevent hepatitis E; however, a recombinant hepatitis E vaccine undergoing Phase II/III study has produced promising preliminary results.[73]

OUTCOME EVALUATION

- Monitoring for efficacy in patients treated for chronic hepatitis B or C includes evaluating aminotransferase levels and viral loads.

Patient Encounter, Part 3

The patient has received treatment for hepatitis C for 4 weeks, and the following laboratory results have just been obtained:

- Sodium 138 mEq/L (mmol/L), potassium 4.0 mEq/L (mmol/L), chloride 98 mEq/L (mmol/L), CO_2 19 mEq/L (mmol/L), BUN 21 mg/dL (7.50 mmol/L), serum creatinine 1.0 mg/dL (88 µmol/L), glucose 103 mg/dL (5.7 mmol/L)

- Hemoglobin 10.1 g/dL (101 g/L or 6.3 mmol/L), hematocrit 30.3% (0.303), WBC 2.2 × 10³/mm³ (× 10⁹/L), platelets 104 × 10³/mm³ (× 10⁹/L), ANC 0.92 × 10³/mm³ (× 10⁹/L)

- AST 41 IU/L (0.68 µKat/L), ALT 32 IU/L (0.53 µKat/L)

- Total bilirubin 1.0 mg/dL (17.1 µmol/L), albumin 3.6 g/dL (36 g/L), alkaline phosphatase 168 IU/L (2.8 µKat/L),

What questions should you ask the patient?

What action should you take at this time?

Patient Encounter, Part 2: Creating a Care Plan

Based on the information presented, create a care plan for this patient's hepatitis. Your plan should include:

(a) a statement of the drug-related needs and/or problems;
(b) the goals of therapy;
(c) a patient-specific detailed therapeutic plan;
(d) a follow-up plan to determine whether the goals have been achieved; and (e) a follow-up plan to identify potential adverse effects of therapy.

Patient Encounter, Part 4

What additional information should you counsel your patient about in addition to the side effects associated with the hepatitis C therapy?

Hepatitis B

- Monitor ALT every 12 weeks and HBV DNA levels every 12 to 24 weeks to determine treatment response in all patients with chronic hepatitis B undergoing HBV therapy.[34,35]

- Monitor HBeAg and anti-HBe every 24 weeks to determine if seroconversion to anti-HBe occurred or HBeAg was lost in patients with HBeAg-positive chronic hepatitis B.[35,74]

- Monitor HBsAg every 6 to 12 months to determine if HBsAg was lost or anti-HBs developed in patients with HBeAg-negative chronic hepatitis B with persistently undetectable serum HBV DNA levels.[35,74]

- Reevaluate the patient at month 6 and add a more potent hepatitis B antiviral agent to the current hepatitis B regimen if the viral count remains 2,000 IU/mL or more.[34]

- Continue treatment in patients who achieved complete virologic response (HBV DNA level less than 60 IU/mL) by week 24.

- Obtain a CBC with differential every 4 weeks and thyroid stimulating hormone and fasting lipid panel evaluated every 12 weeks in patients undergoing pegylated interferon therapy for hepatitis B.[35]

- For patients receiving tenofovir or adefovir, monitor serum creatinine for nephrotoxicity at baseline and every 12 weeks.

- For patients taking telbivudine, monitor creatine kinase at baseline and periodically (e.g., every 12 weeks), as muscle weakness and myopathy have been observed with therapy.[35,50,51,58]

Hepatitis C

- SVR is defined as having an undetectable viral load or HCV RNA level at 6 months post treatment.[61,62]

- Biochemical response is defined as normalization of ALT; monitor ALT levels every 4 weeks.

- Histologic response is defined as improving inflammation and fibrosis as noted by liver biopsy scores. Repeat liver biopsies are conducted primarily in the setting of clinical trials.

- Check the HCV RNA level at week 12 of therapy to determine the effectiveness of treatment. Discontinue treatment if the HCV RNA has not decreased by at least 2 logs or become undetectable by week 12.

- For patient with genotype 1 HCV: If the HCV RNA level is undetectable at week 12 of therapy, continue treatment for at least another 36 weeks (48 weeks total). Obtain an HCV RNA level to determine end-of-treatment response at the end of the 48-week treatment and repeat at 6 months post-therapy to determine SVR.

- For patients with genotype 2 and 3 HCV: Check the HCV RNA level at week 12. If HCV RNA is undetectable, continue treatment for a total of 24 weeks. Repeat the HCV RNA 24 weeks after completion of therapy to determine SVR.

- In patients receiving treatment with pegylated interferon with or without ribavirin, monitor the WBC, ANC, platelets, and hemoglobin levels either weekly or biweekly

Patient Care and Monitoring

1. Evaluate the patient for risk factors for acquiring viral hepatitis (Table 24–1).

2. Educate patients to avoid hepatotoxic agents (e.g., some dietary supplements).

3. Educate patients to avoid consuming any alcohol if viral hepatitis has been diagnosed. Alcohol may further worsen the liver disease and if on treatment, may decrease the effectiveness of therapy.

4. Determine if the patient has been vaccinated against hepatitis A and B. If not, then vaccinate accordingly (Tables 24–3 and 24–4).

5. Obtain a thorough past medical history focusing on psychiatric disorders, cardiac disorders, endocrine disease, and renal insufficiency.

6. Review the liver biopsy report (if available) to determine the severity of liver damage and need for chronic hepatitis B or C treatment.

7. Assess for adverse effects in patients with hepatitis B or C treated with pegylated interferon with or without ribavirin.

8. Encourage medication compliance with viral hepatitis treatments to increase the SVR.

9. Encourage patients to drink at least 8 glasses of water to prevent dehydration while on hepatitis C medications.

10. Educate all women of childbearing age and men who are able to father a child to use two forms of contraception during and 6 months after ribavirin therapy.

11. Provide patient education:

    - How to prevent viral hepatitis transmission

    - Who should be vaccinated against hepatitis A and B

    - Importance of taking all medications at scheduled times

    - Adverse effects of interferon, pegylated interferon, and ribavirin therapy

    - How to self-administer interferon and pegylated interferon injections

    - Importance of appropriate disposal of used needles

during the first month of therapy and monthly thereafter if stable.

- Monitor thyroid stimulating hormone and fasting lipid panel every 12 weeks while on hepatitis C treatment.

- Monitor serum creatinine in patients receiving ribavirin to detect renal insufficiency that may result in ribavirin accumulation and toxicity (e.g., hemolytic anemia).

Abbreviations Introduced in This Chapter

ALT	Alanine aminotransferase
ANC	Absolute neutrophil count
Anti-HAV	Hepatitis A virus antibody
Anti-HBc	Hepatitis B core antibody
Anti-HBe	Hepatitis B envelope antibody
Anti-HBs	Hepatitis B surface antibody
Anti-HCV	Hepatitis C antibody
Anti-HDV	Hepatitis D antibody
Anti-HEV	Hepatitis E antibody
AST	Aspartate aminotransferase
CrCl	Creatinine clearance
ESLD	End-stage liver disease
HAV	Hepatitis A virus
HBcAg	Hepatitis B core antigen
HBeAg	Hepatitis B envelope antigen
HBIG	Hepatitis B immunoglobulin
HBsAg	Hepatitis B surface antigen
HBV	Hepatitis B virus
HBV DNA	Hepatitis B deoxyribonucleic acid
HCV	Hepatitis C virus
HCV RNA	Hepatitis C virus ribonucleic acid
HDV	Hepatitis D virus
HDVAg	Hepatitis D antigen
HDV RNA	Hepatitis D virus ribonucleic acid
HEV	Hepatitis E virus
IgG	Immunoglobulin G
IgG anti-HD	IgG antibodies to hepatitis D virus antigen
IgM	Immunoglobulin M
IgM anti-HD	IgM antibodies to hepatitis D virus antigen
IG	Immune globulin
IGIM	Immune globulin for intramuscular administration
IGIV	Immune globulin for intravenous administration
MMR	Measles, mumps, rubella vaccine
PCR	Polymerase chain reaction
SVR	Sustained virologic response

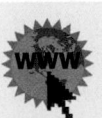

Self-assessment questions and answers are available at *http://www.mhpharmacotherapy. com/pp.html.*

REFERENCES

1. World Health Organization. Department of Communicable Disease Surveillance and Response. WHO/CDS/CSR/EDC/2000.7. *http://www.who.int/csr/disease/hepatitis/whocdscsredc2007/en/index.html.*

2. Centers for Disease Control and Prevention (CDC). Hepatitis A outbreak associated with green onions at a restaurant—Monaca, Pennsylvania, 2003. MMWR Morb Mortal Wkly Rep 2003;52(47):1155–1157.

3. Wasley A, Samandari T, Bell BP. Incidence of hepatitis A in the U.S. in the era of vaccination. JAMA 2005;294:194–201.

4. Advisory Committee on Immunization Practices (ACIP), Fiore AE, Wasley A, Bell BP. Prevention of hepatitis A through active or passive immunization: recommendations of the Advisory Committee on Immunization Practices (ACIP). MMWR Recomm Rep 2006;55(RR-7):1–23.

5. Zhou F, Shefer A, Weinbaum C, et al. Impact of hepatitis A vaccination on health care utilization in the U.S., 1996–2004. Vaccine 2007;25:3581–3587.

6. Fiore AE. Hepatitis A transmitted by food. Clin Infect Dis 2004;38:705–715.

7. Keystone JS, Hershey JH. The underestimated risk of hepatitis A and hepatitis B: Benefits of an accelerated vaccination schedule. Int J Infect Dis 2008;12:3–11.

8. World Health Organization. Hepatitis B. *http://www.who.int/mediacentre/factsheets/fs204/en/.*

9. World Health Organization. Hepatitis B Vaccines. Weekly epidemiological record 2004;79:253–264.

10. Mast EE, Weinbaum CM, Fiore AE, et al. A comprehensive immunization strategy to eliminate transmission of hepatitis B virus infection in the U.S.: Recommendations of the Advisory Committee on Immunization Practices (ACIP) Part II: Immunization of adults. MMWR Recomm Rep 2006;55(RR-16):1–33.

11. Pan CQ, Zhang JX. Natural history and clinical con-sequences of hepatitis B virus infection. Int J Med Sci 2005;2:36–40.

12. McMahon BJ. The natural history of chronic hepatitis B virus infection. Semin Liver Dis 2004;24(suppl 1):17–21.

13. World Health Organization. Department of Communi-cable Disease Surveillance and Response. WHO/CDS/CSR/LYO/2003. Hepatitis C. *http://www.who.int/csr/disease/hepatitis/whocdscsrlyo2003/en/index.html.*

14. Rustgi VK. The epidemiology of hepatitis C infection in the U.S. J Gastroenterol 2007;42:513–521.

15. Missiha SB. Ostrowski M. Heathcote EJ. Disease progression in chronic hepatitis C: Modifiable and nonmodifiable factors. Gastroenterology 2008;134:1699–1714.

16. Lauer GM, Walker BD. Hepatitis C virus infection. N Engl J Med 2001;345:41–52.

17. Centers for Disease Control and Prevention. Recommen-dations for prevention and control of hepatitis C virus (HCV) infection and HCV-related chronic disease. MMWR Recomm Rep 1998;47(RR-19):1–39.

18. World Health Organization, Department of Communicable Disease Surveillance and Response. Hepatitis delta. *http://www.who.int/csr/disease/hepatitis/HepatitisD_whocdscsrncs2001_1.pdf.*

19. Hsieh TH, Liu CJ, Chen DS, Chen PJ. Natural course and treatment of hepatitis D virus infection. J Formos Med Assoc 2006;105:869–881.

20. Shakil AO, Hadziyannis S, Hoofnagle JH, et al. Geographic distribution and genetic variability of hepatitis delta virus genotype I. Virology 1997;160–167.

21. Purcell RH, Emerson SU. Hepatitis E: An emerging awareness of an old disease. J Hepatol 2008;48:494–503.

22. World Health Organization, Department of Communicable Disease Surveillance and Response. Hepatitis E. *http://www.who.int/csr/disease/hepatitis/HepatitisE_whocdscsredc2001_12.pdf.*

23. Martin A, Lemon SM. Hepatitis A Virus: From Discovery to Vaccines. Hepatology 2006;43(2 Suppl 1):S164–S172.

24. Ganem D, Prince AM. Hepatitis B virus infection-natural history and clinical consequences. N Engl J Med 2004;350:1118–1129.

25. EASL Jury. EASL International Consensus Conference on Hepatitis B: September 13–14, 2002: Geneva, Switzerland. Consensus statement (short version). J Hepatol 2003;38:533–540.

26. Lisker-Melman M, Sayuk GS. Defining optimal therapeutic outcomes in chronic hepatitis. Arch Med Res 2007;38:652–660.

27. Centers for Disease Control and Prevention (CDC). Prevention of hepatitis A after exposure to hepatitis A virus and in international travellers. Updated recommendations of the advisory committee on immunization practices (ACIP). MMWR Recomm Rep 2007;56;41:1080–1084.

28. Victor JC, Monto AS, Surdina TY, et al. Hepatitis A vaccine versus immune globulin for postexposure prophylaxis. N Engl J Med 2007;357:1685–1694.

29. Mast EE, Margolis HS, Fiore AE, et al. A comprehensive immunization strategy to eliminate transmission of hepatitis B virus infection in the U.S: Recommendations of the Advisory Committee on Immunization Practices (ACIP) part 1: Immunization of infants, children, and adolescents. MMWR Recomm Rep 2005;54(RR-16):1–31.

30. Gabbuti A, Romanò L, Blanc P, et al. Long-term immunogenicity of hepatitis B vaccination in a cohort of Italian healthy adolescents. Vaccine 2007;25:3129–3132.

31. Bialek SR, Bower WA, Novak R, et al. Persistence of protection against hepatitis B virus infection among adolescents vaccinated with recombinant hepatitis B vaccine beginning at birth: A 15-year follow-up study. Pediatr Infect Dis J 2008;27:881–885.

32. Murdoch DL, Goa K, Figgitt DP. Combined hepatitis A and B vaccines: A review of their immunogenicity and tolerability. Drugs 2003;63:2625–2649.

33. National Institutes Of Health Consensus Development Conference Statement. Management of Hepatitis B. October 20–22, 2008. *http://consensus.nih.gov/2008/hebB%20draft%20statement%20102208_FINAL.pdf.*

34. Keeffe EB, Dieterich DT, Han SH, et al. A treatment algorithm for the management of chronic hepatitis B virus infection in the U.S.: 2008 update. Clin Gastroenterol Hepatol 2008 Aug 23. [Epub ahead of print].

35. Lok AS, McMahon BJ. Chronic hepatitis B. Hepatology 2007;45:507–539.

36. Lau D T-Y, Everhart J, Kleiner DE, et al. Long-term follow-up of patients with chronic hepatitis B treated with interferon alfa. Gastroenterology 1997;113:1660–1667.

37. van Zonneveld M, Honkoop P, Hansen BE, et al. Long-term follow-up of alpha-interferon treatment of patients with chronic hepatitis B. Hepatology 2004;39:804–810.

38. Manesis EK, Hadziyannis SJ. Interferon alpha treatment and retreatment of hepatitis B e antigen-negative chronic hepatitis B. Gastroenterology 2001;121:101–109.

39. Lampertico P, Del Ninno E, Vigano M, et al. Long-term suppression of hepatitis B e antigen-negative chronic hepatitis B by 24-month interferon therapy. Hepatology 2003;37:756–763.

40. Chang TT, Gish RG, de Man R, et al. A comparison of entecavir and lamivudine for HBeAg-positive chronic hepatitis B. N Engl J Med 2006;354:1001–1010.

41. Gish RG, Lok AS, Chang TT, et al. Entecavir therapy for up to 96 weeks in patients with HBeAg-positive chronic hepatitis B. Gastroenterology 2007;133(5):1437–1444.

42. Lai CL, Shouval D, Lok AS, et al. Entecavir versus lamivudine for patients with HBeAg-negative chronic hepatitis B. N Engl J Med 2006;354:1011–1020.

43. Sherman M, Yurdaydin C, Sollano J, et al. Entecavir is superior to continued lamivudine for the treatment of lamivudine-refractory, HBeAg(+) chronic hepatitis B: Results of phase III study ETV-026. Hepatology 2004; 40:664A.

44. McMahon MA, Jilek BL, Brennan TP, et al. The HBV drug entecavir: Effects on HIV-1 replication and resistance. N Engl J Med 2007;356:2614–2621.

45. Heathcote EJ, Gane E, DeMan R, et al. A randomized, double-blind, comparison of tenofovir (TDF) versus adefovir dipivoxil (ADV) for the treatment of HBeAg-positive chronic hepatitis B (CHB): Study GS-US-174-0103. Hepatology 2007;46 (Suppl 1):861A.

46. Marcellin P, Buti M, Krastev Z, et al. A randomized, double-blind, comparison of tenofovir (TDF) versus adefovir dipivoxil (ADV) for the treatment of HBeAg-negative chronic hepatitis B (CHB): Study GS-US-174-0102. Hepatology 2007;46(Suppl 1):290A–291A.

47. Leemans WF, Niesters HG, van der Eijk AA, et al. Selection of an entecavir-resistant mutant despite prolonged hepatitis B virus DNA suppression, in a chronic hepatitis B patient with preexistent lamivudine resistance: Successful rescue therapy with tenofovir. Eur J Gastroenterol Hepatol 2008;20:773–777.

48. Reijnders JG, Janssen HL. Potency of tenofovir in chronic hepatitis B: Mono or combination therapy? J Hepatol 2008;48:383–386.

49. Tan J, Degertekin B, Wong SN, et al. Tenofovir mono-therapy is effective in hepatitis B patients with antiviral treatment failure to adefovir in the absence of adefovir-resistant mutations. J Hepatol 2008;48:391–398.

50. Rifkin BS, Perazella MA. Tenofovir-associated nephrotoxicity: Fanconi syndrome and renal failure. Am J Med 2004;117:282–284.

51. Verhelst D, Monge M, Meynard JL, et al. Fanconi syndrome and renal failure induced by tenofovir: A first case report. Am J Kidney Dis 2002; 40:1331–1333.

52. Marcellin P, Chang TT, Lim SG, et al. Adefovir dipivoxil for the treatment of hepatitis B e antigen-positive chronic hepatitis B. N Engl J Med 2003;348:808–816.

53. Hadziyannis SJ, Tassopoulos NC, Heathcote EJ. Adefovir dipivoxil for the treatment of HBeAg-negative chronic hepatitis B. N Engl J Med 2003;348:800–807.

54. Marcellin P, Chang TT, Lim SG, et al. Long-term efficacy and safety of adefovir dipivoxil for the treatment of hepatitis B e antigen-positive chronic hepatitis B. Hepatology 2008;48:750–758.

55. Hadziyannis SJ, Tassopoulos NC, Heathcote EJ, et al. Long-term therapy with adefovir dipivoxil for HBe Ag-negative chronic hepatitis B for up to 5 years. Gastro-enterology 2006;131:1743–1751.

56. Lai CL, Chien RN, Leung NW, et al. A one-year trial of lamivudine for chronic hepatitis B. Asia Hepatitis Lamivudine Study Group. N Engl J Med 1998;339:61–68.

57. Dienstag JL, Goldin RD, Heathcote EJ, et al. Histological outcome during long-term lamivudine therapy. Gastroenterology 2003;124:105–117.

58. Lai CL, Gane E, Liaw YF, Hsu CW, et al. Telbivudine versus lamivudine in patients with chronic hepatitis B. N Engl J Med 2007;357:2576–2588.

59. Stramer SL. Current risks of transfusion-transmitted agents: A review. Arch Pathol Lab Med 2007;131:702–707.

60. Strickland GT, El-Kamary SS, Klenerman P, Nicosia A. Hepatitis C vaccine: Supply and demand. Lancet Infect Dis 2008;8:379–386.

61. Dienstag JL, McHutchison JG. American Gastro-enterological Association technical review on the management of hepatitis C. Gastroenterology 2006;130:231–264.

62. Strader DB, Wright T, Thomas DL, Seeff LB; American Association for the Study of Liver Diseases. Diagnosis, management, and treatment of hepatitis C. Hepatology 2004;39:1147–1171.

63. Manns MP, McHutchison JG, Gordon SC, et al. Peginterferon alfa-2b plus ribavirin compared with interferon alfa-2b plus ribavirin for initial treatment of chronic hepatitis C: A randomised trial. Lancet 2001;358:958–965.

64. Fried MW, Shiffman ML, Reddy KR, et al. Peginterferon alfa-2a plus ribavirin for chronic hepatitis C virus infection. N Engl J Med 2002;347:975–982.

65. McHutchison JG, Manns M, Patel K, et al. Adherence to combination therapy enhances sustained response in genotype-1-infected patients with chronic hepatitis C. Gastroenterology 2002;123:1061–1069.

66. Fried MW. Side effects of therapy of hepatitis C and their management. Hepatology 2002;36:S237–S244.

67. Afdhal NH, McHutchison JG. Review article: Pharmacological approaches for the treatment of thrombocytopenia in patients with chronic liver disease and hepatitis C infection. Aliment Pharmacol Ther 2007;26 (Suppl 1):29–39.

68. Younossi ZM, Nader FH, Bai C, et al. A phase II dose finding study of darbepoetin alpha and filgrastim for the management of anaemia and neutropenia in chronic hepatitis C treatment. J Viral Hepat 2008;15:370–378.

69. Koirala J, Gandotra SD, Rao S, et al. Granulocyte colony-stimulating factor dosing in pegylated interferon alpha-induced neutropenia and its impact on outcome of anti-HCV therapy. J Viral Hepat 2007;14:782–787.

70. McHutchison JG, Manns MP, Brown RS Jr, et al. Strategies for managing anemia in hepatitis C patients undergoing antiviral therapy. Am J Gastroenterol 2007;102:880–889.

71. Farci P, Chessa L, Balestrieri C, et al. Treatment of chronic hepatitis D. J Viral Hepat 2007;14 (Suppl 1):58–63.

72. Farci P, Roskams T, Chessa L, et al. Long-term benefit of interferon alpha therapy of chronic hepatitis D: regression of advanced hepatic fibrosis. Gastroenterology 2004;126:1740–1749.

73. Shrestha MP, Scott RM, Joshi DM, et al. Safety and efficacy of a recombinant hepatitis E vaccine. N Engl J Med 2007;356:895–903.

74. Hoofnagle JH, Doo E, Liang TJ, et al. Management of hepatitis B: Summary of a clinical research workshop. Hepatology 2007;45:1056–1075.

25 Acute Kidney Injury

Mary K. Stamatakis

LEARNING OBJECTIVES

● **Upon completion of the chapter, the reader will be able to:**

1. Assess a patient's kidney function based on clinical presentation, laboratory results, and urinary indices.

2. Identify pharmacotherapeutic outcomes and endpoints of therapy in a patient with acute kidney injury (AKI).

3. Apply knowledge of the pathophysiology of AKI to the development of a treatment plan.

4. Design a diuretic regimen with consideration to the pharmacokinetic and pharmacodynamic characteristics of the drug.

5. Select pharmacotherapy to treat complications associated with AKI.

6. Develop strategies to minimize the occurrence of AKI.

7. Monitor and evaluate the safety and efficacy of the therapeutic plan.

KEY CONCEPTS

❶ Equations to estimate creatinine clearance (CrCl) which incorporate a single creatinine concentration (e.g., Cockcroft-Gault) may underestimate or overestimate kidney function depending on whether acute kidney injury (AKI) is worsening or resolving.

❷ There is no evidence that drug therapy hastens patient recovery in AKI, decreases length of hospitalization, or improves survival.

❸ Loop diuretics are the diuretics of choice for the management of volume overload in AKI.

❹ There is no indication for the use of low-dose dopamine in the treatment of AKI.

❺ Identifying patients at high risk for development of AKI and implementing preventive methods to decrease its occurrence or severity is critical.

Acute kidney injury (AKI) is a potentially life-threatening clinical syndrome that occurs primarily in hospitalized patients and frequently complicates the course of the critically ill. It is characterized by a rapid decrease in glomerular filtration rate (GFR) and the resultant accumulation of nitrogenous waste products (e.g., creatinine and urea nitrogen), with or without a decrease in urine output. The term acute renal failure (ARF) has traditionally been used to describe this syndrome. However, AKI has emerged as a name that more completely encompasses the entire spectrum of acute injury to the kidney, from mild changes in kidney function to end-stage kidney disease, requiring renal replacement therapy (RRT). Furthermore, the definition of ARF has been inconsistent in the literature and a recent survey showed more than 35 definitions for ARF used in the literature.[1] Efforts to standardize the definition of ARF in recent years has lead to a change in terminology to AKI as well as a consensus definition and severity staging for AKI.[2] The acronym *RIFLE* has been coined to represent the classification scheme of AKI and places patients into categories, dependent on their change in serum creatinine or GFR from baseline and/or decrease in urine output.[3] The categories of kidney dysfunction include patients at risk (R); those with kidney injury (I); and those with kidney failure (F). Two additional categories of clinical outcomes include sustained loss (L), which requires RRT for at least 4 weeks; and end stage (E), which necessitates RRT for at least 3 months. These two outcome classes are defined by the duration of loss of kidney function. The complete schematic for the *RIFLE* classification and the diagnostic criteria are further depicted in Figure 25–1. For example, a patient with a urine output of less than 0.5 mL/kg/h for less than 6 hours would be in the risk (R) category, while a patient with the same decrease in urine output but for 12 hours would be in the injury (I) category. For the purposes of this chapter, the term AKI is used to be consistent with the recent consensus statement.

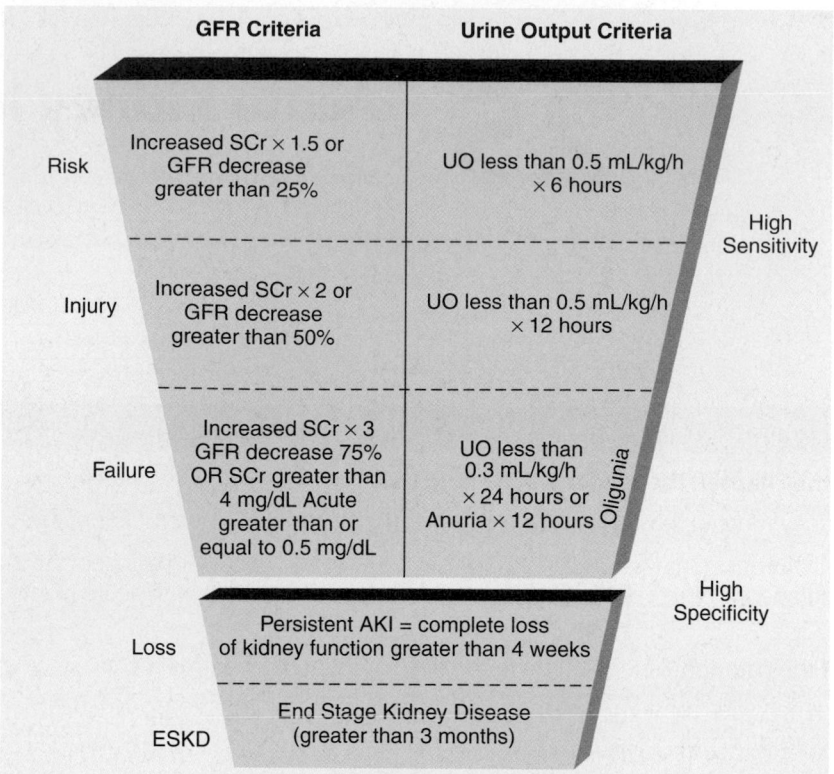

FIGURE 25–1. Alogrithm for classification of acute kidney injury. The classification system includes separate criteria for creatinine and urine output. A patient can fulfill the criteria through changes in serum creatinine or changes in urine output, or both. The criteria that lead to the worst possible classification should be used. Note that the F component of RIFLE (**R**isk of renal dysfunction, **I**njury to the kidney, **F**ailure of kidney function, **L**oss of kidney function and **E**nd-stage kidney disease) is present even if the increase in SCr is under threefold as long as the new SCr is greater than 4.0 mg/dL (350 μmol/L) in the setting of an acute increase of at least 0.5 mg/dL (44 μmol/L). The designation RIFLE-FC should be used in this case to denote "acute-on-chronic" disease. Similarly, when the RIFLE-F classification is achieved by urine output criteria, a designation of RIFLE-FO should be used to denote oliguria. The shape of the figure denotes the fact that more patients (high sensitivity) will be included in the mild category, including some without actually having renal failure (less specificity). In contrast, at the bottom of the figure the criteria are strict and therefore specific, but some patients will be missed. (AKI, acute kidney injury; GFR, glomerular filtration rate; SCr, serum creatinine concentration; UO, urine output.) (From Ref. 2.)

EPIDEMIOLOGY AND ETIOLOGY

Between 5% and 25% of all hospitalized patients develop AKI.[4] A greater prevalence of AKI is found in critically ill patients.[5] Despite improvements in the medical care of individuals with AKI, mortality generally exceeds 50%.[6]

PATHOPHYSIOLOGY

There are typically three categories of AKI: prerenal, intrinsic, and postrenal AKI. The pathophysiologic mechanisms differ for each of the categories.

Prerenal AKI

Prerenal AKI is characterized by reduced blood delivery to the kidney. A common cause is intravascular volume depletion due to conditions such as hemorrhage, dehydration, or GI fluid losses. Prompt correction of volume depletion can restore kidney function to normal because no structural damage to the kidney has occurred.

Conditions of reduced cardiac output (e.g., congestive heart failure [CHF] or myocardial infarction) and hypotension can also reduce renal blood flow, resulting in decreased glomerular perfusion and prerenal AKI. With a mild to moderate decrease in renal blood flow, intraglomerular pressure is maintained by dilation of afferent arterioles (arteries supplying blood to the glomerulus), constriction of efferent arterioles (arteries removing blood from the glomerulus), and redistribution of renal blood flow to the oxygen-sensitive renal medulla.[7] Drugs may cause a functional AKI when these adaptive mechanisms are compromised. Nonsteroidal anti-inflammatory drugs (NSAIDs) impair prostaglandin-mediated dilation of afferent arterioles. Angiotensin-converting enzyme (ACE) inhibitors and angiotensin receptor blockers (ARBs) inhibit angiotensin II–mediated efferent arteriole vasoconstriction. Cyclosporine and tacrolimus, particularly in high doses, are potent renal vasoconstrictors. All of these agents can reduce intraglomerular pressure, with a resultant decrease in GFR. Prompt discontinuation of the offending drug can often return kidney function to normal. Other causes of prerenal AKI are renovascular obstruction (e.g., renal artery stenosis), hyperviscosity syndromes (e.g., multiple myeloma), or systemic vasoconstriction (e.g., hepatorenal syndrome). Prerenal AKI occurs in approximately 10% to 25% of patients diagnosed with AKI.[8]

Intrinsic AKI

Intrinsic renal failure is caused by diseases that can affect the integrity of the tubules, glomerulus, interstitium, or blood vessels. Damage is within the kidney; changes in kidney structure can be seen on microscopy.[9] Acute tubular necrosis (ATN) is a term that is often used synonymously with intrinsic renal failure, but relates more specifically to a pathophysiologic condition that results from toxic (e.g., aminoglycosides, contrast agents, or amphotericin B) or ischemic insult to the kidney only. ATN results in necrosis of the proximal tubule epithelium and basement membrane, decreased glomerular capillary permeability, and backleak of glomerular filtrate into the venous circulation.[10] Maintenance of ATN is mediated by intrarenal vasoconstriction.[10] The most common cause of intrinsic renal failure is due to ATN and it accounts for approximately 50% of all cases of AKI.[8] Glomerular, interstitial, and blood vessel diseases may also lead to intrinsic AKI, but occur with a much lower incidence. Examples include glomerulonephritis, systemic lupus erythematosus, interstitial nephritis, and vasculitis. In addition, prerenal AKI can progress to intrinsic AKI if the underlying condition is not promptly corrected.[9]

Postrenal AKI

Postrenal AKI is due to obstruction of urinary outflow. Causes include benign prostatic hypertrophy, pelvic tumors, and precipitation of renal calculi.[9] Rapid resolution of postrenal AKI without structural damage to the kidney can occur if the underlying obstruction is corrected. Postrenal AKI accounts for less than 10% of cases of AKI.[8]

ASSESSMENT OF KIDNEY FUNCTION

The most common measure of overall kidney function is GFR. It is defined as the volume of plasma filtered across the glomerulus per unit time and correlates well with the filtration, secretion, reabsorption, endocrine, and metabolic functions of the kidney. In addition to aiding in the diagnosis and assessment of the severity of AKI, an accurate estimate of GFR can assist in proper dosing of drugs that undergo renal elimination. In an individual with normal kidney function, GFR ranges from approximately 90 to 120 mL/min. Because GFR is difficult to measure directly, it is routinely estimated by determining the renal clearance of a substance that is filtered at the glomerulus and which does not undergo significant tubular reabsorption or secretion. Creatinine is an endogenous substance that is a normal byproduct of muscle

metabolism. Ninety percent of creatinine is eliminated by glomerular filtration; tubular secretion is responsible for the remaining 10%.

Direct measurement of creatinine clearance (CrCl) requires collection of urine over an extended time interval (usually 24 hours) with measurement of urine volume, urine creatinine concentration, and serum creatinine concentration (SCr) (Table 25–1). Because kidney function can fluctuate significantly during AKI, this method may underestimate or overestimate kidney function depending on whether AKI is worsening or resolving.

Numerous equations have been developed for a quick bedside estimate of CrCl or GFR. They incorporate patient-specific variables such as SCr, body weight, age, and gender. One of the most widely used equations is the Cockcroft-Gault equation (Table 25–1).[11] It is generally considered acceptable in individuals whose renal function is relatively constant, as defined as a daily change in serum creatinine of less than 10% to 15% within 24 hours. ❶ *Because only a single SCr is factored into equations such as Cockcroft-Gault, the calculated CrCl may underestimate or overestimate kidney function depending on whether AKI is worsening or resolving.*

In instances where kidney function is fluctuating, several equations have been developed to assess unstable kidney function.[12-14] These equations estimate CrCl by considering the change in serum creatinine over a specified time period. While they are more mathematically difficult to calculate, they take into consideration a change in serum creatinine compared to an equation that only includes a single creatinine concentration. It should be noted that these methods have not been validated, and drug dosage adjustments based on CrCl estimates from these formulas in patients with AKI have not been evaluated. CrCl estimates in AKI must be viewed as best estimates under variable conditions, and ongoing patient monitoring is necessary to avoid drug toxicity. The Jelliffe equation for changing renal function is listed in Table 25–1.

Estimating CrCl is only one part of evaluating a patient's overall kidney function. Other factors, such as symptomatology, laboratory test results, urinary indices, and results of diagnostic procedures will aid in the diagnosis and assessment of the severity of disease. By monitoring SCr on a routine basis, it can be estimated whether kidney function is improving or worsening. Kidney function can also be evaluated based on urine output. Oliguria and anuria are defined as urine outputs of less than 400 mL and 50 mL over 24 hours, respectively. Patients with reduced urine output often have an increased mortality and may represent a more severe form of AKI. Nonoliguric AKI is defined as a urine output of greater than 400 mL per day. It may still represent severe AKI but may be associated with better patient outcomes.[15]

TREATMENT
Desired Outcomes

A primary goal of therapy is ameliorating any identifiable underlying causes of AKI such as hypovolemia, nephrotoxic

---

Table 25–1

Equations for Estimation of CrCl

Urine Collection Method

$$CrCl\ (mL/min) = \frac{(Ucr)(V)}{(SCr)(T)}$$

Ucr = urine creatinine concentration, mg/dL
V = volume of urine, mL
SCr = serum creatinine concentration, mg/dL
T = time of urine collection, minute
(Note: time equals 1,440 minutes for a 24-hour collection)

Cockcroft-Gault Equation for Adults[11]

$$CrCl\ (mL/min) = \frac{(140 - Age) \times (BW)}{(SCr) \times 72}\ (\times\ 0.85\ if\ women)$$

Age, years
BW = actual body weight, kg[a]
SCr = serum creatinine concentration, mg/dL

Brater Equation for Changing Renal Function[12]

Males
CrCl (mL/min/70 kg) = (293 − 2.03 [age]) × (1.035 − 0.01685 [SCr_1 + SCr_2])
 + 49 (SCr_1 − SCr_2/Δt) (SCr_1 + SCr_2)

Females
CrCl = male value × 0.86

Age, in years
Δt = time in days between measurement of SCr_1 and SCr_2
SCr_1 = first serum creatinine concentration
SCr_2 = second serum creatinine concentration

Jelliffe Equation for Changing Renal Function[13]

Males
E^{SS} = IBW (29.3 − 0.203 [age])
E^{SS}_{corr} = E^{SS} (1.035 − 0.0337 [SCr_2])
E = E^{SS}_{corr} − (4 × IBW × [SCr_2 − SCr_1])/Δt
CrCl (mL/min/1.73 m²) = E/14.4 (SCr)

Females
E^{SS} = IBW (25.1 − 0.175 [age])
E^{SS}_{corr} = E^{SS} (1.035 − 0.0337 (SCr))
E = E^{SS}_{corr} − (4 IBW [SCr_2 − SCr_1])/Δt

E^{SS} = steady state creatinine excretion
Δt = time in days between measurement of SCr_1 and SCr_2
IBW = ideal body weight, kg
Age, years
E^{SS}_{corr} = corrected steady-state creatinine excretion
SCr_1 = first serum creatinine concentration
SCr_2 = second serum creatinine concentration
E = creatinine excretion

Chiou Equation for Changing Renal Function[14]

Males
CrCl (mL/min) = 2(28.0 − 0.2 [age]) × (2[V_d (SCr_2 − SCr_1)] [0.0286(V_d)])
(SCr_1 + SCr_2) (SCr_1 + SCr_2) Δt

Females
CrCl (mL/min) = 2(22.4 − 0.16 (age)) × (2[V_d (SCr_2 − SCr_1)] [.0286(V_d)])
(SCr_1 + SCr_2) (SCr_1 + SCr_2) Δt

V_d = volume of distribution = 0.6 L (IBW)
SCr_1 = first serum creatinine concentration
SCr_2 = second serum creatinine concentration
IBW = ideal body weight, kg
Age, years

---

[a]Typically substituted with ideal body weight, or adjusted body weight when body weight is significantly greater (i.e., greater than 130%) than ideal body weight: Adjusted body weight = Ideal body weight + 0.25(Actual body weight − Ideal body weight).

CrCl, creatinine clearance.

---

drug administration, or ureter obstruction. Prerenal and postrenal AKI can be reversed if the underlying problem is promptly identified and corrected, while treatment of intrinsic renal failure is more supportive in nature. ❷ *There is no evidence that drug therapy hastens patient recovery in AKI, decreases length of hospitalization, or improves survival.*[16] Therefore, options are limited to supportive therapy, such as fluid, electrolyte, and nutritional support, RRT, and treatment of nonrenal complications such as sepsis and GI bleeding while regeneration of the renal epithelium occurs. In addition, prevention of adverse drug reactions

by discontinuing nephrotoxic drugs or adjustment of drug dosages based on the patient's renal function is desired.

Pharmacologic Therapy

▶ Loop Diuretics

There is significant controversy over the role of loop diuretics in the treatment of AKI. Theoretical benefits in hastening recovery of renal function include decreased metabolic oxygen requirements of the kidney, increased resistance to

Clinical Presentation and Diagnosis of AKI

While some clinical and laboratory findings assist in the general diagnosis of AKI, others are used to differentiate among prerenal, intrinsic, and postrenal AKI. For example, patients with prerenal AKI typically demonstrate enhanced sodium reabsorption, which is reflected by a low urine sodium concentration and a low fractional excretion of sodium. Urine is typically more concentrated with prerenal AKI and there is a higher urine osmolality and urine:plasma creatinine ratio compared to intrinsic and postrenal AKI.

Signs and Symptoms of Uremia

- Peripheral edema
- Weight gain
- Nausea/vomiting/diarrhea/anorexia
- Mental status changes
- Fatigue
- Shortness of breath
- Pruritus
- Volume depletion (prerenal AKI)
- Weight loss (prerenal AKI)
- Anuria alternating with polyuria (postrenal AKI)
- Colicky abdominal pain radiating from flank to groin (postrenal AKI)

Physical Examination Findings

- Hypertension
- Jugular venous distention (JVD)
- Pulmonary edema
- Rales
- Asterixis
- Pericardial or pleural friction rub
- Hypotension/orthostatic hypotension (prerenal AKI)
- Rash (acute interstitial nephritis)
- Bladder distention (postrenal bladder outlet obstruction)
- Prostatic enlargement (postrenal AKI)

Laboratory Tests

- Elevated SCr (normal range approximately 0.6–1.2 mg/dL [53 to 106 μmol/L])
- Elevated BUN concentration (normal range approximately 8 to 25 mg/dL [2.9–8.9 mmol/L])
- Decreased CrCl (normal 90–120 mL/min)
- BUN:creatinine ratio (elevated in prerenal AKI)
  Greater than 20:1 for traditional units (prerenal AKI)
  Less than 20:1 for traditional units (intrinsic or postrenal AKI)
- Hyperkalemia
- Metabolic acidosis

Urinalysis

- Sediment
- Scant or bland (prerenal or postrenal AKI)
- Brown, muddy granular casts (highly indicative of ATN)
- Proteinuria (glomerulonephritis or allergic interstitial nephritis)
- Eosinophiluria (acute interstitial nephritis)
- Hematuria/red blood cell casts (glomerular disease or bleeding in urinary tract)
- WBCs or casts (acute interstitial nephritis or severe pyelonephritis)

Urinary Indices	Prerenal AKI	Intrinsic and Postrenal AKI
Urine osmolality (concentration of solutes in the urine in mOsm)	Greater than 500	Less than 350
Urine sodium concentration (mEq/L)	Less than 20	Greater than 40
Fractional excretion of sodium (FENa)	Less than 1%	Greater than 1%
Specific gravity	Greater than 1.020	Less than 1.015
Urine:plasma creatinine ratio	Greater than 40:1	Less than 20:1

$$\text{Fractional excretion of sodium (FENa)} = 100 \times \frac{\left(\begin{array}{c} \text{Urinary sodium concentration} \times \\ \text{Plasma creatinine concentration} \end{array} \right)}{\left(\begin{array}{c} \text{Plasma sodium concentration} \times \\ \text{Plasma creatinine concentration} \end{array} \right)}$$

FENa is a measure of the percentage of sodium excreted by the kidney. A FENa of less than 1% may indicate prerenal AKI as it represents the response of the kidney to decreased renal perfusion by decreasing sodium excretion. Loop diuretics such as furosemide enhance sodium excretion and increase FENa, confounding the interpretation of the test.

Common Diagnostic Procedures

- Urinary catheterization (insertion of a catheter into a patient's bladder; an increase in urine output may occur with postrenal obstruction)
- Renal ultrasound (uses sound waves to assess size, position, and abnormalities of the kidney; dilatation of the urinary tract can be seen with postrenal AKI)
- Renal angiography (administration of IV contrast dye to assess the vasculature of the kidney)
- Retrograde pyelography (injection of contrast dye into the ureters to assess the kidney and collection system)
- Kidney biopsy (collection of a tissue sample of the kidney for the purpose of microscopic evaluation; may aid in the diagnosis of glomerular and interstitial diseases)

Patient Encounter, Part 1

A 73-year-old man with a history of diabetes mellitus, chronic kidney disease, gout, osteoarthritis, and hypertension is hospitalized with pyelonephritis and possible urosepsis. He recently completed a 14-day course of antibiotics and was ready for discharge when his morning labs showed an increase in BUN (42 mg/dL or 15 mmol/L) and SCr (2.9 mg/dL). His serum creatinine 24 hours earlier was 2.4 mg/dL (212 μmol/L). Upon examination, he was found to have 2+ pitting edema, weight gain, nausea, elevated blood pressure, and rales on chest auscultation.

What signs and symptoms does the patient have that may indicate AKI?

What risk factors does he have for the development of AKI?

What additional information do you need to fully assess this patient?

Patient Encounter, Part 2: The Medical History, Physical Examination, and Laboratory Tests

PMH: Type 1 diabetes mellitus since the age of 32; chronic kidney disease (BUN and serum creatinine were 30 mg/dL [10.7 mmol/L] and 2.5 mg/dL [221 μmol/L], respectively, on admission); hypertension; gout; osteoarthritis

FH: Father with a history of type 2 diabetes mellitus, hypertension, and stage 5 chronic kidney disease; he died from a myocardial infarction at age 68; mother with a history of hypertension; she died from injuries sustained in a motor vehicle accident at the age of 52

SH: Retired coal miner; no smoking, occasional alcohol use

Hospital Meds: Gentamicin 120 mg IV piggyback every 12 hours (dose discontinued after 3 days); gentamicin 120 mg IV piggyback every 24 hours (days 4 through 14, discontinued this morning); ampicillin 2 g IV piggyback every 8 hours (14-day course, discontinued this morning); sliding scale insulin; allopurinol 100 mg orally daily; ranitidine 150 mg orally every 12 hours; atenolol 50 mg orally daily; naproxen 275 mg orally every 12 hours; enalapril 2.5 mg orally daily

Home Meds: NPH insulin 20 units in the morning and 10 units in the evening; regular insulin 10 units in the morning and 10 units in the evening; allopurinol 100 mg orally daily; naproxen 275 mg orally every 12 hours; atenolol 50 mg orally daily

ROS: (–) fever or chills, (+) N, (–) V/D

PE:

VS: BP 154/95 mm Hg, pulse 80 bpm, RR 26/min, temperature 37.7°C, current wt 79 kg (admission wt 75 kg), ht 5'10" (178 cm)

Chest: Basilar crackles, inspiratory wheezes

CV: S_1, S_2 normal, no S_3

MS/Exts: 2+ pedal edema

Urinalysis: Color, yellow; character, hazy; glucose (–); ketones (–); specific gravity 1.020; pH 5.0; (+) protein; coarse granular casts, 5 to 10/low-powered field; WBC count, 5 to 10/high-powered field; RBC count, 2 to 5/high-powered field; no bacteria; nitrite (–); blood small; osmolality 325 mOsm; urinary sodium 77 mEq/L (77 mmol/L); urinary creatinine 63 mg/dL (5,569 μmol/L)

Day 3 Labs:

Gentamicin Concentrations:

- 3.4 mcg/mL (7.12 μmol/L) = trough concentration drawn immediately prior to the next dose
- 6.4 mcg/mL (13.38 μmol/L) = peak concentration drawn 1 hour after the end of the infusion
- Urine (+) *Enterococcus* spp.

Given this additional information, what is your assessment of the patient's condition?

Identify your treatment goals for the patient.

---

ischemia, increased urine flow rates that reduce intraluminal obstruction and filtrate backleak, and renal vasodilation.[8] Theoretically, these effects could lead to increased urine output, decreased need for dialysis, improved renal recovery, and ultimately, increased survival. However, there are conflicting reports in the literature over the efficacy of loop diuretics. Most studies demonstrate an improvement in urine output, but with no effect on survival or need for dialysis. There are some reports that loop diuretics may worsen kidney function.[17] This may be due in part to excessive preload reduction that results in renal vasoconstriction. Thus, loop diuretics are limited to instances of volume overload and edema, and are not intended to hasten renal recovery or improve survival.

Loop diuretics (furosemide, bumetanide, torsemide, and ethacrynic acid) are all equally effective when given in equivalent doses. Therefore, selection is based on the side-effect profile, cost, and pharmacokinetics of the agents. The incidence of ototoxicity is significantly higher with ethacrynic acid compared to the other loop diuretics; therefore, its use is limited to patients who are allergic to the sulfa component in the other loop diuretics.[18] While ototoxicity is a well-established side effect of furosemide, its incidence may be greater when administered by the IV route at a rate exceeding 4 mg/min. Torsemide has not been reported to cause ototoxicity.

There are several pharmacokinetic differences between loop diuretics. Fifty percent of a dose of furosemide is excreted unchanged by the kidney with the remainder undergoing glucuronide conjugation in the kidney.[19] In contrast, liver metabolism accounts for 50% and 80% of the elimination of bumetanide and torsemide, respectively.[19] Thus, patients with AKI may have a prolonged half-life of furosemide. The bioavailability of both torsemide and bumetanide is higher than for furosemide. The IV:oral ratio for bumetanide and torsemide is 1:1, bioavailability of oral furosemide is approximately 50%, with a reported range of 10% to 100%.[20]

Furosemide and bumetanide are both available in generic formulations and are generally less expensive than torsemide.

The pharmacodynamic characteristics of loop diuretics are similar when equivalent doses are administered. Because loop diuretics exert their effect from the luminal side of the nephron, urinary excretion correlates with diuretic response. Substances that interfere with the organic acid pathway, such as endogenous organic acids which accumulate in renal disease, competitively inhibit secretion of loop diuretics. Therefore, large doses of loop diuretics may be required to ensure that adequate drug reaches the nephron lumen. In addition, loop diuretics have a ceiling effect where maximal natriuresis occurs.[19,21] Thus, very large doses of furosemide (e.g., 1 g) are generally not considered necessary and may unnecessarily increase the risk of ototoxicity.

Several adaptive mechanisms by the kidney limit effectiveness of loop diuretic therapy. Postdiuretic sodium retention occurs as the concentration of diuretic in the loop of Henle decreases. This effect can be minimized by decreasing the dosage interval (i.e., dosing more frequently) or by administering a continuous infusion.[22] In patients with a CrCl of 25 mL/min or higher, furosemide at a dose of 10 mg/h would be a reasonable starting dose.[19] A starting dose of 20 mg/h would be reasonable in patients with a CrCl of less than 25 mL/min.[19] With a continuous infusion, a loading dose is recommended. Continuous infusion loop diuretics may be easier to titrate than bolus dosing, requires less nursing administration time, and may lead to fewer adverse reactions.

Prolonged administration of loop diuretics can lead to a second type of diuretic resistance. Enhanced delivery of sodium to the distal tubule can result in hypertrophy of distal convoluted cells.[19] Subsequently, increased sodium chloride

absorption occurs in the distal tubule which diminishes the effect of the loop diuretic on sodium excretion. Addition of a distal convoluted tubule diuretic, such as metolazone or hydrochlorothiazide, to a loop diuretic can result in a synergistic increase in urine output. There are no data to support the efficacy of one distal convoluted tubule diuretic over another. The common practice of administering the distal convoluted tubule diuretic 30 to 60 minutes prior to the loop diuretic has not been studied, although this practice may first inhibit sodium reabsorption at the distal convoluted tubule before it is inundated with sodium from the loop of Henle.

A usual starting dose of IV furosemide for the treatment of AKI is 40 mg (Fig. 25–2). Reasonable starting doses for bumetanide and torsemide are 1 mg and 20 mg, respectively.[19] Efficacy of diuretic administration can be determined by comparison of a patient's hourly fluid balance. Other methods to minimize volume overload, such as fluid restriction and concentration of IV medications, should be initiated as needed. If urine output does not increase to about 1 mL/kg/h, the dosage can be increased to a maximum of 160 to 200 mg of furosemide or its equivalent (Fig. 25–2).[20] Dosing frequency is based on the patient's response, the ability to restrict sodium intake, and the duration of action of the diuretic. Other methods to improve diuresis can be initiated sequentially, such as: (a) shortening the dosage interval, (b) adding hydrochlorothiazide or metolazone, and (c) switching to a continuous infusion loop diuretic. A loading dose should be administered prior to both initiating a continuous infusion and increasing the infusion rate. When high doses of loop diuretics are administered, especially in combination with distal convoluted tubule diuretics, the hemodynamic and fluid status of the patient should be monitored every shift, and the electrolyte status of the patient should be monitored at least daily to prevent profound diuresis and electrolyte abnormalities, such as hypokalemia. Patients will not benefit from switching from one loop diuretic to another because of the similarity in mechanisms of action.

▶ *Other Diuretics*

Thiazide diuretics, when used as single agents, are generally not effective for fluid removal. Mannitol is also not recommended for the treatment of volume overload associated with AKI. Mannitol is removed by the body by glomerular filtration. In patients with renal dysfunction, mannitol excretion is decreased, resulting in expanded blood volume and hyperosmolality. Potassium-sparing diuretics, which inhibit sodium reabsorption in the distal nephron and collecting duct, are not sufficiently effective in removing fluid. In addition, they increase the risk of hyperkalemia in patients already at risk. ❸ *Thus, loop diuretics are the diuretics of choice for the management of volume overload in AKI.*

▶ *Dopamine*

Low-dose dopamine (LDD), in doses ranging from 0.5 to 3 mcg/kg/min, predominantly stimulates dopamine-1 receptors, leading to renal vascular vasodilation and

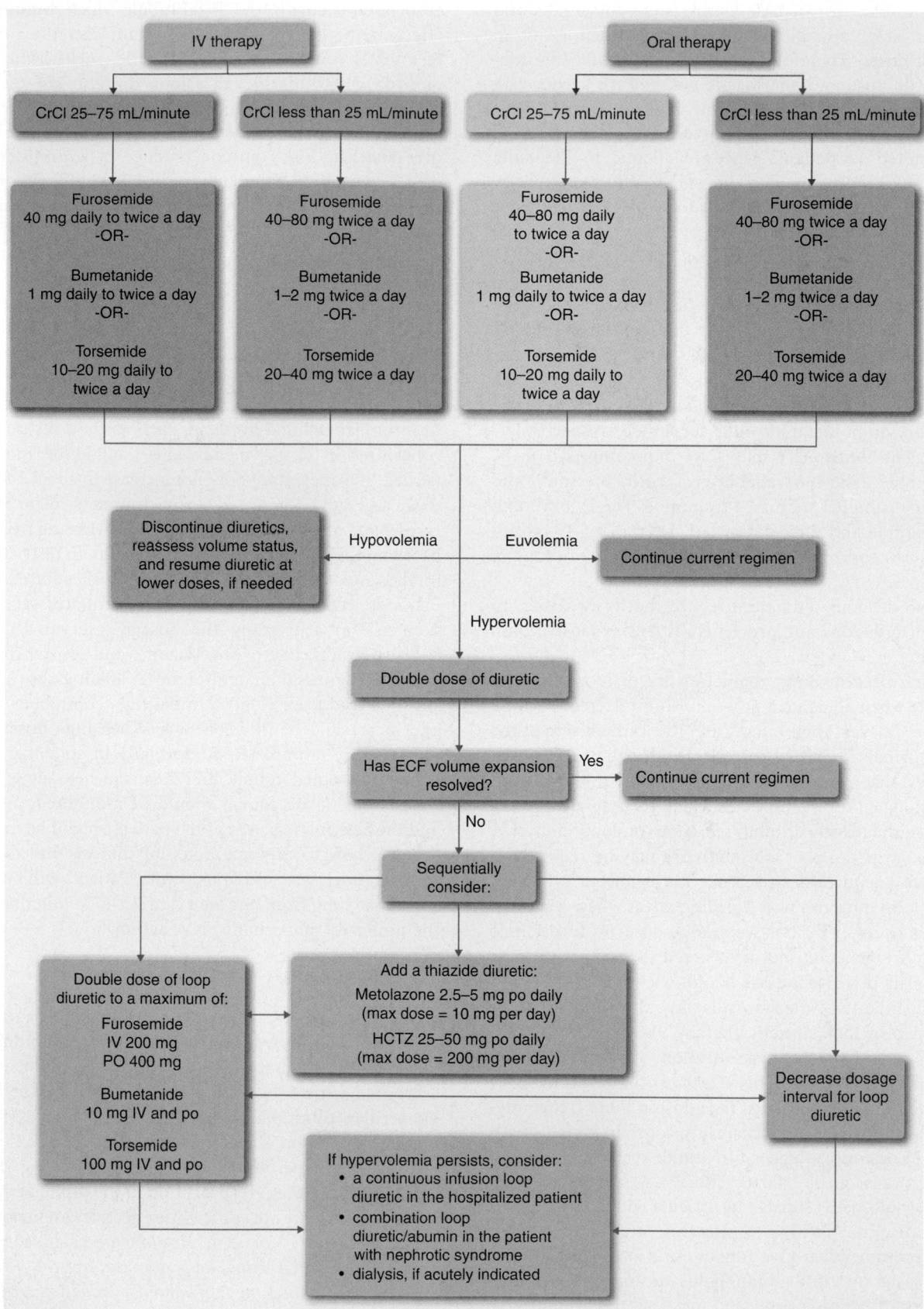

FIGURE 25–2. Algorithm for treatment of extracellular fluid expansion. (CrCl, creatinine clearance; ECF, extracellular fluid; HCTZ, hydrochlorothiazide; po, oral.)

increased renal blood flow. While this effect has been substantiated in healthy, euvolemic individuals with normal kidney function, a lack of efficacy data exists in patients with AKI. The most comprehensive study evaluating efficacy of LDD, the Australian and New Zealand Intensive Care Society (ANZICS) Clinical Trials Group study, did not find that LDD alters peak SCr, need for RRT, duration of stay in the intensive care unit, or survival to discharge compared to placebo.[23] A recent meta-analysis was performed on all published human trials that used LDD in the prevention or treatment of AKI.[24] A total of 61 studies were identified that randomized more than 3,300 patients to LDD or placebo. Results reveal no significant difference between the treatment and control groups for mortality, requirement for RRT, or adverse effects.

LDD is not without adverse reactions and most studies have failed to evaluate its potential toxicities. Adverse reactions that may be associated with LDD include: tachycardia, arrhythmias, myocardial ischemia, depressed respiratory drive, gut ischemia, and impaired resistance to infection. Furthermore, significant overlap in receptor activation occurs. Therefore, doses considered to activate only dopamine receptors may increase cardiac output and blood pressure through dopamine's effect on β- or α-adrenergic receptors.

Based on the results of the ANZICS trial, the lack of conclusive evidence in many earlier studies, and several meta-analyses, ❹ *there is no indication for the use of LDD in the treatment of AKI.*

▶ Fenoldopam

Fenoldopam is a selective dopamine-1 receptor agonist that is approved for short-term management of severe hypertension. Because it does not stimulate dopamine-2, α-adrenergic, and β-adrenergic receptors, fenoldopam causes vasodilation in the renal vasculature with potentially fewer nonrenal effects than dopamine. In normotensive individuals with normal kidney function, IV fenoldopam increases renal blood flow without lowering systemic blood pressure.[25] While preliminary studies in animal models of AKI are encouraging, few studies are available assessing its effectiveness in the treatment of AKI. A prospective randomized study comparing fenoldopam to placebo in early ATN did not find a difference in need for dialysis or mortality.[26] A second prospective, randomized study in septic patients did find less of an increase in SCr in the fenoldopam group compared to placebo, but no difference in survival or need for RRT.[27] Large, prospective trials are needed before fenoldopam can be recommended. Other agents that are under evaluation for the treatment of AKI include atrial natriuretic peptide, urodilatin, and nesiritide.

Nonpharmacologic Treatment

▶ Renal Replacement Therapy

RRT using dialysis may be necessary in patients with established AKI to treat volume overload that is unresponsive to diuretics, to minimize the accumulation of nitrogenous waste products, and to correct electrolyte and acid-base abnormalities while renal function recovers. Five to thirty percent of patients with AKI treated with dialysis will not have recovery of their renal function and will need to remain on long-term dialysis.[28] This may be due in part to underlying illnesses, as AKI is often seen in the setting of multiorgan failure. There are two types of dialysis modalities commonly used in AKI: intermittent hemodialysis (IHD) and continuous renal replacement therapy (CRRT). IHD is a higher-efficiency form of dialysis which is provided for several hours a day at a variable frequency (usually daily or three to five times per week) at a higher blood flow rate. CRRT is a pump-driven form of dialysis which provides slow fluid and solute removal on a continuous, 24-hour basis. The primary advantage of CRRT is hemodynamic stability and better volume control, particularly in patients who are unable to tolerate rapid fluid removal. The primary disadvantages associated with CRRT are continuous nursing requirements, continuous anticoagulation, frequent clotting of the dialyzer, patient immobility, and increased cost. There is no conclusive evidence that one type of dialysis is preferred to another in terms of mortality and recovery of renal function.[29] Thus, selection of CRRT over IHD is often governed by the critical illness of the patient and by the comfort level of the institution with one particular type of dialysis.

With either type of dialysis, studies suggest that recovery of renal function is decreased in AKI patients who undergo dialysis compared with those not requiring dialysis. Decreased recovery of renal function may be due to hemodialysis-induced hypotension causing additional ischemic injury to the kidney. Also, exposure of a patient's blood to bioincompatible dialysis membranes (cuprophane or cellulose acetate) results in complement and leukocyte activation which can lead to neutrophil infiltration into the kidney and release of vasoconstrictive substances that can prolong renal dysfunction.[30] Synthetic membranes composed of substances such as polysulfone, polyacrylonitrile, and polymethylmethacrylate are considered to be more biocompatible and would be less likely to activate complement. Synthetic membranes are generally more expensive than cellulose-based membranes. Several recent metaanalyses found no difference in mortality between biocompatible and bioincompatible membranes. Whether biocompatible membranes lead to better patient outcomes continues to be debated.

▶ Supportive Therapy

Supportive therapy in AKI includes adequate nutrition, correction of electrolyte and acid-base abnormalities (particularly hyperkalemia and metabolic acidosis), fluid management, and correction of any hematologic abnormalities. Because AKI is often associated with multiorgan failure, treatment includes the medical management of infections, cardiovascular and GI conditions, and respiratory failure. Finally, all drugs should be reviewed, and dosage adjustments made based on an estimate of the patient's GFR.

Patient Encounter, Part 3: Creating a Care Plan

Based on the information presented, create a care plan for this patient's AKI. Your plan should include: (a) a statement of the drug-related need and/or problems, (b) the goals of therapy, (c) a detailed patient-specific therapeutic plan, and (d) a plan for follow-up to determine whether the goals have been achieved and adverse effects avoided.

PREVENTION OF ACUTE RENAL FAILURE

Avoidance

The best preventive measure for AKI, especially in individuals at high risk, is to avoid medications that are known to precipitate AKI. Nephrotoxicity is a significant side effect of aminoglycosides, ACE inhibitors, angiotensin receptor antagonists, amphotericin B, NSAIDs, cyclosporine, tacrolimus, and radiographic contrast agents.[8] Unfortunately, an effective, non-nephrotoxic alternative may not always be appropriate for a given patient and the risks and benefits of selecting a drug with nephrotoxic potential must be considered. For example, serious gram-negative infections may require double antibiotic coverage, and based on culture and sensitivity reports, aminoglycoside therapy may be necessary. In cases such as this, other measures to reduce the risk of AKI should be instituted. ❺ *Thus, identifying patients at high risk for development of AKI and implementing preventive methods to decrease its occurrence or severity is critical.*

Drug-Induced ARF

▶ *Aminoglycosides*

Aminoglycosides (gentamicin, tobramycin, and amikacin) can cause nonoliguric intrinsic AKI. Injury is due to binding of aminoglycosides to proximal tubular cells in the renal cortex, and subsequent cellular uptake and cell death.[31] In clinical practice, all aminoglycosides are considered equally nephrotoxic, and similar precautions should be used for all of the agents. High cumulative drug exposure increases the incidence of aminoglycoside-induced AKI. Additional risk factors include a prolonged course of aminoglycoside therapy (typically longer than 7–10 days), pre-existing chronic kidney disease, and increased age.[32] Alternative antibiotics should be considered in individuals with AKI or those who are at a high risk for developing AKI, although resistance of some strains of gram-negative organisms to other antibiotics may necessitate their use.

Methods to minimize drug exposure with conventional (multiple doses per day) dosing include maintaining trough concentrations less than 2 mcg/mL for gentamicin and tobramycin (less than 10 mcg/mL for amikacin), minimizing length of therapy, and avoiding repeated courses of aminoglycosides. Concurrent exposure to other nephrotoxic medications and dehydration may also worsen AKI. There is conflicting evidence as to whether the combination of vancomycin and an aminoglycoside has a higher incidence of AKI than aminoglycoside therapy alone. Aminoglycoside-induced AKI is usually reversible upon drug discontinuation; however, dialysis may be needed in some individuals while kidney function improves.

Another method to minimize toxicity is with extended-interval dosing (e.g., once daily). The goal of extended-interval dosing is to provide greater efficacy against the microorganism with a lower incidence of nephrotoxicity. Aminoglycosides demonstrate concentration-dependent killing and a prolonged postantibiotic effect. The mechanism by which extended-interval aminoglycoside dosing may reduce the incidence of nephrotoxicity is by providing high, transient concentrations of drug which saturate proximal tubule uptake sites. Once saturated, the remaining aminoglycoside molecules pass through the proximal tubule and are excreted in the urine.[33] Thus, less drug is available for cellular uptake during a 24-hour period. A consistent finding in studies is that extended-interval aminoglycoside dosing is as effective as conventional dosing and is not more nephrotoxic, and in some studies is less nephrotoxic than conventional dosing. Aminoglycosides can also cause hearing loss and/or vestibular toxicity, although the incidence of ototoxicity appears to be similar with extended-dosing and conventional dosing. Prolonged exposure to the drug, repeated courses of therapy, and concurrent use of other ototoxic drugs increase toxicity. Extended-interval dosing is not recommended in patients with pre-existing kidney disease, conditions where high concentrations are not needed (e.g., urinary tract infections), hyperdynamic patients that may demonstrate increased drug clearance (e.g., burn patients), and others where you would suspect altered pharmacokinetics or increased risk of ototoxicity.

▶ *Amphotericin B*

Amphotericin B–induced AKI occurs in as many as 49% to 65% of patients treated with the conventional desoxycholate formulation.[34] Nephrotoxicity is due to renal arterial vasoconstriction and distal renal tubule cell damage. Risk factors include high daily dosage, large cumulative dose, pre-existing kidney dysfunction, dehydration, and concomitant use of other nephrotoxic drugs.[34] Three lipid-based formulations of amphotericin B have been developed in an attempt to improve efficacy and limit toxicity, particularly nephrotoxicity: amphotericin B lipid complex, amphotericin B colloidal dispersion, and liposomal amphotericin B. The range of nephrotoxicity reported is 15% to 25% for these formulations. The mechanism for decreased nephrotoxicity has not been completely elucidated, but it is thought to be due to preferential delivery of amphotericin B to the site of infection, with less of an affinity for the kidney.[35] Lipid-based formulations are recommended in individuals with risk factors for development of AKI. Administration of IV normal saline may also attenuate nephrotoxicity associated with amphotericin B.

Whether there are significant differences in nephrotoxicity between the three lipid-based formulations remains unclear. A recent review of the literature from 1997 through 2007 summarized the studies to date comparing lipid-based formulations.[35] Only amphotericin B lipid complex and liposomal amphotericin B have been compared, mainly in observational studies. Nine studies showed a similar incidence of AKI between amphotericin B lipid complex and liposomal amphotericin B. However, in one prospective, randomized study, the incidence of nephrotoxicity was lower with liposomal amphotericin B dosed at 5 mg/kg/day (14.8%) compared to amphotericin B lipid complex dosed at 5 mg/kg/day (42%) in febrile, neutropenic patients.[36] Large, prospective studies comparing the incidence of nephrotoxicity between these agents are needed to ascertain differences in nephrotoxicity.

▶ Radiocontrast Agents

Intravascular radiographic contrast agents are administered during radiologic studies and carry with them the well-documented risk of AKI. Patients at risk for developing AKI include patients with chronic kidney disease, diabetic nephropathy, dehydration, and higher doses of contrast dye.[37] Contrast agents are water-soluble, triiodinated, benzoic acid salts that cause an osmotic diuresis due to their osmolality, which exceeds that of plasma. The mechanism of nephrotoxicity is not fully understood; however, direct tubular toxicity, renal ischemia, and tubular obstruction have been implicated.[38] Diatrizoate and iothalamate are ionic contrast agents. Iohexol, iopamidol, ioversol, and iopromide represent nonionic agents. The incidence of nephrotoxicity with ionic and nonionic agents is similar in patients at low risk for developing AKI; however, in high-risk patients, nephrotoxicity is significantly greater when ionic contrast agents are used. In diabetic patients with chronic kidney disease and an SCr of greater than 1.5 mg/dL (133 µmol/L), nephrotoxicity occurred in 33.3% and 47.7% of patients receiving nonionic and ionic contrast agents, respectively.[39] The cost of nonionic agents is approximately 10-fold higher, which may limit their routine use in all patients undergoing radiographic studies.

Therapeutic measures that have been used to decrease the incidence of contrast-induced nephropathy include extracellular volume expansion, minimization of the amount of contrast administered, and treatment with oral acetylcysteine. Theophylline, fenoldopam, loop diuretics, mannitol, dopamine, and calcium antagonists have no effect or may worsen AKI.

The most effective therapeutic maneuver to decrease the incidence of contrast-induced nephropathy is extracellular volume expansion.[40] Several recent studies have compared the efficacy of isotonic sodium chloride (0.9%) to half normal saline (0.45%) or to oral hydration.[41,42] Isotonic fluid is superior to hypotonic fluid in prevention of nephropathy. A common regimen is IV isotonic sodium chloride (1 mL/kg of body weight/hour) administered for 12 hours before and 12 hours after the procedure. Fluid should be administered cautiously to patients with CHF, left ventricular dysfunction, and significant renal dysfunction. Recent evidence suggests that hydration, plus sodium bicarbonate to alkalize renal tubule fluid, may reduce free radical formation and lead to less oxidant damage, although studies have been conflicting.[43,44] Most studies investigating sodium bicarbonate hydration administered therapy at a rate of 3 mL/kg/h (154 mEq/L) for one before the procedure, and 1 mL/kg/h during and 6-hour postcontrast. A large, randomized clinical trial that provides definitive conclusions is needed.

Minimizing the quantity of contrast media administered may be beneficial in preventing nephropathy. Some studies, but not all, have directly associated dose of contrast media and nephrotoxicity. Avoidance of contrast dye with alternative diagnostic procedures should be considered in high-risk patients, but may not always be feasible. In addition, avoidance of multiple contrast studies in a short time period will allow renal function to return to normal between procedures.

Because production of reactive oxygen species has been implicated in the pathophysiology of contrast-induced AKI, prophylactic administration of the antioxidant acetylcysteine has been investigated. An oral dose of 600 mg twice daily the day before and the day of the procedure decreased the incidence of AKI in one small study, although patient outcomes such as mortality and length of hospitalization were not evaluated.[45] Since then, at least 25 additional studies evaluating the efficacy of oral acetylcysteine have been conducted, with mixed results. In addition, a series of metaanalyses have also analyzed the results of the studies with varying conclusions. The studies were varied in terms of study population, sample size, definition of contrast nephropathy, type of contrast agent used, hydration, and formulation of acetylcysteine administered, thus making collective interpretation of the results difficult. It is routinely used in many hospitals due to its low cost and safe side effect profile at low oral doses, although data are not conclusive that it prevents development of AKI, particularly on patient outcomes such as mortality, need for dialysis, and length of hospitalization. It is noted that acetylcysteine is not considered a replacement for adequate hydration, which remains the standard of care for prevention of contrast nephropathy.

Fenoldopam does not decrease the incidence of contrast nephropathy.[46] Due to its hypotensive effect, it may worsen kidney function.

▶ Cyclosporine and Tacrolimus

Cyclosporine and tacrolimus are calcineurin inhibitors that are administered as part of immunosuppressive regimens in kidney, liver, heart, lung, and bone marrow transplant recipients. In addition, they are used in autoimmune disorders such as psoriasis and multiple sclerosis. The pathophysiologic mechanism for AKI is renal vascular vasoconstriction.[47] It often occurs within the first 6 to

12 months of treatment, and can be reversible with dose reduction or drug discontinuation. Risk factors include high dose, elevated trough blood concentrations, increased age, and concomitant therapy with other nephrotoxic drugs.[47] Cyclosporine and tacrolimus are extensively metabolized by the liver through the cytochrome P450 3A4 pathway and drugs that inhibit their metabolism (e.g., erythromycin, clarithromycin, fluconazole, ketoconazole, verapamil, diltiazem, and nicardipine) can precipitate AKI. Because AKI is dose dependent, careful monitoring of cyclosporine or tacrolimus trough concentrations can minimize its occurrence; however, AKI can develop with normal or low blood concentrations. In addition, there is some evidence that calcium channel blockers have a renoprotective effect through dilation of the afferent arterioles and are often used preferentially as antihypertensive agents in kidney transplant recipients.

It is often difficult to differentiate AKI from acute rejection in the kidney transplant recipient, as both conditions may present with similar symptoms and physical examination findings. However, fever and graft tenderness are more likely to occur with rejection while neurotoxicity is more likely to occur with cyclosporine or tacrolimus toxicity. Kidney biopsy is often needed to confirm the diagnosis of rejection.

▶ ACE Inhibitors and ARBs

In instances of decreased renal blood flow, production of angiotensin II increases, resulting in efferent arteriole vasoconstriction and maintenance of glomerular capillary pressure and GFR (Fig. 25–3). In patients initiated on ACE inhibitors or ARBs, angiotensin II synthesis decreases, thereby dilating efferent arterioles and decreasing glomerular capillary pressure and GFR. Risk factors for developing AKI are pre-existing renal dysfunction, severe atherosclerotic renal artery stenosis, volume depletion, and severe CHF.[48]

AKI often develops within days, with a rapid rise in blood urea nitrogen (BUN) and SCr. Discontinuation of the drug usually results in return of renal function to baseline, although a small decrease in kidney function may be acceptable in patients with severe CHF who would benefit from the hemodynamic effect of ACE inhibitors or ARBs.

▶ Nonsteroidal Anti-Inflammatory Drugs

NSAIDs (e.g., inbuprofen, naproxen, sulindac) can likewise cause prerenal AKI through inhibition of prostaglandin-mediated renal vasodilation. Risk factors are similar to those of ACE inhibitors and ARBs. Additional risk factors include hepatic disease with ascites, systemic lupus erythematosus, and advanced age. The onset is often within days of initiating therapy and patients typically present with oliguria. It is usually reversible with drug discontinuation. Agents that preferentially inhibit cyclooxygenase-2 pose a similar risk as traditional, nonselective NSAIDs.[49]

▶ Other Drugs

Other drugs that are commonly implicated in causing AKI include acyclovir, adefovir, carboplatin, cidofovir, cisplatin, foscarnet, ganciclovir, indinavir, methotrexate, pentamidine, ritonavir, sulfinpyrazone, and tenofovir.[50]

OUTCOME EVALUATION

Goals of therapy are to maintain a state of euvolemia with good urine output (at least 1 mL/kg/h), to return serum creatinine to baseline, and to correct electrolyte and acid-base abnormalities. In addition, appropriate drug dosages based on kidney function and avoidance of nephrotoxic drugs are goals of therapy. Assess vital signs, weight, fluid intake, urine output, BUN, creatinine, and electrolytes daily in the unstable patient.

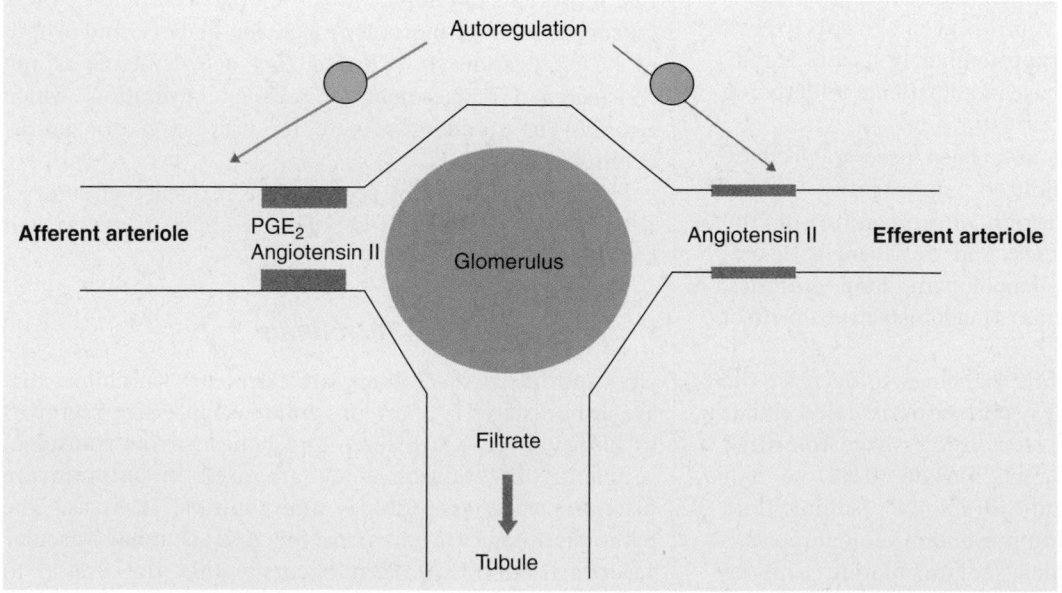

FIGURE 25–3. Normal glomerular autoregulation serves to maintain intraglomerular capillary hydrostatic pressure, glomerular filtration rate, and ultimately, urine output. This is accomplished by modulation of afferent and efferent arterioles. Afferent and efferent arteriolar vasoconstrictions are primarily mediated by angiotensin II, whereas afferent vasodilation is primarily mediated by prostaglandins. (PGE_2, prostaglandin E_2.)

Patient Care and Monitoring

1. Assess kidney function by evaluating a patient's signs and symptoms, laboratory test results, and urinary indices. Calculate a patient's CrCl to evaluate the severity of kidney disease.

2. Obtain a thorough and accurate drug history, including the use of nonprescription drugs such as NSAIDs.

3. Evaluate a patient's current drug regimen to:

   - Determine if drug therapy may be contributing to AKI. Consider not only drugs that can directly cause AKI (e.g., aminoglycosides, amphotericin B, NSAIDs, cyclosporine, tacrolimus, ACE inhibitors, and ARBs), but also drugs that can predispose a patient to nephrotoxicity or prerenal AKI (i.e., diuretics and antihypertensive agents).

   - Determine if any drugs need to be discontinued, or alternate drugs selected, to prevent worsening of renal function.

   - Adjust drug dosages based on the patient's CrCl or evidence of adverse drug reactions or interactions.

4. Develop a plan to provide symptomatic care of complications associated with AKI, such as diuretic therapy to treat volume overload. Monitor the patient's weight, urine output, electrolytes (such as potassium), and blood pressure to assess efficacy of the diuretic regimen.

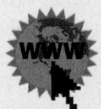

Self-assessment questions and answers are available at *http://www.mhpharmacotherapy.com/pp.html.*

Abbreviations Introduced in This Chapter

ACE	Angiotensin-converting enzyme
AKI	Acute kidney injury
ANZICS	Australian and New Zealand Intensive Care Society
ARB	Angiotensin receptor blocker
ARF	Acute renal failure
ATN	Acute tubular necrosis
BUN	Blood urea nitrogen
CHF	Congestive heart failure
CrCl	Creatinine clearance
CRRT	Continuous renal replacement therapy
DM	Diabetes mellitus
FENa	Fractional excretion of sodium
GFR	Glomerular filtration rate
IHD	Intermittent hemodialysis
JVD	Jugular venous distention
LDD	Low-dose dopamine
NSAIDs	Nonsteroidal anti-inflammatory drugs
PGE_2	Prostaglandin E_2
RRT	Renal replacement therapy
SCr	Serum creatinine concentration

REFERENCES

1. Kellum JA, Levin N, Bouman C, Lameire N. Developing a consensus classification system for acute renal failure. Curr Opin Crit Care 2002;8:509–514.
2. Bellomo R, Ronco C, Kellum, et al. and the ADQI Workgroup. Acute renal failure – definition, outcome measures, animal models, and information technology needs: The Second International Consensus Conference of the Acute Dialysis Quality Initiative (ADQI) Group. Critical Care 2004;8:R204–R212.
3. Kellum JA. Acute kidney injury. Crit Care Med 2008;36:S141–S145.
4. Pruchnicki MC, Dasta JF. Acute renal failure in hospitalized patients: Part I. Ann Pharmacother 2002;36:1261–1267.
5. Joannidis M, Metnitz PGH. Epidemiology and natural history of acute renal failure in the ICU. Crit Care Clin 2005;21:239–249.
6. Ympa YP, Sakr Y, Reinhart K, et al. Has mortality from acute renal failure decreased? A systematic review of the literature. Am J Med 2005;118:827–832.
7. Schetz M. Diuretics in acute renal failure? Contrib Nephrol 2004;144:166–181.
8. Dishart MK, Kellum JA. An evaluation of pharmacological strategies for the prevention and treatment of acute renal failure. Drugs 2000;59:79–91.
9. Bellomo R. Defining, quantifying, and classifying acute renal failure. Crit Care Clin 2005;21:223–237.
10. Nissenson AR. Acute renal failure: Definition and pathogenesis. Kidney Int 1998;53:S7–S10.
11. Cockroft DW, Gault MH. Prediction of creatinine clearance from serum creatinine. Nephron 1976;16:31–41.
12. Brater DC. Drug Use in Renal Disease. Balgowlah, Australia: ADIS Health Science Press, 1983;22–56.
13. Jelliffe R. Estimation of creatinine clearance in patients with unstable renal function, without a urine specimen. Am J Nephrol 2002;22:320–324.
14. Chiou WL, HSU FH. A new simple rapid method to monitor renal function based on pharmacokinetic considerations of endogenous creatinine. Res Commun Chem Pathol Pharmacol 1975;10:315–330.
15. Bellomo R, Kellum JA, Ronco C. Defining acute renal failure: Physiologic principles. Intensive Care Med 2004;30:33–37.
16. Venkataraman R. Prevention of acute renal failure. Crit Care Clin 2005;21:281–289.
17. Mehta RL, Pascual MT, Soroko S, et al. Diuretics, mortality, and nonrecovery of renal function in acute renal failure. JAMA 2002;288:2547–2553.
18. Greenberg A. Diuretic complications. Am J Med Sci 2000;319:10–24.
19. Shankar SS, Brater DC. Loop diuretics: From the Na-K-2Cl transporter to clinical use. Am J Physiol Renal Physiol 2003;284:F11–F21.
20. Brater DC. Pharmacology of diuretics. Am J Med Sci 2000;319:38–50.
21. Rudy DW, Gehr TW, Matzke GR, et al. The pharmcodynamics of intravenous and oral torsemide in patients with chronic renal insufficiency. Clin Pharmacol Ther 1994;56:39–47.
22. Rudy DW, Voelker JR, Greene PK, et al. Loop diuretics for chronic renal insufficiency: A continuous infusion is more efficacious than bolus therapy. Ann Intern Med 1991;115:360–366.
23. Bellomo R, Chapman M, Finfer S, et al. Low-dose dopamine in patients with early renal dysfunction: A placebo-controlled randomized trial. Australian and New Zealand Intensive Care Society (ANZICS) Clinical Trials Group. Lancet 2000;356:2139–2143.

24. Friedrich JO, Adhikari N, Herridge MS, et al. Meta-analysis: Low-dose dopamine increases urine output but does not prevent renal dysfunction or death. Ann Intern Med 2005;142:510–524.

25. Mathur VS, Swam SK, Lambrecht LJ, et al. The effects of fenoldopam, a selective dopamine receptor agonists, on systemic and renal hemodynamics in normotensive subjects. Crit Care Med 1999;27:1832–1837.

26. Tumlin JA, Finkel KW, Murray PT, et al. Fenoldopam mesylate in early acute tubular necrosis: A randomized, double-blind, placebo-controlled clinical trial. Am J Kidney Dis 2005;46:26–34.

27. Morelli A, Ricci Z, Bellomo R, et al. Prophylactic fenoldopam for renal protection in sepsis. A randomized, double-blind, placebo-controlled pilot study. Crit Care Med 2005;33:2451–2456.

28. Silvester W. Outcome studies of continuous renal replacement therapy in the intensive care unit. Kidney Int 1998;66:S138–S141.

29. Tonelli M, Manns B, Feller-Kopman D. Acute renal failure in the intensive care unit: A systematic review of the impact of dialytic modality on mortality and renal recovery. Am J Kidney Dis 2002;40:875–885.

30. Jaber BL, Lau J, Schmid CH, et al. Effect of biocompatibility of hemodialysis membranes on mortality in acute renal failure: A meta-analysis. Clin Nephrol 2002;57:274–282.

31. Mingeot-Leclercq MP, Tulkens PM. Aminoglycosides: Nephrotoxicity. Antimicrob Agents Chemother 1999;43:1003–1012.

32. Streetman DS, Nafziger AN, Destache CJ, et al. Individualized pharmacokinetic monitoring results in less aminoglycoside-associated nephrotoxicity and fewer associated costs. Pharmacotherapy 2001;21:443–451.

33. Pannu N, Nadim M. An overview of drug-induced acute kidney injury. Crit Care Med 2008;36:S216–S223.

34. Deray G. Amphotericin B nephrotoxicity. J Antimicrob Chemother 2002;49:37–41.

35. Saliba F, Dupont B. Renal impairment and Amphotericin B formulations in patients with invasive fungal infections. Med Mycol 2008;46:97–112.

36. Wingard JR, White MH, Anaissie E, et al. A randomized, double-blind comparative trial evaluating the safety of liposomal amphotericin B versus amphotericin B lipid complex in the empirical treatment of febrile neutropenia. Clin Infect Dis 2000;31:1155–1163.

37. Weisbord SD, Palevsky PM. Radiocontrast-induced acute renal failure. J Intensive Care Med 2005;20:63–75.

38. McCullough PA, Soman SS. Contrast-induced nephropathy. Crit Care Clin 2005;21:261–280.

39. Rudnick MR, Goldfarb S, Wexler L, et al. Nephrotoxicity of ionic and nonionic contrast media in 1196 patients: A randomized trial. Kidney Int 1995;47:254–261.

40. Solomon R, Werner C, Mann D, et al. Effects of saline, mannitol, and furosemide on acute decreases in renal function by radiocontrast agents. N Engl J Med 1994;331:1416–1420.

41. Mueller C, Buerkle G, Buettner HJ, et al. Prevention of contrast media-associated nephropathy: Randomized comparison of 2 hydration regimens in 1620 patients undergoing coronary angioplasty. Arch Int Med 2002;162:329–336.

42. Trivedi HS, Moore H, Nasr S, et al. A randomized prospective trial to assess the role of saline hydration on the development of contrast nephrotoxicity. Nephron 2003;93:C29–C34.

43. Merten GJ, Burgess WP, Gray LV, et al. Prevention of contrast-induced nephropathy with sodium bicarbonate: A randomized controlled trial. JAMA 2004;291:2328–2334.

44. Brar SS, Shen AY, Jorgensen MB, et al. Sodium bicarbonate vs sodium chloride for the prevention of contrast medium-induced nephropathy in patients undergoing coronary angiography. JAMA 2008;300:1038–1046.

45. Tepel M, Van der Giet M, Schwarzfeld C, et al. Prevention of radiographic contrast agent-induced reduction in renal function by acetylcysteine. N Engl J Med 2000;343:180–184.

46. Stone GW, McCullough PA, Tumlin JA, et al. Fenoldopam mesylate for the prevention of contrast-induced nephropathy. JAMA 2003;290:2284–2291.

47. De Mattos AM, Olyaei AJ, Bennett WM. Nephrotoxicity of immunosuppressive drugs: Long-term consequences and challenges for the future. Am J Kidney Dis 2000;35:333–346.

48. Perazella MA. Drug-induced renal failure: Update on new medications and unique mechanisms of nephrotoxicity. Am J Med Sci 2003;325:349–362.

49. Brater DC. Effects of nonsteroidal antiinflammatory drugs on renal function; focus on cyclooxygenase-2—selective inhibition. Am J Med 1999;107:S65–S70.

50. Izzedine H, Launay-Vacher V, Deray G. Antiviral drug-induced nephropathy. Am J Kidney Dis 2005;45:804–817.

26 Chronic and End-Stage Kidney Disease

Kristine S. Schonder

LEARNING OBJECTIVES

Upon completion of the chapter, the reader will be able to:

1. List the risk factors for development and progression of chronic kidney disease (CKD).

2. Explain the mechanisms associated with progression of CKD.

3. Outline the desired outcomes for treatment of CKD.

4. Develop a therapeutic approach to slow progression of CKD, including lifestyle modifications and pharmacologic therapies.

5. Identify specific consequences associated with CKD.

6. Design an appropriate therapeutic approach for specific consequences associated with CKD.

7. Recommend an appropriate monitoring plan to assess the effectiveness of pharmacotherapy for CKD and specific consequences.

8. Educate patients with CKD about the disease state, the specific consequences, lifestyle modifications, and pharmacologic therapies used for treatment of CKD.

KEY CONCEPTS

❶ Chronic kidney disease (CKD) is a progressive disease that eventually leads to kidney failure (end-stage kidney disease [ESKD]).

❷ Early detection and treatment of CKD are fundamental factors in minimizing morbidity and mortality associated with CKD.

❸ Declining kidney function disrupts the homeostasis of the systems regulated by the kidney, leading to fluid and electrolyte imbalances, anemia, and metabolic bone disease.

❹ Angiotensin-converting enzyme inhibitors (ACEIs) and angiotensin II receptor blockers decrease protein excretion and are the drugs of choice for hypertension in patients with CKD.

❺ The most common complication of CKD is anemia, which is caused by a decline in erythropoietin production by the kidneys and can lead to cardiovascular disease (CVD).

❻ The goal of anemia management in CKD is to maintain hemoglobin levels between 11 g/dL (110 g/L or 6.8 mmol/L) and 12 g/dL (120 g/L or 7.4 mmol/L), which generally requires a combination of erythropoiesis-stimulating agents (ESAs) and iron supplements.

❼ Bone and mineral metabolism disorders stem from disruptions in calcium, phosphorus, and vitamin D homeostasis through the interaction with the parathyroid hormone.

❽ The management of secondary hyperparathyroidism (sHPT) involves correction of serum calcium and phosphorus levels, and decreasing parathyroid hormone secretion.

❾ Patient education and planning for dialysis should begin at stage 4 CKD, before ESKD is reached, to allow for time to establish appropriate access for dialysis.

❿ Dialysis involves the removal of metabolic waste products and excess fluids and electrolytes by diffusion and ultrafiltration from the bloodstream across a semipermeable membrane into an external dialysate solution.

The kidney is made up of approximately 2 million nephrons that are responsible for filtering, reabsorbing and excreting solutes and water. As the number of functioning nephrons declines, the primary functions of the kidney that are affected include:

- Production and secretion of erythropoietin
- Activation of vitamin D
- Regulation of fluid and electrolyte balance
- Regulation of acid–base balance

Chronic kidney disease (CKD), also known as chronic kidney insufficiency, progressive kidney disease, or nephropathy, is defined as the presence of kidney damage or decreased glomerular filtration rate (GFR) for 3 months or more.[1] Generally, CKD is a progressive decline in kidney function (a decline in the number of functioning nephrons) that occurs over a period of several months to years. A decline in kidney function that occurs more rapidly, over a period of days to weeks, is known as acute kidney injury (AKI), which is discussed in Chapter 25. The decline in kidney function in CKD is often irreversible. Therefore, measures to treat CKD are aimed at slowing the progression to end-stage kidney disease (ESKD).

EPIDEMIOLOGY AND ETIOLOGY

The National Kidney Foundation (NKF) developed a classification system for CKD (Table 26–1).[1] The staging system defines the stages of CKD based on GFR level, but also accounts for evidence of kidney damage in the absence of changes in GFR, as in stage 1 CKD. The GFR is calculated using the abbreviated Modification of Diet in Renal Disease study equation:

$$\text{GFR} = 186 \times (\text{SCr})^{-1.194} \times (\text{age})^{-0.214} \times (0.742 \text{ if female}) \times (1.21 \text{ if African American})$$

Based on the National Health and Nutrition Examination Survey (NHANES) 2003 to 2006, the prevalence of CKD in the United States is 16%, corresponding to more than 31 million people.[2] This number is increased from 12.8% reported with the previous NHANES report from 1988 to 1994,[2] which is attributed to the increased prevalence of diabetes and hypertension, and the aging population.[3]

❶ *CKD is a progressive disease that eventually leads to ESKD.* The prevalence of ESKD has increased more than five-fold since 1980 to more than 500,000 people in 2006 with nearly 111,000 new cases of ESKD diagnosed in 2006.[2] The prevalence of ESKD is related to ethnicity, affecting 3.6 times more African Americans and 1.8 times more Native Americans as Caucasians.[2]

This is likely because these ethnicities have increased risk and prevalence of the causes of CKD, including diabetes mellitus (DM) and hypertension, and other vascular diseases.[1]

Because of the progressive nature of CKD, determination of risk factors for CKD is difficult. Risk factors identified for CKD are classified into three categories (Table 26–2):

- Susceptibility factors, which are associated with an increased risk of developing CKD, but are not directly proven to cause CKD. These factors are generally not modifiable by pharmacologic therapy or lifestyle modifications.

- Initiation factors, which directly cause CKD. These factors are modifiable by pharmacologic therapy.

- Progression factors, which result in a faster decline in kidney function and cause worsening of CKD. These factors may also be modified by pharmacologic therapy or lifestyle modifications to slow the progression of CKD.

Susceptibility Factors

Susceptibility factors can be readily used to develop screening programs for CKD. For example, older patients, those with low kidney mass or birth weight, and those with a family history of kidney disease should be routinely screened for CKD. Minority and low socioeconomic communities may be targets for more widespread CKD screening programs. Other factors, such as hyperlipidemia, are not directly proven to cause CKD, but can be modified by drug therapies.

▶ *Hyperlipidemia*

Patients with CKD have a higher prevalence of dyslipidemia compared to the general population. The dyslipidemia in

---

Table 26–1

NKF-K/DOQI Classification for CKD

State	GFR (mL/min/1.73 m²)
1	90[a] or higher
2	60–89
3	30–59
4	15–29
5	Less than 15 (includes patients on dialysis)

GFR, glomerular filtration rate; NKF-K/DOQI, National Kidney Foundation-Dialysis Outcome Quality Initiative.

[a]CKD can be present with a normal or near normal GFR if other markers of kidney disease are present, such as proteinuria, hematuria, biopsy results showing kidney damage, or anatomic abnormalities (e.g., cysts).

Table 26–2

Risk Factors Associated With CKD

Susceptibility
- Advanced age
- Reduced kidney mass
- Low birth weight
- Racial/ethnic minority
- Family history of kidney disease
- Low income or education
- Systemic inflammation
- Dyslipidemia

Initiation
- Diabetes mellitus
- Hypertension
- Autoimmune disease
- Polycystic kidney disease
- Drug toxicity
- Urinary tract abnormalities (infections, obstruction, stones)

Progression
- Hyperglycemia: Poor blood glucose control (in patients with diabetes)
- Hypertension: Elevated blood pressure
- Proteinuria
- Tobacco smoking

CKD is manifested as an elevation in total cholesterol (TC) levels, low-density lipoprotein cholesterol (LDL-C) levels, triglycerides, and lipoprotein(a) levels, and decreases in high-density lipoprotein cholesterol (HDL-C) levels. The prevalence within the CKD population appears to be related somewhat to the degree of proteinuria. In nephrotic syndrome, with urine protein excretion rates that exceed 3 g/24 hour, almost all patients have some degree of dyslipidemia.[4] Mounting evidence suggests that hyperlipidemia can promote kidney injury and subsequent progression of CKD. The mechanism is similar to that of atherosclerosis, whereby lipid deposition causes activation of macrophages and monocytes, which secrete growth factors that stimulate cell proliferation and oxidation of lipoproteins. These lead to endothelial dysfunction, cellular injury, and fibrosis in the kidney.[5]

Initiation Factors

The three most common causes of CKD in the United States are DM, hypertension, and glomerulonephritis. Together these account for about 75% of the cases of CKD (37% for diabetes, 24% for hypertension, and 14% for glomerulonephritis).[6] These are discussed in further detail below.

▶ Diabetes

DM is the most common cause of CKD, causing 43% of all ESKD, which is increased from 13% in 1980.[6] The risk of developing diabetic kidney disease (DKD) associated with DM is closely linked to hyperglycemia and is similar for both type 1 and type 2, although it is slightly higher in patients with type 2 DM.[7] An estimated 3% of patients with DM will develop ESKD, which is 12 times greater than those without DM.[8]

▶ Hypertension

The second most common cause of CKD is hypertension.[6] It is more difficult to determine the true risk of developing CKD in patients with hypertension because the two are so closely linked, with CKD also being a cause of hypertension. The prevalence of hypertension is correlated with the degree of kidney dysfunction (decreased GFR) with 40% of patients with CKD stage 1, 55% of patients with CKD stage 2, and over 75% of patients with CKD stage 3 presenting with hypertension.[1] The risk of developing ESKD is linked to both systolic and diastolic blood pressure.[9] A blood pressure greater than 210/120 mm Hg is associated with a 22% increased relative risk of developing ESKD, compared with a blood pressure less than 120/80 mm Hg.[9]

▶ Glomerulonephritis

The etiologic and pathophysiologic features of glomerular diseases vary with the specific disease, making it difficult to extrapolate the risk for progression of CKD in patients affected by glomerular diseases. Certain glomerular diseases are known to rapidly progress to ESKD, while others progress more slowly or may be reversible.

Progression Factors

Progression factors can be used as predictors of CKD. The most important predictors of CKD include proteinuria, elevated blood pressure, hyperglycemia, and tobacco smoking.

▶ Proteinuria

The presence of protein in the urine is a marker of glomerular and tubular dysfunction and is recognized as an independent risk factor for the progression of CKD.[10] Furthermore, the degree of proteinuria correlates with the risk for progression of CKD. An increase of 1 g of protein excretion per day is associated with a fivefold increase in the risk of progression of CKD, regardless of the cause of CKD.[11] The mechanisms by which proteinuria potentiates CKD are discussed later. Microalbuminuria (greater than 30 mg albumin excreted per day) is also linked with vascular injury and increased cardiovascular mortality.[12]

▶ Elevated Blood Pressure

Systemic blood pressure correlates with glomerular pressure and elevations in both systemic blood pressure and glomerular pressure contribute to glomerular damage. The rate of GFR decline is related to elevated systolic blood pressure and mean arterial pressure. The decline in GFR is estimated to be 14 mL/min per year with a systolic blood pressure of 180 mm Hg. Conversely, the decline in GFR decreases to 2 mL/min per year with a systolic blood pressure of 135 mm Hg.[13]

▶ Elevated Blood Glucose

The reaction between glucose and protein in the blood produces advanced glycation end products (AGEs), which are metabolized in the proximal tubules. Hyperglycemia increases the synthesis of AGEs in patients with diabetes and the corresponding increase in metabolism is suspected to be a cause of DKD.[14]

▶ Tobacco Smoking

Smoking is an independent risk factor for the development of microalbuminuria in primary hypertension. In patients with CKD, smoking is also an independent and dose-dependent risk factor for development of CKD and microalbuminuria, and progression to ESKD.[15] The risk is more pronounced in men compared to women (odds ratio [OR] 3.59), independent of other risk factors.[15] Smoking increases the risk for progression to ESKD in patients with CKD from any cause, and can increase the risk as much as 10-fold, compared to nonsmokers.[15]

The effects of smoking on the kidney are multifactorial and occur in both healthy individuals and those with CKD. Smoking induces intimal thickening and hyperplasia of the glomerulus, and raises systemic blood pressure.[15] Similar effects were seen with chewing tobacco. These effects are related to the amount of nicotine exposure.[15]

PATHOPHYSIOLOGY

● A number of factors can cause initial damage to the kidney. The resulting sequelae, however, follow a common pathway that promotes progression of CKD and results in irreversible damage leading to ESKD (Fig. 26–1).

The initial damage to the kidney can result from any of the initiation factors listed in Table 26–2. Regardless of the cause, however, the damage results in a decrease in the number of functioning nephrons. The remaining nephrons hypertrophy to increase glomerular filtration and tubular function, both reabsorption and secretion, in attempt to compensate for the loss of kidney function. Initially, these adaptive changes preserve many of the clinical parameters of kidney function, including creatinine and electrolyte excretion. However, as time progresses, angiotensin II is required to maintain the hyperfiltration state of the functioning nephrons. Angiotensin II is a potent vasoconstrictor of both the afferent and efferent arterioles, but has a preferential effect to constrict the efferent arteriole, thereby increasing the pressure in the glomerular capillaries. Increased glomerular capillary pressure expands the pores in the glomerular basement membrane, altering the size-selective barrier and allowing proteins to be filtered through the glomerulus.[16]

Protein excretion through the nephron, or proteinuria, increases nephron loss through various complex mechanisms.

Filtered proteins are reabsorbed in the renal tubules, which activates the tubular cells to produce inflammatory and vasoactive cytokines and triggers complement activation.[16] These cytokines cause interstitial damage and scarring in the renal tubules, leading to damage and loss of more nephrons. Ultimately, the process leads to progressive loss of nephrons to the point where the number of remaining functioning nephrons is too small to maintain clinical stability, and kidney function declines.

ASSESSMENT

Because CKD often presents without symptoms, assessment for CKD relies on appropriate screening strategies in all patients with risk factors for developing CKD (Table 26–2). Evaluation for CKD and the subsequent treatment strategies are dependent on the diagnosis, comorbid conditions, severity and complications of disease, and risk factors for the progression of CKD. ❷ *Early treatment of CKD and the associated complications of CKD are the most important factors to decrease morbidity and mortality associated with CKD.* However, the probability of patients not diagnosed with CKD to have an assessment of serum creatinine (SCr) or urine protein excretion ranges from 0.01 to 0.04, depending on insurance coverage.[17] Screening for CKD

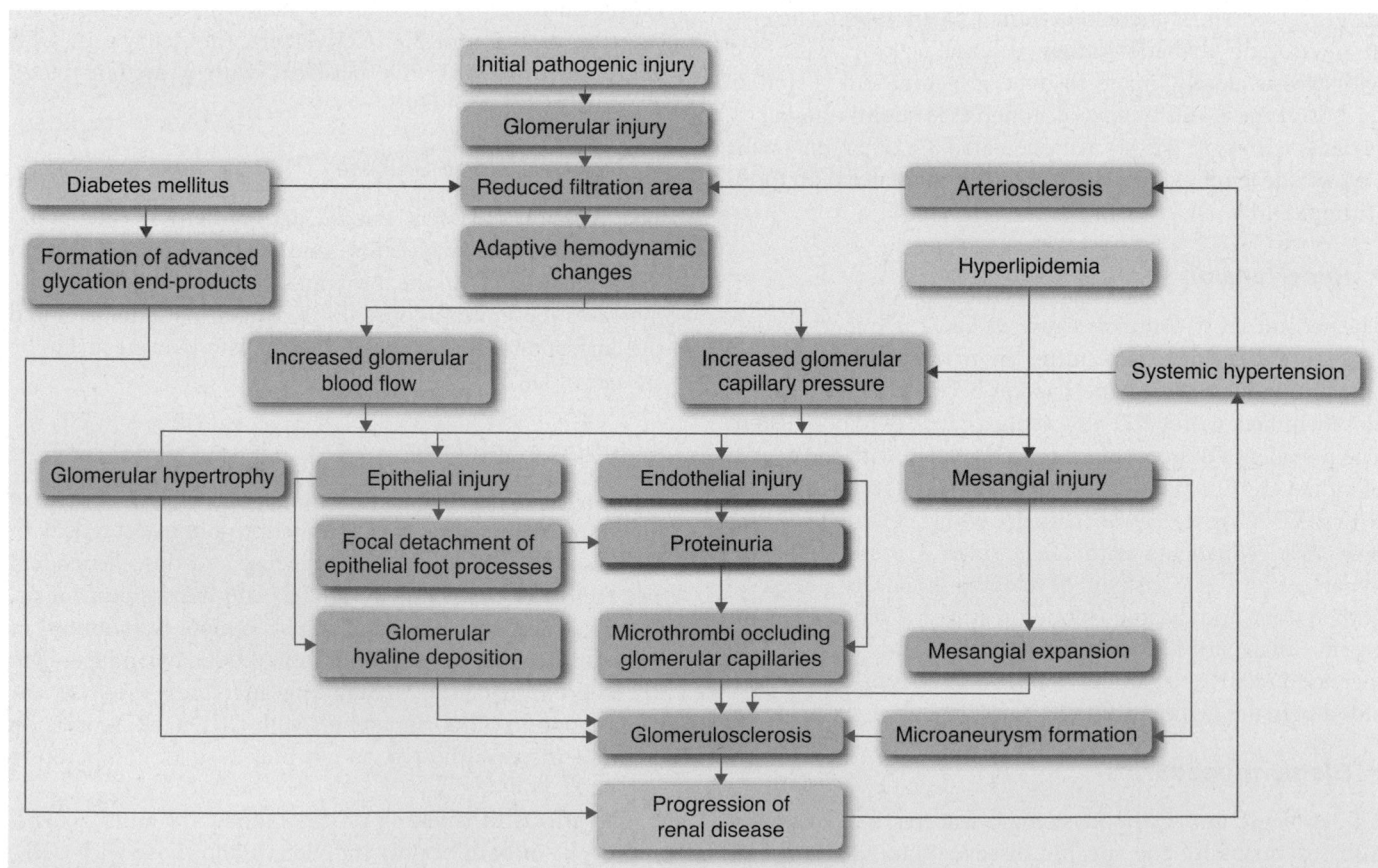

FIGURE 26–1. Proposed mechanisms for progression of kidney disease. (From Joy MS, Kshirsagar A, Franceschini N. Chronic kidney disease: Progression-modifying therapies. In: DiPiro JT, Talbert RL, Yee GC, et al., eds. Pharmacotherapy: A Pathophysiologic Approach, 7th ed. New York: McGraw-Hill; 2008: 749, with permission.)

should be performed in all people with an increased risk for developing CKD, including patients with DM, hypertension, genitourinary abnormalities, autoimmune disease, increased age, or a family history of kidney disease. The assessment for CKD should include measurement of SCr, urinalysis, blood pressure, serum electrolytes, and/or imaging studies.

The primary marker of structural kidney damage is proteinuria, even in patients with normal GFR. Clinically significant proteinuria is defined as urinary protein excretion greater than 300 mg/day or greater than 20 mcg/min in a timed urine collection. Significant proteinuria can also be determined by a spot urine dipstick greater than 30 mg/dL or a urine protein/creatinine ratio greater than 200 mg/g.[1] Microalbuminuria is defined as 30 to 300 mg of albumin excreted in the urine per day or a urine albumin/creatinine ratio greater than 30 mg/day.[1] The NKF recommends routine assessment of proteinuria to detect CKD. A urine dipstick positive for the presence of protein warrants quantification of proteinuria. Patients with a urine protein/creatinine ratio greater than 200 mg/g or urine albumin/creatinine ratio greater than 30 mg/g should undergo diagnostic evaluation; patients with values below these levels should be reevaluated routinely.[1] Assessment of microalbuminuria is particularly important in patients with DM. Screening for microalbu-minuria should be performed 5 years after the diagnosis of type 1 DM and at the time of diagnosis of type 2 DM.[18]

Other markers for structural kidney damage that can be used in place of proteinuria include abnormalities in urinary sediment, such as hematuria, or abnormalities in imaging studies or kidney biopsy.[1]

Complications

❸ The decline in kidney function is associated with a number of complications, which will be discussed later in the chapter, including:

- Fluid and electrolyte disorders
- Anemia
- Metabolic bone disease

TREATMENT

Desired Outcomes

The primary goal is to slow and prevent the progression of CKD. This requires early identification of patients at risk for CKD to initiate interventions early in the course of the disease.

Clinical Presentation and Diagnosis of CKD

General

The development of CKD is usually subtle in onset, often with no noticeable symptoms.

Symptoms

Stages 1 and 2 CKD are generally asymptomatic.

Stages 3 and 4 CKD may be associated with minimal symptoms.

Stage 5 CKD can be associated with pruritus, dysgeusia, nausea, vomiting, constipation, muscle pain, fatigue, and bleeding abnormalities.

Signs

Cardiovascular: Worsening hypertension, edema, dyslipidemia, left ventricular hypertrophy, electrocardiographic changes and chronic heart failure.

Musculoskeletal: Cramping.

Neuropsychiatric: Depression, anxiety, impaired mental cognition.

GI: Gastroesophageal reflux disease, GI bleeding, and abdominal distention.

Genitourinary: Changes in urine volume and consistency, "foaming" of urine (indicative of proteinuria), and sexual dysfunction.

Laboratory Tests

Stages 1 and 2 CKD: Increased blood urea nitrogen (BUN) and serum creatinine (SCr) and decreased GFR.

Stages 3, 4, and 5 CKD: Increased BUN and SCr; decreased GFR.

Advanced stages: Increased potassium, phosphorus, and magnesium; decreased bicarbonate (metabolic acidosis); calcium levels are generally low in earlier stages of CKD and may be elevated in stage 5 CKD, secondary to the use of calcium-containing phosphate binders.

Decreased albumin, if inadequate nutrition intake in advanced stages.

Decreased red blood cell (RBC) count, hemoglobin (Hgb) and hematocrit (Hct); iron metabolism may also be altered (iron level, total iron binding capacity [TIBC], serum ferritin level, and transferrin saturation [TSAT]). Erythropoietin levels are not routinely monitored and are generally normal to low. Urine positive for albumin or protein.

Increased parathyroid hormone (PTH) level; decreased vitamin D levels (stages 4 or 5 CKD).

Stool may be Hemoccult-positive if GI bleeding occurs from uremia.

Other Diagnostic Tests

Structural abnormalities of kidney may be present on diagnostic exams.

Nonpharmacologic Therapy

▶ *Nutritional Management*

Reduction in dietary protein intake has been shown to slow the progression of kidney disease.[10] However, protein restriction must be balanced with the risk of malnutrition in patients with CKD. Patients with a GFR less than 25 mL/min/1.73 m² received the most benefit from protein restriction;[10] therefore, patients with a GFR above this level should not restrict protein intake. The NKF recommends that patients who have a GFR less than 25 mL/min/1.73 m² who are not receiving dialysis, however, should restrict protein intake to 0.6 g/kg/day. If patients are not able to maintain adequate dietary energy intake, protein intake may be increased up to 0.75 g/kg/day.[19] Malnutrition is common in patients with ESKD for various reasons, including decreased appetite, hypercatabolism, and nutrient losses through dialysis. For this reason, patients receiving dialysis should maintain protein intake of 1.2 g/kg/day to 1.3 g/kg/day.

Protein intake can have unique contributions to kidney damage in patients with DM. Dietary protein, particularly protein from animal sources, produces AGEs, which are an important cause of kidney damage in patients with DM.[20] The NKF recommends that patients with DM with CKD stages 1 to 4 should limit protein intake to 0.8 g/kg/day to reduce proteinuria and stabilize kidney function.[18]

Pharmacologic Therapy

▶ *Intensive Blood Glucose Control (for Patients With Diabetes)*

The target glycosylated hemoglobin level (HbA1c) should be less than 7.0% (0.07) for patients with DM to decrease the incidence of proteinuria and albuminuria in patients with and without documented DKD.[18] This generally involves intensive insulin therapy, the administration of insulin three or more times daily to maintain preprandial blood glucose levels between 70 and 120 g/dL (3.9–6.7 mmol/L) and postprandial blood glucose levels less than 180 g/dL (10 mmol/L). This strategy has been proven to be effective in delaying the development and progression of DKD in patients with type 1[21] and type 2 DM.[18] Continued benefits of intensive insulin therapy have been demonstrated up to 8 years in patients with type 1 DM.[21] A decrease in HbA1c levels by 0.9% (0.009) has been shown to decrease the relative risk for microalbuminuria by 30% in patients with type 2 DM.[22]

▶ *Optimal Blood Pressure Control*

Reductions in blood pressure are associated with a decrease in proteinuria, leading to a decrease in the rate of progression of kidney disease. The NKF recommends a goal blood pressure of less than 130/80 mm Hg in patients with stages 1 through 4 CKD.[23]

In patients with stage 5 CKD who are receiving hemodialysis, cardiovascular mortality is affected by blood pressure levels both before and after hemodialysis.[24] Elevated blood pressure levels after hemodialysis increases cardiovascular risk. Both systolic blood pressure greater than 180 mm Hg and diastolic blood pressure greater than 90 mm Hg are independently associated with an increased risk of cardiovascular mortality (relative risk 1.96 and 1.73, respectively).[24] Likewise, low blood pressure levels either before or after hemodialysis are also associated with increased cardiovascular mortality. A systolic blood pressure less than 110 mm Hg before hemodialysis is associated with a four-fold increase in cardiovascular mortality; the same blood pressure at the end of hemodialysis is associated with a 2.62 relative risk.[24] Therefore, the NKF recommends achieving a goal blood pressure less than 140/90 mm Hg before hemodialysis and less than 130/80 mm Hg after hemodialysis.[25] These goals are controversial, however. One recent study demonstrated an increased risk of mortality for patients who achieved the target blood pressure recommended by the guidelines (hazards ratio 1.9).[26]

Because hypertension and kidney dysfunction are linked, blood pressure control can be more difficult to attain in patients with CKD compared to patients with normal kidney function. All antihypertensive agents have similar effects on reducing blood pressure. However, three or more agents are generally required to achieve the blood pressure goal of less than 130/80 mm Hg in CKD patients.[23]

▶ *Reduction in Proteinuria*

The ability of antihypertensive agents to preserve kidney function differs. Angiotensin-converting enzyme inhibitors (ACEIs) and angiotensin receptor blockers (ARBs) decrease glomerular capillary pressure and volume because of their effects on angiotensin II. This, in turn, reduces the amount of protein filtered through the glomerulus, independent of the reduction in blood pressure,[27] which ultimately decreases the progression of CKD. ❹ *The ability of ACEIs and ARBs to reduce proteinuria is greater than that of other antihypertensives, up to 35% to 40%,[23] making ACEIs and ARBs the antihypertensive agents of choice for all patients with CKD, unless contraindicated.* All patients with documented proteinuria should receive an ACE-I or ARB, regardless of blood pressure.[23] Because diabetes is associated with an early onset of microalbuminuria, all patients with diabetes should also receive an ACE-I or ARB, regardless of blood pressure.[23] When initiating ACE-I or ARB therapy, the dose should be titrated to the maximum tolerated dose, even if the blood pressure is less than 130/80 mm Hg. Figure 26–2 depicts an algorithm for the treatment of hypertension in patients with CKD. Patients who do not achieve adequate reductions in blood pressure or protein excretion may benefit from combination therapy with an ACE-I and an ARB.[23] However, the benefits of combination therapy have been questioned by recent studies. Several large clinical trials have demonstrated that combination therapy with an ACE-I and

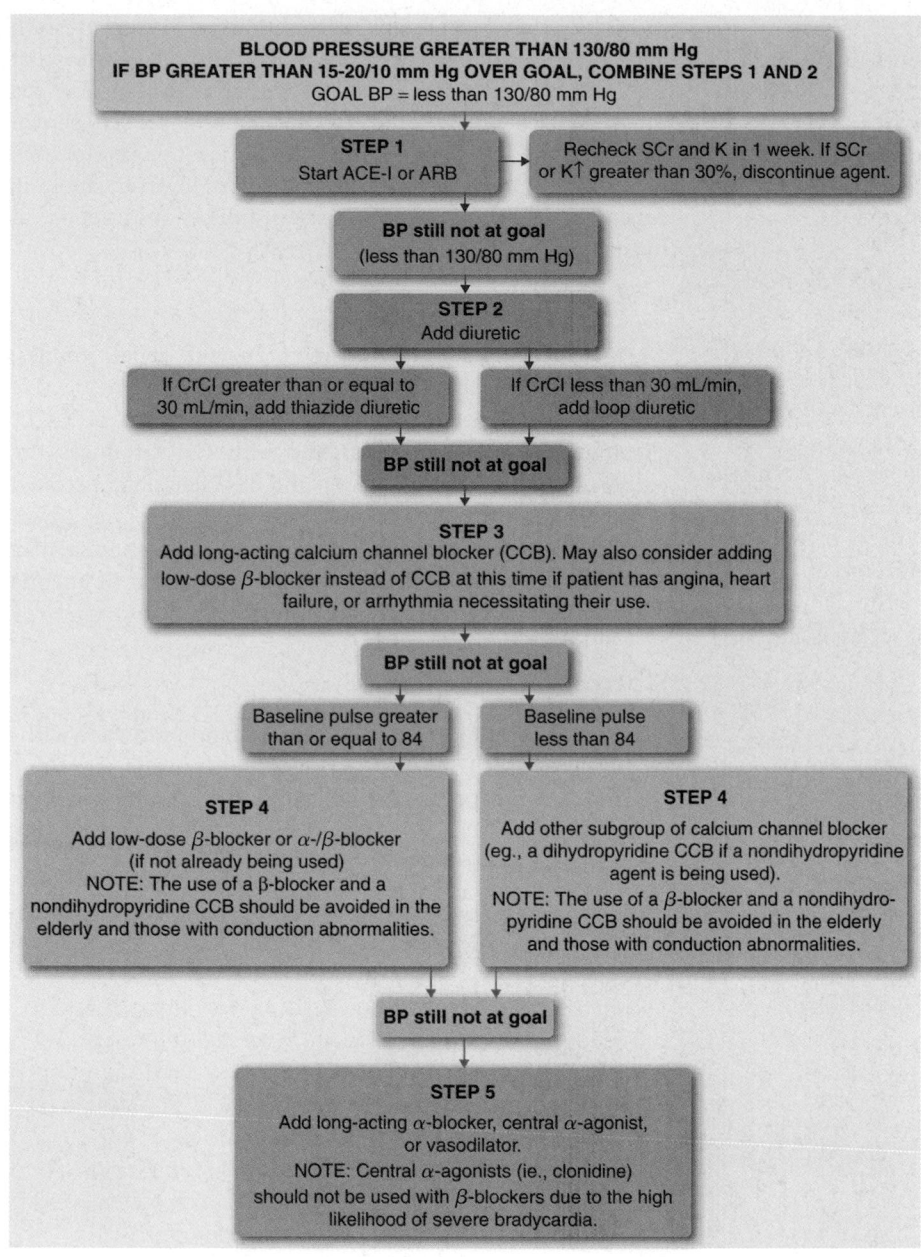

BLOOD PRESSURE GREATER THAN 130/80 mm Hg
IF BP GREATER THAN 15-20/10 mm Hg OVER GOAL, COMBINE STEPS 1 AND 2
GOAL BP = less than 130/80 mm Hg

STEP 1
Start ACE-I or ARB

Recheck SCr and K in 1 week. If SCr or K↑ greater than 30%, discontinue agent.

BP still not at goal
(less than 130/80 mm Hg)

STEP 2
Add diuretic

If CrCl greater than or equal to 30 mL/min, add thiazide diuretic

If CrCl less than 30 mL/min, add loop diuretic

BP still not at goal

STEP 3
Add long-acting calcium channel blocker (CCB). May also consider adding low-dose β-blocker instead of CCB at this time if patient has angina, heart failure, or arrhythmia necessitating their use.

BP still not at goal

Baseline pulse greater than or equal to 84

Baseline pulse less than 84

STEP 4
Add low-dose β-blocker or α-/β-blocker (if not already being used)
NOTE: The use of a β-blocker and a nondihydropyridine CCB should be avoided in the elderly and those with conduction abnormalities.

STEP 4
Add other subgroup of calcium channel blocker (eg., a dihydropyridine CCB if a nondihydropyridine agent is being used).
NOTE: The use of a β-blocker and a nondihydropyridine CCB should be avoided in the elderly and those with conduction abnormalities.

BP still not at goal

STEP 5
Add long-acting α-blocker, central α-agonist, or vasodilator.
NOTE: Central α-agonists (ie., clonidine) should not be used with β-blockers due to the high likelihood of severe bradycardia.

FIGURE 26–2. Hypertension management algorithm for patients with CKD. Dosage adjustments should be made every 2 to 4 weeks as needed. The dose of one agent should be maximized before another is added. (ACE-I, angiotensin-converting enzyme inhibitor; ARB, angiotensin receptor blocker; BP, blood pressure; CrCl, creatinine clearance; K, potassium; Scr, serum creatinine.) (From Joy MS, Kshirsagar A, Franceschini N. Chronic kidney disease: Progression-modifying therapies. In: DiPiro JT, Talbert RL, Yee GC, et al., eds. Pharmacotherapy: A Pathophysiologic Approach, 7th ed. New York: McGraw-Hill; 2008: 752, with permission.)

ARB has been demonstrated to reduce proteinuria more than maximal doses of either agent alone.[28,29] However, one study discovered that progression of kidney disease was worsened with combination therapy compared to either agent alone.[28]

The nondihydropyridine calcium channel blockers (CCBs) have been shown to also decrease protein excretion in patients with and without diabetes,[30] but the reduction in proteinuria appears to be related to the reductions in blood pressure. The maximal effect of nondihydropyridine CCBs on proteinuria is seen with a blood pressure reduction to less than 130/80 mm Hg and no additional benefit is seen with increased doses. Dihydropyridine CCBs, however, do not have the same effects on protein excretion. In fact, dihydropyridine CCBs worsen protein excretion, despite similar reductions in blood pressure as nondihydropyridine CCBs.[30]

Other Interventions to Limit Progression of CKD

▶ *Hyperlipidemia Treatment*

Hyperlipidemia plays a role in the development of cardiovascular disease (CVD) in patients with CKD. The primary goal of treatment of dyslipidemias is to decrease the risk of atherosclerotic CVD. A secondary goal in patients with CKD is to reduce proteinuria and decline in kidney function. Treatment of hyperlipidemia in patients with CKD has been demonstrated to slow the decline in GFR by 1.9 mL/min per year of treatment with antihyperlipidemic agents.[31]

The NKF suggests that CKD should be classified as a coronary heart disease (CHD) risk equivalent and the goal

LDL-C level should be below 100 mg/dL (2.59 mmol/L) in all patients with CKD.[25,32] The most frequently used agents for the treatment of dyslipidemias in patients with CKD are the 3-hydroxy-3-methylglutaryl coenzyme A (HMG-CoA) reductase inhibitors ("statins") and the fibric acid derivatives. However, other treatments have been studied in patients with CKD and should be considered if first-line therapies are contraindicated.

Another important consideration in treating lipid disorders in patients with CKD is management of proteinuria. Protein excretion in the nephrotic range (greater than 3 g/day) is associated with an increase in both total and LDL-C levels.[33] Triglyceride levels can also be elevated in patients with severe proteinuria. Results from clinical trials suggest that the use of ACEIs to reduce proteinuria can decrease TC levels.[34] While the use of ACEIs is unlikely to decrease cholesterol to goal levels, reducing proteinuria can aid in cholesterol reduction, particularly in patients with nephrotic syndrome or severe proteinuria. Conversely, treatment of hyperlipidemia can reduce protein excretion and subsequent progression of CKD.[4]

▶ Smoking Cessation

While the effects of smoking on the development and progression of CKD are well established, as discussed previously, the effect of smoking cessation on CKD progression has not been studied. Data are emerging that suggest that smoking cessation may be a practical approach to slow the progression of CKD. Smoking cessation has been shown to reduce the risk of myocardial infarction by 50% to 70%, regardless of previous nicotine exposure.[15] However, smoking cessation does not reverse existing kidney dysfunction in former smokers.

▶ Anemia Treatment

Anemia decreases oxygen delivery to the renal tubules, promoting the release of inflammatory and vasoactive cytokines, which contribute to the progression of CKD. Treatment of anemia in patients with CKD reduces the cardiovascular effects of anemia and has been demonstrated to decrease morbidity and mortality by as much as 20%.[35] Studies have demonstrated that treatment of anemia may slow the progression of CKD.[36] The management of anemia will be discussed later.

Outcome Evaluation

Monitor SCr and potassium levels and blood pressure within 1 week after initiating ACE-I or ARB therapy. Discontinue the medication and switch to another agent if a sudden

---

Patient Encounter, Part 1

A 62-year-old obese Caucasian female with a history of diabetes and hypertension presents to clinic for routine follow-up. Her fasting blood sugars have been elevated recently, averaging 180 to 250 mg/dL (10–13.9 mmol/L).

PMH: Diabetes mellitus for 8 years, not currently controlled; hypertension for 5 years, not currently controlled; hyperlipidemia, currently managed by diet therapy

FH: Mother is alive at age 87 with coronary artery disease; father is deceased from diabetes; she has no siblings

SH: She does not work; she smokes one pack of cigarettes per day, but denies alcohol or illicit drug use; she is sedentary

Meds: Furosemide 20 mg orally daily; nifedipine XL 30 mg orally daily; glyburide 10 mg orally daily

ROS: Unremarkable

PE:

VS: BP 145/92 mm Hg, P 82 bpm, T 36.9°C (98.4°F), ht 5'4" (163 cm), wt 86.4 kg (190 lb)

CV: RRR, normal S_1, S_2; no murmurs, rubs or gallops; lungs clear

Abd: Obese; no organomegaly, bruits or tenderness, (+) bowel sounds; heme (–) stool

Exts: Trace pedal edema bilaterally; decreased sensation in feet to light touch; no lesions

Labs (Fasting): Sodium 145 mEq/L (145 mmol/L); potassium 3.2 mEq/L (3.2 mmol/L); chloride 112 mEq/L (112 mmol/L); carbon dioxide 26 mEq/L (26 mmol/L); blood urea nitrogen (BUN) 20 mg/dL (7.14 mmol/L urea); serum creatinine (SCr) 1.4 mg/dL (124 μmol/L); glucose 240 mg/dL (13.32 mmol/L); total cholesterol 196 mg/dL (5.07 mmol/L); low-density lipoprotein cholesterol (LDL-C) 112 mg/dL (2.90 mmol/L); high-density lipoprotein cholesterol (HDL-C) 28 mg/dL (0.72 mmol/L); triglycerides 280 mg/dL (3.16 mmol/L); hemoglobin$_{A1c}$ (Hb$_{A1c}$) 10% (0.1); urine microalbumin 270 mg/dL (2.7 g/L)

What risk factors does the patient have for the development of CKD?

What signs and symptoms are consistent with CKD?

How would you classify her CKD?

Identify your treatment goals for the patient.

What lifestyle modifications would you recommend for this patient with CKD?

What pharmacologic alternatives are available for this patient for treatment of CKD?

What other interventions are appropriate to minimize the progression of CKD?

increase in SCr greater than 30% occurs, hyperkalemia develops, or the patient becomes hypotensive. Titrate the dose of the ACE-I or ARB every 1 to 3 months to the maximum tolerable dose. If blood pressure is not reduced to less than 130/80 mm Hg, add another agent to the regimen. Refer the patient to a nephrologist to manage complications associated with CKD. As CKD progresses to stage 4, begin discussion to prepare the patient for renal replacement therapy (RRT).

CONSEQUENCES OF CKD AND ESKD

Impaired Sodium and Water Homeostasis

Sodium and water balance are primarily regulated by the kidney. Reductions in the number of functioning nephrons decrease glomerular filtration and subsequent reabsorption of sodium and water, leading to edema.

▶ *Pathophysiology*

Sodium and water balance can be maintained despite wide variations in intake with normal kidney function. The fractional excretion of sodium (FE_{Na}) is approximately 1% to 3% with normal kidney function, allowing sodium balance to be maintained with a sodium intake of 120 to 150 mEq (120–150 mmol) per day. Urine osmolality can range from 50–1,200 mOsm/L (50 to 1,200 mmol/L) with normal kidney function, allowing for water balance to be maintained with a wide range of fluid intake. As the number of functioning nephrons decreases, the remaining nephrons increase sodium excretion and FE_{Na} may increase up to 10% to 20%.[37] This produces an osmotic diuresis which impairs the ability of the kidneys to concentrate and dilute urine and the urine becomes fixed at an osmolality close to that of the plasma, approximately 300 mOsm/L (300 mmol/L). The inability of the kidney to concentrate the urine results in nocturia in patients with CKD, usually presenting as early as stage 3 CKD.

As the number of functioning nephrons continues to decline, the sodium load overwhelms the remaining nephrons and total sodium excretion is decreased, despite the increase in sodium excretion by the functioning nephrons. Sodium retention causes fluid retention that increases intravascular volume and raises systemic blood pressure. Severe volume overload can lead to pulmonary edema.

▶ *Treatment*

Nonpharmacologic Therapy   The kidney is unable to adjust to abrupt changes in sodium intake in patients with severe CKD. Therefore, patients should be advised to refrain from adding salt to their diet, but should not restrict sodium intake. Changes in sodium intake should occur slowly over a period of several days to allow adequate time for the kidney to adjust urinary sodium content. Sodium restriction produces a negative sodium balance, which causes fluid excretion to restore sodium balance. The resulting volume contraction can decrease perfusion of the kidney and hasten the decline in GFR. Saline-containing IV solutions should be used cautiously in patients with CKD because the salt load may precipitate volume overload.

Fluid restriction is generally unnecessary as long as sodium intake is controlled. The thirst mechanism remains intact in CKD to maintain total body water and plasma osmolality near normal levels. Fluid intake should be maintained at the rate of urine output to replace urine losses, usually fixed at approximately 2 L/day as urine concentrating ability is lost. Significant increases in free water intake orally or IV can precipitate volume overload and hyponatremia. Patients with stage 5 CKD require RRT to maintain normal volume status. Fluid intake is often limited in patients receiving hemodialysis to prevent fluid overload between dialysis sessions.

Pharmacologic Therapy   Diuretic therapy is often necessary to prevent volume overload in patients with CKD in those who still produce urine. Loop diuretics are most frequently used to increase sodium and water excretion. Thiazide diuretics are ineffective when used alone in patients with a GFR less than 30 mL/min/1.73 m².[23,38] As CKD progresses, higher doses, as much as 80 to 1,000 mg/day of furosemide, or continuous infusion of loop diuretics may be needed, or combination therapy with loop and thiazide diuretics to increase sodium and water excretion.[23,38]

▶ *Outcome Evaluation*

Monitor edema after initiation of diuretic therapy. Monitor fluid intake to ensure obligatory losses are being met and avoid dehydration. If adequate diuresis is not attained with a single agent, consider combination therapy with another diuretic.

Clinical Presentation and Diagnosis of Impaired Sodium and Water Homeostasis

General

Alterations in sodium and water balance in CKD manifests as increased edema.

Symptoms

Nocturia can present in stage 3 CKD.

Edema generally presents in stage 4 CKD or later.

Signs

Cardiovascular: Worsening hypertension, edema

Genitourinary: Change in urine volume and consistency

Laboratory Tests

Increased blood pressure

Sodium levels remain within the normal range

Urine osmolality is generally fixed at 300 mOsm/L (300 mmol/L)

Impaired Potassium Homeostasis

Potassium balance is also primarily regulated by the kidney via the distal tubular cells. Reduction in the number of functioning nephrons decreases the overall tubular secretion of potassium, leading to hyperkalemia. Hyperkalemia is estimated to affect more than 50% of patients with stage 5 CKD.[39]

▶ *Pathophysiology*

The distal tubules secrete 90% to 95% of the daily dietary intake of potassium. The fractional excretion of potassium (FE_K) is approximately 25% with normal kidney function.[40] The GI tract excretes the remaining 5% to 10% of dietary potassium intake. Following a large potassium load, extracellular potassium is shifted intracellularly to maintain stable extracellular levels.

As the number of functioning nephrons decreases, both the distal tubular secretion and GI excretion are increased in the functioning nephrons because of aldosterone stimulation. Functioning nephrons increase FE_K up to 100% and GI excretion increases as much as 30% to 70% in CKD,[41] as a result of aldosterone secretion in response to increased potassium levels.[41] This maintains serum potassium concentrations within the normal range through stages 1 to 4 CKD. Hyperkalemia begins to develop when GFR falls below 20% of normal, when the number of functioning nephrons and renal potassium secretion is so low that the capacity of the GI tract to excrete potassium has been exceeded.[41]

Medications can increase the risk of hyperkalemia in patients with CKD, including ACE-I and ARBs, used for the treatment of proteinuria and hypertension. Potassium-sparing diuretics, used for the treatment of edema and chronic heart failure, can also exacerbate the development of hyperkalemia, and should be used with caution in patients with stage 3 CKD or higher.

▶ *Treatment*

Nonpharmacologic Therapy Patients with CKD should avoid abrupt increases in dietary intake of potassium because the kidney is unable to increase potassium excretion with an acute potassium load, particularly in latter stages of the disease. Hyperkalemia resulting from an acute increase in potassium intake can be more severe and prolonged. Patients who develop hyperkalemia should restrict dietary intake of potassium to 50 to 80 mEq (50–80 mmol) per day. Potassium concentrations can also be altered in the dialysate for patients receiving hemodialysis and peritoneal dialysis to manage hyperkalemia. Because GI excretion of potassium plays a large role in potassium homeostasis in patients with stage 5 CKD, a good bowel regimen is essential to minimize constipation, which can occur in 40% of patients receiving hemodialysis.[40] Severe hyperkalemia is most effectively managed by hemodialysis.

Pharmacologic Therapy Patients with acute hyperkalemia usually require other therapies to manage hyperkalemia

---

Clinical Presentation and Diagnosis of Hyperkalemia

General

Hyperkalemia is generally asymptomatic in patients with CKD until serum potassium levels are greater than 5.5 mEq/L (5.5 mmol/L), when cardiac abnormalities present

Symptoms

Mild hyperkalemia is generally not associated with overt symptoms

Symptoms generally appear in stage 4 or 5 CKD

Signs

Cardiovascular: ECG changes (peaked T waves, widened QRS complex, loss of P wave)

Laboratory Tests

Increased serum potassium levels

---

until dialysis can be initiated. Patients who present with hyperkalemia-induced cardiac abnormalities, which manifest as peaked T waves, a widened QRS complex or loss of P waves, should receive calcium gluconate or chloride (1 g IV) to reverse the cardiac effects. Temporary measures can be employed to shift extracellular potassium into the intracellular compartment to stabilize cellular membrane effects of excessive serum potassium levels. Such measures include the use of regular insulin (5–10 units IV) and dextrose (5–50% IV), or nebulized albuterol (salbutamol) (10–20 mg). Sodium bicarbonate should not be used to shift extracellular potassium intracellularly in patients with CKD unless severe metabolic acidosis (pH less than 7.2) is present. These measures will decrease serum potassium levels within 30 to 60 minutes after treatment, but potassium must still be removed from the body. Shifting potassium to the intracellular compartment, however, decreases potassium removal by dialysis. Often, multiple dialysis sessions are required to remove potassium that is redistributed from the intracellular space back into the serum.

Sodium polystyrene sulfonate (SPS, 15–30 g orally or rectally), a sodium-potassium exchange resin, promotes potassium excretion from the GI tract. The onset of action is within 2 hours after administration of SPS, but the maximum effect on potassium levels may not be seen for up to 6 hours, which limits the utility in patients with severe hyperkalemia. Of note, loop diuretics are often used to decrease potassium levels in patients with normal or mildly decreased kidney function, but are not useful in patients with stage 5 CKD to decrease potassium concentrations. Fludrocortisone is a mineralocorticoid that mimics the effects of aldosterone and increases potassium excretion in the distal tubules and through the GI tract. However, fludrocortisone causes significant sodium and water retention, which exacerbates edema and hypertension, and may not be tolerated by many CKD patients.

▶ Outcome Evaluation

Monitor ECG continuously in patients with cardiac abnormalities until serum potassium levels drop below 5 mEq/L (5 mmol/L) or cardiac abnormalities resolve. Evaluate serum potassium and glucose levels within 1 hour in patients who receive insulin and dextrose therapy. Evaluate serum potassium levels within 2 to 4 hours after treatment with SPS or diuretics. Repeat doses of diuretics or SPS if necessary until serum potassium levels fall below 5 mEq/L (5 mmol/L). Monitor blood pressure and serum potassium levels in 1 week in patients who receive fludrocortisone.

Anemia of CKD

The progenitor cells of the kidney produce 90% of the hormone erythropoietin (EPO), which stimulates red blood cell (RBC) production. ❺ *Reduction in the number of functioning nephrons decreases renal production of EPO, which is the primary cause of anemia in patients with CKD. The development of anemia of CKD results in decreased oxygen delivery and utilization, leading to increased cardiac output and left ventricular hypertrophy (LVH), which increase the cardiovascular risk and mortality in patients with CKD.*

▶ Epidemiology and Etiology

Current NKF guidelines define anemia as a hemoglobin (Hgb) level less than 13.5 g/dL (135 g/L or 8.37 mmol/L) in males and less than 12 g/dL (120 g/L or 7.4 mmol/L) in females.[42] A number of factors can contribute to the development of anemia, including deficiencies in vitamin B_{12}

or folate, hemolysis, bleeding, or bone marrow suppression. Many of these can be detected by alterations in RBC indices, which should be included in the evaluation for anemia. A complete blood cell count is also helpful in evaluating anemia to determine overall bone marrow function.

The prevalence of anemia correlates with the degree of kidney dysfunction. More than 26% of patients with a GFR greater than 60 mL/min/1.73 m² are estimated to have Hgb levels less than 12 g/dL (120 g/L or 7.4 mmol/L), and the number increases to 75% in patients with a GFR less than 15 mL/min/1.73 m².[43] The risk of developing anemia also increases as GFR declines, doubling for patients with stage 3 CKD, increasing to 3.8-fold in patients with stage 4 CKD, and to 10.5-fold for patients with stage 5 CKD, compared to stages 1 and 2 CKD.[43]

▶ Pathophysiology

The primary cause of anemia in patients with CKD is a decrease in EPO production. With normal kidney function, as Hgb, hematocrit (Hct), and tissue oxygenation decrease, the plasma concentration of EPO increases exponentially. As the number of functioning nephrons decrease, EPO production also decreases. Thus, as Hgb, Hct, and tissue oxygenation decrease in patients with CKD, plasma EPO levels remain constant within the normal range, but low relative to the degree of hypoxia present. The result is a normochromic, normocytic anemia.

Several other factors also contribute to the development of anemia in patients with CKD. Uremia, the accumulation of toxins that results from declining kidney function, decreases the lifespan of RBCs from a normal of 120 days to as low as

---

Patient Encounter, Part 2

The patient returns to your clinic 2 years later with complaints of "feeling tired all of the time." She had been trying to exercise more, but has not had enough energy to exercise for the past 6 months or so. She also complains that she feels cold all of the time, despite increasing the temperature in her house.

Current Meds: Furosemide 80 mg orally daily; lisinopril 40 mg orally daily; metoprolol tartarate 50 mg orally twice daily; insulin glargine 25 units subcutaneously at bedtime; insulin lispro subcutaneously per sliding scale with meals

ROS: Slightly pale skin color; fatigue daily in the afternoon; otherwise unremarkable

PE:

VS: BP 135/85 mm Hg, P 72 bpm, T 35.9°C (96.6°F); wt 79.5 kg (175 lb)

Chest: RRR, normal S_1, S_3 present.

Abd: Obese; no organomegaly, bruits or tenderness, (+) bowel sounds; heme (–) stool

Exts: 1+ pedal edema bilaterally; decreased sensation in feet; small lesion on left ankle that appears to be healing slowly

Labs: Sodium 142 mEq/L (142 mmol/L); potassium 4.8 mEq/L (4.8 mmol/L); chloride 103 mEq/L (103 mmol/L); carbon dioxide 20 mEq/L (20 mmol/L); BUN 58 mg/dL (20.71 mmol/L urea); SCr 3.2 mg/dL (283 μmol/L); glucose 130 mg/dL (7.28 mmol/L); white blood cell (WBC) count 4.8 × 10³ cells/m³ (4.8 × 10⁹/L); red blood cell (RBC) count 2.5 × 10⁶ cells/m³ (2.5 × 10¹²/L); hemoglobin (Hgb) 8.0 g/dL (80 g/L or 4.96 mmol/L); hematocrit (Hct) 25% (0.25); platelets 250 × 10³ cells/m³ (250 × 10⁹/L); Hb$_{A1c}$ 7.5% (0.075)

What signs and symptoms are consistent with anemia of CKD?

What additional information could you request to determine other causes of anemia in this patient?

60 days in patients with stage 5 CKD. Iron deficiency and blood loss from regular laboratory testing and hemodialysis also contribute to the development of anemia in patients with CKD.

▶ Treatment

General Approach to Therapy   Studies have demonstrated that initiation of treatment for anemia before stage 5 CKD decreases mortality in patients with ESKD receiving dialysis, particularly in the elderly.[44] The treatment of anemia can decrease morbidity, increase exercise capacity and tolerance, and slow the progression of CKD if target Hgb levels are achieved.[45]

Patients with CKD should be evaluated for anemia when the GFR falls below 60 mL/min or if the SCr rises above 2 mg/dL (177 mmol/L). If the Hgb is less than 11 g/dL (110 g/L or 6.8 mmol/L), an anemia workup should be performed. The workup for anemia should rule out other potential causes for anemia (see Chap. 63). Abnormalities found during the anemia workup should be corrected before initiating erythropoiesis-stimulating agents (ESAs), particularly iron deficiency, as iron is an essential component of RBC production. If Hgb is still below the goal level when all other causes of anemia have been corrected, EPO deficiency should be assumed. EPO levels are not routinely measured and have little clinical significance in monitoring progression and treatment of anemia in patients with CKD.

Clinical Presentation and Diagnosis of Anemia of CKD

General

Anemia of CKD generally presents with fatigue and decreased quality of life.

Symptoms

Anemia of CKD is associated with symptoms of cold intolerance, shortness of breath, and decreased exercise capacity.

Signs

Cardiovascular: Left ventricular hypertrophy, ECG changes, congestive heart failure

Neurologic: Impaired mental cognition

Genitourinary: Sexual dysfunction

Laboratory Tests

Decreased RBC count, Hgb, and Hct

Decreased serum iron level, TIBC, serum ferritin, and TSAT

Decreased erythropoietin levels relative to the degree of hypoxia that is present

---

❻ *Generally, treatment for anemia of CKD requires a combination of ESA and iron supplementation.* The goal of treatment is to maintain Hgb levels between 11 g/dL (110 g/L or 6.8 mmol/L) and 12 g/dL (120 g/L or 7.4 mmol/L).[46] The goals for iron supplementation are:

- Serum ferritin levels
  - 100 to 500 ng/mL (225–1,123.5 pmol/L) for patients not receiving hemodialysis
  - 200 to 500 ng/mL (449.4–123.5 pmol/L) for patients receiving hemodialysis
- Transferrin saturation (TSAT): greater than 20% (0.2).[42]

The approach to the management of anemia of CKD with ESA and iron supplementation is illustrated in Figures 26–3 and 26–4.

Nonpharmacologic Therapy   Sufficient dietary iron intake must be maintained in patients with anemia of CKD. Approximately 1 to 2 mg of iron is absorbed daily from the diet. This small amount is generally not adequate to preserve adequate iron stores to promote RBC production. RBC transfusions have been used in the past as the primary means to maintain Hgb and Hct levels in patients with anemia of CKD. This treatment is still utilized today in patients with severe anemia or contraindications to ESAs, but is considered a third-line therapy for anemia of CKD.

Pharmacologic Therapy   The first-line treatment for anemia of CKD involves replacement of erythropoietin with ESAs. Erythropoietin-stimulating agents are synthetic formulations of EPO produced by recombinant human DNA technology. Use of ESAs increases the iron demand for RBC production and iron deficiency is common, requiring iron supplementation to correct and maintain adequate iron stores to promote RBC production. Androgens were used extensively before the availability of ESAs but are no longer recommended for the treatment of anemia[42] primarily because of toxicity, namely, hepatotoxicity.

Erythropoiesis-Stimulating Agents.   Erythropoietin is a growth factor that acts on erythroblasts formed from stem cells in the bone marrow, stimulating proliferation and differentiation into normoblasts, then reticulocytes, which are released into the bloodstream to eventually mature into erythrocytes (mature RBCs). The ESAs currently available in the United States are:

- Epoetin alfa (distributed as Epogen by Amgen, Inc., Thousand Oaks, CA; and Procrit by Ortho Biotech, Johnson & Johnson, Raritan, NJ)
- Darbepoetin alfa (Aranesp by Amgen, Inc.)

Epoetin α and epoetin β, which is available outside the United States, have the same biological activity as endogenous EPO. Darbepoetin alfa differs from epoetin alfa by the addition of carbohydrate side chains that increase the half-life of darbepoetin alfa compared to epoetin alfa and endogenous EPO, allowing for less frequent dosing than that of epoetin alfa. All ESAs are equivalent in their efficacy and have a similar adverse-effect profile.

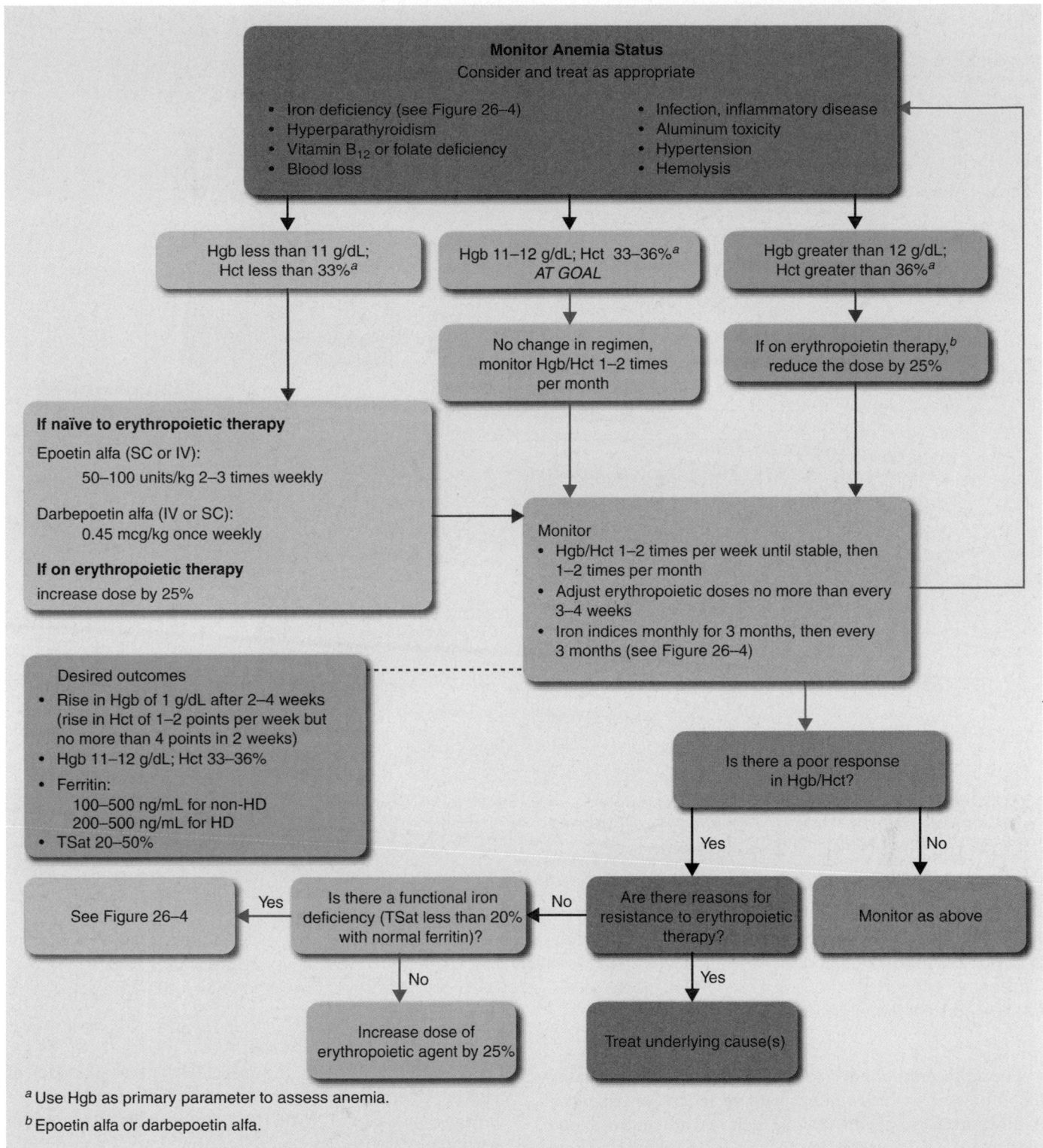

FIGURE 26–3. Guidelines for erythropoietic therapy in the management of anemia of CKD. (Hgb, hemoglobin; SC, subcutaneous; TSat; transferrin saturation.) (Adapted from Hudson JQ. Chronic kidney disease: Management of complications. In: DiPiro JT, Talbert RL, Yee GC, et al., eds. Pharmacotherapy: A Pathophysiologic Approach, 7th ed. New York: McGraw-Hill; 2008: 775, with permission.)

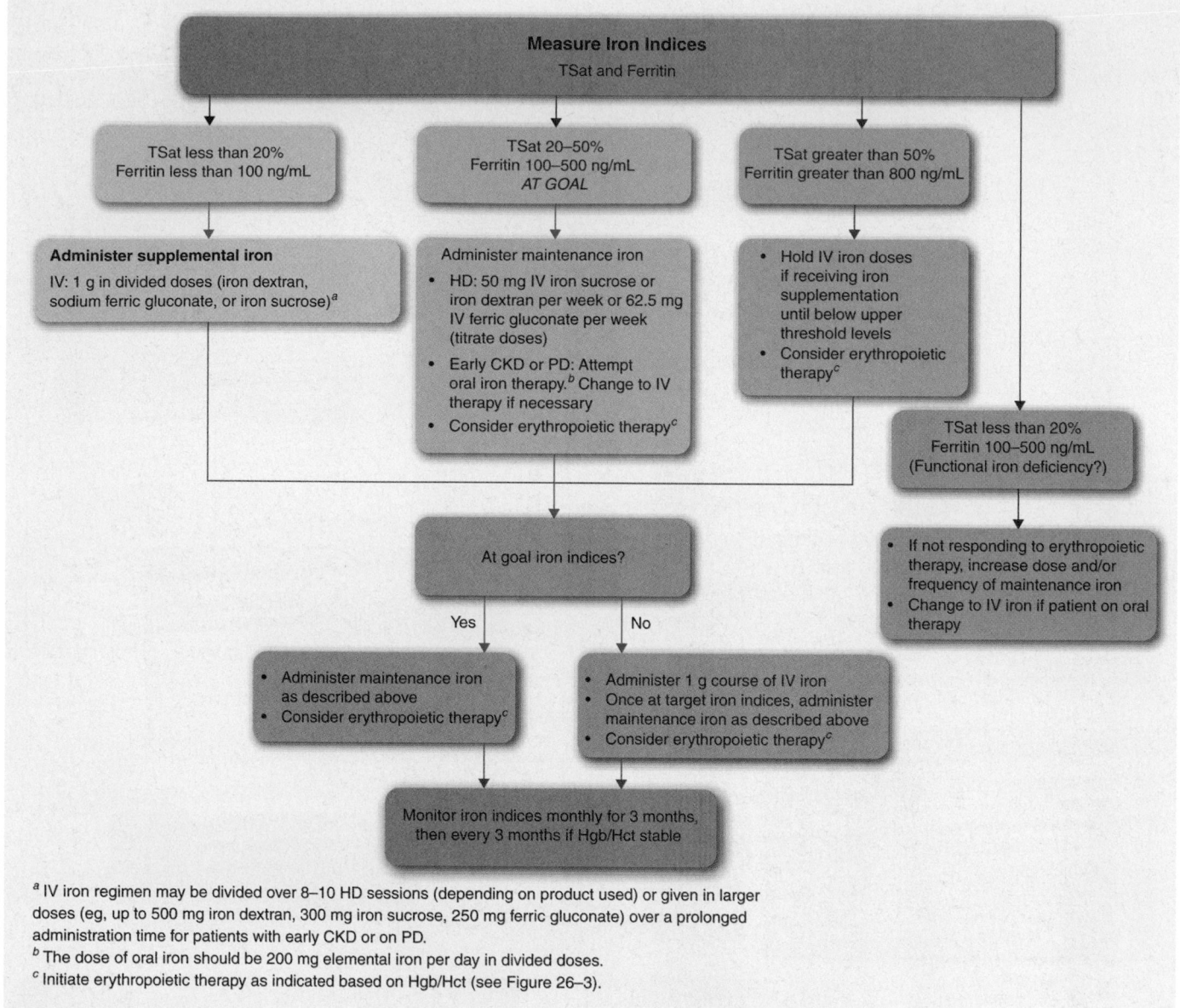

FIGURE 26–4. Guidelines for iron therapy in the management of anemia of CKD. (CKD, chronic kidney disease; HD, hemodialysis; Hgb, hemoglobin; PD, peritoneal dialysis; TSat, transferrin saturation.) (Adapted from Hudson, JQ. Chronic kidney disease: Management of complications. In: DiPiro JT, Talbert RL, Yee GC, et al., eds. Pharmacotherapy: A Pathophysiologic Approach, 7th ed. New York: McGraw-Hill, 2008: 774, with permission.)

The most common adverse effect seen with ESA is increased blood pressure, which can occur in up to 23% of patients.[42] Antihypertensive agents may be required to control blood pressure in patients receiving ESAs. Caution should be used when initiating an ESA in patients with very high blood pressures (greater than 180/100 mm Hg). If blood pressures are refractory to antihypertensive agents, ESAs may need to be withheld.

Subcutaneous (SC) administration of ESA produces a more predictable and sustained response than IV administration, and is therefore the preferred route of administration for both agents. IV administration is often utilized in patients who have established IV access or are receiving hemodialysis. Starting doses of ESAs depend on

the patient's Hgb level, the target Hgb level, the rate of Hgb increase, and clinical circumstances.[42] The initial increase in Hgb should be 1 to 2 g/dL (10–12 g/L or 0.62–1.24 mmol/L) per month. The recommended starting dose of epoetin alfa is 50 to 100 units/kg/dose administered SC or IV 2 to 3 times weekly; the starting dose of darbepoetin alfa is 0.45 mcg/kg administered SC or IV once weekly (Table 26–3).

Two recent clinical trials evaluated the target level of Hgb in patients receiving ESAs. Both studies indicated that targeting Hgb levels greater than 13 g/dL (130 g/L or 8.07 mmol/L) resulted in more cardiovascular complications or death, compared to target Hgb levels less than 11 g/dL (110 g/L or 6.82 mmol/L). The effect of achieving the higher Hgb target on quality of life differed between

Table 26–3

Estimated Starting Doses of Darbepoetin Alfa Based on Previous Epoetin Alfa Dose

Previous Epoetin Alfa Dose (units/week)	Weekly Darbepoetin Alfa Dose (mcg/week)
Less than 2,500	6.25
2,500–4,999	12.5
5,000–10,999	25
11,000–17,999	40
18,000–33,999	60
34,000–59,999	100
60,000–89,999	150
90,000 or more	200

the two studies.[47,48] A secondary analysis of one study indicated that the inability to achieve the target Hgb level was associated with an increased risk of cardiovascular outcomes and death, regardless of the target Hgb level.[49] Further studies are needed to evaluate the appropriate target level for Hgb. Nonetheless, based on the findings of these studies, the FDA recommended a black box warning be added to the product information for all ESAs indicating the maximum target Hgb should be between 10 and 12 g/dL (100 and 120 g/L or 6.21 and 7.45 mmol/L) for patients who are receiving ESAs.

Iron Supplementation. Use of ESAs can lead to iron deficiency if iron stores are not adequately maintained. If serum ferritin and TSAT fall below the goal levels, iron supplementation is required. Oral iron supplements are less costly than IV supplements and are generally the first-line treatment for iron supplementation for patients with CKD not receiving hemodialysis.[42] When administering iron by the oral route, 200 mg of elemental iron should be delivered daily to maintain adequate iron stores.

Oral iron supplementation is generally not effective in maintaining adequate iron stores in patients receiving ESAs because of poor absorption and an increased need for iron with ESA therapy, making the IV route necessary for iron supplementation. The IV iron products currently available are:

- Iron dextran (distributed as INFeD by Watson Pharmaceuticals, Inc., Morristown, NJ, and Dexferrum by American Reagent, Inc., Shirley, NY)
- Sodium ferric gluconate (Ferrlecit by Watson Pharmaceuticals, Inc., Corona, CA)
- Iron sucrose (Venofer by American Reagent, Inc., Shirley, NY)

Initiation of IV iron should be based on evaluation of iron stores. A serum ferritin level less than 100 ng/mL (225 pmol/L) in conjunction with a TSAT level less than 20% (0.2) indicates absolute iron deficiency and is a clear indication for the need for iron replacement.[42] Serum ferritin is an acute phase reactant, which may become elevated with inflammation and stress. Thus, when serum ferritin is normal or elevated in conjunction with TSAT levels less than 20%, treatment should be based on the clinical picture of the patient. Iron

supplementation may be indicated if Hgb levels are below the goal level. One clinical trial evaluated the efficacy of IV iron supplementation in patients with high serum ferritin levels (500–1,200 ng/mL [1,123.5–2,696.4 pmol/L]) and low TSAT levels (less than 25% [0.25]). A significant increase in Hgb was noted in patients who received IV supplementation compared to those who did not. Furthermore, more patients achieved an increase in Hgb and the response rate was faster. The authors concluded that serum ferritin alone is not a good marker for iron deficiency.[50]

When replacing iron stores IV in patients receiving ESA therapy, the general approach to treatment is to give a total of 1 g of IV iron, administered in smaller, sequential doses. Table 26–4 lists the FDA-approved doses of the IV iron products. Because iron stores deplete quickly in patients who do not receive iron supplementation, maintenance doses are often used, particularly in patients receiving hemodialysis. Maintenance doses consist of smaller doses of iron administered weekly or with each dialysis session (e.g., iron dextran or iron sucrose 20–100 mg/week; sodium ferric gluconate 62.5–125 mg/week).

IV iron preparations are equally effective in increasing iron stores. Iron dextran has been associated with side effects, including anaphylactic reactions and delayed reactions, such as arthralgias and myalgias. A test dose of 25 mg iron dextran should be administered 30 minutes before the full dose to monitor for potential anaphylactic reactions. However, patients should be monitored closely when receiving iron dextran, as anaphylactic reactions can occur in patients who safely received prior doses of iron dextran. For this reason, use of iron dextran has decreased dramatically in CKD patients in favor of the newer iron preparations, sodium ferric gluconate and iron sucrose, which are associated with fewer severe reactions. The most common side effects seen with these preparations include hypotension, flushing, nausea, and injection site reactions. A test dose is not required prior to the administration of either sodium ferric gluconate or iron sucrose. Long-term use of IV iron may increase oxidative stress, inflammation, and renal and cardiovascular injury.[51]

Outcome Evaluation Evaluate Hgb every 1 to 2 weeks when ESA therapy is initiated or the dose is adjusted until Hgb is between 11 g/dL (110 g/L or 6.8 mmol/L) and 12 g/dL (120 g/L or 7.4 mmol/L). Once goal Hgb is attained, evaluate Hgb every 2 to 4 weeks thereafter. While the patient is receiving ESA therapy, monitor iron stores monthly in patients who are not receiving iron supplements or every 3 months in patients who are receiving iron supplements. When the goal Hgb is reached, monitor iron stores every 3 months.

Secondary Hyperparathyroidism and Bone and Mineral Metabolism Disorders

▶ Epidemiology and Etiology

Increases in parathyroid hormone (PTH) occur early as kidney function begins to decline. The actions of PTH on bone turnover lead to bone and mineral metabolism

Table 26–4

Intravenous Iron Products

Iron Formulation (Product)	FDA-approved Indications	FDA-Approved Dosing	Warnings	Dose Ranges[a]	How Supplied
Iron dextran (INFeD, DexFerrum)	Patients with iron deficiency in whom oral iron is unsatisfactory	IV push: 100 mg over 2 minutes (25 mg test dose required)	Black box (risk of anaphylactic reactions)	25–1,000 mg	2 mL vials containing 50 mg elemental iron per mL
Ferric gluconate (Ferrlecit)	Adult and pediatric HD patients age 6 years and older receiving ESA therapy	IV push (adult): 125 mg over 10 minutes IV infusion (adult): 125 mg in 100 mL of 0.9% NaCl over 60 minutes IV infusion (pediatric): 1.5 mg/kg in 25 mL of 0.9% NaCl over 60 minutes; maximum dose 125 mg	General	6.25–1,000 mg	5 mL ampules containing 62.5 mg elemental iron (12.5 mg/mL)
Iron sucrose (Venofer)	HD patients with CKD receiving ESA therapy Nondialysis-CKD patients receiving or not receiving ESA therapy PD patients receiving ESA therapy	IV push: 100 mg over 2–5 minutes IV infusion: 100 mg in maximum of 100 mL of 0.9% NaCl over 15 minutes IV push: 200 mg over 2–5 minutes on 5 different occasions within 14-day period IV infusion: 2 infusions 14 days apart, of 300 mg in maximum of 250 mL of 0.9% NaCl over 1.5 hour, followed by 1 infusion 14 days later, of 400 mg in maximum of 250 mL of 0.9% NaCl over 2.5 hour	General	25–1,000 mg	5 mL single-dose vials containing 100 mg elemental iron (20 mg/mL)

CKD, chronic kidney disease; ESA, erythropoietin-stimulating agent; HD, hemodialysis; PD, peritoneal dialysis.

[a]Small dosing ranges (e.g., 25–100 mg/week) generally used for maintenance regimens. Larger doses (e.g., 1 g) should be administered in divided doses.

Patient Encounter, Part 3

The patient returns to your clinic in one week and states that her symptoms have not changed. She is asking about the results from her laboratory studies.

Labs: WBC 4.5×10^3 cells/m³ (4.5×10^9/L); RBC 2.3×10^6 cells/m³ (2.3×10^{12}/L); Hgb 8.1 g/dL (81 g/L or 5 mmol/L); Hct 24% (0.24); mean corpuscular volume (MCV) 88 fL; mean corpuscular hemoglobin concentration (MCHC) 35 g/dL (350 g/L); iron 35 mcg/dL (6.26 μmol/L); total iron binding capacity (TIBC) 450 mcg/dL (80.55 μmol/L); ferritin 75 ng/mL (168 pmol/L); transferrin saturation (TSAT) 15% (0.15); stool guaiac negative × 3

What treatment would you recommend for this patient for treatment of anemia?

How would you evaluate the effectiveness of treatment of anemia?

---

disorders (BMMD). As many as 75% to 100% of patients with stage 3 CKD have BMMD.[52] The type of bone disease can vary based on the degree of bone turnover. High bone turnover is the most common cause of bone abnormalities in patients with CKD, present in as many as 75% of patients receiving dialysis,[52] and is generally mediated by high levels of PTH. Adynamic bone disease, characterized by low bone turnover, is less common, although the prevalence appears to be increasing,[52] which may be related to more aggressive treatment of hyperparathyroidism. The development of BMMD can dramatically affect morbidity in patients with CKD.

▶ *Pathophysiology*

As kidney function declines in patients with CKD, decreased phosphorus excretion disrupts the balance of calcium and phosphorus homeostasis. Decreased vitamin D activation in the kidney also decreases calcium absorption from the GI tract. ❼ *The parathyroid glands release PTH in response to decreased serum calcium and increased serum phosphorus levels. The actions of PTH include the following:*

- Increasing calcium resorption from bone
- Increasing calcium reabsorption from the proximal tubules in the kidney
- Decreasing phosphorus reabsorption in the proximal tubules in the kidney
- Stimulating activation of vitamin D by 1-α-hydroxylase to calcitriol (1,25-dihydroxyvitmin D_3) to promote calcium absorption in the GI tract and increased calcium mobilization from bone

All of these actions are directed at increasing serum calcium levels and decreasing serum phosphorus levels, although the activity of calcitriol also increases phosphorus absorption in the GI tract and mobilization from the bone, which can worsen hyperphosphatemia. Calcitriol also decreases PTH levels through a negative feedback loop. These measures are sufficient to correct serum calcium levels in the earlier stages of CKD.

As kidney function continues to decline and the GFR falls less than 40 mL/min/1.73 m², phosphorus excretion continues to decrease and calcitriol production decreases,[53] causing PTH levels to begin to rise significantly, leading to secondary hyperparathyroidism (sHPT). The excessive production of PTH leads to hyperplasia of the parathyroid glands, which decreases the sensitivity of the parathyroid glands to serum calcium levels and calcitriol feedback, further promoting sHPT.

The most dramatic consequence of sHPT is alterations in bone turnover and the development of BMMD. Other complications of CKD can also promote BMMD. Metabolic acidosis decreases bone formation and excessive aluminum levels cause aluminum uptake into bone in place of calcium, weakening the bone structure. The pathogenesis of sHPT and BMMD are depicted in Figure 26–5.

The increased serum phosphorus binds to calcium in the serum, which leads to deposition of hydroxyapatite crystals throughout the body. The calcium-phosphorus (Ca-P) product reflects serum solubility. A Ca-P product greater than 75 mg²/dL² (5.81 mmol²/L²) promotes crystal deposition in the joints and eye, leading to arthritis and conjunctivitis, respectively. Soft tissue deposition primarily affects the coronary arteries of the heart, lungs, and vascular tissue[53] and is associated with a Ca-P product greater than 55 mg²/dL² (4.44 mmol²/L²).[54] The Ca-P product has been associated with a 40% increase in mortality[54] and is a risk factor for calcification of vascular and soft tissues.[52]

Metabolic acidosis, a common complication of CKD, also contributes to BMMD by altering the solubility of hydroxyapatite, promoting bone dissolution. Additionally, metabolic acidosis inhibits the activity of osteoblasts to decrease bone formation, while stimulating osteoclasts to promote bone resorption. Finally, metabolic acidosis can worsen sHPT by reducing the sensitivity of the parathyroid gland to serum calcium levels.[55]

▶ Treatment

General Approach ⑧ *Diagnosis and management of bone disease in CKD is based on corrected serum levels of calcium and phosphorus, the Ca-P (using corrected calcium levels), and intact PTH levels (iPTH).[56] The target levels of each vary with*

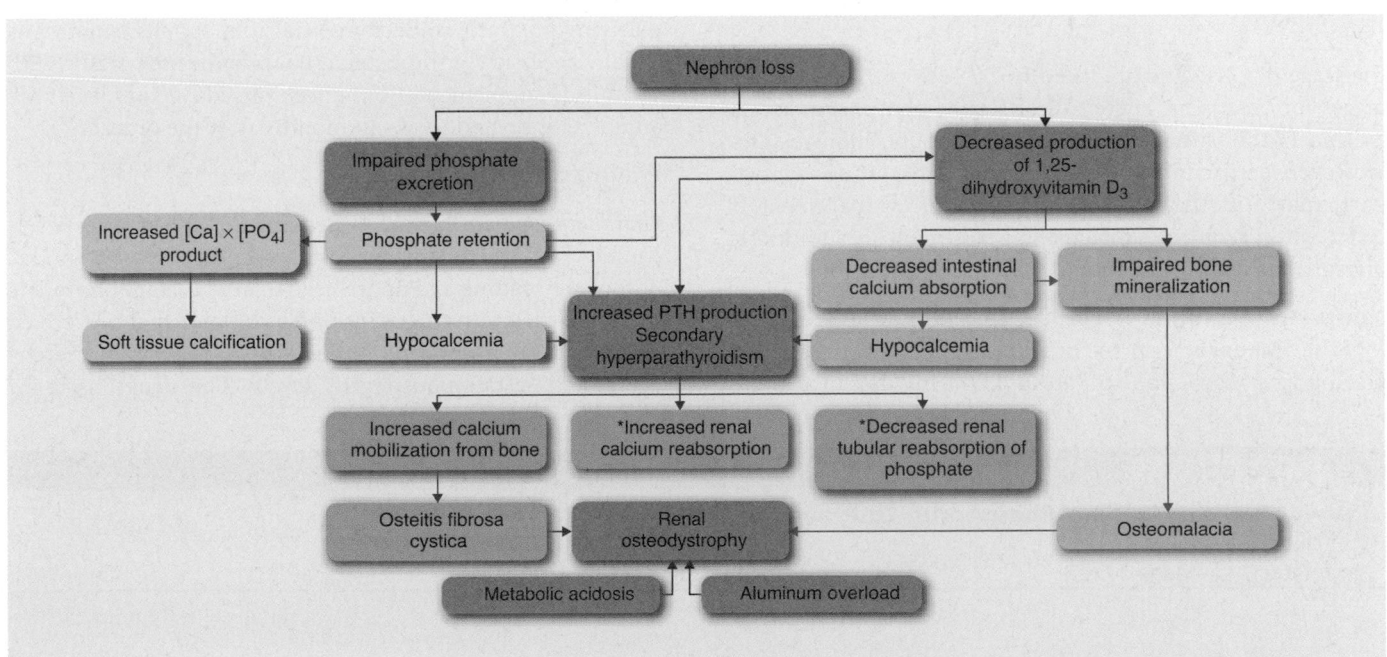

FIGURE 26–5. Pathogenesis of secondary hyperparathyroidism and bone and mineral disorder in patients with CKD. *These adaptations are lost as kidney failure progresses. ([Ca] × [PO₄], calcium-phosphorus product; PTH, parathyroid hormone. (From Hudson JQ. Chronic kidney disease: Management of complications.) In: DiPiro JT, Talbert RL, Yee GC, et al., eds. Pharmacotherapy: A Pathophysiologic Approach, 7th ed. New York: McGraw-Hill, 2008:767, with permission.)

Clinical Presentation and Diagnosis of sHPT and ROD

General

Onset of sHPT and ROD is subtle and may not be associated with symptoms.

Symptoms

sHPT and ROD are usually asymptomatic in early disease. Calcification in the joints can be associated with decreased range of motion.

Conjunctival calcifications are associated with a gritty sensation in the eyes, redness, and inflammation.

Signs

Cardiovascular: Increased stroke index, heart rate, and diastolic and mean arterial pressures

Musculoskeletal: Bone pain, muscle weakness

Dermatologic: Pruritus

Laboratory Tests

Increased serum phosphorus levels

Low to normal serum calcium levels

Increased Ca-P product

Increased PTH levels

Decreased vitamin D levels

Diagnostic Tests

Radiographic studies show calcium-phosphate deposits in joints and/or cardiovascular system

Bone biopsy of the iliac crest

---

the stage of CKD and are listed in Table 26–5. The primary target for treatment is control of serum phosphorus levels, as this is the initial parameter that disrupts homeostasis. However, serum phosphorus can be difficult to control, particularly in the latter stages of CKD. Management of sHPT often requires supplemental treatment in addition to phosphorus management.

Nonpharmacologic Therapy The first-line treatment for the management of hyperphosphatemia is dietary phosphorus restriction to 800 to 1,000 mg/day in patients with stage 3 CKD or higher who have phosphorus levels at the upper limit of the normal range or elevated iPTH levels.[56] Foods high in phosphorus are also high in protein, which can make it difficult to restrict phosphorus intake while maintaining adequate protein intake to avoid malnutrition. Hemodialysis and peritoneal dialysis can remove up to 2 to 3 g of phosphorus per week. However, this is insufficient to control hyperphosphatemia, and pharmacologic therapy is necessary in addition to dialysis treatment.

Other nonpharmacologic strategies to manage sHPT and BMMD in patients with CKD include restriction of aluminum exposure and parathyroidectomy. Ingestion of aluminum-containing antacids and other aluminum-containing products should be avoided in patients with stage 4 CKD or higher (GFR less than 30 mL/min/1.73 m²) because of the risk of aluminum toxicity and potential uptake into the bone. Purification techniques for dialysate solutions also minimize the risk of exposure to aluminum.

Parathyroidectomy is a treatment of last resort for sHPT, but should be considered in patients with persistently elevated iPTH levels above 800 pg/mL (800 ng/L) that is refractory to medical therapy to lower serum calcium and/or phosphorus levels.[56] A portion or all of the parathyroid tissue may be removed, and in some cases a portion of the parathyroid tissue may be transplanted into another site, usually the forearm. Bone turnover can be disrupted in patients undergoing parathyroidectomy whereby bone production outweighs bone resorption. The syndrome, known as "hungry bone syndrome," is characterized by excessive uptake of calcium, phosphorus, and magnesium for bone production, leading to hypocalcemia, hypophosphatemia, and hypomagnesemia. Serum ionized calcium levels should be monitored frequently (every 4–6 hours for the first 48–72 hours) in patients receiving a parathyroidectomy. Calcium supplementation is usually necessary, administered IV initially, then orally (with vitamin D supplementation) once normal calcium levels are attained for several weeks to months after the procedure.

Pharmacologic Therapy

Phosphate-Binding Agents. When serum phosphorus levels cannot be controlled by restriction of dietary intake, phosphate-binding agents are used to bind dietary phosphate in the GI tract to form an insoluble complex that is excreted in the feces. Phosphorus absorption is decreased, thereby decreasing serum phosphorus levels. The drugs used for

---

Table 26–5

Target Levels for Calcium, Phosphorus, Ca-P, and Intact PTH

Parameter	Stage 3 CKD	Stage 4 CKD	Stage 5 CKD
Corrected calcium	"Normal"	"Normal"	8.4–9.5 mg/dL (2.1–2.37 mmol/L)
Phosphorus	2.7–4.6 mg/dL (0.87–1.49 mmol/L)	2.7–4.6 mg/dL (0.87–1.49 mmol/L)	3.5–5.5 mg/dL (1.13–1.78 mmol/L)
Ca-P product	Less than 55 mg²/dL² (4.44 mmol²/L²)	Less than 55 mg²/dL² (4.44 mmol²/L²)	Less than 55 mg²/dL² (4.44 mmol²/L²)
Intact PTH	35–70 pg/mL (35–70 ng/L or 3.7–7.5 pmol/L)	70–110 pg/mL (70–110 ng/L or 7.5–11.8 pmol/L)	150–300 pg/mL (150–300 ng/L or 16–32 pmol/L)

Ca-P, calcium-phosphorus product; CKD, chronic kidney disease; PTH, parathyroid hormone.

binding dietary phosphate are listed in Table 26–6. These agents should be administered with each meal and can be tailored to the amount of phosphorus that is typically ingested during each meal. For example, patients can take a smaller dose with smaller meals or snacks, and a larger dose with larger meals.

Calcium-based phosphate binders, including calcium carbonate and calcium acetate, are effective in decreasing serum phosphate levels, as well as in increasing serum calcium levels. Calcium acetate binds more phosphorus than the carbonate salt, making it a more potent agent for binding dietary phosphate. Calcium citrate is usually not used as a phosphate-binding agent because the citrate salt can increase aluminum absorption. The calcium-containing phosphate binders also aid in the correction of metabolic acidosis, another complication of kidney failure. Caution should be used with these agents if serum calcium levels are near the upper end of the normal range or are elevated because of the risk of increasing the Ca-P product and potentiating vascular and soft tissue calcifications. The dose of calcium-based phosphate binders should not provide more than 1,500 mg of elemental calcium per day, and the total elemental calcium intake per day should not exceed 2,000 mg, including medication and dietary intake.[56] The most common adverse effects of calcium-containing phosphate binders are constipation and hypercalcemia.

Aluminum- and magnesium-containing phosphate-binding agents are not recommended for chronic use in patients with CKD to minimize the risk of aluminum and magnesium accumulation. Aluminum-containing agents may be used for a short course of therapy (less than 4 weeks) if phosphorus levels are significantly elevated greater than 7 mg/dL (2.26 mmol/L), but should be replaced by other phosphate-binding agents after no more than 4 weeks. Excessive aluminum levels lead to aluminum intoxication, causing neurotoxicity that can manifest as encephalopathy or dementia. Other consequences of aluminum intoxication include anemia and bone disease as aluminum is taken up in place of iron in RBCs and calcium in skeletal bones. In addition to the risk of magnesium accumulation, the use of magnesium-containing agents is also limited by the GI side effects, primarily diarrhea.

Phosphate-binding agents that do not contain calcium, magnesium, or aluminum include sevelamer hydrochloride, sevelamer carbonate, and lanthanum carbonate. These agents are particularly useful in patients with hyperphosphatemia who have elevated serum calcium levels or who have vascular or soft tissue calcifications. Sevelamer is a cationic polymer that is not systemically absorbed and binds to phosphate in the GI tract, and prevents absorption and promotes excretion of phosphate through the GI tract via the feces. Sevelamer has an added benefit of reducing LDL-C by up to 30% and increasing HDL-C levels.[56] The most common side effects of sevelamer are GI complaints, including nausea, constipation, and diarrhea. The cost of sevelamer is significantly higher compared to calcium-containing phosphate binders, which often makes sevelamer a second-line agent for controlling phosphorus levels. However, recent studies have demonstrated that sevelamer decreases mortality in patients receiving hemodialysis compared to calcium-containing phosphate binders, primarily by decreasing the occurrence of calcifications in the coronary arteries.[57, 58]

Lanthanum is a naturally occurring trivalent rare earth element (atomic number 57). Lanthanum carbonate quickly dissociates in the acidic environment of the stomach, where the lanthanum ion binds to dietary phosphorus, forming an insoluble compound that is excreted in the feces. Lanthanum has been shown to remove more than 97% of dietary phosphorus from the GI tract.[59] Side effects of lanthanum include nausea, peripheral edema, and myalgias.

Vitamin D Therapy. Exogenous vitamin D compounds that mimic the activity of calcitriol act directly on the parathyroid gland to decrease PTH secretion. This is particularly useful when reduction of serum phosphorus levels does not sufficiently reduce PTH levels. The most active form of vitamin D is calcitriol (1,25-dihydroxyvitamin D). The effects of calcitriol are mediated by upregulation of the vitamin D receptor in the parathyroid gland, which decreases parathyroid gland hyperplasia and PTH synthesis and secretion. However, vitamin D receptor upregulation also occurs in the intestines, which increases calcium and phosphorus absorption, increasing the risk of hypercalcemia and hyperphosphatemia. It is important that serum calcium and phosphorus levels are within the normal range for the stage of CKD and the Ca-P product is less than 55 mg^2/dL^2 (4.44 $mmol^2/L^2$) prior to starting calcitriol therapy.

Vitamin D supplementation can be used to lower serum PTH levels in patients with CKD. Ergocalciferol has been shown to be effective in lowering PTH secretion in patients with stage 3 CKD.[61] However, as CKD progresses to stages 4 and 5, the kidney loses the ability to produce 1α-hydroxylase, which is responsible for renal activation of vitamin D. In these later stages of CKD, activated vitamin D analogs must be used to decrease PTH secretion. Calcitriol (1,25-dihydroxyvitamin D_3) is available commercially as an oral formulation (Rocaltrol by Roche Laboratories, Inc., Nutley, NJ) and an injectable formulation (Calcijex by Abbott Laboratories, North Chicago, IL). This analog has the same biologic activity as endogenous calcitriol. Other vitamin D analogs available in the United States include paricalcitol (19-nor-1,25-dihydroxyvitamin D_2, Zemplar by Abbott Laboratories, North Chicago, IL and doxercalciferol (1-α-hydroxyvitamin D_2, Hectorol by Genzyme Corp., Cambridge, MA), both of which are also available in oral and injectable formations. Alfacalcidiol (1-α-hydroxyvitamin D_3) is only available outside the United States. Paricalcitol has less effect on vitamin D receptors in the intestines, decreasing the effects on intestinal calcium and phosphorus absorption, while retaining the effects on parathyroid gland hyperplasia and PTH synthesis and secretion.[60] This makes paricalcitol more useful in patients with an elevated Ca-P product. Doxercalciferol, on the other hand, has similar effects as calcitriol on vitamin D receptors in the parathyroid glands and intestines. Like calcitriol, calcium and phosphorus levels and the Ca-P product should be within the normal

Table 26–6

Phosphate-Binding Agents Used in the Treatment of Hyperphosphatemia in CKD

Compound	Trade Name	Compound Content (mg)	Elemental Calcium Content (mg)	Starting Dose	Comments
Calcium carbonate (40% elemental calcium)	Tums	500, 750, 1,000; 1,250	200, 300, 400, 500	0.5–1 g (elemental calcium) 3 times a day with meals	First-line agent; dissolution characteristics and phosphorus-binding effect may vary from product to product; try to limit daily intake of elemental calcium to 1,500 mg/day
	Oscal-500	1,250	500		
	Caltrate 600	1,500	600		
	Nephro-Calci	1,500	600		Approximately 39 mg phosphorus bound per 1 g calcium carbonate
	LiquiCal	1,200	480		
	CalciChew	1,250	500		
Calcium acetate (25% elemental calcium)	Phos-Lo	667	167	0.5–1 g (elemental calcium) 3 times a day with meals	First-line agent; comparable efficacy to calcium carbonate with one-half the dose of elemental calcium; do not exceed 1,500 mg elemental calcium intake per day
					Approximately 45 mg phosphorus bound per 1 g calcium acetate
					By prescription only
Sevelamer HCl, sevelamer carbonate	Renagel, Renvela	400, 800	—	800 mg 3 times a day with meals	First-line agent; lowers LDL-C
					More expensive than calcium products; preferred in patients at risk for extraskeletal calcification
					May require large doses to control phosphorus levels
Lanthanum	Fosrenol	250, 500 chewable tablets	—	750–1,500 mg 3 times a day with meals	Second-line agent; more expensive than calcium products; preferred in patients at risk for extraskeletal calcification
					Most patients require 1,500–3,000 mg/day to control phosphorus
Aluminum hydroxide	Alterna GEL Amphojel	600 mg/5 mL 300, 600 (tablet) 320 mg/5 mL (suspension)	—	300–600 mg 3 times a day with meals	Third-line agents; do not use concurrently with citrate-containing products
	Alu-Cap	400			Reserve for short-term use (4 weeks) in patients with hyperphosphatemia not responding to other binders
Aluminum carbonate	Basaljel	500 (tablet, capsule) 400 mg/5 mL (suspension)	—	450–500 mg 3 times a day with meals	Same as for aluminum hydroxide
Magnesium carbonate	Mag-Carb	70 (capsule)	—	70 mg 3 times a day with meals	Third-line agent; diarrhea common; monitor serum magnesium
Magnesium hydroxide	Milk of magnesia	300, 600 (tablet) 400 mg/5 mL, 800 mg/5 mL (suspension)	—	300–400 mg 3 times a day with meals	Same as for magnesium carbonate
Magnesium carbonate/ calcium carbonate	MagneBind 400	400 mg (elemental magnesium)	80	400 mg 3 times a day with meals	Same as for calcium carbonate and magnesium carbonate

LDL-C, low-density lipoprotein cholesterol.

range for the stage of CKD prior to starting doxercalciferol. Recommendations for vitamin D analog therapy depend on the stage of CKD (Table 26–7).[56]

It is important to monitor vitamin D therapy aggressively to assure that PTH levels are not oversuppressed. Oversuppression of PTH levels can induce adynamic bone disease, which manifests as decreased osteoblast and osteoclast activity, decreased bone formation, and low bone turnover.

Calcimimetics   Cinacalcet is a calcimimetic that increases the sensitivity of receptors on the parathyroid gland to serum calcium levels to reduce PTH secretion. In addition to lowering PTH levels, cinacalcet has been shown to reduce serum calcium levels by approximately 5% and serum phosphorus levels by 2.6% to 8.4%.[62] This makes cinacalcet beneficial to use in patients with elevated PTH levels who have an increased Ca-P product and cannot use vitamin D therapy. Because the effects of cinacalcet on PTH can reduce serum calcium levels and result in hypocalcemia, cinacalcet should not be used if serum calcium levels are below 8.4 mg/dL (2.1 mmol/L). Cincalcet should also be used with caution in patients with seizure disorders because low serum calcium levels can lower the seizure threshold.[62]

Reversal of Metabolic Acidosis   Studies have demonstrated that reversal of metabolic acidosis can improve bone disease associated with CKD.[55] Serum bicarbonate levels should be maintained at 22 mEq/L (22 mmol/L) in patients with bone disease associated with CKD.[56] The treatment of metabolic acidosis is described later.

▶ Outcome Evaluation

Monitor serum calcium and phosphorus levels regularly in patients receiving phosphate-binding agents. When initiating therapy, monitor serum levels every 1 to 4 weeks, depending on the severity of hyperphosphatemia. Titrate doses of phosphate binders to achieve the target levels of serum calcium and phosphorus and the Ca-P product (Table 26–5). Once target levels are achieved, monitor serum calcium and phosphorus levels every 1 to 3 months. Monitor intact PTH levels monthly while initiating vitamin D therapy, then every 3 months once stable iPTH levels are achieved. When starting or increasing the dose of cinacalcet, monitor serum calcium and phosphorus levels within 1 week and iPTH levels should be monitored within 1 to 4 weeks. Once target levels are achieved, decrease monitoring to every 3 months.

Metabolic Acidosis

▶ Epidemiology and Etiology

Approximately 80% of patients with a GFR less than 20 to 30 mL/min/1.73 m^2 develop metabolic acidosis.[55] Metabolic acidosis can increase protein catabolism and decrease albumin synthesis, which promote muscle wasting, and alter bone metabolism. Other consequences associated with metabolic acidosis in CKD include worsening cardiac disease, impaired glucose tolerance, altered growth hormone and thyroid function, and inflammation.[55]

Table 26–7				
Dosing Recommendations for Vitamin D in Patients with CKD				
Serum PTH (pg/mL)	Ergocalciferol	Calcitriol Dose	Paricalcitol Dose	Doxercalciferol Dose
Stage 3 or 4 CKD				
70–300[a]	Stage 3 CKD: 50,000 IU orally once or twice weekly 800 IU orally daily	0.25 mcg orally daily	1 mcg orally daily or 2 mcg orally 3 times a week	2.5 mg orally 3 times a week
Stage 5 CKD on Hemodialysis				
70 – 300[b]	N/A	0.25–0.5 mcg orally daily	1–2 mcg orally daily	2.5 mg orally 3 times a week or daily
300–600[b]	N/A	0.5–1.5 mcg po or IV per HD	2.5–5 mcg IV per HD	5 mcg orally per HD 2 mcg IV per HD
600–1,000[b]	N/A	1–4 mcg orally per HD 1–3 mcg IV per HD	6–10 mcg IV per HD	5–10 mcg orally per HD 2–4 mcg IV per HD
Greater than 1,000[c]	N/A	3–7 mcg orally per HD 3–5 mcg IV per HD	10–15 mcg IV per HD	10–20 mcg orally per HD 4–8 mcg IV per HD
Stage 5 CKD on Peritoneal Dialysis				
Greater than 300[b]	N/A	0.25 mcg orally daily 0.5–1 mcg orally 2–3 times a week	Not recommended	2.5–5 mcg orally 2–3 times a week

CKD, chronic kidney disease; HD, hemodialysis; PTH, parathyroid hormone.

[a]If serum calcium less than 9.5 mg/dL (2.37 mmol/L), phosphorus less than 4.6 mg/dL (1.49 mmol/L), and Ca-P product less than 55 mg^2/dL^2

[b]If serum calcium less than 9.5 mg/dL (2.37 mmol/L), phosphorus less than 5.5 mg/dL (1.78 mmol/L), and Ca-P product less than 55 mg^2/dL^2

[c]If serum calcium less than 10 mg/dL (2.5 mmol/L), phosphorus less than 5.5 mg/dL (1.78 mmol/L), and Ca-P product less than 55 mg^2/dL^2

Patient Encounter, Part 4

The patient returns to your clinic 1 year later for routine follow-up. She has no complaints at this time.

Current Meds: Furosemide 80 mg orally daily; lisinopril 40 mg orally daily; metoprolol 75 mg orally twice daily; insulin glargine 28 units subcutaneously at bedtime; insulin lispro subcutaneously per sliding scale with meals; darbepoetin 60 mcg subcutaneously weekly

ROS: Unremarkable

PE:

VS: BP 128/75 mm Hg, P 68 bpm, T 36.5°C (97.9°F); wt 77.3 kg (170 lb)

Chest: RRR, normal S_1, S_2 present

Abd: Obese; no organomegaly, bruits, tenderness, (+) bowel sounds; heme (–) stool

Exts: 2+ edema bilaterally; decreased sensation to light touch in feet; no lesions

Labs: Sodium 144 mEq/L (144 mmol/L); potassium 5.0 mEq/L (5.0 mmol/L); chloride 105 mEq/L (105 mmol/L); carbon dioxide 18 mEq/L (18 mmol/L); BUN 75 mg/dL (26.78 mmol/L urea); SCr 4.8 mg/dL (424 μmol/L); glucose 115 mg/dL (6.38 mmol/L); calcium 8.6 mg/dL (2.15 mmol/L); phosphate 7.8 mg/dL (2.52 mmol/L); albumin 3.0 mg/dL (30 g/L); intact parathyroid hormone (iPTH) 538 pg/mL (538 ng/L or 57.6 pmol/L); WBC 6.0×10^3 cells/mm³ (6.0×10^9/L); RBC 3.5×10^6 cells/mm³ (3.5×10^{12}/L); Hgb 10.5 g/dL (6.51 mmol/L); Hct 32% (0.32); platelets 350×10^3 cells/mm³ (350×10^9/L)

What signs are consistent with secondary hyperparathyroidism (sHPT)?

How would you determine whether treatment is necessary for this patient?

What treatment would you recommend for sHPT?

▶ Pathophysiology

The kidney plays a key role in the management of acid–base homeostasis in the body by regulating excretion of hydrogen ions. With normal kidney function, bicarbonate that is freely filtered through the glomerulus is completely reabsorbed via the renal tubules. Hydrogen ions are generated at a rate of 1 mEq/kg (1 mmol/kg) per day during metabolism of ingested food and are excreted at the same rate by the kidney via buffers in the urine created by ammonia generation and phosphate excretion. As a result, the pH of body fluids is maintained within a very narrow range.

As kidney function declines, bicarbonate reabsorption is maintained, but hydrogen excretion is decreased because the ability of the kidney to generate ammonia is impaired. The positive hydrogen balance leads to metabolic acidosis, which is characterized by a serum bicarbonate level of 15 to 20 mEq/L (15–20 mmol/L). This picture is generally seen when the GFR declines below 20 to 30 mL/min/1.73 m².[55]

▶ Treatment

Serum electrolytes should be monitored in patients with CKD for the development of metabolic acidosis. Metabolic acidosis in patients with CKD is generally characterized by an elevated anion gap greater than 17 mEq/L (17 mmol/L), due to the accumulation of phosphate, sulfate, and other organic anions.

Nonpharmacologic Therapy   Treatment of metabolic acidosis in CKD requires pharmacologic therapy. Other disorders that may contribute to metabolic acidosis should also be addressed. Altering bicarbonate levels in the dialysate fluid in patients receiving dialysis may assist with the treatment of metabolic acidosis, although pharmacologic therapy may still be required.

Pharmacologic Therapy   Pharmacologic therapy with sodium bicarbonate or citrate/citric acid preparations may be needed in patients with stage 3 CKD or higher to replenish body stores of bicarbonate. Calcium carbonate and calcium acetate, used to bind phosphorus in sHPT, also aid in increasing serum bicarbonate levels, in conjunction with other agents.

Sodium bicarbonate tablets are administered in increments of 325 and 650 mg tablets. A 650 mg tablet of sodium bicarbonate contains 7.7 mEq (7.7 mmol) each of sodium and bicarbonate. Sodium retention associated with sodium bicarbonate can cause volume overload, which can exacerbate hypertension and chronic heart failure. Patient tolerability of sodium bicarbonate is low because of carbon dioxide production in the GI tract that occurs during dissolution.

Solutions that contain sodium citrate/citric acid (Shohl's solution and Bicitra) provide 1 mEq/L (1 mmol/L) each of sodium and bicarbonate. Polycitra is a sodium/potassium citrate solution that provides 2 mEq/L (2 mmol/L) of bicarbonate, but contains 1 mEq/L (1 mmol/L) each of sodium and potassium, which can promote hyperkalemia in patients with severe CKD. The citrate portion of these preparations is metabolized in the liver to bicarbonate, while the citric acid portion is metabolized to CO_2 and water, increasing tolerability compared to sodium bicarbonate. Sodium retention is also decreased with these preparations. However, these products are liquid preparations, which may not be palatable to some patients. Citrate can also promote aluminum intoxication by augmenting aluminum absorption in the GI tract.

When determining the dose of bicarbonate replacement, the goal for therapy is to achieve a normal serum bicarbonate level of 24 mEq/L (24 mmol/L). The dose is usually determined by calculating the base deficit: [0.5 L/kg × (body weight)] × [(normal CO_2) – (measured CO_2)]. Because of the risk of volume overload resulting from the sodium load administered with bicarbonate replacement, the total base deficit should be administered over several days. Once the goal serum bicarbonate level is attained, a maintenance dose of bicarbonate is necessary and should be titrated to maintain serum bicarbonate levels.

▶ Outcome Evaluation

Monitor serum electrolytes and arterial blood gases regularly. Correct metabolic acidosis slowly to prevent the development of metabolic alkalosis or other electrolyte abnormalities.

Other Therapeutic Considerations in CKD

▶ Uremic Bleeding

Uremia can lead to a number of alterations in clotting ability, resulting in hemorrhage. Bleeding complications associated with CKD include ecchymoses, prolonged bleeding from mucous membranes and puncture sites used for blood collection and hemodialysis, GI bleeding, intramuscular bleeding, and others. Most bleeding complications associated with CKD are mild. However, serious bleeding events, including GI bleeds and intracranial hemorrhage, can occur.

Pathophysiology Uremia alters a number of mechanisms that contribute to bleeding. Platelet function and aggregation are altered through decreased production of thromboxane.[63] Platelet–vessel wall interactions are also altered in patients with uremia because of decreased activity of von Willebrand's factor[63] and are exacerbated by anemia in CKD patients. With a normal RBC count in the plasma, platelets skim the surface of the endothelial tissue in the blood vessels. In patients with anemia, RBC count is decreased and platelets circulate closer to the center of the vessels, which decreases the interaction with the vessel wall. The risk of bleeding is increased in patients receiving hemodialysis. Anticoagulants administered to prevent or treat clotting during hemodialysis or in vascular access sites, including heparin, warfarin, aspirin, and clopidogrel, exacerbate the risk of bleeding in these patients.

Treatment

Nonpharmacologic Therapy. The incidence and severity of bleeding associated with uremia has decreased since dialysis has become the mainstay of treatment for ESKD. Dialysis initiation improves platelet function and reduces bleeding time.[63] Improved care of the patient with ESKD, with anemia treatment and improvement in nutritional status, are also likely contributors to decreased uremic bleeding.

Pharmacologic Therapy. Treatments used to decrease bleeding time in patients with uremic bleeding include cryoprecipitate, which contains various components important in platelet aggregation and clotting, such as von Willebrand's factor and fibrinogen. Cryoprecipitate decreases bleeding time within 1 hour in 50% of patients. However, cost and the risk of infection have limited the use of cryoprecipitate.

Desmopressin (DDAVP) increases the release of factor VIII (von Willebrand's factor) from endothelial tissue in the vessel wall. Bleeding time is promptly reduced, within 1 hour of administration, and is sustained for 4 to 8 hours.[63] Doses used for uremic bleeding are 0.3 to 0.4 mcg/kg IV over 20 to 30 minutes, 0.3 mcg/kg subcutaneously, or 2 to 3 mcg/kg intranasally. Repeated doses can cause tachyphylaxis by depleting stores of von Willebrand's factor. Side effects of DDAVP include flushing, dizziness, and headache.

Estrogens have also been used to decrease bleeding time. The onset of action is slower than that of DDAVP, but more sustained, and it depends on the route of administration. IV doses of 0.6 mg/kg/day for 4 to 5 days decreases bleeding time within 6 hours of administration, and produces an effect that lasts up to 2 weeks after stopping therapy. The onset of action with oral doses of 50 mg/kg daily is within 2 days of treatment and is sustained for 4 to 5 days after stopping therapy. Transdermal patches providing 50 to 100 mcg/day have also been shown to be effective in decreasing bleeding time.[63] Side effects of estrogen use include hot flashes in both females and males, fluid retention, and hypertension.

▶ Pruritus

Pruritus can affect 25% to 86% of patients with advanced stages of CKD, and is not related to the cause of kidney failure.[64] Pruritus can be significant and has been linked to mortality in patients receiving hemodialysis.[64]

Pathophysiology The cause of pruritus is unknown, although several mechanisms have been proposed. Vitamin A is known to accumulate in the skin and serum of patients with CKD, but a definite correlation with pruritus has not been established. Histamine may also play a role in the development of pruritus, which may be linked to mast cell proliferation in patients receiving hemodialysis. Hyperparathyroidism has also been suggested as a contributor to pruritus, despite the fact that serum PTH levels do not correlate with itching. Accumulation of divalent ions, specifically magnesium and aluminum, may also play a role in pruritus in patients with CKD. Other theories that have been proposed include inadequate dialysis, dry skin, peripheral neuropathy, and opiate accumulation.[64]

Treatment

Nonpharmacologic Therapy. Pruritus associated with CKD is difficult to alleviate. It is important to evaluate other potential dermatologic causes of pruritus to maximize the potential for relief. Adequate dialysis is generally the first line of treatment in patients with pruritus. However, this has not been shown to decrease the incidence of pruritus significantly. Maintaining proper nutritional intake, especially with regard to dietary phosphorus and protein intake, may lessen the degree or occurrence of pruritus. Patients who do not attain relief from other measures may benefit from ultraviolet B phototherapy.

Pharmacologic Therapy. Topical emollients have been used as treatment for pruritus in patients with dry skin, but are often not effective in relieving pruritus associated with CKD. Antihistamines, such as hydroxyzine 25 to 50 mg or diphenhydramine 25 to 50 mg orally or IV, are used as first-line oral agents used to treat pruritus. Cholestyramine has also been used at doses of 5 g twice daily. Oral activated charcoal has also been used in doses of 1 to 1.5 g four times daily with some demonstrated efficacy. Other therapies that are often used in combination with other agents include oral ondansetron or naltrexone and topical capsaicin. Each has been reported to have efficacy in the treatment of pruritus associated with CKD.[64]

▶ *Vitamin Replacement*

Water-soluble vitamins removed by hemodialysis (HD) contribute to malnutrition and vitamin deficiency syndromes. Patients receiving HD often require replacement of water-soluble vitamins to prevent adverse effects. The vitamins that may require replacement are ascorbic acid, thiamine, biotin, folic acid, riboflavin, and pyridoxine. Patients receiving HD should receive a multivitamin B complex with vitamin C supplement, but should not take supplements that include fat-soluble vitamins, such as vitamins A, E, or K, which can accumulate in patients with kidney failure.

RENAL REPLACEMENT THERAPY

Patients who progress to ESKD require RRT. The modalities that are used for RRT are dialysis, including HD and peritoneal dialysis (PD), and kidney transplantation. The United States Renal Data Service (USRDS) reported that the number of patients with ESKD was 506,256, with 110,854 new cases being diagnosed in 2006.[2] The most common form of RRT is dialysis, accounting for 65% of all patients with ESKD.[2] The principles and complications associated with dialysis are discussed below. Chapter 55 discusses the principles of kidney transplantation.

Indications for Dialysis

⑨ *Planning for dialysis should begin when GFR falls less than 30 mL/min/1.73 m² (stage 4 CKD),[1] when progression to ESKD is inevitable, to allow time to educate the patient and family on the treatment modalities and establish the appropriate access for the modality of choice.* Ideally, initiation of dialysis should be done at a point when the patient is ready to undergo treatment, rather than when the patient is in emergent need of dialysis.

Initiation of dialysis is dependent on the patient's clinical status. Symptoms that may indicate the need for dialysis include persistent anorexia, nausea, vomiting, fatigue, and pruritus. Other criteria that indicate the need for dialysis include declining nutritional status, declining serum albumin levels, uncontrolled hypertension, and volume overload, which may manifest as chronic heart failure, and electrolyte abnormalities, particularly hyperkalemia. Blood urea nitrogen (BUN) and SCr levels may be used as a guide for the initiation of dialysis, but should not be the absolute indicator. Dialysis is initiated in most patients when the GFR

falls below 15 mL/min/1.73 m².[1] Patients should determine which modality of dialysis to use based on their own preferences. Advantages and disadvantages of hemodialysis and peritoneal dialysis are listed in Tables 26–8 and 26–9, respectively.

The goals of dialysis are to remove toxic metabolites to decrease uremic symptoms, correct electrolyte abnormalities, restore acid–base status, and maintain volume status to ultimately improve quality of life and decrease the morbidity and mortality associated with ESKD.

Hemodialysis

▶ *Principles of Hemodialysis*

⑩ *Hemodialysis (HD) involves the exposure of blood to a semipermeable membrane (dialyzer) against which a physiologic solution (dialysate) is flowing (Fig. 26–6).* The dialyzer is composed of thousands of capillary fibers made up of the semipermeable membrane, which are enclosed in the dialyzer, to increase the surface area of blood exposure to maximize the efficiency of removing substances. The dialysate is composed of purified water and electrolytes, and is run through the dialyzer countercurrent to the blood on the other side of the semipermeable membrane. The process allows for the removal of several substances from the bloodstream, including water, urea, creatinine, electrolytes, uremic toxins, and drugs. Although the dialysate is not sterilized, the membrane prevents bacteria from entering into the bloodstream. However, if the membrane ruptures

---

Table 26–8

Advantages and Disadvantages of Hemodialysis

Advantages
1. Higher solute clearance allows intermittent treatment
2. Parameters of adequacy of dialysis are better defined and therefore underdialysis can be detected early
3. The technique's failure rate is low
4. Even though intermittent heparinization is required, hemostasis parameters are better corrected with hemodialysis than peritoneal dialysis
5. In-center hemodialysis enables closer monitoring of the patient

Disadvantages
1. Requires multiple visits each week to the hemodialysis center, which translates into loss of control by the patient
2. Dysequilibrium, dialysis, hypotension, and muscle cramps are common. May require months before patient adjusts to hemodialysis
3. Infections in hemodialysis patients may be related to the choice of membranes, the complement-activating membranes being more deleterious
4. Vascular access is frequently associated with infection and thrombosis
5. Decline of residual renal function is more rapid compared to peritoneal dialysis

From Foote EF, Manley HJ. Hemodialysis and peritoneal dialysis. In: DiPiro JT, Talbert RL, Yee GC, et al., (eds.) Pharmacotherapy: A Pathophysiologic Approach. 7th ed. New York: McGraw-Hill; 2008: 0104, with permission.

Table 26–9

Advantages and Disadvantages of Peritoneal Dialysis

Advantages
1. More hemodynamic stability (blood pressure) due to slow ultrafiltration rate
2. Increased clearance of larger solutes, which may explain good clinical status in spite of lower urea clearance
3. Better preservation of residual renal function
4. Convenient intraperitoneal route of administration of drugs such as antibiotics and insulin
5. Suitable for elderly and very young patients who may not tolerate hemodialysis well
6. Freedom from the "machine" gives the patient a sense of independence (for continuous ambulatory peritoneal dialysis)
7. Less blood loss and iron deficiency, resulting in easier management of anemia or reduced requirements for erythropoietin and parenteral iron
8. No systemic heparinization requirement
9. Subcutaneous versus IV erythropoietin or darbepoetin is usual, which may reduce overall doses and be more physiologic

Disadvantages
1. Protein and amino acid losses through the peritoneum and reduced appetite owing to continuous glucose load and sense of abdominal fullness predispose to malnutrition
2. Risk of peritonitis
3. Catheter malfunction, and exit site and tunnel infection
4. Inadequate ultrafiltration and solute dialysis in patients with a large body size, unless large volumes and frequent exchanges are employed
5. Patient burnout and high rate of technique failure
6. Risk of obesity with excessive glucose absorption
7. Mechanical problems such as hernias, dialysate leaks, hemorrhoids, or back pain may occur
8. Extensive abdominal surgery may preclude peritoneal dialysis
9. No convenient access for IV iron administration

From Foote EF, Manley HJ. Hemodialysis and peritoneal dialysis. In: DiPiro JT, Talbert RL, Yee GC, et al., (eds.) Pharmacotherapy: A Pathophysiologic Approach. 7th ed. New York: McGraw-Hill; 2008: O105, with permission.

Patient Encounter, Part 5

The patient presents to clinic several years later and complains that she "feels lousy." She states that she doesn't feel like eating and has lost 9 kg (20 lb) in the last 6 months.

Current Meds: Furosemide 80 mg orally twice daily; metolazone 5 mg orally twice daily; lisinopril 40 mg orally daily; metoprolol 75 mg orally twice daily; insulin glargine 30 units subcutaneously at bedtime; insulin lispro subcutaneously per sliding scale with meals; darbepoetin 100 mcg subcutaneously weekly; iron polysaccharide 150 mg orally daily; sevelamer 800 mg orally three times a day with meals; calcitriol 0.25 mcg orally daily; sodium bicarbonate 1,300 mg orally three times a day

ROS: Unremarkable

PE:

VS: BP 160/85 mm Hg, P 70 bpm, T 36.8°C (98.2°F), wt 68.2 kg (150 lb)

Chest: RRR, normal S_1, S_3, and S_4 both present; slight pericardial friction rub

Exts: 3+ bilateral lower extremity edema which is present half-way up her calf

Labs: Sodium 142 mEq/L (142 mmol/L); potassium 5.8 mEq/L (5.8 mmol/L); chloride 102 mEq/L (102 mmol/L); carbon dioxide 16 mEq/L (16 mmol/L); BUN 85 mg/dL (30.35 mmol/L urea); SCr 9.5 mg/dL (840 μmol/L); glucose 112 mg/dL (6.22 mmol/L); calcium 8.2 mg/dL (2.05 mmol/L); phosphate 5.8 mg/dL (1.87 mmol/L); iPTH 438 pg/mL (438 ng/L or 46.9 pmol/L); WBC 5.3×10^3 cells/mm³ (5.3×10^9/L); RBC 3.2×10^6 cells/mm³ (3.2×10^{12}/L); Hgb 9.8 g/dL (98 g/L or 6.08 mmol/L); Hct 29% (0.29); platelets 390×10^3 cells/mm³ (390×10^9/L)

What indications does the patient have for dialysis?

What alternatives for renal replacement therapy exist for the patient?

What are the advantages and disadvantages of each modality for renal replacement?

---

during hemodialysis, infection becomes a major concern for the patient.

Three types of membranes used for dialysis are classified by the size of the pores and the ability to remove solutes from the bloodstream.

- Conventional (standard) membranes have small pores, which limit solute removal to relatively small molecules, such as creatinine and urea.
- High-efficiency membranes also have small pores, but have a higher surface area that increases removal of small

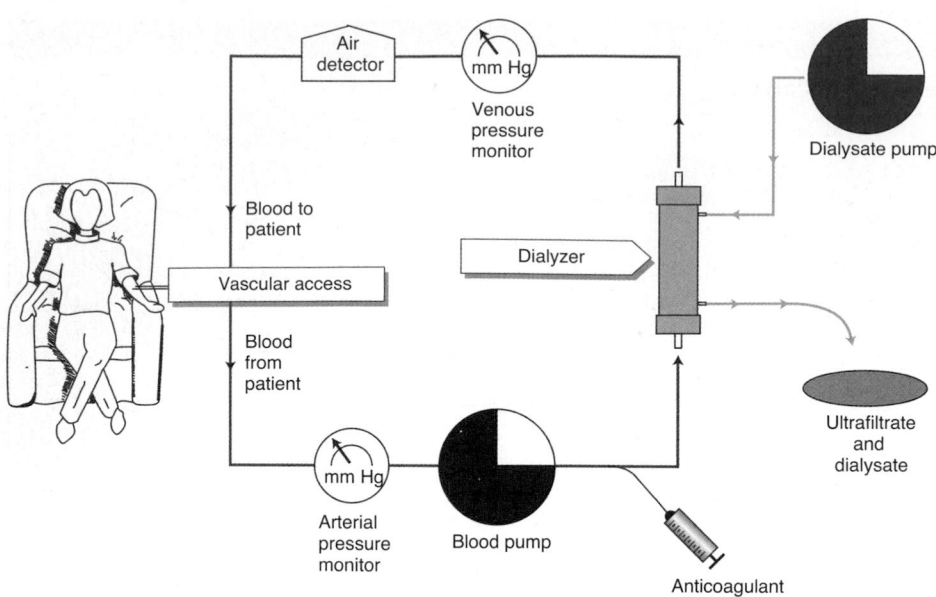

FIGURE 26–6. In hemodialysis, the patient's blood is pumped to the dialyzer at a rate of 300 to 600 mL/min. An anticoagulant (usually heparin) is administered to prevent clotting in the dialyzer. The dialyate is pumped at a rate of 500 to 1,000 mL/min through the dialyzer countercurrent to the flow of blood. The rate of fluid removal from the patient is controlled by adjusting the pressure in the dialysate compartment. (From Foote EF, Manley HJ. Hemodialysis and peritoneal dialysis. In: DiPiro JT, Talbert RL, Yee GC, et al., eds. Pharmacotherapy: A Pathophysiologic Approach, 7th ed. New York: McGraw-Hill, 2008: O106, with permission.)

molecules, such as water, urea, and creatinine from the blood.

- High-flux membranes have larger pores that allow for the removal of substances with higher molecular-weight, including some drugs, such as vancomycin, than conventional membranes.

Three primary processes are utilized for the removal of substances from the blood.

- Diffusion is the movement of a solute across the dialyzer membrane from an area of higher concentration (usually the blood) to a lower concentration (usually the dialysate). This process is the primary means for small molecules, such as electrolytes, to be removed from the bloodstream. At times, solutes can be added to the dialysate that are diffused into the bloodstream. Changing the composition of the dialysate allows for control of the amount of electrolytes that are being removed.

- Ultrafiltration is the movement of solvent (plasma water) across the dialyzer membrane by applying hydrostatic or osmotic pressure, and is the primary means for removing water from the bloodstream. Changing the hydrostatic pressure applied to the dialyzer or the osmotic concentration of the dialysate allows for control of the amount of water being removed.

- Convection is the movement of dissolved solutes across the dialyzer membrane by "dragging" the solutes along a pressure gradient with a fluid transport and is the primary means for larger molecules to be removed from the bloodstream, such as urea. Changing the pore size of the dialyzer membrane alters the efficiency of convection and allows for control of the amount of water removed in relation to the amount of solute being removed.

▶ **Vascular Access**

Long-term permanent access to the bloodstream is a key component of HD. There are three primary techniques used to obtain permanent vascular access in patients receiving HD, including arteriovenous fistulas (AVF), arteriovenous grafts (AVG) and catheters. An AVF is the preferred access method because it has the longest survival rate and the fewest complications.[65] An AVF is made by creating an anastomosis between an artery and a vein, usually in the forearm of the nondominant arm (Fig. 26–7). An AVG results in a similar access site, but uses a synthetic graft, usually made of polytetrafluoroethylene, to connect the artery and vein in the forearm (Fig. 26–7). The advantages of the AVG is that it is able to be used within 2 to 3 weeks, compared to 2 to 3 months for an AVF. However, AVGs are complicated by stenosis, thrombosis, and infections, which lead to a shorter survival time of the graft. Double-lumen venous catheters, placed in the femoral, subclavian, or jugular vein, are often used as temporary access while waiting for the AVF or AVG to mature. The catheters are tunneled beneath the skin to an exit site to reduce the risk of infection. Venous catheters can also be used as permanent access in patients in whom arteriovenous access cannot be established.

▶ **Complications of Hemodialysis**

Complications associated with HD include hypotension, muscle cramping, thrombosis, and infection.

Hypotension Hypotension is the most common complication seen during hemodialysis. It has been reported to occur with approximately 10% to 30% of dialysis sessions, but may be as frequent as 50% of sessions in some patients.[66]

Pathophysiology. Hypotension associated with hemodialysis manifests as a symptomatic sudden drop of more than 30 mm Hg in mean arterial or systolic pressure or a systolic pressure drop to less than 90 mm Hg during the dialysis session. The primary cause is fluid removal from the bloodstream. Ultrafiltration removes fluid from the plasma, which promotes redistribution of fluids from extracellular spaces into the plasma. However, decreased serum albumin levels and removal of solutes from the

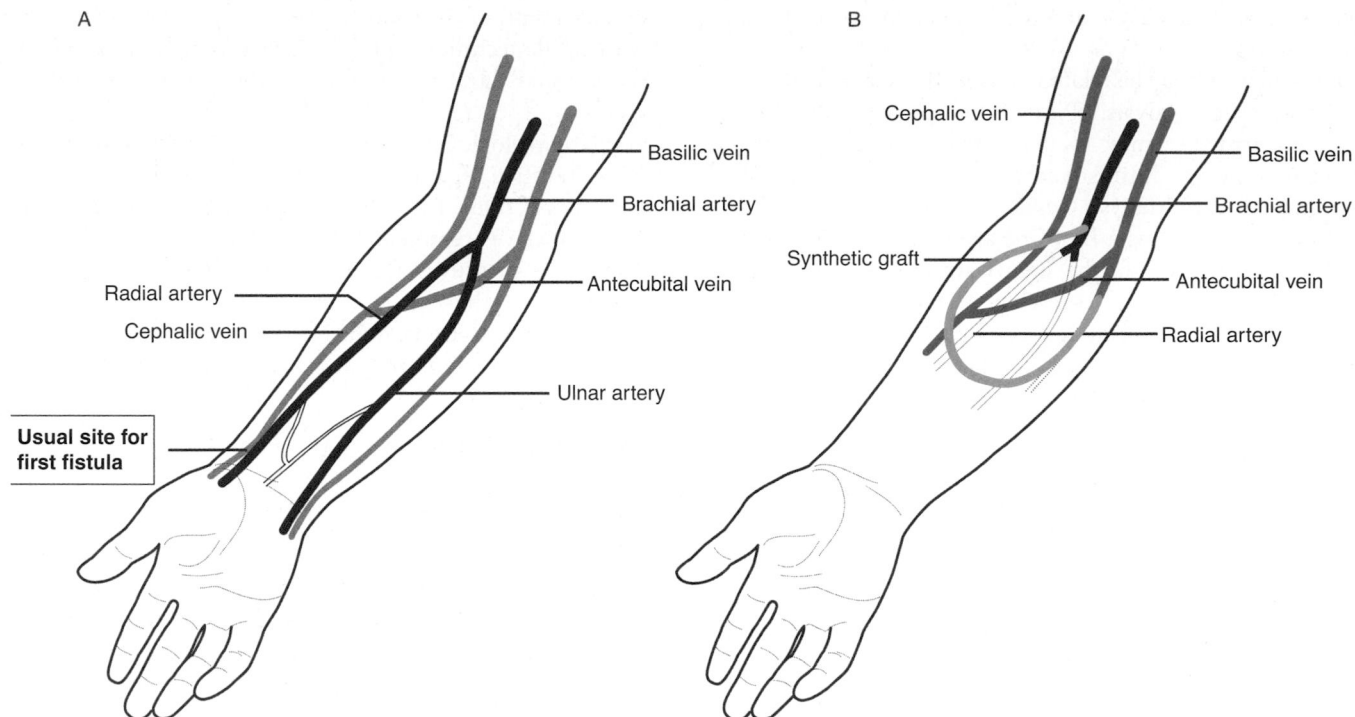

FIGURE 26–7. The predominant types of vascular access for chronic dialysis patients are (**A**) the arteriovenous fistula and (**B**) the synthetic arteriovenous forearm graft. The first primary arteriovenous fistula is usually created by the surgical anastamosis of the cephalic vein with the radial artery. The flow of blood from the higher-pressure arterial system results in hypertrophy of the vein. The most common AV graft (depicted in green) is between the brachial artery and the basilic or cephalic vein. The flow of blood may be diminished in the radial and ulnar arteries because it preferentially flows into the low pressure graft. (From Foote EF, Manley HJ. Hemodialysis and peritoneal dialysis. In: DiPiro JT, Talbert RL, Yee GC, et al., eds. Pharmacotherapy: A Pathophysiologic Approach, 7th ed. New York: McGraw-Hill, 2008: O106, with permission.)

bloodstream decrease the osmotic pressure of the plasma relative to the extracellular spaces, slowing redistribution during hemodialysis.[67] The decreased plasma volume causes hypotension. Other factors that can contribute to hypotension include antihypertensive medications prior to HD, a target "dry weight" (the target weight after HD session is complete) that is too low, diastolic or autonomic dysfunction, low dialysate calcium or sodium, high dialysate temperature, or ingesting meals prior to HD.

Risk factors that may increase the potential for hypotension include elderly age, diabetes, autonomic neuropathy, uremia, and cardiac disease.[66] The symptoms associated with hypotension during dialysis include dizziness, nausea, vomiting, sweating, and chest pain.

Treatment. Nonpharmacologic management of acute hypotension that occurs during dialysis involves placing the patient in the Trendelenburg position (with the head lower than the feet) and decreasing the ultrafiltration rate. Pharmacologic management of acute hypotension during dialysis includes administration of normal saline (100–200 mL), hypertonic saline (23.4%, 10–20 mL), or mannitol (12.5 g) to restore intravascular volume.

Preventive measures for patients who may be prone to hypotension include accurate determination of the "dry weight" and maintaining a constant ultrafiltration rate.

Patient Encounter, Part 6

The patient presents to the dialysis clinic 3 months later for her scheduled hemodialysis session. One hour into the session, she begins to complain of feeling dizzy and faint.

PE:

VS: BP 80/50 mm Hg (was 142/88 mm Hg at the start of hemodialysis), P 92 bpm; T 35.1°C (95.1°F); wt 65.9 kg (145 lb)

Chest: RRR, normal S_1, S_2 present

What are the potential causes of her hypotension?

What are the treatment alternatives for hypotension in the patient?

What are potential alternatives to avoid hypotension in future dialysis sessions?

Midodrine is an α-adrenergic agonist that is effective in reducing hypotension in patients with autonomic dysfunction that is taken with each dialysis session or as chronic therapy. Midodrine can be administered at doses of 2.5 to 10 mg prior to HD or 5 mg twice daily for chronic hypotension. Side effects of midodrine include pruritus and paresthesias.

Hypotension may be related to alterations in levocarnitine levels during dialysis. Patients who have low levels of levocarnitine may benefit from supplementation. Levocarnitine is administered as doses of 20 mg/kg IV at the end of each dialysis session. However, levocarnitine should not be used as a first-line agent for the treatment of hypotension because of the significant cost associated with the treatment. Patients receiving levocarnitine should be evaluated every 3 months for response to therapy.[68] Other preventive measures that have not been well studied include caffeine, sertraline, or fludrocortisone.

Muscle Cramps

Pathophysiology. Muscle cramps can occur with up to 20% of dialysis sessions.[69] The cause is often related to excessive ultrafiltration, which causes hypoperfusion of the muscles. Other contributing factors to the development of muscle cramps include hypotension and electrolyte and acid-base imbalances that occur during hemodialysis sessions.

Treatment. Nonpharmacologic treatments of muscle cramping that occurs during hemodialysis include decreasing the ultrafiltration rate and accurately determining the "dry weight." Pharmacologic measures include vitamin E, which is administered at doses of 400 IU daily. Other options that are not as well studied include oxazepam and prazosin.

Thrombosis Thrombosis associated with hemodialysis most commonly occurs in patients with venous catheter access for dialysis and is a common cause of catheter failure. However, thrombosis can occur in synthetic grafts and less frequently in AV fistulas.

Nonpharmacologic management of thrombosis in a hemodialysis catheter involves saline flushes. Smaller clots may be managed by balloon angioplasty to mechanically open the catheter. In severe cases in whom clots cannot be removed by either mechanical or pharmacologic therapy, the catheter may require replacement.

Pharmacologic management of thrombosis includes local administration of thrombolytic agents. Alteplase (2 mg per port) and reteplase (0.5 unit per port) are the two most commonly used agents today. Urokinase has been used in the past, but after its reintroduction to the U.S. market, the larger dosed vial size makes it less cost effective than the newer agents.

Infection Infections are an important cause of morbidity and mortality in patients receiving hemodialysis. The cause of infection is usually related to organisms found on the skin, namely *Staphylococcus epidermidis* and *S. aureus.* Other organisms have also been found to cause access-related infections. The greatest risk to patients receiving hemodialysis is the development of bacteremia. As with thrombosis, venous catheters are most commonly infected, followed by synthetic AV grafts, and finally AV fistulas.

Blood cultures should be obtained for any patient receiving hemodialysis who develops a fever. Nonpharmacologic management of infections involves preventive measures with sterile technique, proper disinfection, and minimizing the use and duration of venous catheters for hemodialysis access.

Pharmacologic management of infections should cover the Gram-positive organisms that most frequently cause access-related infections. Patients who have positive blood cultures should receive treatment tailored to the organism isolated. Preventive measures for access-related infections include mupirocin at the exit site and povidone-iodine ointment. The recommendations of the NKF for treatment of infections associated with hemodialysis are listed in Table 26–10.

Peritoneal Dialysis

▶ *Principles of PD*

PD utilizes similar principles as hemodialysis in that blood is exposed to a semipermeable membrane against which a physiologic solution is placed. In the case of PD, however, the semipermeable membrane is the peritoneal membrane, and a sterile dialysate is instilled into the peritoneal cavity. The peritoneal membrane is composed of a continuous single layer of mesothelial cells that covers the abdominal and pelvic walls on one side of the peritoneal cavity, and the visceral organs, including the GI tract, liver, spleen, and diaphragm on the other side. The mesothelial cells are covered by microvilli that increase the surface area of the peritoneal membrane to approximate body surface area (1–2 m²). Blood vessels that supply the abdominal organs, muscle, and mesentery serve as the blood component of the system.

The gaps between the mesothelial cells allow for large solutes to pass through into the bloodstream. Both the interstitium and endothelial cells of the blood vessels provide resistance to limit the solute size that is removed from the blood. Diffusion is the most important component of solute transport in PD, which is enhanced by the large surface area and volume of dialysate, as well as contact time with the peritoneal membrane. Ultrafiltration is achieved in PD by creating an osmotic pressure gradient between the dialysate and the blood. Traditionally, glucose has been used to create the osmotic gradient, but the solutions are not biocompatible with the peritoneal membrane, resulting in cytotoxicity of the cells. More recently, polymeric glucose derivatives, such as icodextrin, have been used to create a colloid-driven osmosis that results in ultrafiltration and convection of solute removal.

In PD, prewarmed dialysate is instilled into the peritoneal cavity where it "dwells" for a specified length of time (usually one to several hours, depending on the type of PD) to adequately clear metabolic waste products and excess fluids and electrolytes. At the end of the dwell time, the dialysate is drained and replaced with fresh dialysate. The continuous nature of PD provides for a more physiologic removal of waste products from the bloodstream, which mimics endogenous kidney function by decreasing the fluctuations seen in serum concentrations of the waste

Table 26–10

Management of Hemodialysis Access Infections

AV Fistula	Treat as subacute bacterial endocarditis for 6 weeks
	Initial antibiotic choice should always cover Gram-positive organisms (e.g., vancomycin 20 mg/kg IV with serum concentration monitoring or cefazolin 20 mg/kg IV 3 × per week)
	Gram-negative coverage is indicated for patients with diabetes, HIV infection, prosthetic valves, or those receiving immunosuppressive agents (gentamicin 2 mg/kg IV with serum concentration monitoring)
Synthetic Grafts (AVG)	
Local infection	Empiric antibiotic coverage for Gram-positive, Gram-negative, and *Enterococcus* (e.g., gentamicin plus vancomycin, then individualize after culture results become available); continue for 2–4 weeks
Extensive infection	Antibiotics as above plus total resection
Access less than 1 month old	Antibiotics as above plus removal of the graft
Tunneled Cuffed Catheters (Internal Jugular, Subclavian)	
Infection localized to catheter exit site	No drainage: topical antibiotics (e.g., mupirocin ointment)
	Drainage present: Gram-positive coverage (e.g., cefazolin 20 mg/kg IV 3 × per week)
Bacteremia with or without systemic signs or symptoms	Gram-positive coverage as above
	If stable and asymptomatic, change catheter and provide culture-specific antibiotic coverage for a minimum of 3 weeks

AV, arteriovenous.

products. Similarly, water is removed at a more constant rate, lessening the fluctuations in intravascular fluid balance and providing for more hemodynamic stability.

There are several types of PD that are used:

- Continuous ambulatory peritoneal dialysis (CAPD) is the most common. The patient exchanges 1 to 3 L of dialysate every 4 to 6 hours throughout the day with a longer dwell time overnight.

- Automated peritoneal dialysis (APD) procedures involve the use of a cycler machine that performs sequential exchanges overnight while the patient is sleeping.

- Continuous cycling PD (CCPD) performs three to five exchanges throughout the night. The final exchange remains in the peritoneal cavity to dwell for the duration of the day.

- Nightly intermittent PD (NIPD) performs six to eight exchanges throughout the night. The final exchange of dialysate is drained in the morning and the peritoneal cavity remains empty throughout the day.

- Nocturnal tidal PD (NTPD) is similar to NIPD, with the exception that only a portion of the dialysate is exchanged throughout the night. The final exchange is drained in the morning and the peritoneal cavity remains empty throughout the day.

▶ **Peritoneal Access**

Access to the peritoneal cavity requires placement of an indwelling catheter with the distal end of the catheter resting in the peritoneal cavity. The central portion of the catheter is generally tunneled under the abdominal wall and subcutaneous tissue where it is held in place by cuffs that provide stability and mechanical support

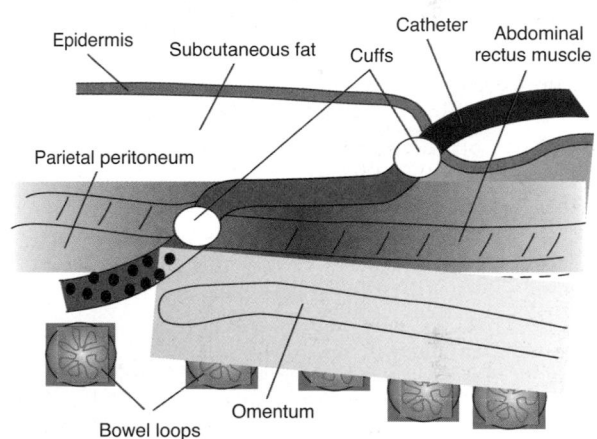

FIGURE 26–8. Diagram of the placement of a peritoneal dialysis catheter through the abdominal wall into the peritoneal cavity. (From Foote EF, Manley HJ. Hemodialysis and peritoneal dialysis. In: DiPiro JT, Talbert RL, Yee GC, et al., eds. Pharmacotherapy: A Pathophysiologic Approach, 7th ed. New York: McGraw-Hill, 2008: O110, with permission.)

to the catheter. The proximal portion of the catheter exits the abdomen near the umbilicus (Fig. 26–8). There are several types of indwelling catheters available; the most common is the Tenckhoff catheter. Placement and handling of the catheter during PD exchanges requires a sterile environment to minimize the risk of infectious complications.

▶ **Complications of Peritoneal Dialysis**

Complications associated with PD include mechanical problems related to the PD catheter, metabolic problems associated with the components of the dialysate fluid, damage to the peritoneal membrane, and infections (Table 26–11). Strategies to manage infectious complications of PD are discussed below.

Peritonitis Peritonitis is a leading cause of morbidity in PD patients, which often leads to loss of the catheter and subsequent change to HD as the treatment modality. However, recent advances with connectors used during instillation and drainage of dialysate and delivery systems have dramatically decreased the incidence of peritonitis. Peritonitis can be caused by chemical irritation or microorganisms.

Pathophysiology. Gram-positive organisms, namely *S. epidermidis*, are the most common cause of peritonitis. Other pathologic organisms include *S. aureus*, streptococcal species, enterococcus species, Gram-negative organisms including *Escherichia coli* and *Pseudomonas* species, and fungal organisms. Peritonitis should be presumed if cloudy fluid is drained from the peritoneal cavity and the fluid should be evaluated by cultures. Antibiotic treatment should be initiated immediately, until cell counts and cultures prove otherwise.[70] Patients with peritonitis may also complain of abdominal pain, although pain may be absent in some cases.

Treatment. The International Society of Peritoneal Dialysis (ISPD) revised the recommendations for the treatment of

---

> **Table 26–11**
>
> ## Common Complications During Peritoneal Dialysis
>
> **Mechanical Complications**
> Kinking in catheter
> Catheter migration
> Catheter adherence to peritoneal tissue
> Excessive movement of catheter at exit site
>
> **Peritoneal Damage**
> Alterations in permeability of the peritoneal membrane
> Sclerosis of the peritoneal membrane
>
> **Pain**
> Impingement of the catheter tip on visceral organs
> Instillation pain
> • Rapid inflow of dialysate
> • Acidic pH of dialysate
> • Chemical irritation from dialysate additives (e.g., antibiotics)
> • Low dialysate temperature
>
> **Infections**
> Peritonitis
> Exit-site infections
> Tunnel infections
>
> **Metabolic Complications**
> Exacerbation of diabetes mellitus from glucose load
> Fluid overload
> • Exacerbation of chronic heart failure
> • Edema
> • Pulmonary congestion
> Electrolyte abnormalities
> Malnutrition
> • Albumin and amino acid loss
> • Muscle wasting
> • Increased adipose tissue
> • Fibrin formation in dialysate

PD-related infections in 2005.[70] Drug selection for empiric treatment of peritonitis should cover both Gram-positive and Gram-negative organisms specific to the dialysis center and be based on the protocols and sensitivity patterns of organisms known to cause peritonitis, as well as the history of infections in the patient. First-generation cephalosporins, such as cefazolin, or vancomycin are recommended for empiric coverage of Gram-positive organisms. Appropriate coverage for Gram-negative organisms includes third- or fourth-generation cephalosporins, such as ceftazidime or cefepime, or aminoglycosides. Alternatives for Gram-negative coverage include oral fluoroquinolones. An example of an appropriate empiric treatment for peritonitis includes cefazolin in combination with ceftazidime, cefepime, or an aminoglycoside. If the patient has a cephalosporin allergy, vancomycin in combination with an aminoglycoside is an alternative empiric treatment.[70]

The preferred route of administration is intraperitoneal (IP) rather than IV to achieve maximum concentrations at the site of infection. Antibiotics can be administered IP intermittently as a single large dose in one exchange per day or continuously as multiple smaller doses with each exchange. Intermittent administration requires at least 6 hours of dwell time in the peritoneal cavity to allow for adequate systemic absorption and provides adequate levels to cover the 24-hour period. However, continuous administration is better suited for PD modalities that require more frequent exchanges (less than 6-hour dwell time). The reader should refer to the ISPD guidelines for dosing recommendations for IP antibiotics in CAPD and automated PD patients.[70] The dose of the antibiotics should be increased by 25% for patients with residual kidney function who are able to produce more than 100 mL urine output per day.

Once the organism has been identified and sensitivities are known, drug selection should be adjusted to reflect the susceptibilities of the organism. Streptococcal, staphylococcal, and enterococcal species sensitive to β-lactam antibiotics should be treated with continuous IP dosing to increase efficacy and minimize resistance.[70] Peritonitis caused by *S. aureus* or *P. aeruginosa* are often associated with catheter-related infections, which are difficult to treat and often require removal of the catheter. Rifampin 600 mg orally daily (in a single or divided dose) may be added to IP vancomycin for the treatment of methicillin-resistant *S. aureus* (MRSA), but should be limited to duration of 1 week to minimize the development of resistance. Two antibiotics are required for treatment of *P. aeruginosa* peritonitis.[70] If multiple organisms are cultured, treatment should cover all of the organisms, including anaerobic organisms, and the patient should be evaluated for other intra-abdominal pathologies.[70]

Peritonitis caused by fungal organisms is associated with mortality in 25% of patients,[70] which can be reduced by removing the catheter after fungal organisms are identified. Empiric treatment should include IP amphotericin B and flucytosine.[70] Although IP amphotericin administration is associated with chemical irritation and pain, penetration of amphotericin into the peritoneal cavity is poor with IV administration. Fluconazole, voriconazole, or caspofungin may be suitable alternatives, depending on culture results.

Catheter-Related Infections   Catheter-related infections generally occur at the exit site or the portion of the catheter that is tunneled in the subcutaneous tissue. Previous infections increase the risk and incidence of catheter-related infections.

Pathophysiology.   The major pathologic organisms responsible for causing catheter-related infections are *S. aureus* and *P. aeruginosa*. These organisms also cause the most serious catheter-related infections. *S. epidermidis* is found in less than 20% of catheter-related infections. Other organisms include diphtheroids, anaerobic bacteria, *Legionella*, and fungi.[70]

Exit-site infections present with purulent drainage at the site. Erythema may or may not be present with an exit-site infection. Tunnel infections are generally an extension of the exit-site infection and rarely occur alone. Symptoms of a tunnel infection may include tenderness, edema, and erythema over the tunnel pathway, but are often asymptomatic. Ultrasound can be used to detect tunnel infections in asymptomatic patients. Exit-site infections caused by *S. aureus* and *P. aeruginosa* often spread to tunnel infections and are the most common causes of catheter-infection–related peritonitis.

Treatment.   Exit-site infections may be treated immediately with empiric coverage, or treatment may be delayed until cultures return. Empiric treatment of catheter-related infections should cover *S. aureus*. Coverage for *P. aeruginosa* should also be included if the patient has a history of infections with this organism.[70] Cultures and sensitivity testing are particularly important in tailoring antibiotic therapy for catheter-related infections to ensure eradication of the organism and prevent recurrence or related peritonitis.

Less severe infections may be treated with topical antibiotic cream, although this practice is controversial. Oral antibiotics are also effective for treatment of catheter-related infections. Empiric or routine use of vancomycin for Gram-positive infections should be avoided unless the infection is caused by MRSA. Rifampin may be added to therapy for severe infections or slowly-resolving *S. aureus* infections, but monotherapy is not recommended.[70] Oral fluoroquinolones are used as first-line agents to treat *P. aeruginosa*, which can be difficult to treat and require prolonged treatment. If the infection is slow to resolve or if it recurs, IP ceftazidime or a second agent should be added.[70] Treatment of catheter-related infections should be continued until the exit site appears normal with no erythema or drainage. Generally, at least 2 weeks of therapy or longer are required to ensure complete eradication of the organism and prevent future recurrence, which is common with *S. aureus* and *P. aeruginosa*. Infections that do not resolve may require replacement of the PD catheter. Catheter-related infections that present in conjunction with or progress to peritonitis with the same organism require removal of the PD catheter until the peritonitis is resolved.[70]

Prophylaxis of Peritonitis and Catheter-Related Infections   Prevention of peritonitis and catheter-related infections starts when the catheter is placed. The exit site should be properly cared for until it is well healed before it can be used for PD. Patients should receive proper instructions for care of the catheter during this time period, which can last up to 2 weeks. Patients should also be instructed on the proper techniques to use for dialysate exchanges to minimize the risk of infections during exchanges, which is the most common cause of peritonitis.

Intranasal *S. aureus* increases the risk of *S. aureus* exit-site infections, tunnel infections, peritonitis, and subsequent catheter loss.[70] Several measures have been used to decrease the risk of peritonitis caused by *S. aureus*, including mupirocin cream applied daily around the exit site, intranasal mupirocin cream twice daily for 5 days each month, or rifampin 300 mg orally twice daily for 5 days, repeated every 3 months.[70] Mupirocin use is preferred over rifampin to prevent the development of resistance to rifampin, although mupirocin resistance has also been reported.[70] Other measures that have been used to decrease both *S. aureus* and *P. aeruginosa* infections include gentamicin cream applied twice daily and ciprofloxacin otic solution applied daily to the exit site.[70]

Outcome Evaluation   Clinical improvement should be seen within 48 hours of initiating treatment for peritonitis or catheter-related infections. Perform daily inspections of peritoneal fluid or the exit site to determine clinical improvement. Peritoneal fluid should become clear with improvement of peritonitis and erythema, and discharge should remit with improvement of catheter-related infections. If no improvement is seen within 48 hours, obtain additional cultures and cell counts to determine the appropriate alterations in therapy.

Abbreviations Introduced in This Chapter

ACE-I	Angiotensin-converting enzyme inhibitor
AGE	Advanced glycosylation end-product
AKI	Acute kidney injury
APD	Automated peritoneal dialysis
ARB	Angiotensin receptor blocker
ARF	Acute renal failure
AVF	Arteriovenous fistula
AVG	Arteriovenous graft
BMMD	Bone and mineral metabolism disorders
BUN	Blood urea nitrogen
Ca-P	Calcium-phosphorus product
CAPD	Continuous ambulatory peritoneal dialysis
CCBs	Calcium channel blockers
CCPD	Continuous cycling peritoneal dialysis
CHD	Coronary heart disease
CKD	Chronic kidney disease
CVD	Cardiovascular disease
DDAVP	Desmopressin
DKD	Diabetic kidney disease
DM	Diabetes mellitus

Patient Care and Monitoring

1. Assess the patient to determine if the patient should be evaluated for CKD. Does the patient have any risk factors for CKD?

2. Review any available laboratory data to determine the staging of CKD.

3. Obtain a thorough medical and medication history from the patient. Does the patient have any concomitant diseases, such as diabetes or hypertension, that should be treated to prevent the progression of CKD?

4. Determine if an ACE-I or ARB is appropriate for the patient. Does the patient have proteinuria?

5. Develop a plan to assess and optimize treatment of CKD.

6. Determine if the patient requires medical treatment for electrolyte imbalances. Does the patient have edema? Does the patient have an arrhythmia?

7. Educate the patient on dietary changes to manage electrolyte imbalances associated with CKD.

8. Assess the patient for the presence of anemia. Do the laboratory tests suggest the patient requires medical treatment?

9. Develop a plan to assess and optimize treatment for anemia.

10. Determine if the patient requires medical intervention to prevent the development of or treatment for sHPT.

11. Develop a plan to assess and optimize treatment for sHPT.

12. Establish if the patient requires RRT.

13. Evaluate the patient for complications associated with dialysis. Does the patient develop hypotension or cramps during hemodialysis? Does the patient have symptoms consistent with peritonitis or a catheter infection?

14. Develop a plan to assess and optimize treatment for complications associated with dialysis.

15. Stress the importance of adherence with the treatments for CKD and associated complications, including lifestyle modifications and medications. Recommend a therapeutic regimen that is easy for the patient to accomplish.

16. Provide patient education with regard to CKD and the associated complications, lifestyle modifications, and drug therapy:

   • What causes CKD and what things to avoid.

   • Possible complications of CKD and symptoms associated with the complications.

   • When to take medications.

   • What potential adverse effects may occur.

   • Which drugs may interact with therapy.

   • Warning signs to report to the physician (edema, irregular heart beat, fatigue, unusual bleeding).

ESA	Erythropoiesis-stimulating agent
ESKD	End-stage kidney disease
ESRD	End-stage renal disease
FE_K	Fractional excretion of potassium
FE_{Na}	Fractional excretion of sodium
GFR	Glomerular filtration rate
Hb_{A1c}	Hemoglobin$_{A1c}$
Hct	Hematocrit
HD	Hemodialysis
HDL-C	High-density lipoprotein cholesterol
Hgb	Hemoglobin
HMG-CoA	3-Hydroxy-3-methylglutaryl coenzyme A
IP	Intraperitoneal
iPTH	Intact parathyroid hormone
ISPD	International Society of Peritoneal Dialysis
LDL-C	Low-density lipoprotein cholesterol
LVH	Left ventricular hypertrophy
MCHC	Mean corpuscular hemoglobin concentration
MCV	Mean corpuscular volume
MRSA	Methicillin-resistant *Staphylococcus aureus*
NHANES	National Health and Nutrition Examination Survey
NIPD	Nightly intermittent peritoneal dialysis
NKF	National Kidney Foundation
NKF-K/DOQI	National Kidney Foundation-Dialysis Outcome Quality Initiative
NTPD	Nocturnal tidal peritoneal dialysis
PD	Peritoneal dialysis
PTH	Parathyroid hormone
ROD	Renal osteodystrophy
RRT	Renal replacement therapy
SCr	Serum creatinine
sHPT	Secondary hyperparathyroidism
SPS	Sodium polystyrene sulfonate
TC	Total cholesterol
TIBC	Total iron binding capacity
TSAT	Transferrin saturation
USRDS	United States Renal Data Service

 Self-assessment questions and answers are available at *http://www.mhpharmacotherapy.com/pp.html*.

REFERENCES

1. National Kidney Foundation. K/DOQI clinical practice guidelines for chronic kidney disease: Evaluation, classification and stratification. Am J Kidney Dis 2002;39(suppl 1):S1–S266.
2. U.S. Renal Data System, USRDS 2008 Annual Data Report: Atlas of Chronic Kidney Disease and End-Stage Renal Disease in the United States, National Institutes of Health, National Institute of Diabetes and Digestive and Kidney Diseases, Bethesda, MD, 2008.
3. Coresh J, Selvin E, Stevens LA, et al. Prevalence of chronic kidney disease in the United States. JAMA 2007;298(17):2038–2047.
4. Kasiske BL. Hyperlipidemia in patients with chronic renal disease. Am J Kidney Dis 1998;32(suppl 30):S142–S156.
5. Agarwal R, Curley TM. The role of statins in chronic kidney disease. Am J Med Sci 2005;333(2):69–81.
6. National Institutes of Health, National Institute of Diabetes and Digestive and Kidney Diseases. U.S. Renal Data System, USRDS 2008 annual data report: Atlas of end-stage renal disease in the United States. Bethesda, MD: Author; 2008.
7. Ritz E, Orth SR. Nephropathy in patients with type 2 diabetes mellitus. N Engl J Med 1999;341(15):1127–1133.
8. Brancati FL, Whelton PK, Randall BL, et al. Risk of end-stage renal disease in diabetes mellitus: Prospective cohort study of men screened for MRFIT. JAMA 1997;278(23):2069–2074.
9. Klag MJ, Whelton PK, Randall BL, et al. Blood pressure and end-stage renal disease in men. N Engl J Med 1996;334(1):13–18.
10. Peterson JC, Adler S, Burkart JM, et al. Blood pressure control, proteinuria, and the progression of renal disease: The modification of diet in renal disease study. Ann Int Med 1995;123(10):754–762.
11. Jafar TH, Stark PC, Schmid CH, et al. Proteinuria as a modifiable risk factor for the progression of non-diabetic renal disease. Kidney Int 2001;60:1131–1140.
12. Taal MW. Proteinuria: New information from an old friend. Curr Opin Nephrol Hyperten 2003;12:615–617.
13. Bakris GL. A practical approach to achieving recommended blood pressure goals in diabetic patients. Arch Int Med 2001;161:2661–2667.
14. Saito A, Tetsuro T, Sato K, et al. Significance of proximal tubular metabolism of advanced glycation end products in kidney diseases. Ann N Y Acad Sci 2005;1043:637–643.
15. Orth SR. Effects of smoking on systemic and intrarenal hemodynamics: Influence on renal function. J Am Soc Nephrol 2004;15(suppl 1):S58–S63.
16. Remuzzi G, Bertani T. Pathophysiology of progressive nephropathies. N Engl J Med 1998;339(20):1448–1456.
17. National Institutes of Health, National Institute of Diabetes and Digestive and Kidney Diseases. U.S. Renal Data System, USRDS 2005 annual data report: Atlas of end-stage renal disease in the United States. Bethesda, MD: Author; 2005.
18. National Kidney Foundation. KDOQI clinical practice guidelines and clinical practice recommendations for diabetes and chronic kidney disease. Am J Kidney Dis 2007;49(2 Suppl 2):S12–S154.
19. National Kidney Foundation. K/DOQI clinical practice guidelines for nutrition in chronic renal failure. Am J Kidney Dis 2000;35(6 suppl 2):S1–S140.
20. Uribarri J, Tuttle KR. Advanced glycation end products and nephrotoxicity of high-protein diets. Clin J Am Soc Nephrol 2006;1:1293–1299.
21. The Writing Team for the Diabetes Control and Complications Trial (DCCT)/Epidemiology of Diabetes Interventions and Complications (EDIC) Research Group. Sustained effect of intensive treatment of type 1 diabetes mellitus on development and progression of diabetic nephropathy: The epidemiology of diabetes interventions and complications (EDIC) study. JAMA 2003;290(16):2159–2167.
22. United Kingdom Prospective Diabetes Study (UKPDS) Group. Intensive blood-glucose control with sulfonylureas or insulin compared with conventional treatment and risk of complications in patients with type 2 diabetes. Lancet 1998;352:837–853.
23. National Kidney Foundation. K/DOQI clinical practice guidelines on hypertension and antihypertensive agents in chronic kidney disease. Am J Kidney Dis 2004;43(suppl 1):S1–S290.
24. Zager PG, Nikolic J, Brown RH, et al. "U" curve association of blood pressure and mortality in hemodialysis patients. Kidney Int 1998;54:561–569.
25. National Kidney Foundation. K/DOQI clinical practice guidelines for cardiovascular disease in dialysis patients. Am J Kidney Dis 2005;45(suppl 4);S1–S153.
26. Tentori F, Hunt WC, Rohrscheib M, et al. Which targets in clinical practice guidelines are associated with improved survival in a large dialysis organization? J Am Soc Nephrol 2007;18:2377–2384.
27. Remuzzi G, Ruggenenti P, Perico N. Chronic renal diseases: Renoprotective benefits of renin-angiotensin system inhibition. Ann Int Med 2002;136(8):604–615.
28. Mann JFE, Schmieder RE, McQueen M, et al. Renal outcomes with telmisartan, ramipril, or both, in people at high vascular risk (the ONTARGET study): A multicenter, randomized, double-blind, controlled trial. Lancet 2008;372:547–553.
29. Acri M, Erdem Y. Dual blockade of the renin-angiotensin system for cardiorenal protection: An update. Am J Kidney Dis 2009;53(2):332–345.
30. Bakris GL, Weir MR, Secic M, et al. Differential effects of calcium antagonist subclasses on markers of nephropathy progression. Kidney Int 2004;65:1991–2002.
31. Fried LF, Orchard TJ, Kasiske BL. Effect of lipid reduction on the progression of renal disease: A meta-analysis. Kidney Int 2001;59:260–269.
32. National Kidney Foundation. K/DOQI clinical practice guidelines for managing dyslipidemias in chronic kidney disease. Am J Kidney Dis 2003;41(suppl 3):S1–S92.
33. Wheeler DC. Lipid abnormalities in the nephrotic syndrome: The therapeutic role of statins. J Nephrol 2001;14(suppl 4):S70–S75.
34. Ravid M, Neumann L, Lishner M. Plasma lipids and the progression of nephropathy in diabetes mellitus type II: Effect of ACE inhibitors. Kidney Int 1995;47:907–910.
35. Tsakiris D. Morbidity and mortality reduction associated with the use of erythropoietin. Nephron 2000;85(suppl 1):2–8.
36. Rossert J, Fouqueray B, Boffa JJ. Anemia management and the delay of chronic renal failure progression. J Am Soc Nephrol 2003;14:S173–S177.
37. Shemin D, Dworkin LD. Sodium balance in renal failure. Curr Opin Nephrol Hyperten 1997;6(2):128–132.
38. Sica DA, Gehr TWB. Diuretic use in stage 5 chronic kidney disease and end-stage renal disease. Curr Opin Nephrol Hypertens 2003;12:483–490.
39. Gennari FJ, Segal AS. Hyperkalemia: An adaptive response in chronic renal insufficiency. Kidney Int 2002;62:1–9.
40. Ahmed J, Weisberg LS. Hyperkalemia in dialysis patients. Semin Dial 2001;14(5):348–356.
41. Musso CG. Potassium metabolism in patients with chronic kidney disease (CKD), part I: Patients not on dialysis (stages 3–4). Int Urol Nephrol 2004;36:465–468.
42. National Kidney Foundation. K/DOQI clinical practice guidelines and clinical practice recommendations for anemia in chronic kidney disease. Am J Kidney Dis 2006;47(suppl 3):S1–S146.
43. McClellan W, Aronoff SL, Bolton WK, et al. The prevalence of anemia in patients with chronic kidney disease. Curr Med Res Opin 2004;20(9):1501–1510.
44. Xue JL, St. Peter WL, Ebben JP, et al. Anemia treatment in the pre-ESRD period and associated mortality in elderly patients. Am J Kidney Dis 2002;40(6):1153–1161.
45. Hudson JQ, Schonder KS. Advances in anemia management in chronic kidney disease. J Pharm Pract 2002;15(6):437–455.
46. National Kidney Foundation. KDOQI clinical practice guideline and clinical practice recommendations for anemia in chronic kidney disease, 2007 update of hemoglobin target. Am J Kid Dis 2007;50(3):471–530.
47. Bishu K, Agarwal R. Acute injury with intravenous iron and concerns regarding long-term safety. Clin J Am Soc Nephrol 2006;1(suppl 1):S19–S23.
48. Drueke TB, Loctelli F, Clyne N, et al. Normalization of hemoglobin level in patients with chronic kidney disease and anemia. New Engl J Med 2006;335(20):2071–2084.

49. Singh AK, Szczech L, Tang KL, et al. Correction of anemia with epoetin alfa in chronic kidney disease. New Engl J Med 2006;335(20):2085–2099.

50. Szczech LA, Barnhart HX, Inrig JK, et al. Secondary analysis of the CHOIR trial epoetin-α dose and achieved hemoglobin outcomes. Kidney Int 2008;74:791–798.

51. Coyne DW, Kapoian T, Suki W, et al. Ferric gluconate is highly efficacious in anemic hemodialysis patients with high serum ferritin and low transferring saturation: Results of the dialysis patients' response to IV iron with elevated ferritin (DRIVE) study. J Am Soc Nephrol 2007;18:975–984.

52. de Francisco ALM. Secondary hyperparathyroidism: Review of the disease and its treatment. Clin Ther 2004;26:1976–1993.

53. Alfrey AC. The role of abnormal phosphorus metabolism in the progression of chronic kidney disease and metastatic calcification. Kidney Int 2004;66(suppl 90):S13–S17.

54. Noordzij M, Korevaar JC, Boeschoten EW, et al. The Kidney Diseae Outcomes Quality Initiative (K/DOQI) guideline for bone metabolism and disease in CKD: Association with mortality in dialysis patients. Am J Kid Dis 2005;46(5):925–932.

55. Kraut JA, Kurtz I. Metabolic acidosis of CKD: Diagnosis, clinical characteristics and treatment. Am J Kidney Dis 2005;45:978–993.

56. National Kidney Foundation. K/DOQI clinical practice guidelines for bone metabolism and disease in chronic kidney disease. Am J Kidney Dis 2003;42(suppl 3):S1–S202.

57. Block GA, Raggi P, Bellasi A, et al. Mortality effect of coronary calcification and phosphate binder choice in incident hemodialysis patients. Kidney Int 2007;71:438–441.

58. Suki WN, Zabaneh R, Cangiano JL, et al. Effects of sevelamer and calcium-based phosphate binders on mortality in hemodialysis patients. Kidney Int 2007;72:1130–1137.

59. Behets GJ, Verberckmoes SC, D'Haese PC, De Broe ME. Lanthanum carbonate: A new phosphate binder. Curr Opin Nephrol Hyperten 2004;13:403–409.

60. Uhlig K, Sarnak MJ, Singh AK. New approaches to the treatment of calcium and phosphorus abnormalities in patients on hemodialysis. Curr Opin Nephrol Hyperten 2001;10:793–798.

61. Al-Aly A, Qazi RA, González EA, et al. Changes in serum 25-hydroxyvitamin D and plasma intact PTH levels following treatment with ergocalciferol in patients with CKD. Am J Kidney Dis 2007;50(1):59–68.

62. Byrnes CA, Shepler BM. Cinacalcet: A new treatment for secondary hyperparathyroidism in patients receiving hemodialysis. Pharmacotherapy 2005;25(5):709–716.

63. Hedges SJ, Dehoney SB, Jooper JS, et al. Evidence-based treatment recommendations for uremic bleeding. Nat Clin Pract Nephrol 2007;3:138–153.

64. Murphy M, Carmichael AJ. Renal itch. Clin Exp Dermatol 2000;25:103–106.

65. National Kidney Foundation. K/DOQI clinical practice guidelines for vascular access: Update 2000. Am J Kidney Dis 2001;37(1 suppl 1):S137–S180.

66. Perazella MA. Clinical dilemmas in dialysis: Managing the hypotensive patient. Am J Kidney Dis 2001;38(4):607–617.

67. Rosner MH. Hemodialysis for the non-nephrologist. S Med J 2005;98(8):785–791.

68. Eknoyan G, Latos DL, Lindberg J. Practice recommendations for the use of L-Carnitine in dialysis-related carnitine disorder: National Kidney Foundation carnitine consensus conference. Am J Kidney Dis 2003;41(4):868–876.

69. Himmelfarb J. Hemodialysis complications. Am J Kidney Dis 2005;45(6):1122–1131.

70. Piraino B, Bailie GR, Bernardini J, et al. ISPD guidelines/recommendations: Peritoneal dialysis-related infections recommendations: 2005 update. Perit Dial Int 2005;25:107–131.

27 Fluids and Electrolytes

Mark A. Malesker and Lee E. Morrow

LEARNING OBJECTIVES

● **Upon completion of the chapter, the reader will be able to:**

1. Estimate the volumes of various body fluid compartments.
2. Calculate the daily maintenance fluid requirement for patients given their weight, and gender.
3. Differentiate among currently available fluids for volume resuscitation.
4. Identify the electrolytes primarily found in the extracellular and intracellular fluid compartments.
5. Describe the unique relationship between serum sodium concentration and total body water (TBW).
6. Review the etiology, clinical presentation, and management for disorders of sodium, potassium, calcium, phosphorus, and magnesium.

KEY CONCEPTS

❶ Total body water (TBW) is approximately 50% of lean body weight in normal females and 60% of lean body weight in males. TBW is comprised of the intracellular fluid (two-thirds of TBW) and the extracellular fluid (one-third of TBW). The extracellular fluid is made up of two major fluid subcompartments: the interstitial fluid and the intravascular fluid.

❷ Therapeutic fluids include crystalloid and colloid solutions. The most commonly used crystalloids include normal saline, hypertonic saline, and lactated Ringer's solution. Examples of colloids include albumin, the dextrans, hetastarch, and fresh-frozen plasma.

❸ The calculated serum osmolality helps determine deviations in TBW content.

❹ Concentrated electrolytes (potassium chloride [KCl], potassium phosphate, and sodium chloride [NaCl] greater than 0.9%) should not be stored in patient care areas as a patient safety measure.

❺ Hyponatremia is a very common finding in hospitalized patients and is defined as a serum sodium concentration below 136 mEq/L (136 mmol/L).

❻ IV potassium infusions running at rates of greater than 10 mEq/h require cardiac monitoring.

❼ Calcium gluconate is the preferred peripherally infused calcium supplement because it is less irritating to the veins. Calcium chloride (CaCl) must be infused via a central line.

❽ Severe hypophosphatemia can result in impaired diaphragmatic contractility and acute respiratory failure.

❾ Serum magnesium concentrations do not correlate well with total body magnesium stores. For this reason, magnesium supplementation is often given empirically to critically ill patients.

BODY FLUID COMPARTMENTS

A thorough understanding of the fundamentals of fluid and electrolyte homeostasis is essential given the frequency with which clinical disturbances are seen and the profound effects these disturbances can have on various aspects of patient care. However, the interplay of body fluids, serum electrolytes, and clinical monitoring is complex, and a thorough command of these issues is a challenging task even for advanced practitioners.[1] Practitioners must be familiar with the key concepts of body compartment volumes, calculation of daily fluid requirements, and the various types of fluid available for replacement. The management of disorders of sodium, potassium, calcium, phosphorus, and magnesium integrates these concepts with issues of dose recognition and patient safety.

The most fundamental concept to grasp is an assessment of total body water (TBW), which is directly related to body weight. ❶ *TBW constitutes approximately 50% of lean body weight in healthy females and 60% of lean body weight in males.* The percentage of TBW decreases as body fat increases and/or with age (75–85% of body weight is water for newborns).

Unless the patient is obese (body weight greater than 120% of ideal body weight [IBW]), clinicians typically use a patient's actual body weight when calculating TBW.[2] In obese patients, it is customary to estimate TBW using lean body weight or IBW as calculated by the Devine–Devine method: males' lean body weight = 50 kg + (2.3 kg/in. × [height in inches – 60]) and females' lean body weight = 45.5 kg + (2.3 kg/in. × [height in inches – 60]).[3–5] Note that 1 kg is equivalent to 2.2 lb, 1 in. is equivalent to 2.54 cm, and 1 L of water weighs 1 kg (2.2 lb).

The intracellular fluid (ICF) represents the water contained within cells and is rich in electrolytes such as potassium, magnesium, phosphates, and proteins. ❶ *The ICF is approximately two-thirds of TBW regardless of gender.* For a 70-kg man, this would mean that the TBW is 42 L and the ICF is approximately 28 L. For a 70-kg woman, these values would be 35 L and 24 L, respectively. Note that ICF represents approximately 40% of total body weight in men and approximately 33% of total body weight in women.

The extracellular fluid (ECF) is the fluid outside the cell and is rich in sodium, chloride, and bicarbonate. ❶ *The ECF is approximately one-third of TBW (14 L in a 70-kg man or 12 L in a 70-kg woman) and is subdivided into two compartments: the interstitial fluid and the intravascular fluid.* The interstitial fluid represents the fluid occupying the spaces between cells, and is about 25% of TBW (10.5 L in a 70-kg man or 8.8 L in a 70-kg woman). The intravascular fluid (also known as plasma) represents the fluid within the blood vessels and is about 8% of TBW (3.4 L in a 70-kg man or 2.8 L in a 70-kg woman). Because the exact percentages are cumbersome to recall, many clinicians accept that the ECF represents roughly 20% of body weight (regardless of gender) with 15% in the interstitial space and 5% in the intravascular space.[6] Note that serum electrolytes are routinely measured from the ECF.

The transcellular fluid includes the viscous components of the peritoneum, pleural space, and pericardium, as well as the cerebrospinal fluid, joint space fluid, and the GI digestive juices. Although the transcellular fluid normally accounts for about 1% of TBW, this amount can increase significantly during various illnesses favoring fluid collection in one of these spaces (e.g., pleural effusions or ascites in the peritoneum). The accumulation of fluid in the transcellular space is often referred to as "third spacing." To review the calculations of the body fluid compartments in a representative patient, see Patient Encounter 1.

Fluid balance is assessed by several means each of which has its limitations. Blood pressure (BP) measurements estimate fluid status relative to the amount of blood volume pumped by the heart but are affected by cardiac function and vascular pliability. Patients with significant volume deficiency may appear hypotensive, but this is a late finding that may require greater than 20% of TBW to be lost. Patients with significant volume excess may appear edematous; however, third spacing may hide this finding until late in the course as well. The physical exam can indicate the presence of fluid deficits (dry mucous membranes) and fluid excess (peripheral edema, coarse breath sounds). More invasive assessments would include the use of an arterial catheter, a pulmonary artery catheter to measure left ventricular function and fluid status, and a central venous catheter, which measures fluid status and right ventricular function. However, the correlation between these measured pressures and their associated volume is an area of debate.

To maintain fluid balance, the total amount of fluid gained throughout the day (input, or "ins") must equal the total amount of fluid lost (output, or "outs"). Although most forms of the body's input and output can be measured, several cannot. For a normal adult on an average diet, ingested fluids are easily measured and average 1,400 mL/day. Other fluid inputs, such as those from ingested foods and the water by-product of oxidation, are not directly measurable. Fluid outputs such as urinary and stool losses are also easily measured and are referred to as sensible losses. Other sources of fluid loss, such as evaporation of fluid through the skin and/or lungs, are not readily measured and are called insensible losses. Table 27–1 shows the estimated ins and outs (I&Os) for a healthy 68-kg (150-lb) man.[6] The measurable I&Os are routinely measured in hospitalized patients and are used to estimate total fluid balance for each 24-hour period. It is important to realize that in hospitalized patients, multiple other forms of fluid loss must be considered. These include losses from enteric suctioning (most commonly, nasogastric [NG] tubes), from surgical drains (e.g., chest tubes, nephrostomy tubes, and pancreatic drains), via fistulous tracts, and enhanced evaporative losses (burns and fever).

TBW depletion (often referred to as "dehydration") is typically a gradual, chronic problem. Because TBW depletion represents a loss of hypotonic fluid (proportionally more water is lost than sodium) from all body compartments, a primary disturbance of osmolality is usually seen. The signs and symptoms of TBW depletion include CNS disturbances (mental status changes, seizures, and coma), excessive thirst, dry mucous membranes, decreased skin turgor, elevated

Patient Encounter 1: Body Fluid Compartments

Calculate the total body water, ICF, and extracellular fluid in a 70-kg male.

Table 27–1

Approximate I&Os for a Healthy 68-kg (150-lb) Man

Input	mL/day	Output	mL/day
Ingested fluid[a]	1,400	Urine[a]	1,500
Fluid in food	850	Skin losses	500
Water of oxidation	350	Respiratory tract losses	400
		Stool	200
Total	2,600	Total	2,600

[a]Readily quantifiable.

serum sodium, increased plasma osmolality, concentrated urine, and acute weight loss. Common causes of TBW depletion include insufficient oral intake, excessive insensible losses, diabetes insipidus, excessive osmotic diuresis, and impaired renal concentrating mechanisms. Long-term care residents are frequently admitted to the acute care hospital with TBW depletion secondary to lack of adequate oral intake, often with concurrent excessive insensible losses.

The volume of fluid required to correct TBW depletion equals the basal fluid requirement plus ongoing exceptional losses plus the fluid deficit. Basal daily fluid requirements are calculated using the formulas in Table 27–2. For an adult, this represents 1,500 mL/day for the first 20 kg of body weight plus 20 mL/day for each additional kilogram. The volume of replacement fluids required for a given patient (the fluid deficit) can be estimated by the acute weight change in the patient (1 kg = 1 L of fluid). Because the precise weight change is not typically known, it is often calculated as follows: fluid deficit = normal TBW − present TBW. Normal TBW is estimated based on the patient's height using the formulas in Table 27–2, and the present TBW is estimated based on the patient's current body weight. The choice of fluids used for replacement is guided by the presence of concurrent electrolyte abnormalities. The adequacy of replacement is guided by each patient's objective response to fluid replacement (improved skin turgor, adequate urine output, normalization of heart rate, BP, etc.).

Once TBW has been restored, the volume of "maintenance" fluid equals the basal fluid requirement plus ongoing exceptional losses. If the pathophysiologic process leading to TBW depletion has not been identified and corrected (or accounted for in the calculation of maintenance fluid requirements), TBW depletion will quickly recur. To review the concepts involved in the calculation of replacement fluids for a representative patient see Patient Encounter 2.

Compared to TBW depletion, ECF depletion tends to occur acutely. In this setting, rapid and aggressive fluid replacement is required to maintain adequate organ perfusion. Because ECF depletion is generally due to the loss of isotonic fluid (proportional losses of sodium and water), major disturbances

of plasma osmolality are not common. ECF depletion manifests clinically as signs and symptoms associated with decreased tissue perfusion: dizziness, orthostasis, tachycardia, decreased urine output, increased hematocrit, decreased central venous pressure, and/or hypovolemic shock. Common causes of ECF depletion include external fluid losses (burns, hemorrhage, diuresis, GI losses, and adrenal insufficiency) and third spacing of fluids (septic shock, anaphylactic shock, or abdominal ascites).

In clinical practice, the most commonly encountered problem is depletion of TBW and ECF. Accordingly, the fluid resuscitation strategy should address both of these compartments. As these compartments are repleted, serum electrolytes must be monitored closely as discussed in subsequent sections of this chapter.

THERAPEUTIC FLUIDS

Crystalloids

❷ *Therapeutic IV fluids include crystalloid solutions, colloidal solutions, and oxygen-carrying resuscitation solutions.* Crystalloids are composed of water and electrolytes, all of which pass freely through semipermeable membranes and remain in the intravascular space for shorter periods of time. As such, these solutions are very useful for correcting electrolyte imbalances, but result in smaller hemodynamic changes for a given unit of volume.

Crystalloids can be classified further according to their tonicity. Isotonic solutions (i.e., normal saline or 0.9% sodium chloride [NaCl]) have a tonicity equal to that of the ICF (approximately 310 mEq/L or 310 mmol/L) and do not shift the distribution of water between the ECF and the ICF. Because hypertonic solutions (i.e., hypertonic saline or 3% NaCl) have greater tonicity than the ICF (greater than 376 mEq/L or 376 mmol/L), they draw water from the ICF into the ECF. In contrast, hypotonic solutions (i.e., 0.45% NaCl) have less tonicity than the ICF (less than 250 mEq/L or 250 mmol/L) leading to osmotic pressure gradient that favors shifts of water from the ECF into the ICF. The tonicity, electrolyte content, and glucose content of selected fluids are shown in Table 27–3.

The tonicity of crystalloid solutions is directly related to their sodium concentration. The most commonly used crystalloids include normal saline, hypertonic saline, and lactated Ringer's solution. Excessive administration of any fluid replacement therapy, regardless of tonicity, can lead to fluid overload, particularly in patients with cardiac or renal insufficiency. Glucose is often added to hypotonic crystalloids in amounts than result in isotonic fluids (D$_5$W, D5½NS, and D5¼NS). These solutions are often used as maintenance fluids to provide basal amounts of calories and water.

▶ Normal Saline (0.9% NaCl or NS)

Normal saline is an isotonic fluid composed of water, sodium, and chloride. It provides primarily ECF replacement and can be used for virtually any cause of TBW depletion. Common uses of normal saline include perioperative fluid

---

Table 27–2

Useful Calculations for the Estimation of Patient Maintenance Fluid Requirements

Neonate (1–10 kg) = 100 mL/kg
Child (10–20 kg) = 1,000 mL + 50 mL for each kilogram greater than 10
Adult (greater than 20 kg) = 1,500 mL + 20 mL for each kilogram greater than 20

Patient Encounter 2: Fluid Requirements

Calculate the daily fluid requirement for a 70-kg adult male.

Table 27–3

Electrolyte and Dextrose Content of Selected Crystalloid Fluids

IV Solution	Osmolarity (mOsm)	Dextrose (g/L) (mmol/L)	Sodium (mEq/L) (mmol/L)	Potassium (mEq/L) (mmol/L)	Calcium (mEq/L) (mmol/L)	Chloride (mEq/L) (mmol/L)	Lactate (mEq/L) (mmol/L)
D5%	250	50 / 2.78					
D10%	505	100 / 5.55					
0.9% NaCl	308		154			154	
0.45% NaCl	154		77			77	
3% NaCl	1,025		512			512	
D5% and 0.45% NaCl	405	50 / 2.78	77			77	
D5% and 0.2% NaCl	329	50 / 2.78	34			34	
Ringer's injection	310		147	4	5 / 2.5	156	
Lactated Ringer's solution	274		130	4	3 / 1.5	109	28
Lactated Ringer's solution and D5%	525	50 / 2.78	130	4	3 / 1.5	109	28

D, dextrose; NaCl, sodium chloride.

administration; volume resuscitation of shock, hemorrhage, or burn patients; fluid challenges in hypotensive or oliguric patients; and hyponatremia. Normal saline can also be used to treat metabolic alkalosis (also known as contraction alkalosis).

▶ Half-Normal Saline (0.45% NaCl or ½ NS)

Half-normal saline is a hypotonic fluid that provides free water in relative excess when compared to the sodium concentration. This crystalloid is typically used to treat patients who are hypertonic due to primary depletion of the ECF. Because half-normal saline is hypotonic, serum sodium must be closely monitored during administration.

▶ Hypertonic Saline (3% NaCl)

Hypertonic saline is obviously hypertonic and provides a significant sodium load to the intravascular space. This solution is used very infrequently given the potential to cause significant shifts in the water balance between the ECF and the ICF. It is typically used to treat patients with severe hyponatremia who have symptoms attributable to low serum sodium. Hypertonic saline in concentrations of 7.5% to 23.4% has been used to acutely lower intracranial pressure in the setting of traumatic brain injury and stroke. The literature is inconsistent for the appropriate hypertonic

concentration, dosing, timing of replacement, and goals for use in this population. Serum sodium and neurologic status must be very closely monitored whenever given.

▶ Ringer's Lactate

This isotonic volume expander contains sodium, potassium, chloride, and lactate in concentrations that approximate the fluid and electrolyte composition of the blood. Ringer's lactate (also known as "lactated Ringer" or LR) provides ECF replacement and is most often used in the perioperative setting, and for patients with lower GI fluid losses, burns, or dehydration. The lactate component of LR works as a buffer to increase the pH. Accordingly, large volumes of LR may cause iatrogenic metabolic alkalosis. Because patients with significant liver disease are unable to metabolize lactate sufficiently, LR administration in this population may lead to accumulation of lactate with iatrogenic lactic acidosis.

▶ 5% Dextrose in Water (D₅W)

D$_5$W is a solution of free water and dextrose that provides a modest amount of calories but no electrolytes. Although it is technically isotonic, it acts as a hypotonic solution in the body. It is commonly used to treat severe hypernatremia. D$_5$W is also used in small volumes (100 mL) to dilute many

IV medications or at a low infusion rate (10–15 mL/h) to "keep the vein open" (KVO) for IV medications.

Colloids

In contrast to crystalloids, colloids do not dissolve into a true solution, and therefore do not pass readily across semipermeable membranes. As such, colloids effectively remain in the intravascular space and increase the oncotic pressure of the plasma. This effectively shifts fluid from the interstitial compartment to the intravascular compartment. In clinical practice, these theoretical benefits are generally short-lived (given metabolism of colloidal proteins/sugars) and for most patients there is little therapeutic advantage of colloids over crystalloids or vice versa. Examples of colloids include 5% albumin, 25% albumin, the dextrans, hetastarch, and fresh-frozen plasma (FFP). Because each of these agents contains a substance (proteins and complex sugars) that will ultimately be metabolized, the oncotic agent will be ultimately lost and only the remaining hypotonic fluid delivery agent will remain. As such, use of large volumes of colloidal agents is more likely to induce fluid overload compared to crystalloids. Although smaller volumes of colloids have equal efficacy as larger volumes of crystalloids, they generally must be infused more slowly. Often the net result is that the time to clinical benefit is the same regardless of which class of fluid is utilized. For example, 500 mL of normal saline is required to increase the systolic BP to the same degree as seen with approximately 250 mL of 5% albumin; however, the normal saline can be administered twice as fast.

▶ Albumin

Albumin is a protein derived from fractionating human plasma. Because albumin infusion is expensive and may be associated with adverse events, it should be used for acute volume expansion and *not* as a supplemental source of protein calories. Historically, albumin was used indiscriminately in the intensive care unit until anecdotal publications suggested that albumin may cause immunosuppression. However, the recently completed Saline Versus Albumin Fluid Evaluation (SAFE) trial randomized nearly 7,000 hypovolemic patients to either albumin or normal saline therapy and found that the mortality for those who received albumin was the same as for those who received normal saline.[7] A subsequent post hoc analysis reported that patients with traumatic brain injury had higher mortality rates when given albumin for fluid resuscitation. These conflicting findings highlight the controversy and confusion surrounding the use of human albumin versus normal saline therapy for resuscitation of critically ill patients.[8–10] Albumin combined with furosemide has been demonstrated to improve fluid balance, oxygenation, and hemodynamics in the subset of patients with acute lung injury who have low serum protein.[11]

Recent events have resulted in an albumin shortage in the United States with ongoing allocation of all albumin products. In brief, albumin is obtained as a by-product of routine intravenous immunoglobulin (IVIG) processing.

As a result, the albumin supply is driven by the amount of plasma fractioning for IVIG. Increased efficiency of the IVIG collection techniques and decreased IVIG consumption has led to an unintended shortage of albumin available for use. Based upon this limited availability, health systems and hospitals have had to define the appropriate albumin indications for their patients and ration albumin accordingly. Evidence-based indications for albumin include plasmaphoresis/apharesis, large volume paracentesis (greater than 4 liters removed), hypotension in hemodialysis, and the need for aggressive diuresis in hypoalbuminemic hypotensive patients. Inappropriate uses of albumin include nutritional supplementation, impending hepatorenal syndrome, pancreatitis, alteration of drug pharmacokinetics, or acute normovolemic hemodilution in surgery. Practitioners can keep up with medication shortages by checking the American Society of Health-System Pharmacists (ASHP) website (*www. ashp.org*).

▶ Hetastarch and Dextran

While albumin is the most commonly used colloid, the other available products are not without their own risks and benefits. Hetastarch (various manufacturers) and Voluven contain 6% starch and 0.9% NaCl. This product has no oxygen-carrying capacity and is administered intravenously as a plasma expander. Limitations of this product include acquisition cost, hypersensitivity reactions, and bleeding. Dosing should be reduced in the presence of renal dysfunction. Hextend is a comparable plasma expander that contains 6% hetastarch in lactated electrolyte solution. Low-molecular-weight dextran (various manufacturers) and high-molecular-weight dextran (various manufacturers) are polysaccharide plasma expanders. Anaphylactic reactions and prolonged bleeding times have limited the use of these products. Potential mechanisms of colloid solution-induced bleeding include platelet inhibition or possible dilution of clotting factors via infusion of a large volume colloid solution. Although FFP has been used as a volume expander in cases of excessive blood loss (surgery or trauma) and to prevent bleeding in the presence of abnormal coagulation studies, it is now rarely used for volume expansion given risks of anaphylaxis, potential for viral transmission, and increased nosocomial infection rates.

Fluid Management Strategies

Classic indications for IV fluid include maintenance of BP, restoring the ICF volume, replacing ongoing renal or insensible losses when oral intake is inadequate, and the need for glucose as a fuel for the brain.[12] Although large volumes of fluid are given during the resuscitation of most trauma patients, a recent analysis reported uncertainty about the use of early large volume fluid replacement in patients with active bleeding, calling into question our understanding of the need for fluids in various patient populations.[13]

When determining the appropriate fluid to be utilized, it is important to first determine the type of fluid problem (TBW versus ECF depletion), and start therapy accordingly. For patients demonstrating signs of impaired tissue perfusion, the immediate therapeutic goal is to increase the intravascular volume and restore tissue perfusion. The standard therapy is normal saline given at 150 to 500 mL/h (for adult patients) until perfusion is optimized. Although LR is a therapeutic alternative, lactic acidosis may arise with massive or prolonged infusions. In severe cases, a colloid or blood transfusion may be indicated to increase oncotic pressure within the vascular space. Once isovolemia is achieved, patients may be switched to a more hypotonic maintenance solution (0.45% NaCl) at a rate that delivers estimated daily needs.

The clinical scenario and the severity of the volume abnormality dictate monitoring parameters during fluid replacement therapy. These may include the subjective sense of thirst, mental status, skin turgor, orthostatic vital signs, pulse rate, weight changes, blood chemistries, fluid input and output, central venous pressure, pulmonary capillary wedge pressure, and cardiac output. Fluid replacement requires particular caution in patient populations at risk of fluid overload, such as those with renal failure, cardiac failure, hepatic failure, or the elderly. Other complications of parenteral fluid therapy include IV site infiltration, infection, phlebitis, thrombophlebitis, and extravasation.

In summary, common settings for fluid resuscitation include hypovolemic patients (e.g., sepsis or pneumonia), hypervolemic patients (e.g., congestive heart failure [CHF], cirrhosis, or renal failure), euvolemic patients who are unable to take oral fluids in proportion to insensible losses (e.g., the perioperative period), and patients with electrolyte abnormalities (see below).

ELECTROLYTES

Normally, the number of anions (negatively charged ions) and cations (positively charged ions) in each fluid compartment are equal. Cell membranes play the critical role of maintaining distinct ICF and ECF spaces, which are biochemically distinct. Serum electrolyte measurements reflect the stores of ECF electrolytes rather than that of ICF electrolytes. Table 27–4 lists the chief cations and anions along with their normal concentrations in the ECF and ICF. The principal cations are sodium, potassium, calcium, and magnesium, while the key anions are chloride, bicarbonate, and phosphate. In the ECF, sodium is the most common cation and chloride is the most abundant anion, while in the ICF, potassium is the primary cation and phosphate is the main anion. Normal serum electrolyte values are listed in Table 27–5.

Osmolality is a measure of the number of osmotically active particles per unit of solution, independent of the weight or nature of the particle. Equimolar concentrations of all substances in the undissociated state exert the same osmotic pressure. Although the normal serum osmolality is 280 to 300 mOsm/kg (280–300 mmol/kg), multiple scenarios

Table 27–4

Normal Cation and Anion Concentrations in the ECF and ICF

Ion Species	ECF Plasma (mEq/L or mmol/L)	Interstitial Fluid (mEq/L or mmol/L)	Ion Species	ICF mEq/L or mmol/L
Cations			Cations	
Na$^+$	142	144	K$^+$	135
K$^+$	4	4	Mg^{2+}	43
Ca^{2+}	5	2.5		
Mg^{2+}	3	1.5		
Total	154	152	Total	178
Anions			Anions	
Cl$^-$	103	114	PO$_4^{2-}$	90
HCO$_3^-$	27	30	Protein	70
PO$_4^{2-}$	2	2	SO$_4^{2-}$	18
SO$_4^{2-}$	1	1		
Organic acid	5	5		
Protein	16	0		
Total	154	152	Total	178

ECF, extracellular fluid; ICF, intracellular fluid.

Table 27–5

Normal Ranges for Serum Electrolyte Concentrations

Sodium	136–145 mEq/L or 136–145 mmol/L
Potassium	3.5–5.0 mEq/L or 3.5–5.0 mmol/L
Chloride	98–106 mEq/L or 98–106 mmol/L
Bicarbonate	21–30 mEq/L or 21–30 mmol/L
Magnesium	1.4–2.2 mEq/L or 0.7–1.1 mmol/L
Calcium:	
Total	4.4–5.2 mEq/L (9–10.5 mg/dL) or 2.25–2.5 mmol/L
Ionized	2.2–2.8 mEq/L (4.5–5.6 mg/dL) or 1.1–1.4 mmol/L
Phosphorus	3–4.5 mg/dL (1.0–1.4 mmol/L)

exist where this value becomes markedly abnormal. ❸ *The calculated serum osmolality helps determine deviations in TBW content.* As such, it is often useful to calculate the serum osmolality as follows:

Serum osmolality (mOsm/L) =
    2 (Na mEq/L) + (glucose [mg/dL])/18
    + (BUN [mg/dL])/2.8.

Note: For glucose, multiply by a factor of 0.055 to convert conventional glucose units (mg/dL) to SI glucose units (mmol/L). To convert SI units of glucose (mmol/L) to conventional glucose units (mg/dL), multiply SI units by a factor of 18.18. For blood urea nitrogen (BUN), multiply by a factor of 0.357 to convert conventional BUN units (mg/dL) to SI BUN units (mmol/L). To convert SI units of BUN (mmol/L) to conventional BUN units (mg/dL), multiply SI units by a factor of 2.8.

Because the body regulates water to maintain osmolality, deviations in serum osmolality are used to estimate TBW stores. Water moves freely across all cell membranes, making serum osmolality an accurate reflection of the osmolality

Patient Encounter 3: Calculate the Plasma Osmolality

A 50-year-old homeless man is brought to the emergency department staggering and smelling like beer. Rapid respiration, tachycardia, and a BP of 90/60 mm Hg were noted. The sodium is 142 mEq/L (142 mmol/L), potassium 3.6 mEq/L (3.6 mmol/L), chloride 100 mEq/L (100 mmol/L), bicarbonate 12 mEq/L (12 mmol/L), glucose 180 mg/dL (9.99 mmol/L), and BUN 28 mg/dL (9.99 mol/L). The measured osmolarity is 360 mOsm/L.

Calculate the osmolality.

Calculate the osmolar gap.

What is the likely cause of an increased gap in this patient?

within all body compartments. An increase in osmolality is equated with a loss of water greater than the loss of solute (TBW depletion). A decrease in serum osmolality is seen when water is retained in excess of solute (CHF or hepatic cirrhosis). The difference between the measured serum osmolality and the calculated serum osmolality, using the equation above, is referred to as the osmolar gap. Under normal circumstances the osmolar gap should be 10 mOsm/L or less. An increased osmolar gap suggests the presence of a small, osmotically active agent and is most commonly seen with the ingestion of alcohols (ethanol, methanol, ethylene glycol, or isopropyl alcohol) or medications such as mannitol or lorazepam. Patient Encounter 3 illustrates the utility of serum osmolality in a clinical setting.

Many of the electrolyte disturbances discussed in the remainder of this chapter represent medical emergencies that call for aggressive interventions including the use of concentrated electrolytes. However, these solutions are a frequent source of medical errors with significant potential for patient harm. ❹ *As such, the 2005 National Patient Safety Goals published by the Joint Commission on Accreditation of Healthcare Organizations (JCAHO) recommends that concentrated electrolyte solutions (KCl, potassium phosphate, and NaCl greater than 0.9%) be removed from patient care areas.* In addition, JCAHO recommends standardizing and limiting the number of drug concentrations available in each institution so as to further reduce the risk of medication errors and improve outcomes.[14]

Sodium

The body's normal daily sodium requirement is 1.0 to 1.5 mEq/kg (80–130 mEq, which is 80–130 mmol) to maintain a normal serum sodium concentration of 136 to 145 mEq/L (136–145 mmol/L).[15] Sodium is the predominant cation of the ECF and largely determines ECF volume. Sodium is also the primary factor in establishing the osmotic pressure relationship between the ICF and ECF. All body fluids are in osmotic equilibrium and changes in serum sodium concentration are associated with shifts of water into and out of body fluid

compartments. When sodium is added to the intravascular fluid compartment, fluid is pulled intravascularly from the interstitial fluid and the ICF until osmotic balance is restored. As such, a patient's measured sodium concentration should *not* be viewed as an index of sodium need because this parameter reflects the balance between total body sodium content and TBW. Disturbances in the sodium concentration most often represent disturbances of TBW. Sodium imbalances cannot be properly assessed without first assessing the body fluid status.

❺ *Hyponatremia is very common in hospitalized patients and is defined as a serum sodium concentration below 136 mEq/L (136 mmol/L).* Clinical signs and symptoms appear at concentrations below 120 mEq/L (120 mmol/L) and typically consist of agitation, fatigue, headache, muscle cramps, and nausea. With profound hyponatremia (less than 110 mEq/L [110 mmol/L]), confusion, seizures, and coma may be seen. Because therapy is also influenced by volume status, hyponatremia is further defined as: (a) hypertonic hyponatremia; (b) hypotonic hyponatremia with an increased ECF volume; (c) hypotonic hyponatremia with a normal ECF volume; and (d) hypotonic hyponatremia with a decreased ECF volume.[16]

Hypertonic hyponatremia is usually associated with significant hyperglycemia. Glucose is an osmotically active agent that leads to an increase in TBW with little change in total body sodium. For every 60 mg/dL (3.33 mmol/L) increase in serum glucose above 200 mg/dL (11.1 mmol/L), the sodium concentration is expected to decrease by approximately 1 mEq/L (1 mmol/L). Appropriate treatment of the hyperglycemia will return the serum sodium concentration to normal.[15]

Hypotonic hyponatremia with an increase in ECF (hypervolemic hyponatremia) is also known as dilutional hyponatremia. In this scenario, patients have an excess of total body sodium and TBW; however, the excess in TBW is greater than the excess in total body sodium. Common causes include CHF, hepatic cirrhosis, and nephrotic syndrome. Treatment includes sodium and fluid restriction in conjunction with treatment of the underlying disorder—for example, salt and water restrictions are used in the setting of CHF along with loop diuretics, angiotensin-converting enzyme inhibitors, and spironolactone.[15]

In hypotonic hyponatremia with a normal ECF volume (euvolemic hyponatremia), patients have an excess of TBW with relatively normal sodium content. In essence, there is a presence of excess free water. This is most frequently seen in patients with the syndrome of inappropriate antidiuretic hormone secretion (SIADH). Common causes of SIADH include carcinomas (e.g., lung or pancreas), pulmonary disorders (e.g., pneumonias or tuberculosis), CNS disorders (e.g., meningitis, stroke, tumor, or trauma), and medications (e.g., sulfonylureas, antineoplastic agents, barbiturates, morphine, antipsychotics, tricyclics, nonsteroidal anti-inflammatory agents, selective serotonin reuptake inhibitors, dopamine agonists, and general anesthetics). These medications stimulate the release of antidiuretic hormone (ADH) from the pituitary gland resulting in water retention and dilution of the body's sodium stores. Treatment generally consists of fluid restriction alone. Hypertonic saline is used only when the sodium concentration is less than 110 mEq/L (110 mmol/L) and/or severe symptoms (e.g., seizures) are present. Refractory SIADH may respond to demeclocycline (Declomycin, ESP Pharma) dosed at 900 to 1,200 mg/day, lithium (various generics), furosemide (various generics), or urea. Given the limitations associated with these treatment strategies (unpredictable therapeutic effects and side effects), the arginine vasopressin antagonist conivaptan (Vaprisol, Astellas) was developed for short-term treatment of euvolemic hyponatremia. While conivaptan can also be used to manage hypervolemic hyponatremia in hospitalized patients, it should not be used for hypovolemic hyponatremia. Conivaptan is dosed 20 mg IV over 30 minutes, followed by a 20 mg continuous infusion over 24 hours for up to 4 days.

In hypotonic hyponatremia with a decreased ECF volume (hypovolemic hyponatremia), patients usually have a deficit of both total body sodium and TBW, but the sodium deficit exceeds the TBW deficit. Common causes include diuretic use, profuse sweating, wound drainage, burns, GI losses (vomiting or diarrhea), hypoadrenalism (low cortisol and low aldosterone), and renal tubular acidosis. Treatment includes the administration of sodium to correct the sodium deficit and water to correct the TBW deficit. The sodium deficit can be calculated with the following equation[2]:

Sodium deficit (mEq) =
(TBW [in liters]) (desired Na+ concentration [mEq/L or mmol/L] − current Na+ concentration).

Although both water and sodium are required in this instance, sodium needs to be provided in excess of water to fully correct this abnormality. As such, hypertonic saline (3% NaCl) is often used. One can estimate the change in serum sodium concentration after 1 L of 3% NaCl infusion using the following equation[16]:

Change in serum Na+ (mEq/L or mmol/L) =
(infusate Na+ − serum Na+)/(TBW + 1).

In this formula, TBW is increased by 1 to account for the addition of the liter of 3% NaCl. Patient Encounters 4 and 5 illustrate the concepts of calculating and correcting the sodium deficit.

Depending on the severity of the hyponatremia and acuity of onset, 0.9%, 3%, or 5% NaCl can be utilized. Most patients can be adequately managed with normal saline rehydration, which is generally the safest agent. Hypertonic saline (3% or 5% NaCl) is generally reserved for patients with severe hyponatremia (less than 120 mEq/L [120 mmol/L]) accompanied by coma, seizures, or high urinary sodium

Patient Encounter 4: Calculation of Sodium Deficit

Calculate the sodium deficit for a 75-kg male with a serum sodium of 123 mEq/L (123 mmol/L).

Patient Encounter 5: Estimate the Anticipated Change in Serum Sodium

Estimate the anticipated change in serum sodium concentration after the infusion of 1 L of 3% NaCl in a 75-kg male with a serum sodium of 123 mEq/L (123 mmol/L).

losses. Roughly one-third of the sodium deficit can be replaced over the first 12 hours as long as the replacement rate is less than 0.5 mEq/h (0.5 mmol/L). The remaining two-thirds of the deficit can be administered over the ensuing days. Overly aggressive correction of symptomatic hyponatremia (greater than 12 mEq/L [12 mmol/L] per day) can result in central pontine myelinolysis.[17] Given the potential for irreversible neurologic damage if untreated or if improperly treated, acute hyponatremia is an urgent condition that should be promptly treated with careful attention to monitoring serial sodium values and adjusting therapeutic infusions accordingly.[18]

Hypernatremia is a serum sodium concentration greater than 145 mEq/L (145 mmol/L) and can occur in the absence of a sodium deficit (pure water loss) or in its presence (hypotonic fluid loss).[19] The signs and symptoms of hypernatremia manifest with a serum sodium concentration of greater than 160 mEq/L (160 mmol/L) and are usually the same as those found in TBW depletion: thirst, mental slowing, and dry mucous membranes. Signs and symptoms become more profound as hypernatremia worsens, with the patient eventually demonstrating confusion, hallucinations, acute weight loss, decreased skin turgor, intracranial bleeding, and/or coma. Many coexisting disorders and medications may complicate the diagnosis.

The classic causes of hypernatremia are associated with TBW depletion. These include dehydration from loss of hypotonic fluid from the respiratory tract or skin, decreased water intake, osmotic diuresis (e.g., mannitol, available as generic), and diabetes insipidus (e.g., decreased ADH; phenytoin, available as generic; lithium, available as generic). Hypernatremia in hospitalized patients occurs secondary to inappropriate fluid management in patients at risk for increased free water losses and impaired thirst or restricted water intake.[20] Iatrogenic hypernatremia is occasionally caused by the administration of excessive hypertonic saline. Treatment of hypernatremia includes calculation of the TBW deficit followed by the administration of hypotonic fluids as previously described. The fluid volume should be replaced over 48 to 72 hours depending on the severity of symptoms and the degree of hypertonicity.[21] For asymptomatic patients, the rate of correction should not exceed 0.5 mEq/L/h (0.5 mmol/L/h). One rule of thumb is to replace half the calculated TBW deficit over 12 to 24 hours and the other half of the deficit over the next 24 to 48 hours.[2,19] Excessively rapid correction of hypernatremia may lead to cerebral edema and death. Patient Encounters 6 and 7 reinforce the concepts

Patient Encounter 6: Calculate Water Deficit

Calculate the water deficit in a 75-kg male with a serum sodium of 154 mEq/L (154 mmol/L).

Patient Encounter 7: Calculate the Anticipated Change in Serum Sodium

Calculate the anticipated change in serum sodium concentration after IV infusion of 1 L of 5% dextrose in a 75-kg male with a serum sodium of 156 mEq/L (156 mmol/L).

of calculating TBW deficit and expected changes in serum sodium concentration with therapy.

Potassium

The body's normal daily potassium requirement is 0.5 to 1 mEq/kg (0.5–1 mmol/kg) or 40 to 80 mEq (40–80 mmol) to maintain a serum potassium concentration of 3.5 to 5 mEq/L (3.5–5 mmol/L). Potassium is the most abundant cation in the ICF, balancing the sodium contained in the ECF and maintaining electroneutrality of bodily fluids. Because the majority of potassium is intracellular, serum potassium concentration is not a good measure of total body potassium; however, clinical manifestations of potassium disorders correlate well with serum potassium. The acid–base balance of the body affects serum potassium concentrations: hyperkalemia is routinely seen in patients with decreased pH (acidosis). Potassium regulation is primarily under the control of the kidneys with excess dietary potassium being excreted in the urine. Although mild abnormalities of serum potassium are considered a nuisance, severe hyperkalemia or hypokalemia can be life-threatening.[22,23,32]

Hypokalemia (serum potassium less than 3.5 mEq/L [3.5 mmol/L]) is a common clinical problem. While generally asymptomatic, signs and symptoms of hypokalemia include cramps, muscle weakness, polyuria, electrocardiogram (ECG) changes (flattened T-waves and presence of U-waves), and cardiac arrhythmias (bradycardia, heart block, atrial flutter, premature ventricular contractions, and ventricular fibrillation). Causes of hypokalemia include GI losses (vomiting, diarrhea, or NG tube suction), renal losses (high aldosterone and low magnesium), inadequate potassium intake (in IV fluids or oral), or alkalosis. Many medications can precipitate hypokalemia. β_2-agonists (e.g., albuterol, available as generic) and insulin (multiple product formulations) lower potassium via cellular redistribution. The use of loop diuretics (furosemide [Lasix], also available as generic), thiazide diuretics (hydrochlorothiazide, available

as generic), high-dose antibiotics (penicillin, available as generic), and corticosteroids (prednisone, available as generic) cause renal potassium wasting. In addition, amphotericin B (available as generic), cisplatin (available as generic), and foscarnet (Foscavir, AstraZeneca) can also produce hypokalemia secondary to depletion of magnesium. Hypomagnesemia diminishes intracellular potassium concentration and produces potassium wasting. Given the potential for significant morbidity and mortality, serum potassium concentrations should be monitored closely for patients with known (or suspected) hypokalemia.[2,24,32] Hypokalemia is a risk factor for digitalis toxicity.

Each 1 mEq/L (1 mmol/L) fall in serum potassium (i.e., from 4 to 3 mEq/L [4 to 3 mmol/L]) represents a loss of approximately 200 mEq (200 mmol) of potassium in the adult. However, when the serum potassium is below 3 mEq/L (3 mmol/L), each 1 mEq/L fall in serum potassium represents a 200 to 400 mEq (200–400 mmol) reduction in serum concentration in the adult patient. Potassium repletion should be guided by close monitoring of serial serum concentrations instead of using empirically chosen amounts. Of the five potassium salts available, potassium acetate (10.2 mEq/K⁺/g or 10.2 mmol/K⁺/g) and KCl (13.4 mEq/K⁺/g or 13.4 mmol/K⁺/g) are the most commonly used forms. When hypokalemia occurs in the setting of alkalosis, KCl is the preferred agent; in acidosis, potassium should be provided in the form of acetate, citrate, bicarbonate, or gluconate salt. Table 27–6 outlines the potassium content of each potassium salt preparation, and Table 27–7 lists each of the oral potassium replacement products. Potassium acetate and chloride are available for IV infusions as premixed solutions. The usual dose of these agents is 10 to 20 mEq (10–20 mmol) diluted in 1,000 mL of normal saline.[2,24,25]

Moderate hypokalemia is defined as a serum potassium of 2.5 to 3.5 mEq/L (2.5–3.5 mmol/L) without ECG changes. In this setting, potassium replacement can usually be given orally at a dose of 40 to 120 mEq/day (40–120 mmol/day). Anecdotally, oral potassium supplementation (see Table 27–7) is often more effective in repleting moderate hypokalemia. For patients with an ongoing source of potassium loss, chronic replacement therapy should be considered. The potassium deficit is a rough approximation of the amount

Table 27–6

Potassium Content in Various Potassium Salt Preparations

Potassium Salt	mEq/g (mmol/L)
Potassium gluconate[a]	4.3
Potassium citrate[a]	9.8
Potassium bicarbonate[a]	10.0
Potassium acetate[a]	10.2
Potassium chloride[b]	13.4

[a]Favored for hypokalemia and concurrent acidosis.

[b]Favored for hypokalemia and concurrent alkalosis.

of potassium needed to be replaced and can be estimated as follows:

$$\text{Potassium deficit (mEq)} =$$
$$(4.0 - \text{current serum potassium}) \times 100$$

Severe hypokalemia is defined as a serum potassium less than 2.5 mEq/L (2.5 mmol/L) or hypokalemia of any magnitude that is associated with ECG changes (e.g., flattening of T-wave or elevation of U-wave) and cardiac arrhythmias. In these situations, IV replacement should be initiated urgently. ❻ *Potassium infusion at rates exceeding 10 mEq/h requires cardiac monitoring given the potential for cardiac arrhythmias.* Although the maximally concentrated solution for potassium replacement is 80 mEq/L (80 mmol/L), the maximum infusion rate is 40 mEq/h (40 mmol/h), and must be administered via a central line. Table 27–8 outlines current IV potassium replacement guidelines.

Caution must be exercised when repleting potassium with IV agents given possible vein irritation and/or thrombophlebitis. The risk of these complications is minimized by using less concentrated solutions and by giving infusions via central access if possible. Administration of potassium in vehicles containing glucose is discouraged, as glucose facilitates the intracellular movement of potassium. Post-therapy improvements in serum potassium may be transient and continuous monitoring is required. Patients with a low serum magnesium will have exaggerated potassium losses from the kidneys and GI tract leading to refractory hypokalemia.

In this situation, the magnesium deficit must be corrected in order to successfully treat the concurrent potassium deficiency. In the hypokalemic patient with concurrent acidosis, potassium is often given as the acetate salt, given that acetate is metabolized to bicarbonate. In the patient with depleted phosphorus and potassium, therapy with potassium phosphate is the natural choice.[22,26,27]

Hyperkalemia is defined as a serum potassium concentration greater than 5 mEq/L (5 mmol/L). Manifestations of hyperkalemia include muscle weakness, paresthesias, hypotension, ECG changes (e.g., peaked T-waves, shortened QT intervals, and wide QRS complexes), cardiac arrhythmias, and a decreased pH. Causes of hyperkalemia fall into three broad categories: (a) increased potassium intake, (b) decreased potassium excretion, and (c) potassium release from the intracellular space.

Increased potassium intake results from excessive dietary potassium (salt substitutes), excess potassium in IV fluids, and other select medications (potassium-sparing diuretics, cyclosporine [available as generic], angiotensin-converting enzyme inhibitors, nonsteroidal anti-inflammatory agents, pentamidine [available as generic], unfractionated heparin, and low-molecular-weight heparins). Decreased potassium excretion results from acute renal failure, chronic renal failure, or Addison's disease. Excess potassium release from cells results from tissue breakdown (surgery, trauma, hemolysis, or rhabdomyolysis), blood transfusions, and metabolic acidosis.

In addition to discontinuing all potassium supplements, potassium-sparing medications, and potassium-rich salt substitutes, management of hyperkalemia addresses three concurrent strategies: (a) agents to antagonize the proarrhythmic effects of hyperkalemia; (b) agents to drive potassium into the intracellular space and acutely lower the serum potassium; and (c) agents that will definitively (but more gradually) lower the total body potassium content.[28] If the serum potassium concentration is greater than 7 mEq/L (7 mmol/L) and/or ECG changes are present, IV calcium is provided to stabilize the myocardium. Depending on the acuity of the situation, 1 g of calcium chloride (13.5 mEq or 6.75 mmol) is administered by direct injection or diluted in 50 mL of D_5W and delivered IV over 15 minutes. Clinical effects are seen within 1 to 2 minutes of infusion and persist for 10 to 30 minutes. Repeat doses may be administered as necessary. Because most patients with clinically significant hyperkalemia receive multiple boluses of calcium directed by ECG findings, iatrogenic hypercalcemia is a potential

Table 27–7

Oral Potassium Replacement Products

Product	Salt	Strength[a]
Extended/controlled release tablets	Chloride	8 mEq (600 mg)
		10 mEq (750 mg)
		15 mEq (1,125 mg)
		20 mEq (1,500 mg)
Effervescent tablets	Chloride and bicarbonate	20 mEq
		25 mEq
		50 mEq
Liquid	Chloride	20 mEq/15 mL (10%)
		30 mEq/15 mL (15%)
		40 mEq/15 mL (20%)
Powder packets	Chloride	15 mEq
		20 mEq
		25 mEq

[a]For potassium, 1 mEq = 1 mmol.

Table 27–8

Recommended Potassium Dosage/Infusion Rate

Clinical Scenario	Maximum Infusion Rate[a]	Maximum Concentration[a]	Maximum 24-Hour Dose[a]
K+ greater than 2.5 mEq/L AND No ECG changes of hypokalemia	10 mEq/h	40 mEq/L	200 mEq
K+ less than 2.5 mEq/L OR ECG changes of hypokalemia	40 mEq/h	80 mEq/L	400 mEq

[a]For potassium, 1 mEq = 1 mmol.

complication of hyperkalemia treatment. As such, total calcium concentration is commonly checked with each potassium concentration measurement. Ionized calcium measurements should be obtained in patients who have comorbid conditions that would lead to inconsistency between total serum calcium and free calcium (abnormal albumin, protein, or immunoglobulin concentrations).

Dextrose and insulin (with or without sodium bicarbonate) are typically given at the time of calcium therapy in order to redistribute potassium into the intracellular space. Dextrose 50% (25 g in 50 mL) can be given by slow IV push over 5 minutes or dextrose 10% with 20 units of regular insulin can be given by continuous IV infusion over 1 to 2 hours. The onset of action for this combination is 30 minutes and the duration of clinical effects is 2 to 6 hours. High-dose inhaled β_2-agonists (e.g., albuterol, available as generic) may also be used to acutely drive potassium into the intracellular space.

It is critically important to recognize that the treatments of hyperkalemia discussed thus far are transient, temporizing measures. They are intended to provide time to institute definitive therapy aimed at removing excess potassium from the body. Agents that increase potassium excretion from the body include sodium polystyrene sulfonate, loop diuretics, and hemodialysis or hemofiltration (used only in patients with renal failure). Sodium polystyrene sulfonate (Kayexalate, various manufacturers) can be given orally, via NG tube, or as a rectal retention enema and is dosed at 15 to 60 g in four divided doses per day.

Calcium

More than 99% of total body calcium is found in bone; the remaining less than 1% is in the ECF and ICF. calcium plays a critical role in the transmission of nerve impulses, skeletal muscle contraction, myocardial contractions, maintenance of normal cellular permeability, and the formation of bones and teeth. There is a reciprocal relationship between the serum calcium concentration (normally 8.6–10.2 mg/dL [2.15–2.55 mmol/L]) and the serum phosphate concentration that is regulated by a complex interaction between parathyroid hormone, vitamin D, and calcitonin. About one-half of the serum calcium is bound to plasma proteins; the other half is free ionized calcium. Given that the serum calcium has significant protein binding, the serum calcium measurement must be corrected in patients who have low albumin concentrations (the major serum protein). The most commonly used formula adds 0.8 mg/dL (0.2 mmol/L) of calcium for each gram of albumin deficiency as follows:

Corrected [Ca] =
    Measured [Ca mg/dL]
    + [0.8 × (4 − measured albumin g/dL)][29–31]

Note: To convert conventional units (mg/dL) to SI calcium units multiply by a factor of 0.25. To convert SI calcium units to conventional calcium units multiply by a factor of 4. To convert conventional albumin units (g/dL) to SI albumin units (g/dL) multiple by a factor of 10. To convert SI albumin units (g/dL) to conventional albumin units (g/dL) divide by a factor of 2.

Hypocalcemia is caused by inadequate intake (vitamin deficiency, poor dietary calcium sources, alcoholism) or excessive losses (hypoparathyroidism, renal failure, alkalosis, pancreatitis). Clinical manifestations of hypocalcemia are seen with total serum concentrations less than 6.5 mg/dL (1.63 mmol/L) or an ionized calcium of less than 1.12 mmol/L and include tetany, circumoral tingling, muscle spasms, hypoactive reflexes, anxiety, hallucinations, hypotension, myocardial infarction, seizures, lethargy, stupor, and Trousseau's sign or Chvostek's sign.[32,37] Trousseau's sign is elicited by inflating a BP cuff on the patient's upper arm, whereby hypocalcemic patients will experience tetany of the wrist and hand as evidenced by thumb adduction, wrist flexion, and metacarpophalangeal joint flexion. Chvostek's sign is elicited by tapping on the proximal distribution of the facial nerve (adjacent to the ear). This will produce a brief spasm of the upper lip, eye, nose, or face in hypocalcemic patients. Ionized calcium concentrations are typically used to assess calcium status in the critically ill patient.

Causes of hypocalcemia include hypoparathyroidism, hypomagnesemia, alcoholism, hyperphosphatemia, blood product infusion (due to chelation by the citrate buffers), chronic renal failure, vitamin D deficiency, acute pancreatitis, alkalosis, and hypoalbuminemia. In the setting of hypocalcemia, magnesium concentration should be checked and corrected if low. Given that hypocalcemia may be caused by hypomagnesemia, clinicians should be aware that the serum calcium concentrations may not normalize until serum magnesium is replaced. Medications that cause hypocalcemia include phosphate replacement products, loop diuretics, phenytoin (Dilantin, available as generic), phenobarbital (available as generic), corticosteroids, aminoglycoside antibiotics, and acetazolamide (available as generic).[34,39,42]

Oral calcium replacement products include calcium carbonate (OsCal, GlaxoSmithKline and various generics; Tums, GlaxoSmithKline and various generics) and calcium citrate (Citrical, Mission Pharmacal, and various generics). IV calcium replacement products include calcium gluconate and calcium chloride (both products available as generic). ❼ *Calcium gluconate is preferred for peripheral use because it is less irritating to the veins; it may also be given intramuscularly.* Each 10 mL of a 10% calcium gluconate solution provides 90 mg (4.5 mEq or 2.25 mmol) of elemental calcium. Calcium chloride is associated with more venous irritation and extravasation and is generally reserved for administration via central line. Each 10 mL of a 10% calcium chloride solution contains 270 mg (13.5 mEq or 6.75 mmol) of elemental calcium. IV calcium products are given as a slow push or added to 500 to 1,000 mL of 0.9% normal saline for slow infusion.[37,42] In addition to hypocalcemia, IV calcium may also be used for massive blood transfusions, calcium channel blocker overdose, and emergent hyperkalemia and hypermagnesemia.

For acute symptomatic hypocalcemia, 200 to 300 mg of elemental calcium is administered IV and repeated until symptoms are fully controlled. This is achieved by infusing 1 g of calcium chloride or 2 to 3 g of calcium gluconate at a rate no faster than 30 to 60 mg of elemental calcium per minute. More rapid administration is associated with hypotension, bradycardia, or cardiac asystole. Total calcium concentration is commonly monitored in critically ill patients. Under normal circumstances, about half of calcium is loosely bound to serum proteins while the other half is free. Total calcium concentration measures bound and free calcium. Ionized calcium measures free calcium only. Under usual circumstances, a normal calcium concentration implies a normal free ionized calcium concentration. Ionized calcium should be obtained in patients with comorbid conditions that would lead to inconsistency between total calcium and free serum calcium (abnormal albumin, protein, or immunoglobulin concentrations). For chronic asymptomatic hypocalcemia, oral calcium supplements are given at doses of 2 to 4 g/day of elemental calcium. Many patients with calcium deficiency have concurrent vitamin D deficiency that must also be corrected in order to restore calcium homeostasis.[2,37,38]

Hypercalcemia is defined as a calcium concentration greater than 10.2 mg/dL (2.55 mmol/L). It may be categorized as mild if total serum calcium is 10.3 to 12 mg/dL (2.575–3 mmol/L), moderate if total serum calcium is 12.1 to 13 mg/dL (3.025–3.25 mmol/L), or severe when serum concentration is greater than 13 mg/dL (3.25 mmol/L). Causes of hyper-calcemia include hyperparathyroidism, malignancy, Paget's disease, Addison's disease, granulomatous diseases (e.g., tuberculosis, sarcoidosis, or histoplasmosis), hyperthyroidism, immobilization, multiple bony fractures, acidosis, and milk-alkali syndrome. Multiple medications cause hypercalcemia and include thiazide diuretics, estrogens, lithium (available as generic), tamoxifen (Nolvadex, available as generic), vitamin A, vitamin D, and calcium supplements.[2,33,37,42]

Because the severity of symptoms and the absolute serum concentration are poorly correlated in some patients, institution of therapy should be dictated by the clinical scenario. All patients with hypercalcemia should be treated with aggressive rehydration: normal saline at 200 to 300 mL/h is a routine initial fluid prescription. For patients with mild hypercalcemia, hydration alone may provide adequate therapy. The moderate and severe forms of hypercalcemia are more likely to have significant manifestations and require prompt initiation of additional therapy. These patients may present with anorexia, confusion, and/or cardiac manifestations (bradycardia and arrhythmias with ECG changes). Total calcium concentrations greater than 13 mg/dL (3.25 mmol/L) are particularly worrisome, as these concentrations can unexpectedly precipitate acute renal failure, ventricular arrhythmias, and sudden death.

Once fluid administration has repleted the ECF, forced diuresis (with associated calcium loss) can be initiated with a loop diuretic. For this approach to be successful, normal kidney function is required. In renal failure patients, the alternative therapy is emergent hemodialysis. Other treatment options include bisphosphonates (zoledronic acid [Zometa, Novartis], pamidronate [Aredia, available as generic]), hydrocortisone (available as generic), mithramycin (Mithracin), calcitonin, and gallium. Given their efficacy and favorable side-effect profile, bisphosphonates are typically the agents of choice. Table 27–9 outlines the treatment options for hypercalcemia including time to onset of effect, duration of effect, and efficacy.[2,34,37,38]

Phosphorus

Phosphorus is primarily found in the bone (80%–85%) and ICF (15%–20%): the remaining less than 1% is found in the ECF. Note that phosphorus is the major anion within the cells. Given this distribution, serum phosphate concentration does not accurately reflect total body phosphorus stores. Phosphorus is expressed in milligrams (mg) or millimoles (mmol), not as milliequivalents (mEq). Because phosphorus is the source of phosphate for adenosine triphosphate (ATP) and phospholipid synthesis, manifestations of phosphorus imbalance are variable.

Dietary intake, parathyroid hormone levels, and renal function are the major determinants of the serum phosphorus concentration, which is normally 2.7 to 4.5 mg/dL (0.87–1.45 mmol/L).[2,35-37] Hypophosphatemia is defined by a serum phosphorus concentration less than 2.5 mg/dL (0.81 mmol/L); severe hypophosphatemia occurs when the phosphorus concentration is less than 1 mg/dL (0.323 mmol/L). Hypophosphatemia can be caused by increased distribution to the ICF (hyperglycemia, insulin therapy, or malnourishment), decreased absorption (starvation, excessive

Table 27–9				
Selected Treatment Options for the Management of Hypercalcemia				
Therapy	**Dose**	**Onset**	**Duration**	**Efficacy**[a]
Normal saline	3–6 L/day	Hours	Hours	1–2 mg/dL
Furosemide (Lasix, available as generic)	80–160 mg/day	Hours	Hours	1–2 mg/dL
Hydrocortisone (available as generic)	200 mg/day	Hours	Days	Mild/unpredictable
Calcitonin (Miacalcin, Novartis)	4–8 units/kg	Hours	Hours	1–2 mg/dL
Mithramycin (Mithracin)	25 mcg/kg	12 hours	Days	1–5 mg/dL
Pamidronate (Aredia, available as generic)	30–90 mg/week	Days	1–4 weeks	1–5 mg/dL
Zoledronic acid (Zometa, available as generic)	4–8 mg	Days	Weeks	1–5 mg/dL
Gallium (Ganite, Genta Inc.)	200 mg/m²	Days	Days–weeks	1–5 mg/dL

[a]Expected decrease in serum Ca^{2+}.

use of phosphorus-binding antacids, vitamin D deficiency, diarrhea, or laxative abuse) or increased renal loss (diuretic use, diabetic ketoacidosis, alcohol abuse, hyperparathyroidism, or burns).[38,39] **❽** *Severe hypophosphatemia can result in impaired diaphragmatic contractility and acute respiratory failure.* Medications that cause hypophosphatemia include diuretics (acetazolamide [Diamox, available as generic], furosemide [Lasix, available as generic], hydrochlorothiazide [Hydrodiuril, available as generic]), sucralfate (Carafate, available as generic), corticosteroids, cisplatin (available as generic), antacids (aluminum carbonate, calcium carbonate, and magnesium oxide [antacids all available as generic]), foscarnet (Foscavir, Astra Zeneca), phenytoin (Dilantin, available as generic), phenobarbital (available as generic), and phosphate binders (sevelamer [Renvela, Genzyme Corp.], and calcium acetate [PhosLo, Nabi]).

Signs and symptoms of hypophosphatemia include paresthesias, muscle weakness, myalgias, bone pain, anorexia, nausea, vomiting, red blood cell breakdown (hemolysis), acute respiratory failure, seizures, and coma.[38,40] For mild hypophosphatemia, patients should be encouraged to eat a high-phosphorus diet including eggs, nuts, whole grains, meat, fish, poultry, and milk products. For moderate hypophosphatemia (1–2.5 mg/dL, 0.323–0.808 mmol/L), oral supplementation of 1.5 to 2 g/day (30–60 mmol/day) is usually adequate. Diarrhea may be a dose-limiting side effect with oral phosphate replacement products. Injectable phosphate products are reserved for patients with severe hypophosphatemia or those in the intensive care unit.[41] The available agents are provided as sodium or potassium salts; however, unless concurrent hypokalemia is present, sodium phosphate is usually used. Empirically, if the serum phosphorus is 2.3 to 2.7 mg/dL (0.74–0.87 mmol/L), the corresponding IV phosphorus dose is 0.08 to 0.16 mmol/kg; for a serum phosphorus of 1.5 to 2.2 mg/dL (0.48–0.71 mmol/L), the replacement dose is 0.16 to 0.32 mmol/kg; and the dose is 0.32 to 0.64 mmol/kg when the serum phosphorus is less than 1.5 mg/dL (0.48 mmol/L).[2] IV phosphorus preparations are usually infused over 4 to 12 hours. Table 27–10 compares the available phosphate replacement products.

Hyperphosphatemia is defined by a serum phosphorus concentration greater than 4.5 mg/dL (1.45 mmol/L). The manifestations of hyperphosphatemia are similar to findings of hypocalcemia (see above), and include paresthesias, ECG changes (prolonged QT interval and prolonged ST segment), and metastatic calcifications. Causes of hyperphosphatemia include impaired phosphorus excretion (hypoparathyroidism

or renal failure), redistribution of phosphorus to the ECF (acid–base imbalance, rhabdomyolysis, muscle necrosis, or tumor lysis during chemotherapy), and increased phosphorus intake (various medications).[38] Medications that can cause hyperphosphatemia include enemas containing phosphorus (e.g., Fleet, Fleet), laxatives containing phosphate or phosphorus, oral or parenteral phosphorus supplements (e.g., Neutra-Phos, Ortho McNeil), vitamin D supplements, and the bisphosphonates (e.g., pamidronate, various manufacturers).[42]

Hyperphosphatemia is generally benign and rarely needs aggressive therapy. Dietary restriction of phosphate and protein is effective for most minor elevations. Phosphate binders such as aluminum-based antacids, calcium carbonate, calcium acetate (PhosLo, Nabi), sevelamer (Renvela, Genzyme), and lanthanum carbonate (Fosrenol, Shire) may be necessary for some patients (typically those with chronic renal failure).[43] If patients exhibit findings of hypocalcemia (tetany), IV calcium should be administered empirically.

Magnesium

The body's normal daily magnesium requirement is 300 to 350 mg/day to maintain a serum magnesium concentration of 1.5 to 2.4 mg/dL (0.75–1.2 mmol/L). Because magnesium is the second most abundant ICF cation, serum concentrations are a relatively poor measure of total body stores. Magnesium catalyzes and/or activates more than 300 enzymes, provides neuromuscular stability, and is involved in myocardial contraction. Magnesium is generally not part of standard chemistry panels, and therefore must be ordered separately.[2,37,42,44,45]

Hypomagnesemia is defined as a serum magnesium less than 1.5 mg/dL (0.75 mmol/L), and is most frequently seen in the intensive care and postoperative settings. Hypomagnesemia results from inadequate intake (alcoholism, dietary restriction, or inadequate magnesium in total parenteral nutrition [TPN]), inadequate absorption (steatorrhea, cancer, malabsorption syndromes, or excess calcium or phosphorus in the GI tract), excessive GI loss of magnesium (diarrhea, laxative abuse, NG tube suctioning, or acute pancreatitis), or excessive urinary loss of magnesium (primary hyperaldosteronism, certain medications, diabetic ketoacidosis, and renal disorders). Hypomagnesemia often occurs in the setting of hypokalemia and hypocalcemia. Clinicians should evaluate the magnesium concentration in these patients and correct if low. In order for calcium and potassium concentrations to normalize, magnesium supplementation is often required. Medications that potentially

Table 27–10					
Phosphate Replacement Products					
Product	**Route**	**mg PO_4^-**	**mmol PO_4^-**	**mEq (mmol) Na^+**	**mEq (mmol) K^+**
Potassium phosphate (KPO_4/mL), available as generic	IV	94	3	0	4.4
Sodium phosphate ($NaPO_4$/mL), available as generic	IV	94	3	4	0
K-Phos, Beach	po	125	4	2.9	1.4
K-Phos Neutral Tablets, Beach	po	250	8	13.1	1.4

can cause hypomagnesemia include aminoglycoside antibiotics, amphotericin B (available as generic), cisplatin (available as generic), insulin, cyclosporine (available as generic), loop diuretics, and thiazide diuretics. There is also a strong correlation between hypokalemia and hypomagnesemia.[38,42,46]

The findings of hypomagnesemia include muscle weakness, cramps, agitation, confusion, tremor, seizures, ECG changes (increased PR interval, prolonged QRS complex, and increased QT interval), findings of hypocalcemia (see above), refractory hypokalemia (see above), metabolic alkalosis, and digoxin toxicity.[42,47,48]

Asymptomatic mild magnesium deficiencies (1.0–1.5 mg/dL) (0.5–0.75 mmol/L) can be managed with increased oral intake of magnesium-containing foods or with oral supplementation. Magnesium oxide (MagOx, Blaine Pharmaceuticals and various manufacturers) 400 mg tablets contain 241 mg (20 mEq or 10 mmol) of magnesium. Diarrhea is often a dose-limiting side effect of oral supplementation. Severely deficient patients (less than 1.0 mg/dL) (0.5 mmol/L) and all deficient critically ill patients should be managed with IV magnesium sulfate. Ten milliliters of a 10% magnesium sulfate solution contains 1 g of magnesium, which is equivalent to 98 mg (8.12 mEq or 4.06 mmol) of elemental magnesium. IV magnesium supplementation may also be used in the setting of status asthmaticus, premature labor, and torsades de pointes. Magnesium concentrations need to be monitored closely in these patients. **❾** *Because magnesium concentration does not correlate well with total body magnesium stores, magnesium is often administered empirically to critically ill patients.*[2,37]

The most common causes of hypermagnesemia are renal failure, often in conjunction with magnesium-containing medications (cathartics, antacids, or magnesium supplements), and lithium therapy (available as generic). Hypermagnesemia is defined as a serum magnesium concentration greater than 2.4 mg/dL (1.2 mmol/L). Mild hypermagnesemia is present if the serum magnesium concentration is between 2.5 and 4 mg/dL (1.25–2 mmol/L) and manifests as nausea, vomiting, cutaneous vasodilation, and bradycardia. Moderate hypermagnesemia is present if the serum magnesium concentration is between 4 and 12 mg/dL (2–6 mmol/L) and may manifest with hyporeflexia, weakness, somnolence, hypotension, and ECG changes (increased QRS interval). Severe hypermagnesemia is present if the serum magnesium concentration is greater than 13 mg/dL (6.5 mmol/L) and can manifest as muscle paralysis, complete heart block, asystole, respiratory failure, refractory hypotension, and death.[2,49]

All patients with hypermagnesemia should have all magnesium supplements or magnesium-containing medications discontinued.[2,37] Iatrogenic hypermagnesemia has been observed after IV magnesium therapy for refractory asthma or pre-eclampsia. Mild hypermagnesemia and moderate hypermagnesemia without cardiac findings can be treated with normal saline infusion and furosemide therapy (assuming the patient has normal renal function). Moderate hypermagnesemia with cardiac irritability and severe hypermagnesemia require concurrent IV calcium gluconate to reverse the neuromuscular and cardiovascular effects. Calcium gluconate given at typical doses of 1 to 2 g IV will have transient effects and can be repeated as clinically indicated. Hemodialysis may be necessary for those with severely compromised renal function.

CONCLUSION

Because disturbances in fluid balance are routinely encountered in clinical medicine, it is essential to have a thorough understanding of body fluid compartments and the therapeutic use of fluids. Similarly, disturbances in serum sodium, potassium, calcium, phosphorus, and

---

Patient Encounter 8: Putting It All Together

TO, a 77-year-old male nursing home resident is admitted to the hospital with a 3-day history of altered mental status. The patient was unable to give a history or review of systems. On physical examination, the vital signs revealed a BP of 100/60 mm Hg, pulse 110 beats per minute, respirations 14 per minute, and a temperature of 38.3°C (101°F). Rales and dullness to percussion were noted at the posterior right base. The cardiac exam was significant for tachycardia. No edema was present. Laboratory studies included sodium 160 mEq/L (160 mmol/L), potassium 4.6 mEq/L (4.6 mmol/L), chloride 120 mEq/L (120 mmol/L), bicarbonate 30 mEq/L (30 mmol/L), glucose 104 mg/dL (5.77 mmol/L), BUN 34 mg/dL (12.14 mmol/L), and creatinine 2.2 mg/dL (194.5 μmol/L). The CBC was within normal limits. Chest x-ray indicated a right lower lobe pneumonia.

The patient is 5 ft 10 in. (152.4 cm) tall and currently weighs 72.6 kg (160 lb). His normal weight is 77.1 kg (170 lb).

What are the likely causes for the increased sodium concentration in this patient?

Calculate the TBW, ICF, and ECF for this patient.

Calculate TO's fluid deficit if one is present.

In the next 24 hours, the medical team wants to replace 50% of the fluid deficit plus an extra 240 mL to account for increased insensible losses in addition to the patient's maintenance needs. Using the equation (1,500 mL + 20 mL for each kilogram greater than 20 kg), calculate the rate of fluid administration for the total fluids needed in this 24-hour period and over the next 48 hours.

Calculate TO's daily maintenance fluids.

Calculate TO's fluid administration rate for the first 24 hours (Hospital day 1).

Calculate TO's fluids for the subsequent 48 hours (hospital days 2 and 3) if the goal is to replete the remaining fluid deficit during that time.

What type of fluid should be used to treat TO's fluid disorder?

magnesium are ubiquitous and must be mastered by all clinicians. Dysregulation of fluid and/or electrolyte status has serious implications regarding the concepts of drug absorption, volumes of distribution, and toxicity. Similarly, many medications can disrupt fluid and/or electrolyte balance as an unintended consequence.

Abbreviations Introduced in This Chapter

ADH	Antidiuretic hormone
ASHP	American Society of Health-System Pharmacists
ATP	Adenosine triphosphate
BUN	Blood urea nitrogen
CaCl	Calcium chloride
CHF	Congestive heart failure
Cl	Chloride
D_5W	Dextrose 5% water
ECF	Extracellular fluid
FFP	Fresh-frozen plasma
I&Os	Ins and outs
IBW	Ideal body weight
ICF	Intracellular fluid
IVIG	Intravenous immune globulin
JCAHO	Joint Commission on Accreditation of Healthcare Organizations
KPO_4	Potassium phosphate
KVO	Keep the vein open
LR	Lactated Ringer's (solution)
NaCl	Sodium chloride
$NaPO_4$	Sodium phosphate
NG	Nasogastric
NS	Normal saline
SAFE	Saline versus Albumin Fluid Evaluation
SIADH	Syndrome of inappropriate antidiuretic hormone secretion
TBW	Total body water
TPN	Total parenteral nutrition

 Self-assessment questions and answers are available at *http://www.mhpharmacotherapy.com/pp.html*.

REFERENCES

1. Faber MD, Kupin WL, Heilig CW, Narins RG. Common fluid–electrolyte and acid–base problems in the intensive care unit: Selected issues. Semin Nephrol 1994;14:8–22.
2. Kraft MD, Btaiche IF, Sacks GS, Kudsk KA. Treatment of electrolyte disorders in adult patients in the intensive care unit. Am J Health Syst Pharm 2005;62:1663–1682.
3. Faubel S, Topf J. The Fluid Electrolyte and Acid–Base Companion. San Diego, CA: Alert and Oriented publishing, 1999.
4. Chenevey B. Overview of fluids and electrolytes. Nurs Clin North Am 1987;22:749–759.
5. Devine BJ. Gentamicin therapy. Drug Intell Clin Pharm 1974;7:650–655.
6. Rose BD, Post TW. Clinical Physiology of Acid–Base and Electrolyte Disorders. New York: McGraw Hill, 2001.
7. The SAFE Study Investigators. A comparison of albumin and saline for fluid resuscitation in the intensive care unit. N Engl J Med 2004;350:2247–2256.
8. The Albumin Reviewers (Alderson P, Bunn F, Lefebvre C, Li Wan Po A, Li L, Roberts I, Schlerhout G). Human albumin solution for resuscitation and volume expansion in critically ill patients. The Cochrane Database of Systematic Reviews 2004, Issue 4. Art. No.: CD001208.pub2. DOI: 10.1002/14651858.CD001208.pub2.
9. Vincent JL, Gerlach H. Fluid resuscitation in severe sepsis and septic shock: An evidence based review. Crit Care Med 2004;32(Suppl):S451–S454.
10. Weil MH, Tang W. Albumin versus crystalloid solutions for the critically ill and injured. Crit Care Med 2004;32:2154–2155.
11. Martiin GS, Mangialardi RJ, Wheeler AP, et al. Albumin and furosemide therapy in hypoproteinemic patients with acute lung injury. Crit Care Med 2002;30:2175–2182.
12. Shafiee MAS, Bohn D, Hoorn EJ, Halperin ML. How to select optimal maintenance intravenous therapy. QJ Med 2003;96:601–610.
13. Kwan I, Bunn F, Roberts I, on behalf of the WHO Pre-Hospital Trauma Care Steering Committee. Timing and volume of fluid administration for patients with bleeding. The Cochrane Database of Systematic Reviews 2003, Issue 3, Art. No.:CD002245. DOI: 10.1002/145651858.CD002245.
14. Joint Commission for the Accreditation of Healthcare Organizations. *http:www.jointcommission.org/GeneralPublic/NPSG/05_gp_npsg.htm*
15. Kumar S, Berl T. Sodium. Lancet 1998;352:220–228.
16. Adrigoue H, Madias NE. Hyponatremia. N Engl J Med 2000;342:1581–1589.
17. Sterns RH. The treatment of hyponatremia: First, do no harm. Am J Med 1990;88:557–560.
18. Cluitmans FHM, Meinders AE. Management of severe hyponatremia: Rapid or slow correction? Am J Med 1990;88:161–166.
19. Adrogue HJ, Madias NE. Hypernatremia. N Engl J Med 2000;342:1493–1499.
20. Palevsky PM, Bhagrath R, Greenberg A. Hypernatremia in hospitalized patients. Ann Intern Med 1996;124:197–203.
21. Kang SK, Kim W, Oh MS. Pathogenesis and treatment of hypernatremia. Nephron 2002;92(Suppl 1):14–17.
22. Mandal AK. Hypokalemia and hyperkalemia. Med Clin North Am 1997;81:611–639.
23. Halperin ML. Potassium. Lancet 1998;352:135–140.
24. Gennari FJ. Hypokalemia. N Engl J Med 1998;339:451–458.
25. Hamil RJ, Robinson LM, Wexler HR, Moote C. Efficacy and safety of potassium infusion therapy in hypokalemic critically ill patients. Crit Care Med 1991;19:694–699.
26. Kruge JA, Carlson RW. Rapid correction of hypokalemia using concentrated intravenous potassium chloride infusions. Arch Intern Med 1990;150:613–617.
27. Cohn JN, Kowey PR, Whelton PK, Prisant M. New guidelines for potassium replacement in clinical practice. Arch Intern Med 2000;160:2429–2436.
28. Williams ME. Hyperkalemia. Crit Care Clin 1991;7:155–174.
29. Carroll MF, Schade DS. A practical approach to hypercalcemia. Am Fam Physician 2003;67:1959–1966.
30. Bushinsky DA, Monk RD. Calcium. Lancet 1998;352:305–311.
31. Zaloga GP. Hypocalcemia in critically ill patients. Crit Care Med 1992;20:251–262.
32. Body JJ, Bouillon R. Emergencies of calcium homeostasis. Rev Endocr Metab Disord 2003;4:167–175.
33. Bilezikian JP. Clinical review 51. Management of hypercalcemia. J Clin Endocrinol Metab 1993;77:1445–1449.
34. Davidson TG. Conventional treatment of hypercalcemia of malignancy. Am J Health-Syst Pharm 2001;58(Suppl 3):S8–S15.
35. Knochel JP. The pathophysiology and clinical characteristics of severe hypophosphatemia. Arch Intern Med 1977;137:203–220.
36. Stoff JS. Phosphate homeostasis and hypophosphatemia. Am J Med 1982;72:489–495.

37. Metheny NM. Fluid and Electrolyte Balance: Nursing Considerations. 4th ed. Lippincott, NY; 2000.

38. Just the Facts: Fluids and Electrolytes. Philadelphia: Lippincott Williams & Wilkins, 2005.

39. Weisinger JR, Bellorin-Font E. Magnesium and phosphorous. Lancet 1998;352:391–396.

40. Aubier M, Murciano D, Lecocguic Y, et al. Effect of hypophosphatemia on diaphragmatic contractility in patients with acute respiratory failure. N Engl J Med 1985;313:420–424.

41. Perreault MM, Ostron NI, Tiemey MG. Efficacy and safety of intravenous phosphate replacement in critically ill patients. Ann Pharmacother 1997;31:683–688.

42. Kee JL, Paulanka BJ, Purnell LD. Fluids and Electrolytes with Clinical Applications. A Programmed Approach. 7th ed. Clifton Park, NY: Delmar Learning, 2000.

43. Schucker JJ, Ward KE. Hyperphosphatemia and phosphate buffers. Am J Health-Syst Pharm 2005;62:2355–2361.

44. Oster JR, Epstein M. Management of magnesium depletion. Am J Nephrol 1988;8:349–354.

45. Al-Ghamdi SMG, Cameron EC, Sutton AL. Magnesium deficiency: Pathophysiologic and clinical overview. Am J Kidney Dis 1994;24:737–752.

46. Salem M, Munoz R, Chernow B. Hypomagnesemia in critical illness: A common and clinically important problem. Crit Care Clin 1991;7:225–252.

47. Zalman SA. Hypomagnesemia. J Am Soc Nephrol 1999;10:1616–1622.

48. Dube L, Granry JC. The therapeutic use of magnesium in anesthesiology, intensive care and emergency medicine: A review. Can J Anesth 2003;50:732–746.

49. Van Hook JW. Hypermagnesemia. Crit Care Clin 1991;7:215–223.

28 Acid–Base Disturbances

Lee E. Morrow and Mark A. Malesker

LEARNING OBJECTIVES

● **Upon completion of the chapter, the reader will be able to:**

1. Define primary acid–base disturbances within the human body.

2. Apply simple formulas in order to determine the etiology of simple acid–base disturbances and the adequacy of compensation.

3. Integrate the supplemental concepts of the anion gap and the excess gap to help assess complex acid–base disturbances.

4. Discuss the most common causes of each primary acid–base irregularity.

5. Determine the appropriate management for patients with acid–base disorders.

KEY CONCEPTS

❶ Acid–base homeostasis is tightly regulated by the complex, but predictable, interactions of the kidneys, the lungs, and various buffer systems. The kidneys control serum bicarbonate (HCO_3^-) concentration through the excretion or reabsorption of filtered HCO_3^-, the excretion of metabolic acids, and synthesis of new HCO_3^-. The lungs control the arterial carbon dioxide (CO_2) concentration through changes in the depth and/or rate of respiration.

❷ Respiratory acidosis and alkalosis result from primary disturbances in the arterial CO_2 concentration. Metabolic compensation of respiratory disturbances is a slow process, requiring days for the serum HCO_3^- to reach the steady state.

❸ Respiratory acidosis is caused by respiratory insufficiency resulting in an increased arterial CO_2 concentration. The compensation for respiratory acidosis (if present for prolonged periods) is an increase in serum HCO_3^-.

❹ Respiratory alkalosis is caused by hyperventilation resulting in a decreased arterial CO_2 concentration. The compensation for respiratory alkalosis (if present for prolonged periods) is a decrease in serum HCO_3^-.

❺ Metabolic acidosis and alkalosis result from primary disturbances in the serum HCO_3^- concentration. Respiratory compensation of metabolic disturbances begins within minutes and is complete within 12 hours.

❻ Metabolic acidosis is characterized by a decrease in serum HCO_3^-. The anion gap is used to narrow the differential diagnosis, as metabolic acidosis may be caused by addition of acids (increased anion gap) or loss of HCO_3^- (normal anion gap). The compensation for metabolic acidosis is an increase in ventilation with a decrease in arterial CO_2.

❼ Metabolic alkalosis is characterized by an increase in serum HCO_3^-. This disorder requires loss of fluid that is low in HCO_3^- from the body or addition of HCO_3^- to the body. The compensation for metabolic alkalosis is a decrease in ventilation with an increase in arterial CO_2.

❽ Arterial blood gases, serum electrolytes, physical examination findings, the clinical history, and the patient's recent medications must be reviewed in order to establish the etiology of a given acid–base disturbance.

❾ It is critical to treat the underlying causative process to effectively resolve most observed acid–base disorders. However, supportive treatment of the pH and electrolytes is often needed until the underlying disease state is improved.

Given its reputation for complexity and the need to memorize innumerable formulas, acid–base analysis intimidates many health care providers. In reality, acid–base disorders always obey well-defined biochemical and physiologic principles. The pH determines a patient's acid–base status and an assessment of the bicarbonate (HCO_3^-) and arterial carbon dioxide ($PaCO_2$) values identifies the underlying process. Rigorous use of a systematic approach to arterial blood gases increases the likelihood that derangements in acid–base physiology are recognized and correctly interpreted. This chapter will outline a clinically useful approach to acid–base abnormalities and then apply this approach in a series of increasingly complex clinical scenarios.

Disturbances of acid–base equilibrium occur in a wide variety of illnesses and are among the most frequently encountered disorders in critical care medicine. The importance of a thorough command of this content cannot be overstated given that acid–base disorders are remarkably common and may result in significant morbidity and mortality. Although severe derangements may affect virtually any organ system, the most serious clinical effects are cardiovascular (arrhythmias and impaired contractility), neurologic (coma and seizures), pulmonary (dyspnea, impaired oxygen delivery, respiratory fatigue, and respiratory failure), and/or renal (hypokalemia). Changes in acid–base status also affect multiple aspects of pharmacokinetics (clearance and protein binding) and pharmacodynamics.

ACID–BASE HOMEOSTASIS

Acid–base homeostasis is responsible for maintaining blood hydrogen ion concentration $[H^+]$ near normal despite the daily acidic and/or alkaline loads derived from the intake and metabolism of foods. Acid–base status is traditionally represented in terms of pH, the negative logarithm of $[H^+]$. Because $[H^+]$ is equal to 24 times the ratio of $PaCO_2$ to HCO_3^-, the pH can be altered by a change in either the bicarbonate concentration or the dissolved carbon dioxide. A critically important concept is that $[H^+]$ is dependent only on the *ratio* of $PaCO_2$ to HCO_3^- and not the absolute amount of either. As such, a normal $PaCO_2$ or HCO_3^- alone does not guarantee that the pH will be normal. Conversely, a normal pH does not imply that either the $PaCO_2$ or HCO_3^- will be normal.[1]

① *Acid–base homeostasis is tightly regulated by the complex, but predictable, interactions of the kidneys, the lungs, and various buffer systems. The kidneys control serum bicarbonate (HCO_3^-) concentration through the excretion or reabsorption of filtered HCO_3^-, the excretion of metabolic acids, and synthesis of new HCO_3^-. The lungs control arterial carbon dioxide (CO_2) concentrations through changes in the depth and/or rate of respiration.* The net result is tight regulation of the blood pH by these three distinct mechanisms working in harmony: extracellular bicarbonate and intracellular protein buffering systems; pulmonary regulation of $PaCO_2$, effectively allowing carbonic acid to be eliminated by the lungs as CO_2; and renal reclamation or excretion of HCO_3^- and excretion of acids such as ammonium.

Because the kidneys excrete less than 1% of the estimated 13,000 mEq of H^+ ions generated in an average day, renal failure can be present for prolonged periods before life-threatening imbalances occur. Conversely, cessation of breathing for minutes results in profound acid–base disturbances.[1]

The best way to assess a patient's acid–base status is to review the results of an arterial blood gas (ABG) specimen. Blood gas analyzers directly measure the pH and $PaCO_2$, while the HCO_3^- value is calculated using the Henderson–Hasselbalch equation. A more direct measure of serum HCO_3^- is obtained by measuring the total venous carbon dioxide (tCO_2). Because dissolved carbon dioxide is almost exclusively in the form of HCO_3^-, tCO_2 is essentially equivalent to the measured serum HCO_3^- concentration. This value (HCO_3^-) is routinely reported on basic chemistry panels. In the remainder of this chapter, the pH and $PaCO_2$ values should be assumed to come from an ABG while HCO_3^- values should be considered to be measured serum concentrations.

BASIC PATHOPHYSIOLOGY

Under normal circumstances, the arterial pH is tightly regulated between 7.35 and 7.45. Acidemia is an abnormally low arterial blood pH (less than 7.35) while acidosis is a pathologic process that acidifies body fluids. Similarly, alkalemia is an abnormally high arterial blood pH (greater than 7.45) while alkalosis is a pathologic process that alkalinizes body fluids. As such, although a patient can simultaneously have acidosis *and* alkalosis, the end result will be acidemia *or* alkalemia.

Changes in the arterial pH are driven by changes in the $PaCO_2$ and/or the serum HCO_3^-. Carbon dioxide is a volatile acid that is regulated by the depth and rate of respiration. Because CO_2 can be either "blown off" or "retained" by the respiratory system, it is referred to as being under respiratory control. **②** *Respiratory acidosis and alkalosis result from primary disturbances in the arterial CO_2 concentration. Metabolic compensation of respiratory disturbances is a slow process, often requiring days for the serum HCO_3^- to reach the steady state.* **③** *Respiratory acidosis is caused by respiratory insufficiency resulting in an increased arterial CO_2 concentration. The compensation for respiratory acidosis (if present for prolonged periods) is an increase in serum HCO_3^-.* **④** *Respiratory alkalosis is caused by hyperventilation resulting in a decreased arterial CO_2 concentration. The compensation for respiratory alkalosis (if present for prolonged periods) is a decrease in serum HCO_3^-.*

A respiratory acid–base disorder is a pH disturbance caused by pathologic alterations of the respiratory system or its central nervous system control. Such an alteration may result in the accumulation of $PaCO_2$ beyond normal limits (greater than 45 mm Hg or 6 kPa), a situation termed respiratory acidosis, or it may result in the loss of $PaCO_2$ beyond normal limits (less than 35 mm Hg or 4.7 kPa), a condition termed respiratory alkalosis. Variations in respiratory rate and/or depth allow the lungs to achieve changes in the $PaCO_2$ very quickly (within minutes).

Bicarbonate is a base that is regulated by renal metabolism via the enzyme carbonic anhydrase. As such, bicarbonate is often referred to as being under metabolic control. **⑤** *Metabolic acidosis and alkalosis result from primary disturbances in the serum HCO_3^- concentration. Respiratory compensation of metabolic disturbances begins within minutes and is complete within 12 hours.* **⑥** *Metabolic acidosis is characterized by a decrease in serum HCO_3^-. The anion gap is used to narrow the differential diagnosis, as metabolic acidosis may be caused by addition of acids (increased anion gap)* or loss of HCO_3^- (normal anion gap). The compensation for metabolic acidosis is an increase in ventilation with a decrease in arterial CO_2. ❼ Metabolic alkalosis is characterized by an increase in serum HCO_3^-. This disorder requires loss of fluid that is low in HCO_3^- from the body or addition of HCO_3^- to the body. The compensation for metabolic alkalosis is a decrease in ventilation with an increase in arterial CO_2.

A metabolic acid–base disorder is a pH disturbance caused by derangement of the pathways responsible for maintaining a normal HCO_3^- concentration. This may result in a pathologic accumulation of HCO_3^- (greater than 26 mEq/L or mmol/L), a condition termed metabolic alkalosis, or it may result in the loss of HCO_3^- beyond normal (less than 22 mEq/L or mmol/L), a condition termed metabolic acidosis. In contrast to the lungs' rapid effects on CO_2, the kidneys change the HCO_3^- very slowly (hours to days).

Respiratory and metabolic derangements can occur in isolation or in combination. If a patient has an isolated primary acid–base disorder that is not accompanied by another primary acid–base disorder, a simple (uncomplicated) disorder is present. The most common clinical disturbances are simple acid–base disorders. If two or three primary acid–base disorders are simultaneously present, the patient has a mixed (complicated) disorder. More complex clinical situations lead to mixed acid–base disturbances. Because CO_2 is a volatile acid, it can rapidly be changed by the respiratory system. If a respiratory acid–base disturbance is present for minutes to hours it is considered an acute disorder, while if it is present for days or longer it is considered a chronic disorder. By definition, the metabolic machinery that regulates HCO_3^- results in slow changes and all metabolic disorders are chronic.

Changes that follow the primary disorder and attempt to restore the blood pH to normal are referred to as compensatory changes. It should be stressed that compensation never normalizes the pH. Because all metabolic acid–base disorders are chronic and the normal respiratory system can quickly alter the $PaCO_2$, essentially all metabolic disorders are accompanied by some degree of respiratory compensation.[2,3] Similarly, chronic respiratory acid–base disorders are typically accompanied by attempts at metabolic compensation.[4,5] However, with acute respiratory acid–base disorders there is insufficient time for the metabolic pathways to compensate significantly.[6] As such, acute respiratory derangements are essentially uncompensated.

The amount of compensation (metabolic or respiratory) can be reliably predicted based on the degree of derangement in the primary disorder. Table 28–1 outlines the simple acid–base disorders and provides formulas for calculating the expected compensatory responses.[7] Although it is not mandatory to memorize these formulas in order to interpret acid–base problems, they can be helpful tools. If the measured values differ markedly from the calculated values (the measured serum HCO_3^- is greater than 2 mEq/L [2 mmol/L] from the calculated value or the measured $PaCO_2$ is more than 4 mm Hg [0.54 kPa] from the calculated value), a second acid–base disorder is present as outlined in Table 28–2.

Table 28–1

The Six Simple Acid–Base Disorders

Type of Disorder	pH	PaCO₂[a]	HCO₃⁻
1. Metabolic acidosis	↓	Decreased[b] $PaCO_2 = (1.5 \times HCO_3^-) + 8$	Decreased[c]
2. Metabolic alkalosis	↑	Increased[b] $PaCO_2 = (0.9 \times HCO_3^-) + 15$	Increased[c]
3. Acute respiratory acidosis	↓	Increased[c]	Approximately normal $\Delta HCO_3^- = 0.1 \times \Delta PaCO_2$[a]
4. Chronic respiratory acidosis	↓	Increased[c]	Increased[d] $\Delta HCO_3^- = 0.35 \times \Delta PaCO_2$[a]
5. Acute respiratory alkalosis	↑	Decreased[c]	Approximately normal $\Delta HCO_3^- = 0.2 \times \Delta PaCO_2$[a]
6. Chronic respiratory alkalosis	↑	Decreased[c]	Decreased[d] $\Delta HCO_3^- = 0.4 \times \Delta PaCO_2$[a]

[a]$PaCO_2$ in mm Hg.
[b]Respiratory compensation: if inappropriate, see Table 28–2.
[c]Primary disorder.
[d]Metabolic compensation: if inappropriate, see Table 28–2.

Table 28–2

Diagnosis of Concurrent Acid–Base Disturbances When Compensation Is Inappropriate

Primary Acid–Base Disturbance	Assessment of Compensation	Concurrent Acid–Base Disturbance
Metabolic acidosis	$PaCO_2$ too low[a] $PaCO_2$ too high[a]	Respiratory alkalosis Respiratory acidosis
Metabolic alkalosis	$PaCO_2$ too low[a] $PaCO_2$ too high[a]	Respiratory alkalosis Respiratory acidosis
Respiratory acidosis	HCO_3^- too low[b] HCO_3^- too high[b]	Metabolic acidosis Metabolic alkalosis
Respiratory alkalosis	HCO_3^- too low[b] HCO_3^- too high[b]	Metabolic acidosis Metabolic alkalosis

[a]Measured $PaCO_2$ more than 4 mm Hg from the calculated value.
[b]Measured HCO_3 more than 2 mEq/L from the calculated value.

APPLICATION OF BASIC PATHOPHYSIOLOGY

When given an ABG for interpretation, it is essential to use an approach that is focused yet comprehensive.[8] An algorithm illustrating this concept is shown in Figure 28–1. Using this algorithm, Step 1 is to identify all abnormalities in the pH, $PaCO_2$, and/or HCO_3^- and then decide which abnormal values are primary and which are compensatory.

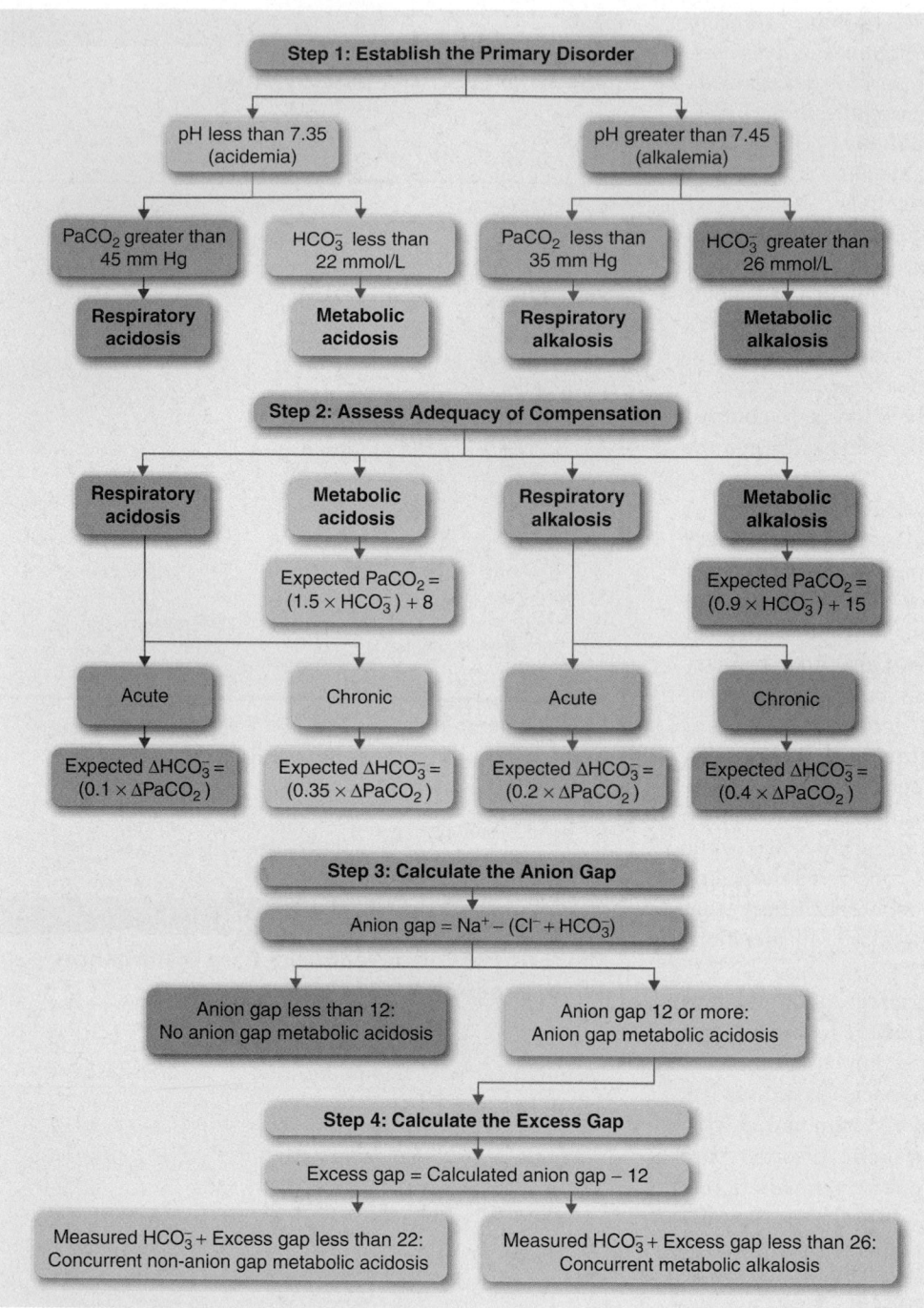

FIGURE 28-1. An algorithmic approach to acid–base disorders. Normal values: pH 7.35 to 7.45, $PaCO_2$ 35 to 45 mm Hg (4.7–6 kPa), HCO_3^- 22 to 26 mEq/L (mmol/L), anion gap less than 12 mEq/L (mmol/L). Note that $PaCO_2$ should be in millimeters of mercury to use the equations in the figure. (Cl^-, chloride ion; HCO_3^-, bicarbonate; Na^+, sodium ion; $PaCO_2$, partial pressure of arterial carbon dioxide.)

This is best done by initially looking at the pH. Whichever side of 7.40 the pH is on, the process that caused it to shift to that side is the primary abnormality. If the arterial pH is lower than 7.40 (acidemia), an elevated $PaCO_2$ (greater than 45 mm Hg or 6 kPa, **respiratory acidosis**) or a lowered HCO_3^- (less than 22 mEq/L or mmol/L, **metabolic acidosis**) would be the primary abnormality. If the arterial pH is higher than 7.40 (alkalemia), a decreased $PaCO_2$ (less than 35 or 4.7 kPa, **respiratory alkalosis**) or an increased HCO_3^- (greater than 25 mEq/L or mmol/L, **metabolic alkalosis**) would be the primary abnormality. Once the primary disorder is established, Step 2 is to apply the formulas from Table 28–1

to assess whether compensation is appropriate and to look for concurrent processes.[7]

An alternative to a diagnostic algorithm is use of a graphic nomogram.[9] Nomograms are plots of the pH, $PaCO_2$, and HCO_3^- that allow the user to rapidly determine whether arterial blood gas values are consistent with one of the six simple primary acid–base disturbances. Although nomograms are commonly used to identify acid–base disturbances in clinical practice, only individuals who fully comprehend the fundamental concepts of acid–base assessment should use these tools. Also, appreciate that nomograms have limited utility when dealing with complex acid–base derangements.

Patient Encounters 1 Through 5: Application of Basic Pathophysiology

Case Study 1

An unconscious 23-year-old man is brought to the emergency department by several friends who quickly disappear without providing any clinical history. On exam the patient has prominent "track marks" consistent with chronic IV drug abuse. The initial ABG has a pH of 7.16, $PaCO_2$ of 70 mm Hg (9.3 kPa), and HCO_3^- of 27 mEq/L (mmol/L).

What is the primary acid–base disorder?

Has compensation occurred?

Given the clinical history, what is the most likely explanation for the ABG findings?

Case Study 2

The next patient is a 72-year-old man with advanced emphysema who requires chronic oxygen therapy. During a routine office visit, an ABG is checked to verify his ongoing need for supplemental oxygen. His blood gas sample has a pH of 7.34, $PaCO_2$ of 60 mm Hg (8.0 kPa), and HCO_3^- of 35 mEq/L (mmol/L).

What is the primary acid–base disorder?

Has compensation occurred?

Given the clinical history, what is the most likely explanation for the ABG findings?

Case Study 3

Now consider a healthy 20-year-old woman who is having labs drawn as part of a research protocol. Her ABG shows a pH of 7.50, $PaCO_2$ of 29 mm Hg (3.86 kPa), and HCO_3^- of 22 mEq/L (mmol/L).

What is the primary acid–base disorder?

Has compensation occurred?

Given the clinical history, what is the most likely explanation for the ABG findings?

Case Study 4

This 59-year-old woman has a long history of ischemic cardiomyopathy and congestive heart failure that requires daily furosemide (Lasix) therapy. An ABG has been drawn because of increasing dyspnea and shows the following: pH of 7.50, $PaCO_2$ of 47 mm Hg (6.3 kPa), and HCO_3^- of 36 mEq/L (mmol/L).

What is the primary acid–base disorder?

Has compensation occurred?

Given the clinical history, what is the most likely explanation for the ABG findings?

Case Study 5

The final patient in this section is a 46-year-old woman with chronic renal insufficiency who is being hospitalized for gastroenteritis with profound diarrhea. Her ABG shows a pH of 7.20, $PaCO_2$ of 20 mm Hg (2.7 kPa), and HCO_3^- of 8 mEq/L (mmol/L).

What is the primary acid–base disorder?

Has compensation occurred?

Given the clinical history, what is the most likely explanation for the ABG findings?

Acid–base disturbances are always manifestations of underlying clinical disorders. It is useful to specifically define the primary acid–base abnormality, as each disorder is caused by a limited number of disease processes. Establishing the specific disease process responsible for the observed acid–base disorder is clinically important because treatment of a given disorder will only be accomplished by correcting the underlying disease process.

ADVANCED PATHOPHYSIOLOGY

The concepts in this section will be used to further expand on Steps 3 and 4 of the diagnostic algorithm shown in Figure 28–1. Under normal circumstances the serum is in the isoelectric state. This means that the positively charged entities reported in a standard chemistry panel (cations: sodium and potassium) should be exactly balanced by the negatively charged entities (anions: chloride and bicarbonate). However, this relationship is consistently incorrect, as the measured cations are higher than the measured anions by 10 to 12 mEq/L (mmol/L). This discrepancy results from the presence of unmeasured anions (e.g., circulating proteins, phosphates, and sulfates). This apparent difference in charges, the serum **anion gap**, is calculated as follows:

$$\text{Anion gap} = Na^+ - (Cl^- + HCO_3^-).$$

Because the serum potassium content is relatively small and is very tightly regulated, it is generally omitted from the calculation.[10]

It is important to realize that the serum HCO_3^- concentration may be affected by the presence of unmeasured endogenous acids (lactic acid or ketoacids). Bicarbonate will attempt to buffer these acids, resulting in a 1 mEq loss of serum HCO_3^- for each 1 mEq of acid titrated. Because the cation side of the equation is not affected by this transaction, the loss of serum HCO_3^- results in an increase in the calculated anion gap. Identification of an increased anion gap is very important as a limited number of clinical scenarios lead to this unique acid–base disorder. A mnemonic to recall the differential diagnosis for an anion gap acidosis is shown in Table 28–3. The concept of the increased anion gap will be applied later in Patient Encounters 6 through 10.

Step 3 in Figure 28–1 suggests that any time an ABG is analyzed it is wise to concurrently inspect the serum chemistry values and to calculate the anion gap. The body does not generate an anion gap to compensate for a primary disorder. As such, if the calculated anion gap exceeds 12 mEq/L (mmol/L) there is a primary metabolic acidosis regardless of the pH or the serum HCO_3^- concentration. The anion gap may be artificially lowered by decreased serum albumin, multiple myeloma, lithium intoxication, or a profound increase in the serum potassium, calcium, or magnesium.[11]

Step 4 in Figure 28–1 shows how calculation of the anion gap also facilitates determination of the excess gap or the degree to which the calculated anion gap exceeds the normal anion gap. The excess gap is calculated as follows:

$$\text{Excess gap} = \text{anion gap} - 12 = [Na^+ - (Cl^- + HCO_3^-)] - 12.$$

The excess gap represents the amount of HCO_3^- that has been lost due to buffering unmeasured cations. The excess gap can be added back to the measured HCO_3^- to determine what the patient's bicarbonate would be if these endogenous acids were not present. This is a very valuable tool that can be used in narrowing the differential diagnosis of certain acid–base disorders as well as in uncovering occult or mixed acid–base disorders.

Patient Encounters 6 Through 10: Application of Advanced Pathophysiology

Case Study 6

A 31-year-old psychiatric facility resident is admitted to the ICU after ingesting an unknown quantity of aspirin tablets. The presenting labs show a pH of 7.50, $PaCO_2$ of 20 mm Hg (2.7 kPa), HCO_3^- of 16 mEq/L (mmol/L), a sodium concentration of 140 mEq/L (mmol/L), and a chloride concentration of 103 mEq/L (mmol/L).

What is the primary acid–base disorder?

Is there a mixed disorder?

Given the clinical history, what is the most likely explanation for the ABG findings?

Case Study 7

A 56-year-old man is brought to the emergency department by his family. He has felt unwell for the past week and did not attend his regular hemodialysis sessions. He began vomiting 36 hours ago but refused medical evaluation. When family members found him unresponsive this morning they sought medical attention. Lab analyses show: pH of 7.40, $PaCO_2$ of 40 mm Hg (5.3 kPa), HCO_3^- of 24 mEq/L (mmol/L), sodium concentration of 145 mEq/L (mmol/L), and chloride concentration of 100 mEq/L (mmol/L).

What is the primary acid–base disorder?

Is there a mixed disorder?

Given the clinical history, what is the most likely explanation for the ABG findings?

Case Study 8

A 39-year-old woman is brought to the emergency department by rescue squad after being found "profoundly intoxicated" in a city park. Shortly after arrival, she has several episodes of emesis with witnessed aspiration. She is transferred to the ICU where she develops progressive hypoxia during the ensuing hours. Following elective intubation her blood work shows a pH of 7.50, $PaCO_2$ of 20 mm Hg (2.7 kPa), HCO_3^- of 15 mEq/L (mmol/L), sodium

concentration of 145 mEq/L (mmol/L), and chloride concentration of 100 mEq/L (mmol/L).

What is the primary acid–base disorder?

Is there a mixed disorder?

Given the clinical history, what is the most likely explanation for the ABG findings?

Case Study 9

A 69-year-old insulin-dependent diabetic man is being evaluated for unresponsiveness. His wife says he had "stomach flu" for several days with frequent bouts of emesis. She thinks he has stopped taking his insulin because he has not been eating. He became somnolent yesterday and she called an ambulance when she noticed his breathing was very slow and shallow. The blood work drawn prior to urgent intubation shows a pH of 7.10, $PaCO_2$ of 50 mm Hg (6.7 kPa), HCO_3^- of 15 mEq/L (mmol/L), sodium concentration of 145 mEq/L (mmol/L), and chloride concentration of 100 mEq/L (mmol/L).

What is the primary acid–base disorder?

Is there a mixed disorder?

Given the clinical history, what is the most likely explanation for the ABG findings?

Case Study 10

The final patient is a 23-year-old woman who was admitted 6 hours ago for diabetic ketoacidosis. With appropriate therapy, her hyperglycemia has improved and her serum ketones are improving. Because she continues to feel poorly, repeat blood work is obtained. Studies show a pH of 7.15, $PaCO_2$ of 15 mm Hg (2 kPa), HCO_3^- of 5 mEq/L (mmol/L), sodium concentration of 140 mEq/L (mmol/L), and chloride concentration of 110 mEq/L (mmol/L).

What is the primary acid–base disorder?

Is there a mixed disorder?

Given the clinical history, what is the most likely explanation for the ABG findings?

Table 28–3

Mnemonics for the Differential Diagnoses of Metabolic Acidosis

Elevated Anion Gap[a]	Normal Anion Gap[a]
M—Methanol, metformin	U—Ureteral diversion
U—Uremia	S—Saline infusion
D—Diabetic (or alcoholic) ketoacidosis	E—Exogenous acid
P—Paraldehyde, phenformin	D—Diarrhea
I—Isoniazid, iron	C—Carbonic anhydrase inhibitors
L—Lactic acidosis	A—Adrenal insufficiency
E—Ethylene glycol, ethanol	R—Renal tubular acidosis
S—Salicylates	

[a]Anion gap = serum sodium concentration – (serum chloride concentration + serum bicarbonate concentration). Under normal circumstances, the anion gap should be 10 mEq/L (mmol/L) or less.

Table 28–4

Common Causes of Metabolic Acidosis

Elevated Anion Gap[a]	Normal Anion Gap[a]
Intoxications	Bowel fistula
Methanol	Diarrhea
Ethylene glycol	Dilutional acidosis
Salicylates	Drugs
Paraldehyde	Acetazolamide[b]
Isoniazid	Ammonium chloride[b]
Ketoacidosis	Amphotericin B[b]
Diabetic	Arginine hydrochloride[c]
Ethanol	Cholestyramine[b]
Starvation	Hydrochloric acid[b]
Lactic acidosis	Lithium[b]
Carbon monoxide poisoning	Parenteral nutrition[b]
Drugs	Topiramate[b]
IV lorazepam (due to vehicle)[c]	Zonisamide[b]
Metformin[b]	Lead poisoning
Nitroprusside (due to cyanide accumulation)[b]	Renal tubular acidosis
Nucleoside reverse transcriptase inhibitors[b]	Surgical drains
Propofol[c]	Ureteral diversion
Seizures	Villous adenomas (some)
Severe hypoxemia	
Shock	
Renal failure	

[a]Anion gap = serum sodium concentration – (serum chloride concentration + serum bicarbonate concentration). Under normal circumstances, the anion gap should be 10 mEq/L (mmol/L) or less.

[b]May be observed with therapeutic doses or overdoses.

[c]Typically observed only with overdoses.

In summary, the approach to assessment of acid–base status involves four key steps as outlined in Figure 28–1: Step 1—initial inspection of the pH, $PaCO_2$, and HCO_3^-; Step 2—assessment of the adequacy of compensation; Step 3—calculation of the anion gap; and Step 4—calculation of the excess gap.

ETIOLOGY AND TREATMENT

8 *Arterial blood gases, serum electrolytes, physical examination findings, the clinical history, and the patient's recent medications must be reviewed in order to establish the etiology of a given acid–base disturbance.* Tables 28–3 through 28–7 outline the most commonly encountered causes for each of the primary acid–base disorders. The therapeutic approach to each of these acid–base derangements should emphasize a search for the cause, as opposed to immediate attempts to normalize the pH.

9 *It is critical to treat the underlying causative process to effectively resolve most observed acid–base disorders. However, supportive treatment of the pH and electrolytes is often needed until the underlying disease state is improved.*[12,13]

All patients with significant disturbances in their acid–base status require continuous cardiovascular and hemodynamic monitoring. Because frequent assessment of the patient's response to treatment is critical, an arterial line is often placed to minimize patient discomfort with serial ABG collections. If the anion gap was initially abnormal, serial chemistries should be followed to ensure that the anion gap resolves with treatment. Specific treatment decisions depend on the underlying pathophysiologic state (e.g., dialysis for renal failure, insulin for diabetic ketoacidosis, or improving tissue perfusion and oxygenation for lactic acidosis).

Metabolic Acidosis

Metabolic acidosis is characterized by a reduced arterial pH, a primary decrease in the HCO_3^- concentration, and a compensatory reduction in the $PaCO_2$. The etiologies of metabolic acidosis are divided into those that lead to an increase in the anion gap and those associated with a normal anion gap and are listed in Table 28–4. Although there are numerous mnemonics to recall the differential diagnosis of the metabolic acidosis, two simple ones are shown in Table 28–3. High anion gap metabolic acidosis is most frequently caused by lactic acidosis, ketoacidosis, and/or renal failure. Although there is considerable variation, the largest anion gaps are caused by ketoacidosis, lactic acidosis, and methanol or ethylene glycol ingestion.[14]

Symptoms of metabolic acidosis are attributable to changes in cardiovascular, musculoskeletal, neurologic, or pulmonary functioning. Respiratory compensation requires marked increases in minute ventilation and may lead to dyspnea, respiratory fatigue, and respiratory failure. Acidemia predisposes to ventricular arrhythmias and reduces cardiac contractility, each of which can result in pulmonary edema and/or systemic hypotension.[15] Neurologic symptoms range from lethargy to coma and are usually proportional to the severity of the pH derangement. Chronic metabolic acidosis leads to a variety of musculoskeletal problems including impaired growth, rickets, osteomalacia, or osteopenia. These changes are believed to be caused by the release of calcium and phosphate during bone buffering of excess H^+ ions.

As previously discussed, in anion gap metabolic acidosis, the isoelectric state is maintained because unmeasured anions are present. With a *normal* anion gap metabolic acidosis, the isoelectric state is maintained by an increase in the measured chloride. Because of this, normal anion gap metabolic acidosis is often referred to as hyperchloremic acidosis.

In patients with a normal anion gap metabolic acidosis, it is often helpful to calculate the urine anion gap (UAG).[16] The UAG is calculated as follows:

$$UAG = (Urine\ Na^+ + Urine\ K^+) - Urine\ Cl^-.$$

The normal UAG ranges from 0 to 5 mEq/L (mmol/L) and represents the presence of unmeasured urinary anions. In metabolic acidosis, the excretion of NH_4^+ and concurrent Cl^- should increase markedly if renal acidification is intact. This results in UAG values from −20 to −50 mEq/L (mmol/L). This occurs because the urinary Cl^- concentration now markedly exceeds the urinary Na^+ and K^+ concentrations. Diagnoses consistent with an excessively negative UAG include proximal (type 2) renal tubular acidosis, diarrhea, or administration of acetazolamide or hydrochloric acid (HCl). Excessively positive values of the UAG suggest a distal (type 1) renal tubular acidosis.

In order to effectively treat metabolic acidosis, the *causative process* must be identified and treated.[17] The precise role of adjunctive therapy with sodium bicarbonate ($NaHCO_3$) is not universally agreed upon. However, most practitioners accept that $NaHCO_3$ is indicated when renal dysfunction precludes adequate regeneration of HCO_3^- or when severe acidemia (pH less than 7.10) is present. The metabolic acidosis seen with lactic acidosis and ketoacidosis generally resolves with therapy targeted at the underlying cause and $NaHCO_3$ may be unnecessary regardless of the pH. The metabolic acidosis of renal failure, renal tubular acidosis, or intoxication with ethylene glycol, methanol, or salicylates is much more likely to require $NaHCO_3$ therapy.

If $NaHCO_3$ is used, the plasma HCO_3^- should not be corrected entirely. Instead, aim at increasing HCO_3^- above an absolute value of 10 mEq/L (10 mmol/L). The total HCO_3^- deficit can be calculated from the current bicarbonate concentration ($HCO_{3\ curr}^-$), the desired bicarbonate concentration ($HCO_{3\ post}^-$), and the body weight (in kilograms) as follows:

$$HCO_3^-\ deficit = [(2.4/HCO_{3\ curr}^-) + 0.4] \times weight \times (HCO_{3\ curr}^- - HCO_{3\ post}^-).$$

No more than half of the calculated HCO_3^- deficit should be given initially to avoid volume overload, hypernatremia, hyperosmolarity, overshoot alkalemia, and/or hypokalemia. The calculated HCO_3^- deficit reflects only the present situation and does not account for ongoing H^+ production and HCO_3^- loss. When giving HCO_3^- therapy, serial blood gases are needed to monitor therapy.

Another option for patients with severe acidemia is tromethamine (THAM).[18] This inert amino alcohol buffers acids and CO_2 through its amine ($-NH_2$) moiety:

$$THAM-NH_2 + H^+ = THAM-NH_3^+$$
$$THAM-NH_2 + H_2O + CO_2 = THAM-NH_3^+ + HCO_3^-.$$

Protonated THAM (with Cl^- or HCO_3^-) is excreted in the urine at a rate that is slightly higher than creatinine

clearance. As such, THAM augments the buffering capacity of the blood without generating excess CO_2. THAM is less effective in patients with renal failure and toxicities may include hyperkalemia, hypoglycemia, and possible respiratory depression.

Chronic metabolic acidosis can successfully be managed using potassium citrate/citric acid (Polycitra-K) or sodium citrate/citric acid (Bicitra).

Metabolic Alkalosis

Metabolic alkalosis is characterized by an increased arterial pH, a primary increase in the HCO_3^- concentration, and a compensatory increase in the $PaCO_2$. Patients will always hypoventilate to compensate for metabolic alkalosis—even if it results in profound hypoxemia. For a metabolic alkalosis to persist, there must concurrently be a process that elevates serum HCO_3^- concentration (gastric or renal loss of acids) and another that impairs renal HCO_3^- excretion (hypovolemia, hypokalemia, or mineralocorticoid excess). The etiologies of metabolic alkalosis are listed in Table 28–5.

Patients with metabolic alkalosis rarely have symptoms attributable to alkalemia. Rather, complaints are usually related to volume depletion (muscle cramps, positional dizziness, weakness) or to hypokalemia (muscle weakness, polyuria, polydipsia).

In order to effectively treat metabolic alkalosis, the *causative process* must be identified and treated. The major causes of metabolic alkalosis are often readily apparent after carefully reviewing the patient's history and medication list. In hospitalized patients always look for administration of compounds such as citrate in blood products and acetate in parenteral nutrition that can raise the HCO_3^- concentration. If the etiology of the metabolic alkalosis is still unclear, measurement of the urinary chloride may be useful. Some processes leading to metabolic alkalosis (vomiting, nasogastric suction losses, factitious diarrhea) will have low

---

Table 28–5	
Common Causes of Metabolic Alkalosis	
Urine Cl⁻ less than 10 mEq/L (less than 10 mmol/L)	**Urine Cl⁻ greater than 10 mEq/L (greater than 10 mmol/L)**
Alkali administration	Drugs[a]
IV bicarbonate therapy	Corticosteroid therapy
Oral alkali therapy	Diuretics
Parenteral nutrition with acetate	Hypokalemia
"Contraction alkalosis"	Mineralocorticoid excess
postdiuretic use	Hyperaldosteronism
Decreased chloride intake	Bartter's syndrome
Loss of gastric acid	Cushing's syndrome
Vomiting	
Nasogastric suction	
Posthypercapnia	
Villous adenomas (some)	

[a]May be observed with therapeutic doses or overdoses.

urinary Cl⁻ concentrations (less than 25 mEq/L or mmol/L), while others (diuretics, hypokalemia, and mineralocorticoid excess) will have higher urinary Cl⁻ concentrations (greater than 40 mEq/L or mmol/L).

In general, contributing factors such as diuretics, nasogastric suction, and corticosteroids should be discontinued if possible. Any fluid deficits should be treated with IV normal saline. Recognize that patients with varieties of metabolic alkalosis with high urine Cl⁻ (though rather uncommon) will be resistant to saline loading. Potassium supplementation should always be given if it is also deficient.

In patients with mild or moderate alkalosis who require ongoing diuresis but have rising HCO_3^- concentrations, the carbonic anhydrase inhibitor acetazolamide can be used to reduce the HCO_3^- concentration. Acetazolamide is typically dosed at 250 mg every 6 to 12 hours as needed to maintain the pH in a clinically acceptable range. This agent results in gradual changes in the serum HCO_3^- and is not used to acutely correct a patient's acid–base status. If alkalosis is profound and potentially life-threatening (due to seizures or ventricular tachyarrhythmias), consideration can be given to hemodialysis or transient HCl infusion. The hydrogen ion deficit (in milliequivalents or millimoles) can be estimated from the current bicarbonate concentration ($HCO_{3\,curr}^-$), the desired bicarbonate concentration ($HCO_{3\,post}^-$), and the body weight (in kilograms) as follows:

$$H^+ \text{ deficit} = 0.4 \times \text{weight} \times (HCO_{3\,curr}^- - HCO_{3\,post}^-).$$

After estimating the H⁺ deficit, 0.1 to 0.2 N HCl is infused at 20 to 50 mEq/h (mmol/h) into a central vein. Arterial pH must be monitored at least hourly and the infusion stopped as soon as clinically feasible. Ammonium chloride and arginine hydrochloride, agents that result in the formation of HCl, are not commonly prescribed, as they may lead to significant toxicity. Ammonium chloride may cause accumulation of ammonia leading to encephalopathy while arginine hydrochloride can induce life-threatening hyperkalemia through unclear mechanisms.

Respiratory Acidosis

Respiratory acidosis is characterized by a reduced arterial pH, a primary increase in the arterial $PaCO_2$ and, when present for sufficient time, a compensatory rise in the HCO_3^- concentration. Because increased CO_2 is a potent respiratory stimulus, respiratory acidosis represents ventilatory failure or impaired central control of ventilation as opposed to an increase in CO_2 production. As such, most patients will have hypoxemia in addition to hypercapnia. The most common etiologies of respiratory acidosis are listed in Table 28–6.

Severe, acute respiratory acidosis produces a variety of neurologic abnormalities. Initially these include headache, blurred vision, restlessness, and anxiety. These may progress to tremors, asterixis, somnolence, and/or delirium. If untreated, terminal manifestations include peripheral vasodilation leading to hypotension and cardiac arrhythmias.

Table 28–6
Common Causes of Respiratory Acidosis

Central nervous system disease	Pneumonia
Brain stem lesions	Pneumonitis
Central sleep apnea	Pulmonary edema
Infection	Restrictive lung disease
Intracranial hypertension	Ascites
Trauma	Chest wall disorder
Tumor	Fibrothorax
Vascular	Kyphoscoliosis
Drugs[a]	Obesity
Aminoglycosides	Pleural effusion
Anesthetics	Pneumoconiosis
β-Blockers	Pneumothorax
Botulism toxin	Progressive systemic
Hypnotics	sclerosis
Narcotics	Pulmonary fibrosis
Neuromuscular blocking agents	Spinal arthritis
Organophosphates	Smoke inhalation
Sedatives	Upper airway obstruction
Neuromuscular disease	Foreign body
Guillain-Barré syndrome	Laryngospasm
Muscular dystrophy	Obstructive sleep apnea
Myasthenia gravis	Others
Polymyositis	Abdominal distention
Pulmonary disease	Altered metabolic rate
Lower airway obstruction	Congestive heart failure
Chronic obstructive pulmonary	Hypokalemia
disease	Hypothyroidism
Foreign body	Inadequate mechanical
Status asthmaticus	ventilation

[a]May be observed with therapeutic doses or overdoses.

Chronic respiratory acidosis is typically associated with cor pulmonale and peripheral edema.

In order to effectively treat respiratory acidosis, the *causative process* must be identified and treated. If a cause is identified, specific therapy should be started. This may include naloxone for opiate-induced hypoventilation or bronchodilator therapy for acute bronchospasm. Because respiratory acidosis represents ventilatory failure, an increase in alveolar ventilation is required. This can often be achieved by controlling the underlying disease (e.g., bronchodilators and corticosteroids in asthma) and/or physically augmenting ventilation.

Although their precise role and mechanisms of action are unclear, agents such as medroxyprogesterone, theophylline, and doxapram stimulate respiration and have been used to treat mild to moderate respiratory acidosis. Moderate or severe respiratory acidosis requires assisted ventilation. This can be provided to spontaneously breathing patients via bilevel positive airway pressure (BiPAP) delivered via a tight-fitting mask, or by intubation followed by mechanical ventilation. In mechanically ventilated patients, respiratory acidosis is treated by increasing the minute ventilation. This is achieved by increasing the respiratory rate and/or tidal volume.

As with the treatment of metabolic acidosis, the role of $NaHCO_3$ therapy is not well defined for respiratory acidosis.

Realize that administration of $NaHCO_3$ can paradoxically result in increased CO_2 generation ($HCO_3^- + H^+ \rightarrow H_2CO_3 \rightarrow H_2O + CO_2$) and worsened acidemia. Careful monitoring of the pH is required if $NaHCO_3$ therapy is started for this indication. The use of tromethamine in respiratory acidosis (see Metabolic Acidosis, above) has unproven safety and benefit.

The goals of therapy in patients with chronic respiratory acidosis are to maintain oxygenation and to improve alveolar ventilation if possible. Because of the presence of renal compensation it is usually not necessary to treat the pH, even in patients with severe hypercapnia. Although the specific treatment varies with the underlying disease, excessive oxygen and sedatives should be avoided as they can worsen CO_2 retention.

Respiratory Alkalosis

Respiratory alkalosis is characterized by an increased arterial pH, a primary decrease in the arterial $PaCO_2$ and, when present for sufficient time, a compensatory fall in the HCO_3^- concentration. Respiratory alkalosis represents hyperventilation and is remarkably common. The most common etiologies of respiratory alkalosis are listed in Table 28–7 and range from benign (anxiety) to life-threatening (pulmonary embolism). Some causes of hyperventilation and respiratory acidosis are remarkably common (hypoxemia or anemia).

The symptoms produced by respiratory alkalosis result from increased irritability of the central and peripheral nervous systems. These include light-headedness, altered consciousness, distal extremity paresthesias, circumoral paresthesia, cramps, carpopedal spasms, and syncope. Various supraventricular and ventricular cardiac arrhythmias may occur in extreme cases, particularly in critically ill patients. An additional finding in many patients with severe respiratory alkalosis is hypophosphatemia, reflecting a shift of phosphate from the extracellular space into the cells. Chronic respiratory alkalosis is generally asymptomatic.

It is imperative to identify serious causes of respiratory alkalosis and institute effective treatment. In spontaneously breathing patients, respiratory alkalosis is typically only mild or moderate in severity and no specific therapy is indicated. Severe alkalosis generally represents respiratory acidosis imposed on metabolic alkalosis and may improve with sedation. Patients receiving mechanical ventilation are treated with reduced minute ventilation achieved by decreasing the respiratory rate and/or tidal volume. If the alkalosis persists in the ventilated patient, high-level sedation or paralysis is effective.

SUMMARY

Acid–base disturbances are common clinical problems that are not difficult to analyze if approached in a consistent manner. The pH, $PaCO_2$, and HCO_3^- should be inspected to identify all abnormal values. This should lead to an assessment of which deviations represent the primary abnormality and which represent compensatory changes. The serum electrolytes should always be used to calculate the anion gap. In cases in which the anion gap is increased, the excess anion gap should be added back to the measured HCO_3^-. The anion gap

---

Table 28–7
Common Causes of Respiratory Alkalosis

Central nervous system disease	Pulmonary disease
Infection	Early restrictive lung disease
Trauma	Infection
Tumor	Pneumothorax
Vascular	Pulmonary edema
Drug- or toxin-induced[a]	Pulmonary embolism
Catecholamines	Tissue hypoxia
Doxapram	Burn injury
Methylphenidate	Excessive mechanical
Methylxanthines	ventilation
Nicotine	Fever
Progesterone	Hepatic failure
Salicylates	Hypoxemia
Psychiatric disease	Pain
Anxiety	Postmetabolic acidosis
Hyperventilation	Pregnancy
Hysteria	Severe anemia
Panic disorder	Thyrotoxicosis

[a]May be observed with therapeutic doses or overdoses.

Patient Care and Monitoring

1. Every patient with a suspected acid–base disturbance should have an arterial blood gas and a serum chemistry panel drawn concurrently. The results of these tests should be reviewed using a systematic approach to ensure proper interpretation.

2. What is the primary disorder? Has compensation occurred?

3. Is the anion gap excessively large? If so, does calculation of the excess gap identify another acid–base disorder?

4. Continuous cardiovascular and hemodynamic monitoring should be used for significant pH disturbances, as the most serious sequelae of acid–base disorders include electrolyte abnormalities, cardiac dysrhythmias, and systemic hypotension.

5. All acid–base abnormalities result from underlying disease processes. Definitive therapy for these disturbances requires treatment of the illness that has disrupted the pH equilibrium.

6. Review each patient's history, physical exam, and current medication list for clues regarding potential causes of the observed acid–base disorder.

7. Serial arterial blood gases and serum chemistries should be compared, as every patient's acid–base status is continuously changing based on the underlying disease state and any therapy initiated.

and the excess gap are useful tools that can identify hidden disorders. This rigorous assessment of the patient's acid–base status, incorporated with the available clinical data, increases the likelihood that the clinician will successfully determine the cause of each identified disorder. Although supportive therapy is often required for profound acid–base disturbances, definitive therapy must target the underlying process that has led to the observed derangements.

Abbreviations Introduced in This Chapter

ABG	Arterial blood gas
BiPAP	Bilevel positive airway pressure
Cl^-	Chloride ion
CO_2	Carbon dioxide
Δ(delta)	Change
H^+	Hydrogen ion
HCl	Hydrochloric acid
HCO_3^-	Bicarbonate
$HCO_{3\ curr}^-$	Current bicarbonate
$HCO_{3\ post}^-$	Post-therapy bicarbonate
Hg	Mercury
K^+	Potassium ion
kg	Kilogram
kPa	Kilopascal
L	Liter
mEq	Milliequivalent
mm	Millimeter
mmol	Millimole
Na^+	Sodium ion
$NaHCO_3$	Sodium bicarbonate
NH_2	Terminal amine group
NH_4^+	Ammonium
pH	Logarithm of the hydrogen ion concentration
$PaCO_2$	Partial pressure of arterial carbon dioxide
tCO_2	Total venous carbon dioxide
UAG	Urine anion gap

 Self-assessment questions and answers are available at *http://www.mhpharmacotherapy. com/pp.html*.

REFERENCES

1. Rose BD, Post TW. Clinical Physiology of Acid–Base and Electrolyte Disorders. 5th ed. New York, NY: McGraw-Hill, 2001: 299.
2. Schlichtig R, Grogono A, Severinghaus J. Human $PaCO_2$ and standard base excess for compensation of acid–base imbalances. Crit Care Med 1998;26:1173–1179.
3. Pierce NF, Fedson DS, Brigham KL, et al. The ventilatory response to acute base deficit in humans. Time course during development and correction of metabolic acidosis. Ann Intern Med 1970;72:633–640.
4. Javaheri S, Kazemi H. Metabolic alkalosis and hypoventilation in humans. Am Rev Respir Dis 1987;136:1011–1016.
5. Polak A, Haynie GD, Hays RM, Schwartz WB. Effects of chronic hypercapnia on electrolyte and acid–base equilibrium. J Clin Invest 1961;40:1223–1237.
6. Gennari FJ, Goldstein MB, Schwartz WB. The nature of the renal adaptation to chronic hypocapnia. J Clin Invest 1972;51:1722–1730.
7. van Yperselle de Striho C, Brasseur L, de Coninck JD. The "carbon dioxide response curve" for chronic hypercapnia in man. N Engl J Med 1966;275:117–122.
8. Haber RJ. A practical approach to acid–base disorders. West J Med 1991;155:146–151.
9. Arbus GS. An in-vivo acid–base nomogram for clinical use. Can Med Assoc J 1973;109:291–293.
10. Narins R. Clinical Disorders of Fluid and Electrolyte Metabolism. 5th ed. New York, NY: McGraw-Hill, 1994: 778.
11. Goodkin DA, Gollapudi GK, Narins RG. The role of the anion gap in detecting and managing mixed metabolic acid–base disorders. Clin Endocrinol Metab 1984;13:333–349.
12. Adrogué HJ, Madias NE. Management of life-threatening acid–base disorders. First of two parts. N Engl J Med 1998;338:26–34.
13. Adrogué HJ, Madias NE. Management of life-threatening acid–base disorders. Second of two parts. N Engl J Med 1998;338:107–111.
14. Abelow B. Understanding Acid–Base. Baltimore, MD: Williams & Wilkins, 1998: 229.
15. Kearns T, Wolfson A. Metabolic acidosis. Emerg Med Clin North Am 1989;7:823–835.
16. Batlle DC, Hizon M, Cohen E, Gutterman C, Gupta R. The use of the urinary anion gap in the diagnosis of hyperchloremic metabolic acidosis. N Engl J Med 1988;318:594–599.
17. Hood FL, Tannen RL. Protection of acid–base balance by pH regulation of acid production. N Engl J Med 1998;339:819–826.
18. Chernow B, ed. The Pharmacologic Approach to the Critically Ill Patient. 3rd ed. Baltimore, MD: Williams & Wilkins, 1994: 965.

29 Multiple Sclerosis

Melody Ryan

LEARNING OBJECTIVES

● **Upon completion of the chapter, the reader will be able to:**

1. Identify risk factors for multiple sclerosis (MS).

2. Describe pathophysiologic findings of MS.

3. Recognize common presenting symptoms of MS.

4. Distinguish between the forms of MS based on patient presentation and course of disease.

5. Compare and contrast MS disease-modifying treatment choices for a specific patient.

6. Determine appropriate symptomatic treatment choices and develop a detailed therapeutic plan for a specific patient.

7. Develop a monitoring plan for a patient placed on specific medications.

KEY CONCEPTS

❶ Multiple sclerosis (MS) symptoms are a function of the location of lesions within the CNS.

❷ The McDonald criteria, utilizing clinical exam in combination with MRI and cerebrospinal fluid (CSF) data, facilitates earlier diagnosis, and thus earlier treatment initiation.

❸ The clinical course of MS has four basic patterns: Relapsing remitting, secondary progressive, primary progressive, and progressive relapsing.

❹ Acute relapses are treated with corticosteroids to speed recovery of the patient.

❺ Disease-modifying therapies decrease the number of relapses, prevent permanent neurologic damage, and prevent disability.

❻ Symptomatic treatment minimizes the impact of MS on quality of life.

❼ Dose–response curves have been observed with the β-interferons.

❽ There is no consensus on the best medication for initial therapy.

❾ Mitoxantrone and natalizumab should be reserved for patients with rapidly advancing disease who have failed other therapies.

❿ MS patients must be treated with agents specific for upper motor neuron spasticity.

Multiple sclerosis (MS) is an inflammatory disease of the CNS, variable in symptoms and presentation. Multiple describes the number of CNS lesions, and sclerosis refers to the demyelinated lesions, today called plaques.

EPIDEMIOLOGY AND ETIOLOGY

Epidemiology

Approximately 400,000 Americans have MS. Diagnosis usually occurs between the ages of 20 and 50. Twice as many women as men develop MS.[1] Risk factors for MS include family history of MS, autoimmune diseases, or migraine; personal history of autoimmune diseases or migraine; and, in women, smoking and exposure to second-hand smoke.[2,3] Prevalence decreases with decreases in latitude.[4]

Etiology

▶ Inheritance Theory

MS probably has a genetic component: family members of MS patients have a 5% risk. Monozygotic twins have highest risk (25–30% concordance).[5] Genetic susceptibility is probably found in the human leukocyte antigen chromosomal region.[5] A straightforward inheritance pattern cannot fully explain the etiology of MS because only a small proportion of patients report a family member with MS.[5]

▶ **Environment Theory**

Over 20 infectious agents have been suggested as etiologic agents. Currently, human herpes virus 6 (HHV-6) is the most likely causative virus. HHV-6 may initiate MS in two ways. First, HHV-6 is structurally similar to myelin basic protein. When T cells become sensitive to HHV-6, the cells may attack myelin basic protein. Second, HHV-6 may directly stimulate the complement cascade, activating autoimmune processes.[6] Infection with HHV-6 cannot fully explain MS, because HHV-6 is found in 75% of the population, but MS is much less common.

PATHOPHYSIOLOGY

While the causative agent of MS is unclear, the result is the development of an autoimmune disorder with areas of CNS demyelination and axonal transection.

Demyelination

An unknown antigen presented by the major histocompatibility complex (MHC) class II molecules causes T cells to become autoreactive (Fig. 29–1). Once activated, T cells penetrate the blood–brain barrier by attachment to upregulated adhesion molecules and production of matrix metalloproteinases (MMP) that cause blood–brain barrier breakdown. In the CNS, the T cells come into contact with antigen-presenting cells (APCs) and proliferate. The T-helper cells differentiate into proinflammatory T-helper-1 cells (Th1 cells) and anti-inflammatory T helper-2 cells (Th2 cells).[8] Th1 cells secrete cytokines that enhance macrophage and microglial cells that attack myelin.[8]

B cells cross previously damaged sections of the blood–brain barrier to arrive in the CNS, an area normally free of B cells. Autoreactive T cells trigger B cells to form myelin autoantibodies. B-cell antibodies also initiate the complement cascade, causing myelin degradation.[8] These inflammatory processes probably cause relapses.[5]

Axonal Transection

Axonal transection disrupts nerve signals completely and irreversibly. There is growing evidence that cytotoxic T cells cause axonal injury.[6] Axonal transection begins as early as 2 weeks after diagnosis and continues throughout the disease.[9] Axonal loss is likely responsible for MS progression.[5]

CLINICAL PRESENTATION, DIAGNOSIS, AND CLINICAL COURSE

Diagnosis

MS diagnostic criteria were revised in 2001 (Fig. 29–2).[17–19] Diagnosis requires that plaques be disseminated in time and space. Previously, diagnosis relied on clinical examination. ❷ *The McDonald criteria, which utilizes the clinical exam in combination with MRI and (cerebrospinal fluid) CSF*

Table 29–1	
Diagnostic Tests for MS	
Test	**Findings in MS**
MRI	
T2 weighted	Demyelinated plaques, both active and inactive
Gadolinium enhanced	Active demyelinating plaques
CSF analysis	**Oligoclonal bands** of immunoglobulin G Elevated **immunoglobulin G index**
Evoked potential testing	Slowed nerve impulse conduction

CSF, cerebrospinal fluid; MS, multiple sclerosis.

From Refs. 17, 20.

data, facilitates earlier diagnosis, and thus earlier treatment initiation (Table 29–1).

Clinical Course

❸ *The clinical course of MS has four basic patterns: Relapsing remitting, secondary progressive, primary progressive, and progressive relapsing (Fig. 29–3).* Relapsing remitting MS develops into secondary progressive MS in 50% of patients within 10 years and in 75% within 25 years of diagnosis.[1] Rating scales are used clinically (Table 29–2). MS reduces overall life expectancy 6 to 7 years.[23] Suicide is disproportionately high in MS patients, accounting for about 15% of MS-related deaths.[24]

TREATMENT

Desired Outcomes and General Approach to Treatment

The overall goal of treatment is preventing permanent neurologic damage. There are three general approaches to treatment. ❹ *First, acute relapses are treated with corticosteroids to speed recovery.* ❺ *Second, disease-modifying therapies decrease the number of relapses, prevent permanent neurologic damage, and prevent disability.* ❻ *Third, symptomatic treatments minimize the impact of MS on quality of life.*

Pharmacologic Treatment

▶ **Treatment of Acute Relapses**

The mechanism of action of corticosteroids is unclear, but may involve:

- Prevention of inflammatory cytokine activation
- Inhibition of T-cell activation
- Prevention of immune cells from entering the CNS
- Increased death of activated immune cells[25]

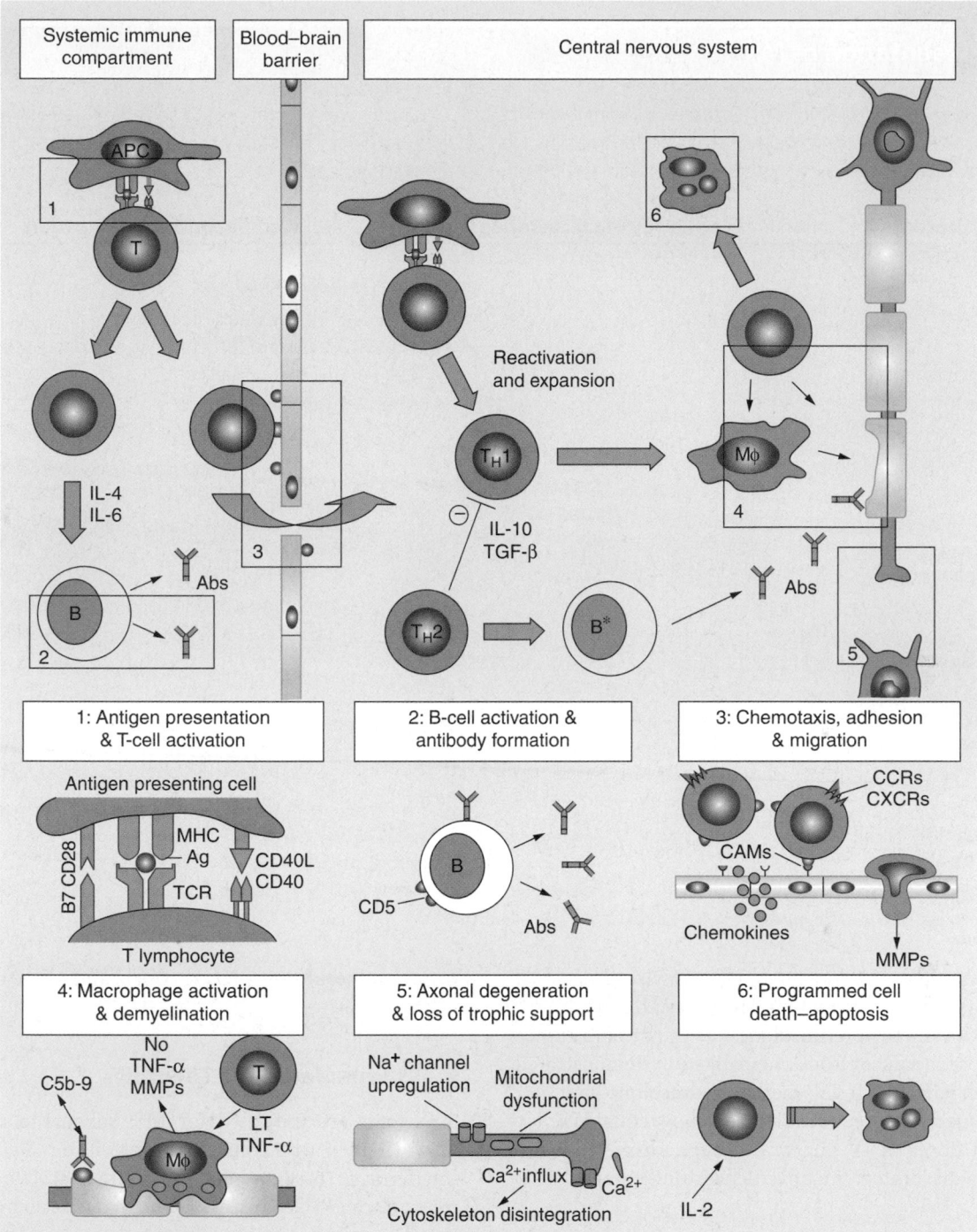

FIGURE 29–1. Synoptic view of the immune response in the pathogenesis of MS. Autoreactive T cells recognize with their TCR a specific autoantigen presented by MHC class II molecules and the simultaneous delivery of costimulatory signals (CD 28, B7, CD40, CD 40L) on the cell surface of APCs, such as macrophages, in the systemic immune compartment (*panel 1*). Activated T lymphocytes can cross the blood–brain barrier in order to enter the CNS. The mechanisms of transendothelial migration is mediated by the complex interplay of CAMs, chemokines, and their receptors (CCRs, CXCRs) and MMPs (*panel 3*). Within the CNS, T cells activate microglia cells/macrophages (Mφ) to enhanced phagocytic activity; production of cytokines, such as TNF-*a* and LT; and the release of toxic mediators, such as NO, propagating demyelination and axonal loss. Abs crossing the blood–brain barrier or locally produced by B cells or mast cells (B*) contribute to this process. Autoantibodies activate the complement cascade resulting in the formation of the membrane-attack complex (C5b-9) and its subsequent lysis of the target structure (*panels 2 and 4*). The upregulation of Na+ and Ca2+ channels on the axon as well as mitochondrial dysfunction and loss of trophic support contribute to axonal disintegration and degeneration (*panel 5*). The inflammatory response is regulated by anti-inflammatory cytokines, such as IL-10 or TGF-*β*, as well as IL-2, inducing programmed cell death (apoptosis) in immunoreactive T lymphocytes (*panel 6*). (Abs, autoantibodies; Ag, antigen; APC, antigen-presenting cells; CAM, cellular adhesion molecule; CNS, central nervous system; IL, interleukin; LT, lymphotoxin; MHC, major histocompatibility complex; MMP, matrix metalloproteinases; NO, nitric oxide; T, T cell; TCR, T-cell receptor; TGF, transforming growth factor; TNF, tumor necrosis factor.) (From Ref. 7.)

Clinical Presentation of MS[10–16]

❶ *MS symptoms are a function of the location of lesions within the CNS.* Because myelin increases the speed of nerve impulse transmission, demyelination slows the speed of transmission. No impulses can be transmitted if the axon is transected. The primary symptoms of MS are caused by this delay or cessation of impulses. Secondary symptoms of MS result from the primary symptoms.

Primary Symptoms	Frequency of Occurrence (%)	Related Secondary Symptoms
Urinary symptoms	90	
Incontinence		Decubitus ulcers
Urinary retention		Urinary tract infections
Spasticity	60	Falls, care difficulties, pain, gait problems
Visual symptoms		
Optic neuritis	55	Falls, care difficulties
Diplopia		
Bowel symptoms		
Incontinence	29–51	Decubitus ulcers
Constipation	35–54	Pain
Depression	50	Suicide
Cognitive deficits	50	Care difficulties
Weakness		Falls, care difficulties, gait problems
Fatigue	76–92	
Uhthoff's phenomenon	80	
Sexual dysfunction		
Erectile dysfunction	70	
Female sexual dysfunction	72	
Tremor	25	
Pain		
Trigeminal neuralgia	2	
Lhermitte's sign	9	
Dysesthetic pain	18	

IV adrenocorticotropic hormone, IV methylprednisolone, or oral prednisone hasten functional recovery after relapses.[26] Traditionally, IV methylprednisolone was the drug of choice for acute relapses because an optic neuritis study demonstrated reduced recurrence with IV methylprednisolone, but not oral prednisone.[27,28] More recent studies show equal efficacy of equivalent doses of IV and oral dosage forms, and oral dosing avoids discomfort, inconvenience, and expense of IV therapy.[29,30]

Adverse Effects Short-term corticosteroid use is not associated with most of the adverse effects of chronic steroid use. The most common adverse effects are GI upset, insomnia, and mood swings.[27]

Dosing and Administration Methylprednisolone is given 1 g/day IV as one dose or in divided doses for 3 to 5 days. Oral prednisone 1,250 mg/day given every other day for five doses provides an equivalent dose.

Clinical improvement usually begins during corticosteroid treatment. Neurologic recovery is equivalent with or without a subsequent oral prednisone taper.[31]

Outcome Evaluation

• Monitor for improvement of symptoms

• Educate regarding adverse effects and reporting directions

▶ *Disease-Modifying Therapies*

Six agents are indicated for MS: subcutaneous interferon β-1a (Rebif); intramuscular interferon β-1a (Avonex); interferon β-1b (Betaseron); glatiramer acetate (Copaxone); mitoxantrone (Novantrone); and natalizumab (Tysabri). A broad look across all studies of these immunomodulators shows about 30% relapse reduction.[32]

β-Interferons

Pharmacology and Mechanism of Action. The mechanism of action of β-interferons is incompletely understood. The following properties are thought to be important:

• Decrease in T-cell activation, decreasing cytokine secretion and preserving myelin

• Prevention of upregulation of adhesion molecules on activated T cells, limiting the number of T cells that can get into the brain

• Suppression of MMPs, maintaining the integrity of the blood–brain barrier

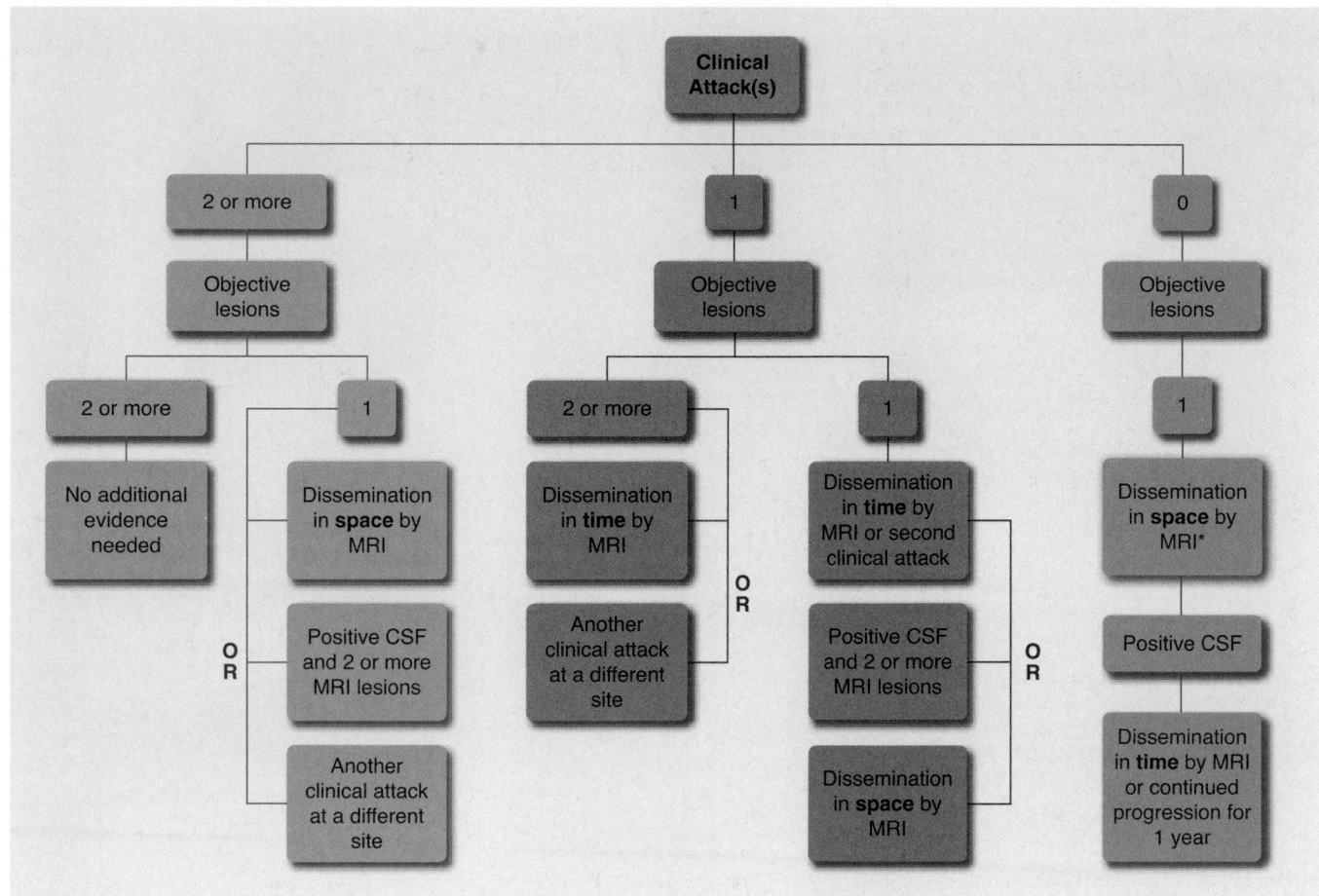

FIGURE 29–2. McDonald diagnostic criteria for MS.[17–19] MRI evidence of dissemination over time is a gadolinium-enhancing lesion on an MRI done at least 3 months following onset of clinical attack at a site different from the initial attack, or a gadolinium-enhancing lesion or new T2-weighted lesion 6 months following onset of clinical attack. Positive CSF is oligoclonal immunoglobulin G bands in CSF but not serum or elevated immunoglobulin G index. Positive evoked potentials are delayed, but maintain a well-preserved waveform. (CSF, cerebrospinal fluid.)

* Dissemination in space by MRI evidence of nine or more T2-weighted brain lesions, or two or more cord lesions, or four to eight brain and one cord lesion, or positive visual evoked potentials with four to eight MRI lesions, or positive visual evoked potentials with less than four brain lesions plus one cord lesion.

- Decrease in microglial proliferation, preserving myelin
- Promotion of formation of Th2 cells rather than Th1 cells, decreasing inflammation
- Inhibition of viruses, important if MS has a viral etiology[8,33]

Efficacy

Patients With Relapsing Remitting MS. A metaanalysis of all β-interferons determined that treated patients were 27% and 19% less likely to have a relapse during the first and second years of treatment, respectively, compared to placebo.[34] Early treatment after a first clinical attack delayed time to a second attack by 9 to 13 months compared to placebo.[35,36] Treating early is also associated with a lower incidence of developing clinically definite MS compared to delaying treatment.[37,38]

Patients With Secondary Progressive Ms Who Experience Relapses. β-Interferons have mixed results for slowing disease progression in secondary progressive MS. Treatment is most likely to be effective if clinical relapses or MRI signs of inflammatory activity are present.[39]

Adverse Effects. Adverse effects are common with the β-interferons (Table 29–3). Flu-like symptoms include fever, fatigue, muscle aches, malaise, and chills. Symptoms begin a few hours postinjection and dissipate within 8 to 24 hours.[40] Preventive measures can be employed (Table 29–4). In temperature-sensitive patients, β-interferon–induced fever can transiently worsen MS symptoms. Injection site reactions range from redness to necrosis. There are preventive and treatment measures for these reactions (Table 29–4). At the threshold laboratory values (Table 29–4), interferon should be suspended. When values normalize, interferon is resumed with gradual dose increases and careful monitoring.[40] α- and γ-interferons are associated with depression. Up to 50% of MS patients experience depression, even without

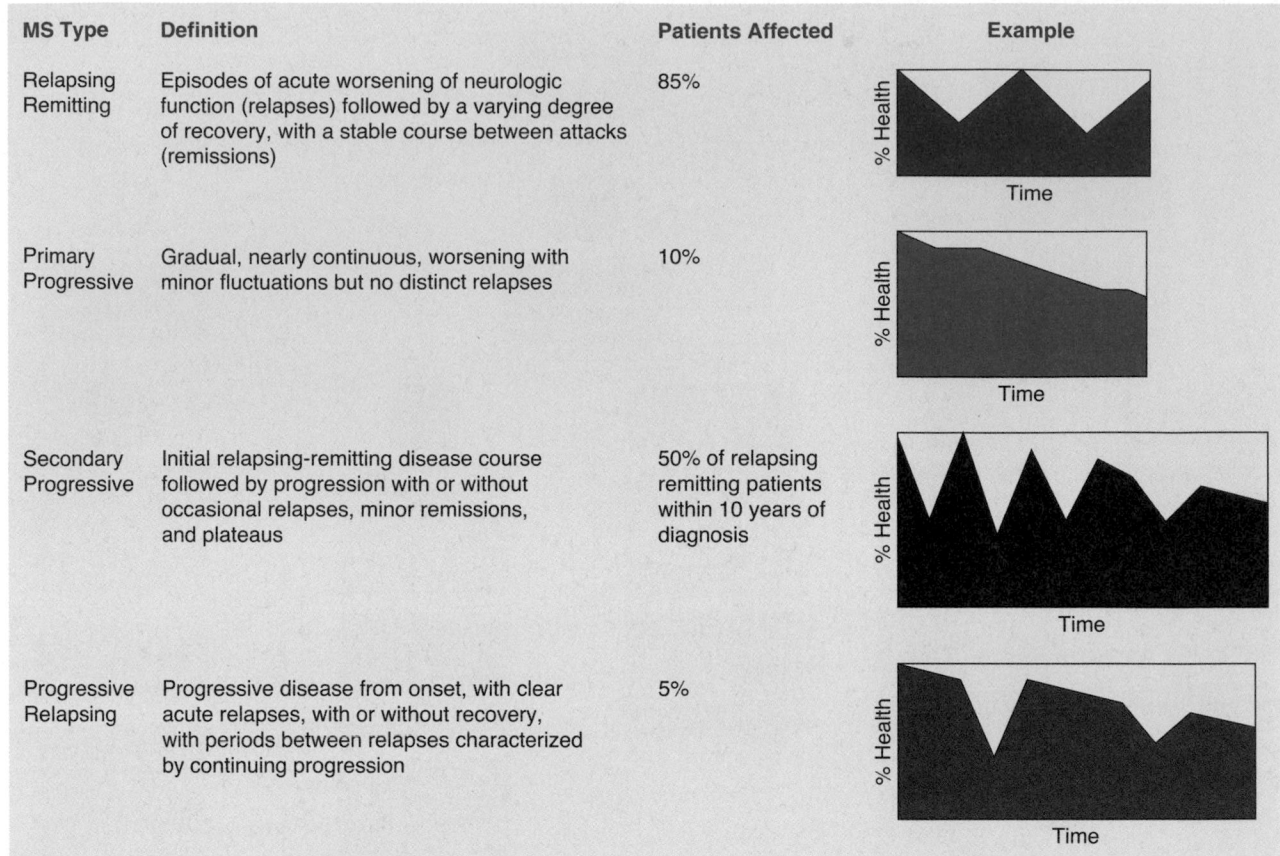

FIGURE 29–3. Comparison of clinical course of MS by type.

Table 29–2
Clinical Rating Scales Used in MS

EDSS

Rates functional systems from 0 (normal) to 10 (death due to MS)
Emphasis is on ambulation over other symptoms

MSFC

Three-part tool rating ambulation, limb function, and cognitive function
Composite score is compared to standardized population
Correlates better with MRI data than EDSS

MS, multiple sclerosis; EDSS, Expanded Disability Status Scale;
MSFC, multiple sclerosis functional composite.

From Refs. 21, 22.

Patient Encounter, Part 1

CN is a 28-year-old woman who complains of a 2-day history of weakness and tingling in her right arm and leg. These symptoms began over a 4-hour period. She also reports an episode 2 years ago of right eye pain and blurred vision that resolved over 1 month. She was diagnosed with **optic neuritis** at that time. Following an MRI, she is diagnosed with relapsing remitting MS today.

Why was her MS classified as relapsing remitting?
How would you treat the episode today?

β-interferon treatment.[14] Because of conflicting data, it is difficult to determine whether β-interferons cause or worsen MS-related depression.[14]

Tests for Responsiveness. Antibodies to β-interferons can reduce their clinical benefit.[41] **Neutralizing antibodies** develop 18 to 24 months after treatment begins.[41] Neutralizing antibodies can form against any β-interferon, but frequency

and route of administration affect neutralizing antibody development: 28% to 47% for subcutaneous interferon β-1b; 12% to 28% for subcutaneous interferon β-1a; and 2% to 6% for intramuscular interferon β-1a.[41]

Issues surround neutralizing antibodies including standardization of the neutralizing antibody assay, testing recommendations, and treatment recommendations for positive tests.[42] Neutralizing antibodies may disappear even

Table 29–3

Comparison of Disease-Modifying Therapies

Drug	Dose	Route	Frequency	Adverse Effects
Interferon β-1a (Avonex)	30 mcg	IM	Weekly	Flu-like symptoms 61% Anemia 8%
Interferon β-1a (Rebif)	44 mcg	SQ	3 × per week	Flu-like symptoms 28% Injection site reactions 66% Leukopenia 22% Increased aspartate aminotransferase/alanine transaminase 17–27%
Interferon β-1b (Betaseron)	0.25 mg	SQ	Every other day	Flu-like symptoms 60–76% Injection site reactions 50–85% Asthenia 49% Menstrual disorder 17% Leukopenia 10–16% Increased aspartate aminotransferase/alanine transaminase 4–19%
Glatiramer acetate (Copaxone)	20 mg	SQ	Daily	Injection site reaction 90% Systemic reaction 15%
Mitoxantrone (Novantrone)	12 mg/m^2 up to 140 mg/m^2 (maximum lifetime dose)	IV	Every 3 months	Nausea 76% Arrhythmia 3–18% Cardiotoxicity Alopecia 61% Menstrual disorders 61% Urinary tract infection 32% Amenorrhea 25% Leukopenia 19% γ-Glutamyl transpeptidase increase 15%
Natalizumab (Tysabri)	300 mg	IV	Every 4 weeks	Headache 38% Fatigue 27% Arthralgia 19% Urinary tract infection 20% Hypersensitivity reaction less than 1%

From Refs. 26, 40, 46, 49, 50.

Table 29–4

Prevention or Treatment Strategies for β-Interferon Adverse Effects

Flu-Like Symptoms	Injection Site Reaction	Laboratory Abnormalities[a]
Inject dose in the evening	Bring medication to room temperature	Hemoglobin less than 9.4 g/dL (94 g/L or 5.8 mmol/L) White blood cells less than 3 × 10^3/mm^3 (less than 3 × 10^9/L)
Begin at ¼–½ dose for 2 weeks of treatment, then increase to a full dose	Ice injection site prior to the injection Rotate injection sites	Absolute neutrophil count less than 1.5 × 10^3/mm^3 (less than 1.5 × 10^9/L)
Use ibuprofen 200 mg before and 6 and 12 hours after injection	If severe, use hydrocortisone 1% cream on the site	Platelets less than 75 × 10^3/mm^3 (less than 75 × 10^9/L) Bilirubin greater than 2.5 × baseline
Alternatives to ibuprofen include acetaminophen, prednisone taper, and pentoxifylline	If necrotic: Temporarily discontinue; consult dermatologist; do not use topical corticosteroids	AST/ALT greater than 5 × baseline Alkaline phosphatase greater than 5 × baseline

ALT, alanine aminotransferase; AST, aspartate aminotransferase.

[a]At these threshold values, β-interferon should be temporarily discontinued and laboratory values monitored.

From Refs. 40, 46.

during continued treatment.[43] Neutralizing antibodies exhibit cross-reactivity with other β-interferons.[42]

β-Interferons induce the expression of interferon-responsive genes, such as myxovirus-resistance-protein A (MxA). The ability of the patient to respond to β-interferons can be determined by testing MxA gene expression. Lack of expression is associated with MS relapses.[44]

Dosing and Administration. Dose, frequency, and route of administration differ between the β-interferon products (Table 29–3). **❼** *Dose–response curves have been observed with the β-interferons.* However, it is unknown if the total weekly dose or the frequency of administration is more important.[39]

Glatiramer Acetate

Pharmacology and Mechanism of Action. The mechanism of action of glatiramer acetate is unknown; the following properties have been observed:

- Binds to MHC class II, blocking the activation of T cells
- Activates Th2 cells, preventing inflammation
- Activated Th2 cells secrete brain-derived neurotrophic factor, which may be neuroprotective.[8,33]

Efficacy. Glatiramer acetate reduces relapses by 28% each year compared to placebo. Additionally, relapses occur later compared to placebo (322 vs 219 days).[45]

Adverse Effects. Patients report pain, redness, itching, swelling, and bruising at injection sites (Table 29–3). Icing the injection site pre- and post-injection improves these reactions; topical anesthetics can also be used. Systemic reactions involve flushing, chest tightness, palpitations, anxiety, and shortness of breath. This reaction usually occurs within 30 minutes of the injection; recurrence is infrequent. Doses may be reduced by 75% for the week following the reaction, then increased by 25% per week to the full dose.[46]

Issues With Self-Injected Disease-Modifying Therapies

Adherence. Adherence to injectable medications is a significant problem; but there is no significant difference in rates of discontinuation between products (17%–41%). Main reasons for discontinuation are adverse effects and lack of efficacy. Realistic expectations regarding therapy and higher educational levels improve adherence rates.[47]

Choosing Therapy. **❽** *There is no consensus on the best medication for initial therapy.* Comparative β-interferon trials indicate better efficacy with more frequent and/or higher dosing.[39] This consideration must be balanced with neutralizing antibody development, patient acceptance, and tolerance.

Patient Education. Refer to Table 29–5 for key components of patient self-injection education.

Mitoxantrone

Pharmacology and Mechanism of Action. Mitoxantrone is an anthracenedione antineoplastic indicated for MS. The

---

Table 29–5
Patient Education for Self-Injection

Keep all nonrefrigerated supplies together and out of the reach of children and pets

If refrigerated, allow medication to warm to room temperature

Wash hands thoroughly

Choose injection site, rotating among sites

Ice area to be injected for no more than 15 minutes, if desired

Clean injection site thoroughly with alcohol or soap and water

Administer injection

Ice injection site for no more than 15 minutes after injection, if desired

---

mechanisms of action thought to be important for MS are as shown below:

- Causes **apoptosis** in T and APCs, preventing initial T cell activation
- Inhibits DNA and RNA synthesis, decreasing the proliferation of T cells, B cells, and macrophages
- Decreases cytokine release, preventing inflammation
- Inhibits macrophages, preventing myelin degradation[48]

Efficacy. Mitoxantrone is indicated for secondary progressive MS, progressive relapsing MS, and for patients with worsening relapsing remitting MS. It reduces the clinical attack rate and attack-related MRI outcome measures in patients with relapsing disease. **❾** *Because of significant potential for toxicities, mitoxantrone should be reserved for patients with rapidly advancing disease who have failed other therapies.*[26]

Adverse Effects. Adverse effects are seen regularly in patients given mitoxantrone (Table 29–3). Bluish discoloration of the sclera and the urine often lasts 24 hours postinfusion.[49] Transient leukopenia and neutropenia are common (nadir 10–14 days after the infusion); exposure to infectious individuals during this time should be avoided.[49] Patients taking mitoxantrone should not receive live virus vaccines; other vaccines should be held for 4 to 6 weeks after a mitoxantrone dose.[49] Amenorrhea may be permanent, an important consideration in women of child-bearing potential.[26]

Arrhythmias may occur shortly after the drug is given. Cardiotoxicity is a serious, rare adverse effect of mitoxantrone. The incidence of congestive heart failure was 0.15% in patients with normal left ventricular ejection fraction and 2.18% in those who had asymptomatic left ventricular ejection fraction of less than 50% at baseline.[49] Therefore, mitoxantrone should not be used in patients with baseline cardiomyopathy, even if asymptomatic. The risk of cardiotoxicity is dose related. The maximum lifetime dose of mitoxantrone is 140 mg/m^2 (about 3 years of therapy). Cyclooxygenase-2 inhibitors should be avoided in patients receiving mitoxantrone because of a potential for worsening cardiac toxicity.[49]

Acute myelogenous leukemia occurred in 0.07% of mitoxantrone-treated patients.[49] This acute leukemia appears within 2 to 4 years of initiating mitoxantrone and is generally responsive to standard antileukemic therapy.

Table 29–6		
Monitoring Disease-Modifying Therapies		
Therapy	**Tests**	**Frequency**
β-Interferons (Avonex, Betaseron, Rebif)	CBC, bilirubin, electrolytes, AST, ALT, γ-glutamyl transferase, alkaline phosphatase	Baseline, 4–6 weeks, 12 weeks, then every 3 months
	EDSS, MSFC, neurologic history and examination	Every 3 months during the first year of therapy then every 6 months
Mitoxantrone (Novantrone)	CBC, bilirubin, AST, ALT, alkaline phosphatase, pregnancy test	Before each infusion
	ECG	Baseline
	Echocardiogram or MUGA scan	Baseline and every 6–12 months; prior to each infusion after 100 mg/m²
	EDSS, MSFC, neurologic history and examination	Every 3 months during the first year of therapy then every 6 months
Glatiramer acetate (Copaxone)	EDSS, MSFC, neurologic history and examination	Every 3 months during the first year of therapy then every 6 months
Natalizumab (Tysabri)	EDSS, MSFC, neurologic history and examination	Every 3 months during the first year of therapy then every 6 months
	MRI, CSF examination for JC virus	At onset of new neurologic symptoms not suggestive of MS
	Preinfusion patient checklist	Prior to every infusion
	Status report and reauthorization questionnaire	Every 6 months

ALT, alanine aminotransferase; AST, aspartate aminotransferase; CBC, complete blood count; CSF, cerebrospinal fluid; EDSS, Expanded Disability Status Scale; MS, multiple sclerosis; MSFC, Multiple Sclerosis Functional Composite; MUGA, multiple gated acquisition.

Dosing and Administration Mitoxantrone is infused intravenously over 30 minutes to reduce the chance of cardiotoxicity.[49] Mitoxantrone is administered every 3 months, if cardiac function and laboratory values are normal (Table 29–6).

Natalizumab

Pharmacology and Mechanism of Action. Natalizumab is a α_4-integrin antagonist indicated for relapsing forms of MS. Its postulated mechanism of action follows:

- Binds to $\alpha_4\beta_1$ and $\alpha_4\beta_7$ integrins, preventing migration of lymphocytes into the CNS and inflammation
- Inhibits binding of α_4-positive leukocytes to fibronectin and osteopontin, decreasing the activation of leukocytes already within the CNS[50]

Efficacy. Treatment with natalizumab reduced relapses by 68% at 1 year and disability by 42% at 2 years compared to placebo.[50]

Adverse Effects. Adverse effects of natalizumab include infection, arthralgia, headache, and fatigue.[50] Hypersensitivity reactions have been observed; symptoms may include itching, dizziness, fever, rash, hypotension, dyspnea, chest pain, and anaphylaxis, usually within 2 hours of administration. A much more serious, but rare, adverse effect is progressive multifocal leukoencephalopathy (PML). PML, caused by the JC polyomavirus virus, is rapidly progressive and usually results in death or permanent disability. Shortly after natalizumab was introduced, three patients developed PML, leading to temporary withdrawal of the medicine. Natalizumab was reintroduced through a restricted distribution program. ❾ These concerns lead to the recommendation that *natalizumab be reserved for patients with rapidly advancing disease who have failed other therapies.* Specific recommendations are to avoid in patients with PML, HIV, immunodeficiency, or hematological malignancy; to carefully assess for immune compromise in patients previously treated with immunosuppression or chemotherapy; and to perform a baseline cranial MRI for later comparison if new neurologic symptoms develop.[51]

Antinatalizumab antibodies develop in 9% to 12% of patients. If patients are persistently antibody-positive, relapse rates and disability increase; antibody development is also associated with hypersensitivity reactions.[52]

Dosing and Administration. Natalizumab should be used as monotherapy for MS.[51] Natalizumab is administered 300 mg in 100 mL normal saline over a 1-hour IV infusion every 4 weeks. Patients have not been treated for more than 2 years with natalizumab.

Outcome Evaluation

- Assess periodically for changes in symptoms.
- In patients taking β-interferons with frequent relapses, testing for neutralizing antibodies and/or MxA gene expression may assist in choosing therapy.
- Monitor the patient for medication-specific adverse effects (Tables 29–3 and 29–6).
- Assess regularly for adherence with all components of therapy.

▶ *Symptomatic Therapies*

MS patients develop many symptoms that require treatment. The symptoms most unique to MS are fatigue and spasticity. Other important symptoms such as urinary incontinence, pain, depression, cognitive impairment, and sexual dysfunction are discussed only briefly (refer to other chapters).

Fatigue There are nonpharmacologic and pharmacologic strategies for decreasing the impact of fatigue on the lifestyle of MS patients (Table 29–7). Pharmacologic management of fatigue includes amantadine or stimulants; however, evidence of efficacy from randomized controlled trials is limited.

Spasticity The goals of treating spasticity are patient-specific. For ambulatory patients, reducing spasticity may improve mobility. For bed-bound patients, treating spasticity may relieve pain and facilitate transfers and care. Physical therapy is a nonpharmacologic treatment for spasticity.[10]

MS patients usually have upper motor neuron spasticity; this type of spasticity cannot be treated with muscle relaxants (i.e., carisoprodol). ❿ *MS patients must be treated with agents specific for upper motor neuron spasticity (Table 29–8).*[10] MS spasticity is classified as focal or generalized. If the spasticity involves only one muscle group, it is focal and may benefit from botulinum toxin administration.[10] Systemic medications are used for generalized spasticity. No clear conclusion can be reached regarding the superiority in efficacy of one agent; medication selection is usually based on adverse effects (see Table 29–8).[10]

Other Symptoms Two types of urinary tract symptoms are commonly seen in MS: Incomplete bladder emptying and incontinence. Incomplete bladder emptying is due to dyscoordination of the external urethral sphincter and detrusor activity.[13] Most patients who develop this condition require intermittent or permanent urinary catheterization.[13] Incontinence in most MS patients is caused by neurogenic detrusor overactivity. First-line treatments are anticholinergics such as oxybutynin, tolterodine, flavoxate, or antimuscarinic tricyclic antidepressants.

Bowel symptoms in MS patients can include both fecal incontinence and constipation. Fecal incontinence is difficult to treat; a regular schedule for emptying the bowel with laxative suppositories or enemas may be helpful. Alternatively, antidiarrheal medications such as loperamide can be used.[13]

Pain may occur in up to 86% of patients with MS. Pain may be neuropathic, related to spasticity, related to treatment, or unrelated to MS. Correct pain type classification is necessary for effective treatment.[16]

Desipramine and sertraline are efficacious for MS-related depression.[14] If β-interferon treatment appears to be causing depression, discontinuation could be considered.

Patient Encounter, Part 2

CN begins to improve after 2 days of methylprednisolone 1 g IV daily. The treatment team wants to begin a disease-modifying treatment.

Do you agree that she should be on a disease-modifying treatment? Why?

If so, which treatment would you choose? Recommend a dosing regimen.

How should the patient be counseled on the chosen treatment?

Table 29–7

Pharmacologic and Nonpharmacologic Treatments for Fatigue

Nonpharmacologic	Pharmacologic	Renal Dosing
Appropriate rest-to-activity ratio Use of assistive devices to conserve energy	*First-line therapy:* Amantadine 100 mg orally every morning and early afternoon	CrCl 30–50 mL/min 100 mg/day CrCl 15–29 mL/min 100 mg every other day CrCl less than 15 mL/min 200 mg every 7 days
Environmental modifications to make activities more energy-efficient		
Cooling strategies to avoid fatigue caused by elevations in core body temperature due to heat, exercise-related exertion, and fever	*Second-line therapy:* Methylphenidate 10–20 mg every morning and noon	
Regular aerobic exercise, geared to the person's ability, to promote cardiovascular health, strength, improved mood, and reduce fatigue		
Stress management techniques		

CrCl, creatinine clearance.

From Refs. 11, 53.

Table 29–8

Comparison of Antispasticity Agents

Place in Therapy	Medication	Mechanism of Action	Dose
First-line	Baclofen	Pre- and post-synaptic γ-aminobutyric acid β-receptor blocker	5 mg orally 3 × daily, increase by 5 mg/dose every 3 days to a maximum of 80 mg/day *Renal dysfunction:* Dose reduction may be necessary
	Tizanidine	Centrally acting a_2-receptor agonist	4 mg orally daily, increase by 2–4 mg 3–4 × daily to a maximum of 36 mg/day *Hepatic and renal dysfunction:* Dose reduction may be necessary
Second-line	Dantrolene	Direct inhibitor of muscle contraction by decreasing the release of calcium from skeletal muscle sarcoplasmic reticulum	25 mg orally daily, increase to 25 mg 3–4 × daily, then increase by 25 mg every 4–7 days to a maximum of 400 mg/day
	Diazepam	γ-Aminobutyric acid agonist	2–10 mg orally 3–4 × daily *Cirrhosis:* Reduce dose by 50%
Third-line	Intrathecal baclofen	Pre- and post-synaptic γ-aminobutyric acid β-receptor blocker	Titrated individually, usual range 62–749 mcg/day
Focal spasticity	Botulinum toxin	Prevents release of acetylcholine in the neuromuscular junction	Individualized

Data from Refs. 10, 54.

Patient Encounter, Part 3

After 3 years of treatment, CN has had one additional relapse, but otherwise is doing fairly well. At her routine clinic appointment, she describes some difficulty walking due to leg spasticity and urinary incontinence episodes that occur about twice a week.

What treatment options are available for spasticity, and which would you choose?

Should this patient's incontinence be treated? If so, what medication would you recommend?

Cognitive impairment and memory dysfunction can be troublesome, affecting 40% to 60% of patients. Treatment with β-interferon has demonstrated improvement. Acetylcholinesterase inhibitors may also be beneficial.[55]

Phosphodiesterase type 5 inhibitors are effective for MS-induced erectile dysfunction.[13] In women, vaginal dryness or dyspareunia may respond to lubricating jellies.

Outcome Evaluation

- Assess for improvement/recurrence of symptoms.
- Monitor for adverse effects of medications.
- Monitor for adherence.

Patient Care and Monitoring

1. Once diagnosed, work with the patient to select either a β-interferon or glatiramer acetate, considering:
   - Route of administration
   - Frequency of administration
   - Adverse-effect profile and other concerns (e.g., neutralizing antibodies and concomitant depression)
2. Obtain the required baseline laboratory studies (Table 29–6).
3. Educate the patient regarding self-injection (Table 29–5).
4. Assess the patient for symptomatic treatment needs.
5. Initiate needed symptomatic treatments.
6. Refer the patient to the National MS Society for information, newsletters, and local support groups (www.nmss.org).
7. Instruct the patient to contact the clinician for any sudden changes in symptoms that may suggest a relapse.
8. Monitor the patient for efficacy and adverse effects of disease-modifying and symptomatic therapies every 3 months for the first year and every 6 months thereafter and as required for selected therapy (Table 29–6).
9. Treat any relapses with methylprednisolone IV or prednisone orally.

Abbreviations Introduced in This Chapter

Abs	Autoantibodies
ALT	Alanine aminotransferase
APC	Antigen-presenting cell
AST	Aspartate aminotransferase
CAM	Cellular adhesion molecule
CSF	Cerebrospinal fluid
EDSS	Expanded Disability Status Scale
HHV-6	Human herpes virus 6
IL	Interleukin
LT	Lymphotoxin
MHC	Major histocompatibility complex
MMP	Matrix metalloproteinase
MS	Multiple sclerosis
MSFC	Multiple Sclerosis Functional Composite
MUGA	Multiple gated acquisition
MxA	Myxovirus-resistance-protein A
NO	Nitric oxide
PML	Progressive multifocal leukoencephalopathy
TCR	T-cell receptor
TGF	Transforming growth factor
Th1	T-helper-1 cells
Th2	T-helper-2 cells
TNF	Tumor necrosis factor

Self-assessment questions and answers are available at *http://www.mhpharmacotherapy.com/pp.html.*

REFERENCES

1. National Multiple Sclerosis Society. Just the facts: 2006–2007. Available at *http://www.nationalmssociety.org/multimedia-library/brochures/general-information/download.aspx?id=22.*
2. Zorzon M, Zivadinov R, Nasuelli D, et al. Risk factors of multiple sclerosis: A case-control study. Neurol Sci 2003;24:242–247.
3. Sundstrom P, Nystrom L, Hallmans G. Smoke exposure increases the risk for multiple sclerosis. Eur J Neurol 2008;15:579–583.
4. Gale CR, Martyn CN. Migrant studies in multiple sclerosis. Prog Neurobiol 1995;47:425–448.
5. Oksenberg JR, Baranzini SE, Sawcer S, Hauser SL. The genetics of multiple sclerosis: SNPs to pathways to pathogenesis. Nature 2008; 9:516–526.
6. Fotheringham J, Jacobson S. Human herpesvirus 6 and multiple sclerosis: Potential mechanisms for virus-induced disease. Herpes 2005; 12:4–9.
7. Wiendl H, Kieseier BC. Disease-modifying therapies in multiple sclerosis: An update on recent and ongoing trials and future strategies. Expert Opin Invest Drugs 2003;12:689–712.
8. Hartung HP, Bar-Or A, Zoukos Y. What do we know about the mechanism of action of disease-modifying treatments in MS? J Neurol 2004;251(Suppl 5):v12–v29.
9. Kuhlmann T, Lingfeld G, Bitsch A, et al. Acute axonal damage in multiple sclerosis is most extensive in early disease stages and decreases over time. Brain 2002;125: 2202–2212.
10. Hasselkorn JK, Balsdon RC, Fry WD, et al. Overview of spasticity management in multiple sclerosis. Evidence-based management strategies for spasticity treatment in multiple sclerosis. J Spinal Cord Med 2005;28:167–199.
11. Lapierre Y, Hum S. Treating fatigue. Int MS J 2007;14: 64–71.
12. Andersson KE, Pehron R. CNS involvement in overactive bladder: Pathophysiology and opportunities for pharmacological intervention. Drugs 2003;63: 2595–2611.
13. DasGupta R, Fowler CJ. Bladder, bowel and sexual dysfunction in multiple sclerosis: Management strategies. Drugs 2003;63:153–166.
14. Goldman Consensus Group. The Goldman Consensus statement on depression in multiple sclerosis. Mult Scler 2005;11:328–337.
15. Pittock SJ, McClelland BL, Mayr WT, et al. Prevalence of tremor in multiple sclerosis and associated disability in the Olmsted County population. Mov Disord 2004;19:1482–1485.
16. Pollmann W, Feneberg W. Current management of pain associated with multiple sclerosis. CNS Drugs 2008; 22:291–324.
17. McDonald WI, Compston A, Edan G, et al. Recommended diagnostic criteria for multiple sclerosis: Guidelines from the international panel on the diagnosis of multiple sclerosis. Ann Neurol 2001;50:121–127.
18. Dalton CM, Brex PA, Miszkiel KA, et al. Application of the new McDonald criteria to patients with clinically isolated syndrome suggestive of multiple sclerosis. Ann Neurol 2002;52:47–53.
19. Tintore M, Rovira A, Rio J, et al. New diagnostic criteria for multiple sclerosis: Application in first demyelinating episode. Neurology 2003;60:27–30.
20. Keegan BM, Noseworthy JH. Multiple sclerosis. Annu Rev Med 2002;53:285–302.
21. Rudick RA, Cutter G, Reingold S. The Multiple Sclerosis Functional Composite: A new clinical outcome measure for multiple sclerosis trials. Mult Scler 2002;8:359–365.
22. Kurtzke JF. Rating neurologic impairment in multiple sclerosis: An expanded disability status scale (EDSS). Neurology 1983;33:1444–1452.
23. Sadovnick AD, Ebers GC, Wilson RW, et al. Life expectancy in patients attending multiple sclerosis clinics. Neurology 1992;42:991–994.
24. Sadovnick AD, Eisen K, Ebers GC, Paty DW. Cause of death in patients attending multiple sclerosis clinics. Neurology 1991;41:1193–1196.
25. Sloka JS, Stefanelli M. The mechanism of action of methylprednisolone in the treatment of multiple sclerosis. Mult Scler 2005;11:425–432.
26. Goodin DS, Frohman EM, Garmany GP, et al. Disease modifying therapies in multiple sclerosis: Report of the Therapeutics and Technology Assessment Subcommittee of the American Academy of Neurology and the MS Council for Clinical Practice Guidelines. Neurology 2002;58:169–178.
27. Filippini G, Brusaferri F, Sibley WA, et al. Corticosteroids or ACTH for acute exacerbations in multiple sclerosis (review). *Cochrane Database Syst Rev* 2000;4: CD001331.
28. Beck RW, Cleary PA, Anderson MM, et al. A randomized, controlled trial of corticosteroids in the treatment of acute optic neuritis. The Optic Neuritis Study Group 1992;326:581–588.
29. Morrow SA, Stoian CA, Dmitrovic J, et al. The bioavailability of IV methylprednisolone and oral prednisone in multiple sclerosis. Neurology 2004;63:1079–1080.
30. Alam SM, Kyriakides T, Lawden M, Newman PK. Methylprednisolone in multiple sclerosis: A comparison of oral with intravenous therapy at equivalent high dose. J Neurol Neurosurg Psychiatry 1993;56:1219–1220.
31. Perumal JS, Caon C, Hreha S, et al. Oral prednisone taper following intravenous steroids fails to improve disability or recovery from relapses in multiple sclerosis. Eur J Neurol 2008;15:677–680.
32. Medical Advisory Board of the National Multiple Sclerosis Society, Changing Therapy Consensus Statement Taskforce. Changing therapy in relapsing multiple sclerosis: Considerations and recommendations of a task force of the National Multiple Sclerosis Society. Available at *http://www.nationalmssociety.org/for-professionals/healthcare-professionals/expert-opinion-papers/download.aspx?id=129.*
33. Dhib-Jalbut S. Mechanisms of action of interferons and glatiramer acetate in multiple sclerosis. *Neurology* 2002;58:S3–S9.

34. Filippini G, Munari L, Incorvaia B, et al. Interferons in relapsing remitting multiple sclerosis: A systematic review. Lancet 2003;361:545–552.

35. Jacobs LD, Beck RW, Simon JH, et al. Intramuscular interferon beta-1a therapy initiated during a first demyelinating event in multiple sclerosis. N Engl J Med 2000;343:898–904.

36. Comi G, Filippi M, Barkhof F, et al. Effect of early interferon treatment on conversion to definite multiple sclerosis: A randomized study. Lancet 2001;357:1576–1582.

37. CHAMPIONS Study Group. IM interferon β-1a delays definite multiple sclerosis 5 years after a first demyelinating event. Neurology 2006;66:678–684.

38. Kappos L, Freedman MS, Polman CH, et al. Effect of early versus delayed interferon beta-1b treatment on disability after a first clinical event suggestive of multiple sclerosis: A 3-year follow-up analysis of the BENEFIT study. Lancet 2007;370:389–397.

39. Multiple Sclerosis Therapy Consensus Group. Escalating immunotherapy of multiple sclerosis: New aspects and practical application. J Neurol 2004;251:1329–1339.

40. Moses H, Brandes DW. Managing adverse effects of disease-modifying agents used for treatment of multiple sclerosis. Curr Med Res Opin 2008;24:2679–2690.

41. Vartanian T, Sorensen PS, Rice G. Impact of neutralizing antibodies on the clinical efficacy of interferon beta in multiple sclerosis. J Neurol 2004;251(Suppl 2):II25–II30.

42. Hartung HP, Munschauer F, Schellekens H. Significance of neutralizing antibodies to interferon beta during treatment of multiple sclerosis: Expert opinions based on the Proceedings of an International Consensus Conference. Eur J Neurol 2005;12:588–601.

43. Soelberg Sorensen P, Koch-Henriksen N, Ross C, et al. Appearance and disappearance of neutralizing antibodies during interferon-beta therapy. Neurology 2005;65:33–39.

44. Malucchi S, Gilli F, Caldano M, et al. Predictive markers for response to interferon therapy in patients with multiple sclerosis. Neurology 2008;70:1119–1127.

45. Boneschi FM, Rovaris M, Johnson KP, et al. Effects of glatiramer acetate on relapse rate and accumulated disability in multiple sclerosis: Meta-analysis of three double-blind, randomized, placebo-controlled clinical trials. Mult Scler 2003;9:349–355.

46. Galetta SL, Markowitz C. U.S. FDA-approved disease-modifying treatments for multiple sclerosis: Review of adverse effect profiles. CNS Drugs 2005;29:239–252.

47. Daugherty KK, Butler JS, Mattingly M, Ryan M. Factors leading patients to discontinue multiple sclerosis therapies. J Am Pharm Assoc 2005;45:371–375.

48. Chofflon M. Mechanisms of action for treatments in multiple sclerosis: Does a heterogeneous disease demand and multi-targeted therapeutic approach? Biodrugs 2005;19:299–308.

49. Cohen BA, Mikol DD. Mitoxantrone treatment of multiple sclerosis: Safety considerations. Neurology 2004;63:S28–S32.

50. Polman CH, O'Connor PW, Havrdova E, et al. A randomized, placebo-controlled trial of natalizumab for relapsing multiple sclerosis. N Eng J Med 2006;354; 899–910.

51. Kappos L, Bates D, Hartung HP, et al. Natalizumab treatment for multiple sclerosis: Recommendations for patient selection and monitoring. Lancet Neurol 2007;6:431–441.

52. Calabresi PA, Giovannoni G, Confavreux C, et al. The incidence and significance of anti-natalizumab antibodies: Results from AFFIRM and SENTINEL. Neurology 2007;69:1391–1403.

53. Lee D, Newell R, Ziegler L, Topping A. Treatment of fatigue in multiple sclerosis: A systematic review of the literature. Int J Nurs Pract 2008;14:81–93.

54. Shakespeare DT, Boggild M, Young C. Anti-spasticity agents for multiple sclerosis. The Cochrane Database of Systematic Reviews 2003; Issue 4. Art. No.: CD001332. DOI: 10.1001/14651858.CD001332.

55. Christodoulou C, Melville P, Scherl WF, et al. Effect of donepezil on memory and cognition in multiple sclerosis. J Neurol Sci 2006;245: 127–136.

30 Epilepsy

Timothy E. Welty and Edward Faught

LEARNING OBJECTIVES

● **Upon completion of the chapter, the reader will be able to:**

1. Describe the epidemiology and social impact of epilepsy.
2. Define terminology related to epilepsy, including seizure, convulsion, and epilepsy.
3. Describe the basic pathophysiology of seizures.
4. Describe the basic pathophysiology of epilepsy.
5. Differentiate and classify seizure types when provided a description of the clinical presentation of the seizure and electroencephalogram.
6. Identify key therapeutic decision points in the treatment of epilepsy.
7. Establish therapeutic goals for pharmacotherapy in a patient with epilepsy.
8. Discuss nonpharmacologic treatments for epilepsy.
9. Recommend an appropriate pharmacotherapeutic regimen for the treatment of epilepsy.
10. Select appropriate monitoring parameters for a pharmacotherapeutic regimen of epilepsy.
11. Devise a plan for switching a patient from one antiepileptic regimen to a different regimen.
12. Recognize complications of pharmacotherapy for epilepsy.
13. Analyze potential drug interactions with antiepileptic drugs (AEDs).
14. Determine when and how to discontinue AED therapy.
15. Educate a patient or caregiver on epilepsy and pharmacotherapy for this disorder.

KEY CONCEPTS

❶ A distinction among convulsions, a single seizure, pseudoseizure, and epilepsy should be made in patients presenting with possible seizures.

❷ Selection of appropriate pharmacotherapy is dependent upon distinguishing, identifying, and understanding different seizure types.

❸ Prior to starting pharmacologic therapy, it is essential to determine the risk of having a subsequent seizure.

❹ Mechanisms of action, effectiveness for specific seizure types, common adverse effects, and potential for drug interactions are key elements in selecting a medication for individual patients.

❺ Antiepileptic drugs (AEDs) therapy should usually be initiated carefully using a titration schedule to minimize adverse events.

❻ Changes in AED regimens should be done in a stepwise fashion, keeping in mind drug interactions that may be present and that may necessitate dosage changes in concomitant drugs.

❼ Discontinuation of AEDs should be done gradually, only after the patient has been seizure-free for 2 to 5 years, and with careful consideration of factors predictive of seizure recurrence.

❽ Children and women with epilepsy have unique problems related to the use of AEDs.

❾ Patients receiving AEDs for seizures should have regular monitoring for seizure frequency, seizure patterns, acute adverse effects, chronic adverse effects, and possible drug interactions.

EPIDEMIOLOGY, SOCIAL IMPACT, AND ETIOLOGY

Epidemiology

● **Epilepsy** is a disorder that afflicts approximately 2 million individuals in the United States, with an age-adjusted prevalence of approximately 4 to 7 cases/1,000 persons.[1] The incidence of epilepsy in the United States is estimated at

35 to 75 cases/100,000 persons per year, which is similar to that of other developed countries.[2,3] In developing countries, the incidence is higher at 100 to 190 cases/100,000 persons per year, possibly related to poor health care and prenatal care, increased risk of neurologic trauma, and increased rates of infections. About 8% of the U.S. population will experience a seizure during their lifetime. New onset seizures occur most frequently in infants less than 1 year of age and in adults after age 55.[4] However, the largest number of patients suffering from epilepsy is between the ages of 15 and 64 years.

Social Impact

Epilepsy is a disorder with profound impact on a patient's life. All states limit driving for individuals who have recently had a seizure with impaired consciousness, and restrictions vary from state to state.[5] Patients who live in communities without adequate public transportation face major impediments to simple activities of life, such as purchasing groceries or getting to a job. Education is also problematic for patients with epilepsy.[6,7] Individuals with persistent seizures have poor school attendance. Fifty percent of patients with epilepsy complain of cognitive difficulties and believe their seizures interfere with learning. Additionally, patients with epilepsy score 50% lower on standardized examinations and have lower graduation rates from high school and college. Transportation and educational difficulties combine with persistent seizures to cause patients with epilepsy to be unemployed or underemployed. Thus, this group of patients faces multiple financial difficulties and often do not have health insurance.

Finally, patients with epilepsy are often dependent upon caregivers to assist with medications, transportation, and ensuring the patient's safety. Caregivers should be informed of the patient's medical needs and how to assist should a seizure occur.

Etiology

For nearly 80% of patients with epilepsy, the underlying etiology is unknown.[8] The most common recognized causes of epilepsy are head trauma and stroke. Developmental and genetic defects are the cause of about 5% of cases of epilepsy. CNS tumors, CNS infections, and neurodegenerative diseases are other common causes. Other important causes of epilepsy are HIV infection or neurocysticercosis infection, primarily occurring in Latin America.

Isolated seizures that are not epilepsy can be caused by stroke, CNS trauma, CNS infections, metabolic disturbances (e.g., hyponatremia, hypoglycemia), and hypoxia. If these underlying causes of seizures are not corrected, they may lead to the development of recurrent seizures or epilepsy. Medications can also cause seizures. Some drugs that are commonly associated with seizures include tramadol, buproprion, theophylline, some antidepressants, some antipsychotics, amphetamines, cocaine, imipenem, lithium, excessive doses of penicillins or cephalosporins, and sympathomimetics or stimulants.

PATHOPHYSIOLOGY

Seizures

Regardless of the underlying etiology, all seizures involve a sudden electrical disturbance of the cerebral cortex. A population of neurons fires rapidly and repetitively for seconds to minutes. Cortical electrical discharges become excessively rapid, rhythmic, and synchronous. This phenomenon is presumably related to an excess of excitatory neurotransmitter action, a failure of inhibitory neurotransmitter action, or a combination of the two. In the individual patient, however, it is usually impossible to identify which neurochemical factors are responsible.

Neurotransmitters

The major excitatory neurotransmitter in the cerebral cortex is glutamate.[9] When glutamate is released from a presynaptic neuron, it attaches to one of several receptor types on the postsynaptic neuron. The result is opening of membrane channels to allow sodium or calcium to flow into the postsynaptic neuron, thus depolarizing it and transmitting the excitatory signal.[10] Many antiepileptic drugs (e.g., phenytoin, carbamazepine, lamotrigine) work by interfering with this mechanism, either by blocking the release of glutamate or by blocking the sodium or calcium channels, thus preventing excessive excitation.[11] These drugs typically do not block normal neuronal signaling, only the excessively rapid firing characteristic of a seizure. For this reason, they do not usually affect normal brain function.

The major inhibitory neurotransmitter in the cerebral cortex is *gamma-aminobutyric acid* (GABA). It attaches to neuronal membranes and opens chloride channels. When chloride flows into the neuron, it becomes hyperpolarized and less excitable. This mechanism is probably critical for shutting off seizure activity by controlling the excessive neuronal firing. Some antiepileptic drugs (AEDs), primarily barbiturates and benzodiazepines, work by enhancing the action of GABA.

Cortical function is modulated by many other neurotransmitters. However, their role in the pathophysiology of epilepsy and in the action of AEDs is not yet well known.

Neuronal Mechanisms

Seizures originate in a group of neurons that do not have normal electrical behavior.[12] Presumably, this is due to an underlying imbalance of neurotransmitter function as described above. At the level of the individual neuron, firing is excessively prolonged and repetitive. Instead of firing a single action potential, these neurons stay depolarized too long, firing a train of many action potentials. This long, abnormal depolarization is called a *paroxysmal depolarizing shift* (PDS).

The excessive electrical discharges can spread to other neurons, either adjacent ones or distant ones connected by fiber tracts. The seizure thus spreads to other areas of the brain, recruiting them into the uncontrolled firing pattern. The neurons involved may not be abnormal themselves, but are diverted from their normal functioning to participate in the wildly excessive discharges. The degree of spread and the location of brain areas involved determine the clinical manifestations of the seizure.

Nearly all seizures stop spontaneously, because after seconds to minutes, brain inhibitory mechanisms become strong enough to shut off the abnormal excitation.

Epilepsy

Epilepsy is the tendency to have seizures on a chronic, recurrent basis. This implies that there is a permanent change in cortical function which renders neurons more likely to participate in a seizure discharge. This process is referred to as epileptogenesis, and the exact way in which it occurs is not known. A process thought to be similar to epileptogenesis in humans occurs after prolonged, intermittent electrical stimulation of animal brains and is known as kindling. Epilepsy may develop days, months, or many years after an insult to the cortex. It may be that an originally small group of abnormal neurons causes adjacent or connected neurons to gradually become abnormal as well, by bombarding them over time with frequent, repeated electrical impulses. When the network of abnormal neurons becomes sufficiently large, it becomes capable of sustaining an excessive firing pattern for at least several seconds: a seizure. This hyperexcitable network of neurons is then the seizure focus.

If the change in cortical electrical characteristics is permanent, why don't seizures occur all the time? This is probably because the occurrence of an individual seizure depends upon an interplay of environmental and internal brain factors that, from time to time, result in loss of the normal mechanisms that contain and control abnormal neuronal firing. Some common factors are sleep loss and fatigue, but it is impossible to determine what sets off a particular seizure in most patients.

Clinical Presentation and Diagnosis of Epilepsy

General

Typically, health care providers are not able to observe a patient's seizures and for most types of seizures the patient has no memory of the event. It is important to obtain a careful history from the patient and any individuals who witness the seizures.

Common Descriptions of Seizures

The clinical presentation of seizures will vary from patient to patient depending on the portion of brain involved in the seizure. Events will tend to be stereotypical for an individual patient.

Patients who experience seizures may complain of paroxysmal spells of

- Blanking out spells, lapses in memory, periods of altered consciousness
- Warnings or auras consisting of various sensations or automatic, uncontrolled movements
- Daydreaming
- Jerks, shoulder shrugs, sudden chills of spine
- Falling out

Associated Symptoms

- Incontinence, usually of urine
- Tongue biting
- Traumatic injuries, usually associated with falling during a seizure

Diagnosis

Description of events: The patient and any witnesses to the seizures should be carefully interviewed to obtain a full and complete description of typical seizures.

Neurologic examination: Usually, the neurologic physical examination is completely normal. Any neurologic deficits that are identified should be fully investigated because seizures do not usually cause permanent, detectable neurologic deficits.

Electroencephalogram (EEG): A routine EEG can be helpful if epileptiform discharges are seen. However, the EEG may be normal between seizures and most routine EEGs are not performed during a seizure. Maneuvers such as sleep deprivation, photic stimulation, hyperventilation, or prolonged monitoring can help expose EEG changes consistent with epilepsy.

Neuroimaging (preferably an MRI of the brain): Imaging of the brain is important to rule out obvious causes of seizures such as stroke or tumors. An MRI scan is also helpful in detecting mesial temporal sclerosis, a finding often associated with mesial temporal epilepsy and predictive of positive surgical outcomes.

Video EEG monitoring: A procedure consisting of continuous video monitoring of the patient with a simultaneous EEG. Usually a patient is monitored in the hospital for 4 to 5 days. This procedure is used to determine if the patient is truly having seizures, to determine the specific type of seizures the patient is having, and to localize the area of the brain that is the origin of the seizures.

In some patients, epilepsy worsens over time, with the seizures becoming more frequent as patients grow older. This does not occur in most patients with epilepsy. In those so affected, it is possible that the seizures themselves may cause some damage to the cortex; loss of neurons, especially inhibitory neurons, has been demonstrated in tissue from seizure foci. Other changes occur in brain areas affected by seizures: reorganization of connections between groups of neurons may strengthen excitatory connections and weaken inhibitory connections, making the occurrence of future seizures more likely. Additionally, epilepsy is associated with an increased mortality rate.[13] For these reasons, an argument can be made for controlling epileptic seizures with medications as early as possible. This may reduce the possibility of permanent changes in brain function, although this hypothesis is unproven.

Genetic Factors

Patients with seizures may be concerned that their children or other family members will inherit epilepsy. This fear is usually unfounded. Patients with acquired causes of seizures, such as head trauma or stroke, will not transmit the problem. There is a group of patients, however, who apparently have epilepsy on a genetic basis. Most of these individuals have primary generalized epilepsy.[14,15] Usually these patients develop seizures during childhood. However, the hereditary tendency is not strong. Complex inheritance patterns are usually seen, indicating the likely involvement of several abnormal genes or other factors for seizures to be clinically expressed in offspring. Thus, most patients can be reassured that their children and siblings are unlikely to develop epilepsy. Increasing numbers of epilepsy syndromes are being identified as being of genetic origin, and once the specific genes are identified it may be possible to target drug therapies more specifically toward individual biochemical defects.

SEIZURE CLASSIFICATION AND PRESENTATION

General Principles

● Careful diagnosis and identification of seizure types is essential to proper treatment of epilepsy. Numerous schemes and descriptions of seizures exist, but the International League Against Epilepsy (ILAE) has established the currently accepted standard for classifying epileptic seizures (Fig. 30–1) and epilepsies or epilepsy syndromes (Table 30–1).[16,17] Classification of epileptic seizures is based upon electroencephalographic (EEG) findings combined with the clinical findings or semiology of the seizure events. Clinical presentations of seizures vary widely depending upon the region and amount of brain involved in the seizure.

Primary Generalized Seizures

If the entire cerebral cortex is involved in the seizure from the onset of the seizure, the seizure is classified as primary generalized. The following are types of primary generalized seizures:

- **Tonic-clonic:** Characterized by a sudden loss of consciousness accompanied by tonic extension and rhythmic clonic contractions of all major muscle groups. The duration of the seizure is usually 1 to 3 minutes. These seizures are often described as "grand mal."

- **Absence:** Characterized by sudden and brief (i.e., several seconds in duration) losses of consciousness without muscle movements. These seizures are often described as daydreaming or blanking out episodes. A common term for these seizures is "petit mal."

- **Myoclonic:** Characterized by single and very brief jerks of all major muscle groups. Patients with these seizures

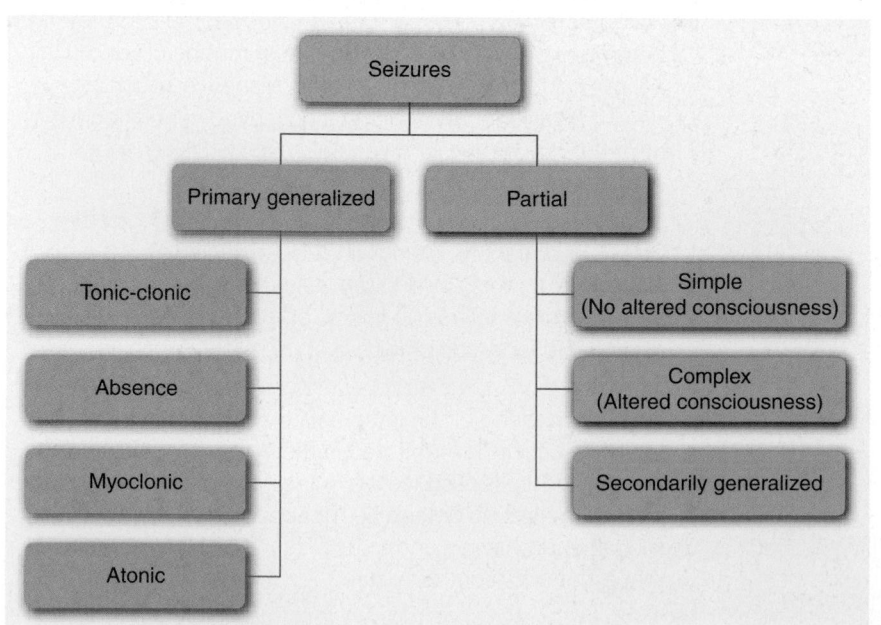

FIGURE 30–1. ILAE classification of epileptic seizures (1981). (From Ref. 16.)

Table 30–1

ILAE Classification Scheme for Epilepsies and Epilepsy Syndromes

I. Localization-related (focal, local, partial) epilepsies and epileptic syndromes
  A. Idiopathic with age-related onset
    1. Benign childhood epilepsy with centrotemporal spikes
    2. Childhood epilepsy with occipital paroxysms
  B. Symptomatic
II. Generalized epilepsies and epileptic syndromes
  A. Idiopathic and age-related onset
    1. Benign neonatal epilepsy
    2. Childhood absence epilepsy (pyknolepsy)
    3. Juvenile myoclonic epilepsy (impulsive petit mal)
    4. Juvenile absence epilepsy with generalized tonic-clonic seizure on awakening
  B. Secondary (idiopathic or symptomatic)
    1. West's syndrome (infantile spasms)
    2. Lennox-Gastaut syndrome
  C. Symptomatic
    1. Nonspecific etiology (early myoclonic encephalopathy)
    2. Specific syndromes (epileptic seizures that may complicate many diseases, e.g., Ramsay-Hunt syndrome, Unverricht's disease)

From Ref. 17.

may not lose consciousness due to the seizure lasting less than 3 to 4 seconds. Patients may describe these seizures as shoulder shrugs or spinal chills. Myoclonic seizures may cluster and build into a generalized tonic-clonic seizure.

- **Atonic:** Characterized by loss of consciousness and muscle tone. No muscle movements are typically noted, and the patient falls if not lying down or sitting in a chair. These seizures may be described as "falling out."

Partial Seizures

When the seizure begins in a localized area of the brain, it is defined as partial. There are three types of partial seizures in the current classification system (Fig. 30–1):

- **Simple:** The patient has a sensation or uncontrolled muscle movement of a portion of their body without an alteration in consciousness. The type of sensation or movement is dependent upon the location of seizure in the brain.
- **Complex:** Although the seizure is localized in a specific area of the brain, like a simple partial seizure, there is an alteration in the patient's level of consciousness.
- **Secondarily generalized:** The seizure starts as a simple or complex partial seizure and spreads to involve the entire brain. Patients may report a warning or aura, and these are actually the start of the seizure.

Epilepsy Syndromes

Classification of epilepsies and epilepsy syndromes is helpful in determining appropriate pharmacotherapy. This classification scheme is based upon the type of seizures a patient has and an attempt to identify the etiology of the epilepsy or epilepsy syndrome:

- **Idiopathic epilepsies:** These syndromes are thought to be due to genetic alterations, but the underlying etiology is not identified. Neurologic functions are completely normal apart from the occurrence of seizures.
- **Symptomatic epilepsies:** There is an identifiable cause for the seizures, such as trauma or hypoxia.
- **Cryptogenic epilepsies:** In these epilepsies the seizures are the result of an underlying neurologic disorder that is often ill-defined or undocumented. Neurologic functions are often abnormal or developmentally delayed in patients with cryptogenic epilepsies.

A complete description of a patient's epilepsy should include the seizure type with the epilepsy or syndrome type (e.g., idiopathic, symptomatic, cryptogenic).

Commonly encountered epilepsy syndromes are:

- **Juvenile myoclonic epilepsy (JME):** A primary generalized epilepsy syndrome that usually starts in the early to middle teenage years and has a strong familial component. Patients have myoclonic jerks and tonic-clonic seizures and may also have absence seizures.
- **Lennox-Gastaut syndrome (LGS):** Patients with this syndrome have cognitive dysfunction and mental retardation. Their seizures usually consist of a combination of tonic-clonic, absence, atonic, and myoclonic seizures.
- **Mesial temporal lobe epilepsy (MTLE):** A type of epilepsy that consists of partial seizures arising from the mesial temporal lobe of the brain. Often this type of epilepsy is associated with an anatomical change described as hippocampal sclerosis. Patients with this type of epilepsy often have excellent surgical outcomes.
- **Infantile spasms:** A seizure syndrome that occurs in infants less than 1 year of age. It is characterized by a specific EEG pattern and spasms or jitters, and is also known as West's syndrome. Infants with infantile spasms often develop other seizure types and epilepsies later in life.

Other Classifications

The ILAE is proposing a new classification system that improves the description of the seizure type and epilepsy.[18,19] The proposed scheme revolves around five axes:

- Axis 1: description of the seizure event
- Axis 2: epileptic seizure type or types
- Axis 3: any syndrome type
- Axis 4: etiology when known
- Axis 5: degree of impairment by the epilepsy

This classification system is undergoing final review and should become the standard in the near future.

DIAGNOSIS

Determining a correct and accurate diagnosis is essential prior to any consideration of pharmacotherapy. ❶ *When a patient complains of paroxysmal, stereotypical spells that may be seizures, it must be determined if the spells are really seizures.* Numerous other disorders, including convulsions, syncope, psychogenic nonepileptic events (i.e., pseudoseizures), anxiety attacks, cardiac arrhythmias, hypoglycemia, transient ischemic attacks, tics, and complicated migraine headaches, are often mistaken as seizures by patients and caregivers. Seizures are typically brief spells, lasting no more than 5 minutes. However, seizures can be prolonged and can last for 15 minutes or more. In this situation the patient is in status epilepticus and requires immediate medical attention.

A proper diagnostic workup of a patient presenting with seizures should include the following elements:

- Thorough neurologic examination
- EEG
- Laboratory tests (complete blood count [CBC], liver function tests [LFTs], serum chemistry)
- Neuroimaging (preferably MRI).

In patients with epilepsy these laboratory findings may be normal. Many of the tests are done to rule out other causes of seizures (e.g., infection, electrolyte imbalance). Often the EEG appears normal between seizures.[20] Several manipulations can be done in an attempt to capture seizure or seizure-like activity on the EEG. These include sleep deprivation, photic stimulation, prolonged (greater than 20 minutes) EEG recording, and 24-hour EEG monitoring with video correlation.

TREATMENT

Desired Outcomes

The ultimate outcome goal for any patient with epilepsy is elimination of all seizures without any adverse effects of the treatment. An effective treatment plan would allow the patient to pursue a normal lifestyle with complete control of seizures. Specifically, the treatment should enable the patient to drive, perform well in school, hold a reasonable job, and function effectively in the family and community. However, due to the intractability of the seizures or sensitivity to AEDs, many patients are not able to achieve these outcomes. In these cases, the goal of therapy is to provide a tolerable balance between reduced seizure severity and/or frequency and medication adverse effects that optimizes the individual's ability to have a lifestyle as nearly normal as possible.

General Approach to Treatment

Once it is concluded that the patient has seizures, the type of seizure and epilepsy syndrome, if any, must be determined. ❷ *Proper identification and classification of the seizure type is essential in selecting appropriate pharmacotherapy.* Without an accurate classification of the seizure type, it is possible to select a medication that is ineffective or even harmful to the patient.

❸ *Additionally, the risk of a subsequent seizure must be determined before starting pharmacotherapy.* If there is an underlying treatable cause, such as hyponatremia or a CNS infection, the risks of another seizure and the development of epilepsy are very small. In these cases, the only pharmacotherapy that is necessary is to correct the underlying problem and possibly short-term use of an AED. Risk factors for repeated seizures in patients without an underlying disorder include

- Structural CNS lesion
- Abnormal EEG
- Partial seizure type
- Positive family history
- Postictal motor paralysis[21]

Patient Encounter 1: New Onset Seizures

AG, a 20-year-old male who is a college student, is seen by his physician 4 days after an apparent seizure during finals week. According to his roommate he suddenly fell to the floor and had a generalized tonic-clonic seizure. This seizure lasted for 1 to 2 minutes. The patient was incontinent for urine during the seizure. He was sleepy and confused when the paramedics arrived 10 minutes later. Due to final examinations he reports being sleep deprived.

His physical exam is completely normal and no focal neurologic deficits were observed.

What diagnostic tests should be done at this time?

Should these tests be performed prior to starting medications?

His MRI is normal, and focal epileptiform activity originating from his left temporal lobe is observed on the EEG.

Should an AED be started at this point?

If you decide to treat, what drug and dose would you use?

How should that drug be monitored?

Three months later he has another seizure, but this time it is characterized by a rising feeling in his stomach followed by confused speech, lip smacking, repetitive movements of his right hand, and unresponsiveness. This episode lasts for 2 to 3 minutes, and it takes 15 minutes for his speech to return to normal.

If he is receiving an AED, should a second AED be started at this time?

What tests and evaluations should you do before starting a second AED?

If a second drug is started, what drug and dose would you use?

If no risk factors are present, the risk of another seizure is 10% to 15%. However, if two or more risk factors are present, the risk of another seizure is 100%.

When sufficient evidence is available to determine the patient has real seizures and is at risk for another seizure, pharmacotherapy is usually started (Fig. 30–2). The patient should be in agreement with the plan, be willing to take the medication, and be able to monitor seizure frequency and adverse drug effects in some way. ❹ *Design of an appropriate pharmacotherapeutic plan is based upon the patient's seizure type, the common adverse effect profile of possible AEDs, potential drug interactions, and economic factors (e.g., cost of the drug, insurance formulary, ability to pay).* Other patient factors such as gender, concomitant drugs, age, and lifestyle also need to be considered.

Nonpharmacologic Therapy

Several nonpharmacologic treatments for epilepsy are available. For some patients, surgery is the treatment approach with the greatest probability of eliminating seizures.[22] The most common surgical approach for epilepsy is temporal lobectomy. When the seizure focus can be localized and it is in a region of the brain that is not too close to critical areas, such as those responsible for speech or muscle control, surgical removal of the focus can result in 80% to 90% of patients becoming seizure free. According to a National Institutes of Health Consensus Conference, three criteria should be met for patients to be candidates for surgery.[23] These criteria are (a) a definite diagnosis of epilepsy; (b) failure of adequate drug therapies; and (c) definition of the electroclinical syndrome (i.e., localization of the seizure focus in the brain). Other surgical procedures that are less likely to make a patient seizure free include corpus callosotomy and extratemporal lesion removal.

Vagal nerve stimulation is another nonpharmacologic approach to treating all types of seizures.[24] In this treatment, a unit that generates an intermittent electrical current is placed under the skin in the chest. A wire is tunneled under the skin to the left vagus nerve in the neck. The unit generates a small electrical current every 5 minutes that stimulates the vagus nerve. Additional stimulations can be initiated by the patient swiping a magnet over the device located in the chest. This treatment approach is essentially

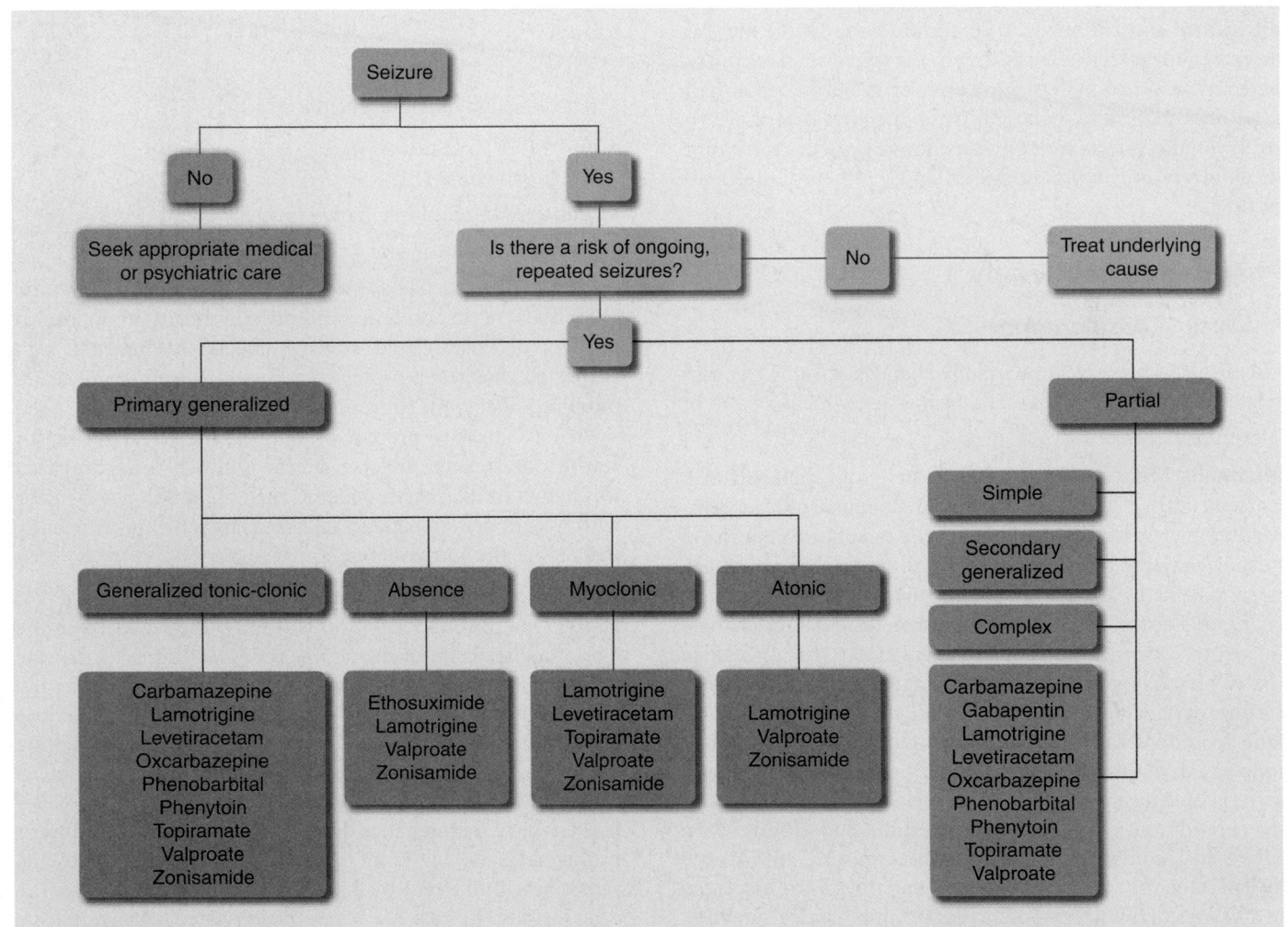

FIGURE 30–2. Treatment algorithm for management of seizure disorders.

equivalent to starting a new medication with regard to efficacy, but the precise mechanism for its effect has not been elucidated. Approximately 25% to 50% of patients who have a vagal nerve stimulator placed will experience at least a 50% reduction in seizure frequency. However, fewer than 10% become seizure free. Adverse effects include hoarseness, swallowing difficulties, tingling or vibration in the neck, infection or bleeding due to surgery, and, rarely, laryngeal spasms. Vagal nerve stimulation is usually reserved for patients who do not respond to several drugs and are not surgical candidates.

One of the oldest nonpharmacologic treatments is the ketogenic diet.[25] Modern use of the diet was started in the 1920s. This diet produces a keto-acidotic state through the elimination of nearly all carbohydrates. To initiate the diet, patients undergo 24 to 48 hours of fasting until ketones are detected in the urine. The diet consisting of dietary fats (e.g., butter, heavy cream, fatty meats) and protein with no added sugar is started. Daily urinalysis for ketones is performed to ensure the patient remains in ketosis. Any inadvertent consumption of sugar results in the diet needing to be reinitiated. Pharmacists have an important role in maintaining the diet, by determining the sugar or carbohydrate content of medications the patient is taking. This diet is typically used only in children with difficult to control seizures. In certain patients the diet can be extremely effective, resulting in complete seizure control and reduction of AEDs. However, it is hard to maintain a ketotic state, and palatability of the diet is a concern. Additionally, there are concerns about growth retardation in children and hypercholesterolemia with prolonged use of the diet.

Pharmacologic Therapy

▶ Special Considerations

Use of AEDs present some unique challenges, some of which relate to their pharmacokinetic properties, which need to be clearly understood.[26]

Michaelis-Menten Metabolism Phenytoin metabolism is capacity limited. Michaelis-Menten metabolism or Michaelis-Menten pharmacokinetics is when the maximum capacity of hepatic enzymes to metabolize the drug is reached within the normal dosage range. The clinical significance is that small changes in doses result in disproportionate and large changes in serum concentrations. The patient is at risk of sudden toxicity if too large a dose increase is made, or a breakthrough seizure may occur if too large a reduction in dose is made. Due to individual differences in metabolism, each patient follows a different curve in the relationship between dose and serum concentrations. These differences can only be defined by careful use of serum concentration and dosing data. There are numerous schemes for determining appropriate dosage adjustments of phenytoin, and these are discussed in pharmacokinetic textbooks. For routine clinical practice, dosage adjustments for adults with normal protein binding

of phenytoin and a steady-state serum concentration can be made using the following plan:

- For serum concentrations less than 7 mcg/mL (28 μmol/L), the total daily dose is increased by 100 mg.
- For serum concentrations of 7 to 12 mcg/mL (28–48 μmol/L), the total daily dose is increased by 50 mg.
- For serum concentrations greater than 12 mcg/mL (48 μmol/L), the total daily dose is increased by no more than 30 mg.[27]

Protein Binding Some AEDs, especially phenytoin and valproate, are highly bound to plasma proteins. When interpreting a reported concentration for these drugs, it is important to remember the value represents the total (i.e., bound and unbound) concentration in the blood. Because of differences in the metabolism of these drugs, the clinical effects of altered protein binding are different for these drugs.

Normally, 88% to 92% of phenytoin is bound to plasma protein, leaving 8% to 12% as unbound. The unbound component is able to leave the blood to produce the clinical effect in the CNS, produce dose-related side effects in the CNS and at other sites, distribute to other peripheral sites, and be metabolized. Certain patient groups are known to have decreased protein binding, resulting in an increased percentage of drug that is unbound. These patient groups include

- Those with kidney failure
- Those with hypoalbuminemia
- Neonates
- Pregnant women
- Those taking multiple highly protein bound drugs
- Patients in critical care

Due to the Michaelis-Menten metabolism of phenytoin, alterations in its protein binding will result in increased severity of dose-related adverse effects. In patients with suspected changes in protein binding, it is useful to measure unbound phenytoin concentrations.

When valproate protein binding is altered, the risk for severe dose-related adverse effects is much less compared to phenytoin. Michaelis-Menten metabolism is not a factor with valproate, so hepatic enzymes are able to efficiently metabolize the additional unbound portion.

Autoinduction Carbamazepine is a potent inducer of hepatic microsomal enzymes. Not only does it increase the rate of metabolism for many other drugs, it increases the rate of its own metabolism. Hepatic enzymes become maximally induced over several weeks, necessitating a small initial dose of carbamazepine that is increased over time to compensate for the enzyme induction (Fig. 30–3). Most dosage regimens for carbamazepine call for a starting dose that is 25% to 30% of the typical maintenance dose of 15 mg/kg/day. The dosage is increased weekly until the target maintenance dose is achieved within 3 to 4 weeks. Titration of the carbamazepine dose lessens the risk for severe dose-related adverse effects when carbamazepine is first started.

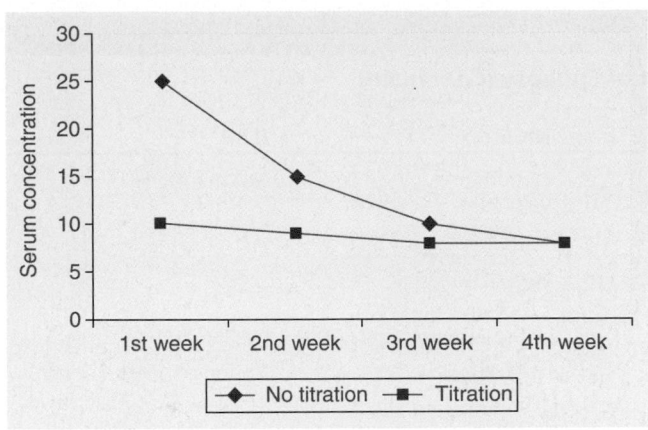

FIGURE 30–3. Serum concentrations of carbamazepine in the presence and absence of appropriate dose titration.

▶ *Drug Selection and Seizure Type*

The key to selecting effective pharmacotherapy is to base the decision on the seizure type. Several consensus treatment guidelines from the Scottish Intercollegiate Guidelines Network (SIGN), the National Institute for Clinical Excellence in the United Kingdom (NICE), the American Academy of Neurology (AAN), and ILAE all use determination of seizure type as the basis for selection of pharmacotherapy (Table 30–2).[28-30] While the guidelines make recommendations for specific drugs to be used in certain seizure types, the consensus recommendations utilize only data available from the medical literature. In many cases, a recommendation is not made because there are no published data on which to make an evidence-based decision. Therefore, a drug may not currently be recommended for a seizure type simply because it has not been studied for that seizure type. Absence of a recommendation should not be taken to mean the drug is ineffective for a specific seizure type.

Outside of the evidence-based guidelines, other pharmacologic treatments are commonly used or avoided. For initial treatment of absence seizures, ethosuximide and valproate are commonly used, not only in the United Kingdom, but also in the United States. Zonisamide may be also used for initial treatment of absence and myoclonic

---

Table 30–2

Evidence-Based Guidelines for Initial Monotherapy Treatment of Epilepsy

Seizure Type	AAN	SIGN	NICE	ILAE
Primary generalized tonic-clonic	Carbamazepine[a] Lamotrigine[a] Oxcarbazepine[a] Phenobarbital[a] Phenytoin[a] Topiramate[a] Valproate[a]	Lamotrigine Valproate	Carbamazepine Lamotrigine Topiramate Valproate *Second-line:* Clobazam[b] Levetiracetam Oxcarbazepine	*Adults:* Carbamazepine[c] Lamotrigine[c] Oxcarbazepine[c] Phenobarbital[c] Phenytoin[c] Topiramate[c] Valproate[c] *Children:* Carbamazepine[c] Phenobarbital[c] Topiramate[c] Valproate[c]
Absence	Lamotrigine (children)	Ethosuximide Lamotrigine Valproate	Ethosuximide Lamotrigine Valproate *Second-line:* Clobazam Clonazepam Topiramate	*Children:* Ethosuximide[c] Lamotrigine[c] Valproate[c]
Myoclonic	Not mentioned	Lamotrigine Valproate	Valproate Topiramate (children with severe myoclonic epilepsy of infancy) *Second-line:* Clobazam[b] Clonazepam Lamotrigine Levetiracetam Piracetam[b] Topiramate	Clonazepam[d] Lamotrigine[d] Levetiracetam[d] Topiramate[d] Valproate[d] Zonisamide[d]

(Continued)

Table 30-2

Evidence-Based Guidelines for Initial Monotherapy Treatment of Epilepsy (Continued)

Seizure Type	AAN	SIGN	NICE	ILAE
Tonic	Not mentioned	Not mentioned	Lamotrigine Valproate *Second-line:* Clobazam[b] Clonazepam Levetiracetam Topiramate	Not mentioned
Atonic	Not mentioned	Not mentioned	Lamotrigine Valproate *Second-line:* Clobazam[b] Clonazepam Levetiracetam Topiramate	Not mentioned
Partial with or without secondary generalization	Carbamazepine Gabapentin Lamotrigine Oxcarbazepine Phenobarbital Phenytoin Topiramate Valproate	Phenytoin Carbamazepine Valproate Lamotrigine Oxcarbazepine	Carbamazepine Lamotrigine Oxcarbazepine Valproate Topiramate *Second-line:* Clobazam[b] Gabapentin Levetiracetam Phenytoin Tiagabine	*Adults:* Carbamazepine[e] Phenytoin[e] Valproate[c] Gabapentin[c] Lamotrigine[c] Oxcarbazepine[c] Phenobarbital[c] Topiramate[c] Vigabatrin[c] *Children:* Oxcarbazepine[e] Carbamazepine[c] Phenobarbital[c] Phenytoin[c] Topiramate[c] Valproate[c] Lamotrigine[c] Vigabatrin[c] *Elderly:* Lamotrigine[e] Gabapentin[e] Carbamazepine[c] Topiramate[c] Valproate[c]

AAN, American Academy of Neurology; ILAE, International League Against Epilepsy; NICE, National Institute for Clinical Excellence in the United Kingdom; SIGN, Scottish Intercollegiate Guidelines Network.

[a]Based upon data from newly diagnosed epilepsy patients of multiple seizure types.

[b]Not currently available in the United States.

[c]Possibly effective.

[d]Probably effective.

[e]Proven effective.

From Refs. 27–30.

seizures. In absence and myoclonic seizures, carbamazepine, oxcarbazepine, gabapentin, tiagabine, and pregabalin should be avoided, as they have been associated with an exacerbation of these types of seizures.

❺ *When an appropriate AED has been chosen, doses are started very low and titrated over several weeks.* Usually a moderate target dose is chosen until the patient's response can be further evaluated in clinic. If seizures continue, the dose should be increased gradually until the patient becomes seizure-free or adverse effects appear. For some drugs like lamotrigine, specific titration guidelines are established by the manufacturer.

Refractory seizure (i.e., unresponsive to at least two first-line AEDs) treatment is somewhat different. According to the AAN Practice Parameter, topiramate is useful as monotherapy for primary generalized tonic-clonic seizures, and there is insufficient evidence to make any recommendation regarding gabapentin, lamotrigine, oxcarbazepine, tiagabine, levetiracetam, or zonisamide.[31] Combinations of drugs are not addressed by the AAN, but may be useful in patients with difficult to control primary generalized seizures. This practice parameter also gives the highest recommendation to oxcarbazepine and topiramate as monotherapy in patients with refractory partial epilepsy. Additionally, lamotrigine is noted to be effective as monotherapy for refractory partial seizures, but was associated with a high dropout rate in the clinical trials. All AEDs, except ethosuximide, are effective in combination therapy for partial seizures.

▶ Complications of Pharmacotherapy

Adverse effects of AEDs are frequently dose limiting or can cause a drug to be discontinued. Two types of adverse effects occur with AEDs: concentration related and idiosyncratic (Table 30–3). Concentration-related adverse effects happen with increasing frequency and severity as the dose or concentration of a drug is increased. For many AEDs, common concentration-related adverse effects include sedation, ataxia, and diplopia. These adverse effects should be carefully considered and used as one of the AED selection criteria. For example, if a patient has a job that requires mental alertness, it is best to choose an AED that is less likely to cause sedation (e.g., lamotrigine).

Idiosyncratic adverse effects are not dose or concentration related and will almost always result in the AED being discontinued. Rash, hepatotoxicity, and hematological toxicities are the most common idiosyncratic reactions seen with AED. Because many of these adverse effects are life threatening or potentially life threatening, the AED should be discontinued immediately when the reaction is observed. Carbamazepine, phenytoin, phenobarbital, valproate, lamotrigine, oxcarbazepine, and felbamate are most likely to cause these types of reactions. Many of these reactions are thought to occur primarily on an immunological basis, which raises the possibility of cross-reactivity. This is especially true for carbamazepine, phenytoin, phenobarbital, and oxcarbazepine, where 15% to 25% of patients who have an idiosyncratic reaction to one drug will have a similar reaction to the other drugs.

Table 30–3
Characteristics of Common AEDs

Drug	Mechanism of Action	Dose	Pharmacokinetic Parameters	Usual Serum Concentration Range	Dose-Related Adverse Effects	Idiosyncratic Adverse Effects
Carbamazepine	Fast sodium channel inactivation	*Loading dose:* Not recommended due to excessive dose-related toxicity *Maintenance dose:* Titrate dosage to target over 3–4 weeks Adults: 10–20 mg/kg/day as a divided dose Children: 20–30 mg/kg/day as a divided dose	*Half-life:* 10–25 hours with chronic dosing *Apparent volume of distribution:* 0.8–1.9 L/kg *Protein binding:* 67–81% *Primary elimination route:* Hepatic	4–12 mcg/mL (17–51 µmol/L)	Diplopia, drowsiness, nausea, sedation	Aplastic anemia, hyponatremia, leucopenia, osteoporosis, rash
Clonazepam	Enhance GABA activity	*Loading dose:* Not recommended due to increased adverse effects *Maintenance dose:* Initiate at 0.5 mg 1–3 times daily, titrate dose to effectiveness, usually 3–5 mg daily in 2 or 3 divided doses	*Half-life:* 30–40 hours *Apparent volume of distribution:* 3.2 L/kg *Protein binding:* 47–80% *Primary elimination route:* Hepatic	Not established	Ataxia, memory impairment, sedation, slowed thinking	

(Continued)

Table 30–3

Characteristics of Common AEDs *(Continued)*

Drug	Mechanism of Action	Dose	Pharmacokinetic Parameters	Usual Serum Concentration Range	Dose-Related Adverse Effects	Idiosyncratic Adverse Effects
Ethosuximide	Modulate calcium channels	*Loading dose:* Not recommended due to increased adverse effects *Maintenance dose:* Initiate at 250 mg twice daily and titrate to 500–1,000 mg twice daily	*Half-life:* 60 hours *Apparent volume of distribution:* 0.6–0.7 L/kg *Protein binding:* None *Primary elimination route:* Hepatic	40–100 mcg/ mL (283–708 µmol/L)	Ataxia, sedation	Hepatotoxicity, neutropenia, rash
Felbamate	Inhibit glutamate activity	*Loading dose:* Not recommended due to increased adverse effects *Maintenance dose:* 1,200–3,600 mg/day in 3 or 4 divided doses	*Half-life:* Monotherapy: 20 hours Concurrent enzyme inducers: 11–16 hours *Apparent volume of distribution:* 0.7–0.8 L/kg *Protein binding:* 25–35% *Primary elimination route:* Hepatic	Not established	Anxiety, insomnia, nausea	Anorexia, aplastic anemia, headache, hepatotoxicity, weight loss
Gabapentin	Modulate calcium channels and enhance GABA activity	*Loading dose:* Not recommended due to short half-life *Maintenance dose:* 900–3,600 mg/day in 3 or 4 divided doses (doses up to 10,000 mg/day have been tolerated)	*Half-life:* 5–7 hours (proportional to creatinine clearance) *Apparent volume of distribution:* 0.6–0.8 L/kg *Protein binding:* less than10% *Primary elimination route:* Renal	Not established	Drowsiness, sedation	Peripheral edema, weight gain
Lacosamide	Slow sodium channel inactivation; modulate collapsin response; mediator protein-2	*Loading dose:* Data unavailable *Maintenance dose:* 200–400 mg/day; Start at 100 mg/ day in 2 divided doses and titrate upward according to response	*Half-life:* Approximately 13 hours *Volume of distribution:* 0.6 L/kg *Protein binding:* less than 15% *Primary elimination route:* 40% renal 60% hepatic	Not established	Ataxia, dizziness, diplopia, headache, nausea, vomiting	PR interval prolongation
Lamotrigine	Fast sodium channel inactivation	*Loading dose:* Not recommended due to increased risk of rash *Maintenance dose:* 150–800 mg/day in 2 or 3 divided doses. Doses should be initiated and titrated according to the manufacturer's recommendations to reduce the risk of rash	*Half-life:* Monotherapy: 24 hours Concurrent enzyme inducers: 12–15 hours Concurrent enzyme inhibitors: 55–60 hours *Apparent volume of distribution:* 1.1 L/kg *Protein binding:* 55% *Primary elimination route:* Hepatic	Not established	Ataxia, drowsiness, headache, insomnia, sedation	Rash

Table 30–3

Characteristics of Common AEDs *(Continued)*

Drug	Mechanism of Action	Dose	Pharmacokinetic Parameters	Usual Serum Concentration Range	Dose-Related Adverse Effects	Idiosyncratic Adverse Effects
Levetiracetam	Modulate synaptic vesicle protein	*Loading dose:* Not recommended due to excessive adverse effects *Maintenance dose:* 1,000–3,000 mg/day. Start at 1,000 mg/day and titrated upward as indicated by response	*Half-life:* 6–8 hours *Apparent volume of distribution:* 0.5–0.7 L/kg *Protein binding:* less than 10% *Primary elimination route:* 70% renal 30% hepatic	Not established	Somnolence, dizziness	Depression
Oxcarbazepine	Fast sodium channel inactivation	*Loading dose:* Not recommended due to excessive adverse effects *Maintenance dose:* 600–1,200 mg/day Start at 300 mg twice daily and titrated upward as indicated by response	*Half-life:* Parent drug Approximately 2 hours; 10-monohydroxy *Metabolite* Approximately 9 hours *Apparent volume of distribution:* 0.5–0.7 L/kg *Protein binding:* 40% *Primary elimination route:* Hepatic	Not established	Diplopia, dizziness, somnolence	Hyponatremia, 25–30% cross sensitivity in patients with hypersensitivity to carbamazepine
Phenobarbital	Fast sodium channel inactivation	*Loading dose:* 10–20 mg/kg as single or divided IV infusion or orally in divided doses over 24–48 hours *Maintenance dose:* Adults: 1–4 mg/kg/day as a single or divided dose Children: 3–6 mg/kg/day as divided dose Neonates: 1–3 mg/kg/day as divided dose	*Half-life:* Adults: 49–120 hours Children: 37–73 hours Neonates: approximately 115 hours *Volume of distribution:* 0.7–1 L/kg *Protein binding:* Approximately 50% *Primary elimination route:* Hepatic	15–40 mcg/mL (65–172 μmol/L)	Ataxia, drowsiness, sedation	Attention deficit, cognitive impairment, hyperactivity, osteoporosis, passive-aggressive behavior
Phenytoin	Fast sodium channel inactivation	*Loading dose:* Adults: 15–20 mg/kg single IV dose or divided oral dose Infants less than 3 months: 10–15 mg/kg single IV dose Neonates: 15–20 mg/kg single IV dose *Maintenance dose:* Adults: 5–7 mg/kg/day, as single or divided dose Children: 6–15 mg/kg/day, as divided dose Neonates: 3–8 mg/kg/day, as divided dose	*Half-life:* Follows capacity-limited or Michaelis-Menten pharmacokinetics. Half-life increases as the dose and serum concentration increases. *Volume of distribution:* Adults: 0.7 L/kg Children: 0.8 L/kg Neonates: 1.2 L/kg *Protein binding:* Adults, children: 88–92% Neonates: 65% *Primary elimination route:* Hepatic	10–20 mcg/mL (40–79 μmol/L) total concentration 1–2 mcg/mL (4–8 μmol/L) unbound concentration	Ataxia, diplopia, drowsiness, sedation	Anemia, gingival hyperplasia, hirsutism, lymphade-nopathy, osteoporosis, rash

(Continued)

Table 30–3

Characteristics of Common AEDs *(Continued)*

Drug	Mechanism of Action	Dose	Pharmacokinetic Parameters	Usual Serum Concentration Range	Dose-Related Adverse Effects	Idiosyncratic Adverse Effects
Pregabalin	Modulate calcium channels	*Loading dose:* Not recommended due to increased adverse effects *Maintenance dose:* Initiate at 150 mg/day in 2 or 3 divided doses and titrate to a maximum dose of 600 mg/day	*Half-life:* 6.3 hours, proportional to creatinine clearance *Apparent volume of distribution:* 0.5 L/kg *Protein binding:* Negligible *Primary elimination route:* Renal	Not established	Ataxia, blurred vision, dizziness, dry mouth, somnolence	Edema, weight gain
Rufinamide	Unknown, may enhance inactivation of sodium channels	*Loading dose:* Data unavailable *Maintenance dose:* Children: 45 mg/kg/day or 3,200 mg/day; start at 10 mg/kg/day in 2 divided doses and titrate upward according to response Adults: 3,200 mg/day; start at 400–800 mg/day in 2 divided doses and titrate upward according to response	*Half-life:* 6–10 hours *Apparent volume of distribution:* Approximately 0.7 L/kg, varies with dose *Protein binding:* 34% (27% to albumin) *Primary elimination route:* Hepatic	Not established	Dizziness, fatigue, headache, nausea, somnolence, vomiting	
Tiagabine	Enhance GABA activity	*Loading dose:* Not recommended due to excessive adverse effects *Maintenance dose:* 32–56 mg/day in 4 divided doses. Doses should be titrated upward over 6 weeks, starting at 4 mg/day	*Half-life:* Monotherapy: 7–9 hours Concurrent enzyme inducers: 2.5–4.5 hours *Apparent volume of distribution:* 0.6–0.8 L/kg *Protein binding:* 96% *Primary elimination route:* Hepatic	Not established	Dizziness, somnolence, irritability, slowed thinking	
Topiramate	Fast sodium channel inactivation, inhibit glutamate activity, enhance GABA activity	*Loading dose:* Not recommended due to excessive adverse effects *Maintenance dose:* 100–400 mg/day in 2 or 3 divided doses. Doses should be started at 25–50 mg/day and gradually titrated upward over 3–6 weeks to avoid excessive adverse effects	*Half-life:* Monotherapy: 21 hours Concurrent enzyme inducers: 11–16 hours *Apparent volume of distribution:* 0.55–0.8 L/kg *Protein binding:* 13–17% *Primary elimination route:* 60% renal 40% hepatic	Not established	Ataxia, dizziness, drowsiness, slowed thinking	Acute glaucoma, metabolic acidosis, oligohidrosis, paresthesia, renal calculi, weight loss

Table 30–3

Characteristics of Common AEDs *(Continued)*

Drug	Mechanism of Action	Dose	Pharmacokinetic Parameters	Usual Serum Concentration Range	Dose-Related Adverse Effects	Idiosyncratic Adverse Effects
Valproic acid/ divalproex sodium	Fast sodium channel inactivation	*Loading dose:* 20–40 mg/kg *Maintenance dose:* Adults: 15–45 mg/kg/day in 2–4 divided doses Children: 5–60 mg/kg/day in 2–4 divided doses	*Half-life:* Adults: 8–15 hours Children: 4–15 hours Infants less than 2 months: 65 hour *Volume of distribution:* 0.1–0.5 L/kg *Protein binding:* 90% (decreases with increasing serum concentrations) *Primary elimination route:* Hepatic	50–100 mcg/mL (346–693 µmol/L). Children may require concentrations up to 150 mcg/mL (1,040 µmol/L)	Drowsiness, nausea, sedation, tremor	Hepatotoxicity, osteoporosis, pancreatitis, weight gain
Vigabatrin	Inhibits GABA transaminase	*Children:* 1 month–2 years: 50 mg/kg/day in 2 divided doses *Adults:* Initiate at 1,000 mg/day in 2 divided doses, titrate up to 3,000 mg/day *Renal failure:* CrCl 50–80 mL/min decrease dose by 25%; CrCl 30–50 mL/min decrease dose by 50%; CrCl 10–30 mL/min decrease dose by 75%	*Half-life:* 7.5 hours, proportional to creatinine clearance *Volume of distribution:* 1.1 L/kg *Protein binding:* negligible *Primary route of elimination:* Renal	Not established	Convulsion, dizziness, headache, nasopharyngitis, somnolence, weight gain	Vision loss and blindness
Zonisamide	Modulate sodium and calcium channels	*Loading dose:* Not recommended due to excessive adverse effects *Maintenance dose:* 100–600 mg/day; start at 100 mg/day and titrated upward as indicated by response	*Half-life:* Approximately 63 hours *Apparent volume of distribution:* 1.45 L/kg *Protein binding:* 40% *Primary elimination route:* Hepatic	Not established	Dizziness, somnolence	Metabolic acidosis, oligohidrosis, paresthesia, renal calculi

GABA, gamma-aminobutyric acid.

From Refs. 25, 35–38.

▶ Chronic Adverse Effects

Because AEDs are administered for long periods of time, adverse effects due to prolonged drug exposure are of concern. Chronic adverse effects tend to be primarily idiosyncratic in nature. Some chronic adverse effects associated with AEDs include peripheral neuropathy and cerebellar atrophy. Other chronic adverse effects are extensions of acute adverse effects, for example, weight gain.

One chronic adverse effect that is of concern is osteoporosis.[32,33] Carbamazepine, phenytoin, phenobarbital, oxcarbazepine, and valproate have all been shown to decrease bone mineral density, even after only 6 months of treatment. Data on the relationship between other AEDs and osteoporosis are not currently available. Multiple studies have shown the risk of osteoporosis due to chronic AED use to be similar to the risk with chronic use of glucocorticosteroids. Patients taking carbamazepine, oxcarbazepine, phenytoin, phenobarbital, or valproate for longer than 6 months should take supplemental calcium and vitamin D. Additionally, routine monitoring for osteoporosis should be performed every 2 years and patients should be instructed on ways to protect themselves from fractures.

▶ Practical Issues

Comorbid Disease States Patients with epilepsy often have comorbid disease states. Disorders such as chronic headaches and asthma are frequent problems. For patients who also have asthma, care must be taken to identify drug interactions between AEDs and medications used for asthma. These interactions may necessitate close monitoring for changes in efficacy or increased toxicity, and dosage changes of other drugs may be necessary when an AED is added or removed. Patients with chronic headaches need special attention in the selection of an AED. Agents known to prevent headache (e.g., valproate and topiramate) may be preferred among several choices, and agents associated with increased headaches (e.g., lamotrigine and felbamate) may be a secondary or tertiary alternative.

Depression is a common problem in patients with epilepsy, with approximately 30% having symptoms of major depression at some point.[34] Patients with epilepsy should be routinely assessed for signs of depression, and treatment should be initiated if necessary. Certain AEDs may exacerbate depression, for example, levetiracetam and phenytoin. Other AEDs (e.g., lamotrigine, carbamazepine, oxcarbazepine) may be useful in treating depression. Changes in mood can be precipitated by the addition or discontinuation of an AED. If treatment for depression is necessary, caution should be exercised in choosing an agent that does not increase seizure frequency and does not interact with AEDs.

Switching Drugs Changing from one AED to another can be a complex process. If the first drug is stopped too abruptly, breakthrough seizures may occur. ❻ *Stopping or adding a drug can introduce various problems such as drug interactions which should be considered in any regimen change.* Typically the new drug is started at a low initial dose and gradually increased over several weeks. Once the new drug is at a minimally effective dose, the drug to be discontinued is gradually tapered while the dose of the new drug continues to be increased to the target dose. During a transition between drugs, patients should be cautioned about the possibility of increased seizures or adverse reactions.

Stopping Therapy Epilepsy is generally considered to be a life-long disorder that requires ongoing treatment. However, many patients who are seizure-free may desire to discontinue their medications.[35] Patients who become seizure free following surgery for their epilepsy may have medications slowly tapered starting 1 to 2 years after their surgery. Many patients will choose to stay on at least one medication, following successful surgery, to ensure they remain seizure free. ❼ *Five criteria must be met before considering the discontinuation of AEDs.[36] They are:*

- *No seizures for 2 to 5 years*
- *Normal neurologic examination*
- *Normal intelligence quotient*
- *Single type of partial or generalized seizure*
- *Normal EEG with treatment*

Individuals who fulfill all of these criteria have a 61% chance of remaining seizure-free after AEDs are discontinued. Additionally, there is a direct relationship between the duration of seizure freedom while taking medications and the chance of being seizure-free after medications are withdrawn. Withdrawal of AEDs is done slowly, usually with a tapering dose over at least 1 to 3 months.

▶ **Dosing**

Dosing of AEDs is determined by general guidelines and response of the patient. Serum concentrations may be helpful in benchmarking a specific response. Therapeutic ranges that are often quoted are broad guidelines for dosing but should never replace careful evaluation of the patient's response. It is not unusual for a patient to be well managed with serum concentrations or doses outside the typical ranges.

▶ **Drug Interactions**

AEDs are associated with many different drug interactions.[37–39] These interactions are primarily in relation to absorption, metabolism, and protein binding. Tube feedings and antacids

---

Patient Encounter 2: Switching a Patient to a Different AED

BC, a 22-year-old woman, was diagnosed 2 years ago with JME. She has been treated with valproate 1,500 mg/day. Since starting valproate she has gained 20.5 kg (45 lb), continues to have occasional myoclonic jerks, had a generalized tonic-clonic seizure 3 months ago, and is sexually active. Additionally, she complains of easily falling asleep during the day. Due to adverse effects, poor seizure control, and the risk of birth defects with valproate, the decision is made to switch to a different AED.

What drug would be the optimal alternative for this patient?

How should the new drug be started and the valproate discontinued?

What instructions should be given to the patient regarding the switch to another drug?

Patient Encounter 3: Discontinuing AED Therapy

The consultant pharmacist is reviewing the care of AN, who is a 79-year-old male resident of a long-term care facility. According to his records, he has received phenytoin and phenobarbital ever since suffering a stroke 12 years ago. There is no record of a seizure in his chart, and the nursing staff has not observed a seizure since he arrived at the facility 2 years ago. His family recalls that he had one seizure around the time of his stroke, but has not had any more seizures.

Can his antiepileptic medications be discontinued?

What additional information would be helpful to determine the possibility of discontinuing his AEDs?

If the AEDs are stopped, how should they be discontinued?

Table 30–4

Cytochrome P450 and AED Interactions

Enzyme	Substrate	Common Inducers	Common Inhibitors
CYP 1A2	Carbamazepine	Carbamazepine Phenytoin Phenobarbital Rifampin	Cimetidine Ciprofloxacin Erythromycin Clarithromycin
CYP 2C9	Phenobarbital[a] Phenytoin[a] Carbamazepine Valproate	Carbamazepine Phenytoin Phenobarbital Rifampin	Amiodarone Cimetidine Fluconazole Valproate
CYP 2C19	Phenobarbital Phenytoin Valproate Lacosamide		Felbamate Ticlopidine Topiramate Zonisamide
CYP 2D6	Zonisamide	Carbamazepine	
CYP 3A4	Carbamazepine[a] Tiagabine[a] Zonisamide[a]	Carbamazepine Phenytoin Phenobarbital Rifampin	Amiodarone Erythromycin Propoxyphene Ketoconazole
Uridine diphosphate glucuronyl-transferase	Lamotrigine[a] Carbamazepine Valproate	Lamotrigine Phenobarbital Phenytoin Hormonal contraceptives	Valproate

[a]Primary route of metabolism.

From Refs. 37–39.

are known to reduce the absorption of phenytoin and carbamazepine. Phenytoin, carbamazepine, and phenobarbital are potent inducers of various CYP 450 isoenzymes, increasing the clearance of other drugs metabolized through these pathways (Table 30–4). In contrast, valproate is a CYP 450 isoenzyme inhibitor and reduces the clearance of some drugs. Phenytoin and valproate are highly protein bound and can be displaced when taken concurrently with other highly protein-bound drugs. For example, when phenytoin and valproate are taken together, there may be increased dose-related adverse effects within several hours of dosing. This can be avoided by staggering doses or giving smaller doses more frequently during the day. Whenever a change in a medication regimen occurs, drug interactions should be considered and appropriate adjustments in dose of AEDs made.

▶ Special Populations

8 *Children and women present special challenges in the management of epilepsy and use of AEDs.* In children, developmental changes occur rapidly, and metabolic rates are greater than those seen in adults. When treating a child it is imperative to control seizures as quickly as possible to avoid interference with development of the brain and cognition. AED doses are increased rapidly, and frequent changes in the regimen are made to maximize control of seizures. Due to the rapid metabolic rates seen in children, doses of AEDs are typically higher on a milligram per kilogram basis compared to adults, and serum concentrations are used more extensively to help ensure an adequate trial of a drug has been given.

For women, the treatment of epilepsy poses challenges, including teratogenicity, interactions between AEDs and hormonal contraceptives, and reduced fertility.[40,41] Recommendations for managing women of child-bearing potential and who are pregnant have been developed (Table 30–5). Several AEDs have been implicated in causing both minor and serious birth defects.[42] Of special concern are neural tube defects (e.g., spina bifida, microcephaly, anencephaly) associated most commonly with valproate and possibly carbamazepine. Additionally, valproate has been associated with impaired cognitive development in children born to women taking valproate during pregnancy. Use of valproate is not absolutely contraindicated in women who

Table 30–5

Management of AEDs During Pregnancy

Give supplemental folic acid 1–4 mg daily to all women of child-bearing potential

Use monotherapy whenever possible

Use lowest doses that control seizures

Continue pharmacotherapy that best controls seizures prior to pregnancy

Monitor AED serum concentrations at start of pregnancy and monthly thereafter

Adjust AED doses to maintain baseline serum concentrations

Administer supplemental vitamin K during eighth month of pregnancy to women receiving enzyme-inducing AEDs

Monitor postpartum AED serum concentrations to guide adjustments of drug doses

Patient Encounter 4: Hormonal Contraceptives and Interactions With AEDs

LJ, a 25-year-old-woman with complex partial seizures, presents a prescription to the pharmacy for a triphasic oral contraceptive containing ethinyl estradiol and norgestimate. A review of her medication profile shows that she is taking carbamazepine extended release 1,200 mg/day. Her last refill for this prescription was 2 weeks ago. She reports that she has not had a seizure for 1 year and that she just became engaged. She is planning to be married in 4 months.

Is there an interaction between carbamazepine and the oral contraceptive?

If so, what is the cause and clinical outcome of the interaction?

If there is an interaction, how should it be managed?

What AEDs interact with hormonal contraceptives?

What are the clinical implications of these interactions? How should they be managed?

may become pregnant, but it is appropriate to use alternative AEDs, if possible, in women of child-bearing potential. All women of child-bearing potential who have epilepsy should take 1 to 4 mg daily of supplemental folic acid to reduce the risk of these defects. Many AEDs are excreted in breast milk. However, infants were exposed to higher concentrations of AED in utero, so it is unclear if drugs in breast milk are harmful to the child. Decisions about breast-feeding should be made on an individual basis.

As noted above, many of the AEDs induce hepatic microsomal enzyme systems and thus reduce the effectiveness of hormonal contraceptives. Women taking AEDs that may reduce the effectiveness of hormonal contraceptives should be encouraged to also use other forms of birth control. In contrast to these interactions, hormonal contraceptives induce glucoronidation of lamotrigine and valproate. Oral contraceptives that cycle hormones cause reductions in serum concentrations of lamotrigine or valproate during days of the cycle when hormones are taken; serum concentrations increase during days when hormones are not taken. Due to induction or inhibition of sex hormone metabolism and changes in binding of hormones to sex hormone binding globulin, some AEDs may reduce fertility. For example, valproate has been associated with a drug-induced polycystic ovarian syndrome. Women who experience difficulties with fertility should seek the advice of health care professionals with expertise in fertility.

OUTCOME EVALUATION

❾ *Regular reporting and monitoring of seizure counts, changes in seizures, adverse events, and drug interactions are essential to proper management of a patient with epilepsy.*

Patient Care and Monitoring

1. *Monitor the patient's seizure frequency and characteristics.* The only objective measure of efficacy for AEDs is a count of seizure frequency. Ask patients to keep seizure calendars, noting the numbers and types of seizures that occur, and have them bring the calendars to clinic at every visit for analysis and documentation of seizure frequency.

2. *Monitor for acute and chronic adverse effects of AED.* Acute adverse effects are best detected by a thorough neurologic examination at clinic visits. Instruct patients to report sedation, ataxia, rash, or other problems immediately. Monitor for chronic adverse effects, including a loss of bone mineral density, which should be measured every 2 years in patients taking phenytoin, phenobarbital, carbamazepine, and valproate.

3. *Monitor for comorbid disease states at each clinic visit.* Evaluate for depression at every clinic visit. Monitor comorbid disease states when a change in AED therapy is made.

4. *Take measures to ensure compliance with medications and access to care.* Compliance with medication regimens is a common problem for patients with epilepsy. Ask patients at every visit how they are taking their medications and whether they miss any doses. Identify barriers to care, such as financial issues or transportation problems.

5. *Instruct patients, family members, and caregivers on first aid for seizures.* First aid for seizures consists primarily of keeping patients from hurting themselves. They should be placed on the floor, if possible, and their head cushioned. First responders to a seizure should never attempt to restrain the patient or force an item into their mouth. If a seizure lasts longer than 5 to 10 minutes, emergency medical assistance should be called.

Efficacy

- Seizure counts are the only reasonable and standard way to evaluate efficacy of treatment.

- Encourage patients to keep a seizure calendar that notes the time and day a seizure occurs and the type of seizure. Compare seizure counts on a monthly basis to determine the level of seizure control.

Toxicity

- Monitor acute toxicity of AEDs at every clinic visit.

- Question patients about common adverse effects of the AEDs they are receiving. Weigh the impact of acute adverse effects against the extent of seizure control achieved from a treatment regimen. If it is determined the adverse effects negatively impact the patient more than the extent of seizure control benefits the patient, adjust the therapeutic regimen. Continuously monitor chronic adverse effects of AEDs.

Abbreviations Introduced in This Chapter

AAN	American Academy of Neurology
AED	Antiepileptic drug
EEG	Electroencephalograph
GABA	Gamma-aminobutyric acid
ILAE	International League Against Epilepsy
JME	Juvenile myoclonic epilepsy
LFTs	Liver function tests
LGS	Lennox-Gastaut syndrome
MTLE	Mesial temporal lobe epilepsy
NICE	National Institute for Clinical Excellence in the United Kingdom
PDS	Paroxysmal depolarizing shift
SIGN	Scottish Intercollegiate Guidelines Network

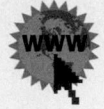

Self-assessment questions and answers are available at *http://www.mhpharmacotherapy.com/pp.html.*

REFERENCES

1. Hauser WA, Kurland LT. The epidemiology of epilepsy in Rochester, Minnesota, 1935 through 1967. Epilepsia 1975;16:143–161.
2. Annegers JF, Hauswer WA, Eleveback LR. Remission of seizures and relapse in patients with epilepsy. Epilepsia 1979;20:729–737.
3. Shamansky SL, Glaser GH. Socioeconomic characteristics of childhood seizure disorders in the New Haven area: An epidemiologic study. Epilepsia 1979;20:457–474.
4. Jallon P, Samdja D, Cabre P, et al. Epileptic seizures epilepsy and risk factors: Experiences with an investigation in Martinique. Epimart Group. Rev Neurol (Paris) 1998;154:408–411.
5. Epilepsy Foundation. Driver information by state. *http://www.epilepsyfoundation.org/living/wellness/transportation/drivinglaws.cfm.* Accessed October 5, 2009.
6. Elger CE, Helmstaedter C, Kurthen M. Chronic epilepsy and cognition. Lancet Neurol 2004;3(11):663–672.
7. Epilepsy Foundation. Education. *http://www.epilepsyfoundation.org/answerplace/Social/education/.* Accessed October 5, 2009.
8. Jallon P, Loiseau P, Loiseau J. Newly diagnosed unprovoked epileptic seizures: Presentation at diagnosis in the CAROLE study. Epilepsia 2001;42:464–475.
9. Najm I, Möddel G, Janigro D. Mechanisms of epileptogenesis and experimental models of seizures. In: Wyllie E, ed. The Treatment of Epilepsy. 4th ed. Philadelphia: Lippincott Williams and Wilkins, 2006.
10. Jones SW. Basic cellular neurophysiology. In Wyllie E, ed. The Treatment of Epilepsy. 4th ed. Philadelphia: Lippincott Williams and Wilkins, 2006.
11. Czapinski P, Blaszczyk B, Czuczwar SJ. Mechanisms of action of antiepileptic drugs. Curr Top Med Chem 2005;5(1):3–14.
12. Abrous DN, Koehl M, Le Moal M. Adult neurogenesis: From precursors to network and physiology. Physiol 2005;85(2):523–569.
13. Gaitatzis A, Sander JW. The mortality of epilepsy revisited. Epileptic Disord 2004;6:3–13.
14. Panayiotopoulos CP. Idiopathic generalized epilepsies: A review and modern approach. Epilepsia 2005;46(Suppl9):1–6.
15. Wong M. Advances in the pathophysiology of developmental epilepsies. Semin Pediatr Neurol 2005; 12:72–87.
16. Commission on Classification and Terminology of the International League Against Epilepsy. Proposal for revised clinical and electroencephalographic classification of epileptic seizures. Epilepsia 1981;22:489–501.
17. Commission on Classification and Terminology of the International League Against Epilepsy. Proposal for revised classification of epilepsies and epileptic syndromes. Epilepsia 1989;30:389–399.
18. Fisher RS, van Emde Boas W, Blume W, et al. Epileptic seizures and epilepsy: Definitions proposed by the International League Against Epilepsy (ILAE) and the International Bureau for Epilepsy (IBE). Epilepsia 2005;46(4):470–472.
19. Engel J Jr. A proposed diagnostic scheme for people with epileptic seizures and with epilepsy: Report of the ILAE Task Force on Classification and Terminology. Epilepsia 2001;42:796–803.
20. Smith SJ. EEG in the diagnosis, classification, and management of patients with epilepsy. J Neurol Neurosurg Psychiatry 2005;76(Suppl 2):ii2–ii7.
21. Hauser WA, Rich SS, Annegers JF, et al. Seizure recurrence after a first unprovoked seizure: An extended follow-up. Neurology 1990;40:1163–1170.
22. Lachhwani DK, Wyllie E. Outcome and complications of epilepsy surgery. In Wyllie E, ed. The Treatment of Epilepsy. 4th ed. Philadelphia: Lippincott Williams and Wilkins, 2006.
23. National Institute of Neurological Disorders and Stroke. Surgical treatment of epilepsy. Proceedings of a Consensus Conference. March 19–21, 1990. Epilepsy Res 1992;5(Suppl):1–250.
24. Wheless JW. Vagus nerve stimulation therapy. In Wyllie E, ed. The Treatment of Epilepsy. 4th ed. Philadelphia: Lippincott Williams and Wilkins, 2006.
25. Nordli DR, DeVivo DC. The ketogenic diet. In Wyllie E, ed. The Treatment of Epilepsy. 4th ed. Philadelphia: Lippincott Williams and Wilkins, 2006.
26. Perruca E. An introduction to antiepileptic drugs. Epilepsia 2005;46(Suppl 4):31–37.
27. Privitera MD. Clinical rules for phenytoin dosing. Ann Pharmacother. 1993 Oct;27(10):1169–1173.
28. Scottish Intercollegiate Guidelines Network. Diagnosis and management of epilepsy in adults. *http://www.sign.ac.uk/pdf/sign70.pdf.* Accessed October 5, 2009.
29. National Institute for Clinical Excellence. The epilepsies: The diagnosis and management of the epilepsies in children and adults in primary and secondary care. *http://www.guidance.nice.org.uk/CG20.* Accessed October 5, 2009.
30. French JA, Kanner AM, Bautista J, et al. Efficacy and tolerability of the new antiepileptic drugs I: Treatment of new onset epilepsy report of the Therapeutics and Technology Assessment Subcommittee and Quality Standards Subcommittee of the American Academy of Neurology and the American Epilepsy Society. Neurology 2005;62:1252–1260.
31. French JA, Kanner AM, Bautista J, et.al. Efficacy and tolerability of the new antiepileptic drugs II: Treatment of refractory epilepsy report of the Therapeutics and Technology Assessment Subcommittee and Quality Standards Subcommittee of the American Academy of Neurology and the American Epilepsy Society. Neurology 2005;62:1261–1273.
32. Vestergaard P. Epilepsy, osteoporosis and fracture risk—A meta-analysis. Acta Neurol Scand. 2005;112:227–286.
33. Koppel BS, Harden CL, Nikolov BG, Labar DR. An analysis of lifetime fractures in women with epilepsy. Acta Neurol Scand 2005;111(4):225–228.
34. Harden CL, Goldstein MA. Mood disorders in patients with epilepsy: Epidemiology and management. CNS Drugs 2002;16:291–302.
35. Schmidt D, Loscher W. Uncontrolled epilepsy following discontinuation of antiepileptic drugs in seizure-free patients: A review of current clinical experience. Acta Neurol Scand 2005;111(5):291–300.

36. Tsur VG, O'Dell C, Shinnar S. Initiation and discontinuation of antiepileptic drugs. In Wyllie E, ed. The Treatment of Epilepsy. 4th ed. Philadelphia: Lippincott Williams and Wilkins, 2006.

37. Perucea E. Clinically relevant drug interactions with antiepileptic drugs. Br J Clin Pharmacol 2006;61(3):246–255.

38. Bailer M. The pharmacokinetics and interactions of new antiepileptic drugs: An overview. Their Drug Monit 2005;27(6):722–726.

39. Anderson GD. Pharmacogenetic and enzyme induction/inhibition properties of antiepileptic drugs. Neurology 2004;63(10 Suppl 4):53–58.

40. Crawford P. Best practice guidelines for the management of women with epilepsy. Epilepsia 2005;46(Suppl 9):117–124.

41. Foldvary-Schaefer N, Morrel MJ. Epilepsy in women: The biological basis for the female experience. Cleve Clin J Med 2004;71(Suppl 2):S1–S8.

42. Artama M, Auvinen A, Raudaskoski T, et al. Antiepileptic drug use of women with epilepsy and congenital malformations in offspring. Neurology 2005;64(11):1874–1878.

31 Status Epilepticus

Gretchen M. Brophy and Eljim P. Tesoro

LEARNING OBJECTIVES

● **Upon completion of the chapter, the reader will be able to:**

1. Discuss the pathophysiology of status epilepticus (SE).
2. Explain the urgency of diagnosis and treatment of SE.
3. Recognize the signs and symptoms of SE.
4. Identify the treatment options available for termination of SE.
5. Formulate an initial treatment strategy for a patient in generalized convulsive SE.
6. Compare the pharmacotherapeutic options for refractory SE.
7. Describe adverse drug events associated with the pharmacotherapy of SE.
8. Recommend monitoring parameters for a patient in SE.

KEY CONCEPTS

❶ Status epilepticus (SE) is a neurologic emergency that can lead to permanent brain damage or death.

❷ SE can be defined as any seizure lasting more than 30 minutes, with or without loss of consciousness, or having recurrent seizures without regaining consciousness between episodes. However, this definition does not provide any guidance for treatment in the clinical setting where interventions begin within a few minutes of seizure onset. A more practical definition would be continuous seizure activity lasting more than 5 minutes, or two or more seizures without complete recovery of consciousness.

❸ It is important to evaluate possible etiologies of SE and treat underlying causes to optimize seizure control.

❹ The goal of therapy is to arrest physical and electroencephalographic evidence of seizures, prevent their recurrence, and minimize adverse drug events.

❺ The first-line treatment for SE is IV benzodiazepines. Lorazepam, diazepam, or midazolam may be used to rapidly control clinical signs of seizures. Lorazepam is currently considered the first-line agent by most clinicians.

❻ Antiepileptic drugs (AEDs) are used to prevent the seizure recurrence. IV phenytoin (or fosphenytoin) and phenobarbital are administered after benzodiazepines.

❼ Refractory status epilepticus (RSE) is seizure activity that is not controlled by first- and second-line therapies, including benzodiazepines and AEDs.

❽ Midazolam, propofol, and pentobarbital infusions can be used for RSE, but intensive monitoring and supportive care are required.

❶ *Status epilepticus (SE) is a neurologic emergency that can lead to permanent brain damage or death.* ❷ *SE can be defined as any seizure lasting more than 30 minutes, with or without a loss of consciousness; or having recurrent seizures without regaining consciousness between episodes.*[1] *However, this definition does not provide any guidance for treatment in the clinical setting where interventions begin within a few minutes of seizure onset. A more practical definition would be continuous seizures lasting more than 5 minutes or two or more seizures without complete recovery of consciousness.*[2] *Refractory status epilepticus (RSE) can be defined as seizure activity that does not respond to first- or second-line antiepileptic therapy.*[3]

SE can present as nonconvulsive status epilepticus (NCSE) or generalized convulsive status epilepticus (GCSE). NCSE is characterized by a persistent state of impaired consciousness and/or motor or sensory seizures without impaired consciousness. For patients with NCSE, electroencephalography (EEG) is essential for diagnosis. GCSE is characterized by full body motor seizures and involves the entire brain. This chapter will focus on GCSE, the most common type of SE, which is associated with the greatest risk of neurologic and physical damage.

Patient Encounter, Part 1

CH, a 42-year-old man, comes into the emergency department after his sister discovered him seizing at home. He has a history of hypertension, diabetes, epilepsy, and rheumatoid arthritis. His medications include hydrochlorothiazide, glyburide, phenytoin, and aspirin. He smokes one pack per day, drinks heavily on the weekends, and has a history of cocaine use. Upon further discussion with his sister, you discover that he stopped taking his phenytoin 4 days ago due to failure to obtain a refill from his doctor. He is currently unarousable since his last seizure 10 minutes ago.

What initial assessments should be performed?

What are some possible etiologies for his seizure?

What interventions need to be performed at this time?

EPIDEMIOLOGY AND ETIOLOGY

There are an estimated 150,000 cases of SE each year in the United States, with approximately 55,000 associated deaths, and an estimated annual direct cost for inpatient admissions of $4 billion.[4,5] SE occurs more frequently in African Americans, children, and the elderly.

❸ *It is important to understand the underlying cause of SE, as this will guide the course of treatment, potentially shortening the duration of SE and improve outcomes.* The causes of SE can be categorized as acute or chronic. Acute changes that cause SE include metabolic disturbances; CNS disorders, infections, or injuries; hypoxia; drug toxicity (e.g., theophylline, isoniazid, cyclosporine, cocaine); or acute illness. Chronic processes that cause SE includes pre-existing epilepsy, chronic alcohol abuse (withdrawal seizures), CNS tumors, and strokes.[3] In epileptics, the common causes of SE are anticonvulsant withdrawal or subtherapeutic anticonvulsant levels. Patients with SE due to chronic processes generally respond well to antiepileptic drug (AED) therapy.

PATHOPHYSIOLOGY

SE occurs when the brain fails to stop an isolated seizure. The exact reason for this failure is unknown and probably involves multiple mechanisms. A seizure is likely to occur due to a mismatch of excitatory and inhibitory neurotransmitters in the brain. The primary excitatory neurotransmitter is glutamate. Glutamate stimulates postsynaptic N-methyl-D-aspartate (NMDA) receptors, causing an influx of calcium into the cells and depolarization of the neuron. Sustained depolarization may maintain SE and eventually cause neuronal injury and death.[6] The primary inhibitory neurotransmitter, γ-aminobutyric acid (GABA), opposes the excitatory response by stimulating $GABA_A$ receptors, enhancing chloride inhibitory currents, producing hyperpolarization, and inhibition of the postsynaptic cell membrane. The inhibitory ability of GABA diminishes as the duration of seizures increases, perhaps due to a mechanistic shift in the functional properties of the $GABA_A$ receptors, which causes a decrease in response to GABA-receptor agonists.[7,8] Seizures lasting more than 30 minutes can cause injury and neuronal loss in the hippocampal, cortical, and thalamic regions. These neurologic sequelae are related to the excessive electrical activity and alterations in cerebral metabolic demand. The clinical impact of the $GABA_A$-receptor changes on treatment response and the worsening degree of neuronal injury with prolongation of seizure activity highlights the urgency of rapid control of SE.

Several systemic changes occur in two phases during the course of SE. Phase I occurs during the first 30 minutes of seizure activity, and phase II occurs after 30 minutes of seizure activity.[9]

Phase I

During phase I, each seizure causes a sharp increase in autonomic activity with elevations in epinephrine, norepinephrine, and steroid plasma concentrations, resulting in hypertension, tachycardia, hyperglycemia, hyperthermia, sweating, and salivation. Cerebral blood flow is also increased to preserve the oxygen supply to the brain during this period of high metabolic demand. Increases in sympathetic and parasympathetic stimulation with muscle hypoxia can lead to ventricular arrhythmias, severe acidosis, and rhabdomyolysis, which could then lead to hypotension, shock, hyperkalemia, and acute tubular necrosis.

Phase II

After approximately 30 minutes of continuous seizure activity, phase II begins with loss of cerebral autoregulation, decreased cerebral blood flow, increased intracranial pressure, and systemic hypotension. Metabolic demand is still high; however, the body is no longer able to compensate. The systemic changes that may occur include hypoglycemia, hyperthermia, respiratory failure, hypoxia, respiratory and metabolic acidosis, hyperkalemia, hyponatremia, and uremia. It is important to note that motor activity may not be clinically evident during prolonged seizures, but the electrical activity may still exist. This is referred to as subclinical seizure activity and needs to be recognized and treated aggressively.

CLINICAL PRESENTATION AND DIAGNOSIS

History

❸ *When a patient presents with seizures, a thorough history is needed to determine the type and duration of the seizure activity. This will help guide therapy and identify which laboratory and diagnostic tests need to be conducted.* A diagnosis of SE will be made when a patient with a history of repeated seizures and impaired consciousness has a seizure witnessed by a health care professional.

Clinical Presentation of SE

General

The patient may present with or without clinically noticeable seizure activity.

Symptoms

- Impaired consciousness ranging from lethargy to coma
- Disorientation after cessation of GCSE
- Pain from associated injuries (e.g., tongue lacerations, dislocated shoulder, head trauma, facial trauma)

Signs

Phase I:

- Generalized convulsions
- Hypertension, tachycardia
- Fever and sweating
- Muscle contractions, spasms
- Respiratory compromise
- Incontinence

Phase II (greater than 30 minutes of SE):

- Respiratory failure with pulmonary edema
- Cardiac failure (arrhythmias, shock)
- Hypotension
- Hyperthermia
- Rhabdomyolysis and multiorgan failure

Laboratory Tests

- Hyperglycemia (phase I) and hypoglycemia (phase II) can occur
- Hyponatremia, hypernatremia, hyperkalemia, hypocalcemia, hypomagnesemia, and hypoglycemia can cause SE
- The WBC count may slightly increase
- Abnormal ABGs due to hypoxia and respiratory or metabolic acidosis
- Elevated serum creatinine will be present in renal failure patients
- Myoglobinuria can occur in patients with continuous seizures

Diagnostic Tests

- EEG will show seizure activity

Physical Examination

Once seizures are controlled, a neurologic examination should be conducted to evaluate level of consciousness (coma, lethargy, or somnolence), motor function and reflexes (rhythmic contractions, rigidity, spasms, or posturing), and pupillary response. A physical examination to identify secondary injuries from SE should also be conducted.

Clinical Symptoms

Patients with SE usually present with generalized, convulsive tonic-clonic seizure activity that is unresponsive to initial AED treatment. They may also be hypertensive, tachycardic, febrile, and diaphoretic; however, these symptoms will resolve soon after the seizure is terminated. A loss of bowel or bladder function, respiratory compromise, and nystagmus may also be observed. When seizure activity is sustained for more than approximately 30 to 60 minutes, muscle contractions may no longer be visible, but the patient remains in SE. Twitching of the face, hands, or feet may be seen in these comatose patients with prolonged seizures. As motor signs diminish, an EEG will be necessary to diagnose SE.

Laboratory Parameters

3 *It is important to obtain a serum chemistry profile to help identify the underlying cause of SE.* Abnormalities that can cause seizures include hypoglycemia, hyponatremia, hypernatremia, hypomagnesemia, hypocalcemia, and renal and liver failure. In a febrile patient with an elevated white blood cell count (WBC), an active infection should be ruled out or treated appropriately. Cultures from the blood, cerebrospinal fluid (CSF), respiratory tract, and urine should be obtained once the seizures are controlled. CT or MRI can be done to rule out CNS abscesses, bleeding, or tumors, all of which may be a source for seizure activity. A blood alcohol level and urine toxicology screen for drugs of abuse should also be conducted to determine if alcohol withdrawal, illicit drug use, or a drug overdose could be the underlying cause of SE. Also, drug levels should be obtained in a drug overdose situation to rule out toxicity as a cause of SE. **3** *Knowing the source of SE will help guide the initial antiepileptic therapy and increase the probability of halting seizure activity.*

In patients who use AEDs, a baseline serum concentration may be useful to determine if the drug concentration is below the desired range and if a loading dose is needed. Albumin levels, renal function tests, and liver function tests can also be utilized when assessing antiepileptic therapy.

Hypoxia and respiratory or metabolic acidosis are common in patients with SE. Therefore, pulse oximetry and arterial blood gas (ABG) measurements are used to assess respiratory status and determine if airway protection or supplemental oxygen is needed. Metabolic acidosis typically corrects on its own after seizure activity stops, so pharmacologic treatment is not required.

Diagnostic Tests

The only way to determine if a comatose patient has SE is by EEG, which should be used in patients who remain unconscious after initial antiepileptic treatment, and for those who receive long-acting paralytic agents or require prolonged therapy for RSE. Treatment should never be delayed while awaiting EEG results. An ECG should be obtained to rule out cardiac dysfunction when hypotension or an abnormal heart rate is observed.

Patient Encounter, Part 2

Physical examination and laboratory studies reveal the following additional information about CH.

PE:

VS: BP 148/87 mm Hg, pulse 115 bpm, RR 23/min, T 39.0°C (102.2°F), ht 180 cm (5'11"), wt 80 kg (176 lb)

CNS: Unresponsive, unarousable

CV: Sinus tachycardia; normal S1, S2; no murmurs, rubs, gallops

Pulmonary: Tachypneic; oxygen saturation 92% on room air; no rhonchi, wheezes, rales

Abdomen: Firm, nontender, nondistended; (+) bowel sounds; no hepatosplenomegaly

Extremities: Rhythmic tonic-clonic movements of all extremities

GU: Incontinent of urine and stool

HEENT: Persistent upward gaze

Labs:

Sodium 130 mEq/L (130 mmol/L)
WBC 12 × 10³/mm³ (12 × 10⁹/L)
Phenytoin 2.1 mcg/mL (8.3 μmol/L)
Albumin 3.5 g/dL (35 g/L)
Potassium 3.5 mEq/L (3.5 mmol/L)
Hemoglobin 14 g/dL (140 g/L or 8.7 mmol/L)
Chloride 100 mEq/L (100 mmol/L)
Hematocrit 42% (0.42 volume fraction)
Carbon dioxide 12 mEq/L (12 mmol/L)
Platelets 235 × 10³/mm³ (235 × 10⁹/L)
Blood urea nitrogen 10 mg/dL (3.6 mmol/L)
Prothrombin time 12 seconds
Serum creatinine 0.9 mg/dL (80 μmol/L)
International Normalized Ratio 1.1
Glucose 189 mg/dL (10.5 mmol/L)
Activated partial thromboplastin time 28 seconds

What is your assessment of the cause of this patient's condition?

Identify your goals of therapy for this patient.

What therapies must be instituted next?

TREATMENT

Desired Outcomes

④ The goals of treatment of SE include the cessation of any seizure activity, both clinical and subclinical, and the prevention of further seizures. Ideally, this is accomplished through directed pharmacotherapy with minimization of any side effects or adverse reactions. Complications of SE should also be treated.

General Approach

The initial approach to SE involves first removing the patient from harmful surroundings and ensuring a safe airway to prevent respiratory collapse or aspiration. Benzodiazepines are the first medications administered, as they are the drugs of choice to stop acute seizure activity, followed by the initiation of an AED. Medications are typically given IV for immediate onset of action, but if no IV access is available, certain medications may be given intramuscularly (IM), rectally, buccally, or via an endotracheal tube. Once the seizures stop, clinicians must identify and treat the underlying cause of the seizures, such as toxins, hypoglycemia, or trauma. Patients with known seizure disorders should be evaluated for abrupt cessation of their medications or for history of noncompliance.

Nonpharmacologic Treatment

Nondrug interventions include administration of oxygen or intubation for mechanical ventilation in cases of hypoxia or body cooling for febrile seizures. Specialists in neurology or epileptology should be consulted as appropriate. Admission to an emergency department or intensive care unit will allow appropriate monitoring during the seizure and postictal period.

Pharmacologic Treatment

▶ Initial Treatment

All patients should receive glucose in case of hypoglycemia-induced SE. In patients with a history of alcohol abuse, thiamine 100 mg should be given prior to the administration of any glucose-containing solutions to prevent encephalopathy.

▶ Benzodiazepines

⑤ Initial drug therapy begins with the administration of an IV benzodiazepine since they are most effective in aborting seizure activity. IV bolus doses of diazepam, lorazepam, and midazolam have all been used in SE because of their rapid effects at inhibitory GABA receptors in the CNS. Lorazepam is now considered the first-line agent by most clinicians. When treating patients on chronic benzodiazepines therapy, clinicians should consider higher doses to overcome the effects of tolerance. Diazepam and lorazepam should be diluted with normal saline in a 1:1 ratio before parenteral administration via peripheral veins to avoid venous irritation from the propylene glycol diluent in the formulation.

Diazepam Being extremely lipophilic, diazepam penetrates quickly into the CNS, but can rapidly redistribute out into the body fat and muscle. This results in a faster decline in CNS levels and early recurrence of seizures. It is dosed at 5 to 10 mg (or 0.15 mg/kg) and infused no faster than 5 mg/min. Repeated doses can be given every 5 minutes until seizure activity stops or toxicities are seen (e.g., respiratory depression). Diazepam can also be administered as a rectal suppository, making it possible for nonmedical personnel to provide rapid therapy for seizures that develop at home or in public areas.[10] The adult dose is 10 mg given rectally and this dose may be repeated once if necessary. Diazepam is erratically absorbed via the IM route; therefore, IM administration is not recommended.

Lorazepam Less lipophilic than diazepam, lorazepam has a longer redistribution half-life, resulting in longer duration of action and a decrease in the need for repeated doses. Both lorazepam and diazepam are effective in stopping seizures,[11] but lorazepam is currently the preferred agent due to a longer duration of action. Lorazepam is given as a single IV dose of 0.1 mg/kg (maximum dose is 4 mg) with a maximum rate of infusion of 2 mg/min. It can be redosed every 10 to 15 minutes (up to a maximum cumulative dose of 8 mg) until seizure activity stops or side effects such as respiratory depression occur. IM administration is not preferred due to slow and unpredictable absorption.

Midazolam Midazolam is water-soluble and can be administered IV, IM,[12] buccally,[13] and nasally.[14] At physiologic pH, it becomes more lipophilic and can diffuse into the CNS. Compared to diazepam and lorazepam, it has fewer effects on the respiratory and cardiovascular systems. Its short half-life requires that it be redosed frequently or administered as a continuous infusion. Midazolam can be given at 0.2 mg/kg either IV or IM as a single dose.[15] The liquid or injectable formulation can be given buccally or intranasally (0.3 mg/kg) when IV access cannot be secured. Nasal administration in SE can be hindered by rapid breathing and increased nasal secretions.

▶ Anticonvulsants

6 *Once the first dose of benzodiazepine is given, an AED should be started to prevent further seizures from occurring.* If the underlying cause of the seizures has been corrected (e.g., hypoglycemia) and seizure activity has ceased, an AED may not be necessary. AEDs must not be given as first-line therapy because they are infused relatively slowly to avoid adverse effects, delaying their onset of action.

Once the loading dose of the AED is administered, it is important to initiate maintenance doses to ensure that therapeutic levels are sustained. Chronic and idiosyncratic side effects as well as potential drug interactions should be considered if the patient will continue AED therapy indefinitely. All drugs should be adjusted for any hepatic or renal disease states. Table 31–1 summarizes the drug doses used in SE, and Table 31–2 provides an example of an algorithm for the

---

Table 31–1

Parenteral Medications Used in SE in Adults

Drug Name (Brand Name)	Loading Dose and RSE Maintenance Dose (If Applicable)	Administration Rate	Therapeutic Level	Side Effects	Comments
Diazepam (Valium)	0.15 mg/kg	5 mg/min (IVP)	N/A	Hypotension, respiratory depression	Rapid redistribution rate; can be given rectally
Lorazepam (Ativan)	0.1 mg/kg	2 mg/min (IVP)	N/A	Hypotension, respiratory depression	May be longer-acting than diazepam
Midazolam (Versed)	0.2 mg/kg RSE: 0.05–2 mg/kg/h	2 mg/min (IVP)	N/A	Sedation, respiratory depression	Can also be given IM, buccally, intranasally; expensive
Phenytoin (Dilantin)	15–20 mg/kg	Up to 50 mg/min	10–20 mcg/mL (39.6–79.2 µmol/L)	Arrhythmias, hypotension,	Hypotension, especially in elderly
Fosphenytoin (Cerebyx)	15–20 mg PE/kg	Up to 150 mg PE/min	10–20 mcg/mL (39.6–79.2 µmol/L)	Paresthesias, hypotension	Can be given IM; less CV side effects than phenytoin
Phenobarbital (Luminal)	20 mg/kg	50–100 mg/min	15–40 mcg/mL (64.7–172.4 µmol/L)	Hypotension, sedation, respiratory depression	Long acting
Valproate sodium (Depacon)	15–20 mg/kg (up to 40 mg/kg)	3–6 mg/kg/min	50–150 mcg/mL (346.5–1,039.5 µmol/L)		Less CV side effects than phenytoin
Propofol (Diprivan)	1–2 mg/kg RSE: 2–15 mg/kg/h	Approximately 40 mg every 10 seconds	N/A (typically titrated to EEG)	Hypotension, respiratory depression	Requires mechanical intubation; high lipid load (increased calories); propofol infusion syndrome
Pentobarbital (Nembutal)	10–15 mg/kg RSE: 0.5–4 mg/kg/h	Up to 50 mg/min	10–20 mcg/mL (typically titrated to EEG)	Hypotension, respiratory depression, cardiac depression, infection, ileus	Requires mechanical intubation, pressors, hemodynamic monitoring

CV, cardiovascular; EEG, electroencephalogram; IM, intramuscular; IVP, intravenous push; N/A, not applicable; PE, phenytoin equivalents.

Table 31–2

Algorithm for Treatment of SE in Adults

Time (Minutes)	Assessment/Monitoring	Treatment
0	Vital signs[a] Assess airway Monitor cardiac function (ECG) Pulse oximeter Check blood glucose Check laboratory tests: CBC Serum chemistries Liver function tests ABG Blood cultures Serum anticonvulsant levels Urine drug/alcohol screen	Stabilize airway (intubate if necessary) Administer oxygen Secure IV access and start fluids Give thiamine (100 mg) + glucose (50 mL of 50% solution) if hypoglycemic
0–10	Vital signs[a] Physical examination Patient history including medications (prescription, OTC, and herbals)	Lorazepam 0.1 mg/kg (maximum 4 mg) IVP at 2 mg/min (may repeat in 10–15 minutes to maximum of 8 mg if no response) If no IV access, can give: diazepam 10 mg PR (may repeat in 10 minutes if no response); midazolam 0.2 mg/kg IM (may repeat in 10 minutes if no response) AED may not be necessary if underlying cause is corrected and seizures have ceased
10–30	Vital signs[a] Review laboratory results and correct any underlying abnormalities CT scan (if seizures controlled)	Phenytoin 15–20 mg/kg IV at a maximum rate of 50 mg/min (or fosphenytoin 15–20 mg PE/kg IV at a maximum rate of 150 mg/min) If no IV access, can give fosphenytoin IM In patients allergic to phenytoin, give valproate sodium 20 mg/kg IV at a maximum rate of 6 mg/kg/min Treat for possible infection
30–60	Vital signs[a] Consult neurologist/epileptologist Consider admission to ICU Consider EEG	If seizures continue: Additional phenytoin bolus 5–10 mg/kg (or fosphenytoin 5–10 mg PE/kg) OR start phenobarbital at 20 mg/kg IV at a maximum rate of 100 mg/min OR start valproate sodium 20 mg/kg IV at a maximum rate of 6 mg/kg/min in patients who are not intubated
Greater than 60: RSE	Vital signs[a] Transfer to ICU Obtain EEG Consider MRI when controlled	Midazolam 2 mg/kg bolus followed by 0.05–2 mg/kg/h CI OR propofol 1 mg/kg bolus followed by 2–15 mg/kg/h CI OR pentobarbital 10–15 mg/kg bolus over 1–2 hours followed by 0.5–4 mg/kg/h Consider intubation and/or pressor support if needed Optimize AED levels: repeat boluses of phenobarbital 10 mg/kg OR valproate sodium 20 mg/kg

CI, continuous infusion; EEG, electroencephalography; IVP, intravenous push; OTC, over-the-counter; PE, phenytoin equivalents; PR, per rectum; RSE, refractory status epilepticus.

[a]Heart rate, respiratory rate, blood pressure, temperature.

Adapted from Phelps SJ, Hovinga CA, Wheless JW. Status epilepticus. In: DiPiro JT, Talbert RL, Yee GC, et al. (eds.) Pharmacotherapy: A Pathophysiologic Approach. 7th ed. New York: McGraw-Hill; 2008: 958, with permission.

treatment of patients in SE. Published studies comparing these treatment strategies are summarized in Table 31–3.

Phenytoin The most widely used AED is phenytoin, which is administered IV as a loading dose (for patients previously not on phenytoin) of 15 to 20 mg/kg. The loading dose must be modified in patients taking phenytoin who have subtherapeutic levels in order to avoid toxic serum concentrations. The loading dose is infused no faster than 50 mg/min due to potential risks of hypotension or arrhythmias. Continuous monitoring of ECG and blood pressure is recommended. Maintenance dosing can be started

12 hours after the loading dose. Phenytoin should not be infused with other medications because of stability concerns (it is soluble in propylene glycol and compatible only in 0.9% sodium chloride solutions). It should not be given via the IM route due to its alkaline nature. **Extravasation** of the drug can cause local discoloration, edema, pain, and sometimes necrosis (purple glove syndrome). Oral loading is not recommended in SE due to the delay in absorption.

Fosphenytoin Fosphenytoin is a water-soluble, phospho-ester prodrug that is rapidly converted to phenytoin in the body. It is compatible with most IV solutions and is well

Table 31–3				
Randomized, Prospective Trials Comparing Treatments for SE in Adults				
Study	**Treatment**	**Outcome**	**Adverse Events**	**Comments**
Leppik (1983)[16]	Diazepam 10 mg Lorazepam 4 mg	Seizure control: 76% 89%	Adverse events: 12% 13%	Onset did not differ between two groups
Shaner (1988)[17] *Goal*: Time to seizure control	Diazepam + phenytoin Phenobarbital +/– phenytoin	Time spent in SE: 9 minutes 5 minutes	Incidence of intubation, hypotension, and arrhythmias similar in both groups	Unblinded study
Treiman (1998)[18] *Goal*: Seizure control within 20 minutes and no recurrence within 60 minutes	Diazepam 0.15 mg/kg + phenytoin 18 mg/kg Lorazepam 0.1 mg/kg Phenobarbital 15 mg/kg Phenytoin 18 mg/kg	Seizure control: 55.8% 64.9% 58.2% 43.6%	Respiratory/cardiac events: 2.1–31.6% 7.2–25.8% 3.3–34.1% 6.9–27%	Patients with subtle GCSE fared worse than patients with overt GCSE
Alldredge (2001)[19] *Goal*: Seizure control on arrival to ED	Lorazepam 2 mg Diazepam 5 mg Placebo	Seizure control: 59.1% 42.6% 21.1%	Respiratory/cardiac events: 10.6% 10.3% 22.5%	Higher doses used in hospital for SE
Misra (2006)[20] *Goal*: Seizure control after infusion	Valproate sodium 30 mg/kg Phenytoin 18 mg/kg	Seizure control: 66% 42%	Respiratory/cardiac events: 4%/0% 14%/14%	As second-line agent, valproate controlled more seizures than phenytoin (79% vs 25%)
Agarwal (2007)[21] *Goal*: Motor or EEG seizure activity controlled within 20 minutes and no recurrence within 12 hours	Valproate sodium 20 mg/kg Phenytoin 20 mg/kg	Seizure control: 88% 84%	Respiratory/cardiac events: 0/0 4%/12%	Improved response seen if treated within 2 hours versus later; also these patients were relatively young (~27years)
Gilad (2008)[22] *Goal*: Seizure cessation within 20 minutes	Valproate sodium 30 mg/kg over 20 minutes Phenytoin 18 mg/kg over 20 minutes	Seizure control: 72.3% 77.8%	Adverse effects: 0% 12%	No benzodiazepine given initially

ED, emergency department; GCSE, generalized convulsive status epilepticus.

tolerated as an IM injection, even with the large volumes associated with loading doses (20–30 mL).[23] It is dosed in phenytoin equivalents (PE), and it can be infused three times as fast as phenytoin, up to 150 mg PE/min. The loading dose for patients not taking phenytoin is 15 to 20 mg PE/kg. It can be an advantage to use IM fosphenytoin when IV access cannot be obtained immediately and in patients without vascular access. Although it has fewer cardiovascular side effects than phenytoin, clinicians should still continuously monitor blood pressure, ECG, and heart rate. Maintenance doses are begun 12 hours after the loading dose. A common side effect is paresthesias, especially around the lips and groin, which typically resolves within a few minutes and should not necessitate stopping the infusion. If a post-load serum level is desired, it should be obtained 2 hours after an IV load or 4 hours after an IM load. Generic fosphenytoin is now available, so increased expense is no longer an issue.

Phenobarbital If phenytoin or fosphenytoin fails to prevent seizure recurrence, phenobarbital can be administered. However, emerging evidence suggests that phenobarbital may not be effective if SE persists after giving benzodiazepines and phenytoin. This may be due to the progressive resistance of the GABA$_A$ receptor, where barbiturates also act.[24] It is dosed as an IV load of 15 to 20 mg/kg with a maximum rate of administration of 100 mg/min. Adverse reactions of phenobarbital include sedation, hypotension, and respiratory depression; therefore, patients who receive a rapid IV loading dose of phenobarbital should have hemodynamic monitoring and be mechanically ventilated. Its long half-life makes it a popular agent for both acute treatment and chronic maintenance therapy.

Valproate Sodium Although valproate sodium is not FDA-approved for SE, its IV use has been documented in various types of SE including generalized tonic-clonic, myoclonic, and nonconvulsive SE.[25,26] One study comparing it to phenytoin found similar efficacy (80% cessation of seizure activity) but with less cardiopulmonary side effects.[21] It can be considered when the use of phenytoin and phenobarbital are precluded due to allergies or intolerance. Valproate sodium can be loaded IV at 15 to 20 mg/kg and infused at a rate of up to

Patient Encounter, Part 3

Treatment Failure

It has been 45 minutes since CH's arrival, and he has been given lorazepam 4 mg twice and loaded with 1,500 mg of phenytoin. He received another 400 mg dose of phenytoin 15 minutes ago, but is still unarousable. His jerking movements have slowed down, but his temperature is now 39.9°C (103.8°F), and his blood pressure has dropped to 124/62 mm Hg. His oxygen saturation is 91% on 4 L oxygen via nasal cannula. Bilateral crackles are heard upon auscultation of his lungs. A CT scan of his head is obtained and shows no evidence of hemorrhage, tumor, or mass effect.

What is your assessment of this patient's condition?

What possible treatment options exist at this time?

How would you optimize this patient's outcome?

6 mg/kg/min. Higher doses (up to 30–40 mg/kg) have also been used to attain serum levels of 100 to 150 mcg/mL (673–1,040 μmol/L), in less responsive cases of SE.[27]

Treatment of RSE

❼ *Seizure activity that does not respond to benzodiazepines (first-line) and antiepileptics (second-line), or persists beyond 60 minutes in duration can be considered RSE.*[28] It can occur in up to 30% of patients with SE and has a mortality rate approaching 50%. Patients in RSE are unlikely to return to their baseline state, even if the seizures are eventually controlled. As RSE progresses, clinical signs may become subtle, and in certain patients, an EEG is required to detect ongoing seizure activity. **❶** *Even SE patients without clinical signs of seizing are at risk for brain damage or even death.*

The optimal therapy for RSE has not been determined. Clinicians must aggressively investigate and treat possible causes including infection, tumors, drugs or toxins, metabolic disorders, liver failure, or fever.[29] In general, patients with RSE are managed in an ICU where hemodynamic and respiratory support are available and frequent monitoring can be performed. Continuous EEG monitoring is desirable to document cessation of seizure activity, but treatment should not be delayed if continuous EEG monitoring is not immediately available or while waiting for results. Any AEDs initiated before treatment for RSE should be continued, and their serum levels optimized in order to minimize any breakthrough or withdrawal seizures. **❽** *Treatment of RSE typically consists of continuous IV infusions of benzodiazepines (midazolam), anesthetic agents (propofol), or barbiturates (pentobarbital) to suppress all clinical and EEG evidence of seizures.*[30] These agents are typically titrated to achieve "burst suppression" on the EEG, although no strong evidence exists to support this as the universal goal.[31] Patients should be intubated and mechanically ventilated before initiating these treatment strategies for RSE. Consultation with a neurologist or epileptologist is highly recommended in these cases.

▶ *Midazolam*

A loading dose of 0.2 mg/kg (repeated up to a maximum of 2 mg/kg) followed by a continuous infusion of 0.05 to 2 mg/kg/h is recommended in RSE.[32-34] The dose must be adjusted during prolonged infusions, especially in patients with renal impairment, as the active metabolite can accumulate.[35] Breakthrough seizures are common with midazolam infusions and usually respond to a bolus and a 20% increase in the rate. Despite this, tachyphylaxis can occur and the patient should be switched to another agent if seizures continue.

▶ *Propofol*

The anesthetic agent propofol can be started with loading doses of 1 mg/kg repeated every 3 to 5 minutes until a clinical response is achieved, after which the infusion can be initiated at 2 to 4 mg/kg/h. Propofol can cause hypotension, especially with loading doses. Long-term, high-dose (greater than 5 mg/kg/h) propofol infusions are associated with rhabdomyolysis, acidosis, and cardiac arrhythmias (propofol infusion syndrome), especially in children.[36] Propofol has a very short serum half-life and should be tapered off slowly to avoid withdrawal seizures. High-dose propofol infusions can also provide a considerable amount of calories (1 kcal/mL [4.2 kJ/mL]) over time, so other sources of nutrition may have to be adjusted accordingly.

▶ *Pentobarbital*

Barbiturate infusions have been reported to be highly successful in treating RSE,[37] but their side effects are considerable. They can cause significant hypotension, myocardial and respiratory depression, ileus, and infection (especially gram-positive organisms). As a result, patients often require mechanical ventilation, IV **vasopressor** therapy, invasive hemodynamic monitoring, and total parenteral nutrition while undergoing "barbiturate coma." On the other hand, barbiturates are beneficial in patients with elevated intracranial pressure (ICP) problems.

Pentobarbital is commonly loaded at a dose of 10 to 15 mg/kg over 1 to 2 hours, followed by a continuous infusion of 0.5 to 4 mg/kg/h. Therapy can be tapered off after 12 to 24 hours of seizure control as evident on the EEG.[38] One meta-analysis reported a lower incidence of treatment failure with pentobarbital (3%) when compared to midazolam (21%) or propofol (20%), although the risk of hypotension requiring vasopressor therapy was higher with pentobarbital.[39] This relative efficacy for pentobarbital must be considered together with its complications when determining which agent to use. Patients who fail midazolam and/or propofol infusions should be switched over to pentobarbital therapy.

▶ *Levetiracetam*

Although not FDA approved for SE, levetiracetam is a newer antiepileptic that has ideal characteristics since it does not have the significant cardiopulmonary, hepatic, and sedative side effects seen with the other agents nor does it have potentially harmful drug interactions. Both IV and oral formulations have been used in RSE patients as add-on therapy with some success, although it is unclear if levetiracetam would be effective as a single agent in these cases.[40] Loading doses of up to 2,000 mg over 15 to 30 minutes in the critically ill have been documented with very little toxicity noted.[41]

▶ Other Agents

Ketamine,[42] topiramate, and inhaled anesthetics have also been used to treat RSE. Ketamine is an NMDA-receptor antagonist that has been given orally[43] and IV[44] for RSE in children. Topiramate is a newer oral antiepileptic agent with multiple mechanisms of action that may have some benefit in RSE. The dose in adults ranges from 300 to 1,600 mg/day.[45] Children have also been administered topiramate at a starting dose of 2 to 3 mg/kg/day and titrated to a maintenance dose of 5 to 6 mg/kg/day.[46] Topiramate can induce metabolic acidosis, and this should be monitored carefully. The inhaled anesthetics, desflurane and isoflurane,[47] are normally delivered in an operating room, and require special equipment for administration in an ICU. Future studies will determine their place in therapy.

Special Populations

Certain patient populations require special considerations due to their altered metabolism, unique volume of distribution, or increased risk for side effects.[48] Although many of these patients are excluded from clinical trials in SE, the standard algorithm for SE still applies in terms of immediate care, assessment, and drugs (see Table 31–2).

▶ Pediatrics

The treatment approach of SE in children is similar to that in adults with a few exceptions (Table 31–4). The doses are also weight-based but are typically higher than those used in adults due to higher clearance by the liver. It may be difficult to rapidly obtain IV access in children, so alternate routes of drug administration have been studied, including intranasal, buccal, rectal, and IM. Early administration of benzodiazepines and reduced time to hospital admission are important factors in decreasing the incidence of prolonged seizures.[49]

▶ Geriatrics

The elderly are prone to injury and toxicity from multiple concomitant disease states and polypharmacy. Seizures in the elderly can easily arise from metabolic disorders, drug interactions, or even incorrect dosing of medications in patients with impaired renal and hepatic function and decreased protein binding. Clinicians treating elderly patients with SE should investigate drug- and disease state–induced causes, since treating these etiologies alone may terminate seizures. Acute treatment with benzodiazepines and AEDs is no different in the elderly, but they may have more pronounced reactions to these medications in terms of their sedative and cardiorespiratory side effects. Phenytoin and fosphenytoin loading doses should be carefully calculated in the elderly, as their weights may be overestimated, and they may not tolerate high doses. They should also be infused

Table 31–4		
Drugs Used in Pediatric SE		
Drug	**Dose**	**Comments**
Diazepam (Valium injection, Diastat rectal gel)	IV: 0.2–0.3 mg/kg over 2–5 minutes PR: 2–5 years: 0.5 mg/kg 6–11 years: 0.3 mg/kg greater than 12 years: 0.2 mg/kg	Maximum dose in children less than 5 years: 5 mg Maximum dose in children greater than 5 years: 15 mg A second rectal dose can be given 4–12 hours after the first dose if necessary
Lorazepam (Ativan)	0.05–0.1 mg/kg IV over 2–4 minutes	May redose twice in 10–15 minutes if necessary
Midazolam (Versed)	0.2 mg/kg IV bolus followed by 0.05–0.6 mg/kg/h continuous infusion	Bolus dose may also be given intranasally, buccally, or intramuscularly
Phenytoin (Dilantin)	15–20 mg/kg IV at 1–3 mg/kg/min *max*	
Fosphenytoin (Cerebyx)	15–20 mg PE/kg IV at 3 mg/kg/min *max*	Dose can be given intramuscularly
Phenobarbital (Luminal)	15–20 mg/kg IV at 100 mg/min *max*	
Valproate sodium (Depacon)	15–20 mg/kg IV at 1.5–3 mg/kg/min	May have fewer cardiovascular side effects than other agents
Propofol (Diprivan)		Not recommended due to adverse events (e.g., propofol infusion syndrome)
Pentobarbital (Nembutal)	10–15 mg/kg IV over 1–2 hours followed by continuous infusion at 1 mg/kg/h	Titrated to EEG

PR, per rectum; EEG, electroencephalograph; PE phenytoin equivalent.

at slower rates to minimize hypotension and arrhythmias. Phenobarbital may cause respiratory depression earlier in the elderly, especially after benzodiazepines are administered. Clinicians should consider using smaller doses and evaluate for renal and hepatic insufficiency if repeated doses are to be given.

▶ *Pregnancy*

The main concern in the treatment of pregnant females in SE is the safety of the fetus that is at risk of hypoxia during periods of prolonged seizures. Although many of the agents used in SE are **teratogenic**, clinicians should still use them as acute measures to stop the seizures and consider alternative agents as maintenance therapy. The volume of distribution and clearance of many drugs are typically increased during pregnancy, and this should be considered when calculating doses.

Patient Care and Monitoring

1. Obtain a seizure history from the patient or family members, including precipitating factors and duration of seizure activity.

2. Identify the underlying cause of the seizures and correct the cause, if possible. Does the patient have any laboratory abnormalities? Is there a positive toxicology screen for alcohol or drugs?

3. Obtain a thorough history of nonprescription, prescription, and alternative or herbal drug use. Determine adherence with the medication regimen and whether barriers to care exist. Does the patient have the financial ability and transportation to obtain their prescriptions?

4. Assess the AED serum concentration and adjust therapy as needed for agents with a defined therapeutic range (e.g., phenytoin, carbamazepine, valproic acid, and phenobarbital). Drug levels can also be used to determine adherence to medication regimens for agents that do not have defined ranges.

5. Evaluate the patient for adverse drug reactions, IV site extravasation, and allergic reactions. What alternative AEDs should be used if a drug allergy is identified?

6. Determine whether there are any drug interactions with the patient's current or home medication regimens. Do you need to adjust the dose of any medications for toxic or subtherapeutic concentrations from the drug interaction?

7. Maintain adequate cardiovascular support, nutrition, and electrolyte and glucose serum concentrations to prevent recurrence of seizure activity.

8. Continue to evaluate the patient for seizure activity and adjust therapy as needed to control seizures and optimize quality of life.

OUTCOME EVALUATION

❹ *The success of treatment is measured by the early termination of seizures, without adverse drug effects or brain injury.* Therefore, start pharmacologic treatment as soon as possible.

- First-line treatment for SE should halt seizure activity within minutes of administration.

- In patients who are unarousable following treatment, an EEG can confirm termination of seizures.

- Perform a physical exam and evaluation of the patient's laboratory results to help determine if the cause or complications of seizure activity are being appropriately treated.

  Once seizure activity has ceased and the patient has stabilized, review the patient's therapeutic regimen.

- Evaluate and monitor serum trough concentrations of AEDs with defined target ranges to determine patient-specific therapeutic goals.

- If there is a known cause of SE, treat it and simplify therapy.

- In patients with RSE on multiple AEDs, slowly decrease the dose of one drug at a time while continuing to evaluate the patient for seizure activity.

- Base the titration schedule on the half-life of the drug and individual patient response.

- Optimize treatment using the fewest medications to prevent seizure recurrence without causing adverse drug reactions.

- Continue to monitor AED serum trough concentrations approximately every 3 to 5 days until the AEDs have reached steady-state concentrations.

- Give additional loading doses or hold doses as needed to maintain target trough concentrations.

- Monitor the patient for signs of drug toxicity and seizures until drug concentrations have stabilized.

- Drug interactions are common in patients taking multiple AEDs; therefore, closely evaluate their medication profiles and change drugs or doses to minimize any interaction, if possible.

Abbreviations Introduced in This Chapter

ABG	Arterial blood gas
AED	Antiepileptic drug
CSF	Cerebrospinal fluid
EEG	Electroencephalography
GABA	γ-Aminobutyric acid
GCSE	Generalized convulsive status epilepticus
HEENT	Head ears eyes nose throat
ICP	Intracranial pressure
IM	Intramuscular
NCSE	Nonconvulsive status epilepticus

NMDA   *N*-Methyl-D-aspartate
PE   Phenytoin equivalent
PR   Per rectum
RSE   Refractory status epilepticus
SE   Status epilepticus

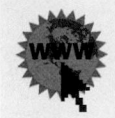 Self-assessment questions and answers are available at *http://www.mhpharmacotherapy. com/pp.html.*

REFERENCES

1. Commission on Classification of Terminology, International League against Epilepsy. Proposal for revised clinical and electroencephalographic classification of epileptic seizures. Epilepsia 1981;22:489–501.
2. Lowenstein D, Bleck T, Macdonald RL. It's time to revise the definition of status epilepticus. Epilepsia 1999;40:120–122.
3. Lowenstein DH, Alldredge BK. Status epilepticus. N Engl J Med 1998;338:970–976.
4. DeLorenzo RJ, Pellock JM, Towne AR, Boggs JG. Epidemiology of status epilepticus. J Clin Neurophysiol 1995;12:316–328.
5. Penberthy LT, Towne A, Garnett LK, et al. Estimating the economic burden of status epilepticus to the health care system. Seizure 2005;14:46–51.
6. Pitkanen A. Efficacy of current antiepileptics to prevent neurodegeneration in epilepsy models. Epilepsy Res 2002;50:141–160.
7. Jones DM, Esmaeil N, Maren S, et al. Characterization of pharmacoresistance to benzodiazepines in the rat Li-pilocarpine model of status epilepticus. Epilepsy Res 2002;50:301–312.
8. Brooks-Kayal A, Shumate M, Rikhter T, Coulter D. Selective changes in single cell GABA A receptor subunit expression and function in temporal lobe epilepsy. Nat Med 1998;4:1166–1172.
9. Lothman E. The biochemical basis and pathophysiology of status epilepticus. Neurology 1990;40:13–23.
10. Fitzgerald BJ, Okos AJ, Miller JW. Treatment of out-of-hospital status epilepticus with diazepam rectal gel. Seizure 2003;12:52–55.
11. Cock HR, Schapira AH. A comparison of lorazepam and diazepam as initial therapy in convulsive status epilepticus. QJM 2002;95:225–231.
12. Towne AR, DeLorenzo RJ. Use of intramuscular midazolam for status epilepticus. J Emerg Med 1999;17:323–328.
13. Kutlu NO, Dogrul M, Yakinci C, Soylu H. Buccal midazolam for treatment of prolonged seizures in children. Brain Dev 2003;25: 275–278.
14. Knoester PD, Jonker DM, Van Der Hoeven RT, et al. Pharmacokinetics and pharmacodynamics of midazolam administered as a concentrated intranasal spray. A study in healthy volunteers. Br J Clin Pharmacol 2002;53(1):501–507.
15. Fountain NB, Adams RE. Midazolam treatment of acute and refractory status epilepticus. Clin Neuropharmacol 1999;22:261–267.
16. Leppik IE, Derivan AT, Homan RW, et al. Double-blind study of lorazepam and diazepam in status epilepticus. JAMA 1983;249: 1452–1454.
17. Shaner DM, McCurdy SA, Herring MO, Gabor AJ. Treatment of status epilepticus: A prospective comparison of diazepam and phenytoin versus phenobarbital and optional phenytoin. Neurology 1988;3(2):202–207.
18. Treiman DM, Meyers PD, Walton NY, et al. A comparison of four treatments for generalized convulsive status epilepticus. N Eng J Med 1998;339:792–798.
19. Alldredge BK, Gelb AM, Isaacs SM, et al. A comparison of lorazepam, diazepam, and placebo for the treatment of out-of-hospital status epilepticus. N Eng J Med 2001;345:631–637.

20. Misra UK, Kalita J, Patel R. Sodium valproate vs phenytoin in status epilepticus: A pilot study. Neurology 2006;67:340–342.
21. Agarwal P, Kumar N, Chandra R, et al. Randomized study of intravenous valproate and phenytoin in status epilepticus. Seizure 2007;16:527–532.
22. Gilad R, Izkovitz N, Dabby R, et al. Treatment of status epilepticus and acute repetitive seizures with i.v. valproic acid vs phenytoin. Acta Neurol Scand 2008;118:296–300.DOI: 10.1111/j.1600-0404.2008.01097.x.
23. Pryor FM, Gidal B, Ramsay RE, et al. Fosphenytoin: Pharmacokinetics and tolerance of intramuscular loading doses. Epilepsia 2001;42(2):245–250.
24. Mazarati AM, Baldwin RA, Sankar R, Wasterlain CG. Time-dependent decrease in the effectiveness of antiepileptic drugs during the course of self-sustaining status epilepticus. Brain Res 1998;814:179–185.
25. Limdi NA, Shimpi AV, Faught E, et al. Efficacy of rapid IV administration of valproic acid for status epilepticus. Neurology 2005;64:353–355.
26. Peters CN, Pohlmann-Eden B. Intravenous valproate as an innovative therapy in seizure emergency situations including status epilepticus—Experience in 102 adult patients. Seizure 2005;14:164–169.
27. Uberall MA, Trollmann R, Wunsiedler U, Wenzel D. Intravenous valproate in pediatric epilepsy patients with refractory status epilepticus. Neurology 2000;54(11):2188–2189.
28. Mayer SA, Claassen J, Lokin J, et al. Refractory status epilepticus. Arch Neurol 2002;59:205–210.
29. Bleck TP. Refractory status epilepticus. Curr Opin Crit Care 2005;11:117–120.
30. Kalviainen R, Eriksson K, Parviainen I. Refractory generalized convulsive status epilepticus—A guide to treatment. CNS Drugs 2005;19(9):759–768.
31. Marik PE, Varon J. The management of status epilepticus. Chest 2004;126:582–591.
32. Parent JM, Lowenstein DH. Treatment of refractory generalized status epilepticus with continuous infusion of midazolam. Neurology 1994;44(10):1837–1840.
33. Claassen J, Hirsch LJ, Emerson RG, et al. Continuous EEG monitoring and midazolam infusion for refractory nonconvulsive status epilepticus. Neurology 2001;57(6):1036–1042.
34. Ulvi H, Yoldas T, Mungen B, Yigiter R. Continuous infusion of midazolam in the treatment of refractory generalized convulsive status epilepticus. Neurol Sci 2002;23(4):177–182.
35. Nantoku DK, Sinha S. Prolongation of midazolam half-life after sustained infusion for status epilepticus. Neurology 2000;54(6):1366–1368.
36. Kang TM. Propofol infusion syndrome in critically ill patients. Ann Pharmacother 2002;36(9):1453–1456.
37. Van Ness PC. Pentobarbital and EEG burst suppression in treatment of status epilepticus refractory to benzodiazepines and phenytoin. Epilepsia 1990;31(1):611–617.
38. Krishnamurthy KB, Drislane FW. Depth of EEG suppression and outcome in barbiturate anesthetic treatment for refractory status epilepticus. Epilepsia 1999;40(6):759–762.
39. Claassen J, Hirsch LJ, Emerson RG, et al. Treatment of refractory status epilepticus with pentobarbital, propofol, or midazolam: A systemic review. Epilepsia 2002;43:146–153.
40. Knake S, Gruener J, Hattemer K, et al. Intravenous levetiracetam in the treatment of benzodiazepine refractory status epilepticus. J Neurol Neurosurg Psychiatry 2008;79:588–589.
41. Ruegg S, Naegelin Y, Hardmeier M, et al. Intravenous levetiracetam: Treatment experience with the first 50 critically ill patients. Epilepsy Behav 2008;12:477–480.
42. Borris DJ, Bertram EH, Kapur J. Ketamine controls prolonged status epilepticus. Epilepsy Res 2000;42(2–3):117–122.
43. Mewasingh LD, Sekhara T, Aeby A, et al. Oral ketamine in paediatric non-convulsive status epilepticus. Seizure 2003;12(7):483–489.
44. Sheth RD, Gidal BE. Refractory status epilepticus: Response to ketamine. Neurology 1998;51(6):1765–1766.

45. Towne AR, Garnett LK, Waterhouse EJ, et al. The use of topiramate in refractory status epilepticus. Neurology 2003;60(2):332–334.

46. Kahriman M, Minecan D, Kutluay E, et al. Efficacy of topiramate in children with refractory status epilepticus. Epilepsia 2003;44(10): 1353–1356.

47. Mirsattari SM, Sharpe MD, Young GB. Treatment of refractory status epilepticus with inhalational anesthetic agents isoflurane and desflurane. Arch Neurol 2004;61(8):1254–1259.

48. Leppik IE. Treatment of epilepsy in 3 specialized populations. Am J Manag Care. 2001;7(Suppl 7):S221–226.

49. Chin RF, Neville BG, Peckham C, et al. Treatment of community-onset, childhood convulsive status epilepticus: A prospective, population-based study. Lancet Neurol 2008;7:696–703.

32 Parkinson's Disease

Mary L. Wagner

LEARNING OBJECTIVES

● **Upon completion of the chapter, the reader will be able to:**

1. Explain the etiology of Parkinson's disease (PD).

2. Explain the pathologic and biochemical changes in patients with PD.

3. Identify motor and nonmotor symptoms of PD as well as symptoms that indicate disease progression.

4. Explain the desired therapeutic goals for patients with PD.

5. Recommend lifestyle modifications and pharmacotherapy interventions for treating motor symptoms of patients with PD.

6. Recommend drug and nondrug interventions for treating the nonmotor symptoms of patients with PD.

7. Develop a monitoring plan to assess effectiveness and adverse effects of nonpharmacologic therapy and pharmacotherapy for PD.

8. Educate patients about the disease state, appropriate lifestyle modifications, and drug therapy required for effective treatment.

KEY CONCEPTS

❶ Patients with Parkinson's disease (PD) display both motor and nonmotor symptoms. The nonmotor symptoms may precede the motor symptoms.

❷ The most useful diagnostic tool is the clinical history, including both presenting symptoms and associated risk factors. The Unified Parkinson's Disease Rating Scale (UPDRS) is used to define the degree of disability.

❸ The goals of treatment are to maintain patient independence, activities of daily living (ADL), and quality of life (QOL) by alleviating the patient's symptoms, minimizing the development of response fluctuations, and limiting medication-related adverse effects.

❹ The treatment of PD is categorized into three phases:

• Lifestyle changes, nutrition, and exercise

• Pharmacologic intervention, primarily with drugs that enhance dopamine concentrations

• Surgical treatments for those who fail pharmacologic interventions

❺ The best time to initiate dopaminergic therapy is controversial and patient-specific. Generally, medication is started when the patient's physical impairment affects QOL. However, some clinicians believe that starting treatment earlier may improve outcomes.

❻ Medication schedules should be individualized. The doses are divided throughout the day to maximize on and minimize off periods.

❼ The treatment of nonmotor symptoms should be based on whether they are worse during an off state or if they could be related to other neurotransmitter dysfunction.

❽ As the disease progresses, most patients develop response fluctuations. Treatment is based on optimizing the pharmacokinetic and pharmacodynamic properties of PD medications.

❾ Patient monitoring should involve a regular systematic evaluation of efficacy and adverse events, referral to appropriate specialists, and patient education.

Parkinson's disease (PD) is a slow, progressive, neurodegenerative disease of the extrapyramidal motor system. Dopamine neurons in the substantia nigra are primarily affected, and degeneration of these neurons causes a disruption in the ability to generate body movements. There is no cure, and treatment is aimed at controlling symptoms and slowing disease progression.

EPIDEMIOLOGY AND ETIOLOGY

PD affects approximately one million Americans (1% of people over 60 years of age). The average age of onset is 60 years of age, and PD is fairly uncommon in those under age 40. About 15% of patients with PD have a first-degree relative with the disease. The pathogenesis of cell death (neuron degeneration) may be due to oxidative stress, mitochondrial dysfunction, increased concentrations of excitotoxic aminoacids and inflammatory cytokines, immune system disorders, trophic factor deficiency, signal-mediated apoptosis, and environmental toxins. Conditions that may promote oxidative stress include increased monoamine oxidase-B metabolism or decreased glutathione clearance of free radicals which can promote cell dysfunction and death. Drugs that deplete central dopamine, such as some antipsychotics, amoxapine, antinausea drugs (e.g., prochlorperazine), and metoclopramide, worsen PD symptoms.[1-4]

In PD there is a loss of pigmented cells in the substantia nigra that make and store dopamine. When patients are diagnosed with PD, they have lost 50% to 60% of their dopamine neurons in the substantia nigra, and the remaining neurons may not function well, as they have lost about 80% of their activity in the striatum. There may be cortical Lewy bodies along with Lewy neurites seen in microscopic samples from the basal ganglia, cortex, brain stem, spinal cord, sympathetic ganglia, cardiac plexus, and GI system that may explain some of the nonmotor symptoms of PD.[2-4]

PATHOPHYSIOLOGY

The extrapyramidal motor system controls muscle movement through a system of pathways and nerve tracts that connect the cerebral cortex, basal ganglia, thalamus, cerebellum, reticular formation, and spinal neurons. Patients with PD lose dopamine neurons in the substantia nigra, which is located in the midbrain within the brain stem. The substantia nigra sends nerve fibers up to the corpus striatum, which is part of the basal ganglia in the cerebrum. The corpus striatum is made up of the caudate nucleus and the lentiform nuclei that consist of the pallidum (globus pallidus) and putamen (Fig. 32–1). As dopamine neurons die, dopamine-relayed messages cannot communicate to other motor centers of the brain, and patients develop motor symptoms. A variety of chemicals are active in the basal ganglia including acetylcholine, histamine, glutamate, serotonin, dopamine, norepinephrine, epinephrine, gamma-aminobutyric acid (GABA), enkephalins, substance P, and adenosine. Some of these neurotransmitters also decrease in concentration as other brain regions degenerate resulting in degeneration of norepinephrine neurons in the locus ceruleus and acetylcholine neurons in the nucleus basalis,

---

Patient Encounter, Part 1

MW, a 65-year-old man with a 2-year history of mild depression, comes for an initial visit to evaluate his symptoms of tremor and slowness. The tremor started in his right hand about 6 months ago, and he does not remember how long he has been slower at completing his tasks. His wife reports that for the last 4 months he has been slower and that he kicks her while they are sleeping.

Identify this patient's motor and nonmotor symptoms of PD.

What additional information would you collect before creating this patient's treatment plan?

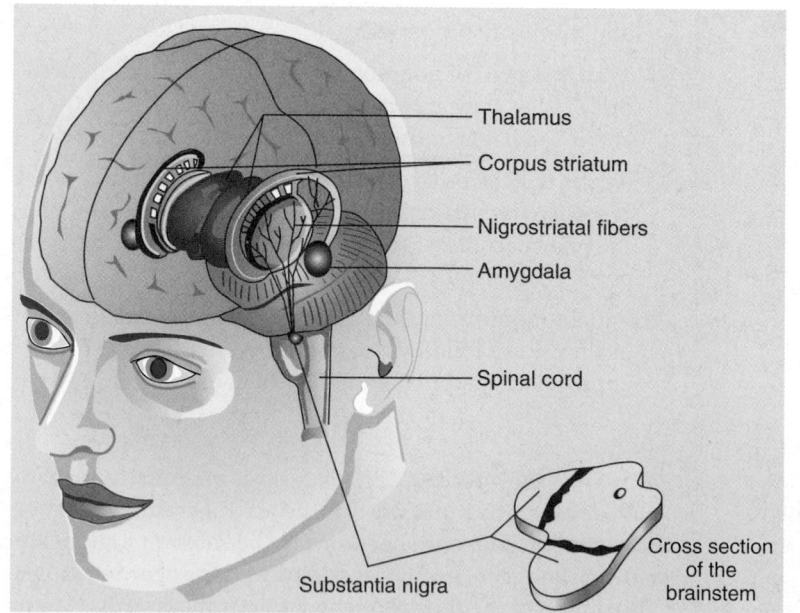

FIGURE 32–1. Anatomy of the extrapyramidal system. The extrapyramidal motor system controls muscle movement through a system of pathways and nerve tracts that connect the cerebral cortex, basal ganglia, thalamus, cerebellum, reticular formation, and spinal neurons. Patients with PD have a loss of dopamine neurons in the substantia nigra in the brainstem that leads to depletion of dopamine in the corpus striatum. The corpus striatum is made up of the caudate nucleus and the lentiform nuclei that are made up of the putamen and the globus pallidus.

Labels in figure: Thalamus · Corpus striatum · Nigrostriatal fibers · Amygdala · Spinal cord · Substantia nigra · Cross section of the brainstem

Clinical Presentation of PD

❶ *Patients with PD display both motor and nonmotor symptoms. The nonmotor symptoms may precede the motor symptoms.*

Motor Symptoms (TRAP)[7]

T = Tremor at rest ("pill rolling")

R = Rigidity (stiffness and cogwheel rigidity)

A = **Akinesia** or **bradykinesia**

P = Postural instability and gait abnormalities

Nonmotor Symptoms (SOAP)

S = Sleep disturbances (insomnia, rapid eye movement sleep behavioral disorder, restless legs syndrome [RLS])

O = Other miscellaneous symptoms (problems with nausea, fatigue, speech, pain, **dysesthesias**, vision, seborrhea)

A = Autonomic symptoms (drooling, constipation, sexual dysfunction, urinary problems, sweating, orthostatic hypotension, dysphagia)

P = Psychological symptoms (anxiety, psychosis, cognitive impairment, depression)

Response Fluctuations (MAD)

M = Motor fluctuations (delayed peak, wearing off, random off, freezing)

A = **Akathisia**

D = **Dyskinesias** (e.g., chorea, dystonia, diphasic dyskinesia)

as well as selected neurons of the dorsal motor nucleus of the vagus, spinal cord, and peripheral autonomic system. Decreases in these neurotransmitters may explain some of the nonmotor symptoms of PD.[3] For example, loss of dopamine and norepinephrine neurons in the limbic system has been associated with depression and anxiety.[5] Loss of acetylcholine, dopamine, norepinephrine, and serotonin, in the substantia nigra, locus coeruleus, nucleus raphe, and limbic system is associated with cognitive impairment.[6]

CLINICAL PRESENTATION AND DIAGNOSIS

❶ *Patients with PD display both motor and nonmotor symptoms. The nonmotor symptoms may precede the motor symptoms.*

Motor Symptoms

The onset of PD is insidious. A thorough patient history including past and present medications, family history, environmental exposure, and a detailed description of symptom onset is essential in making an accurate diagnosis. Patients feel slowed down or trapped in their body unable to move. The tremor of PD occurs during rest and disappears

with purposeful movement. Tremor usually affects the hands or feet, but may occur in other body parts such as in the lip and chin. The hand tremor can appear as if the patient is rolling a pill between their fingers. Patients describe rigidity as stiffness. Upon physical exam, it feels like uniform resistance as the muscles seem to be in a constant state of increased tone. It is defined as cogwheel rigidity when the examiner extends or flexes the patient's extremities and feels as if they are rhythmically hitting a series of teeth on the rim of a wheel, or a gear that is meshing with another gear with teeth. Bradykinesia is noted when there is hesitancy in movement initiation, slowness in movement performance, or rapid fatiguing during movement. Patients may have a decrease in automatic movements, such as blinking, a decrease in facial expressions (often termed masked facies), or a decrease in arm swing while walking. Postural instability is a result of the loss of reflexes necessary to maintain balance when standing or ambulating. Patients may report a feeling of unsteadiness. Gait abnormalities may be evidenced by shuffling, leg dragging, **festination**, propulsion, retropulsion, or freezing. Rigidity and bradykinesia may make handwriting difficult as evidenced by **micrographia**.[2,7,8]

Because of a high diagnostic error rate, patients who are thought to have PD should be referred to a movement disorder specialist before starting medication. The diagnosis can often be made by history and physical. However, special imaging tests such as a MRI or single photon emissions computed tomography (SPECT) may be warranted to rule out stroke, intoxications, or other degenerative disorders.[4,9]

Nonmotor Symptoms

Nonmotor symptoms are due to multiple neurotransmitter abnormalities throughout the brain, and some symptoms may be aggravated by PD medications. Sleep disturbance can affect more than 70% of PD patients and includes insomnia, sleep fragmentation, rapid eye movement sleep behavioral disorder (RBD), vivid dreams, nightmares, night terrors, hallucinations, restless legs syndrome (RLS), and sleep walking. Speech problems may be exhibited as a decrease in normal volume, slurring, monotone speech, rapid speech, or stammering. Visual problems such as reading problems, double vision, perceptual changes, decreased blink, burning eyes, or itchy eyes are the result of impaired function of the muscles that move the eyeball and decreased retinal dopamine.[6–11]

As the autonomic system is disturbed in patients with PD, orthostatic hypotension and GI, urinary, sexual, and dermatologic symptoms are common. Patients with orthostatic hypotension may experience dizziness, lightheadedness, fainting upon standing, or fall-related injuries. GI symptoms include constipation and **dysphagia** due to a slowing of the automatic pattern of contraction and relaxation of the throat muscles. These swallowing difficulties may lead to weight loss, **sialorrhea**, and aspiration. Genitourinary symptoms include urinary incontinence, urgency, and frequency related to over activity of the bladder emptying reflex. Symptoms may be worse at night, causing nocturia. Sexual dysfunction includes decreased libido, erectile dysfunction, and delayed ejaculation. Skin symptoms include sweating and intolerance to heat and cold.[6–8,11,12]

Psychological symptoms may be exaggerated during the patient's off periods and include psychosis, dementia, impaired cognitive function, depression, and anxiety. Psychosis occurs in nearly 30% of PD patients and is exhibited as vivid dreams, hallucinations (usually visual), paranoia, and delusions. Hallucinations may be more common when the patient is in dim light, falling asleep, or upon awakening. Dementia occurs in 20% to 44% of patients. Depression occurs in 30% to 70% of PD patients and may appear as apathy, psychomotor slowing, memory problems, irritability, sadness, agitation, and sleep disturbances. Some features of PD, such as the decreased facial expression and bradykinesia, may make the diagnosis of depression more difficult. Anxiety may present as panic attacks, phobia, or generalized anxiety, and occurs in 30% of patients. Anxiety was noted in 66% of patients with motor fluctuations and is often comorbid with depression.[6–9,11,13,14]

Response Fluctuations

Response fluctuations occur with disease progression, as the patient's dopamine reserves are depleted in the brain, and as a complication of PD treatment. Motor fluctuations include delayed peak response, early wearing off, random unpredictable on-off, and freezing. Dyskinesias include chorea, dystonia, and diphasic dyskinesia. Wearing off can be visualized by imagining the therapeutic window of dopamine narrowing over time. The therapeutic window is defined as the minimum effective concentration of dopamine required to control PD symptoms (on without dyskinesia) and the maximum concentration before experiencing side effects from too much dopamine (on with dyskinesia). Early in the disease, a dose of levodopa is administered, and the plasma concentrations are supplemented by the brain's supply of dopamine. Thus, although the plasma half-life of levodopa is 1.5 to 2 hours, the therapeutic effect lasts about 5 hours, and the patient experiences no dopamine side effects. As the disease progresses over time, the therapeutic window narrows because the brain can no longer supplement each levodopa dose with additional dopamine. Thus, during advanced disease, each dose lasts 2 to 3 hours, and patients experience dopamine side effects in order to be in an on state.[4,15–16]

❷ *The most useful diagnostic tool is the clinical history, including both presenting symptoms and associated risk factors. The Unified Parkinson's Disease Rating Scale (UPDRS) is used to define the degree of disability in motor and some nonmotor symptoms.*

The patient's degree of disability should be evaluated by using the UPDRS which has six parts. The scale combines patient history and a physical examination that is performed on both sides of the body, as symptoms may appear asymmetric in early disease. It evaluates mentation, behavior, and mood (Part 1); activities of daily living (ADL, Part 2); PD motor symptoms (Part 3); complications of therapy (Part 4); modified Hoehn and Yahr stage of disease (Part 5); and Schwab and England ADL (Part 6). The modified Hoehn and Yahr staging scale defines eight stages of PD ranging from no symptoms to wheelchair or bed bound. A copy of the exam

---

Patient Encounter, Part 2: Medical History, Physical Exam, and Diagnostic Tests

Chief Complaint

MW complains of stiffness, slow movements, and mild tremor that worsen his handwriting. The wife says that she took over the tasks that require good handwriting. She also notes that her husband is more apathetic, irritable, and kicks during the night.

PMH: Depression for 2 years

SH: After owning a dry cleaning store for 40 years, he is thinking about retiring because he does not enjoy visiting with the customers anymore; he does not smoke or drink alcohol

Meds: Fluoxetine 10 mg every morning for 2 years

Gen: Pessimistic attitude, apathetic, looks older than stated age, slow movements, thin

PE:

VS: BP: sitting 130/80 mm Hg, standing 110/80 mm Hg (with no orthostatic symptoms); P 78 bpm, RR 16/min, wt 65 kg (143 lb)

CV: RRR, normal S_1, S_2; no murmurs, rubs, gallops

Abd: Soft, nontender, nondistended; (+) bowel sounds, no hepatosplenomegaly

Skin: Scalp itchy, oily, and flaky silverish scales

Exts: Tremor in right hand and foot while sitting, cogwheel rigidity in right elbow

Neuro: Steady gait, sensory function intact, alert, normal mental status,

Rating Scales:

Unified Parkinson's Disease Rating Scale (UPDRS) = 10 while "on"

International Restless Legs Syndrome Scale (IRLS) = 5

Labs: Within normal limits

Given this additional information, what is your assessment of the patient's condition?

Identify treatment goals for the patient.

Describe nonpharmacologic and pharmacologic treatments that are available for the patient.

can be obtained at *http://www.mdvu.org/library/ratingscales/pd/updrs.pdf.*[17]

TREATMENT

Desired Outcomes

❸ *The goals of treatment are to maintain patient independence, ADL, and quality of life (QOL) by alleviating the patient's symptoms, minimizing the development of response fluctuations, and limiting medication-related adverse effects.*

General Approach to Treatment

❹ *The treatment of PD is categorized into three phases:*

- *Lifestyle changes, nutrition, and exercise*
- *Pharmacologic intervention, primarily with drugs that enhance dopamine concentrations*
- *Surgical treatments for those who fail pharmacologic interventions*

The initial therapeutic modality selected depends in part on the patient's age, risk of psychiatric adverse effects, degree of physical impairment, and one's school of thought on the best time to initiate therapy. The 2002 American Academy of Neurology guidelines[18] and 2006 European National Institute for Health and Clinical Excellence guidelines (*http://www.nice.org.uk/nicemedia/pdf/cg035fullguideline.pdf*) suggest that symptomatic treatment should be delayed until the patient experiences functional disability. Preliminary data, however, suggest that earlier treatment may delay the progression of disease. Trials are in progress to compare different classes of PD drugs to determine which drug class is best for initial therapy and which agent is best in various situations.[9]

Nonpharmacologic Therapy

► *Lifestyle Modifications*

Lifestyle modifications should be started early and continued throughout treatment. They may improve ADL, gait, balance, and mental health. The most common interventions include maintaining good nutrition, physical condition, and social interactions. Patients should avoid medications that block central dopamine (e.g., antipsychotics), as they may worsen PD symptoms.[1,19] A multidisciplinary approach using the expertise of nutritionists, speech therapists, physical therapists, occupational therapists, and social workers may optimize care, but may not be covered by insurance. Patients should maintain regular visits with their optometrist/ophthalmologist and dentist. PD medications decrease saliva flow, increasing the risk of dental caries.

Dietary modifications improve constipation, nausea, erratic drug absorption, and minimize the risk of aspiration and weight loss. Nutritionists help with meal selection, products to boost calories, and suggestions for arranging the proper protein content of meals to maximize medication absorption. Speech therapy may improve swallowing, articulation, and the force of speech.

Physical and occupational therapy may improve a patient's confidence, ability to stay active, and reduce the risks of falling. An exercise program and increased activity during the day should minimize daytime sleepiness, possibly improve sleep at night, and may be neuroprotective.[1,8,20] Occupational therapists provide information about adaptive equipment for the home, specialized clothing, and personal training that can maximize independence, safety, and ADLs. They can help improve handwriting and train patients to use communication software.

Social workers help patients and their families handle problems related to disease progression. They provide family counseling to help keep patients engaged in family activities and to minimize family conflicts. They also arrange for special community assistance programs.

Surgery

Surgical treatment is for patients with persistent and disabling rigidity, tremor, or motor fluctuations despite maximizing medications. Symptoms of poor balance, akinesia, speech impairment, and freezing do not improve with surgery. There is an increased risk of depression following surgery, and long-term safety trials are in progress.[9] Deep-brain stimulation, the surgery of choice, involves the implantation of a high-frequency device that provides electrical stimulation of the globus pallidus and subthalamic nucleus. Patients can expect a 40% to 75% decrease in symptoms.[2,21,22]

Pharmacologic Therapy

❺ *The best time to initiate dopaminergic therapy is controversial and patient-specific. Generally, medication is started when the patient's physical impairment affects QOL. However, some clinicians believe that starting treatment earlier may improve outcomes.*

❻ *Medication schedules should be individualized. The doses should be divided throughout the day to maximize on and minimize off periods.*

Pharmacologic options include anticholinergic drugs, amantadine, monoamine oxidase type B (MAO-B) inhibitors, dopamine agonists, levodopa/carbidopa, and catechol-*O*-methyltransferase (COMT) inhibitors. Medications help relieve symptoms, improve QOL, and may lengthen life expectancy, but they are not curative, and treated PD patients still die earlier than controls.[1] Knowing how dopamine is metabolized and how drugs affect dopamine metabolism is important in understanding the pharmacology of PD medications (Fig. 32–2). The American Academy of Neurology and the Movement Disorder Society determined that it is reasonable to start with levodopa or a dopamine agonist. Starting treatment with a dopamine agonist rather than levodopa may help to delay the onset of dyskinesias and the on/off fluctuations commonly seen with long-term levodopa use. However, initiating therapy with a dopamine agonist instead of levodopa/carbidopa may result in less motor benefit and greater risk of hallucinations or somnolence. Levodopa results in greater motor improvement and should

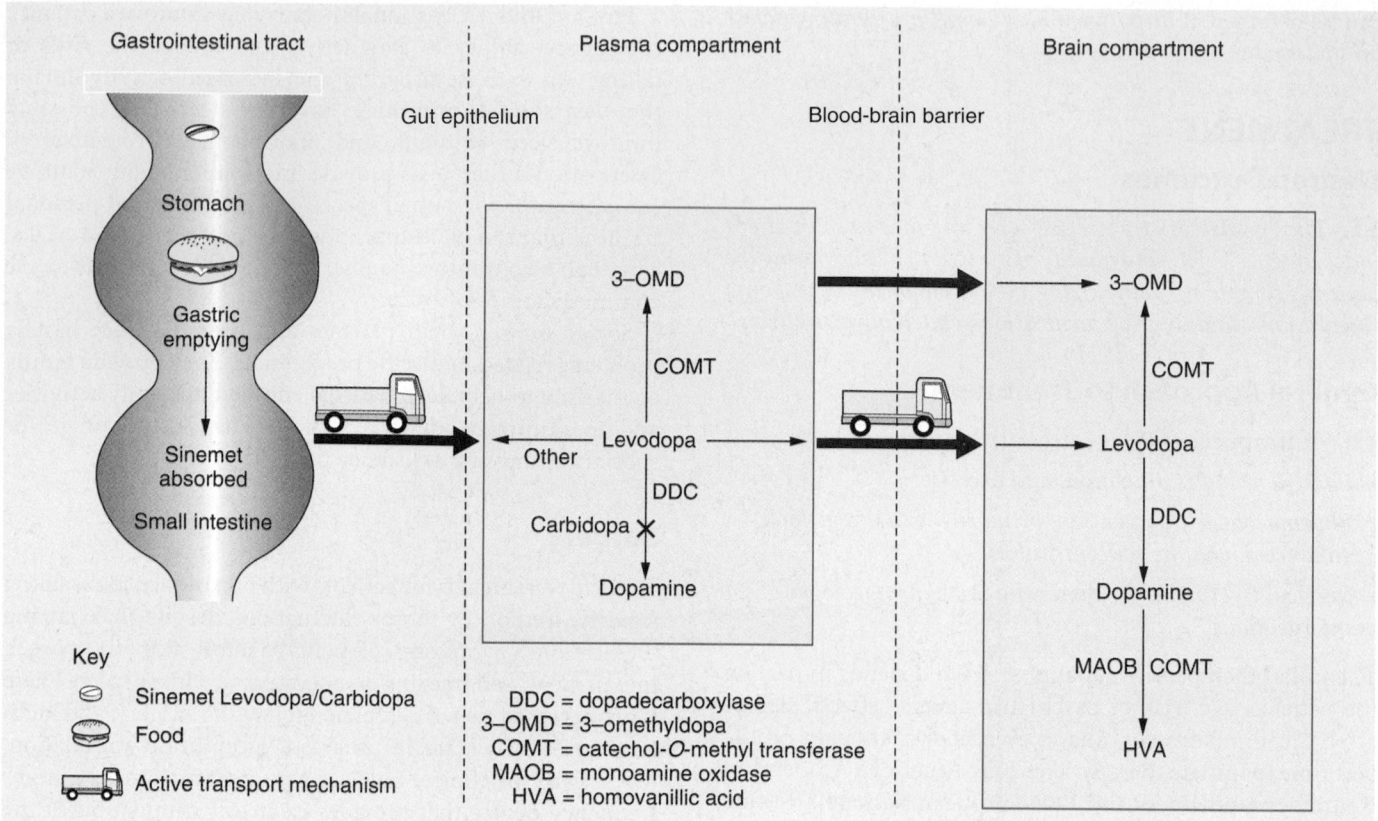

FIGURE 32–2. Levodopa absorption and metabolism. Levodopa is absorbed in the small intestine and is distributed into the plasma and brain compartments by an active transport mechanism. Levodopa is metabolized by dopadecarboxylase, monoamine oxidase, and catechol-O-methyltransferase. Carbidopa does not cross the blood–brain barrier. Large, neutral aminoacids in food compete with levodopa for intestinal absorption (transport across gut endothelium to plasma). They also compete for transport into the brain (plasma compartment to brain compartment). Food and anticholinergics delay gastric emptying resulting in levodopa degradation in the stomach and a decreased amount of levodopa absorbed. If the interaction becomes a problem, administer levodopa 30 minutes before or 60 minutes after meals.

be used as initial therapy in the elderly (greater than 75 years of age) and in those with cognitive impairment. There is no preference for using controlled-release over immediate-release levodopa as initial therapy. There are insufficient data to recommend initiating treatment with both levodopa and a dopamine agonist. Initiating treatment with anticholinergic medications, amantadine, or MAO-B inhibitors is only for patients who have mild symptoms, as they are not as effective as dopamine agonists.[1,18,23–25]

Medications should be started at the lowest dose and increased gradually based on symptoms (Table 32–1). When interviewing patients, ask the following questions for each scheduled dose before adjusting the dose or timing of medications:

- When did the dose start to work and how long did it last?

- How did you feel just before the dose, and during the dosing period?

If the dose did not last long enough, consider adding another dose each day, higher individual doses, an additional agent, or changing to a longer-acting dosage form. If the patient experiences side effects related to excessive dopamine concentrations (e.g., dyskinesia), consider decreasing the dose, increasing the time interval between doses, or decreasing the use of concomitant medications that augment dopamine concentrations.

▶ Anticholinergics

Anticholinergics may minimize resting tremor and drooling, but they are not as good as other agents in controlling rigidity, bradykinesia, and gait problems. Anticholinergics should be discontinued gradually to avoid withdrawal effects or worsening of PD symptoms. Side effects of anticholinergics include dry mouth (decreased saliva), blurred vision, constipation, cognitive impairment (forgetfulness, confusion), hallucinations, urinary retention, orthostatic hypotension, temperature sensitivity, and sedation. They are usually avoided or used with caution in patients older than 70 years of age because of an increased risk of cognitive impairment.[1,2,7–9,21–25] Use of anticholinergics is associated with an increased incidence of amyloid plaques and neurofibrillary tangles in patients with PD that may translate to an increased risk of Alzheimer's disease.[26] Anticholinergics decrease gastric motility which may decrease levodopa drug absorption.[16,19]

Table 32–1

Mechanism of Action and Dosing of Medications to Treat PD

Generic Name (Trade Name)	Mechanism of Action and Receptor Specificity	Dosing
Levodopa with carbidopa (Sinemet)	Standard, immediate-release LD (LD is metabolized to dopamine) CD blocks peripheral conversion of LD to DA and increases LD CNS penetration	Start with (Sinemet) ½ tab (100 mg LD, 25 mg CD) twice daily for 1 week, then ½ tab three times daily; then, increase by ½ tab daily every week; usual MD is 300–2,000 mg daily; since the duration of LD is 2–3 hours, patients may require doses every 2 hours
(Parcopa with phenylalanine)	Rapid-dissolving LD	Same as Sinemet
(Sinemet CR)	Sustained-release LD	Start with 1 tab (100 mg LD, 25 mg CD) 2-3 times daily; as symptoms increase, use 200mg LD tab 2–4 times daily; usual MD is 200–2,200 mg daily
(Duodopa orphan drug on fast track for approval)	Stable gel suspension of LD	Portable pump that continuously delivers LD 20 mg/mL and carbidopa 5 mg/mL via a duodenal tube
Apomorphine (Apokyn)	Activate postsynaptic D1 and D2 DA receptors	Start an antiemetic for 3 days, then give apomorphine 2 mg SC injection (1 mg if outpatient) while monitoring blood pressure; then increase by 1–2 mg every 2 or more hours; usual MD is 2–6 mg 3–5 times daily for off periods
Bromocriptine (Parlodel)	Activate postsynaptic D2 and blocks D1 DA receptors	Start with 1.25 mg daily at bedtime, then 1.25 mg twice daily; on week 2, increase to 2.5 mg twice daily, then increase by 2.5 mg daily every 2–4 weeks up to 15–45 mg daily divided 2–3 times daily
Pramipexole (Mirapex)	Activate postsynaptic D2 DA receptors	Start with 0.125 mg three times daily; increase about weekly by 0.375–0.75 mg/day to a MD of 0.5–1.5 mg three times daily; dosage reduction needed in patients with creatinine clearance less than 60 mL/min
Ropinirole	Activate postsynaptic D2 DA receptors	Start with 0.25 mg three times daily; increase about weekly by 0.75–1.5 mg daily to a MD dose of 3–8 mg three times daily
(Requip)	Immediate release	
(Requip XL)	Extended-release	Start with 2 mg once daily for 1–2 weeks, increase by 2 mg/day in 1 week intervals; maximum dose is 24 mg/day. When switching from immediate-release form, use dose closest to the total daily dose
Selegiline (Eldepryl)	Blocks MAO-B metabolism and presynaptic reuptake of DA in the brain	Start with 5 mg in the morning; if symptoms continue, add 5 mg at noon; 5 mg daily may be as clinically effective as 10 mg daily with fewer side effects
(Zelapar with phenylalanine)	Rapid-dissolving selegiline	Start with 1.25 mg every morning before breakfast; if symptoms continue after 6 weeks, increase dose to 2.5 mg every morning. Avoid food or liquid for 5 minutes before or after the dose
Rasagaline (Azilect)	Blocks MAO-B metabolism	Start with 0.5 mg daily if symptoms continue, increase to 1 mg daily
Tolcapone (Tasmar)	Peripherally blocks COMT metabolism of DA; some central activity	Start with 100 mg with first Sinemet dose once daily; if symptoms continue, increase to 2 and then 3 times daily, then to 200 mg each dose; usual MD is 100–200 mg 3 times daily
Entacapone (Comtan)	Peripherally blocks COMT metabolism of DA	200-mg tab with each Sinemet dose up to 8 tabs daily; usual MD is 200 mg 3–4 times daily; decrease dose by 50% with hepatic impairment
CD/LD/Entacapone (Stalevo)	See CD, LD, and entacapone	Usual MD is 300–1,600 mg LD daily; the largest strength tab contains 150 mg LD and 200-mg entacapone; patients requiring larger LD doses will need additional LD medication; titrate as with LD
Amantadine (Symmetrel)	NMDA-receptor antagonist that blocks glutamate transmission, promotes DA release, and blocks Ach	Start with 100 mg daily at breakfast; after 1 week, add 100 mg daily; decrease dose as creatinine clearance decreases less than 80 mL/minute; usual MD is 200–300 mg daily with last dose in afternoon
Anticholinergics (various, including trihexyphenidyl, benztropine)	Block Ach, decrease Ach: DA ratio	

Ach, acetylcholine; CD, carbidopa; COMT, catechol-O-methyltransferase; D1, a class of dopamine receptors which includes D_1 and D_5 subtypes; D2, a class of dopamine receptors which includes D_2, D_3, and D_4 subtypes; DA, dopamine; LD, levodopa; MAO, monoamine oxidase; MD, maintenance dose; NMDA, N-methyl-D-aspartate.

From Refs. 1, 4, 25.

▶ *Amantadine*

Amantadine improves PD symptoms in mildly affected patients and reduces motor fluctuations and dyskinesias in patients with more advanced disease. It may minimize or delay the development of motor complications, as levodopa's pulsatile stimulation of dopamine receptors is associated with *N*-methyl-D-aspartate (NMDA) receptor changes and resultant motor complications. Patients who develop tolerance to amantadine's effects may benefit from a drug holiday. Doses need to be reduced in patients with renal impairment. When stopping amantadine, it should be gradually discontinued to minimize potential withdrawal effects. Side effects include nausea, dizziness, livedo reticularis (purple mottling of the skin), peripheral edema, orthostatic hypotension, hallucinations, restlessness, and anticholinergic effects. Its stimulant action may worsen insomnia, so amantadine should not be dosed in the evening. It should be avoided in the elderly who cannot tolerate its anticholinergic effects.[1,2,4,7–9,16,18,21–25] It should be used cautiously with memantine, as there may be an increased risk of psychosis and prolonged QT-interval.[19,27]

▶ *MAO-B Inhibitors*

MAO-B inhibitors include selegiline and rasagiline. They may provide mild symptomatic benefit for those patients who choose to delay dopaminergic medications. Combining selegiline or rasagaline with levodopa in early treatment may delay motor complications. In patients with advanced disease, they decrease off time and improve wearing-off symptoms in patients with motor fluctuations.[23,25,28]

Rasagiline may delay the progression of PD, as patients receiving rasagiline monotherapy had higher UPDRS and QOL scores than patients who had delayed starting rasagiline for 6 months. After 1 year, patients in the delayed start group did not catch up with those who received rasagiline earlier.[28,29] Rasagiline may be neuroprotective and neurorestorative because it minimizes apoptosis and increases concentrations of neurotrophic factors.[30] The potential neuroprotective effects of selegiline may be offset by the neurotoxic effects of its amphetamine metabolite.[29]

Selegiline is available in a patch formulation which should be avoided in patients with PD. The orally disintegrating tablet formulation avoids first pass metabolism which improves bioavailability and decreases serum concentrations of the amphetamine metabolite. Side effects of selegiline are minimal but include nausea, confusion, hallucinations, headache, jitteriness, and orthostatic hypotension. The amphetamines metabolite may improve fatigue but cause insomnia. Thus, selegeline should not be dosed in the late afternoon or evening. Doses are limited to 10 mg daily, as MAO-B selectivity may be lost at higher doses increasing the risk of adverse effects and drug interactions.[1,23–25,28]

Rasagiline is not metabolized to amphetamine; thus, there is less risk of insomnia. Side effects are primarily GI with no increased risk of vasoreactive or psychiatric effects.[28] The manufacturer recommends that patients restrict the intake of tyramine-containing foods and medications that contain amines, however a recent abstract suggests that 2 mg or less of rasagiline a day may safely be administered without dietary tyramine restrictions.[31] In addition, several trials were conducted without restriction of tyramine-containing foods without any reactions.[28]

Dyskinesias can be minimized by decreasing the levodopa dose when adding either of these agents. Patients should avoid or use these medications cautiously with narcotic analgesics, antidepressants, or sympathomimetic amines (cold and weight loss products). Rasagiline is metabolized by the CYP1A2 pathway, thus drugs that inhibit CYP1A2 (e.g., ciprofloxacin or cimetidine) increase rasagiline concentrations, and inducers (e.g., omeprazole) may reduce rasagiline concentrations. Rasagline does not induce or inhibit enzymes in the P450 system. Selegiline is metabolized by CYP2B6 and CYP3A4. It does not inhibit P450 enzymes, but CYP3A4 inducers (e.g., phenytoin and carbamazepine) could reduce selegiline concentrations.[1,2,7,8,16,22–25,28]

▶ *Dopamine Agonists*

Dopamine agonists are useful as initial therapy, as they can delay the need to start levodopa and can decrease the risk of developing motor fluctuations by two- to three-fold during the first 4 to 5 years of treatment. After a few years, dopamine agonists inadequately control the patient's symptoms, and levodopa needs to be started. In advanced disease, dopamine agonists can be added to levodopa because they have a longer duration of action, minimize fluctuations in dopamine blood concentrations, decrease off time, improve wearing-off symptoms, allow a reduction in levodopa dose, and improve ADLs.[1–4,16,23–25,28,31]

Dopamine agonists include the ergot derivatives (bromocriptine) and the nonergot derivatives (rotigotine, pramipexole, ropinirole, and apomorphine). Generally, all are equally effective except bromocriptine, which is the least effective. There are five subtypes of dopamine receptors that are divided into two classes called D1 (D_1 and D_5 subtypes) and D2 (D_2, D_3, and D_4 subtypes). Receptor selectivity may result in subtle differences between the products, as pramipexole is thought to have an antidepressant effect, because it has greater D_3 receptor affinity. Ropinirole may have higher D_3 specificity, but less than pramipexole. Rotigotine is a once-daily skin patch that is available in Europe but has been withdrawn in the United States, until stability problems are resolved. If patients fail one dopamine agonist, another can be tried. Although not well established, it appears that bromocriptine 30 mg, ropinirole 15 mg, and pramipexole 4.5 mg are equivalent and this relationship can be a guide when switching agents.[1,4,16,23–25,28,31]

Common side effects include nausea, vomiting, sedation (highest with apomorphine), pedal edema, orthostatic hypotension (highest with pramipexole and cabergoline), and psychiatric effects that are greater than with levodopa (nightmares, confusion, and hallucinations). Ergot side effects are uncommon but include painful reddish discoloration of the skin over the shins and pleuropulmonary, retroperitoneal, and cardiac fibrosis.[1,16,23–25,31] Obsessive-compulsive behaviors such as pathologically excessive gambling, shopping, sexual desire, or eating may occur. Reducing or eliminating the agonist usually resolves these problems.[32] A questionnaire is available to help clarify potential psychiatric complications in patients with PD.[33]

Excessive daytime sleepiness occurs in 15% to 20% of PD patients and can be aggravated by all dopaminergic drugs potentially compromising the ability to drive. Sleep attacks without warning may occur in up to 6% of patients. Patients at greatest risk of sleep attacks are those with an Epworth Sleepiness Scale[34] score more than 10, long duration of PD, and those taking dopamine agonists with levodopa.[10,11,35,36] Adding modafinil (100–200 mg twice daily) or possibly selegiline can improve alertness.[37]

All dopamine agonists are metabolized by the liver except pramipexole, which is eliminated unchanged in the urine by active tubular secretion and requires dose reduction when creatinine clearance is less than 60 mL/min. Drug interactions may occur if it is given concurrently with other agents that are eliminated by active tubular secretion, such as verapamil and cimetidine. Ropinirole is metabolized by cytochrome P450 oxidation in the liver and subject to drug–drug interactions with drugs that induce (smoking) or inhibit (ciprofloxacin, fluvoxamine, and mexiletine) CYP1Λ2.[23–25,28]

Apomorphine is approved for acute off episodes in patients with advanced stages of PD. The onset of effect is within 10 to 20 minutes, and the duration of effect is about 60 minutes. It requires premedication with an antiemetic because it causes nausea and vomiting. Patients who are allergic to sulfites may be allergic to apomorphine.[23–25,38]

▶ Levodopa/Carbidopa

Although, levodopa, a dopamine precursor, is the most effective agent for PD, when to initiate therapy remains controversial. Patients experience a 40% to 50% improvement in motor function with levodopa versus 30% with dopamine agonists.[1] However, some feel it best to delay starting treatment because about one-half of patients develop motor fluctuations and dyskinesias after 5 years of levodopa.[1,16,25] Others feel levodopa should be started sooner because it may normalize basal ganglia dysfunction.[39] In support of this idea, patients from the prelevodopa era who delayed starting levodopa until it became available developed dykinesias sooner than modern era patients. In addition, patients who had a longer delay in starting levodopa treatment developed dyskinesias sooner than those who had a shorter delay.[1,8,16,23–25]

Levodopa is absorbed in the small intestine and peaks in the plasma in 30 to 120 minutes. A stomach with excess acid, food, or anticholinergic medications will delay gastric emptying time and decrease the amount of levodopa absorbed. Antacids decrease stomach acidity and improve levodopa absorption. Levodopa absorption requires active transport by a large, neutral aminoacid transporter protein (Fig. 32–2). Levodopa competes with other aminoacids, such as those contained in food, for this transport mechanism. Thus, in advanced disease, adjusting the timing of protein-rich meals in relationship to

levodopa doses may be helpful. Levodopa also binds to iron supplements, and administration of iron products should be spaced by at least 2 hours from the levodopa dose.[1,8,23–25]

The controlled-release (CR) formulation (labeled as sustained-release or extended-release depending on brand) is more slowly absorbed and longer acting than immediate-release tablets. With these dosage forms the total daily dose should be increased by 30%, as it is not as bioavailable as the immediate-release levodopa/carbidopa. The CR formulation has a delayed onset (45–60 minutes) compared to the standard formulation (15–30 minutes). Thus, patients may also need to take immediate-release tablets or even a liquid formulation when they want a quicker onset of effect, such as with the first morning dose.[1,8,23–25]

Levodopa is usually administered as a combination product with carbidopa, a dopa-decarboxylase inhibitor, in order to decrease the peripheral conversion of levodopa to dopamine. Carbidopa does not cross the blood–brain barrier and does not interfere with levodopa conversion in the brain. Concomitant administration of carbidopa and levodopa allows for lower levodopa doses and minimizes levodopa peripheral side effects such as nausea, vomiting, anorexia, and hypotension. Generally 75 to 100 mg daily of carbidopa is required to adequately block peripheral dopamine decarboxylase. Taking extra carbidopa may reduce nausea related to initiating levodopa.[8,23–25]

Initial levodopa side effects include orthostatic hypotension, dizziness, anorexia, nausea, vomiting, and discoloration of urine/sweat. Most of these effects can be minimized by taking levodopa with food and using a slow dose titration. Postural hypotension may worsen as the autonomic symptoms of PD worsen, or with coadministration of other medications that lower blood pressure. Side effects that develop later in therapy include dyskinesias, sleep attacks, impulse control disorders, and psychiatric effects (confusion, hallucinations, nightmares, and altered behavior). Dyskinesias caused by adding other PD drugs to levodopa may be improved by decreasing the levodopa dose.[1,8,23–25]

Patients with severe dyskinesias and off periods may achieve more constant blood concentrations (lower peak and higher trough concentrations) by taking a liquid formulation of levodopa with carbidopa. Each day patients may make a 1 mg/mL levodopa solution made with water and ascorbic acid or with a carbonated beverage, which allows patients to take a precisely adjusted dose every 30 to 90 minutes.[23–25,40]

▶ COMT Inhibitors

COMT inhibitors are used in conjunction with levodopa/carbidopa. They minimize peak and trough levodopa fluctuations by prolonging the half-life and area under the curve of levodopa. They may allow for a decrease in daily levodopa doses while increasing on time by 1 to 2 hours, decreasing wearing off, and improving ADLs in patients with motor fluctuations. Some clinicians believe that a COMT inhibitor should be added when levodopa is first introduced in an effort to promote more continuous dopamine stimulation, potentially minimizing long-term complications associated with the more pulsatile effect of intermittent levodopa administration. However, starting multiple drugs at the same time increases the risk of side effects. Side effects include diarrhea (worse with tolcapone), nausea, vomiting, anorexia, dyskinesias, urine discoloration, daytime sleepiness, sleep attacks, orthostatic hypotension, and hallucinations. Dyskinesias should improve with a decrease in the levodopa dose.[23–25,28,31] Entacapone inhibits P4502C9; thus drugs like warfarin may have increased effects.[19]

Tolcapone is associated with three cases of severe liver failure, including fatalities, and has been removed from the market in some countries. Thus, it should be used only in patients who cannot take or do not respond to entacapone. When starting therapy, patient informed consent should be documented. Serum alanine aminotransferase and aspartate aminotransferase concentrations should be monitored at baseline, then every 2 to 4 weeks for 6 months, and then periodically for the remainder of therapy. Patients who fail to show symptomatic benefit after 3 weeks should discontinue tolcapone. Entacapone has not been associated with liver damage, so monitoring of liver enzymes is not currently recommended.[23–25,28,31]

▶ Herbs and Supplements

Clinicians should ask patients if they take any herbs and supplements. There is very little support for using creatine, gingko, ginseng, green tea, ginger, yohimbine, or St John's wort in patients with PD. Patients should be cautioned that supplements and herbs are not well controlled by the FDA and may not contain the active ingredient or amounts indicated on the label. Melatonin and valerian may improve insomnia, but there are insufficient data on their use in PD patients.[41]

Patients should eat a balanced diet and take a multivitamin with minerals, but there is generally no need to supplement with specific vitamins. Some clinicians recommend vitamins C and E for their antioxidant properties; however, no significant improvements have been documented. Encourage patients to eat a diet rich in vitamin C and E (i.e., bright colored fruits and vegetables, nuts, and whole grains). Metabolism of levodopa may elevate homocysteine concentrations that may be associated with an increased risk of vascular disease, dementia, and depression. Administering levodopa with a COMT inhibitor may minimize the increase in homocysteine. Vitamin B is involved in maintaining normal homocysteine concentrations; thus PD patients may have a greater requirement for B vitamins than patients not receiving levodopa. Eating foods rich in B vitamins (i.e., wheat gram, beans, and whole grains) should be sufficient; however, B vitamin supplements may be warranted in patients with elevated homocysteine concentrations. Excess pyridoxine (vitamin B_6) may decrease the effect of levodopa, so limit doses to less than 50 mg per day.[8,42,43]

Coenzyme Q_{10} is an antioxidant essential for mitochondrial function. Patients taking 1,200 mg daily had a slower decline in UPDRS scores than patients not receiving coenzyme Q_{10}. Lower doses were no better than placebo. Many formulations contain vitamin E, and patients should not exceed recommended daily allowances of this vitamin, as bleeding times may be prolonged.[44,45]

⬥ TREATMENT OF NONMOTOR SYMPTOMS

❼ *The treatment of nonmotor symptoms should be based on whether they are worse during an off state or if they could be related to other neurotransmitter dysfunction.*

The treatment of nonmotor symptoms, such as psychological conditions, sleep disorders, and autonomic dysfunction, should include both pharmacologic and nonpharmacologic approaches. Patients should be given suggestions for maintaining ADLs, a positive self-image, family communication, and a safe environment.

Psychological Symptoms

Vivid dreams or nightmares may herald psychosis. Other potential causes of psychosis, dementia, or depression, such as infections, metabolic changes, electrolyte disturbances, or toxic exposures should be ruled out. Confusion may be alleviated by the presence of a night light or correction of vision and hearing deficits. PD therapy should be adjusted to decrease off periods when depression and anxiety may be more likely to occur. Low-efficacy PD medications should be gradually decreased and stopped in patients with psychosis. Patients should be encouraged to participate in tasks that improve cognition, such as puzzles or reading. Some patients and their families may benefit from professional counseling. Some antidepressants may be used for anxiety, panic, or depression. Low-dose quetiapine (12.5–200 mg) at bedtime can improve psychosis. Dementia symptoms may improve with an acetylcholinesterase inhibitor or memantine. Consider electroconvulsive therapy in depressed patients who fail medications.[2,7–9,11,13,14,46,47]

Sleep Problems

Sleep problems and fatigue are common in PD and may be due to medications, uncontrolled PD symptoms, or many other medical and psychological causes. The patient's bed partner can provide useful information on the patient's quality of sleep. Patients may benefit from instruction on good sleep hygiene, adjustment of therapy to control nighttime PD symptoms, or cognitive behavioral therapy. Referral to a sleep specialist may be necessary. Amantadine and selegiline may worsen insomnia; selegiline and tricyclic antidepressants may worsen RBD; and some antidepressants and antipsychotics may worsen RLS. Short-acting benzodiazepines (e.g., zaleplon, zolpidem), and sedating antidepressants (e.g., trazodone) are used for short periods to improve insomnia. However, benzodiazepines may increase the risk of falling. Antidepressants may worsen cognition and hypotension. Ramelteon may prove beneficial in patients with circadian sleep disorders (study in progress).

Pramipexole, melatonin, and clonazepam are recommended for RBD. In addition to dopaminergic medications, iron and gabapentin are recommended for RLS. However, iron may decrease the absorption of levodopa and increase constipation. A nighttime dose of a COMT inhibitor may help RLS.[2,6,10,11,46,47]

Autonomic and Other Problems

Drooling may be accompanied by speech problems and dysphagia. Anticholinergics, botulinum toxin injections, and sublingual atropine can decrease drooling. Speech therapists perform swallowing studies to assess the risk of aspiration, and nutritionists optimize diet. Patients at high risk of aspiration or poor nutrition may require placement of a percutaneous endoscopic gastrostomy tube. Nausea improves if patients take their PD medications with meals or pharmacologic therapy (domperidone [in Canada] or trimethobenzamide). Sexual dysfunction or urinary problems may require a urologic evaluation. Adjustment of PD therapy to increase on time, removal of drugs that decrease sexual response, and pharmacologic therapy (sildenafil or yohimbine) may help treat sexual dysfunction. Patients with urinary frequency may find a bedside urinal along with a decrease in evening fluids helpful. Improvement in PD symptom control can improve urinary frequency, but worsening symptoms may require catheterization or pharmacologic measures (oxybutynin, tolterodine, propantheline, imipramine, hyoscyamine, or nocturnal intranasal desmopressin). Anticholinergic drugs could cause urinary retention and constipation. Constipation can be improved by increased fluid intake, a fiber-rich diet, and physical activity. Patients should generally avoid cathartic laxatives and use stool softeners, osmotic or bulk-forming laxatives, glycerin suppositories, or enemas. Dyskinesia-related sweating may respond to PD therapy adjustment or β-blockers. Orthostasis may respond to removal of offending drugs (tricyclic antidepressants, PD medications, alcohol, and antihypertensives) increasing carbidopa doses, or addition of salt or fluids to the diet, compression stockings, fludrocortisone, indomethacin, or mitodrine. Seborrhea usually responds to over-the-counter dandruff shampoos or topical steroids.[2,6–8,11,12,46,47]

Treatment of Response Fluctuations

❽ *As the disease progresses, most patients develop response fluctuations. Treatment is based on optimizing the pharmacokinetic and pharmacodynamic properties of Parkinson's disease medications.*

Treatment includes adjusting or adding medications to maximize the patient's on time, minimize the time on with dyskinesia, and minimize off time (Table 32–2). Use various dosage plans to minimize suboptimal or delayed peak levodopa concentrations by adding longer-acting medications to minimize wearing-off periods, adding or adjusting medications to stop an unpredicted off period, and providing treatments that decrease freezing episodes.

Table 32–2

Management of Motor Complications in Advanced PD

I. Motor fluctuations
A. Suboptimal or delayed peak response
  1. Take Sinemet on an empty stomach
  2. Decrease dietary protein and fat around the dose that is delayed
  2. Use rapid-dissolving tablet (Parcopa), crush Sinemet, or make liquid Sinemet
  3. Substitute standard Sinemet for some of the Sinemet CR
  4. Minimize constipation
  5. Withdraw drugs with anticholinergic properties
  6. Add intermittent subcutaneous apomorphine
B. Optimal peak but early wearing off
  1. Decrease dose and increase frequency of standard Sinemet
  2. Substitute Sinemet CR for some of the standard Sinemet
  3. Add other PD medications (dopamine agonist, MAO-B inhibitor, amantadine, or COMT inhibitor)
C. Optimal peak but unpredictable offs
  1. Adjust time of medications with meals and avoid high-protein meals or redistribute the amount of protein in diet
  2. Substitute or add rapid-dissolving tablet form or liquid form of Sinemet
  3. Add COMT inhibitor
  4. Add or try a different dopamine agonist
  5. Consider continuous infusion of levodopa (Duodopa), apomorphine, or lisuride
  6. Deep-brain stimulation procedure
D. Freezing
  1. Gait modifications (use visual cues such as walk-over lines, tapping, rhythmic commands, rocking; use rolling walker)
  2. Difficult to treat, so adjust current medication up or down based on other PD symptoms
    a. On freezing—reduce dopamine medications, inject botulinum toxin
    b. Off freezing, increase Sinemet dose or add dopamine agonists
  3. Treat anxiety if present

II. Dyskinesias
A. Peak dose chorea
  1. Evaluate the value of adjunctive PD medications
  2. Decrease risk by lowering Sinemet dose when adding other PD medications
  3. Adjust levodopa formulation, dose, or frequency
  4. Add amantadine
  5. Add propranolol, fluoxetine, buspirone, or clozapine
  6. Deep-brain stimulation
B. Off period dystonia in the early morning (e.g., foot cramping)
  1. Add Sinemet CR or dopamine agonist at bedtime if having nighttime offs
  2. Morning Sinemet dose should be immediate-release with or without CR
  3. Selective denervation with botulinum toxin
  4. Add lithium or baclofen
C. Diphasic dyskinesia
  1. Avoid controlled-release preparations; consider liquid Sinemet
  2. Add dopamine agonist, amantadine, or COMT inhibitor
  3. Increase Sinemet dose and frequency
  4. Deep brain stimulation

III. Akathisia
  1. Benzodiazepine
  2. Propranolol
  3. Dopamine agonists
  4. Gabapentin

COMT, catechol-O-methyltransferase.

From Refs. 2, 15, 16, 44–46.

Patient Encounter, Part 3: Creating a Care Plan

Considering the goals of therapy, treatment options, and your assessment of each of the patient's problems in part 2, create a care plan for MW that includes:

a. Nondrug and drug therapy for each problem

b. A protocol for monitoring efficacy and adverse effects

When the disease progresses, describe how you would help a family member make the decision to hire more home help versus move the patient into an assisted living facility or nursing home.

Patient Encounter, Part 4: Evaluation of the Outcomes

At the last visit, MW's fluoxetine was changed to bupropion, pramipexole was started and gradually increased to 0.5 mg three times daily, and a dandruff shampoo was started. Since that time, his skin condition, attitude, apathy, stiffness, rigidity, handwriting, tremor, slowness, and kicking have improved. The UPDRS is 5 while "on".

Do you agree with this therapeutic plan?

Have therapeutic goals been achieved?

It also involves adjusting or adding medications to decrease chorea, dystonia, diphasic dyskinesias, or akathisia. Patients should schedule activities when they are on. Patients can also keep an extra dose of medication with them when they are away from home in case their medication wears off.[2,6,15,16,46–48]

OUTCOME EVALUATION

❾ *Patient monitoring should involve a regular systematic evaluation of efficacy and adverse events, referral to appropriate specialists, and patient education.*

Evaluate the clinical outcomes of treatment by using the UPDRS. In addition, periodically ask patients to record the amount of on and off time they have with and without dyskinesias in a diary. There are a variety of scales that can be used to assess QOL, depression, anxiety, and sleep disorders. Patients with PD cannot be cured; but treatment can delay the progression of symptoms and improve QOL. Delaying the patient's admission into a nursing home is a good outcome.

Patient Care and Monitoring

❾ *Patient monitoring should involve a regular systematic evaluation of efficacy and adverse events, referral to appropriate specialists, and patient education.*

1. Determine type of symptoms, frequency, and exacerbating factors. Assess for PD treatment-related complications? Assess the patient's symptoms to determine if therapy should be adjusted or maintained, or if referral for more extensive evaluation is needed.

2. Review any available diagnostic data to determine status, motor ability, dyskinesias, and nonmotor symptoms.

3. Obtain a thorough history of prescription, nonprescription, and complementary/alternative medication use. Determine what treatments have been helpful to the patient in the past. Is the patient taking any medications that may increase PD symptoms?

4. Educate the patient about lifestyle modifications that will improve symptoms and sustain independence.

5. Is the patient taking the appropriate dose of PD medication to maximize on time and minimize adverse effects? If not, why?

6. Determine if polytherapy treatment is necessary and/or adequate.

7. Assess improvement in QOL measures.

8. Evaluate the patient for the presence of drug adverse reactions, allergies, and interactions.

9. Recommend a therapeutic regimen that is easy for the patient to follow. Educate the patient on how to use medications, and allow the patient to adjust medications for fluctuations in response.

10. Educate patients regarding PD, including lifestyle modifications and drug therapy, including:
    - When and how to take medications
    - The potential adverse effects that may occur
    - Which drugs may interact with therapy (give patients a list)
    - Warning signs to report to the physician
    - Where they can obtain further information such as books and Web sites (e.g., http://www.apdaparkinson.org; http://www.parkinson.org)

11. Refer patients to a local PD support group where they can obtain educational materials as well as empathy and social support from fellow PD patients. Support groups that include patients with advanced disease may upset patients with early disease; therefore, the advantages and disadvantages of attending should be explained to the patient.

Abbreviations Introduced in This Chapter

ADL   Activities of daily living
COMT   Catechol-*O*-methyltransferase
CR   Controlled-release
GABA   *γ*-Aminobutyric acid
MAO   Monoamine oxidase
NMDA   *N*-Methyl-D-aspartate
PD   Parkinson's disease
QOL   Quality of life
RBD   Rapid eye movement sleep behavior disorder
RLS   Restless legs syndrome
SPECT   Single photon emission computerized tomography
UPDRS   Unified Parkinson's Disease Rating Scale

 Self-assessment questions and answers are available at *http://www.mhpharmacotherapy.com/pp.html.*

REFERENCES

1. Nutt JG, Wooten GF. Diagnosis and initial management of Parkinson's disease. N Engl J Med 2005;353:1021–1027.
2. Samii A, Nutt JG, Ransom BR. Parkinson's disease. Lancet 2004;363:1783–1793.
3. Halbig TD, Winona Tse, Olanow CW. Neuroprotective agents in Parkinson's disease: Clinical evidence and caveats. Neurol Clin 2004;22:S1–S17.
4. Goetz CG. Hypokinetic Movement Disorders in Textbook of Clinical Neurology. 3rd ed. Philadelphia, PA, Saunders, an imprint of Elsevier Inc., 2007. Available online at *http://www.mdconsult.com*
5. Remy P, Doder M, Lees A, et al. Depression in Parkinson's disease: Loss of dopamine and noradrenaline innervation in the limbic system. Brain 2005;128:1314–1322.
6. Truong DD, Bhidayasiri R, Wolters E. Management of nonmotor symptoms in advanced Parkinson disease. J Neurol Sci 2008;266:216–228.
7. Weiner WJ, Shulman LM, Lang AE. Parkinson's Disease. A Complete Guide for Patients and Families. Baltimore: The John Hopkins University Press; 2001.
8. Duvoisin RC, Sage J. Parkinson's Disease: A Guide for Patient and Family. 5th ed. Philadelphia: Lippincott Williams & Wilkins; 2001.
9. Clarke CE. Parkinson's disease. BMJ 2007;335:441–445.
10. Simuni T. Somnolence and other sleep disorders in Parkinson's disease: The challenge for the practicing neurologist. Neurol Clin 2004;22:S107–S126.
11. Adler CH. Nonmotor complications in Parkinson's disease. Mov Disord 2005;20(Suppl 11):S23–S29.
12. Dewey RB. Autonomic dysfunction in Parkinson's disease. Neurol Clin 2004;22:S127–S140.
13. Chen JJ. Anxiety, depression, and psychosis in Parkinson's disease: Unmet needs and treatment challenges. Neurol Clin 2004;22:S63–S89.
14. Elmer L. Cognitive issues in Parkinson's disease. Neurol Clin 2004;22:S91–S106.
15. Pahwa R, Lyons KE. Options in the treatment of motor fluctuations and dyskinesias in Parkinson's disease: a brief review. Neurol Clin 2004;22:S35–S52.
16. Bhidayasiri R, Truong DD. Motor complications in Parkinson disease: Clinical manifestations and management. J Neurol Sci 2008;266:204–215.
17. Fahn S, Elton R, Members of the UPDRS Development Committee. In: Fahn S, Marsden CD, Calne DB, Goldstein M, eds. Recent Developments in Parkinson's Disease. Vol. 2. Florham Park, NJ: Macmillan Health Care Information, 1987:153–163, 293–304.
18. Miyasaki JM, Martin W, Suchowersky O, et al. Practice parameter: Initiation of treatment for Parkinson's disease: An evidence-based review. Report of the quality standards subcommittee of the American Academy of Neurology. Neurology 2002;58:11–17.
19. Jost WH, Bruck C. Drug interactions in the treatment of Parkinson's disease. J Neurol 2002;249(Suppl 3):24–29.
20. Keus SHJ, Bloem BR, Hendriks EJM, et al. Evidence-based analysis of physical therapy in Parkinson's disease with recommendations for practice and research. Mov Disord 2007;22:451–460.
21. Esselink RA, de Bie RM, de Haan RJ, et al. Unilateral pallidotomy versus bilateral subthalamic nucleus stimulation in PD: A randomized trial. Neurology 2004;62(2):201–207.
22. The deep-brain stimulation for Parkinson's disease study group. Deep-brain stimulation of the subthalamic nucleus or the pars internal of the globus pallidus in Parkinson's disease. N Engl J Med 2001;345:956–963.
23. Chen JJ, Swope DM. Pharmacotherapy for Parkinson's disease. Pharmacotherapy. 2007;27(12 Pt2):161S–173S.
24. Olanow CW, Watts RI, Koller WC. An algorithm (decision tree) for the management of Parkinson's diseases (2001): Treatment-guidelines. Neurology 2001;56(Suppl 5):S1–S88.
25. Anonymous. Treatment guidelines from the medical letter. Drugs Parkinson's Dis. 2007;5(62):89–94.
26. Perry EK, Kilford L, Lees AJ, et al. Increased Alzheimer's pathology in Parkinson's disease related to antimuscarinic drugs. Ann Neurol. 2003;54:235–238.
27. Factor SA, Molho ES, Brown DL. Acute delirium after withdrawal of amantadine in Parkinson's disease. Neurology 1998;50:1456–1458.
28. Fernandez HH, Chen JJ. Monoamine oxidase-B inhibition in the treatment of Parkinson's disease. Pharmacotherapy 2007;27:174S–185S.
29. Hughes B. New hope for Parkinson's disease progression delay. Nat Rev 2008;7:791.
30. Guillaume M. Thebault J, Cohen S. Assessment of potential pharmacodynamic interaction between rasagiline and oral tyramine in healthy subjects. AAN 59th annual meeting poster session. Boston, May 1, 2007. *http://www.abstracts2view.com/aan2007boston/view.php?nu=AAN07L_P02.040.*
31. Widnell KL, Comella C. Role of COMT inhibitors and dopamine agonists in the treatment of motor fluctuations. Mov Disord 2005;20(Suppl 11):S30–S37.
32. Stamey W, Jankovic J. Impulse control disorders and pathological gambling in patients with Parkinson disease. Neurologist 2008;14:89–99.
33. Visser M, Verbaan D, van Rooden SM. Assessment of psychiatric complications in Parkinson's disease: The SCOPA-PC. Mov Disord 2007;22:2221–2228.
34. Banergee D. The Epworth sleepiness scale. Occup Med 2007;57:232.
35. Paus S, Brecht HM, Koster J, et al. Sleep attacks, daytime sleepiness, and dopamine agonists in Parkinson's disease. Mov Disord 2003;18:659-667.
36. Arnulf I, Konofal E, Merino-Andreu M, et al. Parkinson's disease and sleepiness: an integral part of PD. Neurology 2002;58:1019–1024.
37. Nieves AV, Lang AE. Treatment of excessive daytime sleepiness in patients with Parkinson's disease with modafinil. Clin Neuropharmacol 2002;25:111–114.
38. Anonymous. Apomorphine (Apokyn) for advanced Parkinson's disease. Med Lett 2005;47(1200):7–8.
40. Pappert EJ, Goetz CG, Niederman F, et al. Liquid levodopa/carbidopa produces significant improvement in motor function without dyskinesia exacerbation. Neurology 1996;47:1493–1495.
41. Stevinson C, Ernst E. Valerian for insomnia: A systemic review of randomized clinical trials. Sleep Med 2000;1:91–99.

42. Rogers JD, Sanchez-Saffon A, et al. Elevated plasma homocysteine levels in patients treated with levodopa: association with vascular disease. Arch Neurol 2003;60:59–64.

43. Miller JW, Selhub J, Nadeau MR, et al. Effect of L-dopa on plasma homocysteine in PD patients' relationship to B-vitamin status. Neurology 2003;60:1125–1129.

44. Shults CW, Oakes D, Kieburtz K, et al. Parkinson Study Group. Effects of coenzyme Q10 in early Parkinson disease: Evidence of slowing of the functional decline. Arch Neurol 2002;59(10):1541–1550.

45. Shults CW, Flint Beal M, Song D, Fontaine D. Pilot trial of high dosages of coenzyme Q10 in patients with Parkinson's disease. Exp Neurol 2004;188(2):491–494.

46. Sharma N, Richman E. Parkinson's Disease and the Family. A New Guide. Baltimore: Harvard University Press, 2005.

47. Ahlskog JE. The Parkinson's Disease Treatment Book. Partnering with Your Doctor to Get the Most from Your Medications. New York: Oxford University Press, 2005.

48. Panisset M. Freezing and gait in Parkinson's disease. Neurol Clin. 2004;22:S53–S62.

33 Pain Management

Christine K. O'Neil

LEARNING OBJECTIVES

Upon completion of the chapter, the reader will be able to:

1. Identify characteristics of the types of pain—nociceptive, inflammatory, neuropathic, and functional.

2. Explain the mechanisms involved in pain transmission.

3. Select an appropriate method of pain assessment.

4. Recommend an appropriate choice of analgesic, dose, and monitoring plan for a patient based on type and severity of pain and other patient-specific parameters.

5. Perform calculations involving equianalgesic doses, conversion of one opioid to another, rescue doses, and conversion to a continuous infusion.

6. Educate patients and caregivers about effective pain management, dealing with chronic pain, and the use of nonpharmacologic measures.

KEY CONCEPTS

❶ Pain is an unpleasant, subjective experience that is the net effect of a complex interaction of the ascending and descending neurons involving biochemical, physiologic, psychological, and neocortical processes.

❷ Following initial assessment of pain, reassessment should be done as needed based on medication choice and the clinical situation.

❸ Effective treatment involves an evaluation of the cause, duration, and intensity of the pain and selection of an appropriate treatment modality for the pain situation.

❹ Whenever possible, the least potent oral analgesic should be selected.

❺ Equianalgesic doses should be used when converting from one opioid to another.

INTRODUCTION

Pain is defined by the International Association for the Study of Pain (IASP) as "an unpleasant sensory and emotional experience associated with actual or potential tissue damage, or described in terms of such damage."[1] ❶ *Pain is an unpleasant subjective experience that is the net effect of a complex interaction of the ascending and descending neurons involving biochemical, physiologic, psychological, and neocortical processes.* Pain can affect all areas of a person's life including sleep, thought, emotion, and activities of daily living. Because there are no reliable objective markers for pain, the patient is the only person who can describe the intensity and quality of their pain.

Pain is the most common symptom prompting patients to seek medical attention and is reported by more than 80% of individuals who visit their primary care provider.[1] Despite the frequency of pain symptoms, individuals often do not obtain satisfactory relief of pain. This has led to recent initiatives in health care to make pain the fifth vital sign, thus making pain assessment equal in importance to obtaining a patient's temperature, pulse, blood pressure, and respiratory rate.

EPIDEMIOLOGY AND ETIOLOGY

Prevalence of Pain

Most people experience pain at some time in their lives, and pain is a symptom of a variety of diseases. For some, pain might be mild to moderate, intermittent, easily managed, and have minimal effect on daily activities. For others, pain might be chronic, severe or disabling, all consuming, and treatment resistant. Thus, identifying the exact prevalence of pain is a difficult task. According to the American Pain Foundation, more than 76 million people in the United States suffer from chronic pain, and an additional 25 million experience acute pain from injury or surgery.[2] About 26% of the adults, mostly women and the elderly, experience chronic pain such as back pain, headache, and joint pain.

Prevalence rates for a variety of different types of pain have been described. Approximately one quarter of U.S. adults reported having low back pain lasting at least 1 day in the past 3 months.[3] Migraine affects more than 28 million Americans, and 78% of Americans experience a tension headache during their lifetime.[4] Pain resulting from fibromyalgia affects 10 million Americans.[5] Pain ranges in prevalence from 14% to 100% among cancer patients. Cancer is commonly associated with both acute and chronic pain and about 50% to 70% of those in active treatment will experience significant pain.[6]

The prevalence of neuropathic pain is unknown because of the lack of epidemiologic studies. Current estimates suggest that approximately 1.5% of the population in the United States might be affected by neuropathic pain.[7] However, this figure is probably an underestimate and will likely increase due to the increase in disorders associated with neuropathic pain in the ever-growing older population. Approximately 25% to 50% of all pain clinic visits are related to neuropathic pain.[8] Central neuropathic pain is estimated to occur in 2% to 8% of all stroke patients.[9]

The elderly, defined as people 65 years of age and over, bear a significant burden of pain, and pain continues to be under-recognized and undertreated in this population. The prevalence of pain in people older than 60 years is twice that in those younger than 60 years.[10] Studies suggest that 25% to 50% of community-dwelling elderly suffer pain. Pain is quite common among nursing home residents. It is estimated that pain in 45% to 80% of nursing home patients contributes to functional impairment and a decreased quality of life.[11]

The financial impact of pain is considered to be significant. Low back pain alone is responsible for direct medical costs of more than $26 billion annually in 1998 and as much as $50 billion per year in indirect costs.[12] The American Productivity Audit of the U.S. workforce, conducted from 2001 to 2002, revealed that the cost of lost productivity due to arthritis, back pain, headache, and other musculoskeletal pain was approximately $80 billion per year.[13]

Undertreatment of Pain

Despite the growing emphasis on pain management, pain often remains undertreated and continues to be a problem in hospitals, long-term care facilities, and the community. In one series of reports, 50% of seriously ill hospitalized patients reported pain; however, 15% were dissatisfied with pain control, and some remained in pain after hospitalization.[14, 15]

Misconceptions about pain management, both from patients and health care providers, are among the most common causes of analgesic failure. Some clinicians might be hesitant to treat pain because either they do not believe the patient's reports of pain or feel the patient is exaggerating symptoms in order to obtain medications. Inadequate clinical knowledge of available pain management strategies, including pharmacologic, nonpharmacologic, and alternative therapy options, also often leads to suboptimal pain management. In one survey, approximately three-fourths of physicians cited low competence in pain assessment as the major barrier to effective pain management.[16] Concerns about opiate misuse,

abuse, and diversion also contribute to less than optimal pain management and cause providers to exercise caution when prescribing opiates for pain. Misunderstandings about the terms addiction, physical dependence, tolerance, and pseudoaddiction are additional obstacles to optimal pain management.

Patients might present barriers to pain management by not reporting pain symptoms because of fear of becoming addicted or because of cultural beliefs. Elderly patients might not report pain for a variety of reasons including belief that pain is something they must live with, fear of consequences (e.g., hospitalization, loss of independence), or fear that the pain might be forecasting impending illness, inability to understand terminology used by health care providers, or a belief that showing pain is unacceptable behavior.

PATHOPHYSIOLOGY

Types of Pain

Several distinct types of pain have been described, for example, nociceptive, inflammatory, neuropathic, and functional.[17] Nociceptive pain is a transient pain in response to a noxious stimulus at nociceptors that are located in cutaneous tissue, bone, muscle, connective tissue, vessels, and viscera. Nociceptors are classified as thermal, chemical, or mechanical. The nociceptive system extends from the receptors in the periphery to the spinal cord, brain stem, to the cerebral cortex where pain sensation is perceived. This system is a key physiologic function that prevents further tissue damage due to the body's autonomic withdrawal reflex.

When tissue damage occurs despite the nociceptive defense system, inflammatory pain ensues. The body now changes focus from protecting against painful stimuli to protecting the injured tissue. The inflammatory response contributes to pain hypersensitivity that serves to prevent contact or movement of the injured part until healing is complete, thus reducing further damage.

Neuropathic pain is defined as spontaneous pain and hypersensitivity to pain associated with damage to or pathologic changes in the peripheral nervous system as in painful diabetic peripheral neuropathy (DPN), AIDS, polyneuropathy, postherpetic neuralgia (PHN), or in the CNS, that which occurs with spinal cord injury, multiple sclerosis, and stroke. Functional pain, a relatively newer concept, is pain sensitivity due to an abnormal processing or functioning of the CNS in response to normal stimuli. Several conditions considered to have this abnormal sensitivity or hyper-responsiveness include fibromyalgia and irritable bowel syndrome.

Mechanisms of Pain

▶ Pain Transmission

The mechanisms of nociceptive pain are well-defined and provide a foundation for the understanding of other types of pain.[18] Following nociceptor stimulation, tissue injury causes the release of substances (bradykinin, serotonin, potassium, histamine, prostaglandins, and substance P) that might further sensitize and/or activate nociceptors. Nociceptor activation produces action potentials (transduction) that are transmitted along myelinated Aδ-fibers and unmyelinated C-fibers to the spinal cord. The Aδ-fibers are responsible for first, fast, sharp pain and release excitatory amino acids that activate α-amino-3-hydroxy-5-methylisoxazole-4-propionic acid (AMPA) receptors in the dorsal horn. The C-fibers produce second pain, which is described as dull, aching, burning, and diffuse. These nerve fibers synapse in the dorsal horn of the spinal cord, where several neurotransmitters are released including glutamate, substance P, and calcitonin gene-related peptide. Transmission of pain signals continues along the spinal cord to the thalamus, which serves as the pain relay center, and eventually to the cortical regions of the brain where pain is perceived.

▶ Pain Modulation

Modulation of pain (inhibition of nociceptive impulses) can occur by a number of processes. Based on the gate-control theory, pain modulation might occur at the level of the dorsal horn.[19] Because the brain can process only a limited number of signals at one time, other sensory stimuli at nociceptors might alter pain perception. This theory supports the effectiveness of counterirritants and transcutaneous electrical nerve stimulation (TENS) in pain management. Pain modulation can occur through several other complex processes. The endogenous opiate system consists of endorphins (enkephalins, dynorphins, and β-endorphins) that interact with μ-, δ-, and κ-receptors throughout the CNS to inhibit pain impulses and alter perception. The CNS also includes inhibitory descending pathways from the brain that can attenuate pain transmission in the dorsal horn. Neurotransmitters involved in this descending system include endogenous opioids, serotonin, norepinephrine, γ-aminobutyric acid (GABA), and neurotensin. The perception of pain involves not only nociceptive stimulation but physiologic and emotional input that contributes to the perception of pain. Consequently, cognitive behavioral treatments such as distraction, relaxation, and guided imagery can reduce pain perception by altering pain processing in the cortex.

▶ Peripheral Sensitization, Central Sensitization, and Wind-Up

Under normal conditions, a balance generally exists between excitatory and inhibitory neurotransmission. Changes in this balance can occur both peripherally and centrally, resulting in exaggerated responses and sensitization such as that observed in inflammatory, neuropathic, or functional chronic pain. Pain in these settings might occur spontaneously without any stimulus or might be evoked by a stimulus. Evoked pain might arise from a stimulus that normally does not cause pain (allodynia) such as a light touch in neuropathic pain. Hyperalgesia, an exaggerated and/or prolonged pain response to a stimulus that normally causes pain, can also occur as a result of increased sensitivity in the CNS.

During normal pain transmission, the AMPA receptors are activated, but the N-methyl-D-aspartate (NMDA) receptor is blocked by magnesium.[16] Repeated nerve depolarization causes release of the magnesium block, allowing the influx of calcium and sodium, and results in excessive excitability and amplification of signals. Continued input from C-fibers and subsequent increases in substance P and glutamate causes the activation of the NMDA receptor, a process referred to as wind-up. Wind-up increases the number and responsiveness of neuron in the dorsal horn irrespective of the input from the periphery. Recruitment of neurons not normally involved in pain transmission or spread occurs, leading to allodynia, hyperalgesia, and spread to uninjured tissues.[20] The wind-up phenomenon supports the observation that untreated acute pain can lead to chronic pain and the belief that pain processes are plastic and not static.

CLINICAL PRESENTATION AND DIAGNOSIS

Classification of Pain

Pain has always been described as a symptom. However, recent advances in the understanding of neural mechanisms have demonstrated that unrelieved pain might lead to changes in the nervous system known as neural plasticity. Because these changes reflect a process that influences a physiologic response, pain, particularly chronic pain, might be considered a disease unto itself.

Pain can be divided into two broad categories, acute and chronic pain. Acute pain is also referred to as adaptive pain since it serves to protect the individual from further injury or promote healing.[17] However, chronic pain has been called maladaptive, a pathologic function of the nervous system or pain as a disease.

▶ Acute Pain

Acute pain is pain that occurs as a result of injury or surgery and is usually self-limited, subsiding when the injury heals. Untreated acute pain can produce physiologic symptoms including tachypnea, tachycardia, and increased sympathetic nervous system activity, such as pallor, diaphoresis, and pupil dilation. Furthermore, poorly treated pain can cause psychological stress and compromise the immune system due to the release of endogenous corticosteroids. Somatic acute pain arises from injury to skin, bone, joint, muscle, and connective tissue, and it is generally localized to the site of injury. Visceral pain involves injury to nerves on internal organs (e.g., intestines, liver) and can present as diffuse, poorly differentiated, and often referred pain. Acute pain should be treated aggressively, even before the diagnosis is established, except in conditions of head or abdominal injury where pain might assist in the differential diagnosis.

▶ Chronic Pain

Chronic pain persists beyond the expected normal time for healing and serves no useful physiologic purpose. Chronic pain might be nociceptive, inflammatory, neuropathic, or functional in origin; however, all forms share some common characteristics. Chronic pain can be intermittent or persistent, or both. Physiologic responses observed in acute pain are often absent in chronic pain; however, other symptoms might predominate. There are four main effects of chronic pain, and these include: (a) effects on the physical function, (b) psychological changes, (c) social consequences, and (d) societal consequences. Effects of chronic pain on physical function include impaired activities of daily living and sleep disturbances. Psychological components of chronic pain might include depression, anxiety, anger, and loss of self-esteem. As a result of physical and psychological changes, social consequences might ensue, such as changes in relationships with friends and family, intimacy, and isolation. On a societal level, chronic pain contributes to increased health care costs, disability, and lost productivity. Management of chronic pain should be multimodal and might involve cognitive interventions, physical manipulations, pharmacologic agents, surgical intervention, and regional or spinal anesthesia.

Chronic Malignant Pain Chronic malignant pain is associated with a progressive disease that is usually life-threatening such as cancer, AIDS, progressive neurologic diseases, end-stage organ failure, and dementia.[21] The goal is pain alleviation and prevention, often through a systematic and stepwise approach. Tolerance, dependence, and addiction are often not a concern due to the terminal nature of the illness.

Chronic Nonmalignant Pain Pain not associated with a life-threatening disease and lasting longer than 6 months beyond the healing period is referred to as chronic nonmalignant pain. Pain associated with low back pain, osteoarthritis, previous bone fractures, peripheral vascular disease, genitourinary infection, rheumatoid arthritis, and coronary heart disease is considered nonmalignant. The numerous causes of this type of chronic pain make treatment complex and involves a multidisciplinary approach. Treatment is initially conservative but might involve the use of more potent analgesics including opiates in psychologically healthy patients.[22]

Neuropathic Pain Neuropathic pain is considered to be a type of chronic nonmalignant pain involving disease of the central and peripheral nervous systems. Neuropathic pain might be broadly categorized as peripheral or central in nature. Examples of neuropathic pain include PHN, which is pain associated with acute herpetic neuralgia or an acute shingles outbreak. Peripheral or polyneuropathic pain is associated with the distal polyneuropathies of diabetes, human immunodeficiency virus (HIV), and chemotherapeutic agents. Types of central pain include central stroke pain, trigeminal neuralgia, and a complex of syndromes known as complex regional pain syndrome (CRPS). CRPS includes both reflex sympathetic dystrophy and causalgia, both of which are neuropathic pain associated with abnormal functioning of the autonomic nervous

system. One of the newest categories of neuropathic pain is neuropathic low back pain.

The symptoms of neuropathic pain are characterized as tingling, burning, shooting, stabbing, electric shock–like quality, or radiating pain. The patient might describe either a constant dull throbbing or burning pain, or an intermittent pain that is stabbing or shooting. Damage to the peripheral nerves might frequently be referred to the body region innervated by those nerves.

Pain Assessment

Effective pain management begins with a thorough and accurate assessment of the patient. Even though pain is a common presenting complaint, lack of regular assessment and reassessment of pain remains a problem and contributes to the undertreatment of pain.[23]

▶ Pain Assessment Guidelines/Regulations for Specific Practice Settings

Screening for pain should be a part of a routine assessment, and this has led several organizations such as the Veterans Health Administration (VHA) and the American Pain Society (APS) to declare pain as the fifth vital sign. Many states have adopted a bill of rights for patients in pain. In 2001, the Joint Commission on Accreditation of Health Care Organizations (JCAHO) incorporated pain as the fifth vital sign in its accreditation standards.[24] According to the JCAHO, patients have a right to appropriate assessment and management of their pain and education regarding their pain. ❷ *Following initial assessment of pain, reassessment should be done as needed based on medication choice and the clinical situation.*

Clinical Presentation and Diagnosis of Pain Management

General

Patients may be in acute distress (acute pain) or have no signs or symptoms of suffering (chronic pain).

Symptoms

Pain is described based on the following characteristics: onset, duration, location, quality, severity, and intensity. Other symptoms may include anxiety, depression, fatigue, anger, fear, and insomnia.

Signs

Acute pain may cause hypertension, tachycardia, diaphoresis, mydriasis, and pallor.

Diagnosis

The patient is the only person who can describe the intensity and quality of their pain. There are no laboratory tests that can diagnose pain.

► Methods of Pain Assessment

A patient-oriented approach to pain is essential, and methods do not differ greatly from those used in other medical conditions. A comprehensive history (medical, family, and psychological) and physical are necessary to evaluate underlying disease processes for the source of pain and other factors contributing to the pain.[20] A thorough assessment of the characteristics of the pain should be completed, including questions about the pain (onset, duration, location, quality, severity, and intensity), pain relief efforts, and efficacy and side effects of current and past treatments for pain. A common mnemonic for pain assessment is PQRST (Palliative/precipitating, Quality, Radiation, Severity, and Time).[25] Some clinicians have suggested the addition of U (you) to this mnemonic.[26] During the pain interview, the impact of the pain on the patient's functional status, behavior, and psychological states should also be assessed. Evaluation of psychological status is especially important in patients with chronic pain since depression and affective disorders might be common comorbid conditions. A history of drug and alcohol should be elicited due to the potential for addiction in patients who might require opiates or other pain medications with a potential for abuse. Other conditions, such as renal or hepatic dysfunction, diabetes, and conditions that effect bowel function, can influence therapy choices and goals. A discussion of the patient's expectations and goals with respect to pain management (level of pain relief, functional status, and quality of life) should also be part of any pain interview.

► Pain Assessment Tools

Pain, particularly acute pain, might be accompanied by physiologic signs and symptoms, but there are no reliable objective markers for pain. Many tools have been designed for assessing the severity of pain including rating scales and multidimensional pain assessment tools.

Rating scales provide a simple way to classify the intensity of pain, and should be selected based on the patient's ability to communicate (Fig. 33–1).[27] Numeric scales are widely used and ask patients to rate their pain on a scale of 0 to 10, with 0 indicating no pain and 10 being the worst pain possible. Using this type of scale, 1 to 3 is considered mild pain, 4 to 6 is moderate pain, and 8 to 10 is severe pain. The visual analog scale (VAS) is similar to the numerical scale in that it requires patients to place a mark on a 10-cm line where one end is no pain, and the worst possible pain is on the other end. For patients who have difficulty assigning a number to their pain, a categorical scale might be an option to communicate the intensity of the pain experience. Examples of this include a simple descriptive list of words and the Wong-Baker FACES of Pain Rating Scale.[28]

Multidimensional assessment tools obtain information about the pain and impact on quality of life, but are often more time-consuming to complete. Examples of these types of tools include the Initial Pain Assessment Tool, Brief Pain Inventory, McGill Pain Questionnaire, the Neuropathic Pain Scale, and the Oswestry Disability Index.[29–33]

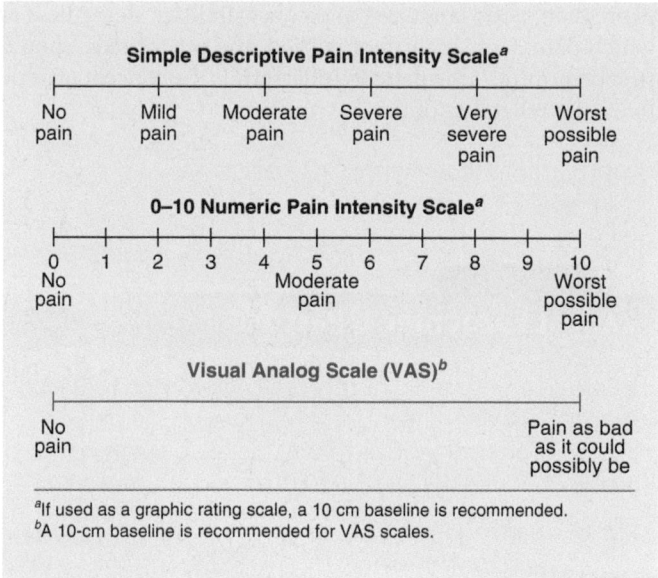

FIGURE 33–1. Pain rating scales. (From Ref. 27.)

Pain Assessment in Challenging Populations

Children. Pain interviews can be conducted with children as young as 3 or 4 years of age; however, communication might be limited by vocabulary.[34] Terms familiar to children such as hurt, owie, or boo boo might be used to describe pain. The VAS is best used with children older than 7 years. Other scales based on numbers of objects (e.g., pokers chips), increasing color intensity, or faces of pain might be helpful for children between 4 and 7 years of age. In children younger than 3 to 4 years, behavioral or physiologic measures, such as pulse or respiratory rate, might be more appropriate. Pain assessment in newborns and infants relies on behavioral observation for such clues as vocalizations (crying and fussing), facial expressions, body movements (flailing of limbs and pulling legs in), withdrawal, and change in eating and sleeping habits.[35] Preschool children experiencing pain might become clingy, lose motor and verbal skills, and start to deny pain because treatment might be linked to discomfort or punishment. School-age children might exhibit aggressiveness, nightmares, anxiety, and withdrawal when in pain, while adolescents might respond to pain with oppositional behavior and depression.

Elderly. Most of the previously discussed pain scales can be used in older persons who are cognitively intact or with mild dementia. The pain thermometer and FACES of pain have been studied in older persons. In persons with moderate-to-severe dementia or those who are nonverbal, observation of pain behaviors, such as guarding or grimacing, provides an alternative for pain assessment. The Pain Assessment in Advanced Dementia (PAINAD) tool might be used to quantify signs of pain and involves observing the older adult for 15 minutes for breathing, negative vocalizations, facial expression, body language, and consolability.[36] Regardless of which pain assessment tool is used, the practitioner should first determine if the patient understands the concept of scale to ensure reliability of the instrument.

Patient Encounter 1, Part 1

HPI: BA is a 58-year-old male recently diagnosed with lung cancer. Following surgery he was placed on morphine patient-controlled analgesia (PCA). He has been using 80 mg of morphine/24 hours with adequate pain control.

PMH: Hypertension × 18 years

FH: Noncontributory

SH: Lives with wife; has four grown children; smoked two packs of cigarettes per day × 40 years (quit with diagnosis of lung cancer)

Meds: Hydrochlorothiazide 25 mg every day

Pain assessment: Patient rates pain as 8 on a scale of 1 to 10.

The physician would like to convert him to a combination preparation of oxycodone and APAP. What dosing regimen would you suggest?

Six months later, BA's pain is controlled with the escalating doses of the combination product; however, he has exceeded the maximum daily dose of APAP. What would you suggest at this time?

TREATMENT

General Approach to Treatment

❸ *Effective treatment involves an evaluation of the cause, duration and intensity of the pain and selection of an appropriate treatment modality for the pain situation.* Depending on the type of pain, treatment might involve pharmacologic and nonpharmacologic therapy or both. General principles for the pharmacologic management of pain are listed in the section: Patient Care and Monitoring. Two common approaches to the selection of treatment are based on severity of pain and the mechanism responsible for the pain (Fig. 33–2). Clinical practice guidelines for pain management are available from the APS, the Agency for Health care Research and Quality (AHRQ), the American Geriatrics Society (AGS), and the American Society of Anesthesiologists (ASA).

▶ Selection of Agent Based on Severity of Pain

❹ *Whenever possible, the least potent, oral analgesic should be selected.* Guidelines for the selection of therapeutic agents based on pain intensity are derived from the World Health Organization (WHO) analgesic ladder for the management of cancer pain (Table 33–1).[37] Mild-to-moderate pain is generally treated with nonopioid analgesics. Combinations of medium-potency opioids and acetaminophen (APAP) or nonsteroidal anti-inflammatory drugs (NSAIDs) are often used for moderate pain. Potent opioids are recommended for severe pain. Throughout this progression, adjuvant medications are added, as needed, to manage side effects and to augment analgesia. While these guidelines can be useful for initial therapy, the clinical situation (type of pain), cost and pharmacokinetic profile of available drugs, and patient-specific factors (age, concomitant illnesses, previous response, and other medications) must also be considered.

Table 33–1

Selection of Analgesics Based on Intensity of Pain

Pain Intensity	Corresponding Numerical Rating	WHO Therapeutic Recommendations	Examples of Initial Therapy	Comments
Mild	1–3/10	Nonopioid analgesic; regular scheduled dosing	Acetaminophen 1,000 mg every 6 hours; ibuprofen 600 mg every 6 hours	Consider adding an adjunct or using an alternate regimen if pain is not reduced in 1–2 days
Moderate	4–6/10	Add an opioid to the nonopioid for moderate pain; regular scheduled dosing	Acetaminophen 325 mg + codeine 60 mg every 4 hours; acetaminophen 325 mg + oxycodone 5 mg every 4 hours	Consider step-up therapy if pain is not relieved by two or more different drugs
Severe	7–10/10	Switch to a high-potency opioid; regular scheduled dosing	Morphine 10 mg every 4 hours; hydromorphone 4 mg every 4 hours	

WHO, World Health Organization.

From Ref. 37.

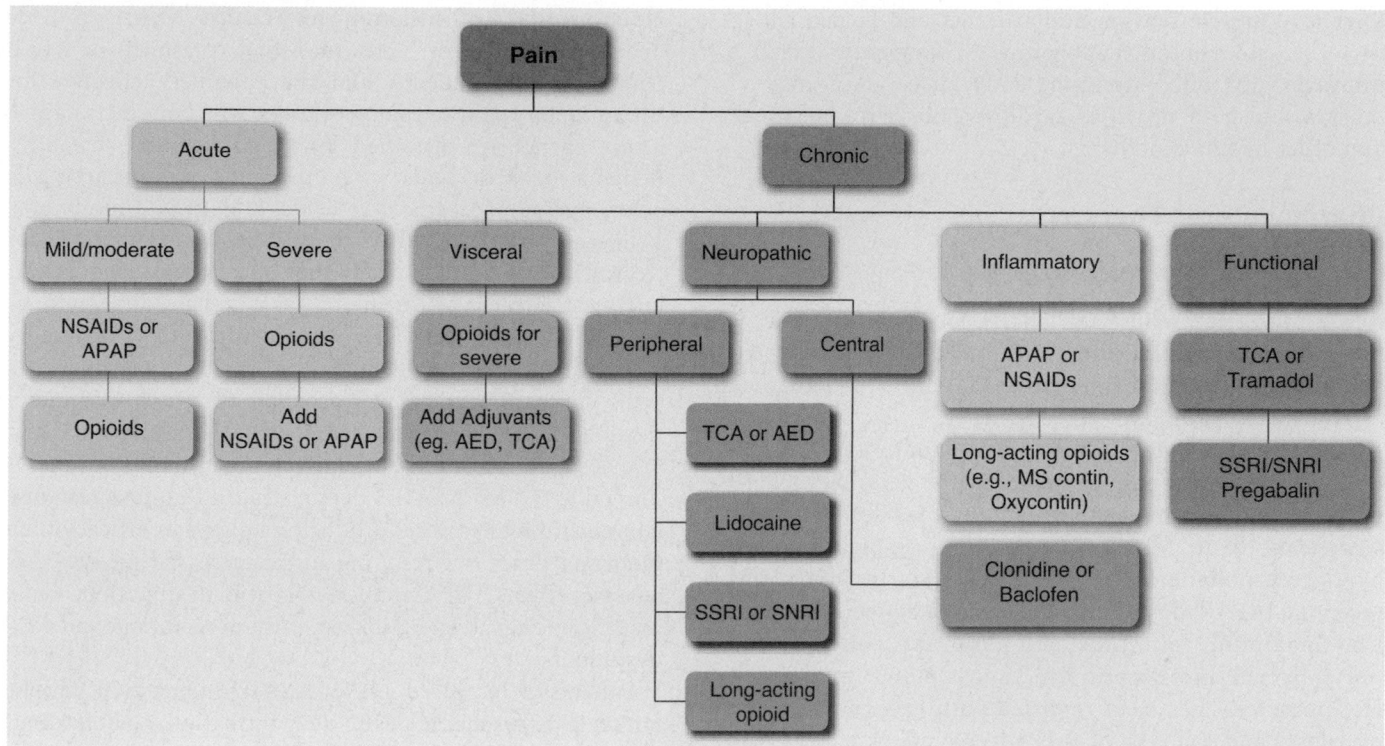

FIGURE 33–2. Pain algorithm.

Pain medications might also be used in the absence of pain in anticipation of a painful event such as surgery to minimize peripheral and central sensitization.

▶ *Mechanistic Approach to Therapy*

Current analgesic therapy is aimed at controlling or blunting pain symptoms. However, diverse mechanisms contributing to the various types of pain continue to be further elucidated. An understanding of these new mechanisms of pain transmission might lead to improvement in pain management, as pharmacologic management of pain becomes more mechanism-specific. Use of NSAIDs for inflammatory types of pain is an example of a mechanistic approach. Since several mechanisms of pain often coexist, a polypharmacy approach seems rational to target each mechanism.

Two current foci in pain management are to identify the mechanisms that are responsible for pain hypersensitivity and to prevent this initial hypersensitivity. Therefore, the goal of pain therapy is to reduce peripheral sensitization and subsequent central stimulation and amplification associated with wind-up, spread, and central sensitization.[17]

Nonpharmacologic Therapy

Nonpharmacologic therapies (psychological interventions and physical therapy) might be used in both acute and chronic pain. Psychological interventions can reduce pain as well as the anxiety, depression, fear, and anger associated with pain. Psychological interventions helpful in management of acute pain are imagery (picturing oneself in a safe, peaceful place) and distraction (listening to music or focusing on breathing). Chronic pain patients might benefit from relaxation, biofeedback, cognitive behavioral therapy, psychotherapy, support groups, and spiritual counseling. Biofeedback teaches patients to control physiological responses to pain and has been effective in headache and chronic low back pain. Cognitive therapy encourages patients to monitor their perceptions of pain, reducing stress and negativism. Psychotherapy is very useful for patients with chronic pain; it can also assist in treatment of psychiatric comorbidities and help patients to deal with terminal illness.[38] The patient should be educated about what to expect regarding pain and its treatment, whether pain is acute pain (i.e., preoperative explanations of expected postsurgic pain) or chronic (i.e., patient and family education in hospice care).

Physical therapy is an essential part of many types of pain situations. Treatment modalities include heat, cold, water, ultrasound therapy, TENS, massage, and therapeutic exercise. Heat and cold therapy are utilized in a variety of musculoskeletal conditions (muscle spasms, low back pain, fibromyalgia, sprains, and strains). Heating modalities include local hot packs, paraffin wrap, hydrotherapy, and deep-heating methods (ultrasound). Cold treatments might be delivered via cold packs, ice massage, cold water immersion, or coolant sprays. TENS therapy is based on the theory that electrical stimulation of a nerve in a particular area can block pain impulses originating from that area. TENS is also believed to release endogenous endorphins and enkephalins. Massage therapy is used to relieve muscle tension and stiffness and is also felt to increase endogenous endorphins. Therapeutic exercise improves not only strength, endurance, and range of motion, but also provides cardiovascular, psychological, and other health benefits.

Pharmacologic Therapy

▶ Nonopioid Analgesics

Acetaminophen APAP, an analgesic and antipyretic, is often selected as initial therapy for mild-to-moderate pain and is considered first-line in several pain situations such as low back pain and osteoarthritis.[39] Mechanistically, APAP is believed to inhibit prostaglandin synthesis in the CNS and block pain impulses in the periphery. APAP is well tolerated at usual doses and has few clinically significant drug interactions except causing increased hypoprothrombinemic response to warfarin in patients receiving APAP doses of more than 2,000 mg per day. The maximum recommended dose for patients with normal renal and hepatic function is 4,000 mg per day. Hepatotoxicity has been reported with excessive use and overdose, and the risk of this adverse effect increases in those with hepatitis or chronic alcohol use, as well as those who binge drink or are in a fasting state. Regular chronic use of APAP has been associated with chronic renal failure, but reports are conflicting. For these reasons, the maximum dose should be reduced by 50% to 75% in patients with renal dysfunction or hepatic disease and in those who engage in excessive alcohol use.

Aspirin and Other Salicylates Aspirin, nonacetylated salicylates, and other NSAIDs have analgesic, antipyretic, and anti-inflammatory actions. These agents inhibit cyclo-oxygenase (COX-1 and COX-2) enzymes, thereby preventing prostaglandin synthesis, which results in reduced nociceptor sensitization and an increased pain threshold. NSAIDs are the preferred agents for mild-to-moderate pain in situations that are mediated by prostaglandins (rheumatoid arthritis, menstrual cramps, and postsurgical pain) and in the management of pain from bony metastasis, but they are of minimal use in neuropathic pain.

Aspirin is effective for mild-to-moderate pain; however, the risk of GI irritation and bleeding limits frequent use of this drug for pain management. Direct effects of aspirin on the GI mucosa and irreversible platelet inhibition contribute to this risk, which can occur even at low doses. Hypersensitivity reactions are also possible and might occur in 25% of patients with coexsiting asthma, nasal polyps, or chronic urticaria. Of additional concern is the potential for cross-sensitivity of other NSAIDs in this group of patients. Nonacetylated salicylates (choline magnesium salicylate and sodium salicylate) have a reduced risk of GI effects and platelet inhibition and might be used in aspirin-sensitive patients. Diflunisal, a salicylic acid derivative, is associated with fewer GI complaints compared to aspirin, but platelet inhibition does increase the risk of GI bleeding.

Nonsteroidal Anti-inflammatory Drugs NSAIDs provide analgesia equal to or better than that of aspirin or APAP combined with codeine, and they are very effective for inflammatory pain and pain associated with bone metastasis.[18] These agents are classified by their chemical structures (fenamates, acetic acids, propionic acids, pyranocarboxylic acids, pyrrolizine carboxylic acids, and COX-2 inhibitors). While only some members of this class have approval for treatment of pain, it is likely that all of them have similar analgesic effects. All members of this class appear to be equally effective, but there is great intrapatient variability in response. After an adequate trial of 2 to 3 weeks with a particular oral agent, it is reasonable to switch to another member of the class. Ketorolac is available in parenteral and oral dosage forms; unlike other NSAIDs, its duration of use is limited to 5 days. NSAIDs demonstrate a flat-dose response curve, with higher doses producing no greater efficacy than moderate doses but resulting in an increased incidence of adverse effects (GI irritation, hepatic dysfunction, renal insufficiency, platelet inhibition, sodium retention, and CNS dysfunction).

Patients at increased risk of NSAID-induced GI adverse effects (e.g., dyspepsia, peptic ulcer formation, and bleeding) include the elderly, those with peptic ulcer disease, coagulopathy, and patients receiving high doses of concurrent corticosteroids. Nephrotoxicity is more common in the elderly, patients with creatinine clearance values less than 50 mL/min, and those with volume depletion or on diuretic therapy. NSAIDs should be used with caution in patients with reduced cardiac output due to sodium retention and in patients receiving antihypertensives, warfarin, and lithium.

NSAIDs are classified as nonselective (they inhibit COX-1 and COX-2) or selective (inhibit only COX-2) based on degree of COX inhibition. COX-2 inhibition is responsible for anti-inflammatory effects, while COX-1 inhibition contributes to increased GI and renal toxicity associated with nonselective agents. Because the antiplatelet effect of nonselective NSAIDs is reversible, concurrent use might reduce the cardioprotective effect of aspirin due to competitive inhibition of COX-1. For this reason, administration of aspirin prior to the NSAID is recommended.[40] The cardiovascular safety of the COX-2 inhibitors has been questioned due to increased risk of myocardial infarction (MI) and stroke noted in several trials.[41-43] The FDA Committees on Arthritis and Drug Safety and Risk Management convened in February 2005 to evaluate the published studies and manufacturer information about the cardiovascular adverse events associated with COX-2 inhibitors.[44] As a follow-up to the committee's recommendations, the FDA took regulatory action in April 2005 announcing that the increased risk of cardiovascular events was likely a class effect of NSAIDs. A boxed warning highlighting the potential for increased risk of cardiovascular events and GI bleeding is now required for all prescription nonselective NSAIDs and celecoxib. Stronger warnings about these adverse events are also required on nonprescription NSAIDs. As a result of the data and subsequent events, two members of this class, rofecoxib and valdecoxib, have been withdrawn from the market. Future COX-2 inhibitors and nonselective NSAIDs will likely have to undergo cardiovascular safety studies before receiving FDA approval. When a NSAID is needed in a patient with cardiovascular risk, the benefits of therapy must outweigh the risks, and the lowest effective dose of NSAID is recommended.

▶ Opioid Analgesics

Opioids are considered the agents of choice for the treatment of severe acute pain and moderate-to-severe pain associated with cancer.[45] For chronic pain, their use was once highly controversial, however, use of opioids in chronic pain is now gaining acceptance.[46] Opioids are classified by their activity at the receptor site, usual pain intensity treated, and duration of action (short- vs. long-acting).

Selection and Dosing The opioids exert their analgesic efficacy by stimulating opioid receptors (μ, κ, and δ) in the CNS. There is a wide variety of potencies among the opioids, with some used for moderate pain (codeine, hydrocodone, tramadol, and partial agonists) and others reserved for severe pain (morphine and hydromorphone). Pure agonists (morphine) bind to μ-receptors to produce analgesia that increases with dose without a ceiling effect. Pure agonists are divided into three chemical classes, phenanthrenes or morphine-like, phenylpiperidine or meperidine-like, and diphenylheptane or methadone-like. Partial agonists/antagonists (butorphanol, pentazocine, and nalbuphine) partially stimulate the μ-receptor and antagonize the κ-receptors. This activity results in reduced analgesic efficacy with a ceiling dose, reduced side effects at the μ-receptor, psychotomimetic side effects due to κ-receptor antagonism, and possible withdrawal symptoms in patients who are dependent on pure agonists.

Selection of the agent and route depend on individual patient-related factors including severity of pain, individual perceptions, weight, age, opioid tolerance, and concomitant disease (renal or hepatic dysfunction). Because pure agonists are pharmacologically similar, choice of agent might be also guided by pharmacokinetic parameters and other drug characteristics. Hepatic impairment can decrease the metabolism of most opioids, particularly methadone, meperidine, pentazocine, and propoxyphene. Furthermore, the clearance of meperidine, propoxyphene, and morphine and their metabolites is reduced in renal dysfunction.

Table 33–2 provides a summary of opiate options, but several drugs warrant further discussion. Normeperidine, the active metabolite of meperidine, can produce tremors, myoclonus, delirium, and seizures. Due to the potential for accumulation of normeperidine, meperidine should not be used in the elderly, those with renal impairment, in patients using patient-controlled analgesia (PCA) devices, or for more than 1 to 2 days of intermittent dosing. Propoxyphene also

---

Patient Encounter 1, Part 2: Converting to Different Drugs and Adjusting Doses

Two years following his diagnosis of lung cancer, BA has been diagnosed as having bone metastases. Pain has been controlled with the following medications: hydromorphone (Dilaudid) 10 mg IV every hour and levorphanol (Levo-Dromoran) 10 mg orally every 4 hours. He is currently receiving hydrochlorothiazide 25 mg daily, senna 2 tablets twice daily, and docusate sodium 100 mg twice daily. As the home care pharmacist, you are asked to convert this patient's pain medications to a morphine infusion.

Morphine equivalents (based on 10 mg parenteral morphine) (Table 33–2)

Parenteral hydromorphone 1.5 mg is equivalent to 10 mg of parenteral morphine.

Levorphanol 4 mg orally is equivalent to 10 mg of parenteral morphine.

Based on BA's opioid requirement, recommend an initial infusion rate (in milligrams per hour) of parenteral morphine.

Which adjuvant therapy could be considered for BA?

Recommend a monitoring plan for this patient.

How would you assess pain response?

Table 33–2

Equianalgesic Doses of Selected Opioids

Opioid (Brand Name)	Dose Equianalgesic to 10 mg of Parenteral Morphine (mg)	
	Parenteral (mg)	Oral (mg)
Mild–Moderate Pain		
Codeine (generic, various)	120	200
Hydrocodone (Vicodin, Lorcet)	N/A	30
Oxycodone (OxyContin, OxyFast, Oxy IR)	N/A	20
Meperidine (Demerol)	100	400
Propoxyphene (Darvon)	N/A	65–130
Moderate–Severe Pain		
Morphine (Roxanol, MS Contin, Kadian, Avinza)	10	30
Hydromorphone (Dilaudid)	1.5	7.5
Oxymorphone (Opana, Opana SR, Numorphan)	1	N/A
Levorphanol (Levo-Dromoran)	2	4
Fentanyl (Duragesic)	0.1–0.2	N/A[a]
Methadone (Dolophine)	10[b]	3–5[b]

[a]Transdermal: 100 mcg/h = 2–4 mg/h of IV morphine.

[b]Dosage calculations when converting from morphine to methadone are not linear. The equianalgesic dose of methadone will decrease progressively as the morphine equivalents increase (Table 33–4).

From Refs. 26, 45, 49, 51.

has an increased risk of seizures and cardiac conduction abnormalities and should be avoided in the elderly. Despite its popularity, propoxyphene has proven to be no more effective than APAP, aspirin, or codeine alone.[18] Methadone is unique among the opiates as it has several mechanisms (μ-agonist, NMDA-receptor antagonist, and inhibition of reuptake of serotonin and norepinephrine) that make it an interesting choice for chronic pain. The long-half of methadone (30 hours) permits extended dosing intervals; however, the potential for accumulation with repeated dosing often results in challenging dose conversion. Tramadol is a synthetic opioid with a dual mechanism of action (μ-agonist and inhibition of serotonin and norepinephrine reuptake) and efficacy and safety similar to that of equianalgesic doses of codeine plus APAP. Tramadol has been evaluated in several types of neuropathic pain and might have a role in the treatment of chronic pain. Tramadol is associated with an increased risk of seizures in patients with a seizure disorder, those at risk for seizures, and those taking medications that can lower the seizure threshold. Doses greater than 500 mg have also been associated with seizures. The use of tramadol with other serotonergic drugs (e.g., selective serotonin reuptake inhibitors [SSRI]) might precipitate serotonin syndrome. While originally thought to be nonhabit forming, dependence can occur with tramadol.

About 70% of individuals will experience significant analgesia from 10 mg/70 kg of body weight of IV morphine or its equivalent.[18] For severe pain in opiate-naive patients, a usual starting dose is 5 to 10 mg of morphine every 4 hours. In the initial stages of severe pain, medication should be given around the clock. Rescue doses should be made available for breakthrough pain in doses equivalent to 10% to 20% of the total daily opioid requirement and administered every 2 to 6 hours if needed. Alternatively 1/6 of the total daily dose or 1/3 of the 12-hourly dose might be used. Scheduled doses should be titrated based on the degree of pain. One method involves adjustment of the maintenance dose based on the total 24-hour rescue dose requirement. Alternatively, utilizing dose escalation, doses could be increased by 50% to 100% or 30% to 50% of the current dose, for those in severe and moderate pain, respectively. Once pain relief is achieved, and if treatment is necessary for more than a few days, conversion to a controlled-release or long-acting opioid should be made with an equal amount of agent. Several sustained-release products are available containing morphine, oxycodone, and fentanyl. Some clinicians will reduce the total daily dose of the long-acting dosage form by 25% when initiating a sustained-release product to reduce the likelihood of oversedation. The dose of a pure agonist is limited only by tolerability to side effects. Tolerance might develop to analgesic effects, necessitating increasing doses to achieve the same level of pain relief. Physical dependence will also occur with long-term use of opioids. However, addiction or psychological dependence is unlikely in legitimate pain patients unless there are predisposing risk factors. Pain patients who are undertreated might appear to be drug-seeking (pseudoaddiction), however effective pain management resolves the behaviors. When opioids are used for chronic pain, use of informed consent for chronic opioid therapy, medication management agreements, or pain contracts might be appropriate to monitor the use (prescribing and dispensing) of controlled substances.

Opioids are administered by a variety of routes, including oral (tablet and liquid), sublingual, rectal, transdermal, transmucosal, IV, subcutaneous, and intraspinal. While the oral and transdermal routes are most common, the method of administration is based on patient needs (severity of pain) and characteristics (swallowing difficulty and preference). Oral opioids have an onset of effect of 45 minutes, so IV or subcutaneous administration might be preferred if more rapid relief is desired. Intramuscular (IM) injections are not recommended because of pain at the injection site and wide fluctuations in drug absorption and peak plasma concentrations achieved. More invasive routes of administration such as PCA and intraspinal (epidural and intrathecal) are primarily used postoperatively, but might also be used in refractory chronic pain situations. PCA delivers a self-administered dose via an infusion pump with a preprogrammed dose, minimum dosing interval, and a maximum hourly dose. Morphine, fentanyl, and hydromorphone are commonly administered via PCA pumps by the IV route, but less frequently by the subcutaneous or epidural route.

Epidural analgesia is frequently used for lower extremity procedures and pain (e.g., knee surgery, labor pain, and some abdominal procedures). Intermittent bolus or continuous infusion of preservative-free opioids (morphine, hydromorphone, or fentanyl) and local anesthetics (bupivacaine) might be used for epidural analgesia. Opiates given by this route might cause pruritus that is relieved by naloxone. Adverse effects including respiratory depression, hypotension, and urinary retention might occur. When epidural routes are used in narcotic-dependent patients, systemic analgesics must also be used to prevent withdrawal since the opioid is not absorbed and remains in the epidural space. Doses of opioids used in epidural analgesia are 10 times less than IV doses, and intrathecal doses are 10 times less than epidural doses (i.e., 10 mg of IV morphine is equivalent to 1 mg epidural morphine and 0.1 mg of intrathecally administered morphine).[45]

Combination Analgesics Combinations of opioids and nonopioids often result in enhanced analgesia and lower dose of each. Combination analgesics are frequently used in moderate pain. However, in severe pain, the nonopioid component reaches maximum dosage, and thus the usefulness of nonopioids in this situation is limited. Additionally, the combination products are short acting and often not suitable for chronic therapy. Single agents offer greater dosing flexibility than combination products.

Opioid Allergy True narcotic allergies are rare and should not be confused with pruritus associated with opiate use. Cross-sensitivity between morphine-like, meperidine-like, and methadone-like agents is unlikely. Therefore, when an individual is allergic to one drug in a chemical class of opioids, it is reasonable to select an agent in another chemical class. For the purpose of drug selection in patients with allergies, mixed agonists/antagonists should be treated as morphine-like agents.

Tapering of Opioids Tapering of opioids might be necessary once the painful situation has resolved in patients receiving doses greater than 160 mg/day of oral morphine (or the equivalent) or in those with prolonged opioid use. In these situations the dose should be reduced by 15% to 20% each day to avoid withdrawal symptoms.

Managing Opioid Side Effects and Drug Interactions

Side effects common to all opioids include sedation, hallucinations, constipation, nausea and vomiting, urinary retention, myoclonus, and respiratory depression. Table 33–3 shows side-effect management strategies. In terms of medication management, the most frequent are sedation, nausea, and constipation. Sedation and nausea are common when initiating therapy and when increasing doses. Nausea can be prevented with a centrally acting antiemetic. Sedation usually improves with continued therapy but might become intractable at high doses, and stimulants, such as methylphenidate might be needed. Respiratory depression is a serious adverse effect, and usually occurs after acute administration in opioid-naive patients. Tolerance to respiratory depression develops rapidly with repeated doses, and respiratory depression is rarely a clinically significant problem in pain patients even those with respiratory impairment. Constipation is a significant adverse effect to which tolerance does develop, and prophylaxis with stimulant laxatives (e.g., senna or bisacodyl) and stool softeners, such as docusate, is recommended.

Codeine, hydrocodone, morphine, methadone, and oxycodone are substrates of the cytochrome P450 (CYP) enzyme—CYP2D6.[47] Inhibition of CYP2D6 results in decreased analgesia of codeine and hydrocodone due to decreased conversion to the active metabolites (e.g., morphine and hydromorphone, respectively) and increased effects of morphine, methadone, and oxycodone. Methadone is also a substrate of CYP3A4, and its metabolism is increased by phenytoin and decreased by cimetidine. CNS depressants might potentiate the sedative effects of opiates.

Opioid Rotation Opioid rotation is the switch from one opioid to another to achieve a better balance between analgesia and treatment limiting adverse effects. This practice is often used when escalating doses (greater than 1 gram of morphine/day) become ineffective. In some settings, opioid rotation is utilized routinely to prevent the development of analgesic tolerance.[48]

Equianalgesic Dosing of Opioid Analgesics Conversion from one dosage form to another or from one opioid to another might be necessary in situations such as ineffective pain control, emergence of side effects, change in patient status, and in formulary restrictions. ❺ *Equianalgesic doses should be used when converting from one opioid to another.* Clinicians should be familiar with the equianalgesic dosing and conversion strategies to avoid analgesic failure. Equianalgesic tables serve as a guide for selection of the dosage of the new opioid, but have limitations as they are often based

Table 33–3

Managing Opioid Side Effects

Adverse Effects	Drug Treatment/Management
Excessive sedation	Reduce dose by 25% or increase dosing interval
Constipation	Casanthranol-docusate 1 cap at bedtime or twice daily; senna 1–2 tabs at bedtime or twice daily; bisacodyl 5–10 mg daily + docusate 100 mg twice daily
Nausea and vomiting	Prevention: Hydroxyzine 25–100 mg (po/IM) every 4–6 hours as needed; diphenhydramine 25–50 mg (po/IM) every 6 hours as needed; ondansetron 4 mg IV or 16 mg po
	Treatment: Prochlorperazine 5–10 mg (po/IM) every 3–4 hours as needed or 25 mg PR twice daily; ondansetron 4–8 mg IV every 8 hours as needed
Gastroparesis	Metoclopramide 10 mg (po/IV) every 6–8 hours
Vertigo	Meclizine 12.5–25 mg po every 6 hours as needed
Urticaria/itching	Hydroxyzine 25–100 mg (po/IM) every 4–6 hours as needed; diphenhydramine 25–50 mg (po/IM) every 6 hours as needed
Respiratory depression	Mild: Reduce dose by 25%
	Moderate–severe: Naloxone 0.4–2 mg IV every 2–3 minutes (up to 10 mg) for complete reversal; 0.1–0.2 mg IV every 2–3 minutes until desired reversal for partial reversal; may need to repeat in 1–2 hours depending on narcotic half-life
CNS irritability	Discontinue opioid; treat with benzodiazepine

IM, intramuscular; po, orally; PR, per rectum.

From Refs. 27, 45, 49.

on single-dose studies and clinical observations.[49] Opioid potency is compared using a reference standard of 10 mg of parenteral morphine. Switching from one dosage form to another of the same opioid (i.e., IV to oral) is relatively simple. The current total daily dose is calculated and the total of the new dosage form is determined using a ratio of the equianalgesic doses. This result is then adjusted based on the usual dosing frequency of the new form. When converting to a sustained-release form of the same opioid, dosage may be reduced by 25% to avoid initial sedation; however, the specific product literature should also be consulted.

The first step in an opioid rotation is to calculate the patient's total daily dose of opioid based on the regularly scheduled dose and the total amount of rescue dose needed in 24 hours. This total is then converted to morphine-dosing equivalents using equianalgesic doses (Table 33–2). The total daily morphine dose is then used to calculate the daily dose of the new opioid using dosing equivalents from an equianalgesic table. Because cross-tolerance may not be complete between opioids, some references suggest that the calculated equianalgesic dose be reduced by 25% to 50%.[49] If the opioid switch is due to uncontrolled pain, a dosage reduction may not be needed. The calculated equianalgesic dose may need to be reduced more in the medically frail and when converting to methadone.[50,51] Methadone appears to be much more potent than once believed, and morphine to methadone ratios vary according to the total dose of morphine taken at the time of making the conversion to methadone (Table 33–4).[52,53] Conversion to methadone is a complex process, and several different strategies have been proposed including a switch of the entire dose in one day or a gradual conversion over 3 days.

▶ Adjuvant Agents for Chronic Pain

The role of NSAIDs and opioids in chronic nonmalignant pain has been discussed; however, a review of adjuvant agents for chronic pain, particularly neuropathic pain, is warranted. Adjuvant analgesics are drugs that have indications other than pain but are useful as monotherapy or in combination with nonopioids and opioids. Common adjuvants include antiepileptic drugs (AEDs), antidepressants, antiarrhythmic drugs, local anesthetics, topical agents (e.g., capsaicin), and a variety of other drugs (e.g., NMDA antagonists, clonidine, and muscle relaxants).

There is little consensus on the optimal management of neuropathic pain, because much of the evidence for treatment effectiveness consists of anecdotal reports or poorly designed trials. Published guidelines have been suggested for the general management of neuropathic pain.[54] Suggestions for first-line therapy include gabapentin or pregabalin, transdermal lidocaine, or tricyclic antidepressants (TCAs) (Table 33–5).[54-58] Newer antidepressants, such as the SSRIs, have fewer side effects but appear to be less effective than the TCAs for neuropathic pain. However, serotonin–norepinephrine reuptake inhibitors (SNRIs), (e.g., duloxetine and venlafaxine) have been used successfully for painful DPN. A stepwise approach is suggested for managing the patient with neuropathic pain beginning with the least-invasive effective therapeutic choice and proceeding to the rational use of multiple drug regimens. To guide choice of pharmacologic agents, patients might be identified as candidates for AEDs, TCAs, or opioids based on the presence of peripheral or central nerve pain and description of symptoms (Fig. 33–2).

Choice of agent might also depend on dosing frequency and comorbidities. Data on combination therapy are lacking, and the use of combined treatment is empirical based on additive therapeutic benefit. Scheduled medication regimens instead of "as-needed" dosing should be employed when treating chronic pain, and the effectiveness of therapy should be reassessed regularly. If patients are managed on a multiple drug regimen and changes are indicated, changing only one drug at a time is suggested. Topical agents (e.g., capsaicin) might be added to a regimen to reduce the oral medication load, particularly if adverse effects are a problem or if pain is not relieved.

Table 33–5

Selected Adjuvant Analgesics and Suggested Dosing

Agent	Dosing Guidelines	FDA-Approved Indication
Amitriptyline (Elavil)	10–25 mg at bedtime with weekly increments to a target dose of 25–150 mg of amitriptyline or an equivalent dose of another TCA	
Duloxetine (Cymbalta)	DPN: 60 mg daily Fibromyalgia: 30 mg daily, may be increased by 30 mg increments to a maximum of 120 mg daily	DPN, fibromylagia
Gabapentin (Neurontin)	Initially, 300 mg three times a day up to a maximum of 3,600 mg daily, in divided doses[a]	PHN
Pregabalin (Lyrica)	DPN: Initially, 50 mg three times a day; may be increased to 100 mg three times a day within 1 week based on efficacy and tolerability[a]	DPN, PHN, and fibromyalgia
	PHN: Initially 75 mg twice a day or 50 mg three times a day; may be increased to 100 mg three times a day within 1 week based on efficacy and tolerability[a] Fibromyalgia: Initially 75 mg twice a day, increase to 300 mg daily over 7 days	
Lidocaine 5% (Lidoderm patch)	Up to 3 patches may be applied directly over the painful site once daily; patches are applied using a regimen of 12 hours on and 12 hours off	PHN

DPN, diabetic peripheral neuropathy; PHN, postherpetic neuralgia; TCA, tricyclic antidepressant.

[a]Dosing for creatinine clearance of 60 mL/min or greater.

From Refs. 54–58.

Table 33–4

Methadone Dose Conversions

Total Daily Dose of Oral Morphine	Morphine: Methadone Factor
Less than 100 mg	3:1
	3 mg morphine:1 mg methadone
101–300 mg	5:1
301–600 mg	10:1
601–800 mg	12:1
801–1,000 mg	15:1
Greater than 1,000 mg	20:1

From Ref. 53.

▶ *Complementary and Alternative Medicine*

Complementary and alternative medicine (CAM) is a term used to encompass a variety of therapies (e.g., acupuncture, chiropractic, botanical and nonbotanical dietary supplements, and homeopathy). Painful conditions are among the most common reasons individuals seek relief from CAM. In a recent survey, neck pain, joint pain, arthritis, and headache were among the top ten reasons for use of CAM, and low back pain ranked the number one reason for CAM therapies. Of the CAM therapies, chiropractic and acupuncture are the most accepted and utilized modalities. A variety of dietary supplements have been suggested for painful conditions such as *S*-adenosylmethionine (SAM-e), ginger, fish oil, feverfew, *γ*-linoleic acid, glucosamine, and chondroitin. Of these, glucosamine and chondroitin are the most popular and have the most evidence supporting their efficacy. Glucosamine in doses of 1,500 mg/day has been shown to be effective in reducing pain of osteoarthritis by fostering repair of cartilage, and it is recommended by the Osteoarthritis Research Society International (OARSI).[59]

OUTCOME EVALUATION

Individualize the treatment goals at the beginning of treatment. Utilize information obtained during the pain interview to create goals that are consistent with the patient's expectations. Prevention, reduction, or elimination of pain are important goals for treatment of acute pain. With chronic pain, elimination of pain might not be possible, and goals might focus on improvement or maintenance of functional capacity and quality of life. Thus, for example, pain goals might include "pain scale less than three," or "be able to play a game with grandchildren," or "be able to knit again." Assess patients periodically, depending on the method of analgesia and pain condition, for achievement of pain goals. Evaluate the patient for the presence of adverse drug reactions, drug allergies, and drug interactions.

Abbreviations Introduced in This Chapter

AED	Antiepileptic drug
AGS	American Geriatrics Society
AHRQ	Agency for Health care Research and Quality
AMPA	α-amino-3-hydroxy-5-methylisoxazole-4-propionic acid
APAP	Acetaminophen
APS	American Pain Society
ASA	American Society of Anesthesiologists
CAM	Complementary and alternative medicine
CHF	Congestive heart failure
COX	Cyclo-oxygenase
CRPS	Complex regional pain syndrome
CYP	Cytochrome P450 enzyme
DPN	Diabetic peripheral neuropathy
GABA	Gama-aminobutyric acid
HTN	Hypertension
IASP	International Association for the Study of Pain
IM	Intramuscular
JCAHO	Joint Commission on Accreditation of Healthcare Organizations
MI	Myocardial infarction
NMDA	*N*-methyl-D-aspartate
NSAID	Nonsteroidal anti-inflammatory drug
OARSI	Osteoarthritis Research Society International
PAINAD	Pain Assessment in Advanced Dementia (tool)
PCA	Patient-controlled analgesia
PHN	Postherpetic neuralgia
PQRST	Palliative/precipitating, Quality, Radiation, Severity, and Time
SAM-e	*S*-adenosylmethionine
SNRI	Serotonin-norepinephrine reuptake inhibitor
SSRI	Selective serotonin reuptake inhibitor
TCA	Tricyclic antidepressant
TENS	Iranscutaneous electrical nerve stimulation
VAS	Visual analog scale
VHA	Veterans Health Administration
WHO	World Health Organization

Patient Care and Monitoring

1. Identify the source of pain.

2. Assess the level of pain using a pain intensity scale.

3. Base the initial choice of analgesic on the severity and type of pain, as well as on the patient's medical condition and concurrent medications.

4. Use the least potent oral analgesic that provides adequate pain relief and causes the fewest side effects.

5. Titrate the dose to one that achieves an adequate level of pain control.

6. Use a dosing schedule versus as-needed dosing.

7. Assess the patient for analgesic effectiveness and for side effects at each visit or more frequently, depending on the acuity of the patient's condition.

8. Avoid excessive sedation.

9. Adjust the route of administration if the patient is unable to take oral medications.

10. Use equianalgesic doses as a guide when switching opioids.

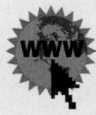

Self-assessment questions and answers are available at *http://www.mhpharmacotherapy.com/pp.html.*

REFERENCES

1. Nagda J, Bajwa ZH. Definitions of the classification of pain. In: Warfield CA, Bajwa ZH, eds. Principles and Practice of Pain Medicine. 2nd ed. New York: McGraw-Hill, 2004:51–54.
2. American Pain Foundation. Fast Facts. *http://www.painfoundation. org/page.asp?file=Newsroom/PainFacts.htm.*
3. Deyo RA, Mirza SK, Martin BL. Back pain prevalence and visit rates: Estimates from U.S. national surveys, 2002. Spine 2006;31:2724–2727.
4. American Council for Headache Education. What you should know about headache. *http://www.achenet.org/education/patients/ TypesofHeadaches.asp.*
5. National Fibromyalgia Association. Who is affected? *http://www. fmaware.org/site/PageServer?pagename=fibromyalgia_affected.*
6. Christo PJ, Mazloomdoost D. Cancer pain and analgesia. Ann N Y Acad Sci 2008;1138:278–298.
7. Carter GT, Galer BS. Advances in the management of neuropathic pain. Phys Med Rehabil Clin N Am 2001;12:447–459.
8. Wallace MS. Diagnosis and treatment of neuropathic pain. Curr Opin Anaesthesiol 2005;18:548–554.
9. Sadosky A, McDermott AM, Brandenburg NA, Strauss M. A review of the epidemiology of painful diabetic peripheral neuropathy, postherpetic neuralgia, and less commonly studied neuropathic pain conditions. Pain Pract 2008;8:45–56.
10. American Geriatrics Society Panel on Persistent Pain in Older Persons. The management of persistent pain in older persons. J Am Geriatr Soc 2002;50(6):1–20.
11. Ferrell BA. The management of pain in long-term care. Clin J Pain 2004;20:240–243.
12. Luo X, Pietrobon R, Sun SX, et al. Estimates and patterns of direct health care expenditures among individuals with back pain in the United States. Spine 2004;29:79–86.
13. Stewart W, Ricci J, Chee E, Lipton R. Work-related cost of pain in the U.S.: Results from the American Productivity Audit. International Association for the Study of Pain, 10th World Congress on Pain; August 19–22, 2002; San Diego, CA. Abstract 697:331.
14. Desbiens NA, Wu AW, Broste SK, et al. Pain and satisfaction with pain control in seriously ill hospitalized adults: Findings from the SUPPORT research investigations. Crit Care Med 1996;24:1953–1961.
15. Desbiens NA, Wu AW. Pain and suffering in seriously ill hospitalized patients. J Am Geriatr Soc 2000;48:S183–S186.
16. Von Roenn JH, Cleeland CS, Gonin R, et al. Physician attitudes and practice in cancer pain management. A survey from the Eastern Cooperative Oncology Group. Ann Intern Med 1993;119:121–126.
17. Woolf CJ. Pain: moving from symptom control toward mechanism-specific pharmacologic management. Ann Intern Med 2004;140:441–451.
18. Reisner L, Koo PJS. Pain and its management. In: Koda-Kimble MA, Young LY, Kradjan WA, et al, eds. Applied Therapeutics: The Clinical Use of Drugs. 8th ed. Philadelphia: Lippincott Williams & Wilkins, 2005:9-1–9-40.
19. Renn CL, Doresy SG. The physiology and processing of pain. A review. AACN Clin Issues 2005;16:277–290.
20. National Pharmaceutical Council. Pain: Current understanding of assessment, management, and treatments. Reston, VA: National Pharmaceutical Council, 2001. *http://www.npcnow.org/resources/PDFs/ painmonograph.pdf.*
21. Ashburn MA, Lipman AG. Pain in society. In: Lipman AG, ed. Pain Management for Primary Care Clinicians. Bethesda, MD: American Society of Health-System Pharmacists; 2004:1–12.
22. Rowbotham MC, Twilling L, Davies PS, et al. Oral opioid therapy for chronic peripheral and central neuropathic pain. N Engl J Med 2003;348:1223–1232.
23. Curtiss CP, McKee AL. Assessment of the person with pain. In: Lipman AG, ed. Pain Management for Primary Care Clinicians. Bethesda, MD: American Society of Health-System Pharmacists, 2004:27–42.
24. Joint Commission on Accreditation of Health care Organizations. Pain assessment and management an organizational approach. Oakbrook Terrace, IL: JCAHO, 2000:1–6.
25. Twycross RG. Pain and analgesics. Curr Med Res Opin 1978;5:497–505.
26. Gammaitoni AR, Fine P, Alvarez N, et al. Clinical application of opioid equianalgesic data. Clin J Pain 2003;19:286–297.
27. U.S. Department of Health and Human Services, Agency for Health Care Policy and Research. Clinical practice guideline, cancer pain management. Rockville, MD: AHCPR, 1994. *http://www.ncbi.nlm.nih. gov/books/bookres.fcgi/hstat6/f37_capcf4.gif.*
28. Wong D, Baker C. Pain in children: comparison of assessment scales. Pediatr Nurs 1988;14:9–17.
29. Brief Pain Inventory. *http://www.cityofhope.org/prc/pdf/BPI%20 Long%20Version.pdf.*
30. Initial Pain Assessment Tool. *http://www.stratishealth.org/health-care/ documents/1McCaffreyBeebe.pdf.*
31. McGill Pain Questionnaire. *http://www.hsrd.ann-arbor.med.va.gov/ creme(section2).pdf.*
32. Galer BS, Jensen MP. Development and preliminary validation of a pain measure specific to neuropathic pain: The Neuropathic Pain Scale. Neurology 1997;48:332–338.
33. Oswestry Disability Index. *http://www.drridgway.ca/pdfs/Oswestry.pdf.*
34. American Academy of Pediatrics. Committee on Psychosocial Aspects of Child and Family Health; Task Force on Pain in Infant, Children, and Adolescents. The assessment and management of acute pain in infants, children, and adolescents. Pediatrics 2001;108:793–797.
35. Mathew PJ, Mathew JL. Assessment and management of pain in infants. Postgrad Med J 2003;79:438–443.
36. Warden V, Hurley AC, Volicer L. Development and psychometric evaluation of the Pain Assessment in Advanced Dementia (PAINAD) scale. J Am Med Dir Assoc 2003;4:9–15.
37. World Health Organization. WHO's pain ladder. *http://www.who.int/ cancer/palliative/painladder/en/.*
38. Gallagher RM. Rational integration of pharmacologic, behavioral, and rehabilitation strategies in the treatment of chronic pain. Am J Phys Med Rehabil 2005;84(suppl):S64–S76.
39. American College of Rheumatology Subcommittee on Osteoarthritis. Recommendations for the medical management of osteoarthritis of the hip and knee. Arthritis Rheum 2000;43:1905–1915.
40. Kurth T. Glynn RJ, Walker AM, et al. Inhibition of clinical benefits of aspirin on first myocardial infarction by nonsteroidal anti-inflammatory drugs. Circulation 2003;108:1191–1195.
41. Bombardier C, Laine L, Reicin A, et al. Comparison of upper gastrointestinal toxicity of rofecoxib and naproxen in patients with rheumatoid arthritis. VIGOR Study Group. N Engl J Med 2000;343:1520–1528.
42. Silverstein FE, Faich G, Goldstein JL, et al. Gastrointestinal toxicity with celecoxib vs nonsteroidal anti-inflammatory drugs for osteoarthritis and rheumatoid arthritis: The CLASS study: A randomized controlled trial. Celecoxib Long-term Arthritis Safety Study. JAMA 2000;284:1247–1255.
43. FitzGerald GA. Coxibs and cardiovascular disease. N Engl J Med 2004;351:1709–1711.
44. Food and Drug Administration. Arthritis Advisory Committee and the Drug Safety and Risk Management Advisory Committee Briefing Information. *http://www.fda.gov.ohrms/dockets/ac/05/ briefing/2005-4090bl.htm.*
45. American Pain Society. Principles of analgesic use in the treatment of acute pain and cancer pain. 5th ed. Glenview, IL: American Pain Society, 2003:13–41.
46. Ballantyne JC, Mao J. Medical progress: Opioid therapy for chronic pain. N Engl J Med 2003;349(20):1943–1953.
47. Barkin RL, Barkin D. Pharmacologic management of acute and chronic pain: Focus on drug interactions and patient-specific pharmacotherapeutic selection. South Med J 2001;94:756–812.
48. Cleary JF. The pharmacologic management of cancer pain. J Palliat Med 2007;10:1369–1394.
49. Pereira J, Lawlor P, Vigrano A, et al. Equianalgesic dose ratios for opioids: A critical review and proposals for long-term dosing. J Pain Symptom Manage 2001;22:672–687.

50. Ripamonti C, Groff L, Brunelli C, et al. Switching from morphine to oral methadone in treating cancer pain: What is the equianalgesic dose ratio? J Clin Oncol 1998;16:3216–3221.

51. Mancini I, Lossignol D, Body JJ. Opioid switch to oral methadone in cancer pain. Curr Opin Oncol 2000;12:308–313.

52. Ripamonti C, Bianchi M. The use of methadone for cancer pain. Hematol Oncol Clin North Am 2002;16:543–555.

53. Gazelle G, Fine PG. Fast fact and concepts #75. Methadone for the treatment of pain. End-of-life Physician Education Resource Center. *http://www.eperc.mcw.edu*.

54. Gilron I, Watson CP, Cahill CM, Moulin DE. Neuropathic pain: a practical guide for the clinician. CMAJ 2006;175:265–275.

55. Backonja M, Beydoun A, Edwards KR, et al. Gabapentin for the treatment of painful neuropathy in patients with diabetes mellitus: A randomized controlled trial. JAMA 1998;280:1831–1836.

56. Rowbotham M, Harden N, Stacey B, et al. Gabapentin for the treatment of postherpetic neuralgia: A randomized controlled trial. JAMA 1998;280:1837–1842.

57. Zin CS, Nissen LM, Smith MT, et al. An update on the pharmacological management of post-herpetic neuralgia and painful diabetic neuropathy. CNS Drugs 2008;22:417–442.

58. Dworkin RH, O'Connor AB, Backonja M, et al. Pharmacologic management of neuropathic pain: Evidence-based recommendations. Pain 2007;132:237–251.

59. Zhang W, Moskowitz RW, Nuki G, et al. OARSI recommendations for the management of hip and knee osteoarthritis, part II: OARSI evidence-based, expert consensus guidelines. Osteoarthritis Cartilage 2008;16:137–162.

34 Headache

Leigh Ann Ross and Brendan S. Ross

LEARNING OBJECTIVES

● **Upon completion of this chapter, the reader will be able to:**

1. Differentiate among types of headaches based on symptoms and signs.

2. List underlying causes and precipitating factors of different types of headache disorders.

3. Recommend appropriate nonpharmacologic measures for headache treatment and prevention of headache.

4. Based on patient-specific data; determine when pharmacologic therapy is indicated for headache.

5. Propose individualized pharmacologic treatment regimens for the acute and chronic management of headache syndromes.

6. Construct therapeutic and adverse effect monitoring plans for patients with headache.

7. Discuss pertinent patient education points for patients with headache disorders.

KEY CONCEPTS

❶ Headache may be a primary condition, or a secondary disorder due to an underlying medical condition.

❷ Primary headaches are classified as migraine, tension-type, or cluster and other trigeminal autonomic cephalalgias.

❸ The pain experienced with headaches is likely due to overactivity in the trigeminovascular system of the brain.

❹ Migraine is further classified as migraine with aura and migraine without aura.

❺ The short-term goal of headache therapy is pain relief and a return to normal activities.

❻ The long-term goal of therapy is the prevention of headache recurrence.

❼ Pharmacologic treatment of acute headache should be started early to improve the response to therapy.

❽ Prophylaxis is indicated if headaches are frequent or severe, lead to significant disability, or require the use of pain-relieving medications two or more times per week.

❾ Regimens for headache disorders should be individualized based on the pattern of occurrence, response to therapy, medication tolerability, and comorbid medical conditions.

H eadaches are common and have a significant impact on quality of life. ❶ *They can be classified as primary or secondary; the latter are causally related to an underlying medical disorder*. Primary headaches are more common and will be the focus of this chapter. Patients may seek evaluation of headache from a variety of health care providers. Therefore, all clinicians must be familiar with the types of headache, their diagnostic criteria, red flags indicating need for urgent intervention or specialist referral, and nonpharmacologic and pharmacologic options for treatment. ❷ *The International Headache Society (IHS) classifies primary headaches as migraine, tension-type, or cluster and other trigeminal autonomic cephalalgias.*[1] Tension-type headaches (TTHs) are more common than migraine, and both are more common in women than men. Cluster is a less common chronic headache syndrome that affects predominantly men.

EPIDEMIOLOGY OF HEADACHE DISORDERS

Migraine Headache

Migraine is a primary headache disorder that is estimated to affect 10% to 15% of adults in the United States.[2] Less than one-half of headaches meeting the diagnostic criteria for migraine are appropriately diagnosed. Migraine prevalence depends upon age and gender. In children younger than 12 years of age, migraines are more prevalent in males. After age 12, this prevalence shifts markedly to women. The evolution in this gender difference is brought on by the hormonal changes of menarche.[3] Onset typically occurs between the ages of 10 and 30 years, but the prevalence is highest in the age range of 35 to 45 years.[4] Migraines significantly impact patient function with over one-half of sufferers reporting severe disability requiring bed rest during an attack. The economic burden of migraine due to direct and indirect costs is substantial. Migraines are the leading cause of employee absenteeism and decreased workplace productivity.[5]

Tension-Type Headache

TTH is the most common primary headache disorder. It is often under-represented in clinical practice, as many patients do not present for care.[6] The term TTH is used to describe all headache syndromes in which muscle contraction is the most significant factor in the pathogenesis of pain. The 1-year prevalence of TTH in the population ranges from 30% to 90%.[6] It is more common in adult females. Environmental factors, as opposed to genetic predisposition, play a central role in the development of TTH. TTHs can be further divided into episodic or chronic. The mean frequency of attacks is 3 days per month in episodic disorders, and chronic TTH is defined as 15 or more attacks in a one-month period.[7] The estimated prevalence of chronic TTH is less than 5%.[6] Some researchers believe that chronic TTHs represent a continuum of headache severity with migraine headache.[8] When severe headaches are difficult to differentiate clinically, treatment should initially target TTH.

Cluster Headache and Other Trigeminal Autonomic Cephalalgias

Cluster headache disorders are the most uncommon and severe primary headache syndromes.[9] The estimated point prevalence is less than 0.5% to 1%. Unlike migraine and TTH, cluster headaches occur more frequently in men. Onset commonly occurs prior to age 30.[6] A genetic predisposition is apparent, although affected individuals often provide a history of tobacco use and alcohol abuse.[6] Attacks consist of debilitating, unilateral head pains that occur in series lasting up to months at a time, but which remit over months to years between occurrences. In rare instances, cluster headache can be a chronic disorder without remissions.[4]

ETIOLOGY AND PATHOPHYSIOLOGY OF HEADACHE DISORDERS

Migraine Headache

The mechanism by which headache occurs in migraineurs is not confirmed, and competing pathoetiologic theories exist: tissue pain generated by vascular reactivity and pain induced by neuronal imbalances accompanied by trigeminovascular system overactivity.[10] The vascular hypothesis suggests that intracerebral vasoconstriction leads to neural ischemia, which is followed by reflex extracranial vasodilation and pain. Recent neuroimaging evidence and the effectiveness of medications with no vascular properties do not support this

Patient Encounter, Part 1

A 28-year-old woman complains of a "terrible headache that won't go away." She describes the pain as "on one side and throbbing." The pain began yesterday morning and caused her to have to leave work. She reports a history of similar headaches since the age of 16, but none lasted this long. In the past, her headaches were relieved with the use of over-the-counter (OTC) nonsteroidal anti-inflammatory drugs. She often has to take them multiple times per week.

What type of headache is the patient most likely experiencing?

What characteristics of the headache support this diagnosis?

What are possible causes or triggers of headache in this patient?

What additional information is needed to formulate a treatment plan?

theory, and vascular changes alone are no longer accepted as the primary cause of migraine distress.[6] A neuronal etiology has emerged as the leading mechanism for the development of migraine.[11] Depressed neuronal electrical activity spreads across the brain, producing transitory neural dysfunction.[12] ❸ *Headache pain is likely due to compensatory overactivity in the trigeminovascular system of the brain.* Activation of trigeminal sensory nerves leads to the release of vasoactive peptides (e.g., calcitonin gene-related peptide [CGRP], neurokinin A, substance P) that can produce a sterile inflammatory response around vascular structures in the meninges of the brain, which provokes a sensation of pain.[11] Continued sensitization of CNS sensory neurons can potentiate and intensify headache pain as an attack progresses.[12] Bioamine pathways projecting from the brain stem regulate activity within the trigeminovascular system. Thus, the pathogenesis of migraine may be due to an imbalance in the modulation of nociception and blood vessel tone by serotonergic and noradrenergic neurons.[13]

Tension-Type Headache

The pathophysiologic mechanisms of TTH are not clearly understood. The pain is thought to originate in the myofascial tissues of the head, but central brain processing is believed to be an important modulator of pain perception.[14] Chronic TTH syndromes may evolve from recurrent episodic headaches as central nociception is sensitized.[15]

Cluster Headache and Other Trigeminal Autonomic Cephalalgias

Cluster headache is one of a group of disorders referred to as trigeminal autonomic cephalalgias.[16] The autonomic dysfunction is characterized by sympathetic underactivity and parasympathetic activation. Similar to migraine, the

Patient Encounter, Part 2: Medical History, Physical Examination, and Diagnostic Tests

PMH: Asthma, mild persistent; gastroesophageal reflux disease (GERD); generalized anxiety disorder

FH: Father living, age 58 years; hypertension, diabetes mellitus, dyslipidemia; mother living, age 57 years; chronic daily "sick" headaches; no siblings; paternal grandparents, died at ages 58 and 65 years, both of ischemic stroke; maternal grandparents, living, ages 73 and 84 years; hypertension, osteoarthritis

SH: Married; employed as an account officer in a local bank; no tobacco use, "social" alcohol intake (1–2 glasses of wine on weekends), drinks three to four caffeinated beverages per day

Meds: Advair 250/50 mg one inhalation twice daily; albuterol (salbutamol) two inhalations by MDI when necessary for bronchospasm; esomeprazole 20 mg orally daily; desvenlafaxine 50 mg orally daily; combination ethinyl estradiol/norgestimate oral contraceptive; naproxen sodium 220 mg, two tablets orally twice daily as needed headache

Review of Systems: Headache, severe in intensity; sensitivity to light; no chest pain or palpitations; no shortness of breath or wheezing; nauseated, anorectic; dizzy, difficulty concentrating

PE:

VS: BP 138/82, P 88, RR 16, T 37.0°C (98.6°F), oral

HEENT: No papilledema, no neck stiffness

CV: RRR, normal S1, S2, no MRG

Chest: CTA

Abd: Benign, bowel sounds positive

Neuro: Nonfocal

Labs: CBC and chemistry panel within normal limit

What is your assessment of this patient's condition?

What medical comorbidities or drug therapies may be contributing to her distress?

Identify treatment goals for this patient.

What nonpharmacologic options are needed at present, and what options are appropriate in the long-term for this patient?

What pharmacologic therapy would you recommend for this patient in the acute setting?

Does this patient require long-term pharmacologic prophylaxis against recurrent headaches?

---

pain of a cluster headache is believed to be the result of vasoactive peptide release and neurogenic inflammation. The exact cause of trigeminal activation is not clear.[9] One hypothesis is that hypothalamic dysfunction, occasioned by diurnal or seasonal changes in neurohumoral balance, are responsible for headache periodicity.[6] Serotonin affects neuronal activity in the hypothalamus and trigeminal system and may play a role in the pathophysiology of cluster headache. The precipitation of cluster headache by high-altitude exposure also implicates hypoxemia in the pathogenesis of trigeminal autonomic cephalalgias.[17]

CLINICAL PRESENTATION OF HEADACHES

Migraine Headache

Migraine presents as a recurrent headache that is severe enough to interfere with daily functioning. ❹ *Migraine headaches are classified as migraine with aura and migraine without aura.*[6] The correlating terms of "classic" and "common" migraine are no longer employed. Aura is defined as a transient focal neurologic symptom that can be positive or negative, which can occur prior to or during an attack.[18] Examples of positive symptoms include the visual perception of flickering lights, spots, or wavy lines, whereas a partial loss of vision, a scotoma, is considered a negative finding characteristic of migraine aura. The International

Classification of Headache Disorders (ICHD) outlines diagnostic criteria that differentiate migraine without and with aura.[6] The pain of a migraine headache is typically described as moderate to severe, throbbing, unilateral and retro-orbital in location. The pain is accompanied by nausea, sensitivity to light and sound, and difficulty in concentrating.[19] Untreated migraines can last from 4 to 72 hours. Migraines occurring 15 days per month or more for 3 months or longer, without the overuse of analgesic medications, are classified as chronic migraines.[6] Severe and debilitating migraine pain lasting greater than 72 hours is termed status migrainosus.[19] Even in the absence of neurologic focality, brain imaging is mandated in patients with frequent, severe, and prolonged attacks or attacks, which are atypical for a migraineur's stereotyped presentation.[20]

Tension-Type Headache

TTH pain differs from migraine pain in that it is usually reported to be mild-to-moderate, nonpulsating, and bilateral.[6] The pain is described by sufferers as a band-like tightness or pressure around the head. No transient neurologic deficits are noted, and systemic symptoms are rare.[4] TTHs infrequently disrupt normal activity. Muscle palpation in the frontotemporal and parietooccipital may identify localized tender points.[4] Neuroimaging and laboratory testing are unrevealing, and such tests are

Clinical Presentation and Diagnosis of Migraine Without Aura

Patients experiencing "migraine without aura" display the following headache symptoms and characteristics:

Two or more of the following are present:

1. Pain interrupts or worsens with physical activity
2. Unilateral pain
3. Pulsating pain
4. Moderate to severe pain intensity

Two or more of the following are present during headache:

1. Nausea
2. Vomiting

3. Photophobia
4. Phonophobia
5. Osmophobia

Duration: 4 to 72 hours (treated or not treated)

Criteria for diagnosis: five or more attacks fulfilling above criteria are necessary for diagnosis

Laboratory assessments that may be helpful in excluding medical comorbidities: CBC, chemistry panel, thyroid function tests, erythrocyte sedimentation rate (ESR)

Clinical Presentation and Diagnosis of Migraine With Aura

Patients experiencing "migraine with aura" may display the following headache symptoms and characteristics:

One or more of the following present with no motor weakness:

1. Visual symptoms (positive and/or negative; reversible)
2. Sensory symptoms (positive and/or negative; reversible)
3. Dysphasic speech (reversible)
4. Moderate or severe pain intensity

Two or more of the following:

1. Homonymous visual symptoms and/or unilateral sensory symptoms
2. One aura symptom develops at least 5 minutes prior and/or a second aura symptom develops in 5 minutes or more after headache
3. Duration of each symptom 4 to 60 minutes

Criteria for diagnosis: two or more attacks fulfilling above criteria are necessary for diagnosis

unnecessary if the presentation and clinical history is classic for TTHs.

Cluster Headache

Pain associated with cluster headache differs from migraine and TTH in that it is severe, intermittent, and short in duration.[6] Headaches typically occur at night, but attacks may occur multiple times per day.[9] The pain is usually unilateral, but, unlike migraine, it is not described as pulsatile.[6] Aura is not a feature, and pain intensity peaks early after onset and may persist for hours.[6] The headache is described as explosive and excruciating. A constellation of features, ascribed to parasympathetic overactivity, can be seen, such as ipsilateral conjunctival injection, lacrimation, rhinorrhea, and sweating.[9] Unlike the migraineurs, cluster headache disorder patients tend to become excited and restless during attacks, rather than seeking quiet and solitude.[16]

TREATMENT OF HEADACHE DISORDERS
Desired Outcomes

5 *The primary short-term treatment goal of migraine is to achieve rapid pain relief allowing the patient to resume normal*

activities.[21] **6** *The long-term goal of therapy is to prevent headache recurrences and to diminish headache severity. Similarly, the goal of TTH is to lessen headache pain, while the long-term goal is to avoid analgesic dependence.*[22] *The short-term goal in cluster headache therapy is to achieve rapid pain relief.* Prophylactic therapy may be necessary to obtain the intermediate-term outcome of reducing the frequency and severity of headaches within a periodic cluster series, as well as to achieve the long-term goal of delaying or eliminating recurrent periods.[23]

General Approach to Treatment

The most important goal of acute headache management is pain relief. First-line pharmacologic agents include nonsteroidal and opiate analgesics, and serotonin-receptor agonists (triptans).[24] Despite the availability of targeted prescription therapies, most headache patients rely on OTC products for pain relief and so are not treated adequately.[25] **7** *Pharmacologic treatment of acute headache should be started early to abort the intensification of pain and to improve response to therapy.* The long-term management of headache syndromes focuses on lifestyle modification and other nonpharmacologic therapeutic options; if the headaches are severe and frequent, then prophylactic

Clinical Presentation and Diagnosis of TTH

Patients experiencing TTH may display the following headache symptoms and characteristics:

Two or more of the following present:

1. Bilateral pain

2. Nonpulsating pain

3. Mild or moderate pain intensity

Both of the following:

1. No nausea or vomiting (anorexia possible)

2. Either photophobia or phonophobia (not both)

Duration: 30 minutes to 7 days

Criteria for diagnosis: 10 or more attacks fulfilling above criteria occurring on average less than 1 day per month are necessary for diagnosis

Clinical Presentation and Diagnosis of Cluster Headache

Patients experiencing "cluster headache" may display the following headache symptoms and characteristics:

1. Unilateral pain

2. Orbital, supraorbital, or temporal pain

3. Sharp and stabbing pain

One or more of the following present:

1. Conjunctival injection and/or lacrimation

2. Nasal congestion and/or rhinorrhea

3. Eyelid edema

Duration of pain: 2 seconds to 10 minutes

Frequency of attacks: One or more per day more than half of the time

Criteria for diagnosis: 20 or more attacks fulfilling above criteria are necessary for diagnosis

---

pharmacologic therapy is needed.[26] Several clinical markers, so-called "red flags," have been identified that warrant urgent physician referral and further diagnostic evaluation (Table 34–1).

Nonpharmacologic Therapy

Comprehensive patient education is key to the successful management of headache disorders. Recording headache frequency, duration, and severity in a "headache diary" provides beneficial information for the patient regarding headache precipitants and useful insights for the clinician selecting appropriate management strategies.[27] To prevent future occurrences, exposure to headache triggers (Table 34–2) should be limited. In the acute setting, environmental control can lessen the severity of a migraine attack, so patients may benefit from resting in a dark, quiet area.[28] Behavioral interventions, such as biofeedback therapy, relaxation training, and cognitive-behavioral training, are effective and can be recommended for headache prevention.[17] TTHs may also be managed through stress management training.[17] Acupuncture has yielded inconsistent benefits in clinical trials.[22] Cluster headache patients should be advised to moderate alcohol use and curtail tobacco abuse.[23] Emotional distress may compound headache pain through the outward displacement of inner conflicts: somatization. Psychological interventions are urged in such instances, and should be considered in all headache sufferers resistant to standard medication treatments.[29] All such nonprescription therapies may be useful in augmenting pharmacologic response.

Table 34–1

Headache Red Flags Indicating Need for Urgent Medical Evaluation

New onset sudden and/or severe pain
Onset after 40 years of age
Stereotyped pattern worsens
Systemic signs (e.g., fever, weight loss, and accelerated hypertension)
Focal neurologic symptoms (i.e., other than typical visual or sensory aura)
Papilledema
Cough, exertion, or valsalva-triggered headache
Pregnancy or postpartum state
Patients with cancer, HIV, and other infectious and immunodeficiency disorders
Seizures

Pharmacologic Therapy

▶ Migraine

Analgesics, such as nonsteroidal anti-inflammatory drugs (NSAIDs) and acetaminophen, without or with an opioid, are the initial pharmacologic option for the acute management of migraine headache. If these analgesics prove to be ineffective, then migraine-specific medications, such as triptans, are administered.[30] Early, abortive treatment should be the rule. If the orally administered route is selected for medication administration, then larger doses

Table 34–2
Migraine Triggers

Behavioral:
Fatigue
Menstruation or menopause
Sleep excess or deficit
Stress
Vigorous physical activity

Environmental:
Flickering lights
High altitude
Loud noises
Strong smells
Tobacco smoke
Weather changes

Food:
Alcohol
Caffeine intake or withdrawal
Chocolate
Citrus fruits, bananas, figs, raisins
Dairy products
Fermented or pickled products

Food containing:
Monosodium glutamate (MSG): Asian food, seasoned salt
Nitrites: processed meats
Saccharin/aspartame: diet soda or diet food
Sulfites: shrimp
Tyramine: cheese, wine, organ meats
Yeast: breads

Medications:
Cimetidine
Estrogen or oral contraceptives
Indomethacin
Nifedipine
Nitrates
Reserpine
Theophylline
Withdrawal due to overuse of analgesics, benzodiazepines, decongestants, or ergotamines

than otherwise required to produce pain relief may need to be provided, due to the enteric stasis and poor drug absorption accompanying migraine attacks.[20] Intranasal, parenteral, and rectal administration can circumvent this complication.

Clinical trial evidence supports many NSAID medications in the acute treatment of migraines with and without aura.[30] The currently marketed cyclooxygenase-2 (COX-2) selective drugs are not clearly supported for migraine use, but are likely acceptable. Acetaminophen alone, or in proprietary combinations with aspirin, opioids, caffeine, or the barbiturate butalbital is also effective.[28] Although deemed to have a benign adverse effect profile on gastric mucosal integrity and renal blood flow, overwhelming clinical experience supports the observation that the overuse of acetaminophen may lead to tolerance or dependence clinically manifested as acute withdrawal headaches.[31] These so-called "rebound" headaches are the result of poor attention to prevention therapies, and thus the chronic use of

daily analgesics.[32] A proprietary fixed-dose combination of the anti-inflammatory analgesic naproxen sodium with oral sumatriptan was recently approved for the acute management of migraine with and without aura in adults.

The triptans are considered specific therapies in that they target the pathophysiology underlying migraine.[33] They abort headache through beneficial effects on neuronal imbalances.[11] Triptans inhibit neurotransmission in the trigeminal complex and activate serotonin 1B/1D pathways in the brainstem, which modulate nociception. They also decrease the release of vasoactive peptides leading to vascular reactivity and to pain.[34] The triptans are a welcome addition to the therapeutic armamentarium in that they are available in intranasal, subcutaneous, and oral dosage forms. The available agents differ in their dosing and pharmacokinetic properties, but all are effective treatments to abort or diminish migraine headache (Table 34–3).[43] Patient responses can be variable. If a patient does not respond to one agent, then another is selected before a patient is prematurely labeled as triptan-unresponsive.[44] The initial severity of headache correlates with symptomatic response, thus administration should be prompt. Relief is usually experienced within 2 to 4 hours. Treatment delay may lead to decreased analgesia through the development of refractory central pain sensitization. Efficacy tends to be dose related, though adverse effects are less so.[45] These medications are well-tolerated; the most common side effects are dizziness, a sensation of warmth, chest fullness, and nausea. Rarely, ischemic vascular events may be precipitated by the vasoconstrictive nature of these drugs.[34] An initial dose under direct practitioner supervision is indicated for patients presumed at cardiovascular risk. Triptans are avoided in patients with migraine associated with neurologic focality, a history of previous stroke, poorly controlled hypertension, or unstable angina. Triptans are relatively contraindicated for routine use in pregnancy.[30] Triptans should not be used with concurrent ergotamine administration.[34]

Ergotamine derivatives produce salutary effects on serotonin receptors similar to triptans. They also impact adrenergic and dopaminergic receptors. Ergotamine tartrate and dihydroergotamine (DHE) are the most commonly employed agents.[20] The latter is not available in an oral dosage form. Analgesic onset is within 4 hours, though additional dosing is required if an acceptable response is not achieved. When dosed parenterally, these drugs are usually provided with an antiemetic, due to their potential to worsen the nausea associated with migraine. Metoclopramide and chlorpromazine are the drugs of choice in such instances. Intranasal DHE can be self-administered to abort an attack.[20] The outpatient use of subcutaneous ergotamines is limited by the lack of a prefilled syringe form. The same cautions associated with triptan use are also applicable to ergot use in patients at risk for vascular events.

The choice of initial therapy for acute migraine attacks is a subject of debate among specialists.[46] Some believe that nonspecific analgesics should be used first-line, while others believe migraine-specific drugs should be the choice for patients with severe pain or a history of significant

Table 34–3

Comparison of Serotonin Receptor Agonists (Triptans)

Medication (Brand Name)	Dosage Forms	Strength (mg)	Usual Dosage (mg)	May Repeat in (hours)	Potential Drug Interactions
Almotriptan (Axert)	Oral tablets	6.25 12.5	6.25–12.5		Ergot derivatives
Eletriptan (Relpax)	Oral tablets	20 40	20–40		Substrate: CYP 3A4, CYP 2D6; ergot derivatives
Frovatriptan (Frova)	Oral tablets	2.5	2.5	2	Substrate: CYP 1A2; ergot derivatives
Naratriptan (Amerge)	Oral tablets	1 2.5	2.5	4	Substrate: CYP (various); ergot derivatives
Rizatriptan (Maxalt and Maxalt MLT)	Oral tablets Disintegrating tablets	5 10	5–10	2	Ergot derivatives; MAO-A inhibitors
Sumatriptan (Imitrex)	Subcutaneous injection Oral tablets	6 25, 50, 100	6 50	1 2	Ergot derivatives; MAO-A Inhibitors
Sumatriptan/naproxen sodium (Treximet)	Nasal spray Oral tablets	5, 20 85/500	5–20 85/500	2 12	
Zolmitriptan (Zomig and Zomig-ZMT)	Oral tablets Disintegrating tablets Nasal spray	2.5, 5 5	2.5 5	2 2	Substrate: CYP 1A2; ergot derivatives; MAO-A inhibitors

CYP, cytochrome P450 enzyme; MAO-A, monoamine oxidase type A inhibitor.

From Refs. 35–42.

disability.[47] A stepped-care approach within attacks from less-to-more specific drugs is usually recommended. Once a history of headache refractory to common analgesics is established, triptans should be utilized as initial therapy. In patients who present to the hospital with intractable pain, intravenous metoclopramide supplemented with DHE may be needed. Oral medications in this setting are not utilized, as nausea and vomiting limit their bioavailability. Migraneurs with frequent and severe attacks are candidates for prophylactic treatment.

▶ Tension-Type Headache

Most individuals who experience episodic TTHs will not seek medical attention.[22] Instead, they will find relief with the use of widely available OTC analgesics. Acetaminophen products and NSAIDs are commonly utilized. An individual patient may benefit from topical analgesics (e.g., ice packs) or physical manipulation (e.g., massage) during an acute attack, but the evidence supporting nonpharmacologic therapies is inconsistent.[6] Relaxation techniques can often reduce headache frequency and severity. When pain is unrelieved, prescription-strength NSAID use is required or the combination of acetaminophen with an opioid analgesic may be necessary. The frequency of use of these more potent analgesics should be limited so as to prevent the development of dependency. Use for more than 2 days per week suggests the need for prophylactic therapy.[48] In those sufferers who do not seek expedient medical attention, but rely instead on the frequent use of unprescribed analgesics, medication-overuse

headache may supervene. This chronic daily-headache syndrome requires physician referral to desensitize patient-initiated analgesic tolerance and dependence.[49]

▶ Cluster Headache

Cluster headache also responds to many of the treatment modalities used in acute migraine; however, initial prophylactic therapy is required to limit the frequency of recurrent headaches within a periodic series. A unique therapy specific to cluster headaches is the administration of high-flow-rate oxygen: 100% at 5 to 10 L/min by nonrebreather face mask for approximately 15 minutes.[50] In case the pain is not aborted, retreatment is indicated. No side effects are seen with short-term oxygen use. If oxygen therapy is not wholly effective, then pharmaceuticals are useful as an adjunctive therapy. Drug therapy is also used when supplemental oxygen is not readily available. The triptan class is safe and effective. Intranasal or subcutaneous sumatriptan has demonstrated efficacy in decreasing cluster headache pain.[51] Oral triptans are also effective, but their delayed onset of action may limit their applicability in acute cluster headache treatment.[52] Cluster headache is rapid in onset and achieves peak intensity quickly, but can be of short duration. Oral agents may have utility in limiting the recurrence of cluster attacks. Intranasal, intramuscular, or IV ergotamine agents are an alternative to triptan use.[6] Repeated dosing may break a cluster series. For those patients in whom triptans and ergotamine derivatives are contraindicated due to ischemic vascular disease, octreotide may be helpful to relieve pain.[53] Octreotide is a somatostatin analogue that has a shorter half-life and may be administered subcutaneously. Unlike the other abortive agents, it has no vasoconstrictive effects. The most prominent treatment emergent adverse effect is gastrointestinal upset. Glucocorticoids, provided intravenously and later tapered orally, are effective when cluster headache attacks are not satisfactorily controlled.[9]

Pharmacologic Therapy for Headache Prophylaxis

❽ *Prophylaxis for headache disorders is indicated if headaches are frequent or severe, if significant disability occurs, or if pain-relieving medications are used two or more times per week.*

▶ Migraine Prophylaxis

Migraine headaches that are severe, frequent, or lead to significant disability will require long-term medication therapy. Prophylactic therapy is also recommended for migraines associated with neurologic focality, as it may prevent permanent sequelae. Although multiple medication classes have garnered FDA labeling for migraine prevention, there is no consensus on the best initial therapy (Table 34–4). The choice of pharmacologic agent is individually tailored to patient tolerability and medical comorbidities.

The β-blockers propranolol and timolol are FDA-approved for migraine prophylaxis, but others in the class are also as effective.[57] Cautious dosage titration is advised for those patients who do not have other indications for β-blocker use. Rizatriptan interacts with propranolol, and thus dosages must be downward titrated, or another triptan should be chosen for abortive therapy.[44] Comorbid reactive airway disease is a relative contraindication to β-blocker prophylaxis, and patients with cardiac conduction disturbances should be closely monitored. Calcium-channel antagonists are often used when patients cannot tolerate β-blockers. They are purported to beneficially impact aura as well as pain. Different calcium-blocker drugs are variably effective, and none carries an FDA indication. Moreover, even in responsive patients, tachyphylaxis may develop. Recently, rennin-angiotensin antagonists have been noted to decrease headache frequency and severity in migraine sufferers.[58] Consensus recommendations for hypertension treatment often advocate multidrug regimens to achieve tight control[59]; combination therapies with the antihypertensive agents noted above are ideal combinations for migraneurs.

Low-dose amitriptyline or other tricyclic antidepressants (TCAs) are also of proven efficacy in migraine prevention.[27] Due to sedation, these medications are commonly administered at night. The use of later generation tricyclic medications (e.g., nortriptyline) or heterocyclic compounds (e.g., trazodone) decreases the dose-limiting adverse effects of TCAs, especially those attributable to their anticholinergic properties (e.g., dry mouth, constipation, and urinary retention). Whether the various selective serotonin reuptake inhibitors (SSRIs) can yield consistent efficacy in the majority

of migraneurs is questionable.[21] Although they affect serotonin balance in the brain, their utility may be derived from their beneficial impact on mood and anxiety, rather than through serotonergic effects on migraine generation. Concurrent TCA and triptan administration may be rarely precipitate the serotonin syndrome, a serious and potentially life-threatening drug–drug interaction, which presents clinically with confusion, GI upset, symptomatic BP changes, and muscle rigidity.[20]

The antiepileptics valproic acid and topiramate are approved for migraine prophylaxis. Gabapentin and lamotrigine are anecdotally reported to be efficacious as well. In patients whose migraine headaches are believed to be related to trigeminal neuralgia, carbamazepine is employed as prevention for both disorders. The precise mechanism of benefit of these agents is unclear, but enhancement

Table 34–4

Medications for Prophylaxis of Migraines

Medication (Brand Name)	Usual Dosage (mg/day)	Main Adverse Effects
Antiepileptics:		
Gabapentin (Neurontin)	1,200–2,400	Paresthesias, dizziness, fatigue, nausea
Lamotrigine (Lamictal)	50–200	
Topiramate[a] (Topamax)	50–200	
Valproic acid (Depakene)	500–1,500	
Divalproex sodium[a] (Depakote)	500–1,500	
β-Blockers:		
Atenolol (Tenormin)	50–200	Fatigue, exercise intolerance
Metoprolol (Lopressor)	50–200	
Nadolol (Corgard)	20–160	
Propranolol[a] (Inderal)	80–240	
Timolol[a] (Blocadren)	20–30	
Calcium-Channel Blockers:		
Amlodipine (Norvasc)	2.5–10	Constipation
Verapamil (Calan)	120–320	
Tricyclic Antidepressants:		
Amitriptyline (Elavil)	10–150	Weight gain, dry mouth, sedation
Nortriptyline (Pamelor)	10–150	
Ergot Alkaloids:		
Ergotamine tartrate (Cafergot)	1	
Methysergide (Sansert)	2–6	
Others:		
Hormones (various)	Varies per agent	
Muscle Relaxants (various)	Varies per agent	
Trazodone (Desyrel)	25–150	

[a]FDA-approved for migraine prophylaxis.[67–69]

From Refs. 54–56.

of γ-aminobutyric acid (GABA) neuroinhibition and modulation of the neuroexcitatory amino acid glutamate is likely.[60] Divalproex sodium doses are gradually titrated to 1,000 mg/day; topiramate is titrated to a maximum of 100 mg twice per day. At these doses, serum drug level monitoring is infrequently needed. These medications are as effective as propranolol at reducing the frequency and severity of migraines and are preferred for prevention in patients intolerant to β-blockers.[61] Topiramate is especially useful in metabolic syndrome, diabetes, and dyslipidemic patients, as it is unlikely to lead to the weight gain often seen with valproic acid use. Patients prescribed topiramate should be advised to stay well hydrated to prevent dysgeusia, disordered taste, and, more seriously, hyperthermia.

Methysergide is an ergotamine derivative that impacts central serotonin balance. Inflammatory fibrosis is a rare, but serious, adverse reaction associated with prolonged use of methysergide. Retroperitoneal fibrosis, pulmonary fibrosis, or fibrosis in cardiac tissue can occur. These conditions may resolve upon drug withdrawal, but cardiac valvular damage can be irreversible. Some experts believe it is the best choice for refractory migraine with frequent attacks, but due to its significant adverse effect profile, it is not marketed in the United States.[62]

▶ Tension-Type Headache Prophylaxis

The prevention of chronic TTHs employs the same pharmacologic strategies as for migraine prophylaxis. TCAs are a mainstay of chronic therapy. The efficacy of serotonergic agonists remains in question. Although there is little need for muscle relaxants (e.g., methocarbamol) in the treatment of acute TTH, they are often provided as a preventive intervention.[6] Combination prophylactic therapies may be needed to wean patients from daily analgesic abuse. Stress reduction techniques may be particularly effective in this setting. The injection of botulinum toxin into cranial muscles has demonstrated prophylactic efficacy for severe TTHs.[49]

▶ Cluster Headache Prophylaxis

The calcium channel blocker verapamil is the mainstay of cluster attack prevention and chronic prophylaxis.[6] Within an attack period, it is dosed at 240 to 360 mg/day. Higher doses may be necessary to stave off recurrent cluster periods. Beneficial effects may be appreciated after 1 week of treatment, but 4 to 6 weeks is usually needed. Adverse effects include smooth muscle relaxation with the subsequent exacerbation of gastroesophageal reflux and the development of constipation. Caution should be exercised in patients with myocardial disease, as verapamil is an inotropic and chronotropic cardiac suppressant. Pharmacokinetic drug–drug interactions must be considered, as verapamil is a potent inhibitor of oxidative metabolism through cytochrome P450 (CYP) enzyme 3A4. Eletriptan is a CYP 3A4 substrate and should not be administered concurrently with verapamil.[44] Lithium is another effective therapy

Patient Encounter, Part 3: Creating a Care Plan

Based on the information presented, create a care plan for acute and chronic management of this patient's headache. Your plan should include:

(a) a statement of the drug-related needs and/or problems,
(b) goals of therapy,
(c) patient-specific detailed therapeutic plan, and (d) plan for follow-up to determine whether the goals have been achieved and adverse effects avoided.

to reduce headache frequency in a cluster series and to limit recurrences.[9] The dose administered should be individualized to achieve a low serum concentration (0.4–0.8 mEq/L [mmol/L]). Dose adjustments in the setting of renal disease or congestive heart failure (CHF) are required.[6] Lithium is contraindicated in patients concurrently prescribed thiazide diuretics and angiotensin-converting enzyme inhibitors (ACEIs) or angiotensin receptor blockers (ARBs). Patient persistence with long-term lithium therapy may be hindered by the emergence of tremor, GI distress, and lethargy. Verapamil and lithium doses can be lowered when used in combination with ergotamine. If possible, bedtime dosing is recommended, given the nocturnal predilection of cluster headache attacks.[16] Methysergide can shorten the course of cluster attacks, but long-term use should be avoided.

SPECIAL POPULATIONS

Migraine Headache in Children and Adolescents

Migraine headaches are common in children and their prevalence increases in the adolescent years.[2,3] The diagnosis and evaluation of headaches is especially difficult in children, given their decreased ability to articulate symptoms. Treatment presents another challenge to the practitioner, because medications used for headache management in adults have not been fully evaluated for efficacy and safety in children. Consensus panel recommendations identify ibuprofen as effective and acetaminophen as probably effective in the acute treatment of headache in patients older than 6 years.[26] Aspirin use is avoided due to the risk of precipitating Reye's syndrome. Antiemetic therapy can be used alone or in combination with analgesics; promethazine is usually prescribed, as it is less prone to cause extrapyramidal reactions than other antiemetics. For adolescents older than 12, triptans are effective and are beneficial for abortive migraine therapy.[26] Medication prophylaxis for migraines in children and adolescents is understudied. The data are conflicting, and no consensus recommendation for the use of preventive drug therapy exists.[26] Nonpharmacologic interventions and trigger identification and avoidance are advised.

Pregnancy

Headaches are more common in women than in men. Fluctuations in estrogen levels are believed to account for this gender discrepancy.[63] Hence, headaches are common in pregnancy. TTHs predominate; migraine attacks may increase in frequency, but more usually they decrease in frequency during pregnancy.[64] Recommendations for headache care during pregnancy are based on an insufficient evidence base and are largely anecdotal. As headaches are not associated with fetal harm, reflexive pharmacologic therapy should be avoided and drug treatment choices considered carefully. Standard nonpharmacologic therapies are often sufficient. Acetaminophen is safe for the pregnant woman and her fetus.[65] NSAIDs are avoided late in the third trimester to prevent detrimental prostaglandin alterations, leading to premature ductus arteriosus closure. Opioids are second-line agents. They are not to be used chronically, as they can lead to dependence in the mother and to acute withdrawal in the baby after birth. Centrally acting antiemetic agents are safe and may be useful as adjunctive agents. Corticosteroids may be needed for intractable headache relief. Prednisone and methylprednisone are preferred, as they are metabolized in the placenta and do not expose the fetus. In pregnant women with migraine, vasoconstrictive agents such as triptans are relatively contraindicated, even though maternal registry data reveal little teratogenicity.[66] Ergot compounds are strictly avoided, as they may precipitate uterine contractions and consequent ischemia leading to hypoxemia in the fetus. Migraine prophylaxis is considered cautiously, as β-blockers and calcium-channel antagonists may lead to maternal hypotension and diminished placental blood flow or fetal bradycardia. Antiepileptic drug use in this setting has not been sufficiently studied to allow definitive recommendations.

Some headache disorders are specific to the pregnant state. These include postprocedure headache and those associated with pre-eclampsia. The former are the result of dural puncture with cerebrospinal fluid (CSF) leak after spinal anesthesia.[67] Puncture headache generally responds to bed rest in the supine position, though analgesics may be needed

---

Patient Care and Monitoring

❾ *Regimens for headache disorders should be individualized based on headache type, pattern of occurrence, response to therapy, medication tolerability, and comorbid medical conditions.*

1. Assess the patient complaint to yield a detailed description of headache: precipitating factors; presence or absence of prodromal symptoms; location, intensity, and duration of pain; changes in sensory acuity, and; neurologic alterations.

2. Determine if immediate referral for emergency or specialist care is necessary.

3. Identify medication allergies, and obtain a thorough history of nonprescription and prescription drug use and complementary and alternative therapies utilized.

4. Identify the presence of drug–drug interactions that may guide therapeutic decision making in regard to selecting acute and prophylactic headache treatments.

5. Obtain a complete medical and social history, and identify any potential drug–disease interactions or social factors that may influence treatment choices.

6. Obtain a family medical history, focusing on headache or mental health disorders in first degree relatives.

7. Complete a review of systems and physical examination to identify causes or complications of headache.

8. Determine the type of headache disorder and rule out acute complications.

9. Recommend appropriate pharmacologic therapy to abort headache based on type, patient characteristics, current medication profile, and comorbid conditions.

10. Educate the patient on administration, maximum dosage, and anticipated adverse effects of the prescribed medication.

11. Recommend appropriate nonpharmacologic therapy to abort headache and to prevent future headaches.

12. Determine if the patient is a candidate for prophylactic pharmacologic therapy.

13. Recommend appropriate pharmacologic treatment for the prevention of future headaches.

14. Assess response to therapy indicated by the absence of pain and a return to normal activities. Assess response to prophylactic therapy by improvements in headache frequency and severity.

15. Instruct the patient to keep a headache diary to identify potential causes of headaches and responses to therapy.

16. Provide the patient specific information regarding actions to take, if therapy is ineffective or adverse effects develop.

17. Educate the patient on the importance of adherence to their individualized pharmacologic regimen to prevent headache and to diminish pain upon recurrence.

18. Educate the patient on the warning symptoms and signs of headache complications, and when to seek emergency medical attention.

as well. The latter are seen in the third trimester accompanied by the clinical triad of hypertension, edema, and proteinuria. Pre-eclamptic headache is believed to result from alterations in cerebral blood flow.[68] Headaches experienced in pre-eclamptic women herald eclampsia, and urgent delivery is indicated.[69] Antihypertensives are administered to prevent intracranial thrombosis or hemorrhage, and prophylactic anticonvulsants are provided to prevent eclamptic seizures.

Abbreviations Introduced in This Chapter

ACEI	Angiotensin-converting enzyme inhibitor
AMI	Acute myocardial infarction
ARB	Angiotensin receptor blocker
CCU	Coronary care unit
CGRP	Calcitonin gene-related peptide
CHF	Congestive heart failure
COX-2	Cyclooxygenase type 2 inhibitor
CSF	Cerebrospinal fluid
CT	Computed tomography
CTA	Clear to auscultation
CYP	Cytochrome P450 isoenzyme system
DHE	Dihydroergotamine
ESR	Erythrocyte sedimentation rate
GABA	γ-Aminobutyric acid
GERD	Gastroesophageal reflux disease
ICHD	International Classification of Headache Disorders
IHS	International Headache Society
MAO-A	Monoamine oxidase type A
MRG	Murmur, rub, gallop
NSAID	Nonsteroidal anti-inflammatory drug
OTC	Over-the-counter
RR	Respiratory rate
SNRI	Serotonin-norepinephrine reuptake inhibitor
SSRI	Selective serotonin reuptake inhibitors
TCA	Tricyclic antidepressant
TTH	Tension-type headache

 Self-assessment questions and answers are available at *http://www.mhpharmacotherapy.com/pp.html.*

REFERENCES

1. Silberstein SD, Lipton RB, Dalessio DJ. Overview, diagnosis, and classification of headache. In: Silberstein SD, Lipton, RB, Dalessio DJ, eds. Wolff's Headache and Other Head Pain, 7th ed. New York: Oxford University Press, 2001:6–26.
2. Lipton RB, Stewart WF, Diamond S, et al. Prevalence and burden of migraine in the United States: Data from the American Migraine Study II. Headache 2001;41:646–657.
3. Loder E. Menstrual migraine: Timing is everything. Neurology 2004;63:202.
4. Headache Classification Committee of the International Headache Society. The international classification of headache disorders, 2nd ed. Cephalalgia 2004;24(supp 1):1–160.
5. Hu XH, Markson LE, Lipton RB, et al. Burden of migraine in the United States. Arch Intern Med 1999;159:813–818.
6. Silberstein SD, Lipton RB, Goadsby PJ. Headache in Clinical Practice. London: Martin Dunitz, 2002;21–33:69–128.
7. Lipton RB, Bigal ME, Steiner MB, et al. Classification of primary headaches. Neurology 2004;63:427–435.
8. Ruoff G, Urban G. Treatment of primary headache: episodic tension-type headache. In: Standards of Care for Headache Diagnosis and Treatment. Chicago IL: National Headache Foundation, 2004:53–58.
9. Bahra A, May A, Goadsby PJ. Cluster headache: a prospective clinical study with diagnostic implications. Neurology 2002;58:354–361.
10. Goadsby PJ, Lipton RB, Ferrari MD. Migraine—current understanding and treatment. N Engl J Med 2002;346:257–270.
11. Hargreaves RJ, Shepheard SL. Pathophysiology of migraine: New insights. Can J Neurol Sci 1999;26(Suppl 3):S12–S19.
12. Edvinsson L. On migraine pathophysiology. In: Edvinsson OL, ed. Migraine and Headache Pathophysiology. London: Martin Dunitz, 1999:3–15.
13. MacGregor EA, Brandes J, Eikermann A. Migraine prevalence and treatment patterns: The global migraine and zolmitriptan evaluation survey. Headache 2003;43:19–26.
14. Jenson R. Pathophysiological mechanisms of tension-type headache: A review of epidemiological and experimental studies. Cephalalgia 1999;19:602–621.
15. Dodick PW. Chronic daily headache. N Engl J Med 2006;354(2):158–165.
16. Matharu MS, Boees CJ, Goadsby PJ. Management of trigeminal autonomic cephalalgias and hemicrania continua. Drugs 2003;63:1637–1677.
17. King DS, Wofford MR. Headache Disorders. In: DiPiro JT, Talbert RL, Yee GC, et al., eds. Pharmacotherapy: A Pathophysiologic Approach. 7th ed. New York City: McGraw-Hill, 2008:1105–1121.
18. Silberstein SD. Migraine. Lancet 2004;363:381–391.
19. Solomon S. Migraine variants. Curr Pain Headache Rep 2001;5:165–169.
20. Silberstein SD. Practice parameter: Evidence-based guidelines for migraine headache (an evidence-based review). Neurology 2000;55:754–763.
21. Silberstein SD, Goadsby PJ, Lipton RB. Management of migraine: An algorithmic approach. Neurology 2000;55(Suppl 2):S46–S52.
22. Mueller L. Tension-type, the forgotten headache. Postgrad Med 2002;111:25–50.
23. Biondi D, Mendes P. Treatment of primary headache: Cluster headache. In: Standards of Care for Headache Diagnosis and Treatment. Chicago IL: National Headache Foundation, 2004:59–72.
24. Peters M, Abu-Saad HH, Vydelingum V, et al. Migraine and chronic daily headache management: A qualitative study of patients' perceptions. Scand J Caring Sci 2004;18:294–303.
25. Wenzel RG, Schommer JC, Marks TG. Morbidity and medication preferences of individuals with headache presenting to a community pharmacy. Headache 2004;44:90–94.
26. Lewis D, Ashwal S, Hershey A, et al. Practice parameter: Pharmacological treatment of migraine headache in children and adolescents. Report of the American Academy of Neurology Quality Standards Subcommittee and the Practice Committee of the Child Neurology Society. Neurology 2004;63:2215–2224.
27. Silberstein SD, Goadsby PJ. Migraine: Preventive treatment. Cephalalgia 2002;22:491–512.
28. Snow V, Weiss K, Wall EM, Mottur-Pilson C. Pharmacologic management of acute attacks of migraine and prevention of migraine headache. Ann Intern Med 2002;137:840–849.
29. Rollnik JD, Karst M, Piepenbrock S, et al. Gender differences in coping with tension-type headaches. Eur Neurol 2003;50:73–77.
30. del Rio MS, Silberstein SD. How to pick optimal acute treatment for migraine headache. Curr Pain Headache Rep 2001;5:170–178.
31. Lipton RB, Stewart WF, Ryan RE, et al. Efficacy and safety of acetaminophen, aspirin, and caffeine in alleviating migraine headache

pain: Three double-blind, randomized, placebo-controlled trials. Arch Neurol 1998;55:210–217.

32. Relja G, Granato A, Antonello RM, Zorzon M. Headache induced by chronic substance use: Analysis of medication overused and minimum dose required to induce headache. Headache 2004;44:148–153.

33. Goldstein J, Silberstein SD, Saper JR, et al. Acetaminophen, aspirin, and caffeine versus sumatriptan succinate in the early treatment of migraine: Results from the ASSET trial. Headache 2005;45(8):973–982.

34. Ferrari MD. Migraine. Lancet 1998;351:1043–1051.

35. Axert [package insert]. Raritan, NJ: Ortho-McNeil Pharmaceuticals, Inc.; 2005.

36. Relpax [package insert]. New York, NY: Pfizer Inc.; 2003.

37. Frova [package insert]. Chadds Ford, PA: Endo Pharmaceuticals Inc.; 2005.

38. Amerge [package insert]. Research Triangle Park, NC: GlaxoSmithKline; 2003.

39. Maxalt [package insert]. Whitehouse Station, NJ: Merck & Co., Inc.; 2003.

40. Imitrex [package insert]. Research Triangle Park, NC: GlaxoSmithKline; 2005.

41. Zomig [package insert]. Wilmington, DE: AstraZeneca Pharmaceuticals; 2005.

42. Treximet [package insert]. Research Triangle Park, NC: GlaxoSmithKline; 2008.

43. Ferrari MD, Roon KI, Lipton RB, Goadsby PJ. Oral triptans (serotonin 5-HT1B/1D agonists) in acute migraine treatment: A meta-analysis of 53 trials. Lancet 2001;358:1558–1575.

44. Pringsheim T, Gawel M. Triptans: Are they all the same? Curr Pain Headache Rep 2002;6:140–146.

45. Deleu D, Hanssens Y. Current and emerging second-generation triptans in acute migraine therapy: A comparative review. J Clin Pharmacol 2000;40:687–700.

46. Dahlof CGH. Current concepts of migraine and its treatment. Neurology 1999;14:67–77.

47. Pascual J, Cabarrocas X. Within-patient early versus delayed treatment of migraine attacks with almotriptan: The sooner the better. Headache 2002;42:28–31.

48. Lipton RB, Stewart WF, Stone AM, et al. Stratified care vs step care strategies for migraine: The Disability in Strategies of Care (DISC) Study: A randomized trial. JAMA 2000;284:2599–2606.

49. Jenson R, Olesen J. Tension-type headache: An update on mechanisms and treatment. Curr Opin Neurol 2000;13:285–289.

50. Rozen TD. High oxygen flow rates for cluster headache. Neurology 2004;63(3):593.

51. Gobel H, Lindner V, Heinz A, et al. Acute therapy for cluster headache with sumatriptan: Findings of a one-year long-term study. Neurology 1998;51:430–435.

52. Bahra A, Gawel MJ, Hardebo JE, et al. Oral zolmitriptan is effective in the acute treatment of cluster headache. Neurology 2000;54:291–296.

53. Goadsby PJ. New targets in the acute treatment of headache. Curr Opin Neurol 2005;18(3):283–288.

54. Topamax [package insert]. Titusville, NJ: Ortho-McNeil Neurologics, Inc.; 2005.

55. Depakote [package insert]. North Chicago, IL: Abbott Laboratories; 2006.

56. Inderal [package insert]. Philadelphia, PA: Wyeth Pharmaceuticals Inc; 2004.

57. Linde K, Rossnagel K. Propranolol for migraine prophylaxis. Cochrane Database Syst Rev 2004;2:CD003225.

58. Tronvik E, Stovener LJ, Helde G, et al. Prophylactic treatment of migraine with angiotensin II receptor blocker: A randomized, controlled trial. JAMA 2003;289:65–69.

59. Joint National Committee on Prevention, Detection, Evaluation, and Treatment of High Blood Pressure. The Seventh Report of the Joint National Committee on Prevention, Detection, Evaluation, and Treatment of High Blood Pressure: The JNC 7 Report. JAMA 2003;289:2560–2572.

60. Cutrer FM. Antiepileptic drugs: How they work in headache. Headache 2001;41(Suppl):S3–S10.

61. Bigal ME, Krymchantowski AV, Rapoport AM. New developments in migraine prophylaxis. Expert Opin Pharmacother 2003;4:433–443.

62. Silberstein SD. Methysergide. Cephalalgia 1998;18:421–435.

63. Winner P, Rothner AD, Saper J, Nett R. A randomized double-blind, placebo-controlled study of sumatriptan nasal spray in the treatment of acute migraine in adolescents. Pediatrics 2000;106:989.

64. Maggioni F, Alessi C, Maggino T, Zanchin G. Headache during pregnancy. Cephalalgia 1997;17:765.

65. Scharff L, Marcus DA, Turk DC. Headache during pregnancy and in the postpartum: A prospective study. Headache 1997;37:203.

66. Lipton RB, Baggish JS, Stewart WF, et al. Efficacy and safety of acetaminophen in the treatment of migraine: Results of a randomized, double-blind, placebo-controlled, population-based study. Arch Intern Med 2000;160:3486.

67. Olesen C, Steffensen FH, Sorensen HT, et al. Pregnancy outcome following prescription for sumatriptan. Headache 2000;40:20.

68. Evans RW, Armon C, Frohman EM, Goodin DS. Assessment: Prevention of post-lumbar puncture headaches. Report of the Therapeutics and Technology Assessment Subcommittee of the American Academy of Neurology. Neurology 2000;55:909.

69. Belfort MA, Saade GR, Grunewald C, et al. Association of cerebral perfusion pressure with headache in women with pre-eclampsia. Br J Obstet Gynaecol 1999;106:814.

35 Alzheimer's Disease

Megan J. Ehret, Gary M. Levin, and
Toya M. Bowles

LEARNING OBJECTIVES

● **Upon completion of the chapter, the reader will be able to:**

1. Describe the epidemiology of Alzheimer's disease (AD) and its effects on society.

2. Describe the pathophysiology including genetic and environmental factors that may be associated with the disease.

3. Detail the clinical presentation of the typical patient with AD.

4. Describe the clinical course of the disease and typical patient outcomes.

5. Describe how nonpharmacologic therapy is combined with pharmacologic therapy for patients with AD.

6. Recognize and recommend treatment options for disease-specific symptoms as well as behavioral/noncognitive symptoms associated with the disease.

7. Develop an alternative treatment plan for patients with AD.

8. Educate patients and/or caregivers about the expected outcomes for patients with AD, and provide contact information for support/advocacy agencies.

KEY CONCEPTS

❶ Alzheimer's disease (AD) is characterized by progressive cognitive decline including memory loss, disorientation, and impaired judgment and learning.

❷ Pathologic hallmarks of the disease in the brain include *neurofibrillary tangles* and *neuritic plaques (senile plaques)* made up of various proteins, which result in a shortage of the neurotransmitter acetylcholine.

❸ A diagnosis can be made only at autopsy; therefore, the diagnosis is established following an extensive history and physical examination, and by ruling out other potential causes of dementia.

❹ Treatment is focused on delaying disease progression and preservation of functioning as long as possible.

❺ The current gold standard of treatment for cognitive symptoms includes pharmacologic management with a cholinesterase inhibitor and/or an *N*-methyl-D-aspartate (NMDA) receptor antagonist.

❻ Future therapies for AD may be based on disease-modifying therapies.

❼ The general approach to treatment of cognitive symptoms includes both pharmacologic and nonpharmacologic management.

❽ Treatment of behavioral symptoms should begin with nonpharmacologic treatments, but may also include antipsychotic agents and/or antidepressants.

❾ Therapeutic response in AD is genotype-specific depending on the genes associated with pathogenesis and/or genes responsible for drug metabolism.

INTRODUCTION

❶ *Alzheimer's disease (AD) is a nonreversible, progressive dementia manifested by gradual deterioration in cognition and behavioral disturbances.* AD is primarily diagnosed by exclusion of other potential causes for dementias. There is no single symptom unique to AD; therefore, diagnosis relies on a thorough patient history. The exact pathophysiologic mechanism underlying AD is not entirely known, although certain genetic and environmental factors may be associated with the disease. There is currently no cure for AD; however, drug treatment can slow symptom progression over time.

Family members of AD patients are profoundly affected by the increased dependence of their loved ones as the disease progresses. Referral to an advocacy organization, such as the Alzheimer's Association, can provide early education and social support of both the patient and family, which is also important treatment. The Alzheimer's Association has developed a checklist of common symptoms (Table 35–1).[1]

Table 35–1

Ten Warning Signs of AD

1. Memory loss: more than typical forgetfulness without remembering later
2. Difficulty performing familiar everyday tasks (e.g., preparing a meal and grooming)
3. Problems with language: forgetting simple words or substituting unusual words
4. Disorientation to time and place: may forget where they are and/or how they got there
5. Poor or decreased judgment: dress without regard to weather or falling prey to scam artists
6. Problems with abstract thinking: not just difficulty balancing a checkbook, but forgetting what the numbers represent
7. Misplacing things in unusual places: such as placing an iron in a freezer
8. Changes in mood or behavior: rapid mood swings with no apparent reason
9. Changes in personality: extreme confusion, suspicion, or fearfulness
10. Loss of initiative: passivity and loss of interest in usual activities

From Ref. 1.

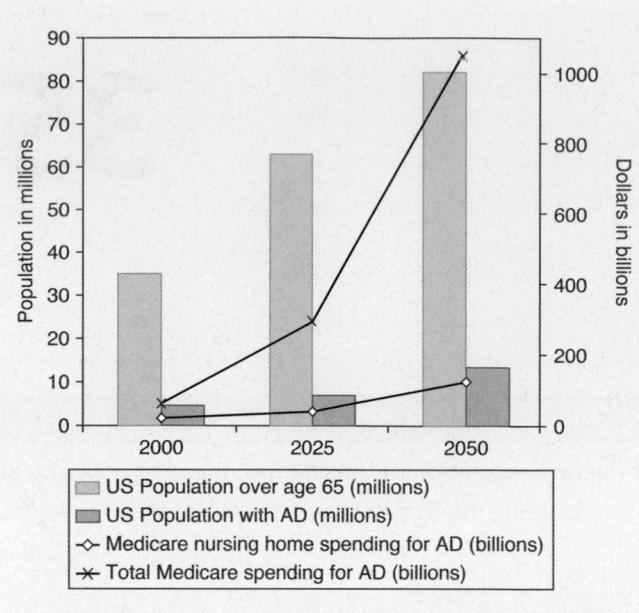

FIGURE 35–1. Projected increases in the population of patients with AD, Medicare nursing home spending, and total Medicare spending. (AD, Alzheimer's disease.) (From Refs. 4 and 5.)

EPIDEMIOLOGY AND ETIOLOGY

AD is the most common type of dementia, affecting approximately 4.5 million Americans in the year 2000.[2] Various classifications of dementia include dementia of the Alzheimer's type, vascular dementia, and dementia due to HIV disease, head trauma, Parkinson's disease, Huntington's disease, Pick's disease, or Creutzfeldt-Jakob disease.[3] This chapter will address only dementia of the Alzheimer's type.

The prevalence of AD increases with age, and it is most prevalent in persons aged 65 years and older. In the year 2000, it was estimated that there were 4.5 million people with AD in the United States. Of those affected, 7% were 65 to 74 years of age, 53% were between 75 and 84 years of age, and 40% were persons over 85 years of age.[2] It is projected that by the year 2050, there will be a threefold increase in prevalence yielding potentially 13.4 million AD patients due to a population increase in persons over 65 years of age. It is projected that three out of five individuals greater than or equal to 85 years of age will have AD. Additionally, the cost to society due to rising Medicare spending for AD is projected to increase from $62 billion in 2000 to over $1 trillion in 2050. Furthermore, the costs associated with nursing home care alone are projected to increase from $19 billion in 2000 to $118 billion in 2050 (Fig. 35–1).[4,5] The severity of AD also correlates with increasing age and is classified as mild, moderate, or severe. Other risk factors associated with AD besides age include family history, female gender, and vascular risk factors such as diabetes, hypertension, heart disease, and current smoking.[6,7] However, it is unknown how other factors such

as environment contribute and interact with the genetic predisposition for AD.

The mean survival time of persons with AD is reported to be approximately 6 years from the onset of symptoms until death. However, age at diagnosis, severity of AD, and other medical conditions affect survival time.[8] Although AD does not directly cause death, it is associated with an increase in various risk factors which often contribute to death such as senility, sepsis, stroke, pneumonia, dehydration, and decubitus ulcers.

The exact etiology of AD is unknown; however, it has been suggested that genetic factors may contribute to errors in protein synthesis resulting in the formation of abnormal proteins involved in the pathogenesis of AD.[9] Early onset, which is defined as AD prior to age 60, accounts for approximately 1% of all AD. This type is usually familial and follows an autosomal dominant pattern in approximately 50% of cases of early-onset AD. Mutations in three genes, presenilin 1 on chromosome 14, amyloid precursor protein (APP) on chromosome 21, and presenilin 2 on chromosome 1, lead to an increase in the accumulation of amyloid beta (Aβ) in the brain, resulting in oxidative stress, neuronal destruction, and the clinical syndrome of AD.[10,11]

The genetic basis for the more common late-onset AD appears more complex. Genetic susceptibility is more sporadic and it may be more dependent on environmental factors.[9] The apolipoprotein E (apo E) gene on chromosome 19 has been identified as a strong risk factor for late-onset AD. There are three variants of apo E; however, carriers of two or more of the apo E4 allele have an earlier onset of AD (approximately 6 years earlier) compared with noncarriers.[9] Only 50% of AD patients have the apo E4 allele, thus indicating it is only a susceptibility marker.

PATHOPHYSIOLOGY

❷ *The pathologic hallmarks of the disease in the brain include neurofibrillary tangles and neuritic plaques made up of various proteins, which result in a shortage of the neurotransmitter acetylcholine (Ach).* These are primarily located in brain regions involved in learning, memory, and emotional behaviors such as the cerebral cortex, hippocampus, basal forebrain, and amygdala.[12]

Tangles

Neurofibrillary tangles are intracellular and consist of abnormally phosphorylated τ protein, which is involved in microtubule assembly. Tangles interfere with neuronal function, resulting in cell damage, and their presence has been correlated with the severity of dementia.[13] Unfortunately, these tangles are insoluble even after the cell dies, and they cannot be removed once established. The neurons that provide most of the cholinergic innervation to the cortex are most prominently affected.[14] Therefore, prevention is the key to targeted therapy of these tangles.

Plaques

Neuritic or senile plaques are extracellular protein deposits of fibrils and amorphous aggregates of β-amyloid protein.[12] This formed protein is central to the pathogenesis of AD. The β-amyloid protein is present in a nontoxic, soluble form in human brains. In AD, conformational changes occur that render it insoluble and cause it to deposit into amorphous diffuse plaques associated with dystrophic neuritis.[15] Over time, these deposits become compacted into plaques and the β-amyloid protein becomes fibrillar and neurotoxic. Inflammation occurs secondary to clusters of astrocytes and microglia surrounding these plaques.

Acetylcholine

The neurotransmitter Ach is responsible for transmitting messages between certain nerve cells in the brain. In AD, the plaques and tangles damage these pathways, leading to a shortage of Ach, resulting in learning and memory impairment.[16] The loss of Ach activity correlates with the severity of AD. The basis of pharmacologic treatment of AD has been to improve cholinergic neurotransmission in the brain. Acetylcholinesterase is the enzyme that degrades Ach in the synaptic cleft. Blocking this enzyme leads to an increased level of Ach with a goal of stabilizing neurotransmission.[17]

Glutamate

Glutamate is the primary excitatory neurotransmitter in the CNS involved in memory, learning, and neuronal plasticity. It acts by providing information from one brain area to another and affects cognition through facilitation of connections with cholinergic neurons in the cerebral cortex and basal forebrain.[18] In AD, one type of glutamate receptor, N-methyl-D-aspartate (NMDA), is less prevalent than normal. There also appears to be overactivation of unregulated glutamate signaling. This results in a rise in calcium ions that induces secondary cascades, which lead to neuronal death and an increased production of APP.[17] The increased production of APP is associated with higher rates of plaque development and hyperphosphorylation of τ protein.[19] Memantine is a noncompetitive NMDA antagonist that targets this pathophysiologic mechanism.[20]

Cholesterol

Increased cholesterol concentrations have been associated with AD. The cholesterol increases β-amyloid protein synthesis which can lead to plaque formation.[17] Also, the apo E4 allele is thought to be involved in cholesterol metabolism and is associated with higher cholesterol levels.[17]

Estrogen

Estrogen appears to have properties that protect against memory loss associated with normal aging. It has been suggested that estrogen may block β-amyloid protein production and even trigger nerve growth in cholinergic nerve terminals.[21,22] Estrogen is also an antioxidant and helps prevent oxidative cell damage.[21] It is important to note, however, that the Women's Health Initiative Memory Study reported that hormone replacement with either estrogen alone or estrogen plus medroxyprogesterone resulted in negative effects on memory.[23]

CLINICAL PRESENTATION AND DIAGNOSIS

❸ *Diagnosing AD relies on a thorough medical and psychological history, mental status testing, and laboratory data to exclude other possible causes of dementia. There are no biological markers other than those pathophysiologic changes found at autopsy that can confirm AD.*

The American Academy of Neurology has adopted practice guidelines for the diagnosis and management of AD.[24] The diagnostic criteria are based on the *Diagnostic and Statistical Manual of Mental Disorders*, Fourth Edition, Text Revision (*DSM-IV-TR*) (Table 35–2)[25] or the National Institute of Neurological and Communicative Diseases and Stroke/ Alzheimer's Disease and Related Disorders Association (NINCDS-ADRDA).

AD is a progressive disease that, over time, affects multiple areas of cognition. The symptoms of AD can be divided into cognitive symptoms, noncognitive symptoms, and functional symptoms for assessment and treatment purposes. Table 35–3 describes the stages of cognitive decline.[26,27]

Clinical Presentation and Diagnosis of AD

General

The diagnosis of AD relies on thorough mental status testing and neuropsychological tests, medical and psychiatric history, neurologic examination, interview of caregivers and family members, and laboratory and imaging data to support the diagnosis and exclude other causes.

Signs and Symptoms

- Cognitive: memory loss, problems with language, disorientation to time and place, poor or decreased judgment, problems with learning and abstract thinking, misplacing things
- Noncognitive: changes in mood or behavior, changes in personality, or loss of initiative
- Functional: difficulty performing familiar tasks

Laboratory Tests

- MRI or CT is used to measure changes in brain size and volume and rule out stroke, brain tumor, or cerebral edema.
- Tests to exclude possible causes of dementia include a depression screen, vitamin B_{12} deficiency, thyroid function tests (thyroid-stimulating hormone and free triiodothyronine and thyroxine), CBC, and chemistry panel.[21]
- Other diagnostic tests to consider for differential diagnosis: erythrocyte sedimentation rate, urinalysis, toxicology, chest x-ray, heavy metal screen, HIV testing, CSF examination, electroencephalography, and neuropsychological tests such as the Folstein Mini Mental Status Examination.

Table 35–2

Diagnostic Criteria for AD Based on *DSM-IV-TR*

Dementia of the Alzheimer's type
A. The development of multiple cognitive deficits manifested by both
 1. Memory impairment (impaired ability to learn new information or to recall previously learned information)
 2. One or more of the following cognitive disturbances:
  (a) Aphasia (language disturbance)
  (b) Apraxia (impaired ability to carry out motor activities despite intact motor function)
  (c) Agnosia (failure to recognize or identify objects despite intact sensory function)
  (d) Disturbance in executive funning (e.g., planning, organizing, sequencing, abstracting)
B. The cognitive deficits in criteria A1 and A2 each cause significant impairment in social or occupational functioning and represent a significant decline from a previous level of functioning
C. The course is characterized by gradual onset and continuing cognitive decline
D. The cognitive deficits in criteria A1 and A2 are not due to any of the following:
 1. Other CNS conditions that cause progressive deficits in memory and cognition
 2. Systemic conditions that are known to cause dementia
 3. Substance-induced conditions
E. The deficits do not occur exclusively during the course of delirium
F. The disturbance is not better accounted for by another **Axis I** disorder

From Ref. 3.

TREATMENT

Desired and Expected Outcomes

Although there are currently five agents approved for the treatment of AD, none of these agents are curative or are known to directly reverse the disease process.

❹ Consequently, the primary desired outcome of treatment of AD is to symptomatically treat the cognitive symptoms of the patient and preserve the patient's functioning for as long as possible. Secondary goals include treating psychiatric and behavioral symptoms that may occur during the course of the disease.

General Approach to Treatment

❺ The current gold standard of treatment for cognitive symptoms includes pharmacologic management with a cholinesterase (ChE) inhibitor and/or an NMDA antagonist. The following are four ChE inhibitors: tacrine, donepezil, rivastigmine, and galantamine. The use of tacrine is limited due to its propensity for hepatotoxicity, difficult titration schedule, four times daily dosing, poor bioavailability, and increased adverse events of nausea, diarrhea, and urinary incontinence. There is only one NMDA antagonist, memantine. Psychiatric and behavioral symptoms that occur during the course of the disease should be treated as they occur.

Essential elements in the treatment of AD include education, communication, and planning with the family/caregiver of the patient. Treatment options, legal and financial decisions, and course of the illness need to be discussed with the patient and family members. In this regard, the clinician's emphasis should be on helping to maintain a therapeutic living environment while minimizing the burden of care resulting from the disease.

Nonpharmacologic Treatment

Treatment of AD involves both pharmacologic and nonpharmacologic methods. Upon the initial diagnosis, the patient and family should be counseled on the course of the illness, prognosis, available treatments, legal decisions,

Table 35–3		
Stages of Cognitive Decline		
Stage	**Clinical Attribute**	**Pathology and Clinical Picture**
Stage 1	No cognitive impairment	No memory problems and no impairment is evident to a health care professional
Stage 2	Very mild decline	Lapses of memory; forgetting familiar names or locations of personal objects (e.g., keys or glasses); problems not evident to friends, family, coworkers, or health care professionals
Stage 3	Mild cognitive decline	Friends, family, and coworkers begin to notice deficiencies; problems with names or words become evident; performance issues become evident; retention of reading material declines; losing valuable objects; decline in planning and organizational abilities
Stage 4	Moderate cognitive decline (mild or early-stage AD)	Medical interview detects clear-cut deficiencies; decreased knowledge of current events; impaired ability to perform difficult mathematical problems (e.g., serial 7s); decreased ability to perform complex tasks (managing finances); decreased recall of personal history; individuals may become withdrawn and subdued
Stage 5	Moderately severe cognitive decline (moderate AD)	Major gaps in memory appear and assistance with day-to-day activities is necessary; inability to recall details such as current address and telephone number may begin; difficulty with orientation to place and time; less challenging mathematical problems may become difficult (e.g., serial 4s or 2s); can still recall their own name and those of spouse and children
Stage 6	Severe cognitive decline (moderately severe AD)	Significant personality and behavioral symptoms may emerge (delusions, suspiciousness, hallucinations, compulsions) and extensive help with ADLs becomes necessary (e.g., toileting); loss of awareness of recent experiences and surroundings; may still recall their own name, but recall of other personal history is decreasing; need help in getting dressed properly; disruptions of sleep/wake cycle occur; increase in urinary and fecal incontinence; wandering and getting lost become common
Stage 7	Very severe cognitive decline (severe AD)	Final stage of illness; loss of ability to respond to surroundings; inability to speak and control movement; help is required for eating, walking, and toileting; movements become abnormal and rigid, and swallowing is impaired

AD, Alzheimer's disease; ADLs, activities of daily living.

From Ref. 27.

Patient Encounter, Part 1

A woman arrives at the clinic with her 80-year-old mother, LB, complaining that her mother is becoming increasingly forgetful and confused with old age. The woman complains that her mother sometimes takes her diabetes and hypertension medications at a frequency greater than that prescribed. This has become more frequent in the last 6 months and the mother has been getting very agitated when her daughter confronts her. The woman asks for a pill organizer and if any of the over-the-counter drugs claiming to help with memory would help her mother.

What information is suggestive of AD?

Does the mother have any risk factors for AD?

How would you approach and address the daughter's question?

---

and quality-of-life issues. The life of a patient with AD must become progressively more simple and structured as the disease progresses, and the caregiver must learn to keep requests and demands on the patient simple. The family of the patient will need to be prepared to face changes in life that will occur as the disease becomes worse. Basic principles in the treatment of patients with AD are shown in Table 35–4.

Table 35–4
Basic Principles in the Treatment of Patients With AD
• Using a gentle, calm approach to the patient
• Giving reassurance when needed
• Empathizing with the patient's concerns
• Using distraction and redirection
• Maintaining daily routines
• Providing a safe environment
• Providing daytime activities
• Avoiding overstimulation
• Using familiar decorative items in the living area
• Bringing abrupt declines in function and the appearance of new symptoms to professional attention

Conventional Pharmacologic Treatment for Cognitive Symptoms

► *ChE Inhibitors (Donepezil, Rivastigmine, and Galantamine)*

⑥ *The ChE inhibitors all have the indication for the treatment of dementia of the Alzheimer's type.* Guidelines for the treatment of AD recommend the use of ChE inhibitors as a valuable treatment for AD and the use of memantine for moderate-to-severe AD.[28–30] None of the ChE inhibitors have been compared in head-to-head studies, so the decision to use one over another is based on differences in mechanisms of action, adverse reactions, and titration schedules.

Treatment should begin as early as possible in patients with a diagnosis of AD.[31] Figure 35–2 provides a recommended treatment algorithm for AD.[32] Patients should be switched to another ChE inhibitor from their initial ChE inhibitor if they show an initial lack of efficacy, initially respond to treatment but lose clinical benefit, or experience safety/tolerability issues. This switch should not be attempted until the patient has been on a maximally tolerated dose for a period of 3 to 6 months. The switch should also be based on realistic expectations of the patient and/or caregiver.[33] ChE inhibitor therapy should be discontinued in patients who experience poor tolerance or adherence, who show a lack of clinical improvement after 3 to 6 months at optimal dosing, who continue to deteriorate at the pretreatment rate, or who demonstrate dramatic clinical deterioration following initiation of treatment.[34]

▶ Donepezil

❼ *Donepezil is a piperidine ChE inhibitor, which reversibly and noncompetitively inhibits centrally active acetylcholinesterase.*[35]

Donepezil is approved for the treatment of dementia of the Alzheimer's type at a dose of 5 mg/day. This dose should be increased to 10 mg/day if needed after 4 to 6 weeks. Efficacy has been demonstrated in patients with mild-to-moderate and -severe AD. Table 35–5 describes the dosing strategies for all of the approved agents for AD.[35–39]

Adverse reactions with donepezil include nausea, vomiting, and diarrhea. Table 35–6 compares the major side effects for all of the approved agents for AD.[35–39]

Only a small number of drug interactions have been reported with donepezil. In vitro studies show a low rate of binding of donepezil to cytochrome P450 (CYP)3A4 or 2D6. Whether donepezil has the potential for enzyme induction is not known. Monitoring for possible increased peripheral side effects is advised when adding a CYP2D6 or 3A3/4 inhibitor to donepezil treatment. Also, inducers of CYP2D6 and 3A4 could increase the rate of elimination of donepezil.[35]

▶ Rivastigmine

❽ *Rivastigmine has central activity for both the acetylcholinesterase and butyrylcholinesterase enzymes.*[37] Acetylcholinesterase is found in two forms: globular 4 and globular 1. In postmortem studies, globular 4 is significantly depleted, while globular 1 is still abundant. Thus, blocking metabolism of globular 1 may lead to higher concentrations of Ach. Rivastigmine has higher activity at globular 1 than at globular 4. Theoretically this may be advantageous, as rivastigmine prevents the degradation of Ach via the acetylcholinesterase globular 1 over the course of the disease as compared to the other ChE inhibitors.

The dual inhibition of acetylcholinesterase and butyrylcholinesterase may lead to broader efficacy. As acetylcholinesterase activity decreases with disease progression, the acetylcholinesterase-selective agents may lose their effect, while the dual inhibitors may still be effective due to the

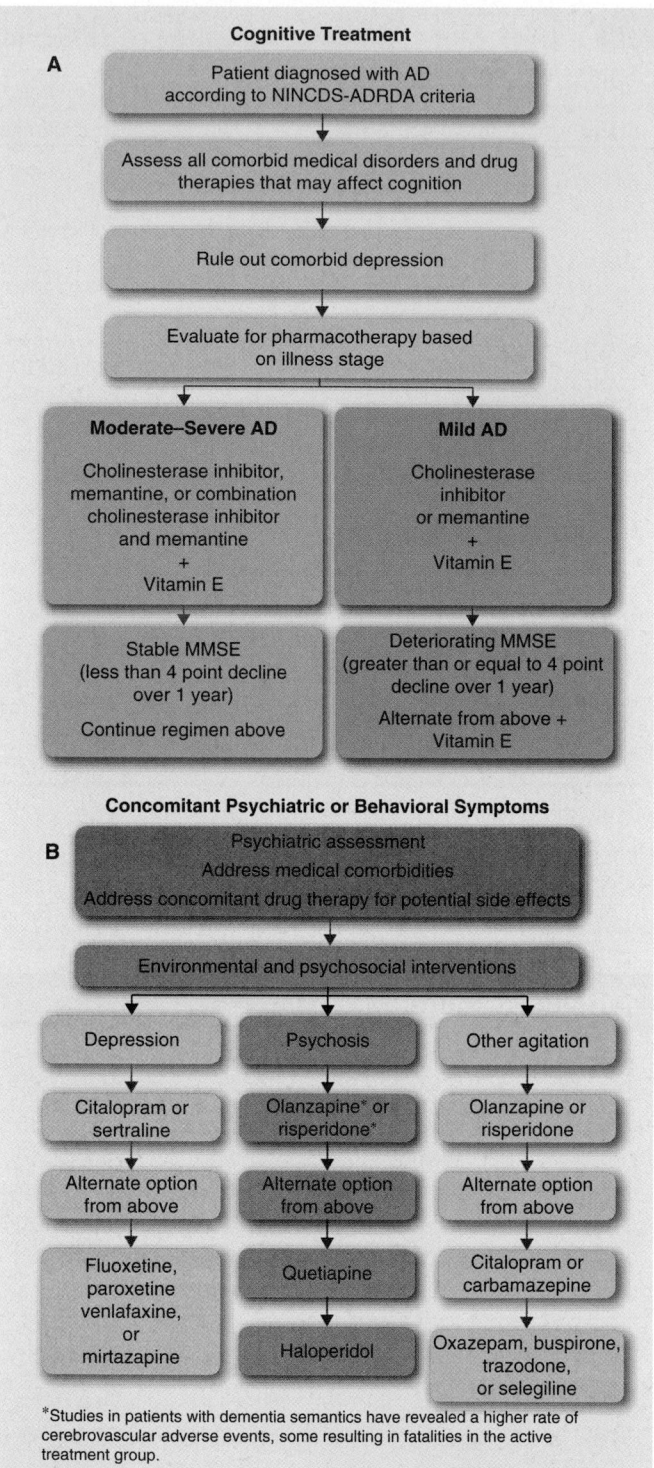

FIGURE 35–2. Treatment algorithm for AD. *A.* Cognitive treatment. *B.* Treatment of psychiatric or behavioral symptoms. (AD, Alzheimer's disease; MMSE, Mini Mental Status Examination; NINCDS-ADRDA, National Institute of Neurological and Communicative Disorders and Stroke-Alzheimer's Disease and Related Disorders Association.) (From Faulkner JD, Bartlett J, Hicks P. Alzheimer's disease. In: DiPiro JT, Talbert RL, Yee GC, et al., eds. Pharmacotherapy: A Pathophysiologic Approach, 6th ed. New York: McGraw-Hill, 2005:1164, with permission.)

Table 35–5

Dosing Strategies for Cognitive Agents

	Tacrine (Cognex)	Donepezil (Aricept)	Rivastigmine (Exelon)	Galantamine (Razadyne)	Memantine (Namenda)
Starting dose	10 mg 4 × daily	5 mg daily	1.5 mg 2 × daily or 4.2 mg/24 hours applied daily (patch)	4 mg 2 × daily or 8 mg daily	5 mg daily
Maintenance dose	20–40 mg 4 × daily	5–10 mg daily	3–6 mg 2 × daily or 9.5 mg/24 hours applied daily (patch)	8–12 mg 2 × daily or 16–24 mg daily	10 mg 2 × daily
Time between dose adjustments	4–6 weeks	4–6 weeks	2 weeks for oral and 4 weeks for patch	4 weeks	1 week
Dosage adjustments for renal or hepatic impairment	Do not administer in hepatic impairment	None	None	Do not exceed 16 mg for moderately impaired hepatic or renal function; do not administer in severe renal or hepatic impairment	Caution should be taken in patients with severe hepatic impairment

From Refs. 35–39.

Table 35–6

Comparative Common Adverse Effects of AD Medications From Clinical Trial Data[a]

Adverse Event	Tacrine (%) (n = 634)	Donepezil (%) (n = 747)	Rivastigmine (%) (n = 1,189)	Galantamine (%) (n = 1,040)	Memantine (%) (n = 940)
Elevated liver function tests	29	NR	NR	NR	NR
Nausea or vomiting	28	NR	NR	NR	NR
Nausea	NR	11	47	24	NR
Vomiting	NR	5	31	13	3
Diarrhea	16	10	19	9	NR
Headache	11	10	17	8	6
Dizziness	12	8	21	9	7
Muscle cramps	9	6	NR	NR	NR
Insomnia	6	9	9	5	NR
Fatigue	4	5	9	5	2
Anorexia	9	4	17	9	NR
Depression	4	3	6	7	NR
Abnormal dreams	NR	3	NR	NR	NR
Weight decrease	3	3	3	7	NR
Abdominal pain	8	NR	13	5	NR
Agitation	7	NR	NR	NR	NR
Rhinitis	8	NR	4	4	NR

NR, not reported.

[a]Caution is urged in making comparisons between drugs based on these data, as different clinical trials often collect adverse event data using different methodologies.

From Refs. 35–39.

added inhibition of butyrylcholinesterase. However, this has not been demonstrated clinically.

Rivastigmine is approved for the treatment of mild-to-moderate dementia of AD at an initial dose of 1.5 mg twice daily; if this dose is tolerated for at least 2 weeks, then the dose can be increased to 3 mg twice daily. Increases to 4.5 mg twice daily and 6 mg twice daily should be attempted only after at least 2 weeks at the previous dose. Tolerability and absorption are improved when the dose is given with food.

Rivastigmine is also available in a patch formulation, with an initial dose of 4.2 mg/24 hours applied once daily. The maintenance dose of the patch is 9.5 mg/24 hours applied once daily. A minimum of 4 weeks of treatment and good tolerability with the previous dose should be observed before consideration of an increase in dose. When switching from the oral formulation to the patch, if the patient is taking less than 6 mg/day of oral, then the 4.2 mg/24 hours patch is recommended. If the patient is taking 6 to 12 mg/day of oral, then the 9.5 mg/24 hours patch is recommended. The first patch should be applied on the day following the last oral dose.[37]

Cholinergic side effects are common with rivastigmine, but are usually well tolerated if the recommended dosing schedule is followed. If side effects cause intolerance, several doses can be held, then dosing can be restarted at the same or next lower dose. There are no pharmacokinetic drug interactions with drugs metabolized via CYP1A2, 2D6, 3A4/5, 2E1, 2C9, 2C8, or 2C19. Drugs that induce or inhibit CYP450 metabolism are not expected to alter the metabolism of rivastigmine.[37]

▶ Galantamine

⑨ *Galantamine is a ChE inhibitor, which elevates Ach in the cerebral cortex by slowing the degradation of Ach.*[38] It also modulates the nicotinic Ach receptors to increase Ach release from surviving presynaptic nerve terminals. In addition, it may increase glutamate and serotonin levels. The clinical benefit of action of these additional neurotransmitters is unknown.

Galantamine is approved for the treatment of mild-to-moderate dementia of AD. It can be dosed once or twice daily (if using the immediate-release tablet or extended-release capsule). The initial dose is 8 mg daily (or 4 mg twice daily) for 4 weeks. If tolerated the dose can be increased if needed to 16 mg daily (or 8 mg twice daily) for at least 4 weeks. Again, if this dose is tolerated, the dose can be increased if needed to 24 mg daily (or 12 mg twice daily).

The adverse reactions associated with galantamine are similar to that observed with the ChE inhibitors.

CYP3A4 and 2D6 are the major enzymes involved in the metabolism of galantamine. Pharmacokinetic studies with inhibitors of this system have resulted in increased galantamine concentrations or reductions in clearance. Similarly to donepezil, if inhibitors are given concurrently with galantamine, monitoring for increased cholinergic side effects should be done.[38]

▶ NMDA Receptor Antagonist

Memantine ⑩ *Memantine is a noncompetitive antagonist of the NMDA type of glutamate receptors, which are located ubiquitously throughout the brain.* It regulates activity throughout the brain by controlling the amount of calcium that enters the nerve cell, a process essential for establishing an environment required for information storage. Overstimulation of the NMDA receptor by excessive glutamate allows too much calcium into the cell, disrupting information processing. Blocking NMDA receptors with memantine may protect neurons from the effects of excessive glutamate without disrupting normal neurotransmission.[39]

Memantine is indicated for the treatment of moderate-to-severe dementia of the Alzheimer's type. The initial dose is 5 mg/day with increases to 20 mg/day if needed, with a minimum of 1 week between dosage increases. Doses greater than 5 mg/day should be given in two divided doses. A suggested titration is: 5 mg/day for at least 1 week, 5 mg twice daily for at least 1 week, 15 mg/day (5 mg in the morning and 10 mg in the evening) for at least 1 week, then 10 mg

twice daily. If the patient has a creatinine clearance of 5 to 29 mL/min, then the target dose should be 5 mg twice daily. It is likely to be given as monotherapy, but can be given in combination with ChE inhibitors.

Adverse reactions associated with memantine include constipation, confusion, dizziness, headache, coughing, and hypertension. Extra monitoring should be done if memantine is given concurrently with a ChE inhibitor.

In vitro studies have shown that memantine produces minimal inhibition of CYP450 enzymes CYP1A2, 2A6, 2C9, 2D6, 2E1, and 3A4. These data indicate that no pharmacokinetic interactions with drugs metabolized by these enzymes should be expected.[39]

▶ Future Therapies

⑪ *Future therapies for AD may be based on disease-modifying therapies.* Current investigations involving the amyloid hypothesis are reviewing various compounds in the secondary prevention of AD. Mechanisms by which these compounds are thought to work include[10]:

- Decreasing the production of Aβ
- Stimulation of clearance of Aβ formed
- Prevention of aggregation of Aβ into amyloid plaques
- Prevention of neuronal damage by limiting inflammation and neurotoxicity caused by Aβ

Nonconventional Pharmacologic Treatment

⑫ *Many other nonconventional treatments have been used as adjunctive treatments during the course of AD.* Vitamin E has often been recommended for use as an adjunctive treatment because of its antioxidant properties.[40] It has potential effectiveness, a favorable side-effect profile, and low cost. The maintenance dose of vitamin E should be titrated to 1,000 IU twice daily. However, a recent meta-analysis suggests that high doses (greater than 400 IU/day) of vitamin E should be avoided due to an increased all-cause mortality.[41] Estrogen has been investigated for use in AD, but as mentioned previously, was associated with an increased risk of dementia. Nonsteroidal anti-inflammatory drugs (NSAIDs) have also been investigated for their place in the therapy of AD. There is a lack of convincing data and significant adverse effects (gastritis and GI bleeds) associated with their use, so they are not recommended for general use in the treatment or prevention of AD at this time.[42] Statins (3-hydroxy-3-methylglutaryl-CoA reductase inhibitors) should be reserved for those patients who have other indications for their use.[43] Ginkgo biloba has also been studied for its potential use in AD. Until this product has a more standardized manufacturing process and until its long-term safety and efficacy are established, it should be recommended with caution.[44]

Treatment for Behavioral Symptoms

⑬ *Treatment of behavioral symptoms should begin with nonpharmacologic treatments, but may also include*

Patient Encounter, Part 2: Medical History, Physical Examination, and Diagnostic Tests

HPI: LB has seen a neurologist to address her cognitive decline and behavioral issues and is at the clinic for follow-up after obtaining her assessments and labs

PMH

- Diabetes mellitus since age 55; it was well controlled until last year when it worsened because of increased confusion of when to take her medication
- Hypertension treated for 20 years and well controlled; has been hypotensive on a few occasions recently during physicals
- Insomnia which is getting worse

FH: Father died of myocardial infarction at age 76; mother died of breast cancer at age 79

SH: Lives alone; denies drinking alcohol or smoking

Meds

- Hydrochlorothiazide 25 mg orally once daily
- Losartan 50 mg orally twice daily
- Metformin 1,000 mg orally twice daily
- Lorazepam 1 mg orally at bedtime

ROS: (+) weight loss of 5.5 kg (12 lb); (−) N/V/D, change in appetite, heartburn, chest pain, or shortness of breath

PE:

VS: BP 128/62 mm Hg supine, P 77 bpm, RR 15/min, T 37°C (98.6°F)

Gen: Poorly groomed, thin woman looks stated age

Neuro: Folstein Mini Mental Status Exam score 16/30; disoriented to month, date, and day of week, clinic name and floor; poor registration with impaired attention and short-term memory; recalled zero out of three items; good language skills but problems with commands

CT scan: Mild-to-moderate generalized cerebral atrophy

Based on the new information, what is your assessment of the patient?

What nonpharmacologic and pharmacologic interventions could be recommended?

What are the short-term and long-term treatment goals?

---

antipsychotic agents and/or antidepressants. Nonpharmacologic recommendations for treatment include[45]:

- Music
- Videotapes of family members
- Audio tapes of the voices of caregivers
- Walking and light exercise
- Sensory stimulation and relaxation

The atypical antipsychotics are the preferred agents for the treatment of psychosis (hallucinations, delusions, and suspiciousness) and the disruptive behaviors (agitation and aggression) of AD. Double-blind, controlled trials support the efficacy of risperidone and olanzapine in reducing the rate of psychosis and agitation.[46–48] Risperidone should be initiated at 0.25 mg/day and titrated in 0.25 to 0.5 mg/day increments to 1 mg/day, with a maximum dose of 2 mg/day.[46,47,49] Olanzapine has been studied with modest results at doses of 5 to 10 mg/day, and 15 mg/day has not been shown to be any better than placebo.[48]

In April 2005, the FDA issued a statement requesting black-box warnings on all atypical antipsychotics stating that elderly people with dementia-related psychosis treated with an atypical antipsychotic are at an increased risk of death compared to those treated with placebo. Of a total of 17 placebo-controlled trials investigating olanzapine, aripiprazole, quetiapine, and risperidone in elderly demented patients with behavioral disorders, 15 showed a numerical increase in mortality in the drug-treated group compared to the placebo-treated groups (1.6–1.7 times increased risk of death). Specific causes for these deaths were heart-related events (heart failure and sudden death) and infections (mostly pneumonia). The atypical antipsychotics are not currently approved for the treatment of elderly patients with dementia-related psychosis. Therefore, it is important to individually assess and balance the risk versus benefit of antipsychotic use in this population.

Differentiating between depression and dementia can be difficult, so symptoms of depression should be documented for several weeks prior to initiating therapy for the treatment of depression with AD. Citalopram and sertraline are recommended as first-line agents because of their efficacy in placebo-controlled trials.[50] Indications for the use of antidepressants include depression characterized by poor appetite, insomnia, hopelessness, anhedonia, withdrawal, suicidal thoughts, and agitation.

Other miscellaneous therapies for AD include benzodiazepines for anxiety, agitation, and aggression. However, their routine use is not advised.[29] Additionally, benzodiazepines have been associated with an increase in falls leading to the potential for hip fractures in the elderly.[51] Buspirone has shown benefit in treating agitation and aggression in a limited number of patients with minimal adverse effects.[52,53] In open-label and controlled studies, selegiline decreased anxiety, depression, and agitation.[54,55] Finally, trazodone has been shown to decrease insomnia, agitation, and dysphoria, and has been used to treat sundowning in Alzheimer's patients. Figure 35–2 also provides a treatment algorithm for the behavioral symptoms of AD.[32]

GENOMICS

⑭ *Therapeutic response in AD is genotype-specific depending upon the genes associated with pathogenesis and/or genes responsible for drug metabolism.* Recent investigations have demonstrated that the therapeutic response in AD is genotype-specific, depending upon genes associated with AD pathogenesis and/or genes responsible for drug metabolism. apo E-4/4 carriers tend to show a faster disease progression and a poorer therapeutic response to all available treatments than any other polymorphic variant associated with AD. Extensive and intermediate metabolizers of CYP450 enzymes are the best responders to pharmacotherapy, while poor and ultrarapid metabolizers are the worst responders. The pharmacogenetic response in AD may depend upon the interaction of genes involved in drug metabolism and the genes associated with AD pathogenesis.[56]

OUTCOME EVALUATION

- The success of therapy is measured by the degree to which the care plan decreases the pretreatment deterioration rate, preserves the patients' functioning, and treats psychiatric and behavioral symptoms. The primary outcome measure is thus subjective information from the patient and the caregiver, although the Mini Mental Status Examination (MMSE) can be a helpful tool. There are no physical examination or laboratory parameters that are used to evaluate the success of therapy.

- Once a tolerated agent is found, continue that therapy until poor tolerance or poor adherence occurs, no clinical improvement is seen with 3 to 6 months of optimal dosing, or the pretreatment deterioration rate continues. Inform the patient and the caregiver that the treatments available for AD are not curative, but may slow the deterioration rate of the patient.

- Treat behavioral and psychiatric issues as they arise. Consider the patient's choices of nonpharmacologic and pharmacologic options before recommending a treatment. Discontinue the pharmacologic treatments periodically to reevaluate the need for continued treatment.

- Develop a plan to assess the effectiveness of the ChE inhibitor in slowing the deterioration of cognitive functioning after an appropriate interval (3–6 months). Assess improvement in quality-of-life measures such as ability to function independently and for slowing of memory deterioration. Evaluate the patient for the presence of adverse drug reactions, drug allergies, and drug interactions at appropriate intervals. Continue to be a resource for the patient and caregiver throughout the long course of the disease.

Patient Care and Monitoring

1. Assess the frequency and duration of the patient's cognitive and noncognitive symptoms. Could the patient be depressed?

2. Review any available diagnostic data from the medical and psychiatric history including interviews from family, neuropsychologic testing, and other labs.

3. Obtain a thorough history of prescription, nonprescription, and natural drug product use. Is the patient taking any medications that could contribute to cognitive changes in the elderly?

4. Educate both the patient and caregivers about lifestyle modification and refer them to support when needed.

5. Monitor pharmacotherapy initiation. Is it titrated correctly?

6. Develop a plan to monitor cognitive response to treatment over time.

7. Routinely assess medication adherence.

8. Educate patient and caregivers on what to expect from pharmacotherapy.

9. Regularly evaluate the patient for the presence of adverse drug reactions, drug allergies, and drug–drug and drug–disease interactions.

10. Be a resource and give continuous support to the patient and caregivers throughout the long course of the disease.

Table 35–7

Living With AD: Ten Quick Tips

1. Carry with you a book of important notes and photos
2. Enroll in Alzheimer's Association Safe Return
3. Be open to accepting help from others
4. Keep doing the things you most enjoy
5. Talk to others who have AD
6. Find ways to laugh as often as you can
7. Maintain your physical health
8. Take steps to make your home safe
9. Extend the time you can live safely in your home with help from your family and friends
10. Put plans in place now for your future

From Ref. 57.

SUMMARY

AD is a progressive deterioration of cognitive abilities, and patients are likely to have behavioral disturbances and personality changes in the later stages of the disease. In an effort to help prepare patients and their caregivers for the inevitable, the Alzheimer's Association has developed ten quick tips on "Living with Alzheimer's disease" (Table 35–7).[57] The Alzheimer's Association can provide many resources as well as facilitate contacts with other organizations. Contact the association at:

Alzheimer's Association
Contact Center: 1.800.272.3900
TDD Access: 1.312.335.8882
Website: www.alz.org
E-mail: info@alz.org
National Office: 225 N. Michigan Ave., Fl. 17
Chicago, IL 60601–7633

Abbreviations Introduced in This Chapter

Ach	Acetylcholine
AD	Alzheimer's disease
apo E	Apolipoprotein E
APP	Amyloid precursor protein
ChE	Cholinesterase
CYP	Cytochrome P450
DSM-IV-TR	*Diagnostic and Statistical Manual of Mental Disorders*, Fourth Edition, Text Revision
MMSE	Mini Mental Status Examination
NINCDS-ADRDA	National Institute of Neurological and Communicative Disorders and Stroke-Alzheimer's Disease and Related Disorders Association
NMDA	*N*-Methyl-D-aspartate
NSAID	Nonsteroidal anti-inflammatory drug

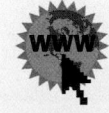

Self-assessment questions and answers are available at *http://www.mhpharmacotherapy. com/pp.html.*

REFERENCES

1. Alzheimer's Association. Available at: *www.alz.org/alzheimers_disease_symptoms_of_alzheimers.asp.*
2. Hebert LE, Scherr PA, Bienias JL, et al. Alzheimer disease in the U.S. population: Prevalence estimates using the 2000 census. Arch Neurol 2003;60:1119–1122.
3. American Psychiatric Association. Diagnostic and Statistical Manual of Mental Disorders, 4th ed. Text revision. Washington, DC: American Psychiatric Association, 2000:147–154.
4. U.S. Census Bureau. Available at: http://*www.census.gov/population/projections/nation/summary/np-t3-g.pdf.*
5. Report of the Lewin Group to the Alzheimer's Association. Available at *www.alz.org/news_and_events_alzheimers_news_12-5-2005.asp.*
6. Luchsinger JA, Reitz C, Honig LS, et al. Aggregation of vascular risk factors and risk of incident Alzheimer disease. Neurology 2005;65: 545–551.
7. Gorelick PB. Risk factors for vascular dementia and Alzheimer disease. Stroke 2004;35:S2620–S2622.
8. Ganguli M, Dodge HH, Shen C, et al. Alzheimer disease and mortality. Arch Neurol 2005;62:779–784.
9. Kamboh MI. Molecular genetics of late-onset Alzheimer's disease. Ann Hum Genet 2004;68:381–404.
10. van Marum RJ. Current and future therapy in Alzheimer's disease. Fundam Clin Pharmacol 2008;22:265–274.
11. Holmes C. Genotype and phenotype in Alzheimer's disease. Br J Psychiatry 2002;180:131–134.
12. Mattson MP. Pathways towards and away from Alzheimer's disease. Nature 2004;430:631–639.
13. DeKosky ST. Pathology and pathways of Alzheimer's disease with an update on new developments in treatment. J Am Geriatr Soc 2003;51:S314–S320.
14. Munoz DG, Feldman H. Causes of Alzheimer's disease. Can Med Assoc J 2000;162:65–72.
15. Yanker BA, Lu T. Amyloid β-protein toxicity and the pathogenesis of Alzheimer's disease. J Biol Chem Epub Nov 13, 2008.
16. Gauthier S. Advances in the pharmacotherapy of Alzheimer's disease. Can Med Assoc J 2002;166:616–623.
17. Pietrzik C, Behl C. Concepts for the treatment of Alzheimer's disease: Molecular mechanisms and clinical application. Int J Exp Path 2005;86:173–185.
18. Sze C, Bi H, Kleinschmidt-DeMasters BK, et al. N-Methyl-D-aspartate receptor subunit proteins and their phosphorylation status are altered selectively in Alzheimer's disease. J Neurol Sci 2001;182: 151–159.
19. Parsons CG, Danysz W, Quack G. Glutamate in CNS disorders as a target for drug development: An update. Drug News Perspect 1998; 11:523–569.
20. Parsons CG, Stoffler A, Danysz W. Memantine: A NMDA receptor antagonist that improves memory by restoration of homeostasis in the glutamatergic system—too little activation is bad, too much is even worse. Neuropharmacology 2007;53:699–723.
21. Czlonkowaka A, Ciesielska A, Joniec I. Influence of estrogens on neurodegenerative processes. Med Sci Monit 2003;10:247–256.
22. Simpkins JW, Singh M, Bishop J. The potential role for estrogen replacement therapy in the treatment of the cognitive decline and neurodegeneration associated with Alzheimer's disease. Neurobiol Aging 1994;15:S195–S197.
23. Shumaker SA, Legault C, Kuller L, et al. Conjugated equine estrogens and incidence of probable dementia and mild cognitive impairment in postmenopausal women (Women's Health Initiative Memory Study). JAMA 2004;291:2947–2958.
24. Knopman DS, DeKosky ST, Cummings JL, et al. Practice parameter: diagnosis of dementia (an evidence-based review). Report of the quality standards subcommittee of the American Academy of Neurology. Neurology 2001;56:1143–1153.
25. American Psychiatric Association. Diagnostic and Statistical Manual of Mental Disorders, 4th ed. Text revision. Washington, DC: American Psychiatric Association, 2000:154–157.
26. Alzheimer's Association. Available at www.alz.org/alzheimers_disease_causes_risk_factors.asp.
27. Reisberg B. Alzheimer's disease. Stages of cognitive decline. Am J Nurs 1984;84:225–228.
28. Doody RS, Stevens JC, Beck C, et al. Practice parameter: Management of dementia (an evidence-based review). Neurology 2001;56: 1154–1166.
29. APA Working Group on Alzheimer's Disease and other Dementias, Rabins PV, Blacker D, et al. American Psychiatric Association practice guideline for the treatment of patients with Alzheimer's disease and other dementias, 2nd ed. Am J Psychiatry 2007;164:5–56.
30. Small GW, Rabins PV, Barry PP, et al. Diagnosis and treatment of Alzheimer's disease and related disorders: consensus statement of the American Association for Geriatric Psychiatry, the Alzheimer's Association, and the American Geriatrics Society. JAMA 1997;278: 1363-1371.
31. Cummings JL. Use of cholinesterase inhibitors in clinical practice: Evidence-based recommendations. Am J Geriatr Psych 2003;11: 131–145.
32. Slattum PW, Swerdlow RH, Massey Hill A. Alzheimer's disease. In: DiPiro JT, Talbert RL, Yee GC, et al., eds. Pharmacotherapy: A Pathophysiologic Approach, 6th ed. New York: McGraw-Hill, 2008: 1051–1065.

33. Gauthier S, Emre M, Farlow MR, et al. Strategies for continued successful treatment of Alzheimer's disease: Switching cholinesterase inhibitors. Curr Med Res Opin 2003;19(8):707–714.

34. Swanwick GR, Lawlor BA. Initiating and monitoring cholinesterase inhibitor treatment for Alzheimer's disease. Int J Geriatr Psych 1999; 14:244–248.

35. Product Information. Aricept (donepezil hydrochloride). Teaneck, NJ: Eisai; 2006 (Nov).

36. West-ward Pharmaceutical Corp. Cognex (tacrine hydrochloride) [product information]. Eatontown, NJ: Author; 2002 (Jan).

37. Novartis. Exelon (rivastigmine tartrate) [product information]. East Hanover, NJ: Author; 2007 (July).

38. Ortho-McNeil Neurologics. Razadyne ER/Razadyne (galantamine hydrobromide) [product information]. Titusville, NJ: Author; 2007 (April).

39. Forest Pharmaceutica, Inc. Namenda (memantine hydrochloride) [product information]. St. Louis, MO: Author; 2007 (April).

40. Sano M, Ernest C, Thomas RG, et al. A controlled trial of selegiline, alpha-tocopherol, or both as treatment for Alzheimer's disease. N Engl J Med 1997;336:1216–1222.

41. Miller ER, Pastor-Barriuso R, Dalal D, et al. Meta-analysis: High-dosage vitamin E supplementation may increase all-cause mortality. Ann Intern Med 2005;142:37–46.

42. Aisen PS, Schafer KA, Grundman M, et al. Effects of rofecoxib or naproxen versus placebo on Alzheimer's disease progression. JAMA 2003;289:2819–2826.

43. Cooper JL. Dietary lipids in the etiology of Alzheimer's disease. Drugs Aging 2003;20:399–418.

44. Dekosky ST, Williamson JD, Fitzpatrick AL, et al. Ginkgo biloba for prevention of dementia: a randomized controlled trial. JAMA 2008;300:2253–2262.

45. Cummings J. Drug therapy: Alzheimer's disease. N Engl J Med 2004;351:56–67.

46. Katz IR, Jeste DV, Mintzer JE, et al. Comparison of risperidone and placebo for psychosis and behavioral disturbances associated with dementia: A randomized, double-blind trial. J Clin Psych 1999;60: 107–115.

47. De Deyn PP, Rabheru K, Rasmussen A, et al. A randomized trial of risperidone, placebo, and haloperidol for behavioral symptoms of dementia. Neurology 1999;53:946–955.

48. Street JS, Clark WS, Gannon KS, et al. Olanzapine treatment of psychotic and behavioral symptoms in patients with Alzheimer's disease in nursing care facilities: A double-blind, randomized, placebo-controlled trial. Arch Gen Psych 2000;57:968–976.

49. Brodaty H, Ames D, Snowdon J, et al. A randomized placebo-controlled trial of risperidone for the treatment of aggression, agitation, and psychosis of dementia. J Clin Psych 2003;64:134–143.

50. Lyketsos CG, Olin J. Depression in Alzheimer's disease: Overview and treatment. Biol Psychiatry 2002;52:243–252.

51. Allain H, Bentue-Ferrer D, Polard E, et al. Postural instability and consequent falls and hip fractures associated with use of hypnotics in the elderly: A comparative review. Drugs Aging 2005;22:749–765.

52. Sakuye KM, Camp CJ, Ford PA. Effects of buspirone on agitation associated with dementia. Am J Geriatr Psych 1993;1:82–84.

53. Hermann N, Eryavec G. Buspirone in the management of agitation and aggression associated with dementia. Am J Geriatr Psych 1993;1: 249–253.

54. Tariot PN, Cohen RM, Sunderland T, et al. L-deprenyl in Alzheimer's disease. Arch Gen Psych 1987;44:427–433.

55. Schneider LS, Pollock VE, Zemansky MF, et al. A pilot study of low dose L-deprenyl in Alzheimer's disease. J Geriatr Psych Neurol 1991;4:143–148.

56. Cacabelos R. Pharmacogenomics and therapeutic prospects in dementia. Eur Arch Psychiatry Clin Neurosci 2008;258:28–47.

57. Alzheimer's Association. 10 quick tips: Living with Alzheimer's. Available at *www.alz.org/espanol_11842.asp.*

36 Substance-Related Disorders

Sally K. Guthrie and Theadia L. Carey

LEARNING OBJECTIVES

● **Upon completion of the chapter, the reader will be able to:**

1. Identify the extent of abuse of and dependence on commonly used drugs in different segments of the U.S. population.

2. Explain the commonalities of action of abused substances on the reward system in the brain.

3. Identify the typical signs and symptoms of intoxication associated with the use of alcohol, opioids, cocaine/amphetamines, and cannabis, and determine the appropriate treatment measures to produce a desired outcome following episodes of intoxication.

4. Determine when a patient meets criteria for substance dependence.

5. Describe the different approaches to treating drug withdrawal, and identify the circumstances in which each of these different approaches would be most appropriate.

6. Recognize when long-term maintenance therapy is indicated for an opioid addict, and describe how to choose and initiate a maintenance regimen.

7. Determine which nonpharmacologic therapies should be used, either alone or in combination with pharmacologic treatments, to foster a recovery from addiction.

8. Recommend a comprehensive treatment and monitoring program to establish lifestyle changes that help maintain sobriety and prevent relapse.

KEY CONCEPTS

❶ Virtually all abused substances appear to activate the same brain reward pathway.

❷ While activation of the reward pathways explains the pleasurable sensations associated with acute substance use, chronic use of abused substances, resulting in both addiction and withdrawal, may be related to neuroadaptive effects occurring within the brain.

❸ Individuals with a pattern of chronic use of commonly abused substances should be assessed to determine if they meet the *Diagnostic and Statistical Manual, Fourth Edition, Text Revision* (*DSM-IV-TR*) criteria for substance dependence (addiction).

❹ The treatment goals for acute intoxication of ethanol, cocaine/amphetamines, and opioids include (a) management of psychological manifestations of intoxication, such as aggression, hostility, or psychosis and (b) management of medical manifestations of intoxication, such as respiratory depression, hyperthermia, hypertension, cardiac arrhythmias, or stroke.

❺ The treatment goals for withdrawal from ethanol, cocaine/amphetamines, and opioids include (a) a determination if pharmacologic treatment of withdrawal symptoms is necessary, (b) management of medical manifestations of withdrawal, such as hypertension, seizures, arthralgias, and nausea, and (c) referral to the appropriate program for substance abuse treatment.

❻ To facilitate recovery from addiction it is necessary to utilize a comprehensive biopsychosocial assessment that includes the motivation for change. Pharmacologic treatments are always adjunctive to psychosocial therapy.

❼ While pharmacologic agents may help prevent relapse, psychotherapy should be the core therapeutic intervention. Motivational enhancement therapy (MET), cognitive-behavioral therapy (CBT), 12-step facilitation (TSF), behavioral couples therapy (BCT), community reinforcement approaches, and contingency management are the best-studied forms of psychotherapy in this group of patients.

❽ Certain pharmacologic agents have been helpful in the treatment of withdrawal and drug maintenance programs.

⑨ A major component of successful treatment of addiction is to continue monitoring the use of medications designed to decrease craving or to block the hedonic effects of abused substances, such as disulfiram, naltrexone, or acamprosate. Also, it is important to identify a mechanism for long-term support of sobriety that might be appropriate for a specific individual, such as Alcoholics Anonymous (AA), a spiritual group, or professional recovery programs for professionals, such as doctors, nurses, police officers, or other professionals.

Substance abuse and dependence are highly prevalent problems in the United States and in the world. In the United States, the use of all substances of abuse has undergone a series of periodic cycles of societal tolerance or condemnation. As an example, cocaine was first isolated from coca leaves in 1860 by a chemistry graduate student in Germany. Its use was advocated by many in the medical establishment until around the mid-1890s when it became evident that chronic use of cocaine might be addictive in some individuals and could be associated with deleterious physiologic effects. Its use decreased following restriction of prescribing and dispensing of cocaine in the early 20th century. Cocaine continued to be abused by a small segment of the population, but much of the medical community seemed to forget the earlier cocaine epidemic. By the late 1970s, at least one pharmacology textbook indicated that cocaine was not addicting. Unfortunately, in the 1980s, a smokeable formulation of cocaine (crack) became available, and cocaine use again became an epidemic. The cyclic nature of substance abuse is common to many drugs, including heroin and marijuana, in addition to cocaine.

The abused substances covered in this chapter include: nicotine, alcohol, cocaine, amphetamines, cannabis, and opioids. While many more substances can be and have been abused, these drugs are among the most popular.

EPIDEMIOLOGY

In the United States, the federal government annually conducts the National Survey on Drug Use and Health, using a sample of persons who are 12 years of age or older to determine the prevalence of licit and illicit drug use.[1] In 2006, 8.3% of the American population (12 and older) had used an illicit drug within the previous month. Fifty percent of the population currently used alcohol, and 6.9% were heavy users. Tobacco use in Americans has stabilized, in recent years, to a rate of 29.6%. Unfortunately, use in the younger age groups remains high. In 2006, 35.6% of Americans in the 18- to 20-year-old range and 40.2% in the 21- to 25-year-old range reported using cigarettes within the previous month. The trends in prevalence of use for eighth, tenth, and twelfth graders are shown in Figure 36–1. The uses of any illicit drug and of marijuana have both decreased since 1999, but still remain higher than the minimum use recorded in 1992.[2]

While initiation of the use of substances is often in middle and high school, chronic use may be established in young

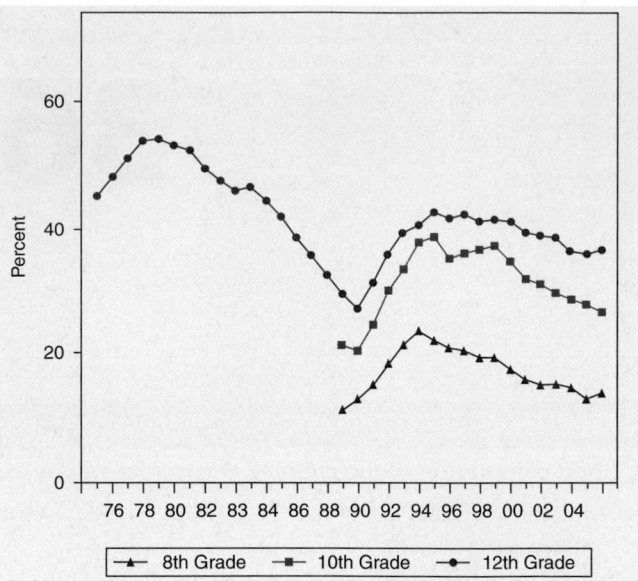

FIGURE 36–1. Trends in illicit drug use in eighth, tenth, and twelfth graders from the Monitoring the Future survey showing the percent that used any illicit drug in lifetime. (From Ref. 2.)

adulthood. The National Alcohol Epidemiologic Survey reported that 9.2% of its 18- to 29-year-old sample met criteria for alcohol dependence.[3]

The association of substance abuse with emergency department (ED) visits in the United States is reported by the Drug Abuse Warning Network (DAWN). This survey notes ED visits that are due to a condition induced by or related to drug use. Included in the data, are ED visits associated with alcohol, alone and in combination with other substances of abuse including cocaine, heroin, marijuana, and major stimulants. Figure 36–2 presents 2006 data depicting the number of ED visits per 100,000 people in the population that are associated with illicit drugs. Alcohol in combination with other substances ranged from 219 to 268 per 100,000 in each 4-year-age subpopulation from the ages of 18 to 44. The rate dropped to 173 per 100,000 for the 45- to 54-year-old group, and down to 51 for the 55 to 64 and further to 12 per 100,000 population for the 65 and over group.[4]

The results of these surveys indicate that substance abuse is wide ranging, begins early, and is associated with a considerable number of medical emergencies.

PATHOPHYSIOLOGY
Reward Pathway

Abused drugs generally produce pleasant effects that are desired by the user. However, while most individuals will experience pleasant effects, not everyone abuses these drugs, and not everyone who abuses them becomes dependent on them. Why some persons abuse drugs while most people do not is a complex area of research. It appears that genetic, environmental, and cultural factors may all interact

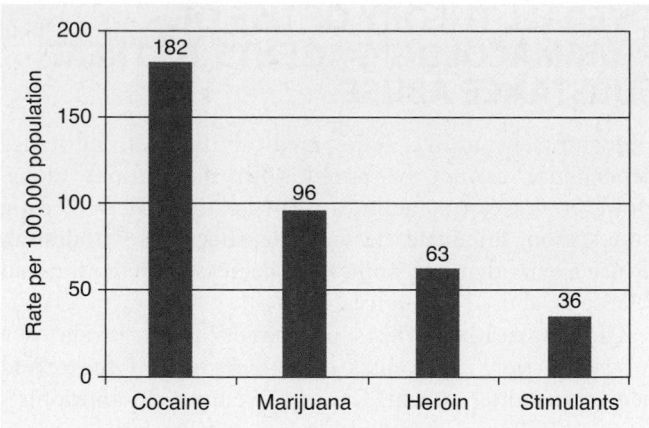

FIGURE 36–2. Rates of emergency department visits involving selected illicit drugs: 2006. (From Ref. 4.)

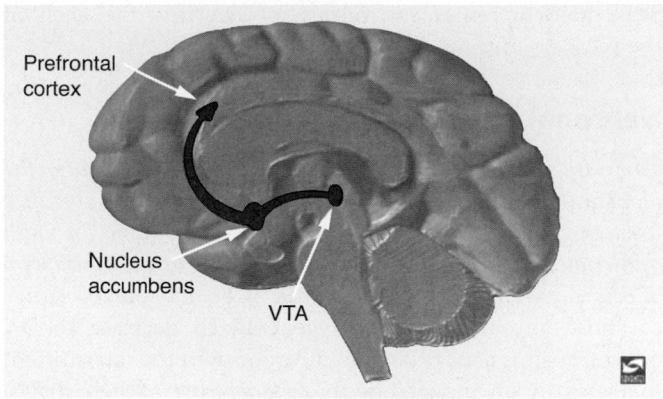

FIGURE 36–3. Location of the dopamine neural tracts associated with the reward system in the brain. (From Ref. 5.)

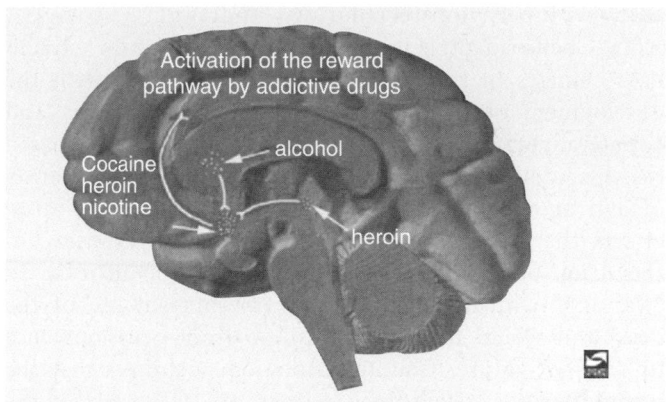

FIGURE 36–4. Locations where different abused substances interact with the reward system in the brain. (From Ref. 5.)

to predispose some individuals to substance abuse and subsequent dependence. The initial hedonic experiences secondary to use of drugs appear to be primarily due to their ability to activate the primary reward circuits in the brain. These same reward circuits operate under normal circumstances to reinforce certain activities that promote survival, such as food, social affiliation, or sexual activity.

❶ *Virtually all abused substances appear to activate the same brain reward pathway.* Key components of the reward pathway are the dopamine (DA) **mesocorticolimbic** system that projects from the **ventral tegmental area** (VTA) and the **nucleus accumbens** (NA) to the prefrontal cortex, the **amygdala**, and the **olfactory tubercle** (see Figs. 36–3 and 36–4).[5] Animal studies indicate that ablation of DA neurons in the NA results in decreases in cocaine self-administration. Although many other neurotransmitters can be involved in activation of the reward system, DA appears to be a final common neurotransmitter of this pathway.[6]

Cocaine and stimulants, such as amphetamines, probably activate reward circuits by blocking the DA reuptake transporter. Additionally, amphetamines also cause the reverse transport of DA into the extracellular space.[6] Although opioids eventually utilize the same circuitry as stimulants, initially they activate μ-opioid receptors, in the NA or VTA, which ultimately results in an increase DA release in the NA. However, reinforcement of opioid use may derive from two mechanisms because in animal studies, when the DA fibers are destroyed, the reinforcing effects of opioids remain.[6] Ethanol probably produces its effects through multiple neurotransmitter pathways. Antagonists of γ-amino butyric acid (GABA) reverse some of the behavioral effects of ethanol, suggesting that there may be cross-reactivity between benzodiazepines and alcohol, and that alcohol may somehow modulate GABA receptors. Ethanol may activate the DA system indirectly by facilitating the activity of GABA neurons in the pars reticulata, ultimately disinhibiting the VTA DA neurons, resulting in an increase in DA in the NA.[6] There also may be an interaction between serotonin (5-HT) and the reinforcing effects of ethanol, because both

5-HT reuptake inhibitors and $5-HT_{2C}$ receptor antagonists decrease ethanol intake in animals. However, studies of these drugs in alcohol-dependent humans have not been very promising. Animal studies indicated that when opioid antagonists were administered to the central nucleus of the amygdala, oral ethanol self-administration decreased. Studies in humans showed a modest decrease in alcohol consumption in alcoholics who took a long-acting opioid antagonist (naltrexone) following detoxification. Finally, small doses of ethanol inhibit N-methyl-D-aspartate (NMDA) glutamate receptors, and animals will substitute glutamate receptor antagonists for ethanol, suggesting that they find the effects of the two drugs to be similar. Nicotine also affects the reward pathways by more than one mechanism. In animal studies, either DA antagonists or destruction of DA neurons in the NA decreased nicotine self-administration. Nicotine also interacts with the opioid pathway, because opioid antagonists can precipitate nicotine withdrawal in animals. Finally, marijuana's main active component, tetrahydrocannabinol (THC), binds to cannabinoid-1 (CB_1) receptors resulting in activation of DA neurons in the mesocorticolimbic system.

THC also increases the release of DA into the shell of the NA.[6]

Neuronal Adaptation

❷ *While activation of the reward pathways explains the pleasurable sensations associated with acute substance use, chronic use of abused substances resulting in both addiction and withdrawal may be related to neuroadaptive effects occurring within the brain.* Chronic use of drugs of abuse appears to cause a generalized decrease in DA neurotransmission, probably in response to the intermittent increases in DA induced by the frequent use of these drugs. Additionally, with chronic drug use, release of corticotropin releasing factor (CRF) is increased, indicating an activation of central stress pathways. In vivo microdialysis studies in rats withdrawing from ethanol, cocaine, or THC all showed an increase in extracellular CRF. Also, microinjections of a CRF antagonist into the amygdala reversed some of the anxiogenic behaviors seen during withdrawal.[7]

Two neuroadaptive models have been used to explain how changes in reward function are associated with the development of substance dependence: sensitization and counteradaptation.[7] Sensitization refers to the increased response following repeated intermittent administration of a drug. This is in contrast to the tolerance to drug effects that occurs secondary to continuous exposure to the drug. Sensitization may be akin to the increase in "wanting" a drug after repeated intermittent use of the drug and would facilitate transition from occasional use to compulsive use. Counteradaptation postulates that the initial positive rewarding feelings are followed by the opposing development of tolerance. Because tolerance takes longer to dissipate than the positive rewarding effects, a cycle of escalating drug use ensues. Ultimately, chronic activation of the reward system may result in a depletion of neurotransmitter systems that are overactivated in an effort to maintain response to drugs of abuse. During withdrawal, microdialysis experiments have documented decreases in dopaminergic and serotonergic transmission in the NA. Also seen during alcohol withdrawal are an increase in opioid receptor sensitivity combined with decreased GABAergic and increased NMDA glutamatergic transmission in the accumbens–amygdala pathway. The increase in CRF and concomitant decrease in neuropeptide Y during withdrawal are associated with increases in anxiety, and an activation of norepinephrine (NE) pathways, which in turn also activates more CRF release, possibly resulting in an amplification of arousal and stress and maybe even neurotoxicity if these actions are long-lasting.[7]

With regard to relapse, multiple factors are associated with an increased risk including the availability of the abused drug, an increase in psychological stressors, and a triggering of conditioning factors (cues) such as seeing a white powder or going to a location where drugs were often previously used or obtained. These factors may be acting to trigger residual adaptive changes that occurred in the brain during the period of drug addiction.

OVERALL THEORY OF USE OF PHARMACOLOGIC AGENTS TO TREAT SUBSTANCE ABUSE

Unfortunately, unlike some medical diseases, substance dependence cannot be cured with medications alone. However, we can sometimes alleviate the effects of drug intoxication, attenuate the adverse effects of withdrawal, or use agents that may somewhat decrease craving for, and relapse to, abused substances.

The intoxicating effects of opioids appear to be due to their action as agonists on μ-receptors of the opioid neurotransmitter system. Competitive μ-opioid antagonists such as naloxone and naltrexone, acutely reverse many of the adverse effects of opioids. To date, we do not have specific antagonists for most other abused substances, so rapid pharmacologic reversal of intoxication is usually not possible.

Similarly, reversal of withdrawal syndromes caused by abused substances is not always possible. One pharmacologic solution for reversing a drug withdrawal syndrome, most commonly employed by dependent individuals, is to readminister the drug that caused the physiologic dependence. The more commonly used clinical method is to administer a medication that has some cross-dependence with the abused drug, but also has fewer of the reinforcing effects and a more predictable pharmacokinetic profile. A good example is the use of benzodiazepines for the withdrawal of ethanol. While benzodiazepines can cause dependence, they are rated as less desirable than ethanol by substance abusers, they cause fewer of the long-term adverse health effects of ethanol, and they are easier to manage medically.

In the case of heroin addiction, maintaining the addict on a regimen of medically managed, orally administered opioids may be preferred over rapidly detoxifying the patient who has a high likelihood of returning to heroin use when extensive strategies for rehabilitation have not been put in place. In order to allow time for psychosocial strategies to help the addicted individual change his or her overall lifestyle, a period of opioid agonist treatment may be indicated. This strategy has been used to maintain addicts on either orally administered μ opioid agonists such as methadone, or partial agonists such as buprenorphine.

No matter which method has been used to facilitate detoxification from the abused substance, addicts have a high risk for reusing substances and manifesting their dependence again. In the long term, the most effective mechanisms for maintaining sobriety are psychosocial strategies rather than pharmacologic ones.

CLINICAL PRESENTATION AND DIAGNOSIS

❸ *Individuals with a pattern of chronic use of commonly abused substances should be assessed to determine if they meet the DSM-IV-TR criteria for substance dependence (addiction).*[8] Criteria are not defined for each separate abused substance,

Patient Encounter 1

BB, a 48-year-old man with a history of hypertension, presents to your clinic for follow-up evaluation of his hypertension. You notice that he admits to drinking between one-half to one pint of whiskey daily. He says he drinks more on the weekends, but he drinks every day. When you question him about his drinking, he says that he does not think that it is a problem but admits that his wife has told him he needs to "cut down." He does not believe that he is alcohol dependent because on work days he never drinks before 5 PM. He admits to having had occasional blackouts.

What information would suggest that this patient might be alcohol dependent?

What additional information would you need to determine if he meets the criteria for alcohol dependence?

rather a pattern of behavior common to the abuse or dependence of all drugs of abuse is established.

The criteria for abuse indicate an established pattern of using a substance that has resulted in undesirable family, job, or legal consequences, such as recurrent instances of neglecting school, work, or family responsibilities, or being arrested for driving under the influence. However, abuse becomes dependence when tolerance to the drug, withdrawal from the drug, or an inability to discontinue use of the drug is apparent or there is a loss of control over its use or the use has become compulsive. The criteria for substance dependence from the *DSM-IV-TR* are listed in Table 36–1.[8]

Intoxication Signs and Symptoms

Euphoria is the one symptom that most drugs of abuse (with the exception of tobacco) have in common. Other signs and symptoms are specific to the particular drug or class of drugs involved. Table 36–2 lists the psychological/behavioral and physiologic effects of intoxication with ethanol, cocaine and amphetamines, opioids, and cannabis.[9–11]

Withdrawal Signs and Symptoms

Although most abused drugs can cause some degree of physiologic dependence, the severity of withdrawal varies considerably among these drugs. Table 36–3 lists the common withdrawal symptoms seen upon abstinence from drug use.[9–12]

TREATMENT OF INTOXICATION SYNDROMES

❹ The treatment goals for acute intoxication of ethanol, cocaine/amphetamines, and opioids include (a) management of psychological manifestations of intoxication, such as

Table 36–1

DSM-IV-TR Criteria for Diagnosis of Substance Dependence

A maladaptive pattern of substance use, leading to clinically significant impairment or distress, as manifested by three (or more) of the following, occurring at any time in the same 12-month period:

(1) Tolerance, as defined by either of the following:
   (a) a need for markedly increased amounts of the substance to achieve intoxication or desired effect
   (b) a markedly diminished effect with continued use of the same amount of the substance
(2) Withdrawal, as manifested by either of the following:
   (a) the characteristic withdrawal syndrome for the substance
   (b) the same (or a closely related) substance is taken to relieve or avoid withdrawal symptoms
(3) The substance is often taken in larger amounts or over a longer period than was intended
(4) There is a persistent desire or unsuccessful efforts to cut down or control substance use
(5) A great deal of time is spent in obtaining the substance (e.g., visiting multiple doctors or driving long distances), using the substance (e.g., chain-smoking), or recovering from its effects
(6) Important social, occupational, or recreational activities are given up or reduced because of substance use
(7) The substance use is continued despite knowledge of having a persistent or recurrent physical or psychological problem that is likely to have been caused or exacerbated by the substance (e.g., current cocaine use despite recognition of cocaine-induced depression, or continued drinking despite recognition that an ulcer was made worse by alcohol consumption)

Specify if:
- With physiologic dependence: Evidence of tolerance or withdrawal (i.e., either Item 1 or 2 is present)
- Without physiologic dependence: No evidence of tolerance or withdrawal (i.e., neither Item 1 nor 2 is present)

From Ref. 8.

Patient Encounter 2

KI, a 27-year-old woman, was admitted to the cardiology unit from the emergency department (ED) after she called 911 claiming that she had severe chest pain. Upon arrival in the ED it was noted that her blood pressure was slightly elevated at 143/92, and that she was diaphoretic. She was in otherwise good physical condition, with no previous cardiac history. After a urine toxicology screen was positive for cocaine she admitted that she had smoked several rocks of crack 1 hour prior to having the chest pain. She said she almost never uses crack, but she's currently really depressed because she has lost her job.

What are the possible physical signs and symptoms of cocaine use?

What are the possible psychiatric symptoms associated with cocaine use?

Table 36-2

Signs and Symptoms of Drug Intoxication

Drug	Behavioral Effects	Physiologic Effects
Ethanol	Mood lability, inappropriate aggressive or sexual behavior, giddiness or verbally loud, impaired judgment; possibly progressing to somnolence and coma as the blood level increases	At blood levels of 0.02–0.09% (20–90 mg/dL or 4.34–19.5 mmol/L): May see some prolonged reaction time and muscular incoordination
		At blood levels from 0.1% to 0.2% (100–200 mg/dL or 21.7–43.4 mmol/L): May see obvious prolonged reaction time, obvious incoordination and ataxia, and mental impairment
		At blood levels from 0.2% to 0.3% (200–300 mg/dL or 43.4–65.1 mmol/L): Marked ataxia, some dysarthria, and possible nausea and vomiting
		At blood levels from 0.3% to 0.4% (300–400 mg/dL or 61.5–86.8 mmol/L): Severe dysarthria, amnesia, and hypothermia
		At blood levels from 0.4% to 0.6% (400–600 mg/dL or 86.8–130.2 mmol/L): Alcoholic coma often occurs, accompanied by decreased respiration, blood pressure, and body temperature
		Blood levels between 0.6% and 0.8% (600–800 mg/dL or 130.2–173.6 mmol/L): Are often fatal resulting from respiratory arrest, aspiration of gastric contents, or airway obstruction due to flaccid tongue
Cocaine/ stimulants	Initially, most prominent effect is elated mood, although depression may occur; hypervigilance and anxiety that may progress to panic; with high doses or chronic use, may see impairment of judgment, violence to others or self, paranoia or psychosis with delusions and hallucinations (hallucinations are generally tactile or auditory, rarely visual); an increase in motor activity is common; compulsive or stereotyped behavior (e.g., skin picking) may be seen; severe intoxication may result in a self-limited delirium	Neurologic: Pupillary dilation, headache, tremor, hyper-reflexia, muscle twitching, flushing, hyperthermia or cold sweats, seizures, coma, and possible cerebral hemorrhage
		Cardiovascular: Increased pulse and blood pressure, peripheral vasoconstriction, arrhythmias, and myocardial infarction
		GI: Nausea and vomiting
		Renal: Possible incontinence or renal failure
		Neuromuscular: **Rhabdomyolysis**, possibly resulting in renal failure
Opioids	Euphoria and sedation are the most prominent effects; analgesia is also prominent; slurred speech, and impaired memory and attention can be seen along with psychomotor retardation	Nausea and vomiting; respiratory depression that is dose-related and may progress to coma; constipation is very common in chronic users, itching, and miosis (pinpoint pupils)
Cannabis	Euphoria or giddiness and increase in appetite may occur; depending on the social setting and the amount ingested, may see panic, paranoia, hallucinations, and depersonalization or delirium	Ocular: Conjunctival reddening, a slight miosis, and decreased intraocular pressure
		Cardiovascular: Tachycardia and vasodilation combined with orthostatic hypotension in high doses
		Neuromuscular: Decreased muscular coordination may be seen
		GI/genitourinary: Dry mouth is common and urinary retention may occur in some persons

From Refs. 9–11.

aggression, hostility, or psychosis and (b) management of medical manifestations of intoxication such as respiratory depression, hyperthermia, hypertension, cardiac arrhythmias, or stroke. In all cases of intoxication associated with a substance use disorder (abuse or dependence), referral to and participation in substance abuse treatment following acute treatment for intoxication is desirable.

Alcohol Intoxication

Most cases of mild to moderate intoxication with alcohol, as well as cases in which blood alcohol levels (BALs) are at the lower limits of legal intoxication, do not require formal treatment. Such intoxications are characterized by mood lability, loud or inappropriate behavior, slurred speech, incoordination, or unsteady gait. Providing a safe environment and supportive reassurance until the effects of alcohol have worn off is sufficient in most cases. At more severe levels of intoxication, confusion, stupor, coma, and death may be observed. In nontolerant individuals, confusion, impaired consciousness, and vomiting are observed at BALs of 200 to 300 mg/dL (0.2–0.3% or 43.4–65.1 mmol/L); stupor and coma are seen with BALs exceeding 300 to 400 mg/dL (0.3–0.4% or 65.1–86.8 mmol/L). Death may occur at levels of 400 mg/dL (0.4% or 86.8 mmol/L) or higher from cardiac arrhythmias or respiratory depression. Thus, the

Table 36–3		
Signs and Symptoms of Drug Withdrawal		
Drug	**Duration**	**Symptoms**
Ethanol	As ethanol level decreases	Vivid dreams, insomnia
	Within 6–24 hours	Tremor, nausea and vomiting, tachycardia (greater than 110 bpm), and hypertension (greater than 140/90 mm Hg)
	6–48 hours	Convulsions (usually one or two of the grand mal–type, but they can be more numerous and possibly fatal)
	Days 3–5	Delirium tremens
	Onset at any time	Hallucinations, usually visual
Cocaine/amphetamine	Immediately following binge	Stimulant craving, accompanied by intense dysphoria, depression, anxiety, and agitation
	Within 1–4 hours	Desire for sleep, dysphoria continues
	Days 3–4	Hypersomnia, increased appetite, craving may dissipate slightly, but returns strongly later
Opioids	For shorter-acting opioids (e.g., heroin, morphine, hydrocodone, oxycodone) withdrawal may begin within 6–24 hours following the last dose and last for about 1 week; with longer-action opioids (e.g., methadone) it may take up to 2–4 days for withdrawal to emerge, and it will last longer	GI: Nausea and vomiting, diarrhea, and dehydration Neurologic/psychological: Irritability, restlessness, yawning, tremulousness, and twitching Cardiovascular: Increase in heart rate and blood pressure Musculoskeletal: Chills, increased body temperature, piloerection, and rhinorrhea Ocular: Lacrimation and dilated pupils
Nicotine	Within 24 hours of cessation of use	The severity of symptoms reflects the degree and duration of nicotine use; symptoms include anxiety, irritability, frustration, anger, craving, difficulty concentrating, decreased heart rate, and increased appetite
Cannabis	Withdrawal is not usually noticeable, except in heavy, chronic marijuana users; withdrawal occurs within 24 hours, peaks in 2–4 days and resolves in 1–2 weeks	Symptoms are generally mild and reflect the degree and duration of dependence; symptoms include irritability, insomnia, restlessness, anorexia, diaphoresis, diarrhea, and muscle twitches; mild increases in heart rate and blood pressure may also occur

From Refs. 9–12.

most important physiologic goal of treating high levels of intoxication is maintaining cardiopulmonary functioning, including the prevention of aspiration. Accordingly, vital signs must be monitored regularly. Serial BALs at least hourly are strongly recommended, and patients should not be allowed to leave the treatment setting on their own while legally intoxicated (greater than or equal to 80 mg/dL [0.08% or 17.4 mmol/L]). Initially, BALs may continue to rise if GI absorption is still occurring. Otherwise, the BAL generally decreases at a rate of 15 to 20 mg/dL (0.015–0.02% or 3.3–4.3 mmol/L) per hour. Although more tolerant individuals may not show the same level of symptoms for a given BAL as nontolerant individuals, behavioral tolerance and tolerance for vital physiologic functions may differ. Thus, alcoholic patients who are awake and alert at a BAL greater than or equal to 400 mg/dL (0.4% or 86.8 mmol/L) may still be at risk for cardiopulmonary instability and collapse.

Other causes of confusion, stupor, or coma must be ruled out, because alcohol-intoxicated individuals commonly combine alcohol with other substances, sustain head and other injuries, and have vitamin deficiencies and electrolyte abnormalities. If consciousness is impaired, then thiamine should be given IV or intramuscularly (IM) at 100 mg

daily for at least 3 days. Patients may also develop adverse interactions between alcohol and medications that have been prescribed including disulfiram. See Table 36–4 for a listing of drug–drug interactions.[13-15] If hypoglycemia is suspected, then thiamine administration should precede administration of glucose-containing fluids to prevent precipitation of an acute Wernicke's syndrome.

Behaviorally, patients may insist on driving, become physically aggressive and agitated, or otherwise become a danger to self or others. Indeed, most suicidal behaviors among alcohol-dependent individuals occur while intoxicated. In such cases, the desired outcomes are appropriate management of medical problems, prevention of harmful behaviors, and stabilization of mood. Antipsychotics may lower seizure threshold and are best avoided. However, in some instances, agitation may require treatment with haloperidol such as 5 to 10 mg by mouth every 2 to 4 hours, or 5 mg either IV or IM every 1 to 2 hours. Sedation with benzodiazepines has been used in some cases, but the risk of respiratory depression when mixed with the alcohol already in the patient's system can be dangerous if not fatal.

There are no available medications that can fully reverse the effects of alcohol intoxication. Caffeine and other stimulants

Table 36–4

Drug Interactions With Abused Drugs or Drugs Used to Treat Drug Abuse

Drug	Interacting Drug	Type of Interaction and Appropriate Action
Amphetamine	MAOIs (phenelzine, tranylcypromine, possibly linezolid)	Pharmacodynamic interaction resulting in an increase in blood pressure; possibly resulting in a hypertensive emergency or stroke; avoid this combination
	Sodium bicarbonate	Sodium bicarbonate increases renal tubular reabsorption of amphetamine, resulting in a prolonged amphetamine elimination half-life; be aware of this combination
Buprenorphine	There are currently no reported drug interactions with buprenorphine; however, buprenorphine is metabolized primarily by CYP3A4	Theoretically buprenorphine metabolism could be inhibited by itraconazole, ketoconazole, grapefruit juice, and erythromycin or any other CYP3A4 inhibitor; the effects may be greater than expected for the dose of buprenorphine being given; may need to decrease buprenorphine dose
		Conversely, buprenorphine metabolism could by increased by carbamazepine, phenytoin, St. John's wort efavirenz, and nevirapine, or any other CYP3A4 inducer; the effects may be less than expected; may need to increase buprenorphine dose
Cigarette smoking	Clozapine	Cigarette smoking induces CYP1A2; increasing the metabolism of clozapine; may need to increase usual clozapine dose when a patient begins to smoke, or decrease clozapine dose if smoking is stopped or nicotine replacement is used instead of smoking
	Olanzapine	Similar interactions as clozapine; may need to increase the usual olanzapine dose when a patient begins to smoke, or decrease olanzapine dose if smoking is stopped or nicotine replacement is used instead of smoking
	Theophylline	Theophylline is also a CYP1A2 substrate; may need to increase the usual theophylline dose when a patient begins to smoke, or decrease the theophylline dose if smoking is stopped or nicotine replacement is used instead of smoking
Clonidine	Amitriptyline, imipramine, desipramine (also likely with nortriptyline, doxepin, protriptyline, and trimipramine)	Pharmacodynamic interaction; clonidine acts as an agonist at α_2-receptors, and these TCAs block this receptor to varying degrees; the result is an increase in blood pressure; either avoid this interaction by choosing another antidepressant or increase the dose of clonidine
	Cyclosporine	Clonidine may increase cyclosporine blood levels; although only a single case report supports this, it would be prudent to monitor cyclosporine blood levels in a patient receiving clonidine
	Mirtazapine	This interaction is the same as the one when clonidine is combined with TCAs; however, mirtazapine is a more potent α_2-receptor blocker than the TCAs; avoid this interaction and choose an alternative antidepressant without α_2-blocking effects
Disulfiram	Benzodiazepines (including alprazolam, chlordiazepoxide, diazepam, flurazepam, halzepam, prazepam, triazolam)	Disulfiram inhibits CYP enzymes 1A2, 2C9, and 3A4; many benzodiazepines are metabolized via these pathways; lorazepam, temazepam, and oxazepam are NOT metabolized via the CYP450 system and are reasonable alternatives
		Otherwise, if benzodiazepines are combined with disulfiram the pharmacologic effect may be greater than expected, and the dose of benzodiazepine may need to be lowered
	Cocaine	Disulfiram decreases the clearance of cocaine from the body; may see increased or prolonged cocaine effects with this combination
	Isoniazid	The addition of disulfiram to isoniazid therapy has resulted in changes in affect and behavior and decreased coordination; avoid the combination if possible; if they must be given concomitantly, monitor closely
	Phenytoin	Disulfiram decreases the metabolism of phenytoin, resulting in higher phenytoin levels; the dose of phenytoin will need to be reduced; since phenytoin undergoes nonlinear metabolism it is difficult to predict the magnitude of increase in blood levels that could be seen; it is best to avoid this interaction if possible; otherwise, closely monitor phenytoin blood levels
	Theophylline	Disulfiram inhibits CYP1A2, resulting in an increase in theophylline blood levels; monitor theophylline blood concentration; may need to decrease theophylline dose
	Warfarin	Disulfiram inhibits several of the enzymes responsible for warfarin metabolism; increased PT/INR have been noted; if disulfiram is added to warfarin therapy, carefully monitor PT/INR; the warfarin dose will probably have to be decreased
Ethanol	Acetaminophen	Chronic ethanol use increases the risk of hepatotoxicity when acetaminophen is used in high doses; however, acute ingestion of alcohol along with an acetaminophen overdose decreases the toxicity of acetaminophen
	Cefamandole, cefoperazone, cefotetan, and moxalactam, metronidazole	A disulfiram-type reaction may occur when these anti-infectives are combined with alcohol; the reaction includes flushing, diaphoresis, tachycardia, headache, and increases in blood pressure; avoid alcohol if these drugs are used
	Isoniazid	Hepatotoxicity is a higher risk when isoniazid is given to those who chronically drink large amounts of alcohol; avoid isoniazid in this group if possible, otherwise monitor LFTs
	Methotrexate	Hepatotoxicity is a higher risk when methotrexate is given to those who chronically drink large amounts of alcohol; avoid methotrexate in this group if possible; otherwise monitor LFTs

(Continued)

Table 36–4

Drug Interactions with Abused Drugs or Drugs Used to Treat Drug Abuse *(Continued)*

Drug	Interacting Drug	Type of Interaction and Appropriate Action
	MAOIs	Ethanol DOES NOT interact with MAOIs; however, tyramine may be a component of some aged alcoholic drinks, such as red wines or tap beers; if a reaction occurs, hypertension and a pounding headache are the most likely symptoms; usually white wine is fine (in moderation) and most widely available domestic canned beers do not contain significant amounts of tyramine
Methadone	Carbamazepine	Carbamazepine is an inducer of CYP3A4 and methadone is primarily metabolized via CYP3A4; if carbamazepine is added to a drug regimen containing methadone, the methadone dose will probably need to be adjusted upward to avoid withdrawal
	Didanosine	Methadone decreases the amount of didanosine (a reverse transcriptase inhibitor) that is orally absorbed by about 40%. It is likely that the oral didanosine dose should be increased when it is given with methadone
	Efavirenz	This HIV drug is a CYP3A4 inducer; efavirenz decreases methadone blood levels and has precipitated withdrawal in opioid-dependent individuals; may need to increase methadone dose
	Fluconazole	Fluconazole is an antifungal agent that moderately inhibits CYP3A4; when added to a drug regimen containing methadone, higher blood levels have been noted; adjustment of methadone dose should be based on clinical judgment, but a decrease of dose may be necessary. NOTE: Both itraconazole and ketoconazole are more potent inhibitors of CYP3A4, although interactions have not yet been reported, theoretically, they are very likely to occur, resulting in elevated methadone concentrations
	Nevirapine	Nervirapine is an HIV drug that is a CYP3A4 inducer; in a small sample, nevirapine caused a 50% reduction in methadone blood levels, resulting in complaints of methadone withdrawal symptoms in patients receiving methadone maintenance; may need to increase methadone dose in patients who have nevirapine added to their drug regimen
	Phenobarbital	An inducer of many CYP450 enzymes; may result in complaints of withdrawal symptoms in methadone maintenance patients when added to their drug regimen; may need to increase methadone dose
	Phenytoin	Similar to phenobarbital; may need to increase methadone dose when phenytoin is added to a methadone maintenance drug regimen to avoid withdrawal symptoms
	Stavudine	Methadone decreases the amount of stavudine (a reverse transcriptase inhibitor) by about 25%. Although this may not be clinically significant in some cases, the clinician should be aware of the possibility of this interaction
	St. John's wort	This herbal remedy may induce CYP3A4; the certainty of an interaction probably rests on the specific preparation being used, but caution would dictate that this herbal product should be avoided in those receiving methadone treatment; withdrawal symptoms have been noted in patients taking methadone maintenance who have added St. John's wort to their drug regimen
	Zidovudine	Methadone increases the blood level of this anti-HIV drug, probably via methadone inhibition of both metabolic and renal clearance of zidovudine; may need to decrease zidovudine dose to avoid toxicity
Naltrexone	Acamprosate	Naltrexone increases oral bioavailability of acamprosate. However, clinical implications appear to be minor. If tolerability of acamprosate decreases when naltrexone is added to the drug regimen, a decrease of acamprosate dose may be considered

CYP, cytochrome P450 isoenzyme; HIV, human immunodeficiency virus; INR, International Normalized Ratio; LFTs, liver function tests; MAOI, monoamine oxidase inhibitor; PT, prothrombin time; TCA, tricyclic antidepressant.

From Refs. 13–15.

can induce arousal and alertness, but they are less effective at reversing poor judgment and motor incoordination, that are vital for complex tasks such as driving. Thus, stimulants are neither indicated nor considered a viable option to make driving safe. Flumazenil (Romazicon) reverses the effects of benzodiazepine agonists at GABA receptors, which mediate some of alcohol's effects, but alcohol also acts on many other neurotransmitter systems making flumazenil generally ineffective in reversing alcohol intoxication.

Stimulant Intoxication (Cocaine and Amphetamines)

The desired outcomes of stimulant intoxication are appropriate management of medical and psychiatric problems. Medical problems include hyperthermia, hypertension, cardiac arrhythmias, stroke, and seizures. Some medical problems are related to route of administration such as nosebleeds with intranasal administration and infections with IV administration. Psychiatric effects include anxiety, irritability and aggression, and psychosis. Psychosis may take the form of tactile hallucinations (such as the sensation of bugs crawling under one's skin, i.e., formication), visual hallucinations (usually simple geometric shapes), and most commonly, auditory hallucinations, as well as delusions of paranoia or grandeur. Cocaine is short acting, and a single dose of a benzodiazepine sedative-hypnotic may be sufficient treatment for anxiety reactions. Depending on the half-life of the benzodiazepine, one or more sequential doses may be required for amphetamine intoxication. Because stimulants are commonly used in combination with alcohol or opioids, benzodiazepines could increase sedation and respiratory depressant effects, so a comprehensive drug history and urine drug screen should be obtained. In a small percentage of patients, benzodiazepines can cause paradoxical activation and aggression. Thus, antipsychotics may be needed. Antipsychotics are definitely indicated when psychosis is present, and the psychosis usually responds quite rapidly in the absence of other co-occurring psychiatric disorders.

Opioid Intoxication

The word "opioid" is used to refer to the overall class including the semisynthetic and fully synthetic agents, but the word "opiate" only refers to the naturally occurring opioids, such as heroin, opium, and morphine.

Patients who are acutely intoxicated with an opioid usually present with miosis, euphoria, slow breathing and slow heart rate, low blood pressure, and constipation. Seizures may occur with certain agents, such as meperidine (Demerol). It is critically important to monitor patients carefully to avoid cardiac/respiratory depression and death from an excessive dose of opioids. One strategy is to reverse the intoxication by utilizing naloxone (Narcan) 0.4 to 2 mg IV every 2 to 3 minutes up to 10 mg. Alternatively, the IM or subcutaneous (SC) route may be used if an IV access is not available. Because naloxone is shorter acting than most abused opioids, it may need to be readministered at periodic intervals; otherwise the patients could lapse into cardiopulmonary arrest after a symptom-free interval of reversed intoxication. In addition, naloxone can induce withdrawal symptoms in opioid-dependent patients, so patients may awaken feeling quite distressed and agitated. The other critical issue is to secure the airway and breathing of a patient. In some cases, intubation and manual/mechanical ventilation might be required. This is a necessary measure to avoid oxygen desaturation leading to brain hypoxia or anoxia that may cause brain damage or death.

Overall, intoxication with any of the substances discussed above is evidence of substance abuse and is strongly suggestive of substance dependence. In all cases, it is important to strongly emphasize to the patient that this is an issue that needs to be addressed, and that entry into a treatment program could be very beneficial.

TREATMENT OF WITHDRAWAL SYNDROMES

❺ *The treatment goals for withdrawal from ethanol, cocaine/ amphetamines, and opioids include (a) a determination if pharmacologic treatment of withdrawal symptoms is necessary, (b) management of medical manifestations of withdrawal, such as hypertension, seizures, arthralgias, and nausea, and (c) referral to the appropriate program for substance abuse treatment.* The desired outcomes in the treatment of withdrawal syndromes are to ensure patient safety, comfort, and successful transition from treatment of withdrawal to treatment of dependence. Referral to specialized treatment for substance dependence is strongly recommended following treatment for withdrawal syndromes, because treatment of withdrawal is not sufficient treatment to prevent relapse to problematic substance use. Achieving a drug-free state by detoxification and then rehabilitation with a focus on total abstinence is the ideal outcome.

Alcohol Withdrawal

There are four different alcohol withdrawal syndromes, which differ in terms of their pharmacologic treatment and need for hospitalization.

▶ *Uncomplicated Alcohol Withdrawal*

This is the most commonly observed syndrome, and as the name denotes, is not complicated by seizures, delirium tremens (DTs), or hallucinosis. Symptoms are typically rated using a validated scale such as the Clinical Institute Withdrawal Assessment Scale for Alcohol—Revised (CIWA-Ar, Table 36–5).[16] The recommended CIWA-Ar threshold score for treating uncomplicated alcohol withdrawal with medications on an outpatient basis is between 8 and 10. For patients who score greater than or equal to 15, inpatient treatment should be strongly considered. Patients who score 20 or higher on the CIWA-Ar should always be treated with medications. The risks of not treating high-scoring patients with medications are seizures and DTs, and those with a prior history of seizures or DTs have an increased risk for subsequent episodes. Therefore, when a history of seizures or DTs is positive, the lower threshold of eight is recommended, and hospitalization is safer than outpatient detoxification. There is some evidence for "kindling" during successive episodes of alcohol withdrawal, such that symptom severity and complications increase with additional withdrawal episodes. Thus, some authors recommend routinely using medications when the CIWA-Ar score is in the 8 to 10 range.

Benzodiazepines are the evidence-based treatment of choice for uncomplicated alcohol withdrawal.[17] Barbiturates are not recommended because of their low therapeutic index due to respiratory depression. Some of the anticonvulsants have also been used to treat uncomplicated withdrawal (particularly carbamazepine and sodium valproate). Although anticonvulsants provide an alternative to benzodiazepines,

Table 36–5

Clinical Institute Withdrawal Assessment for Alcohol—Revised (CIWA-Ar)

Patient name _____

Date: _____ Time: _____

Pulse: _____ Blood pressure: _____

Nausea and vomiting: Ask "Do you feel sick to your stomach? Have you vomited?" Observation
0 No nausea and no vomiting
1 Mild nausea with no vomiting
2
3
4 Intermittent nausea with dry heaves
5
6
7 Constant nausea, frequent dry heaves and vomiting

Tremor: Arms extended and fingers spread apart. Observation.
0 No tremor
1 Not visible, but can be felt fingertip to fingertip
2
3
4 Moderate, with patient's arms extended
5
6
7 Severe, even with arms not extended

Paroxysmal sweats: Observation.
0 No sweat visible
1 Barely perceptible sweating, palms moist
2
3
4 Beads of sweat obvious on forehead
5
6
7 Drenching sweats

Anxiety: Ask, "Do you feel nervous?" Observation.
0 No anxiety, at ease
1 Mildly anxious
2
3
4 Moderately anxious or guarded, so anxiety is inferred.
5
6
7 Equivalent to acute panic states, as seen in severe delirium or acute schizophrenic reactions

Agitation: Observation.
0 Normal activity
1 Somewhat more than normal activity
2
3
4 Moderately fidgety and restless
5
6
7 Paces back and forth during most of the interview, or constantly thrashes about

Tactile disturbances: Ask "Have you any itching, pins and needles sensations, any burning, any numbness, or do you feel bugs crawling on or under your skin?" Observation

0 None
1 Very mild itching, pins and needles, burning, or numbness
2 Mild itching, pins and needles, burning, or numbness
3 Moderate itching, pins and needles, burning, or numbness
4 Moderately severe hallucinations
5 Severe hallucinations
6 Extremely severe hallucinations
7 Continuous hallucinations

Auditory disturbances: Ask "Are you more aware of sounds around you? Are they harsh? Do they frighten you? Are you hearing anything that is disturbing to you? Are you hearing things you know are not there?" Observation
0 Not present
1 Very mild harshness or ability to frighten
2 Mild harshness or ability to frighten
3 Moderate harshness or ability to frighten
4 Moderately severe hallucinations
5 Severe hallucinations
6 Extremely severe hallucinations
7 Continuous hallucinations

Visual disturbances: Ask, "Does the light appear to be too bright? Is the color different? Does it hurt your eyes? Are you seeing anything that is disturbing to you? Are you seeing things you know are not there?" Observation
0 Not present
1 Very mild sensitivity
2 Mild sensitivity
3 Moderate sensitivity
4 Moderately severe hallucinations
5 Severe hallucinations
6 Extremely severe hallucinations
7 Continuous hallucinations

Headache, fullness in head: Ask "Does your head feel different? Does it feel like there is a band around your head?" Do not rate dizziness or lightheadedness. Otherwise, rate severity
0 Not present
1 Very mild
2 Mild
3 Moderate
4 Moderately severe
5 Severe
6 Very severe
7 Extremely severe

Orientation and clouding of sensorium: Ask, "What day is this? Where are you? Who am I?" Observation
0 Oriented and can do serial additions
1 Cannot do serial additions or is uncertain about date
2 Disoriented for date by no more than 2 calendar days
3 Disoriented for date by more than 2 calendar days
4 Disoriented for place and/or person
Total Score: _____
Rater: _____

Maximum Possible Score: 67

From Ref. 16.

they are not as well studied and are less commonly used. The most commonly employed benzodiazepines are lorazepam, oxazepam, diazepam, and chlordiazepoxide. They differ in three major ways: (a) their pharmacokinetic properties, (b) the available routes for their administration, and (c) the rapidity of their onset of action due to the rate of GI absorption and rate of crossing the blood–brain barrier.

Benzodiazepines can be administered using a symptom-triggered approach when withdrawal signs and symptoms are already present.[18] In this approach, medication is administered every hour when the CIWA-Ar is greater than or equal to eight. For the shorter-acting agents, oxazepam (15–60 mg orally) or lorazepam (1–4 mg orally), the CIWA-Ar is repeated hourly after each administration during the first 24 hours until the patient is comfortably sedated. Because of their short half-life, dosing of lorazepam or oxazepam on subsequent days may be needed, and the risk of seizures may possibly (although not definitively proven) be higher. For the longer-acting agents, chlordiazepoxide and diazepam, the symptom-triggered approach is used in combination with another technique known as loading. With the loading technique, chlordiazepoxide at doses of 50 to 100 mg or diazepam (10–20 mg) is administered orally at 1-hour intervals during the first 24 hours until the patient is comfortably sedated and the CIWA-Ar score is lower than four. Then loading is stopped, and for the next 24 hours the benzodiazepine is used as needed only if the CIWA-Ar score is greater than or equal to eight, although the long half-lives of these drugs and their active metabolites usually provide a natural taper without further drug administration. The loading technique is especially useful in the hospital where patients can be medically monitored throughout the day. If vital signs are elevated in the absence of high CIWA-Ar scores, then antiadrenergic drugs like clonidine or propanolol may be used if there are no contraindications (see Chap. 5 Hypertension).

In contrast to chlordiazepoxide and diazepam, lorazepam and oxazepam are not metabolized into active compounds in the liver. Instead, they are excreted by the kidneys following glucuronidation. This is important because many alcohol-dependent patients have compromised liver function. Therefore, when treatment is initiated before the results of blood tests for liver function are known, as is often the case in outpatient clinics, lorazepam and oxazepam may be preferred. Patients with liver disease may still be treated with diazepam or chlordiazepoxide, but at lower doses. This can be accommodated with the loading technique, although hourly dosing with 5 mg of diazepam or 25 mg of chlordiazepoxide may be sufficient.

Oxazepam is available in oral form only, so it is useful only for uncomplicated withdrawal. Other benzodiazepines are available in injectable form and will be further described below. Diazepam and lorazepam are more lipophilic than chlordiazepoxide and oxazepam, resulting in quicker GI absorption and passage across the blood–brain barrier, which makes them valuable in an inpatient setting, especially to treat or prevent seizures. However, their faster onset of action may be associated with feeling high, which can be a disadvantage of their use.

▶ Alcohol Withdrawal Seizures

Alcohol withdrawal seizures (AWS) are a medical emergency and should be treated in an inpatient setting. Withdrawal seizures are usually few in number and generalized. The occurrence of focal seizures or status epilepticus may suggest another etiology. Management consists of keeping the airway open and preventing self-injury during convulsions. Benzodiazepines are the treatment of choice. IV diazepam 5 to 10 mg is preferred to terminate a seizure in progress if IV access is available. The dose may be repeated in 5 minutes if seizures persist. Alternatively, lorazepam 4 mg may be given IM, followed by insertion of an IV line when convulsive movements have subsided. In the event of a recurrent seizure, lorazepam 2 mg IV may be administered if the patient already received IM lorazepam. IM use of diazepam or chlordiazepoxide should be avoided because of erratic absorption that complicates the timing of subsequent doses and can result in delayed oversedation. IV benzodiazepines may depress respiration, so they should be administered only when and where advanced cardiopulmonary support is readily available. When the patient becomes conscious enough to take medication orally, then treatment may continue using the loading procedure for diazepam or the symptom-triggered technique for lorazepam as described above. Electrolyte imbalances can contribute to seizures and should be corrected if they exist. IV magnesium sulfate should be given in addition to benzodiazepine treatment. As with alcohol intoxication, thiamine should be given IV or IM at 100 mg daily for at least 3 days to prevent precipitation of an acute Wernicke's encephalopathy, although some guidelines recommend higher doses (250 mg daily parenterally for 3–5 days) for patients with signs of malnutrition or a history of not eating properly.[19] Still higher doses of thiamine (500 mg three times daily parenterally for at least 2 days followed by 250 mg IM or IV daily for 5 days) have been recommended to treat suspected or diagnosed cases of Wernicke's encephalopathy and to prevent the development of Korsakoff's syndrome.[19] In addition, thiamine administration should always precede administration of any dextrose-containing IV fluids.

▶ Alcohol Withdrawal Delirium (Delirium Tremens)

DTs are another medical emergency that require hospitalization in order to prevent mortality. Parenterally administered benzodiazepines are the treatment of choice.[20] DTs are characterized by hallucinations, delirium, severe agitation, fever, elevations of blood pressure and heart rate, and possible cardiac arrhythmias. A sample regimen consists of diazepam 5 mg IV (at 2.5 mg/min) every 5 to 10 minutes until "light somnolence" is achieved, referring to a tendency to fall asleep without stimulation or a light stage of sleep from which the patient is easily awakened. If the first two doses of diazepam are not effective, then 10 mg IV every 5 to 10 minutes can be administered for the third and fourth doses. If still not effective, then up to 20 mg IV may be used thereafter. Once a state of light somnolence is induced, then it should be maintained with diazepam 5 to 20 mg IV every 1 hour as needed. Similarly, lorazepam 1 to 4 mg IV every

5 to 10 minutes or lorazepam 1 to 4 mg IM every 30 to 60 minutes may be given to achieve light somnolence, which is then maintained by similar doses every hour as needed. The antipsychotic, haloperidol, is given only for severe agitation that is unresponsive to benzodiazepine therapy. The evidence does not support the use of an antipsychotic as a single agent.[20] Haloperidol may be given as 0.5 to 5 mg IV or IM every 30 to 60 minutes as needed or 0.5 to 5 mg orally every 4 hours as needed. The newer generation antipsychotic agents have not been studied yet for the treatment of DTs. Thiamine should be given according to the same guidelines described above for AWS.

▶ Alcohol Hallucinosis

Alcohol hallucinosis refers to auditory hallucinations that occur during a clear sensorium, which distinguishes it from DTs, during which hallucinations are associated with a reduced clarity of awareness of the environment. Alcohol hallucinosis is generally treated with oral antipsychotics at usual therapeutic dosages for psychosis.

Stimulant Withdrawal (Cocaine Withdrawal and Amphetamine Withdrawal)

Cocaine and amphetamine withdrawal are grouped together because their symptom profiles as described in *DSM-IV-TR*[8] are identical, and the physiologic basis of their withdrawal syndromes involves the DA neurotransmitter system. Stimulants of this group also include methylphenidate, but not nicotine and caffeine, which have different neurophysiologic mechanisms of action. Although neurophysiologic alterations underlie the syndrome of stimulant withdrawal, its symptoms are manifested psychologically for the most part as a depressed or dysphoric mood. Consequently, the major adverse complication of stimulant withdrawal is profound depression with suicidal thoughts, and the major goal of treatment is to prevent suicide. Other symptoms that are commonly associated with the mood disturbance include fatigue, sleep disturbance, increased appetite, psychomotor retardation or agitation, and/or vivid dreaming—although these symptoms are neither life-threatening nor require pharmacologic treatment. Therefore, unless suicidality warrants hospitalization, stimulant withdrawal can be treated on an outpatient basis with psychological support and reassurance.

A number of medications have been studied to alleviate symptoms of stimulant withdrawal and the intense craving that may accompany it, but inconsistent results across controlled trials preclude any recommendations for their routine use. Patients with stimulant use disorders should be referred for substance abuse treatment because of the high risk for continued use either during or immediately following stimulant withdrawal.

Opioid Withdrawal

Almost no one dies from opioid withdrawal per se, however underlying medical complications (e.g., hypertension, recent myocardial infarction, etc.) increase the risk of complications and death. Therefore, it is important to manage and stabilize any medical issues (e.g., uncontrolled blood pressure, diabetes, among others), and then determine if hospitalization is appropriate. Patients with underlying medical problems should be evaluated for possible triage to an inpatient detoxification program, to be followed up with substance abuse treatment on either the inpatient or outpatient level. Rapid referral for substance abuse treatment will help "seize the moment" and introduce patients to the concept of recovery while they still vividly remember the negative consequences from using substances. Withdrawal from opioids is commonly described by patients as resembling "a bad case of the flu" and symptoms include: nausea, vomiting, diarrhea, anxiety, headaches, mydriasis, rhinorrhea, lacrimation, muscle/bone/joint pain, piloerection, yawning, fever, increased heart rate, and hypertension. The use of clinical withdrawal scales such as Clinical Opiate Withdrawal Scale (COWS),[21] provides high inter-rater reliability and clinical utility since it is an objective measurement of withdrawal severity. See Table 36–6 for a copy of the COWS. The baseline score helps to make the decision to treat pharmacologically or to observe. A score of less than or equal to five is considered very mild, and these patients usually do not require pharmacologic intervention, although they benefit from a supportive environment and observation. A score of greater than 5 to 12 is considered mild and 13 to 24 is moderate. Patients with scores in these ranges should be managed with a "symptoms-based approach" (see Table 36–7) or initiation of buprenorphine induction/detoxification. A score of 25 to 36 is moderately severe, and a score greater than 36 is considered severe withdrawal. In severe withdrawal, either buprenorphine or a full μ agonist is recommended for detoxification. Methadone is the most commonly used full μ-agonist but under current U.S. law, methadone detoxification requires referral to a federally approved methadone detoxification program. The two possible options for the treatment of opioid withdrawal in regular clinical settings are symptomatic treatment and μ opioid agonists.

Symptomatic treatment focuses on minimizing the withdrawal symptoms to help patients be as comfortable as possible (see Tables 36–7 through 36–9). This is combined with the use of methadone or buprenorphine (Suboxone or Subutex) to suppress the withdrawal symptoms by providing a μ-opioid full or partial agonist in a tapering dose schedule within a controlled environment.

Treatment with a μ-opioid agonist is accomplished with either buprenorphine or methadone. Buprenorphine is a partial agonist at the μ-opioid receptors that can be used sublingually. It is available in three formulations in the United States, two of which are indicated for the treatment of addiction. Buprenorphine plus naloxone (Suboxone) in ratio of 4:1 (2 mg:0.5 mg or 8 mg:2 mg) is the recommended formulation unless the patient is pregnant or hypersensitive to naloxone, in which case buprenorphine without naloxone (Subutex) is recommended. Naloxone was added to the Suboxone formulation to secure FDA approval in the United States. Because naloxone is poorly absorbed when used

---

Table 36–6

Clinical Opiate Withdrawal Scale

Patient's name:_____   Date: __/__/____   Time: ____

Reason for assessment:_____

Resting pulse rate: _____beats/min
Measured after patient is sitting or lying for 1 minute
0 Pulse rate 80 or below
1 Pulse rate 81–100
2 Pulse rate 101–120
4 Pulse rate greater than 120

Sweating: Over past 1/2 hour not accounted for by room
  temperature or patient activity
0 No report of chills or flushing
1 Subjective report of chills or flushing
2 Flushed or observable moistness on face
3 Beads of sweat on brow or face
4 Sweat streaming off face

Restlessness: Observation during assessment
0 Able to sit still
1 Reports difficulty sitting still, but is able to do so
3 Frequent shifting or extraneous movements of legs/arms
5 Unable to sit still for more than a few seconds

Pupil size:
0 Pupils pinned or normal size for room light
1 Pupils possibly larger than normal for room light
2 Pupils moderately dilated
5 Pupils so dilated that only the rim of the iris is visible

Bone or joint aches: If patient was having pain previously, only the
  additional component attributed to opiates withdrawal is scored
0 Not present
1 Mild diffuse discomfort
2 Patient reports severe diffuse aching of joints/muscles
4 Patient is rubbing joints or muscles and is unable to sit still because of
  discomfort

Runny nose or tearing: Not accounted for by cold symptoms or
  allergies
0 Not present

1 Nasal stuffiness or unusually moist eyes
2 Nose running or tearing
4 Nose constantly running or tears streaming down cheeks

GI upset: Over last 1/2 hour
0 No GI symptoms
1 Stomach cramps
2 Nausea or loose stool
3 Vomiting or diarrhea
5 Multiple episodes of diarrhea or vomiting

Tremor: Observation of outstretched hands
0 No tremor
1 Tremor can be felt, but not observed
2 Slight tremor observable
4 Gross tremor or muscle twitching

Yawning: Observation during assessment
0 No yawning
1 Yawning once or twice during assessment
2 Yawning three or more times during assessment
4 Yawning several times/min

Anxiety or irritability:
0 None
1 Patient reports increasing irritability or anxiousness
2 Patient obviously irritable or anxious
4 Patient so irritable or anxious that participation in the assessment
  is difficult

Gooseflesh skin:
0 Skin is smooth
3 Piloerection of skin can be felt or hairs standing up on arms
5 Prominent piloerection

Total score:_____

The total score is the sum of all 11 items

Initials of person completing assessment:_____

From Center for Substance Abuse Treatment. Clinical Guidelines for the Use of Buprenorphine in the Treatment of Opioid Addiction. Treatment Improvement Protocol (TIP) Series 40. DHHS Publication no. (SMA) 04–3939. Rockville MD: Substance Abuse and Mental Health Services Administration, 2004.

---

sublingually but blocks opioid receptors if injected, this combination is designed to minimize diversion of the drug to the street for IV use. Only 10% of buprenorphine is bioavailable if it is swallowed but 50% is bioavailable via the sublingual route. An IM/IV preparation of buprenorphine is available in the United States (Buprenex), and its bioavailability reaches 80% if used IM and 100% if used IV. The Buprenex formulation is indicated only for anesthesia and operative pain use, but not detoxification or maintenance of opioid dependence, due to the high risk for abuse and diversion.

To initiate a buprenorphine induction, a patient has to be suffering moderate or severe withdrawal, and the last opioid use should be at least 12 to 24 hours earlier, depending on the half-life of the particular opioid (the longer the half-life, the longer a clinician should wait before initiating buprenorphine induction). The score on the COWS should be greater than or equal to five, otherwise buprenorphine likely will induce withdrawal since it has high affinity for μ-receptors and it will displace any other μ-opioid agonist that is present. Also, buprenorphine should not be used in those taking greater than 60 to 80 mg/day of methadone because buprenorphine would have low efficacy; the methadone dose should be decreased below this amount prior to induction of buprenorphine detoxification. Once withdrawal is established, buprenorphine can be started at 2 to 4 mg every 2 hours with a maximum recommended dose of 8 mg the first day. See Table 36–10. The next day, if the patient is still in withdrawal, the first buprenorphine dose should be the total amount required in the previous 24-hour period. Then the dose can be increased gradually every 2 hours up to a maximum of 16 mg. By the third day, the dose can be increased up to 32 mg/day to achieve maximum relief of withdrawal symptoms (see Table 36–10 for a typical induction regimen). Then the dose is tapered down gradually to zero within 1 to 2 weeks (a 25% reduction per day

Table 36–7

A "Symptoms-Based" Treatment Approach for Opioid Withdrawal

This approach includes the use of any single or a combination of two or more of the following agents, depending on the symptoms reported:

(a) Clonidine (Catapres) 0.1–0.2 mg every 6–8 hours blocks the peripheral response and reduces anxiety (shaking, sweating, and piloerection). Patients may be given as-needed doses, maximum dosage not to exceed 1.2 mg in 24 hours. Blood pressure should be monitored prior to each clonidine dose in the clinic. Hold if systolic blood pressure is below 85 mm Hg or diastolic is below 55 mm Hg

   Advantages and limitations: Clonidine is a non-narcotic agent that effectively reduces opioid withdrawal. However, lethargy, craving, insomnia, and muscle pains are not as well treated as other withdrawal symptoms, and supplemental medications are often necessary. Patients with low blood pressure may require inpatient treatment. Avoid in pregnant patients; they can be treated with buprenorphine (Subutex, NOT Suboxone) or methadone in a government-licensed program

(b) Dicyclomine (Bentyl) at 20 mg orally every 8–12 hours up to 80 mg/day as needed for abdominal cramps

(c) Loperamide (Imodium) 2-mg capsules; use two capsules by mouth initially, and then one capsule by mouth as needed for diarrhea (max dose 4 capsules/day)

(d) Trimethobenzamide (Tigan) suppository 200 mg; one per rectum daily as needed for nausea or vomiting to help with stomach contractions and cramping

(e) Nonsteroidal anti-inflammatory or analgesic medications (acetaminophen 500 mg–1 g by mouth every 6 hours or ibuprofen 600 mg by mouth every 8 hours or naproxen 600 mg by mouth every 12 hours) for general pain

(f) Benzodiazepines such as lorazepam (Ativan) by mouth 1 mg every 6–8 hours or oxazepam (Serax) 15–30 mg every 6–8 hours to help with anxiety and sleep

Developed by K. Brower and M. Karam-Hage.

Table 36–8

Sample Regimen of Clonidine for Withdrawal From All Opioids except Methadone and Fentanyl (Duragesic) Patches

Day	Clonidine Oral Dosage
1	0.1 mg 4 × daily
2	0.1 mg 4 × daily to 0.2 mg 3 × daily
3–5	Maintain day 2 dose as tolerated
6+	Decrease dose by 0.1–0.2 mg/day; reduce nighttime dose last

Developed by K. Brower and M. Karam-Hage.

Table 36–9

Sample Regimen of Clonidine for Withdrawal From Methadone (Up to 20–30 mg/Day) or Equivalent Fentanyl (Duragesic) Patches

Day	Clonidine Oral Dosage
1	0.1 mg 4 × daily
2	0.1 mg 4 × daily to 0.2 mg 3 × daily
3	0.1 mg 4 × daily to 0.2 mg 4 × daily
4–10	Maintain on day 3 dose
11+	Decrease by 0.2 mg/day; reduce nighttime dose last

Developed by K. Brower and M. Karam-Hage.

Table 36–10

Sample Regimen[a] for Buprenorphine Induction Treatment of Opioid Withdrawal

Day	Buprenorphine Oral Dosage
1	2 mg every 2 hours (max 8 mg on first day)
2	Start by total dose of day 1, with additional 2 mg every 2 hours (max 16 mg)
3	Start by total dose of day 2, with additional 4 mg every 2 hours (max 32 mg)
4–5	Maintain on dose required to alleviate withdrawal symptoms
6+	Decrease dose by 25% each day (or less if patient does not tolerate 25%)

[a]For withdrawal from any opioid including fentanyl (Duragesic) patches.

From Ref. 21.

▶ General Patient Guidelines for Outpatient Opioid Detoxification

When treating opioid withdrawal with pharmacologic agents, patient safety is the highest priority. The first step is to educate patients about the course of withdrawal. Symptoms peak at around 5 to 7 days and may last up to 2 weeks. Patients also should be advised regarding the side effects of the drugs used to detoxify. For instance, clonidine causes dizziness from low blood pressure, sedation (which may impair driving or operating heavy machinery), and dry mouth. There is also an overdose potential if clonidine is mixed with opioids or other CNS sedatives or antihypertensives. The risk of these adverse events needs to be balanced with potential benefits. The side effects of buprenorphine include constipation (most commonly), sedation, and headaches. It should also be noted that there is a potential for serious overdose when buprenorphine is mixed with benzodiazepines or other sedative-hypnotics. The risk of developing physiologic tolerance to buprenorphine is high if it is used for prolonged periods. In this case, buprenorphine should be slowly tapered to discontinuation. However, withdrawal from buprenorphine is easier and less severe than withdrawal from a pure agonist, such as methadone.

is a general rule of thumb). Methadone, can also be used for opioid detoxification, however, in the United States, this can be done only at a federally approved methadone clinic. Because this drug cannot legally be used for opioid detoxification by the general clinician, methadone detoxification regimens will not be covered here, as they are available elsewhere.[22]

Successful transition from treatment of withdrawal to treatment of opioid dependence in a rehabilitation setting is the most important challenge for a clinician. Patients often think that all they need is detoxification, but this is not the case because a successful outcome is tied to successful rehabilitation and acquiring recovery skills after detoxification. This goal can be accomplished by either achieving detoxification on site during rehabilitation or by quick and seamless transition of the patient from detoxification to a rehabilitation program. The more time that elapses between the two, the greater the likelihood of failure and return to drug use. This transition is especially important for patients who have engaged in ultrarapid opioid detoxification using naltrexone or naloxone under conscious sedation. These opioid detoxification regimens are experimental and controversial and they are currently considered to be risky procedures due to several reported deaths mainly due to pulmonary edema.[23]

Nicotine Withdrawal

Smoking cessation counseling should be provided to all smokers, and those interested should be directed and assisted to achieve cessation (Surgeon General Report, July 2000). Furthermore, it is now a standard of practice for clinicians to screen for smoking and provide all smokers with brief advice and assistance with appropriate medications to quit or provide referral to specialized services when needed.[24]

Symptomatic detoxification from nicotine is achieved with any single or combination of the currently available nicotine replacement therapies (NRTs).[25] Several CNS neurotransmitters, are affected by nicotine including: DA, NE, 5-HT, glutamate, GABA, and endogenous opioid peptides. In the brain, nicotine activates nicotinic acetylcholine (nACh) receptors, which are part of the neurotransmitter-gated ion channel family and have crucial neuromodulatory roles in the CNS.[26] Nicotine dependence is assessed using the Fagerström test for nicotine dependence, and a score of greater than or equal to 4 is indicative of physical dependence on nicotine.[27] Nicotine withdrawal can be measured using any of the available scales (e.g., the Wisconsin scale for nicotine withdrawal). In the United States, the FDA does not have the authority to regulate tobacco products; however, it does regulate all NRT formulations. Some of the NRTs are prescription-only (Rx), and some are available without prescription; others are available in both forms. The FDA has approved the following NRTs: polacrilex gum (nonprescription), patches (16- or 24-hour; Rx and nonprescription), nasal spray (Rx), buccal inhaler (puffer; Rx), flavored gum (nonprescription), and lozenges (nonprescription). Table 36–11 shows NRT and other smoking cessation products. Non-nicotine medications that are thought to be helpful for craving and maybe even withdrawal from nicotine include sustained release bupropion (Zyban or Wellbutrin-SR), varenicline (Chantix or Champix), nortriptyline (Pamelor or Aventyl), and clonidine (Catapres) (see Table 36–11 for specific details and dosing). The sustained release form of the antidepressant bupropion was approved by the FDA with a new name (Zyban) for the treatment of tobacco dependence. It is started 1 to 2 weeks before the quit date. It is begun at 150 mg/day for 3 to 7 days and then increased to 300 mg/day (divided into two doses). Bupropion blocks reuptake of DA and NE. Additionally, it acts as a noncompetitive antagonist on a high-affinity nACh receptor. It reduces nicotine reinforcement, withdrawal, and craving.[28] Doubling up the NRTs, i.e., double patch or adding NRTs to each other, is a more effective strategy for certain refractory smokers than either strategy used alone.[29] Studies have also suggested that NRTs are safe in certain high-risk patients, such as those with cardiac diseases (i.e., postmyocardial infarction) and pregnant smokers, as long as the risk-to-benefit ratio is favorable. The FDA has approved varenicline, (Chantix), which is a $\alpha_4\beta_2$ nACh partial agonist. Varenicline decreases withdrawal and craving and prevents reinforcing effects of nicotine if the patient relapses, and is at least as effective as bupropion in clinical trials.[30] It is started 1 week before the quit date. It is begun at 0.5 mg daily for days 1 to 3, then 0.5 mg twice daily for days 4 to 7, then 1 mg twice daily.

Second-line pharmacotherapies include nortriptyline and clonidine. Clonidine exhibits modest efficacy in smoking cessation trials; two meta-analyses that included a total of 13 placebo-controlled clinical trials indicate that it is superior to placebo, with odds ratios of 2.4 (1.7–32.8) and 2.0 (1.3–3.0).[31] Several tricyclic antidepressants (TCAs) that inhibit the reuptake of NE and 5-HT, such as nortriptyline, might facilitate smoking cessation, either alone or in combination with behavioral treatment. However, TCAs have significant disadvantages, including a significant anticholinergic burden, cardiac side effects, and possible lethality in overdose.[32]

Table 36–11

Pharmacotherapies for Smoking Cessation

Medication	Dose Range and Use
Nicotine patch (transdermal)	7–22 mg/day (started at 21 mg/day × 2 weeks then 14 mg/day × 2 weeks then 7 mg/day)
Nicotine gum (buccal)	20–40 mg/day; 2 or 4 mg/piece; one piece every 2 hours up to 10 × daily
Nicotine lozenge (buccal)	20–40 mg/day; 2–4 mg/lozenge; one lozenge every 2 hours, up to 10 × daily
Nicotine nasal spray (intranasal)	16–32 mg/day; 1–2 mg/spray, one in each nostril up to 16 × daily
Nicotine vapor inhaler (buccal)	6–16 mg/day; continuous puffing up to 10 puffs per cartridge maximum of 12 cartridges daily (approx. 120 puffs)
Bupropion (oral tablets)	Begin at 150 mg/day × 3–7 days then 300 mg/day in twice-per-day dosing
Clonidine (oral tablets)	0.6–1.2 mg/day, 2–3 × daily
Tricyclic antidepressants: Nortriptyline Doxepin	Given by mouth once daily or in two divided doses 75–150 mg/day 150–250 mg/day

From Ref. 25.

Nonpharmacologic Treatments for Tobacco Cessation

Behavioral treatment delivered by a variety of clinicians (e.g., physician, psychologist, nurse, pharmacist, and dentist) increases abstinence rates. The five As should be applied by all clinicians.[24]

- Ask if they smoke
- Advise to quit
- Assess motivation for change
- Assist if willing to change
- Arrange for follow-up

The Department of Health and Human Services, in concert with other public health and federal government agencies, has provided general guidelines for smoking cessation (Table 36–12).[24]

There are in excess of 100 studies validating the use of multimodal behavioral therapies for smoking cessation, either alone or in combination with pharmacologic therapies. Multimodal behavioral therapies without pharmacologic agents achieve double the quit rates compared with controls, and the 6-month efficacy ranges between 20% and 25%. Not every smoker requires the same amount of intervention.

One of the possible future directions in smoking cessation is the controversial notion of substituting smokeless tobacco for cigarettes. The idea is based on the premise that the exposure to most carcinogens in tobacco is a result of formation by pyrolysis during the combustion of tobacco. This approach has not been embraced widely by public health and antitobacco advocates because certain diseases are more prevalent in users of smokeless tobacco, such as gum disease (i.e., gingivitis) and oral (mouth and lip) cancers. Some types of smokeless tobacco products may be safer than others, such as the Swedish Snus (widely available in Sweden and available without prescription in some states in the United States). These contain air-dried and processed tobacco that eliminates most nitrosamines that are produced by bacterial fermentation of tobacco and constitute a major group of carcinogenic substances present in tobacco. Other

---

Table 36–12

General Guidelines on How to Assist if a Patient Wants to Quit Smoking

Start bupropion-SR (Zyban or Wellbutrin SR) 1–2 weeks before quit date
Help patient set a quit date (one of the most important strategies).
Remove all tobacco products the night before the quit date
Follow-up with patient on the quit date or next day to support self-efficacy
Provide nicotine replacement: patch, nasal spray or mouth inhaler, gum, or lozenge
Identify and help educate a support person (best if ex-smoker).
Educate about the high risk for relapse and how to cope with it: "don't quit quitting"

From Ref. 24.

---

potentially promising developments in different phases of testing[25] include:

- CB$_1$-blockers, rimonabant (under FDA review)
- Combination of nicotine antagonist mecamylamine and bupropion (Quitpack)
- Nicotine vaccine

GENERAL APPROACH TO THE TREATMENT OF SUBSTANCE DEPENDENCE

The overall goals in recovery from addiction are the same for all substances, and they consist of:

- Developing coping skills—establish a balanced lifestyle between stressors and positive healthy rewards
- Developing a sober social network—this can be through 12-step programs or other mutual self-help resources
- Relapse prevention skills and strategies—the recovering addict should develop a menu of options, a toolbox of coping skills
- Addressing and beginning to process prior histories of interpersonal problems/conflicts/abuse
- Searching for a spiritual meaning for one's life

All of the above correlate with better long-term outcomes. ⑥ *To facilitate recovery from addiction, it is necessary to utilize a comprehensive biopsychosocial assessment that includes the motivation for change. Pharmacologic treatments are always adjunctive to psychosocial therapy.* It is important to remember that mere treatment of withdrawal is not sufficient treatment of *DSM*-IV-TR dependence (addiction), and that medications are always adjunctive to psychosocial therapy. Comorbid psychiatric conditions such as anxiety, depression, insomnia, pain, and continued smoking should be addressed. All of these conditions increase the risk of relapse to use of drugs. Special precautions are needed when treating dual diagnosis and chronic pain patients with controlled substances.

Nonpharmacologic Therapy

⑦ *While pharmacologic agents may help prevent relapse, psychotherapy should be the core therapeutic intervention. MET, CBT, TSF, and contingency management are the best-studied forms of psychotherapy in this group of patients.*

▶ Individual Therapy

Traditional psychodynamic therapy in the treatment of addiction often fails, however, the principles of psychodynamic therapy are still valuable and important for a clinician in order to understand patients and help them work through their mechanisms of defense, attachment difficulties, processing grief, and coping with internal and external drives.[33] Among the validated and thoroughly studied approaches are the following:

- Enhancing motivation, known as motivational interviewing therapy or MET, is designed to engage patients with basic principles like expressing empathy, highlighting the discrepancy between patient's ideals and their current behavior, working within the framework of a specific patient's defenses.

- The development of coping skills is designed to help patients cope with life events, daily stressors, and managing painful affects.
- CBT has the specific goal of learning relapse prevention techniques, such a having a ready "toolbox" to deal with cravings and avoidance of triggers that have lead to relapses in the past.
- Contingency management consists of providing positive rewards for desirable behavior and setting limits and consequences for undesirable behavior.
- Improving interpersonal functioning and enhancing social supports can be accomplished through TSF, or any other mechanism for developing a sober social network.
- Finally, engaging the spouse or significant other, as well as the nuclear family, is a very important aspect in the initial stages, as well as in consolidating recovery. One such therapy is BCT.

▶ Group Therapy

Group therapy for substance abuse/dependence includes more than three people (ideally eight to ten) who interact in the same room for 90 to 120 minutes. Group therapy provides patients with the opportunity to bond with others and the advantages of this can be mutual identification, dealing with shame and guilt, minimizing isolation and the provision of peer acceptance and role modeling, realistic feedback, and optimism and hope for future. The disadvantages are: a lack of focus on a particular person's problem, the discussion is not always pertinent to every member, and scheduling times are inflexible. It is also not very successful in small communities where people might know each other prior to formation of the group, and or for people with certain personality disorders such as borderline, schizoid, avoidant, or paranoid.[33]

Pharmacologic Therapy

▶ Maintenance Treatment

8 *Certain pharmacologic agents have been helpful in the treatment of withdrawal and in drug maintenance programs.* Remaining sober following the treatment of withdrawal is extremely difficult. This is probably related to a complex interaction of biological factors (craving), social factors (lack of employment, lack of a sober social network), and psychological factors (lack of the ability to cope with negative emotions without resorting to drug use). Long-term use of medications to help achieve a reduction in drug craving or to maintain a steady state of legally supervised and predictable drug use may have a better long-term outcome than immediate abstinence. The ultimate goal is always abstinence, but these strategies may allow time to develop new behavioral strategies and a social network within which the patient will be more likely to achieve long-term sobriety.

▶ Alcohol Dependence

Currently the three FDA-approved medications that are indicated to treat alcohol dependence are disulfiram, naltrexone, and acamprosate. Both disulfiram and acamprosate are indicated in patients who have already achieved initial abstinence. Only naltrexone may be initiated without regard to abstinence status.

Disulfiram First marketed in the United States in the 1950s, disulfiram works by irreversibly blocking the enzyme aldehyde dehydrogenase, a step in the metabolism of alcohol, resulting in increased blood levels of the toxic metabolite acetaldehyde. As levels of acetaldehyde increase, the patient experiences decreased blood pressure, increased heart rate, chest pain, palpitations, dizziness, flushing, sweating, weakness, nausea and vomiting, headache, shortness of breath, blurred vision, and syncope. These effects are commonly referred to as the disulfiram–ethanol reaction. Their severity increases with the amount of alcohol that is consumed, and they may warrant emergency treatment. Disulfiram is contraindicated in patients who have cardiovascular or cerebrovascular disease or in combination with antihypertensive medications, because the hypotensive effects of the disulfiram–alcohol reaction could be fatal in such patients. Disulfiram is relatively contraindicated in patients with diabetes, hypothyroidism, epilepsy, liver disease, and kidney disease, as well as impulsively suicidal patients.

Psychologically, disulfiram works through negative reinforcement, and drinking is avoided to prevent the aversive disulfiram–ethanol reaction. The classic study by Fuller et al. demonstrated that the efficacy of disulfiram was compromised by noncompliance.[34] Although that randomized controlled trial is widely cited as a negative study, because no difference between the three groups (disulfiram 250 mg daily, disulfiram 1 mg daily, and no disulfiram) was found for continuous abstinence rates over a 1-year follow-up period, the 250 mg group drank on significantly fewer days (49 days) during that 1-year period than the other groups (75.4 and 86.5 days for the 1-mg disulfiram and no disulfiram groups, respectively). Other controlled trials have demonstrated that disulfiram can be highly effective when procedures for enhancing compliance are employed, such as supervised administration.[35] This may be particularly true when supervised administration is coupled with receiving incentives, such as described above for contingency management techniques, BCT, and the community reinforcement approach.

The usual starting dose of disulfiram is 250 mg/day orally, and the range is 125 to 500 mg daily. Compared to 250 mg daily, the larger dose is recommended in the absence of a disulfiram–ethanol reaction, and the smaller dose is given when intolerable side effects are experienced. Dosing begins only after the BAL is zero (usually 12–24 hours after the last drink) and after the patient understands the consequences of the disulfiram–ethanol reaction. The most common side effects are rash, drowsiness, metallic or garlic-like taste, and headache. If drowsiness occurs, the dose may be lowered or given at night. Other adverse effects include optic neuritis and peripheral neuropathy. Because of potential hepatotoxicity with disulfiram including rare cases of fulminant liver failure, estimated at 1 in 25,000 treated patients,[35] baseline liver function tests (LFTs) and periodic monitoring are recommended. If serum levels of alanine aminotransferase (ALT) or aspartate aminotransferase (AST) are greater than three times normal values, then disulfiram should be withheld and the tests repeated every 1 to 2 weeks until they are normal. Once LFTs are within prescribing range, they may be repeated every 1 to 6 months. Although elevated LFTs may signal disulfiram-induced hepatotoxicity, the more likely cause in clinical practice is noncompliance and ethanol-induced hepatotoxicity. Alcohol-dependent patients are also at high risk for viral hepatitis. Another uncommon side effect of disulfiram is psychosis, which has been reported in doses exceeding 500 mg daily, especially in predisposed patients. Nevertheless, alcohol-dependent patients with schizophrenia and other cooccurring mental disorders have received disulfiram at usual therapeutic doses without difficulties.[36]

Drug Interactions. The disulfiram–ethanol interaction is described above. Depending on the dose of disulfiram, sensitivity to disulfiram, amount of alcohol consumed, and metabolism, patients may be at risk for an adverse interaction with alcohol for 2 to 14 days after stopping disulfiram (5 days on average) and should be warned accordingly. See Table 36–4 for additional drug–drug interactions with disulfiram.

Naltrexone Naltrexone is a competitive opioid antagonist, especially at μ-opioid receptors, that decreases alcohol intake in both animals and humans. There is evidence that it works by decreasing both craving for alcohol and alcohol-induced euphoria. The large majority of over 15 double-blind randomized controlled trials of naltrexone versus placebo demonstrate its moderate efficacy for decreasing relapse to heavy drinking,[37] but not for decreasing rates of total continuous abstinence. Both oral and sustained release injections of naltrexone are approved in the United States for the treatment of alcohol dependence. The usual therapeutic dose of oral naltrexone is 50 mg/day, with a range from 25 to 100 mg. The 25-mg dose is commonly given initially as a test dose to minimize side effects, especially nausea, and then increased to 50 mg daily as tolerated. An alternate dosing regimen is 100 mg on Mondays, 100 mg on Wednesdays, and 150 mg on Fridays, which is most conducive for patients taking naltrexone under conditions of supervised observation. Adherence to daily doses of naltrexone strongly affects both the days to relapse to heavy drinking and days of continuous abstinence. Because of this, a sustained release IM injection of naltrexone, designed to be given once monthly, has been marketed. A 380-mg monthly injection of naltrexone (Vivitrol) resulted in a significantly greater reduction in heavy drinking days compared to placebo injection.[38] The major disadvantage of injectable naltrexone at this time is the high cost (approximately $700 per month).

Because naltrexone can precipitate withdrawal in patients dependent on opioids, the first dose should be withheld for 7 to 10 days following the last use of opioids and given only when the urine drug screen for opioids is negative. Also, naltrexone can be hepatotoxic, albeit typically not at oral doses less than 250 mg daily or at the recommended injectable dose of 380 mg per month. Nevertheless, the same guidelines for monitoring LFTs as with disulfiram (described above) are recommended. The most common side effects are nausea, headache, fatigue, and nervousness. Injectable naltrexone is also associated with injection site pain or reactions. It is important for patients to carry a pocket warning card or wear a warning bracelet because, in the event that emergency treatment is needed, they will be insensitive to opioid analgesia unless usually toxic doses are administered. Patients need to be warned of the potential for an opioid overdose under two different conditions. First, dosing with opioids to reverse opioid insensitivity (i.e., naltrexone's competitive blockade of opioid receptors) requires very high doses of opioids that can cause respiratory depression and death. Second, chronic antagonist therapy with naltrexone may cause patients to become hypersensitive to opioid drugs after stopping naltrexone, thereby facilitating respiratory depression and death when opioids are used.

Reported predictors of naltrexone efficacy include, a family history of alcoholism, early age at onset of drinking problems, high levels of the active metabolite, β-naltrexol, and medication adherence.[39] Combining naltrexone with disulfiram had no advantage over either medication alone in one study of alcohol-dependent patients with comorbid psychiatric disorders.[36] Combining naltrexone with acamprosate is discussed below in the section on acamprosate. Combining naltrexone with CBT possibly may have an advantage over combining naltrexone with other psychotherapies.[40]

Drug Interactions. Naltrexone can theoretically increase the risk of hepatotoxicity if combined with disulfiram, although in practice this was not demonstrated.[36] As mentioned above, it can reverse the effects of opioid receptor agonists, rendering them therapeutically ineffective. Finally, somnolence and lethargy have been reported in combination with the antipsychotic, thioridazine. See Table 36–4 for drug–drug interactions.

Acamprosate Acamprosate is an NMDA receptor antagonist that was approved by the FDA in 2004, but it has been available in Europe for nearly 20 years and is also available in Canada. Alcohol use acutely inhibits NMDA receptors and chronically causes upregulation of NMDA receptors. During alcohol withdrawal and postacute alcohol withdrawal, increased activity of the NMDA system is caused by upregulation of receptors and the absence of alcohol-related inhibition. Acamprosate is believed to modulate and normalize the NMDA receptor system, although it is ineffective in diminishing acute withdrawal symptoms. It may also have some GABA-enhancing activity.

The efficacy of acamprosate has been extensively reviewed.[41] In contrast to both disulfiram and naltrexone, acamprosate increases continuous abstinence rates in alcohol-dependent patients for periods of 3 to 12 months.[41] Project COMBINE used a large-scale, randomized, controlled trial to compare acamprosate and naltrexone to each other and to a combination of both drugs.[42] Medical management alone was also compared to medical management in combination with a "combined behavior intervention" (consisting of elements from CBT, MET, and TSF). In this study naltrexone alone was more effective than placebo, and the addition of combined behavior intervention to naltrexone significantly increased efficacy. However, in this study, acamprosate alone or with combined behavior intervention was no more effective than placebo, nor did the addition of acamprosate to naltrexone increase time to first heavy drinking day. A recent meta-analysis concluded that acamprosate may be more effective at promoting complete abstinence, whereas naltrexone may more effectively prevent relapses to heavy drinking.[43]

The therapeutic dose of acamprosate is 666 mg orally three times daily, and it is supplied as a 333-mg tablet. It can be started at the full dose in most patients without titration. It is not metabolized by the liver and is excreted unchanged by the kidneys. Consequently, it is contraindicated in patients with severe renal impairment (creatinine clearance less than or equal to 30 mL/min), and dose reduction is necessary when the creatinine clearance is between 30 and 50 mL/min. The most common side effects are GI and include nausea and diarrhea. Rates of suicidal thoughts were also increased in patients treated for 1 year with acamprosate (2.4%) versus placebo (0.8%). If necessary, the dose may be decreased by 333 to 999 mg/day to alleviate side effects.

Drug Interactions. Naltrexone can increase blood levels of acamprosate by increasing its absorption, but the clinical significance of this is not known.

Other Agents   Anticonvulsants, especially topiramate, and serotonergic drugs, especially ondansetron, showed promise in initial, well-designed, randomized, controlled trials.[44] Further studies are needed. Buspirone is well-studied, but results are inconsistent. Finally, a recent metaanalysis of antidepressants to treat alcohol dependence with or without comorbid depression, concluded that any beneficial effects were modest at best.[45]

▶ Stimulant Dependence

There are no proven pharmacotherapies for treatment of cocaine or amphetamine dependence. Disulfiram, however, shows some promise in randomized, controlled trials for treating cocaine dependence at doses of 250 mg daily, especially in combination with CBT.[46] Its mechanism of action for treating cocaine dependence is not known, but may be due to its inhibition of the dopamine β-hydroxylase enzyme that converts DA to NE in the brain. The resulting increase in DA levels may counter the DA deficiency state that is believed to underlie cocaine withdrawal and craving.

▶ Opioid Dependence

In certain patients who have failed one or more abstinence-based treatments for opioid dependence, maintenance treatment might be the best possible option.

After the conclusion of withdrawal, some patients still do not feel their usual selves for a long time and may relapse to using opioids again, just to "feel normal." Long-term use of opioids results in changes in the brain, and the brain might not readily return to its prior homeostasis. Since the goal of treatment is to encourage stability, both in the body and in the patient's life, if an individual is not successful in tapering off of opioids because of a reemergence of severe withdrawal or a return to opioid use then maintenance treatment should be considered.

Opioid Agonists   The time-honored opioid agonist treatment for opioid dependence is methadone maintenance, which is beyond the scope of this chapter. Methadone maintenance can be provided only in officially designated and approved methadone clinics. The Office-Based Opioid Treatment (OBOT) exclusively utilizes buprenorphine, a partial μ agonist.[21] The effective maintenance dose of buprenorphine (Suboxone) is usually between 8 and 16 mg/day, with maximum reported efficacy at 64 mg/day. Patients receiving buprenorphine maintenance should sign a treatment contract requiring full compliance, financial responsibility for treatment, adherence to office policies, respectful behavior to staff, agreement to provide random urine samples for drug screens, and patients should bring their bottles for pill counts at every visit. In the event of failure of OBOT, the alternative to buprenorphine maintenance is a referral to an approved methadone clinic where methadone is used at minimal effective doses of 80 mg/day or higher. Under the provisions of the OBOT law, physicians may prescribe buprenorphine (Suboxone or Subutex) in their office if they meet requirements of expertise in the area of substance abuse or if they receive 8 hours of approved training.[21] In either case a registration with the Drug Enforcement Administration (DEA) to obtain a specially designated DEA number is needed after receiving a "waiver."

Opioid Antagonists   Naloxone, naltrexone, and nalmefene (not available yet in the United States for clinical use) can be used to reinforce abstinence. The long-acting naltrexone is especially ideal for health professionals or others who are highly motivated or face major consequences if they do not maintain their abstinence. It is important not to initiate an antagonist until the withdrawal period is over and after 7 to 12 days from the last use of opioid agonists. This is necessary to avoid precipitating more severe withdrawal due to hypersensitive or upregulated opioid receptors as a result of prior long-term or heavy use of opioid agonists. Naloxone can be used 0.2 to 0.4 mg SC (naloxone challenge) to test if an individual is indeed abstinent and to make sure it does not induce withdrawal before giving the longer-acting oral naltrexone, although this technique is rarely used in actual practice. Most opioid-dependent patients will be honest about how recently they have used when (a) they understand that severe withdrawal is a consequence of premature naltrexone administration, and (b) a urine drug test is obtained.

Patient Encounter 3

A 19-year-old man has undergone detoxification of his three-bags-per-day addiction to heroin. The detoxification regimen began when he had been heroin-free for 24 hours and was undergoing some mild withdrawal symptoms. He was begun on 8 mg daily of sublingual buprenorphine and the dose of buprenorphine was slowly tapered off during the next 4 weeks. He had begun snorting heroin at about 15 years of age and eventually had progressed to injecting his daily heroin. He dropped out of high school at 17 years of age, prior to graduation, and has never worked, except once in a fast-food restaurant for a 2-week period. Since achieving abstinence he has come to realize that he has no legal means of earning a living and he is reluctant to return home to his parents because they have recently divorced. He feels he is worthless and has wasted his life up to now.

What are the most immediate concerns regarding this young man's newly achieved abstinence?

How can he be helped to maintain abstinence?

OUTCOME EVALUATION

To determine immediate treatment outcomes for patients with intoxication and withdrawal syndromes, evaluate parameters such as blood pressure, heart rate, respirations, and body temperature as well as mental state. Choose from a number of validated and standardized rating scales to monitor the responsiveness of withdrawal syndromes to medical treatment. To determine the overall effectiveness of your health system for the treatment of substance abuse and dependence, you could monitor outcomes using sentinel events such as the rates of cardiopulmonary arrest, seizures, discharges against medical advice, patient violence, and use of physical restraints. The ultimate goal should be to enable the transition of patients to formal substance abuse treatment when indicated because this is the optimal outcome of treatment for substance-induced intoxications and withdrawals.

⑨ *A major component of successful treatment of addiction is to continue monitoring the use of medications designed to decrease craving or to block the hedonic effects of abused substances, such as disulfiram, naltrexone, or acamprosate. Also, it is important to identify a mechanism for long-term support of sobriety that might be appropriate for a specific individual such as AA, a spiritual group, or professional recovery programs for professionals such as doctors, nurses, police officers, etc.*

Important outcome indicators to evaluate postintoxication and/or postwithdrawal treatment can be divided into three major groups: decreased consumption of substances, decreased problems associated with substance use, and improved psychosocial functioning. Although it is less commonly employed, a quality of life scale can help determine how substance abuse/dependence treatment has affected your patients' lives. If you are involved in the cost-justification of services, a cost–benefit analysis could also become important, although this is more often used at the administrative level, than the patient care level. In cases where complete abstinence has not been achieved, quantify the consumption of substances using: quantity–frequency measures, rates of abstinence, and time to first relapse as determined by interviews and self-report, and by biological markers such as urine and blood tests. One example of an instrument to measure alcohol-related problems is the drinker inventory of consequences.[47] Another scale that you could use to determine the severity of alcohol-related problems is the addiction severity index, which measures problems associated with any type of substance dependence across a variety of dimensions, including legal, family, psychiatric, medical, and social.[48] If you are concerned about the effects of substance abuse or dependence on cognitive abilities in an older adult, the mini-mental state examination is a commonly used scale. Scores of 26 and higher are generally considered to indicate acceptable cognitive ability with regard to every day functioning.[49] Quantify overall psychosocial functioning using the global assessment of functioning scale, which is readily accessible in *DSM*-IV-TR.[8]

Abbreviations Introduced in This Chapter

AA	Alcoholics Anonymous
ALT	Alanine aminotransferase
AST	Aspartate aminotransferase
AWS	Alcohol withdrawal seizures
BAL	Blood alcohol level
BCT	Behavioral couples therapy
CB_1	Cannabinoid-1 receptor
CBT	Cognitive-behavioral therapy
CIWA-Ar	Clinical Institute Withdrawal Assessment for Alcohol—Revised
COWS	Clinical Opiate Withdrawal Scale
CRF	Corticotropin-releasing factor
DA	Dopamine
DAWN	Drug Abuse Warning Network
DEA	Drug Enforcement Administration
DSM-IV-TR	*Diagnostic and Statistical Manual of Mental Disorders*, 4th Ed., Text Revision
DTs	Delirium tremens
ED	Emergency department
GABA	γ-aminobutyric acid
5-HT	Serotonin
IM	Intramuscular
LFT	Liver function test
MET	Motivational enhancement therapy
NA	Nucleus accumbens
nACh	Nicotinic acetylcholine

Patient Care and Monitoring

1. By evaluating the patient's history and symptoms, determine if substance intoxication, or withdrawal are likely.

2. If drug intoxication is the likely scenario:

   • Conduct a physical exam, and obtain blood pressure, heart and respiratory rate, and body temperature.

   • In most cases, management of intoxication is supportive. The most important goal is to maintain cardiopulmonary function. If consciousness is impaired, obtain blood chemistries and administer IV glucose and thiamine (100–250 mg).

   • Cocaine or stimulant intoxication may require administration of a small dose of a short-acting benzodiazepine (e.g., lorazepam 1–2 mg) for agitation or severe anxiety. Antipsychotics (e.g., haloperidol 2–5 mg) should be used only if psychosis is present. If hyperthermia is present, initiate cooling measures.

   • Observe the patient until the intoxication has resolved (if alcohol, the BAL should be less than 80 mg/dL [0.08% or 17.4 mmol/L]). Encourage the patient to consider treatment for substance abuse, especially if this is not the first episode of intoxication.

3. If substance withdrawal is the likely scenario:

   • Determine from which substance or substances the patient is withdrawing.

   • Conduct a physical exam to determine if medical problems are present.

   • If withdrawal is from alcohol administer the CIWA-Ar to determine withdrawal severity. A score of 8 to 10 denotes relatively mind withdrawal, and the patient can be treated as an outpatient with supportive care only. A patient with score from 11 to 14 can be treated on either an outpatient or inpatient basis, with either supportive care or with benzodiazepines, depending on the presence of underlying medical problems and the prior history of the severity of withdrawal. A score greater than or equal to 15 merits strong consideration of inpatient treatment combined with medications. Those with a score of 20 or greater should always be treated in an inpatient setting with medications.

   • Always treat AWS or DTs in the inpatient setting. The drug of choice for both is a benzodiazepine.

   • Withdrawal from opioids is uncomfortable but unlikely to be fatal unless the patient has underlying medical problems. Administer the COWS to determine the severity of withdrawal. Those with a score of 5 or less require no pharmacologic intervention, while those with scores from 6 to 24 are likely to benefit from either a symptoms-based approach or the initiation of buprenorphine. Those with scores greater than 25 should receive either buprenorphine or an alternative full μ agonist.

4. Withdrawal from nicotine is treated in the outpatient setting. Symptomatic detoxification from nicotine is achieved with any single or combination of NRTs. Additional non-nicotine medications, such as bupropion, varenicline, nortriptyline, or clonidine may be helpful to reduce craving and various other withdrawal symptoms. Combining behavioral therapy with sobriety, utilizes both nonpharmacologic and pharmacologic means. pharmacologic treatment increases the abstinence rate.

5. The overall goals in recovery from addiction are the same for all substances and include improved coping skills and relapse prevention. To achieve long-term recovery:

   • Consider initiation of buprenorphine or methadone maintenance treatment for opioid dependence. In the United States, buprenorphine is easier to arrange since physicians can be approved to prescribe buprenorphine following a short course of federally approved training.

   • Disulfiram (250 mg/day) can be used to promote abstinence from alcohol. Acamprosate and naltrexone can be used to decrease craving for alcohol but are not likely to result in complete abstinence from alcohol use.

NE	Norepinephrine
NMDA	*N*-Methyl-D-aspartate
NRT	Nicotine replacement therapy
OBOT	Office-Based Opioid Treatment
OTC	Over the counter
Rx	Prescription medication
SC	Subcutaneous
TCA	Tricyclic antidepressant
THC	Tetrahydrocannabinol
TSF	12-Step facilitation
VTA	Ventral tegmental area

Self-assessment questions and answers are available at *http://www.mhpharmacotherapy.com/pp.html.*

REFERENCES

1. Substance Abuse and Mental Health Services Administration. Results from the 2006 National Survey on Drug Use and Health: National Findings (Office of Applied Studies, NSDUH Series H-32, DHHS Publication No. SMA 07–4293). Rockville, MD, 2007.

2. Johnston LD, O'Malley PM, Bachman JG, Schulenberg JE. Monitoring the Future national study results on adolescent drug use: Overview of key findings, 2007. (NIH Publication No. 08–6418) Bethesda, MD: National Institute on Drug Abuse, 2008:11.

3. *http://www.niaaa.nih.gov/Resources/DatabaseResources/QuickFacts/AlcoholDependence/abusdep2.htm*

4. Substance Abuse and Mental Health Services Administration, Office of Applied Studies. Drug Abuse Warning Network, 2006: National Estimates of Drug-Related Emergency Department Visits. DAWN Series D-30, DHHS Publication No. (SMA) 08–4339. Rockville, MD, 2008.

5. The National Institute on Drug Abuse. The Neurobiology of Drug Addiction. *http://www.drugabuse.gov/pubs/Teaching/*

6. Kelly AE, Berridge KC. The neuroscience of natural rewards: Relevance to addictive drugs. J Neurosci 2002;22:3306–3311.

7. Koob GF, Ahmed SH, Boutrel B, et al. Neurobiological mechanisms in transition from drug use to drug dependence. Neurosci Behav Rev 2004;27:739–749.

8. Diagnostic and Statistical Manual of Mental Disorders, 4th ed. Text Revision. Arlington: American Psychiatric Publishing, 2000.

9. Rastegar DA, Fingerhood MI. Addiction Medicine: An Evidence-based Handbook. Chapter 5. Alcohol. Philadelphia, PA: Lippincott Williams & Wilkins, 2005:36–75.

10. Knapp CM, Ciraulo DA, Jaffe J. Opiates: Clinical aspects. In: Lowinson JH, Ruiz P, Millman RB, Langrod JG, eds. Substance Abuse, A Comprehensive Textbook, 4th ed. Philadelphia, PA: Lippincott Williams & Wilkins, 2005:180–195.

11. Gold MS, Jacobs WS. Cocaine and crack: Clinical aspects. In: Lowinson JH, Ruiz P, Millman RB, Langrod JG, eds. Substance Abuse: A Comprehensive Textbook, 4th ed. Philadelphia, PA: Lippincott Williams & Wilkins, 2005:218–251.

12. Rustin TA. Management of nicotine withdrawal. In: Graham AW, Schultz TK, eds. Principles of Addiction Medicine, 2nd ed. Chevy Chase: American Society of Addiction Medicine 1998:487–495.

13. Hansten PD, Horn JR. Drug Interactions, Analysis and Management. St. Louis: Wolters Kluwer Health, 2008:1–1015.

14. Henderson L, Yue QY, Bergquist C, et al. St. John's wort (hypericum perforatum): Drug interactions and clinical outcomes. Br J Clin Pharmacol 2002;54:349–356.

15. Michalets E. Update: Clinically significant cytochrome p-450 drug interactions. Pharmacotherapy 1998;18:84–112.

16. Sullivan JT, Sykora K, Schneiderman J, et al. Assessment of alcohol withdrawal: The revised Clinical Institute Withdrawal Assessment for Alcohol scale (CIWA-Ar). Addiction 1989;84:1353–1357.

17. Chang G, Kosten TR. Detoxification. In: Lowinson JH, Ruiz P, Millman RB, Langrod JG, eds. Substance Abuse: A Comprehensive Textbook, 4th ed. Philadelphia, PA: Lippincott Williams & Wilkins, 2005:579–587.

18. Daeppen JB, Gache P, Landry U, et al. Symptom-triggered vs fixed-schedule doses of benzodiazepine for alcohol withdrawal: A randomized treatment trial. Arch Intern Med 2002;162:1117–1121.

19. Lingford-Hughes AR, Welch S, Nutt DJ. Evidence-based guidelines for the pharmacological management of substance misuse, addiction and comorbidity: Recommendations from the British Association for Psychopharmacology. J Psychopharmacol 2004;18:293–335.

20. Mayo-Smith MF, Beecher LH, Fischer TL, et al. Management of alcohol withdrawal delirium. An evidence-based practice guideline. Arch Intern Med 2004;164:1405–1412.

21. Center for Substance Abuse Treatment. Clinical Guidelines for the Use of Buprenorphine in the Treatment of Opioid Addiction. Treatment Improvement Protocol (TIP) Series 40. DHHS Publication no. (SMA) 04–3939. Rockville MD: Substance Abuse and Mental Health Services Administration, 2004.

22. Dole VP, Nyswander ME. A medical treatment for diacetyl-morphine (heroin) addiction. JAMA 1965;193:646–650.

23. O'Connor PG, Fiellin DA. Pharmacologic treatment of heroin-dependent patients. Ann Int Med 2000;133:40–54.

24. The Tobacco Use and Dependence Clinical Practice Guidelines Panel, Staff, and Consortium Representatives. A clinical practice guideline for treating tobacco use and dependence. A US public health service report. JAMA 2000;283:3244–3254.

25. Nides, M. Update on pharmacologic options for smoking cessation treatment. Am J Med 2008;121:S20–S31.

26. Picciotto MR, Caldarone BJ, King SL, Zachariou V. Nicotinic receptors in the brain: Links between molecular biology and behavior. Neuropsychopharmacology 2000;22:451–465.

27. Heatherton TF, Kozlowski LT, Fecker RC, Fägerstrom KO. The Fägerstrom test for nicotine dependence: A revision of the Fägerstrom tolerance questionnaire. Br J Addict 1991;86:1119–1127.

28. Slemmer JE, Martin BR, Damaj MI. Bupropion is a nicotinic antagonist. J Pharmacol Exp Ther 2000;295:321–327.

29. Sweeney CT, Fant RV, Fägerstrom KO, et al. Combination nicotine replacement therapy for smoking cessation: Rationale, efficacy and tolerability. CNS Drugs 2001;15:453–467.

30. Hays, JT, Ebbert, JO, Sood, A. Efficacy and safety of varenicline for smoking cessation. Am J Med 2008;121:S32–S42.

31. Covey LS, Glassman AH. A meta-analysis of double-blind placebo-controlled trials of clonidine for smoking cessation. Br J Addict 1991;86:991–998.

32. Henningfield JE, Fant RV, Buchhalter AR, Stitzer ML. Pharmacotherapy for nicotine dependence. CA Cancer J Clin 2005;55:281–299.

33. Galanter M, Kleber HD: Textbook of Substance Abuse Treatment, 4th ed. Washington, DC: American Psychiatric Publishing, 2008.

34. Fuller RK, Branchey L, Brightwell DR, et al. Disulfiram treatment of alcoholism. A veterans administration cooperative study. JAMA 1986;256:1449–1455.

35. Fuller RK, Gordis E. Does disulfiram have a role in alcoholism treatment today? Addiction 2004;99:21–24.

36. Petrakis IL, Poling J, Levinson C, et al. Naltrexone and disulfiram in patients with alcohol dependence and comorbid psychiatric disorders. Biol Psychiatry 2005;57:1128–1137.

37. Srisurapanont M, Jarusuraisin N. Naltrexone for the treatment of alcoholism: A meta-analysis of randomized controlled trials. Int J Neuropsychopharmacol 2005;8:267–280.

38. Garbutt JC, Kranzler HR, O'Malley SS, et al. Efficacy and tolerability of long-acting injectable naltrexone for alcohol dependence: A randomized controlled trial. JAMA 2005;293:1617–1625.

39. Rubio G, Ponce G, Rodriguez-Jimenez R, et al. Clinical predictors of response to naltrexone in alcoholic patients: Who benefits most from treatment with naltrexone? Alcohol Alcohol 2005;40:227–233.

40. Anton RF, Moak DH, Latham P, et al. Naltrexone combined with either cognitive behavioral or motivational enhancement therapy for alcohol dependence. J Clin Psychopharmacol 2005;25:349–357.

41. Mann K, Lehert P, Morgan MY. The efficacy of acamprosate in the maintenance of abstinence in alcohol-dependent individuals: Results of a meta-analysis. Alcohol Clin Exp Res 2004;28:51–63.

42. COMBINE Study Research Group. Combined pharmacotherapies and behavior interventions for alcohol dependence, the COMBINE study: A randomized controlled trial. JAMA 2006;295:2003–2017.

43. Rösner S, Leucht S, Ehert P, Soyka M. Acamprosate supports abstinence, naltrexone prevents excessive drinking: Evidence from a meta-analysis with unreported outcomes. J Psychopharmacol 2008;22:11–23.

44. Johnson BA. An overview of the development of medications including novel anticonvulsants for the treatment of alcohol dependence. Expert Opin Pharmacother 2004;5:1943–1955.

45. Nunes EV, Levin FR. Treatment of depression in patients with alcohol or other drug dependence: A meta-analysis. JAMA 2004;291:1887–1896.

46. Carroll KM, Fenton LR, Ball SA, et al. Efficacy of disulfiram and cognitive behavior therapy in cocaine-dependent outpatients: A randomized placebo-controlled trial. Arch Gen Psychiatry 2004;61:264–272.

47. Miller WR, Tonigan JS, Longabaugh R. The drinker inventory of consequences (DrInc): An instrument for assessing adverse consequences of alcohol abuse. National Institute on Alcohol Abuse and Alcoholism Project MATCH Monograph Series, Vol. 4. Rockville, MD: National Institutes of Health (Publication No. 95–3911), 1995.

48. McLellan AT, Kushner H, Metzger D, et al. The fifth edition of the addiction severity index. J Subst Abuse Treat 1992;9:199–213.

49. Crum RM, Anthony JC, Bassett SS, Folstein MF. Population-based norms for the Mini-Mental State Examination by age and educational level. JAMA 1993;269:2386–2391.

37 Schizophrenia

Deanna L. Kelly, Elaine Weiner, and
Heidi J. Wehring

LEARNING OBJECTIVES

● **Upon completion of the chapter, the reader will be able to:**

1. Explain the pathophysiologic mechanisms that are thought to underlie schizophrenia.

2. Recognize the signs and symptoms of schizophrenia and be able to distinguish among positive, negative, and cognitive symptoms of the illness.

3. Identify the treatment goals for a patient with schizophrenia.

4. Recommend appropriate antipsychotic medications based on patient-specific data.

5. Compare the side-effect profiles of individual antipsychotics.

6. Describe the components of a monitoring plan to assess the effectiveness and safety of antipsychotic medications.

7. Educate patients and families about schizophrenia, treatments, and the importance of adherence to antipsychotic treatment.

KEY CONCEPTS

❶ A diagnosis of schizophrenia is made clinically, as there are no psychological assessments, brain imaging, or laboratory examinations that confirm the diagnosis.

❷ The goals of treatment are to reduce symptomatology, decrease psychotic relapses, and improve patient functioning and social outcomes.

❸ Patients presenting with odd behaviors, illogical thought processes, bizarre beliefs, and hallucinations should be assessed for schizophrenia.

❹ The cornerstone of treatment is antipsychotic medications. Because most patients with schizophrenia relapse when not medicated, long-term treatment is usually necessary.

❺ Psychosocial support is needed to help improve functional outcomes.

❻ Compared to the older antipsychotics (first-generation antipsychotics [FGAs]), the more recently developed second-generation antipsychotics (SGAs) are associated with a lower risk of motor side effects (tremor, stiffness, restlessness, and dyskinesia); may offer greater benefits for affective, negative, and cognitive symptoms; and may prolong the time to psychotic relapse.

❼ SGAs as a class are heterogeneous with regard to side-effect profiles. Many SGAs carry an increased risk for weight gain and for the development of glucose and lipid abnormalities; therefore careful monitoring is essential.

❽ Education of the patient and family regarding the benefits and risks of antipsychotic medications and the importance of adherence to their therapeutic regimens must be integrated into pharmacologic management.

In most cases schizophrenia is a chronically debilitating disorder and is likely one of the most devastating of chronic medical illnesses. Conceptually, schizophrenia might better be thought of as a clinical syndrome, comprising several disease entities that manifest with psychotic symptoms, including hallucinations, delusions, and disordered thinking. Commonly, these more flagrant symptoms are accompanied by more insidious ones, including cognitive impairment (abnormalities in thinking, reasoning, attention, memory, and perception), impaired insight and judgment, loss of motivation (avolition), loss of emotional range (restricted affect), and a decrease in spontaneous speech (poverty of speech). The latter three symptoms are termed negative symptoms, and when taken together, are frequently called the deficit syndrome. Cognitive impairments and negative symptoms account for much of the poor social and functional outcomes observed in schizophrenia. Schizophrenia is the

Patient Encounter, Part 1

AC Is a 28-year-old, single African American male with an approximately 3-year history of paranoia, increasing use of marijuana and cocaine, and poor work performance. His symptoms seemed to intensify around his being caught taking money from his girlfriend's bank account to buy cocaine. Since then he has become suspicious that the police were watching his movements and that people on the street knew personal information about him. He has left several jobs one after another due to his belief that other employees were sabotaging him and that people were talking behind his back. He occasionally hears his father speaking to him but has not seen him in 10 years. He is sad and hopeless about the state of his life and very guilty about his substance abuse and stealing from his girlfriend. Though supportive of him, the patient's girlfriend is feeling somewhat frustrated by the patient's withdrawal from her and reluctance to socialize to the extent that they had in the past.

What diagnoses are suggested by this presentation?

What additional information would help to clarify the diagnosis?

fourth leading cause of disability among adults and is associated with substantially lower rates of employment, marriage, and independent living compared to population norms. Approximately 10% of people with schizophrenia die by suicide.[1] However, earlier diagnosis and treatment, as well as advances in research and newer treatment developments, have led to better outcomes for people who suffer from this complex and challenging illness.

EPIDEMIOLOGY AND ETIOLOGY

One percent of the world's population suffers from schizophrenia, and symptoms usually first present in late adolescence or early adulthood.[1] While equally prevalent between genders, symptoms generally appear earlier in males, and males have a younger age at first hospitalization (15–24 years) compared to females (25–34 years).

The etiology of schizophrenia remains largely unknown, though the evidence strongly supports a genetic basis for the disorder. First-degree relatives of patients with schizophrenia carry a 10% risk of developing the disorder. When both parents have the diagnosis, the risk to their offspring is 40%. For monozygotic twins, the likelihood of one twin developing the illness if the other twin has schizophrenia is about 50%. Many genes have been weakly associated with the development of schizophrenia; however, no clear association exists for any one gene. There is probably no single "schizophrenic gene," but research continues in the hopes of more fully exploring candidate genes.[2] Environmental stimuli or triggers along with genetic liability may contribute to the expression of the

illness. Some data suggest that intrauterine exposure to viral or bacterial infections may be a risk factor; however, more research is needed in this area.

PATHOPHYSIOLOGY

The oldest theory associated with the pathophysiology of schizophrenia is the dopamine hypothesis, which proposes that psychosis is due to excessive dopamine in the brain. This hypothesis was formed in the late 1950s, following the discovery that chlorpromazine, the first antipsychotic drug, acted as a postsynaptic dopamine antagonist. Studies have also shown that drugs which cause an increase in dopamine (e.g., cocaine and amphetamines) increase psychotic symptoms, while drugs that decrease dopamine (as do all current antipsychotic medications) decrease psychotic symptoms. A wide array of scientific work over the last several decades has revealed a more complicated picture with both hyperdopaminergic, as well as hypodopaminergic brain regions. Hypodopaminergic activity observed in the prefrontal lobe is thought to relate to the core negative symptoms associated with schizophrenia. Thus, a more modern reworking of the dopamine hypothesis is the "dysregulation hypothesis" which takes these findings into account.[3] It is possible, however, that the dopamine abnormalities hypothesized to underlie the etiology of schizophrenia may represent compensatory changes that occur secondary to other pathophysiologic abnormalities intrinsic to the illness. Other neurotransmitter systems have also been implicated in schizophrenia. Some investigators have suggested that a combined dysfunction of the dopamine and glutamate transmitter systems may better explain the disorder.[4] In particular, it is hypothesized that glutamate, possibly through malfunctioning N-methyl-D-aspartate (NMDA) receptors, interacts to impact dopaminergic activity in areas of the brain such as the mesolimbic and mesocortical pathways. NMDA antagonists such as phencyclidine (PCP) and ketamine can elicit a state resembling the psychotic symptoms of schizophrenia, including positive, negative, and cognitive symptoms. There has also been a great deal of speculation regarding a role for serotonin receptor antagonism in antipsychotic efficacy,[5] as many second-generation antipsychotics (SGAs) are active at serotonin receptors. Serotonin receptor binding may be important to drug action, possibly by modulating dopamine activity in mesocortical pathways. However, a compelling pathophysiologic theory relating to dopamine and serotonin receptor affinities does not yet exist. It is important to note that to date, antipsychotics without any primary or secondary dopamine-modulating properties have been ineffective for the treatment of positive symptoms of schizophrenia.

CLINICAL PRESENTATION AND DIAGNOSIS

People with schizophrenia may appear uncooperative, suspicious, hostile, anxious, or aggressive due to their misinterpretation of reality. They may have poor hygiene and

Clinical Presentation of Schizophrenia

General

❶ *Schizophrenia is a chronic disorder of thought and affect, causing a significant disturbance in the individual's ability to function vocationally and interpersonally.* The onset of symptoms in most cases is insidious, usually preceded by a prodromal phase characterized by gradual social withdrawal, diminished interests, changes in appearance and hygiene, changes in cognition, and bizarre or odd behaviors. Despite the tendency of the media to portray a stereotype, the clinical presentation of a person with schizophrenia is extremely varied. Hallmark symptoms include psychotic symptoms, negative symptoms, and cognitive impairments that last for at least 6 months.

Symptoms

Psychotic symptoms: These symptoms are sometimes called positive symptoms, as they are "added on to" a person's normal experience. They may include hallucinations (distortions or exaggeration of perception), delusions (fixed false beliefs), and thought disorder (illogical thought and speech). Hallucinations, most frequently auditory, can also be visual, olfactory, gustatory, and tactile. Auditory hallucinations may be experienced as voices or as thoughts that feel distinct from the person's own thoughts. The content of the hallucinations is variable but often they are threatening or commanding (i.e., commanding the person to perform a particular action). Patients may feel compelled to perform the commanded task or may experience much anxiety when they do not. Delusions frequently involve fixed false beliefs despite invalidating evidence, and may be bizarre in nature. Often

they have paranoid themes, which may make the patient suspicious of others. The characteristic thought disorder of schizophrenia includes loosening of associations, tangentiality, thought blocking, concreteness, circumstantiality, and perseveration. Thinking and speech may be incomprehensible and illogical. Subtle disturbances in associative thinking may develop years before disorganized thinking (formal thought disorder).

Negative symptoms: So called because they are qualities "taken away" from the personality, include impoverished speech and thinking, lack of social drive, flatness of emotional expression, and apathy. Though quite ubiquitous, these symptoms are difficult to evaluate because they occur in a continuum with normality, and can be due to secondary causes, including medication side effects, mood disorder, environmental understimulation, or demoralization. When due to schizophrenia itself, they are termed primary negative symptoms or deficit symptoms. The best strategy for differentiating primary from secondary negative symptoms is to observe for their persistence over time, despite efforts at resolving the other causes. Approximately 10% to 15% of people with schizophrenia may present primarily with negative symptoms; these people may be referred to as having a deficit syndrome.

Cognitive symptoms: Neuropsychological research shows that patients with schizophrenia show abnormalities in the areas of attention, processing speed, verbal and visual memory, working memory, and problem solving. There is a loss of, on average, one standard deviation of preillness IQ, with the average IQ between 80 and 84.

appear unkempt, as psychosis, as well as depressive symptoms, may lead to impaired self-care. Sleep and appetite are often disturbed. People with schizophrenia often have difficulty living independently in the community and have difficulty forming close relationships with others. Additionally, they have problems with initiating or maintaining employment. Comorbid medical disorders, such as type 2 diabetes and chronic obstructive pulmonary disease, are prevalent in schizophrenia due to sedentary lifestyles, poor dietary habits leading to obesity, and/or heavy cigarette smoking. Approximately 85% of people with schizophrenia smoke, and approximately 50% use drugs and alcohol, rates that are much higher than in the general population.[6]

❶ *A diagnosis of schizophrenia is made clinically, as there are no psychological assessments, brain imaging, or laboratory examinations that confirm the diagnosis.*

Biological markers are being investigated, but currently, the diagnosis is made by ruling out other causes of psychosis and meeting specified diagnostic criteria that are based on symptoms and functioning. Family history of psychiatric

disorders is helpful in supporting the diagnosis. The commonly accepted diagnostic criteria for schizophrenia are from the *Diagnostic and Statistical Manual of Mental Disorders*, Fourth Edition, Text Revision (*DSM*-IV-TR)[7] (Table 37–1).

COURSE AND PROGNOSIS

The onset of psychosis, whether insidious or acute, is marked by difficulties for patients, families, and clinicians. The severity of symptoms may be denied, and the nature of behavioral disturbances may be misunderstood. Patients may try to keep symptoms hidden from family and friends; they may also isolate themselves from social support networks. The gradual development of psychosis, combined with the frequent misunderstanding of symptoms, generally leads to a substantial time period between symptom onset and diagnosis and treatment. While not unequivocal, recent data suggest that people with fewer episodes of acute psychosis and those treated early on in their illness may have a better

---

Table 37–1

Diagnostic Criteria for Schizophrenia

A. *Characteristic symptoms*: Two (or more) of the following, each present for a significant portion of time during a 1-month period (or less if successfully treated):[a]
  • Delusions
  • Hallucinations
  • Disorganized speech (e.g., frequent derailment/incoherence)
  • Grossly disorganized/catatonic behavior
  • Negative symptoms (e.g., flat affect, alogia, avolition)
B. *Social/occupational dysfunction*: For a significant portion of the time since the onset of the disturbance, one or more major areas of functioning such as work, interpersonal relations, or self-care are markedly below the level achieved prior to onset (or when onset is in childhood or adolescence, failure to achieve the expected level of interpersonal, academic, or occupational achievement)
C. *Duration*: Continuous signs of disturbance persist for at least 6 months. This 6-month period must include at least 1 month of symptoms (or less if successfully treated) that meet criterion A (i.e., active-phase symptoms), and may include periods of prodromal or residual symptoms. During these prodromal or residual periods, the signs of disturbance may be manifested by only negative symptoms, or by two or more symptoms listed in category A present in an attenuated form (e.g., odd beliefs, unusual perceptual experiences)
D. *Ruling out other disorders*:
  • Schizoaffective and mood disorder exclusion: Schizoaffective disorder and mood disorder with psychotic features have been ruled out because either (a) no major depressive, manic, or mixed episodes have occurred concurrently with the active-phase symptoms; or (b) if mood episodes have occurred during active-phase symptoms, their total duration has been brief relative to the duration of the active and residual periods
  • Substance/general medical condition exclusion: The disturbance is not due to the direct physiologic effects of a substance (e.g., drug of abuse or medication) or a general medical condition
  • Pervasive developmental disorder: If there is a history of autistic disorder or another pervasive developmental disorder, the additional diagnosis of schizophrenia is made only if prominent delusions or hallucinations are also present for at least a month (or less if successfully treated)

---

[a]Only one symptom from category A is required if delusions are bizarre or hallucinations consist of a voice maintaining a running commentary on the person's behavior or thoughts, or two or more voices conversing. Adapted from Ref. 7.

prognosis. Therefore, the first challenge of optimal therapy is to move treatment initiation closer to the onset of psychosis.

Although the course of schizophrenia is variable, the long-term prognosis for independent function is often poor. The course of illness is marked by intermittent acute psychotic episodes with a downward decline in psychosocial functioning. Over time, a patient may become more withdrawn, bizarre, and nonfunctional. Complete return to full premorbid functioning is uncommon. Many of the more dramatic and acute symptoms fade with time, but severe residual symptoms may persist. Family and friends often find this illness difficult to interpret and understand. Involvement with the law is fairly common for misdemeanors such as vagrancy, loitering, and disturbing the peace. The overall life expectancy is shortened primarily due to suicide, accidents, and the inability of self-care. The lifetime risk of suicide for people with schizophrenia is about 10%.[8] Persistent compliance with a tolerable drug regimen improves prognosis, though relapse without medication exceeds 50% annually.

TREATMENT

Desired Outcomes

❷ *The goal is for people with schizophrenia to receive, as early in their course as possible, comprehensive treatment designed to achieve functional outcomes. While in the past, the primary* *treatment goal was to decrease positive symptoms and the associated hostile and aggressive behaviors, newer approaches to treatment have a wider focus, including positive, negative, depressive, and anxious symptoms, as well as preserving cognition. The aim is to not only reduce symptomatology and psychotic relapses, but also to improve functional and social outcomes.*[9] It is important to keep in mind that some symptoms respond earlier than others. Combativeness, hostility, sleep disturbances, appetite, and hallucinations may be some of the first symptoms to improve. Improvements in negative symptoms, cognitive functioning, social skills, and judgment generally require a longer period to improve.

Over the past few years, partial recovery and remission have become an increasingly prominent paradigm for treatment of schizophrenia. A range of interventions must be incorporated into long-term treatment strategies, including pharmacologic interventions and psychosocial therapies. Current treatment planning is increasingly focused on functional outcomes by providing treatment and recovery-oriented services to people with schizophrenia. Also, implementation of evidence-based practice, whereby new information from the published literature gets incorporated into clinicians' prescribing behavior, has led to the use of interventions that promote a remission or recovery attitude.[10] Moreover, recent attempts have been made to address and measure patient satisfaction with treatments and instill hope and optimism in order to attempt to empower patients. Unfortunately, this new paradigm is in the earliest stages of implementation, and

Patient Encounter, Part 2

Past Psychiatric History: Though AC describes himself as being depressed "all my life" and remembers that he felt able to read peoples' minds in high school, he denied prior psychiatric treatment until his first hospitalization 2 years ago at the height of his paranoia. At that time, he believed there was a conspiracy against him. He lived in constant fear that his phone was tapped and his home was bugged. He felt he was being watched in public places, and therefore he began avoiding going out. He experienced voices commenting on his behavior and believed the television was talking to him and that shows were about him. At times he felt his "brain was being squeezed" for information, so that his mind was being read. He believed his girlfriend was having affairs, and he could not be reassured. He reported decreased appetite, difficulty sleeping, and suicidal ideation. His toxicology screen and blood alcohol test in the emergency department were negative. In the hospital he was given a diagnosis of major depressive disorder with psychotic features. He was started on olanzapine 10 mg/day for psychosis and fluoxetine 20 mg/day for depression, with some improvement.

Past Medical History: He has no history of medical illness, head trauma, or seizure disorder.

Social History: He grew up in an upper middle class family, completed high school, and entered the Navy where he was discharged dishonorably due to not following rules. He began using alcohol in high school and continued to use other substances intermittently since then. He has held several jobs, the longest for 6 months. He thinks he might apply for disability.

Family Psychiatric History: His father had an alcohol problem.

Mental Status Exam

Appearance: Nicely dressed and groomed. No abnormal movements. Poor eye contact
Speech: Quiet and somewhat monotonous
Mood: Nervous
Affect: Guarded and mildly anxious with restricted range
Thought content: Adequate historian but with a tendency to leave out detail. Experiences hearing others call his name, and interpreting the car lights coming down his street as meaning people are out to get him. He denies suicidal or homicidal thoughts
Thought processes: Logical but vague
Cognition: Grossly intact
Insight and judgment: Mixed, as he can at times question his thinking, but at other times has full conviction of his beliefs. He is currently taking his medication and cooperating with the evaluation appointments

Given this additional information, how has your differential diagnosis changed?

What are the goals of outpatient treatment?

What pitfalls are likely to occur during outpatient treatment?

---

despite these advances and recent treatment improvements, long-term outcomes currently remain poor, and many patients fail to receive comprehensive care.

General Approach to Treatment

❸ *Patients presenting with odd behaviors, illogical thought processes, bizarre beliefs, and hallucinations should be assessed for schizophrenia.*

A person presenting with the initial episode of psychosis requires a comprehensive assessment and careful diagnosis, as psychosis is not pathognomonic for schizophrenia. The differential diagnosis includes a wide array of neurologic, psychiatric, and general medical conditions (Table 37–2). Often, people present with a short history of psychopathology and cannot recall historical information accurately. This lack of information, along with frequent comorbid substance abuse, medical illnesses, and psychosocial stressors often confound the case. Patients presenting with psychotic symptoms, particularly those in their initial episode, should have a thorough medical and laboratory (electrolytes, blood urea nitrogen, serum creatinine, urinalysis, liver and thyroid function profile, syphilis serology, serum pregnancy test, and urine toxicology) evaluation, including a careful review of systems and a physical exam that includes a neurologic evaluation. At the minimum, in accordance with the American Psychiatric Association Practice Guidelines[11] and

Table 37–2

Disorders That May Present With Psychotic Symptoms

Addison's disease	Huntington's disease
Asperger's disorder	Major depression
Autism	Post-traumatic stress disorder
Bipolar disorder	Sarcoidosis
Cancer	Seizure disorder
Cushing's disease	Substance abuse
Delirium	Syphilis
Dementia	Thyrotoxicosis
Head trauma	Viral encephalitis

the Expert Consensus Guideline Series for Schizophrenia,[12] psychotic patients should have a medical workup at the time of admission to rule out other diagnoses or contributing factors.

❹ *Because early detection and intervention in schizophrenia is important for maximizing outcomes, treatment with antipsychotic medications should begin as soon as psychotic symptoms are recognized. Antipsychotic medications are the cornerstone of therapy for people with schizophrenia, and most patients are on lifelong therapy as nonadherence and discontinuation of antipsychotics are associated with high relapse rates.* If other symptoms are present such as depression and anxiety, these symptoms should also be aggressively treated. Additionally, psychosocial treatments should be used concomitantly to improve patient outcomes.

Nonpharmacologic Therapy

❺ *Psychosocial support is needed to help improve functional outcomes.* Only 30% of patients respond robustly to antipsychotics, another 30% respond partially, and another 30% have a minimal response. Patients who do respond often continue to have residual symptoms such as amotivation, isolation, and impaired social functioning, thus limiting their participation in social, vocational, and educational endeavors. Psychosocial interventions are based on the premise that increased psychosocial functioning will lead to improvements in subjective feelings of self-esteem and life satisfaction. A few of the best-supported and most promising approaches to psychosocial rehabilitation are social skills training (SST), cognitive-behavioral therapy (CBT), and cognitive remediation (CR). These treatments are mainly utilized as targeted treatments for social and cognitive impairments and as adjuncts to pharmacotherapy for psychotic symptoms.[13] Most psychosocial studies have been carried out in the United Kingdom, and findings are not yet widely utilized in the United States. Nonetheless, there are substantial data to support that family education and vocational support help to improve long-term functional outcomes.

Pharmacologic Therapy

● Generally, all people with schizophrenia should be treated with antipsychotics, and adjunctive medications should be used when necessary to treat specific symptoms or comorbid diagnoses. Medications specifically targeting negative symptoms and cognitive deficits are actively being investigated. Because each schizophrenic patient presents differently, each treatment regimen should be individually tailored. After a period of nearly 20 years during which only first-generation antipsychotics (FGAs; typical antipsychotics) were available, nine new antipsychotics have been marketed in the United States since 1990. These agents, known as SGAs (atypical antipsychotics), include risperidone (Risperdal), olanzapine (Zyprexa), quetiapine (Seroquel), ziprasidone (Geodon; Zeldox), aripiprazole (Abilify), paliperidone (Invega), iloperidone (Fanapt), asenapine (Saphris), and clozapine (Clozaril). Clozapine, the prototype of this class of medications, is reserved as second-line therapy due to its

unusual side-effect profile (see below). ❻ *Compared to the older FGAs, the more recently developed SGAs are associated with a lower risk of motor side effects (tremor, stiffness, restlessness, and dyskinesia); may offer greater benefits for affective, negative, and cognitive symptoms; and may prolong the time to psychotic relapse.*

Since the introduction of SGAs the use of FGAs has been progressively decreasing, and the current market share for these agents in treatment of schizophrenia is less than 10%. This occurred due to the touted lower side-effect profile and other benefits of SGAs in several domains of the illness. Early comparative studies used high dose, high-potency FGAs such as haloperidol and concluded that SGAs were more effective in some domains. More recently, a large multisite clinical trial ($N =$ greater than 1,400 patients) was designed to examine the effectiveness of SGAs relative to a midpotency FGA, perphenazine (the Clinical Antipsychotics Trials of Intervention Effectiveness; CATIE trial). This study demonstrated that FGAs may be as effective as SGAs when using the primary endpoint of time to discontinuation of medication.[14] Thus, while these results suggest that midpotency FGAs may be similar in efficacy to SGAs, the CATIE trial had several limitations, and other evidence suggests SGAs may be more effective in some illness domains, such as relapse prevention, affective and negative symptoms, and cognitive function. The SGAs have historically been much more expensive than the FGAs, however risperidone and clozapine are now available in lower cost generic formulations, and other SGAs will lose patent protection in the next 5 years. In conclusion, when selecting among the various agents, the risk benefit profile becomes fundamental, as all the antipsychotics are associated with somewhat different side-effect profiles.

Second-Generation (Atypical) Antipsychotics

While FGAs exert most of their effect through dopamine-receptor blockade at the dopamine$_2$ (D_2) receptor, the SGAs may work through a more complicated mechanism, as SGAs have greater affinity for serotonin receptors than for dopamine receptors (Fig. 37–1). Despite being very heterogeneous with regard to receptor binding, the overall efficacy among the SGAs is similar.[14] Recently new comparative data among SGAs and FGAs (lower doses) have reported that overall efficacy is similar between groups, which suggests a reevaluation of the place of FGAs in therapy is needed.[14] Only clozapine, however, has demonstrated superior efficacy for some patients (see the section on treatment-resistant patients). An important distinction of the SGAs as a class is their lower propensity to cause extrapyramidal symptoms (EPS) and tardive dyskinesia (TD). The annual risk of TD is considered to be less than 1.5% per year in adults (less than 54 years old) taking SGAs compared to approximately a 5% per year risk in those taking FGAs.[15] Pharmacologic profiles and side-effect profiles, however, are very different among the agents. ❼ *SGAs as a class are heterogeneous with regard to side-effect profiles. Many SGAs carry an increased risk for weight gain and for the development of glucose and lipid abnormalities; therefore, careful monitoring*

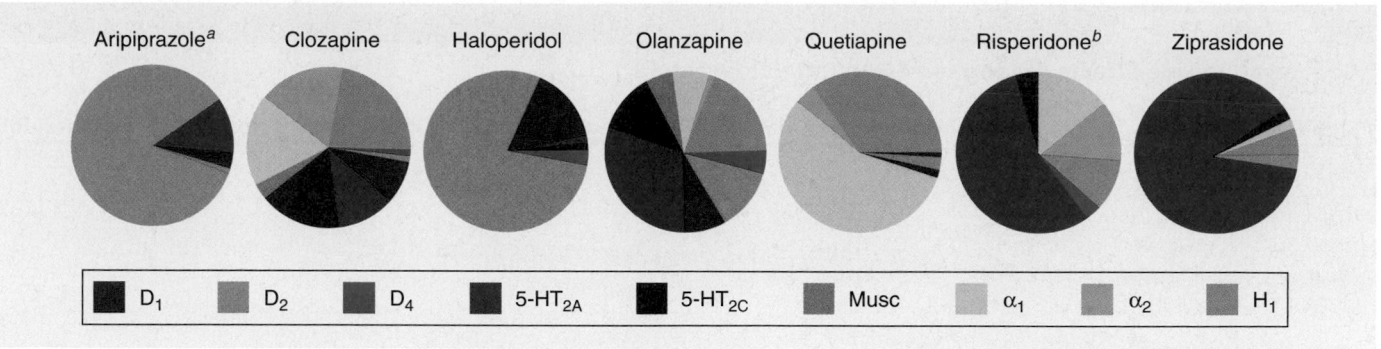

FIGURE 37–1. Profiles for receptor binding of second-generation antipsychotics and haloperidol. [a]Partial agonist activity at D_2 receptors, whereas all others are D_2 antagonists. [b]Paliperidone data are unavailable, but would be expected to be similar to risperidone. Iloperidone and asenapine are not shown here due to recency of approval. (D, dopamine receptor; H_1, histamine receptor; 5-HT, serotonin receptor; Musc, muscarinic receptor; α_1 and α_2, receptors.) Adapted from The Journal of Clinical Psychiatry and Physicians Post Graduate Press. Collaborative Working Group on Clinical Trial Evaluations. J Clin Psychiatry 1998; 59[Suppl 12]:7, and Pharmacologic Treatment of Schizophrenia. Caddo, OK. Professional Communications, Inc, 2003:52, with permission.

Table 37–3

Second-Generation (Atypical) Antipsychotics

Second-Generation Antipsychotic	Usual Target Dose (mg/day)	Maximal Dose Likely to Be Beneficial (mg/day)	Available Dosage Forms
Aripiprazole (Abilify)	15–30	30	• 2, 5, 10, 15, 20, and 30 mg tablets • 1 mg/mL oral solution • 10 and 15 mg discmelt orally disintegrating tablets • IM 9.75 mg/1.3 mL
Asenapine (Saphris)	10	10–20	• 5 and 10 mg sublingual tablets
Clozapine (Clozaril, also available generically)	400	500–800	• 12.5, 25 50, 100, and 200 mg tablets • FazaClo (orally disintegrating tablets) 12.5, 25, and 100 mg
Iloperidone (Fanapt)	12–24	24	• 1, 2, 4, 6, 8, 10, 12 mg tablets
Olanzapine (Zyprexa)	15–20	30–40[a]	• 2.5, 5, 7.5, 10, 15, and 20 mg tablets • Zyprexa Zydis (orally disintegrating tablets) 5, 10, 15, and 20 mg • IM 10 mg vial (after reconstitution, approx. 5 mg/mL)
Paliperidone (Invega)	6	6–12	• 1.5, 3, 6, 9 mg tablets • Invega sustenna 39, 78, 117, 156, 234 mg prefilled syringes
Quetiapine (Seroquel)	300–800	800	• 25, 50, 100, 200, 300, 400 mg tablets • Seroquel XR (extended release tablets) 50, 150, 200, 300, and 400 mg
Risperidone (Risperdal, also available generically)	3–6	6–8	• 0.25, 0.5, 1, 2, 3, and 4 mg tablets • 1 mg/mL (30 mL) solution • Risperdal M-tab (orally disintegrating tablets) 0.5, 1, 2, 3, and 4 mg • Risperdal Consta long-acting injectable 12.5, 25, 37.5, and 50 mg vial/kit
Ziprasidone (Geodon)	100–120	160–240[a]	• 20, 40, 60, and 80 mg capsules • IM 20 mg/mL

[a]Outside product labeling guidelines.

is essential. Table 37–3 lists the SGA agents, recommended dosing, and dosage forms available. Table 37–4 lists the side-effect profiles of the SGAs and haloperidol. Clozapine is discussed in the section on treatment-resistant patients.

▶ *Risperidone*

Risperidone, a benzisoxazole derivative, was the first SGA to be marketed following the release of clozapine. Risperidone is the only SGA available for administration

Table 37–4							
Comparative Side Effects Among the SGAs and Haloperidol[a]							
Side Effect	**Clozapine**	**Risperidone**[b]	**Olanzapine**	**Quetiapine**	**Ziprasidone**	**Aripiprazole**	**Haloperidol**
Anticholinergic side effects (dry mouth, constipation, blurred vision, urinary hesitancy)	+++	±	++ (higher doses)	+	±	±	±
EPS at clinical doses	+	+	±	±	±	±	++
Dose-dependent EPS	0	++	+	0	+	±	+++
Orthostatic hypotension	+++	++	+	++	+	+	++
Prolactin elevation	0	+++	+	±	+	0	+
QTc prolongation	+	±	±	±	+	±	±
Sedation	+++	+	+	++	+	+	+
Seizures	++	±	±	±	±	±	±
Weight gain	+++	++	+++	++	+	+	±
Glucose dysregulation	++	+	++	+	±	±	±
Lipid abnormalities	+++	+	+++	++	±	±	±

0, absent; ±, minimal; +, mild or low risk; ++, moderate; +++, severe; EPS, extrapyramidal side effects; SGAs, second-generation antipsychotics.

[a]Iloperidone and asenapine are not included due to recency of approval.

[b]Side effects similar for paliperidone.

as a long-acting injection in the United States, and is also the only first-line oral SGA to become available generically. It has high binding affinity to both serotonin 2_A (5-HT$_{2A}$) and D$_2$ receptors and binds to α_1 and α_2 receptors, with very little blockade of cholinergic receptors.[16] Multicenter registry trials found 6 to 16 mg of risperidone at least as equally efficacious as haloperidol (20 mg), while 6 mg of risperidone produced EPS at a rate no different than placebo.[17] Risperidone is also approved for relapse prevention and is associated with significantly lower relapse rates than long-term haloperidol treatment.[18] At clinically effective doses (less than or equal to 6 mg/day), EPSs are low, although higher doses are clearly associated with a greater incidence of EPS. Risperidone is associated with serum prolactin elevations that are similar to or greater than those seen with the FGAs. Elevated prolactin levels can, but do not always, lead to clinical symptoms such as hormonal problems (e.g., amenorrhea, galactorrhea, and gynecomastia) or sexual dysfunction. Risperidone is associated with mild to moderate weight gain, and mild elevations in lipid and glucose may occur. However, patients chronically treated with other antipsychotics such as olanzapine may experience a decline in cholesterol and triglyceride levels when changed to risperidone monotherapy.[14]

▶ Olanzapine

Olanzapine has greater affinity for 5-HT$_{2A}$ than for D$_2$ receptors. In addition, the compound has affinity at the binding sites of D$_4$, D$_3$, 5-HT$_3$, 5-HT$_6$, α_1-adrenergic, muscarinic$_{1-5}$ (M$_{1-5}$), and histamine$_1$ (H$_1$) receptors.[19] Multicenter clinical trials have reported that the effectiveness of olanzapine is at least equal to that of haloperidol for the treatment of positive symptoms[20,21] and equal or superior to haloperidol for the treatment of negative symptoms. The premarketing clinical trials reported no significant differences in efficacy among dosage groups. However, the higher dose range appeared to offer the greatest

benefits for both positive and negative symptoms when compared to haloperidol (20 mg). In one study, olanzapine (16.3 mg/day mean modal dose) was superior to haloperidol (16.4 mg/day) for the treatment of negative symptoms,[20] while another study found that 13.2 mg olanzapine was superior for both positive and negative symptoms compared to 11.8 mg haloperidol.[21] Among the first-line antipsychotic agents, olanzapine is associated with the longest time to treatment discontinuation,[14] a finding that suggests that olanzapine may somewhat differ from the other SGAs in effectiveness. Olanzapine has a low rate of EPS and causes slight, transient prolactin elevations. However, clinically significant weight gain occurs with olanzapine across the dosage range. The degree of weight gain is similar to that seen with clozapine and greater than that observed with the other SGAs. Olanzapine is also associated with hypertriglyceridemia, increased fasting glucose, and new-onset type 2 diabetes (i.e., metabolic syndrome), and among the first-line SGAs, it is associated with the greatest elevations in these metabolic parameters.[14]

▶ Quetiapine

Structurally quetiapine is related to clozapine and olanzapine. Quetiapine has high affinity for 5-HT$_{2A}$ receptors and lower affinity for D$_2$ and D$_1$ receptors. This drug has some affinity for α_1, α_2, and H$_1$ receptors, and very little for muscarinic receptors. The efficacy of quetiapine for psychosis was established in two controlled trials, which found that maximum benefits occurred at 300 mg per day or greater.[22,23] The most effective doses of quetiapine may be higher than 500 mg/day. Quetiapine may have beneficial effects for anxious and depressive symptoms. Because of its low D$_2$ occupancy, motor side effects and prolactin elevations are usually not seen with quetiapine. Orthostasis occurred in 4% of subjects in clinical trials. Sedation may occur but is generally transient. Mild weight gain and minor elevations in triglycerides can occur.

► Ziprasidone

Ziprasidone was developed specifically to be a compound that blocks D_2 receptors, but also binds with even greater affinity to central 5-HT_{2A} receptors. As a result, ziprasidone has a binding affinity ratio of 11:1 for 5-HT_{2A}:D_2 receptors. Ziprasidone also has a relatively high affinity for 5-HT_{2C}, 5-HT_{1D}, α_1-adrenergic, and D_1 receptors.[24] Several short-term, placebo-controlled, premarketing clinical trials led to the recommended dose range of 40 to 160 mg daily with food.[25,26] Current dosing suggests that efficacy may be greater at doses over 200 mg/day. Liability for EPS, weight gain, and lipid elevations were very low in the clinical trials. Ziprasidone is associated with some prolongation of the QT interval corrected for heartrate (QTc) interval in adults. However, drug overdose data and studies of pharmacokinetic interactions have thus far shown little evidence that significant QTc prolongation may occur. It is advised to utilize caution, however, when using medications that may affect ziprasidone metabolism and when it is prescribed along with other medications known to prolong QTc. Please see the Pharmacokinetics section of this chapter for further discussion of this topic. Caution should also be used when prescribing ziprasidone in situations that have increased risk for prolongation of QTc including comorbid diabetes, electrolyte disturbances (e.g., low serum sodium and potassium concentrations), heavy alcohol consumption, female gender, and congenital QTc disorder.

► Aripiprazole

Aripiprazole was formulated in the early 1980s to function as a potential dopamine modulator, with both antagonist and agonist activity at the D_2 receptor. It is the first D_2 partial agonist available for the treatment of schizophrenia and is sometimes referred to as a third-generation antipsychotic. This novel mechanism is termed a "dopamine system stabilizer," functioning as an antagonist in a hyperdopaminergic state and as an agonist when in a hypodopaminergic state. Aripiprazole is also a partial agonist at 5-HT_{1A} receptors, an antagonist at 5-HT_{2A} receptors, and also has affinity for D_3 receptors. Additionally, it has a moderate affinity for α_1 and H_1 receptors with no appreciable affinity for the M_1 receptor.[27] The recommended starting dose is 10 to 15 mg daily given without regard to meals. No titration is required, as the starting dose is an effective dose. The recommended dosing range is 10 to 30 mg/day; doses greater than 30 mg have not been systematically evaluated. Side effects are low with sedation and nausea and vomiting occurring most frequently. Elevations in weight, lipids, and glucose are generally negligible, and due to its partial dopamine receptor agonism, it does not usually cause elevations in prolactin. In fact, patients switched to aripiprazole from other antipsychotic agents may experience decreases in prolactin levels.

► Paliperidone

Paliperidone is the separately marketed 9-hydroxy metabolite of risperidone. The effects of risperidone and paliperidone

---

Patient Encounter, Part 3

Soon after his discharge from the hospital, AC stopped taking his olanzapine. He had gained a lot of weight, and he didn't believe the medication was helping. He continued to have difficulties maintaining employment and being involved socially. With encouragement from his girlfriend, AC sought treatment again and was started on risperidone 2.5 mg a day. He continued to experience paranoia, still feeling unable to function up to his potential at work, and still tending to be reclusive. A new therapist supported his involvement in Alcoholics Anonymous, and AC began to question the depression diagnosis. She referred him to a center specializing in schizophrenia where the diagnosis was established to be schizophrenia, paranoid type, continuous with depressive episode, single episode, alcohol dependence, early full remission; and polysubstance abuse, early full remission.

Why was risperidone selected as the next antipsychotic choice for AC?

Describe nonpharmacologic treatment strategies that may be appropriate for AC.

Discuss a risperidone dosing plan, and list side effects AC may experience on this medication.

in the body are expected to be similar, as the effects of risperidone are thought to be a result of both the parent drug and the 9-hydroxy metabolite. The neurotransmitter receptor binding affinity is also similar between the two agents, with paliperidone having a greater affinity at 5-HT_{2A} compared to D_2 receptors. Unlike many other antipsychotic medications, the majority of paliperidone is excreted unchanged. Paliperidone is available as an extended release tablet, given once daily. Patients may be told to expect to see the shell of the tablet in the stool, as it does not dissolve in the digestive tract. For adults with schizophrenia, the recommended dose is 6 mg every morning. No dose titration is required; however if needed, the dose can be adjusted at five day intervals to doses of 3 to 12 mg once daily. Side effects of paliperidone are expected to be similar to those of risperidone, including the potential for dose related EPS and prolactin elevation.[28] A long-acting injectible form of paliperidone has been recently approved.

► Iloperidone (Fenapt)

Iloperidone was approved in the United States in 2009 and is indicated for acute treatment of adults with schizophrenia. Iloperidone exhibits high affinity for 5HT_{2a} and dopamine D_2 and D_3 receptors and acts as an antagonist at these receptors, as well as the 5HT_{1a} and norepinephrine α_1/α_{2c} receptors. Doses must be titrated due to the risk of orthostatic hypotension and starts at 1 mg twice daily, titrating daily up to a close of 24 mg total daily dose (12 mg twice daily). Iloperidone has the potential to prolong the QT interval, so

Table 37–5

First-Generation (Typical) Antipsychotics

Class	Agent (Brand Name)	Dosage Range (mg/day)	Chlorpromazine Equivalents (mg)	Available Formulations
Butryphenone	Haloperidol (Haldol)	5–30	2	T, LC, I
Dibenzoxazepine	Loxapine (Loxitane)	25–100	10	C
Diphenylbutylpiperidone	Pimozide (Orap)	1–10	1–2	T
Indole	Molindone (Moban)	25–100	10	T
Phenothiazines	Chlorpromazine (Thorazine)	300–800	100	T, LC, I, R
	Fluphenazine (Prolixin)	2–40	2	T, L, I
	Perphenazine (Trilafon)	8–64	10	T, LC
	Thioridazine (Mellaril)	300–800	100	T, LC
	Trifluoperazine (Stelazine)	15–30	5	T
Thioxanthenes	Thiothixene (Navane)	5–40	4	C

C, capsule; C-SR, controlled- or sustained-release; I, injection; L, liquid solution, elixir, or suspension; LC, liquid concentrate, R, rectal suppository; T, tablet.

Low-potency antipsychotics include thioridazine, mesoridazine, and chlorpromazine.

High-potency antipsychotics include haloperidol, fluphenazine, thiothixene, and pimozide.

clinicians should consider using other drugs first. Common adverse reactions include dizziness, dry mouth, fatigue, orthostatic hypotension, tachycardia, and weight gain.

▶ Asenapine (Saphris)

Asenapine was approved in the United States in 2009 and is indicated for the acute treatment of schizophrenia in adults. Asenapine's mechanism of action is thought to be associated with antagonistic activity at $5HT_{2a}$ and D_2 receptors. Asenapine also exhibits a high affinity for other serotonerigic and dopaminergic receptors, as well as α_1 and α_2 adrenergic receptors and H_1 receptors. The recommended starting and target dose for the treatment of symptoms of schizophrenia is 5 mg sublingually twice a day. Tablets must be placed under the tongue and allowed to be dissolved completely; the tablets should not be chewed or swallowed. Patients should refrain from drinking or eating for 10 minutes post administration. In controlled trials no added benefit was seen with doses above 10 mg twice daily, but there was an increase in adverse effects. Adverse effects commonly seen with asenapine may include somnolence, dizziness, and akathisia.

First-Generation (Typical) Antipsychotics

FGAs are high-affinity D_2 receptor antagonists. During chronic treatment, these agents block 65% to 80% of D_2 receptors in the striatum and block dopamine receptors in the other dopamine tracts in the brain as well.[29] Clinical response is generally associated with 60% D_2-receptor blockade, while 70% and 80% are associated with hyperprolactinemia and EPS, respectively. This group of antipsychotics was widely used from the 1950s to the 1990s, when the SGAs began to replace these agents as first-line therapy.

Dosages for these agents are frequently given as chlorpromazine equivalent dosages, which are defined as the dosage of any of the FGAs equipotent with 100 mg

of chlorpromazine. The target dose recommendation for acute psychosis is 400 to 600 chlorpromazine equivalents, unless the patient's history indicates that this dose may result in intolerable side effects. Generally maintenance therapy should provide a dose of 300 to 600 chlorpromazine equivalents for maximum efficacy. Information on dosing and available dosage forms is provided in Table 37–5. All FGAs are equally efficacious in groups of patients when used in equipotent doses. However, individual variation does occur, such that a patient may not respond equally to each antipsychotic. Selection of a particular antipsychotic should be based on patient variables, such as the need to avoid certain side effects or interactions with concomitant medications. Previous patient or family history of response is also helpful in the selection of a particular agent.

▶ Decanoates

Long-acting, depot preparations are available for two FGAs (fluphenazine decanoate and haloperidol decanoate) in the United States. These compounds are esterified antipsychotics formulated in sesame seed oil for deep intramuscular (IM) injection. Because these are long-acting preparations, patients should be exposed to the oral form of the drug first to ensure tolerability. With initial dosing of haloperidol decanoate, oral supplementation may temporarily be necessary, as the drug accumulates over many weeks, not reaching steady state until 4 to 5 dosing intervals have elapsed. The pharmacokinetic profiles of the depot agents are useful parameters for strategic dosing. Patients may be dosed with fluphenazine decanoate on a 1- to 3-week interval, while haloperidol decanoate is usually dosed once a month. Conversion from oral to depot and maintenance dosing recommendations are shown in Table 37–6. Based on these recommendations, a reasonable estimate is that 12.5 mg (0.5 mL) of fluphenazine decanoate given every 2 weeks is approximately equivalent to 10 mg/day of fluphenazine orally. A maintenance haloperidol decanoate

Table 37–6

Antipsychotic Dosing of Long-Acting Preparations

Drug	Starting Dose	Maintenance Dose	Comments
Haloperidol decanoate	20 × oral haloperidol daily dose; in the elderly use 10–15 × oral haloperidol daily dose Generally 100–450 mg/month Initial dose should not exceed 100 mg regardless of previous dose requirements (if greater than 100 mg give 3–7 days apart)	10–15 × oral haloperidol daily dose, generally 50–300 mg/month	With initial dosing, oral supplementation may temporarily be necessary; deep IM injection generally with 21-gauge needle; maximum volume per injection site should not exceed 3 mL Available in 50 mg/mL and 100 mg/mL (5-mL vials and 1-mL ampules)
Fluphenazine decanoate	1.2 × oral fluphenazine daily dose, generally 12.5–mg/2–3 weeks	Based on starting dose and clinical response Generally 12.5–25 mg dosed at 2–4 week intervals (may be up to 6 weeks in some cases)	Can be administered IM or SC; 21-gauge needle, must be dry Should not exceed 100 mg; when dosing above 50 mg, should increase in increments of 12.5 mg Available in 25 mg/mL (5-mL vials)
Paliperidone (Invega sustenna)	Initiate with 234 mg on day 1 and 156 mg 1 week later, both in deltoid muscle	Recommended monthly maintenance dose is 117 mg (range 39–234 mg)	First two doses must be given in the deltoid muscle; following that, monthly doses given in either deltoid or gluteal muscle. Available as 39–, 78–, 117–, 156–, 234–mg prefilled syringes
Risperidone long-acting injection (Risperdal Consta)	25 mg every 2 weeks	25–50 mg every 2 weeks	Previous antipsychotics should be continued for 3 weeks following initial dose of risperidone long-acting injection Recommended to establish tolerability with oral risperidone prior to initiation of long-acting injection Available in 12.5-, 25-, 37.5-, and 50- mg vial/kit; must use needle supplied with kit, administer IM

IM, intramuscular, SC, subcutaneous.

dose of 150 mg every 4 weeks is approximately equivalent to 10 mg/day of oral haloperidol. Initial decanoate injections should be preceded by a small test dose.

Side Effects of FGAs

The FGAs are associated with a host of side effects that largely differ between high- and low-potency agents. In general, the low-potency agents are less likely to cause EPS than the high-potency agents. Of note, lower doses and midpotency agents may be associated with less EPS than once believed and similar to SGAs in clinical trials.[14]

FGAs are associated with EPS, which includes akathisia (motor and/or subjective restlessness), dystonia (muscle spasm), and pseudoparkinsonism (akinesia, tremor, and rigidity). These fairly common motor side effects are caused by dopamine antagonism in the nigrostriatal pathways. Akathisia is the most frequently occurring motor side effect, with approximately 20% to 40% of people treated with FGA drugs experiencing an objective or subjective feeling of restlessness. Roughly half of the cases of akathisia present within one month of antipsychotic initiation although the onset of akathisia many times may be within 5 to 10 days after the first dose or increase in dosage. Younger people and those taking high doses of high-potency antipsychotics are at greater risk for the development of akathisia. Acute dystonic reactions are abrupt in onset and are usually seen within 24 to 96 hours after a first dose or increase in dosage. Characteristic signs and symptoms include abnormal positioning or spasm of the muscles of the head, neck, limbs, or trunk. Dystonia may occur in 10% to 20% of patients. There is higher risk for dystonia in young male patients and those taking high-potency FGAs. Pseudoparkinsonism resembles idiopathic Parkinson's disease, and features may be present in up to 30% to 60% of people treated with FGAs. The onset of symptoms is usually seen within 1 to 2 weeks following initiation of dosing or a dose increase. Risk factors include older age, female gender, high doses, and possibly those with depressive symptoms.[30]

TD is a movement disorder characterized by abnormal choreiform (rapid, objectively purposeless, irregular, and spontaneous movement) and athetoid (slow and irregular) movements occurring late in onset in relation to initiation of antipsychotic therapy. This adverse effect usually develops

Table 37–7
Side Effects of FGAs

	EPS	Sedation	Anticholinergic Side Effects	Cardiovascular Side Effects	Seizure Effects/ QTc Prolongation
Chlorpromazine	++	++++	+++	++++	++
Thioridazine	++	++++	++++	++++	+++
Loxapine	+++	+++	++	+++	+
Trifluoperazine	+++	++	++	++	+
Molindone	++	+	++	++	+
Perphenazine	+++	++	++	++	+
Thiothixene	+++	++	++	++	+
Fluphenazine	++++	++	++	++	+
Haloperidol	++++	+	+	+	+

+, very low; ++, low; +++, moderate; ++++, high; EPS, extrapyramidal side effects; FGAs, first-generation antipsychotics.

over several months or after at least 3 months of cumulative exposure to neuroleptic medications. Severity of TD can range from mild and barely noticeable to severe. In some cases TD may be severe enough to interfere with ambulation, and may stigmatize persons taking antipsychotics if symptoms are visible to others. The estimated average prevalence of TD is 20% with a range of 13% to 36%. The incidence of new cases per treatment year with FGAs is approximately 5%.[31] TD is reversible in one-third to one-half of cases with the cessation of the antipsychotic.[32] When the antipsychotic is tapered or discontinued, there is typically initial worsening of abnormal movements. Risk factors for TD include older age, longer duration of antipsychotic treatment, and presence of EPS, substance abuse, and mood disorders. SGAs carry a lower risk of TD than FGAs. A pooled analysis of studies indicated that new onset TD incidence was 0.8% with SGA treatment versus 5.4% for FGAs.[15] A more recent review of studies published from 2004 to 2008 reported a smaller difference in incidence of TD between agents, at 3.9% for SGAs and 5.5% for FGAs.[33]

Neuroleptic malignant syndrome (NMS), a life-threatening emergency characterized by severe muscular rigidity, autonomic instability, and altered consciousness, can occur uncommonly with all the FGAs, and may also occur with SGAs. Rapid dose escalation, the use of high-potency FGAs at higher doses, and younger patients are associated with a higher risk of NMS. When NMS is diagnosed or suspected, antipsychotics should be discontinued and supportive and symptomatic treatment begun (e.g., antipyretics, cooling blanket, IV fluids, oxygen, monitoring of liver enzymes, and complete blood cell count). Dopamine agonists (e.g., bromocriptine) should be considered in moderate to severe cases.

Additionally, dermatologic side effects, photosensitivity, and cataracts may occur with the phenothiazine agents. Sedation is caused from H_1-receptor antagonism; anticholinergic side effects (constipation, blurred vision, dry mouth, and urinary retention) are caused from M_1-receptor antagonism; and α_1-receptor blockade is associated with orthostatic hypotension and tachycardia (Table 37–7). QTc prolongation may occur with lower-potency FGAs, and thioridazine has a black box warning for QTc prolongation.

Treatment Guidelines and Algorithms

Due to the plethora of choices and the rising costs of SGAs, algorithms and treatment/consensus guidelines have been developed for the treatment of schizophrenia. The most widely accepted algorithm in the United States was developed as part of the Texas Implementation of Medication Algorithms (TIMA). A national panel of experts developed this algorithm, most recently updated in 2006.[34] Algorithms go beyond guidelines, providing a framework for clinical decision making at critical decision points. According to the TIMA schizophrenia algorithm, SGAs (except clozapine) should be utilized as first-line treatment. The choice of SGA is guided by consideration of the side-effect profiles and the clinical characteristics of the patient. Treatment with a given drug should be continued for 4 to 6 weeks in order to assess response. If only partial response or nonresponse is noted, a trial of a second SGA should be initiated (Fig. 37–2). Other similar guidelines include the American Psychiatric Association Practice Guidelines for schizophrenia,[11] The Expert Consensus Guideline Series,[12] and the Schizophrenia Patient Outcomes Research Team (PORT) Treatment Recommendations.[35] In contrast to the TIMA guidelines, the PORT recommends either the use of FGAs or SGAs as first-line therapy.

Treatment Adherence

Medication nonadherence in schizophrenia is common and often associated with symptom relapse.[36] Estimates of nonadherence to antipsychotics range from approximately 24% to 88% with a mean of approximately 50%. Subjects

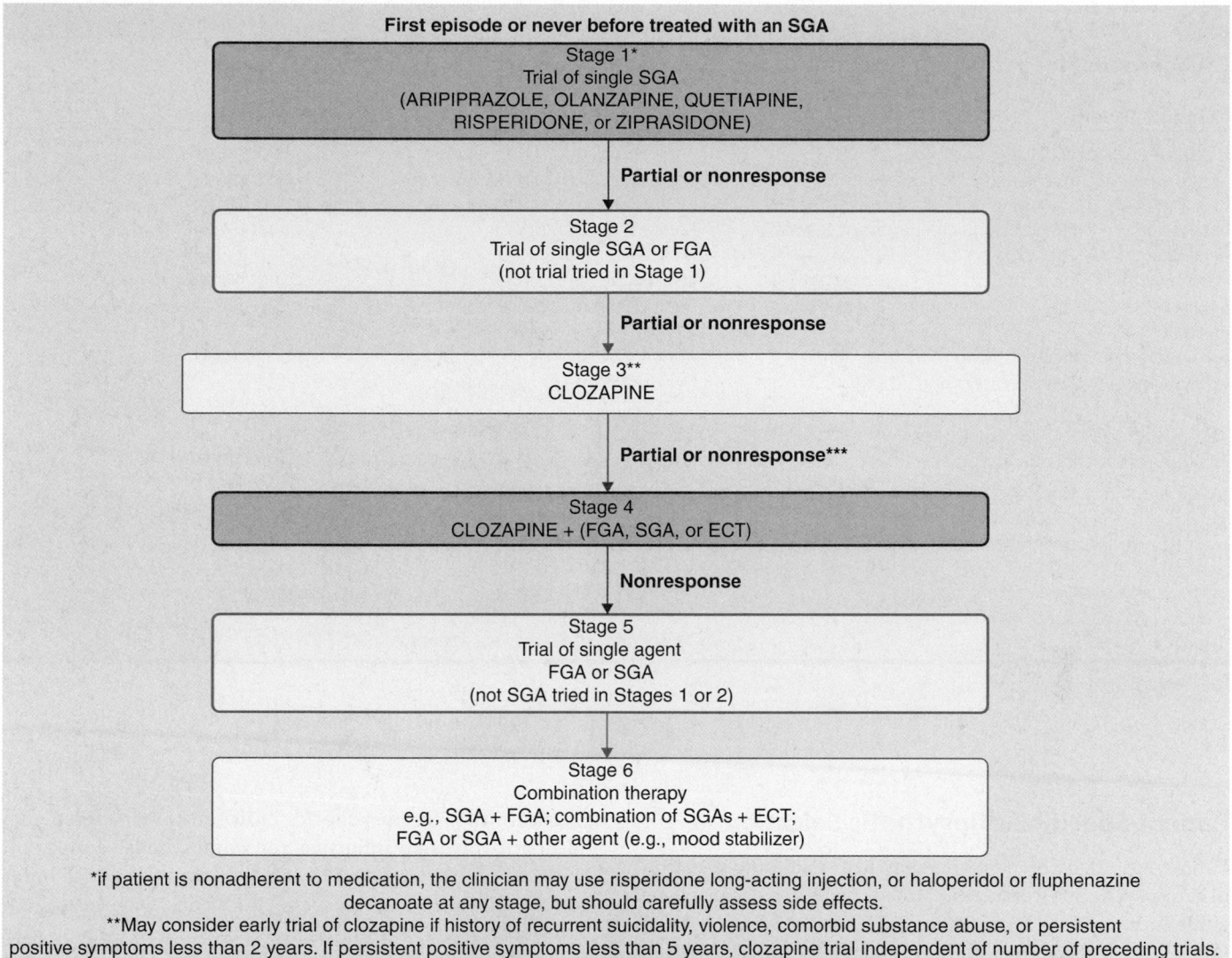

First episode or never before treated with an SGA

Stage 1*
Trial of single SGA
(ARIPIPRAZOLE, OLANZAPINE, QUETIAPINE,
RISPERIDONE, or ZIPRASIDONE)

↓ **Partial or nonresponse**

Stage 2
Trial of single SGA or FGA
(not trial tried in Stage 1)

↓ **Partial or nonresponse**

Stage 3**
CLOZAPINE

↓ **Partial or nonresponse*****

Stage 4
CLOZAPINE + (FGA, SGA, or ECT)

↓ **Nonresponse**

Stage 5
Trial of single agent
FGA or SGA
(not SGA tried in Stages 1 or 2)

Stage 6
Combination therapy
e.g., SGA + FGA; combination of SGAs + ECT;
FGA or SGA + other agent (e.g., mood stabilizer)

*if patient is nonadherent to medication, the clinician may use risperidone long-acting injection, or haloperidol or fluphenazine
decanoate at any stage, but should carefully assess side effects.
**May consider early trial of clozapine if history of recurrent suicidality, violence, comorbid substance abuse, or persistent
positive symptoms less than 2 years. If persistent positive symptoms less than 5 years, clozapine trial independent of number of preceding trials.
***Evaluate patient for other underlying or concomitant factors;
consider adding cognitive behavioral therapy and other psychosocial intervention.

FIGURE 37–2. TIMA algorithm for antipsychotic treatment in schizophrenia. Choice of antipsychotic should be guided by considering the clinical characteristics of the patient and the efficacy and side-effect profiles of the medication. Any stage may be skipped depending on the clinical picture or history of antipsychotic failures. (ECT, electroconvulsive therapy; FGA, first-generation antipsychotic; SGA, second-generation antipsychotic.) (Adapted from the Texas Department of State Health Services.)

who are nonadherent have approximately a fourfold greater risk of a relapse than those who are adherent. Adherence to antipsychotic regimens is problematic for many reasons. Neurocognitive deficits and paranoid symptoms may hamper adherence to the therapeutic regimen, and identification of nonadherence by caretakers and providers can be challenging. Frequently, there is no obvious connection between nonadherence and symptom exacerbation, as there may be no immediate consequences of missing a dose, and patients may relapse suddenly after only several weeks or months of nonadherence. Antipsychotic side effects such as EPS, weight gain, and sexual dysfunction are also a major contributing factor to treatment nonadherence, with 25% to

66% of subjects citing adverse effects as the primary reason for nonadherence.[37] Several other factors are associated with nonadherence, including younger age, delusions, substance abuse, and deficit symptoms. For patients who have relapsed several times due to nonadherence, have a history of dangerous behavior, or risk a significant loss of social/vocational gains when relapsed, treatment with long-acting formulations should be encouraged. Risperidone is currently the only SGA with a long-acting formulation available. It uses a microsphere technology that maintains stable blood levels for about 2 weeks. Dosing is generally 25 to 50 mg every 2 weeks with oral supplementation in the first 3 weeks.

Table 37–8		
Suggestions for First-Line Antipsychotic Therapy in Specific Patients		
Clinical Condition	**First-Line Treatment**	**Other Options**
Diabetes or family history of diabetes	Aripiprazole, quetiapine, ziprasidone	Risperidone
Hyperlipidemia or significant family history of hyperlipidemia	Aripiprazole, ziprasidone	Risperidone, quetiapine
Hypertriglyceridemia or significant family history of elevated triglycerides	Aripiprazole, ziprasidone	Risperidone, quetiapine
Overweight or obese, or concerns about weight	Aripiprazole, ziprasidone	Risperidone, quetiapine
Current sexual dysfunction or concerns about sexual dysfunction	Aripiprazole, quetiapine, clozapine	Olanzapine, ziprasidone
Amenorrhea or problems with menstrual period	Aripiprazole, quetiapine, clozapine	Olanzapine, ziprasidone
Cardiac arrhythmias or current antiarrhythmic treatment	*Not* ziprasidone or clozapine	
Suicidal or history of frequent suicide attempts	Clozapine	
Current or past anticholinergic side effects	Risperidone, quetiapine, aripiprazole ziprasidone	Olanzapine (low dose)
EPS or severe EPS in the past	Quetiapine, aripiprazole, clozapine	Ziprasidone
Current tardive dyskinesia	Clozapine, quetiapine	Risperidone, olanzapine, ziprasidone
History of nonadherence	Long-acting risperidone	
Difficulty swallowing tablets/capsules	Risperidone or aripiprazole liquid, orally-disintegrating tablets (risperidone, olanzapine, clozapine)	Long-acting risperidone

EPS, extrapyramidal symptoms.

From Refs. 11, 12, 35, 53.

Patient-Specific Antipsychotic Selection

Patient-specific characteristics may help guide the selection of antipsychotic treatment. Based on expert consensus guidelines, Table 37–8 provides evidence-based suggestions for SGA selection to aid the clinician in individualizing treatment. FGAs continue to have a place in therapy for patients who cannot afford the SGAs or for those who have responded favorably to these agents in the past. However, in the next few years several of the SGAs will be available generically, and cost may become less of an advantage for FGAs. New data suggest that the efficacy of FGAs is comparable to SGAs,[14] however clinicians must evaluate the risk to benefit profile on an individualized basis.

Special Populations

▶ Adolescents

Epidemiologic data show that 10% to 30% of patients with schizophrenia develop their first psychotic symptoms prior to their 18th birthday. The diagnosis of schizophrenia in children and adolescents is often difficult to make, and the differential diagnosis includes pervasive developmental disorders, attention-deficit/hyperactivity disorder, and language or communication disorders. The existence of prominent hallucinations or delusions, however, helps make the diagnosis, as they are not a prominent part of the other disorders. Fifty-four percent to 90% of patients developing schizophrenia before age 18 have premorbid abnormalities such as withdrawal, odd traits, and isolation.[38]

Treatment for psychotic children and adolescents ideally involves an intensive and comprehensive program with a highly structured environment that includes special education and psychoeducation. Day treatment, hospitalization, or long-term residential treatment may be necessary. Pharmacologic treatment is indicated if psychotic symptoms cause significant impairments or interfere with other interventions. Children and adolescents are more vulnerable to EPS, particularly dystonias, than are adults. Due to concerns about EPS and TD, it has been recommended that pharmacotherapy in children and adolescents should be initiated with SGAs. Aripiprazole and risperidone are both FDA-indicated for the treatment of schizophrenia in adolescents aged 13 to 17. Recommended initiation and target dosing is lower for adolescents than adults.

Agents with significant sedation and anticholinergic side effects are not preferred, as they can cause attention difficulties and cognitive dulling that may interfere with optimal school performance. Compared to adults, children and adolescents tend to gain more weight on these agents. Young patients should be started on lower doses than adults and should be titrated at a slower rate. Side effects should be monitored closely during initiation and throughout maintenance therapy. Informed consent, addressing the rationale for treatment, and potential risks and benefits of therapy, should be obtained from the parents or guardians prior to treatment with any antipsychotic medication, and assent should be obtained from the child as well.

► Elderly

Psychotic symptoms in late life (greater than 65 years of age) are generally a result of an ongoing chronic illness carried over from younger life; however, a small percentage of patients develop psychotic symptoms de novo, defined as late-life schizophrenia. However, other illnesses presenting with psychotic symptoms are common in this population, as approximately one-third of patients with Alzheimer's disease, Parkinson's disease, and vascular dementia experience psychotic symptoms. The majority of data for antipsychotic use in the elderly comes from experience treating these other disease states.

Antipsychotics can be safe and effective for the treatment of psychosis in the elderly, if used at lower doses than those commonly used in younger adults. Older adults are particularly vulnerable to the side effects of FGAs. Parkinsonian symptoms reportedly occur in over 50% of all elderly patients receiving these agents, and the cumulative annual incidence of TD in middle-aged and elderly patients is over 25%. With the SGAs, the risk appears to be approximately 4%. However, these data are based on a limited number of studies, and future investigations are likely to yield more specific information regarding TD risk with the SGAs.[39] The likelihood of reversing this potentially debilitating condition diminishes with age. Orthostasis, estimated to occur in 5% to 30% of geriatric patients, is a major contributing factor to the occurrence of falls that often leads to fractures, injuries, and loss of independence. Low-potency antipsychotics and clozapine are more likely to cause significant drops in orthostatic blood pressure. Antipsychotics may cause or worsen anticholinergic effects including constipation, dry mouth, urinary retention, and cognitive impairment. Cognitive impairment may lead to decreased independence, and a more rapid decline in cognitive functioning may occur in the elderly treated with antipsychotics than the younger adult population. As a result of data showing a statistically significant increase in mortality rate in elderly dementia patients who are treated with SGAs, all SGAs now carry a warning, and patients and families should be informed of this risk prior to treatment with these agents. Dosing in the elderly is initiated lower and titration is slower than in adults. Maximum doses are often one-half of adult doses.

► Dually Diagnosed

The prevalence of substance dependence and abuse among persons with schizophrenia is significantly higher than in the general population. Conservative estimates of the proportion of schizophrenic patients abusing alcohol and/or illicit drugs range from one-third to as many as one-half.[40] The most common drugs of abuse are cannabis and cocaine and alcohol abuse. Unfortunately, substance use often worsens the course and complicates the treatment of schizophrenia. Dually-diagnosed patients are more likely to be nonadherent with treatment. Characteristically, they have a poorer response rate to FGAs, have more severe psychosis, and have higher rates of relapse and rehospitalization compared to patients who are not abusing substances. Some studies have found that EPS may occur more frequently in substance-abusing patients, and alcohol use is a risk factor for developing TD. There is a growing body of literature indicating that SGAs are effective in this population, and some studies have shown a reduction in the use of drugs and alcohol with SGAs.[41]

► Treatment-Resistant Patients

For approximately 20% to 30% of people with schizophrenia, drug treatment is ineffective. A standard definition of treatment resistance is persistent positive symptoms despite treatment with at least two different antipsychotics given at adequate doses (at least 600 chlorpromazine equivalents) for an adequate duration (4–6 weeks). In addition, patients must have a moderately severe illness as defined by rating instruments, and have a persistence of illness for at least 5 years.[42] These patients are often highly symptomatic and require extensive periods of hospital care.

Clozapine To date, clozapine remains the only drug with proven and superior efficacy in treatment-resistant patients, and it is currently the only drug approved for the treatment-resistant schizophrenic. Studies have shown a response of approximately 30% to 50% in these well-defined treatment-resistant patients. Clinical trials have consistently found clozapine to be superior to traditional antipsychotics for treatment-refractory patients, and it is efficacious even after nonresponse to other SGAs and in partially responsive patients. It is often effective even in those who have had a poor response to other medication for years. Recent studies have demonstrated that it has a beneficial effect for aggression and suicidality, which led to the FDA approval for the treatment of suicidal behavior in people with psychosis.[43]

A great deal of interest has been generated in understanding what pharmacologic properties of clozapine contribute to its superior efficacy, but to date this has not been clearly elucidated. Clozapine has a low affinity for D_2 receptors, also blocks D_1 receptors, and is a 5-HT_{2A} antagonist. Its unsurpassed efficacy suggests that there is a neuropharmacologic effect associated with clozapine that is to date unique to this agent.

Clozapine's use is limited by its association with the rare but life-threatening risk of agranulocytosis. Other side effects include seizures, as well as common unpleasant side effects including sedation, enuresis, anticholinergic effects, weight gain, and hypersalivation. The long-term hematologic monitoring (see monitoring section) required for prevention of agranulocytosis can represent a barrier to both patients and care providers. The optimal plasma level of clozapine is a minimum trough level of 300 to 350 ng/mL (300–350 mcg/L or 0.92 to 1.07 μmol/L or 918–1,071 nmol/L), usually corresponding to a daily dose of 200 to 400 mg, although dosage must be individualized. According to published guidelines and recommendations, clozapine should be considered after two failed antipsychotic trials, but may be considered sooner if the individual patient situation warrants.[34]

Other Strategies Approximately 30% of patients treated with clozapine will not respond, and another 30% will have only a partial response to the drug. Treatment options with other medications are limited after clozapine nonresponse. For these patients, the best evidence points to augmentation using an FGA, SGA, or electroconvulsive therapy (ECT). The only available data support the combination of clozapine with risperidone; however, controlled trial results are mixed. Other potential strategies include combining antipsychotics with mood stabilizers (e.g., lithium, lamotrigine, valproate, and topiramate).[34]

▶ Acutely Psychotic Patients

Psychiatric emergencies occur in a variety of settings, including emergency departments, psychiatric units, medical facilities, and outpatient settings. Although verbal interventions are recommended as initial interventions, most psychiatric emergencies require both pharmacologic and psychological interventions. Often, the psychiatrist must make decisions based on limited information and history. IM formulations are available for a number of FGAs and three SGAs (aripiprazole, ziprasidone, and olanzapine). These formulations are safe and effective in treating acute psychosis. These SGAs are now recommended as first-line therapy in agitated schizophrenia patients; however, IM lorazepam with or without concomitant oral (tablets, liquid, or disintegrating tablets) SGAs are also used. Concomitant olanzapine and benzodiazepines may cause orthostasis. High dosing of FGAs, termed rapid neuroleptization, is no longer recommended.

▶ Pregnancy and Lactation

When to use antipsychotics in pregnancy and during lactation remains a complicated decision based on a careful analysis of risks and benefits. Women with schizophrenia, even those who are unmedicated have a significantly greater risk for stillbirth, infant death, preterm delivery, low infant birth weight, and infants that are small for gestational age. Furthermore, women who experience a relapse in psychotic symptoms during pregnancy are at the greatest risk for birth complications.[44] Because risks related to psychotic relapse may be more detrimental than antipsychotic treatment to both mother and baby, antipsychotics are often continued during this period.

Essentially all antipsychotic medications pass through the placenta. High-potency FGAs are associated with a low risk for congenital abnormalities; however, limb defects and dyskinesias have been reported.[45] Low-potency phenothiazine antipsychotics may increase the risk of congenital abnormalities when used in the first trimester. According to the relevant literature published to date, there appears to be little risk associated with the first-line SGAs.[46] Long-term neurobehavioral studies of children exposed to SGA in utero have not yet been done, however. On the basis of available data, generalization is impossible, and each case and specific antipsychotic should be weighed on an individual basis. While SGAs are excreted in breast milk, most case reports have reported a low frequency of deleterious effects on the infant. Women taking SGAs may have enhanced fertility compared to women taking FGAs, as SGAs (except risperidone and paliperidone) are less likely to cause prolactin elevations leading to anovulation. Therefore, careful discussion with patients, including education about birth control, must occur.

Pharmacokinetics

Pharmacokinetic and pharmacodynamic issues are not generally a major concern with antipsychotic treatment; however, additive side effects may occur with combined treatment, and a few clinically significant drug interactions

---

Table 37–9

Metabolism and Drug Interactions With Antipsychotics

Antipsychotic	Major CYP450 Metabolic Enzyme	Other CYP450 Metabolic Pathways	Increase Antipsychotic Concentrations	Decrease Antipsychotic Concentrations
Clozapine	1A2	3A3/4, 2D6, 2C19	Fluvoxamine, ciprofloxacin, paroxetine	Cigarette smoking
Risperidone	2D6	3A3/4	Fluoxetine, paroxetine	Carbamazepine
Olanzapine	1A2	2D6	Fluvoxamine, ciprofloxacin, paroxetine	Cigarette smoking
Quetiapine	3A3/4	2D6	Fluvoxamine, ketoconazole	Carbamazepine
Ziprasidone	3A3/4		Fluvoxamine, ketoconazole	Carbamazepine
Aripiprazole	3A3/4	2D6	Fluvoxamine, ketoconazole	Carbamazepine
Iloperidone	2D6, 3A4		Ketoconazole, fluoxetine, paroxetine	
Asenapine	1A2	3A4, 2D6	Fluvoxamine	
Haloperidol	2D6, 3A3/4		Fluvoxamine, fluoxetine, ketoconazole	Carbamazepine
Thioridazine	2D6	1A2	Fluvoxamine	Cigarette smoking
Perphenazine	2D6		Fluvoxamine, fluoxetine, paroxetine	

CYP450, cytochrome P-450 isoenzyme.

are notable (Table 37–9). All of the antipsychotics are highly protein-bound; however, protein-binding interactions are generally not clinically significant. Absorption of most antipsychotics is not affected by food, with the exception of ziprasidone, the absorption of which is increased by 60% to 70% when given with meals.

All antipsychotics are, at least to some extent, metabolized by hepatic microsomal enzymes to water-soluble compounds that are excreted by the kidneys. Table 37–9 lists the primary metabolic enzymes and some potential drug interactions for the antipsychotic medications. Clinicians should assess the clinical impact of the addition or discontinuation of these drugs in individual patients and should make appropriate adjustments when necessary. Unlike the other antipsychotics, ziprasidone is mostly metabolized by aldehyde oxidase, a metabolic system independent of the CYP450 system. Paliperidone, the 9-hydroxy metabolite of risperidone, is mostly excreted unchanged in the urine, although up to one-third may be metabolized. Another recent discovery in metabolism of antipsychotics and their distribution involves the transmembrane energy-dependent efflux transporter, P-glycoprotein. This may limit the ability of a number of drugs to penetrate the blood–brain barrier and therefore impact pharmacologic activity in the brain.[47] Antipsychotics currently known to use this pathway include perphenazine, haloperidol, fluphenazine, quetiapine, risperidone, and olanzapine.[48]

Due to its propensity to cause prolongation of the QTc interval, the use of ziprasidone with other agents that prolong the QTc interval should be avoided. These other agents include, but are not limited to, antiarrhythmic medications such as quinidine and sotalol, certain FGAs (chlorpromazine, droperidol, mesoridazine, pimozide, and thioridazine), and certain antibiotics (e.g., gatifloxacin, halofantrine, mefloquine, moxifloxacin, and pentamidine). Ziprasidone has not been shown to have clinically significant drug interactions with the CYP4503A3/4 inhibitors regarding increasing the QTc; however, higher doses, especially given with inhibitors of CYP4503A3/4 (e.g., ketoconazole and erythromycin), should be used cautiously. Clinicians should also be vigilant to avoid pharmacodynamic interactions with any of the antipsychotics involving additive side effects from combination therapies. Side effects that may be worsened with combination therapies include sedation, hypotension, anticholinergic symptoms, and weight gain or metabolic abnormalities.

Adjunct Pharmacologic Treatments

The judicious use of pharmacologic therapies other than antipsychotics is often necessary in the treatment of patients with schizophrenia. Concomitant medications may be indicated for the treatment of motor side effects, anxiety, depression, mood elevation, and possibly refractory psychotic symptoms. Anticholinergic medications (e.g., benztropine, 1–2 mg two times daily; trihexyphenidyl, 1–3 mg three times daily; and diphenhydramine, 25–50 mg two times daily) are used to effectively treat EPS,

thereby improving the tolerability of these medications. They may be prescribed prophylactically with high-D_2-binding agents or in patients at risk for EPS, or for treatment of EPS. β-Blockers (e.g., propranolol in doses of 30–120 mg/day) are sometimes effective for patients who develop akathisia. In some situations, such as on an inpatient unit, the concomitant use of benzodiazepines (e.g., lorazepam in doses of 1–3 mg/day) with the SGAs may be necessary for agitation and insomnia.

Antidepressants may be useful for patients with depressive symptoms that are not due to negative symptomatology or emotional blunting secondary to parkinsonian-type side effects. Since suicide and depression are linked, aggressive treatment is necessary when depression is present. Selective serotonin reuptake inhibitors (SSRIs) are the preferred agents, but may inhibit the CYP450 enzymes, thus raising plasma concentrations of clozapine, olanzapine, and haloperidol. Mood stabilizers, such as lithium and the anticonvulsants, have long been used adjunctively with antipsychotics to treat the affective component of schizoaffective disorder. Lastly, much research is currently underway to develop better treatments for primary negative symptoms and cognitive impairment; however, no approved treatments are yet available.

OUTCOME EVALUATION

Patient Education

8 *Education of the patient and family regarding the benefits and risks of antipsychotic medications and the importance of adherence to their therapeutic regimens must be integrated into pharmacologic management.* Too often, patients receive little education about schizophrenia and may not have a good understanding of their diagnosis. Meetings for purposes of medication management offer an opportunity to provide some education on the general illness. Discuss the nature and course of schizophrenia and be prepared to accept that the patient might have a different understanding of the nature of his or her illness. Key points to cover include:

- Involve families in the education and treatment plans, since family psychoeducation may decrease relapse, improve symptomatology, and enhance psychosocial and family outcomes.[49]

- Be clear that there is no cure for schizophrenia and that medications only help to decrease the symptoms.

- Explain common side effects of medications.

- Discuss rare but dangerous side effects that may also occur.

- Stress the importance of medication and treatment adherence for improving long-term outcomes in schizophrenia.

Symptom Monitoring

Develop a good working alliance with the patient. When a solid therapeutic foundation is not formed, patients are

---

Table 37–10

Monitoring Protocol for Patients on SGAs

	Baseline	4 Weeks	8 Weeks	12 Weeks	Quarterly	Annually	Every 5 Years
Personal/family history[a]	X					X	
Weight	X	X	X	X	X		
Waist circumference	X					X	
Blood pressure	X			X		X	
Fasting plasma glucose	X			X		X	
Fasting plasma lipids	X			X			X

[a]Of obesity, diabetes, dyslipidemia, hypertension, or cardiovascular disease.

From Ref. 52.

Table 37–11

Monitoring of WBC and Absolute Neutrophil Count During Clozapine Treatment

	Hematologic Values	Frequency of WBC and ANC Monitoring
Prior to clozapine initiation	Recommended levels: WBC greater than or equal to $3.5 \times 10^3/mm^3$ and ANC greater than or equal to $2 \times 10^3/mm^3$ No history of a myeloproliferative disorder or clozapine-induced agranulocytosis	
Initiation to 6 months	WBC greater than or equal to $3.5 \times 10^3/mm^3$ and ANC greater than or equal to $2 \times 10^3/mm^3$	Weekly for 6 months
6–12 months	WBC greater than or equal to $3.5 \times 10^3/mm^3$ and ANC greater than or equal to $2 \times 10^3/mm^3$	Every 2 weeks for 6 months
After 12 months of therapy	WBC greater than or equal to $3.5 \times 10^3/mm^3$ and ANC greater than or equal to $2 \times 10^3/mm^3$	Every 4 weeks
Whenever clozapine is discontinued		Weekly for at least 4 weeks from day of discontinuation
Mild leukopenia or granulocytopenia	WBC value lies between $3 \times 10^3/mm^3$ and $3.5 \times 10^3/mm^3$ and/or ANC lies between $1.5 \times 10^3/mm^3$ and $2 \times 10^3/mm^3$	Twice weekly until returned to recommended levels
Moderate leukopenia or granulocytopenia	WBC value lies between $2 \times 10^3/mm^3$ and $3 \times 10^3/mm^3$ and/or ANC value lies between $1 \times 10^3/mm^3$ and $1.5 \times 10^3/mm^3$	Interrupt therapy; monitor daily until WBC greater than $3 \times 10^3/mm^3$ and ANC greater than $1.5 \times 10^3/mm^3$, then twice weekly until back to recommended levels
Severe leukopenia or granulocytopenia or agranulocytosis	WBC less than $2 \times 10^3/mm^3$ and/or ANC less than $1 \times 10^3/mm^3$ ANC less than or equal to $0.5 \times 10^3/mm^3$	Discontinue treatment and do not rechallenge; monitor daily until WBC greater than $3 \times 10^3/mm^3$ and ANC greater than $1.5 \times 10^3/mm^3$, then twice weekly until back to recommended levels

ANC, absolute neutrophil count; WBC, white blood cell count.

$3.5 \times 10^3/mm^3 = 3.5 \times 10^9/L$; $3 \times 10^3/mm^3 = 3 \times 10^9/L$; $2 \times 10^3/mm^3 = 2 \times 10^9/L$; $1.5 \times 10^3/mm^3 = 1.5 \times 10^9/L$; $1 \times 10^3/mm^3 = 1 \times 10^9/L$; $0.5 \times 10^3/mm^3 = 0.5 \times 10^9/L$.

---

frequently reluctant to share their psychotic experiences. Once a solid working relationship and some knowledge of the patient's psychotic experiences exist, perform a more structured interview. Many assessments are available to more objectively rate positive and negative symptoms, level of function, and life satisfaction. The most commonly used scales include:

- Positive and Negative Symptom Scale (PANSS)
- Brief Psychiatric Rating Scale (BPRS)
- Clinical Global Impression (CGI) Scale

Using these scales on a regular basis, particularly when switching medications or changing doses, is a more reliable means of monitoring for improvement. Certainly symptom assessments cannot capture the full range of possible improvements a patient may experience, but they can be useful in deciding whether a medication is having substantial benefit.

Patient Encounter, Part 4

With his care providers, AC discussed several possible medication choices. Because there had been improvement of auditory hallucinations on risperidone, the initial choice was made to increase the dose to target the ongoing paranoid thinking. AC was seen weekly to monitor for emergence of EPS or akathisia. He was able to tolerate an increase to 4 mg of risperidone daily with improvement in his paranoid thinking. He went on several job interviews and accepted part-time employment at a coffee shop. When he complained of emergence of sexual dysfunction, his prolactin level was determined to be 42 ng/mL (42 mcg/L) (normal prolactin levels are less than or equal to 18–20 ng/mL [18–20 mcg/L] in men and less than or equal to 24 ng/mL [24 mcg/L] in women). He discussed risks and benefits of therapy with his clinicians and decided to continue risperidone for now, as he had improved in his ability to work and get out more in the community. He remains interested in having an aripiprazole trial in the future, as he hopes he might more easily lose the weight he gained while taking olanzapine and resume normal sexual functioning. He is no longer taking an antidepressant, and though he has some low days, he does not meet the criteria for diagnosis of depressive episode. He continues to be free of substance abuse, and his girlfriend continues to support his treatment. He still hopes to return to work in his field of expertise someday.

Based on the information above, create a care plan for this patient's treatment. Your plan should include: (a) a statement of the drug-related concerns and/or problems, (b) the goals of therapy, and (c) a plan for monitoring and follow-up to determine whether the goals have been achieved and adverse effects minimized.

Patient Care and Monitoring

1. Assess the patient's symptoms, review patient and family history, and obtain initial medical evaluation to rule out other causes of psychosis.

2. Periodically review patient data for consistency with diagnostic criteria, and regularly monitor changes in symptomatology.

3. Obtain a thorough history of prescription medication use, and determine what treatments have been helpful in the past, which treatments the patient is currently receiving, and previous side effects experienced.

4. Determine whether the patient is taking an appropriate antipsychotic drug and dose and whether the patient has other symptoms that may need to be treated.

5. Educate the patient, and the family if possible, about the disease state, medication treatments, possible side effects, and goals of treatment.

6. Develop a plan to assess the effectiveness of the current treatment regimen. Also, consider alternative treatments if current treatment is ineffective.

7. Encourage a healthy lifestyle, including eliminating or decreasing substance abuse and cigarette use, as well as appropriate nutritional counseling and exercise suggestions.

8. Determine the role of psychosocial treatments.

9. Evaluate the patient for the presence of adverse drug reactions, drug interactions, and allergies.

10. Monitor the appropriate laboratory measures to prevent or minimize metabolic abnormalities and other side effects.

11. Stress the importance of adherence with the treatment regimen and maintain treatment even if the patient is feeling well.

Side Effect Monitoring

❼ *Regularly monitor patients for side effects and overall health status while taking antipsychotic medications.*[50,51] Perform orthostatic blood pressure measurements before initiating antipsychotics and throughout treatment. Ask about impaired menstruation, libido, and sexual performance regularly. Encourage patients to have annual eye exams, as several of the antipsychotic medications have been associated with the premature development of cataracts. Check body weight, fasting glucose, glycosylated hemoglobin, and lipid profile at baseline, at 4 months after initiation of medication, and then yearly.[52] For patients who are at higher risk of developing diabetes and those who gain weight, check body weight more often (Table 37–10). Encourage patients to act proactively against weight gain through healthier eating and exercise. Perform a baseline

ECG for patients with pre-existing cardiovascular disease and risk for arrhythmia. With clozapine therapy there is a risk for the development of agranulocytosis, which is greatest in the first 6 months of treatment. Current guidelines require the monitoring of white blood cell counts (WBCs) prior to drug dispensing (Table 37–11).

Commonly used rating scales to monitor for EPS include the Simpson Angus Scale (SAS) and the Extrapyramidal Symptom Rating Scale (ESRS). Akathisia is commonly monitored by the Barnes Akathisia Scale (BAS). The emergence of dyskinesias (writhing or involuntary movements) could represent the emergence of TD. Monitor for TD at least annually, and if FGAs are used, patients should be evaluated at each visit. The most commonly used instrument to measure these symptoms is the Abnormal Involuntary Movement Scale (AIMS).

Abbreviations Introduced in This Chapter

5-HT	Serotonin
AIMS	Abnormal Involuntary Movement Scale
ANC	Absolute neutrophil count
BAS	Barnes Akathisia Scale
BPRS	Brief Psychiatric Rating Scale
CATIE	Clinical Antipsychotics Trials of Intervention Effectiveness
CBT	Cognitive-behavioral therapy
CGI	Clinical Global Impression Scale
CR	Cognitive remediation
CYP450	Cytochrome P-450 isoenzyme
D	Dopamine
DSM-IV-TR	*Diagnostic and Statistical Manual of Mental Disorders*, 4th Edition, Text Revision
ECT	Electroconvulsive therapy
EPS	Extrapyramidal side effects
ESRS	Extrapyramidal Symptom Rating Scale
FGA	First-generation antipsychotic
H	Histamine
IM	Intramuscular
M	Muscarinic
NMDA	N-methyl-D-aspartate
NMS	Neuroleptic malignant syndrome
PCP	Phencyclidine
PANSS	Positive and Negative Symptom Scale
PORT	Schizophrenia Patient Research Outcomes Team
SAS	Simpson Angus Scale
SGA	Second-generation antipsychotic
SSRI	Selective serotonin reuptake inhibitor
SST	Social skills training
TD	Tardive dyskinesia
TIMA	Texas Implementation of Medication Algorithms

Self-assessment questions and answers are available at *http://www.mhpharmacotherapy.com/pp.html*.

REFERENCES

1. Schultz SK, Andreasen NC. Schizophrenia. Lancet 1999;353(9162):1425–1430.
2. Abdolmaleky HM, Thiagalingam S, Wilcox M. Genetics and epigenetics in major psychiatric disorders: Dilemmas, achievements, applications, and future scope. Am J Pharmacogenomics 2005;5(3):149–160.
3. Abi-Dargham A. Do we still believe in the dopamine hypothesis? New data bring new evidence. Int J Neuropsychopharmacol 2004;7(Suppl 1):S1–S5.
4. Laruelle M, Kegeles LS, Abi-Dargham A. Glutamate, dopamine, and schizophrenia: From pathophysiology to treatment. Ann N Y Acad Sci 2003;1003:138–158.
5. Meltzer HY, Li Z, Kaneda Y, Ichikawa J. Serotonin receptors: Their key role in drugs to treat schizophrenia. Prog Neuropsychopharmacol Biol Psychiatry 2003;27(7):1159–1172.
6. Goff DC, Cather C, Evins AE, et al. Medical morbidity and mortality in schizophrenia: guidelines for psychiatrists. J Clin Psychiatry 2005;66(2):183–194.
7. American Psychiatric Association. Diagnostic and Statistical Manual of Mental Disorders. 4th ed. Text rev. Washington, DC: American Psychiatric Association, 2000.
8. Pompili M, Girardi P, Ruberto A, Taterelli R. Toward a new prevention of suicide in schizophrenia. World J Biol Psychiatry 2004;5(4):201–210.
9. Casey DE. Long-term treatment goals: Enhancing healthy outcomes. CNS Spectr 2003;8(11 Suppl 2):26–28.
10. Resnick SG, Fontana A, Lehman AF, Rosenheck RA. An empirical conceptualization of the recovery orientation. Schizophr Res 2005;75(1):119–128.
11. American Psychiatric Association. Practice guidelines for the treatment of patients with schizophrenia. Am J Psychiatry 2004;161(2 Suppl):1–56.
12. The expert consensus guideline series: treatment of schizophrenia. J Clin Psychiatry 1996;57(Suppl 12B):31.
13. Bellack AS. Skills training for people with severe mental illness. Psychiatr Rehabil 2004;27(4):375–391.
14. Lieberman JA, Stroup TS, McEvoy JP, et al. For the Clinical Antipsychotic Trials of Intervention Effectiveness (CATIE) Investigators. Effectiveness of antipsychotic drugs in people with chronic schizophrenia. N Engl J Med 2005;353(12):1209–1223.
15. Correll CU, Leucht S, Kane JM. Lower risk for tardive dyskinesia associated with second-generation antipsychotics: A systematic review of 1-year studies. Am J Psychiatry 2004;161(3):414–425.
16. Schotte A, Janssen PFM, Gommeren W, et al. Risperidone compared with new and reference antipsychotic drugs: In vitro and in vivo receptor binding. Psychopharmacology 1996;124(1–2):57–73.
17. Marder SR, Meibach RC. Risperidone in the treatment of schizophrenia. Am J Psychiatry 1994;151(6):825–835.
18. Csernansky JG, Mahmoud R, Brenner R, Risperidone-USA-79 Study Group. A comparison of risperidone and haloperidol for the prevention of relapse in patients with schizophrenia. N Engl J Med 2002;346(1):16–22.
19. Richelson E. Receptor pharmacology of neuroleptics: Relation to clinical effects. J Clin Psychiatry 1999;60(Suppl 10):5–14.
20. Beasley CM, Tollefson G, Tran P, et al. Olanzapine versus placebo and haloperidol: Acute phase results of the North American double-blind olanzapine trial. Neuropsychopharmacology 1996;14(2):111–123.
21. Tollefson GD, Beasley CM, Tran PV, et al. Olanzapine versus haloperidol in the treatment of schizophrenia and schizoaffective and schizophreniform disorders: Results of an international collaborative trial. Am J Psychiatry 1997;154(4):457–465.
22. Arvanitis LA, Miller BG, the Seroquel Trial 13 Study Group. Multiple fixed doses of Seroquel (quetiapine) in patients with acute exacerbation of schizophrenia: A comparison with haloperidol and placebo. Biol Psychiatry 1997;42(4):233–246.
23. Small JG, Hirsch SR, Arvenitis LA, et al. Quetiapine in patients with schizophrenia: a high- and low-dose double-blind comparison with placebo. Arch Gen Psychiatry 1997;54(6):549–557.
24. Seeger TF, Seymour PA, Schmidt AW, et al. Ziprasidone (CP-88,059): A new antipsychotic with combined dopamine and serotonin receptor antagonist activity. J Pharmacol Exp Ther 1995;275(1):101–113.
25. Keck P, Buffenstein A, Ferguson J, et al. Ziprasidone 40 and 120 mg/day in the acute exacerbation of schizophrenia and schizoaffective disorder: A 4-week placebo-controlled trial. Psychopharmacology 1998;140(2):173–184.
26. Daniel DG, Zimbroff DL, Potkin SG, et al. Ziprasidone 80 mg/day and 160 mg/day in the acute exacerbation of schizophrenia and schizoaffective disorder: A 6-week placebo-controlled trial. Neuropsychopharmacology 1999;20(5):491–505.
27. Shapiro DA, Renock S, Arrington E, et al. Aripiprazole, a novel atypical antipsychotic drug with a unique and robust pharmacology. Neuropsychopharmacology 2003;28(8):1400–1411.

28. Dolder C, Nelson M, Deyo Z. Paliperidone for schizophrenia. Am J Health Syst Pharm 2008;65(5):403–413.

29. Kapur S, Seeman P. Does fast dissociation from the dopamine d(2) receptor explain the action of atypical antipsychotics? A new hypothesis. Am J Psychiatry 2001;158(3):360–369.

30. Wirshing WC. Movement disorders associated with neuroleptic treatment. J Clin Psychiatry 2001;62:Suppl 21:15–18.

31. Margolese HC, Chouinard G, Kolivakis TT, et al. Tardive dyskinesia in the era of typical and atypical antipsychotics. Part 2: Incidence and management strategies in patients with schizophrenia. Can J Psychiatry 2005;50(11):703–714.

32. Egan MF, Apud J, Wyatt RJ. Treatment of tardive dyskinesia. Schizophr Bull 1997;23(4):583–609.

33. Correll CU, Schenk EM. Tardive dyskinesia and new antipsychotics. Curr Opin Psychiatry 2008;21:151–156.

34. Moore TA, Buchanan RW, Buckley PF, et al. The Texas Medication Algorithm Project antipsychotic algorithm for schizophrenia: 2006 update. J Clin Psychiatry 2007;68(11):1751–1762.

35. Lehman AF, Kreyenbuhl J, Buchanan RW, et al. The schizophrenia patient outcomes research team (PORT): Updated treatment recommendations 2003. Schizophr Bull 2004;30(2):193–217.

36. Byerly MJ, Nakonezny PA, Lescouflair E. Antipsychotic medication adherence in schizophrenia. Psychiatr Clin N Am 2007;30(3):437–452.

37. Perkins DO. Predictors of noncompliance in patients with schizophrenia. J Clin Psychiatry 2002;63:1121–1128.

38. Remschmidt H. Early-onset schizophrenia as a progressive-deteriorating developmental disorder: Evidence from child psychiatry. J Neural Transm 2002;109:101–117.

39. Jeste DV, Caligiuri MP, Paulsen JS, et al. Risk of tardive dyskinesia in older patients. A prospective longitudinal study of 266 outpatients. Arch Gen Psychiatry 1995;52:756–765.

40. Tsuang J, Fong TW. Treatment of patients with schizophrenia and substance abuse disorders. Curr Pharm Des 2004;10(18):2249–2261.

41. Wobrock T, Soyka M. Wobrock T, Soyka M. Pharmacotherapy of schizophrenia with comorbid substance use disorder-reviewing the evidence and clinical research. Prog Neuropsychopharmacol Biol Psychiatry 2008;32(6):1375–1385.

42. Conley RR, Kelly DL. Management of treatment resistance in schizophrenia. Biol Psychiatry 2001;50(11):898–911.

43. Meltzer HY. Suicide in schizophrenia, clozapine and adoption of evidence-based medicine. J Clin Psychiatry 2005;60(Suppl 12):47–50.

44. Nilsson E, Lichtenstein P, Cnattingius S, et al. Women with schizophrenia: pregnancy outcome and infant death among their offspring. Schizophr Res 2002;58(2–3):221–229.

45. Diav-Citrin O, Schechtman S, Ornoy S, et al. Safety of haloperidol and penfluridol in pregnancy: a multicenter, prospective, controlled study. J Clin Psychiatry 2005;66(3):317–322.

46. McKenna K, Koren G, Tetelbaum M, et al. Pregnancy outcome of women using atypical antipsychotic drugs: a prospective comparative study. J Clin Psychiatry 2005;66(4):444–449.

47. Wang JS, Taylor R, Ruan Y, et al. Olanzapine penetration into brain is greater in transgenic Abcb1a P-glycoprotein-deficient mice and FVB1 (wild type) animals. Neuropsychopharmacology 2004;29(3):551–557.

48. Sandson NB, Armstrong SC, Cozza KL. An overview of psychotropic drug-drug interactions. Psychosomatics 2005;46(5):464–494.

49. Murray-Swank AB, Dixon L. Family psychoeducation as evidence-based practice. CNS Spect 2004;9(12):905–912.

50. Marder SR, Essock SM, Miller AL, et al. The Mount Sinai conference on the pharmacotherapy of schizophrenia. Schizophr Bull 2002;28(1):5–16.

51. Marder SR, Essock SM, Miller AL, et al. Physical health monitoring of patients with schizophrenia. Am J Psychiatry 2004;161(8):1334–1349.

52. American Diabetes Association, American Psychiatric Association, American Association of Clinical Endocrinologists, North American Association for the Study of Obesity. Consensus development conference on antipsychotic drugs and obesity and diabetes. Diabetes Care 2004;27(2):596–601.

53. Love RC, Mackowick M, Carpenter D, Burks EJ. Expert consensus-based medication-use evaluation criteria for atypical antipsychotic drugs. Am J Health Syst Pharm 2003;60:2455–2470.

38 Major Depressive Disorder

Cherry W. Jackson, Marshall E. Cates, and Jacqueline M. Feldman

LEARNING OBJECTIVES

● **Upon completion of the chapter, the reader will be able to:**

1. Explain the etiology and pathophysiology of major depressive disorder (MDD).

2. Identify symptoms and clinical features of MDD.

3. Differentiate antidepressants according to pharmacologic properties, adverse-effect profiles, pharmacokinetic profiles, drug interaction profiles, and dosing features.

4. Predict adverse-effect profiles of antidepressants based on pharmacology.

5. State the goals of pharmacotherapy in MDD.

6. Educate patients and caregivers on the proper use of antidepressants.

KEY CONCEPTS

❶ Classic views as to the cause of major depressive disorder (MDD) focus on the monoamine neurotransmitters norepinephrine (NE), serotonin (5-HT), and to a lesser extent, dopamine (DA) in terms of both synaptic concentrations and receptor functioning.

❷ It is not uncommon for a patient to experience only a single major depressive episode, but most patients with MDD will experience multiple episodes.

❸ One extremely important goal in the treatment of MDD is the prevention of suicidal attempts.

❹ Sexual dysfunction is common and challenging to manage and often leads to noncompliance with serotonergic medications.

❺ Each antidepressant has a response rate of approximately 60% to 80%, and no antidepressant medication or class has been reliably shown to be more efficacious than another.

❻ It is widely accepted that approximately 2 to 4 weeks of treatment are required before improvement is seen in emotional symptoms of depression, such as sadness and anhedonia. Furthermore, as long as 6 to 8 weeks of treatment may be required to see the full effects of antidepressant therapy.

❼ Because the typical major depressive episode lasts 6 months or longer, if antidepressant therapy is interrupted for any reason following the acute phase, the patient may relapse into the depressive episode. When treating the first depressive episode, antidepressants must be given for an additional 4 to 9 months in the continuation phase for the purpose of preventing relapse.

❽ Pediatric patients and young adults should be observed closely for suicidality, worsened depression, agitation, irritability, and unusual changes in behavior, especially during the initial few months of therapy or at times of dosage changes. Furthermore, families and caregivers should be advised to monitor patients for such symptoms.

❾ Lack of patient understanding concerning optimal antidepressant drug therapy frequently leads to partial compliance or noncompliance with therapy; thus, the primary purpose of antidepressant counseling is to enhance compliance and improve outcomes.

My spirit is broken, my days are cut short, the grave awaits me.

—Job 17:1

Contrary to popular belief, major depression is not a fleeting "bad day," is not the result of personal weaknesses or character flaws, and does not respond to volitional efforts simply to feel better. Major depressive disorder (MDD) is a serious medical condition with a biological foundation, and it responds to biological and psychological treatments. Individuals who suffer from MDD experience significant and pervasive symptoms that can affect mood, thinking, physical health, work, and relationships. Unfortunately, suicide is often the result of MDD that has not been diagnosed and treated adequately.

The last two decades have seen improvements in the screening, diagnosis, and treatment of MDD. The willingness of general practitioners to involve themselves in the identification and treatment of MDD is noteworthy. To that end, antidepressants have become some of the most commonly prescribed drugs, and they account for 10 of the top 100 prescription drugs dispensed in the United States.[1] Inadequate treatment remains a serious concern.[2]

EPIDEMIOLOGY

MDD is quite common; lifetime and 12-month prevalence estimates are 16.2% and 6.6%, respectively.[2] Females are approximately twice as likely as males to experience MDD.[2] The average age at onset is the mid-twenties.[3] Interestingly, MDD appears to occur earlier in life in people born in more recent decades.[2] Most patients with MDD also suffer from comorbid psychiatric disorders, especially anxiety disorders and substance-use disorders.[2]

According to the World Health Organization (WHO), depression is the leading cause of disability (based on years lived with disability) and the fourth leading contributor to the global burden of disease (based on disability adjusted life years).[4]

ETIOLOGY/PATHOPHYSIOLOGY

● The exact cause of MDD remains unknown, but it is probably multifactorial. Biological, psychological, and social theories abound, and many practitioners suggest that the development of depression often is predicated on the complex synthesis of genetic predisposition, psychological stressors, and biological pathophysiology. At present, there are currently no accepted unifying theories that explain these various factors adequately.

Patient Encounter 1, Part 1

PT is a 34-year-old male who was brought into the hospital by friends after telling them that he was considering taking an overdose of pain killers. He lost his job 2 months ago, followed by the loss of his home to foreclosure. In addition, he lost most of his 401-K and children's college fund due to the downturn in the market. On questioning, he is tearful and describes overwhelming feelings of sadness and guilt. He also states that he has not been sleeping or eating and that he has experienced a 6.8 kg (15 lb) weight loss over the last 6 weeks. He states that he drinks three or four beers per night in order to relax and fall asleep

What information is suggestive of MDD?

What medical or psychiatric issues could be contributing to his symptoms?

Does he have risk factors for depression?

What additional information do you need to know before creating a treatment plan for this patient?

Genetics

First-degree relatives of MDD patients are about three times more likely to develop MDD compared with first-degree relatives of normal control individuals. Adoption studies and twin studies reveal that the familial aggregation of MDD is due to genetic influences.[5]

Life Stress

Depression can occur in the absence of major life stressors, and conversely, major life stressors do not invariably cause depression. Nevertheless, there is an undeniable association between life stressors and depression, and there appears to be a significant interaction between life stressors and genetic liability in causing depression.[6] Although acute stressors may precipitate depression, chronic stressors have a longer risk period, cause longer episodes, and are more likely to lead to relapse and recurrence.[6]

Monoamine Neurotransmitter and Receptor Hypotheses

❶ *Classic views as to the cause of MDD focus on the monoamine neurotransmitters norepinephrine (NE), serotonin (5-HT), and to a lesser extent, dopamine (DA) in terms of both synaptic concentrations and receptor functioning.* The monoamine hypothesis asserts that depression is due to a deficiency of monoamine neurotransmitters. The major supporting evidence for this hypothesis is that existing antidepressants increase synaptic monoamine concentrations through various mechanisms (see Pharmacologic Therapy). One argument against the monoamine hypothesis is that depressed patients do not consistently exhibit decreased monoamine concentrations. In addition, monoamine levels are altered within hours of the initiation of antidepressant therapy, but there is a latency period of weeks before the actual antidepressant effect is typically evident.[7–9]

The neurotransmitter receptor hypothesis suggests that depression is related to abnormal functioning of neurotransmitter receptors. In this model, antidepressants presumably exert therapeutic effects by altering receptor sensitivity. In fact, chronic administration of antidepressants has been shown to cause desensitization, or downregulation, of β-adrenergic receptors and various 5-HT receptors. Importantly, the time required for changes in receptor sensitivity corresponds to the onset of antidepressant effects.[7–9]

Such models of the pathophysiology of depression are assuredly an oversimplification. Depression probably involves a complex dysregulation of monoamine systems, and these systems, in turn, modulate and are modulated by other neurobiological systems.[10]

Other Neurobiological Hypotheses

Various other pathophysiological hypotheses are proposed. These hypotheses include the role of nonmonoamine neurotransmitters (e.g., glutamate and γ-aminobutyric acid), neuroendocrine systems (e.g., the hypothalamic-pituitary-adrenal axis), neurosteroids (e.g., allopregnanolone),

Clinical Presentation of MDD

Patients typically present with a combination of emotional, physical, and cognitive symptoms:

- Emotional
  - Sadness
  - Anhedonia
  - Pessimism
  - Feeling of emptiness
  - Irritability
  - Anxiety
  - Worthlessness
  - Thoughts of death/suicidal ideation (SI)
- Physical
  - Disturbed sleep
  - Change in appetite/weight
  - Psychomotor changes
  - Decreased energy
  - Fatigue
  - Bodily aches and pain

- Cognitive
  - Impaired concentration
  - Indecisiveness
  - Poor memory

Occasionally, severely depressed patients also will present with psychotic symptoms:

- Hallucinations
- Delusions

Some patients present with "atypical features" of depression:

- Reactive mood (i.e., mood improves in response to positive events)
- Significant increase in appetite/weight gain
- Hypersomnia
- Heavy feelings in arms or legs
- Sensitivity to interpersonal rejection

---

neuronal plasticity (e.g., brain-derived neurotrophic factor),[11] messenger cascades, and gene expression.[12]

CLINICAL PRESENTATION AND DIAGNOSIS

The diagnosis of a major depressive episode requires the presence of a certain number of depressive symptoms (five) for a minimum specified duration (2 weeks) that cause clinically significant effects (Table 38–1).[3]

HINT: In order to remember the nine diagnostic symptoms for a major depressive episode, learn the following mnemonic: Depression = SIG E CAPS (depression, sleep, interest, guilt, energy, concentration, appetite, psychomotor, suicide).

In turn, the diagnosis of MDD is based on the presence of one or more major depressive episodes during a person's lifetime.[3]

Differential Diagnosis

Major depressive episodes also occur in patients with bipolar disorder. Persons with bipolar disorder also experience manic, hypomanic, and/or mixed episodes (see Chap. 39) during the course of their illness, whereas persons with MDD do not.[3]

The presence of a significant medical disorder can produce depressive symptoms via either psychological or physiological mechanisms. Examples include hypothyroidism, neoplasms, anemia, infections, electrolyte disturbances, cardiovascular

Table 38–1

Diagnostic Criteria for Major Depressive Episode

At least five of the following symptoms have been present during the same 2-week period and represent a change from previous functioning:

- Depressed mood[a]
- Markedly diminished interest or pleasure in usual activities[a]
- Increase or decrease in appetite or weight
- Increase or decrease in amount of sleep
- Increase or decrease in psychomotor activity
- Fatigue or loss of energy
- Feelings of worthlessness or guilt
- Diminished ability to think, concentrate, or make decisions
- Recurrent thoughts of death, suicidal ideation, or suicide attempt

The symptoms cause clinically significant distress or impairment in functioning

The symptoms are not due to the direct physiological effects of a substance or medical condition

[a]One of these two symptoms must be present.
From Ref. 3.

diseases, neurologic disorders, and many others.[9] Various psychiatric conditions, such as substance-use disorders and anxiety disorders, have been associated with depression as well.[9] The use of CNS depressants, such as benzodiazepines and narcotics, is associated with increased propensity for depression.[13] Drugs that reportedly cause depressive symptoms or depressive-like side effects include corticosteroids, contraceptives, gonadotropin-releasing hormone agonists, interferon-α, interleukin-2, mefloquine, isotretinoin, propranolol, and sotalol.[14]

Dysthymia is a condition that must be differentiated from depression. Many of the symptoms of dysthymia are similar to those of depression, but in dysthymia, symptoms are chronic and milder. Symptoms of dysthymia must be present for at least 2 years and may include sleep and appetite disturbances, a loss of energy, a lack of interest in things that would usually be enjoyable, and poor self-image. Patients with dysthymia often have family members with a history of depression or dysthymia. It occurs more frequently in women, and patients with dysthymia are more likely to develop major depression than the general population.[3]

COURSE/PROGNOSIS

Symptoms of a major depressive episode usually develop over days to weeks, but mild depressive and anxiety symptoms may last for weeks to months prior to the onset of the full syndrome. Left untreated, major depressive episodes typically last 6 months or more, but a minority of patients experience chronic episodes that last at least 2 years. Approximately two-thirds of patients recover fully from major depressive episodes and return to normal mood and full functioning, whereas the other one-third have only partial remission.[3]

The course of MDD varies markedly from patient to patient. ❷ *It is not uncommon for a patient to experience only a single major depressive episode, but most patients with MDD will experience multiple episodes.* Some patients experience isolated episodes separated by many years, others have clusters of episodes, and still others suffer more frequent episodes as they age. The number of prior episodes predicts the likelihood of developing subsequent episodes. A patient experiencing a third major depressive episode has about a 90% chance of having a fourth one. MDD is associated with a high mortality rate because about 15% of patients ultimately commit suicide.[3]

☙ TREATMENT

Desired Outcomes

The goals of therapy for the depressed patient are the resolution of depressive symptoms, a return to euthymia, and prevention of relapse and recurrence of depressive symptoms. ❸ *One extremely important goal in the treatment of MDD is the prevention of suicidal attempts.* Other desired outcomes include improvement of the patient's quality of life, normalization of functioning in areas such as work and relationships, avoidance or minimization of adverse effects, and reduction of health care costs.[15]

Nonpharmacologic Therapy

Interpersonal therapy and cognitive behavioral therapy are psychotherapies that have well-documented efficacy for the treatment of MDD. Psychotherapy alone is an initial treatment option for mild-to-moderate depression, and it

---

Patient Encounter, Part 2: Medical History, Physical Exam, and Diagnostic Tests

The workup on PT reveals:

PMH: Chronic back pain since motor vehicle accident 3 years ago.

PPH: Noncontributory

FH: Mother with diabetes mellitus and MDD; father is alive and well with no medical problems; brother is a recovered alcoholic

SH: Worked for a construction company, but job ended 2 months ago. For the last several months he has been drinking three to four beers per night. He denies smoking cigarettes or using illicit substances

Current Meds: Ranitidine 150 mg twice daily; oxycontin 10 mg twice daily

ROS: Decreased energy; decreased sleep; all others noncontributory

PE:

Ht 5 ft 10 in. (178 cm); wt 66 kg (146 lb); weight loss of 6.8 kg (15 lb) over last 6 weeks

MSE: Depressed mood; decreased concentration; positive SI with plan

Labs: Within normal limits

Given this additional information, what is your assessment of the patient's condition?

Identify your treatment goals for the patient.

What nonphamacologic and pharmacologic alternatives are available for this patient?

---

may be useful when combined with pharmacotherapy in the treatment of more severe cases. The combination of psychotherapy and pharmacotherapy can be more effective than either treatment modality alone in severe or recurrent MDD. It may be especially helpful for patients with significant psychosocial stressors, interpersonal difficulties, or comorbid personality disorders.[16]

Electroconvulsive therapy (ECT) is a highly efficacious treatment for MDD. The response rate is about 80% to 90%, and it exceeds 50% for patients who have failed pharmacotherapy.[16,17] ECT may be particularly beneficial for MDD that is complicated by psychotic features, severe suicidality, refusal to eat, pregnancy, or contraindication/nonresponse to pharmacotherapy.[16,17] Around 6 to 12 treatments are typically necessary with response occurring in 10 to 14 days. Once ECT is discontinued, antidepressants are initiated to help maintain the response. ECT is typically a very safe treatment alternative, but various cautions do exist. Side effects include confusion and memory impairment.[16]

Light therapy is an alternative treatment for depression associated with seasonal (e.g., winter) exacerbations. Side effects include eye strain, headache, insomnia, and hypomania.[16,17] Potentially vulnerable patients, such as those with photosensitivity or a history of skin cancer, should be evaluated carefully prior to therapy.[16,17]

Vagus nerve stimulation (VNS) may be used for adult patients with treatment-resistant depression. A pulse generator is surgically implanted under the skin of the left chest, and an electrical lead connects the generator to the left vagus nerve. Stimulation of this nerve sends signals to the brain. This therapy is used along with traditional therapies such as pharmacotherapy and ECT.[18] Adverse effects of VNS include alterations in patients' voice, coughing, pharyngitis, sore throat, hoarseness, headache, nausea, vomiting, dyspnea, and paresthesias.[18]

Transcranial magnetic stimulation is a noninvasive and well-tolerated procedure that is FDA approved for use after one failed trial of an antidepressant.[19] Some data suggest that physical exercise may reduce depressive symptoms, but well-controlled studies are needed to document efficacy.[20]

Pharmacologic Therapy

▶ Clinical Distinctions

Each antidepressant has its unique blend of characteristics, and in fact, even individual drugs within the same class have important differences.[21]

▶ General Pharmacology

Table 38-2 demonstrates the differing pharmacologic properties of the antidepressant medications,[7–9] whereas Table 38-3 delineates the results of those pharmacologic actions.[7,8] Monoamine oxidase inhibitors (MAOIs) inhibit the enzyme responsible for the intraneuronal breakdown of 5-HT, NE, and DA. Tricyclic antidepressants (TCAs) possess both 5-HT (serotonin) reuptake inhibition (SRI) and NE reuptake inhibition (NRI) properties but unfortunately also block the so-called "dirty receptors," including α_1-adrenergic, histamine-1, and muscarinic cholinergic receptors, which contribute to side effects but not efficacy. The selective serotonin reuptake inhibitors (SSRIs) are classified as such because SRI is the predominant effect. Bupropion is an NE and DA reuptake inhibitor (NDRI). Venlafaxine, desvenlafaxine, and duloxetine are 5-HT and NE reuptake inhibitors (SNRIs) but are also weak inhibitors of DA reuptake. Compared with venlafaxine and desvenlafaxine, which have primarily SRI activity, duloxetine has more balanced SRI and NRI activities and has a higher affinity for the reuptake sites. Nefazodone and trazodone are 5-HT antagonists/reuptake inhibitors. Their SRI activity is not as pronounced as that of SSRIs, but they potently block 5-HT$_{2A}$ receptors, which allows more 5-HT to interact at postsynaptic 5-HT$_{1A}$ sites. In addition, trazodone blocks histaminergic and α-adrenergic receptors, whereas nefazodone possesses weak NRI and α-adrenergic blocking properties. Finally, mirtazapine is a noradrenergic and specific serotonergic

---

Table 38-2
Primary Pharmacologic Actions of Antidepressants

Action	MAOIs	TCAs	SSRIs	Bupropion	Venlafaxine and Desvenlafaxine	Duloxetine	Trazodone	Nefazodone	Mirtazapine
Monoamine oxidase inhibition	X								
Serotonin reuptake inhibition		X	X		X X	X	X	X	
Norepinephrine reuptake inhibition		X		X	X X	X			
Dopamine reuptake inhibition				X					
α_2-Adrenergic receptor blockade									X
Serotonin-2A receptor blockade							X	X	X
Serotonin-2C receptor blockade									X
Serotonin-3 receptor blockade									X
α_1-Adrenergic receptor blockade		X					X	X	
Histamine-1 receptor blockade		X					X		X
Muscarinic cholinergic receptor blockade		X							

MAOI, monoamine oxidase inhibitor; SSRI, selective serotonin reuptake inhibitor; TCA, tricyclic antidepressant.

See text for discussion of more secondary pharmacologic actions.

From Refs. 7–9.

Table 38–3

Efficacy and Adverse-Effect Profiles Based on Pharmacology

Pharmacologic Action	Result
SRI	Antidepressant and antianxiety efficacy (via interaction of 5-HT at 5HT-1A receptors)
	Anxiety, insomnia, sexual dysfunction (via interaction of 5-HT at 5HT-2A receptors)
	Anxiety, anorexia (via interaction of 5-HT at 5HT-2C receptors)
	Nausea, GI problems (via interaction of 5-HT at 5HT-3 receptors)
NRI	Antidepressant efficacy
	Tremor, tachycardia, sweating, jitteriness, increased blood pressure
Dopamine reuptake inhibition	Antidepressant efficacy
	Euphoria, psychomotor activation, aggravation of psychosis
a_2-Adrenergic receptor blockade	Increase in serotonergic and noradrenergic activity—see actions of SRI and NRI above
Serotonin-2A receptor blockade	Antianxiety efficacy
	Increased REM sleep, decreased sexual dysfunction
Serotonin-2C receptor blockade	Antianxiety efficacy
	Increased appetite/weight gain
Serotonin-3 receptor blockade	Antinauseant, decreased GI problems
a_1-Adrenergic receptor blockade	Orthostatic hypotension, dizziness, reflex tachycardia
Histamine-1 receptor blockade	Sedation, weight gain
Muscarinic cholinergic receptor blockade	Dry mouth, blurred vision, constipation, urinary hesitancy, sinus tachycardia, memory problems

NRI, Norepinephrine reuptake inhibition; SRI, serotonin reuptake inhibition.

From Refs. 7 and 8.

antidepressant. It blocks presynaptic α_2 receptors, both autoreceptors on noradrenergic neurons and heteroreceptors on serotonergic neurons, with resulting increases in NE and 5-HT synaptic concentrations, respectively. Mirtazapine also blocks various postsynaptic serotonergic receptors and histamine-1 receptors.[7–9]

St. John's wort (*Hypericum perforatum*) is a herbal medication that has shown some efficacy in mild-to-moderate depression but minimal efficacy for moderate-to-severe depression.[20] Many patients believe that herbal medications, being "natural" products, are devoid of adverse effects and drug interactions; however, St. John's wort can cause GI irritation, headache, fatigue, and nervousness,[17] and it triggers drug interactions through induction of CYP3A4 enzymes, as well as other potential mechanisms.[22] The safety and efficacy of St. John's wort combined with standard antidepressant medications remain unknown.[16]

▶ Adverse Effects

The important adverse effects of the various antidepressants are often a function of their underlying pharmacologic profiles[7,8] (Table 38–3). TCAs cause problematic sedative, anticholinergic, and cardiovascular adverse effects owing to their interaction with "dirty receptors." While these adverse effects generally are considered to be common and bothersome, they can be quite serious in some cases. For example, constipation in its extreme form can lead to paralytic ileus. The tertiary amines (e.g., amitriptyline, imipramine) are more sedative and anticholinergic than secondary amines (e.g., desipramine, nortriptyline). TCAs have a quinidine-like effect on the heart, which makes them quite toxic on overdose. The average lethal dose in a young adult is only 30 mg/kg, which is typically less than a 1 month's supply.[7,9,21,23]

The adverse-effect profile of the SSRIs includes sexual dysfunction (e.g., delayed or absent orgasms), CNS stimulation (e.g., nervousness and insomnia), and GI disturbances (e.g., nausea and diarrhea).[7,9,21,23] ❹ *Sexual dysfunction is common and challenging to manage and often leads to noncompliance.*[24] Various strategies to deal with antidepressant-induced sexual dysfunction include waiting for symptoms to subside, reducing the dosage, permitting periodic "drug holidays," prescribing adjunctive therapy, and switching antidepressants.[25] However, waiting for symptoms to subside usually does not work because sexual dysfunction may very well persist throughout the duration of therapy. Reducing the dose and using drug holidays may weaken the antidepressant effects. Thus, clinicians often prescribe adjunctive therapy such as dopaminergic drugs (e.g., bupropion or amantadine), 5-HT$_2$ antagonists (e.g., cyproheptadine or nefazodone), and phosphodiesterase inhibitors (e.g., sildenafil), or simply switch to antidepressants with less likelihood of causing these effects, such as bupropion, mirtazapine, or nefazodone.[24,25]

Bupropion causes insomnia, nightmares, decreased appetite, anxiety, and tremors, but the most concerning adverse effect is seizures. Because of the risk for seizures, patients with a CNS lesion, history of seizures, head trauma, or bulimia should not receive the drug. The daily dose of bupropion should not exceed 450 mg/day, and any single dose of the immediate-release formulation should not exceed 150 mg. Occurrences of insomnia and/or nightmares often respond to moving the last daily dose from bedtime to late afternoon.[7,9,21,23]

Table 38–4

Relative Incidence of Adverse Effects of Various Newer Antidepressants

Drug	Sedation	Activation	Weight Gain	Weight Loss	GI Upset	Sexual Dysfunction
Bupropion	+	++++	+	++	+++	+
Citalopram	+	+	+	+	++++	++++
Fluoxetine	+	++++	+	+	++++	++++
Mirtazapine	+++	+	++	+	+	+
Nefazodone	++	+	+	+	++	+
Paroxetine	++	++	+	+	++++	++++
Sertraline	+	+++	+	+	++++	++++
Venlafaxine	++	+++	+	+	++++	++++
Desvenlafaxine	++	+++	+	+	++++	++++

+, minimal; ++, low; +++, moderate; ++++, high.

From Refs. 9, 13, 28.

The adverse effects of SNRIs are similar to those of SSRIs. Nausea can be particularly troublesome with venlafaxine and desvenlafaxine, which sometimes necessitates using lower starting dosages than usual and giving the medication with food. A dose-related elevation in blood pressure can occur at higher doses, probably owing to the NRI effects. Blood pressure monitoring should be conducted for patients receiving venlafaxine and desvenlafaxine therapy. As a rule, duloxetine should not be prescribed to patients with extensive alcohol use or evidence of chronic liver disease owing to the potential for hepatic injury.[9,21,26,27]

Trazodone routinely causes sedation, which is why it is used far more often as an adjunct with other antidepressants for sleep than as an antidepressant. Priapism is a rare but serious adverse effect in males who take trazodone. In addition, orthostatic hypotension and dizziness are more common with trazodone than with nefazodone because the latter agent has a weaker effect at α-adrenergic receptors and also has a balancing of adrenergic effects owing to weak NRI activity. Unfortunately, nefazodone has been associated with development of hepatotoxicity, which has led to a black-box warning and a great reduction in its use. It has been discontinued in some countries.[7,9,21,23]

Mirtazapine can cause sedation and weight gain by virtue of blocking histamine-1 receptors. Despite being partially a serotonergic drug, it rarely causes serotonergic-related adverse effects because it blocks the various postsynaptic 5-HT receptors. Although it carries a bolded warning for neutropenia owing to a handful of cases reported during clinical trials, it is questionable whether neutropenia is any more problematic with this agent than other antidepressants.[9,21,23]

The relative incidence of adverse effects among some of the newer antidepressant agents are shown in Table 38–4.[9,13,28]

▶ Pharmacokinetic Parameters

Pharmacokinetic parameters of the newer antidepressants are shown in Table 38–5.[9,29] Several antidepressants are not

Table 38–5

Pharmacokinetic Parameters of Newer Antidepressants

Drug	Protein Binding (%)	Elimination Half-Life (hours)	Active Metabolite(s)
Bupropion	84	10–21	Yes
Citalopram	80	33	Yes
Duloxetine	90	9–19	No
Escitalopram	56	27–32	No
Fluoxetine	94	4–6 days with chronic dosing; 4–16 days (active metabolite)	Yes
Fluvoxamine	77	15–26	No
Mirtazapine	85	20–40	No
Nefazodone	99	2–4	Yes
Paroxetine	95	21	No
Sertraline	98	27	Yes
Venlafaxine	27	5	Yes
Desvenlafaxine	30	7.5	No

From Refs. 9, 29.

highly protein-bound, and the most notable of these are venlafaxine and desvenlafaxine. The elimination half-lives of nefazodone and venlafaxine are relatively short compared with the other agents. Conversely, fluoxetine has a very long half-life (i.e., 5–9 days) with chronic dosing, and its active metabolite (norfluoxetine) has an even longer half-life. Owing to the extremely long half-life of fluoxetine and its active metabolite, a 5-week washout of fluoxetine is required before starting an MAOI. Sertraline and citalopram are the other SSRIs with active metabolites, but these metabolites (desmethylsertraline and desmethylcitalopram, respectively) are only about one-eighth as potent as the parent compounds in terms of SRI activity.

▶ Drug Interactions

The major drug interactions of antidepressants are shown in Table 38–6.[9,22,30] The usual pharmacodynamic drug interactions involve the "dirty receptors" blocked by some antidepressants. Hence, especially TCAs can cause significant additive effects with drugs that cause sedation, hypotension, or anticholinergic effects. Similarly, nefazodone and mirtazapine can interact with other drugs that cause hypotensive and sedative effects, respectively. By far, the most concerning pharmacodynamic interactions are hypertensive crisis and 5-HT syndrome, which are both potentially life-threatening when they occur. Hypertensive crisis is characterized by sharply elevated blood pressure, occipital headache, stiff or sore neck, nausea, vomiting, and sweating. It may result during MAOI therapy if the patient takes a sympathomimetic drug, such as ephedrine, pseudoephedrine, phenylephrine, or phenylpropanolamine, or if the patient consumes foods rich in tyramine, such as tap beers, aged cheeses, fava beans, yeast extracts, liver, dry sausage, sauerkraut, or tofu.[23] There are extensive lists of foods and drinks that are permitted and not permitted during therapy with MAOIs, and these always should be provided to patients. Since many over-the-counter products contain sympathomimetics, patients always should be told to consult with their clinician and/or pharmacist prior to using these drugs. 5-HT syndrome is characterized by confusion, restlessness, fever, abnormal muscle movements, hyper-reflexia, sweating, diarrhea, and shivering.[31] It may result when a serotonergic agent is added to any serotonergic antidepressant, but the MAOIs are strongly associated with severe cases of 5-HT syndrome.[31] 5-HT syndrome is complicated by (a) an unawareness by clinicians of the diagnosis[31] and (b) the fact that many implicated drugs are not obviously serotonergic in nature, such as dextromethorphan, meperidine, and tramadol.

Several antidepressants, including most of the SSRIs, nefazodone, and duloxetine, are known to inhibit various cytochrome P450 isoenzymes, thereby elevating plasma levels of substrates for those isoenzymes and thus potentially leading to increased adverse effects or toxicity. The propensity to cause these drug interactions will vary with the particular antidepressant and the precise isoenzyme[9,22,30] (Table 38–6).

▶ Dosing

Dosing is summarized in Table 38–7.[13,16,17,20,29,32] The extended-release formulations of venlafaxine and bupropion allow for once-daily dosing. The delayed-release capsule of fluoxetine can be given once weekly, which can be started 7 days after the last regular-release capsule or tablet. Selegiline is available as a transdermal patch and a dose of 6 mg/24 hours can be used without the usual dietary restrictions associated with MAOI use, although patients on the higher doses (9 and 12 mg/24 hours) should follow the usual dietary restrictions. Liquid dosage forms and disintegrating tablets of various antidepressants are ideal for patients who have difficulty swallowing tablets or capsules or those who otherwise may attempt to "cheek" their medication.

The starting dose is the usual therapeutic dose for most of the SSRIs, desvenlafaxine, duloxetine, and mirtazapine,

---

Table 38–6

Drug Interactions of Antidepressants[a]

Antidepressants	Type of Interaction	Examples of Interacting Drugs
TCAs, trazodone, mirtazapine	Pharmacodynamic—additive sedation	Benzodiazepines, alcohol, antihistamines
TCAs, trazodone	Pharmacodynamic—additive hypotensive effects	Prazosin, antipsychotics
TCAs	Pharmacodynamic—additive anticholinergic effects	Phenothiazines, benztropine
TCAs	Pharmacodynamic—additive cardiac toxicity	Thioridazine, quinidine
TCAs	Pharmacodynamic—decreased antihypertensive effect	Guanethidine, clonidine, methyldopa
Bupropion	Pharmacodynamic—increased seizure risk	TCAs, phenothiazines
MAOIs	Pharmacodynamic—hypertensive crisis	Tyramine-rich foods, sympathomimetics
MAOIs, TCAs, SSRIs, SNRIs, SARIs	Pharmacodynamic—5-HT syndrome	Serotonergic antidepressants, meperidine, dextromethorphan, tramadol
Fluvoxamine	Pharmacokinetic—CYP1A2 inhibition	TCAs, clozapine, theophylline
Fluoxetine, fluvoxamine, sertraline	Pharmacokinetic—CYP2C inhibition	TCAs, phenytoin, warfarin, tolbutamide
Fluoxetine, paroxetine, duloxetine, sertraline	Pharmacokinetic—CYP2D6 inhibition	TCAs, haloperidol, risperidone, codeine, propranolol, propafenone
Nefazodone, fluoxetine, fluvoxamine	Pharmacokinetic—CYP3A4 inhibition	TCAs, alprazolam, verapamil, carbamazepine, lovastatin

MAOI, monoamine oxidase inhibitor; SARI, serotonin antagonist and reuptake inhibitor; SNRI, serotonin and norepinephrine reuptake inhibitor; SSRI, selective serotonin reuptake inhibitor; TCA, tricyclic antidepressant.

[a]Not an all-inclusive list.

From Refs. 9, 22, 30.

Table 38–7

Dosing of Antidepressants in Adult Patients

Generic Name	Brand Name	Generic	Dosage Forms	Initial Dose (mg/day)	Usual Dosage Range (mg/day)	Usual Dosing Schedule
MAOIs						
Phenelzine	Nardil	No	Tablet	15–30	15–90	Twice daily
Tranylcypromine	Parnate	No	Tablet	10–20	30–60	Twice daily
Selegiline	Emsam	No	Patch	6	6–12	Once daily
TCAs and Tetracyclics						
Amitriptyline	Elavil[a]	Yes	Tablet	25–50	100–300	Once daily
Amoxapine	Asendin[a]	Yes	Tablet	25–50	100–400	Once to twice daily
Clomipramine	Anafranil	Yes	Capsule	25	100–250	Once daily
Desipramine	Norpramin	Yes	Tablet	25–50	100–300	Once daily
Doxepin	Sinequan	Yes	Capsule, solution	25–50	100–300	Once daily
Imipramine	Tofranil	Yes	Tablet, capsule (PM)	25–50	100–300	Once daily
Maprotiline	Ludiomil[a]	Yes	Tablet	50–75	100–225	Once to twice daily
Nortriptyline	Pamelor	Yes	Capsule, solution	25	50–150	Once daily
Protriptyline	Vivactil	No	Tablet	5–10	15–60	Once daily
Trimipramine	Surmontil	No	Capsule	25–50	100–300	Once daily
SSRIs						
Citalopram	Celexa	Yes	Tablet, solution	20	20–60	Once daily
Escitalopram	Lexapro	No	Tablet, solution	10	10–20	Once daily
Fluoxetine	Prozac	Yes	Tablet, capsule; solution	10–20	20–80	Once daily
	Prozac weekly	No	Delayed-release capsule	—	90	Once weekly
Fluvoxamine	Luvox	Yes	Tablet	50	50–300	Twice daily
Paroxetine	Paxil	Yes	Tablet, suspension	10–20	20–50	Once daily
	Paxil CR	Yes	Controlled-release tablet	12.5–25	25–62.5	Once daily
Sertraline	Zoloft	Yes	Tablet, concentrate	25–50	50–200	Once daily
NDRI						
Bupropion	Wellbutrin	Yes	Tablet	150–200	300–450	Twice to thrice daily
	Wellbutrin SR	Yes	Sustained-release tablet	150	300–400	Twice daily
	Wellbutrin XL	Yes	Extended-release tablet	150	300–450	Once daily
SNRIs						
Duloxetine	Cymbalta	Yes	Capsule	40–60	40–60	Once to twice daily
Venlafaxine	Effexor	Yes	Tablet	37.5–75	75–375	Twice daily
	Effexor XR	Yes	Extended-release capsule	37.5–75	75–225	Once daily
Desvenlafaxine	Pristiq	No	Extended-release tablet	50	50–100	Once daily
SARIs						
Nefazodone	Serzone[a]	Yes	Tablet	100–200	300–600	Twice daily
Trazodone	Desyrel	Yes	Tablet	50–150	200–600	Twice daily
NaSSA						
Mirtazapine	Remeron	Yes	Tablet, disintegrating tablet (SolTab)	15	15–45	Once daily

MAOI, monoamine oxidase inhibitor; NaSSA, noradrenergic and specific serotonergic antidepressant; NDRI, norepinephrine and dopamine reuptake inhibitor; SARI, serotonin antagonist and reuptake inhibitor; SNRI, serotonin and norepinephrine reuptake inhibitor; SSRI, selective serotonin reuptake inhibitor; TCA, tricyclic antidepressant.

[a]Brand no longer available in the United States.

From Refs. 13, 16, 17, 20, 29, 32.

whereas there is usually need for at least some upward titration of venlafaxine, bupropion, and nefazodone. A particular disadvantage of TCAs is that the customary way of dosing them involves meticulous upward titration from a small starting dose to a wide usual therapeutic dosage range. On the contrary, one advantage of some TCAs is that plasma levels may be used to help guide dosing, especially for those that have well-defined therapeutic plasma level ranges, including nortriptyline (50–150 ng/mL or mcg/L, or 190–570 nmol/L), desipramine (100–160 ng/mL or mcg/L, or 375–600 nmol/L), amitriptyline (75–175 ng/mL or mcg/L, 255–595 nmol/L), and imipramine (200–300 ng/mL or mcg/L, or 714–1,071 nmol/L).[28]

▶ Efficacy of Pharmacotherapy

❺ *Each antidepressant has a response rate of approximately 60% to 80%, and no antidepressant medication or class has been reliably shown to be more efficacious than another.*[7,21] MAOIs may be the most effective therapy for atypical depression, but MAOI use continues to wane because of problematic adverse effects, dietary and drug restrictions, and possibility of fatal drug interactions.[21,28] There is some evidence that dual-action antidepressants, such as TCAs and SNRIs, may be more effective for inpatients with severe depression than are the single-action drugs such as SSRIs,[21,28] but the more general assertion that multiple mechanisms of action confer efficacy advantages is quite controversial.[33]

▶ Selection of Medication

Figure 38–1 depicts a well-known algorithm for the pharmacologic treatment of nonpsychotic MDD—the Texas Medication Algorithm Project.[34] Notable aspects of this algorithm include the preferential use of newer antidepressants in the earlier stages of treatment and sequential trials of antidepressant monotherapy prior to the use of combination therapy (see Managing Partial Response or Nonresponse). It has been shown that patients undergoing treatment guided by this algorithm fared better than those who received treatment not guided by the algorithm during a 1-year period, as measured by clinician-rated symptoms, self-reported symptoms, and overall mental functioning.[35] Antipsychotic medication should be combined with antidepressant medication in cases of depression with psychotic features.[16]

Various factors must be taken into account when selecting antidepressant therapy for a particular patient. The most reliable predictor of response is the patient's history of response (e.g., efficacy, side effects, and overall satisfaction) to antidepressants. To a lesser extent, the history of a first-degree relative's response to antidepressants may be used to predict a patient's response. Adverse-effect profiles should be considered because compliance is influenced greatly by tolerability. In this regard, a frank discussion should occur with the patient in order to determine which adverse effects are acceptable and which are not and how to deal with side effects (i.e., using chewing gum, hard candy, or ice chips for dry mouth). The clinician must be careful to contemplate potential drug–drug interactions and disease-state interactions. For instance, a patient with seizure disorder would be an inappropriate candidate for bupropion therapy. The presence of comorbid psychiatric conditions can help the clinician to determine the best antidepressant to choose for a patient. For example, an SSRI can treat both MDD and panic disorder, obviating the need for separate medication therapy. The patient must be willing and able to comply with dosing schedules (e.g., upward titration of TCAs or twice-daily dosing of nefazodone) and special instructions (e.g., dietary restrictions with MAOI therapy) associated with certain antidepressants. Another patient-specific factor is the potential for accidental or intentional overdosing because certain antidepressants (e.g., TCAs) are quite toxic and potentially lethal in overdose situations. Finally, the patient should be able to comfortably afford the chosen medication or else compliance is at risk.[21]

Time Course of Response

Unfortunately, antidepressants do not produce a clinical response immediately. Improvement in physical symptoms, such as sleep, appetite, and energy, can occur within the first week or so of treatment. Although a recent metaanalysis suggests earlier effects of antidepressant treatment,[36] ❻ *it is widely accepted that approximately 2 to 4 weeks of treatment are required before improvement is seen in emotional symptoms of depression, such as sadness and anhedonia. Furthermore, as long as 6 to 8 weeks of treatment may be required to see the full effects of antidepressant therapy.*[7,21,23]

Managing Partial Response or Nonresponse

Approximately one-third of patients with MDD do not respond satisfactorily to their first antidepressant medication.[37] In such cases, the clinician must evaluate the adequacy of antidepressant therapy, including dosage, duration, and patient compliance.[17] Treatment reappraisal should also include verification of the patient's diagnosis and reconsideration of clinical factors that could be impeding successful therapy, such as concurrent medical conditions (e.g., thyroid disorder), comorbid psychiatric conditions (e.g., alcohol abuse), and psychosocial issues (e.g., marital stress).[16]

A series of reports from the Sequenced Treatment Alternatives to Relieve Depression (STAR*D) trial revealed that remission is associated with a better overall prognosis for patients than is improvement alone. STAR*D also established that in patients with a greater level of resistance, clinicians are less likely to push the patient to achieve remission, and in addition, those patients with the greatest levels of resistance had the highest rates of relapse. In these cases, STAR*D established some successful treatment recommendations.[37]

For patients who have experienced a partial response, extending the medication trial and/or using higher doses within the recommended dosage range of the antidepressant may be helpful.[16] Another option is to employ augmentation therapy, that is, adding another medication that generally is not used as an antidepressant.[38] Augmenting agents with clear efficacy include lithium and triiodothyronine, whereas initial enthusiasm has lessened to some extent for the serotonergic drugs buspirone and pindolol owing to negative findings in controlled trials.[39] Aripiprazole, a second-generation antipsychotic was recently FDA approved for augmenting partial response to antidepressants. Efficacy has been suggested for dopaminergic drugs (e.g., pramipexole), psychostimulants (e.g., methylphenidate), and atypical antipsychotics (e.g., olanzapine), whereas various other medications such as anticonvulsants (e.g., valproic acid), modafinil, and estrogen have anecdotal evidence to support their use.[39] A third option is to make use of combination therapy, whereby another antidepressant, typically from a different pharmacologic class, is added to the first antidepressant medication. Examples include combining bupropion and SSRIs and combining TCAs and SSRIs.[39,40]

Switching to a different antidepressant is a common strategy for patients who have had no response to initial

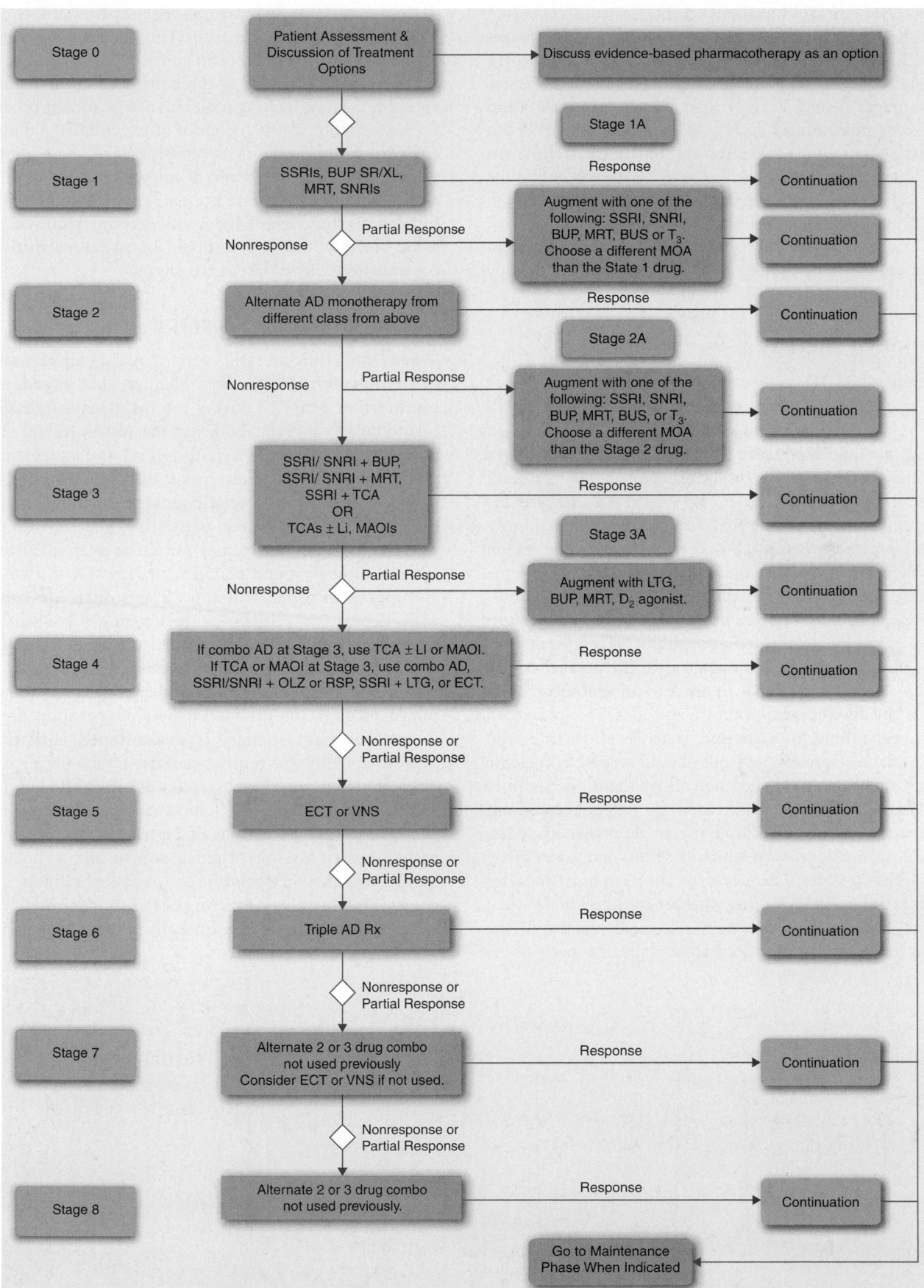

FIGURE 38–1. Strategies for the treatment of nonpsychotic major depression. Redrawn with permission from the Texas Medication Algorithm Project. (AD, antidepressant; BUP, Bupropion; BUS, Buspirone; ECT, electroconvulsive therapy; Li, lithium; T$_3$, liothyronine; LTG, lamotrigine; MAOI, monoamine oxidase inhibitor; MOA, Mechanism of action; MRT, Mirtazapine; OLZ, Olanzapine; RSP, risperidone; SNRI, serotonin and norepinephrine reuptake inhibitor; SSRI, selective serotonin reuptake inhibitor; TCA, tricyclic antidepressant; VNS, vagus nerve stimulation.

antidepressant therapy but also is acceptable in cases of partial response.[16] Relative to augmentation/combination, advantages of switching include improved compliance, decreased costs, and less concern over drug–drug interactions, whereas disadvantages include loss of time ("reset the clock") and loss of any improvement seen with the initial drug.[40] When switching from one antidepressant to another, clinicians may choose to stay within the same class (e.g., sertraline to fluoxetine) or go outside of the class (e.g., paroxetine to venlafaxine).[38,40]

Nonpharmacologic interventions in cases of treatment nonresponse include adding or changing to psychotherapy or initiating ECT.[16]

Duration of Therapy

Treatment of MDD can be conceptualized as a series of three phases: acute, continuation, and maintenance[7,8,16] (Fig. 38–2). During a major depressive episode, a clinician will initiate antidepressant therapy for the purpose of attaining **remission** of symptoms. This acute phase of treatment typically lasts 6 to 12 weeks. ❼ *Because the typical major depressive episode lasts 6 months or longer, if antidepressant therapy is interrupted for any reason following the acute phase, the patient may relapse into the depressive episode. When treating the first depressive episode, antidepressants must be given for an additional 4 to 9 months in the continuation phase for the purpose of preventing relapse.* Maintenance treatment takes place after the normal course of a major depressive episode in order to prevent recurrence, which is the development of future episodes. This phase can last for years, if not for a lifetime. Whereas all patients who suffer a major depressive episode should receive both acute and continuation treatment, not all of them will require maintenance treatment. The reason for this is because not all patients experience multiple major depressive episodes, and even in many cases in which they do, many years may separate the episodes. Therefore, the clinician must consider various factors in determining whether an individual patient requires maintenance treatment. A major factor is the number of prior episodes experienced by the patient. As

discussed earlier, the more episodes experienced, the more likely future episodes will occur. This has led many clinicians to adopt the "three strikes and you're on" approach, whereby a patient with a history of three or more major depressive episodes is given lifelong maintenance treatment because of the very high (i.e., 90%) chance of experiencing additional episodes. Other factors to consider are the severity of previous episodes, especially if suicide attempts were made or psychotic features were present, and patient preference.[16] In general, the dose of the antidepressant required in the acute phase of treatment should be sustained during the continuation and maintenance phases.[16]

Discontinuation of Therapy

When the clinician and patient are ready to attempt discontinuation of therapy, whether at the end of the continuation phase or during the maintenance phase, it is best to do so via gradual taper of the antidepressant. This is done for two reasons. First, almost all antidepressants can produce withdrawal syndromes if discontinued abruptly or tapered too rapidly, especially antidepressants with shorter half-lives (e.g., venlafaxine, paroxetine, and fluvoxamine).[17] These withdrawal syndromes can cause sleep disturbances, anxiety, fatigue, mood changes, malaise, GI disturbances, and a host of other symptoms,[17] and often are confused with depressive relapse or recurrence.[16] In general, a tapering schedule involving a small dosage decrement (e.g., paroxetine 5 mg) every 3 to 5 days should prevent significant withdrawal symptoms.[17] Second, depressive symptoms may return on taper or discontinuation of the antidepressant. If antidepressant therapy is discontinued abruptly and depressive symptoms return weeks later, then the lag time to onset of action must be observed once the antidepressant is restarted ("reset the clock"); however, if gradual tapering is carried out, then early signs of depression can be countered with a return to the original dosage and a potentially quicker response.[16] Depending on the patient's illness and the clinical circumstances, tapering of the antidepressant can be extended for weeks or even months because of the concern over relapse or recurrence.

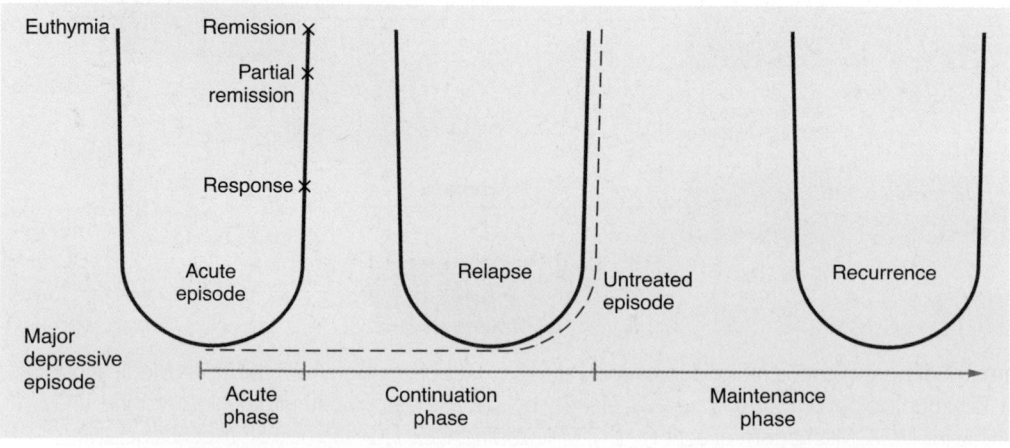

FIGURE 38–2. The course of depression and phases of treatment. (From Refs. 7, 8.)

Patient Encounter, Part 3: Creating a Care Plan

On the basis of information presented, create a care plan for PT. Your plan should include:

(a) a statement of the drug-related needs and/or problems,
(b) the goals of therapy,
(c) a patient-specific detailed therapeutic plan, and
(d) a plan for follow-up to determine whether the goals have been achieved.

Special Considerations

▶ Pregnant/Breast-Feeding Patients

It is a common misconception that pregnancy protects against depression (i.e., the "glow" of pregnancy). Depression actually is quite common in pregnancy, especially for women with a history of recurrent depression. Both maternal and fetal well-being must be taken into account when weighing the benefits and risks of using antidepressant therapy during pregnancy.[41] In general, studies have not demonstrated an increased risk of miscarriage or congenital malformations with antidepressant use,[41] but the prescribing information for paroxetine was changed recently to reflect the findings of epidemiological studies in which an increased risk of congenital malformations, in particular atrial or ventricular septal defects, was seen in infants born to women taking the drug during the first trimester of pregnancy.[42] Sertraline and citalopram have also been associated with causing septal heart defects when taken during the first trimester. In addition, the incidence of having a baby with a septal heart defect was four times higher for mothers taking more than one SSRI in the first trimester.[43] Antidepressants have been reported occasionally to cause perinatal sequelae, such as poor neonatal adaptation, respiratory distress, feeding problems, and jitteriness.[41] Data concerning the long-term neurobehavioral effects of in utero antidepressant exposure remain quite limited.[41] Fluoxetine, citalopram, and TCAs have the greatest reproductive safety data and should be considered first-line treatments when pharmacotherapy is indicated.[41]

There will be at least some drug exposure to the infant from nursing mothers taking antidepressant medications. Although there have been rare anecdotal reports of adverse effects (i.e., respiratory depression and seizure-like episodes) in infants exposed to antidepressants through breast milk, no rigorous study has confirmed adverse effects of these drugs, and it is generally accepted that the benefits of breast-feeding outweigh the risks to the infant of antidepressant exposure. However, the decision needs to be made on an individual basis.[44]

▶ Geriatric Patients

It is generally agreed that depression in older adults is under-recognized and undertreated.[45] Although not uncommon in community samples, MDD is particularly prevalent among those living in long-term care facilities.[15,45] Barriers to recognition of geriatric depression include the tendency toward "masked" presentations, that is, complaints of physical symptoms (e.g., pain and GI problems) instead of mood symptoms, the frequent presence of medical illnesses, and the overlap of mood and cognitive symptoms with those of dementia.[15,45] Age-related pharmacokinetic and pharmacodynamic changes cause geriatric patients to be more sensitive to the effects of antidepressant medications.[15] Thus, lower starting doses of antidepressants with slow upward titrations as tolerated are recommended for geriatric patients.[13,16,45] SSRIs are chosen frequently to treat geriatric depression because of their overall favorable adverse-effect profiles and low toxicity, whereas most TCAs are avoided owing to problematic anticholinergic, cardiovascular, and sedative properties.[45] Desipramine and nortriptyline are two TCAs that are more tolerable in terms of these adverse effects and thus may be used in geriatric depression.[45] Other newer antidepressants, such as bupropion, venlafaxine, nefazodone, and mirtazapine, are alternatives for the treatment of geriatric patients as well.[45]

▶ Pediatric Patients

Antidepressant medications appear to be useful for certain children and adolescents, particularly those who have severe or psychotic depression, fail psychotherapeutic measures, or experience chronic or recurrent depression. SSRIs generally are considered the initial antidepressants of choice, although comorbid conditions may favor alternative agents. Clinicians should be aware of the possibility of "behavioral activation" with the SSRIs, including such symptoms as impulsivity, silliness, daring conduct, and agitation.[46] Desipramine should be used with caution in this population because of several reports of sudden death, and a baseline and follow-up ECG may be warranted when this medication is used to treat pediatric patients.[9]

The FDA has warned that antidepressants increase the risk of suicidality (i.e., suicidal thinking and behavior) in children and young adults. A large analysis of clinical trials revealed that the risk of such events was 4% for antidepressant medications versus 2% for placebo, although no completed suicides occurred in the trials. Because of this increased risk, antidepressants have black-box warnings concerning the matter, and patient medication guides are required to be distributed with each prescription or refill of antidepressant medications. **❽** *Pediatric patients should be observed closely for suicidality, worsened depression, agitation, irritability, and unusual changes in behavior, especially during the initial few months of therapy or at times of dosage changes. Furthermore, families and caregivers should be advised to monitor patients for such symptoms.*[47]

▶ Suicidal Patients

The FDA is in the process of analyzing data to determine whether there is an increased risk of suicidality in adult patients similar to that seen in pediatric patients (see above). Even though the suicidality risk for adults taking antidepressant medications is currently unknown, similar monitoring for suicidality and clinical worsening that is mandated for pediatric patients should be followed for adult patients.[48]

Table 38–8

Patient Counseling

Counseling Point	Clinical Rationale
Mechanism of action—The medication works by affecting certain chemicals in the brain	Patient may feel that depression is a character weakness or personality flaw instead of a biological disorder
Lack of addiction potential—Although the medication affects certain chemicals in the brain, it is not addicting	Patient may worry that because the antidepressant is psychoactive, it must be addicting
Need for routine use—The medication will only work if it is taken as prescribed every day	Patient may try taking the medication on an as-needed basis
Delayed onset of action—It may take several weeks to see significant improvement in symptoms	Patient may prematurely discontinue therapy prior to onset of beneficial effects
Prolonged duration of therapy—The medication should be taken for at least 6–12 months; do not discontinue it without consulting with the prescriber	Patient may prematurely discontinue therapy after symptoms have remitted, which could lead to relapse or recurrence
Adverse effects—Mention common and expected adverse effects as well as what to do should they occur	Patient may be more likely to discontinue therapy and distrust the prescriber if adverse effects occur without forewarning
Avoidance of alcohol/CNS depressants—Use of alcohol or other CNS depressants could cause worsened depression and additive adverse effects with the medicine	Patient may be unaware of the possible consequences of drinking alcohol or taking other drugs with antidepressants
Risk of suicidality—Be alert to symptoms of worsening depression and suicidality	Patient may become suicidal or have suicidal thinking while taking the antidepressant

From Refs. 28, 49.

The clinician should bear in mind the toxic potential for the various antidepressant medications when patients already have or develop suicidality. The TCAs and MAOIs have narrow therapeutic indices, whereas the SSRIs, SNRIs, nefazodone, and mirtazapine have wide therapeutic indices.[21]

Patient Counseling

Major counseling points and the clinical rationale behind them are outlined in Table 38–8.[28,49] ❾ *Lack of patient understanding concerning optimal antidepressant drug therapy frequently leads to partial compliance or noncompliance with therapy; thus, the primary purpose of antidepressant counseling is to enhance compliance and improve outcomes.*[49]

OUTCOME EVALUATION

- Review the patient's medication profile to ensure that there are no potential/actual pharmacotherapy problems related to dosing, disease-state precautions or contraindications, drug–drug interactions, or unnecessary therapeutic duplication.
- Verify the extent of compliance with pharmacotherapy.
- Assess the response to pharmacotherapy, especially with regard to suicidality and those symptoms that cause significant subjective distress and/or functional impairment.
- Determine whether the patient is experiencing adverse effects of pharmacotherapy. Although general questioning (e.g., "Are you having any side effects?") may reveal some problems with therapy, it is better to use direct questioning concerning adverse effects that are

most common and/or most problematic (e.g., "Have you noticed any change in your sexual functioning?").
- Provide counseling to enhance patient understanding of MDD and its pharmacotherapy.

Abbreviations Introduced in This Chapter

DA	Dopamine
DRI	Dopamine reuptake inhibitor
DSM-IV-TR	*Diagnostic and Statistical Manual of Mental Disorders*, 4th Ed., Text Revision
ECT	Electroconvulsive therapy
5-HT	Serotonin
MAOI	Monoamine oxidase inhibitor
MDD	Major depressive disorder
NaSSA	Noradrenergic and specific serotonergic antidepressant
NDRI	Norepinephrine and dopamine reuptake inhibitor
NE	Norepinephrine
NRI	Norepinephrine reuptake inhibitor
SARI	Serotonin antagonist and reuptake inhibitor
SI	Suicidal ideation
SARI	Serotonin antagonist and reuptake inhibitor
SNRI	Serotonin and norepinephrine reuptake inhibitor
SRI	Serotonin reuptake inhibition
SSRI	Selective serotonin reuptake inhibitor
TCA	Tricyclic antidepressant
VNS	Vagus nerve stimulation

Patient Care and Monitoring

1. Assess the patient's severity of symptoms to determine if patient-directed therapy is appropriate or whether a psychiatrist should evaluate the patient.

2. Obtain a thorough history of prescription, nonprescription, natural, and illicit drug use. Rule out medications or medical disorders that may cause or mimic depressive symptoms.

3. Review *Diagnostic and Statistical Manual of Mental Disorders*, 4th Edition, Text Revision (*DSM-IV-TR*) criteria to determine an appropriate diagnosis.

4. Determine appropriate pharmacologic and psychological treatments (e.g., cognitive-behavioral therapy), including what has been helpful to the patient in the past.

5. Educate patient and/or caretaker about the disease state, lifestyle modifications, and medication therapy.

   - What risk factors are present that could contribute to depression?
   - What lifestyle modifications could be made to improve condition (e.g., exercise)?
   - How the medication should be taken?
   - What potential adverse effects may occur?
   - Which drugs may interact with their therapy?
   - Warning signs and prevention of suicidal and/or homicidal ideation.

6. Develop a plan to assess effectiveness of pharmacologic therapy after 4 weeks of being on a clinically effective dose.

7. Evaluate the patient for the presence of adverse drug reactions, drug allergies, and drug interactions.

8. Assess improvement in quality-of-life measures such as physical, psychological, and social functioning and well-being.

9. If the patient does not respond, determine if the patient is taking the appropriate medication and dose.

10. Recommend changes in therapy if the patient does not respond.

11. Determine long-term maintenance therapy.

 Self-assessment questions and answers are available at *http://www.mhpharmacotherapy.com/pp.html*.

REFERENCES

1. The top 300 prescriptions for 2005 by number of U.S. prescriptions dispensed. *http://www.rxlist.com/top200.htm*.
2. Kessler RC, Berglund P, Demler O, et al. The epidemiology of major depressive disorder: Results from the National Comorbidity Survey Replication (NCS-R). JAMA 2003;289:3095–3105.
3. American Psychiatric Association. Diagnostic and Statistical Manual of Mental Disorders, 4th ed. Text revision. Washington, DC: American Psychiatric Association, 2000.
4. World Health Organization. Depression. *http://www.who.int/mental_health/management/depression/definition/en/print.html*.
5. Levinson DF. The genetics of depression: A review. Biol Psych 2006;60:84–92.
6. Tennant C. Life events, stress and depression: a review of recent findings. Aust N Z J Psychiatry 2002;36:173–182.
7. Boland RJ, Keller MB. Antidepressants. In: Tasman A, Kay J, Lieberman JA, eds. Psychiatry Therapeutics, 2nd ed. Hoboken, NJ: Wiley, 2003:292–334.
8. Stahl SM. Essential psychopharmacology: Neuroscientific basis and practical applications, 3rd ed. New York: Cambridge University Press, 2008:135–295.
9. Kando JC, Wells BG, Hayes PE. Depressive disorders. In: DiPiro JT, Talbert RL, Yee GC, et al, eds. Pharmacotherapy: A Pathophysiologic Approach, 7th ed. New York: McGraw-Hill, 2008:1235–1255.
10. Belmaker RH, Agam G. Major Depressive Disorder. New Engl J Med 2008;358:55–68.
11. Wolkowitz OM, Reus VI. Neurotransmitters, neurosteroids, and neurotrophins: New models of the pathophysiology and treatment of depression. World J Biol Psychiatry 2002;4:98–102.
12. Vaidya VA, Duman RS. Depression—emerging insights from neurobiology. Br Med Bull 2001;57:61–79.
13. Peveler R, Carson A, Rodin G. Depression in medical patients. BMJ 2002;325:149–152.
14. Patten SB, Barbui C. Drug-induced depression: A systematic review to inform clinical practice. Psychother Psychosom 2004;73:207–215.
15. Raj A. Depression in the elderly. Tailoring medical therapy to their special needs. Postgrad Med 2004;115:26–28, 37–42.
16. Kaiser Permanente Care Management Institute. Depression Clinical Practice Guidelines Oakland (CA). Kaiser Permanente Care Management Institute, 2006; 1–196.
17. Trivedi M, Kleider BA. Algorithm for the treatment of chronic depression. J Clin Psychiatry 2001;22–29.
18. VNS therapy system. *http://www.fda.gov/cdrh/mda/docs/p970003s050.html*.
19. Gershon AA, Dannon PN, Grunhaus L. Transcranial magnetic stimulation in the treatment of depression. Am J Psychiatry 2003;160:835–845.
20. Sutherland JE, Sutherland SJ, Hoehns JD. Achieving the best outcome in treatment of depression. J Fam Pract 2003;52:201–209.
21. Cates M. Selecting antidepressant therapy for patients with major depression. Am J Pharm Educ 2001;65: 190–194.
22. Spina E, Scordo MG. Clinically significant drug interactions with antidepressants in the elderly. Drugs Aging 2002;19:299–320.
23. Maxmen JS, Ward NG. Psychotropic Drugs Fast Facts. 3rd ed. New York: WW Norton, 2002:95–214.
24. Cassano P, Fava M. Tolerability issues during long-term treatment with antidepressants. Ann Clin Psychiatry 2004;16:15–25.
25. Worthington JJ, Peters PM. Treatment of antidepressant-induced sexual dysfunction. Drugs Today 2003;39: 887–896.
26. Westanmo AD, Gayken J, Haight R. Duloxetine: A balanced and selective norepinephrine- and serotonin-reuptake inhibitor. Am J Health-Syst Pharm 2005;62:2481–2490.
27. Eli Lilly and Company. Manufacturer's Information. Prozac. Indianapolis, IN, 2007.
28. Stimmel GL. Mood disorders. In: Helms RA, Quan DJ, eds. Textbook of Therapeutics: Drug and Disease Management, 8th ed. Philadelphia: Lippincott Williams & Wilkins, 2006:1416–1431.
29. Clinical Pharmacology. *http://cpip.gsm.com/*.
30. Devane CL. Antidepressant-drug interactions are potentially but rarely significant. Neuropsychopharmacology 2006;31:1594–1604.
31. Boyer EW, Shannon M. The serotonin syndrome. N Engl J Med 2005;352:1112–1120.
32. To SE, Zepf RA, Woods AG. The symptoms, neurobiology, and current pharmacological treatment of depression. J Neurosci Nurs 2005;37:102–107.

33. Burke WJ. Selective versus multi-transmitter antidepressants: Are two mechanisms better than one? J Clin Psychiatry 2004;65(suppl 4):37–45.

34. Texas Medication Algorithm Project—nonpsychotic depression algorithm. *http://www.dshs.state.tx.us/mhprograms/disclaimer.shtm.*

35. Trivedi MH, Rush AJ, Crismon ML, et al. Clinical results for patients with major depressive disorder in the Texas Medication Algorithm Project. Arch Gen Psychiatry 2004;61:669–680.

36. Posternak MA, Zimmerman M. Is there a delay in the antidepressant effect? A meta-analysis. J Clin Psychiatry 2005;66:148–158.

37. Rush JA. STAR*D: What have we learned? Am J Psych 2007;164: 201–204.

38. Klein N, Sacher J, Wallner H, et al. Therapy of treatment resistant depression: Focus on the management of TRD with atypical antipsychotics. CNS Spectr 2004;9: 823–832.

39. Fava M. Augmentation and combination strategies in treatment-resistant depression. J Clin Psychiatry 2001;62(suppl 18):4–11.

40. Nelson JC. Managing treatment-resistant major depression. J Clin Psychiatry 2003;64(suppl 1):5–12.

41. Cohen LS, Nonacs R, Viguera AC, Reminick A. Diagnosis and treatment of depression during pregnancy. CNS Spectr 2004;9:209–216.

42. FDA public health advisory—paroxetine. *http://www.fda.gov/cder/drug/advisory/paroxetine200512.htm.*

43. Pedersen LH, Henriksen TB, Vestergaard M, et al. Selective serotonin reuptake inhibitors in pregnancy and congenital malformations: Population based cohort study. BMJ 2009;339:b3569.

44. Gentile S. The use of contemporary antidepressants during breastfeeding: A proposal for a specific safety index. Drug Safety 2007;30:107–121.

45. Doraiswamy PM. Contemporary management of comorbid anxiety and depression in geriatric patients. J Clin Psychiatry 2001:62(Suppl 12):30–35.

46. Ryan ND. Treatment of depression in children and adolescents. Lancet. 2005;366:933–940.

47. FDA public health advisory—suicidality in children and adolescents being treated with antidepressant medications. *http://www.fda.gov/cder/drug/antidepressants/SSRIPHA200410.htm.*

48. FDA public health advisory—suicidality in adults being treated with antidepressant medications. *http://www.fda.gov/cder/drug/advisory/SSRI200507.htm.*

49. Bollini P, Pampallona S, Kupelnick B, et al. Improving compliance in depression: A systematic review of narrative reviews. J Clin Pharm Ther 2006;31:253–260.

39 Bipolar Disorder

Brian L. Crabtree and Martha J. Faulkner

LEARNING OBJECTIVES

● **Upon completion of the chapter, the reader will be able to:**

1. Explain the pathophysiologic mechanisms underlying bipolar disorder.

2. Recognize the symptoms of a manic episode and depressive episode in patients with bipolar disorder.

3. Identify common comorbidities of bipolar disorder.

4. Recognize the *Diagnostic and Statistical Manual of Mental Disorders*, Fourth Edition, Text Revision (*DSM*-IV-TR) criteria for bipolar disorder as well as the subtypes of bipolar I disorder, bipolar II disorder, and cyclothymic disorder.

5. List the desired therapeutic outcomes for patients with bipolar disorder.

6. Explain the use of drugs as first-line therapy in bipolar disorder, including appropriate dosing, expected therapeutic effects, potential adverse effects, and important drug–drug interactions.

7. Recommend individualized drug therapy for acute treatment and relapse prevention based on patient-specific data.

8. Recommend monitoring methods for assessment of therapeutic and adverse effects of drugs used in the treatment of bipolar disorder.

9. Recommend treatment approaches for special populations of patients with bipolar disorder, including pediatric patients, geriatric patients, and pregnant patients.

10. Educate patients with bipolar disorder about their illness, drug therapy required for effective treatment, and the importance of adherence.

KEY CONCEPTS

❶ Patients presenting with depressive or elevated mood features and a history of abnormal or unusual mood swings should be assessed for bipolar disorder.

❷ The diagnosis of bipolar disorder is made based on clinical presentation, a careful diagnostic interview, and review of the history. There are no laboratory examinations, brain imaging studies, or other procedures that confirm the diagnosis.

❸ Goals of treatment are to reduce symptoms, induce remission, prevent relapse, improve patient functioning, and minimize adverse effects of drug therapy.

❹ Psychotherapy improves functional outcomes and may help treat or prevent mood episodes.

❺ The primary treatment modality for manic episodes is mood stabilizing agents, often combined with antipsychotic drugs.

❻ The primary treatment for depressive episodes in bipolar disorder is mood stabilizing agents or certain antipsychotic drugs, sometimes combined with antidepressant drugs.

❼ The primary treatment for relapse prevention is mood stabilizing agents, often combined with antipsychotic drugs.

❽ Education of the patient regarding benefits and risks of drug therapy and the importance of adherence to treatment must be integrated into pharmacologic management.

INTRODUCTION

Bipolar disorder is a mood disorder characterized by one or more episodes of mania or hypomania, often with a history of one or more major depressive episodes.[1] It is a chronic illness with a course characterized by relapses and improvements or remissions. Mood episodes can be manic, depressed, or mixed. They can be separated by long periods of stability or can cycle rapidly. They occur with or without psychosis. Disability and other consequences (i.e., increased risk of

Patient Encounter, Part 1

MW, a 43-year-old Caucasian female, is a married mother of two boys and is moderately obese. She is dressed in a short skirt, low-cut blouse, heavy makeup, and is somewhat disheveled. Motorically, she is mildly agitated, speaking rapidly, has fair eye contact, and appears tired and anxious.

Chief complaint: "I am about to get fired from my job, and I can't seem to get any sleep."

What diagnoses are suggested by this patient's presentation?

What additional information is needed to clarify the diagnosis?

suicide) of bipolar disorder can be devastating to patients. Correct diagnosis and treatment are essential as early as possible in the course of the illness to prevent complications and maximize response to treatment.

EPIDEMIOLOGY AND ETIOLOGY

Epidemiology

Bipolar disorders have been categorized into bipolar I disorder, bipolar II disorder, and bipolar disorder not otherwise specified (NOS). Bipolar I disorder is characterized by one or more manic or mixed mood episodes. Bipolar II disorder is characterized by one or more major depressive episodes and at least one hypomanic episode. Hypomania is an abnormally and persistently elevated, expansive, or irritable mood, but not of sufficient severity to cause significant impairment in social or occupational function and does not require hospitalization. The lifetime prevalence of bipolar I disorder is estimated to be between 0.3% and 2.4%. The lifetime prevalence of bipolar II disorder ranges from 0.2% to 5%. When including the bipolar spectrum, the lifetime prevalence is between 3% and 6.5%.[1]

Bipolar I disorder affects men and women equally. Bipolar II is more common in women. Rapid cycling and mixed mood episodes occur more often in women. In all, 78% to 85% of individuals with bipolar disorder report having another *Diagnostic and Statistical Manual*, Fourth Edition, Text Revision (*DSM*-IV-TR) diagnosis during their lifetime. The most common comorbid conditions include anxiety, substance abuse, and eating disorders.[2]

The mean age of onset of bipolar disorder is 20, although onset may occur in early childhood to the mid-40s.[1] If the onset of symptoms occurs after age 60, the condition is probably secondary to medical causes. Early onset of bipolar disorder is associated with greater comorbidities, more mood episodes, a greater proportion of days depressed, and greater lifetime risk of suicide attempts, compared to bipolar disorder with a later onset. Substance abuse and anxiety disorders are more common in patients with an early onset. Patients with bipolar disorder also have higher rates of suicidal thinking, suicide attempts, and completed suicides.

Etiology

The precise etiology of bipolar disorder is unknown. Thought to be genetically based, bipolar disorder is influenced by a variety of factors that may enhance gene expression. These include trauma, environmental factors, anatomical abnormalities, exposure to chemicals or drugs, and others.[3-5] Neurochemical abnormalities in bipolar disorder may be caused by these factors, discussed further in the pathophysiology section.

PATHOPHYSIOLOGY

Neurochemical

The pathophysiology of bipolar disorder remains incompletely understood. Imaging techniques such as positron emission tomography (PET) scans and functional MRI (fMRI) are being used to elucidate the cause. Research in the 1970s focused on neurotransmitters such as norepinephrine (NE), dopamine (DA), and serotonin. One hypothesis was that bipolar disorder is caused by an imbalance of cholinergic and catecholaminergic neuronal activity. Serotonin (5-HT) has been suggested to modulate catecholamine activity. Dysregulation of this relationship could cause a mood disturbance.[6] An early theory was that elevation of NE and DA caused mania, and a reduction caused depression, but this theory is now considered overly simplistic.[3] Other neurotransmitters are involved and interact with multiple neurochemical and neuroanatomic mechanisms and pathways. The pathophysiology of bipolar disorder has also been hypothesized from the mechanisms of action of lithium and other mood stabilizers. Lithium, valproate, and carbamazepine all have similar effects on neuronal growth that are reversible by inositol, supporting the hypothesis that bipolar disorder is related to inositol disturbance.[7] Evidence has shown that brain-derived neurotrophic factor (BDNF) may also play a role in bipolar disorder. Serum BDNF is low in mania and improves with response to treatment.[8]

Genetic

Results of family and twin studies suggest a genetic basis for bipolar disorder.[4] The lifetime risk of bipolar disorder in relatives of a bipolar patient is 40% to 70% for a monozygotic twin and 5% to 10% for another first-degree relative.

CLINICAL PRESENTATION AND DIAGNOSIS

Diagnosis of Bipolar Disorder

Bipolar disorder can be conceptualized as a continuum or spectrum of mood disorders.[9] They include four subtypes: bipolar I (periods of major depressive, manic, and/or mixed episodes); bipolar II (periods of major depression and

Patient Encounter, Part 2: Medical History, Physical Exam, Laboratory Exam

The interview reveals the following additional information about MW.

PMH: Para 2, gravida 2.

Hx: STD (unspecified) as a teen and in her 20s, but has been monogamous since last marriage at 34 years of age. She states, "It has not always been easy to stay with my husband." She feels sexually attracted to many men.

Past Psychiatric Hx: Hospitalized at age 15 for physical aggression toward parents, suicidality, and running away. Does not remember if she was placed on medication or if she was given a diagnosis. Admits history of sleep disturbance that alternates between hyposomnia and hypersomnia and moodiness, when she shifts from feeling "on top of the world" to very depressed, "like I'm a nobody."

FH: Father was an alcoholic and died at 55 years of age of cirrhosis. Mother is alive, has an anxiety disorder and emphysema. Brother was incarcerated for attempted murder and drug trafficking. Sister has an anxiety disorder and self-medicates with marijuana.

SH: Obtained general education diploma (GED). Smokes two packs of cigarettes per day (PPD). Multiple jobs and two previous marriages. Currently works as a salesperson in an auto parts store. Lives with husband who is a mechanic and two elementary school-aged sons.

SA Hx: In late teens into mid-20s, heavy abuse of stimulants, barbiturates, and alcohol. Currently smokes marijuana three times per week and states "it calms me down and helps me sleep." Occasionally drinks beer on weekends.

Meds: Antacids as needed for heartburn, ibuprofen as needed for headache

ROS: (+) increased energy, irritability and anger outbursts, racing thoughts, decreased need for sleep; (–) heart palpitations, weight loss, nausea, vomiting, diarrhea

PE:

VS: BP 130/88, P 88, RR 20, T 37.0°C (98.6°F)

HEENT: Neck supple, thyroid smooth, symmetrical, nontender, moveable

CV: RRR, normal S1, S2; no murmurs, rubs, gallops, or heaves

Abd: Soft, nontender, nondistended; (+) bowel sounds, no hepatosplenomegaly

Labs: Within normal limits (WNL) except + tetrahydrocannabinol (THC)

Considering this additional information, what is the most likely diagnosis?

What are the key pieces of information leading you to this conclusion?

hypomania); cyclothymic disorder (periods of hypomanic episodes and depressive episodes that do not meet all criteria for diagnosis of a major depressive episode), and bipolar disorder NOS. The defining feature of bipolar disorders is one or more manic or hypomanic episodes in addition to depressive episodes that are not caused by a medical condition, substance abuse, or other psychiatric disorder.[1]

Initial and subsequent episodes of bipolar disorder are mostly depressive.[10] Studies that followed patients with bipolar disorder over an average of about 13 years show that bipolar I patients spend about 32% of weeks with depressive symptoms compared to 9% of weeks with manic or hypomanic symptoms.[11] Patients with bipolar II disorder spend 50% of weeks symptomatic for depression and only 1% with hypomanic symptoms.[12] Because patients may present with depression and spend more time with symptoms of depression than mood elevation, bipolar disorder is often misdiagnosed or underdiagnosed. It is helpful to utilize a screening tool such as the mood disorder questionnaire.[13]

DSM-IV-TR criteria for the diagnosis of bipolar disorder are summarized in Table 39–1.

▶ *Bipolar I Disorder*

- The diagnosis of bipolar I disorder requires at least one episode of mania, for at least 1 week or longer, with a persistently elevated, expansive, or irritable mood with related symptoms of decreased need for sleep, excessive energy, racing thoughts, a propensity to be involved in high-risk activities, and excessive talkativeness.[1] Bipolar I depression can be misdiagnosed as major depressive disorder (MDD); therefore, it is essential to rule out past episodes of hypomania or mania. If bipolar depression is mistaken for MDD and the patient is treated with antidepressants, this can precipitate a manic episode or induce rapid cycling of depression and mania.

▶ *Bipolar II Disorder*

- The distinguishing feature of bipolar II disorder is depression with past hypomanic episodes that often are not recalled by the individual as being unusual. Irritability and anger episodes are also common. There cannot have been a prior full-manic episode.[1,14]

▶ *Cyclothymic Disorder*

- Cyclothymic disorder is a chronic mood disturbance generally lasting at least 2 years (1 year in children and adolescents) and characterized by mood swings including periods of hypomania and depressive symptoms. Hypomanic symptoms include inflated self-esteem or grandiosity (nondelusional), decreased need for sleep, pressure of speech, flight of ideas (FOI), distractibility, and increased involvement in goal-directed activities, not causing severe impairment in social or occupational functioning or requiring hospitalization. Psychotic features are not found in cyclothymic disorder.[1]

❶ Clinical Presentation and Diagnosis

General

The patient may present in a hypomanic, manic, depressed, or mixed state and may or may not be in acute distress.

Symptoms

Mood and Affect:

- Mood elevation
- Expansive mood
- Irritable mood
- Depression
- Hopelessness
- Suicidality

Physical/Behavioral:

- Agitation
- Impulsivity
- Aggression
- Rapid, pressured speech
- Decreased need for sleep
- Insomnia (sometimes for days or weeks)
- Hypersexuality
- Increased physical energy
- Inflated self-esteem, boasting, grandiosity
- Heightened interest in pleasurable activities with high risk of negative consequences (spending sprees, promiscuity, etc.)
- Fatigue
- Hypersomnia

Thought Processes, Content, and Perceptions:

- Racing thoughts, FOI, distractibility
- Delusions of grandeur, ideas of reference, persecution, wealth, religion
- Psychosocial
- Substance use
- Disrupted relationships
- Job loss

Laboratory and Other Diagnostic Assessments

❷ *There are no objective laboratory tests or procedures to diagnose bipolar disorder, but such testing can be done to rule out other medical diagnoses.*

- Urinalysis, urine toxicology, thyroid function, and white blood cell count in the elderly to rule out urinary tract infection
- Mood disorder questionnaire, completed by the patient, asks about common symptoms of bipolar disorder, problems caused by the symptoms, and family history in a "yes" or "no" answer format. It is then scored by the clinician.

Suicidality risk is increased in the presence of:

- Substance abuse
- Prior suicide attempts and lethality of attempts
- Access to a means of suicide
- Command hallucinations/psychosis
- Severe anxiety
- Family history of attempted or completed suicide

_____

Compiled from Refs. 1, 3, 4.

▶ Suicide

Patients with bipolar disorder have a high risk of suicide. Factors that increase that risk are early age at disease onset, high number of depressive episodes, comorbid alcohol abuse, personal history of antidepressant-induced mania, and family history of suicidal behavior.[15] In those with bipolar disorder, one of five suicide attempts is fatal, in contrast to one of 10 to one of 20 in the general population.

▶ Differential Diagnosis

Schizophrenia and bipolar disorder share certain symptoms, including psychosis in some patients. The prominence of mood symptoms and the history of mood episodes distinguish bipolar disorder and schizophrenia. In addition, the psychosis of schizophrenia occurs in the absence of prominent mood symptoms.

Personality disorders are inflexible and maladaptive patterns of behavior that deviate markedly from expectations of society beginning in adolescence or early adulthood.[1] Personality disorders and bipolar disorder may be comorbid, and patients with personality disorders may have mood symptoms. The two diagnoses are distinguished by the predominance of mood symptoms and the episodic course of bipolar disorder, in contrast to the stability and persistence of the behavioral patterns of personality disorders.

Delirium is characterized by a disturbance of consciousness and a change in cognition that develops over a short period of time, usually hours or days. The course can fluctuate over the course of the day, usually worsening in the evening. Underlying medical problems such as urinary tract infections in the elderly, substance abuse, or withdrawal symptoms in adults may precipitate delirium.[1]

Dementia is the loss of function in multiple cognitive domains that occurs over a longer period of time, usually months to years. Diagnostic features include memory impairment and at least one of the following: aphasia (deterioration of speech), apraxia (impaired ability to execute motor activities despite intact motor abilities, sensory function, and comprehension of the required task), agnosia (failure to recognize or identify objects despite intact sensory function), or disturbances in executive functioning.[1]

Table 39–1

Evaluation and Diagnostic Criteria of Mood Episodes

Diagnostic workup depends on clinical presentation and findings		• Mental status examination • Psychiatric, medical, and medication history • Physical and neurologic examination • Basic laboratory tests: CBC, blood chemistry screen, thyroid function, urinalysis, urine drug screen • Psychological testing • Brain imaging: MRI and fMRI; alternative: CT, PET • Lumbar puncture • Electroencephalogram
Diagnosis episode	Impairment of functioning or need for hospitalization[a]	*DSM*-IV-TR criteria[b]
Major depressive	Yes	Greater than or equal to 2-week period of either depressed mood or loss of interest or pleasure in normal activities, associated with at least five of the following symptoms: • Depressed, sad mood (adults); can be irritable mood in children • Decreased interest and pleasure in normal activities • Decreased appetite, weight loss • Insomnia or hypersomnia • Psychomotor retardation or agitation • Decreased energy or fatigue • Feelings of guilt or worthlessness • Impaired concentration and decision making • Suicidal thoughts or attempts
Manic	Yes	Greater than or equal to 1-week period of abnormal and persistent elevated mood (expansive or irritable), associated with at least three of the following symptoms (four if the mood is only irritable): • Inflated self-esteem (grandiosity) • Racing thoughts (FOI) • Distractible (poor attention) • Increased activity (either socially, at work, or sexually) or increased motor activity or agitation • Excessive involvement in activities that are pleasurable but have a high risk for serious consequences (buying sprees, sexual indiscretions, poor judgment in business ventures)
Hypomanic	No	At least 4 days of abnormal and persistent elevated mood (expansive or irritable); associated with at least three of the following symptoms (four if the mood is only irritable): • Inflated self-esteem (grandiosity) • Decreased need for sleep • Increased talking (pressure of speech) • Racing thoughts (FOI) • Increased activity (either socially, at work, or sexually) or increased motor activity or agitation • Excessive involvement in activities that are pleasurable but have a high risk for serious consequences (buying sprees, sexual indiscretions, poor judgment in business ventures)
Mixed	Yes	Criteria for both a major depressive episode and manic episode (except for duration) occur nearly every day for at least a 1-week period
Rapid cycling	Yes	More than four major depressive or manic episodes (manic, mixed, or hypomanic) in 12 months

[a]Impairment in social or occupational functioning; need for hospitalization because of potential self-harm, harm to others, or psychotic symptoms.

[b]The disorder is not caused by a medical condition (e.g., hypothyroidism) or substance-induced disorder (e.g., antidepressant treatment, medications, electroconvulsive therapy).

Reprinted from DiPiro JT, Talbert RL, Yee GC, et al. (eds.) Pharmacotherapy: A Pathophysiologic Approach. 7th ed. New York, McGraw-Hill, 2008:1145.

Patient Encounter, Part 3: Creating a Care Plan

Based on all information presented, create a care plan for this patient's bipolar disorder. Your plan should include (a) a statement of the drug-related needs and/or problems, (b) the goals of therapy, (c) a patient-specific therapeutic plan, and (d) a plan for follow-up to assess therapeutic response and adverse effects.

▶ Comorbid Psychiatric and Medical Conditions

Psychiatric Lifetime prevalence rates of psychiatric comorbidity with bipolar disorder are 42% to 50%.[16] Comorbidities, especially substance abuse, make establishing a definitive diagnosis more difficult and complicate treatment. Comorbidities also place the patient at risk for a poorer outcome, high rates of suicidality, and onset of depression.[2] Psychiatric comorbidities include:

- Personality disorders
- Alcohol and substance abuse or dependence
- Anxiety disorders
  - Panic disorder
  - Obsessive-compulsive disorder
  - Social phobia
  - Eating disorders
- Attention deficit hyperactivity disorder

Medical comorbidities include:

- Migraine
- Multiple sclerosis
- Cushing's syndrome
- Brain tumor
- Head trauma

TREATMENT

Desired Outcomes

❸ Desired outcomes for the treatment of bipolar disorder are to:

- reduce the symptoms of mania.
- reduce the symptoms of bipolar depression.
- prevent the recurrence of manic and depressive episodes.
- avoid or minimize adverse treatment effects.
- promote treatment adherence.
- maintain or improve quality of life and improve functioning.

General Approach to Treatment

Treatment guidelines for manic and depressive episodes of bipolar disorder are included in Table 39–2.

Although not all patients achieve asymptomatic remission, this is a goal of treatment. The mainstay of drug therapy has been mood stabilizing drugs, but studies increasingly support the use of antipsychotic drugs as monotherapy or adjunctively with mood stabilizing drugs, discussed below. A person entering treatment for a first mood episode in bipolar disorder must have a complete assessment and careful diagnosis to rule out nonpsychiatric causes. A variety of conditions can cause similar symptoms (Table 39–3). Since early and accurate diagnosis is essential to maximizing response to treatment, pharmacologic and nonpharmacologic therapy should begin as soon as possible. Treatment is often lifelong. Comorbid conditions should also be addressed aggressively.

▶ Suicidality Risk

Patients should be assessed for their potential for violence and harm to others. Friends or family can be asked to remove from home, guns, caustic chemicals, medications, and objects which the person might use to harm self or others. Risk factors for suicide include severity of depression, feelings of hopelessness, comorbid personality disorder, and a history of a previous suicide attempt.[18]

▶ Nonpharmacologic Therapy

❹ *Interpersonal, family, or group therapy with a licensed psychiatric nurse practitioner/clinical nurse specialist, psychologist, social worker, or counselor assists individuals with bipolar disorder to establish and maintain a daily routine and sleep schedule and to improve interpersonal relationships.*[19,20] These therapies may help treat and protect against manic episodes.

Cognitive behavioral therapy (CBT) is a type of psychotherapy that combines cognitive and behavioral theories. It stresses the importance of recognizing patterns of cognition (thought) and how thoughts influence subsequent feelings and behaviors. Other people, situations, and events external to the individual are not seen as the sources of thoughts and behaviors. With CBT, patients are taught self-management skills to change their negative thoughts even if external circumstances do not change.

Electroconvulsive therapy (ECT) is the application of prescribed electrical impulses to the brain for the treatment of severe depression, mixed states, psychotic depression, and treatment refractory mania. It also may be used in pregnant women who cannot take carbamazepine, lithium, or divalproex (DVP).

Psychoeducation for patients, their families, and groups regarding chronicity of bipolar disorders, self-management through sleep hygiene, nutrition, exercise, stress reduction, and abstinence from alcohol or drugs is critical to the success of supporting the individual in managing bipolar disorder. The development of a crisis intervention plan is essential.

The following websites provide additional information:

- National Association of Cognitive Behavioral Therapists—*http://www.nacbt.org/*

Table 39–2

Guidelines for the Acute Treatment of Mood Episodes in Patients With Bipolar I Disorder

Acute Manic or Mixed Episode	Acute Depressive Episode
General guidelines	General guidelines
Assess for secondary causes of mania or mixed states (e.g., alcohol or drug use)	Assess for secondary causes of depression (e.g., alcohol or drug use)
Taper off antidepressants, stimulants, and caffeine if possible	Taper off antipsychotics, benzodiazepines or sedative-hypnotic agents if possible
Treat substance abuse	Treat substance abuse
Encourage good nutrition (with regular protein and essential fatty acid intake), exercise, adequate sleep, stress reduction, and psychosocial therapy	Encourage good nutrition (with regular protein and essential fatty acid intake), exercise, adequate sleep, stress reduction, and psychosocial therapy
Optimize the dose of mood stabilizing medication(s) before adding on benzodiazepines; if psychotic features are present, add on antipsychotic; ECT used for severe or treatment-resistant manic/mixed episodes or features	Optimize the dose of mood stabilizing medication(s) before adding on lithium lamotrigine, or antidepressant (e.g., bupropion or an SSRI); if psychotic features are present, add on antipsychotic; ECT used for severe or treatment-resistant depressive episodes or for psychotic catatonia

Hypomania	Mania	Mild to Moderate Depressive Episode	Severe Depressive Episode
First, optimize current mood stabilizer or initiate mood-stabilizing medication: lithium,[a] valproate,[a] or carbamazepine.[a] Consider adding a benzodiazepine (lorazepam or clonazepam) for short-term adjunctive treatment of agitation or insomnia if needed	First, two or three drug combinations: lithium or valproate plus a benzodiazepine (lorazepam or clonazepam) for short-term adjunctive treatment of agitation or insomnia; lorazepam is recommended for catatonia. If psychosis is present initiate atypical antipsychotic in combination with above	First, initiate and/or optimize mood-stabilizing medication: lithium[a] or lamotrigtine[b]	First, two or three drug combinations: lithium[a] or lamotrigine[b] plus an antidepressant[c]; lithium plus lamotrigine. If psychosis is present, initiate atypical antipsychotic in combination with above
Alternative medication treatment options: carbamazepine[a]; If patient does not respond or tolerate, consider atypical antipsychotic (e.g., olanzapine, quetiapine, risperidone) or oxcarbazepine	Alternative medication treatment options: carbamazepine[a]; If patient does not respond or tolerate, consider oxcarbazepine	Alternative anticonvulsants: valproate,[a] carbamazepine,[a] or oxcarbazepine	Alternative anticonvulsants: valproate;[a] carbamazepine,[a] or oxcarbazepine. Second, if response is inadequate, consider adding an atypical antipsychotic (quetiapine). Third, if response is inadequate, consider a three drug combination:
Second, if response is inadequate, consider a two-drug combination: • Lithium[a] plus an anticonvulsant or an atypical antipsychotic • Anticonvulsant plus an anticonvulsant or atypical antipsychotic	Second, if response is inadequate, consider a three-drug combination: • Lithium[a] plus an anticonvulsant plus an atypical antipsychotic • Anticonvulsant plus an anticonvulsant plus an atypical antipsychotic Third, if response is inadequate consider ECT for mania with psychosis or catatonia[a]; or add clozapine for treatment-refractory illness		• Lamotrigine[b] plus an anticonvulsant plus an antidepressant • Lamotrigine[b] plus lithium[a] plus an antidepressant Fourth, if response is inadequate, consider ECT for treatment-refractory illness and depression with psychosis or catatonia[d]

ECT, electroconvulsive therapy; MAOI, manoamine oxidase inhibitor, SNRI, serotonin-norepinephrine reuptake inhibitor; SSRI, selective serotonin reuptake inhibitor; TCA, tricyclic antidepressant.

[a]Use standard therapeutic serum concentration ranges if clinically indicated; if partial response or breakthrough episode, adjust dose to achieve higher serum concentrations without causing intolerable adverse effects; valproate is preferred over lithium for mixed episodes and rapid cycling; lithium and/or lamotrigine is preferred over valproate for bipolar depression.

[b]Lamotrigine is not approved for the acute treatment of depression, and the dose must be started low and slowly titrated to decrease adverse effects if used for maintenance therapy of bipolar I disorder. A drug interaction and a severe dermatologic rash can occur when lamotrigine is combined with valproate (i.e., lamotrigine doses must be halved from standard dosing titration).

[c]Antidepressant monotherapy is not recommended for bipolar depression. Bupropion, SSRIs (e.g., citalopram, escitalopram, or sertraline), and SNRIs (e.g., venlafaxine) have shown good efficacy and fewer adverse effects in the treatment of unipolar depression; MAOIs and TCAs have more adverse effects (e.g., weight gain) and can have a higher risk of causing antidepressant-induced mania; fluoxetine, fluvoxamine, nefazodone, and paroxetine inhibit liver metabolism and should be used with caution in patients on concomitant medications that require cytochrome P450 clearance; paroxetine and venlafaxine have a higher risk for a discontinuation syndrome.

[d]ECT is used for severe mania or depression during pregnancy and for mixed episodes; prior to treatment, anticonvulsants, lithium, benzodiazepines should be tapered off to maximize therapy and minimize adverse effects.

Reprinted from DiPiro JT, Talbert RL, Yee GC, et al. (eds.) Pharmacotherapy: A Pathophysiologic Approach. 7th ed. New York, McGraw-Hill, 2008:1148.

Table 39–3
Secondary Causes of Mania

General Medical Conditions

Alzheimer's disease
Cerebral infarction
Cerebral tumors
Closed head injury
Cushing's syndrome
Hemodialysis
Hepatic encephalopathy
Huntington's disease
Hyperthyroidism
Ictal or postictal mania
Multiple sclerosis
Neurosyphilis
Systemic lupus erythematosus
Vitamin B deficiency

Medications

Corticosteroids
Diltiazem
Levodopa
Oral contraceptives
Zidovudine

Illicit Substances

Anabolic steroids
Hallucinogens
Stimulants (cocaine, amphetamines)

From Ref. 17.

- National Association for the Mentally Ill—*http://www. nami.org/*
- National Institutes for Mental Health, Bipolar Disorder—*http://www.nimh.nih.gov/healthinformation/bipolarmenu. cfm*

▶ *Pharmacologic Therapy*

⑤ *Pharmacotherapy is the cornerstone of acute and maintenance treatment of bipolar disorder.* Mood stabilizing drugs are first-line treatments and include lithium, DVP, carbamazepine, and lamotrigine. Atypical antipsychotics other than clozapine and paliperidone are also approved for treatment of acute mania. Lithium, lamotrigine, aripiprazole, olanzapine, and quetiapine are approved for maintenance therapy. Quetiapine's maintenance therapy indication is adjunctive with lithium or DVP. Drugs used with less research support and without FDA approval include topiramate and oxcarbazepine. Benzodiazepines are used adjunctively for mania.

⑥ *Mood stabilizing drugs are the primary treatment for bipolar depression.* Among antipsychotic drugs, quetiapine as monotherapy and olanzapine in combination with fluoxetine are approved for bipolar depression. Antidepressants can be used, but usually along with a mood stabilizing agent to prevent a mood switch to mania and after the patient has failed to respond adequately to optimal mood stabilizing therapy.[21] Combinations of two mood stabilizing drugs or a mood stabilizing drug and either an antipsychotic or antidepressant drug are common, especially in acute mood episodes.

⑦ *Mood stabilizer drugs are considered the primary pharmacotherapy for relapse prevention, and they are often combined with antipsychotic drugs. Aripiprazole, olanzapine, and quetiapine are approved for maintenance therapy.*

Table 39–4 includes a summary of current drug therapy for bipolar disorder. An algorithm for treatment of bipolar mania is shown in Table 39–2.

▶ *Mood Stabilizing Drugs*

The ideal mood stabilizing drug has four desired effects: treatment of acute mania, treatment of acute bipolar depression, prevention of manic relapse, and prevention of bipolar depression relapse. All currently approved mood stabilizing drugs have demonstrated efficacy over placebo for one or more of these effects, but there are differences among them with regard to specific patient populations. Choice of treatment is dictated by individual patient characteristics and history. Few studies have compared mood stabilizing drugs to each other in systematic clinical trials. Effect sizes across placebo-controlled trials of individual agents are generally similar. Lithium is often considered the first-choice drug for the classic presentation of bipolar disorder. Treatment of childhood bipolar disorder is less well researched. Lithium is FDA approved in children and adolescents as young as age 12. Among antipsychotic drugs, aripiprazole and risperidone are FDA approved in children and adolescents as young as age 10. Treatment of bipolar disorder during pregnancy and during breast-feeding is a challenge because of the risks of drug exposure in utero and transmission of drugs via breast milk.

Lithium Lithium was the first approved mood stabilizing drug. It remains a first-line agent and sets the standard for efficacy against which other drugs are usually measured. It has antimanic efficacy, prevents bipolar disorder relapse, and more modest efficacy for bipolar depression.[22] It remains the only drug classified as a mood stabilizer that is supported by multiple controlled trials in mania, depression, and relapse prevention. In most studies, lithium's efficacy is equivalent to that of the anticonvulsant mood stabilizers and the atypical antipsychotic drugs.[23] It is most effective for patients with few previous episodes, symptom-free interepisode remission, and a family history of bipolar disorder with good response to lithium. Patients with rapid cycling bipolar disorder are less responsive to lithium, however, than to other mood stabilizing drugs such as DVP.[24] Additionally, its efficacy for bipolar depression is less robust than for mania.[25] It may also be less effective in patients with mixed mood episodes (symptoms of mania and depression occurring simultaneously) and in mania secondary to nonpsychiatric illness.

Table 39–4

Product Formulation, Dose, and Clinical Use of Agents Used in the Treatment of Bipolar Disorder

Generic Name	Brand Names	Formulations	Dosages	Clinical Use
Lithium Salts				
FDA approved for use in bipolar disorder				
Lithium carbonate Lithium citrate	Eskalith Eskalith CR Lithobid, generic	Capsule: 300 mg, ER tablet: 450 mg ER tablet: 300 mg Tablet: 300 mg Capsule: 150, 300, 600 mg 300 mg/5 mL (8 mEq or mmol per 5 mL)	900–2,400 mg/day in 2–4 divided doses, preferably with meals. There is wide variation in the dosage needed to achieve therapeutic response and 12-hour serum lithium concentration (i.e., 0.6–1.2 mEq/L (mmol/L) for maintenance therapy and 1–1.5 mEq/L (mmol/L) for acute mood episodes taken 12 hours after last dose). Single daily dosing is effective and causes fewer renal effects	Monotherapy or in combination with other drugs for the acute treatment of mania and for maintenance treatment
Anticonvulsants				
FDA approved for use in bipolar disorder				
Carbamazepine	Equetro Tegretol Tegretol XR Carbatrol	Capsule: 100 mg, 200 mg, 300 mg SR; may open capsule but do not crush or chew beads; take with food Tablet: 200 mg Chewable tablet: 100 mg Suspension: 100 mg/5 mL ER tablet: 100, 200, 400 mg ER capsule: 200, 300 mg	Start at 100–200 mg twice a day; increase by 200 mg every 3–4 days 200–1,800 mg/day in 2–4 divided doses. Target serum concentration is 4–12 mcg/mL (17–51 μmoles/L)	Monotherapy or in combination with other drugs for the acute treatment of mania or mixed episodes for bipolar I disorder
DVP sodium	Depakote, generic Depakote ER	Enteric-coated, delayed-release tablet: 125, 250, 500 mg Sprinkle capsule: 125 mg ER tablet: 250, 500 mg	750–3,000 mg/day (20–60 mg/kg/day) in 2–3 divided doses for delayed-release DVP or VPA ER DVP may be given once daily A loading dose of 20–30 mg/kg/day can be given, then 20 mg/kg/day and titrated to a serum concentration of 50–125 mcg/mL (347–866 μmoles/L)	Monotherapy or in combination with other drugs for the acute treatment of mania. Although commonly used for relapse prevention, maintenance treatment is not FDA approved
VPA VPA syrup	Depakene, generic Depakene, generic	Capsule: 250 mg 250 mg/5 mL		
Lamotrigine	Lamictal	Tablet: 25, 100, 150, 200 mg Chewable tablets: 2, 5, 25 mg Orally disintegrating tablet: 25, 50, 100, 200 mg	50–400 mg/day in divided doses. Dosage should be slowly increased by following prescribing information. If DVP is added to lamotrigine, the lamotrigine dosage should be reduced by half	Monotherapy or in combination with other drugs for the long-term maintenance treatment of bipolar depression
Anticonvulsants and Other Drugs Not FDA Approved for Use in Bipolar Disorder				
Clonazepam	Klonopin, generic	Tablet: 0.5, 1, 2 mg	0.5–20 mg/day in divided doses or one dose at bedtime Dosage should be slowly adjusted up and down according to response and adverse effects	Use in combination with other drugs for the acute treatment of mania or mixed episodes. Use as a short-term adjunctive sedative-hypnotic agent
Lorazepam	Ativan, generic	Tablet: 0.5, 1, 2 mg Oral solution: 2 mg/mL Injection: 2, 4 mg/mL	2–10 mg/day in divided doses or one dose at bedtime Dosage should be slowly adjusted up and down according to response and adverse effects	

(Continued)

Table 39–4

Product Formulation, Dose, and Clinical Use of Agents Used in the Treatment of Bipolar Disorder (*Continued*)

Generic Name	Brand Names	Formulations	Dosages	Clinical Use
Anticonvulsants and Other Drugs Not FDA Approved for Use in Bipolar Disorder				
Oxcarbazepine	Trileptal, generic	Tablet: 150, 300, 600 mg Suspension: 300 mg/ 5 mL	300–1,200 mg/day in two divided doses Doses should be slowly adjusted up and down according to response and adverse effects (e.g., 150–300 mg twice daily and increase by 300–600 mg/day at weekly intervals)	May cause fewer adverse drug–drug interactions than carbamazepine, but causes more GI side effects and hyponatremia. Evidence is limited regarding efficacy
Topiramate	Topamax	Tablet: 25, 100, 200 mg Sprinkle capsule: 15, 25 mg	50–200 mg/day in divided doses Dosage should be slowly increased to minimize adverse effects (e.g., 25 mg at bedtime for 1 week, then 25–50 mg/day increments at weekly intervals	Not recommended for the acute treatment of mania or mixed episodes due to lack of efficacy; used as an adjunctive agent with established mood stabilizers
Atypical Antipsychotics				
FDA approved for bipolar disorder				
Aripiprazole	Abilify Abilify Discmelt	Tablet: 2, 5, 10, 15, 20, 30 mg Oral solution: 5 mg/5 mL Tablet, orally disintegrating: 10, 15 mg	10–30 mg/day once daily	Used as monotherapy or in combination with lithium or valproate for the acute treatment of mania or mixed states for bipolar I disorder and prevention of manic relapse
Olanzapine	Zyprexa Zyprexa Zydis	Tablet: 2.5, 5, 7.5, 10, 15, 20 mg Tablet, orally disintegrating: 5, 10, 15, 20 mg	5–20 mg/day in one or two doses	Used as monotherapy or in combination with lithium or valproate for acute treatment of mania or mixed states for bipolar I disorder and prevention of manic relapse. Used in combination with fluoxetine (OFC) for treatment of bipolar depression
Quetiapine	Seroquel Seroquel XR	Tablet: 25, 50, 100, 200, 300, 400 mg ER tablet: 50, 150, 200, 300, 400 mg	50–800 mg/day in divided doses or once daily when stabilized	Used as monotherapy or in combination with lithium or DVP for acute treatment of mania, mixed states for bipolar I disorder, and depression of bipolar I and bipolar II disorder. Used adjunctively with lithium or DVP for relapse prevention of bipolar mania and depression
Risperidone	Risperdal, generic Risperdal M-Tabs Risperdal Consta	Tablet: 0.25, 0.5, 1, 2, 3, 4 mg Oral solution: 1 mg/mL Tablet, orally disintegrating: 0.5, 1, 2, 3, 4 mg Long-acting injectable: 12.5, 25, 37.5, 50 mg	0.5–6 mg/day in one or two doses	Used as monotherapy or adjunctively with lithium or DVP for acute mania or mixed episodes of bipolar I disorder Risperidone microspheres is not FDA approved for bipolar disorder
Ziprasidone	Geodon	Capsule: 20, 40, 60, 80 mg	40–160 mg/day in divided doses	Used as monotherapy or adjunctively with lithium or DVP for acute mania or mixed episodes of bipolar I disorder

VPA, Valproic acid; DVP, divalproex.

From Refs. 23, 28, 30, 33, 34–36, 42, 43.

Evidence shows lithium's effect on suicidal behavior is superior to that of other mood stabilizing drugs.[26] Lithium reduces the risk of deliberate self-harm or suicide by about 70%.

Mechanism of Action. Lithium's pharmacologic mechanism of action is not well understood and involves multiple effects. Possibilities include altered ion transport, effects on neurotransmitter signaling, blocking adenyl cyclase systems, effects on inositol, neuroprotection or increased BDNF, and inhibition of second messenger systems.[27]

Dosing and Monitoring. Lithium is usually initiated at a dosage of 600 to 900 mg/day. Although it is most commonly given in a divided dosage, once-daily dosing is acceptable, especially with sustained-release formulations, and once-daily dosing can improve patient adherence and reduce some side effects. Lithium has a narrow therapeutic index, meaning the toxic dosage is not much greater than the therapeutic dosage. Lithium requires regular serum concentration monitoring as a guide to dosage titration and to minimize adverse effects. At least weekly monitoring is recommended until the patient is stabilized, then the frequency can be decreased. Well-maintained patients who tolerate lithium without difficulty can be monitored by serum concentration as infrequently as twice yearly. Dosage is titrated to achieve a serum lithium concentration of 0.6 to 1.4 mEq/L (mmol/L). Higher serum concentrations are usually required to treat an acute episode than to prevent relapse. Serum lithium maintained above 0.8 mEq/L (mmol/L) may be more effective at preventing relapse, however, than lower serum concentrations. The suggested therapeutic serum concentration range is based on a 12-hour postdose sample collection, usually a morning trough in patients taking more than one dose per day. At least 2 weeks at a suggested therapeutic serum concentration is required for an adequate trial of lithium. Table 39–5 shows pharmacokinetic parameters and desired serum concentrations of mood stabilizing drugs used for bipolar disorder. It is common for lithium to be combined with other mood stabilizing drugs or antipsychotic drugs, if necessary, in order to achieve more complete remission of symptoms.

Adverse Effects. The most common adverse effects are GI upset, tremor, and polyuria,[28] which are dose related. Nausea, dyspepsia, and diarrhea can be minimized by coadministration with food, use of sustained-release formulations, and giving smaller doses more frequently to reduce the amount of drug in the GI tract at a given time. Tremor is present in up to 50% of patients. In addition to the approaches above, low-dose β-blocker therapy such as propranolol 20 to 60 mg/day often reduces the tremor.

Lithium impairs the kidney's ability to concentrate urine due to its inhibitory effect on vasopressin. This causes an increase in urine volume and urinary frequency and a consequent increase in thirst. Polyuria and polydipsia occur in up to 70% of patients. A severe form of polyuria, when urine volume exceeds 3 L/day, is known as nephrogenic lithium-induced diabetes insipidus. It can be treated with hydrochlorothiazide or amiloride. If the former is used, the lithium dosage should be reduced by 33% to 50% to account for the drug–drug interaction that could increase serum lithium concentrations and cause toxicity. Long-term lithium therapy can cause structural kidney changes such as glomerular sclerosis or tubular atrophy. Once-daily dosing of lithium is less likely to cause renal adverse effects than divided-daily dosing.

Lithium is concentrated in the thyroid gland and can impair thyroid hormone synthesis. Although goiter is uncommon, as many as 30% of patients develop at least transiently elevated thyroid stimulating hormone (TSH) values. Lithium-induced hypothyroidism is not usually an indication to discontinue the drug. Patients can be supplemented with levothyroxine if continuation of lithium is desired.[28]

Other common adverse effects include poor concentration, acneiform rash, alopecia, worsening of psoriasis, weight gain, metallic taste, and glucose dysfunction. Lithium causes ECG. Less commonly, it can cause or worsen arrhythmias. Cardiologic evaluation is recommended for patients with pre-existing cardiac disease who are candidates for lithium therapy. A benign leukocytosis is also common.[28]

Lithium and other mood stabilizing drugs require baseline and routine laboratory monitoring to help determine medical appropriateness for initiation of therapy and monitoring of potential adverse effects. Guidelines for such monitoring are outlined in Table 39–6.

Acute lithium toxicity, which can occur at serum concentrations over 2 mEq/L (mmol/L), can be severe and life-threatening, necessitating emergency medical treatment. Symptoms include worsening of GI distress to include severe vomiting and diarrhea; deterioration in motor coordination including a coarse tremor, ataxia, and dysarthria; and impaired cognition. In its most severe form, seizures, cardiac arrhythmias, coma, and kidney damage have been reported. Treatment includes discontinuation of lithium, IV fluids to correct fluid and electrolyte imbalance, and osmotic diuresis or hemodialysis. In case of overdose, gastric lavage is indicated. Clinical symptoms can continue well after the serum concentration is lowered, as clearance from the CNS is slower than from the serum. Factors predisposing to lithium toxicity include fluid and sodium loss due to hot weather or exercise or drug interactions that increase serum lithium.[28]

Drug Interactions. Drug interactions involving lithium are common. Because lithium is not metabolized or protein bound, however, it is not associated with metabolic drug interactions that occur with other mood stabilizing drugs. Common and significant drug interactions involve thiazide diuretics, nonsteroidal anti-inflammatory drugs, and angiotensin-converting enzyme (ACE) inhibitor drugs. If a diuretic must be used with lithium and a thiazide is not required, loop diuretics such as furosemide are less likely to increase lithium retention. The ACE inhibitors can abruptly increase serum lithium with the potential of acute and fatal toxicity, even after months of no change in the

Table 39–5

Pharmacokinetics and Therapeutic Serum Concentrations of Lithium and Anticonvulsants Used in the Treatment of Bipolar Disorder

	Lithium	Carbamazepine	Oxcarbazepine	DVP Sodium/VPA	Lamotrigine
GI Absorption					
Regular release	Rapid: 95–100% within 1–6 hours	Slow and erratic: 85–90%	Slow and complete: 100%	Rapid and complete (VPA)	Rapid: 98%
Syrup/suspension/ solution	Faster rate of absorption: 100%	Faster rate of absorption	Unknown	Faster rate of absorption than tablets	NA
Extended-release/ enteric-coated tablets	Delayed absorption: 60–90%	Delayed absorption: 89% of the suspension; and less than regular-release tablets	NA	Delayed absorption with delayed-release tablets; valproate is rapidly converted to VPA in the intestine, then is rapidly and almost completely absorbed from the GI tract Extended-release bioavailability is approximately 15% less than delayed release	NA
Delay in absorption by food	Yes	No; reports of increased rate of absorption with fatty meals (extended-release capsule)	Unknown	Yes; food slows the rate of absorption but not the extent for DVP	Bioavailability not affected by food
Time to reach peak serum concentrations	0.5–3 hours (regular release) 4–12 hours (extended release) 0.25–1 hour (oral solution)	4–5 hours (regular-release); 1.5 hours (suspension); 3–12 hours (extended-release tablets); 4.1–7.7 hours (extended-release capsules); higher peak concentrations with chewable tablets	4.5 hours (range of 3–13 hours)	1–4 hours (VPA) 3–5 hours (DVP single dose) 7–14 hours (DVP extended-release multiple dosing)	1–4 hours
Distribution					
Volume of distribution	Initial: 0.3–0.4 L/kg Steady-state: 0.7–1 L/kg	0.6–2 L/kg (adults)	10-monohydroxy carbazepine (metabolite): 49 L/kg	11 L/1.73 m² (total valproate); 92 L/1.73 m² (free valproate)	0.9–1.3 L/kg
Crosses the placenta	Yes; pregnancy risk category: D Risk of cardiac defects: 0.1–0.5%	Yes; pregnancy risk category: D	Yes; pregnancy risk category: C	Yes: pregnancy risk category: D Risk of neural tube defects: 1–5%	Yes; pregnancy risk category: C
Crosses into breast milk	Yes: 35–50% of mother's serum concentration; breast-feeding not recommended	Yes: ratio of concentration in breast milk to plasma is 0.4 for drug and 0.5 for epoxide metabolite; considered compatible with breast-feeding	Yes: both drug and active metabolite; breast-feeding not recommended	Yes: considered compatible with breast-feeding	Yes; breast-feeding not recommended
Protein binding	No	75–90%	40% of active metabolite	80–90% (dose dependent)	55%
Renal clearance	Yes: 10–40 mL/min with 90–98% of dose excreted in urine; 80% of lithium that is filtered by the renal glomeruli is reabsorbed	Yes; 1–3% excreted unchanged in urine	Yes; 95% excreted in the urine less than 1% excreted unchanged	Yes: 30–50% excreted as glucuronide conjugate; less than 3% excreted unchanged	Yes; 94% excreted as glucuronide conjugate

(Continued)

Table 39–5

Pharmacokinetics and Therapeutic Serum Concentrations of Lithium and Anticonvulsants Used in the Treatment of Bipolar Disorder *(Continued)*

	Lithium	Carbamazepine	Oxcarbazepine	DVP Sodium/VPA	Lamotrigine
Metabolism					
Hepatic metabolism	No	Yes: oxidation and hydroxylation; induces liver enzymes to increase its own metabolism and metabolism of other drugs	Yes: oxidation and conjugation	Yes: oxidation and glucuronide conjugation	Yes: glucuronic acid conjugation induces its own metabolism in normal volunteers
Metabolites	No	Yes: 10, 11-epoxide (active)	Yes: 10-mono-hydroxy carbazepine (active)	Yes (not active)	No
Kinetics	First-order	First-order after initial enzyme induction phase	First-order	First-order	First-order
Half-life (t½)	18–27 hours (adult); more than 36 hours (elderly or patients with renal impairment)	t½ decreases over time due to autoinduction: 25–65 hours (initial) 12–17 hours (adult multiple dosing) 8–14 hours (children multiple dosing)	2 hours (parent) 9 hours (metabolite)	5–20 hours (adults)	25 hours; increases to 59 hours with concomitant VPA therapy
Cytochrome P450 (CYP450) Isoenzyme					
CYP450 substrate	No	2C8 and 3A3/4	Unknown	2C19	Unknown
CYP450 inhibitor	No	No	2C19	2C9, 2D6, and 3A3/4	Unknown
CYP450 inducer	No	1A2, 2C9/10, and 3A3/4	3A3/4	No	Unknown
Therapeutic Serum/Plasma Concentrations					
Obtain blood level 10–12 hours postdose	1–1.5 mEq/L (mmol/L): for adult, acute mania 0.4–0.6 mEq/L (mmol/L): for elderly or medically ill 0.6–1.2 mEq/L (mmol/L): for adult, maintenance	4–12 mcg/mL (17–51 µmol/L): for adult, acute mania and maintenance 4–8 mcg/mL: for elderly or medically ill	No established therapeutic range; 12–30 mcg/mL for 10-hydroxy carbazepine based on epilepsy trials	50–125 mcg/mL (347–866 µmol/L): adult, acute mania and maintenance 40–75 mcg/mL: elderly or medically ill	No established therapeutic range: 4–20 mcg/mL (16–80 µmol/L) based on epilepsy trials

DVP, divalproex; NA, not applicable; VPA, valproic acid.

From Refs. 28, 30, 33–35.

serum lithium concentration. This combination is strongly discouraged.[29]

DVP Sodium and Valproic Acid DVP sodium is comprised of sodium valproate and VPA. The delayed-release and extended-release formulations are converted in the small intestine into VPA, which is the systemically absorbed form. It was developed as an anticonvulsant, but also has efficacy for mood stabilization and migraine headaches. It is FDA approved for the treatment of the manic phase of bipolar disorder. It is generally equal in efficacy to lithium and some

other drugs for bipolar mania. It has particular utility in bipolar disorder patients with rapid cycling, mixed mood features, and substance abuse comorbidity. Although not FDA approved for relapse prevention, studies support this use, and it is widely prescribed for maintenance therapy. DVP can be used as monotherapy or in combination with lithium or an antipsychotic drug.[30]

Mechanism of Action. The mechanism of action of DVP is not well understood. It is known to affect ion transport and enhances the activity of gamma-aminobutyric acid (GABA).

Table 39–6

Guidelines for Baseline and Routine Laboratory Tests and Monitoring for Agents Used in the Treatment of Bipolar Disorder

	Baseline: Physical Examination and General Chemistry[a]	Hematologic Tests[b]		Metabolic Tests[c]		Liver Function Tests[d]		Renal Function Tests[e]		Thyroid Function Tests[f]		Serum Electrolytes[g]		Dermatologic[h]	
	Baseline	Baseline	6–12 Months	Baseline	6–12 Months	Baseline	6–12 Months	Baseline	6–12 Months	Baseline	6–12 Months	Baseline	6–12 Months	Baseline	3–6 Months
Atypical antipsychotics[i]	X			X	X										
Carbamazepine[j]	X	X	X			X	X	X				X	X	X	X
Lamotrigine[k]	X													X	X
Lithium[l]	X	X	X	X	X			X	X	X	X			X	X
Oxcarbazepine[m]	X	X	X									X	X		
Valproate[n]	X	X	X	X	X	X	X							X	

[a]Screen for drug abuse and serum pregnancy

[b]CBC with differential and platelets.

[c]Fasting glucose, serum lipids, weight.

[d]Lactate dehydrogenase, aspartate aminotransferase, alanine aminotransferase, total bilirubin, alkaline phosphatase.

[e]Serum creatinine, blood urea nitrogen, urinalysis, urine osmolality, specific gravity.

[f]Triiodothyronine, total thyroxine, thyroxine uptake, and thyroid-stimulating hormone.

[g]Serum sodium.

[h]Rashes, hair thinning, alopecia.

[i]Atypical antipsychotic: Monitor for increased appetite with weight gain (primarily in patients with initial low or normal body mass index); monitor closely if rapid or significant weight gain occurs during early therapy; cases of hyperlipidemia and diabetes reported.

[j]Carbamazepine: Manufacturer recommends CBC and platelets (and possibly reticulocyte counts and serum iron) at baseline, and that subsequent monitoring be individualized by the clinician (e.g., CBC, platelet counts, and liver function tests every 2 weeks during the first 2 months of treatment, then every 3 months if normal). Monitor more closely if patient exhibits hematologic or hepatic abnormalities or if the patient is receiving a myelotoxic drug; discontinue if platelets are less than 100,000/mm^3, if WBC is less than 3,000/mm^3 or if there is evidence of bone marrow suppression or liver dysfunction. Serum electrolyte levels should be monitored in the elderly or those at risk for hyponatremia. Carbamazepine interferes with some pregnancy tests.

[k]Lamotrigine: If renal or hepatic impairment, monitor closely and adjust dosage according to manufacturer's guidelines. Serious dermatologic reactions have occurred within 2 to 8 weeks of initiating treatment and are more likely to occur in patients receiving concomitant valproate, with rapid dose escalation, or using doses exceeding the recommended titration schedule.

[l]Lithium: Obtain baseline ECG for patients older than 40 years or if pre-existing cardiac disease (benign, reversible T-wave depression can occur). Renal function tests should be obtained every 2 to 3 months during the first 6 months, then every 6 to 12 months; if impaired renal function, monitor 24-hour urine volume and creatinine every 3 months; if urine volume more than 3 L/day, monitor urinalysis, osmolality, and specific gravity every 3 months. Thyroid function tests should be obtained once or twice during the first 6 months, then every 6 to 12 months; monitor for signs and symptoms of hypothyroidism; if supplemental thyroid therapy is required, monitor thyroid function tests and adjust thyroid dose every 1 to 2 months until thyroid function indices are within normal range, then monitor every 3 to 6 months.

[m]Oxcarbazepine: Hyponatremia (serum sodium concentrations less than 125 mEq/L) has been reported and occurs more frequently during the first 3 months of therapy; serum sodium concentrations should be monitored in patients receiving drugs that lower serum sodium concentrations (e.g., diuretics or drugs that cause inappropriate antidiuretic hormone secretion) or in patients with symptoms of hyponatremia (e.g., confusion, headache, lethargy, and malaise). Hypersensitivity reactions have occurred in approximately 25% to 30% of patients with a history of carbamazepine hypersensitivity and requires immediate discontinuation.

[n]Valproate: Weight gain reported in patients with low or normal body mass index. Monitor platelets and liver function during first 3 to 6 months if evidence of increased bruising or bleeding. Monitor closely if patients exhibit hematologic or hepatic abnormalities or in patients receiving drugs that affect coagulation, such as aspirin or warfarin; discontinue if platelets are less than 100,000/mm^3/L or if prolonged bleeding time. Pancreatitis, hyperammonemic encephalopathy, polycystic ovary syndrome, increased testosterone, and menstrual irregularities have been reported; not recommended during first trimester of pregnancy due to risk of neural tube defects.

From DiPiro JT, Talbert RL, Yee GC, et al., (eds.) Pharmacotherapy: A Pathophysiologic Approach. 7th ed. New York, McGraw-Hill, 2008:1153.

Like lithium, it also has possible neuroprotective effects through enhancement of BDNF.[31]

Dosing and Monitoring. DVP is usually initiated at 500 to 1,000 mg/day, but studies indicate a therapeutic serum VPA concentration can be reached more quickly through a loading dose approach of 20 to 30 mg/kg/day. Using this approach, patients may respond with a significant reduction in symptoms within the first few days of treatment. The dosage is then titrated according to response, tolerability, and serum concentration. The most often referenced desired VPA serum concentration is 50 to 125 mcg/mL (347–866 μmoles/L), but it is not unusual for patients to require more than 100 mcg/mL (693 μmoles/L) for optimal efficacy. Some patients require high milligram dosages in order to reach a desired serum concentration. The suggested serum concentration range is based on morning sampling, which is a trough value for patients taking divided daily dosing. Serum concentration monitoring is recommended at least every 2 weeks until stabilized, then less frequently, sometimes as infrequently as twice yearly. The extended-release formulation can be taken once daily (see Table 39–4). If administered at night, a morning blood sampling is not an actual trough. The drug could be given in the morning so that blood sampling the following day would be a trough value and more easily interpreted. The systemic bioavailability of extended-release DVP is about 15% less than that of the delayed-release formulation. Patients who have difficulty swallowing large tablets can use the sprinkle formulation. The immediate-release formulation, either capsules or syrup, is generally given three or four times per day.[30]

Adverse Effects. The most common adverse effects of DVP are GI (loss of appetite, nausea, dyspepsia, diarrhea), tremor, and drowsiness. GI distress can be reduced by coadministration with food. The delayed-release and extended-release formulations are less likely to cause gastric distress than the immediate-release VPA. This is an advantage for DVP, along with fewer daily doses, which can improve patient adherence to treatment. Dosage reduction can reduce all of the common DVP side effects. As with lithium, a low-dose β-blocker may alleviate the tremor. Weight gain is also common, occurring in up to 50% of patients on maintenance therapy.[30]

Other adverse effects that are less common include alopecia or a change in hair color or texture. Hair loss can be minimized by supplementation with a vitamin containing selenium and zinc. Polycystic ovarian syndrome associated with increased androgen production has been reported. Thrombocytopenia is not uncommon, and the platelet count should be monitored periodically. It is a dose-related adverse effect and usually asymptomatic, but the drug is usually stopped if the platelet count decreases to less than 100 × 10³/mm³ (100 × 10⁹/L). More rare are hepatic toxicity and pancreatitis, which are not always dose related. Severe GI symptoms of hepatic or pancreatic toxicity include vomiting, pain, and loss of appetite. When these occur the patient should be evaluated for possible hepatitis or pancreatitis.

DVP has a wide therapeutic index. Acute toxicity for high dosages or overdosage is not life-threatening.[30]

Drug Interactions. Drug interactions involving DVP are common. It is a weak inhibitor of some of the drug metabolizing liver enzymes and can affect the metabolism of other drugs. These include other anticonvulsants and tricyclic antidepressants. The interaction between DVP and lamotrigine is particularly important. The risk of a dangerous rash due to lamotrigine is increased when given concurrently with DVP. When lamotrigine is added to DVP, the initial lamotrigine dosage should be half the typical starting dosage, and lamotrigine should be titrated more slowly than usual. When DVP is added to lamotrigine, the lamotrigine dosage should be reduced by 50%. Conversely, the metabolism of DVP can be increased by enzyme-inducing drugs such as carbamazepine and phenytoin, while DVP may simultaneously slow metabolism of the other agents.[29]

Carbamazepine Although long utilized as a mood stabilizing drug, only the extended-release formulation of carbamazepine has received FDA approval for treatment of bipolar disorder. Like DVP, it also has efficacy for mood stabilization, but is considered possibly less desirable as a first-line agent because of safety and drug interactions. It is sometimes reserved for patients who fail to respond to lithium or for patients with rapid cycling or mixed bipolar disorder. Carbamazepine can be used as monotherapy or in combination with lithium or an antipsychotic drug.[32,33]

Mechanism of Action. The mechanism of action of carbamazepine is not well understood. It blocks ion channels and inhibits sustained repetitive neuronal excitation, but whether this explains its efficacy as a mood stabilizing drug is not known.[32]

Dosing and Monitoring. Carbamazepine is usually initiated at 400 to 600 mg/day. The sustained-release formulation can be given in two divided doses. In addition to a formulation that is completely sustained-release, an additional extended-release formulation contains a matrix of 25% immediate-release, 40% extended-release, and 35% enteric-release beads.[33] The suggested therapeutic serum concentration is 4 to 12 mcg/mL (17–51 μmol/L). As with DVP, some patients require high milligram dosages to achieve a desired serum concentration and therapeutic effect. The dosage can be increased by 200 to 400 mg/day as often as every 2 to 4 days to achieve the desired effect. Serum concentration monitoring is suggested at least every 2 weeks until stabilized, then less frequently.[32]

Adverse Effects. The most common adverse effects are drowsiness, dizziness, ataxia, lethargy, and confusion. At mildly toxic serum concentrations, it also causes diplopia and dysarthria. These effects can be minimized through dosage adjustments, use of sustained-release formulations, and giving more of the drug late in the day. GI upset is also common. Carbamazepine has an antidiuretic effect similar to the syndrome of inappropriate antidiuretic hormone secretion and can cause hyponatremia. Mild elevations in liver enzymes can occur, but hepatitis is less common.

Mild, dose-related leukopenia is not unusual and not usually an indication for stopping the drug. More serious blood count abnormalities such as aplastic anemia and agranulocytosis are rare, but life-threatening.[33] Suggested baseline and routine laboratory monitoring is reviewed in Table 39–6.

Drug Interactions. Carbamazepine induces the hepatic metabolism of many drugs, including other anticonvulsants, antipsychotics, some antidepressants, oral contraceptives, and antiretroviral agents. Carbamazepine is also an autoinducer, i.e., it induces its own metabolism. The dosage may require an increase after 1 month or so of therapy because of this effect. Conversely, the metabolism of carbamazepine can be slowed by enzyme inhibiting drugs such as some antidepressants, macrolide antibiotics including erythromycin and clarithromycin, azole antifungal drugs including ketoconazole and itraconazole, and grapefruit juice. Carbamazepine should not be given concurrently with clozapine because of the additive risk of agranulocytosis.[29]

Lamotrigine Lamotrigine is effective for the maintenance treatment of bipolar disorder. It is more effective for depression relapse prevention than for mania relapse. Its primary limitation as an acute treatment is the time required for titration to an effective dosage. In addition to maintenance monotherapy, it is sometimes used in combination with lithium or DVP, although combination with DVP increases the risk of rash, and lamotrigine dosage adjustment is required.[34]

Mechanism of Action. The mechanism of action of lamotrigine appears to involve blockage of ion channels and effects on glutamate transmission, although the precise mechanism in bipolar disorder is not clear.[34]

Dosing and Monitoring. Lamotrigine is usually initiated at 25 mg daily for the first 1 to 2 weeks, then increasing in a dose-doubling fashion every 1 to 2 weeks to a target dosage of 200 to 400 mg/day. If lamotrigine is added to DVP, the starting dosage is 25 mg every other day with a slower titration to reduce the risk of rash. If DVP is added to lamotrigine, the lamotrigine dosage should be reduced by 50% for the same reason. If lamotrigine therapy is interrupted for more than a few days, it should be restarted at the initial dosage. Serum concentration monitoring is not routinely recommended for patients with bipolar disorder.[34]

Adverse Effects. The lamotrigine adverse effect of greatest significance is a maculopapular rash, occurring in up to 10% of patients.[34] Although usually benign and temporary, some rashes can progress to life-threatening Stevens–Johnson syndrome. The risk of rash is greater with a rapid dosage titration and when given concurrently with DVP or other metabolic enzyme inhibitors. The risk is minimal when the dosage titration schedule is slow. Other side effects include dizziness, drowsiness, headache, blurred vision, and nausea. In contrast to other mood stabilizing drugs such as lithium and DVP, lamotrigine does not significantly influence body weight.

Drug Interactions. Drug interactions involving lamotrigine are usually due to induction or inhibition of its metabolism by other drugs. It does not affect drug metabolizing hepatic enzymes on its own, but other drugs that affect these pathways can have a significant effect on lamotrigine's clearance. In particular, DVP slows the rate of elimination of lamotrigine by about half, necessitating dosage reduction. Conversely, carbamazepine increases the rate of lamotrigine metabolism. Upward adjustment in the lamotrigine dosage may be needed as a result.[29]

Oxcarbazepine Oxcarbazepine is an analogue of carbamazepine, developed as an anticonvulsant. An advantage over carbamazepine is that routine monitoring of hematology profiles and serum concentrations are not indicated as the drug is less likely to cause hematologic abnormalities.[35] Additionally, drug interactions are less significant, although it is at least a mild inducer of certain metabolic pathways, and vigilance for drug interactions is needed, especially with oral contraceptives. Oxcarbazepine appears in the most recent treatment algorithms for bipolar disorder,[36] but clinical trial data are limited. A systematic review concluded that there are insufficient data from well-designed clinical trials to provide guidance on its use.[37]

Adverse Effects. Adverse effects due to oxcarbazepine include drowsiness, dizziness, GI upset, and hyponatremia, the latter two of which may be more likely than with carbamazepine.[35]

Others High potency benzodiazepine agents such as clonazepam and lorazepam have been used as adjunctive therapy, especially during acute mania episodes, to reduce anxiety and improve sleep.[38] Topiramate is commonly used for its putative mood stabilizing effects, but unpublished, well-designed, randomized, controlled trials sponsored by the manufacturer showed no difference between topiramate and placebo for treatment of bipolar disorder. Uncontrolled, open-label data suggest possible use as an adjunctive agent.[39] Gabapentin has shown no efficacy over placebo and is not recommended for patients with bipolar disorder. One of the few randomized, placebo-controlled trials of gabapentin in bipolar disorder actually showed a statistical inferiority compared to placebo.[40] As complementary or alternative medicines gain wider usage, omega-3 fatty acids have been used in mood disorders. Insufficient well-designed studies exist to support a recommendation of routine use or to establish a place in therapy relative to usual therapies.

▶ Antipsychotic Drugs

Conventional antipsychotic drugs such as chlorpromazine and haloperidol have long been used in the treatment of acute mania. Atypical antipsychotic drugs including aripiprazole, olanzapine, quetiapine, risperidone, and ziprasidone have been approved for the treatment of bipolar mania or mixed mood episodes as monotherapy or in combination with mood stabilizing drugs.[23] Aripiprazole, olanzapine, and quetiapine are also approved for maintenance therapy for prevention of manic relapse. The combination of olanzapine and fluoxetine is approved for treatment of acute bipolar depression. Quetiapine is approved as monotherapy for acute bipolar depression and as adjunctive therapy with lithium or DVP for prevention of bipolar depression relapse. Approval of antipsychotic drugs in bipolar disorder patients applies without regard to the presence of psychotic symptoms. In comparative studies, atypical antipsychotic drugs are equivalent in efficacy to lithium and DVP for treatment of acute mania. Treatment guidelines include antipsychotic drugs as first-line therapy.[36] Of interest is evidence that the combination of mood stabilizing drugs and antipsychotic drugs is more likely to achieve remission of acute manic episodes than monotherapy with either.[23] The quetiapine data in relapse prevention of both manic and bipolar depression episodes likewise favored combination therapy over mood stabilizing drug monotherapy.[41]

The mechanisms of action, usual dosages, pharmacokinetics, adverse effects, and drug interactions involving antipsychotic drugs are discussed in detail in the chapter on schizophrenia. Dosages in bipolar disorder are similar to those used in schizophrenia. Higher dosages are often required to treat an acute episode than to prevent relapse. The recommended dosage of aripiprazole for bipolar disorder is 20 to 30 mg/day, somewhat higher than the average dosage used in schizophrenia.[42] The recommended dosage for quetiapine in treatment of acute bipolar depression is 300 mg/day, less than the 600 mg/day recommended in acute mania.[43]

Atypical antipsychotic drugs are less likely than conventional antipsychotics to cause neurologic side effects, especially movement abnormalities. As a group, however, they are more likely to cause metabolic side effects, such as weight gain, glucose dysregulation, and dyslipidemia.[44] Among the atypical antipsychotic drugs approved for treatment of bipolar disorder, olanzapine is more likely to cause metabolic side effects. Quetiapine and risperidone cause less metabolic effects than olanzapine. Aripiprazole and ziprasidone are least associated with effects on weight, glucose, and lipids. Metabolic adverse effects data regarding paliperidone in acute and limited long-term studies show mild weight gain and little effect on glucose and lipids.[45] More experience is needed to fully understand paliperidone's profile. Paliperidone is not FDA approved for bipolar disorder at present. The chapter on schizophrenia discusses adverse effects of antipsychotic drugs in more detail.

▶ Antidepressants

Treatment of depressive episodes in bipolar disorder patients presents a particular challenge because of the risk of a drug-induced mood switch to mania, although there is not complete agreement about such risk. The FDA requires the product label of all antidepressant drugs to contain language about the potential risk of inducing a mood switch to mania. Randomized, controlled data show no advantage for adjunctive antidepressant use compared to mood stabilizer therapy alone.[46] Treatment guidelines suggest lithium or lamotrigine as first-line

therapy.[36,47] However, the guidelines do not reflect the more recent data on olanzapine and quetiapine, discussed above. When usual treatment fails, efficacy data support use of antidepressants.[21]

Guidelines agree that when antidepressants must be used, they should be combined with a mood stabilizing drug to reduce the risk of mood switch to hypomania or mania.[36,47] The question of which antidepressant drugs are less likely to cause a mood switch is not resolved, but tricyclic antidepressants are thought to carry a greater risk of treatment-emergent mania. A randomized comparison of venlafaxine, sertraline, and bupropion as adjunctive therapy to a mood stabilizer showed venlafaxine with the highest risk of a mood switch to mania or hypomania and bupropion with the least.[48]

Special Populations

Assessment and management by appropriate psychiatric specialists is important for special populations such as pediatrics, geriatrics, pregnancy, and others.

▶ Pediatrics

Evidence regarding treatment of bipolar disorder in children and adolescents is more limited than in adults. Children and adolescents appear to be particularly sensitive to medication side effects. With these caveats, an increasing body of evidence supports the use of mood stabilizing drugs and atypical antipsychotic drugs in children and adolescents with bipolar disorder. Lithium is FDA approved for treatment of bipolar disorder in children and adolescents as young as age 12. Aripiprazole and risperidone are FDA approved in children and adolescents as young as age 10. The guidelines additionally support DVP, carbamazepine, olanzapine, quetiapine, and risperidone.[49]

Initial dosages of drug therapy in the pediatric population are lower than in adults. Metabolic elimination rates of many drugs are increased in children, however, so they may actually require higher dosages on a weight-adjusted basis. Dosages are titrated carefully according to response and tolerability. For lithium, DVP, and carbamazepine, serum concentration monitoring is recommended as a guide to dosage adjustment and minimizing adverse effects.

Children and adolescent patients are often more sensitive to drug side effects than adults. In particular, they are likely to experience significant weight gain due to atypical antipsychotic drugs.[50] Cognitive toxicity, manifested as confusion, memory or concentration impairment, or impaired learning, is often difficult to detect and is a special consideration in the pediatric population so that intellectual and educational development is not hindered by drug therapy.

Comorbid conditions must be addressed in order to maximize desired outcomes. For comorbid bipolar disorder and attention deficit hyperactivity disorder when stimulant therapy is indicated, treatment of mania is recommended before starting the stimulant in order to avoid exacerbation of mood symptoms by the stimulant.

▶ Geriatrics

Treatment of elderly patients with bipolar disorder requires special care because of increased risks associated with concurrent medical conditions and drug–drug interactions. General medical conditions including endocrine, metabolic, or infectious diseases can mimic mood disorders. Patients should be evaluated for such medical illnesses that may cause or worsen mood symptoms. As physiologic systems change with aging, elimination of drugs is often slowed. Examples are slowed renal elimination of lithium and slowed hepatic metabolism of carbamazepine and VPA. As a result, dosages of drugs required for therapeutic effect are generally lower in geriatric patients. Also, changes in membrane permeability with aging increase risk of CNS side effects. Increased frequency of patient monitoring is often required, including serum drug concentration monitoring.

Vigilance for drug–drug interactions is required because of the greater number of medications prescribed to elderly patients and enhanced sensitivity to adverse effects. Pharmacokinetic interactions include metabolic enzyme induction or inhibition and protein binding displacement interactions, for example, DVP and warfarin. Pharmacodynamic interactions include additive sedation and cognitive toxicity, which increase risk of falls and other impairments.

▶ Pregnancy and Postpartum

Treatment of bipolar disorder during pregnancy is fraught with controversy and conflicting recommendations. The key issue is the relative risk of teratogenicity with drug use during pregnancy versus risk of bipolar relapse without treatment with consequent potential harm to both the pregnant patient and the fetus. Therapeutic judgments depend on the history of the patient and whether the pregnancy is planned or unplanned. Treatment is best managed when the pregnancy is planned. Clinicians should discuss the issue with every patient with bipolar disorder who is of childbearing potential. A pregnancy test should be obtained prior to initiating drug therapy. For a patient with severe bipolar disorder, a history of multiple mood episodes, rapid cycling, or suicide attempts, discontinuing treatment, even for a planned pregnancy, is unwise. For a patient with a remote history of a single mood episode with subsequent long stability and who is contemplating pregnancy, the answer is less clear. Patients should be provided clear and reliable information about risks versus benefits of stopping or continuing therapy in order to make an informed decision. Patients who decide to discontinue drug therapy prior to pregnancy should taper medications slowly in order to reduce risk of relapse.[51]

Lithium administration during the first trimester is associated with Ebstein's anomaly in the infant, a downward displacement of the tricuspid valve into the right ventricle. Although more likely to occur in children of patients who took lithium during pregnancy, the absolute risk is considered small, around 0.1%. Pharmacokinetic handling of lithium changes as pregnancy progresses. Renal lithium clearance increases, which requires a dosage increase to maintain a therapeutic serum concentration. It may be advisable to decrease or discontinue lithium at term or the onset of labor to avoid toxicity postpartum when there is a large reduction in fluid volume.[52]

Lithium can cause hypotonicity and cyanosis in the neonate, usually termed the "floppy baby" syndrome. Most data indicate normal neurobehavioral development once these symptoms resolve. Lithium is readily transferred via breast milk. Breast-feeding is not advised for patients who are taking lithium.[28]

VPA and carbamazepine are human teratogens. Neural tube defects such as spina bifida occur in up to 9% of infants exposed during the first trimester. The risk of neural tube defects is related to exposure during the third and fourth weeks following conception. As such, women with unplanned pregnancies may not know they are pregnant until after the risk of exposure has occurred. Carbamazepine can cause fetal vitamin K deficiency. Vitamin K is important for facial growth and for clotting factors. Risk of facial abnormalities is increased with carbamazepine and VPA, and neonatal bleeding is increased in infants of mothers who are treated with carbamazepine during pregnancy.[51,52]

Less data are available on other anticonvulsant mood stabilizing drugs. Lamotrigine may be associated with an increased risk of oral clefts in association with first trimester exposure.[51]

Conventional antipsychotic drugs have been available for many years, and more data are available on their use in pregnancy compared to atypical antipsychotic drugs, but treatment guidelines for bipolar disorder do not otherwise support conventional antipsychotics as an initial choice in treatment.

Patient Encounter, Part 4: Outcome Evaluation

Following initial assessment, including evaluation of potential suicidality, support systems, and need for inpatient versus outpatient treatment, MW was hospitalized briefly, then followed in the community on medication along with psychotherapy. She has abstained from illicit substances and has returned to her job. She has responded well to treatment with sustained-release lithium carbonate 900 mg once daily at bedtime with a snack. Steady-state 12-hour serum lithium concentrations have stabilized at 0.9 mEq/L (mmol/L). She now returns to clinic for routine follow-up. She has tolerated the lithium except for a mild tremor and a gain of 3.2 kg (7 lb). She is willing to accept these side effects for now, but asks about how long she must take medication since she is now feeling well.

How would you assess therapeutic and adverse effects of treatment for this patient?

How would you educate the patient regarding the need for continued maintenance treatment?

Use of antidepressant drugs during pregnancy is discussed in the chapter on depression.

OUTCOME EVALUATION
Assessment of Therapeutic Effects

Effective interviewing skills and a therapeutic relationship with the patient are essential to assessing response to treatment. Understand the particular symptom profile and needs of individual patients. These become the primary therapeutic monitoring parameters. In addition to the clinical interview, some clinicians utilize symptom rating scales such as the Young Mania Rating Scale (YMRS) for mania and the Hamilton Depression Rating Scale (Ham-D, discussed in the chapter on depression). Check serum concentrations of

---

Patient Care and Monitoring

1. Assess the patient's symptoms and review the past history. Review the family history, including the history of response to treatment by family members.

2. Obtain an initial medical evaluation to rule out other causes of mood episodes.

3. Obtain a thorough medication-use history, including present and past drugs, prescription and nonprescription drugs, the patient's self-assessment of response and side effect problems, alcohol, tobacco, caffeine, illicit substances, herbal products, dietary supplements, allergies, and adherence.

4. Assess potential drug–disease, drug–drug, and drug–food interactions.

5. Evaluate physiologic parameters that may influence pharmacokinetics.

6. Develop a plan for monitoring therapeutic outcomes, focusing on the individual symptom profile, and level of function of each patient. Include a plan for dosage adjustments or alternate therapy if the patient fails to respond adequately. Include serum drug concentration monitoring as appropriate.

7. Develop a monitoring plan for drug side effects. Include measures to prevent side effects as well as management if they occur. Include appropriate laboratory measures.

8. Determine the role of nonpharmacologic therapy and how it is to be integrated with drug therapy.

9. Educate the patient on the nature of bipolar disorder, its treatment, what to expect with regard to response and side effects, and stress the need for adherence to treatment, even when feeling well.

10. Encourage a healthy lifestyle, including eliminating or stopping substance abuse, smoking cessation, and encouraging proper nutrition and exercise.

---

mood stabilizing drugs as a guide to dosage adjustment for optimal efficacy. The frequency of follow-up visits depends on response, tolerability, adherence, and other factors.

Assessment of Adverse Effects

Adverse effects cause more nonadherence to prescribed therapy than any other factor. Monitor patients regularly for adverse effects and health status, especially since mood stabilizing drugs and antipsychotic drugs commonly cause metabolic side effects such as weight gain. Repeat laboratory tests for renal and thyroid function for patients taking lithium and hematology and liver function for patients taking carbamazepine or DVP. Annual measurement of serum lipase may be advisable for patients taking DVP. More specific discussion of metabolic side effect monitoring of patients taking atypical antipsychotic drugs is discussed in the chapter on schizophrenia.

Patient Education

8 *Patient education improves adherence to treatment, which reduces risk of relapse.* This is especially important because responsiveness to treatment declines as the number of mood episodes increases. Discuss the nature and chronic course of bipolar disorder and the risks of repeated relapses. Help patients understand that treatment of bipolar disorder is not a cure, but many patients can enjoy symptom-free or nearly symptom-free function. Make clear that long-term recovery is dependent on adherence to both pharmacologic and nonpharmacologic treatment. Explain the purpose of medication, common side effects to expect, and how to respond to them. Provide the patient and family with written information about medication indications, benefits, risks, and side effects. Discuss less frequent but more dangerous side effects of drugs, and give written instructions on seeking medical attention immediately should they occur.

Abbreviations Introduced in This Chapter

5-HT	5-hydroxytryptamine
ACE	Angiotensin-converting enzyme
BDNF	Brain-derived neurotrophic factor
CBT	Cognitive behavioral therapy
DA	Dopamine
DSM-IV-TR	*Diagnostic and Statistical Manual of Mental Disorders*, Fourth Edition, Text Revision
DVP	Divalproex
ECT	Electroconvulsive therapy
fMRI	Functional magnetic resonance imaging
FOI	Flight of ideas
GABA	Gamma-aminobutyric acid
Ham-D	Hamilton Depression Rating Scale
MAOI	Manoamine oxidase inhibitor
MDD	Major depressive disorder
NE	Norepinephrine
PPD	Packs per day
SA Hx	Substance abuse history

SNRI	Serotonin-nornepinephrine reuptake inhibitor
SSRI	Selective serotonin reuptake inhibitor
THC	Tetrahydrocannabinol, psychoactive substance in marijuana
TCA	Tricyclic antidepressant
TSH	Thyroid stimulating hormone
VPA	Valproic acid
WNL	Within normal limits
YMRS	Young Mania Rating Scale

 Self-assessment questions and answers are available at *http://www.mhpharmacotherapy. com/pp.html.*

REFERENCES

1. American Psychiatric Association. DSM-IV-TR: Diagnostic and Statistical Manual of Mental Disorders, Text Revision, 4th ed. Washington, DC: American Psychiatric Association, 2000.
2. Krishnan KR. Psychiatric and medical comorbidities of bipolar disorder. Psychosom Med 2005;67:1–8.
3. Thase ME. Mood disorders: Neurobiology. In: Sadock BJ, Sadock VA, eds. Kaplan and Sadock's Comprehensive Textbook of Psychiatry, 8th ed. Philadelphia: Lippincott Williams & Wilkins, 2005:1594–1603.
4. Shih RA, Belmonte PL, Zandi PP. A review of the evidence from family, twin and adoption studies for a genetic contribution to adult psychiatric disorders. Int Rev Psychiatry 2004;16:260–283.
5. Hajek T, Carrey N, Alda M. Neuroanatomical abnormalities as risk factors for bipolar disorder. Bipolar Disord 2005;7:393–403.
6. Mahmood T, Silverstone T. Serotonin and bipolar disorder. J Affect Disord 2001;66:1–11.
7. Kim H, McGrath BM, Silverstone PH. A review of the possible relevance of inositol and the phosphatidylinositol second messenger system (PI-cycle) to psychiatric disorders—Focus on magnetic resonance spectroscopy (MRS) studies. Hum Psychopharmacol 2005;20:309–326.
8. Post RM. Role of BDNF in bipolar and unipolar disorder: Clinical and theoretical implications. J Psychiatr Res 2007;41:979–990.
9. Hirschfeld RM. Bipolar spectrum disorder: Improving its recognition and diagnosis. J Clin Psychiatry 2001;62(Suppl 14):5–9.
10. Perugi G, Micheli C, Akiskal HS, et al. Polarity of the first episode, clinical characteristics, and course of manic depressive illness: A systematic retrospective investigation of 320 bipolar I patients. Compr Psychiatry 2000;41:13–18.
11. Judd LL, Akiskal HS, Schettler PJ, et al. The long-term natural history of the weekly symptomatic status of bipolar I disorder. Arch Gen Psychiatry 2002;59:530–537.
12. Judd LL, Akiskal HS, Schettler PJ, et al. A prospective investigation of the natural history of the long-term weekly symptomatic status of bipolar II disorder. Arch Gen Psychiatry 2003;60:261–269.
13. Hirschfeld RM, Holzer C, Calabrese JR, et al. Validity of the mood disorder questionnaire: A general population study. Am J Psychiatry 2003;160:178–180.
14. Berk M, Dodd S. Bipolar II disorder: A review. Bipolar Disord 2005;7:11–21.
15. Slama F, Bellivier F, Henry C, et al. Bipolar patients with suicidal behavior: Toward the identification of a clinical subgroup. J Clin Psychiatry 2004;65:1035–1039.
16. McElroy SL, Altshuler LL, Suppes T, et al. Axis I psychiatric comorbidity and its relationship to historical illness variables in 288 patients with bipolar disorder. Am J Psychiatry 2001;158:420–426.
17. Akiskal HS. Mood disorders: Clinical features. In: Sadock BJ, Sadock VA, eds. Kaplan and Sadock's Comprehensive Textbook of Psychiatry, 8th ed. Philadelphia, PA: Lippincott Williams & Wilkins, 2005:1611–1651.
18. Valtonen H, Suominen K, Matere O, et al. Suicidal ideation and attempts in bipolar I and II disorders. J Clin Psychiatry 2005;66:1456–1462.
19. Otto MW, Reilly-Harrington N, Sachs GS. Psychoeducational and cognitive-behavioral strategies in the management of bipolar disorder. J Affect Disord 2003;73:171–181.
20. Miklowitz DJ. Adjunctive psychotherapy for bipolar disorder: State of the evidence. Am J Psychiatry 2008;165:1408–1419.
21. Salvi V, Fagiolini A, Swartz HA, et al. The use of antidepressants in bipolar disorder. J Clin Psychiatry 2008;69:1307–1318.
22. Geddes JR, Burgess S, Hawton K, et al. Long-term lithium therapy for bipolar disorder: Systematic review and meta-analysis of randomized controlled trials. Am J Psychiatry 2004;161:217–222.
23. Scherk H, Pajonk FG, Leucht S. Second-generation antipsychotic agents in the treatment of acute mania. A systematic review and meta-analysis of randomized controlled trials. Arch Gen Psychiatry 2007;64:442–455.
24. Schneck CD. Treatment of rapid-cycling bipolar disorder. J Clin Psychiatry 2006;67(Suppl 11):22–27.
25. Bowden CL, Calabrese JR, Sachs G, et al. A placebo-controlled 18-month trial of lamotrigine and lithium maintenance treatment in recently manic or hypomanic patients with bipolar I disorder. Arch Gen Psychiatry 2003;60:392–400.
26. Cipriani A, Pretty H, Hawton K, Geddes JR. Lithium in the prevention of suicidal behavior and all-cause mortality in patients with mood disorders: A systematic review of randomized trials. Am J Psychiatry 2005;162:1805–1819.
27. Marmol F. Lithium: Bipolar disorder and neurodegenerative diseases. Possible cellular mechanisms of the therapeutic effects of lithium. Prog Neuropsychopharmacol Biol Psychiatry 2008;32:1761–1771.
28. Lithium package insert. Roxane Laboratories. Columbus, OH, 2007.
29. Sandson NB, Armstrong SC, Cozza KL. An overview of psychotropic drug-drug interactions. Psychosomatics 2005;46:464–494.
30. Divalproex package insert. Abbott Laboratories. North Chicago, IL, 2008.
31. Walz JC, Frey BN, Andreazza AC, et al. Effects of lithium and valproate on serum and hippocampal neurotrophin-3 levels in an animal model of mania. J Psychiatr Res 2008;42:416–421.
32. Harrison TS, Keating GM. Extended-release carbamazepine capsules in bipolar I disorder. CNS Drugs 2005;19:709–716.
33. Carbamazepine extended-release capsules package insert. Validus Pharmaceuticals. Parsippany, NJ, 2007.
34. Lamotrigine package insert. GlaxoSmithKline. Research Triangle Park, NC, 2007.
35. Oxcarbazepine package insert. Novartis Pharmaceuticals. East Hanover, NJ, 2007.
36. Suppes T, Dennehy DB, Hirschfeld RMA, et al. The Texas implementation of medication algorithms: Update to the algorithms for treatment of bipolar I disorder. J Clin Psychiatry 2005;66:870–886.
37. Vasudev A, Macritchie K, Watson S, et al. Oxcarbazepine in the maintenance treatment of bipolar disorder. Cochrane Database Syst Rev 2008, issue 1:CD005171.
38. Nardi AE, Perna G. Clonazepam in the treatment of psychiatric disorders: An update. Int Clin Psychopharmacol 2006;21:131–142.
39. Goodnick PJ. Anticonvulsants in the treatment of bipolar mania. Expert Opin Pharmacother 2006;7:401–410.
40. Pande AC, Crockatt JG, Janney CA, et al. Gabapentin in bipolar disorder: A placebo-controlled trial of adjunctive therapy. Bipolar Disord 2000;2:249–255.
41. Vieta E, Suppes T, Eggens I, et al. Efficacy and safety of quetiapine in combination with lithium or divalproex for maintenance of patients with bipolar I disorder (international trial 126). J Affect Disord 2008;109:251–263.
42. Keck PE, Marcus R, Tourkodimitris S, et al. A placebo-controlled, double-blind study of the efficacy and safety of aripiprazole in patients with acute bipolar mania. Am J Psychiatry 2003;160:1651–1658.

43. Thase ME, Macfadden W, Weisler RH, et al. Efficacy of quetiapine monotherapy in bipolar I and II depression. J Clin Psychopharmacol 2006;26:600–609.

44. American Diabetes Association, American Psychiatric Association, American Association of Clinical Endocrinologists, North American Association for the Study of Obesity. Consensus development conference on antipsychotic drugs and obesity and diabetes. Diabetes Care 2004;27:596–601.

45. Kramer M, Simpson G, Maciulis V, et al. Paliperidone extended-release tablets for prevention of symptom recurrence in patients with schizophrenia. A randomized, double-blind, placebo-controlled study. J Clin Psychopharmacol 2007;27:6–14.

46. Sachs GS, Nierenberg AA, Calabrese JR, et al. Effectiveness of adjunctive antidepressant treatment for bipolar depression. N Engl J Med 2007;356:1711–1722.

47. International Consensus Group on Bipolar I Depression Treatment Guidelines. J Clin Psychiatry 2004;65:569–579.

48. Leverich GS, Altshuler LL, Frye MA, et al. Risk of switch in mood polarity to hypomania or mania in patients with bipolar depression during acute and continuation trials of venlafaxine, sertraline, and bupropion as adjuncts to mood stabilizers. Am J Psychiatry 2006;163:232–239.

49. Kowatch RA, Fristad M, Birmaher B, et al. Treatment guidelines for children and adolescents with bipolar disorder. J Am Acad Child Adolesc Psychiatry 2005;44:213–235.

50. McIntyre RS, Jerrell JM. Metabolic and cardiovascular adverse events associated with antipsychotic treatment in children and adolescents. Arch Pediatr Adolesc Med 2008;162:929–935.

51. Cohen LS. Treatment of bipolar disorder during pregnancy. J Clin Psychiatry 2007;68(Suppl 9):4–9.

52. Yonkers KA, Wisner KL, Stowe Z, et al. Management of bipolar disorder during pregnancy and the postpartum period. Am J Psychiatry 2004;161:608–620.

40 Generalized Anxiety Disorder, Panic Disorder, and Social Anxiety Disorder

Sheila Botts, Anna Lockwood, and Timothy Allen

LEARNING OBJECTIVES

Upon completion of the chapter, the reader will be able to:

1. Describe pathophysiologic findings in generalized anxiety, panic, and social anxiety disorder patients.

2. List common presenting symptoms of generalized anxiety, panic, and social anxiety disorders.

3. Identify the desired therapeutic outcomes for patients with generalized anxiety, panic, and social anxiety disorders.

4. Discuss appropriate lifestyle modifications and nonprescription medication use.

5. Recommend psychotherapy and pharmacotherapy interventions for patients with generalized anxiety, panic, and social anxiety disorders.

6. Develop a monitoring plan for anxiety patients placed on specific medications.

7. Educate patients about their disease state and appropriate lifestyle modifications, as well as psychotherapy and pharmacotherapy for effective treatment.

KEY CONCEPTS

❶ The goals of therapy for generalized anxiety disorder (GAD) are to acutely reduce the severity and duration of anxiety symptoms and restore overall functioning. The long-term goal in GAD is to achieve and maintain remission.

❷ Antidepressants are considered first-line agents in the management of chronic GAD.

❸ Benzodiazepines are recommended for acute treatment of GAD when short-term relief is needed, as an adjunct during initiation of antidepressant therapy, or to improve sleep.

❹ The acute phase of panic disorder (PD) treatment lasts about 12 weeks and should result in marked reduction in panic attacks (ideally total elimination) and minimal anticipatory anxiety and phobic avoidance. Treatment should be continued to prevent relapse for an additional 12 to 18 months before attempting discontinuation.

❺ PD patients are more likely to experience stimulant-like side effects of antidepressants than patients with major depression. Antidepressants should be initiated at lower doses in PD patients than in depressed patients or those with other anxiety disorders.

❻ Antidepressants should be tapered when treatment is discontinued to avoid withdrawal symptoms, which include dysphoric mood, irritability, and agitation.

❼ The dose of benzodiazepine required for improvement in PD generally is higher than that used in other anxiety disorders.

❽ Based on their tolerability and efficacy, selective serotonin reuptake inhibitors are considered the drugs of choice for social anxiety disorder.

❾ The onset of response to antidepressants in social anxiety disorder is delayed and may be as long as 8 to 12 weeks. Patients responding to medication should be continued on treatment for at least 1 year.

❿ Pharmacotherapy of social anxiety disorder should lead to improvement in physiologic symptoms of anxiety and fear, functionality, and overall well-being.

Anxiety is a normal response to stressful or fearful circumstances. Most people experience some degree of anxiety in reaction to stressful situations. This allows an individual to adapt to or manage the stressful/threatening situation. Anxiety symptoms generally are short-lived and do not necessarily impair function. Anxiety that becomes excessive, causes irrational thinking or behavior, and impairs a person's functioning is considered an anxiety disorder.

The diagnosis is often missed or attributed incorrectly to medical illnesses, and most patients are treated inadequately.[1] The burden of detection and diagnosis most often falls to primary care clinicians. Untreated anxiety disorders may result in increased health care utilization, morbidity and mortality, and poorer quality of life.

EPIDEMIOLOGY AND ETIOLOGY
Epidemiology

▶ *Prevalence*

With a lifetime prevalence of 28.8%, anxiety disorders collectively represent the most prevalent psychiatric disorders,[2] with specific phobia (12.5%) and social anxiety disorder (SAD) (12.1%) being the most common.[3] Recent reports from the National Comorbidity Survey Revised (NCS-R) estimate the lifetime prevalence of generalized anxiety disorder (GAD) for those 18 years of age and older to be 5.7%.[3,4] Rates for panic disorder (PD) are slightly lower, with an estimated lifetime prevalence of 4.7%.

Most studies report higher rates of anxiety disorders among women (2:1, female:male) and older adults.[5] Prevalence rates across the anxiety spectrum increase from the younger age group (18–29) to older age groups (30–44 and 45–59); however, rates are substantially lower for those older than 59 years of age.[3]

▶ *Course of Illness*

PD and GAD have a median age of onset of 24 and 31 years, respectively, whereas specific phobia and SAD tend to develop much earlier (median age of onset 7 and 13 years, respectively).[3] As many as half of adult anxiety patients report subthreshold symptoms during childhood.[6]

Anxiety disorders are chronic, and symptoms tend to wax and wane, with less than a third of patients experiencing spontaneous symptom remission.[7] The risk for relapse and recurrence of symptoms is also high for anxiety disorders. In a 12-year follow-up study of anxiety disorder patients, recurrence rates ranged from 58% of PD and GAD patients to 39% of SAD patients.[8] Remission, if achieved with treatment, is most likely to occur within the first 2 years of an index episode.[9] Similarly, the highest rates of relapse are seen within the same timeframe; thus, many patients need ongoing maintenance treatment. Rates of remission and relapse do not appear to vary by gender;[9] however, one study reported that women with PD without agoraphobia were three times more likely than men to experience a relapse of symptoms. Patients with anxiety disorders spend a significant portion of time "being ill" during a particular episode, ranging from 41% to 80% of the time.[8] Expectedly, anxiety disorders are associated with impaired psychosocial functioning and a compromised quality of life.[10] Appropriate treatment improves the patient's overall quality of life and psychosocial functioning.[10]

▶ *Comorbidity*

More than 90% of individuals with an anxiety disorder have a lifetime history of one or more other psychiatric disorders.[11]

Depression is the most common lifetime comorbid illness, followed by alcohol or substance use disorders, and other co-occurring anxiety disorders, especially GAD and PD.[11] Generally, the onset of SAD and GAD symptoms precedes major depressive disorder (MDD), whereas there is an equal chance of PD onset before, during, or after MDD. Comorbid psychiatric illness is associated with lower rates of remission and higher rates of relapse. It is essential that both disorders are treated appropriately.

Etiology

Both genetic and psychosocial factors appear to play a role in the initiation and expression of anxiety disorders.[12] Moderate genetic risk has been documented for all anxiety disorders. Currently, no definitive gene or set of genes has been identified as being the causative factor for a specific anxiety disorder. It is unclear if anxiety disorders share common genetic risk factors. Genetic overlap may exist between GAD and PD and, to a lesser extent, SAD.[12]

Genetics may create a vulnerable phenotype for an anxiety disorder, and an individual's life stressors and means of coping with the stress may also play a role in precipitation and continuation of the anxiety disorder.[13] Some researchers believe that stressful life events may play a strong role in the onset of anxiety disorders, especially in GAD and PD.[12] It has been reported that those experiencing one or more negative life events have a threefold increased chance of developing GAD.[5] Similar findings have been reported with PD.[13]

PATHOPHYSIOLOGY

The thalamus and amygdala are important in the generation of a normal fear response and play a central role in most anxiety disorders. The thalamus provides the first real processing region to organize sensory data obtained from the environment. It passes information to higher cortical centers for finer processing and to the amygdala for rapid assessment of highly charged emotional information. The amygdala provides the emotional importance of the information. This helps the organism to act quickly on ambiguous but vital events. The cortex then performs a more detailed analysis, and sends updates to the amygdala for comparison and any needed course corrections, thus enabling a decision on a course of action.

Anxiety can become independent of stimuli as in PD, be associated with benign stimuli as in phobias, or continue beyond the stimulus duration as in GAD. The precise mechanism by which these changes occur is unknown, but much has been discovered regarding how this may be regulated by treatment (Fig. 40–1).

Direct and indirect connections to the reticular activating system (RAS), a region spanning the medulla, pons, and midbrain, help to regulate arousal, vigilance, and fear. These connections are modulated by serotonin and norepinephrine, which have their primary origins in the RAS.[14] The amygdala sends projections to the hypothalamus, thus influencing the autonomic nervous system to affect heart rate, blood pressure, and stress-associated changes. It also influences

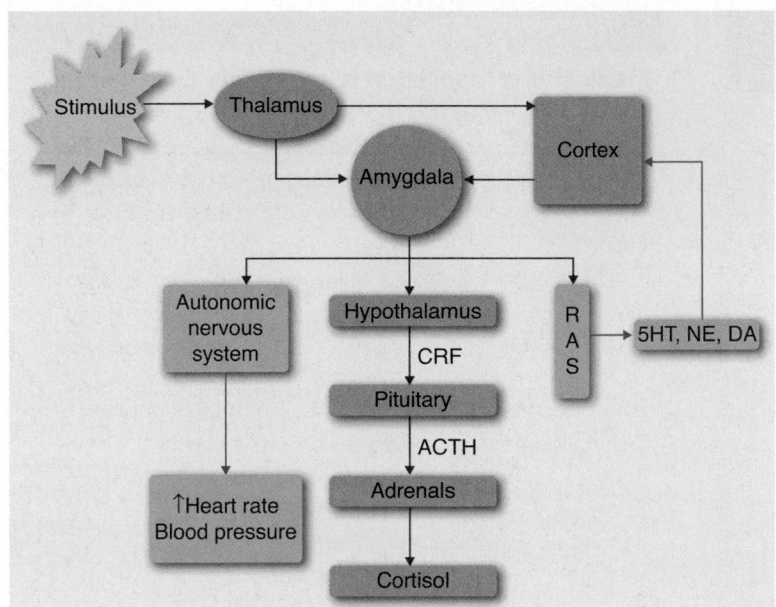

FIGURE 40–1. Neurocircuitry and key neurotransmitters involved in mediating anxiety disorders.

the **hypothalamic–pituitary–adrenal** (HPA) **axis,** leading to a cascade of stress hormones.[15] One such hormone is cortisol, which, if elevated for prolonged periods, can damage the brain and other organs. These are important targets in our understanding of how the amygdala regulates the fear response.

Noradrenergic System

Norepinephrine (NE)-producing cells reside primarily in a region of the brain called the **locus ceruleus** (LC). Increased activity in this region is associated with an increase in arousal, anxiety, and panic. Drugs such as yohimbine that increase activity in the LC can be anxiogenic, whereas drugs that decrease activity in the LC appear to improve anxiety symptoms. Furthermore, dysregulation of this region is implicated by elevated levels of NE or its metabolites in subjects with GAD, PD, and specific phobias.[15]

Serotonergic System

The **raphe nuclei** and the resident cell bodies of serotonin (5-HT)-producing neurons over time inhibit firing of noradrenergic cells in the LC. They also regulate cells in the prefrontal cortex and amygdala. Perhaps the strongest evidence for the involvement of the serotonergic system is the success of serotonin reuptake inhibitors in treatment of anxiety disorders.[15]

γ-Aminobutyric Acid

γ-Aminobutyric acid (GABA) is an inhibitory neurotransmitter. The effects of GABA are nonspecific, and its role is complex. GABAergic drugs are used for acute anxiety reduction, but the lack of a specific target for their effect leads to multiple undesirable effects. Current research is focused on defining receptor subtypes that may allow for greater specificity in targeting anxiety symptoms.[16]

Hypothalamic–Pituitary–Adrenal Axis

The HPA axis provides a critical mechanism for regulation of the stress response and its effects on the brain and other organ systems. Several important hormones, including corticotropin-releasing hormone and cortisol regulate the effects of anxiety on the body and provide positive feedback to the brain.[15] A cycle of anxiety and sensitization by such feedback could, if unchecked, result in escalation of symptoms. Neuropeptides may provide one mechanism to balance positive and negative feedback, helping to minimize such escalation.

Neuropeptides

Several neuropeptides are under investigation for their role in anxiety disorders. Important neuropeptides include neuropeptide Y (NPY), substance P, and cholecystokinin. NPY appears to reduce the effect of stress hormones and inhibits activity of the LC. Both mechanisms may contribute to the anxiolytic properties seen experimentally. Substance P may have anxiolytic and antidepressant properties due in part to its effects on corticotropin-releasing hormone.[17]

GENERALIZED ANXIETY DISORDER

TREATMENT

Desired Outcomes

❶ *The goals of therapy for GAD are to acutely reduce the severity and duration of anxiety symptoms and restore overall functioning. The long-term goal in GAD is to achieve and maintain remission.* With a positive response to treatment, patients with GAD and comorbid depression should have minimal depressive symptoms.

Clinical Presentation and Diagnosis of GAD

General

Onset is typically in early adulthood. Anxiety emerges and dissipates more gradually than in PD. Laboratory evaluation usually is reserved for later onset, atypical presentation, or poor response to treatment.

Symptoms[2]

Excessive anxiety or worry involving multiple events or activities occurring more days than not for at least 6 months and associated with at least three of the following:

- Restlessness
- Easily fatigued
- Poor concentration
- Irritability
- Muscle tension
- Insomnia or unsatisfying sleep

Differential Diagnosis

Rule out underlying medical or psychiatric disorders and medications that may cause anxiety (Tables 40–1 and 40–2)

Laboratory Evaluation

- Basic metabolic panel
- Thyroid-stimulating hormone (TSH)
- Polysomnogram

Table 40–1

Medical Conditions That Can Cause Anxiety

Psychiatric Disorders
Mood disorders, hypochondriasis, personality disorders, alcohol/substance abuse, alcohol/substance withdrawal, other anxiety disorders

Neurologic Disorders
CVA, seizure disorders, dementia, stroke, migraine, encephalitis, vestibular dysfunction

Cardiovascular Disorders
Angina, arrhythmias, congestive heart failure, mitral valve prolapse, myocardial infarction

Endocrine and Metabolic Disorders
Hypo/hyperthyroidism, hypoglycemia, Cushing's disease, Addison's disease, pheochromocytoma, hyperadrenocorticism, hyponatremia, hyperkalemia, vitamin B_{12} deficiency

Respiratory Disorders
Asthma, COPD, pulmonary embolism, pneumonia, hyperventilation

Other
Carcinoid syndrome, anemias, systemic lupus erythematosus

COPD, chronic obstructive pulmonary disease; CVA, cerebrovascular accident.

From Refs. 2, 18, 19.

Table 40–2

Medications Associated With Anxiety Symptoms

Category	Examples
Anticonvulsants	Carbamazepine, ethosuximide
Antidepressants	Bupropion, SSRIs, SNRIs, TCAs
Antihypertensives	Felodipine
Antimicrobials	Cephalosporins, ofloxacin, isoniazid
Antiparkinson drugs	Levodopa
Bronchodilators	Albuterol (salbutamol), isoproterenol, theophylline
Corticosteroids	Prednisone, methylprednisolone
Decongestants	Pseudoephedrine, phenylephrine
Herbals	Ma huang, St. John's wort, ginseng, guarana, belladonna
NSAIDs	Ibuprofen, indomethacin
Stimulants	Amphetamines, caffeine, cocaine, methylphenidate
Thyroid hormones	Levothyroxine
Toxicity	Anticholinergics, antihistamines, digoxin
Withdrawal of CNS depressants (abrupt)	Alcohol, barbiturates, benzodiazepines

NSAIDs, nonsteroidal anti-inflammatory drugs; SNRIs serotonin-norepinephrine reuptake inhibitors; SSRIs, selective serotonin reuptake inhibitors; TCAs, tricyclic antidepressants.

From Refs. 2, 18–20.

Patient Encounter 1, Part 1

AX, a 27-year-old African American woman, presents to your clinic with GI complaints (e.g., constipation, bloating, and cramping) and fatigue. She is a single mother of three (ages 2, 3, and 6 years) and is a full-time college student. She states that she worries about everything: her grades, finances, the 6-year-old riding the school bus, etc. She states that "even if it's not important, I still worry." She has difficulty sleeping and says that she often feels like she might jump out of her skin. On one occasion she felt like she might be having a "heart attack or something."

What manifestations described above are suggestive of an anxiety disorder?

What additional information do you need to establish a diagnosis and develop a treatment plan?

General Approach to Treatment

Patients with GAD may be managed with psychotherapy, pharmacotherapy, or both. The treatment plan should be individualized based on symptom severity, comorbid illnesses, medical status, age, and patient preference. Patients with severe symptoms resulting in functional impairment should receive antianxiety medication.

Patient Encounter 1, Part 2

AX returns to your clinic 4 months later stating that despite meeting with the school psychologist a few times, she continues to have problems. In addition to worrying and feeling nervous, she feels down a lot. "I don't have the energy to play with my children. I obsess over everything. My grades have really gone downhill. I cry a lot and feel hopeless."

PMH: IBS, GAD

FH: Mother treated for depression; father, ethanol dependence

SH: Drinks ethanol occasionally; cigarettes one pack a day; lives independently with three children

Meds: Centrum multivitamin

Given this information, what is your assessment of this patient?

Develop a treatment plan, including nonpharmacologic and pharmacologic recommendations, duration of therapy, and monitoring plan.

Nonpharmacologic Therapy

Nonpharmacologic therapy includes psychoeducation, exercise, stress management, and psychotherapy. Psychoeducation should include instructing patients to avoid stimulating agents such as caffeine, decongestants, diet pills, and excessive alcohol use. Regular exercise is also recommended. Cognitive-behavioral therapy (CBT), the most effective psychological therapy for GAD patients, helps patients to recognize and alter patterns of distorted thinking and dysfunctional behavior. Some trials suggest that treatment gains with CBT may be maintained for up to 1 year.[21] The combination of CBT and an antidepressant may be more effective than either treatment alone. In a recent study, 80.7% of children were much improved on the combination of CBT and an antidepressant, versus 54.9% with sertraline and 59.7% with CBT alone.[22]

Pharmacologic Therapy

Antidepressants, benzodiazepines, buspirone, hydroxyzine, pregabalin, and the second-generation antipsychotics (SGAs), olanzapine and risperidone, have controlled clinical trial data supporting their use in GAD. Antidepressants have replaced benzodiazepines as the drugs of choice for chronic GAD owing to a tolerable side-effect profile, no risk for dependency, and efficacy in common comorbid conditions including depression, panic, obsessive–compulsive disorder (OCD), and SAD. Benzodiazepines remain the most effective and commonly used treatment for short-term management of anxiety where immediate relief of symptoms is desired.

They are also recommended for intermittent or adjunctive use during GAD exacerbation or for sleep disturbance during the initiation of antidepressant treatment.[27] Buspirone and pregabalin are alternative agents for patients with GAD without depression. Hydroxyzine is usually adjunctive and is less desirable for long-term treatment owing to side effects including sedation and anticholinergic effects.

Patients with GAD should be treated to remission of symptoms. Most guidelines recommend continuing treatment for an additional 3 to 10 months.[21,23–25] An algorithm for the pharmacologic management of GAD is shown in Figure 40–2.

▶ *Antidepressants*

② *Antidepressants* (*Table 40–3*) *are considered first-line agents in the management of chronic GAD.* These agents reduce the psychic symptoms (e.g., worry and apprehension) of anxiety with a modest effect on autonomic or somatic

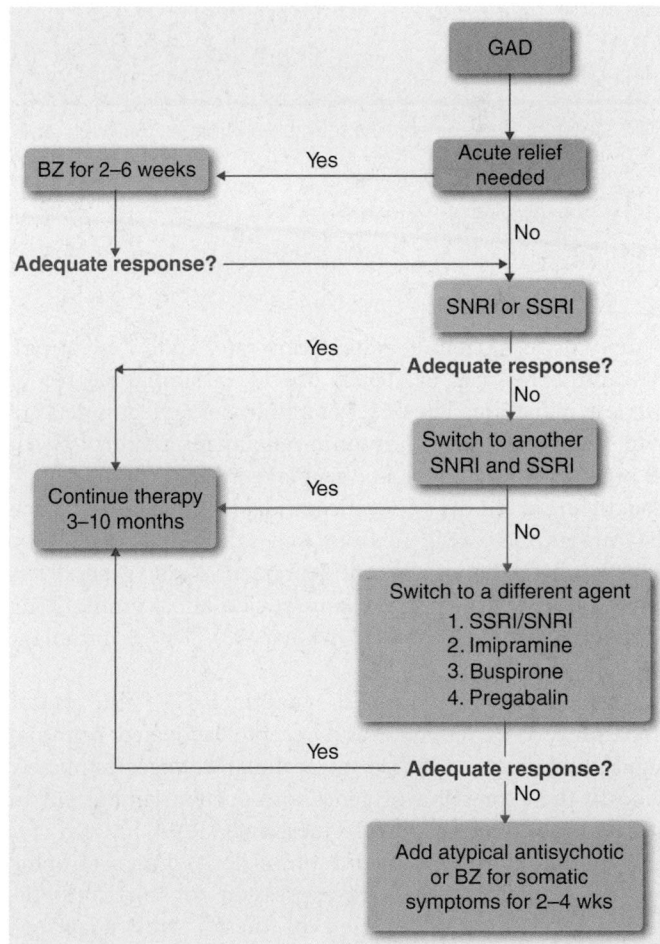

FIGURE 40–2. Treatment algorithm for GAD. BZ, benzodiazepine; SSRI, selective serotonin reuptake inhibitor; SNRI, serotonin and norepinephrine reuptake inhibitor. (Adapted, from Kirkwood CK, Melton ST. Anxiety disorders: I. Generalized anxiety, panic and social anxiety disorders. In: DiPiro JT, Talbert RL, Yee GC, Matzke GR, et al., eds. Pharmacotherapy: A Pathophysiologic Approach, 7th ed. New York: McGraw-Hill, 2008:1163–1178.)

Table 40-3

Antidepressants Used in the Treatment of GAD

Medication Class	Recommended Starting Dose (mg/day)	Usual Therapeutic Dosage Range (mg/day)	Hepatic Insufficiency	Renal Insufficiency
SSRIs				
Citalopram (Celexa)	20	20–50	Max 40 mg/day	
Escitalopram[a] (Lexapro)	10	10–20	Max 10 mg /day	
Fluoxetine (Prozac)	20	20–80	Titrate with caution	
Fluvoxamine (Luvox)	50	100–300	Titrate with caution	
Paroxetine	20	20–50	Titrate with caution	
Paroxetine CR (Paxil, Paxil CR)	25	25–62.5	Max 50 mg/day	Max 50 mg/day
Sertraline (Zoloft)	50–100	50–200	Reduce dose	
SNRI				
Venlafaxine XR[a] (Effexor XR)	75	75–300	Reduce dose 50%	Reduce dose 25–50%
Duloxetine (Cymbalta)	30	60–120	Use not recommended	Use is not recommended[b]
TCAs				
Imipramine (Tofranil)	50–75	75–200	Titrate with caution	

SNRIs, serotonin-norepinephrine reuptake inhibitors; SSRIs, selective serotonin reuptake inhibitors; TCAs, tricyclic antidepressants.

[a]FDA approved for use in GAD.

[b]Duloxetine use not recommended in severe renal impairment (CrCl less than 30 mL/min).

From Refs. 20, 26.

symptoms (e.g., tremor, rapid heart rate, and/or sweating). All antidepressants evaluated provide a similar degree of anxiety reduction. The onset of antianxiety effect is delayed 2 to 4 weeks. Selective serotonin reuptake inhibitors (SSRIs) or serotonin-norepinephrine reuptake inhibitors (SNRIs) are usually preferred over tricyclic antidepressants (TCAs) such as imipramine owing to improved safety and tolerability. Selection of a particular antidepressant agent generally is based on history of prior response, side-effect profile, drug interaction profile (discussed in Chap. 38), cost, or formulary availability.

Antidepressants modulate synaptic 5-HT, NE, and/or dopamine (DA) reuptake and receptor-activated neuronal signal transduction. These intracellular changes ultimately modify the expression of genes and proteins important in stress response (e.g., increase messenger RNA [mRNA] for glucocorticoid receptors and brain-derived neurotrophic factor and decrease mRNA expression for corticotropin-releasing factor).[26] Activation of these "stress-adapting" pathways is thought to improve both somatic and psychic symptoms of anxiety.[27]

Serotonin-Norepinephrine Reuptake Inhibitors Venlafaxine and duloxetine alleviate anxiety in GAD patients with and without depression. Venlafaxine was shown to reduce anxiety effectively at doses 75 to 225 mg/day, and response was maintained over an additional 6 months of treatment.[28] Venlafaxine has more favorable safety and side-effect profiles than TCAs. The most common venlafaxine

side effects reported by GAD patients are nausea, somnolence, dry mouth, dizziness, sweating, constipation, and anorexia.[28]

Duloxetine is effective for the treatment of GAD as well, but long-term efficacy has not yet been established. At 60 to 120 mg/day, its efficacy is noninferior to venlafaxine, and tolerability is similar.[29] For patients with concurrent pain syndromes, duloxetine has been found to improve anxiety, pain, and functional impairment when compared to placebo.[30]

Selective Serotonin Reuptake Inhibitors The SSRIs paroxetine, escitalopram, and sertraline have been shown to be significantly more effective than placebo in reducing anxiety symptoms. Paroxetine at doses of 20 and 40 mg/day achieved response in 62% and 68% of patients, respectively, over 8 weeks of treatment.[31] Remission occurred in 30% and 36%, respectively. In a 24-week relapse-prevention study, paroxetine was more effective than placebo at maintaining response, and patients were more likely to achieve remission with continued treatment (42.5% at 8 weeks versus 73% at 24 weeks).[32] In GAD trials, paroxetine was associated with a high rate of somnolence, nausea, abnormal ejaculation, dry mouth, decreased libido, and asthenia compared with placebo.[31]

Escitalopram, in a dose range of 10 to 20 mg/day, was more effective than placebo in patients with GAD without depression. Fifty-eight percent of patients on escitalopram achieved response versus 38% on placebo over the 8 weeks of treatment.[30] Side effects included headache, nausea, somnolence, upper respiratory tract infection, decreased libido, ejaculation disorder, and anorgasmia.[33]

Sertraline was more efficacious than placebo in patients with GAD being treated for 12 weeks. Sertraline treatment resulted in 56% of patients achieving response, whereas 31% achieved remission.[34] Side effects included increased rates of nausea, insomnia, sweating, decreased libido, diarrhea, fatigue, and ejaculation disorder.[34] Citalopram has been shown to be efficacious in the treatment of GAD in the elderly.[35] Limited comparative trial data suggest comparable outcomes between these SSRIs.[36,37] SSRI therapy is better tolerated than TCAs, and tolerability is similar to that with venlafaxine.

Tricyclic Antidepressants Imipramine provided a higher rate of remission of anxiety symptoms than trazodone, diazepam, or placebo (e.g., 73% versus 69% versus 66% versus 47%) in an 8-week controlled trial of GAD patients.[38] Antidepressants were more effective than diazepam or placebo in reducing psychic symptoms of anxiety. The use of TCAs generally is limited by bothersome adverse effects (e.g., sedation, orthostatic hypotension, anticholinergic effects, and weight gain). TCAs have a narrow therapeutic index and are lethal in overdose due to atrioventricular (AV) heart block.

Novel Antidepressants Mirtazapine, an α-2 adrenergic antagonist and postsynaptic serotonin (5-HT$_2$, 5-HT$_3$) receptor antagonist, is an effective antidepressant but has not been extensively evaluated in anxiety disorders. One open-label study found treatment of GAD for 12 weeks with mirtazapine 30 mg to be efficacious and well tolerated.[39] Mirtazapine is not associated with sexual dysfunction, a common antidepressant side effect, but does have a greater propensity to cause sedation and weight gain. Bupropion, a dopamine and norepinephrine reuptake inhibitor, lacks the common antidepressant side effects of weight gain and sexual dysfunction. Bupropion has not been studied or used extensively in anxiety disorders owing to its stimulating effects that would be expected to worsen anxiety symptoms. However, a pilot-controlled trial comparing bupropion XL to escitalopram found buproprion to have comparable anxiolytic efficacy and tolerability.[40]

▶ Benzodiazepines

❸ *Benzodiazepines are recommended for acute treatment of GAD when short-term relief is needed, as an adjunct during initiation of antidepressant therapy, or to improve sleep.*[21,23] Benzodiazepine treatment results in a significant improvement in 65% to 75% of GAD patients, with most of the improvement occurring in the initial 2 weeks of therapy.[38] They are more effective in reducing somatic symptoms of anxiety than psychic symptoms. The major disadvantages of benzodiazepines are their lack of effectiveness in treating depression, the risk for dependency and abuse, and potential interdose rebound anxiety especially with short-acting formulations. Benzodiazepines should be avoided in patients with chemical dependency.

Benzodiazepines exert their effects by enhancing transmission of the inhibitory neurotransmitter GABA through interaction with the GABA$_A$ receptor complex.[41] Although all benzodiazepines possess anxiolytic properties, only 7 of the 13 currently marketed agents are approved by the FDA for the treatment of anxiety disorders (Table 40–4). All benzodiazepines are expected to provide equivalent benefit when given in comparable doses. Benzodiazpines differ substantially in their pharmacokinetic properties and potency for the GABA$_A$ receptor site.

Benzodiazepines are metabolized by hepatic oxidation (cytochrome P450 3A4) and glucuronide conjugation. Because lorazepam and oxazepam bypass hepatic oxidation and are conjugated only, they are preferred agents for patients with reduced hepatic function secondary to aging or disease (e.g., cirrhosis commonly seen in patients abusing alcohol or with Hepatitis B/C from IV drug use). Many benzodiazepines are metabolized to long-acting metabolites (Table 40–4) that provide long-lasting anxiety relief. Drugs that either inhibit or induce CYP450 isozymes or glucuronidation are the major source of drug interactions (Table 40–5).

The most common side effects associated with benzodiazepine therapy include CNS depressive effects (e.g., drowsiness, sedation, psychomotor impairment, and ataxia) and cognitive effects (e.g., poor recall and anterograde amnesia). Anterograde amnesia is more likely to occur with high-potency benzodiazepines, such as lorazepam or alprazolam.[42] Some patients also may be disinhibited with benzodiazepine treatment and experience confusion, irritability, aggression, and excitement.[42] Discontinuation of benzodiazepines may be associated with withdrawal, rebound anxiety, and a high rate of relapse. Higher doses of benzodiazepines and longer duration of therapy increase the severity of withdrawal and risk of seizures after abrupt or rapid discontinuation. Patients should be tapered rather than discontinued abruptly from benzodiazepine therapy to avoid withdrawal symptoms. The duration of the taper should increase with extended duration of benzodiazepine therapy.[24] For example, patients on benzodiazepine therapy over 2 to 6 months should be tapered over 2 to 8 weeks, whereas patients receiving 12 months of treatment should be tapered over 2 to 4 months. A general approach to the taper is to reduce the dose by 25% every 5 to 7 days until reaching half the original dose and then decreasing by 10% to 12% per week until discontinued. Patients should expect minor withdrawal symptoms and discomfort even when tapering. Rebound symptoms (e.g., return of original symptoms at increased intensity) are transient. The patient should be counseled so that rebound anxiety is not interpreted as a relapse. Relapse or recurrence of anxiety may occur in as many as 50% of patients discontinuing benzodiazepine treatment.[38] It is unclear if this relapse rate represents an inferiority of benzodiazepines or supports the chronic nature of GAD.

▶ Buspirone

Buspirone, a 5-HT$_{1A}$ partial agonist, is thought to exert its anxiolytic effects by reducing presynaptic 5-HT firing.[43]

Table 40–4

Benzodiazepine Comparison Chart

Drug Name (Brand Name) Active Metabolites	Time to Peak Concentration (hour)	Half-Life Range (hour)	Approved Dosage Range (mg/day)	Dose Equivalent (mg)
Alprazolam[a,b] (Xanax)	1–2	12–15	1–4 (GAD)	0.5
			1–10 (PD)	
Chlordiazepoxide[a] (Librium)	1–4	5–30	25–100	10
Desmethylchlordiazepoxide		18		
Demoxepam		14–95		
Desmethyldiazepam		40–120		
Oxazepam		5–15		
Clonazepam[b] (Klonopin)	1–4	18–50	1–4	0.25
Clorazepate[a] (Tranzene)	1–2		7.5–60	7.5
Desmethyldiazepam		40–120		
Oxazepam		5–15		
Diazepam[a] (Valium)	0.5–2	20–80	2–40	5
Desmethyldiazepam		40–120[c]		
Temazepam		8–15		
Oxazepam		5–15		
Lorazepam[a] (Ativan)	2–4	10–20	0.5–10	0.75–1
Oxazepam[a] (Serax)	2–4	5–15	30–120	15

GAD, generalized anxiety disorder; PD, panic disorder.

[a]FDA approved for use in GAD.

[b]FDA approved for use in PD.

[c]CYP2C19 genetic polymorphisms resulting in little or no enzyme activity are present in 15% to 20% of Asians and 3% to 5% of Blacks and Caucasians resulting in reduced clearance of desmethyldiazepam.[48]

From Refs. 24, 26.

Unlike benzodiazepines, it does not have abuse potential, cause withdrawal reactions, or potentiate alcohol and sedative-hypnotic effects. However, it has a gradual onset of action (i.e., 2 weeks) and does not provide immediate anxiety relief. Buspirone is considered a second-line agent for GAD owing to inconsistent data regarding its efficacy in chronic GAD or GAD with comorbid depression.[21,23] Some research suggests that buspirone is less effective in patients who have been treated previously (4 weeks to 5 years) with benzodiazepines.[44]

Buspirone should be initiated at a dose of 7.5 mg twice daily and titrated in 5 mg/day increments (every 2–3 days) to a usual target dose of 20 to 30 mg/day.[44] The maximum daily dose is considered to be 60 mg/day.

Buspirone generally is well tolerated and does not cause sedation. The most common side effects include dizziness, nausea, and headaches. Drugs that inhibit CYP3A4 (e.g., verapamil, diltiazem, itraconazole, fluvoxamine, nefazodone, and erythromycin) can increase buspirone levels. Likewise, enzyme inducers such as rifampin can reduce buspirone levels significantly. Bupirone may increase blood pressure when coadministered with a monoamine oxidase inhibitor (MAOI).

▶ Alternative Agents

Hydroxyzine, pregabalin, and adjunctive SGAs are alternative agents. Hydroxyzine may be effective for acute reduction of somatic symptoms of anxiety.[23] It does not improve psychic features of anxiety and does not treat depression or other common comorbid anxiety disorders.

Pregabalin is mechanistically unique for an anxiolytic. It is a presynaptic modulator of excessive excitatory neurotransmitter release. It accomplishes this by selectively binding to the α_2-δ subunit of voltage-gated calcium channels. In a 4-week controlled trial versus alprazolam and placebo, pregabalin was effective for both somatic and psychic symptoms of anxiety with an onset of effect similar to that of alprazolam.[45] Compared to venlafaxine and placebo, pregabalin was found to be safe, well-tolerated, and efficacious in GAD, and results were seen 1 week sooner than with venlafaxine.[46] Pregabalin has an elimination half-life of approximately 6 hours and must be dosed two to three times daily. It is excreted renally and has a low risk of drug–drug interactions. Pregabalin is a schedule V controlled substance owing to a propensity to cause euphoria and risk of withdrawal symptoms when discontinued abruptly. Pregabalin should be used with caution

Table 40–5

Pharmacokinetic Drug Interactions With Benzodiazepines

Drug	Effect
Alcohol (chronic)	Increased CL of BZs
Carbamazepine	Increased CL of alprazolam
Cimetidine	Decreased CL of alprazolam, diazepam, chlordiazepoxide, and clorazepate and increased $t_{1/2}$
Disulfiram	Decreased CL of alprazolam and diazepam
Erythromycin	Decreased CL of alprazolam
Fluoxetine	Decreased CL of alprazolam and diazepam
Fluvoxamine	Decreased CL of alprazolam and prolonged $t_{1/2}$
Itraconazole	Potentially decreased CL of alprazolam and diazepam
Ketaconazole	Potentially decreased CL of alprazolam
Nefazodone	Decreased CL of alprazolam, AUC doubled, and $t_{1/2}$ prolonged
Omeprazole	Decreased CL of diazepam
Oral contraceptives	Increased free concentration of chlordiazepoxide and slightly decreased CL; decreased CL and increased $t_{1/2}$ of diazepam and alprazolam
Paroxetine	Decreased CL of alprazolam
Phenobarbital	Increased CL of clonazepam and reduced $t_{1/2}$
Phenytoin	Increased CL of clonazepam and reduced $t_{1/2}$
Probenecid	Decreased CL of lorazepam and prolonged $t_{1/2}$
Propranolol	Decreased CL of diazepam and prolonged $t_{1/2}$
Ranitidine	Decreased absorption of diazepam
Rifampin	Increased metabolism of diazepam
Theophylline	Decreased alprazolam concentrations
Valproate	Decreased CL of lorazepam

AUC, area under the plasma concentration curve; BZ, benzodiazepine; CL, clearance; $t_{1/2}$, elimination half-life.

From Kirkwood CK, Melton ST. Anxiety disorders: I. Generalized anxiety, panic, and social anxiety disorders. In: DiPiro JT, Talbert RL, Yee GC, et al., eds. Pharmacotherapy: A Pathophysiologic Approach, 7th ed. New York: McGraw Hill, 2008:1169.

in patients with a current or past history of substance abuse. It is not beneficial for depression or other anxiety disorders, and long-term effectiveness in GAD is not established.

Atypical antipsychotics have recently been evaluated for anxiety. Both quetiapine and aripiprazole were effective in reducing anxiety symptoms when added to an antidepressant.[47,48] However, several other studies of SGAs have failed to demonstrate a significant improvement in anxiety symptoms in poorly responsive patients. Given their risk for metabolic side effects including weight gain, increased triglycerides, and diabetes, compelling effectiveness data are needed to consider these agents as first- or second-line treatment options.

Outcome Evaluation

Assess patients for improvement of anxiety symptoms and for return to baseline occupational, social, and interpersonal functioning. With effective treatment, the patient should have no or minimal symptoms of anxiety or depression. While drug therapy is being initiated, evaluate patients more frequently to ensure tolerability and response. Increase the dose in patients exhibiting a partial response after 2 to 4 weeks on an antidepressant or 2 weeks on a benzodiazepine. Individualize the duration of treatment because some patients require up to 1 year of treatment.[24]

PANIC DISORDER

TREATMENT

Desired Outcomes

● The main objectives of treatment are to reduce the severity and frequency of panic attacks, reduce anticipatory anxiety and agoraphobic behavior, and minimize symptoms of depression or other comorbid disorders.[49] The long-term goal is to achieve and sustain remission.

General Approach to Treatment

Treatment options include medication, psychotherapy (e.g., CBT preferred), or a combination of both. In some cases, pharmacotherapy will follow psychotherapy treatments when full response is not realized. Patients with panic symptoms without agoraphobia may respond to pharmacotherapy alone. Agoraphobic symptoms generally take longer to respond than panic symptoms. ❹ *The acute phase of PD treatment lasts about 12 weeks and should result in marked reduction in panic attacks (ideally total elimination), minimal anticipatory anxiety, and phobic avoidance. Treatment should be continued to prevent relapse for an additional 12 to 18*

Clinical Presentation and Diagnosis of PD

General

Typically presents in late adolescence or early adulthood. Onset in older adults increases suspicion of relationship to medical disorders or substance use. Laboratory evaluation must be driven by history and physical examination.

Symptoms[2]

Recurrent, discrete episodes that typically develop rapidly and peak within 10 minutes involving at least four of the following symptoms:

- Palpitations or rapid heart rate
- Sweating
- Trembling or shaking
- Sensation of shortness of breath or smothering
- Feeling of choking
- Chest pain or discomfort
- Feeling dizzy or lightheaded
- Feelings of unreality or being detached from oneself
- Fear of dying
- Numbness or tingling sensation
- Chills or hot flushes

Differential Diagnosis

Rule out underlying medical or psychiatric disorders and medications that may cause anxiety (Tables 40–1 and 40–2).

Laboratory Evaluation

- Urine drug screen
- Basic metabolic panel
- TSH
- Electrocardiogram
- Holter monitor
- Electroencephalogram
- Urine vanillylmandelic acid (VMA)

---

months before attempting discontinuation.[49,50] Patients who relapse following discontinuation of medication should have therapy resumed.[49,50]

Nonpharmacologic Therapy

Patients with PD should be counseled to avoid stimulant agents (e.g., decongestants, diet pills, and caffeine) that may precipitate a panic attack. CBT consists of psychoeducation, continuous panic monitoring, breathing retraining, cognitive restructuring, and exposure to fear cues.[50] CBT may involve these features to varying degree. Panic-focused psychodynamic psychotherapy (PFPP) focuses on underlying meaning of panic symptoms (e.g., they have a specific emotional significance) and on current social and emotional functioning.[50] PFPP may be used alone or with other modalities. Exposure therapy is useful for patients with phobic avoidance. CBT is considered a first-line treatment of PD, with efficacy similar to that of pharmacotherapy. In a large placebo-controlled trial comparing CBT with imipramine or combination (CBT + imipramine), CBT was as effective as the antidepressant after 12 weeks. Patients receiving CBT were less likely to relapse during the 6 months after treatment discontinuation.[51,52] In a recent trial of PD with or without agoraphobia, SSRI plus CBT therapy was more effective than SSRI or CBT monotherapy after 9 months of treatment.[53]

Pharmacologic Therapy

PD may be treated successfully with TCAs, SSRIs, SNRIs, or MAOIs, as well as benzodiazepines[50,52] (Table 40–6). While all these agents are similarly effective, SSRIs have become the treatment of choice in PD. Benzodiazepines often are used concomitantly with antidepressants, especially early in treatment, or as monotherapy to acutely reduce panic symptoms. Benzodiazepines are not preferred for long-term treatment but may be used when patients fail several antidepressant trials.[49,50] PD patients with comorbid depression should be treated with an antidepressant. An algorithm for pharmacologic management of PD appears in Figure 40–3.

▶ Antidepressants

Antidepressants have a delayed onset of antipanic effect, typically 4 weeks, with optimal response at 6 to 12 weeks. Reduction of anticipatory anxiety and phobic avoidance generally follows improvement in panic symptoms. ❺ *PD patients are more likely to experience stimulant-like side effects of antidepressants than patients with major depression. Antidepressants should be initiated at lower doses (Table 40–6) in PD patients than in depressed patients or those with other anxiety disorders. Target doses are similar to those used in depression.* ❻ *Antidepressants should be tapered when treatment is discontinued to avoid withdrawal symptoms including irritability, agitation, and dysphoria.*

Tricyclic Antidepressants Treatment with imipramine, the most studied TCA, leaves 45% to 70% of patients panic-free. Both desipramine and clomipramine have demonstrated effectiveness in PD as well. Despite their efficacy, TCAs are rendered second-line pharmacotherapy due to poorer tolerability, patient acceptance, and toxicity on overdose.[49,50] TCAs are associated with a greater rate of discontinuation from treatment than SSRIs.[54] PD patients taking TCAs may experience anticholinergic effects, orthostatic hypotension,

Table 40–6

Antidepressants Used in the Treatment of PD

Medication Class	Recommended Starting Dose (mg/day)	Usual Therapeutic Dosage Range (mg/day)	Advantages	Disadvantages
SSRIs/SNRIs			*SSRIs (in general)*	*SSRIs (in general)*
Citalopram	10	20–60	Antidepressant activity; antianxiety activity; single daily dosing (all but fluvoxamine); low toxicity; some available in generic	Activation; delayed onset of action; may precipitate mania; sexual side effects; GI side effects
Escitalopram	5–10	10–20		
Fluoxetine[a]	5–10	20–60		
Fluvoxamine	25	100–300		
Paroxetine[a]	10	20–60		
Sertraline[a]	25	50–200		
Venlafaxine XR[a]	37.5	75–225		
TCAs			*TCAs (in general)*	*TCAs (in general)*
Clomipramine	25 mg (2 × day)	75–250	Established efficacy; available in generic	Activation; sedation; anticholinergic effects; cardiovascular effects; delayed onset of action; may precipitate mania; sexual side effects; toxic in overdose; weight gain
Imipramine[a]	10–25	75–250		
MAOI				
Phenelzine	15	45–90	Antidepressant effects; available in generic	Dietary restrictions; drug interactions; weight gain; orthostasis; may precipitate mania

SSRIs, selective serotonin reuptake inhibitors; SNRIs, serotonin-norepinephrine reuptake inhibitors; TCAs, tricyclic antidepressants; MAOI, monoamine oxidase inhibitor.

[a]FDA approved for use in panic disorder.

From Refs. 24, 26, 52.

sweating, sleep disturbances, dizziness, fatigue, sexual dysfunction, and weight gain. Stimulant-like side effects occur in up to 40% of patients.[49,50]

Selective Serotonin Reuptake Inhibitors SSRIs are the drugs of choice for PD. All SSRIs have demonstrated effectiveness in controlled trials, with 60% to 80% of patients achieving a panic-free state.[25,49,50] With similar efficacy reported and no trials comparing different SSRIs, selection generally is based on pharmacokinetics, drug interactions, side effects, and cost differences (see Chap. 38). The most common side effects of SSRIs include headaches, irritability, nausea and other GI complaints, insomnia, sexual dysfunction, increased anxiety, drowsiness, and tremor.[49,50]

Serotonin-Norepinephrine Reuptake Inhibitors Venlafaxine is FDA approved for the treatment of PD. In doses of 75 to 225 mg/day, it reduced panic and anticipatory anxiety in short-term controlled trials, and it prevents relapse with extended treatment over 6 months.[55,56] The most common side effects include anorexia, dry mouth, constipation, somnolence, tremor, abnormal ejaculation, and sweating.

Monoamine Oxidase Inhibitors MAOIs have not been evaluated systematically for treatment of PD under the current diagnostic classification and generally are reserved for patients who are refractory to other treatments.[49,50] They have significant side effects that limit adherence. Additionally, patients must adhere to dietary restriction of tyramine and avoid sympathomimetic drugs to avoid hypertensive crisis (see Chap. 38).

The reversible inhibitors of monoamine oxidase A (RIMAs) (brofaromine and meclobemide) have been studied with mixed results.[49] Neither is approved for use in the United States, but they are available in Canada.

Other Drugs Bupropion, trazodone, and nefazodone are not recommended for treatment of PD.[50]

▶ *Benzodiazepines*

Benzodiazepines are effective antipanic agents with significant effects on anticipatory anxiety and phobic behaviors. Alprazolam, the one studied most extensively, is associated with significant panic reduction after 1 week of therapy (e.g., 55–75% panic-free).[49,50] Benzodiazepines achieve similar outcomes to antidepressants over extended treatment, but benzodiazepine-treated patients are more likely to relapse when the drug is discontinued.[49,50] The risk for dependence and withdrawal and lack of efficacy for depression are significant concerns for long-term treatment of PD. There is no evidence that tolerance to therapeutic effect does

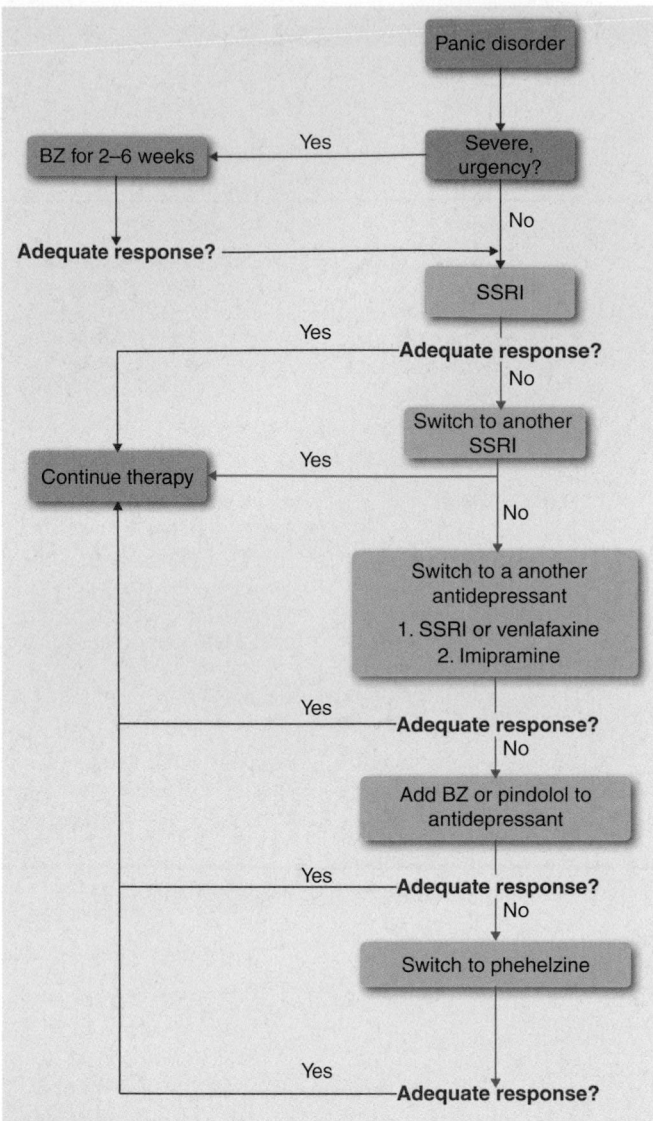

FIGURE 40–3. Algorithm for the pharmacotherapy of panic disorder. BZ, benzodiazepines; SSRIs, selective serotonin reuptake inhibitors (Adapted from Kirkwood CK, Melton ST. Anxiety disorders: I. Generalized anxiety, panic and social anxiety disorders. In: DiPiro JT, Talbert RL, Yee GC, Matzke GR, et al., eds. Pharmacotherapy: A Pathophysiologic Approach, 7th ed. New York: McGraw-Hill, 2008:1163–1178.)

occur. In fact, patients do not require dose escalation during extended treatment. Patients with PD do experience greater rebound anxiety and relapse when discontinuing benzodiazepines than do GAD patients. Tapering should be done at a slower rate and over a more extended period of time than with other anxiety disorders.[25,49,50]

❼ *The dose of benzodiazepine required for improvement generally is higher than that used in other anxiety disorders,* and this may explain why high-potency agents such as alprazolam and clonazepam generally are preferred. Lorazepam and diazepam, when given in equivalent doses, produce similar treatment benefits.[49] Doses should be titrated to response (Table 40–4). The use of extended-release alprazolam or clonazepam will

minimize breakthrough panic symptoms that are sometimes observed with immediate-release alprazolam.[57]

Side effects associated with benzodiazepines in PD patients are similar to those observed in other disorders. Sedation, fatigue, and cognitive impairment are the most commonly reported side effects.[49] Benzodiazepines should be avoided in patients with current or past substance abuse/dependence or sleep apnea. Additionally, caution should be used in older adults because they have more pronounced psychomotor and cognitive effects.

▶ *β-Blockers*

❺ *Pindolol 25 mg three times a day has been shown effective as an adjunctive treatment for PD when used with an SSRI.[58] Propranolol 120 to 240 mg/day has been found equivalent to alprazolam in reduction of panic attacks.[59]* β-Blockers are not expected to reduce psychic anxiety or avoidance behavior. Additionally, heart rate and blood pressure reduction are dose-related adverse events that may limit use.

Outcome Evaluation

Evaluate patients for symptom improvement frequently (e.g., weekly) during the first 4 weeks of therapy. The goal is to alleviate panic attacks and reduce anticipatory anxiety and phobic avoidance with resumption of normal activities. Alter the therapy of patients who do not achieve a significant reduction in panic symptoms after 6 to 8 weeks of an adequate dose of antidepressant or 3 weeks of a benzodiazepine. Strategies may include augmentation (e.g., add CBT if already on medication) or switch to another medication or treatment modality. Regularly evaluate patients for adverse effects, and educate them about appropriate expectations of drug therapy.

Once the patient has achieved a significant response, continue therapy for at least 1 year. Evaluate for symptom relapse as well as adverse effects that may emerge with continued treatment (e.g., weight gain and sexual dysfunction). During drug discontinuation, monitor frequently for withdrawal, rebound anxiety, and relapse.

SOCIAL ANXIETY DISORDER

TREATMENT

Desired Outcomes

SAD is a chronic disorder that begins in adolescence and occurs with significant functional impairment and high rates of comorbidity. The goal of acute treatment is to reduce physiologic symptoms of anxiety, fear of social situations, and phobic behaviors. Patients with comorbid depression should have a significant reduction in depressive symptoms. The long-term goal is to restore social functioning and improve the patient's quality of life.

General Approach to Treatment

Patients with SAD may be managed with pharmacotherapy or psychotherapy. There is insufficient evidence to

Clinical Presentation and Diagnosis of SAD

General

Often occurs in context of other anxiety disorders. The feared social or performance situation can be limited to a specific social interaction (e.g., public speaking) or generalized to most any social interaction. Differs from specific phobia, in which the fear and anxiety are limited to a particular object or situation (e.g., insects, heights, public transportation).

Symptoms[2]

- Persistent fear of social interactions, during which time the individual is concerned about being embarrassed or being under scrutiny.

- Engaging in the feared activities can lead to extreme anxiety and panic.
- The fear leads to distress or avoidance of the situation sufficient enough to cause trouble in the patient's life.

Differential Diagnosis

Rule out underlying medical or psychiatric disorders and medications that may cause anxiety (Tables 40–1 and 40–2).

Laboratory Evaluation

Laboratory investigation is of limited value and should be pursued only in context of other history or physical examination findings.

---

recommend one treatment over the other, and data are lacking on the benefits of combining treatment modalities. Pharmacotherapy often is the first choice of treatment owing to relative greater access and reduced cost compared with psychotherapy.[60] Patients with SAD generally respond slowly to treatment, and many will not achieve a full response. Relapse is common when patients are discontinued after effective short-term treatment. Patients generally are continued on treatment for at least 1 year before attempting discontinuation.

Nonpharmacologic Therapy

Patient education on disease course, treatment options, and expectations is essential given the chronic nature and functional impairment of SAD. Support groups may be beneficial for some patients. CBT targets avoidance-learning and negative-thinking patterns associated with social anxiety by exposing the patient to a feared situation. CBT is effective for reducing anxiety and phobic avoidance and leads to a greater likelihood of maintaining response after treatment discontinuation than does pharmacotherapy.[60]

Pharmacologic Therapy

Several pharmacologic agents have demonstrated effectiveness in SAD, including SSRIs, venlafaxine, phenelzine, RIMAs, benzodiazepines, gabapentin, and pregabalin. **8** *SSRIs are considered the drugs of choice based on their tolerability and efficacy for SAD and comorbid depression if present.* **9** *The onset of response for antidepressants may be as long as 8 to 12 weeks.*[25,61] *Patients responding to medication should be continued on treatment for at least 1 year.* Many will relapse when medication is discontinued, and there are no clear predictive factors for who will maintain response.[61] Some patients may elect more long-term treatment owing to fear of relapse. A suggested treatment algorithm is shown in **Figure 40–4**.

Patient Encounter 2

BB, a 34-year-old white woman with generalized SAD is transferring her care to your clinic. She has been maintained on diazepam 10 mg twice daily for the past 4 years for her SAD. She states that her current therapy has her anxiety under control, and she is performing her duties as an office manager without problems. She has joined a gym recently and is attending a church social for single women once monthly. She has noticed she has difficulty thinking "sharply" and is more forgetful. She occasionally feels sad and becomes tearful but is usually able to "pick herself up." She is moderately overweight (BMI 29) with no other current medical problems. Denies ethanol or other substance use.

Develop a treatment plan for this patient. Include (a) goals of therapy, (b) a detailed therapeutic plan, and (c) a monitoring plan for recommended therapy.

▶ *Selective Serotonin Reuptake Inhibitors and Venlafaxine*

The efficacy of paroxetine, sertraline, and escitalopram was established in large controlled trials.[60-63] SSRIs improve social anxiety and phobic avoidance and reduce overall disability. Approximately 50% of patients achieve response during acute treatment. Limited data suggest that both fluvoxamine and citalopram are effective in SAD. Fluoxetine is not effective.[60,61]

The initial dose of SSRI is similar to that used in depression. Patients should be titrated as tolerated to response. Many patients will require maximum recommended daily doses. Patients with comorbid PD should be started on lower doses (Table 40–6). When discontinuing SSRIs, the dose should be tapered slowly to avoid withdrawal symptoms. Relapse rates

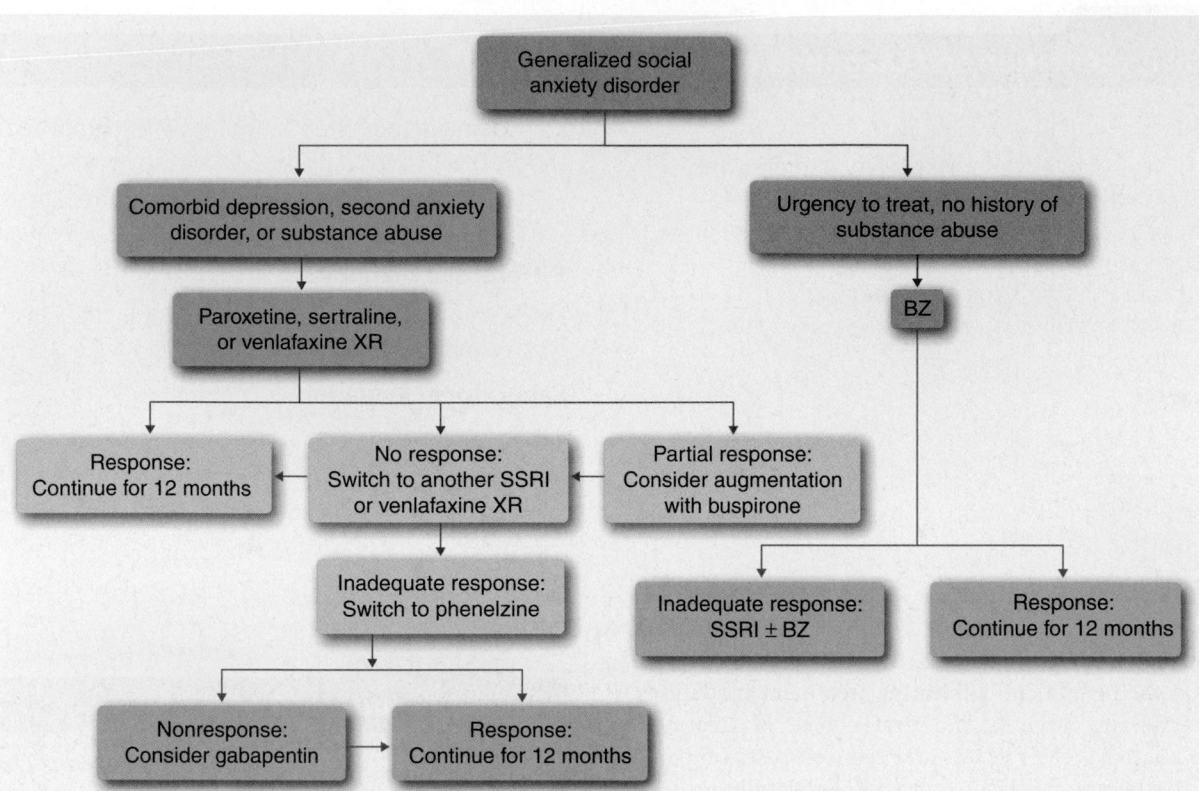

FIGURE 40–4. Algorithm for the pharmacotherapy of SAD. BZ, benzodiazepines; SSRI, selective serotonin reuptake inhibitor (Adapted from Kirkwood CK, Melton ST. Anxiety disorders: I. Generalized anxiety, panic and social anxiety disorders. In: DiPiro JT, Talbert RL, Yee GC, Matzke GR, et al., eds. Pharmacotherapy: A Pathophysiologic Approach, 7th ed. New York: McGraw-Hill, 2008:1163–1178.)

may be as high as 50%, and patients should be monitored closely for several weeks.[60,61] Side effects of SSRIs in SAD patients are similar to those seen in depression and most commonly include nausea, sexual dysfunction, somnolence, and sweating.

Venlafaxine extended release, in doses of 75 to 225 mg/ day, improves social anxiety, performance, and avoidance behavior with a reduction in disability.[64] Treatment with venlafaxine results in response rates similar to those seen with paroxetine.[64] Venlafaxine may be effective in SSRI nonresponders.[65] As with SSRIs, doses should be tapered slowly when discontinuing therapy. Tolerability is similar to that observed in depression trials with venlafaxine extended release. Common side effects are anorexia, dry mouth, nausea, insomnia, and sexual dysfunction.

▶ *MAOIs/Reversible Inhibitors of MAO-A*

Phenelzine is effective in 64% to 69% of SAD patients.[61] It is generally reserved for treatment-refractory patients owing to dietary restrictions,[66] drug interactions, and side effects. The RIMAs brofaromine and meclobemide are effective in SAD. Neither is currently available in the United States, but they are available in Canada.

▶ *Alternative Agents*

Benzodiazepines Benzodiazepines are used commonly in SAD; however, there are limited data supporting their use. Clonazepam has been effective for social anxiety, fear, and phobic avoidance, and it reduced social and work disability during acute treatment.[61] Long-term treatment is not desirable for many SAD patients owing to the risk of withdrawal and difficulty with discontinuation, cognitive side effects, and lack of effect on depressive symptoms. Benzodiazepines may be useful for acute relief of physiologic symptoms of anxiety when used concomitantly with antidepressants or psychotherapy. Benzodiazepines are contraindicated in SAD patients with alcohol or substance abuse or history of such.

Anticonvulsants (Gabapentin, Pregabalin) Gabapentin, a nonbenzodiazapine GABA analog, was modestly effective in a 14-week controlled trial in SAD. Most patients were titrated to a maximal dose of 3,600 mg/day.[61] Pregabalin 600 mg/day was effective for social anxiety, fear, and avoidance behavior in a 10-week controlled trial.[67] Pregabalin was well tolerated, and the most common side effects were somnolence and dizziness.

β-Blockers β-Blockers decrease physiologic symptoms of anxiety and are useful for reducing performance anxiety.

Patient Care and Monitoring

1. Review medical and laboratory data to rule out contributing causes of anxiety.

2. Assess the patient's symptoms and level of functional impairment to determine if pharmacotherapy is appropriate for the anxiety disorder.

3. Obtain a thorough history of prescription, nonprescription, and natural product use.

4. Determine what treatments have been tried or were useful in the past. Is the patient taking medication that may cause anxiety?

5. Educate the patient about lifestyle changes that will improve symptoms of anxiety. These include adequate sleep and exercise, stress management, meditation, and coping skills.

6. Inform patients of treatment options for anxiety disorders and the expected benefits of each (e.g., pharmacotherapy, psychotherapy, and combination treatment).

7. Develop a plan to assess the effectiveness of drug therapy during the first 12 weeks.

8. Determine an appropriate duration of treatment. Is long-term maintenance treatment needed?

9. Assess improvement in academic, social, interpersonal, and occupational functioning; quality of life, and well-being.

10. Evaluate the patient for the presence of adverse drug effects, drug–drug interactions, and drug allergies.

11. Stress the importance of adherence to medications to achieve and maintain response.

12. Provide patient education regarding disease state, lifestyle modifications, and pharmacotherapy:

    - What differentiates anxiety from an anxiety disorder? How should it be treated?

    - What are potential complications of an untreated anxiety disorder?

    - What potential adverse effects may occur? Is there a risk of dependence?

    - Which drugs may interact with therapy?

    - How to record symptoms (e.g., fears, panic attacks, avoidance behaviors) and report back to their clinician.

Propranolol or atenolol should be administered 1 hour before a performance situation. β-Blockers are not useful in generalized SAD.[61]

Outcome Evaluation

❿ *Pharmacotherapy of SAD should lead to improvement in physiologic symptoms of anxiety and fear, functionality, and overall well-being.*[23] Many patients may not achieve full remission of symptoms, but they should have significant improvement. Monitor patients weekly during acute treatment (e.g., initiation and titration of pharmacotherapy). Once patients are stabilized, monitor monthly. Inquire about adverse effects and SAD symptoms at each visit. To aid in assessing improvement, ask patients to keep a diary to record fears, anxiety levels, and behaviors in social situations.[23] You may administer the Leibowitz Social Anxiety Scale (LSAS) to rate SAD severity and change, and the Social Phobia Inventory can be used as a "self-assessment" tool for SAD patients. Lastly, counsel patients on appropriate expectations of pharmacotherapy in SAD, including the gradual onset of effect and the need for extended treatment of at least 1 year.

Abbreviations Introduced in This Chapter

AV	Atrioventricular
BUN	Blood urea nitrogen
CBT	Cognitive-behavioral therapy
DA	Dopamine
GABA	γ-Aminobutyric acid
GAD	Generalized anxiety disorder
HPA	Hypothalamic–pituitary–adrenal
5-HT	Serotonin
IBS	Irritable bowel syndrome
LC	Locus ceruleus
LSAS	Liebowitz Social Anxiety Scale
MAOI	Monoamine oxidase inhibitor
MDD	Major depressive disorder
mRNA	Messenger RNA
NCS-R	National Comorbidity Survey, Revised
NE	Norepinephrine
NPY	Neuropeptide Y
OCD	Obsessive–compulsive disorder
PD	Panic disorder
PFPP	Panic-focused psychodynamic psychotherapy
RAS	Reticular activating system
RIMA	Reversible inhibitors of monoamine oxidase A
SAD	Social anxiety disorder
SCr	Serum creatinine
SGA	Second-generation antipsychotic
SNRI	Serotonin-norepinephrine reuptake inhibitor
SSRI	Selective serotonin reuptake inhibitor
TCA	Tricyclic antidepressant
TSH	Thyroid-stimulating hormone
VMA	Vanillylmandelic acid

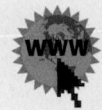

Self-assessment questions and answers are available at *http://www.mhpharmacotherapy. com/pp.html.*

REFERENCES

1. Young AS, Klap R, Sherbourne CD, Wells KB. The quality of care for depressive and anxiety disorders in the United States. Arch Gen Psychiatry 2001;58:55–61.
2. Diagnostic and Statistical Manual of Mental Disorders, 4th ed, Text revision. Washington, DC: American Psychiatric Association, 2000:429–484.
3. Kessler RC, Berglund P, Demler O, et al. Lifetime prevalence and age-of-onset distributions of the DSM-IV disorders in the National Comorbidity Survey Replication. Arch Gen Psychiatry 2005a;62:593–602.
4. Kessler RC, Chiu WT, Demler O, et al. Prevalence, severity, and comorbidity of 12-month DSM-IV disorders in the National Comorbidity Survey Replication. Arch Gen Psychiatry 2005;62(6):617–627.
5. Kessler RS, Keller MB, Wittchen HU. The epidemiology of generalized anxiety disorder. Psychiatr Clin North Am 2001;13:78–88.
6. Pollack MH. The pharmacotherapy of panic disorder. J Clin Psychiatry 2005;66(Suppl 4):23–27.
7. Wittchen HU, Hoyer J. Generalized anxiety disorder: Nature and course. J Clin Psychiatry 2001;62(Suppl 11):15–19.
8. Bruce SE, Yonkers SE, Otto MW, et al. Influence of psychiatric comorbidity on recovery and recurrence in generalized anxiety disorder, social phobia, and panic disorder: A 12-year prospective study. Am J Psychiatry 2005;162:1179–1187.
9. Yonkers KA, Bruce SE, Dyck IR, Keller MB. Chronicity, relapse, and illness-course of panic disorder, social phobia, and generalized anxiety disorder: Findings in men and women from 8 years of follow-up. Depress Anxiety 2003;17:173–179.
10. Cramer V, Torgersen S, Kringlen E. Quality of life and anxiety disorders: A population study. J Nerv Ment Dis 2005;193:196–202.
11. Kaufman J, Charney D. Comorbidity of mood and anxiety disorders. Depress Anxiety 2000;12(Suppl 1):69–76.
12. Hettema JM, Prescott CA, Myers JM, et al. The structure of genetic and environmental risk factors for anxiety disorders in men and women. Arch Gen Psychiatry 2005;62:182–189.
13. Ninan PT, Dunlop BW. Neurobiology and etiology of panic disorder. J Clin Psychiatry 2005;66(Suppl 4):3–7.
14. Pierii JN, Lewis DA. Functional neuroanatomy. In: Sadock BJ, Sadock VA, eds. Kaplan & Sadock's Comprehensive Textbook of Psychiatry, 8th ed. Philadelphia: Lippincott Williams & Wilkins, 2005:3–32.
15. Gould TD, Gray NA, Manji HK. Cellular neurobiology of severe mood and anxiety disorders: Implications for development of novel therapeutics. In: Charney DS, ed. Molecular Neurobiology for the Clinician (Review of Psychiatry Series. Vol. 22. Number 3; Oldham JM, and Riba MB, series eds). Washington, DC: American Psychiatric Publishing, 2003:123–200.
16. Plata-Salaman CR, Shank RP, Smith-Swintosky VL. Amino acids as neurotransmitters. In: Sadock BJ, Sadock VA, eds. Kaplan & Sadock's Comprehensive Textbook of Psychiatry, 8th ed. Philadelphia: Lippincott Williams & Wilkins, 2005:60–72.
17. Young LJ, Owens MJ, Nemeroff CB. Neuropeptides: Biology, regulation, and role in neuropsychiatric disorders. In: Sadock BJ, Sadock VA, eds. Kaplan & Sadock's Comprehensive Textbook of Psychiatry, 8th ed. Philadelphia: Lippincott Williams & Wilkins, 2005:3–32.
18. Papp LA, Kleber MS. Phenomenology of generalized anxiety disorder. In: Stein DJ, Hollander E, eds. Textbook of Anxiety Disorders, 5th ed. Washington, DC: American Psychiatric Publishing, 2002.
19. House A, Stark D. Anxiety in medical patients. BMJ 2002;325:207–209.

20. Kirkwood CK, Melton ST. Anxiety disorders: I. Generalized anxiety, panic and social anxiety disorders. In: DiPiro JT, Talbert RL, Yee GC, Matzke GR, et al., eds. Pharmacotherapy: A Pathophysiologic Approach, 7th ed. New York: McGraw-Hill, 2008:1163–1178.
21. Allgulander C, Bandelow B, Hollander E, et al. WCA recommendations for the long-term treatment of generalized anxiety disorder. CNS Spectr 2003 Aug;8(Suppl 1):53–61.
22. Walkup JT, Albano AM, Piacentini J, et al. Cognitive behavioral therapy, sertraline or a combination in childhood anxiety. N Engl J Med 2008;359(26):2753–2766.
23. Ballanger JC, Davidson JR, Lecrubier Y, et al. Consensus statement on generalized anxiety disorder from the international consensus group on depression and anxiety. J Clin Psychiatry 2001;62(Suppl 11):53–58.
24. Rickels R, Ryan M. Pharmacotherapy of generalized anxiety disorder. J Clin Psychiatry 2002;63(Suppl 14):9–16.
25. Bandelow B, Zohar J, Hollander E, et al. Guidelines for the pharmacological treatment of anxiety, obsessive-compulsive and post-traumatic stress disorders. World J Biol Psychiatry 2002;3:171–199.
26. Micromedex Healthcare Series. Drugdex Evaluations, 2005.
27. Shelton RC, Brown LL. Mechanisms of action in the treatment of anxiety. J Clin Psychiatry 2001;62(Suppl 12):10–15.
28. Allgulander C, Hackett D, Salinas E. Venlafaxine extended release (ER) in the treatment of generalized anxiety disorder: 24-Week, placebo-controlled dose-ranging study. Br J Psychiatry 2001;179:15–22.
29. Allgulander C, Nutt D, Detke M, et al. A non-inferiority comparison of duloxetine and venlafaxine in the treatment of adult patients with generalized anxiety disorder. J Psychopharmacol 2008;22(4):417–425.
30. Hartford JT, Endicott J, Kornstein SG, et al. Implications of pain in generalized anxiety disorder: Efficacy of duloxetine. Prim Care Companion J Clin Psychiatry 2008;10(3):197–204.
31. Rickels K, Zaninelli R, McCafferty J, et al. Paroxetine treatment of generalized anxiety disorder: A double-blind, placebo-controlled study. Am J Psychiatry 2003;160:749–756.
32. Stocchi F, Nordera G, Jokinen R, et al. Efficacy and tolerability of paroxetine for the long-term treatment of generalized anxiety disorder (GAD). J Clin Psychiatry 2003;64(3):250–258.
33. Davidson JR, Bose A, Korotzer A, Zheng H. Escitalopram in the treatment of generalized anxiety disorder: Double-blind, placebo-controlled, flexible-dose study. Depress Anxiety 2004;19(4):234–240.
34. Allgulander C, Dahl AA, Austin C, et al. Efficacy of sertraline in a 12-week trial for generalized anxiety disorder. Am J Psychiatry 2004;161(9):1642–1649.
35. Lenze EJ, Mulsant BH, Shear MK, et al. Efficacy and tolerability of citalopram in the treatment of late-life anxiety disorders: Results from an 8-week randomized, placebo-controlled trial. Am J Psychiatry 2005;162(1):146–150.
36. Ball SG, Kuhn A, Wall D, et al. Selective serotonin reuptake inhibitor treatment for generalized anxiety disorder: A double blind, prospective comparison between paroxetine and sertraline. J Clin Psychiatry 2005;66:94–99.
37. Bielski RJ, Bose A, Chang CC. A double-blind comparison of escitalopram and paroxetine in the long-term treatment of generalized anxiety disorder. Ann Clin Psychiatry 2005;17(2):65–69.
38. Sramek JJ, Zarotsky V, Cutler NR. Generalised anxiety disorder. Drugs 2002;62:1635–1648.
39. Gambi F, De Berardis D, Campanella D, et al. Mirtazapine treatment of generalized anxiety disorder: A fixed dose, open label study. J Psychopharmacol 2005;19(5):483–487.
40. Bystritsky A, Kerwin L, Feusner JD, and Vapnik T. A pilot controlled trial of bupropion XL versus escitalopram in generalized anxiety disorder. Psychopharmacol Bull 2008;41(1):46–51.
41. US Food and Drug Administration. *http://www.fda.gov/cder/genomics/ genomic_biomarkers_table.htm.*
42. Longo LP, Johnson B. Benzodiazepines: Side effects, abuse risk and alternatives (addiction part 1). Am Fam Physician 2000;61:2121–2128.
43. Gorman JM. Treating Generalized anxiety disorder. J Clin Psychiatry 2003;64(Suppl 2):24–29.
44. Chessick CA, Allen MH, Thase M, et al. Azapirones for generalized anxiety disorder. Cochrane Database Syst Rev 2006;3:CD006115.

45. Rickels K, Pollack MH, Feltner DE, et al. Pregabalin for the treatment of generalized anxiety disorder: A 4-week, multicenter, double-blind, placebo-controlled trial of pregabalin and alprazolam. Arch Gen Psychiatry 2005;62:1022–1030.

46. Montgomery SA, Tobias K, Zornberg GL, et al. Pregabalin and venlafaxine improve symptoms of generalised anxiety disorder. Evid Based Ment Health 2007;10:23.

47. Katzman MA, Vermani M, Jacobs L, et al. Quetiapine as an adjunctive pharmacotherapy for the treatment of non-remitting generalized anxiety disorder: A flexible-dose, open-label pilot trial. J Anxiety Disord 2008;22(8):1480–1486.

48. Hoge EA, Worthington JJ 3rd, Kaufman RE, et al. Aripiprazole as augmentation treatment of refractory generalized anxiety and panic disorder. CNS Spectr 2008;13(6):522–527.

49. Pollack MH, Allgulander C, Bandelow B, et al. WCA recommendations for the long-term treatment of panic disorder. CNS Spectr 2003;8(Suppl 1): 17–30.

50. American Psychiatric Association. Practice Guideline for the Treatment of Patients with Panic Disorder, 2nd ed. 2009, *http://www.psychiatryonline.com/pracGuide/pracGuideTopic_9.aspx*. DOI: 10.1176/appi.books.9780890423905.154688

51. Barlow DH, Gorman JM, Shear MK, et al. Cognitive-behavioral therapy, imipramine, or their combination for panic disorder: A randomized controlled trial. JAMA 2000;283:2529–2536.

52. Lydiard B. Pharmacotherapy for panic disorder. In: Stein DJ, Hollander E, eds. Textbook of Anxiety Disorders, 5th ed. Washington, DC: American Psychiatric Publishing, 2002.

53. van Apeldoorn FJ, van Hout WJ, Mersch PP, et al. Is a combined therapy more effective than either CBT or SSRI alone? Results of a multicenter trial on panic disorder with or without agoraphobia. Acta Psychiatr Scand 2008 Apr;117(4):260–270.

54. Bakker A, von Balkom AJ, Spinhoven P. SSRIs vs. TCAs in the treatment of panic disorder: A meta-analysis. Acta Psychiatr Scand 2002;106:163–167.

55. Bradwejn L, Ahokas A, Stein DJ, et al. Venlafaxine extended release capsules in panic disorder: Flexible-dose, double-blind, placebo-controlled study. Br J Psychiatry 2005;187:352–359.

56. Ferguson JM, Khan A, Mangano R, et al. Relapse prevention of panic disorder in adult outpatient responders to treatment with venlafaxine extended release. J Clin Psychiatry 2007;68(1):58–68.

57. Rickels K. Alprazolam extended release in panic disorder. Expert Opin Pharmacother 2004;5(7):1599–1611.

58. Hirschmann S, Dannon PN, Iancu I et al. Pindolol augmentation in patients with treatment-resistant panic disorder: A double-blind, placebo-controlled trial. J Clin Psychopharmacol, 2000;20(5):556–559.

59. Ravaris CL, Friedman MJ, Hauri PJ, McHugo GJ. A controlled study of alprazolam and propranolol in panic-disordered and agoraphobic outpatients. J Clin Psychopharmacol 1991;11(6):344–350.

60. Van Ameringen M, Allgulander C, Bandelow B, et al. WCA recommendations for the long-term treatment of social phobia. CNS Spectr 2003;8(Suppl 1):40–52.

61. Stein DJ, Ipser JC, Balkom AJ. Pharmacotherapy of social anxiety disorder (review). Cochrane Library 2005;4:1–51.

62. Lader M, Stender K, Burger V, Nil R. Efficacy and tolerability of escitalopram in 12 and 24-week treatment of social anxiety disorder: Randomized, double-blind, placebo-controlled, fixed-dose study. Depress Anxiety 2004;19(4):241–248.

63. Kasper S, Stein DJ, Loft H, Nil R. Escitalopram in the treatment of social anxiety disorder: Randomized, placebo-controlled, flexible-dosage study. Br J Psychiatry 2005;186:222–226.

64. Rickels K, Mangano R, Khan A. A double-blind, placebo-controlled study of flexible dose of venlafaxine ER in adult outpatients with generalized social anxiety disorder. J Clin Psychopharmacol 2004;24(5):488–496.

65. Altamura AC, Pioli R, Vitto M, et al. Venlafaxine in social phobia: A study in selective serotonin reuptake non-responders. Int Clin Psychopharmacol 1999;14:239–245.

66. Gardner DM, Shulman KI, Walker SE, Tailor SA. The making of a user friendly MAOI diet. J Clin Psychiatry 1996;57(3):99–104.

67. Pande AC, Feltner DE, Jefferson JW, et al. Efficacy of the novel anxiolytic pregabalin in social anxiety disorder: A placebo-controlled, multicenter study. J Clin Psychopharmacol 2004;24(2):141–149.

41 Sleep Disorders

John M. Dopp and Bradley G. Phillips

LEARNING OBJECTIVES

● **Upon completion of this chapter, the reader will be able to:**

1. Articulate the incidence and prevalence of sleep disorders, list the sequelae of undiagnosed or untreated sleep disorders, and appreciate the importance of successful treatment of sleep disorders.

2. Describe the pathophysiology and characteristic features of the sleep disorders covered in this chapter including: insomnia, narcolepsy, restless legs syndrome (RLS), obstructive sleep apnea (OSA), and parasomnias.

3. Assess patient sleep complaints, conduct sleep histories, and evaluate sleep studies to recognize daytime and nighttime symptoms and characteristics of common sleep disorders.

4. Recommend and optimize appropriate sleep hygiene and nonpharmacologic therapies for the management and prevention of sleep disorders.

5. Recommend and optimize appropriate pharmacotherapy for sleep disorders.

6. Describe the components of a monitoring plan to assess safety and efficacy of pharmacotherapy for common sleep disorders.

7. Educate patients about preventive behavior, appropriate lifestyle modifications, and drug therapy required for effective treatment and control of sleep disorders.

KEY CONCEPTS

❶ Insomnia is most frequently a symptom or manifestation of an underlying disorder (comorbid insomnia) but may occur in the absence of contributing factors (primary insomnia). Early treatment of insomnia may prevent the development of persistent psychophysiologic insomnia.

❷ Patients with sleep complaints should have a careful sleep history performed to assess for possible sleep disorders and to guide diagnostic and therapeutic decisions.

❸ Although clinical history guides diagnosis and therapy, only overnight polysomnography and multiple sleep latency tests (MSLTs) can definitively diagnose and/or guide therapy for obstructive sleep apnea (OSA), narcolepsy, and periodic limb movements of sleep.

❹ Treatment goals vary between different sleep disorders but generally include restoration of normal sleep patterns, elimination of daytime sequelae, improvement in quality of life, and prevention of complications and adverse effects from therapy.

❺ Benzodiazepine receptor agonists, including traditional benzodiazepines, zolpidem, zaleplon, and eszopiclone, are approved by the FDA for the treatment of insomnia and are first-line therapies.

❻ Treatment of excessive daytime sleepiness in narcolepsy and other sleep disorders may require the use of sustained- and immediate-release stimulants to effectively promote wakefulness throughout the day and at key times that require alertness.

❼ Restless-legs syndrome (RLS) treatment involves suppression of abnormal sensations and leg movements, and consolidation of sleep. Dopaminergic and sedative-hypnotic medications are commonly prescribed.

❽ The primary therapy for OSA is nasal continuous positive airway pressure (CPAP) therapy because of its effectiveness.

❾ It is important to review patient medication profiles for drugs that may aggravate sleep disorders. Patients should be monitored for adverse drug reactions, potential drug–drug interactions, and adherence to their therapeutic regimens.

Normal humans sleep up to one-third of their lives and spend more time sleeping compared with any other single activity. Despite this, our understanding of the full purpose of sleep and the mechanisms regulating sleep homeostasis remains incomplete. Sleep is necessary to maintain wakefulness, health, and welfare. Unfortunately, disruption of normal sleep is prevalent and represents a major cause of societal morbidity, lost productivity, and reduced quality of life.[1] The link between adequate sleep and optimal health is becoming increasingly apparent, and sleep disturbances may contribute to the development and progression of comorbid medical conditions.

Sleep is governed and paced by the suprachiasmic nucleus in the brain that regulates circadian rhythm. Environmental cues and amount of previous sleep also influence sleep on a daily basis. There are two main types of sleep: rapid-eye-movement (REM) sleep, where eye movements and dreaming occur but the body is mostly paralyzed, and non-REM sleep, which consists of four substages (stages 1–4). Stage 1 serves as a transition between wake and sleep. Most of the time asleep is spent in stage 2 non-REM sleep. Stage 3 and stage 4 sleep often are grouped together and referred to as *deep sleep,* or *delta sleep,* because prominent delta waves are seen on the electroencephalogram (EEG) during these sleep stages.

EPIDEMIOLOGY AND ETIOLOGY

Sleep disorders are common. Approximately 50% of adults will report a sleep complaint over the course of their lives.[2] In general, sleep disturbances increase with age, and each disorder may have gender differences. The full extent and impact of disordered sleep on our society are not known because many patients' sleep disorders remain undiagnosed. Normal sleep, by definition, is "a reversible behavioral state of perceptual disengagement from and unresponsiveness to the environment."[3] As a result, individuals with sleep disorders will exhibit or complain about consequent symptoms (e.g., daytime sleepiness), or a bed partner will observe hallmark characteristics of the sleep disorder. Insomnia, restless legs syndrome (RLS), and sleep-related breathing disorders are the most common sleep disorders.

Insomnia

The prevalence of insomnia increases with age and is nearly 1.5 times greater in females than in males. Approximately one-third of patients older than age 65 have persistent insomnia.[4,5] In the adult population, about 10% will experience chronic insomnia and slightly more will experience short-term insomnia. ❶ *Insomnia is most frequently a symptom or manifestation of an underlying disorder (comorbid insomnia) but may occur in the absence of contributing factors (primary insomnia). Early treatment of insomnia may prevent the development of persistent psychophysiologic insomnia.* Forty percent of patients with psychiatric conditions will have accompanying insomnia.[6] Comorbid insomnia may be triggered by acute stress and disappears when the

stress resolves. Numerous coexisting medical conditions, such as pain, thyroid abnormalities, asthma, and reflux, and medications, including selective serotonin reuptake inhibitors (SSRIs), steroids, stimulants, and β-agonists, can interfere with sleep and cause comorbid insomnia. In cases of comorbid insomnia, the clinician should treat the underlying primary cause along with insomnia symptoms.

Narcolepsy

Although difficult to estimate, the prevalence of narcolepsy is between 0.03% and 0.06%.[7] Significant differences have been reported for various ethnic groups. Narcolepsy has a higher prevalence in the Japanese and a lower prevalence in the Israeli populations.[8,9] Cataplexy is not required for diagnosis, however, between 50% and 80% of patients with narcolepsy have accompanying cataplexy.[10]

Restless Legs Syndrome

RLS occurs in 6% to 12% of the population, making it a common sleep disorder.[11,12] The prevalence of RLS increases with age and in various medical conditions such as end-stage renal disease (ESRD), pregnancy, and iron deficiency.[13] RLS appears to be more common in women than in men and has a genetic link. The majority of patients (63–92%) report a positive family history for RLS.[14]

Obstructive Sleep Apnea

Obstructive sleep apnea (OSA) is a common disorder that is often unrecognized, affecting 4% of middle-aged white men and 2% of middle-aged white women.[15] In women, the frequency of OSA increases after menopause. OSA is as common or more common in African Americans and less common in Asian populations. The risk of OSA increases with age and obesity. Individuals with OSA experience repetitive upper airway collapse during sleep, which decreases or stops airflow, with subsequent arousal from sleep to resume breathing. The severity is determined by nocturnal polysomnography (NPSG) and is graded by the number of episodes of apnea (total cessation of airflow) and hypopnea (partial airway closure with blood oxygen desaturation) experienced during sleep. The severity is expressed as the respiratory disturbance index (RDI), quantified in events per hour. Mild sleep apneics have an RDI of between 5 and 15 episodes per hour; moderate, 15 and 30; and individuals with severe OSA can exhibit more than 30 episodes per hour.

Parasomnias

Non-REM parasomnias have variable prevalence rates depending on patient age and comorbid diagnoses. Sleep talking, bruxism, sleepwalking, sleep terrors, and enuresis occur more frequently in childhood than in adulthood. Nightmares appear to occur with similar frequency in adults and children. REM behavior disorder (RBD), an REM-sleep parasomnia, has a reported prevalence of 0.5% and frequently is associated with concomitant neurologic conditions.[16] Chronic RBD is more common in elderly men and may have a familial disposition.

PATHOPHYSIOLOGY

Although the neurophysiology of sleep is complex, certain neurotransmitters promote sleep and wakefulness in different areas of the central nervous system (CNS). Serotonin is thought to control non-REM sleep, whereas cholinergic and adrenergic transmitters mediate REM sleep. Dopamine, norepinephrine, hypocretin, substance P, and histamine all play a role in wakefulness. Perturbations of various neurotransmitters are responsible for some sleep disorders and explain why various treatment modalities are beneficial.

Insomnia

Because insomnia is a complex and multifaceted disorder, there is no single pathophysiologic explanation for its various manifestations. Current hypotheses focus on a combination of possible models that incorporate physiologic, cognitive, and cortical arousal. Most insomnia models focus on hyperarousal and its interference with the initiation or maintenance of sleep.

Narcolepsy

The onset of narcolepsy–cataplexy is typically in adolescence and not at birth, suggesting that the disease may require environmental influence to develop. Currently, it is believed that narcolepsy results from autoimmune insult to the CNS because it is associated with HLA (major histocompatibility complex) DQB1*0602 and DQ1A1*0102.[17,18] Concentrations of hypocretin (a wake-promoting neuropeptide) in the cerebrospinal fluid (CSF) of narcolepsy patients are reduced significantly, suggesting that the autoimmune attack is against hypocretin-producing cells in the hypothalamus.[19] Intact hypocretin neurons normally stimulate arousal and wake-promoting neurons to stimulate cortical activation and behavioral arousal.

RLS and Periodic Limb Movements of Sleep

RLS is a neurologic medical condition characterized by an irresistible desire to move the limbs. It is thought that these abnormal sensations are a result of iron deficiency in the brain and iron-handling abnormalities in the CNS. Iron and H-ferritin concentrations, along with transferrin receptor and iron transporter numbers, are reduced in the substantia nigra of patients with RLS.[20] These iron abnormalities lead to dysfunction of dopaminergic transmission in the substantia nigra.

Obstructive Sleep Apnea

At least 20 muscles and soft-tissue structures control patency of the upper airway. Patients with OSA may have differences in upper airway muscle activity during sleep and may have smaller airways, predisposing them to upper airway collapse

and consequent apneic episodes during sleep. The inability of the upper airway to contend with factors that promote collapse, including fat deposition in the neck, negative pressure in the airway during inspiration, and a smaller lower jawbone, also may play a role in the pathogenesis of OSA. Hallmarks of OSA include witnessed apneas, gasping, or both.

Poor sleep architecture and fragmented sleep secondary to OSA can cause excessive daytime sleepiness (EDS) and neurocognitive deficits. These sequelae can affect quality of life and work performance, and may be linked to occupational and motor vehicle accidents. OSA is also associated with systemic disease such as hypertension, heart failure, and stroke.[21,22] OSA is likely an independent risk factor for the development of hypertension.[23] Further, when hypertension is present, it is often resistant to antihypertensive therapy. Fatal and nonfatal cardiovascular events are two- to threefold higher in male patients with severe OSA.[24] OSA is associated with or aggravates biomarkers for cardiovascular disease, including C-reactive protein and leptin.[25,26] Patients with sleep apnea often are obese and may be predisposed to weight gain. Hence, obesity may further contribute to cardiovascular disease in this patient population.

Several factors suggest an association between OSA and systemic disease. Breathing against a closed upper airway during sleep causes intermittent and repetitive episodes of hypoxemia and hypercapnia, dramatic changes in intrathoracic pressure, and activation of the sympathetic nervous system. These responses can produce acute hemodynamic and humoral responses. Blood pressure can increase to 220/120 mm Hg with each apneic episode.[27] Concentrations of circulating vasoconstrictors, such as endothelin-1 and

---

Patient Encounter, Part 1

CH, a 53-year-old man with a history of hypertension, comes to your clinic complaining of sleepiness in the daytime, "crawly legs" at bedtime, and frequent awakenings at night. After further questioning, he explains that for the last hour or so before bedtime he cannot keep his legs still. He reports that he falls asleep relatively easily during the day. The symptoms have been gradually worsening over the past year and occur nightly. His wife reports that he kicks his legs the first part of the night, snores, and occasionally gasps for air after a breathing pause. His body mass index (BMI) is 30 kg/m², and he has experienced recent weight gain and complains about morning headaches.

What sleep disorders do his symptoms suggest?

What sleep disorders could you diagnose subjectively? What is your initial recommendation?

What additional information do you need to know before creating a treatment plan for this patient?

norepinephrine, are increased during OSA.[28] These acute responses to OSA may predispose to and enhance the progression of vascular disease in the longer term. This is supported by studies showing impaired endothelium-dependent vasodilation, an early marker for vascular disease, in patients with untreated moderate to severe OSA.[29]

Parasomnias

The pathogenesis of parasomnias (e.g., sleepwalking, enuresis, sleep talking) is variable and not well described and involves state dissociation, whereby two states of being overlap simultaneously. For example, abnormal activation of the central pattern generator of the spinal cord that produces motor movements is hypothesized to underlie sleepwalking behavior. In RBD, active inhibition of motor activity in the perilocus coeruleus region is lost, resulting in loss of paralysis and dream enactment.

Clinical Presentation and Diagnosis of Sleep Disorders

Patients with sleep disorders may complain about daytime symptoms. A bed partner may witness hallmark characteristics of the sleep disorder. ❷ *Patients with sleep complaints should have a careful sleep history performed to assess their possible sleep disorder in order to guide diagnostic and therapeutic decisions.*

Daytime Symptoms and Associated Characteristics— EDS is the primary symptom described by patients with sleep disorders. It is usually described as not waking up refreshed in the morning, or falling asleep or fighting the urge to sleep during the day despite a night of sleep. Other daytime characteristics of sleep disorders include:

- Irritability, fatigue, or depression
- Confusion, or impaired performance at work or school
- Cataplexy (associated with narcolepsy)
- Hypertension (associated with OSA)

Nighttime Sleep Complaints—Depending on the sleep disorder, patients may exhibit or experience various nocturnal complaints during sleep hours. Some of these complaints can be uncovered by clinical history alone (e.g., hallucinations, RLS, snoring), while others can be diagnosed during sleep studies (e.g., OSA, nighttime awakenings, somnambulism, PLMS, etc.). Frequent complaints include:

- Inability to fall asleep, nighttime awakenings
- Sleep walking (somnambulism), sleep talking (somniloquy)
- Cessation of breathing (apnea), snoring
- Sleep paralysis and/or hallucinations when waking or falling asleep
- Restlessness (PLMS or RLS)

CLINICAL PRESENTATION AND DIAGNOSIS

❸ *Although clinical history guides diagnosis and therapy, only overnight polysomnography and/or multiple sleep latency tests (MSLTs) can definitively diagnose and guide therapy for OSA, narcolepsy, and periodic limb movements of sleep.*

Insomnia (Difficulty Initiating or Maintaining Sleep)

Insomnia is often characterized by difficulty falling asleep, frequent nocturnal awakenings, and early-morning awakenings, which may result in daytime impairments in concentration and school or work performance. In comorbid insomnia, social factors (e.g., family difficulties, bereavement), medications (e.g., antidepressants, β-agonists, corticosteroids, decongestants), and coexisting medical or psychiatric conditions (e.g., depression, bipolar disorder) may help to explain difficulties in initiating and maintaining sleep. Insomnia may be described as transient (a few days), short term (less than 3 weeks), or chronic (greater than 1 month) in duration.

Narcolepsy

The hallmark of narcolepsy is EDS and the need for unwanted episodes of sleep during the day. Patients with narcolepsy may experience repeated nighttime awakenings and terrifying dreams, along with difficulty falling asleep. Narcoleptics frequently experience abnormal manifestations of REM sleep, including hallucinations and sleep paralysis that occur on falling asleep and/or awakening. Cataplexy is a weakness or loss of skeletal muscle tone in the jaw, legs, or arms that is elicited by emotion (e.g., anger, surprise, laughter, or sadness).

Obstructive Sleep Apnea

Common characteristics of OSA include snoring, choking, gasping for air, nocturnal reflux symptoms, and morning headaches. A bed partner or roommate may observe these characteristics and witness episodes where the patient stops breathing during sleep. Obesity predisposes to and can worsen OSA. Patients with large neck sizes (greater than 45 cm [about 18 in.] neck circumference) and a body mass index (BMI) of 30 kg/m² or greater are at higher risk for OSA. Hypertension, depression, and hypothyroidism are found frequently in patients with OSA.

PLMS and RLS

Although RLS symptoms can vary, patients commonly report creepy-crawly, burning, tingling, or achy feelings in the legs or arms. These sensations create a desire to move the limbs and may produce motor restlessness. Symptoms are worse in the evening and are worse or exclusively present at rest, with temporary relief with movement. Symptoms also can occur during sleep and often lead to semirhythmic (periodic) limb movements during sleep (PLMS). PLMS are objective findings during overnight polysomnography recorded by leg electrodes. PLMS are present in most patients with RLS but can occur independently. PLMS frequently are described by a bed partner as restlessness, or repeated kicking of legs or thrashing of arms during sleep.

Parasomnias

Parasomnias are characterized by undesirable physical or behavioral phenomena that occur during sleep (e.g., sleepwalking, sleep talking, bruxism [grinding of teeth], enuresis, night terrors, and RBD). RBD patients act out their dreams during sleep, often in a violent manner.

Circadian Rhythm Disorders

The most common circadian rhythm disorders (CRDs) include jet lag, shift-work sleep disruption, delayed sleep-phase disorder, and advanced sleep-phase disorder. Jet lag occurs when a person travels across time zones, and the external environmental time is mismatched with the internal circadian clock. Delayed and advanced sleep-phase disorders occur when bed and wake times are delayed or advanced (by 3 or more hours) compared with socially prescribed bed and wake times.

Sleep Diagnostics

Complete overnight polysomnography is the "gold standard" for diagnosing and identifying sleep-disordered breathing, PLMS, parasomnias, and nocturnal sleep irregularities related to narcolepsy. Sleep is observed and monitored in a controlled setting using an EEG, electro-oculogram, electromyogram, ECG, air thermistors, abdominal and thoracic strain belts, and an oxygen saturation monitor. This setup assesses and records sleep onset, arousals, sleep stages, eye movements, leg and jaw movements, heart rhythm, arrhythmias, airflow during sleep, respiratory effort, and oxygen desaturations.

Evaluations of Daytime Sleepiness

The two most commonly performed objective evaluations to assess daytime sleepiness are the MSLT and the maintenance of wakefulness test (MWT). During the MSLT, the patient attempts to take a 20-minute nap every 2 hours during the day beginning 2 hours after morning awakening (following a normal night's sleep) to evaluate physiologic sleepiness. The patient is instructed not to resist the urge to fall asleep. Sleep latency of less than 5 or 6 minutes is considered pathologically sleepy. The occurrence of an REM onset period during two naps is indicative of a diagnosis of narcolepsy. The MWT is performed to assess a patient's ability to avoid succumbing to sleepiness (manifest sleepiness). Similar

---

Patient Encounter, Part 2: Medical History, Physical Exam, and Diagnostic Test

CH undergoes nocturnal polysomnography and returns to your clinic for follow-up.

PMH: Hypertension poorly controlled since 1999

FH: Father died at age 70 from stroke; mother is still alive with history of RLS and hypothyroidism.

SH: Married, works as an accountant, has never smoked, two drinks/night on the weekends

Meds: Hydrochlorothiazide 25 mg orally once daily; amlodipine 10 mg orally once daily

ROS: (+) daytime sleepiness (Epworth sleepiness score: 18/24)

PE:

VS: BP 154/84, P 78, RR 16, T 37°C (98.6°F)

Mouth: Airway crowded, large tonsils and uvula

Labs: Within normal limits

Overnight polysomnogram: Frequent obstructive apneas, hypopneas, and leg movements:

- RDI 12 events/h
- 310 leg movements, mostly occurring in first half of the night
- Successful alleviation of apneas and hypopneas with CPAP

Given this additional information, summarize the patient's diagnosis.

Identify your treatment goals and recommendations for the patient.

What nonpharmacologic and pharmacologic alternatives are available for this patient if prescribed therapy is not successful or not tolerated?

---

nap opportunities are set up for the MWT, with the exception that the patient is instructed to lie down in bed and attempt to stay awake. A subjective assessment of sleepiness can be completed using the Epworth Sleepiness Scale (ESS). The ESS is a validated questionnaire that is easy to use and reliably predicts subjective sleepiness. The maximum score is 24, and any patient with a score greater than 10 is considered sleepy.

TREATMENT

❹ *Treatment goals vary among different sleep disorders but generally include restoration of normal sleep patterns, elimination of daytime sequelae, improved quality of life, and prevention of complications and adverse effects from therapy.* All patients presenting with sleep complaints

---

Table 41-1
Nonpharmacologic Therapies for Insomnia

Sleep Hygiene
- Keep a regular sleep schedule
- Exercise frequently but not immediately before bedtime
- Avoid alcohol and stimulants (caffeine, nicotine) in the late afternoon and evening
- Maintain a comfortable sleeping environment that is dark, quiet, and free of intrusions
- Avoid consuming large quantities of food or liquids immediately before bedtime

Stimulus Control
- Go to bed only when sleepy
- Avoid daytime naps
- If you cannot sleep, get out of bed and go to another room—only return to your bed when you feel the need to sleep
- Bed is for sleep and intimacy only (no eating or watching TV in bed)
- Always wake up at the same time each day

Relaxation Training
- Reduce somatic arousal (muscle relaxation)
- Reduce mental arousal (attention focusing procedures, imagery training, meditation, etc.)
- Biofeedback (use of visual or auditory feedback to reduce tension)

Cognitive Therapy
- Alter beliefs, attitudes, and expectations about sleep

---

should have a thorough inventory of their sleep habits and sleep hygiene investigated during the interview and history taking. Nonpharmacologic interventions for insomnia are outlined in Table 41-1. Sleep hygiene should be reinforced in all patients, and behavioral, cognitive, and stimulus-control interventions are used mainly for patients with insomnia-type complaints. Both pharmacologic and nonpharmacologic therapies are effective at improving sleep and reducing insomnia complaints. An algorithm for the initial assessment and first treatment step of EDS is provided in Figure 41-1.

Insomnia

The ideal hypnotic drug would be effective at reducing sleep latency and increasing total sleep time and would be free of unwanted side effects. ❺ *Benzodiazepine receptor agonists, including traditional benzodiazepines, zolpidem, zaleplon, and eszopiclone, are approved by the FDA for the treatment of insomnia and are first-line therapies.*[30,31] Not all products are available in all countries. Pharmacologic treatment of insomnia is recommended for transient and short-term insomnia. Long-term use of hypnotics is not contraindicated unless the patient has another contraindication to their use. Eszopiclone is the only sedative hypnotic approved by the FDA for chronic use up to 6 months.[32] Although not first-line agents for insomnia, sedating antidepressants are prescribed commonly, and the number of prescriptions for antidepressants for this purpose has increased dramatically

over the last 20 years.[33] These and other therapies, detailed below, are used to treat insomnia.

▶ *Benzodiazepine Receptor Agonists*

There are currently eight benzodiazepine receptor agonists (BZDRAs) approved for insomnia, and the pharmacokinetic differences between these agents help to guide selection depending on patient considerations and specific sleep complaints (Table 41-2). These agents occupy the benzodiazepine receptors on the gamma-aminobutyric acid (GABA) type A receptor complex, resulting in opening of chloride channels that facilitate GABA inhibition and promote sleepiness.[34] BZDRAs have become the first-line agents for treating insomnia and sleep-maintenance problems because they are all efficacious, have wide therapeutic indices, and in clinical use have a low incidence of abuse.[30,34]

Patients should be instructed to take BZDRAs at bedtime and to avoid engaging in activities requiring alertness after ingestion. The BZDRAs come closer to the "ideal hypnotic" compared with other agents because they increase total sleep time (except for zaleplon) and reduce sleep latency with fewer adverse effects. Although BZDRAs generally are well-tolerated and have good safety profiles, mild to moderate side effects can occur, and precautions are warranted, especially in high-risk populations.

Precautions and Safety The most common side effects associated with BZDRAs include residual sedation (a prolongation of the sedative effects into the waking hours after sleep), grogginess, and psychomotor impairment.[35] Careful selection of a hypnotic agent with a duration of action matching the patient's budgeted sleep time can help minimize the risk of residual sedation. BZDRAs should be initiated at low doses, and agents with active metabolites (Table 41-2) should be avoided in elderly patients. BZDRAs may cause anterograde amnesia, defined as memory loss of activities and interactions after ingestion of the drug. All hypnotics can cause anterograde amnesia, and higher doses increase the extent of amnesia.[36,37]

On discontinuation of hypnotic BZDRAs, patients can experience rebound effects, specifically rebound insomnia that may last for one to two nights. Rebound insomnia occurs more frequently after discontinuation of shorter-duration BZDRAs (e.g., triazolam) compared with long-duration BZDRAs. Intermittent hypnotic therapy with the lowest dose possible reduces the likelihood of tolerance, dependence, and withdrawal when therapy is stopped. Patients should be counseled that rebound insomnia is not necessarily a return of their original symptoms, and it may take a few nights for rebound symptoms to subside.

▶ *Sedating Antidepressants*

The increasing popularity of sedating antidepressants for the treatment of insomnia resulted in trazodone being the most prescribed drug in 2002.[38] Other common antidepressants also prescribed for insomnia include amitriptyline, mirtazapine, nefazadone, and doxepin. Antidepressants may be an

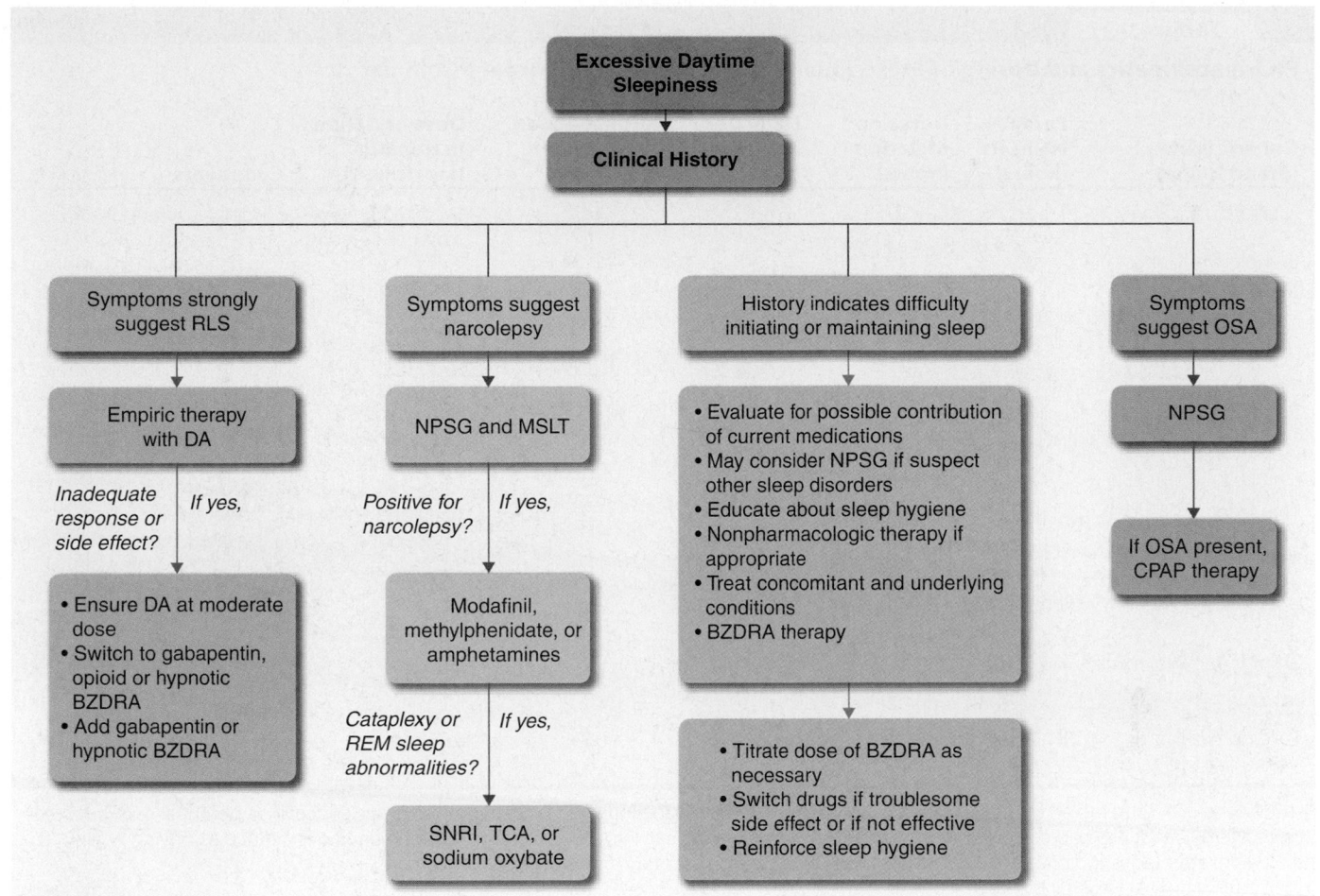

FIGURE 41–1. Primary assessment and initial treatment for complaint of excessive daytime sleepiness. (BZDRA, benzodiazepine receptor agonist; CPAP, continuous positive airway pressure; DA, dopamine agonist; MSLT, multiple sleep latency test; OSA, obstructive sleep apnea; RLS, restless legs syndrome; SNRI, serotonin and norepinephrine reuptake inhibitor; NPSG, nocturnal polysomnography; TCA, tricyclic antidepressant.)

appealing option for insomnia in patients with concomitant depression. However, at the doses frequently used for sleep, only mirtazapine exhibits significant antidepressant activity. Further, quality clinical studies demonstrating efficacy for treating insomnia are lacking. Side effects from antidepressants can be frequent and often are unpleasant, including carryover sedation, grogginess, anticholinergic effects, and weight gain. Tricyclic antidepressants (TCAs) should be used with caution in the elderly and patients with cardiovascular and hepatic impairment. Mirtazapine can cause daytime sedation, dizziness, and weight gain, a side effect that may worsen concomitant OSA.[39] Trazodone can cause hypotension and dizziness, and should be used with caution in patients with heart disease or hypertension and those taking cardiovascular agents.[40,41]

▶ Over-the-Counter and Miscellaneous Agents

Over-the-counter antihistamines such as diphenhydramine are frequently used (usual doses 25 to 50 mg) for difficulty sleeping. Diphenhydramine is approved by the FDA for the treatment of insomnia and can be effective at reducing sleep latency and increasing sleep time.[42] However, diphenhydramine produces undesirable anticholinergic effects and carryover sedation that limit its use. As with TCAs and BZDRAs, diphenhydramine should be used with caution in the elderly. Valerian root is a herbal sleep remedy that has inconsistent effects on sleep but may reduce sleep latency and efficiency at commonly used doses of 400 to 900 mg valerian extract. Ramelteon, a new melatonin receptor agonist, is indicated for insomnia characterized by difficulty with sleep onset. The recommended dose is 8 mg at bedtime. Ramelteon is not a controlled substance, and thus is a viable option for patients with a history of substance abuse.[43]

Narcolepsy

Therapy for narcolepsy involves two key principles: (a) treatment of EDS with scheduled naps and CNS stimulants, and (b) suppression of cataplexy and REM-sleep abnormalities with aminergic signaling drugs. Modafinil, methylphenidate, and amphetamines are effective FDA-approved drugs for the treatment of EDS with narcolepsy.[44]

Table 41–2

Pharmacokinetics and Dosing of Prescription Medications[a] Used to Treat Insomnia

Generic Name (Brand Name)	Parent Half-Life (hours)	Duration of Action (hours)	Daily Dose Range (mg)	Recommended Daily Dose in Elderly (mg)[b]	Dose or Action in Hepatic Impairment	Comments
Estazolam (Prosom)	2	12–15	1–2	0.5	Dose reduction may be needed	Moderate duration
Eszopiclone (Lunesta)	6	8	2–3	1–2	1 mg in severe impairment	Can be used up to 6 months for chronic insomnia
Flurazepam (Dalmane)	8	10–30	15–30	15	No change necessary	High risk of hangover and residual effects
Quazepam (Doral)	2	25–41	7.5–15	7.5–15	Dose reduction may be needed	High risk of hangover and residual effects
Ramelteon (Rozerem)	1–2.6	Unpublished[c]	8	No specific recommendations	Do not use in severe hepatic impairment	Noncontrolled substance, may be useful in patients with history of substance abuse
Temazepam (Restoril)	10–15	7	7.5–30	7.5	No change necessary	Moderate duration, well-tolerated, inexpensive
Triazolam (Halcion)	2	6–7	0.125–0.25	0.125	0.125 mg	Short-acting, little residual hangover
Zaleplon (Sonata)	1	6	5–10	5	5 mg	Short-acting, only for difficulty falling asleep
Zolpidem (Ambien)	2–2.6	6–8	5–10	5	5 mg	Short–moderate duration, no effects on sleep architecture
Zolpidem CR (Ambien CR)	2.8	7–8	6.25–12.5	6.25	6.25 mg	

[a]In 2007, the FDA required additional information added to the safety labeling of sedative-hypnotic drugs concerning potential risks, including severe allergic reactions and complex sleep-related behaviors, which may include sleep-driving. Sleep driving is defined as driving while not fully awake after ingestion of a sedative-hypnotic product, with no memory of the event.

[b]If a dosing range is displayed, the first dose listed should be the starting dose.

[c]Data not available.

From DiPiro JT, Talbert RL, Yee GC, et al. (eds.) Pharmacotherapy: A Pathophysiologic Approach. 7th ed. New York: McGraw Hill; 2008:1194.

Modafinil is potentially advantageous in part because it is a schedule IV medication in contrast to CNS stimulants, which are schedule II. Modafinil is renewable for 6 months at a time and may have fewer peripheral and cardiovascular effects than traditional stimulants. Selegiline, a selective monoamine oxidase B enzyme inhibitor, is metabolized to amphetamines and can be successful at reducing daytime sleepiness. In an individual patient, one wake-promoting agent may work better than another, and if the first drug selected is not successful at adequate doses, a trial with another agent should be attempted. ❻ *Treatment of EDS in narcolepsy and other sleep disorders may require the use of sustained- and immediate-release stimulants to effectively promote wakefulness throughout the day and at key times that require alertness.* One potential treatment regimen includes a sustained-release preparation first thing in the morning and again at noon, followed by an immediate-release preparation as needed in the late afternoon or prior to driving to maintain wakefulness. One advantage of traditional CNS stimulants over modafinil is their ability to suppress REM sleep, which also may help to control cataplexy and REM-sleep abnormalities.

Traditional CNS stimulants have the potential to increase blood pressure and heart rate when used long term. In addition, excessive CNS stimulation can cause tremors and tics and can carry over into evening hours, where initiation of normal nighttime sleep can be disrupted. Caution should be used in patients with underlying cardiovascular or cerebrovascular disease and in patients with a history of seizures because stimulants may lower the seizure threshold.

▶ **Cataplexy**

Traditionally, aminergic signaling antidepressants have been used effectively to control symptoms of cataplexy, sleep paralysis, and other REM-sleep manifestations of narcolepsy. These include TCAs and certain selective serotonin and serotonin/norepinephrine reuptake inhibitors (SSRIs and SNRIs). Clomipramine, protriptyline, imipramine, venlafaxine, and fluoxetine are the agents that have been used most frequently. In addition, low-dose selegiline also has been effective at reducing cataplexy. Although these drugs are not approved by the FDA for treatment of cataplexy, they effectively suppress REM sleep and have been the mainstay of anticataplectic therapy for years. Sodium oxybate, a potent sedative with a very short duration of action, is FDA approved for the treatment of narcolepsy with cataplexy. The mechanism whereby it reduces cataplexy is unknown. Two doses per night are taken, one at bedtime and one follow-up dose taken 2½ to 4 hours later. Patients frequently need to set an alarm to wake up to take their second dose. Sodium oxybate is tightly regulated and is only available from one central pharmacy owing to the high abuse potential of its active ingredient (γ-hydroxybutyrate).

Restless Legs Syndrome

❼ *RLS treatment involves suppression of abnormal sensations and leg movements and consolidation of sleep. Dopaminergic and sedative-hypnotic medications are prescribed commonly.* In the last few years, dopamine agonists (DAs) have become the therapy of choice for the treatment of RLS, replacing levodopa/carbidopa as first-line agents. The DAs offer many advantages over levodopa/carbidopa, including longer half-lives to cover overnight symptoms, flexible dosing, and a reduced incidence of symptom augmentation. Up to 80% of patients who take levodopa/carbidopa eventually will experience symptom augmentation: RLS symptoms appear earlier in the day, previously unaffected body parts become involved, and higher doses of medication are required to control symptoms.[45] Ropinirole (Requip) and pramipexole (Mirapex) are FDA approved for the treatment of RLS, and ropinirole is available in a sustained-release product.[46,47]

Gabapentin is an effective treatment for RLS, particularly in patients with painful symptoms.[48] BZDRAs such as temazepam, clonazepam, zolpidem, and zaleplon effectively reduce arousals associated with PLMS in patients with RLS.[49] Their main benefit is derived from improving sleep continuity in patients with RLS, particularly as adjunct treatment with other pharmacologic therapies. Opioids are effective for some patients' RLS symptoms, with oxycodone, propoxyphene, hydrocodone, and codeine being used most frequently. For both BZDRAs and opioids, caution should be used in the elderly, in patients who snore and are at risk for sleep apnea, and in patients with a history of substance abuse. Low iron levels frequently exacerbate RLS symptoms. Iron supplementation should be prescribed in patients who are iron-deficient. Iron supplementation in patients with serum ferritin concentrations of less than 50 mcg/L improves RLS symptoms. Medications frequently used for RLS are shown in Table 41–3.

Obstructive Sleep Apnea

❽ *The main therapy for OSA is nasal continuous positive airway pressure (CPAP) therapy.* CPAP alleviates sleep-disordered breathing by producing a positive pressure column in the upper airway using room air. The CPAP machine is small enough to be transportable and sits at the bedside. A flexible tube connects the CPAP machine to a mask that covers the nose. During overnight polysomnography, the

---

Table 41–3			
Frequently Used Medications for RLS			
Generic Name (Brand Name)	**Half-Life (hours)**	**Dose Range (mg/day)[a]**	**Potential Side Effect or Disadvantage**
Dopaminergic Agents[b]			
Levodopa/carbidopa (Sinemet)	1.5–2	100–200 of levodopa	Nausea/vomiting, high incidence of symptom augmentation
Pramipexole (Mirapex)	8–12[c]	0.125–1.5	Nausea/vomiting, risk of compulsive behaviors[d]
Ropinirole (Requip)	6[e]	0.25–3	Nausea/vomiting, risk of compulsive behaviors[d]
Anticonvulsants			
Gabapentin (Neurontin)	5–7[c]	300–3,600	Dizziness, ataxia
Hypnotic Agents			
Clonazepam (Klonopin)	30–40	0.5–2	Tolerance, carryover sedation
Temazepam (Restoril)	10–15	7.5–30	Tolerance, carryover sedation
Zolpidem (Ambien)	2–2.6[e]	5–10	Tolerance
Zaleplon (Sonata)	1[e]	5–10	Tolerance, may not last entire night
Opioids			
Hydrocodone	3.8–4.5[e]	5–10	Constipation, nausea, sedation
Codeine	2.5–3.5[e]	30–60	Constipation, nausea, sedation
Propoxyphene	6–12[e]	100–600	Constipation, nausea, sedation
Oxycodone	3.2–12[c,e]	5–30	Constipation, nausea, sedation

[a]Usual range, all medications (other than dopaminergic agents) are dosed at bedtime.

[b]Dopaminergic agents are frequently given at bedtime or 2 hours prior to bedtime or the anticipated onset of RLS symptoms.

[c]May be longer in patients with renal dysfunction.

[d]Compulsive behaviors such as gambling, shopping, sexual behaviors and eating have been reported in patients taking DAs.

[e]May be longer in patients with hepatic dysfunction.

From Ref. 49.

pressure setting is increased until sleep-disordered breathing is eliminated. CPAP therapy has been shown to have a favorable impact on blood pressure and to attenuate some of the potential hemodynamic and neurohumoral responses that may link OSA to systemic disease.

Not all individuals tolerate CPAP therapy in part because it requires wearing a mask during sleep, and therapy can dry and irritate the upper airway. In some individuals, these barriers for adherence may be lessened or eliminated by properly fitting the mask, adding humidity or heat to therapy, or using bilevel positive airway pressure (BiPAP) therapy. BiPAP therapy applies a variable pressure into the airway during the inspiratory phase of respiration but, unlike CPAP, reduces the applied pressure during the expiratory phase of respiration.

There are other therapies for OSA. Obesity can worsen sleep apnea, and weight management should be implemented for all overweight patients with OSA. In obese patients with mild OSA, weight loss alone can be effective, and studies have reported improvement in severity of OSA with gastric stapling. For those patients who cannot tolerate CPAP, oral appliances can be used to advance the lower jawbone and to keep the tongue forward to enlarge the upper airway. For individuals who suffer OSA only during certain positions (e.g., when on their back) during sleep, positional therapies may be effective. Surgical therapy (uvulopalatopharyngoplasty) opens the upper airway by removing the tonsils, trimming and reorienting the posterior and anterior tonsillar pillars, and removing the uvula and posterior portion of the palate. This is not a first-line option because of its invasiveness. In very severe cases, tracheostomy may be necessary. This procedure may be indicated in selected individuals who are morbidly obese, have severe facial skeletal deformity, experience severe drops in oxygen saturation (e.g., SaO_2 less than 70%), or have significant cardiac arrhythmias associated with their OSA.

There is no drug therapy for OSA. Drug therapy for symptoms of OSA may be considered in selected patients. For example, modafinil (Provigil) is a wake-promoting medication that is approved by the FDA to improve wakefulness in patients who have residual daytime sleepiness while treated with CPAP. Initiation of wake-promoting medications should be attempted only after patients are using optimal CPAP therapy to alleviate sleep-disordered breathing. Other therapies used in the past (e.g., medroxyprogesterone) are not effective and may worsen OSA. Untreated or inadequately treated sleep apnea may hinder achieving blood pressure control in hypertensive patients. OSA should be considered and evaluated in hypertensive patients who are resistant to therapy or have signs and symptoms of OSA.

Parasomnias

Non-REM parasomnias usually do not require treatment. If needed, low-dose benzodiazepines such as clonazepam can be prescribed for bothersome episodes. Clonazepam reduces the amount of sleep time spent in stages 3 and 4 of non-REM sleep, where most non-REM parasomnias occur. For treating RBD, clonazepam 0.5 to 2 mg at bedtime is the drug of choice, although melatonin 3 to 12 mg at bedtime also may be effective. Patients with RBD also should have dangerous objects removed from the bedroom and cushions placed on the floor to reduce the chance of injury from breakthrough episodes.

Circadian Rhythm Disorders

Melatonin at doses of 0.5 to 5 mg taken at appropriate target bedtimes for east or west travel is becoming the drug of choice for jet lag. Melatonin significantly reduces jet lag and shortens sleep latency in travelers.[50] Hypnotic agents with relatively short durations of action (3 to 5 hours) also may be used to sustain sleep during the initial adaptation to the new time zone.

Drug–Disease and Drug–Drug Interactions

❾ *It is important to review patient medication profiles for drugs that may aggravate sleep disorders. Patients should be monitored for adverse drug reactions and potential drug–drug interactions. They should be assessed for adherence to their therapeutic regimens. Pharmacotherapy for sleep disorders should be individualized.* Medications can be used commonly to treat several concomitant sleep disorders. Conversely, drug therapy may be effective for one sleep disorder and exacerbate another. For example, antidepressants may alleviate depressive symptoms but exacerbate symptoms of RLS. Medications that block dopaminergic transmission may worsen RLS symptoms. Smoking can worsen OSA, presumably by increasing upper airway edema. Alcohol and CNS depressants, including opiate analgesics, sedatives, and muscle relaxants, can worsen OSA, even in small

---

Patient Encounter, Part 3: Modifying Treatment Plan

CH returns to the clinic 3 months later. The physician previously diagnosed him with OSA and RLS. He received a prescription for CPAPs for OSA and ropinirole 0.5 mg at bedtime for RLS at his last visit. Via phone calls, his ropinirole dose has been increased to 3 mg at bedtime. He has received moderate relief of his RLS symptoms, but on occasion, he still awakens and cannot fall back asleep. His sleepiness and RLS symptoms are improved: ESS 13/24.

Based on the information presented, recommend additional therapy for the patient.

What medications would you consider adding to reduce RLS symptoms and awakenings?

How would you assess the patient's CPAP therapy and adherence?

What precautions would you want to counsel the patient on about his therapy?

Patient Care and Monitoring

Insomnia

1. Ideally limit hypnotic therapy to short-term use, and reevaluate after 2 to 3 weeks of therapy.

2. Evaluate improvement in the specific sleep complaint (e.g., how has therapy affected sleep latency or sleep maintenance?).

3. Inquire about carryover sedation and other side effects associated with the selected agent. Use a lower dose or select a drug with a shorter duration of action if the patient experiences carryover sedation.

4. Address other psychiatric and medical conditions that frequently coexist with insomnia and medications which can worsen symptoms.

Narcolepsy

1. Administer the ESS at each visit to monitor progress with modafinil or stimulant therapy. Unfortunately, EDS in narcolepsy patients rarely is fully reversed.

2. Evaluate how sleepiness changes throughout the day to best determine how to use sustained- and immediate-release stimulants to maintain wakefulness. If the patient complains of sleep disruption from stimulant therapy, move the dosing time a few hours earlier until sleep disruption is avoided.

3. Review patient's sleep diaries to track the number of cataplexy, sleep paralysis, and hallucinatory events and when they occur.

RLS

1. Carefully assess both the patient's and bed partner's reports of the patient's nighttime limb movements.

2. Measure sleepiness (via ESS) and RLS symptoms at each visit to track progress with therapy.

3. Evaluate potential side effects of therapy, including nausea, drowsiness, sleep attacks, compulsive behaviors, and headaches for the DA agents.

4. Review the sleep diaries and timing of RLS symptoms to screen for possible symptom augmentation.

5. If symptoms are not resolved, increase the dose of DA agent or add another agent such as gabapentin or a short–moderate duration sedative hypnotic.

OSA

1. Evaluate CPAP therapy annually or at any time individuals experience symptoms (e.g., daytime sleepiness) despite CPAP therapy. For example, change in pressure settings to alleviate OSA may be needed if weight gain occurs.

2. Monitor compliance with CPAP therapy. CPAP machines have a built-in compliance meter to measure the hours used at effective pressure. Patients should use CPAP therapy for at least 5 hours each night. In addition to alleviating sleep-disordered breathing, CPAP therapy may improve cardiovascular outcomes.

Parasomnias

1. Ask patients and family members about any bothersome or dangerous sleepwalking episodes since the last visit and if therapy has reduced the frequency of these events.

2. For RBD, review the sleep diaries and interview bed partners to determine the number and nature of episodes.

3. Inquire about carryover sedation and anterograde amnesia from therapy.

---

doses, by reducing respiratory drive and relaxing the upper airway muscles responsible for maintaining patency. CNS depressants should be avoided, and if they are necessary, they should not be administered before sleep. Drug therapy for sleep disorders should be patient specific, and careful consideration should be given to coexisting diseases, concomitant medications, and potential drug–drug and drug–disease interactions to optimize patient care and treatment.

OUTCOME EVALUATION

To determine the success of treatment, evaluate whether the treatment plan restored normal sleep patterns, reduced daytime sequelae, and improved quality of life without causing adverse effects. Schedule patients for follow-up within 3 weeks for insomnia and within 3 months for other sleep disorders. Perform a detailed clinical history to determine the patient's perception of treatment progress and symptoms along with medication effectiveness and side effects.

Instruct patients to keep sleep diaries of nightly sleep (number of hours, number of awakenings, and worsening or improved sleep) and daytime symptoms, along with documentation of episodes such as cataplexy or RBD. Increase medication to effective doses, and if necessary, start additional therapy to control symptoms. Patients with sleep disorders should experience relief of symptoms the first night of drug therapy but may not receive maximal benefit (effect on daytime symptoms) for a few weeks. Perform a detailed history of prescription, nonprescription, and complementary or alternative medications, and review the patient's sleep diary, daytime symptoms, and nonpharmacologic therapies on a regular basis.

Abbreviations Introduced in This Chapter

BiPAP	Bilevel positive airway pressure
BMI	Body mass index
BZDRA	Benzodiazepine receptor agonist
CNS	Central nervous system
CPAP	Continuous positive airway pressure

CRD	Circadian rhythm disorder
CSF	Cerebrospinal fluid
DA	Dopamine agonist
EDS	Excessive daytime sleepiness
EEG	Electroencephalogram
ESRD	End-stage renal disease
ESS	Epworth Sleepiness Scale
GABA	Gamma-aminobutyric acid
HLA	Histocompatibility leukocyte antigen
MSLT	Multiple sleep latency test
MWT	Maintenance of wakefulness test
NPSG	Nocturnal polysomnography
OSA	Obstructive sleep apnea
PLMS	Periodic limb movements of sleep
RBD	REM behavior disorder
RDI	Respiratory disturbance index
REM	Rapid eye movement
RLS	Restless legs syndrome
SNRI	Serotonin and norepinephrine reuptake inhibitor
SSRI	Selective serotonin reuptake inhibitor
TCA	Tricyclic antidepressant

 Self-assessment questions and answers are available at *http://www.mhpharmacotherapy.com/pp.html*.

REFERENCES

1. Malow B. Approach to the patient with disordered sleep. In: Kryger M, Roth T, Dement W, eds. Principles and Practice of Sleep Medicine, 4th ed. Philadelphia: Elsevier Saunders, 2005:589–593.
2. NIH State-of-the-Science Conference Statement on Manifestations and Management of Chronic Insomnia in Adults. 2005, *http://consensus.nih.gov/2005/2005InsomniaSOS026html.htm*.
3. Carskadon MA, Dement WC. Normal human sleep: An overview. In: Kryger M, Roth T, Dement W, eds. Principles and Practice of Sleep Medicine, 4th ed. Philadelphia: Elsevier Saunders, 2005:13–23.
4. Dodge R, Cline MG, Quan SF. The natural history of insomnia and its relationship to respiratory symptoms. Arch Intern Med 1995;155:1797–1800.
5. Kim K, Uchiyama M, Okawa M, et al. An epidemiological study of insomnia among the Japanese general population. Sleep 2000;23:41–47.
6. Shocat T, Umphress J, Isreal AG, et al. Insomnia in primary care patients. Sleep 1999;22:S359–S365.
7. Silber MH, Krahn LE, Olson EJ, et al. The epidemiology of narcolepsy in Olmsted County, Minnesota: A population-based study. Sleep 2002;25:197–202.
8. Tashiro T, Kambayashi T, Hishikawa Y. An epidemiological study of narcolepsy in Japanese. Proceedings of the 4th International Symposium on Narcolepsy. Tokyo, Japan. June 16–17, 1994:13.
9. Lavie P, Peled R, Narcolepsy is a rare disease in Israel. Sleep 1987;10:608–609.
10. Mignot E, Hayduk R, Black J, et al. HLA DQB1*0602 is associated with cataplexy in 509 narcoleptic patients. Sleep 1997;20:1012–1020.
11. Berger K, Kurth T. RLS epidemiology—Frequencies, risk factors and methods in population studies. Mov Disord 2007;22:S420–S423.
12. Phillips B, Young T, Finn L, et al. Epidemiology of restless legs symptoms in adults. Arch Intern Med 2000;160:2137–2141.
13. Lee KA, Zaffke ME, Baratte-Beebe K. Restless legs syndrome and sleep disturbance during pregnancy: The role of folate and iron. J Womens Health Gend Based Med 2001;10:335–341.
14. Bonati MT, Ferini-Strambi L, Aridon P, et al. Autosomal dominant restless legs syndrome maps on chromosome 14q. Brain 2003;126:1485–1492.
15. Young T, Palta M, Dempsey J, et al. The occurrence of sleep-disordered breathing among middle-aged adults. N Engl J Med 1993;328:1230–1235.
16. Ohayon MM, Caulet M, Priest RG. Violent behavior during sleep. J Clin Psychiatry 1997;58:369–376.
17. Mignot E, Lin X, Arrigoni J, et al. DQB1*0602 and DQA1*0102(DQ1) are better markers than DR2 for narcolepsy in Caucasian and black Americans. Sleep 1994;17:S60–S67.
18. Mignot E, Kimura A, Lattermann A, et al. Extensive HLA class II studies in 58 non-DRB1*15(DR2) narcoleptic patients with cataplexy. Tissue Antigens 1997;49:329–341.
19. Nishino S, Ripley B, Overeem S, et al. Hypocretin (orexin) deficiency in human narcolepsy. Lancet 2000;355:39–40.
20. Connor JR, Boyer PJ, Menzies SL, et al. Neuropathological examination suggests impaired brain iron acquisition in restless legs syndrome. Neurology 2003;61:304–309.
21. Somers VK, White DP, Amin R, et al. Sleep apnea and cardiovascular disease: An American Heart Association/American College of Cardiology Foundation Scientific Statement from the American Heart Association Council for High Blood Pressure Research Professional Education Committee, Council on Clinical Cardiology, Stroke Council, and Council on Cardiovascular Nursing. In collaboration with the National Heart, Lung, and Blood Institute, National Center on Sleep Disorders Research (National Institutes of Health). Circulation 2008;118:1080–1111.
22. Sahlin C, Sandberg O, Gustafson Y, et al. Obstructive sleep apnea is a risk factor for death in patients with stroke. Arch Intern Med 2008;168:297–301.
23. Peppard PE, Young T, Palta M, et al. Prospective study of the association between sleep-disordered breathing and hypertension. N Engl J Med 2000;342:1378–1384.
24. Marin JM, Carrizo SJ, Vicente E, et al. Long-term cardiovascular outcomes in men with obstructive sleep apnoea-hypopnoea with or without treatment with continuous positive airway pressure: An observational study. Lancet 2005;365:1046–1053.
25. Shamsuzzaman AS, Winnicki M, Lanfranchi P, et al. Elevated C-reactive protein in patients with obstructive sleep apnea. Circulation 2002;105:2462–2464.
26. Phillips BG, Kato M, Narkiewicz K, et al. Increases in leptin levels, sympathetic drive and weight gain in obstructive sleep apnea. Am J Physiol 2000;279:234–237.
27. Somers VK, Dyken ME, Clary MP, et al. Sympathetic neural mechanisms in obstructive sleep apnea. J Clin Invest 1995;96:1897–1904.
28. Phillips BG, Krzysztof N, Pesek CA, et al. Effects of obstructive sleep apnea on endothelin-1 and blood pressure. J Hypertens 1999;17:61–66.
29. Kato M, Roberts-Thomson P, Phillips BG, et al. Impairment of endothelium dependent vasodilation of resistance vessels in patients with obstructive sleep apnea. Circulation 2000;102:2607–2610.
30. Nowell PD, Mazumdar S, Buysse DJ, et al. Benzodiazepines and zolpidem for chronic insomnia: A meta-analysis of treatment efficacy. JAMA 1997;278:2170–2177.
31. Roehrs T, Roth T. Hypnotics: An update. Curr Neurol Neurosci Rep 2003;3:181–184.
32. Krystal AD, Walsh JK, Laska E, et al. Sustained efficacy of eszopiclone over 6 months of nightly treatment: Results of a randomized, double-blind, placebo-controlled study in adults with chronic insomnia. Sleep 2003;26:793–799.
33. Walsh JK, Schweitzer PK. Ten-year trends in the pharmacological treatment of insomnia. Sleep 1999;22:371–375.
34. Greenblatt DJ, Shader RI. Benzodiazepines in Clinical Practice. New York: Raven Press, 1974.
35. Roth T, Roehrs T. Issues in the use of benzodiazepine therapy. J Clin Psychiatry 1992;53:S14–S18.

36. Roth T, Roehrs TA, Stepanski EJ, et al. Hypnotics and behavior. Am J Med 1990;8:43S–46S.
37. Greenblatt D, Harmatz JS, Shapiro L, et al. Sensitivity to triazolam in eldery. N Engl J Med 1991;324:1691–1698.
38. Compton-McBride S, Schweitzer PK, Walsh JK. Most commonly used drugs to treat insomnia in 2002. Sleep 2004;27:A255.
39. Flores BH, Schatzberg AF. Mirtazepine. In: Schatzberg AF, Nemeroff CB, eds. The American Psychiatric Publishing Textbook of Psychopharmacology. ASCN. Washington, DC: American Psychiatric Publishing, 2004:341–347.
40. Golden RN, Dawkins K, Nicholas L. The American Psychiatric Textbook of Psychopharmacology. Trazadone and nefazodone, ed. Schatzberg A, Nemeroff C. 2004, Washington, DC: American Psychiatric Publishing. 315–325.
41. Bucknall C, Brooks D, Curry PV, et al. Mianserin and trazodone for cardiac patients with depression. Eur J Clin Pharmacol 1988;33:565–569.
42. Kudo Y, Kurihara M. Clinical evaluation of diphenhydramine hydrochloride for the treatment of insomnia in psychiatric patients. J Clin Pharmacol 1990;30:1041–1048.
43. Johnson MW, Suess PE, Griffiths RR. A novel hypnotic lacking abuse liability and sedative adverse effects. Arch Gen Psychiatry 2006;63:1149–1157.
44. Littner M, Johnson SF, McCall WV, et al. Practice parameters for the treatment of narcolepsy: An update for 2000. Sleep 2001;24:451–455.
45. Earley CJ, Allen RP. Pergolide and carbidopa/levodopa treatment of the restless legs syndrome and periodic leg movements in sleep in a consecutive series of patients. Sleep 1996;19:801–810.
46. Product Information: Requip, ropinirole. GlaxoSmithKline Pharmaceuticals, Research Triangle Park, NC, 2006.
47. Hening WA, Allen RP, Earley CJ, et al. Restless Legs Syndrome Task Force of the Standards of Practice Committee of the American Academy of Sleep Medicine. An update on the dopaminergic treatment of restless legs syndrome and periodic limb movement disorder. Sleep 2004;27:560–583.
48. Garcia-Borreguero D, Larrosa O, de la Llave Y, et al. Treatment of restless legs syndrome with gabapentin: A double-blind, cross-over study. Neurology 2002;59:1573–1579.
49. Earley CJ. Restless legs syndrome. N Engl J Med 2003;348:2103–2109.
50. Herxheimer A, Petrie KJ. Melatonin for the prevention and treatment of jet lag. [Systematic review] Cochrane Depression, Anxiety and Neurosis Group. Cochrane Database Syst Rev 2005;4.

42 Attention-Deficit Hyperactivity Disorder

John Erramouspe and Kevin W. Cleveland

LEARNING OBJECTIVES

● **Upon completion of the chapter, the reader will be able to:**

1. Explain accepted criteria necessary for the diagnosis of attention-deficit hyperactivity disorder (ADHD).

2. Recommend a therapeutic plan, including initial doses, dosage forms, and monitoring parameters, for a patient with ADHD.

3. Differentiate between the available pharmacotherapy used for ADHD with respect to pharmacology and pharmaceutical formulation.

4. Recommend second-line and/or adjunctive agents that can be effective alternatives in the treatment of ADHD when stimulant therapy is less than adequate.

5. Address potential cost-benefit issues associated with pharmacotherapy of ADHD.

6. Recommend strategies for minimizing adverse effects of ADHD medications.

KEY CONCEPTS

❶ To meet present attention-deficit hyperactive disorder (ADHD) diagnostic criteria, patients need to display hyperactivity, impulsivity, and/or inattentiveness before 7 years of age.

❷ The exact cause of ADHD is unknown, but dysfunction in neurotransmitters norepinephrine and dopamine has been implicated as a key component.

❸ ADHD is rarely encountered without comorbid conditions.

❹ Treatment goals for ADHD are to improve behavior, increase attention/**response inhibition**, and minimize side effects associated with pharmacotherapy.

❺ Pharmacotherapy is superior to behavioral therapy in the treatment of ADHD, but both should be emphasized in order to maximize outcomes.

❻ **Stimulants** are first-line agents for the treatment of ADHD. If the initial trial of a stimulant fails, then a trial of an alternative stimulant should be tried. On failure of the second stimulant, it is rational to attempt a third trial with a different stimulant formulation or select a nonstimulant agent such as bupropion, atomoxetine, or imipramine.

Attention-deficit hyperactivity disorder (ADHD) is the most common mental disorder that occurs in the pediatric population.[1-3] This disorder must begin in childhood before 7 years of age and may continue into adulthood. ADHD is characterized by a core triad of symptoms: hyperactivity, impulsivity, and inattention. It can have a severe impact on a patient's ability to function in both academic and social environments. The exact cause of ADHD is unknown, but twin studies strongly suggest a genetic etiology.[3-5] Early diagnosis and appropriate treatment are essential to compensate for areas of deficit.

EPIDEMIOLOGY AND ETIOLOGY

❶ *This disorder usually begins by 3 years of age but must occur prior to 7 years of age to meet diagnostic criteria.* In the United States, ADHD is the most common neurobehavioral disorder that affects children.[1-3,6] ADHD has been estimated to occur in 4.3% to 12% of school-aged children.[6,7] ADHD tends to occur at a greater incidence in males than in females by approximately 3:1 in school-aged children.[7]

Although ADHD generally is considered a childhood disorder, symptoms can persist into adolescence and adulthood. The prevalence of adult ADHD is estimated to be 4%, with 60% of these adults having manifested symptoms of ADHD from childhood.[8,9] Further, problems associated with ADHD (e.g., social, marital, academic, career, anxiety, depression, smoking, and substance-abuse problems) increase with the transition of patients into adulthood.

PATHOPHYSIOLOGY

❷ *The exact pathologic cause of ADHD has not been identified.* ADHD is generally thought of as a disorder of self-regulation or response inhibition. Patients who meet the criteria for ADHD have difficulty maintaining self-control, resisting distractions, and concentrating on ideas.[4,6] Further, children with ADHD often alternate between inattentiveness to monotonous tasks and overexcitement. Multiple brain studies have failed to elucidate any pathophysiologic basis for ADHD.

❷ *Dysfunction of the neurotransmitters norepinephrine and dopamine is thought to be key in the pathology of ADHD.* Norepinephrine is responsible for maintaining alertness and attention, whereas dopamine is responsible for regulating learning, motivation, goal setting, and memory. Both these neurotransmitters predominate in the frontal subcortical system, an area of the brain responsible for maintaining attention and memory. Genetics appears to play a role with a 50% chance of developing ADHD in a child who has a parent who is also affected. An association has been made between the development of ADHD and fetal alcohol syndrome, lead poisoning, maternal smoking, and hypoxia.[4,6]

CLINICAL PRESENTATION AND DIAGNOSIS

❸ *ADHD is rarely encountered without comorbid conditions, and often is underdiagnosed.* Between 40% and 75% of patients with ADHD will have one or more comorbidities (e.g., learning disabilities, oppositional defiant, conduct, anxiety, or depressive disorders).[10] It is important to identify other coexisting conditions in patients with ADHD to select initial and modify ongoing treatment.

When a patient presents with inattention, hyperactivity, academic underachievement, and/or relational problems, additional information about behavior in various settings should be gathered from the patient, family, and teachers/supervisors. The age of onset, frequency, severity, and duration of symptoms should be documented.[10]

The most useful diagnostic criteria for ADHD is the *Diagnostic and Statistical Manual of Mental Health Disorders*, 4th edition, Text Revision (*DSM*-IV-TR) (Table 42–1). The *DSM*-IV-TR defines three subtypes of ADHD: (a) predominately inattentive, (b) predominantly hyperactive/impulsive, and (c) combined, in which both inattentive and hyperactive symptoms are evident.[11] Neuroimaging, electroencephalograms, and continuous performance examinations are investigational and not used clinically for diagnosis. It is recommended that parents and teachers complete a standardized rating scale based on the *DSM*-IV-TR criteria that measures various behaviors of ADHD.[12] These rating scales do not by themselves diagnose ADHD but are aids to a careful history and interview in securing the diagnosis.[12]

Although ADHD is considered a childhood disorder, signs and symptoms persist into adolescence in 40% to 80% of cases and into adulthood in approximately 60% of cases.[1,9]

Clinical Presentation and Diagnosis of ADHD

General

Patients with ADHD can present with inattention and/or hyperactivity–impulsivity. ADHD is rarely encountered without comorbid conditions.

Symptoms

- Inattention; difficulty paying attention to details in school, work, and social activities; difficulty completing tasks that require a lot of mental effort; easily distracted; forgetful
- Hyperactivity–impulsivity; difficulty sitting still, fidgets; has trouble playing quietly and waiting turns; frequently interrupts
- Combined; exhibits both inattention and hyperactivity–impulsivity

Diagnostic Criteria

- Must exhibit symptoms before 7 years of age that persist for more than 7 months
- Symptoms must be present in two or more settings and adversely affect functioning in social situations, school, or work
- Must meet the diagnostic criteria in *DSM*-IV-TR (Table 42–1)
- Symptoms cannot be better explained by another mental disorder (e.g., autism)

Patient Encounter, Part 1

A single mother and her rambunctious 6-year-old boy, AD, come to your clinic. The mother is concerned because her neighbor, who watches AD after school for no charge, has complained about the problems he is causing among her own children (4½- and 6-year-old boys). AD refuses to wait for his turn in games and frequently hits the younger boy. The neighbor has said that unless AD becomes more manageable, she will not watch him after school. This is very distressing to AD's mother, who barely provides for her son and herself by working at the local convenience store for minimum wage. She cannot afford a professional babysitter for AD. She does not qualify for medical assistance. Further, she explains that his performance at school is getting worse, and he is becoming unmanageable in the classroom.

Which of the patient's symptoms are suggestive of ADHD?

What other information do you need to assess for ADHD?

What help/suggestions could you offer to AD's mother?

<table>
<tr><td colspan="1">

Table 42–1

</td></tr>
</table>

***DSM*-IV-TR Diagnostic Criteria for ADHD**

I. Either A or B:
   A. ***Inattention***. Must have at least six or more of the following symptoms of inattention for at least 6 months:
      1. Does not pay close attention to details in schoolwork, work, or other activities.
      2. Has trouble maintaining attention to tasks or activities.
      3. Has trouble actively listening when directly spoken to.
      4. Has difficulty following instructions and fails to finish important daily tasks (i.e., homework, chores, and responsibilities at work).
      5. Demonstrates difficulty in organizing tasks/activities.
      6. Tends to avoid or put off activities that require concentration.
      7. Tends to misplace items needed to complete tasks or activities.
      8. Is easily distracted from current tasks or activities.
      9. Forgetful.
   B. ***Hyperactivity/impulsivity***. Must have at least six or more of the following symptoms of hyperactivity/impulsivity for at least 6 months:
   Hyperactivity
      1. Fidgets and is restless in a sitting position.
      2. Cannot sit still for extended periods.
      3. Runs around when it is not appropriate.
      4. Cannot play quietly.
      5. Often "on the move."
      6. Talks excessively.
   Impulsivity
      1. Answers questions prematurely.
      2. Difficulty waiting one's turn.
      3. Interruptive or intrudes on others.
II. Above symptoms were present before 7 years of age.
III. Above symptoms are present in two or more settings.
IV. Impairment is clearly evident in social, school, or work functioning.
V. Symptoms cannot be attributed to another mental disorder (e.g., anxiety, depression, autism, or a personality disorder).
Based on the above criteria, ADHD can be divided into three types:
      1. ADHD combined type: Both 1A and 1B.
      2. ADHD inattentive type: 1A criteria are met.
      3. ADHD hyperactive-impulsive type: 1B criteria are met.

From Ref. 11.

Adult ADHD is difficult to assess, and diagnosis is always suspect in patients failing to display clear symptoms prior to 7 years of age.[4] Adults with ADHD have higher rates of psychopathology, substance abuse, social dysfunction, and occupational underachievement.

TREATMENT
Desired Outcomes

❹ *The primary therapeutic objectives in ADHD are to improve behavior and increase attention/response inhibition; secondary goals of treatment are to:*

- Improve relationships with family, teachers, and peers
- Decrease disruptive behavior in academic and social settings

- Improve academic performance
- Increase independence in activities
- Minimize undesirable adverse effects of therapy

Nonpharmacologic (Behavioral) Therapy

Behavioral therapy can be used to treat patients with ADHD; however, it is generally not recommended as first-line monotherapy.[8] ❺ *Several studies have demonstrated that treatment with medication alone is superior to behavioral intervention alone in improving attention.*[13] *However, behavioral therapy in combination with stimulant therapy is better at improving oppositional and aggressive behaviors.*[13] Behavioral modification involves training parents, teachers, and caregivers to change the physical and social environment and establish a reward/consequence system.[10] Success of behavioral modifications depends on the cooperation and involvement of the patient's parents and teachers.

Pharmacologic Therapy

The proposed mechanism of ADHD pharmacotherapy is to modulate neurotransmitter function in order to improve academic and social functioning. Pharmacologic therapy can be divided into two categories: stimulants and nonstimulants. Stimulant medications include methylphenidate, dexmethylphenidate, amphetamine salts, and dextroamphetamine; whereas, nonstimulant medications include atomoxetine, bupropion, tricyclic antidepressants (TCAs) (e.g., imipramine), clonidine, and guanfacine.

▶ Stimulants

❻ *Psychostimulants (e.g., methylphenidate and dextroamphetamine with or without amphetamine) are the most effective agents in treating ADHD. Once the diagnosis of ADHD has been made, a stimulant medication should be considered first-line in treating ADHD* (Fig. 42–1). Stimulants are safe and effective and have a response rate of 70% to 90% in patients with ADHD.[3,10,14] Generally, a trial of at least 3 months on a stimulant is appropriate, and this includes dose titration to response while balancing side effects.[8,10] ❻ *If treatment with the first stimulant formulation fails, it is recommended to switch to a different stimulant formulation.*[10] For example, if the patient was started on methylphenidate but could not tolerate the side effects, switching to dextroamphetamine with or without amphetamine is rational. The majority of patients who fail one stimulant will respond to an alternative stimulant.[10] ❻ *If the patient fails two appropriate trials of different stimulant medications, a third stimulant formulation or second-line nonstimulant such as bupropion, atomoxetine, or imipramine can be considered.* The diagnosis of ADHD should be revalidated as well.

Stimulants theoretically exert their primary effect by blocking the reuptake of dopamine and norepinephrine. Stimulants have been shown to decrease fidgeting and finger tapping, increase on-task classroom behavior and

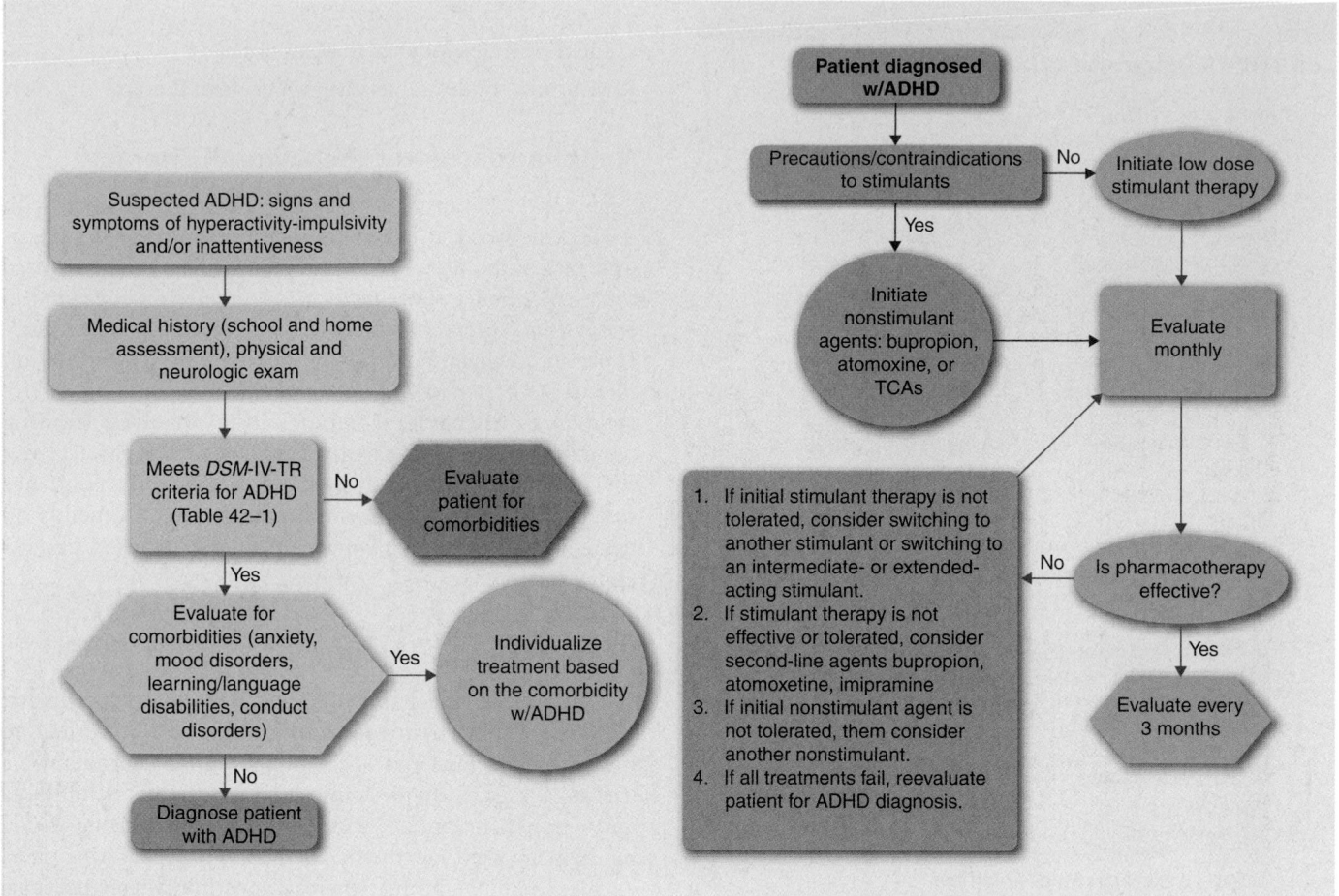

FIGURE 42–1. ADHD diagnosis and treatment algorithm.[8,10,16]

positive interactions at home and in social environments, and ameliorate conduct and anxiety disorders.[14]

Stimulants should be initiated at recommended starting doses and titrated up with a consistent dosing schedule to the appropriate response while minimizing side effects (Table 42–2). Generally, stimulants should not be used in patients who have glaucoma, severe hypertension or cardiovascular disease, hyperthyroidism, severe anxiety, or previous illicit or stimulant drug abuse. Further, stimulants can be used, albeit cautiously, in patients with seizure disorders, Tourette's syndrome, and motor tics.[14]

Stimulant drug formulations can be divided into short-, intermediate-, and extended-acting preparations (Table 42–2). Initial response to short-acting stimulant formulations (e.g., methylphenidate and dextroamphetamine) is seen within 30 minutes and can last for 4 to 6 hours.[10,14] This short duration of effect frequently requires that short-acting stimulant formulations be dosed at least twice daily, thus increasing the chance of missed doses and noncompliance. Further, patients using any stimulant formulation, but especially short-acting formulations, can experience a rebound effect of ADHD symptoms as the stimulant wears off.[14]

Most intermediate-acting stimulants release the medication in a slow, continuous fashion without any early release (except Dexedrine Spansules). The onset of action for this category of stimulants (typically 60–90 minutes) may be inadequate for some patients. Some practitioners prescribe a short-acting stimulant concurrently with an intermediate-acting stimulant in order to curtail the delay in onset of action of the intermediate-acting stimulant.

To minimize rebound problems associated with short-acting formulations and still maintain early stimulant release, extended-acting formulations with rapid onsets have been developed. These formulations have an early release of medication and deliver a delayed release of stimulant in either a pulsed (Adderall XR, Focalin XR, Metadate CD, and Ritalin LA) or continuous manner (Concerta). Formulations available as capsules contain coated beads that can be opened and sprinkled on semisolid food. Concerta tablets have an immediate-release overcoat and then an oral osmotic controlled-release which delivers methylphenidate in an extended manner. Further, patients should be counseled that the empty tablet shell of Concerta can be detected in the stool.

Two extended-acting stimulants with slower-onsets have recently been developed, Daytrana and Vyvanse. Daytrana transdermal patches are to be applied for only 9 hours per day, have a delayed onset of 2 hours, and their effects persist for 3 hours once removed. Skin sensitization and irritation have been reported in some patients. Vyvanse is a prodrug

Table 42–2

Selected Medications in Treating ADHD[a]

Drug, Generic (Brand Name)	Initial Dose	Titration Schedule	Typical Dosing Range (Maximum Dose)
Stimulants			
Short Acting			
Methylphenidate[b] (Methylin, Ritalin)	5 mg 2 × daily	Increase 5–10 mg/day in weekly intervals	5–20 mg 2–3 × daily (60 mg/day)
Dexmethylphenidate[b] (Focalin)	2.5 mg 2 × daily	Increase 2.5–5 mg/day in weekly intervals	5–10 mg twice daily (20 mg/day)
Dextroamphetamine[b] (Dexedrine)	2.5–5 mg every morning	Increase 2.5–5 mg/day in weekly intervals	5–20 mg twice daily (40 mg/day)
Intermediate Acting			
Methylphenidate[b] (Ritalin SR, Metadate ER, Methylin ER)	10 mg once daily	Increase 10 mg/day in weekly intervals	20–40 mg daily in the morning (60 mg/day)
Dextroamphetamine/ amphetamine[b] (Adderall)	2.5–5 mg once to twice daily	Increase 2.5–5 mg/day in weekly intervals	10–30 mg every morning or 5–20 mg twice daily (40 mg/day)
Dextroamphetamine[b] (Dexedrine Spansule)	5 mg every morning	Increase 5 mg/day in weekly intervals	5–30 mg daily or 5–15 mg twice daily (40 mg/day)
Extended Acting			
Methylphenidate[b] (Concerta)	18 mg every morning	Increase 9–18 mg/day in weekly intervals	18–54 mg every morning (54 mg/day)
(Metadate CD)	20 mg every morning	Increase 10–20 mg/day in weekly intervals	20–40 mg daily in the morning (60 mg/day)
(Ritalin LA)	20 mg every morning	Increase 10 mg/day in weekly intervals	20–40 mg daily in the morning (60 mg/day)
Dextroamphetamine/ amphetamine[b] (Adderall XR)	5–10 mg every morning (children); 20 mg once daily (adults)	Increase 5–10 mg/day in weekly intervals	10–30 mg every morning or 5–15 mg twice daily (30 mg/day, children) (60 mg/day, adult)
Dexmethylphenidate[b] (Focalin XR)	5 mg every morning (children); 10 mg every morning (adults)	Increase 5 mg/day in weekly intervals	10–20 mg daily in the morning (20 mg/day)
Lisdexamfetamine[b] (Vyvanse)	30 mg every morning (children and adults)	Increase 10–20 mg/day in weekly intervals	30–70 mg daily in the morning (70 mg/day)
Nonstimulants			
Atomoxetine[b] (Strattera)	Less than or equal to 70 kg: 0.5 mg/kg/day divided once to twice daily	Increase to target dose of 1.2 mg/kg /day after 3 days	40–60 mg/day (1.4 mg/kg or 100 mg/day, whichever is less)
	Greater than 70 kg: 40 mg once daily	Increase 40 mg/day after 3 days (may ↑ to total of 100 mg/day after 2–3 weeks)	40–80 mg/day divided once to twice daily (100 mg/day)
Imipramine (Tofranil)	1.5 mg/kg/day in one or two divided doses	Increase 1 mg/kg/day every 3–4 days	1.5–3 mg/kg/day in one or two divided doses (5 mg/kg/day, child) 100–300 mg/day in one or two divided doses (300 mg/day, adult)
Clonidine (Catapres)	0.05 mg once daily	Increase 0.05 mg/day every 3–7 days	0.1 mg 1 to 4 times daily (0.4 mg/day)
Guanfacine (Tenex)	0.5 mg at bedtime	Increase 0.5 mg every 3–14 days	1.5–3 mg/day divided into 2–3 × daily (4 mg/day)
Bupropion (Wellbutrin, Wellbutrin SR, Wellbutrin XL)	3 mg/kg/day for 7 days (children); 150 mg once daily of SR or XL (adults)	Increase 3 mg/kg/day in weekly intervals (children); increase 150–300 mg/day in weekly intervals (adults)	6 mg/kg/day or 400 mg/ day—whichever is smaller (children); 150–450 mg/day (400 mg/day SR; 450 mg/ day XL—adults)

[a]Pediatric dosing except where adult dosing specified.

[b]FDA approved for treatment of ADHD.

requiring oral ingestion to be hydrolyzed to its active form, dextroamphetamine. Inhalation or injection abuse potential is minimized due to impeded hydrolysis by these routes. Onset of action for Vyvanse has been reported as soon as 2 hours.[15]

Adverse effects of stimulants can be generalized to the whole class (Table 42–3). Most of these side effects can be managed by changing dosing routine (i.e., giving with food, dividing daily dose, or giving the dose earlier in the day). Serious side effects such as hallucinations and abnormal movements require discontinuation of medication.[10,14]

Growth suppression or delay is a major concern for parents of children taking stimulants. However, the evidence of this side effect is not clear. At present, growth delay

---

Table 42–3

ADHD Medication Side-Effect Profiles, Management, and Monitoring

Drug	Side Effects	Management	Monitoring
Stimulants			
Methylphenidate, dextroamphetamine, dextroamphetamine/ amphetamine (mixed-salts amphetamine, dexmethylphenidate, lisdexamfetamine)	GI upset, nausea, decreased appetite, potential growth delay	Administer after meals Encourage high-calorie meals Divide dose Give snacks in the evening Change to shorter-acting stimulant Use drug holiday or different medication if severe growth delay	Height, weight, blood pressure, pulse ECG if warranted Eating and sleeping patterns Evaluate every 2–4 weeks until stable dose is achieved; then evaluate every 3 months
	Sleep disturbance	Move dose(s) earlier in the day, and discontinue later day dose if problem persists Give clonidine or guanfacine at bedtime Change to a shorter-acting stimulant	
	Rebound symptoms	Change to longer-acting stimulant Overlap stimulant dosing	
	Moodiness	Decrease dose or change to longer-acting stimulant Verify diagnosis/comorbidity	
	Irritability	Evaluate time of occurrence Early onset: Decrease dose or change to longer-acting stimulant Late onset: Switch to longer-acting stimulant Evaluate for comorbidity	
	Increased blood pressure and pulse	Decrease dose or change to longer-acting stimulant	
	Tics	Discountinue or change to a different stimulant Give clonidine or guanfacine	
Nonstimulants			
Atomoxetine	Increased blood pressure and pulse, nausea, vomiting, fatigue, and insomia	Decrease dose or change to another medication	Same as above but with baseline and routine liver function tests for hepatotoxicity
	Hepatotoxicity, suicidal thoughts	Discountinue or change to a another medication	
TCAs (imipramine)	Sedation	Administer later in the day	Blood pressure, pulse, sleeping pattern, ECG Evaluate every 3 days until stable dose is achieved; then evaluate every 3 months
	Cardiac conduction delay, dizziness, increased pulse	Decrease dose or change medication	
	Anticholinergic effects (constipation, dry mouth, difficult urinating, blurry vision)	Decrease dose or change medication	
Clonidine and guanfacine	Sedation, arrhythmia, constipation, dizziness (decreased blood pressure)	Sedation: administer later in the day Decrease dose or change medication	Same as above
Bupropion	GI upset, restlessness, sleep disturbances, rash, tics, risk of seizures, tremor	Decrease Dose or change medication Tics, rash, and seizures: discontinue medication	Height, weight, blood pressure, pulse every month Eating and sleeping patterns

appears to be transient and to resolve by midadolescence, but more data are needed to firmly resolve this issue.[10] Another concern is the risk of substance abuse with stimulant use. A diagnosis of ADHD alone increases the risk of substance abuse in adolescents and adults. However, stimulant use has not been shown to further increase this risk but actually may decrease this risk, provided ADHD is treated adequately.[16]

The choice of ADHD medication should be made based on the patient's condition, the prescriber's familiarity with the medications, the ease of administration, and cost. Stimulants should be used first-line in most ADHD patients, although studies in groups of patients have shown no clear advantage of using one stimulant over another.[17]

▶ Nonstimulants

Atomoxetine Atomoxetine is approved in both children and adults. In clinical studies, atomoxetine has demonstrated superior efficacy over placebo and either equivalent or inferior efficacy when compared with a suboptimal immediate-release methylphenidate dose or Concerta (18 to 54 mg given once daily), respectively.[18-23] ❻ *Atomoxetine may be used as a second- or third-line medication for ADHD.*

Atomoxetine selectively inhibits the reuptake of adrenergic neurotransmitters, principally norepinephrine.[18-21] Atomoxetine is metabolized through the cytochrome P450 (CYP) 2D6 pathway. Concurrent use of certain antidepressants (i.e., fluoxetine, paroxetine) may inhibit this enzyme and necessitate slower dose titration of atomoxetine. Approximately 5% to 10% of the population are CYP2D6 poor metabolizers, and atomoxetine half-life is increased significantly in this population.[24] The recommended dosing for atomoxetine depends on the weight of the patient and is given daily in either a single or two divided doses[24] (Table 42–2). In poor metabolizers, atomoxetine should be dosed once daily at 25% to 50% of the dose typically used in normal metabolizers.[24] The maximum therapeutic effect of atomoxetine may take up to 4 weeks to be seen, which is significantly longer than what is required with stimulants. Common side effects of atomoxetine are similar to those of stimulants: dyspepsia, nausea, vomiting, somnolence, and decreased appetite. Some studies have reported an increase in blood pressure and heart rate.[19-21] There is evidence that atomoxetine can slow growth rate and cause weight loss; thus, height and weight should be monitored routinely in pediatric patients[19-21] (Table 42–3). Further, atomoxetine labeling includes strong warnings about severe hepatotoxicity and increased association with suicidal thinking.

Atomoxetine is similar to extended-acting stimulants in that it can be given once daily in many patients. It appears to lack any abuse potential and is not a controlled substance.[25] One big disadvantage of atomoxetine is cost compared with other ADHD medications (Table 42–4).

Due to the high cost, lack of long-term efficacy data, and few comparison studies with stimulants, atomoxetine should be advocated only if the patient has failed or is intolerant to the standard stimulant therapy (Fig. 42–1).

Bupropion Bupropion is a monocyclic antidepressant that weakly inhibits the reuptake of norepinephrine and dopamine. Bupropion is effective for relieving symptoms of ADHD in children but is not as effective as stimulants.[26,27] Similar results have been shown in adults.[26] Specific dosing recommendations are outlined in Table 42–2. Bupropion is well tolerated with minimal side effects (e.g., insomnia, headache, nausea, and tremor). Side effects typically disappear with continuation of therapy and are minimized with slow titration of dose. Bupropion can worsen tics and movement disorders. It is a rational choice in an ADHD patient with comorbid depression.[26] However, seizures have been associated with bupropion doses greater than 6 mg/kg/day.[28] Seizures related to high doses can be minimized by reducing the dose or switching to a longer-acting formulation. Owing to the propensity of seizures with bupropion, its use is contraindicated in patients with seizure and eating disorders.

Tricyclic Antidepressants The TCAs, such as imipramine, can alleviate symptoms of ADHD, but they are less effective than stimulants. Like bupropion, TCAs likely will improve symptoms associated with comorbid anxiety and depression. Although TCAs block the reuptake of serotonin, it is the blockade of norepinephrine that is felt to be responsible for their anti-ADHD effects. TCA use in ADHD has declined owing to case reports of sudden death and anticholinergic side effects[6,10] (Table 42–3). If a TCA is prescribed for a child or an

---

Patient Encounter, Part 2: Medical History, Physical Exam, and ADHD Evaluation

AD's baseline physical examination is unremarkable. Family history is negative for cardiovascular disease, and there is no documented history of ADHD in the family.

Wt: 20 kg (44 lb)

Allergies: None known

Ht: 45 in. (114 cm)

BP: 96/55 mm Hg

P: 80 bpm

AD's mother does not qualify for medical assistance, and she can hardly afford their monthly expenses.

What stimulants and/or nonstimulants are available that might control AD's symptoms?

Which medications will maximize efficacy, facilitate adherence, minimize potential side effects, and offer an acceptable cost for AD's mother?

What other information do you need before starting stimulant therapy?

What are important counseling points to discuss with AD's mother?

Table 42-4

30-Day Cost[a] of Selected ADHD Medication Regimens

Generic (Brand)	Regimen (Brand)	Cost[a]
Short-Acting Rapid-Onset Stimulants		
Methylphenidate		
Generic	5-, 10-, or 20-mg tablet twice daily	$
Methylin	5 mg/5 mL solution twice daily	$$$$
Dexmethylphenidate		
Generic	2.5-mg tablet twice daily	$
Generic	5- or 10-mg tablet twice daily	$$
Dextroamphetamine		
Generic	5- or 10-mg tablet twice daily	$
Intermediate-Acting Slower-Onset Stimulants		
Methylphenidate		
Methylin ER	10- or 20-mg ER tablet daily	$
Dextroamphetamine[c]		
Generic	5-, 10-, or 15-mg capsule daily	$$
Dextroamphetamine/amphetamine		
Generic	5-, 7.5-, 10-, 12.5-, 15-, 20-, or 30-mg tablet daily	$
Extended-Acting Rapid-Onset Stimulants		
Methylphenidate		
Concerta[c]	18-, 27-, 36-, or 54-mg tablet daily	$$$$
Metadate CD[b]	10-, 20-, or 30-mg capsule daily	$$$
Ritalin LA[b]	10-, 20-mg capsule daily	$$$
Dextroamphetamine/amphetamine		
Adderall XR[b]	5-, 10-, 15-, 20-, 25-, or 30-mg capsule daily	$$$$
Dexmethylphenidate		
Focalin XR[b]	5-, 10-, 15-, or 20-mg capsule daily	$$$$
Extended-Acting Slower-Onset Stimulants		
Lisdexamfetamine		
Vyvanse	20-, 30-, 40-, 50-, 60-, or 70-mg capsule daily	$$$$
Methylphenidate		
Daytrana transdermal patch	10-, 15-, 20-, or 30-mg patch daily	$$$$
Nonstimulants		
Atomoxetine		
Strattera	10-, 18-, 25-, 40-, 60-, 80-, or 100-mg capsule daily	$$$$
Imipramine		
Generic	10-, 25-, or 50-mg tablet twice daily	$
Clonidine		
Generic	0.1-, 0.2-, or 0.3-mg tablet twice daily	$
Guanfacine		
Generic	1-mg tablet twice daily	$
Generic	2-mg tablet twice daily	$$
Bupropion		
Generic	75- or 100-mg tablet twice daily	$
Generic	100- or 150-mg SR tablet twice daily	$$
Generic	200-mg SR tablet twice daily	$$$
Generic	150-mg or 300-mg XL tablet daily	$$

Chew tablet, chewable tablet; CD, extended release (biphasic immediate release with extended release); ER, extended release; LA, long-acting; SR, sustain release; XL, extended release.

[a]Cost based on brand regimen specified without a dispensing fee or discount for a 30-day supply. Costs are current as of September 2009.

[b]Bimodal release (early then late; mimics twice daily dosing of shorter-acting stimulant counterpart).

[c]Ascending release (early then gradual/continuous). $, less than $40; $$, $40–$79; $$$, $80–$120; $$$$, greater than $120.

adolescent, desipramine should be avoided due to a higher case fatality rate compared with other TCAs.[29] Further, TCAs may lower seizure threshold and increase the risk of cardiotoxicity (e.g., arrhythmia). Patients starting on TCAs should have a baseline and routine ECGs.

Clonidine and Guanfacine Clonidine and guanfacine are central α_2-adrenergic agonists that inhibit the release of norepinephrine presynaptically. Both these agents are less effective than stimulants in treating symptoms of ADHD but typically are used as adjuncts to stimulants to control disruptive or aggressive behavior and alleviate insomnia.[30] Guanfacine will last 3 to 4 hours longer than clonidine and requires less frequent dosing. Common side effects with clonidine and guanfacine are low blood pressure and sedation. Sedation is transient and generally subsides after 2 to 3 weeks of therapy.[30] Rarely, severe side effects such as bradycardia, rebound hypertension, irregular heart beats, and sudden death have been reported.

Pharmacoeconomic and Treatment Adherence Considerations

Proper ADHD treatment is a substantial financial burden.[31,32] Annual health care costs of patients with ADHD are more than double those of patients without ADHD ($1,343 versus $503, respectively).[31] The financial burden of ADHD can be attributed to the direct cost of pharmacotherapy, office visits, diagnostic measurements, therapy monitoring, and indirect costs (e.g., lost work time and productivity). When selecting a treatment for an ADHD patient, the cost burden to the patient's family should be considered. Immediate-release stimulants may be more cost-effective in many patients compared with longer-acting stimulant formulations (Table 42–4), but in certain circumstances, longer-acting stimulant formulations may provide a greater benefit owing to increased adherence to the medication and prolonged control of symptoms of ADHD. Some nonstimulant ADHD medications (e.g., bupropion, TCAs, and α_2-adrenergic agonists) appear to be less costly than many stimulant formulations; however, these agents have not been proven to have superior efficacy over stimulants in treating ADHD. Decisions on selection of specific ADHD medications should not be based solely on cost, but on efficacy and safety, along with adherence to the prescribed regimen, should be considered foremost.

OUTCOME EVALUATION

It is important to carefully document core ADHD symptoms at baseline to provide a reference point from which to evaluate effectiveness of treatment. Improvement in individualized patient outcomes are desired, such as (a) family and social relationships, (b) disruptive behavior, (c) completing required tasks, (d) self-motivation, (e) appearance, and (f) self-esteem. It is very important to elicit evaluations of the patient's behavior from family, school, and social environments in order to assess these outcomes. Using standardized rating scales (e.g., Conners Rating Scales—Revised, Brown Attention-Deficit Disorder Scale, and Inattentive-Overactive With Aggression [IOWA] Conners Scale) in both children and adults with ADHD helps to minimize variability in evaluation.[33] After initiation of therapy, evaluate every 2 to 4 weeks to determine efficacy of treatment and potential effects on height, weight, pulse, and blood pressure. Use physical examinations or liver function tests as appropriate to monitor for adverse effects. In children being considered for ADHD pharmacotherapy, obtain baseline ECGs when known or suspected cardiac disease exists or the clinician judges it necessary.[34–36] Typically, therapeutic benefits will be seen within days of initiating

Patient Care and Monitoring

1. Assess the patient's symptoms and parent/teacher evaluations to determine whether they meet the *DSM*-IV-TR diagnostic criteria for ADHD. Evaluate whether the symptoms can be explained by another disorder.

2. Interview the patient and/or caregivers to obtain a complete medical history, which should include family medical history, current and past prescription and nonprescription medications, and dietary intake. Determine whether the patient is taking medication/supplements that could interfere with the therapy.

3. Educate the patient's parents and/or caregivers that behavioral therapy is not as effective as stimulant therapy. Educate parents regarding the issues of growth delay and substance-abuse risks with stimulants.

4. Perform a baseline physical examination before starting stimulant therapy. Include blood pressure, pulse, and height and weight measurements. In patients taking stimulants, perform a general physical examination yearly, and monitor blood pressure quarterly in adults. In children, baseline ECGs should be obtained when known cardiac disease exists or if the patient history, family history, or physical exam suggests cardiac disease. ECGs for other patients are not mandatory but should be considered according to the clinician's judgment. Patients beginning a TCA are an exception, requiring baseline and routine ECGs.

5. Start patients on a low initial dose of a stimulant and titrate up to the desired response in order to minimize side effects and costs.

6. If the patient is not responding to therapy after an adequate trial, assess compliance with the prescribed regimen. If the patient is not compliant, counsel the patient and caregivers and explore reasons for noncompliance. In some cases, switching to another stimulant formulation may improve compliance.

7. Important counseling points to convey to the patient and/or caregiver:
   - What is ADHD?
   - What are the complications of untreated ADHD?
   - When to take medications and what to expect with therapy.
   - What side effects to expect and what to do if these occur.
   - Controversy over substance abuse and growth delay with stimulant therapy.
   - What prescription and nonprescription medications to avoid.

stimulants and within a month or two of starting bupropion and atomoxetine. Once a maintenance dose has been achieved, schedule follow-up visits every 3 months. At these visits, assess height and weight, and screen for possible adverse drug effects. If a patient has failed to respond to multiple agents, reevaluate for other possible causes of behavior dysfunction. Counsel patients and their families that treatment generally is long term. Typically, appropriately treated patients learn to better control their ADHD symptoms as adults.

Abbreviations Introduced in This Chapter

ADHD	Attention-deficit hyperactivity disorder
CYP	Cytochrome P450
DSM-IV-TR	*Diagnostic and Statistical Manual of Mental Disorders,* Fourth Edition, Text Revision
GABA	Gamma aminobutyric acid
IOWA	Inattentive-Overactive With Aggression
TCA	Tricyclic antidepressant

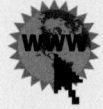 Self-assessment questions and answers are available at *http://www.mhpharmacotherapy. com/pp.html.*

REFERENCES

1. Wolraich ML, Wibbelsman CJ, Brown TE, et al. Attention-deficit/ hyperactivity disorder among adolescents: A review of the diagnosis, treatment, and clinical implications. Pediatrics 2005;115(6):1734–1746.
2. Zametkin AJ, Ernst M. Problems in the management of attention-deficit-hyperactivity disorder. N Engl J Med 1999;340(1):40–46.
3. Elia J, Ambrosini PJ, Rapoport JL. Treatment of attention-deficit-hyperactivity disorder. N Engl J Med 1999;340(10):780–788.
4. Voeller KKS. Attention-deficit hyperactivity disorder (ADHD). J Child Neurol 2004;19:798–814.
5. Herrerias CT, Perrin JM, Stein MT. The child with ADHD: Using the AAP clinical practice guideline. Am Fam Physician 2001;63(9):1803–1810.
6. Biederman J, Faraone S. Attention-deficit hyperactivity disorder. Lancet 2005;366:237–248.
7. Centers for Disease Control and Prevention. Prevalence of diagnosis and medication treatment for attention-deficit/hyperactivity disorder—United States, 2003. MMWR 2005;54:842–847.
8. Rappley MD. Attention deficit-hyperactivity disorder. N Engl J Med 2005;352:165–173.
9. Elliott H. Attention deficit hyperactivity disorder in adults: A guide for the primary care physician. South Med J 2002;95:736–742.
10. American Academy of Pediatrics. Subcommittee on Attention-Deficit/ Hyperactivity Disorder and Committee on Quality Improvement. Clinical practice guideline: Treatment of the school-aged child with attention-deficit/hyperactivity disorder. Pediatrics 2001;108:1033–1044.
11. American Psychiatric Association. Diagnostic and Statistical Manual of Mental Disorders. 4th ed. Text Rev. Washington, DC: American Psychiatric Press, 2000:39–134.
12. Pliszka S. AACAP Work Group on Quality Issues. Practice parameter for the assessment and treatment of children and adolescents with attention-deficit/hyperactivity disorder. J Am Acad Child Adolesc Psychiatry. 2007;46:894–921.
13. MTA Cooperative Group. A 14-month randomized clinical trial of treatment strategies for attention-deficit/hyperactivity disorder. Arch Gen Psychiatry 1999(Dec);56(12):1073–1086.
14. Greenhill LL, Pliszka S, Dulcan MK, et al. Practice parameter for the use of stimulant medications in the treatment of children, adolescents, and adults. J Am Acad Child Adolesc Psychiatry 2002;41(Suppl 2):26S–49S.
15. Biederman J, Boellner SW, Childress A, et al. Lisdexamfetamine dimesylate and mixed amphetamine salts extended-release in children with ADHD: A double-blind, placebo-controlled, crossover analog classroom study. Biol Psychiatry 2007;62:970–976.
16. Wilens TE, Faraone SV, Biederman J, et al. Does stimulant therapy of attention-deficit/hyperactivity disorder beget later substance abuse? A meta-analytic review of the literature. Pediatrics 2003;111:179–185.
17. Brown RT, Amler RW, Freeman WS, et al. Treatment of attention-deficit/hyperactivity disorder: Overview of the evidence. Pediatrics 2005;115:749–757.
18. Michelson D, Faries D, Wernicke J, et al. Atomoxetine in the treatment of children and adolescents with attention-deficit/hyperactivity disorder: A randomized, placebo-controlled, dose-response study. Pediatrics 2001;108(5):E83.
19. Kratochvil CJ, Heiligenstein JH, Dittmann R, et al. Atomoxetine and methylphenidate treatment in children with ADHD: A prospective, randomized, open-label trial. J Am Acad Child Adolesc Psychiatry 2002;41(7):776–784.
20. Michelson D, Allen AJ, Busner J, et al. Once-daily atomoxetine treatment for children and adolescents with attention deficit hyperactivity disorder: A randomized, placebo-controlled study. Am J Psychiatry 2002;159:1896–1901.
21. Biederman J, Heiligenstein JH, Faries DE, et al. Efficacy of atomoxetine versus placebo in school-age girls with attention-deficit/hyperactivity disorder. Pediatrics 2002;110(6):E75.
22. Newcorn JH, Kratochvil CJ, Allen AJ, et al. Atomoxetine and osmotically released methylphenidate for the treatment of attention deficit hyperactivity disorder: Acute comparison and differential response. Am J Psychiatry 2008;165(6):721–730.
23. Wang Y, Zheng Y, Du Y, et al. Atomoxetine versus methylphenidate in paediatric outpatients with attention deficit hyperactivity disorder: A randomized, double-blind comparison trial. Aust N Z J Psychiatry 2007;41(3):222–230.
24. Belle DJ, Ernest S, Sauer J, et al. Effect of potent CYP2D6 inhibition by paroxetine on atomoxetine pharmacokinetics. J Clin Pharmacol 2002;42:1219–1227.
25. Heil SH, Holmes HW, Bickel WK, et al. Comparison of the subjective physiological, and psychomotor effects of atomoxetine and methylphenidate in light drug users. Drug Alcohol Depend 2002;67(2):149–156.
26. Daviss WB, Bentivoglio P, Racusin R, et al. Bupropion sustained release in adolescents with comorbid attention-deficit/hyperactivity disorder and depression. J Am Acad Child Adolesc Psychiatry 2001;40(3):307–314.
27. Wilens TE, Spencer TJ, Biederman J, et al. A controlled clinical trial of bupropion for attention deficit hyperactivity disorder in adults. Am J Psychiatry 2001;158:282–288.
28. Tallian K. Pharmacotherapy of ADHD. In: Schumock G, Brundage D, Chapman M, et al., eds. Pharmacotherapy Self-Assessment Program, 5th ed. Pediatrics II. Kansas City, MO: American College of Clinical Pharmacy, 2006:275–297.
29. Amitai Y, Frischer H. Excess fatality from desipramine in children and adolescents. J Am Acad Child Adolesc Psychiatry 2006;45:54–60.
30. Hazell PL, Stuart JE. A randomized controlled trial of clonidine added to psychostimulant medication for hyperactive and aggressive children. J Am Acad Child Adolesc Psychiatry 2003;42:886–894.

31. Matza LS, Paramore C, Prasad M. A review of the economic burden of ADHD. Cost Eff Resour Alloc 2005;3:5.

32. Birnbaum HG, Kessler RC, Lowe SW, et al. Costs of attention deficit-hyperactivity disorder (ADHD) in the U.S.: Excess costs of persons with ADHD and their family members in 2000. Curr Med Res Opin 2005;21(2):195–205.

33. Collett BR, Ohan JL, Myers KM. Ten-year review of rating scales. V: Scales assessing attention-deficit/hyperactivity disorder. J Am Acad Child Adolesc Psychiatry 2003;42(9):1015–1037.

34. Vetter VL, Elia J, Erickson C, et al. Cardiovascular monitoring of children and adolescents with heart disease receiving medications for Attention Deficit/Hyperactivity Disorder: A scientific statement from the American Heart Association Council on Cardiovascular Disease in the Young Congenital Cardiac Defects Committee and the Council on Cardiovascular Nursing. Circulation. 2008;117:2407–2423.

35. Perrin JM, Friedman RA, Knilans TK, et al. Cardiovascular monitoring and stimulant drugs for Attention-Deficit/Hyperactivity Disorder. Pediatrics 2008; 122:451–453.

36. ECGs before stimulants in children. Med Lett Drugs Ther 2008 Jul 28;50(1291):60.

43 Diabetes Mellitus

John T. Johnson, Susan Cornell, and
William E. Wade

LEARNING OBJECTIVES

● **Upon completion of the chapter, the reader will be able to:**

1. Discuss the incidence and economic impact of diabetes.

2. Distinguish clinical differences in type 1 (T1DM), type 2 (T2DM), and gestational diabetes.

3. List screening and diagnostic criteria for diabetes.

4. Discuss therapeutic goals for blood glucose, blood pressure, and lipids for a patient with diabetes.

5. Recommend nonpharmacologic therapies, including meal planning and physical activity, for patients with diabetes.

6. Compare oral agents used in treating diabetes by their mechanisms of action, time of action, side effects, contraindications, and effectiveness.

7. Select appropriate insulin therapy based on onset, peak, and duration of action.

8. Develop a comprehensive therapeutic monitoring plan for a patient with diabetes based on patient-specific factors.

KEY CONCEPTS

❶ Diabetes mellitus (DM) describes a group of chronic metabolic disorders that are characterized by hyperglycemia and associated with long-term microvascular, macrovascular, and neuropathic complications.

❷ Type 1 DM (T1DM) is usually diagnosed before the age of 30, but can develop at any age. The autoimmune destruction of the β-cells causes insulin deficiency.

❸ Type 2 DM (T2DM) accounts for approximately 90% to 95% of all diagnosed cases, is progressive in its development, and is often preceded by prediabetes. A combination of insulin deficiency, insulin resistance, and other hormonal irregularities, primarily glucagon, are key problems with T2DM. The majority of people with T2DM are overweight, and an increasing number of cases in children have been observed.

❹ Glycemic control remains the primary objective in managing diabetes and its complications, but hypertension and hyperlipidemia are significant comorbidities.

❺ Patients and clinicians can evaluate control of the patient's diabetes by monitoring daily blood glucose values, hemoglobin A_{1c} or estimated average blood glucose values, blood pressure, and lipid levels.

❻ Oral and injectable agents are available to treat patients with T2DM who are unable to achieve glycemic control through meal planning and physical activity.

❼ Insulin is the primary treatment to lower blood glucose levels for patients with T1DM and the addition of injected amylin may decrease fluctuations in blood glucose levels.

❽ Uncontrolled blood pressure plays a major role in the development of macrovascular events and nephropathy in patients with DM. The American Diabetes Association recommends that blood pressure goals for patients with DM be less than 130/80 mm Hg.

❾ Peripheral neuropathy is the most common complication reported in T2DM. This complication generally presents as pain, tingling, or numbness in the extremities.

❿ Lower extremity amputations are one of the most feared and disabling sequelae of long-term uncontrolled DM. A foot ulcer is an open sore that develops and penetrates to the subcutaneous tissues. Complications of the feet develop primarily as a result of peripheral vascular disease, neuropathies, and foot deformations.

INTRODUCTION

❶ *Diabetes mellitus (DM) describes a group of chronic metabolic disorders characterized by hyperglycemia that may result in long-term* microvascular, macrovascular, and *neuropathic complications.* These complications contribute to diabetes being the leading cause of: (a) new cases of blindness among adults, (b) end-stage renal disease, and (c) nontraumatic lower limb amputations. While prevention and treatment of DM remain a challenge, several studies have shown that complications associated with DM such as retinopathy and neuropathy can be delayed or prevented through proper blood glucose management.[1,2]

The increased cardiovascular risk associated with DM contributes to it being the sixth leading cause of death in the United States. In 2007, diabetes caused approximately 284,000 deaths, accounted for more than 15 million workdays absent and an additional 107 million workdays lost due to unemployment disability. The financial impact of DM in 2007 was approximately $174 billion, or one of every five dollars spent on health care in the United States.[3]

EPIDEMIOLOGY AND ETIOLOGY

DM is characterized by a complete lack of insulin, a relative lack of insulin, or insulin resistance as well as disorders of other hormones. These defects result in an inability to use glucose for energy. DM affects an estimated 23.6 million persons in the United States, or 7% of the population. While an estimated 17.9 million persons have been diagnosed, another 5.7 million people have DM but are unaware they have the disease. Worldwide, the number of people with DM is expected to rise to 35% by the year 2025.[3] The increasing prevalence of DM is due in part to three influences: lifestyle, ethnicity, and age.

Lifestyle

Sedentary lifestyle coupled with greater consumption of high-fat foods and larger portion sizes have resulted in increasing rates of persons being overweight or obese. Current estimates indicate that 65% of the U.S. population is overweight and of those, 30% are obese. Overweight is defined as a body mass index (BMI) of greater than 25 kg/m², whereas a BMI of greater than 30 kg/m² constitutes obesity. The Centers for Disease Control and Prevention (CDC) estimates that 25% to 33% of Americans do not engage in an adequate amount of daily activity.[4]

Ethnicity

In addition to current lifestyle trends and increased body weight, certain ethnic groups are at a disproportionately high risk for developing DM. Individuals of Native American, Native Alaskan, African American, and Hispanic/Latino American descent have 1.7 to 2.2 times greater risk of developing DM when compared with non-Hispanic whites.[3] In addition, African American and Hispanic/Latino American populations are growing at a faster rate than the general U.S. population. This is a contributing factor to the rising U.S. population who has DM.

Age

The third factor contributing to the increased prevalence of diabetes is age. The prevalence of DM increases with age from approximately 2% of individuals 20 to 39 years of age to 20.9% of individuals older than 60 years of age.[3] As the population ages, the incidence of DM is expected to increase.

❷ *Type 1 DM (T1DM) usually is diagnosed before the age of 30, but can develop at any age. The autoimmune destruction of the β-cells causes insulin deficiency.* ❸ *Type 2 DM (T2DM) accounts for approximately 90% to 95% of all diagnosed cases, is progressive in its development, and is often preceded by prediabetes. A combination of insulin deficiency, insulin resistance, and other hormonal irregularities, primarily glucagon, are key problems with T2DM. The majority of people with T2DM are overweight and an increasing number of cases in children have been observed.*

T1DM is an autoimmune disease in which insulin-producing β-cells in the pancreas are destroyed, leaving the individual insulin-deficient. This is usually precipitated through genetic susceptibility and/or an environmental trigger. Certain genetic markers can be measured to determine if a person is at risk of diabetes. The presence of human leukocyte antigens (HLAs), especially HLA-DR, is strongly associated with the development of T1DM. Over 95% of people with T1DM have HLA-DR3 and HLA-DR4 present. In addition, these individuals often develop islet cell antibodies, insulin autoantibodies, or glutamic acid decarboxylase autoantibodies. More than 90% of persons with T1DM have at least one diabetes-related antibody present. As more β-cells are destroyed, glucose metabolism becomes compromised due to reduced insulin release following a glucose load. At the time of diagnosis, most patients have a 90% loss of β-cell function. The remaining 10% of β-cell function at diagnosis creates a "honeymoon period" during which blood glucose levels are easier to control and smaller amounts of insulin are required. Once this remaining β-cell function is lost, patients become completely insulin-deficient and require more exogenous insulin. Diagnosis of T1DM occurs before the age of 30 in approximately 70% of patients. Approximately one in 400 people under the age of 20 are diagnosed with T1DM.

Latent autoimmune diabetes in adults (LADA), slow-onset type 1 or type 1.5 DM, is a form of autoimmune T1DM that occurs in individuals older (over 30 years of age) than the usual age of T1DM onset. Patients often are mistakenly thought to have T2DM because the person is older and may respond initially to treatment with oral blood glucose lowering agents. These patients do not have insulin resistance, but antibodies are present in the blood that are known to destroy pancreatic β-cells.

Measurement of C-peptide levels, insulin levels, and autoantibodies can be used to distinguish between T1DM and T2DM. It has been suggested that the easiest way to differentiate between T1DM and T2DM is by measuring C-peptide levels.[5] People with T1DM have C-peptide levels below 1 ng/mL

(0.33 nmol/L), whereas those with T2DM will have values greater than 1 ng/mL (0.33 nmol/L). Although different institutions may have varying reference ranges for C-peptide, according to the literature, the standard "normal" range for C-peptide in patients without diabetes is 0.5 to 2 ng/mL (0.17–0.66 nmol/L).[5]

Prediabetes is defined as having either a fasting and/or a postprandial blood glucose level higher than normal but not high enough to be classified as DM. A fasting blood glucose level greater than 100 mg/dL, but less than 126 mg/dL, or a postprandial blood glucose level greater than 140 mg/dL, but less than 200 mg/dL indicates prediabetes. It is currently estimated that 57 million persons in the United States have prediabetes. The development of prediabetes places the individual at high risk of eventually developing diabetes. Because progression from prediabetes to diabetes is not predictable, interventions during prediabetes are gaining popularity.

T2DM is usually slow and progressive in its development and is often preceded by prediabetes. Risk factors for T2DM include:

- First-degree family history of DM (i.e., parents or siblings)
- Overweight or obese
- Habitual physical inactivity
- Race or ethnicity (Native American, Latino/Hispanic American, Asian American, African American, and Pacific Islanders)
- Prediabetes (i.e., previously identified with impaired glucose tolerance [IGT] or impaired fasting glucose [IFG])
- Hypertension (greater than or equal to 140/90 mm Hg)

- High-density lipoprotein (HDL) less than 35 mg/dL (0.91 mmol/L) and/or a triglyceride level greater than 250 mg/dL (2.83 mmol/L)
- History of gestational diabetes or delivery of a baby weighing greater than 4 kg (9 lb)
- History of vascular disease
- History of polycystic ovary disease
- Other conditions associated with insulin resistance (e.g., acanthosis nigricans)[6]

Gestational diabetes mellitus (GDM) is defined as glucose intolerance in women during pregnancy. This complication develops in approximately 7% of all pregnancies. Women who have GDM have a 40% to 60% chance of developing T2DM.[7] Risk factors for GDM include obesity, glycosuria, strong family history of DM, age greater than 35 years, prediabetes detected before pregnancy, previous delivery of babies with birth weights greater than 4 kg (9 lb), and ethnicity (African American, Hispanic/Latino American, or Native American).[7] Clinical detection of and therapy for GDM are important because blood sugar control produces significant reductions in perinatal morbidity and mortality.

Rare forms of DM have been reported and account for 1% to 5% of all diagnosed cases. Causes of these conditions include specific genetic conditions, surgery, drugs, malnutrition, infections, and other illnesses. Table 43–1 contains a list of medications that may affect glycemic control. While the use of these medications is not contraindicated in persons with DM, caution and awareness of the effects on blood glucose should be taken into account when managing these patients.

Table 43–1
Medications That May Affect Glycemic Control

Drug	Effect on Glucose	Mechanism/Comment
Angiotensin-converting enzyme inhibitors	Slight reduction	Improves insulin sensitivity
Alcohol	Reduction	Reduces hepatic glucose production
α-Interferon	Increase	Unclear
Diuretics	Increase	May increase insulin resistance
Glucocorticoids	Increase	Impairs insulin action
Nicotinic acid	Increase	Impairs insulin action, increases insulin resistance
Oral contraceptives	Increase	Unclear
Pentamidine	Decrease, then increase	Toxic to β-cells; initial release of stored insulin, then depletion
Phenytoin	Increase	Decreases insulin secretion
β-Blockers	May increase	Decreases insulin secretion
Salicylates	Decrease	Inhibition of I-kappa-B kinase-β (IKK-β) (only high doses, e.g., 4–6 g/day)
Sympathomimetics	Slight increase	Increased glycogenolysis and gluconeogenesis
Clozapine and olanzapine	Increase	Decreases insulin sensitivity; weight gain

This list is not inclusive of all medications reported to cause glucose changes.

From DiPiro JT, Talbert RL, Yee GC, et al., (eds.) Pharmacotherapy: A Pathophysiologic Approach, 7th ed. New York: McGraw-Hill; 2008: Table 77–11, p. 1219.

PATHOPHYSIOLOGY

Normal Carbohydrate Metabolism

The body's main fuel source is glucose. Cells metabolize glucose completely through glycolysis and the Kreb cycle, producing adenosine triphosphate (ATP) as energy. Glucose is stored in the liver and muscles as glycogen. When energy is required, glycogenolysis converts stored glycogen back to glucose. Excess glucose also may be converted to triglycerides and stored in fat cells. Triglycerides subsequently undergo lipolysis, yielding glycerol and free fatty acids. While usually reserved for other functions, proteins also can be converted to glucose through gluconeogenesis. Normal homeostasis is achieved through a balance of the metabolism of glucose, free fatty acids, and amino acids to maintain a blood glucose level sufficient to provide an uninterrupted supply of glucose to the brain.

Insulin and glucagon are produced in the pancreas by cells in the islets of Langerhans. β-Cells make up 70% to 90% of the islets and produce insulin and **amylin**, whereas α-cells produce glucagon. The main function of insulin is to decrease blood glucose levels, whereas glucagon, along with other counterregulatory hormones such as growth factor, cortisol, and epinephrine, increases blood glucose levels. While blood glucose levels vary, the opposing actions of insulin and glucagon, along with the counterregulatory hormones, maintain these values between 70 and 120 mg/dL (3.9–6.7 mmol/L).[8–10]

▶ Normal Insulin Action

Insulin secretion during fasting periods is a low, steady basal rate of 0.5 to 1 unit/h. After food is consumed, blood glucose levels rise, and the insulin-secretion response occurs in two phases.[11] An initial burst, known as *first phase insulin response,* lasts approximately 10 minutes and serves to suppress hepatic glucose production. This bolus of insulin minimizes hyperglycemia during meals and during the postprandial period. The loss of this first phase insulin response is an early event in the progression from glucose intolerance to DM. The *second phase of insulin response* is characterized by a gradual increase in insulin secretion, which stimulates glucose uptake by peripheral insulin-dependent tissues. Approximately 80% to 85% of glucose metabolism during this time occurs in muscle.[12] Slower release of insulin allows the body to respond to the new glucose entering from digestion while maintaining blood glucose levels.

Amylin is a naturally occurring hormone that is cosecreted from β-cells with insulin. People with diabetes have either a relative or complete lack of amylin. Amylin has three major mechanisms of action: suppression of postmeal glucagon secretion, regulation of the rate of gastric emptying from the stomach to the small intestine, and the suppression of appetite.

▶ Impaired Insulin Secretion

A pancreas with normal β-cell function is able to adjust insulin production to maintain normal blood glucose levels.

Hyperinsulinemia, or high blood levels of insulin, is an early finding in the development of T2DM. More insulin is secreted to maintain normal blood glucose levels until eventually the pancreas can no longer produce sufficient insulin. The resulting hyperglycemia is enhanced by extremely high insulin resistance, pancreatic burnout in which β-cells lose functional capacity, or both. Patients with T2DM typically have approximately 40% β-cell function at diagnosis. Impaired β-cell function results in a reduced ability to produce a first-phase insulin response sufficient to signal the liver to stop producing glucose after a meal. As DM progresses, large numbers of patients with T2DM eventually lose all β-cell function and require exogenous insulin to maintain blood glucose control.[13]

▶ Insulin Resistance

Insulin resistance is the primary factor that differentiates T2DM from other forms of diabetes. Insulin resistance may be present up to 10 years prior to the diagnosis of DM and can continue to progress throughout the course of the disease. Resistance to insulin occurs most significantly in skeletal muscle and the liver. Insulin resistance in the liver poses a double threat since the liver becomes nonresponsive to insulin for glucose uptake, and hepatic production of glucose after a meal does not cease, which leads to elevated fasting and postmeal blood glucose levels.

▶ Impaired Glucagon Secretion

The release of glucagon is impaired in people with T1DM and T2DM. Glucagon is a counterregulatory hormone released by the α-cells that raises blood glucose levels. The release of insulin and the inhibition of glucagon is glucose-stimulated, meaning that as glucose is consumed, the release of insulin increases and the release of glucagon decreases in people without diabetes.[14] Most patients with a 10- to 20-year history of T1DM have lost their ability to release glucagon, which increases their risk for hypoglycemic unawareness. People with T2DM have impaired phase 1 and phase 2 insulin release, and some have impaired glucagon-like peptide 1 (GLP-1) and gastric inhibitory polypeptide (GIP) release, which further reduces the release of insulin. This leads to the liver producing and releasing glucose even in the postprandial state.[15]

▶ Metabolic Syndrome

Insulin resistance has been associated with a number of other cardiovascular risks, including abdominal obesity, hypertension, dyslipidemia, hypercoagulation, and hyperinsulinemia. The clustering of these risk factors has been termed metabolic syndrome. It is estimated that 50% of the U.S. population older than 60 years of age have metabolic syndrome. The most widely used criteria to define metabolic syndrome were established by the National Cholesterol Education Program Adult Treatment Panel III Guidelines[16] (summarized in Table 43–2). Patients having these additional risk factors have been found to be at a much

Table 43–2
Five Components of Metabolic Syndrome

Risk Factor	Defining Level
1. Abdominal obesity	
• Men	Waist circumference greater than 102 cm (40 inches)
• Women	Waist circumference greater than 89 cm (35 inches)
2. Triglycerides	Greater than or equal to 150 mg/dL (1.70 mmol/L)
3. HDL cholesterol	
• Men	Less than 40 mg/dL (1.04 mmol/L)
• Women	Less than 50 mg/dL (1.3 mmol/L)
4. Blood pressure	Greater than or equal to 130/85 mm Hg
5. Fasting glucose	Greater than or equal to 100 mg/dL (5.55 mmol/L)

Individuals having at least three of the five above meet the diagnostic criteria for metabolic syndrome.

From Ref. 16.

higher cardiovascular risk than would be expected from the individual components of the syndrome. Therefore, it is important to assume a more aggressive treatment plan for each of the individual abnormal components. As a result, a patient with prediabetes or DM having a convergence of other risk factors should be treated more aggressively than a patient having prediabetes or DM alone.

▶ Incretin Effect

A great deal of research is occurring today to develop compounds that enhance the incretin effect, either by mimicking its action or by enabling incretin hormones to remain physiologically active for longer periods of time.[15,17–19] As early as the late 1960s, Perley and others observed that insulin's response to oral glucose exceeded that of IV glucose administration.[19] It was concluded that factors in the gut, or incretins, affected the release of insulin after a meal is consumed. When nutrients enter the stomach and intestines, incretin hormones are released which stimulates insulin secretion. This was validated by measuring C-peptide and insulin response to the IV and oral glucose loads. GLP-1 and GIP are the two major incretin hormones, with GLP-1 being studied the most. GLP-1 is secreted by the L cells of the ileum and colon primarily, and GIP is secreted by the K cells.

GLP-1 was identified in the early 1980s. It is a 30/31 amino acid peptide that is a product of the glucagons gene. GLP-1 secretion is caused by endocrine and neural signals started when nutrients enter the GI tract. Within minutes of food ingestion, GLP-1 levels rise rapidly. A glucose-dependent release of insulin occurs and dipeptidyl peptidase-IV (DPP-IV) cleaves GLP-1 rapidly to an inactive metabolite. Much of the research on glucose lowering products involves prolonging the action of GLP-1. Other glucose lowering effects of GLP-1 include suppression of glucagons, slowing gastric emptying, and increasing satiety.[15,17–19]

CLINICAL PRESENTATION AND DIAGNOSIS
Screening

● Currently, the American Diabetes Association (ADA) recommends routine screening for T2DM every 3 years in all adults starting at 45 years of age. Earlier and more frequent screening should be reserved for patients who are at higher risk. The ADA does not recommend screening for T1DM due to the low incidence and acute presentation of symptoms.[20] See Table 43–3[20] for complete screening guidelines.

Gestational Diabetes

● Risk assessment for GDM should be performed early in pregnancy with a random glucose test. If the normal diagnostic threshold for diabetes is exceeded during the first

Clinical Presentation and Diagnosis of Diabetes Mellitus

Characteristic	T1DM	T2DM
Age of onset	Childhood or adolescence	Greater than 40 years of age
Speed of onset	Abrupt	Gradual
Family history	Negative	Positive
Body type	Thin	Obese or history of obesity
Metabolic syndrome	No	Often
Autoantibodies	Present	Rare
Symptoms	Polyuria, polydipsia, polyphagia, rapid weight loss	Asymptomatic
Ketones at diagnosis	Present	Uncommon
Acute complications	Diabetic keto acidosis	Rare
Microvascular complications at diagnosis	Rare	Common
Macrovascular complications at or before diagnosis	Rare	Common

Table 43–3

ADA Screening Recommendations for Diabetes

Asymptomatic type 1
The ADA does not recommend screening for T1DM due to the low incidence in the general population and to the acute presentation of symptoms

Asymptomatic type 2
1. The ADA recommends screening for T2DM every 3 years in all adults beginning at 45 years of age, particularly in those with a BMI greater than or equal to 25 kg/m²
2. Testing should be considered for persons younger than 45 years of age or more frequently in individuals who are overweight (BMI greater than or equal to 25 kg/m²) and have additional risk factors:
   • Habitually inactive
   • First-degree relative with diabetes
   • Member of a high-risk ethnic population (e.g., African American, Latino, Native American, Asian American, Pacific Islander)
   • Delivered a baby weighing greater than 4.1 kg (9 lb) or previous diagnosis of GDM
   • Hypertensive (greater than or equal to 140/90 mm Hg)
   • High-density lipoprotein (HDL) cholesterol level less than 35 mg/dL (0.91 mmol/L) and/or a triglyceride level greater than 250 mg/dL (2.83 mmol/L)
   • Polycystic ovary syndrome
   • Previous IGT or IFG
   • Other clinical conditions associated with insulin resistance (e.g., acanthosis nigricans)
   • History of vascular disease

Type 2 in children and adolescents
Criteria:
   • Overweight (BMI greater than 85th percentile for age and sex, weight for height greater than 85th percentile, or weight greater than 120% of ideal for height)
Plus any two of the following risk factors:
   • Family history of T2DM in first- or second-degree relatives
   • Race/ethnicity (Native American, African American, Latino/Hispanic American, Asian American, Pacific Islander)
   • Signs of insulin resistance or conditions associated with insulin resistance (acanthosis nigricans, hypertension, dyslipidemia, or polycystic ovary disease)
Age of initiation:
   Age 10 or at onset of puberty, if puberty occurs at a younger age
   Frequency of testing: Every 2 years
   Test method: FPG preferred
Clinical judgment should be used to test for diabetes in high-risk patients who do not meet these criteria

Gestational diabetes
1. Risk assessment performed at first prenatal visit with random glucose screen
2. All women should be screened with an OGTT between weeks 24 and 28 of gestation unless they are in the low-risk category

ADA, American Diabetes Association; BMI, body mass index; FPG, fasting plasma glucose; GDM, gestational diabetes mellitus; IFG, impaired fasting glucose; IGT, impaired fasting glucose; OGTT, oral glucose tolerance test; T1DM, type 1 diabetes mellitus; T2DM, type 2 diabetes mellitus.

From Ref. 20.

test and confirmed on a subsequent day, a diagnosis of GDM can be made. Otherwise, all women should be screened with an oral glucose tolerance test (OGTT) between weeks 24 and 28 of gestation unless they are in the low-risk category. The diagnostic criteria for OGTT are listed in Table 43–4.[21] Women considered low risk include those of normal weight before pregnancy; younger than 25 years of age; without first-degree relatives with diabetes; non-Hispanic, non–African American, or non–Native American ethnicity; and no prior history of glucose intolerance or poor obstetric outcome.[7,21]

Any woman diagnosed with GDM should be retested at 6 weeks postpartum. If the fasting plasma glucose (FPG) level is normal, then reassessment for DM should occur every 3 years. Family planning for subsequent pregnancies should be discussed, and monitoring for the development of symptoms of DM should be undertaken.

Diagnostic Criteria

Diagnosis of DM includes glycemic outcomes exceeding threshold values with one of three testing options (Table 43–5).[21] Confirmation of abnormal values must be made on a subsequent day for diagnosis unless unequivocal symptoms of hyperglycemia exist, such as polydipsia, polyuria, and polyphagia. The ADA recommends FPG determination as the principal tool for diagnosis of DM in nonpregnant adults owing to ease of use, acceptability to patients, and lower cost.[20] While the OGTT is more sensitive

Table 43–4		
Diagnosis of Gestational Diabetes With a 100 or 75 g Glucose Load		
	Plasma Glucose	
Time	**mg/dL**	**mmol/L**
100 g glucose load		
Fasting	95	5.3
1 hour	180	10
2 hours	155	8.6
3 hours	140	7.8
75 g glucose load		
Fasting	95	5.3
1 hour	180	10
2 hours	155	8.6

Two or more venous plasma concentrations must be met or exceeded for a positive diagnosis of diabetes to be made. The test should be done in the morning after an 8- to 14-hour fast and after at least 3 days of unrestricted diet and unlimited physical activity. The patient should remain seated and should not smoke during the test.

From Ref. 21.

Table 43–6		
Categorization of Glucose Status		
	mg/dL	**Mmol/L**
FPG		
• Normal	Less than 100	Less than 5.6
• IFG (prediabetes)	100–125	5.6–6.9
• Diabetes	Greater than or equal to 126	7
2-hour postload plasma glucose (OGTT)		
• Normal	Less than 140	7.8
• IGT (prediabetes)	140–199	7.8–11
• Diabetes	Greater than or equal to 200	11.1

FPG, fasting plasma glucose; IFG, impaired fasting glucose; IGT, impaired glucose tolerance; OGTT, oral glucose tolerance test.

From Ref. 22.

and modestly more specific than FPG determination, it is more costly and difficult to reproduce the results and is rarely performed in practice today.

The ADA categorizes patients demonstrating IFG or IGT as having prediabetes.[21] The categorization thresholds of glucose status for FPG determination and the OGTT are listed in Table 43–6.[22] These two conditions may coexist or may be identified independently. FPG level represents hepatic glucose production during the fasting state, whereas postprandial glucose levels in the OGTT may reflect glucose uptake in peripheral tissues, insulin sensitivity, or a decreased first-phase insulin response.

Table 43–5
Criteria for the Diagnosis of Diabetes
1. Symptoms of diabetes plus a casual plasma glucose concentration greater than or equal to 200 mg/dL (11.1 mmol/L). *Casual* is defined as any time of day without regard to time since last meal. The classic symptoms of diabetes include polyuria, polydipsia, and unexplained weight loss
or
2. *FPG* greater than or equal to 126 mg/dL (7 mmol/L). *Fasting* is defined as no caloric intake for at least 8 hours
or
3. 2-hours postload glucose greater than or equal to 200 mg/dL (11.1 mmol/L) during an OGTT. The test should be performed as described by the WHO, using a glucose load containing the equivalent of 75 g anhydrous glucose dissolved in water

FPG, fasting plasma glucose; OGTT, oral glucose tolerance test; WHO, World Health Organization.

In the absence of hyperglycemia, these criteria should be confirmed by repeat testing on a different day. The OGTT is not recommended for routine clinical use.

From Ref. 21.

TREATMENT

Goals of Therapy

DM treatment goals include reducing long-term microvascular and macrovascular complications, preventing acute complications from high blood glucose levels, minimizing hypoglycemic episodes, and maintaining the patient's overall quality of life. To achieve these goals, near-normal blood glucose levels are fundamental, thus ❹ *glycemic control remains the primary objective in diabetes management.* Two landmark trials, the Diabetes Control and Complications Trial[2] and the United Kingdom Prospective Diabetes Study,[3] showed that lowering blood glucose levels decreased the risk of developing chronic complications. A near-normal blood glucose level can be achieved with appropriate patient education, lifestyle modification, and medications.

Proper care of DM requires goal setting and assessment for glycemic control, self-monitoring of blood glucose (SMBG), monitoring of blood pressure and lipid levels, regular monitoring for the development of complications, dietary and exercise lifestyle modifications, and proper medication use. The complexity of proper DM self-care principles has a dramatic impact on a patient's lifestyle and requires a highly disciplined and dedicated person to maintain long-term control.

▶ *Setting and Assessing Glycemic Targets*

❺ *Patients and clinicians can evaluate control of the patient's diabetes by monitoring daily blood glucose values, hemoglobin A_{1c} (A_{1c}) or estimated average glucose (eAG) values, blood pressure, and lipid levels.* SMBG enables patients to obtain their current blood glucose level at any time easily and relatively inexpensively. The A_{1c} test provides a weighted-mean blood glucose level from the previous 3 months.

Self-Monitoring of Blood Glucose SMBG is the standard method for routinely checking blood glucose levels. Each reading provides a point-in-time evaluation of glucose control that can vary widely depending on numerous factors including food, exercise, stress, and time of day.

By examining multiple individual points of data, patterns of control can be established. Therapy can be evaluated from these patterns, and adjustments can be made to improve overall blood glucose control. The ADA premeal plasma glucose goals are 70 to 130 mg/dL (3.9–7.2 mmol/L), and peak postprandial plasma glucose goals are less than 180 mg/dL (10 mmol/L).[7] The American Association of Clinical Endocrinologists (AACE) supports tighter SMBG controls, with premeal goals of less than 110 mg/dL (6.1 mmol/L) and peak postmeal goals of less than 140 mg/dL (7.8 mmol/L).[23] For patients with T1DM, the ADA recommends that SMBG be performed at least three times daily. The frequency of testing in patients with T2DM is still controversial. The ADA recommends testing frequently enough to gain and maintain blood glucose control. While the majority of practitioners recommend SMBG to their patients with T1DM, the role of SMBG in improving glucose control in T2DM is unproven.[24]

Typically, in SMBG, a drop of blood is placed on a test strip that is then read by a blood glucose monitor. Recent technological advancements have decreased the blood sample size required to as small as 0.3 microliters, provide the capability of alternate site testing, and deliver readings in as few as 5 seconds. Many SMBG devices can download or transfer information to a computer program that can summarize and produce graphs of the data. Identifying patterns in the patient's blood glucose data can aid practitioners in modifying treatment for better glucose control. Specific therapy adjustments can be made for patterns found at certain times of the day, on certain days, or with large day-to-day variances.

While most testing occurs by lancing the fingertip to produce a blood droplet, alternate-site testing has been approved for testing the palm, arm, leg, and abdomen. Alternate-site testing was developed as a means to decrease the pain encountered with repeated fingersticks by using body locations that have a lower concentration of nerve endings.

In choosing a glucose meter for a patient, several additional factors may aid in the best selection for the patient. Larger display areas or units with audible instructions and results may be better suited for older individuals and those with visual impairment. Patients with arthritis or other conditions that decrease dexterity may prefer larger meters with little or no handling of glucose strips. Younger patients or busy professionals may prefer smaller meters with features such as faster results, larger memories, reminder alarms, and downloading capabilities. Several continuous glucose sensors are now available that work with or independently of insulin pumps. These monitors provide blood glucose readings, primarily through interstitial fluid (ISF). A small sterile disposable glucose-sensing device called a sensor is inserted into the subcutaneous tissues. This sensor measures the change in glucose in ISF, and sends the information to a monitor which stores the results. The monitor must be calibrated daily by entering several blood glucose readings obtained at different times using a standard blood glucose meter.

Hemoglobin A$_{1c}$ Glucose interacts spontaneously with hemoglobin in red blood cells to form glycosylated derivatives. The most prevalent derivative is A$_{1c}$. Greater amounts of glycosylation occur when blood glucose levels increase. Because hemoglobin has a life span of approximately 120 days, levels of A$_{1c}$ provide a marker reflecting the average glucose levels over this timeframe.[25] The ADA goal for persons with DM is less than 7%, whereas the AACE supports a goal of less than 6.5%. Testing A$_{1c}$ levels should occur at least twice a year for patients who are meeting treatment goals and four times per year for patients not meeting goals or those who have had recent changes in therapy.

Estimated Average Glucose Recently the ADA and several other organizations have introduced replacing the use of A$_{1c}$ with eAG. This value more closely correlates with readings that patients obtain from their home glucose monitors. The equation to convert from A$_{1c}$ to eAG is: eAG = 28.7 × A$_{1c}$ – 46.7.[26] The goal eAG would be 154 mg/dL (8.55 mmol/L) instead of an A$_{1c}$ of less than 7%, and an eAG of 240 mg/dL (13.32 mmol/L) would be equivalent to an A$_{1c}$ of 10%.

Ketone Monitoring Urine/blood ketone testing is important in people with T1DM, in pregnancy with preexisting diabetes, and in GDM. People with T2DM may have positive ketones and develop diabetic ketoacidosis (DKA) if they are ill.

The presence of ketones may indicate a lack of insulin or ketoacidosis, a condition that requires immediate medical attention. When there is a lack of insulin, peripheral tissues cannot take up and store glucose. This causes the body to think it is starving and excessive lipolysis and ketones, primarily β-hydroxybutric and acetoacetic acid, are produced as byproducts of free fatty acid metabolism in the liver. Glucose and ketones are osmotically active, and when an excessive amount of ketones are formed, the body gets rid of them through urine leading to dehydration. Patients with T1DM should test for ketones during acute illness or stress or when blood glucose levels are consistently elevated above 300 mg/dL (16.65 mmol/L). This commonly occurs when insulin is omitted. Women with pre-existing diabetes before pregnancy or with GDM should check ketones using their first morning urine sample or when any symptoms of ketoacidosis such as nausea, vomiting, or abdominal pain are present. Positive ketone readings are found in normal individuals during fasting and in up to 30% of first morning urine specimens from pregnant women. Urine ketone tests using nitroprusside containing reagents can give false-positive results in the presence of several medications including captopril. False-negative readings have been reported when test strips have been exposed to air for an extended period of time or when

Table 43-7

ADA Recommended Goals of Therapy

Area	Goals
Glycemia	
A_{1c}	Less than 7%
	Evaluate every 3 months until in goal; then every 6 months
eAG	Less than 154 mg/dL (8.5 mmol/L)
Preprandial plasma glucose	70–130 mg/dL (3.9–7.2 mmol/L)
Peak postprandial plasma glucose[a]	Less than 180 mg/dL (less than 10 mmol/L)
Blood Pressure	Less than 130/80 mm Hg
	Evaluate at every visit
Lipids	Evaluate at least yearly
LDL	Less than 100 mg/dL (2.59 mmol/L) or less than 70 mg/dL (1.81 mmol/L) if high risk
HDL	Greater than 40 mg/dL (1.04 mmol/L) for males; greater than 50 mg/dL (1.3 mmol/L) for females
Triglycerides	Less than 150 mg/dL (1.70 mmol/L)
Monitoring for Complications	
Eyes	Dilated eye exam yearly
Feet	Feet should be examined at every visit
Urinary microalbumin	Yearly

A_{1c}, hemoglobin A_{1c}; eAG, estimated average glucose; HDL, high-density lipoprotein; LDL, low-density lipoprotein.

[a]Peak postprandial glucose measurements should be made 1 to 2 hours after the beginning of the meal.

urine specimens have been highly acidic, such as after large intakes of ascorbic acid. Currently, available urine ketone tests are not reliable for diagnosing or monitoring treatment of ketoacidosis. Blood ketone testing methods that quantify β-hydroxybutyric acid, the predominant ketone body, are available and are the preferred way to diagnose and monitor ketoacidosis.

Home tests for β-hydroxybutyric acid are available. The specific treatment of DKA may differ at institutions but includes rehydration, correction of electrolyte imbalances, and insulin administration.

▶ Blood Pressure, Lipids, and Monitoring for Complications

The ADA standards of medical care address many of the common comorbid conditions, as well as complications that result from the progression of DM. Table 43–7 presents goals for blood pressure measurements, lipids values, and monitoring parameters for complications associated with diabetes.

General Approach to Therapy

▶ Type 1 Diabetes Mellitus

Treatment of T1DM requires providing exogenous insulin to replace the endogenous loss of insulin from the nonfunctional pancreas. Ideal insulin therapy mimics normal insulin physiology. The basal-bolus approach attempts to reproduce basal insulin response using intermediate- or long-acting insulin, whereas short- or rapid-acting insulin replicates bolus release of insulin physiologically seen around a meal

in nondiabetics. A number of different regimens have been used through the years to more closely follow natural insulin patterns. As a rule, basal insulin makes up approximately 50% of the total daily dose. The remaining half is provided with bolus doses around three daily meals.

Exact doses are individualized to the patient and the amount of food consumed. T1DM patients frequently are started on about 0.6 unit/kg/day, and then doses are titrated until glycemic goals are reached. Most people with T1DM use between 0.6 and 1 unit/kg/day.

Currently, the most advanced form of insulin delivery is the insulin pump, also referred to as continuous subcutaneous insulin infusion (CSII). Using rapid-acting insulin only, these pumps are programmed to provide a slow release of small amounts of insulin as the basal portion of therapy, and larger boluses of insulin are injected by the patient to account for the consumption of food. Pramlintide, a synthetic analog of the naturally occurring hormone amylin, is another injectable blood glucose lowering medication that can be used in people with T1DM or in people with T2DM using insulin for treatment. A more in-depth description is listed in the pharmacologic treatment section.

▶ Type 2 Diabetes Mellitus

Treatment of T2DM has changed dramatically over the past decade with the addition of a number of new drugs and the ADA recommendations to maintain tighter glycemic control. Figures 43–1 and 43–2 summarize updated treatment algorithms for T2DM.[27] Algorithms from AACE for T2DM can be found at *www.aace.com/pub*.[28] Lifestyle modifications including education, nutrition, and exercise

Patient Encounter, Part 1

You have developed a collaborative practice with a group of family practice practitioners and run a small apothecary in the same office as theirs. You have established a patient education and monitoring center in conjunction with a registered dietician, nurse practitioner, and physician's assistant at the office.

EP is a 58-year-old Caucasian male who is 6 ft, 0 in. (183 cm) tall and weighs 118 kg (260 lb). He comes in today for his annual physical. He has a 10-year history of hypertension and elevated cholesterol. His fasting blood sugar today was 190 mg/dL (10.5 mmol/L). He is asked to have fasting labs done and then return to the office in 3 days for a reevaluation. His fasting blood sugar at the return visit is 165 mg/dL (9.2 mmol/L) and additional information from his return visit and labs are listed below.

Labs:

Fasting glucose: 190 mg/dL (10.5 mmol/L) and 165 mg/dL (9.2 mmol/L); **BP:** 148/86 mm Hg; **BUN:** 123 mg/dL (43.9 mmol/L); **creatinine:** 0.9 mg/dL (80 µmol/L); **GFR** (Modified Diet in Renal Disease [MDRD]) 90.8; **AST/SGOT:** 19 IU/L (0.32 µKat/L); **ALT/SGPT:** 20 IU/L (0.33 µKat/L); **TSH:** 1.26 microunits/mL (1.26 mU/L); **total cholesterol:** 202 mg/dL (5.23 mmol/L); **LDL:** 118 mg/dL (3.05 mmol/L); **HDL:** 43 mg/dL (1.11 mmol/L); **triglycerides:** 205 mg/dL (2.32 mmol/L); A_{1c}: 7.9%; **body fat:** 42.8%; **waist circumference:** 44 inches (112 cm).

PMH: History of hypertension × 10 years; history of elevated cholesterol × 10 years; occasional cold symptoms over the last several years; reports last eye examination about 20 years ago; believes he could use glasses

FH: Father 84 years of age—history of hypertension, stroke, and myocardial infarction; mother 78 years of age—history of T2DM, hypertension, and obesity; sister 56 years of age—history of gestational diabetes mellitus (GDM), T2DM, and obesity

SH: Drinks six packs of beer on weekends and self-reports that he does not smoke or use tobacco products or illegal substances

Meds: Atenolol 50 mg (takes one tablet daily to lower BP); hydrochlorothiazide 25 mg (takes one tablet daily to lower BP); simvastatin 40 mg (takes one tablet daily to lower cholesterol)

Meal History: Fast food for morning and evening meal that is high in carbohydrate and saturated fat. Jelly donuts and coffee for breakfast and peanut butter and banana sandwiches for lunch on other days. High fat meats, starchy vegetables, rolls and sweet tea for supper most nights

PH: No outside work activity. Dances some on stage when performs.

What information is suggestive of diabetes?

What criteria must be met before a diagnosis of diabetes can be made?

What type of diabetes do you think EP has based on his clinical characteristics?

What challenges can you identify for optimal clinical outcomes through the initial assessment of EP?

What additional information do you need to obtain before creating a treatment plan and goals with EP?

---

are paramount to managing the disease successfully. Many patients assume that once pharmacologic therapy is initiated, lifestyle modifications are no longer necessary. Practitioners should educate patients regarding this misconception. Because T2DM generally tends to be a progressive disease, blood glucose levels will eventually increase, making insulin therapy and lifestyle modifications the eventual required therapy in many patients. It may be necessary for patients to inject insulin to lower their blood glucose levels. Figure 43–2 is an illustration of a way to start insulin therapy, while keeping the patient on some oral medications. This is usually done when several oral agents have been used with inadequate glucose lowering results.[27]

▶ *Gestational Diabetes*

An individualized meal plan consisting of three meals and three snacks per day is commonly recommended in GDM. Preventing ketosis, promoting adequate growth of the fetus, maintaining satisfactory blood glucose levels, and preventing nausea and other undesired GI side effects are desired goals in these patients. Controlling blood sugar levels is important to prevent harm to the baby. An abundance of glucose causes excessive insulin production by the fetus which, if left uncontrolled, can lead to the development of an abnormally large fetus. Infant hypoglycemia at delivery, hyperbilirubinemia, and complications associated with delivery of a large baby also may occur when blood glucose levels are not controlled adequately.

Insulin should be used when blood glucose levels are not maintained adequately at target levels by diet and physical activity. Even though there have been small studies showing the safety of using glyburide, metformin, and insulin glargine during pregnancy, the use of these agents is not recommended as a general rule. In women who develop GDM and cannot control blood glucose levels with lifestyle modifications, the use of insulin aspart, lispro, or regular insulin have category B safety ratings.

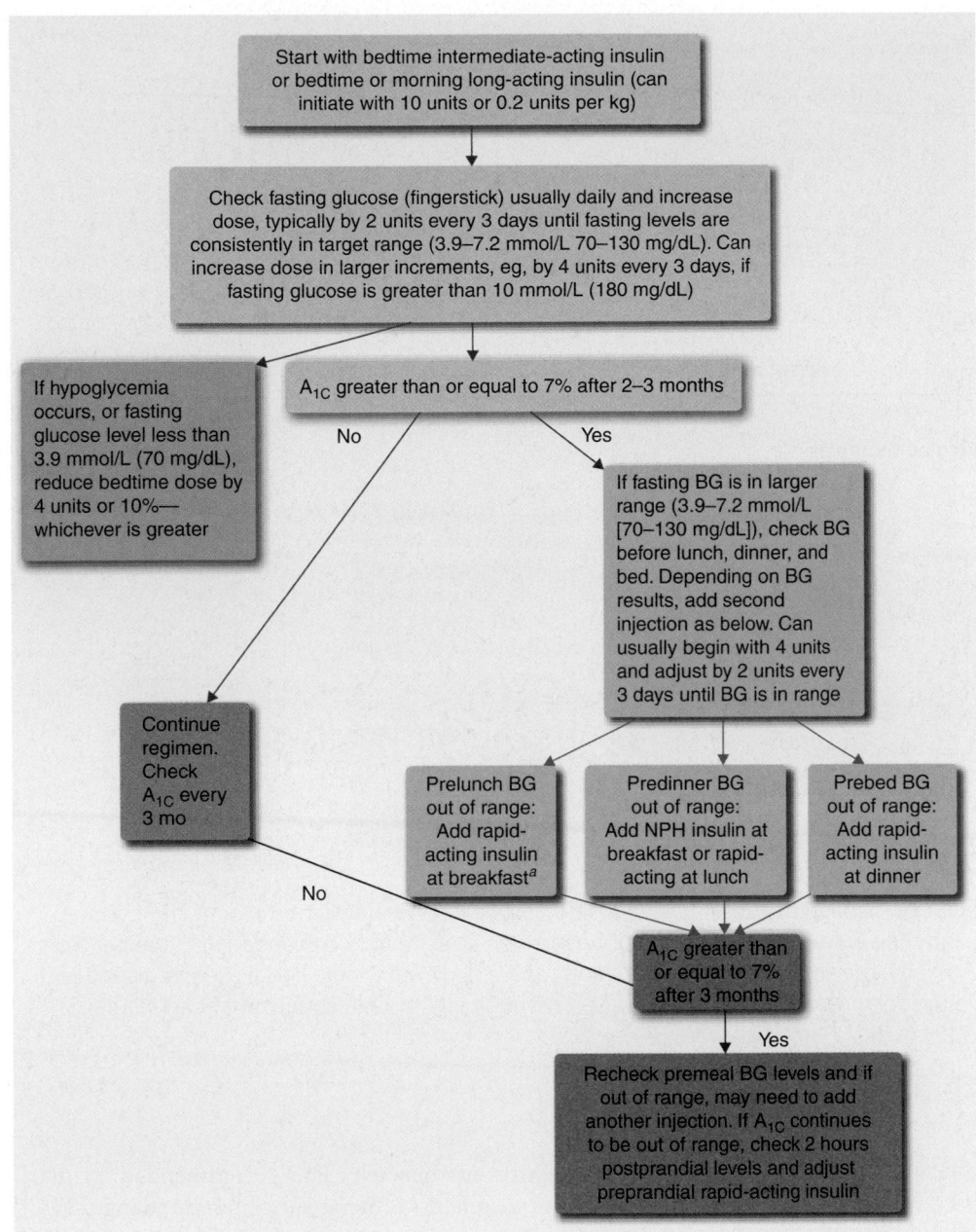

FIGURE 43–1. Initiation and adjustment of insulin regimens. Insulin regimens should be designed taking lifestyle and meal schedule into account. The algorithm can only provide basic guidelines for initiation and adjustment of insulin. [a]Premixed insulins not recommended during adjustment of doses; however, they can be used conveniently, usually before breakfast and/ or dinner, if proportion of rapid- and intermediate-acting insulins is similar to the fixed proportions available. (A_{1c}, hemoglobin A_{1c}; BG, blood glucose; NPH, neutral protamine Hagedorn.) (From Ref. 27.)

Nonpharmacologic Therapy

▶ *Medical Nutrition Therapy*

Despite the popular notion, there is not a "diabetic diet," and the recommended meal plan for patients with diabetes should be low in fat, high in fiber, low to moderate in calories, and achieve a balance of the various components and nutrients needed.[27] Medical nutrition therapy (MNT) is considered an integral component of diabetes management and diabetes self-management education. People with DM should receive individualized MNT, preferably by a registered dietitian. As part of the diabetes management plan, MNT should not be a single education session, but rather an ongoing dialog. MNT should be customized to take into account cultural, lifestyle, and financial considerations. MNT plans should integrate a variety of foods that the patient enjoys and allow for flexibility to encourage patient empowerment and improve patient adherence.

During these MNT educational and planning sessions, patients receive instructions on appropriate food selection, preparation, and proper portion control. The primary focus of MNT for patients with T1DM is matching optimal insulin dosing to carbohydrate consumption. In T2DM, the primary focus is portion control and controlling blood glucose, blood pressure and lipids through individualizing limits of carbohydrates, saturated fats, sodium, and calories.

Carbohydrates are the primary contributor to postmeal glucose levels. There have been recent studies showing the benefit of low carbohydrate meal plans, especially to enhance weight loss. Total daily carbohydrate levels should

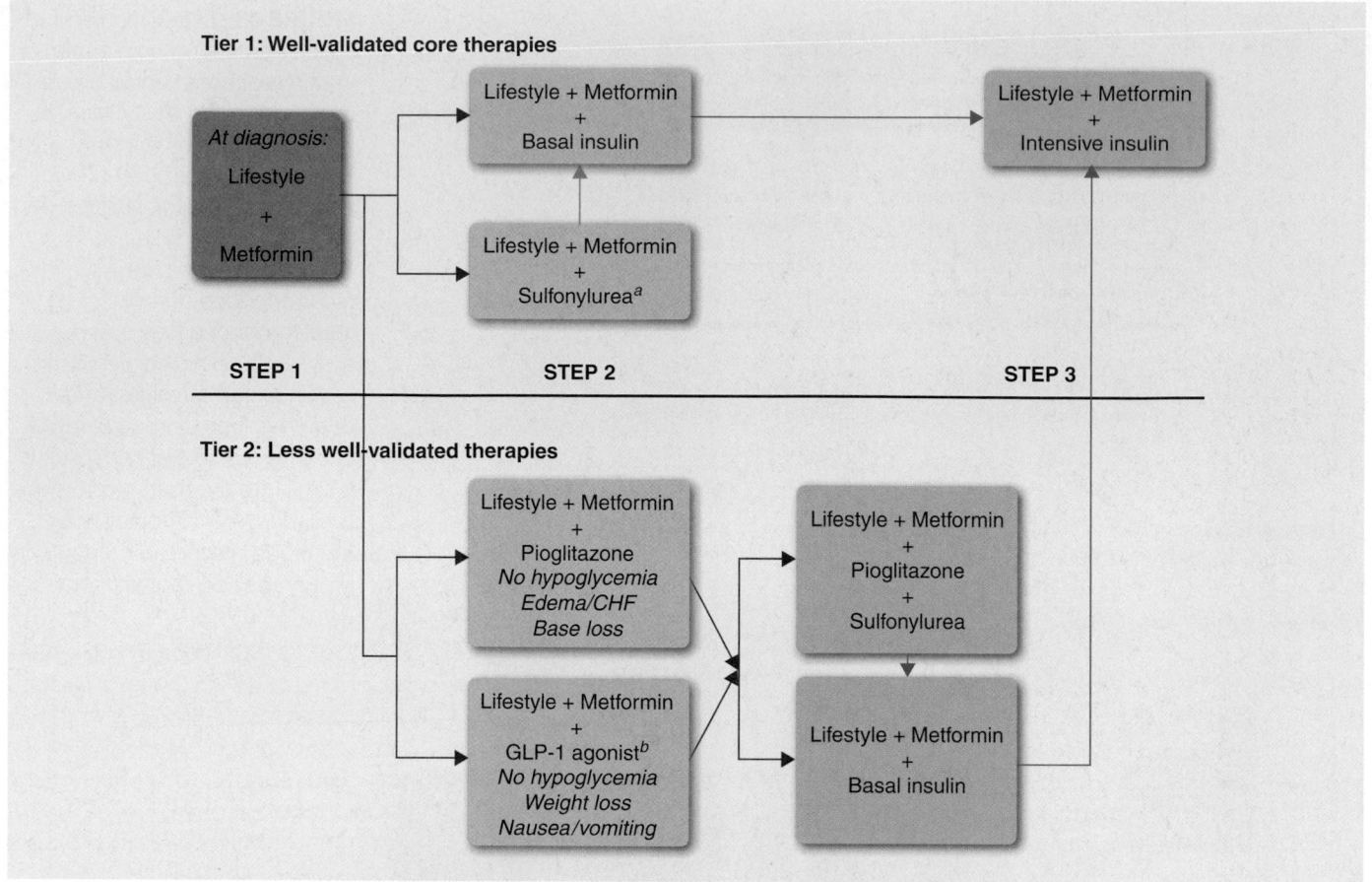

FIGURE 43–2. Algorithm for the metabolic management of T2DM; reinforce lifestyle interventions at every visit and check A_{1c} every 3 months until A_{1c} less than 7% and then at least every 6 months. The interventions should be changed if A_{1c} greater than or equal to 7%. [a]Sulfonylureas other than glybenclamide (glyburide) or chlorpropamide. [b]Insufficient clinical use to be confident regarding safety. See Figure 43–1 for initiation and adjustment of insulin. (A_{1c}, hemoglobin A_{1c}; CHF, congestive heart failure; GLP-1, glucagon-like peptide-1.) (From Ref. 27.)

not be less than 135 g for most patients and should make up approximately 40% of calories. The percentage of fat, protein, and other components of the meal should be individualized based on the specific goals of the patient.

▶ Dietary Supplements

Many patients with diabetes may seek and utilize dietary supplements in the treatment of diabetes. Commonly used products include α-lipoic acid, omega-3 fatty acids, and chromium. Current clinical evidence regarding dietary supplements is limited and does not support the use of these agents as treatment. Nevertheless, patients will inquire and use dietary supplements. It is important that pharmacists respect the patient's health beliefs, address their questions and concerns, and educate patients on the differences between dietary supplements and prescribed therapies.[29]

▶ Weight Management

Moderate weight loss has been shown to reduce cardio-vascular risk, as well as delay or prevent the onset of DM

in those with prediabetes. The recommended primary approach to weight loss is therapeutic lifestyle change (TLC), which integrates a 500 to 1,000 kcal/day (about 2,100–4,200 kJ/day) reduction in calorie intake and an increase in physical activity.[30] A slow but progressive weight loss of 0.45 to 0.91 kg (1–2 lb) per week is preferred. While individual target caloric goals should be set, a general rule for weight loss diets is that they should supply at least 1,000 to 1,200 kcal/day (about 4,200–5,000 kJ/day) for women and 1,200 to 1,600 kcal/day (about 5,000–6,700 kJ/day) for men. Because 80% of patients with T2DM are overweight, this strategy works best for these patients.

▶ Physical Activity

Physical activity is also an important component of a comprehensive DM management program. Regular physical activity has been shown to improve blood glucose control and reduce cardiovascular risk factors such as hypertension and elevated serum lipid levels. Physical activity is also a primary factor associated with long-term maintenance of weight loss and overall weight control. Regular physical activity also may prevent the onset of T2DM in high-risk persons.

Prior to initiating a physical activity program, several considerations should be made. Patients should undergo a detailed physical examination, including screening for microvascular or macrovascular complications that may be worsened by a particular activity. Initiation of physical activities in an individual with a history of a sedentary lifestyle should begin with a modest increase in activity. Walking, swimming, and cycling are examples of low-impact exercises that could be encouraged. At the same time, gardening and usual housecleaning tasks are good exercises as well. Long-term goals are to perform at least 30 minutes of aerobic activity as many days a week as possible.[22]

▶ Psychological Assessment and Care

Mental health and social state have been shown to have an impact on a patient's ability to carry out DM management care tasks. Approximately one in four patients with DM experience episodes of major depression. Clinicians should incorporate psychological assessment and treatment into routine care. The ADA guidelines recommend psychological screening, which includes determining the patient's attitudes regarding DM, expectations of medical management and outcomes, mood and affect, general and diabetes-related quality of life, and financial, social, and emotional resources. Patients demonstrating nonadherence, depression, an eating disorder, and/or cognitive functioning that impairs judgment should be referred to a mental health specialist familiar with DM.[7]

▶ Immunizations

Influenza and pneumonia are common preventable infectious diseases that increase mortality and morbidity in persons with chronic diseases including DM.[7] Yearly influenza vaccinations, commonly called flu shots, are recommended for patients with DM. Pneumococcal vaccination is also recommended for patients with DM as a one-time vaccination for most patients.

Pharmacologic Therapy

❻ *Oral and injectable agents are available to treat patients with T2DM who are unable to achieve glycemic control through meal planning and physical activity.* Currently there are 10 classes of blood glucose lowering agents available for the treatment of diabetes: seven classes of oral agents and three injectable classes. Figure 43–1 shows a way to start insulin therapy for people with T2DM who are going to continue to take oral glucose lowering medications.[27] Table 43–8[31–34] lists the oral agents, and Figure 43–2 displays the ADA Treatment Algorithm for Patients with T2DM.[27] The various classes of blood glucose lowering agents target different organs and have different mechanisms of action. Each of these agents may be used individually or in combination with other medications that target different organs for synergistic effects.

▶ Sulfonylureas

Sulfonylureas represent the first class of oral blood glucose lowering agents approved for use in the United States. These drugs are classified as being either first- or second-generation agents. Both classes of sulfonylureas are equally effective when given at equipotent doses. Today, the vast majority of patients receiving a sulfonylurea are prescribed a second-generation agent.

Sulfonylureas enhance insulin secretion by blocking ATP-sensitive potassium channels in the cell membranes of pancreatic β-cells. This action results in membrane depolarization, allowing an influx of calcium to cause the translocation of secretory granules of insulin to the cell surface, and enhances insulin secretion. The extent of insulin secretion depends on the blood glucose level. More insulin is released in response to higher blood glucose levels, whereas the additional insulin secretion from sulfonylureas is less at near-normal glucose levels. Insulin is then transported through the portal vein to the liver, suppressing hepatic glucose production.[12]

All sulfonylureas undergo hepatic biotransformation, with most agents being metabolized by the cytochrome P450 2C9 pathway. First-generation sulfonylureas are more likely to cause drug interactions than second-generation agents. All sulfonylureas except tolbutamide require a dosage adjustment or are not recommended in renal impairment. In elderly patients or those with compromised renal or hepatic function, lower starting dosages are necessary.

Sulfonylureas' blood glucose lowering effects can be observed in both fasting and postprandial levels. Monotherapy with these agents generally produce a 1.5% to 2% decline in A_{1c} concentrations and a 60 to 70 mg/dL (3.3–3.9 mmol/L) reduction in fasting blood glucose (FBG) levels. Secondary failure with these drugs occurs at a rate of 5% to 7% per year as a result of continued pancreatic β-cell destruction. One limitation of sulfonylurea therapy is the inability of these products to stimulate insulin release from β-cells at extremely high glucose levels, a phenomenon called glucose toxicity. Common adverse effects include hypoglycemia and weight gain. There may be some cross sensitivity in patients with sulfa allergy.

▶ Nonsulfonylurea Secretagogues (Glitinides)

While producing the same effect as sulfonylureas, non-sulfonylurea secretagogues, also referred to as meglitinides, have a much shorter onset and duration of action. Glitinide secretagogues also produce a pharmacologic effect by interacting with ATP-sensitive potassium channels on the β-cells; however, this binding is to a receptor adjacent to those to which sulfonylureas bind.

The primary benefit of nonsulfonylurea secretagogues is in reducing postmeal glucose levels by about 40 mg/dL (2.2 mmol/L). These agents have demonstrated a reduction in A_{1c} levels between 0.6% and 1%. Since they have a rapid onset and short duration of action, they are to be taken within 15 minutes of a meal.

Table 43–8

Oral Agents for the Treatment of T2DM

Drug Class	Target Organ	Blood Glucose Affected	Adjustment for Renal Impairment CrCl 30–50 mL/min	Adjustments for Renal impairment CrCl Less Than 30 mL/min	Adjustments for Hepatic Impairment	Common Adverse Drug Reactions	Drugs Trade	Generic/ Commercially Available	Dosing Strategy (All Agents Are Taken Orally)
α-Glucosidase Inhibitors	Brush border of small intestine	Postprandial	No dosage adjustment necessary	25 mL/min: Acarbose not recommended	None	GI (bloating, flatulence)	Precose	Acarbose/N	25 mg at start of meals Advance weekly to max of 100 mg 3 × daily (To be taken only if eating)
			No dosage adjustment necessary	25 mL/min: Acarbose not recommended	None		Glyset	Miglitol/N	25 mg 3 × daily at start of meals Advance weekly to max of 100 mg 3 × daily
Glitinides (should not be used in combination with insulin or other insulin secretagogues)	Pancreas	Postprandial	No dosage adjustment necessary	No dosage adjustment necessary	Possible increased hypoglycemia when combined with gemfibrozil due to inhibition of CYP2C8 by gemfibrozil and increased glucoronidation leading to prolonged action of repaglinide	Hypoglycemia	Prandin	Repaglinide/N	0.5 mg, 15–30 minutes before each meal Double preprandial dose every 7 days to max of 4 mg/ dose or 16 mg/ day (To be taken only if eating)
			No dosage adjustment necessary	No dosage adjustment necessary			Starlix	Nateglinide/N	120 mg 3 × day before meals (To be taken only if eating)
2nd Generation sulfonylureas	Pancreas	Fasting and postprandial	Not recommended	Not recommended	Dose adjustments may be necessary due to metabolism in the liver to prevent hypoglycemia		Micronase	Glyburide/Y	2.5–5 mg daily with breakfast Increase by 2.5–5 mg weekly to max of 20 mg daily
				Less than 10 mL/min: Not recommended			DiaBeta	Glyburide/Y	2.5–5 mg daily with breakfast Increase by 2.5–5 mg weekly to max of 20 mg daily

	Site of action	Glucose effect				Side effects	Brand name	Generic/Hypoglycemia	Dosage
				No dosage adjustment necessary			Glucatrol	Glipizide/Y	5 mg daily, 30 minutes before a meal. Increase by 5 mg weekly to max of 40 mg daily. Divide dose if greater than 15 mg/day
							Glucatrol XL	glipizide extended release/Y	5 mg once daily before a meal. Increase by 5 mg weekly to max of 20 mg daily
							Amaryl	Glimeperide/Y	
Biguanides	Liver	Fasting	Avoid	Avoid	Dosage adjustments not necessary	GI (bloating, diarrhea)	Glucophage Fortamet Riomet	Metformin/Y	500 mg daily with dinner. Advance weekly to max of 1,000 mg twice a day
							Glucophage ER, Glumetza	Metformin, extended release/Y	
Thiazolidinediones	Peripheral tissue	Fasting and postprandial	No dosage adjustment necessary	No dosage adjustment necessary	No dosage adjustments necessary	Edema (exacerbation of CHF) Weight gain	Avandia	Rosiglitazone/N	4 mg daily (or 2 mg twice a day). Increase after 12 weeks to a max of 8 mg daily if alone or combined with other OAD and max of 4 mg daily if combined with insulin
							Actos	Pioglitazone/N	15–30 mg daily. Increase after 12 weeks to a max of 45 mg daily
Dipeptidyl peptidase-4 inhibitors	GI tract (increases GLP-1)	Postprandial	50 mg once daily	25 mg once daily	No dosage adjustment necessary	Upper respiratory	Januvia	Sitagliptin/N	25 mg daily. Advance weekly to max of 100 mg daily
	Increases GLP-1	Postprandial	2.5 mg once daily	2.5 mg once daily	No dose adjustment	Upper respiratory/headache	Onglyza	Saxagliptin	2.5 or 5 mg once daily
Dopamine receptor agonist	Hypothalamus	Postprandial	No dosage adjustment	No dosage adjustment	No dosage adjustment	Nausea, headache	Cycloset	Bromocriptine mesylate	1.6 to 4.8 mg once daily within 2 hours of waking

A1c, hemoglobin A1c; BUN, blood urea nitrogen; CHF, congestive heart failure; eAG, estimated average glucose; GLP-1, glucagon-like peptide-1; OAD, oral agent.

From Refs. 31–34, 44.

They also may be used in combination therapy with other drugs to achieve synergistic effects. Combinations with biguanides are most commonly seen.

▶ *Biguanides*

The only biguanide approved by the FDA and currently available in the United States is metformin. Metformin was approved in the United States in 1995. This agent is thought to lower blood glucose by decreasing hepatic glucose production and increasing insulin sensitivity in both hepatic and peripheral muscle tissues; however, the exact mechanism of action remains unknown. Metformin has been shown to reduce A_{1c} levels by 1.5% to 2% and FPG levels by 60 to 80 mg/dL (3.3–4.4 mmol/L) when used as monotherapy. The response to metformin can vary according to the baseline blood glucose levels. Larger effects can be seen in patients with a higher initial A_{1c} level (e.g., greater than 10%) than in patients beginning therapy with a relatively lower value (e.g., less than 8%). Metformin lowers both fasting blood sugar (FBS) and postmeal blood glucose. The ADA treatment algorithm (Fig. 43–2) considers lifestyle modification and metformin as first-line therapy.[27] Metformin does not affect insulin release from β-cells of the pancreas, so hypoglycemia is not a common side effect. Metformin has been shown to produce beneficial effects on serum lipid levels, and has become a first-line agent for T2DM patients with metabolic syndrome.

Triglyceride and low-density lipoprotein (LDL) cholesterol levels often are reduced by 8% to 15%, whereas high-density lipoprotein (HDL) cholesterol improves by approximately 2%.[31] Metformin is often used in combination with a sulfonylurea or a thiazolidinedione (TZD) for synergistic effects.

Metformin does not undergo significant protein binding and is eliminated from the body unchanged in the urine. Elderly patients with a calculated creatinine clearance of less than 70 to 80 mL/min should not receive this product. It is contraindicated in patients with a serum creatinine level greater than or equal to 1.4 mg/dL (124 μmol/L) in women and 1.5 mg/dL (133 μmol/L) in men. Additionally, therapy with metformin should be withheld in patients undergoing radiographic procedures in which a nephrotoxic dye is used. Therapy should be withheld the day of the procedure, and renal function should be assessed 48 hours after the procedure. If normal, therapy can be resumed.

Primary side effects associated with metformin therapy are GI in nature, including decreased appetite, nausea, and diarrhea. These side effects can be minimized through slow titration of the dose and often subside within 2 weeks.

Biguanides such as metformin are thought to inhibit mitochondrial oxidation of lactic acid, thereby increasing the chance of lactic acidosis occurring. Fortunately, the incidence of lactic acidosis in clinical practice is rare. Patients at greatest risk for developing lactic acidosis include those with liver disease or heavy alcohol use, severe infection, heart failure, and shock. Thus, it is common practice to evaluate liver function prior to initiation of metformin.

▶ *Thiazolidinediones*

Commonly referred to as TZDs or glitazones, thiazolidinediones have established a significant role in T2DM therapy. TZDs are known to increase insulin sensitivity by stimulating peroxisome proliferator-activated receptor gamma (PPAR-γ). Stimulation of PPAR-γ results in a number of intracellular and extracellular changes including an increased number of insulin receptors, increased insulin receptor sensitivity, decreased plasma fatty acid levels, and an increase in a host of intracellular signaling proteins that enhance glucose uptake.

As monotherapy, both rosiglitazone and pioglitazone reduce FPG levels by 30 to 50 mg/dL (1.7–2.8 mmol/L), and the overall effect on A_{1c} is a 1% to 1.5% reduction. Onset of action for TZDs is delayed for several weeks and may require up to 12 weeks before maximum effects are observed. Combining a sulfonylurea, nonsulfonylurea secretagogue, metformin, or insulin with a thiazolidinedione can improve A_{1c} reductions to 2% to 2.5%.

Additional effects of TZDs are seen in the lipid profile. Both pioglitazone and rosiglitazone increase HDL cholesterol by 3 to 9 mg/dL (0.08–0.23 mmol/L). Pioglitazone has been shown to decrease serum triglycerides by 10% to 20%, whereas no substantial effect is observed with rosiglitazone. LDL cholesterol concentrations increase by 5% to 15% with rosiglitazone, whereas no significant increase has been reported for pioglitazone.

TZDs may produce fluid retention and edema; the mechanism by which this occurs is not completely understood. It is known that blood volume increases approximately 10% with these agents, resulting in approximately 6% of patients developing edema. Thus, these drugs are contraindicated in situations in which an increased fluid volume is detrimental such as heart failure. Fluid retention appears to be dose-related and increases when combined with insulin therapy.

A few cases of hepatotoxicity have been reported with rosiglitazone and pioglitazone, but no serious complications have been reported, and symptoms typically reverse within several weeks of discontinuing therapy. Periodic liver function tests should be performed at baseline and periodically. Patients with a baseline alanine aminotransferase (ALT) level greater than 2.5 times the upper limit of normal should not receive a TZD. If ALT levels rise to greater than three times the upper limit of normal in patients receiving a TZD, the medication should be discontinued.

The results of several recent studies have posed questions on the benefit or harm of using these agents. Both agents require a black box warning of increased risk of heart failure.[35] Although the results of meta-analyses were not conclusive regarding possible cardiovascular risks related to rosiglitazone, the ADA no longer recommends the use of this agent.[27]

▶ *α-Glucosidase Inhibitors*

Acarbose and miglitol are α-glucosidase inhibitors currently approved in the United States. An enzyme that is along the brush boarder of the intestine cells called α-glucosidase breaks down complex carbohydrates into simple sugars, resulting in absorption. The α-glucosidase inhibitors work by delaying the absorption of carbohydrates from the intestinal tract, which reduces the rise in postprandial blood glucose concentrations. As monotherapy, α-glucosidase inhibitors primarily reduce postprandial glucose excursions. FPG concentrations have been decreased by between 40 and 50 mg/dL (2.2–2.8 mmol/L); however, A_{1c} reductions range only from 0.3% to 1%. While these agents have been popular in Europe and other parts of the world, they have failed to gain widespread use in the United States. High incidences of GI side effects including flatulence (41.5%), abdominal discomfort (11.7%), and diarrhea (28.7%) have limited their use. GI side effects occur as the result of intestinal bacteria in the distal gut metabolizing undigested carbohydrates and producing carbon dioxide and methane gas. Low initial doses followed by gradual titration may minimize GI side effects. The α-glucosidase inhibitors are contraindicated in patients with short-bowel syndrome or inflammatory bowel disease. In addition, neither drug in this class is recommended for patients with a creatinine clearance of less than 25 mL/min.

Because GI motility is increased in prediabetes and newly diagnosed patients, the α-glucosidase inhibitors are particularly useful when used early in the disease.

▶ Dipeptidyl Peptidase-4 Inhibitors

Sitagliptin, the first in a new class of diabetic drugs called dipeptidyl peptidase-4 (DPP-4) inhibitors, was approved in October 2006 as an adjunct to diet and exercise to improve glycemic control in adults with T2DM. These agents lower blood glucose concentrations by inhibiting DPP-4, the enzyme found in the intestinal K cells that degrades endogenous GLP-1 within 2 minutes of secretion. DPP-4 inhibitors increase the amount of endogenous GLP-1. The blood glucose lowering effect of the gliptins is primarily on postprandial levels. A modest reduction in FPG concentration can be observed because glucagon suppression will result in decreased hepatic gluconeogenesis. Because DPP-4 inhibitors can affect the regulation of GI motility, their greatest effects are noted in recently diagnosed T2DM, but they have been shown to be moderately effective in people with long-standing diabetes. Typical A_{1c} reductions are 0.6% to 0.8%. Common adverse effects include diarrhea, nasopharyngitis, upper respiratory tract infections, and headache. Hypoglycemia is not a common adverse effect with these agents because insulin secretion results from GLP-1 activation due to meal-related glucose detection and not from direct pancreatic β-cell stimulation. Dosage adjustments to 50 and 25 mg daily are recommended for patients with moderate (creatinine clearance 30–49 mL/min) and severe (creatinine clearance less than 30 mL/min) renal impairment, respectively. Renal function monitoring is recommended prior to initiation and periodically thereafter.

The U.S. Food and Drug Administration (FDA) is revising the prescribing information for sitagliptin and sitagliptin/metformin to include information on reported cases of acute pancreatitis in patients using these products after 88 postmarketing cases of acute pancreatitis, including two cases of hemorrhagic or necrotizing pancreatitis, were reported between October 2006 and February 2009 in patients taking sitagliptin.

A second agent, saxagliptin, was recently approved and dosing information can be found in Table 43–8.

▶ Central Acting Dopamine Agonist

A quick release formulation of a central acting dopamine agonist, bromocriptine, has been approved by the FDA in May 2009 for the treatment of T2DM. It has the potential of being used as monotherapy or combination therapy with existing oral agents. Available evidence indicates that the therapy acts centrally to reset hypothalamic centers, regulating postprandial insulin-mediated glucose and lipid metabolism to thereby reduce postprandial hyperglycemia and hyperlipidemia. It should be taken 2 hours after waking in the morning with food. The initial dose used in clinical trials was 0.8 mg, titrated up weekly until a maximum dose of 1.6 to 4.8 mg daily is achieved. It will be available as a 0.8-mg tablet and is currently not on the market. The main side effects during clinical trials included headache and nausea. Several contraindications include hypotension, syncopal migranes, and women that are nursing.

▶ Insulin

Insulin is the one agent that can be used in all types of DM with the most effectiveness for blood sugar control.[33] ❼ *Insulin is the primary treatment to lower blood glucose levels for patients with T1DM and injected amylin can be added to decrease fluctuations in blood glucose levels.* An insulin treatment algorithm for T2DM is found in Figure 43–2.[27]

Insulin is available commercially in various formulations that vary markedly in terms of onset and duration of action. Insulin can be divided into two main classes, basal and bolus, based on their length of action to mimic endogenous insulin physiology. Most formulations are available as U-100, indicating a concentration of 100 unit/mL. Insulin is typically refrigerated, and most vials are good for 28 days at room temperature. Insulin detemir can be stored at room temperature for 42 days. Specific details of insulin products are listed in Table 43–9.[32,33]

The most common route of administration for insulin is subcutaneous injection using a syringe or pen device. Patients should be educated to rotate their injection sites to minimize lipohypertrophy, a build up of fat that decreases or prevents proper insulin absorption. Additionally, patients should understand that the absorption rate may vary among injection sites (abdomen, thigh, arm, and buttocks) due to differences in blood flow, with absorption occurring fastest in the abdomen and slowest in the buttocks. Differences in absorption of insulin based on site of injection do not appear to be significant when analog insulins such as aspart, detemir, glargine, glulisine, and lispro are administered.

Insulin syringes are distinguished according to the syringe capacity, syringe markings, and needle gauge, and length.

Table 43-9

Insulin Agents for the Treatment of T1DM and T2DM

Generic Name (Insulin)	Brand/Rx Only	Manufacturer	Strength	Onset (minutes)	Peak (hours)	Duration (hours)	Administration Options
Rapid-Acting Insulin							
Lispro	Humalog/yes	Eli Lilly	U-100	15–30	0.5–2.5	3–4	10 mL vial, 3 mL cartridge and disposable pen
Aspart	Novolog/yes	Novo-Nordisk	U-100	15–30	1–3	3–5	10 mL vial, 3 mL cartridge and disposable pen
Glulisine	Apidra/yes	Aventis	U-100	15–30	1–2	3–4	10 mL vial, 3 mL cartridge and disposable pen
Short-Acting Insulin							
Regular	Humulin R/no	Eli Lilly	U-100, U-500	30–60	2–3	3–6	U-100 10 mL vial; U-500 20 mL vial
	Novolin R/no	Novo-Nordisk	U-100				10 mL vial, 3 mL cartridge, 3 mL *InnoLet*
Intermediate-Acting Insulin							
Neutral protamine Hagedorn	Humulin N/no	Eli Lilly	U-100	2–4 hours	4–6	8–12	10 mL vial, 3 mL cartridge
	Novolin N/no	Novo-Nordisk	U-100				10 mL vial, 3 mL cartridge, 3 mL *InnoLet*
Long-Acting Insulin							
Glargine	Lantus/yes	Aventis	U-100	4–5 hours	Flat	22–24	10 mL vial, 3 mL cartridge for *Opticlik* Available in SoloSTAR disposable pen
Detemir	Levemir/yes	Novo-Nordisk	U-100	3–4 hours	Flat	Up to 24	10 mL vial, 3 mL cartridge, 3 mL *InnoLet*, 3 mL disposable *FlexPen*
Combination Insulin Products							
Neutral protamine Hagedorn and regular	Humulin 70/30/no	Eli Lilly	U-100	30–60	1.5–16	10–16	10 mL vial, 3 mL disposable pen
	Novolin 70/30/no	Novo Nordisk	U-100	30–60	2–12	10–16	10 mL vial, 3 mL cartridge, 3 mL *InnoLet*
	Humulin 50/50/no	Eli Lilly	U-100	30–60	2–5.5	10–16	10 mL vial
Neutral protamine lispro and lispro	Humalog Mix 75/25/yes	Eli Lilly	U-100	15–30	1–6.5	15–18	10 mL vial, 3 mL disposable pen
Neutral protamine aspart and aspart	Novolog Mix 70/30/yes	Novo Nordisk	U-100	15–30	1–4	Up to 24	10 mL vial, 3 mL cartridge, 3 mL disposable *FlexPen*

From Refs. 32, 33.

Insulin pens are self-contained systems of insulin delivery. The primary advantage of the pen system is that the patient does not have to draw up the dose from the insulin vial.

Bolus Insulins

Regular Insulin. Regular insulin is unmodified crystalline insulin commonly referred to as natural or human insulin. It is a clear solution that has a relatively short onset and duration of action and is designed to cover insulin response to meals. On subcutaneous injection, regular insulin forms small aggregates called hexamers that undergo conversion to dimers followed by monomers before systemic absorption can occur. Patients should be counseled to inject regular insulin subcutaneously 30 minutes prior to consuming a meal. Regular insulin is the only insulin that can be administered IV.

Rapid-Acting Insulin. Three rapid-acting insulins have been approved in the United States: aspart, glulisine, and lispro. Substitution of one or two amino acids in regular insulin results in the unique pharmacokinetic properties characteristic of these agents. Onset of action of rapid-acting insulins varies from 15 to 30 minutes, with peak effects occurring 1 to 2 hours following administration and is dosed prior to or with meals.

Basal Insulins

Intermediate-Duration Insulin. Neutral protamine Hagedorn, better known as NPH insulin, is prepared by a process in which protamine is conjugated with regular insulin, rendering a product with a delayed onset but extended duration of action, and is designed to cover insulin requirements in between meals and/or overnight. With the advent of the long-acting insulins, NPH insulin use has declined due to: (a) an inability to predict accurately when peak effects occur and (b) a duration of action of less than 24 hours. Additionally, protamine is a foreign protein that may increase the possibility of an allergic reaction.

NPH insulin can be mixed with regular insulin and used immediately, or stored for future use up to 1 month at room temperature or 3 months in refrigeration. NPH insulin can be mixed with either aspart or lispro insulins, but it must be injected immediately after mixing. Whenever mixing insulin products with NPH insulin, the shorter-acting insulin should be drawn into the syringe first.

Long-Duration Insulin. Two long-duration insulin preparations are approved for use in the United States. Glargine and detemir are designed as once-daily-dosing basal insulins. Insulin glargine differs from regular insulin by three amino acids, resulting in a low solubility at physiologic pH. The clear solution is supplied at a pH of 4, which precipitates on subcutaneous administration.

Detemir binds to albumin in the plasma which gives it sustained action. Neither glargine nor detemir can be administered IV or mixed with other insulin products. Neither glargine or detemir produce peak serum concentrations, and both can be administered irrespective of meals or time of day.[36]

Combination Insulin Products

A number of combination insulin products are available commercially. NPH is available in combinations of 70/30 (70% NPH and 30% regular insulin) and 50/50 (50% NPH and 50% regular insulin). Two short-acting insulin analog mixtures are also available. Humalog mix 75/25 contains 75% insulin lispro protamine suspension and 25% insulin lispro. Novolog mix 70/30 contains 70% insulin aspart protamine suspension and 30% insulin aspart. The lispro and aspart insulin protamine suspensions were developed specifically for these mixture products and will not be commercially available separately.

▶ *Insulin Pump Therapy*

Insulin pump therapy consists of a programmable infusion device that allows for basal infusion of insulin 24 hours daily (Fig. 43–3), as well as bolus administration prior to meals and snacks. Currently there are seven commercially available

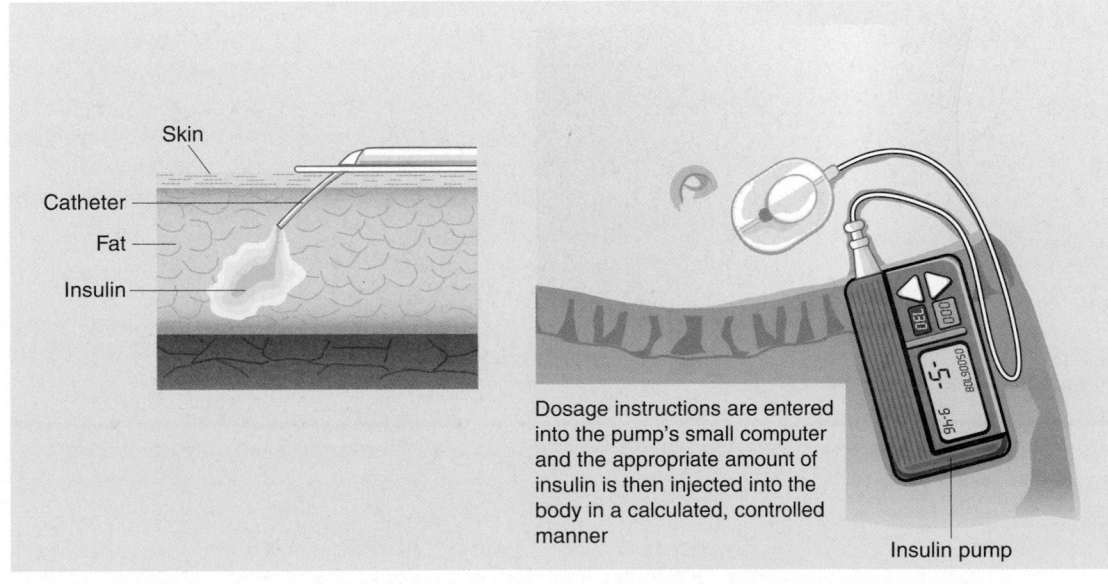

FIGURE 43–3. Insulin pump and placement.

Skin

Catheter

Fat

Insulin

Dosage instructions are entered into the pump's small computer and the appropriate amount of insulin is then injected into the body in a calculated, controlled manner

Insulin pump

insulin pumps in the United States. Insulin is delivered from a reservoir either by infusion set tubing or through a small canula. Most pump infusion sets are inserted in the abdomen, arm, or other infusion site by a small needle. Most patients prefer insertion in abdominal tissue because this site provides optimal insulin absorption. Infusion sets should be changed every 2 to 3 days to reduce the possibility of infection.

Patients use a carbohydrate-to-insulin ratio to determine how many units of insulin are required. More specifically, an individual's ratio is calculated to determine how many units of the specific insulin being used in the pump "covers" for a certain amount of carbohydrates to be ingested at a particular meal. The 450 rule or 500 rule is commonly used. To calculate the ratio using the 500 rule, the patient would divide 500 by his or her total daily dose of insulin. For example, if a patient were using 25 units of insulin daily, his or her carbohydrate-to-insulin ratio would be 500:25, or 20:1. This ratio theoretically means that 1 unit of rapid-acting insulin should cover 20 g of carbohydrate. If blood sugar levels are below or above the desired blood glucose target, the amount of insulin can be adjusted. Once this ratio is determined, patients can eat more or fewer carbohydrates at a given meal and adjust the bolus dose accordingly.

Insulin pump therapy may be used to lower blood glucose levels in any type of DM; however, patients with T1DM are the most likely candidates to use these devices. Use of an insulin pump may improve blood glucose control, reduce wide fluctuations in blood glucose levels, and allow individuals to have more flexibility in timing and content of meals and exercise schedules. Insulin pump therapy is not for everyone and the complexity associated with its use, cost, increased need for blood glucose monitoring, and psychological factors may prevent individuals from using this technology optimally.

▶ *Incretin Mimetics*

Incretin mimetics are agents with biologic activities similar to incretin hormones but have longer durations of action. Incretin hormones are substances produced by the GI tract in response to food that stimulates insulin secretion. It is thought that obese, insulin-resistant patients with T2DM have lower levels of incretin hormones. This may or may not be true. Exenatide (Byetta), is the first incretin mimetic approved by the FDA and is indicated as adjunct therapy in T2DM in which adequate blood glucose control has not been achieved with sulfonylureas, metformin, or both (Table 43–10).[37] A_{1c} reductions ranging from 0.5% to 1% have

Table 43–10

Noninsulin Injectable Agents for the Treatment of Diabetes

Generic Name (Brand)	Type of Diabetes	Dosage Strengths (mcg)[a]	Starting Dosage	Doses/ Day	Titration Interval	Maximum Dose (mcg)	Time to Effect (minutes)	Comments/Cautions
Pramlintide[b] (Symlin)	1	15, 30, 45, 60	15	3	3–7 days	60	20	Take just before major meals; reduce insulin by 50% Maintenance dose 30–60 mcg
	2	60, 120	60	3	3–7 days	120	20	Side effects: Hypoglycemia, nausea, vomiting Available in SymlinPen 60 and 120
Exanatide[b] (Byetta)	2	5, 10	5	2	1 month	10	15–30	Inject 15–20 minutes before 2 meals of the day with 6 hours separating the meals; prefilled disposable pen. May delay absorption of oral drugs; separate doses by 1 hour Side effects: Nausea, vomiting, diarrhea, increased hypoglycemia with sulfonylureas

[a]Pramlintide supplied as 0.6 mg/mL in 5-mL vials. Exanatide supplied as 250 mcg/mL, 1.2 mL for the 5-mcg prefilled pen, and 2.4 mL for the 10-mcg per dose prefilled pen.

[b]Generic not available in United States.

From Ref. 37.

been observed with this agent, whereas FPG concentrations decrease by 8 to 10 mg/dL (0.44–0.56 mmol/L). Postprandial glucose values decline by 60 to 70 mg/dL (3.3–3.9 mmol/L).

Exenatide lowers blood glucose levels by: (a) producing glucose-dependent insulin secretion; (b) reducing postmeal glucagon secretion which decreases postmeal glucose output; (c) increasing satiety which decreases food intake; and (d) regulating gastric emptying which allows nutrients to be absorbed into the circulation more smoothly. Serum levels peak approximately 2 hours after subcutaneous administration. Exenatide is eliminated renally and is not recommended in patients with a creatinine clearance of less than 30 mL/min.

An increased risk of hypoglycemia occurs when exenatide is used in combination with a sulfonylurea, and the dose of the sulfonylurea may need to be reduced or discontinued once blood glucose control improves. Hypoglycemia is not encountered when used as monotherapy or in conjunction with metformin and/or thiazolidinedione therapy. Side effects include nausea (44%), vomiting (13%), and diarrhea (13%). No major drug interactions have been found with exenatide. The extent and rate of absorption of orally administered drugs may be affected with concomitant use of exenatide; however, no clinical significance has been established to date.

Exenatide is available in 5 and 10 mcg injectable prefilled disposable pens. Initial therapy is 5 mcg twice daily, injected before the two largest meals of the day. Meals should be separated by at least 5 to 6 hours. Doses are then increased after a month to 10 mcg if the patient's blood glucose is improving and nausea is limited. Exenatide can be given up to 60 minutes before a meal, but practical use indicates that injection 15 to 20 minutes before a meal may decrease nausea. An average weight loss of 1.4 to 2.3 kg (3–5 lb) commonly occurs with the 5 mcg dose, whereas a weight loss of 2.3 to 4.6 kg (5–10 lb) is observed with the 10 mcg dose.

Amylin Pramlintide acetate was approved for use in the United States in March 2005 (Table 43–10).[35] This agent is a synthetic analog of human amylin, which is a naturally occurring neuroendocrine peptide that is cosecreted by the β-cells of the pancreas in response to food. Amylin secretion is completely deficient in patients with T1DM, or relatively deficient in patients with T2DM. Pramlintide is given by subcutaneous injection before meals to lower postprandial blood glucose elevations. Pramlintide generally results in an average weight loss of 1 to 2 kg (2.2–4.4 lb).

Pramlintide is indicated as combination therapy with insulin in patients with types 1 or 2 DM. It has been shown to decrease A_{1c} by an additional 0.4% to 0.5%. Pramlintide slows gastric emptying without altering absorption of nutrients, suppresses glucagon secretion, and leads to a reduction in food intake by increasing satiety. By slowing gastric emptying, the normal initial postmeal spike in blood glucose is reduced.

Hypoglycemia, nausea, and vomiting are the most common side effects encountered with pramlintide therapy, although pramlintide itself does not produce hypoglycemia. To decrease the risk of hypoglycemia, doses of short-acting, rapid-acting, or premixed insulins should be reduced by 50% before pramlintide is initiated. Some practitioners will not decrease the premeal insulin dose this much because of fear of loss of glucose control. Primarily, the kidneys metabolize pramlintide, but dosage adjustments in liver or kidney impairment are not required.

Pramlintide has the potential to delay the absorption of orally administered medications. When rapid absorption is needed for efficacy of an agent, pramlintide should be administered 2 hours before or 1 hour after this drug. Pramlintide should not be used in patients receiving medications that alter GI motility, such as anticholinergic agents, or drugs that slow the absorption of nutrients such as α-glucosidase inhibitors. A disposable pen formulation is now on the market and available as SymlinPen 60 for patients with T1DM and SymlinPen 120 for people with T2DM. The number of days the pen will last will vary depending on the daily dose. The amount of medication is 1.5 mL in the SymlinPen 60 and 2.7 mL in the SymlinPen 120.

Treatment of Concomitant Conditions

▶ *Glucose Control and Cardiovascular Health*

The results of three trials have recently been released showing the relationship between glucose control and cardiovascular health. The Action to Control Cardiovascular Risk in Diabetes (ACCORD),[38] Action in Diabetes and Vascular Disease (ADVANCE),[39] and Veterans Affairs Diabetes Trial (VADT)[40] examined if cardiovascular risks could be decreased or prevented with intensive glucose lowering. Other variables were evaluated in these trials, but the results indicated a decrease in cardiovascular events with tighter glycemic control.

At the same time, there was an increase in mortality reported in the ACCORD trial, but not in the ADVANCE or VADT trials. Additionally, these studies demonstrated that controlling blood pressure and cholesterol in these patients were beneficial. For more detailed results of these trials, the reader is referred to the references indicated above.

▶ *Coronary Heart Disease*

Nearly two-thirds of patients with DM will die of coronary heart disease (CHD). Interventions targeting smoking cessation, glycemic control, blood pressure control, lipid management, antiplatelet therapy, and lifestyle changes, including diet and exercise, can reduce the risk of cardiovascular events. Patients with diabetes should receive at least an 81 mg aspirin daily unless contraindicated.

▶ *Hyperlipidemia*

The National Cholesterol Education Program Adult Treatment Panel III guidelines classify the presence of DM to be of the same risk equivalence as CHD.[16] The primary target for lipid-lowering treatment of LDL cholesterol is less than 100 mg/dL (2.59 mmol/L). For patients at high cardiovascular risk, the LDL target is 70 mg/dL (1.81 mmol/L). Treatment with a HMG-CoA reductase inhibitor, commonly called a *statin,* is often required to achieve these goals. After LDL cholesterol goals are reached, triglyceride and HDL goals also should be achieved. Treatments including niacin or fibrate therapy may be used to reach these secondary goals. However, caution should be used with statin and fibrate combination therapy because a higher risk of adverse events has been reported (refer to Chap. 12: Dyslipidemias).

▶ Hypertension

❽ *Uncontrolled blood pressure plays a major role in the development of macrovascular events and nephropathy in patients with DM. The ADA recommends that blood pressure goals for patients with DM be less than 130/80 mm Hg.* In addition, there are several general principles regarding the treatment of hypertension in diabetes patients. Angiotensin-converting enzyme (ACE) inhibitors, angiotensin II receptor blockers, and calcium channel blockers are recommended as initial therapy because of their beneficial effects on renal function. Low-dose thiazide diuretics also can be used as either first- or second-line therapy.

The most common use of thiazide diuretics for patients with DM is in synergistic combination with other agents. Another choice of treatment is β-blockers which can also be used as either first- or second-line therapies. While β-blockers may mask the symptoms of hypoglycemia, it is generally believed that the benefit of β-blockers outweighs the low risk of hypoglycemia in patients with T2DM. In order to achieve blood pressure goals, most patients require combination therapy with two or three antihypertensive agents.

Treatment of Acute Complications

▶ Hypoglycemia

Hypoglycemia, or low blood sugar, can be defined clinically as a blood glucose level of less than 50 mg/dL (2.8 mmol/L). Individuals with DM can experience symptoms of hypoglycemia at varying blood glucose levels. Patients who have regular blood glucose levels as high as 300 to 400 mg/dL (16.7–22.2 mmol/L) may experience symptoms of hypoglycemia once blood glucose levels are lowered to the middle to upper 100 mg/dL (5.55 mmol/L) range. Most people whose blood glucose levels are controlled adequately may experience symptoms when levels fall below 70 mg/dL (3.9 mmol/L). Symptoms of hypoglycemia include shakiness, sweating, fatigue, hunger, headaches, and confusion.

Common causes of hypoglycemia include delayed or inadequate amounts of food intake, especially carbohydrates, excessive doses of medications (e.g., sulfonylureas and insulin), exercising when insulin doses are reaching peak effect, or inadequately adjusted drug therapy in patients with impaired renal or hepatic function. Patients experiencing symptoms of hypoglycemia should check their blood glucose level, consume 15 g of carbohydrate, and wait 10 to 15 minutes for symptom resolution. Examples of acceptable treatments may include a small box of raisins, 4 oz (approximately 120 mL) of orange juice, 8 oz (approximately 240 mL) of skim milk, or three to six glucose tablets. In patients receiving an

α-glucosidase inhibitor in combination with a sulfonylurea or insulin, hypoglycemia should be treated with glucose tablets or skim milk owing to the mechanism of action of the α-glucosidase inhibitors.

For those patients whose blood glucose levels have dropped below 50 mg/dL (2.8 mmol/L), as much as 30 g of carbohydrate may be necessary to raise blood glucose levels adequately. For patients with hypoglycemia experiencing a loss of consciousness, a glucagon emergency kit should be administered by intramuscular or subcutaneous route. It is important to contact emergency medical personnel in this particular situation. The patient should be rolled onto his or her side to prevent aspiration, as many patients receiving the glucagon injection will vomit.

▶ Diabetic Ketoacidosis

DKA is a reversible but potentially life-threatening medical emergency that results from a relative or absolute deficiency in insulin. Without insulin, the body cannot use glucose as an energy source and must obtain energy via lipolysis. This process produces ketones and leads to acidosis. While DKA occurs frequently in young patients with T1DM on initial presentation, it can occur in adults as well as with patients who have T2DM. Often, precipitating factors such as infection or errors in administration of insulin or oral diabetes medications can cause DKA. Signs and symptoms develop rapidly over a few hours and commonly include fruity or acetone breath, nausea, vomiting, dehydration, polydipsia, polyuria, and deep, rapid breathing. Nonspecific symptoms include lethargy, headache, and weakness.

Hallmark diagnostic criteria for DKA include hyperglycemia (greater than 250 mg/dL, 13.9 mmol/L), ketosis (anion gap greater than 10), and acidosis (arterial pH less than or equal to 7.25). Typical fluid deficit is 6 L or more, and major deficits of serum sodium and potassium are common.

The severity of DKA depends on the magnitude of the decrease in arterial pH, serum bicarbonate levels, and the mental state rather than the magnitude of the hyperglycemia. Treatment goals of DKA consist of reversing the underlying metabolic abnormalities, rehydrating the patient, and normalizing the serum glucose. Fluid replacement with normal saline at 1 L/h is recommended to rehydrate the patient and to ensure that the kidneys are perfused.

Potassium and other electrolytes are supplemented as indicated by laboratory assessment. The use of sodium bicarbonate in DKA is controversial and generally not recommended when the pH is greater than or equal to 7.1. Regular insulin at 0.1 to 0.2 unit/kg/h by continuous IV infusion is the preferred treatment in DKA to regain metabolic control rapidly. Once plasma glucose values drop below 250 mg/dL (13.9 mmol/L), the insulin infusion may be decreased, and dextrose 5% to 10% can be added to the IV fluids. During the recovery period, it is recommended to continue administering insulin and to allow patients to eat as soon as possible. Dietary carbohydrates combined with insulin assist in the clearance of ketones.

Resolution of DKA is indicated by a blood glucose level of less than 200 mg/dL (11.1 mmol/L), a bicarbonate level of

Table 43–11

Management of DKA

1. Confirm diagnosis (increased plasma glucose, positive serum ketones, metabolic acidosis)
2. Admit to hospital; intensive-care setting may be necessary for frequent monitoring or if pH less than 7 or unconscious
3. Assess: Serum electrolytes (K^+, Na^+, Mg^{2+}, Cl^-, bicarbonate, phosphate), acid–base status—pH, HCO_3^-, Pco_2, β-hydroxybutyrate, renal function (creatinine, urine output)
4. Replace fluids: 2–3 L of 0.9% saline over first 1–3 hours (5–10 mL/kg/h); subsequently, 0.45% saline at 150–300 mL/h; change to 5% glucose and 0.45% saline at 100–200 mL/h when plasma glucose reaches 250 mg/dL (14 mmol/L)
5. Administer regular insulin: IV (0.1 unit/kg) or IM (0.4 unit/kg), then 0.1 unit/kg/h by continuous IV infusion; increase 2- to 10-fold if no response by 2–4 hours. If initial serum potassium is less than 3.3 mmol/L (3.3 mEq/L), do not administer insulin until the potassium is corrected to greater than 3.3 mmol/L (3.3 mEq/L)
6. Assess patient: What precipitated the episode (e.g., nonadherence, infection, trauma, infarction, cocaine)? Initiate appropriate workup for precipitating event (cultures, chest x-ray, ECG)
7. Measure capillary glucose every 1–2 hours; measure electrolytes (especially K^+, bicarbonate, phosphate) and anion gap every 4 hours for first 24 hours
8. Monitor blood pressure, pulse, respirations, mental status, and fluid intake and output every 1–4 hours
9. Replace K^+: 10 mEq/h when plasma K^+ less than 5.5 mEq/L (5.5 mmol/L), ECG normal, urine flow and normal creatinine documented; administer 40–80 mEq/h when plasma K^+ less than 3.5 mEq/L (3.5 mmol/L) or if bicarbonate is given
10. Continue above until patient is stable, glucose goal is 150–250 mg/dL (8.3–14 mmol/L), and acidosis is resolved. Insulin infusion may be decreased to 0.05–0.1 unit/kg/h
11. Administer intermediate or long-acting insulin as soon as patient is eating. Allow for overlap in insulin infusion and subcutaneous insulin injection

Cl, chloride; HCO_3, serum bicarbonate; IM, intramuscular; K, potassium; Mg, magnesium; Na, sodium; Pco_2, partial pressure of carbon dioxide in the arterial blood.

From Refs. 41, 42.

greater than or equal to 10 mEq/L (10 mmol/L), and a venous pH of greater than 7.3. See Table 43–11 for the management of DKA.[41,42]

▶ Hyperosmolar Hyperglycemic State

Hyperosmolar hyperglycemic state (HHS) is a life-threatening condition similar to DKA that also arises from inadequate insulin, but HHS occurs primarily in older patients with T2DM. DKA and HHS also differ in that HHS lacks the lipolysis, ketonemia, and acidosis associated with DKA. Patients with hyperglycemia and dehydration lasting several days to weeks are at the greatest risk of developing HHS. Illness and infection are common precipitating causes of HHS. Two main diagnostic criteria for HHS are a plasma glucose value of greater than 600 mg/dL (33.3 mmol/L) and a serum osmolality of greater than 320 mOsm/kg. The extreme hyperglycemia and large fluid deficits resulting from osmotic diuresis are major challenges to overcome with this condition. Similar to DKA, the treatment of HHS consists of aggressive rehydration, correction of electrolyte imbalances, and continuous insulin infusion to normalize serum glucose. However, in patients with HHS, blood glucose levels should be reduced gradually to minimize the risk of cerebral edema.

Treatment of Long-Term Complications

▶ Retinopathy

Diabetic retinopathy occurs when the microvasculature that supplies blood to the retina becomes damaged. This damage permits leakage of blood components through the vessel walls. Diabetic retinopathy is the leading cause of blindness in adults 20 to 74 years of age in the United States. Retinopathy is staged as either nonproliferative or proliferative.

Nonproliferative retinopathy often causes no visual disturbances and may remain asymptomatic for years. Proliferative retinopathy occurs when new retinal vessels form as a result of retinal ischemia in a process called neovascularization. Vision loss from proliferative retinopathy may range from mild blurring to obstruction of vision to complete blindness. Blurred vision is the presenting symptom for many patients who are diagnosed with diabetes. The ADA recommends that patients with DM receive a dilated eye examination annually by an ophthalmologist or optometrist. Glycemic control is the best prevention for slowing the progression of retinopathy. Early retinopathy may be reversed with improved glucose control.

▶ Neuropathy

❾ Peripheral neuropathy is the most common complication reported in T2DM. This complication generally presents as pain, tingling, or numbness in the extremities. The feet are affected more often than the hands and fingers. A number of treatment options have been tried with mixed success. Current options include pregabalin, gabapentin, low-dose tricyclic antidepressants, duloxetine, venlafaxine, topiramate, nonsteroidal anti-inflammatory drugs, and topical capsaicin.

Autonomic neuropathy is also a common complication as DM progresses. Clinical presentation of autonomic neuropathy may include gastroparesis, resting tachycardia, orthostatic hypotension, impotence, constipation, and hypoglycemic autonomic failure. Therapy for each individual autonomic complication is addressed separately.

▶ *Microalbuminuria and Nephropathy*

DM is the leading contributor to end-stage renal disease. Early evidence of nephropathy is the presence of albumin in the urine. Therefore, as the disease progresses, larger amounts of protein spill into the urine. The ADA recommends urine protein tests annually in T2DM patients. For children with T1DM, annual urine protein testing should begin with the onset of puberty or 5 years after the diagnosis of diabetes. The most common form of screening for protein in the urine is a random collection for measurement of the urine albumin/creatinine ratio. The desirable value is less than 30 mcg of albumin per mg of creatinine.

Microalbuminuria is defined as between 30 and 300 mcg of albumin per mg of creatinine. The presence of micro-albuminuria is a strong risk factor for future kidney disease in T1DM patients. In T2DM patients, microalbuminuria has been found to be a strong risk factor for macrovascular disease.

Glycemic control and blood pressure control are primary measures for the prevention of progression of nephropathy. ACE inhibitors and angiotensin II receptor blockers prevent the progression of renal disease in T2DM patients. Treatment of advanced nephropathy includes dialysis and kidney transplantation.

▶ *Foot Ulcers*

🔟 *Lower extremity amputations are one of the most feared and disabling sequelae of long-term uncontrolled DM. A foot ulcer is an open sore that develops and penetrates to the subcutaneous tissues. Complications of the feet develop primarily as a result of peripheral vascular disease, neuropathies, and foot deformations.*

Peripheral vascular disease causes ischemia to the lower limbs. This decreased blood flow deprives the tissues of oxygen and nutrients, and impairs the ability of the immune system to function adequately. Symptoms of peripheral vascular disease include intermittent claudication, cold feet, pain at rest, and loss of hair on the feet and toes. Smoking cessation is the single most important treatment for peripheral vascular disease. In addition, exercising by walking to the point of pain, and then resting and resuming can be a vital therapy to maintain or improve the symptoms of peripheral vascular disease. Pharmacologic intervention with pentoxifylline or cilostazol also may be useful to improve blood flow and reduce the symptoms of peripheral vascular disease.

Neuropathies play a large part in the development of foot ulcers. Loss of sensation in the feet allows trauma to go unnoticed. Autonomic neuropathy can cause changes in the blood flow, perspiration, skin hydration, and possibly bone composition of the foot. Motor neuropathy can lead to muscle atrophy, resulting in weakness and changes in the shape of the foot. To prevent foot complications, the ADA

Patient Encounter, Part 2: Follow-Up Visit

EP comes in 1 week later for more education and brings in his blood glucose readings for you to download and review with him. See below. Readings are in units of mg/dL (mmol/L)

	Before Breakfast	After Breakfast	Before Lunch	After Lunch	Before Supper	After Supper	Bedtime
Mon	118 (6.5)					168 (9.3)	
Tue	122 (6.8)					187 (10.4)	
Wed	134 (7.4)					140 (7.8)	
Thur	110 (6.1)					244 (13.5)	
Fri	98 (5.4)					257 (14.3)	
Sat	128 (7.1)					297 (16.5)	
Sun	116 (6.4)					240 (13.3)	

Are his blood glucose readings within target? What questions would you ask EP? Has a pattern been established?

You ask EP to remove his shoes and socks and you perform a foot screening. Why did you do this? Why is it important to record the results of the foot screening?

Does EP need to be referred to any specialists? If so, what type?

What nonpharmacologic interventions would you recommend for EP?

Are his blood pressure and lipids under control? Would you make any adjustments to therapy, and if so, specifically what?

---

recommends daily visual examination of the feet and a foot check performed at every physician visit. Sensory testing with a 10-gauge monofilament can detect areas of neuropathy. Treatment consists of glycemic control, preventing infection, debriding dead tissues, applying dressings, treating edema, and limiting ambulation. Untreated foot problems may develop gangrene, necessitating surgical intervention.

Special Situations

▶ *Hospitalized Care*

Aggressive treatment of hyperglycemia in hospitalized patients can prevent unnecessary cost to patients and health care systems. When patients are either physically or emotionally stressed, counterregulatory hormones are released, increasing blood glucose levels.

Insulin drip therapy for patients with blood glucose levels greater than 140 mg/dL (7.8 mmol/L) is considered superior to sliding-scale insulin. Sliding-scale insulin therapy typically lags the blood glucose level instead of proactively addressing the increased blood glucose levels. Blood glucose levels can be measured by several methods. Arterial samples are usually 5 mg/dL (0.28 mmol/L) higher than capillary values and 10 mg/dL (0.56 mmol/L) greater than venous values.

When preparing an insulin infusion for a patient, several factors must be considered. Insulin will absorb to glass and plastic, reducing the amount of insulin actually delivered by 20% to 30%. Priming the tubing will decrease variability of insulin infused. Therefore, when patients can be converted safely from infusion to needle and syringe therapy, the total daily dose should be reduced by 20% to 50% of the daily infusion amount.

When transferring someone from IV insulin drip to subcutaneous insulin, basal insulin should be administered several hours before the drip is discontinued to prevent loss of glycemic control. IV drip protocols are institution specific and will not be discussed. Hospitals may apply to receive a Certificate of Distinction for Inpatient Diabetes Care sponsored by the Joint Commission and the ADA.[43]

▶ Sick Days

Patients should monitor their blood glucose levels more frequently during sick days because it is common for illness to increase blood glucose values. Patients with T1DM should check ketones when their blood glucose levels are greater than 300 mg/dL or higher. This may need to be done every 1 to 2 hours and additional insulin coverage may be necessary to prevent DKA.[39] Sugar and electrolyte solutions such as sports drinks may be used by T1DM patients to prevent dehydration, electrolyte depletion, and hypoglycemia. Insulin treated patients with longstanding T2DM may also require ketone testing on sick days. Patients with T2DM may require sugar-free products if blood glucose levels are elevated consistently. Patients should be advised to eat smaller meals if possible during sick days to decrease nausea and maintain blood glucose control. With proper management, patients can decrease their chance of illness-induced hospitalization.

OUTCOME EVALUATION

- The success of therapy for DM is measured by the ability of the patient to manage his or her disease appropriately between health care provider visits.

- Appropriate therapy necessitates adequate patient education about the disease, development of a meal plan to which patients can comply, and integration of a regular exercise program.

Patient Encounter, Part 3: Follow-Up

It has been 3 years since EP was diagnosed with diabetes. His weight is now 123 kg (270 lb) and additional information can be found below about today's visit.

Fasting glucose: 190 mg/dL (10.5 mmol/L); **BP**: 142/84 mm Hg; **BUN**: 13 mg/dL (4.64 mmol/L); **creatinine**: 0.9 mg/dL (80 μmol/L); **AST/SGOT**: 19 IU/L (0.34 μKat/L); **ALT/SGPT**: 20 IU/L (0.33 μKat/L); **TSH**: 1.26 microunits/mL (1.26 mU/L); **total cholesterol**: 236 mg/dL (6.1 mmol/L); **LDL**: 152 mg/dL (3.93 mmol/L); **HDL**: 29 mg/dL (0.75 mmol/L); **triglycerides**: 223 mg/dL (2.52 mmol/L); A_{1c}: 10.6%; **body fat**: 48%; **waist circumference**: 48 inches (122 cm).

Blood Glucose Results (Units of mg/dL [mmol/L])

	Before Breakfast	After Breakfast	Before Lunch	After Lunch	Before Supper	After Supper	Bedtime
Mon				206 (11.4)			
Tue				227 (12.6)			
Wed	235 (13)				201 (11.2)		
Thur			300 (16.7)				260 (14.4)
Fri						233 (12.9)	
Sat	220 (12.2)			285 (15.8)			269 (14.9)
Sun	240 (13.3)						273 (15.2)

Current Meds:

- Metformin 1,000 mg (take one tablet twice daily to lower blood sugars)

- Glipizide 10 mg (take two tablets 30 minutes before breakfast daily to lower blood sugars)

- Diovan 320 mg (take one tablet daily to lower blood pressure)

- Chlorthalidone 25 mg (take one tablet daily to lower blood pressure)

- Simvastatin 80 mg (take one tablet daily to lower cholesterol)

- Cymbalta 60 mg (take one capsule once daily for peripheral neuropathy)

Meal History: EP says he is following his meal plan of 2,200 calories (9,205 kJ) (60 g carbohydrates at each meal and 30 g for bedtime snack). He also says he is limiting saturated fat to 17 g/day and sodium to 2,000 mg/day.

Physical Activity: Started walking 4 days/week for 30 minutes at moderate intensity

Plan—Next Steps

What are your treatment goals for EP regarding blood glucose, blood pressure, and lipids?

What therapeutic options would you consider if you determine that lifestyle or stress is not the cause of the changes in his results?

When would you want to see EP back in the office?

Patient Encounter, Part 4: Insulin Therapy

EP comes in 3 months later to assess the effectiveness of the changes that you suggested. His blood glucose, blood pressure, and lipids have been doing better. It is now 8 years since he was diagnosed, and he brings his readings in. He is discouraged because, although he has been taking his medication, following his meal plan, and is still physically active, he weighs 109 kg (240 lb). What therapeutic changes would you make and how would you teach EP to use the therapy suggested?

Fasting glucose: 180 mg/dL (10 mmol/L); **BUN:** 13 mg/dL (4.64 mmol/L); **creatinine:** 1 mg/dL (88 μmol/L); **AST/SGOT:** 26 IU/L (0.43 μKat/L); **ALT/SGPT:** 26 IU/L (0.43 μKat/L); **TSH:** 1.26 microunits/mL (1.26 mU/L); **total cholesterol:** 180 mg/dL (4.65 mmol/L); **LDL:** 98 mg/dL (2.53 mmol/L); **HDL:** 46 mg/dL (1.19 mmol/L); **triglycerides:** 130 mg/dL (1.47 mmol/L); **A$_{1c}$:** 8.6%; **body fat:** 42%; **waist circumference:** 42 inches (107 cm)

Blood Glucose Results (units of mg/dL [mmol/L])

	Before Breakfast	After Breakfast	Before Lunch	After Lunch	Before Supper	After Supper	Bedtime
Mon				206 (11.4)			
Tue				233 (12.9)			
Wed	203 (11.3)					299 (16.6)	
Thur			300 (16.7)				276 (15.3)
Fri						159 (8.82)	
Sat	285 (15.8)			285 (15.8)			221 (12.3)
Sun	240 (13.3)						321 (17.8)

Current Medications

- Metformin 1,000 mg (take one tablet twice daily to lower blood sugars)
- Glipizide 10 mg (take two tablets 30 minutes before breakfast daily to lower blood sugars)
- Byetta 10 mg (inject twice daily to lower blood sugars)
- Diovan 320 mg (take one tablet daily to lower blood pressure)
- Chlorthalidone 25 mg (take one tablet daily to lower blood pressure)
- Lipitor 40 mg (take one tablet daily to lower cholesterol)
- Tricor 145 mg (take one tablet daily to lower cholesterol)
- Cymbalta 60 mg (take one capsule once daily for peripheral neuropathy)

Meal History: EP says he is following a meal plan of 2,000 calories (8,368 kJ) (60 g carbohydrates at each meal and 20 g for bedtime snack). He also says he is limiting saturated fat to 15 g/day and sodium to 2,000 mg/day.

Physical Activity: Increased walking to 5 days/week for 45 minutes at moderate intensity.

Plan—Next Steps

What are your treatment goals for EP regarding blood glucose, blood pressure, and lipids?

Are his readings within target? What questions would you ask EP? Has a pattern been established?

What therapeutic options would you consider if you determine that lifestyle or stress is not the cause of the changes in his results?

Should insulin therapy be considered for EP?

What type of insulin and dose would you recommend, and how would you transition EP to insulin?

What does EP need to know about insulin therapy before he leaves, and when should he return?

- Patient care plans should include a number of daily evaluations to be performed by the patient, such as examination of the feet for any sores, cuts, or abrasions; checking the skin for dryness to prevent cracking and chafing; and monitoring blood glucose values as directed. Weekly appraisals of weight and blood pressure are also advised.

- Until A$_{1c}$ levels are at goal, quarterly visits with the patient's primary health care provider are recommended. Table 43–7 summarizes the specific ADA goals for therapy. The practitioner should review SMBG data and a current A$_{1c}$ level for progress, and address any therapeutic or educational issues.

- At minimum, yearly laboratory evaluation of serum lipids, urinary microalbumin, and serum creatinine should be performed.

Abbreviations Introduced in This Chapter

A$_{1c}$	Hemoglobin A$_{1c}$
AACE	American Association of Clinical Endocrinologists
ACCORD	Action to Control Cardiovascular Risk in Diabetes
ACE	Angiotensin-converting enzyme inhibitors
ADA	American Diabetes Association
ADVANCE	Action in Diabetes and Vascular Disease
ALT	Alanine aminotransferase
AST	Aspartate aminotransferase
ATP	Adenosine triphosphate
BMI	Body mass index
BUN	Blood urea nitrogen

Patient Care and Monitoring

1. Assess the patient for development or progression of DM and DM-related complications.

2. Evaluate SMBG for glycemic control, including FPG and postprandial levels.
   - Are the blood glucose values too high or low?
   - Are there specific times of day or specific days not in control?
   - Is hypoglycemia occurring?

3. Assess the patient for changes in quality-of-life measures such as physical, psychological, and social functioning and well-being.

4. Perform a thorough medication history of prescription, over-the-counter, and herbal product use.
   - Are there any medication problems, including presence of adverse drug reactions, drug allergies, and drug interactions?
   - Is the patient taking any medications that may affect blood glucose control?

5. Review all available laboratory data (some settings may have only patient-reported values) for attainment of ADA goals (Table 43–7). What therapy goals are not being met? What tests or referrals to other members of the health care team are needed?

6. Recommend appropriate therapy and develop a plan to assess effectiveness.

7. Stress adherence to prescribed lifestyle and medication regimen.

8. Provide patient education on diabetes, lifestyle modifications, appropriate monitoring, and drug therapy:
   - Causes of DM complications and how to prevent them.
   - How lifestyle changes including diet and exercise can affect diabetes.
   - How to perform SMBG and what to do with the results.
   - When to take medications and what to expect.
   - What adverse effects may occur?
   - What warning sign(s) should be reported to the physician?

CHD	Coronary heart disease
CHF	Congestive heart failure
Cl	Chloride
CSII	Continuous subcutaneous insulin infusion
DKA	Diabetic ketoacidosis
DM	Diabetes mellitus
DPP-4	Dipeptidyl peptidase-4
DPP	Diabetes Prevention Program
eAG	Estimated average glucose
FBG	Fasting blood glucose
FBS	Fasting blood sugar
FDA	Food and Drug Administration

FPG	Fasting plasma glucose
GDM	Gestational diabetes mellitus
GFR	Glomerular filtration rate
GIP	Glucose-dependent insulinotropic Polypeptide
GLP-1	Glucagon-like peptide-1
HCO_3	Serum bicarbonate
HDL	High-density lipoprotein cholesterol
HHS	Hyperosmolar hyperglycemic state
HLA	Human leukocyte antigen
IDPP	Indian Diabetes Prevention Programme
IFG	Impaired fasting glucose
IGT	Impaired glucose tolerance
IKK-β	I-kappa-B kinase-β
IM	Intramuscular
ISF	Interstitial fluid
K	Potassium
LADA	Latent autoimmune diabetes in adults
LDL	Low-density lipoprotein cholesterol
MDRD	Modified Diet in Renal Disease
Mg	Magnesium
MNT	Medical nutrition therapy
Na	Sodium
NNH	Number needed to cause harm in one patient
NPH	Neutral Protamine Hagedorn
OGTT	Oral glucose tolerance test
Pco_2	Partial pressure of carbon dioxide in arterial blood
PPAR-γ	Peroxisome proliferator activator receptor gamma
SGOT	Serum glutamic oxolacetic transaminase
SGPT	Serum glutamic pyruvic transaminase
SMBG	Self-monitoring of blood glucose
STOP-NIDDM	Study to Prevent Non-Insulin Dependent Diabetes Mellitus
T1DM	Type 1 diabetes mellitus
T2DM	Type 2 diabetes mellitus
TLC	Therapeutic lifestyle change
TSH	Thyroid-stimulating hormone
TZDs	Thiazolidinediones
VADT	Veterans Affairs Diabetes Trial
WHO	World Health Organization

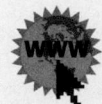 Self-assessment questions and answers are available at *http://www.mhpharmacotherapy.com/pp.html.*

REFERENCES

1. The Diabetes Control and Complications Trial Research Group. The effect of intensive treatment of diabetes on the development and progression of long-term complications in insulin-dependent diabetes mellitus. N Engl J Med 1993;329(14):977–986.
2. UK Prospective Diabetes Study (UKPDS) Group. Intensive blood-glucose control with sulfonylureas or insulin compared with

conventional treatment and risk of complications in patients with type 2 diabetes (UKPDS 33). Lancet 1998; 352(9131):837–853.

3. American Diabetes Association. Diabetes facts and figures. *http://www.diabetes.org/diabetes-statistics.jsp*.

4. Centers for Disease Control and Prevention. Overweight and obesity trends, *http://www.cdc.gov/nccdphp/dnpa/obesity/index.htm*.

5. DeFelippes M, Frank B, Chance R, et al. Insulin chemistry and pharmacokinetics. In: Porte DS, Baron A, eds. Ellenberg's and Rifkin's Diabetes Mellitus, 6th ed. New York: McGraw-Hill, 2003:481.

6. American Diabetes Association. Standards of medical care in diabetes—2008. Diabetes Care 2008;31(Suppl 1):S12–S54.

7. Delahanty L, Wylie-Rosett J. Lifestyle for prevention: Choices, changes, challenges. In: Mensing C, ed. The Art and Science of Diabetes Self-Management Education. A Desk Reference for Healthcare Professionals, 1st ed. Chicago, IL: American Association of Diabetes Educators, 2006:24.

8. Chipkin SR, Kelly KL, Ruderman NB. Hormone-fuel interrelationships: Fed state, starvation, and diabetes mellitus. In: Kahn CR, Weir GC, eds. Joslin's Diabetes Mellitus, 13th ed. Malvern, PA: Lea and Febiger, 1994:97–115.

9. Kaiser N, Leibowitz G, Nesher R. Glucotoxicity and beta-cell failure in type 2 diabetes mellitus. J Pediatr Endocrinol Metab 2003;16(1):5–22.

10. Role of Alpha Cells in Diabetes, *http://www.medscape.com/viewarticle/452112*.

11. Shulman GI, Barrett EJ, Sherwin RS. Integrated fuel metabolism. In: Porte D Jr, Sherwin RS, eds. Ellenberg's and Rifkin's Diabetes Mellitus, 5th ed. Stamford, CT: Appleton & Lange, 1997:1–17.

12. Triplett CL, Reasner CA, Isley WL. Diabetes mellitus. In: DiPiro JT, Talbert RL, Yee GC, et al., eds. Pharmacotherapy: A Pathophysiologic Approach, 7th ed. New York: McGraw-Hill, 2008:1205–1241.

13. Klinke D. Extent of beta cell destruction is important but insufficient to predict the onset of type 1 diabetes mellitus. Plos One v.2008;3(1).

14. Vinik A, Vinik E. Diabetic neuropathies. In: Mensing C, ed. The Art and Science of Diabetes Self-Management Education—A Desk Reference for Healthcare Professionals, 1st ed. Chicago, IL: American Association of Diabetes Educators, 2006:564.

15. Aronoff S, Berkowitz K, Shreiner B, Want L. Glucose metabolism and regulation: Beyond insulin and glucagon. Diabetes Spectr 2004;17:183–190.

16. Executive summary of the third report of the National Cholesterol Education Program (NCEP) expert panel on detection, evaluation, and treatment of high blood cholesterol in adults (Adult Treatment Panel III). JAMA 2001;285(19):2486–2497.

17. Uwaifo GI, Ratner RE. Novel pharmacologic agents for type 2 diabetes. Endocrino Meta Clin North Am 2005;34:155–197.

18. DeFronzo RA. New concepts in pathophysiology: Incretins in type 2 diabetes. Clinical Highlights Newsletter: The Role of Incretin Mimetics and Potentiating Agents in the Prevention and Treatment of Type 2 Diabetes, 2004;1:3–4.

19. Perley MJ, Kipnis DM. Plasma insulin responses to oral and intravenous glucose: Studies in normal and diabetic subjects. J Clin Invest 1967;46:1954–1962.

20. American Diabetes Association. Screening for type 2 diabetes. Diabetes Care 2008;31(Suppl 1):S12–S54.

21. American Diabetes Association. Diagnosis and classification of diabetes mellitus. Diabetes Care 2008;31(Suppl 1):S5–S10.

22. Zinman B, Ruderman N, Campaigne BN, et al. Physical activity/exercise and diabetes. Diabetes Care 2004;27(Suppl 1):S58–S62.

23. American Association of Clinical Endocrinologists. Medical guidelines for the management of diabetes mellitus: The AACE system of intensive diabetes self-management—2002 update. Endocr Pract 2002; 8(Suppl 1):40–82.

24. Kennedy L. Self-monitoring of blood glucose in type 2 diabetes: Time for evidence of efficacy. Diabetes Care 2001;24(6):977–978.

25. American Diabetes Association. Diabetes Care 2008;31(Suppl 1):S18.

26. Nathan D, Kuenen J, Borg R, et al. For the A1c Derived Average Glucose (ADAG) study group. Translating the A1c assay into estimated average glucose values. Diabetes Care 2008;31:1473–1478.

27. Nathan DM, Buse JB, Davidson MB, et al. Medical management of hyperglycemia in type 2 diabetes: A consensus algorithm for the initiation and adjustment of therapy: A consensus statement from the American Diabetes Association and the European Association for the Study of Diabetes. Diabetes Care 2009;32:1–11.

28. American Association of Clinical Endocrinologist. *http://www.aace.com/pub*.

29. Shane-McWhorter, L. Biological complementary therapies in diabetes. In: Mensing C, ed. The Art and Science of Diabetes Self-Management Education. A Desk Reference for Healthcare Professionals, 1st ed. Chicago, IL: American Association of Diabetes Educators, 2006:431–460.

30. Franz MJ, Bantle JP, Beebe CA, et al. Nutrition principles and recommendations in diabetes. Diabetes Care 2004;27(Suppl 1):S36–S46.

31. Inzucchi SE. Oral antihyperglycemic therapy for type 2 diabetes: Scientific review. JAMA 2002;287(3):360–372.

32. Lacy C, Armstrong L, Goldman M, Lance, L. LexiComp's Drug Information Handbook, 12th ed. Hudson, OH: Lexi-Comp, 2004.

33. Drug Facts and Comparisons Pocket Version, 8th ed. Lippincott, Williams & Wilkins, 2003.

34. National Diabetes Education Program. Diabetes medications: Section A. In working together to manage diabetes: Diabetes medications supplement. *NDEP* May 2007(Suppl 1):2–5.

35. Prospective pioglitazone clinical trial in microvascular events. *http://www.proactiveresults.org*.

36. Takiya L, Dougherty T. Pharmacist's guide to insulin preparations: A comprehensive review. Pharm Times 2005;71:90.

37. Amori R, Lau J, Pittas AG. Efficacy and safety of incretin therapy in type 2 diabetes: Systematic review and meta-analysis. JAMA 2007;298:194–206.

38. Accord Study Group. Effects of intensive glucose lowering in type 2 diabetes. N Engl J Med 2008;358:2545–2559.

39. Advance Study Group. *http:// www.advance-trial.com*.

40. Abraira C, Moritz TE, Reaven P, et al. Glycemic control and cardiovascular outcomes—The VA Diabetes Trial. Presented at ADA 68th Scientific Sessions; June 6–10, 2008; San Francisco.

41. Davidson MB. Diabetic ketoacidosis and hyperosmolar nonketotic coma. In: Davidson MB, ed. Diabetes Mellitus: Diagnosis and Treatment, 4th ed. New York: WB Saunders, 1998:159–194.

42. Ilag LL, Kronick S, Ernst RD, et al. Impact of a critical pathway on inpatient management of diabetic ketoacidosis. Diabetes Res Clin Pract 2003;62:23–32.

43. Joint Commission on Accreditation of Health Care Organizations. *http:http://www.jointcommission.org/CertificationPrograms/Inpatient+Diabetes/*.

44. Drug interactions of medications commonly used in diabetes. Diabetes Spectrum 2006;19:202–211.

44 Thyroid Disorders

Michael D. Katz

LEARNING OBJECTIVES

● **Upon completion of the chapter, the reader will be able to:**

1. Explain the major components of the hypothalamic–pituitary–thyroid axis and the interaction among these components.

2. Discuss the prevalence of thyroid disorders, including subclinical (mild) and overt (typical signs and/or symptoms present) hypothyroidism and hyperthyroidism.

3. Discuss the relationship between serum thyroid-stimulating hormone (TSH) levels and primary thyroid disease and the advantages for the use of TSH levels over other tests such as serum T_4 (thyroxine) and T_3 (triiodothyronine) levels.

4. Identify the typical signs and symptoms of hypothyroidism and the consequences of inadequate treatment.

5. Discuss the issues regarding levothyroxine (LT_4) product bioequivalence and the advantages of maintaining patients on the same product.

6. Describe the clinical use of LT_4 in the treatment of hypothyroidism.

7. Describe the management of hypothyroidism and hyperthyroidism in pregnant women.

8. Identify the typical signs and symptoms of Graves' disease and the consequences of inadequate treatment.

9. Discuss the pharmacotherapy of Graves' disease, including the advantages and disadvantages of antithyroid drugs versus radioactive iodine, adverse effects, and patient monitoring.

10. Describe the potential effects of amiodarone, lithium, and interferon-α on thyroid function.

KEY CONCEPTS

❶ In most patients with thyroid hormone disorders, the measurement of a serum thyroid-stimulating hormone (TSH) level is adequate for the initial screening and diagnosis of hypothyroidism and hyperthyroidism. Serum free thyroxine (T_4) and triiodothyronine (T_3) levels may be helpful in distinguishing subclinical (mild) thyroid disease from overt disease. The target TSH for most patients being treated for thyroid disorders should be the mean normal value of 1.4 milliunits/L (mU/L) or 1.4 microunits/mL (μU/mL) (target range 0.5–2.5 milliunits/L or 0.5–2.5 microunits/mL). The target TSH may be different in patients being treated with levothyroxine (LT_4) for thyroid cancer.

❷ Hypothyroidism can affect virtually any tissue or organ in the body. The most common symptoms, such as fatigue, lethargy, sleepiness, cold intolerance, and dry skin, are nonspecific and are seen with many other disorders. The classic overt signs, such as myxedema and delayed deep tendon reflexes, are seen uncommonly now because more patients are screened or seek earlier medical attention. Patients with mild hypothyroidism may have subtle symptoms that progress so slowly that they are not noticed easily by the patient or family. The lack of overt or specific signs and symptoms emphasizes the importance of using the serum TSH level to identify patients with hypothyroidism.

❸ There are three major goals in the treatment of hypothyroidism: replace the missing hormones, relieve symptoms, and achieve a stable biochemical euthyroid state.

❹ Despite the availability of a wide array of thyroid hormone products, it is clear that synthetic LT_4 is the treatment of choice for almost all patients with hypothyroidism. LT_4 mimics the normal physiology of the thyroid gland, which secretes mostly T_4 as a prohormone. As needed, based on metabolic demands, peripheral tissues convert thyroxine (T_4) to triiodothyronine (T_3). If T_3 is used to treat hypothyroidism, the peripheral tissues lose their ability to control local metabolic rates. LT_4 also has distinct pharmacokinetic advantages over T_3. With a 7- to 10-day half-life, LT_4 provides a very smooth dose-response curve with little peak and trough effect. In a small number of patients who have impairment of conversion of T_4 to T_3, addition of T_3 may be warranted.

5 There is no evidence that one LT_4 product is better than another. However, given the evidence that these products have different bioavailabilities, patients should be maintained on the same specific LT_4 product. Given the generic substitution regulations of most U.S. states, this is best accomplished by prescribing a brand-name product or otherwise ensuring that the product remains constant. The prescriber should not allow substitution in the way mandated by state regulations.

6 The goals of treating hyperthyroidism are to relieve symptoms, to reduce thyroid hormone production to normal levels, to achieve biochemical euthyroidism, and to prevent long-term adverse sequelae.

7 Agranulocytosis is one of the most serious adverse effects of antithyroid drug therapy.

8 The growth and spread of thyroid carcinoma are stimulated by TSH. An important component of thyroid carcinoma management is the use of LT_4 to suppress TSH secretion. Early in therapy, patients receive the lowest LT_4 dose sufficient to fully suppress TSH to undetectable levels. Controlled trials show that suppressive LT_4 therapy reduces tumor growth and improves survival.

9 Patients receiving amiodarone must receive monitoring for thyroid abnormalities. Baseline measurements of serum TSH, FT_4, FT_3, antithyroid peroxidase antibody (anti-TPOAb), and TSH receptor-stimulating antibodies (TSHR-SAb) should be performed. TSH, FT_4, and FT_3 should be checked 3 months after initiation of amiodarone and then at least a TSH every 3 to 6 months.

Thyroid disorders are common. Over 2 billion people, or 38% of the world's population, have iodine deficiency, resulting in 74 million people with goiters. While iodine deficiency is not a significant problem in developed countries, a number of common thyroid conditions exist. The most common conditions are hypothyroidism and hyperthyroidism, which often require long-term pharmacotherapy. Undetected or improperly treated thyroid disease can result in long-term adverse sequelae, including increased mortality. It is important that clinicians are aware of the prevalence of thyroid disorders, the methods of identifying thyroid disorders, and the appropriate therapy.

This chapter focuses on the most common pharmacologically treated thyroid disorders.

THYROID HORMONE PHYSIOLOGY AND BIOSYNTHESIS

The thyroid gland is the largest endocrine gland in the body, residing in the neck, anterior to the trachea, between the cricoid cartilage and the suprasternal notch. The thyroid gland produces two biologically active hormones, thyroxine (T_4) and triiodothyronine (T_3). Thyroid hormones are essential for proper fetal growth and development, particularly of the CNS. After delivery, the primary role of thyroid hormone is in the regulation of energy metabolism. These hormones can affect the function of virtually every organ in the body. The parafollicular C cells of the thyroid gland produce calcitonin. The function of calcitonin and its therapeutic use are discussed in other chapters in this book.

T_4 and T_3 are produced by the organification (binding of iodine to tyrosine residues of thyroglobulin) of iodine in the thyroid gland. Iodine is actively transported into the thyroid follicular cells. This inorganic iodine is oxidized by thyroid peroxidase and covalently bound to tyrosine residues of thyroglobulin. These iodinated tyrosine residues monoiodotyrosine and diiodotyrosine couple to form T_4 and T_3. Eighty percent of thyroid hormone is synthesized as T_4 and is stored in the thyroid bound to thyroglobulin. Thyroid hormones are released from the gland when needed, primarily under the influence of TSH (thyroid stimulating hormone, thyrotropin) from the anterior pituitary. T_4 and T_3 are transported in the blood by three proteins, 70% to thyroid-binding globulin (TBG), 15% to transthyretin (thyroid-binding prealbumin), and 15% to albumin. T_4 is 99.97% protein-bound, and T_3 is 99.7% protein-bound, with only the unbound or free fractions physiologically active. The high degree of protein-binding results in a long half-life of these hormones: approximately 7 to 10 days for T_4 and 24 hours for T_3.

Most of the physiologic activity of thyroid hormones is from the actions of T_3. T_4 can be thought of primarily as a prohormone. Eighty percent of needed T_3 is derived from the conversion of T_4 to T_3 in peripheral tissue under the influence of tissue deiodinases. These deiodinases allow end organs to produce the amount of T_3 needed to control local metabolic functions. These enzymes also catabolize T_3 and T_4 to biologically inactive metabolites.

The production and release of thyroid hormones are regulated by the hypothalamic–pituitary–thyroid axis (Fig. 44–1). Hypothalamic thyrotropin-releasing hormone (TRH) stimulates the release of TSH (thyrotropin) when there are physiologically inadequate levels of thyroid hormones. TSH promotes the production and release of thyroid hormones from the gland. As circulating thyroid hormone levels rise to needed levels, negative feedback results in decreased release of TSH and TRH. The release of TRH is inhibited by somatostatin and its analogs, and the release of TSH can be inhibited by dopamine, dopamine agonists, and high levels of glucocorticoids.

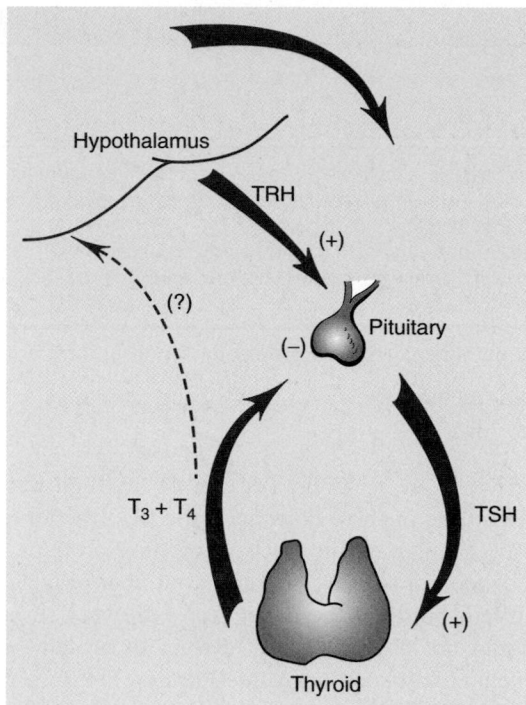

FIGURE 44–1. Hypothalamic–pituitary–thyroid axis. Thyrotropin-releasing hormone (TRH) is synthesized in the neurons within the paraventricular nucleus of the hypothalamus. TRH is released into the hypothalamic–pituitary portal circulation and carried to the pituitary, where it activates the pituitary to synthesize and release thyrotropin (TSH). TSH activates the thyroid to stimulate the synthesis and secretion of thyroxine (T_4) and triiodothyronine (T_3). T_4 and T_3 inhibit TRH and TSH secretion, closing the feedback loop.

SPECTRUM OF THYROID DISEASE

There are two general modes of presentation for thyroid disorders: changes in the size or shape of the gland and changes in secretion of hormone from the gland. In some cases, structural changes can result in changes in hormone secretion. Thyroid nodules and goiters in euthyroid patients are common problems. Patients with a goiter who are biochemically euthyroid often require no specific pharmacotherapy, unless the goiter is due to iodine deficiency. In developing countries, iodized salt is the primary therapy in treating goiter. Thyroid nodules, seen in 4% to 7% of adults, may be malignant or may autonomously secrete thyroid hormones. A discussion of thyroid nodules is beyond the scope of this chapter; however, thyroid cancer will be discussed briefly in the context of levothyroxine (LT_4) suppressive therapy. Refer to other resources for a more extensive review of thyroid cancer management.

Changes in hormone secretion can result in hormone deficiency or excess. While patients with overt hypothyroidism and hyperthyroidism may have dramatic signs and symptoms, most patients have subtle signs and symptoms that progress slowly over time. The availability of sensitive

and specific biochemical tests for the diagnosis of thyroid hormone disorders has facilitated screening and earlier diagnosis, including those with subclinical thyroid disorders. Screening of newborns for congenital hypothyroidism has reduced the incidence of mental retardation and cretinism dramatically in the United States. However, congenital hypothyroidism owing to iodine deficiency remains a significant worldwide public health problem.

EPIDEMIOLOGY OF THYROID DISEASE

A number of studies have assessed the epidemiology of thyroid hormone abnormalities. The 1999 to 2002 National Health and Nutrition Examination Survey (NHANES)[1] reported the prevalence of thyroid hormone disorders in 4,392 people 12 years of age and over in a sample representing the geographic and ethnic distribution of the U.S. population. Hypothyroidism was found in 3.7% (3.4% mild) and hyperthyroidism in 0.5% of the sample. The prevalence of hypothyroidism was higher in older age groups and in whites and Hispanics, whereas blacks had a lower prevalence of hypothyroidism. The prevalence of hypothyroidism correlated with age. Compared to the total population, people of age 50 to 79 had an almost twofold higher prevalence, and those age 80 and older had a fivefold higher prevalence. Pregnant women also had a higher prevalence of hypothyroidism. The Colorado Thyroid Health Survey[2] assessed thyroid function in 25,862 subjects attending a health fair. The overall prevalence of an abnormal TSH level was 11.7% of the study population, with 9.4% hypothyroid (9% subclinical) and 2.2% hyperthyroid (2.1% subclinical). Of the 916 subjects taking thyroid medication, 60% were euthyroid, with an equal distribution between subclinical hypothyroidism and hyperthyroidism. The NHANES study also found that many patients receiving thyroid medications had an abnormal TSH. These findings imply that many patients who are receiving thyroid medications are not being managed successfully.

PATIENT ASSESSMENT AND MONITORING

The assessment of patients for thyroid disorders entails a history and physical examination. In many patients with subclinical or mild thyroid disease, there may be an absence of specific signs and symptoms, and the physical examination may be normal. Various diagnostic tests can be used, including serum thyroid hormone(s), TSH, thyroid antibody levels, and imaging techniques to evaluate patients for thyroid disorders. Reference ranges for selected laboratory tests are given in Table 44–1.

TSH Levels

❶ *In most patients with thyroid hormone disorders, the measurement of a serum TSH level is adequate for the initial screening and diagnosis of hypothyroidism and hyperthyroidism. Serum free T_4 and T_3 levels may be helpful in distinguishing subclinical (mild) thyroid disease from overt*

Table 44–1		
Selected Thyroid Tests for Adults		
Test	**Reference Range**	**Comments**
TSH	0.5–4.5 milliunits/L (0.5–4.5 microunits/mL)[a]	Gold standard; may be lowered by dopamine, dopamine agonists, glucocorticoids, octreotide, recovery from severe nonthyroidal illness
FT_4	0.7–1.9 ng/dL (9.0–24.5 pmol/L)	May be normal in mild thyroid disease
Anti-TPOAb	Less than 100 units/mL	Present in autoimmune hypothyroidism; predicts more rapid progression from subclinical to overt hypothyroidism
TSHR-SAb	Undetectable	Confirms Graves' disease

Anti-TPOAb, antithyroid peroxidase antibody; T_4, thyroxine; TSH, thyroid-stimulating hormone; TSH-SAb, TSH receptor-stimulating antibodies.

[a]Milliunits/L (mU/L) = microunits/mL (μU/mL); clinical laboratories use either unit of measurement.

disease. The target TSH for most patients being treated for thyroid disorders should be the mean normal value of 1.4 milliunits/L (mU/L) or 1.4 microunits/mL (μU/mL) (target range 0.5–2.5 milliunits/L or 0.5–2.5 microunits/mL). The target TSH may be different in patients being treated with LT_4 for thyroid cancer.

TSH is a highly sensitive bioassay of the thyroid axis. A two-fold change in serum free T_4 levels will result in a 100-fold change in TSH levels. This biologic magnification by TSH allows the TSH to be used in early diagnosis as well as in closely titrating therapy in hypothyroidism and hyperthyroidism. In patients with primary hypothyroidism or hyperthyroidism resulting from gland dysfunction, there is an inverse relationship between the TSH level and thyroid function. High TSH signifies hypothyroidism (or iatrogenic under-replacement), and low TSH signifies hyperthyroidism (or iatrogenic over-replacement). There is controversy regarding the normal or laboratory reference ranges for TSH. NHANES[3] showed that the mean TSH level in a normal population was 1.46 milliunits/L (milliunits/L = microunits/mL; clinical laboratories use either unit of measurement, usually expressed as mU/L or μU/mL), but the values were not normally distributed. While most laboratories quote the upper limit of normal for TSH as 4.5 milliunits/L based on NHANES data, 95% of subjects had a TSH level of between 0.5 and 2.5 milliunits/L. The population of subjects whose TSH level was 2.5 to 4.5 milliunits/L may have had mild hypothyroidism and should not have been included as part of the normal reference range for TSH. However, the mean normal TSH in the elderly appears to be higher, even in people with no clinical evidence of hypothyroidism.[4] It has been proposed that the reference TSH range be redefined with an upper limit of normal of 2.5 or 3 milliunits/L.[5] However, it is not clear what the clinical impact would be with such a change. The target TSH for most patients being treated for thyroid disorders is not the same as the reference range. Ideally, the TSH should be the mean normal value of 1.4 milliunits/L or 1.4 microunits/mL (target range 0.5–2.5 milliunits/L or 0.5–2.5 microunits/mL).

Serum Hormone Levels

Serum T_4 and T_3 levels were used commonly to assess thyroid function. Screening thyroid function tests measure total serum T_4 or T_3 levels. Because of the high degree of protein binding of these hormones, the free fraction can be altered by changes in the levels of binding proteins or the degree of protein binding. Because a number of factors can alter protein binding, the older assays are very insensitive and should no longer be used, even with protein-binding adjustment factors such as the free T_4 index. Free or unbound T_4 (FT_4) and T_3 (FT_3) assays are readily available and are more sensitive in identifying thyroid dysfunction than the older total assays.[6] However, patients with mild hypothyroidism or hyperthyroidism will have a normal FT_4 level despite an abnormal TSH level.

The laboratory assessment of patients with suspected thyroid disorders must be based on the continuum of disease from subclinical or mild to overt (Fig. 44–2).

Other Diagnostic Tests

Global tests of thyroid gland function can be performed to assess the rate of hormone synthesis. The radioactive iodine uptake (RAIU) will be elevated in hyperthyroidism and can aid in identifying thyrotoxicosis owing to nonthyroid gland sources. Radionuclide thyroid scans are used in the evaluation of thyroid nodules. Because many thyroid disorders are autoimmune, measurement of various serum antithyroid antibodies can be performed. Antithyroid peroxidase (anti-TPOAb) and antithyroglobulin antibodies (anti-TGAb) are present in many patients with hypothyroidism. Most patients with Graves' disease will have TSH receptor-stimulating antibodies (TSHR-SAb) as well as elevated anti-TPOAb and antimicrosomal antibodies.

HYPOTHYROIDISM

Hypothyroidism is the most common clinical disorder of thyroid function. It is the clinical syndrome that results from inadequate secretion of thyroid hormones from the thyroid gland. The vast majority of hypothyroid patients have primary gland failure, whereas rare patients have pituitary or hypothalamic failure. Most studies define hypothyroidism based on a serum TSH level above the upper limit of the laboratory reference range. In adults, 1.4% of women and 0.1% of men are biochemically hypothyroid. However, the incidence is highly age-dependent. In the

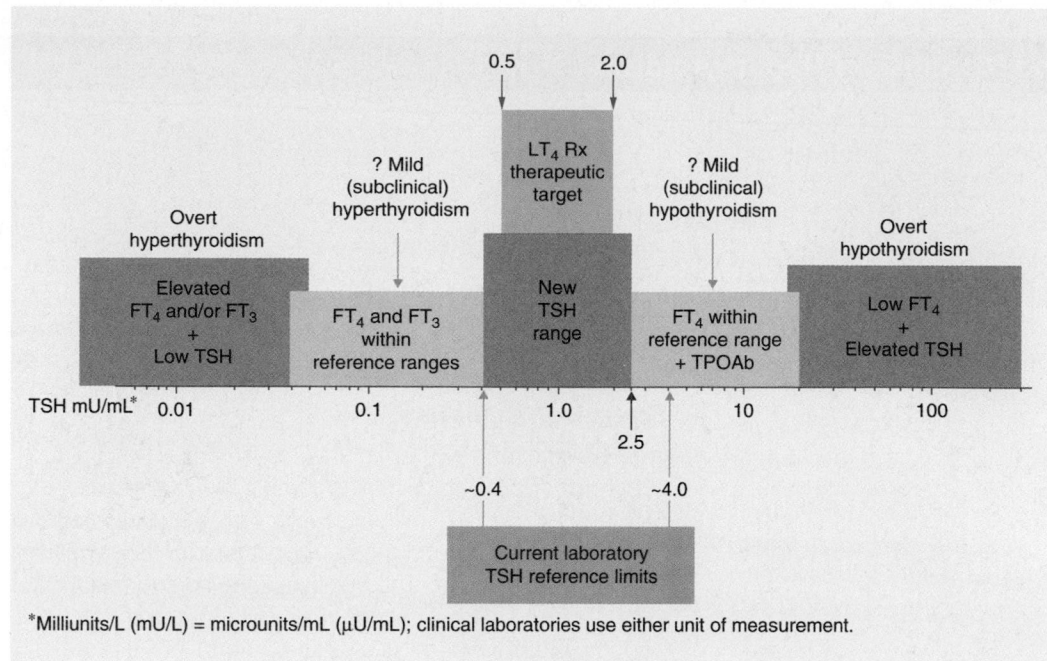

FIGURE 44-2. TSH and the continuum of thyroid disorders. (FT_3, free T_3; FT_4, free T_4; LT_4, levothyroxine; TPOAb, thyroid peroxidase antibody; TSH, thyroid-stimulating hormone.) (From Ref. 5.)

*Milliunits/L (mU/L) = microunits/mL (µU/mL); clinical laboratories use either unit of measurement.

Colorado Thyroid Health Study,[2] by age 64, 12% of women and 5% of men were hypothyroid, and in the over 74 year age group, the incidence in men approached that of women. Most epidemiologic studies of hypothyroidism in the elderly show a prevalence of 6% to 12%. There is a strong correlation between the presence of anti-TPOAb or anti-TGAb and the risk of developing hypothyroidism. In patients with subclinical hypothyroidism and positive anti-TPOAb, 5% per year will progress to overt hypothyroidism.[7] Other risk factors for the development of hypothyroidism include postpartum state, family history of autoimmune thyroid disorders, a previous history of head and neck or thyroid surgery, head and neck irradiation, other autoimmune endocrine disorders such as type 1 diabetes and Addison's disease, other nonendocrine autoimmune diseases such as celiac disease and pernicious anemia, prior history of treatment for hyperthyroidism, treatment with amiodarone or lithium, and an iodine-deficient diet.

Screening for Hypothyroidism

Because the prevalence of hypothyroidism is high in certain populations, screening may be useful. Screening for hypothyroidism in women over age 35 is as cost effective as screening for breast cancer and hypertension,[8] although some organizations recommend screening of adults over the ages of 50 or 60. Others advocate a case-finding approach, defined as performing a TSH determination in patients based on risk factors or the presence of signs and symptoms.[9,10] Refer to Clinical Presentation and Diagnosis of Hypothyroidism for more information regarding screening and diagnosis.

Causes of Hypothyroidism

The most common causes of hypothyroidism are listed in Table 44–2.[11,12] Up to 90% of patients with autoimmune thyroiditis have circulating anti-TPOAbs. The autoimmune inflammatory response results in a lymphocytic infiltration of the thyroid gland and its eventual destruction.

Iatrogenic hypothyroidism can follow thyroid irradiation or surgery and excessive doses of antithyroid drugs. Several drugs can cause hypothyroidism, including iodine-containing drugs such as amiodarone and iodinated radiocontrast media, lithium, interferon-α, sunitinib, p-aminosalicylic acid, ethionamide, sulfonylureas, valproic acid, and aminoglutethimide.[13] Iodine deficiency is a common worldwide cause of hypothyroidism, including congenital

Table 44–2
Common Causes of Hypothyroidism

Primary Hypothyroidism
Autoimmune thyroiditis (Hashimoto's disease)
Iatrogenic (irradiation, surgery)
Drugs (amiodarone, radiocontrast media, lithium, α-interferon, sunitinib)
Silent thyroiditis (including postpartum)
Iodine deficiency and excess

Secondary Hypothyroidism
Pituitary disease
Hypothalamic disease

From Refs. 11, 12.

Clinical Presentation and Diagnosis of Hypothyroidism

Symptoms

- Fatigue
- Lethargy
- Sleepiness
- Mental impairment
- Depression
- Cold intolerance
- Hoarseness
- Dry skin
- Decreased perspiration
- Weight gain
- Decreased appetite
- Constipation
- Menstrual disturbances
- Arthralgia
- Paresthesia

Signs

- Slow movements
- Slow speech
- Hoarseness
- Bradycardia
- Dry skin
- Nonpitting edema (myxedema)
- Hyporeflexia
- Delayed relaxation of reflexes

Screening/Diagnosis

A TSH level of 4.5 to 10 milliunits/L constitutes mild or subclinical hypothyroidism, and some patients with a TSH level of 2.5 to 4.5 milliunits/L also may be mildly hypothyroid. A TSH level greater than 10 milliunits/L signifies overt hypothyroidism.[a] The free T_4 level will be normal (0.7–1.9 ng/dL or 9.0–24.5 pmol/L) in mild or subclinical hypothyroidism and low (less than 0.7 ng/dL or 9.0 pmol/L) in patients with obvious signs and/or symptoms.

---

[a]Milliunits/L (mU/L) = microunits/mL (µU/mL); clinical laboratories use either unit of measurement.

From Refs. 11, 12.

---

hypothyroidism in newborns. Patients with hypothalamic or pituitary disease often have other signs of piuitary disease, such as hypogonadism, and the TSH level will be low.

Signs and Symptoms of Hypothyroidism

❷ *Hypothyroidism can affect virtually any tissue or organ in the body. The most common symptoms, such as fatigue, lethargy, sleepiness, cold intolerance, and dry skin, are nonspecific and can be seen with many other disorders. The classic overt signs, such as myxedema and delayed deep tendon reflexes, are seen uncommonly now because more patients are screened or seek medical attention earlier. Patients with mild hypothyroidism may have subtle symptoms that progress so slowly that they are not noticed easily by the patient or family. The lack of overt or specific signs and symptoms emphasizes the importance of using the serum TSH level to identify patients with hypothyroidism.*

Sequelae of Hypothyroidism

Hypothyroidism is a chronic disease that may result in significant long-term sequelae. Hypercholesterolemia is associated with hypothyroidism, increasing the long-term risk of cardiovascular disease and cardiovascular mortality.[14] Between 4% and 14% of patients with hypercholesterolemia are found to be hypothyroid. The Colorado Thyroid Health Study[2] showed a direct correlation

between the degree of TSH elevation and the rise in serum cholesterol. Hypothyroidism also may result in increased systemic vascular resistance, decreased cardiac output, and increased diastolic blood pressure. Hypothyroidism can cause significant neuropsychiatric problems, including a dementia-like state in the elderly that is reversible with LT_4 therapy. Maternal hypothyroidism can have dire consequences for the developing fetus. The fetus is almost completely dependent on maternal thyroid hormones during the first trimester, a time crucial for development of the CNS. Inadequately treated maternal hypothyroidism results in increased risk of miscarriage and developmental impairment in the child.[15]

Myxedema coma is seen in advanced hypothyroidism. These patients develop CNS depression, respiratory depression, cardiovascular instability, and fluid and electrolyte disturbances. Myxedema coma often is triggered by an underlying acute medical condition such as infection, stroke, trauma, or administration of CNS depressant drugs.

Treatment of Hypothyroidism

❸ *There are three major goals in the treatment of hypothyroidism: replace the missing hormones, relieve symptoms, and achieve a stable biochemical euthyroid state.* While these goals should not be difficult to achieve, 20% to 40% of treated patients are not receiving optimal pharmacotherapy.

▶ Thyroid Hormone Products

A number of thyroid hormone products are marketed in the United States (Table 44–3). These products include synthetic LT_4 and T_3, combinations of synthetic LT_4 and T_3, and animal-derived products. ❹ *Despite the availability of a wide array of thyroid hormone products, it is clear that synthetic LT_4 is the treatment of choice for almost all patients with hypothyroidism.*[11,12] *Using LT_4 mimics the normal physiology of the thyroid gland, which secretes mostly T_4 as a prohormone. Peripheral tissues convert T_4 to T_3 as needed, based on metabolic demands. If T_3 is used to treat hypothyroidism, the peripheral tissues lose their ability to control local metabolic rates. LT_4 also has distinct pharmacokinetic advantages over T_3. With a 7 to 10 day half-life, LT_4 provides a very smooth dose-response curve with little peak and trough effect. In a small number of patients who have impairment of conversion of T_4 to T_3, addition of T_3 may be warranted. T_3, with a 24-hour half-life, provides a significant peak and trough effect, and many patients will have symptoms of thyrotoxicosis after each dose is administered. For patients who have difficulty adhering to a once-daily regimen, a once-weekly LT_4 regimen is safe and effective.*[11]

Animal-derived products such as desiccated thyroid and thyroglobulin are obtained from cow and pig thyroid and have various degrees of purity. These products contain both LT_4 and T_3, but the amount of T_3 is much higher (T_4:T_3 = 4:1) than what would be found in the human thyroid gland (T_4:T_3 = 14:1). With the desiccated thyroid products, there are concerns about standardizing the amount of hormone and lot-to-lot variability. While some patients want to use these agents because they are "natural," they are not natural for humans. With the strong evidence supporting the safety and efficacy of LT_4 in the treatment of hypothyroidism, there is no rationale for the use of these animal-derived products.

Patients who are being treated with these agents should be strongly encouraged to switch to synthetic LT_4. Also, patients should be encouraged not to purchase thyroid hormone- or iodine-containing products from health food stores or from questionable Internet sites.

Several studies have been published that evaluate the use of LT_4 and T_3 combinations in ratios that mimic human physiology. A meta-analysis of 11 randomized, controlled clinical trials comparing LT_4 and T_3 combinations with LT_4 monotherapy show no outcome benefit with combination therapy.[16] Except in rare circumstances (such as patients with impaired T_4-to-T_3 conversion), there is no rationale for using combinations of LT_4 and T_3 to treat hypothyroidism.

▶ Bioequivalence and LT_4 Product Selection

LT_4 products have a long history of bioavailability problems.[17] Over the years, LT_4 bioavailability has increased, so maintenance doses today are significantly lower than those seen in the 1970s and early 1980s. Currently, the average bioavailability of LT_4 products is about 80%. Because of long-standing concerns about LT_4 bioequivalence, and because LT_4 products had never undergone formal approval by the FDA under the 1938 Food, Drug, and Cosmetics Act, the FDA mandated that all manufacturers of LT_4 products submit an Abbreviated New Drug Application (ANDA) to keep their products on the U.S. market after 2001.[18] Products approved under this process would have to comply with FDA manufacturing and bioequivalence standards. This FDA action has resulted in many changes in the U.S. LT_4 market, as well as renewed interest in LT_4 bioequivalence. By 2009, a variety of brand and generic products had been approved by the FDA. Some of the generic products carry AB ratings (bioequivalence) to certain brand products.[19]

Table 44–3

Thyroid Preparations

Drug/Brand Name	Content	Relative Dose	Comments
LT_4 (Synthroid, Levoxyl, Unithroid), other brands, and generics	Synthetic LT_4; 25, 50, 75, 88, 100, 112, 125, 137, 150, 175, 200, and 300 mcg tablets; 500 mcg vial for injection	60 mcg	Gold standard for treating hypothyroidism; products not therapeutically equivalent; full replacement dose 1–1.6 mcg/kg/day; when switching from animal product, lower calculated daily dose by 25–50 mcg; IV form rarely needed
Liothyronine (Cytomel)	Synthetic T_3; 5, 25, and 50 mcg tablets	15 mcg	Rarely needed in treatment of hypothyroidism; rapid absorption and pharmacologic effect; increased toxicity versus LT_4; no outcome benefit to combining with LT_4
Thyroid (desiccated) USP (Armour, others)	Desiccated pork or beef thyroid glands; contains T_3 and T_4; 0.25, 0.5, 1, 1.5, 2, 3, 4, and 5 grain tablets	1 grain (65 mg)	Nonphysiologic for humans; unpredictable hormone content and stability; T_3 content may cause toxicity
Thyroglobulin (Proloid)	Partially purified pork thyroglobulin; 32, 65, 100, 130, and 200 mg tablets	65 mg	Nonphysiologic T_4: T_3 ratio; T_3 content may cause toxicity; removed from U.S. market
Liotrix (Thyrolar)	Synthetic T_4, T_3 in fixed 4:1 ratio; $\frac{1}{4}$, $\frac{1}{2}$, 1, 2, 3 strength tablets	12.5/50 mcg T_3: T_4 (1 strength)	Nonphysiologic T_4: T_3 ratio; T_3 content may cause toxicity

LT_4, levothyroxine; T_3, triiodothyronine; T_4, thyroxine.

For many years, there have been concerns regarding the FDA bioequivalence methodology for LT_4 products. FDA bioequivalence standards allow a −20% to +25% variance in pharmacokinetic parameters between the test and reference products. Many people feel that this degree of allowed variance is not appropriate for a narrow-therapeutic-index (NTI) drug such as LT_4.[20] Also, there are unique challenges to performing bioequivalence studies with an endogenous hormone such as LT_4. Because these single-dose pharmacokinetic studies are done in healthy volunteers, the pharmacokinetic data are a combination of endogenous and exogenous LT_4. Seventy percent of the area under the curve (AUC) in these studies consists of the subjects' endogenous T_4. Thus, it is doubtful that bioavailability differences among products could be detected. Blakesley and colleagues[21] showed that the standard FDA bioequivalence methodology would rate 600, 450, and 400 mcg LT_4 doses as bioequivalent. This study also showed that mathematically removing the subjects' endogenous T_4 level (baseline correction) improves the sensitivity of the analysis, allowing a distinction between 33% and 25% but not 12.5% dose differences. Based on these data, the FDA, since 2003, has required that LT_4 bioequivalence data undergo baseline correction. While this method has improved the ability to identify large differences in LT_4 bioequivalence, small but clinically significant differences will not be identified.

More important than bioequivalence is the therapeutic equivalence of LT_4 products. Will patients have the same outcomes if bioequivalent products are used? The study by Dong and colleagues[22] helps to answer this question. Twenty-two well-controlled hypothyroid women were randomly switched to the same dose of four different products every 6 weeks. Nonbaseline corrected bioequivalence data showed these products to be bioequivalent. However, as each product switch occurred, more of the subjects had an abnormal TSH level.[23] By the end of the third product switch, 52% had an abnormal TSH level. This is strong evidence that LT_4 products are not therapeutically equivalent even if they are rated as bioequivalent by the FDA.

Evidence does exist that small differences in the LT_4 dose can result in large changes in TSH. The impact on TSH of small changes in LT_4 dose was assessed in 21 adult therapeutically optimized hypothyroid patients.[24] When the daily dose was reduced by 25 mcg, 78% had an elevated TSH level. When the daily dose was increased by 25 mcg, 55% had a low TSH level. Clearly, differences in the LT_4 dose or bioavailability within the FDA-allowed variance for bioequivalent products can cause significant changes in TSH.

❺ *There is no evidence that one LT_4 product is better than another. However, given the evidence that these products do have different bioavailabilities, patients should be maintained on the same LT_4 product. Given the generic substitution regulations of most states, this is best accomplished by prescribing a brand-name product or otherwise assuring that the product remains constant, and not allowing substitution in the way mandated by state regulations.* While practitioners are pressured by managed-care organizations and employers to substitute LT_4 products as a cost-saving measure, such switching is not in the best interest of the patient and should

not be allowed. If patients are switched to a different product, a TSH determination should be done in 6 to 8 weeks to allow retitration. The economic impact of retitration must be considered when formularies are changed to reduce the drug acquisition cost.

▶ *Therapeutic Use of LT_4*

❶ LT_4 is indicated for patients with overt hypothyroidism.[25] However, the need for treatment is controversial in patients with mild or subclinical disease (TSH less than 10 milliunits/L or 10 microunits/mL and normal free T_4). There is some evidence that mild or subclinical hypothyroidism is associated with increased cardiovascular morbidity and mortality,[26,27] though there are conflicting data.[28] There are no large clinical trials that show an outcome benefit with treating these patients, and the therapeutic decision must be individualized. Many patients with "subclinical" hypothyroidism do, in fact, have subtle symptoms that improve with LT_4 replacement. In patients without symptoms who have high cardiovascular risk, goiter, positive anti-TPOAb, and/or are infertile or pregnant, LT_4 replacement should be considered.[29]

Patient Encounter 1, Part 1

HT, a 34-year-old woman, comes to the clinic complaining of fatigue, lethargy, and having a "fuzzy head" for the past 6 months. She thought it was because she was working too hard, but the symptoms have not improved despite a better work schedule. She has noticed a 2.3-kg (5-lb) weight gain over the past 6 months, her menses have become heavier, she feels cold all the time, and her skin is drier. She takes no medications other than occasional acetaminophen for headache and milk of magnesia for constipation. Her vital signs and physical examination, including pelvic examination are normal.

Labs

Serum cholesterol: 220 mg/dL (5.7 mmol/L; normal less than 200 mg/dL, or 5.2 mmol/L)

TSH: 9.7 milliunits/L (normal 0.5–2.5 milliunits/L)*

Free T_4: 0.6 ng/dL (7.7 pmol/L; normal 0.7–1.9 ng/dL, or 9–24.5 pmol/L)

PE: Wt: 66 kg (145 lb), ht: 5 ft, 7 in. (170 cm).

Why should HT receive LT_4 therapy?

What initial dose of LT_4 would you choose?

How would you monitor and titrate her therapy?

What would you tell HT regarding the significance of her symptoms, elevated TSH level, and risk versus benefits of LT_4 therapy?

---

*Milliunits/L (mU/L) = microunits/mL; (μU/mL); clinical laboratories use either unit of measurement.

In patients younger than age 65 with overt hypothyroidism, the average LT$_4$ replacement dose is 1.6 mcg/kg/day (use ideal body weight in obese patients[30]). If there is no history of cardiac disease, these patients may be started on the full replacement dose. The full replacement dose in patients over age 75 is lower, about 1 mcg/kg/day.[11] In the elderly, the starting dose is 25 to 50 mcg/day, and the dose is titrated to the full replacement dose.[31] In patients with ischemic heart disease, start with 12.5 to 25 mcg/day and slowly titrate to the full replacement dose. If the patient develops angina or other forms of myocardial ischemia, lower the dose and titrate more slowly. At the start of therapy and with each change in dose, recheck the TSH in 6- to 8-week intervals. If the TSH is not in the target range (0.5–2.5 milliunits/L or microunits/mL), change the dose by 10% to 20% and then recheck the TSH 6 to 8 weeks later. As the dose is titrated, assess the patient's symptoms. Many patients will improve quickly, and many patients will feel the best if the TSH is titrated to low-normal to middle-normal levels (0.5–1.5 milliunits/L or microunits/mL).

Patients with mild or subclinical hypothyroidism do not need to be started on the full replacement dose because they still have some endogenous hormone production. Start these patients on 25 to 50 mcg/day, and titrate every 6 to 8 weeks based on TSH levels. Over time, it is likely that the LT$_4$ dose will need to be increased slowly as the patient's thyroid gland loses residual function.

▶ Risks of Over- and Undertreatment

Patients receiving LT$_4$ therapy who are not maintained in a euthyroid state are at risk for long-term adverse sequelae. In general, overtreatment and a suppressed TSH is more common than undertreatment with an elevated TSH.[32] Patients with long-term overtreatment are at higher risk for atrial fibrillation and other cardiovascular morbidities, depression or mental status changes, and postmenopausal osteoporosis. Patients who are undertreated are at higher risk for hypercholesterolemia and other cardiovascular problems, depression or mental status changes, and obstetric complications.

▶ Alterations in LT$_4$ Dose Requirements

A number of factors can alter LT$_4$ dose requirements (Table 44–4). The most common cause of increased dose requirement is the coadministration of LT$_4$ with calcium or iron supplements (including prenatal vitamins). Counsel patients that they should take the LT$_4$ dose at least 2 hours before or 6 hours after the calcium or iron dose. The most common cause of decreased dose requirement is aging.

▶ Patient Monitoring

Patients on stable LT$_4$ therapy do not need frequent monitoring. In most patients, measuring a TSH every 6 to 12 months, along with an assessment of clinical status, is adequate (Table 44–5). If the patient's clinical status changes

(e.g., pregnancy, etc.), more frequent monitoring may be necessary. LT$_4$ prescriptions should be written as microgram doses to avoid potential errors when written as milligram doses.

Table 44–4

Factors That Alter LT$_4$ Dose Requirements

Increased Dose Requirement	Decreased Dose Requirement
Decreased LT$_4$ absorption	Aging
Malabsorption syndromes	Delivery of pregnancy
Drugs diet	Withdrawal of interacting substance
Calcium	
Iron	
Aluminum	
Fiber	
Soy	
Cholestyramine/colestipol	
Sucralfate	
Sodium polystyrene sulfonate	
Phosphate binders	
Increased TBG	
Pregnancy	
Cirrhosis	
Estrogen therapy	
Tamoxifen, raloxifene therapy	
Hereditary	
Increased clearance	
Rifampin	
Carbamazepine	
Phenytoin	
Phenobarbital	
Impaired deiodination	
Amiodarone	
Mechanism unknown	
Sertraline	
Lovastatin	

LT$_4$, levothyroxine; TBG, thyroxine-binding globulin.

Table 44–5

Monitoring LT$_4$ Therapy

- Serum TSH:
  - Every 6–12 months or if change in clinical status
  - 6–8 weeks after any dose or product change
  - In first trimester pregnancy, then monthly
- Same product prescribed/dispensed with every refill
- Watch for mg/mcg dosing errors
- Assess patient's understanding of disease, therapy, and need for adherence and tight control
- Assess for signs/symptoms of over- and undertreatment
- Identify potential interactions between LT$_4$, and foods and/or drugs

LT$_4$, levothyroxine; TSH, thyroid-stimulating hormone.

Patient education is an important component of care. Treatment adherence rates (at least 80% of doses available) in hypothyroid patients are 68%, slightly less than adherence rates seen in hypertensive patients.[33] Educate patients about the benefits of proper therapy, the importance of adherence, consistency in time and method of administration, and the importance of receiving a consistent LT_4 product. Some patients will take excessive amounts of LT_4 in an effort to "feel better" or as a weight-loss treatment. Explain to patients that excessive amounts of LT_4 will not improve symptoms more than therapeutic doses will, can cause serious problems, and that this drug is not an effective treatment for obesity.

► *Special Populations and Conditions*

Hypothyroidism and Pregnancy Hypothyroidism during pregnancy has a variety of maternal and fetal adverse effects.[15,34] During pregnancy, β-human chorionic gonadotropin (β-hCG) acts as a TSH receptor agonist, increasing the amount of thyroid hormone available for fetal growth and development. Maternal hypothyroidism results in an increased rate of miscarriage and decreased intellectual capacity of the child. Endocrinologists recommend a TSH measurement as soon as the pregnancy is confirmed. Most hypothyroid women who become pregnant will quickly need an increased dose of LT_4, averaging 50% above the prepregnancy dose.[34,35] The increased dose should be maintained throughout the pregnancy, with monthly TSH monitoring to keep the TSH in the middle- to low-normal range. After delivery, the LT_4 dose can be reduced to prepregnancy levels. Since prenatal vitamins contain significant amounts of calcium and iron, remind these patients to take the LT_4 dose at least 2 hours before or 6 hours after the vitamin.

Patient Encounter 1, Part 2

One year later, HT comes to you and excitedly states that she is pregnant. She just saw her obstetrician, who started her on a prenatal vitamin. She has felt very well since starting her LT_4 and that she is amazed at how much better she feels ("I didn't know how bad I felt until I started the thyroid medicine"). The most recent TSH determination, obtained 6 months ago, was 1.5 milliunits/L (normal 0.5–2.5 milliunits/L).* Her current LT_4 dose is 88 mcg/day.

How will pregnancy affect HT's LT_4 dose requirement?

What would you recommend regarding her LT_4 dose and monitoring?

What would you tell HT regarding the potential impact of her pregnancy on her LT_4 therapy and the potential risks to her baby if she is not given an adequate dose of LT_4 during her pregnancy?

*Milliunits/L (mU/L) = microunits/mL (µU/mL); clinical laboratories use either unit of measurement.

Children Congenital hypothyroidism is still seen in the United States, and all newborns in the United States undergo screening with a TSH level. As soon as the hypothyroid state is identified, the newborn should receive the full LT_4 replacement dose. The replacement dose of LT_4 in children is age-dependent. In newborns, the usual dose is 10 to 17 mcg/kg/day. LT_4 tablets may be crushed and mixed with breast milk or formula. Serum FT_4 levels (target 1.6–2.2 ng/dL or 20.59–28.31 pmol/L) are used for dose titration in infants because the TSH level may not respond to treatment as it does in older children and adults. By 6 months of age, the required dose is reduced to 5 to 7 mcg/kg/day, and from ages 1 to 10 years, the dose is 3 to 6 mcg/kg/day. After age 12, adult doses can be given.

Myxedema Coma This is a life-threatening condition owing to severe, long standing hypothyroidism and has a mortality rate of 60% to 70%. These patients are given 300 to 500 mcg IV LT_4 initially, using caution in patients with underlying cardiac disease. While administration of T_3 would provide a more rapid onset of action, there is no evidence that T_3 improves outcomes in myxedema coma. Historically, glucocorticoids, such as hydrocortisone 50 to 100 mg every 6 hours, are administered owing to concern about simultaneous adrenal insufficiency. While there is no strong evidence for an outcome benefit, the use of glucocorticoids is reasonable because such treatment may be lifesaving, and the risks of a short course of corticosteroids at this dose are low. As patients improve, the LT_4 dose can be given orally in a typical full replacement dose.

HYPERTHYROIDISM/THYROTOXICOSIS

Hyperthyroidism is much less common than hypothyroidism. In NHANES,[1] 0.5% of the population was hyperthyroid, with the highest incidences in women overall and in men and women in the over 80 years of age groups. The Colorado Thyroid Health Study[2] showed a hyperthyroid incidence of 2.2% (2.1% subclinical).

Causes of Thyrotoxicosis/Hyperthyroidism

Thyrotoxicosis is any syndrome caused by excess thyroid hormone. Hyperthyroidism is related to excess thyroid hormone secreted by the thyroid gland. Thyrotoxicosis can be related to the presence or absence of excess hormone production (hyperthyroidism). The common causes of thyrotoxicosis are shown in Table 44–6.[36–38] Graves' disease is the most common cause of hyperthyroidism. Thyrotoxicosis in the elderly is more likely due to toxic thyroid nodules or multinodular goiter than to Graves' disease. Excessive intake of thyroid hormone may be due to overtreatment with prescribed therapy. Surreptitious use of thyroid hormones also may occur, especially in health professionals or as a self-remedy for obesity. Thyroid hormones can be obtained easily without a prescription from health food stores or Internet sources. Refer to Clinical Presentation and Diagnosis of Hyperthyroidism for information regarding screening and diagnosis.

Patient Care and Monitoring: Hypothyroidism

1. Use serum TSH to identify patients with hypothyroidism and to monitor LT$_4$ replacement therapy.

2. Use synthetic LT$_4$ as the treatment of choice for hypothyroidism.

3. Provide LT$_4$ replacement to patients with overt hypothyroidism.

4. Consider replacement therapy in patients with a TSH level of greater than 2.5 but less than 10 milliunits/L* who have subtle symptoms (e.g., mild fatigue, lethargy, etc.), elevated cholesterol, or positive anti-TPOAbs.

5. Provide the calculated full replacement LT$_4$ dose (1.6 mcg/kg/day based on ideal body weight if obese) to patients with overt hypothyroidism who are older than 12 and younger than 65 years of age and who do not have cardiac disease.

6. Patients with mild hypothyroidism may be started at 25 to 50 mcg/day of LT$_4$.

7. Elderly patients or those with cardiac disease should be started at a lower LT$_4$ dose (e.g., 12.5–25 mcg/day).

8. Measure serum TSH 6 to 8 weeks after starting or any dose change. If the TSH level is not in the target range, alter the dose by 10% to 20% increments.

9. The target TSH for patients on LT$_4$ replacement therapy for hypothyroidism is 0.5 to 2.5 milliunits/L. Most patients feel best at a TSH level in the low- to middle-normal range (i.e., 0.5–1.5 milliunits/L).*

10. Provide a brand-name LT$_4$ product, and do not allow the patient to be switched to different products. If the product is switched, check a TSH in 6 weeks and retitrate the dose.

11. Write LT$_4$ prescriptions as microgram not milligram doses to avoid errors.

12. Check a TSH every 6 to 12 months in stable patients receiving LT$_4$ replacement.

13. Make sure that patients understand the importance of adherence and the risks of over- and underuse of LT$_4$.

14. At each visit, assess the patient for signs and symptoms of over- and undertreatment.

15. Monitor for drug interactions, such as LT$_4$ absorption problems caused by calcium and iron.

16. Check a TSH in pregnant women as soon as the pregnancy is diagnosed. In hypothyroid pregnant women, check the TSH monthly, and expect to raise the LT$_4$ dose during the first trimester. Maintain the TSH in the low- to middle-normal range. After delivery, reduce the LT$_4$ dose to the prepregnancy dose.

*Milliunits/L (mU/L) = microunits/mL (μU/mL); clinical laboratories use either unit of measurement.

Clinical Presentation and Diagnosis of Hyperthyroidism

Symptoms

- Nervousness
- Fatigue
- Weakness
- Increased perspiration
- Heat intolerance
- Tremor
- Hyperactivity, irritability
- Palpitations
- Appetite change (usually increased)
- Weight change (usually weight loss)
- Menstrual disturbances (often oligomenorrhea)
- Diarrhea

Signs

- Hyperactivity
- Tachycardia

- Atrial fibrillation (especially in elderly)
- Hyper-reflexia
- Warm, moist skin
- Ophthalmopathy, dermopathy (Graves' disease)
- Goiter
- Muscle weakness

Screening/Diagnosis

- Low TSH level (less than 0.5 milliunit/L) will signify thyrotoxicosis.
- Free T$_4$ is elevated in overt hyperthyroidism.
- Increased radioiodine uptake in the thyroid indicates increased hormone production by the thyroid gland.
- Almost all patients with Graves' disease will have positive TSHR-SAbs and positive anti-TPOAbs.

From Refs. 36–38.

Table 44–6

Causes of Thyrotoxicosis

Primary hyperthyroidism
    Graves' disease
    Toxic multinodular goiter
    Toxic adenoma
    Thyroid cancer
    Struma ovarii
    Iodine excess (including radiocontrast, amiodarone)
Thyrotoxicosis without hyperthyroidism
    Subacute thyroiditis
    Silent (painless) thyroiditis
    Excess thyroid hormone intake (thyrotoxicosis factitia)
    Drug-induced (amiodarone, iodine, lithium, interferons)
Secondary hyperthyroidism
    TSH-secreting pituitary tumors
    Trophoblastic (hCG-secreting) tumors
    Gestational thyrotoxicosis

hCG, human chorionic gonadotropin; TSH, thyroid-stimulating hormone.

From Refs. 36–38.

Clinical Manifestations of Thyrotoxicosis

Many of the signs and symptoms seem to be related to autonomic hyperactivity. As with hypothyroidism, the clinical manifestations may be subtle initially and slowly progressive. Screening of patients for thyroid disease may identify patients with subclinical or mild thyrotoxicosis. Patients may seek medical attention only after a long period of thyrotoxicosis or owing to an acute complication such as atrial fibrillation. The clinical manifestations of thyrotoxicosis in the elderly may be blunted or atypical. These patients may present only with atrial fibrillation, depression, or altered mental status or cognition.

Subclinical Hyperthyroidism

Subclinical or mild hyperthyroidism is defined as a low TSH with a normal FT_4 level. While there may be few or no symptoms in these patients, there are several areas of concern.[29] Many patients will progress to overt thyrotoxicosis. Patients with subclinical hyperthyroidism have been shown to suffer long-term cardiovascular and bone sequelae. The impact of subclinical hyperthyroidism on cardiovascular mortality is not clear.[26-29] Several studies have shown that prolonged subclinical thyrotoxicosis speeds the loss of bone mineral density and increases fracture rates in postmenopausal women.[29] Treatment of patients with subclinical hyperthyroidism is controversial, but should be considered in postmenopausal women and in patients with underlying cardiovascular disease.[29]

Graves' Disease

Graves' disease[36] is an autoimmune syndrome that includes hyperthyroidism, diffuse thyroid enlargement, exophthalmos and other eye findings, and skin findings.

The prevalence of Graves' disease in the United States is approximately 0.4% in women and 0.1% in men. The peak age of incidence is 20 to 49 years, with a second peak after 80 years of age. Hyperthyroidism results from the production of TSHR-SAbs in at least 80% of patients with clinical Graves' disease. These antibodies have TSH agonist activity, thereby stimulating hormone synthesis and release. These antibodies cross-react with orbital and fibroblastic tissue, resulting in ophthalmopathy and dermopathy. While the underlying cause of Graves' disease is not known, heredity seems to play a role. Subclinical Graves' disease may become acutely overt in the presence of iodine excess, infection, stress, parturition, smoking, and lithium and cytokine therapy.

There are several features of Graves' disease that are distinct from other forms of thyrotoxicosis. Clinically apparent ophthalmopathic changes are seen in 20% to 40% of patients and include exophthalmos, proptosis, chemosis, conjunctival injection, and periorbital edema. Lid retraction causes a typical staring or startled appearance (Fig. 44–3). Patients may complain of vague eye discomfort and excess tearing. In severe cases, the eyelids are unable to close completely, resulting in corneal damage. In very severe cases, the optic nerve can be compressed, resulting in permanent vision loss. All patients with suspected or known Graves' disease must be evaluated and monitored by an ophthalmologist.

Dermopathy occurs in 5% to 10% of patients with Graves' disease and usually is associated with severe ophthalmopathy. Skin findings include hyperpigmented, nonpitting induration of the skin, typically over the pretibial area (pretibial myxedema), the dorsa of the feet, and shoulder areas. Clubbing of the digits (thyroid acropachy) is associated with long-standing thyrotoxicosis.

Treatment of Hyperthyroidism

Treatment of thyrotoxicosis due to hyperthyroidism is similar, regardless of the underlying cause. ⑥ *The goals of treating hyperthyroidism are to relieve symptoms, to reduce thyroid hormone production to normal levels and achieve biochemical euthyroidism, and to prevent long-term adverse sequelae.*

▶ *β-Blockers*

Because many of the manifestations of hyperthyroidism appear to be mediated by the β-adrenergic system, β-adrenergic blockers are used to rapidly relieve palpitations, tremor, anxiety, and heat intolerance.[38] Because β-blockers do not reduce the synthesis of thyroid hormones, they are used only until more specific antithyroid therapy is effective. Since nonselective agents can impair the conversion of T_4 to T_3, propranolol and nadolol are used. An initial propranolol dose of 20 to 40 mg four times daily should be titrated to relieve signs and symptoms. β-Blockers should not be used in patients with decompensated heart failure or asthma. When a contraindication to β-blockers exists, clonidine or diltiazem may be used.

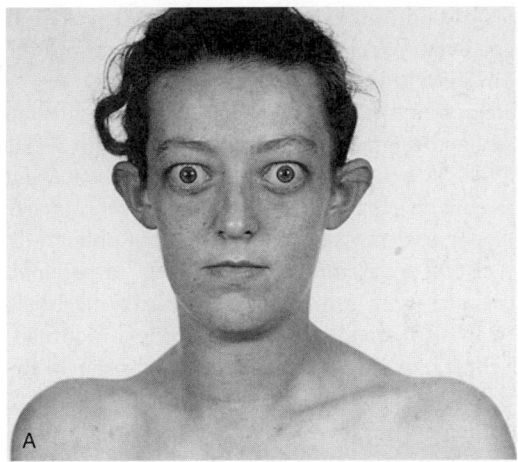

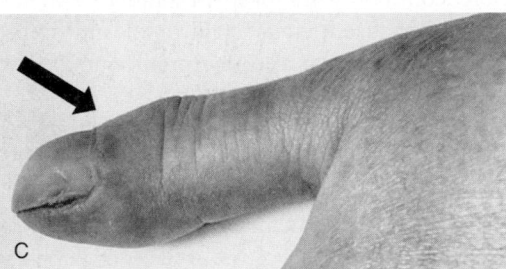

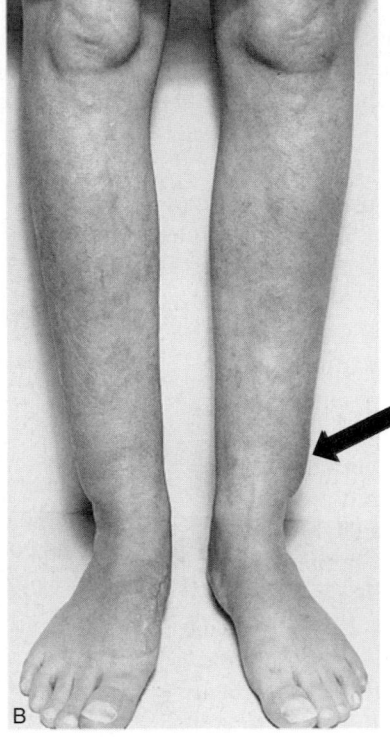

FIGURE 44–3. Features of Graves' disease. (A) Facial appearance: exophthalmos, lid retraction, periorbital edema, and proptosis. (B) Thyroid dermopathy over lateral aspects of shins. (C) Thyroid clubbing (acropachy). (From Jameson JL, Weetman AP. Disorders of the thyroid gland. In: Kasper DL, Braunwald E, Fauci AS, et al., eds. Harrison's Principles of Internal Medicine, 16th ed. New York: McGraw-Hill, 2004:2114.)

Patient Encounter 2, Part 1

GD is a 24-year-old woman who comes to the clinic stating, "I'm so nervous and hungry, and I'm losing weight. What is wrong with me?" She first noticed these symptoms 2 months ago, and they have worsened steadily. She feels anxious for no reason and has trouble sleeping. She has noticed that her appetite has increased, although she has lost about 4.6 kg (10 lb) over the past 2 months. Sometimes she can feel her heart beating in her chest, but she denies chest pain or syncope. She also has noticed that she is always sweaty and that her menses have become very light. Her only medications are a hormonal oral contraceptive and occasional naproxen for dysmenorrhea. She thinks that her mother had some kind of thyroid problem when she was pregnant.

PE:

VS: Pulse 112 bpm, blood pressure 108/72, RR 12, temperature 37.4°C (99.3°F)

HEENT: Diffusely enlarged thyroid; mild exophthalmos

CV: Tachycardic, RRR

Exts: Fine tremor

Skin: Warm and moist

ECG: Sinus tachycardia

Labs:

Electrolytes, complete blood count normal. Urine hCG negative. TSH less than 0.5 milliunit/L (normal 0.5–2.5 milliunits/L);* free T_4 (FT_4) 3.1 ng/dL (39.9 pmol/L; normal 0.7–1.9 ng/dL, or 9.0–24.5 pmol/L); +TSHR-SAbs

What therapeutic options exist for GD's Graves' disease?

What would you recommend?

How would you initiate and titrate therapy?

What would you tell GD regarding the cause of her signs and symptoms, significance of her abnormal thyroid function tests, and therapeutic options?

*Milliunits/L (mU/L) = microunits/mL (μU/mL); clinical laboratories use either unit of measurement.

▶ Methods to Reduce Thyroid Hormone Synthesis

Excess production of thyroid hormone can be reduced in four ways: iodides, antithyroid drugs, radioactive iodine, and surgery.[37–41]

Iodide Large doses of iodide inhibit the synthesis and release of thyroid hormones. Serum T_4 levels may be reduced within 24 hours, and the effects may last for 2 to 3 weeks. Iodides are used most commonly in Graves' disease patients prior to surgery and to quickly reduce hormone release in patients with thyroid storm. Potassium iodide is administered either as a saturated solution (SSKI) that contains 38 mg iodide per drop or as Lugol's solution, which contains 6.3 mg iodide per drop. The typical starting dose is 120 to

400 mg/day. Iodide therapy should start 7 to 14 days prior to surgery. Iodide should not be given prior to radioactive iodine treatment because the iodide will inhibit concentration of the radioactivity in the thyroid. Iodides also are used to protect the thyroid from radioactive iodine fallout after a nuclear accident or attack. Daily administration of 30 to 100 mg iodide will markedly reduce thyroid gland uptake of radioactive iodine. The most frequent toxic effects with iodide therapy are hypersensitivity reactions, "iodism" (characterized by palpitations, depression, weight loss, and pustular skin eruptions), and gynecomastia.

Antithyroid Drugs The thionamide agents propylthiouracil and methimazole are used in the United States to treat hyperthyroidism.[40–42] Carbimazole, a methimazole prodrug, is available in Europe. These drugs inhibit thyroid hormone synthesis by interfering with thyroid peroxidase–mediated iodination of tyrosine residues in thyroglobulin. Propylthiouracil has the added effect of inhibiting the conversion of T_4 to T_3. The thionamides also have immunosuppressant effects. In patients with Graves' disease treated with thionamides, TSHR-SAb levels and other immune mediators decrease over time. Both drugs are well absorbed from the GI tract. Propylthiouracil has a half-life of 1 to 2.5 hours, whereas the half-life of methimazole is 6 to 9 hours.

Antithyroid drugs are used as primary therapy for Graves' disease or as preparative therapy before surgery or radioactive iodine administration. The decision to use antithyroid drugs as primary therapy must be weighed against the risks and benefits of radioiodine or surgery. Patient preference must be considered.

In most patients, there is no clear advantage of one thionamide over the other. While propylthiouracil has the advantage of inhibiting T_4-to-T_3 conversion, methimazole can be given as a single daily dose. Methimazole is preferred to normalize thyroid function prior to radioactive iodine therapy, though both thionamides increase the failure rate of radioactive iodine therapy.[43] The usual starting dose of methimazole is 15 to 30 mg/day, and the usual starting dose of propylthiouracil is 100 mg three times daily. Thyroid hormone levels drop in 2 to 3 weeks, and after 6 weeks, 90% of patients with Graves' disease will be euthyroid. Thyroid function testing should be performed every 4 to 6 weeks until stable. After the patient becomes euthyroid, the antithyroid drug dose often can be decreased (5–10 mg/day methimazole, 100–200 mg/day propylthiouracil) to maintain the euthyroid state. Excessive doses of antithyroid drugs will result in hypothyroidism.

Remission of Graves' disease occurs in 40% to 60% of patients after 1 to 2 years of therapy. Antithyroid therapy may be stopped or tapered after 12 to 24 months. Relapse usually occurs in the first 3 to 6 months after stopping antithyroid therapy. Levels of TSHR-SAb after a course of treatment may have predictive value for the risk of relapse in that antibody-positive patients almost always will relapse. However, antibody-negative patients also may relapse after therapy is stopped. About 75% of women in remission who become pregnant will have a postpartum relapse.

When therapy is discontinued, a therapeutic strategy should be in place in the event of relapse. Many patients will opt for radioactive iodine as a long-term solution.

Antithyroid drugs are associated with a low rate of adverse effects. Skin rash, arthralgias, and GI upset are seen in 5% of patients. While the drug can be continued in the presence of a minor skin rash, the development of arthralgia warrants discontinuation. Hepatotoxicity is an uncommon but potentially serious adverse effect, occurring in 0.1% to 0.2% of patients. However, transient rises in aminotransferase enzyme levels are seen in up to 30% of patients treated with propylthiouracil. Severe hepatocellular damage can occur from propylthiouracil, whereas methimazole can cause cholestatic jaundice. Vasculitis is another potentially serious but uncommon reaction that is more common with propylthiouracil. Patients may develop a drug-induced lupus syndrome, and some, particularly Asians, can develop antineutrophil cytoplasmic antibody-positive vasculitis.

❼ *Agranulocytosis is one of the most serious adverse effects of antithyroid drug therapy.* Agranulocytosis must be distinguished from a transient decrease in white blood cell count seen in up to 12% of adults and 25% of children with Graves' disease. Agranulocytosis occurs in 0.3% of patients, and the incidence may be the same with propylthiouracil and methimazole therapy. Agranulocytosis almost always occurs within the first 3 months of therapy, and it occurs suddenly and unpredictably. Patients will present with fever, malaise, and sore throat, and the absolute neutrophil count will be less than 1,000/mm³. Patients may develop sepsis and die rapidly.

Patient Encounter 2, Part 2

One month later, GD is back for a follow-up visit. She notes that her thyrotoxic symptoms are gone, and overall, she feels great. She is receiving propylthiouracil 100 mg three times daily. Her most recent TSH was 0.9 milliunit/L (normal 0.5–2.5 milliunits/L)* and her free T_4 was 1.6 ng/dL (20.6 pmol/L; normal 0.7–1.9 ng/dL, or 9.0–24.5 pmol/L). However, over the past few days she has developed a sore throat and feels achy. She wonders if she has the flu. Her vital signs show a pulse of 92 bpm and a temperature of 38.3°C (101°F). A CBC reveals a total WBC of 0.1 × 10³/mm³ or 0.1 × 10⁹/L (normal 4–10 × 10³/mm³ or 4–10 × 10⁹/L) with 15 neutrophils (absolute neutrophil count 150).

What has happened to GD?

What are you concerned about?

How will you manage this problem?

What will you tell GD regarding the possible cause of her new symptoms, the significance of her low WBC, and recommended actions?

---

*Milliunits/L (mU/L) = microunits/mL (μU/mL); clinical laboratories use either unit of measurement.

Agranulocytosis is thought to be autoimmune-mediated. If agranulocytosis occurs, discontinue the antithyroid drug immediately, administer broad-spectrum antibiotics if the patient is febrile, and consider the administration of granulocyte colony-stimulating factor. The white blood cell count should recover in a week or two. Patients who develop agranulocytosis should not be switched to another thionamide drug. Monitoring for agranulocytosis is controversial owing to its sudden and unpredictable nature. Most practitioners do not recommend routine monitoring of the complete blood count, although early detection could improve patient outcomes. Patients initiating thionamide therapy must be informed about the signs and symptoms of agranulocytosis, and other serious side effects. Patients should be asked to report signs and symptoms suggestive of infection, such as fever and sore throat lasting more than 2 or 3 days, or any bruising.

Radioactive Iodine Radioactive iodine, typically ^{131}I, produces thyroid ablation without surgery. ^{131}I is well absorbed after oral administration. The iodine is concentrated in the thyroid gland and has a half-life of 8 days. Over a period of weeks, thyroid cells that have taken up the ^{131}I begin to develop abnormalities and necrosis. Eventually, thyroid cells are destroyed, and hormone production is reduced. After a single dose, 40% to 70% of patients will be euthyroid in 6 to 8 weeks, and 80% will be cured. In most patients, hypothyroidism will develop, and long-term LT$_4$ replacement will be necessary. Because ^{131}I has a slow onset of action, most patients are treated initially with β-blockers and antithyroid drugs. Thionamide drugs must be withdrawn for at least 4 to 6 days prior to ^{131}I administration to allow adequate accumulation of the radioactive iodine in the gland. β-Blockers can be continued during ^{131}I therapy. The dose of ^{131}I is based on the estimated weight of the patient's thyroid gland. Radioactive iodine therapy is contraindicated during pregnancy and breast-feeding. Radioactive iodine therapy may acutely worsen Graves' ophthalmopathy. Patients with prominent eye disease may be started on prednisone 40 mg/day, with the dose tapered over 2 to 3 months. Radioactive iodine also may cause a painful thyroiditis, which may necessitate anti-inflammatory therapy. Any long-term carcinogenic effect of ^{131}I has not been demonstrated in long-term clinical trials.

Surgery Subtotal thyroidectomy is indicated in patients with very large goiters and thyroid malignancies and those who do not respond or cannot tolerate other therapies. Patients must be euthyroid prior to surgery, and patients often are administered iodide preoperatively to reduce gland vascularity. The overall surgical complication rate is 2.7%. Postoperative hypothyroidism occurs in 10% of patients who undergo subtotal thyroidectomy.

▶ Special Conditions and Populations

Graves' Disease and Pregnancy[34,35,44] Pregnancy may worsen or precipitate thyrotoxicosis in women with underlying Graves' disease owing to the TSH agonist effect of β-hCG. Untreated maternal thyrotoxicosis may result in increased rates of miscarriage, premature delivery, eclampsia, and low-birth-weight infants. Fetal and neonatal hyperthyroidism may occur as a result of transplacental passage of TSHR-SAbs. Because radioactive iodine is contraindicated and surgery is best avoided during pregnancy, most patients are treated with antithyroid drugs. Propylthiouracil is considered the treatment of choice, and the lowest possible dose to maintain maternal euthyroidism should be used. Antithyroid therapy in excessive doses may suppress fetal thyroid function.

Neonatal and Pediatric Hyperthyroidism Some neonates born to mothers with Graves' disease will be hyperthyroid at delivery. Antithyroid drug therapy (propylthiouracil 5–10 mg/kg/day or methimazole 0.5–1 mg/kg/day) may be required for up to 12 weeks. One drop per day of SSKI may be used in the first few days to rapidly reduce thyroid hormone synthesis and release.

Thyroid Storm Thyroid storm is a life-threatening condition caused by severe thyrotoxicosis.[45] Signs and symptoms include high fever, tachycardia, tachypnea, dehydration, delirium, coma, and GI disturbances. Thyroid storm is precipitated in a previously hyperthyroid patient by infection, trauma, surgery, radioactive iodine treatment, and sudden withdrawal from antithyroid drugs. Patients are treated with a short-acting β-blocker such as IV esmolol, IV or oral iodide, and large doses of propylthiouracil (900–1,200 mg/day in three to four divided doses). Supportive care with acetaminophen to suppress fever, fluid and electrolyte management, and antiarrhythmic agents are important components of therapy. IV hydrocortisone 100 mg every 8 hours is used often due to the potential presence of adrenal insufficiency.

NONTHYROIDAL ILLNESS (EUTHYROID SICK SYNDROME)

A number of changes in the hypothalamic–pituitary–thyroid axis occur during acute illness.[46,47] These changes are termed nonthyroidal illness or euthyroid sick syndrome. The type and degree of abnormalities depend on the severity of illness. Mild to moderate medical illness, surgery, or starvation causes a decrease in serum T$_3$ levels owing to decreased peripheral conversion of T$_4$ to T$_3$. The reduced T$_3$ levels do not correlate with ultimate mortality and are thought to be an adaptive response to stress. Patients with more severe illness, especially those in the intensive-care unit, frequently have reduced total T$_4$ levels, although FT$_4$ levels usually are normal. In the critically ill, there is a correlation between the degree of serum T$_4$ reduction and mortality. In most acutely ill patients who are euthyroid, the TSH level is normal. However, administration of dopamine, octreotide, or high doses of glucocorticoids can reduce TSH levels. During recovery from acute illness, the TSH level may become modestly elevated to renormalize serum T$_4$ levels. During this time, thyroid function tests may be misinterpreted to indicate hypothyroidism. Despite the sometimes very low T$_4$ levels, there is no evidence that LT$_4$ administration has any benefit. Patients with possible thyroid abnormalities during acute illness should be evaluated by an endocrinologist.

Patient Care and Monitoring: Hyperthyroidism

1. A low or undetectable TSH level identifies thyrotoxicosis.

2. Refer the patient for a diagnostic assessment to identify the underlying cause. Identify Graves' disease by the presence of eye and/or skin findings and the presence of TSHR-SAbs.

3. Refer patients with Graves' disease to an ophthalmologist for assessment and monitoring.

4. Treat severe or troublesome autonomic signs and symptoms with a nonselective β-blocker such as propranolol 20 to 40 mg four times daily. Titrate the β-blocker dose based on signs and symptoms.

5. In patients with excess thyroid hormone production, reduce hormone production with an antithyroid drug and/or radioactive iodine. Choose therapy based on patient-specific factors and preference.

6. Antithyroid drugs have a delayed effect. After 2 to 4 weeks of therapy, adjust the dose if the TSH is not in the target range (0.5–2.5 milliunits/L).* Once the patient is

euthyroid, consider reducing the dose of antithyroid drug to avoid hypothyroidism.

7. Consider stopping antithyroid therapy in Graves' disease after 12 to 18 months to see if remission has occurred.

8. Monitor patients on antithyroid drugs for signs and symptoms of adverse effects.

9. Monitor for symptoms of neutropenia (e.g., fever or sore throat), and check white blood cell count if symptoms occur.

10. If radioactive iodine is given, make sure that antithyroid drugs are stopped 4 to 6 days prior to treatment.

11. Several months after radioactive iodine, expect that the patient will require permanent LT_4 replacement.

12. Treat pregnant hyperthyroid women with propylthiouracil.

---

*Milliunits/L (mU/L) = microunits/mL (μU/mL); clinical laboratories use either unit of measurement.

THYROID CANCER AND LT_4 SUPPRESSION

❽ *The growth and spread of thyroid carcinoma is stimulated by TSH. An important component of thyroid carcinoma management is the use of LT_4 to suppress TSH secretion. Early in therapy, patients receive the lowest LT_4 dose sufficient to fully suppress TSH to undetectable levels. Controlled trials show that suppressive LT_4 therapy reduces tumor growth and improves survival.* These patients are purposefully "overtreated" with LT_4, sometimes to a fully-suppressed TSH level and rendered subclinically hyperthyroid. Postmenopausal women should receive aggressive osteoporosis therapy to prevent LT_4-induced bone loss. Other thyrotoxic complications, such as atrial fibrillation, should be monitored and managed appropriately.

DRUG-INDUCED THYROID ABNORMALITIES

Drugs can affect thyroid function in a number of ways.[13,48] Effects of drugs on thyroid hormone protein binding, LT_4 absorption, and metabolism have been discussed previously. Several commonly used medications can alter thyroid hormone secretion.

Amiodarone

Amiodarone[49] is a commonly prescribed antiarrhythmic drug that contains two iodide atoms, constituting 38% of its mass. Each 200-mg dose of amiodarone provides 75 mg iodide. Amiodarone deiodination releases about 6 mg of free iodine

daily, 20 to 40 times more than the average daily intake of iodine in the United States. Amiodarone blocks conversion of T_4 to T_3, inhibits entry of T_3 into cells, and decreases T_3 receptor binding. Amiodarone causes rapid reduction in serum T_3 levels, increases free and total T_4 levels, and increases TSH level. After 3 months of therapy, TSH levels usually return to normal, although the serum T_3 and T_4 level changes may remain. Most of these patients are euthyroid because the free T_3 levels are in the low-normal range. Amiodarone can cause thyroid abnormalities frequently in previously euthyroid patients. In a study of amiodarone treatment of persistent atrial fibrillation,[50] 25.8% of patients developed subclinical hypothyroidism, and 5% developed overt hypothyroidism. Hyperthyroidism occurred in 5.3%. Thyroid abnormalities, when they occurred, were seen within 6 months of initiation of amiodarone therapy in almost all patients. Amiodarone-induced hypothyroidism is more common in iodine-sufficient areas of the world. Patients with underlying autoimmune thyroiditis are much more likely to develop amiodarone-induced hypothyroidism. Amiodarone-induced hypothyroidism occurs most commonly within the first year of therapy. If amiodarone cannot be discontinued, LT_4 therapy will be effective in most patients. If amiodarone can be stopped, thyroid function will return to normal in 2 to 4 months.

Amiodarone is more likely to cause thyrotoxicosis in iodine-deficient areas. Type 1 amiodarone-induced thyrotoxicosis is caused by iodine excess, and typically occurs in patients with pre-existing multinodular goiter or subclinical Graves' disease. Type 2 amiodarone-induced thyrotoxicosis is a destructive thyroiditis that occurs in patients with no underlying thyroid disease. Amiodarone-induced thyrotoxicosis is more common in men. Because amiodarone has β-blocking activity, palpitations and tachycardia may be absent. In type 1 thyrotoxicosis, amiodarone should be discontinued. If amiodarone therapy cannot be stopped, larger doses of antithyroid drugs may be needed to control thyrotoxicosis. In type 2 thyroiditis, stopping amiodarone may not be necessary because spontaneous resolution may occur. Prednisone 40 to 60 mg/day will quickly improve thyrotoxic symptoms. Prednisone may be tapered after 1 to 2 months of therapy.

⑨ *Patients receiving amiodarone must receive monitoring for thyroid abnormalities. Baseline measurements of serum TSH, FT_4, FT_3, anti-TPOAbs, and TSHR-SAbs should be performed. TSH, FT_4, and FT_3 should be checked 3 months after initiation of amiodarone and then at least a TSH every 3 to 6 months.*

Lithium

- Lithium is associated with hypothyroidism in up to 34% of patients, and hypothyroidism may occur after years of therapy. Lithium appears to inhibit thyroid hormone synthesis and secretion. Patients with underlying autoimmune thyroiditis are more likely to develop lithium-induced hypothyroidism. Patients may require LT_4 replacement even if lithium is discontinued.

Interferon-α

- Interferon-α causes hypothyroidism in up to 39% of patients being treated for hepatitis C infection. Patients may develop a transient thyroiditis with hyperthyroidism prior to becoming hypothyroid. The hypothyroidism may be transient as well. Asians and patients with pre-existing anti-TPOAbs are more likely to develop interferon-induced hypothyroidism. The mechanism of interferon-induced hypothyroidism is not known. If LT_4 replacement is initiated, it should be stopped after 6 months to reevaluate the need for replacement therapy.

OUTCOME EVALUATION

- Desired outcomes include relieving signs and symptoms and achieving a euthyroid state.

- Success of therapy for thyroid disorders must be based not only on short-term improvement of the patient's clinical status and abnormal laboratory values but also on achievement of a long-term euthyroid state. Maintaining the TSH level in the normal range improves symptoms and reduces the risk of long-term complications.

- Because pharmacotherapy often is lifelong, especially in patients with hypothyroidism, patients must undergo periodic monitoring to avoid the long-term complications of hypothyroidism and hyperthyroidism. In the hypothyroid patient, such monitoring may involve simply asking the patient about signs and symptoms, and a yearly measurement of the TSH level.

- Any change in the patient's clinical status, such as a new pregnancy or a major change in body weight, necessitates a reevaluation of therapy. Patients at high risk for complications, such as pregnant women, the elderly, and patients with underlying cardiac disease, must be monitored more closely.

- Patients should be educated and periodically reminded about the importance of adherence and long-term tight control, the need for periodic clinical and laboratory monitoring, and the importance of staying on one LT_4 product.

- In the hyperthyroid patient, relieving signs and symptoms, and achieving a euthyroid state are the desired outcomes. The method of achieving these outcomes may change over time with the use of antithyroid drugs versus radioactive iodine.

- Patients with hyperthyroidism also must undergo periodic clinical and laboratory monitoring, with more frequent monitoring if there is a change in the patient's clinical status.

- Patients who receive antithyroid drugs must be monitored for adverse drug events such as agranulocytosis.

- Patients who receive radioactive iodine must be monitored for the development of hypothyroidism.

- In patients with thyroid cancer, the desired outcomes with LT_4 therapy often are different from those in the hypothyroid patient.

- LT_4 doses sufficient to suppress tumor growth may result in a suppressed TSH and mild hyperthyroidism. These patients must be monitored closely for complications of the mild hyperthyroid state, such as bone mineral loss and development of atrial fibrillation.

Abbreviations Introduced in This Chapter

ANDA	Abbreviated New Drug Application
Anti-TGAb	Antithyroglobulin antibody
Anti-TPOAb	Antithyroid peroxidase antibody
AUC	Area under the (time-concentration) curve
β-hCG	β-Human chorionic gonadotropin
FT_3	Free T_3
FT_4	Free T_4
hCG	Human chorionic gonadotropin
LT_4	Levothyroxine
NHANES	National Health and Nutrition Examination Survey
NTI	Narrow therapeutic index
RAIU	Radioactive iodine uptake
SSKI	Saturated solution of potassium iodide
T_3	Triiodothyronine
T_4	Thyroxine
TBG	Thyroxine-binding globulin
TPOAb	Thyroid peroxidase antibody
TRH	Thyrotropin-releasing hormone
TSH	Thyroid-stimulating hormone
TSHR-SAb	TSH receptor-stimulating antibodies

Self-assessment questions and answers are available at *http://www.mhpharmacotherapy.com/pp.html*.

REFERENCES

1. Aoki Y, Belin RM, Clickner R, et al. Serum TSH and total T$_4$ in the United States population and their association with participant characteristics: National Health and Nutrition Examination Survey (NHANES 1999–2002). Thyroid 2007;17:1211–1223.

2. Canaris GJ, Manowitz NR, Mayor G, Ridgeway EC. The Colorado thyroid disease prevalence study. Arch Int Med 2000;160:526–534.

3. Spencer CA, Hollowell JG, Karazosyan M, Braverman LE. National Health and Nutrition Examination Survey III thyroid-stimulating hormone (TSH)-thyroperoxidase antibody relationships demonstrate that TSH upper reference limits may be skewed by occult thyroid dysfunction. J Clin Endocrinol Metb 2007;92:4236–4240.

4. Surks MI, Hollowell JG. Age-specific distribution of serum thyrotropin and antithyroid antibodies in the U.S. population: Implications for the prevalence of subclinical hypothyroidism. J Clin Endocrinol Metab 2007;92:4575–4582.

5. Wartofsky L, Dickey RA. The evidence for a narrower thyrotropin reference range is compelling. J Clin Endocrinol Metab 2005;90:5483–5488.

6. Toft AD, Beckett GJ. Measuring serum thyrotropin and thyroid hormone and assessing thyroid hormone transport. In: Braverman LE, Utiger RD, eds. Werner & Ingbar's The Thyroid. A Fundamental and Clinical Text, 9th ed. Philadelphia: Lippincott Williams & Wilkins, 2005:329–344.

7. Vanderpump MPJ, Tunbridge WMG, French JM, et al. The incidence of thyroid disorders in the community: A twenty year follow-up of the Whickham survey. Clin Endocrinol (Oxf) 1995;43:55–69.

8. Danese MD, Powe NR, Sawin CT, Ladenson PW. Screening for mild thyroid failure at the periodic health examination. A decision and cost-effectiveness analysis. JAMA 1996;276:285–292.

9. Ladenson PW, Singer PA, Ain KB, Bagchi N, et al. American Thyroid Association guidelines for detection of thyroid dysfunction. Arch Int Med 2000;160: 1573–1575.

10. U.S. Preventative Services Task Force. Screening for thyroid disease: Recommendation statement. Ann Int Med 2004;140:125–127.

11. Devdhar M, Ousman YH, Burman KD. Hypothyroidism. Endocrinol Metab Clin North Amer 2007;36:595–615.

12. Vaidya B, Pearce SHS. Management of hypothyroidism in adults. BMJ 2008;337:284–289.

13. Ma RCW, Kong APS, Chan N, et al. Drug-induced endocrine and metabolic disorders. Drug Safety 2007;30:215–245.

14. Volzke H, Schwann C, Wallaschofski H, Dorr M. Review: The association of thyroid dysfunction with all-cause and circulatory mortality: Is there a causal relationship? J Clin Endocrinol Metab 2007;92:2421–2429.

15. Glinder D. Thyroid disease during pregnancy. In: Braverman LE, Utiger RD, eds. Werner & Ingbar's The Thyroid. A Fundamental and Clinical Text, 9th ed. Philadelphia: Lippincott Williams & Wilkins, 2005:1086–1108.

16. Grozinsky-Glasberg S, Fraser A, Nahshoni E, et al. Thyroxine-triiodothyronine combination therapy versus thyroxine monotherapy for clinical hypothyroidism: Meta-analysis of randomized controlled trials. J Clin Endocrinol Metab 2006;91:2592–2599.

17. Hennessey JV. Levothyroxine a new drug? Since when? How could that be? Thyroid 2003;13:279–282.

18. U.S. Department of Health and Human Services, Food and Drug Administration Center for Drug Evaluation and Research Guidance for Industry. Levothyroxine Sodium Products Enforcement of August 14, 2001 Compliance Date and Submission of New Applications. *www.fda.gov/cder/guidance/index.htm*.

19. Food and Drug Administration Center for Drug Evaluation and Research Electronic Orange Book. Approved Drug Products with Therapeutic Equivalence Evaluations. *www.fda.gov/cder/ob/default.htm*.

20. Benet LZ, Goyan JE. Bioequivalence and narrow therapeutic index drugs. Pharmacother 1995;15:433–440.

21. Blakesley V, Awni W, Locke C, Ludden T, et al. Are bioequivalence studies of levothyroxine sodium formulations in euthyroid volunteers reliable? Thyroid 2004;14:191–200.

22. Dong BJ, Hauck WW, Gambertoglio JG, Gee L, et al. Bioequivalence of generic and brand-name levothyroxine products in the treatment of hypothyroidism. JAMA 1997;277:1205–1213.

23. Mayor GH, Orlando T, Kurtz NM. Limitations of levothyroxine bioequivalence evaluation: An analysis of an attempted study. Am J Ther 1995;2:417–432.

24. Carr D, McLeod DT, Parry G, Thornes HM. Fine adjustment of thyroxine replacement dosage: Comparison of the thyrotrophin releasing hormone test using a sensitive thyrotrophin assay with measurement of free thyroid hormones and clinical assessment. Clin Endocrinol 1988;28:325–333.

25. Toft AD. Thyroxine therapy. New Engl J Med 1994;331:174–180.

26. Singh S, Duggal J, Molnar J, et al. Impact of subclinical thyroid disorders on coronary heart disease, cardiovascular and all-cause mortality: A meta-analysis. Int J Cardiol 2008;125:41–48.

27. Ochs N, Auer R, Bauer DC, et al. Meta-analysis: Subclinical thyroid dysfunction and the risk for coronary heart disease and mortlity. Ann Int Med 2008;148: 832–845.

28. Cappola AR, Fried LP, Arnold AM, et al. Thyroid status, cardiovascular risk and mortality in older adults. JAMA 2006;295:1033–1041.

29. Biondi B, Cooper DS. The clinical significance of subclinical thyroid dysfunction. Endocrine Rev 2008;29:76–131.

30. Santini F, Pinchera A, Marsili A, et al. Lean body mass is a major determinant of levothyroxine dosage in the treatment of thyroid diseases. J Clin Endocrinol Metab 2005;90:124–127.

31. Laurberg P, Andersen S, Pedersen IB, Carle A. Hypothyroidism in the elderly: Pathophysiology, diagnosis and treatment. Drugs Aging 2005;22:23–38.

32. Helfand M, Crapo LM. Monitoring therapy in patients taking levothyroxine. Ann Int Med 1990;113:450–454.

33. Briesacher BA, Andrade SE, Fouayzi H, Chan A. Comparison of drug adherence rates among patients with seven different medical conditions. Pharmacother 2008;28:437–443.

34. LeBeau SO, Mandel SJ. Thyroid disorders during pregnancy. Endocrinol Clin North Amer 2006;35:117–136.

35. Abalovich M, Amino N, Barbour LA, et al. Management of thyroid dysfunction during pregnancy and postpartum: An Endocrine Society clinical practice guideline. J Clin Endocrinol Metab 2007;92(suppl):S1–S47.

36. Braverman LE, Utiger RD. Introduction to thyrotoxicosis. In: Braverman LE, Utiger RD, eds. Werner & Ingbar's The Thyroid. A Fundamental and Clincal Text, 9th ed. Philadelphia: Lippincott Williams & Wilkins, 2005:453–455.

37. Cooper DS. Hyperthyroidism. Lancet 2005;362:459–468.

38. Nayak B, Hodak SP. Hyperythyroidism. Endocrinol Metab Clin North Amer 2007;36:617–656.

39. Cooper DS. Approach to the patient with subclinical hyperthyroidism. J Clin Endocrinol Metab 2007;92:3–9.

40. Farwell BP, Braverman LE. Thyroid and antithyroid drugs. In: Brunton L, Lazo J, Parker K, eds. Goodman & Gilman's The Pharmacological Basis of Therapeutics, 11th ed. New York: McGraw-Hill, 2006:1511–1540.

41. Cooper DS. Treatment of thyrotoxicosis. In: Braverman LE, Utiger RD, eds. Werner & Ingbar's The Thyroid. A Fundamental and Clinical Text, 9th ed. Philadelphia: Lippincott Williams & Wilkins, 2005:665–694.

42. Cooper DS. Drug therapy: Antithyroid drugs. New Engl J Med 2005;352:905–917.

43. Walker MA, Briel M, Chrit-Crain M, et al. Effects of antithyroid drugs on radioiodine treatment: Systematic review and meta-analysis of randomized controlled trials. BMJ 2007;335:1–7.

44. Marx H, Amin P, Lazarus JH. Hyperthyroidism and pregnancy. BMJ 2008;336:663–667.

45. Nayak B, Burman K. Thyrotoxicosis and thyroid storm. Endocrinol Metab Clin North Amer 2006;35:663–867.

46. Mebis L, Debaveye Y, Visser TJ, Van den Berghe G. Changes with the thyroid axis during the course of critical illness. Endocrinol Metab Clin North Amer 2006;35:807–821.

47. Langton JE, Brent GA. Nonthyroidal illness syndrome: Evaluation of thyroid function in sick patients. Endocrinol Metab Clin North Am 2002;31:159–172.

48. Surks MI, Sievert R. Drugs and thyroid function. New Engl J Med 1995;333:1688–1694.

49. Basaria S, Cooper DS. Amiodarone and the thyroid. Am J Med 2005;118:706–714.

50. Batcher EL, Tang C, Singh BN, et al. Thyroid function abnormalities during amiodarone therapy for persistent atrial fibrillation. Am J Med 2007;120:880–885.

45 Adrenal Gland Disorders

Devra K. Dang, Judy T. Chen, Frank Pucino Jr., and Karim Anton Calis

LEARNING OBJECTIVES

● **Upon completion of the chapter, the reader will be able to:**

1. Explain the regulation and physiologic roles of hormones produced by the adrenal glands.

2. Recognize the clinical presentation of patients with adrenal insufficiency.

3. Describe the pharmacologic management of patients with acute and chronic adrenal insufficiency.

4. Recommend therapy monitoring parameters for patients with adrenal insufficiency.

5. Recognize the clinical presentation of Cushing's syndrome and the physiologic consequences of cortisol excess.

6. Describe the pharmacologic and nonpharmacologic management of patients with Cushing's syndrome.

7. Recommend strategies to prevent the development of Cushing's syndrome associated with exogenous glucocorticoid administration.

8. Recommend therapy monitoring parameters for patients with Cushing's syndrome.

KEY CONCEPTS

❶ Signs and symptoms of adrenal insufficiency reflect the disturbance of normal physiologic carbohydrate, fat, and protein homeostasis caused by inadequate cortisol production and inadequate cortisol action.

❷ Lifelong glucocorticoid replacement therapy may be necessary for patients with adrenal insufficiency, and mineralocorticoid replacement therapy is usually required for those with Addison's disease.

❸ During an acute adrenal crisis, the immediate treatment goals are to correct volume depletion, manage hypoglycemia, and provide glucocorticoid replacement.

❹ Patients with known adrenal insufficiency should be educated regarding the need for additional glucocorticoid replacement and prompt medical attention during periods of excessive physiologic stress.

❺ Patients with Cushing's syndrome due to endogenous or exogenous glucocorticoid excess typically present with similar clinical manifestations.

❻ Surgical resection is considered the treatment of choice for Cushing's syndrome from endogenous causes if the tumor can be localized and if there are no contraindications.

❼ Pharmacotherapy is generally reserved for patients: (a) in whom the ectopic adrenocorticotropic hormone (ACTH)-secreting tumor cannot be localized, (b) who are not surgical candidates, (c) who have failed surgery, (d) who have had a relapse after surgery, or (e) in whom adjunctive therapy is required to achieve complete remission.

❽ In drug-induced Cushing's syndrome, discontinuation of the offending agent is the best management option. However, abrupt withdrawal of the glucocorticoid can result in adrenal insufficiency or exacerbation of the underlying disease.

❾ Glucocorticoid doses less than 7.5 mg/day of prednisone or its equivalent for less than 3 weeks generally would not be expected to lead to suppression of the hypothalamic–pituitary–adrenal (HPA) axis.

INTRODUCTION

The adrenal glands are important in the synthesis and regulation of key human hormones. They play a crucial role in water and electrolyte homeostasis, as well as regulation of blood pressure, carbohydrate and fat metabolism, physiologic response to stress, and sexual development and differentiation. This chapter focuses on pharmacologic and nonpharmacologic management of the two most common conditions associated with adrenal gland dysfunction: glucocorticoid insufficiency (e.g., Addison's disease) and glucocorticoid excess (Cushing's syndrome). Other adrenal disorders such as congenital adrenal hyperplasia, pheochromocytoma, hypoaldosteronism, and hyperaldosteronism are beyond the scope of this chapter.

PHYSIOLOGY, ANATOMY, AND BIOCHEMISTRY OF THE ADRENAL GLAND

The adrenal gland is located on the upper segment of the kidney (Fig. 45–1).[1] It consists of an outer cortex and an inner medulla. The adrenal medulla secretes the catecholamines epinephrine (also called adrenaline) and norepinephrine (also called noradrenaline), which are involved in the regulation of the sympathetic nervous system. The adrenal cortex consists of three histologically distinct zones: the zona glomerulosa, zona fasciculata, and an innermost layer called the zona reticularis. Each zone is responsible for production of different hormones (Fig. 45–2).

The zona glomerulosa is responsible for the production of the mineralocorticoids aldosterone, deoxycorticosterone, and 18-hydroxy-deoxycorticosterone. Aldosterone promotes renal sodium retention and potassium excretion. Its synthesis and release are regulated by renin in response to decreased vascular volume and renal perfusion. Adrenal aldosterone production is regulated by the renin-angiotensin-aldosterone system.

The zona fasciculata produces the glucocorticoid hormone cortisol. Cortisol is responsible for maintaining homeostasis of carbohydrate, protein, and fat metabolism. Its secretion follows a circadian rhythm, generally beginning to rise at approximately 4 AM and peaking around 6 to 8 AM. Thereafter, cortisol levels decrease throughout the day, approach 50% of the peak value by 4 PM, and reach their nadir around midnight.[2] The normal rate of cortisol production is approximately 8 to 15 mg/day.[3] Cortisol plays a key role in the body's response to stress. Its production increases markedly during physiologic stress such as during acute illness, surgery, or trauma. In addition, certain conditions such as alcoholism, depression, anxiety disorder, obsessive-compulsive disorder, poorly controlled diabetes, morbid obesity, starvation, anorexia nervosa, and chronic renal failure are associated with increased cortisol levels. High total cortisol levels are also observed in the presence of increased cortisol binding globulin (the carrier protein for 80% of circulating cortisol molecules), which is seen in pregnancy or other high-estrogen states (e.g., exogenous estrogen administration).[2] Cortisol is converted in the liver to an inactive metabolite known as cortisone.

The zona reticularis produces the androgens androstenedione, dehydroepiandrosterone (DHEA), and the sulfated form of dehydroepiandrosterone (DHEA-S). Only a small amount of testosterone and estrogen are produced in the adrenal glands. Androstenedione and DHEA are converted in the periphery, largely to testosterone and estrogen.

Adrenal hormone production is controlled by the hypothalamus and pituitary. Corticotropin-releasing hormone (CRH) is secreted by the hypothalamus and stimulates secretion of adrenocorticotropic hormone (ACTH; also known as corticotropin) from the anterior pituitary. ACTH in turn stimulates the adrenal cortex to produce cortisol. When sufficient or excessive cortisol levels are reached, a negative feedback is exerted on the secretion of CRH and ACTH, thereby decreasing overall cortisol production. The control of adrenal androgen synthesis also follows a similar negative feedback mechanism. Figure 46–1 in the Pituitary Gland Disorders chapter depicts the hormonal regulation with the hypothalamic–pituitary–adrenal axis.

ADRENAL INSUFFICIENCY

EPIDEMIOLOGY AND ETIOLOGY

Adrenal insufficiency generally refers to the inability of the adrenal glands to produce adequate amounts of cortisol for normal physiologic functioning or in times of stress. The condition is usually classified as primary, secondary, or tertiary, depending on the etiology (Table 45–1).[2,4–8] The estimated prevalences of primary adrenal insufficiency and secondary adrenal insufficiency are approximately 60 to 143 and 150 to 280 cases per one million persons, respectively. Primary adrenal insufficiency is usually diagnosed in the third to fifth decade of life, whereas secondary adrenal insufficiency is commonly detected during the sixth decade.[2,9] Adrenal insufficiency is more prevalent in women than in men, with a ratio of 2.6:1.[2] Chronic adrenal insufficiency is rare.

PATHOPHYSIOLOGY

Primary adrenal insufficiency, also known as Addison's disease, occurs when the adrenal glands are unable to produce cortisol. It occurs from destruction of the adrenal

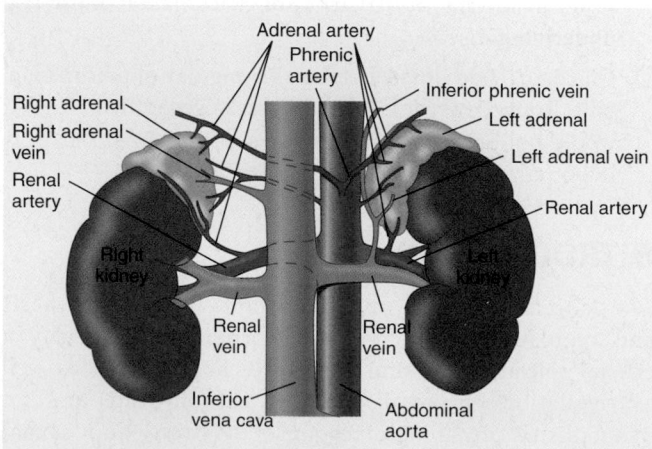

FIGURE 45–1. Anatomy of the adrenal gland. (From Ref. 1.)

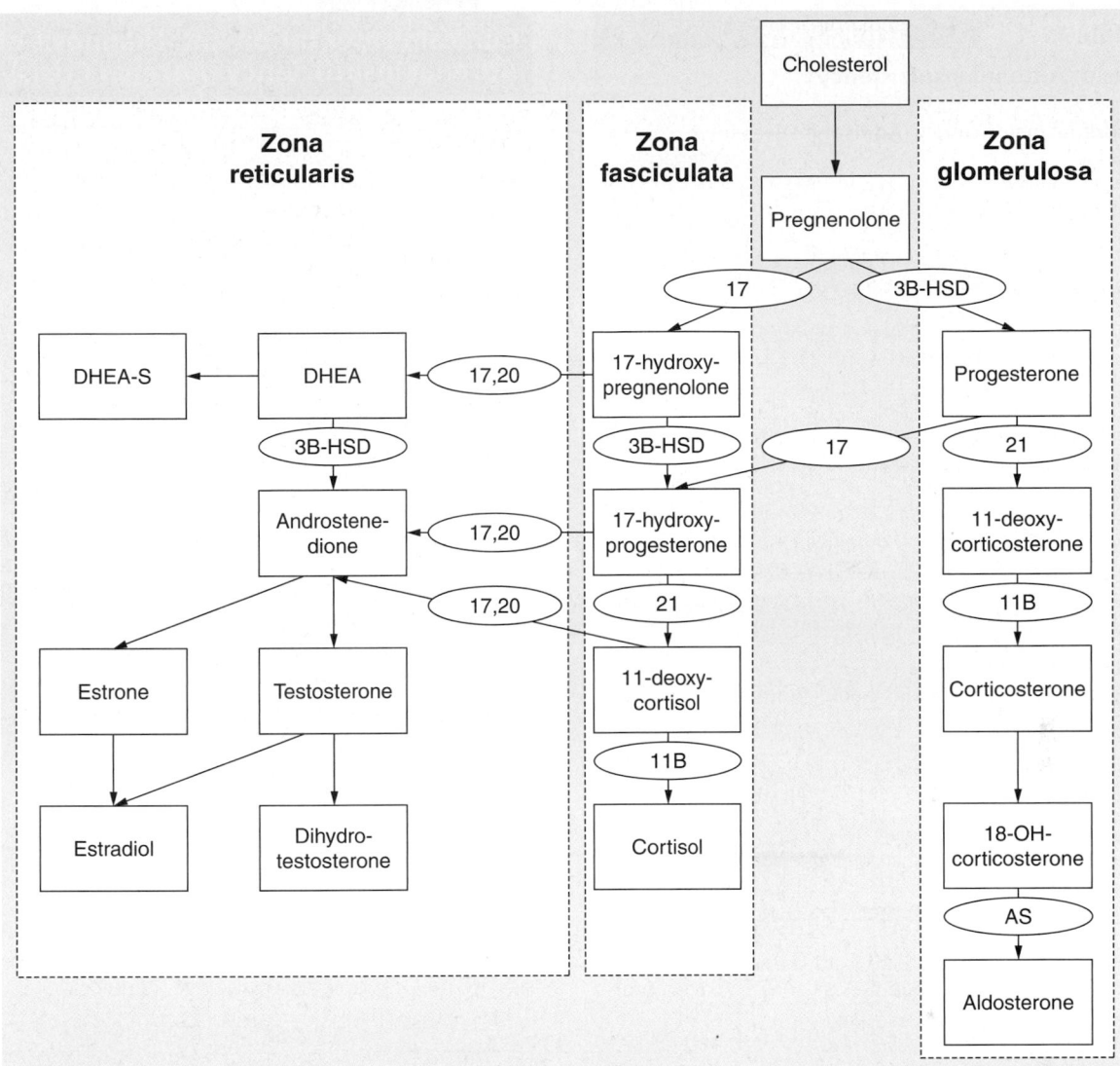

FIGURE 45–2. Adrenal steroid synthesis. The adrenal cortex consists of three histologically distinct zones: The zona glomerulosa, zona fasciculata, and an innermost layer called the zona reticularis. Each zone is responsible for production of different hormones. (17, 17-hydroxylase; 3B-HSD, 3β-hydroxysteroid dehydrogenase; 21, 21α-hydroxylase; 17,20, 17,20-lyase; 11B, 11β-hydroxylase; AS, aldosterone synthase; DHEA, dehydroepiandrosterone; DHEA-S, sulfated form of dehydroepiandrosterone.)

cortex, usually from an autoimmune process. In general, the clinical manifestations are observed when destruction of the cortex exceeds 90%.[4] **❶** *Signs and symptoms of adrenal insufficiency reflect the disturbance of normal physiologic carbohydrate, fat, and protein homeostasis caused by inadequate cortisol production and inadequate cortisol action.* Primary adrenal insufficiency usually develops gradually. Patients may remain asymptomatic in the early stages, with signs and symptoms present only during times of physiologic stress. Persistent signs and symptoms of hypocortisolism typically occur with disease progression. Additionally, primary adrenal insufficiency may be accompanied by a reduction in aldosterone and androgen production. See Clinical Presentation and Diagnosis of Chronic Adrenal Insufficiency and Clinical Presentation and Diagnosis of Acute Adrenal Insufficiency (Adrenal Crisis) textboxes.

Secondary adrenal insufficiency occurs as a result of a pituitary gland dysfunction, whereby decreased production and secretion of ACTH leads to a decrease in cortisol synthesis. Tertiary adrenal insufficiency is a disorder of the hypothalamus that results in decreased production and release of CRH, which in turn decreases pituitary ACTH production and release. In contrast to Addison's disease (i.e., primary adrenal insufficiency), aldosterone production is unaffected in the secondary and tertiary forms of the disease. Chronic adrenal insufficiency often has a good prognosis if diagnosed early and treated appropriately.

Acute adrenal insufficiency (i.e., adrenal crisis) results from the body's inability to sufficiently increase endogenous cortisol during periods of excessive physiologic stress. Adrenal crisis can occur when patients with chronic adrenal insufficiency do not receive adequate glucocorticoid replacement during stressful conditions such as those

Table 45–1

Etiologies of Adrenal Insufficiency

Primary Adrenal Insufficiency (Addison's Disease)
- Autoimmune—accounts for 70–90% of all cases of primary adrenal insufficiency
- Infectious or granulomatous diseases
  - Cytomegalovirus
  - Fungal (histoplasmosis, coccidioidomycosis, cryptococcosis, *Blastomyces dermatitidis* infection)
  - HIV, AIDS
    - Mycobacterial, cytomegaloviral, *Pneumocystic jiroveci*, and *Toxoplasma gondii* infection
  - Sarcoidosis
  - Tuberculosis
- Medications—inhibitors of steroidogenesis (etomidate, ketoconazole, metyrapone, mitotane)
- Hemorrhagic
  - Bilateral adrenal hemorrhage or infarction—usually due to anticoagulant therapy, coagulopathy, thromboembolic disease, or meningococcal infection. Causes acute adrenal insufficiency
- Adrenalectomy
- Adrenoleukodystrophy (in males)
- Adrenomyeloneuropathy
- Infiltrative disorders—amyloidosis, hemochromatosis
- Genetic causes
  - Congenital adrenal hyperplasia
  - Familial glucocorticoid deficiency and hypoplasia
- Metastatic malignancy

Secondary Adrenal Insufficiency
- Drug-induced (most common cause of secondary adrenal insufficiency)
  - Chronic glucocorticoid administration at supraphysiologic doses
  - Megestrol acetate—has glucocorticoid-like activity
  - Mifepristone (RU 486)—antagonizes glucocorticoid receptors
- Cushing's syndrome
- Panhypopituitarism
- Pituitary tumor
- Transsphenoidal pituitary microsurgery
- Pituitary irradiation
- Traumatic brain injury

Tertiary Adrenal Insufficiency
- Hypothalamic failure
- Drug-induced—chronic glucocorticoid administration at supraphysiologic doses

From Refs. 1, 4–8.

Clinical Presentation and Diagnosis of Acute Adrenal Insufficiency (Adrenal Crisis)

General
- Onset of symptoms is acute and precipitated by excessive physiologic stress.

Symptoms
- Severe weakness and fatigue
- Abdominal or flank pain

Signs
- Severe dehydration leading to hypotension and shock (circulatory collapse). Hypovolemia may not be responsive to IV hydration and may require the use of vasopressors.
- Tachycardia
- Nausea, vomiting
- Fever
- Confusion
- Hypoglycemia
- Laboratory abnormalities are similar to those observed in chronic adrenal insufficiency.

Laboratory Tests
- The unstimulated serum cortisol and rapid ACTH stimulation tests are useful in the diagnosis of adrenal crisis (Table 45–2). The insulin tolerance test is contraindicated due to pre-existing hypoglycemia. The metyrapone test is also contraindicated since metyrapone inhibits cortisol production.

Note: Due to the life-threatening nature of this condition, empiric treatment should be started before laboratory confirmation in patients who present with the clinical picture of an acute adrenal crisis.

From Refs. 2, 4, 9.

---

experienced during surgery, infection, acute illness, invasive medical procedures, or trauma. Acute adrenal insufficiency can also result from bilateral adrenal infarction due to hemorrhage, embolus, sepsis, or adrenal vein thrombosis. Additionally, abrupt discontinuation or rapid tapering of glucocorticoids, given chronically in supraphysiologic doses, may lead to adrenal crisis. This condition results from prolonged suppression of the hypothalamic–pituitary–adrenal (HPA) axis and subsequent adrenal gland atrophy and hypocortisolemia. Other drugs associated with adrenal insufficiency include those that inhibit production (e.g., ketoconazole) or increase metabolism (e.g., the cytochrome P-450 subfamily IIIA polypeptide 4 [CYP450 3A4] inducer rifampin) of cortisol.[4] Regardless of etiology, patients experiencing an adrenal crisis require immediate glucocorticoid treatment because manifestations such as circulatory collapse can lead to life-threatening sequelae.

TREATMENT AND OUTCOME EVALUATION

Chronic Adrenal Insufficiency

The general goals of treatment are to manage symptoms and prevent development of adrenal crisis. ❷ *Lifelong glucocorticoid replacement therapy may be necessary for patients with adrenal insufficiency, and mineralocorticoid replacement therapy is usually required for those with Addison's disease. Glucocorticoids with sufficient mineralocorticoid activity are generally required.* However, the addition of a potent mineralocorticoid such as fludrocortisone, along with adequate salt intake, is

Clinical Presentation and Diagnosis of Chronic Adrenal Insufficiency

General

- The symptoms develop gradually (especially in the early stages), may be vague, and may mimic those of other medical conditions.
- The cardinal symptoms and signs are weakness and fatigue requiring rest periods, GI symptoms, weight loss, and hypotension. These symptoms are due to cortisol deficiency.
- Patients with autoimmune adrenal insufficiency may have other autoimmune disorders such as type 1 diabetes mellitus and autoimmune thyroiditis.

Symptoms (Percentage Prevalence)

- Weakness and fatigue are the most common (99%).
- Anorexia, nausea, and diarrhea (56–90%). These may range from mild to severe with vomiting and abdominal pain.
- Hypoglycemia may occur in some patients.
- Amenorrhea may occur in some women.
- Salt craving may occur in some (approximately 22%) patients with primary adrenal insufficiency due to aldosterone deficiency.

Signs

- Weight loss (97%)
- Hypotension (less than 110/70 mm Hg) and orthostasis (87%)
- Dehydration, hypovolemia, and hyperkalemia (in primary adrenal insufficiency only) due to aldosterone deficiency.
- Decreased serum sodium and chloride levels due to aldosterone deficiency. Hyponatremia can also be present in secondary adrenal insufficiency due to cortisol deficiency and increased antidiuretic hormone secretion leading to subsequent water retention.
- Increased serum blood urea nitrogen and creatinine due to dehydration.
- Hyperpigmentation of skin and mucous membranes (92%). This is usually observed around creases, pressure areas, areolas, genitalia, and new scars. Dark freckles and patches of vitiligo may be present. Hyperpigmentation, due to increased ACTH levels, occurs in most patients with primary adrenal insufficiency but does not occur in secondary or tertiary adrenal insufficiency.
- Personality changes (irritability and restlessness) due to cortisol deficiency.
- Loss of axillary and pubic hair in women due to decreased androgen production.
- Blood count abnormalities (normocytic, normochromic anemia, relative lymphocytosis, neutrophilia, eosinophilia) due to cortisol and androgen deficiency.

Laboratory Tests (Also See Table 45–2)

- Decreased basal and stress-induced cortisol levels.
- Decreased aldosterone level (in primary adrenal insufficiency only).
- Lack of increase in cortisol and aldosterone levels after ACTH stimulation.

Other Diagnostic Tests (Also See Table 45–2)

- CT or MRI of the adrenal glands, pituitary, and/or hypothalamus can aid in determining the etiology.
- The presence of antiadrenal antibodies is suggestive of an autoimmune etiology.

From Refs. 2, 4, 5, 9.

---

sometimes needed to prevent sodium loss, hyperkalemia, and intravascular volume depletion. Mineralocorticoid supplementation typically is not indicated for the treatment of secondary or tertiary adrenal insufficiency because aldosterone production is often unaffected. Moreover, patients with secondary or tertiary adrenal insufficiency may only require replacement therapy until the HPA axis recovers. Hydrocortisone is often prescribed because it most closely resembles endogenous cortisol with its relatively high mineralocorticoid activity and short half-life, and allows the design of regimens that simulate the normal circadian cycle.[5] Other glucocorticoids, however, can be used. The pharmacologic characteristics of commonly used glucocorticoids are presented in Table 45–3.[4] Since patients with primary adrenal insufficiency can experience DHEA deficiency, DHEA replacement also has been tried. Several small clinical studies, consisting mostly of women, suggest that treatment with DHEA can improve mood and fatigue and provide a general sense of well-being.[10–13] Nonetheless, use of DHEA remains controversial and requires further study. The specific management strategies for chronic adrenal insufficiency are as follows[2,5,9]:

- For the treatment of primary adrenal insufficiency (Addison's disease), oral hydrocortisone 12 to 15 mg/m^2 is typically administered in two divided doses, with two-thirds of the dose given in the morning upon awakening to mimic the early morning rise in endogenous cortisol, and the remaining one-third of the dose given in the late afternoon to avoid insomnia and allow for the lowest concentration in the blood at around midnight. Hydrocortisone may also be given in three doses but this may decrease adherence. The longer-acting glucocorticoids (e.g., prednisone, dexamethasone) may provide a more prolonged clinical response thereby avoiding symptom recurrence that can occur at the end of the dosing interval with short-acting agents such as hydrocortisone. Longer-acting agents also may improve adherence in some patients. Patients should be monitored for weight, blood pressure, serum electrolytes, and symptom resolution and feeling of general well-being, and dosages should

Table 45–2

Tests for Diagnosing Adrenal Insufficiency

Test	Procedure	Rationale	Finding in Adrenal Insufficiency	Comments
Screening and Diagnostic Tests for Adrenal Insufficiency				
Unstimulated serum cortisol measurement	Measure serum cortisol at 6–8 AM	Serum cortisol level peaks in the early morning	Serum cortisol greater than 18 mcg/dL (497 nmol/L) is normal. Serum cortisol less than 3 mcg/dL (83 nmol/L) is indicative of adrenal insufficiency	Used as a general initial screening test for the presence of adrenal insufficiency. Evaluate result in conjunction with those from the other tests
Rapid ACTH stimulation test (also called cosyntropin stimulation test)	Measure serum cortisol 30–60 minutes after administering cosyntropin 250 mcg IV	Increased cortisol secretion in normal individuals in response to ACTH stimulation but not in adrenal insufficiency	Serum cortisol concentration less than 18 mcg/dL (497 nmol/L)	Used as the gold standard test for diagnosing primary adrenal insufficiency. False negative results may occur if the ACTH deficiency is of recent onset (less than 1 month). Although not widely accepted, a low-dose (1 mcg) ACTH stimulation test has been useful for the diagnosis of partial adrenal insufficiency. If measured serum cortisol concentration is low, measure plasma ACTH, aldosterone, and renin concentrations to differentiate between primary and secondary or tertiary adrenal insufficiency (see below)
Insulin tolerance test (insulin-induced hypoglycemia test)	Administer insulin IV to induce hypoglycemia then measure serum cortisol during symptomatic hypoglycemia (confirm that blood glucose is less than 40 mg/dL [2.22 mmol/L])	Evaluates ability of entire HPA axis to respond to stress (hypoglycemia)	Serum cortisol concentration less than 18 mcg/dL (497 nmol/L) is indicative of secondary adrenal insufficiency	If the result of the rapid ACTH stimulation test is normal, either this or the overnight metyrapone test is still needed to evaluate for secondary adrenal insufficiency. The insulin tolerance test is considered the gold standard. Contraindicated in patients with a seizure history, older than 60 years, or with cardiovascular or cerebrovascular disease. Requires close medical supervision. Contraindicated in adrenal crisis
Overnight metyrapone test	Administer metyrapone at midnight then measure serum cortisol at 8 AM the next day	Metyrapone inhibits cortisol synthesis. Its administration leads to rise in levels of ACTH and the precursor of cortisol. Patients with adrenal insufficiency do not exhibit this	Normal response is a decrease in serum cortisol to less than 5 mcg/dL (138 nmol/L) and an increase in the cortisol precursor to more than 7 mcg/dL (193 nmol/L). Response not seen in secondary adrenal insufficiency	Distinguishes between normal individuals and patients with secondary adrenal insufficiency. Contraindicated in adrenal crisis
Tests for Differential Diagnosis of Primary, Secondary, and Tertiary Adrenal Insufficiency				
Plasma ACTH concentration	Measure plasma ACTH	In primary adrenal insufficiency, hypocortisolism leads to elevated plasma ACTH concentration via positive HPA axis feedback	Primary adrenal insufficiency: elevated plasma ACTH. Secondary or tertiary adrenal insufficiency: plasma ACTH low or inappropriately normal	Evaluate result of test in combination with those from the plasma aldosterone and plasma renin tests

(Continued)

Table 45–2

Tests for Diagnosing Adrenal Insufficiency (*Continued*)

Test	Procedure	Rationale	Finding in Adrenal Insufficiency	Comments
Plasma aldosterone concentration	Measure plasma aldosterone from same blood samples as those used in ACTH stimulation test	Patients with primary adrenal insufficiency may experience a reduction in aldosterone production	Primary adrenal insufficiency: low plasma aldosterone Secondary or tertiary adrenal insufficiency: aldosterone concentration is usually normal (greater than or equal to 5 ng/dL [139 pmol/L])	Evaluate result of test in combination with those from the plasma ACTH and plasma renin tests
Plasma renin concentration or activity	Measure plasma renin concentration or activity	Mineralocorticoid deficiency occurs in primary adrenal insufficiency but is usually not present in secondary or tertiary adrenal insufficiency	Primary adrenal insufficiency: elevated plasma renin. Secondary or tertiary adrenal insufficiency: plasma renin concentration or activity is usually normal	Evaluate result of test in combination with those from the plasma ACTH and plasma aldosterone concentration tests

ACTH, adrenocorticotropic hormone or corticotropin; CRH, corticotropin-releasing hormone; HPA, hypothalamic–pituitary–adrenal.

From Refs. 4, 5.

Table 45–3

Pharmacologic Characteristics of Commonly Used Glucocorticoids

Glucocorticoid	Estimated Potency Relative to Hydrocortisone		Equivalent Dose (mg)
	Glucocorticoid (Anti-inflammatory) Activity	Mineralocorticoid (Sodium-Retaining) Activity	
Short Acting (Half-Life Less than 12 hours)			
Hydrocortisone	1	1	20
Cortisone	0.8	0.8	25
Intermediate Acting (Half-Life 12–36 hours)			
Prednisone	4	0.25	5
Prednisolone	4	0.25	5
Methylprednisolone	5	Less than 0.01	4
Triamcinolone	5	Less than 0.01	4
Long Acting (Half-Life Greater Than 48 hours)			
Betamethasone	25	Less than 0.01	0.6–0.75
Dexamethasone	30–40	Less than 0.01	0.75

From Ref. 4.

be adjusted accordingly. Doses of hydrocortisone, dexamethasone, prednisone, and other glucocorticoids may need to be increased or decreased in patients taking CYP450 3A4 inducers (e.g., phenytoin, rifampin, barbiturates) or inhibitors (e.g., protease inhibitors), respectively. Adverse drug reactions from glucocorticoid administration should be monitored. Glucocorticoid therapy at physiologic replacement doses should not lead to the development of Cushing's syndrome; however, careful monitoring should still be performed, and the smallest effective dose used. Patients should receive education regarding the need for increased glucocorticoid dosage during excessive physiologic stress. In addition, oral fludrocortisone at a daily dose of approximately

Patient Encounter 1, Part 1: Presentation and Medical History

AB is a 58-year-old female presenting to the clinic with a chief complaint of fatigue and weakness. She has noticed a gradual increase in symptoms over the past year but attributed this to "old age." Recently, she has required more frequent rest breaks than before. Upon further questioning, she complained of intermittent nausea leading to decreased appetite and a 4.6-kg (10-lb) weight loss over the past year. She also reported darkening of a recent scar and denies recent or past use of glucocorticoids.

PMH: Type 1 diabetes mellitus since age 5, currently controlled; hypothyroidism, currently controlled; osteoarthritis (knees) for 5 years

FH: Unknown

SH: Retired secretary, denies smoking, alcohol use, or illicit drug use

Current Meds: Insulin glargine 30 units at bedtime; lispro insulin three times daily with meals—practices carbohydrate counting; levothyroxine 75 mcg once daily; acetaminophen 1,000 mg every 8 hours as needed for joint pain; capsaicin 0.075% cream three times a day for joint pain

PE:

VS: Sitting BP 108/70 mm Hg, sitting P 74 bpm, RR 14 breaths/min, standing BP 96/68, standing P 86, wt 68 kg (150 lb), ht 5'5" (165 cm)

Skin: Hyperpigmentation on creases of palms and around breast nipples, darkening of scar of left leg

CV: RRR, normal S_1, S_2; no murmurs, rubs, or gallops

Labs: Serum electrolytes: sodium 132 mEq/L (132 mmol/L), potassium 5.2 mEq/L (5.2 mmol/L), chloride 98 mEq/L (98 mmol/L), bicarb 30 mEq/L (30 mmol/L), blood urea nitrogen (BUN) 25 mg/dL (8.9 mmol/L), creatinine 1.2 mg/dL (106 μmol/L), glucose 120 mg/dL (6.7 mmol/L).

Which signs or symptoms of adrenal insufficiency does AB exhibit?

Does AB's presentation offer any clues as to the etiology or classification of adrenal insufficiency?

Which tests would be most useful for determining the etiology and confirming the diagnosis of adrenal insufficiency?

0.05 mg to 0.2 mg in the morning should be administered. Monitoring for resolution of hypotension, dizziness, dehydration, hyponatremia, and hyperkalemia should occur, and the dose can be increased if needed. Conversely, consider decreasing the dose if adverse reactions from mineralocorticoid administration such as hypertension, hypokalemia, fluid retention and other significant adverse events occur. In patients receiving hydrocortisone, it should be kept in mind that this drug also possesses mineralocorticoid activity. All patients with primary adrenal insufficiency should also maintain an adequate sodium intake (about 3–4 g/day). Lastly, although controversial, consider giving DHEA 50 mg/day (in the morning) to female patients who do not experience an improvement in mood and well-being even with adequate glucocorticoid and mineralocorticoid replacement. In these patients, monitor serum DHEA-S (aim for the middle range of normal levels in healthy young people) and free testosterone level.

- Patients with secondary and tertiary adrenal insufficiency are treated with oral hydrocortisone or a longer-acting glucocorticoid in the same manner as previously described for primary adrenal insufficiency. However, patients with secondary and tertiary adrenal insufficiency may require a lower dose. Some patients will only require glucocorticoid replacement temporarily, which can be discontinued after recovery of the HPA axis (e.g., patients with drug-induced adrenal insufficiency or adrenal insufficiency following treatment for Cushing's syndrome). Progression of the underlying etiology for the adrenal insufficiency should be monitored. Fludrocortisone therapy is generally not needed.

Acute Adrenal Insufficiency

❸ *During an acute adrenal crisis, the immediate treatment goals are to correct volume depletion, manage hypoglycemia, and provide glucocorticoid replacement.* Volume depletion and hypoglycemia can be corrected by giving large volumes (approximately 2–3 L) of IV normal saline and 5% dextrose solution.[2] Glucocorticoid replacement can be accomplished by administering IV hydrocortisone, starting at a dose of 100 mg every 6 to 8 hours for 24 hours, increasing to 200 mg to 400 mg/day if complications occur, or decreasing to 50 mg every 6 to 8 hours after achieving hemodynamic stability. The hydrocortisone dose can then be tapered to a maintenance dose by the fourth or fifth day and fludrocortisone can be added if needed.[2]

❹ *Patients with known adrenal insufficiency should be educated regarding the need for additional glucocorticoid replacement and prompt medical attention during periods of excessive physiologic stress.* Although the dosage of glucocorticoid is generally individualized, a common recommendation is to double the maintenance dose of hydrocortisone if the patient experiences fever, or undergoes invasive dental or diagnostic procedures.[5] Patients who experience vomiting or diarrhea may not adequately absorb oral glucocorticoids and may benefit from parenteral therapy until symptoms resolve. Prior to major surgery, additional glucocorticoid replacement (higher dose and parenteral route) must be given to prevent adrenal crisis. A sample protocol is as follows[2]:

- Correct electrolytes, blood pressure, and fluid status as necessary.
- Give 100 mg of hydrocortisone sodium phosphate or hydrocortisone sodium succinate intramuscularly (also, make sure this is readily available to the operating room).
- Give 50 mg of hydrocortisone intramuscularly or IV in the recovery room and then every 6 hours for the first 24 hours.
- If the patient is hemodynamically stable, reduce dosage to 25 mg every 6 hours for 24 hours and then taper to maintenance dosage over 3 to 5 days.
- Resume previous fludrocortisone dose when the patient is taking oral medications.
- Maintain or increase hydrocortisone dosage to 200 mg to 400 mg/day if fever, hypotension, or other complications occur.

Patient Encounter 1, Part 2: Treatment

After appropriate laboratory and diagnostic tests are performed, AB is diagnosed with Addison's disease.

How should her chronic primary adrenal insufficiency be treated?

What monitoring parameters (therapeutic and toxic) should be implemented?

HYPERCORTISOLISM (CUSHING'S SYNDROME)

EPIDEMIOLOGY AND ETIOLOGY

Cushing's syndrome refers to the pathophysiologic changes associated with exposure to supraphysiologic cortisol concentrations (endogenous hypercortisolism) or pharmacologic doses of glucocorticoids (exogenous hypercortisolism). Cushing's syndrome from endogenous causes is a rare condition, with an estimated incidence of two to five cases per 1 million persons per year.[14] Patients receiving chronic supraphysiologic doses of glucocorticoids,

---

Patient Care and Monitoring: Adrenal Insufficiency

1. Evaluate patients presenting with the typical clinical manifestations for chronic or acute adrenal insufficiency.

2. Perform initial screening tests to confirm the presence of adrenal insufficiency.

3. Once diagnosis is confirmed, perform further testing to differentiate between primary, secondary, and tertiary adrenal insufficiency.

4. In patients presenting with acute adrenal crisis who have not been previously diagnosed with adrenal insufficiency, immediate treatment with injectable hydrocortisone and IV saline and dextrose solutions should be initiated prior to confirmation of the diagnosis because of the life-threatening nature of this condition. Determine and correct the underlying cause of the acute adrenal crisis (e.g., infection).

5. Glucocorticoid replacement therapy is necessary for patients with adrenal insufficiency, and mineralocorticoid replacement therapy is required for those with Addison's disease.

6. In patients with chronic adrenal insufficiency, when excessive physiologic stress is anticipated (e.g., pending surgery), devise a strategy to give supplemental doses of glucocorticoid during this period. Monitor the patient for signs of an acute adrenal crisis and develop a plan to treat this emergency condition.

7. Monitor the patient for adequacy of treatment as well as adverse reactions from glucocorticoid and/or mineralocorticoid therapy.

8. Determine the duration of treatment for patients with secondary and tertiary adrenal insufficiency.

9. Provide patient education regarding disease state and its treatment:
   - Causes of adrenal insufficiency, including drug-induced etiologies.
   - How to recognize the clinical manifestations.
   - How to prevent an acute adrenal crisis (adhere to therapy and do not abruptly stop glucocorticoid treatment). There may be a need to increase the dose of glucocorticoid during excessive physiologic stress.
   - Administration of parenteral glucocorticoid during an acute adrenal crisis.
   - Need to notify all health care providers of condition.
   - Encourage wearing or carrying a medical alert (e.g., bracelet, card).
   - Counsel on dietary and pharmacologic therapy, including duration of treatment and potential adverse consequences of glucocorticoid and mineralocorticoid replacement.

such as those with rheumatologic disorders, are at high risk of developing Cushing's syndrome.

PATHOPHYSIOLOGY

Cushing's syndrome can be classified as ACTH-dependent or ACTH-independent (Table 45–4).[2,15–17] ACTH-dependent Cushing's syndrome results from ACTH-secreting (or rarely CRH-secreting) adenomas. ACTH-independent Cushing's syndrome is due either to excessive cortisol secretion by the adrenal glands (independent of ACTH stimulation) or to exogenous glucocorticoid administration. ❺ *Patients with Cushing's syndrome due to endogenous or exogenous glucocorticoid excess typically present with similar clinical manifestations.* The term *Cushing's disease* refers specifically to Cushing's syndrome from an ACTH-secreting pituitary adenoma. The plasma ACTH concentration is elevated in ACTH-dependent conditions but not in ACTH-independent causes because elevated cortisol concentrations suppress pituitary ACTH secretion via negative feedback. ACTH and cortisol concentrations are elevated episodically in ACTH-dependent disease due to random hypersecretion of ACTH.[4] Other major differences among the vast etiologies of Cushing's syndrome are shown in Table 45–5.[1,4,12,18]

Physiologic cortisol secretion follows a circadian pattern, with cortisol levels rising in the early morning, peaking at approximately 6 to 8 AM, and then declining steadily throughout the remainder of the day until they reach a nadir at midnight. This circadian rhythm is lost in most patients with Cushing's syndrome. As such, detection of elevated midnight cortisol concentrations can be useful in the diagnosis of Cushing's syndrome.

Cushing's disease and adrenal carcinomas cause adrenal androgen hypersecretion in high enough concentrations to result in signs of androgen excess such as acne, menstrual irregularities, and hirsutism, and cause virilization in women.[4] Drug-induced Cushing's syndrome from glucocorticoid administration occurs most commonly in patients receiving oral therapy, but other routes such as inhalation, dermal, nasal, and intra-articular have also been implicated.[15] Nonprescription products, including dietary supplements, should also be evaluated since they may contain corticosteroids. Drug-induced Cushing's syndrome has been reported with the use of Chinese herbal products that contain corticosteroids.[19,20] The risk of glucocorticoid-induced Cushing's syndrome appears to increase with higher doses and/or longer treatment durations.[15]

Left untreated, patients with Cushing's syndrome may experience severe complications of hypercortisolism, resulting in up to a nearly fourfold increase in mortality.[18] Mortality in patients with Cushing's syndrome is mostly attributed to cardiovascular disease. Hypertension, hyperglycemia, and hyperlipidemia are common findings and can be associated with cardiac hypertrophy, atherosclerosis, and hypercoagulability. Osteopenia, osteoporosis, and increased fractures also have been reported.[18] Children may experience linear growth retardation from reduced growth hormone secretion and inhibition of epiphysial cartilage development in long bones.[14,18]

TREATMENT

The goal of treatment in patients with Cushing's syndrome is reversal of hypercortisolism and management of the associated comorbidities, including the potential for long-term sequelae such as cardiac hypertrophy. ❻ *Surgical resection is considered the treatment of choice for Cushing's syndrome from endogenous causes if the tumor can be*

Table 45–4

Etiologies of Cushing's Syndrome

ACTH-Dependent
- ACTH-secreting pituitary tumor (Cushing's disease)—70% of cases of endogenous Cushing's syndrome
- ACTH-secreting nonpituitary tumors (ectopic ACTH syndrome)—15% of cases of endogenous Cushing's syndrome; usually from small cell lung carcinoma, bronchial carcinoids, pheochromocytoma, or from thymus, pancreatic, ovarian, or thyroid tumor. The tumor is usually disseminated (difficult to localize)
- CRH-secreting nonpituitary tumors (ectopic CRH syndrome)—rare

ACTH-Independent—15% of cases of endogenous Cushing's syndrome
- Unilateral adrenal adenoma
- Adrenal carcinoma
- Bilateral nodular adrenal hyperplasia—rare (less than 1%)

Drug-Induced Cushing's Syndrome (ACTH-independent)—most common cause of Cushing's syndrome
- Prescription glucocorticoid preparations (most routes of administration)
- Nonprescription and natural health products with glucocorticoid activity (e.g., nonprescription anti-itch products with hydrocortisone, natural health products with magnolia bark or those claiming to contain adrenal cortex extracts or other by-products)
- Other drugs with glucocorticoid activity (e.g., megestrol acetate, medroxyprogesterone)

ACTH, adrenocorticotropic hormone or corticotropin; CRH, corticotropin-releasing hormone.

From Refs. 2, 15–17.

Table 45–5					
Differences Among the Major Etiologies of Cushing's Syndrome					
	ACTH DEPENDENT		**ACTH INDEPENDENT**		
	Pituitary Dependent (Cushing's Disease)	**Ectopic ACTH Syndrome**	**Exogenous Glucocorticoid Administration**	**Adrenal Adenoma**	**Adrenal Carcinoma**
Onset of signs and symptoms	Gradual	Rapid	Gradual to rapid	Gradual	Rapid
Symptoms severity	Mild to moderate	Atypical	Mild to severe	Mild to moderate	Severe
Dominant sex/age	Female; 20–40 years (range childhood to 70 years)	Male; adults	Female and male; all ages	Female	Female; children
Virilization	+	+	+	+	+++
Abdominal mass	0	0	0	0	++
Plasma ACTH concentration	Slightly elevated	Elevated	Low	Low	Low
CRH stimulation test	Response	Rare response	Decreased or no response	No response	No response
High-dose dexamethasone suppression test	Between 50% and 80% cortisol suppression	Less cortisol suppression	No cortisol suppression	No cortisol suppression	No cortisol suppression
Pituitary MRI	Tumor	Normal	Normal	Normal	Normal
Adrenal gland CT or MRI	Normal or bilateral hyperplasia	Normal or bilateral hyperplasia	No change	Mass(es)	Mass(es)

0, none; +, mild; ++, moderate; +++, pronounced; ACTH, adrenocorticotropic hormone or corticotropin; CRH, corticotropin-releasing hormone.

From Refs. 1, 4, 12, 18.

localized and if there are no contraindications. The treatment of choice for Cushing's syndrome from exogenous causes is gradual discontinuation of the offending agent.

Nonpharmacologic Therapy

Transsphenoidal pituitary microsurgery is the treatment of choice for Cushing's disease. Removal of the pituitary tumor can bring about complete remission or cure in 78% to 97% of cases. HPA axis suppression associated with chronic hypercortisolism can result in prolonged adrenal insufficiency lasting for months after surgery and requiring exogenous glucocorticoid administration. Pituitary irradiation or bilateral adrenalectomy is usually reserved for patients who are not surgical candidates or for those who relapse or do not achieve complete remission following pituitary surgery. Because the response to pituitary irradiation can be delayed (several months to years), concomitant treatment with cortisol-lowering medication may be necessary. Bilateral adrenalectomy is also used for the management of adrenal carcinoma and in patients with poorly controlled ectopic Cushing's disease in whom the ACTH-producing lesion cannot be localized. Bilateral laparoscopic adrenalectomy achieves an immediate and total remission (nearly 100% cure rate), but these patients will require lifelong glucocorticoid and mineralocorticoid supplementation.[21,22] **Nelson's syndrome**

may develop in nearly 20% to 50% of patients who undergo bilateral adrenalectomy without pituitary irradiation. This condition presumably results from persistent hypersecretion of ACTH by the intact pituitary adenoma, which continues to grow because of the loss of feedback inhibition by cortisol. Treatment of Nelson's syndrome may involve pituitary irradiation or surgery.[4]

The treatment of choice in patients with adrenal adenomas is unilateral laparoscopic adrenalectomy. These patients require glucocorticoid supplementation during and after surgery due to atrophy of the contralateral adrenal gland and suppression of the HPA axis. Glucocorticoid therapy is continued until recovery of the remaining adrenal gland is achieved. Patients with adrenal carcinomas have a poor prognosis, with a 5-year survival of 20% to 58%, due to the advanced nature of the condition (metastatic disease). Surgical resection to reduce tumor burden and size, pharmacologic therapy, or bilateral laparoscopic adrenalectomy are the treatment options commonly utilized to manage this condition.[1,22]

Pharmacologic Therapy

❼ *Pharmacotherapy is generally reserved for patients: (a) in whom the ectopic ACTH-secreting tumor cannot be localized, (b) who are not surgical candidates, (c) have failed surgery, (d) who have had a relapse after surgery, or (e) in whom adjunctive therapy is required to achieve complete remission.*[23] The drugs

Clinical Presentation and Diagnosis of Cushing's Syndrome

General

- Patients with Cushing's syndrome due either to endogenous or exogenous glucocorticoid excess typically present with similar clinical manifestations.

- Differential diagnoses include diabetes mellitus and the metabolic syndrome, as patients with these conditions share several similar characteristics with Cushing's syndrome patients (e.g., obesity, hypertension, hyperlipidemia, hyperglycemia, and insulin resistance). In women, the presentations of hirsutism, menstrual abnormalities, and insulin resistance are similar to those of polycystic ovary syndrome. Cushing's syndrome can be differentiated from these conditions by identifying the classic signs and symptoms of truncal obesity, "moon facies" with facial plethora, a "buffalo hump" and supraclavicular fat pads, red-purple skin striae, and proximal muscle weakness.

- True Cushing's syndrome also must be distinguished from other conditions that share some clinical presentations (as well as elevated plasma cortisol concentrations) such as depression, alcoholism, obesity, and chronic illness—the so-called pseudo-Cushing's states.

Signs and Symptoms (Percentage Prevalence)

General Appearance

- Weight gain and obesity, manifesting as truncal obesity (90%)

- A rounded and puffy face ("moon facies") (75%)

- Dorsocervical ("buffalo hump") and supraclavicular fat accumulation

- Hirsutism (excessive hair growth) (75%)

Skin Changes—From Atrophy of Dermis and Connective Tissue

- Thin skin

- Facial plethora (70%)

- Skin striae ("stretch marks" that are usually red or purple in appearance and greater than 1 cm) (50%)

- Acne (35%)

- Easy bruising (40%)

- Hyperpigmentation

Metabolic

- Hyperglycemia that can range from impaired glucose tolerance (75%) to diabetes mellitus (20–50%)

- Hyperlipidemia (70%)

- Polyuria (30%)

- Kidney stones (15–50%)

- Hypokalemic alkalosis (from mineralocorticoid effect of cortisol)

Cardiovascular

- Hypertension (from mineralocorticoid effect of cortisol) (85%)

- Patients are at risk of the cardiovascular complications of hypertension, hyperlipidemia, and hyperglycemia

- Peripheral edema

Genitourinary

- Menstrual irregularities (the most typical presentation is amenorrhea) (70%)

- Erectile dysfunction (85%)

Other

- Psychiatric changes such as depression, emotional lability, psychosis, euphoria, anxiety, and decreased cognition (85%)

- Sleep disturbances

- Osteopenia (80%) and osteoporosis—usually affecting trabecular bone

- Linear growth impairment in children

- Proximal muscle weakness (65%)

- Avascular necrosis—more common in iatrogenic cases

- Glaucoma and cataracts

- Impaired wound healing and susceptibility to opportunistic infections

- Hypothyroidism

Laboratory Tests

- The diagnosis of Cushing's syndrome and its etiology is often complex and generally requires the involvement of endocrinologists and specialized testing centers.

- Initial screening tests to confirm the presence of hypercortisolism and differentiate Cushing's syndrome from conditions with similar presentations include 24-hour urinary free cortisol and overnight low-dose dexamethasone suppression test (DST; Table 45–6).

- The midnight plasma cortisol or combined dexamethasone suppression plus CRH test are less commonly used.

- Typically, a combination of at least two screening tests is used to establish the preliminary diagnosis.

- Once the diagnosis is confirmed, additional tests can be performed to determine the etiology.

Other Diagnostic Tests

- Imaging studies may be used to distinguish among pituitary, ectopic, and adrenal tumors (Table 45–5).

From Refs. 2, 14, 15.

Table 45–6

First-Line Screening Tests in Patients With Characteristics of Cushing's Syndrome

Test	Test Procedure and Measurement	Rationale	Typical Finding in Cushing's Syndrome	Comments
24-Hour urinary free cortisol	Collect urine over 24 hours and measure unbound cortisol excreted by kidneys	Urinary cortisol is elevated in hypercortisolic states	Urinary free cortisol greater than 4 times the upper reference limit is indicative of Cushing's syndrome Values between 1 and 4 times the upper reference limit suggest either Cushing's syndrome or pseudo-Cushing's syndrome	Easy to perform but should not be used alone since sensitivity and specificity depend on the assay used To exclude periodic hypercortisolism, 3 or more samples should be obtained (with urinary creatinine measurement to assess completeness of the collection) Distinguishes Cushing's syndrome from obesity (no elevation). However, false positive if other pseudo-Cushing's states, physiologic stress, or pregnancy False negative if decreased renal function, or subclinical hypercortisolism
Overnight low-dose dexa-methasone suppression test (DST)	Give 1 mg oral dexamethasone at 11 PM, then measure plasma cortisol at 8–9 AM the next morning	Dexamethasone administration suppresses morning plasma cortisol in normal individuals	Plasma cortisol greater than 14.3 mcg/dL (395 nmol/L) is diagnostic for Cushing's syndrome Plasma cortisol less than 1.2 mcg/dL (33 nmol/L) is not suggestive of Cushing's syndrome	Simple to perform and inexpensive Can be used in conjunction with, or instead of, the urinary free cortisol test Can also use the 2-day 2-mg DST False positive if pseudo-Cushing's states, physiologic stress, pregnancy, estrogen treatment, uremia, taking inducers of dexamethasone metabolism (phenytoin, etc.), or decreased dexamethasone absorption False negative if subclinical hypercortisolism or slow metabolism of dexamethasone
Late-night salivary cortisol	Collect salivary cortisol concentration at 11 PM	Loss of circadian rhythm of cortisol secretion (no nadir at night) in Cushing's syndrome but not in pseudo-Cushing's states	Elevated late-night salivary cortisol	Diagnostic criteria need further validation Easiest screening test to perform (sample can be collected at home by patient) Can be used in conjunction with, or instead of, the urinary free cortisol test

DST, dexamethasone suppression test.

From Refs. 2, 14, 18.

used are classified according to their mechanism and site of action (Table 45–7).[21,24–26] The most widely used therapeutic class is the adrenal steroidogenesis inhibitors.[23] Agents in this class include ketoconazole, etomidate, and metyrapone. Steroidogenesis inhibitors can treat hypercortisolism by inhibiting enzymes involved in the biosynthesis of cortisol. Because of their potential to cause adrenal suppression, temporary glucocorticoid replacement, and in some cases mineralocorticoid supplementation, may be needed during and after treatment. Centrally-acting neuromodulators of ACTH release such as bromocriptine, cyproheptadine, octreotide, ritanserin, and valproic acid are generally ineffective.

❽ *In drug-induced Cushing's syndrome, discontinuation of the offending agent is the best management option.*

However, abrupt withdrawal of the glucocorticoid can result in adrenal insufficiency or exacerbation of the underlying disease.[15] ❾ *Glucocorticoid doses less than 7.5 mg/day of prednisone or its equivalent for less than 3 weeks generally would not be expected to lead to suppression of the HPA axis.*[2,22] However, in patients receiving pharmacologic doses of glucocorticoids for prolonged periods, gradual tapering to near physiologic levels (5–7.5 mg/day of prednisone or its equivalent) should precede drug discontinuation. Administration of a short-acting glucocorticoid in the morning and use of alternate-day dosing may reduce the risk of adrenal suppression. Testing of the HPA axis may be useful in assessing adrenal reserve. In some cases, supplemental glucocorticoid administration during excessive physiologic

Table 45–7

Pharmacologic Treatments for Cushing's Syndrome

Drug	Mechanism of Action	Dosage[a]: Initial, Usual, Maximum, Dosing Adjustment for Renal and/or Hepatic Failure	Common and/or Major Adverse Reactions	Comment
Inhibitors of Adrenal Steroidogenesis				
Ketoconazole[b] (oral administration)	Inhibits several cytochrome P450 enzymes including 17,20-lyase, 17-hydroxylase, and 11β-hydroxylase. Also inhibits cholesterol synthesis	*Adults:* 200 mg twice daily; 600–800 mg/day in two divided doses; NTE 1,200 mg/day in 2–3 divided doses *Pediatric:* Safety and effectiveness have not been established Extensively metabolized by liver and dosing adjustment should be considered in severe liver disease. Dosing adjustment not needed in renal disease	Generally well-tolerated. Transaminase elevations, GI intolerance, and rash. Gynecomastia, testicular function impairment, and adrenal insufficiency at high doses (more than 600 mg/day)	Effective in a majority of cases; rapid clinical improvement seen Monitor efficacy with urinary cortisol Monitor liver transaminases for hepatotoxicity Useful in women with hirsutism and patients with hyperlipidemia Requires gastric acidity for dissolution and absorption, and therefore not useful in patients with achlorhydria and those taking proton pump inhibitors or round-the-clock antacids or histamine-2 receptor blockers
Metyrapone[b] (oral administration)	Inhibits 11-hydroxylase. Also suppresses aldosterone synthesis	*Adults:* 750 mg/day; 500–4,000 mg/day in four divided doses; NTE 6 g/day *Pediatric:* Safety and effectiveness have not been established Dosages in special populations (liver and kidney disease, elderly patients) have not been established	Generally well-tolerated Hirsutism, acne, adrenal insufficiency, GI intolerance, rash, hypokalemia, edema, hypertension	Used in Cushing's disease, ectopic ACTH syndrome, and adrenal carcinoma Also used as a test to diagnose adrenal insufficiency
Etomidate[b] (IV administration)	Inhibits 17,20-lyase, 17-hydroxylase, and 11β- hydroxylase	*Adults:* Limited clinical experience, 1.6–4.2 mg/h intermittently *Pediatric:* Safety and effectiveness have not been established Extensively metabolized in the liver to inactive metabolites. Due to changes in protein binding, dosing adjustment may be needed in kidney and liver disease	Injection site pain, nausea, vomiting, myoclonus	IV route of administration limits use

Adrenolytic Agent

Agent	Mechanism	Dosing	Adverse Effects	Comments
Mitotane[b] (oral administration)	Inhibits steroidogenesis at lower doses and is adrenolytic at higher doses. Inhibits 11β-hydroxylase and cholesterol side-chain cleavage. Reduces aldosterone synthesis	*Adults:* 2–6 g/day in 3–4 divided doses; 9–10 g/day in 3–4 divided doses; NTE 16 g/day in 3–4 divided doses. Elderly patients may require a dose decrease. *Pediatric:* Safety and effectiveness have not been established. Primarily metabolized by the liver and dosing adjustment may be needed in liver disease	GI intolerance (high incidence), fatigue, dizziness, somnolence, gynecomastia. Hyperlipidemia requiring lipid-lowering treatment. Adrenal insufficiency requiring glucocorticoid replacement therapy	Used primarily for adrenal carcinoma but can be used in other types of Cushing's syndrome. Efficacy takes several weeks. Lower rate of relapse when used with pituitary radiation. Also enables lower doses and therefore lower rate of adverse reactions

Peripheral Glucocorticoid Antagonist

Agent	Mechanism	Dosing	Adverse Effects	Comments
Mifepristone (RU 486)[b] (oral administration)	Antagonizes glucocorticoid receptors	*Adults and children:* Up to 20 mg/kg/day. Metabolized by the liver, and therefore dosing adjustment may be required in liver disease. Dose adjustment in renal dysfunction not established	GI intolerance, rash, drowsiness, gynecomastia, hypoadrenalism. Has abortifacient and embryotoxic properties	Requires cautious use since few clinical experiences and no biochemical markers available to monitor efficacy of treatment. Increases cortisol level via antagonism of negative feedback of ACTH secretion

ACTH, adrenocorticotropic hormone or corticotropin; NTE, not to exceed.

[a]Dosing guidelines (including age ranges) for children have not been definitively established.

[b]These medications do not have FDA-approved indications for the treatment of Cushing's syndrome in either adults or children.

From Refs. 21, 24–26.

Table 45–8

Principles of Glucocorticoid Administration to Avoid Hypercortisolism or Hypocortisolism

To Prevent Hypercortisolism and Development of Cushing's Syndrome:
- Give the lowest glucocorticoid dose that will manage the disease being treated and for the shortest possible duration
- If feasible, give glucocorticoid via administration routes that minimize systemic absorption (such as inhalation or dermal)
- If feasible, administer glucocorticoid treatment every other day (calculate the total 48-hour dose and give as a single dose of intermediate-acting glucocorticoid in the morning)[4]
- Avoid concurrent administration of drugs that can inhibit glucocorticoid metabolism

To Prevent Hypocortisolism and Development of Adrenal Insufficiency or Adrenal Crisis:
- Assess patients at risk for adrenal insufficiency with screening tests (serum cortisol, plasma ACTH stimulation, etc.)
- If the patient requires discontinuation from chronic treatment with supraphysiologic doses of glucocorticoid, the following discontinuation protocol can be used[4]:
  - Gradually taper the dose to approximately 20 mg of prednisone or equivalent per day, given in the morning, then
  - Change glucocorticoid to every other day administration, in the morning
  - Stop the glucocorticoid when the equivalent physiologic dose is reached (20 mg/day of hydrocortisone or 5–7.5 mg/day of prednisone or equivalent)
  - Understand that recovery of the HPA axis may take up to a year after glucocorticoid discontinuation during which the patient may require supplementation therapy during periods of physiologic stress
- Evaluate patients at risk for adrenal insufficiency as a result of treatment(s) of Cushing's syndrome and initiate glucocorticoid and mineralocorticoid replacement therapy as appropriate
- Avoid concurrent administration of drugs that can induce glucocorticoid metabolism
- Educate patients about:
  - The need for replacement or supplemental glucocorticoid and mineralocorticoid therapy
  - How to administer parenteral glucocorticoid if unable to immediately access medical care during an emergency
  - Need to wear or carry medical identification regarding their condition (e.g., card, bracelet)

ACTH, adrenocorticotropic hormone or corticotropin; HPA, hypothalamic–pituitary–adrenal.

Patient Encounter 2

EF is a 45-year-old woman who presents to the dermatologist for evaluation of facial acne. She has a history of a 11.4-kg (25-lb) weight gain, irregular menses, and frequent vaginal yeast infections over the past 2 years. During the review of systems, she also complains of increased facial hair growth and lower extremity muscle weakness. Physical exam reveals facial acne, facial hirsutism, truncal obesity, thin skin, and purple abdominal striae. Her past medical history is significant for hypertension, type 2 diabetes mellitus, hyperlipidemia, and lupus.

Which findings are suggestive of Cushing's syndrome?

Is there anything in the patient's history that would suggest an exogenous cause of the patient's presumed Cushing's syndrome?

hypercortisolism. Symptoms often improve immediately after surgery and soon after initiation of drug therapy. However, it may take months for symptoms to resolve following radiation therapy.

- Monitor for normalization of serum cortisol concentrations.

- The Patient Care and Monitoring textbox discusses additional evaluation strategies.

Abbreviations Introduced in This Chapter

ACTH	Adrenocorticotropic hormone or corticotropin
AS	Aldosterone synthase
CRH	Corticotropin-releasing hormone
DHEA	Dehydroepiandrosterone
DHEA-S	Sulfated form of dehydroepiandrosterone
DST	Dexamethasone suppression test
HPA	Hypothalamic–pituitary–adrenal

stress may be needed for up to 1 year after glucocorticoid discontinuation.[15] Table 45–8 lists strategies to prevent the development of hypercortisolism and hypocortisolism.

Outcome Evaluation

- Monitor patients receiving surgical, medical, or radiation therapy for resolution of the clinical manifestations of

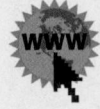

Self-assessment questions and answers are available at *http://www.mhpharmacotherapy. com/pp.html*.

Patient Care and Monitoring: Cushing's Syndrome

1. Patient evaluation should include a thorough history of all medications and herbal or dietary supplements.

2. Perform initial screening tests to confirm Cushing's syndrome and rule out those with pseudo-Cushing's conditions.

3. Once diagnosis is confirmed, perform further testing to determine etiology of Cushing's syndrome.

4. Attempt to taper glucocorticoid if Cushing's syndrome is from exogenous administration.

5. If endogenous Cushing's syndrome, determine if patient is an appropriate candidate for surgical resection of the tumor. Does the patient have any conditions that contraindicate surgical resection such as advanced disease (metastatic adrenal carcinoma)?

6. Develop a formal plan to assess the response and complications associated with surgery[21]:

   - Measure plasma cortisol post surgery to determine if the patient displays persistent hypercortisolism (surgical treatment failure) or hypocortisolism (adrenal insufficiency requiring steroid replacement therapy).

   - In patients demonstrating hypocortisolism:

     - Monitor for signs and symptoms of glucocorticoid withdrawal (headache, fatigue, malaise, myalgia).

     - Monitor for signs and symptoms of adrenal insufficiency.

     - Monitor morning cortisol or response to ACTH stimulation every 3 to 6 months to assess for HPA axis recovery. Discontinue glucocorticoid replacement therapy when cortisol concentrations are greater than 19 mcg/dL (524 nmol/L) on either test.

     - Monitor cortisol, ACTH, low-dose dexamethasone suppression, or other tests to assess for risk of relapse of hypercortisolism.

   - Monitor for development of pituitary hormone deficiency

7. If surgical resection does not achieve satisfactory disease control or is not indicated, evaluate patient for pituitary radiation or bilateral adrenalectomy with concomitant pituitary radiation.

   - Monitor patients treated with pituitary radiation for development of pituitary hormone deficiency.

8. Evaluate patients with adrenal adenomas for unilateral adrenalectomy.

9. Give glucocorticoid and mineralocorticoid replacement to patients who undergo adrenalectomy (permanently in the case of bilateral adrenalectomy).

10. Evaluate patient for appropriateness of pharmacologic therapy depending on etiology of Cushing's syndrome.

11. Monitor patient for response to therapy, need for dose adjustments, and presence of adverse drug reactions.

12. Once disease control is achieved, continue to monitor biochemical markers and patient for development of complications of Cushing's syndrome, as relapse may occur.

13. Provide patient education regarding disease state and treatment:

    - Causes of Cushing's syndrome, including drug-induced etiologies.

    - How to recognize the clinical manifestations of Cushing's syndrome.

    - Possible sequelae of Cushing's syndrome.

    - How to reduce modifiable cardiovascular and metabolic complications.

    - Advantages and disadvantages of potential treatment options.

    - Possible adverse consequences of treatment.

    - Need for glucocorticoid and mineralocorticoid replacement after treatment, if appropriate.

    - Importance of adherence to therapy.

REFERENCES

1. Gums JG, Anderson S. Adrenal gland disorders. In: DiPiro JT, Talbert RL, Yee GC, Matzke GR, Wells BG, Posey LM, eds. Pharmacotherapy: A Pathophysiologic Approach, 7th ed. New York City: McGraw-Hill, 2008:1265–1280.

2. Aron DC, Findling JW, Tyrrell JB. Glucocorticoids and adrenal androgens. In: Greenspan FS, Gardner DG, eds. Basic and Clinical Endocrinology. New York City: Lange Medical Books/McGraw-Hill, 2004:362–413.

3. Cooper MS, Stewart PM. Corticosteroid insufficiency in acutely ill patients. N Engl J Med 2003;348:727–734.

4. Williams GH, Dluhy RG. Disorders of the adrenal cortex. In: Kasper DL, Braunwald E, Fauci A, Hauser S, Longo D, Jameson JL, eds. Harrison's Principles of Internal Medicine. New York City: McGraw-Hill, 2005.

5. Salvatori R. Adrenal insufficiency. JAMA 2005;294:2481–2488.

6. Coursin DB, Wood KE. Corticosteroid supplementation for adrenal insufficiency. JAMA 2002;287:236–240.

7. Alevritis EM, Sarubbi FA, Jordan RM, Peiris AN. Infectious causes of adrenal insufficiency. South Med J 2003;96:888–890.

8. Raedler TJ, Jahn H, Goedeken B, Gescher DM, Kellner M, Wiedemann K. Acute effects of megestrol on the hypothalamic-pituitary-adrenal axis. Cancer Chemother Pharmacol 2003;52:482–486.

9. Arlt W, Allolio B. Adrenal insufficiency. Lancet 2003;361:1881–1893.

10. Hunt PJ, Gurnell EM, Huppert FA, et al. Improvement in mood and fatigue after dehydroepiandrosterone replacement in Addison's disease in a randomized, double blind trial. J Clin Endocrinol Metab 2000;85:4650–4656.

11. Johannsson G, Burman P, Wiren L, et al. Low dose dehydroepiandrosterone affects behavior in hypopituitary androgen-deficient women: A placebo-controlled trial. J Clin Endocrinol Metab 2002;87:2046–2052.

12. Arlt W, Callies F, van Vlijmen JC, et al. Dehydroepiandrosterone replacement in women with adrenal insufficiency. N Engl J Med 1999;341:1013–1020.

13. Gurnell EM, Hunt PJ, Curran SE, et al. Long-term DHEA replacement in primary adrenal insufficiency: A randomized, controlled trial. J Clin Endocrinol Metab 2008;93:400–409.

14. Findling JW, Raff H. Screening and diagnosis of Cushing's syndrome. Endocrinol Metab Clin North Am 2005;34:385–402, ix–x.

15. Hopkins RL, Leinung MC. Exogenous Cushing's syndrome and glucocorticoid withdrawal. Endocrinol Metab Clin North Am 2005;34:371–384, ix.

16. Raff H, Findling JW. A physiologic approach to diagnosis of the Cushing syndrome. Ann Intern Med 2003;138:980–991.

17. Lacroix A, Bourdeau I. Bilateral adrenal Cushing's syndrome: Macronodular adrenal hyperplasia and primary pigmented nodular adrenocortical disease. Endocrinol Metab Clin North Am 2005;34:441–458, x.

18. Arnaldi G, Angeli A, Atkinson AB, et al. Diagnosis and complications of Cushing's syndrome: A consensus statement. J Clin Endocrinol Metab 2003;88:5593–5602.

19. Goldman JA, Myerson G. Chinese herbal medicine: Camouflaged prescription antiinflammatory drugs, corticosteroids, and lead. Arthritis Rheum 1991;34:1207.

20. Keane FM, Munn SE, du Vivier AW, Taylor NF, Higgins EM. Analysis of Chinese herbal creams prescribed for dermatological conditions. BMJ 1999;318:563–564.

21. Utz AL, Swearingen B, Biller BM. Pituitary surgery and postoperative management in Cushing's disease. Endocrinol Metab Clin North Am 2005;34:459–478, xi.

22. Young WF, Jr., Thompson GB. Laparoscopic adrenalectomy for patients who have Cushing's syndrome. Endocrinol Metab Clin North Am 2005;34:489–499, xi.

23. Morris D, Grossman A. The medical management of Cushing's syndrome. Ann N Y Acad Sci 2002;970:119–133.

24. Package insert. Mifeprex (mifepristone). New York, NY: Danco Laboratories; 2005 July.

25. Chu JW, Matthias DF, Belanoff J, Schatzberg A, Hoffman AR, Feldman D. Successful long-term treatment of refractory Cushing's disease with high-dose mifepristone (RU 486). J Clin Endocrinol Metab 2001;86:3568–3573.

26. Sonino N, Boscaro M. Medical therapy for Cushing's disease. Endocrinol Metab Clin North Am 1999;28:211–222.

46 Pituitary Gland Disorders

Judy T. Chen, Devra K. Dang, Frank Pucino Jr., and Karim Anton Calis

LEARNING OBJECTIVES

● **Upon completion of the chapter, the reader will be able to:**

1. List the mediators and primary effects of pituitary hormones.

2. Identify clinical features of patients with acromegaly.

3. Discuss the role of surgery and radiation therapy for patients with acromegaly.

4. Select appropriate pharmacotherapy for patients with acromegaly based on patient-specific factors.

5. Identify clinical features of children and adults with growth hormone (GH) deficiency and select appropriate pharmacotherapy for these patients.

6. Recommend monitoring parameters necessary to assess therapeutic outcomes and adverse effects in patients receiving GH therapy.

7. List common etiologies of hyperprolactinemia.

8. Identify clinical features of patients with hyperprolactinemia.

9. Select appropriate pharmacologic and nonpharmacologic treatments for patients with hyperprolactinemia based on patient-specific factors.

KEY CONCEPTS

❶ Surgical resection of the pituitary tumor through transsphenoidal pituitary microsurgery is the treatment of choice for most patients with growth hormone (GH)-producing pituitary adenomas.

❷ Somatostatin analogs are the mainstay of pharmacotherapy for the treatment of acromegaly when surgery is contraindicated or has failed.

❸ Pegvisomant is indicated for patients who do not tolerate or fail other treatments, or for those with extremely elevated insulin-like growth factor (IGF) I levels.

❹ Dopamine agonists may be appropriate for patients with mildly elevated IGF-I levels who have GH and prolactin cosecreting tumors.

❺ Prolonged exposure to elevated GH and IGF-I levels can lead to serious complications in patients with acromegaly. Aggressively manage comorbid conditions such as hypertension, diabetes, dysrhythmias, coronary artery disease, and heart failure to prevent vascular and/or neuropathic complications.

❻ Recombinant GH therapy is the main pharmacologic treatment for GH deficiency in both children and adults.

❼ Although comparative trials have not been conducted, recombinant GH products appear to have similar efficacy for treating GH deficiency.

❽ Dopamine agonists are the first-line treatment of choice for all patients with hyperprolactinemia; transsphenoidal surgery and radiation therapy are reserved for patients who are resistant to or severely intolerant of pharmacologic therapy.

❾ Women who become pregnant while on a dopamine agonist should discontinue treatment immediately to minimize fetal exposure. Because cabergoline has a long half-life, women who plan to become pregnant should discontinue the drug at least 1 month before planned conception.

PHYSIOLOGY OF THE PITUITARY GLAND

The pituitary gland, located at the base of the brain in proximity to the nasal cavity, is a small endocrine gland about the size of a pea weighing approximately 600 mg. The pituitary gland is referred to as the "master gland" because it is responsible for the regulation of many other endocrine glands and body systems. Growth, development, metabolism, reproduction, and stress homeostasis are among the functions influenced by

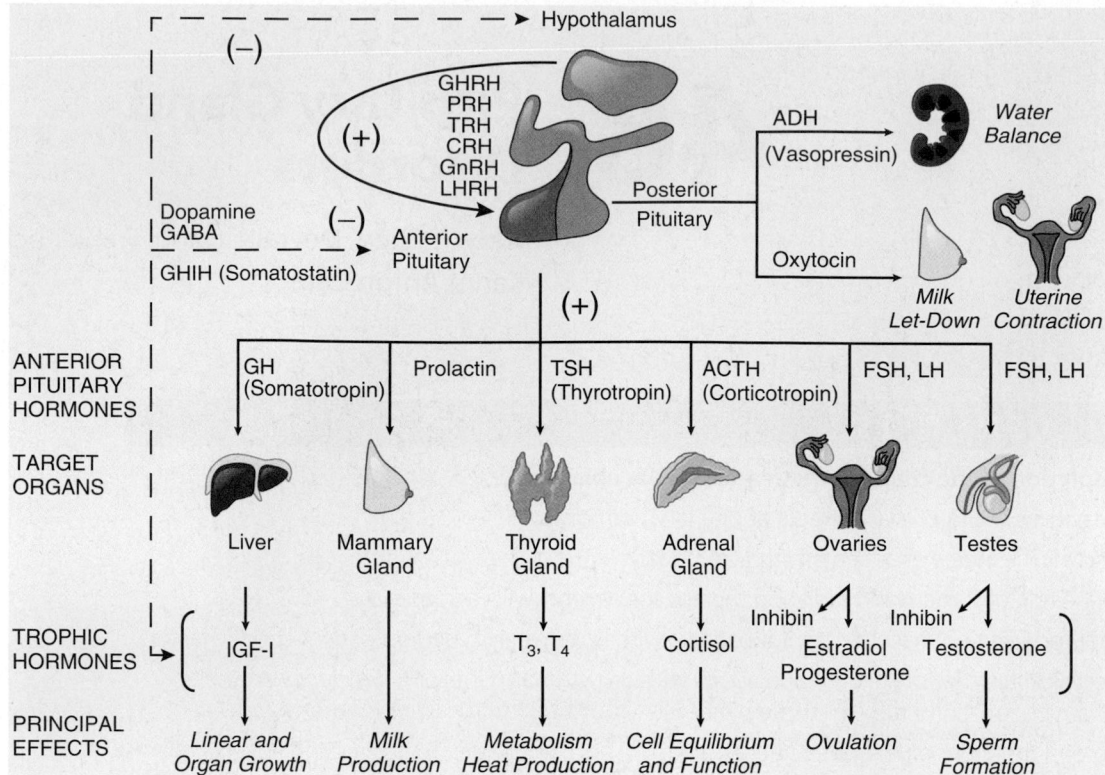

FIGURE 46–1. Hypothalamic–pituitary–target-organ axis. The hypothalamic hormones regulate the biosynthesis and release of eight pituitary hormones. Stimulation of each of these pituitary hormones produces and releases trophic hormones from their associated target organs to exert their principal effects. These trophic hormones regulate the activity of endocrine glands. Subsequently, increased serum concentration of the trophic hormones released from the target organs can inhibit both the hypothalamus and the anterior pituitary gland to maintain homeostasis (negative feedback). Inhibin is produced by the testes in the male and ovaries in the female during pregnancy. Inhibin directly inhibits pituitary production of follicle-stimulating hormone (FSH) through a negative feedback mechanism. Melanocyte-stimulating hormone (MSH) produced by the anterior pituitary is not illustrated in the figure [(–), inhibit; (+), stimulate; ACTH, adrenocorticotropic hormone (corticotropin); ADH, antidiuretic hormone (vasopressin); CRH, corticotropin-releasing hormone; FSH, follicle-stimulating hormone; GABA, γ-aminobutyric acid; GH, growth hormone (somatotropin); GHIH, growth hormone–inhibiting hormone (somatostatin); GHRH, growth hormone–releasing hormone; GnRH, gonadotropin-releasing hormone; IGF-I, insulin-like growth factor I; LH, luteinizing hormone; LHRH, luteinizing hormone–releasing hormone; PRH, prolactin-releasing hormone; T$_3$, triiodothyronine; T$_4$, thyroxine; TRH, thyrotropin-releasing hormone; TSH, thyroid-stimulating hormone (thyrotropin).]

the pituitary. Functionally, the gland consists of two distinct sections: the anterior pituitary lobe (adenohypophysis) and the posterior pituitary lobe (neurohypophysis). The pituitary receives neural and hormonal input from the inferior hypothalamus via blood vessels and neurons contained in the pituitary stalk (infundibulum).

The posterior pituitary is innervated by nervous stimulation from the hypothalamus, resulting in the release of specific hormones to exert direct tissue effects. The hypothalamus synthesizes two hormones, oxytocin and vasopressin. These hormones are stored in and released from the posterior pituitary lobe. Oxytocin exerts two actions, it: (a) promotes uterine contractions during labor and (b) contracts the smooth muscles in the breast to stimulate the release of milk from the mammary gland during lactation. Vasopressin is an antidiuretic hormone essential for proper fluid and electrolyte balance in the body. Specifically, vasopressin increases the permeability of the distal convoluted tubules

and collecting ducts of the nephrons to water. This causes the kidney to excrete less water in the urine. Consequently, the urine becomes more concentrated as water is conserved.

In contrast to the posterior pituitary lobe, the anterior pituitary lobe is under the control of several releasing and inhibiting hormones secreted from the hypothalamus via a portal vein system. The anterior pituitary, in turn, synthesizes and secretes six major hormones. Figure 46–1 summarizes the physiologic mediators and effects of each of these hormones.

Hormonal Feedback Regulatory Systems

The hypothalamus is responsible for the synthesis and release of hormones that regulate the pituitary gland. Stimulation or inhibition of the pituitary hormones elicits a specific cascade of responses in peripheral target glands. In response, these glands secrete hormones that exert a negative feedback on other hormones in the hypothalamic–pituitary axis (Fig. 46–1). This negative feedback serves to maintain body system homeostasis. High circulating hormone levels inhibit the release of hypothalamic and anterior pituitary hormones.

Damage and destruction of the pituitary gland may result in secondary hypothyroidism, **hypogonadism**, adrenal insufficiency, growth hormone (GH) deficiency, hypoprolactinemia, or insufficiency or absence of all anterior pituitary hormones (i.e., **panhypopituitarism**). A tumor (adenoma) located in the pituitary gland may result in excess secretion of a hormone or may physically compress the gland and suppress adequate hormone release. The type, location, and size of a pituitary tumor often determine a patient's clinical presentation. This chapter discusses the pathophysiology and role of pharmacotherapy in the treatment of **acromegaly**, GH deficiency, and **hyperprolactinemia**. The following hormones are discussed elsewhere in this textbook: adrenocorticotropic hormone (ACTH or corticotropin), thyroid-stimulating hormone (TSH or thyrotropin), luteinizing hormone (LH), follicle-stimulating hormone (FSH), vasopressin (antidiuretic hormone), and oxytocin.

GH (SOMATOTROPIN)

Somatotropin or GH is the most abundant hormone produced by the anterior pituitary lobe. The GH-secreting **somatotropes** account for 50% of hormone–secreting cells in the anterior pituitary. GH is regulated primarily by the hypothalamic-pituitary axis. The hypothalamus releases growth hormone–releasing hormone (GHRH) to stimulate GH synthesis and secretion, whereas somatostatin inhibits it.[1] Upon stimulation by GHRH, somatotropes release GH into the circulation, thereby stimulating the liver and other peripheral target tissues to produce insulin-like growth factors (IGFs). These IGFs, also known as somatomedins, are the peripheral GH targets. There are two types of IGFs: **IGF-I** and IGF-II. IGF-II is responsible primarily for regulating fetal growth, whereas IGF-I is the hormone responsible for growth of bone and other tissues. High levels of IGF-I inhibit GH secretion through somatostatin, thereby inhibiting GHRH secretion.[1] The hypothalamus also may stimulate the release of somatostatin to inhibit GH secretion. Effects of IGF-I in peripheral tissues are both GH-dependent and GH-independent.[2] GH is an anabolic hormone with direct "anti-insulin" metabolic effects. By stimulating protein synthesis and shifting the body's energy source from carbohydrates to fats, GH promotes a diabetic state (Table 46–1).[2] GH controls somatic growth and has a critical role in the development of normal skeletal muscle, myocardial muscle, and bone.

In healthy individuals, GH is secreted in a pulsatile pattern throughout a 24-hour period, with several short bursts occurring mostly during the night. The most intense period of GH secretion occurs within the first 1 to 2 hours of slow-wave sleep (stage 3 or 4 deep sleep).[1] In between these bursts, basal concentration of GH falls to very low or undetectable levels because of its short half-life in the blood (approximately 19 minutes). The amount of GH secretion fluctuates throughout a person's lifetime. Secretion of GH

Table 46–1

Effects of Growth Hormone

	Action(s)	Effect(s)
Lipid metabolism	Increases the use of fat by stimulating triglyceride breakdown and oxidation of adipocytes	Increases breakdown of fat (lipolysis) Increases circulating fatty acid levels Increases lean body mass
Protein metabolism	Stimulates protein anabolism by increasing amino acid uptake and protein synthesis and decreasing oxidation of proteins	Increases muscle mass
Carbohydrate metabolism	Suppresses the ability of insulin to stimulate uptake of glucose in peripheral tissues	Decreases glucose utilization
	Decreases insulin receptor sensitivity	Insulin resistance
	Impairs postreceptor insulin action	Hyperglycemia
	Stimulates glucose synthesis in the liver (gluconeogenesis)	Increases hepatic glucose output

From Ref. 2.

is lowest during infancy, increases during childhood, peaks during adolescence, and then declines gradually during the middle years.[1] These changes are parallel to an age-related decline in lean muscle mass.

GH Excess

▶ *Epidemiology and Etiology*

Acromegaly affects both genders equally, and the average age of presentation is 44 years. Approximately 50 to 70 people per 1 million population are affected, with an estimated annual incidence of 3 to 4 cases per 1 million people.[3–5] In more than 95% of the cases, overproduction of GH is due to a benign pituitary tumor (adenoma), whereas malignant tumors occur in less than 1%.[3] Most pituitary adenomas occur spontaneously as a result of a genetic mutation acquired during life. Depending on the size of the tumor, pituitary adenomas are classified as: (a) microadenomas if they are 10 mm or less in diameter; or (b) macroadenomas if they are greater than 10 mm. Rarely, nonpituitary tumors cause acromegaly. These tumors can produce GH, but more commonly they secrete GHRH and result in excessive GH and IGF-I production.

▶ *Pathophysiology*

Acromegaly is a rare, insidious disorder that manifests gradually over time. It is caused by an adenoma of the pituitary that overproduces GH and stimulates excessive production of IGF-I during adulthood. This typically occurs after fusion of the epiphyses (growth plates) of the long bones.[3] The facial features of an acromegalic patient are depicted in Figure 46–2. Gigantism refers to GH excess that occurs during childhood before epiphyseal closure and results in excessive linear growth.

Diagnosis of acromegaly is based on both clinical and biochemical findings. Because secretion of GH fluctuates throughout the day, a single random measurement is never reliable for diagnosing GH excess.[1] However, GH-mediated IGF-I production results in relatively stable serum IGF-I concentrations during the day, which correlate positively with 24-hour mean GH levels.[1] This makes elevated IGF-I levels an ideal screening test for acromegaly and a reliable monitoring biochemical marker to assess disease activity and response to therapy.[6,7] Because IGF-I levels may fluctuate with age and gender, it is important to compare IGF-I levels with age- and sex-matched population values.[6,7] Other conditions such as nutritional status, liver dysfunction, insulin levels, and illness also can affect IGF-I levels. The measurement of serum GH secreted by the pituitary in response to an oral glucose tolerance test (OGTT) is the primary biochemical test for diagnosing acromegaly. GH is suppressed after administration of a 75 g oral glucose challenge because postprandial hyperglycemia inhibits secretion of GH for at least 1 hour. If the GH level does not decline to less than 1 ng/mL (1 mcg/L) during the test, the patient is diagnosed with acromegaly.[3] In addition to clinical presentation, elevated IGF-I serum concentration helps to confirm the diagnosis.

▶ Acromegaly Treatment Goals

Patients with untreated acromegaly experience a twofold increase in mortality rate primarily due to cardiovascular and pulmonary diseases.[10] Normalization of GH and IGF-I levels reverses the mortality risk and alleviates significant comorbid complications, especially cardiovascular, pulmonary, metabolic, and respiratory abnormalities.[11] Reduction of IGF-I levels alone does not appear to be a reliable predictor of long-term outcome.[6,12] The goals of therapy are as follows[3,13–15]:

- Normalize biochemical markers.
  - Reduce GH to less than 1 ng/mL (1 mcg/L) after OGTT. When using the older GH assay, suppression of GH levels to less than 1 ng/mL (1 mcg/L) after OGTT is the biochemical target. Lower cut off levels have been suggested using the more sensitive GH assays.[13–15]
  - Normalize IGF-I levels to age- and sex-matched control values.
- Ablate or reduce tumor size to relieve tumor mass effect.
- Prevent tumor recurrence and control tumor size.
- Preserve normal pituitary function.
- Improve clinical signs and symptoms.
- Alleviate significant morbidities.
- Reduce mortality rates to that of the general population.

▶ General Approaches to Treatment

The American Association of Clinical Endocrinologists published medical guidelines for the diagnosis and treatment of acromegaly (Fig. 46–3). According to these guidelines, ❶ *surgical resection of the pituitary tumor through trans-sphenoidal pituitary microsurgery is the treatment of choice for most patients with GH-producing pituitary adenomas.*[3] When performed by experienced surgeons, approximately 70% to 80% of patients with microadenomas and less than 50% of patients with macroadenomas achieve biochemical control.[10] Complete resection of a macroadenoma may be difficult if the tumor has already invaded the surrounding nerves and tissues. In such cases, debulking of the tumor along with adjunctive radiation and/or pharmacotherapy may improve treatment outcome. Infrequent surgical complications include meningitis, serious visual impairment, cerebrospinal fluid leakage, diabetes insipidus, and permanent hypopituitarism.[3] Relative contraindications to surgery include patient frailty, acromegaly-associated comorbidities, and medically unstable conditions such as

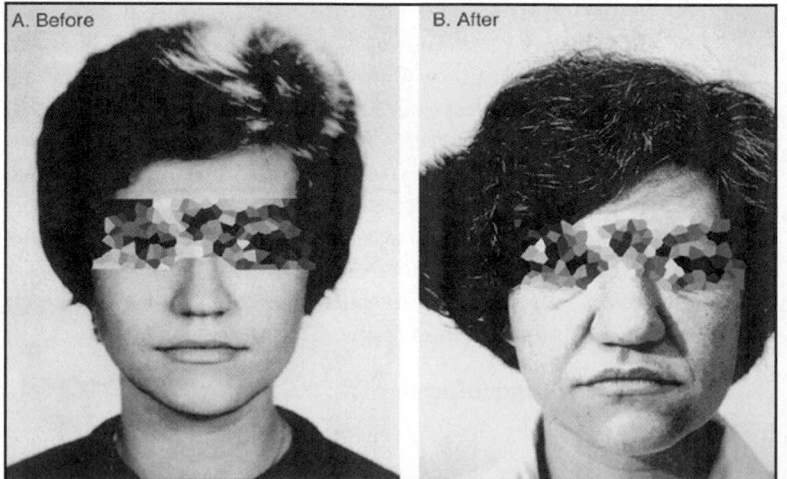

FIGURE 46–2. Before and after photographs of an acromegalic patient. Compare the photographs of an acromegalic woman (A) before the onset of acromegaly and (B) after approximately 20 years, when the diagnosis was well established. Notice the coarsening of facial features, with enlarged nose, lips, and forehead.

Clinical Presentation and Diagnosis of Acromegaly

General

The patient will experience slow development of soft-tissue overgrowth affecting many body systems. Signs and symptoms may progress gradually over 7 to 10 years.

Symptoms

- Headache and compromised visual function (loss of peripheral vision and blurred vision) caused by the actual tumor mass and its close proximity to the optic structures.
- Loss of other hormonal functions (i.e., LH, FSH, TSH, and ACTH) caused by massive tumor size compressing the anterior pituitary lobe.
- Absence of regular menstrual periods (amenorrhea), impotence, and decreased libido caused by disruption of the gonadotropin secretion.
- Excessive sweating, joint pain, nerve pain, and abnormal neurologic sensations (paresthesias) related to elevated GH and IGF-I levels.

Signs

- Coarsening of facial features
- Increased hand volume
- Increased ring and shoe size
- Increased spacing between teeth
- Increased acne/oily skin
- Enlarged tongue
- Deepening of voice
- Thick, irregular, patchy skin discoloration
- Enlarged nose, lips, and forehead (frontal bossing)
- Abnormal protrusion of the mandible (prognathia)
- Inappropriate secretion of breast milk (galactorrhea)
- Abnormal enlargement of various organs (organomegaly) such as liver, spleen, and heart

- Carpal tunnel syndrome caused by nerve compression from the swollen tissue

Laboratory Tests

- GH level greater than 1 ng/mL (1 mcg/L) following an OGTT and elevated IGF-I level compared with age- and sex-matched control values
- Glucose intolerance may be present in up to 50% of patients

Additional Clinical Sequelae

- Cardiovascular diseases: hypertension, coronary heart disease, cardiomyopathy, left ventricular hypertrophy, and arrhythmia
- Osteoarthritis and joint damage develop in up to 90% of patients
- Respiratory disorders and sleep apnea occur in up to 60% of patients
- Type 2 diabetes mellitus develops in 25% of patients
- Increased risk for the development of esophageal, colon, and stomach cancer

Other Diagnostic Tests

- Perform MRI examination and CT of the pituitary to locate the tumor and validate the diagnosis.
- Without obvious pituitary tumor but proven acromegaly, measurement of GHRH may be helpful to detect ectopic tumors.

Adapted, from Sheehan AH, Yanovski JA, Calis KA. Pituitary Gland Disorders. In: Dipiro JT, Talbert RL, Yee GC, et al., eds. Pharmacotherapy. A Pathophysiologic Approach. 7th ed. New York: McGraw Hill, 2008:1284.

From Refs. 4, 8, 9.

---

airway difficulties, severe hypertension, or uncontrolled diabetes.

▶ Pharmacologic Therapy

Pharmacologic therapy is often necessary for patients in whom surgery is not an option. Somatostatin analogs, GH receptor antagonists, and dopamine agonists are the primary pharmacologic therapies used for the management of acromegaly (Table 46–2).[3] Pharmacologic therapy avoids hypopituitarism and other surgical risks.

▶ Somatostatin Analog (GH-Inhibiting Hormone)

❷ *Somatostatin analogs are the mainstay of pharmacotherapy for the treatment of acromegaly when surgery is contraindicated or has failed.* These agents mimic endogenous somatostatins and bind to the somatostatin receptors in the pituitary to cause potent inhibition of GH, insulin, and glucagon secretion. Long-term treatment can sustain hormone suppression, alleviate soft-tissue manifestations, and reduce tumor size. Use of the first-generation somatostatin analog, octreotide, is limited by its extremely short duration of action which necessitates frequent injections of at least three times per day. The long-acting preparations of octreotide and lanreotide are considered the cornerstone of therapy due to improved patient adherence and acceptability. Typically, at least a 2-week trial of short-acting octreotide is recommended to determine efficacy and tolerance before switching to a long-acting preparation. The long-acting formulations can be administered every 14 to 28 days. Their efficacy and safety have been demonstrated in long-term studies (up to 9 years with octreotide and 4 years with lanreotide).[16–18] Long-acting octreotide effectively suppresses

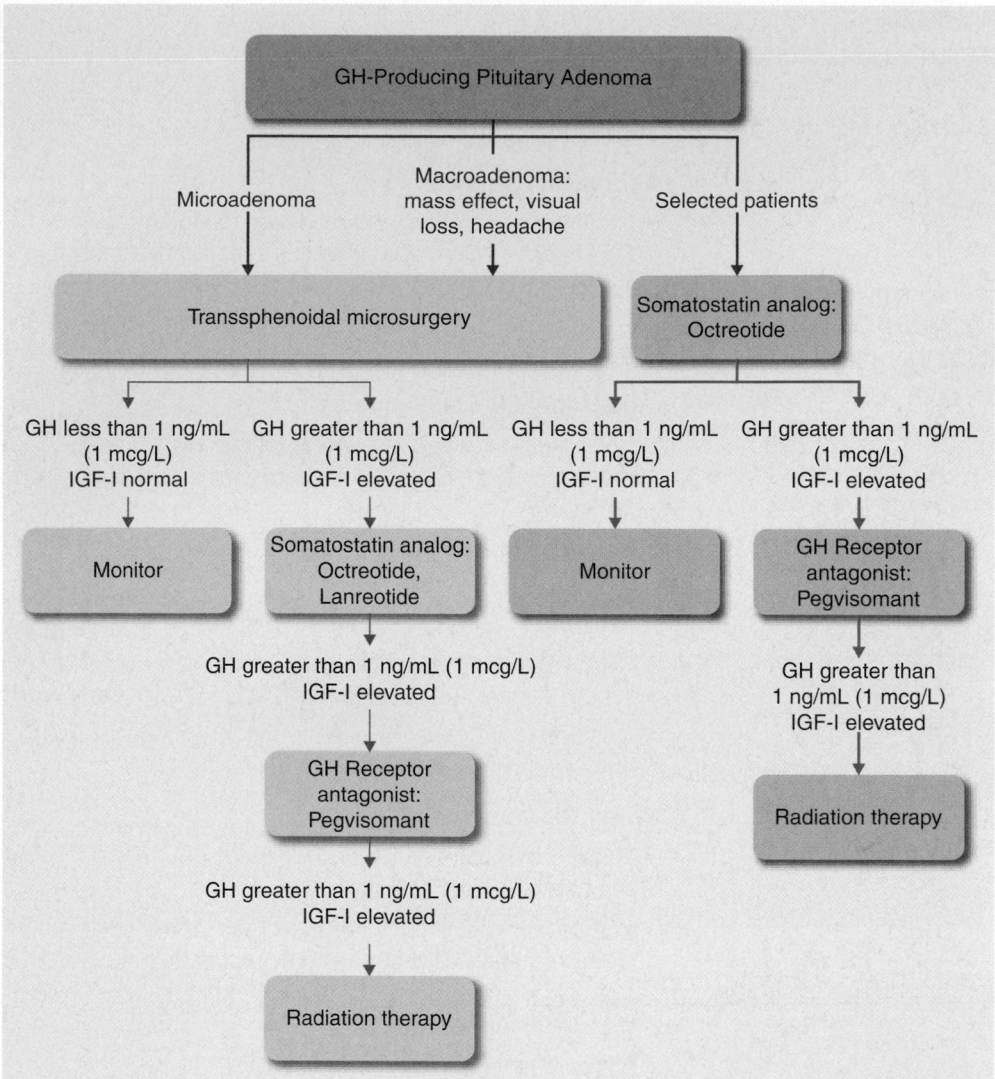

FIGURE 46–3. Management of growth hormone–producing adenomas (GH, growth hormone; IGF-I, insulin-like growth factor I.) (Adapted from Ref. 3.)

GH levels and achieves normal IGF-I levels in 67% and 57% of patients, while lanreotide slow-release formulation achieved lower response rates of 48% and 47%, respectively.[19] However, the response rate of long-acting octreotide may be overestimated due to differences in subject selection.[19] Recent limited data suggested treatment with lanreotide autogel is comparable to lanreotide slow-release and as effective as long-acting octreotide.[18] Since somatostatin analogs can achieve substantial relief of clinical symptoms with significant reduction in tumor size,[19,20] it is important to monitor patients for tumor recurrence if treatment is discontinued. Due to lack of sufficient data, routine use of presurgical somatostatin analogs is currently not recommended unless a delay in surgery is anticipated.[18]

Somatostatin analogs are generally well tolerated. Common adverse effects include transient GI disturbances such as diarrhea, abdominal pain, flatulence, constipation, and nausea.[18] These adverse GI effects usually subside within the first 3 months of therapy.[5] Somatostatin analogs inhibit gallbladder contractility and decrease bile secretion; therefore, their major adverse effect is development of biliary sludge and asymptomatic gallstones (cholelithiasis). Biliary sludge is a predisposing factor for the high incidence of cholelithiasis observed in up to 20% of patients.[5] Development of gallstones typically occurs in patients treated for 12 months or longer and is unrelated to age, gender, or dose. Somatostatin analog-induced gallstones should be managed according to standard guidelines.[5] Additionally, somatostatin analogs may alter the balance of counterregulatory hormones (i.e., glucagon, insulin, and GH), resulting in either hypoglycemia or hyperglycemia.[18] Octreotide also may suppress pituitary release of TSH, leading to decreased thyroid hormone secretion and subsequent hypothyroidism in 12% of treated patients. Close monitoring of thyroid function and glucose metabolism is recommended. Sinus bradycardia, conduction abnormalities, and arrhythmias have been reported with octreotide and lanreotide. Due to the potential adverse effects of the somatostatin analogs, concomitant use with insulin, oral hypoglycemic agents, β-blockers, or calcium channel blockers may require careful dosage adjustment. Somatostatin analogs also may alter the bioavailability and

Table 46–2

Comparison of Various Drugs for Treatment of Acromegaly

Drug Type	Dopamine Agonist	Somatostatin Analog				GH Receptor Antagonist
Agent	Cabergoline	Octreotide (Sandostatin)	Octreotide LAR (Sandostatin LAR)	Lanreotide SR	Lanreotide Autogel (Somatuline Depot)	Pegvisomant (Somavert)
Preferred indication	GH and prolactin cosecreting tumors	Somatostatin analog-responsive	Somatostatin analog-responsive	Somatostatin analog-responsive	Somatostatin analog-responsive	High IGF-I levels not responsive to somatostatin analog-therapy
Starting dose	0.5–1 mg/week orally	50 mcg SC 3 × daily	20 mg IM every 4 weeks	60 mg IM every 2 weeks	90 mg deep SC every 4 weeks[a]	10 mg SQ daily after initial loading dose of 40 mg
Maximal dose	4 mg/week orally	200 mcg SC 3 × daily	40 mg IM every 4 weeks[b]	120 mg IM every 7 days	120 mg deep SC every 4 weeks	40 mg SQ daily
Dosage in hepatic insufficiency	Dosage reduction may be recommended for patients with severe hepatic failure		Cirrhosis: 10 mg IM every 4 weeks	Dosage reduction may be necessary. No guidelines available	Moderate to severe impairment: starting dose 60 mg every 4 weeks	Discontinue therapy if liver function tests are elevated at least 5 × the upper limit of normal or transaminase at least 3 × upper limit of normal with any increase in serum total bilirubin
Dosage in renal failure	None	Dialysis-dependent: adjustment may be necessary. No guidelines available	Dialysis-dependent renal impairment: 10 mg IM every 4 weeks	Dosage reduction may be necessary. No guidelines available	Moderate to severe impairment: starting dose 60 mg every 4 weeks	None
Side effects	Nausea, GI cramps, headache	Nausea, GI cramps, gallstones	Nausea, GI cramps, gallstones	Nausea, GI cramps, gallstones	Nausea, GI cramps, gallstones	Headache, fatigue, abnormal liver enzymes
Monitoring suggestions	GH, IGF-I	GH, IGF-I, ultrasonography of gallbladder (if symptoms)	GH, IGF-I, ultrasonography of gallbladder (if symptoms)	GH, IGF-I, ultrasonography of gallbladder (if symptoms)	GH, IGF-I, ultrasonography of gallbladder (if symptoms)	Liver function tests monthly for 6 months, then every 6 months, then biannually for the next year; MRI every 6 months. IGF-I (not GH) after first year, then yearly

GH, growth hormone; IGF-I, insulin-like growth factor I; IM, intramuscularly; LAR, long-acting release; SC, subcutaneously; SR, slow release.

[a]In the United States, initiate lanreotide at 90 mg every 28 days for 3 months then titrate accordingly based on patient response. Different labeled dosing guidelines exist for the United Kingdom and Canada.

[b]Product labeling recommends a maximum of 30 mg IM every 4 weeks.

Adapted from Ref. 3. by permission of publisher, AACE Corp.

elimination of cyclosporine, and monitoring of cyclosporine serum concentration is necessary.

GH-Receptor Antagonist GH-receptor antagonist represents a novel approach to the treatment of acromegaly. Pegvisomant is the only genetically engineered GH-receptor antagonist that blocks the action of GH. The effects of pegvisomant work independently of tumor characteristics, somatostatin, and dopamine receptors.[21] Up to 97% of acromegalic patients treated with pegvisomant (10–20 mg/day) achieved normal age-related IGF-I levels and experienced significant improvement in clinical symptoms of GH excess by 1 year of therapy.[22,23] In patients previously resistant to somatostatin analog therapy, normal IGF-I concentrations were achieved in 75% of patients treated with pegvisomant[24] and in 69% to 100% of patients treated with pegvisomant and somatostatin analog therapy.[25–27] Pegvisomant therapy may have favorable effects on glucose tolerance (the body's ability to metabolize glucose) and insulin sensitivity (capacity of cells to respond to insulin).[24] However, use of pegvisomant is associated with significant dose-dependent increases in GH despite the declining IGF-I levels.[22,23] The dose-dependent increase in GH is troubling because it has been suggested that persistent elevation of GH levels may be indicative of tumor growth. Thus, careful monitoring with periodic imaging scans is indicated, especially when administering pegvisomant to patients at risk for visual damage from large tumors that may impinge on the optic chiasm. ❸ *Pegvisomant is indicated for patients who do not tolerate or fail other treatment options, or for those with extremely elevated IGF-I levels (greater than 900 ng/mL or 900 mcg/L).[3]* Long-term efficacy and safety profiles of pegvisomant in acromegaly remain to be established. Available data suggest that pegvisomant appears well-tolerated with minimal adverse effects such as self-limiting injection-site reactions, nausea, diarrhea, infection, and flu-like symptoms. Approximately 17% of patients who receive pegvisomant develop non-neutralizing anti-GH antibodies. Although the long-term consequences are unknown, the presence of antibodies does not appear to affect the efficacy of pegvisomant. Cases of hepatotoxicity have been reported in clinical trials,[22,23] with a higher risk observed in diabetics receiving combined pegvisomant and somatostatin analogs.[27] Therefore, obtain baseline levels of transaminases, total bilirubin, and alkaline phosphatase prior to initiating therapy and periodically thereafter. Caution should be used when administering pegvisomant to patients with elevated liver function tests, and therapy should be discontinued in the presence of clinical signs and symptoms of hepatic injury.

Dopamine Agonists Dopamine is one of the neurotransmitters that can increase GH secretion in healthy adults. However, dopamine agonists administered to patients with acromegaly exert the opposite effect and suppress GH release from the tumor. The first dopamine agonist for acromegaly, bromocriptine, achieved normal IGF-I levels in fewer than 10% of patients and was associated with significant adverse effects, including nausea, dizziness, and headaches.[10] The large doses of bromocriptine required to achieve the desired response often are associated with dose-limiting toxicity, such as GI discomfort and orthostatic hypotension. Cabergoline, the selective long-acting agonist with improved tolerability, effectively can normalize IGF-I levels in 35% of patients and reduce GH levels in 44% of patients.[28] Acromegalic patients with coexisting hyperprolactinemia also had a more favorable response to cabergoline, with 50% of patients achieving normal IGF-I levels, 56% GH suppression, and 65% tumor shrinkage.[28] Although orally administered dopamine agonists are the least expensive medical therapy for managing acromegaly, the major disadvantage is their relative lack of efficacy compared with existing therapeutic options. ❹ *Dopamine agonists may be appropriate for patients with mildly elevated IGF-I levels who have GH and prolactin cosecreting tumors.[3]*

▶ Radiation Therapy

Radiation therapy is an important adjunctive therapy in patients with residual GH excess following surgery or pharmacologic therapy. Treatment involves the use of radiation to destroy rapidly growing tumor cells and often results in a reduction in tumor size. A major complication resulting from radiation therapy is hypopituitarism, requiring lifelong hormone replacement.[3] There is also the potential for optic nerve damage if the pituitary tumor is near the optic tracts. Radiation therapy may take 10 to 20 years before its full effects become evident.[10] Owing to delay in onset of radiation effectiveness, pharmacologic therapy often is indicated as bridge therapy.[3] Men and women who desire to have children should be warned that pituitary irradiation therapy may impair fertility.[3]

▶ Outcome Evaluation

- Following a baseline evaluation, monitor patients regularly for symptom relief. See Acromegaly: Patient Care and Monitoring text Box

- Lifelong biochemical assessment is critical for determining therapeutic outcomes. Although some patients may experience a rapid decline in GH levels following transsphenoidal microsurgery, stabilization of IGF-I levels usually occurs 3 months following surgery but rarely may be delayed for up to 12 months. Measure GH and IGF-I levels 3 months postoperatively to assess treatment response.[6]

- Because up to 10% of pituitary tumors may recur within 15 years following surgery,[6] continual postoperative monitoring is recommended.

- For patients treated with somatostatin analogs, assess baseline fasting blood glucose, thyroid function tests, and heart rate. Thereafter, periodically monitor patients for adverse reactions such as GI disturbances, glucose intolerance, signs and symptoms of thyroid abnormalities, bradycardia, and arrhythmias in patients receiving long-term somatostatin analogs. Reevaluate IGF-I and GH levels at 3-month intervals

Acromegaly: Patient Encounter 1: Medical History, Physical Examination, and Diagnostic Tests

EB, a 48-year-old woman, presents to a new primary care clinic. EB's chief complaints are chronic pain of the knee and "pins and needles" and "numbness" in both hands. Over the past few years, she feels that her body has been changing. EB reports increased urinary frequency, excessive sweating, worsening headaches, an increase of two shoe sizes, and facial hair that she shaves once a week. She says that her hands have enlarged to the point that "my wedding band won't fit anymore."

PMH: Hypertension for 12 years, currently controlled; hyperlipidemia for 10 years, currently controlled; osteoarthritis for 5 years

FH: Mother died of colon cancer at age of 58 years. Father died of myocardial infarction at an unknown age

SH: Married, a nurse practitioner, highly educated, and physically active (bikes four times per week)

Meds: Lisinopril/hydrochlorothiazide 20/12.5 mg once daily; atorvastatin 10 mg once daily; acetaminophen 500 mg every 8 hours as needed for joint pain

ROS: (+) Coarse facial hair. Deepening of voice

PE:

VS: BP 118/76 mm Hg, P 78 bpm, RR 18 breaths/min, T 37.5°C (99.5°F)

HEENT: Ophthalmic examination reveals normal visual acuity and fields. (+) Protruding jaw and large fleshy nose

CV: RRR, normal S_1, S_2; no murmurs, rubs, gallops

Abd: Soft, nontender, nondistended; (+) bowel sounds, no hepatosplenomegaly

Rectal: Heme (–) stool

Labs: Electrolytes and renal function are within normal limits. Fasting blood glucose level is 206 mg/dL (11.43 mmol/L), HbA$_{1c}$ is 8.5%, and (–) microalbumin. GH level following an OGTT is 8 ng/mL (8 mcg/L). Elevated IGF-I level at 790 ng/mL (790 mcg/L)

MRI and CT: Both reveal a pituitary tumor approximately 5 mm in diameter.

Given this information, what signs and symptoms of acromegaly does EB exhibit?

Identify your treatment goals for EB.

What nonpharmacologic and pharmacologic treatment options are available for EB?

---

to determine therapeutic response. Because the frequency of symptomatic gallstones associated with somatostatin analogs varies among studies, the need for routine ultrasound evaluation remains controversial. However, ultrasonography of the gallbladder would be indicated if the patient develops symptoms of biliary abnormalities.

- For patients treated with a GH receptor antagonist, GH levels are not measured because pegvisomant is a modified GH molecule that is detected in commercial GH assays, resulting in falsely elevated GH levels. Therefore, IGF-I level is the principal biochemical marker used to assess response to pegvisomant therapy. After appropriate dose titration, monitor IGF-I levels every 6 months.[6] Concern for tumor growth requires careful monitoring of tumor size; therefore, performing MRI every 6 months during the first year of therapy and annually thereafter is recommended.[6] Because of abnormal liver function associated with pegvisomant therapy, it is mandatory to monitor all patients' liver function tests prior to initiation of therapy, monthly during the first 6 months, and every 6 months thereafter.[6]

- For patients receiving dopamine agonists, the maximal suppression of GH and IGF-I levels may take up to 3 months to achieve. Once stable control of biochemical markers is achieved with dopamine agonists or somatostatin analogs, monitor GH and IGF-I levels annually.[6]

- With conventional multidose radiation therapy, the most rapid decline in GH serum levels occurs within the first 2 years; monitor GH levels at the second year and annually thereafter.[6] Patients who receive single-dose radiation therapy should be evaluated at 6-month intervals because response is observed earlier.

- For patients receiving concurrent pharmacologic therapy with radiation therapy, withdraw therapies every 6 to 12 months to evaluate endogenous GH secretion and assess the development of hypopituitarism.[6]

- ⑤ *Prolonged exposure to elevated GH and IGF-I can lead to serious complications in patients with acromegaly. Aggressively manage comorbid conditions such as hypertension, diabetes, dysrhythmias, coronary artery disease, and heart failure to prevent vascular and/or neuropathic complications* (Table 46–3).[29]

GH Deficiency

▶ *Epidemiology and Etiology*

In the United States, GH deficiency affects approximately 50,000 adults, with around 6,000 new cases diagnosed annually.[30] Approximately 10,000 to 15,000 children have growth failure owing to GH deficiency. Children may present with GH deficiency at any time during their developmental stages. The evaluation for GH deficiency in a short child

Table 46–3

Assessment of Acromegaly Complications at Diagnosis and Follow-Up

At the Time of Diagnosis	During Long-Term Follow-Up
Glucose tolerance test (with concurrent GH sampling)	Fasting blood glucose, HbA$_{1c}$ if diabetes present (as appropriate)
Serum cholesterol and lipid profile	Annually
Echocardiography	Annually
ECG	Annually
Exercise ECG	If angina present
Colonoscopy	Every 2–3 years
DEXA (hypogonadal only)	Every 2–3 years
Sleep assessment	Annually (if altered at diagnosis)
Blood pressure monitoring	Annually or change of treatment (if hypertensive)
Echo-Doppler of carotid artery	As indicated by clinical features

DEXA, dual-energy x-ray absorptiometry; GH, growth hormone; HbA$_{1c}$, glycosylated hemoglobin A$_{1c}$.

From Ref. 29.

should be deferred until appropriate exclusion of other identifiable causes of growth failure, such as hypothyroidism, chronic illness, malnutrition, genetic syndromes, and skeletal disorders. Also, several medications, such as methoxamine, isoproterenol, glucocorticoids, cimetidine, methylphenidate, and amphetamines, may induce GH insufficiency.[31]

▶ *Pathophysiology*

GH deficiency exists when GH is absent or produced in inadequate amounts. GH deficiency may be congenital, acquired, or result from disruption of the hypothalamus–pituitary axis. GH deficiency may be an isolated condition or occasionally be accompanied by other endocrine disorder (e.g., panhypopituitarism). The diagnosis of GH deficiency remains a clinical challenge because no "gold standard" currently exists. Because GH is frequently undetectable with random sampling, a stimulation or provocative test usually is performed to confirm the diagnosis in both adults and children in whom GH deficiency is suspected. Numerous pharmacologic agents such as insulin-induced hypoglycemia, levodopa, arginine, arginine plus levodopa, arginine plus GHRH, clonidine, and glucagon have been used to stimulate the pituitary to produce GH.[32] However, no single test perfectly predicts GH deficiency or displays 100% sensitivity and specificity.[33] Additionally, administration of each of these tests is associated with adverse effects requiring close medical supervision. Further, current abnormal cutoffs to determine diagnosis are arbitrarily defined and lack universal consensus.[32,33] With further studies, these diagnostic criteria are likely to evolve and become more

Acromegaly: Patient Care and Monitoring

1. Assess patient's clinical signs and symptoms to determine severity of acromegaly.

2. Review the biochemical disease markers to assess severity of acromegaly.

3. Review the available diagnostic data to determine pituitary tumor size and location. Determine if the patient has a coexisting prolactin secreting tumor. Determine if the tumor extends toward the optic chiasm or if it is continuous on the optic tracts.

4. Assess presence of acromegaly complications. Identify any significant comorbidities associated with acromegaly that require immediate treatment or early diagnosis.

5. Determine what treatment options the patient has tried in the past.

6. Evaluate patient for presence of surgical contraindications to transsphenoidal microsurgery. Determine if the patient is able or willing to undergo surgical intervention.

7. Develop a formal plan to assess patient's response and complications to surgical intervention. Measure both GH and IGF-I levels.

8. If surgical intervention does not achieve satisfactory disease control, select subsequent appropriate pharmacologic therapy based on patient-specific factors. In selecting therapy, be sure to consider if the patient has any contraindications or allergies to therapies.

9. Evaluate patient for presence of adverse drug reactions, drug allergies, and drug interactions.

10. Develop a plan to assess efficacy of pharmacologic therapy. Also consider if the patient's therapy requires any dose adjustments.

11. Assess biochemical markers annually once disease control is achieved.

12. Routinely assess acromegaly complications; include blood pressure, glucose tolerance, fasting lipid profile, cardiac evaluations (if clinically indicated), colonoscopy, dual energy x-ray absorptiometry (DEXA) scan (hypogonadal only), evaluation of residual pituitary function, and evaluation of sleep apnea.

13. Provide patient education in regards to disease state, nondrug and drug therapy. Discuss with the patient:

    • Possible complications of acromegaly,

    • How to reduce the modifiable cardiovascular and metabolic risk factors,

    • Potential effectiveness and disadvantages of existing treatment options,

    • Importance of adherence to therapy, and

    • Potential adverse effects that may occur.

accurate. In prepubertal children, measurement of IGF-I concentrations may be useful in evaluating GH deficiency, with 100% specificity and 70% to 90% sensitivity.[34] In children, the diagnosis of GH deficiency is further supported if height is more than two standard deviations below the population mean (age- and sex-matched).[30] Failure of linear growth is an almost universal presenting feature of childhood GH deficiency.

Childhood GH deficiency may or may not continue into adulthood. Most adults with GH deficiency have overt pituitary disease and present with nonspecific clinical disorders distinct from pediatric GH deficiency, thereby making diagnosis of GH deficiency in adults more difficult than in children. Additionally, adult GH deficiency presumably is associated with increased risk of death from cardiovascular diseases.[35]

▶ Treatment Goals

The goal of treatment for GH deficiency is to correct associated clinical symptoms.[30] In children, prompt diagnosis and early initiation of treatment are important to maximize final adult height. In adults, efforts should be made to achieve normal physiologic GH levels in an attempt to reverse the metabolic, functional, and psychological abnormalities.[32]

▶ Pharmacologic Therapy

GH Therapy ❻ *Recombinant GH therapy is the main pharmacologic treatment for GH deficiency in both children and adults.* It promotes skeletal, visceral, and general body growth; stimulates protein anabolism; and affects bone, fat, and mineral metabolism[2] (Table 46–1). GH therapy requires subcutaneous or intramuscular administrations. Since two-thirds of GH secretion normally occurs during sleep, it is recommended to administer injections in the evening.[36] Many preparations of synthetic GH are available with a variety of injection devices to make administration more appealing and easier. Protropin (somatrem) and Tev-Tropin (somatropin) are approved by the FDA for use in children, whereas other somatropin products such as Nutropin, Nutropin AQ, Humatrope, Norditropin, Genotropin, Omnitrope, and Saizen are FDA approved in both children and adults.

❼ *Although comparative trials have not been conducted to date, recombinant GH products appear to have similar efficacy for treating GH deficiency as long as the regimen follows currently approved guidelines.* GH secretion decreases with age. Therefore, older adults with GH deficiency often require substantially lower replacement doses than younger individuals. The optimal therapeutic approach is to initiate GH therapy with lower doses. The recommended initial GH dose is 0.2 mg/day for young men, 0.3 mg/day for young women, and 0.1 mg/day for older adults.[32] Conventional weight-based regimens are not recommended in adults due to the lack of evidence supporting higher dosages in heavier individuals and greater potential for adverse effects.[32,35] Maintenance doses may be lower with chronic GH therapy.[37] For elderly patients, lower GH replacement doses often are adequate because of increased GH sensitivity.[32] Carefully monitor patients requiring replacement therapy with estrogens, thyroid hormones, or glucocorticoids due to potential interactions with GH therapy.[32] In prepubertal children, the recommended replacement dose is 25 to 50 mcg/kg/day.[38] Replacement doses should be titrated based on clinical and biochemical responses. The conversion of international units (IU or mU) to mg is a 3:1 ratio.[30] Selection of an injection device depends on patient preference because there is currently no difference in clinical outcomes among the various injection systems.[38]

Evidence has suggested that GH treatment in GH-deficient children can increase short-term growth and improve final

Clinical Presentation and Diagnosis of GH Deficiency in Children

General
The patient will have a physical height that is greater than two standard deviations below the population mean for a given age and gender.

Signs
- The patient will present with reduced growth velocity and delayed skeletal maturation.
- Children with GH-deficient or GH-insufficient short stature also may present with abdominal obesity, prominence of the forehead, and immaturity of the face.

Laboratory Tests
- Patients will exhibit a peak GH level of less than 10 ng/mL (10 mcg/L) following a GH stimulation test.
- Reduced IGF-I concentration also may be present.

- Because GH deficiency may be accompanied by the loss of other pituitary hormones, hypoglycemia and hypothyroidism also may be noted.

Other Diagnostic Tests
- Perform MRI or CT of the hypothalamic–pituitary region to detect structural or developmental anomaly.
- Perform x-ray of left wrist and hand for children over 1 year of age to estimate bone age (knee and ankle for children younger than 1 year of age).

Adapted from Sheehan AH, Yanovski JA, Calis KA. Pituitary Gland Disorders. In: Dipiro JT, Talbert RL, Yee GC, et al., eds. Pharmacotherapy. A Pathophysiologic Approach. 7th ed. New York: McGraw Hill, 2008:1288.

From Refs. 8, 30.

Clinical Presentation and Diagnosis of GH Deficiency in Adults

General

The patient likely will have a history of childhood-onset GH deficiency, hypothalamic or pituitary disorder, or the presence of three or four other pituitary hormone deficiencies caused by head trauma, tumor, infiltrative diseases, surgery, or radiation therapy.

Symptoms

- Reduced strength and exercise capacity
- Defective sweating
- Psychological problems
- Low self-esteem
- Depression
- Fatigue/listlessness
- Sleep disturbance
- Anxiety
- Social isolation
- Emotional lability and impaired self-control
- Poor marital and socioeconomic performance

Signs

- Increased fat mass (especially abdominal obesity)
- Reduced lean body mass
- Reduced muscle strength
- Reduced exercise performance
- Thin, dry skin; cool peripheries; poor venous access
- Depressed affect, labile emotions
- Impaired cardiac function

Laboratory Tests

- Patients will exhibit a peak GH level of less than 5 ng/mL (5 mcg/L) following a GH stimulation test.
- Low or low-normal IGF-I level also may be present.
- Increased low-density lipoprotein cholesterol, total cholesterol, triglycerides; decreased high-density lipoprotein cholesterol.
- Reduced bone mineral density associated with an increased risk of fracture.
- Increased insulin resistance and increased prevalence of impaired glucose tolerance.
- GH deficiency may be accompanied by the loss of other pituitary hormones.

From Refs. 32, 35, 36.

adult height.[30] Beneficial effects of GH therapy in adults with GH deficiency have been demonstrated in subsequent studies to normalize body composition and metabolic process; improve cardiac risk profile, bone mineral density, quality of life and psychological well-being; and increase muscle strength, and exercise capacity.[35] Although long-term efficacy of GH replacement in adults has been demonstrated in a 10-year prospective study,[37] overall reduction in mortality with GH therapy remains to be established.

Begin GH therapy as soon as possible to optimize long-term growth, especially for young children in whom GH deficiency is complicated by fasting hypoglycemia.[30] Selection of the optimal GH replacement dose will need to be individualized depending on response, financial resources, and product availability. Although the appropriate time to discontinue therapy remains controversial in childhood GH deficiency, it is reasonable to continue GH replacement until either the child has reached satisfactory adult height, achieved documented epiphyseal closure, or failed to respond to therapy.[30] Management of the transition between pediatric and adult GH replacement remains a challenge because there are no current data to indicate the correct approach. Starting GH therapy at a low dose and gradually titrating upward may decrease the potential for adverse effects. The need for GH replacement therapy may be lifelong.

Children treated with GH replacement therapy rarely experience significant adverse effects, whereas adults are more susceptible to dose-related adverse effects. Treatment with GH may mask underlying central hypothyroidism and adrenal insufficiency. GH-induced symptoms, such as edema, arthralgia, myalgia, and carpal tunnel syndrome, are common and necessitate dose reductions in up to 40% of adults. Benign increases in intracranial pressure may occur with GH therapy and generally are reversible with discontinuation of treatment. Often, GH therapy can be restarted with smaller doses without symptom recurrence.

In rapidly growing children, a slipped capital femoral epiphysis may occur when the head of the femur shifts in a backward direction.[38] There is no evidence that this problem is caused by GH therapy, but any child who experiences a change in gait during treatment should be evaluated by an orthopedic surgeon.[38] Treatment with GH may induce insulin resistance and lead to the development of glucose intolerance in patients with pre-existing risk factors. Presently, there is no compelling evidence that GH replacement therapy is associated with an increased risk of leukemia, solid tumor, or tumor recurrence.[30,32] However, in children with a history of malignancies, it would be prudent to wait for a 1-year tumor-free period (5 years for adults) before initiating GH therapy.[30] Any patients treated for a prior malignancy may be at risk for a second malignancy and should be monitored carefully for tumor recurrence.[30] Other rare findings associated with GH replacement therapy include breast development, pancreatitis, juvenile osteochondritis (inflammation of a bone and its cartilage), worsening of scoliosis, and increased pigmentation.[38] Because deaths have been reported with use of GH in children with Prader-Willi syndrome who are severely obese or suffer from respiratory impairments, use of GH is contraindicated in these individuals.

Insulin-Like Growth Factor I Therapy Mecasermin (Increlex) is the only recombinant IGF-I replacement therapy for the treatment of growth failure in children with severe primary IGF-I deficiency or with GH gene deletions who have developed neutralizing antibodies to GH. This product has not been evaluated in patients with GH deficiency aside from the genetic abnormalities.

▶ *Outcome Evaluation*

- Children with GH deficiency should be evaluated by a pediatric endocrinologist every 3 to 6 months. Monitor for an increase in height and change in height velocity to assess response to GH therapy.[30,38] Every effort should be made to maximize height before the onset of puberty. Once final adult height is reached and GH is discontinued for at least 1 month, retest and reevaluate the patient using the adult GH-deficiency diagnostic criteria.[38]

- Assess patients with scoliosis for further curvature of the spine.

- Although GH and IGF-I levels do not always correlate with growth response, measure IGF-I levels yearly to assess adherence to therapy and patient response. If the IGF-I levels are substantially above the normal range 2 years after GH replacement therapy, the dose should be reduced.[38] IGF-I level may be used as a guide to gradually reduce replacement dose after epiphyseal closure.

- Routine monitoring of fasting lipid profile, bone mineral density, and body composition in children is not typically required during GH replacement but should be done before and after discontinuation of therapy.[30,38]

- In adults, measurement of serum IGF-I, along with careful clinical evaluation, appears to be the most reliable way to assess the appropriateness of the GH dose. Measure IGF-I serum concentrations annually and 6 weeks following dosage adjustments.[35]

- Continuously monitor for dose-related adverse effects such as edema, arthralgia, myalgia, and carpal tunnel syndrome.

- Evaluate psychological well-being. Assess patient's bone mineral density every 2 years. Measure body composition, metabolic status, and cardiac risks (e.g., fasting lipid profile) yearly.[32]

- Patients with a history of cancer or those at risk for malignancy should be monitored closely.

- Measure a free thyroxine serum concentration at baseline and at 6- to 12-month intervals thereafter.[30]

- Measure fasting blood glucose levels at baseline and annually to assess for glucose intolerance.[35]

PROLACTIN

Prolactin is an essential hormone for normal production of breast milk following childbirth. It also plays a pivotal role in a variety of reproductive functions. Prolactin is regulated primarily by the hypothalamus-pituitary axis and secreted solely by the lactotroph cells of the anterior pituitary gland. Under normal conditions, secretion of prolactin is predominantly under inhibitory control by dopamine and acts on the D_2 receptors located on the lactotroph cells.

GH Deficiency in Children: Patient Care and Monitoring

1. Assess child's growth characteristics, and compare physical height with a population standard (e.g., Centers for Disease Control and Prevention Growth Charts).

2. Obtain a thorough history and physical examination that may indicate the possible presence of GH deficiency. Exclude other identifiable causes of growth failure, such as hypothyroidism, chronic illness, malnutrition, genetic syndromes, and skeletal disorders.

3. Perform imaging tests of the hypothalamic–pituitary region to detect structural or developmental anomalies. Perform x-ray of the wrist and hand to estimate bone age.

4. Perform a provocative test to measure GH and IGF-I levels.

5. Initiate GH replacement therapy based on patient preference. Make sure that the child does not have any contraindications to GH therapy.

6. Develop a formal plan to assess response (increase in height and change in height velocity) and adverse effects

of GH replacement therapy. Make dosage adjustments when appropriate.

7. May continue GH replacement therapy until child reaches satisfactory adult height, achieves documented epiphyseal closure, or fails to respond to treatment.

8. Review and retest the child using adult GH deficiency diagnostic criteria once the child reaches final adult height.

9. Provide patient education in regard to disease state and drug therapy. Discuss with the child and parents:

   - GH deficiency
   - Potential effectiveness and disadvantages of existing GH replacement therapy
   - Importance of adherence to therapy
   - Potential for adverse effects or need for lifelong replacement

GH Deficiency in Adults: Patient Care and Monitoring

1. Assess patient's clinical signs and symptoms to determine severity of GH deficiency.

2. Perform a provocative test to measure GH and IGF-I levels.

3. Evaluate the patient for the presence of metabolic abnormalities and cardiovascular and fracture risks.

4. Initiate GH replacement therapy based on patient preference. Make sure that the patient does not have any contraindications to GH therapy.

5. Develop a plan to assess the efficacy and adverse effects of GH therapy, and consider if the patient's therapy requires any dose adjustments based on IGF-I level, patient response, and adverse effects.

6. Provide patient education in regard to disease state and drug therapy. Discuss with the patient:

   - Possible complications of GH deficiency
   - How to reduce the modifiable cardiovascular and metabolic risk factors
   - Potential disadvantages and effectiveness of existing GH replacement therapy
   - Importance of adherence to therapy
   - Potential for adverse effects or need for lifelong replacement

Increase of hypothalamic thyrotropin-releasing hormone in primary hypothyroidism can stimulate the release of prolactin.

Hyperprolactinemia

▶ Epidemiology and Etiology

Hyperprolactinemia affects women of reproductive age more than men. Although this disorder occurs in less than 1% of the general population, the estimated prevalence in women with reproductive disorders (e.g., amenorrhea) is as high as 15% to 43%.[39] Numerous etiologies of hyperprolactinemia are presented in Table 46–4.[39] Any medications that antagonize dopamine or stimulate prolactin release can induce hyperprolactinemia.[8,31,39,40] Therefore, it is important to exclude medication-induced hyperprolactinemia from other common causes such as pregnancy, primary hypothyroidism, benign prolactin-secreting pituitary adenoma (prolactinoma), and renal insufficiency. Prolactinomas are the most common pituitary tumors. They are classified as microprolactinomas if they are less than 10 mm in diameter and as macroprolactinomas if they are 10 mm or greater in diameter.[40] In general, microprolactinomas rarely increase in size, whereas macroprolactinomas have the potential to enlarge and invade the surrounding tissues.[41]

▶ Pathophysiology

Hyperprolactinemia is a condition of elevated serum prolactin.[40] It is the most common endocrine disorder of the hypothalamic–pituitary axis. High prolactin levels inhibit the release of gonadotropin-releasing hormone by the hypothalamus and subsequently suppress secretion of LH and FSH from the

Table 46–4

Causes of Hyperprolactinemia

Physiologic Causes
Pregnancy
Stress (including exercise and hypoglycemia)
Breast stimulation
Breast-feeding
Coitus
Sleep
Meal

Increased Prolactin Production
Ovarian: polycystic ovarian syndrome
Oophorectomy (removal of an ovary)
Pituitary tumors:
   Adenomas
   Microprolactinoma (less than 10 mm diameter)
   Macroprolactinoma (greater than or equal to 10 mm diameter)
Hypothalamic stalk interruption (prevent dopamine from reaching the pituitary)
Hypophysitis (inflammation)
Ectopic tumors

Hypothalamic Prolactin Stimulation
Primary hypothyroidism
Adrenal insufficiency

Reduced Prolactin Elimination
Chronic renal failure
Hepatic cirrhosis

Neurogenic Causes
Chest-wall injury (e.g., surgery, herpes zoster)
Spinal cord lesions

Abnormal Molecules
Macroprolactinemia

Medications
Dopamine antagonists: antipsychotics[a]; phenothiazines; metoclopramide; domperidone
Dopamine-depleting agents: reserpine; α-methyldopa
Prolactin stimulators: serotonin reuptake inhibitors; dexfenfluramine; estrogens; progestins; antiandrogens; gonadotropin-releasing hormone analogs; benzodiazepines; tricyclic antidepressants; monoamine oxidase inhibitors; protease inhibitors; histamine$_2$ receptor antagonists
Other: isoniazid; cocaine; opioids; verapamil

Seizures

Idiopathic (Unknown)

[a]Atypicals (olanzapine and clozapine) other than risperidone may cause an early but transient elevation in prolactin.

Adapted in part, with permission, from Sheehan AH, Yanovski JA, Calis KA. Pituitary gland disorders. In: Dipiro JT, Talbert RL, Yee GC, et al., eds. Pharmacotherapy. A Pathophysiologic Approach. 7th ed. New York: McGraw Hill, 2008:1291.

From Refs. 8, 31, 39, 40, 42.

anterior pituitary. High prolactin levels result in reduced gonadal hormone levels, often leading to reproductive dysfunction and galactorrhea (inappropriate breast milk production).

In combination with clinical symptoms, at least three repeated measures of serum prolactin levels greater than 20 ng mL (20 mcg/L) are needed to confirm the diagnosis. A number of physiologic factors such as eating, exercise, and stress can transiently elevate prolactin levels.[8] Therefore, prolactin measurements should be obtained at rest, preferably in the morning under fasting conditions.[39] If an IV line is present or planned, it is prudent to wait at least 2 hours after line insertion before measuring serum prolactin to decrease detecting transient physiologic increases in prolactin level[39,42] (Table 46–4). Medication-induced hyperprolactinemia typically is associated with prolactin levels of less than 150 ng/mL (150 mcg/L), whereas prolactin levels greater than 250 ng/mL (250 mcg/L) are almost always associated with macroprolactinoma.[43]

▶ Treatment Goals for Hyperprolactinemia

Because hyperprolactinemia is often associated with hypogonadism, the goals for management of hyperprolactinemia are to restore the clinical consequences of hypogonadism and reduce its associated risk for osteoporosis, as follows[42]:

- Normalize prolactin level
- Improve clinical symptoms
- Restore normal fertility
- Restore and maintain normal gonadal function
- Protect against development of osteoporosis
- Prevent disease recurrence
- If a pituitary tumor is present:
  - Ablate or reduce tumor size to relieve tumor mass effect
  - Preserve normal pituitary function

Clinical Presentation and Diagnosis of Hyperprolactinemia

General

Hyperprolactinemia most commonly affects women of reproductive age and is very rare in men.

Signs and Symptoms

Premenopausal women:

- Headache and compromised or loss of vision caused by the prolactin-secreting tumor and its close proximity to the optic structures.
- Clinical presentation is associated with the degree of prolactin elevation:
  - Prolactin greater than 100 ng/mL (100 mcg/L): hypogonadism, galactorrhea, and amenorrhea
  - Prolactin 51 to 75 ng/mL (51–75 mcg/L): oligomenorrhea (infrequent menstruation).
  - Prolactin 31 to 50 ng/mL (31–50 mcg/L): decreased libido and infertility.
- Increased body weight may be associated with prolactin-secreting pituitary tumor.
- The degree of hypogonadism generally is proportionate to the degree of prolactin elevation.
- Excessive hair growth (hirsutism) and acne also may be present owing to relative androgen excess compared with low estrogen levels.

Men:

- Decreased libido, decreased energy, erectile dysfunction, impotence, decreased sperm production, infertility, gynecomastia, and rarely, galactorrhea.
- Impotence is unresponsive to treatment and is associated with reduced muscle mass, loss of pubic hair, and osteoporosis.

Laboratory Tests

- Prolactin serum concentrations at rest will be greater than 20 ng/mL (20 mcg/L) in men or 25 ng/mL (25 mcg/L) in women with at least three measurements.
- Obtain β-human chorionic gonadotropin level to exclude pregnancy.
- Obtain TSH level to exclude primary hypothyroidism.
- Obtain blood urea nitrogen and serum creatinine tests to exclude renal failure.

Other Diagnostic Tests

- Perform MRI to locate the tumor, exclude a pseudoprolactinoma, and validate the diagnosis.
- Consider a bone mineral density test in patients with long-term hypogonadism.

Additional Clinical Sequelae

- The prolonged suppression of estrogen in premenopausal women with hyperprolactinemia leads to decreases in bone mineral density and significant risk for the development of osteoporosis.
- Risk for ischemic heart disease may be increased with untreated hyperprolactinemia.

Adapted, with permission, from Sheehan AH, Yanovski JA, Calis KA. Pituitary gland disorders. In: Dipiro JT, Talbert RL, Yee GC, et al., eds. Pharmacotherapy. A Pathophysiologic Approach. 7th ed. New York: McGraw Hill, 2008:1291.

From Refs. 8, 40, 42.

- Prevent progression of pituitary tumor or hypothalamic disease

▶ *General Approaches to Treatment*

Management of drug-induced hyperprolactinemia is to discontinue the offending agent, if possible, and start an appropriate therapeutic alternative. In situations where the offending agent cannot be discontinued, cautious use of hormone replacement, biphosphonate therapy, and/or dopamine agonists may be considered depending on the patient's clinical circumstances.[44] Treatment options for the management of hyperprolactinemia include: (a) clinical observation; (b) pharmacologic therapy with dopamine agonists; (c) transsphenoidal pituitary adenomectomy; and (d) radiation therapy. Figure 46–4 outlines an approach to the management of hyperprolactinemia after excluding drug-induced causes and other etiologies (e.g., hypothyroidism, renal failure, hepatic dysfunction).[42] Clinical observation and close monitoring are justifiable in patients with asymptomatic elevation of prolactin. ❽ *Dopamine agonists are the first-line treatment of choice for all patients with hyperprolactinemia; transsphenoidal surgery and radiation therapy are reserved for patients who are resistant to or severely intolerant of pharmacologic therapy.*[39]

▶ *Pharmacologic Therapy*

Dopamine is the principal neurotransmitter responsible for the inhibition of prolactin secretion from the anterior pituitary. Thus, dopamine agonists are the main pharmacologic therapy used for management of hyperprolactinemia.[40] Treatment with dopamine agonists has proven to be extremely effective in normalizing serum prolactin level, restoring gonadal function, decreasing tumor size, and improving visual fields.[40] Patients with macroprolactinomas generally require a higher dose to normalize prolactin levels compared with patients with microprolactinomas.[43]

Two dopamine agonists are used for the management of hyperprolactinemia, bromocriptine, and cabergoline (Table 46–5).[39,45] Because these two dopamine agonists are ergot derivatives, they are contraindicated in combination with potent cytochrome P-450 subfamily IIIA polypeptide 4 (CYP3A4) inhibitors, including protease inhibitors (e.g., ritonavir and indinavir), azole antifungals (e.g., ketoconazole and itraconazole), and some macrolide antibiotics (e.g., erythromycin and clarithromycin). Furthermore, ergot derivatives can cause constriction of peripheral and cranial blood vessels. These medications are also contraindicated in patients with uncontrolled hypertension, severe ischemic heart disease, or peripheral vascular disorders. Caution should be exercised with concomitant use of other ergot derivates and in patients with impaired renal or hepatic function, dementia, concurrent antihypertensive therapy, or a history of psychosis, peptic ulcer disease, or cardiovascular disease.

Bromocriptine Bromocriptine directly binds to the D_2 receptors on the lactotroph cells to exert its effect. Bromocriptine normalizes prolactin level in more than 90% of patients, restores menstrual cycles, and reduces tumor size in 62% of patients.[39] Adverse effects such as nausea, dizziness, and orthostatic hypotension often limit 5% to 10% of patients from continuing treatment. Thus, start bromocriptine at a low dose (e.g., 0.625–1.25 mg) at bedtime (taken with a snack) to decrease adverse effects.[41] Slowly titrate up to the optimal therapeutic dose (2.5–15 mg/day) because most adverse effects subside with continual treatment.[43] If the adverse GI effects are not tolerable, bromocriptine can be administered vaginally at a reduced dose (2.5 mg/day).[46] Owing to its short half-life of only 6 hours, bromocriptine must be administered in divided doses, which may compromise patient adherence.

Cabergoline Cabergoline has a higher affinity for D_2 receptors than bromocriptine. It is a long-acting dopamine agonist capable of inhibiting pituitary prolactin secretion for at least 7 days after a single oral dose.[45] The prolonged duration of action allows for once- or twice-weekly administration. Cabergoline appears to be significantly better tolerated than bromocriptine.[39] Transient elevations of serum alkaline phosphatase, bilirubin, and aminotransferases have been reported in a few patients treated with cabergoline. Cabergoline is more effective in normalizing prolactin levels and restoring menses than bromocriptine.[45] It also may be effective in treating hyperprolactinemia in patients who are resistant to or intolerant of bromocriptine and in men and women with micro- and macroprolactinomas.[39] Given its favorable safety and efficacy profile and ease of administration, cabergoline has replaced bromocriptine as first-line therapy for the management of hyperprolactinemia.[40] Withdrawal of pergolide from the U.S. market due to increased risk for valvular heart disease raised concerns about the safety of cabergoline. In patients with prolactinomas, tricuspid regurgitation was associated with higher cabergoline cumulative dose of more than 280 mg.[47] However, recent studies suggest the lower doses of cabergoline commonly used in the management of hyperprolactinemia do not appear to increase the risk of clinically significant valvular heart diseases.[48,49]

▶ *Nonpharmacologic Therapy*

In a small number of patients who have failed or are intolerant of dopamine agonists, transsphenoidal adenomectomy may be necessary. Surgical treatment is also considered in patients with nonprolactin-secreting tumors or macroprolactinomas that jeopardize the optic chiasm.[40] Nonetheless, surgical intervention does not reliably lead to long-term cure and may cause permanent complications.[42] Radiation therapy is reserved for failures of both pharmacologic therapy and surgery.[40] However, normalization of prolactin levels with radiation therapy may take 10 years to show full benefit, and radiation-induced hypopituitarism may require lifelong hormone replacement.

▶ *Management of Hyperprolactinemia in Pregnancy*

Most women with hyperprolactinemia require dopamine agonist therapy to achieve regular ovulatory cycles and

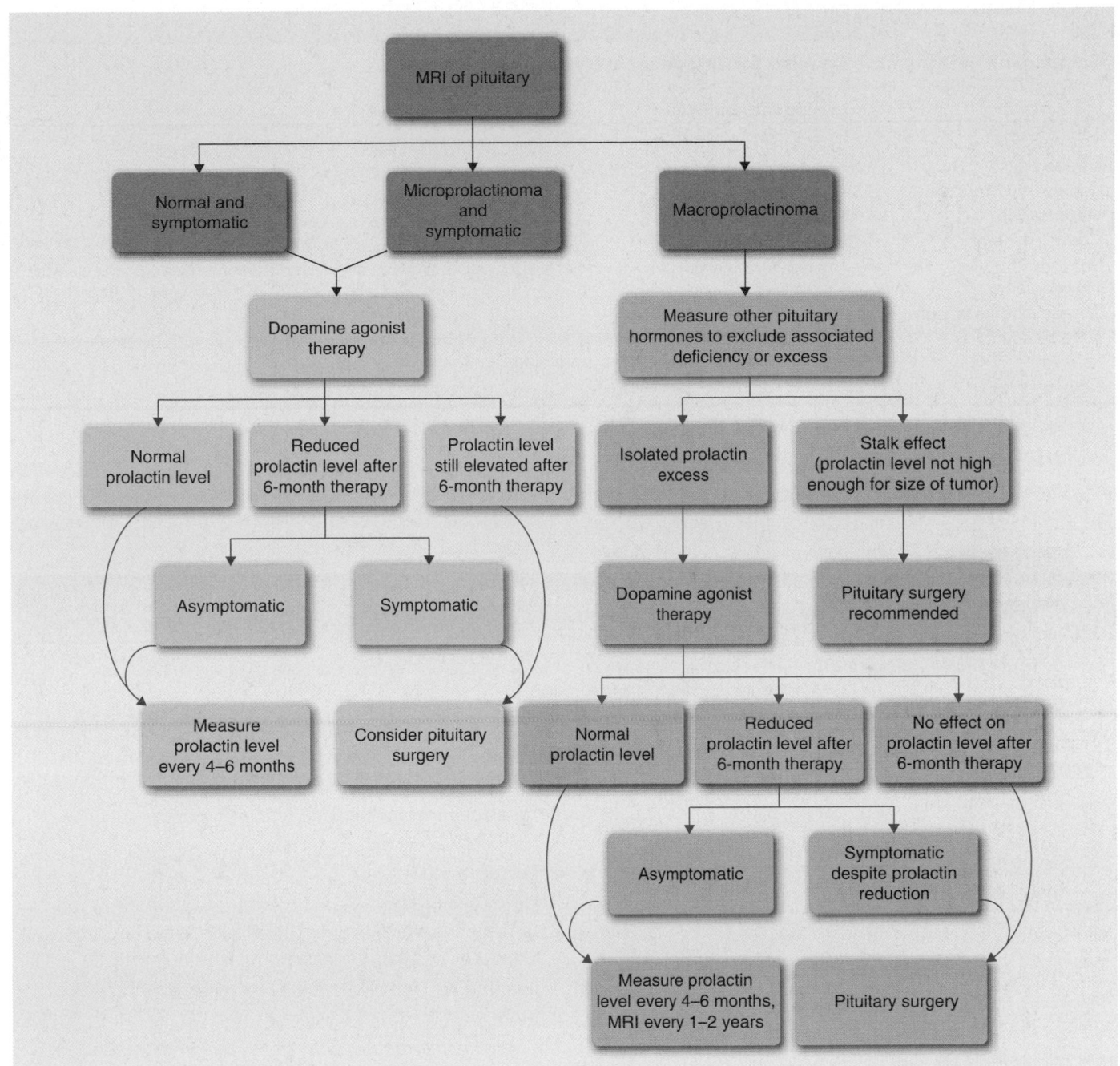

FIGURE 46–4. Management of hyperprolactinemia. (From Ref. 42.)

pregnancy. Since restoration of the ovulatory cycle may occur within 1 week of initiating therapy, it is necessary to caution patients regarding their potential to become pregnant.[50]

Overall, there is reassuring worldwide experience that bromocriptine use during pregnancy does not increase fetal malformations, spontaneous miscarriage, ectopic pregnancy, or multiple births.[39,41] Furthermore, no teratogenic effects have been reported in women who received cabergoline during the first and second trimesters of pregnancy.[41,45] Despite these data, ❾ *women who become pregnant while on a dopamine agonist should discontinue treatment immediately to minimize fetal exposure. Because cabergoline has a prolonged half-life, women who plan to become pregnant*

should discontinue the drug at least 1 month before planned conception.[45]

Microadenomas rarely cause complications during pregnancy. However, untreated macroprolactinomas carry about 15% to 35% risk of tumor enlargement and potentially can jeopardize vision.[43] Therefore, monitor women with macroprolactinomas closely for the development of headache and visual impairments. Baseline and routine visual field examinations are essential. Evidence of abnormal visual fields may indicate tumor growth and should be followed by an MRI. Should tumors enlarge, bromocriptine is the preferred choice over cabergoline because of greater experience with this drug during pregnancy.[41,50]

Table 46–5

Comparison of Dopamine Agonists for Treatment of Hyperprolactemia

	Bromocriptine (Parlodel)	Cabergoline
Starting dose	0.625–1.25 mg/day at bedtime	0.5 mg/week, or 0.25 mg twice/week
Titrating dose	1.25 mg increments at 1-week interval	0.5 mg increment at 4-week intervals
Usually effective dose	2.5–15 mg/day	1–2 mg/week
Maximal dose	40 mg/day	4.5 mg/week
Dosing frequency	2–3 divided doses per day	Once or twice weekly
Dosage in hepatic insufficiency	May be required in acute hepatitis or cirrhosis. No guidelines are available	Dose reductions may be recommended for patients with severe hepatic failure (Child-Pugh scores of 10 or higher)
Dosage in renal failure	None	None
Adverse effects	Dizziness, headache, syncope, nausea, vomiting, GI cramps, orthostatic hypotension	Similar but orthostatic hypotension less common
Cost	$	$$

$, moderately expensive; $$, more expensive.

From Refs. 39, 45.

Hyperprolactinemia: Patient Encounter 2: Medical History, Physical Examination, and Diagnostic Tests

WB, a 27-year-old woman, presents to the Women's Health Clinic. Her chief complaint is milky fluid discharge from both breasts. WB also mentions that her menstrual periods have stopped since she stopped taking her oral contraceptive 8 months ago with the hope of conceiving. Her menstrual cycle was regular before starting the oral contraceptive. WB does not have recent weight change, excessive hair growth, or acne. She also does not exercise excessively and is otherwise healthy. She took a home pregnancy test 1 week ago, which was negative.

PMH: None

FM: Both parents are still alive and healthy.

SH: Married, works as a high school teacher, and is physically active (walks 3 miles twice a week)

Meds: NuvaRing use as directed (discontinued 8 months ago); acetaminophen 325 mg two tablets every 4 to 6 hours as needed for mild headaches

ROS: Negative, other than in history of present illness.

PE:

HEENT: Ophthalmic examination reveals normal visual acuity and fields. (–) goiter

VS: BP 100/62 mm Hg, P 82 bpm, RR 18 breaths/min, T 37.1°C (98.8°F)

CV: RRR, normal S_1, S_2; no murmurs, rubs, or gallops

Breasts: (+) bilateral expressible galactorrhea with no other abnormality

Abd: Soft, nontender, nondistended; (+) bowel sounds; no hepatosplenomegaly

Rectal: Heme (–) stool

Labs: Electrolytes, renal and thyroid function, FSH, LH, and testosterone are within normal limits. Elevated prolactin at 115 ng/mL (115 mcg/L). Pregnancy test is negative.

Imaging: MRI reveals a pituitary tumor approximately 9 mm in diameter.

Given this information, what signs and symptoms does WB have for hyperprolactinemia?

Identify your treatment goals for WB.

What nonpharmacologic and pharmacologic treatment options are available for WB?

Outcome Evaluation

- Assess patients for tolerability to dopamine agonists.
- Monitor clinical symptoms associated with hyperprolactinemia every month for the first 3 months to assess therapeutic efficacy and assist with dose titration.

- Evaluate the patient for symptoms, such as headache, visual disturbances, menstrual cycles in women, and sexual function in men, to assess clinical response to therapy.
- Once the prolactin level is normalized and clinical symptoms of hyperprolactinemia have resolved, monitor prolactin level every 6 to 12 months.[42,43]

Hyperprolactinemia: Patient Care and Monitoring

1. Assess patient's clinical signs and symptoms of hyperprolactinemia.

2. Review the available diagnostic data to determine severity and exclude other common causes of hyperprolactinemia.

3. Obtain a thorough medication history to exclude medication-induced hyperprolactinemia.

4. Determine patient's plan regarding pregnancy because this influences treatment.

5. Educate patient about safety and efficacy of dopamine agonists. Make sure that the patient does not have any contraindications or allergies to drug therapies.

6. Develop a formal plan to assess response and adverse effects of dopamine agonists. When appropriate, be sure to make dose adjustments.

7. If the prolactin level remains normal for 2 years, reassess the need to continue treatment. Make sure that the patient is taking the lowest effective dose for management of hyperprolactinemia.

8. Provide patient education in regard to disease state and nondrug and drug therapy. Discuss with the patient:

   - Risk factors associated with hyperprolactinemia
   - Potential disadvantages and effectiveness of existing dopamine agonist therapy
   - Potential disadvantages and effectiveness of surgery and radiation treatment
   - Importance of adherence to therapy
   - Potential for adverse effects or long-term complications

---

- Evaluate visual fields in pregnant patients every 2 to 3 months.[40]

- If the prolactin level is well controlled with dopamine agonist therapy for 2 to 3 years, gradually taper therapy to the lowest effective dose.[40] Check prolactin levels after each dose reduction.

- If the prolactin levels remain unchanged for 1 year at the reduced dose, dopamine agonist therapy may be discontinued.

- It is essential to monitor prolactin levels every 6 months or annually to detect the possibility of permanent remission of pituitary disease.[42]

- The need to continue dopamine agonists in postmenopausal women with microprolactinomas must be reassessed because these patients have a higher probability of maintaining normal prolactin levels after treatment is discontinued.[40]

- In patients with macroprolactinomas, monitor visual field at baseline and repeat the test 1 month after initiation of a dopamine agonist.

- Repeat the MRI 6 months after initiating therapy, or if an increase in symptoms, or rise in prolactin levels suggests the presence of tumor growth.[43]

- Discontinuation of therapy in patients with macroprolactinomas usually leads to tumor regrowth and recurrence of hyperprolactinemia. This decision warrants careful consideration.

Abbreviations Introduced in This Chapter

ACTH   Adrenocorticotropic hormone or corticotropin
DEXA   Dual energy x-ray absorptiometry

FSH   Follicle-stimulating hormone
GH   Growth hormone or somatotropin
GHRH   Growth hormone-releasing hormone
IGF   Insulin-like growth factor
LH   Luteinizing hormone
OGTT   Oral glucose tolerance test
TSH   Thyroid-stimulating hormone or thyrotropin

 Self-assessment questions and answers are available at *http://www.mhpharmacotherapy.com/pp.html.*

REFERENCES

1. Muller EE, Locatelli V, Cocchi D. Neuroendocrine control of growth hormone secretion. Physiol Rev 1999;79:511–607.

2. Le Roith D, Bondy C, Yakar S, et al. The somatomedin hypothesis: 2001. Endocr Rev 2001;22:53–74.

3. AACE Medical Guidelines for Clinical Practice for the diagnosis and treatment of acromegaly. Endocr Pract 2004;10:213–225.

4. Ferone D, Resmini E, Bocca L, et al. Current diagnostic guidelines for biochemical diagnosis of acromegaly. Minerva Endocrinol 2004;29:207–223.

5. Melmed S. Medical progress: Acromegaly. N Engl J Med 2006;355:2558–2573.

6. Biochemical assessment and long-term monitoring in patients with acromegaly: Statement from a joint consensus conference of the Growth Hormone Research Society and the Pituitary Society. J Clin Endocrinol Metab 2004;89:3099–3102.

7. Clemmons DR. Role of insulin-like growth factor-I in diagnosis and management of acromegaly. Endocr Pract 2004;10:362–371.

8. Sheehan AH, Yanovski JA, Calis KA. Pituitary gland disorders. In: DiPiro JT, Talbert RL, Yee GC, et al., eds. Pharmacotherapy: A Pathophysiologic Approach. 6th ed. New York City: McGraw-Hill Companies, 2008:1281–1295.

9. Colao A, Ferone D, Marzullo P, et al. Systemic complications of acromegaly: Epidemiology, pathogenesis, and management. Endocr Rev 2004;25:102–152.

10. Katznelson L. An update on treatment strategies for acromegaly. Expert Opin Pharmacother 2008;9:2273–2280.

11. Colao A, Auriemma RS, Pivonello R, et al. Medical consequences of acromegaly: What are the effects of biochemical control? Rev Endocr Metab Disord 2008;9:21–31.

12. Ayuk J, Clayton RN, Holder G, et al. Growth hormone and pituitary radiotherapy, but not serum insulin-like growth factor-I concentrations, predict excess mortality in patients with acromegaly. J Clin Endocrinol Metab 2004;89:1613–1617.

13. Bonadonna S, Doga M, Gola M, et al. Diagnosis and treatment of acromegaly and its complications: Consensus guidelines. J Endocrinol Invest 2005;28:43–47.

14. Freda PU, Nuruzzaman AT, Reyes CM, et al. Significance of "abnormal" nadir growth hormone levels after oral glucose in postoperative patients with acromegaly in remission with normal insulin-like growth factor-I levels. J Clin Endocrinol Metab 2004;89:495–500.

15. Giustina A, Melmed S. Acromegaly consensus: The next steps. J Clin Endocrinol Metab 2003;88:1913–1914.

16. Cozzi R, Montini M, Attanasio R, et al. Primary treatment of acromegaly with octreotide LAR: A long-term (up to nine years) prospective study of its efficacy in the control of disease activity and tumor shrinkage. J Clin Endocrinol Metab 2006;91:1397–1403.

17. Ronchi CL, Varca V, Beck-Peccoz P, et al. Comparison between six-year therapy with long-acting somatostatin analogs and successful surgery in acromegaly: Effects on cardiovascular risk factors. J Clin Endocrinol Metab 2006;91:121–128.

18. Bush ZM, Vance ML. Management of acromegaly: Is there a role for primary medical therapy? Rev Endocr Metab Disord 2008;9:83–94.

19. Freda PU, Katznelson L, van der Lely AJ, et al. Long-acting somatostatin analog therapy of acromegaly: A meta-analysis. J Clin Endocrinol Metab 2005;90:4465–4473.

20. Melmed S, Sternberg R, Cook D, et al. A critical analysis of pituitary tumor shrinkage during primary medical therapy in acromegaly. J Clin Endocrinol Metab 2005;90:4405–4410.

21. Paisley AN, Trainer P, Drake W. Pegvisomant: A novel pharmacotherapy for the treatment of acromegaly. Expert Opin Biol Ther 2004;4: 421–425.

22. Trainer PJ, Drake WM, Katznelson L, et al. Treatment of acromegaly with the growth hormone-receptor antagonist pegvisomant. N Engl J Med 2000;342:1171–1177.

23. Van der Lely AJ, Hutson RK, Trainer PJ, et al. Long-term treatment of acromegaly with pegvisomant, a growth hormone receptor antagonist. Lancet 2001;358:1754–1759.

24. Colao A, Pivonello R, Auriemma RS, et al. Efficacy of 12-month treatment with the GH receptor antagonist pegvisomant in patients with acromegaly resistant to long-term, high-dose somatostatin analog treatment: Effect on IGF-I levels, tumor mass, hypertension and glucose tolerance. Eur J Endocrinol 2006;154:467–477.

25. Feenstra J, de Herder WW, ten Have SM, et al. Combined therapy with somatostatin analogues and weekly pegvisomant in active acromegaly. Lancet 2005;365:1644–1646.

26. Jorgensen JO, Feldt-Rasmussen U, Frystyk J, et al. Cotreatment of acromegaly with a somatostatin analog and a growth hormone receptor antagonist. J Clin Endocrinol Metab 2005;90:5627–5631.

27. Neggers SJ, van Aken MO, Janssen JA, et al. Long-term efficacy and safety of combined treatment of somatostatin analogs and pegvisomant in acromegaly. J Clin Endocrinol Metab 2007;92:4598–4601.

28. Abs R, Verhelst J, Maiter D, et al. Cabergoline in the treatment of acromegaly: A study in 64 patients. J Clin Endocrinol Metab 1998; 83:374–378.

29. Giustina A, Casanueva FF, Cavagnini F, et al. Diagnosis and treatment of acromegaly complications. J Endocrinol Invest 2003;26:1242–1247.

30. Gharib H, Cook DM, Saenger PH, et al. American Association of Clinical Endocrinologists medical guidelines for clinical practice for growth hormone use in adults and children-2003 update. Endocr Pract 2003;9:64–76.

31. Tovar JM, Gums JG. Hypothalamic, pituitary, and adrenal disorders. In: Tisdale JE, Miller DA, eds. Drug-Induced Diseases: Prevention, Detection, and Management. 1st ed. Bethesda, MD: American Society of Health-System Pharmacists, 2005:393–408.

32. Ho KK. Consensus guidelines for the diagnosis and treatment of adults with GH deficiency II: A statement of the GH Research Society in association with the European Society for Pediatric Endocrinology, Lawson Wilkins Society, European Society of Endocrinology, Japan Endocrine Society, and Endocrine Society of Australia. Eur J Endocrinol 2007;157:695–700.

33. Gandrud LM, Wilson DM. Is growth hormone stimulation testing in children still appropriate? Growth Horm IGF Res 2004;14: 185–194.

34. Federico G, Street ME, Maghnie M, et al. Assessment of serum IGF-I concentrations in the diagnosis of isolated childhood-onset GH deficiency: A proposal of the Italian Society for Pediatric Endocrinology and Diabetes (SIEDP/ISPED). J Endocrinol Invest 2006;29:732–737.

35. Nilsson AG, Svensson J, Johannsson G. Management of growth hormone deficiency in adults. Growth Horm IGF Res 2007;17: 441–462.

36. Cummings DE, Merriam GR. Growth hormone therapy in adults. Annu Rev Med 2003;54:513–533.

37. Gotherstrom G, Bengtsson BA, Bosaeus I, et al. A 10-year, prospective study of the metabolic effects of growth hormone replacement in adults. J Clin Endocrinol Metab 2007;92:1442–1445.

38. Wilson TA, Rose SR, Cohen P, et al. Update of guidelines for the use of growth hormone in children: The Lawson Wilkins Pediatric Endocrinology Society Drug and Therapeutics Committee. J Pediatr 2003;143:415–421.

39. Crosignani PG. Current treatment issues in female hyperprolactinaemia. Eur J Obstet Gynecol Reprod Biol 2006;125:152–164.

40. Brue T, Delemer B. Diagnosis and management of hyperprolactinemia: Expert consensus—French Society of Endocrinology. Ann Endocrinol 2007;68:58–64.

41. Gillam MP, Molitch ME, Lombardi G, et al. Advances in the treatment of prolactinomas. Endocr Rev 2006;27:485–534.

42. Serri O, Chik CL, Ur E, et al. Diagnosis and management of hyperprolactinemia. CMAJ 2003;169:575–581.

43. Schlechte JA. Clinical practice. Prolactinoma. N Engl J Med 2003;349:2035–2041.

44. Molitch ME. Medication-induced hyperprolactinemia. Mayo Clin Proc 2005;80:1050–1057.

45. Bankowski BJ, Zacur HA. Dopamine agonist therapy for hyperprolactinemia. Clin Obstet Gynecol 2003;46:349–362.

46. Darwish AM, Farah E, Gadallah WA, et al. Superiority of newly developed vaginal suppositories over vaginal use of commercial bromocriptine tablets: A randomized controlled clinical trial. Reprod Sci 2007;14:280–285.

47. Colao A, Galderisi M, Di Sarno A, et al. Increased prevalence of tricuspid regurgitation in patients with prolactinomas chronically treated with cabergoline. J Clin Endocrinol Metab 2008;93: 3777–3784.

48. Bogazzi F, Buralli S, Manetti L, et al. Treatment with low doses of cabergoline is not associated with increased prevalence of cardiac valve regurgitation in patients with hyperprolactinaemia. Int J Clin Pract 2008;62:1864–1869.

49. Wakil A, Rigby AS, Clark AL, et al. Low dose cabergoline for hyperprolactinaemia is not associated with clinically significant valvular heart disease. Eur J Endocrinol 2008;159:R11–R14.

50. Davis JR. Prolactin and reproductive medicine. Curr Opin Obstet Gynecol 2004;16:331–337.

47 Pregnancy and Lactation: Therapeutic Considerations

Ema Ferreira, Évelyne Rey, and Caroline Morin

LEARNING OBJECTIVES

Upon completion of the chapter, the reader will be able to:

1. Explain the principles of embryology and teratology.
2. Identify known teratogens and drugs of concerns during lactation.
3. Compare the main sources of drug information during pregnancy and lactation.
4. Evaluate the risks of a drug when taken during pregnancy or lactation.
5. Apply a systematic approach to counseling on the use of drugs during pregnancy and lactation.
6. Recommend the appropriate dose of folic acid to prevent congenital anomalies.
7. Describe physiologic changes during pregnancy and their impact on pharmacokinetics.
8. Choose an appropriate treatment for common conditions in a pregnant or lactating woman.

KEY CONCEPTS

❶ Although the risk of drug-induced teratogenicity is of concern, the actual risk of birth defects from most drug exposures is small.

❷ The risk of birth defects is higher during organogenesis.

❸ Counsel all women of childbearing age on the use of folic-acid containing multivitamins to prevent congenital anomalies.

❹ Most drugs are safe during breast-feeding.

❺ When possible, treat conditions occurring during pregnancy with nonpharmacologic treatments instead of drug therapy.

❻ Evaluate the need for treatment, including benefits and risks. Avoid treatments that do not show evidence of benefit or that can be delayed until after pregnancy or breast-feeding.

Medication use during pregnancy and lactation is a great challenge for health professionals as pregnant and breast-feeding women are usually excluded from clinical trials. In general, medications should not be used in these populations unless benefits outweigh risks. Therefore, it is important to know on which information sources to rely, how to interpret the data retrieved from these sources, and how to communicate this information to patients. This chapter will review the available resources that help to guide therapy, general strategies to reduce risks of drug use in pregnant and lactating women, and specific recommendations for some common conditions treated during pregnancy and lactation.

EPIDEMIOLOGY AND ETIOLOGY

Use of Medications During Pregnancy and Lactation

Recent studies conducted in the United States have estimated that a woman takes a mean of two nonprescribed medications and two prescribed medications (multivitamins excluded) during pregnancy.[1,2] Moreover, since approximately one-half of pregnancies are unplanned, many women are exposed to medications before being aware of their pregnancy.[3]

The most popular medications are vitamins and minerals, analgesics, antacids, antibiotics, antiemetics, laxatives, asthma medication, cold and flu medications, and medications for topical administration (e.g., antifungals, antibiotics, corticosteroids).[1,2]

One study from the Netherlands indicated that 65.9% of breast-feeding women took at least one medication (53% after exclusion of vitamins and minerals) over a 6-month period. The most popular medications were vitamins, analgesics, iron, antimicrobials, homeopathic remedies, oral contraceptives, cold and flu medications, and laxatives.[4]

▶ *Background Risks of Anomalies in Pregnancy*

Table 47–1 describes the baseline risks of congenital anomalies and some obstetrical complications observed in the general population. This will be important when evaluating the risks associated with drugs, and in order to counsel pregnant women.[6]

▶ Causes of Congenital Anomalies

1 *Although the risk of drug-induced teratogenicity is of concern, the actual risk of birth defects from most drug exposures is small.* Medications are associated with less than 1% of all congenital anomalies. As it is a modifiable cause of anomalies, it is important to evaluate and manage drug use in pregnant women and women planning a pregnancy. Causes of anomalies are monogenetic conditions (8–18%), chromosomal disorders (7–10%), maternal infections (1%), maternal conditions (1–3%; e.g., maternal diabetes), multifactorial heredity (23–50%), and unknown causes (34–43%).[5]

PATHOPHYSIOLOGY

Age of Pregnancy

The age of pregnancy can be defined as gestational or postconceptional ages. Gestational age (GA) is calculated from the first day of the last menstruation (or by ultrasound dating if menstrual cycles are irregular or if dates are unknown).

Postconceptional age (PCA) is calculated from the day of conception (plus or minus 2 days of ovulation).

Principles of Embryology

Pregnancy is usually divided into three trimesters of 13 weeks. However, it can be divided more precisely into three phases: implantation and predifferentiation, organogenesis (or embryogenesis), and fetogenesis. Table 47–2 describes these phases and the effects that drugs could have if taken during these phases. **2** *The risk of birth defects is higher during organogenesis.*

▶ Teratogens

A **teratogen** is an exogenous agent that can modify normal embryonic or fetal development. Teratogenicity can manifest as structural anomalies, a functional deficit,

---

Table 47–1

Occurrence of Some Obstetrical Complications and Risk of Congenital Anomalies in the General Population

	Risk of Occurrence in Population (%)
Abortion during the *all-or-none* period (pregnancy loss before a woman knows she is pregnant)	50
Spontaneous abortion/miscarriage (pregnancy loss that occurs after the pregnancy is known and before 20 weeks of GA)	15
Fetal loss or stillbirth (pregnancy loss after 20 weeks of GA)	0.5
Prematurity (less than 37 completed weeks of gestation)	12.7
Congenital anomalies (percentage of live births):	
• Minor malformations (recognized at birth or during childhood)	10–15
• Major malformations at birth	3
• Major malformations at 1-year-old	6–7
Low birth weight (less than 2,500 g)	8.2

GA, gestational age.
From Refs. 6, 49–52.

Table 47–2

Phases of Embryonic and Fetal Development

Phase of Development	Stage of Pregnancy	What Happens During This Phase of Development	Potential Teratogenic Effect
Implantation and predifferentiation	0–14 days after conception	*All-or-none period* Very little contact between the blastocyst and the mother's blood Cells are pluripotent, capacity to repair a damage remains Cells are fragile at this moment. If too many are killed, a miscarriage will occur before the pregnancy is detected	Spontaneous abortion or miscarriage Even if stopped during this period, prolonged half-life drugs could cause organogenesis problems
Organogenesis (embryogenesis)	From day 14 until the 9th week after conception	Organs are formed; most critical period for structural anomalies Organs are formed at different times; period of sensitivity for a potential teratogen could be different for each organ Refer to Figure 47–1 for the time frame of organ formation	Major or minor structural anomalies
Fetogenesis	After the organogenesis and until birth	The fetus grows and organs begin to function (e.g., kidneys are formed during the organogenesis, but glomerular filtration begins during fetogenesis) Active cell growth, proliferation, and migration, particularly in the CNS	Fetal growth retardation Functional deficit (e.g., renal insufficiency, pulmonary hypertension, neurologic impairment)

From Refs. 6, 8.

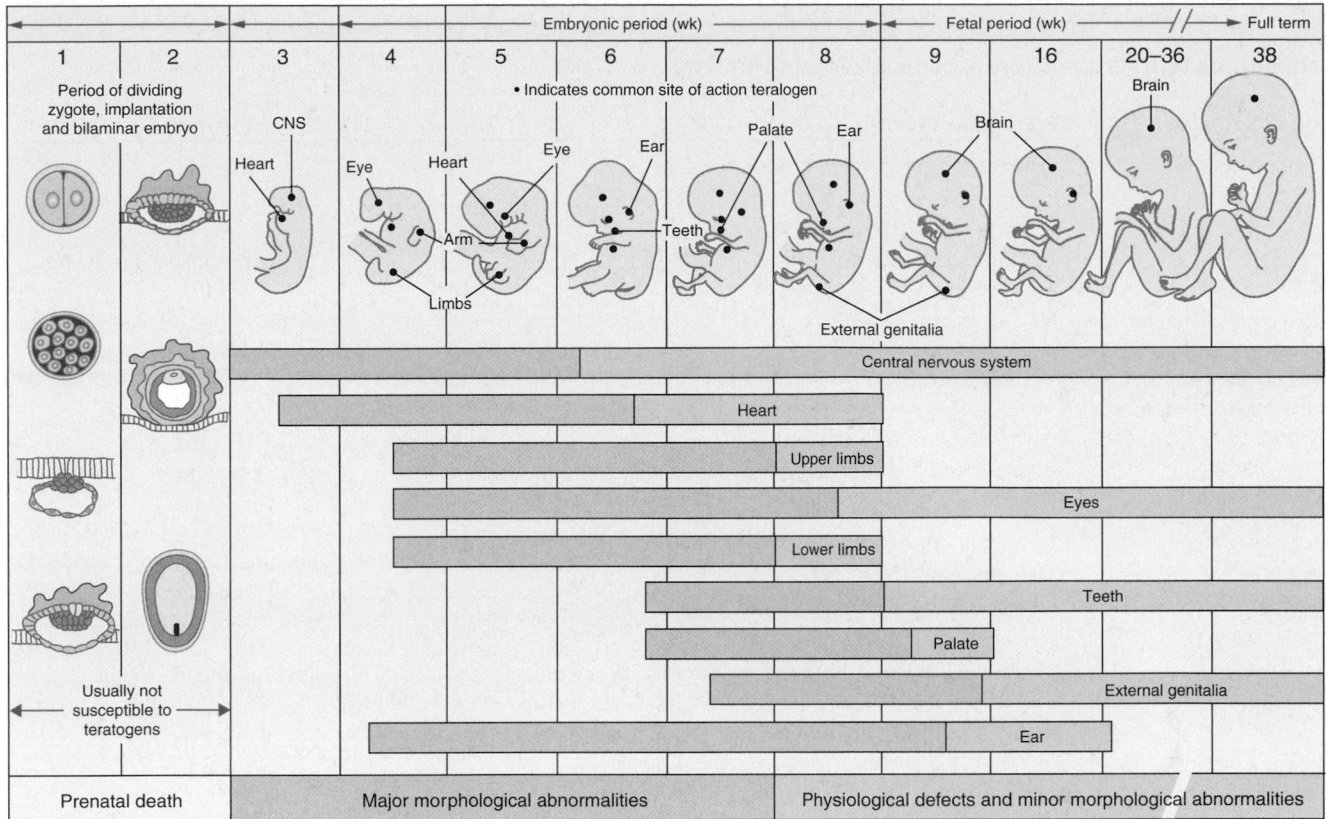

FIGURE 47–1. Embryonic development. The horizontal bars represent potential sensitivity to teratogens. The colored areas represent the more critical times. (Reprinted, with permission, from Moore KL. The Developing Human. New York: Elsevier; p 96; copyright 1974.)

cancer, growth retardation, and death (spontaneous abortion, stillbirth).

Criteria have been proposed to determine if a causal relationship between congenital anomalies and a medication is plausible (teratogenic effect).[3] Four essential criteria have been identified. First, exposure to the medication during the critical period of development for a defect is essential. In addition, two out of three of the following criteria must be present: pattern of anomalies or syndrome AND consistent effect in at least two epidemiological studies OR rare anomaly associated to a rare exposure.

Other criteria yield a stronger causal effect but are not essential:

- Same effects observed in animal studies
- Biological plausibility based on pharmacologic effect
- Higher incidence of the anomaly in the population with the use of the medication followed by a diminished incidence of the anomaly in the absence of the medication.

Using these criteria, there are approximately 30 medications established to be teratogens. They are shown in Table 47–3. Some medications have been associated with a higher risk of anomalies; however, they do not have all the criteria to be classified as teratogens.

RISK EVALUATION

Desired Outcomes

The primary goal for drug use during pregnancy and lactation is to effectively treat maternal or fetal conditions when necessary while minimizing risk to the developing fetus or the neonate.

Medication and Pregnancy

To study the efficacy and side effects of medications, researchers conduct randomized controlled trials. For unethical reasons pregnant women are excluded from these studies, thus most available data come from postmarketing reports.

Case reports and case series provide the first data on the use of medications during pregnancy. A causal relationship between a single case report and an anomaly cannot usually be established unless a rare anomaly is repeatedly associated with the use of a specific medication.

Cohort studies and company registries try to compare the risks observed following exposure to a medication to the risk observed in a control group or in the general population. When studying structural anomalies, it is important to select women exposed to medication during

Table 47–3

Medications With Proven Teratogenic Effects in Humans

Drug or Drug Class	Teratogenic Effects	Critical Period
Alkylating agents	Malformations of many different organs	Organogenesis
Amiodarone	Transitory hypothyroidism (17%, goitre in 18% of these cases) or hyperthyroidism (3%)	From 10th week after conception
Androgens (danazol, testosterone)	Masculinization of genital organs in female fetus	Danazol: from 6th week after conception
		Testosterone: Not defined
Angiotensin conversion enzyme inhibitors/ Angiotensin II receptor antagonists	Renal failure, anuria, oligohydramnios, pulmonary hypoplasia, intrauterine growth restriction, limbs contracture, skull hypoplasia	After the first trimester
Anticonvulsants • Carbamazepine • Phenytoin • Phenobarbital • Valproic acid	Neural tube defects (for carbamazepine and valproic acid); oral cleft, skeletal, urogenital, craniofacial, digital, and cardiac malformation; microcephalia	Organogenesis
	Risk estimated at 5–10% depending on the agent used (until 14% for valproic acid)	
Systemic corticosteroids	Oral cleft (risk of 3–4/1,000 versus 1/1,000 in general population)	Organogenesis
Diethylstilbestrol	Girls: Cervical or vaginal adenocarcinoma, indidence of less than 1.4/1,000 exposures. Structural genital anomalies (e.g., of cervix, vagina) in 25% of cases	First and second trimesters
	Boys: Genital anomalies, spermatogenesis anomalies	
Fluconazole	Skeletal and craniofacial malformations, cleft palate (with chronic dose of greater than 400 mg/day; not reported with one dose of 150 mg)	Not defined, but cases are reported where exposure was for most parts of pregnancy
Isotretinoin, acitretin, etretinate, and vitamin A	CNS, skull, eyes and ears malformations, micrognatia, oral cleft, cardiac malformation, thymus anomalies, mental retardation: estimated at 25–30%	Organogenesis
	Contraindicated throughout pregnancy	
	Isotretinoin: discontinue 1 month before pregnancy, prescribed under a special program called iPLEDGE	
	Acitretin, etretinate: discontinue 2–3 years before pregnancy	
Lithium	Cardiac malformations: risk of 0.9–6.8% versus risk of approximately 1% in general population	Cardiac organogenesis
	Includes Ebstein's anomaly: risk estimated at 0.05–0.1%	
Methimazole / Propylthiouracil	Methimazole: aplasia cutis, syndrome including choanes atresia, esophageal atresia, facial anomalies, developmental delay; risk probably low	Organogenesis
	Methimazole/propylthiouracil: fetal hypothyroidism in 2–10% of infants whose mother was treated for Graves' disease or goitre	Second and third trimesters
Methotrexate	Contraindicated during pregnancy	Organogenesis
	CNS and cranial malformations, oral cleft, skeletal and limb malformations	
	It is recommended to stop the medication 3 months before pregnancy	
Misoprostol	Moebius syndrome ± limb anomalies ± CNS anomalies	Organogenesis
Nonsteroidal anti-inflammatory drugs	In utero closure of ductus arteriosus (constriction is rare before 25 week, 50–70% at 30 week and 100% at 32 weeks (gestational age) and pulmonary hypertension	Third trimester
Penicillamine	Cutis laxis	Not defined
Tetracyclines	Teeth discoloration	14 weeks postconceptional
Thalidomide	Limb anomalies	20–36 days after conception
	Cardiac, urogenital, GI, and ear malformations	
	Prescribed under a special program called STEPS (System for Thalidomide Education and Prescribing Safety)	
Trimethoprim	Cardiac and urogenital malformations, neural tube defects, oral cleft	Organogenesis
Warfarin	Warfarin embryopathy including nasal hypoplasia, epiphysis dysplasia, vertebral malformation	Between 4th and 7th week postconception

From Refs. 3, 6, 8, 28.

Clinical Presentation and Diagnosis of Pregnancy and Lactation

Confirmation of Pregnancy

Positive urine human chorionic gonadotropin followed by positive ultrasound, fetal heart sounds, and/or fetal movement.

Pregnancy Dating and Gestational Age

Calculated from the first day of the last menstrual period.

Due dates typically are estimated at 40 weeks of gestation; however, infants delivered between 38 and 42 weeks are considered full term.

Pregnancy Symptoms

First trimester: Menstrual spotting, missed menses, fatigue, breast tenderness, increased urination, mood swings, nausea/vomiting, headache, heartburn, constipation

Second trimester: Frequent urination, heartburn, constipation, dry skin, edema, linea nigra, melasma

Third trimester: Backache, edema, shortness of breath

Routine Pregnancy Visits

In a normal, uncomplicated pregnancy, visits should occur monthly until 28 weeks of gestation, every 2 to 3 weeks from 28 to 36 weeks of gestation, and then weekly until birth.

Examination for each of the following is performed at each visit:

- Blood pressure
- Weight
- Urine for protein and glucose
- Uterine size
- Fetal heart rate
- Fetal movement

Routine Lab Testing for Normal Pregnancies (First Trimester Unless Otherwise Indicated)

- Human immunodeficiency virus
- Purified protein derivative (PPD) test for tuberculosis
- Venereal Disease Research Laboratory (VDRL) slide test for syphilis
- Rubella immunity
- Cervical cytology
- Blood and Rh type
- Hepatitis B surface antigen
- Hepatitis C antibodies (if high risk)
- Bacterial vaginosis testing if symptomatic or at high risk (previous preterm labor)
- Antibody screen for Rh antibodies
- Hemoglobin and hematocrit for anemia (repeated at 26–32 weeks)
- Urinalysis with culture for asymptomatic bacteriuria
- Gonorrhea and chlamydia
- Screens for Down's syndrome and neural tube defects (at 15–20 weeks)
- Gestational diabetes screening (at 24–28 weeks)
- Group B *Streptococcus* screening (at 35–37 weeks)

Assessing Suitability of the Cervix for Labor Induction

Suitability is based on cervical dilation, length, consistency, and position. These findings are translated to a numerical rating called the Bishop score. A Bishop score of less than 6 indicates that pharmacologic therapy is needed to ripen the cervix prior to delivery.

Select Problems Experienced During Pregnancy or Lactation

Hyperemesis gravidarum. Severe, persistent nausea and vomiting during pregnancy accompanied by dehydration, electrolyte disturbance, ketonuria, and/or weight loss.

Bacteriuria. Often asymptomatic in pregnancy. Diagnosed by positive urine culture.

Bacterial vaginosis. Clinically diagnosed by presence of three of the following:

- White, noninflammatory discharge
- Clue cells on microscopic examination
- Vaginal pH greater than 4.5
- A fishy odor before or after addition of 10% potassium hydroxide (i.e., "whiff" test)

Vulvovaginal candidiasis. Typical symptoms include vaginal itching and discharge. Clinical characteristics include:

- Vaginal pH less than 4.5
- Observation of yeast on Gram stain or wet preparation
- Thick, white, "cottage cheese–like" discharge

Chlamydia and gonorrhea. Typically asymptomatic. Diagnosed by positive culture.

Genital herpes simplex virus. Characterized by vesicular or ulcerative lesions. Diagnosis confirmed by virologic or serologic testing. Prodrome manifests as pain, burning, or itching at the site where lesions will develop.

Pelvic inflammatory disease. Difficult to diagnose in pregnancy. Symptoms may include:

- Uterine/ovarian tenderness
- Cervical motion tenderness
- Fever
- Abnormal cervical or vaginal discharge
- Presence of white blood cells in vaginal secretions
- Elevated erythrocyte sedimentation rate
- Elevated C-reactive protein

(Continued)

Clinical Presentation and Diagnosis of Pregnancy and Lactation (*Continued*)

Syphilis. Early disease may be characterized by a single genital lesion. Diagnosed by positive serologic testing (e.g., VDRL or rapid plasma reagin [RPR] test).

Trichomoniasis. Symptoms may include vulvar irritation and yellow-green discharge. Diagnosed after microscopic visualization of the organism.

Preterm labor. Onset of labor prior to 37 weeks of gestation.

Group B streptococcus. Diagnosed by positive culture on vaginal and rectal swab.

Mastitis. Characterized by localized redness, tenderness, and warmth on one breast accompanied by fever and flulike symptoms. Although uncommon, symptoms also may be bilateral.

Nipple candidiasis. Typical symptoms include nipple pain, itching, burning, and/or breast pain that persist after feeding.

Gestational diabetes. See Chapter 40.

Hypertension in pregnancy. Categorized as one of the following:

- Chronic hypertension (blood pressure greater than or equal to 140/90 mm Hg prior to pregnancy or prior to 20 weeks of gestation that lasts more than 12 weeks postpartum)
- Pre-eclampsia (blood pressure greater than or equal to 140/90 mm Hg after 20 weeks of gestation accompanied by proteinuria)
- Chronic hypertension with superimposed pre-eclampsia (onset of proteinuria after 20 weeks of gestation in a woman with chronic hypertension)
- Gestational hypertension (hypertension without proteinuria after 20 weeks of gestation)
- Transient hypertension (diagnosis made retrospectively when blood pressure returns to normal before 12 weeks postpartum)

organogenesis (often reported as exposure during first trimester). Cohort studies usually evaluate the general risk of malformations and are not designed to evaluate the risk associated with a specific anomaly. When a signal of association between an anomaly and a drug exposure is observed, a case-control study can be conducted to clarify the relationship. A case-control study also has more power to detect rare anomalies. When several studies have been published using very similar methodologies, a meta-analysis can be conducted to reach higher statistical power.[6]

Usually, older medications have been studied more extensively. When interpreting data retrieved from medical literature, it is important to keep in mind the principles of embryology and teratology (period of sensitivity, background risks, other causes of anomalies) and adapt the information to the patient who is being counseled.

▶ Sources of Information on the Use of Drugs During Pregnancy

Specialized information sources provide data on the use of medications during pregnancy. Some of these sources are listed in Table 47–4.

The 1979 FDA regulations establishing pregnancy categories for drugs are well known to health care professionals (Table 47–5). For many years, this system of categorization has been criticized by teratologists, genetic counselors, and other experts in the field who recommend relying on other information sources.[7] They assert that the FDA categories are too simplistic, can lead to a misperception of the risk, and do not take into account other important information such as expected incidence, severity of anomalies, degree of risk, gestational timing

---

Table 47–4

Sources of Information on Drug Use in Pregnancy and Lactation

Books

- Briggs GG, Freeman RK, Yaffe SJ. Drugs in Pregnancy and Lactation, 8th ed. Philadelphia : Lippincott Williams & Wilkins, 2008
- Schaefer CE, Peters PW, Miller RK. Drugs during Pregnancy and Lactation, Treatment Options and Risk Assessment, 2nd ed. Amsterdam: Elsevier, 2007
- Hale TW. Medications and Mother's Milk, 13th ed. Amarillo, TX: Pharmasoft, 2008

Database

- *www.reprotox.org*
- Teris: *http://depts.washington.edu/terisweb/teris/index.html*

Websites

- *www.otispregnancy.org*
- *www.motherisk.org*
- *www.marchofdimes.com*
- *www.cdc.gov*
- *www.pubmed.com*
- List of pregnancy registries: *http://www.fda.gov/womens/registries/registries.html*
- Lactmed: *http://toxnet.nlm.nih.gov/cgi-bin/sis/htmlgen?LACT*

Teratology Information Service

- Organization of Teratology Information Specialists (OTIS): Go to *www.otispregnancy.org* to find your local Teratogen Information Service, or call at the National Toll-Free Number: (866) 626-OTIS

of exposure, and route of administration.[7] In May 2008, the FDA proposed that the categories be removed and replaced by a short statement. This statement includes the description and the risk of fetal defects, the sources of data

Table 47-5

FDA Pregnancy Categories

Category A	Adequate, well-controlled studies in pregnant women have not shown an increased risk of fetal abnormalities
Category B	Animal studies have revealed no evidence of harm to the fetus; however, there are no adequate and well-controlled studies in pregnant women, *OR* animal studies have shown an adverse effect, but adequate and well-controlled studies in pregnant women have failed to demonstrate a risk to the fetus
Category C	Animal studies have shown an adverse effect, and there are no adequate and well-controlled studies in pregnant women, *OR* no animal studies have been conducted and there are no adequate and well-controlled studies in pregnant women
Category D	Studies, adequate well-controlled or observational, in pregnant women have demonstrated a risk to the fetus. However, the benefits of therapy may outweigh the potential risk
Category X	Studies, adequate well-controlled or observational, in animals or pregnant women have demonstrated positive evidence of fetal abnormalities. The use of the product is contraindicated in women who are or may become pregnant

(animal or human data), a comparison with the population baseline risk of birth defects, and the relationship with the dosage. An equivalent section for drug use during lactation will be inserted.[7] This new regulation will not be available for several years. Meanwhile, clinicians should rely on other information sources to evaluate the risk of a medication during pregnancy and lactation.

▶ Communication of the Information

To determine a woman's risk of birth defects, it is important to obtain a good medical, obstetrical, and pharmacologic history (including nonprescribed medication) and to take into account exposure to alcohol, tobacco, and other recreational drugs.[8] All these elements can influence the risk and the perception of risk.

The goal in the process of risk communication is to offer guidance and support while providing all the pertinent information to the woman to allow her to make an informed decision. The information given should include a well-grounded assessment of risks, including baseline risks in the general population, risks associated with the medication, and the underlying pathology. Women often have misconceptions and misperceptions about use of medications during pregnancy. They overestimate their risk of having an affected child after an exposure to a medication and underestimate the risks associated with chronic medical conditions.[3,8]

▶ Folic Acid

● Folic acid is an essential vitamin that plays an important role in the prevention of congenital anomalies, particularly neural tube defects. Recent data indicate that folic acid may also be involved in the reduction of other congenital anomalies including cardiovascular, oral clefts, limb deformities, and urinary malformations.[9] ❸ *All women of childbearing age should be counseled on the appropriate dose of folic acid to prevent congenital anomalies.* The American College of Obstetricians and Gynecologists (ACOG) recommends that every woman of childbearing age take 0.4 to 1 mg of folic acid daily, beginning 3 months before pregnancy, because nutritional sources alone are not sufficient.[10] Women at higher risk of neural tube defects (e.g., those who have had a previous child with a neural tube defect, those with prepregnancy diabetes, or epilepsy, or those taking carbamazepine or valproic acid) are counseled to take 4 mg of folic acid per day.[10] The Society of Obstetricians and Gynecology of Canada advocates the use of higher doses of folic acid for a broader range of women including obese women, Sikh, Celtic, and Northern Chinese women, who are at higher risk of having a child with a neural tube defect.[11]

▶ Iron Supplements

Anemia is a common problem during pregnancy. Up to 27% of women are anemic in the third trimester.[12] Maternal symptoms of anemia include fatigue, palpitations, and decreased resistance to exercise and infections. Fetal risks are prematurity, low birth weight, and fetal death. Recommendations are that all pregnant women be screened for anemia, and those with iron deficiency should be treated with oral iron preparations in addition to prenatal vitamins.[12] Iron supplementation decreases the prevalence of maternal anemia at delivery. It is unclear if supplementing nonanemic pregnant women will improve perinatal outcomes.[12]

▶ Impact of Physiologic Changes During Pregnancy on Pharmacokinetics

Absorption Drug absorption is affected in several ways during pregnancy, and it is difficult to predict the final

Patient Encounter, Part 1

LC, a 28-year-old woman thinks that she is pregnant. She has not had a period in 9 weeks. A few days ago, she used a home pregnancy test which was positive. In your office, a repeat urine pregnancy test confirms that the patient is pregnant.

What counseling would be appropriate at this time?

What are the estimated postconceptional age (PCA) and gestational age (GA) of the embryo?

What prenatal screening would you perform at this time?

repercussion on drug efficacy. Decreased GI transit can result in a delay in drug peak effect, prolonging the time of contact of drugs with the intestinal mucosa, and possibly enhancing absorption of certain drugs. The higher gastric pH may affect the absorption of weak bases or acids. Skin, tissue, and lung absorption might also be increased by physiologic changes during pregnancy.[13]

Distribution The volume of distribution increases for most drugs during pregnancy due to plasma volume expansion and the presence of amniotic fluid, the placenta, and the fetus. This results in a decrease in maximal concentrations of drugs and in their half-life. In addition, hypoalbuminemia and decreased protein binding of drugs increases free fraction of some medications.[13,14]

Metabolism During pregnancy the activity of some isoenzymes is increased (e.g., CYP3A4, CYP2A6, CYP2D6, CYP2C9), and the activity of others is decreased (e.g., CYP1A2, CYP2C19). It is difficult to predict the net impact on drug effect since there is a wide interindividual variability and since some drugs are metabolized by several isoenzymes.[13-15] The activity of uridine diphosphate glucuronosyltransferase (UGT) is also increased during pregnancy.[13-15]

Renal Elimination Renal blood flow and glomerular filtration are increased significantly during pregnancy. The impact of this increase is more important for drugs that are eliminated unchanged in the urine.[14]

Table 47–6 shows clinical recommendations based on pharmacokinetic changes during pregnancy for several drugs.

Medication and Lactation

According to a 2005 policy statement from the American Academy of Pediatrics (AAP), new mothers should breast-feed exclusively for 6 months.

Approximately 46% of new mothers report that they breast-feed exclusively at birth. However, this figure drops to 17% at 6 months, as many new mothers supplement breast-feeding with other foods or quit entirely by this point.[46]

For the breast-feeding mother it is important to balance the need for treatment against the potential toxicity to the infant.

▶ Drug Transfer Into Breast Milk

To study drug effects in a breast-fed infant, serum drug levels could be measured to help evaluate safety in the infant; however, that is often not possible. Therefore, in

---

Table 47–6

Altered Pharmacokinetics During Pregnancy: Clinical Implications and Management

Drugs	Pharmacokinetic Changes	Recommendations and Monitoring
Antiretrovirals	Cl and C_{max} variable	Monitor clinical response; drug levels can be useful to adjust drug dosage of some antiretrovirals
Caffeine	↑ $t_{1/2}$ ↓ Cl (T_1, T_2, T_3)	Risk of more frequent and prolonged side effects; decrease caffeine consumption
Carbamazepine	↑ Cl ↓ $t_{1/2}$	Measure free fraction (preferably); increase dose according to clinical response and levels
Digoxin	↑ maternal Cl ↓ maternal C_{max}	Follow plasma levels; increase doses if necessary; to treat fetal disease, higher doses might be required
Fluoxetine	↑ Cl (T_3)	Increase dose according to clinical response
Heparin LMWH	↑ Cl (T_1, T_2, T_3)	Consider increasing the frequency of administration
Lamotrigine	↑ Cl (T_1, T_2, T_3)	Measure drug levels at least every trimester; increase dose according to clinical response and levels; decrease dose to prepregnancy dosage after delivery
Levothyroxine (T4)	↓ff	Increase dose at the beginning of pregnancy; follow TSH levels at least every trimester; decrease dose after delivery
Lithium	↑ Cl (T_1, T_2, T_3) ↓ $t_{1/2}$	Measure drug levels at least every trimester; increase dose according to levels if necessary; decrease dose to prepregnancy dosage after delivery
Nicotine	↓ $t_{1/2}$ ↑ Cl (T_2, T_3)	Higher doses might be required (smoking cessation) at T_2 and T_3; however, increased transdermal absorption might lead to higher nicotine plasma levels
Nifedipine	↑ Cl (T_3)	Monitor clinical effect; increase doses/frequency of administration if necessary
Phenytoin	↓ C_{total}, ↑ ff ↑ Cl (T_3) ↓ $t_{1/2}$	Measure free fraction; increase dose according to clinical response and levels
Valproic acid	↓ C_{total} ↑ ff	Measure free fraction if a prepregnancy reference level is available; dose will remain the same in most cases. Increase dose according to clinical response and levels

↑, increase; ↓, decrease; ↔, unchanged; C_{max}, maximum serum concentration; Cl, clearance; ff, free fraction; T, trimester; $t_{1/2}$, elimination half-life; LMWH, low molecular weight heparins; C_{total}, total concentration.

Adapted and translated from Ref. 6.

most instances, the approximate quantity of drug ingested by the breast-fed infant is estimated using published measured drug concentrations in breast milk. With these data, one can calculate the percentage of pediatric dose or the relative infant dose (percentage of maternal dose adjusted by weight) (assuming an average of 150 mL/kg/day of milk ingested by a breast-fed infant). Usually, a percentage of less than 10% of the pediatric dose, or when a pediatric dose is not available, a percentage of less than 10% of maternal dose adjusted by weight is acceptable in full term infants.[47]

▶ Drug Pharmacokinetics

If clinical data are not available on drug transfer into breast milk, choose drugs that are highly protein bound, have a high molecular weight, have a short half-life, have no active metabolites, and are well tolerated by children.[47]

▶ Milk/Plasma Ratio

The milk/plasma ratio is reported in several references but does not take into account the absolute amount of drugs ingested by the infant. For example, propranolol has a milk to plasma ratio of 1.65, indicating that it concentrates into milk; however, it is estimated that the breast-fed infant will ingest less than 1% of the neonatal dose.[47]

▶ AAP Tables

Since 1983, the AAP has been publishing their position on the compatibility of drug during breast-feeding. Although useful, these tables do not take into consideration the dose, infant characteristics, and maternal conditions.[19]

▶ Drugs of Concern During Breast-Feeding

❹ *Most drugs are safe during breast-feeding.* However, use of some drugs creates some concern and requires a more thorough assessment by the clinicians (Table 47–7).

CONDITIONS PREVALENT IN PREGNANCY AND LACTATION

Nausea and Vomiting

As many as 80% of pregnant women suffer from nausea or vomiting.[16]

Nonpharmacologic measures, such as lifestyle (rest, avoidance of nausea triggers such as strong odors) and dietary changes (small and frequent meals, fluid restriction during meals) should be used as first-line management. Acupuncture and acupressure can be also helpful.[16]

The combination of pyridoxine (vitamin B$_6$) and doxylamine is well studied during pregnancy and is the first-line pharmacologic treatment of nausea and vomiting during pregnancy (Table 47–8).[16,17] This combination is not available in the United States, and the ingredients have to be administered separately. When the combination of pyridoxine/doxylamine is insufficient, other drugs such as

Table 47–7	
Drugs of Concern During Breast-Feeding	
Drug or Class	**Comments**
Acebutolol	Neonatal β-blockade reported
Amiodarone	May accumulate because of long half-life; possible neonatal thyroid and cardiovascular toxicity
Antineoplastics	Neonatal myelosuppression possible
Atenolol	Neonatal β-blockade reported
Bromocriptine	Lactation suppression
Cabergoline	Lactation suppression
Ergotamine	Symptoms of ergotism (vomiting and diarrhea) reported; inhibition of prolactin secretion possible
Illicit drugs	Unknown contents and effects
Lamotrigine	A breast-fed infant will receive a dose estimated between 10% and 50% of the lowest pediatric dose; serum concentrations reported in breast-fed infants were between 3% and 50% of maternal serum levels; potential for rash and CNS side effects
Lithium	Up to 50% of maternal serum levels have been measured in infants; cases of infant toxicity have been reported
Radioactive iodine-131	Long radioactive half-life (21–42 days)
Tetracyclines	Chronic use may lead to dental staining or decreased epiphyseal bone growth

From Refs. 6, 47.

metoclopramide or diphenhydramine can be prescribed; ondansetron is another alternative.[16,17]

Constipation and Hemorrhoids

Nonpharmacologic treatment is the mainstay of constipation and hemorrhoids treatment in pregnant patients. Pregnant women should be counseled to eat a high-fiber diet, drink plenty of fluids, exercise regularly, and avoid prolonged time on the toilet. To relieve hemorrhoids, pregnant women may soak in warm sitz baths and apply ice to the area. Bulk-forming laxatives, such as psyllium and calcium polycarbophil are first-line agents (Table 47–8).[18] If these methods fail, stimulant laxatives, such as bisacodyl and senna, are acceptable second-line agents for short-term or intermittent use.[6,18] During lactation, bulk-forming laxatives and the stimulant laxatives are safe for use.[19]

Studies are lacking on safe and effective approaches for management of hemorrhoids during pregnancy.[20] Acetaminophen and topical analgesics agents may be used for pain. Surgical resection or banding can also be performed during pregnancy, but it is generally preferable to delay the surgery until after delivery.

Heartburn

Nonpharmacologic recommendations for the treatment of heartburn during pregnancy do not differ from recommendations for nonpregnant patients. Small and

Table 47–8

Medication Dosing Recommendations During Pregnancy and Lactation

Drug	Dosage	Comments
Micronutrients and Vitamins		
Calcium	1,000–1,300 (elemental calcium) mg/day	To be taken in combination with vitamin D
Folic acid	0.4 mg orally daily	
	4 mg orally daily	Higher dose recommended for women at higher risk of having a child with NTD, e.g., personal or family history (FH) of NTD, medication known to cause NTD, or prepregnancy diabetes
Iron	27 mg (elemental iron) orally daily (contained in a prenatal vitamin)	Daily requirements during pregnancy
	60–120 mg (elemental iron) orally per day	Higher doses to treat iron-deficiency anemia
Vitamin D	200 IU orally daily	Daily requirement during pregnancy
	400 IU orally daily	Dose recommended for breast-fed infants
Nausea and Vomiting		
Diphenhydramine or dimenhydrinate	25–50 mg orally 4 × daily	
Doxylamine	12.5 mg orally 3–4 × daily	Can be taken with pyridoxine
Metoclopramide	5–15 mg orally 3–4 × daily	
Meclizine	12.5–50 mg orally daily	
Pyridoxine	25 mg orally 3 × daily	Can be taken with doxylamine
Heartburn		
Antacids (calcium carbonate, magnesium hydroxide)	Product specific dosing, 15–30 mL or 250 mg to 1.5 g up to 4 × daily	
Ranitidine	150 mg orally twice daily	
Metoclopramide	5–10 mg orally 3–4 × daily	
Omeprazole	20 mg orally daily	
Sucralfate	1 g orally 4 × daily	
Constipation		
Polycarbophil	2 tablets 1–4 × daily	
Psyllium	Product specific dosing, usually 1 packet/scoopful in water up to 3 × daily	
Docusate	100–400 mg orally per day (given in 1 or 2 doses)	
Bisacodyl	5–10 mg orally (tablets) or rectally (suppositories) as needed	
Senna	17.2 mg orally (tablets or syrup) once or twice daily or rectally (suppositories) as needed	
Lactulose	15–30 mL daily or twice daily	
Nasal Congestion and Cough		
Decongestants		
Oxymetazoline	0.05% spray, 2–3 sprays in each nostril twice daily for 3–5 days	Avoid using more than 3–5 days to prevent rebound congestion
Pseudoephedrine	60 mg orally every 4–6 hours	Second and third trimesters only
		Short term (3–5 days) only
Antihistamines		
Chlorpheniramine	4 mg every 4–6 hours	
Cetirizine	10 mg orally daily	
Loratadine	10 mg orally daily	
Sodium cromolyn	2.6 mg spray, 3–4 × daily	
Nasal Corticosteroids		
Budesonide	32 mcg spray, 1–4 sprays daily	First-line agents for chronic congestion
Beclomethasone	50–100 mcg spray, twice daily	
Fluticasone	100 mcg spray daily	
Cough		
Dextromethorphan	30 mg orally every 6–8 hours	
Codeine	10–20 mg orally every 6–8 hours	

(Continued)

Table 47–8

Medication Dosing Recommendations During Pregnancy and Lactation (*Continued*)

Drug	Dosage	Comments
Bacterial Vaginosis		
Metronidazole	250 mg 3 × daily for 7 days or 500 mg twice a day for 7 days	
Clindamycin	300 mg orally twice daily for 7 days in pregnancy	
	100 mg cream or suppository intravaginally at bedtime for 3–7 days	Use oral formulation during pregnancy and intravaginal formulation for breast-feeding mothers
	37.5 mg gel intravaginally at bedtime for 5 days	
Vulvovaginal Candidiasis		
Butoconazole	2% cream, 5 g intravaginally for 3–6 days	
Clotrimazole	1% cream, 5 g intravaginally for 7 days	
	100-mg vaginal tablet daily for 7 days	
Miconazole	2% cream, 5 g intravaginally for 7 days	
	100-mg vaginal suppository daily for 7 days	
Terconazole	0.4% cream, 5 g intravaginally for 7 days	
Nystatin	100,000-unit vaginal tablet, 1 tablet for 14 days	
Chlamydia		
Azithromycin	1 g orally (1 dose only)	
Amoxicillin	500 mg 3 × daily for 7 days	
Erythromycin base	500 mg orally 4 × daily for 7 days or 250 mg orally 4 × daily for 14 days	
Doxycycline	100 mg orally twice daily for 7 days	Breast-feeding only
Gonorrhea (Uncomplicated)		
Cefixime	400 mg orally once	
Ceftriaxone	125 mg intramuscularly once	
Spectinomycin	2 g intramuscularly once	For cephalosporin-allergic patients
Ciprofloxacin	500 mg orally once	During lactation only; check for resistance with the CDC
Genital Herpes Simplex Virus (Uncomplicated)		
Acyclovir	*First episode*: 400 mg orally 3 × daily for 7–10 days, or 200 mg 5 × daily for 7–10 days	
	Recurrent episode: 400 mg orally 3 × daily for 5 days, or 800 mg twice daily for 5 days, or 800 mg 3 × daily for 2 days	
	Suppressive therapy: 400 mg orally 3× daily	From 36 weeks until delivery
Valacyclovir	*First episode*: 1 g once daily for 7–10 days	
	Recurrent episode: 500 mg twice daily for 3 days, or 1 g daily for 5 days	
	Suppressive therapy: 500 mg twice daily	From 36 weeks until delivery
Syphilis		
Benzathine penicillin G	Primary, secondary, or early latent: 2.4 million units intramuscularly once	Desensitize penicillin-allergic patients during pregnancy; also first-line agent during lactation
	Late latent or of unknown duration or tertiary: 2.4 million units intramuscularly 3 × at 1-week interval	
Trichomoniasis		
Metronidazole	2 g orally for 1 dose	During lactation, temporarily stop breast-feeding for 12–24 hours (most important for premature or very young infants)

(Continued)

Table 47–8

Medication Dosing Recommendations During Pregnancy and Lactation (*Continued*)

Drug	Dosage	Comments
Premature Rupture of Membranes		
Ampicillin	2 g IV initially, then 1 g IV every 6 hours for 48 hours followed by amoxicillin	Ampicillin/amoxicillin are used with erythromycin
Amoxicillin	250–500 mg 3 × daily for 5 days	Ampicillin/amoxicillin are used with erythromycin
Erythromycin base	333 mg 3 × daily for 7 days	Ampicillin/amoxicillin are used with erythromycin
Fetal Lung Maturation		
Betamethasone	12 mg intramuscularly every 24 hours for 2 doses	
Dexamethasone	6 mg intramuscularly or IV every 12 hours for 4 doses	
Preterm Labor		
Nifedipine (short acting)	30 mg oral load, then 10–20 mg every 4–6 hours for 48 hours	
Magnesium sulfate	4–6 g IV bolus over 20 minutes, then 2–3 g/h IV drip	
Indomethacin	50–100 mg oral load, then 25–50 mg orally every 6 hours × 48 hours	
Terbutaline	0.25 mg subcutaneously every 20 minutes to 3 hours	
Glyceriltrinitrate (nitric oxide donor)	10 mg patch for every 12 hours until contractions cease up to 48 hours	
Atosiban	6.75 mg IV load (over 1 minute), then infusion of 18 mg/h for 3 hours, then 6 mg/h for up to 45 hours	
Group B *Streptococcus*		
Penicillin G	5 million units IV initially, then 2.5 million units IV every 4 hours until delivery	
Ampicillin	2 g IV initially, then 1 g IV every 4 hours until delivery	
Cefazolin	2 g IV initially, then 1 g IV every 8 hours until delivery	
Clindamycin	900 mg IV every 8 hours until delivery	
Erythromycin base	500 mg IV every 6 hours until delivery	
Vancomycin	1 g IV every 12 hours until delivery	
Thyroid Diseases		
Hypothyroidism		
T4	1–2 mcg/kg according to thyroxin stimulating hormone (TSH) level	
Hyperthyroidism		
Propylthiouracil	50–100 mg 1–3 × daily according to T4 levels	Use the lowest dose to avoid fetal effects
Mastitis		
Outpatient Treatment		
Dicloxacillin	500 mg orally 4 × daily	Treat for 10–14 days
Cephalexin	500 mg orally 4 × daily	
Amoxicillin 875 mg + 125 mg clavulanate	1 tablet orally 2 × daily	
Inpatient Treatment for More Severe Cases		
Oxacillin	2 g IV every 4 hours	Treat IV for 24–48 hours until afebrile then continue with outpatient treatment
Nafcillin	2 g IV every 4 hours	
Clindamycin	600–900 mg IV every 6–8 hours	
Vancomycin	1,000 mg IV every 12 hours	If allergic to penicillin and MRSA
Breast Candidiasis		
Mother		
Clotrimazole, miconazole, or nystatine	Topical cream	After each feeding and for 1 week after symptoms have resolved. Treat also infant even if asymptomatic

(Continued)

Table 47–8		
Medication Dosing Recommendations During Pregnancy and Lactation (*Continued*)		
Drug	**Dosage**	**Comments**
Fluconazole	200–400 mg orally for 1 dose followed by 100–200 mg orally daily	If topical treatment not efficacious, add fluconazole until 1 week after symptoms have resolved (minimum of 2 weeks of treatment). Also treat infant even if asymptomatic
Infant		
Nystatin oral solution	100,000–200,000 units (1–2 mL) to be swabbed into infant's mouth 4 × daily, after feedings	
Clotrimazole or miconazole topical cream	Apply in a thin layer in infant's mouth 4 × daily, after feedings	
Other Treatments for Candidiasis		
Gentian violet 0.5–1% solution	To be swabbed into infant's mouth once daily for 5 days before a feeding	To be used if other options fail. Can stain clothes and skin
		If nipples or mouth are not violet after application and the feeding, reapply the treatment

CDC, Centers for Disease Control and Prevention; MRSA, methicillin-resistant *Staphylococcus aureus*; NTD, neural tube defect; T4, levothyroxine; TSH, thyroxine stimulating hormone.

From Refs. 5, 6, 12, 16–18, 20, 24, 25, 27, 30–32, 34, 36, 39, 40, 44, 45, 53, 54.

frequent meals, remaining upright after eating, elevating the head of the bed, and avoiding foods known to decrease lower esophageal sphincter tone (such as chocolate, coffee, fatty foods, and peppermint) are recommended.

Calcium- or magnesium-containing antacids are first-line therapies. If antacids fail to improve symptoms, ranitidine can be recommended, as it is the drug with the best safety data among the H[2] blockers (Table 47–8).[21] Omeprazole, sucralfate, and metoclopramide are also safe in pregnancy (Table 47–8).[22]

All the drugs used for heartburn during pregnancy are acceptable during lactation.[19]

Nasal Congestion and Cough

Do not underestimate the impact of nasal congestion, especially if it is chronic and associated with snoring and sleep disorders. Rest, fluids, humidified air, nasal saline, and acetaminophen are the mainstays of therapy for the common cold. Recommend avoiding irritants and known allergens, raising the head of the bed at 30 to 45 degrees. Nasal strips might be helpful.

Treat nasal congestion as in the nonpregnant population, reminding that: (a) Avoid oral decongestants during the first trimester owing to the risk of fetal gastroschisis (incidence 4–6 per 10,000 treated women). Pseudoephedrine is the preferred agent.[23] (b) Stop topical decongestants after 3 to 5 days in order to minimize the incidence of rebound congestion. (c) Most first- and second-generation antihistamines are safe in pregnancy at recommended dosages.[23] (d) Nasal corticosteroids are the best drugs for chronic rhinitis.[23,24]

Treat cough with oral dextromethorphan or codeine (Table 47–8). Maintain ongoing allergen immunotherapy, but do not initiate it.

During lactation, all the drugs previously used during pregnancy can be continued.[19,24]

Bacteriuria

Bacteriuria during pregnancy, including asymptomatic disease, is associated with higher risk of pyelonephritis (compared to the risk in nonpregnant women) and of some obstetrical complications, such as low birth weight and preterm delivery. Treatment reduced these risks.[25] All women testing positive for bacteriuria should be treated empirically with antimicrobial therapy targeted at *Escherichia coli* infection.[26] Safe agents for empirical therapy include penicillins, cephalosporins, and nitrofurantoin[27] (Table 47–8). Sulfonamides and ampicillin or amoxicillin also have been used, but increasing bacterial resistance to these agents renders them second-line choices.[27] Avoid quinolones owing to the theoretical risk of bone and cartilage malformations. Avoid trimethoprim and sulfamethoxazole during organogenesis (since antifolate drugs have been associated with congenital malformations) and near term due to theoretical risk of neonatal jaundice.[28] Once culture and sensitivity results are available, change the antimicrobial regimen if necessary. Recommend standard 3-day or longer antimicrobial therapy because there is insufficient evidence among pregnant women to support 1-day regimens.[29] Repeat urine culture 10 days after completion of therapy for bacteriuria.

Bacterial Vaginosis

Bacterial vaginosis is associated with adverse pregnancy outcomes such as premature rupture of the membranes, chorioamnionitis, and preterm labor and delivery. Treatment is recommended in symptomatic women or in asymptomatic

Patient Encounter, Part 2

During your first encounter with LC, you collected the following data:

PMH: Seasonal allergic rhinitis

FH: Patient's mother delivered two preterm infants

SH: Works as a librarian. Denies use of alcohol, tobacco, or illicit substances

Meds: Loratadine 10 mg orally daily; ibuprofen 400 mg orally as needed for headache (uses approximately once weekly); ortho-Tri-Cyclen Lo daily; multivitamin (generic for Centrum) daily

ROS: (+) Nausea with occasional vomiting on awakening in the morning × 2 weeks. Nausea lasts for 1 to 2 hours. Has missed 3 days of work because of nausea. Remainder of ROS within normal limits.

VS: BP 118/62, P 72 bpm, RR 12, T 37°C (98.6°F)

The patient expresses concern over the medications she has been using over the last 9 weeks. She states that neither she nor her husband could handle having a "deformed" baby, and she asks you if she should consider terminating the pregnancy.

What resources can you use to help determine the risk of her drug exposures?

What do you recommend for her morning sickness?

women at high risk for preterm delivery. The Centers for Disease Control and Prevention (CDC) recommends oral metronidazole for the treatment of bacterial vaginosis in pregnant women (Table 47–8).[30] Metronidazole is deemed safe for use by the CDC during all stages of pregnancy despite package labeling listing a contraindication in the first trimester.[28–30] Oral clindamycin is an option for women who do not tolerate metronidazole, but its efficacy is lower than that of metronidazole in nonpregnant populations.[30] Avoid clindamycin vaginal cream due to association with low birth weight and neonatal infection.[30]

During lactation, clindamycin or metronidazole vaginal formulations are the preferred therapies for bacterial vaginosis (Table 47–8). Counsel patients that clindamycin cream weakens latex condoms and diaphragms, potentially rendering them ineffective.

Since the cure rate is expected to be around 70%, it is important to do a culture 1 month after completion of therapy.[31]

Vulvovaginal Candidiasis

Only symptomatic vulvovaginal candidiasis should be treated in pregnant or lactating women. First-line treatment is topical azole therapy for 7 days in pregnant women; shorter courses can be used during lactation. Oral fluconazole is not a first-line treatment during pregnancy (Table 47–8).[30] Women should be counseled that using topical azoles weakens latex condoms and diaphragms, potentially rendering them ineffective.

Sexually Transmitted Infections

► Chlamydia

Chlamydia infections during pregnancy, including those that are asymptomatic, can be treated with azithromycin, amoxicillin, or erythromycin to reduce the risk of preterm labor and neonatal infection (Table 47–8).[28–30] Doxycycline should be avoided in pregnant women owing to known teratogenic effects when used after 16 weeks of gestational age. Erythromycin estolate should also be avoided because of drug related hepatotoxicity.[28]

During lactation, azithromycin and doxycycline are first-line choices (Table 47–8).[13,31] Nucleic acid amplification tests should be repeated 3 to 4 weeks after completion of therapy.[30]

► Gonorrhea

Gonorrheal infections, including those that are asymptomatic, should be treated during pregnancy with cefixime or ceftriaxone to reduce the risk of preterm labor and neonatal infection (Table 47–8).[30] Spectinomycin is an alternative for penicillin- or cephalosporin-allergic women.[30] Tetracycline should be avoided during pregnancy owing to tooth and bone malformations, and quinolones should be avoided because of the theoretical risk of bone or cartilage malformations (Table 47–8).[28]

All CDC recommended first-line therapies for gonorrhea are deemed compatible with breast-feeding by the AAP.[19] Since the number of quinolone-resistant species is increasing, the CDC recommendations should be consulted before prescribing a quinolone.[30] Perform an endocervical swab culture for gonorrhea 3 weeks after completion of therapy.

► Herpes Simplex

Herpes simplex virus may be transmitted to the neonate at birth. The risk of transmission is more likely if the mother acquired genital herpes near the time of delivery (30–50%). Prevention of neonatal herpes includes preventing acquisition of herpes infection during late pregnancy and avoiding fetal exposure to active herpetic lesions during delivery.

The majority of obstetricians recommend cesarean section for women with active genital herpetic lesions at the onset of labor, even though caesarean section does not completely eliminate the risk of neonate transmission. Oral acyclovir is recommended for treatment of herpes episodes. Acyclovir or valacyclovir is recommended to decrease the risk of a recurrence at term (Table 47–8).[32,33] IV therapy may be indicated for severe episodes. Surveillance data do not suggest an increased risk of teratogenic effects with acyclovir.[28,32] Acyclovir is preferred over valacyclovir or famciclovir because experience with the latter agents during organogenesis is limited.

Acyclovir and valacyclovir are deemed compatible with breast-feeding, but no recommendation can be made regarding the safety of famciclovir during lactation.[19] Infants born to mothers with active disease at birth should be monitored for signs and symptoms of disease.

▶ Syphilis

Treponema pallidum can cross the placenta and cause fetal infection with severe consequences. All women should be screened serologically for syphilis at the beginning of pregnancy. Serologic testing should be repeated at 28 to 32 weeks of pregnancy and at delivery in populations in which the prevalence of syphilis is high or in women at high risk, such as those who were previously untested or had a positive serology in the first trimester.[30]

Benzathine penicillin G administered to the mother is effective to prevent transmission and to cure the disease in the fetus (Table 47–8).[30] Penicillin-allergic women must undergo desensitization to the drug since alternative therapies used in nonpregnant patients are either teratogenic (e.g., tetracycline and doxycycline) or will not cure disease in the fetus (e.g., erythromycin).[30] The intensity of the treatment should be adjusted to the stage of syphilis.

Syphilis in lactating women should be treated with benzathine penicillin G or any of the CDC-recommended alternatives for penicillin-allergic patients (Table 47–8).[13,30]

▶ Trichomoniasis

Vaginal trichomoniasis is associated with maternal symptoms, premature rupture of the membranes, preterm delivery, low birth weight, and respiratory or genital infection of the neonate. However, treatment does not reduce perinatal morbidity.[19] Thus, treatment is reserved to alleviate maternal symptoms, and asymptomatic disease should not be treated.[19] Recommended treatment is oral metronidazole (Table 47–8).[19]

Women requiring single-dose metronidazole during lactation should discontinue breast-feeding for 12 hours in order to minimize the infant's exposure to the drug.[19,30] During this time, women should pump and discard breast milk in order to avoid engorgement.

Women taking metronidazole should avoid drinking alcohol or using alcohol-containing substances to avoid having a disulfiram-like reaction.

Preterm Labor

Preterm birth, especially before 32 weeks of pregnancy, is the major cause of short- and long-term neonatal mortality and morbidity. The underlying pathophysiologic conditions are diverse, and most are unknown. There is a wide variation in management, diagnosis, and treatment of preterm labor across the world.

▶ Antenatal Corticosteroids

The most beneficial intervention in preterm labor is the administration of antepartum corticosteroids. A single course of antenatal corticosteroids should be administered between 24 and 34 weeks' gestation to women at risk of preterm delivery within 7 days (Table 47–8). This approach decreases the incidence and severity of neonatal respiratory distress syndrome, intraventricular hemorrhage, necrotizing enterocolitis, and death.[33–36] Current guidelines do not support the use of repeat courses of corticosteroids, as the effectiveness of repeat doses has not been clearly established.[34,37]

▶ Tocolytic Agents

Tocolytic therapy is used to buy time to complete a course of corticosteroids, transfer the patient to a center with neonatal intensive care unit facilities, and to delay delivery. Agents commonly used as tocolytics in the United States include magnesium sulfate, terbutaline, indomethacin, and nifedipine (Table 47–8).[34] Nitric oxide donors and atosiban (an oxytocin receptor antagonist) are used in other countries.[36] Few head-to-head comparisons have been made between tocolytic agents. All have limited benefit. Agent selection is based on maternal status and potential adverse drug reactions, as there is no clear first-line tocolytic drug.[34] Combined tocolytics and prolonged or repeated tocolytic therapy should not be used as it may lead to increased fetal risk without evidence of efficacy.[34]

All tocolytic agents expose the mother and the fetus to serious side effects. A systematic review concludes that nifedipine offers the best benefit-to-risk ratio, but some authors opine that this conclusion is based upon studies of poor quality.[36,38] Potential maternal adverse reactions of nifedipine include headache, flushing, dizziness, transient hypotension, and maternal pulmonary edema.[34,37]

Data proving that magnesium sulfate prolongs pregnancy are lacking. It is contraindicated for use in women with myasthenia gravis, and serious complications such as maternal pulmonary edema and cardiac arrest have been reported.[34] More benign side effects such as flushing, headache, and nausea often cause discontinuation of magnesium sulfate therapy.[34]

Terbutaline has been shown to prolong pregnancy but has not decreased neonatal morbidity.[34,39] It is contraindicated in women with pre-existing cardiac arrhythmia. Common adverse effects include hyperglycemia, palpitations, tremor, nausea, headache, and chest pain. Potentially serious maternal adverse effects include pulmonary edema, cardiac arrhythmia, and myocardial ischemia. Reported fetal and neonatal adverse effects include tachycardia, hyperglycemia, and hyperinsulinemia.[34]

Indomethacin also prolongs pregnancy, but it has not been independently associated with decreased neonatal morbidity.[34] It may be of particular benefit in women with hydramnios.[34] Indomethacin should be avoided in women with a history of renal or hepatic impairment, aspirin or nonsteroidal anti-inflammatory drug (NSAID) allergy, peptic ulcer disease, other bleeding disorders, or after 32 weeks of pregnancy. Reports of increased risk of maternal postpartum hemorrhage, and neonatal complications (e.g., premature closure of the ductus arteriosus, necrotizing enterocolitis, bronchopulmonary dysplasia, renal insufficiency, and intraventricular hemorrhage) are worrisome.[34]

▶ Antibiotics

The administration of a 7-day course of parenteral (48 hours) and oral therapy with ampicillin or amoxicillin and erythromycin in the presence of premature rupture of the membranes is associated with a delay in delivery and a reduction in maternal and neonatal morbidity.[40]

Group B *Streptococcus* Infection

Maternal transmission of group B *Streptococcus* during the intrapartum period is a cause of neonatal sepsis and death. All pregnant women should be screened for group B *Streptococcus* disease using vaginal and rectal swabs between 35 and 37 weeks of gestation. Antibiotic therapy has been proven to reduce the incidence of early-onset neonatal group B *Streptococcus* infection when administered to high-risk groups of women. Empirical treatment should be started for group B *Streptococcus* at the time of membrane rupture and continued until delivery (Table 47–8). The antibiotic of choice for group B streptococcal disease is penicillin G, although ampicillin, erythromycin, or clindamycin are good alternatives.[41] Resistance has developed with the use of some alternative choices for penicillin-allergic patients.

The neonate should be observed for signs and symptoms of sepsis until 48 hours after birth. If present, a full diagnostic workup (including complete blood cell count and blood culture) should be initiated and empirical antibiotic therapy started.[41]

Thyroid Disorders

Pregnant and lactating women need more iodine intake (250 mcg/day) than other women. Milk products and prenatal vitamins are a good source of iodine. Iodine deficiency is a major cause of fetal neurologic damage. Pregnancy induces significant changes in thyroid function. Maternal thyroid disorders, even if subclinical, may have adverse effects on the pregnancy and the fetus/neonate. Maternal hypothyroidism is associated with a higher risk of miscarriage, preterm delivery, and damage to fetal neurologic development.

Screening for thyroid disorders is recommended only in women with personal or FH of thyroid disease, immunological disease (e.g., diabetes mellitus type 1) or presenting suspicious symptoms (e.g., fatigue, constipation, excessive weight gain).[38]

It is important to maintain euthyroidism during pregnancy. For women already on chronic thyroid replacement therapy, the dose should be increased at diagnosis of pregnancy, and thyroxine-stimulating hormone (TSH) levels should be monitored every 4 to 6 weeks. Thyroid replacement therapy can be titrated to maintain a TSH level below 2.5 microunits/mL [μU/mL] (2.5 milliunits/L [mU/L]) in the first trimester and below 3 microunits/mL [μU/mL] (3 milliunits/L

[mU/L]) in the second and third trimesters.[45] The Endocrine Society recommends treating subclinical hypothyroidism in pregnant women, although there are no data on the impact of thyroid replacement therapy on long-term infant neurologic outcomes.[45]

The presence of antibodies to thyroid peroxidase increases the risk of hypothyroidism during and after pregnancy and miscarriage. The appropriate management of this condition is unknown.[45]

A low TSH level early in pregnancy can be due to normal physiology, hyperemesis, hyperfunctioning nodule, or Graves' disease. Gestational hyperthyroidism associated with *hyperemesis gravidarum* is self-remitting and does not require antithyroid treatment. Overt maternal hyperthyroidism is associated with a higher risk of miscarriage, intrauterine death, small growth, and fetal/neonatal hyperthyroidism (transplacental passage of TSH receptor antibodies in Graves' disease). Treatment of the mother with antithyroid drugs can induce fetal/neonatal hypothyroidism.

Propylthiouracil is the first-line agent for treatment of hyperthyroidism, as methimazole can be associated with fetal anomalies (Table 47–8).[45] The lowest dose necessary to keep T4 levels in the upper range of the normal should be used. I[131] should not be used in pregnancy. If surgery is required, it should be done in the second trimester.[45]

After delivery, the dose of thyroid replacement therapy should be reduced to prepregnancy levels. TSH should be evaluated 6 to 12 weeks after delivery. All newborns must be evaluated for thyroid dysfunction. Thyroid replacement drugs and antithyroid drugs can be used during lactation.[19]

Enhancement of Lactation

Optimization of breast-feeding techniques is the first approach when decreased lactation is suspected. No drugs are currently approved by the FDA for lactation enhancement, but dopamine antagonists, metoclopramide and domperidone, are sometimes used for this purpose. The efficacy of metoclopramide is controversial.[42] Maternal side effects include fatigue, irritability, abdominal pain, extrapyramidal symptoms, and depression (with long-term use). No side effects in the infant have been reported. Increased milk production should be observed within 2 to 5 days. The drug should be taken for 1 to 2 weeks and then tapered by 10 mg/day at weekly intervals. The efficacy of domperidone is also controversial, but side effects are infrequent, as domperidone does not cross the blood–brain barrier. However, domperidone is not available in the United States, and the FDA issued a warning against domperidone use in 2004 owing to reports of cardiac arrhythmia,

---

Patient Encounter, Part 3

LC had an uneventful pregnancy before arriving at the hospital in labor at 31 weeks of gestation.

What do you recommend at this time?

myocardial infarction, and sudden death associated with high IV doses prescribed for gastric disorders in patients with electrolyte disturbances and complex disease states.[43]

Mastitis

Bacterial mastitis presents with fever or shivering and the presence of two local signs of inflammation (redness, swelling, heat, or pain), most often localized to the external superior quadrant of one breast. The most commonly encountered bacteria are *Staphylococcus aureus*, followed by *Streptococcus*, *Staphylococcus epidermidis*, and *E. coli*. In rare circumstances, a culture of the abscess liquid is performed, but generally, treatment is empirical.

Nonpharmacologic measures, such as cold or warm compresses and more frequent breast-feeding should be encouraged. If a woman is not breast-feeding, it is important to empty the infected breast with a pump to prevent milk stasis. Several antibiotics can be used (Table 47–8). Analgesics (e.g., acetaminophen, ibuprofen, or naproxen) can be used to relieve pain.[44]

Breast Candidiasis

Candidiasis presents with severe and persistent nipple pain which can be throbbing and radiating to the breasts and back. The pain is usually more intense during and immediately after breast-feeding. The infant can be symptomatic or asymptomatic. *Candida albicans* is the most commonly found type of *Candida* species. It is recommended to breast-feed more frequently than usual for a shorter period of time. Milk does not have to be discarded; however, clothes and towels

---

Patient Care and Monitoring[48]

1. Provide prenatal counseling regarding lifestyle modifications (healthy diet, exercise, avoidance of tobacco, alcohol, and illicit or unnecessary drugs) and medication use during pregnancy. When possible, attain good control of maternal conditions prior to conception. Identify patients at risk of psychosocial problems. Immunize as needed.

2. Perform routine screening at first appointment during pregnancy
   - Hematocrit or hemoglobin levels
   - Urinalysis and urine culture
   - Determination of blood group and Rhesus type
   - Determination of immunity to rubella virus
   - Syphilis and sexually transmitted diseases
   - Cervical cytology (if needed)
   - Hepatitis B surface antigen
   - HIV antibody testing

3. Recommend appropriate folic acid and multivitamins prior to conception.

4. After pregnancy is achieved, encourage lifestyle modifications, routine pregnancy monitoring and care, and medication adherence.

5. ❺ *When possible, treat pregnancy conditions with nonpharmacologic treatments instead of using drug therapy.*

6. When considering pharmacologic treatment, evaluate the following:
   - ❻ *Evaluate the need for treatment, including benefits and risks. Avoid treatments that do not show evidence of benefit or that can be delayed until after pregnancy of breast-feeding.*

   - Are the symptoms related to benign conditions of pregnancy? (e.g., palpitations); how bothersome are the symptoms? (e.g., nausea and vomiting); in case of chronic treatment, does it need to be continued during pregnancy? (e.g., dyslipidemia); is the condition interfering with other pathologies? (e.g., nausea and diabetes); could starting/continuing/stopping the treatment pose a risk for the fetus/neonate?

   - Is an effective treatment available?
   - What are the maternal side effects of the drug?
   - Which is the best drug when used alone?
   - Which is the drug with the best safety data in pregnancy/lactation?

7. Encourage breast-feeding. If maternal drug therapy is required during breast-feeding, try to choose short-acting agents with the longest history of safe use in lactation, and administer immediately after feedings.

   - Avoid treatments that show no evidence of benefit or that can be delayed until after breast-feeding.

   - If possible, select drugs that are used in neonates or children and that are well tolerated.

   - When possible, select drugs that yield low percentages of pediatric or relative infant doses (preferably less than 10%).

   - Consider infant age when analyzing safety of a drug during breast-feeding. Premature or very young children will be more sensitive to drug effects than older children.

   - Avoid drugs that can hinder breast milk production.

8. Monitor infants for birth defects and/or unusual reactions that may be due to maternal drug use. Report suspected drug-related reactions to the FDA or pharmaceutical companies.

in contact with the breasts and the baby's mouth should be washed in hot water. Antifungal treatment must to be given to the mother and the baby simultaneously (Table 47–8). If no improvement is seen within 24 to 48 hours, the treatment should be reevaluated. Analgesics (e.g., acetaminophen, ibuprofen, or naproxen) can be used to relieve pain.

Abbreviations Introduced in This Chapter

AAP	American Academy of Pediatrics
ACOG	American College of Obstetricians and Gynecologists
CNS	Central nervous system
GA	Gestational age
NSAID	Nonsteroidal anti-inflammatory drug
OTIS	Organization of Teratology Information Specialists
PCA	Postconceptional age
STEPS	System for Thalidomide Education and Prescribing Safety
T4	Levothyroxine
TSH	Thyroxine-stimulating hormone
UGT	Uridine diphosphate glucuronosyltransferase

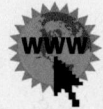 Self-assessment questions and answers are available at *http://www.mhpharmacotherapy. com/pp.html.*

REFERENCES

1. Refuerzo JS, Blackwell SC, Sokol RJ, et al. Use of over-the-counter medications and herbal remedies in pregnancy. Am J Perinatol 2005;22(6):321–324.
2. Andrade SE, Gurwitz JH, Davis RL, et al. Prescription drug use in pregnancy. Am J Obstet Gynecol 2004;191(2):398–407.
3. Briggs GG. Drug effects on the fetus and breast-fed infant. Clin Obstet Gynecol 2002;45(1):6–21.
4. Schirm E, Schwagermann MP, Tobi H, de Jong-van den Berg LT. Drug use during breast-feeding. A survey from the Netherlands. Eur J Clin Nutr 2004;58(2):386–390.
5. Miller R, Peters P, Schaefer C. General commentary on drug therapy and drug risks in pregnancy. In: Schaefer C, Peters P, Miller RK, eds. Drugs during pregnancy and lactation, treatment options and risk assessment, 2nd ed. Amsterdam: Elsevier, 2007:1–26.
6. Ferreira E. Grossesse et allaitement: guide thérapeutique. Montreal: Éditions CHU-Ste-Justine, 2007.
7. Kweder SL. Drugs and biologics in pregnancy and breast-feeding: FDA in the 21st century. Birth Defects Res A Clin Mol Teratol 2008;82(9):605–609.
8. Polifka JE, Friedman JM. Medical genetics: 1. Clinical teratology in the age of genomics. CMAJ 2002;167(3):265–273.
9. Goh YI, Koren G. Folic acid in pregnancy and fetal outcomes. J Obstet Gynecol 2008;28(1):3–13.
10. Cheschier N. ACOG practice bulletin. Neural tube defects. Number 44, July 2003. (Replaces committee opinion number 252, March 2001.) Int J Gynecol Obstet 2003;83(1):123–133.
11. Wilson RD, Johnson JA, Wyatt P, et al. Pre-conceptional vitamin/folic acid supplementation 2007: The use of folic acid in combination with a multivitamin supplement for the prevention of neural tube defects and other congenital anomalies. J Obstet Gynecol Can 2007;29(12):1003–1026.

12. ACOG Practice Bulletin. ACOG practice bulletin No. 95: Anemia in pregnancy. Obstet Gynecol 2008;112(1):201–207.
13. Dawes M, Chowienczyk PJ. Drugs in pregnancy. Pharmacokinetics in pregnancy. Best Pract Res Clin Obstet Gynecol 2001;15(6):819–826.
14. Anderson GD. Pregnancy-induced changes in pharmacokinetics: A mechanistic-based approach. Clin Pharmacokinet 2005;44(10):989–1008.
15. Frederiksen MC. Physiologic changes in pregnancy and their effect on drug disposition. Semin Perinatol 2001;25(3):120–123.
16. Arsenault MY, Lane CA, MacKinnon CJ, et al. The management of nausea and vomiting of pregnancy. J Obstet Gynecol Can 2002;24(10):817–831.
17. ACOG Practice Bulletin. Nausea and vomiting of pregnancy. Obstet Gynecol 2004;103(4):803–814.
18. Jewell DJ, Young G. Interventions for treating constipation in pregnancy. Cochrane Database Syst Rev 2001(2):CD001142.
19. Committee on Drugs, American Academy of Pediatrics. Transfer of drugs and other chemicals into human milk. Pediatrics 2001;108(3):776–789.
20. Quijano CE, Abalos E. Conservative management of symptomatic and/or complicated haemorrhoids in pregnancy and the puerperum. Cochrane Database Syst Rev 2005(3):CD004077.
21. Tytgat GN, Heading RC, Muller-Lissner S, et al. Contemporary understanding and management of reflux and constipation in the general population and pregnancy: A consensus meeting. Aliment Pharmacol Ther 2003;18(3):291–301.
22. Diav-Citrin O, Arnon J, Shechtman S, et al. The safety of proton pump inhibitors in pregnancy: A multicentre prospective controlled study. Aliment Pharmacol Ther 2005;21(3):269–275.
23. Wallace DV, Dykewicz MS, Bernstein DI, et al. The diagnosis and management of rhinitis: An updated practice parameter. J Allergy Clin Immunol 2008;122(2 Suppl):S1–S84.
24. Incaudo GA, Takach P. The diagnosis and treatment of allergic rhinitis during pregnancy and lactation. Immunol Allergy Clin North Am 2006;26(1):137–154.
25. Smaill F, Vazquez JC. Antibiotics for asymptomatic bacteriuria in pregnancy. Cochrane Database Syst Rev 2007(2):CD000490.
26. U.S. Preventive Services Task Force. Screening for Asymptomatic Bacteriuria in Adults: U.S. Preventive Services Task Force Reaffirmation Recommendation Statement. Ann Intern Med 2008;149:43–47.
27. Le J, Briggs GG, McKeown A, Bustillo G. Urinary tract infections during pregnancy. Ann Pharmacother 2004;38(10):1692–1701.
28. Briggs GG, Freeman RK, Yaffe SJ. Drugs in Pregnancy and Lactation, 8th ed. Philadephia: Lippincott Williams & Wilkins, 2008.
29. Villar J, Lydon-Rochelle MT, Gulmezoglu AM, Roganti A. Duration of treatment for asymptomatic bacteriuria during pregnancy. Cochrane Database Syst Rev 2000(2):CD000491.
30. Workowski KA, Berman SM. Sexually transmitted diseases treatment guidelines, 2006. MMWR Recomm Rep 2006;55(RR-11):1–94.
31. Centers for Disease Control and Prevention. Sexually transmitted diseases treatment guidelines 2002. MMWR Recomm Rep 2002;51(RR-6):1–78.
32. ACOG Practice Bulletin. ACOG practice bulletin No. 82: Clinical management guidelines for obstetrician-gynecologists, June 2007. Management of herpes in pregnancy. Obstet Gynecol 2007;109(6):1489–1498.
33. Committee on Obstetric Practice. ACOG committee opinion: Antenatal corticosteroid therapy for fetal maturation. Obstet Gynecol 2002;99(5 Pt 1):871–873.
34. ACOG Practice Bulletin. ACOG practice bulletin No. 43: Management of preterm labor, May 2003. Int J Gynecol Obstet 2003;82(1):127–135.
35. Crowley P. Prophylactic corticosteroids for preterm birth. Cochrane Database Syst Rev 2000(2):CD000065.
36. Di Renzo GC, Roura LC. Guidelines for the management of spontaneous preterm labor. J Perinat Med 2006;34(5):359–366.
37. King JF, Flenady VJ, Papatsonis DN, et al. Calcium channel blockers for inhibiting preterm labour. Cochrane Database Syst Rev 2003(1):CD002255.

38. Lamont RF, Khan KS, Beattie B, et al. The quality of nifedipine studies used to assess tocolytic efficacy: A systematic review. J Perinat Med 2005;33(4):287–295.

39. Anotayanonth S, Subhedar NV, Garner P, et al. Betamimetics for inhibiting preterm labour. Cochrane Database Syst Rev 2004(4):CD004352.

40. ACOG Practice Bulletin. ACOG practice bulletin No. 80: Premature rupture of membranes. Clinical management guidelines for obstetrician-gynecologists. Obstet Gynecol 2007;109(4):1007–1019.

41. Schrag S, Gorwitz R, Fultz-Butts K, Schuchat A. Prevention of perinatal group B streptococcal disease. Revised guidelines from CDC. MMWR Recomm Rep 2002;51(RR-11):1–22.

42. Ilett KF, Kristensen JH. Drug use and breast-feeding. Expert Opin Drug Saf 2005;4(4):745–768.

43. Hampton T. FDA warns against breast milk drug. JAMA 2004; 292(3):322.

44. Betzold CM. An update on the recognition and management of lactational breast inflammation. J Midwifery Womens Health 2007; 52(6):595–605.

45. Abalovich M, Amino N, Barbour LA, et al. Management of thyroid dysfunction during pregnancy and postpartum: An Endocrine Society Clinical Practice Guideline. J Clin Endocrinol Metab 2007; 92(8 Suppl):S1–S47.

46. Gartner LM, Morton J, Lawrence RA, et al. Breast-feeding and the use of human milk. Pediatrics 2005;115(2):496–506.

47. Hale T. Medications and Mothers' Milk, 13th ed. Amarillo: Hale, 2008.

48. Gilstrap LC, Oh W. Guidelines for Perinatal Care, 5th ed. Washington, DC: American Academy of Pediatrics and American College of Obstetricians and Gynecologists, 2002.

49. March of Dimes Foundation. Miscarriage. Quick reference and fact sheets. June 2005. *http://www.marchofdimes.com/ printableArticles/14332_1192.asp.* Accessed September 29, 2008.

50. March of Dimes Foundation. Stillbirth. Quick reference and fact sheets. April 2008. *http://www.marchofdimes.com/printableArticles/ 14332_1198.asp.* Accessed September 29, 2008.

51. March of Dimes Foundation. Perinatal data snapshots: United States. September 2008. *http://www.marchofdimes.com/peristats/pdflib/999/ pds_99_all.pdf.* Accessed September 29, 2008.

52. Schardein J. Chemically Induced Birth Defects, 3rd ed. New York: Marcel Dekker, 2000.

53. Update to CDC's sexually transmitted diseases treatment guidelines, 2006: Fluoroquinolones no longer recommended for treatment of gonococcal infections. MMWR Morb Mortal Wkly Rep 2007;56(14): 332–336.

54. Jewell D, Young G. Interventions for nausea and vomiting in early pregnancy. Cochrane Database Syst Rev 2003(4):CD000145.

48 Contraception

Julia M. Koehler and Kathleen B. Haynes

LEARNING OBJECTIVES

● **Upon completion of the chapter, the reader will be able to:**

1. Discuss the physiology of the normal female reproductive system.

2. Compare the efficacy of oral contraceptives with that of other methods of contraception.

3. State the mechanism of action of hormonal contraceptives.

4. Discuss the risks associated with the use of contraceptives, and state absolute and relative contraindications to their use.

5. List side effects associated with the use of various contraceptives, and recommend strategies for minimizing or eliminating such side effects.

6. Describe advantages and disadvantages of various contraceptives, including both oral and nonoral formulations.

7. Cite important drug interactions that may occur with oral contraceptives.

8. Provide appropriate patient education regarding the important differences between various barrier methods of contraception.

9. Discuss how emergency contraception (EC) may be employed to prevent accidental pregnancy.

10. Provide appropriate patient education regarding the use of oral contraceptives, and recommend and discuss the use of nonoral contraceptives when appropriate.

KEY CONCEPTS

❶ Heavy smokers (greater than or equal to 15 cigarettes per day) over the age of 35, as well as patients with a history of thromboembolic disease, stroke, coronary artery disease, any estrogen-dependent neoplasm, or undiagnosed abnormal uterine bleeding, should not take estrogen-containing contraceptives.

❷ Side effects associated with the use of combination oral contraceptives may be minimized by appropriately adjusting either the total estrogen or progestin content.

❸ Antibiotic administration during contraceptive use may decrease the efficacy of many hormonal contraceptives.

❹ Nonoral forms of contraceptives, such as the transdermal patch and the transvaginal ring, avoid the need for daily administration and, as such, may enhance patient convenience and compliance.

❺ Oral, transdermal, and transvaginal contraceptives, as well as intrauterine devices (IUDs) and most barrier contraceptives, do not protect against sexually transmitted diseases (STDs).

❻ When a contraceptive dose is missed, the risk of accidental pregnancy may be increased. Depending on how many doses were missed, the contraceptive formulation being used, and the phase of the cycle during which doses were missed, counseling regarding the use of additional methods of contraception may be warranted.

Historically, the 1950s represented an important time in the control of human fertility. It was during that decade that the first combination oral contraceptives were developed. Shortly after the discovery that the exogenous administration of hormones such as progesterone successfully blocked ovulation, the use of hormonal steroids quickly became the most popular method of contraception worldwide. Specifically, combination oral contraceptives represent the most commonly used reversible form of contraception today, and it is estimated that nearly 100 million women worldwide take oral contraceptives.[1] Further, in the United States, it is estimated that at some time during their lives, more than 80% of women born since 1945 have used oral contraceptives.[1,2]

Since the introduction of oral contraceptives, many newer forms of contraceptives have been developed and are available for use in the United States. New hormone delivery systems, such as transdermal systems, transvaginal systems, and intrauterine devices (IUDs), offer women effective and more convenient alternatives to oral contraceptives.

EPIDEMIOLOGY

According to the National Survey of Family Growth, approximately 6.3 million pregnancies occur annually in the United States.[3] Of these pregnancies, it is estimated that nearly 3.15 million are unintended.[3,4] Contributing to the risk of unintended pregnancy is the fact that approximately 7.5% of all women who are at risk of becoming pregnant do not use any form of contraception.[3,4] In addition, many women who do use contraceptives use their chosen method of contraception imperfectly, and this also increases the risk of undesired pregnancy. Given these statistics, the provision of appropriate and adequate instruction to patients regarding how to use contraceptive methods effectively is essential in order to reduce the risk of unwanted pregnancy.

Exposure to sexually transmitted diseases (STDs) is also a concern for women who are sexually active. It is estimated that 15 million people in the United States become newly infected annually with an STD.[5] Given that not all methods of contraception protect the user against STDs, the provision of proper patient education by health care professionals regarding this risk is absolutely essential.

PHYSIOLOGY

The female menstrual cycle is divided into four functional phases: follicular, ovulatory, luteal, and menstrual.[6] The

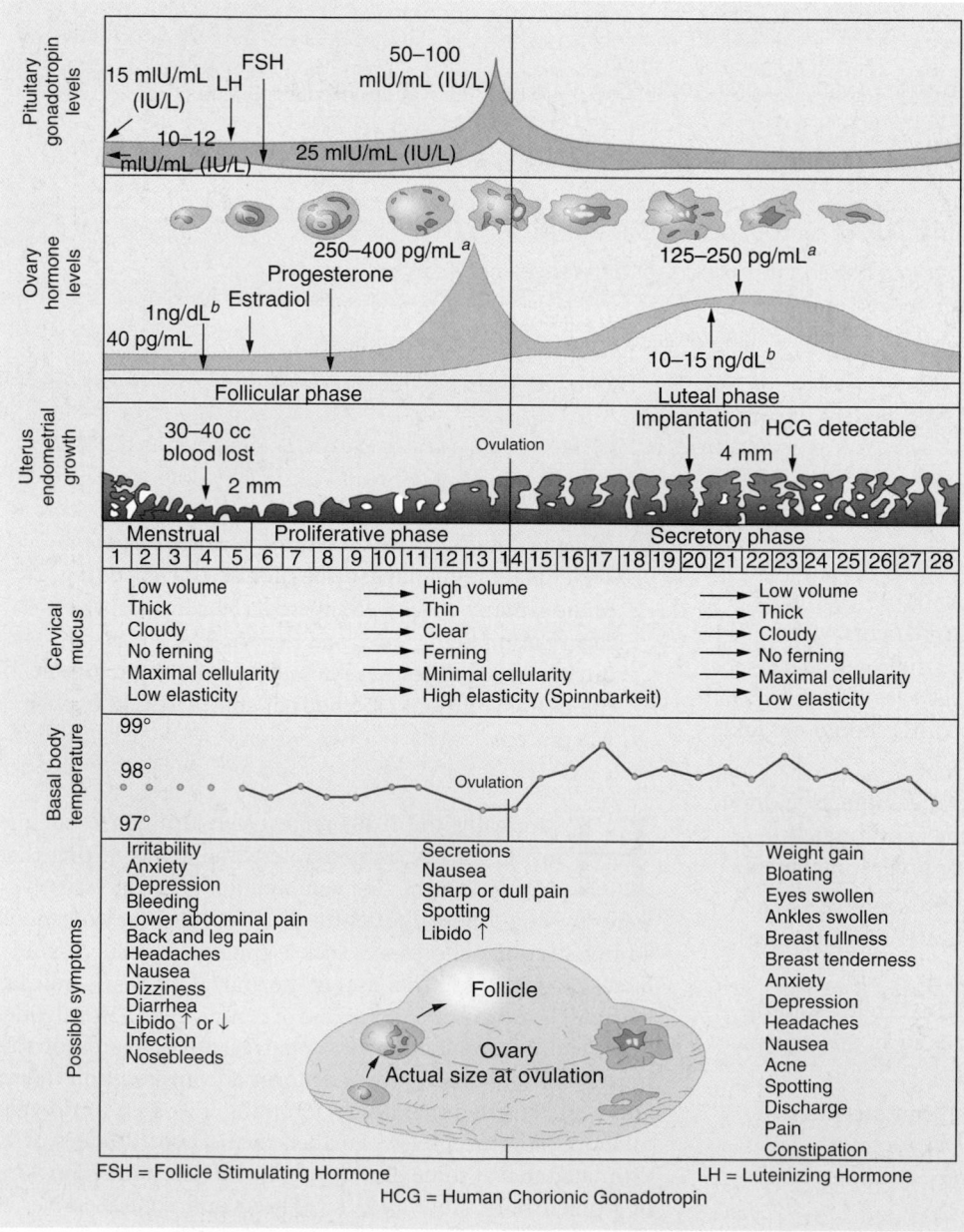

FIGURE 48–1. Menstrual cycle events. [a]Estradiol: 40 pg/mL = 147 pmol/L; 250 to 400 pg/mL = 918 to 1,468 pmol/L; 125 to 250 pg/mL = 459 to 918 pmol/L. [b]Progesterone: 1 ng/dL = 0.032 nmol/L; 10 to 15 ng/dL = 0.32 to 0.48 nmol/L. (Adapted from Ref. 6.)

follicular phase begins the cycle, and ovulation generally occurs around day 14. The luteal phase then begins and continues until menstruation occurs.[6] The menstrual cycle is regulated by a negative-feedback hormone loop between the hypothalamus, anterior pituitary gland, and ovaries.[6] (Fig. 48–1).

Initially, the hypothalamus releases gonadotropin-releasing hormone (GnRH), which stimulates the anterior pituitary to produce follicle-stimulating hormone (FSH) and luteinizing hormone (LH). The levels of FSH and LH released vary depending on the phase of the menstrual cycle. Just prior to ovulation, FSH and LH both are at their peak levels. The FSH helps to promote growth of the follicle in preparation for ovulation by causing granulosa cells lining the follicle to grow and produce estrogen. The LH promotes androgen production by theca cells in the follicle, promotes ovulation and oocyte maturation, and converts granulosa cells to cells that secrete progesterone after ovulation.

Conception is most likely to occur when viable sperm are present in the upper region of the reproductive tract at the time of ovulation. Fertilization occurs when a spermatozoan penetrates an ovum. Approximately 6 to 8 days after ovulation, attachment of the early embryo to the lining of the uterine cavity—implantation—occurs.

PREVENTION OF PREGNANCY: CONTRACEPTIVES AND DEVICES

Goals of Contraception/Desired Outcome

The most common goal of contraception is the prevention of pregnancy. However, some patients use contraceptive methods for other benefits, such as menstrual cycle regulation, reduction of premenstrual symptoms, or treatment of acne.

Choice of Contraceptives: Important Considerations

When helping a patient decide on a contraceptive, the most important goal is to find an option that the patient is comfortable with and that the clinician feels will be beneficial for the patient. It is imperative to explain the side effects, safety concerns, and noncontraceptive benefits of each alternative to the patient so that she may make an informed decision. Fertility goals vary for each patient. It must be determined if the goal is to postpone contraception, space out the next pregnancy, or avoid further pregnancy altogether. Also, a clinician must understand the patient's desire to have or not have a regular bleeding pattern, because many contraceptives will affect menses.

As discussed later in this chapter, contraindications exist for various forms of contraception. Patients must be evaluated completely by a health care professional to rule out any medical contraindications to certain contraceptives. The physical examination also will allow health care professionals to determine if there are other medical concerns, such as hypertension, diabetes, or liver disease, that need to be considered when selecting an appropriate contraceptive agent. Clinicians also should review family history for potential risks with certain forms of birth control.

Sexual behavior of the female must be determined to understand the risk for STDs. Women who are not in a monogamous relationship must consider their risk of STDs as a factor in their contraceptive decision. Some barrier methods protect against STDs, but hormonal contraceptives do not prevent STDs if used alone.

Personal preference plays a large role when determining the best contraceptive option. For instance, if a woman is not interested in using a method that interrupts sexual activity, then a diaphragm would be an inappropriate choice. Preference of the sexual partner may be important as well. Certain agents such as male condoms require the male partner to play an active role in contraception.

Cost is also another related issue for patients. Insurance may not cover all forms of contraception, and patients may have to bear the entire cost for certain options.

Efficacy of Contraceptives

The accidental pregnancy rate for women who do not use any form of contraception is unknown. Therefore, it is difficult to determine the true efficacy of contraceptives in preventing unwanted pregnancy. Table 48–1 shows the percentage of women who experience unintended pregnancy within 1 year of contraceptive use with ongoing sexual activity.[7]

Oral Contraceptives (Combination)

Combination oral contraceptives contain a combination of a synthetic estrogen and one of several steroids with progestational activity. Most oral contraceptives contain one of two types of estrogen: ethinyl estradiol, which is pharmacologically active, or mestranol, which is converted by the liver to ethinyl estradiol. Many different progestins are found in the various oral contraceptives. These include norethindrone, norethindrone acetate, ethynodiol diacetate, norgestrel, levonorgestrel, desogestrel, norgestimate, and drospirenone.

The primary mechanism by which combination oral contraceptives prevent pregnancy is through inhibition of ovulation. FSH and LH regulate the production of estrogen and progesterone by the ovaries. Secretion of estrogen and progesterone by the ovaries occurs in a cyclic manner, which, in turn, determines the regular hormonal changes that occur in the uterus, vagina, and cervix associated with the menstrual cycle. Cyclic changes in the levels of estrogen and progesterone in the blood, together with FSH and LH, modulate the development of ova and the occurrence of ovulation. The estrogen component of combination oral contraceptives is most active in inhibiting FSH release.[1] However, at sufficiently high doses, estrogens also may cause inhibition of LH release. In low-dose combination oral contraceptives, the progestin component causes suppression of LH.[1] Ovulation is prevented by suppression of the midcycle surge of both FSH and LH,[1] and this suppression, which is induced by combination oral contraceptives, mimics the physiologic changes that occur during pregnancy.

Table 48–1

Unintended Pregnancy Rates

Method	Percentage of Women Experiencing Unintended Pregnancy Within First Year of Use		Percentage of Women Continuing Use at 1 Year[c]
	Typical Use[a]	Perfect Use[b]	
No method	85	85	
Spermicides	29	18	42
Withdrawal	27	4	43
Fertility awareness-based methods	25		51
Standard days method		5	
Two-day method		4	
Sponge			
Parous women	32	20	46
Nulliparous women	16	9	57
Diaphragm	16	6	57
Condom			
Female (reality)	21	5	49
Male	15	2	53
Combination pill and mini-pill	8	0.3	68
Ortho Evra patch	8	0.3	68
NuvaRing	8	0.3	68
Depo-Provera	3	0.3	56
IUD			
ParaGard (copper T)	0.8	0.6	78
Mirena (LNG-IUS)	0.2	0.2	80
Implanon	0.05	0.05	
Female sterilization	0.5	0.5	100
Male sterilization	0.15	0.1	100

[a]Among *typical* couples who initiate use of a method (not necessarily for the first time), the percentage who experience an accidental pregnancy during the first year if they do not stop use for any other reason. Estimates of the probability of pregnancy during the first year of typical use for spermicides, withdrawal, periodic abstinence, the diaphragm, the male condom, the pill, and Depo-Provera are taken from the 1995 National Survey of Family Growth corrected for under-reporting of abortion.

[b]Among couples who initiate use of a method (not necessarily for the first time) and who use it *perfectly* (both consistently and correctly), the percentage who experience an accidental pregnancy during the first year if they do not stop use for any other reason.

[c]Among couples attempting to avoid pregnancy, the percentage who continue to use a method for 1 year.

Adapted from Ref. 7.

Although suppression of FSH and LH is the primary mechanism by which combination oral contraceptives prevent ovulation, there are other mechanisms by which these hormones work to prevent pregnancy. Other mechanisms include reduced penetration of the egg by sperm, reduced implantation of fertilized eggs, thickening of cervical mucus to prevent sperm penetration into the upper genital tract, and slowed tubal motility, which may delay transport of sperm.[1] Thus, in addition to inhibition of ovulation, combination oral contraceptives induce changes in the cervical mucus and endometrium that make sperm transport and implantation of the embryo unlikely.[1]

Table 48–2 contains a partial listing of the many oral contraceptives available in the United States today.[8] Although the efficacy of combination oral contraceptives was quickly demonstrated following their introduction into the market, it took longer to determine their safety and acceptability for patients. Since the mid-1960s, ethinyl estradiol has been the primary estrogen used in most combination oral contraceptives. However, the amount of ethinyl estradiol used in combination oral contraceptives has decreased progressively since that time, and most pills now contain 35 mcg or less of ethinyl estradiol. In addition, to reduce side effects and improve tolerability associated with oral contraceptive use, new progestins and different routes of administration have been explored. In an attempt to minimize the undesirable androgenic side effects associated with the progestins of combination oral contraceptives, the synthetic progestins were modified to create "third generation" progestins (e.g., desogestrel and norgestimate). These synthetic progestins are extremely potent in their ability to inhibit ovulation and prevent pregnancy.

Combination oral contraceptives are available in monophasic, biphasic, and triphasic preparations. Monophasic preparations contain fixed doses of estrogen and progestin in each active pill. Although all three preparations contain both estrogens and progestins, biphasic and triphasic preparations differ from monophasic preparations in that they contain varying proportions of one or both hormones during the pill cycle. These preparations were introduced to reduce a patient's cumulative exposure to progestins, as well as to mimic more closely the hormonal changes of the menstrual cycle. However, there is no evidence to suggest that biphasic and triphasic preparations offer any clinical advantage over monophasic pills.[8]

▶ Noncontraceptive Benefits of Combination Oral Contraceptives

In addition to preventing pregnancy, there are several noncontraceptive benefits associated with the use of combination oral contraceptive pills. Some of the potential noncontraceptive benefits are highlighted below.

Reduction in the Risk of Endometrial Cancer The risk of endometrial cancer among women who have used oral contraceptives for at least 1 year is approximately 40% less than the risk in women who have never used oral contraceptives.[9] There is additional evidence to suggest that the benefit of reduced risk for endometrial cancer is detectable within 1 year of use[10–12] and that the benefit may persist for years following discontinuation of oral contraceptives.[9]

Reduction in the Risk of Ovarian Cancer When compared with women who have never used oral contraceptives, women who have used oral contraceptives for 4 years or less are 30% less likely to develop ovarian cancer. There is also additional evidence to suggest that the longer the duration of oral contraceptive use, the greater the reduction in the risk of

Table 48–2

Some Available Oral Contraceptives

Brand Name	Estrogen (mcg/Tablet)	Progestin (mg/Tablet)
Monophasic Preparations		
Loestrin 21 1/20	EE (20)	Norethindrone (1)
Loestrin Fe 1/20	EE (20)	Norethindrone (1)
Loestrin 24 Fe	EE (20)	Norethindrone (1)
Microgestin Fe 1/20	EE (20)	Norethindrone (1)
Alesse	EE (20)	Levonorgestrel (0.1)
Lybrel	EE (20)	Levonorgestrel (0.09)
Yaz	EE (20)	Drospirenone (3)
Desogen	EE (30)	Desogestrel (0.15)
Ortho-Cept	EE (30)	Desogestrel (0.15)
Levlen	EE (30)	Levonorgestrel (0.15)
Nordette	EE (30)	Levonorgestrel (0.15)
Seasonale	EE (30)	Levonorgestrel (0.15)
Yasmin	EE (30)	Drospirenone (3)
Lo/Ovral	EE (30)	Norgestrel (0.3)
Loestrin 21 1.5/30	EE (30)	Norethindrone (1.5)
Loestrin Fe 1.5/30	EE (30)	Norethindrone (1.5)
Microgestin Fe 1.5/30	EE (30)	Norethindrone (1.5)
Ortho-Cyclen	EE (35)	Norgestimate (0.25)
Ovcon-35	EE (35)	Norethindrone (0.4)
Brevicon	EE (35)	Norethindrone (0.5)
Necon 0.5/35	EE (35)	Norethindrone (0.5)
Necon 1/35	EE (35)	Norethindrone (1)
Ortho-Novum 1/35	EE (35)	Norethindrone (1)
Demulen 1/35	EE (35)	Ethynodiol diacetate (1)
Zovia 1/35E	EE (35)	Ethynodiol diacetate (1)
Ovral	EE (50)	Norgestrel (0.5)
Ovcon-50	EE (50)	Norethindrone (1)
Demulen 1/50	EE (50)	Ethynodiol diacetate (1)
Zovia 1/50E	EE (50)	Ethynodiol diacetate (1)
Necon 1/50	Mestranol (50)	Norethindrone (1)
Norinyl 1 + 50	Mestranol (50)	Norethindrone (1)
Ortho-Novum 1/50	Mestranol (50)	Norethindrone (1)
Biphasic Preparations		
Mircette	EE (20, 0,10)	Desogestrel (0.15)
Kariva	EE (20, 0,10)	Desogestrel (0.15)
Ortho-Novum 10/11	EE (35)	Norethindrone (0.5,1)
Necon 10/11	EE (35)	Norethindrone (0.5,1)
Triphasic Preparations		
Estrostep Fe	EE (20, 30, 35)	Norethindrone (1)
Tri-Levlen	EE (30, 40, 30)	Levonorgestrel (0.05, 0.075, 0.125)
Triphasil	EE (30, 40, 30)	Levonorgestrel (0.05, 0.075, 0.125)
Ortho Tri-Cyclen	EE (35)	Noregestimate (0.18, 0.215, 0.25)
Tri-Norinyl	EE (35)	Norethindrone (0.5, 1, 0.5)
Ortho-Novum 7/7/7	EE (35)	Norethindrone (0.5, 0.75, 1)
Ortho Tri-Cyclen Lo	EE (25)	Norgestimate (0.18, 0.215, 0.25)
Velivet	EE (25)	Desogestrel (0.1, 0.125, 0.15)
Cyclessa	EE (25)	Desogestrel (0.1, 0.125, 0.15)

EE, ethinyl estradiol.

From Refs. 8, 19.

ovarian cancer. Women who have taken oral contraceptives for 5 to 11 years are 60% less likely to develop ovarian cancer, and women who have taken oral contraceptives for more than 12 years are 80% less likely to develop ovarian cancer than those who have never used oral contraceptives. As with the reduced risk of endometrial cancer, there is evidence to suggest that the reduced risk of ovarian cancer may persist for years following discontinuation of oral contraceptives.[10–12]

Improved Regulation of Menstruation Women who take oral contraceptives typically experience more regular menstrual cycles. In general, oral contraceptive use is associated with less cramping and dysmenorrhea.[1,8] Also, women who take oral contraceptives have a smaller volume of menstruum and experience fewer days of menstruation each month and consequently experience less blood loss with each menstrual period.[1,13] Some studies suggest that oral contraceptive use decreases overall monthly menstrual flow by 60% or more, which may be particularly beneficial in women who are anemic.[1]

Relief of Benign Breast Disease Women who use oral contraceptives are less likely to develop benign breast cysts or fibroadenomas.[1,8]

Prevention of Ovarian Cysts Because oral contraceptives suppress ovarian stimulation, women who take them are less likely to develop ovarian cysts.[8]

Reduction in the Risk of Symptomatic Pelvic Inflammatory Disease The risk of hospitalization owing to symptomatic pelvic inflammatory disease caused by gonorrheal infection is reduced in oral contraceptive users.[14] While the exact protective mechanism is unknown, it is believed that thickening of the cervical mucus and/or reduction in the ability of pathogens to enter the fallopian tubes may contribute to the lower incidence of pelvic inflammatory disease experienced by oral contraceptive users.[1]

Improvement in Acne Control All combination oral contraceptives can improve acne by increasing the quantity of sex hormone–binding globulin and thereby decreasing free testosterone concentrations.[8] Third generation progestins, such as desogestrel and norgestimate, are believed to have less androgenic activity.[8] However, it is not clear that combination oral contraceptives containing these progestins confer any advantage over other combination oral contraceptives with respect to their ability to improve acne control. Only Ortho Tri-Cyclen (ethinyl estradiol and norgestimate) and Estrostep Fe (ethinyl estradiol and norethindrone acetate) are approved by the FDA for the treatment of acne.[1,8]

► Potential Risks of Combination Oral Contraceptives

● While there are many noncontraceptive benefits associated with the use of combination oral contraceptives, their use is not without risk or potential for adverse effects.

● **Sexually Transmitted Diseases** Because the use of combination oral contraceptives may decrease the use of selected barrier contraceptive methods that do protect against STDs (e.g., latex condoms), one of the most common risks associated with the use of oral contraceptives is the increased risk of acquiring an STD.[8]

Cardiovascular Events and Hypertension A WHO collaborative study found that high-dose (50 mcg or more of ethinyl estradiol) oral contraceptive users with uncontrolled hypertension have an increased risk of experiencing a myocardial infarction or stroke.[8,15] In this study, women who had the lowest risk for experiencing a myocardial infarction or stroke were those who did not smoke, took low-dose oral contraceptives, and had their blood pressure checked prior to beginning oral contraceptives.[16–18] Hypertension secondary to oral contraceptive use is thought to occur in up to 1% to 3% of women, and this is believed to be attributed to the effect that estrogens and progestins can have on aldosterone activity.[1] Given this and the risk for cardiovascular events, women should have their blood pressure checked prior to initiating oral contraceptives, as well as periodically throughout oral contraceptive use. If significant elevations in blood pressure are noted, oral contraceptives should be discontinued. Estrogen-containing contraceptives are not recommended for smokers who are older than 35 years of age, for women with hypertension, or for women who experience migraine headaches (especially those with focal neurologic symptoms).[8,19]

Venous Thromboembolism It is believed that the estrogen component of combination oral contraceptives stimulates the liver to produce higher levels of clotting factors. Lower-dose estrogen pills (less than 50 mcg estrogen) have been associated with a threefold to fourfold increase in the risk of venous thromboembolism compared with women who do not use oral contraceptives.[8] Contraceptive users at greatest risk for the development of venous thromboembolism include those who are obese, those who smoke, those who have hypertension, and those with diabetes complicated by end-organ damage. It is important to note, however, that the increase in risk of venous thromboembolism in oral contraceptive users is lower than that of pregnant women.[8] Newer progestins, such as desogestrel, were reported initially to be associated with a higher risk of venous thromboembolism.[20,21] However, prospective studies validating this risk are lacking. In general, progestin-only contraceptives are preferred for women who are at increased risk of cardiovascular or thromboembolic complications, including women with a prior history of thromboembolic disease.[8]

Glucose Intolerance Older oral contraceptive formulations containing higher doses of hormones were shown in some cases to induce hyperglycemia.[1] Because estrogens may inhibit the release of insulin from islet cells of the pancreas, low-dose estrogen formulations may be preferred in patients with diabetes. Progesterone competes with insulin for binding to its receptor. Although it is thought that progestins may increase insulin resistance, the newer progestins are thought to be less androgenic and have little effect on carbohydrate and lipid metabolism. In general, the use of combination oral contraceptives is relatively contraindicated in patients with diabetes.

Gallbladder Disease In women with pre-existing gallstones, low-dose estrogen-containing oral contraceptives may enhance the potential for the development of symptomatic gallbladder disease.[1] Although this risk has not been demonstrated with the use of higher-dose oral contraceptives, combination oral contraceptives containing estrogen should be used with caution in patients with a history of gallbladder disease.

Hepatic Tumors Although the use of oral contraceptives is not associated with an increased risk for the development of hepatocellular carcinoma, long-term use of high-dose oral contraceptives has been associated with the development of benign liver tumors.[1] Because even benign liver tumors may pose significant risk to the patient, oral contraceptives should be discontinued if liver enlargement is noted on physical examination.

Cervical Cancer There appears to be an increased risk for the development of cervical cancer among long-term users of oral contraceptives.[1] Whether or not this increase in risk can be attributed directly to the use of oral contraceptives is uncertain, however. Data suggest that oral contraceptive users, on average, tend to have more sexual partners and use condoms less frequently, and as a result, this may increase their susceptibility to becoming infected with human papilloma virus (HPV), a known risk factor for cervical cancer.

Breast Cancer While a history of breast cancer traditionally has been considered an absolute contraindication to the use of oral contraceptives, most recent studies evaluating the relationship between oral contraceptive use and the risk for breast cancer suggest little, if any, association between the two. A recent study illustrated that current or past use of oral contraceptives among women between the ages of 35 and 64 was not associated with an increased risk for the development of breast cancer.[22] In older studies of patients using combination oral contraceptives containing 50 to 80 mcg ethinyl estradiol per pill, a link between oral contraceptive use and breast cancer was suggested. The cancers diagnosed in those studies were found to be more localized.[23] Although the relationship between oral contraceptive use and the potential for breast cancer in older patients is becoming better understood, still the question of risk for breast cancer diagnosis in oral contraceptive users under age 35 is less clear.[1] ❶ *Absolute and relative contraindications to the use of oral contraceptives are listed in Table 48–3.*[1]

▶ Adverse Effects of Oral Contraceptives and Their Management

As with all medications, there are potential adverse effects with combination oral contraceptives (COCs). ❷ *Many side effects can be minimized or avoided by adjusting the estrogen and/or progestin content of the oral contraceptive.*

Patient Encounter, Part 1

RC, a 22-year-old nulliparous woman, presents to your clinic requesting information on contraception. You begin to take a history and determine that the patient is currently sexually active and is not using any method of birth control. Her past medical history is significant only for acne, and she takes no medications except occasional ibuprofen for menstrual cramps. On further questioning, you discover that she has a positive family history of hypertension and coronary artery disease. As you discuss various contraceptive options with the patient, it is clear that she has a preference for an oral contraceptive agent.

What additional information do you need to know before recommending a contraceptive for this patient?

Based on the information provided by the patient, what oral contraceptive agent would you recommend for the patient and why?

What education would you provide to this patient regarding risks associated with oral contraceptive use?

Table 48–3

① Contraindications to the Use of Combined Oral Contraceptives (COCs)

Absolute Contraindications

History of thromboembolic disease
History of stroke (or current cerebrovascular disease)
History of (or current) coronary artery disease
History of carcinoma of the breast (known or suspected)
History of any estrogen-dependent neoplasm
Undiagnosed abnormal uterine bleeding
Pregnancy (known or suspected)
Heavy smokers (15 cigarettes or more per day) who are greater than 35 years of age
History of hepatic tumors (benign or malignant)
Active liver disease

Relative Contraindications

Smoking (less than 15 cigarettes per day) at any age
History of migraine headache disorder
Hypertension
Fibroid tumors of the uterus
Breast-feeding
Diabetes

From Refs. 1, 19.

It is also important to individualize the selection of oral contraceptives, because some women are at increased risk for potentially serious side effects.

Women stop their oral contraceptives owing to side effects such as headaches, nausea, vomiting, or weight gain that occur during oral contraceptive use. Package labeling reports a higher incidence of these side effects, although it cannot be determined if they occurred because of the pill or just happened when the women were on the pill.[1] One double-blind trial compared women taking oral contraceptives with women taking placebo for 6 months. A similar percentage of patients in each group experienced headaches, nausea, vomiting, mastalgia, and weight gain, and there were no significant differences in the traditional "hormone-related" side effects.[24] Given that oral contraceptives often are discontinued owing to side effects, proper counseling before initiation of COCs is necessary.

Between 30% and 50% of women complain of breakthrough bleeding or spotting when oral contraceptives are initiated. These side effects tend to resolve by the third or fourth cycle.[1] Before changing formulations, other more serious causes of bleeding or spotting, such as pregnancy, infection, poor absorption of the oral contraceptive owing to drug interaction, or GI problems should be ruled out. Once these causes have been ruled out, the timing of the spotting must be determined in order to adjust the formulation appropriately.

Women who have spotting or bleeding before they finish their active pills need a higher progestin content to increase endometrial support. Either a monophasic formulation with a higher progestin or a triphasic formulation with an increasing dose of progestin would be appropriate. Women with continued bleeding after menses need more estrogen support. Either increasing the estrogen component or having a lower early progestin component (in triphasic pills) should be sufficient. If midcycle bleeding occurs, it is more difficult to determine the cause. It may be best to increase both the estrogen and progestin component for such women.[1]

Hormonal methods of contraception usually decrease the amount of withdrawal bleeding quite significantly, and patients need to be made aware of this. Lower-dose estrogen formulations may increase the risk of breakthrough bleeding. Switching to a higher estrogen formulation or to a triphasic formulation will help to minimize breakthrough bleeding and will increase the amount of withdrawal bleeding.

Acne, oily skin, and hirsutism are all side effects from progestins with increased androgenicity. Older progestins such as norgestrel and levonorgestrel have more androgenic effects, whereas agents containing norgestimate or desogestrel are less likely to have such side effects. If patients are complaining of such side effects, switching to a product with a lower risk of androgenic effects is appropriate.

GI complaints are seen often with oral contraceptives. Estrogen can induce nausea and vomiting via the CNS, whereas progesterone slows peristalsis, causing constipation and feelings of bloating and distention.[1] Most women will adjust to the symptoms, and the symptoms often will resolve within 1 to 3 months. Taking the pill at bedtime or with food may be a good strategy to help cope with nausea. If women are unable to tolerate the GI side effects, then either a decrease in ethinyl estradiol to a low-dose 20 mcg formulation may minimize nausea or a decrease in progestin may minimize bloating and constipation. Progestin-only products may be considered if even low-dose ethinyl estradiol causes nausea.

Headaches are a common occurrence for women, and they must be evaluated because they can be a major warning sign for stroke. If headaches begin or become worse after initiation of COCs, all differential diagnoses must be considered. Blood pressure should be evaluated to rule out hypertension. If any neurologic symptoms or blurred vision occur with the headache, the oral contraceptive should be stopped immediately. Migraine headaches with aura showed a significant increase in the risk for ischemic stroke in one WHO study.[17] If the headaches are not serious but still are troublesome to the patient, the following changes are suggested: (a) discontinue the oral contraceptive, (b) lower the dose of estrogen, (c) lower the dose of progestin, or (d) eliminate the pill-free interval for two to three consecutive cycles (for women with headaches during the pill-free interval only).[1]

Although rare, some women may complain of a decrease in libido. This often is found to coincide with feelings of depression. Alterations to vaginal lubrication and free testosterone levels may occur with some COCs, and both can relate to decreased libido.[25] Low levels of estrogen can decrease vaginal lubrication as well and make intercourse painful. Use of the vaginal hormonal ring (NuvaRing) may help with lubrication problems.[1]

Dyslipidemias can occur from hormone therapy. Estrogen is known to cause an increase in high-density lipoprotein cholesterol (HDL-C), triglycerides, and total cholesterol levels and to decrease low-density lipoprotein cholesterol (LDL-C). Androgenic progestins are more likely to decrease HDL-C and triglycerides and increase LDL-C. Depending on the ratio of estrogen to progestin content, the HDL-C, LDL-C, and triglyceride levels may fluctuate up or down. In women with no risk factors for dyslipidemias (e.g., women who do not smoke, have hypertension, or have a family history of heart disease), it is not necessary to obtain a baseline lipid panel. However, if the lipid panel is monitored, and if dyslipidemia occurs, then it is recommended to replace an androgenic progestin with a more estrogenic progestin. In women with triglyceride levels greater than 350 mg/dL (3.96 mmol/L) at baseline, estrogen-containing formulations should be used only with caution, and low doses of 20 to 25 mcg ethinyl estradiol or a progestin-only formulation might be preferred.[1]

Mastalgia can occur in up to 30% of women taking oral contraceptives and is most likely due to the estrogen component. The average woman has a 20% increase in breast volume in the luteal phase owing to venous and lymphatic engorgement. Estrogen also causes adipose cell hypertrophy in the breast.[1] Lower-dose pills (20 mcg) produce less mastalgia than those with 35 mcg of ethinyl estradiol.[26] If tenderness occurs prior to menses, switching to a contraceptive that offers extended cycle length (see Unique Oral Contraceptives below) may minimize problems as well.

Women often are concerned about using oral contraceptives for fear of gaining weight. It has been proven that oral contraceptives containing less than or equal to 35 mcg ethinyl estradiol do not increase the risk of weight gain in women compared with placebo.[24] Estrogen can cause hypertrophy of adipose cells, and therefore, women see an increase in measurement of their breasts, hips, and thighs.[1] Decreasing the estrogen content of the COCs will minimize this effect. Weight gain associated with premenstrual fluid

retention may occur with the combination of estrogen and a higher androgenic progestin. Switching to a lower-dose estrogen and a progestin with less androgenic activity may be beneficial in this situation.[1]

Additional side effects have been noted in some women. Women wearing contact lenses may have visual changes and more disturbances with lenses. If normal saline eye drops do not help, referral to an ophthalmologist is recommended. Melasma and chloasma can occur secondary to estrogen stimulation of melanocyte production. Women with darker pigmentation are more susceptible to hyperpigmentation effects. The melasma may not be completely reversible on discontinuation. Progestin-only products may be preferable, and sunscreen use is highly recommended.[1]

As described earlier, many of the side effects of COCs may be minimized by adjusting the estrogen or progestin content of the preparation. However, while low- and ultra-low-dose COCs may cause fewer side effects, it is important to note that in the event that doses are missed, such COCs may be more likely to result in contraceptive failure.

Progestin-Only Pills

For women unable to take estrogen-containing oral contraceptives, there is an alternative—oral contraceptives containing only progestin (previously called mini-pills). There are two active ingredients used in this form of contraception, norethindrone and norgestrel. These agents are slightly less effective than COCs but have other advantages over COCs. Progestin-only products have not shown the same risk of thromboembolic events as products containing estrogen have. Therefore, women at increased risk for or with a history of thromboembolism may be good candidates for progestin-only oral contraceptives. Also, these products can minimize menses, and many women have amenorrhea after six to nine cycles. Spotting does not subside in some women, and this is a common cause for discontinuation. These products should be taken at the same time every day, and there is no pill-free or hormone-free period.

Unique Oral Contraceptives

Along with varying doses of ethinyl estradiol and different progestins, there are also formulation modifications that may benefit various patient situations. In the United States, these formulations include products such as Loestrin-24 Fe, Seasonale, Seasonique, Ortho Tri-Cyclen, Estrostep Fe, Yasmin, Yaz, Mircette, Ovcon 35, and Lybrel. Each of these products may show benefit in certain women owing to their unique characteristics.

Loestrin-24 Fe (norethindrone/ethinyl estradiol) is an extended cycle preparation which contains a low-dose estrogen, a high amount of progestin, and medium androgenic activity. Similar to other low-dose estrogen combination OCs, Loestrin-24 Fe may offer a smaller margin of error when pills are missed but offers the potential advantage of fewer estrogen-related side effects (e.g., nausea and breast tenderness). Unlike the typical 28 pill packs which contain 21 active tablets and seven placebo tablets, Loestrin-24 Fe contains 24 active tablets and 4 placebo tablets, allowing for shorter menstrual periods and fewer menstrual-related symptoms, such as menstrual-related headaches, menorrhagia, and anemia.

Seasonale (levonorgestrel/ethinyl estradiol) is a monophasic combination that is packaged as a 91-day treatment cycle with 84 active tablets that are taken consecutively followed by seven placebo tablets. The extended cycle length of this product allows for one menstrual cycle per "season," or four per year. This formulation may be appealing to women with perimenstrual side effects or those at higher risk for anemia with menstrual bleeding. Seasonale may improve anxiety, headache, fluid retention, dysmenorrhea, breast tenderness, bloating, and menstrual migraines. However, in the SEA 301 clinical trial comparing the efficacy of Seasonale with that of an equivalent-dosage 28-day cycle regimen, 7.7% versus 1.8% of women discontinued prematurely for unacceptable bleeding.[27] The risk of intermenstrual bleeding and/or spotting is higher for patients taking Seasonale than for patients taking 28-day-regimen COCs.[27]

Seasonique (levonorgestrel/ethinyl estradiol) is also an extended cycle preparation which is similar to Seasonale, but instead contains seven tablets with low-dose estrogen rather than placebo. Menstruation-related problems which may improve with Seasonique include menstrual-related headaches, menorrhagia, and anemia. In addition, endometriosis-related menstrual pain may be relieved by providing a continuous regimen without a pill-free interval.[28]

Ortho Tri-Cyclen (norgestimate/ethinyl estradiol) and Estrostep Fe (norethindrone acetate/ethinyl estradiol) both have an approved indication for treatment of moderate acne vulgaris in females 15 years of age or older desiring contraception who have not responded adequately to conventional antiacne medication. This can help clinicians to streamline medications by serving dual purposes.

Yasmin and Yaz (drospirenone/ethinyl estradiol) are the only oral contraceptives that contain the progestin drospirenone. This hormone not only has antiandrogenic properties but also showed antimineralcorticoid activity in preclinical trials. It has a unique application in young women who experience problems associated with producing too much androgen. Drospirenone is a spironolactone analog, and the 3 mg dose available in Yasmin and Yaz has antimineralocorticoid activity equal to 25 mg spironolactone. It can affect the sodium and water balance in the body, although it has not shown superior efficacy for side effects such as bloating compared with other oral contraceptives. Caution should be used in women with chronic conditions or other medications that may affect serum potassium.[29] It is advised to check a baseline potassium level in patients at risk for hyperkalemia, such as those taking angiotensin-converting enzyme inhibitors or angiotensin II receptor blockers. Yaz (drospirenone/ethinyl estradiol) is an extended cycle preparation which contains a low-dose estrogen and antimineralocorticoid and antiandrogenic activity. Like Loestrin-24 Fe, Yaz contains 24 active tablets and four placebo tablets, allowing for shorter menstrual periods

and fewer menstrual-related symptoms, such as menstrual-related headaches, menorrhagia, and anemia.

Mircette (desogestrel/ethinyl estradiol) has a unique dosing schedule. After the usual 21 active tablets, there are only two tablets with inert ingredients. The last five tablets in the package have 10 mcg of ethinyl estradiol. In theory, this may minimize bleeding during the menstrual cycle, although the clinical significance of this dosing schedule has not been established.[30] It is important to counsel patients to complete the entire pack and not to discard the last 7 days of medication.

Another unique formulation is a chewable tablet available to women who have difficulty swallowing medications. Ovcon 35 (norethindrone/ethinyl estradiol) has all 28 tablets in chewable form and has added spearmint flavoring.[31]

Finally, Lybrel (levonorgestrel/ethinyl estradiol) is the first continuous cycle OC approved by the FDA. Active pills are taken every day throughout the year with no pill-free interval. The major advantage of this product is elimination of menstrual periods, resulting in improvement in or elimination of menstrual-related symptoms (e.g., headaches, menorrhagia, anemia, and endometriosis-related menstrual pain). The most bothersome side effect associated with Lybrel is a high incidence of spotting and breakthrough bleeding during the initial months of use. It appears as though the incidence of breakthrough bleeding with Lybrel decreases with continued use.[32]

Drug Interactions with Oral Contraceptives

Ethinyl estradiol is metabolized in the liver primarily via cytochrome P450 (CYP450) 3A4. When reviewing drug interactions of oral contraceptives, ❸ *it is important to keep in mind that antibiotic administration during contraceptive use may decrease the efficacy of many combination oral contraceptives.* Refer to Table 48–4 for a list of common drug interactions seen with oral contraceptives.[1,33]

Patient Encounter, Part 2: Adverse Effects

After 10 weeks of taking Microgestin 1/20, RC returns to your clinic complaining of breakthrough bleeding during her third week of active pills. The patient also reports a 1.4-kg (3-lb) weight gain since starting Microgestin 1/20. Because she has heard that birth control pills cause weight gain, she expresses concern and wants to discuss other birth control options.

What are some potential causes of the breakthrough bleeding that the patient has been experiencing?

What information can you provide to the patient regarding the potential association between weight gain and oral contraceptive use?

What strategy would you recommend to eliminate or minimize the potential adverse effects experienced by the patient?

Table 48–4

Commonly Seen Drug Interactions With COCs

Medication	Mechanism	Clinical Effect
Anticonvulsants (carbamazepine, oxcarbazepine, phenytoin, phenobarbital, primidone, topiramate, and felbamate)	Increase metabolism of COCs via induction of various cytochrome P450 enzymes	Decrease efficacy of OCs (EE doses less than 35 mcg are not recommended in women on these medications)
Benzodiazepines (alprazolam)	COCs may inhibit oxidative metabolism	Increase side effects of benzodiazepines
Corticosteroids (hydrocortisone, methylprednisolone, prednisone)	COCs may inhibit metabolism of corticosteroids	Increase side effects of corticosteroids
Griseofulvin	Increase metabolism of COCs	Decrease efficacy of COCs; backup method of contraception is recommended
Modafinil	Increase metabolism of COCs	Decrease efficacy of COCs; alternative method of contraception is recommended
Penicillins (amoxicillin, ampicillin); tetracyclines (doxycycline, minocycline, tetracycline)	Broad-spectrum antibiotics may alter intestinal flora, reducing enterohepatic circulation of estrogen metabolites; although the drop in estrogen levels has been shown to be only statistically significant, rather than clinically significant	Decrease efficacy of COCs, although the recommendation of a backup method of contraception is controversial
Protease inhibitors (amprenavir, nelfinavir, lopinavir, saquinavir, ritonavir)	Increase or decrease serum levels of estrogen and progestins	Decrease efficacy of COCs or increase side effects of COCs
Rifampin, rifabutin	Increase metabolism of COCs	Decrease efficacy of COCs; backup method of contraception is recommended
Selegiline	COCs decrease metabolism of selegiline	Increase side effects of selegiline; may adjust dose of selegiline if needed
St. John's wort	Increase metabolism of COCs via induction of various cytochrome P450 enzymes	Decrease efficacy of COCs; avoid use with COCs
Theophylline	COCs decrease theophylline clearance by 34% and increase half-life by 33%	Increase side effects of theophylline

From Refs. 1, 33.

Nonoral Hormonal Contraceptives

❹ *As an alternative to oral contraceptive pills, which must be taken daily in order to reliably prevent pregnancy, nonoral contraceptives in the form of transdermal, transvaginal, and injectable preparations are available and offer patients safe and effective alternatives to the pills for prevention of pregnancy. These formulations also do not require daily administration, making them more convenient than the pill formulations.*

Ortho-Evra is a transdermal patch that contains both an estrogen (20 mcg of ethinyl estradiol) and a progestin (150 mcg of norelgestromin). A new patch is applied to the abdomen, buttocks, upper torso, or upper (outer) arm once weekly for 3 weeks, followed by seven patch-free days.[8] Although some women have noted irregular bleeding during the first two cycles of patch use, the patch has been demonstrated to provide similar menstrual cycle control and contraceptive efficacy to that of COCs.[34] It is important to note, however, that higher contraceptive failure rates are seen when the patch is used in women weighing more than 90 kg (about 200 lb).[8,34] Further, the manufacturer prescriber information for the product indicates that women who take Ortho-Evra are exposed to approximately 60% more estrogen than women who take COCs with 35 mcg estrogen.[35] While the clinical significance of this is not well defined, recent studies have suggested a link between the use of the patch and an increased risk for venous thromboembolism. A slightly higher reported incidence of breast discomfort and local skin irritation has also been reported with the patch.[8,36]

NuvaRing is a unique transvaginal delivery system that provides 15 mcg ethinyl estradiol and 120 mcg etonogestrel for the prevention of ovulation. NuvaRing is inserted into the vagina on or before day 5 of the menstrual cycle and is removed from the vagina 3 weeks later.[8] Seven days after the ring is removed, a new ring should be inserted. In clinical trials, NuvaRing demonstrated comparable efficacy and cycle control to that of COCs.[8] Side effects seen with NuvaRing are similar to those observed in women taking COCs.[8,37] NuvaRing should not be removed during intercourse. If the ring is dislodged or removed for more than 3 hours, efficacy could be compromised, and a backup method of contraception is recommended until a new ring has been in place for 7 days.

Depo-Provera is a progestin-only injectable contraceptive that contains depot medroxyprogesterone acetate. Depo-Provera is administered intramuscularly as a 150-mg injection once every 3 months. An advantage of Depo-Provera is that it provides an estrogen-free method of contraception either for women in whom estrogens are contraindicated or for women who cannot tolerate estrogen-containing preparations. Depo-Provera is extremely effective in preventing pregnancy. However, the incidence of menstrual irregularities (including amenorrhea) and weight gain appears to be much greater than that seen with COCs. The use of Depo-Provera also has been demonstrated to result in significant loss of bone mineral density (BMD).[38] Although it is not known whether the use of Depo-Provera will increase the risk for osteoporotic fracture, a black-box warning within the product labeling cautions against the risk of potentially irreversible BMD loss associated with long-term use (e.g., greater than 2 years) of the injectable product. While the extended duration of activity of this product may offer women the advantage of less frequent administration, it is important to note that on discontinuation of Depo-Provera, the return of fertility can be delayed by approximately 10 to 12 months (range 4–31 months).[8]

Depo-SubQ Provera 104 is also an injectable contraceptive product that contains only a progestin (depot medroxyprogesterone acetate). This product, which was approved by the FDA in 2005, is different from Depo-Provera in that it is given subcutaneously rather than intramuscularly, and it contains only 104 mg medroxyprogesterone acetate (approximately 30% less hormone) every 3 months for the prevention of pregnancy.[39] Clinical trials have demonstrated that the subcutaneous formulation of depot medroxyprogesterone acetate is as effective as the intramuscular formulation in the prevention of pregnancy.[40] Although this product carries the same warning in its package labeling regarding possible effects on BMD as DepoProvera,[39] it is not yet known if the lower progestin dose will lessen the potential for long-term side effects.

Implantable Devices

There are currently three implantable contraceptive devices available, two containing a progestin and one nonhormonal device. After insertion, Mirena, a levonorgestrel-releasing IUD, can provide contraceptive protection for up to 5 years. Paragard T 380A, a copper IUD, can provide contraceptive protection for up to 10 years. Implanon, the newest of the implantable devices, is an etonogestrel-releasing system that is surgically implanted under the skin of the upper arm and is effective for up to 3 years. Surveys have shown that IUDs have the highest satisfaction rate among patients using reversible contraceptives.

Although the mechanism of action for IUDs is not completely understood, several theories have been suggested. The original theory is that the presence of a foreign body in the uterus causes an inflammatory response that interferes with implantation. It is believed that copper-containing IUDs may have a direct toxic effect on spermatozoa. Progestin-containing implantable contraceptives can have direct effects on the uterus, such as thickening of cervical mucus and alterations to the endometrial lining. Mirena and Implanon can inhibit ovulation because they contain a progestin, but Paragard T 380A does not prevent ovulation.

It is important to evaluate a patient to determine if she is an appropriate candidate for an implantable contraceptive. Implantable contraceptives are recommended for women with at least one child, in a monogamous relationship, who have no history of pelvic inflammatory disease (PID) and no

history or risk of ectopic pregnancy. There are also multiple contraindications to IUD use. Evaluation of the patient is essential because IUDs cannot be used in the following situations: (a) pregnancy or suspected pregnancy, (b) anatomically abnormal or distorted uterine cavity, (c) acute PID or history of PID, unless there has been a subsequent intrauterine pregnancy, (d) postpartum endometritis or infected abortion in the past 3 months, (e) known or suspected uterine or cervical neoplasia or unresolved abnormal pap smear, (f) genital bleeding of unknown etiology, (g) untreated acute cervicitis or vaginitis, (h) acute liver disease or liver tumor, (i) woman or her partner has multiple sexual partners, (j) previously inserted IUD still in place, (k) conditions associated with increased susceptibility to infections (e.g., leukemia or acquired immune deficiency syndrome), (l) genital actinomycosis, (m) hypersensitivity to any component of the IUD, (n) known or suspected carcinoma of the breast, (o) history of ectopic pregnancy or a condition that would predispose to ectopic pregnancy, and (p) Wilson's disease.[41,42]

There are potential side effects of IUD use. The most common adverse effects are cramping, abnormal uterine bleeding, and expulsion of the device. Other side effects seen are ectopic pregnancy, sepsis, PID, embedment of the device, uterine or cervical perforation, and ovarian cysts.[41,42]

Nonpharmacologic Contraceptive Methods

▶ Barrier Contraceptives

As an alternative to hormonal contraceptives, several barrier contraceptive options are available for the prevention of pregnancy. While barrier contraceptives are associated with far fewer adverse effects compared with hormonal contraceptives, their efficacy is highly user-dependent. Overall, compared with both hormonal contraceptives and IUDs, barrier contraceptives are associated with much higher accidental pregnancy rates.[8] (Table 48–1).

Diaphragms and Cervical Caps Diaphragms and cervical caps are dome-shaped rubber caps that are placed over the cervix to provide barrier protection during intercourse. Both diaphragms and cervical caps require fitting by a health care professional, and they must be refitted in the event of weight gain or weight loss. Diaphragms or cervical caps typically can be placed over the cervix as much as 6 hours prior to intercourse. They must be left in place for at least 6 hours after intercourse before they can be removed. Diaphragms should not be left in place longer than 24 hours, and smaller cervical caps should not be left in place longer than 48 hours owing to the risk of toxic shock syndrome (TSS). Diaphragms and cervical caps are used along with spermicides to prevent pregnancy. When sexual intercourse is repeated with the diaphragm, reapplication of the spermicide is necessary. However, when sexual intercourse is repeated with a cervical cap, reapplication of the spermicide typically is not necessary.[8] Whether or not diaphragms or cervical caps provide adequate protection against STDs remains unclear.[43]

Spermicides Nonoxynol-9, a surfactant that destroys the cell membranes of sperm, is the most commonly used spermicide in the United States.[8,44] Nonoxynol-9 is available in a variety of forms, including a cream, foam, film, gel, suppository, and tablet. Spermicides may be used alone, with a barrier method, or adjunctively with other forms of contraceptives to provide additional protection against unwanted pregnancy.[44] To be used most effectively, spermicides must be placed in the vagina not more than 1 hour prior to sexual intercourse, and they must come in contact with the cervix.[8] While the efficacy of spermicides depends largely on how consistently and correctly they are used, their efficacy is enhanced when they are used in combination with a barrier contraceptive device.[44] Clinical trials assessing the ability of spermicides to protect against STDs have failed to produce positive results.[44] Further, there exists some evidence to suggest that frequent use of spermicides actually may increase risk for transmission of HIV secondary to vaginal mucosal tissue breakdown, which may allow a portal of entry for the virus.[8] In December 2007, the FDA issued a statement requiring manufacturers of nonoxynol-9 products to include a warning on the product label indicating that the spermicide does not provide protection against infection from HIV or other STDs.

Condoms Condoms, which are available for both male and female use, act as physical barriers to prevent sperm from coming into contact with ova.[45] Condoms are easy to use, available without a prescription, and inexpensive. Most condoms are made of latex. When used correctly, condoms can be very effective in prevention of unwanted pregnancy. Condoms should be stored in a cool, dry place, away from exposure to direct sunlight. When stored improperly or when used with oil-based lubricants, however, latex condoms can break during intercourse, increasing the risk of pregnancy.[8] For latex-sensitive individuals, condoms made from lamb intestine ("natural membrane" condoms) and synthetic polyurethane condoms are available. Unlike latex condoms, condoms made from lamb intestine contain small pores that may permit the passage of viruses and therefore do not provide adequate protection against STDs.[45] ❺ *Both latex and synthetic condoms can provide some protection against many STDs. Data from one metaanalysis suggested that HIV transmission can be reduced by as much as 90% when condoms are consistently used.[46] This is in contrast to hormonal contraceptives (oral, transdermal, or vaginal), IUDs, and most other barrier contraceptives, which do not protect against STDs.* Relative to male condoms, female condoms may offer even better protection against STDs because they provide more extensive barrier coverage of external genitalia, including the labia and the base of the penis.[44] It is important to note that the male and female condoms are not recommended to be used together because they may adhere to one another, causing displacement of one or both condoms.[44]

Sponge The Today sponge is a small, pillow-shaped polyurethane sponge impregnated with nonoxynol-9.[44] It is an over-the-counter barrier contraceptive that has been shown to be generally less effective at preventing pregnancy than diaphragms.[47] The sponge is moistened with water and then is inserted and placed over the cervix for up to 6 hours prior to sexual intercourse. The sponge then is left in place for at least 6 hours following intercourse.[44] Although the sponge maintains efficacy for 24 hours (even if intercourse is repeated), as with diaphragms, the sponge should be removed after 24 hours owing to the risk of TSS.[8]

▶ *Fertility Awareness–Based Methods*

Fertility awareness–based methods (natural methods) represent another nonpharmacologic means of pregnancy prevention. Although failure rates of such methods can be high, some couples still prefer these types of approaches. Fertility awareness–based methods depend on the ability of the couple to identify the woman's "fertile window," or the period of time in which pregnancy is most likely to occur as a result of sexual intercourse.[48] During the fertile window, the couple practices abstinence, or avoidance of intercourse, in order to prevent pregnancy. In some cases, rather than practicing abstinence during the fertile period, some couples may prefer to employ barrier methods or spermicides as a means of preventing pregnancy rather than to avoid intercourse altogether.[8] In order to identify the fertile window, a number of different fertility awareness–based methods may be tried. The calendar (rhythm) method involves counting the days in the menstrual cycle and then using a mathematical equation to determine the fertile window.[48] The temperature method involves monitoring changes in the woman's basal body temperature using a basal thermometer.[48] The cervical mucus (or Billings ovulation) method involves observing changes in the characteristics of cervical secretions throughout the cycle.[48] Around ovulation, the mucus becomes watery. The symptothermal method, which is considered to be the most difficult to learn but potentially the most effective, is a combination of both

---

Patient Encounter, Part 3: Missed Doses

RC calls your clinic in a panic today because she forgot to start a new package of oral contraceptives. Three days have elapsed since she took her last placebo pill, and she reports having had unprotected sexual intercourse last night. The patient is very concerned about her risk of pregnancy, and she would like to discuss her options for prevention of pregnancy. ❻ *When a contraceptive dose is missed, the risk of accidental pregnancy may be increased. Depending on how many doses were missed, the contraceptive formulation being used, and the phase of the cycle during which doses were missed, counseling regarding the use of additional methods of contraception may be warranted.*

Given this patient's reported imperfect use of her oral contraceptive, what information can you provide to the patient regarding her risk of pregnancy?

Provide appropriate patient education regarding the use of Plan B.

Patient Care and Monitoring

1. Obtain a thorough medical and family history and carefully evaluate each patient's risk factors prior to prescribing contraceptives.

2. Educate all women taking hormonal contraceptives to prevent pregnancy regarding self-monitoring for early warning signs that may precede adverse events. Health care professionals can easily recall the major warning signs by using the two simple pneumonics highlighted below:

   ACHES—for women taking hormonal contraceptives

   A = Abdominal pain. This may be an early warning sign of the presence of an abdominal thromboembolism, liver adenoma, or gallbladder disease.

   C = Chest pain. The presence of chest pain may indicate pulmonary embolism, angina, or myocardial infarction.

   H = Headaches. Headaches (particularly those associated with focal neurologic symptoms, such as blurred vision, speech impairment, and/or weakness) may represent strokelike symptoms. Headaches also may indicate poorly controlled blood pressure.

   E = Eye problems. Blurred vision and/or ocular pain may be early warning signs for stroke and/or blood clots. In addition, visual changes may occur in patients wearing contact lenses (secondary to changes in corneal shape).

   S = Severe leg pain. Patients taking hormonal contraceptives who complain of severe leg pain should be evaluated for the presence of venous thromboembolism.

   PAINS—for women with an IUD

   P = Period late

   A = Abdominal pain, pain with intercourse

   I = Infection, abnormal or odorous vaginal discharge

   N = Not feeling well, fever, chills

   S = String (missing, shorter, longer)

3. In addition to the preceding, monitor patients taking hormonal contraceptives for missed periods, signs of pregnancy, appearance of jaundice, and/or severe mood changes. Instruct patients to consult a health care professional upon noticing or experiencing any of these warning signs.[1]

4. Stress the importance of adherence to the patient's chosen method of contraception in order to reliably prevent pregnancy. Educate the patient on what to do in the event of missed doses with hormonal contraception.

cycles or who have difficulty interpreting their fertility signs correctly.[48]

Emergency Contraception

Emergency contraception (EC) is used to prevent pregnancy after known or suspected unprotected sexual intercourse. Previously, the *Yuzpe regimen*, named after Alfred Yuzpe who discovered it in 1974, using ethinyl estradiol and levonorgestrel, was a widely used EC option for women. This regimen had an increased risk of side effects and no difference in efficacy compared to the use of levonorgestrel alone; thus, it is no longer marketed for this use. Plan B is an FDA-approved emergency contraceptive currently available. With this formulation, patients take one tablet of 0.75 mg levonorgestrel within 72 hours of unprotected intercourse and then a second dose 12 hours later. In 2009, the FDA approved Plan B for nonprescription sale to patients 17 years of age and older. It is important to note that EC is more effective the earlier it is used after unprotected intercourse. This progestin-only formulation has shown decreased risk of side effects such as nausea and vomiting compared to the Yuzpe method, which decreases the risk of EC failure.

OUTCOME EVALUATION/MONITORING

Side effects of contraceptives tend to occur in the first few months of therapy. Thus, schedule a follow-up visit 3 to 6 months after initiating a new contraceptive. Yearly checkups usually are sufficient for patients who are doing well on a particular product.[1] At each follow-up visit, assess blood pressure, headache frequency, and menstrual bleeding patterns, as well as compliance with the prescribed regimen.

Abbreviations Introduced in This Chapter

BMD	Bone mineral density
COC	Combined oral contraceptive
CYP450	Cytochrome P450
EC	Emergency contraception
FSH	Follicle-stimulating hormone
GnRH	Gonadotropin-releasing hormone
HDL	High-density lipoprotein
HPV	Human papilloma virus
IUD	Intrauterine device
LDL	Low-density lipoprotein
LH	Luteinizing hormone
PID	Pelvic inflammatory disease
STD	Sexually transmitted disease
TSS	Toxic shock syndrome

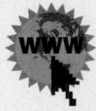

Self-assessment questions and answers are available at *http://www.mhpharmacotherapy. com/pp.html.*

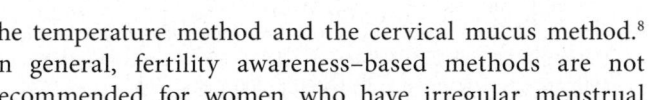

the temperature method and the cervical mucus method.[8] In general, fertility awareness–based methods are not recommended for women who have irregular menstrual

REFERENCES

1. Nelson A. Combined oral contraceptives. In: Hatcher RA, Trussel J, Nelson AL, et al. Contraceptive Technology, 19th rev. ed. New York: Ardent Media, 2007:193–270.

2. Blackburn RD, Cunkelman A, Zlidar VM. Oral contraceptives—An update. Popul Rep A 2000;28:1–32.

3. Abma JC, Chandra A, Mosher WD, et al. Fertility, family planning, and women's health: New data from the 1995 National Survey of Family Growth. Vital Health Stat 1997;19:series 23.

4. Henshaw SK. Unintended pregnancy in the United States. Fam Plann Perspect 1998;30:24–29.

5. Cates W Jr, and the American Social Health Association Panel. Estimates of the incidence and prevalence of sexually transmitted diseases in the United States. Sex Transm Dis 1999;26:S2–S7.

6. Hatcher RA, Namnoum AB. The menstrual cycle. In: Hatcher RA, Trussel J, Nelson AL, et al. Contraceptive Technology, 19th rev. ed. New York: Ardent Media, 2007:7–18.

7. Trussel J. Choosing a contraceptive: Efficacy, safety, and personal considerations. In: Hatcher RA, Trussel J, Nelson AL, et al. Contraceptive Technology, 19th rev. ed. New York: Ardent Media, 2007:19–48.

8. Anonymous. Choice of contraceptives: Treatment Guidelines from The Medical Letter. Med Lett 2007;64:101–108.

9. Vessey MP, Painter R. Endometrial and ovarian cancer and oral contraceptives—Findings in a large cohort study. Br J Cancer 1995;71:1340–1342.

10. Ness RB, Grisso JA, Klapper J, et al., for the SHARE Study Group. Risk of ovarian cancer in relation to estrogen and progestin dose and use characteristics of oral contraceptives. Steroid hormones and reproduction. Am J Epidemiol 2000;152:233–241.

11. Burkman RT. Oral contraceptives: Current status. Clin Obstet Gynecol 2001;44:62–72.

12. Schildkraut JM, Calingaert B, Marchbanks PA, et al. Impact of progestin and estrogen potency in oral contraceptives on ovarian cancer risk. J Natl Cancer Inst 2002;94:32–38.

13. Iyer V, Farquhar C, Jepson R. Oral contraceptive pills for heavy menstrual bleeding. Cochrane Database Syst Rev 2000;2:CD000154.

14. Panser LA, Phipps WR. Type of oral contraceptive in relation to acute, initial episodes of pelvic inflammatory disease. Contraception 1991;43:91–99.

15. Tanis BC, van den Bosch MA, Kemmeren JM, et al. Oral contraceptives and the risk of myocardial infarction. Arch Intern Med 2001;161:1065–1070.

16. Schwingl PJ, Ory HW, Visness CM. Estimates of the risk of cardiovascular death attributable to low-dose oral contraceptives in the United States. Am J Obstet Gynecol 1999;180:241–249.

17. Chang CL, Donaghy M, Poulter N. Migraine and stroke in young women: Case-control study. The World Health Organization Collaborative Study of Cardiovascular Disease and Steroid Hormone Contraception. BMJ 1999;318:13–18.

18. Curtis KM, Chrisman CE, Peterson HB, WHO Programme for Mapping Best Practices in Reproductive Health. Contraception for women in selected circumstances. Obstet Gynecol 2002;99:1100–1112.

19. Petitti DB. Clinical practice. Combination estrogen-progestin oral contraceptives. N Engl J Med 2003;349:1443–1450.

20. Hennessy S, Berlin JA, Kinman JL, et al. Risk of venous thromboembolism from oral contraceptives containing gestodene and desogestrel versus levonorgestrel: A meta-analysis and formal sensitivity analysis. Contraception 2001;64:125–133.

21. Kemmeren JM, Algra A, Grobbee DE. Third generation oral contraceptives and risk of venous thrombosis: Meta-analysis. BMJ 2001;323:131–134.

22. Marchbanks PA, McDonald JA, Wilson HG, et al. Oral contraceptives and the risk of breast cancer. N Engl J Med 2002;346:2025–2032.

23. Collaborative Group on Hormonal Factors in Breast Cancer. Breast cancer and hormonal contraceptives: Collaborative reanalysis of individual data on 53,297 women with breast cancer and 100,239 women without breast cancer from 54 epidemiological studies. Lancet 1996;347:1713–1727.

24. Redmond G, Godwin AJ, Olson W, Lippman JS. Use of placebo controls in an oral contraceptive trial: Methodological issues and adverse event incidence. Contraception 1999;60:81–85.

25. Graham CA, Ramos R, Bancroft J, et al. The effects of steroidal contraceptives on the well-being and sexuality of women: A double-blind, placebo-controlled, two-centre study of combined and progestogen-only methods. Contraception 1995;52:363–369.

26. Rosenberg MJ, Meyers A, Roy V. Efficacy, cycle control, and side effects of low- and lower-dose oral contraceptives: A randomized trial of 20 micrograms and 35 micrograms estrogen preparations. Contraception 1999;60:321–329.

27. Duramed Pharmaceuticals. Product information for Seasonale. Pomona, NY: Duramed Pharmaceuticals, Inc; 2003(Sep).

28. Vercellini P, Frontino G, De Giorgi O, et al. Continuous use of an oral contraceptive for endometriosis-associated recurrent dysmenorrhea that does not respond to a cyclic pill regimen. Fertil Steril 2003;80: 560–563.

29. Berlex, Inc. Product information for Yasmin. Montville, NJ: Berlex, Inc; 2005(Feb).

30. Mircette Patient Information Guide. *http://www.mircette.com/guide.html.*

31. Bristol-Myers Squibb Co. Product information for Ovcon 35. Princeton, NJ: Bristol-Myers Squibb Co; 2003(Nov).

32. Wyeth Pharmaceuticals, Inc. Product information for levonorgestrel 90 mcg and ethinyl estradiol 20 mc (Lybrel). Philadelphia, PA: Wyeth Pharmaceuticals; 2007(May).

33. Tom W. Oral contraceptive drug interactions. Pharmacist's Letter/Prescriber's Letter 2005;21:210903.

34. Anonymous. Ortho Evra—A contraceptive patch. Med Lett Drugs Ther 2002;1122:8.

35. Anonymous. An update on Ortho Evra and the risk of thromboembolism. Pharmacist's Letter/Prescribers Letter 2005;21:211202.

36. Smallwood GH, Meador ML, Lenihan JP, et al. for the Ortho Evra/Evra 002 Study Group. Efficacy and safety of a transdermal contraceptive system. Obstet Gynecol 2001;98:799–805.

37. Dieben TO, Roumen FJ, Apter D. Efficacy, cycle control, and user acceptability of a novel combined contraceptive vaginal ring. Obstet Gynecol 2002;100:585–593.

38. Westhoff C. Bone mineral density and DMPA. J Reprod Med 2002;47:795–799.

39. Pharmacia and Upjohn. Product information for Depo-subQ Provera 104. New York: Pharmacia and Upjohn; 2005(Mar).

40. Toh YC, Jain J, Rahnny MH, et al. Suppression of ovulation by a new subcutaneous depot medroxyprogesterone acetate (104 mg/0.65 mL) contraceptive formulation in Asian women. Clin Ther 2004;26:1845–1854.

41. Berlex, Inc. Product information for Mirena. Montville, NJ: Berlex; 2004(Sep).

42. FEI Products LLC. Product information for Paragard T 380A. N. Tonawanda, NY: FEI Products LLC; 2003(Oct).

43. Moench TR, Chipato T, Padian NS. Preventing disease by protecting the cervix: The unexplored promise of internal vaginal barrier devices. AIDS 2001;15:1595–1602.

44. Cates W Jr, Raymond EG. Vaginal barriers and spermicides. In: Hatcher RA, Trussel J, Nelson AL, et al. Contraceptive Technology, 19th rev. ed. New York: Ardent Media, 2007:317–336.

45. Warner L, Steiner MJ. Male condoms. In: Hatcher RA, Trussel J, Nelson AL, et al. Contraceptive Technology, 19th rev. ed. New York: Ardent Media, 2007:297–316.

46. Davis KR, Weller SC. The effectiveness of condoms in reducing heterosexual transmission of HIV. Fam Plann Perspect 1999;31:272–279.

47. Kuyoh MA, Toroitich-Ruto C, Grimes DA, et al. Sponge versus diaphragm for contraception: A Cochrane review. Contraception 2003;67:15–18.

48. Jennings VH, Arevalo M. Fertility awareness-based methods. In: Hatcher RA, Trussel J, Nelson, AL, et al. Contraceptive Technology, 19th rev. ed. New York: Ardent Media, 2007:343–360.

49

Menstruation-Related Disorders

Elena M. Umland, Lara C. Weinstein, and Edward Buchanan

LEARNING OBJECTIVES

● **Upon completion of the chapter, the reader will be able to:**

1. Describe the underlying etiology and pathophysiology of amenorrhea, menorrhagia, dysmenorrhea, and anovulatory bleeding and how they relate to selection of effective treatment modalities.

2. Describe the clinical presentation of amenorrhea, menorrhagia, dysmenorrhea, and anovulatory bleeding.

3. Recommend appropriate lifestyle and dietary modifications and pharmacotherapeutic interventions for patients with amenorrhea, menorrhagia, dysmenorrhea, and anovulatory bleeding.

4. Identify the desired therapeutic outcomes for patients with amenorrhea, menorrhagia, dysmenorrhea, and anovulatory bleeding.

5. Design a monitoring plan to assess the effectiveness and adverse effects of pharmacotherapy for amenorrhea, menorrhagia, dysmenorrhea, and anovulatory bleeding.

KEY CONCEPTS

❶ Unrecognized pregnancy remains the most common cause of amenorrhea, and a urine pregnancy test should be one of the first steps in the evaluation of this disorder.

❷ For most conditions associated with primary and secondary amenorrhea, estrogen treatment (along with a progestin to minimize the risk of endometrial hyperplasia) is utilized.

❸ Causes of menorrhagia can be divided into systemic disorders and specific uterine abnormalities.

❹ Intrauterine pregnancy, ectopic pregnancy, and miscarriage must be at the top of the differential diagnosis list for any woman presenting with heavy menses.

❺ The reduction in menorrhagia-related blood loss with the use of nonsteroidal anti-inflammatory drugs (NSAIDs) and oral contraceptives (OCs) is directly proportional to the amount of pretreatment blood loss.

❻ The most significant mechanism for primary dysmenorrhea is the release of prostanoids and possible eicosanoids in the menstrual fluid; given their impact on inhibiting prostaglandins as well as their ability to provide direct analgesia, NSAIDs are the treatment of choice.

❼ Intrauterine devices (IUDs) are considered therapeutic options in a variety of menstrual-related disorders. Guidelines from the American College of Obstetricians and Gynecologists (ACOG) indicate that any woman (regardless of parity) at low risk of sexually transmitted diseases is a good candidate for IUD use.

❽ Anovulatory bleeding, also referred to as dysfunctional uterine bleeding, is secondary to the effects of unopposed estrogen and does not include bleeding owing to an anatomic lesion of the uterus.

❾ The use of metformin and thiazolidinediones for anovulatory bleeding associated with polycystic ovary syndrome (PCOS) is beneficial for anovulatory bleeding and fertility and also improves glucose tolerance and decreases overall cardiovascular risk.

Problems related to the menstrual cycle are common in women of reproductive age. The issues considered in this chapter are the most frequently encountered menstrual-related difficulties and include amenorrhea, menorrhagia, dysmenorrhea, and dysfunctional uterine bleeding. The need for effective treatments for these disorders stems from their impact on any or all of the following: A reduced quality of life, negative effects on reproductive health, and the potential for long-term detrimental health effects, such as osteoporosis in the case of amenorrhea and cardiovascular disease in the case of polycystic ovary disease.

AMENORRHEA

Amenorrhea is described as either primary or secondary in nature. Primary amenorrhea is the absence of menses by age 16 in the presence of normal secondary sexual development or the absence of menses by age 14 in the absence of normal secondary sexual development. Secondary amenorrhea is the absence of menses for three cycles or 6 months in a previously menstruating woman. However, in clinical practice, there is a significant amount of overlap. The initial evaluation of amenorrhea is often the same regardless of age of onset, except in unusual clinical situations.[1]

EPIDEMIOLOGY AND ETIOLOGY

❶ *Unrecognized pregnancy remains the most common cause of amenorrhea, and a urine pregnancy test should be one of the first steps in the evaluation of this disorder.* To help organize an approach to diagnosis and treatment, it is helpful to consider the organs involved in the menstrual cycle, which include the uterus, ovaries, anterior pituitary, and hypothalamus. After pregnancy, the five most common causes of secondary amenorrhea, in descending order of prevalence, include[2]:

- Hypothalamic suppression (33%)
- Chronic anovulation (28%)
- Hyperprolactinemia (14%)
- Ovarian failure (12%)
- Uterine disorders (7%)

PATHOPHYSIOLOGY

The physiology of the normal menstrual cycle depends on a coordinated system of hormonal interactions involving the hypothalamus, anterior pituitary gland, ovary, and endometrium. Figures 49–1 and 49–2 summarize these points. Pulsatile gonadotropin-releasing hormone (GnRH)

secretion from the hypothalamus stimulates the anterior pituitary to secrete follicle-stimulating hormone (FSH) and luteinizing hormone (LH). In the specialized cells of the ovarian follicle, FSH and LH stimulate the release of estradiol. Estradiol stimulates endometrial growth during the follicular phase of the cycle. Following the LH surge and ovulation, the follicle is transformed into the corpus luteum. Progesterone that is secreted by the corpus luteum during the luteal phase of the cycle causes endometrial "organization." If conception does not occur, the drop in estrogen and progesterone stimulates the shedding of the endometrium.[3]

Table 49–1 illustrates the pathophysiology of amenorrhea relative to the organ system(s) involved, as well as the related condition(s) that result in amenorrhea. Amenorrhea is also an expected, potential side effect resulting from the use of low-dose oral contraceptives (OCs), extended-cycle OC pill use, or depo medroxyprogesterone acetate (MPA) use.[8] Many women may experience delayed return of menses after discontinuation of OCs. Postpill amenorrhea usually

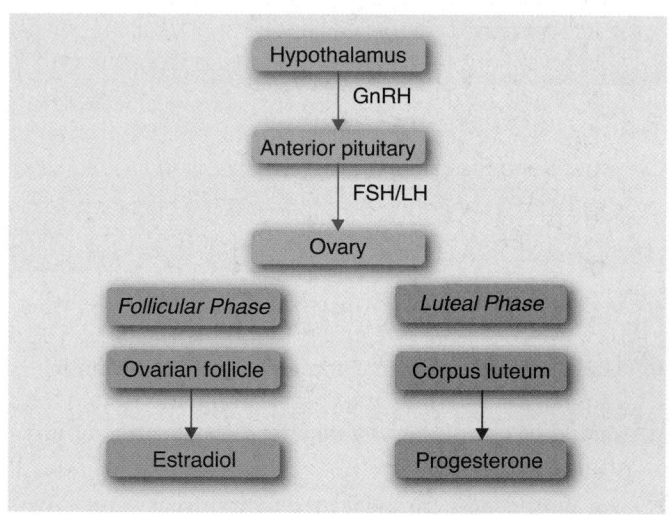

FIGURE 49–1. Summary of the normal menstrual cycle.

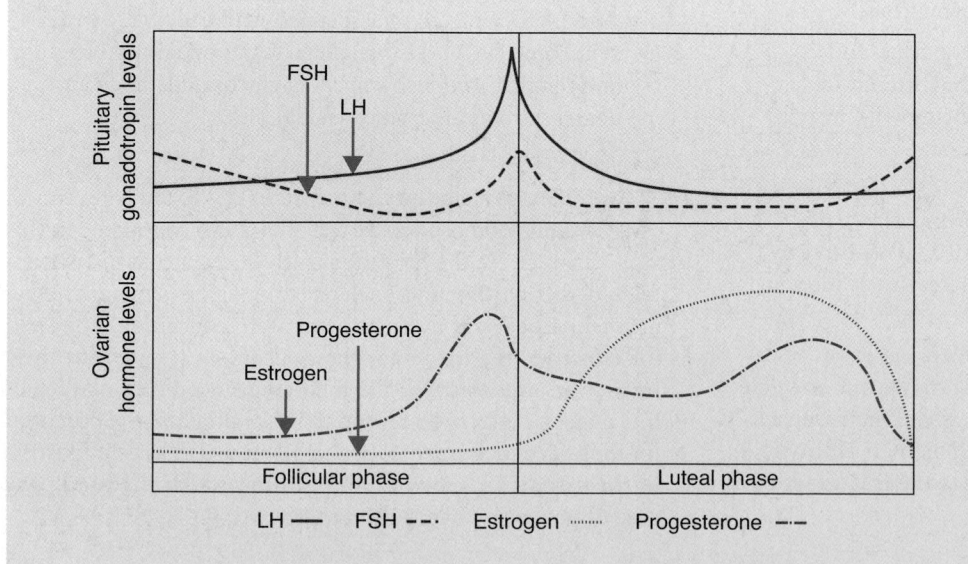

FIGURE 49–2. Hormonal fluctuations with the normal menstrual cycle. (From DiPiro JT, Talbert RL, Yee GC, et al., (eds.) Pharmacotherapy: A Pathophysiologic Approach. 7th ed. New York: McGraw-Hill, 2008.)

Table 49–1

Pathophysiology of Selected Menstrual Bleeding Disorders

Organ System	Condition	Pathophysiology/Laboratory Findings
Amenorrhea		
Uterus	Asherman's syndrome	Postcurettage/postsurgical uterine adhesions
	Congenital uterine abnormalities	Abnormal uterine development
Ovaries	Turner's syndrome	Lack of ovarian follicles
	Gonadal dysgenesis	Other genetic anomalies
	Premature ovarian failure	Early loss of follicles
	Chemotherapy/radiation	Gonadal toxins
Anterior pituitary	Pituitary prolactin-secreting adenoma	↑ Prolactin suppresses HPO axis
	Hypothyroidism	TRH causing ↑ prolactin, other abnormalities
	Medications—antipsychotics, verapamil	↑ Prolactin suppresses HPO axis
Hypothalamus	"Functional" hypothalamic amenorrhea	↓ Pulsatile GnRH secretion in the absence of other abnormalities
	Disordered eating	↓ Pulsatile GnRH secretion, ↓ FSH and LH secondary to weight loss
	Exercise	↓ Pulsatile GnRH secretion, ↓ FSH and LH secondary to low body fat
	Anovulation/PCOS	Asynchronous gonadotropin and estrogen production, abnormal endometrial growth
Anovulatory bleeding		
Physiologic causes	Adolescence	Immaturity of the hypothalamic–pituitary–ovarian axis: No LH surge
	Perimenopause	Declining ovarian function
Pathologic causes	Hyperandrogenic anovulation—PCOS	Hyperandrogenism: High testosterone, high LH, hyperinsulinemia, and insulin resistance
	Hypothalamic dysfunction (physical or emotional stress, exercise, weight loss)	Suppression of pulsatile GnRH secretion and estrogen deficiency: Low LH, low FSH
	Hyperprolactinemia (pituitary gland tumor, psychiatric medications)	High prolactin
	Hypothyroidism	High TSH
	Premature ovarian failure	High FSH
Menorrhagia		
Hematologic	von Willebrand's disease	Factor VII defect causing impaired platelet adhesion and increased bleeding time
	Idiopathic thrombocytopenic purpura	Decrease in circulating platelets—can be acute or chronic
Hepatic	Cirrhosis	Decreased estrogen metabolism, underlying coagulopathy
Endocrine	Hypothyroidism	Alterations in HPO axis
Uterine	Fibroids	Alteration of endometrium, changes in uterine contractility
	Adenomyosis	Alteration of endometrium, changes in uterine contractility
	Endometrial polyps	Alteration of endometrium
	Gynecologic cancers	Various dysplastic alterations of endometrium, uterus, cervix

↑, high; ↓, low; FSH, follicle-stimulating hormone; GnRH, gonadotropin-releasing hormone; HPO, hypothalamic–pituitary–ovarian axis; LH, luteinizing hormone; PCOS, polycystic ovary disease; TRH, thyrotropin-releasing hormone; TSH, thyroid-stimulating hormone.

From Refs. 1, 4–7.

is a self-limited condition. Further evaluation for other unrecognized conditions, such as polycystic ovary syndrome (PCOS), should be considered if spontaneous resolution of the amenorrhea does not occur within 3 to 6 months following discontinuation of the OCs.

TREATMENT

Desired Outcomes

Therapeutic modalities for amenorrhea are targeted at restoring the normal menstrual cycle. The goals of treatment are to preserve bone density, prevent bone loss, and restore ovulation,

thus improving fertility as desired. Amenorrhea resulting from conditions contributing to hypoestrogenism also may affect quality of life via the induction of hot flashes (premature ovarian failure), dyspareunia, and in prepubertal females, lack of secondary sexual characteristics, and absence of menarche.

Nonpharmacologic Therapy

Nonpharmacologic therapy for amenorrhea varies depending on its underlying cause. Amenorrhea secondary to anorexia may respond to weight gain. Such patients would also benefit from psychotherapy. In young women for whom excessive exercise is an underlying cause, a reduction in exercise is recommended.

Clinical Presentation and Diagnosis of Amenorrhea

General

Patients may be concerned about cessation of menses and fertility implications but generally are not in acute distress

Symptoms

- Cessation of menses
- Possible complaints of infertility, vaginal dryness, decreased libido

Signs

- Cessation of menses for longer than 6 months in women with established menstruation, or absence of menses by age 16 in the presence of normal secondary sexual development, or absence of menses by age 14 in the absence of normal secondary sexual development
- Recent significant weight loss or weight gain
- Presence of acne, hirsutism, hair loss, or **acanthosis nigricans** may suggest androgen excess

Laboratory Tests

- Pregnancy test
- TSH
- Prolactin
- If PCOS is suspected, consider free or total testosterone, 17-hydroxyprogesterone, fasting glucose, and fasting lipid panel
- If premature ovarian failure is suspected, consider FSH and LH measurements

Other Diagnostic Tests

- Progesterone challenge
- Pelvic ultrasound to evaluate for polycystic ovaries

Patient Encounter 1, Part 1

JK is an 18-year-old African American woman who presents to her physician with complaints of no menses for 8 months. She is sexually active and has been with the same male partner for the last 5 months. She is not using any form of contraception. She has recently begun college. In addition, she has been active in cross-country training for the past 4 years.

What menstruation-related disorder does this patient have?

What are the potential etiologies for this condition?

Pharmacologic Therapy

▶ *Estrogen/Progestin Replacement Therapy*

❷ *For most conditions associated with primary or secondary amenorrhea, estrogen treatment (along with a progestin to minimize the risk of endometrial hyperplasia) is utilized. The purpose of estrogen therapy in this patient population is twofold: To reduce the risk of osteoporosis and to improve quality of life.[9,10] Table 49–2 identifies a variety of therapeutic options for amenorrhea, including recommended doses. Figure 49–3 illustrates a treatment algorithm for the management of amenorrhea.*

▶ *Bromocriptine*

If hyperprolactinemia is identified as the cause of amenorrhea, the use of bromocriptine, a dopamine agonist, results in a reduction in prolactin concentrations and the resumption of menses.

Amenorrhea related to anovulation resulting from PCOS may respond to the use of agents that reduce insulin resistance. The use of metformin for this purpose will be discussed in the anovulatory bleeding section that follows.

▶ *Progesterone*

Progestins have long been used to induce withdrawal bleeding in women with secondary amenorrhea. Several factors predict the efficacy of progesterone for this purpose.[15] These factors include estrogen concentrations greater than or equal to 35 pg/mL (128 pmol/L) and endometrial thickness (the greater it is, the greater is the amount of withdrawal bleeding).

The efficacy of progestins for secondary amenorrhea also varies depending on the formulation used. For example, progesterone in oil administered intramuscularly results in withdrawal bleeding in 70% of treated patients, whereas oral MPA induces withdrawal bleeding in 95% of treated patients.[15] Table 49–2 identifies the types and doses of progesterones used for inducing withdrawal bleeding in women with secondary amenorrhea. Figure 49–3 illustrates when to consider the use of progesterone for the treatment of amenorrhea.

For all patients experiencing amenorrhea, owing to the negative impact this has on bone health, it is essential that a diet rich in calcium and vitamin D be followed.

AMENORRHEA IN ADOLESCENTS

Amenorrhea in the adolescent population is of great importance because this is the time in the female life cycle when peak bone mass is achieved. The cause of amenorrhea and appropriate treatment must be identified promptly in this population because hypoestrogenism contributes negatively to bone development. Estrogen replacement, typically via an OC, is important. In addition, ensuring that the patient is receiving adequate amounts of calcium and vitamin D is imperative.

Table 49–2

Therapeutic Agents for Selected Menstrual Disorders

Specific Menstrual Disorder(s)	Agent(s)	Dose Recommended	Common Adverse Effects
Amenorrhea (primary or secondary)	CEE	0.625–1.25 mg by mouth daily on days 1–25 of the cycle[10]	Thromboembolism, breast enlargement, breast tenderness, bloating, nausea, GI upset, headache, peripheral edema
	Ethinyl estradiol patch Combination OC	50 mcg/24 hours 30–40 mcg formulations[9]	
Amenorrhea (secondary)	Oral MPA	5–10 mg by mouth on days 14–25 of the cycle[10]	Edema, anorexia, depression, insomnia, weight gain or loss, increase in serum total and LDL cholesterol, may reduce HDL cholesterol
Amenorrhea related to hyperprolactinemia	Bromocriptine	2.5 mg by mouth 2–3 × daily	Hypotension, nausea, constipation, anorexia, Raynaud's phenomenon
Anovulatory bleeding	Combination OC	Optimal dose unknown[7] For acute bleeding, product containing 35 mcg ethinyl estradiol; take one tablet by mouth 3 × daily × 1 week; then one tablet by mouth daily × 3 weeks[13]	As noted above for CEE, ethinyl estradiol, and combination OC (progesterone side effects with the OC depend on agent chosen)
	Oral MPA	For acute bleeding, 20 mg by mouth 3 × daily × 1 week; then 20 mg by mouth once daily × 3 weeks[13]	As noted above for oral MPA
Dysmenorrhea	Combination OC	Less than 35 mcg formulations + norgestrel or levonorgestrel[14]; use of extended-cycle formulations are beneficial for this indication	As noted above for CEE, ethinyl estradiol, and combination OC (progesterone side effects with the OC depend on agent chosen)
	Depo MPA	150 mg intramuscularly every 12 weeks	Irregular menses, amenorrhea
	Levonorgestrel IUD[12]	20 mcg released daily	Irregular menses, amenorrhea
	NSAIDs—any are acceptable; the most commonly studied/cited are included in this table	Diclofenac 50 mg by mouth 3 × daily	GI upset, stomach ulcer, nausea, vomiting, heartburn, indigestion, rash, dizziness
		Ibuprofen 800 mg by mouth 3 × daily Mefenamic acid 500 mg by mouth as a loading dose, then 250 mg by mouth up to 4 × daily as needed[11] Naproxen 550 mg loading dose by mouth started 1–2 days prior to menses, followed by 275 mg by mouth every 6–12 hours as needed[14] Treatment should begin 1–2 days prior to the suspected onset of menses[11]	
Menorrhagia	Combination OC	Optimal dose unknown	As noted above
	Levonorgestrel IUD	20 mcg released daily	As noted above
	MPA (oral)	5–10 mg by mouth on days 5–26 of the cycle *or* during the luteal phase[12]	As noted above
	NSAIDs	Doses as recommended for above; therapy should be initiated with the onset of menses[12]	As noted above
PCOS-related amenorrhea and/or anovulatory bleeding	Clomiphene[8]	50 mg by mouth daily × 5 days starting 3–5 days after the start of menses; doses up to 100 mg by mouth daily have been used in significantly obese patients	Hot flashes, ovarian enlargement, thromboembolism, blurred vision, breast discomfort
	Depo MPA	150 mg intramuscularly every 12 weeks	As noted above
	MPA (oral)	10 mg by mouth × 10 days[7]	As noted above
	Metformin	1,500–2,000 mg by mouth daily in 2–3 divided doses[7]	Anorexia, nausea, vomiting, diarrhea, flatulence, lactic acidosis
	Thiazolidinediones[7]	Pioglitazone 15–45 mg by mouth daily; rosiglitazone 4–8 mg by mouth daily	Weight gain; increase in total, LDL, and HDL cholesterol; edema; headache; fatigue; hepatic injury (rare)

CEE, conjugated equine estrogen; HDL, high-density lipoprotein; IUD, intrauterine device; LDL, low-density lipoprotein; OC, oral contraceptive; NSAIDs, nonsteroidal anti-inflammatory drugs; MPA, medroxyprogesterone acetate.

From Refs. 7, 9–14.

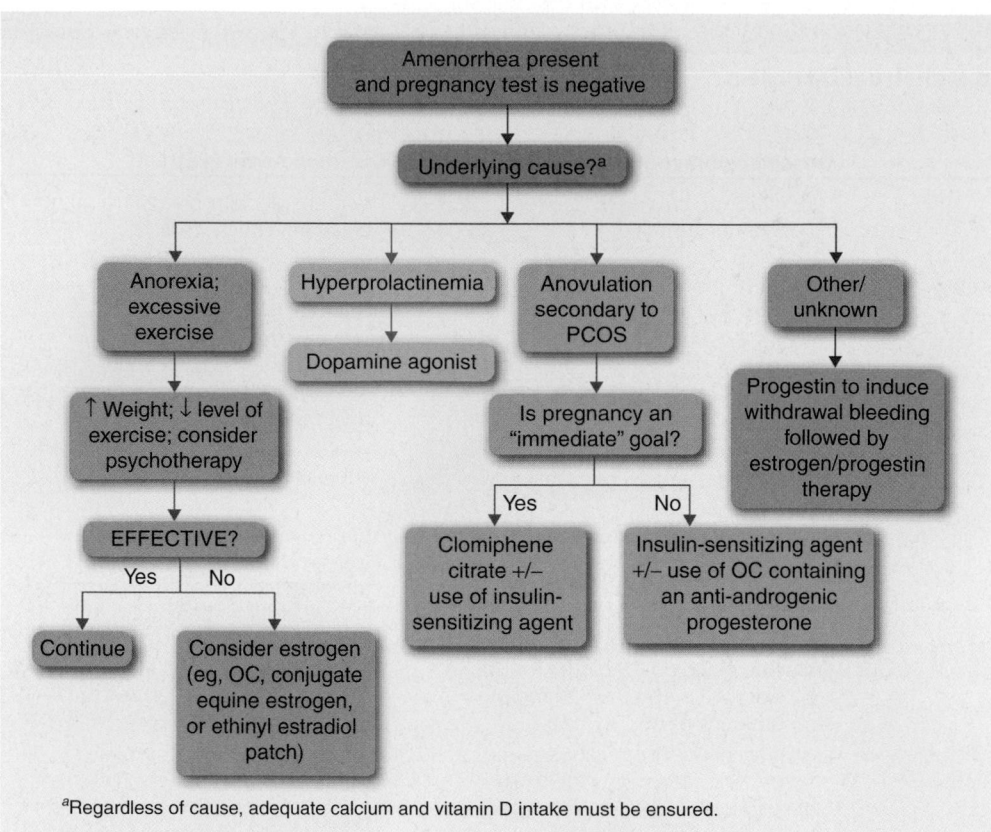

FIGURE 49–3. Treatment algorithm for amenorrhea.

aRegardless of cause, adequate calcium and vitamin D intake must be ensured.

Patient Encounter 1, Part 2

Additional Workup of JK Reveals:

PMH: Seasonal allergic rhinitis

PSH: None

FH: Mother and father are alive and well. She has two younger siblings (ages 12 and 15) who are alive and well

SH: The patient works part-time as a waitress. She has participated in cross-country running throughout high school and now into college. She denies smoking cigarettes or drinking alcohol.

Meds: Loratadine 10 mg daily

Past Gynecologic Hx: Never pregnant and never on contraception; (–) history of abnormal pap smears; (–) history of sexually transmitted infections; (+) history of irregular menses each year during track season

ROS: (–) restrictive eating patterns or self-induced vomiting; (–) galactorrhea, headaches, change in vision; (–) abnormal hair growth; (–) acne

PE:

Gen: Thin appearing African American female, no acute distress

VS: BP 118/62, P 74, RR 16, wt 56 kg (123 lb), ht 5'6" (168 cm), BMI: 19.9 kg/m²

HEENT: (–) hirsutism

Breasts: (–) galactorrhea

Pelvic: Normal appearance of external genitalia and vagina, cervix without lesions, uterus midposition without masses, adnexa without masses

Labs:

Urine HCG: Negative

TSH: 1.8 μIU/mL (1.8 mIU/L) (within normal limits)

Prolactin: 10 ng/mL (10 mcg/L) (within normal limits)

Progesterone challenge: No withdrawal bleeding

FSH: 7.4 mIU/mL or mU/mL (7.4 U/L) (within normal limits)

LH: 0.4 mIU/mL or mU/mL (0.4 U/L) (within normal limits)

Head MRI: Normal

Given this information what is your assessment of this patient's condition?

Identify your treatment goals for this patient.

What therapeutic options exist for this patient? Identify those that would be most appropriate.

What monitoring parameters are necessary to employ in assessing efficacy and safety of the therapeutic options?

MENORRHAGIA

The traditional definition of menorrhagia is a menstrual blood loss of more than 80 mL per cycle. This definition has been questioned for several reasons, including difficulty with quantifying menstrual blood loss in clinical practice. Many women are with "heavy menses" but who experience blood loss of less than 80 mL merit consideration for treatment because of problems with containment of flow, unpredictable heavy flow days, and other associated symptoms such as dysmenorrhea.[16,17]

Epidemiology and Etiology

Rates of menorrhagia in healthy women range from 9% to 14%.[4] ❸ *Causes of menorrhagia can be divided into systemic disorders and specific uterine abnormalities.* ❹ *Intrauterine pregnancy, ectopic pregnancy, and miscarriage, must be at the top of the differential diagnosis list for any woman presenting with heavy menses.* In several studies of adolescents with acute menorrhagia, underlying bleeding disorders accounted for 3% to 13% of emergency department visits. von Willebrand's disease has an incidence of 1% in the general population and may present initially as heavy menses

Clinical Presentation and Diagnosis of Menorrhagia

General

Patient may or may not be in acute distress

Symptoms

Complaints of heavy/prolonged menstrual flow and fatigue and light-headedness in the case of severe blood loss. These symptoms may or may not occur with dysmenorrhea

Signs

Orthostasis, tachycardia, and pallor may be noted, especially in cases of significant acute blood loss

Laboratory Tests

Complete blood count (CBC) and ferritin levels; hemoglobin and hematocrit results may be low

If the history dictates, testing may be done to identify coagulation disorder(s) as a cause

Other Diagnostic Tests

- Pelvic ultrasound
- Pelvic MRI
- Pap smear
- Endometrial biopsy
- Hysteroscopy
- Sonohysterogram

in an adolescent.[8] Hypothyroidism also may be associated with heavy menses. Specific uterine causes of menorrhagia are more common in older childbearing women, and they include fibroids, adenomyosis, endometrial polyps, and gynecologic malignancies.

PATHOPHYSIOLOGY

Table 49–1 illustrates the pathophysiology of menorrhagia relative to the organ system(s) involved, as well as the specific conditions that result in menorrhagia.

TREATMENT

Desired Outcomes

Menorrhagia therapy should focus on reducing menstrual blood flow, improving the patient's quality of life, and deferring the need for surgical intervention. Table 49–2 identifies the various agents used in the management of menorrhagia. It also includes their dosing and common side effects. Figure 49–4 illustrates how to decide which treatment(s) to use and when.

▶ Nonpharmacologic Therapy

Nonpharmacologic interventions for menorrhagia include surgical interventions that are reserved for patients not responding to pharmacologic treatment. These interventions may vary from conservative endometrial ablation to hysterectomy.[18]

Pharmacologic Therapy

▶ Nonsteroidal Anti-Inflammatory Drugs

Nonsteroidal anti-inflammatory drugs (NSAIDs) are first-line treatments for menorrhagia associated with ovulatory cycles.[19] *They have the advantage of being taken only during menses, and their use is associated with a significant reduction in menstrual blood loss. A 20% to 50% reduction in blood loss has been observed in 75% of treated women.*[12] *In some patients, as much as an 80% reduction has been observed.* ❺ *This reduction is directly proportional to the amount of pretreatment blood loss.*[12]

▶ Combination OCs

The use of OCs is beneficial to women with menorrhagia who do not desire pregnancy. A 43% to 53% reduction in menstrual blood loss has been observed in 68% of patients treated with OCs containing greater than or equal to 35 mcg estradiol for the treatment of menorrhagia.[12] As with the use of NSAIDs, ❺ *the reduction in blood loss is proportional to pretreatment blood loss.*

▶ Progesterone

Menorrhagia also may be treated with the levonorgestrel-releasing intrauterine devices (IUD). This is a very effective

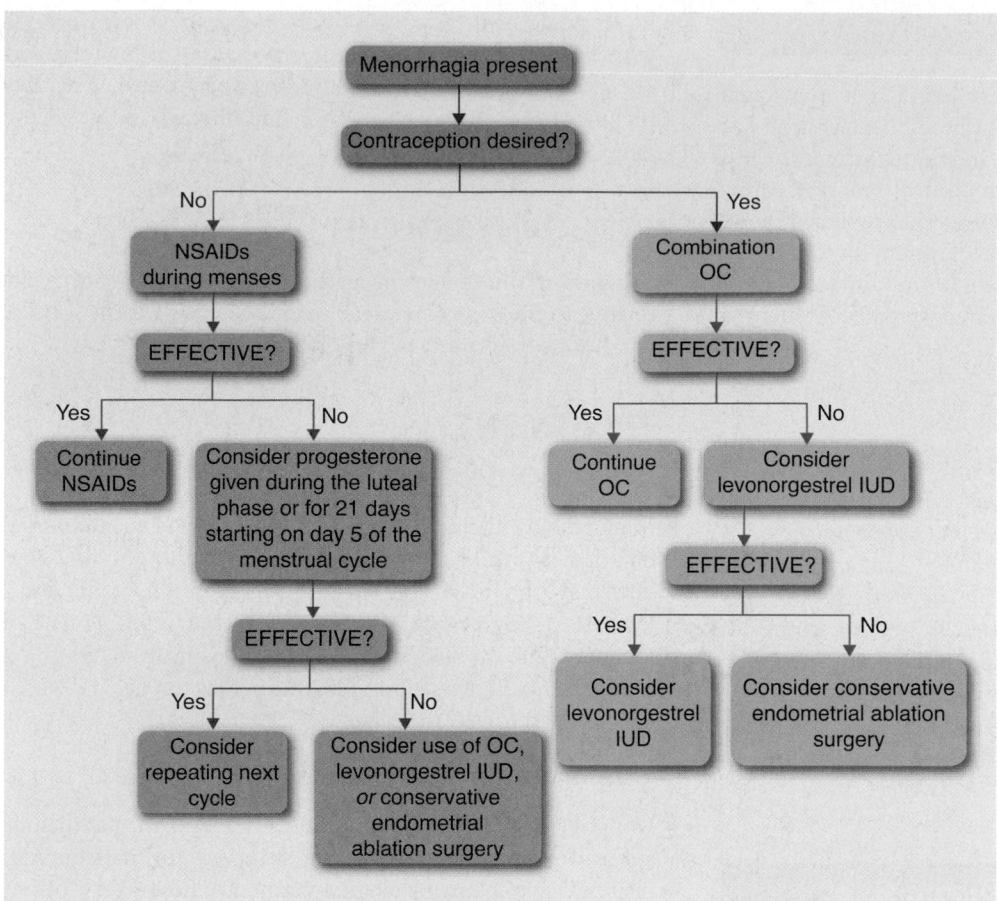

FIGURE 49–4. Treatment algorithm for menorrhagia.

treatment that consistently reduces menstrual flow by 90% or greater.[12,20–22] Its use has resulted in the postponement or cancellation of scheduled endometrial resection surgery or hysterectomy. Specifically, 60% of treated patients have been able to avoid hysterectomy.[22–24]

Progesterone therapy either during the luteal phase of the menstrual cycle or for 21 days starting on day 5 after the onset of menses results in a 32% to 50% reduction in menstrual blood loss.[12] Its use has not been shown to be superior to other medical treatments, including NSAIDs.[12] In addition, it is not associated with any contraceptive benefit.[19]

DYSMENORRHEA

Dysmenorrhea is commonly defined as crampy pelvic pain occurring with or just prior to menses. Primary dysmenorrhea implies pain in the setting of normal pelvic anatomy and physiology, whereas secondary dysmenorrhea is associated with underlying pelvic pathology.[11]

EPIDEMIOLOGY AND ETIOLOGY

Rates of dysmenorrhea range from 20% to 90%.[11,25] Dysmenorrhea can be associated with significant interference in attendance at work and school for 15% of women affected by the most severe form.[25] Risk factors for dysmenorrhea include young age, heavy menses, and nulliparity.[11] Causes of secondary dysmenorrhea may include cervical stenosis, endometriosis, pelvic infections,

---

Clinical Presentation and Diagnosis of Dysmenorrhea

General

Patient may or may not be in acute distress depending on the level of menstrual pain experienced

Symptoms

Complaints of crampy pelvic pain beginning shortly before or at the onset of menses. Symptoms typically last from 1 to 3 days

Laboratory Tests

- Sexually active females should have a pelvic examination to screen for sexually transmitted diseases
- Gonorrhea, chlamydia cultures or PCR, wet mount

Other Diagnostic Tests

Pelvic ultrasound may be used to identify anatomic abnormalities such as masses/lesions or to detect ovarian cysts and endometriomas

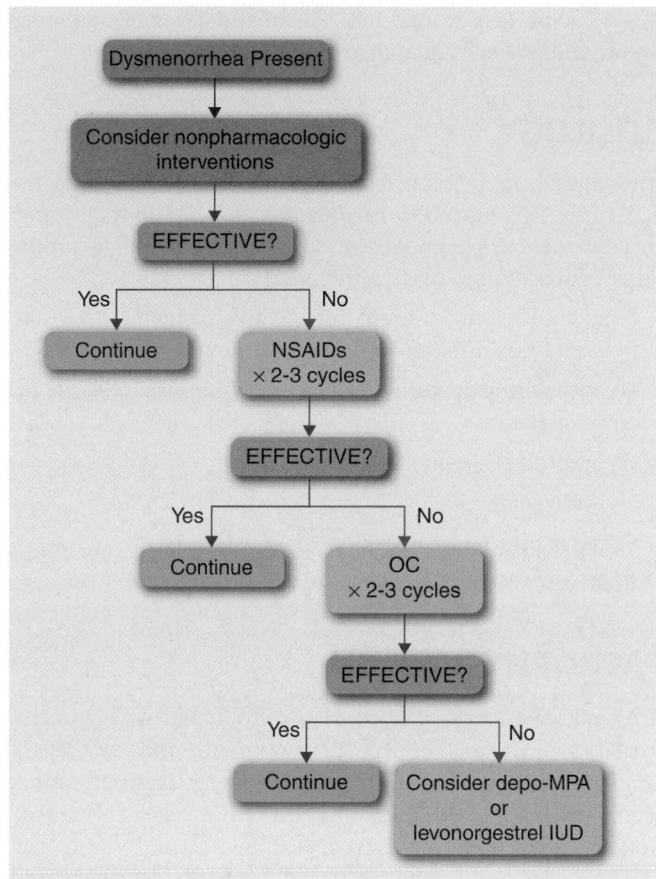

FIGURE 49–5. Treatment algorithm for dysmenorrhea.

pelvic congestion syndrome, uterine or cervical polyps, and uterine fibroids.[26]

PATHOPHYSIOLOGY

❻ *The most significant mechanism for primary dysmenorrhea is the release of prostanoids and possibly eicosanoids in the menstrual fluid* inducing uterine contractions, reducing uterine blood flow, and causing uterine hypoxia.[25] Vasopressin-mediated vasoconstriction may also contribute to the resulting symptoms.[8,11,25]

TREATMENT

Desired Outcomes

The medical management of dysmenorrhea should relieve the related pelvic pain and result in a reduction in lost school and work days. Table 49–2 identifies the agents used in the management of dysmenorrhea, their recommended doses, and their common side effects. Figure 49–5 is a treatment algorithm for the management of dysmenorrhea.

Nonpharmacologic Therapy

Several nonpharmacologic interventions exist for the management of dysmenorrhea. Among these, topical heat therapy, exercise, and following a low-fat vegetarian diet all have been shown to reduce the intensity of the

dysmenorrhea.[11,14] Dietary changes also may shorten the duration of dysmenorrhea. These interventions require little time and minimal cost and are associated with little risk. Other nonpharmacologic options that may be considered before or, in most cases, after a trial of pharmacologic interventions include the use of transcutaneous electrical nerve stimulation (TENS), acupressure, and acupuncture.[11]

Pharmacologic Therapy

▶ *Nonsteroidal Anti-Inflammatory Drugs*

❻ *Given their impact on inhibiting prostaglandins as well as their ability to provide direct analgesia, NSAIDs are the treatment of choice for dysmenorrhea.* There does not appear to be a difference between agents in efficacy. Choice of one agent over another may be based on cost, convenience, and patient preference.[11,25] The most commonly used agents are naproxen and ibuprofen.

It has been suggested that a loading dose (twice the usual single dose) of the NSAID be taken, followed by the usually recommended dose until symptoms resolve.[14] An alternate recommendation is to begin the NSAID at the onset of menses or perhaps even the day prior and to continue treatment around the clock instead of waiting until the onset of symptoms. For patients in whom NSAID use is contraindicated, the agents discussed below should be considered. The use of acetaminophen has been proven inferior to the use of NSAIDs for the treatment of this disorder.[11]

▶ *Oral Contraceptives*

OCs help to improve dysmenorrhea by inhibiting the proliferation of endometrial tissue. This reduction in tissue translates into a reduction in endometrial-derived prostaglandins that are thought to contribute to the pelvic pain experienced.[14,25] A trial of 2 to 3 months of OC dosing is required to establish whether the patient is a responder or a nonresponder. Significant improvements in mild, moderate, and severe dysmenorrhea have been noted with the use of OCs. These agents have other benefits, such as the prevention of pregnancy, improving acne, and reducing ovarian cancer risk. While monophasic formulations may be more efficacious for this indication, the supporting evidence for this is limited.[11]

▶ *Progesterone*

The benefit of depo MPA in dysmenorrhea is related to its ability to render most patients amenorrheic within 1 year of use.[11] This is an expected side effect. Since the pelvic pain of dysmenorrhea is related to the prostaglandins released during menses, in the setting of amenorrhea, the underlying cause of dysmenorrhea is removed.

Observational data illustrate a reduction in dysmenorrhea from 60% to 29% with the levonorgestrel-releasing IUD after 3 years.[11] As observed with depo MPA, this reduction is likely secondary to the increasing incidence of amenorrhea in users of this contraceptive device.

DYSMENORRHEA IN ADOLESCENTS

Dysmenorrhea is very common in adolescent females. Any of the treatment measures discussed earlier for other patients would be appropriate in the adolescent population. While NSAIDs and OCs are among the top choices, use of the levonorgestrel IUD is also an option.[22] It had been thought previously that nulliparous females should avoid the use of IUDs secondary to an increased risk of pelvic inflammatory disease (PID) and a subsequent increased risk of infertility. **❼** *Guidelines from the American College of Obstetricians and Gynecologists (ACOG) state that any woman (regardless of parity) at low risk of sexually transmitted diseases and thus PID is a good candidate for IUD use.*[22]

ANOVULATORY BLEEDING

Anovulatory bleeding is irregular menstrual blood flow from the uterine endometrium that ranges from light spotting to heavy blood flow.[5] **❽** *Anovulatory bleeding, also referred to as dysfunctional uterine bleeding, is secondary to the effects of unopposed estrogen and does not include bleeding owing to an anatomic lesion of the uterus.* Anovulatory bleeding includes PCOS, which typically presents with irregular menstrual bleeding, hirsutism, obesity, or infertility.

EPIDEMIOLOGY

Anovulatory bleeding is the most common form of noncyclic uterine bleeding.[5] Patients often seek medical care to regulate their menstrual cycle or improve fertility. All women of reproductive age should have a pregnancy test when presenting with irregular menstrual bleeding. Anovulation may be secondary to physiologic or pathologic causes. It is common at menarche and in the perimenopausal period. During adolescence, ovulatory menstrual cycles may not be regular for a year or more after menarche.[5] Overall, the frequency of ovulation is related to the time since menarche and the age at menarche.[27] In the year following menarche, there may be an immature feedback mechanism in the hypothalamic–pituitary–ovarian (HPO) axis whereby the LH surge needed for ovulation does not occur. During perimenopause, anovulatory cycles may occur owing to a declining quality and quantity of ovarian follicles. As ovarian function declines, estrogen secretion continues and progesterone secretion decreases. Chronic anovulatory cycles and unopposed estrogen secretion lead to endometrial proliferation and increased risk of polyps, endometrial hyperplasia, and carcinoma.

Anovulation also may occur at any time during the reproductive years due to a pathologic cause. The most common causes of nonphysiologic ovulatory dysfunction and their prevalence rates[5] are:

- PCOS (70%)
- Hypothalamic amenorrhea (10%)
- Hyperprolactinemia (10%)
- Premature ovarian failure (10%)

PCOS, while responsible for 70% of the cases of ovulatory dysfunction, occurs in approximately 4% of women.[28]

ETIOLOGY

Anovulation may result from a problem at any level of the HPO axis. In addition to various physiologic life stages such as adolescence, perimenopause, pregnancy, and lactation, other causes of anovulation include:[5,27]

- Hyperandrogenic anovulation (PCOS, congenital adrenal hyperplasia, androgen-producing tumors)
- Hypothalamic dysfunction (anorexia nervosa, physical or emotional stress)
- Hyperprolactinemia
- Hypothyroidism
- Primary pituitary disease
- Premature ovarian failure

PATHOPHYSIOLOGY

A normal ovulatory cycle consists of follicular development, ovulation, corpus luteum development, and luteolysis. During the cycle, the endometrium undergoes proliferation, secretory change, and desquamation. This cycle is influenced first by the effects of estrogen alone, then by estrogen and progesterone, and culminates with estrogen and progesterone withdrawal. Progesterone stops the growth of the endometrium and stimulates its differentiation. In patients with anovulation, a corpus luteum is not formed, and the ovary does not secrete progesterone. Without progesterone, there is no desquamation or differentiation of the endometrium.

Clinical Presentation and Diagnosis of Anovulatory Bleeding

General

May or may not be in acute distress

Symptoms

Irregular, heavy, or prolonged vaginal bleeding, perimenopausal symptoms (hot flashes, etc.)

Signs

Acne, hirsutism, obesity

Laboratory Tests

- If suspect PCOS, consider free or total testosterone, fasting glucose, fasting lipid panel
- If suspect perimenopause, FSH

Other Diagnostic Tests

Pelvic ultrasound to evaluate for polycystic ovaries

Patient Encounter 2, Part 1

TP, a 22-year-old woman, presents to your office for a routine gynecologic examination. She entered menarche at the age of 12. Her last menstrual period was 3 months ago. Her periods are often irregular and occur about every 2 to 3 months. She has had all normal Pap smears in the past and no history of sexually transmitted infections. She is currently in a monogamous relationship with a male partner. She has had four sexual partners. She is not taking OCs and does not routinely use condoms. She has never been pregnant in the past, but she plans to start a family in the near future. As you examine the patient, you note facial and chest acne, increased facial and abdominal hair, and obesity.

What anovulatory disorder is most likely present?

What signs/symptoms support this conclusion?

What diagnostic tests should be done?

Chronic unopposed estrogen causes continuous endometrial proliferation, and the endometrium becomes vascular and fragile, resulting in noncyclic menstrual bleeding. In addition, the endometrium may become hyperplastic and progress to a precancerous state, placing the patient at increased risk of endometrial cancer.[6] See Table 49–1 for the pathophysiology of anovulatory bleeding relative to the specific conditions that contribute to it.

The most common pathologic cause of anovulation is PCOS. It is a syndrome of ovarian dysfunction diagnosed by the presence of two of the following three characteristics: Oligoanovulation or anovulation, clinical or laboratory evidence of hyperandrogenism, and polycystic ovary morphology on ultrasound.[29] No gene or environmental substance has been found to cause PCOS.[7] However, the observance of familial clustering of cases suggests that genetics plays a role.[30] It is thought that insulin resistance, hyperandrogenism, and changes in gonadotropins also influence the development of PCOS.[28] The underlying cause for increased androgens is unknown.[30]

PCOS is associated with a three to seven times increased risk of developing type 2 diabetes.[29] Patients diagnosed with PCOS should be screened for impaired glucose tolerance, diabetes, hypertension, and dyslipidemia.[28] If any of these conditions are present, there is an increased risk of cardiovascular events.

TREATMENT

Desired Outcomes

In the short term, the desired outcome is to stop acute bleeding. The long-term goals of therapy include preventing future episodes of noncyclic bleeding, decreasing the long-term complications of anovulation (e.g., osteopenia and infertility), and improving overall quality of life.[5] Table 49–2 identifies the agents used in the management of anovulatory bleeding, their doses, and common side effects.

Nonpharmacologic Therapy

Nonpharmacologic treatment options for anovulatory bleeding depend on the underlying cause. In a woman of reproductive age with PCOS, weight loss may be beneficial. In women who have completed childbearing or who have failed medical management, endometrial ablation or resection and hysterectomy are surgical options. It is unclear as to which procedure is preferred. Short term, it appears that ablation or resection results in less morbidity and shorter recovery periods.[18] However, a significant number of these women eventually undergo hysterectomy in the 5 years that follow.[5]

Pharmacologic Therapy

▶ Estrogen

Estrogen is the recommended treatment for managing acute bleeding episodes because it promotes endometrial growth and stabilization.[5] Further, its use (via OC regimens) has been observed to avert emergency surgical procedures in 95% of treated patients.[13] Following its initial use for controlling acute bleeding episodes, it is necessary to continue therapy to prevent future occurrences. The use of OCs fulfills this role.

In addition to controlling acute bleeding, the use of OCs also aids in the prevention of recurrent anovulatory bleeding. They suppress ovarian hormones and adrenal androgen production. They also, indirectly, increase sex hormone–binding globulin (SHBG). This, in turn, binds and reduces circulating androgen. For women with high androgen levels and related signs (e.g., hirsutism), low-dose OCs (less than or equal to 35 mcg ethinyl estradiol) are the treatment of choice.[5] In theory, one may consider the use of an OC with a progesterone such as drospirenone that has a larger impact on increasing SHBG and antiandrogenic effects.[31] However, to date there is no consensus as to the best OC choice for these women (e.g., those with PCOS).[7]

▶ Medroxyprogesterone Acetate

Specifically, for women with PCOS, the use of depot and intermittent oral MPA suppresses pituitary gonadotropins and circulating androgens.[7] Further, the use of cyclic progesterone may benefit women over age 40 with anovulatory bleeding.[5] Similar to the use of OCs, the use of oral MPA has been observed to avert emergency surgical procedures in 100% of patients for acute uterine bleeding justifying immediate medical attention.[13]

▶ Insulin-Sensitizing Agents

The use of metformin and the thiazolidinediones pioglitazone and rosiglitazone results in improved insulin sensitivity. In patients with PCOS, this is associated with reduced circulating androgen concentrations, increasing ovulation rates, and improving glucose tolerance.[7] These improvements can be attributed to the increase in SHBG that occurs via

Patient Encounter 2, Part 2

PMH: (+) Obesity and acne

FH: Father is living and has hypertension. Mother is living and has diabetes mellitus and hypercholesterolemia. Both parents are obese.

SH: The patient works as a secretary. She lives with her fiancé. She denies any tobacco or recreational drug use. She drinks about five alcoholic beverages per week. She is sedentary

Meds: None

ROS: (+) acne, (+) hirsutism, (−) dysmenorrhea, (−) breast tenderness, (−) vaginal discharge

PE:

VS: BP 128/82, P 80 bpm, RR 18 bpm, wt 123 kg (270 lb), ht 5 ft, 3 in. (160 cm), BMI 47.9 kg/m²

Abd: Obese, soft, nontender, nondistended, (+) bowel sounds, no hepatosplenomegaly

Gyn: Normal external appearance of labia minora and majora, vaginal walls within normal limits, cervix well visualized and without lesions, midposition uterus, no cervical motion tenderness, no adnexal masses palpated

Labs: Urine HCG negative, free testosterone 100 ng/dL (3.47 nmol/L) (elevated), TSH 2.1 μU/mL (2.1 mU/L) (within normal limits), prolactin 9 ng/mL (9 mcg/L) (within normal limits), fasting glucose 120 mg/dL (6.66 mmol/L). Fasting lipid panel: Total cholesterol 181 mg/dL (4.69 mmol/L), HDL cholesterol 58 mg/dL (1.50 mmol/L), triglycerides 65 mg/dL (0.73 mmol/L), LDL cholesterol 110 mg/dL (2.85 mmol/L)

Pelvic Ultrasound: 15 follicles in right ovary, 14 follicles in left ovary, increased ovarian volume of 12 mL

What treatment options are available for this patient?

Will this patient have fertility problems in the future?

Table 49–3

Expected Outcome Measures for Selected Menstrual Bleeding Disorders

Menstrual Disorder	Expected Outcome Measures
Amenorrhea	*Efficacy:* Normal breast development (especially primary amenorrhea in adolescents); preservation/improvement of BMD; return of menses *Time to relief/effect:* Menses should occur within 1–2 months of therapy
Menorrhagia	*Efficacy:* Decline in the amount of blood lost with menses (monitor a decline in the number of times feminine hygiene products such as pads and tampons require changing during menses); monitor for an increase in hemoglobin/hematocrit if anemia was present as a result of menorrhagia *Time to relief/effect:* A decline in menstrual blood loss should be realized within 1–2 cycles of initiation of therapy
Anovulatory bleeding	*Efficacy:* Alleviation of acute bleeding when present; ovulation and subsequent pregnancy in women desiring this; reduced risk of developing the long-term complications of, for example, PCOS (e.g., diabetes and cardiovascular disease); improved quality of life *Time to relief/effect:* The acute treatment of heavy bleeding should result in a decline in bleeding within 10 days of therapy onset; the return of ovulation may require several months of therapy; when OCs are used, control of abnormal bleeding can be expected within 1–2 cycles of therapy
Dysmenorrhea	*Efficacy:* Reduction in/absence of pelvic pain related to menses; reduction in time lost from work/school; improved quality of life *Time to relief/effect:* Improvement in pain may be observed within hours of NSAID therapy; improvement with other options such as OCs may be observed after a full 1–3 cycles of their use

BMD, bone mineral density; NSAID, nonsteroidal anti-inflammatory drug; OCs, oral contraceptives; PCOS, polycystic ovary syndrome.

From Refs. 5, 6, 8, 17, 20, 27.

---

increased insulin sensitivity. ❾ *These agents are of benefit not only for anovulatory bleeding and fertility but also because they improve glucose tolerance and decrease overall cardiovascular risk.*[7] If pregnancy is a desired outcome, it is important to note that metformin is a pregnancy category B agent, whereas pioglitazone and rosiglitazone are category C.

Although the use of insulin-sensitizing agents may improve fertility, if the goal of treatment is to improve fertility via ovulation induction, then the treatment of choice is combination therapy with an insulin-sensitizing agent such as metformin plus clomiphene citrate.[32,33] Treatment with clomiphene citrate 50 mg/day for 5 days can be initiated between days 3 and 5 of the menstrual cycle. This often may occur following the induction of withdrawal bleeding with a progesterone such as MPA at 10 mg/day by mouth for 10 days.

ANOVULATORY BLEEDING IN ADOLESCENTS

Anovulatory cycles are not unusual in the perimenarchal reproductive years. Ovulation typically is established a year or more following menarche. When anovulatory bleeding

Patient Care and Monitoring

1. Assess symptoms to determine if patient-directed therapy is appropriate (e.g., NSAIDs for dysmenorrhea) or whether the patient should be evaluated by a physician (e.g., amenorrhea, menorrhagia, anovulatory bleeding, or premenstrual dysphoric disorder (PMDD). Does the patient have any related complications, such as symptoms of anemia in patients presenting with menorrhagia or complaints of difficulty conceiving in women with amenorrhea or anovulatory bleeding?

2. Review any available diagnostic data, as appropriate, to determine hormonal, reproductive, and pregnancy status.

3. Obtain a thorough history of prescription, nonprescription, and natural drug product use. Determine which treatments have been helpful to the patient in the past.

4. Educate the patient on lifestyle modifications that will improve symptoms and prevent complications.

5. Is the patient taking the appropriate dose of the prescribed medication? If not, why not?

6. Develop a plan to assess effectiveness of the prescribed medication after 1 to 2 months of therapy.

7. Determine if long-term maintenance treatment is necessary.

8. Assess improvement in quality-of-life measures such as physical, psychological, social functioning, and well-being.

9. Evaluate for adverse drug reactions, drug allergies, and drug interactions.

10. Stress the importance of adherence with the therapeutic regimen, including lifestyle modifications. Recommend a therapeutic regimen that is easy for the patient to adhere to.

11. Provide patient education regarding disease state, lifestyle modifications, and drug therapy by noting the following:
    - What causes the menstruation-related disorder?
    - What are the possible complications of the menstruation-related disorder?
    - What lifestyle modifications may help to reduce the risk associated with these complications?
    - When and how should patients take their medications?
    - What potential adverse effects may occur?
    - Which drugs may interact with their therapy?

occurs in this population, it may be excessive. If the bleeding is excessive, the patient should be evaluated for blood dyscrasias. The prevalence of blood dyscrasias, including von Willebrand's disease and prothrombin deficiency, and the prevalence of idiopathic thrombocytopenia purpura in this population ranges from 5% to 20%.[5]

In the adolescent population, specific blood dyscrasias should be treated. In addition, acute, severe bleeding may be managed with high-dose estrogen. Low-dose OCs (less than or equal to 35 mcg ethinyl estradiol) are the treatment of choice in adolescents with chronic anovulation.[5]

OUTCOME EVALUATION

Measure the treatment success for the various menstruation-related disorders by the degree to which the care plan (a) relieves or reverses symptoms of the disorder, (b) prevents or reverses the complications of the disorder (e.g., osteoporosis, anemia, and infertility), and (c) minimizes side effects. The return of a regular menstrual cycle with minimal premenstrual symptoms or symptoms of dysmenorrhea should occur. Depending on the desire for conception and subsequent therapy, this cycle may be ovulatory or anovulatory.

Assess the effectiveness of therapy in resuming normal menstrual cycles with minimal related pain after an appropriate treatment interval (1–2 months). Assess improvement in

quality-of-life measures such as physical, psychological, and social functioning and well-being. Evaluate the patient for adverse drug reactions, drug allergies, and drug interactions. Table 49–2 illustrates the common side effects that may occur for which monitoring is required. Table 49–3 illustrates the specific expected outcome measures for each of the menstruation-related disorders discussed in this chapter.

Abbreviations Introduced in This chapter

ACOG	American College of Obstetricians and Gynecologists
CEE	Conjugated equine estrogen
FSH	Follicle-stimulating hormone
GnRH	Gonadotropin-releasing hormone
HCG	Human chorionic gonadotropin
HDL	High-density lipoprotein
HPO	Hypothalamic–pituitary–ovarian
IUD	Intrauterine device
LDL	Low-density lipoprotein
LH	Luteinizing hormone
MPA	Medroxyprogesterone acetate
NSAID	Nonsteroidal anti-inflammatory drug
OC	Oral contraceptive

PCOS   Polycystic ovary syndrome
PID   Pelvic inflammatory disease
PMH   Past medical history
ROS   Review of systems
SH   Social history
SHBG   Sex hormone–binding globulin
TENS   Transcutaneous electrical nerve stimulation
TSH   Thyroid-stimulating hormone

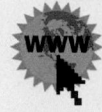 Self-assessment questions and answers are available at *http://www.mhpharmacotherapy.com/pp/html.*

REFERENCES

1. Speroff L, Fritz MA. Clinical Gynecologic Endocrinology and Infertility. 7th ed. Philadelphia: Lippincott Williams & Wilkins, 2005:187–232, 401–463.
2. Reindollar RH, Novak M, Tho SP, McDonough PG. Adult-onset amenorrhea: A study of 262 patients. Am J Obstet Gynecol 1986;155(3):531–543.
3. Barbeiri RL, Ryan KJ. The menstrual cycle. In: Ryan Kistner's Gynecology and Women's Health. 7th ed. St. Louis, MO: Mosby, 1999:23–57.
4. Stenchever MA, Droegemueller W, Herbst AL, Mishell DR. Abnormal uterine bleeding: Ovulatory and anovulatory dysfunctional uterine bleeding, management of acute and chronic excessive bleeding. In: Comprehensive Gynecology. 4th ed. St. Louis, MO: Mosby, 2001:1079–1097.
5. American College of Obstetricians and Gynecologists. Management of anovulatory bleeding. ACOG Practice Bulletin Number 14. Obstet Gynecol 2000(Mar):495–502.
6. Speroff L, Glass RH, Kase NG. Clinical gynecologic endocrinology and infertility. 6th ed. Baltimore, MD: Lippincott Williams & Wilkins, 1999:487–511.
7. American College of Obstetricians and Gynecologists. Polycystic ovary syndrome. ACOG Practice Bulletin Number 41. Obstet Gynecol 2002;100:1389–1402.
8. Adams Hillard PJ, Deitch HR. Menstrual disorders in the college age female. Pediatr Clin N Am 2005;52(1):179–197.
9. Gordon CM, Nelson LM. Amenorrhea and bone health in adolescents and young women. Curr Opin Obstet Gynecol 2003;15:377–384.
10. Pletcher JR, Slap GB. Menstrual disorders—Amenorrhea. Pediatr Clin N Am 1999;46(3):505–518.
11. French L. Dysmenorrhea. Am Fam Physician 2005;71:285–292.
12. Roy SN, Bhattacharya S. Benefits and risks of pharmacological agents used for the treatment of menorrhagia. Drug Safety 2004;27(2):75–90.
13. Munro MG, Mainor N, Basu R, et al. Oral medroxyprogesterone acetate and combination oral contraceptives for acute uterine bleeding: A randomized clinical trial. Obstet Gynecol 2006;108:924–929.
14. Harel Z. A contemporary approach to dysmenorrhea in adolescents. Pediatr Drugs 2002;4(12):797–805.
15. Simon JA. Progestogens in the treatment of secondary amenorrhea. J Reprod Med 1999;44:185–189.
16. Warner PE, Critchley HO, Lumsden MA, et al. Menorrhagia I: Measured blood loss, clinical features, and outcome in women with heavy periods: A survey with follow-up data. Am J Obstet Gynecol 2004;190(5):1216–1223.
17. Warner PE, Critchley HO, Lumsden MA, et al. Menorrhagia II: Is the 80-mL blood loss criterion useful in management of complaint of menorrhagia? Am J Obstet Gynecol 2004;190(5):1224–1229.
18. Dickersin K, Munro MG, Clark M, et al. Hysterectomy compared with endometrial ablation for dysfunctional uterine bleeding: A randomized controlled trial. Obstet Gynecol 2007;110(6):1279–1289.
19. Prentice A. Fortnightly review: Medical management of menorrhagia. BMJ 1999;319(7221):1343–1345.
20. Reid PC, Virtanen-Kari S. Randomized comparative trial of levonorgestrel intrauterine system and mefenamic acid for the treatment of idiopathic menorrhagia: A multiple analysis using total menstrual fluid loss, menstrual blood loss and pictorial blood loss assessment charts. Br J Obstet Gynecol 2005;112:1121–1125.
21. American College of Obstetricians and Gynecologists. Noncontraceptive uses of the levonorgestrel intrauterine system. ACOG Committee Opinion Number 337. Obstet Gynecol 2006(June);107:1479–1482.
22. American College of Obstetricians and Gynecologists. Intrauterine device. ACOG Practice Bulletin No. 59. Obstet Gynecol 2005;105:223–232.
23. Hurskainen R, Paavonen J. Levonorgestrel-releasing intrauterine system in the treatment of heavy menstrual bleeding. Curr Opin Obstet Gynecol 2004;16:487–490.
24. Hurskainen R, Teperi J, Rissanen P, et al. Clinical outcomes and costs with the levonorgestrel-releasing intrauterine system or hysterectomy for treatment of menorrhagia: Randomized trial 5-year follow-up. JAMA 2004;291(12):1456–1463.
25. Dawood MY. Primary dysmenorrhea: Advances in pathogenesis and management. Obstet Gynecol 2006;108:428–441.
26. Stenchever MA, Droegemueller W, Herbst AL, Mishell DR. Primary and secondary dysmenorrhea and premenstrual syndrome etiology, diagnosis, and management. In: Stenchever MA, ed. Comprehensive Gynecology. 4th ed. St. Louis, MO: Mosby, 2001:1065–1078.
27. American College of Obstetricians and Gynecologists. Menstruation in girls and adolescents: Using the menstrual cycle as a vital sign. ACOG Committee Opinion Number 349. American Academy of Pediatrics; American College of Obstetricians and Gynecologists. Obstet Gynecol 2006(Nov);108:1323–1328.
28. Guzick DS. Polycystic ovary syndrome. Am J Obstet Gynecol 2004;103(1):181–192.
29. Rotterdam ESHRE/ASRM-Sponsored PCOS Consensus Workshop Group. Revised 2003 consensus on diagnostic criteria and long-term health risks related to polycystic ovary syndrome. Fertil Steril 2004;81(1):19–25.
30. Buggs C, Rosenfield, RL. Polycystic ovary syndrome in adolescence. Endocrinol Metab Clin N Am 2005;34:677–705.
31. Mathur R, Levin O, Azziz R. Use of ethinylestradiol/drospirenone combination in patients with the polycystic ovary syndrome. Ther Clin Risk Manag 2008;4(2):487–492.
32. Creanga AA, Bradley HM, McCormick C, et al. Use of metformin in polycystic ovary syndrome: A meta-analysis. Obstet Gynecol 2008;111(4):959–968.
33. Khorram O, Helliwell JP, Katz S, et al. Two weeks of metformin improves clomiphene citrate-induced ovulation and metabolic profiles in women with polycystic ovary syndrome. Fertil Steril 2006;85(5):1448–1451.

50 Hormone Therapy in Menopause

Nicole S. Culhane and Kelly R. Ragucci

LEARNING OBJECTIVES

● **Upon completion of the chapter, the reader will be able to:**

1. Explain the pathophysiologic changes associated with menopause.
2. Identify the signs and symptoms associated with menopause.
3. Determine the desired therapeutic outcomes for a patient taking hormone therapy (HT).
4. Explain how to evaluate a patient for the appropriate use of HT.
5. Recommend nonpharmacologic therapy for menopausal symptoms.
6. List the adverse effects of and contraindications to HT.
7. Differentiate between topical and systemic forms of HT.
8. Explain the risks and benefits associated with HT.
9. Educate a patient regarding the proper use and potential adverse effects of HT.
10. Monitor a patient taking HT for efficacy and toxicity.
11. Recognize that alternative, nonhormonal therapies for menopausal symptoms exist and should be considered in some circumstances for women unable to take HT.

KEY CONCEPTS

❶ Common symptoms of menopause include hot flashes, night sweats, vulvovaginal atrophy, and vaginal dryness. Women less commonly may experience mood swings, depression, insomnia, arthralgia, myalgia, and urinary frequency.

❷ Hormone therapy (HT) remains the most effective treatment for vasomotor symptoms and vulvovaginal atrophy and should be considered for women experiencing these symptoms.

❸ Women should receive a thorough history and physical examination, including assessing for coronary heart disease (CHD) and breast cancer risk factors, before HT is considered. They should be informed of the risks and the benefits of HT and should be encouraged to be involved in the decision-making process. If a woman does not have any contraindications to HT, including CHD or significant CHD risk factors, and also does not have a personal history of breast cancer, HT may be an appropriate therapy option.

❹ Oral or transdermal estrogen products should be prescribed at the lowest effective dose and for the shortest duration possible to provide relief of vasomotor symptoms. Topical products in the form of creams, tablets, or rings should be prescribed for women exclusively experiencing vulvovaginal atrophy.

❺ Women who have an intact uterus should be prescribed a progestogen in addition to estrogen in order to decrease the risk of endometrial hyperplasia and endometrial cancer.

❻ HT is also indicated for the prevention of osteoporosis but is not recommended for long-term use. Alternative osteoporosis therapies should be considered as first-line therapy for the prevention of osteoporosis, in addition to appropriate doses of calcium and vitamin D.

❼ Combined estrogen plus progestogen should not be used in the prevention of chronic diseases because it increases the risk of CHD, stroke, breast cancer, and venous thromboembolism (VTE). However, colorectal cancer and rates of fracture were reduced with combined hormonal treatment.

❽ HT improves overall well-being and mood in women with vasomotor symptoms but has not demonstrated an improvement in quality of life (QoL) in women without vasomotor symptoms.

⑨ In appropriately selected women, HT should be recommended at the lowest dose for the shortest duration and should be tapered before discontinuation in order to prevent the recurrence of hot flashes.

⑩ Since the publication of the Women's Health Initiative (WHI) study, there has been an increase in the use of alternative and nonhormonal therapies for the management of menopausal symptoms. Particularly for women with CHD and/or breast cancer risk factors, these therapies may offer another option to assist with symptom management. A wide range of therapies, both prescription and herbal, have been studied with varying degrees of success. In choosing a particular therapy, it is important to match patient symptoms with a therapy that is not only effective but also safe.

Menopause is the permanent cessation of menses following the loss of ovarian follicular activity. The diagnosis of menopause is primarily a clinical one and is made after a woman experiences amenorrhea for 12 consecutive months. The loss of ovarian follicular activity leads to an increase in follicle-stimulating hormone (FSH), which, on laboratory examination, may help to confirm the diagnosis.

Many women seek medical treatment for the relief of menopausal symptoms, primarily hot flashes; however, the role of hormone therapy (HT) has changed dramatically over the years. HT has long been prescribed for relief of menopausal symptoms and, until recent years, has been purported to protect women from coronary heart disease (CHD). The original reason behind recommending HT in postmenopausal women revolved around a simple theory: If the hormones lost during menopause were replaced through drug therapy, women would be protected from both menopausal symptoms and chronic diseases that often follow after a woman experiences menopause. Recent studies have disproved this theory.

In 1996, the United States Preventive Services Task Force first published its recommendations that not all postmenopausal women should be prescribed HT, but rather, therapy should be individualized based on risk factors. This recommendation was further supported with publication of the Heart and Estrogen/Progestin Replacement Study (HERS) in 1998, which demonstrated that women who had established CHD were at an increased risk of experiencing a myocardial infarction within the first year of HT use compared with a similar group of women without CHD risk factors. As a result, the authors concluded that HT is not recommended for the secondary prevention of CHD.[1] Then, in 2002, the Women's Health Initiative (WHI) study was published. This trial demonstrated that HT was not protective against CHD but rather could increase the risk in women with underlying CHD risk factors. The risk of breast cancer was also increased after a woman was on therapy for approximately 3 years. As a result of this study, the FDA issued a statement that HT should not be initiated or continued for the primary prevention of CHD.[2]

This series of trials, and many more, has led to the dramatic change in how HT is currently prescribed and greater understanding of the associated risks. HT, once thought of as a cure-all for menopausal symptoms, is now a therapy that should be used primarily to reduce the frequency and severity of vasomotor symptoms associated with menopause in women without risk factors for CHD or breast cancer. The changes that have occurred over the years in the use of HT further support the importance of evidence-based practice and judicious medication use.

EPIDEMIOLOGY AND ETIOLOGY

Menopause is a period of time marked by the cessation of menses. It occurs in all women either naturally or surgically and usually occurs between the ages of 40 and 58 years. The median age for a woman to experience menopause is 52 years. However, women who have undergone a total abdominal hysterectomy (surgical menopause) generally experience menopause earlier compared with women who experience natural menopause. Some other factors that may be associated with early menopause include low body weight, increased menstrual cycle length, nulliparity, and smoking. Smokers generally experience menopause approximately 2 years earlier than nonsmokers.[3]

The usual transitional period prior to menopause, known as perimenopause or the *climacteric,* is a period when hormonal and biologic changes begin to occur. These changes may begin 2 to 8 years prior to menopause and eventually lead to irregular menstrual cycles, an increase in cycle interval, and a decrease in the length of menses. During this time, women also may experience physical symptoms similar to menopausal symptoms, primarily vasomotor symptoms, and they may require treatment depending on symptom severity.[3,4]

Because the perimenopausal and postmenopausal periods are marked by many biologic and endocrinologic changes, women should inform their health care provider when they experience any signs and symptoms in order to discuss the most appropriate therapeutic approach.

PATHOPHYSIOLOGY

Reproductive physiology is regulated primarily by the hypothalamic-pituitary-ovarian axis. The hypothalamus secretes gonadotropin-releasing hormone (GnRH), which stimulates the anterior pituitary to secrete FSH and luteinizing hormone (LH). FSH and LH regulate ovarian function and stimulate the ovary to produce sex steroids. All of these hormones are influenced by a negative-feedback system and will increase or decrease based on the levels of estradiol and progesterone.

The pathophysiologic changes that occur during the perimenopausal and menopausal periods are caused by the decrease and eventual loss of ovarian follicular activity. As women age, the number of ovarian follicles decreases, and the remaining follicles require higher levels of FSH for maturation and ovulation. During perimenopause, FSH concentrations rise during some menstrual cycles but can fall again during subsequent menstrual cycles, leading to irregular and unpredictable menses. During menopause, FSH concentrations increase 10- to 15-fold, LH concentrations increase fivefold, and levels of circulating estradiol decrease by over 90%.[5]

❶ *Vasomotor symptoms (hot flashes, night sweats), as well as other menopausal symptoms such as vulvovaginal atrophy, vaginal dryness, mood swings, and insomnia, occur in over 50% of perimenopausal women and over 80% of menopausal women.*[4] Menopausal symptoms tend to be more severe in women who undergo surgical menopause compared with natural menopause because of the more rapid decline in estrogen concentrations. Women who seek medical treatment should undergo laboratory evaluation to rule out other conditions that may present with similar symptoms, such as abnormal thyroid function or pituitary adenoma. Once symptoms have been evaluated and other conditions have been excluded, HT should be considered.

vaginal dryness, or mood swings. HT should be considered for these women, but is not the most appropriate choice for all women. ❸ *Women should receive a thorough history and physical examination, including assessing for CHD and breast cancer risk factors, before HT is considered. They should be informed of the risks and the benefits of HT and encouraged to be involved in the decision-making process. If a woman does not have any contraindications to HT, including CHD or significant CHD risk factors, and also does not have a personal history of breast cancer, HT would be an appropriate therapy option (Fig. 50–1).* Women who have undergone a hysterectomy need only be prescribed estrogen. A progestogen should be added to the estrogen only for women with an intact uterus. Alternative and nonhormonal treatment options are available for women who are not candidates for HT, but they

TREATMENT

Desired Outcomes

❷ *HT remains the most effective treatment for vasomotor symptoms and vulvovaginal atrophy and should be considered for women experiencing these symptoms.* The goals of treatment are to alleviate or reduce menopausal symptoms and to improve the patient's quality of life (QoL) while minimizing adverse effects of therapy. The appropriate route of administration should be chosen based on individual patient symptoms, and therapy should be continued at the lowest dose for the shortest duration consistent with treatment goals for each patient.

General Approach to Treatment

Women suffering from vasomotor symptoms should attempt lifestyle or behavioral modifications before seeking medical treatment. Women who seek medical treatment usually suffer from symptoms that diminish their QoL, such as multiple hot flashes per day or week, sleep disturbances,

---

Patient Encounter, Part 1

BW, a 50-year-old woman with a history of osteoarthritis and hypothyroidism, presents to the clinic complaining of hot flashes, vaginal dryness, and insomnia. She states that she experiences approximately two hot flashes per day and is awakened from sleep at least three to four times a week in a "pool of sweat" requiring her to change her clothes and bed linens. Her symptoms began about 3 months ago, and over that time, they have worsened to the point where they have become very bothersome. On questioning, she states her last menstrual period was 1 year ago.

Which of the patient's symptoms and past medical history are consistent with menopause?

What additional information do you need to know in order to make an appropriate therapeutic plan for this patient?

Clinical Presentation and Diagnosis of HT in Menopause

❶ **Menopausal Symptoms**

- *Vasomotor symptoms (**hot flashes**, night sweats)*
- *Irregular menses*
- *Episodic amenorrhea*
- *Sleep disturbances*
- *Mood swings*
- *Vaginal dryness*
- *Depression*

Less Common Symptoms

- Fatigue

- Irritability
- Migraine
- Arthralgia
- Myalgia

Diagnosis

- Amenorrhea for 1 year
- FSH greater than 40 mIU/mL (40 IU/L)
- Fivefold increase in LH

Patient Encounter, Part 2: Medical History, Physical Exam, and Diagnostic Tests

BW's work-up reveals the following additional information:

PMH: Osteoarthritis of the lower back for 5 years controlled on acetaminophen 500 mg two tablets by mouth 3 to 4 times daily; hypothyroidism since age 25, currently controlled

FH: Father: Alive with HTN and CHD (MI at age 60). Mother: Alive with hypothyroidism and GERD. Siblings: Two sisters alive and well

SH: Occupation: nurse; nonsmoker; drinks one to two glasses of red wine with dinner on the weekends; denies illicit drug use

Meds: Acetaminophen 500 mg two tablets by mouth 3 to 4 times daily; synthroid 0.075 mg by mouth once daily; multivitamin by mouth once daily

ROS: (+) hot flashes, night sweats, vaginal dryness and itching; (+) insomnia, myalgias, bowel changes, weight gain, constipation

PE:

VS: BP 128/82, P 78, RR 16, T 37.0°C (98.6°F), wt 74.5 kg (164 lb)

HEENT: WNL

Neck: Supple; no bruits, no adenopathy, no thyromegaly

Breasts: Supple; no masses

CV: RRR, normal S_1 and S_2; no murmurs, rubs, or gallops

Abd: Soft, nontender, nondistended; (+) BS, no masses

Genitourinary: Pelvic examination normal except (+) mucosal atrophy

Labs:

FSH: 76 mIU/mL (76 IU/L)

TSH: 2.5 μU/mL (2.5 mIU/L)

Chem-7: Na 135 mEq/L (135 mmol/L), K 4.5 mEq/L (4.5 mmol/L), Cl 109 mEq/L (109 mmol/L), CO_2 25 mEq/L (25 mmol/L), BUN 9 mg/dL (3.21 mmol/L), SCr 0.9 mg/dL (80 μmol/L), Glucose 98 mg/dL (5.44 mmol/L)

CBC: Hgb 13 g/dL (130 g/L or 8.06 mmol/L), Hct 39% (0.39 volume fraction), WBC 5.5×10^3/mm³ (5.5×10^9/L), platelets 234×10^3/mm³ (234×10^9/L)

Fasting lipid levels: TC 232 mg/dL (6 mmol/L), low-density lipoprotein (LDL) 145 mg/dL (3.76 mmol/L), high-density lipoprotein (HDL) 45 mg/dL (1.17 mmol/L), Triglycerides (TG) 200 mg/dL (2.26 mmol/L)

Assess the patient's condition based on this additional information.

What are the goals of treatment for this patient?

Assess the patient's risk factors for heart disease and breast cancer.

Recommend nonpharmacologic and pharmacologic treatment for this patient. Justify your recommendations.

---

are less efficacious than hormonal therapies. These treatments should be chosen based on the efficacy and safety profile of the treatment and the patient's past medical history and current medications.

Nonpharmacologic Therapy

Nonpharmacologic therapies for menopause-related symptoms have not been studied in large randomized trials, and evidence of benefit is not well documented. Owing to minimal adverse effects with these types of interventions, it is prudent for patients to try lifestyle or behavioral modifications before and in addition to pharmacologic therapy. The most common nonpharmacologic interventions for vasomotor symptoms include the following:[3,8,9]

- Smoking cessation
- Limit alcohol and caffeine
- Limit hot beverages (e.g., coffee/tea, soups)
- Limit spicy foods
- Keep cool, and dress in layers
- Stress reduction (e.g., meditation, relaxation exercises)
- Increase exercise
- Paced respiration

Exercise demonstrated an improvement in QoL but did not improve vasomotor symptoms. Paced respiration, a form of deep, slow breathing, improved vasomotor symptoms in a small group of patients.

Dyspareunia may result from vaginal dryness. Water-based lubricants may provide relief for several hours after application. Moisturizers may provide relief for a longer period of time and potentially can prevent infections by maintaining the acidic environment in the vagina. Both these treatments require frequent application.

A decline in estrogen concentrations also may be associated with urinary stress incontinence. Kegel exercises

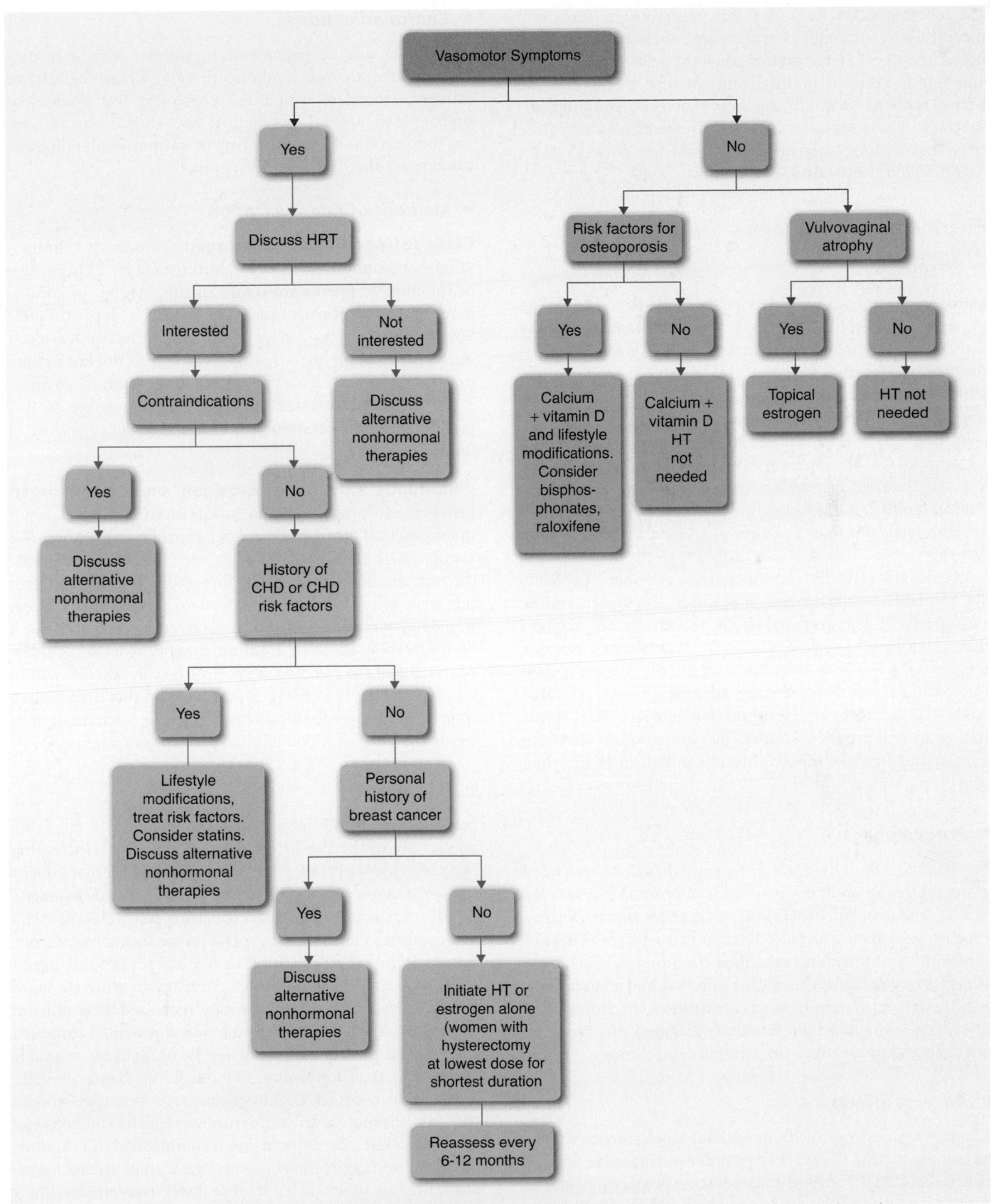

FIGURE 50–1. Treatment algorithm for postmenopausal women. (From Refs. 2, 6, 7.)

are recommended as a first-line intervention for stress incontinence, although pharmacologic therapy also may be necessary. Kegel exercises strengthen the pelvic floor muscles and help to keep the urethra from opening at inappropriate times, such as when lifting heavy objects, coughing, or sneezing. These exercises have no adverse effects, take little time, may be done inconspicuously, and when done correctly, may help to restore normal urine flow.

Pharmacologic Therapy

▶ Estrogens

Estrogen currently is indicated for the treatment of moderate to severe vasomotor symptoms and vulvovaginal atrophy associated with menopause. In addition, it is indicated for the prevention of postmenopausal osteoporosis in women with significant risk; however, it is recommended that nonestrogen medications receive consideration for long-term use. ❹ *Oral or transdermal estrogen products should be prescribed at the lowest effective dose and for the shortest duration possible to provide relief of vasomotor symptoms. Topical products in the form of creams, tablets, or rings should be prescribed for women exclusively experiencing vulvovaginal atrophy.*

Many systemically administered estrogen products are available in the United States, but conjugated equine estrogens (CEEs), prepared from the urine of pregnant mares, is the most widely prescribed. Transdermal estrogen preparations are also available and usually are prescribed for patients who experience adverse effects, elevated triglycerides (TG), or liver function abnormalities while taking an oral product. Transdermal preparations also have a lower incidence of venous thromboembolism (VTE) than oral preparations.[10]

▶ Progestogens

❺ *Women who have an intact uterus should be prescribed a progestogen in addition to estrogen in order to decrease the risk of endometrial hyperplasia and endometrial cancer.*[11] Progestogens should be prescribed for at least 12 to 14 days of the month and often are prescribed continuously. Low doses of oral estrogen therapy, as well as some vaginal preparations, require daily or intermittent administration of a progestogen in order to provide endometrial protection. Table 50–1 lists estrogen and progestogen preparations and dosages.

▶ Adverse Effects

Therapy with estrogen with or without a progestogen should be initiated at the lowest dose in order to minimize adverse effects. Because the adverse effects of these preparations can be similar, it may be difficult to assess whether the estrogen or the progestogen is the cause. Changing preparations, particularly the progestogen, or changing the method of administration may help to alleviate adverse effects. Table 50–2 lists the adverse effects that may be associated with estrogen and progestogen preparations.

▶ Contraindications

● HT should not be prescribed to women with a history of or active thromboembolic disease, breast cancer or estrogen-dependent neoplasm, pregnancy, liver disease, or undiagnosed vaginal bleeding. It also should not be used for the prevention or treatment of cardiovascular disease, cerebrovascular disease, or dementia.[4]

▶ Methods of Administration

Cyclic Estrogen and Progestogen Estrogen is administered daily, and progestogen is administered for 12 to 14 days of the month. The disadvantage of this method of administration is the return of monthly menses in approximately 90% of women 1 to 2 days following the last progestogen dose. However, the withdrawal bleeding does not last as long or is not as heavy as a typical menstrual period. Women may view this scheduled bleeding as an advantage to this method of administration as it limits spotting or soiling of undergarments.

Continuous Combined Estrogen and Progestogen Estrogen and progestogen are administered daily and result in endometrial atrophy. Therefore, women do not experience a withdrawal bleed but may experience unanticipated breakthrough bleeding or spotting during the month. Although this may sound more appealing than a withdrawal bleed, women may view the unpredictable bleeding or spotting as a disadvantage to this type of administration. Women should be educated that the bleeding or spotting usually resolves within 6 to 12 months. If bleeding persists beyond this time period, women should seek medical attention to rule out more serious conditions such as endometrial hypertrophy or carcinoma.

▶ Low-Dose HT

Lower doses of HT have become more popular following publication of the WHI study results. There is an increasing body of evidence proving the effectiveness of these regimens in the management of menopausal symptoms. The Women's Health, Osteoporosis, Progestin/Estrogen (HOPE) trial demonstrated that lower doses of CEE ± medroxyprogesterone acetate (MPA) (CEE 0.45 mg or 0.3 mg ± MPA 2.5 mg or 1.5 mg) decreased hot flashes comparable with standard HT, improved vulvovaginal atrophy, increased bone mineral density (BMD) at the spine and hip, and provided sufficient endometrial protection.[14-18] Currently, no data are available on the effects of lower-dose HT on the incidence of VTE, breast cancer, or CHD. Lower-dose HT provides women with an alternative to standard-dose HT for menopausal symptoms but also should be recommended for a short duration. Although many women have switched to lower-dose HT, only time will tell if lower doses translate into lower risks.

▶ Bioidentical HT

Bioidentical hormones are exogenous hormones that are identical to those produced in a woman's body (e.g.,

Table 50–1

Estrogen and Progestogen Formulations and Dosages

Product	Available Strengths	Common Dosages
Oral estrogens		
CEE (Premarin)	0.3–1.25 mg	0.3–0.625 mg/day
Synthetic conjugated estrogens (Cenestin; Enjuvia)	0.3–1.25 mg	0.3–0.625 mg/day
Esterified estrogens (Menest)	0.3–2.5 mg	0.3–0.625 mg/day
Estradiol (Estrace[a]/Gynodiol[a]; Femtrace[a])	0.5–2 mg; 0.45–1.8 mg	0.5–1 mg/day
Estropipate (Ogen[a]; Ortho-Est[a])	0.625–5 mg; 0.625–1.25 mg	0.625 mg/day
Transdermal estrogens		
Estradiol patch	0.025–0.1 mg/24 hours	0.025–0.05 mg, changed weekly (Climara) or changed twice weekly
(Alora, Climara, Esclim, Estraderm, FemPatch, Vivelle, Vivelle Dot)		
Menostar[b]	14 mcg/24 hours	14 mcg once weekly[b]
Estradiol gel	0.06%	0.87 g/day; 1.25 g/day
(Elestrin, Estrogel) (Divigel)	0.1%	0.25, 0.5, 1 mg packets/day
Estradiol spray (Evamist)	1.53 mg/actuation	1–3 sprays/day
Topical estrogens		
Vaginal creams		
CEE (Premarin)	0.625 mg/g	0.5–2 g/day
Estradiol (Estrace)	0.01% estradiol	1g 1–3 times/week
Estropipate (Ortho-Est)	1.5 mg/g	2–4 g/day
Vaginal rings		
Estradiol (Estring; Femring)	0.0075 mg/24 hours; 0.05–0.1 mg/24 hours	1 ring every 3 months
Vaginal tablet		
Estradiol (Vagifem)	25 mcg estradiol	1 tablet 2 times/week
Emulsions		
Estradiol (Estrasorb)	0.25%	3.84 g applied daily
Oral progestogens[c,d]		
MPA (Provera)	2.5–10 mg	
Micronized progesterone	100–200 mg	
Transdermal Progestogens[c,d]		
Levonorgestrel	0.015 mg	
Norethindrone acetate	0.25–1 mg	
Norgestimate	0.09 mg	
Combination products		
Oral		
CEE + MPA (Prempro; Premphase)	0.3 mg/1.5 mg–0.625 mg/5 mg; 0.625/5 mg	0.3–0.625/2.5–5 mg/day
Estradiol + norethindrone (Activella)	1/0.5 mg	1 tablet daily
Estradiol + drospirenone (Angeliq)	1/0.5 mg	1 tablet daily
Ethynyl estradiol + norethindrone (FemHRT)	2.5 mcg/0.5 mg; 5 mcg/1 mg	55 mcg/1 mg/day
Estradiol + norgestimate (Ortho-Prefest)	1/0.09 mg	1 tablet daily
Transdermal		
Estradiol + norethindrone (Combipatch)	0.05/0.14–0.05/0.25 mg/24 hours	Apply one patch twice weekly
Estradiol + levonorgestrel (Climara Pro)	0.45/0.015 mg/24 hours	Apply one patch once weekly

CEE, conjugated equine estrogens; MPA, medroxyprogesterone acetate.

[a]FDA commercially available bioidentical product.

[b]Indicated for the prevention of postmenopausal osteoporosis only.

[c]May be administered cyclically or continuously.

[d]Dose varies based on daily or weekly administration.

From Refs. 6, 12–14.

Table 50–2

Adverse Effects of Estrogens and Progestogens

Estrogens
Common adverse effects
 Nausea
 Headache
 Bloating
 Breast tenderness
 Bleeding
Serious adverse effects
 Coronary heart disease
 Stroke
 Venous thromboembolism
 Breast cancer
 Gallbladder disease

Progestogens
Common adverse effects
 Nausea
 Headache
 Weight gain
 Bleeding
 Irritability
 Depression
Serious adverse effects
 Venous thromboembolism
 Decreased bone mineral density

From Refs. 5, 6, 13, 14.

estradiol, estrone, estriol, and progesterone). They are either commercially manufactured or chemically compounded in pharmacies into formulations such as topical creams, gels, and suppositories. The commercially manufactured prescription products are subject to regulation by the FDA and have been tested for potency, purity, efficacy and safety (Table 50–1). Conversely, pharmacist-compounded formulations are not subject to the same regulations and therefore, the efficacy and safety is questionable. Some patients view bioidentical hormones, particularly the pharmacist-compounded formulations, as "natural" and assume these formulations are safer than currently marketed prescription hormone products. However, due to a lack of regulation, these products could potentially cause more harm than benefit. There is little evidence comparing the safety and efficacy of conventional HT to prescription bioidentical HT and thus, the same risks and benefits should be assumed.[19,20]

▶ Benefits of HT

Vasomotor Symptoms HT is indicated primarily for the relief of moderate to severe vasomotor symptoms. It remains the most effective treatment for vasomotor symptoms and should be considered only in women experiencing those symptoms. Women with mild vasomotor symptoms may benefit from nonpharmacologic therapy alone; however, many women will seek medical treatment for these symptoms. The benefits of HT outweigh the risks in women who do not have CHD or CHD and breast cancer risk factors; however, careful consideration should be given to alternative and nonhormonal therapies for the relief of menopausal symptoms in women with these risks. Women should be involved in the decision and may choose to use HT due to the severity of their symptoms despite having some risk factors. Regardless of the situation, HT should be prescribed at the lowest dose that relieves or reduces menopausal symptoms and should be recommended only for short-term use. Women should be reassessed every 6 to 12 months, and discontinuation of therapy should be considered.

Vulvovaginal Atrophy HT is indicated for the treatment of vulvovaginal atrophy. Approximately 50% of postmenopausal women experience vulvovaginal atrophy and seek medical attention for relief. Vulvovaginal atrophy is associated with vaginal dryness and dyspareunia and also may be associated with recurrent urinary tract infections, urethritis, and urinary urgency and frequency. Topical preparations generally should be prescribed as first-line therapy unless the patient is also experiencing vasomotor symptoms. Topical estrogen has demonstrated increased efficacy over systemic estrogen and generally does not require supplementation with a progestogen in women with an intact uterus using low doses of micronized 17β-estradiol.[21] Women using regular or high doses of topical estrogen products do require intermittent treatment with a progestogen. Although few data are available on the appropriate progestogen dose, some data indicate that 10 days every 12 weeks may be sufficient to prevent endometrial hyperplasia.[22] Estradiol in the form of a tablet or a ring is not significantly absorbed systemically and may be used safely in a woman with contraindications to estrogen therapy and symptoms of vulvovaginal atrophy.[23]

Osteoporosis Prevention Postmenopausal osteoporosis is a condition that affects millions of women and is characterized by low bone mass with microarchitectural deterioration of bone tissue that can lead to fractures.[24] Fractures, particularly hip fractures, are associated with a high incidence of morbidity and mortality and a decrease in QoL. Before the WHI study, only observational data were available regarding the association of HT and the reduction of fractures. The WHI was the first randomized controlled trial (RCT) that demonstrated a reduction in total fractures, including the hip, spine, and wrist.[2,25]

❻ *Because HT should be maintained only for the short-term, alternative therapies such as bisphosphonates or raloxifene should be considered as first-line therapy for the prevention of postmenopausal osteoporosis, in addition to appropriate doses of calcium and vitamin D. Because of the associated risks, HT should not be prescribed solely for the prevention of osteoporosis.*

Colon Cancer Retrospective observational studies suggested that HT was associated with lower rates of colorectal cancer. The WHI was the first and largest RCT to confirm that HT decreases the risk of colorectal cancer.[2] However, in the WHI estrogen alone arm, the cases of colorectal cancer were not lower in the estrogen group compared with the placebo group.[26] Unfortunately, these data are inconsistent and are not compelling enough to justify long-term use of estrogen therapy to prevent colon cancer.

Risks of HT

Cardiovascular Disease   CHD is the leading cause of death among women in the United States. Retrospective data indicated that HT was associated with a decrease in risk of CHD by 30% to 50%.[26] However, the results of recent RCTs demonstrate that HT does not prevent or treat CHD in women and that it actually may cause an increase in CHD events. The HERS, published in 1998, was the first RCT conducted in women with established CHD. This trial demonstrated an increased incidence of CHD events within the first year of treatment with HT and an increased risk of VTE and gallbladder disease. There was a trend of decreasing incidence of CHD death in years 3 to 5 that prompted a continuation of the study.[1] The HERS II was an open-label continuation of the HERS for an additional 2.7 years. No difference was found in CHD events between the HT and placebo groups; however, there was an increased risk of VTE and biliary tract surgery in the HT group.[27]

The WHI was the first RCT conducted in women without established CHD. Women aged 50 to 79 years with an intact uterus were assigned to receive HT (CEE 0.625 mg + MPA 2.5 mg) daily for 8.5 years. The trial was stopped after only 5.2 years owing to an increased incidence of breast cancer in women taking HT compared with placebo. The WHI demonstrated an increased risk of CHD within the first year of treatment of 0.37% in the HT group compared with 0.3% in the placebo group (hazard ratio [HR] 1.29, 95% confidence interval [CI]) 1.02–1.63). This translates into a number needed to treat to harm (NNTH) of 1,428. There also was an increased risk of stroke in the HT group (0.29%) compared with placebo (0.21%) (HR 1.41, 95% CI 1.07–1.85), with an NNTH of 1,250. Therefore, for every 10,000 women treated per year with HT, there would be seven more CHD deaths and eight more strokes.[3]

The estrogen alone arm of the WHI, which included women aged 50 to 79 years with a history of hysterectomy, continued for another 1.6 years (average follow-up 6.8 years). This arm of the study did not demonstrate an increased risk of CHD compared with placebo. However, there was an increased risk of stroke in the estrogen alone group (0.44%) compared with placebo (0.32%) (HR 1.39, 95% CI 1.10–1.77). This translates into an NNTH of 833 and 12 more strokes for every 10,000 women treated per year with estrogen therapy.[26]

The results of these trials demonstrate that HT should not be prescribed for the prevention of CHD or in patients with pre-existing CHD. For women suffering from vasomotor symptoms with a history of CHD, including CHD risk factors, alternative nonhormonal therapies should be considered. Additionally, lifestyle modifications should be implemented, and therapies to treat risk factors such as hypertension and hyperlipidemia should be prescribed. It is important to note that the average age of women included in the HERS and the WHI trials was 67 and 63 years, respectively, and they started HT a mean of 10 years after menopause. Therefore, these trials were unable to assess the true risk in younger, potentially healthier women with fewer cardiovascular risk factors.[21]

Breast Cancer   Breast cancer is the most common cancer in women in the United States. Observational data indicated an association between HT and breast cancer risk. The WHI was the first RCT to demonstrate an increased risk of invasive breast cancer among women taking HT. In fact, the trial was stopped early owing to an increased incidence of breast cancer in women taking HT (0.38%) compared with placebo (0.3%) (HR 1.26, 95% CI 1–1.59). This translates into an NNTH of 1,250 and 8 more cases of invasive breast cancer for every 10,000 women treated per year with HT. The risk of breast cancer was evident after only 3 years of treatment and continued throughout the study duration.[2]

Breast cancer was not increased in the estrogen-alone arm of the WHI, and in fact, the risk was nonsignificantly lower in this group than in the placebo group.[26] These conflicting data point to a possible link of progestogen with breast cancer risk; however, this theory needs to be studied further.

Because the WHI is the best evidence to date linking HT with breast cancer, women with a personal history of breast cancer and possibly even a strong family history of breast cancer should avoid the use of HT and consider some alternative and nonhormonal therapies for the treatment of vasomotor symptoms.

Venous Thromboembolism   The WHI demonstrated an increased risk for venous thromboembolic disease in the HT group (0.34%) compared with placebo (0.16%) (HR 2.11, 95% CI 1.58–2.82). This translates into an NNTH of approximately 555 and 18 more cases of venous thromboembolic events for every 10,000 women treated per year with HT.[2] The risk for deep vein thrombosis was also increased in the estrogen alone arm of the WHI, but pulmonary embolism was not increased significantly.[26]

⑦   *In summary, combined estrogen plus progestogen should not be used for the prevention of chronic diseases because it increases the risk of CHD, stroke, breast cancer, and VTE. However, colorectal cancer and rates of fracture were reduced with combined hormonal treatment.*

Other Effects of HT

QoL and Cognition   Although women generally consider QoL measures when deciding whether to use HT, the effects of HT on overall QoL have been inconsistent. HT did not demonstrate a clinically meaningful effect on QoL; however, women taking HT did have a small improvement in sleep disturbances, physical functioning, and bodily pain after 1 year of therapy.[28] Results from the HERS demonstrated that HT did improve emotional measures such as depressive symptoms, but only if women suffered from flushing at trial entry. QoL improvement scores declined significantly in women without flushing symptoms.[29]

The prevalence of age-associated memory impairment is approximately 17% to 34% in the general population.[30] Observational studies have suggested a potential benefit of HT on cognitive functioning and dementia. However, the WHI Memory Study (WHIMS), conducted in postmenopausal women aged 65 years or older, failed to demonstrate an improvement in cognitive function and demonstrated a dementia rate, including Alzheimer's disease, two times greater than with placebo.[30,31] The estrogen alone arm of the WHIMS also demonstrated similar results.[32,33]

⑧ *HT improves overall well-being and mood in women with vasomotor symptoms, but it has not demonstrated an improvement in QoL in women without vasomotor symptoms.*

▶ Discontinuation of HT

⑨ *In appropriately selected women, HT should be recommended at the lowest dose for the shortest duration and should be tapered before discontinuation in order to prevent the recurrence of hot flashes.* Although vasomotor symptoms in most women will subside within 4 years, approximately 10% of women continue to experience symptoms that interfere with their QoL. Therefore, it is important to continually reassess a woman's vasomotor symptoms while taking HT and to try to taper the therapy after 1 year. Literature suggests that one of every four women needs to be reinitiated on HT due to persistent and bothersome symptoms.[34–36]

Limited evidence is available to guide health care providers regarding the most effective, safe, and least disruptive way to taper HT. Slowly discontinuing HT over time may be associated with less risk of symptom return. The time frame for tapering HT is unknown but can take up to 3 to 6 months or longer in some cases. Tapering HT may be done in one of two ways: dose taper or day taper. The dose taper involves decreasing the dose of estrogen over several weeks to months and monitoring closely for a return of symptoms. If symptoms recur, the next reduction in dose should not occur until symptoms resolve or at least stabilize on the current dose. The day taper involves decreasing the number of days of the week that a woman takes the HT dose, for example, decreasing a daily dose of 0.3 mg estrogen to 0.3 mg estrogen 5 days a week. Again, if symptoms recur, continue on the current dose until symptoms resolve or stabilize before trying a subsequent decrease. These tapering regimens have not been studied in clinical trials and may not prove to be beneficial in individual women.[36]

▶ Nonhormonal and Alternative Treatments

⑩ *Since publication of the WHI study, there has been an increase in the use of alternative and nonhormonal therapies for the management of menopausal symptoms. Particularly for women with CHD and/or breast cancer risk factors, these therapies may offer another option to assist with symptom management. A wide range of therapies, both prescription and herbal, have been studied with varying degrees of success. In choosing a particular therapy, it is important to match patient symptoms with a therapy that is not only effective but also safe.*

A variety of nonhormonal and alternative therapies (Table 50–3) have been studied for symptomatic management of vasomotor symptoms, including antidepressants (e.g., selective serotonin reuptake inhibitors [SSRIs] and venlafaxine), herbal products (e.g., soy/isoflavones, black

cohosh, evening primrose oil and dong quai), and a group of miscellaneous agents (e.g., gabapentin, clonidine).[37,38] The limited and often conflicting evidence demonstrates that these agents are only modestly effective. It is also widely assumed that these agents are safer than HT, when in reality, few have been evaluated in randomized trials.

SSRIs and venlafaxine are theorized to reduce the frequency of hot flashes by increasing serotonin in the central nervous system and by decreasing LH. Of the SSRIs, fluoxetine, citalopram, paroxetine, and sertraline have been studied and demonstrated a reduction in hot flashes while treating other symptomatic complaints such as depression and anxiety.[37] It is important to note that many of these trials were conducted in women with breast cancer who were also on antiestrogen therapy. Overall, these antidepressant medications offer a reasonable option for women who are unwilling or cannot take hormonal therapies, particularly those who suffer from depression or anxiety.

Alternative therapies used for the relief of menopausal symptoms are purported to act by a number of different mechanisms. Phytoestrogens are plant sterols that are structurally similar to human and animal estrogen. Soy protein is a common source of phytoestrogens.[37–39] There has been conflicting results as to the efficacy of phytoestrogens in treating hot flashes and if used, at least 45 to 60 g/day of isoflavone content is necessary for any possible benefit. Because the effect of isoflavones on breast cancer and other female-related cancers, bone mass, and vaginal dryness is unknown, phytoestrogens should not be considered in women with a history of estrogen-dependent cancers.[41]

Black cohosh has been one of the most studied alternative therapies for vasomotor symptoms, but it has not demonstrated a substantial benefit over placebo. The mechanism of action, safety profile, drug-drug interactions, and adverse effects of black cohosh remain unknown. In non–placebo-controlled trials conducted for 6 months or less, black cohosh (40–80 mg/day) demonstrated a small, nonstatistically significant reduction in vasomotor symptoms.[37,38,40] In addition, there have been case reports of hepatotoxicity with the use of black cohosh.[42] Caution should be exercised when considering the use of this product, especially in patients with liver dysfunction. There is insufficient evidence to determine the effectiveness of black cohosh and due to safety concerns, it should not be recommended at this time.[41,43]

Dong quai, evening primrose oil and several other alternative therapies, including passion flower, sage, valerian root, flaxseed, and wild yam, have not demonstrated efficacy with regard to the relief of vasomotor symptoms, and the safety of these products is also questionable.[37,38,40] Therefore, these products should not be recommended for the relief of vasomotor symptoms in postmenopausal women.

There are a number of other prescription products that have been studied for the management of menopausal symptoms. Gabapentin is thought to exert its effect by affecting the thermoregulatory process of the pituitary-hypothalamic region through modulation of calcium currents that, in turn, affect adrenergic and serotonergic pathways. In RCTs,

Table 50–3

Nonhormonal Therapies for Menopause

Agent	Demonstrated Efficacy	Dosing	Adverse Effects/Precautions
Citalopram	Nonrandomized trial demonstrated efficacy in hot flash reduction	20–60 mg daily	Nausea, dizziness, somnolence
Fluoxetine	One RCT demonstrated significant reduction in hot flashes; one RCT found drug no better than placebo	20 mg daily	Nausea, insomnia, nervousness, fatigue
Paroxetine	Two RCTs demonstrated significant reduction in and severity of hot flashes (approximately 30%)	10–20 mg daily	Headache, nausea, insomnia
Sertraline	Case series demonstrating efficacy in hot flash reduction	25–50 mg daily	Nausea, dizziness, somnolence
Venlafaxine	Two RCTs reported short-term significant reductions in and severity of hot flashes	12.5 mg twice daily	Nausea, dry mouth
Soy protein	Eighteen small RCTs demonstrate conflicting evidence; systematic reviews demonstrate no clinical superiority over placebo	45–60 mg isoflavones daily	GI upset; other adverse effects unknown; do not use in those with history of or high risk of estrogen-dependent cancer
Black cohosh	Seven small, short-term RCTs demonstrated benefit in mild-moderate hot flashes, especially when associated with sleep and mood disturbances	Varied dosing based on herbal product combination; most studied: Reminfemin 40–80 mg twice daily	GI upset (take with food); potential hepatoxicity; not recommended to be taken over a 6-month period of time
Gabapentin	Four RCTs concluded that drug was significantly more effective than placebo at reducing the frequency and severity of hot flashes (approximately 50%), including those with breast cancer	900 mg daily	Dizziness and somnolence
Clonidine	Eleven studies, seven of which demonstrated significant reductions in frequency and severity of hot flashes	0.1–0.4 mg daily	Dry mouth, blood pressure lowering; monitor blood pressure
Dong quai	No demonstrated efficacy in one RCT	Not recommended	Structurally similar to coumarins—avoid with warfarin because INR can increase
Evening primrose oil, passion flowers, sage, valerian root, and wild yam	No demonstrated efficacy for any product in RCTs	Not recommended	Caution with all plant products in women with hay fever and plant allergies

RCT, randomized controlled trial.

From Refs. 37–40.

gabapentin at doses of 900 mg/day demonstrated significant reductions in severity and frequency of hot flashes compared to placebo. Clonidine is thought to work by reducing small-vessel response, both centrally and peripherally, to various stimuli. It has been studied in several small RCTs at doses of 0.1 to 0.4 mg/day and has demonstrated statistically significant reductions in hot flashes.[40] This agent may be considered in women with a history of hypertension, but the adverse effects may outweigh the benefits.

Overall, alternative and nonhormonal therapies are less effective in treating vasomotor symptoms than HT but do offer another option for women experiencing menopausal symptoms who cannot or are unwilling to take HT. SSRIs and clonidine have the best evidence for efficacy, however, health care providers should weigh the benefits and risks of all therapies, and women should be advised to discuss their options with physicians and pharmacists.

OUTCOME EVALUATION

Evaluating the outcomes of any therapy for menopausal symptoms focuses primarily on the woman's report of symptom resolution. Ask women to report the resolution or reduction of hot flashes, night sweats, and vaginal dryness, and any improvement or change in sleep patterns. Also ask women taking hormonal therapies to report any breakthrough bleeding or spotting. If abnormal or heavy bleeding occurs, refer the woman to her primary care provider. Monitor subjective parameters such as adverse effects and adherence to the therapy regimen, as well as monthly breast self-examinations. In addition, monitor objective parameters, including blood pressure, at every outpatient visit; encourage yearly clinical breast examinations, mammograms, and thyroid-stimulating hormone (TSH) determination, particularly for women with hypothyroidism on thyroid

Patient Care and Monitoring

1. Assess the patient for use of HT by evaluating for the presence of vasomotor symptoms. If the patient is experiencing bothersome vasomotor symptoms, consider the use of HT only after assessing for risk factors for heart disease and breast cancer. If vasomotor symptoms are tolerable and/or the patient has risk factors for heart disease and/or breast cancer, consider alternative, nonhormonal treatments for vasomotor symptoms.

2. Obtain a thorough medication history, including the use of over-the-counter and herbal products.

3. Educate the patient on lifestyle or behavioral interventions that may help to alleviate vasomotor symptoms.

4. Discuss methods of HT administration, and have the patient decide in conjunction with the health care provider which one she feels will work best for her.

5. Recommend the appropriate dose of HT, and use the lowest effective dose for the shortest duration possible.

6. Educate the patient regarding the proper administration, potential adverse effects, and expectations of HT.

7. Monitor the patient for a reduction in vasomotor symptoms, vaginal dryness, and improvement in sleep.

Also monitor for breakthrough bleeding and spotting, adverse effects of HT, and improvement in QOL.

8. Monitor the following objective parameters:
   - Blood pressure at every outpatient visit
   - Yearly lipoprotein panels
   - Yearly fasting plasma glucose determinations
   - Yearly breast examinations and mammograms
   - Yearly TSH determinations, particularly for women with hypothyroidism on thyroid therapy
   - Endometrial studies in women with undiagnosed vaginal bleeding

9. Educate the patient regarding the importance of adhering to the medication regimen.

10. Educate the patient regarding the importance of obtaining a yearly mammogram and Papanicolaou (Pap) smear (if applicable), as well as performing a monthly breast self-examination.

11. Assess patient symptoms every 6 to 12 months, and consider tapering the HT dose and discontinuing treatment after 1 year. If vasomotor symptoms return, determine if a longer tapering schedule is warranted or if long-term treatment is necessary.

Patient Encounter, Part 3: Creating a Care Plan

Based on the information presented, create a care plan for BW's hot flashes and vaginal dryness. The plan should include:

(a) a statement identifying the patient problem and its severity,
(b) goals of therapy,
(c) a therapeutic plan based on individual patient-specific factors,
(d) subjective and objective monitoring parameters, and
(e) a follow-up evaluation to assess for adverse effects and adherence and to determine if the goals of therapy have been achieved.

Abbreviations Introduced in This Chapter

BMD	Bone mineral density
CEEs	Conjugated equine estrogen
CI	Confidence interval
CHD	Coronary heart disease
FSH	Follicle-stimulating hormone
GnRH	Gonadotropin-releasing hormone
HR	Hazard ratio
HDL	High-density lipoprotein
HERS	Heart and Estrogen/Progestin Replacement Study
HOPE	Women's Health, Osteoporosis, Progestin/Estrogen trial
HT	Hormone therapy
LDL	Low-density lipoprotein
LH	Luteinizing hormone
MPA	Medroxyprogesterone acetate
NNTH	Number needed to treat to harm
QoL	Quality of life
RCT	Randomized controlled trial
SSRI	Selective serotonin reuptake inhibitor
TG	Triglycerides
TSH	Thyroid-stimulating hormone
VTE	Venous thromboembolism
WHI	Women's Health Initiative
WHIMS	Women's Health Initiative Memory Study

therapy, and conduct a BMD test every 5 years. Also perform endometrial studies, as necessary, in women with undiagnosed vaginal bleeding. Lastly, evaluate the patient's overall QOL. Because the management of menopause is largely symptomatic, it is important to document symptoms at the beginning of therapy and monitor symptom improvement and potential adverse effects at each visit. Frequent follow-up, proper monitoring, and education will help to ensure that the woman achieves optimal results from any therapy chosen to treat menopausal symptoms.

Self-assessment questions and answers are available at *http://www.mhpharmacotherapy.com/pp.html*.

REFERENCES

1. Hulley S, Grady D, Bush T, et al. for the Heart and Estrogen/progestin Replacement Study (HERS) Research Group. Randomized trial of estrogen plus progestin for secondary prevention of coronary heart disease in postmenopausal women. JAMA 1998;280(7):605–613.

2. Rossouw JE, Anderson GL, Prentice RL, et al. Risks and benefits of estrogen plus progestin in healthy postmenopausal women: Principal results from the Women's Health Initiative randomized controlled trial. JAMA 2002;288(3):321–333.

3. National Institutes of Health State-of-the-Science Conference statement: Management of menopause-related symptoms. Ann Intern Med 2005;142(12 pt 1):1003–1013.

4. Nelson HD. Menopause. Lancet 2008;371;760–770.

5. Burger HG. The endocrinology of the menopause. J Steroid Biochem Mol Biol 1999;69(1–6):31–35.

6. Kalantaridou SN, Davis SR, Anton Calis K. Hormone therapy in women. In: Dipiro JT, Talbert RL, Yee GC et al., eds. Pharmacotherapy: A Pathophysiologic Approach, 7th ed. New York: McGraw-Hill, 2008:1351–1368.

7. Rymer J, Wilson R, Ballard K. Making decisions about hormone replacement therapy. BMJ 2003;326(7384):322–326.

8. McKee J, Warber SL. Integrative therapies for menopause. South Med J 2005;98(3):319–326.

9. Sikon A, Thacker HL. Treatment options for menopausal hot flashes. Cleve Clin J Med 2004;71(7):578–582.

10. Scarabin PY, Oger E, Plu-Bureau G. Differential association of oral and transdermal oestrogen-replacement therapy with venous thromboembolism risk. Lancet 2003;362(9382):428–432.

11. Lethaby A, Suckling J, Barlow D, et al. Hormone replacement therapy in postmenopausal women: Endometrial hyperplasia and irregular bleeding. Cochrane Database Syst Rev 2004;(3):CD000402.

12. Ragucci KR, Carson DS. Women's health. In: Hansen LB, Kelly W, eds. Pharmacotherapy Self-Assessment Program: Geriatrics/Special Populations, 5th ed. Kansas City: American College of Clinical Pharmacy, 2006:133–161.

13. Klasco RK e. Estrogens. DrugDex 2006. Available at: *http://www.thomsonhc.com/*

14. Klasco RK e. Medroxyprogesterone. DrugDex 2006. Available at: *http://www.thomsonhc.com/*

15. Archer DF, Dorin M, Lewis V, et al. Effects of lower doses of conjugated equine estrogens and medroxyprogester-one acetate on endometrial bleeding. Fertil Steril 2001;75(6):1080–1087.

16. Lindsay R, Gallagher JC, Kleerekoper M, et al. Effect of lower doses of conjugated equine estrogens with and without medroxyprogesterone acetate on bone in early postmenopausal women. JAMA 2002;287(20):2668–2676.

17. Pickar JH, Yeh I, Wheeler JE, et al. Endometrial effects of lower doses of conjugated equine estrogens and medroxyprogesterone acetate. Fertil Steril 2001;76(1):25–31.

18. Utian WH, Shoupe D, Bachmann G, et al. Relief of vaso-motor symptoms and vaginal atrophy with lower doses of conjugated equine estrogens and medroxyprogesterone acetate. Fertil Steril 2001;75(6):1065–1079.

19. Boothby LA, Doering PL, Kipersztok S. Bioidentical hormone therapy: A review. Menopause 2004;11:356–367.

20. Utian WH. Bioidentical hormones: Separating science from marketing. The Female Patient. *http://www.femalepatient.com/html/arc/sig/meno/articles/030_10_021.asp.*

21. The North American Menopause Society. Estrogen and progestogen use in peri- and postmenopausal women: March 2007 position statement of The North American Menopause Society. Menopause 2007;14:168–182.

22. Davis S. Hormone replacement therapy. Indications, benefits and risk. Aust Fam Physician 1999;28(5):437–445.

23. Notelovitz M. Urogenital atrophy and low-dose vaginal estrogen therapy. Menopause 2000;7(3):140–142.

24. The North American Menopause Society. Management of postmenopausal osteoporosis: Position statement of The North American Menopause Society. Menopause 2002;9:84–101.

25. Cauley JA, Robbins J, Chen Z, et al. Effects of estrogen plus progestin on risk of fracture and bone mineral density: The Women's Health Initiative randomized trial. JAMA 2003;290(13):1729–1738.

26. Anderson GL, Limacher M, Assaf AR, et al. Effects of conjugated equine estrogen in postmenopausal women with hysterectomy: The Women's Health Initiative randomized controlled trial. JAMA 2004;291(14):1701–1712.

27. Grady D, Herrington D, Bittner V, et al. Cardiovascular disease outcomes during 6.8 years of hormone therapy: Heart and Estrogen/Progestin Replacement Study followup (HERS II). JAMA 2002;288(1):49–57.

28. Hays J, Ockene JK, Brunner RL, et al. Effects of estrogen plus progestin on health-related quality of life. N Engl J Med 2003;348(19):1839–1854.

29. Hlatky MA, Boothroyd D, Vittinghoff E, et al. Quality-of-life and depressive symptoms in postmenopausal women after receiving hormone therapy: Results from the Heart and Estrogen/Progestin Replacement Study (HERS) trial. JAMA 2002;287(5):591–597.

30. Rapp SR, Espeland MA, Shumaker SA, et al. Effect of estrogen plus progestin on global cognitive function in postmenopausal women: The Women's Health Initiative Memory Study: A randomized controlled trial. JAMA 2003;289(20):2663–2672.

31. Shumaker SA, Legault C, Rapp SR, et al. Estrogen plus progestin and the incidence of dementia and mild cognitive impairment in postmenopausal women: The Women's Health Initiative Memory Study: A randomized controlled trial. JAMA 2003;289(20):2651–2662.

32. Espeland MA, Rapp SR, Shumaker SA, et al. Conjugated equine estrogens and global cognitive function in postmenopausal women: Women's Health Initiative Memory Study. JAMA 2004;291(24):2959–2968.

33. Shumaker SA, Legault C, Kuller L, et al. Conjugated equine estrogens and incidence of probable dementia and mild cognitive impairment in postmenopausal women: Women's Health Initiative Memory Study. JAMA 2004;291(24):2947–2958.

34. Stephenson J. FDA orders estrogen safety warnings: Agency offers guidance for HRT use. JAMA 2003;289(5):537–538.

35. Executive summary. Hormone therapy. Obstet Gynecol 2004;104(4 suppl):1S–4S.

36. Grady D. A 60-year-old woman trying to discontinue hormone replacement therapy. JAMA 2002;287(16):2130–2137.

37. Nelson HD, Vesco KK, Haney E, et al. Nonhormonal therapies for menopausal hot flashes: Systematic review and meta-analysis. JAMA 2006;295:2057–2071.

38. Newton KM, Reed SD, LaCroix AZ, et al. Treatment of vasomotor symptoms of menopause with black cohosh, multibotanicals, soy, hormone therapy or placebo: A randomized trial. Ann Intern Med 2006;145(12):869–879.

39. Glazier MG, Bowman MA. A review of the evidence for the use of phytoestrogens as a replacement for traditional estrogen replacement therapy. Arch Intern Med 2001;161(9):1161–1172.

40. Cheema D, Coomarasamy A, El-Toukhy T. Non-hormonal therapy of postmenopausal vasomotor symptoms: A structured evidence-based review. Arch Gynecol Obstet 2007;276(5):463–469.

41. American College of Obstetricians and Gynecologists Committee on Practice Bulletins—Gynecology. ACOG Practice Bulletin. Clinical Management Guidelines for Obstetrician-Gynecologists. Use of botanicals for management of menopausal symptoms. Obstet Gynecol 2001;97(6):suppl 1–11.

42. Lontos S, Jones RM, Angus PW, et al. Acute liver failure associated with the use of herbal preparations containing black cohosh. Med J Aust 2003;179(7):390–391.

43. The North American Menopause Society. Treatment of menopause-associated vasomotor symptoms: Position statement of The North American Menopause Society. Menopause 2004;11(1):11–33.

51   Erectile Dysfunction

Cara Liday and Catherine Heyneman

LEARNING OBJECTIVES

● **Upon completion of the chapter, the reader will be able to:**

1. Identify the structures of the male reproductive system and describe the physiology of a penile erection.

2. Differentiate between organic and psychogenic erectile dysfunction (ED) and describe the etiology and pathophysiology of each.

3. Identify the drug classes most likely to contribute to ED.

4. Define the essential components of history, physical examination, and laboratory data needed to evaluate the patient presenting with ED.

5. Describe current nonpharmacologic and pharmacologic options for treating ED and determine an appropriate first-line therapy for a specific patient.

6. Compare and contrast the benefits and risks for the current phosphodiesterase (PDE) inhibitors.

7. Identify patients with significant cardiovascular risk and recommend an appropriate treatment approach for their ED.

KEY CONCEPTS

❶ Erectile dysfunction (ED) can be classified as organic, psychogenic, or mixed. Many patients may initially have organic dysfunction, but develop a psychogenic component as they cope with their inability to achieve an erection.

❷ In addition to a physical exam, a thorough medical, social, and medication history with emphasis on cardiac disease must be taken before starting any treatment for ED to assess for ability to safely perform sexual activity and to assess for possible drug interactions.

❸ A wide range of treatment options is now available for men with ED. These include medical devices, pharmacologic treatments, lifestyle modifications, surgery, and psychotherapy.

❹ When determining the best treatment for an individual, the role of the clinician is to inform the patient and his partner of all available options while understanding his medical history, desires, and goals. The choice of treatment is primarily left up to the couple, but most often treatment is initiated with the least invasive option and then progresses to more invasive options if needed.

❺ Vacuum section devices (VEDs) and intracavernosal injections are highly effective for many patients, but side effects, lack of spontaneity, and fear of needles limit their widespread use as first-line therapy.

❻ Effectiveness of the three available phosphodiesterase (PDE) inhibitors is essentially comparable, but differences exist in duration of action and, to a small degree, incidence of side effects and drug interactions.

❼ Androgens are important for general sexual function and libido, but testosterone supplementation is only effective in patients with documented low serum testosterone levels.

INTRODUCTION

Erectile dysfunction (ED) is defined as the inability to achieve or maintain an erection sufficient for sexual intercourse. The definition is very subjective due to differences in desired or needed rigidity in patients of different ages and in different types of relationships. Patients may refer to their dysfunction as "impotence," but the National Institutes of Health Consensus Development Conference recommends that the term "erectile dysfunction" replace the term "impotence" due to confusion with other forms of sexual dysfunction and the negative connotation associated with the term "impotence."[1] Patients may also develop libido or ejaculatory disorders, but these are not considered ED.

EPIDEMIOLOGY AND ETIOLOGY

ED becomes increasingly frequent as men age. Few men report erection problems before the age of 40, but the percentage of men experiencing ED increases to 26% in men aged 50 to 59 years and 40% in men aged 60 to 69 years.[2] The increase in incidence could be due to physiologic changes that occur with aging, the onset of chronic disease states associated with ED, increased medication use, lifestyle factors, or a combination of the above.

PATHOPHYSIOLOGY

The penis consists of three components, two dorsolateral corpora cavernosa and a ventral corpus spongiosum that surrounds the penile urethra and distally forms the glans penis. The corpora cavernosa consist of blood-filled sinusoidal or lacunar spaces, which are lined with endothelial cells, supported by trabecular smooth muscle, and surrounded by a thick fibrous sheath called the tunica albuginea. The cavernosal arteries, which are branches of the penile artery, penetrate the tunica albuginea and supply blood flow to the penis.

Sympathetic and parasympathetic nerves innervate the penis. In the flaccid state, α_2-adrenergic receptors mediate tonic contraction of the arterial and corporal smooth muscles. This maintains high penile arterial resistance and a balance exists between blood flow into and out of the corpora. With sexual stimulation, nerve impulses from the brain travel down the spinal cord to the thoracolumbar ganglia.[3] A decrease in sympathetic tone and an increase in parasympathetic activity then occurs, causing a net increase in blood flow into the

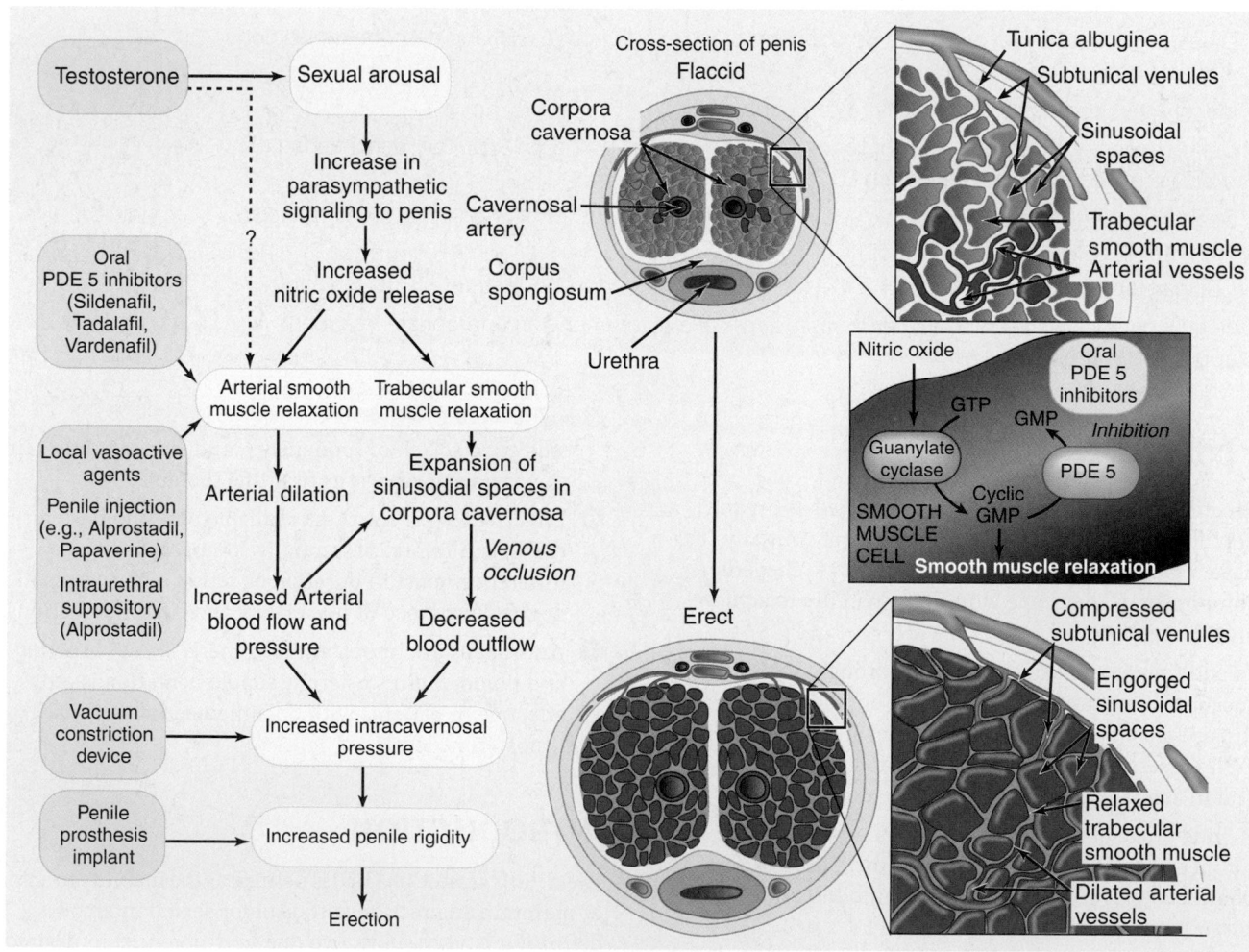

FIGURE 51-1. Mechanism of erection and sites of action of various treatment modalities for erectile dysfunction (ED). Penile erection is achieved through relaxation of smooth muscle cells lining arterial vessels and sinusoidal spaces in the corpora cavernosa, which leads to increased arterial inflow and pressure, decreased venous outflow, and increased intracavernosal pressure. Smooth muscle relaxation is mediated by intracellular generation of cyclic guanosine monophosphate (cGMP) from guanosine triphosphate (GTP) via activation of guanylate cyclase by nitric oxide. Treatment modalities for ED (shown in blue) include oral phosphodiesterase type 5 (PDE-5) inhibitors, which inhibit the breakdown of cGMP, and local vasoactive agents. A link between testosterone and nitric oxide synthase has been demonstrated experimentally, but the significance of this observation in humans has not been established (indicated by the dashed line and question mark). Psychotherapy (not shown) may also be effective in selected individuals with ED. (From Ref. 4.)

erectile tissue. Erections may also occur as a result of a sacral nerve reflex arc while patients are sleeping (nocturnal erections). Acetylcholine-mediated parasympathetic activity leads to production of the nonadrenergic–noncholinergic transmitter nitric oxide (NO). By enhancing the activity of guanylate cyclase, NO increases the production of cyclic guanosine monophosphate (cGMP). Vasoactive peptide and prostaglandins E_1 and E_2 stimulate increased production of cyclic adenosine monophosphate (cAMP). Both cAMP and cGMP ultimately lead to a decrease in calcium concentration within smooth muscle cells of the penile arteries and the sinusoidal spaces, leading to smooth muscle relaxation and increased blood flow. As the sinusoidal spaces become engorged, intracavernosal pressure increases, subtunical venules are compressed, and the penis becomes rigid and elongated (Fig. 51–1).

Detumescence occurs with sympathetic discharge after ejaculation. Sympathetic activity induces smooth muscle contraction of arterioles and vascular spaces leading to a reduction in blood inflow, decompression of the sinusoidal spaces, and enhanced outflow.

Testosterone also plays a significant albeit complex role in erectile function. Testosterone is responsible for much of a man's libido. With low serum concentrations, libido declines. Additionally, testosterone helps with stabilization of intracavernosal levels of NO synthase, the enzyme responsible for triggering the NO cascade. Interestingly, some patients with low or borderline low serum concentrations of testosterone will have normal erectile function, while some with normal levels will have dysfunction.

Normal penile erections are complex events that require the full function of the vascular, neurologic, and hormonal systems. Anything that affects the function of these systems may lead to ED. ❶ *ED can be classified as organic, psychogenic, or a mixture of these.* Organic dysfunction includes abnormalities in the three systems responsible for a normal erection or may be medication-induced (Tables 51–1 and 51–2). Note that many of the risk factors for ED are the same as risk factors for cardiovascular (CV) disease. In many patients, ED is the first indication of the endothelial dysfunction associated with cardiovascular disease.[7] The presence of ED risk factors leads to the assumption that the patient has organic dysfunction. Most commonly, medical conditions that impair arterial flow into or out of the erectile tissue or affect the innervation will be strongly associated with ED. Patients with diabetes mellitus have exceptionally high rates of ED as a result of vascular disease and neuropathy. Additionally, a relationship has been found between low testosterone levels and an increased incidence of metabolic syndrome and type 2 diabetes.[8]

Psychogenic dysfunction occurs if a patient does not respond to psychological arousal. It occurs in up to 30% of all cases of ED. Common causes include performance anxiety, strained relationships, lack of sexual arousability, and overt psychiatric disorders such as depression and schizophrenia.[9]

❶ *Many patients may initially have organic dysfunction, but develop a psychogenic component as they try to cope with their*

Table 51–1
Factors Associated With ED

Chronic medical conditions
- Hypertension
- Diabetes mellitus
- Inflammatory conditions of the prostate
- Coronary and peripheral vascular disease
- Neurologic disorders (e.g., Parkinson's disease and multiple sclerosis)
- Endocrine disorders (hypogonadism and pituitary, adrenal, and thyroid disorders)
- Psychiatric disorders (depression, anxiety, and schizophrenia)
- Hyperlipidemia
- Renal failure
- Liver disease
- Penile disease (Peyronie's disease or anatomic abnormalities)

Surgical procedures
- Perineal surgery
- Radical prostatectomy
- Vascular surgery

Lifestyle
- Age
- Smoking
- Excessive alcohol consumption
- Obesity
- Poor overall health and reduced physical activity

Trauma
- Pelvic fractures
- Spinal cord injuries

Table 51–2
Medication Classes Associated With ED

Antihypertensives
- β-Blockers (particularly nonselective)
- Thiazide diuretics
- Centrally acting agents (clonidine, methyldopa, and reserpine)
- Spironolactone
- α-Blockers

Lipid medications
- Gemfibrozil

Antidepressants
- Tricyclic antidepressants
- Monoamine oxidase inhibitors
- Selective serotonin reuptake inhibitors/serotonin-norepinephrine reuptake inhibitors

Antipsychotics
- Phenothiazines
- Risperidone
- Lithium

Anticonvulsants
- Carbamazepine
- Phenytoin

Histamine antagonists
- Cimetidine

Antiandrogens and hormones
- 5α-Reductase inhibitors
- Progesterone and estrogen

Recreational drugs
- Ethanol
- Cocaine
- Marijuana
- Opiates

From Refs. 3, 5, 6.

inability to achieve an erection. It has been estimated that up to 80% of ED cases have an organic cause, with many having a psychogenic component as well.[1]

TREATMENT

Desired Outcomes

ED is not a life-threatening condition, but left untreated it can be associated with depression, loss of self-esteem, poor self-image, and marital discord.[13] The primary goal of therapy is achievement of erections suitable for intercourse and improvement in patient quality of life. Additionally, the ideal therapy should have minimal side effects, be convenient to administer, have a quick onset of action, and have few or no drug interactions.[10] ❷ *In addition to a physical exam, a thorough medical, social, and medication history with emphasis on cardiac disease must be taken before starting any treatment for ED to assess for ability to safely perform sexual activity and to assess for possible drug interactions.*

General Approach to Treatment

After determining whether the ED is organic or psychogenic, the initial step in management is to identify associated disease states and lifestyle activities that adversely affect erectile function and treat them optimally. Medications suspected to

---

Clinical Presentation and Diagnosis of ED[10,11]

The introduction of oral medications and direct-to-consumer advertising has made patients feel more comfortable approaching practitioners for treatment advice. Despite this, some patients may only discuss their dysfunction when questioned directly by their provider or if their partner initiates the interaction. Patients may still feel that a loss in erectile function translates into a loss of masculinity.

Possible Signs and Symptoms

- Embarrassment
- Anxiousness
- Anger
- Marital problems
- Low self-confidence or morale
- Full inability to achieve erections
- Ability to achieve partial erections, but not suitable for intercourse
- Erections sufficient for intercourse, but early detumescence
- The problem may have a slow or acute onset, or may wax and wane

Diagnosis

ED may be the presenting symptom of other chronic disease states.

Full medical, social, and medication histories should be taken to determine areas that can cause or exacerbate ED and to assess the patient's ability to safely perform intercourse.

- Medical history with emphasis on cardiovascular and psychiatric disorders, diabetes, trauma, and surgical procedures
- Social history: smoking, recreational drug use, exercise, and alcohol consumption

- Medication history including prescription, nonprescription, and dietary supplements

PE

- Review for hypogonadism (gynecomastia, testicular atrophy, reduced body hair, increase in body fat)
- Digital rectal exam to determine if prostate is enlarged
- Vital signs
- Abnormalities of the penis or impaired vasculature and nerve function to the penis

Labs

- Thyroid function
- HbA1c
- Serum testosterone
- Fasting lipid panel
- Metabolic panel
- Further cardiac testing if warranted

Determine severity

- Sexual health inventory for men[12]:
  - How do you rate your confidence that you could get and keep an erection?
  - When you had erections with sexual stimulation, how often were your erections hard enough for penetration?
  - During sexual intercourse, how often were you able to maintain your erection after you had penetrated (entered) your partner?
  - During sexual intercourse, how difficult was it to maintain your erection to completion of intercourse?
  - When you attempted sexual intercourse, how often was it satisfactory for you?
  - Questions scored 1 to 5, very low to very high respectively. Score of 21 or less indicates ED likely.

Table 51–3

Common Drug Treatment Regimens for ED

Route of Administration	Generic Name	Brand Name	Typical Dosing Range[a]	Maximum Dosing Frequency
Oral	Sildenafil	Viagra	25–100 mg 1 hour prior to intercourse	Once daily
	Tadalafil	Cialis	5–20 mg prior to intercourse	Once daily
	Vardenafil	Levitra	5–20 mg 1 hour prior to intercourse	Once daily
	Yohimbine[b]	Aphrodyne, Yocon	5.4 mg 3 times daily	N/A
Intracavernosal	Alprostadil	Caverject, Caverject Impulse, Edex	1.25–60 mcg 5–20 minutes prior to intercourse[c]	3 times weekly, 24 hours between injections
	Papaverine	N/A	Typically used in combination at variable doses	3 times weekly, 24 hours between injections
	Phentolamine	N/A	Typically used in combination at variable doses	3 times weekly, 24 hours between injections
Intraurethral	Alprostadil	MUSE	125–1,000 mcg 5–10 minutes prior to intercourse[c]	2 times daily
Intramuscular	Testosterone cypionate	Depo-Testosterone	50–400 mg every 2–4 weeks	Once weekly
	Testosterone enanthate	Delatestryl	50–400 mg every 2–4 weeks	Once weekly
Topical	Testosterone patches	Testoderm	4–6 mg/day applied to scrotum	Once daily
		Testoderm TTS	4–6 mg/day applied to arm, back, or upper buttocks	Once daily
		Androderm	2.5–5 mg/day applied to back, abdomen, upper arms, or thighs	Once daily
	Testosterone gel	AndroGel 1%, Testim	5–10 g daily to shoulders, upper arms, or abdomen (AndroGel only)	Once daily
Buccal	Testosterone	Striant	30 mg every 12 hours to gum region above incisor; rotate to alternate sides with each dose	Twice daily
Subcutaneous implantable pellet	Testosterone	Testopel	150–450 mg (150 mg for every 25 mg testosterone propionate required weekly)	Every 3 to 6 months

MUSE, medicated urethral system for erection.

[a]Use the lowest effective dose to limit adverse effects.

[b]Not FDA-approved for this indication.

[c]Initial dose must be titrated in physician's office.

cause or worsen ED should also be discontinued if possible. In patients with intermediate or high cardiovascular risk, additional testing should occur to determine if sexual activity is safe.

❸ A wide range of treatment options is now available for men with ED. These include medical devices, pharmacologic treatments, lifestyle modifications, surgery, and psychotherapy.

❹ When determining the best treatment for an individual, the role of the clinician is to inform the patient and his partner of all available options while understanding his medical history, desires, and goals. Most often treatment is initiated with the least invasive option and then treatment progresses to more invasive options if needed. Ultimately, the choice of therapy should be individualized, taking into account patient and partner preferences, concomitant disease states, response, administration route, cost, tolerability, and safety. Common drug treatment regimens for ED are listed in Table 51–3.

Patient Encounter, Part 1

A 52-year-old man with type 2 diabetes, hypertension, and dyslipidemia returns to your clinic for follow-up on his chronic disease states. When reviewing his history, he describes problems having satisfactory sexual intercourse. After further questioning, you determine that his dysfunction has progressively gotten worse over the last year. He is quite emotional and states that the problem is distressing and has caused significant marital discord. He wonders about "those ads on television" suggesting a pill.

Based on the available information, how would you classify his ED?

What additional information do you need to determine his ability to safely perform intercourse?

What additional information do you need before establishing an appropriate treatment regimen?

▶ *Nonpharmacologic Therapy*

Lifestyle Modifications Lifestyle modifications should always be addressed in the management of ED. A healthy diet, increase in regular physical activity and weight loss are associated with higher International Index of Erectile Dysfunction (IIED) scores and an improvement in erectile function.[14] The clinician should recommend smoking cessation, reduction in excessive alcohol intake, and discontinuation of illicit drug use.

Psychotherapy Psychotherapy is an appropriate treatment approach for patients with psychogenic or mixed dysfunction. It should address immediate causes of dysfunction, and if possible the partner should attend sessions as well. Effectiveness is not well documented for organic dysfunction unless combined with other therapies. Advantages include noninvasiveness and partner participation, while disadvantages include increased cost and time commitment.

Vacuum Erection Devices Vacuum erection devices (VEDs) induce erections by creating a vacuum around the penis; the negative pressure draws blood into the penis by passively dilating arteries and engorging the corpora cavernosa. The erection is maintained with a constriction band placed at the base of the penis to reduce venous outflow (Fig. 51–2). They may be used as often as desired, but it is recommended that the constriction band not be left in place longer than 30 minutes at a time.

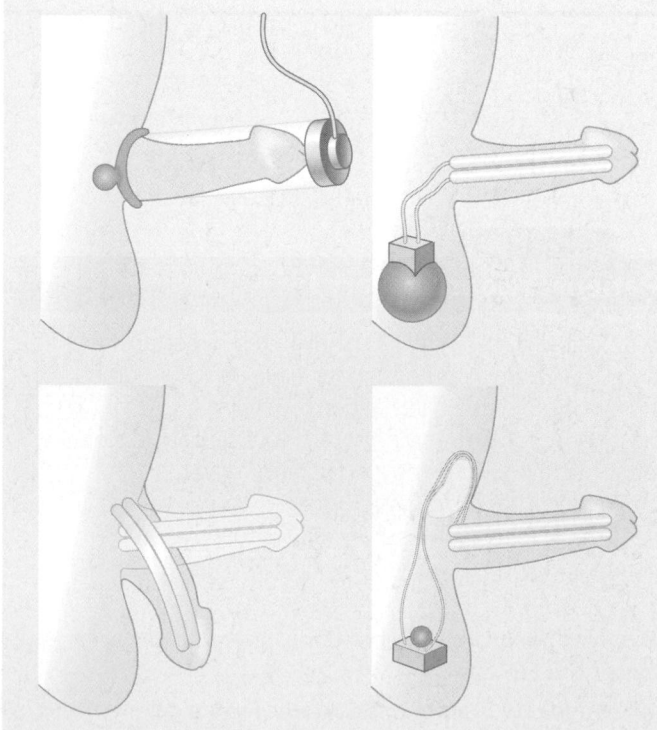

FIGURE 51–2. Available devices and prostheses used to treat ED. (From Ref. 15.)

⑤ *VEDs are one of the most effective treatment modalities for ED. They have a success rate of greater than 90% in obtaining an erection sufficient for coitus and are considered a first-line noninvasive therapy.*[16] Rigidity may be improved by using a double pump technique in which the vacuum is applied for a couple of minutes, removed, then reapplied for another few minutes. Higher efficacy rates can also be achieved by combining VEDs with other therapies.

Onset of action is slow at around 30 minutes, which limits spontaneity. In addition, patients and partners may complain of a cold, lifeless, discolored penis that has a hinge-like feel. Painful ejaculation or inability to ejaculate are additional adverse effects. VEDs are contraindicated in persons with sickle cell disease and should be used with caution in patients on oral anticoagulants or who have bleeding disorders due to the increased possibility of priapism.

Prostheses Penile prostheses are semi-rigid malleable or inflatable rods, which are inserted surgically into the corpus cavernosa to allow erections (Fig. 51–2). The malleable rods are rigid at all times, but may be bent into position by the patient when desired. The inflatable prostheses remain flaccid until the pump within the scrotum moves fluid from a reservoir to the cylinders within the penis. Detumescence is achieved when the fluid is then transferred back to the reservoir by activating a release button.

Because prostheses are the most invasive treatment available, they are only considered in patients who do not respond to medications or external devices, or those who have significant adverse effects from other therapies. Patient satisfaction rates can be as high as 95% with partner satisfaction rates just slightly lower.[17] The primary risk of insertion is infection, although this only happens in 3% of first-time prostheses. Semi-rigid malleable rods may interfere with urination, are difficult to conceal, and have a higher likelihood of erosion.[17] Most devices need replacement after 10 to 15 years.

▶ *Pharmacologic Therapy*

Phosphodiesterase Type 5 Inhibitors Sildenafil (Viagra), tadalafil (Cialis), and vardenafil (Levitra) act by selectively inhibiting phosphodiesterase (PDE) type 5, an enzyme that breaks down cGMP. By inhibiting the breakdown of cGMP, smooth muscle relaxation is induced, leading to an erection (Fig. 51–1). However, the PDE inhibitors are only effective in the presence of sexual stimulation to drive the NO/cGMP system, making them facilitators of an erection, not initiators. Patients must be informed of the need for sexual stimulation to induce an erection, as it will not occur spontaneously.

⑥ *Effectiveness of the three available PDE inhibitors is essentially comparable, but differences exist in duration of action and, to a small degree, incidence of side effects and drug interactions (Table 51–4).* Review of available data for each individual agent shows a 50% to 80% response rate depending on the dose of agent used and the etiology of dysfunction. Response rates tend to be lower in patients with radical prostatectomy as well as those with diabetes, severe

Table 51–4

Comparison of PDE Inhibitors

	Sildenafil (Viagra)	Tadalafil (Cialis)	Vardenafil (Levitra)
Available strengths	25-, 50-, 100-mg tabs	2.5-, 5-, 10-, 20-mg tabs	2.5-, 5-, 10-, 20-mg tabs
Initial dosage in healthy adults (mg)	50 mg up to once daily taken 1 hour prior to sexual activity	10 mg up to once daily taken 1 hour prior to sexual activity or 2.5 mg daily at the same time each day	10 mg up to once daily taken 1 hour prior to sexual activity
Dosing range for healthy adults (mg)	25–100	5–20	5–20
Dosage in the elderly	25 mg every day	10 mg every day	5 mg every day
Dosage in renal impairment	50 mg every day (moderate[a]) 25 mg every day (severe[b])	5 mg every day (moderate[a] and severe[b])	5–20 mg every day
Dosage in hepatic impairment	25 mg every day	10 mg[c]	5–10 mg[d]
Time to onset	30 minutes	15 minutes	Less than 1 hour
Onset delayed by high-fat meal?	Yes	No	Yes
Duration of effect	Up to 4 hours	Up to 36 hours	Up to 4 hours
Half-life	3–4 hours	18 hours	3–4 hours
Metabolism	CYP3A4 (major) CYP2C9 (minor)	CYP3A4	CYP3A4 (major) CYP3A5 (minor) CYP2C (minor)
Clinically relevant drug interactions	Nitrates, protease inhibitors, azole antifungals, erythromyin	Nitrates, a_1-blockers[e], azole antifungals, erythromycin	Nitrates, antiarrhythmic agents,[f] a_1-blockers, erythromycin

CYP, cytochrome P450 isoenzyme.

[a]Moderate renal impairment = creatinine clearance (CrCl) 31 to 50 mL/min.

[b]Severe renal impairment = CrCl less than 30 mL/min.

[c]Mild to moderate only—contraindicated in severe liver disease.

[d]Mild to moderate only—not yet evaluated in severe liver disease.

[e]Selective a_1-blockers (such as 0.4 mg tamsulosin every day) are appropriate in combination with tadalafil.

[f]Vardenafil can cause QT-interval prolongation; this effect in combination with certain antiarrhythmic agents can lead to life-threatening arrhythmias.

nerve damage, or severe vascular disease.[18] While efficacy rates appear to be similar between agents, there are some data to suggest continuation rates are higher and patient preference greater with tadalafil.[19] The PDE inhibitors are considered first-line therapies due to high efficacy rates, convenience of dosing, and minimal severe adverse effects.

The most dramatic difference among the three agents is tadalafil's extended duration of action, earning it the nickname "the weekender drug." While sildenafil and vardenafil have average half-lives of 3 to 4 hours, tadalafil's half-life is approximately 18 hours.[20] The extended half-life allows for more spontaneous sexual activity over a couple of days, but may increase the duration of adverse effects and likelihood of drug interactions. Tadalafil has been approved for use as a daily medication at a lower dose (2.5–5 mg) than the as-needed dose. The dosing efficacy appears to be similar to as-needed dosing, but cost will be prohibitive for many patients.

The most common side effects experienced with PDE inhibitors include headache, facial flushing, nasal congestion, dyspepsia, myalgia, back pain, and, rarely, priapism. Vardenafil

and sildenafil may also cause difficulty in discriminating blue from green, bluish tones in vision, or difficulty seeing in dim light due to cross-reactivity with PDE 6 in the retina. Labeling for all PDE inhibitors includes a warning about nonarteritic ischemic optic neuropathy (NAION) in a small number of patients. This is a condition in which blood flow is blocked to the optic nerve. If patients experience sudden or decreased vision loss they should call a health care provider immediately.

Concern exists about the safety of renewing sexual activity and using PDE inhibitors in patients with cardiovascular disease. Because of the numerous adverse cardiovascular events reported after the release of sildenafil, a management approach was developed to give recommendations for the use of PDE inhibitors as well as to determine the safety of intercourse in patients with cardiovascular disease[21,22] (Table 51–5). In addition to the inherent risk of renewing sexual activity, PDE inhibitors can lead to significant hypotension. Patients taking organic nitrates are the most at risk, as these drugs potentiate the drop in blood pressure. All three PDE inhibitors are absolutely contraindicated in

Table 51–5

Recommendations of the Second Princeton Consensus Conference for Cardiovascular Risk Stratification of Patients Being Considered for PDE Inhibitor Therapy

Risk Category	Description of Patients' Conditions	Management Approach
Low risk	Has asymptomatic CV disease with less than three risk factors for CV disease Has well-controlled hypertension Has mild, stable angina Has mild congestive heart failure (NYHA Class I) Has mild valvular heart disease Had a myocardial infarction 6 weeks ago	Patient can be started on PDE inhibitor
Moderate risk	Has greater than or equal to three risk factors for CV disease Has moderate, stable angina Had a recent myocardial infarction or stroke within the past 6 weeks Has moderate congestive heart failure (NYHA Class II)	Patient should undergo complete cardiovascular workup and treadmill stress test to determine tolerance to increased myocardial energy consumption associated with increased sexual activity
High risk	Has unstable or symptomatic angina, despite treatment Has uncontrolled hypertension Has severe congestive heart failure (NYHA Class III or IV) Had a recent myocardial infarction or stroke within the past 2 weeks Has moderate or severe valvular heart disease Has high risk cardiac arrhythmias Has obstructive hypertrophic cardiomyopathy	PDE inhibitor is contraindicated; sexual intercourse should be deferred

CV, cardiovascular; NYHA, New York Heart Association; PDE, phosphodiesters.

From Ref. 11.

patients taking any form of nitrate, whether scheduled or sublingual for acute situations. Caution should be used when using a PDE inhibitor in patients taking α-blockers due to an increased risk of hypotension. In addition, the labeling for vardenafil contains a precautionary statement about the possibility of QT prolongation with the use of the drug. Other drug interactions and cautions vary slightly between agents and are described in Table 51–4.

The introduction of the oral PDE inhibitors has dramatically changed the treatment of ED. Direct-to-consumer advertising has informed patients of the availability of oral drugs for treatment. However, patients must be fully informed of side effects, drug interactions, mechanism of action, and dosing before being prescribed the medication. In addition, they need to understand the need for sexual stimulation to achieve the desired result and that a single trial is not adequate. It is estimated that six to eight attempts with a medication and specific dose may be needed before successful intercourse results.[23]

Alprostadil Alprostadil is a prostaglandin E_1 analog that induces an erection by stimulating adenyl cyclase, which leads to an increase in smooth muscle relaxation, rapid arterial inflow, and increased penile rigidity. Alprostadil is available as an intracavernosal injection (Caverject or Edex) or a transurethral suppository (MUSE, medicated urethral system for erection), but the injectable form is more effective

(Fig. 51–3). Both forms of alprostadil are considered more invasive than oral medications or VEDs, and are therefore second-line therapies.

MUSE consists of a urethral pellet of alprostadil with an applicator. Onset of action is within 5 to 10 minutes and it is effective for 30 to 60 minutes. Initial dose titration should occur in a physician's office to ensure correct dose and prevent adverse events. Although effectiveness rates in clinical trials have been as high as 65%,[24] its success in practice has been lower.[25] Aching in the penis, testicles, legs, and perineum; warmth or burning sensation in the urethra, minor urethral bleeding or spotting, priapism, and lightheadedness are all possible adverse effects. In addition, partners may experience vaginal burning or itching. Disadvantages include lower effectiveness, high cost, adverse effects, complicated insertion technique, and a contraindication against use with a pregnant partner unless using a condom.

Alprostadil injected into the corpus cavernosum is the more effective route and is the only FDA-approved injection for ED. The onset of action is similar to transurethral alprostadil, but duration varies with dose and must be titrated in a physician's office to achieve an erection lasting no more than 1 hour. Injections should be done into one side of the penis directly into the corpus cavernosum, and then the penis should be massaged to distribute the drug. Because of cross-circulation, both corpora will become erect when massaging. Education is extremely important with intracavernosal injections. Patients

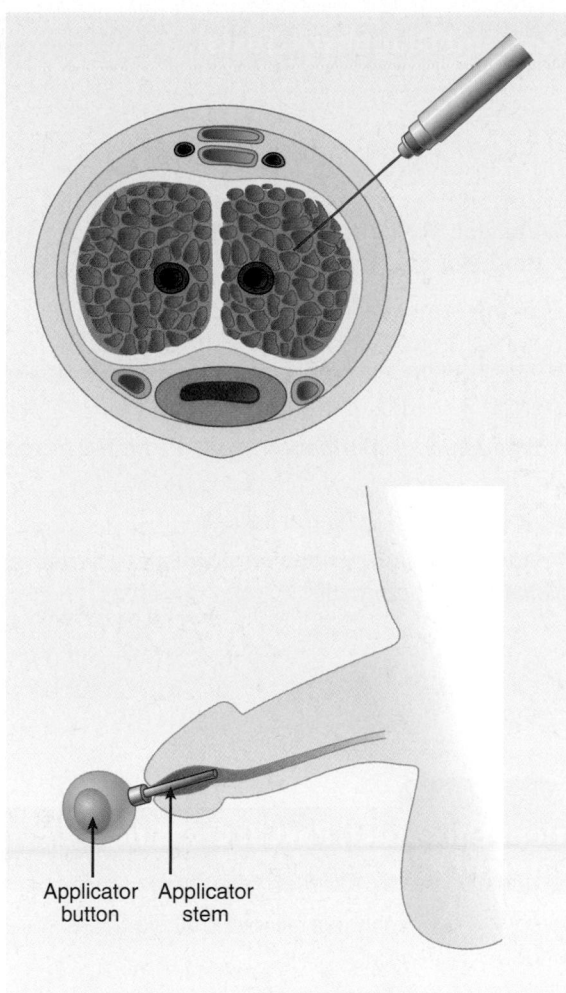

FIGURE 51–3. Intraurethral and intracavernosal administration of alprostadil. (From Ref. 15.)

Applicator button   Applicator stem

must be adequately informed of technique, expectations, side effects, and when to seek help. ❻ *Intracavernosal injections are effective in up to 90% of patients, but side effects, lack of spontaneity, and fear of needles limit their widespread use as first-line therapy,* and therefore this therapy is most appropriate for patients in long-term stable relationships. Adverse effects include pain with injection, bleeding or bruising at the injection site, fibrosis, or priapism. Use with caution in patients with sickle cell disease, those on anticoagulants, or those who have bleeding disorders, due to an increased risk of priapism and bleeding.

Papaverine and Phentolamine Papaverine and phentolamine are non–FDA-approved agents used for intracavernosal injection. Papaverine is a nonselective PDE inhibitor that induces an erection by relaxing smooth muscle and increasing blood flow. Phentolamine is a competitive α-adrenergic receptor antagonist that increases arterial inflow by opposing arterial constriction. Both drugs are rarely used alone, and are most often mixed in various concentrations

with alprostadil for increased effectiveness and in an effort to reduce adverse effects with smaller doses of each medication. Patients typically must see a specialist for use of these medications in mixtures, as the providers are the most likely to compound them and adjust dosages.

Yohimbine Yohimbine is an indole alkaloid produced in the bark of yohimbe trees. It selectively inhibits α_2-adrenergic receptors in the brain that are associated with libido and penile erection. Because there are only limited data supporting its efficacy, yohimbine is not a recommended treatment for any form of ED.[26] Adverse effects of the drug include nausea, irritability, headaches, anxiety, tachycardia, and hypertension.

Testosterone Supplementation ❼ *Androgens are important for general sexual function and libido, but testosterone supplementation is only effective in patients with documented low serum testosterone levels.* In patients with hypogonadism, testosterone replacement is the initial treatment of choice, as it corrects decreased libido, fatigue, muscle loss, sleep disturbances, and depressed mood. Improvements in ED may occur, but they should not be expected to occur in all patients. The initial trial should be for 3 months. At that time, re-evaluation and the addition of another ED therapy is warranted. Dosage forms include oral, intramuscular, topical patches or gel, an implanted pellet, and a buccal tablet.

Injectable esters of testosterone offer the most inexpensive replacement option. Testosterone cypionate and enanthate have the longest duration of action and are therefore the preferred agents. There are several drawbacks associated with parenteral testosterone including the need to administer deep intramuscular injections every 2 to 4 weeks. In addition, levels of hormone are well above physiologic values within the first few days. Concentrations then decline and eventually dip below physiologic levels just before the next dose. These extreme changes in concentration lead to mood swings and a reduced sense of well-being.[5]

Treatment with topical products is attractive to patients due to convenience, but they tend to be more expensive than the injections. Testosterone patches and gels are administered daily and result in serum levels within the physiologic range during the 24-hour dosing period.[5] Most patients prefer the nonscrotal patch or the gel because the scrotal patch requires shaving of the area, and the patch has a tendency to fall off. Care must be taken with the use of the gel to wash hands thoroughly after use and avoid baths or showers within 5 to 6 hours of application. The most common side effects of topical testosterone are dermatologic reactions caused by the absorption enhancers.

Oral testosterone products are also available for supplementation. Unfortunately, testosterone has poor oral bioavailability and undergoes extensive first-pass metabolism. Alkylated derivatives such as methyltestosterone and fluoxymesterone have been formulated to compensate for these problems, but this modification makes them considerably more hepatotoxic. This adverse effect makes

Patient Encounter, Part 2: Medical History, Physical Exam, and Diagnostic Tests

PMH: Type 2 diabetes for 15 years; not controlled due to his stressful profession; he often works late, eats on the run, and has no time for exercise. Hypertension for 8 years, currently uncontrolled. Dyslipidemia for 8 years, currently controlled

FH: Father had type 2 diabetes and died of myocardial infarction at the age of 50 years; mother is alive at 75, with no major illnesses

SH: Works long hours as a business executive; drinks alcohol only occasionally, but smokes half a pack of cigarettes per day; has a 20-pack per year history

Meds: Metformin 1,000 mg orally twice daily; metoprolol XL 50 mg orally once daily; simvastatin 20 mg orally once daily

ROS: (–) Morning, nocturnal, or spontaneous erections suitable for intercourse; (–) nocturia, urgency, symptoms of prostatitis; (+) significant life stressors; (+) mild pain in feet

PE:

VS: BP 148/90 mm Hg, p 85 bpm, RR 18/min, T 37°C (98.6°F)

CV: Normal exam

Genital/Rectal: Normal scrotum and testicles w/o masses; penis without discharge or curvature

Labs: Complete metabolic panel, CBC, and thyroid panel within normal limits; lipid panel: total cholesterol, LDL, HDL, triglycerides within normal limits; hemoglobin A1c 8% (0.08), testosterone 700 ng/dL (24 nmol/L)

Given this additional information, what are his risk factors for ED?

Identify treatment goals for this patient.

What pharmacologic and nonpharmacologic alternatives are available for this patient?

---

oral replacement undesirable and this route of administration should not be used.

An alternative to the oral route is the buccal mucoadhesive system. The Striantbuccal system adheres to the inside of the mouth and the testosterone is absorbed through the oral mucosa and delivered to the systemic circulation. There is no first-pass effect, as the liver is bypassed by this route of administration. Patients apply a 30-mg tablet to the upper gum twice daily. The cost is similar to that of the patch or gel. Side effects unique to this dosage form include oral irritation, bitter taste, and gum edema.

General side effects of testosterone include gynecomastia, dyslipidemia, polycythemia, and acne. Weight gain, hypertension, edema, and exacerbations of congestive heart failure also occur due to sodium retention. Before initiating testosterone, the patient should undergo evaluation for benign prostatic hypertrophy and prostate cancer. Routine follow-up includes yearly prostate-specific antigen, digital rectal exam, hemoglobin and liver function, in addition to assessment of response.

OUTCOME EVALUATION

Successful therapy for ED results in an increase in erections suitable for intercourse, and most importantly in an improvement in the patient's quality of life. Ideally, the therapy chosen is free of significant adverse effects, discomfort, and inconvenience. Laboratory evaluation and a physical exam are not necessary for evaluation of effectiveness, but may be necessary to determine if adverse events are occurring.

Evaluate satisfaction and effectiveness after a 4-week trial unless the patient initiates follow-up sooner. Some therapies

Patient Encounter, Part 3: Creating a Treatment Plan

Based on the information available, create a treatment plan for this patient's ED.

Which of the available options will be your treatments of choice based on degree of invasiveness, ease of use, and side-effect profile?

Perform a cardiovascular risk assessment to determine risk.

What are the safety and efficacy monitoring parameters for the chosen treatment?

Patient Encounter, Part 4

The patient now presents with new-onset chest pain for which his provider has given him a prescription of sublingual nitroglycerin.

What is your treatment of choice based on this new information?

What are the safety and efficacy monitoring parameters for the chosen treatment?

---

such as intracavernosal injections will require multiple visits over the long term to determine the correct dose and to detect adverse effects. If the initial therapy is not effective, the patient must be further evaluated to determine if the initial assessment of comorbid disease states, type of dysfunction, and patient goals were correct. After ensuring that patient goals are realistic and providing further counseling, providers will then increase the dose of drug if not at maximum, switch to another therapy, or add a therapy if indicated.

Abbreviations Introduced in This Chapter

cAMP   Cyclic adenosine monophosphate
cGMP   Cyclic guanosine monophosphate

CHF	Congestive heart failure
ED	Erectile dysfunction
GTP	Guanosine triphosphate
IIED	International Index of Erectile Dysfunction
MUSE	Medicated urethral system for erection
NAION	Nonarteritic ischemic optic neuropathy
NO	Nitric oxide
PDE	Phosphodiesterase
VED	Vacuum erection device

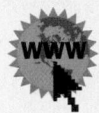 Self-assessment questions and answers are available at *http://www.mhpharmacotherapy.com/pp.html.*

Patient Care and Monitoring

1. Assess the patient's specific symptoms to determine the type of dysfunction. Does the patient have ED or an ejaculatory or libido disorder?

2. If problems are with erectile ability, ask specific questions related to onset, frequency, and sexual relationships. Does the patient history imply psychogenic, organic, or mixed dysfunction?

3. Perform a thorough medical and social history as well as a physical exam to diagnose ED and to determine potential causes that may be treatable.

4. Perform a thorough history of prescription and nonprescription medications. Are any of the patient's medications associated with ED or are they contraindicated with possible ED therapies?

5. Generally treatment is started with the least invasive option and then progresses to more invasive options, but ultimately patient preference determines the initial therapy.

6. Discontinue medications that may cause ED if possible and optimally treat associated disease states.

7. If the patient is not satisfied, provide further counseling to ensure that they are using the therapy appropriately and that they have realistic goals.

8. Provide patient education with regard to disease state, lifestyle modifications, drug therapy, and device technique:

   - The causes of ED
   - The fact that therapy will not cure ED, but may be helpful in improving erections; it is important to have realistic expectations
   - The appropriate use of medications and devices
   - Typical adverse effects
   - Drug interactions
   - Warning signs and their management (e.g., vision changes, fibrosis, pain, priapism, or hypotension)
   - The importance of frequent follow-up with the provider

REFERENCES

1. NIH Consensus Conference. NIH Consensus Development Panel on Impotence. JAMA 1993;270:83–90.
2. Bacon CG, Mittleman MA, Kawachi I, et al. Sexual function in men older than 50 years of age: Results from the health professionals follow-up study. Ann Int Med 2003;139:161–168.
3. AACE Male Sexual Dysfunction Task Force. American association of clinical endocrinologists medical guidelines for clinical practice for the evaluation and treatment of male sexual dysfunction: A couple's problem, 2003 update. Endocr Pract 2003;9:77–95.
4. Morgentaler A. A 66-year-old man with sexual dysfunction. JAMA 2004;291:2994–3003.
5. Morales A. Testosterone replacement: When is there a role? Int J Impot Res 2000;12(Suppl 4):S112–S118.
6. Hafez ESE, Hafez SD. Erectile dysfunction: Anatomical parameters, etiology, diagnosis, and therapy. Arch Androl 2005;51:15–31.
7. Billups KL. Sexual dysfunction and cardiovascular disease: Integrative concepts and strategies. Am J Cardiol 2005;96(Suppl):57M–61M.
8. Shabsigh R, Arver S, Channer KS, et al. The triad of erectile dysfunction, hypogonadism and the metabolic syndrome. Int J Clin Pract 2008;62:791–798.
9. Deveci S, O'Brien K, Ahmed A, et al. Can the International Index of Erectile Function distinguish between organic and psychogenic erectile function? BJU Int 2008;102:354–356.
10. Mikhail N. Management of erectile dysfunction by the primary care physician. Clev Clin J Med 2005;293–294, 296–297, 301–305.
11. Lee M. Erectile dysfunction. In: Dipiro JT, Talbert RL, Yee GC, et al., eds. Pharmacotherapy: A Pathophysiologic Approach, 7th ed. New York: McGraw-Hill, 2008:1369–1385.
12. Rosen RC, Cappelleri JC, Smith MD, et al. Development and evaluation of an abridged, 5-item version of the International Index of Erectile Dysfunction (IIEF-5) as a diagnostic tool for erectile dysfunction. Int J Impot Res 1999;11:319–326.
13. Paige NM, Hays RD, Litwin MS, et al. Improvement in emotional well-being and relationships of users of sildenafil. J Urol 2001;166:1774–1778.
14. Esposito K, Giugliano F, DiPalo C, et al. Effect of lifestyle changes on erectile dysfunction in obese men. JAMA 2004;291:2978–2984.
15. Wagner G, Saenz de Tejada I. Update on male erectile dysfunction. BMJ 1998;316:678–682.
16. Montague DK. Nonpharmacologic treatment of erectile dysfunction. Rev Urol 2002;4(Suppl 3):S9–S16.
17. Brant WO, Bella AJ, Lue TF. Treatment options for erectile dysfunction. Endocrinol Metab Clin N Am 2007;36:465–479.
18. De Tejada IS. Therapeutic strategies for optimizing PDE-5 inhibitor therapy in patients with erectile dysfunction considered difficult or challenging to treat. Int J Impot Res 2004;16(Suppl 1):S40–S42.

19. Doggrell SA. Comparison of clinical trials with sildenafil, vardenafil and tadalafil in erectile dysfunction. Expert Opin Pharmaother 2005;6:75–84.

20. Gresser U, Gleiter CH. Erectile dysfunction: Comparison of efficacy and side effects of the PDE-5 inhibitors sildenafil, vardenafil and tadalafil: Review of the literature. Eur J Med Res 2002;7:435–446.

21. Rosen RC, Jackson G, Kostis JB. Erectile dysfunction and cardiac disease: Recommendations of the Second Princeton Conference. Curr Urol Rep 2006;7:490–496.

22. Kostis JB, Jackson G, Rosen R, et al. Sexual dysfunction and cardiac risk (the Second Princeton Consensus Conference). Am J Cardiol 2005;96:313–321.

23. Steers WD. Pharmacologic treatment of erectile dysfunction. Rev Urol 2002;4(Suppl 3):S17–S25.

24. Padma-Nathan H, Hellstrom WJ, Kaiser FE, et al., for the Medicated Urethral System for Erection (MUSE) Study Group. Treatment of men with erectile dysfunction with transurethral alprostadil. N Engl J Med 1997;336:1–7.

25. Guay AT, Perez JB, Velasquez E, et al. Clinical experience with intraurethral alprostadil (MUSE) in the treatment of men with erectile dysfunction. A retrospective study. Medicated urethral system for erection. Eur Urol. 2000;38:671–676.

26. American Urological Association. The management of erectile dysfunction: An update, 2006. Available at: www.auanet.org/guidelines/edmgmt.cfm.

52 Benign Prostatic Hyperplasia

Mary Lee and Roohollah Sharifi

Upon completion of the chapter, the reader will be able to:

1. Explain the pathophysiologic mechanisms underlying the symptoms and signs of benign prostatic hyperplasia (BPH).
2. Recognize the symptoms and signs of BPH in individual patients.
3. List the desired treatment outcomes for a patient with BPH.
4. Identify factors that guide selection of a particular α-adrenergic antagonist for an individual patient.
5. Compare and contrast α-adrenergic antagonists versus 5α-reductase inhibitors in terms of mechanism of action, treatment outcomes, adverse effects, and interactions when used for management of BPH.
6. Describe the indications for combination drug treatment of BPH.
7. Describe the indications for surgical intervention of BPH.
8. Formulate a monitoring plan for a patient on a given drug treatment regimen based on patient specific information.
9. Formulate appropriate counseling information for patients receiving drug treatment for BPH.

KEY CONCEPTS

❶ The lower urinary tract symptoms (LUTS) and signs of benign prostatic hyperplasia (BPH) are due to static, dynamic, or detrusor factors. The static factor refers to anatomic obstruction of the bladder neck caused by an enlarged prostate gland. The dynamic factor refers to excessive stimulation of α-adrenergic receptors in the smooth muscle of the prostate, urethra, and bladder neck. The detrusor factor refers to irritability of hypertrophied detrusor muscle as a result of long-standing bladder outlet obstruction.

❷ Drug treatment goals for BPH include relieving obstructive and irritative voiding symptoms, preventing complications of disease, and reducing the need for surgical intervention.

❸ Watchful waiting is indicated for patients with mild symptoms that are not bothersome.

❹ Single-drug treatment with an α-adrenergic antagonist is preferred for patients with moderate or severe symptoms of BPH. Single-drug treatment with a 5α-reductase inhibitor should be reserved for patients with moderate or severe symptoms and significantly enlarged prostates of at least 30 g (1.05 oz).

❺ Surgical intervention should be reserved for patients with severe LUTS due to BPH and those with complications of disease, such as recurrent urinary tract infections, recurrent severe gross hematuria, renal failure, and bladder calculi.

❻ α-Adrenergic antagonists reduce the dynamic factor. They competitively antagonize α-adrenergic receptors, thereby causing relaxation of the bladder neck, prostatic urethra, and prostate smooth muscle. They do not shrink an enlarged prostate. The onset of action is days to weeks, depending on the need for up-titration of the daily dose to achieve a therapeutic response. Dose limiting adverse effects include hypotension and syncope. In addition, delayed or retrograde ejaculation has been reported. Combined use with antihypertensives, diuretics, or phosphodiesterase inhibitors can increase the risk of hypotensive episodes.

❼ Among the α-adrenergic antagonists, modified-release alfuzosin is considered functionally uroselective because usual therapeutic doses produce relaxation of the bladder neck and prostatic smooth muscle with minimal peripheral vascular relaxation. Although alfuzosin appears to produce less hypotension than immediate-release formulations of terazosin and doxazosin, it is not clear if it has the same cardiovascular profile as tamsulosin. Although not uroselective, controlled-release doxazosin produces less hypotension than the immediate release formulation. Tamsulosin and silodosin are pharmacologically uroselective and exert greater antagonism of α_{1A}- and α_{1D}-receptors, which predominate in prostatic and bladder detrusor muscle, respectively, as compared to vascular α_{1B}-receptors. Therefore, tamsulosin and silodosin can be initiated with a full therapeutic dose, which achieves peak effects sooner than with immediate-release formulations of terazosin and doxazosin, which must be up-titrated. Tamsulosin appears to have the lowest potential to cause hypotension. In various clinical trials, tamsulosin is well tolerated in the elderly and in patients taking diuretics and antihypertensives. It is also commercially available in a controlled-release dosage formulation. Therefore, with chronic use, tamsulosin can be taken once daily at the patient's convenience.

❽ 5α-Reductase inhibitors shrink enlarged prostates, reducing symptoms caused by the static factor. They do so by inhibiting 5α-reductase that is responsible for intraprostatic conversion of testosterone to dihydrotestosterone, the active androgen that stimulates prostate tissue growth. The onset of action is slow with peak shrinkage of the prostate taking up to 6 months. Unlike treatment with α-adrenergic antagonists, 5α-reductase inhibitors have been shown to reduce the incidence of acute urinary retention and need for prostate surgery in patients with significantly enlarged prostate glands (more than 30 g), and those with **prostate-specific antigen (PSA) serum levels of 1.5 ng/mL (1.5 mcg/L) or more**. Because 5α-reductase inhibitors do not produce cardiovascular adverse effects, they are preferred for treatment of moderate to severe symptoms of BPH when the patient is at risk of hypotension, but wants to be treated medically. Adverse effects include gynecomastia, decreased libido, erectile dysfunction, and ejaculation disorders. Drug interactions are uncommon.

❾ When monitoring efficacy of drug treatment for BPH, subjective end points include relief of obstructive and irritative voiding symptoms. Objective end points include improvements of urinary flow rates, decreased postvoid residual urinary volume, and decreased complications of disease.

INTRODUCTION

The prostate is a heart-shaped, chestnut-sized organ that encircles the portion of the proximal urethra that is located at the base of the urinary bladder. The prostate produces secretions, which are part of the ejaculate.

Benign prostatic hyperplasia (BPH) is the most common benign neoplasm in males who are at least 40 years of age. BPH can produce lower urinary tract voiding symptoms that are consistent with impaired emptying of urine from and storage of urine in the bladder. Medications are a common mode of treatment to reduce symptoms and/or delay complications of the disease. For this reason, clinicians should be knowledgeable about the medical management of this disease.

EPIDEMIOLOGY AND ETIOLOGY

BPH is present as microscopic disease in many elderly males.[1] The prevalence increases with advancing patient age. However, only about 50% and 25% of patients with microscopic BPH disease develop an enlarged prostate on palpation and clinical voiding symptoms, respectively.[2] It is estimated that 25% of males 40 years of age or more have voiding symptoms consistent with BPH, and 20% to 30% of all male patients who live to the age of 80 years will require a **prostatectomy** for severe voiding symptoms of BPH.[2]

Two etiologic factors for BPH include advanced patient age and the stimulatory effect of androgens.

- Prior to 40 years of age, the prostate in the adult male stays the same size, approximately 15 to 20 g. However, in males who have reached 40 years of age, the prostate undergoes a growth spurt, which continues as the male advances in age. Enlargement of the prostate can result in clinically symptomatic BPH.

- The testes and adrenal glands produce 90% and 10%, respectively, of circulating testosterone. Testosterone enters prostate cells, where predominantly type II 5α-reductase activates testosterone to dihydrotestosterone, which combines with a cytoplasmic receptor. The complex enters the nucleus and induces changes in protein synthesis which promote glandular tissue growth of the prostate. Thus, 5α-reductase inhibitors (e.g., finasteride and dutasteride) directly interfere with one of the major etiologic factors of BPH.

- The prostate is composed of two types of tissue: (a) glandular or epithelial tissue, which produces prostatic secretions, including prostate-specific antigen (PSA) and (b) muscle or stromal tissue, which can contract around the urethra when stimulated. Whereas androgens stimulate glandular tissue growth, androgens have no direct effect on stromal tissue. It has been postulated that stromal tissue growth may be stimulated by estrogen. Since testosterone is converted to estrogen in peripheral tissues in males, testosterone may be associated indirectly with stromal hyperplasia. Stromal tissue is innervated by α_{1A}-receptors. When stimulated, prostatic stroma contracts around the urethra, narrowing the urethra and causing obstructive voiding symptoms.

PATHOPHYSIOLOGY

❶ *The symptoms and signs of BPH are due to static, dynamic, and/or detrusor factors. The static factor refers to anatomic obstruction of the bladder neck caused by an enlarged prostate gland. As the gland grows around the urethra, the prostate* *occludes the urethral lumen. The dynamic factor refers to excessive stimulation of* α_{1A}-*adrenergic receptors in the smooth muscle of the prostate and urethra, which results in smooth muscle contraction. This reduces the caliber of the urethral lumen. The detrusor factor refers to bladder detrusor muscle instability, in which bladder muscle fibers have decompensated as a result of excessive, prolonged hypertrophy in response to prolonged bladder outlet obstruction.* Patients with detrusor muscle instability will develop irritative voiding symptoms, such as urinary urgency and frequency.[1] Detrusor muscle fibers are embedded with α_{1D}-receptors. Therefore, it has been proposed that some α_{1D}-adrenergic antagonists may be particularly useful for controlling these symptoms.[3,4]

In an enlarged gland, the epithelial/stromal tissue ratio is 1:5.[1] Androgens stimulate epithelial, but not stromal tissue hyperplasia. Hence, androgen antagonism does not induce a complete reduction in prostate size to normal. This explains one of the limitations of the clinical effect of 5α-reductase inhibitors.

Stromal tissue is the primary locus of α_1-adrenergic receptors in the prostate. An estimated 98% of the α-adrenergic receptors in the prostate are found in prostatic stromal tissue. Of the α_1-receptors found in the prostate, 70% of them are of the α_{1A}-subtype.[4] This explains why α-adrenergic antagonists are effective for managing symptoms of BPH.

Symptoms of BPH are classified as obstructive or irritative. Obstructive symptoms result from failure of the urinary bladder to empty urine when the bladder is full. The patient will complain of reduced force of the urinary stream, urinary hesitation, dribbling, and straining to empty the bladder. Irritative symptoms result from the failure of the urinary bladder to store urine until the bladder is full. With long-standing bladder outlet obstruction, detrusor muscle fibers undergo hypertrophy so that the bladder can generate higher pressure to overcome the bladder outlet obstruction and empty urine from the bladder. Once maximal bladder muscle hypertrophy occurs, the muscle decompensates. The detrusor becomes irritable, contracting abnormally in response to small amounts of urine in the bladder. As a result, the patient complains of urinary frequency and urgency.

The natural history of untreated BPH is unclear in patients with mild symptoms. It is estimated that up to 38% of untreated men with mild symptoms will have symptom improvement over a 2.5- to 5-year period.[5] It may be that such patients attribute their symptoms to aging, grow tolerant of their symptoms, or adopt behavioral changes in their lifestyle that minimize their voiding symptoms. On the other hand, a significant portion of patients with mild symptoms will likely experience disease progression. In one Veterans Affairs study, approximately one-third of men with mild BPH symptoms, who were initially randomized to watchful waiting, developed progressive symptoms and required surgical intervention within 5 years of initial diagnosis.[6] Patients with moderate to severe symptoms can experience a decreased quality of life as daily activities are adjusted because of urinary incontinence. Also, such patients may develop complications of BPH, which include acute refractory urinary retention, renal failure, urinary tract infection, urinary incontinence, bladder stones, large bladder diverticuli, and recurrent gross hematuria. Predictors of disease progression include an enlarged prostate of at least 30 g (1.05 oz) or PSA of at least 1.5 ng/mL (1.5 mcg/L).[7–9]

Clinical Presentation and Diagnosis of BPH

General

Patients may or may not be in acute distress. In early stages of disease, the patient may complain of obstructive voiding symptoms. If untreated, in late stages of disease the patient may complain of irritative voiding symptoms, or acute urinary retention, which is painful due to maximal distention of the urinary bladder. Also, the patient may be symptomatic of disease complications, including urosepsis, pyelonephritis, cystitis, or overflow urinary incontinence.

Symptoms

Patients may complain of obstructive voiding symptoms (e.g., urinary hesitancy, decreased force of urinary stream, straining to void, incomplete bladder emptying, dribbling, and intermittency) and/or irritative voiding symptoms (e.g., urinary frequency, nocturia, dysuria, urgency, and urinary incontinence). Severity of symptoms should be assessed by the patient using a standardized instrument (e.g., the American Urological Association [AUA] Symptom Scoring Index; Table 52–1). However, it is important to recognize that a patient's perception of the bothersomeness of his voiding symptoms may not match with the AUA Symptom Score. In this case, after thorough evaluation of the signs and complications of BPH disease, if present, the physician and patient should discuss the bothersomeness of the patient's symptoms and decide together on the most appropriate course of treatment for the patient.[1,10] Lower urinary tract symptoms (LUTS) is a term that refers to the collection of obstructive and irritative voiding symptoms characteristic of, but not specific for, BPH. That is, other urologic diseases (e.g., urinary tract infection, prostate cancer, prostatitis, or neurogenic bladder) can also cause LUTS.

Signs

- Enlarged prostate on digital rectal exam (DRE); check for prostate nodules or induration, which would suggest prostate cancer instead of BPH as the cause of the patient's voiding symptoms

- Distended urinary bladder

- Rule out meatal stenosis or urethral masses, which could cause voiding symptoms similar to LUTS

(Continued)

Clinical Presentation and Diagnosis of BPH (*Continued*)

- Check anal sphincter tone as an indirect assessment of peripheral innervation to the detrusor muscle of the bladder

Complications of Untreated BPH

Upper and lower urinary tract infection, urosepsis, urinary incontinence refractory urinary retention, chronic renal failure, bladder diverticuli, bladder stones, or recurrent gross hematuria.

Medical History

- Check the patient's general health including previous surgery, presence of diabetes mellitus, or medications that may cause or worsen voiding symptoms.
- Have the patient provide a diary of his voiding pattern for the past week: date and time of each voiding, volume voided, and whether or not the patient had urinary leakage during the day.

Laboratory Tests

- Serum PSA: The combination of PSA and DRE of the prostate is used to screen for prostate cancer, which could also cause an enlarged prostate. Also PSA is a surrogate marker for an enlarged prostate due to BPH. Using a PSA greater than 1.5 ng/mL (1.5 mg/L) suggests that a patient has a prostate volume greater than 30 mm^3 (30 g or 1.05 oz).[11]
- Urinalysis to rule out infection as a cause of the patient's voiding symptoms; also check urinalysis for microscopic hematuria, which typically accompanies BPH.
- Plasma blood urea nitrogen (BUN) and serum creatinine may be increased as a result of long-standing bladder outlet obstruction. These tests are not routinely performed but rather are reserved for those patients in whom renal dysfunction is suspected.

Other Diagnostic Tests (Table 52–2)

- Decreased peak and mean urinary flow rate (less than 10–15 mL/s) on uroflowmetry; decreased urinary flow rate is not specific for BPH; it can also be due to other urologic disorders (e.g., urethral stricture, meatal stenosis, or bladder hypotonicity)
- Increased postvoid residual urine volume (PVR) (more than 50 mL)
- DRE to check for an enlarged prostate (more than 15–20 g) (0.5–0.7 oz)
- Transurethral cytoscopy reveals an enlarged prostate, which decreases urethral lumen caliber; information from this procedure helps the surgeon decide on the best surgical approach
- Transrectal ultrasound of the prostate; a transrectal probe is inserted to evaluate prostate size and best surgical approach
- Transrectal prostate needle biopsy to be done if the patient has areas of nodularity or induration on DRE; tissue biopsy can document the presence of prostate cancer, which can also cause enlargement of the prostate
- IV pyelogram (IVP) will show retention of radiocontrast in the bladder if the patient has bladder outlet obstruction due to an enlarged prostate; only indicated in patients with recurrent hematuria, recurrent urinary tract infection, renal insufficiency, and urolithiasis
- Filling cystometry provides information on bladder capacity, detrusor contractility, and the presence of uninhibited bladder contractions, which could also cause LUTS

Patient Encounter 1, Part 1

AA is a 65-year-old male patient with an AUA symptom score of 19, urinary hesitancy, a slow urinary stream, urinary frequency, and nocturia. He wakes up three times every night to void. A DRE reveals an enlarged prostate of approximately 40 g (1.4 oz). His PSA is 4 ng/mL (4 mcg/L).

What stage of BPH does this patient have?

TREATMENT

Desired Outcomes

- ❷ *Reducing or eliminating obstructive and irritative voiding symptoms. An improvement in the AUA Symptom*

Score should be observed. Drug treatment with an α-adrenergic antagonist or 5α-reductase inhibitor is expected to reduce the AUA Symptom Score by 30% to 50%, improve peak and mean urinary flow rate by 1 to 3 mL/s, and decrease PVR to normal (less than 50 mL total) when compared to pretreatment baseline values. The AUA Symptom Score may not correlate with response to therapy.

- Slowing disease progression. When compared to baseline, symptoms and serum BUN and creatinine should improve, stabilize, or decrease to the normal range with treatment.
- Preventing disease complications and reducing the need for surgical intervention.
- Avoiding or minimizing adverse treatment effects.
- Providing economical therapy.
- Maintaining or improving quality of life.

Table 52–1

Questions to Determine the AUA Symptom Score

Directions for the patient: The patient should be asked to respond to each question based on the absence or presence of symptoms over the past month. For each question, the patient can respond using a 1–5 scale, where 0 = not at all or none; 1 = less than 1 time in 5; 2 = less than half of the time; 3 = about half of the time; 4 = more than half of the time; and 5 = almost always

Directions for the clinician: After the patient completes the questionnaire, the scores for individual items should be tallied for a final score. Scores of 0–7 = mild symptoms; scores of 8–19 = moderate symptoms; scores more than 20 = severe symptoms

Questions to Assess Obstructive Voiding Symptoms
1. How often have you had a sensation of not emptying your bladder completely after you finished urinating?
2. How often have you found you stopped and started again several times when you urinated?
3. How often have you had a weak urinary stream?
4. How often have you had to push or strain to begin urinating?

Questions to Assess Irritative Voiding Symptoms
5. How often have you found it difficult to postpone urination?
6. How often have you had to urinate again less than 2 hours after you finished urinating?
7. How many times did you most typically get up to urinate from the time you went to bed at night until the time you got up in the morning?

From Ref. 10.

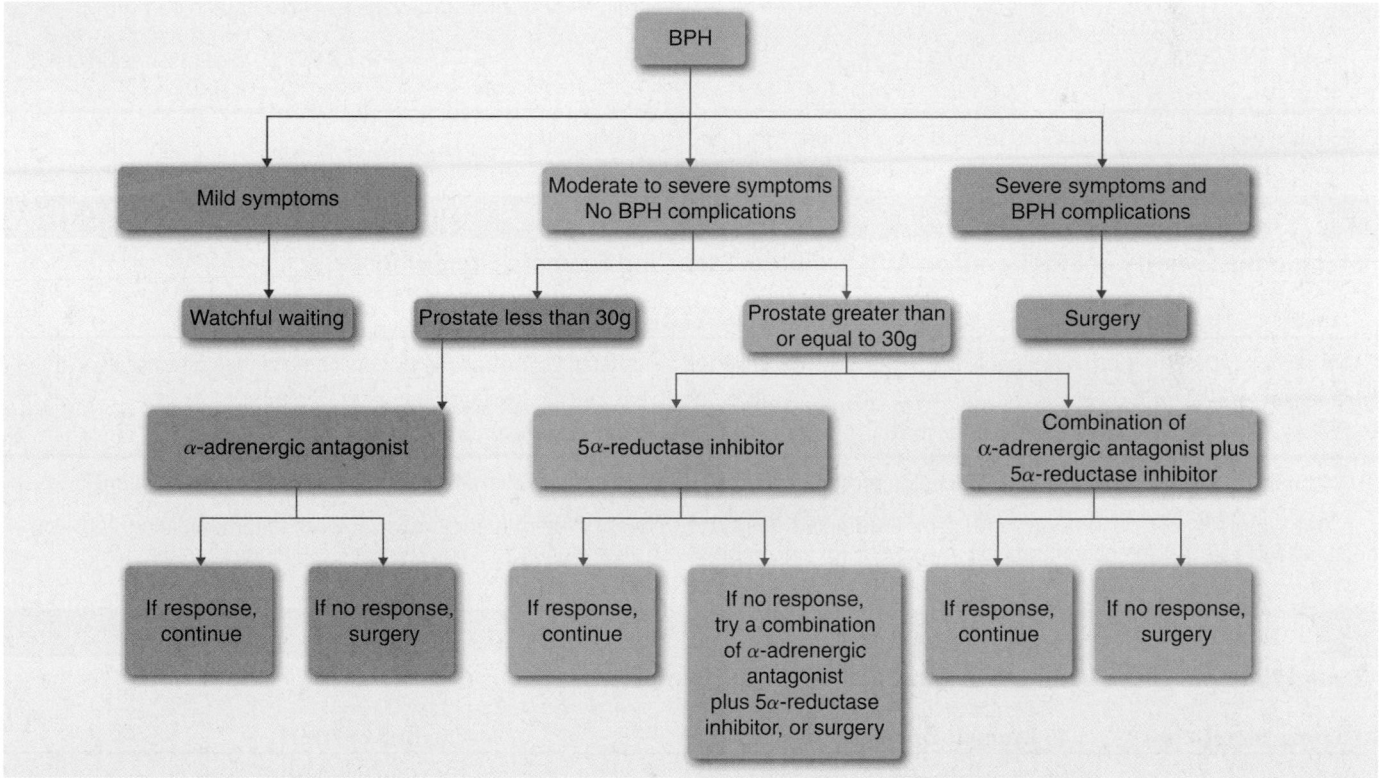

FIGURE 52–1. Algorithm for selection of treatment for BPH based on symptom severity and presence of disease complications.

General Approach to Treatment

Until recently, the principal approach to treatment focused on reducing BPH symptoms (Fig. 52–1, Tables 52–1, 52–2, and 52–3). However, treatment should also slow disease progression and decrease complications of BPH.

❸ *For patients with mild symptoms, which the patient does not consider to be bothersome, watchful waiting is a reasonable approach to treatment.* The patient is instructed to schedule return visits to the clinician every 3 to 6 months. At each visit, the patient's symptoms are reassessed using the AUA Symptom Scoring Index, and results are compared to baseline (Table 52–1). In addition, the patient is educated about avoiding factors that worsen obstructive and irritative voiding symptoms (Table 52–4). The DRE is repeated annually. If the patient's symptoms are unchanged, then watchful waiting is continued. If the patient's symptoms worsen, then specific treatment is initiated.[10]

Table 52–2

Objective Tests Used to Assess the Size of the Prostate and Complications of BPH

Test	How the Test Is Performed	Normal Test Result	Test Result in Patients With BPH
DRE of the prostate	Prostate is palpated through the rectal mucosa; the physician inserts an index finger into the patient's rectum	Prostate is soft, symmetric, mobile; size is 15–20 g (0.5–0.7 oz)	Prostate is enlarged, more than 20 g (0.5 oz); no areas of induration or nodularity
Peak and mean urinary flow rate	Patient drinks water until bladder is full; patient empties bladder; volume of urine output and time to empty the bladder are measured; the flow rate (mL/s) is calculated	Peak and mean urinary flow rate are at least 10 mL/s	Peak and mean urinary flow rates are less than 10 mL/s
PVR	Measurement of urine left in the bladder after the patient has tried to empty out his bladder; assessed by urethral catheterization or ultrasonography	PVR should be 0 mL	PVR greater than 50 mL is a significant amount of retained urine; this is associated with recurrent urinary tract infection
Urinalysis	Midstream urine is analyzed microscopically for white blood cells and bacteria	Urine should have no white cells or bacteria in it	Urine with white blood cells and bacteria is suggestive of inflammation and infection; if positive, urine is sent for bacteriologic culture
Prostate needle biopsy	Transrectally, a biopsy needle is inserted into the prostate; tissue core is sent to a pathologist for analysis	A normal prostate should have no evidence of BPH or prostate cancer	The biopsy is consistent with BPH
PSA	Blood test for this chemical, which is secreted by the prostate	Less than 4 ng/mL (4 mcg/L)	A PSA greater than 1.5 ng/mL (1.5 mcg/L) is a surrogate marker for an enlarged prostate greater than 30 g (1.05 oz)

DRE, digital rectal exam; PVR, postvoid residual urine volume; PSA, prostate-specific antigen.

Table 52–3

Staging the Severity of BPH Based on AUA Symptom Score and Example Signs of Disease

	AUA Symptom Score	Signs of Disease
Mild	Less than or equal to 7	Enlarged prostate on DRE, peak urinary flow rate less than or equal to 10 mL/s
Moderate	8–19	All of the above, PVR greater than 50 mL, irritative symptoms
Severe	Greater than or equal to 20	All of the above plus one or more complications of BPH

AUA, American Urological Association; BPH, benign prostatic hyperplasia; DRE, digital rectal exam; PVR, postvoid residual urine volume.

The AUA Symptom Score focuses on seven items (incomplete emptying, frequency, intermittency, urgency, weak stream, straining, and nocturia) and asks that the patient quantify the severity of his complaints on a scale of 0 to 5. Thus, the score can range from 0 to 35.

Table 52–4

Drugs That Can Cause Irritative or Obstructive Voiding Symptoms

Pharmacologic Class	Example Drugs	Mechanism of Effect
Androgens	Testosterone	Stimulate prostate enlargement
α-Adrenergic agonists	Phenylephrine, pseudoephedrine	Stimulate contraction of prostatic and bladder neck smooth muscle
Anticholinergic agents	Antihistamines, phenothiazines, tricyclic antidepressants, antiparkinsonian agents	Block bladder detrusor muscle contraction, thereby impairing bladder emptying
Diuretics	Thiazides diuretics, loop diuretics	Produce polyuria

---

❹ For patients with moderate to severe symptoms, the patient is usually offered drug treatment first. α-Adrenergic antagonists are preferred over 5α-reductase inhibitors because the former have a faster onset of action (days to a few weeks) and improve symptoms independent of prostate size. 5α-reductase inhibitors have a delayed onset of action (i.e., peak effect may be delayed for up to 6 months) and are seldom effective in patients with smaller size prostate glands (less than 30 g or 1.05 oz). Drug treatment must be continued as long as the patient responds (Table 52–5).[10]

Table 52–5

Comparison of α-Adrenergic Antagonists and 5α-Reductase Inhibitors for Treatment of BPH

Characteristic	α-Adrenergic Antagonists	5α-Reductase Inhibitors
Relaxes prostatic smooth muscle	Yes	No
Reduces size of enlarged prostate	No	Yes
Useful in patients with enlarged prostates	No (works independent of the size of the prostate)	Yes
Efficacy in relieving voiding symptoms and improving flow rate	++	+
Frequency of daily dosing	Once or twice daily, depending on the agent and the dosage formulation	Once daily
Requirement for up-titration of dose	Yes (for terazosin and doxazosin immediate-release); No (for alfuzosin or silodosin; possibly for doxazosin extended-release and tamsulosin)	No
Peak onset of action	Days–6 weeks, depending on need for dose titration	6 months
Decreases PSA	No	Yes
Cardiovascular adverse effects	Yes	No
Drug-induced sexual dysfunction	Ejaculation disorders	Decreased libido, erectile dysfunction, ejaculation disorders

PSA, prostate-specific antigen.

⑤ *For patients with complications of BPH disease (e.g., recurrent urinary tract infection, urosepsis, urinary incontinence, refractory urinary retention, chronic renal failure, large bladder diverticuli, recurrent severe gross hematuria, or bladder calculi secondary to prolonged urinary retention), surgery is indicated.* Although it is potentially curative, surgery can result in significant morbidity, including erectile dysfunction, retrograde ejaculation, urinary incontinence, bleeding, or urinary tract infection.[12] The gold standard is a prostatectomy, which can be performed transurethrally or as an open surgical procedure, which can be performed suprapubically or retropubically. To avoid complications of prostatectomy, minimally invasive surgical procedures, such as transurethral incision of the prostate, transurethral needle ablation, or transurethral microwave thermotherapy, are options.[10,12,13] Drug treatment is used in patients with severe disease when the patient refuses surgery or when the patient is not a surgical candidate because of concomitant diseases.

In the Multiple Treatment of Prostate Symptoms Study, it was found that selected patients with moderate to severe symptoms will benefit from a combination of α-adrenergic antagonist plus 5α-reductase inhibitor drug therapy.[14] Specifically, the use of doxazosin plus finasteride is more effective than doxazosin alone or finasteride alone in relieving symptoms, reducing the need for prostatectomy, and decreasing the incidence of BPH complications in patients at highest risk of developing disease complications (i.e., those with prostate size of at least 40 g [1.4 oz]). Combination therapy is more expensive than monotherapy and also produces more adverse effects. Therefore, the clinician should discuss the advantages and disadvantages of combination therapy with a patient before deciding on a final treatment regimen.

Nonpharmacologic Therapy

To reduce nocturia, patients should be instructed to stop drinking fluids several hours before going to bed, and then voiding before going to sleep. During the day, patients should avoid excessive caffeine and alcohol intake, as these may cause urinary frequency. Patients should avoid taking nonprescription medications that can worsen obstructive voiding symptoms (e.g., antihistamines or decongestants) (Table 52–4). In addition, toilet mapping (knowing the location of toilets on the way to and from various destinations) may help reassure the patient that he can still continue with many of his routine daily activities. Patients are also advised to lose weight, if overweight. Because testosterone is converted to estrogen in fat tissue, an alteration in the testosterone:estrogen ratio occurs in overweight men, similar to that which occurs in elderly males, which may contribute to the development of BPH.[15–17]

Although a variety of herbal agents are used for symptomatic management, including pygeum (African plum), secale cereale (rye pollen), and hypoxis rooperi (South African star grass), objective evidence of efficacy is lacking.[18,19] Also, in a randomized, double-blind, and placebo-controlled clinical trial, saw palmetto was no different than placebo in improving symptoms or increasing peak urinary flow rate.[20]

Pharmacologic Therapy

▶ α-Adrenergic Antagonist Monotherapy[21]

⑥ *α-Adrenergic antagonists reduce the dynamic factor causing BPH symptoms. These drugs competitively antagonize α-adrenergic receptors, thereby causing relaxation of the bladder neck, prostatic urethra, and prostate smooth muscle.* A secondary mechanism of action may be that α-adrenergic antagonists induce prostatic apoptosis,[22] which suggests that these agents may cause some shrinkage of an enlarged prostate. However, the clinical importance of this remains to be elucidated.

All α-adrenergic antagonists are considered equally effective in relieving symptoms.[10] In various clinical trials, 30% to 80% of patients experience improvement in AUA Symptom Score by 30% to 45% and 20% to 40% of patients experience urinary flow rate increases of 2 to 3 mL/s.[15] The onset of action is days to weeks, depending on the need for titration of the dose from a subtherapeutic starting dose to a therapeutic dose. An adequate clinical trial is considered to be at least 1 to 2 weeks of continuous treatment at a full maintenance dose with any of these agents.[10] Durable responses have been demonstrated for up to 5 years of continuous use of terazosin,[23] 10 years with doxazosin,[24] and 6 years with tamsulosin.[25] However, some patients will develop disease progression despite treatment. α-Adrenergic antagonists are hepatically catabolized. Therefore, in patients with significant hepatic dysfunction, these drugs should be used in the lowest possible dose. With the exception of silodosin, these drugs do not require dosage modification in patients with renal dysfunction. These agents can be differentiated by their adverse effect profile. Dose limiting adverse effects include hypotension and syncope, which are more common with immediate-release terazosin and doxazosin, less frequent with extended-release doxazosin and alfuzosin, and least frequent with uroselective α-adrenergic antagonists.[26,27] Delayed or retrograde ejaculation has been reported most often with tamsulosin 0.8 mg orally once a day. Combined use with antihypertensives, diuretics, or phosphodiesterase inhibitors can lead to additive blood pressure–lowering effects; however, this appears to be less of a problem with tamsulosin.[26,27]

α-Adrenergic antagonists are recommended as first-line treatment for moderate to severe BPH. The agents in this pharmacologic class can be classified by several characteristics (Table 52–6):

- *Generation of α-adrenergic antagonist.* First-generation agents (e.g., phenoxybenzamine) block presynaptic and postsynaptic α-adrenergic receptors. Whereas blockade of postsynaptic α-adrenergic receptors is desirable for BPH management, blockade of presynaptic α-adrenergic receptors is undesirable, as it results in release of catecholamines and tachycardia. Thus, first-generation α-adrenergic antagonists are not used for treatment of BPH.[28] Second-generation α-adrenergic antagonists block postsynaptic α-adrenergic receptors in the bladder neck, prostate, and peripheral vasculature. Hypotensive adverse effects are dose-related and common. Examples include terazosin, doxazosin, and alfuzosin. Third-generation α-adrenergic antagonists (e.g., tamsulosin, silodosin) selectively block postsynaptic α_{1A}-receptors, which concentrate in the prostate. As a result, hypotensive adverse effects are less common than with second-generation agents.

- ❼ *Uroselectivity.* Pharmacologic uroselectivity refers to preferential inhibition of α_{1A}-and α_{1D}-receptors, which

predominate in the prostatic stroma and bladder detrusor muscle, respectively.[21] Pharmacologically uroselective α_{1A}-adrenergic antagonists have the potential to produce less hypotension, as they have a lower propensity to antagonize α_{1B}-adrenergic receptors in the peripheral vasculature. Tamsulosin and silodosin are the only commercially available α-adrenergic antagonists with pharmacologic uroselectivity. In contrast, despite the potential of inhibiting α-adrenergic receptors in both the prostate and peripheral vasculature, functionally uroselective α-adrenergic antagonists in usually-prescribed doses, produce effective relaxation of prostatic smooth muscle with minimal vascular vasodilation. Thus, blood pressure–lowering effects are mild or absent. The only functionally uroselective α-adrenergic antagonist is alfuzosin extended-release tablets. The mechanism of functional uroselectivity is unclear. It may be related to a drug formulation which produces a higher concentration in target tissues than in nontarget tissues.[28] Both pharmacologically and functionally uroselective agents appear to be clinically uroselective, in that they improve BPH symptoms without causing cardiovascular adverse effects in humans.[21]

Pharmacologic and functional uroselectivity are dose-related phenomena. Large daily doses of tamsulosin or alfuzosin may cause loss of uroselectivity with resultant hypotension and dizziness in some patients.

- *Need for up-titration of daily dose.* Up-titration is required for immediate-release terazosin and doxazosin. It is minimally required for extended-release doxazosin and tamsulosin. It is not required for extended-release alfuzosin or silodosin.

- *Plasma half-life.* α-Adrenergic receptors with short plasma half-lives (e.g., prazosin) require multiple doses during the day. This is challenging for most patients, and, thus, prazosin is not recommended for BPH.[10]

- *Dosage formulation.* Immediate-release formulations of terazosin and doxazosin are quickly absorbed and produce high peak plasma levels. Modified- or extended-release formulations of doxazosin, alfuzosin, and tamsulosin produce lower peak levels, but more sustained therapeutic plasma levels, than immediate-release formulations and have less potential for producing hypotensive episodes. This allows for initiation of treatment with a therapeutic dose and once daily dosing.[29-31]

- *Adverse effects.* Hypotensive adverse effects of α-adrenergic antagonists can range from asymptomatic blood pressure reductions to dizziness and syncope. This adverse effect is most commonly associated with immediate-release terazosin and doxazosin; is less commonly associated with extended-release alfuzosin and extended-release doxazosin, and silodosin; and least commonly associated with tamsulosin.[26,27] To minimize first-dose syncope from terazosin and doxazosin immediate-release, a slow up-titration from a subtherapeutic dose of 1 mg/day to a therapeutic dose is essential. The first dose should be given

Table 52–6

Comparison of Pharmacologic Properties of α-Adrenergic Antagonists

	Terazosin	Doxazosin	Alfuzosin	Tamsulosin	Silodosin
Brand name	Hytrin	Cardura	Uroxatral	Flomax	Rapaflo
Generation	Second	Second	Second	Third	Third
Uroselective	No	No	Functionally and clinically uroselective	Pharmacologically and clinically uroselective	Pharmacologically and clinically uroselective
Need for up-titration	Yes	Yes (with immediate-release); possibly (with extended-release)	No	Minimal	No
Daily oral dose (mg)	5–20	2–8, immediate-release; 4–8, extended-release	10	0.4–0.8; 0.8 mg/day (dose has not consistently produced clinical improvement over 0.4 mg/day[20])	8
Recommended dose reduction in patients with renal dysfunction	None needed	None needed	None needed	If creatinine clearance greater than 10 mL/min, none needed. Tamsulosin has not been studied in patients with creatinine clearance less than 10 mL/min	If creatinine clearance 30–50 mL/min, use 4 mg/day. Contraindicated in patients with creatinine clearance less than 30 mL/min
Recommended dose reduction in patients with hepatic dysfunction	Manufacturer provides no specific recommendation. Terazosin should be used cautiously as it undergoes extensive hepatic metabolism	Manufacturer provides no specific recommendation. Doxazosin should be used cautiously as it undergoes extensive hepatic metabolism	Contraindicated in patients with moderate/severe hepatic impairment. Alfuzosin should be used cautiously in patients with mild hepatic impairment	Patients with mild/moderate hepatic impairment require no dosage adjustment. Tamsulosin has not been studied in patients with severe hepatic impairment	Patients with mild/moderate hepatic impairment require no dosage adjustment. Contraindicated in patients with severe hepatic impairment
Best time to take doses	At bedtime	Immediate-release: anytime during the day; however, it is typically given at bedtime. Extended-release: anytime during the day	After meals for best oral absorption	On an empty stomach for best oral absorption; if taken 30 minutes after a meal, as recommended by the manufacturer, extent of absorption is reduced, thereby further reducing the potential for hypotensive adverse effects	Take with a meal, which decreases extent of absorption. Theoretically, this would help decrease hypotensive adverse effects
Half-life (hours)	12	22	5	10	13
Formulation	Immediate-release	Immediate-release and extended-release	Extended-release	Modified-release	Immediate-release
Cardiovascular adverse effects	++	++	+	0 to +	0 to +
Ejaculation disorders	+	+	+	++	++
Rhinitis	+	+	+	+	+
Malaise	+	+	+	+	+

at bedtime so that the patient can sleep through the peak serum concentration of the drug when the adverse effect is most likely to occur. A 3- to 7-day interval between each dosage increase should be allowed, and the patient should be maintained on the lowest effective dose of α-adrenergic antagonist. If the patient is noncompliant with his regimen of terazosin or doxazosin, and he skips or interrupts treatment, the α-adrenergic antagonist should be restarted using the usual starting dose and then retitrated up. He should not be instructed to simply double up on missed doses or resume treatment with his currently prescribed daily dose, as this can lead to significant hypotension.

Ejaculation disorders, including delayed and retrograde ejaculation, occur with all adrenergic antagonists. Although largely thought to be due to pharmacologic blockade of peripheral α-adrenergic receptors at the bladder neck (i.e., the bladder neck is unable to close during ejaculation in the presence of α-adrenergic blockade), a CNS mechanism of action cannot be discounted.[32] The incidence appears to be dose-related and highest with tamsulosin 0.8 mg daily, occurring in up to 26% of treated patients.[33] Ejaculation disorders generally do not necessitate discontinuation of treatment. Although they may decrease the patient's satisfaction with the quality of sexual intercourse, ejaculation disorders are not harmful to the patient.

Rhinitis and malaise occur with α-adrenergic antagonists and are an extension of the pharmacologic blockade of α-adrenergic receptors in the vasculature of the nasal mucosa and in the CNS, respectively. Tolerance often develops to these adverse effects and they rarely require discontinuation of treatment. Avoid use of topical or oral decongestants, as these may exacerbate obstructive voiding symptoms. Cautious use of antihistamines with anticholinergic adverse effects is also recommended in patients with BPH, as these drugs may cause acute urinary retention in patients with an obstructed bladder neck.

Floppy iris syndrome has been reported with α-adrenergic antagonists, most often with tamsulosin. In response to tamsulosin, the iris dilator muscle relaxes. As a result, in a tamsulosin-treated patient who is undergoing cataract surgery, the iris can become flaccid, billow out, or become floppy. This can interfere with the surgical procedure and increase the risk of intraoperative and postoperative complications. A patient who plans to undergo cataract surgery is advised to inform his ophthalmologist that he is taking an α-adrenergic antagonist. Although the drug will not need to be held or discontinued, the ophthalmologist can plan to use certain surgical techniques, for example, iris hooks or iris expansion rings, to deal with the drug's effect on the iris dilator muscle.[34,35]

Alfuzosin has been linked to two cases of hepatitis.[36,37] The cause-effect relationship remains to be elucidated.

- *Potential for drug interactions.* Hypotensive adverse effects of terazosin and doxazosin can be additive with those of diuretics, antihypertensives, and phosphodiesterase inhibitors (e.g., sildenafil). In patients at greatest risk for hypotension, or in those patients who tolerate hypotension poorly, including those with poorly controlled coronary artery disease or severe orthostatic hypotension, tamsulosin 0.4 mg appears to be the safest choice.[38,39] In patients who cannot tolerate tamsulosin, a 5α-reductase inhibitor or prostatectomy should be considered. When initiating sildenafil, tadalafil, or vardenafil, patients who are taking α-adrenergic antagonists should be stabilized first on a fixed dose of the α-adrenergic antagonist, and patients should be instructed to allow a 4-hour interval between the α-adrenergic antagonist and the phosphodiesterase inhibitor to minimize the likelihood of hypotensive effects.

❼ *Among the α-adrenergic antagonists, tamsulosin and silodosin are unique in that they are third-generation α-adrenergic antagonists. They are pharmacologically uroselective and exert greater antagonism of α_{1A}- and α_{1D}- receptors, which predominate in prostatic and bladder detrusor muscle. Tamsulosin exerts comparatively low antagonism of vascular α_{1B}-receptors. Therefore, tamsulosin can be started with a therapeutic dose, which achieves peak effects sooner than terazosin and doxazosin immediate-release, which must be up-titrated. Tamsulosin appears to have the lowest potential to cause hypotension.[26,27] In various clinical trials, tamsulosin has minimal hypotensive adverse effects and is well tolerated in the elderly, as well as in patients taking diuretics, antihypertensives, or phosphodiesterase inhibitors.*

Patient Encounter 2, Part I

BB has moderate BPH symptoms and is started on tamsulosin 0.4 mg orally once a day. After 2 to 3 weeks, BB states that his symptoms have not improved. He is not experiencing any drug-related adverse effects.

What should be the next step in management of this patient?

It is also commercially available in a modified-release dosage formulation, which is dosed at 0.4 mg orally once a day. With chronic use, tamsulosin can be taken at any time of the day and at the patient's convenience. Although the package insert states that the dose can be increased to 0.8 mg daily, no consistent improvement in clinical efficacy has been observed in patients taking the higher dose.[26] It is not clear at this time whether silodosin has the same clinical cardiovascular safety profile as tamsulosin.

In patients with BPH and hypertension, it is not recommended to use an α-adrenergic antagonist alone to treat both disorders. In the ALLHAT study, where doxazosin was compared to other agents for treatment of essential hypertension, doxazosin was associated with a higher incidence of congestive heart failure. Therefore, in patients with hypertension and BPH, it is recommended that an appropriate antihypertensive be added to an α-adrenergic antagonist.[26]

▶ 5α-Reductase Inhibitor Monotherapy

❽ *5α-Reductase inhibitors reduce the static factor, which results in shrinkage of an enlarged prostate. They do so by inhibiting 5α-reductase, which is responsible for intraprostatic conversion of testosterone to dihydrotestosterone, the active androgen that stimulates prostate tissue growth. In the prostate, there are two subtypes of 5α-reductase; the majority is the type II isoenzyme type and the minority is the type I isoenzyme type. In addition, 5α-reductase inhibitors induce apoptosis of prostatic epithelial cells.[40] The onset of action is slow with peak shrinkage of the prostate taking up to 6 months.[10] Unlike α-adrenergic antagonists, 5α-reductase inhibitors are used to prevent BPH-related complications and disease progression. Finasteride has been shown to reduce the incidence of acute urinary retention and need for prostate surgery in patients with significantly enlarged prostate glands (greater than 40 g [1.4 oz]),[14] and those with serum levels of PSA of at least 1.5 ng/mL (1.5 mcg/L).[11] Because 5α-reductase inhibitors do not produce cardiovascular adverse effects, they are preferred for men with moderate to severe BPH who are at risk of developing complications of BPH (i.e., the patient has an enlarged prostate of at least 30 g [1.05 oz]), and has a PSA of greater than 1.5 ng/mL (1.5 mg/L).[8,11,41]*

With regard to their use for the symptomatic treatment of BPH, 5α-reductase inhibitors relieve BPH symptoms in 30% to 70% of patients and increase urinary flow rate by 1 to 2 mL/s, which is less improvement than that seen with α-adrenergic antagonists.[10,14] A minimum of 6 months is required to evaluate the effectiveness of treatment. This is a disadvantage in patients with moderate to severe symptoms, as it will take that long to determine if the drug is or is not effective. Durable responses have been demonstrated in responding patients treated up to 6 years with finasteride and 4 years with dutasteride.[42,43] These agents are hepatically metabolized. No specific recommendations for dosage modification are currently available in patients with significant hepatic dysfunction; however, due to drug specificity for its enzyme target, it is unlikely that any dosage adjustment will be required. No dosage adjustment is needed in patients with renal impairment. Adverse effects include decreased libido, erectile dysfunction, and ejaculation disorders, which generally decrease in frequency with continued use, and gynecomastia and breast tenderness.[33,40] Serum testosterone levels increase by 10% to 20% in treated patients; however, the clinical significance of this is not clear at this time.[10] Drug interactions are uncommon. These drugs do produce a mean 50% decrease in serum levels of PSA. Therefore, to preserve the usefulness of this laboratory test as a diagnostic and monitoring tool, it is recommended that prescribers obtain a baseline PSA prior to the start of treatment and repeat it at least annually during treatment. A significantly elevated PSA in treated patients is an indicator for further diagnostic workup.[44] Exposure to 5α-reductase inhibitors is contraindicated in pregnant females, as the drugs may cause feminization of a male fetus. Pregnant females should not handle these drugs unless they are wearing gloves.

5α-Reductase inhibitors include finasteride and dutasteride. Finasteride is a selective type II 5α-reductase inhibitor, whereas dutasteride is a nonselective type I and II 5α-reductase inhibitor. When compared to finasteride, dutasteride produces a faster and more complete inhibition of 5α-reductase in prostate cells. However, no difference in clinical efficacy or adverse effects has been demonstrated between these two agents. Thus, finasteride and dutasteride are considered therapeutically interchangeable (Table 52–7).[45]

By reducing serum levels of dihydrotestosterone, which is linked to the development of prostate cancer, it has been hypothesized that 5α-reductase inhibitors may prevent the development of prostate cancer. The Predict Trial reported that finasteride reduced the detection of prostate cancer with prostatic needle biopsy by 25%; however, higher-grade tumors were more common in treated patients.[46] This finding is likely due to the fact that the drug-induced shrinkage of the prostate increased the probability that the prostate needle biopsy procedure was able to obtain cancerous tissue.[46] The ongoing Reduce Trial, which will follow dutasteride-treated patients for 4 years, may provide more clarification on this issue.[47]

▶ Combination Therapy

A combination of an α-adrenergic antagonist and 5α-reductase inhibitor may be considered in symptomatic patients at high risk of BPH complications, which are defined as those with an enlarged prostate of at least 30 g (1.05 oz) and a PSA of at

---

Patient Encounter 1, Part 2

AA is started on finasteride 5 mg orally once a day. Four weeks later the patient returns for a follow-up visit and complains that he is not experiencing any symptom improvement.

What should be the next step in management of this patient?

---

least 1.5 ng/mL (1.5 mcg/L). In such patients, combination therapy will relieve voiding symptoms and also may reduce the risk of developing BPH-related complications and reduce the need for prostatectomy by 67%.[12,14] Because combination therapy is more expensive and associated with the array of adverse effects associated with each drug in the combination,

---

Table 52–7

Comparison of Pharmacologic Properties of 5α-Reductase Inhibitors

	Finasteride	Dutasteride
Brand name	Proscar	Avodart
Subtype inhibition of the 5α-reductase enzyme	Type II	Types I and II
Percentage of inhibition of serum dihydrotestosterone level	70–76	90–95
Percentage of patients with reduction in serum dihydrotestosterone	49	Greater than 85
Time to peak onset of reduction in serum dihydrotestosterone level	6 months	1 month
Percentage of inhibition of intraprostatic dihydrotestosterone	85–90	Greater than 95
Half-life	6.2 hours	3–5 hours
Daily dosage (mg)	5	0.5
Recommended dose reduction in patients with renal dysfunction	None needed	None needed
Recommended dose reduction in patients with hepatic dysfunction	Manufacturer provides no specific recommendation. Finasteride should be used cautiously as it undergoes extensive hepatic metabolism	Manufacturer provides no specific recommendation. Dutasteride should be used cautiously as it undergoes extensive hepatic metabolism

From Refs. 41, 44.

clinicians should discuss the advantages and disadvantages of each treatment regimen with the patient before a final decision is made.[10]

To streamline and reduce the cost of treatment regimens, it has been suggested that the α-adrenergic antagonist may be discontinued after the first 6 to 12 months of combination therapy. However, long-term treatment is required to determine if such a regimen is as effective as continuous combination therapy.[48,49]

Another enhancement to BPH symptom management is the addition of an anticholinergic agent to an α-adrenergic antagonist. The rationale for the anticholinergic agent is that irritative symptoms (e.g., urinary urgency and frequency) are thought to be due to hyper-reactive bladder detrusor muscle contraction, which can be ameliorated by blockade of acetylcholine receptors.[49,50] Also, α_{1D}-adrenergic receptors in the detrusor muscle, which cause muscle contraction when stimulated, can be blocked by α-adrenergic antagonists. As a result, use of an α-adrenergic antagonist may also decrease involuntary bladder muscle contraction and increase the bladder's compliance. Thus, the combination may have an additive pharmacologic effect on relieving irritative voiding symptoms.[51,52] A recent study documenting the addition of tolterodine to tamsulosin showed significant irritative symptom improvement, more than what was observed with tamsulosin alone. No cases of urinary retention were reported.[51]

OUTCOME EVALUATION

❾ *Once the peak effects of drug treatment are expected to occur, monitor the drug for effectiveness. Assess symptom improvement using the AUA Symptom Scoring Index. A reduction in symptom score is anticipated with symptom improvement. However, it should be noted that the AUA Symptom Score may not match the patient's perception of the bothersomeness of his voiding symptoms. If the patient perceives his symptoms as bothersome, independent of the AUA Symptom Score, consideration should be given to modifying the patient's treatment regimen. Similarly, a patient may regard his symptoms as not bothersome even though the AUA symptom score is high. In this case, the physician should objectively assess symptoms at baseline and during treatment by performing a repeat uroflowmetry, which can detect an improvement in peak and mean urinary flow rate. If the patient shows a response to treatment, instruct the patient to continue the drug regimen and have the patient return at 6-month intervals for monitoring. If the patient shows an inadequate response to treatment, the dose of α-adrenergic antagonist can be increased (except for extended-release alfuzosin) until the patient's symptoms improve or until the patient experiences adverse drug effects.*

For the α-adrenergic antagonists, the severity of hypotensive-related adverse effects, which may manifest as dizziness or syncope, may require a dosage reduction or a slower up-titration of immediate-release terazosin or doxazosin, or halting the up-titration of the α-adrenergic

antagonist. If the patient develops adverse effects at this dose, the drug should be discontinued. Other adverse effects of α-adrenergic antagonists are nasal congestion, malaise, headache, and ejaculation disorders. None of these generally require discontinuation of treatment and these often improve as treatment continues. For the 5α-reductase inhibitors,

---

Table 52–8

Summary of Adverse Effects of α-Adrenergic Antagonists and 5α-Reductase Inhibitors and Management Suggestions

Drug Class	Adverse Reaction	Management Suggestion
α-Adrenergic antagonist	Hypotension	Start with lowest effective dose, give doses at bedtime, and slowly up-titrate at 0.5- to 1-week intervals to a full therapeutic dose, if using immediate-release terazosin or doxazosin Use tamsulosin, silodosin, extended-release doxazosin, or alfuzosin, as alternatives to immediate-release products, particularly in patients taking other antihypertensives
	Malaise	Educate the patient that this is a common adverse effect; tolerance may develop to malaise. Usually it is not so severe that it requires discontinuation of treatment
	Rhinitis	Educate the patient that this is a common adverse effect; tolerance may develop to rhinitis. Usually it is not so severe that it requires discontinuation of treatment
	Retrograde ejaculation	Educate the patient that this is a common adverse effect and it is not harmful
5α-Reductase inhibitor	Gynecomastia	Educate the patient that this may be bothersome, but not harmful
	Decreased libido	If the patient is sexually active, sexual counseling may be helpful. May be reversible despite continued use of the 5α-reductase inhibitor
	Erectile dysfunction	The addition of sildenafil or another erectogenic drug may be helpful. May be reversible despite continued use of the 5α-reductase inhibitor
	Ejaculation disorders	Educate the patient that this may occur but it is not harmful. May be reversible despite continued use of the 5α-reductase inhibitor

the most bothersome adverse effects are decreased libido, erectile dysfunction, and ejaculation disorders. In sexually active males, erectile dysfunction may be improved with erectogenic drugs; however, this adverse effect may necessitate discontinuation of treatment.

During continuing treatment of BPH, the patient should undergo an annual repeat PSA and DRE. A rising PSA level suggests that the patient has worsening BPH, new-onset prostate cancer, or that the patient is noncompliant with his regimen of 5α-reductase inhibitor. An abnormal DRE suggestive of prostate cancer would reveal a nodule or area of induration on the prostate, or a gland that is fixed in place. In such a case, a prostate biopsy is required to rule out prostate cancer.

Drug treatment failures may result from a variety of factors. Initial failure to respond to α-adrenergic antagonists occurs in 20% to 70% of treated patients. It is likely in these patients that the static factor may predominate as the cause of symptoms in these patients. In these patients, adding a 5α-reductase inhibitor may be helpful. Initial failure to respond to 5α-reductase inhibitors occurs in 30% to 70% of treated patients. It is likely that the dynamic factor may predominate as the cause of symptoms in these patients. In these patients, switching to or adding an α-adrenergic antagonist may be helpful. In contrast, drug treatment failures after an initial good response to drug therapy will likely be an indication of progressive BPH disease. In such patients, surgical intervention may be indicated.

Table 52–8 summarizes the adverse effects of the agents used to treat BPH and includes management suggestions for these situations.

Abbreviations Introduced in This Chapter

AUA	American Urological Association
BPH	Benign prostatic hyperplasia
BUN	Blood urea nitrogen
DRE	Digital rectal exam
IVP	Intravenous pyelogram
LUTS	Lower urinary tract (voiding) symptoms
PSA	Prostate-specific antigen
PVR	Postvoid residual urine volume

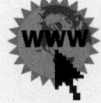 Self-assessment questions and answers are available at *http://www.mhpharmacotherapy.com/pp.html.*

REFERENCES

1. Beckman TJ, Mynderse LA. Evaluation and medical management of benign prostatic hyperplasia. Mayo Clin Proc 2005;80:1356–1362.
2. Berry SJ, Coffey DS, Walsh PC, et al. The development of human benign prostatic hyperplasia with age. J Urol 1984;132:474–479.
3. Ruggieri MR, Braverman AS, Pontari MA. Combined use of α-adrenergic and muscarinic antagonists for the treatment of voiding dysfunction. J Urol 2005;174:1743–1748.
4. Pool JL, Kirby RS. Clinical significance of α₁-adrenoceptor selectivity in the management of benign prostatic hyperplasia. Int Urol Nephrol 2001;33:407–412.
5. Isaacs JT. Importance of the natural history of benign prostatic hyperplasia in the evaluation of pharmacologic intervention. Prostate 1990;3(Suppl):1–7.
6. Flanigan RC, Reda DJ, Wasson JHM, et al. 5 year outcome of surgical resection and watchful waiting for men with moderately symptomatic benign prostatic hyperplasia: A Department of Veterans Affairs cooperative study. J Urol 1998;160:12–17.
7. Jacobsen SJ, Girman CJ, Lieber MM. Natural history of benign prostatic hyperplasia. Urology 2001;58(Suppl 6A):5–16.
8. Marks LS, Roehrborn CG, Andriole GL. Prevention of benign prostatic hyperplasia disease. J Urol 2006;176:1299–1306.
9. Patel A, Chapple C. Acute urinary retention: Who is at risk and how best to manage it. Curr Urol Rep 2006;7:252–259.
10. AUA Practice Guidelines Committee. AUA guideline on the management of benign prostatic hyperplasia (2003). Chapter 1: Diagnosis and treatment recommendations. J Urol 2003;170:530–547.
11. Roehrborn CG, Boyle P, Gould AL, et al. Serum prostate-specific antigen as a predictor of prostate volume in men with benign prostatic hyperplasia. Urology 1999;53:581–589.
12. Rassweiler J, Teber D, Kuntz R, et al. Complications of transurethral resection of the prostate (TURP)-incidence, management, and prevention. Eur Urol 2006;50:969–980.
13. Kaminetsky JC. Comorbid LUTS and erectile dysfunction: Optimizing their management. Curr Med Res Opin 2006;22:2497–2506.
14. McConnell JD, Roehrborn CG, Bautista OM, et al. The long-term effect of doxazosin, finasteride, and combination therapy on the

---

Patient Care and Monitoring

- Monitor the patient for the drug's effectiveness in relieving symptoms by using the AUA Symptom Scoring Index. Monitor to ensure that the score improves and that the patient subjectively feels that symptoms have improved. If the patient has no improvement after several weeks of a therapeutic dose of α-adrenergic antagonist or after 6 months of a 5α-reductase inhibitor, consider surgical intervention. Alternatively, if the patient was on a 5α-reductase inhibitor alone, it may be reasonable to consider adding an α-adrenergic antagonist.

- If the patient is started on an α-adrenergic antagonist, monitor the patient for hypotension, dizziness, or syncope. If present, assess the severity of each symptom. Reduce the drug dose, switch to a uroselective α-adrenergic antagonist, or discontinue the drug, as necessary. If the patient has malaise or rhinitis, reassure the patient that these are usual, but bothersome, adverse effect, that often improve with continued therapy.

- If the patient is started on a 5α-reductase inhibitor, monitor the patient for drug-induced decreased libido, erectile dysfunction, or ejaculation disorders. If severe, discontinue the drug.

clinical progression of benign prostatic hyperplasia. N Engl J Med 2003;349:2389–2398.

15. Parsons JK. Modifiable risk factors for benign prostatic hyperplasia and lower urinary tract symptoms: New approaches to old problems. J Urol 2007;178:395–401.

16. Ranjan P, Dalela D, Sankhwar SN. Diet and benign prostatic hyperplasia: Implications for prevention. Urology 2006;68:470–476.

17. Kristal AR, Arnold KB, Schenk JM, et al. Race/ethnicity, obesity, health-related behaviors and the risk of symptomatic benign prostatic hyperplasia: Results from the prostate cancer prevention trial. J Urol 2007;177:1395–1400.

18. Avins AL, Bent S. Saw palmetto and lower urinary tract symptoms: What is the latest evidence? Curr Urol Rep 2006;7:260–265.

19. Dedhia RC, McVary KT. Phytotherapy for lower urinary tract symptoms secondary to benign prostatic hyperplasia. J Urol 2006;179:2119–2125.

20. Bent S, Kane C, Shinohara K, et al. Saw palmetto for benign prostatic hyperplasia. N Engl J Med 2006;354:557–566.

21. Schwinn DA, Price DT, Narayan P. Alpha 1-adrenoceptor subtype selectivity and lower urinary tract symptoms. Mayo Clin Proc 2004;79:1423–1434.

22. Chon JK, Borkowsky A, Partin AW, et al. Alpha 1-adrenoceptor antagonists terazosin and doxazosin induce prostate apoptosis without affecting cell proliferation in patients with benign prostatic hyperplasia. J Urol 1999;161:2002–2008.

23. Lowe F. Alpha-1-adrenceptor blockade in the treatment of benign prostatic hyperplasia. Prostate Cancer Prostatic Dis 1999;2:2110–2119.

24. Dutkiewicz S. Long term treatment with doxazosin in men with benign prostatic hyperplasia: 10 year follow up. Intern Urol Nephrol 2004;36:169–173.

25. Narayan P, Evans CP, Moon T. Long term safety and efficacy of tamsulosin for the treatment of lower urinary tract symptoms associated with benign prostatic hyperplasia. J Urol 2003;170:498–502.

26. Kaplan SA, Neutel J. Vasodilatory factors in treatment of older men with symptomatic benign prostatic hyperplasia. Urology 2006;67:225–231.

27. Milani S, Djavan B. Lower urinary tract symptoms suggestive of benign prostatic hyperplasia: Latest update on α_1-adrenoceptor antagonist. BJU Int 2005;95(Suppl 4):29–36.

28. Lowe FC. Role of the newer alpha$_1$ adrenergic receptor antagonists in the treatment of benign prostatic hyperplasia-related lower urinary tract symptoms. Clin Ther 2004;26:1701–1713.

29. Kirby RS, Andersen M, Gratzke P, et al. A combined analysis of double blind trials of the efficacy and tolerability of doxazosin gastrointestinal therapeutic system, doxazosin standard and placebo in patients with benign prostatic hyperplasia. BJU Int 2001;87:192–200.

30. Elhilali MM. Alfuzosin: An α_1-receptor blocker for the treatment of lower urinary tract symptoms associated with benign prostatic hyperplasia. Expert Opin Pharmacother 2006;7(5):583–596.

31. Goldsmith DR, Plosker GL. Doxazosin gastrointestinal therapeutic system. Drugs 2005;65(14):2037–2047.

32. Hellstrom WJ, Sikka SC. Effects of acute treatment with tamsulosin versus alfuzosin on ejaculatory function in normal volunteers. J Urol 2007;177:1587–1588.

33. Larson TR. Current treatment options for benign prostatic hyperplasia and their impact on sexual function. Urology 2003;61:692–698.

34. Lawrentschuk N, Bylsma GW. Intraoperative floppy iris syndrome and its relationship to tamsulosin: A urologist's guide. BJU Int 2006;97:2–4.

35. Schwinn DA, Afshari NA. Alpha(1)-Adrenergic receptor antagonists and the iris: New mechanistic insights into floppy iris syndrome. Surv Ophthalmol 2006;51:501–512.

36. Zabala S, Thomson C, Valdearcos S, Gascon A, Pina MA. Alfuzosin-induced hepatotoxicity. J Clin Pharm Ther 2000;25:73–74.

37. Yolcu OF, Koklu S, Koksal AS, et al. Alfuzosin-induced acute hepatitis in a patient with chronic liver disease. Ann Pharmacother 2004;38:1443–1445.

38. Lowe FC. Coadministration of tamsulosin and three antihypertensive agents in patients with benign prostatic hyperplasia: Pharmacodynamic effect. Clin Ther 1997;19:730–742.

39. Nieminen T, Tammela TLJ, Koobi T, et al. The effects of tamsulosin and sildenafil in separate and combined regimens on detailed hemodynamics in patients with benign prostatic enlargement. J Urol 2006;176:2551–2556.

40. Chapple CR. Pharmacological therapy of benign prostatic hyperplasia/lower urinary tract symptoms: An overview for the practicing clinician. BJU Int 2004;94:738–744.

41. Marks LS. Use of 5α-reductase inhibitors to prevent benign prostatic hyperplasia disease. Curr Urol Rep 2006;4:293–303.

42. Roehrborn CG, Marks LS, Fenter T, et al. Efficacy and safety of dutasteride in the four-year treatment of men with benign prostatic hyperplasia. Urology 2004;63:709–715.

43. Roehrborn CG, Bruskewitz R, Nickel JC, et al. Sustained decrease in incidence of acute urinary retention and surgery with finasteride for 6 years in men with benign prostatic hyperplasia. J Urol 2004;171:1194–1198.

44. Evans HC, Goa KL. Dutasteride. Drugs Aging 2003;20:905–916.

45. Anon. Dutasteride (Avodart) for benign prostatic hyperplasia. Med Letter 2002;44:109–110.

46. Thompson IM, Goodman PJ, Tangen CM, et al. The influence of finasteride on the development of prostate cancer. N Engl J Med 2003;349:215–224.

47. Musquera M, Fleshner NE, Finelli A, Zlotta AR. The REDUCE trial: Chemoprevention in prostate cancer using a dual 5-alpha reductase inhibitor, dutasteride. Expert Rev Anticancer Ther 2008;8:1073–1079.

48. Baldwin KC, Ginsberg PC, Roehrborn CG, Harkaway RC. Discontinuation of α blockade after initial treatment with finasteride and doxazosin for bladder outlet obstruction. Urol Int 2001;55:84–88.

49. Barkin J, Guimares M, Jacobi G, et al. Alpha blocker therapy can be withdrawn in the majority of men following initial combination therapy with the dual 5α reductase inhibitor dutasteride. Eur Urol 2003;44:461–466.

50. Reynard JM. Does anticholinergic medication have a role for men with lower urinary tract symptoms/benign prostatic hyperplasia either alone or in combination with other agents? Curr Opin Urol 2004;14:13–16.

51. Kaplan SA, Roehrborn CG, Rovner ES, et al. Tolterodine and tamsulosin for treatment of men with lower urinary tract symptoms and overactive bladder. JAMA 2006;296:2319–2328.

52. Lee JY, Kim HW, Lee SJ, et al. Comparison of doxazosin with or without tolterodine in men with symptomatic bladder outlet obstruction and an overactive bladder. BJU Int 2004;94:817–820.

53 Urinary Incontinence and Pediatric Enuresis

David R.P. Guay

LEARNING OBJECTIVES

Upon completion of the chapter, the reader will be able to:

1. Explain the pathophysiology of the major types of urinary incontinence (UI; urge, stress, overflow, and functional) and pediatric enuresis.

2. Recognize the signs and symptoms of the major types of UI and pediatric enuresis in individual patients.

3. List the treatment goals for a patient with UI or pediatric enuresis.

4. Compare and contrast anticholinergics/antispasmodics, α-adrenoceptor agonists, dual serotonin-norepinephrine reuptake inhibitors, vaginal estrogens, cholinomimetics, tricyclic antidepressants (TCAs), and vasopressin analogues in terms of mechanism of action, treatment outcomes, adverse effects, and drug–drug interaction potential when used to manage UI or pediatric enuresis.

5. Identify factors that guide drug selection for an individual patient.

6. Formulate a monitoring plan for a patient on a given treatment regimen based on patient-specific information.

7. Describe indicators for combination drug therapy of UI or pediatric enuresis.

8. Describe nonpharmacologic treatment approaches (including surgery) for UI or pediatric enuresis.

9. Formulate appropriate patient counseling information for patients undergoing drug therapy for UI or pediatric enuresis.

KEY CONCEPTS

① Accurate diagnosis and classification of urinary incontinence (UI) type is critical to the selection of appropriate drug therapy.

② Many medications can influence the lower urinary tract, including those not used for managing genitourinary disorders, and can precipitate new onset or aggravate existing voiding dysfunction and UI.

③ Patient-specific treatment goals should be identified. This frequently requires reaching a compromise between efficacy and tolerability of drug therapy. These goals are not static and may change with time.

④ Nonpharmacologic treatment can allow the use of lower drug doses. The combination of both therapies may have at least an additive effect on UI signs and symptoms.

⑤ The anticholinergic/antispasmodic drugs are the pharmacologic first-line treatments for urge UI. They are the most effective agents in suppressing premature detrusor contractions, enhancing bladder storage, and relieving symptoms.

⑥ Patient characteristics (e.g., age, comorbidities, concurrent drug therapies, and ability to adhere to the prescribed regimen) can also influence drug therapy selection.

⑦ Careful dose titration is necessary to maximize efficacy and tolerability.

⑧ If therapeutic goals are not achieved, a switch to an alternative agent should be made.

⑨ Vaginally administered estrogen plays only a modest role in managing stress urinary incontinence (SUI; urethral underactivity), unless it is accompanied by local signs of estrogen deficiency (e.g., atrophic urethritis or vaginitis).

⑩ The major impediment to using the α-adrenoceptor agonist class is the extensive list of contraindications.

⑪ The use of duloxetine in SUI is complicated by: (a) the potential for multiple clinically relevant drug–drug interactions with cytochrome P-450 2D6 and 1A2 inhibitors; (b) withdrawal reactions if abruptly discontinued; (c) high rates of nausea and other side effects; (d) hepatotoxicity that contraindicates its use in patients with any degree of hepatic impairment; and (e) its mild hypertensive effect. Another disconcerting finding is the high discontinuation rate when duloxetine is used in a "usual use" clinic environment (68%, two-thirds due to adverse events and one-third due to lack of efficacy).

⑫ In overflow UI due to atonic bladder, a trial of bethanecol may be reasonable if contraindications do not exist.

⑬ In overflow UI due to obstruction, the goal of treatment is to relieve the obstruction.

⑭ Considering that pharmacotherapy is inferior to select nonpharmacologic treatment modalities in pediatric enuresis, pharmacotherapy will be most valuable in patients who are not candidates for nonpharmacologic therapy due to nonadherence or who do not achieve the desired outcomes on nonpharmacologic therapy alone.

⑮ Desmopressin (DDAVP) is the first-line drug choice in pediatric enuresis.

URINARY INCONTINENCE

INTRODUCTION

Urinary incontinence (UI) is defined as the complaint of involuntary leakage of urine.[1] It is often associated with other bothersome lower urinary tract symptoms such as urgency, increased daytime frequency, and nocturia. Despite its prevalence across the lifespan and in both sexes, it remains an underdetected and underreported health problem that can have significant negative consequences for the individual's quality of life. Patients with UI may be depressed due to a perceived loss of self-control, loss of independence, and lack of self-esteem, and often curtail or substantially modify their activities for fear of an "accident." Serious medical and economic consequences may also occur in untreated or undertreated patients, including perineal dermatitis and

infections, worsening or lack of healing of pressure ulcers, urinary tract infections (UTIs), falls, and the need for long-term institutionalization in extended care facilities (including skilled nursing facilities (SNFs), or nursing homes).

EPIDEMIOLOGY AND ETIOLOGY

The true prevalence of UI has been difficult to determine because of methodologic issues such as varying definitions of UI and reporting bias.[2] Although the condition occurs across the lifespan, the peak prevalence, at least in women, is around the age of menopause (approximately 50 years), which is followed by a slight decrease in the 55- to 60-year-old age group, and then a steadily increasing prevalence after age 65. In general, the median prevalences of UI are as follows[3]:

- 20% to 30% in young females
- 30% to 40% in middle-aged females
- 30% to 50% in elderly females (50–75% in female SNF residents)
- 10% in adult males (in excess of 50% in elderly male SNF residents)

UI can result from abnormalities within (intrinsic to) and outside of (extrinsic to) the urinary tract. Within the urinary tract, abnormalities may occur in the urethra (including the bladder outlet and urinary sphincters), the bladder, or a combination of both structures. Focusing on abnormalities in these two structures, a simple classification scheme emerges for all but the rarest intrinsic causes of UI. **❶** *Accurate diagnosis and classification of UI type is critical to the selection of appropriate drug therapy.*

PATHOPHYSIOLOGY

Stress Urinary Incontinence Related to Urethral Underactivity[4]

In stress urinary incontinence (SUI), the urethra and/or urethral sphincters cannot generate enough resistance to impede urine flow from the bladder when intra-abdominal pressures (that are transmitted to the bladder, which is an intra-abdominal organ) are elevated. Intra-abdominal pressures are elevated by exertional activities like exercise, running, lifting, coughing, and sneezing. The amount of urine lost is generally small with each episode. Nocturia and enuresis are rarely seen. The factors responsible for urethral underactivity are incompletely understood, although the loss of the trophic effects of estrogen on the uroepithelium at menopause is thought to be important. The peak of SUI prevalence in the perimenopausal years supports this hypothesis. Clearly established risk factors for SUI include[5]:

- Pregnancy (increased risk with increased parity)
- Childbirth (vaginal delivery)
- Menopause
- Cognitive impairment
- Obesity
- Increasing age

Patient Encounter 1, Part 1

A 50-year-old woman with hypertension and diabetes comes into your clinic seeking advice about which incontinence pads work best. After questioning her, you determine that she has multiple issues of low volume urine loss daily, which is a significant change (increase) from 1 year ago. All episodes occur at times of physical activity. She's a single mother of three grown children, all delivered vaginally. Her last menstrual period was 11 months ago.

What information suggests that she has UI?

Does she have risk factors for UI?

What additional information do you need to know before creating a treatment plan for this patient?

Clinical Presentation of SUI Related to Urethral Underactivity[4]

General

The patient usually notes UI during activities like exercise, running, lifting, coughing, or sneezing. This type of UI is much more common in females (seen only in males with lower urinary tract surgery or injury compromising the sphincter).

Symptoms

Urine leakage with physical activity (volume is proportional to activity level). No UI with physical inactivity, especially when supine (no nocturia). May develop urgency and frequency as a compensatory mechanism (or independently as a separate component of bladder overactivity).

Diagnostic Tests

Observation of urethral meatus (opening) while patient coughs or strains

Unless the sphincter mechanism is compromised by surgery or trauma, SUI is exceedingly rare in males. The most common surgeries predisposing to SUI in males are radical prostatectomy for prostate cancer and transurethral resection of the prostate for benign prostatic hyperplasia (BPH).

Urge Urinary Incontinence Related to Bladder Overactivity[4]

In urge urinary incontinence (UUI), the detrusor (bladder) muscle is overactive and contracts inappropriately during the filling phase. The amount of urine lost per episode can be as large as the entire contents of the bladder may empty. Sleep may be disrupted by nocturia and enuresis.

Clinical Presentation of UUI Related to Bladder Overactivity[4]

General

Can have bladder overactivity and UI without urgency, if sensory input from the lower urinary tract is absent.

Symptoms

Urinary frequency (greater than 8 micturitions/day); urgency with or without urge incontinence; nocturia (greater than or equal to 2 micturitions/night) and enuresis may be present as well.

Diagnostic Tests

Urodynamic studies are the gold standard for diagnosis. Also urinalysis and urine culture should be negative (rule out urinary tract infection (UTI) as cause of frequency).

In most patients, the cause of bladder overactivity is unknown (idiopathic). Clearly established risk factors for UUI include:

- Increasing age
- Neurologic disorders (e.g., stroke, Parkinson's disease, multiple sclerosis, and spinal cord injury)
- Bladder outlet obstruction (e.g., benign or malignant prostatic enlargement or hyperplasia)
- Hysterectomy
- Recurrent UTIs

Overactivity may be myogenic or neurogenic in origin or a combination of both. These etiologies appear to be interconnected and complementary.

Overflow Urinary Incontinence Related to Urethral Overactivity and/or Bladder Underactivity[4]

In overflow urinary incontinence (OUI), an important but uncommon form of UI in both sexes, the bladder is filled to capacity at all times but cannot empty, causing urine to leak out episodically. If caused by bladder underactivity, the detrusor muscle has weakened, in some cases enough to lose the ability to voluntarily contract. In this case, the bladder cannot be emptied completely and large volumes of residual urine remain after micturition. Clinically, this is most commonly seen in the setting of long-term chronic bladder outlet obstruction due to benign or malignant prostatic enlargement. However, this may also be a manifestation of neurogenic bladder, frequently being seen in patients with diabetes, lower spinal cord injury, multiple sclerosis, or following radical pelvic surgery.

Clinical Presentation of OUI Related to Urethral Overactivity and/or Bladder Underactivity[4]

General

Important but rare type of UI in both sexes. Urethral overactivity usually due to prostatic enlargement (males) or cystocele formation or surgical overcorrection following antiurethral underactivity (SUI) surgery (females).

Symptoms

Lower abdominal fullness, hesitancy, straining to void, decreased force of stream, interrupted stream, sense of incomplete bladder emptying. May have urinary frequency and urgency, too. Abdominal pain if acute urinary retention is also present

Signs

Increased postvoid residual urine volume

If due to urethral overactivity, the resistance of the urethra and/or sphincters cannot be overcome by detrusor contractility. This functional or anatomic obstruction results in incomplete bladder emptying. Clinically, in males this most frequently occurs in the context of long-term chronic bladder outlet obstruction as outlined previously. In females, urethral overactivity is rare but may result from cystocele formation or surgical overcorrection during anti-SUI surgery. In both sexes, systemic neurologic diseases such as multiple sclerosis or spinal cord injury may be the etiology.

Functional UI[4]

● Functional UI is not generally caused by intrinsic urinary tract pathology. It is usually caused by factors extrinsic to the urinary tract. Examples of factors predisposing to functional incontinence include:

- Immobility (due to pain, traction, or use of nonportable medical devices)
- Lack of or slowed access to toileting facilities
- Cognitive impairment (difficulty with recognition of the urinary urge and proper response to it)
- UTIs
- Postmenopausal atrophic urethritis and/or vaginitis
- Diabetes mellitus (glucosuria leading to polyuria)
- Diabetes insipidus (polyuria due to decreased antidiuretic hormone [ADH])
- Pelvic malignancy (extrinsic pressure on urinary tract structures causing obstruction)
- Constipation or fecal impaction
- Congenital malformations
- CNS disorder resulting in a decreased level of consciousness
- Depression (apathy leading to recognition and response difficulties)

Mixed and Drug-Induced UI[4]

Frequently, two or more types of UI may coexist in a given patient, combinations termed mixed UI. This can lead to diagnostic and therapeutic difficulties due to the confusing array of presenting signs and symptoms and the opposing effects that a given treatment can have in different types of UI (i.e., a given drug may reduce the signs and symptoms of one type of UI but worsen those of other types). Another interesting type of mixed UI is coexisting bladder overactivity (UUI) and impaired bladder contractility (OUI). Most common in the elderly, this combination is called *detrusor hyperactivity with impaired contractility* (DHIC).

❷ *Many medications can influence the lower urinary tract, including those not used for managing genitourinary disorders, and can precipitate new onset or aggravate existing voiding dysfunction and UI* (Table 53–1).

Table 53–1
Medications Influencing Lower Urinary Tract Function

Medication	Effect
Diuretics	Polyuria, frequency, urgency
α-Adrenoceptor antagonists	Urethral relaxation: may relieve obstruction in males, induces/worsens SUI in females
α-Adrenoceptor agonists	Urethral constriction: aggravates obstruction in males (may cause urinary retention), potential SUI treatment in females
Calcium channel blockers (dihydropyridines)	Urethral constriction (may cause urinary retention), especially in males
Opioid analgesics	Impaired bladder contractility (may cause urinary retention)
Sedative-hypnotics	Functional UI due to immobility, delirium, sedation
Psychotherapeutics with anticholinergic properties; anticholinergics	Urinary retention due to impaired bladder contractility or potential UUI treatment
TCAs	Combination of anticholinergic and α-adrenoceptor blocking activities can lead to unpredictable effects on UI
Ethanol	Polyuria and frequency (via effects on ADH), functional UI (delirium, sedation), urgency
ACEIs	Cough leading to SUI (ARBs do not induce cough)
Cyclophosphamide	Hemorrhagic cystitis due to acrolein metabolite (prevent with MESNA)

ACEI, angiotensin-converting enzyme inhibitor; ADH, antidiuretic hormone (or vasopressin); ARB, angiotensin II receptor blocker, MESNA, sodium 2-mercaptoethanesulfonate; SUI, stress urinary incontinence; TCA, tricyclic antidepressant; UI, urinary incontinence; UUI, urge urinary incontinence.

CLINICAL PRESENTATION AND DIAGNOSIS

The clinical presentation of UI depends on the underlying pathophysiology. The literature evaluating the prevalences of different UI types by age and sex has produced widely varying results due to a number of factors. The clinician should thus consider a given patient as having virtually any type of UI until ruled out during diagnostic evaluation.

A complete medical history and targeted physical examination are essential to correctly classify the type(s) of UI present. It is important to assess the degree of annoyance of the patient due to UI signs and symptoms. The degree of annoyance of the patient may not correlate well with the results of quantitative tests such as symptom frequency/severity, use of absorbent products, frequency/severity of neurologic signs, and postvoid residual urine volume. This is especially the case in "hypersensitive" and "stoic" individuals. Items to address during the evaluation

Table 53–2

Items Which Should Be Addressed During Diagnostic Evaluation of UI

Item	Comments
Urine leakage	
Use of absorbent products	Yes/no, type(s), quantity, times of day worn
	Quantity may relate more to personal preference and hygiene than to UI type and severity (e.g., use of large number of pads by a fastidiously hygienic patient with low volume loss)
Quantity lost per episode	Dribbling versus small volumes intermittently versus large volumes
	Consistent or varied quantities
Precipitants	Yes/no, physical activity, excessive fluid intake, drug(s)
Times of day	Daytime/nighttime/both
Symptoms	
Urgency	Yes/no, how often, how severe, duration from urge onset to micturition
Frequency	Yes/no, daytime/nighttime/both, how often
Nocturia	Yes/no, how often, proportion associated with UI
Obstructive symptoms	Yes/no, type(s) (hesitancy, strain to void, decreased force of stream, start and stop stream, sense of incomplete emptying), severity
Lower abdominal fullness	Yes/no, how often, how severe
Comorbidities	
Current medication use	See Table 53–1. Remember CAMs, OTCs
Evidence of pre-existing or new-onset:	
Diabetes mellitus	
Metastatic or genitourinary malignancy	
Multiple sclerosis or other neurologic disease	
CNS disease above the pons	Usually UUI
Spinal cord injury	UUI or OUI, depending on level and degree of completeness of injury
Recent nongenitourinary surgery	Functional UI
Previous local surgery/radiation	Prostate surgery, lower abdominal cavity surgery (direct injury versus denervation), radiation (direct injury)
Gynecologic history	Childbirth (vaginal versus cesarean section), prior gynecologic surgery, hormonal status (pre- versus peri- versus postmenopausal)
Pelvic floor disease	Constipation, diarrhea, fecal incontinence, dyspareunia, sexual dysfunction, pelvic pain
UTI	**Dysuria**, CVA tenderness, frequency
Gross hematuria	Possible bladder or other genitourinary cancer

CAM, complementary and alternative medications; CVA, costovertebral angle; OTC, over-the-counter; OUI, overflow urinary incontinence; SUI, stress urinary incontinence; UTI, urinary tract infection; UUI, urge urinary incontinence.

are illustrated in Table 53–2. Components of the physical examination include[4]:

- Abdominal examination (look for distended bladder, organomegaly and masses).

- Neurologic evaluation of perineum and lower extremities to evaluate lumbosacral nerve function (includes digital rectal exam to check rectal tone, reflexes, ability to perform a voluntary pelvic muscle contraction in females and size and surface quality of prostate in males)

- Pelvic exam (females) (look for evidence of prolapse of bladder, small bowel, rectum, or uterus, or estrogen deficiency)

- Genital/prostate exam (men)

- Direct observation of urethral meatus (opening) when patient coughs/strains (urine spurt consistent with SUI)

- Perineal exam (looking for skin maceration, redness, breakdown, ulceration and evidence of fungal skin infection)

TREATMENT

❸ *Patient-specific treatment goals should be identified. This frequently requires reaching a compromise between efficacy and tolerability of drug therapy. These goals are not static and may change with time.*

Desired Outcomes

- Restoration of continence
- Reduction of the number of UI episodes (daytime and nighttime) and frequency of nocturia
- Prevention of disease complications (e.g., dermatologic infections and skin breakdown, delay institutionalization)

Patient Encounter 1, Part 2: Medical History, Physical Examination, and Diagnostic Tests

PMH: Insulin-dependent diabetes mellitus since age 7; it is "reasonably well-controlled" per patient; hypertension for 2 years, currently "controlled" per patient

FH: Mother had diabetes and died of a myocardial infarction at 62 years of age; father smoked 1 to 3 packs of cigarettes per day and developed fatal lung cancer at age 57

SH: Works two jobs as a waitress; denies alcohol use or smoking

Meds: NPH insulin 20 units before breakfast and 5 units before supper; enalapril 10 mg twice daily; aspirin 325 mg once daily

ROS: (+) Recurrent coughing, UI, dyspareunia, vaginal itching, multiple UTIs; (−) nocturia, enuresis, urgency, dysuria, frequency, lower abdominal fullness, decreased force of stream

PE:

VS: BP 124/70 mm Hg, P 80 bpm, RR 16/min, T 37.0°C (98.6°F)

CV: RRR; normal S_1, S_2; no murmurs, rubs, gallops

Abd: Soft, nontender, nondistended; (+) bowel sounds; bladder not palpable

Neuro: Within normal limits (gross sensory, motor, reflexes)

GU: Valsalva caused urine spurt; friable, bleeding vaginal lining on pelvic exam

Labs: Hemoglobin A_{1c} 8.2% (0.082); rest within normal limits

Given this additional information, what is your assessment of the patient's condition?

Identify your treatment goals for the patient.

What nonpharmacologic and pharmacologic alternatives are available to the patient?

- Avoidance or minimization of adverse consequences of treatment
- Minimization of treatment costs
- Improvement in patient's quality of life

Nonpharmacologic Treatment

At the primary care level, nonpharmacologic treatment of UI constitutes the chief approach to UI management. In patients in whom pharmacologic or surgical management is inappropriate or undesirable or refused, nonsurgical nonpharmacologic treatment is the only option. Examples of patients fitting this scenario include:

- Those not medically fit for surgery

- Those who plan future pregnancies (as pregnancy/childbirth can compromise the long-term results of certain types of continence surgery)
- Those with OUI whose condition is not amenable to surgical or drug treatment
- Those with comorbidities which place them at high-risk for significant side effects to drug therapy
- Those who wish to delay or avoid surgery
- Those with mild to moderate symptoms who do not wish to undergo surgery or take medication

Nonpharmacologic approaches include lifestyle modifications, scheduled voiding regimens, pelvic floor muscle rehabilitation (PFMR), anti-incontinence devices, and supportive interventions.[4,6] Many of these are best utilized through attendance at multidisciplinary UI clinics staffed by specialist nurses and/or physical therapists in addition to physicians. Behavioral interventions are among the first-line treatment approaches for SUI, UUI, and mixed UI. However, these lifestyle modifications, scheduling regimens, and PFMR methods require a motivated patient and/or caregiver who can play an active role in developing the treatment plan. Anything that interferes with active participation (including cognitive dysfunction) will render these approaches suboptimal. Patients/caregivers also must attend regular follow-up visits to monitor outcomes. Of interest, nonpharmacologic treatment may even be superior to pharmacologic treatment in select cases. For example, the short-term (6 months) and long-term (21 months) results of a combination of PFMR plus behavioral training produced statistically superior results compared to anticholinergic therapy in women with UUI.[7,8] Even if the results of nonpharmacologic treatment have not fully achieved the desired outcomes, if it has provided at least some improvement in UI signs and symptoms, it should be continued during pharmacologic treatment. ❹ *Nonpharmacologic treatment can allow the use of lower drug doses. The combination of both therapies may have at least an additive effect on UI signs and symptoms.*

In the recent systematic review of nonsurgical treatments for UI by Shamliyan et al., the only nonpharmacologic treatment for which true objective evidence of benefit exists is the combination of PFMR plus behavioral training (restored continence with an **effect size** of 0.13 (95% CI, 0.07–0.20) but improvement in continence was not consistent between trials). Although PFMR alone or combined with biofeedback restored and improved continence, the effect size was not consistent between trials.[9] Weight loss of 5% to 10% in overweight or obese women has an efficacy similar to that of other nonpharmacologic treatments.

Surgery is rarely a first-line treatment for UI. Surgery is generally considered only when the degree of bother or lifestyle compromise is sufficient and other nonoperative therapies are either undesired or have been ineffective. Surgery can be used to manage urethral overactivity due to benign prostatic enlargement and bladder outlet obstruction (via endoscopic incision using a cystoscope). Bladder underactivity cannot be managed surgically and rarely is surgery considered for UUI. Surgery is most effective in the management of SUI. Surgery for SUI is directed toward stabilizing the urethra and bladder neck and/or augmenting urethral resistance using periurethral collagen and other injectables. In males, SUI is best treated by implanting an artificial urinary sphincter.[4]

Pharmacologic Treatment

▶ *Urge Urinary Incontinence*

❺ *The anticholinergic/antispasmodic drugs are the first-line pharmacologic treatment for UUI. They are the most effective agents in suppressing premature detrusor contractions, enhancing bladder storage, and relieving symptoms.* It must be emphasized that the improvements in clinical and urodynamic parameters are modest at best, although still considered by experts in the field to be positive.[10] In the recent systematic review/meta-analysis of 50 clinical trials in UUI by Novava et al., there were no clinically important or relevant differences found among different anticholinergics.[10]

The major problem with existing agents is their lack of selectivity to bladder muscarinic receptors, thus leading to dose-limiting side effects outside of the urinary tract. These include dry mouth, constipation, blurred vision, confusion, cognitive dysfunction, and tachycardia. With oxybutynin, orthostasis due to α-receptor blockade and sedation and weight gain due to histamine-1 receptor blockade may also occur. Dry mouth is the most problematic of the anticholinergic side effects and is frequently dose limiting. In the systematic review and meta-analysis cited previously, in terms of tolerability, only the difference between tolterodine immediate-release (IR) and oxybutynin IR (wherein the former was better and tolerable than the latter) was statistically and clinically significant. With regard to IR formulations, dose escalation might yield some limited improvements in efficacy, but at the cost of significant increases in the rates of adverse events. Comparing extended-release (ER) and IR formulations, the former demonstrated advantages in terms of efficacy and safety. Lastly, with regard to route of administration, the dermal route of administration did not provide a significant advantage over the oral route. Thus, oral ER formulations should probably be preferred over IR and/or dermal (i.e., transdermal or gel) ones. More clinical trials are necessary to identify first-, second-, and third-line agents.[11] In terms of urinary retention, relative safety of at least one anticholinergic has been suggested. In a preliminary open-label trial in males with UUI and presumed nonobstructive BPH (where maximum urine flow rates were at least 15 mL/s), tolterodine LA (as monotherapy or combined with prior unsuccessful α-adrenoceptor antagonist therapy) produced significant objective and subjective benefits versus UUI and BPH. Mean postvoid residual urine volume did not increase and urinary retention occurred at a rate of only 0.3%.[12]

Details regarding the pharmacokinetics, contraindications/precautions, and dosing of the six recommended agents (oxybutynin, tolterodine, trospium chloride, solifenacin,

darifenacin, and fesoterodine) are illustrated in Table 53–3.[13–21] A current clinical controversy is which of these agents should be considered first line in UUI, and in the case of oxybutynin, tolterodine, and trospium chloride which formulations should be recommended. There are few head-to-head clinical trials to assist in decision making and those few that exist have demonstrated either broad equivalence or clinically unimportant differences in efficacy. In the recent systematic review of Shamliyan et al., data for analysis were adequate only for oxybutynin IR (5–10 mg/day) and tolterodine LA (4 mg/day). Both of these agents restored continence with an effect size of 0.18 (95% CI, 0.13–0.22). The authors could not claim one as being superior to the other.[9] **❻** *Patient characteristics (e.g., age, comorbidities, concurrent drug therapies, and ability to adhere to the prescribed regimen) can also influence drug therapy selection.* Drug selection frequently will be based on differences in tolerability (wherein the ER oral, or gel TD formulations are better tolerated than the IR formulations) and cost. **❼** *Careful dose titration is necessary to maximize efficacy and tolerability.* The selected agent should be titrated to the maximum tolerated dose and maintained there for at least 4 weeks in order to assure an adequate therapeutic trial. **❽** *If therapeutic goals are not achieved, a switch to an alternative agent should be made.* There is no rationale for use of two or more anticholinergics concurrently at low doses. Another clinical controversy is the relevance of the pharmacologic antagonism between anticholinergics and cholinesterase inhibitors when used concurrently.[22]

Other drugs, such as propantheline, flavoxate, tricyclic antidepressants (TCA; especially imipramine), dicyclomine, and scopolamine, are less effective, no safer, and/or have not been adequately studied; therefore, their use is not recommended.[6]

Women with mixed UI (UUI plus SUI) or UUI plus atrophic vaginitis and/or urethritis may also benefit from the addition of a locally administered (per vagina [PV]) estrogen to anticholinergic therapy. Preliminary data suggest that desmopressin (DDAVP) may reduce daytime UUI symptoms (i.e., for up to approximately 8 hours after morning dosing) when used on both regular and "as needed" bases.[23] An intriguing pilot placebo-controlled trial of duloxetine in UUI in individuals with bladder capacities below 400 mL suggests at least short-term (12 weeks) benefit.[24]

▶ *Stress Urinary Incontinence*

The goal of pharmacologic therapy of urethral underactivity is to improve the urethral closure mechanism by one or more of the following:

- Stimulating α-adrenoceptors in the smooth muscle of the proximal urethra and bladder neck
- Enhancing the supportive structures underlying the urethral mucosa
- Enhancing the positive effects of serotonin and norepinephrine in the afferent and efferent pathways of the micturition reflex

Table 53–3

Anticholinergic/Antispasmodic Drugs Recommended for UUI

Parameter	Oxybutynin	Tolterodine	Trospium Chloride	Solifenacin	Darifenacin	Festerodine
Dosage forms	IR tablets, solution; SR-ER tablets, SR-TD patch, topical gel	IR tablets; SR-LA capsules	IR tablets; ER tablets	IR tablets	ER tablets	ER tablets
Dosing	IR: 2.5–5 mg 2–4 × daily 0.3–0.5 mg/kg/day thrice daily; SR (oral): 5–30 mg once daily (pediatrics: 0.3–0.5 mg/kg/day thrice daily (IR)); SR (TD): 3.9 mg/day patch applied twice weekly; SR (gel): 1 sachet applied once daily	IR: 1 or 2 mg twice daily (pediatrics: 1 mg twice daily); SR: 2 or 4 mg once daily (pediatrics: 2 mg once daily)	IR: 20 mg twice daily; ER: 60 mg once daily	5–10 mg once daily	7.5–15 mg once daily	4–8 mg once daily
Kinetics	Active metabolite (N-desethyl) Not altered in renal or hepatic disease or advanced age	Active metabolite (5-hydroxymethyl) Polymorphic metabolism (CYP4502D6) Not altered in advanced age. Significantly altered in hepatic disease (decreased CL in cirrhosis) and renal disease (decreased CL)	Food: decreased BA by 70–80% Significantly altered in renal disease (decreased CL) but not in hepatic disease or advanced age	Metabolized via CYP4503A4 but only one active metabolite (4-hydroxy) Significantly altered in severe renal impairment, moderate hepatic impairment (Child-Pugh B), and advanced age (decreased CL in all)	Complex metabolism (polymorphic CYP4502D6, CYP4503A4) Not altered in advanced age, renal impairment, mild hepatic impairment (Child-Pugh A) Significantly altered in moderate hepatic impairment (Child-Pugh B) (decreased CL)	Prodrug (for 5-hydroxymethyl tolterodine) Inactive metabolites Not altered in advanced age Significantly altered in renal disease (decreased CL) and moderate hepatic impairment (Child-Pugh B) (decreased CL)
Contraindications and precautions	Use caution if CYP4503A4 inhibitors are also being taken (decreased oxybutynin CL)	Reduce dose 50% in those taking CYP4503A4 inhibitor(s) or with hepatic cirrhosis or with CrCl less than 30 mL/min Antacid-SR (oral) prep, interaction (dose-dumping) (not seen with PPI)	Give on empty stomach Decrease dose 50% when CrCl less than 30 mL/min and use IR formulation	Do not exceed 5 mg/day if CrCl less than 30 mL/min, patient has moderate hepatic impairment, or patient is taking CYP4503A4 inhibitor(s) If severe hepatic impairment, do not use	Do not exceed 7.5 mg/day if patient is taking potent CYP4503A4 inhibitor(s) Use caution if patient is taking moderate CYP4503A4 inhibitor(s) or CYP4503A4 or 2D6 substrate(s) Do not chew, divide, or crush the ER tablets	Do not exceed 4 mg/day if CrCl less than 30 mL/min or patient is taking potent CYP450 3A4 inhibitor(s) If severe hepatic impairment, do not use

BA, bioavailability; CL, total body clearance; CrCl, creatinine clearance; CYP450, cytochrome P450; TD, transdermal; ER, extended release; IR, immediate release; LA, long acting; PPI, proton pump inhibitor; SR, sustained release.

It is generally felt that there is no role for pharmacologic therapy in SUI in males resulting from surgery or trauma.[25] Initial data, however, suggest a possible role for duloxetine added to nonpharmacologic treatment (PFMR), rather than PFMR alone, in males postradical prostatectomy, at least over the first 4 to 6 months.[26] It should be kept in mind that SUI (in contrast to UUI) is frequently curable by surgery, thus obviating years of drug therapy that may be incompletely effective in symptom relief.

Estrogens[4] ❾ *Vaginally administered estrogen plays only a modest role in managing SUI (urethral underactivity), unless it is accompanied by local signs of estrogen deficiency (e.g., atrophic urethritis or vaginitis).*

Although not supported by rigorous clinical trial evidence, local (PV) and systemic estrogens have been considered mainstays of pharmacologic management since the 1940s. They are believed to work by a trophic effect on uroepithelial cells and underlying collagenous subcutaneous tissue, enhancement of local microcirculation by increasing the number of periurethral blood vessels, and enhancement of the number and/or sensitivity of α-adrenoceptors. Open trials have supported the use of estrogens administered by the oral, TD, and local routes of administration. However, randomized controlled trials have found no significant clinical or urodynamic effects of oral estrogen compared to placebo in SUI. In fact, most trials have found that oral estrogen/hormone replacement therapy actually increases the risk of new-onset UI (SUI, UUI, mixed UI).[9] Systemic estrogen therapy also carries numerous short- and long-term side effect risks (mastodynia, uterine bleeding, nausea, thromboembolism, cardiac and cerebrovascular ischemic events, and enhanced breast and endometrial cancer risks). If estrogens are to be used in SUI management, only locally administered products should be used (Table 53–4). Even with locally administered products, improvement of continence has been inconsistent between trials.[9]

α-Adrenoceptor Agonists[4] Open and randomized controlled trials utilizing clinical and urodynamic endpoints have supported the use of a variety of α-adrenoceptor agonists, including phenylpropanolamine, ephedrine, and pseudoephedrine, in the therapy of mild and moderate SUI. In addition, several studies have demonstrated clinical and urodynamic benefits for combination estrogen–α-adrenoceptor agonist use over those of the individual agents. However, in the recent systematic review of Shamliyan et al., monotherapy with this class failed to restore continence or improve incontinence compared with placebo or PFMR.[9] Phenylpropanolamine was removed from the U.S. market in late 2000 due to the risk of ischemic stroke in women taking this drug.[27] However, this drug is still available via the Internet, so clinicians need to monitor and discourage its use. Although still available by prescription, ephedrine is considerably more toxic than other α-adrenoceptor agonists and its use is not recommended. Although phenylephrine is now available in oral formulations, the lack of data regarding its use in SUI and the reported lack of efficacy in maximum recommended

doses for rhinitis suggest that this agent should be avoided at present.

This leaves the clinician with only one practical agent to use pseudoephedrine: (Table 53–4). Side effects include hypertension, headache, dry mouth, nausea, insomnia, and restlessness.[28] ❿ *The major impediment to using the α-adrenoceptor agonist class is the extensive list of contraindications (Table 53–4).* In the past, α-adrenoceptor agonist therapy was generally added to estrogen therapy in those insufficiently improved with estrogen alone and in whom its use was not contraindicated. With the recent availability of duloxetine, treatment is now available for estrogen non or hyporesponders whether they can or cannot take α-adrenoceptor agonists.

Duloxetine[29] Duloxetine is a selective serotonin-norepinephrine reuptake inhibitor similar pharmacologically to venlafaxine. Approved for the treatment of major depression, painful diabetic peripheral neuropathy, fibromyalgia, and generalized anxiety disorder,, its use in SUI is off-label in the United States. Duloxetine enhances central serotonergic and adrenergic tone which is involved in ascending and descending control of urethral smooth muscle and the internal urinary sphincter. Urethral and urinary sphincter smooth muscle tone during the filling phase are thus enhanced.[30,31] The pharmacokinetics, contraindications/precautions, and dosing of duloxetine are illustrated in Table 53–4.[29,32] Clearly, duloxetine has demonstrated modest efficacy in SUI and a major question is its role in SUI compared to estrogen and α-adrenoceptor agonists as well as potentially curative surgery. In the absence of head-to-head clinical trial data, this is a difficult question to answer, at least for the comparison of duloxetine to α-adrenoceptor agonists. In the recent systematic review of Shamliyan et al., duloxetine improved incontinence with an effect size of 0.11 (95% CI, 0.07–0.14) but failed to restore continence.[9] One controlled trial has demonstrated modest, although significant, benefit from duloxetine in the treatment of SUI in males after radical prostatectomy.[33] ⓫ *The use of duloxetine in stress UI is complicated by (a) the potential for multiple clinically relevant drug drug interactions with cytochrome P450 (CYP450) 2D6 and 1A2 inhibitors, (b) withdrawal reactions if abruptly discontinued, (c) high rates of nausea and other side effects, (d) hepatotoxicity contraindicating its use in patients with any degree of hepatic impairment, and (e) its mild hypertensive effect. Another disconcerting finding is the high discontinuation rate when duloxetine is used in a "usual use" clinic environment (68%, two-thirds due to adverse events and one-third due to lack of efficacy).*[34]

▶ Overflow Incontinence Due to Bladder Underactivity[4]

⓬ *In overflow UI due to atonic bladder, a trial of bethanecol may be reasonable if contraindications do not exist.* There is no established effective pharmacologic therapy for OUI due to poor bladder contractility (atonic bladder). The efficacy of the cholinomimetic bethanecol (25–50 mg three or four times daily) is uncertain and, in well done clinical trials,

Table 53–4

Drugs Used for SUI

Parameter	Estrogens	Pseudoephedrine	Duloxetine
Dosage forms	Avoid systemic (parenteral, oral, TD); use vaginal: tablet, cream, intravaginal ring	Tablets, solution	DR capsules
Dosing	Estradiol 25 mcg vaginal tablets (insert one PV daily × 14 days, then one PV twice weekly) CEE vaginal cream (1/2–2 g daily PV; consider 3 weeks on, 1 week off; may be able to decrease frequency of use over time) Estradiol 2 mg vaginal ring (1 ring PV every 3 months)	15–60 mg 3 × daily	40–80 mg/day in one or two doses (optimal regimen from a tolerability perspective is 20 mg twice daily × 2 weeks → 40 mg twice daily)
Kinetics	Use local route to minimize systemic BA and side effects	Less than 1% of dose is metabolized (inactive metabolites) Primarily renal elimination of unchanged drug Would not expect hepatic impairment to have an effect (no data) Expect significant effect if renal impairment and no effect if advanced age (beyond decreased CrCl with age) (no data)	Extensive metabolism via CYP4502D6 and 1A2 (inactive metabolites) Not altered in advanced age, mild to moderate renal impairment, mild hepatic impairment (Child-Pugh A) Significantly altered in severe renal disease and moderate hepatic impairment (Child-Pugh B) Systemic exposure to duloxetine decreased by 1/3 in smokers (dose change not recommended)
Contraindications/ precautions	Contraindications include known or suspected breast or endometrial cancer Abnormal genitourinary bleeding of unknown etiology Active thromboembolism (or history of TE associated with previous estrogen use)	Contraindications include hypertension, tachyarrhythmias, coronary artery disease, MI, cor pulmonale, hyperthyroidism, renal failure, narrow-angle glaucoma	Multiple drug–drug interactions possible with CYP4502D6 and 1A2 substrates/inhibitors Avoid if CrCl less than 30 mL/min and in all patients with hepatic disease Can raise BP Do not discontinue abruptly (withdrawal syndrome) Suicide risk even in patients without psychiatric disease Avoid in uncontrolled narrow-angle glaucoma (causes mydriasis) Hepatotoxic; avoid in alcoholics even if signs/symptoms of hepatic disease are absent

BA, bioavailability; BP, blood pressure; CEE, conjugated equine estrogens; CrCl, creatinine clearance; CYP450, cytochrome P-450; DR, delayed-release; MI, myocardial infarction; PV, per vagina; TD, transdermal; TE, thromboembolism.

it has had mixed results. In addition, its cholinomimetic effect is not urospecific and its side effects are bothersome, including muscle and abdominal cramping, hypersalivation, diarrhea, and potentially life-threatening bradycardia and bronchospasm. α-adrenoceptor antagonists such as silodosin, prazosin, terazosin, doxazosin, tamsulosin, and alfuzosin may benefit this condition by relaxing the bladder outflow tract and hence reducing outflow resistance. If pharmacologic therapy fails, intermittent urethral catheterization by the patient or caregiver three or four times per day is recommended. Less satisfactory alternatives include indwelling urethral or suprapubic catheters or urinary diversion.

▶ Overflow Incontinence Due to Obstruction

⓭ In overflow UI due to obstruction, the goal of treatment is to relieve the obstruction.

Patient Encounter 1, Part 3: Creating a Care Plan

Based on the information presented, create a care plan for this patient's UI. Your plan should include:

(a) a statement of the drug-related needs and/or problems, (b) the goals of therapy, (c) a patient-specific detailed therapeutic plan, and (d) a plan for follow-up to determine whether or not the goals have been achieved and adverse events avoided.

OUTCOME EVALUATION

- Monitor the patient for symptom relief. Have the desired outcomes jointly developed by the health care team and the patient/caregiver been achieved and to what degree. Inspect the daily diary completed by the patient/caregiver since the last clinic visit and quantitate the clinical response (e.g., number of micturitions, number of incontinence episodes, and pad use). If a diary has not been used, ask the patient how many incontinence pads have been used and how they have been doing in terms of "accidents" since the last visit. If appropriate, administer a short-form instrument used to measure symptom impact and condition-specific quality of life and compare to previous result(s).

- Elicit adverse effects of drug therapy using a nonleading approach and ask the patient/caregiver to judge their severity and what measures, if any, the patient/caregiver used to ameliorate them. Assess adherence (ask patient/caregiver about missed doses or do a pill count if the prescription container was brought to the visit).

- The balance of clinical response and tolerability will dictate the approach to adjusting drug dosage. Potential approaches include dosage increase, maintenance, or decrease. If adverse effects are quite bothersome to the patient and patient safety and/or adherence are compromised, stop, or taper, the offender and initiate another drug option.

PEDIATRIC ENURESIS

INTRODUCTION

Pediatric enuresis is not a disease but a symptom, which can present alone or at the same time as other disorders, in children and adolescents. It is defined as the repeated voiding of urine into bed or clothes at least twice a week for at least three consecutive months in a child at least 5-years-old (per the *Diagnostic and Statistical Manual of Mental Disorders*, 4th ed., Text Revision).[35,36] Enuresis can still be present even if the above frequency and duration parameters are not met, provided that associated distress or functional impairment exists. The terms "nocturnal" and "diurnal" refer to periods during sleep and while awake, respectively. Primary enuresis

Patient Care and Monitoring: UI

1. Assess the patient's symptoms to determine if patient-directed therapy is appropriate or whether or not the patient should be evaluated by a physician. Assessment includes the types and severities of symptoms and the presence or absence of exacerbating factors. Does the patient have any UI-related complications?

2. Review any available diagnostic data to determine disease status.

3. Obtain a thorough medication history, including use of prescription, nonprescription, and complementary and alternative drug products. Determine which, if any, treatments in the past had been helpful as judged by the patient. Could any of the patient's current medications be contributing to UI?

4. Educate the patient on lifestyle modifications that may improve symptoms, including but not limited to, smoking cessation (for patients with cough-induced SUI), weight reduction for those patients with SUI and UUI, prevention of constipation in patients at risk, caffeine reduction, and modification of diet and fluid intake (e.g., timing and quantity of fluid intake and avoidance of foods or beverages that worsen UI).

5. Is the patient taking the appropriate drug(s) for his or her type(s) of UI? Are the dose(s) appropriate? If no (to either question), why?

6. Develop a plan to assess efficacy after a minimum of 4 weeks.

7. Assess changes in quality of life (physical, psychological, social functioning, and well-being).

8. Evaluate the patient for drug-related adverse events, allergies, and interactions (drug–drug and drug–disease).

9. In cognitively intact elderly patients, focus communications to elicit the preferences of the patient, not those of potential proxies.

10. Stress the importance of adherence with the prescribed regimen, including lifestyle modifications. Recommend the most "patient-friendly" treatment regimen possible.

11. Provide patient education regarding the disease state, lifestyle modifications, and drug therapy:
    - Causes of UI and what things to avoid (see 3 and 4 above)
    - Possible UI complications
    - Timing of medication intake
    - Potential adverse events (limit to most frequent and/or clinically relevant)
    - Potential drug-drug interactions

refers to a process wherein the patient has never been consistently dry throughout the night. Secondary enuresis refers to a process wherein the patient has resumed wetting after a period of dryness of at least 6 months in duration. Lastly, monosymptomatic and polysymptomatic enuresis should be differentiated. Monosymptomatic enuresis refers to wetting at nighttime with no other urinary tract and no daytime symptoms. Polysymptomatic enuresis refers to wetting at nighttime associated with other urinary tract symptoms (e.g., urge or frequency without any other urinary symptoms) and daytime symptoms as well.

Enuresis is not a benign disorder that children will just "grow out of." Emotional and/or physical abuse of the child by adult caregivers lead to secondary problems such as chronic anxiety, low self-esteem, and delayed developmental milestones such as attending camp or going on "sleepovers" at the homes of friends. The emotional and developmental damage produced by enuresis may be more significant to the child than the enuresis itself.

EPIDEMIOLOGY AND ETIOLOGY

Five to seven million children and adolescents in the United States suffer from nocturnal enuresis. Primary enuresis is twice as common as secondary enuresis. Enuresis is twice as common in boys as compared to girls. The incidence of enuresis varies as a function of age[35,36]:

- 40% in 3-year-olds
- 12% to 25% in 4-year-olds
- 15% to 20% in 5-year-olds
- 10% in 6-year-olds
- 6% to 10% in 7- and 8-year-olds
- 5% in 10-year-olds
- 2% to 3% in 12-year-olds
- 1% to 3% in adolescents
- 0.5% in adults

Five to ten percent of children with enuresis will suffer the condition as adults. It may also predispose to UUI in adults. In the enuretic population, 80% to 85% are monosymptomatic, 5% to 10% are polysymptomatic, and under 5% have an organic cause. The spontaneous annual cure rate (i.e., restoration of continence) ranges from 14% to 16% (exception: at about 4 or 5 years of age, it may be as high as 30%).

The etiology of enuresis is poorly understood, but there is a clear genetic link. The incidence in children from families in whom there are no members with enuresis, where one parent had enuresis as a child, and where both parents had enuresis as children are 14%, 44%, and 77%, respectively. Loci for enuresis have been located on chromosomes 12, 13, and 22. Sleep disorders are not considered major contributors with the exception of sleep apnea. Enuresis occurs in all sleep stages in proportion to the time spent in each stage. However, a small proportion of individuals are not aroused from sleep by bladder distention and have uninhibited bladder contractions preceding enuresis.

PATHOPHYSIOLOGY

The vast majority of children with enuresis have normal urodynamics, including nocturnal bladder capacity. Functional bladder capacity can be estimated using the formula: age in years +2 equals to the ounces of capacity. In some children, there appears to be a relationship between developmental immaturity (motor and language milestones) and enuresis, but the mechanism is unknown. There is evidence that affected individuals have an attenuated vasopressin circadian rhythm (females more so than males) with lower vasopressin plasma concentrations.[37] Drugs like lithium, clozapine, risperidone, valproic acid, selective serotonin reuptake inhibitors, and theophylline can rarely cause and aggravate enuresis. Psychological factors are clearly contributory in only a minority of individuals. The most frequent example of this is secondary enuresis precipitated by a stressor such as divorce, school trauma, sexual abuse, or hospitalization. In rare cases, the family may be so dysfunctional that the child has never been properly toilet-trained.

CLINICAL PRESENTATION AND DIAGNOSIS

Clinical Presentation and Diagnosis: Pediatric Enuresis

Proper assessment of the child or adolescent with enuresis should explore every aspect of UI, especially the genitourinary and nervous systems. The minimum assessment should include[34,35]:

- Interview of child and parent(s), being sensitive to the emotional consequences of the enuresis

- Direct physical examination, looking for enlarged adenoids/tonsils, bladder distention, fecal impaction, abnormal genitalia, spinal cord anomalies, and abnormal neurologic signs (look for an organic cause amenable to surgery or drugs; see Table 53–5)

- Obtain a urinalysis (consider a urine culture at the same time)

- A 2-week diary of wet and dry nights prior to intervention is useful in that it can be used to monitor the response to treatment. A first-morning urine specific gravity may help to predict response to DDAVP therapy. Polysymptomatic presentation may require a more elaborate workup, including voiding cystourethrogram, renal and/or bladder ultrasound, urodynamics, and sleep studies.

Patient Encounter 2, Part 1

A 7-year-old female is brought into your clinic, her mother seeking advice about how to prevent her daughter's nighttime bedwetting. She asks about the suitability of any OTC or complementary and alternative medications. After questioning both individuals, you determine that her daughter has been wetting the bed for several months, which has caused some ill-defined "family disharmony." No obvious precipitating event is apparent.

What should you do at this point?

Table 53–5

Major Potentially Treatable Organic Causes of Enuresis

Potentially Treatable by Surgery
- Ectopic ureter
- Lower UTI (correct congenital anomalies)
- Neurogenic bladder
- Bladder calculus (stone) or foreign body
- Obstructive sleep apnea

Potentially Treatable by Drugs
- UTI
- Diabetes mellitus
- Diabetes insipidus
- Fecal impaction
- Constipation

UTI, urinary tract infection.

TREATMENT

Desired Outcomes

- Restoration of continence, which may not initially be a realistic outcome
- Reduction in the number of enuresis episodes
- Prevention or amelioration of disease complications including adverse psychological effects on the patient and caregivers or delay in developmental milestones
- Avoidance or prevention of adverse treatment effects
- Minimization of treatment costs
- Improvement in the patient's and caregivers' quality of life

General Approach to Treatment

Treatment is guided by the findings of the patient assessment. Daytime wetting, abnormal voiding such as unusual posturing, discomfort, straining, or poor stream, history of recurrent UTIs, and abnormalities of the genitalia suggest the need for referral to a urologist. In the rare circumstance of a true psychological cause, individual and/or family psychotherapy and crisis intervention are recommended.

Patient Encounter 2, Part 2: Medical History, Physical Examination, Diagnostic Tests, and Creating a Care Plan

PMH: Unremarkable pregnancy/delivery. All developmental milestones within normal limits. Two episodes of AOM treated with no sequelae. Current on all immunizations

FH, SH: Noncontributary

Meds: None

ROS: (+) nocturnal incontinence 5 nights/week or more; (–) vaginal itching, UTIs, urgency, frequency, dysuria, lower abdominal fullness

PE:

VS: BP ___/___ mm Hg, P ___ bpm, RR ___/min, T 37.0°C (98.6°F)

Resp: Within normal limits

CV: Within normal limits

Abd: Soft, nontender, nondistended; (+) bowel sounds; bladder not palpable

Neuro: Within normal limits (gross sensory, motor, reflexes)

GU: Within normal limits per inspection only

Rectal: Deferred

Labs: Urinalysis within normal limits

Given this additional information, what is your assessment of this patient's condition?

Identify your treatment goals for this patient.

What nonpharmacologic and pharmacologic alternatives are available to the patient?

What initial treatment would you suggest?

In the absence of an identified cause and comorbidities, monosymptomatic nocturnal enuresis is present which can be amenable to nonpharmacologic and pharmacologic therapies (Fig. 53–1). Nonpharmacologic therapy should be utilized initially, provided that the patient and family are sufficiently motivated. Use of one nonpharmacologic method at a time is reasonable, provided that each is given an adequate trial period. If response is suboptimal after 6 months, a different method should be substituted or added. There is some evidence to justify combination therapy. There is no consensus as to when pharmacologic therapy should be added to or substituted for nonpharmacologic therapy. ⓮ *Considering that pharmacotherapy is inferior to select nonpharmacologic treatment modalities in pediatric enuresis, pharmacotherapy will be most valuable in patients who are not candidates for nonpharmacologic therapy due to nonadherence or who do not achieve the desired outcomes on nonpharmacologic therapy alone.*

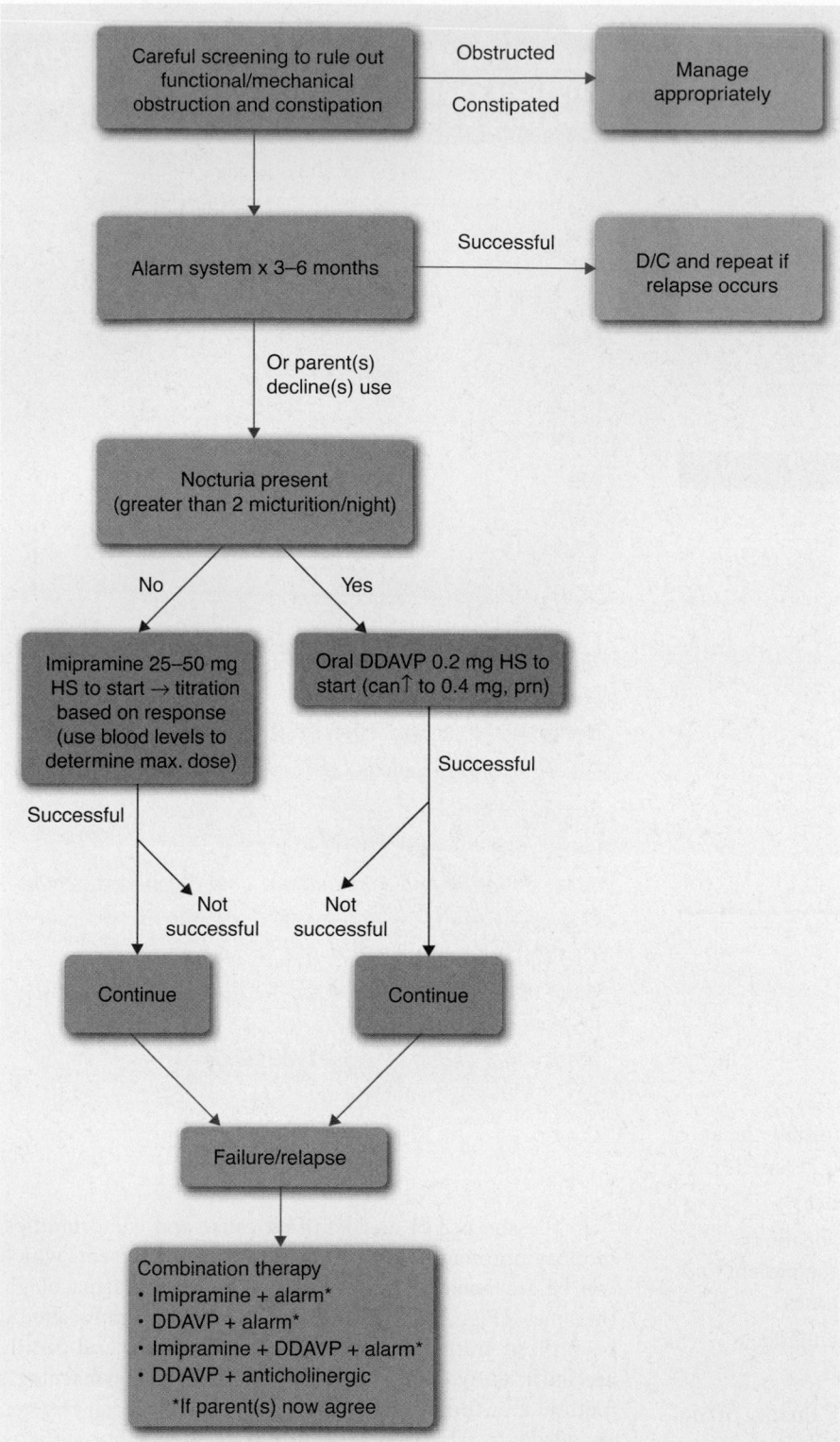

FIGURE 53–1. Enuresis treatment protocol. (DDAVP, desmopressin; HS, at bedtime; D/C, discontinue; prn, as needed.)

▶ *Nonpharmacologic Treatment*[38]

The standard first-line therapy is supportive in nature. This involves education about the condition, demystification, and assurance that the parents do not punish the child for enuresis. Journal keeping, fluid restriction, and nighttime awakenings of the child to pre-empt "accidents" make for a high level of caregiver involvement. The behavioral treatments of enuresis are explained in Table 53–6. Alarms, overlearning, and dry-bed training are the most complex and effective nonpharmacologic treatments available and compare favorably to pharmacologic therapy. A 3- to 6-month trial is recommended. Once dryness is achieved, relapse rates are low.

Measures that *do not* help include:

- Bladder stretching exercises (done by delaying voiding despite the urge to do so)
- Hypnotherapy

Table 53–6

Behavioral Treatments for Enuresis

Lifting	Procedure wherein the caregiver takes the child to the toilet at regular intervals during the night to urinate without fully awakening him or her
Night awakening	Procedure wherein the caregiver fully awakens the child to void shortly before he or she would usually have wet the bed; once the child is consistently dry, the frequency of awakening drops or (for single awakenings) the time of awakening is gradually moved to earlier in the night (i.e., closer to bedtime) until the child is dry when awakened 1 hour after going to bed
Alarm	An alarm device and a moisture-sensitive sensor are used in combination, with the sensor being placed under the sheets, or more commonly, attached to the child's pajamas or underwear near the urethra
Overlearning	This is commenced at a minimum of 2 weeks after the alarm has rendered the child dry; the child drinks 500 mL (about 16 oz.) during the hour before going to bed; alarm use is continued until he or she is dry for 14 consecutive nights with the extra fluid intake; is used to reduce relapse rates seen with alarm use alone
Dry-bed training	This begins with an intensive first night of training which involves increased fluid consumption, hourly awakenings, praise when the bed is dry at hourly awakenings, and, when the alarm goes off, a mild reprimand and cleanliness training (child changes wet clothes and bed linens, remakes the bed, resets the alarm); before going to bed and after each wetting, the child engages in 20 practice trials of appropriate toileting (i.e., positive practice): for each practice trial, the child lies in bed, counts to 50, arises and attempts to urinate in the toilet, then returns to bed; on subsequent nights, child is woken only once, usually about 3 hours after the child has gone to bed; after a dry night, the night awakening moves up 30 minutes earlier; it is discontinued when it is scheduled to occur 1 hour after bedtime; after 7 consecutive dry nights, the alarm is discontinued, but is reinstated if two episodes of wetting occur in a 1-week period

- Dietary changes
- Desensitization to allergens
- Acupuncture[39]
- Chiropractic

▶ *Pharmacologic Treatment*

The two primary agents used to treat enuresis are DDAVP and imipramine (Table 53–7). ⑮ *DDAVP is the drug of choice in pediatric enuresis.* Anticholinergics have a limited role (Table 53–7). Other agents have been studied with inconclusive results.[40]

Desmopressin[41,42] A synthetic analogue of ADH, DDAVP was first studied in enuresis in the 1970s. It was approved by the FDA in 1990 for the treatment of nocturnal enuresis in children at least 6 years of age. It decreases the number of wet nights per week by a mean of 1.34. The between-study variability in response to DDAVP is quite large, with a frequency of wetting ranging from 10% to 91% of patients, but only 25% become completely dry on the drug. Response is dose-independent for the nasal formulation (20 = 40 = 60 mcg); however, 20 mcg is the minimum dose resulting in therapeutic benefit. Response is dose-dependent for the oral formulation (e.g., the number of wet nights fell 27%, 30%, and 40% with 0.2-, 0.4-, and 0.6-mg doses, compared to 10% with placebo in one study). Benefit exists only as long as the patient takes DDAVP, with relapse rates of up to 94% after discontinuation. Insufficient data are available to judge the relative efficacies of the two formulations. DDAVP appears to work better with monosymptomatic versus polysymptomatic enuresis. The oral route is generally preferred since nasal congestion and sinusitis can reduce the bioavailability (BA) of the nasal formulation. DDAVP is an ideal agent for rapid-onset,

Table 53–7

Dosing of Pharmacologic Treatments of Enuresis

Desmopressin	Nasal: Start with 10 mcg 1 hour before bedtime and titrate upward in 10 mcg increments every week to a maximum of 40 mcg/day
	Oral: Start with 0.2 mg 1 hour before bedtime and titrate upward in 0.1 mg increments every week to a maximum of 0.6 mg/day
Imipramine	Start with 1 mg/kg/day (approximately 25 mg in 5- to 8-year-olds and 50 mg in older children and adolescents) and titrate in 0.5 mg/kg/day increments every 2 weeks to a maximum of 2.5 mg/kg/day
Anticholinergics	Refer to Table 53–3

short-term use such as attendance at camp or going on a "sleepover." If the desire is for long-term therapy and if it is sufficiently effective short-term, a 3- to 6-month trial is reasonable. At the end of this period, the drug should be tapered off by 0.1 mg (oral) or 10 mcg (nasal) per month. Relapse is less likely with a tapered withdrawal compared to an abrupt discontinuation. The following factors should be considered in individuals with partial responses to DDAVP: suboptimal dosing, poor adherence, poor BA (change nasal to oral preparation), and poor fluid/dietary habits (i.e., fluid restriction and high protein intake during the day and liberal salt and fluid intake after suppertime).[43] In individuals with presumed DDAVP resistance (i.e., poor response to usual doses or deterioration after a good response has been established), oral furosemide 0.5 mg/kg in the early morning may be useful. Furosemide works by reversing the abnormal circadian rhythm of renal tubular sodium handling which is common in such individuals.[44] In 12 patients with DDAVP-resistant enuresis, furosemide 0.5 mg/kg once daily in the morning was added to DDAVP therapy. In 9/12 (75%), enuresis events were reduced to less than one wet night per month. In the remaining three patients, although events were reduced from baseline (7 wet nights/week), they were still wet 2, 3, and 6 nights per week. Two of these three patients exhibited signs/symptoms of overactive bladder and one of the two patients had to discontinue furosemide therapy due to the increased frequency of daytime symptoms.[44] Side effects to DDAVP are minor and infrequent.[45] The most serious complication, water intoxication, is extremely uncommon when DDAVP is used to treat enuresis, with only 48 reported cases, all due to the nasal formulation.[45] However, electrolyte monitoring is recommended if intercurrent illness complicates the situation. Children should also not drink more than 8 ounces (about 240 mL) of fluid at suppertime, 8 ounces (240 mL) in the evening, and none in the 2 hours prior to bed in order to reduce the risk of water intoxication.

Imipramine[46]   The TCA imipramine was first used in the treatment of enuresis in the 1960s. Although trials involving other TCAs have been performed over the years, there is insufficient evidence to assess the relative performance of these agents versus imipramine and the latter is considered the gold standard TCA in enuresis management. Its mechanism of action is unclear, although it is an anticholinergic and antispasmodic and may increase plasma ADH concentrations. Up to 80% of treated patients may respond, although the long-term continence rate is only about 25%. A patient can expect approximately one fewer wet night per week with imipramine use. As with DDAVP, benefit only occurs as long as the drug is being taken, with relapse rates after discontinuation of therapy of up to 50%. There is no significant correlation of drug concentration with response. If sufficiently effective short-term, a 4- to 6-months trial is reasonable, followed by a weaning-off period of 3 to 4 weeks. There is a high frequency of neurologic side effects in children, including lethargy, dizziness, and headache in 5%; irritability in 11%; anxiety in 10%; and sleep disturbances in 16%.[45] GI symptoms occur in about 25% of pediatric patients.[45]

Anticholinergics   Oxybutynin and tolterodine monotherapies have no significant effect in monosymptomatic nocturnal enuresis. Oxybutynin and related agents (see adult UI section of this chapter) should be used only if the patient has concurrent daytime urgency or frequency. Combination therapy with DDAVP may also be worthwhile in patients refractory to combinations incorporating alarm therapy, DDAVP, and/or imipramine.

Comparison of Therapies   Most of the comparisons between treatments have been made by means of meta-analyses conducted by the Cochrane Enuresis Collaborative.[40,42,46–48] Unfortunately, most enuresis treatment studies have been so poorly designed they compromise the ability

to pool studies for meta-analysis. With this in mind, the comparative efficacies of monotherapy and combination therapies using the best data available follow.

The most effective nonpharmacologic method is the use of bed alarms. Defining success as less than 1 wet night per month, the initial success rate for alarms is 66%, with long-term success after discontinuation occurring in 45% (versus 1% with no treatment). However, this method requires highly motivated families and the development of improvement is slow (over 4 to 12 or more weeks). Data are inadequate to compare the various commercial brands of alarms available to consumers or to compare alarms to other behavioral interventions. Supplementing this method with either overlearning or dry-bed training significantly reduces the already low relapse rates seen with alarms. Alarm therapy is also significantly more effective than DDAVP, evaluated at both the end of therapy and long-term. Similar findings are noted for the alarm-versus-imipramine comparison. There are conflicting data regarding the value of supplementing the alarm method with DDAVP.

The American Academy of Child and Adolescent Psychiatry and the International Children's Continence Society (ICCS) published preliminary practice guidelines for the assessment and treatment of pediatric enuresis in 2004.[35,36] However, the modified algorithm of Reiner is inclusive of all potentially useful treatments and distinguishes approaches based on nocturnal urine output (nocturia), an important distinction not considered in previous recommendations.[49–51]

OUTCOME EVALUATION

- Monitor the patient for symptom relief. Have the desired outcomes jointly developed by the health care team, the patient, and his or her parents/guardians been achieved and to what degree? Evaluate the daily diary completed by the patient or parents/guardians since the last clinic visit and quantitate the clinical response (the number of dry nights versus the total number of nights, and the frequency of nights with greater than or equal to two enuresis episodes). If a diary has not been used, elicit the clinical response, in general terms, since the last visit.

- Elicit adverse events of therapy in a nonleading manner and ask the patient to judge their severity. Ask the patient or parents/guardians what measures if any were used to ameliorate them. Assess adherence (ask patient or parents/guardians about missed doses; do pill counts if the prescription vial is available).

- The balance of clinical response, tolerability, and burden on the family will dictate the approach to management. As most nonpharmacologic approaches are "all or none" and drug dosages after an initial titration period are fixed, the major decision process involves either changing therapy if clinical results are inadequate, or beginning or continuing tapering-off and discontinuation of therapy after success. There is no consensus on which

Patient Care and Monitoring: Pediatric Enuresis

1. Assess the patient's symptoms to determine if patient-directed therapy is appropriate or whether the patient should be evaluated by a physician. Assessment includes the types and severities of symptoms and the presence or absence of exacerbating factors. Does the patient have any enuresis-related complications?

2. Review any available diagnostic data to determine disease status.

3. Obtain a thorough medication history, including use of prescription, nonprescription, and complementary and alternative drug products. Determine which, if any, treatments in the past had been helpful as judged by the patient and/or caregiver(s). Could any of the patient's current medications be contributing to enuresis?

4. Educate the patient and/or caregiver(s) on lifestyle modifications that may improve symptoms or assist the clinician in monitoring the responses to therapy, including but not limited to, fluid restriction and journal keeping. The patient and/or caregiver(s) should be referred to local enuresis clinics (if available) for training in nonpharmacologic treatments such as use of bed alarms, overlearning, and dry-bed training.

5. Assess if the patient is taking the appropriate drug(s) for his or her enuresis? Are the doses appropriate? If no (to either question), why?

6. Develop a plan to assess efficacy after a minimum of 3 months.

7. Assess changes in quality of life (physical, psychological, and social functioning and well-being).

8. Evaluate the patient for drug-related adverse events, allergies, and interactions (drug–drug and drug–disease).

9. Stress the importance of adherence with the prescribed regimen, including lifestyle modifications and nonpharmacologic treatment. Recommend the most "patient-friendly" treatment regimen possible.

10. Provide the patient and/or caregiver(s) with education regarding the disease state, lifestyle modifications, and drug therapy:

    - The causes of enuresis and what things the patient and/or caregiver(s) can do to reduce its frequency
    - Possible enuresis complications
    - Timing of medication intake
    - Potential adverse events (limit to most frequent and/or clinically relevant)
    - Potential drug–drug interactions.

treatment approach to withdraw first, although the ICCS recommends the nonpharmacologic (alarm) therapy first, then pharmacologic (DDAVP) therapy.

Abbreviations Introduced in This Chapter

ADH	Antidiuretic hormone
BA	Bioavailability
CAM	Complementary and alternative medicine
CL	Total body clearance
CrCl	Creatinine clearance
CVA	Costovertebral angle
CYP450	Cytochrome P-450
DDAVP	Desmopressin
DHIC	Detrusor hyperactivity with impaired contractility
ER	Extended release
ICCS	International Children's Continence Society
IR	Immediate release
LA	Long acting
MESNA	Sodium 2-mercaptoethanesulfonate
OTC	Over the counter
OUI	Overflow urinary incontinence
PV	Per vagina
SNF	Skilled nursing facility
SR	Sustained release
SUI	Stress urinary incontinence
TCA	Tricyclic antidepressant
TD	Transdermal
UI	Urinary incontinence
UTI	Urinary tract infection
UUI	Urge urinary incontinence

 Self-assessment questions and answers are available at *http://www.mhpharmacotherapy.com/pp.html.*

REFERENCES

1. Abrams P, Cardozo L, Fall M, et al. The standardization of terminology of lower urinary tract function: Report from the standardization sub-committee of the International Continence Society. Neurourol Urodyn 2002;21:167–178.
2. Arnold EP, Burgio K, Diokno AC, et al. Epidemiology and natural history of urinary incontinence (UI). In: Abrams P, Khoury S, Wein AJ, eds. Incontinence. Plymouth, UK: Plymbridge Distributors; 1999:199–226.

3. Brown JS, Nyberg LM, Kusek JW, et al. Proceedings of the National Institute of Diabetes, Digestive and Kidney Diseases International Symposium on Epidemiologic Issues in Urinary Incontinence in Women. Am J Obstet Gynecol 2003;188:S77–S88.

4. Rovner ES, Wyman J, Lackner T, Guay DRP. Urinary Incontinence. In: DiPiro J, Talbert R, Hayes P, Yee G, Matzke G, Posey LM, eds. Pharmacotherapy: A Pathophysiologic Approach. 7th ed. New York: McGraw-Hill, 2008:1399–1415.

5. Groutz A, Gordon D, Keidar R, et al. Stress urinary incontinence: Prevalence among nulliparous compared with primiparous and grand multiparous premenopausal women. Neurourol Urodyn 1999;18:419–425.

6. Abrams P, Cardozo L, Khoury S, Wein A, eds. Incontinence. Second International Consultation on Incontinence. 2nd ed. Plymouth, UK: Health Publications Ltd, 2002.

7. Kafri R, Langer R, Dvir Z, et al. Rehabilitation vs drug therapy for urge urinary incontinence: Short-term outcome. Int Urogynecol J 2007;18:407–411.

8. Kafri R, Shames J, Raz M, et al. Rehabilitation versus drug therapy for urge urinary incontinence: Long-term outcomes. Int Urogynecol J Pelvic Floor Dyfunet 2008;19:47–52.

9. Shamliyan TA, Kane RL, Wyman J, et al. Systematic review: Randomized, controlled trials of nonsurgical treatments for urinary incontinence in women. Ann Intern Med 2008;148:459–473.

10. Chapple C, Khullar V, Gabriel Z, Dooley JA. The effects of antimuscarinic treatments in overactive bladder: A systematic review and meta-analysis. Eur Urol 2005;48:5–26.

11. Novara G, Balfano A, Secco S, et al. A systematic review and meta-analysis of randomized controlled trials with antiimmunocarcinic drugs for overactive bladder. Eur Urol 2008;54:740–763.

12. Hofner K, Burkart M, Jacob G, et al. Safety and efficacy of tolterodine extended release in men with overactive bladder symptoms and presumed non-obstructive benign prostatic hyperplasia. World J Urol 2007;25:627–633.

13. Ortho-McNeil Pharmaceutical. Ditropan XL (oxybutynin) package insert. Raritan, NJ: Ortho-McNeil Pharmaceutical, 2008.

14. Pharmacia & Upjohn. Detrol and Detrol LA (tolterodine) package inserts. New York: Pharmacia & Upjohn, 2005.

15. Watson Pharma. Oxytrol (oxybutynin transdermal system) package insert. Corona, CA: Watson Pharma, 2003.

16. Odyssey/Indevus Pharmaceuticals. Sanctura (trospium chloride) package insert. East Hanover, NJ/Lexington, MA: Odyssey/Indevus Pharmaceuticals, 2004.

17. Astellas Pharma U.S. VESIcare (solifenacin) package insert. Deerfield, IL: Astellas Pharma U.S., 2004.

18. Novartis. Enablex (darifenacin) package insert. East Hanover, NJ: Novartis, 2004.

19. Guay DRP. Drug forecast: Solifenacin (VESIcare): An investigational anticholinergic for overactive bladder. Consult Pharm 2004;19:437–444.

20. Guay DRP. Trospium chloride: An update on a quaternary anticholinergic for treatment of urge urinary incontinence. Ther Clin Risk Manag 2005;1:157–166.

21. Guay DRP. Darifenacin: Another antimuscarinic for overactive bladder. Consult Pharm 2005;20:424–431.

22. Sink KM, Thomas J 3rd, Xu H, et al. Dual use of bladder anticholinergics and cholinesterase inhibitors: Long-term functional and cognitive outcomes. J Am Geriatr Soc 2008;56:847–853.

23. Hashim H, Abrams P. Novel uses for antidiuresis. Int J Clin Pract 2007;(Suppl 155):32–36.

24. Steers WD, Herschorn S, Kreder KJ, et al. Duloxetine compared with placebo for treating women with symptoms of overactive bladder. BJU Int 2007;100:337–345.

25. Peyromaure M, Ravery V, Boccon-Gibod L. The management of stress urinary incontinence after radical prostatectomy. BJU Int 2002;90:155–161.

26. Filcamo MT, LiMarzi V, DelPopolo G, et al. Pharmacologic treatment in postprostatectomy stress urinary incontinence. Eur Urol 2007;51:1559–1564.

27. Kernan WN, Viscoli CM, Brass LM, et al. Phenylpropanolamine and the risk of hemorrhagic stroke. N Engl J Med 2000;343:1826–1832.

28. Owens RG, Karram MM. Comparative tolerability of drug therapies used to treat incontinence and enuresis. Drug Saf 1998;2:123–139.

29. Guay DRP. Duloxetine. The first therapy licensed for stress urinary incontinence. Am J Geriatr Pharmacother 2005;3:25–38.

30. Fraser MO, Chancellor MB. Neural control of the urethra and development of pharmacotherapy for stress urinary incontinence. BJU Int 2003;91:743–748.

31. Burgard EC, Fraser MO, Thor KB. Serotonergic modulation of bladder afferent pathways. Urology 2003;62(Suppl 1):10–15.

32. Eli Lilly & Co. Cymbalta (duloxetine) package insert. Indianapolis, IN: Eli Lilly & Co, 2004.

33. Filocamo MT, LiMarzi V, Del Popolo G, et al. Pharmacologic treatment in postprostatectomy stress urinary incontinence. Eur Urol 2007; 51: 1559–1564.

34. Duckett JR, Vella M, Kavalakuntla G, et al. Tolerability and efficacy of duloxetine in a nontrial situation. BJOG 2007;114:543–547.

35. Fritz G, Rockney R, Bernet W, et al. Practice parameter for the assessment and treatment of children and adolescents with enuresis. J Am Acad Child Adolesc Psychiatry 2004;43:1540–1550.

36. Hjalmar K, Arnold T, Bower W, et al. Nocturnal enuresis: An international evidence based management strategy. J Urol 2004;171(6 pt 2):2545–2561.

37. Rittig S, Schaumberg HL, Siggaard C, et al. The circadian effect in plasma vasopressin and urine output is related to desmopressin response and enuresis status in children with nocturnal enuresis. J Urol 2008;179:2389–2395.

38. Blum NJ. Nocturnal enuresis: Behavioral treatments. Urol Clin North Am 2004;31:499–507.

39. Bower WF, Diao M, Tang JL, Yeung CK. Acupuncture for nocturnal enuresis in children: A systematic review and exploration of rationale. Neurourol Urodyn 2005;24:267–272.

40. Glazener CM, Evans JH, Peto RE. Drugs for nocturnal enuresis in children (other than desmopressin and tricyclics). Cochrane Database Syst Rev 2003;(4):CD002238.

41. Aventis Pharmaceuticals. DDAVP (desmopressin) package inserts. Bridgewater, NJ: Aventis Pharmaceuticals, 2002.

42. Glazener CM, Evans JH. Desmopressin for nocturnal enuresis in children. Cochrane Database Syst Rev 2002;(3):CD002112.

43. Raes A, Dehoorne J, Van Laecke E, et al. Partial response to intranasal desmopressin in children with monosymptomatic nocturnal enuresis is related to persistent nocturnal polyuria on wet nights. J Urol 2007;178:1048–1052.

44. DeGuchtenaere A, Vande Walle C, Van Sintjan P, et al. Desmopressin resistant nocturnal polyuria may benefit from furosemide therapy administered in the morning. J Urol 2007;178:2635–2639.

45. Muller D, Roehr CC, Eggert P. Comparative tolerability of drug treatment for nocturnal enuresis in children. Drug Saf 2004;27:717–727.

46. Glazener CM, Evans JH, Peto RE. Tricyclic and related drugs for nocturnal enuresis in children. Cochrane Database Syst Rev 2003;(3):CD002117.

47. Glazener CM, Evans JH. Simple behavioural and physical interventions for nocturnal enuresis in children. Cochrane Database Syst Rev 2004;(2):CD003637.

48. Glazener CM, Evans JH, Peto RE. Complex behavioural and educational interventions for nocturnal enuresis in children. Cochrane Database Syst Rev 2004;(1):CD004668.

49. Reiner WG. Pharmacotherapy in the management of voiding and storage disorders, including enuresis and encopresis. J Am Acad Child Adolesc Psychiatry 2008;47:491–498.

50. Neveus T. The dilemmas of refractory nocturnal enuresis. J Urol 2008;179:817–818.

51. Neveus T, Tullus K. Tolterodine and imipramine in refractory enuresis: A placebo-controlled crossover study. Pediatr Nephrol 2008;23:263–267.

54 Allergic and Pseudoallergic Drug Reactions

J. Russell May and Philip H. Smith

LEARNING OBJECTIVES

● **Upon completion of the chapter, the reader will be able to:**

1. Describe the potential incidence of allergic and pseudoallergic reactions and why it is difficult to obtain accurate numbers.

2. Describe the Gell and Coombs categories of reactions.

3. Identify the classes of drugs most commonly associated with allergic and pseudoallergic reactions.

4. Recommend specific treatment for a patient experiencing anaphylaxis.

5. Recommend an approach to drug selection in patients with multiple drug allergies.

6. Describe drug desensitization procedures for selected drugs.

KEY CONCEPTS

❶ Allergic and pseudoallergic reactions represent 24% of reported adverse drug reactions, are costly, and cause considerable morbidity and mortality.

❷ Drug allergy is an adverse immune response to a stimulus; such responses are traditionally placed in the Gell and Coombs categories: type I (immediate hypersensitivity), type II (complement-mediated antibody reactions), type III (immune complex reactions), and type IV (cellular or delayed-type hypersensitivity). However, drug exposures may stimulate several or all of these types of reactions. To complicate the picture further, drug reactions do not always fit the categories.

❸ Reactions that clinically resemble allergic reactions but lack an immune basis have been referred to as "pseudoallergic." They include almost the entire range of immediate hypersensitivity clinical patterns and range in significance from the alarming but trivial anxiety or vasovagal reactions caused by local dental anesthetics to the potentially fatal reactions to ionic radiocontrast media.

❹ Penicillins and cephalosporins both have a β-lactam ring joined to an S-containing ring structure (penicillins: a thiazolidine ring, cephalosporins: a dihydrothiazine ring). Because of this structural difference, the extent of cross-allergenicity appears to be relatively low. Cross-allergenicity is less likely with newer generation cephalosporins compared to the first generation agents.

❺ Reactions to sulfonamide antibiotics, ranging from mild (most common) to life-threatening (rare), occur in 2% to 4% of healthy patients, with rates as high as 60% in patients with AIDS.

❻ IgE-mediated urticarial/angioedema reactions and anaphylaxis are associated with aspirin and nonsteroidal anti-inflammatory drugs (NSAIDs). Urticaria is the most common form of IgE-mediated reaction. However, most reactions are the result of metabolic idiosyncracies, such as aspirin-induced respiratory disease which may produce severe and even fatal bronchospasm. This class is second, only to β-lactams, in causing anaphylaxis.

❼ Radiocontrast media may cause serious immediate pseudoallergic reactions such as urticaria/angioedema, bronchospasm, shock, and death. These reactions have been reduced with the introduction of nonionic, lower osmolality products.

❽ Opiates (morphine, meperidine, codeine, hydrocodone, and others) stimulate mast cell release directly, resulting in pruritis and urticaria with occasional mild wheezing. Though these reactions are not allergic, many patients state that they are "allergic" to one or more of the opiates. Pretreatment with an antihistamine may reduce these reactions. These pseudoallergic reactions are rarely, if ever, life threatening.

❾ Drug desensitization is a potentially life-threatening procedure, and requires continuous monitoring in a hospital setting, with suitable access to emergency treatment and intubation. It should only be undertaken under the direction of a physician with suitable training and experience and only when a suitable alternative is not available. In such hands, desensitization may present less risk than treatment failure with a less effective alternative medication.

INTRODUCTION

Allergic and pseudoallergic drug reactions are reported together. They are rarely confirmed by testing, making statistical analysis imprecise, with both over-reporting and under-reporting. But there is no doubt they are costly and cause considerable morbidity and mortality. ❶ *Allergic reactions may represent as many as 24% of reported adverse drug reactions.*[1] Between 10% and 20% of hospitalized patients incur drug reactions (7% in the general population), with about one-third possibly due to hypersensitivity; however, most of these reactions are not reported, especially in pediatrics.[1-3] Patients experiencing an allergic drug reaction in the hospital result in increased costs of $275 to $600 million annually.[4] This financial burden can occur due to several reasons including increased indirect cost of: (a) time and lost labor, (b) the use of costlier alternative medications, and (c) treatment failures. Outpatient rates are not well studied and much harder to collect. Relying on a patient's history without an attempt to verify the relationships between drugs taken and symptoms experienced results in confusion. Health care professionals and patients use the term "drug allergy" in such a general way that it is not medically useful and, further, perpetuates a level of fear and concern in the public and in medical practice that is inappropriate and costly. This same confusion and anxiety sometimes leads medical personnel to ignore or forget "drug allergy" with potentially catastrophic results. Clearly, an understanding of how allergic and pseudoallergic reactions occur and how they might be managed or prevented is important to health care professionals and their patients.

PATHOPHYSIOLOGY

Drug allergies are immune responses resulting from different mechanisms of immunologic recognition and activation, and reactions are produced by multiple physiologic pathways. This produces a confusing spectrum of clinical pictures and complex pathophysiologic mechanisms. ❷ *Allergy is an adverse immune response to a stimulus and is traditionally placed in the Gell and Coombs categories: type I (immediate hypersensitivity), type II (complement-mediated antibody reactions), type III (immune complex reactions), and type IV (cellular or delayed-type hypersensitivity). Drug exposures often stimulate several or all of these types of reactions, and clinical symptoms do not always fit neatly into the categories.*

The immune system uses many tools such as blood vessel dilation or constriction, causing fluid to flood an infected area, or even producing special cells to kill bacteria or the infected cells in which they harbor. The pattern of these responses is either inborn (the innate immune response) or learned from previous infections and injuries (the adaptive immune response). Most drug reactions involve the adaptive response and certainly, in the sense that they cause more harm than good, are "mistakes."

T cells control these "learned" responses and decide which "tools" to use in the reaction. Sometimes they choose several different "tools" at once, and multiple reactions ensue, as when a person becomes sensitized to penicillin and has not only anaphylaxis but hemolytic anemia and serum sickness, as well. There are different types of T cells, and they communicate either directly with other cells or by chemical messages, called "cytokines." The pattern of cytokines released is one way T cells have of determining which kind of response will occur. They are broadly called Th1 and Th2 responses, with Th1 mostly responding to infections and Th2 sometimes producing allergy or asthma.

Immunologic drug reactions generally represent T-cell activation. The type of T cell activated determines the type of reaction to the drug. Th1 cytokines (largely interferon-γ) produce many more chronic (and at times serious) skin reactions and destruction of cells (as in hemolytic anemia or thrombocytopenia). Sometimes these responses can damage tissues, such as the kidney (interstitial nephritis). Th2 cytokines tend to cause the antibodies produced to be switched to the immune globulin E (IgE) or allergic antibody class, which can result in hives or anaphylaxis. Other classes of antibodies are often made, and these can produce serum sickness or indirect destruction of cells (thrombocytopenia). T-cell receptors respond to one peptide only, which makes each activation response exclusive to the original stimulus (drug) or to chemical structures with very close resemblance.

Antigens

Antigen-presenting cells recognize complex, three-dimensional protein molecules of at least 1,000 Daltons (Da) in size. Most drugs are much smaller than this, and cannot be recognized on their own. Only proteins such as insulin or exogenous sera are identified and their peptides presented directly to T cells.

Drugs that are chemically reactive may bond covalently to body proteins, altering them and forming large enough molecules for antigen-presenting cells to recognize. This process is called haptenation, and the smaller reactive molecule, a hapten. Some other drugs are inert until they are partially metabolized (prohaptens), and their breakdown products bind native proteins to serve as antigens. Metabolic variations in some patients may produce more active haptens, or prevent these fragments from being detoxified, causing them to accumulate and make binding proteins more likely.

Gell and Coombs

Type I reactions occur when the drug or its bound hapten incites an IgE antibody response. IgE binds to high-affinity receptors on mast cells and basophils. When the original antigen cross-links cell-bound IgE, the effector cell releases enormous amounts of preformed mediators, producing the well-known symptoms of immediate hypersensitivity: urticaria, rhinitis, bronchoconstriction, and anaphylaxis.

Type II reactions are produced by IgG (or IgM) antibody. The drug or hapten that elicited the antibody response binds to target cells. When antibody binds the drug, complement activation destroys the cell. Blood dyscrasias like thrombocytopenia or hemolytic anemia are the most common examples of type II reactions.

Type III or immune complex reactions also involve IgG antibody production. In this case, when the concentration of the sensitizing drug or hapten is in slight excess to the antibody, the two combine in the serum, producing lattices of antigen–antibody complexes. These are deposited, particularly in vessel walls. They activate complement, causing vasculitis. The classic forms of type III reaction are serum sickness (usually including arthralgias, fever, malaise, and urticaria that develop 7 to 14 days after exposure to the causative antigen) and the localized Arthus reaction, a local inflammatory response due to deposition of immune complexes in tissues.

Type IV reactions are mediated by T cells themselves. "Delayed-type hypersensitivity" reactions from positive tuberculin tests to contact dermatitis are typical type IV reactions, but understanding T-cell function allows us to further define this category as shown in Table 54–1.[5,6]

Pseudoallergic Drug Reactions

❸ *Reactions that clinically resemble allergic reactions but lack an immune basis have been referred to as "pseudoallergic." They include almost the entire range of immediate hypersensitivity clinical patterns. Pseudoallergic reactions range in significance from the alarming but trivial anxiety or vasovagal reactions* caused by local dental anesthetics to sometimes fatal reactions to ionic radiocontrast media. However, cytotoxic reactions, serum sickness, and severe dermatologic reactions (e.g., Stevens-Johnson syndrome and toxic epidermal necrolysis) are immunologic processes that are not likely to be mimicked by nonimmune processes seen with pseudoallergic reactions.

Pseudoallergic reactions are important in patient counseling and management considerations. The reactions represent common biological functions (direct histamine release by vancomycin, opiates), whereas immunologic (allergic) reactions are based on the structure of the drug. Even a mild drug allergy may carry significant potential for anaphylaxis on readministration. In contrast, pseudoallergic reactions tend to remain constant whether mild or severe and are dose-related.

Pseudoallergic reactions, then, are reactions where the tools of the immune system are used in exactly the same way, but without the "learning" response by T cells and generally without the much greater danger that true immunologic sensitization implies. Pseudoallergic reactions may be thought of as a subtype of idiopathic reactions, rather than an activation of the patient's immune system. The pathophysiology of pseudoallergic reactions is generally unknown, but indicators of immune activation are not seen when they occur.

PROBLEMATIC DRUG CLASSES AND TREATMENT OPTIONS

The first priority is to avoid doing serious harm by administering a drug that the patient cannot tolerate. We can generally establish the likelihood of a relationship between the suspected drug and the observed reaction and, also, whether it is likely to be an immune or idiopathic reaction by

Table 54–1
Reaction Classification, Clinical Symptoms, and Potential Causative Drugs

Gell and Coombs Classification	Immune Response	Clinical Symptoms	Potential Causative Drugs[a]
Type I	IgE	Anaphylaxis, urticaria	β-Lactam antibiotics penicillins (primarily), cephalosporins, carbapenems Non-β-lactam antibiotics: sulfonamides, vancomycin Others: insulins, heparin
Type II	IgG	Hemolytic anemia, thrombocytopenia	Quinidine, methyldopa, penicillins, heparin
Type III	IgG and IgM	Vasculitis, serum sickness, lupus	Penicillins, sulfonamides, radiocontrast agents, phenytoin
Type IV			β-Lactam antibiotics, sulfonamides, and phenytoin
IVa	Th1 cytokines	Tuberculin reaction, eczema	See text for examples
IVb[b]	Th2 cytokines	Maculopapular and bullous exanthema	
IVc[b]	Cytotoxic T cells (CD4 and CD8)	Same as IVb, also eczema, pustular exanthema	
IVd	T cells (IL-8)	Pustular exanthema	

[a]These drugs represent a list of causative agents. Many drugs can cause these reactions

[b]IVb and IVc reactions may combine to produce erythema multiforme, Stevens-Johnson's syndrome, and toxic epidermal necrolysis

From Refs. 5, 6.

Clinical Presentation and Diagnosis of Allergic and Pseudoallergic Drug Reactions

The clinical presentation of a patient experiencing an allergic reaction varies greatly. The primary reactions are described below:

- **Anaphylaxis**: Anaphylaxis is an acute life-threatening allergic reaction. Signs and symptoms involve the skin (e.g., pruritis, urticaria), respiratory tract (e.g., dyspnea, wheezing), gastrointestinal tract (e.g., nausea, cramping), and cardiovascular system (e.g., hypotension, tachycardia). Onset is usually within 30 minutes, but can be as long as 2 hours. Treatment must begin immediately. Anaphylaxis may recur 6 to 8 hours after exposure so patients experiencing anaphylaxis should be observed for at least 12 hours.

- **Cytotoxic reactions**: These reactions usually take the form of hemolytic anemia, thrombocytopenia, granulocytopenia, or agranulocytosis.

- **Immune complex reactions**: These reactions usually involve a serum sickness-like syndrome (e.g., arthralgias, fever, malaise, and urticaria) that usually develops 7 to 14 days after exposure to the causative antigen.

- **Dermatologic reactions**: Rashes may range from mild to life-threatening
  - *Urticaria*: These are itchy, raised, swollen areas on the skin. Also known as hives.
  - *Maculopapular rash*: A rash that contains both macules and papules. A macule is a flat discolored area of the skin, and a papule is a small raised bump. A maculopapular rash is usually a large area that is red, and has small, bumps.
  - *Erythema multiforme*: A rash characterized by papular (small raised bump) or vesicular lesions (blisters), and reddening or discoloration of the skin often in concentric zones about the lesion.
  - *Stevens-Johnson syndrome*: A severe expression of erythema multiforme (also known as erythema multiforme major). It typically involves the skin and the mucous membranes with the potential for severe morbidity and even death.
  - *Toxic epidermal necrolysis*: A life-threatening skin disorder characterized by blistering and peeling of the top layer of skin.

examining the time-course and specific signs and symptoms as precisely and objectively as possible. Reevaluating the patient's physical findings and laboratory values (taking into account pre-existing diseases) allows further clarification of the need to change treatments and to add therapy for the reaction itself.

Reviewing the original indications for the treatment that caused the reaction is important. For example, in many respiratory illnesses, a prescribed antibiotic may be unnecessary. If the disease persists and indications for some treatment are established, alternatives must be sought, either by adjusting dose or administration rate, finding effective and unrelated alternative medication, or desensitizing the patient to the original drug.

When adverse drug reactions occur, the health care provider should carefully describe all aspects of the reaction and assess the potential for it to reoccur. Many patients have frightening associations of the term "allergy" with severe and unpredictable anaphylaxis. It is difficult to undo fears created by injudiciously labeling a patient as allergic in the medical record. Labeling a person "allergic" may hamper future medical care, as patients may refuse treatment or fail to adhere to medication regimens. If the original reaction is clearly documented, health care providers can appropriately counsel patients about any true dangers.

Anaphylaxis is a true medical emergency and must be treated promptly. Otherwise, managing allergic reactions begins with stopping the offending agent. Understanding the allergic reaction and potential for **cross-allergenicity** between similar drugs will assist in selecting an alternative

medication. Desensitization is a management option if the patient truly needs the medication and alternative drugs are not available. While any drug may cause an allergic or pseudoallergic reaction, several drugs and drug classes are strongly associated with such reactions (Table 54–2). These classes will be discussed individually.

β-Lactam Antibiotics

Hypersensitivity reactions with β-lactam antibiotics, especially penicillin, may encompass any of the Type I through IV Gell-Coombs classifications. The most common reactions are **maculopapular** and urticarial eruptions.[7] While rare (lesser than 0.05%), anaphylaxis to penicillins cause the greatest concern, as they are responsible for the majority of all drug-induced anaphylaxis deaths in patients, accounting for 75% of all anaphylaxis cases in the United States.[5,8] The treatment of anaphylaxis is given in Table 54–3.[9]

Table 54–2
Problematic Drug Classes
β-Lactam antibiotics
Sulfonamide antibiotics
Aspirin and nonsteroidal anti-inflammatory drugs
Radiocontrast media
Opiates
Chemotherapy
Insulin
Anticonvulsants

Table 54–3

Pharmacologic Management of Anaphylactic Reactions

Immediate Intervention
Epinephrine 1:1,000 (1 mg/mL)
- Adults: Give 0.2–0.5 mg intramuscular (IM) or subcutaneous (SC); repeat every 5 minutes as needed
- Pediatrics: 0.01 mg/kg (maximum 0.3 mg) IM or SC, repeat every 5 minutes as needed

Subsequent Interventions
Normal Saline Infusion
- Adults: 1–2 L at a rate of 5–10 mL/kg in the first 5 minutes, followed by slow infusion
- Pediatrics: up to 30 mL/kg in the first hour
Epinephrine Infusion
If patient is NOT responding to epinephrine injections and volume resuscitation:
- Adults: epinephrine infusion (1 mg in 250 mL dextrose 5% in water [D$_5$W]): 1–4 mcg/min, titrating based on clinical response or side effects
- Pediatrics: epinephrine 1:10,000 (0.1 mg/mL): 0.01 mg/kg (up to 0.3 mg) over several minutes

Other Considerations after Epinephrine and Fluids
Diphenhydramine
- Adults: 25–50 mg intravenous (IV) or IM
- Pediatrics: 1–1.25 mg/kg (maximum of 300 mg/24 hour)
Ranitidine
- Adults: 50 mg in D$_5$W 20 mL IV over 5 minutes
- Pediatrics: 1 mg/kg (up to 50 mg) in D$_5$W 20 mL IV over 5 minutes
Inhaled β-agonist (bronchospasm resistant to epinephrine)
2–5 mg in 3 mL of normal saline, nebulized, repeat as needed
Dopamine (hypotension refractory to fluids and epinephrine)
2–20 mcg/kg/min titrated to maintain systolic blood pressure greater than 90 mm Hg
Hydrocortisone (severe or prolonged anaphylaxis)
- Adults: 250 mg IV (prednisone 20 mg can be given orally in mild cases)
- Pediatrics: 2.5–10 mg/kg/24 hours

From Ref. 9.

Patient Encounter 1

A 44-year-old male is admitted to the hospital for treatment of a cellulitis. He states that he has no known allergies. He is prescribed IV nafcillin for his infection. During the first infusion, he notices that his ears are itching and he calls for a nurse. Upon the nurse's arrival, the patient appears nervous and is having difficulty breathing.

What type allergic reaction is the patient most likely having?

What is the first action this nurse should take?

Outline the medical treatment for this reaction and how fast should it be started?

The health care professional is faced with a difficult task when approaching a patient who claims a history of penicillin allergy. While as many as 12% of hospital patients state they have an allergy to penicillin, about 90% will have negative skins tests.[10] Table 54–4 shows the traditional protocol for penicillin skin testing.[11] This test only evaluates IgE-mediated reactions. A patient with a history of other serious reactions such as erythema multiforme, Stevens-Johnson syndrome, or toxic epidermal necrolysis should not receive penicillins and should not be tested.

❹ *Penicillins and cephalosporins both have a β-lactam ring joined to an S-containing ring structure (penicillins: a thiazolidine ring, cephalosporins: a dihydrothiazine ring). The extent of cross-allergenicity appears to be relatively low, with an estimate of around 4%.[12]* *Cross-allergenicity is less likely with newer generation cephalosporins compared to the first generation agents.* Anaphylactic reactions to cephalosporins are rare, with a predicted range of 0.0001% to 0.1%. Minor skin reactions including urticaria, **exanthem**, and pruritis are the most common allergic reactions with

Table 54–4

Procedure for Performing Penicillin Skin Testing

A. Percutaneous (Prick) Skin testing

Materials	Volume (in Drops)
Pre-Pen 6 × 10^6 M	1
Penicillin G 10,000 units/mL	1
β-Lactam drug 3 mg/mL	1
0.03% albumin-saline control	1
Histamine control (1 mg/mL)	1

Place a drop of each test material on the volar surface of the forearm
Prick the skin with a sharp needle inserted through the drop at a 45° angle gently tenting the skin in an upward motion
Interpret skin responses after 15 minutes
A wheal at least 2 × 2 mm with erythema is considered positive
If the prick test is nonreactive, proceed to the intradermal test
If the histamine control is nonreactive, the test is considered uninterruptible

B. Intradermal Skin Testing

Materials	Volume (mL)
Pre-Pen 6 × 10^{6}M	0.02
Penicillin G 10,000 Units/mL	0.02
β-Lactam drug 3 mg/mL	0.02
0.03% Albumin-saline control	0.02
Histamine control (0.1 mg/mL)	0.02

Inject 0.02–0.03 mL of each test material intradermally (amount sufficient to produce a small bleb)
Interpret skin responses after 15 minutes
A wheal at least 6 × 6 mm with erythema and at least 3 mm greater than the negative control is considered positive
If the histamine control is nonreactive, the test is considered uninterruptible
Antihistamines may blunt the response and cause false-negative reactions

cephalosporins, showing severe reactions less often than with penicillins.[13]

For other β-lactam agents, the recommendations are fairly straightforward.[9] Carbapenems should be considered cross-reactive with penicillins. Monobactams (e.g., aztreonam) do not cross react with any β-lactam drugs except ceftazidime because they share an identical R-group side chain.

Sulfonamide Antibiotics

Sulfonamides are compounds that contain a sulfonamide moiety (i.e., SO_2NH_2). This group includes sulfonamide antibiotics, furosemide, thiazide diuretics, sulfonylureas, and celecoxib. The sulfonamide antibiotics contain an aromatic amine at the N4 position and a substituted ring at the N1 position. Because of this different chemical structure, cross-allergenicity with the other sulfonamides may not occur. Predisposition to allergic reactions is a more likely reason than cross-reactivity between these differing molecules.[14] The sulfonamide antibiotics are significant because they account for the largest percentage of antibiotic-induced toxic epidermal necrolysis and Stevens-Johnson syndrome cases.[15]

❺ *Reactions to sulfonamide antibiotics, ranging from mild (most common) to life-threatening (rare), occur in 2% to 4% of healthy patients, with rates as high as 60% in patients with AIDS.*[7] Anaphylaxis or anaphylactoid reactions almost always occur within 30 minutes but may be up to 90 minutes after exposure, most commonly after parenteral administration. Isolated angioedema or urticaria can occur within minutes to days. Serum sickness occurs within 1 to 2 weeks. Fixed drug eruptions (lesions) occur within a half-hour to 8 hours. These lesions resolve within 2 to 3 weeks after drug removal. The more severe conditions of Stevens-Johnson syndrome and toxic epidermal necrolysis tend to occur 1 to 2 weeks after initiation of therapy. Because trimethoprim-sulfamethoxazole is the drug of choice for patients infected with *Pneumocystis carinii*, desensitization may be necessary. A history of Stevens-Johnson syndrome or toxic epidermal necrolysis is an absolute contraindication for the desensitization procedure.

▶ Patients With Multiple Antibiotic Allergies

Dealing with patients who claim to have multiple antibiotic allergies can be challenging. Combining knowledge of cross-allergenicity with a careful assessment of patient history may be helpful in designing an antimicrobial regimen. Table 54–5 outlines a series of questions that can be useful in developing an effective treatment plan.[16] If available and indicated, skin testing may be useful to complete the puzzle. Often with careful assessment, an antibiotic of choice may be used when the patient's initial history would have ruled it out. Based on data gathered, the patient's record should reflect: antibiotics safe to use if needed; antibiotics to be avoided; and antibiotics that can be used only after desensitization. While this table was designed with antibiotics in mind, it can be modified for any multiple allergy situations.

Table 54–5
Multiple Antibiotic Allergies: Obtaining Background Information
For each antibiotic to which the patient claims to be allergic, gather the following information: What type of infection was being treated? Have you ever received the drug without experiencing a reaction? How many times have you received the drug and experienced a reaction? What was the drug dose and route of administration with the last reaction? How many doses did you take before the onset of the last reaction? How many doses did you take after the last reaction? Can you describe the adverse reaction? What was the duration of the reaction? What treatment was given for the reaction? Was there any permanent damage? **For each antibiotic that the patient has received and does not claim allergy, gather the following information:** What was the last type of infection being treated? What was the drug dose and route of administration? Have you received this drug more than once without reactions? **Other information to be gathered:** Have you had adverse reactions to any other drugs? If so, give dates and describe the reaction Document any risk factors for allergic reactions such as chronic urticaria, liver or kidney disease, HIV (human immunodeficiency virus), or any other immune deficiencies

From Ref. 15.

Aspirin and Nonsteroidal Anti-inflammatory Drugs

Aspirin and the nonsteroidal anti-inflammatory drugs (NSAIDs) can induce allergic and pseudoallergic reactions. Because these drugs are so widely used, with much over-the-counter use, the health care professional must have a basic understanding of the types of reactions that can occur and how to prevent them. Three types of reactions occur: bronchospasm with rhinoconjunctivitis, urticaria/angioedema, and anaphylaxis. Remember that patients with gastric discomfort or bruising from these agents may describe themselves as being allergic, however these are not allergic or pseudoallergic reactions.

Two specific conditions: aspirin-exacerbated respiratory disease (AERD) and chronic idiopathic urticaria, are important because they are commonly seen. AERD may include asthma, rhinitis with nasal polyps, and aspirin sensitivity.[17] Upon exposure to aspirin or a NSAID, patients with AERD experience rhinorrhea, nasal congestion, conjunctivitis, laryngospasm, and asthma. Chronic idiopathic urticaria may also be seen with aspirin or NSAID-induced pseudoallergic reactions.[18] Patients with a history of chronic idiopathic urticaria are likely to see a flare of urticaria if aspirin or a cyclooxygenase (COX)-1 inhibiting NSAID is given. Cross-reactions between aspirin and older COX-1 inhibiting NSAIDs exist in patients with AERD and chronic idiopathic urticaria. Even though product warning labels for COX-2 inhibitors state that these agents should not be used in these two conditions, there are no reports of cross-reactivity in AERD and only rare reports in patients with chronic idiopathic urticaria.[19]

❻ *IgE-mediated urticarial/angioedema reactions and anaphylaxis are associated with aspirin and NSAIDs. Urticaria is the most common form of IgE-mediated reaction. However, most reactions are the result of metabolic idiosyncracies, such as aspirin-induced respiratory disease which may produce severe and even fatal bronchospasm. This class is second only to β-lactams in causing anaphylaxis.* Most reactions in this class are due to a complex metabolic pattern which causes increasingly recurrent and severe nasal polyps and often refractory asthma. The metabolic problem is constant, once it emerges, accounting for the persistence and difficulty of these clinical problems, but is also capable of causing severe, sometimes fatal acute reactions to aspirin or many if not all the other NSAIDs as well. Rare reports of non-cross-reactive severe reactions suggest possible specific IgE-mediated reactions to individual NSAIDs, and there are some occurrences of urticaria related to NSAIDs as well. Because aspirin therapy is highly beneficial in primary and secondary prevention in coronary artery disease (CAD), aspirin desensitization should be considered in patients who have had reactions to aspirin. Desensitization is contraindicated in patients who have experienced aspirin-induced anaphylactoid reaction, hypotension, tachypnea, or altered consciousness. Alternate agents must be used. A comprehensive approach to aspirin-sensitive patients with CAD has been described.[20]

Radiocontrast Media

❼ *Radiocontrast media may cause serious, immediate pseudoallergic reactions such as urticaria/angioedema, bronchospasm, shock, and death. These reactions have been reduced with the introduction of nonionic, lower osmolality products.* Because a small percentage of patients who have reacted previously to radiocontrast media will react if reexposed, several steps (listed below) should be taken to prevent reactions in these patients. These steps should also be followed in patients with high risk factors: asthmatic patients, patients on β-blockers, and patients with cardiovascular disease.[5]

- Determine if the study is essential
- Be sure the patient understands the risks
- Ensure adequate hydration
- Use nonionic, lower osmolar agents
- Pretreat with prednisone 50 mg orally 13, 7, and 1 hour(s) before the procedure and diphenhydramine 50 mg orally 1 hour before the procedure

Delayed reactions with these agents occur in 1% to 3% of patients.[21] Although reactions are occasionally severe, most are mild and manifest as maculopapular rashes, fixed eruptions, erythema multiforme, and urticarial eruptions.

Opiates

❽ *Opiates (morphine, meperidine, codeine, hydrocodone, and others) stimulate mast cell release directly, resulting in pruritis and urticaria with occasional mild wheezing. Though these reactions are not allergic, many patients state that they are "allergic" to one or more of the opiates. Pretreatment with an antihistamine may reduce these reactions. These pseudoallergic reactions are rarely, if ever, life threatening.*[5] Avoiding other mast cell degranulating medications while patients require opiates also reduces the chances of frightening and uncomfortable reactions. Patients may state they are allergic if they have experienced gastrointestinal upset, a common side effect to opiates, with previous exposures. Obtaining a thorough history from the patient will prove useful. If a more serious reaction has occurred, a non-narcotic analgesic should be selected.

Chemotherapy

Hypersensitivity reactions have occurred with all chemotherapy agents. Reactions are most common with the taxanes, platinum compounds, asparaginases, and epipodophyllotoxins.[7] Reactions range from mild (flushing and rashes) to severe (dyspnea, bronchospasm, urticaria, and hypotension). IgE-mediated type I reactions are the most common. To reduce the risk, patients are routinely premedicated with corticosteroids and H_1 and H_2 receptor antagonists. The platinum compounds have produced anemia, probably via a cytotoxic immunologic mechanism.

Insulin

Insulin is one of a very few medications which is itself a whole protein, and can induce IgE sensitivity directly. This can result in anaphylaxis. Adverse reactions to insulin also include erythema, pruritis, and indurations,[22] which are usually transient and may be injection site-related. For the sensitivity reactions, treatment options include dexamethasone or desensitization. If the reaction is injection site-related, a change in delivery system (i.e., insulin pump or inhaled insulin) may be helpful.

Anticonvulsants

A life-threatening syndrome can occur following a few weeks of therapy with anticonvulsants, such as phenytoin, phenobarbital, and carbamazepine. Symptoms include fever, a maculopapular rash, generalized lymphadenopathy and varying degrees of internal organ dysfunction. The rash may be mild at first but can progress to exfoliative dermatitis, erythema multiforme, Stevens-Johnson syndrome, or toxic epidermal necrolysis. The causative agent should be withdrawn immediately. Valproic acid, gabapentin, and lamotrigine may be acceptable alternatives for seizure control.[5]

Drug Desensitization

Drug desensitization may be undertaken for some drugs in the absence of useful alternative medications. The risk of

Patient Encounter 2

A 55-year-old female is admitted to the hospital with an intra-abdominal infection. During the patient interview, she states that she is allergic to aspirin, codeine, sulfa drugs, penicillin, levofloxacin, and vancomycin. The reactions are described as follows:

Aspirin: Easy bruising

Codeine: Upset stomach and itching after one dose

Sulfa drugs: Mild rash occurred 2 hours after taking a double strength trimethoprim-sulfamethoxazole tablet prescribed for a urinary tract infection

Penicillin: Rash, itching, and shortness of breath

Levofloxacin: Upset stomach

Vancomycin: Burning sensation when the drug was infused

Based on the patient's descriptions, which of the reactions represent an allergic or pseudoallergic reaction?

Which medications would you want to avoid based on this history?

What further questions would be useful to ask before developing a care plan?

If narcotic analgesics are required to treat this patient, what medication may be helpful as a pretreatment?

severe systemic reactions and anaphylaxis associated with desensitization must be compared to the risk of not treating the patient. Thorough evaluation should establish that the drug probably caused the reaction by an allergic mechanism. Because of the dangers involved with drug desensitization, an expert review of the patient's indication for the drug should be conducted. Consider the possibility that the patient does not really need the drug.

❾ *Desensitization is a potentially life-threatening procedure, and requires continuous monitoring in a hospital setting, with suitable access to emergency treatment and intubation if required. It should only be undertaken under the direction of a physician with suitable training and experience. In such hands, desensitization may present less risk than treatment failure with a less effective alternative medication.*

The possibility of readministering a suspected drug may be safely tested by gradual dose escalation in some cases, and there are certainly many more patients who are harmed by inappropriately withholding medications than there are those who suffer significant harm from testing and desensitization.[23]

Only type I IgE-mediated allergy may be treated by classical desensitization. Desensitization may occur within hours to several weeks, unlike specific immunotherapy injections for inhalant allergy (i.e., "allergy shots" which may take months of therapy before a patient realizes any benefit and years to complete). The mechanism of drug desensitization is poorly understood, but produces temporary drug-specific tolerance of the offending drug. Any interruption of therapy of 24 hours or more requires full repeat desensitization, and abrupt significant increases of dosage have been reported to break through the tolerance with some drugs.

The process probably involves either: (a) cross-linking small subthreshold numbers of bound IgE molecules gradually depleting mast cells of their mediators, or (b) binding of the IgE by monomers or hapten-protein entities which cannot cross-link the antibody. The low doses used at the beginning of all protocols would provide small amounts of antigen, favoring these mechanisms. Both drug-specific IgE and IgG serum concentrations increase after successful desensitization, but skin test positivity generally decreases.[24]

Oral and intravenous protocols are available for most drugs in this category, with the oral route producing somewhat milder reactions, but the intravenous route providing more precision in dosing. Intravenous administration can also be used in unresponsive patients where the oral route is not feasible. Protocols generally begin at about 1% of the therapeutic dose and increase in intervals defined by the patient's reaction and the distribution and metabolism of the drug itself. Half-$\log_{10}$ dose increases (about threefold) are often tolerated.

Penicillin desensitization is the most common drug desensitization protocol, and is required for penicillin-allergic patients when penicillin is clearly the only treatment option, for example when syphilis is present in pregnancy. Protocols have been adapted to most antibiotics. Tables 54–6 and 54–7 describe procedures for intravenous and oral penicillin desensitization.[25]

Table 54–6

Protocol for Oral Penicillin Desensitization

Phenoxymethyl Penicillin

Step	Concentration (units/mL)	Volume (mL)	Dose (Units)	Cumulative Dose (Units)
1	1,000	0.1	100	100
2	1,000	0.2	200	300
3	1,000	0.4	400	700
4	1,000	0.8	800	1,500
5	1,000	1.6	1,600	3,100
6	1,000	3.2	3,200	6,300
7	1,000	6.4	6,400	12,700
8	10,000	1.2	12,000	24,700
9	10,000	2.4	24,000	48,700
10	10,000	4.8	48,000	96,700
11	80,000	1.0	80,000	176,700
12	80,000	2.0	160,000	336,700
13	80,000	4.0	320,000	656,700
14	80,000	8.0	640,000	1,296,700
Observe for 30 minutes				
15	500,000	0.25	125,000	
16	500,000	0.5	250,000	
17	500,000	1.0	500,000	
18	500,000	2.25	1,125,000	

From Ref. 25.

Aspirin desensitization is useful in diseases where low-level antiplatelet action is needed and in the care of patients with aspirin sensitivity and intractable nasal polyps. Lysine aspirin availability in Europe allows desensitization by inhalation at greatly reduced risk. New procedures utilizing ketorolac as a nasal topical application may allow similar reduction of risk in the United States.[26] As with all desensitizations, constant daily administration must be maintained once the desired dose is reached. Table 54–8 summarizes several similar aspirin desensitization protocols.[27] Table 54–9 depicts a 2-day alternative protocol.[28]

All desensitization procedures are expected to produce mild symptoms in the patient at some point, and the patient must be made to understand this before doses are started. Mild sensitivity to the drug still remains, and large dose increases as well as missing doses should be avoided. Late complications, such as urticaria, may occur with Type I desensitization, and serum sickness or hemolytic anemia may also occur with high-dose therapy in allergic, desensitized patients.

Some regimens are designed for outpatient administration over much longer time periods and have been used, for example with allopurinol dermal reactions. Such late-onset morbilliform reactions, sometimes overlapping with erythema multiforme minor, are difficult to evaluate as it is often unclear to what extent the patients were at risk for recurrent reaction.

Severe life-threatening reactions not mediated by IgE, such as Stevens-Johnson syndrome and toxic epidermal necrolysis, are absolute contraindications to testing, desensitization attempts, and readministration.

Table 54–7

Parenteral Penicillin Desensitization Protocol

| Injection No. | Benzylpencillin | | |
	Concentration (Units)	Volume (mL)	(Route)
1	100	0.1	ID
2	100	0.2	SC
3	100	0.4	SC
4	100	0.8	SC
5	1,000	0.1	ID
6	1,000	0.3	SC
7	1,000	0.6	SC
8	10,000	0.1	ID
9	10,000	0.2	SC
10	10,000	0.4	SC
11	10,000	0.8	SC
12	100,000	0.1	ID
13	100,000	0.3	SC
14	100,000	0.6	SC
15	1,000,000	0.1	ID
16	1,000,000	0.2	SC
17	1,000,000	0.2	IM
18	1,000,000	0.4	IM
19	Continuous IV infusion at 1,000,000 units/h		

ID, intradermal; IM, intramuscular; SC, subcutaneous.

From Ref. 25.

Table 54–8

Oral Aspirin Desensitization Protocols

Dose Increments (mg)	Dose Interval	Cumulative Dose (mg)
30, 60, 100, 325, 600	2 hours	1,115
1, 10, 50, 100, 300	30–40 minutes	461
1, 10, 50, 100, 500	60 minutes	661
30, 60, 120, 300, 600	2 hours	1,110
10, 20, 50, 80, 150, 300	30 minutes	610
30, 60, 125, 250, 500	60 minutes	965

From Ref. 27.

Table 54–9

Oral Aspirin Desensitization Protocol

| Day 1 | | Day 2 | |
Doses (mg)[a]	Cumulative Dose (mg)	Doses	Cumulative Dose (mg)
30	30	150	330
60	90	325	655
90	180	650	1,305

[a]Doses administered every 3 hours, patient observed for 3 hours after final dose.

From Ref. 28.

Patient Encounter 3

A 50-year-old male is visiting the clinic for a routine checkup. Pertinent findings are below:

PMH: Hypertension diagnosed 5 years ago, currently controlled; seasonal allergic rhinitis

FH: Father died of myocardial infarction at age 59; grandfather died of a stroke at age 62

SH: Smokes less than one pack a day; drinks one glass of red wine daily

Meds: Hydrochlorothiazide 25 mg orally once daily; atenolol 50 mg once daily; fluticasone nasal spray, one spray in each nostril daily during allergy season; loratadine 10 mg daily during allergy season

Allergies: History of an anaphylactoid reaction after taking aspirin one year ago for headache

Development of a Care Plan

Based on the patient's history, is he a candidate for daily aspirin therapy?

If so, is the patient a candidate for aspirin desensitization? Why or why not?

OUTCOME EVALUATION

To successfully treat a patient with a drug allergy or pseudoallergy, several goals must be accomplished:

- If a reaction occurs, it must be identified and managed quickly.
- The patient should be educated about the reaction.
- True drug contraindications should be avoided if at all possible.
- Patients should receive the medications they need or a suitable alternative. If this is not possible due to an allergy, desensitization should be considered.
- Patients should always be monitored for adverse drug reactions.

CONCLUSION

Allergic and pseudoallergic reactions may be mild or life threatening. Efforts to manage these reactions or change the patient's treatment due to the reactions may increase costs and prevent best therapeutic outcomes. The health care professional should carefully explore all available information to accurately assess potential risks from drugs after an apparent reaction to guide both avoidance and alternative treatments. The health care professional should partner with the patient to document reactions so the patient can avoid drugs that present dangers to them if possible and receive the best drug choices when needed.

Patient Care and Monitoring

1. Before administering any medication, take a thorough drug history to establish any past allergic or adverse reactions experienced by the patient.

2. For any reaction, use questions given in Table 54–5 to establish the nature of the reaction and the likelihood it was caused by the suspected drug. For nonantibiotics, the first question regarding infection type is not needed.

3. Document the reaction, in detail, in the patient's medical record.

4. Recommend an alternative choice if the prescribed drug is contraindicated, and develop a plan to assess safety and effectiveness.

5. Consult with a physician trained in desensitization if the patient has a true allergy and no acceptable alternative medication is available.

6. Educate the patient about the allergy or pseudoallergy so they are able to work with health care providers to avoid the reaction in the future.

Abbreviations Introduced in This Chapter

AERD	Aspirin-exacerbated respiratory disease
COX	Cyclooxygenase
D_5W	Dextrose 5% in water
ID	Intradermal
Ig	Immune globulin (followed by the specific Type of immune globulin: E, G, or M)
NSAIDs	Nonsteroidal anti-inflammatory drugs

 Self-assessment questions and answers are available at *http://www.mhpharmacotherapy.com/pp.html.*

REFERENCES

1. Lazarou J, Pomeranz BH, Corey PN. Incidence of adverse drug reactions in hospitalized patients. A meta-analysis of prospective studies. JAMA 1998;269:1200–1205.
2. Gomes ER, Demoly P. Epidemiology of hypersensitivity reactions. Curr Opin Allergy Clin Immunol 2005;5(4):309–316.
3. Impicciatore P, Choonara I, Clarkson A, et al. Incidence of adverse drug reactions in paediatric in/out patients: A systematic review and meta-analysis of prospective studies. Br J Clin Pharmacol 2001;52:77–83.
4. Adkinson NF, Essayan D, Gruchalla R, et al. Task force report: Future research needs for the prevention and management of immune-mediated drug hypersensitivity reactions. J Allergy Clin Immunol 2002;109(3):S461–S478.
5. Anon, Part 1: Executive summary of disease management of drug hypersensitivity: A practice parameter. Ann Allergy Asthma Immunol 1999;83:665–700.
6. Pichler WJ. Delayed drug hypersensitivity reactions. Ann Intern Med 2003;139:683–690.
7. Gruchalla RS. Allergic disorders. J Allergy Clin Immunol 2003:111(2):S548–S559.
8. Neugut A, Ghatak A, Miller R. Anaphylaxis in the United States: An investigation into its epidemiology. Arch Intern Med 2001;161:15–21.
9. Lieberman P, Kemp SF, Oppenheimer J, et al. The diagnosis and management of anaphylaxis: An updated practice parameter. J Allergy Clin Immunol 2005;115(3):S483–S523.
10. Thethi AK and Van Dellen RG. Dilemmas and controversies in penicillin allergy. Immunol Allergy Clin North Am 2004;24:445–461.
11. Sullivan TJ. Current Therapy in Allergy. St. Louis, MO: Mosby, 1985:57–61.
12. Kelkar PS, Li JT. Cephalosporin allergy. N Engl J Med 2001;345:804–809.
13. Madaan A, Li JT. Cephalosporin allergy. Immunol Allergy Clin North Am 2004;24:463–476.
14. Strom BL, Schinnar R, Apter AJ, et al. Absence of cross-reactivity between sulfonamide antibiotics and sulfonamide nonantibiotics. N Engl J Med 2003;349(17):1628–1635.
15. Slatore CG, Tilles SA. Sulfonamide hypersensitivity. Immunol Allergy Clin North Am 2004;24:477–490.
16. Macy E. Multiple antibiotic allergy syndrome. Immunol Allergy Clin North Am 2004;24:533–543.
17. Fahrenholz J. Natural history and clinical features of aspirin-exacerbated respiratory disease. Clin Rev Allergy Immunol 2003;24:113–24.
18. Sanchez-Borges M, Caprilles-Hulett A, Caballero-Fonseca F. Cutaneous reactions to aspirin and NSAIDs. Clin Rev Allergy Immunol 2003;24:125–135.

19. Stevenson DD. Aspirin and NSAID sensitivity. Immunol Allergy Clin North Am 2004;24:491–505.

20. Ramanuja S, Breall JA, Kalaria VG. Approach to "Aspirin allergy" in cardiovascular patients. Circulation 2004;110:e1–e4.

21. Christiansen C. X-ray contrast media—An overview. Toxicology 2005;209:185–187.

22. Richardson T, Kerr D. Skin-related complications of insulin therapy: Epidemiology and emerging management strategies. Am J Clin Dermatol 2003;4(10):661–667.

23. Adkinson NF Jr, "Drug Allergy," Middleton's Allergy Principles & Practice, 6th ed. Philadelphia, PA: Mosby, 2003:1690.

24. Schmitz-Schumann M, Juhl E, et al. Analgesic asthma-provocation challenge with acetylsalicylic acid. Atemw Lungenkrkh Jahrgang 1985;10:479–485.

25. Weiss ME, Adkinson NF. Diagnostic testing for drug hypersensitivity. Immunol Allerg Clin North Am 1998;18:731–734.

26. White A, Bigby T, Stevenson D. Intranasal ketorolac challenge for the diagnosis of aspirin exacerbated respiratory disease. Ann Allergy Asthma Immunol 2006;97:190–195.

27. Melillo G, Balzano G, Bianco S, et al. Report of the INTERASMA Working Group on Standardization of Inhalation Provocation Tests in Aspirin-induced Asthma. Oral and inhalation provocation tests for the diagnosis of aspirin-induced asthma. Allergy 2001;56(9):899–911.

28. Stevenson DD and Simon R, Sensitivity to aspirin and non-steroidal anti-inflammatory drugs. In: Middleton E et al., eds. Allergy Principles and Practice. St. Louis, MO: Mosby, 1998:1225.

55 Solid Organ Transplantation

Steven Gabardi and Ali J. Olyaei

LEARNING OBJECTIVES

● **Upon completion of the chapter, the reader will be able to:**

1. Describe the reasons for solid-organ transplantation.

2. Differentiate between the functions of cell-mediated and humoral immunity and how they relate to organ transplant.

3. Describe the roles of the antigen-presenting cells (APCs) in initiating the immune response.

4. Compare and contrast the types of rejection including hyperacute, acute, chronic, and humoral rejection.

5. Define the terms "host-graft adaptation" and "tolerance," paying close attention to their differences.

6. Discuss the desired therapeutic outcomes and appropriate pharmacotherapy utilized to avoid allograft rejection.

7. Compare and contrast the currently available immunosuppressive agents in terms of mechanisms of action, adverse events, and drug–drug interactions (DDIs).

8. Design an appropriate therapeutic regimen for the management of immunosuppressive drug complications based on patient-specific information.

9. Develop a therapeutic drug-monitoring plan to assess effectiveness and adverse events of the immunosuppressive drugs.

10. Write appropriate patient education instructions and identify methods to improve patient adherence following transplantation.

KEY CONCEPTS

❶ T cells are the chief component initiating the immune response against the allograft. The activity of T cells is mediated largely through the synthesis and release of interleukin-2 (IL-2).

❷ Antigen-presenting cells (APCs) are vital in initiation of the immune response and play a role in both direct and indirect allorecognition.

❸ The goal of pharmacotherapy in transplantation is to induce immunosuppression with a multidrug approach to target various points of the immune system with resultant long-term allograft and patient survival, while minimizing the complications of suppressing the immune system.

❹ The goals of induction therapy are to improve short-term allograft and patient survival, and to reduce the incidence of acute rejection in the immediate post-transplant period.

❺ The calcineurin inhibitors, cyclosporine and tacrolimus, block T-cell activation by inhibiting the production of IL-2. They are associated with significant adverse events, such as nephrotoxicity, cardiovascular disease, post-transplant diabetes, and neurotoxicity.

❻ The antiproliferatives, azathioprine, and the mycophenolic acid derivatives inhibit T-cell proliferation. Myelosuppression is the most significant adverse event associated with these agents.

❼ Sirolimus, a target of rapamycin inhibitor, works by decreasing the ability of T cells to respond to IL-2. The major adverse events associated with this agent are decreased wound healing, hyperlipidemia and myelosuppression. This agent appears to have promising effects in allowing for calcineurin inhibitor withdrawal in some patient populations.

❽ Corticosteroids induce a nonspecific immuno-suppression. Due to their overwhelming incidence of adverse events, many practitioners attempt to use

939

low-dose maintenance therapy or, in some cases, complete steroid withdrawal. These agents are also effective in reversing acute rejection.

❾ Long-term patient and allograft survival is complicated by several factors, including drug–drug interactions (DDIs) with the immunosuppressive agents, infectious disease, cardiovascular disease, new onset diabetes after transplant, and malignancy. The goals of treating these complications are to prevent allograft damage and improve patient survival.

INTRODUCTION

The earliest recorded attempts at organ transplant date back thousands of years.[1] More than a few apocryphal descriptions exist from ancient Egypt, China, India, and Rome describing experimentation with transplantation. For example, an Indian text from 2nd century BC describes the procedure for nasal reconstruction surgery with the use of autografted skin. Also, Roman Catholic lore has saints Damian and Cosmas replacing the gangrenous leg of a man with the leg of a recently deceased man in the third century AD.[1]

French surgeon, Alexis Carrel, pioneered the art of surgical techniques for transplantation in the early 1900s.[1] Together with Charles Guthrie, Carrel experimented in artery and vein transplantation. Using revolutionary methods in anastomosis operations and suturing techniques, Carrel laid the groundwork for modern transplant surgery. He was one of the first to identify the dilemma of rejection, an issue that remained nearly impossible to circumvent for nearly half a century.[1]

Prior to the work of Alexis Carrel, malnourishment was the prevailing theory regarding the mechanism of allograft rejection.[1] However, in 1910, Carrel noted that tissue damage in the transplanted organ was likely caused by multiple, circulating biological factors. It was not until the late 1940s with the work of Peter Medawar that we began to gain a better understanding of transplant immunology. Medawar was able to define the immunologic nature of rejection using skin allografts. In addition, George Snell observed that grafts shared between inbred animals were accepted but were rejected when transplanted between animals of different strains.[1]

The seminal work by early transplant researchers eventually led to the concept of histocompatibility.[1,2] Histocompatibility describes the process where polymorphic genes encode cell membrane antigens that serve as targets for immune response, even within a species. Further research in transplant immunobiology has led to an accurate understanding of the immune response after transplantation.[1,2]

Joseph Murray performed the first successful organ transplant in 1954.[1] It was a kidney transplant between identical twins. This was a success in large part because no immunosuppression was necessary due to the fact that the donor and recipient were genetically identical. Murray's success led to attempts with other organs (Table 55–1).

EPIDEMIOLOGY AND ETIOLOGY

Heart

Nearly five million Americans are afflicted with heart failure.[1,3] Cardiac transplantation is one option for patients with severe congestive heart failure. Candidates for cardiac transplantation generally present with New York Heart Association (NYHA) class III or IV symptoms and have an ejection fraction of less than 20%. The general indications for cardiac transplantation include rapidly declining cardiac function and having a projected 1-year mortality rate of greater than 75%. Mechanical support with an implantable left ventricular assist device may be appropriate as bridge therapy while patients await the availability of a viable organ.[1,3] Indications for heart transplant include:

- Cardiomyopathy (i.e., dilated myopathy, hypertrophic cardiomyopathy, restrictive myopathy)
- Congenital heart disease
- Coronary artery disease
- Valvular heart disease

Most heart transplants are orthotopic; however, in certain situations, heterotopic cardiac transplants have been performed. There have been a handful of cardiac transplants that involved living donation. Although this seems strange, this occurs when one patient receives a simultaneous heart-lung transplant, but their native heart is well functioning and may be subsequently transplanted into another recipient. This procedure is referred to as a "domino" heart transplant. There were 1,852 heart transplant procedures done in 2009.[3]

Intestine

An intestine transplant may involve the use of an entire intestine or just a shortened segment. The majority of intestine transplants completed in the United States have involved the transplant of the full organ and are often performed in conjunction with a liver transplant. Although most intestine transplants involve organs harvested from a deceased donor, recent advances in the field have made it possible for living donor intestinal segment transplants.

Table 55–1

Solid Organ Transplant History

Year	Event
1963	First successful deceased donor kidney transplant
1966	First successful pancreas transplant
1967	First successful liver transplant
1967	First successful heart transplant
1981	First successful heart-lung transplant
1983	First successful single-lung transplant
1987	First successful double-lung transplant
1987	First successful intestine transplant
1989	First successful living donor liver transplant
1990	First successful living donor lung transplant
1998	First successful live-donor partial pancreas transplant

There were 155 intestine transplants (152 deceased donors, 2 living donors) done in 2009.[3] Reasons for intestine transplant include:

- Functional bowel problems (i.e., Hirschsprung's disease, neuronal intestinal dysplasia, pseudoobstruction, protein-losing enteropathy, microvillous inclusion disease)
- Short gut syndrome (i.e., intestinal artresia, necrotizing enterocolitis, intestinal volvulus, massive resection secondary to inflammatory bowel disease, tumors, mesenteric thrombosis)

Kidneys

Over 20 million Americans have chronic kidney disease (CKD), with another 20 million more considered to be at increased risk for the development of kidney disease. End-stage renal disease (ESRD) only constitutes a small portion of those patients with CKD, with over 450,000 patients currently diagnosed with ESRD throughout the United States. However, the ESRD population continues to increase, with projections estimating that more than 660,000 people will carry a diagnosis of ESRD by 2010. All patients with ESRD should be considered for renal transplantation if they are healthy enough to undergo the transplant surgery. A successful kidney transplant offers advantages in terms of both quality and duration of life compared to other renal replacement therapies (i.e., hemodialysis, peritoneal dialysis). It is also more effective than dialysis from a medical and economic perspective. Reasons for kidney transplant include:

- Congenital, familial, and metabolic disorders (i.e., congenital obstructive uropathy, Fabry's disease, medullary cystic disease, nephrolithiasis)
- Diabetes mellitus (DM)
- Glomerular diseases (i.e., antiglomerular basement membrane disease, focal segmental glomerularsclerosis, IgA nephropathy, hemolytic uremic syndrome, systemic lupus erythematosus, Alport's syndrome, amyloidosis, membranous nephropathy, Goodpasture's syndrome)
- Hypertension
- Neoplasm (i.e., renal cell carcinoma, Wilms' tumor)
- Polycystic kidney disease (PKD)
- Renovascular disease
- Tubular and interstitial diseases (i.e., analgesic nephropathy, drug-induced nephritis, oxalate nephropathy, radiation nephritis, acute tubular necrosis, sarcoidosis)

Most kidney transplant procedures are heterotopic, where the kidney is implanted above the pelvic bone and attached to the patient's iliac artery and vein. The ureter of the transplant kidney is attached directly to the recipient's bladder or native ureter. The native kidneys are usually not removed, and data have shown that under most circumstances, removal of the native kidneys does not influence patient and **allograft survival**. However, special circumstances, such as renal cell carcinoma and PKD, may necessitate native kidney removal.[1,3] There were 14,059 (8,812 deceased donors, 5,247 living donors) kidney transplants done in 2009.[3]

Liver

A liver transplant may involve the use of the entire organ or a segment of the liver. The majority of cases involve utilizing the full organ (deceased donor); however, segmental transplants are gaining popularity. In recent years, segmental transplants have been conducted using living donors. This procedure requires donation of the left hepatic lobe, which accounts for nearly 60% of the overall liver mass. This type of procedure is possible because the liver can regenerate; therefore, both the donor and recipient, in theory, will have normal liver function shortly after the transplant procedure.[1,3] There were 5,316 (5,124 deceased donors, 192 partial lobe-living donors) liver transplants done in 2009.[3] Reasons for liver transplant include:

- Acute hepatic necrosis (i.e., chronic or acute hepatitis B or C)
- Biliary atresia
- Cholestatic liver disease/cirrhosis (i.e., primary biliary cirrhosis)
- Metabolic disease (i.e., Wilson's disease, primary oxalosis, hyperlipidemia)
- Neoplasms (i.e., hepatoma, cholangiocarcinoma, hepatoblastoma, bile duct cancer)
- Noncholestatic cirrhosis (i.e., alcoholic cirrhosis, postnecrotic cirrhosis, drug-induced cirrhosis)

Lungs

Lung transplants may involve deceased donation of two lungs or a single lung. More recently, lobar transplants from blood group compatible living donors have been performed for a small segment of the population. Most of the lobar transplants have been performed on cystic fibrosis patients. On rare occasions, a simultaneous heart-lung transplant occurs. This type of procedure is reserved for patients with severe pulmonary and cardiac disease. There were 1,392 (1,391 deceased donors, 1 living donor) lung transplants and 23 simultaneous heart-lung transplant procedures done in 2009.[3] Reasons for lung transplant include:

- α-1-Antitrypsin deficiency
- Congenital disease (i.e., Eisenmenger's syndrome)
- Cystic fibrosis
- Emphysema/chronic obstructive pulmonary disease
- Idiopathic pulmonary fibrosis
- Primary pulmonary hypertension

Pancreas

The exact nationwide prevalence of all diseases of the pancreas has not been fully quantified; however DM, both types 1 and 2, affects nearly 21 million people in the United States alone.

Some people suffering from DM may also be afflicted with ESRD. A small percentage of these patients may undergo a simultaneous pancreas-kidney (SPK) transplant, which may be accomplished using organs from deceased or living donors. There were 325 pancreas transplants and 724 SPK procedures done in 2009.[3] Reasons for pancreas transplants include:

- DM (i.e., type 1 and 2, DM secondary to chronic pancreatitis, DM secondary to cystic fibrosis)
- Pancreatic cancer

Transplant of a pancreas may involve either the entire organ or a pancreas segment. Currently, whole organ transplant is the most common procedure, with a portion of the duodenum often transplanted along with the pancreas. Living donors are often the source of segmental transplants. In recent years, isolation and transplantation of β islet cells alone have been completed. Islet transplantation is intended to treat organ dysfunction by replacing nonfunctioning islet cells with new ones. In most cases no surgery is needed, and islet cells from a deceased donor's pancreas are removed and infused into a portal vein of the patient. Islet transplants are still considered experimental, and long-term benefit and/or risk of this procedure needs to be studied extensively.

PATHOPHYSIOLOGY

Major Histocompatibility Complex

The primary target of the immune response against a transplanted organ is the major histocompatibility complex (MHC).[1,2] The MHC is a region of highly polymorphic genes located on the short arm of chromosome six. The human MHC is referred to as human leukocyte antigen (HLA). HLA are a set of glycoproteins that are expressed on the surface of most cells. These proteins are involved in immune recognition, which is the discrimination of self from nonself, but are also the principal antigenic determinants of allograft rejection.[1,2]

The protein products of the HLA have been classified into two major groups, Class I and II:

- Class I: these molecules are expressed on the surfaces of all nucleated cells and are recognized by CD8+ cells, also known as cytotoxic T cells.
  - The three subclasses of MHC Class I are HLA-A, HLA-B, and HLA-C.
- Class II: these molecules are expressed solely on the surfaces of antigen-presenting cells (APCs). The APCs serve to stimulate CD4+ cells, also known as helper T cells.
  - The three subclasses of MHC Class II are HLA-DP, HLA-DQ, and HLA-DR.

T and B Lymphocytes

Lymphocytes are one of the five kinds of white blood cells. Mature lymphocytes are astonishingly diverse in their functions. The most abundant of the lymphocytes are T lymphocytes (also called T cells) and B lymphocytes (also called B cells).

T Lymphocytes

❶ *T cells play a major role in the cell-mediated immune response.* These cells are produced in the bone marrow but their final stage of development occurs in the thymus, hence the abbreviation "T." There are three recognized subclasses of T cells.

- Cytotoxic T cells (CD8+) promote target cell destruction by activating cellular **apoptosis** or aggressively killing the target cell via the release of cytotoxic proteins.
- Helper T cells (CD4+) are the great communicators of the immune response. Once activated, they proliferate and secrete cytokines that regulate **effector cell** function. Some helper T cells secrete cytokines that recruit cytotoxic T cells, B cells, or APCs, while others secrete cytokines that turn off the immune response once an antigen has been destroyed.
- Regulatory T cells, or suppressor T cells, suppress the activation of an immune response. The activity of these cells in organ transplant is not well elucidated.

B Lymphocytes

B cells play a large role in the humoral immune response. In humans, B cells are produced and mature in the bone marrow. The human body produces several types of B cells. Each B cell is unique, with a distinctive cell surface receptor protein that binds to only one particular antigen. Once B cells encounter their antigen and receive a cytokine signal from helper T cells, they can further differentiate into one of two cells, plasma B cells or memory B cells. Plasma B cells secrete antibodies that induce the destruction of target antigens through a process known as **opsonization**. Memory B cells play an important role in long-term immunity. Once formed to a specific antigen, memory B cells are capable of rapidly responding to subsequent exposures to their target antigen.

Antigen-Presenting Cells

❷ *APCs are vital in initiation of the immune response. An APC is a cell that displays a foreign antigen complexed with MHC on its cell surface.* Its major responsibility is to present these foreign antigens to T cells. T cells can identify this complex using their T-cell receptors (TCRs). There are three main types of APCs: dendritic cells (DCs), macrophages, and activated B cells. DC are present in tissues that are in contact with the environment, such as the skin and the lining of the nose, lungs, stomach, and intestines. They are responsible for antigen **phagocytosis**. After phagocytosis, they express the foreign antigen on their cell surface and then migrate to the lymphoid tissues to interact with T and B cells to initiate the immune response. Macrophages' main role is in the removal of pathogens and necrotic debris. However, like DCs, macrophages also phagocytize antigens and express them on their cell membranes to present to T cells in order to initiate an immune response. The first time an antigen is encountered, the DCs and macrophages act as the primary APCs. However, if the same antigen is encountered again, memory B cells become the most important APC because they initiate the immune response quickly after antigen presentation. It appears that both the DCs and macrophages have the most activity in terms of allorecognition.

Allorecognition

1 2 *Recognition of the antigens displayed by the transplanted organ (alloantigens) is the prime event that initiates the immune response against the allograft.* There are currently two accepted pathways for T-cell allorecognition, direct and indirect pathways:

- Direct pathway: donor APCs migrate out of the allograft into the recipient's lymph nodes and present donor MHC molecules to the TCR of the recipient's T cells.

- Indirect pathway: recipient APCs migrate into the graft and phagocytize alloantigens. The donor MHC molecules are then expressed on the cell surface of the recipient's APCs and presented to recipient T cells in the lymph nodes.

T-cell activation

1 *Whether it is by the direct or indirect pathway, in order for a T cell to become activated against the transplanted organ, two interactions, or signals must take place between the APCs and the recipient's T cells*[1,2]:

- Signal 1 is the interaction of the TCR with the foreign antigens presented by the APCs.

- A second, costimulatory signal, known as Signal 2, must also take place for T-cell activation. This signal is an interaction between one of several costimulatory receptors and paired ligands on the cell surfaces of the APCs and T cells, respectively. This interaction is of the utmost importance, as Signal 1 in the absence of Signal 2 induces T-cell anergy.

Once activated, T cells undergo clonal expansion under the influence of cytokines, specifically interleukin-2 (IL-2). These steps elicit an antidonor T-cell response that results in graft destruction.

Mechanisms of Acute Rejection

After activation, cytotoxic T cells emerge from lymphoid organs to infiltrate the graft and trigger the immune response. These cells have been shown to induce graft destruction via two mechanisms: (a) secretion of the cytotoxic proteins perforin and granzyme B and (b) induction of cellular apoptosis through interaction with various cell surface receptors. Besides the cytotoxic T cells, several other cell lines may play a role in allograft destruction including B cells, granulocytes, and natural killer cells.

Types of Rejection

▶ *Hyperacute Rejection*

Hyperacute rejection is an immediate recipient immune response against the allograft due to the presence of preformed recipient antibodies directed against the donor's HLA. This type of reaction generally occurs within minutes of the transplant. The organ must be removed immediately to prevent a severe systemic response. Those patients at highest risk for hyperacute rejection include any patients that have preformed HLA or ABO blood group antibodies, including patients with a history of a previous organ transplant, or multiple blood transfusions, as well as mothers receiving transplanted organs from their children. Hyperacute rejection has been largely eliminated due to routine surveillance testing completed prior to the transplant.

▶ *Acute Rejection*

Acute rejection is a cell-mediated process that generally occurs within 5 to 90 days after the transplant procedure; however, it can occur at any time post-transplant. This reaction is mediated through alloreactive T cells as discussed previously in the Mechanisms of Acute Rejection section. Organ specific signs and symptoms of acute rejection can be seen in Table 55–2.[1,3]

To avoid acute or chronic rejection, assessment of pretransplant immune risk factors of recipients plays an important role in the prevention of immune-mediated allograft injuries. Evaluation of the presence or absence of alloantibodies and T cell activities to HLA antigens plays a significant role in individualization of immunosuppressive therapy. Patients with a high panel of reactive antibodies (PRA) have a greater risk of immune mediated injuries to the transplanted allograft. The PRA test measures the recipient's mismatches and preformed antibodies against 50 to 60 different individuals (not donor).[4] If 25 cells react, it is considered 50% reactive (PRA of 50%). Patients with higher PRAs and preformed antibodies have lower long-term allograft survival. Although PRA is a sensitive test and has predictive value, lymphocytes directly obtained from donor is a superior method of immune monitoring before and early after transplant.[4] The assay is aimed to detect the presence of antibodies directed against the HLA antigens of the donor. In this setting, presence of donor-specific antibodies (DSA) are identified. In one study, the allograft survival was significantly lower in patients with DSA. Thus, detecting DSA and presence of high PRA may indicate the need to enhance immunosuppression to improve post-transplant long-term outcomes and allograft survival rate.

▶ *Humoral Rejection*

Also known as antibody-mediated rejection, humoral rejection is the process of creating graft-specific antibodies.[1,5] This type of rejection occurs less frequently than cell-mediated acute rejection. Humoral rejection is characterized by deposition of immunoglobulins and complement in

Table 55–2

Organ-Specific Signs and Symptoms of an Acute Rejection Episode

Organ	Clinical Symptoms	Laboratory Signs
Heart	Fever, lethargy, weakness, SOB, DOE, hypotension, tachycardia, atrial flutter, ventricular arrhythmias	Leukocytosis, endomyocardial biopsy positive for mononuclear infiltrates
Kidney	Fever, graft tenderness and swelling, decreased urine output, malaise, hypertension, weight gain, edema	Increased SCr, BUN, leukocytosis, renal biopsy positive for lymphocytic infiltration
Intestine	Fever and GI symptoms (i.e., bloating, cramping, diarrhea, increased stomal output)	There are no reliable biochemical markers for intestine transplant rejection, but biopsies may be helpful.
Liver	Fever, lethargy, change in color or quantity of bile in patients with biliary T-tube, graft tenderness and swelling, back pain, anorexia, ileus, tachycardia, jaundice, ascites, encephalopathy	Abnormal LFTs, increased bilirubin, alkaline phosphate, transaminases, biopsy positive for mononuclear cell infiltrate with evidence of tissue damage
Lung	Fever, impaired gas exchange, SOB, malaise, anxiety	Decreased FEV, infiltrate on CXR, biopsy positive for lymphocytic infiltration
Pancreas	Fever, graft tenderness and swelling, abdominal pain, ileus, and malaise	Increased FBS, leukocytosis, decreased human C-peptide and urinary amylase levels

BUN, blood urea nitrogen; CXR, chest x-ray; DOE, dyspnea on exertion; FBS, fasting blood sugar; FEV, forced expiratory volume; LFTs, liver function tests; SCr, serum creatinine; SOB, shortness of breath

From Refs. 1, 3.

allograft tissues. Treatment for this type of rejection is not well defined; yet several reports have shown that treatments such as plasmapheresis, immunoglobulin therapy, rituximab and/or antithymocyte globulin, or other B cell targeted agents may be effective.

▶ Chronic Rejection

Chronic rejection has traditionally been thought of as a slow, insidious form of acute rejection, resulting in worsening organ function over time. The exact immunologic processes of chronic rejection are poorly understood; however, many believe that both the cell-mediated and humoral immune systems and drug-induced toxicities play a vital role in its development. Currently, retransplantation is the only effective treatment option.[1,6]

Host-Graft Adaptation

The term host-graft adaptation describes the decreased immune response against the allograft over time.[2] This phenomenon is evident by the reduced incidence of acute rejection episodes seen months after the transplant procedure. In theory, host-graft adaptation is thought to be secondary to a weakened T-cell response to the donor antigens when patients are receiving maintenance immunosuppression.[2]

Tolerance

Tolerance is the process that allows organ-specific antigens to be accepted as self.[2,7] This would mean that the immune system would cease to respond to the allograft and immunosuppressive medications would not be required. Immune tolerance has been achieved in the lab, but has yet to be successfully accomplished in humans.[2,7] The definition of "achieved tolerance" is highly variable and subjective.

Currently, a number of protocols focusing on testing clinically-safe regimens to achieve chimerism or tolerance are being studied.

TREATMENT

Desired Outcome

❸ *The major focus of transplant practitioners is to achieve long-term patient and allograft survival.*[2,8] Short-term outcomes (e.g., acute rejection rates, 1-year graft survival) have improved significantly since the first successful transplant due to an improved understanding of the immune system and enhancements in surgical techniques, organ procurement, immunosuppression, and post-transplant care. Despite the success in improving short-term outcomes, the overall frequency of graft loss remains higher than desired.[1,2]

It is imperative that transplant practitioners be aware of the specific advantages and disadvantages of the available immunosuppressants, as well as their adverse drug reaction and drug–drug interaction (DDI) profiles. There are generally considered to be three stages of medical immunosuppression: (a) induction therapy, (b) maintenance therapy, and (c) treatment of acute rejection episodes. ❸ *Overall, the immunosuppressive regimens utilize multiple medications that work on different targets of the immune system.* Please refer to Table 55–3 for a list of all currently available immunosuppressive agents.[2,8,9]

Immunosuppressive Therapies— Induction Therapy

❹ *The goal of induction therapy is to provide a high level of immunosuppression in the critical early post-transplant period,*

Table 55–3

Currently Available Immunosuppressive Agents

Generic Name (Brand Name)	Common Dosage	Common Adverse Effects	AWP (Per Dose or Dosage Form)
Induction Therapy Agents			
Alemtuzumab (Campath)	20–30 mg × 1–2 doses	Flu-like symptoms, chills, rigors, fever, rash, myelosuppression	$1,230.60–$3,682.36
Antithymocyte globulin equine (ATGAM)	15 mg/kg IV × 3–14 days	Flu-like symptoms, chills, rigors, fever, rash, myelosuppression	$21,797.24–$101,720.47
Antithymocyte globulin rabbit (Thymoglobulin)	1.5 mg/kg IV × 3–14 days	Flu-like symptoms, chills, rigors, fever, rash, myelosuppression	$5,433.75–$25,357.50
OKT-3 (Orthoclone OKT-3)	5 mg IV × 7–14 days	Headache, hypertension, pulmonary edema, tremor, fever, aseptic meningitis	$6,935.46–$13,870.92
Daclizumab (Zenapax)	1 mg/kg IV × 5 doses	Hyperglycemia (only after infusion)	$6,906.76
Basiliximab (Simulect)	20 mg IV × 2 doses	None reported compared to placebo	$3,400.72
Maintenance Immunosuppressants			
Cyclosporine (Sandimmune, Neoral, Gengraf)	4–5 mg/kg by mouth twice a day	Neurotoxicity, gingival hyperplasia, hirsutism, hypertension, hyperlipidemia, glucose intolerance, nephrotoxicity, electrolyte abnormalities	Sandimmune 25 mg = $1.74 100 mg = $6.93 Neoral 25 mg = $1.53 100 mg = $6.11 Gengraf 25 mg = $1.38 100 mg = $5.50
Tacrolimus (Prograf)	0.05–0.075 mg/kg by mouth twice a day	Neurotoxicity, alopecia, hypertension, hyperlipidemia, glucose intolerance, nephrotoxicity, electrolyte abnormalities	1 mg = $3.97 5 mg = $19.74
Azathioprine (Imuran)	1–2.5 mg/kg by mouth once a day	Myelosuppression, GI disturbances, pancreatitis	50 mg = $1.30
Mycophenolate mofetil (CellCept)	0.5–1.5 gm by mouth twice a day	Myelosuppression, GI disturbances	250 mg = $3.11 500 mg = $6.21
Enteric-coated MPA (Myfortic)	720 mg by mouth twice a day	Myelosuppression, GI disturbances	180 mg = $2.53 360 mg = $5.05
Sirolimus (Rapamune)	1–10 mg by mouth once a day	Hypertriglyceridemia, myelosuppression, mouth sores, hypercholesterolemia, GI disturbances, impaired wound healing, lymphocele, pneumonitis	1 mg = $6.57 2 mg = $13.15
Prednisone (Deltasone)	Maintenance: 2.5–20 mg by mouth once a day	Mood disturbances, psychosis, cataracts, hypertension, fluid retention, peptic ulcers, osteoporosis, muscle weakness, impaired wound healing, glucose intolerance, weight gain, hyperlipidemia	2.5 mg = $0.07 5 mg = $0.04 10 mg = $0.06 20 mg = $0.11

AWP, average wholesale price; MPA, mycophenolic acid.

From Refs. 2, 8, 9.

when the risk of acute rejection is highest.[2,8,10–12] This stage of immunosuppression is often initiated intraoperatively or immediately postoperatively and is generally concluded within the first 7 to 10 days after transplantation. Induction therapy is not a mandatory stage of recipient immunosuppression. However, since acute rejection is a major concern in solid organ transplant recipients and its impact on chronic rejection is undeniable, induction therapy is often considered essential to optimize outcomes.[2,8,10–12]

▶ Goals of Induction Therapy

❹ First, the induction agents are highly immunosuppressive, allowing for significant reductions in acute rejection episodes and improved 1-year graft survival. Second, due to their unique pharmacologic effect, these agents are often considered essential for use in patients at high risk for poor short-term outcomes, such as those patients with preformed antibodies, history of previous organ transplants, multiple HLA mismatches, or transplantation of organs with prolonged cold ischemic time, or from expanded criteria donors. Specifically in renal transplant recipients, induction therapy plays an important role in preventing early onset calcineurin inhibitor-induced nephrotoxicity. With the use of induction agents, initiation of calcineurin inhibitors can be delayed until the graft regains a modicum of function.[8,11,12]

The improved short-term outcomes gained from induction therapy come with a degree of risk. By using these highly immunosuppressive agents, particularly the antilymphocyte antibodies (ALA; Muronomab-CD3 [OKT-3], the antithymocyte antibodies, and alemtuzumab), the body loses much of its innate ability to mount a cell-mediated immune response, which increases the risk of opportunistic infections and malignancy.[8,12] Cytokine release syndrome is a common complication of T-cell depleting agents following first two doses and require methylprednisolone, diphenhydramine, and acetaminophen 30 to 60 minutes before infusion.

▶ Currently Available Induction Therapies

Please note that declining worldwide use and the expense associated with manufacturing both muromonab-CD3 and daclizumab have led the makers of these agents to decide to discontinue their production. At the time of this publication, it is expected that the current supply of muromonab-CD3 will last through the end of 2010 and the current supply of daclizumab will last through 2011. Once these supplies have been exhausted, these agents will no longer be available for clinical use.

Basiliximab and Daclizumab Both of these agents are monoclonal antibodies. Daclizumab is a humanized antibody that is approximately 10% murine and 90% human, while basiliximab is a chimeric antibody that is approximately 30% murine and 70% human.[8,10] These agents bind with high affinity to the IL-2 receptor where they act as receptor antagonists. These receptors are present on almost all activated T cells. Their role in induction therapy involves inhibiting IL-2 mediated activation of lymphocytes, which is an important step for the clonal expansion of T cells.

The dose of basiliximab is 20 mg IV given within 2 hours prior to the transplant, followed by a second 20 mg dose on postop day 4.[8,9,11] This dosing schedule can be used for both children greater than or equal to 35 kg (77 lb) and adults. Two 10 mg doses with the same dosing schedule should be used for children less than 35 kg (77 lb). There is no specific dosage adjustments needed in renal or hepatic impairment.[8,9,11]

The FDA-approved dose of daclizumab is 1 mg/kg within 24 hours of transplant surgery and then 1 mg/kg administered every 2 weeks after surgery for a total of five doses.[8,9,11] No dose adjustment is necessary in renal impairment but no data are available for dose adjustments in hepatic dysfunction. Several trials have shown that a shorter dosing regimen of daclizumab, two doses given in a similar manner as basiliximab, may be as safe and effective as the full, five-dose course.[13,14]

Safety is one of the most evident benefits of induction therapy with the IL-2 receptor antibodies. The most common adverse reaction with daclizumab is hyperglycemia, with clinical studies showing that a total of 32% of patients developed hyperglycemia.[9,11] The majority of the high glucose levels occurred the day after transplant or in patients with pre-existing DM. All other adverse events in the daclizumab clinical trials showed no statistically significant difference compared to placebo. The incidence of all adverse reactions with basiliximab was similar to placebo in clinical trials.[10,12]

Antithymocyte Globulin Equine Antithymocyte globulin equine (eATG) contains antibodies against several T-cell surface markers, including CD2, CD3, CD4, CD8, CD11a, and CD18. After binding to these cell surface markers, eATG promotes T-cell depletion through opsonization and complement-mediated T-cell lysis.[8-10] The common dosing strategy for eATG when used for induction therapy is 10 to 30 mg/kg/day IV for 3 to 14 days. The first dose usually begins shortly before or after transplantation.[8-10]

After T-cell lysis there is a cytokine release. Due to this phenomenon, eATG is associated with several adverse reactions.[8-10] The most common of these include fever (63%), chills (43.2%), headache (34.6%), back pain (43.2%), nausea (28.4%), diarrhea (32.1%), dizziness (24.7%), malaise (3.7%), and myelosuppression (leukopenia [29.6%] and thrombocytopenia [44.4%]). The overall incidence of opportunistic infections is 27.2%, with cytomegalovirus (CMV) disease occurring in 11.1% of patients. There are currently no reported pharmacokinetic DDIs with this agent.[8-10]

Antithymocyte Globulin Rabbit (Thymoglobulin)

Thymoglobulin induces T-cell clearance, but more importantly, it alters T-cell activation, homing, and cytotoxic activities. Compared to eATG, thymoglobulin causes less T-cell lysis due to its multiple mechanisms of immunosuppression. It is also believed that thymoglobulin plays a role in inducing T-cell apoptosis. Thymoglobulin has been dosed between 1 and 4 mg/kg/day (typically dosed at 1.5 mg/kg/day) and is usually administered for 3 to 10 days after transplantation.[8-10] Many renal transplant centers aim to initiate the first dose intraoperatively to help reduce organ reperfusion injury.

Adverse reactions are common and may include fever (63.4%), chills (57.3%), headache (40.2%), nausea (36.6%), diarrhea (36.6%), malaise (13.4%), dizziness (8.5%), leukopenia (57.3%), thrombocytopenia (36.6%), and generalized pain (46.3%).[8,10] The incidence of infection is 36.6%, with CMV disease occurring in 13.4% of patients. There are no reported DDIs with the use of thymoglobulin at this time.[8-10]

Muronomab-CD3 OKT-3 is a murine monoclonal antibody that targets the CD3 receptor. The CD3 receptor is only found on activated T cells and medullary thymocytes.[9,12,15] Binding of this agent to the CD3 receptor inactivates the adjacent TCR portion of the T lymphocyte cell membrane, preventing the activation of T lymphocytes. After the first dose of OKT-3, lymphocytes are removed from circulation via opsonization. The lymphocyte count falls precipitously within a few hours of administration of OKT-3.

This agent is dosed at 5 mg/day and is given daily for 10 to 14 days. Lower doses have been used successfully in all organ transplant recipients (2 mg IV/day).[15]

Due to its ability to cause widespread T-cell lysis after the first dose, OKT-3 has several severe adverse events that manifest within a few hours after administration.[9,12,15] These adverse reactions are often referred to as the "first-dose effect" and are usually secondary to cytokine release. The adverse reaction profile of OKT-3 includes fever (77%), chills (43%), dyspnea (16%), nausea (32%), vomiting (25%), diarrhea (37%), and tachycardia (26%). Due to a number of severe and potentially fatal reactions, today the role of OKT-3 is limited to the treatment of severe acute rejection refractory to other T cell depleting agents. One of the major complications of OKT-3 is the development of severe pulmonary edema.[9,16,17] In reported cases of this complication, most patients were fluid overloaded at the time of the initial dose. Thus, chest X-ray to rule out any evidence of fluid overload is a must before administration of OKT-3 for the treatment of acute cellular rejection. Another problematic adverse reaction is the development of cytokine nephropathy.[9,18] The herbal product echinacea has been theorized to interact with OKT-3, due to echinacea's proposed ability to stimulate the immune system.[9]

Alemtuzumab Alemtuzumab is a recombinant DNA-derived monoclonal antibody that binds to CD52. CD52 is present on the surface of almost all B and T lymphocytes, many macrophages, NK cells, and a subpopulation of granulocytes. This agent's mechanism of action is believed to be antibody-dependent cell lysis following its binding to CD52 cell surface markers. When used for induction therapy, alemtuzumab produces a rapid and extensive lymphocyte depletion that may take several months to return to pretransplant levels. Although it is not FDA-approved for use in organ transplantation, studies have demonstrated a dose of 20 to 30 mg on day zero and again on either postoperative day 1 or 4 to be effective in preventing acute rejection. However, current studies are evaluating the use of a single 30 mg dose given on postoperative day zero (i.e., the hours immediately following surgery), which has been shown to be as effective but better tolerated than ATG induction.

Alemtuzumab has been associated with serious adverse reactions that include anemia (47%), neutropenia (70%), thrombocytopenia (52%), headache (24%), dysthesias (15%), dizziness (12%), nausea (54%), vomiting (41%), diarrhea (22%), autoimmune hemolytic anemia (rare), infusion-related reactions (15–89%), and infection (37%; CMV viremia occurred in 15% of patients). The FDA recommends that premedication with acetaminophen and oral antihistamines are advisable to reduce the incidence of infusion-related reactions.

Comparative Efficacy—Induction Therapy Agents The improvements in short-term outcomes gained from the use of induction therapies cannot be denied. However, despite these advances, use of induction therapy has not impacted long-

term allograft function or survival. There are a few studies that help to delineate the ideal induction therapy agent. For example, studies comparing thymoglobulin and eATG, show that thymoglobulin is more effective in lowering acute rejection rates and improving 1-year allograft survival.[19] Conversely, studies evaluating the use of basiliximab versus antithymocyte globulin demonstrate similar short-term efficacy between both groups.[20] However, a more recent analysis of these two agents demonstrated similar results for allograft and patient survival, but a benefit for thymoglobulin in lowering the incidence of acute allograft rejection.[21] When choosing an agent for induction therapy, one must weigh the risks versus the benefits. For the most part, the ALAs are considered to be most effective, but are associated with a higher incidence of infectious disease and cancer.

Patient Encounter, Part 1: Medical History, Physical Exam, and Diagnostic Tests

JJ is a 52-year-old woman who presents to your transplant center for a living-related renal transplant.

PMH:

- ESRD—secondary to PKD and failed previous transplant
- One prior renal transplant from husband in 1995, which failed secondary to chronic allograft nephropathy in 2004 (presumably from multiple rejection episodes within the first few years after transplant).
- For the previous transplant the patient was maintained on cyclosporine, mycophenolate, and prednisone.
- Hypertension; hyperlipidemia; insomnia

FH: Father died of a myocardial infarction at age 53, while her mother is alive and living with hypertension, systemic lupus erythematosus, DM, and osteoporosis at the age of 75.

SH: The patient works as a secretary. Was a heavy tobacco user (45 pack years), but quit 3 years ago. She denies alcohol and IV drug use.

Admission Meds: Calcitriol 0.25 mg by mouth once a day; calcium acetate 1,334 mg by mouth three times a day; ferrous sulfate 325 mg by mouth once a day; epo 4,000 units IV every hemodialysis session; zocor 20 mg by mouth once a day at bedtime; metoprolol 100 mg by mouth twice a day; ASA 81 mg by mouth once a day; zolpidem 10 mg by mouth once a day at bedtime

Allergies: Codeine (upset stomach); penicillin (hives); sulfa (rash)

Misc:

- CMV serostatus: Donor is CMV immunoglobulin G (IgG) positive
- CMV serostatus: Recipient is CMV IgG positive

Identify your treatment goals for this patient.

Create a plan for induction therapy (i.e., would you recommend induction therapy, if so, which agent?).

Immunosuppressive Therapies— Maintenance Therapy

The goals of maintenance immunosuppression are to prevent acute and chronic rejection episodes and to optimize patient and graft survival. Antirejection medications require careful selection and dosage titration to balance the risks of rejection with the risks of toxicities.

Common maintenance immunosuppressive agents can be divided into four basic medication classes:

- Calcineurin inhibitors (cyclosporine and tacrolimus);
- Antiproliferatives (azathioprine and the mycophenolic acid [MPA] derivatives);
- Target of Rapamycin (ToR) inhibitors (sirolimus); and
- Corticosteroids (prednisolone derivatives and dexamethasone).

Maintenance immunosuppression is generally achieved by combining two or more medications from the different classes to maximize efficacy by specifically targeting unique components of the immune response. Please refer to Figure 55–1 for a schematic representation of these different drug mechanisms and Figure 55–2 for an example protocol for administration of immunosuppressive medications post-transplant. This method of medication selection also helps to minimize toxicities by choosing agents with different adverse event profiles. Immunosuppressive regimens vary between organ types and transplant centers, but most often they include a calcineurin inhibitor with an adjuvant agent, plus or minus corticosteroids. Selection of appropriate immunosuppressive regimens should be patient-specific. In doing so, the transplant practitioner must take into account patients' pre-existing disease states, medication regimens, and preferences.

▶ Calcineurin Inhibitors

⑤ *Cyclosporine and tacrolimus belong to a class of immunosuppressants called the calcineurin inhibitors.* These agents are considered by many to be the cornerstone of immunosuppression protocols. The calcineurin inhibitors work by complexing with cytoplasmic proteins (cyclosporine with cyclophylin and tacrolimus with FK binding protein-12).[8,9,22,23] These complexes then inhibit calcineurin phosphatase, which results in reduced IL-2 gene transcription. The final outcome is a decrease in IL-2 synthesis and a subsequent reduction in T-cell activation.[8,9,22,23]

Cyclosporine Cyclosporine USP was first approved by the FDA in 1983, but was associated with a variable oral absorption. The development of a newer formulation, cyclosporine microemulsion USP introduced in 1994, allowed

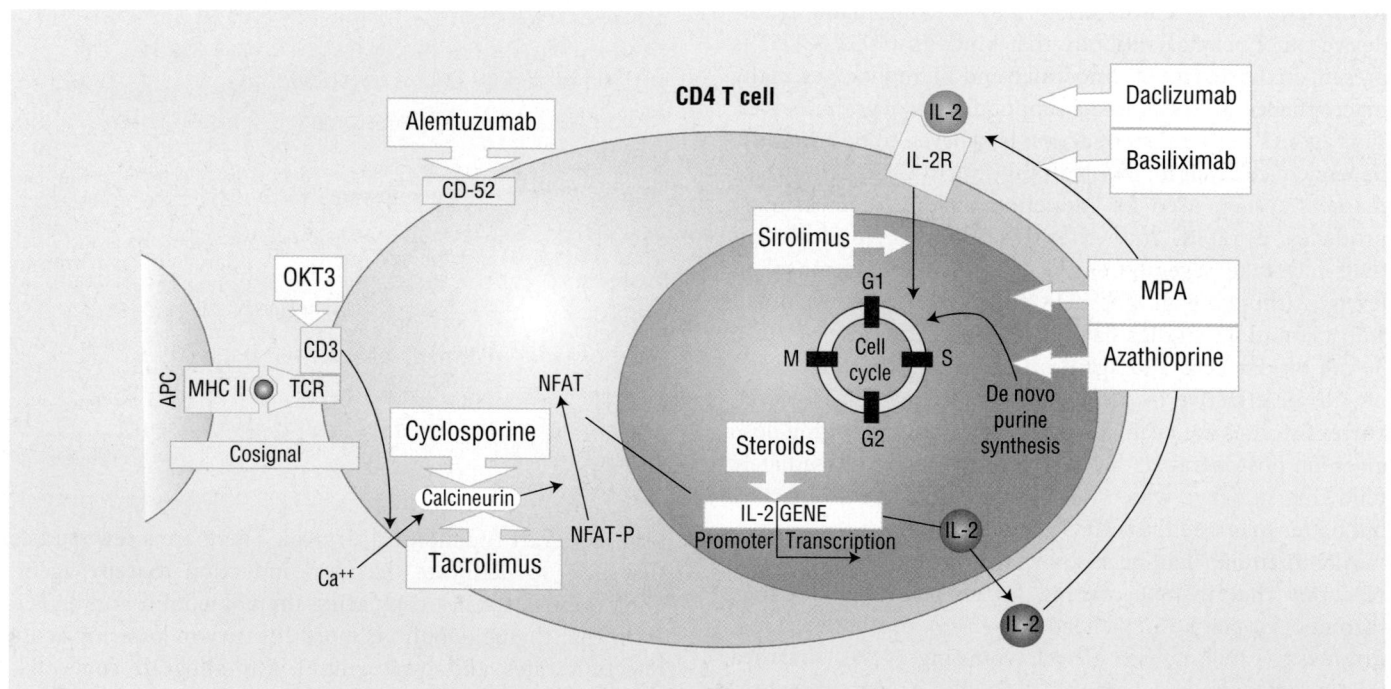

FIGURE 55–1. Identification of the sites of action of the various immunosuppressive medications. Antigen-major histocompatibility complex (MHC) II molecule complexes are responsible for initiating the activation of CD4 T cells. These MHC-peptide complexes are recognized by the T-cell recognition complex (TCR). A costimulatory signal initiates signal transduction with activation of second messengers, one of which is calcineurin. Calcineurin removes phosphates from the nuclear factors (NFAT-P), allowing them to enter the nucleus. These nuclear factors specifically bind to interleukin-2 (IL-2) promoter gene facilitating IL-2 gene transcription. Interaction of IL-2 with the IL-2 receptor (IL-2R) on the cell membrane surface induces cell proliferation and production of cytokines specific to the T cell. (APCs, antigen producing cells; MPA, myophenolic acid; OKT-3, muronomab-CD3.) (From Schonder KS, Johnson HJ. Solid organ transplantation. In: DiPiro JT, Talbert RL, Yee GC, et al., eds. Pharmacotherapy: A Pathophysiologic Approach, 7th ed. New York: McGraw-Hill, 2008:1463.)

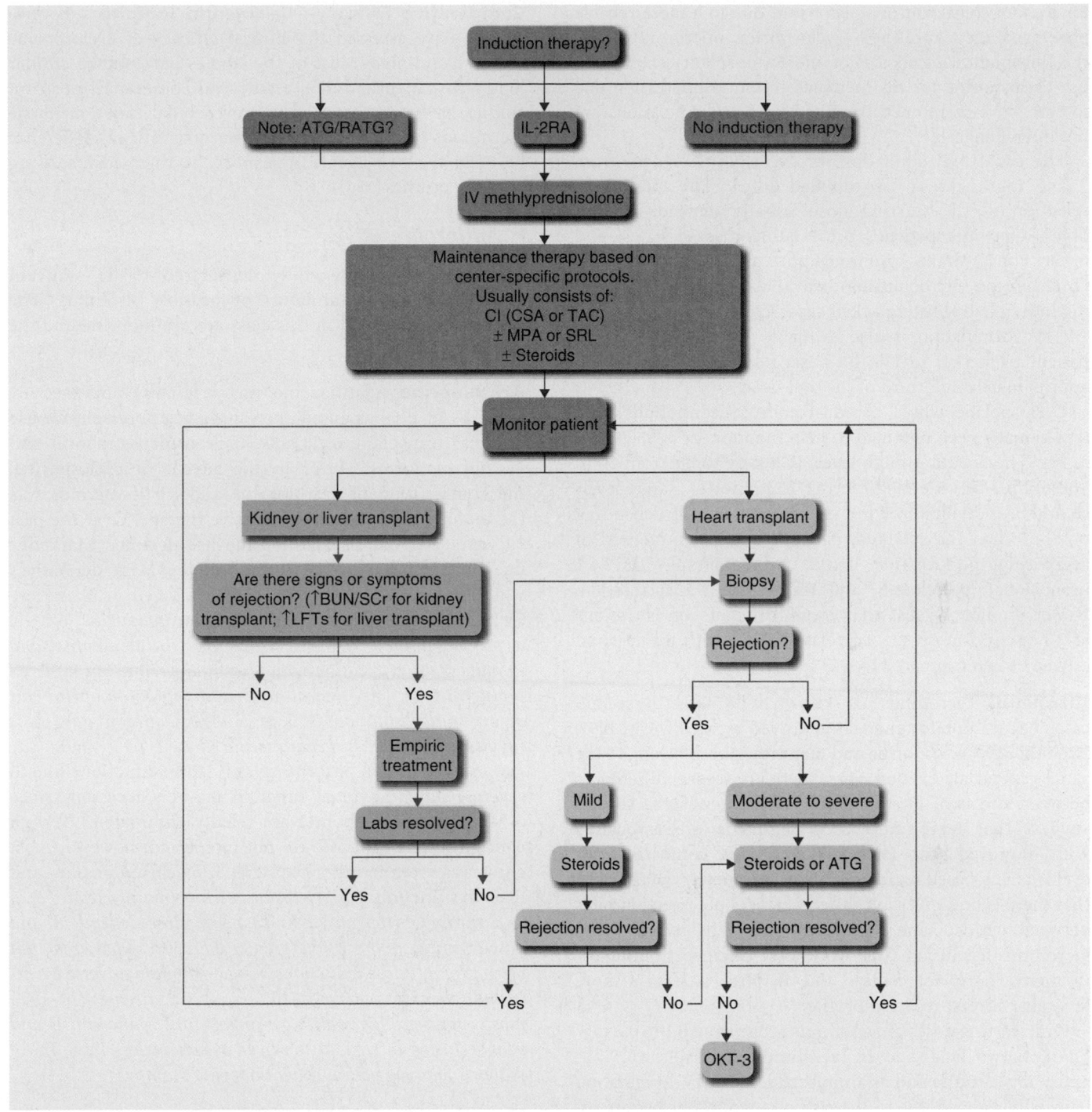

FIGURE 55–2. **Example protocol of immunosuppressive medication use in organ transplantation.** Center-specific protocols may use rabbit antithymocyte immunoglobulin (RATG), an interleukin 2 receptor antagonist (IL-2RA), or no induction therapy. In any situation, patients receive IV methylprednisone prior to, during, or immediately following the transplant operation. The patient then will begin the maintenance immunosuppressive regimen. The center-specific protocol will specify which calcineurin inhibitor (cyclosporine or tacrolimus) is used in combination with mycophenolate mofetil or sirolimus with or without steroids. Patients then are monitored for signs and symptoms of rejection. If rejection is suspected, a biopsy can be done for definitive diagnosis, or the patient may be treated empirically for rejection. Empirical treatment generally involves administration of corticosteroids. If signs and symptoms of rejection are resolved with empirical therapy, the patient will continue to be monitored according to the center-specific protocol. If rejection is confirmed by biopsy, treatment may be based on the severity of rejection. High-dose corticosteroids are used most frequently for mild to moderate rejection. RATG can be used for moderate to severe rejections or steroid-resistant rejections. Severe rejection episodes that are not resolved with steroids or RATG are treated with OKT-3. (BUN, blood urea nitrogen; CI, calcineurin inhibitor; CSA, cyclosporine; IL2RA, interleukin 2 receptor antagonist; LFT, liver function test; MPA, mycophenolic acid; OKT-3, moronomab-CD3; SCr, serum creatinine; SRL, sirolimus; TAC, tacrolimus.) (From Schonder KS, Johnson HJ. Solid Organ Transplantation. In: DiPiro JT, Talbert RL, Yee GC, et al., eds. Pharmacotherapy: A Pathophysiologic Approach, 7th ed. New York: McGraw-Hill, 2008:1466.)

for a more consistent drug exposure due to a more reliable pharmacokinetic profile.[24] Cyclosporine microemulsion is the formulation of choice for most transplant centers that use cyclosporine for maintenance immunosuppression due to the above mentioned benefit. The two formulations are not interchangeable.

The usual oral adult dose of cyclosporine ranges from 3 to 7 mg/kg/day in two divided doses.[9] The appropriate selection of the starting dose usually depends on the organ type, the patient's pre-existing disease states, and other concomitant immunosuppressive agents utilized. Cyclosporine microemulsion is available as 25 mg and 100 mg individually blister packed capsules and an oral solution. An IV formulation is also available. When converting a patient from oral to IV, the dosage should be reduced to approximately one-third of the oral dose.[9]

Cyclosporine whole blood trough concentrations have traditionally been obtained to help monitor for efficacy and safety. Therapeutic trough levels (C_0) may range from 50 to 400 ng/mL (50–400 mcg/L or 42–333 nmol/L). Target levels should be individualized for each patient, usually depending on the organ transplanted, patient's condition, method of assay (high-performance liquid chromatography [HPLC], monoclonal, polyclonal), and time since transplantation. Newer studies suggest that monitoring of concentrations at 2 hours postdose (C_2) correlates better with toxicity and efficacy when compared to C_0.[25]

Tacrolimus Tacrolimus (also known as FK506) is the second calcineurin inhibitor and was approved by the FDA in 1997. Even though cyclosporine and tacrolimus both belong to the same general medication class, there are several differences between the two. First, looking at efficacy, some studies suggest that tacrolimus-based regimens are associated with improved short-term survival when compared with cyclosporine-based regimens.[26] However, newer data suggest that there is no significant difference in acute rejection rates between cyclosporine and tacrolimus.[27] In recent years, tacrolimus has become the workhorse calcineurin inhibitor in many transplant centers, due in large part to a more favorable adverse reaction profile.[23]

Oral starting doses of tacrolimus range from 0.1 to 0.2 mg/kg/day in two divided doses. Tacrolimus is available in 0.5-, 1-, and 5-mg capsules and as an injectable.[9] The IV formulation is usually avoided due to the risk of anaphylaxis because of its castor oil component and nephrotoxicity. Tacrolimus C_0 whole blood levels should be monitored (12 hours after the last administered dose) and maintained between 5 and 15 ng/mL (5–15 mcg/L), again depending on the transplanted organ, patient's condition, and time since transplant.[9]

Adverse Drug Reactions ⑤ *One of the major drawbacks of the calcineurin inhibitors is their ability to cause acute and chronic nephrotoxicity.* Acute nephrotoxicity has been correlated with high doses and is usually reversible. Chronic calcineurin inhibitor toxicity, however, is typically irreversible and is linked to chronic drug exposure. Table 55–4 expands upon the more common calcineurin inhibitor-induced adverse events.

Comparative Efficacy—Calcineurin Inhibitors Several studies have assessed the clinical efficacy of cyclosporine versus tacrolimus. Most of the studies have shown similar long-term patient and allograft survival. Some renal transplant studies have demonstrated improved renal function in the tacrolimus treated patients. The most significant difference between the two agents appears to be their adverse drug reaction profiles.[1–3]

▶ Antiproliferatives

These agents are generally considered to be adjuvant to the calcineurin inhibitors or possibly sirolimus. The medications included in this class are azathioprine and the MPA derivatives.

Azathioprine Azathioprine was originally approved by the FDA in 1968 as an adjunct immunosuppressant for use in renal transplant recipients. It is available in oral and IV dosage forms.[9] Prior to the advent of cyclosporine, the combination of azathioprine and corticosteroids was the mainstay of immunosuppressive therapy. Over the past 10 years, the use of azathioprine has declined markedly, due in large part to the success of the MPA derivatives which are more specific inhibitors of T-cell proliferation. ⑥ *Azathioprine is a prodrug for 6-mercaptopurine (6-MP), a purine analog. 6-MP acts as an antimetabolite and inhibits DNA replication with a resultant reduction in T-cell proliferation.*[9] *The typical oral dose of azathioprine for organ transplantation is 3 to 5 mg/kg once a day.*[9] *The maintenance dose is usually reduced to 1 to 2 mg/kg/day within a few weeks post-transplant.* Dose reductions due to severely impaired renal function may be necessary since 6-MP and its metabolites are renally eliminated.[9] Trough concentrations of 6-MP are not monitored; however, most clinicians often monitor for signs of myelosuppression and liver dysfunction. ⑥ *Myelosuppression (mainly leukopenia and thrombocytopenia) is a frequent, dose-dependent and dose-limiting complication (greater than 50% of patients) that often prompts dose reductions.*[9] *Other common adverse events include hepatotoxicity (2–10%) and GI disease (10–15%; mostly nausea and vomiting). Importantly, pancreatitis and venoocclusive disease of the liver occurs in less than 1% of patients following chronic azathioprine therapy.*[9]

Mycophenolic Acid Derivatives Mycophenolate mofetil was approved by the FDA in 1995 and enteric-coated MPA in 2004. Both agents are considered to be adjunctive immunosuppressants. ⑥ *Both mycophenolate mofetil and enteric-coated MPA are prodrugs for MPA. MPA acts by inhibiting inosine monophosphate dehydrogenase, a vital enzyme in the de novo pathway of purine synthesis. Inhibition of this enzyme prevents the proliferation of most cells that are dependent upon the de novo pathway for purine synthesis including T cells.*[8,9,28–30]

Mycophenolate mofetil is available in 250 mg and 500 mg capsules, an oral suspension (100 mg/mL; in cherry syrup) and as an injectable.[9] Usual doses of mycophenolate mofetil range from 1,000 to 3,000 mg/day in two to four divided doses.

Table 55–4

Management of Common Adverse Effects of Calcineurin Inhibitors

Adverse Event	Most Likely Offending CI	Monitoring Parameters	Therapeutic Management Options
Nephrotoxicity	Either	Serum creatinine BUN Urine output Biopsy-proven CI-induced nephrotoxicity	Reduce CI dose (if possible) Use of CCB for HTN control Modify regimen (add or change to non-CI containing regimen)
Hypertension[a]	Cyclosporine	Blood pressure Heart rate	Initiate patient-specific antihypertensive therapy Reduce cyclosporine dose (if possible) Change from cyclosporine to tacrolimus or sirolimus
Hyperlipidemia[a]	Cyclosporine	Fasting lipid panel	Initiate patient-specific cholesterol-lowering therapy Reduce cyclosporine dose (if possible) Change from cyclosporine to tacrolimus or sirolimus
Hyperglycemia[b]	Tacrolimus	Blood glucose (fasting and nonfasting) Hemoglobin A_{1c}	Diet modifications Reduce tacrolimus dose (if possible) Reduce steroids (if patient is taking them and if possible) Initiate patient-specific glucose-lowering therapy (insulin or oral therapy) Change from tacrolimus to cyclosporine or sirolimus
CNS toxicities[b]	Tacrolimus	Fine hand tremor Headache Mental status changes	Reduce tacrolimus dose (if possible) Change from tacrolimus to cyclosporine or sirolimus
Hematologic	Either	WBC Platelets Hemoglobin Hematocrit Symptoms of anemia	Reduce CI dose (if possible) Modify regimen (add or change to non-CI containing regimen; although hematologic risk is high for all meds except steroids)
Hepatotoxicity	Either	Liver function tests	Reduce CI dose (if possible) Modify regimen (add or change to non-CI containing regimen)
Electrolyte Imbalance	Either	K (usually ↑) Mg (usually ↓) PO_4 (usually ↓)	Treat electrolyte imbalance (i.e., Mg replacement) Reduce CI dose (if possible) Modify regimen (add or change to non-CI containing regimen)
Hirsutism	Cyclosporine	Patient complains of excessive hair growth or male-pattern hair growth	Reduce cyclosporine dose (if possible) Cosmetic hair removal Change from cyclosporine to tacrolimus or sirolimus
Alopecia	Tacrolimus	Patient complains of excessive hair loss	Reduce tacrolimus dose (if possible) Hair growth treatments (i.e., minoxidil, finasteride—males only) Change from tacrolimus to cyclosporine or sirolimus
Gingival Hyperplasia	Cyclosporine	Patient complains of excessive gum growth Recommendations for therapy from the patient's dentist	Reduce cyclosporine dose (if possible) Oral surgery (gum resection) Change from cyclosporine to tacrolimus or sirolimus

BUN, blood urea nitrogen; CCB, calcium channel blocker; CI, calcineurin inhibitor; CNS, central nervous system; HTN, hypertension; K, potassium; Mg, magnesium; PO_4, phosphate.

[a]Tacrolimus is also associated with hypertension and hyperlipidemia, but to a much lower extent compared to cyclosporine

[b]Cyclosporine is also associated with hyperglycemia and CNS toxicities, but to a much lower extent compared to tacrolimus

From Refs. 1, 8, 9.

The conversion between oral and IV mycophenolate mofetil is 1:1. Enteric-coated MPA is available in 180-mg and 360-mg tablets. The appropriate equimolar conversion between mycophenolate mofetil and enteric-coated MPA is 1,000 mg of mycophenolate mofetil to 720 mg of enteric-coated-MPA.[28,31] The recommended starting dose of enteric-coated MPA is 720 mg given twice daily.[12] It appears that conversion of mycophenolate mofetil to enteric-coated MPA is safe, but more studies are needed to determine the exact role of enteric-coated MPA in the immunosuppressive armamentarium.

MPA trough concentrations can be monitored; however, they are not routinely recommended.

❻ *The most common adverse events associated with these agents are GI (18–54%; diarrhea, nausea, vomiting, and gastritis) and myelosuppression (20–40%).*[8,12,28–30] Despite being enteric-coated, enteric-coated MPA has produced the same degree of GI adverse events as mycophenolate mofetil.[28] However, recent data suggest that there is a benefit in converting patients with documented mycophenolate-induced GI disease from mycophenolate mofetil to enteric-coated MPA.

Comparative Efficacy—Antiproliferatives Due to the results of several studies, the MPA derivatives have replaced azathioprine as the antiproliferative agent of choice in most organ transplant centers. The MPA derivatives are generally considered to provide a more specific immunosuppressive effect compared to azathioprine. Mycophenolate mofetil and enteric-coated mycophenolate acid have similar safety and efficacy data in renal transplant recipients. The decision to choose one agent over another is a purely practitioner-dependent preference.

▶ *Target of Rapamycin Inhibitors*

Sirolimus Sirolimus is currently the only FDA-approved ToR inhibitor. One of its derivatives, everolimus, is in phase III clinical trials and has been approved for use in some European countries.[32] Sirolimus is a macrolide antibiotic that has no affect on calcineurin phosphatase.[8,33,34] Studies have shown that sirolimus may be used safely and effectively with either cyclosporine or tacrolimus as a replacement for either azathioprine or mycophenolate mofetil.[35] Sirolimus can also be used as an alternative agent for patients who do not tolerate calcineurin inhibitors due to nephrotoxicity or other adverse events.[36] ❼ *At this time, the most exciting data for sirolimus point to its ability to prevent long-term allograft dysfunction when used as a substitute for the calcineurin inhibitors in renal transplant recipients.*[33,35,36]

❼ *Sirolimus inhibits T-cell activation and proliferation by binding to and inhibiting the activation of the mammalian ToR, which suppresses cellular response to IL-2 and other cytokines (i.e., IL-4, IL-15).*[9,33]

Sirolimus is available in a 1-mg and 2-mg tablet and a 1 mg/mL oral solution. The current FDA approved dosing regimen for sirolimus is a 6 mg loading dose followed by a 2 mg/day maintenance dose.[9] It was recommended that this agent does not require therapeutic drug monitoring. However, most centers do check trough concentrations and adjust doses to reach goal concentrations.[37] Most clinicians who use sirolimus utilize a loading dose of 5 to 15 mg/day for 1 to 3 days to more rapidly achieve adequate immunosuppression.[33,35,36] Maintenance doses of sirolimus usually range from 1 to 10 mg/day given once daily. Sirolimus blood C_0 levels should be obtained and maintained between 5 and 20 ng/mL, depending on the institution-specific protocols.[37] Switching between immunoassays may produce different results that may be clinically significant. Of note, sirolimus has a half-life of approximately 62 hours, which means that it will not reach steady state after dosage changes for several days.[9]

❼ *The most common adverse events reported with sirolimus are leukopenia (20%), thrombocytopenia (13–30%), and hyperlipidemia (38–57%).*[9,33] Other adverse effects include delayed wound healing, anemia, diarrhea, arthralgias, rash, hyperglycemia, pneumonitis, and mouth ulcers. Sirolimus has a FDA black-box warning in newly transplanted liver and lung recipients.[9] In liver transplant recipients, use of sirolimus immediately after transplant is associated with an increased risk of hepatic artery thrombosis, graft loss, and death. In lung transplant recipients, bronchial anastomotic dehiscence, including some fatal cases, has been noted in patients treated with sirolimus, tacrolimus, and corticosteroids.

▶ *Corticosteroids*

Traditional triple-therapy immunosuppressive regimens have consisted of a calcineurin inhibitor, an antiproliferative or ToR inhibitor, and corticosteroids. In recent years, many protocols have focused on corticosteroid sparing or avoidance. Avoidance or sparing of corticosteroids has been supported in the literature, although more studies are needed to help better characterize which patients should follow these protocols.[38–41] A typical taper includes a bolus of IV methylprednisolone 100 to 500 mg at the time of transplant, then tapered over 5 to 7 days to a maintenance low dose of prednisone 5 to 10 mg/day. Although most centers still use low dose steroids for immunologically high risk patients, a number of programs have developed an immunosuppression protocol that completely avoids or withdraws corticosteroids at some point post-transplantation.[2,8] At most transplant centers, therapeutic drug monitoring of corticosteroids is not employed. ❽ *Corticosteroids are associated with a variety of acute and chronic toxicities.* The most common adverse events have been summarized in Table 55–5.[9]

❽ *Corticosteroids have various effects on immune and inflammatory response systems, although their exact mechanism of immunosuppression is not fully understood.* It is generally believed that at high doses, the agents are directly lymphotoxic and at lower doses, the corticosteroids act by inhibiting the production of various cytokines that are necessary to amplify the immune response.[12]

The most commonly used corticosteroids are methylprednisolone (IV and oral) and prednisone (oral), although prednisolone and dexamethasone have also been shown to be effective for organ transplantation. Corticosteroid doses vary by center-specific protocols, organ type, and patient characteristics.

Immunosuppressive Therapies—Future Immunosuppressive Agents

The immunosuppressant armamentarium is expanding with novel small molecules (i.e., AEB, bortezimibe, and the Janus-Kinase 3 inhibitors) and biological agents (i.e., costimulatory pathway blockers) currently in clinical development. These newer agents appear promising and may represent the emergence of novel immunosuppressive agents that can deliver immunosuppression without the long-term toxicities. Some currently marketed immunosuppressants may also have beneficial effects in organ transplantation.

Table 55–5	
Common Adverse Events Associated With Corticosteroids	
Body System	**Adverse Event**
Cardiovascular	Hyperlipidemia
	Hypertension
Central nervous system	Anxiety
	Insomnia
	Mood changes
	Psychosis
Dermatologic	Acne
	Diaphoresis
	Ecchymosis
	Hirsutism
	Impaired wound healing
	Petechiae
	Thin skin
Endocrine/metabolic	Cushing's syndrome
	Hyperglycemia
	Sodium and water retention
Gastrointestinal	Gastritis
	Increased appetite
	Nausea, vomiting, diarrhea
	Peptic ulcers
Hematologic	Leukocytosis
Neuromuscular/skeletal	Arthralgia
	Impaired growth
	Osteoporosis
	Skeletal muscle weakness
Ocular	Cataracts
	Glaucoma
Respiratory	Epistaxis

From Ref. 9.

Several agents, including alefacept, bortezimibe, alemtuzumab (discussed previously), efalizumab, leflunomide, and rituximab, have already been used successfully in renal transplantation.

Immunosuppressive Therapies—Treatment of Acute Rejection Episodes

Acute rejection is generally treated with a course of high-dose methylprednisolone (250–1,000 mg/day IV for 3 days), which is usually sufficient to ameliorate the rejection episode. If the acute rejection episode is resistant to the initial course of steroids, a second course may be administered or the patient may begin therapy with antithymocyte globulin (1.5 mg/kg/day for 3–14 days). Acute rejection refractory to these treatments may require OKT-3. However, the use of this agent has fallen out of favor due to the severe short- and long-term adverse events associated with its use.

Maintenance Immunosuppressive Therapies—Common Drug–Drug Interactions

❾ *As the number of medications that a patient takes increases, so does the potential for DDIs.* Disease severity, patient age, and organ dysfunction are all risk factors for increased DDIs. In general, DDIs can be broken down into two categories: (a) pharmacokinetic interactions, and (b) pharmacodynamic interactions.

- Pharmacokinetic interactions result when one drug alters the absorption, distribution, metabolism, or elimination of another drug.
- Pharmacodynamic interactions include additive, synergistic, or antagonistic interactions that can affect efficacy or toxicity.

▶ *Pharmacokinetic Interactions*

Given the large number of medications consumed by transplant recipients, it is no surprise that this patient population is at high risk for DDIs. Pharmacokinetic DDIs pose a major dilemma with the maintenance immunosuppressants. Pharmacokinetic interactions can either result in increased concentrations of one or more agents with an increased risk for drug-induced toxicities, or lowered (i.e., subtherapeutic) drug concentrations, possibly leading to allograft rejection. As mentioned above, pharmacokinetic DDIs can be further categorized into interactions of absorption, distribution, metabolism, and elimination.

Interactions of Absorption Most DDIs due to altered absorption occur within the intestines. There are a variety of potential mechanisms through which the absorption of the maintenance immunosuppressants is altered, including:

- Drug metabolism within the gut ("Interactions of Metabolism" will be discussed below)
- Alterations in the active transport process
- Changes in intestinal motility
- Chelation interactions

Active transporters (i.e., P-glycoprotein [P-gp]) play an important role in drug-interactions. P-gp, a plasma membrane transport protein, is present in the gut, brain, liver, and kidneys.[42,43] This protein provides a biological barrier, eliminating toxic substances and xenobiotics that may accumulate in these organ systems. P-gp plays an important role in the absorption and distribution of many medications. In the GI tract, P-gp is located in the brush borders of mature enterocytes. The colon has the largest percentage of P-gp, while the stomach and jejunum-ileum contain the lowest percentage. P-gp affects the absorption of cyclosporine, tacrolimus, and sirolimus. Some medications can alter the activity of P-gp (inhibit or induce its activity). Medications that are cytochrome P450 (CYP) 3A4 substrates, inhibitors or inducers, also tend to affect P-gp; therefore, the potential exists for several DDIs with the immunosuppressants by this mechanism.[42,43] For example, medications that inhibit P-gp activity will increase concentrations of cyclosporine, tacrolimus, and sirolimus due to a reduction in P-gp-dependent drug elimination from the hepatic circulation.

When looking at the ability of drugs that change intestinal motility and their effects on the maintenance immunosuppressants, you can see notable interactions between the prokinetic agents and the calcineurin inhibitors. Metoclopramide has been shown to increase the absorption of cyclosporine and tacrolimus by enhancing gastric mobility and emptying.[44]

Most of the interactions with mycophenolate mofetil and enteric-coated MPA are due to reductions in intestinal absorption. Aluminum, magnesium, and calcium containing products decrease the peak level of MPA.[9] If a patient requires aluminum, magnesium, or calcium, it should be administered at least 4 hours before or after MPA. Of note, iron does not interact with the MPA preparations.[45]

Interactions of Distribution Interactions of distribution tend to occur with drugs that are highly protein bound. A drug that is extensively bound to plasma proteins can be displaced from its binding site by another agent that has greater affinity for the same binding site, thereby raising free concentrations of the displaced drug. MPA is the only highly protein bound (97% bound to albumin) maintenance immunosuppressant with a reported DDI by this mechanism. It has been shown that concomitant administration of MPA with salicylates increases the free concentrations of MPA.[9] The adverse sequelae of this drug interaction have not been assessed. DDIs studies have not been completed evaluating the MPA derivatives, or the other highly protein bound maintenance immunosuppressants, when used with other highly protein bound drugs.

Interactions of Metabolism Oxidative metabolism by CYP isozymes is the primary method of drug metabolism.[46] The purpose of drug metabolism is to make drugs more water-soluble so they can be more easily eliminated. Cyclosporine, tacrolimus, and sirolimus are all substrates of the CYP3A isozyme system. The majority of CYP-mediated metabolism takes place in the liver; however, CYP is also expressed in the intestine, lungs, kidneys, and brain. Two types of interactions usually occur with medications metabolized via the CYP enzyme system, inhibitory interactions and inducing interactions. Enzyme inhibition occurs when there is enzyme inactivation or mutual competition of substrates at a catalytic site. This usually results in a reduction of drug metabolism leading to increased concentrations of all medications involved. Enzyme induction interactions are just the opposite and occur when there is increased synthesis or decreased degradation of CYP enzymes. This type of interaction can produce decreased concentrations of medications.[46] Being CYP3A substrates, it would be anticipated that cyclosporine, tacrolimus, and sirolimus would all experience similar pharmacokinetic DDIs. Table 55–6 details the clinically relevant DDIs that occur with the calcineurin inhibitors and sirolimus due to inhibition or induction of the CYP isozyme system.

One of the most often overlooked DDIs in transplant recipients is the effect corticosteroids have on drug metabolism. Dexamethasone is a CYP3A isozyme inducer, meaning that it may increase the whole blood trough concentrations of cyclosporine, tacrolimus, and sirolimus.[9,47] Conversely, methylprednisolone is a CYP3A isozyme inhibitor, and it may reduce the whole blood trough concentrations of

cyclosporine, tacrolimus, and sirolimus.[9,47] This is usually not a noteworthy interaction, since doses of cyclosporine, tacrolimus, and sirolimus are titrated to achieve target concentrations in patients maintained on stable doses of corticosteroids. However, these DDIs may be problematic after pulse dose steroids for treatment of acute rejection or during steroid withdrawal.

Not all metabolic DDIs occur through the CYP system. Azathioprine has a considerable interaction with allopurinol that is not mediated through CYP.[48,49] Allopurinol inhibits xanthine oxidase, which is the enzyme responsible for metabolizing 6-MP to inactive 6-thiouricate. Combining these agents can result in 6-MP accumulation and severe toxicities, particularly myelosuppression. It is recommended that concomitant therapy with azathioprine and allopurinol be avoided, but if necessary, azathioprine doses must be reduced to one-third or one-fourth of the current dose.[49]

Interactions of Elimination There are very few interactions of elimination with the maintenance immunosuppressants. However, the major interaction through this process involves MPA. MPA is metabolized to MPA-glucuronide (MPAG) via hepatic glucuronosyltransferase.[9,28] MPAG is excreted in the bile for elimination in the gut. Deconjugation of MPAG back to MPA by intestinal flora results in a secondary absorption of MPA several hours after its administration.[9,28] Several medications have been shown to interfere with the biliary excretion of MPAG, thereby eliminating its reabsorption in the intestines and lowering the overall exposure to MPA. Cyclosporine has been shown to reduce the overall exposure to the MPA derivatives through competitive inhibition of MPAG enterohepatic recirculation.[50] MPA levels are lower when it is administered in cyclosporine-based immunosuppression regimens compared to tacrolimus-based regimens. The bile acid sequestrants (i.e., cholestyramine, colestipol, colesevelam) have also been shown to decrease overall MPA exposure through a similar mechanism.[51,52]

▶ **Pharmacodynamic Interactions**

In addition to the numerous pharmacokinetic interactions seen with the maintenance immunosuppressants, there also exists the possibility for pharmacodynamic interactions. An in-depth review of pharmacodynamic interactions with maintenance immunosuppressive agents goes beyond the scope of this chapter. However, some common pharmacodynamic DDIs will be discussed. Pharmacodynamic interactions are the backbone of modern immunosuppressive therapies that employ multiple medications with different mechanisms of action resulting in additive immunosuppression. Unfortunately, pharmacodynamic interactions can also be problematic, such as when medications with similar adverse events are used concomitantly. For example, nephrotoxic agents, such as amphotericin B, aminoglysides (i.e., gentamicin, tobramycin, amikacin) and non-steroidal anti-inflammatory drugs (NSAIDs; i.e., naproxen, ibuprofen, ketorolac) may potentiate the nephrotoxic effects of the calcineurin inhibitors.[9] The use of myelosuppressive

Table 55–6

Potential DDIs With the Calcineurin Inhibitors and Sirolimus Mediated Through the Cytochrome P-450 System 3A (CYP3A4) Isozyme

Substrates[a]		Inducers[b]	Inhibitors[c]
Alfentanil	Lidocaine	Carbamazepine	Cimetidine
Alprazolam	Loratadine	Dexamethasone	Clarithromycin
Amiodarone	Lovastatin	Ethosuximide	Clotrimazole
Amlodipine	Nevirapine	Isoniazid	Delavirdine
Atorvastatin	Nicardipine	Nevirapine	Diltiazem
Cilostazol	Nifedipine	Phenobarbital	Erythromycin
Cisapride	Omeprazole	Phenytoin	Fluconazole
Chlorpromazine	Paclitaxel	Prednisone	Fluoxetine
Clonazepam	Propafenone	Rifabutin	Fluvoxamine
Cocaine	Progesterone	Rifampin	Grapefruit juice
Cortisol	Quetiapine	St. John's wort	Indinavir
Cyclophosphamide	Quinidine		Itraconazole
Dantrolene	Sertraline		Ketoconazole
Dapsone	Simvastatin		Miconazole
Diazepam	Tamoxifen		Nefazodone
Disopyramide	Testosterone		Nelfinavir
Enalapril	Triazolam		Ritonavir
Estradiol	Venlafaxine		Saquinavir
Estrogen	Vinblastine		Troleandomycin
Etoposide	Warfarin		Verapamil
Felodipine	Zolpidem		Voriconazole
Flutamide			Zafirlukast

[a]Substrates of the CYP3A4 isozyme will compete with cyclosporine, tacrolimus, and sirolimus for metabolism; therefore, concentrations of both medications will be increased (usually by less than or equal to 20%).

[b]Inducers of the CYP3A4 isozyme will enhance the metabolism of cyclosporine, tacrolimus, and sirolimus; therefore, concentrations of these medications will be decreased.

[c]Inhibitors of the CYP3A4 isozyme will decrease the metabolism of cyclosporine, tacrolimus, and sirolimus; therefore, concentrations of these medications will be increased.

From Ref. 9.

agents, such as cotrimoxazole and valganciclovir, could enhance the myelosuppressive effects of induction therapy and the maintenance immunosuppressants.[9]

The potential exists for multiple DDIs in transplant recipients due to the complexity of their medication regimens. Practitioners must be diligent in reviewing all medications for potential DDIs. In addition to reviewing prescription medications, it is essential to question patients about the use of both nonprescription and complementary and alternative medicines, as these products also have the potential for significant interactions.

Immunosuppressive Therapies—Management of Immunosuppressive Drug Complications

▶ Opportunistic Infections

❾ *Solid organ transplant recipients are at increased risk of infectious diseases, which are a chief cause of early*

Patient Encounter, Part 2

Identify your treatment goals for JJ in terms of maintenance immunosuppressants.

Create a plan for maintenance therapy for JJ, making sure to compare and contrast the pros and cons of the different maintenance immunosuppressants.

Identify the potential DDIs that may exist with the addition of the maintenance immunosuppressants and the medications that JJ is currently taking.

morbidity and mortality. The prevalence of post-transplant infection depends on several factors, including clinical risk factors, environmental exposures and the degree of immunosuppression. Anti-infectives are universally prescribed in this population and their use can be split into three different categories:

- Prophylaxis: antimicrobials given to prevent an infection;
- Empiric: preemptive therapy given based on clinical suspicion of an active infection; and
- Treatment: antimicrobials given to manage a documented infection.

Post-transplant infections generally occur in a standard pattern; therefore, prevention is a key management strategy. The information in this section is designed to only highlight prophylaxis options routinely used in organ transplant recipients. Please refer to Table 55–7 for a list of agents used for the prevention of *Pneumocystis jiroveci* pneumonia and CMV disease.

▶ **Pneumocystis jiroveci *Pneumonia***

❾ *Without prophylaxis, P. jiroveci (formerly Pneumocystis carinii) pneumonia occurs in 5% to 15% of transplant recipients.*[53] Antipneumocystis prophylaxis is enormously helpful and is generally used in all organ transplant recipients. The duration of prophylaxis is usually 6 to 12 months after transplant, but may be prolonged in highly immunosuppressed patients (i.e., active CMV disease, treatment for rejection) or liver or lung recipients.[54] Sulfamethoxazole-trimethoprim is the preferred agent for prophylaxis. One of its major advantages is its relatively broad spectrum of activity. Not only is it effective against *Pneumocystis pneumonia*, but it also has activity against toxoplasmosis and other common bacterial infections. Patients who have sulfa allergies, glucose-6 phosphate dehydrogenase (G6PD) deficiency, or are

---

Table 55–7

Prophylactic Options for *Pneumocystis jiroveci* Pneumonia and CMV

Medication	Dosing	Common Adverse Events
Antipneumocystis Prophylaxis		
Sulfamethoxazole-trimethoprim (Bactrim, Septra, SMZ-TMP, cotrimoxazole)	One SS tablet by mouth once a day[a] One DS tablet by mouth once a day[a] One DS tablet by mouth every M/W/F[a]	Hyperkalemia Myelosuppression Nephrotoxicity Neutropenia Photosensitivity Rash
Pentamadine (NebuPent)	300 mg inhaled every 3–4 weeks	Bronchospasm Cough Hypo- or hyperglycemia
Dapsone (Avlosulfon)	50–100 mg tablet by mouth once a day	Hepatotoxicity Myelosuppression Nephritis
Atovaquone (Mepron)	1,500 mg suspension by mouth once a day	Elevated liver transaminases Nausea Rash
Antivirals		
Valganciclovir (Valcyte)	450–900 mg by mouth once a day[a]	Stomach upset (8–41%) Myelosuppression (2–27%) Headache (9–22%)
Ganciclovir (Cytovene)	5 mg/kg IV everyday; or 1,000 mg by mouth three times a day[a]	Stomach upset (13–40%) Myelosuppression (5–40%) Rash (10–15%)
Valacyclovir (Valtrex)	1–2 grams by mouth four times a day[a]	Stomach upset (1–15%) Myelosuppression (less than 1%) Headache (14–35%)
CMV IgG (CytoGam) and polyvalent IVIG	The maximum recommended total dosage per infusion is 150 mg/kg beginning within 72 hours of transplantation. Follow-up doses and time intervals depend on the type or organ transplanted.	Stomach upset (1–6%) Fevers and chills (1–6%) Flushing (1–6%)

CMV, cytomegalovirus; DS, double-strength (800 mg SMZ, 160 mg TMP); M/W/F, Monday, Wednesday and Friday; SS, single-strength (400 mg SMZ, 80 mg TMP); SMZ, sulfamethoxazole; TMP, trimethoprim.

[a]Dose adjustment required in renal insufficiency.

From Refs. 54, 55.

unable to tolerate sulfamethoxazole-trimethoprim should be given one of the second-line treatments.[9] Unfortunately, the second-line agents are antiparasitics and have no meaningful activity against common bacteria. These agents include dapsone, atovaquone, and pentamidine.

▶ Cytomegalovirus

CMV is the most concerning opportunistic pathogen in transplantation due to its association with poor outcomes.[55] CMV infection is present in 30% to 97% of the general population, but CMV disease is typically restricted to immunocompromised hosts.[56] The risk of CMV disease is highest among CMV-naive recipients who receive a CMV-positive organ (Donor +/Recipient –).[55] Other factors that augment the risk of CMV disease include organ type (lung and pancreas recipients are highest risk) and immunosuppressive agents (ALA use increases risk). CMV disease characteristically occurs within the first 3 to 6 months post-transplantation, but delayed onset disease has been seen in patients receiving antiviral prophylaxis.[55]

❾ *Several antivirals have proven efficacy in preventing and treating CMV.*[55] Valacyclovir and valganciclovir, prodrugs of acyclovir and ganciclovir, respectively, have improved bioavailability compared to their parent compounds and offer the advantage of less frequent dosing. CMV prophylaxis is classically continued for the first 100 days, or longer, after transplantation.[56,57] Both IV ganciclovir and oral valganciclovir may be used for preemptive therapy or for treatment of established CMV disease. The adverse events are similar among these agents and include myelosuppression and GI effects.[9]

Clinical Presentation and Diagnosis of *Pneumocystis jiroveci* Pneumonia

General
- Patients may not be in acute distress or they may feel tired (malaise)—symptoms vary from patient to patient.

Symptoms
- Patients may complain of fever, cough, and progressive dyspnea.

Signs
- The most common findings are fever and tachypnea.
- Chest examination may reveal crackles and rhonchi.

Radiographic Tests
- Chest radiographs may be normal in up to 25% of patients.
- The most common radiographic abnormalities are diffuse, bilateral, interstitial, or alveolar infiltrates.

▶ Fungal Infections

Fungal infections are an important cause of morbidity and mortality in solid organ transplant recipients. Immunologic (i.e., immunosuppressants, CMV infection), anatomic (i.e., tissue ischemia and damage), and surgical (i.e., duration of surgery, transfusion requirements) factors contribute to the risk for invasive fungal infections. Mucocutaneous candidiasis (i.e., oral thrush, esophagitis) is associated with corticosteroid and ALA use. ❾ *Oral nystatin or clotrimazole troches are effective prophylactic options for the prevention of thrush.* However, clotrimazole inhibits the CYP3A system in the gut and can alter immunosuppressive levels.[9] The use of systemic fungal prophylaxis, such as oral fluconazole, is controversial due to the potential for DDIs and the risk of developing resistance. The American Society of Transplantation and the American Society of Transplant Surgeons have recommended antifungal prophylaxis in liver, lung, and intestine transplantation.[58] The choice of agents depends on the fungal risk in that particular population. For example, liver and intestine transplant recipients are at high risk for candidiasis; therefore, the use of medications that cover *Candida* spp. is crucial, such as the triazole antifungals (i.e., fluconazole, itraconazole) or the echinocandins (i.e., caspofungin, micafungin). Lung transplant recipients are at high risk for aspergillosis; therefore, it is imperative to use antifungal prophylaxis that covers *Aspergillus* spp., such as the echinocandins or polyenes (i.e., amphotericin B, lipid-based amphotericin B products).[58]

▶ Hypertension

❾ *Cardiovascular disease has been identified as one of the leading causes of death in organ transplant recipients.*[59] Post-transplant hypertension is associated with an increase in cardiac morbidity and patient mortality in all transplant patients and is also an independent risk factor for chronic allograft dysfunction and loss.[60] Based on all of the available post-transplant morbidity and mortality data, it is imperative that post-transplant hypertension be identified and managed appropriately.

There are several underlying mechanisms responsible for post-transplant hypertension. Some causes of hypertension in transplant recipients may include renal dysfunction, increased sensitivity to endothelin-1 and angiotensin, increased density of glucocorticoid receptors in the vascular smooth muscle, and decreased production of vasodilatory prostaglandins.[61] However, one of the most easily

---

Patient Encounter, Part 3

Identify your treatment goals for JJ in terms of antimicrobial prophylaxis.

Create a plan for JJ's antimicrobial prophylaxis, making sure to compare and contrast the pros and cons of the different agents.

recognized causes of post-transplant hypertension is the use of corticosteroids and the calcineurin inhibitors.[62,63] Corticosteroids usually cause sodium and water retention,[61] thus increasing blood pressure, whereas calcineurin inhibitors are associated with a number of effects that may result in hypertension, including reduced glomerular filtration rate (GFR) and renal blood flow (RBF), increased systemic and intrarenal vascular resistance, sodium retention, reduced concentrations of systemic vasodilators (i.e., prostacyclin, nitric oxide), and increased concentrations of vasoconstrictive thromboxanes.[64] When compared with cyclosporine in clinical trials, tacrolimus displayed significantly less severe hypertension, and patients taking tacrolimus required significantly fewer antihypertensive medications at both 24 and 60 months post-transplant.[65–67]

Treatment ❾ *Controlling hypertension post-transplant is essential in preventing cardiac morbidity and mortality and prolonging graft survival.* The target blood pressure in kidney transplant recipients should be less than 130/80 mm Hg. This goal blood pressure may not be suitable for all organ transplant recipients. In such cases, the Joint National Committee Seventh Report (JNC7) guidelines should be followed.

Lifestyle Modifications In order to achieve a goal blood pressure, lifestyle modifications including diet, exercise, sodium restriction, and smoking cessation are recommended.[67] Unfortunately, lifestyle modifications alone are often inadequate to control hypertension in this high-risk population and antihypertensive medications are usually initiated early after transplant.

Immunosuppressive Regimen Modification Because tacrolimus has shown the propensity to cause less severe hypertension when compared to cyclosporine, conversion from cyclosporine-based immunosuppression to tacrolimus-based immunosuppression may be one way to help reduce the severity of hypertension in transplant recipients. Conversion to sirolimus, which is not associated with increases in blood pressure, may also be an alternative to the calcineurin inhibitors in patients with difficult-to-treat hypertension. Corticosteroid taper or withdrawal are effective strategies for lowering blood pressure, but are not warranted in all clinical situations.

Antihypertensive Agents There is no single class of antihypertensive medications recognized as the ideal agent. Numerous factors must be considered when determining appropriate treatment for a given patient, including the safety and efficacy data of the available agents, patient-specific situations, and potential comorbidities, and medication cost. A large majority of patients often require multiple medications to achieve their goal blood pressure. This conclusion is supported by the recommendations of JNC-VII, where combination therapy is regarded as an appropriate first-line therapy.

β-Blockers and thiazide diuretics have proven benefits in reducing cardiovascular disease-associated morbidity and mortality.[59] Tolerability permitting, these agents are to be considered first-line therapies in most transplant recipients.

The angiotensin converting enzyme (ACE) inhibitors and angiotensin receptor blockers (ARB) have definite benefits in patients with nephropathy and are believed to have renoprotective effects in most patients. However, due to their ability to cause an initial increase in serum creatinine, these agents should be used cautiously when used in combination with the calcineurin inhibitors. The dihydropyridine calcium channel blockers have demonstrated an ability to reverse the nephrotoxicity associated with cyclosporine and tacrolimus. In general, antihypertensive therapy should focus on agents with proven benefit in reducing the progression of cardiovascular disease and should be chosen on a patient-specific basis.[59]

▶ *Hyperlipidemia*

❾ *Hyperlipidemia is seen in up to 60% of heart, lung, and renal transplant patients and greater than 30% of liver transplant patients.*[68–70] As a result of elevated cholesterol levels, transplant recipients are not only at an increased risk of atherosclerotic events, but emerging evidence also shows an association between hyperlipidemia and allograft vasculopathy.[70] Hyperlipidemia, along with other types of cardiovascular disease, is now one of the primary causes of morbidity and mortality in long-term transplant survivors.[71]

Elevated cholesterol levels in transplant patients are due to a culmination of factors such as age, genetic disposition, renal dysfunction, DM, proteinuria, body weight, and immunosuppressive therapy. Many of the immunosuppressive agents can produce elevations in serum lipid levels.

Treatment ❾ *Lowering cholesterol has shown to significantly decrease severe rejection and transplant vasculopathy, and improve 1-year survival in heart transplant recipients.*[72] Although these results cannot be extrapolated to the other transplant populations, they do demonstrate the potential benefits of aggressive cholesterol lowering in organ transplant recipients. Due to high prevalence of cardiovascular disease among organ transplant recipients, most health care practitioners consider these patients to fall in the highest risk category for lipid lowering as established by the National Cholesterol Education Panel (NCEP) III guidelines. These guidelines call for a calculated LDL (LDL-C) target level of less than 100 mg/dL (2.59 mmol/L).[73]

Lifestyle Modifications Generally, lowering cholesterol in patients begins with therapeutic lifestyle changes. These changes are initiated either alone or in conjunction with lipid-lowering drug therapy depending on baseline cholesterol levels and other risk factors. Therapeutic lifestyle changes entail a reduction in saturated fat and cholesterol intake and an increase in moderate physical activity.[73] As with hypertension, lifestyle modifications alone rarely are effective enough to achieve a goal LDL-C level.[70] Modifications of the immunosuppressive regimen and use of cholesterol-lowering medications are often warranted in this patient population.

Immunosuppressive Regimen Modifications Tacrolimus has shown the propensity to cause less severe hyperlipidemia when compared to cyclosporine. Conversion from cyclosporine-based immunosuppression to tacrolimus-based immunosuppression may be one way to counteract this disease in transplant recipients.[70]

In past studies, steroid withdrawal in renal transplant patients did lower total cholesterol by 17% and LDL cholesterol by 16%; unfortunately, an 18% decrease in high-density lipoproteins (HDL) levels was also noted in these patients.[70]

Cholesterol-Lowering Agents 3-Hydroxy-3-methylglutaryl coenzyme A (HMG-CoA) reductase inhibitors or statins, are considered to be first-line therapy for hyperlipidemia in the general population.[70,74–77] However, there is some uncertainty about the pathogenesis of cardiovascular disease in transplant recipients and whether statin therapy will have similar effectiveness in organ transplant recipients. Statins have shown definite advantages when used in heart transplantation, including a reduction in LDL-C and major adverse cardiac outcomes (MACE), as well as an apparent cardioprotective effect. In renal transplant recipients, statins are known to lower LDL-C levels and reduce the incidence of some cardiac events, however, the ability to lower MACE may not be evident in this patient population. Despite these mixed results, statins are still considered the primary therapeutic option for hyperlipidemia in all organ transplant recipients.[70]

Fibric acid derivatives are an excellent choice for lowering triglycerides, but are not as effective as statins at lowering the LDL-C.[70] These agents may play a role in conjunction with statins in patients with both elevated cholesterol and triglycerides. Nicotinic acid is very effective at improving the lipid panel, with excellent results in lowering LDL-C, as well as increasing HDL. However, patient tolerability issues are of concern with this agent. The bile acid sequestrants should be avoided in organ transplant recipients due to their high incidence of GI adverse events, as well as their propensity for pharmacokinetic DDIs with the immunosuppressants. Future studies are needed to establish ideal regimens involving the antihyperlipidemic and immunosuppressive medications in order to decrease morbidity and mortality, and ultimately prevent cardiovascular events.[70]

▶ New-Onset DM After Transplantation

❾ *New-onset DM after transplantation (NODAT) is a serious complication that is often underestimated by transplant practitioners.*[78] Kasiske and colleagues attempted to quantify the cumulative incidence of NODAT in renal transplant recipients and found that 8.3% of patients developed NODAT at 3 months post-transplant, 12.9% at 12 months, and 22.3% at 36 months.[78] Even more alarming is that recent studies have revealed an overwhelming prevalence of impaired glucose tolerance, which is also accepted as a risk factor for long-term morbidity and mortality.[78] NODAT is associated with increases in cardiovascular events, with an approximately 22% higher risk of mortality. Patients with NODAT are also more likely to suffer acute rejection episodes and infectious complications than patients without this complication.[78]

Prevention ❾ *NODAT prevention mainly consists of identifying patients at risk pretransplant and controlling modifiable risk factors both pre- and post-transplantation.*[78] The major modifiable risk factors are choice of immunosuppressive therapy and body mass index. For example:

- Immunosuppressive medications: steroid minimization and possibly withdrawal are effective strategies for the prevention of NODAT. Also, patients with worsening blood sugars after transplantation who are receiving tacrolimus may benefit from conversion to cyclosporine.[78]

- Body mass index: a reduction in body weight is always recommended in obese patients prior to the transplant procedure to help lower their NODAT risks.[78]

Treatment ❾ *Lifestyle modifications are always in order in patients who have developed or those who are at increased risk of developing NODAT.*[78] Insulin therapy and oral hypoglycemic agents are often utilized in those patients where lifestyle modifications alone have not controlled blood glucose. Please refer to the chapter on DM for proper instruction on choosing the appropriate treatment regimens in patients with DM.

▶ Neoplasia

Skin Cancer Skin cancer remains the most common malignancy after organ transplantation. The rate of skin cancers occurs from as low as 3.4-fold (melanoma) up to as high as 84-fold (Kaposi's sarcoma) higher in organ transplant recipients when compared to the general population.[79] The incidence of these types of cancers increases with time post-transplant, with one study showing a prevalence rate of 35% among patients within 10 years after transplant.[80] More alarming than the high prevalence is the activity of these cancers in the patient on maintenance immunosuppression. Skin cancers in transplant recipients tend to grow more rapidly and are more likely to metastasize.[79]

The most common risk factors for skin cancer development after transplant include increased age, excessive UV light exposure, high degree of immunosuppression, Fitzpatrick skin types I, II, and III, history of skin cancers, and infection by human papillomavirus.[79]

It is of the utmost importance that transplant practitioners be vigilant about educating their patients about excessive exposure to the sun.[79] Patients should be warned about the risk of skin cancer and be advised on simple methods to limit their risk:

- Use of protective clothing (i.e., long-sleeved shirts and long pants, dark-colored clothing)

- Use of sunscreen daily that is applied to all sun-exposed skin

  - Sun protection factor (SPF) 30 or higher is recommended

Patient Encounter, Part 4

JJ has recovered from her transplant procedure and is now doing relatively well. She returns to your clinic one month after the transplant:

Labs:

Na: 141 mEq/L (141 mmol/L)

K: 4.9 mEq/L (4.9 mmol/L)

Cl: 100 mEq/L (100 mmol/L)

CO_2: 22 mEq/L (22 mmol/L)

BUN: 22 mg/dL (7.9 mmol/L)

SCr: 1.2 mg/dL (106 μmol/L)

Glucose: 89 mg/dL (4.9 mmol/L)

Lipid panel: Total cholesterol = 271 mg/dL (7.0 mmol/L); LDL-C = 180 mg/dL (4.7 mmol/L); HDL = 30 mg/dL (0.8 mmol/L); triglycerides = 325 mg/dL (3.7 mmol/L)

Tacrolimus: 10.1 mg/dL (10.1 mcg/L)

VS: BP 154/95 mm Hg (152/88 mm Hg repeated); HR 60 bpm

Meds: Tacrolimus 3 mg by mouth twice a day; mycophenolate mofetil 1,000 mg by mouth twice a day; prednisone 10 mg by mouth once a day; atovaquone 1,500 mg by mouth once a day; valganciclovir 450 mg by mouth once a day; vitamin D 800 IU by mouth once a day; calcium carbonate 1,250 mg by mouth twice a day separated from food and mycophenolate; simvastatin 20 mg by mouth once a day at bedtime; metoprolol 100 mg by mouth twice a day; amlodipine 10 mg by mouth once a day; ASA 81 mg by mouth once a day; zolpidem 10 mg by mouth once a day at bedtime

Identify why JJ is taking each agent listed.

What are some treatment options, in addition to Metoprolol 100 mg twice daily and Amlodipine 10 mg daily, for JJ's elevated blood pressure?

Design a monitoring plan for JJ's therapy.

▶ *Post-transplant Lymphoproliferative Disorders*

9 *Post-transplant lymphoproliferative disorders (PTLD) are a major complication in patients following organ transplantation.*[81] Large series of case reports have demonstrated that the incidence of PTLD is 1% for renal patients, 1.8% for cardiac patients, 2.2% for liver patients, and 9.4% for heart-lung patients. The risk of developing non-Hodgkin's lymphoma is 28- to 49-fold higher in solid organ transplant recipients compared with the general population. Another independent risk factor is the presence of the Epstein-Barr virus (EBV).[81-83] Lymphomas are the most common form of lymphoproliferative disease found in transplant recipients.[81]

The incidence of disease depends on certain factors. These factors include the type of organ transplanted, the age of the transplant recipient, the degree of immunosuppression, the type of immunosuppression, and exposure to EBV.[81,83] The mortality rate in these patients is about 50%, with most patients dying shortly after diagnosis. It has also been demonstrated that the risk of developing PTLD is greater in the population of EBV seronegative patients at the time of transplant.[83]

Another risk factor for the development of PTLD is the type of immunosuppressive regimens used. ALAs have come to be widely used in the prevention and treatment of acute rejection. These agents work by causing widespread T-cell lysis. Immunosuppressive regimens utilizing the ALAs have been proven to increase the risk of PTLD.[81]

Treatment **9** *Treatment for PTLD is still controversial; however, the most common treatment options include reduction of immunosuppression, chemotherapy,*[84] *and anti-B cell monoclonal antibodies.*[81] PTLD continues to be a long-term complication of prolonged immunosuppression. Current treatment options are all associated with certain risks. Prevention is the most effective treatment for PTLD. A better understanding in future of the disease process and the risk factors involved with the development of PTLD will aid in the prophylaxis and treatment of this disorder.

OUTCOME EVALUATION

Successful outcomes in solid organ transplantation are generally measured in terms of several separate end points: (a) preventing acute rejection, (b) increasing 1-year graft survival, (c) preventing immunosuppressive drug complications, and (d) improving long-term allograft and patient survival.

The short-term goals after organ transplantation revolve around reducing the incidence of acute rejection episodes and attaining a high graft survival rate. By accomplishing these goals, transplant clinicians hope to attain good allograft function to allow for an improved quality of life. These goals can be achieved through the appropriate use of medical immunosuppression and scrutinizing over the therapeutic and toxic monitoring parameters associated with each medication employed. In addition, transplant recipients should be monitored for adverse drug reactions, DDIs, and adherence with their therapeutic regimen.

The long-term goals after organ transplant are to maximize the functionality of the allograft and prevent the complications of immunosuppression, which lead to improved patient survival. Clinicians must play multiple roles in the long-term care of transplant recipients as, not only must the patient be followed from an immunologic perspective, but practitioners must be focused in identifying and treating the adverse sequelae associated with lifelong immunosuppression including cardiovascular disease, malignancy, infection, and osteoporosis among others. Again, limiting drug misadventures and assuring adherence with the therapeutic regimen is important and should be stressed.

Patient Care and Monitoring

Early Management of Transplant Recipients

- Review any available diagnostic and laboratory data to evaluate the function of the allograft and the health of the recipient.
- Assess the patient's current medication regimen, including:
  - Induction therapy agent:
    - Assess for appropriate dose and duration of therapy
    - Therapeutic monitoring parameters (organ function)
    - Toxic monitoring parameters
  - Maintenance immunosuppressive agents:
    - Assess for appropriate dose and duration of therapy
    - Therapeutic monitoring parameters (organ function)
    - Toxic monitoring parameters
  - Anti-infective prophylaxis:
    - Assess suitability of chosen prophylactic agents (i.e., drug allergies, CMV donor and recipient serostatus)
    - Therapeutic monitoring parameters
    - Toxic monitoring parameters
  - Medications used for comorbidities:
    - Assess appropriate selection of these medications for pharmacokinetic and pharmacodynamic DDIs, need (i.e., do renal transplant recipients need to continue to take erythropoietin?), and efficacy.
    - Therapeutic monitoring parameters
    - Toxic monitoring parameters
- Evaluate the patient for the presence of adverse drug reactions, drug allergies or DDIs.
- Develop patient-specific short-term and long-term therapeutic goals.
- Provide patient education regarding the organ transplant, the complications associated with transplantation, the need for lifestyle modifications to reduce risk of complications (i.e., wear sunscreen, low-sodium diet) and drug therapy.
- Stress importance of adherence with therapeutic regimen.

Outpatient Management of Transplant Recipients

- Obtain a thorough history of prescription, nonprescription, and complimentary and alternative medication use.
  - Maintenance immunosuppressive agents:
    - Assess for appropriate dose and duration of therapy
    - Therapeutic monitoring parameters (organ function)
    - Toxic monitoring parameters
  - Anti-infective prophylaxis:
    - Assess suitability of chosen prophylactic agents (i.e., drug allergies, CMV donor and recipient serostatus)
      - Does the patient need continued prophylaxis therapy?
      - When do you stop prophylaxis?
    - Therapeutic monitoring parameters
    - Toxic monitoring parameters
  - Medications used for comorbidities:
    - Assess appropriate selection of these medications for pharmacokinetic and pharmacodynamic DDIs, need and efficacy
    - Therapeutic monitoring parameters (drug- and disease-specific)
    - Toxic monitoring parameters (drug-specific)
- Evaluate the patient for the presence of adverse drug reactions, drug allergies, or DDIs.
- Reassess your patient-specific short-term and long-term therapeutic goals.
- Continue with patient education in regards to the complications associated with transplantation, the need for lifestyle modifications to reduce risk of the complications (i.e., wear sunscreen, low-sodium diet) and drug therapy.
- Re-emphasize the importance of adherence with their therapeutic regimen.
- Assess improvement in quality of life measures such as physical, psychological and social functioning, and well-being.

Abbreviations Introduced in This Chapter

6-MP	6-Mercaptopurine
ACE	Angiotensin converting enzyme
ALA	Antilymphocyte antibodies (includes OKT-3, eATG, and antithymocyte globulin)
ANF	Atrial natriuretic factor
APC	Antigen-presenting cell
ARB	Angiotensin receptor blocker
AWP	Average wholesale price
BMI	Body mass index
BUN	Blood urea nitrogen
C_0	Trough concentration
C_2	Drug concentration 2 hours postdose
CD4+	Helper T cells
CD8+	Cytotoxic T cells
CKD	Chronic kidney disease
CMV	Cytomegalovirus
CSA	Cyclosporine

CYP	Cytochrome P-450 system
CYP3A	Cytochrome P-450 system 3A isozyme
DC	Dendritic cell
DDI	Drug–drug interaction
DM	Diabetes mellitus
DOE	Dyspnea on exertion
DS	Double strength
eATG	Antithymoglobulin equine
EBV	Epstein-Barr virus
ESRD	End-stage renal disease
FBS	Fasting blood sugar
FEV	Forced expiratory volume
G6PD	Glucose-6-phosphate-dehydrogenase
GFR	Glomerular filtration rate
HDL	High-density lipoproteins
HgA_{1c}	Hemoglobin A_{1c}
HLA	Human leukocyte antigen
HMG-CoA	3-Hydroxy-3-methylglutaryl coenzyme A reductase
HPLC	High-performance liquid chromatography
HTN	Hypertension
IgG	Immunoglobulin G
IL-2	Interleukin-2
IL-2RA	Interleukin-2 receptor antagonist
IL-2R	Interleukin-2 receptor
JNC7	Joint National Committee Seventh Report
K	Potassium
LDL	Low-density lipoproteins
LDL-C	Calculated low-density lipoproteins
LFT	Liver function test
MACE	Major adverse cardiovascular events
Mg	Magnesium
MHC	Major histocompatibility complex
MMF	Mycophenolate mofetil
MPA	Mycophenolic acid
MPAG	mAP-glucorinide
NCEP	National Cholesterol Education Program
NFAT (NFAT-P)	Nuclear factors
NODAT	New-onset diabetes mellitus after transplantation
NSAID	Nonsteroidal anti-inflammatory drug
NYHA	New York Heart Association
OKT-3	Muronomab-CD3
P-gp	P-glycoprotein
PKD	Polycystic kidney disease
PO_4	Phosphate
PRA	Panal of reactive antibodies
PTLD	Post-transplant lymphoproliferative disorders
RATG	Rabbit antithymocyte immunoglobulin
RBF	Renal blood flow
SCr	Serum creatinine
SOB	Shortness of breath
SRL	Sirolimus
SPK	Simultaneous pancreas-kidney
SS	Single strength
TAC	Tacrolimus

TCR	T-cell receptor
ToR	Target of Rapamycin

 Self-assessment questions and answers are available at *http://www.mhpharmacotherapy. com/pp.html.*

REFERENCES

1. Calne RY. Transplantation: Current developments and future directions. Front Biosci 2007;12:3727–3733.
2. Halloran PF. Immunosuppressive drugs for kidney transplantation. N Engl J Med 2004;351(26):2715–2729.
3. The Organ Procurement and Transplant Network (OPTN). Available at *http://www.optn.org/latestData/viewDataReports.asp.*
4. Remuzzi G, Chiaramonte S, Perico N, Ronco C (eds): Humoral immunity in kidney transplantation. What clinicians need to know. Contrib Nephrol 2009;162:1–12
5. Michaels PJ, Fishbein MC, Colvin RB. Humoral rejection of human organ transplants. Springer Semin Immunopathol 2003;25(2):119–140.
6. Joosten SA, Sijpkens YW, van Kooten C, Paul LC. Chronic renal allograft rejection: Pathophysiologic considerations. Kidney Int 2005;68(1):1–13.
7. Monaco AP. The beginning of clinical tolerance in solid organ allografts. Exp Clin Transplant 2004;2(1):153–161.
8. Hardinger KL, Koch MJ, Brennan DC. Current and future immunosuppressive strategies in renal transplantation. Pharmacotherapy 2004;24(9):1159–1176.
9. Micromedex Healthcare Series, (electronic version). Greenwood Village, CO: Thomson Healthcare, Inc., 2008.
10. Mohty M, Gaugler B. Mechanisms of action of antithymocyte globulin: Old dogs with new tricks! Leuk Lymphoma 2008;49(9):1664–1667.
11. Mottershead M, Neuberger J. Daclizumab. Expert Opin Biol Ther 2007;7(10):1583–1596.
12. Nashan B. Antibody induction therapy in renal transplant patients receiving calcineurin-inhibitor immunosuppressive regimens: A comparative review. BioDrugs 2005;19(1):39–46.
13. Vincenti F, Pace D, Birnbaum J, Lantz M. Pharmacokinetic and pharmacodynamic studies of one or two doses of daclizumab in renal transplantation. Am J Transplant 2003;3(1):50–52.
14. Soltero L, Carbajal H, Sarkissian N, et al. A truncated-dose regimen of daclizumab for prevention of acute rejection in kidney transplant recipients: A single-center experience. Transplantation 2004;78(10):1560–1563.
15. Whiting JF, Fecteau A, Martin J, Bejarano PA, Hanto DW. Use of low-dose OKT3 as induction therapy in liver transplantation. Transplantation 1998;65(4):577–580.
16. Hooks MA, Wade CS, Millikan WJ, Jr. Muromonab CD-3: A review of its pharmacology, pharmacokinetics, and clinical use in transplantation. Pharmacotherapy 1991;11(1):26–37.
17. Wilde MI, Goa KL. Muromonab CD3: A reappraisal of its pharmacology and use as prophylaxis of solid organ transplant rejection. Drugs 1996;51(5):865–894.
18. Abramowicz D, De Pauw L, Le Moine A, et al. Prevention of OKT3 nephrotoxicity after kidney transplantation. Kidney Int Suppl 1996;53:S39–S43.
19. Brennan DC, Flavin K, Lowell JA, et al. A randomized, double-blinded comparison of Thymoglobulin versus Atgam for induction immunosuppressive therapy in adult renal transplant recipients. Transplantation 1999;67(7):1011–1018.
20. Lebranchu Y, Bridoux F, Buchler M, et al. Immunoprophylaxis with basiliximab compared with antithymocyte globulin in renal transplant patients receiving MMF-containing triple therapy. Am J Transplant 2002;2(1):48–56.

21. Brennan DC, Daller JA, Lake KD, Cibrik D, Del Castillo D. Rabbit antithymocyte globulin versus basiliximab in renal transplantation. N Engl J Med 2006;355(19):1967–1977.

22. Beaty CA, Cymet T. Organ transplantation for the primary care provider: What you need to know to get your patient a new liver or kidney. Compr Ther 2008;34(2):69–76.

23. Golshayan D, Buhler L, Lechler RI, Pascual M. From current immunosuppressive strategies to clinical tolerance of allografts. Transpl Int 2007;20(1):12–24.

24. Cyclosporine microemulsion (Neoral) absorption profiling and sparse-sample predictors during the first 3 months after renal transplantation. Am J Transplant 2002;2(2):148–156.

25. Citterio F, Scata MC, Romagnoli J, Nanni G, Castagneto M. Results of a three-year prospective study of C2 monitoring in long-term renal transplant recipients receiving cyclosporine microemulsion. Transplantation 2005;79(7):802–806.

26. Mayer AD, Dmitrewski J, Squifflet JP, et al. Multicenter randomized trial comparing tacrolimus (FK506) and cyclosporine in the prevention of renal allograft rejection: A report of the European Tacrolimus Multicenter Renal Study Group. Transplantation 1997;64(3):436–443.

27. Levy G, Villamil F, Samuel D, et al. Results of lis2t, a multicenter, randomized study comparing cyclosporine microemulsion with C2 monitoring and tacrolimus with C0 monitoring in de novo liver transplantation. Transplantation 2004;77(11):1632–1638.

28. Gabardi S, Tran JL, Clarkson MR. Enteric-coated mycophenolate sodium. Ann Pharmacother 2003;37(11):1685–1693.

29. Sollinger HW. Mycophenolates in transplantation. Clin Transplant 2004;18(5):485–492.

30. Buell C, Koo J. Long-term safety of mycophenolate mofetil and cyclosporine: A review. J Drugs Dermatol 2008;7(8):741–748.

31. Sollinger H. Enteric-coated mycophenolate sodium: Therapeutic equivalence to mycophenolate mofetil in de novo renal transplant patients. Transplant Proc 2004;36(2 Suppl):517S–520S.

32. Gabardi S, Cerio J. Future immunosuppressive agents in solid-organ transplantation. Prog Transplant 2004;14(2):148–156.

33. Augustine JJ, Bodziak KA, Hricik DE. Use of sirolimus in solid organ transplantation. Drugs 2007;67(3):369–391.

34. Marder W, McCune WJ. Advances in immunosuppressive therapy. Semin Respir Crit Care Med 2007;28(4):398–417.

35. MacDonald AS. A worldwide, phase III, randomized, controlled, safety and efficacy study of a sirolimus/cyclosporine regimen for prevention of acute rejection in recipients of primary mismatched renal allografts. Transplantation 2001;71(2):271–280.

36. Kreis H, Oberbauer R, Campistol JM, et al. Long-term benefits with sirolimus-based therapy after early cyclosporine withdrawal. J Am Soc Nephrol 2004;15(3):809–817.

37. Holt DW. Therapeutic drug monitoring of immunosuppressive drugs in kidney transplantation. Curr Opin Nephrol Hypertens 2002;11(6):657–663.

38. Ahsan N, Hricik D, Matas A, et al. Prednisone withdrawal in kidney transplant recipients on cyclosporine and mycophenolate mofetil—A prospective randomized study. Steroid Withdrawal Study Group. Transplantation 1999;68(12):1865–1874.

39. Liu CL, Fan ST, Lo CM, et al. Interleukin-2 receptor antibody (basiliximab) for immunosuppressive induction therapy after liver transplantation: A protocol with early elimination of steroids and reduction of tacrolimus dosage. Liver Transpl 2004;10(6):728–733.

40. Laftavi MR, Stephan R, Stefanick B, et al. Randomized prospective trial of early steroid withdrawal compared with low-dose steroids in renal transplant recipients using serial protocol biopsies to assess efficacy and safety. Surgery 2005;137(3):364–371.

41. Kaufman DB, Leventhal JR, Koffron AJ, et al. A prospective study of rapid corticosteroid elimination in simultaneous pancreas-kidney transplantation: Comparison of two maintenance immunosuppression protocols: Tacrolimus/mycophenolate mofetil versus tacrolimus/sirolimus. Transplantation 2002;73(2):169–177.

42. Elbarbry FA, Marfleet T, Shoker AS. Drug-drug interactions with immunosuppressive agents: Review of the in vitro functional assays and role of cytochrome P450 enzymes. Transplantation 2008;85(9):1222–1229.

43. DuBuske LM. The role of P-glycoprotein and organic anion-transporting polypeptides in drug interactions. Drug Saf 2005;28(9):789–801.

44. Prescott WA, Jr, Callahan BL, Park JM. Tacrolimus toxicity associated with concomitant metoclopramide therapy. Pharmacotherapy 2004;24(4):532–537.

45. Gelone DK, Park JM, Lake KD. Lack of an effect of oral iron administration on mycophenolic acid pharmacokinetics in stable renal transplant recipients. Pharmacotherapy 2007;27(9):1272–1278.

46. Lynch T, Price A. The effect of cytochrome P450 metabolism on drug response, interactions, and adverse effects. Am Fam Physician 2007;76(3):391–396.

47. van Duijnhoven EM, Boots JM, Christiaans MH, Stolk LM, Undre NA, van Hooff JP. Increase in tacrolimus trough levels after steroid withdrawal. Transpl Int 2003;16(10):721–725.

48. Aronson J. Serious drug interactions. Practitioner 1993;237(1531):789–791.

49. Baroletti S, Bencivenga GA, Gabardi S. Treating gout in kidney transplant recipients. Prog Transplant 2004;14(2):143–147.

50. Gregoor PJ, de Sevaux RG, Hene RJ, et al. Effect of cyclosporine on mycophenolic acid trough levels in kidney transplant recipients. Transplantation 1999;68(10):1603–1606.

51. Ekbal NJ, Holt DW, Macphee IA. Pharmacogenetics of immunosuppressive drugs: Prospect of individual therapy for transplant patients. Pharmacogenomics 2008;9(5):585–596.

52. Anglicheau D, Legendre C, Beaune P, Thervet E. Cytochrome P450 3A polymorphisms and immunosuppressive drugs: An update. Pharmacogenomics 2007;8(7):835–849.

53. Fishman JA. Infection in solid-organ transplant recipients. N Engl J Med 2007;357(25):2601–2614.

54. Pneumocystis jiroveci (formerly Pneumocystis carinii). Am J Transplant 2004;(4 Suppl)10:135–141.

55. Egli A, Binggeli S, Bodaghi S, et al. Cytomegalovirus and polyomavirus BK posttransplant. Nephrol Dial Transplant 2007;(22 Suppl)8:viii72–viii82.

56. Gabardi S, Magee CC, Baroletti SA, Powelson JA, Cina JL, Chandraker AK. Efficacy and safety of low-dose valganciclovir for prevention of cytomegalovirus disease in renal transplant recipients: A single-center, retrospective analysis. Pharmacotherapy 2004;24(10):1323–1330.

57. Paya C, Humar A, Dominguez E, et al. Efficacy and safety of valganciclovir vs. oral ganciclovir for prevention of cytomegalovirus disease in solid organ transplant recipients. Am J Transplant 2004;4(4):611–620.

58. Kethireddy S, Andes D. CNS pharmacokinetics of antifungal agents. Expert Opin Drug Metab Toxicol 2007;3(4):573–581.

59. Beaty CA, Cymet T. Organ transplantation for the primary care provider: What you need to know to get your patient a new liver or kidney. Compr Ther 2008;34(2):69–76.

60. Taylor DO, Edwards LB, Mohacsi PJ, et al. The registry of the International Society for Heart and Lung Transplantation: Twentieth official adult heart transplant report—2003. J Heart Lung Transplant 2003;22(6):616–624.

61. Knoll G. Trends in kidney transplantation over the past decade. Drugs 2008;(68 Suppl)1:3–10.

62. Taler SJ, Textor SC, Canzanello VJ, et al. Role of steroid dose in hypertension early after liver transplantation with tacrolimus (FK506) and cyclosporine. Transplantation 1996;62(11):1588–1592.

63. Salifu MO, Tedla F, Aytug S, Hayat A, McFarlane SI. Posttransplant diabetes and hypertension: Pathophysiologic insights and therapeutic rationale. Curr Diab Rep 2008;8(3):221–227.

64. Perico N, Benigni A, Zoja C, Delaini F, Remuzzi G. Functional significance of exaggerated renal thromboxane A2 synthesis induced by cyclosporin A. Am J Physiol 1986;251(4 Pt 2):F581–F587.

65. Tang IY, Meier-Kriesche HU, Kaplan B. Immunosuppressive strategies to improve outcomes of kidney transplantation. Semin Nephrol 2007;27(4):377–392.

66. Jensik SC. Tacrolimus (FK 506) in kidney transplantation: Three-year survival results of the US multicenter, randomized, comparative trial. FK 506 Kidney Transplant Study Group. Transplant Proc 1998;30(4):1216–1218.

67. Sacks FM, Svetkey LP, Vollmer WM, et al. Effects on blood pressure of reduced dietary sodium and the Dietary Approaches to Stop Hypertension (DASH) diet. DASH-Sodium Collaborative Research Group. N Engl J Med 2001;344(1):3–10.

68. Kasiske BL. Hyperlipidemia in patients with chronic renal disease. Am J Kidney Dis 1998;32(5 Suppl 3):S142–S156.

69. Tannock LR, Reynolds LR. Management of dyslipidemia in patients after solid organ transplantation. Postgrad Med 2008;120(1):43–49.

70. Mathis AS, Dave N, Knipp GT, Friedman GS. Drug-related dyslipidemia after renal transplantation. Am J Health Syst Pharm 2004;61(6):565–585; quiz 86–87.

71. Kobashigawa JA, Kasiske BL. Hyperlipidemia in solid organ transplantation. Transplantation 1997;63(3):331–338.

72. Kobashigawa JA, Katznelson S, Laks H, et al. Effect of pravastatin on outcomes after cardiac transplantation. N Engl J Med 1995;333(10):621–627.

73. Executive Summary of The Third Report of The National Cholesterol Education Program (NCEP) Expert Panel on Detection, Evaluation, and Treatment of High Blood Cholesterol in Adults (Adult Treatment Panel III). JAMA 2001;285(19):2486–2497.

74. Kasiske BL, Heim-Duthoy KL, Singer GG, Watschinger B, Germain MJ, Bastani B. The effects of lipid-lowering agents on acute renal allograft rejection. Transplantation 2001;72(2):223–227.

75. Downs JR, Clearfield M, Weis S, et al. Primary prevention of acute coronary events with lovastatin in men and women with average cholesterol levels: Results of AFCAPS/TexCAPS. Air Force/Texas Coronary Atherosclerosis Prevention Study. JAMA 1998;279(20):1615–1622.

76. Wenke K, Meiser B, Thiery J, et al. Simvastatin reduces graft vessel disease and mortality after heart transplantation: A four-year randomized trial. Circulation 1997;96(5):1398–1402.

77. Katznelson S, Wilkinson AH, Kobashigawa JA, et al. The effect of pravastatin on acute rejection after kidney transplantation—A pilot study. Transplantation 1996;61(10):1469–1474.

78. Davidson J, Wilkinson A, Dantal J, et al. New-onset diabetes after transplantation: 2003 International consensus guidelines. Proceedings of an international expert panel meeting. Barcelona, Spain, February 19, 2003. Transplantation 2003;75(10 Suppl):SS3–SS24.

79. Traywick C, O'Reilly FM. Management of skin cancer in solid organ transplant recipients. Dermatol Ther 2005;18(1):12–18.

80. Navarro MD, Lopez-Andreu M, Rodriguez-Benot A, Aguera ML, Del Castillo D, Aljama P. Cancer incidence and survival in kidney transplant patients. Transplant Proc 2008;40(9):2936–2940.

81. Gottschalk S, Rooney CM, Heslop HE. Post-transplant lymphoproliferative disorders. Annu Rev Med 2005;56:29–44.

82. Markert E, Siebolts U, Habbig S, et al. Evolution of PTLD following renal transplantation in a child. Pediatr Transplant 2009;13(3):379–383.

83. Marques E, Jimenez C, Manrique A, Vallejo GH, Clemares M, Ortega P, et al. Development of lymphoproliferative disease after liver transplantation. Transplant Proc 2008;40(9):2988–2989.

84. Garrett TJ, Chadburn A, Barr ML, et al. Posttransplantation lymphoproliferative disorders treated with cyclophosphamide-doxorubicin-vincristine-prednisone chemotherapy. Cancer 1993;72(9):2782–2785.

56 Osteoporosis

Beth Bryles Phillips

LEARNING OBJECTIVES

● Upon completion of the chapter, the reader will be able to:

1. Explain the association between osteoporosis and morbidity and mortality.
2. Identify risk factors that predispose patients to osteoporosis.
3. Describe the pathogenesis of fractures.
4. List the criteria for diagnosis of osteoporosis.
5. Recommend appropriate lifestyle modifications to prevent bone loss.
6. Compare and contrast the effect of available treatment options on reduction of fracture risk.
7. Recommend an appropriate treatment regimen for a patient with osteoporosis and develop a monitoring plan for the selected regimen.
8. Educate patients on osteoporosis and drug treatment, including appropriate use, administration, and adverse effects.

KEY CONCEPTS

❶ Major risk factors for osteoporotic fracture include low bone mineral density, personal history of adult fracture, age, family history of osteoporotic fracture, current cigarette smoking, low body mass index, excessive alcohol use, and chronic glucocorticoid use.

❷ A standardized approach for diagnosing osteoporosis is recommended using central dual-energy x-ray absorptiometry (DXA) measurements.

❸ Both pharmacologic and nonpharmacologic therapies for osteoporosis are aimed at preventing fractures and their complications, maintaining or increasing bone mineral density, preventing secondary causes of bone loss, and improving morbidity and mortality.

❹ All men and women over age 50 be should be considered for pharmacologic treatment if they meet any of the following criteria: history of hip or vertebral fracture, *T*-score less than or equal to –2.5 at femoral neck or spine, or osteopenia and at least a 3% 10-year probability of hip fracture or at least a 20% 10-year probability of major osteoporosis-related fracture as determined by FRAX.

❺ Adequate calcium and vitamin D intake is essential in prevention and treatment of osteoporosis. Calcium and vitamin D supplements to meet requirements should be added to all drug therapy regimens for osteoporosis.

❻ Bisphosphonates are first-line therapy for postmenopausal osteoporosis due to established efficacy in preventing hip and vertebral fractures.

❼ Alendronate should be considered first-line treatment for primary osteoporosis in men due to proven benefit in reducing fractures and relative safety.

❽ For prevention of glucocorticoid-induced osteoporosis, bisphosphonate therapy is recommended in all patients who are starting treatment with glucocorticoids (prednisone 5 mg or more daily or equivalent) for at least 3 months. For patients receiving chronic glucocorticoids (prednisone 5 mg or more daily or equivalent), bisphosphonate therapy is also recommended if the bone mineral density is low or if there is a history of fracture.

INTRODUCTION

Osteoporosis is a common and often silent disorder causing significant morbidity and mortality and reduced quality of life. It is associated with increased risk and rate of bone fracture and is responsible for over 1.5 million fractures in the United States annually resulting in direct health care costs of over $17 billion.[1] As the population ages, these numbers are expected to increase by two- to threefold. It is estimated that postmenopausal Caucasian women have a

50% lifetime chance of developing an osteoporosis-related fracture, whereas men have a 20% lifetime chance.[1] Common sites of fracture include the spine, hip, and wrist, although almost all sites can be affected. Only a fraction of patients with osteoporosis receive optimal treatment.

The fractures associated with osteoporosis have an enormous impact on individual patients. In addition to the initial pain associated with a new fracture, several adverse long-term complications can occur, including chronic pain, loss of mobility, depression, nursing home placement, and death. Patients with vertebral fractures may experience chronic pain, height loss, kyphosis, and decreased mobility due to limitations in bending and reaching. Multiple vertebral fractures may lead to restrictive lung disease and alter abdominal anatomy. Patients with hip fractures have added risks associated with surgical intervention to repair the fracture. Some patients never fully recover or regain preinjury independence; mortality is common within one year of hip fracture.

Due to the widespread impact of osteoporosis on the population as a whole, several societies and governmental agencies have published clinical guidelines with recommendations for appropriate evaluation, screening, prevention and treatment of these patients. These groups include the American Association of Clinical Endocrinologists (AACE),[2] American College of Physicians (ACP),[3,4] International Society for Clinical Densitometry,[5] National Osteoporosis Foundation (NOF),[1] North American Menopause Society (NAMS),[6] and United States Preventive Services Task Force (USPSTF).[7] The most recent guidelines were published in 2008 by the National Osteoporosis Foundation. The recommendations of these groups are represented throughout the chapter.

EPIDEMIOLOGY AND ETIOLOGY

Osteoporosis is the most common skeletal disorder, affecting over 10 million Americans. Additionally, over 30 million Americans have low bone mass. The prevalence of vertebral fracture in postmenopausal women is greater than 20%.[2] Only one in three patients with osteoporosis has been diagnosed, and only one in seven will receive treatment.[2]

Osteoporosis can be classified as either primary (no known cause) or secondary (caused by drugs or other diseases). Primary osteoporosis is most often found in postmenopausal women and aging men, but it can occur in other age groups as well.

The prevalence of osteoporosis varies by age, gender, and race/ethnicity. The risk of fracture increases exponentially with each decade in age over 50.[8] Residents of nursing homes may be at an even higher risk of fracture. Both men and women lose bone as they age. However, women have accelerated bone loss surrounding menopause due to loss of estrogen. Men have some protection from osteoporosis due to their large bone mass and size and the absence of menopause. Fragility fractures of the hip and spine are common among men, especially as age increases. Men comprise 20% of the Americans with osteoporosis. Secondary causes of osteoporosis are found more commonly in men with fragility fractures.

Table 56-1
Risk Factors for Osteoporosis

General Risk Factors	American College of Physicians Risk Factors for Men
Low bone mineral density[a]	Age greater than 70 years
History of low trauma fracture as an adult[a]	Low body weight (BMI less than 20–25 kg/m²)
Current cigarette smoking[a]	Weight loss (greater than 10% compared to adult weight or weight loss in recent years)
Low body weight or body mass index[a]	Physical inactivity
Advanced age[a]	Corticosteroid use
Alcohol in amounts more than 2 drinks/day[a]	Androgen deprivation therapy
Systemic glucocorticoid therapy[a]	Previous fragility fracture
Female sex	
Osteoporotic fracture in a first-degree relative (especially hip fracture)[a]	
Secondary osteoporosis (especially rheumatoid arthritis[a])	
Low calcium intake	
Low physical activity	
Poor health/frailty	
Minimal sun exposure	
Recent falls	
Cognitive impairment	
Estrogen deficiency before 45 years of age	
Impaired vision	
Caucasian ethnicity	

[a]Major risk factors used in the WHO fracture risk model.

Adapted from DiPiro JT et al., eds. Pharmacotherapy: A pathophysiologic approach. 7th ed. McGraw-Hill: New York, 2008, Table 93–1, page 1486, with permission.

Most hip fractures occur in postmenopausal Caucasian women; this group also has the highest incidence of fracture when adjusted for age.[9] The incidence of osteoporosis and low bone mass is highest in Caucasian women, followed by Asian, Hispanic, and African American women, respectively.[9]

Many of the risk factors for osteoporosis and osteoporotic fractures are predictors of low bone mineral density, such as age and ethnicity (see Table 56–1). ❶ *Major risk factors for osteoporotic fracture include low bone mineral density, personal history of adult fracture, age, family history of osteoporotic fracture, current cigarette smoking, low body mass index, excessive alcohol use, and chronic glucocorticoid use.*[1] As bone mineral density decreases, the risk of fracture increases. However, the threshold at which individual patients develop a fracture varies, and other factors may play a role in fracture susceptibility. One such factor that can influence the development of fracture is falling.

Osteoporosis can also develop from secondary causes such as concurrent disease states and drugs (see Table 56–2). Approximately one-third to one-half of osteoporosis cases in men and half of all cases in perimenopausal women are

Table 56–2	

Medical Conditions and Drugs Associated With Osteoporosis or Low Bone Mass

Medical Conditions	Drugs
Alcoholism	Anticonvulsants (phenytoin, phenobarbital)
Chronic renal disease	
Cushing's syndrome	Aromatase inhibitors (anastrazole, exemestane, letrozole)
Cystic fibrosis	
Diabetes mellitus	
Eating disorders	Cytotoxic drugs (e.g., methotrexate, cisplatin)
GI disorders (e.g., gastrectomy, malabsorption syndromes)	Glucocorticoids (5 mg or more of prednisone daily or equivalent for at least 3 months)
Hematologic disorders (e.g., hemophilia)	
Hyperparathyroidism	Gonadotropin-releasing hormone analogs (leuprolide acetate, nafarelin, gosarelin)
Hyperthyroidism	
Hypogonadal states	Heparin
Organ transplantation	Immunosuppressants (e.g., tacrolimus)
Skeletal cancer (e.g., myeloma)	Lithium
	Medroxyprogesterone acetate
	Thyroid supplements (due to over-replacement)
	Total parenteral nutrition

due to secondary causes.[9] Common secondary causes in men include hypogonadism, glucocorticoid use, and alcoholism. The most common cause of drug-induced osteoporosis is glucocorticoid use.

PATHOPHYSIOLOGY

The human skeleton is comprised of both cortical and trabecular bone. Cortical bone is dense and compact and is responsible for much of bone strength. It is the most common type of bone and accounts for approximately 80% of the skeleton. It is generally found on the surfaces of long and flat bones. Trabecular or cancellous bone has a sponge-like appearance and is generally found along the inner surfaces of long bones and throughout the vertebrae, pelvis, and ribs.

Under normal circumstances, the skeleton undergoes a dynamic process of bone remodeling. Bone tissue responds to stress and injury through continuous replacement and repair. This process is completed by the basic multicellular unit, which includes both osteoblasts and osteoclasts. Osteoclasts are involved with resorption or breakdown of bone and continuously create microscopic cavities in bone tissue. Osteoblasts are involved in bone formation and continuously mineralize new bone in the cavities created by osteoclasts. Until peak bone mass is achieved between the ages of 25 and 35, bone formation exceeds bone resorption for an overall increase in bone mass. Trabecular bone is more susceptible to bone remodeling in part due to its larger surface area.

Patient Encounter 1, Part 1: Patient History

A 74-year-old Caucasian woman with a history of chronic obstructive pulmonary disease (COPD) and gastroesophageal reflux disease (GERD) presents to the clinic for follow-up. She reports intermittent daytime and nighttime sweating that comes on suddenly. She reports soaking her bed sheets when this occurs. She had a hysterectomy at age 20 and has never taken estrogen replacement. She reports good relief of reflux symptoms on her current regimen. She started taking a calcium supplement approximately 2 years ago on the suggestion of her friend because she has never gotten much calcium in her diet. She states she does not like milk and never drank it even as a child. She occasionally eats some dairy products such as cheese and ice cream approximately once a week.

PMH: COPD; GERD; S/P total abdominal hysterectomy and bilateral salpingoophorectomy at age 20; nicotine dependence

FH: Father died at age 85 with Alzheimer's dementia; mother died at age 86 with history of colon cancer and osteoporotic fractures of the hip and spine; brother alive and well at age 71

SH: Retired elementary school teacher; smoked one pack per day for the last 50 years; does not drink alcohol

Meds: Albuterol/ipratropium inhaler two puffs as needed (note: albuterol is known as salbutamol outside the United States); formoterol inhaler 12 mcg twice daily; omeprazole 20 mg daily; calcium carbonate 500 mg daily; multivitamin daily

Do any symptoms suggest the presence of osteoporosis?

What risk factors for osteoporosis does this patient have?

What are her calcium and vitamin D requirements?

How could she incorporate more calcium into her diet?

In osteoporosis, an imbalance in bone remodeling occurs. Most commonly, osteoclastic activity is enhanced resulting in overall bone loss. However, a reduction in osteoblastic activity and reduced bone formation can also occur in certain types of osteoporosis. Due to a decrease in endogenous estrogen, bone remodeling accelerates during menopause and up to 15% of bone is lost during the first 5 years after menopause. After this initial decline, bone loss continues to occur but at a much slower rate of up to 1% per year. The resultant bone loss and change in bone quality predispose patients to low-impact or fragility fractures.

CLINICAL PRESENTATION AND DIAGNOSIS

Diagnosis

Osteoporosis has been defined by the WHO as a disease characterized by low bone density and weakening of bone tissue associated with an increase in fragility and vulnerability to fracture.[10] Because bone strength cannot be measured directly, an assessment of bone mineral density is used, which represents 70% of bone strength. Low bone mineral density has been associated with an increased risk of fractures. X-rays are useful only in identifying patients suspected of sustaining a fracture and are not recommended for diagnosis of osteoporosis.

▶ Measurement of Bone Mineral Density

Bone mineral density can be measured at various sites throughout the skeletal system and by various methods. The site of measurement can be either central (hip and/or spine) or peripheral (heel, forearm, or hand). Dual-energy x-ray absorptiometry (DXA) can be used to measure central and peripheral sites of bone mineral density. Quantitative ultrasound, peripheral quantitative computed tomography, radiographic absorptiometry, and single-energy x-ray absorptiometry are used to measure peripheral sites.

❷ *The WHO recommends a standardized approach to measuring bone mineral density for diagnosis of osteoporosis using central measurement of bone mineral density by DXA.*[9] Central DXA is recommended for diagnosis due to inconsistencies in *T*-scores measured between different sites and by different methods.[1,2] Current standards of practice consist of measuring bone mineral density at the lumbar spine and hip, although the WHO suggests the hip is the preferred site for diagnosis.[8,10]

Peripheral bone mineral density measurements cannot be used for diagnosis because they do not correlate with central measurements. However, they are useful in identifying patients who are candidates for central DXA and who are at increased risk of fracture.[6] They may also be useful in patients who have had multiple fractures or in low-risk patients. Additionally, peripheral measurement of bone mineral density is generally less expensive than central DXA and is easily accessible. Instruments used for peripheral bone densitometry are portable, which allows bone density to be measured in pharmacies and health-fair screening booths.

Once the bone mineral density report is available, *T*-scores and *Z*-scores are useful tools in interpreting the data. The *T*-score is the number of standard deviations from the mean bone mineral density in healthy young white women. Osteoporosis is defined as a *T*-score at least –2.5 standard deviations below the mean (Table 56–3). Osteopenia, or low bone mass that may eventually lead to osteoporosis, is defined as a *T*-score between –2.5 and –1.0 standard deviations below the mean. The International Society for Clinical Densitometry recommends use of the WHO definition and *T*-scores for diagnosis of osteoporosis in postmenopausal women and men over the age of 65, and in men between the ages of 50 and 65 if other risk factors are present.[5]

The *Z*-score is a similar measure that is corrected for age and gender of the patient. The *Z*-score is defined as the number of standard deviations from the mean bone mineral density of age- and sex-matched controls. In premenopausal women, men under the age of 50, and patients who may have secondary causes for low bone mineral density, *Z*-scores may be more clinically relevant in evaluating bone mineral density.

▶ Screening and Risk Factor Assessment

Screening for low bone density is an effective way to identify individuals at risk for osteoporotic fracture. A number of published osteoporosis guidelines provide recommendations for screening based on age and risk factors.[1-7] Routine bone mineral density screening is generally recommended for all women over the age of 65 and men over the age of 70.[1-3,6,7,11] Many guidelines also recommend screening in individuals under these ages but over the age of 50 with specific risk factors such as previous fragility fracture, glucocorticoid use or other high-risk medication, or secondary cause of osteoporosis.

An additional tool, FRAX, was developed by the WHO to evaluate an individual's 10-year risk for hip and major osteoporotic fracture.[1] This probability is calculated based on BMD *T*-score, age, and other risk factors. Its intended use is for men and women over the age of 50 and may be accessed at *www.shef.ac.uk/FRAX*. Although the *T*-score is

---

Clinical Presentation and Diagnosis of Osteoporosis

General

Many patients with osteoporosis are asymptomatic unless they experience a fragility fracture.

Symptoms

Symptoms of fragility fracture include pain at the site of the fracture or immobility.

Signs

Height loss (greater than 2 cm), spinal kyphosis ("dowager's hump"), fragility fracture especially of the hip or spine.

Laboratory Tests

Lab tests are only useful to rule out secondary causes of osteoporosis.

Diagnostic Tests

Bone densitometry using DXA reveals a *T*-score at least –2.5 SD below the mean.

TABLE 56–3	
WHO Definition of Osteoporosis	
Skeletal Disorder	***T*-Score**[a]
Normal	Greater than or equal to –1
Osteopenia	Less than –1 to greater than or equal to –2.5
Osteoporosis	Less than –2.5

[a]*T*-score is the number of standard deviations above or below the mean bone mineral density in young adults.

helpful in calculating risk of fracture with FRAX, fracture risk may be calculated without it.

▶ Laboratory Evaluation

Laboratory assessment has little value in diagnosing osteoporosis, but it can be beneficial in identifying or excluding secondary causes of bone loss, such as hyperparathyroidism, low 25-hydroxyvitamin D levels, hyperthyroidism, hypogonadism, or cancer.[8] Biochemical markers of bone turnover such as pyridinoline, deoxypyridinoline, N-telopeptides, and C-telopeptides of Type I collagen cross-links have been associated with an increased fracture risk in some trials. Variations in the normal ranges of these tests may be related to age, gender, food, and diurnal variation, making interpretation of these tests difficult.[2] For these reasons, biochemical markers of bone turnover are not recommended for diagnosis of osteoporosis.

TREATMENT

Desired Outcomes

❸ *Pharmacologic and nonpharmacologic therapies are aimed at the following goals: (a) preventing fractures and their complications; (b) maintaining or increasing bone mineral density; (c) preventing secondary causes of bone loss; and (d) reducing morbidity and mortality associated with osteoporosis.*

Nonpharmacologic Therapy

The primary goal of nonpharmacologic therapy for osteoporosis is to prevent fractures. Strategies include maximizing peak bone mass, reducing bone loss, and using precautions to prevent falls leading to fragility fractures (Fig. 56–1).

▶ Modification of Risk Factors

Some osteoporosis risk factors (see Tables 56–1 and 56–2) are nonmodifiable, including family history, age, ethnicity, gender, and concomitant disease states. However, certain risk factors for bone loss may be minimized or prevented by early intervention, including smoking, low calcium intake, poor nutrition, inactivity, heavy alcohol use, and vitamin D deficiency. In order to avoid certain risk factors and maximize peak bone mass, efforts must be directed toward osteoporosis prevention at an early age.

▶ Nutrition

Good nutrition is essential for intake of sufficient nutrients and maintenance of appropriate weight. Dietary calcium intake is important for achieving peak bone mass and maintaining bone density. Adequate dietary intake of vitamin D is essential for calcium absorption. Table 56–4 lists calcium and vitamin D requirements for different age groups. Good dietary sources of calcium include dairy products, fortified juice, cruciferous vegetables (e.g., broccoli, kale), salmon, and sardines (see Table 56–5). The most common source of vitamin

D comes from exposure to sunlight. Ultraviolet rays from the sun promote synthesis of vitamin D_3 (cholecalciferol) in the skin. This generally occurs within 15 minutes of sunlight exposure. It is recommended that individuals receive twice weekly sun exposure to ensure optimal synthesis. Vitamin D may also be found in some dietary sources, including fortified milk, egg yolks, salt-water fish, and liver.

▶ Exercise

Exercise can be beneficial in preventing fragility fractures. Weight-bearing exercise such as walking, jogging, dancing, and climbing stairs can help build and maintain bone strength. Muscle-strengthening or resistance exercises can

---

Table 56–4

Recommended Daily Calcium and Vitamin D Intake

	Elemental Calcium (mg)	Vitamin D (IU)	
Adolescents/Young Adults		**Men and Women**	
Age 11–24	1,200–1,500	Age less than 50	200
Men			
Age 25–65	1,000	Age 50 or greater[a]	800–1,000
Age greater than 65	1,500		
Women			
Age 25–50	1,000		
Age 51–65 (postmenopausal)			
On estrogens	1,000		
Not on estrogens	1,500		
Age greater than 65	1,500		
Pregnant and nursing	1,200–1,500		

[a]National Osteoporosis Foundation 2008 recommendations.

From Refs. 1, 12, 13.

Table 56–5

Calcium-Rich Foods[a]

1 cup skim milk
1 cup soy milk (calcium-fortified)
1 cup yogurt
1½ ounces cheddar cheese
1½ ounces jack cheese
1½ ounces Swiss cheese
1½ ounces part-skim mozzarella
4 tablespoonfuls grated Parmesan cheese
8 ounces tofu
1 cup greens (collards, kale)
2 cups broccoli
4 ounces almonds
2 cups low-fat cottage cheese
3 ounces sardines with bones
5 ounces canned salmon
1 cup orange juice (calcium-fortified)

[a]Foods containing approximately 300 mg of elemental calcium.

help improve and maintain strength, agility, and balance, which can reduce falls.[1] It is important to develop and maintain a lifelong routine of weight-bearing and resistance exercise as the benefits on bone can be lost after cessation of the exercise program.[1]

▶ *Falls Prevention*

Another crucial step in avoiding fragility fractures is prevention of falls. Patients with frailty, poor vision, hearing loss, or those taking medications affecting balance are at higher risk for falling and subsequent fragility fractures.[1,2]

A number of medications have been associated with an increased risk of falling, including drugs affecting mental status such as antipsychotics, benzodiazepines, tricyclic antidepressants, sedative/hypnotics, anticholinergics, and corti-costeroids. Some cardiovascular and antihypertensive drugs can also contribute to falls, especially those causing orthostatic hypotension.[1]

Efforts to decrease the risk of falling include balance training, muscle strengthening, removal of hazards in the home, installation of fall reduction measures such as handrails in the home, and discontinuation of predisposing medications.[1,2,14] Use of hip protectors also helps prevent hip fractures, although adherence to this measure may be problematic.[14]

Pharmacologic Treatment (Fig. 56–1)

❹ *The NOF recommends that all men and women over age 50 be considered for pharmacologic treatment if they meet any of the following criteria: history of hip or vertebral fracture, T-score less than or equal to –2.5 at femoral neck or spine, or*

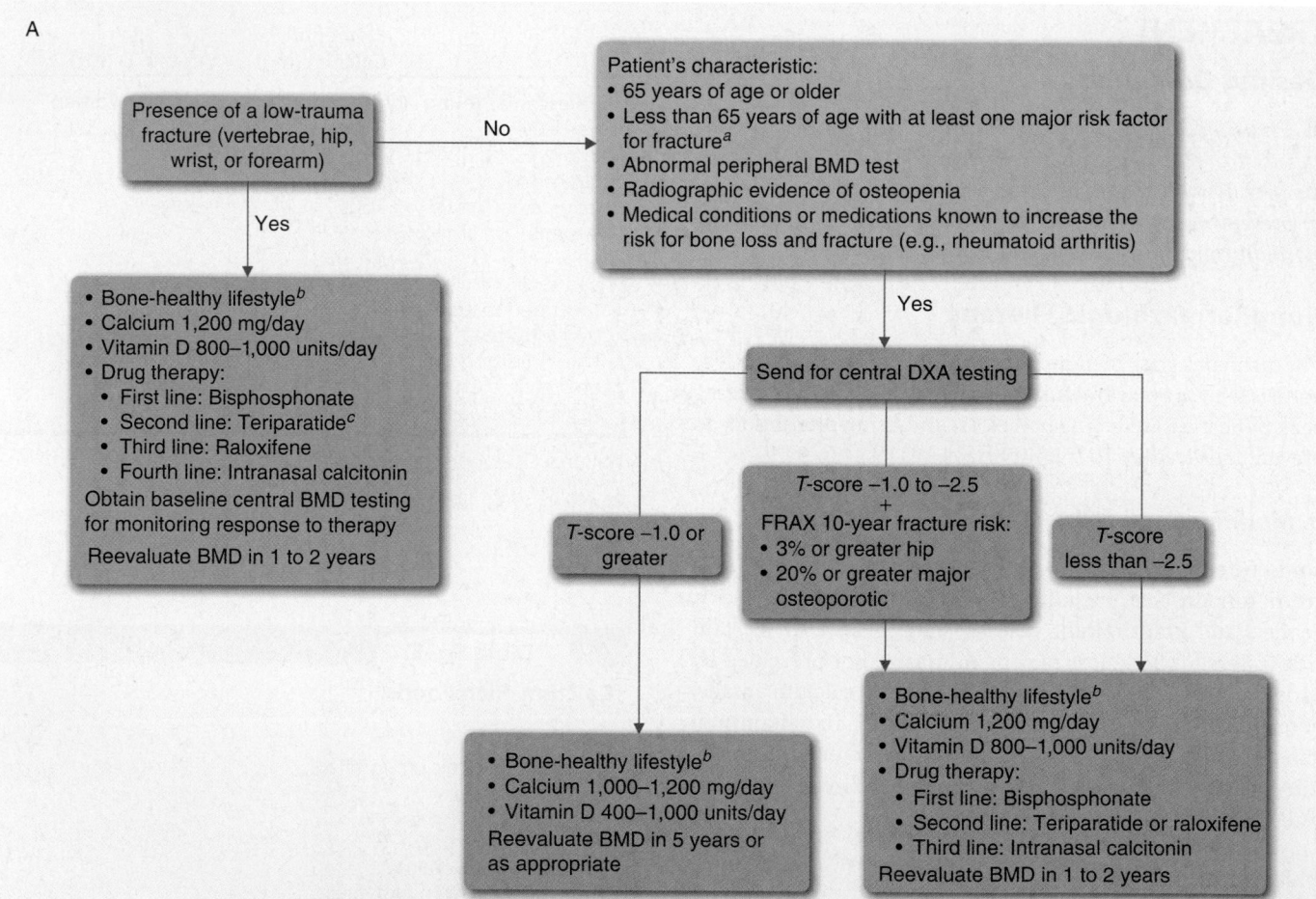

ᵃMajor risk factors: low body weight, personal history of fracture as an adult (after age 45 years), history of low-trauma fracture in a first-degree relative, and rheumatoid arthritis.
ᵇBone-healthy lifestyle: smoking cessation, well-balanced diet, resistance exercise, and fall prevention for seniors.
ᶜTeriparatide can be considered first-line option in patients with a T-score less than –3.5.

FIGURE 56–1. Algorithm for management of osteoporosis in postmenopausal women (A) and in men (B). (BMD, bone mineral density; DXA, dual-energy x-ray absorptiometry.) (Adapted from DiPiro JT, et al., eds. Pharmacotherapy: A Pathophysiologic Approach, 7th ed. New York: McGraw-Hill, 2008:1490–1491, Figure 93–3, with permission; updated with information from Ref. 1.)

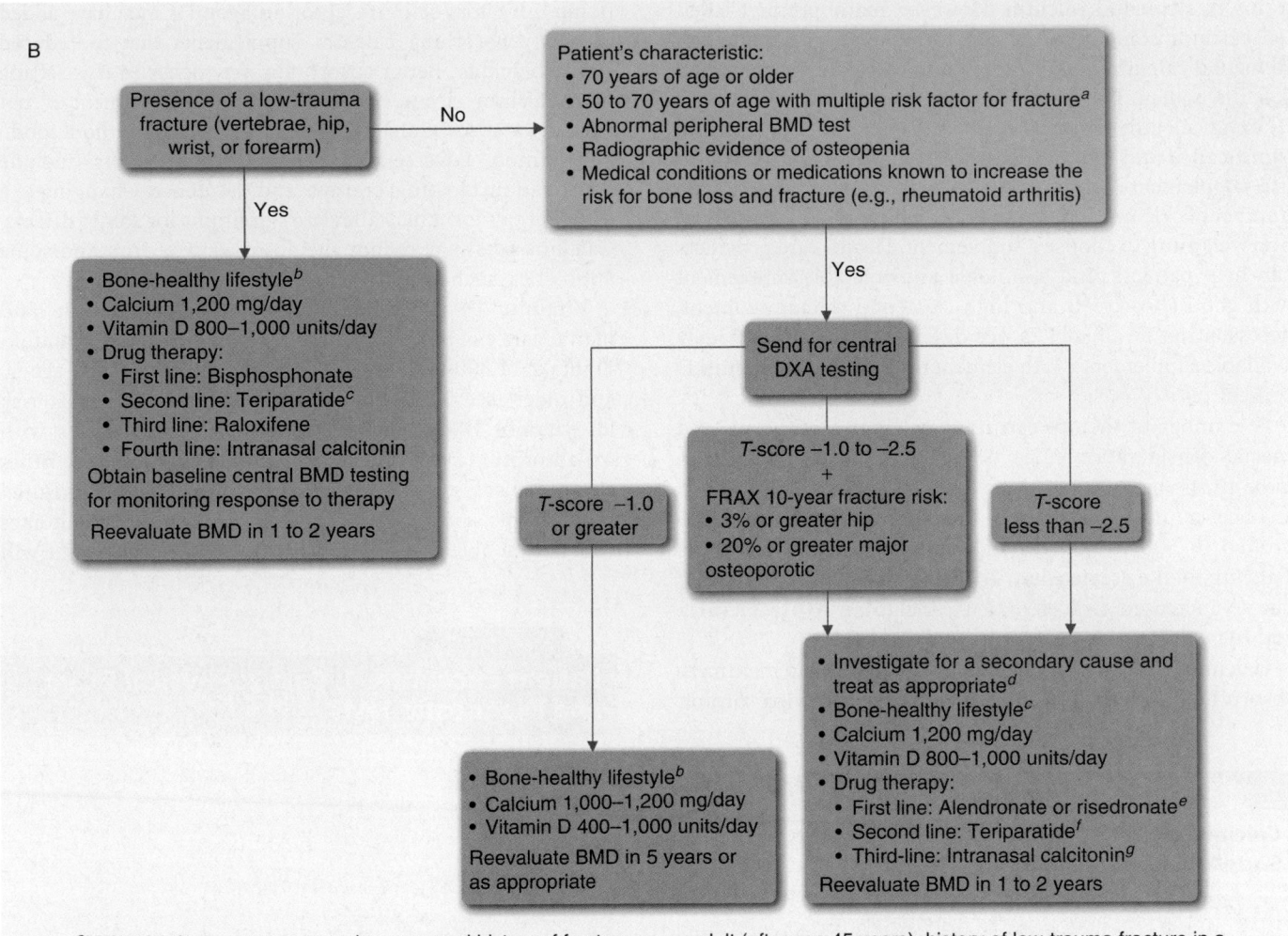

B

Presence of a low-trauma fracture (vertebrae, hip, wrist, or forearm)

→ No →

Patient's characteristic:
- 70 years of age or older
- 50 to 70 years of age with multiple risk factor for fracture[a]
- Abnormal peripheral BMD test
- Radiographic evidence of osteopenia
- Medical conditions or medications known to increase the risk for bone loss and fracture (e.g., rheumatoid arthritis)

Yes ↓ (from fracture box)

- Bone-healthy lifestyle[b]
- Calcium 1,200 mg/day
- Vitamin D 800–1,000 units/day
- Drug therapy:
  - First line: Bisphosphonate
  - Second line: Teriparatide[c]
  - Third line: Raloxifene
  - Fourth line: Intranasal calcitonin

Obtain baseline central BMD testing for monitoring response to therapy

Reevaluate BMD in 1 to 2 years

Yes ↓

Send for central DXA testing

T-score –1.0 or greater

T-score –1.0 to –2.5
+
FRAX 10-year fracture risk:
- 3% or greater hip
- 20% or greater major osteoporotic

T-score less than –2.5

- Bone-healthy lifestyle[b]
- Calcium 1,000–1,200 mg/day
- Vitamin D 400–1,000 units/day

Reevaluate BMD in 5 years or as appropriate

- Investigate for a secondary cause and treat as appropriate[d]
- Bone-healthy lifestyle[c]
- Calcium 1,200 mg/day
- Vitamin D 800–1,000 units/day
- Drug therapy:
  - First line: Alendronate or risedronate[e]
  - Second line: Teriparatide[f]
  - Third-line: Intranasal calcitonin[g]

Reevaluate BMD in 1 to 2 years

[a]Major risk factors: current smoker, personal history of fracture as an adult (after age 45 years), history of low-trauma fracture in a first-degree relative, and rheumatoid arthritis.
[b]Based on a normal male reference database.
[c]Bone-healthy lifestyle: smoking cessation, well-balanced diet, resistance exercise, and fall prevention for seniors.
[d]Examples of secondary causes include hypogonadism, rheumatoid arthritis, chronic obstructive pulmonary disease, systemic glucocorticoids.
[e]Alendronate and risedronate are FDA approved in men. IV bisphosphonates are an option if patient cannot tolerate oral bisphosphonates or has significant adherence problems.
[f]Teriparatide is FDA approved for use in men and can be considered a first-line option in men with a T-score less than –3.5.
[g]Calcitonin is not FDA approved for use in men.

FIGURE 56–1. *(Continued)*

osteopenia and at least a 3% 10-year probability of hip fracture or at least a 20% 10-year probability of major osteoporosis-related fracture as determined by FRAX.[1]

▶ Calcium and Vitamin D

⑤ *Adequate calcium and vitamin D intake are essential for preventing and treating osteoporosis. Calcium and vitamin D supplements to meet requirements should be added to all drug therapy regimens for osteoporosis.* Calcium and vitamin D supplementation increases bone mineral density, and the combination decreases the risk of hip and vertebral fractures. Additionally, vitamin D supplementation decreases nonvertebral fractures in older men and women living independently.[15]

Calcium plays an important role in maximizing peak bone mass and decreasing bone turnover, thereby slowing bone loss. When the calcium supply is insufficient, calcium is taken from bone stores to maintain the serum calcium level. Adequate calcium consumption is essential to prevent this from occurring. Calcium supplementation may also correct hyperparathyroidism in elderly patients.

The highest daily elemental calcium requirements of 1,500 mg are recommended for postmenopausal women and elderly men over age 65. When these requirements cannot be achieved by diet alone, appropriate calcium supplementation is recommended.

Calcium supplements are available in a variety of calcium salts and dosage forms. Calcium requirements are listed in terms of elemental calcium. However, many product labels list calcium content in the salt form, so the percentage of elemental calcium must be known to calculate the elemental calcium content per tablet.

Some calcium products contain lead.[16] While the clinical significance and long-term risks are unknown, it is best to use supplements without a high lead content. Due to the number of calcium supplements available, patients may find it overwhelming to choose a supplement. Health care providers can help patients find a suitable and tolerable supplement with good absorption and high elemental calcium content, necessitating fewer tablets per day. Table 56–6 lists widely available supplements with elemental calcium and vitamin D content.

A number of factors can limit calcium absorption, and special consideration must be given to calcium dosing to maximize absorption. Large amounts of calcium taken at once cannot be absorbed. Supplement doses should be limited to 500 to 600 mg of elemental calcium per dose. Calcium intake greater than 2,500 mg/day should be avoided due to increased risk of toxicity, including hypercalciuria and hypercalcemia.[6]

Calcium carbonate should be taken with food to maximize absorption. Elderly patients or patients receiving proton pump inhibitors or H_2-receptor antagonists may have added difficulty absorbing calcium supplements due to reduced stomach acidity. Better absorption may occur in this setting with calcium citrate because an acid environment is not needed for absorption; it may be taken with or without food.

Common adverse effects of calcium salts include constipation, bloating, cramps, and flatulence. Changing to a different salt form may alleviate symptoms for some patients. Calcium salts may reduce the absorption of iron and some antibiotics, such as tetracycline and fluoroquinolones.

Vitamin D is crucial for calcium absorption and maintenance of bone. The NOF recommends a daily vitamin D intake of 800 to 1,000 mg for all men and women age 50 and older (see Table 56–4).[1] Some individuals are at risk for vitamin D deficiency, including elderly patients with malabsorption syndromes, chronic renal insufficiency, other chronic diseases and those with limited sun exposure.[1] For example, most elderly patients living in nursing homes will not be able to meet vitamin D requirements and will

Table 56–6

Calcium and Vitamin D Content of Common Supplements[a]

Product (% Elemental Calcium)	Elemental Calcium per Tablet (mg)	Vitamin D per Tablet (IU)
Calcium Carbonate (40%)		
Tums 500 mg	200	—
Tums E-X 750 mg	300	—
Tums ULTRA 1,000 mg	400	—
Os-Cal 500	500	—
Os-Cal 500 + D	500	200
Os-Cal Ultra	600	200
Caltrate 600	600	—
Caltrate 600 + D	600	200
Caltrate 600 + Soy	600	200
One-A-Day Women's Multivitamin	450	400
Rolaids 550 mg	220	—
Viactiv	500	100
Calcium Citrate (24%)		
Citracal	200	—
Citracal 250 mg + D	250	62.5
Citracal + D	315	200
Calcium Phosphate, Tribasic (39%)		
Posture – D	600	125
Calcium Lactate (13%)	85	—
Calcium Gluconate (9%)	60	—

[a]Some calcium supplements may contain lead, and many products have not been tested. Tums E-X and Tums Ultra do not contain appreciable amounts of lead.

From Ref. 15.

Patient Encounter 1, Part 2: Physical Exam and Diagnostic Tests

ROS: (+) hot flushes, 5-cm height loss since middle age; (–) back pain

PE:

Gen: Well developed Caucasian woman in no acute distress

VS: BP 122/66, P 77, RR 16, T 36.3°C (97.3°F), wt 55.4 kg (122 lb), ht 5'3½" (161 cm)

Chest: Decreased breath sounds bilaterally, air movement decreased; no rales or rhonchi

CV: RRR, normal S_1, S_2; no murmurs, rubs, or gallops

Abd: Soft, nontender, nondistended; normal bowel sounds, no hepatosplenomegaly

Ext: No clubbing, cyanosis, or edema

Labs: Within normal limits

Bone Densitometry by DXA

- BMD of left hip: 0.544 g/cm²; *T*-score: –3.3
- BMD of lumbar spine: 0.683 g/cm²; *T*-score: –3.3

What additional risk factor and signs of osteoporosis are present in this patient?

What are the goals of pharmacologic and nonpharmacologic therapy?

List at least three nonpharmacologic interventions important in her treatment plan.

What factors support pharmacotherapy for osteoporosis in this patient?

What type of calcium supplement would you recommend for this patient? Why?

need supplementation. Vitamin D deficiency is common in elderly patients due to decreased exposure to sunlight and subsequent decreased vitamin D synthesis in the skin, decreased GI absorption of vitamin D, and reduction in vitamin D_3 synthesis. Individuals living in northern climates also have decreased exposure to sunlight and are less likely to achieve vitamin D requirements.

Vitamin D is often combined in varying amounts with calcium salts. A multiple vitamin is another good source of vitamin D. Most multivitamins contain 400 IU per tablet. Vitamin D is also available as a single entity. To avoid hypercalciuria and hypercalcemia, the maximum recommended dose for most patients is 2,000 IU/day. Ergocalciferol (vitamin D_2) and cholecalciferol (vitamin D_3) are available in higher doses and are generally reserved for patients with vitamin D deficiency.

▶ Bisphosphonates

6 *Bisphosphonates are first-line therapy for osteoporosis due to established efficacy in preventing hip and vertebral fractures.* They are also the most commonly prescribed therapy for osteoporosis. They decrease bone resorption by binding to the bone matrix and inhibiting osteoclast activity. They remain in the bone for a prolonged period and are released very slowly. These effects increase bone mineral density. Although several bisphosphonates are currently available, only alendronate, ibandronate, risedronate, and zoledronic acid are currently approved by the FDA for use in osteoporosis. Table 56–7 contains comparative dosing and cost information for these bisphosphonates.

In placebo-controlled clinical trials, bisphosphonates increased bone mineral density by up to 5% to 8% in the

Table 56–7

Dosage Regimens and Cost of Prescription Agents for Osteoporosis

Drug	Product Size	Usual Dose	Administration	Monthly Cost[a]
Bisphosphonates				
Alendronate	5-, 10-, 35-, 70-mg tablets; 70-mg with cholecalciferol 2,800 IU; 70-mg with cholecalciferol 5,600 IU; 70-mg oral solution	Postmenopausal osteoporosis or osteoporosis in men: 10 mg orally once daily or 70 mg orally once weekly. Glucocorticoid-induced osteoporosis: 5 mg orally once daily for men and women; 10 mg once daily for postmenopausal women not on estrogen. Avoid when CrCl less than 35 mL/min	Take after an overnight fast with 6–8 oz plain water while sitting or standing upright at least 30 minutes prior to morning meal. Do not lie down for 30 minutes after administration. Do not take with other medications or fluids. Do not chew or suck on the tablet	As low as $4 for 70-mg weekly tablet[b]
Ibandronate	2.5-, 150-mg tablets; 3-mg/3 mL injection	Treatment or prevention of postmenopausal osteoporosis: 2.5 mg orally daily or 150 mg orally once monthly; 3 mg IV push over 15–30 seconds every 3 months. Avoid when CrCl less than 35 mL/min	Same as alendronate except administer at least 1 hour prior to morning meal and refrain from lying down for 1 hour after administration	$92 for 150-mg tablet
Risedronate	5-, 35-, 75-, 150-mg tablets; 35-mg with 1,250-mg calcium carbonate tablets	Osteoporosis: 5 mg orally daily, 35 mg orally once weekly, 75 mg on two consecutive days each month, or 150 mg once monthly. Glucocorticoid-induced osteoporosis: 5 mg orally daily. Avoid when CrCl less than 30 mL/min	Same as alendronate	$91 for 35-mg weekly tablet
Zoledronic acid	5 mg/100 mL IV infusion	Osteoporosis: 5 mg infused IV over 15 minutes or longer every 12 months. Avoid when CrCl less than 35 mL/min	Infuse over at least 15 minutes. May premedicate with acetaminophen	$350 for 5-mg dose
Selective Estrogen Receptor Modulators				
Raloxifene	60-mg tablets	60 mg daily	May be taken with or without food	$108 for 60-mg tablet
Calcitonin				
Calcitonin salmon	200 IU/0.9 mL, 3.75-mL nasal spray	Nasal spray: 200 IU daily	Nasal spray: Alternate nostrils on a daily basis	$123 per 3.75-mL nasal spray
Recombinant Human Parathyroid Hormone				
Teriparatide	250 mcg/mL, 3-mL prefilled pen	20 mcg SC daily	Inject into thigh or abdominal wall. Keep pen refrigerated	$899 per prefilled pen

CrCl, creatinine clearance; IM, intramuscularly; SC, subcutaneously.

[a]Monthly cost from drugstore.com.

[b]Wal-Mart $4 prescription drug plan (*www.wal-mart.com*).

lumbar spine, and up to 3% to 6% in the hip.[17-20] Additional data with oral bisphosphonates suggest that bone mineral density continues to increase with long-term therapy of 7 to 10 years.[21,22] Although increases in bone mineral density have been reported at other sites, most of the clinically significant fractures occur in the hip or spine, and these sites have become clinically important measures in the trials. These increases in bone mineral density at the hip and spine are an important marker of treatment effects and are probably related to the decreases in fracture risk found in larger trials.

Large, well-designed trials have proven the benefits of bisphosphonate therapy in preventing vertebral and nonvertebral fractures. Several studies have found decreases in vertebral fracture risk by as much as 40% to 50% with oral bisphosphonates and up to 70% with zoledronic acid.[1,17,23] Although data suggest a similar reduction on vertebral fractures with ibandronate, only alendronate, risedronate, and zoledronic acid have been shown to decrease the incidence of hip and nonvertebral fractures as well by as much as 25% to 40%.[19,20,23,24] In addition to benefits in fracture reduction, the Horizon Recurrent Fracture Trial found a 28% decrease in mortality associated with hip fracture in patients treated with IV zoledronic acid.[20]

Several studies have evaluated the long-term efficacy and safety of bisphosphonates in postmenopausal women. One study evaluated the use of alendronate over a 10-year period and found no difference in adverse effects between women who received alendronate for 10 years compared to women who discontinued alendronate after 5 years. Women who discontinued alendronate after 5 years continued to experience sustained increases in bone mineral density compared to baseline values and reduction in fracture rates.[21] Another study found sustained increases in bone mineral density after discontinuation of alendronate, albeit less than in those who continued longer-term alendronate therapy.[25] A 7-year follow-up study with risedronate found continued increases in bone mineral density and no increase in adverse effects in women receiving risedronate for 7 years compared to women receiving risedronate for 2 years.[22]

The safety of long-term bisphosphonates observed in clinical trials has been challenged by a number of case reports. Concern exists over the use of chronic bisphosphonate therapy due to reports of nonvertebral atraumatic fractures and osteonecrosis of the jaw (ONJ).[26-28] One report described nonvertebral atraumatic fractures in nine patients and delayed fracture healing in four of those patients while receiving alendronate therapy for 3 to 8 years. Bone biopsies in all patients revealed severely suppressed bone turnover, which may have caused bone weakening due to suppression of osteoclastic activity.[26,27] Another report described 63 cases of ONJ resistant to conservative measures and requiring surgical intervention in most cases.[28] A majority of the cases were reported in cancer patients who had received an IV bisphosphonate and only a small number of cases were reported in women who had received oral bisphosphonates for osteoporosis.[28] Risk factors for development of ONJ include chemotherapy, radiotherapy, corticosteroids, infection or pre-existing dental disease.

The most notable adverse effects associated with the bisphosphonates are GI, ranging from relatively mild nausea, vomiting, and diarrhea to more severe esophageal irritation, and esophagitis. However, the most common adverse reactions reported in clinical trials include dyspepsia, abdominal pain, nausea, and esophageal reflux. Clinically significant adverse events include esophageal ulceration, erosions with bleeding, perforation, stricture, and esophagitis. Upper GI adverse effects can occur in up to 20% of patients taking these medications and are often related to inappropriate administration. Other factors that increase risk for GI adverse events include advanced age, previous upper GI tract disease, and use of nonsteroidal anti-inflammatory drugs. Along with appropriate administration, once-weekly administration of oral bisphosphonates may decrease the risk of adverse GI effects.

In addition to the adverse effects associated with oral bisphosphonates, a number of adverse effects have been noted with injectable bisphosphonates, specifically zoledronic acid. Patients in osteoporosis clinical trials experienced a higher rate of atrial fibrillation, increases in serum creatinine, and infusion-related reactions. Pretreatment with acetaminophen may alleviate the influenza-like symptoms of headache, arthralgia, myalgia, and fever.[1,20] Laboratory monitoring, including serum creatinine, alkaline phosphatase, phosphate, magnesium, and calcium, is recommended prior to administration of each dose.

Oral bisphosphonates are poorly absorbed (less than 5%). Taking them in the presence of food or calcium supplementation further reduces absorption. After absorption, bisphosphonate uptake to the primary site of action is rapid and sustained. Once attached to bone tissue, bisphosphonates are released very slowly. They are not recommended for use in patients with renal insufficiency as they are renally excreted and not metabolized.

Proper drug administration is important for optimal absorption and prevention of adverse effects. Oral bisphosphonates should be taken 30 to 60 minutes prior to the first meal or food in the morning after an overnight fast with 6 to 8 ounces (about 180–240 mL) of water (or 2 ounces [60 mL] with the oral solution). Patients should remain upright and refrain from lying down for 30 to 60 minutes after administration. The tablets should be swallowed whole without chewing or sucking. Administration should be with water only and not combined with other fluids. Bisphosphonates should not be taken with other medications or dietary supplements. Bisphosphonates are not recommended for use in patients with esophageal abnormalities, hypocalcemia, renal insufficiency or failure (creatinine clearance less than 30–35 mL/min). For patients unable to tolerate oral bisphosphonates, options exist for IV administration with ibandronate or zoledronic acid.

▶ Selective Estrogen Receptor Modulators

Raloxifene is a selective estrogen receptor modulator (SERM) that has estrogen-like activity on bones and cholesterol metabolism and estrogen antagonist activity in breast and endometrium. These drugs reduce bone resorption and decrease overall bone turnover. The related SERMs tamoxifen and toremifene have partial agonist and antagonist activity at various estrogen receptors. However, the latter agents are limited to the treatment of breast cancer; potential adverse effects preclude further study for long-term use in osteoporosis.

Raloxifene increases bone mineral density and reduces fracture rates. In trials of 1 to 3 years, raloxifene increased vertebral and hip bone mineral density by 2% to 3% and 1% to 2%, respectively.[29] In the Multiple Outcomes for Raloxifene Evaluation (MORE) trial, raloxifene decreased the risk of vertebral fractures by 30% in postmenopausal women with at least one prior fracture.[29] No significant reduction in nonvertebral fractures was reported.

Additional beneficial effects of raloxifene relate to its antagonistic activity in breast tissue. The Raloxifene Use for the Heart (RUTH) study found a significant decrease in estrogen receptor positive invasive breast cancers in postmenopausal women who took raloxifene for more than 5 years.[30] Raloxifene's beneficial effects on the lipid profile prompted the RUTH trial, which sought to determine raloxifene's impact on cardiovascular disease. This study did not find a difference in cardiovascular events but did reveal an increased risk of fatal stroke in women treated with raloxifene.[30]

Adverse effects of raloxifene include hot flushes, leg cramps, and increased risk of venous thromboembolism. Hot flushes are very common and may be intolerable in postmenopausal women who are already predisposed to experiencing them. A more serious adverse effect is the significantly increased risk of venous thromboembolism that has been found in clinical trials.[30] A previous history of venous thromboembolism is a contraindication to therapy.

▶ Hormone Therapy

Estrogen, either alone or in combination with a progestin as hormone replacement therapy (HRT), has a long history as an effective treatment of osteoporosis. The Women's Health Initiative (WHI) trial found a 33% reduction in both vertebral and hip fractures and a 23% reduction in other fractures in postmenopausal women receiving conjugated estrogen and medroxyprogesterone.[31] However, data from the WHI and another well-designed trial, the Hormone and Estrogen/progestin Replacement Study (HERS), found significant risks associated with HRT, including a higher incidence of breast cancer and venous thromboembolism.[31,32] For these reasons, the AACE no longer recommends estrogen or hormone replacement therapy for the treatment of osteoporosis.

▶ Calcitonin

Calcitonin is a naturally occurring mammalian hormone that plays a major role in regulation of calcium levels. It inhibits bone resorption by binding to osteoclast receptors. Compared to mammalian calcitonin, salmon calcitonin has high potency and extended duration of action. Although commercial formulations of calcitonin-salmon are actually synthetic and not derived from salmon, they contain the same amino acid sequence as calcitonin of salmon origin.

Calcitonin salmon is available in injectable and intranasal formulations. It cannot be administered orally due to inactivation by gastric fluids. The parenteral formulation must be administered either subcutaneously or intramuscularly every other day. It is associated with significant adverse effects including flushing, urinary frequency, nausea, vomiting, abdominal cramping, and irritation at the injection site. Additionally, the benefits of the parenteral formulation on bone may diminish over time due to the formation of neutralizing antibodies.

The intranasal formulation is the preferred route of administration due to ease of administration and fewer adverse effects, which are mainly local in nature. Adverse effects associated with the intranasal formulation include rhinitis, nasal irritation, and dryness. Hypersensitivity can develop with either formulation and should be considered before administering to patients with suspected risk of hypersensitivity.

Perhaps the most benefit of calcitonin salmon is in patients with or at risk for vertebral fractures. Nasal calcitonin increases vertebral bone mineral density by 1% to 3%.[33] One 5-year study found a 30% decrease in the risk of vertebral fractures.[33] However, increases in hip bone mineral density and reductions in nonvertebral fractures have not been demonstrated.[33] Calcitonin may have analgesic effects in women with back pain from vertebral fractures. However, enthusiasm for using calcitonin in this setting has waned in favor of managing fracture risk and pain separately.[12]

▶ Anabolic Agents

Teriparatide, recombinant human parathyroid hormone (1–34), is the first anabolic agent approved by the FDA for treatment of osteoporosis. It is generally reserved for patients with moderate to severe osteoporosis. This agent differs from antiresorptive therapies in that it stimulates osteoblastic activity to form new bone when administered once daily. Teriparatide also has many actions that are similar to endogenous parathyroid hormone, and continuous infusions actually stimulate osteoclastic activity and increase bone resorption. In one study, its bone-forming properties increased bone mineral density in the spine and hip by 9% and 3%, respectively. After 21 months of therapy, these increases led to 65% and 35% reductions in vertebral and nonvertebral fractures, respectively.[34]

The dose of teriparatide is 20 mcg given by subcutaneous injection once daily. It is available in a prefilled multiple-dose pen delivery system. Common adverse effects include nausea, headache, leg cramps, dizziness, injection site discomfort, and hypercalcemia. Patients may also experience orthostatic hypotension. For this reason, patients should be seated after the first several doses until drug response is predictable. Osteosarcoma has been observed in animal studies, but no cases have been reported in humans. However, this potential concern has led to the inclusion of a "black-box warning" in the product labeling. The warning states that teriparatide should not be used in patients at increased risk for osteosarcoma, including patients with Paget's disease of bone, unexplained elevations of alkaline phosphatase, prior radiation therapy involving the skeleton, and/ or children and young adults with open epiphyses. Additionally, teriparatide should not be used in patients with pre-existing hypercalcemia. Patient-related concerns regarding the use of teriparatide include cost of therapy and need for subcutaneous injections. The labeling recommends treatment for a maximum of 2 years because it has not been studied for longer periods.

▶ Combination and Sequential Therapy

Interest in combination antiresorptive therapies developed from the hope that using two agents with differing mechanisms for inhibiting bone resorption would result in greater increases in bone mineral density and reductions in fracture rates. Studies have evaluated the combination of bisphosphonates plus estrogen or raloxifene, or estrogen plus calcitonin. Combination therapy produced greater increases in bone mineral density than single agents in some trials, but there was no further reduction in fracture risk. Combination therapy is also more expensive, and concern has been raised that significant reductions in bone turnover may promote bone that is more brittle.[35] The AACE does not recommend combination antiresorptive therapy for treating osteoporosis.

The combination of a bisphosphonate with anabolic therapy (teriparatide) should not be used because a well-controlled trial showed that women receiving the combination actually had smaller increases in bone mineral density than women receiving teriparatide alone.[36] However, sequential therapy with these agents may be more promising. In one study, women who received parathyroid hormone for 1 year followed by alendronate for 1 year had greater increases in bone mineral density than those receiving combination alendronate plus parathyroid hormone, alendronate monotherapy, or parathyroid hormone for one year followed by placebo for 1 year. Additionally, patients who received no therapy after 1 year of parathyroid hormone experienced decreases in bone mineral density.[37] Whether sequential therapy leads to reductions in fracture risk remains to be seen.

▶ Other Therapies

Investigational Agents Several agents, including anabolic and antiresorptive therapies, are currently under investigation for treatment of osteoporosis. A number of SERMs (ospemifene, lasofoxifene, bazedoxifene, and arzoxifene) are undergoing phase 2 and 3 clinical trials for treatment of osteoporosis.[38]

Strontium ranelate is an oral agent possessing bone-forming and antiresorptive properties. Some data suggest significant reductions in vertebral fractures.[39] However, the benefit in nonvertebral fractures is unclear.

Denosumab is a human monoclonal antibody that inhibits receptor activator of nuclear factor-kappa B ligand (RANKL) action. The resultant antiresorptive effects are fully reversible, which may be advantageous in patients who experience adverse events. In clinical trials, denosumab was administered subcutaneously at 3- and 6-month intervals.[40]

PTH (1–84) is an injectable parathyroid hormone that is currently being investigated for use in osteoporosis. It is an 84 amino acid peptide and is known as full-length parathyroid hormone. This is in contrast to teriparatide (PTH 1–34), which is an N-terminal parathyroid hormone analog. It is thought that the full-length parathyroid hormone has additional biologic functions on the bone.[41] PTH (1–84) has shown mixed results in vertebral and hip fracture reduction.[38]

Alternative Therapies Several studies have evaluated dietary supplements such as isoflavones, which are found in soy products and red clover. A well-controlled trial in more than 400 postmenopausal women evaluating a specific isoflavone, ipriflavone, found no benefits on bone mineral density or fracture rates after 3 years.[42] Nevertheless, because these therapies are available without prescription and are not regulated by the FDA, patients may choose to self medicate with isoflavones. Lymphocytopenia appeared in several patients treated with ipriflavone in clinical trials. Additionally, ipriflavone should be used with caution in immunocompromised patients or those with renal disease. It may inhibit CYP 1A2 and 2C9 and may interact with drugs metabolized by those pathways, such as warfarin.

Treatment of Special Populations

▶ Premenopausal Women

The NOF recommends measuring bone mineral density in premenopausal women with specific risk factors for osteoporosis, such as medical condition or medication, in whom treatment would be considered.[1] Premenopausal women at risk for osteoporosis should follow all nonpharmacologic recommendations for exercise and adequate calcium and vitamin D intake. Currently, no good data are available regarding pharmacologic therapy on fracture reduction in this population. Bisphosphonates should be used with caution in this population due to pregnancy risks and uncertain long-term effects.

▶ Men

Compared to postmenopausal osteoporosis, few clinical trials have been conducted evaluating therapies in men. Although alendronate and calcitonin have both been studied, only alendronate reduces fracture rates in men. Teriparatide has also been studied, but no data are yet available on fracture rates. At this time, alendronate and teriparatide are FDA-approved for the treatment of osteoporosis in men. ❼ *Due to proven benefit in reducing fractures and relative safety, alendronate should be considered first-line treatment for primary osteoporosis in men.* Teriparatide should be reserved as alternate therapy in this population. Because secondary osteoporosis causes play a significant role in men, any secondary cause (e.g., hypogonadism) should be excluded or treated before considering other drug therapy.

▶ Glucocorticoid-Induced Osteoporosis

Glucocorticoids play a significant role in bone remodeling. Exogenous glucocorticoid administration results in an increase in bone resorption, inhibition of bone formation, and change in bone quality. Glucocorticoids (e.g., prednisone, hydrocortisone, methylprednisolone, and dexamethasone) promote bone resorption through reduced calcium absorption from the GI tract and increased renal calcium excretion. Bone formation is reduced through inhibition of osteoblasts. They also decrease estrogen and testosterone production.

Patients receiving long-term glucocorticoids are at increased risk of fracture. This risk is greater with higher doses and longer-term therapy. Most bone is lost during the initial 6 to 12 months of therapy, and bone mass continues to decline thereafter. Due to the risk of bone loss and fractures, therapy is recommended for patients receiving long-term supraphysiologic doses of glucocorticoids.

In addition to nonpharmacologic measures, the American College of Rheumatology (ACR) has specific recommendations for preventing and treating patients receiving glucocorticoids.[43] Recommendations for optimal calcium and vitamin D intake are higher for patients receiving glucocorticoids. These recommendations include 1,500 mg daily of elemental calcium and 800 IU daily of vitamin D for all adults receiving glucocorticoids. Patients should take a vitamin D–containing supplement to ensure these requirements are being met.

❽ *The ACR recommends bisphosphonate therapy for all patients who are starting treatment with glucocorticoids (prednisone 5 mg or more daily or equivalent) that will continue for 3 months or longer. For patients receiving chronic glucocorticoids (prednisone 5 mg or more daily or equivalent), bisphosphonate therapy is also recommended if the bone mineral density is low or there is a history of fracture.*[43] Calcitonin may be used in patients who are intolerant of bisphosphonates.

GI Disease

Various GI disorders, including inflammatory bowel disease, celiac disease, and postgastrectomy states, are associated with osteoporosis due to impairment of calcium and vitamin D absorption, corticosteroid-induced bone changes, and chronic inflammatory states. The American Gastroenterological Association recommends bone mineral density measurement in high-risk patients and consideration of treatment for patients with a *T*-score below –2.5, history of vertebral compression fracture, or who are receiving long-term glucocorticoids.[44]

OUTCOME EVALUATION

- Evaluate patients for progression of osteoporosis, including signs and symptoms of new fragility fracture (e.g., localized pain), loss of height, and physical deformity (e.g., kyphosis). Assess patients on an annual basis or more often if new symptoms present.

Patient Care and Monitoring

1. Assess patient risk factors for osteoporosis, with special attention to age, menopausal status, previous history of osteoporotic fracture, smoking status, low body weight, family history of osteoporotic fracture in first-degree relatives, and presence of secondary causes of osteoporosis.

2. Perform a thorough medication history, including prescription, over-the-counter, and alternative therapies. Pay special attention to any vitamins and calcium and vitamin D supplements the patient is taking.

3. Assess nonpharmacologic interventions for preventing osteoporotic fractures, including nutrition, weight-bearing and muscle-strengthening exercise regimens, and fall risk.

4. Determine average calcium intake from diet (Table 56–5) and supplements (Table 56–6). Compare to age-adjusted recommendations (Table 56–4). Evaluate the patient's sources of vitamin D. Recommend appropriate calcium and vitamin D supplementation.

5. Review bone densitometry (i.e., central DXA) for presence of low bone mass (i.e., *T*-score below –2.5 in the spine or hip. If *T*-score is between –1.0 and –2.5, use the FRAX risk calculator to estimate fracture risk.

6. Educate the patient about nonpharmacologic measures to prevent osteoporotic fractures.

7. If drug therapy is indicated, assess the patient for contraindications (e.g., esophageal disease or severe renal impairment for bisphosphonate therapy).

8. Educate the patient on the drug therapy selected, including drug name, dose, method of administration, common or serious adverse reactions, adherence and monitoring. Pay special attention to administration instructions and monitoring for adverse effects. Include a discussion about the therapeutic goals and expectations (e.g., changes in individual *T*-scores may not necessarily correlate with benefit in fracture risk reduction).

9. Develop a monitoring plan, including assessment of efficacy, adverse effects, nonpharmacologic measures to prevent fractures and appropriate drug administration.

Patient Encounter 1, Part 3: Development of a Treatment Plan

Considering all of the information presented, develop a treatment plan for this patient. Include the following information:

(a) recommendations for patient-specific drug therapy including dose and frequency; (b) patient education about the chosen regimen; (c) monitoring plan for efficacy and adverse effects; and (d) consideration of alternative therapies if the initial therapy fails or is intolerable.

- Monitor for beneficial effects on bone density. The NOF recommends a follow-up DXA scan every 2 years to monitor the effects of therapy.
- Assess patients for adverse effects of therapy:
  - Bisphosphonates: Dyspepsia, esophageal reflux, esophageal pain, or burning
  - Zoledronic acid: Influenza-type symptoms related to infusion, ONJ (rare)
  - SERMs: Hot flushes, signs or symptoms of thromboembolic disease (e.g., pain, redness, or swelling in one extremity, chest pain, and shortness of breath)
  - Calcitonin salmon: Nasal irritation or burning
  - Teriparatide: Nausea, headache, leg cramps, hypercalcemia

Abbreviations Introduced in This Chapter

AACE	American Association of Clinical Endocrinologists
ACP	American College of Physicians
ACR	American College of Rheumatology
BMD	Bone mineral density
COPD	Chronic obstructive pulmonary disease
DXA	Dual-energy x-ray absorptiometry
GERD	Gastroesophageal reflux disease
HRT	Hormone replacement therapy
NIH	National Institutes of Health
NOF	National Osteoporosis Foundation
ONJ	Osteonecrosis of the jaw
RUTH	Raloxifene Use for the Heart study
SD	Standard deviation
SERM	Selective estrogen receptor modulator
USPSTF	United States Preventative Services Task Force
WHI	Women's Health Initiative

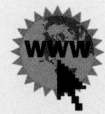

Self-assessment questions and answers are available at *http://www.mhpharmacotherapy.com/pp.html.*

REFERENCES

1. National Osteoporosis Foundation. Clinician's Guide to Prevention and Treatment of Osteoporosis. Washington, DC, 2008, *www.nof.org.*
2. AACE Osteoporosis Task Force. American Association of Clinical Endocrinologists medical guidelines for clinical practice for the prevention and treatment of postmenopausal osteoporosis: 2001 edition, with selected updates for 2003. Endocr Pract 2003;9:545–564.
3. Qaseem A, Snow V, Shekelle P, et al., for the Clinical Efficacy Assessment Subcommittee of the American College of Physicians. Screening for osteoporosis in men: A clinical practice guideline from the American College of Physicians. Ann Intern Med 2008;148:680–684.
4. Qaseem A, Snow V, Shekelle P et al., for the Clinical Efficacy Assessment Subcommittee of the American College of Physicians. Pharmacologic treatment of low bone density or osteoporosis to prevent fractures: A clinical practice guideline from the American College of Physicians. Ann Intern Med 2008;149:404–415.
5. Leib ES, Lewiecki EM, Binkley N, Handy RC. Official positions of the International Society for Clinical Densitometry. J Clin Densitom 2004;7:1–6.
6. NAMS Position Statement. Management of osteoporosis in postmenopausal women: 2006 position statement of the North American Menopause Society. Menopause 2006;13:340–367.
7. US Preventative Services Task Force. Screening for osteoporosis in postmenopausal women: Recommendations and rationale. Ann Intern Med 2002;137:526–528.
8. Raisz LG. Screening for osteoporosis. N Engl J Med 2005;353:164–171.
9. NIH Consensus Development Panel on Osteoporosis Prevention, Diagnosis, and Therapy. Osteoporosis prevention, diagnosis, and therapy. JAMA 2001;285:785–795.
10. Genant HK, Cooper C, Poor G, et al. Interim report and recommendations of the World Health Organization Task-Force for Osteoporosis. Osteoporos Int 1999;10:259–264.
11. Khan AA, Bachrach L, Brown JP, et al. Standards and guidelines for performing central dual-energy x-ray absorptiometry in premenopausal women, men and children. J Clin Densitom 2004;7:51–63.
12. NIH Consensus Development Panel on Optimal Calcium Intake. NIH Consensus Conference: Optimal Calcium Intake. JAMA 1994;272:1942–1948.
13. Institute of Medicine. Dietary Reference Intakes: Calcium, Phosphorus, Magnesium, Vitamin D, and Fluoride. Washington, DC: National Academy Press, 1997.
14. Rosen CJ. Postmenopausal osteoporosis. N Engl J Med 2005;353:595–503.
15. Trivedi DP, Doll R, Khaw KT. Effect of four monthly oral vitamin D_3 (cholecalciferol) supplementation on fractures and mortality in men and women living in the community: Randomized double blind controlled trial. BMJ 2003;326:469.
16. Ross EA, Szabo NJ, Tebbett IR. Lead content of calcium supplements. JAMA 2000;284:1425–1429.
17. Liberman UA, Weiss SR, Broll J, et al. Effect of oral alendronate on bone mineral density and the incidence of fractures in postmenopausal osteoporosis. N Engl J Med 1995;333:1437–1443.
18. Brown JP, Kendler DL, McClung MR, et al. The efficacy and tolerability of risedronate once a week for the treatment of postmenopausal osteoporosis. Calcif Tissue Int 2002;71:103–111.
19. Chestnut CH, Skag A, Christiansen C, et al. Effects of oral ibandronate administered daily or intermittently on fracture risk in postmenopausal osteoporosis. J Bone Miner Res 2004;19:1241–1249.
20. Lyles KW, Colón-Emeric CS, Magaziner JS, et al. Zoledronic acid and clinical fractures and mortality after hip fracture. N Engl J Med 2007;357:1799–1809.
21. Bone HG, Hosking D, Devogelaer JP, et al. Ten years' experience with alendronate for osteoporosis in postmenopausal women. N Engl J Med 2004;350:1189–1199.
22. Mellström DD, Sörensen OH, Goemaere S, et al. Seven years of treatment with risedronate in women with postmenopausal osteoporosis. Calcif Tissue Int 2004;75:462–468.
23. Bone DM, Delmas PD, Eastell R, et al. Once-yearly zoledronic acid for treatment of postmenopausal osteoporosis. N Engl J Med 2007;356:1809–1822.
24. Delmas PD, Recker RR, Chesnut CH, et al. Daily and intermittent oral ibandronate normalize bone turnover and provide significant reduction in vertebral fracture risk: Results from the BONE study. Osteoporos Int 2004;14:792–798.
25. Ensrud KE, Barrett-Connor EL, Schwartz A, et al. Randomized trial of effect of alendronate continuation versus discontinuation in women with low bone mineral density: Results from the Fracture Intervention Trial long-term extension. J Bone Miner Res 2004;19:1259–1269.
26. Odvina CV, Zerwekh JE, Rao DS, et al. Severely suppressed bone turnover: A potential complication of alendronate therapy. J Clin Endocrinol Metab 2005;90:1294–1301.
27. Ott SM. Long-term safety of bisphosphonates. J Clin Endocrinol Metab 2005;90:1897–1899.

28. Ruggiero SL, Mehrotra B, Rosenberg TJ, Engroff SL. Osteonecrosis of the jaws associated with the use of bisphosphonates: A review of 63 cases. J Oral Maxillofac Surg 2004;62:527–534.

29. Ettinger B, Black DM, Mitlak BH, et al. Reduction of vertebral fracture risk in postmenopausal women with osteoporosis treated with raloxifene: Results from a 3-year randomized clinical trial. JAMA 1999;282:637–645.

30. Barrett-Connor E, Mosca L, Collins P, et al., for the Raloxifene Use for the Heart (RUTH) Study Investigators. Effects of raloxifene on cardiovascular events and breast cancer in postmenopausal women. N Engl J Med 2006;355:125–137.

31. Rossouw JE, Anderson GL, Prentice RL, et al. Risks and benefits of estrogen plus progestin in healthy postmenopausal women: Principal results from the Women's Health Initiative randomized controlled trial. JAMA 2002;288:321–333.

32. Hulley S, Grady D, Bush T, et al. Randomized trial of estrogen plus progestin for secondary prevention of coronary heart disease in postmenopausal women. JAMA 1998;280:605–613.

33. Chestnut CH, Silverman S, Andriano K, et al. A randomized trial of nasal spray salmon calcitonin in postmenopausal women with established osteoporosis: The prevent recurrence of osteoporotic fractures study. Am J Med 2000;109:267–276.

34. Neer RM, Arnaud CD, Zanchetta JR, et al. Effect of parathyroid hormone (1–34) on fractures and bone mineral density in postmenopausal women with osteoporosis. N Engl J Med 2001;344:1434–1441.

35. Lecart MP, Bruyere OB, Reginster JY. Combination/sequential therapy in osteoporosis. Curr Osteoporos Rep 2004;2:123–130.

36. Black DM, Greenspan SL, Ensrud KE, et al. The effects of parathyroid hormone and alendronate alone or in combination in postmenopausal osteoporosis. N Engl J Med 2003;349:1207–1215.

37. Black DM, Bilezikian JP, Ensrud KE, et al. One year of alendronate after one year of parathyroid hormone (1–84) for osteoporosis. N Engl J Med 2005;363:555–565.

38. Maxwell AE, Maclayton D, Nguyen H. Current and emerging treatment options for postmenopausal osteoporosis. Formulary 2008;43:166–179.

39. Meunier PJ, Roux C, Seeman E, et al. The effects of strontium ranelate on the risk of vertebral fracture in women with postmenopausal osteoporosis. N Engl J Med 2004;350:459–468.

40. McClug MR, Lewiecki EM, Cohen SB, et al. Denosumab in postmenopausal women with low bone mineral density. N Engl J Med 2006;354:821–831.

41. Hodsman AB, Hanley DA, Ettinger MP, et al. Efficacy and safety of human parathyroid hormone (1–84) in increasing bone mineral density in postmenopausal women. J Clin Endocrinol Metab 2003;88:5212–5220.

42. Alexandersen P, Toussaint A, Christiansen C, et al., for the Ipriflavone Multicenter European Fracture Study. Ipriflavone in the treatment of postmenopausal osteoporosis: A randomized controlled trial. JAMA 2001;285:1482–1488.

43. American College of Rheumatology Ad Hoc Committee on Glucocorticoid-Induced Osteoporosis. Recommendations for the prevention and treatment of glucocorticoid-induced osteoporosis. 2001 update. Arthritis Rheum 2001;44:1496–1503.

44. Anon. American Gastroenterological Association medical position statement: Guidelines on osteoporosis in gastrointestinal diseases. Gastroenterology 2003;124:791–794.

57 Rheumatoid Arthritis

Susan P. Bruce

LEARNING OBJECTIVES

Upon completion of the chapter, the reader will be able to:

1. Identify risk factors for developing rheumatoid arthritis (RA).
2. Describe the pathophysiology of RA, with emphasis on the specific immunologic components.
3. Discuss the comorbidities associated with RA.
4. Recognize the typical clinical presentation of RA.
5. Create treatment goals for a patient with RA.
6. Compare and contrast the available pharmacotherapeutic options, selecting the most appropriate regimen for a given patient.
7. Propose a patient education plan that includes nonpharmacologic and pharmacologic treatment measures.
8. Formulate a monitoring plan to evaluate the safety and efficacy of a therapeutic regimen designed for an individual patient with RA.

KEY CONCEPTS

❶ Comorbidities with the greatest impact on morbidity and mortality associated with rheumatoid arthritis (RA) are: (a) cardiovascular disease; (b) infections; (c) malignancy; and (d) osteoporosis.

❷ Both osteoarthritis and RA are prevalent in the U.S. population, but they differ significantly in presentation.

❸ The most clinically important features associated with poor long-term outcomes include: (a) functional limitation (defined by use of standard measurement scales such as the Health Assessment Questionnaire [HAQ] score); (b) extraarticular disease; (c) positive rheumatoid factor; (d) positive anticyclic citrullinated peptide (anti-CCP) antibodies; and/or (e) bony erosions by radiography.

❹ The goals of treatment for RA are to: (a) reduce or eliminate pain; (b) protect articular structures; (c) control systemic complications; (d) prevent loss of joint function; and (e) improve or maintain quality of life.

❺ It is imperative that the initiation of one or more disease-modifying antirheumatic drugs (DMARDs) occurs in all patients within the first 3 months of diagnosis to reduce joint erosion.

❻ Most clinicians favor the "step-down" approach to slow or reverse the early articular damage as soon as possible.

❼ Methotrexate is the nonbiologic DMARD of choice because of its documented efficacy and safety profile when monitored appropriately.

❽ The risk of infection in patients treated with biologic DMARDs must be considered when selecting and monitoring therapy.

❾ Women of childbearing potential and their partners must be counseled to: (a) use proper birth control while undergoing treatment for RA; and (b) discontinue medications at least 3 months before conception.

❿ In addition to designing an individualized therapeutic regimen to control the progression of RA, the clinician must evaluate the presence of comorbidities and implement measures to control the increased risk.

Introduction

Rheumatoid arthritis (RA) is a complex systemic inflammatory condition manifesting initially as symmetric swollen and tender joints of the hands and/or feet. Some patients may experience mild **articular** (joint) disease, whereas others may present with aggressive disease and/or extraarticular manifestations. The systemic inflammation of

RA leads to joint destruction, disability, and premature death. Juvenile idiopathic arthritis (JIA), formerly known as juvenile rheumatoid arthritis (JRA), is the most common form of arthritis in children.

EPIDEMIOLOGY AND ETIOLOGY

RA affects approximately 1% of the U.S population and 1% to 2% of the world's population.[1,2] RA arises from an immunologic reaction, and there is speculation that it is in response to a genetic or infectious antigen. Risk factors associated with the development of RA include the following:

- Female gender (3:1 females to males)
- Increasing age (peak onset 35–50 years of age)
- Current tobacco smoking. Studies have identified a direct relationship between tobacco use and RA disease severity.[3] Tobacco users also have an increased risk of pulmonary manifestations of RA. This risk is reduced when a patient has remained tobacco-free for at least 10 years.
- Family history of RA. Genetic studies demonstrate a strong correlation between RA and the presence of major histocompatibility complex class II human leukocyte antigens (HLA), specifically HLA-DR1 and HLA-DR4.[4,5] HLA is a molecule associated with the presentation of antigens to T lymphocytes.
- Potential environmental exposures. The number of RA cases has increased during industrialization, although a specific link to environmental factors has not been determined.[6]
- Oral contraceptive use and high ingestion of vitamin D and tea are associated with a decreased risk of RA.[7]
- Fewer than 300,000 children in the United States under age 16 are affected by JIA.[8] There are no known risk factors for JIA.

PATHOPHYSIOLOGY

The characteristics of a synovium affected by RA are: (a) the presence of a thickened, inflamed membrane lining called pannus; (b) the development of new blood vessels; and (c) an influx of inflammatory cells in the synovial fluid, predominantly T lymphocytes. The pathogenesis of RA is driven by T lymphocytes, but the initial catalyst causing this response is unknown. Understanding specific components of the immune system and their involvement in the pathogenesis of RA will facilitate understanding of current and emerging treatment options for RA. The components of most significance are T lymphocytes, cytokines, and B lymphocytes.[4,9]

T Lymphocytes

The development and activation of T lymphocytes are important to maintain protection from infection without causing harm to the host.[9] Activation of mature T lymphocytes requires two signals. The first is the presentation of an antigen by antigen-presenting cells to the T-lymphocyte receptor. Second, a ligand-receptor complex (i.e., CD80/CD86) on antigen-presenting cells binds to CD28 receptors on T lymphocytes. Once a cell successfully passes through all stages, the inflammatory cascade is activated.[10] Activation of T lymphocytes: (a) stimulates the release of macrophages or monocytes, which subsequently causes the release of inflammatory cytokines; (b) activates osteoclasts; (c) activates the release of matrix metalloproteinases or enzymes responsible for the degradation of connective tissue; and (d) stimulates B lymphocytes and the production of antibodies.[4,9]

Cytokines

Cytokines are proteins secreted by cells that serve as intercellular mediators (see Table 57–1). An imbalance of proinflammatory and anti-inflammatory cytokines in the

---

Table 57–1

Cytokines Involved in the Pathogenesis of RA

Cytokine	Source	Activity
Proinflammatory		
TNF-α	Macrophages, monocytes, B lymphocytes, T lymphocytes, fibroblasts	Induces IL-1, IL-6, IL-8, GM-CSF; stimulates fibroblasts to release adhesion molecules
IL-1	Macrophages, monocytes, endothelial cells, B lymphocytes, activated T lymphocytes	Stimulates fibroblasts and chondrocytes to release matrix metalloproteinases
IL-6	T lymphocytes, monocytes, macrophages, synovial fibroblasts	Activates T lymphocytes, induces acute-phase response, stimulates growth and differentiation of hematopoietic precursor cells; stimulates synovial fibroblasts
IL-17	T lymphocytes in synovium	Synergistic effect with IL-1 and TNF leading to increased production of proinflammatory cytokines
Anti-Inflammatory		
IL-4	CD4+ type 2 helper T lymphocytes	Inhibits activation of type 1 helper T lymphocytes, decreases production of IL-1, TNF-α, IL-6, IL-8
IL-10	Monocytes, macrophages, B lymphocytes, T lymphocytes	Inhibits production of IL-1, TNF-α, and proliferation of T lymphocytes

From Refs. 4, 6, 9.

synovium leads to inflammation and joint destruction. The proinflammatory cytokines interleukin 1 (IL-1), tumor necrosis factor-α (TNF-α), IL-6, and IL-17 are found in high concentration in synovial fluid. These proinflammatory cytokines cause the activation of other cytokines and adhesion molecules responsible for the recruitment of lymphocytes to the site of inflammation. Anti-inflammatory cytokines and mediators (IL-4, IL-10, and IL-1 receptor antagonist) are present in the synovium, although concentrations are not high enough to overcome the effects of the proinflammatory cytokines.[4,9]

B Lymphocytes

In addition to serving as antigen-presenting cells to T lymphocytes, B lymphocytes may produce proinflammatory cytokines and antibodies.[5,9] Antibodies of significance in RA are rheumatoid factors (antibodies reactive with the Fc region of IgG) and antibodies against cyclic citrullinated peptide (CCP).[5] Rheumatoid factors are not present in all patients with RA, but their presence is indicative of disease severity, likelihood of extra-articular manifestations, and increased mortality.[10] CCPs are produced early in the course of disease. High levels of anti-CCP antibodies are indicative of aggressive disease and a greater likelihood of poor outcomes. Monitoring anti-CCP antibodies may be useful to predict the severity of disease and match aggressive treatment appropriately.

Comorbidities Associated With RA

RA reduces a patient's average life expectancy by 5 to 10 years, but RA alone rarely causes death.[11,12] Instead, specific comorbidities contribute to premature death independent of safety issues surrounding the use of immunomodulating medications. ❶ *The comorbidities with the greatest impact on morbidity and mortality associated with RA are: (a) cardiovascular disease; (b) infections; (c) malignancy; and (d) osteoporosis.*[11,12]

▶ Cardiovascular Disease

Half of all deaths in RA patients are cardiovascular related.[11] Because a patient with RA experiences inflammation and swelling in his or her joints, it is likely that there is inflammation elsewhere, such as in the blood vessels, termed **vasculitis**. C-reactive protein (CRP), a nonspecific marker of inflammation, is associated with an increased risk of cardiovascular disease; CRP is elevated in patients with RA. Chronic systemic inflammation may contribute to the relationship between RA and cardiovascular disease, but the exact mechanism is still under investigation.[11,12] Uncontrolled hypertension is common in patients with RA. Clinicians should screen for and aggressively treat elevated blood pressure in this population.[13]

▶ Infections

RA itself leads to changes in cellular immunity and causes a disproportionate increase in pulmonary infection

and sepsis.[12] Because medications that alter the immune system are linked to an increased risk of infection, it is difficult to distinguish between an increased risk of infection secondary to RA and the medications used to treat RA. Patients and clinicians must pay close attention to signs and symptoms of infection because of this increased risk.[12]

▶ Malignancy

Patients with RA have an increased risk of developing lymphoproliferative malignancy (e.g., lymphoma, leukemia, and multiple myeloma) and a decreased risk of developing cancer of the digestive tract.[12,14,15] The relationship between RA and cancer is not clear. To confound the issue, medications for the treatment of RA may contribute to increased cancer risk. Patients presenting with new onset of symptoms (e.g., fevers, night sweats, chills, or anorexia) out of proportion with disease activity and patients not responding to conventional RA treatment should be evaluated further for lymphoproliferative malignancy.[12,15]

▶ Osteoporosis

Osteoporosis associated with RA follows a multifaceted pathogenesis, but the primary mechanism likely is mediated by increased **osteoclast** activity.[12] The cytokines involved in the inflammatory process directly stimulate osteoclast and inhibit **osteoblast** activity. Additionally, arthritis medications can lead to increased bone loss. Bone mineral density should be evaluated at baseline and routinely using dual-energy x-ray absorptiometry.[12]

CLINICAL PRESENTATION AND DIAGNOSIS

❷ *Both osteoarthritis and RA are prevalent in the American population, but they differ significantly in presentation* (Table 57–2). Figure 57–1 illustrates the typical joint involvement for patients with RA and osteoarthritis.

Diagnosis

Seven criteria must be met to diagnose RA appropriately:[1]

1. Morning joint stiffness lasting more than 1 hour before disappearing
2. Involvement of three or more joint areas
3. Arthritis of hand joints
4. Symmetric joint involvement
5. Presence of rheumatoid nodules
6. Elevated rheumatoid factor
7. Radiographic changes

A patient may be diagnosed with RA if four or more of these are present. Criteria 1 through 4 must be present for at least 6 weeks. Criteria 2 through 5 must be observed by a clinician.

Table 57–2

Comparison of RA and Osteoarthritis

Characteristic	RA	Osteoarthritis
Gender prevalence (women:men)	3:1	1:1
Peak age of onset	35–50	Greater than 65
Risk factor of obesity	No	Yes
Morning stiffness	Usually 60 minutes or longer	Usually less than 30 minutes
Involved joint distribution	Symmetric	Symmetric or asymmetric
Presence of inflammation	Local and systemic	None or mild, local
ESR	Elevated	Normal
Synovial fluid	Leukocytosis, slightly cloudy	Mild leukocytosis
Systemic manifestations	Yes	No

ESR, erythrocyte sedimentation rate.

From Ref. 6.

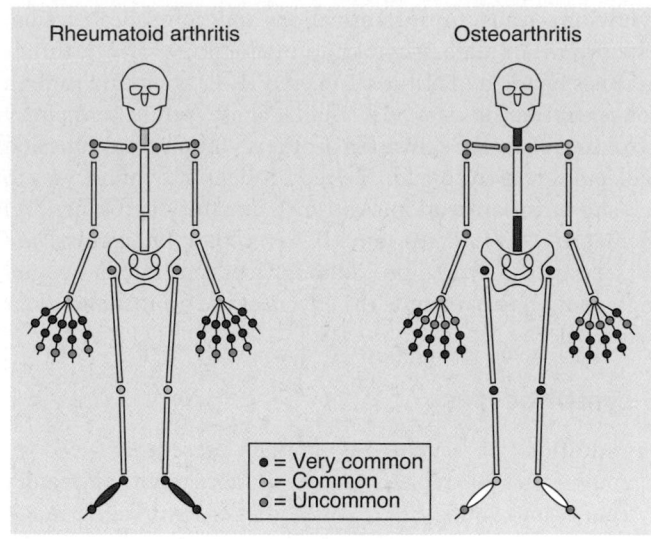

FIGURE 57–1. Patterns of joint involvement in rheumatoid arthritis and osteoarthritis. (From DiPiro JT, Talbert RL, Yee GC, et al., eds. Pharmacotherapy, 7th ed. New York: McGraw-Hill; 2008, Fig. 92–3, p. 1507, with permission.)

Clinical Presentation and Diagnosis of RA

General

- About 60% of patients develop symptoms gradually over several weeks to months.
- Patients may present with systemic findings, joint findings, or both.

Symptoms

- Nonspecific systemic symptoms may include fatigue, weakness, anorexia, and diffuse musculoskeletal pain.
- Patients complain of pain in involved joints and prolonged morning joint stiffness.

Signs

- The metacarpophalangeal (MCP), proximal interphalangeal (PIP), metatarsophalangeal (MTP), and wrist joints are involved frequently.
- Joint involvement is usually symmetric.
- There is often limited joint function.
- Signs of joint inflammation are present (tenderness, warmth, swelling, and erythema).
- Low-grade fever may be present.
- Extraarticular manifestations:
  - *Skin*: Subcutaneous nodules
  - *Ocular*: Keratoconjunctivitis sicca, scleritis
  - *Pulmonary*: Interstitial fibrosis, pulmonary nodules, pleuritis, pleural effusions
  - *Vasculitis*: ischemic ulcers, skin lesions, leukocytoclastic vasculitis
  - *Neurologic*: Peripheral neuropathy, Felty's syndrome
  - *Hematologic:* Anemia, thrombocytosis

Laboratory Tests

- Positive rheumatoid factor (the test is negative in up to 30% of patients)
- Elevated ESR (Westergren ESR: greater than 20 mm/h in men; greater than 30 mm/h in women)
- Elevated C-reactive protein (CRP) (greater than 0.7 mg/dL or / mg/L)
- CBC: Slight elevation in WBC count with a normal differential; slight anemia; thrombocytosis
- Positive anti-CCP antibodies

Other Diagnostic Tests

- *Synovial fluid analysis*: Straw colored, slightly cloudy, WBC 5 to $25 \times 10^3/mm^3$ ($5–25 \times 10^9/L$), no bacterial growth if cultured.
- *Joint x-rays*: To establish baseline and evaluate joint damage.
- *MRI*: May detect erosions earlier in the course of disease than x-rays but is not required for diagnosis.

Several clinical features of RA are associated with a worse long-term prognosis. The presence of these poor prognostic features should be considered at the time initial treatment decisions are made; more aggressive treatment may be warranted if these features are present. ❸ *The most clinically important features associated with poor long-term outcomes include: (a) functional limitation (defined by use of standard measurement scales such as the Health Assessment Questionnaire [HAQ] score); (b) extra-articular disease; (c) positive rheumatoid factor; (d) positive anti-CCP antibodies; and/or (e) bony erosions by radiography.*

Diagnostic criteria for JIA include: (a) age less than 16 years at disease onset; (b) arthritis in one or more joints for more than 6 weeks; (c) exclusion of other types of arthritis. JIA can be divided into three types:

1. *Systemic (approximately 10% of cases)*: occurs equally in girls and boys. There are characteristic fever spikes twice daily (greater than 38.3°C or 101°F) and the presence of a pale, pink, transient rash. The peak onset is between ages 1 and 6 years.

2. *Polyarticular (approximately 40% of cases)*: more likely to affect girls than boys (3:1). Arthritis is present in five or more joints. The disorder resembles adult RA more than the other types of JIA.

3. *Pauciarticular (approximately 50% of cases)*: more likely to affect girls than boys (5:1). Uveitis is more likely to be present. Arthritis is present in four or fewer joints. Categories are further divided into early onset and late onset. Early onset is more likely to occur in girls, whereas late onset is more common in boys.[16]

Patient Encounter, Part 1

AL is a 46-year-old woman who speaks only Spanish. She presents to her physician with a 2-month history of pain and inflammation in her hands and feet. She is accompanied by her daughter, who serves as her interpreter. On questioning, the patient indicates that she experiences joint pain, stiffness, and swelling for at least an hour in the morning. AL is an artist and avid runner, and she wonders if her activities are causing this pain.

What information is suggestive of RA?

What risk factors does she have for RA?

What additional information is necessary to differentiate between osteoarthritis and RA?

What additional information do you need before creating a treatment plan for this patient?

What are the advantages and disadvantages of having a family member serve as an interpreter for the patient?

TREATMENT

Desired Outcomes

❹ *The goals of treatment in RA are to: (a) reduce or eliminate pain; (b) protect articular structures; (c) control systemic complications; (d) prevent loss of joint function; and (e) improve or maintain quality of life.*[1,7] The goals for JIA are the same with the added goals of maintaining normal growth, development, and activity level.[17] It is a common misconception that patients with JIA grow out of the disease. Many children with JIA become adults with JIA. Knowing this, it is essential that early, aggressive treatment is initiated to achieve the goals of therapy.

General Approach to Treatment

The clinician must evaluate patient-specific factors and select appropriate treatment to maximize the care of an individual patient. Thirty percent of all patients with RA have radiographic evidence of erosions at the time of diagnosis; therefore, all patients should be treated early and aggressively to reduce disease progression and to prevent joint erosions.[1] Aggressive treatment is defined as one or more disease-modifying antirheumatic drugs (DMARDs) at effective doses. Delaying treatment will result in more destructive disease that is very difficult to delay or reverse to preserve joint function. Specialty care by a rheumatologist may reduce the likelihood of disease progression and joint damage.[1]

❺ *It is imperative that the initiation of one or more DMARDs occurs in all patients within the first 3 months of diagnosis to reduce joint erosion.* Depending on disease severity and whether poor prognostic features are present, combination therapy may be initiated at the time of diagnosis or after an adequate trial of a DMARD initiated as monotherapy. Starting combination therapy initially is referred to as the *step-down approach*, wherein one or more agents are discontinued once the disease is controlled. Adding a second or third agent after an adequate trial of DMARD monotherapy is considered a *step-up approach*. ❻ *Most clinicians favor the "step-down" approach to slow or reverse the early articular damage as soon as possible.*[7] The following medication classes are prescribed commonly for the treatment of RA: (a) nonsteroidal anti-inflammatory drugs (NSAIDs); (b) glucocorticoids; (c) nonbiologic DMARDs; and (d) biologic DMARDs. Table 57–3 highlights dosing, safety, monitoring, and patient counseling information for the common nonbiologic and biologic DMARDs.

Figures 57–2 and 57–3 outline the course of treatment according to the American College of Rheumatology (ACR) 2008 Recommendations.[18] The recommendations are based on the activity level of the patient's disease, the presence or absence of poor prognostic features, and the duration of disease activity. Figures 57–2 and 57–3 apply to patients who have had RA for less than 6 months. Please consult the ACR guidelines[18] for treatment recommendations for patients having RA for 6 months or longer.

Table 57-3

FDA-Approved Nonbiologic and Biologic DMARDs for Treatment of RA

Drug	Dose[a]	Route	Time to Effect (weeks)	ADRs	Dosing in Hepatic Impairment	Dosing in Renal Impairment	Monitoring	Counseling Points
Methotrexate	Adults: 7.5–20 mg once weekly Polyarticular-course JIA: Recommended starting dose: 10 mg/m² once weekly; usual max dose: 20 mg/m² once weekly	Oral or IM	4–8	N, D, hepatotoxicity, alopecia, new-onset cough or SOB, MYL	CI	CrCl (mL/min): 61–80: 75% of dose 51–60: 70% of dose 10–50: 50% of dose Less than 10: Avoid use	CBC, creatinine, LFTs every 4–8 weeks; monitor for signs of infection	Use of folic acid concomitantly Avoid alcohol Use contraception if childbearing potential
Hydroxy-chloroquine	Adults: 200 mg twice daily Pediatrics: 3–5 mg/kg/day (as sulfate) divided 1–2 times/day to a maximum of 400 mg/day (as sulfate); max 7 mg/kg/day	Oral	8–24	N, D, HA, vision changes, skin pigmentation	Use with caution	No change	Eye exam every 12 months	Sunscreen use
Sulfasalazine	Adults: 1,000 mg 2–3 × daily Pediatrics: Initial: 10 mg/kg/day; increase weekly by 10 mg/kg/day; usual dose: 30–50 mg/kg/day in 2 divided doses; max 2 g/day	Oral	8–12	N, D, rash, yellow-orange discoloration, photosensitivity, MYL	Avoid use	CrCl (mL/min): 10–30: Give twice daily; Less than 10: Give once daily	CBC every 2–4 weeks for 3 months, then every 3 months	
Leflunomide (Arava)	Adults: 100 mg daily for 3 days; then 20 mg daily	Oral	4–12	Hepatotoxicity, D, N, HTN, rash, HA, abdominal pain	Avoid use	Guidelines not available	CBC, creatinine, LFTs every months for 6 months; then every 4–8 weeks Monitor for signs of infection	Avoid alcohol Use contraception if childbearing potential
Etanercept (Enbrel)	Adults: 25 mg twice weekly or 50 mg once weekly Children ages 2–17: 0.8 mg/kg once weekly; max 50 mg/week	SC injection	1–4	ISR	No change	No change	Monitor for infection	ISR—topical corticosteroids, antipruritics, analgesics, rotate injection sites Screen for tuberculosis
Infliximab (Remicade)	Adults: 3–10 mg/kg at 0, 2, and 6 weeks; then every 8 weeks Pediatrics: 3 mg/kg; repeat 3 mg/kg/dose at 2 and 6 weeks after first infusion, then every 8 weeks thereafter	IV infusion	1–4	IR (rash, urticaria, flushing, HA, fever, chills, nausea, tachycardia, dyspnea)	No change	No change	Monitor for infection	Screen for tuberculosis

Drug	Dose	Route		Adverse effects			Monitoring	Screening
Adalimumab (Humira)	Adults: 40 mg every other week; Children older than 4 years and weighing 15–29 kg: 20 mg every other week; Children weighing 30 kg or more: 40 mg every other week	SC injection	1–4	ISR	No change	No change	Monitor for infection	Screen for tuberculosis
Golimumab (Symponi)	Adults: 50 mg once monthly; Children: Safety and efficacy has not been established	SC injection	1–4	ISR	No change	No change	Monitor for infection	Screen for tuberculosis
Certolizumab (Cimzia)	Adults: 400 mg initially, at 2 weeks, 4 weeks, then every 4 weeks thereafter; Children: Safety and efficacy has not been established	SC injection	1–4	ISR	No change	No change	Monitor for infection	Screen for tuberculosis
Anakinra (Kineret)	Adults: 100–150 mg daily	SC injection	2–4	HA, N, V, D, ISR	No data available	CrCl less than 30 mL/min: consider 100 mg every other day	Monitor for infection	
Abatacept (Orencia)	Adults less than 60 kg, 500 mg; 60–100 kg, 750 mg; Adults greater than 100 kg, 1,000 mg on days 1, 15 and every 28 days thereafter	IV infusion	2	HA, infection, IR	No change	No change	Monitor for infection	
Rituximab (Rituxan)	Adults: Two 1,000 mg infusions separated by 2 weeks	IV infusion	4	IR	No change	No change	Monitor for infection	
Tocilizumab (Actemra)	Adults: 8 mg/kg every 4 weeks	IV infusion		Elevated LFTs, total cholesterol, triglycerides and high density lipoprotein; nasopharyngitis, infection	No data available	No data available	Monitor for infection; LFTs	

CI, contraindicated; D, diarrhea; HA, headache; HTN, hypertension; IR, infusion reactions; ISR, injection-site reactions; LFTs, liver function tests; MYL, myelosuppression (watch for fever, symptoms of infection, easy bruisability, and bleeding); N, nausea; SOB, shortness of breath.

[a]Geriatric patients should receive the usual adult dose unless renal or hepatic impairment is present. Pediatric doses are provided for drugs that have FDA-approved indications for juvenile idiopathic arthritis (JIA).

From Refs. 1, 2, 7, 18–20.

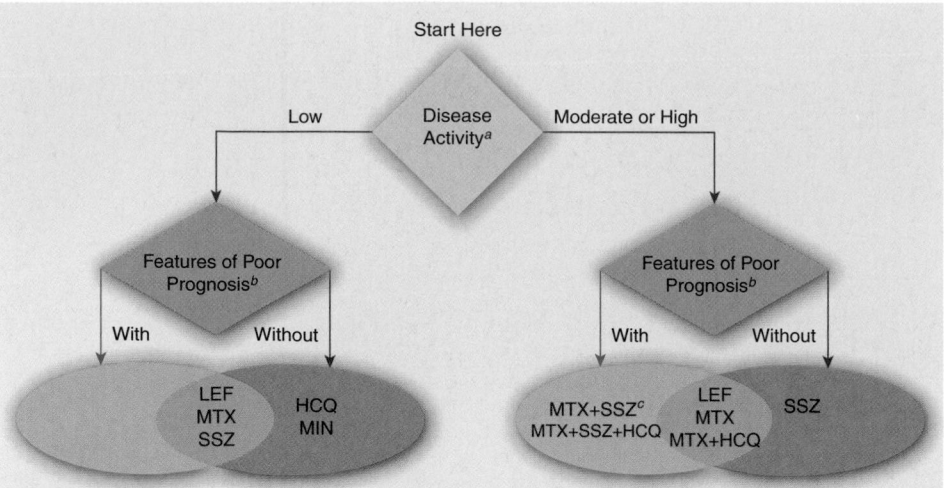

FIGURE 57–2. Recommendations for the use of nonbiologic disease-modifying antirheumatic drugs (DMARDs) in RA patients who have never received DMARDs *and* who have had RA for less than 6 months. These recommendations do not specifically include the potential role of glucocorticoids or NSAIDs in the management of patients with RA. [a]See Ref. 18 for definitions of disease activity. [b]Includes functional limitation (defined using standard measurement scales such as HAQ score or variations of this scale), extraarticular disease (e.g., presence of rheumatoid nodules, secondary Sjogren's syndrome, RA vasculitis, Felty's syndrome, and RA lung disease), rheumatoid factor positivity, positive anti-CCP antibodies, or bony erosions by radiography. [c]Only recommended for patients with high disease activity with features of poor prognosis. (HCQ, hydroxychloroquine; LEF, leflunomide; MIN, minocycline; MTX, methotrexate; SSZ, sulfasalazine.) (From Ref. 18.)

Patients who have had RA for less than 6 months and have been determined to have low disease activity and no poor prognostic features may be treated with a single-agent nonbiologic DMARD (hydroxychloroquine, minocycline, leflunomide, methotrexate, or sulfasalazine) (Fig. 57–2). If patients with low disease activity do have poor prognostic features, treatment should be started with leflunomide, methotrexate, or sulfasalazine. Patients with moderate or high disease activity but without poor prognostic features may receive initial treatment with sulfasalazine, leflunomide, methotrexate, or the combination of methotrexate and hydroxychloroquine. Patients with moderate or high disease activity and evidence of poor prognostic features may receive initial single-drug therapy with leflunomide or methotrexate; however, combination therapy may also be started initially in these patients using methotrexate/hydroxychloroquine, methotrexate/sulfasalazine, or methotrexate/sulfasalazine/hydroxychloroquine.

Biologic DMARDs are usually considered after failure of nonbiologic DMARDs. Patients with early RA (less than 6 months) and low or moderate disease activity are generally not candidates for biologic DMARDs. In contrast, patients who have had RA for less than 6 months but have had high disease activity for less than 3 months and features of poor prognosis should be considered for treatment with a TNF antagonist (etanercept, infliximab, adalimumab, golimumab, or certolizumab pegol) plus methotrexate (Fig. 57–3). Because of treatment expense, this option should be considered only in patients who have no limitations due to cost or insurance coverage. Other biologic DMARDs may be considered under certain circumstances.

Nonpharmacologic Therapy

All patients should receive education about the nonpharmacologic and pharmacologic measures to help manage RA and JIA. Empowered patients take an active role in care by participating in therapy-related decisions. Certain forms of nonpharmacologic therapy benefit all levels of severity, whereas others (i.e., surgery) are reserved for severe cases only.

Occupational and physical therapy may help patients preserve joint function, extend joint range of motion, and strengthen joints and muscles through strengthening exercises. Patients with joint deformities may benefit from the use of mobility or assistive devices that help to minimize disability and allow continued activities of daily living. In situations where the disease has progressed to a severe form with extensive joint erosions, surgery to replace or reconstruct the joint may be necessary.[1]

Pharmacologic Therapy

▶ *Nonsteroidal Anti-Inflammatory Drugs*

NSAIDs provide analgesic and anti-inflammatory benefits for joint pain and swelling. However, they do not prevent joint damage or change the underlying disease.[1] It is appropriate for a patient to begin taking an NSAID along with a DMARD for "bridge therapy" to provide symptomatic relief until the therapeutic effect of the DMARD is observed. Because of interpatient variability in response, patients may find relief from one NSAID and not another. For this reason, if a patient does not receive relief from one NSAID, it is acceptable to

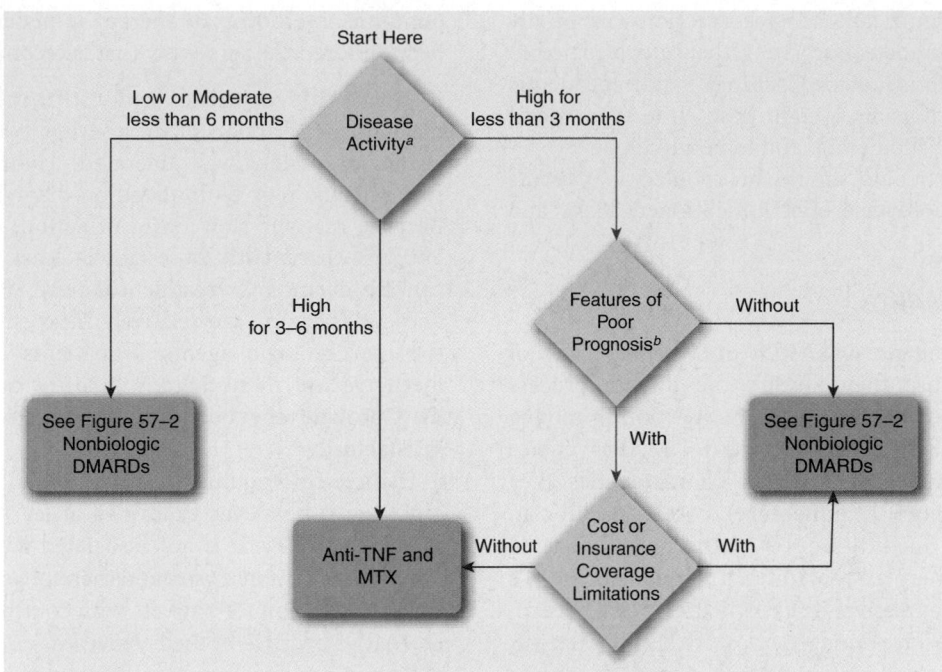

FIGURE 57–3. Recommendations for the use of biologic DMARDs in patients who have had RA for less than 6 months. These recommendations do not specifically include the potential role of glucocorticoids or NSAIDs in the management of patients with RA. [a]See Ref. 18 for definitions of disease activity. [b]Includes functional limitation (defined using standard measurement scales such as HAQ score or variations of this scale), extraarticular disease (e.g., presence of rheumatoid nodules, secondary Sjogren's syndrome, RA vasculitis, Felty's syndrome, and RA lung disease), rheumatoid factor positivity, positive anti-CCP antibodies, or bony erosions by radiography. (DMARD, disease-modifying antirheumatic drug; MTX, methotrexate; TNF, tumor necrosis factor.) (From Ref. 18.)

try a second one. Selecting another NSAID depends on multiple patient-specific factors including cardiovascular risk, potential for GI-related adverse events, adherence to medication regimens, and insurance coverage or lack thereof. Clinicians must weigh these factors carefully to determine if the patient will benefit from another NSAID, if he or she should receive a cyclooxygenase-2 (COX-2) inhibitor, or if another medication class should be considered.

NSAID use is associated with an increased risk of GI ulcers or hemorrhage, fluid retention, exacerbation of existing hypertension, and decreased renal function in certain patient populations.[7,19] Factors that place a patient at a higher risk of GI-related adverse reactions include: (a) history of peptic ulcer disease, (b) high doses of NSAIDs, (c) concomitant use of other medications with an increased risk of GI hemorrhage or ulcers (e.g., anticoagulants, corticosteroids, use of multiple NSAIDs), (d) age greater than 75 years, and (e) serious underlying diseases.[1] If a patient has an increased risk of NSAID-induced adverse reactions, gastroprotection should be considered by coinitiation of a proton pump inhibitor, histamine-2 receptor blocker, or misoprostol. Misoprostol is effective in reducing the occurrence of gastric and duodenal ulcers. However, its tolerability is limited by adverse effects, specifically diarrhea. Histamine-2 receptor blockers effectively prevent duodenal ulcers (but not gastric ulcers) that occur more readily as a result of NSAID therapy. Proton pump inhibitors are the preferred gastroprotective agents due to greater acid suppression, prevention of both

gastric and duodenal ulcers, and a tolerable adverse-effect profile.[20] Changing treatment to low-dose prednisone, a nonacetylated salicylate, or a COX-2 inhibitor are additional options.[1]

NSAIDs may accentuate the increased risk of cardiovascular events inherent in patients with RA. Increases in blood pressure and fluid retention may exacerbate existing cardiovascular disease. With the evidence associating COX-2 inhibitors with cardiovascular disease, clinicians must carefully evaluate the potential risks of NSAID therapy against the potential benefits.[2] See Chapter 58 for additional discussion of NSAID therapy.

NSAIDs are the treatment of choice in children with JIA of mild severity. As in adults, adverse effects of NSAID therapy should be anticipated and treated accordingly in pediatrics.

▶ Glucocorticoids

Low-dose glucocorticoid treatment (equivalent to prednisone 10 mg/day or less) effectively reduces inflammation through inhibition of cytokines and inflammatory mediators and prevents disease progression.[19,21] The goal of glucocorticoid use is to minimize adverse drug events by keeping doses low and using the drugs as infrequently as possible. Patients may receive glucocorticoids for a brief time as "bridge therapy" following DMARD initiation or via intra-articular injections to relieve symptoms of active disease. Patients taking more than 10 mg/day prednisone or equivalent are at an increased risk for clinically significant adverse reactions, especially bone loss leading to osteoporosis. Other glucocorticoid-related adverse reactions include Cushing's syndrome, peptic ulcer disease, hypertension, weight gain, infection, mood changes, cataracts, dyslipidemia, and hyperglycemia.[2,21]

Systemic glucocorticoids should be avoided in patients with JIA due to the adverse effects mentioned above and growth suppression.

► Nonbiologic DMARDs

Nonbiologic and biologic DMARDs are the mainstay of RA treatment because they modify the disease process and prevent or reduce joint damage. In addition to relying on safety and efficacy data, the initial DMARD choice depends on disease severity, patient characteristics (i.e., comorbidities, likelihood of adherence), cost, and clinician experience with the medication.[1,7,18] Methotrexate alone or in combination therapy is the initial treatment of choice for patients with aggressive disease. Patients with early, mild disease may receive monotherapy with sulfasalazine, leflunomide or hydroxychloroquine. Agents such as azathioprine, D-penicillamine, gold salts, and anakinra are used rarely today because of concerns about toxicity and reduced efficacy.[1,18,19]

Methotrexate ❼ *Methotrexate is the nonbiologic DMARD of choice in RA because of its documented efficacy and safety profile when monitored appropriately.*[1,22] Methotrexate exerts its anti-inflammatory effect through inhibition of dihydrofolate reductase, which causes the inhibition of purines and thymidylic acid, and by inhibiting the production of certain cytokines.[2] Unless the patient has contraindications to methotrexate, once-weekly doses should be initiated within 3 months of diagnosis and increased steadily until the patient has symptomatic improvement or a maximum dose of 20 mg/week is reached. Concomitant folic acid is given routinely to reduce the risk of folate-depleting reactions induced by methotrexate therapy (e.g., stomatitis, diarrhea, nausea, alopecia, myelosuppression, and elevations in liver function tests).[1,23]

Serious adverse reactions include pulmonary fibrosis and hepatotoxicity. Patients should be counseled to avoid the use of alcohol, take folic acid as directed, adhere to the laboratory monitoring schedule, and immediately report symptoms of pulmonary fibrosis (e.g., cough or dyspnea) and hepatotoxicity (e.g., jaundice or abdominal pain). If monotherapy does not produce complete resolution of symptoms, methotrexate may be used in combination with other nonbiologic or biologic DMARDs. In situations where the clinician suspects RA but a diagnosis has not yet been made, initiation of methotrexate was found to delay the diagnosis and halt joint damage without untoward adverse effects.[24]

Methotrexate is considered a second-line treatment of JIA. The usual dose is 5 to 15 mg/m² (based on body surface area) once weekly. There are insufficient published data to assess the risk of serious toxicity in children receiving doses greater than 20 mg/m²/wk. Patients will begin to notice a response in 3 to 4 weeks with maximal response in 3 to 6 months. Methotrexate therapy in pediatric patients should be monitored the same way that is recommended in adults.[25]

Hydroxychloroquine and Sulfasalazine The exact mechanism of action of these drugs is unknown, but both agents are fairly well tolerated. Hydroxychloroquine or sulfasalazine may be initiated on diagnosis of mild disease. Because of their slow onset of action, each drug must be given at therapeutic doses for at least 6 months before it can be deemed a treatment failure. Hydroxychloroquine and sulfasalazine are relatively inexpensive compared with the new biologic agents. If patients do not respond to methotrexate monotherapy, adding one of these agents may provide the benefit necessary to reduce symptoms satisfactorily.[2,18]

Hydroxychloroquine may cause retinal toxicity, and patients must have their eyes examined at least annually to detect this abnormality. It is not associated with renal, hepatic, or bone marrow suppression and therefore may be an acceptable treatment option for patients with contraindications to other DMARDs because of their toxicities.

Starting sulfasalazine at low doses and titrating slowly will minimize the nausea and abdominal discomfort caused by the drug. Patients receiving sulfasalazine must undergo routine blood work to monitor for leukopenia.[1] Patients with a sulfa allergy should not receive sulfasalazine.

Hydroxychloroquine and sulfasalazine can be used to treat JIA if methotrexate is not appropriate for the patient.[17] The pediatric dose of hydroxychloroquine is 3 to 5 mg/kg/day divided in 1 to 2 doses. The dose of sulfasalazine for children older than 6 years is 30 to 50 mg/kg/day in two divided doses.

Leflunomide Leflunomide inhibits dihydroorotate dehydrogenase, an enzyme within the mitochondria that supplies T lymphocytes with the necessary components to respond to cytokine stimulation.[26] Thus, leflunomide inhibits the T-lymphocyte response to various stimuli and halts the cell cycle. Its efficacy is similar to that of moderate doses of methotrexate or sulfasalazine.[19] Because of its extended half-life, leflunomide therapy begins with a loading dose followed by a maintenance dose. Patients with pre-existing hepatic disease or a history of heavy alcohol ingestion should not receive leflunomide.[26] Leflunomide may be used in combination with methotrexate, but the added efficacy comes with a dramatic rise in the risk of hepatotoxicity. Liver function tests must be followed closely to prevent or minimize liver damage.[1] If therapy requires abrupt discontinuation (e.g., due to toxicity or pregnancy), administering cholestyramine will accelerate removal of leflunomide from the body.

Leflunomide was shown to effectively treat JIA in clinical trials, but it does not have an FDA-approved indication for this use.[17]

► Biologic DMARDs

Biologic DMARDs are indicated in patients who have failed an adequate trial of DMARD therapy or in combination with nonbiologic DMARDs in patients with early, aggressive disease.[1] These agents may be added to nonbiologic DMARD monotherapy (e.g., methotrexate) or replace ineffective nonbiologic DMARD therapy.[18] The decision to select a particular agent generally is based on the prescriber's comfort level with monitoring the safety and efficacy of the medications, severity of disease activity, presence of factors suggestive of poor prognosis, the frequency and route of administration, the patient's comfort level or manual dexterity to self-administer subcutaneous injections, the cost, and the availability of insurance coverage.[18,27] In general, biologic DMARDs should be avoided in patients with serious infections, demyelinating disorders (e.g., multiple sclerosis or optic neuritis) or hepatitis. TNF antagonists should be avoided in patients with heart failure.[18]

Tumor Necrosis Factor Antagonists Etanercept is a recombinant form of human T receptor.[28] Etanercept provides a therapeutic effect by binding to soluble TNF and preventing its binding with TNF receptors. It is administered subcutaneously once or twice weekly; noticeable symptomatic improvement is seen in 1 to 4 weeks. Etanercept is very effective as monotherapy or in combination with other DMARDs, except anakinra.[28] There is no evidence to suggest a benefit to combination with anakinra, and there is an increased infection risk. The most common adverse reactions with etanercept are injection-site reactions. If such reactions are bothersome, patients should be advised to place ice on the injection-site before and after administration or apply a topical anesthetic or corticosteroid to the affected area.[29] Etanercept has an FDA-approved indication for treatment of JIA. The pediatric dose of etanercept is 0.8 mg/kg subcutaneously once weekly.

Infliximab is a chimeric IgGl monoclonal antibody that binds to soluble and bound TNF-α.[30] Methotrexate typically is given with it to suppress antibody production against the mouse-derived portion of the molecule. Infliximab is delivered via IV infusion every 4 to 8 weeks; however, patients may notice benefit within 1 to 4 weeks of receiving the first infusion. Infusion-related reactions including rash, urticaria, flushing, headache, fever, chills, nausea, tachycardia, and dyspnea may occur during treatment. Qualified health care personnel must be present during the infusion to respond to the infusion-related reactions, if they occur. If patients experience any of these symptoms, the reaction may be treated by: (a) temporarily discontinuing the infusion, (b) slowing the infusion rate, or (c) administering corticosteroids or antihistamines.[29] Clinicians may prescribe pretreatment regimens with corticosteroids or antihistamines if the patient continues to experience infusion reactions.[29] Infliximab was shown in clinical trials to be effective for treatment of JIA, but it has not yet received FDA approval for this indication.

Adalimumab is a recombinant human IgG1 monoclonal antibody specific for human TNF.[31] Adalimumab binds to soluble and bound TNF-α. Patients may experience symptomatic relief in as early as 1 week. Adalimumab can be administered in combination with methotrexate or other DMARDs.[2] Adalimumab has an FDA-approved indication for JIA.

Golimumab is a human monoclonal antibody that binds to membrane-bound and soluble TNF. Golimumab can be administered in combination with methotrexate in patients with moderate to severe RA. One advantage of this agent over others in the class may be the once-monthly dosing. Golimumab is not FDA-approved for use in JIA.

Certolizumab is a humanized antibody Fab fragment conjugated to polyethylene glycol, which delays the metabolism and elimination of the medication. Certolizumab can be administered as monotherapy or in combination with methotrexate in patients with moderate to severe RA. Certolizumab is not FDA-approved for use in JIA.

Interleukin 1 Receptor Antagonist Anakinra is a recombinant form of human IL-1 receptor antagonist. Anakinra inhibits the activity of IL-1 by binding to it and preventing cell signaling. It is indicated for adults with RA who have failed one or more nonbiologic DMARDs. Patients must administer a subcutaneous injection every day, which may be less desirable than other treatment options. Anakinra may be used in combination with other nonbiologic DMARDs in patients not responding to or unable to tolerate nonbiologic DMARDs or TNF antagonists. Anakinra should not be used in combination with TNF antagonists due to the increased risk of infection. Anakinra is not included in the algorithms outlined in the 2008 treatment guidelines due to its infrequent use in RA.

Costimulation Modulators Abatacept is the first agent in this class of medications. It interferes with T-cell signaling, ultimately blocking T-cell activation and leading to anergy, or lack of response to an antigen.[32] Trials conducted in patients refractory to methotrexate and anti-TNF therapy demonstrated significant clinical benefit after administration of abatacept every 28 days with a dose approximating 10 mg/kg.[32] Adverse reactions reported in clinical trials were low and similar to those of placebo, with the exception of an increased incidence of headache, infections, and infusion-related reactions in the treatment group.[32] Abatacept is indicated as monotherapy or in combination with nonbiologic DMARDs. Its exact place in therapy is not yet clear; however, clinicians see a window of opportunity for patients who were intolerant to or did not receive therapeutic benefit from other nonbiologic or biologic DMARDs or developed antibodies to adequate trials of anti-TNF agents, specifically infliximab.[32]

Anti-CD20 Monoclonal Antibody Rituximab is a genetically engineered chimeric anti-CD20 monoclonal antibody that causes B-lymphocyte depletion.[33] Although the exact role of B lymphocytes in the pathogenesis of RA is not clear, a small study in patients with RA demonstrated noticeable efficacy. Further clinical trials showed a sustained therapeutic effect lasting for at least 48 weeks after the initial treatment.[33-35] Adverse effects occurring during or up to 24 hours after the first infusion included changes in blood pressure (increases or decreases), cough, rash, and pruritus. The infusion-related reactions subsided with subsequent infusions. Serious infections occurred in a small number of rituximab-treated patients.

The exact role of rituximab in RA is not clearly defined, but it is indicated for patients with moderate to severe active RA and a history of inadequate response to one or more TNF antagonist therapies. Rituximab carries a black-box warning of fatal infusion reactions and severe mucocutaneous reactions even though these events did not occur during the RA clinical trials. The benefits of rituximab must be tempered against the safety concerns reported with use of rituximab in the oncology setting. Fully humanized anti-CD20 monoclonal antibodies are under development.

Anti-interleukin-6 Receptor Antibody Interleukin-6 (IL-6) is produced in high amounts in patients with RA. High levels are indicative of joint damage and disease activity. In addition, IL-6 plays a significant role in the pathogenesis of anemia of chronic disease.[36] Tocilizumab, an anti-IL-6 receptor monoclonal antibody, inhibits the binding of IL-6 to the IL-6 receptor.[22] Studies in patients not responding to methotrexate or TNF antagonists have demonstrated safety and efficacy of tocilizumab administration.[2,22,37] The tocilizumab dose is 8 mg/kg IV every 4 weeks. Adverse reactions include nasopharyngitis, infection, and elevated lab values including liver function tests and cholesterol parameters. The exact place in therapy of tocilizumab is not yet known. Tocilizumab is not included in the 2008 recommendations from the ACR because the drug was still investigational at the time of writing.

▶ **Selecting a Biologic DMARD**

Developments in the treatment of RA are tempered by the lack of evidence of the long-term safety and efficacy of the biologic DMARDs. In addition, high costs can be a deterrent to use. Longer term data are emerging that suggest that patients receiving therapy with these agents early in the course of disease (within 3 years) for a defined time period have reduced disease activity and less joint destruction. If additional evidence proves this to be true, concerns regarding the cost of biologic DMARDs may be alleviated. Cost analyses may indicate that the increased expenses associated with these drugs are offset by the costs avoided for treatment of advanced RA.

❽ *The risk of infection in patients treated with biologic DMARDs must be considered when selecting and monitoring therapy.*[18,38,39] Influencing the immune response to reduce symptoms of RA may influence the body's response to pathogens. Of particular concern is the use of TNF antagonists in patients with a history of tuberculosis exposure. TNF is important in the formation of granulomas that wall off tuberculosis infection. In theory, if TNF is inhibited, patients with latent tuberculosis may have a reactivated infection. Patients receiving biologic DMARD therapy should be screened for tuberculosis and other infections. Prophylaxis should be initiated in patients with previous tuberculosis exposure or in patients at high risk of developing tuberculosis.[18] Biologic DMARDs should not be initiated

---

Patient Encounter, Part 2: Medical History, Physical Examination, and Laboratory Tests

PMH: Exercise-induced asthma; allergic rhinitis; carpal tunnel syndrome

FH: Father has hypertension, diabetes, dyslipidemia; mother has RA and a history of MI; two siblings (one brother, one sister) alive and well.

SH: She is a successful artist and works from home. She drinks alcohol occasionally and does not smoke or use illicit drugs.

Allergies: NKDA

Meds: Albuterol (salbutamol) 2 puffs 15 to 20 minutes before exercise; ortho Tri-Cyclen by mouth once daily; budesonide nasal spray one spray each nostril daily; calcium (with vitamin D) 600 mg orally twice daily; ibuprofen 400 mg by mouth every 4 hours daily as needed

ROS: (+) fatigue, (–) N/V/D, HA, SOB, chest pain, cough

PE:

VS: BP 126/74, P 70, RR 18, T 38°C (100.4°F); ht 5'6" (168 cm), wt 72.3 kg (159 lb)

Skin: Warm, dry

HEENT: NC/AT, PERRLA, TMs intact

CV: RRR, normal S1 and S2, no m/r/g

Chest: CTA

Abd: Soft, NT/ND

Neuro: A & O × 3; CN II to XII intact

Ext: Bilateral tender and swollen PIPs, MCPs, and MTPs (symmetric)

Labs: ESR 66 mm/h, RF (+), HLA-DR4 (+), anti-CCP (+)

Synovial fluid analysis: Yellow, cloudy, decreased viscosity.

Hand x-rays: Soft-tissue swelling, joint space narrowing, no evidence of erosions.

Given this additional information, what is your assessment of the patient's condition?

Identify your treatment goals for this patient.

What nonpharmacologic and pharmacologic alternatives are available for this patient?

during an acute, serious infection and should be discontinued temporarily during times of infection.[39]

Use of biologic DMARDs is associated with an increased risk of malignancy, specifically lymphoma and skin cancer.[14,40] Patients should be monitored closely for signs and symptoms suggestive of malignancy. Therapy should be discontinued once the risks outweigh the potential benefits of treatment.

▶ *Fertility, Pregnancy, and Fetal Development*

Women of childbearing age should be counseled about the impact of antirheumatic drugs on fertility, pregnancy, fetal development, and lactation. Some women may experience a reduction in disease symptoms during pregnancy; however, many agents used to treat RA are known teratogens. Women desiring motherhood must consult with their physicians to carefully plan for the pregnancy and reduce risks to the developing fetus.[41] Low-dose corticosteroids generally are safe and effective. Certain NSAIDs, hydroxychloroquine, and azathioprine may be considered in severe disease.

Methotrexate use (FDA pregnancy category X) is associated with spontaneous abortion, fetal myelosuppression, limb defects, and CNS abnormalities; therefore, pregnancy must be avoided.[41] Sulfasalazine, on the other hand, may be the drug of choice in women who are pregnant or planning to become pregnant due to its safety profile.[41] There is limited evidence of safety and long-term effects of the use of biologic DMARDs in pregnant women. Case reports of pregnancy during biologic DMARD therapy show no increased risk of fetal toxicity, but long-term data are needed.[28,41]

Male patients with RA must receive counseling about the effects of certain medications on their fertility and potential harm to the fetus. It is difficult to establish causality between use of a medication by a male and the effect on fertility or fetal development; therefore, a conservative approach must be taken. ❾ *Women of childbearing potential and their partners must be counseled to: (a) use proper birth control while undergoing treatment for RA; and (b) discontinue medications at least 3 months before conception.*[41]

OUTCOME EVALUATION

- Rheumatologists rely on standardized criteria to assess treatment interventions through measurement of disease activity. The ACR uses criteria for improvement based on percentage improvement in tender and swollen joint count and the presence of at least three or more of the following measures: (a) pain; (b) patient global assessment; (c) physician global assessment; (d) self-assessed physical disability; and (e) acute-phase reactants.[42] ACR20, ACR50, and ACR70 are common efficacy endpoints in clinical trials. The number corresponds with the percentage improvement. As drug discovery continues to evolve, the acceptable criteria for 20% improvement may be too low. For example, if a patient has 10 tender and swollen joints, reducing that by 20% to 8 tender and swollen joints is, by definition,

an improvement by ACR20 criteria. However, further reduction in symptoms or disease remission may have greater clinical significance and effect on the patient's quality of life.

- Physical disability from RA can be measured through the Stanford HAQ.[43,44] This patient self-assessment tool was developed to evaluate patient outcomes in five dimensions of chronic conditions: (a) disability; (b) discomfort; (c) drug adverse effects; (d) dollar costs; and (e) death. Clinicians and clinical studies in rheumatology use HAQ to assess longitudinally changes that influence the patient's quality of life.[43,44]

- Disease activity can be measured through the Disease Activity Score in 28 joints (DAS 28). Components involved in the calculation are the number of swollen and tender joints, ESR or CRP, and a subjective measure of the patient's general health. A DAS 28 score of 3.2 or less indicates low disease activity, between 3.2 and 5.1 is considered moderate activity, and 5.1 or more is considered to be high activity.[18,45] Remission is defined as a DAS 28 score of less than 2.6.

- Before starting treatment for RA, assess the subjective and objective evidence of disease. For joint findings, this includes the number of tender and swollen joints, pain, limitations on use, duration of morning stiffness, and presence of joint erosions. Systemic findings may include fatigue and the presence of extraarticular manifestations. Obtain laboratory measurements of CRP and ESR. The impact of the disease on quality of life and functional status is also important.

- At follow-up visits, compare the patient's status to baseline or previous visits using standardized criteria for improvement of disease activity and the HAQ to assess longitudinally the influence on quality of life.

- Assess the patient's response to initiation of nonbiologic or biologic DMARD therapy after allowing adequate time for the medication to achieve its therapeutic effect.

- Determine whether any adverse reactions associated with each antirheumatic medication are present.

Patient Encounter, Part 3: Creating a Care Plan

Based on the information available, create a care plan for this patient's RA. The plan should include:
(a) a statement of the drug-related needs and/or problems; (b) the goals of therapy; (c) a patient-specific detailed therapeutic plan; and (d) monitoring parameters to assess safety and efficacy.

Six months later, the patient comes back and mentions that she would like to become pregnant.

Does this change your treatment plan?

If yes, devise a new treatment plan for AL.

Patient Care and Monitoring

1. Assess the patient's symptoms to determine if they are consistent with RA. Evaluate the duration of symptoms and their impact on daily living.

2. Review available diagnostic data to determine the severity of disease and whether the patient is at risk of experiencing poor outcomes.

3. Obtain a thorough medication history, including prescription drugs, over-the-counter drugs, and dietary supplement use.

4. Educate the patient on nonpharmacologic measures that will improve symptoms.

5. Formulate a therapeutic plan, taking into consideration patient-specific factors.

6. Evaluate the patient for the presence of adverse drug reactions, drug allergies, and drug interactions.

7. Develop a plan to assess safety and efficacy of the pharmacologic treatment plan. Determine if the appropriate doses of antirheumatic medications were used and if all medication were given a sufficient trial to achieve therapeutic benefit.

8. Stress importance of adherence with the therapeutic regimen, including required laboratory monitoring, medication dosing and administration. Recommend a therapeutic regimen that is convenient and consistent with the patient's lifestyle.

9. Longitudinally evaluate the patient's clinical response to therapy and the impact on quality of life and mobility.

10. Evaluate the presence of comorbidities and implement measures to control the increased risk.

    - *Cardiovascular*: Keep doses of NSAIDs and glucocorticoids low, consider initiation of folic acid to reduce homocysteine level elevations induced by methotrexate, consider initiation of low-dose aspirin and/or HMG-CoA reductase inhibitors (statins), and encourage smokers to discontinue tobacco use and assist with the development of a tobacco-cessation plan.[11,12] Screen and aggressively treat elevated blood pressure.[13]

    - *Infection*: Wash hands routinely, limit contact with individuals who are ill, and report signs and symptoms of infection immediately (e.g., fever, weight loss, and night sweats).

    - *Malignancy*: Report new onset of signs and symptoms (e.g., fever, chills, anorexia, and night sweats) immediately.[15]

    - *Osteoporosis*: Encourage patients to ingest adequate amounts of calcium and vitamin D, encourage smokers to discontinue tobacco use, and consider initiation of medications for osteoporosis (e.g., bisphosphonates, calcitonin, and parathyroid hormone) if the patient is taking glucocorticoids chronically or if the patient has evidence of low bone mineral density.[19,46]

11. Provide patient education with regard to RA, lifestyle modifications, and drug therapy:

    - What causes RA?
    - What are the comorbidities associated with RA?
    - How will lifestyle modifications affect RA?
    - What are the goals of therapy in the treatment of RA?
    - When and how should the medications be administered?
    - What potential adverse drug reactions may occur?
    - Which drugs may interact with therapy?
    - What are the warning signs to report to the physician?

- Monitor laboratory parameters to ensure patient safety and reduce the risk of adverse reactions.

❿ *In addition to designing an individualized therapeutic regimen to control the progression of RA, the clinician must evaluate the presence of comorbidities and implement measures to control the increased risk.*

Abbreviations Introduced in This Chapter

ACR	American College of Rheumatology
CCP	Cyclic citrullinated peptide
COX-2	Cyclooxygenase-2
CRP	C-Reactive protein
DAS	Disease Activity Score
DMARD	Disease-modifying antirheumatic drug
ESR	Erythrocyte sedimentation rate
HAQ	Health Assessment Questionnaire
HLA	Human leukocyte antigen
IL	Interleukin
JIA	Juvenile idiopathic arthritis
JRA	Juvenile rheumatoid arthritis
MCP	Metacarpophalangeal joint
MTP	Metatarsophalangeal joint
NKDA	No known drug allergies
NSAID	Nonsteroidal anti-inflammatory drug
PIP	Proximal interphalangeal joint
RA	Rheumatoid arthritis
TNF	Tumor necrosis factor

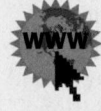 Self-assessment questions and answers are available at *http://www.mhpharmacotherapy.com/pp.html.*

REFERENCES

1. Guidelines for the management of rheumatoid arthritis: 2002 update. Arthritis Rheum 2002;46(2):328–346.

2. Majithia V, Geraci SA. Rheumatoid arthritis: Diagnosis and management. Am J Med 2007;120:936–939.

3. Wolfe F. The effect of smoking on clinical, laboratory, and radiographic status in rheumatoid arthritis. J Rheumatol 2000;27(3):630–637.

4. Choy EH, Panayi GS. Cytokine pathways and joint inflammation in rheumatoid arthritis. N Engl J Med 2001;344:907–916.

5. Kotzin BL. The role of B cells in the pathogenesis of rheumatoid arthritis. J Rheumatol 2005;73(Suppl):14–18.

6. Lipsky PE. Rheumatoid arthritis. In: Kasper DL, Braunwald E, Fauci AS, et al., eds. Harrison's Online, 16th ed. New York: McGraw-Hill, 2005.

7. Rindfleisch JA, Muller D. Diagnosis and management of rheumatoid arthritis. Am Fam Physician 2005;72(6):1037–1047.

8. Juvenile Arthritis Fact Sheet. Arthritis Foundation. www.arthritis.org/ja-fact-sheet.php.

9. Vital EM, Emery P. The development of targeted therapies in rheumatoid arthritis. J Autoimmun 2008;31:219–227.

10. Gonzalez A, Icen M, Kremers HM, et al. Mortality trends in rheumatoid arthritis: The role of rheumatoid factor. J Rheumatol 2008;35:1009–1014.

11. Dhawan SS, Quyyumi AA. Rheumatoid arthritis and cardiovascular disease. Curr Atheroscler Rep 2008;10(2):128–133.

12. Magnano MD, Genovese MC. Management of co-morbidities and general medical conditions in patients with rheumatoid arthritis. Curr Rheumatol Rep 2005;7(5):407–415.

13. Panoulas VF, Metsios GS, Pace AV, et al. Hypertension in rheumatoid arthritis. Rheumatology (Oxford) 2008;47(9):1286–1298.

14. Wolfe F, Michaud K. Biologic treatment of rheumatoid arthritis and the risk of malignancy: Analysis from a large US observational study. Arthritis Rheum 2007;56:2886–2895.

15. Chakravarty EF, Genovese MC. Associations between rheumatoid arthritis and malignancy. Rheum Dis Clin North Am 2004;30(2):271–284.

16. Hashkes PJ, Laxer RM. Medical treatment of juvenile idiopathic arthritis. JAMA 2005;294:1671–1684.

17. Wallace CA. Current management of juvenile idiopathic arthritis. Best Pract Res Clin Rheumatol 2006;20:279–300.

18. Saag KG, Teng GG, Patkar NM, et al. American College of Rheumatology 2008 recommendations for the use of nonbiologic and disease-modifying antirheumatic drugs in rheumatoid arthritis. Arthritis Rheum 2008;59(6):762–784.

19. O'Dell JR. Therapeutic strategies for rheumatoid arthritis. N Engl J Med 2004;350:2591–2602.

20. Naesdal J, Brown K. NSAID-associated adverse effects and acid control aids to prevent them. A review of current treatment options. Drug Saf 2006;29(2):119–132.

21. Rhen T, Cidlowski JA. Antiinflammatory action of glucocorticoids—New mechanisms for old drugs. N Engl J Med 2005;353:1711–1723.

22. Ohsugi Y, Kishimoto T. The recombinant humanized anti-IL-6 receptor antibody tocilizumab, an innovative drug for the treatment of rheumatoid arthritis. Expert Opin Biol Ther 2008;8(5):669–681.

23. Cronstein BN. Low-dose methotrexate: A mainstay in the treatment of rheumatoid arthritis. Pharmacol Rev 2005;57(2):163–172.

24. van Dongen H, van Aken J, Lard LR, et al. Efficacy of methotrexate treatment in patients with probable rheumatoid arthritis: A double blind, randomized, placebo-controlled trial. Arthritis Rheum 2007;56(5):1424–1432.

25. Niehues T, Lankisch P. Recommendations for the use of methotrexate in juvenile idiopathic arthritis. Paediatr Drugs 2006;8:347–356.

26. Cannon GW, Kremer JM. Leflunomide. Rheum Dis Clin North Am 2004;30(2):295–309.

27. Hochberg MC, Tracy JK, Hawkins-Holt M, Flores RH. Comparison of the efficacy of the tumour necrosis factor alpha blocking agents adalimumab, etanercept, and infliximab when added to methotrexate in patients with active rheumatoid arthritis. Ann Rheum Dis 2003;62(Suppl 2):ii13–ii16.

28. Genovese MC, Kremer JM. Treatment of rheumatoid arthritis with etanercept. Rheum Dis Clin North Am 2004;30(2):311–328.

29. Cush JJ. Safety overview of new disease-modifying antirheumatic drugs. Rheum Dis Clin North Am 2004;30(2):237–255.

30. Maini SR. Infliximab treatment of rheumatoid arthritis. Rheum Dis Clin North Am 2004;30(2):329–347.

31. Keystone E, Haraoui B. Adalimumab therapy in rheumatoid arthritis. Rheum Dis Clin North Am 2004;30(2):349–364.

32. Todd DJ, Costenbader KH, Weinblatt ME. Abatacept in the treatment of rheumatoid arthritis. Int J Clin Pract 2007;61(3):494–500.

33. Panayi GS. B cell-directed therapy in rheumatoid arthritis—Clinical experience. J Rheumatol 2005;32(Suppl 73):19–24.

34. Smolen JS, Keystone EC, Emery P, et al. Consensus statement on the use of rituximab in patients with rheumatoid arthritis. Ann Rheum Dis 2007;66(2):143–150.

35. Keystone E, Fleischmann R, Emery P, et al. Safety and efficacy of additional courses of rituximab in patients with active rheumatoid arthritis: An open-label extension analysis. Arthritis Rheum 2007;56(12):3896–3908.

36. Raj DS. Role of interleukin-6 in the anemia of chronic disease. Semin Arthritis Rheum 2009;38:382–388.

37. Emery P, Keystone E, Tony HP, et al. IL-6 receptor inhibition with tocilizumab improves treatment outcomes in patients with rheumatoid arthritis refractory to anti-TNF biologics: Results from a 24-week multicentre randomised placebo controlled trial. Ann Rheum Dis 2008;67:1516–1523.

38. Rychly DJ, DiPiro JT. Infections associated with tumor necrosis factor-alpha antagonists. Pharmacotherapy 2005;25:1181–1192.

39. Curtis JR, Patkar N, Xie A, et al. Risk of serious bacterial infections among rheumatoid arthritis patients exposed to tumor necrosis factor alpha antagonists. Arthritis Rheum 2007;56(4):1125–1133.

40. Bongartz T, Sutton AJ, Sweeting MJ, et al. Anti-TNF antibody therapy in rheumatoid arthritis and the risk of serious infections and malignancies: Systematic review and meta-analysis of rare harmful effects in randomized controlled trials. JAMA 2006;295:2275–2285.

41. Janssen NM, Genta MS. The effects of immunosuppressive and anti-inflammatory medications on fertility, pregnancy, and lactation. Arch Intern Med 2000;160:610–619.

42. Felson DT, Anderson JJ, Boers M, et al. American College of Rheumatology. Preliminary definition of improvement in rheumatoid arthritis. Arthritis Rheum 1995;38:727–735.

43. Bruce B, Fries JF. The Stanford Health Assessment Questionnaire: A review of its history, issues, progress, and documentation. J Rheumatol 2003;30(1):167–178.

44. Bruce B, Fries JF. The Stanford Health Assessment Questionnaire: Dimensions and practical applications. Health Qual Life Outcomes 2003;1(1):20.

45. van der Heijde D, van 't Hof MA, van Riel PL, et al. Judging disease activity in clinical practice in rheumatoid arthritis: First step in the development of a disease activity score. Ann Rheum Dis 1990;49(11):916–920.

46. Recommendations for the prevention and treatment of glucocorticoids-induced osteoporosis: 2001 update. American College of Rheumatology Ad Hoc Committee in Glucocorticoid-Induced Osteoporosis. Arthritis Rheum 2001;44:1496–1503.

58 Osteoarthritis

Steven M. Smith, Benjamin J. Epstein, and John G. Gums

LEARNING OBJECTIVES

Upon completion of the chapter, the reader will be able to:

1. Identify risk factors associated with osteoarthritis (OA).
2. Recognize the signs and symptoms of OA.
3. Determine the goals of therapy for individual patients with OA.
4. Formulate a nonpharmacologic plan for patients with OA.
5. Recommend a pharmacologic plan for OA that considers individual patient factors.
6. Modify an unsuccessful treatment strategy for OA.
7. Develop monitoring parameters to assess effectiveness and adverse effects of pharmacotherapy for OA.
8. Deliver effective disease-state counseling, including lifestyle modifications and drug therapy, to facilitate effective and safe management of OA.

KEY CONCEPTS

❶ Osteoarthritis (OA) is the most common form of arthritis and is most prevalent in the middle to later years of life.

❷ The most common symptoms are joint pain, reduced range of motion, and brief joint stiffness after periods of inactivity.

❸ Treatment goals are to educate the patient and caregivers, relieve pain, maintain or restore mobility, minimize functional impairment, preserve joint integrity, and improve quality of life.

❹ Nonpharmacologic therapy is the cornerstone of treatment; education, exercise, weight loss, and cognitive behavioral intervention are integral components.

❺ Acetaminophen is the initial drug of choice; an adequate dose and duration of therapy should be used before resorting to other drug classes.

❻ Nonsteroidal anti-inflammatory drugs (NSAIDs) may be initiated if acetaminophen therapy fails. At equipotent doses, all NSAIDs elicit similar analgesic and anti-inflammatory responses. Selection is based on patient preference, dosing frequency, tolerability, and cost.

❼ Patients who do not respond adequately to one NSAID may respond to a different NSAID.

❽ NSAIDs are associated with GI, renal, hepatic, and CNS toxicity and may increase blood pressure.

❾ NSAIDs that are selective for the cyclooxygenase-2 (COX-2) isozyme are less likely to cause GI complications but may increase the risk of cardiovascular events. They are no more effective than nonselective NSAIDs and should be reserved for patients at high risk of GI complications and low risk for cardiovascular events.

❿ Glucosamine, tramadol, opioids, topical capsaicin, topical NSAIDs, intra-articular corticosteroids, hyaluronic acid, and surgery may be beneficial in certain situations.

INTRODUCTION

❶ *Osteoarthritis (OA) is the most common form of arthritis.* Weight-bearing joints (e.g., hips and knees) are most susceptible, but nonweight–bearing joints, especially the hands, may also be involved. Because of its high prevalence and involvement of joints critical for daily functioning, the disease causes tremendous morbidity and financial burden.[1] OA is the leading cause of chronic disability and the most common reason for total-hip and total-knee replacement.[2] ❶ *OA is strongly related to age; thus, its incidence and the cost of care will increase dramatically in the coming years due to a burgeoning senior citizenry.* The National Arthritis Data Workgroup predicts that by the year 2020, the number of Americans affected by OA will double from current estimates.

EPIDEMIOLOGY AND ETIOLOGY

The National Arthritis Data Workgroup estimates that 27 million Americans have signs and symptoms of OA.[3] The true extent of the disease is much larger; nearly everyone has radiographic evidence of OA by the eighth decade of life, but individuals without symptoms often go undiagnosed. Approximately 6% of U.S. adults have daily symptomatic knee OA, and 3% report daily symptoms affecting the hip.[4] After age 60, 10% to 15% of persons report such symptoms.

The prevalence of OA is higher in women, and they have more generalized disease. Women are also more likely to have inflammation of the proximal and distal interphalangeal joints of the hands, which manifest as Bouchard's nodes and Heberden's nodes, respectively. OA of the hip occurs more frequently in men.

The prevalence of OA in Caucasians approximates the rate in African Americans, but the latter may experience more severe and disabling disease. Persons of Chinese descent rarely have hip OA; they are also less likely to develop hand OA but more likely to develop knee OA.[5]

PATHOPHYSIOLOGY

OA is characterized by damage to diarthrodial joints and joint structures. In the past, OA was referred to as *degenerative joint disease* (DJD), *hypertrophic arthritis*, or *osteoarthrosis*. However, such nomenclature fails to appreciate the multiple metabolic and pathologic derangements that comprise OA (Fig. 58–1). OA is a multifactorial disease typified by progressive destruction of joint cartilage, erratic new bone formation, thickening of subchondral bone and the joint capsule, bony remodeling, development of osteophytes, variable degrees of mild synovitis, and other changes.[6]

The earliest stages of OA are characterized by increasing water content and softening of cartilage in weight-bearing joints. As the disease progresses, proteoglycan content of cartilage declines, and eventually, cartilage becomes hypocellular. Increasing levels of protease enzymes, such as matrix metalloproteinases (MMPs), occur before changes in cartilage, suggesting that these catabolic proteinases play an important role in the initiation and progression of OA.

Subchondral bone undergoes metabolic changes, including increased bone turnover, that appear to be precursors to tissue destruction. The normally contiguous bony surface becomes fissured. Persistent use of the joint eventually results in loss of cartilage, permitting bone-to-bone contact that ultimately promotes thickening and eburnation of exposed bone. Microfractures may appear in subchondral bone, and osteonecrosis may develop beneath the surface.

New bone is formed haphazardly, leading to the formation of osteophytes that extend into the joint capsule and ligament attachments and may encroach on the joint space. Progressive loss of joint cartilage, subchondral damage, narrowing of joint spaces, and changes in the underlying bone and soft tissues may culminate in deformed, painful joints.[7]

Classification

OA is often divided into primary (idiopathic) and secondary disease (Table 58–1). *Primary OA* is the predominant form and occurs in the absence of a precipitating event. It

Table 58–1
Classification of OA

Primary OA
Localized (involving one or two sites)
Generalized (involving three or more sites)
Erosive

Secondary OA
Mechanical incongruity of joint
Congenital or developmental defect
Posttraumatic
Prior inflammatory disease (rheumatoid arthritis, chronic gouty arthritis, pseudogout, infectious arthritis)
Metabolic disorder (hemochromatosis, ochronosis, Wilson's disease, chondrocalcinosis, Paget's disease)
Endocrinopathies (diabetes mellitus, obesity, acromegaly, iatrogenic hyperadrenocorticism, sex-hormone abnormalities)
Neuropathic disorders
Intra-articular corticosteroid overuse
Avascular necrosis
Bone dysplasia

OA, osteoarthritis.

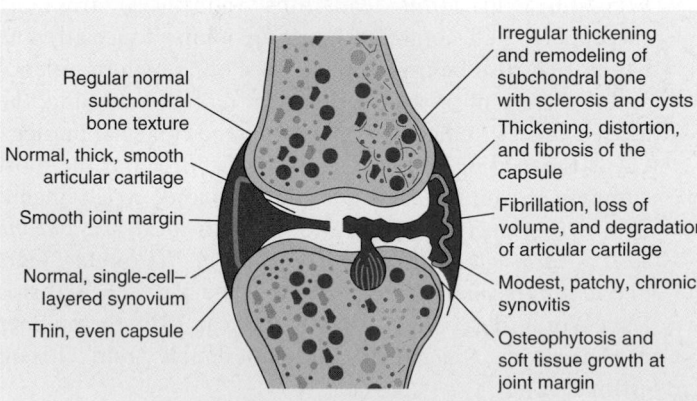

FIGURE 58–1. Characteristics of osteoarthritis in the diarthrodial joint. (From DiPiro JT, Talbert RL, Yee GC, et al., eds. Pharmacotherapy: A Pathophysiologic Approach. 7th ed. New York: McGraw-Hill; 2008: 1521, Figure 95–2, with permission.)

may assume a localized, generalized, or erosive pattern. Localized OA is distinguished from generalized disease by the number of sites involved, whereas erosive disease is characterized by an erosive pattern of bone destruction and marked proliferation of interphalangeal joints of the hands. *Secondary OA* results from congenital or developmental disorders or inflammatory, metabolic, or endocrine diseases.

Risk Factors

OA develops when systemic factors and biomechanical vulnerabilities combine. Systemic factors include age, gender, genetic predisposition, and nutritional status. Age is the strongest predictor of OA, although advanced age alone is insufficient to cause OA.

Joints exposed to biomechanical factors are at increased risk. Occupational and recreational activities involving repetitive motion or injury can provoke OA, although most daily activities do not produce enough joint trauma to cause OA, even after decades of repeated use. However, daily activities may lead to OA if a joint is susceptible because of previous injury, joint deformity, muscle weakness, or systemic factors. Heavy physical activity is a stronger predictor of subsequent OA than light to moderate activities.[8] This is especially true for older individuals, in whom the joint structure is less capable of coping with highly stressful activities. Obesity increases loadbearing stresses on hip and knee joints. The risk of OA increases by 10% for each kilogram of body weight above ideal body weight.[9]

TREATMENT
Desired Outcomes

❸ *Goals of therapy include: (a) educating the patient and caregivers; (b) relieving pain; (c) maintaining or restoring*

Clinical Presentation and Diagnosis of OA

General

- Patients are generally over the age of 50.
- Presentations encompass a spectrum ranging from asymptomatic to severe joint pain and stiffness with functional limitations.
- Joint involvement has an asymmetric local distribution without systemic manifestations.
- In contrast with some other forms of arthritis (e.g., rheumatoid arthritis, gout), inflammation usually is absent or mild and localized when present.

Symptoms

- **❷** *The cardinal symptoms are use-related joint pain, typically described as deep and aching in character, and stiffness. In advanced cases, pain also may be present during rest.*
- Weight-bearing joints may be hindered by instability.
- **❷** *Joint stiffness ("gelling") abates with motion and recurs with rest.*
- **❷** *Joint stiffness generally lasts less than 30 minutes after periods of inactivity, limits the range of joint motion, impairs daily activities, and may be related to weather.*

Signs

- One or more joints may be involved, usually in an asymmetric pattern.
- The following sites are most often involved in primary OA:
  - Distal interphalangeal finger joints (Heberden's nodes)
  - Proximal interphalangeal finger joints (Bouchard's nodes)
  - First carpometacarpal joint
  - Knees, hips, and cervicolumbar spine

- Metatarsophalangeal joint of the great toe
- The following sites are involved most often in secondary OA:
  - Metacarpophalangeal joints
  - Wrists
  - Elbows
  - Glenohumeral joints
  - Ankles
- Joint examination may reveal local tenderness, bony proliferation, soft tissue swelling, crepitus, muscle atrophy, limited motion with passive/active movement, and effusion.

Laboratory Tests

- No specific laboratory test or value is diagnostic for OA.
- The erythrocyte sedimentation rate (ESR) and hematologic and chemistry panels are usually unremarkable.
- Aspirated synovial fluid (if obtained) often displays leukocytosis (WBC less than $2.0 \times 10^3/mm^3$ [$2.0 \times 10^9/L$]) and high viscosity.

Other Diagnostic Tests

- Radiologic evidence may be misleading because structural evidence of OA correlates poorly with symptoms.
- Radiographic changes are often absent in early OA.
- As the disease progresses, joint-space narrowing, subchondral bone sclerosis, and osteophytes may be detected.
- In late severe OA, there may be gross joint deformity and joint effusions.

Patient Encounter, Part 1

CS is a 62-year-old obese woman who presents to your family medicine clinic complaining of deep, aching pain localized to her right knee. The pain is provoked by walking and subsides with rest. She also notes that her knee is difficult to bend for 15 minutes after rising in the morning. The symptoms have worsened over the last several years. Your interview also reveals that she injured her knee several years ago in a minor motor vehicle accident.

What information is suggestive of OA?

What risk factors for OA does CS have?

What other information will you need to differentiate between OA and RA?

What other information will you need before formulating a treatment plan for this patient?

mobility; (d) minimizing functional impairment; (e) preserving joint integrity; and (f) improving quality of life.

General Approach to Treatment

Treatment is individualized and should consider medical history, physical examination, radiographic findings, distribution and severity of joint involvement, and response to previous treatment. Comorbid diseases, concomitant medications, and allergies are integrated into a holistic treatment approach.

A comprehensive treatment algorithm for OA is given in Figure 58–2. Nonpharmacologic treatment is integral to achieving optimal outcomes in patients with OA. Pharmacologic therapy is used as an adjunctive measure to relieve pain; most treatments do not modify the disease course. Surgical intervention generally is reserved for patients with advanced disease complicated by unremitting pain or severely compromised function.

Nonpharmacologic Therapy

Nondrug therapy consists of a three-pronged approach of education, lifestyle modification, and physical therapy. ❹ *Educational programs include a set of systematic educational activities designed to improve health behaviors and health status, thereby slowing OA progression.* The goal is to increase patient knowledge and self-confidence in adjusting daily activities in the face of evolving symptoms. Effective programs produce positive behavioral changes, decreased pain and disability, and improved functioning. In addition to physical outcomes, psychological outcomes such as depression, self-efficacy, and life satisfaction are positively influenced. Patients can be referred to the Arthritis Foundation (*www.arthritis.org*) for educational materials and information on support groups.

❹ *Lifestyle modification should be employed in all patients at risk for OA and in those with established disease.* Aerobic exercise and strength-training programs improve functional capacity in older adults with OA. Stretching and strengthening exercises should target affected and vulnerable joints. Isometric exercises performed three to four times weekly improve physicalfunctioning and decrease disability, pain, and analgesic use. Some patients have the misconception that increased activity will exacerbate joint symptoms, but controlled clinical trials have invalidated this belief.[10] The American Geriatrics Society issued guidelines on the implementation of exercise in OA patients.[11] In general, it is advisable to recommend performing low-impact exercise routinely.

Obesity's association with both the onset and progression of OA make weight loss a pivotal treatment strategy in overweight and obese patients. Women who lose an average of 5 kg (11 lb) lower their risk of knee OA by more than 50%. Symptomatic relief from knee OA and improved quality of life occur in people with knee OA who reduce their body weight. Weight loss should be pursued through dietary modification and increased physical activity (see Chap. 102). It is important to consider the patient's physical capabilities when implementing an exercise program.

❹ *Application of heat or cold treatments to involved joints improves range of motion, reduces pain, and decreases muscle spasms. Practical applications of heat therapy include warm baths or warm water soaks.* Heating pads should be used with caution, especially in the elderly, and patients must be warned of the potential for burns if used inappropriately.

Referral to a physical or occupational therapist may be helpful, particularly in patients with functional disabilities. Physical therapy is tailored to the patient and may include assessment of muscle strength, joint stability, and mobility; use of heat (especially prior to episodes of increased physical activity); structured exercise regimens; and implementation of assistive devices, such as canes, crutches, and walkers. The occupational therapist ensures optimal joint protection and function, energy conservation, and use of splints and other assistive devices.

Pharmacologic Therapy

Simple analgesics such as acetaminophen and nonsteroidal anti-inflammatory drugs (NSAIDs) are first-line agents for treating OA (Table 58–2).

▶ Acetaminophen

Acetaminophen is a centrally acting analgesic that produces analgesia by inhibiting prostaglandin production in the brain and spinal cord. ❺ *It is an effective and inexpensive analgesic with a favorable risk–benefit profile.*[12] *For treatment of mild to moderate pain, acetaminophen should be tried initially at an adequate dose and duration before considering an NSAID.*[13–15] Acetaminophen is generally considered to be as effective as NSAIDs for mild to moderate joint pain with a superior safety profile.[16,17]

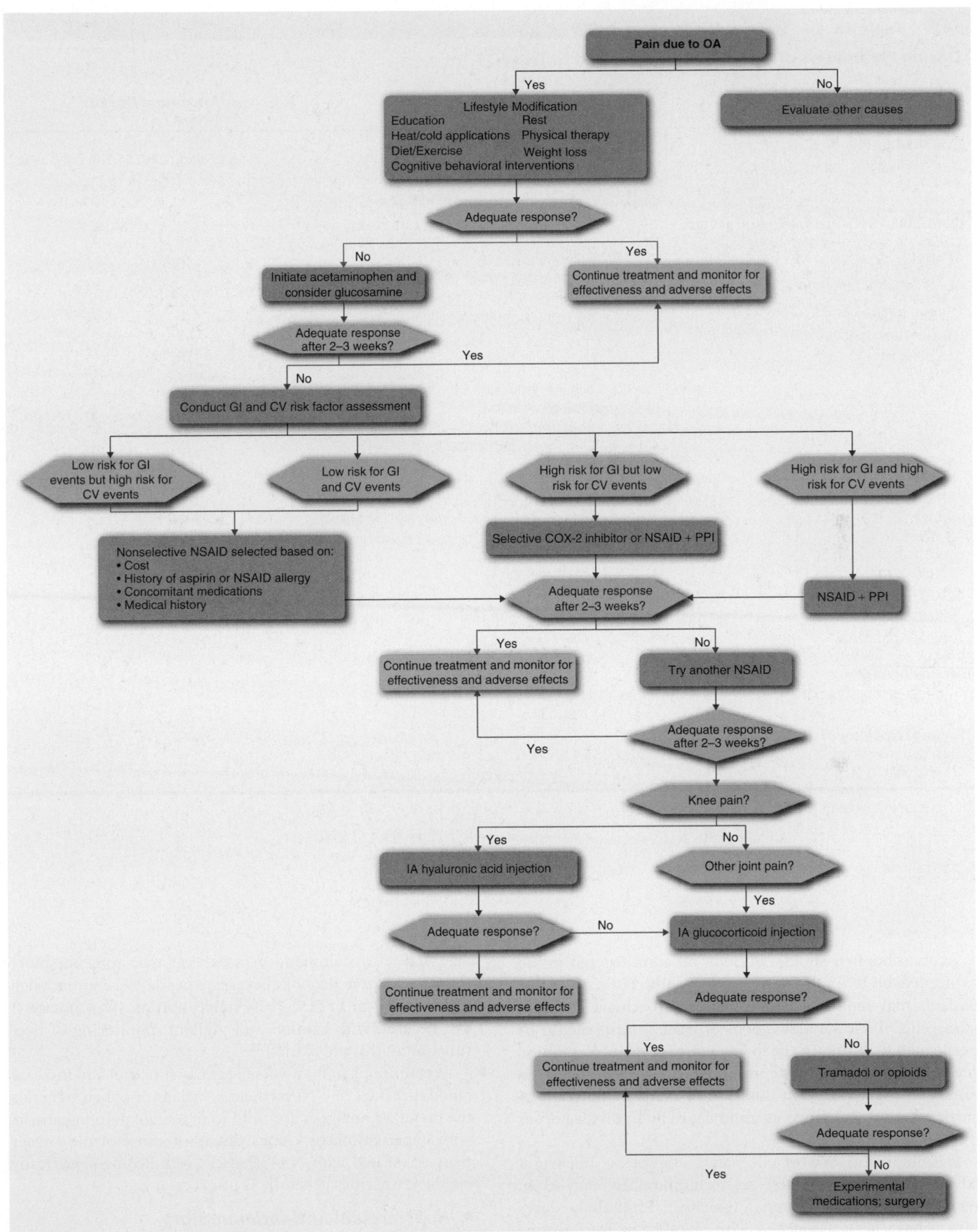

FIGURE 58–2. Treatment of osteoarthritis. (COX-2, cyclooxygenase-2; CV, cardiovascular; IA, intra-articular; NSAID, nonsteroidal anti-inflammatory drug; OA, osteoarthritis; PPI, proton pump inhibitor.)

Table 58–2

Dosing Parameters of Agents Commonly Used to Treat OA

Medication	Dosage and Frequency	Maximum Dosage (mg/day)
Oral Analgesics		
Acetaminophen	325 mg every 4–6 hours or 1 g every 6–8 hours	4,000
Tramadol	50–100 mg every 4–6 hours	400 (300 in elderly)
	CrCl less than30 mL/min: 50–100 mg every 12 hours	200
Nonselective NSAIDs by Chemical Class		
Carboxylic acid (salicylates)		
Aspirin	325–650 mg every 4–6 hours	3,600[a]
Salsalate	500–1,000 mg 2–3 times daily	3,000[a]
Acetic acid		
Etodolac	300–600 mg twice daily	1,200
	400–1,000 mg once daily (extended release)	
Diclofenac	50 mg 2–3 times daily	150
	75 mg twice daily (delayed release)	
	100 mg once daily (extended release)	
Indomethacin	25 mg 2–3 times daily	200
	75 mg 1–2 times daily (sustained release)	
Nabumetone	500–1,000 mg 1–2 times daily	2,000
Propionic acid		
Ibuprofen	400–800 mg 3–4 times daily	3,200
Naproxen	250–500 mg twice daily	1,500
	750–1,000 mg once daily (controlled release)	
	275–550 mg twice daily (naproxen sodium)	1,650
Enolic acid		
Meloxicam	7.5–15 mg once daily	15
COX-2-Selective Agents		
Celecoxib	100 mg twice daily or 200 mg once daily	200
Topical Analgesics		
Capsaicin cream 0.025% or 0.075%	Apply to affected joint every 6–8 hours	
Diclofenac 1% gel		
Lower extremity joints	4 g 4 times daily	16 g[b]
Upper extremity joints	2 g 4 times daily	8 g[b]
Dietary Supplements		
Glucosamine sulfate	500 mg 3 times daily or 1,500 mg once daily	
Chondroitin	400–800 mg 3 times daily with glucosamine	

CrCl, creatinine clearance.

[a]Serum salicylate levels should be monitored for doses greater than 3 g/day.

[b]Total daily dose of diclofenac 1% gel should not exceed 32 g for all affected joints.

Acetaminophen should initially be administered on an as-needed basis in doses up to 4 g daily. However, some patients may require scheduled dosing to achieve adequate pain relief. Periodic assessment of pain control should be performed to maintain the lowest effective dose. A common reason for an inadequate response to acetaminophen is failure to use a sufficient dose for an adequate duration. A sufficient trial is defined as up to 4 g daily in divided doses for 4 to 6 weeks.

Despite being one of the safest analgesics, important adverse effects attributable to acetaminophen can occur, including hepatic and renal toxicity.[18] Total daily doses of 4 g have been associated with significant liver enzyme elevations.[19] Doses greater than 4 g are associated with an increased risk of hepatotoxicity. Concomitant use of alcohol may increase this risk; a maximum acetaminophen dose of 2.5 g daily is recommended in patients who consume more than two to three alcoholic beverages per day. Acetaminophen does not appear to exacerbate stable, chronic liver disease; it can be used with caution and vigilant monitoring of liver function in this population.[18]

Acetaminophen may worsen kidney function and increase blood pressure.[20,21] Nevertheless, acetaminophen remains the preferred analgesic for mild to moderate pain in patients with hypertension or kidney disease because of the greater risks associated with NSAID use.[22] Monitoring specifically for these toxicities generally is unnecessary.

▶ *Nonsteroidal Anti-inflammatory Drugs*

Prostaglandins play an important role in the function of several organ systems. These compounds are synthesized

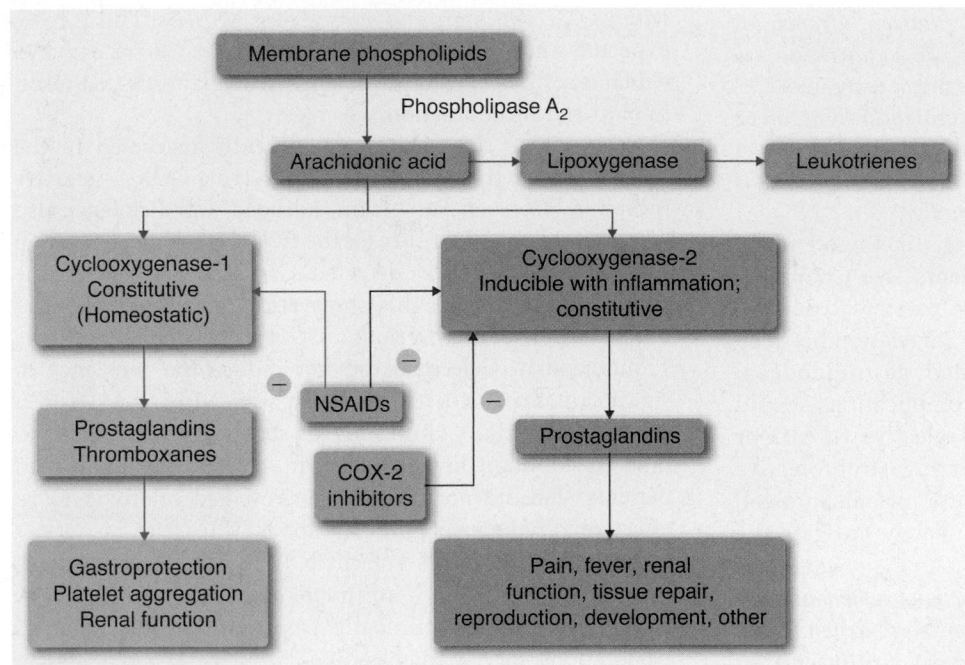

FIGURE 58–3. Synthesis pathway for prostaglandins and leukotrienes. (COX-2, cyclooxygenase enzyme 2; NSAIDs, nonsteroidal anti-inflammatory drugs.) (From DiPiro JT, Talbert RL, Yee GC, et al., eds. *Pharmacotherapy: A Pathophysiologic Approach.* 7th ed. New York: McGraw-Hill; 2008: 1528, Figure 95–6, with permission.)

via the interaction of two isoforms of the cyclooxygenase enzyme (COX-1 and COX-2) with their substrate, arachidonic acid (Fig. 58–3).

The COX-1 enzyme is produced normally in various body tissues (e.g., gastric mucosa, kidney, and platelets). Prostaglandins produced by the actions of the COX-1 enzyme in the GI tract preserve the integrity of the GI mucosa by increasing mucus and bicarbonate secretion, maintaining mucosal blood flow, and decreasing gastric acid secretion. COX-1-associated prostaglandins also promote normal platelet activity and function. In the kidney, COX-1-mediated prostaglandins dilate the afferent arteriole, thereby maintaining intraglomerular pressure and glomerular filtration rate when renal blood flow is reduced.

In contrast, the COX-2 enzyme is not produced normally in most tissues, but its production is increased rapidly in the presence of inflammation and local tissue injury. This leads to the synthesis of prostaglandins involved in pain and inflammation. Consequently, blocking the COX-2 enzyme results in analgesic and anti-inflammatory effects. The beneficial effects of NSAIDs in reducing pain, decreasing joint stiffness, and improving function in patients with OA are thought to be due to inhibition of the COX-2 isoenzyme.

Most NSAIDs (e.g., ibuprofen, naproxen, and others) inhibit both COX-1 and COX-2 isoforms. That is, they are nonselective inhibitors of the COX enzyme system. Inhibition of COX-2 is responsible for analgesic effects, whereas inhibition of COX-1 is responsible for the most common adverse effects of NSAIDs. COX-2-selective inhibitors were developed in attempts to preserve the beneficial effects of COX-2 inhibition while avoiding the deleterious effects associated with inhibition of the COX-1 enzyme. This

approach has not been entirely successful, as discussed below.

❻ *NSAIDs are a reasonable alternative when acetaminophen fails to provide an acceptable analgesic response.* Some authorities recommend NSAIDs over acetaminophen for patients presenting with severe pain or signs and symptoms of inflammation, but this is a matter of much contention. The rationale for this recommendation is that acetaminophen's central mechanism of action renders it ineffective against peripheral joint inflammation, and therefore less effective.[23] Consensus guidelines support the use of NSAIDs as an alternative to acetaminophen if clinical features of peripheral inflammation or severe pain are present.[14,15] Unfortunately, there is no validated mechanism to identify patients who are more likely to respond to NSAIDs than acetaminophen.

❻ *At equipotent doses, the analgesic and anti-inflammatory activity of all NSAIDs and aspirin are similar. The selection of a specific NSAID should be based on tolerability, previous response, and cost.* ❼ *Some patients respond to one NSAID better than to another. If an insufficient response is achieved with one NSAID, another agent from the same or a different chemical class should be tried.* There is no convincing evidence that changing to an NSAID from a different chemical class is more likely to be effective than selecting another drug from the same chemical class. Pain relief occurs rapidly (within hours), but anti-inflammatory benefits are not realized until after 2 to 3 weeks of continuous therapy. This period is the minimal duration that should be considered an adequate NSAID trial.

Inhibition of the COX-1 isoenzyme is thought to be responsible primarily for the adverse effects of NSAIDs on the gastric mucosa, kidney, and platelets. Direct irritant effects also may contribute to adverse GI events.

❽ *Minor GI complaints, including nausea, dyspepsia, anorexia, abdominal pain, flatulence, and diarrhea, are reported by 10% to 60% of patients treated with NSAIDs. Asymptomatic gastric and duodenal mucosal ulceration can be detected in 15% to 45% of patients.*[24] *Perforation, gastric outlet obstruction, and GI bleeding are the most severe complications and occur in 1.5% to 4% of patients annually.*[24]

Several risk factors predict a greater likelihood of GI complications in NSAID-treated patients (see Chap. 18). It is not possible to detect high-risk patients based on symptoms alone because there is poor correlation between the presence of symptoms and actual gastroduodenal damage. Patients at high risk for GI complications should be evaluated for the use of a COX-2-selective NSAID or concomitant treatment with a prophylactic gastroprotective agent such as a proton pump inhibitor or misoprostol. However, these strategies do not completely mitigate the risk of GI complications.

❽ *NSAIDs can cause renal insufficiency when administered to patients whose renal function depends on prostaglandins. Patients with chronic renal insufficiency or left ventricular dysfunction, the elderly, and those receiving diuretics or drugs that interfere with the renin-angiotensin system are particularly susceptible. Decreased glomerular filtration also may cause hyperkalemia. NSAIDs rarely cause* tubulointerstitial *nephropathy and renal papillary necrosis.*

Caution is warranted in pregnant women and women of childbearing age because the risk of bleeding may be increased if the fetus is subjected to the antiplatelet activity of NSAIDs. Ibuprofen and naproxen are rated FDA pregnancy category B in the first and second trimesters. Indomethacin and sulindac have not been rated, whereas celecoxib and etodolac are category C. NSAIDs are contraindicated during the third trimester because they may promote premature closure of the ductus arteriosus in the fetus.

NSAIDs are prone to drug interactions due to high protein binding, detrimental renal effects, and antiplatelet activity. Interactions are encountered frequently with aspirin, warfarin, oral hypoglycemics, antihypertensives, angiotensin-converting enzyme (ACE) inhibitors, angiotensin-receptor blockers (ARBs), β-blockers, diuretics, and lithium. When an interaction with an NSAID is present, vigilant monitoring is warranted for therapeutic efficacy (e.g., NSAIDs blunt the antihypertensive efficacy of diuretics) and adverse effects (e.g., NSAIDs increase the risk of bleeding in anticoagulated patients).

▶ *Selective COX-2 Inhibitors*

Elucidation of the activities of individual COX isoforms led to the development of drugs that selectively inhibit the inducible form of the enzyme, COX-2. Thus COX-2 inhibitors were expected to minimize NSAID GI toxicity and antiplatelet effects (see Fig. 58–3).[25] **❾** *A common misconception is that COX-2 inhibitors are more effective than nonselective NSAIDs in relieving pain and inflammation. In clinical trials, patients experienced similar levels of pain relief* with COX-2 inhibitors and nonselective NSAIDs. This is to be expected since both drug classes inhibit the COX-2 enzyme, which is responsible for producing prostaglandins that result in pain and inflammation.

Celecoxib is the only agent currently marketed in the United States that is considered a true COX-2-selective inhibitor. However, meloxicam, sulindac, and diclofenac also display preferential affinity for the COX-2 isozyme. Celecoxib reduces endoscopically detected GI lesions. However, the clinical importance of this observation has been challenged because many of these lesions are clinically silent and resolve spontaneously. Celecoxib did not reduce the incidence of significant upper GI toxicity compared with NSAIDs in a large clinical trial.[26] However, this study allowed patients to take concomitant low-dose aspirin. A *post hoc* analysis in patients who did not take aspirin revealed celecoxib to be effective in reducing significant upper GI toxicity.

The selective agents rofecoxib (removed from the U.S. market in 2004) and lumiracoxib (not currently FDA approved) decrease clinically important events such as perforations, ulcers, and bleeding.[27,28]

The advent of COX-2-selective inhibitors has led to unexpected results. **❾** *By selectively inhibiting the COX-2 isoform, COX-2-selective NSAIDs may increase the risk of cardiovascular events in certain patients.*[29] COX-2 is responsible for the production of prostacyclin, a vasodilatory and antiplatelet substance. In contrast, COX-1 controls the production of thromboxane A_2, a vasoconstrictor and platelet aggregator. Selective inhibition of COX-2 results in decreased prostacyclin levels in the face of stable thromboxane A_2 levels. An imbalance in the thromboxane A_2: prostacyclin ratio ensues, which creates an environment that favors thrombosis.

As a consequence, COX-2-selective inhibitors may offer enhanced GI safety but compromised cardiovascular safety. Increased cardiovascular risk associated with COX-2 inhibitors is likely multifactorial in nature and may be attributable primarily to selectivity, dosage, and potency of selective agents. This relationship can be explained in part by the mechanism of theses drugs—greater inhibition of COX-2 results in a larger decrease in prostacyclin relative to thromboxane A_2 (favoring thrombosis) but also less GI ulceration because of the greater preservation of mucosal protective factors. Other mechanisms for increasing cardiovascular risk have been proposed for various agents.[30]

Concomitant use of low-dose aspirin mitigates some of the increased cardiovascular risk but also obliterates the GI safety of COX-2 selectivity.[26–28] Patients treated with a COX-2-selective agent plus aspirin experience GI complications at a rate commensurate with that of patients given traditional nonselective agents. Use of less selective agents (e.g., meloxicam) to avoid cardiovascular concerns with COX-2 inhibitors may not be justified because neither GI nor cardiovascular safety is optimized. In patients at risk for cardiovascular disease, a nonselective NSAID plus a proton pump inhibitor is a reasonable option (Table 58–3). Naproxen appears to have the least cardiovascular risk of

Table 58–3

Treatment Options Based on CV and GI Risk

	High CV Risk	Low CV Risk
High GI Risk	NS-NSAID[a] plus PPI or misoprostol	COX-2 or NS-NSAID + gastroprotection
Low GI Risk	NS-NSAID[a]	NS-NSAID

COX-2, selective cyclooxygenase-2 inhibitor; CV, cardiovascular; NS-NSAID, nonsteroidal anti-inflammatory drug; PPI, proton pump inhibitor.

[a]Naproxen may be considered initially due to potentially lower CV risk compared with other NS-NSAIDs.

the nonselective NSAIDs and should generally be considered first.[16]

The COX-2 enzyme is also produced normally in the kidney; thus COX-2 inhibitors exert renal effects similar to those of conventional NSAIDs. Both drug classes may increase sodium reabsorption and fluid retention and can provoke renal insufficiency and hyperkalemia. COX-2 inhibitors should be used with caution in patients with heart failure or hypertension.

COX-2 inhibitors are susceptible to the same drug interactions as nonselective agents. However, the interaction with warfarin is less pronounced because platelet function is affected to a lesser degree.

▶ *Glucosamine and Chondroitin*

Glucosamine is believed to function as a "chondroprotective" agent, stimulating the cartilage matrix and protecting against oxidative chemical damage. Chondroitin is administered often in conjunction with glucosamine. It is thought to inhibit degradative enzymes and serve as a substrate for the production of proteoglycans. Numerous clinical trials have evaluated the efficacy of these substances for the treatment of OA. However, results vary widely and the quality of several of these studies has been questioned. Of the two available glucosamine salts, glucosamine hydrochloride has consistently demonstrated poor efficacy, whereas glucosamine sulfate may provide benefit.[31] ❿ *In the context of such limitations, glucosamine and chondroitin reduce pain and improve mobility by 20% to 35%.*[31,32] *They also may slow disease progression by decreasing the rate of cartilage destruction, although the clinical impact of this effect is not clear.*[33] Glucosamine is not effective for treating acute pain; beneficial effects often mature over a period of weeks. Because these agents are loosely regulated in the United States as dietary supplements, product standards are inconsistent, and the constituents are not validated by any regulatory agency.

In the landmark GAIT trial conducted by the National Institutes of Health (NIH), glucosamine, chondroitin, and their combination were no more effective than placebo

in decreasing pain symptoms in patients with knee OA after 24 weeks.[34] Celecoxib was significantly more effective than placebo. In the subgroup of patients with moderate to severe OA pain, the combination of glucosamine and chondroitin appeared to have a moderate effect, although this subgroup analysis must be interpreted with caution. Analysis of radiologic changes after 2 years of treatment showed no significant benefit of glucosamine, chondroitin sulfate, or the combination over placebo.[35]

In contrast, a European study (the GUIDE trial) that compared a prescription glucosamine product with acetaminophen and placebo in patients with knee OA found that glucosamine performed better versus placebo than did acetaminophen.[36]

Interpretation of these results is challenging given the inconsistencies in study design, differences in end points applied, preparations of glucosamine tested (glucosamine hydrochloride versus sulfate), and the comparator agents (celecoxib versus acetaminophen). Based on the available data, it appears that glucosamine and chondroitin may be effective for some patients with OA of the knee.

The use of glucosamine (derived from crab, lobster or shrimp shells) and/or chondroitin (derived from cattle or shark cartilage) may warrant caution in patients with shellfish allergies, but preliminary evidence suggests little drug-allergy interaction.[37] Additionally, glucosamine may alter cellular glucose uptake, thus elevating blood glucose levels in diabetic patients. A randomized, placebo-controlled trial of 38 diabetic participants failed to detect any significant alteration in hemoglobin A_{1c} levels after 3 months of glucosamine/chondroitin therapy; however, a relatively short study period and low number of participants may account for these negative findings.[38] Blood glucose levels in diabetic patients should be monitored closely after glucosamine initiation or dosage adjustments. Given the favorable safety profile of glucosamine and chondroitin, it is reasonable to present these agents as a treatment option to patients with symptomatic knee OA in the absence of contraindicating factors.

▶ *Intra-articular Therapy*

❿ *Intra-articular injection of corticosteroids or hyaluronan represents an alternative to oral agents for the treatment of joint pain.*[39] These modalities usually are reserved for patients unresponsive to other treatments because of the relative invasiveness of intra-articular injections compared with oral drugs, the small risk of infection, and the cost of the procedure.

Hyaluronan (or Hyaluronic Acid) The mechanism of action of hyaluronan is not fully understood. Healthy cartilage and synovial fluid are replete with hyaluronic acid, a viscous substance believed to facilitate lubrication and shock absorbency under varying conditions of load bearing. Patients with OA demonstrate an absolute and functional decline in hyaluronic acid; thus exogenous administration is referred to as *viscosupplementation*. In responders, the benefit of hyaluronan administration persists for periods that exceed its residence time in the synovium, suggesting that benefits beyond viscoelasticity are involved. Inhibition of inflammatory mediators and cartilage degradation, stimulation of the cartilage matrix, neuroprotective actions, and the ability of hyaluronan to induce its own synthesis may account in part for the benefit.

Pain and joint function have been evaluated frequently in clinical trials administering hyaluronan to patients with OA. Results are conflicting, with some suggesting dramatic improvements and others indicating no effect. In one controlled trial, hyaluronan injections relieved pain to a similar extent as oral NSAIDs.[40] Hyaluronan provides greater pain relief for a longer time than intra-articular corticosteroids, but corticosteroids work more rapidly.[40]

Several formulations of hyaluronan are available for the treatment of knee pain in patients with OA who are unresponsive to other measures. Administration typically consists of weekly injections for 3 to 5 weeks and is well tolerated, although some patients may report local reactions. Rarely, postinjection flares and anaphylaxis have been reported. Intra-articular injection is associated with a low risk of infection (approximately 1 joint in 50,000 injections). Patients should be counseled to minimize activity and stress on the joint for several days after each injection.

Corticosteroids Use of systemic corticosteroids is discouraged in patients with OA. ❿ *However, in a subset of patients with an inflammatory component or knee effusion involving one or two joints, intra-articular corticosteroids can be useful as monotherapy or as an adjunct to analgesics.* The affected joint can be aspirated and subsequently injected with a corticosteroid. The aspirate should be examined for the presence of crystalline formation and infection. A single joint should not be injected more than three to five times per year.

The crystalline nature of corticosteroid suspensions can provoke a postinjection flare in some patients. The ensuing flare mimics the flare of arthritis and inflammation that accompanies infection. Cold compresses and analgesics are recommended to treat symptoms in affected patients.

▶ Tramadol

Use of opioid analgesics may be warranted when pain is unresponsive to other pharmacologic agents or when such agents are contraindicated. Tramadol is a centrally acting synthetic opioid oral analgesic that also weakly inhibits the reuptake of serotonin and norepinephrine. It is effective for treatment of moderate pain but is devoid of anti-inflammatory activity. There is a low potential for abuse compared with conventional opioid analgesics, and tramadol is not scheduled as a controlled substance in the United States.

Tramadol is a reasonable option for patients with contraindications to NSAIDs or failure to respond to other oral therapies. ❿ *For the treatment of hip or knee OA, tramadol is as effective as NSAIDs. The addition of tramadol to NSAIDs or acetaminophen may augment the analgesic effects of a failing regimen, thereby securing sufficient pain relief in some patients.* Moreover, concomitant tramadol may permit the use of lower NSAID doses.

Dizziness, vertigo, nausea, vomiting, constipation, and lethargy are all relatively common adverse events. These effects are more pronounced for several days after initiation and following upward dose titration. Seizures have been reported rarely; the risk is dose-related and appears to increase with concomitant use of antidepressants, such as tricyclic antidepressants or selective serotonin reuptake inhibitors. Tramadol should be avoided in patients receiving monoamine oxidase (MAO) inhibitors because tramadol inhibits the uptake of norepinephrine and serotonin.

▶ Other Opioid Analgesics

Opioids decrease pain, improve sleep patterns, and increase functioning in patients with OA who are unresponsive to nonpharmacologic therapy and nonnarcotic analgesics. Use of opioid analgesics for nonmalignant pain is becoming more acceptable. Emerging evidence suggests that patients can achieve satisfactory analgesia by using nonescalating doses of opioids with a minimal risk of addiction.[41] Opioid analgesics should be reserved for patients who experience moderate to severe pain and do not respond to or are not candidates for other pharmacologic and nonpharmacologic strategies.[42] Opioids also may be useful in patients with conditions that preclude the use of NSAIDs, such as renal failure, heart failure, or anticoagulation.

Opioid analgesics should be initiated at low doses in combination with acetaminophen or an NSAID when possible. Combining opioids with other analgesics reduces the opioid requirement, thereby minimizing adverse events. Conservative initial doses are warranted, with the dose titrated to adequate response with minimal side effects.

Oxycodone is the most extensively studied of the opioids recommended for OA. However, other agents such as morphine, hydromorphone, methadone, and transdermal fentanyl are also effective.[43] The American Pain Society (APS) recommends against using codeine and propoxyphene for OA because of the high incidence of adverse effects and limited analgesic effectiveness.

If opioid therapy is considered, there should be an initial comprehensive medical history and physical examination, firm documentation that nonopioid therapy has failed, clearly defined treatment goals, an understanding between the provider and the patient of the true benefits and risks of long-term opioids, use of a single provider and pharmacy whenever possible, and comprehensive follow-up.

▶ Topical Analgesics

Topical analgesics sometimes are used for mild pain or as an adjunct to systemic therapy. There are limited data to support the use of salicylate-containing rubefacients (e.g., methyl salicylate and trolamine salicylate) or other counterirritants (e.g., menthol, camphor, and methyl nicotinate) in OA.[44] See Chapter 60 for more information on these products when used for musculoskeletal disorders.

Capsaicin achieves pain relief by depleting substance P from sensory neurons in the spine, thereby decreasing pain transmission. Capsaicin is not effective for acute pain; up to

2 weeks may be necessary before pain relief is appreciated. Most patients experience a local burning sensation at the site of application. The discomfort usually does not result in discontinuation and often abates within the first week. Patients should be cautioned not to allow capsaicin to come into contact with eyes or mucous membranes and to wash their hands after each application.

⑩ *Topical NSAID preparations are effective for treating OA involving the superficial joints of the hands, wrists, elbows, knees, ankles, or feet.* Administration via a topical vehicle targets the joints involved and decreases systemic exposure. This may be an attractive option for patients at risk of developing adverse events from oral NSAIDs.

Diclofenac sodium topical gel 1% (Voltaren Gel) is available in the United States; its approval was based on two clinical trials that found decreased pain and improved joint function in patients with hand or knee OA.[45,46] Systemic absorption of topical diclofenac sodium is ~17 times lower than that seen with oral diclofenac. Thus, GI, cardiovascular and renal adverse effects would not be expected with proper administration. The most common adverse effects include application site dermatitis, pruritus, and phototoxicity.

Surgery

⑩ *Surgery generally is reserved for patients who fail to respond to medical therapy and have progressive limitations in activities of daily living (ADL).* In joint replacement surgery (arthroplasty), the damaged joint surfaces are replaced with metal or plastic prosthetic devices. Hip and knee joints are most commonly replaced, but arthroplasty may also be performed on shoulders, elbows, fingers, and ankles. Most patients achieve significant pain relief and functional restoration after arthroplasty, and it is a reasonable option in carefully selected refractory patients.[47]

Surgical debridement may be performed arthroscopically. With this procedure, a tiny video camera is inserted into the affected joint through a small incision, and the surgeon removes torn cartilage or other debris from the joint. The long-term benefits of arthroscopic surgery for OA are unclear, and it may be no better than optimized physical and medical therapy.[48,49]

OUTCOME EVALUATION

- At baseline, quantify the patient's pain using a visual analogue scale, assess range of motion of affected joints, and identify activities of daily living that are impaired.
- In patients treated with acetaminophen or oral NSAIDs, assess pain control after 2 to 3 weeks. It may take longer for the full anti-inflammatory effect of NSAIDs to occur.
- Incorporate other measures to track disease progress. Use radiography to assess severity of joint destruction, determine 50-ft walking time and grip strength,

---

Patient Encounter, Part 2: Medical History, Physical Examination, and Diagnostic Tests

PMH: Obesity (BMI = 34 kg/m²); hypertension for 7 years; type 2 diabetes mellitus; hyperlipidemia, currently at goal; gastroesophageal reflux disease

FH: Father died of stroke at age 72; mother had OA of the hands.

SH: Works as a secretary. Denies alcohol, tobacco, and illicit drug use.

Allergies: NKDA

Meds: Hydrochlorothiazide 12.5 mg once daily; enalapril 10 mg twice daily; metformin 1,000 mg twice daily; atorvastatin 10 mg once daily; pantoprazole 40 mg every morning; enteric-coated aspirin 81 mg once daily; ibuprofen 200 mg as needed for pain

Labs: Within normal limits.

Radiology: Radiography of the affected knee shows joint space narrowing and subchondral bone sclerosis.

Which parameters are consistent with a diagnosis of OA?

What are the treatment goals for this patient?

What nonpharmacologic options are available to treat this patient?

What pharmacologic options are available to treat this patient?

What factors are important to consider when selecting medications for this patient?

Patient Encounter, Part 3: Creating a Care Plan

Based on the information available, create a care plan for this patient's OA. The plan should include:
(a) a statement of the drug-related needs and/or problems;
(b) an individualized, detailed therapeutic plan; and
(c) a plan for follow-up monitoring to document the patient's response and identify adverse reactions.

---

and administer the Western Ontario and McMaster Universities Osteoarthritis Index (WOMAC) and the Stanford Health Assessment Questionnaire, where appropriate, to assess activities of daily living.

- Ask patients if they are experiencing side effects or other problems with their medications and follow-up with more specific questions.
- In patients taking oral NSAIDs, monitor for increases in blood pressure, weight gain, edema, skin rash, and CNS adverse effects such as headaches and drowsiness.

Patient Care and Monitoring

1. Determine whether the patient's symptoms are consistent with OA. Review the medical history to determine whether other rheumatologic diseases may be involved.

2. Assess symptoms to determine if pain warrants additional attention. Does the pain affect quality of life or interfere with activities of daily living?

3. Evaluate symptoms to determine what nonpharmacologic interventions can be recommended and whether pharmacologic treatment is warranted.

4. Obtain a thorough history of previous drug use, including prescription drugs, over-the-counter drugs, and dietary supplements. Determine whether any of these treatments have been effective. Ask the patient about the dose and frequency of previous pharmacologic agents to determine if an adequate trial was given.

5. Educate the patient about appropriate use of nonpharmacologic treatments for OA.

6. Formulate a drug therapy plan, taking into consideration the patient's medical history, concomitant medications, and previous use of medications.

7. Develop a plan to monitor the patient's response to therapy.

8. Evaluate for the presence of adverse drug reactions, drug hypersensitivity, and drug interactions.

9. Document whether the patient has had improvements in quality-of-life measures, such as improved functioning, increased ability to perform activities of daily living, and improved well-being.

10. Emphasize the value of adherence to medication regimens and lifestyle modifications. Facilitate adherence by implementing medication regimens and lifestyle plans that are simple and consistent with the patient's lifestyle.

11. Educate the patient about OA, lifestyle modifications, and medications:

    • What causes OA?

    • How will lifestyle modifications affect the disease?

    • What are the expectations of treatment?

    • When and how should medications be taken?

    • What adverse effects are most common, do they decrease during therapy, and what are the warning signs of more severe complications?

    • What prescription and over-the-counter medications should be avoided to prevent drug-drug, drug-food, or drug-disease interactions?

    • What options are available if the current regimen fails?

• Evaluate serum creatinine, complete blood count, and serum transaminases at baseline and at every 6 to 12 months in patients treated with oral NSAIDs or acetaminophen.

• Perform stool guaiac in patients taking oral NSAIDs when clinically indicated.

• Monitor for drug interactions, including alcohol, at every visit.

Abbreviations Introduced in This Chapter

ACR	American College of Rheumatology
APS	American Pain Society
COX	Cyclooxygenase
DJD	Degenerative joint disease
MMP	Matrix metalloproteinases
NSAID	Nonsteroidal anti-inflammatory drug
OA	Osteoarthritis
WOMAC	Western Ontario and McMaster Universities Osteoarthritis Index

 Self-assessment questions and answers are available at *http://www.mhpharmacotherapy.com/pp.html*.

REFERENCES

1. Centers for Disease Control and Prevention. National and state medical expenditures and lost earnings attributable to arthritis and other rheumatic conditions—United States, 2003. MMWR Morb Mortal Wkly Rep 2007;56(1):4–7.

2. CDC. Prevalence of disabilities and associated health conditions among adults—United States, 1999. MMWR Morb Mortal Wkly Rep 2001;50:120–125.

3. The National Arthritis Data Workgroup. Estimates of the prevalence of arthritis and other rheumatic conditions in the United States: Part II. Arthritis Rheum 2008;58:26–35.

4. Felson DT, Lawrence RC, Dieppe PA, et al. Osteoarthritis: New insights. Part 1: The disease and its risk factors. Ann Intern Med 2000;133:635–646.

5. Felson DT. An update on the pathogenesis and epidemiology of osteoarthritis. Radiol Clin North Am 2004;42:1–9.

6. Brandt KD. Osteoarthritis. In: Kasper DL, Braunwald E, Fauci AS, et al., eds. Harrison's Principles of Internal Medicine, 16th ed. New York: McGraw-Hill, 2005:1692–1698.

7. Lane NE, Schnitzer TJ. Osteoarthritis. In: Goldman L, Ausiello DA, eds. Cecil Medicine, 23rd ed. (Philadelphia, PA: Saunders Elsevier;). 2007, http://www.mdconsult.com/das/book/0/view/1492/1009.html

8. McAlindon TE, Wilson PW, Aliabadi P, et al. Level of physical activity and the risk of radiographic and symptomatic knee osteoarthritis in the elderly: The Framingham Study. Am J Med 1999;106:151–157.

9. Fife RS. Epidemiology, pathology, and pathogenesis. In: Klippel JH, ed. Primer on Rheumatic Diseases, 11th ed. Atlanta, GA: Arthritis Foundation; 1997:216–217.

10. Bennell K, Hinman R. Exercise as a treatment for osteoarthritis. Curr Opin Rheumatol 2005;17:634–640.

11. American Geriatrics Society Panel on Exercise and Osteoarthritis. Exercise prescription for older adults with osteoarthritis pain: Consensus practice recommendations. J Am Geriatr Soc 2001;49:808–823.

12. Nikles CJ, Yelland M, Del Mar C, Wilkinson D. The role of paracetamol in chronic pain: An evidence-based approach. Am J Ther 2005;12:80–91.

13. Felson DT, Lawrence RC, Hochberg MC, et al. Osteoarthritis: New insights. Part 2: Treatment approaches. Ann Intern Med 2000;133:726–737.

14. American College of Rheumatology Subcommittee on Osteoarthritis Guidelines. Recommendations for the medical management of osteoarthritis of the hip and knee: 2000 update. Arthritis Rheum 2000;43:1905–1915.

15. American Pain Society. Guideline for the management of pain in osteoarthritis, rheumatoid arthritis, and juvenile chronic arthritis. American Pain Society 2002;2:43–74.

16. Towheed TE, Maxwell L, Judd MG, et al. Acetaminophen for osteoarthritis. Cochrane Database Syst Rev 2006;(1): CD004257.

17. Courtney P, Doherty M. Key questions concerning paracetamol and NSAIDs for osteoarthritis. Ann Rheum Dis 2002;61:767–773.

18. Graham GG, Scott KF, Day RO. Tolerability of paracetamol. Drug Saf 2005;28:227–240.

19. Watkins PB, Kaplowitz N, Slattery JT, et al. Aminotransferase elevations in healthy adults receiving 4 grams of acetaminophen daily. JAMA 2006;296:87–93.

20. Fored CM, Ejerblad E, Lindblad P, et al. Acetaminophen, aspirin, and chronic renal failure. N Engl J Med 2001;345:1801–1808.

21. Curhan GC, Knight EL, Rosner B, et al. Lifetime non-narcotic analgesic use and decline in renal function in women. Arch Intern Med 2004;164:1519–1524.

22. Forman JP, Stampfer MJ, Curhan GC. Non-narcotic analgesic dose and risk of incident hypertension in U.S. women. Hypertension 2005; 46:500–507.

23. Henrich WL, Agodoa LE, Barrett B, et al. Analgesics and the kidney: Summary and recommendations to the Scientific Advisory Board of the National Kidney Foundation from an Ad Hoc Committee of the National Kidney Foundation. Am J Kidney Dis 1996;27:162–165.

24. Laine L. Approaches to nonsteroidal anti-inflammatory drug use in the high-risk patient. Gastroenterology 2001;120:594–606.

25. Felson DT. The verdict favors nonsteroidal anti-inflammatory drugs for treatment of osteoarthritis and a plea for more evidence on other treatments. Arthritis Rheum 2001;44:1477–1480.

26. Silverstein FE, Faich G, Goldstein JL, et al. Gastrointestinal toxicity with celecoxib vs nonsteroidal anti-inflammatory drugs for osteoarthritis and rheumatoid arthritis: The CLASS study: A randomized controlled trial. Celecoxib Long-term Arthritis Safety Study. JAMA 2000;284: 1247–1255.

27. Bombardier C, Laine L, Reicin A, et al. VIGOR Study Group. Comparison of upper gastrointestinal toxicity of rofecoxib and naproxen in patients with rheumatoid arthritis. N Engl J Med 2000;343: 1520–1528.

28. Schnitzer TJ, Burmester GR, Mysler E, et al. Comparison of lumiracoxib with naproxen and ibuprofen in the Therapeutic Arthritis Research and Gastrointestinal Event Trial (TARGET), reduction in ulcer complications: Randomised controlled trial. Lancet. 2004;364: 665–674.

29. Howard PA, Delafontaine P. Nonsteroidal anti-inflammatory drugs and cardiovascular risk. J Am Coll Cardiol 2004;43:519–525.

30. Zarraga IG, Schwarz ER. Coxibs and heart disease: What we have learned and what else we need to know. J Am Coll Cardiol 2007;49: 1–14.

31. Richy F, Bruyere O, Ethgen O, et al. Structural and symptomatic efficacy of glucosamine and chondroitin in knee osteoarthritis: A comprehensive meta-analysis. Arch Intern Med 2003;163:1514–1522.

32. Vlad SC, LaValley MP, McAlindon TE, Felson DT. Glucosamine for pain in osteoarthritis: Why do trial results differ? Arthritis Rheum 2007;56:2267–2277.

33. Reginster JY, Deroisy R, Rovati LC, et al. Long-term effects of glucosamine sulphate on osteoarthritis progression: A randomised, placebo-controlled clinical trial. Lancet 2001;357:251–256.

34. Clegg DO, Reda DJ, Harris CL, et al. Glucosamine, chondroitin sulfate, and the two in combination for painful knee osteoarthritis. N Engl J Med 2006;354: 795–808.

35. Sawitzke AD, Shi H, Finco MF, et al. The effect of glucosamine and/or chondroitin sulfate on the progression of knee osteoarthritis. Arthritis Rheum 2008;58:3183–3191.

36. Herrero-Beaumont G, Ivorra JA, Del Carmen Trabado M, et al. Glucosamine sulfate in the treatment of knee osteoarthritis symptoms: A randomized, double-blind, placebo-controlled study using acetaminophen as a side comparator. Arthritis Rheum 2007;56: 555–567.

37. Gray HC, Hutcheson PS, Gray RG. Is glucosamine safe in patients with seafood allergy? J Allergy Clin Immunol 2004;114:459–460.

38. Scroggie DA, Albright A, Harris MD. The effect of glucosamine-chondroitin supplementation on glycosylated hemoglobin levels in patients with type 2 diabetes mellitus. Arch Intern Med 2003;163:1587–1590.

39. Gossec L, Dougados M. Intraarticular treatments in osteoarthritis: From the symptomatic to the structure modifying. Ann Rheum Dis 2004;63:478–482.

40. Petrella RJ, DiSilvestro MD, Hildebrand C. Effects of hyaluronate sodium on pain and physical functioning in osteoarthritis of the knee: A randomized, double-blind, placebo-controlled clinical trial. Arch Intern Med 2002;162:292–298.

41. Ballantyne JC, Mao J. Opioid therapy for chronic pain. N Engl J Med 2003;349:1943–1953.

42. The American Academy of Pain Medicine, the American Pain Society: The use of opioids for the treatment of chronic pain: A consensus statement from the American Academy of Pain Medicine and the American Pain Society. Clin J Pain 1997;13:6–8.

43. Avouac J, Gossec L, Dougados M. Efficacy and safety of opioids for osteoarthritis: A meta-analysis of randomized controlled trials. Osteoarthritis Cartilage 2007;15:957–965.

44. Mason L, Moore RA, Edwards JE, et al. Systematic review of efficacy of topical rubefacients containing salicylates for the treatment of acute and chronic pain. BMJ 2004;328:995–998.

45. FDA Center for Drug Evaluation and Research (CDER). Summary Review: Voltaren Gel. http://www.accessdata.fda.gov/drugsatfda_docs/nda/2007/Voltaren_022122.cfm.

46. Altman RD, Dreiser RL, Fisher CL. Diclofenac sodium gel in patients with primary hand osteoarthritis: A randomized, double-blind, placebo-controlled trial. J Rheumatol 2009;36(9):1991–1999.

47. Dieppe P, Basler HD, Chard J, et al. Knee replacement surgery for osteoarthritis: Effectiveness, practice variations, indications and possible determinants of utilization. Rheumatology 1999;38:73–83.

48. Mosely JB, O'Malley K, Peterson NJ, et al. A controlled trial of arthroscopic surgery for osteoarthritis of the knee. N Engl J Med 2002; 347:81–88.

49. Kirkley A, Birmingham TB, Litchfield RB, et al. A randomized trial of arthroscopic surgery for osteoarthritis of the knee. N Engl J Med 2008;359: 1097–1107.

59 Gout and Hyperuricemia

Geoffrey C. Wall

LEARNING OBJECTIVES

Upon completion of the chapter, the reader will be able to:

1. Recognize major risk factors for developing gout in a given person.

2. Develop a pharmacotherapeutic plan for a patient with acute gouty arthritis or uric acid nephropathy that includes individualized drug selection and monitoring for efficacy and safety.

3. Identify patients in whom maintenance therapy for gout and hyperuricemia is warranted.

4. Select an appropriate drug to reduce serum uric acid (SUA) levels in patients with gout, and outline a plan for monitoring efficacy and toxicity.

5. Educate patients on appropriate lifestyle modifications to help prevent gouty arthritis attacks.

KEY CONCEPTS

❶ Gout results from deposition of uric acid crystals in joint spaces, leading to an inflammatory reaction that causes intense pain, erythema, and joint swelling.

❷ Some drugs can cause hyperuricemia and gout, such as thiazide diuretics, niacin, pyrazinamide, cyclosporine, and occasionally, low-dose aspirin.

❸ Long-term consequences of gout and hyperuricemia include joint destruction, tophi, and nephrolithiasis.

❹ Treatment of gout involves: (a) acute relief of a gouty arthritis attack; and (b) in some patients long-term maintenance treatment to prevent future attacks.

❺ Nonsteroidal anti-inflammatory drugs, colchicine, or corticosteroids are used for acute attacks. Selection depends on several patient factors, especially renal function.

❻ Asymptomatic hyperuricemia usually does not require treatment.

❼ Patients with recurrent gout attacks, evidence of tophi or joint destruction, or uric acid nephrolithiasis are candidates for maintenance therapy with allopurinol or probenecid to lower serum uric acid (SUA) levels.

❽ Tumor lysis syndrome (TLS) is a metabolic disorder caused by rapid cell destruction (usually during chemotherapy treatment for cancer) and is associated with several electrolyte disturbances, notably hyperuricemia.

EPIDEMIOLOGY AND ETIOLOGY

Gout is the most common inflammatory arthritis in the United States and western Europe.[1] The annual incidence is approximately 62 cases per 100,000 persons in the United States.[2] The incidence increases with age and appears to be rising, probably because of a larger number of patients with risk factors for gout.[3]

PATHOPHYSIOLOGY

Gout is caused by an abnormality in uric acid metabolism. Uric acid is a waste product of the breakdown of purines contained in the DNA of degraded body cells and dietary protein. Uric acid is water soluble and excreted primarily by the kidneys, although some is broken down by colonic bacteria and excreted via the GI tract.[4,5]

The solubility of uric acid depends on concentration and temperature. At high serum concentrations, lower body temperature causes the precipitation of monosodium urate (MSU) crystals. Collections of these crystals (called microtophi) can form in joint spaces in the distal extremities.

❶ *Gout results from deposition of uric acid crystals in joint spaces, leading to an inflammatory reaction that causes intense pain, erythema, and joint swelling.* Free urate crystals can activate several proinflammatory mediators, including tumor necrosis factor α (TNF-α), interleukin 1 (IL-1), and IL-8. Activation of these mediators signals chemotactic movement of neutrophils into the joint space that "ingest" MSU crystals via phagocytosis. These neutrophils then are lysed and release proteolytic enzymes that trigger the clinical manifestations of an acute gout attack, such as pain and swelling. These inflammatory mechanisms in gout, especially in untreated disease, can lead to cartilage and joint destruction.

The increased serum uric acid (SUA) involves either the underexcretion of uric acid (80% of patients) or its overproduction. The cause of overproduction or underexcretion of uric acid in most gout patients is unknown; this is referred to as *primary gout*.[2]

The reference range for SUA is 3.6 to 8.3 mg/dL (214–494 μmol/L). The risk of gout increases as the SUA concentration increases. Approximately 30% of patients with levels greater than 10 mg/dL (595 μmol/L) develop symptoms of gout within 5 years. However, most patients with hyperuricemia are asymptomatic. Other risk factors for gout include male gender, obesity, ethanol use, hypertension, and dyslipidemia.[6,7] Gout is seen frequently in patients with type 2 diabetes mellitus and coronary artery disease, but a causal relationship has not been established.

Uric acid excretion is reduced in patients with chronic kidney disease, putting them at risk for hyperuricemia. In patients with persistently acidic urine and hyperuricemia, uric acid **nephrolithiasis** can occur in up to 25% of patients; in severe cases, uric acid stones can cause nephropathy and renal failure.[8] Extreme hyperuricemia can occur because of rapid tumor cell destruction in patients undergoing chemotherapy for certain types of cancer. This phenomenon is known as **tumor lysis syndrome (TLS)**.

❷ *Some drugs can cause hyperuricemia and gout, such as thiazide diuretics, niacin, pyrazinamide, cyclosporine, and occasionally, low-dose aspirin. In most cases, these drugs block uric acid secretion in the kidney.* ❸ *Long-term consequences of gout and hyperuricemia include joint destruction, tophi, and nephrolithiasis.*

CLINICAL PRESENTATION AND DIAGNOSIS

Aspiration of affected joint fluid is essential for a definitive diagnosis. Joint fluid containing negatively birefringent MSU crystals confirms the diagnosis. Joint fluid has an elevated WBC count with neutrophils predominating (Fig. 59–1).[9]

Although rarely performed, a 24-hour urine collection can be obtained to determine if the patient is an overproducer or an underexcretor of uric acid. Individuals who excrete more than 800 mg of uric acid in this collection are considered overproducers. Patients with hyperuricemia who excrete less than 600 mg/day are classified as underexcretors of uric acid.

Radiographs of affected joints may have characteristic appearances of gout, including cystic changes, punched-out lytic lesions with overhanging bony edges, and soft-tissue calcified masses. These signs may appear in other arthropathies as well.[10]

Clinical Presentation and Diagnosis of Acute Gouty Arthritis

General

Patients are usually in acute distress.

Symptoms

- Severe pain, swelling, and warmth in the affected joint(s).
- The attack is usually monoarticular; the most common sites are the metatarsophalangeal and knee joints.
- In elderly patients, gouty attacks may be atypical with insidious and polyarticular onset, often involving hand or wrist joints.

Signs

- Affected joint(s) are warm, erythematous, and swollen.
- Mild fever may be present.
- Tophi (usually on hands, wrists, elbows, or knees) may be present in chronic, severe disease.

Laboratory Tests

- The peripheral WBC count may be only mildly elevated.
- The serum uric acid level often is elevated but may be normal during an acute attack.
- Other laboratory markers of inflammation (e.g., increased erythrocyte sedimentation rate) are often present.

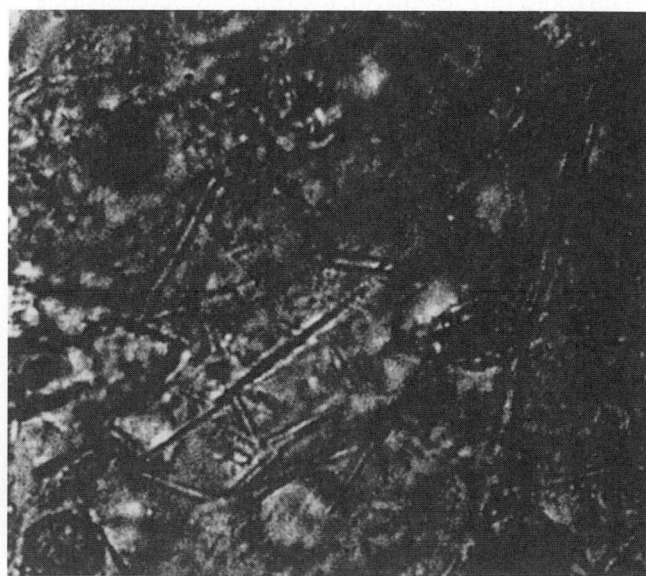

FIGURE 59–1. Synovial fluid containing extracellular and intracellular monosodium urate crystals. (From Schumacher HR, Chen LX . Gout and other crystal arthropathies. In: Fauci AS, Braunwald E, Kasper DL, et al., eds. Harrison's Principles of Internal Medicine, 17th ed. New York: McGraw-Hill; 2008, Fig. 327–1, page 2166, with permission.)

TREATMENT

❹ *Treatment of gout involves: (a) acute relief of a gouty arthritis attack; and (b) in some patients long-term maintenance treatment to prevent future attacks.*

Desired Outcomes

● The goals of therapy of an acute attack are: (a) achieving rapid and effective pain relief; (b) maintaining joint function; (c) preventing disease complications; (d) avoiding treatment-related adverse effects; (e) providing cost-effective therapy; and (f) improving quality of life.[11] Infrequent gouty arthritis is a self-limited disease, and treatment usually focuses on symptom relief.

Nonpharmacologic Therapy

Nondrug modalities play an adjunctive role and usually are not effective when used alone. Immobilization of the affected extremity speeds resolution of the attack. Applying ice packs to the joint also decreases pain and swelling, but heat application may be detrimental.[12]

Pharmacologic Therapy

❺ *Nonsteroidal anti-inflammatory drugs (NSAIDs), colchicine, and corticosteroids are used for acute attacks. Selection depends on several patient factors, especially renal function* (Fig. 59–2). Each drug class has a unique safety and efficacy profile in gout that should be considered carefully before choosing a specific agent (Table 59–1). Generally, the earlier in the course of the arthritic attack these agents are employed, the better the outcome.

▶ *Nonsteroidal Anti-inflammatory Drugs*

The NSAIDs largely have supplanted colchicine as the treatment of choice, and many NSAIDs have been used successfully. These agents are most effective when given within the first 24 hours of the onset of pain. Most studies have shown similar results among agents, and all NSAIDs are considered to be effective. Doses at the higher end of the therapeutic range are often needed.[13]

Indomethacin was used traditionally, but its relative cyclooxygenase-1 (COX-1) selectivity theoretically increases its gastropathy risk. Thus other generic NSAIDs may be preferred. Adverse effects of NSAIDs include gastropathy (primarily peptic ulcers), renal dysfunction, and fluid retention.[14] NSAIDs generally should be avoided in patients at risk for peptic ulcers, those taking warfarin, and those with renal insufficiency or uncontrolled hypertension or heart failure.

Cyclooxygenase-2 (COX-2)-selective inhibitors produce results comparable with those of traditional NSAIDs. However, cardiovascular safety concerns and the high cost of COX-2 inhibitors argue against their use for this disorder. NSAIDs are usually continued until 24 hours after symptoms subside.

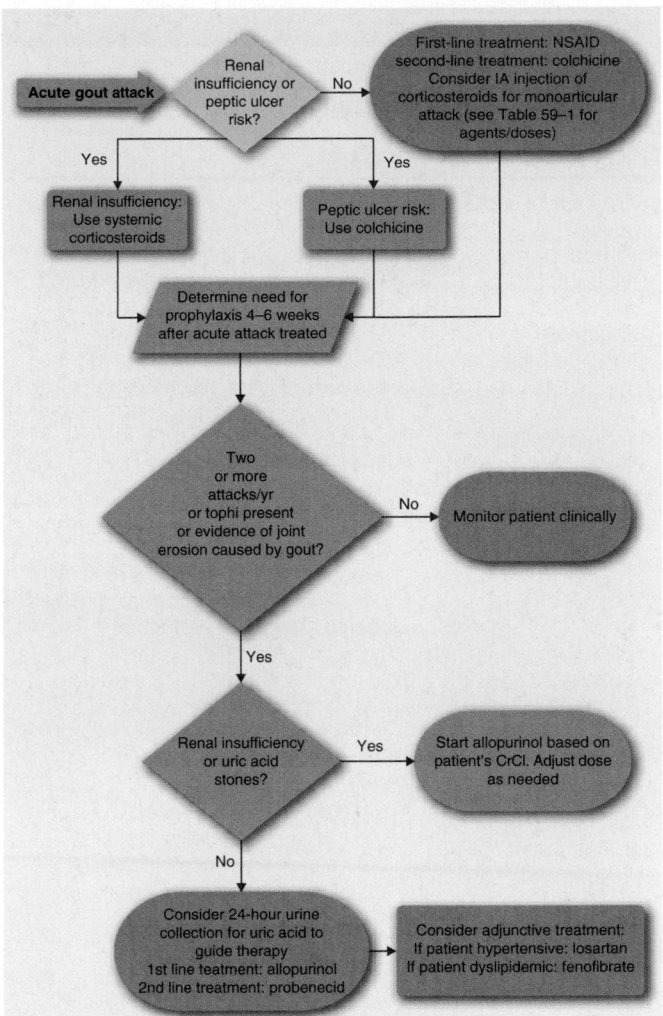

FIGURE 59–2. Treatment algorithm for gout and hyperuricemia. Renal insufficiency is defined as an estimated creatinine clearance (CrCl) of less than 30 mL/min. (IA, intra-articular; NSAID, nonsteroidal anti-inflammatory drug.)

▶ *Colchicine*

Colchicine has a long history of successful use and was the treatment of choice for many years. It is used infrequently today because of its low therapeutic index. Colchicine is thought to exert its anti-inflammatory effects by interfering with the function of mitotic spindles in neutrophils by binding of tubulin dimers; this inhibits phagocytic activity.[15]

Oral colchicine is absorbed rapidly from the GI tract and metabolized extensively in the liver. About two-thirds of patients with acute gout respond favorably if it is given within the first 24 hours of symptom onset. Unfortunately, more than 80% of patients experience adverse effects. GI effects (e.g., nausea, vomiting, diarrhea, and abdominal pain) are most common and are considered a forerunner of more serious systemic toxicity, including myopathy and bone marrow suppression (usually neutropenia). Some clinicians still use the strategy of continuous dosing until either pain relief or GI side effects occur. However, systemic toxicity can

Table 59–1

Dosage Regimens for Acute Gout and Antihyperuricemic Treatment

Drug	Dose
Drugs for Treatment of Acute Gout	
NSAIDs[a]	
Fenoprofen	800 mg po every 6 hours
Flurbiprofen	100 mg po four times a day for 1 day, then 50 mg po four times a day
Ibuprofen	600–800 mg po four times a day
Indomethacin*	150–200 mg po daily (in 3 divided doses) for 3 days, then 100 mg po daily (in 2 divided doses) for 4–7 days
Indomethacin*	50 mg po three times a day
Ketoprofen	50 mg po four times a day or 75 mg po three times a day
Meclofenamate	100 mg po three times a day to four times a day
Naproxen*	1,000 mg daily × 3 days, then 500 mg daily × 7 days or 750 mg po initially, then 250 mg po every 8 hours
Piroxicam	40 mg po once daily
Sulindac*	200 mg two times a day × 7–10 days
Tolmetin	400 mg po three times a day to four times a day
Celecoxib	200 mg po two times a day
Meloxicam	7.5–15 mg po once daily
Colchicine	0.6 mg po every hour for up to 3 doses, then 0.6 mg 1–2 × daily if desired before antihyperuricemic therapy is started; may occasionally use in low doses for prophylaxis
Colcrys* (colchicine)	1.2 mg po at the onset of attack, then 0.6 mg 1 hour later
Local corticosteroids: Methylprednisolone (example)	10–40 mg × 1 dose by intra-articular injection
Systemic corticosteroids: Prednisone (example)	40–60 mg po once daily × 3 days, then decrease by 10 mg every 3 days
Triamcinolone acetonide	60 mg × 1 dose by IM injection
Antihyperuricemic Treatment	
Allopurinol	Starting dose: CrCl greater than 90 mL/min = 300 mg po daily
	CrCl 60–90 mL/min = 200 mg po daily
	CrCl 30–60 mL/min = 100 mg po daily
	CrCl less than 30 mL/min = 50 mg po daily Adjust dosage based on follow-up uric acid levels; maximum 800 mg po daily
Febuxostat*	Starting dose 40 mg orally once daily; increase to 80 mg once daily if serum uric acid does not decline to 6.0 mg/dL or lower after 2 weeks of treatment
Probenecid	Starting dose 250 mg po two times a day; may increase to 1,000 mg po two times a day

CrCl, creatinine clearance; IM, intramuscular; NSAIDs, nonsteroidal anti-inflammatory drugs.

[a]Drugs that are FDA approved for treatment of gout are indicated with an asterisk.

Adapted with permission from Ref. 9. Copyright 2003 Massachusetts Medical Society. All rights reserved. Drug regimens derived from various sources.

occur with oral colchicine without prior GI effects, especially in patients with renal insufficiency.[16,17] Because of these problems, oral colchicine should be reserved for patients who are at risk for NSAID-induced gastropathy or who have failed NSAID therapy. IV colchicine was removed from the U.S. market due to an increased risk of serious and potentially fatal systemic effects when administered by this route.[18]

In July 2009, the FDA approved Colcrys, a single-ingredient colchicine product for treatment of acute gout attacks. As part of the approval process, a dosing study showed that one dose initially and a single additional dose after 1 hour was just as effective and less toxic than continued hourly colchicine dosing. As a result, the approved dosage regimen is 1.2 mg (two 0.6-mg tablets) at the onset of an acute flare, followed by 0.6 mg 1 hour later.

▶ Corticosteroids

When only one or two joints are affected, **intra-articular** corticosteroid injection can provide rapid relief with a relatively low incidence of side effects. Joint fluid obtained by **arthrocentesis** should be examined for evidence of joint space infection and crystal identification. If uric acid crystals are present and there is no infection, intra-articular injection can proceed.

Systemic corticosteroids are a useful option in patients with contraindications to NSAIDs or colchicine (primarily renal impairment) or polyarticular attacks, especially in elderly patients. A single intramuscular injection of a long-acting corticosteroid such as triamcinolone hexacetonide may be used. Oral agents may be needed, especially for severe attacks. Prednisone 40 to 60 mg (or an equivalent dose of another agent) is given daily, with a gradual taper over 2 weeks.

Patient Encounter 1, Part 1

A 48-year-old man with a history of hypertension, peptic ulcer disease (gastric ulcer 1 year ago), and morbid obesity presents to the emergency department complaining of excruciating pain in his left big toe and both ankles. This is similar to a painful episode he had with his left toe and ankle 6 months ago. On examination, his left great toe and both ankles are red, swollen, and warm to the touch. He describes the pain as throbbing and rates it as a 10/10 (where 10 is the worst pain he has ever experienced). He admits to drinking a six pack of beer on weekends. He weighs 150 kg (330 lb) and is 5 ft, 9 in. (175 cm) tall. Medications include chlorthalidone 25 mg/day and pantoprazole 40 mg/day. Serum creatinine is 1.0 mg/dL (88 μmol/L).

What information suggests gout as the cause of his symptoms?

What risk factors for gout does he have?

If the diagnosis is an acute attack of gouty arthritis, what treatment plan would you recommend for this patient?

A recent study found that oral methylprednisolone and naproxen are equivalent in treating acute gout attacks.[19,20]

Too rapid tapering of corticosteroids can cause a rebound gouty flare. To prevent this flare, low-dose colchicine (0.6 mg orally daily) sometimes is added to systemic corticosteroid regimens. This is probably unnecessary if an adequate taper is prescribed.

Short-term adverse effects from corticosteroids include fluid retention, hyperglycemia, CNS stimulation, weight gain, and increased risk of infection. Patients with diabetes should have blood glucose levels monitored carefully during the corticosteroid course.

Corticotrophin (adrenocorticotropic hormone [ACTH]) has been used for acute gouty flares. Worldwide supply problems and the possible superiority of traditional corticosteroids have resulted in decreased use.[21]

ANTIHYPERURICEMIC GOUT PROPHYLAXIS

Gout is an episodic disease, and the number of attacks varies widely from patient to patient. Thus, the benefit of long-term prophylaxis against acute gout flares must be weighed against the cost and potential toxicity of therapy that may not be necessary in all patients.

❻ *Asymptomatic hyperuricemia usually does not require treatment.*

Nonpharmacologic Therapy

Lifestyle modifications alone usually are insufficient for lowering SUA levels in gout patients. Patients should be advised to lose weight if obese and to discontinue ethanol consumption. Low-purine diets are not well tolerated; instead, dietary recommendations should focus on general nutrition principles. Drugs that may cause or aggravate hyperuricemia should be discontinued if possible. Few patients adhere to lifestyle modifications long term, and pharmacologic therapy usually is needed to treat hyperuricemia adequately.[22]

Pharmacologic Therapy

❼ *Patients with recurrent attacks, evidence of tophi or joint destruction, or uric acid nephrolithiasis are candidates for maintenance therapy with allopurinol, febuxostat, or probenecid to lower SUA levels.* Because hyperuricemia is the strongest modifiable risk factor for acute gout, prophylactic therapy involves either decreasing uric acid production or increasing its excretion (Table 59–1). The goal of therapy is to decrease SUA levels significantly, leaving less uric acid available for conversion to MSU crystals.[11]

Ideally, the selection of long-term prophylactic therapy involves determining the cause of hyperuricemia (primarily by analyzing a 24-hour urine collection for uric acid) and tailoring therapy appropriately. If less than 600 mg of uric acid is found in the 24-hour sample, the patient is considered an underexcretor. However, this approach is not used commonly for several reasons. The urine collection is inconvenient for patients and clinicians and does not identify patients who may be both overproducers and underexcretors of uric acid. Also, drugs used to increase uric acid excretion (uricosurics) generally are not as well tolerated as drugs that decrease production, and uricosurics increase the risk of uric acid nephrolithiasis.[23]

Because allopurinol (which reduces uric acid production) is effective in both overproducers and underexcretors and is generally well tolerated, many clinicians forego the 24-hour urine collection and treat patients empirically with it.

▶ Allopurinol

Most patients in the United States are treated with allopurinol, which usually is effective if the dosage is titrated appropriately. The drug and its primary active metabolite, oxypurinol, reduce SUA concentrations by inhibiting the enzyme xanthine oxidase, thereby blocking the oxidation of hypoxanthine and xanthine to uric acid.[11]

Allopurinol is well absorbed with a short half-life of 2 to 3 hours. The half-life of oxypurinol approaches 24 hours, allowing allopurinol to be dosed once daily. Oxypurinol is cleared primarily renally and can accumulate in patients with reduced kidney function. Allopurinol should not be started during an acute gout attack because sudden shifts in SUA levels may precipitate or exacerbate gouty arthritis. Rapid shifts in SUA can change the concentration of MSU crystals in synovial fluid, causing more crystals to precipitate. Thus some clinicians advocate a prophylactic dose of colchicine (0.6 mg/day) during initiation of antihyperuricemic therapy. This is continued until uric acid levels return to normal or maximum of 3 to 6 months. Acute episodes should be treated appropriately before maintenance treatment is started.

The initial dose of allopurinol is based on the patient's renal function. Patients with a creatinine clearance (CrCl) of 50 mL/min or less should receive a starting dose of less than 300 mg/day, although the product literature and other sources list alternative dosing regimens for those with renal insufficiency. The relationship between dose of allopurinol and its most severe side effects is controversial.[24] However, the dose can be adjusted upward as needed and tolerated. It is reasonable to reduce the dose temporarily in patients who develop reversible acute renal failure.

SUA levels must be monitored periodically, with the first follow-up level obtained 6 months (or sooner) after starting therapy. The target SUA level is less than 6 mg/dL (357 μmol/L). The dose should be titrated upward (to a maximum of 800 mg/day) or downward as these levels dictate.

Allopurinol generally is well tolerated; nausea and diarrhea occur in a small percentage of patients. A generalized, maculopapular rash occurs in about 2% of patients.[25] Although usually mild, this can progress to severe skin reactions such as Stevens-Johnson syndrome. Perhaps the most feared side effect is the allopurinol hypersensitivity syndrome, which may involve severe desquamating skin lesions, high fever (usually greater than 39°C [102.2°F]), hepatic dysfunction, leukocytosis with predominant eosinophilia, and renal failure. Although rare, this severe reaction has a 20% mortality rate.[26] Patients with a history of the syndrome should never again receive allopurinol (including desensitization) or oxypurinol (which is available outside the United States). Patients with a mild skin rash who require allopurinol can be desensitized to it using published protocols.[27,28]

There are several important drug–drug interactions with allopurinol. The effects of both theophylline and warfarin may be potentiated by allopurinol. Azathioprine and 6-mercaptopurine are purines whose metabolism is inhibited by concomitant allopurinol therapy; the dose of these drugs must be reduced by 75% with allopurinol cotherapy. Patients taking allopurinol who receive ampicillin are at increased risk of skin rashes.

▶ Febuxostat

In 2009, the FDA approved febuxostat (Uloric), a nonpurine xanthine oxidase inhibitor structurally distinct from allopurinol, for chronic hyperuricemia associated with gout. The initial dose is 40 mg orally once daily. The dose may be increased to 80 mg orally once daily if the SUA does not decrease to 6.0 mg/dL (357 μmol/L) or less after 2 weeks of treatment. No dosage adjustment is necessary in patients with mild or moderate renal impairment. Because of its potency and rapid reduction of SUA levels, prophylactic low-dose colchicine or an NSAID is recommended for 3 to 6 months during initiation of therapy.

Data from phase III trials suggest that febuxostat may be more effective than allopurinol in achieving target SUA levels of 6.0 mg/dL (357 μmol/L) or less and may be more effective in reducing the number of acute gouty flares.[29] However, fixed allopurinol doses were used rather than titrating the allopurinol dose to reach the target SUA level, which may confound these findings.

Adverse effects of febuxostat include nausea, arthralgias, rash, and transient elevation of hepatic transaminases. Periodic liver function tests are recommended (e.g., at baseline, 2 and 4 months after starting therapy, and then periodically thereafter). Due to structural differences, febuxostat would not be expected to crossreact in patients with a history of allopurinol hypersensitivity syndrome. The place of febuxostat in therapy of hyperuricemia has not been fully determined.

▶ Probenecid

Probenecid is a uricosuric agent that blocks the tubular reabsorption of uric acid, increasing its excretion. Because of its mechanism of action, probenecid is contraindicated in patients with a history of uric acid stones or nephropathy. Probenecid loses its effectiveness as renal function declines and should be avoided when the CrCl is 50 mL/min or less. Its uricosuric effect is counteracted by low aspirin doses, which many patients receive for prophylaxis of coronary heart disease.[2,11]

Although generally well tolerated, probenecid can cause GI side effects such as nausea and other adverse reactions including fever, rash, and rarely, hepatic toxicity. Patients should be instructed to maintain adequate fluid intake and urine output to decrease the risk of uric acid stone formation.

Patient Encounter 1, Part 2

The patient returns for a follow-up visit at your clinic 6 weeks later. He reports no pain or swelling in the joints affected previously. The emergency department physician had instructed him to stop the chlorthalidone, so he is currently taking only pantoprazole.

PE:

VS: BP 164/84, P 72, RR 15, T 37.2°C (99°F)

Ext: Trace edema in both ankles

Labs: Serum uric acid 11.5 mg/dL (684 μmol/L); serum creatinine 0.9 mg/dL (80 μmol/L); uric acid crystals were identified on arthrocentesis of the ankle 6 weeks ago.

Given this additional information, what is your assessment of the patient's condition?

Is the patient a candidate for antihyperuricemic therapy? If so, which agent would you choose?

Some experts advocate alkalinizing the urine to decrease this risk.

▶ Other Uricosuric Agents

Sulfinpyrazone was used in the past; it is no longer available in the United States. Several other medications have mild uricosuric effects and may be appropriate adjunctive therapy in some patients. Losartan increases both uric acid excretion and urine pH and may be an option in hypertensive patients with gout.[30] Fenofibrate is also a uricosuric and may be appropriate in selected dyslipidemic patients with gout.

Tumor Lysis Syndrome

❽ *TLS is a metabolic disorder caused by rapid cell destruction (usually during chemotherapy treatment for cancer) and associated with several electrolyte disturbances, notably hyperuricemia.*

TLS is most commonly associated with the chemotherapeutic treatment of cancers, such as leukemias and lymphomas. These types of cancers have a large tumor cell burden and are highly sensitive to destruction by chemotherapy. Massive lysis of intracellular contents occurs including the breakdown of nucleotides into hypoxanthine, xanthine and, eventually, uric acid. These large amounts of uric acid overwhelm normal urinary excretion capacities and can undergo crystalline precipitation. This can lead to acute renal failure and a host of electrolyte disturbances including hyperkalemia and hyperphosphatemia.[31] If not prevented or treated early, TLS can lead to acute kidney damage and perhaps death; thus TLS is considered an oncologic emergency. The incidence of TLS varies according to definition, tumor type, and patient characteristics but is thought to be approximately 5% in high-risk cancers.

Due to the potential severity of TLS, strategies to prevent this disorder are mandatory in susceptible patients. Aggressive hydration (usually with isotonic fluids such as 0.9% saline) and diuresis are the cornerstones of TLS prevention. This strategy promotes the excretion of uric acid before crystallization occurs. Some authors also recommend alkalinization of the urine, which increases the solubility of uric acid. However, investigations of this modality have failed to show a clear benefit, and recent practice guidelines do not recommend its routine use.[32]

Allopurinol has a crucial role in the prevention of TLS. The IV formulation reduces uric acid levels in high-risk patients by as much as 57% and can prevent hyperuricemia in up to 90% of patients treated.[33] Unfortunately, allopurinol does not reduce levels of uric acid formed before treatment, and the IV formulation can cause adverse effects similar to the oral form.

Rasburicase is a recombinant form of urate oxidase indicated for the prevention and treatment of TLS in pediatric patients. This enzyme converts uric acid to the more soluble compound allantoin. This potent agent can dramatically reduce uric acid levels in patients at high risk.[34] Rasburicase is well tolerated; mild cutaneous hypersensitivity reactions are the most common adverse effect. It can also cause hemolysis, especially in patients with glucose 6-phosphate dehydrogenase (G6PD) deficiency. Rasburicase has a higher acquisition cost than IV allopurinol, and some investigators have studied lower doses of the drug or use it preferentially in patients with existing renal insufficiency or uric acid levels greater than 10 mg/dL (590 μmol/L).

OUTCOME EVALUATION

Acute Gout

- Monitor the patient for pain relief and decreased swelling of the affected joints. Both parameters should be improved significantly within 48 hours of starting acute gout therapy.

- Assess the patient's subjective complaints and objective information for adverse effects. For NSAID therapy, be alert for new-onset epigastric pain, dark or tarry stools, blood in vomitus, dizziness or lightheadedness, development of edema, decreased urine output by more than 50% over a 24-hour period, or shortness of breath. For colchicine, monitor for nausea or vomiting, diarrhea, easy bruising, cold or flulike symptoms, lightheadedness, muscle weakness, or pain. Counsel the patient to inform you of any new medications started or stopped while taking colchicine.

- Monitor patients receiving intra-articular corticosteroid injections for increased swelling or pain at the injection site.

Patient Care and Monitoring

1. Assess the patient's symptoms to determine the time of attack onset, which joints are affected, the level of pain, and other symptoms.

2. Review the patient history for contributing lifestyle factors and other disease states that may help guide therapy.

3. Obtain a thorough medication history for prescription drug, nonprescription drug, and dietary supplement use. Determine if any of these products may be contributing to hyperuricemia.

4. Educate the patient on lifestyle modifications that will improve symptoms, including weight loss, if appropriate, and avoidance of ethanol.

5. If the diagnosis of gout has not been confirmed previously, consider aspiration of an affected joint to identify uric acid crystals.

6. Initiate therapy to treat the acute gout attack without delay. Develop a plan to assess this therapy after 24 and 48 hours.

7. Select therapy based on comorbidities and potential for adverse effects. In patients with no other disease states, NSAIDs are the preferred drug class.

8. Assess the need for continuous antihyperuricemic therapy. Use patient factors such as comorbidities to select an agent. Allopurinol is the standard prophylactic agent used in the United States.

9. Do not start antihyperuricemic therapy within 4 weeks of an acute attack.

10. Evaluate the patient for the presence of adverse drug reactions, drug allergies, and drug interactions.

11. Stress the importance of adherence with the therapeutic regimen, including lifestyle modifications, to prevent future gout attacks and long-term complications.

12. Provide patient education about the disease state, lifestyle modifications, and drug therapy.

- Assess patients receiving systemic corticosteroids for mental status changes, fluid retention, increased blood glucose, muscle weakness, or development of new infections.

Antihyperuricemic Therapy

- Assess for new gouty arthritis attacks or the development of tophi. If neither one develops, continue antihyperuricemic therapy as prescribed.

- Obtain the first follow-up SUA level within 6 months of starting therapy. Then monitor levels at least every 6 to 12 months, and adjust the dose to achieve a target SUA level of less than 6 mg/dL (357 μmol/L).

- Evaluate patients taking allopurinol for development of rash, nausea, or new fever. These symptoms usually appear within the first 3 months of therapy but can occur anytime.

- Assess patients receiving probenecid for fever, nausea, or skin rash. Reevaluate therapy if a significant decrease in urine output occurs (greater than 50% in a 24-hour period).

Abbreviations Introduced in This Chapter

ACTH	Adrenocorticotropic hormone
COX	Cyclooxygenase
CrCl	Creatinine clearance
G6PD	Glucose 6-phosphate dehydrogenase
IL	Interleukin
MSU	Monosodium urate
SUA	Serum uric acid
TLS	Tumor lysis syndrome
TNF	Tumor necrosis factor

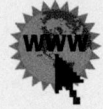 Self-assessment questions and answers are available at *http://www.mhpharmacotherapy.com/pp.html.*

REFERENCES

1. Mikuls TR, MacLean CH, Olivieri J, et al. Quality of care indicators for gout management. Arthritis Rheum 2004;50:937–943.
2. Rott KT, Agudelo CA. Gout. JAMA 2003;289:2857–2860.
3. Arromdee E, Michet CJ, Crowson CS, et al. Epidemiology of gout: Is the incidence rising? J Rheumatol 2002;29:2403–2406.
4. Cassetta M, Gorevic PD. Crystal arthritis: Gout and pseudogout in the geriatric patient. Geriatrics 2004;59:25–31.
5. Agudelo CA, Wise CM. Crystal-associated arthritis. Clin Geriatr Med 1998;14:495–513.
6. Johnson RJ, Kang DH, Feig D, et al. Is there a pathogenetic role for uric acid in hypertension and cardiovascular and renal disease? Hypertension 2003;41:1183–1190.
7. Cardona F, Tinahones FJ, Collantes E, et al. Contribution of polymorphisms in the apolipoprotein AI-CIII-AIV cluster to hyperlipidaemia in patients with gout. Ann Rheum Dis 2005;64:85–88.
8. Shekarriz B, Stoller ML. Uric acid nephrolithiasis: Current concepts and controversies. J Urol 2002;168(4 Pt 1):1307–1314.
9. Terkeltaub RA. Gout. N Engl J Med 2003;349:1647–1655.
10. Schumacher Jr HR. Crystal induced arthritis: An overview. Am J Med 1996;100 (Suppl 2A):46–52.
11. Zhang W, Doherty M, Bardin T, et al. EULAR evidence based recommendations for gout. Part II: Management. Report of a task force of the EULAR Standing Committee for International Clinical Studies Including Therapeutics (ESCISIT). Ann Rheum Dis 2006;65:1312–1324.
12. Schlesinger N, Baker DK, Beutler AM, et al. Local ice therapy during bouts of acute gouty arthritis. J Rheumatol 2002;29:331–334.
13. Schlesinger N. Management of acute and chronic gouty arthritis. Drugs 2004;64:2399–2416.
14. Conaghan PG, Day RO. Risks and benefits of drugs used in the management and prevention of gout. Drug Saf 1994;11:252–258.
15. Smallwood JI, Malawista SE. Colchicine, crystals, and neutrophils tyrosine phosphorylation. J Clin Invest 1993;92:1602–1603.
16. Wallace SL, Singer JZ, Duncan GJ, et al. Renal function predicts colchicine toxicity: Guidelines for the prophylactic use of colchicine in gout. J Rheumatol 1991;18:264–269.
17. Dixon AJ, Wall GC. Probable colchicine-induced neutropenia not related to intentional overdose. Ann Pharmacother 2001;35:192–195.
18. Bonnel RA, Villalba ML, Karwoski CB, Beitz J. Deaths associated with inappropriate intravenous colchicine administration. J Emerg Med 2002;22:385–387.
19. Kim KY, Ralph Schumacher H, et al. A literature review of the epidemiology and treatment of acute gout. Clin Ther 2003;25:1593–1617.
20. Janssens HJ, Janssen M, van de Lisdonk EH, et al. Use of oral prednisolone or naproxen for the treatment of gout arthritis: A double-blind, randomised equivalence trial. Lancet 2008;371:1854–1860.
21. Siegel LB, Alloway JA, Nashel DJ. Comparison of adrenocorticotropic hormone and triamcinolone acetonide in the treatment of acute gouty arthritis. J Rheumatol 1994;21:1325–1327.
22. de Klerk E, van der Heijde D, Landewe R, et al. Patient compliance in rheumatoid arthritis, polymyalgia rheumatica, and gout. J Rheumatol 2003;30:44–54.
23. Pal B, Foxall M, Dysart T, et al. How is gout managed in primary care? A review of current practice and proposed guidelines. Clin Rheumatol 2000;19:21–25.
24. Vazquez-Mellado J, Morales EM, Pacheco-Tena C, Burgos-Vargas R. Relation between adverse events associated with allopurinol and renal function in patients with gout. Ann Rheum Dis 2001;60:981–983.
25. Khoo BP, Leow YH. A review of inpatients with adverse drug reactions to allopurinol. Singapore Med J 2000;41:156–160.
26. Arellano F, Sacristan JA. Allopurinol hypersensitivity syndrome: A review. Ann Pharmacother 1993;27:337–343.
27. Bardin T. Current Management of gout in patients unresponsive or allergic to allopurinol. Joint Bone Spine 2004;71:481–485.
28. Fam AG, Dunne SM, Iazzetta J, Paton TW. Efficacy and safety of desensitization to allopurinol following cutaneous reactions. Arthritis Rheum 2001;44:231–238.
29. Becker MA, Schumacher HR Jr., Wortmann RL, et al. Febuxostat compared with allopurinol in patients with hyperuricemia and gout. N Engl J Med 2005;353:2450–2461.
30. Takahashi S, Moriwaki Y, Yamamoto T, et al. Effects of combination treatment using anti-hyperuricaemic agents with fenofibrate and/or losartan on uric acid metabolism. Ann Rheum Dis 2003;62:572–575.
31. Tiu RV, Mountantonakis SE, Dunbar AJ, Schreiber MJ Jr. Tumor lysis syndrome. Semin Thromb Hemost 2007;33:397–407.
32. Coiffier B, Altman A, Pui CH, et al. Guidelines for the management of pediatric and adult tumor lysis syndrome: An evidence-based review. J Clin Oncol 2008;26:2767–2778.
33. Holdsworth MT, Nguyen P. Role of i.v. allopurinol and rasburicase in tumor lysis syndrome. Am J Health Syst Pharm 2003;60:2213–2222.
34. Cammalleri L, Malaguarnera M. Rasburicase represents a new tool for hyperuricemia in tumor lysis syndrome and in gout. Int J Med Sci 2007;4:83–93.

60 Musculoskeletal Disorders

Jill S. Burkiewicz

LEARNING OBJECTIVES

Upon completion of the chapter, the reader will be able to:

1. Describe the pathophysiological principles associated with tissue injury and inflammation.

2. Identify the desired therapeutic goals and outcomes for a patient with musculoskeletal injury or pain.

3. Identify the factors that guide selection of an analgesic or counterirritant for a particular patient.

4. Recommend appropriate nonpharmacologic and pharmacologic therapy for a patient with musculoskeletal injury or pain.

5. Design a patient education plan including nonpharmacologic therapy and preventative strategies.

6. Develop a monitoring plan to assess treatment of a patient with musculoskeletal disorders.

KEY CONCEPTS

1 The two primary goals of treatment of musculoskeletal disorders are to: (a) relieve pain, and (b) maintain functionality.

2 The cornerstone of nonpharmacologic therapy for acute injury in the first 48 to 72 hours is known by the acronym *RICE: r*est, *i*ce, *c*ompression, and *e*levation.

3 Heat should not be applied during the acute injury phase (the first 48 hours) because it promotes swelling and inflammation.

4 There are two main approaches to pharmacologic intervention for pain relief: oral (systemic) and topical agents.

5 Localized pain may be treated effectively with local topical therapy, whereas generalized pain is best treated with systemic agents.

6 Acetaminophen is the drug of choice for mild-to-moderate regional musculoskeletal pain without inflammation.

7 Aspirin is not more effective than acetaminophen, and it is not recommended for treatment of acute musculoskeletal pain because its adverse effects may be more common and severe.

8 Nonsteroidal anti-inflammatory drugs (NSAIDs) are preferred over acetaminophen in musculoskeletal disorders where inflammation is evident.

9 Patient education on proper use of counterirritants is essential to therapeutic success.

10 Patients using capsaicin should be advised to apply it regularly and consistently three to four times daily and that full effect may take 2 to 3 weeks or longer.

INTRODUCTION

The musculoskeletal system consists of the muscles, bones, joints, tendons, and ligaments. Disorders related to the musculoskeletal system often are classified by etiology. Acute soft-tissue injuries include strains and sprains of muscles and ligaments. Repeated movements in sports, exercise, work, or activities of daily living can lead to repetitive strain injury, where cumulative damage occurs to the muscles, ligaments, or tendons.[1,2] While tendonitis and bursitis can arise from acute injury, more commonly these conditions occur as a result of chronic stress.[2,3] Other forms of chronic musculoskeletal pain, such as pain from rheumatoid arthritis (see Chap. 57) or osteoarthritis (see Chap. 58), are discussed elsewhere in this textbook.

EPIDEMIOLOGY

Musculoskeletal disorders are commonly self-treated, so true estimates of the incidence of both acute and chronic injury are difficult to obtain. Musculoskeletal disorders are among the top 10 causes of ambulatory care visits in the United

States for all age groups.[4] These disorders account for a large portion of medical care expenditures[5] and are a leading cause of work absenteeism and disability, resulting in a substantial economic burden from lost productivity and lost wages.[6]

In addition to chronic conditions such as arthritis and low back pain, some musculoskeletal disorders are induced by trauma at the workplace either via repetition and cumulative trauma or a one-time overexertion.[7] For each reported incident, it is likely that there are at least 10 unreported work-related musculoskeletal events related to repetitive stress to the bones and joints.[8] In the elderly, these injuries may not be related to work but to daily life. Instability combined with activities of daily living such as stair climbing and lifting objects may lead to strains and sprains. In pediatrics, fractures are more common than muscle and tendon injuries since the bones are weaker than the muscle–tendon unit in children and adolescents.[9]

Muscle injuries comprise the majority of sports-related injuries, and roughly half are related to overuse.[2,10] The ankle and the knee are common sites of sports injuries.[9,11] Soccer, football, basketball, track and field, and other sports that require rapid acceleration or higher speeds pose a greater risk of muscle strain.[9,12] *Overuse musculoskeletal injury* is the phrase used to describe disorders arising from repetitive motion. This injury is common in activities such as running, particularly during periods of increased intensity or duration of training.[2] It also can occur in the workplace with repeated, unvaried motion.[13]

PATHOPHYSIOLOGY

Skeletal muscle consists of muscle fibers linked together by connective tissue. Tendons and ligaments are composed of collagenous fibers that have a restricted capability to stretch. Tendons connect the muscle to the bone, whereas ligaments connect bone to bone (Fig. 60–1).

Muscle Strains and Sprains

A **sprain** is an overstretching of supporting ligaments that results in a partial or complete tear of the ligament.[11] While a **strain** also arises from an overstretching of the muscle–tendon unit, it is marked by damage to the muscle fibers or muscle sheath without tearing of the ligament.[9,14] The key difference between a sprain and a strain is that a sprain involves damage to ligaments, whereas a strain involves damage primarily to muscle. One common example of muscle strain and sprain is low back pain.[15]

Overloading the muscle and connective tissue results in complete or partial tears of the skeletal muscle, tendons, or ligaments.[9,14] This usually occurs when the muscle is activated in an *eccentric contraction,* defined as a contraction in which the muscle is being lengthened.[14] Examples of this type of contraction include putting down a large, heavy laundry basket or lowering oneself from a chin-up bar. Small tears can occur in the muscle because it is lengthening while also trying to contract to support the load. This leads to rupture of blood vessels at the site of the injury, resulting

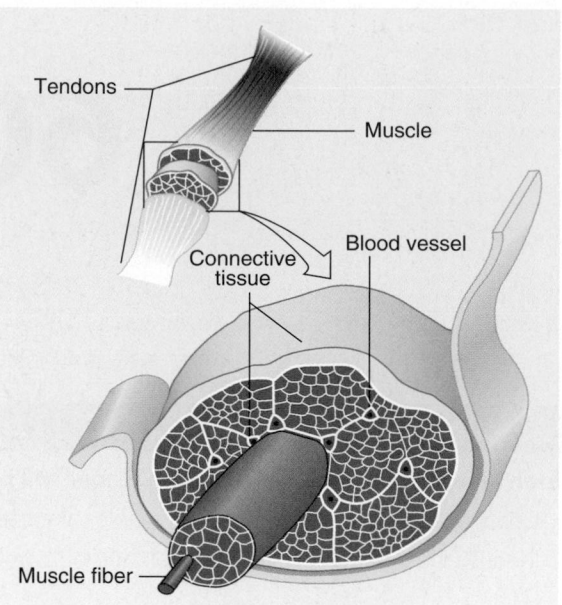

FIGURE 60–1. Skeletal muscle fiber organization. Tendons attach muscle to bone. (From Widmaier EP, Raff H, Strang KT, et al., eds. Vander, Sherman, & Luciano's Human Physiology: The Mechanisms of Body Function. 9th ed. New York: McGraw-Hill; 2004: Fig. 9–1.)

in the formation of a hematoma. Within 24 to 48 hours, an inflammatory response develops. In the inflammatory stage, macrophages remove necrotic fibers.[10] However, there is some evidence that activated neutrophils also release free radicals and proteases that cause further damage to the area.[16] Finally, capillaries grow into the area, and muscle fibers regenerate during the repair and remodeling phases of healing.[10]

Bursitis and Tendonitis

Bursitis is an inflammation of the bursa, the fluid-filled sac near the joint where the tendons and muscles pass over the bone. The bursa assists with movement by reducing friction between joints. **Tendonitis** (also known as *tendinitis*) is an inflammation of the tendon or, more specifically, the fibrous sheath that attaches muscle to bone.[2] **Tenosynovitis** is an inflammation of the tendon sheath.

Repetitive overuse of a tendon can cause cellular changes in the tissues. Specifically, collagenous tendon tissue is replaced with tissue that lacks the longitudinal structure of a normal tendon.[17] As a result; the tendon progressively loses elasticity and its ability to handle stress or weight. This makes the tendon vulnerable to rupture or inflammation (tendonitis and tenosynovitis).

Repeated use also can cause degradation of collagen.[18] In fact, many patients diagnosed with chronic tendonitis may not have inflammation but instead have tendinosis, a condition marked by these collagen changes. Overuse of a joint also can result in an inflamed bursa. Since the bursa serves to reduce friction within the joint space, bursitis causes stiffness and pain.

Inflammation and Peripheral Pain Sensation

Inflammation is a common pathway in soft-tissue injury of musculoskeletal disorders. Inflammatory processes lead to two outcomes: swelling and pain. Inflammatory processes traditionally are considered to be a necessary part of the remodeling process because inflammatory cells remove damaged tissue.[19,20] However, inflammation also contributes to continued pain and swelling that limits range of motion.

The initial injury exposes membrane phospholipids to phospholipase A_2, leading to the formation of arachidonic acid (Fig. 60–2).[19,20] Next, arachidonic acid is transformed by cyclooxygenase (COX) to thromboxanes and prostaglandins (PGs), including prostaglandin E_2 (PGE_2). PGE_2 is the most potent inflammatory mediator; it increases vascular permeability, leading to redness, warmth, and swelling of the affected area. The increased permeability also increases proteolysis, or the breakdown of proteins in the damaged tissue.

Neutrophils, lymphocytes, and monocytes are attracted to the area, and monocytes are converted to macrophages.[19,20] The macrophages then stimulate additional PG production. Phagocytic cells and other players in the immune system release cytokines, including interleukins, interferon, and tumor necrosis factor.

In addition to increasing vascular permeability, PGs also induce pain by sensitizing pain receptors to other substances such as bradykinin. Bradykinin, PGs, leukotrienes, and other inflammatory mediators lower the pain threshold through peripheral pain sensitization. These substances make nerve endings more excitable, and the nerve fibers are more reactive to serotonin, heat, and mechanical stimuli.[20] The increased sensitization in the damaged tissue causes tenderness, soreness, and hyperalgesia or an exaggerated intensity of pain sensation.[21] The process also facilitates production of additional PGs. In a cyclic fashion, the PGs then sensitize the nerves to bradykinin action.

Without interruption, the neurochemicals ultimately lead to a firing of the unmyelinated or thinly myelinated afferent neurons. This sends messages along the pain pathway in the periphery and communicates the pain message to the CNS. Interruption of this cycle occurs via anti-inflammatory agents such as aspirin and nonsteroidal anti-inflammatory drugs (NSAIDs).

Nerve receptors, or nociceptors, release substance P, a peptide that causes vasodilation when released.[20,22] This dilation occurs mainly through substance P-mediated activation of neurokinin receptors. This receptor activation also increases the sensitivity of nociceptors to painful stimuli. Capsaicin relieves pain by stimulating the release of substance P from sensory nerve fibers, which ultimately depletes stores of substance P.

CLINICAL PRESENTATION AND DIAGNOSIS

See next page for information on the clinical presentation and diagnosis of musculoskeletal disorders.

TREATMENT

Desired Outcomes

❶ *The primary goals of treatment of musculoskeletal disorders are to: (a) relieve pain, and (b) maintain functionality.* This is accomplished by decreasing the severity and duration of pain, shortening the recovery period, and preventing acute injury pain from becoming chronic pain. Prevention of swelling and inflammation are initial goals in acute injury because the degree of swelling is directly related to range of motion.[11] If these goals are achieved, functional limitations are decreased. Ideally, a patient should be able to continue to perform activities of daily living (e.g., eating, dressing, cooking, and doing laundry) and maintain normal functions in the workplace. Children ideally should be able to maintain usual play activities and sports schedules.

Further goals include a return to usual activity and prevention of future injury. It is also important to minimize the potential for adverse drug events during treatment.

General Approach to Treatment

Treatment of musculoskeletal disorders involves three phases: (a) therapy of an acute injury using the rest, ice, compression, and elevation (RICE) principle; (b) pain relief using oral or topical agents; and (c) lifestyle and behavioral modifications

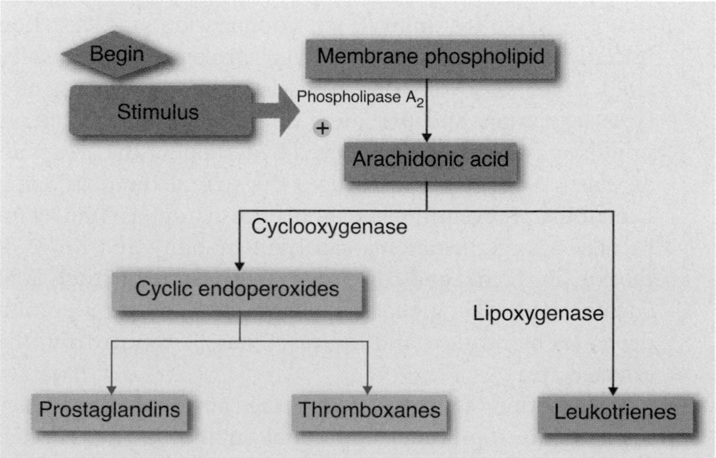

FIGURE 60–2. Eicosanoid synthesis pathway. Cyclooxygenase is inhibited by nonsteroidal anti-inflammatory drugs and aspirin. (From Widmaier EP, Raff H, Strang KT, et al., eds. Vander, Sherman, & Luciano's Human Physiology: The Mechanisms of Body Function. 9th ed. New York: McGraw-Hill; 2004: Fig. 5–11.)

Clinical Presentation and Diagnosis of Musculoskeletal Disorders

General[11]

- Clinical presentation varies based on the etiology of the disorder.
- Repetitive strain or overuse injuries may have a gradual onset.
- Musculoskeletal disorders due to acute injury may be associated with other signs of the injury such as abrasion.
- Low back pain is often more chronic in nature.

Signs and Symptoms of Acute Soft-Tissue Injury (Strains, Sprains)[11]

- Discomfort ranging from tenderness to pain; it may occur at rest or with motion
- Swelling and inflammation of the affected area
- Bruising
- Loss of motion
- Mechanical instability

Signs and Symptoms of Repetitive Strain or Overuse Injury (Tendonitis, Bursitis)[3,23,24]

- Pain and stiffness that occurs either at rest or with motion
- Localized tenderness on palpation

- Mild swelling of the affected area
- Decreased range of motion
- Muscle atrophy

Other Diagnostic Tests and Assessments[25]

- *Radiograph (x-ray):* Evaluate bony structures to rule out fracture, malalignment, or joint erosion as the primary cause of pain.
- *MRI:* Soft-tissue imaging to evaluate for tendon or ligament tears.
- *Ultrasound:* Superficial soft-tissue imaging to evaluate for tears in tendons or ligaments. Ultrasound does not penetrate bone, so it is of limited usefulness for assessing tendons or ligaments deep within joints.
- *Pain scale:* Patient self-rating of pain on a scale of zero (no pain) to 10 (worst possible pain). Used to assess pain both at rest and with movement. Determined at baseline and to assess response to therapy.

Patient Encounter 1, Part 1

A 32-year-old man presents with left ankle pain. He was playing football with friends earlier today and twisted his ankle. The pain occurs at rest and is worsened by movement and weight-bearing activities. There is moderate swelling and mild bruising of the left ankle. He states "I don't like to take pills" and asks for a recommendation to cool the affected area.

What information is suggestive of a musculoskeletal disorder?

What is your assessment of the patient's ankle pain?

What additional information do you need to formulate a treatment plan?

---

for rehabilitation and to prevent recurrent injury or chronic pain (Fig. 60–3).

In many cases, musculoskeletal disorders are self-treated with over-the-counter (OTC) oral or topical agents. However, further evaluation may be warranted if acute pain persists longer than 7 to 10 days, symptoms worsen or subside and then return, or there are signs of a more serious condition.[11,24–26] Warning signs of more serious conditions include joint deformity, dislocation, or lack of movement in a joint. Low back pain accompanied by burning, radiating pain, or difficulty urinating requires further evaluation.

In children and adolescents, treatment practices are similar to the approach in adults with a focus on nonpharmacologic therapy and oral analgesics. Children younger than 2 years of age, elderly persons, and pregnant women also may need special care. Elderly patients may be more prone to systemic effects because of thinning of the skin and increased absorption of topical agents and drug interactions from polypharmacy.

Nonpharmacologic Therapy: RICE

❷ *The cornerstone of nonpharmacologic therapy for acute injury in the first 48 to 72 hours is known by the acronym RICE: rest, ice, compression, and elevation*[10] (Table 60–1). Rest eases pressure on the affected area and promotes pain control during the acute inflammatory phase (the first 1–5 days after injury). Ice, compression, and elevation initially minimize bleeding from broken blood vessels. Cold causes vasoconstriction, assisting in prevention of a large hematoma and providing analgesia by slowing nerve impulses. Compression, achieved by wrapping the area with an elastic bandage, also reduces the size of the developing hematoma. Preventing hematoma formation is important because a large hematoma can limit mobility and range of motion. Both cold and compression also decrease interstitial edema and swelling that accompany the injury. Elevation decreases blood flow and increases venous return from the affected area.

In addition to minimizing the acute inflammatory response, rest prevents additional injury to the affected

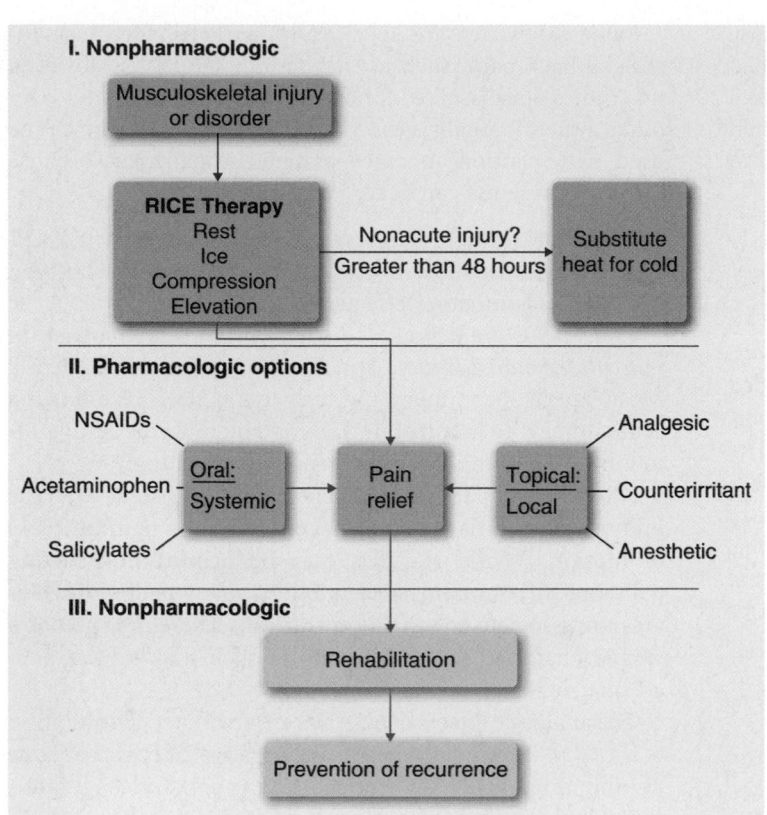

FIGURE 60–3. Treatment plan for musculoskeletal injury or disorder.

Table 60–1		
RICE Therapy		
Therapy	**General Guidelines**	**Therapeutic Benefit**
*R*est	Rest the affected area Use supports such as slings and crutches as necessary Employ during the acute inflammatory phase, 1–5 days after injury	Analgesia Anti-inflammatory Prevent further injury
*I*ce	Cool the affected area by submersion in cool water (13°C [55°F]) or by application of crushed ice in a plastic bag covered with a thin cloth Cool the affected area for 15–20 minutes; repeat every 2 hours for the first 48 hours	Analgesia Anti-inflammatory
*C*ompression	Compress the affected area with an elastic bandage or support Begin wrapping the bandage at the point most distal to the injury (e.g., at the toes for an ankle injury); bind firmly but not tightly If the area distal to the injury (e.g., fingers, toes) throbs or turns cold or blue, the bandage is too tight and should be loosened	Anti-inflammatory Adjunctive analgesia
*E*levation	Elevate the area (especially the extremities) above heart level	Anti-inflammatory

area.[14] The properties of the muscle–tendon unit are altered during the acute injury, with limitations on the ability of the muscles and tendons to stretch. Early activity predisposes a patient to further injury, but prolonged inactivity can lengthen recovery times.

Clinicians should instruct patients to use crushed ice or ice chips because the area will cool more evenly than with large pieces of ice. Patients should not apply ice directly to the affected area or leave it on for longer than the recommended 20 minutes because frostbite can occur.[11] A thin sheet or napkin will protect the skin and also allow for better cold transfer than thicker material such as a towel. Alternatively, soaking the area for 20 minutes in a cool bath (13°C [55°F]) provides effective cooling.

For small areas, an ice massage for 5 to 10 minutes can cool the area and add relief.[23] This is accomplished by freezing water in a paper cup and removing the top part of the cup to expose the ice. The exposed ice is rubbed on the affected area. Any ice application should be stopped if the area becomes white or blue.

❸ *Heat should not be applied during the acute injury phase (the first 48 hours) because it promotes swelling and inflammation.*[11] After the first 48 hours, many patients find that heat decreases pain and eases muscle stiffness associated with immobility. A heating pad, heat wrap, or warm bath can be used on day three or later as long as no swelling develops after heat is applied. Heat should be discontinued if increased swelling occurs. Clinicians should educate patients to avoid sleeping with, or sitting or lying on heating pads because this can result in burns. Low-level heat, such as that supplied by therapeutic heat wraps (e.g., ThermaCare) may provide a safer means of heat application.[27] However, the elderly should still be cautioned about the risk of burns and be advised to wear the wrap over thin clothing.

Pharmacologic Therapy

❹ *There are two main approaches to pharmacologic intervention for pain relief: oral (systemic) and topical agents.* The choice between systemic or topical options is often guided by patient preference. For example, many topical products have a medicinal odor and require frequent applications. The extent of musculoskeletal pain also guides treatment choice.
❺ *Localized pain may be treated effectively with local topical therapy, whereas generalized pain is best treated with systemic agents.* Factors such as alcohol use, liver function, renal function, allergies, age, and comorbid conditions should be considered when choosing among therapeutic options.

▶ *Oral Analgesics*

Nonopioid analgesics, including acetaminophen, aspirin, and NSAIDs, are used commonly for musculoskeletal disorders. All these agents provide analgesia, but aspirin and NSAIDs also work peripherally to decrease production of the principal mediator of acute inflammation, PGE_2.[19] NSAIDs and aspirin inhibit the enzyme COX. While the mechanism of action of acetaminophen is less clear, it appears that acetaminophen acts as a weak inhibitor of PG production. In contrast to aspirin and NSAIDs that inhibit PG production peripherally, acetaminophen exerts its effect centrally with little or no anti-inflammatory effect.[28]

Acetaminophen ❻ *Acetaminophen is the drug of choice for mild-to-moderate regional musculoskeletal pain without inflammation.*[29,30] Comparative trials between acetaminophen and oral NSAIDs demonstrate equivalent analgesia in some situations, but NSAIDs may be preferred in others.[30] Therefore, if adequate analgesia is not achieved with acetaminophen, switching to an NSAID is a reasonable approach. Acetaminophen offers the advantage of less GI toxicity than NSAIDs. While tolerability of acetaminophen is high at therapeutic doses, hepatotoxicity has been reported after overdose and at therapeutic doses, especially in combination with other factors.[31] Acetaminophen should be used with caution in patients who have liver disease or consume alcohol because of the risk of hepatotoxicity.[25]

Salicylates ❼ *Aspirin is not more effective than acetaminophen, and it is not recommended for treatment of acute musculoskeletal pain because its adverse effects may be more common and severe.*[30] Gastric irritation is more common with aspirin, and bleeding risk is increased because aspirin irreversibly inhibits platelet aggregation.[30] Patients with aspirin-induced asthma should avoid aspirin and other salicylates.[31] Aspirin should be avoided in children younger than age 16 due to the risk of Reye's syndrome.

Some salicylates are specifically marketed for musculoskeletal back pain, such as magnesium salicylate. However, no studies specifically support use of these salicylates over other systemic analgesics. Magnesium salicylate should be used with caution in cases of renal impairment because hypermagnesemia can occur.[32]

NSAIDs Oral NSAIDs are used commonly for musculoskeletal pain because of their availability without a prescription and anti-inflammatory effects.[21,32]
❽ *NSAIDs are a preferred choice over acetaminophen in musculoskeletal disorders where inflammation is evident.*[29] Most experts recommend the early use of NSAIDs following acute injury to control inflammation and the range-of-motion limitations that may accompany swelling.[29]

NSAIDs are particularly beneficial for chronic overuse injury, where inflammation is central to the pain and loss of motion. While NSAIDs may be helpful in relieving pain and inflammation in tendonitis, many tendonopathies are not associated with inflammation. Therefore, use of a simple analgesic such as acetaminophen may relieve pain adequately.[24, 32]

The analgesic effects of NSAIDs are attributed to inhibition of the COX-2 enzyme, whereas the negative GI effects are due to inhibition of COX-1.[30] Patients taking oral anticoagulants, those with a history of peptic ulcer disease, or others at high risk for GI complications may be considered candidates for a COX-2 inhibitor (e.g., celecoxib) or a combination of a nonselective NSAID with a gastroprotective agent such as a proton pump inhibitor (see Chap. 58).

COX-2 inhibitors are associated with adverse effects such as nephrotoxicity and a potential increased risk of myocardial infarction (see Chap. 58). Combination of COX-2 inhibitors with alcohol can increase GI adverse effects. All NSAIDs should be used with caution in patients with aspirin-induced asthma.[32]

Opioids Opioid analgesics can be used for patients not responding adequately to nonopioid analgesics or for moderate-to-severe pain.[30] These agents generally are given alone or in combination with simple analgesics such as acetaminophen. Tolerance and physical dependence are considerations but less of a concern when treating acute pain. When used in equivalent doses, opioids produce similar pain relief and adverse effects such as sedation, nausea, constipation, and respiratory depression (see Chap. 33).

Topical (External) Analgesics Topically (or externally) applied drugs that exert a local analgesic, anesthetic, or antipruritic effect by either suppressing cutaneous sensory receptors or by stimulating these receptors in a counterirritant fashion are termed *external analgesics*.[26] These medications are applied directly to the affected area to create high local concentrations of the drug.[33,34] Formulations include gel, cream, lotion, patch, liquid, liniment, or aerosol spray. Negligible systemic concentrations are achieved with intact skin, minimizing systemic adverse effects. Topical application should not be confused with transdermal delivery, where drug absorption into the bloodstream produces a systemic effect. Musculoskeletal disorders often are treated with topical (but not transdermal) medications.

After application, the topical medication penetrates the skin to the soft tissue and peripheral nerves.[26] Here, the drug suppresses the sensitization of pain receptors, thus reducing pain and burning. Examples include topical NSAIDs and local anesthetics, such as lidocaine. External analgesics also include counterirritant products that, in contrast, stimulate cutaneous sensory receptors, producing a burning, warming, or cooling sensation that masks the underlying pain. In effect, the irritation or inflammation caused by the counterirritant distracts from the underlying pain. For example, counterirritants include menthol and capsaicin.

Some patients prefer external analgesics to systemic analgesics because the rubbing during application can be comforting. External analgesics are useful adjuvants to nonpharmacologic therapy and systemic analgesic therapy to provide additional relief.[35] These agents also offer a therapeutic option in patients who cannot tolerate systemic analgesics. Because these agents are not in pill form and many are available without a prescription, they may be overused or misused. This prompted the FDA to issue a warning to consumers.[36] Clinicians should advise patients to always read and follow directions on the labels of OTC products.

Topical NSAIDs Topical NSAIDs have been available commercially in Canada and Europe, and topical diclofenac is now available in gel and patch form in the United States.[37,38] These agents exert a local anti-inflammatory and analgesic effect.[39,40] In soft-tissue injury such as strains and sprains, topical NSAIDs have efficacy that is superior to placebo and similar to oral NSAIDs. Tissue concentrations of topical NSAIDs are high enough to produce anti-inflammatory effects, but systemic concentrations after application remain low.[37-40]

Diclofenac gel (Voltaren Gel) is indicated for joint pain in the knees and hands secondary to osteoarthritis; it is applied up to four times daily. Diclofenac patch (Flector Patch) is indicated specifically for the topical treatment of acute pain from minor sprains and strains.[37,38] The patch is applied to the most painful area twice daily. Patient education for topical NSAIDs is outlined in Table 60–2.

Theoretically, the risk of serious GI adverse events should be less than with oral NSAIDs, but long-term studies evaluating these events are lacking.[39,40] Like oral NSAIDs, topical NSAIDs should be used with caution in patients with a history of GI bleeding or ulcer.[37,38] Studies comparing topical NSAIDs with other topical products, including counterirritants, are also needed. Local cutaneous adverse reactions (e.g., erythema, pruritus, and irritation) occur in up to 4% of the patients and may be due in part to the vehicle used.[37-40]

Local Anesthetics Nonprescription topical anesthetics such as lidocaine and benzocaine are available in many types of products. Local anesthetics decrease discharges in superficial somatic nerves and cause numbness on the skin surface but do not penetrate deeper structures such as muscle where the pain often lies.

However, local anesthetics are helpful when abrasion accompanies the injury.[41] Application of an OTC antibiotic ointment containing an anesthetic provides soothing relief, promotes healing of abrasions, and prevents soft-tissue infection. Minor abrasions should be cleansed thoroughly with mild soap and water before application. More severe abrasions may require removal of debris or foreign bodies by a clinician followed by irrigation with normal saline.

Counterirritants Counterirritants are categorized by the FDA into four groups (groups A–D) based on their primary actions (Table 60–3). They produce a feeling of warmth, cooling, or irritation that diverts sensation from the primary source of pain. Because these irritant effects are central to the beneficial actions, counterirritants should not be combined with topical anesthetics or topical analgesics.

Counterirritants are indicated for the temporary relief of minor aches and pains related to muscles and joints.[26] These symptoms may be associated with simple backache, arthritis, strains, sprains, or bruises. Many are available commercially as combination products with ingredients from different counterirritant groups. Active ingredients in marketed products sometimes change; clinicians should be aware of the current ingredients before providing a product recommendation. ❾ *Patient education on proper use of counterirritants is essential to therapeutic success* (Table 60–4).

Rubefacients (group A) are counterirritants that produce redness on application. Topical rubefacients containing

---

Table 60–2

Patient Education for Topical NSAIDs

All Topical NSAIDs	Gel-Specific	Patch-Specific
Do not apply to damaged or nonintact skin	Use enclosed dosing card to determine amount for application	Apply to skin at the most painful area
Wash hands after application and/or removal	Avoid bathing or showering for 1 hour after application	Do not wear during bathing or showering
Discontinue use if rash or irritation develops	Avoid sun exposure or tanning beds	Tape patch in place if it begins to peel off
Do not use with oral NSAIDs	Do not use with other topical agents (e.g., sunscreens, lotions, moisturizers, and insect repellants)	Discard used patches away from children and pets

From Refs. 37, 38.

Table 60–3

Nonprescription Counterirritant External Analgesics

Group and Effect	Agents and Concentration	Example Products (If Applicable)	Comments
Group A Rubefacients: Produce redness	Allyl isothiocyanate 0.5–5%		Mustard derivative; pungent odor; avoid inhalation
	Ammonia water 1–2.5%		More concentrated solutions are highly caustic; avoid inhalation
	Methyl salicylate 10–60%	BenGay Ultra Strength[a] Flexall Plus[a] Icy Hot Stick[a]	Caution in aspirin sensitivity May produce systemic concentrations May increase INR with warfarin
Group B Produce cooling	Camphor 3–11% Menthol 1.25–16%	JointFlex BenGay Patch Icy Hot Patch Mineral Ice	Medicinal odor Sensation of heat follows cooling Mild anesthetic effects at low concentrations
Group C Produce vasodilation	Methyl nicotinate 0.25–1%		May produce systemic vasodilation
Group D Irritate without redness	Capsaicin 0.025–0.25%	Capzasin-HP	Must use regularly
	Capsicum oleoresin 0.025–0.25%	Zostrix	Burning effect subsides with regular use

INR, International Normalized Ratio.

[a]Included in combination products that also contain menthol and/or camphor.

---

salicylates (e.g., methyl salicylate) are used most commonly. Turpentine oil is no longer judged as either safe or effective but remains in a few products.[26] Clinical trial data evaluating the effect of rubefacients on acute pain from strains, sprains, sports injuries, and chronic musculoskeletal pain are lacking.[42] A systematic review of available evidence concluded that topical salicylates are effective for acute pain but have limited effectiveness in chronic pain.[42]

Methyl salicylate and trolamine salicylate are topical salicylates. Methyl salicylate is considered a counterirritant, but trolamine salicylate is not considered a counterirritant because it does not produce localized irritation after application. Application of both topical salicylates can lead to systemic effects, especially if the product is applied liberally.[43] Repeated application and occlusion with a wrap or bandage also can increase systemic concentrations. Salicylate-containing products should be used with caution in patients in whom systemic salicylates are contraindicated, such as patients with severe asthma or aspirin allergy.[43] Topical salicylates have been reported to increase prothrombin time in patients on warfarin and should be used with caution in patients on oral anticoagulants.[43] Methyl salicylate, including oil of wintergreen, is one of the most common sources of pediatric poisonings.[44] Clinicians should advise patients to keep products out of the reach of children.

The FDA advises that there is insufficient evidence to support the effectiveness of trolamine salicylate contained in products such as Aspercreme.[26] However, many patients choose trolamine products because of the lack of medicinal odor.

Table 60–4

Patient Education for Counterirritants

Apply up to 3–5 times daily to affected area
Only for external use on the skin; do not ingest
Do not apply to broken or damaged skin or cover large areas
Wash hands immediately after application
Avoid contact with the eyes and mouth
Do not use with heating pads or other methods of heat application, because burning or blistering can occur
Do not wrap or bandage the area tightly after application
Consult a physician if:
- Symptoms worsen
- Symptoms persist for more than 7 days[a]
- Symptoms resolve but then recur

[a]Capsaicin may be used for chronic pain and must be applied consistently for efficacy.

From Ref. 26.

The group B counterirritants menthol and camphor exert a sensation of cooling through direct action on sensory nerve endings.[43,45] A sensation of warmth follows the cooling effect. The agents also have mild anesthetic activity at low concentrations.[45] In higher concentrations, they act as counterirritants and cause a burning sensation by stimulating cutaneous nociceptors. Menthol and camphor are used often in combination with rubefacients.

Menthol, also known as peppermint oil, is used widely in toothpastes, mouthwashes, gum, sore-throat lozenges, lip balms, and nasal decongestants. For topical analgesic use, it is available in creams, lotions, ointment, and patches. The patches can be trimmed to fit the affected area.

Menthol and camphor have caused respiratory distress in infants and should not be used in children under 2 years of age. Despite limits on the concentration of available products, camphor can be toxic to children even in small amounts.[46] Patients should be advised to keep the products out of the reach of children.

The group C counterirritants methyl nicotinate and histamine dihydrochloride produce vasodilation.[26] Methyl nicotinate is a nicotinic acid derivative that produces PG-mediated vasodilation.[47] NSAIDs and aspirin block the production of PGs and decrease methyl nicotinate–induced vasodilation. Application over a large area has been reported to cause systemic symptoms and syncope, possibly due to vasodilation and a decrease in blood pressure.[48] Patients should be educated to apply only scant amounts to the affected area to avoid this effect.

The primary counterirritant in group D is capsaicin, a natural substance found in red chili peppers and responsible for the hot, spicy characteristic when used in foods.[33,34,49] Capsaicin stimulates the release of substance P from local sensory nerve fibers, depleting substance P stores over time. A period of reduced sensitivity to painful stimuli follows, and transmission of pain impulses to the CNS is reduced.[33]

As with other counterirritants, capsaicin and its derivatives (i.e., capsicum and capsicum oleoresin) exert a warming or burning sensation. With repeated application, desensitization occurs, and the burning sensation subsides. This typically occurs within the first 1 to 2 weeks. After discontinuation, resensitization occurs gradually and returns completely within a few weeks.[49]

Because of the lag time between initiation and effect, capsaicin is not used for treatment of acute pain from injury. Instead, topical capsaicin is used for chronic pain from musculoskeletal and neuropathic disorders. Capsaicin preparations have been studied in the treatment of pain from diabetic neuropathy, osteoarthritis, rheumatoid arthritis, postherpetic neuralgia, and other disorders.[49] It is often used as an adjuvant to systemic analgesics in these chronic pain conditions.

While systemic adverse effects to capsaicin are rare, local adverse effects are expected and common.[50] Patient education regarding consistent use of capsaicin products is essential to achieving desired outcomes. Product should be applied in a thin layer and rubbed into the skin thoroughly until little remains on the surface.[43] **❿** *Patients using capsaicin should be advised to apply it regularly and consistently three to four times daily and that full effect may take 1 to 2 weeks or longer.* Patients should be assured that the burning effects will diminish with repeated application. Adherence to therapy is essential because the burning sensation persists if applications are less frequent than recommended. Because the burning sensation is enhanced with heat, patients should avoid hot showers or baths immediately before or after application. Wearing gloves during application can decrease the potential for unintended contact with eyes or mucous membranes.[50] Dried product residue has been reported

---

Patient Encounter 1, Part 2: Medical History, Physical Examination, and Diagnostic Tests

PMH: Asthma, well controlled with current medication regimen; allergic rhinitis

SH: Denies smoking; drinks alcoholic beverages on most days

Meds: Fluticasone 220 mcg one puff twice daily; albuterol (salbutamol) two to four puffs 4 times daily as needed

Allergies: Aspirin (difficulty breathing)

Diagnostic Tests: Radiographs of left ankle show no evidence of fracture

What are your treatment goals and desired outcomes?

What nonpharmacologic and pharmacologic treatments options are available? Are there treatment options that should be avoided? If so, which options and why?

---

to cause respiratory effects on inhalation,[49] and caution should be used in patients with asthma or other respiratory illnesses.

▶ *Muscle Relaxants*

Where pain is worsened by muscle spasm, oral muscle relaxants serve as a useful adjunct to therapy.[51] These agents include baclofen, metaxalone, methocarbamol, carisoprodol, and cyclobenzaprine. Muscle relaxants decrease spasm and stiffness associated with either acute or chronic musculoskeletal disorders. These agents should be used with caution because they all may cause sedation, especially in combination with alcohol or narcotic analgesics.

Lifestyle and Behavioral Modifications

After treatment of the acute injury with RICE and pharmacologic therapy, the final phase of therapy is rehabilitation and prevention of future injury. For most injuries, prolonged immobilization can lengthen the recovery time by causing wasting of the healthy muscle fibers.[10,52] Rehabilitation starts with the development of range of motion via stretching exercises. Patient should warm the muscle first with light activity or moderate heat.[10] Warmth produces relaxation and increases elasticity. Next, the patient should start general strengthening exercises.[11,52] Resistance exercises using resistance bands available at sporting goods stores are an effective method of strengthening.[11] Strengthening exercises should be continued beyond the healing phase to prevent future injury.

After rehabilitation, the patient should be educated about behavior changes to prevent reinjury or the development of chronic pain.[2,9,25] The warm-up and strengthening routines learned in the rehabilitation phase should be continued. For overuse injury, correction of

Patient Encounter 1, Part 3: Creating a Care Plan

Based on the information presented, create a care plan to treat this patient's ankle injury. Your plan should include:

(a) the goals of therapy and desired outcomes,
(b) a patient-specific therapeutic plan, including nonpharmacologic therapy, and (c) a plan to monitor the outcome of therapy to determine if goals of therapy have been met and adverse effects avoided.

Patient Encounter 2

A 40-year-old woman presents with right elbow pain. On questioning, you determine that she works in a factory performing repetitive tasks with her right arm. She reports the gradual onset of pain over the last few months. When she wakes in the morning, she has minimal pain after rest, but the pain intensifies after a few hours at work. She tends to have less pain on weekends. She reports decreased range of motion compared with the left side. She is a nonsmoker and does not drink. She has no significant past medical history or allergies. She takes no medications.

Given this information, what is your assessment of the patient's elbow pain?

What is the likely etiology of the pain?

What nonpharmacologic and pharmacologic treatments options should be considered?

Based on the information presented, create a care plan for this patient's elbow injury. Your plan should include: (a) the goals of therapy and desired outcomes, (b) a patient-specific therapeutic plan, including nonpharmacologic therapy, and (c) a monitoring plan to determine if goals of therapy have been met and adverse effects avoided.

biomechanical abnormalities with proper footwear and changes in technique may correct misalignments and imbalances.[2] Repetitive trauma can be decreased with proper training (e.g., by implementing a gradual increase in mileage in a running plan).

Proper lifting techniques can decrease low back pain.[15] Lifting methods include standing with legs shoulder-width apart, lifting with the legs and not the back, and keeping the object close to the body. In the workplace, repetitive motion can be decreased through proper ergonomic design and diversification of job tasks.[13] In pain of the lower extremity, weight loss in overweight or obese patients can assist in reduction of further inflammation and help to

Patient Care and Monitoring

1. Assess the patient's symptoms to determine if empirical care is appropriate or whether diagnostic evaluation is warranted. Determine the timing of injury (if applicable), duration of pain, type and degree of pain, and exacerbating factors. Determine if the musculoskeletal disorder interferes with usual activities or range of motion.

2. Assess exacerbating or alleviating factors. Ask if the patient has tried any nonpharmacologic or pharmacologic treatments.

3. Obtain a complete medication history, including history of prescription drug, nonprescription drug, and dietary supplement use. Determine if the patient has used any successful or unsuccessful treatments for this condition in the past.

4. Gather patient history. Assess factors involved in drug selection. Inquire about social history and alcohol use. Ask the patient about drug allergies and chronic health problems such as asthma.

5. Educate the patient on nonpharmacologic therapy, including each of the steps in RICE. If injury is the source of the pain and it occurred more than 48 hours ago, consider heat instead of ice.

6. Assess patient preference for systemic (oral) or local (topical) therapy. Would frequent application of topical medications be possible? Would the patient accept topical medications with a medicinal odor?

7. Recommend appropriate pharmacologic therapy and educate on proper use. If a counterirritant is recommended, counsel patients on the irritant effect of the product and recommend washing hands immediately after use and to avoid heating pads. For patients using a capsaicin product, emphasize that adherence to regular application is required for effectiveness.

8. Develop a plan to assess effectiveness of pharmacologic therapy. If pain is from an acute injury, assess effectiveness within 7 to 10 days. For chronic pain treated with capsaicin, begin to assess pain control in 2 weeks.

9. Evaluate for adverse effects and drug interactions. For patients on topical therapy, evaluate for local adverse effects. For patients on acetaminophen or NSAIDs, inquire about alcohol use.

10. Stress lifestyle modifications for rehabilitation and prevention. Recommend strength training, range-of-motion exercises, and a warm-up period before exercise. In repetitive-motion injury, recommend methods to correct biomechanical abnormalities and vary work tasks as applicable. Refer to a physical therapist or sports trainer as needed.

prevent reinjury or repetitive strain injuries.[23] Nonweight-bearing activities, such as swimming or bicycling, can be recommended for initial return to activity.[25]

OUTCOME EVALUATION

- Use a pain scale to monitor treatment interventions to ensure that pain relief is achieved. Ask the patient to rate pain on a scale of zero (no pain) to 10 (worst possible pain) both at rest and with movement. Compare the results with baseline pain assessment to monitor the response to therapy. In pediatric patients, use a visual pain scale with facial expressions depicting various degrees of pain.

- Assess range of motion at baseline and after treatment by comparing movement with the unaffected limb and functionality before the injury. Assess functionality by asking patients if they are able to perform activities of daily living or participate in exercise as desired.

- If pain from acute injury does not decrease greatly within 7 to 10 days, further diagnostic evaluation is warranted.

- For patients using capsaicin products, assess adherence to regular application for therapeutic benefit. Assess chronic pain control in 2 weeks.

- Assess medication adverse effects on a regular basis. When NSAIDs and aspirin are used, ask about GI tolerability, bruising, and bleeding. Inquire about local adverse effects, such as burning, when topical counterirritants are used for treatment.

- Evaluate adherence to preventative rehabilitation measures such as proper footwear, warm-up before activity, strength training, and proper lifting technique.

Abbreviations Introduced in This Chapter

COX	Cyclooxygenase
INR	International Normalized Ratio
NSAIDs	Nonsteroidal anti-inflammatory drugs
OTC	Over-the-counter
PG	Prostaglandin

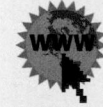
Self-assessment questions and answers are available at *http://www.mhpharmacotherapy. com/pp.html.*

REFERENCES

1. Abasolo L, Blanco M, Bachiller J, et al. A health system program to reduce work disability related to musculoskeletal disorders. Ann Intern Med 2005; 143:404–414.
2. Wilder RP, Sethi S. Overuse injuries: Tendinopathies, stress fractures, compartment syndrome, and shin splints. Clin Sports Med 2004;23:55–81.
3. Biundo Jr. JJ, Irwin RW, Umpierre E. Sports and other soft tissue injuries, tendinitis, bursitis, and occupation-related syndromes. Curr Opin Rheumatol 2001;13:146–149.
4. Schappert SM, Burt CW. Ambulatory care visits to physician offices, hospital outpatient departments, and emergency departments: United States, 2001–02. Vital Health Stat 13. 2006;159:1–66.
5. Yellin E, Herrndorf A, Trupin L, Sonneborn D. A national study of medical care expenditures for musculoskeletal conditions. Arthritis Rheum 2001;44:1160–1169.
6. National Research Council, The Institute of Medicine. Musculoskeletal Disorders and the Workplace: Low Back and Upper Extremities. Washington, DC: National Academy Press, 2001.
7. Mani L, Gerr F. Work-related upper extremity musculoskeletal disorders. Prim Care 2000;27:845–864.
8. Morse T, Dillon C, Kenta-Bibi E, et al. Trends in work-related musculoskeletal disorder reports by year, type, and industrial sector: A capture-recapture analysis. Am J Ind Med 2005;48:40–49.
9. Audette J, Frotera W. Assessment and treatment of pain in sports injuries. In: Warfield CA, Bajwa ZH, eds. Principles and Practice of Pain Medicine, 2nd ed. New York: McGraw-Hill, 2004:35–48.
10. Jarvinen TA, Kaariainen M, Jarvinen M, et al. Muscle strain injuries. Curr Opin Rheumatol 2000;12:155–161.
11. Wolfe MW, Uhl TL, Mattacola CG, et al. Management of ankle sprains. Am Fam Physician 2001;63:93–104.
12. Ivins D. Acute ankle sprain: An update. Am Fam Physician 2006; 74:1714–1720, 1723–1726.
13. Amell T, Kumar S. Work-related musculoskeletal disorders: Design as a prevention strategy: A review. J Occup Rehabil 2001;11:255–265.
14. Noonan TJ, Garrett WE Jr. Muscle strain injury: Diagnosis and treatment. J Am Acad Orthop Surg 1999;7:262–269.
15. Patel AT, Ogle AA. Diagnosis and management of acute low back pain. Am Fam Physician, 2000;61:1779–1786, 1789–1790.
16. Toumi H, Best TM. The inflammatory response: Friend or enemy for muscle injury? Br J Sports Med 2003;37:284–286.
17. Murrell GA. Understanding tendinopathies. Br J Sports Med 2002;36:392–393.
18. Wilson JJ, Best TM. Common overuse tendon problems: A review and recommendations for treatment. Am Fam Physician 2005;72:881–888.
19. Baldwin Lanier A. Use of nonsteroidal anti-inflammatory drugs following exercise-induced muscle injury. Sports Med 2003;33:177–185.
20. Cohen SA. Pathophysiology of pain. In: Warfield CA, Bajwa ZH, eds. Principles and Practice of Pain Medicine, 2nd ed. New York: McGraw-Hill, 2004:35–48.
21. Fields HL, Martin JB. Pain: Pathophysiology and management. In: Kasper DL, Fauci AS, Braunwald E, et al., eds. Harrison's Principles of Internal Medicine, 17th ed. New York City: McGraw-Hill, 2008:81–87.
22. DeVane CL. Substance P: A new era, a new role. Pharmacotherapy 2001; 21:1061–1069.
23. Mazzone MF, McCue T. Common conditions of the Achilles tendon. Am Fam Physician 2002;65:1805–1810.
24. Wilson JJ, Best TM. Common overuse tendon problems: A review and recommendations for treatment. Am Fam Physician 2005;72:811–818.
25. Palmer T, Toombs JD. Managing joint pain in primary care. J Am Board Fam Pract 2004;17(suppl):S32–S42.

26. External analgesics drug products for over-the-counter human use: Tentative final monograph. Fed Regist 1983;48:5851–5869.

27. Pray WS. Treating sore muscles and tendons. US Pharm 2006;5:18–24.

28. Graham GG, Scott KF. Mechanism of action of paracetamol. Am J Ther 2005;12:46–55.

29. Kvien TK, Viktil K. Pharmacotherapy for regional musculoskeletal pain. Best Pract Res Clin Rheumatol 2003;17:137–150.

30. Sachs CJ. Oral analgesics for acute nonspecific pain. Am Fam Physician 2005;71:913–918.

31. Graham GG, Scott KF, Day RO. Tolerability of paracetamol. Drug Saf 2005;28:227–240.

32. Peterson GM. Selecting nonprescription analgesics. Am J Ther 2005;12:67–79.

33. Galer BS. Topical medications. In: Loeser JD, Bonica JJ, eds. Bonica's Management of Pain, 3rd ed. Philadelphia: Lippincott Williams & Wilkins, 2001:1736–1741.

34. Sawynok J. Topical and peripherally acting analgesics. Pharmacol Rev 2003;55:1–20.

35. Tramer MR. It's not just about rubbing—Topical capsaicin and topical salicylates may be useful as adjuvants to conventional pain treatment. BMJ 2004;328:998.

36. FDA Consumer Health Information. Use Caution with Over-the-Counter Creams, Ointments. *http://www.fda.gov/consumer/updates/otc_creams040108.html.*

37. Voltaren Gel (diclofenac sodium topical gel 1%) product information. Novartis Consumer Health. Parsippany, NJ: October 2007.

38. Flector Patch (diclofenac epolamine patch 1.3%). Alpharma Pharmaceuticals. Piscataway, NJ: November 2007.

39. Zacher J, Altman R, Bellamy N, et al. Topical diclofenac and its role in pain and inflammation: An evidence-based review. Curr Med Res Opin 2008;24:925–950.

40. Mason L, Moore RA, Edwards JE, et al. Topical NSAIDs for acute pain: A meta-analysis. BMC Fam Pract 2004;5:10.

41. Blasen LS. Soft tissue injuries. Management of common presentations. Adv Nurse Pract 2000;8:65–66, 84.

42. Mason L, Moore RA, Edwards JE, et al. Systematic review of efficacy of topical rubefacients containing salicylates for the treatment of acute and chronic pain. BMJ 2004;328:995.

43. Martindale: The complete drug reference. London: Pharma-ceutical Press. Electronic version, Thomson Healthcare, Greenwood Village, CO. *http://www.thomsonhc.com.*

44. Davis JE. Are one or two dangerous? Methyl salicylate exposure in toddlers. J Emerg Med 2007;32:63–69.

45. Patel T, Ishiuji Y, Yosipovitch G. Menthol: A refreshing look at this ancient compound. J Am Acad Dermatol 2007;57:873–878.

46. Michael JB, Sztajnkrycer MD. Deadly pediatric poisons: Nine common agents that kill at low doses. Emerg Med Clin North Am 2004;22:1019–1050.

47. Wilkin JK, Fortner G, Reinhardt LA, et al. Prostaglandins and nicotinate-provoked increase in cutaneous blood flow. Clin Pharmacol Ther 1985;38:273–277.

48. Fergusson DA. Systemic symptoms associated with a rubefacient. BMJ 1988;297:1339.

49. Mason L, Moore RA, Derry S, et al. Systematic review of topical capsaicin for the treatment of chronic pain. BMJ 2004;328:991.

50. Rosenstein ED. Topical agents in the treatment of rheumatic disorders. Rheum Dis Clin North Am 1999;25:899–918.

51. Beebe FA, Barkin RL, Barkin S. A clinical and pharmacologic review of skeletal muscle relaxants for musculoskeletal conditions. Am J Ther 2005;12:151–171.

52. Schramm-Bloodworth D, Grabois M. Physical medicine and rehabilitation. In: Warfield CA, Bajwa ZH, eds. Principles and Practice of Pain Medicine, 2nd ed. New York: McGraw-Hill; 2004:35–48.

61 Glaucoma

Mikael D. Jones

LEARNING OBJECTIVES

Upon completion of the chapter, the reader will be able to:

1. Identify risk factors for the development of primary open-angle glaucoma (POAG) and acute angle-closure glaucoma.

2. Recommend a frequency for glaucoma screening based upon patient-specific risk factors.

3. Compare and contrast the pathophysiologic mechanisms responsible for open-angle glaucoma and acute angle-closure glaucoma.

4. Compare and contrast the clinical presentation of chronic open-angle glaucoma and acute angle-closure glaucoma.

5. List the goals of treatment for patients with POAG suspect, POAG, and acute angle-closure glaucoma.

6. Choose the most appropriate therapy based upon patient-specific data for open-angle glaucoma, glaucoma suspect, and acute angle-closure glaucoma.

7. Develop a monitoring plan for patients on specific pharmacologic regimens.

8. Counsel patients about glaucoma, drug therapy options, ophthalmic administration techniques, and the importance of adherence to the prescribed regimen.

KEY CONCEPTS

❶ Practitioners can play an important role in eye care by assessing patients for risk factors and referring to an ophthalmologist for appropriate screening and evaluation.

❷ Acute primary angle-closure glaucoma (PACG) is a medical emergency and requires laser or surgical intervention.

❸ Patients with primary open-angle glaucoma (POAG) typically have a slow, insidious loss of vision. This is contrasted by the course of acute PACG, which can lead to rapid vision loss that develops over hours to days.

❹ The goals of therapy are to prevent further loss of visual function; minimize adverse effects of therapy and its impact on the patient's vision, preserve general health and quality of life; control intraocular pressure (IOP) to reduce or prevent further optic nerve damage; and educate and involve the patient in the management of their disease.

❺ Current therapy is directed at altering the flow and production of aqueous humor, which is the major determinant of IOP.

❻ Because POAG is a chronic, often asymptomatic condition, the decision of when and how to treat patients is difficult because the treatment modalities are often expensive and have potential adverse effects or complications. Therefore the clinician should evaluate the potential effectiveness, toxicity, and the likelihood of patient adherence for each therapeutic modality.

❼ An initial target IOP should be set at 20% lower than the patient's baseline IOP. The target IOP can be set lower (30–50% of baseline IOP) for patients who already have severe disease or have normal-tension glaucoma (NTG).

❽ It is important to review the patient's medication history for potential drug–drug and drug–glaucoma interactions, adherence, presence of systemic and ocular adverse drug reactions, and ability to use ophthalmic preparations.

INTRODUCTION

Glaucoma refers to a spectrum of ophthalmic disorders characterized by neuropathy of the optic nerve and loss of retinal ganglion cells, which leads to permanent deterioration of the visual field and potentially total vision loss. Glaucoma can be classified as primary and secondary. Primary glaucoma refers to glaucoma that cannot be attributed to a pre-existing ocular or systemic disease while, secondary glaucoma refers to glaucoma that can be attributed to pre-existing ocular or systemic disease. Examples of primary glaucoma include open angle, closed angle, and congenital. Examples of secondary glaucoma include pigmentary glaucoma, neovascular glaucoma, traumatic glaucoma, and pseudoexfoliative glaucoma.

Primary open-angle glaucoma (POAG) is characterized by normal anterior-chamber angles, glaucomatous changes of the optic disc, and peripheral visual field loss. Patients with elevated intraocular pressure (IOP), without glaucomatous changes, are considered to have ocular hypertension.[1,2] Patients with ocular hypertension that have normal appearing anterior-chamber angles and an eye exam suspicious of early glaucomatous damage are classified as POAG suspects. Primary angle-closure glaucoma (PACG) is the obstruction of the anterior angle by the iris causing moderate to high elevations in IOP. POAG and PACG represent the most common types of glaucoma and therefore will be the focus of this chapter.

EPIDEMIOLOGY AND ETIOLOGY

Over 66.8 million people worldwide have glaucoma making it the second leading cause of blindness worldwide.[3] In the United States it is estimated that 2.22 million people are affected by POAG, and by 2020 this number will increase to 3.36 million. The prevalence varies with race and ethnicity and it is three to five times more prevalent in African Americans than Caucasian Americans. The prevalence of POAG increases with age and is rarely seen in patients less than 40 years of age.[1,4,5] Of patients diagnosed with POAG, 15% to 40% actually meet the criteria for normal-tension glaucoma (NTG).[1,2] Ocular hypertension is present in about 3 to 6 million of the U.S. population, however, less than 10% will have progression to POAG within 5 years.[6]

The prevalence of PACG is lower than POAG and varies significantly by race and ethnicity. It is low in patients of European descent (0.09–0.16%) but higher in patients of Chinese (1.3%), Eskimo (2.9–5%), and Asian Indian (4.33%) descent. PACG is also more prevalent with increasing age and among females.[7,8]

RISK FACTORS

Primary Open-Angle Glaucoma

❶ *Practitioners can play an important role in eye care by assessing patients for risk factors and referring to an eye care specialist for appropriate screening and evaluation.* Risk factor evaluation is essential in determining the frequency of comprehensive eye exams for patients (Table 61–1). It is also useful in deciding when to start therapy and determining the sequence of pharmacotherapeutic or surgical treatment modalities.[1]

Table 61–1
Recommended Frequency of Comprehensive Adult Medical Eye Evaluation

Age (Years)	With Risk Factors for Glaucoma	No Known Risk Factors
65 or above	6–12 months	1–2 years
55–65	1–2 years	1–3 years
40–54	1–3 years	2–4 years
Under 40	2–4 years	5–10 years

From Ref. 32.

Table 61–2
Risk Factors for Glaucoma

POAG	PACG
Main Risk Factors Elevated IOP African or Hispanic descent Family history of glaucoma Older age Thinner CCT	**Risk Factors** Advancing age Asian or Eskimo ethnicity Female gender Hyperopia Shallow anterior chamber Family history of angle-closure glaucoma
Possible Risk Factors Systemic hypertension Diabetes Myopia Low diastolic perfusion pressures	

CCT, central corneal thickness; IOP, intraocular pressure; POAG, primary open-angle glaucoma; PACG, primary angle-closure glaucoma.

From Refs. 1, 10, 32.

The five primary risk factors associated with POAG are family history, age, race, central corneal thickness (CCT), and elevated IOP (Table 61–2). Patients who have first-degree relatives with POAG are at a higher risk of developing glaucoma than patients with no family history of POAG. Even though IOP is no longer a diagnostic criterion, it is associated with an increased prevalence and progression of the disease.[1,5,7] CCT has recently been recognized as a risk factor for POAG. The Ocular Hypertension Study (OHTS) found patients with ocular hypertension and thinner CCT (less than 555 μm) had a greater risk of progressing to POAG.[1,6,9]

The five major risk factors identified for PACG are hyperopia, family history of PACG, age (greater than 30 years), gender, and Eskimo or Asian ethnicity (Table 61–2). Patients who are hyperopic, female, or of Eskimo or Asian ethnicity tend to have more shallow anterior angles which predispose the eye to angle closure. Advancing age is associated with a decrease in the depth of the anterior angles because the lens becomes thickened and is displaced toward the anterior portion of the eye. Patients who have first-degree relatives with glaucoma are at greater risk for developing PACG with a prevalence of 1% to 12% for Caucasians.[7,8,10]

PATHOPHYSIOLOGY

The pathophysiologic alterations seen with POAG optic neuropathy are not fully understood. Elevated IOP is clearly associated with damage and eventual death of optic nerves; however, optic neuropathy can still occur in patients with normal IOP. Optic nerve degeneration without elevated IOP indicates the presence of independent factors that contribute to the death of the optic nerve. The key to understanding the pathophysiology and treatment of POAG relies on an understanding of aqueous humor dynamics, IOP, and optic nerve anatomy and physiology.[5,7,11]

Aqueous Humor

The eye is separated into two segments by the lens: the anterior segment and the posterior segment (Figs. 61–1 and 61–2). The anterior segment of the eye is separated by the iris into the posterior and anterior chambers. The ciliary body, a ring-like structure that surrounds and supports the lens, produces and secretes an optically neutral fluid called aqueous humor through the diffusion and ultrafiltration of plasma. The nonpigmented epithelium of the ciliary body secretes the aqueous humor into the posterior chamber. Aqueous humor formation can be modified pharmacologically through the α- and β-adrenoceptors, carbonic anhydrase, and sodium and potassium adenosine triphosphatase of the nonpigmented ciliary epithelium.

After the transport of aqueous humor into the posterior chamber, it flows through the pupil into the anterior chamber where it provides oxygen and nutrition to the avascular lens and cornea. Aqueous humor then exits the anterior chamber through the trabecular meshwork and drains into the Schlemm's Canal, which drains aqueous humor into the episcleral venous system.

Eighty percent of aqueous humor drains through the trabecular meshwork which is a lattice of connective tissue that surrounds the anterior chamber. The size of the trabecular meshwork can be altered by the contraction or the relaxation of the ciliary muscle. Stimulation of muscarinic receptors on the ciliary muscle causes contraction which in turn causes the pores of the trabecular meshwork to open, increasing aqueous humor outflow.

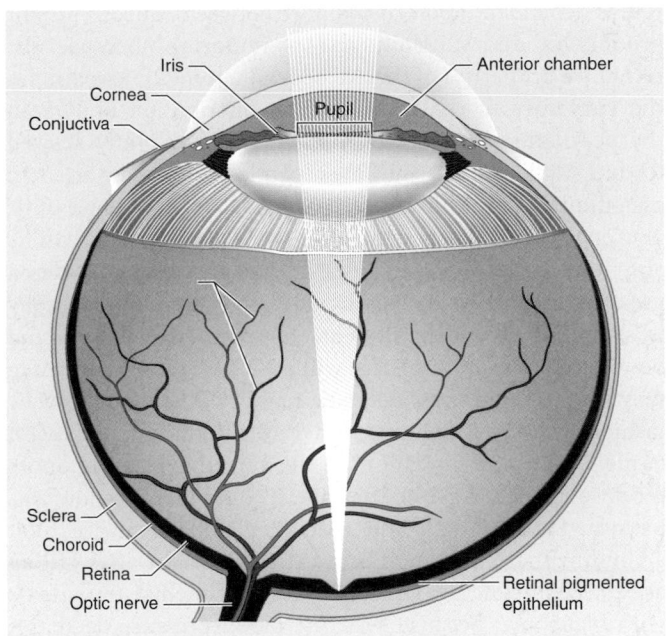

FIGURE 61–1. Anatomy of the eye. (From Lesar TS, Fiscella RG, Edward D. Glaucoma. In: DiPiro JT, Talbert RL, Yee GC, et al., eds. Pharmacotheraphy: A Pathophysiologic Approach, 7th ed. New York: McGraw-Hill, 2008:1552.)

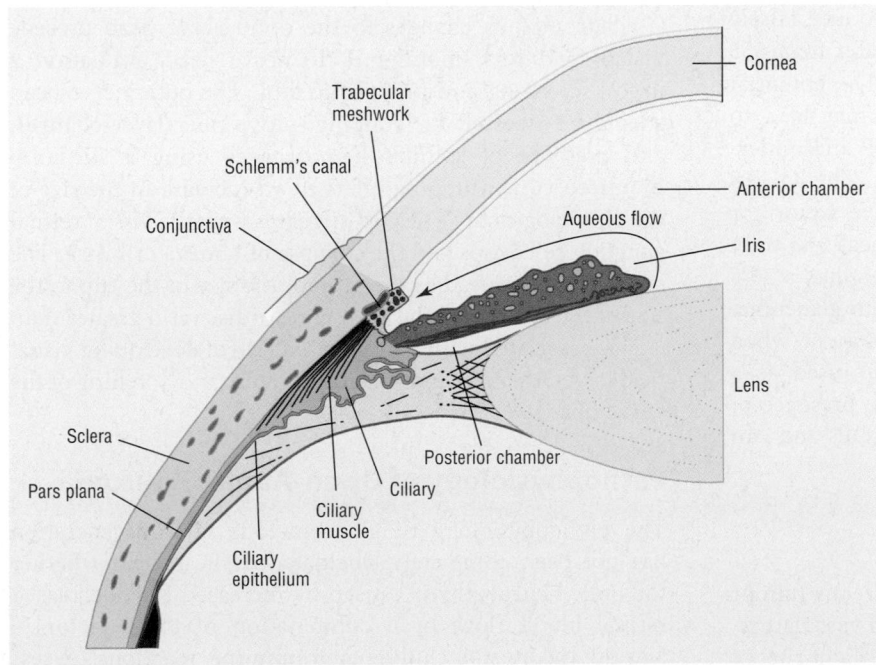

FIGURE 61–2. Anterior chamber of the eye and aqueous humor flow. (From Lesar TS, Fiscella RG, Edward D. Glaucoma. In: DiPiro JT, Talbert RL, Yee GC, et al., eds. Pharmacotheraphy: A Pathophysiologic Approach, 7th ed. New York: McGraw-Hill, 2008:1552.)

A second pathway, uveoscleral outflow, comprises the other 20% of aqueous humor drainage. In the uveoscleral pathway, aqueous humor exits the anterior chamber through the iris root and through spaces in the ciliary muscles which then drains into suprachoroidal space. Uveoscleral outflow can be pharmacologically modulated by adrenoceptors, prostanoid receptors, and prostamide receptors. [5,11–15]

Intraocular Pressure

IOP is dependent upon the balance between aqueous humor production and outflow, and is important because the refractive properties of the eye depend upon IOP to maintain the curvature of the cornea.[16] The distribution of IOP in the population is 10 to 21 mm Hg and is slightly skewed toward higher values; however, caution should be used in assigning this range as being "normal" for IOP because optic neuropathy can be present in the normal range and can be absent at higher IOPs. Elevated IOP is generally considered greater than 21 mm Hg. Optic nerve damage generally is slow and takes several years for noticeable progression between 20 and 30 mm Hg, while IOP of 40 to 50 mm Hg may lead to rapid optic nerve damage. IOP varies in a cyclic fashion over the 24-hour day. IOP was thought to be lowest at night and at its maximum in the morning; however, more recent evidence suggests that not all individuals follow this pattern. Patients with and without glaucoma may exhibit a rhythm that consists of a peak in IOP right after falling asleep. Nighttime peaks in IOP are detrimental to patients with glaucoma, because systemic blood pressure decreases during the night leading to a low ocular perfusion pressure. Decreased ocular perfusion pressure can lead to further optic nerve damage, therefore highlighting the importance of IOP control throughout a 24-hour period.[17–19]

IOP is clinically measured by tonometry and can be performed via applanation, indentation, and indirect tonometry.[20] CCT affects the accuracy of IOP measurements. Thin corneas (less than 540 microns) can produce falsely low IOP readings, whereas thick corneas (greater than 555 microns) may produce falsely high readings. The potential consequences of this error in measurement may lead to overtreatment of patients with falsely high IOP and undertreatment of patients with falsely low IOP. The OHTS demonstrated that CCT is a strong predictive factor for the development of POAG. Patients with corneas less than 555 microns and IOP greater than 25.75 mm Hg had a 36% risk of progressing from ocular hypertension to glaucoma. The CCT of patient should be taken into account when evaluating a patient's IOP.[6] IOP is no longer used as a diagnostic criterion for glaucoma, because the presence of glaucomatous changes can be absent at high IOPs and can be present at lower IOPs.

Optic Nerve

The posterior segment of the eye contains vitreous humor (a clear "jellylike" substance), the retina, retinal vasculature, and the optic nerve head. The retina transforms light energy

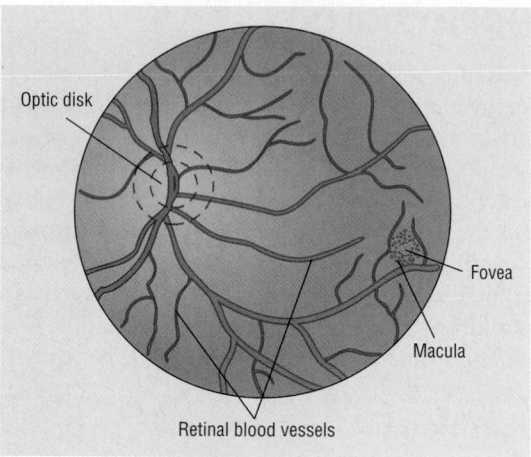

FIGURE 61–3. Normal fundus of the eye and optic disk and cup. (Reprinted with permission from Lesar TS, Fiscella RG, Edward D. Glaucoma. In: DiPiro JT, Talbert RL, Yee GC, et al., eds. Pharmacotherapy: A Pathophysiologic Approach, 7th ed. New York: McGraw-Hill, 2008:1553.)

into neural signals, which are transmitted out of the eye by the retinal ganglion cells. The axons of the retinal ganglion cells converge and exit at the optic nerve head (optic disc) to form the optic nerve (Fig. 61–3). The optic nerve contains 1 million nerve fibers and synapses at the lateral geniculate nucleus of the brain. The optic nerve head is the portion of the optic nerve that is susceptible to elevations in IOP and is visible on fundoscopic examination. The optic nerve head is vertically oval and pale yellow with a depression in the center of the optic nerve, called a physiologic cup which is formed by convergence of the axons. The area surrounding the optic nerve head is the nerve fiber layer which consists of converging retinal ganglion cell axons. Retinal nutrition is dependent upon the transport of trophic factors from the retinal cell ganglion axon to their cell bodies.

Glaucomatous changes to the optic nerve head precede visual field loss, making optic nerve head evaluation a useful screening and prognostic tool. The optic nerve head should be assessed for cupping, nerve fiber layer changes, and presence of splinter hemorrhages using a slit-lamp biomicroscope. Cupping refers to an increase in the size of the physiologic cup. The cup increases with the loss of retinal ganglion cell axons and the collapse of lamina cribrosa. The cup size is expressed as the ratio of the size of the cup to the size of the optic nerve head. A cup-to-disc ratio greater than 0.55 is associated with an increased risk of developing visual field loss. Other findings include atrophy and notching of the nerve fiber layer.[5,7,20,21]

Pathophysiology of Open-Angle Glaucoma

The pathophysiology of glaucomatous neurodegeneration has not been completely elucidated. It is unclear whether the optic neuropathy is caused by increased IOP, decreased retinal blood flow, or a combination of these factors.[5,7] Several theories, including autoimmune reactions, excess nitric oxide, and glutamate toxicity have been proposed as to what ultimately causes the retinal ganglion cells to undergo apoptosis.[5,7]

The level of IOP is related to the death of retinal ganglion cell and optic nerve fibers. As optic neurodegeneration progresses over time, the optic nerve becomes more susceptible to high IOP. Increased IOP causes the retinal ganglion cell axons to undergo mechanical stress, alters axonal protein transport, and decreases blood supply to the retina and the optic nerve leading to tissue ischemia.[5,21,22] Glaucomatous optic neuropathy may also occur independent of increased IOP. Pressure independent causes of optic neuropathy include abnormal blood flow, systemic hypotension, and abnormal blood coagulability.[19] Current glaucoma therapies fail to target IOP-independent glaucoma pathophysiologic factors. However, IOP reduction may still be beneficial as the rate of visual field progression is decreased in some patients who receive IOP reduction via medical or surgical modalities.[23,24]

Pathophysiology of Angle-Closure Glaucoma

PACG involves a mechanical obstruction of aqueous humor outflow through the trabecular meshwork by the peripheral iris. Two major mechanisms of trabecular meshwork obstruction by the peripheral iris include pupillary block and an abnormality of the iris called iris plateau. Pupillary block is the more common mechanism of obstruction and results from a complete or functional apposition of the central iris to the anterior lens and is associated with mid-dilation. The trapped aqueous humor increases pressure behind the iris causing the peripheral iris to bow forward and obstruct the trabecular meshwork. Plateau iris refers to an anterior displacement of the peripheral iris caused by anteriorly positioned ciliary processes. In this configuration the peripheral iris bunches as the eye dilates. Both of these mechanisms result in the occlusion of aqueous humor outflow causing IOP elevation at extreme levels that can lead to vision loss in hours to days.[7,10,20,25,26] The degree of obstruction or angle closure can be determined by **gonioscopy**.

The development of PACG is associated with several anatomical risk factors that lead to shallow anterior chambers. PACG patients may have a thick, anteriorly displaced lens that results from myopia or old age. The axial length of the eye is smaller in individuals with PACG which leads to a lens that is situated more anteriorly than those without PACG.[25,26]

Medications with anticholinergic properties induce mydriasis, which can lead to angle closure in pupillary block and plateau iris. Pupillary block may also be induced by drugs that cause miosis.[12]

PACG can be separated into three categories: acute primary angle closure, subacute primary angle closure, and chronic primary angle closure. Acute PACG is the sudden obstruction of the trabecular meshwork which leads to rapid increases in IOP resulting in pressure-induced optic neuropathy if left untreated. ❷ *Acute PACG is a medical emergency and requires laser or surgical intervention.* Subacute PACG is characterized by self-limiting angle closure that resolves spontaneously. Recurrent attacks or a prolonged acute attack can lead to the development of peripheral anterior **synechia**. Chronic PACG is characterized by the presence of peripheral anterior synechia that partially obstruct the flow of aqueous humor through the trabecular meshwork resulting in an elevated IOP that is similar to what is seen in POAG.[10,25,26]

Clinical Presentation and Diagnosis of POAG

General
- Adult onset (usually greater than 40 years of age)
- Patients may be unaware that they have glaucoma and may be diagnosed during routine eye evaluation
- POAG is usually bilateral with asymmetric disease progression

Symptoms
- Patients with severe disease progression may report loss of peripheral vision and may describe the presence of scotomata (blind spots) in their field of vision

Signs
- Ophthalmoscopic examination may reveal
  - Optic nerve head (optic disc) cupping
  - Large cup-to-disc ratio
  - Diffuse thinning, focal narrowing, or notching of the optic nerve head rim
- Splinter hemorrhages
- Optic nerve head/nerve fiber layer changes occur before visual field changes can be detected

Diagnostic Tests
- Gonioscopy—anterior-chamber angles are to be open
- Applanation tonometry—elevated IOP (greater than 21 mm Hg) may be present. However, patient can have signs of optic neuropathy without elevated IOP
- Pachymetry—measures central corneal thickness. Thin corneas (less than 540 μm) are considered a glaucoma risk factor
- Automated static threshold perimetry—evaluates visual fields. Useful in diagnosis and determining if there is progression
- Other diagnostic tests—scanning laser polarimetry, confocal scanning laser ophthalmoscopy, and optical coherence tomography

Clinical Presentation and Diagnosis of PACG

General

- Medical emergency due to high risk of vision loss
- Unilateral in presentation, but fellow eye is at risk

Symptoms

- Ocular pain
- Red eye
- Blurry vision
- Halos around lights
- Systemic symptoms may develop
  - Nausea/vomiting
  - Abdominal pain
  - Headache
  - Diaphoresis

Signs

- Cloudy cornea caused by corneal edema
- Conjunctival hyperemia
- Pupil semidilated and fixed to light
- Eye will be harder on palpation through closed eye

Diagnostic Tests

- Gonioscopy—anterior-chamber angles will be closed. Peripheral anterior synechiae may be present
- Applanation tonometry—elevated IOP (greater than 21 mm Hg but when symptoms are present IOP may be greater than 30 mm Hg)
- Slit-lamp biomicroscopy—reveals shallow anterior-chamber depth. Signs of previous attacks include Peripheral anterior synechiae, iris atrophy, glaukomflecken, and pupillary dysfunction

Clinical Course

❸ *Patients with POAG typically have a slow, insidious loss of vision. This is contrasted by the course of acute PACG which can lead to rapid vision loss that develops over hours to days.* For POAG, only 4% to 8% of patients may progress to legal blindness. It may take 13 to 16 years for a patient to go blind from glaucoma. A patient's quality of life may not be affected until significant visual field loss is present and the patient can no longer perform the activities of daily living.[27] Vision loss does not occur until there has been significant loss of the retinal ganglion cells. Peripheral vision is the most susceptible to glaucomatous damage, with central vision being preserved until advanced disease progression has occurred. Visual field abnormalities include paracentral scotoma, nasal scotoma, and arcuate scotoma. Patients may also have problems with depth perception and contrast sensitivity. Peripheral vision may worsen until the patient has tunnel vision and ultimately total field loss. Visual fields can be measured by perimetry and can detect defects in the visual field before a patient may notice.[5,7]

TREATMENT

Primary Open-Angle Glaucoma

▶ Desired Outcomes and Goals

❹ *The goals of therapy are to prevent further loss of visual function; minimize adverse effects of therapy and impact on the patient's vision, general health, and quality of life; maintain IOP at or below a pressure at which further optic nerve damage is unlikely to occur; and educate and involve the patient in the*

Patient Encounter 1, Part 1: Risk Factor Evaluation and Recommended Frequency of Eye Care

A 65-year-old African American female with a history of type 2 diabetes, mild intermittent asthma, and hypertension presents to your clinic for her yearly checkup. She states that she is concerned about losing her eyesight because her sister has started losing her vision from glaucoma. She denies any changes in her vision.

Meds: Metformin 1,000 mg orally twice a day, albuterol two puffs every 6 hours as needed for wheezing, lisinopril 10 mg orally daily

What risk factors does this patient have for glaucoma?

Based on the available information, how often would you recommend that this patient receive a comprehensive eye evaluation?

management of their disease. ❺ *Current therapy is directed at altering the flow and production of aqueous humor, which is the major determinant of IOP.*

▶ General Approach

❻ *Because POAG is a chronic, often asymptomatic condition, the decision of when and how to treat patients is difficult, as the treatment modalities are often expensive and have potential adverse effects or complications. The clinician should evaluate the potential effectiveness, toxicity, and the likelihood of patient adherence for each therapeutic modality. The ideal therapeutic regimen should have maximal effectiveness and patient tolerance to achieve the desired therapeutic response.* The American Academy of Ophthalmology (AAO) publishes Preferred Practice Patterns for POAG and POAG Suspect.[1]

Before the selection of a therapeutic modality, the target IOP should be determined for each patient. The target IOP ideally represents an IOP range that will slow the progression of optic neuropathy and not simply obtaining an IOP in the range of 10 to 21 mm Hg. Currently, the initial target IOP is an estimate, but it should be modified based on the progression of the disease at each follow-up visit. ❼ *The AAO recommends an initial target IOP to be set at 20% lower than the patient's baseline IOP. The target IOP can be set lower (30–50% of baseline IOP) for patients who already have severe disease or have NTG.*[1,23,24]

Initial IOP control can be achieved by medical, laser, surgical, or combination of these therapies. The AAO guidelines do not provide a specific recommendation on which therapeutic modality should be selected first, but patients in the early stages of glaucoma should receive treatment. The Early Manifest Glaucoma Trial evaluated the effectiveness of reducing IOP in early untreated POAG. The trial demonstrated that patients who received a topical medication combined with laser therapy had slower progression of glaucoma by an average of 18 months.[28] Initial therapy with laser trabeculoplasty is at least as effective as treatment with topical β-adrenergic antagonist in preserving visual function and optic nerve head status and can be considered as initial treatment.[1] Even though initial treatment of POAG with surgical trabeculectomy compared to medical therapy has similar visual field outcomes at 5 years, surgical intervention is associated with more eye discomfort and increased risk of cataract development.[2,23,24] Surgical therapy is typically not considered as a first-line therapy.[5] Laser or surgical candidates may require additional procedures or medical therapy to main long-term IOP control.[1,5] Table 61–3 describes nonpharmacologic treatment modalities for POAG.

Medical treatment is the most commonly selected therapeutic modality. A well-tolerated ocular antihypertensive, at the lowest concentration, should be selected as the initial mediation (Table 61–4). If monotherapy alone lowers IOP but does not reach target pressure, then combination therapy or switching to another agent is appropriate. Increasing the concentration or dose frequency can also be tried when possible. A uniocular trial can be used to assess the safety and effectiveness of a topical medication before initiation in both eyes; however uniocular drug trials do not always predict the IOP response of the second eye. The lack of correlation between IOP of fellow eyes may be explained by asymmetric IOP in each eye or the potential for contralateral IOP lowering of a uniocular applied medication. Uniocular trials may be more predictive of fellow eye response to a medication in POAG suspects than POAG patients. Ideally, the effect of a medication should be assessed independently using baseline IOP measurements.[29,30]

Table 61–3	
Select Nonpharmacologic Treatment Options for POAG	
	Description
Laser trabeculoplasty	Laser energy aimed at trabecular meshwork
	Improves aqueous humor outflow
Trabeculectomy	Surgical removal of a portion of the trabecular meshwork
	Improves aqueous humor outflow
	Mitomycin C and fluorouracil are used to decrease scarring
Cyclodestructive surgery	Trans-scleral laser reduce rate of aqueous humor production
	Reserved for patients who have failed other options

From Refs. 1, 5, 10.

Treatment Considerations for POAG Suspects POAG suspects should be considered for topical medication therapy if they can be expected to develop optic nerve damage or they may already have early glaucomatous nerve damage that cannot reliably be diagnosed because of inconclusive exam findings. The Ocular Hypertension Treatment Study demonstrated that a 20% decrease in IOP can reduce the progression from ocular hypertension to POAG over a 5-year period. The incidence of progression to POAG in the treatment (4.4%) and control (9.5%) groups was small which underscores the importance of selecting patients at high risk of progressing to POAG.[31] When medical therapy is indicated, a well-tolerated agent should be selected and optimized following the POAG algorithm (Fig. 61–4). The risk to benefit of therapy should be reassessed in patients who may require third or fourth line agents to control IOP. Surgical or laser intervention are rarely indicated in the treatment of glaucoma suspects.[32]

Primary Angle-Closure Glaucoma

▶ Desired Outcomes and Goals

Therapeutic modalities for PACG are targeted at decreasing IOP. The goals of therapy are to preserve visual function by controlling the elevation in IOP; manage an acute attack of angle closure; reverse or prevent angle closure using a laser and/or surgical intervention; educate and involve the patient in the management of the disease.[10]

▶ General Approach

The treatment of choice for PACG is laser iridotomy. Medical therapy is used to lower IOP, reduce pain, and reverse corneal edema before the iridotomy. Laser iridotomy uses laser energy to cut a hole into the iris to alleviate the aqueous humor buildup behind the iris resulting in reversal of appositional angle closure. IOP should first be lowered

Table 61–4

Topical Drugs Used in the Treatment of Glaucoma

Drug	Pharmacologic Properties	Common Brand Names	Dose Form	Strength (%)	Usual Dose[a]	Mechanism of Action
β-Adrenergic Blocking Agents						
Betaxolol	Relative $β_1$-selective	Generic	Solution	0.5	1 drop twice a day	All reduce aqueous production of ciliary body
		Betoptic-S	Suspension	0.25	1 drop twice a day	
Carteolol	Nonselective, intrinsic sympathomimetic activity	Generic	Solution	1	1 drop twice a day	
Levobunolol	Nonselective	Betagan	Solution	0.25, 0.5	1 drop twice a day	
Metipranolol	Nonselective	OptiPranolol	Solution	0.3	1 drop twice a day	
Timolol	Nonselective	Timoptic, Betimol, Istalol	Solution	0.25, 0.5	1 drop every day— 1–2 times a day	
		Timoptic-XE	Gelling solution	0.25, 0.5	1 drop every day[a]	
Nonspecific Adrenergic Agonists						
Dipivefrin	Prodrug	Propine	Solution	0.1	1 drop twice a day	Increased aqueous humor outflow
$α_2$-Adrenergic Agonists						
Apraclonidine	Specific a_2-agonists	Iopidine	Solution	0.5, 1	1 drop 2–3 times a day	Both reduce aqueous humor production; brimonidine known to also increase uveoscleral outflow
Brimonidine		Alphagan P	Solution	0.15, 0.1	1 drop 2–3 times a day	
Cholinergic Agonists Direct Acting						
Carbachol	Irreversible	Carboptic, Isopto Carbachol	Solution	1.5, 3	1 drop 2–3 times a day	All increase aqueous humor outflow through trabecular meshwork
Pilocarpine	Irreversible	Isopto Carpine Pilocar	Solution	0.25, 0.5, 1, 2, 4, 6, 8, 10	1 drop 2–3 times a day	
		Pilopine HS	Gel	4	1 drop 4 times a day Every 24 hours at bedtime	
Cholinesterase Inhibitors						
Echothiophate		Phospholine Iodide	Solution	0.125	Once or twice a day	
Carbonic Anhydrase Inhibitors						
Topical Brinzolamide	Carbonic anhydrase type II inhibition	Azopt	Suspension	1	2–3 times a day	All reduce aqueous humor production of ciliary body
Dorzolamide		Trusopt	Solution	2	2–3 times a day	
Systemic Acetazolamide		Generic	Tablet	125 mg, 250 mg	125–250 mg 2–4 times a day	
			Injection	500 mg/vial	250–500 mg	
Methazolamide		Diamox Sequels	Capsule	500 mg	500 mg twice a day	
		Generic	Tablet	25 mg, 50 mg	25–50 mg 2–3 times a day	
Prostaglandin Analogs						
Latanoprost	Prostaglandin $F_{2α}$ analog	Xalatan	Solution	0.005	1 drop every night	Increases aqueous uveoscleral outflow and, to a lesser extent, trabecular outflow
Bimatoprost	Prostamide analog	Lumigan	Solution	0.03	1 drop every night	
Travoprost		Travatan, Travatan Z	Solution	0.004	1 drop every night	
Combinations						
Timolol-dorzolamide		Cosopt	Solution		Timolol 0.5% dorzolamide 2%	1 drop twice daily
Timolol-brimonidine		Combigan	Solution		Timolol 0.5% brimonide 0.2%	1 drop twice daily

[a]Use of nasolacrimal occlusion will increase the number of patients sucessfully treated with longer dosing intervals.

From DiPiro JT, Talbert RL, Yee GC, et al., (eds.) Pharmacotherapy: A Pathophysiologic Approach. 7th ed. New York: McGraw-Hill; 2008.

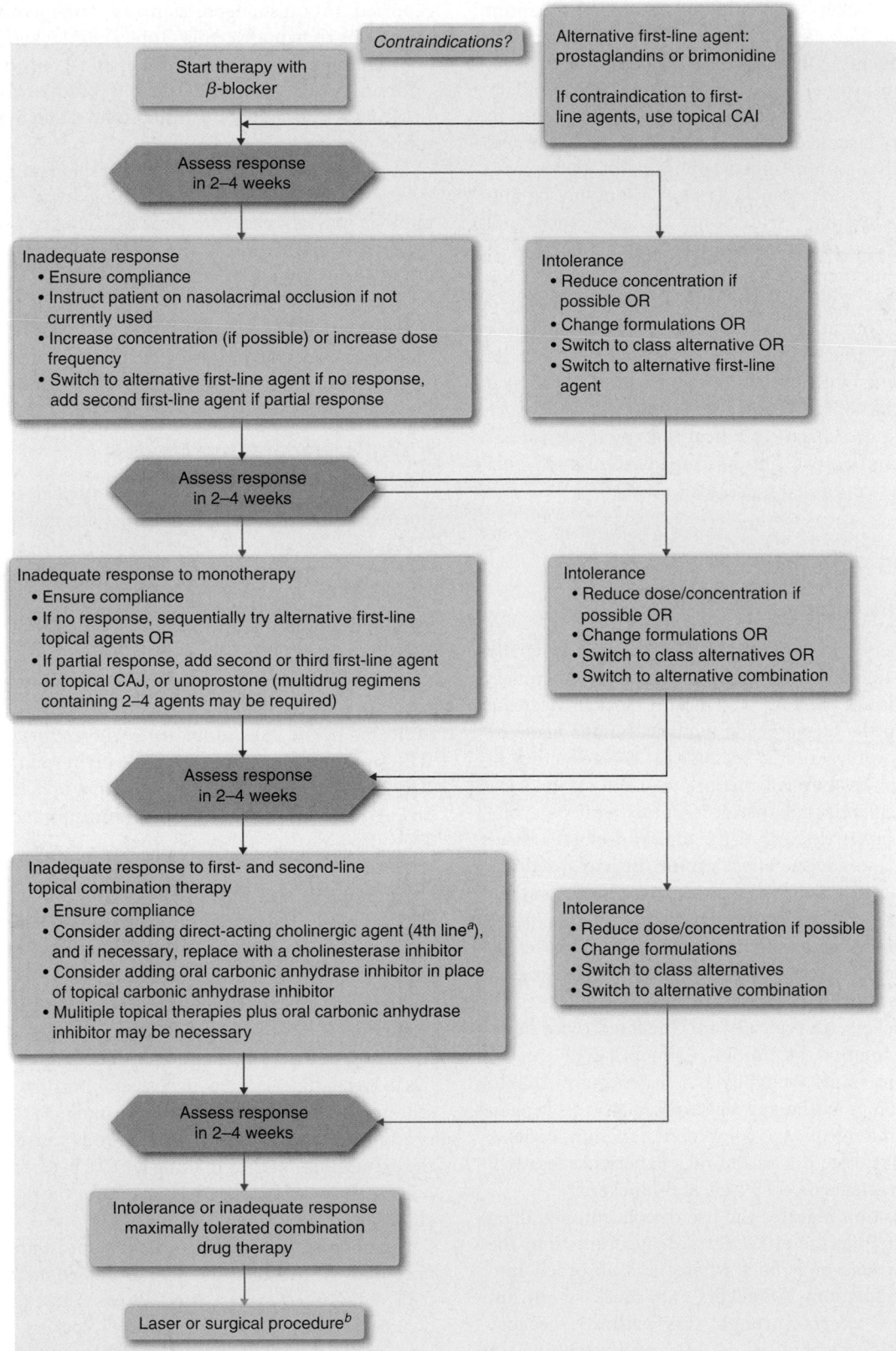

FIGURE 61–4. Algorithm for the pharmacotherapy of open-angle glaucoma. [a]Fourth-line agents not commonly used any longer. [b]Most clinicians believe laser procedures should be performed earlier (e.g., after three-drug maximum, poorly adherent patient). CAI, carbonic anhydrase inhibitor. (From Lesar TS, Fiscella RG, Edward D. Glaucoma. In: DiPiro JT, Talbert RL, Yee GC, et al., eds. Pharmacotherapy: A Pathophysiologic Approach, 7th ed. New York: McGraw-Hill, 2008:1557.)

with topical β-blockers, topical α-agonist, prostaglandin $F_{2\alpha}$ analog, systemic carbonic anhydrase inhibitors, or hyperosmotic agents. Once the IOP has been controlled, miotics (i.e., pilocarpine) can be used to break the pupillary block. A topical IOP-lowering agent should be continued to control IOP until laser iridotomy can be performed. Corneal indentation with a cotton-tipped applicator or gonioscopic lens may break pupillary block. If laser iridotomy cannot be performed incisional iridectomy is used. Incisional iridectomy is the surgical removal of a small portion of the iris to allow drainage of aqueous humor trapped in the posterior chamber. Topical corticosteroid may be employed to decrease inflammation. The fellow eye is at high risk of having acute attack and should receive prophylactic iridotomy. Patients with chronic angle closure should also receive laser iridotomy. Acute and chronic angle-closure patients may require chronic medical therapy if the patient has PACG superimposed on pre-existing POAG or if synechia formation causes continued increases in IOP.[7,10,33]

Pharmacologic Therapy

▶ β-Adrenergic Antagonists

Topical β-adrenergic antagonists (β-blockers) are generally considered first-line agents for the treatment of POAG unless contraindications are present.[11,13] Topical β-blockers decrease IOP by reducing the formation of aqueous humor made by the ciliary body which results in 20% to 35% reduction in IOP.[11,13,34] Timolol, levobunolol, metipranolol and carteolol are nonselective for β_1- and β_2-adrenergic receptors, while betaxolol has β_1-selective properties. All of the topical β-blockers have similar efficacy and adverse effect profile. Betaxolol reduces IOP to a lesser extent than the nonselective β-blockers, but may cause less exacerbation of pulmonary disease. Despite the intrinsic sympathomimetic activity demonstrated by carteolol, this does not translate to a clinically significant decrease in pulmonary or cardiovascular adverse effects.

Topical β-blockers are typically administered twice daily. A gel-forming solution of timolol (Timoptic-XE) can be administered once daily. Tachyphylaxis may occur in 20% to 50% of patients on monotherapy with a β-blocker resulting in the need for a different agent or combination therapy. Patients on concurrent systemic β-blockers may experience less IOP reduction than patients on only topical β-blockers.[11,35]

Ocular medication requires the use of concentrated drug solutions to penetrate the eye. Excess drug drains into the nose via the nasolacrimal duct where it is absorbed into the systemic circulation. β-Blockers can cause significant systemic adverse effects through this pathway, because first-pass hepatic metabolism is bypassed resulting in pharmacologically significant serum drug concentrations.[36] Bronchospasm is the most common pulmonary effect of topical β-blockers. Pulmonary edema, *status asthmaticus,* and respiratory arrest have been reported with β-blockers as well. Cardiovascular effects include bradycardia, hypotension, and congestive heart failure exacerbation. As with systemic β-blockers, topical β-blockers have also been reported to cause depression, hyperlipidemia, and mask symptoms of hypoglycemia. Topical β-blockers are generally contraindicated in patients with asthma, chronic obstructive pulmonary disease (COPD), sinus bradycardia, second or third degree heart block, cardiac failure, and hypersensitivity to the product.[11,36,37]

Local side effects are usually tolerable and may be caused by preservatives, therefore switching from one product to another may alleviate the local side effects. Stinging of the eyes upon instillation is the most common adverse effect. Other local adverse effects include conjunctivitis, keratitis, dry eyes, and uveitis.[11,13]

Patients prescribed topical β-blockers should be counseled on the nasolacrimal occlusion technique to decrease systemic absorption.

▶ Ocular Hypotensive Lipids

The ocular hypotensive lipids in typical ophthalmology practice are considered first-line alternatives to topical β-blockers because of their superior efficacy and safety profiles. Many clinicians may choose to use the ocular hypotensive lipids as first line, especially in patients who have an initial requirement to lower IOP by greater than 25%, or in patients who have relative or absolute contraindications to topical β-blockers.[11,35] Bimatoprost and latanoprost currently have an FDA indication for first-line therapy. Travoprost is indicated by the FDA for patients who are intolerant of other IOP-lowering therapy or insufficiently responsive to another IOP-lowering medication. Latanoprost and travoprost have dosing aids that help patients administer each medication. Travoprost dosing aid is electronic and allows practitioners to track usage of travoprost.

Latanoprost and travoprost are analogs of prostaglandin $F_{2\alpha}$ and are agonists of the prostanoid FP receptor which appears to lower IOP by increasing aqueous humor outflow through the uveoscleral pathway. Bimatoprost is a prostamide analog and appears to lower IOP by activating prostamide receptors in the uveoscleral pathway and possibly through increasing outflow through the trabecular meshwork. The exact mechanism of how uveoscleral outflow is increased is still unclear but stimulation of prostanoid FP receptors and prostamide receptors in the ciliary body cause remodeling of the extracelluar matrix making it more permeable to aqueous humor, thus increasing aqueous humor outflow through the ciliary muscles.[14,15,38]

Latanoprost, travoprost, and bimatoprost are administered once daily at bedtime and should not be increased to twice daily, as this may decrease effectiveness. These agents lower IOP by 25% to 35% and, unlike topical β-blockers, can effectively lower nocturnal IOP, providing IOP control throughout a 24-hour period. The prostaglandin analogs can be used as mono- or combination therapy.[11,35] For patients nonresponsive to latanoprost, switching to brimatoprost may allow some patients to reach their IOP goal presumably because of the proposed difference in the site of action of each drug.[39,40]

The ocular hypotensive lipids are well tolerated and rarely cause systemic side effects (headache has been reported).

Local effects include conjunctival hyperemia, stinging on instillation, increase in iris pigmentation, hypertrichosis, and darkening of the eyelashes. Increases in iris pigmentation occur most commonly in patients with multicolored irides on long-term prostaglandin analog therapy. The mechanism of this effect is by its action on melanocytes of the iris, in which the irides become darker because of increased production of melanin in the iris.[41,42] The 12-month incidence of iris pigmentation varies among the agents. Latanoprost appears to have the highest incidence of iris pigmentation after 12 months of therapy (5.2–25%) compared to travoprost (3.1%) and bimatoprost (1–5.5%).[43–48] The increase in pigmentation may be irreversible or may reverse at a very slow rate. Increased iris pigmentation appears to be only a cosmetic effect but may affect your product selection especially when choosing monocular therapy. Conjunctival hyperemia or engorgement of conjunctival blood vessels is a common adverse effect caused by a vasodilatory effect on scleral blood vessels. It is most prominent early in therapy and usually subsides over time. While generally a benign adverse effect, patients may have a concern if it affects their cosmetic appearance.[43–48] The ocular hypotensive lipids should be used with caution in patients, since they may worsen anterior uveitis and herpetic keratitis. Cystoid macular edema has been reported during treatment with the ocular hypotensive lipids, therefore, use caution in patients with intraocular inflammation, aphakic patients, pseudophakic patients with a torn posterior lens capsule, or in patients with risk factors for macular edema.[11,35]

Patients prescribed ocular hypotensive lipids should be counseled on potential adverse effects and appropriate administration. Patients receiving latanoprost therapy should be instructed to refrigerate the dropper bottle until opened. After the bottle has been opened it can be stored at room temperature for 6 weeks.

▶ α_2-Adrenergic Agonists

Brimonidine and apraclonidine are α_2-adrenergic agonists that decrease IOP by reducing aqueous humor production. Brimonidine has a higher selectivity to the α_2-receptor than apraclonidine and has a dual mechanism of action by increasing uveoscleral outflow.[11,14] Apraclonidine is often used for the prevention and treatment of postsurgical IOP elevations and no longer commonly used for long-term treatment of POAG because of tachyphylaxis and high rate of blepharoconjunctivitis. Brimonidine lowers IOP by 14% to 28%. Peak IOP-lowering effect is similar to that of timolol, but the trough IOP-lowering effect is less than timolol. Brimonidine is usually administered every 8 hours. A 12-hour dosing schedule may be employed by using nasolacrimal occlusion when instilling the drops. Brimonidine-purite 0.1% and 0.15% solution (Alphagan-P) has similar efficacy compared to the brimondine 0.2% solution, because the purite solution's higher pH allows for more drug to penetrate the cornea.[11,13,14]

Apraclonidine and brimonidine cause both local and systemic effects. Local effects of apraclonidine include blepharoconjunctivitis, foreign body sensation, pupillary mydrasis and eyelid retraction. Brimonidine does not cause the α_1-mediated mydrasis and eyelid retraction but does cause blepharoconjunctivitis though at a lesser rate than apraclonidine. The brimonidine-purite solution has a lower incidence of ocular allergy. Systemic effects of both agents include headache, dry mouth, and fatigue.

Brimonidine is typically used as an adjunctive agent in combination with other agents but could be used as a first-line agent as well. The frequency of dosing and local adverse effects may lead to nonadherence in some patients. Patients prescribed brimonidine should be counseled on the nasolacrimal occlusion technique to reduce systemic adverse effects and to improve efficacy.[11,13] A combination product of brimonidine (0.2%) and timolol (0.5%) (Combigan) is available and can be administered twice daily.

▶ Carbonic Anhydrase Inhibitors

Carbonic anhydrase inhibitors decrease aqueous humor production by inhibition of the carbonic anydrase isoenzyme II located in the ciliary body. In the eye, carbonic anhydrase catalyzes the conversion of H_2O and CO_2 to HCO_3^- and H^+, which is a significant step in aqueous humor production. Carbonic anhydrase inhibitors are available in systemic and topical preparations.[11,13,14]

Topical Carbonic Anhydrase Inhibitors Dorzolamide and brinzolamide are the only topical carbonic anhydrase inhibitors available on the market and lower IOP by 15% to 24%. Both medications are administered every 8 hours and are used as adjunctive therapy or as monotherapy for patients who cannot tolerate first-line therapies. Nasolacrimal occlusion may allow for an every 12-hour dosing interval.[11,13] Recently the European Glaucoma Prevention Study found that dorzolamide did not prevent the progression of patients with ocular hypertension to POAG despite a 15% to 22% reduction of IOP over 5 years. Unlike the Ocular Hypertension Treatment Study, a goal IOP reduction of at least 20% was not required for treatment and surprisingly, the placebo treatment had a clinically significant effect on IOP.[49]

Local side effects include burning, stinging, itching foreign body sensation, dry eyes, and conjunctivitis. Brinzolamide may have fewer incidences of these side effects since the drug is in a neutral pH solution. Dorzolamide has been reported to cause irreversible corneal decompensation. Taste abnormalities have been reported with each agent. Both topical carbonic anhydrase inhibitors are sulfonamides and are contraindicated in patients with history of sulfonamide hypersensitivity.[11,13]

A combination product of timolol (0.5%) and dorzolamide (2%) (Cosopt) is available, can be administered twice daily, and provides an additive reduction in IOP.

Systemic Carbonic Anhydrase Inhibitors There are three systemic carbonic anhydrase inhibitors: acetazolamide, dichlorphenamide, and methazolamide. These agents effectively lower IOP by 20% to 30% but are reserved as third-line agents because of their significant adverse effects. They

Patient Encounter 1, Part 2

The patient was referred to an ophthalmologist for a comprehensive eye evaluation. The ophthalmology report reveals the patient has an IOP (as assessed by applanation tonometry) of 26 mm Hg. Gonioscopic examination reveals open anterior angles in both eyes. Pachymetry reveals a corneal thickness of 510 microns. Ophthalmoscopy reveals cupping of the optic discs in both eyes. Visual field examination reveals a nerve fiber bundle defect consistent with glaucoma.

Given this additional information, what additional risk factors does this patient have for glaucoma?

What is your assessment of this patient's glaucoma type?

What pharmacologic and nonpharmacologic treatment modalities are available for the patient?

are typically used as bridge therapy from maximal medical therapy to laser or surgical intervention. The systemic carbonic anhydrase inhibitors can also be used to lower IOP in acute angle-closure glaucoma. Acetazolamide has an IV formulation that can be used in patients having nausea due to the angle-closure attack. Acetazolamide and methazolamide are the best tolerated of the three agents.

The systemic carbonic anhydrase inhibitors are associated with significant adverse effects that include paresthesias of the hands and feet, nausea, vomiting, and weight loss. Patients can develop systemic acidosis, hypokalemia, hyponatremia, and nephrolithiasis due to the inhibition of renal carbonic anhydrase. Sulfonamide allergy, renal failure, hepatic insufficiency, COPD, and decreased serum potassium and sodium levels are all contraindications of systemic carbonic anhydrase inhibitor therapy. Blood dyscrasias from bone marrow suppression have been reported and include agranulocytosis, aplastic anemia, neutropenia, and thrombocytopenia.[11,13]

▶ Cholinergic Agents

Cholinergic agents (also called parasympathomimetics or miotics) were the first class of agents to treat glaucoma. The class can be divided into direct-acting cholinergic agents and indirect-acting cholinergic agents.

Direct-Acting Cholinergic Agents Pilocarpine directly stimulates the muscarinic (M_3) receptors of the ciliary body which causes contraction of the ciliary muscle. This results in widening of the spaces in the trabecular meshwork, which causes an increase in aqueous humor outflow and reduces IOP by 20% to 30%.

Pilocarpine requires administration four times daily, since the IOP-lowering effect lasts only 6 hours. Pilocarpine is available in 1%, 2%, 4%, 6%, and 8% concentrations. Higher concentrations may be needed for patients with dark irides to obtain adequate IOP reduction. A pilocarpine 4% gel is

available and allows for once daily dosing at bedtime.[11,13] In the treatment of PACG, it is important to delay use until IOP has been controlled, because pilocarpine could worsen angle closure by causing anterior displacement of the lens. Once IOP is controlled pilocarpine can be given to break pupillary block by instilling one drop applied twice in an hour.

The adverse effects of pilocarpine are caused by the induction of miosis. The contraction of the ciliary muscle causes the lens to displace forward, which can lead to accommodation spasm and myopia, and can lead to brow ache. Pupillary constriction can also affect night vision. Pilocarpine should be avoided in patients with severe myopia as it increases the risk of developing retinal detachment. Systemic effects may occur at higher concentrations and include nausea, vomiting and diarrhea, and bradycardia.

Carbachol stimulates the same muscarinic receptor as pilocarpine and also inhibits acetylcholinesterase, the enzyme that metabolizes acetylcholine. Carbachol is more potent than pilocarpine, but it causes more accommodation spasm and brow ache and may also cause anterior uveitis. Carbachol is rarely used today because of the side effect profile.

Indirect-Acting Cholinergic Agents Echothiophate iodide and demecarium bromide inhibit acetylcholinesterase. Inhibition of this enzyme increases the availability of acetylcholine at the nerve junction, thus increasing the stimulation of the muscarinic (M_3) receptors of the ciliary body. These products are given twice daily and have similar efficacy to pilocarpine in the degree of IOP reduction. The side effect profile is similar to pilocarpine, however, they can deplete systemic cholinesterases and pseudocholinesterases and may cause the formation of cataracts. These agents should be discontinued at least 1 week before general surgical procedures. Succinylcholine and some local anesthetics are metabolized by pseudocholinesterases, therefore, depletion of this enzyme by echothiopate or demecarium may lead to toxic effects. These agents are typically used when other topical agents have failed and are limited to patients who have had their lenses removed or who have artificial lenses.[11,13]

▶ Hyperosmotics

Glycerin, isosorbide, and mannitol are hyperosmotic agents that increase the osmolality of blood. These agents create an osmotic gradient that draws water from the vitreous humor thus decreasing IOP. The resulting dehydration of the vitreous humor may cause posterior movement of the lens, which then causes the anterior chamber to deepen, thus opening the anterior angle. If the patient is not vomiting, glycerin (1–1.5 g/kg of a 50%) solution and isosorbide (1.5–2 g/kg) can be given orally. Isosorbide is preferred in patients with diabetes because it is not metabolized into glucose. If the patient has nausea or vomiting, mannitol (20%) can be given IV at a dose of 1 to 2 g/kg over 45 minutes. The hyperosmotic agents are rapid acting, reaching peak effect in 30 to 60 minutes. Headache and thirst are common complaints. Patients who are already dehydrated are at risk of developing CNS dehydration, which can lead to coma. These agents should be used with caution in patients with renal or cardiovascular disease as extracellular water is increased.[33]

▶ Nonselective Adrenergic Agonists

Epinephrine and its prodrug, dipivefrine, are rarely used for the treatment of glaucoma and are considered last line agents because of their systemic side effect profile. Dipivefrine increases the corneal penetration. Once it is absorbed through the cornea, it is enzymatically cleaved to epinephrine. Epinephrine has α and β-agonist activity and is thought to increase the outflow of aqueous humor through the trabecular meshwork and the uveoscleral pathway. Both products are instilled twice daily and reduce IOP by 15% to 25%. Local adverse effects include mydriasis, conjunctival hyperemia, and ocular irritation. Aphakic patients should not use these medications because they cause a reversible cystoid macular edema. Epinephrine and dipivefrine should not be used in patients with narrow angles since these agents can cause acute angle closure. Systemic side effects include palpitations, increased blood pressure, and arrhythmia and, therefore, these drugs should be used with caution in patients with cardiovascular disease, cerebrovascular disease, and hyperthyroidism. Using the nasolacrimal technique may decrease systemic effects.[11,13]

SPECIAL CONSIDERATIONS: DRUG-INDUCED GLAUCOMAS

Medications have the potential to cause or exacerbate both POAG and PACG; however, PACG is more likely to be exacerbated by medications than POAG. The use of medications with anticholinergic or sympathomimetics properties can precipitate angle closure. Sulfa-based drugs cause swelling of the ciliary body, which causes an anterior displacement of the lens resulting in a decrease in anterior-chamber depth. Controlled POAG is rarely exacerbated by anticholinergics, sympathomometics, and sulfa-based drugs unless the patient is concomitantly at risk for angle closure. For uncontrolled or untreated POAG, the risk-benefit should be considered before employing these agents. POAG can be exacerbated by corticosteroids. Corticosteroids increase

IOP by causing obstruction of the trabecular meshwork with extracellular material. The increase in IOP appears to increase with potency and intraocular penetration. Ophthalmic corticosteroid preparations carry the highest risk of increasing IOP.[12]

OUTCOME EVALUATION

Primary Open-Angle Glaucoma

Evaluate patients 2 to 4 weeks after the initiation or alteration of medical therapy. The clinician should elicit the status of ocular health since the last visit, systemic medical history, medication history, and presence of local and ocular adverse effects of medications. IOP measurement, visual acuity assessment, and slit-lamp biomicroscopy at every POAG follow-up visit is necessary. The frequency of visual fields and optic nerve evaluation depends on whether IOP is controlled, the length of time IOP has been controlled, and whether there is progression of the disease. Patients who are at target IOP and have no disease progression should have optic nerve head evaluation and visual field testing every 6 to 18 months. Patients with disease progression or who are not at target IOP should receive optic nerve head evaluation every 2 to 12 months and visual field testing every 1 to 6 months.[1] Assess the patient's ability to use topical eye drops.[1,32] (See Application of Ophthalmic Solutions of Suspensions textbox.) Finally, evaluate the patient's adherence to their medical regimen. Nonadherence among patients on topical medical therapy

---

Patient Encounter 1, Part 3

The practitioner and patient agree to start medication therapy. Develop a patient-specific care plan.

Address the patient's (a) drug-related needs, (b) goals of therapy, (c) potential pharmacologic therapies, and (d) plan for follow-up therapy.

List the monitoring parameters for effectiveness and safety for the chosen therapy.

Explain how you would counsel the patient on the chosen therapy, including the administration of an ophthalmic preparation.

Application of Ophthalmic Solutions or Suspensions

1. Clean hands with soap and water.
2. Avoid touching the dropper tip with your fingers or against your eye to maintain sterility of product; shake dropper bottle if product is a suspension.
3. Tilt head back; pull down the lower eye lid with index finger.
4. Hold the dropper bottle with other hand as close as possible without touching the eye. The dropper should be pointing toward the eye with remaining fingers bracing against the face.
5. Gently squeeze the bottle so that one drop is placed into the pocket.
6. Close your eye for 2 to 3 minutes to allow for the maximum corneal penetration of drug
7. Use a tissue to wipe away any excess liquid.
8. Replace and retighten the cap to the dropper bottle.
9. Wait at least 5 minutes before instilling another ophthalmic drug preparation
10. Application of some ophthalmic preparations (suspension and gels) may cause blurring of vision.

ranges from 5% to 80%. Suspect nonadherence in patients who have visual field and optic nerve progression despite a low IOP measurement, as patients may be more adherent to their medical regimen before their visit. Specific patient factors related to the risk of nonadherence have yet to be established, therefore there are few objective measures of adherence. Pharmacy refill histories may be useful in assessing adherence but do not confirm that the patient is actually taking the regimen as prescribed. Using adherence aids, prescribing the least complex regimen, and educating patients about their glaucoma are ways to reduce nonadherence.[50]

Adjust therapy if patients fail to reach their target IOP. Patients who have achieved target IOP yet have progressive damage of the optic nerve or who have worsening of their visual fields should have further adjustment of their therapy. Evaluate these patients further for possible reasons of continued disease progression. Consider determining the diurnal pattern of IOP and looking for signs of poor ocular perfusion pressure. Establish a lower target IOP. Adjust therapy in patients who are intolerant, nonadherent, or develop contraindications to their drug therapy regimen. Consider increasing the target IOP and reducing drug therapy for patients who have stable disease and who have maintained a low IOP; closely follow these patients to assess their response.[1,32]

Primary Angle-Closure Glaucoma

Follow-up of PACG occurs in the postoperative period. Evaluate the patency of the iridotomy and IOP in the postoperative period. Perform gonioscopy and optic nerve head evaluation if not already performed. Treat patients according to POAG guidelines if they have underlying POAG or areas of peripheral anterior synechia with the presence of optic neuropathy.[10]

Abbreviations Introduced in This Chapter

AAO	American Academy of Ophthalmology
CCT	Central corneal thickness
IOP	Intraocular pressure
NTG	Normal-tension glaucoma
OHTS	The Ocular Hypertension Study
PACG	Primary angle-closure glaucoma
POAG	Primary open-angle glaucoma

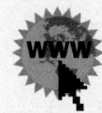 Self-assessment questions and answers are available at http://www.mhpharmacotherapy.com/pp.html.

Patient Care and Monitoring

1. In undiagnosed patients assess their risk factors for glaucoma and their recommended interval of glaucoma screening

2. Obtain a thorough history of the patient's prescription, nonprescription, and natural product use. Review for potential drug–drug and drug–glaucoma interactions

3. Evaluate diagnostic tests (IOP, visual fields, optic nerve evaluations, etc.) to determine if patient's current glaucoma therapy is effective

4. Assess the patient's ability to use ophthalmic preparations

5. Determine patient's adherence level to prescribed medication regimen and factors contributing to poor adherence

6. Evaluate the patient for systemic and ocular adverse drug reactions and drug allergy

7. Provide patient education regarding disease state, drug therapy, and surgical/laser therapy:

   - What causes glaucoma or puts people at risk for glaucoma

   - Possible complications of glaucoma

   - How to use ophthalmic preparations appropriately

   - When to take medications

   - Potential adverse drug reactions of medical therapy

   - Potential benefits and complications of laser or surgical procedures

REFERENCES

1. Panel AAoOG. Primary Open Angle. San Francisco: American Academy of Opthalmology, 2005.
2. Sycha T, Vass C, Findl O, et al. Interventions for normal tension glaucoma. Cochrane Database Syst Rev 2003;(4):CD002222.
3. Resnikoff S, Pascolini D, Etya'ale D, et al. Global data on visual impairment in the year 2002. Bull World Health Organ 2004;82(11): 844–851.
4. Friedman DS, Wolfs RC, O'Colmain BJ, et al. Prevalence of open-angle glaucoma among adults in the United States. Arch Ophthalmol 2004;122(4):532–538.
5. Weinreb RN, Khaw PT. Primary open-angle glaucoma. Lancet 2004 May 22;363(9422):1711–1720.
6. Gordon MO, Beiser JA, Brandt JD, et al. The ocular hypertension treatment study: Baseline factors that predict the onset of primary open-angle glaucoma. Arch Ophthalmol 2002;120(6):714–720; discussion 829–830.
7. Coleman AL. Glaucoma. Lancet 1999;354(9192):1803–1810.
8. Bonomi L. Epidemiology of angle-closure glaucoma. Acta Ophthalmol Scand Suppl 2002;236:11–13.
9. Herndon LW, Weizer JS, Stinnett SS. Central corneal thickness as a risk factor for advanced glaucoma damage. Arch Ophthalmol 2004;122(1):17–21.
10. Panel AAoOG. Primary Angle Closure. San Francisco: American Academy of Ophthalmology, 2005.
11. Marquis RE, Whitson JT. Management of glaucoma: Focus on pharmacological therapy. Drugs Aging 2005; 22(1):1–21.
12. Tripathi RC, Tripathi BJ, Haggerty C. Drug-induced glaucomas: Mechanism and management. Drug Saf 2003;26(11):749–767.

13. Hoyng PF, van Beek LM. Pharmacological therapy for glaucoma: A review. Drugs 2000;59(3):411–434.
14. Woodward DF, Gil DW. The inflow and outflow of anti-glaucoma drugs. Trends Pharmacol Sci 2004;25(5):238–241.
15. Krauss AH, Woodward DF. Update on the mechanism of action of bimatoprost: A review and discussion of new evidence. Surv Ophthalmol 2004;49(Suppl 1):S5–S11.
16. Civan MM, Macknight AD. The ins and outs of aqueous humour secretion. Exp Eye Res 2004;78(3):625–631.
17. Gherghel D, Hosking SL, Orgul S. Autonomic nervous system, circadian rhythms, and primary open-angle glaucoma. Surv Ophthalmol 2004;49(5):491–508.
18. Wax MB, Camras CB, Fiscella RG, Girkin C, Singh K, Weinreb RN. Emerging perspectives in glaucoma: Optimizing 24-hour control of intraocular pressure. Am J Ophthalmol 2002;133 (Suppl):S1–10.
19. Shields MB. Normal-tension glaucoma: Is it different from primary open-angle glaucoma? Curr Opin Ophthalmol 2008;19(2):85–88.
20. Khaw PT, Shah P, Elkington AR. Glaucoma—1: Diagnosis. BMJ 2004;328(7431):97–99.
21. Morrison JC, Johnson EC, Cepurna W, Jia L. Understanding mechanisms of pressure-induced optic nerve damage. Prog Retin Eye Res 2005;24(2):217–240.
22. Flammer J, Orgul S, Costa VP, et al. The impact of ocular blood flow in glaucoma. Prog Retin Eye Res 2002;21(4):359–393.
23. Collaborative Normal-Tension Glaucoma Study Group. Comparison of glaucomatous progression between untreated patients with normal-tension glaucoma and patients with therapeutically reduced intraocular pressures. Am J Ophthalmol 1998;126(4):487–497.
24. Collaborative Normal-Tension Glaucoma Study Group. The effectiveness of intraocular pressure reduction in the treatment of normal-tension glaucoma. Am J Ophthalmol 1998;126(4):498–505.
25. Quigley HA, Friedman DS, Congdon NG. Possible mechanisms of primary angle-closure and malignant glaucoma. J Glaucoma 2003;12(2):167–180.
26. Salmon JF, Sharma T. Chronic angle-closure glaucoma. Ophthalmology 2005;112(10):1844.
27. Robin AL, Frick KD, Katz J, et al. The ocular hypertension treatment study: Intraocular pressure lowering prevents the development of glaucoma, but does that mean we should treat before the onset of disease? Arch Ophthalmol 2004;122(3):376–378.
28. Heijl A, Leske MC, Bengtsson B, et al. Reduction of intraocular pressure and glaucoma progression: Results from the Early Manifest Glaucoma Trial. Arch Ophthalmol 2002;120(10):1268–1279.
29. Chaudhary O, Adelman RA, Shields MB. Predicting response to glaucoma therapy in one eye based on response in the fellow eye: The monocular trial. Arch Ophthalmol 2008;126(9):1216–1220.
30. Realini T, Fechtner RD, Atreides SP, Gollance S. The uniocular drug trial and second-eye response to glaucoma medications. Ophthalmology 2004;111(3):421–426.
31. Kass MA, Heuer DK, Higginbotham EJ, et al. The ocular hypertension treatment study: A randomized trial determines that topical ocular hypotensive medication delays or prevents the onset of primary open-angle glaucoma. Arch Ophthalmol 2002;120(6):701–713; discussion 829–830.
32. Panel A AoOG. Primary Open-Angle Glaucoma Suspect. San Francisco: American Academy of Ophthalmology, 2005:26.
33. Hoh ST, Aung T, Chew PT. Medical management of angle closure glaucoma. Semin Ophthalmol 2002;17(2):79–83.
34. van der Valk R, Webers CA, Schouten JS, et al. Intraocular pressure-lowering effects of all commonly used glaucoma drugs: A meta-analysis of randomized clinical trials. Ophthalmology 2005;112(7):1177–1185.
35. Cantor L. Achieving low target pressures with today's glaucoma medications. Surv Ophthalmol 2003;48(Suppl 1):S8–S16.
36. Vander Zanden JA, Valuck RJ, Bunch CL, et al. Systemic adverse effects of ophthalmic beta-blockers. Ann Pharmacother 2001;35(12):1633–1637.
37. Singh A. Medical therapy of glaucoma. Ophthalmol Clin North Am 2005;18(3):397–408, vi.
38. Eisenberg DL, Toris CB, Camras CB. Bimatoprost and travoprost: A review of recent studies of two new glaucoma drugs. Surv Ophthalmol 2002;47(Suppl 1):S105–S115.
39. Bournias TE, Lee D, Gross R, Mattox C. Ocular hypotensive efficacy of bimatoprost when used as a replacement for latanoprost in the treatment of glaucoma and ocular hypertension. J Ocul Pharmacol Ther 2003;19(3):193–203.
40. Gandolfi SA, Cimino L. Effect of bimatoprost on patients with primary open-angle glaucoma or ocular hypertension who are nonresponders to latanoprost. Ophthalmology 2003;110(3):609–614.
41. Grierson I, Jonsson M, Cracknell K. Latanoprost and pigmentation. Jpn J Ophthalmol 2004;48(6):602–612.
42. Stjernschantz JW, Albert DM, Hu DN, et al. Mechanism and clinical significance of prostaglandin-induced iris pigmentation. Surv Ophthalmol 2002;47(Suppl 1):S162–S175.
43. Cohen JS, Gross RL, Cheetham JK, et al. Two-year double-masked comparison of bimatoprost with timolol in patients with glaucoma or ocular hypertension. Surv Ophthalmol 2004;49(Suppl 1):S45–S52.
44. Easthope SE, Perry CM. Topical bimatoprost: A review of its use in open-angle glaucoma and ocular hypertension. Drugs Aging 2002;19(3):231–248.
45. Higginbotham EJ, Schuman JS, Goldberg I, et al. One-year, randomized study comparing bimatoprost and timolol in glaucoma and ocular hypertension. Arch Ophthalmol 2002;120(10):1286–1293.
46. Netland PA, Landry T, Sullivan EK, et al. Travoprost compared with latanoprost and timolol in patients with open-angle glaucoma or ocular hypertension. Am J Ophthalmol 2001;132(4):472–484.
47. Perry CM, McGavin JK, Culy CR, et al. Latanoprost: An update of its use in glaucoma and ocular hypertension. Drugs Aging 2003;20(8):597–630.
48. Wistrand PJ, Stjernschantz J, Olsson K. The incidence and time-course of latanoprost-induced iridial pigmentation as a function of eye color. Surv Ophthalmol 1997;41(Suppl 2):S129–S138.
49. Miglior S, Zeyen T, Pfeiffer N, et al. Results of the European Glaucoma Prevention Study. Ophthalmology 2005;112(3):366–375.
50. Olthoff CM, Schouten JS, van de Borne BW, Webers CA. Noncompliance with ocular hypotensive treatment in patients with glaucoma or ocular hypertension an evidence-based review. Ophthalmology 2005;112(6):953–961.

62 Allergic Rhinitis

David A. Apgar

LEARNING OBJECTIVES

● **Upon completion of the chapter, the reader will be able to:**

1. Describe two different systems for categorizing allergic rhinitis (AR).
2. Describe the basic pathophysiology of AR.
3. List the typical symptoms of AR and identify the most troublesome one.
4. List the reasons for referral to an allergy specialist.
5. Discuss the categories of pharmacotherapy choices for treatment of AR.
6. Rank the pharmacotherapy choices for efficacy in treating nasal congestion.
7. Describe an approach for treatment of mild AR with over-the-counter (OTC) drugs.
8. Create a therapy plan for treatment of moderate–severe AR.
9. Describe how to monitor patients treated for AR.
10. Identify the differences in approach to the treatment of AR for children, pregnant women, and the elderly, compared to the routine approach in adults.

KEY CONCEPTS

❶ Allergic rhinitis (AR) is an allergen-induced and immunoglobulin E (IgE)-mediated inflammatory condition of the lining of the nose and upper respiratory tract.

❷ AR can be categorized in different ways.

❸ AR is a common disorder that can negatively impact quality of life, yet it has been trivialized in the past.

❹ The goals of treatment of AR are to reduce or minimize the frequency and severity of symptoms; prevent comorbid disorders and complications; improve the patient's quality of life; improve work attendance and productivity and/or school attendance and performance; and minimize adverse effects of therapy.

❺ The general approach for treatment of AR is fourfold: avoidance of allergen triggers, pharmacotherapy, immunotherapy, and patient/family education.

❻ Routine first-line agents for the treatment of AR are intranasal corticosteroids and antihistamines (oral and/or intranasal, depending on the patient). Adjunctive or secondary choice agents, each of which may have a first-line role in selected patients, include decongestants, cromolyn, montelukast, ipratropium, and intranasal saline irrigation.

❼ Intranasal corticosteroids are the most effective therapy for AR, especially for nasal congestion. They are first-line agents for severe manifestations and are also used for those with moderate disease not controlled with oral and/or intranasal antihistamines. Their anti-inflammatory mechanism of action probably contributes to this superiority.

❽ Second-generation antihistamines are first-line agents, especially for mild or intermittent AR. They are preferred over first-generation antihistamines because of their improved side-effect profile. While effective for most symptoms of AR, they are less effective than intranasal corticosteroids for nasal congestion (intranasal administration is better than oral administration).

❾ The best application of decongestants in AR is short-term to overcome severe nasal congestion, including facilitating improved efficacy of intranasal agents. The intranasal administration of decongestants should usually not exceed three consecutive days.

❿ Generally speaking, the treatment of AR in children is the same as it is for adults, except for limitations in terms of FDA-approved products for some age groups and route of administration issues with some products.

INTRODUCTION[1-3]

Rhinitis is inflammation of the lining of the nose and other parts of the upper respiratory tract. Allergy is only one cause of rhinitis. While there are several other types of rhinitis (see Table 62–1), and some patients can manifest a mixed form (both allergic and nonallergic rhinitis), allergic rhinitis (AR) will be the focus of this chapter. Because ocular symptoms frequently occur in association with AR, another term used is allergic rhinoconjunctivitis. This acknowledges involvement of the bulbar and palpebral conjunctivae in the allergic process. ❶ *AR is an allergen-induced and immunoglobulin E (IgE)-mediated inflammatory condition of the lining of the nose and upper respiratory tract.*

❷ *AR has traditionally been categorized as either seasonal or perennial.* Seasonal allergic rhinitis (SAR) is attributed to inhaled allergens (aeroallergens) that have a seasonal variation. These allergens are usually encountered outdoors and are most often plant pollens and substances from molds and fungi. Perennial allergic rhinitis (PAR) is attributed to aeroallergens that are present in the patient's environment almost continuously throughout the year and are usually encountered indoors. Common perennial allergens are the house dust mite, indoor molds and fungi, insects (especially

---

Table 62–1

Types of Rhinitis

Allergic (see Table 62–2 for details)
Nonallergic
   Vasomotor (triggered by irritants, cold air, exercise/running, or unidentified factors)
   Food/meal related (gustatory)
   Infectious
   NARES
Occupational
   Caused by protein allergens (IgE-mediated) or by irritants/sensitizers (probably non-IgE-mediated)
Other rhinitis syndromes
   Hormonally related (pregnancy and menstrual cycle related)
   Drug-related
      Rhinitis medicamentosa (rebound from overuse of intranasal decongestants)
   Drug-induced
      Angiotensin-converting enzyme inhibitor (ACEI)
      a-Antagonists (used for treatment of BPH and HT)
      Phosphodiesterase-5 inhibitors (used for treatment of ED)
      Aspirin and other NSAIDs (as an isolated side effect of AERD)
      Oral contraceptives (controversial)
   Atrophic rhinitis
   Rhinitis associated with inflammatory or immunologic diseases (e.g., granulomatous infections, RA, SLE, Wegener's granulomatosis, sarcoidosis, Churg–Strauss syndrome, and others)

ACEI, angiotensin-converting enzyme inhibitor; AERD, aspirin-exacerbated respiratory disease; BPH, benign prostatic hyperplasia; ED, erectile dysfunction; HT, hypertension; NARES, nonallergic rhinitis with esinophilia [on nasal smear] syndrome; NSAIDs, nonsteroidal anti-inflammatory drugs; RA, rheumatoid arthritis; SLE, systemic lupus erythematosus.

From Refs. 1–3.

---

cockroaches), and companion animals (pets). Some patients are affected year round, but have seasonal exacerbations. These people are probably allergic to both seasonal and perennial aeroallergens. Other patients have only episodic manifestations. These people are probably allergic to aeroallergens that are only occasionally (episodically) encountered. The Joint Task Force on Practice Parameters (representing the American Academy of Allergy, Asthma and Immunology [AAAAI], the American College of Allergy, Asthma and Immunology [ACAAI], and the Joint Council of Allergy, Asthma and Immunology) published practice parameters for the diagnosis and management of AR in August 2008.[1] This document also introduces the term "episodic" AR, as a category in addition to SAR and PAR.

Recognizing that the traditional categories of seasonal and perennial AR are imperfect, another system for categorizing AR has been suggested by the international group Allergic Rhinitis and its Impact on Asthma (ARIA).[2] ❷ *This alternative system categorizes the manifestations by a combination of frequency and severity.* There are two divisions of frequency: intermittent and persistent. Intermittent frequency is defined as AR manifestations occurring less often than 4 days per week or for fewer than four consecutive weeks. Persistent frequency is defined as AR manifestations occurring for four or more days per week *and* for four or more consecutive weeks. Severity is categorized either as mild or as moderate–severe. Mild manifestations are those that do *not* cause interference with sleep, daily activities, or work or school performance and which are not "troublesome." Moderate–severe manifestations were combined because distinction between moderate and severe was not clinically practical. This category includes those patients with manifestations of AR that *do* cause interference with sleep, impairment of daily activities, problems at work or school, or are "troublesome." The ARIA document uses IAR (for intermittent) and PER (for persistent) for the two frequency categories. It is important to realize that IAR and PER are not synonymous with the classical categories of SAR and PAR, respectively. The ARIA system results in four categories: mild intermittent, mild persistent, moderate–severe intermittent, or moderate–severe persistent. The ARIA approach was updated in early 2008.[2] See Table 62–2 for a summary of these categories of AR.

EPIDEMIOLOGY

❸ *AR is one of the most common chronic disorders in the United States.*[4] One source indicates that it ranks fifth in this category.[5] It is estimated that up to 30% of adults and up to 40% of children in the United States are affected.[1,4,6–8] The total direct and indirect costs of AR in the United States for 2002 have been estimated to be in excess of 11 billion dollars.[1] AR is the most common allergic disease in children.[9] ❸ *Despite this, the disease has historically been trivialized.*

The major risk factors for AR are: a family history of allergic disorder; elevated serum IgE levels, especially before the age of 6 years; higher socioeconomic class; positive skin test results; and emigration into a Western industrialized environment.[1,2]

Table 62–2

Categories of AR

Based on AAAAI/ACAAI Practice Parameter
Seasonal—symptoms present only during specific portions of the year
Perennial—symptoms present throughout the year
Episodic—symptoms present only during intermittent exposure to allergen trigger

Based on ARIA 2008 Update
Mild versus moderate–severe
  Mild means no interference with sleep, daily activities, work or school function and attendance, and no troublesome symptoms
  Moderate–severe means the presence of any one of the following: abnormal sleep, impairment of daily activities, impairment of work or school function, troublesome symptoms
Intermittent versus persistent
  Intermittent means that symptoms are present for less than 4 days/week, or for less than 4 consecutive weeks
  Persistent means that symptoms are present for more than 4 days/week and for more than 4 consecutive weeks
  Any one of the four possibilities of these variables can occur: mild intermittent, mild persistent, moderate–severe intermittent, and moderate–severe persistent

From Refs. 1–3.

Certain disorders occur commonly with AR. The most important example is asthma. Some sources consider AR and asthma as two manifestations on a spectrum within the same disease. As many as 78% of patients with asthma have AR, and up to 38% of patients with AR have asthma.[4,8,10] There is evidence that AR can predispose to the development of asthma.[1,4,8,10] Other conditions that can occur with AR include sinusitis, obstructive sleep apnea, otitis media with effusion, and nasal polyposis.[1]

PATHOPHYSIOLOGY[1–3,5,10–12]

AR is an IgE-mediated disorder of people who are allergy prone. Initial contact is required to sensitize the patient to subsequent exposures. Patients with an inherited tendency to allergic disorders produce T-helper lymphocyte type 2 (Th-2)-directed responses, including production of specific IgE antibodies, to one or more allergens. The details of the process are complex, and still are being defined. Many cell types, intermediate substances (including cytokines) and mediators are involved. In response to subsequent exposures to the trigger antigen(s), there is an early phase and often a late phase allergic response. The distinction has therapeutic implications.

During the early phase, the trigger allergen becomes bound to IgE that is fixed to mast cells in the nasal mucosa. This occurs within minutes of subsequent exposure to the antigen and causes the mast cells to degranulate. This degranulation results in release of preformed mediators, the most important of which is histamine. This step stimulates more mast cells, as well as macrophages, eosinophils, and basophils to produce more substances, including cysteine leukotrienes and prostaglandin

D_2. These newly produced mediators bind to receptors in the nose and facilitate many of the manifestations of AR. The resultant vasodilation, mucosal edema, and hypertrophy all contribute to nasal congestion. Clear, watery, and often profuse rhinorrhea is also characteristic in this phase, a combined result of mucous secretion and increased vascular permeability. Sneezing and nasal itch are other prominent features of the early phase. Many patients also have ocular symptoms.

The late phase occurs in up to 50% of AR sufferers. It can begin as soon as 2 hours after the early phase and usually peaks within 12 hours. The late phase involves a second release of many of the mediators of the early phase. In addition, the late phase is characterized by an inflammatory component caused by infiltration of several cell types (e.g., mast cells, eosinophils, basophils, neutrophils, and T lymphocytes) into the nasal mucosa. The most significant manifestation during the late phase is nasal congestion that is often severe and long lasting.

A phenomenon known as the priming response is also of importance. This simply means that prolonged and/or repeated allergen exposure makes it easier to stimulate the process resulting in mediator release and symptoms. The inflammatory component that characterizes the late phase probably contributes to this effect. A vicious cycle results in which smaller doses of allergen can create symptoms (i.e., the threshold is lowered). Thus, even when pollen exposure is decreased, symptoms may continue. In some patients, the threshold is lowered to the degree that even irritant substances (e.g., formaldehyde, tobacco smoke, perfumes, automobile exhaust, and other environmental pollutants) may cause symptoms, on a nonallergic basis.

TREATMENT
Desired Outcomes

❹ *The goals of treatment of AR are to reduce or minimize the frequency and severity of symptoms; prevent comorbid disorders and complications; improve the patient's quality of life; improve work attendance and productivity and/or school attendance and performance; and minimize adverse effects of therapy.* Until a cure is established, these are the only realistic goals.

Nonpharmacologic Therapy

❺ *The general approach for treatment of AR is fourfold: avoidance of allergen triggers, pharmacotherapy, immunotherapy, and patient/family education.* Three of these four are nonpharmacologic.

Avoidance of allergen triggers, to the extent they have been identified and to the extent such avoidance is possible, underlies the treatment for all patients with AR (see Table 62–3).[1,2] Immunotherapy must be administered by a physician. The initial evaluation includes identification of specific allergens to determine individualized therapy. The role of a pharmacist in immunotherapy is appropriate referral of patients to an allergist or immunologist. See Clinical Presentation and Diagnosis for considerations for referral. At the time of this writing, in the United States, subcutaneous injection

Clinical Presentation and Diagnosis of AR[1–4,8]

Typical Symptoms

Rhinorrhea (usually clear and bilateral; primarily anterior but may have posterior [postnasal drip])

Sneezing

Itching (affecting mostly the nose, but also the palate, throat, eyes, and ears)

Nasal congestion (usually the most troublesome symptom)

Other Symptoms

Sleep disturbances

Headache, mild facial or ear pain or fullness

Cough (especially in those with concurrent asthma)

Fatigue, asthenia, malaise, and irritability

Ocular manifestations (itch, redness, tearing, chemosis, periorbital edema)

Presenteeism (impaired performance at work or school)

Absenteeism from work or school

Quality of life impairment (including social function)

Children (especially): rubbing the nose, snorting, sniffling, clearing the throat, learning or attention problems, poor appetite

Signs (Especially Common in Children)

Rubbing the nose (especially with the back of the hand or the palm; so-called allergic salute, which may create a horizontal crease just above the tip of the nose)

Rubbing/scratching at the eyes

Mouth breathing

Dark circles under the eyes

Dennie-Morgan lines or folds

Diagnosis

Typical symptoms, especially in association with exposure to allergen triggers

Other diagnostic testing usually optional, but may be necessary to rule out nonallergic causes of rhinitis or if immunotherapy is a consideration (physical exam, especially of the upper respiratory tract with emphasis on the nose, specific IgE antibody testing by either skin testing or in vitro serum testing, other specialized testing).

Considerations for Referral

Unilateral rhinitis, nasal obstruction without other typical symptoms of AR

Purulent rhinitis, fever, marked facial or ear pain, or recurrent nose bleeds

Ocular symptoms without typical symptoms of AR

Unilateral ocular symptoms, photophobia, or vision changes

Severe symptoms

Failure of therapy (nonresponse or adherence limiting side effects or intolerance)

Desire to have specific allergen triggers identified (e.g., by skin testing)

Candidates for immunotherapy

Concurrent asthma, nasal polyposis, sinusitis, or otitis media with effusion

---

immunotherapy is the only option.[1–3,13,14] In other parts of the world, sublingual immunotherapy is an alternative.[9,15–18] Proposed advantages are mostly ease of administration. Questions remain about comparative efficacy, and the details of optimal dosage, frequency of administration, and duration of therapy. Education of the patient as well as the patient's support system is essential.[1] They need to understand the potential seriousness of AR (including complications such as asthma) and the chronic and/or recurrent nature of the disorder. The patient and significant others should be told about the various treatment options, including their relative advantages and disadvantages. Proper understanding and use of current medication in the patient's regimen should be assured. A better educated patient and support system will result in a better relationship with health care providers and hopefully will optimize patient outcomes.

Pharmacologic Therapy

There are three guideline documents, all published in 2008, that are the basis for the summary that follows.[1–3] Other sources provide additional information for the treatment of AR.[8–10,13,19–27] The recommended approaches begin with allergen avoidance, emphasize patient/family education, and include immunotherapy as an option in selected patients.

The most reasonable plan may include considerations from several of these documents. ⑥ *Routine first-line agents are intranasal corticosteroids and antihistamines (oral and/or intranasal, depending on the patient). Adjunctive or secondary choice agents, each of which may have a first-line role in selected patients, include decongestants, the mast cell stabilizer/cromone (cromolyn), the leukotriene receptor antagonist (LTRA) (montelukast), the antimuscarinic/anticholinergic (ipratropium) and intranasal saline.* In all cases, therapy must be individualized, in cooperation with the patient. Considerations include frequency and severity of specific symptoms, realistic avoidance measures, patient age, patient preferences for route of administration, tolerance of side effects, adherence issues, comorbid disorders, and concurrent therapy. See Table 62–4 of intranasal and oral medications for the treatment of AR.

Table 62–3

Allergen Avoidance Measures

Allergen avoidance underlies all other treatments of AR
There are several limitations to implementing allergen avoidance:
- Identification of allergens is necessary to successfully employ avoidance strategies
- Literature support for a clinically significant impact on symptoms from allergen avoidance, especially any single measure, is meager
- Quality of life may be negatively impacted by forced removal of a pet from the household

Outdoor plant pollen and mold/fungi parts:
- Limit outdoor exposure, especially during high pollen conditions (warm sunny days with wind and low humidity) and during mold/fungi spore release (shortly after rains)
- Wear a face mask during activities that disturb the earth and decaying vegetation
- Keep windows and doors closed
- Use air-conditioning when possible, but maintain clean equipment

Indoor allergens (house dust mite, mold/fungi, cockroaches, and pets):
- Use air-conditioning, as above
- Maintain humidity below 50% if possible, and maintain clean equipment
- Clean frequently and thoroughly to prevent mold growth (dilute bleach with detergent)
- Avoid exposed food and garbage to deter insects, especially in the kitchen
- Clean kitchen frequently and thoroughly
- Use roach traps that facilitate removal of allergen-containing bodies
- Vacuum frequently, and consider use of a high-efficiency particulate air (HEPA) filter
- Minimize carpeting, fabric covered furniture, and fabric wall/window coverings
- Cover bedding (pillow, mattresses, box springs) with allergen-proof, zippered cases
- Launder bedding frequently, in hot water (greater than 130°F or 60°C) if possible, to kill mite ova
- Consider acaricide (e.g., benzyl benzoate) treatment of carpets to kill mites and ova
- Put items that cannot be laundered (e.g., soft toys) in a plastic bag and freeze
- Keep pets out of bedroom and bath cats weekly, if possible

Irritants:
- Avoid to the degree possible, all exposure to smoke, chlorine fumes, formaldehyde fumes, and other substances identified as irritant triggers in the patient (e.g., perfumes, newspaper ink)

From Refs. 1, 2.

Table 62–4

Intranasal and Oral Medications for AR

Corticosteroids
Intranasal[a] (budesonide, beclomethasone, ciclesonide, flunisolide, fluticasone [propionate and furoate], mometasone, triamcinolone)
Oral (rarely used)
Parenteral (not recommended)
Antihistamines
Intranasal[a] (azelastine, olopatadine)
Oral[b]
- First generation/sedating (cautious use in selected patients) (most OTC depending on strength: diphenhydramine, chlorpheniramine, clemastine, and others)
- Second generation/low- or nonsedating[a] (desloratadine, fexofenadine, levocetirizine; OTC: loratadine, cetirizine)
Mast cell stabilizer/cromone
Intranasal (OTC: cromolyn)
Decongestant
Intranasal (short-term use) (tetrahydrozoline; OTC: phenylephrine, naphazoline, oxymetazoline)
Oral[b] (OTC: phenylephrine; BTC[c]: pseudoephedrine)
LTRA
Oral (montelukast is only one indicated)
Antimuscarinic
Intranasal (ipratropium)

Note: All products are Rx unless indicated OTC.

[a]First-line choices.

[b]Some products combine an antihistamine with a decongestant, sometimes with other ingredients.

[c]Behind the counter (OTC plus other requirements necessary; see the **Decongestants** section of text).

From Refs. 1–3, 24–28.

▶ *First-Line Agents*

Corticosteroids Corticosteroids are usually administered by the intranasal route for the treatment of AR. Occasionally, a short course of oral therapy (burst and taper) is necessary. This oral use of corticosteroids is best applied to overcome severe nasal congestion, particularly that due to rhinitis medicamentosa from intranasal decongestants (see **Decongestant** section below). Parenteral administration of corticosteroids in the management of AR is discouraged.[1]

❼ *Intranasal corticosteroids are considered the most effective therapy for AR. They are recommended as the drugs of choice for severe manifestations, and for those with moderate disease not controlled with oral and/or intranasal antihistamines.* They provide very good relief for sneezing, itching, rhinorrhea, as well as nasal congestion and even ocular symptoms. Nasal congestion is often the most bothersome symptom of AR, and the most difficult to control. This is probably because it results from inflammation that predominates in the late phase of the allergic response in AR. **❼** *Intranasal corticosteroids are the best agents for nasal congestion, probably because of their anti-inflammatory mechanism of action.*[1,13,21] Systemic corticosteroids (i.e., orally administered) are also effective, but they are used only as a last resort due to systemic side effects.

The guideline document on AR published in August 2008 by the Joint Task Force (for AAAAI and ACAAI) includes an action plan (similar to what is used for asthma). The entire article, with the action plan, is available on the AAAAI website (*http://www.aaaai.org/professionals/resources/pdf/rhinitis2008.pdf*) in the public domain, for universal access.[1] The application of the differently colored zones on the action plan is explained at the bottom of the form, which is on page S25 of the document. Many patients will benefit from having an action plan.

Several meta-analyses have evaluated the relative efficacy of intranasal corticosteroids in comparison with other types of pharmacologic therapy of AR. The majority (but not all) of the literature suggests that intranasal corticosteroids are superior to intranasal antihistamines, to oral antihistamines, even when combined with a leukotriene antagonist, and to a leukotriene antagonist alone.[1,13]

There are currently eight intranasal corticosteroid products available in the United States, including two different salt forms of fluticasone. Most (e.g., budesonide, ciclesonide, fluticasone furoate, mometasone, and triamcinolone) are usually given in a single daily dose. However, fluticasone propionate may be given either once or twice daily; beclomethasone is usually given twice daily; and flunisolide is given two or three times daily. Despite some differences in formulation, potency, chemistry, and pharmacokinetic and pharmacodynamic properties among the products, there is no good evidence that any single product is superior in efficacy. Intranasal corticosteroids are best given regularly, as the onset of action usually takes up to 12 hours and the maximum effects may be delayed up to 7 to 14 days.[1,8,10] However, there is evidence that in some people the onset is within 3 to 4 hours, so these agents may even be used on an as needed basis.[1,29] When nasal congestion is severe, intranasal administration may not be effective due to limited exposure to the nasal mucosa. In that situation, short-term intranasal decongestants may facilitate better exposure. See Table 62–5 for intranasal corticosteroid products.

The correct technique for administration of intranasal medication is important for optimum efficacy. Consult the individual product labeling for specific instructions. However, also see Table 62–6 for general instructions for the optimal administration of intranasal medications. The technique described maximizes exposure of the drug to the nasal mucosa to optimize efficacy, and minimizes both exposure to the nasal septum and loss of medication down the esophagus. See later for instructions about preparation and use of intranasal saline irrigations.

Most patients tolerate intranasal corticosteroids very well. Local side effects include nasal burning, irritation, and dryness, which may occur in up to 12% of patients.[1,8,10,13,22] Also, up to 10% to 12% of patients may experience mild epistaxis.[13,23] This may be partly due to the administration technique. Sore throat and headache may be noted by some patients.[24] Perforation of the nasal septum is a very rare side effect. This can be minimized by proper administration technique (see Table 62–6), specifically, directing the spray laterally (away) from the (medial) nasal septum.[1,10]

The older intranasal corticosteroids (beclomethasone, flunisolide, and budesonide) have significant absorption, while the newer products (fluticasone, mometasone, and ciclesonide) have bioavailability of no more than 1% to 2%.[13] The decreased absorption minimizes systemic side effects. However, there is still some concern for growth suppression, other manifestations of hypothalamic–pituitary–adrenal (HPA) axis suppression, bone, and ocular effects.[13] Several studies have evaluated the effects of intranasal and inhaled corticosteroids on HPA axis suppression and growth.[1,13] Most have shown little or no clinically significant effects. The product most implicated with growth suppression is beclomethasone. One study demonstrated suppression in children using the drug for 1 year, but at twice the usual recommended dose.[1] There is no confirmation of a causal effect of intranasal corticosteroids on posterior subcapsular cataracts, increased intraocular pressure, or decreased bone density; however, those with risk factors for any of these conditions should be monitored carefully for their development. Ultimately, patient preference for a specific intranasal corticosteroid may be determined more by cost and by formulation differences that affect odor and aftertaste.

Antihistamines Antihistamines used for the treatment of AR are administered by either the oral or the intranasal

Table 62–5			
Intranasal Corticosteroids			
Generic (Brand) Name	mcg/Spray	Usual Adult Dosage (Each Nostril)	Usual Pediatric Dosage (Each Nostril)
Beclomethasone dipropionate (Beconase AQ)	42	1–2 sprays twice daily	6 yo or more: 1–2 sprays twice daily
Budesonide (Rhinocort Aqua)	32	1–4 sprays once daily	6–11 yo or more: 1–2 sprays once daily
Ciclesonide (Omnaris)	50	2 sprays once daily	12 yo or more: 2 sprays once daily
Flunisolide (Nasarel)	25	2 sprays two or three times daily	6–14 yo or more: 1 spray three times daily or 2 sprays twice daily
Fluticasone furoate (Veramyst)	50	2 sprays once daily	2–11 yo or more: 1 spray once daily
Fluticasone propionate (Flonase)	50	1–2 sprays once daily or 1 spray twice daily	4–11 yo or more: 1–2 sprays once daily
Mometasone (Nasonex)	50	2 sprays once daily	2–11 yo or more: 1 spray once daily
Triamcinolone acetonide (Nasacort AQ)	55	1–2 sprays once daily	2–11 yo or more: 1–2 sprays once daily

mcg, micro grams; yo, years old.

All products are FDA Pregnancy category C except budesonide, which is B.

From Refs. 1, 10, 24–26, 28.

Table 62–6

Administration Instructions for Intranasal Medications

1. Clear the nose of mucus and debris to the extent possible
2. Consult product labeling for preadministration instructions (e.g., shaking the container, priming the spray pump)
3. If seated or standing, do not just tilt head backward. This increases the amount of the dosage lost down the esophagus. This decreases efficacy and increases the potential for systemic absorption and thus systemic side effects
4. If standing, bend the head forward (flex the chin onto the chest) so that the nose is the lowest portion of the head. This is best for nasal sprays

   If possible, lie in the prone position with the stomach (ventral side) on a flat surface or kneel down. Then, flex chin onto neck, so that the open nostrils are pointing as far upward, toward the ceiling as possible. This position may be best for nose drops (more volume than sprays)

   An alternate position is to lie supine (on the back) on a flat surface, then bend the head backward (extend the head), again, so that the open nostrils point upward toward the ceiling
5. Use the contralateral hand to insert the spray nozzle or dropper into one nostril (i.e., the left hand for right nostril)
6. Use the other hand to occlude the opposite nostril (the one not being medicated)
7. Aim the spray or drops toward the outer (lateral) internal surface of each nostril, and away from the nasal septum (which is the inner or medial surface)
8. Breath in slowly but deeply through the medicated nostril
9. Repeat this procedure to apply medication to the other nostril
10. Consult the product labeling for cleaning instructions
11. See the text for information about preparation and use of saline irrigation

From Refs. 3, 8.

route. These agents interact with the H_1 (histamine type 1) receptor. Histamine is involved with both the early and the late phases of AR. Activation of H_1 receptors in the nose, upper airway mucosa, and the eye produces the common manifestations of AR (sneezing, itching, rhinorrhea, nasal congestion, and ocular symptoms). ❽ *The antihistamines are very effective for the sneezing, itching, and rhinorrhea of AR. There is some effect to improve nasal congestion, but less so than for the other symptoms. There is also benefit for the ocular symptoms (e.g., itch, redness, tearing). Intranasal administration is more effective than oral administration for the nasal congestion, but less effective for the ocular symptoms.* The onset of action by oral administration is usually within 1 to 2 hours, and that for intranasal administration within 30 minutes.[1,8,13] All antihistamines probably provide better relief if used continuously (during symptomatic periods of seasonal AR, or for perennial or persistent AR), but they are also effective used only when needed.

Antihistamine drugs used for AR are technically inverse agonists, not competitive antagonists; however, there may be little clinical significance to the difference.[10,13,21] These drugs bind to the H_1 receptor, changing its three-dimensional conformation such that it is kept in the inactive state. This results in downregulation of H_1 receptor activity and a decrease in end organ effects. These agents do not prevent release of histamine.

The oral agents are divided into first- and second-generation drugs. The first-generation agents are distributed among six chemical classes, including the more sedating ethanolamine class (e.g., diphenhydramine) and the least sedating alkylamine class (e.g., chlorpheniramine). ❽ *Most sources now discourage the routine use of the first-generation agents for AR. This is due to their CNS and anticholinergic side effects.* The CNS effects are primarily sedation, as well as impairment of cognitive function and performance of tasks. Studies have shown that decision making and driving or work performance are impaired even when the patient is unaware of any overt effects.[1] There is also evidence of decreased performance at school and impaired learning, among pediatric patients.[1] Some controversy remains, however, about how common these problems truly are.[23] The major anticholinergic (perhaps more accurately stated as antimuscarinic) effects include blurred vision, dry mouth, urinary retention, and constipation. The only possible advantage of the antimuscarinic properties is an additional effect to decrease rhinorrhea. However, some patients complain about the increased thickness of the secretions.[21] Another disadvantage of the first-generation antihistamines is that most must be administered three to four times daily. If first-generation antihistamines are recommended by a health care practitioner, care must be taken to educate the patient about these CNS and anticholinergic side effects. Patients who take other sedative substances are prone to an additive effect from the antihistamine. Those taking any other medications with anticholinergic or antimuscarinic properties may experience additive effects from the antihistamine. The elderly are, in general, more sensitive to both types of adverse effects.

Currently available oral second-generation H_1 antihistamines are cetirizine, levocetirizine, loratadine, desloratadine, fexofenadine, and acrivastine. All except acrivastine are available alone, and some are marketed in combination with the decongestant pseudoephedrine. At the time of this writing, only cetirizine and loratadine are available OTC. The second-generation antihistamines do not have the anticholinergic effects of the first-generation agents. Based on current literature, no single H_1 antihistamine (first or second generation) is clearly superior in efficacy; however, very few head to head comparative studies have been conducted. The oral second-generation antihistamines are effective for the sneezing, itching, and rhinorrhea of AR, but less effective for the nasal congestion. They also improve ocular symptoms. Intranasal antihistamines are better for nasal congestion.

Fexofenadine has virtually no sedative effects, even at doses higher than usually recommended. Loratadine and desloratadine are not sedative at recommended doses, but can be at higher doses. Cetirizine, levocetirizine, and acrivastine have some sedative effects, even at recommended doses.[1] All the oral second-generation agents require some dosage reduction with impaired renal function, although the specific recommendations vary with creatinine clearance.[30] To date, none of the currently available oral second-generation antihistamines have been reported to cause QT prolongation or torsade de pointes, as were associated with the two agents that have been removed from the U.S. market (terfenadine and astemizole).[13] Most of the oral second-generation antihistamines can be administered once daily (except for the lower dosage forms of fexofenadine), which probably improves adherence.

There are only two intranasal antihistamine products available in the U.S. market at the time of this writing. Both azelastine and olopatadine are considered second-generation agents, although they also have some mast cell stabilizing effects.[24] Both are available only by prescription. The most common side effect of these products is a bitter taste. This occurs in up to 20% of patients on azelastine, and probably somewhat fewer on olopatadine.[1] Also, there is enough systemic absorption to cause sedation in some patients using azelastine (about 10%) and perhaps somewhat fewer on olopatadine.[1] However, there are no direct comparisons of the two agents, so definitive statements regarding their relative efficacy and side-effect incidence cannot be made. See Table 62–7 for the single-agent second-generation antihistamine products.

8 *Many patients with mild to moderate AR are adequately treated with an OTC oral first- or (preferably) second-generation antihistamine alone.* Others may prefer the intranasal administration of an antihistamine, but these require a prescription. Still others may prefer fexofenadine by prescription due to the absence of sedation. Some patients will need or prefer combination therapy. If nasal congestion is not relieved by the above regimens, addition of a decongestant is reasonable, either alone or as a combination product (see **Decongestant** section below). Perhaps even the combination of an oral with an intranasal antihistamine is reasonable for some patients, depending on their preferences. Other pharmacologic agents can be combined with oral and/or intranasal antihistamines, as necessary for optimal control of symptoms (see below).

Patient Encounter, Part 1

AW is a 26-year-old woman who presents to your clinic or store. She moved to this part of the country with her husband and 2-year-old son about 3 months ago. She complains of sneezing and runny nose, which began for the first time as an adult about 2 months ago. Her symptoms are worse when she is outdoors, especially if the weather is windy. She has symptoms almost every day, and the symptoms interfere with her sleep. She awakens tired and feels that way most of the day. She indicates that she has no other medical problems and is taking no chronic medications. She asks your recommendation for OTC treatment.

What symptoms are consistent with AR?

How would you categorize this patient's condition?

What would you suggest for initial management?

Table 62–7

Single-Agent Second-Generation Antihistamine Products (Oral and Intranasal)

Oral

Generic (Brand) Name	Formulation	Usual Adult Dosage	Usual Pediatric Dosage
Cetirizine[a,b] (Zyrtec, generic)	5, 10 mg tabs/chew tabs; 5 mg/mL syrup	5–10 mg once daily	6–11 mo; 2.5 mg once daily 12–23 mo; 2.5 mg once or twice daily 2–5 yo; 2.5–5 mg once daily or 2.5 mg twice daily 6 yo or more; adult dosage
Desloratadine[b] (Clarinex)	5 mg tabs; 0.5 mg/mL syrup 2.5, 5 mg disintegrating tabs	5 mg once daily	6–11 mo; 1 mg once daily 1–5 yo; 1.25 mg once daily 6–11 yo; 2.5 mg once daily
Fexofenadine[b] (Allegra)	30, 60, 80 mg tabs 30 mg/5 mL suspension	60 mg twice daily or 180 mg once daily	6–23 mo; 15 mg twice daily[c] 2–11 yo; 30 mg twice daily
Levocetirizine (Xyzal)	5 mg tabs 2.5 mg/5 mL solution	5 mg once daily	6–11 yo; 2.5 mg once daily 6 mo–5 yo; 1.25 mg once daily
Loratadine[a,b] (Claritin; Alavert, generic)	10 mg tabs; 1 mg/mL syrup/susp; 5, 10 mg disintegrating tabs	10 mg once daily	2–5 yo; 5 mg once daily 6 yo or more; adult dosage

Intranasal Spray

Generic (Brand) Name	mcg/Spray	Usual Adult Dosage (Each Nostril)	Usual Pediatric Dosage (Each Nostril)
Azelastine (Astelin)	137	1–2 sprays twice daily	5–11 yo; 1 spray twice daily
Olopatadine (Patanase)	665	2 sprays twice daily	Not approved for children less than 12 yo

Note: acrivastine is available only with pseudoephedrine and so is not included in this table.

mo, months old; yo, years old.

[a]Available OTC.

[b]Available in combination with pseudoephedrine (consult labeling for pediatric dosage).

[c]Only approved for idiopathic urticaria, not AR.

From Refs. 1, 24–26, 28.

▶ *Adjunctive or Secondary Choice Agents*

Decongestants Decongestant drugs are useful to relieve the nasal congestion component of AR.[1-3,10,13] This is due to their α_1 adrenergic agonist activity, which results in constriction of the vasculature in the nasal mucosa. They do not prevent release of any of the mediators involved in AR. Thus, they do not provide any benefit for the sneezing, itching, rhinorrhea, or the ocular manifestations. Decongestants can be given alone, either by the oral or by the intranasal route. Also, numerous combination products, consisting of a decongestant with an antihistamine (and sometimes other ingredients), are available as oral medications. There are some special considerations for use of decongestants in pediatric and pregnant patients (see the Special Populations section later).

Oral decongestant products are currently limited to pseudoephedrine and phenylephrine (phenylpropanolamine was removed from the market in 2000).[10] Pseudoephedrine has been changed from truly OTC to a more controlled status because it is an ingredient in the illicit manufacture of methamphetamine. The new, so-called behind-the-counter (BTC) status, established by the federal Combat Methaphetamine Act of 2005, requires special storage; photo identification of purchasers; a log book of sales, which must be signed by purchasers; and specific limitations on daily and monthly quantities.[31,32] Subsequent to this change in status of pseudoephedrine, some manufacturers changed the ingredients of their products by replacing psuedoephedrine with phenylephrine. This was probably to maintain shelf presence in the OTC sales area. However, much controversy surrounds the efficacy of oral phenylephrine. At the time of this writing, the clinical literature suggests that the currently recommended adult dose is minimally effective as a nasal decongestant.[33-35]

The side effects of orally administered decongestants most often affect cardiovascular function or the CNS. The side effects are primarily due to sympathetic stimulation, and are usually dose-related. Some elevation of blood pressure may occur, but in normotensive and well-controlled hypertensive patients, the elevation is usually small. It is not of clinical significance in most situations, especially considering that these drugs are most appropriately used only briefly or intermittently. Insomnia, nervousness, irritability, and anxiety are relatively common CNS side effects. Some patients may have decreased appetite, tremors, headache, and even hallucinations. Men with benign prostatic hyperplasia (BPH) and other patients with disorders causing bladder outlet obstruction may have increased urinary retention due to α_1 stimulation of the urethral sphincter. Theoretically, there may be some differences in the side effects between pseudoephedrine and phenylephrine. This is due to their effects on sympathetic nervous system receptors. Pseudoephedrine stimulates both α and β receptors, whereas the effects of recommended oral doses of phenylephrine are essentially limited to stimulation of α receptors. Comparative studies are not available to confirm these differences in the clinical setting.

The intranasal agents currently available include the OTC products phenylephrine, oxymetazoline, and naphazoline, and the prescription product tetrahydrozoline. Product labeling should be followed for dosage, but it is noteworthy that oxymetazoline is the longest acting of these agents, and is usually given only twice daily. Intranasal application of decongestants provides rapid and effective relief of nasal congestion. This therapy may provide relief for nasal congestion, even for those patients already on intranasal corticosteroids.[36] However, the continuous use of intranasal decongestants often causes a paradoxical rebound phenomenon of persistent nasal congestion, called *rhinitis medicamentosa*.[1-3,10,37] ❾ *While some patients do not develop rhinitis medicamentosa even after several weeks of continuous use of intranasal decongestants, the usual recommendation is to use them for no more than three consecutive days.*[1] Intranasal decongestants can cause local side effects, including stinging, burning, dryness, and even sneezing. These are usually mild and well tolerated. Due to very limited absorption, the intranasal route rarely causes systemic side effects.[1,8,10] Administration technique should be optimized as described in Table 62–6. Should rhinitis medicamentosa occur, the best management is first to discontinue the decongestant, possibly with a taper to minimize worsening the situation. However, the response to withdrawal is often delayed for days. Therefore, it may be necessary to start intranasal corticosteroids, and/or (especially if intranasal corticosteroids are already part of the patient's regimen) begin a short course of oral corticosteroid.[37]

Despite the usual good tolerance of recommended doses of oral decongestants, caution is warranted when they are used in patients with cardiac disease (dysrhythmias, angina pectoris, heart failure), hypertension, cerebrovascular disease, bladder outlet obstruction (including BPH), glaucoma (especially closed angle), hyperthyroidism, and possibly diabetes.[1,10,13] ❾ *The best application of decongestants in AR is short-term to overcome severe nasal congestion, especially to facilitate improved efficacy of (other) intranasal agents (e.g., corticosteroids and antihistamines).* The choice between the two routes of administration is based on several considerations, including cost, convenience, patient preference, speed of onset (within 30 minutes orally, within 5–10 minutes for intranasal), and side effects.[1,8,38]

Mast Cell Stabilizer/Cromone[1,10,21,22,38] Cromolyn is the only agent in the cromone class that is approved in the United States for treatment of AR. It is available as an OTC

Patient Encounter, Part 2

AW returns after 3 weeks of the OTC therapy that you suggested. There is some improvement in her symptoms, but nasal congestion still interferes with her sleep.

What additional information do you want?

What can you offer her in the way of additional OTC therapy?

intranasal product. The mechanism of action in AR is mast cell stabilization. The drug binds to mast cells, and prevents release of the mediators of AR that would otherwise result from allergen exposure. The drug is moderately effective, but less so than both intranasal corticosteroids and oral or intranasal antihistamines. It does have effects on both early and late phases of AR. Its effects begin within 4 to 7 days of use, but may not be maximal for up to 2 weeks.[1] However, it can be used effectively on an as needed basis for episodic exposures to allergen.[1] As with all intranasal products, if there is severe nasal congestion, exposure will be limited. Short-term use of a decongestant or an intranasal antihistamine may solve this problem. Cromolyn is very well-tolerated. The most common side effects are mild local stinging and/or burning, sneezing, unpleasant taste, and possibly nose bleed. A disadvantage is the frequency of administration. At least initially, it should be used four times daily. Some patients may need only two or three daily doses when used continuously after the first few weeks at four times daily. It is most useful for patients with mild or intermittent symptoms, in the pediatric population and in pregnant women.

Leukotriene Receptor Antagonist Leukotrienes are involved in the pathophysiology of AR, and in particular contribute to the nasal congestion in the late phase.[1] They contribute little if anything to nasal itch and sneezing.[38] Leukotriene antagonists have been shown to be effective for some of the manifestations of AR. Montelukast is the only agent in this class with FDA approval for treatment of AR. It is marketed as oral granules, and as both chewable and swallow tablets. The majority of clinical studies published to date indicate that montelukast is inferior to intranasal corticosteroids.[1,10,13,38] Montelukast is either equivalent or slightly inferior to oral H$_1$ antihistamines.[1,10,24,38] The combination of montelukast with an oral antihistamine shows improved efficacy over either agent alone.[13] However, even the combination is probably not better than intranasal corticosteroids.[1] The onset of action of montelukast is delayed for a day or more.[1] The drug is usually considered to be very well-tolerated with minimal side effects. However, in March 2008, based on reports to the manufacturer, the FDA issued a preliminary report concerning an investigation into cases of behavior change and suicidal ideation in association with the drug.[39] It is administered once daily, considered safe (FDA Pregnancy category B and indicated for children as young as 6 months of age), and particularly well-suited to those patients who have concurrent asthma and AR.

Antimuscarinic (Anticholinergic) Agent[1] Ipratropium is currently the only antimuscarinic (or anticholinergic) agent indicated for treatment of AR. It is a quaternary ammonium structure, so systemic absorption is minimal. The product is available by prescription as an intranasal spray. Its use is limited to those patients whose rhinorrhea has not been controlled by other therapy (antihistamines and/or intranasal corticosteroids). There are two strengths available. The 0.03% product is approved for AR in children as young as 6 years of age. The 0.06% product is indicated for rhinorrhea associated with the common cold, in children as young as 5 years old.

Patient Encounter, Part 3

AW returns to talk with you 6 months after your first encounter with her. Since talking with you last, her symptoms almost went away completely, until about 1 month ago. Now she notices sneezing, runny nose, itchy nose, and watery itchy eyes even if she is indoors. The symptoms are present every day. She again has trouble sleeping due to nasal congestion. She still has some of the OTC medications you recommended, but they are not working as well now as previously.

How would you characterize her problem now?

What could you suggest now to help her?

Local side effects are essentially limited to mild epistaxis and nasal dryness.

Saline[1,40,41] Nasal administration of saline is an alternative for treatment of AR. This therapy may benefit any patient with AR. Saline may be administered as drops or a spray, but the irrigation mode of administration is popularly known by several terms, including neti pot, nasal wash, nasal douche, nose bidet, as well as nasal irrigation.[40] While less effective than intranasal corticosteroids, it has been shown to improve sneezing and nasal congestion. It can be used either alone or as add-on therapy. It is best to use canning or pickling salt, which has no iodine, preservatives, or other additives, all of which can be irritating. It appears that isotonic saline is as effective as hypertonic solutions.

An approximate isotonic concentration can be made by dissolution of one teaspoonful of noniodized salt (sodium chloride) in one pint of water. The AAAAI has another recipe.[41] Their instructions start with preparation of the dry powder component. This is done by combining three heaping teaspoonfuls of pickling salt with one rounded teaspoonful of baking soda, and mixing thoroughly. Then, one teaspoonful of the dry powder mixture is dissolved in one cup (8 oz) of lukewarm water. It is best if the water is distilled or has been boiled. About 4 oz of this solution will be used to irrigate each side of the nose. Application can be accomplished while the patient is in the shower or leaning over a sink. The head is bent forward and downward, then tilted to the side opposite the treated nostril. That is, the head is tilted to the left if the right nostril will be irrigated. Then, with a bulb syringe or similar device, slowly introduce about 4 oz of the warm saline solution into one side. Soon, the solution will run out of the opposite nostril. The position of the head should be adjusted as necessary to avoid the solution running into the ears or down the throat. Another source has slightly different instructions for preparation and use.[40]

Nasal irrigation is one delivery method, although the optimal method (spray, drops, nebulizer, or irrigation) is not known. Optimal frequency of administration is also not known. Nasal irrigation is usually given twice daily, but use of smaller volumes as spray products may be given up to four times daily. Local side effects are usually limited to minor nasal irritation. Nausea has been reported.

Patient Encounter, Part 4

AW returns about 1 year later (she is now 27 years old), and asks what you can recommend for her (now 3-year-old) son, who seems to have developed the same AR that she has. Junior is fussy during the day, constantly rubs his nose, sniffles, and sneezes. He does not sleep through the night because of runny nose and congestion. He even snores because his nose is so stuffed up that he has to breathe through his mouth. She notices dark circles and some lines under his eyes. A neighbor gave her some Benadryl-D Children's Allergy and Sinus and her mother-in-law gave her some Allerfrim. Junior is otherwise healthy, up to date on immunizations and weighs about 16 kg (35 lb). According to the medication labels, the dosage for Junior would be ½ teaspoonful up to four times a day. So, mom has been giving that dose of both medications for the last 2 days. It helps some, but Junior is even more fussy.

What information suggests that Junior also has AR?

What more information do you need?

What would you recommend at this time?

Omalizumab[1,22,38] Omalizumab is a monoclonal antibody that binds to IgE. The product is approved for asthma, but not for AR. It is administered by subcutaneous injection. Dosage is determined by the patient's circulating IgE levels. The cost is high compared to other commonly used modes of therapy for both asthma and AR. Investigational use has demonstrated efficacy in AR, although relative efficacy compared to other modes of therapy for AR is unknown. Its use is best limited to those with concurrent asthma and AR, pending specific approval for AR.

Complementary and Alternative Medicine Therapy
While some would consider saline in the category of complementary and alternative agents, this monograph considers it as an adjunctive mode. Complementary and alternative therapy for AR has been reviewed.[42] Consistent evidence for efficacy has not been established and there are some safety concerns.

▶ *Special Populations*

Children ❿ *Generally speaking, the treatment of AR in children is the same as it is for adults. There are, however, limitations in terms of FDA-approved products for different age groups. Also, depending on the age of the patient, there may be administration issues with some products.* Most children affected by AR are more than 2 years old, although the disease may begin in children as young as 6 months of age.[1]

There has been concern about use of combination cough and cold products (many contain an antihistamine and a decongestant) in children. In October 2007, the Nonprescription Drug Advisory Committee of the FDA recommended that OTC combination cough and cold products be limited to children 6 years of age and older. This was based on reports of over 100 deaths in association with these combination products.[1] Most of these bad outcomes seem to have resulted from inadvertent overdosage, often by giving doses of the same medication from different combination products. In October 2008, the FDA notified consumers and health care providers that the Consumer Health Protection Agency (CHPA) decided to voluntarily modify the labeling of combination cough and cold products to indicate that they should not be used in children less than 4 years old.[43] The CHPA is an association comprised of most of the manufacturers of these products. The announcement indicated that the FDA supports this decision.

First-generation H_1 antihistamines are discouraged for children as they are for adults, due to the possible detrimental effects on school performance and learning. Second-generation (less sedating) H_1 antihistamines (primarily for mild or intermittent symptoms) or intranasal corticosteroids (for moderate–severe or persistent manifestations) are first-line modes of therapy. Antihistamines may need to be used even for more severe and/or persistent symptoms in those children who have difficulty with use of intranasal products. If necessary, these two classes can be combined.

See Table 62–7 for dosages of second-generation antihistamines by age groups for which they are indicated. If first-generation antihistamines are used, the health care practitioner should guarantee that the family members or caretakers are carefully and thoroughly educated to read and use the dosage recommendations appropriate for age or weight of the patient, as indicated on the product labeling. They should also be warned about the possibility of a paradoxical CNS stimulant side effect. Special care should be given to avoid administration of the same medication from different (especially combination) products. The most common side effects of second-generation antihistamines in children are similar to those for adults.

See Table 62–5 for dosages of intranasal corticosteroids by age groups for which they are indicated. The consensus of opinion about intranasal corticosteroids and systemic side effects, especially delay in growth, is that most products are safe. The greatest potential for problems may exist with beclomethasone.[1] Several products have been studied in children and have not been shown to delay growth. However, not every product has been studied carefully in all age groups. Some of the conclusions about safety are extrapolated from data with inhaled corticosteroids, used for asthma. The local side effects of intranasal corticosteroids are the same in children as for adults.

Other therapy options may be worth consideration for some pediatric patients. Montelukast provides an oral alternative, especially for those who are too young to cooperate with intranasal administration of corticosteroids. It may be used in combination with an oral antihistamine in hopes of providing some additional efficacy. Another advantage of montelukast is that it is indicated for children as young as 6 months. Another option for mild or intermittent symptoms is intranasal cromolyn, primarily due to its excellent safety. This OTC product is labeled for use in children 2 years

Table 62–8

Intraocular Medications

Category	Generic (Brand) Name	Formulation	Frequency	Age
Decongestant/vasoconstrictor	Naphazoline[a] (Naphcon, Privine, others)	0.012% + 0.025%	Four times daily	Adult
Decongestant/vasoconstrictor + antihistamine	Naphazoline + pheniramine[a] (Visine A)	0.025%/0.3%	Four times daily	6 yo or more
Antihistamine	Emedastine (Emadine)	0.05%	Four times daily	3 yo or more
Mast cell stabilizer	Cromolyn (generic)	4%	Every 4–6 hours	4 yo or more
	Lodoxamide (Alomide)	0.1%	Four times daily	2 yo or more
	Nedocromil (Alocril)	2%	Twice daily	3 yo or more
	Pemirolast (Alamast)	0.1%	Four times daily	3 yo or more
Antihistamine + mast cell stabilizer	Azelastine (Optivar)	0.05%	Twice daily	3 yo or more
	Epinastine (Elestat)	0.05%	Twice daily	3 yo or more
	Ketotifen[a] (Zaditor, Alaway, Claritin, Zyrtee, generic)	0.025%	Every 8–12 hours	3 yo or more
	Olopatadine (Patanol/Pataday)	0.1%/0.2%	Twice daily/once daily	3 yo or more
	Bepotastine (Bepreve)	1.5%	Twice daily	2 yo or more
NSAIDs	Ketorolac (Acular)	0.5%	Four times daily	3 yo or more
Corticosteroid	Loteprednol (Alrex)	0.2%	Four times daily	Adult

NSAID, nonsteroidal anti-inflammatory drug; yo, years old.

[a]Available OTC.

From Refs. 1, 24, 25, 28.

Table 62–9

Routine Approach to Therapy of AR

All patients should practice avoidance of identified allergens to the extent possible

Mild intermittent (including many patients with what some would call seasonal AR)
    First line:
        Oral antihistamine (OTC, initially; preferably second generation)
    Adjunctive/secondary (may use more than one):
        Add OTC oral decongestant for nasal congestion
        Add short-term OTC intranasal decongestant for refractory nasal congestion
        Add nasal irrigation
        Consider prescription therapy for inadequate response (see below)
    Possibly consider referral for immunotherapy
Persistent or moderate–severe
    First line:
        Intranasal corticosteroid
        Add oral antihistamine for possible additional benefit if necessary
    Adjunctive/secondary (may use more than one):
        Add short-term intranasal decongestant for refractory nasal congestion
        Add nasal irrigation
        Add ipratropium for inadequately controlled rhinorrhea
        Consider replacement of one first-line agent, if poorly tolerated, with montelukast
    Consider referral for immunotherapy
Episodic (no order of preference intended)
    Intranasal cromolyn (OTC)
    Intranasal antihistamine
    Intranasal corticosteroid
Special situations (children, pregnant women, elderly, athletes, ocular symptoms)
    See Special Populations section of text

From Refs. 1–3, 8, 10, 19–21, 23, 24, 38.

of age and older. Intranasal ipratropium is indicated for patients 6 years of age or older and may benefit unresponsive rhinorrhea.

Pregnant Women[1,44] Women who have AR may suffer an exacerbation of symptoms during pregnancy. However, only minor changes in the routine approach to therapy are necessary as a result of the pregnancy. Second-generation antihistamines are generally considered safe, based on an increasing number of studies and experience.[1] The same generalization applies to intranasal corticosteroids. However, the products with the best documented safety record are beclomethasone, budesonide, and fluticasone propionate.[1] If an intranasal product is started during pregnancy, the wisest choice might be to use budesonide, based on the fact that it is FDA Pregnancy category of B. Cromolyn is also FDA Pregnancy category B, and is considered safe. The disadvantages, however, are frequent administration and lesser efficacy than antihistamines and intranasal corticosteroids. Montelukast is also FDA Pregnancy category B, but some recommend it be used primarily in those with concurrent asthma or in those who have demonstrated a good response prior to pregnancy.[1] Ipratropium is FDA Pregnancy category B, despite limited data.[44] The decongestants are not considered safe, especially in the first trimester. If nasal congestion is severe enough to warrant consideration for a decongestant, the intranasal route of administration is preferable, due to decreased systemic exposure and the short-term duration of therapy.[1]

Elderly[1,8] Elderly patients can be treated for AR according to the approach for (younger) adults.[1,8] However, the elderly may be more sensitive to the sedative and antimuscarinic effects of antihistamines and to the cardiovascular and CNS stimulant effects of decongestants. Also, the aging process can affect the manifestations of AR. Generalized atrophy of nasal tissues can result in more nasal congestion. An increase in cholinergic activity may result in more rhinorrhea.

Athletes[1] The use of certain medications is prohibited during national and international athletic competition. The list of prohibited drugs changes each year, and may not always be consistent among organizations. The most up-to-date information is available from the World Anti-Doping Agency (WADA).[45] Additional information may be obtained from the United States Anti-Doping Agency (USADA).[46] The USADA website has a "drug reference online" section that is useful.[47]

▶ Ocular Symptoms[1,24,28]

Several products are available for instillation directly into the eyes for those patients with predominant or unresponsive ocular manifestations. They may be appropriate for occasional moderate–severe flares or episodic AR when other modes of therapy are not optimally effective. The combination (antihistamine and mast cell stabilizing) agents may be the most effective, and they have the advantages of rapid onset of action and (usually) only twice daily administration. See Table 62–8 for these products.

Summary of Treatment

Once an agent appropriate for initial therapy is chosen, ongoing management requires repeated checks to ascertain response and freedom from intolerable or adherence limiting side effects. Either "step-up" or "step-down" therapy may be appropriate depending on the individual patient's response. See Table 62–9 for a summary of the approach to treatment of AR. Table 62–10 attempts to rank the relative effectiveness of the classes of agents for treatment of AR by specific symptoms.

OUTCOME EVALUATION

AR is a common condition that can have a profoundly negative effect on quality of life. It has been trivialized in the past, but is increasingly recognized as a significant health problem. There are several modes of management that can improve patient function.

- Educate patients and their families about the disorder (see **Clinical Presentation and Diagnosis**).
- Educate patients and their families about allergen avoidance measures (see **Table 62–3**).
- Assess the patient's symptom response, tolerance, and adherence at each visit.
- Assess the patient's administration technique with intranasal products when symptom response or tolerance is not optimal.

Patient Encounter, Part 5

After one more year passes, AW returns to your clinic to ask for advice about her father. He has recently moved into town, because he has just retired. He will be living independently. He is 65 years old and has hypertension, and BPH. The daughter (AW) thinks he is taking two medications for his blood pressure, one of which is also partly for his prostate. He has had AR on and off in the past. That is all she knows about his medical history. Since he has moved to town 6 weeks ago, he notices increasing symptoms of AR. His most bothersome symptom right now is a runny nose that is worse than ever before. He bought some OTC diphenhydramine because he ran out of his previous prescription of intranasal triamcinolone. The diphenhydramine has helped some, but incompletely, and it makes him sleepy. She asks for your advice for additional OTC medication until they can get an appointment with a primary care provider for him.

What additional information would you like?

What can you recommend at this time?

Table 62–10

Relative Efficacy (Semiquantitative) by Classes of Agents for Specific Symptoms of AR

Drug Class	Nasal Congestion	Sneezing	Rhinorrhea	Nasal Itch	Ocular Symptoms
Nasal corticosteroids	3	3	3	3	2
Oral antihistamines[a]	1	2	2	3	2
Nasal antihistamines	2	2	2	3	0
Oral decongestants[a]	1½	0	0	0	0
Nasal decongestants[a,b]	3	0	0	0	0
Oral leukotriene antagonist	2	½	2	½	2
Nasal mast cell stabilizer[a]	1½	1½	1½	1½	1½
Nasal antimuscarinic	0	0	2	0	0

The information in this table is a composite from numerous sources. There are different opinions about some of the rankings, partly due to inadequate study. Individual variation may create different relative efficacy in some patients.

Higher number equals greater activity.

[a]Some products in these classes are available OTC.

[b]Nasal decongestants are best used for severe, unresponsive nasal congestion or to facilitate mucosal contact of other intranasal medications, but in either case, should usually be limited to no more than 3 days.

From Refs. 1, 8, 10, 20–22.

Patient Care and Monitoring

1. Determine the patient's manifestations

   What is the most troublesome symptom?

   What is the frequency and severity of symptoms?

   How do symptoms affect quality of life, work/school performance, and sleep?

   What allergen or irritant triggers have been identified?

2. Attempt to rule out complications or comorbid conditions that preclude self-care (asthma, sinusitis, otitis media with effusion, and possibly nasal polyposis) and/or warrant referral to a physician (see **Clinical Presentation and Diagnosis**).

3. Determine past attempts at therapy

   What has the patient tried previously for these symptoms (including prescription and all nonprescription [OTC, herbal, other complementary] forms)?

   What was the response to all previous treatments (efficacy and side effects)?

4. Determine other current disorders and treatments

   What conditions are medications taken for on a regular basis?

   What medications are currently being taken regularly?

5. Assess patient's understanding of AR and its management

   What does the patient currently do to avoid triggers?

   How does/did the patient administer and adhere to current or past treatments?

6. Fill in gaps in patient's knowledge

   Manifestations of AR and its complications

   Principles of management (allergen/trigger avoidance, pharmacologic modes, immunotherapy)

   Choices for pharmacologic therapy (OTC and prescription) and determinates (previous experience, ease of use, tolerability, cost, patient preference, and age)

   Discuss realistic goals, which may not be complete elimination of all symptoms

7. Establish a plan appropriate for and with input from the patient

   Recommend initial OTC regimen or refer for evaluation for need for prescription therapy

   Fill in gaps in patient's knowledge about allergen avoidance and optimal adherence and administration technique (where applicable)

8. Reevaluate the patient at appropriate intervals, that will vary with the individual, but will usually be every 1 to 3 months

   Evaluate for efficacy of therapy, including improvement in symptoms, quality of life, work/school performance and sleep pattern

   Evaluate for tolerance of side effects

   Modify the plan as needed (to increase efficacy or modify side effects) including recommendations for a change in medication and/or referral to a physician

- Use or recommend second-generation oral antihistamine therapy for most patients with mild or intermittent (especially seasonal) symptoms (see Clinical Presentation and Diagnosis and Table 62–9).

- Recommend intranasal corticosteroid therapy for moderate–severe or persistent (especially perennial) symptoms. Advise additional adjunctive therapy for those with less than optimal control (see Clinical Presentation and Diagnosis and Table 62–9).

- Consider step-up therapy for exacerbations or less than optimal response.

- Consider step-down therapy if symptoms have been minimal or stable for several months (especially if the disorder is primarily seasonal).

- Consider referral to rule out nonallergic causes of rhinitis in nonresponding patients or those with an atypical presentation (see Clinical Presentation and Diagnosis).

- Consider referral for patients who request immunotherapy.

- Consider referral for patients with comorbid conditions, especially asthma.

Abbreviations Introduced in This Chapter

AAAAI	American Academy of Allergy, Asthma and Immunology
ACAAI	American College of Allergy, Asthma and Immunology
ACEI	Angiotensin-converting enzyme inhibitor
AERD	Aspirin-exacerbated respiratory disease
AR	Allergic rhinitis
ARIA	Allergic Rhinitis and its Impact on Asthma
BPH	Benign prostatic hyperplasia/hypertrophy
BTC	Behind-the-counter
CHPA	Consumer Health Protection Agency
H_1	Histamine type 1 (receptor)
HEPA	High-efficiency particulate air (filter)
HPA	Hypothalamic–pituitary–adrenal (axis)
HT	(essential or primary) hypertension
IAR	Intermittent allergic rhinitis (ARIA system)
IgE	Immunoglobulin E
LTRA	Leukotriene receptor antagonist
NARES	Nonallergic rhinitis with eosinophilia [on nasal smear] syndrome
NSAID	Nonsteroidal anti-inflammatory drug
OTC	Over-the-counter
PAR	Perennial allergic rhinitis (AAAAI/ACAAI system)
PDE-5	Phosphodiesterase (isoenzyme)-5
PER	Persistent allergic rhinitis (ARIA system)
QT	Interval between the Q and T waves in an ECG
SAR	Seasonal allergic rhinitis (AAAAI/ACAAI system)

USADA	United States Anti-Doping Agency
WADA	World Anti-Doping Agency

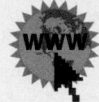 Self-assessment questions and answers are available at *http://www.mhpharmacotherapy. com/pp.html.*

REFERENCES

1. Wallace DV, Dykewicz MS, Bernstein DI, et al. The diagnosis and management of rhinitis: An updated practice parameter. J Allergy Clin Immunol 2008;122(2):S1–S84. [US AAAAI/ACAAAI].
2. Bousquet J, Khaltaev N, Cruzz AA, et al. Allergic rhinitis and its impact on asthma (ARIA) 2008 update. Allergy 2008;63(Suppl 86):S8–S160.
3. Scadding GK, Durham SR, Mirakian R, et al. BSACI guidelines for the management of allergic and nonallergic rhinitis. Clin Exp Allergy 2008;38:19–42.
4. Nathan RA. The burden of allergic rhinitis. Allergy Asthma Proc 2007;28(1):3–9.
5. Broide DH. The pathophysiology of allergic rhinoconjunctivitis. Allergy Asthma Proc 2007;28(4):398–403.
6. Blaiss MS. Allergic rhinoconjunctivitis: Burden of disease. Allergy Asthma Proc 2007;28:393–397.
7. Fletcher RH. An overview of rhinitis. In: Rose BD, ed. UpToDate. Waltham, MA: UpToDate, 2008.
8. Hur SY. Allergic rhinitis. The Rx Consultant 2007;16(3):1–8.
9. Carr WW. Pediatric allergic rhinitis: Current and future state of the art. Allergy Asthma Proc 2008;29(1):14–23.
10. de Bittner MR, Sulli MM, Williams DM. The role of nonprescription antihistamines in the treatment of allergic rhinitis [continuing education monograph on the Internet]. Washington, DC: American Pharmacists Association, 2008.
11. Rosenwasser L. New insights into the pathophysiology of allergic rhinitis. Allergy Asthma Proc 2007;28(1):10–15.
12. deShazo RD, Kemp SF. Pathogenesis of allergic rhinitis (rhinosinusitis). In: Rose BD, ed. UpToDate. Waltham, MA: UpToDate, 2008.
13. deShazo RD, Kemp SF. Management of allergic rhinitis. In: Rose BD, ed. UpToDate. Waltham, MA: UpToDate, 2008.
14. Calderon MA, Alves B, Jacobson M, et al. Allergen injection immunotherapy for seasonal allergic rhinitis [review]. Cochrane Database Syst Rev 2007;Issue 1. Art. No.: CD001936. DOI: 10.1002/14651858.CD001936.pub2.
15. Cox LS, Linnemann DL, Nolte H, et al. Sublingual immunotherapy: A comprehensive review. J Allergy Clin Immunol 2006;117:1021–1035.
16. Pajno GB. Sublingual immunotherapy: The optimism and the issues. J Allergy Clin Immunol 2007;119:796–801.
17. Wilson DR, Torres Lima M, Durham SR. Sublingual immunotherapy for allergic rhinitis [review]. Cochrane Database of Systematic Reviews. 2003, Issue 2. Art. No.: CD002893. DOI: 10.1002/14651858.CD002893.
18. Leatherman BD, Owen S, Parker M, et al. Sublingual immunotherapy: Past, present, paradigm for the future? Otolaryngol Head Neck Surg 2007;136:S1–S20.
19. Carr WW, Nelson MR, Hadley JA. Managing rhinitis: Strategies for improved patient outcomes. Allergy Asthma Proc 2008;29(4):349–357.
20. Lanier B. Allergic rhinitis: Selective comparisons of the pharmaceutical options for management. Allergy Asthma Proc 2007;28(1):16–19.
21. Krouse JH. Allergic rhinitis—Current pharmacotherapy. Otolaryngol Clin North Am 2008;41:347–358.
22. Marple BF, Fornadley JA, Patel AA, et al. Keys to successful management of patients with allergic rhinitis: Focus on patient

confidence, compliance, and satisfaction. Otolaryngol Head Neck Surg 2007;136:S107–S124.

23. Plaut M, Valentine MD. Allergic rhinitis. N Engl J Med 2005; 353(18):1934–1944.

24. Drugs for allergic disorders. Treat Guidel Med Lett 2007;5(60):71–80.

25. Drugs@FDA. U.S. Food and Drug Administration. Center for Drug Evaluation and Research. *http://www.accessdata.fda.gov/scripts/cder/drugsatfda/.*

26. Fluticasone furoate (Veramyst) for allergic rhinitis. Med Lett Drugs Ther 2007;49(1273):90–92.

27. Olopatadine (Patanase) nasal spray for allergic rhinitis. Med Lett Drugs Ther 2007;50(1289):51.

28. Lacy CF, Armstrong L, Goldman MP, et al., eds. Drug Information Handbook 2008–2009. 17th ed. Hudson, OH: LexiComp, 2008.

29. Kirtsreesakul V, Chansaksung P, Ruttanaphol S. Dose-related effect of intranasal corticosteroids on treatment outcome of persistent allergic rhinitis. Otolaryngol Head Neck Surg 2008;139(4):565–569.

30. Aranoff GR, Bennett WM, Berns JS, et al. Drug Prescribing in Renal Failure—Dosing Guidelines for Adults and Children, 5th ed. Philadelphia, PA: American College of Physicians, 2007.

31. American Pharmacists Association (APhA). DEA interim final regulation: Ephedrine, pseudoephedrine, and phenylpropanolamine requirements. September 2006, *http://www.pswi.org/government/Pseudoephedrine093006.pdf.*

32. U.S. Department of Justice. Drug Enforcement Administration. Office of Diversion Control. Combat Methamphetamine Epidemic Act 2005 (Title VII of Public Law 109–177). *http://www.deadiversion.usdoj.gov/meth/index.html.*

33. Kollar C, Schneider H, Waksman J, et al. Meta-analysis of the efficacy of a single dose of phenylephrine 10 mg compared with placebo in adults with acute nasal congestion due to the common cold. Clin Therap 2007;29(6):1057–1070.

34. Hendeles L, Hatton RC. Oral phenylephrine: An ineffective replacement for pseudoephedrine? J Allergy Clin Immunol 2006;118(1):279–280.

35. Hatton RC, Winterstein AG, McKelvey RP, et al. Efficacy and safety of oral phenylephrine: Systematic review and meta-analysis. Ann Pharmacother 2007;41:381–390.

36. Barnes ML, Biallosterski BT, Gray RD, et al. Decongestant effects of nasal xylometazoline and mometasone furoate in persistent allergic rhinitis. Rhinology 2005;43(4):291–295.

37. Lockey RF. Rhinitis medicamentosa and the stuffy nose. J Allergy Clin Immunol 2006;118:1017–1018.

38. Greiner AN, Meltzer EO. Pharmacologic rationale for treating allergic and nonallergic rhinitis. J Allergy Clin Immunol 2006;118:985–996.

39. U.S. Food and Drug Administration. Center for Drug Evaluation and Research. Early communication about an ongoing safety review of montelukast (Singulair). *http://www.fda.gov/cder/drug/early_comm/montelukast.htm.*

40. Rabago D. The use of saline nasal irrigation in common upper respiratory conditions. [continuing education monograph on the Internet]. US Pharmacist. 2008, *http://www.uspharmacist.com/oldformat.asp?url=ce/105757/default.htm.*

41. AAAAI Rhinosinusitis Committee. Saline sinus rinse recipe. American Association of Allergy Asthma & Immunology. *http://www.aaaai.org/patients/publicedmat/sinusitis/rinse_recipe.pdf.*

42. Passalacqua G, Bousquet PJ, Kai-Hakon C, et al. ARIA update: I-systematic review of complementary and alternative medicine for rhinitis and asthma. J Allergy Clin Immunol 2006;117:1054–1062.

43. Food and Drug Administration. FDA statement. FDA statement following CHPA's announcement on nonprescription over-the-counter cough and cold medicines in children. *http://www.fda.gov/bbs/topics/NEWS/2008/NEW01899.html.*

44. Briggs GG, Freeman RK, Yaffe SJ. Drugs in Pregnancy and Lactation., 8th ed. Philadelphia, PA: Lippincott Williams & Wilkins, 2008.

45. World Anti-Doping Agency (WADA) [homepage on the Internet]. Montreal, Quebec. *http://www.wada-ama.org/.*

46. U.S. Anti-Doping Agency (USADA) [homepage on the Internet]. Colorado Springs. *http://www.usantidoping.org/.*

47. U.S. Anti-Doping Agency (USADA) [homepage on the Internet]. Colorado Springs. Drug Reference Online™ (DRO). *http://www.usantidoping.org/dro/.*

63 Ophthalmic Disorders

Kendra J. Grande

LEARNING OBJECTIVES

● Upon completion of the chapter, the reader will be able to:

1. Differentiate between the various ophthalmic disorders based on patient-specific information.

2. Choose an appropriate treatment regimen for an ophthalmic disorder.

3. Discuss the product differences that direct the selection of ophthalmic medications.

4. Assess when further treatment is required based on patient-specific information.

5. Recommend an ophthalmic monitoring plan given patient-specific information, a diagnosis, and a treatment regimen.

6. Educate patients about ophthalmic disease states and appropriate drug and nondrug therapies.

KEY CONCEPTS

❶ The clinician must be able to distinguish ophthalmic conditions that lead to significant morbidity, including blindness.

❷ The choice of topical antibiotic in patients who wear contact lenses must cover *Pseudomonas aeruginosa*.

❸ Both acute and chronic bacterial conjunctivitis are self-limiting, except if caused by staphylococci.

❹ Viral conjunctivitis is usually self-limiting, worsening after 4 to 7 days, but then resolving within 2 to 4 weeks.

❺ Nonpharmacologic measures are critical to prevent the spread of viral conjunctivitis.

❻ Use a step-care approach for treatment of allergic conjunctivitis.

❼ Untreated bacterial keratitis is associated with corneal scarring and potential loss of vision. Corneal perforation may cause the loss of the eye.

❽ There is no cure for age-related macular degeneration (AMD) and the efficacy of most treatments is low.

❾ Dry eye is a chronic condition in which symptoms can be improved with treatment, but it is not usually curable. Patient education is critical.

INTRODUCTION

This chapter provides an overview of common ophthalmic disorders and their treatments. ❶ *Many ophthalmic disorders are benign or self-limited, but the practitioner must be able to distinguish conditions that lead to serious morbidity,* *including blindness.* Preserving both visual function and cosmetic appearance must be done whenever possible.[1] The clinician must understand when referral is appropriate and the appropriate time frame for follow-up. These vary greatly by condition.

OCULAR EMERGENCIES

ETIOLOGY AND EPIDEMIOLOGY

Ophthalmic problems encompass 3% to 10% of all emergency department visits.[1] Falls are a frequent cause of traumatic eye injury in the elderly.[2] Corneal abrasions are the most common eye injury in children and are often due to fingernail scratches or objects swung near the eye. Even aggressive eye rubbing may damage the cornea. Accidental cigarette burns are common in children, but may be a sign of child abuse.[3,4]

Health care practitioners must know the proper treatment for ocular emergencies and the time frame for follow-up in order to prevent further morbidity (Table 63–1).

CORNEAL ABRASIONS

Treatment

▶ *Desired Outcomes*

- Complete healing of the corneal abrasion with no scarring or vision impairment

- Prevent infection and pain

- Prevent corneal loss or corneal transplant

Clinical Presentation and Diagnosis of Corneal Abrasions[3]

Symptoms
- Photophobia
- Pain with extraocular muscle movement
- Foreign body sensation
- Recent ocular trauma
- Gritty feeling
- Headache

Signs
- Excessive tearing
- Blepharospasm
- Blurred vision

Diagnostic Test
Use sterile fluorescein dye strips and visualize the cornea under a cobalt-blue filtered light; abrasions appear green; ensure that no foreign body remains in the eye

---

Table 63–1

Ophthalmic Emergencies: Time to Follow-Up by Ophthalmologist

Immediate Consult Required	Within 24 Hours
Foreign body in eye	Acute angle-closure glaucoma
Acute, painless loss of vision	Orbital cellulitis
Acute chemical burn	Blood in the eye (hyphema)
Blunt trauma to eye	Macular edema
	Retinal detachment
	Sudden congestive proptosis (bulging of eye forward)
	Corneal ulcer
	Corneal abrasion

From Ref. 1.

▶ *General Approach to Treatment*

The five layers of the cornea contain no blood vessels but are nourished by tears, oxygen, and aqueous humor. Minor corneal abrasions heal quickly. Moderate abrasions take 24 to 72 hours to heal. Deep scratches may scar the cornea and require corneal transplant if vision is impaired. Do not use eye patches to treat corneal abrasion, as they decrease oxygen delivery, increase pain, and increase the chance of infection.[3]

Corneal Abrasion Prevention[3]
- Wear eye protection during sports
- Wear industrial safety lenses
- Clip fingernails of infants and children
- Remove low-hanging branches and objects

Patient Encounter 1

A 12-year-old boy presents with a swollen, watery left eye that he cannot open. His mom says he was outside playing when it happened. You question the boy and he says he was sword-fighting with long sticks and was poked in the eye. He says it feels as though a piece of stick might still be in the eye. He rubbed it hard to try and improve it but now it hurts to even open the eye.

What is the proper time frame for follow-up for this injury?

What are the desired outcomes for this patient?

What pharmacologic therapy might be used after the foreign body is removed?

- Tape the eyelids closed or use gels or soft contacts during general anesthesia to prevent lag-ophthalmos
- Carefully fit and place contact lenses

Pharmacologic Therapy

▶ *Topical NSAIDs*

Topical nonsteroidal anti-inflammatory drugs (NSAIDs) decrease pain from corneal abrasion. Available ocular NSAIDs are diclofenac 0.1%, ketorolac 0.5%, nepafenac 0.1%, and bromfenac 0.09%. The usual dose for diclofenac and ketorolac is one drop four times daily; nepafenac is dosed three times daily and bromfenac is dosed twice daily. Use topical NSAIDs with caution in patients with clotting disorders or those who are on systemic NSAIDs or warfarin therapy. Topical administration of NSAIDs may delay wound healing, especially with concurrent topical corticosteroid use.[3,5] Oral analgesics are not well studied for use in corneal abrasion; they may have decreased efficacy. They are less expensive than topical NSAIDs and may be an option for some patients.[3]

▶ *Topical Antibiotics*

Because an infection slows the healing of a corneal abrasion, prophylactic antibiotics are often used. Studies on the efficacy of this are mixed. Discontinue the use of contact lenses until the abrasion is healed and the antibiotic course complete. ❷ *In contact lens wearers, choose an antibiotic that covers* Pseudomonas aeruginosa, *like gentamicin ointment or solution or a fluoroquinolone.*[3] Antibiotic resistance is an increasing problem. Resistance occurs primarily with older antibiotics, but has been reported for fluoroquinolones as well. Two newer fluoroquinolones, gatifloxacin and moxifloxacin, do not yet have reports of resistance. These agents are more expensive.[6]

Outcome Evaluation
1. Reevaluate patients in 24 hours.
2. If symptoms worsen, recheck for foreign bodies.
3. If not fully healed, evaluate again in 3 to 4 days.

4. Refer to ophthalmologist if[3]:
- No improvement in 3 days
- Worsening symptoms
- Symptoms do not improve daily
- Symptoms do not improve within a few hours of contact lens removal

OTHER OCULAR EMERGENCIES: TREATMENT

Traumatic Injuries

Attempt to remove loose foreign bodies by gentle irrigation with artificial tears or sterile saline. If removal is successful, a topical broad-spectrum antibiotic, such as erythromycin, will prevent infection. Some patients may need a short-acting cycloplegic mydriatic-like cyclopentolate or tropicamide to help with pain.[7] Do not use cycloplegic mydriatics in children.[8] If irrigation is unsuccessful, mechanical removal of foreign objects should be completed only by ophthalmologists using a slitlamp. Protect the eye with a metal eye shield or a paper cup taped over the eye while awaiting the ophthalmologist.[7]

Splash Injuries and Chemical Exposure

Instruct patients by phone to irrigate the eye immediately with water or saline continuously for at least 15 minutes before seeking a clinician. Irrigation dilutes and removes the chemical agent, and is the best way to decrease ocular tissue damage. Patients should then seek immediate care from an ophthalmologist or emergency facility.[7]

Loss of Vision

A variety of disorders may lead to rapid, painless, monocular or binocular vision loss. These include central retinal artery occlusion, acute narrow-angle glaucoma, trauma, and others. The differential diagnosis is complex and needs to be undertaken by an emergency department or ophthalmologist.[9]

CONJUNCTIVITIS

While no exact numbers are available, conjunctivitis, also known as red eye, is one of the most common ophthalmic complaints seen by general clinicians. An inflamed conjunctiva is the most common cause of red eye.[10] Use the differential diagnosis algorithm shown in Figure 63–1 to determine the proper treatment or need for referral.

BACTERIAL CONJUNCTIVITIS

Etiology

The vast majority of conjunctivitis cases are viral in nature. For acute bacterial conjunctivitis, the cause is primarily gram-positive organisms.[11] The primary pathogens in acute bacterial conjunctivitis are *Streptococcus pneumoniae*, *Staphylococcus aureus*, or *Haemophilus influenzae*.[12]

Staphylococcus, *Moraxella*, or other opportunistic bacteria typically cause chronic conjunctivitis.[10] *Moraxella* infections may cluster in groups of women who share makeup.[12] ❸ *Both acute and chronic bacterial conjunctivitis are self-limiting except if caused by staphylococci.*[13] Because of this, the pathogens are rarely cultured unless the case is unresponsive to treatment. While infection typically begins in one eye, it will often spread to both within 48 hours.[11]

Hyperacute bacterial conjunctivitis is associated with gonococcal infections in sexually active patients. The causative agents are *Neisseria gonorrhoeae* or *N. meningitidis*. Prompt

FIGURE 63–1. Differential diagnosis for red eye.

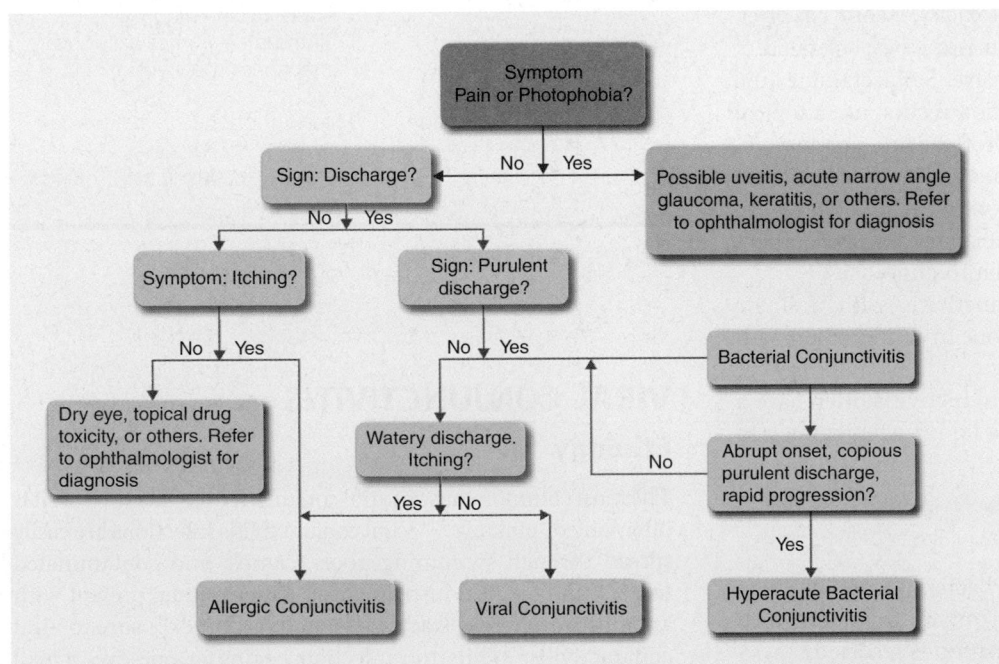

workup and treatment is required, as corneal perforation occurs in 10% of cases within 48 hours.[12] An ophthalmologist should complete a conjunctival scraping and susceptibility testing.[10]

Treatment

▶ Desired Outcomes

- Complete resolution of the bacterial conjunctivitis
- Prevent adverse consequences of the infection
- Preserve functionality of the eye

▶ General Approach to Treatment

Treat acute bacterial conjunctivitis with broad-spectrum antibiotics. Although the condition is usually self-limiting, antibiotic treatment decreases the spread of disease to other people and prevents extraocular infection. Additionally, treatment may help decrease the risk of corneal ulceration or other complications that affect sight. Finally, treatment speeds recovery.[14]

▶ Pharmacologic Therapy

The choice of an antibiotic agent for acute bacterial conjunctivitis is largely empiric. The initial treatment needs to include *Staphylococcus* coverage, but also may be chosen on the basis of cost and side-effect profile.[13,14] In general, ointments are a good dosage form for children. Adults may prefer drops because they do not interfere with vision.[14]

Many broad-spectrum topical antibiotics are approved to treat acute bacterial conjunctivitis (Tables 63–2 and 63–3). Polymyxin B/trimethoprim solution, polymyxin B with bacitracin ointment, or erythromycin ointment are cost-effective, first-line treatments. The aminoglycosides (tobramycin, neomycin, and gentamicin) are alternatives but have incomplete gram-positive coverage.[14] The aminoglycosides can cause corneal epithelial toxicity. Neomycin often causes allergic reactions. Tobramycin is the best tolerated of the class, but is also the most expensive. Sulfacetamide 10% shows increasing resistance. If infection recurs, use a topical fluoroquinolone like ofloxacin, ciprofloxacin, norfloxacin, gatifloxacin, moxifloxacin, or levofloxacin.[12] Fluoroquinolones are not used first-line for conjunctivitis because they have poor *Streptococcus* coverage and are expensive. Development of resistance is also a concern with fluoroquinolones.[14]

Treat hyperacute bacterial conjunctivitis with a single dose of 1 g of intramuscular ceftriaxone in combination with topical antibiotics.[11]

Patients with chronic bacterial conjunctivitis often have a concurrent case of blepharitis. Add a lid hygiene regimen to topical antibiotic treatment.[12]

Outcome Evaluation

Significant improvement of acute bacterial conjunctivitis should be seen within 1 week.[11] Terminate treatment with topical antibiotics when the inflammation is resolved.[12]

Table 63–2
Adult Bacterial Conjunctivitis Dosing Guidelines for Topical Ophthalmic Antibiotics

Azithromycin 1% solution	Days 1 and 2: 1 drop twice daily, 8–12 hours apart
	Days 3–7: 1 drop once daily
Ciprofloxacin 3.5 mg/mL solution	Days 1 and 2: 1–2 drops every 2 hours while awake
	Days 3–7: 1–2 drops every 4 hours while awake
Ciprofloxacin 0.3% ointment	Apply a ½ in. ribbon of ointment 3 times daily for 2 days, then twice daily for next 5 days
Erythromycin 0.5% ointment	Apply a ½ in. ribbon of ointment up to 6 times daily
Gatifloxacin 0.3% solution	Days 1 and 2: 1 drop every 2 hours while awake up to 8 times daily
	Days 3–7: 1 drop every 4 hours while awake
Gentamicin 0.3% solution	1–2 drops every 4 hours. In severe infections, may use up to 2 drops every hour
Levofloxacin 0.5% solution	Days 1 and 2: 1–2 drops every 2 hours while awake, up to 8 times per day
	Days 3–7: 1–2 drops every 4 hours while awake, up to 4 times daily
Moxifloxacin 0.5% solution	1 drop 3 times a day for 7 days
Ofloxacin 0.3% solution	Days 1 and 2: 1–2 drops every 2–4 hours while awake
	Days 3–7: 1–2 drops 4 times daily
Polymyxin B with bacitracin ointment	Apply a ½ in. ribbon of ointment every 3–4 hours for 7–10 days
Polymyxin B/trimethoprim solution	1 drop every 3 hours for 7–10 days
Sulfacetamide 10% ointment	Apply a ½ in. ribbon of ointment every 3–4 hours and at bedtime
Sulfacetamide 10% solution	1–2 drops every 2–3 hours for 7–10 days
Tobramycin 0.3% ointment	Mild-to-moderate infections: Apply a ½ in. ribbon of ointment 2–3 times daily Severe infections: Apply every 3–4 hours
Tobramycin 0.3% solution	Mild-to-moderate infections: 1–2 drops every 4 hours Severe infections: initially, 2 drops every hour

From Refs. 5, 15, 16.

VIRAL CONJUNCTIVITIS

Etiology

The most common cause of viral conjunctivitis is adenovirus. It is often called "pink-eye."[10] Viral conjunctivitis infections are easily spread through swimming pools, camps, and contaminated fingers, and medical instruments.[14] Patients often present with an upper respiratory tract infection or recent exposure to viral conjunctivitis. While the infection begins in one eye, it will

Table 63–3

Pediatric Dosing Guidelines for Bacterial Conjunctivitis for Topical Ophthalmic Antibiotics

Azithromycin 1% solution	Children 1 year of age or older: Days 1 and 2: 1 drop twice daily, 8–12 hours apart Days 3–7: 1 drop once daily
Ciprofloxacin 3.5 mg/mL solution	Children 1 year of age or older, days 1 and 2: 1–2 drops every 2 hours while awake Days 3–7: 1–2 drops every 4 hours while awake
Ciprofloxacin 0.3% ointment	Children 2 years of age or older: Apply a ½ in. ribbon of ointment 3 times daily for 2 days, then twice daily for next 5 days
Erythromycin 0.5% ointment	Apply a ½ in. ribbon of ointment up to 6 times daily
Gatifloxacin 0.3% solution	Children 1 year of age or older, days 1 and 2: 1 drop every 2 hours while awake up to 8 times daily Days 3–7: 1 drop every 4 hours while awake
Gentamicin 0.3% solution	Infants and children 28 days of age or older: 1–2 drops every 4 hours. In severe infections, may use up to 2 drops every hour
Levofloxacin 0.5% solution	Children 1 year of age or older, days 1 and 2: 1–2 drops every 2 hours while awake, up to 8 times daily Days 3–7: 1–2 drops every 4 hours while awake, up to 4 times daily
Moxifloxacin 0.5% solution	Children 1 year of age or older: 1 drop 3 times a day for 7 days
Ofloxacin 0.3% solution	Children 1 year of age or older, days 1 and 2: 1–2 drops every 2–4 hours while awake Days 3–7: 1–2 drops 4 times daily
Polymyxin B with bacitracin ointment	Apply a ½ in. ribbon of ointment every 3–4 hours for 7–10 days
Polymyxin B/ trimethoprim solution	Infants and children 2 months of age or older: 1 drop every 3 hours for 7–10 days
Sulfacetamide 10% ointment	Apply a ½ in. ribbon of ointment every 3–4 hours and at bedtime
Sulfacetamide 10% solution	1–2 drops every 2–3 hours for 7–10 days
Tobramycin 0.3% ointment	Infants and children 2 months of age or older: Mild-to-moderate infections: Apply an approximately ½ in. ribbon 2–3 times daily Severe infections: Apply every 3–4 hours
Tobramycin 0.3% solution	Mild-to-moderate infections: 1–2 drops every 4 hours Severe infections: initially, 2 drops every hour

From Refs. 15, 16.

spread to both eyes 50% of the time. ❹ *Viral conjunctivitis is usually self-limiting, worsening after 4 to 7 days but then resolving within 2 to 4 weeks.*[10] Five percentage of patients remain contagious 16 days after the appearance of symptoms.[11]

Patient Encounter 2

A 40-year-old woman presents complaining of irritation, redness, and stickiness of the right eye for the past 48 hours. Today she woke up with the lids of the right eye stuck together and it took a warm washcloth to get her eye open. Examination reveals a whitish discharge from the right eye and a redness of the left eye. She has worn contact lenses for 6 years.

What is the probable diagnosis?

On physical assessment, how do you differentiate between bacterial, hyperacute bacterial, viral, and allergic causes?

What is a reasonable treatment regimen for her?

Treatment

▶ Desired Outcomes

- Complete resolution of the viral conjunctivitis
- Prevent adverse consequences of the infection
- Avoid spreading infection to other patients

▶ Nonpharmacologic Therapy

❺ *Nonpharmacologic measures are critical to prevent the spread of viral conjunctivitis.* Patients should not share towels or other contaminated objects, should avoid close contact with other people, and avoid swimming for 2 weeks.[10] The virus remains viable on dry surfaces for more than 2 weeks.[13] Take care in the medical setting to thoroughly decontaminate instruments and wash hands.[11]

Patients may obtain symptomatic relief by using cold compresses and artificial tears.[10] If artificial tear solutions sting, recommend a preservative-free formula.

▶ Pharmacologic Therapy

Topical antivirals are not used to treat adenovirus conjunctivitis. Topical antibiotics are often prescribed for viral conjunctivitis, ostensibly to prevent bacterial superinfection. In reality, this is a case of the patient insisting on a medication to speed healing.[11] Avoid the use of antibiotics for a viral infection.[12] Eliminating superfluous antibiotic use also helps prevent the development of antibiotic resistance.

If patients have a severe subepithelial infiltration, a topical steroid may be required. However, topical steroids may cause serious ocular complications and may worsen herpetic conjunctivitis, which has similar symptoms as viral conjunctivitis. Additionally, the period of virus shedding may be prolonged by up to 50% by topical prednisolone. Only ophthalmologists should prescribe topical steroids.[10]

Outcome Evaluation

Refer patients that do not see improvement within 7 to 10 days to an ophthalmologist to rule out herpetic and other infectious processes.[11] If pain or photophobia occurs, suspect corneal involvement and refer the patient. This typically occurs 10 to 14 days after the onset of conjunctivitis.[13]

ALLERGIC CONJUNCTIVITIS

Etiology

Ocular allergy is a broad term that includes several diseases with the hallmark symptom of itching, often accompanied by tearing, conjunctival swelling, and nasal congestion.[14] Seasonal ocular allergy is the most common type of allergic conjunctivitis. This is an IgE-mediated hypersensitivity to pollen or other airborne allergens.[11] Often, the patient's history is positive for atopic conditions such as allergic rhinitis, asthma, or eczema.[14] Perennial allergic conjunctivitis has similar but less severe symptoms and may not be tied to a specific time of year. Finally, conjunctivitis medicamentosa is a contact allergy to a topical medication, often an antibiotic.[11]

Pathophysiology

The conjunctiva of the eye is often the first site of contact with an environmental allergen. Mast cell degranulation occurs, resulting in the release of mediators. The earliest mediator is histamine, which causes itching, redness, and swelling. Leukotrienes and prostaglandins cause increased mucus secretion and cellular infiltration along with chemosis, resulting in conjunctival vasodilation. The mast cells also release cytokines, chemokines, and growth factors which trigger inflammatory processes.[17]

Treatment of ocular allergy is aimed at slowing or stopping these processes. Antihistamines block the histamine receptors and some prevent histamine production and/or inhibit mediator release from the mast cells.[17] Mast cell stabilizers inhibit the degranulation of mast cells, preventing mediator release. Some topical agents have multiple mechanisms of action, combining antihistaminic, mast cell stabilization, and anti-inflammatory properties (Tables 63–4, 63–5, and 63–6).[18]

Treatment

▶ Desired Outcomes

- Relief of current allergic symptoms
- Prevention of future allergic symptoms
- No adverse effects from treatment

▶ Nonpharmacologic Therapy

The primary treatment for ocular allergy is removal and avoidance of the allergen.[19] For conjunctivitis medicamentosa, discontinue the offending medication.[11] Apply cold compresses three to four times daily to reduce redness and itching and to provide symptomatic relief.[20]

▶ Pharmacologic Therapy

❻ Use a step-care approach for the treatment of allergic conjunctivitis. The first step is a nonmedicated, artificial tears solution. The solution dilutes or removes the allergen, providing relief while lubricating the eye. Solutions are applied two to four times daily as needed. Ointments may be used in the evenings to further moisturize the surface of the eye.[19] There are many products on the market. Try a preservative-free formulation if other products sting or burn. Unit-dose preservative-free products are more expensive. Some newer multidose products, such as sodium perborate

---

Table 63–4		
Mechanisms of Action of Ocular Allergy Drugs		
Drug	**Mechanisms**	**Notes**
Antazoline	H_1-receptor antagonist	Available only in combination with naphazoline
Azelastine	H_1-receptor antagonist, mast cell stabilizer	May inhibit cytokine release
Cromolyn sodium	Mast cell stabilizer	
Emedastine	H_1-receptor antagonist; inhibits eosinophil chemotaxis	Superior H_1-receptor binding ability
Epinastine	H_1- and H_2-receptor antagonist, mast cell stabilizer, anti-inflammatory	
Ketorolac	Prostaglandin inhibitor	
Ketotifen	H_1-receptor antagonist, mast cell stabilizer, eosinophil inhibitor, platelet-activating factor inhibitor	May inhibit eosinophil chemotaxis
Levocabastine	H_1-receptor antagonist	Downregulates intracellular adhesion molecules, decreasing the inflammatory response; may be used for up to 2 weeks
Lodoxamide	Mast cell stabilizer	May be used for up to 3 months
Loteprednol	Corticosteroid	Only 0.2% approved for seasonal allergic conjunctivitis
Nedocromil	Mast cell stabilizer, H_1-receptor antagonist	May inhibit eosinophils
Olopatadine	Antihistaminic, mast cell stabilizer	
Pemirolast	Mast cell stabilizer	
Pheniramine	H_1-receptor antagonist	Available only in combination with naphazoline

From Refs. 17–19.

Table 63–5

Adult Dosing and Common Side Effects of Ocular Allergy Drugs

Drug	Dosing[a]	Common Side Effects[b]
Antazoline	Varies by manufacturer and product	Ocular stinging
Azelastine 0.05%	1 drop in affected eye(s) twice daily	Ocular stinging, headache, bitter taste
Cromolyn sodium 4%	1–2 drops in each eye 4–6 times daily	Ocular stinging
Emedastine 0.05%	1 drop in affected eye up to 4 times daily	Headache
Epinastine 0.05%	1 drop in each eye twice daily	Ocular stinging, cold symptoms
Ketorolac 0.4–0.5%	1 drop 4 times a day	Ocular stinging, irritation
Ketotifen 0.025%	1 drop in affected eye(s) twice daily	Red eyes (conjunctival injection), headache
Levocabastine 0.05%	1 drop in affected eye(s) 4 times daily	Ocular stinging, headache
Lodoxamide 0.1%	1–2 drops in affected eye(s) 4 times daily	Ocular stinging, foreign body sensation
Loteprednol 0.2%	1 drop in affected eye(s) 4 times daily	Elevated intraocular pressure, cataracts, decreased wound healing, secondary ocular infections, systemic side effects possible
Nedocromil 2%	1–2 drops in each eye twice daily	Ocular stinging, bitter taste
Olopatadine 0.1%	1–2 drops in affected eye(s) 2 times daily at 6- to 8-hour intervals	Headache
Pemirolast 0.1%	1–2 drops in affected eye(s) 4 times daily	Headache, cold symptoms
Pheniramine	Varies by manufacturer and product	Ocular stinging

[a]From Refs. 5, 15.

[b]From Ref. 19.

Table 63–6

Pediatric Dosing of Ocular Allergy Drugs

Drug	Dosing
Antazoline	Varies by manufacturer and product
Azelastine 0.05%	Children 3 years of age or older: 1 drop in affected eye(s) twice daily
Cromolyn sodium 4%	Children 4 years of age or older: 1–2 drops in each eye 4–6 times daily
Emedastine 0.05%	Children 3 years of age or older: 1 drop in affected eye up to 4 times daily
Epinastine 0.05%	Children 3 years of age or older: 1 drop in each eye twice daily for up to 8 weeks
Ketorolac 0.5%	Children 3 years of age or older: 1 drop in affected eye(s) 4 times a day
Ketotifen 0.025%	Children 3 years of age or older: 1 drop in affected eye(s) twice daily
Levocabastine 0.05%	Children 12 years of age or older: 1 drop in affected eye(s) 4 times daily
Lodoxamide 0.1%	Children 2 years of age or older: 1–2 drops in affected eye(s) 4 times daily
Nedocromil 2%	Children 3 years of age or older: 1–2 drops in each eye twice daily
Olopatadine 0.1%	Children 3 years of age or older: 1–2 drops in affected eye(s) 2 times daily at 6- to 8- hour intervals
Pemirolast 0.1%	Children 3 years of age or older: 1–2 drops in affected eye(s) 4 times daily
Pheniramine	Varies by manufacturer and product

From Ref. 5.

(Purite), have rapidly dissociating preservatives and are more cost-effective.

If artificial tears are insufficient, the second treatment step is a topical antihistamine or antihistamine/decongestant combination. The antihistamine/decongestant combination is more effective than either agent alone. Decongestants are vasoconstrictors that reduce redness and seem to have a small synergistic effect with the antihistamine. The only topical decongestant used in combination products is naphazoline. Topical decongestants burn and sting on instillation and commonly cause mydriasis, especially in patients with lighter-colored eyes. Long-term use leads to rebound congestion. Topical decongestant use should be limited to less than 10 days.[19]

There is still debate whether oral antihistamines control ocular allergy as well as topical antihistamines. Topical antihistamines are recommended before oral agents in step therapy because of the increased risk of systemic side effects with oral drugs. Additionally, topical antihistamines provide faster relief of ocular symptoms. Consider oral antihistamines when systemic symptoms are present.[17]

If insufficient relief is obtained from these products, either a mast cell stabilizer or a multiple-action agent is appropriate.[19] Use mast cell stabilizers prophylactically throughout the allergy season. Full response may take 4 to 6 weeks.

If mast cell stabilizers or multiple-action agents are not successful, a trial of a topical NSAID is appropriate. Ketorolac is the only approved topical agent for ocular itching. NSAIDs do not mask ocular infections, affect wound healing, increase intraocular pressure, or contribute to cataract formation like the topical corticosteroids. However, in clinical trials, for allergic conjunctivitis topical ketorolac was not as effective as olopatadine or emedastine.[17] Full efficacy of ketorolac may take up to 2 weeks.[19]

If all these avenues are ineffective, short-term topical corticosteroids and immunotherapy are the third-line treatments for ocular allergy.[19]

Outcome Evaluation

Monitor patients for relief of symptoms. Ensure an adequate trial of the agent. If no improvement is seen, follow a stepped-care approach to treatment. Refer severe cases that do not respond to an ophthalmologist for short-term topical corticosteroids.

BACTERIAL KERATITIS

EPIDEMIOLOGY

Thirty thousand cases of microbial keratitis occur annually in the United States.[21] Microbial keratitis encompasses bacterial, fungal, and *Acanthamoeba* keratitis.[21] Only bacterial keratitis, the most common form, is discussed here.

PATHOPHYSIOLOGY

Bacterial keratitis is a broad term for a bacterial infection of the cornea. This includes corneal ulcers and corneal abscesses.

Clinical Presentation and Diagnosis of Bacterial Keratitis[10,21]

General

The rate of progression of signs and symptoms varies depending on the infecting organism. A differential diagnosis for keratitis must include viral, fungal, and nematodal infections in addition to bacterial causes.

Symptoms

- Photophobia
- Rapid onset of ocular pain

Signs

- Red eye
- Conjunctival discharge
- Decreased vision

Laboratory Tests

Culture if keratitis is severe or sight-threatening. Otherwise, culture or smear only if the corneal infiltrate is chronic or unresponsive to broad-spectrum antimicrobial therapy.

The cornea in a healthy eye has natural resistance to infection, making bacterial keratitis rare. However, many factors may predispose a patient to bacterial infection by compromising the defense mechanisms of the eye (Table 63–7).[21]

The most common pathogens in bacterial keratitis are *Pseudomonas* (including *Pseudomonas aeruginosa*) and other gram-negative rods, Staphylococci, and Streptococci.[21] If the keratitis is related to the use of contacts, *Pseudomonas* and *Serratia marcescens* are the most common pathogens.[21] For hospitalized infants and adults on respirators, *Pseudomonas* is the most common.[21]

❼ *Untreated bacterial keratitis is associated with corneal scarring and potential loss of vision.*[21] *Corneal perforation may occur and the patient may lose the eye.*[21] In virulent organisms, this destruction may occur within 24 hours.[21] Central corneal scarring may result in vision loss even after successful eradication of the organism.[21]

TREATMENT

Desired Outcomes[21]

- Resolution of infection
- Resolution of corneal inflammation

Table 63–7

Risk Factors for Bacterial Keratitis

Exogenous Factors
Contact lenses
Loose sutures
Previous corneal surgery
Previous ocular or eyelid surgery
Trauma

Ocular Surface Disease
Abnormal lid anatomy or function
Misdirection of eyelashes
Ocular infection (e.g., conjunctivitis, blepharitis)
Tear film deficiencies

Systemic Conditions
Atopic dermatitis
Connective tissue disease
Debilitating illness (e.g., malnourishment or respirator dependence)
Diabetes mellitus
Factitious disease (including anesthetic abuse)
Gonococcal infection
Immunocompromised
Stevens-Johnson syndrome
Substance abuse
Vitamin A deficiency

Medications
Anesthetics
Antimicrobials
Contaminated ocular medications
Glaucoma medications
Preservatives
Steroids
Topical NSAIDs

Corneal Epithelial Abnormalities
Corneal epithelial edema
Predisposition to recurrent erosion of the cornea
Viral keratitis (e.g., herpes simplex or zoster keratitis)

From Ref. 21.

- Reduced corneal pain
- Restored corneal integrity with minimal scarring
- Restored visual function

General Approach to Treatment

All cases of suspected bacterial keratitis require prompt ophthalmology consultation to prevent permanent vision loss.[10]

Pharmacologic Therapy

▶ *Dosage Considerations*

Topical antibiotic drops are preferred. Consider subconjunctival antibiotics if compliance is a concern. Systemic therapy is useful in cases of systemic infection (e.g., gonorrhea) or if the sclera is infected. Reserve ointments for minor cases or adjunctive nighttime therapy.[21]

▶ *Drug Choice*

Start topical broad-spectrum antibiotics empirically. Use a loading dose for severe keratitis (Table 63–8). Single-drug therapy with a fluoroquinolone is as effective as combination therapy. Resistance is seen with some fluoroquinolones. Because of this, choose a newer fluoroquinolone such as

moxifloxacin or gatifloxacin in severe keratitis cases.[6,21] Fortified antibiotic therapy is an option for severe or unresponsive infections, but may increase toxicity to the cornea and surrounding tissues. Fortified antibiotics must be compounded.[21] All compounded formulations must comply with governmental 797 regulations concerning compounding of drug preparations.

Topical corticosteroids are employed in some cases of bacterial keratitis. The suppression of inflammation may reduce corneal scarring. However, local immunosuppression, increased ocular pressure, and reappearance of the infection are disadvantages to their use. There is no conclusive evidence that they alter clinical outcomes. If the patient is already on topical corticosteroids when the keratitis occurs, discontinue use until the infection is eliminated.[21]

Outcome Evaluation[21]

- Monitor patient symptoms for improvement to determine therapeutic efficacy
- Modify treatment regimen based on results of culture and sensitivity testing, if necessary
- Modify the treatment regimen if the patient does not show improvement within 48 hours
- Gram-negative keratitis will have increased inflammation in the first 24 to 48 hours, even on appropriate therapy
- Taper therapy based on clinical response
- Reculture or biopsy if negative clinical response; to improve culture results, discontinue antibiotics for 12 to 24 hours before culturing.

Table 63–8

Pharmacologic Therapies for Bacterial Keratitis

Organism	Drug
Unknown or multiple types of organisms	Cefazolin 50 mg/mL *and* tobramycin/gentamicin 9–14 mg/mL *or* Fluoroquinolones various strengths
Gram-positive cocci	Cefazolin 50 mg/mL *or* Vancomycin[a] 15–50 mg/mL *or* Bacitracin[a] 10,000 international unit *or* Moxifloxacin or Gatifloxacin various strengths
Gram-negative rods	Tobramycin 9–14 mg/mL *or* Gentamicin 9–14 mg/mL *or* Ceftazidime 50 mg/mL *or* Fluoroquinolones various strengths
Gram-negative cocci	Ceftriaxone 50 mg/mL *or* Ceftazidime 50 mg/mL *or* Fluoroquinolones various strengths
Nontuberculous mycobacteria	Amikacin 20–40 mg/mL *or* Oral clarithromycin, adults: 500 mg every 12 hours Fluoroquinolones various strengths
Nocardia	Amikacin 20–40 mg/mL *or* Trimethoprim 16 mg/mL *and* sulfamethoxazole 80 mg/mL

Adult Topical Dosing

Severe keratitis: loading dose every 5–15 minutes for the first hour, then every 15 minutes to 1 hour around the clock. Less severe keratitis may use less frequent dosing

[a]Use for resistant *Enterococcus* and *Staphylococcus* species and penicillin allergy. No gram-negative activity, do not use vancomycin or bacitracin for single agent empiric therapy in bacterial keratitis.

From Ref. 21.

MACULAR DEGENERATION

EPIDEMIOLOGY AND ETIOLOGY

Age-related macular degeneration (AMD) is the primary cause of severe, irreversible vision impairment in developed countries (Figs. 63–2 and 63–3). The prevalence increases with age.[22] In the United States, 1.75 million people age 40 or older have advanced AMD, and another 7 million people may have intermediate AMD.[22] Because of the rapid aging of the U.S. population, it is projected that almost 3 million people will develop AMD by 2020.[23] The causes of AMD are not completely known (Table 63–9).[22]

PATHOPHYSIOLOGY

AMD is a deterioration of the **macula**, the central portion of the retina. The macula facilitates central vision and high-resolution visual acuity because it has the highest concentration of photoreceptors in the retina. The loss of central vision leads to irreversible loss of the ability to drive, read, and perform other fine visual tasks like recognize faces.[25] Peripheral vision is preserved, allowing mobility.[22] AMD is characterized by one or more of the following: **drusen** formation, retinal pigment

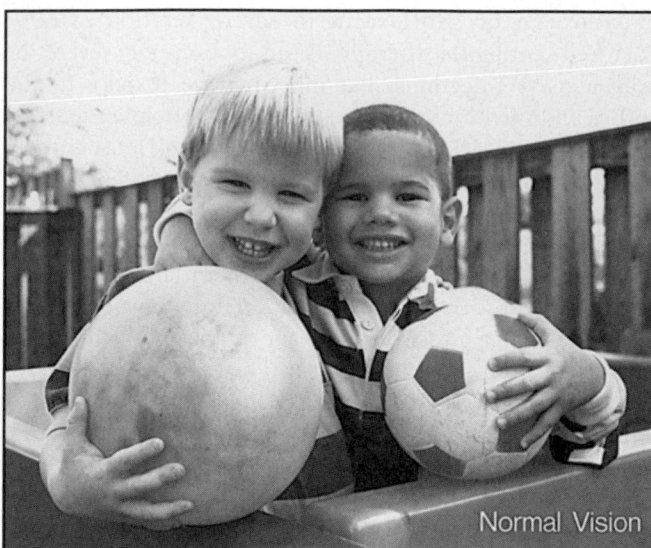

FIGURE 63–2. Normal vision. (From the National Eye Institute, National Institutes of Health Ref. No. EDS01. Accessed online at: *http://www.nei.nih.gov/photo/*)

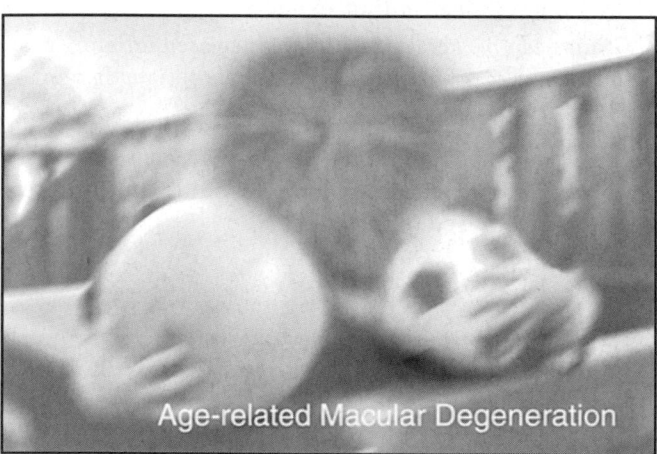

FIGURE 63–3. The scene in Figure 63–2 as it might be viewed by a person with age-related macular degeneration. (From the National Eye Institute, National Institutes of Health Ref. No. EDS05. Accessed online at: *http://www.nei.nih.gov/photo/*)

Table 63–9	
Risk Factors for AMD	
Definite Risk Factors	**Potential Risk Factors**
Advancing age	Cardiovascular disease
Light pigmentation (white ethnicity)	Hypertension
	Low dietary intake of antioxidant vitamins or zinc
Cigarette smoking	Increased body mass index
Family history	Higher dietary fat intake

From Ref. 22, 24.

Clinical Presentation and Diagnosis of AMD[20,23]

Symptoms
- Mild blurry central vision
- Difficulty reading
- Trouble with color and contrast
- Painless, progressive, moderate to severe blurring of central vision
- Sudden loss or distortion of vision possible

Signs
- Drusen
- Retinal pigment epithelial mottling

Other Diagnostic Tests
- Amsler's grid abnormalities indicate fluid in subretinal space (Figs. 63–4 and 63–5)
- Dilated fundus examination shows drusen and pigmentary abnormalities in the macula
- Rapid sequence fluorescein angiography shows leakage in the neovascular form

Patient Encounter 3, Part 1

ET, a 60-year-old white male, presents with difficulty reading and says he is having trouble differentiating between red and orange.

PMH: Hypertension, diabetes mellitus for 12 years, congestive heart failure

SH: Smokes half a pack daily; denies any alcohol or drug use; married, one adult child who lives nearby

FH: Father died at age 57 from heart failure; mother blind from age 50, died at 62 from breast cancer

PE:

BP 140/98, ht 6' 0" (182 cm), wt 120 kg (264 lb)

What risk factors and potential risk factors for age-related macular degeneration does the patient have?

abnormalities (e.g., hypo- or hyperpigmentation), geographic atrophy, and **neovascular maculopathy**.[20]

Based on clinical presentation, AMD is classified as early, intermediate, or advanced.[20] Early AMD is characterized by small or intermediate drusen and minimal macular pigment abnormalities.[20] These patients generally have normal central vision.[20] Intermediate AMD patients have medium or large drusen in one or both eyes.[20] Approximately 18% of these patients will progress to advanced AMD within 5 years.[20]

Advanced AMD is classified as non-neovascular (also called the atropic, nonexudative, or dry form) or neovascular (the exudative or wet form).[22,25] In the non-neovascular form, the retina and other layers atrophy.[25] In the neovascular form, new blood vessels appear.[22,25] Generally, vision is already affected when patients progress to advanced AMD; vision loss is seen in both forms.[22] Ten to twenty percentage of patients with the non-neovascular form will progress to the neovascular form.[26] Once one eye develops advanced AMD, 43% of patients will develop neovascular changes or atrophy in the other eye within 5 years.[22]

TREATMENT

Desired Outcomes

The primary goal of treatment for AMD is to slow the disease progression. This includes slowing the loss of visual acuity and the progression to legal blindness, along with maintaining contrast sensitivity and slowing the rate of progression to late AMD. The secondary goals are maintaining quality of life for the patient and minimizing the adverse effects of treatment.[25]

General Approach to Treatment

8 *There is no cure for AMD and the efficacy of most treatments is low. Newer drug developments show promise but no treatment can reverse damage that has already occurred.*[26] Early diagnosis is critical. High-risk patients need periodic eye examinations because some patients do not notice any changes, even when neovascularization has occurred.[22]

Nonpharmacologic Therapy

▶ *Non-neovascular AMD*

Advise patients to stop smoking as observational data support a causal relationship between smoking and AMD.[22]

Drusen ablation by laser has been used in non-neovascular AMD. However, it is not clear if the treatment reduces progression to neovascular AMD.[26] There is a possibility that the treatments may induce neovascularization and retinal atrophy.[25] Other nonpharmacologic therapies are in trials but there is insufficient evidence for experts to recommend these procedures at this time.[22]

▶ *Neovascular AMD*

Thermal laser photocoagulation reduces severe visual loss 2 to 5 years after the procedure, but leads to an immediate and permanent reduction in central vision. There is a 50% chance that leakage will recur in the next 2 years after the procedure.[25]

Photodynamic therapy uses nonthermal red light to activate verteporfin, which produces reactive oxygen species that locally damage the neovascular endothelium.[27] Verteporfin treatment reduces the risk of loss of visual acuity and legal blindness over 1 to 2 years. Long-term results are not yet available. Severe photosensitivity for 3 to 5 days after the procedure is common and some patients experience a severe loss of vision. Eventually, most patients have some visual recovery. This procedure requires multiple treatments over time.[25] Other nonpharmacologic therapies are in trials but there is insufficient evidence for experts to recommend these procedures at this time.[22]

Pharmacologic Therapy

There are no approved pharmacologic treatments for non-neovascular AMD.[28] The Age-Related Eye Disease Study showed that a supplement containing ascorbic acid 500 mg, vitamin E 400 IU, β-carotene 15 mg, zinc oxide 80 mg, and cupric oxide 2 mg reduced the rate of clinical progression of all types of AMD by 28% in patients with at least intermediate macular degeneration.[28] No benefit was seen in patients with earlier stages of AMD; however, the duration of the study may have been insufficient to detect this benefit.[28] Currently, experts recommend antioxidant supplementation for intermediate AMD or advanced AMD in one eye.[22] Supplementation is not without risk.[26] For example, β-carotene supplementation in smokers may increase the risk of developing lung cancer.[22,26] At this time, it is not clear from the evidence if a patient at a high risk but without symptoms of AMD would benefit from supplementation.[29]

Vascular endothelial growth factor induces angiogenesis, increases vascular permeability, and increases inflammation, all of which are thought to contribute to neovascular AMD.[30] Pegaptanib, a vascular endothelial growth factor antagonist, binds to these growth factors in an attempt to suppress neovascularization.[22,30] In clinical studies, patients treated with pegaptanib experienced a slower rate of visual decline than patients treated with a sham injection.[31] Vision loss

---

Patient Encounter 3, Part 2

ET is diagnosed with non-neovascular intermediate AMD.

What nonpharmacologic treatment options does this patient have?

What pharmacologic treatment options does this patient have? What are the risks and benefits of each option?

What monitoring is appropriate for this patient?

Patient Encounter 3, Part 3

Two years have passed. ET (now 62 years of age) has progressed to advanced neovascular AMD. His central vision continues to deteriorate and he recently gave up driving after several near-accidents. His wife and son help him with his daily routine now.

What treatment options does this patient have? What are the risks and benefits of each option?

continued to occur in patients and the drug was less effective in the second year of treatment.[30] Long-term efficacy studies are not available yet.[30]

Another drug, ranibizumab, binds to and inhibits the activity of VEGF-A, a critical protein in angiogenesis.[22] In one clinical study, 95% of patients treated with ranibizumab maintained visual acuity after 12 months compared with 62% of control patients.[22] Both pegaptanib and ranibizumab are administered by intravitreous injection.[22,30]

Outcome Evaluation

Monitor patients for acute and chronic vision changes or loss. The Amsler's grid (Figs. 63–4 and 63–5) and frequent eye examinations may detect changes more quickly. The long-term prognosis for AMD is poor. Monitor patients for inability to drive and remove driving privileges as appropriate. Work with patients and family members to plan for lifestyle changes as vision decreases.[22]

DRY EYE

EPIDEMIOLOGY

Dry eye is a frequent cause of eye irritation. A lack of a single diagnostic test for the condition limits the available epidemiologic data. One study estimated the prevalence of

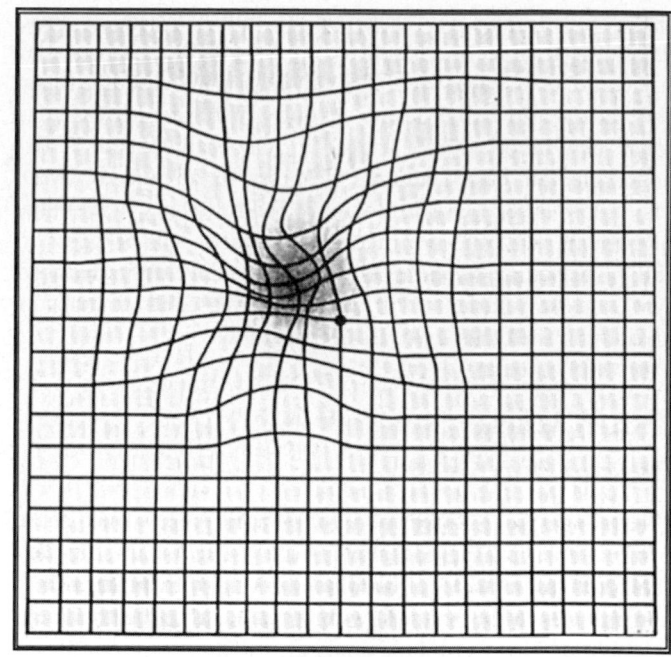

FIGURE 63–5. Amsler's grid as it might appear to someone with AMD. (From the National Eye Institute, National Institutes of Health Ref. No. EC04. Accessed online at: *http://www.nei.nih.gov/photo/*)

dry eye in the U.S. population age 65 and older at 14.6%, which is approximately 4.3 million Americans.[32]

The risk factors for dry eye are listed in Table 63–10. Of interest, the use of caffeine is associated with a decreased risk of dry eye. Dry eye that is left untreated can cause loss of vision or other morbidities over time.[33]

PATHOPHYSIOLOGY

The ocular surface and the tear-secreting glands of the eye function as an integrated unit. This unit refreshes the tear supply and clears away used tears. An autonomic neural reflex loop stimulates secretion of tear fluid and proteins by the lacrimal glands. The sensitivity of the ocular surface decreases with the decrease of aqueous tear production and tear clearance. This results in a decrease in sensory-stimulated reflex tearing which exacerbates dry eye.[32,33] Over time, wearing contact lenses also desensitizes the cornea by constant stimulation.[12]

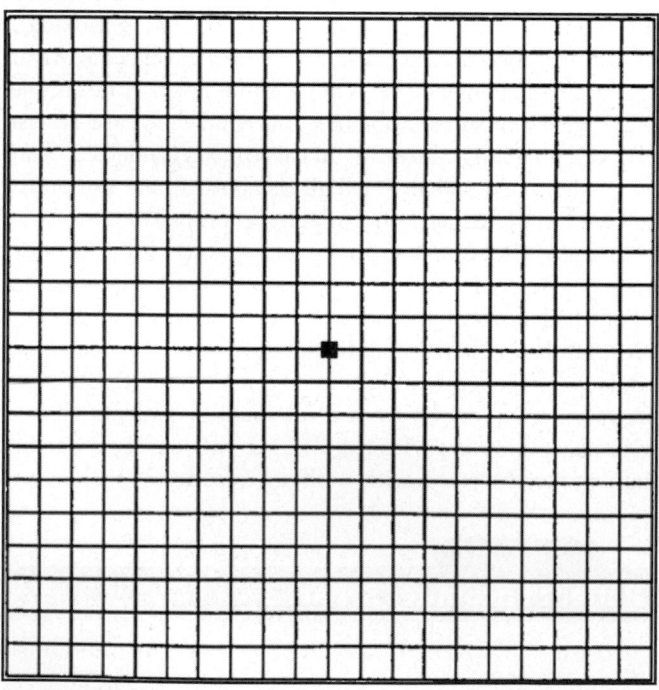

FIGURE 63–4. Amsler's grid distortions in the lines of the grid may be caused by subtle changes in central vision due to fluid in the subretinal space. This is the Amsler's grid as it appears to someone with normal vision. (From the National Eye Institute, National Institutes of Health Ref. No. EC03. Accessed online at: http://www.nei.nih.gov/photo/)

Table 63–10
Risk Factors for Dry Eye
Older age
Female gender
Arthritis
Smoking
Multivitamin use
Estrogen replacement therapy

From Ref. 33.

Table 63–11

Associated Conditions That Cause or Worsen Dry Eye

Ocular Conditions
Blepharitis
Meibomian gland dysfunction

Systemic Diseases
Sjögren's syndrome
Rosacea
Lymphoma
Sarcoidosis
Hemochromatosis
Amyloidosis
HIV
Hepatitis C
Epstein-Barr virus
Graft-versus-host disease
Rheumatoid arthritis
Systemic lupus erythematosus
Scleroderma
Neuromuscular diseases
Bell's palsy
Parkinson's disease

Environmental Factors
Wind
Reduced humidity
Air conditioning or heating
Exogenous irritants or allergens
Prolonged use of computer or reading
Contact lenses
Air travel
Smoke exposure

Local Trauma
Orbital surgery
Radiation
Injury
Chemical exposure

Systemic Medications
Diuretics
Antihistamines
Anticholinergics
Antidepressants
Systemic retinoids
Isotretinoin
Hormones
Hormone therapy
Cardiac antiarrhythmic
Diphenoxylate/atropine
β-Blockers
Chemotherapy agents

From Ref. 33.

Dysfunction may be caused by aging, systemic inflammatory diseases, a decrease in androgen hormones, surgery, ocular surface diseases (such as herpes zoster), systemic diseases, or medications that affect the efferent cholinergic nerves. Decreased tear secretion produces an inflammatory response on the ocular surface called **keratoconjunctivitis sicca**. This inflammation is a target for new medications that treat dry eye.[32,33]

Conditions that increase the evaporative loss of tears also worsen dry eye. In addition to environmental causes (Table 63–11), an abnormal blink reflex is a common cause of increased evaporative loss.[33]

TREATMENT

Desired Outcomes

- Relief of the symptoms of dry eye
- Prevention of recurrence
- Prevention of long-term adverse effects from dry eye

General Approach to Treatment

9 *Dry eye is a chronic condition. Symptoms can be improved with treatment but unless dry eye is secondary to a disease, it is not usually curable. Because of this, patient education is critical and a periodic reassessment of the efficacy of the*

Clinical Presentation and Diagnosis of Dry Eye[33]

General
Many other ocular diseases have similar symptoms. Patients with suggestive symptoms without signs should be placed on a treatment trial. Repeated observations over time may be required for a clinical diagnosis.

Symptoms
- Dry or foreign body sensation
- Mild itching
- Burning
- Stinging
- Photophobia
- Ocular irritation or soreness
- Blurry vision
- Contact lens intolerance
- Diurnal fluctuation
- Symptoms that worsen later in the day

Signs
- Redness
- Mucus discharge
- Increased blink frequency
- Tearing

Other Diagnostic Tests
- The tear break-up time test assesses the stability of precorneal tear film. Break-up times of less than 10 seconds are considered abnormal.
- Ocular surface dye staining assesses the ocular surface and will show blotchy or exposure-zone punctate areas in the dry eye.
- Schirmer's test evaluates aqueous tear production but is not diagnostic for dry eye. Results of 5 mm or less are considered abnormal.
- Assess corneal sensation if trigeminal nerve dysfunction is suspected.
- Evaluate for an autoimmune disorder if significant dry eyes or other signs and symptoms or family history are present.

treatment is appropriate. If the patient is unresponsive to treatment, refer to an ophthalmologist for additional options. If the dry eye is secondary to a systemic disease, the disease should be managed by the appropriate medical specialist.[33]

Nonpharmacologic Therapy

Behavioral and environmental modifications may significantly improve dry eye, especially in mild cases.

Evaluate the patient's environment for air drafts. Consider adding a humidifier in low-humidity areas. Schedule regular breaks from computer work or reading. Lower the computer screen to below eye level to decrease lid aperture. Evaluate medication profile and therapeutically substitute medications that do not exacerbate dry eye. Spectacle sideshields or goggles may reduce tear evaporation.[33]

If pharmacologic and other therapies are not sufficient, punctal occlusion or lateral tarsorrhaphy may be an option. Punctal occlusion is the plugging of the punctal drainage sites with collagen (temporary) or Silastic (permanent) plugs. Lateral tarsorrhaphy sutures portions of the lid margins together to decrease evaporative tear loss. These procedures are reserved for severe cases of dry eye secondary to other diseases.[12]

Pharmacologic Therapy

Regardless of the cause, the mainstay of treatment for dry eye is artificial tears. Artificial tears augment the tear film topically and provide relief. If a patient uses artificial tears more than four times daily, recommend a preservative-free formulation. Preservative-free formulations are also appropriate if the patient develops an allergy to ophthalmic preservatives. Artificial tears are available in gel, ointment, and emulsion forms that provide a longer duration of relief and may allow for less frequent instillation. Ointment use is appropriate at bedtime.[33]

Anti-inflammatory agents may be used in conjunction with artificial tears. The only approved agent is cyclosporine emulsion. Administered topically, the exact mechanism is unknown but it is thought to act as a partial immunomodulator suppressing ocular inflammation. Cyclosporine emulsion increases tear production in some patients. Fifteen minutes should elapse after instillation of cyclosporine before artificial tears are instilled.[34] Use of topical corticosteroids for short periods (e.g., 2 weeks) may suppress inflammation and ocular irritation symptoms. No topical corticosteroid is approved for this indication, however.[33]

The oral cholinergic agonists pilocarpine and cevimeline are used for patients with combined dry eye and dry mouth (e.g., Sjögren's syndrome) or severe dry eye. By binding to muscarinic receptors, the cholinergic agonists may increase tear production. Excessive sweating is a common side effect with pilocarpine and may limit its use (Table 63–12).

Outcome Evaluation[32]

- Monitor patient for relief of symptoms
- Periodically reassess the patient's compliance and understanding of the disease
- It may take 6 weeks before improvement is seen with pilocarpine therapy
- Cyclosporine therapy may take up to 6 months for full efficacy
- If a patient presents with visual loss, moderate or severe pain, corneal ulceration, or a lack of response to therapy, refer the patient to an ophthalmologist for prompt evaluation.

Patient Encounter 4

A 60-year-old woman presents with complaints of redness, burning, and watering of both eyes, which worsen as the day progresses. She does not have any itching of the eyes or other visible discharge. She has had the symptoms for several years but the symptoms have worsened recently. Your physical examination reveals red and teary eyes.

Her medical history includes osteoarthritis, mild osteoporosis, and hypertension. She also has recurrent sinus infections associated with seasonal allergic rhinitis. She has a new job as a medical transcriptionist.

Meds: Metoprolol 100 mg daily; conjugated estrogens 0.3 mg daily; calcium carbonate tablets 1,200 mg daily; ibuprofen 600 mg as needed for joint pain; loratadine 10 mg as needed for allergies; senior nonprescribed multivitamin daily

What is the probable diagnosis?

What are the other contributing factors that may be worsening her condition?

What nonpharmacologic interventions might she benefit from?

What pharmacologic treatment option is best for her?

Table 63–12

Pharmacologic Therapies for Dry Eye

Drug (Brand Name)	Dosing
Pilocarpine 5 mg tablet (Salagen)	5 mg orally 4 times daily
Cevimeline 30 mg capsule (Evoxac)	30 mg orally 3 times daily
Cyclosporine ophthalmic emulsion 0.05% (Restasis)	One drop in each eye twice daily

From Refs. 5, 35.

Patient Care and Monitoring: Nasolacrimal Occlusion[36]

Use of nasolacrimal occlusion decreases systemic absorption up to 60% and may increase ocular bioavailability of the drug. After instilling the eye drop, the patient should close the eye and press a finger gently against the nasolacrimal duct (tear duct) for 2 to 3 minutes.

Table 63–13

Selected Drug-Induced Ocular Changes

Miosis	**Mydriasis**
Narcotics	Anticholinergics
Barbiturates	Tricyclic antidepressants
Phenothiazines	Sympathomimetics

Decreased Tear Volume	**Corneal Deposits**
Anticholinergics	Amiodarone
Diuretics	Chloroquine and
β-Blockers	hydroxychloroquine
Tricyclic antidepressants	Tamoxifen
	Gold
Nystagmus	Ibuprofen, naproxen, and
Phenytoin	indomethacin
Barbiturates	Phenothiazines

Increased Tear Volume	**Cause or Worsen Cataracts**
Cholinergic agents	Corticosteroids
Benzodiazepines	
Phenothiazines	**Decreased Blink Rate**
Induce Uveitis	Sedative-hypnotics
Rifabutin	Ethanol
Bisphosphonates	**Lid or Corneal Edema**
Sulfonamides	Chlorthalidone
Cidofovir	Oral contraceptives
Topical metipranolol	Ibuprofen
Topical corticosteroids	Digoxin
Latanoprost	Phenothiazines

From Refs. 37–39.

DRUG-INDUCED OCULAR DISORDERS

Table 63–13 shows some ocular changes due to the use of certain drugs.

Abbreviations Introduced in This Chapter

AMD   Age-related macular degeneration
NSAID   Nonsteroidal anti-inflammatory drug

Self-assessment questions and answers are available at *http://www.mhpharmacotherapy. com/pp.html.*

REFERENCES

1. Handler JA, Ghezzi KT. General ophthalmologic examination. Emerg Med Clin North Am 1995;13(3):521–538.
2. Harlan JB Jr, Pieramici DJ. Evaluation of patients with ocular trauma. Ophthalmol Clin North Am 2002;15(2):153–161.
3. Wilson SA, Last A. Management of corneal abrasions. Am Fam Physician 2004;70(1):123–128.
4. Deutsch TA. Ocular emergencies in childhood. Pediatrician 1990;17(3):173–176.
5. McEvoy GK, ed. AHFS drug information 2008. Bethesda, MD: American Society of Health-System Pharmacists; 2008.
6. Mino de Kaspar H, Koss MJ, He L, Blumenkranz MS, Ta CN. Antibiotic susceptibility of preoperative normal conjunctival bacteria. Am J Ophthalmol 2005;139(4):730–733.
7. Garcia GE. Management of ocular emergencies and urgent eye problems. Am Fam Physician 1996;53(2):565–574.
8. Barish RA, Naradzay JF. Ophthalmologic therapeutics. Emerg Med Clin North Am 1995;13(3):649–667.
9. LaVene D, Halpern J, Jagoda A. Loss of vision. Emerg Med Clin North Am 1995;13(3):539–560.
10. Donahue SP, Khoury JM, Kowalski RP. Common ocular infections. A prescriber's guide. Drugs 1996;52(4):526–540.
11. Leibowitz HM. The red eye. N Engl J Med 2000;343(5):345–351.
12. Thielen TL, Castle SS, Terry JE. Anterior ocular infections: An overview of pathophysiology and treatment. Ann Pharmacother 2000;34(2):235–246.
13. Baum J. Infections of the eye. Clin Infect Dis 1995;21(3):479–486; quiz 487–488.
14. Morrow GL, Abbott RL. Conjunctivitis. Am Fam Physician 1998;57(4):735–746.
15. McEvoy GK, ed. AHFS drug information Essentials 2008. Bethesda, MD: American Society of Health-System Pharmacists; 2008.
16. Inspire Pharmaceuticals Inc. Azasite (azithromycin 1%) ophthalmic solution prescribing information. Durham NC; 2007 Jul.
17. Bielory L, Lien KW, Bigelsen S. Efficacy and tolerability of newer antihistamines in the treatment of allergic conjunctivitis. Drugs 2005;65(2):215–228.
18. Cook EB, Stahl JL, Barney NP, Graziano FM. Mechanisms of antihistamines and mast cell stabilizers in ocular allergic inflammation. Curr Drug Targets Inflamm Allergy 2002;1(2):167–180.
19. Bielory L. Ocular allergy guidelines: A practical treatment algorithm. Drugs 2002;62(11):1611–1634.
20. Titi JM. A critical look at ocular allergy drugs. Am Fam Physician 1996;53(8):2637–2642, 2645–2646.
21. Rapuano CJ, Feder RS, Jones MR, et al. American Academy of Ophthalmology. Bacterial keratitis, preferred practice pattern. San Francisco: American Academy of Ophthalmology; 2005.
22. Chew EY, Benson WE, Boldt, HC, et al. American Academy of Ophthalmology. Age-related macular degeneration, preferred practice pattern. San Francisco: American Academy of Ophthalmology; 2006.
23. Friedman DS, O'Colmain BJ, Munoz B, et al. Prevalence of age-related macular degeneration in the United States. Arch Ophthalmol 2004;122(4):564–572.
24. Hyman L, Neborsky R. Risk factors for age-related macular degeneration: An update. Curr Opin Ophthalmol 2002;13(3):171–175.
25. Arnold J, Sarks S. Age related macular degeneration. Clin Evid 2004;(11):819–834.
26. Comer GM, Ciulla TA, Criswell MH, Tolentino M. Current and future treatment options for nonexudative and exudative age-related macular degeneration. Drugs Aging 2004;21(15):967–992.
27. Novartis. Visudyne (verteporfin) for injection prescribing information. East Hanover, NJ; 2004.
28. Ferris FL, Chew EY, Sperduto R for the age-related eye disease study group. A randomized, placebo-controlled, clinical trial of high-dose supplementation with vitamins C and E and beta carotene for age-related cataract and vision loss: AREDS report no. 9. Arch Ophthalmol 2001;119(10):1439–1452.
29. Mares JA, La Rowe TL, Blodi BA. Doctor, what vitamins should I take for my eyes? Arch Ophthalmol 2004;122(4):628–635.
30. Eyetech Pharmaceuticals, Inc. Macugen (pegaptanib sodium) injection product information. New York; 2004.
31. Gragoudas ES, Adamis AP, Cunningham ET Jr, et al. Pegaptanib for neovascular age-related macular degeneration. N Engl J Med 2004;351(27):2805–2816.

32. Perry HD, Donnenfeld ED. Dry eye diagnosis and management in 2004. Curr Opin Ophthalmol 2004;15(4):299–304.

33. Matoba AY, Harris DJ, Meisler DM, et al. American Academy of Ophthalmology. Dry eye syndrome, preferred practice pattern; San Francisco: American Academy of Ophthalmology; 2003.

34. Allergan, Inc. Restasis (cyclosporine 0.05%) ophthalmic emulsion prescribing information. Irvine, CA; 2004.

35. Roxane Laboratories. Pilocarpine hydrochloride tablets prescribing information. Columbus, OH; 2007 Sept.

36. Zimmerman TJ, Kooner KS, Kandarakis AS, Ziegler LP. Improving the therapeutic index of topically applied ocular drugs. Arch Ophthalmol 1984;102(4):551–553.

37. Roy FH. Ocular Differential Diagnosis. 7th ed. Philadelphia: Lippincott Williams & Wilkins; 2002.

38. Hollander DA, Aldave AJ. Drug-induced corneal complications. Curr Opin Ophthalmol 2004;15(6):541–548.

39. Moorthy RS, Valluri S. Ocular toxicity associated with systemic drug therapy. Curr Opin Ophthalmol 1999;10(6):438–446.

64 Psoriasis

Rebecca M.T. Law

LEARNING OBJECTIVES

● Upon completion of this chapter, the reader will be able to:

1. Discuss the etiology of psoriasis including genetic and immune changes.

2. Describe the pathophysiology of psoriasis including the types of psoriasis and clinical presentations.

3. Describe the comorbidities and risks in patients with psoriasis.

4. Compare and contrast the treatment modalities for psoriasis, that is, topical therapies, systemic therapies including biologics, and phototherapies.

5. Recommend an appropriate treatment plan for a patient with psoriasis.

6. Recommend appropriate monitoring parameters for a patient with psoriasis.

7. Provide appropriate counseling information to a patient with psoriasis.

KEY CONCEPTS

❶ Patients with psoriasis have a lifelong illness that may be very visible and emotionally distressing. There is a strong need for empathy and a caring attitude in interactions with these patients.

❷ Psoriasis is a T-lymphocyte–mediated inflammatory disease that results from a complex interplay between multiple genetic factors and environmental influences. Genetic predisposition coupled with some precipitating factor triggers an abnormal immune response, resulting in the initial psoriatic skin lesions. Keratinocyte proliferation is central to the clinical presentation of psoriasis.

❸ Diagnosis of psoriasis is usually based on recognition of the characteristic plaque lesion, and not based on lab tests.

❹ Treatment goals for patients with psoriasis are to minimize signs such as plaques and scales, alleviate symptoms such as pruritus, reduce the frequency of flare-ups, and ensure appropriate treatment of associated conditions such as psoriatic arthritis or clinical depression, and minimize treatment-related morbidity.

❺ Management of patients with psoriasis generally involves both nonpharmacologic and pharmacologic therapies.

❻ Nonpharmacologic alternatives such as stress reduction and the liberal use of moisturizers may be extremely beneficial and should always be considered and initiated when appropriate.

❼ Pharmacologic alternatives for psoriasis include topical agents, phototherapy, and systemic agents including the use of biologic response modifiers (BRMs).

❽ In initiating pharmacologic treatment, the choice of therapy is generally guided by the severity of disease: topical agents would be appropriate for mild to moderate disease while a systemic agent would be a more appropriate choice for moderate to severe disease. Phototherapy or photochemotherapy are used for patients with moderate to severe psoriasis, generally when topical therapies alone are inadequate. Patient-specific concerns such as existing comorbid conditions (e.g., renal impairment or hepatic disease) must also be taken into consideration in the choice of therapy. Once the disease is under control, it would be important to step down to the least potent, least toxic agent(s) that maintain control.

❾ Rotational therapy (i.e., rotating systemic drug interventions in a sequential manner) is a means to minimize drug-associated toxicities, since systemic agents for psoriasis often have differing toxicities. This may be considered for psoriasis patients who require systemic treatments long-term to manage their condition.

❿ Some BRMs have proven efficacy for psoriasis; however, there are differences among these agents, including mechanism of action, duration of remission, and adverse-effect profile. In general, due to their immunosuppressive effects, there is an increased risk of infection with most of these agents. The use of live or live-attenuated vaccines during therapy is generally not recommended. Currently, BRMs are often considered for patients with moderate to severe psoriasis when other systemic agents are inadequate or relatively contraindicated. It has also been recommended that BRMs be considered as first-line therapy, alongside conventional systemic agents, for patients with moderate to severe psoriasis; however, in practice, cost may be a limiting factor. They may be appropriate if comorbidities exist.

INTRODUCTION

Psoriasis is a disease that waxes and wanes. It is a chronic illness that is never cured; however, the signs and symptoms of psoriasis may subside totally (go into remission) and then return again (flare-up, exacerbation, or reactivation). Remission may last for years in some patients, while in others exacerbations may occur every few weeks. Triggers include stress, seasonal changes, and some drugs. Disease flare-ups may also occur at times of life crises. Disease severity may vary from mild to disabling. Thus, management of this condition is necessarily long-term, and management modalities may change according to the severity of illness at the time.

❶ *Patients with psoriasis have a lifelong illness that may be very visible and emotionally distressing. There is a strong need for empathy and a caring attitude in interactions with these patients.*

EPIDEMIOLOGY AND ETIOLOGY

Psoriasis is a common inflammatory skin disorder which is estimated to affect 1.5% to 3% of the Caucasian population.[1,2] It may present at any age.[3,4] Ethnic factors influence disease prevalence. In the United States, prevalence among blacks (0.45% to 0.7%) is lower than in the remainder of the U.S. population (1.4% to 4.6%).[1] Between 10% and 30% of patients with psoriasis will also have psoriatic arthritis.[5] In 10% to 15% of psoriatic patients with arthritis, joint symptoms actually appear prior to skin involvement.[3] Our understanding about comorbidities associated with psoriasis is growing. Associated conditions include well known psychiatric/psychological comorbidities such as depression, anxiety and poor self-esteem; as well as more recently found medical comorbidities, such as inflammatory bowel disease, diabetes, cardiovascular disease, and lymphoma.[6] In 2008 the National Psoriasis Foundation published a clinical consensus on psoriasis comorbidities and recommendations for screening, addressing issues such as cardiovascular risk, metabolic syndrome, and obesity.[7]

Clinical depression may be present in up to 60% of patients with psoriasis.[6] The depression may be severe enough that patients contemplate suicide; one study showed that 10% reported a wish to be dead and 5% reported active suicidal ideation. Other psychopathologies include poor self-esteem, anxiety and sexual dysfunction. The emotional and psychological impact of psoriasis may not be reflected by the severity of the psoriatic skin condition, and it is

important to ensure that the psychosocial aspects of the disease is always considered for the patient.[6]

The incidence of inflammatory bowel diseases, such as Crohn's and ulcerative colitis, may be 3.8 to 7.5 times higher in psoriatic patients than in the general population.[6] This has been attributed to shared or closely linked genetic susceptibility traits, with individual susceptibility localized to a similar region of chromosome 16, among others.[6] There may also be a link to multiple sclerosis.[6]

Recent research has shown that psoriatic patients have an increased risk of cardiovascular diseases.[7,8] There is a higher than normal incidence of myocardial infarction. The risk is increased in patients with both mild and severe psoriasis, with the highest risk in younger patients with severe disease.[8] These findings persist even when corrected for the cardiovascular risk factors of smoking, diabetes, obesity, hypertension, and hyperlipidemia.[6,8] Psoriatic patients also have an increased incidence of diabetes, obesity, hypertension, and an atherogenic lipid profile.[6–8] In a recent study in hospitalized patients, the metabolic syndrome is significantly more prevalent in patients with psoriasis than those without.[6,7] Several large epidemiologic studies have shown an increased Body Mass Index (BMI) in psoriatic patients, with the relative risk of developing psoriasis highest in those with the highest BMIs.[6]

With regard to increased cancer risk, although there is ongoing controversy, some studies are showing an increased risk of lymphoma, with one study demonstrating a significantly increased risk of cutaneous T-cell lymphoma (relative risk of 10.75) or Hodgkin's lymphoma (relative risk of 3.18) in patients with severe disease.[6] Some psoriatic treatments with a known lymphoma risk may be confounding factors. Increased cancer risk may be limited to subpopulations: Caucasian with more than 250 PUVA (psoralens + UVA) treatments have a 14-fold greater risk of cutaneous squamous cell carcinoma than those with fewer treatments.[6] However, the risk of melanoma and nonmelanoma skin cancer appears to be equivalent to the general population.[6]

❷ *Psoriasis is a T-lymphocyte–mediated inflammatory disease that results from a complex interplay between multiple genetic factors and environmental influences.*[1] *Genetic predisposition coupled with some precipitating factor triggers an abnormal immune response, resulting in the initial psoriatic skin lesions.* Other risk factors may exacerbate pre-existing psoriasis and cause disease flare-ups. Precipitating factors include skin trauma such as a horse-fly bite (known as the Koebner phenomenon),[6] an environmental change such as cold weather, stress, a viral or streptococcal infection, or use of a β-adrenergic blocker.[2] Factors exacerbating psoriasis include drugs (e.g., lithium, nonsteroidal anti-inflammatory drugs, antimalarials, β-adrenergic blockers, and withdrawal of corticosteroids), and psoriatic patients commonly have exacerbations during times of stress.[2]

There is a polygenic inheritance pattern which may account for disease susceptibility and expression.[9] Family linkage studies have identified several genetic loci that are potentially responsible: the *PSOR1* gene on chromosome 6p21.3, the *PSOR2* gene on chromosome 17q25, the *PSOR3* gene on chromosome 4q34, the *PSOR4* gene on chromosome

1q21, the *PSOR5* gene on chromosome 3q21, the *PSOR6* gene on chromosome 19p13, the *PSOR7* gene on chromosome 1p, the *PSOR8* gene on chromosome 16q12–13 (which links to both psoriasis and Crohn's disease), and the *PSOR9* gene on chromosome 4q31.[1,4,6,8] There are possibly other genetic loci. *PSOR1* (the HLA-Cw6 allele)[6] has been considered the major gene locus for psoriasis;[1,4,6] it appears to be associated with up to 50% of cases of psoriasis.[1]

Studies conducted in twins show a threefold increased risk of psoriasis in monozygotic twins versus fraternal twins.[9] In addition, based on a study in 3,095 families with psoriasis, the calculated lifetime risk of developing psoriasis if no parent, one parent, or both parents have psoriasis was found to be 0.04, 0.28, and 0.65, respectively. If there was already one affected child in the family, the risks were increased to 0.24, 0.51, and 0.83, respectively.[9] As many as 71% of patients with psoriasis during childhood have some positive family history.[1] Similarly, psoriatic arthritis is heritable, with a prevalence 19 times higher in first-degree relatives of patients with psoriatic arthritis than in the general population.[9]

PATHOPHYSIOLOGY

❷ *Keratinocyte proliferation is central to the clinical presentation of psoriasis.* Keratinocytes are skin cells producing keratin which act as a skin barrier. Increased keratinocyte cell turnover (hyperkeratosis) results in the characteristic thick scaly skin lesions seen in patients with psoriasis.[10] Hyperkeratosis results from immune derangements.

The abnormal immune response seen in psoriasis is mediated primarily by T lymphocytes (T cells).[1] In patients with psoriasis, certain types of T cells are overactive and migrate to the skin in large numbers. T cells access the skin by binding to activated endothelial cells via intracellular cell adhesion molecules (ICAM-1).[1,11] These naïve T cells then encounter antigens in the skin, which are presented to the T cells by antigen-presenting cells (APCs), and become activated. There is an LFA-3–CD2 signal which plays an important part in T-cell activation: LFA-3 is the leukocyte function–associated antigen type 3 found on APCs; CD2 is a cell-surface glycoprotein expressed on T-cell subtypes.[1]

When LFA-3 interacts with CD2, there is an increased proliferation of T cells.[12]

Activated T cells begin releasing cytokines including interleukin-2 (IL-2), interferon-γ (IFN-γ), tumor necrosis factor-α (TNF-α), and others.[4,12] Cytokine activity leads to a rapid proliferation and turnover of skin cells, triggering the inflammatory process and the development of psoriatic skin lesions.[4,12,13] TNF-α may have a role in disease severity; it upregulates endothelial and keratinocyte expression of ICAM-1, activates T cells, enhances T-cell infiltration, and augments keratinocyte proliferation.[11]

Treatment of psoriasis is based on an understanding of the underlying pathophysiology. Agents that modulate the abnormal immune response, such as corticosteroids and biologic response modifiers (BRMs), are important treatment strategies for psoriasis. In addition, topical therapies that affect cell turnover are effective for psoriasis. Clinically, a treatment regimen should always be individualized, taking into consideration severity of disease, patient responses, and tolerability of various interventions.

CLINICAL PRESENTATION

❸ *Diagnosis of psoriasis is usually based on recognition of the characteristic plaque lesion, and not based on lab tests.*

Patient Encounter, Part 1

A 25-year-old Caucasian man presents with itchy lesions on his scalp, chest, back, elbows, and knees. He says these lesions started about a month ago, and seem to be spreading. Upon examination, the lesions are well demarcated and are reddish-violet in color—easily distinguished from normal skin. They appeared raised and are covered with loose scales. Scales are silvery in color. Removing the scales caused pinpoints of bleeding to show up. There are signs of excoriation on the patient's chest.

What information is consistent with psoriasis in this patient?

Clinical Presentation and Diagnosis of Plaque Psoriasis

General
- Patients have small discrete to generalized confluent lesions over the entire body.

Symptoms
- Patients may complain of severe itching.

Signs
- Lesions are raised and are red to violet in color (commonly known as plaques).
- Lesions have sharply demarcated borders except where confluent.

- Lesions are loosely covered with silvery-white scales, which if lifted off, show small pinpoints of bleeding (Auspitz's sign).
- Plaques appear most commonly on the elbows, knees, scalp, umbilicus, and lumbar areas, and often extend to involve the trunk, arms, legs, face, ears, palms, soles, and nails.
- Nail involvement presents as pitting, discoloration ("oil spots"), crumbling, splinter hemorrhages, growth arrest lines, or tissue build-up around the nails.

Clinical Presentation and Diagnosis of Other Types of Psoriasis

Inverse psoriasis spares the areas commonly involved in plaque psoriasis and instead appears in intertriginous areas, where scaling is minimal.

Guttate psoriasis presents as a sudden eruption of small, disseminated erythematosquamous papules and plaques, and is often preceded by a streptococcal infection 2 to 3 weeks prior.

Pustular psoriasis may be localized or generalized and may be an acute emergency requiring systemic therapy.

Generalized pustular psoriasis is characterized by disseminated deep-red erythematous areas and pustules, which may merge to become "lakes of pus."

Erythrodermic psoriasis is a generalized, life-threatening condition that presents with erythema, desquamation, and edema, and may require life support measures as well as systemic therapy.

Psoriatic diaper rash is the most common type of psoriasis in children under 2 years old. This usually affects inguinal folds and greater than 90% of psoriatic diaper rash cases may have involvement outside the diaper area.

Patient Encounter, Part 2

Additional relevant information was obtained from the patient, including the following history.

FH: His father and one of his brothers have psoriasis; his only sister has atopic dermatitis

SH: He works as an assistant copywriter in a busy publishing house, and is constantly struggling with multiple deadlines; he is an occasional social drinker and nonsmoker; he is a single father to a 6-year-old boy with asthma

PE:

He appears anxious and embarrassed about the lesions

VS: BP 125/70 mm Hg, P 72 bpm, RR 16/min, T 37°C (98.6°F)

Abd: Soft, nontender; bowel sounds present

Exts: Within normal limits; no joint pains

Skin: Multiple lesions on the scalp, chest, back, elbows, and knees; evidence of excoriation on the chest.

What risk factors does he have for psoriasis?

Identify your treatment goals for the patient.

TREATMENT

Desired Outcomes and Goals

④ *Since psoriasis is a chronic illness with no known cure, the goals of treatment focus on controlling the signs and symptoms of disease, including:*

- Minimizing or eliminating the signs of psoriasis such as plaques and scales.
- Alleviating pruritus and minimizing excoriations.
- Reducing the frequency of flare-ups.
- Ensuring appropriate treatment of associated conditions such as psoriatic arthritis, clinical depression, or itching.
- Avoiding or minimizing adverse effects from topical or systemic treatments used.
- Providing cost-effective therapy.
- Providing guidance or counseling as needed (e.g., stress-reduction techniques).
- Maintaining or improving the patient's quality of life.

General Approach to Treatment

⑤ *Management of patients with psoriasis generally involves both nonpharmacologic and pharmacologic therapies.* Pharmacologic alternatives for plaque psoriasis include topical treatments, **phototherapy**, **photochemotherapy**, and systemic therapies alone (orally or by injection). The choice of treatment is usually dictated by the severity of disease.[14,15]

In some cases, a combination of treatment options may be preferred. Topical therapies can be used in patients with limited or mild to moderately severe disease. Phototherapy and photochemotherapy are used in moderate to severe disease. Systemic therapies are used for patients with extensive or moderate to severe disease. To minimize drug toxicities in these patients, systemic therapies are often used in rotation, or used in conjunction with topical or phototherapy.[14,15] BRMs are becoming incorporated into the same category as other systemic agents and are currently recommended for consideration as first-line therapies alongside conventional systemic agents for moderate to severe disease.[15] However, since there is a significant cost difference, biologic agents are often reserved for cases in which traditional systemic agents provide inadequate control or for patients with comorbidities (e.g., where traditional systemic agents may be inappropriate due to potential adverse effects). There are four recently published treatment guidelines including a 2008 guidelines of care for the management of psoriasis and psoriatic arthritis[6] and a 2003 general consensus on psoriasis treatments,[14] both by the American Academy of Dermatology, a 2009 Canadian Guidelines for the Management of Plaque Psoriasis endorsed by the Canadian Dermatology Association at www.dermatology.ca/psoriasisguidelines.html and a consensus on moderate to severe psoriasis by the Canadian Psoriasis Expert Panel.[15] In addition, it would be important to ensure appropriate screening and treatment of any comorbid illnesses such as depression or diabetes,[7] and to ensure appropriate management of symptoms such as itching.

▶ Efficacy Assessment

Although there are tools to evaluate the efficacy of a psoriasis treatment, these are used primarily in clinical trials and rarely in clinical practice. These include the Psoriasis Area and Severity Index (PASI), the Physician's Global Assessment (PGA), and the National Psoriasis Foundation—Psoriasis Score (NPF-PS). The PASI is the most well known and measures the overall extent and severity of psoriasis, assessing areas of coverage, erythema, induration, and scaling. Clinical efficacy will be reported as a decrease in the PASI score, or an improvement (e.g., 75% improvement or PASI-75).[6]

In clinical practice, subjective qualitative assessments of disease severity is generally used to determine the efficacy of a treatment. In addition, an assessment of the patient's quality of life (QOL) is important in the management of psoriasis. The impact of psoriasis on a patient's psychological well-being may differ substantially from the severity of disease. Various QOL instruments validated for dermatologic diseases include the Dermatology Quality of Life Scales, Dermatology Life Quality Index (DLQI), Dermatology Specific Quality of Life Instrument, and Skindex-29.

▶ Nonpharmacologic Treatment

❻ *Nonpharmacologic alternatives may be extremely beneficial in the patient with psoriasis and complement pharmacologic therapies; thus should always be considered and initiated when appropriate.* These include the following management strategies:[10]

- *Stress reduction techniques.* Psychotherapy including stress management, guided imagery, and relaxation techniques are being used more frequently as adjunctive therapies for patients with psoriasis. Stress reduction has been shown to improve both the extent and severity of psoriasis.
- *Oatmeal baths.* Regular use of oatmeal baths in tepid water may help soothe the itching associated with psoriasis and reduce the need for systemic antipruritic agents.
- *Nonmedicated moisturizers.* Maintaining adequate skin moisture helps to control the scaling associated with psoriasis. Emollients restore skin pliability, reduce skin shedding, reduce pruritus, and help prevent painful cracking and bleeding.[2] Nonmedicated moisturizers may be liberally applied several times daily to help prevent skin dryness. Fragrance-free products should be selected when available.
- *Avoid irritant chemicals on the skin.* Harsh soaps or detergents should not be used. Cleansing should be done with tepid water, preferably using lipid-free and fragrance-free cleansers.
- *Avoid skin trauma.* Sunburns can induce a flare-up of psoriasis. Sunscreens with a sun protection factor of at least 15 should be routinely used when outdoors; often a sun protection factor of 30 is recommended. Avoid scratching the skin, which could lead to excoriations and exacerbate psoriasis. Loose-fitting cotton garments should be worn to minimize skin irritation.

Patient Encounter, Part 3

The diagnosis is that the patient has new-onset mild to moderate plaque psoriasis.

What are the drug-related problems in this patient?

What nonpharmacologic alternatives are appropriate for this patient?

What pharmacologic treatments would be appropriate as initial therapy for this patient?

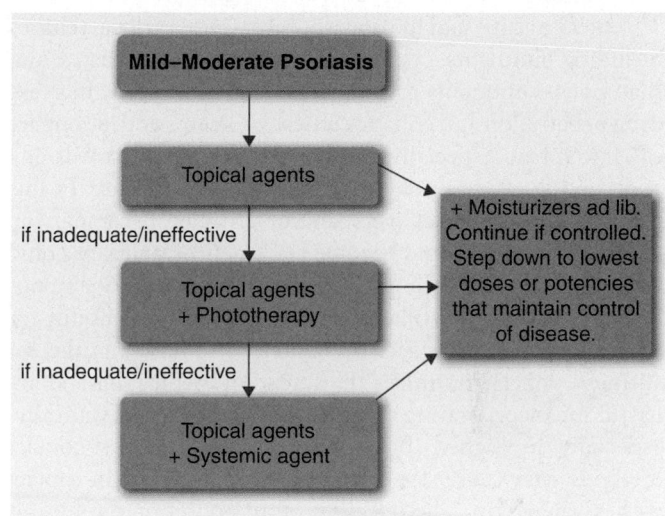

FIGURE 64–1. Treatment algorithm for mild to moderate psoriasis.

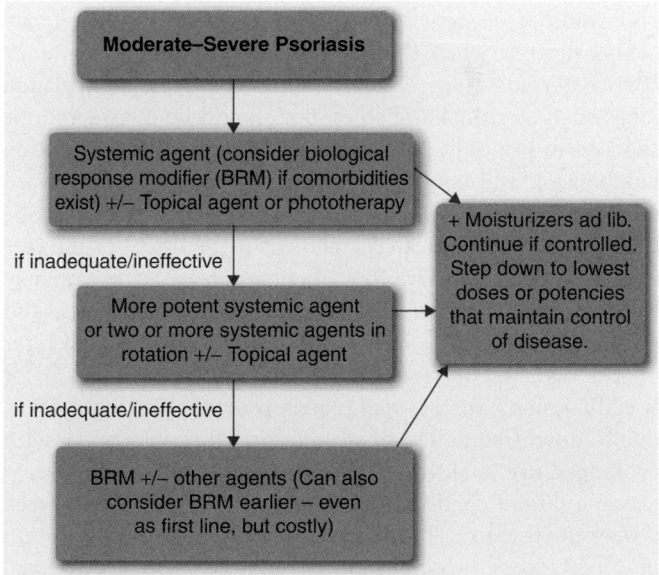

FIGURE 64–2. Treatment algorithm for moderate to severe psoriasis.

▶ Pharmacologic Treatment

❼ *Pharmacologic alternatives for psoriasis include topical agents, phototherapy, and systemic agents including the use of BRMs.* See Figures 64–1 and 64–2 for treatment algorithms.

Topical Therapy for Psoriasis ⑧ *Topical therapy is the initial drug treatment strategy for patients with mild to moderate psoriasis.* It is estimated that approximately 70% to 80% of all patients with psoriasis can be treated adequately with use of topical therapy.[1] Topical therapies include corticosteroids, coal tar products, anthralin, vitamin D_3 analogues such as calcipotriol, retinoids such as tazarotene, and topical immunomodulators such as tacrolimus and pimecrolimus.[16] Vitamin D_3 analogues and topical retinoids all affect keratinocyte functions and the immune response. Currently, these are in wider use than is either anthralin or coal tar preparations.

Topical agents may be incorporated into various vehicles including ointments, creams, gels, lotions, foams, pastes, and shampoos. Ointments provide occlusion, which may increase drug penetration and enhance efficacy. Creams and lotions are easier to spread, especially in hairy areas. Gels may have drying and cooling effects in addition to easy spreadability. Foams may have enhanced delivery and/or efficacy in comparison to lotions or creams and become a cosmetically elegant liquid upon skin contact, with good patient acceptance.[16] Shampoos incorporating tar distillates or salicylic acid are useful for scalp psoriasis. Pastes such as Lasar's paste have an inherent stiffness, which minimizes the spread of medication and are useful for incorporating drugs, such as anthralin. Anthralin, especially in higher concentrations used in short-contact methods, may cause skin irritation and burning if in contact with normal skin. The selection of an appropriate vehicle is often an important consideration.

For mild to moderate psoriasis, mid-potency corticosteroids such as betamethasone valerate (0.05% to 1%) are most frequently selected first, with escalation to higher-potency corticosteroids, if needed, and stepping down to lower-potency corticosteroids when the psoriasis improves. High-potency corticosteroids may be used initially in thicker plaque areas such as palms and soles, but should be considered for short-term use only. These include fluocinonide, clobetasol, halobetasol, and betamethasone dipropionate in optimized base. Low-potency corticosteroids such as hydrocortisone (0.5% to 2%) are appropriate choices if treatment of the face or flexures is necessary. Topical corticosteroids are available as ointments, creams, lotions including scalp lotions, and a few foam products, and should be applied in a thin layer on the skin. Intralesional triamcinolone may be useful for specific lesions, such as nail matrix psoriasis. Tachyphylaxis, due to down-regulation of steroid receptors, can occur with prolonged use, making the treatment regimen ineffective.[2,16] Using a potent corticosteroid for only 1 to 2 days per week ("weekend therapy") has been shown to lengthen the duration of effectiveness.[16] Combining this regimen with calcipotriol used during the week may provide greater efficacy.[16]

It is important to remember that adverse effects of *topical* corticosteroids may be *systemic* in nature and hypothalamic–pituitary–adrenal axis suppression can occur, especially when high-potency corticosteroids are used. Infants and small children may be more susceptible due to their increased skin surface:body mass ratio.[16] Topical corticosteroids may also cause striae, skin atrophy, acne, telangiectasias, and rosacea.[2,10,16] Atrophy can result in thin, fragile, easily lacerated skin. Striae are caused by tearing of dermal connective tissue and are irreversible.[16] Due to their significant adverse-effect profile, it has been recommended that no topical corticosteroid be used regularly for more than 4 weeks without review and reassessment.[2]

Vitamin D analogues (calcipotriol, calcitriol, and tacalcitol) are also frequently selected as initial pharmacotherapy in the management of mild to moderate psoriasis.[2] These inhibit keratinocyte differentiation and proliferation and may be anti-inflammatory.[2] Unlike corticosteroids, tachyphylaxis does not occur with prolonged use. Clearance of lesions should occur after 4 to 6 weeks of treatment.[2] Lack of response by 8 weeks indicates treatment failure.[2] These analogues may cause skin irritation leading to erythema, dryness, stinging, or burning. They may also cause hypercalcemia secondary to excessive absorption or use.[2,10,16] Calcipotriol (50 mcg/g) is currently available in the United States and Canada as ointment, cream, and solution. Topical calcitriol has been studied for treatment of psoriasis and appears almost as effective as betamethasone dipropionate in clearance of lesions, with a longer remission period.[2] It is less irritating than calcipotriol and can be used for the face and flexures.[2] Calcipotriol plus betamethasone is available as a combination product in Canada.[10] In contrast, salicylic acid can completely inactivate calcipotriol on contact.[16] Tacalcitol is a newer vitamin D_3 analogue available in the UK.[1]

Keratolytic agents, such as salicylic acid, are often added to bath oil or shampoos (typically 3% to 4%) for scalp psoriasis.[10] Salicylic acid can also be added to topical corticosteroid preparations to enhance steroid penetration (salicylic acid breaks down keratin).

Coal tar is keratolytic and may have antiproliferative and anti-inflammatory effects.[2] Coal tar products include crude coal tar and tar distillates (liquor carbonis detergens) available as ointments, creams, and shampoos in various strengths. Preparations containing coal tar may precipitate folliculitis,[10] will stain clothing, and have an unpleasant odor. They are also photosensitizing and can be combined with ultraviolet B (UVB) phototherapy (Goekermann's regimen) to increase treatment response.[17]

Anthralin (dithranol) has a direct antiproliferative effect on epidermal keratinocytes[2] and is generally used only on thick plaque areas. It can be used continuously or as short-contact anthralin therapy (SCAT): 1% to 4% applied for minutes to up to 2 hours.[16] Anthralin, including SCAT with high anthralin concentrations, may be highly irritating, especially if SCAT treatments are misused or used continuously.[10] It is important to remember when compounding anthralin preparations that prescribed concentrations can range from 0.1% (meant for continuous use) to 1% to 4% (meant for short-contact use).[16] Normal skin surrounding the psoriasis plaques should be protected by using nonmedicated paste or zinc oxide. People who handle the dry anthralin powder should avoid skin contact (e.g., by wearing gloves while compounding).

Tazarotene is a topical retinoid used for mild to moderate psoriasis and is also effective for acne. It normalizes keratinocyte differentiation and has antiproliferative and anti-inflammatory effects.[2] Tazarotene is available commercially as a 0.05% or 0.1% gel. It may cause significant skin irritation including erythema, pruritus, and burning, especially upon initial use.[2,10,16] Combining tazarotene use with a topical corticosteroid in an alternate-day regimen or morning corticosteroid–evening tazarotene dosing fashion may minimize skin irritation and steroid-induced skin atrophy, and enhance efficacy.[16] Avoid its use in women of child-bearing age unless effective contraception is being used; there is a potential risk of systemic drug absorption[2] and systemic retinoids are known teratogens. Concomitant use of other topical preparations or cosmetics with a strong drying effect should be avoided when possible.[10]

Phototherapy for Psoriasis ❽ *Phototherapy or photo-chemotherapy is used for patients with moderate to severe psoriasis, generally when topical therapies alone are inadequate.* Photochemotherapy is the concurrent use of phototherapy together with topical agents[16,18] or systemic drugs.[1,18] Phototherapy of psoriasis involves the use of either ultraviolet A (UVA) or UVB. UVA is a longer wavelength, and therapy with UVA is always combined with psoralens (e.g., methoxsalen or trioxsalen), which are used as photosensitizers to increase efficacy. There may be an increased risk of skin cancers after prolonged use of phototherapy and risks are greater with PUVA than UVB.[10,18] In particular, long-term PUVA treatments in Caucasians is associated with an increased risk of squamous cell carcinoma and possibly malignant melanoma.[6]

There is a bath PUVA and an oral PUVA. Bath PUVA therapies involve soaking in a bath of psoralens liquid for 15 minutes prior to UVA treatment. Oral PUVA involves taking an oral psoralens capsule the day prior to a UVA treatment. Oral psoralens, such as methoxsalen, cause nausea in many patients.[6] Other adverse effects of PUVA include photosensitivity, which necessitates the use of eye protection and UVA-blocking sunscreen for 24 hours after a PUVA treatment; macular melanosis at exposed sites (PUVA lentigines); and increased risk of skin cancers, especially squamous cell carcinoma.[18]

PUVA has been used in conjunction with other topical agents to increase treatment efficacy. Calcipotriol when added to a regimen of PUVA may reduce the number of PUVA treatments and the total UVA dosage needed for clearing lesions.[16,19,20] The rate ratio for marked improvement in patients receiving PUVA plus calcipotriol versus PUVA alone was 1.2 in a recent meta-analysis of 11 controlled studies.[21] If calcipotriol and PUVA are used together, calcipotriol must be applied *after* PUVA, since irradiation with UVA will inactivate calcipotriol.[22] Use with other topical agents has been limited. One small study of PUVA with tazarotene in 12 patients with extensive plaque psoriasis showed a statistically significant improvement after 3 weeks;[23] however, UVA doses should be reduced by at least one-third if tazarotene is added, since it increases the risk for immediate pigment darkening caused by UVA.[24] Coal tars are photosensitizing[16] and are not generally used with PUVA,[18] and PUVA plus topical corticosteroids have yielded conflicting results.[18]

Patient Encounter, Part 4

The patient's psoriatic condition remains well controlled with topical treatments for about 10 years, then flare-ups become a frequent occurrence. Phototherapy with NB-UVB was initiated. The patient did not respond well to NB-UVB therapy used alone. He is currently presenting with fairly extensive plaque psoriasis, affecting about two-thirds of his body surface area. There are signs of excoriation as well.

What are the drug-related problems in this patient?

What pharmacologic treatments would be appropriate for this patient now?

UVA can be used with other systemic agents including oral retinoids (RePUVA) and methotrexate. This will be discussed later in greater detail.

UVB treatments are often used alone and are effective and cost-effective.[6] Narrowband UVB (NB-UVB) is more effective than broadband UVB and avoids some of the adverse effects of PUVA, but is slightly less effective than PUVA.[6] UVB treatments have also been given in combination with topical or systemic agents to increase treatment efficacy. Topical regimens include UVB with tazarotene,[18] UVB with crude coal tar (Goekermann's regimen),[17,18] UVB with anthralin (Ingram's regimen),[18] and UVB with calcipotriol.[18] UVB with tazarotene (a retinoid) may be synergistic; the effect of each agent seems to be enhanced when used together. However, all retinoids can cause skin thinning, which may allow for easier burning to occur. The erythema induction threshold is lowered by about 25%.[18] Therefore, doses of UVB should be reduced by at least one-third when tazarotene is added.[16,18] UVB with crude coal tar is a regimen developed early in the twentieth century that is still considered one of the most effective regimens available.[18] However, many patients consider it messy and time-consuming. UVB with SCAT may not be consistently effective, and UVB with topical steroids may actually shorten the remission period.[19,25]

Several UVB and systemic therapy combinations have shown efficacy. These include UVB with acitretin (ReUVB) and UVB with methotrexate, and will be discussed later.

Systemic Therapy for Psoriasis ❽ *Systemic therapies are seldom used for mild to moderate psoriasis, and are generally reserved for patients with moderate to severe psoriasis.*[15,26] Oral agents include sulfasalazine, acitretin, methotrexate, cyclosporine, mycophenolate mofetil, azathioprine, tacrolimus, and hydroxyurea. Parenteral agents include the BRMs alefacept, etanercept, infliximab, and many others, currently at various stages of research or approval for psoriasis.

❾ *Rotational therapy (i.e., rotating systemic drug interventions in a sequential manner) is a means to minimize drug-associated toxicities, since systemic agents for psoriasis often have differing toxicities. This may be considered for psoriasis patients who require systemic treatments long-term to manage their condition.* Systemic therapies are optimally used in a rotating fashion to minimize drug toxicities (e.g., methotrexate–acitretin–cyclosporine or methotrexate–PUVA–acitretin).[10] Sequential therapy (i.e., starting with systemic therapy followed by topical therapy) is another method that minimizes toxicities.

Sulfasalazine has variable efficacy and is of limited potency. However, its side-effect profile is better than other systemic therapies and it is sometimes tried as an initial systemic agent for moderate to severe psoriasis. Usual doses are 2 to 4 g/day in divided doses.[10]

Acitretin is an oral retinoid that is likely safer than methotrexate or cyclosporine, especially when considering continuous use over many years.[18] It has the advantage of not being immunosuppressive.[6] The initial dose is 25 mg/day which can be increased to a maximum of 75 mg/day if needed.[15] When acitretin is used concurrently with phototherapy (ReUVB or RePUVA), there appears to be a synergistic treatment effect, and the number and duration of phototherapy sessions needed to achieve clearance is reduced.[18] RePUVA is a well-established treatment regimen for psoriasis.[1,6] When acitretin is used with calcipotriol, improvement and clearance of lesions may be achieved with significantly lower cumulative acitretin dosages.[18,27] However, acitretin is teratogenic and relatively contraindicated in women of childbearing potential. It must not be used in pregnant women, those with unreliable contraception, or those who intend to become pregnant at any time during or for 3 years after discontinuation of therapy.[6,10,26] Ethanol should be avoided during therapy and for 2 months after drug discontinuation, since it causes the transesterification of acitretin to etretinate, which has a much longer elimination half-life.[10,26] Other side effects include ophthalmologic, neuromuscular, hyperlipidemic, and hepatic enzyme changes.[10,26] Long-term continuous use has caused a syndrome of disseminated idiopathic skeletal hyperostosis and mild osteoporosis, found in a few case reports.[18,28]

Methotrexate used in low doses is one of the mainstays of systemic therapy in the treatment of psoriasis. An initial test dose of 2.5 to 5 mg (single dose once weekly) is recommended.[15] If lab values are normal after 1 week, the dose can be increased to a range of 7.5 to 30 mg once weekly.[15] This dosage can be given as a single dose or split into two or three doses given 12 hours apart to minimize GI side effects. Always titrate to the lowest effective dosage for maintenance. Methotrexate is contraindicated in pregnancy, individuals with renal impairment, hepatitis, cirrhosis, alcoholics, unreliable patients, and patients with leukemia or thrombocytopenia.[6] There is a significant risk of hepatotoxicity which is greater than that seen in patients with rheumatoid arthritis given similar cumulative doses of methotrexate.[26] In psoriatic patients with no hepatic risk factors, a liver biopsy is suggested when the cumulative dose of methotrexate reaches 1.5 g.[6] In high-risk psoriatic patients, it is preferable to also perform a biopsy during initial therapy with methotrexate.[10,15,26,29] Monitoring PIIINP (the aminoterminal propeptide of type III procollagen) at least three times yearly may reduce the number of repeat liver biopsies required.[10,26] Liver biopsies are not recommended

in the elderly, those with limited life expectancy, or those with significant medical problems.[26] Besides hepatotoxicity, methotrexate, even in low doses used in psoriasis, may cause leukopenia, megaloblastic anemia, pneumonitis and pulmonary fibrosis. Periodic complete blood cell counts (CBCs), renal and liver function tests (LFTs), and pulmonary toxicity testing should also be conducted.[10,26]

The combination of methotrexate and UVB seems to be synergistic; responses may occur with lower cumulative doses of both methotrexate and UVB. However, stopping methotrexate may cause rebound[18,30] and there is some concern about photosensitivity.[18] Methotrexate and PUVA have been used together in patients refractory to other treatments; however, there is additive carcinogenesis (especially increasing the risk of squamous cell cancer) and subacute phototoxicity.[18]

Methotrexate has been used successfully with cyclosporine, either concurrently[31] or in rotation. Rotational therapy is particularly effective since it minimizes the serious adverse effects of both agents: hepatotoxicity from methotrexate and hypertension and nephrotoxicity from cyclosporine. Having an overlapping treatment period may not be necessary and patients have been successfully switched after a 1-week washout period.[18,32] This is a very useful combination of systemic agents in the long-term management of this chronic disease.

Cyclosporine is used in low doses whether alone or in combination with other agents. The usual dose range is 2 to 2.5 mg/kg/day, given orally in two divided doses, for patients with stable generalized psoriasis or for moderate to severe disease. For patients with severe inflammatory flares of psoriasis, or recalcitrant cases who fail to respond to numerous other therapies, or for a highly distressed patient in a crisis situation, the starting dose is higher at 5 mg/kg/day in two divided doses.[26] This dose should not be exceeded[15] and, once there is a clear response, should be decreased by 0.5 to 1 mg/kg/day at weekly or longer periods, to the lowest effective maintenance dose. If started at 2.5 mg/kg/day, and the response is inadequate, it is recommended to wait at least 1 month before considering a dosage increase. If necessary, the dosage may be increased by 0.5 to 1 mg/kg per day[9,25,32] monthly[15] to a maximum of 5 mg/kg/day.[15] Always titrate to the lowest effective dose for maintenance.[15] Cyclosporine is contraindicated in psoriatic patients with abnormal renal function, uncontrolled hypertension, malignancy (except nonmelanoma skin cancer), uncontrolled infection, primary or secondary immunodeficiency excluding autoimmune disease.

Blood pressure and serum creatinine (SCr) should be assessed prior to beginning cyclosporine therapy to obtain accurate baselines, and should be reassessed biweekly once therapy is started for at least the first 12 weeks of therapy (until values stabilize), and then closely monitored during therapy (bimonthly for doses up to 2.5 mg/kg/day, and monthly for patients receiving higher doses). If SCr increases to 30% above the patient's baseline, the cyclosporine dosage needs to be decreased and SCr rechecked in a month. If the SCr is still above 30% of the patient's baseline, cyclosporine should be discontinued and only resumed when the SCr returns to within 10% of the patient's baseline. Cyclosporine should also be discontinued for inadequate response after 3 months' use at the maximum dose.[10,33] Besides impaired renal function and hypertension, cyclosporine may increase the risk of lymphomas and cutaneous malignancies after long term treatment.[6] Patients should have a careful physical exam for tumors prior to initiation of therapy.

The combination of cyclosporine with calcipotriol may be more efficacious than either agent used alone.[18,34] Cyclosporine and SCAT may also be effective.[18,35] However, cyclosporine *should not* be used concurrently with PUVA; there is a well-documented increased risk of squamous cell cancer and the combination may have a negative effect on lesion clearance.[18] The combination of cyclosporine with methotrexate is extremely effective and minimizes toxicity from either agent as discussed. Cyclosporine has also been used successfully with mycophenolate mofetil[35] and etanercept.[26]

Mycophenolate mofetil in doses of 1 to 1.5 g twice daily (maximum dose 3 g/day) is effective as adjunctive therapy in patients with resistant psoriasis on cyclosporine.[26,35] As monotherapy, there may be some benefit in patients with moderate psoriasis and psoriatic arthritis, but not in severe psoriasis.[26]

Hydroxyurea is an older agent still used occasionally today for patients with psoriasis; however, there have been recent precautions about its use in the elderly and cutaneous vasculitic toxicities in patients with myeloproliferative disorders.[26] Toxicity associated with tacrolimus has limited its use in psoriasis. Azathioprine has a slow onset and significant toxicity.[26] Oral corticosteroids are reserved for severe or life-threatening conditions such as severe psoriatic arthritis or exfoliative psoriasis; prolonged oral steroid use should be avoided.[10]

Biologic Response Modifiers Based on the recent advances in our understanding of the pathogenesis and pathophysiology of psoriasis, there was accompanying research into the development and use of BRMs for psoriasis and psoriatic arthritis. ⑩ *Some BRMs have proven efficacy for psoriasis; however, there are differences among these agents, including mechanism of action, duration of remission, and adverse-effect profile. Currently, BRMs are often considered for patients with moderate to severe psoriasis when other systemic agents are inadequate or relatively contraindicated. It has also been recommended that BRMs be considered as first-line therapy, alongside conventional systemic agents, for patients with moderate to severe psoriasis;*[15] *however, in practice, cost may be a limiting factor. They may be appropriate if comorbidities exist.* BRMs with proven efficacy for psoriasis include alefacept, etanercept, adalimumab, and infliximab.[6] These agents employ the following targeted immunosuppressive strategies: alefacept inhibits T-cell activation by targeting LFA-3–CD2 and inducing apoptosis in memory T cells;[1] etanercept, adalimumab, and infliximab are all TNF-α inhibitors and efalizumab inhibits T-cell activation by targeting CD11a, the α subunit of LFA-1 (ICAM-1).[1,6,10,36] Other biologic agents in clinical trials for psoriasis include HuMax-CD4, siplizumab, daclizumab, and denileukin

diftitox.[10,36] ⑩ *In general, due to their immunosuppressive effects, there is an increased risk of infection with most of these agents.* In particular, efalizumab has recently been suspended from use in Canada and has been voluntarily withdrawn in the United States by the company (in consultation with the FDA) due to serious adverse CNS effects from viral causes. ⑩ *The use of live or live-attenuated vaccines during therapy is generally not recommended.*

The most promising types of BRMs are monoclonal antibodies, cytokines, and fusion proteins.[1] Monoclonal antibodies may be chimeric (fused mouse and human segments; designated "-ximab"), humanized with intermittent murine sequences (designated "-zumab"), human backbone with monkey sequences, or fully human.[37]

Alefacept is a recombinant dimeric fusion protein composed of the extracellular CD2-binding portion of lymphocyte function–associated antigen (LFA)-3 linked to the constant portion of human IgG.[6,37,38] Alefacept inhibits T-cell activation by binding to their CD2 sites, thus impairing costimulatory signals; and alefacept also interacts with natural killer cells to destroy already activated T cells.[1,10] This agent is useful for moderate to severe chronic plaque psoriasis. About one-third of alefacept-treated patients enter prolonged remissions ranging from 6 to 18 months. Alefacept appears to spare helper T-cell function and does not significantly impair primary or secondary antibody responses (e.g., the ability to combat infections or respond to vaccinations). There is a significant risk of malignancy and common side effects include lymphopenia, myalgias and chills, pharyngitis, cough, nausea, and for IM injections pain and inflammation at the injection site.[10,39] The dosage recommended is 15 mg IM once weekly for 12 weeks provided the CD4+ T-cell count is normal (defined as greater than or equal to 250 cells/mm³).[10] Biweekly monitoring of CD4 counts is required during treatment.[6] Dosing should be held for counts less than 250 cells/mm³ and discontinued if the CD4+ count remains below 250 cells/mm³ for four consecutive weeks.[6] The maximum response to alefacept generally occurred 6 to 8 weeks after the last IM injection of the 12-week course.[6,40] The regimen may be repeated in 12 weeks if needed and CD4 counts are normal.[10] Patients who responded to alefacept may achieve additional benefit from successive 12-week treatment courses.[6] Although predictive markers for which patients will respond are currently unknown, those who achieve a PASI-75 or greater tend to maintain a 50% of greater reduction in PASI for a median duration of 10 months.[6] Alefacept is contraindicated in HIV+ve patients due to the potential for accelerating disease progression from CD4 count reduction.[6]

Etanercept is a fully human dimeric fusion protein composed of human TNF-α p75 receptor fused to the Fc portion of human IgG1.[38] It acts as a TNF-α inhibitor by binding to and inactivating soluble and membrane-bound TNF-α, thus preventing interactions with its cell surface receptors.[6,38] This agent is useful for chronic moderate to severe plaque psoriasis and for psoriatic arthritis. Dosing in psoriasis is different from its other indications (rheumatoid arthritis, juvenile rheumatoid arthritis, and ankylosing spondylitis).[6] The approved regimen in psoriasis is 50 mg subcutaneously twice weekly for the first 12 weeks followed by 50 mg weekly thereafter, dosing being continuous.[6] In clinical trials, 49% of patients given 50 mg subcutaneously twice weekly achieved a 75% improvement in PASI by 12 weeks.[10,41] Clinical responses continue to improve with longer treatment,[6,41] but some patients will show a loss of response after 12 weeks when the dose is reduced to once weekly.[6] The drug appears to be well tolerated; common side effects include mild injection site reactions, headache, increased respiratory tract infections (colds and sinusitis), and GI symptoms.[6,10,41] There is an increased risk of tuberculosis[6] and hepatitis B reactivation. Serious infections including fatalities have been reported with etanercept and there were reports of worsening congestive heart failure (CHF) and new-onset CHF.[10] Due to rare reports of blood disorders (anemia, aplastic anemia, leukopenia, neutropenia, pancytopenia, and thrombocytopenia), patients are advised to contact their doctor if they experience persistent fever, bruising, bleeding, or paleness.[10] A systemic lupus erythematosus (SLE)-like syndrome without renal or CNS complications has been rarely reported.[6] Monitoring includes a baseline tuberculin purified protein derivative (PPD) skin test, LFTs, and CBC. Yearly PPD and periodic CBC and LFTs are recommended while on treatment.[6]

Etanercept has been found to be effective in children and adolescents (aged 4–17) with plaque psoriasis. 57% of patients receiving etanercept 0.8 mg/kg once weekly (to a maximum of 50 mg) achieved PASI-75.[6,42]

Efalizumab provides an example of a drug where serious toxicity has been discovered in the postmarketing phase, leading to product withdrawal. Efalizumab is a recombinant humanized murine monoclonal IgG antibody directed against CD11a, the α subunit of leukocyte function–associated antigen type 1 (LFA-1). This inhibits T-cell activation, cutaneous T-cell trafficking, and T-cell adhesion to keratinocytes. Efalizumab is effective for patients with moderate to severe plaque psoriasis and is self-administered subcutaneously by the patient.[6] It is not effective for psoriatic arthritis; and psoriatic arthritis may develop or recur in a small percentage of patients during efalizumab treatment of psoriasis.[6] Recommended dose prior to drug withdrawal was 0.7 mg/kg for the initiation dose followed by weekly 1 mg/kg doses thereafter.[6] Efalizumab has a rapid onset of action with symptom improvement seen in about 4 weeks. About 25% of psoriatic patients receiving either 1 or 2 mg/kg/week improved by at least 75% at 12 weeks of treatment.[11,43,44] Treatment needed to be continued; with cessation of therapy, the median time to relapse is 60 to 80 days. Although with continued therapy patients will continue to improve, with 44% to 50% of patients achieving and maintaining PASI-75 after 6 to 36 months of continuous efalizumab therapy,[6,45] the possibility for serious adverse effects outweighed the benefits. Efalizumab has recently been suspended from use in Canada, and on April 8, 2009, the FDA issued a statement that efalizumab has been voluntarily withdrawn by the company in the United States. This withdrawal is due to reports of progressive multifocal leukoencephalopathy (PML).

There have been 3 confirmed cases and one possible case of PML in patients 47 to 73 years of age with moderate to severe plaque psoriasis who had been using efalizumab continuously for over three years. PML is a rare, serious, progressive neurologic disease caused by a virus that affects the CNS and there is no known effective treatment. The reader is directed to the following FDA website for further information about the issue and the phased-in withdrawal process: http://www.fda.gov/NewsEvents/Newsroom/PressAnnouncements/ucm149561.htm

Common side effects include headache, fever, chills, nausea, and myalgias, which usually diminish after the third week of treatment.[6] Thrombocytopenia, hemolytic anemia, pancytopenia, and peripheral demyelination have also been reported; and a CBC is recommended monthly for the first 3 months and every 3 months during therapy.[6] Worsening psoriasis may occur during treatment or after drug discontinuation and it was recommended that treatment not be discontinued abruptly unless it is essential as rebound may develop.[6] There is an increased risk of infections (other than viral leading to PML) and caution should be exercised in patients at risk for or have a history of malignancy or infection.[6,43,44]

Infliximab is a chimeric human/murine monoclonal antibody against TNF-α which binds to both soluble and transmembrane TNF-α molecules. It is approved for both psoriasis and psoriatic arthritis. Dosing for these patients is 5 mg/kg IV over 2 to 3 hours at weeks 0, 2, and 6 and continued every 8 weeks thereafter.[6] Approximately 80% of patients achieved PASI-75 by 10 weeks (after 3 doses of inflixamab) however by week 50 only about 60% of patients maintained PASI-75.[46,47] Infliximab is also approved for rheumatoid arthritis, ankylosing spondylitis, Crohn's disease, and ulcerative colitis. Significant adverse effects from postmarketing experience and clinical trials have included hematologic abnormalities (leukopenia, neutropenia, thrombocytopenia, and pancytopenia), hepatotoxicity (rarely: acute liver failure, jaundice, hepatitis, and cholestasis), hypersensitivity reactions (anaphylaxis, urticaria, and serum sickness), ocular toxicity (optic neuritis and optic neuropathy), CHF exacerbation and new onset CHF, and increased infections (tuberculosis, hepatitis B reactivation, *Listeria monocytogenes* infections, fungal infections, and sepsis). There is an increased risk of infection by live vaccines and vaccination with live vaccines while receiving infliximab therapy is not recommended. Patients should be evaluated for active or latent tuberculosis (tuberculin PPD skin test) prior to therapy.[6] Recommended baseline and ongoing monitoring include yearly PPD, LFTs, and CBC.[6]

Adalimumab is a fully human TNF-α inhibitor initially approved for the treatment of rheumatoid arthritis in 2003. It is approved for treatment of psoriasis and psoriatic arthritis. Other approved indications include juvenile rheumatoid arthritis, ankylosing spondylitis, adult rheumatoid arthritis, and Crohn's disease.[6] The dosage in psoriasis is 80 mg subcutaneously in the first week, followed by 40 mg the following week, and 40 mg subcutaneously every 2 weeks

Patient Encounter, Part 5

It was decided to begin systemic therapy with either methotrexate or cyclosporine to control the flare ups. Both alternatives were presented to the patient and discussed with the patient.

What lab tests or other measurements would be important to perform prior to starting therapy with methotrexate? With cyclosporine?

What dosage regimen would be appropriate for methotrexate? For cyclosporine?

What monitoring plan would be appropriate for methotrexate? For cyclosporine?

thereafter continuously.[6] With this regimen, 71% of patients achieved PASI-75 by 16 weeks of treatment.[48] Patients should be evaluated for active or latent TB infection (tuberculin PPD skin test) prior to therapy. There is an increased risk of serious infections (in particular, respiratory infections including pneumonia and tuberculosis, and hepatitis B reactivation), of exacerbation in patients with heart failure, and increased risk of lymphoma. Hematologic abnormalities (pancytopenia, thrombocytopenia, and leukopenia) have been rarely reported. Positive antinuclear antibody titers and a lupus syndrome have been reported. Anti-ds DNA antibody determinations are recommended in patients presenting with lupus-like symptoms during adalimumab therapy. A pruritic urticarial eruption that lessens in severity with each subsequent injection has been reported. Rebound does not usually occur.[6]

Natural Health Products There are several natural health products which are considered possibly effective for psoriasis. The most promising is Mahonia aquifolium (Oregon grape). This is not a grape, but a plant with blue-violet berries which is native to southern British Columbia, western Oregon and northern Idaho, and is the state flower of Oregon. An extract from the medicinal part of the plant, the rhisome and root, has been formulated into a 10% topical cream/lotion (Relieva, Apollo Pharmaceuticals) and is marketed in Canada for the treatment of psoriasis. This product has been shown in several recent clinical trials to modestly decrease the severity of psoriasis and improve the quality of life for patients with mild to moderate psoriasis.[49] Preliminary research suggests that it is as effective as calcipotriene cream for some patients.[49] Adverse effects include a burning sensation, irritation, redness and itching, and possible allergic reactions.

Other natural health products which are possibly effective include an aloe vera extract 0.5% hydrophilic cream applied topically three times daily, and an omega-3 fatty acid based lipid infusion (with both DHA and EPA) given intravenously. Oral supplementation with dietary fish oils containing DHA and EPA did not appear to be effective. More research into these natural health products is required before they can be recommended for use in psoriasis.

OUTCOME EVALUATION

- Monitor the patient for clearance of skin lesions. Depending on the agent(s) used and site of lesions it may take 2 to 6 weeks or longer to see a response. Complete clearance may not be achieved for all patients.

- Monitor the patient for specific adverse effects, depending on agent(s) used. Some agents are discussed below, and others are discussed earlier in this chapter.

- Methotrexate: Monitor CBC and liver function tests at baseline and regularly, and consider liver biopsy prior to treatment and at a cumulative dose of 1.5 g. If available, monitor PIIINP at least three times yearly.

- Cyclosporine: Monitor SCr, blood urea nitrogen, and blood pressure at baseline and reassess biweekly for at least 12 weeks (or longer until values stabilize), then regularly. Adjust doses when needed in response to SCr changes as discussed above.[9,32]

- Acitretin: Monitor serum lipids and liver function tests.

Patient Care and Monitoring

With respect to pharmacologic therapies, it is important to:

- Provide patients with an approximate time frame for improvement based on the patient's areas of involvement and type of drug therapy. For example, a statement such as: "There should be less scaling and redness of your scalp lesions and a reduction in the thickly crusted areas within 1 to 2 weeks. You should notice a general improvement in your condition by 6 to 12 weeks. Your palms, soles, elbows, and knees may take longer to clear."[9]

- Provide appropriate advice about drug regimens including how to apply a specific topical agent, how to use a specific systemic agent, and precautions and possible toxicities of any drug therapy, remembering that topical therapies can have significant systemic adverse effects.

- Check the patient profile and talk with the patient to ensure that there are no significant drug interactions with other concurrent medications and therapies.

- Reinforce the importance of adherence to therapies and specific drug regimens.

- Reinforce the importance of regular follow-up with the patient's health care providers including all appointments for follow-up care and lab work (if any).

- Interact with the patient's other health care providers as needed to discuss patient concerns or issues detected including drug interactions, nonadherence, and adverse effects.

- Topical corticosteroids: Monitor for skin thinning, telangiectasias, and possible hypothalamic–pituitary–adrenal axis suppression.
- Interact with the patient's other health care providers as needed to discuss patient concerns or issues.

SUMMARY

It is important to remember that psoriasis is a lifelong illness with no known cure and often has a significant psychosocial component. Author John Updike has said about his own psoriatic condition, that "my torture is skin deep" and that "we hate to look upon ourselves," calling himself a "leper."[50] This disease may be very visible and emotionally distressing, and can cause significant disability both physically and psychologically, affecting psychosocial functioning and quality of life. Empathy and a caring attitude can go a long way in the care of these patients.[50]

Abbreviations Introduced in This Chapter

AAD	American Academy of Dermatology
APC	Antigen-presenting cells
BAD	British Academy of Dermatology
BMI	Body mass index
BRM	Biologic response modifier
BS	Bowel sounds
CHF	Congestive heart failure
DHA	Docosahexaenoic acid
EPA	Eicosapentaenoic acid
ICAM-1	Intracellular cell adhesion molecules
IF-γ	Interferon-*gamma*
IL-2	Interleukin-2
LFA-3	Leukocyte function–associated antigen type 3
LFT	Liver function test
NB-UVB	Narrowband ultraviolet B
PIIINP	The aminoterminal propeptide of type III procollagen
PML	Progressive multifocal leukoencephalopathy
PPD	Purified protein derivative
PUVA	Psoralens + ultraviolet A
RePUVA	Oral retinoid + PUVA
ReUVB	Acitretin + ultraviolet B
RRR	Regular rate and rhythm
SCAT	Short-contact anthralin therapy
TNF	Tumor necrosis factor
UVB	Ultraviolet B

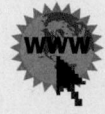
Self-assessment questions and answers are available at *http://www.mhpharmacotherapy.com/pp.html.*

ACKNOWLEDGMENTS

In the first edition, portions of this chapter had been adapted from the following article: Law RM. Psoriasis: An update. Pharmacy Practice 2005:21(12):CE 1–7. With permission from the publisher.

REFERENCES

1. Schon MP, Boehncke WH. Psoriasis. N Engl J Med 2005;352: 1899–1912.
2. Clarke C. Psoriasis—First-line treatments. Pharm J 2005;274:623–626.
3. Christophers E. Psoriasis—Epidemiology and clinical spectrum. Clin Exp Dermatol 2001;26:314–320.
4. Godic A. New approaches to psoriasis treatment. A review. Acta Dermatovenerol Alp Panonica Adriat 2004;13(2):50–57.
5. Kruger JG, Bowcock A. Psoriasis pathophysiology: Current concepts of pathogenesis. Ann Rheum Dis 2005;64(suppl II):ii30–ii36.
6. Menter A. Gottlieb A, Feldman SR et al. Guidelines of care for the management of psoriasis and psoriatic arthritis. Section 1. Overview of psoriasis and guidelines of care for the treatment of psoriasis with biologics. J Am Acad Dermatol 2008;58:826–850.
7. Kimball AB, Gladman D, Gelfand JM et al. National Psoriasis Foundation clinical consensus on psoriasis comorbidities and recommendations for screening. J Am Acad Dermatol 2008;58: 1031–1042.
8. Kremers HM, McEvoy MT, Dann FJ et al. Heart disease in psoriasis. J Am Acad Dermatol 2007;57:347–354.
9. Rahman R, Elder JT. Genetic epidemiology of psoriasis and psoriatic arthritis. Ann Rheum Dis 2005;64(suppl II):ii37–ii39.
10. Law RM, Gulliver WP. Psoriasis: The harried school teacher. Section 14: Dermatologic disorders, no. 100. In: Schwinghammer TL, ed. Pharmacotherapy Casebook: A Patient-Focused Approach. 6th ed: 271–273. And in: Instructor's Guide [to accompany] Pharmacotherapy Casebook: A Patient-Focused Approach. 6th ed: 1183–1194. New York: McGraw-Hill;2005.
11. Veale DJ, Ritchlin C, FitzGerald O. Immunopathology of psoriasis and psoriatic arthritis. Ann Rheum Dis 2005;64(suppl II):ii26-ii29.
12. Ellis CN, Krueger GG. Treatment of chronic plaque psoriasis by selective targeting of memory effector T lymphocytes. N Engl J Med 2001;345:248–255.
13. Lui H, Langley R, Poulin Y, et al. Incorporating biologics into the treatment of psoriasis. J Cutan Med Surg 2004;8(suppl):8–13.
14. Callen JP, Krueger GG, Lebwohl M, et al. AAD consensus statement on psoriasis therapies. J Am Acad Dermatol 2003;49:897–899.
15. Guenther L, Langley RG, Shear NH, et al. Integrating biologic agents into management of moderate-to-severe psoriasis: A consensus of the Canadian Psoriasis Expert Panel. J Cutaneous Med Surg 2004; 8:321–337. *http://www.springerlink.com/content/p30qnput52xh1648/fulltext.pdf* .
16. Lebwohl M, Ali S. Treatment of psoriasis. Part 1. Topical therapy and phototherapy. J Am Acad Dermatol 2001;45:487–498.
17. Lebwohl M. Innovations in the treatment of psoriasis. J Am Acad Dermatol 2004;51(1):S40–S41.
18. Lebwohl M, Menter A, Koo J, Feldman SR. Combination therapy to treat moderate to severe psoriasis. J Am Acad Dermatol 2004;50: 416–430.
19. Speight EL, Farr PM. Calcipotriol improves the response of psoriasis to PUVA. Br J Dermatol 1994;130:79–82.
20. Frappaz A, Thivolet J. Calcipotriol in combination with PUVA: A randomized double blind placebo study in severe psoriasis. Eur J Dermatol 1993;3:351–354.
21. Ashcroft DM, Li WPA, Williams HC, Griffiths CE. Combination regimens of topical calcipotriene in chronic plaque psoriasis: Systematic review of efficacy and tolerability. Arch Dermatol 2000;136: 1536–1543.

22. Lebwohl M, Hecker D, Martinez J, et al. Interactions between calcipotriene and ultraviolet light. J Am Acad Dermatol 1997;37: 93–95.

23. Behrens S, Grundmann-Kollmann M, Peter RU, et al. Combination treatment of psoriasis with photochemotherapy and tazarotene gel, a receptor-selective topical retinoid. Br J Dermatol 1999;141:177.

24. Hecker D, Worsley J, Yueh G, et al. Interactions between tazarotene and ultraviolet light. J Am Acad Dermatol 1999;41:927–930.

25. Horwitz SN, Johnson RA, Sefton J, et al. Addition of a topically applied corticosteroid to a modified Goeckerman regimen for treatment of psoriasis: Effect on duration of remission. J Am Acad Dermatol 1985;13:784–791.

26. Yamauchi PS, Rizk D, Kormeili T, et al. Current systemic therapies for psoriasis: Where are we now? J Am Acad Dermatol 2003;49:S66–S77.

27. van de Kerkhof PC, Cambazard F, Hutchinson PE, et al. The effect of addition of calcipotriol ointment (50 micrograms/g) to acitretin therapy in psoriasis. Br J Dermatol 1998;138:84–89.

28. Saurat JH. Side effects of systemic retinoids and their clinical management. J Am Acad Dermatol 1992;27(6 pt 2):S23–S28.

29. Zachariae H. Liver biopsies and methotrexate: A time for reconsideration? J Am Acad Dermatol 2000;42:531–534.

30. Paul BS, Momtaz K, Stern RS, et al. Combined methotrexate—ultraviolet B therapy in the treatment of psoriasis. J Am Acad Dermatol 1982;7:758–762.

31. Clark CM, Kirby B, Morris AD, et al. Combination treatment with methotrexate and cyclosporin for severe recalcitrant psoriasis. Br J Dermatol 1999;141:279–282.

32. Koo J, Liao W. Update on psoriasis therapy: A perspective from the USA. Keio J Med 2000;49:20–25.

33. Lebwohl M, Ellis C, Gottlieb A, et al. Cyclosporine consensus conference: With emphasis on the treatment of psoriasis. J Am Acad Dermatol 1998;39:464–475.

34. Grossman RM, Thivolet J, Claudy A, et al. A novel therapeutic approach to psoriasis with combination calcipotriol ointment and very low-dose cyclosporine: Results of a multicenter placebo-controlled study. J Am Acad Dermatol 1994;31:68–74.

35. Ameen M, Smith HR, Barker JN. Combined mycophenolate mofetil and cyclosporin therapy for severe recalcitrant psoriasis. Clin Exp Dermatol 2001;26:480–483.

36. Gottlieb A. Immunobiologic agents for the treatment of psoriasis. Arch Dermatol 2003;139:791–793.

37. Walsh SRA, Shear NH. Psoriasis and the new biologic agents: Interrupting a T-AP dance. Can Med Assoc J 2004;170(13):1933–1941.

38. Kormeili T, Lowe NJ, Yamauchi PS. Psoriasis: Immunopathogenesis and evolving immunomodulators and systemic therapies; U.S. experiences. Br J Dermatol 2004;151:3–15.

39. Gottlieb G, Casale TB, Frankel E, et al. CD4+ T-cell-directed antibody responses are maintained in patients with psoriasis receiving alefacept: Results of a randomized study. J Am Acad Dermatol 2003(Nov);49: 816–825.

40. Menter A, Cather JC, Baker D et al. The efficacy of multiple courses of alefacept in patients with moderate to severe chronic plaque psoriasis. J Am Acad Dermatol 2006;54:61–63.

41. Leonardi CL, Powers JL, Matheson RT, et al. Etanercept as monotherapy in patients with psoriasis. N Engl J Med 2003;349:2014–2022.

42. Paller AS, Siegfried EC, Langley RG et al. Etanercept treatment for children and adolescents with plaque psoriasis. N Engl J Med 2008;358:241–251.

43. Lebwohl M, Tyring SK, Hamilton TK, et al. A novel targeted T-cell modulator, efalizumab, for plaque psoriasis. N Engl J Med 2003;349:2004–2013.

44. Gordon KB, Papp KA, Hamilton TK, et al. Efalizumab for patients with moderate to severe plaque psoriasis: A randomized controlled trial. J Am Med Assoc 2003;290:3073–3080.

45. Gottlieb AB, Hamilton T, Caro I et al. Long-term continuous efalizumab therapy in patients with moderate to severe chronic plaque psoriasis: Updated results from an ongoing trial. J Am Acad Dermatol 2006;54(Suppl):S154-S163.

46. Reich K, Nestle FO, Papp K et al. Infliximab induction and maintenance therapy for moderate-to-severe psoriasis: A phase III, multicenter, double-blind trial. Lancet 2005;366:1367–1374.

47. Menter A, Feldman SR, Weinstein GD et al. A randomized comparison of continuous vs intermittent infliximab maintenance regimens over 1 year in the treatment of moderate-to-severe plaque psoriasis. J Am Acad Dermatol 2007;56(31):e1–e15.

48. Menter A, Tyring SK, Gordon K et al. Adalimumab therapy for moderate to severe psoriasis: A randomized, controlled phase III trial. J Am Acad Dermatol 2007;58:106–115.

49. Gulliver WP, Donsky HJ. A report on three recent clinical trials using Mahonia aquifolium 10% topical cream and a review of the worldwide clinical experience with Mahonia aquifolium for the treatment of plaque psoriasis. Am J Ther 2005;12:398–406.

50. Updike J. From the journal of a leper. Northridge, CA: Lord John Press; 1978:21.

65 Common Skin Disorders

Angie L. Goeser

LEARNING OBJECTIVES

● **Upon completion of the chapter, the reader will be able to:**

1. Describe the pathophysiology of common skin disorders.

2. Assess the signs and symptoms of common skin disorders in a presenting patient.

3. List the goals of treatment for patients with common skin disorders.

4. Select appropriate nonpharmacologic and pharmacologic treatment regimens for patients presenting with common skin disorders.

5. Identify adverse effects that may result from pharmacologic agents used in the treatment of common skin disorders.

6. Develop a monitoring plan which will assess the safety and efficacy of the overall disease state management of common skin disorders.

7. Create educational information for patients about common skin disorders, including appropriate self-management, available drug treatment options and anticipated therapeutic responses.

KEY CONCEPTS

❶ The development of acne lesions results from four pathogenic factors which include excess sebum production, keratinization, bacterial growth, and inflammation.

❷ The treatment goals for acne vulgaris are to eliminate existing lesions and prevent new lesions from developing, as well as to decrease discomfort and the incidence of scarring.

❸ Acne is categorized as mild, moderate, or severe based on lesion type and severity and successful treatment approaches are developed based on these categories.

❹ Irritant contact dermatitis results from first-time exposures to irritating substances such as soaps, plants, cleaning solutions, or solvents. Allergic contact dermatitis occurs after an initial sensitivity and further exposure to allergenic substances, including poison ivy, latex and certain types of metals.

❺ The initial treatment goal of contact dermatitis is identifying the causative substance and eliminating its exposure. The second treatment goal is symptom relief.

❻ Although many factors contribute to the etiology of diaper rash, it is most likely the result of prolonged contact of the skin with urine and feces in the diaper.

❼ The primary goal in the treatment of diaper rash is prevention and is most often accomplished through frequent diaper changes.

❽ When a diaper rash is already present, repairing the damaged skin, relieving discomfort and preventing infection are important factors to consider when developing an effective treatment regimen.

INTRODUCTION

The skin is the largest organ of the human body. One of its most important functions is to assist the immune system by serving as a barrier that protects underlying structures from trauma, infection and exposure to harmful environmental elements. The skin also holds in place essential organs and fluids necessary for life. Any significant injury to this outer protective layer may potentially compromise an individual's overall health.

Several thousand skin disorders are currently documented, and many patients will seek the assistance of a health care provider when a complication with their skin develops. Others will utilize methods of self-care to effectively treat their symptoms. Some skin problems, such as mild acne or diaper rash, may be successfully treated with over-the-counter medications and lifestyle modifications. However, if left untreated or treated inadequately, these seemingly simple disorders can worsen and require more advanced care.

As health care providers, it is important to be familiar with the diagnosis and treatment of skin disorders. This chapter discusses acne vulgaris, contact dermatitis (irritant and allergic), and diaper dermatitis; other common skin and soft tissue infections and superficial fungal infections are discussed in Chapters 73 and 83, respectively. Providing patients with appropriate therapy options, as well as patient education on methods of treatment and prevention, will assist the successful resolution of many common skin disorders.

ACNE VULGARIS

Acne vulgaris, an inflammatory skin disorder of the pilosebaceous units of the skin, is the most common dermatologic reason for physician visits in the United States.[1] Although most commonly seen on the face, acne can also present on the chest, back, neck and shoulders (See Fig. 65–1).[2] While generally a self-limiting condition, long-term physical complications of acne may include extensive scarring and psychological distress.[1,3]

EPIDEMIOLOGY AND ETIOLOGY

With an estimated 40 to 50 million people affected, acne vulgaris is the number one skin disease in the United States.[3,4] While acne affects approximately 85% of adolescents

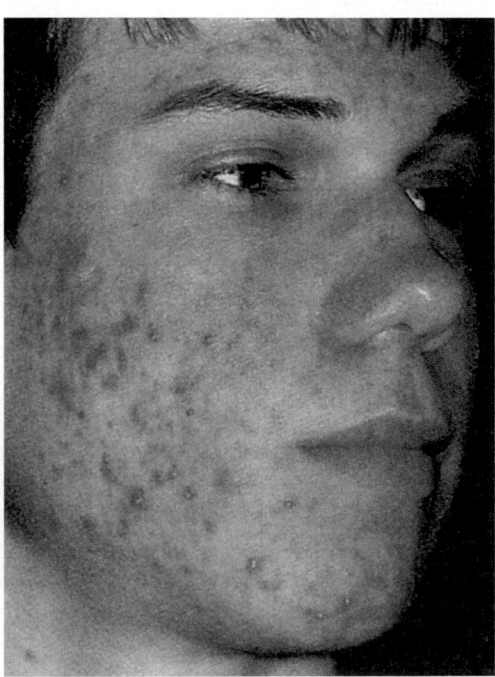

FIGURE 65–1. A spectrum of acne lesions is seen on the face of a 17-year-old male: comedones, papules, pustules, and erythematous macules and scars at the site of resolving lesions. The patient was successfully treated with a 4-month course of isotretinoin; there was no recurrence over the next 5 years. (From Wolff K, Johnson RA. Disorders of sebaceous and apocrine glands. Fitzpatrick's Color Atlas & Synopsis of Clinical Dermatology. 5th ed. New York: McGraw-Hill, 2005: 5.) (From Ref. 2.)

and adults aged 12 to 25 years, the disease can develop or recur in adults aged 30 to 50 years.[5] The prevalence of acne among Whites, African Americans, Hispanics, and Asians is similar, with acne occurring more often in males during adolescence and females during adulthood.[6,7]

PATHOPHYSIOLOGY

① *The development of acne lesions results from four pathogenic factors: excess sebum production, keratinization, bacterial growth and inflammation.*[3,7]

The pilosebaceous unit of the skin consists of a hair follicle and the surrounding sebaceous glands. An initial acne lesion called a comedo forms when there is a blockage in the pilosebaceous unit.[8]

Sebum is released by the sebaceous glands and naturally maintains hair and skin hydration. An increase in androgen levels, especially during puberty, can cause an increase in the size of the sebaceous gland and the production of abnormally high levels of sebum within those glands. This excess sebum can result in plugged follicles and acne formation.

Keratinization, the sloughing of epithelial cells in the hair follicle, is also a natural process. In acne, however, *hyper*keratinization occurs and causes increased adhesiveness of the sloughed cells. Accumulation of these cells clogs the hair follicle, blocks the flow of sebum and forms an acne lesion called an open comedo or "blackhead."

Propionobacterium acnes (*P. acnes*), an anaerobic organism, is also found in the normal flora of the skin. This bacteria proliferates in the mixture of sebum and keratinocytes and can result in an inflammatory response producing a closed comedo or "whitehead." More severe acne lesions such as pustules, papules, and nodules also form with inflammatory acne and result in significant scarring if treated inadequately (see Fig. 65–2 for various stages of acne development).

TREATMENT

Desired Outcomes and Goals

② *While eliminating existing lesions and preventing the development of new lesions are primary goals of acne therapy, secondary goals include relieving pain or discomfort and preventing permanent scarring.*[8] In addition, acne can cause patients a significant amount of stress, anxiety, frustration, embarrassment, and even depression.[10] Because of these psychological symptoms, treatment compliance and patient education on both physical and psychological aspects of this skin disorder are also imperative.

General Approach to Treatment

③ *Acne is categorized as mild, moderate, or severe based on the lesion type and lesion severity* (see Table 65–1). *Successful treatment approaches are developed based on these categories, as well as any previous treatment information presented by the patient.* Improvement of symptoms following treatment occurs gradually, sometimes taking 6 to 8 weeks for results

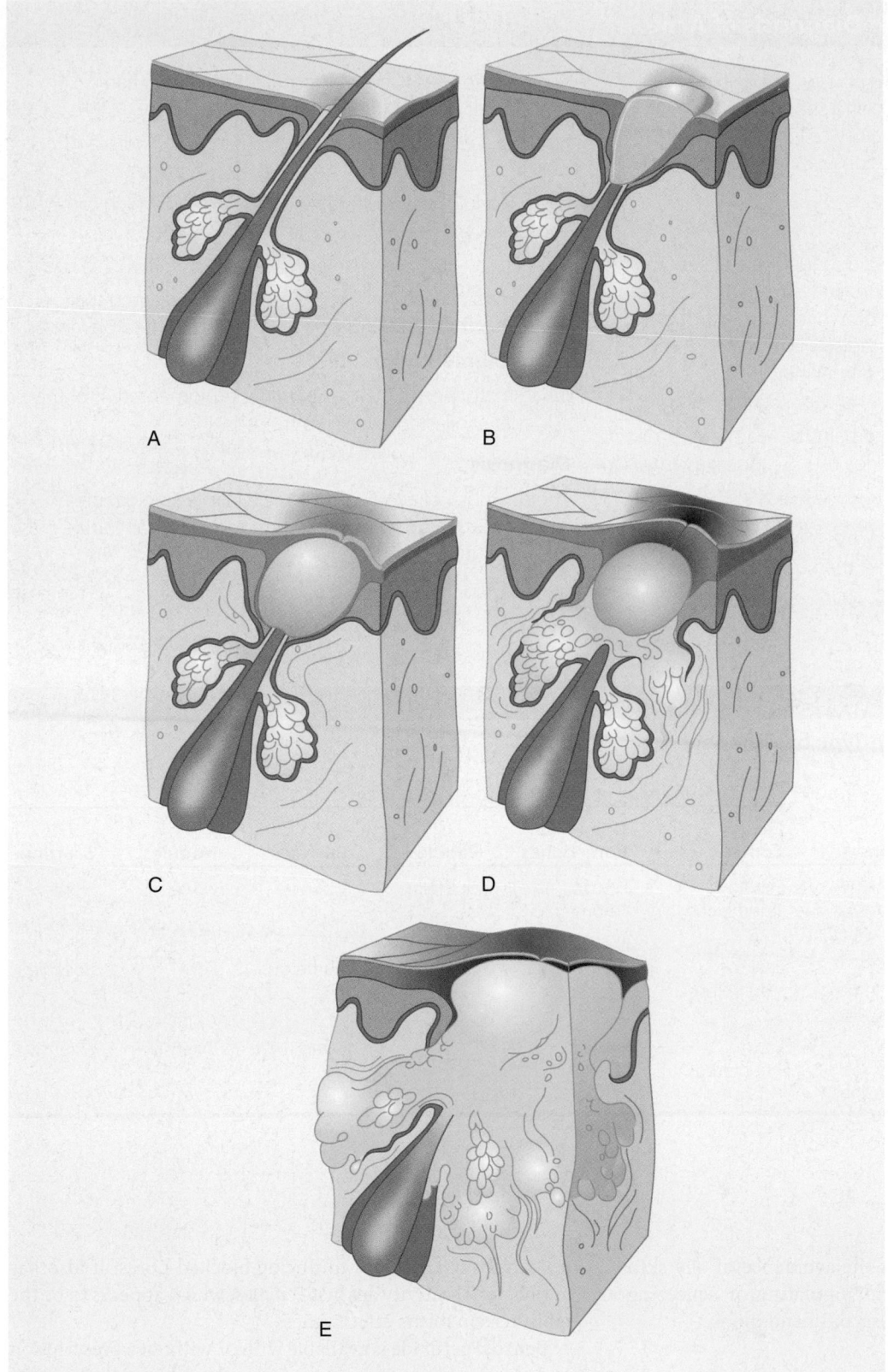

FIGURE 65–2. Stages of acne. A. Normal follicle; B. open comedo (blackhead); C. closed comedo (whitehead); D. papule; E. pustule. (From Ref. 9. Copyright "Hartsock M. Medical illustrations. Cincinnati, OH: The Medical Art Company.")

to be physically apparent.[8] Patients need to be educated on continual treatment compliance during this time and not get discouraged if acne lesions appear to worsen before getting better during the initial 2 to 3 weeks of therapy.[11]

Nonpharmacologic Therapy

There is significant variance in the clinical benefit of many nonpharmacologic interventions for acne vulgaris. Among nondrug treatment alternatives, mild, noncomedogenic facial

Clinical Presentation and Diagnosis of Acne

Acne lesions are most often seen on the face, but can also present on the chest, back, neck, and shoulders and are described as either noninflammatory or inflammatory. In addition, severe inflammatory lesions can lead to scarring and hyperpigmentation.

Noninflammatory Lesions

Open comedo or "blackhead": a plugged follicle of sebum, keratinocytes, and bacteria that protrudes from the surface of the skin and appears black or brown in color. Although dark in color, blackheads do not indicate the presence of dirt, but rather, an accumulation of melanin.

Closed comedo or "whitehead": a plugged follicle of sebum, keratinocytes, and bacteria that remains beneath the surface of the skin. Closed comedos usually appear as small white bumps about 1 to 2 mm in diameter.

Inflammatory Lesions

Papules: Solid, elevated lesion less than 0.5 cm in diameter

Pustules: Vesicles filled with purulent fluid less than 0.5 cm in diameter

Nodules: Lesions greater than 0.5 cm in both width and depth

Cysts: Nodules filled with a fluid or semisolid which can be expressed

Scars

Inflammatory acne can result in permanent scarring that ranges from small depressed pits to large elevated blemishes.

Hyperpigmentation

Inflammatory acne may result in hyperpigmentation of the skin that can last for weeks to months.

Diagnosis

The diagnosis of acne vulgaris is clinical. Lesion cultures may be warranted when treatment regimens fail to rule out other skin infections.

Table 65–1

Predominance of Acne Lesion Type by Acne Severity

Acne Severity	Predominant Lesions	Typical Frequency of Lesion Type					
		Closed Comedones	Open Comedones	Papules	Pustules	Nodules	Scarring
Mild	Noninflammatory lesions (open and closed comedones)	Few to numerous	Few to numerous	Possible	Possible	None	None
Moderate	Inflammatory papules and pustules with some noninflammatory lesions	Few to numerous	Few to numerous	Numerous	Numerous	Few	Possible
Severe	Inflammatory lesions and scarring with some noninflammatory lesions	Few to numerous	Few to numerous	Extensive	Extensive	Extensive	Extensive

From Ref. 3.

---

soap used twice daily, as well as the avoidance of oily skin products and the avoidance of manipulating or squeezing lesions are helpful self-treatment recommendations.

Pharmacologic Therapy

▶ Topical Agents

Benzoyl Peroxide Benzoyl peroxide is easy to use and recommended as first-line therapy in the treatment of mild to moderate noninflammatory acne. Benzoyl peroxide has a comedolytic effect that increases the rate of epithelial cell turnover and helps to unclog blocked pores. It also has antibacterial activity against *P. acnes*, which appears to be the main reason for its effectiveness.[13]

Benzoyl peroxide is available with or without a prescription and remains the most commonly purchased over-the-counter topical treatment for acne.[12] It is available in concentrations ranging from 1% to 10% in various formulations including creams, lotions, gels, and facial washes.

Adverse effects commonly reported with benzoyl peroxide are dryness, irritation, redness, and stinging of the skin. Reducing the incidence of these effects can be achieved by beginning a treatment regimen with the lowest strength and titrating up to higher effective strengths over several weeks if needed. In addition, newer formulations of benzoyl peroxide are combined with moisturizers to help decrease skin redness and irritation.[13] A disadvantage of the agent is that it can bleach and discolor hair and fabrics that come into contact.[12]

A typical regimen for benzoyl peroxide is to apply the product to clean, dry skin no more than two times a day. The strength and dosage form selected may vary from patient to patient depending on acne severity and the sensitivity of the patient's skin. Since gel preparations are the most potent dosage form, patients with dry or overly sensitive skin should be recommended a milder cream, lotion, or facial wash.[3] If severe irritation or allergic reaction develops, benzoyl peroxide use should be discontinued.

Retinoids Retinoids, which are highly effective in the treatment of acne, stimulate epithelial cell turnover and aid in unclogging blocked pores. Retinoids also exhibit anti-inflammatory properties through the inhibition of neutrophil and monocyte chemotaxis.[8] Because of these comedolytic and anti-inflammatory effects, topical retinoids are recommended as first-line treatment for mild to moderate comedonal and inflammatory acne.[3] While success is seen with monotherapy, using a retinoid in combination with benzoyl peroxide or topical antibacterials is also an appropriate and effective therapeutic treatment option.[3] Tretinoin, adapalene, and tazarotene are topical retinoids available for use in the treatment of acne. Table 65–2 describes the strengths and formulations of these agents.

Transient erythema, irritation, dryness, and peeling at the site of application are all common adverse effects. Newer retinoids formulated in either a microsphere gel (Retin-A Micro) or an aqueous-based gel (Atralin) appear to cause less initial skin discomfort than older agents in this class.[13] Photosensitivity can also occur with retinoid use, causing increased skin irritation and redness.[14]

The topical retinoid selected should be applied once daily at bedtime, beginning with a low potency formulation. Increased strengths are then initiated according to treatment results and tolerance. Patients should be advised that a worsening of acne symptoms generally occurs in the first few weeks of therapy, with lesion improvement occurring in 3 to 4 months.[16] The use of topical retinoids should be avoided in children less than 12 years old and in pregnant women.[14]

Antibacterials Topical antibacterials directly suppress *P. acnes* and are also first-line agents used in the treatment of mild to moderate inflammatory acne.[3,16]

Clindamycin 1% and erythromycin 2% preparations, applied once or twice daily, have similar effects and are the most commonly prescribed topical antibacterial agents.[17] These agents, as well as sodium sulfacetamide, are available in various formulations for the treatment of acne.

Adverse effects are generally mild and include dryness, erythema, and itching.[18] Although rare and seen most often with oral therapy, pseudomembranous colitis can occur with the prolonged use of topical clindamycin.[19] As with any antibacterial agent, the possibility of resistance exists with the use of topical antibiotics. However, coadministration of clindamycin or erythromycin and benzoyl peroxide has shown to decrease the incidence of resistance, as well as to improve symptoms of mild to moderate inflammatory acne.[7,20]

Azelaic Acid With antibacterial and anti-inflammatory properties, and the ability to stabilize keratinization, azelaic acid is an effective alternative in the treatment of mild to moderate acne in patients who cannot tolerate benzoyl peroxide or topical retinoids.[3,21] It can also even out skin tone that may prove effective in patients who are prone to postinflammatory hyperpigmentation resulting from acne.[22]

Adverse effects are minimal and transient with erythema and skin irritation most common.[16,21]

Azelaic acid 20% cream should be applied twice daily with improvement of symptoms seen in 1 to 2 months.[21]

Keratolytics Sulfur, resorcinol, and salicylic acid are not as effective as other topical agents, but can be used as second-line therapies in the treatment of mild to moderate acne.[12]

Table 65–2				
Topical Retinoids Available for the Treatment of Acne				
Agent	Brand Name	Dosage Form	Dosage	Side Effects
Tretinoin	Retin-A	0.025%, 0.05%, and 0.1% cream 0.01%, 0.025% gel	Apply small amount once daily before bedtime	Skin irritation, dryness, photosensitivity, initially may worsen acne
	Retin-A Micro	0.04% and 0.1% gel	Apply small amount once daily before bedtime	Skin irritation, dryness, photosensitivity, initially may worsen acne
	Atralin	0.05% gel	Apply small amount once daily before bedtime	Skin irritation, dryness, peeling/flaking skin
Adapalene	Differin	0.1% cream 0.1% and 0.3% gel	Apply small amount once daily before bedtime	Same as tretinoin but may be *less* severe
Tazarotene	Tazorac	0.05% and 0.1% cream 0.05% and 0.1% gel	Apply small amount once daily before bedtime	Same as tretinoin but may be *more* severe

From Ref. 15.

While these agents may cause less skin irritation than benzoyl peroxide or the topical retinoids, several disadvantages exist. Sulfur preparations produce an unpleasant odor when applied to the skin, while resorcinol may cause brown scaling. And although rare, the possibility of salicylism exists with continual salicylic acid use.[3,12]

▶ Oral Agents

Antibacterials Moderate to severe acne can be effectively treated with oral antibiotics, especially when treatment with topical therapy has failed. Because of their ability to decrease *P. acnes* colonization, oral antibiotics can prevent acne lesions from developing.[8] Improvement of symptoms is generally evident at 6 to 10 weeks, with maximum benefits occurring after 6 months of therapy.[23]

Tetracycline, doxycycline, and minocycline are the most commonly prescribed oral antibiotics for acne. Erythromycin and clindamycin are appropriate second-line agents for use when patients cannot tolerate or have developed resistance to tetracycline or its derivatives.[3] Other antibiotics, including trimethoprim (± sulfamethoxazole) and azithromycin are also effective agents to use when patients fail or are unable to tolerate conventional treatment.[7] (See Table 65–3 for antibiotic dosing guidelines.)

Adverse effects with the tetracyclines include GI upset, drug interactions with dairy products, antacids and iron, and phototoxicity. Minocycline can also cause vestibular complications (headache, dizziness) and skin discoloration that is not typical with tetracycline and doxycycline.[16]

Although their effectiveness is similar to the tetracyclines, erythromycin, and clindamycin use is often limited due to their potential adverse outcomes. Erythromycin has increased resistance to *P. acnes* and a high incidence of GI intolerance, while clindamycin causes diarrhea and the risk of developing pseudomembranous colitis with long term use.[3,8]

Isotretinoin Isotretinoin is effective in up to 80% of patients with severe nodulocystic acne who are unresponsive to other topical and oral treatment regimens.[8,23,24] Isotretinoin works on the four pathogenic factors that contribute to acne development and can produce acne remission rates of up to several years.

Adverse effects with the use of isotretinoin are frequent and generally dose-related. About 90% of patients experience drying of the mucosa of the mouth, eyes, and nose.[3] Drying, peeling, and pruritus of the facial skin is also likely. Increases in cholesterol and triglyceride levels have been reported with isotretinoin use; therefore, it is recommended to monitor liver function and serum lipids at baseline, 4 and 8 weeks of therapy to identify any complications. Other serious adverse effects from this medication include increased creatine phosphokinase, increased blood glucose, teratogenicity, photosensitivity, muscle pain, suicidality, and depression.[3] Table 65–4 lists the common adverse effects from isotretinoin therapy and management strategies for those symptoms.

Because it is teratogenic and classified as pregnancy category X, the FDA mandates an online registry program called iPledge to ensure that females do not become pregnant while taking isotretinoin. Wholesalers, pharmacies, doctors, and patients must be registered in the iPledge computer-based system in order to control the distribution, prescribing, and dispensing of isotretinoin. Two negative pregnancy tests prior to initiating therapy and one negative pregnancy test each month thereafter must be obtained and confirmed in the system before a prescription can be dispensed to female patients of child-bearing potential. These patients must also commit to effective measures of birth control during

---

Table 65–3

Oral Agents Used in the Treatment of Moderate to Severe Acne

Drug	Dosage Form	Strength (mg)	Regimen	Side Effects
Tetracycline	Tablets, capsules	250 500	500 mg twice daily before meals. Maintenance dose: 500 mg daily	GI upset, phototoxicity, tooth discoloration, drug and food interactions
Doxycycline	Tablets, capsules	50 100	100–200 mg daily before meals. Maintenance dose: 50 mg daily	GI upset, phototoxicity, drug and food interactions
Minocycline	Tablets, capsules	50 75 100	50 mg twice daily or 100 mg once daily Maintenance dose: 50 mg daily	GI upset, phototoxicity, drug and food interactions, vestibular toxicity, skin discoloration
Erythromycin	Tablets	250 500	500 mg twice daily with food. Maintenance dose: 500 mg daily	GI intolerance, drug interactions
Clindamycin	Capsules	75 150 300	150–300 mg daily Maintenance dose: 150 mg daily	Diarrhea, pseudomembranous colitis
Isotretinoin	Capsules	10 20 40	0.5–1 mg/kg/day in two divided doses Maximum dose: 2 mg/kg/day Cumulative dose: 120–150 mg/day	Dry skin and mucous membranes, muscle and joint pain, elevated liver enzymes and triglycerides, depression, teratogenicity

From Ref. 15.

Table 65–4

Principle Adverse Effects of Oral Isotretinoin

Adverse Effect	Response
Teratogenicity	Contraindicated during pregnancy
Depression	Patient monitoring and counseling; antidepressants
Dryness	
Mouth	Hard candy
Eyes	Eyedrops; avoid contact lenses if possible during treatment course
Nose	Lubricant
Skin	Nondrying gentle skin cleansers; noncomedolytic moisturizers
Lips	Lip moisturizer with sunscreen
Muscle and joint pain	Nonsteroidal anti-inflammatory drugs
Alopecia	Reversible when drug discontinued or dose decreased
Hypertriglyceridemia	Reversible when drug discontinued or dose decreased
Acne flare at start of therapy	Continue therapy
Photosensitivity	Use sunscreens (moisturizing), protective clothing, and sun avoidance

From Ref. 3.

the course of isotretinoin therapy. Contact the program at their website: *https://www.ipledgeprogram.com/* for further details.

Initial dose ranges for treatment are 0.5 to 1 mg/kg daily in two divided doses, with beneficial results generally reported at total daily doses of 120 to 150 mg/day.[3]

Oral Contraceptives Oral contraceptives are a valuable second-line treatment option for moderate to severe acne in female patients. While many contraceptives are effective, three agents (*Yaz*, *Estrostep*, and *Ortho Tri-Cyclen*) have been FDA approved for the treatment of acne.[25] Oral contraceptives decrease the production of androgens by the ovaries, which in turn leads to a decrease in sebum production.[3,16]

Adverse effects include nausea, weight gain, breast tenderness and breakthrough bleeding. Oral contraceptives have also been associated with an increased incidence of thromboembolic disease, particularly in women who use tobacco products or have other risk factors for thromboembolism. The development of these complications is significantly reduced when low dose estrogen formulations of oral contraceptives are used.[3]

Other Agents Although use is infrequent, several other agents are available as second- or third-line treatment options for acne when first-line therapies fail and include the following[3,7]:

- Corticosteroids
- Chemical peels

Patient Encounter 1

A 14-year-old female high school student presents to your clinic with complaints of worsening acne. Upon visual examination, you see that she has four pustules on her chin, two pustules on her forehead, and numerous open and closed comedones on her nose and cheeks. After interviewing the patient, you conclude that her acne lesions are moderately painful and make her feel embarrassed about going to school with so many "zits." She says that she began to have occasional acne at the age of 12, but over the past 6 months symptoms have worsened and states that she always has four to six lesions present on her face. The patient appears to be a healthy teenager who says that she eats well and is very athletic.

What reported symptoms support the diagnosis of acne?

What other information would you obtain from this patient before creating a treatment plan for her?

Describe your treatment goals for this patient.

What nonpharmacologic and pharmacologic treatment options are available for this patient?

Given the information presented, develop a treatment regimen for this patient including (a) a statement of the problem, (b) a patient-specific therapeutic plan, and (c) monitoring parameters to assess efficacy and safety.

Patient Care and Monitoring: Acne

1. Assess patient symptoms and the presence of acne lesions. Determine severity of acne: mild, moderate or severe.

2. Review patient history to determine treatment regimens that have been used in the past, including nonprescription, prescription, and herbal medications.

3. Obtain patient's allergy status.

4. Develop a treatment plan appropriate for improvement of acne.

5. Discuss any monitoring parameters that may be necessary throughout the course of therapy.

6. Provide patient education on acne and its treatment:

   a. What is acne and how does it develop?

   b. Physical and psychological complications that can result from acne.

   c. What drug and nondrug therapies are available for treatment?

   d. Describe the possible side effects of drug therapy.

   e. Emphasize the importance of treatment regimen compliance to ensure positive results.

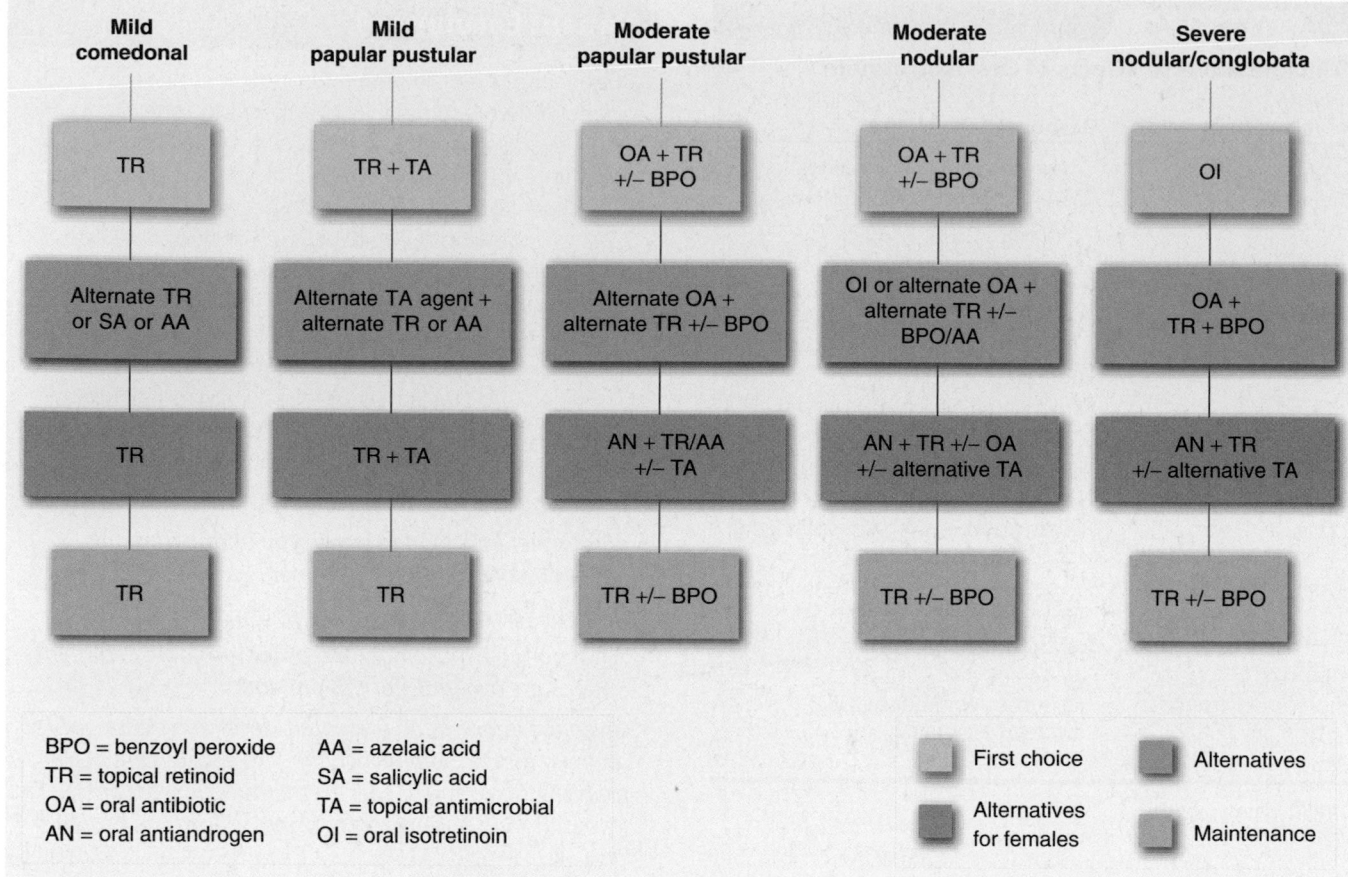

FIGURE 65–3. Algorithms for acne treatment. (From Ref. 3.)

- Surgical extraction
- Phototherapy/photodynamic therapy
- Laser treatments

Figure 65–3 shows useful algorithms for the effective treatment of the various stages of acne.

OUTCOME EVALUATION

Depending on severity, complete resolution of acne may take weeks to months. Monitor patients after 6 weeks of pharmacologic therapy for any improvement of signs and symptoms[12]:

- Decreased number of lesions
- Decreased severity of lesions
- Relief of pain/irritation

If no improvement is reported or symptoms have worsened, patients should be reevaluated and a change in the current treatment regimen may be necessary.

Educate patients on the possibility of adverse effects. Consider a change in therapy if a patient experiences effects that are not tolerated or are considered a compromise to their health.

CONTACT DERMATITIS

Contact dermatitis is a condition in which exposure to an offending substance produces inflammation, erythema, and pruritus of the skin.[26] More specifically, contact dermatitis can be divided into either irritant or allergic forms.[26,27]

❹ *Irritant contact dermatitis results from first-time exposure to irritating substances such as soaps, plants, cleaning solutions, or solvents. Allergic contact dermatitis occurs after an initial sensitivity and further exposure to allergenic substances, including poison ivy, latex, and certain types of metal.*[28] (See Figs. 65–4 and 65–5.) Table 65–5 lists agents commonly responsible for irritant and allergic contact dermatitis. While generally occurring on the exposed skin, such as the hands and face, contact dermatitis can appear anywhere on the body.[26] Although most cases are easily treated, contact dermatitis remains an uncomfortable and sometimes embarrassing skin condition.

EPIDEMIOLOGY AND ETIOLOGY

Contact dermatitis is a common reason for dermatology referrals and constitutes up to 90% of all workers' compensation claims for dermatologic conditions. Although

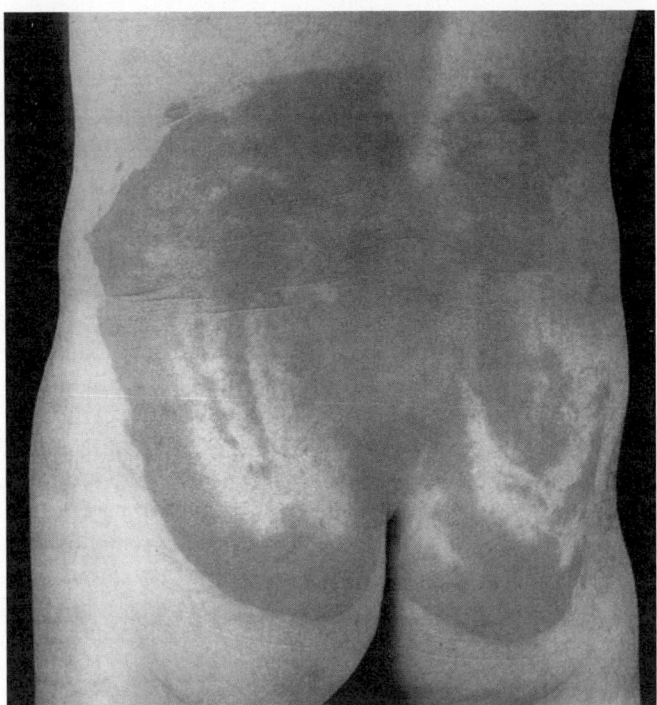

FIGURE 65–4. Irritant contact dermatitis. Erythema and edema with spared areas on the back at sites in contact with an irritant in a 30-year-old male. (From Wolff K, Johnson RA. Eczema/dermatitis. Fitzpatrick's Color Atlas & Synopsis of Clinical Dermatology. 5th ed. New York: McGraw-Hill, 2005: 20.)

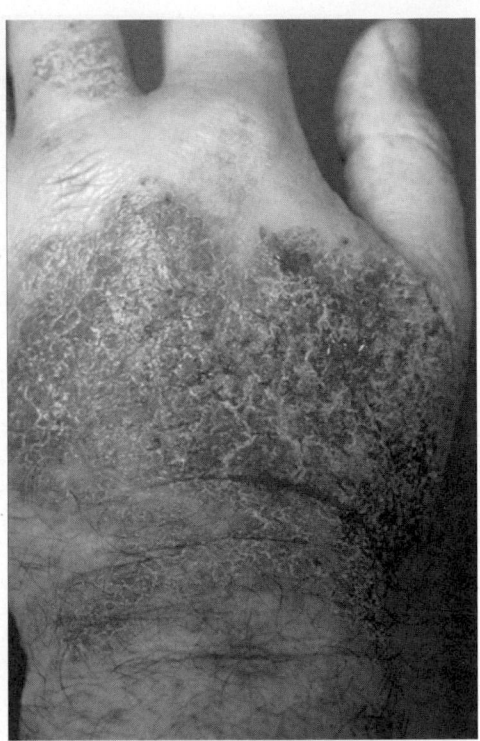

FIGURE 65–5. Allergic contact dermatitis of the hand: chromates. Confluent papules, vesicles, erosions, and crusts on the dorsum of the left hand in a construction worker who was allergic to chromates. (From Wolff K, Johnson RA. Eczema/dermatitis. Fitzpatrick's Color Atlas & Synopsis of Clinical Dermatology. 5th ed. New York: McGraw-Hill, 2005: 27.)

most often seen in adults, contact dermatitis can affect all age groups, with females at slightly greater risk than males.[29]

PATHOPHYSIOLOGY

Irritant contact dermatitis is not the result of an immunologic process, but rather occurs from direct injury to the skin. An irritating agent comes into contact with the skin, damages the protective layers of the epidermis and can cause erythema, the formation of vesicles and pruritus.[26,30,31] Symptoms occur within minutes to hours of exposure and begin to heal soon after removal of the offending substance.[28]

Allergic contact dermatitis is a delayed hypersensitivity reaction.[31] Upon initial exposure, a substance penetrates the skin, binds to a protein and develops into sensitizing antigens. Subsequent exposures to that substance will then elicit an allergic reaction.[26,30,31] Symptoms of allergic contact dermatitis are similar to those of the irritant type, but may take several hours to several days to develop following reexposure.[26,27]

TREATMENT

Desired Outcomes and Goals

⑤ *Identifying the causative substance and eliminating its exposure is the initial treatment goal for contact dermatitis.* Although physical symptoms can develop almost immediately

after contact, removal of the offending agent will improve existing symptoms and prevent the occurrence of further complications. **⑤** *The second treatment goal is symptom relief.* Since inflammation and pruritus, as well as lesion formation, are likely to result from contact dermatitis, appropriate selection of nonpharmacologic and pharmacologic agents for these symptoms is necessary.

Table 65–5
Common Agents Causing Contact Dermatitis

Irritant Contact Dermatitis
Soaps
Detergents
Cosmetics
Solvents
Acid, mild or strong
Alkali, mild, or strong

Allergic Contact Dermatitis
Plant resins, poison ivy, poison oak, sumac
Metals (nickel or gold in jewelry)
Latex and rubber
Cigarette smoke
Local anesthetics (lidocaine, benzocaine)

Clinical Presentation and Diagnosis of Contact Dermatitis

Contact dermatitis is generally confined to the area of contact, but in a highly sensitive person, a widespread or even generalized eruption may occur. Contact dermatitis is divided into two forms—irritant and allergic. Both forms may include, but are not limited to:

- Erythema
- Pruritus
- Vesicles
- Papules
- Crusts
- Burning

Irritant Form

The irritant form usually presents within hours of exposure and the rash is often localized. Irritant contact dermatitis may also result in fissuring and scaling.

Allergic Form

The allergic form can take several days to present and the condition may extend beyond the borders of the region exposed. Allergic contact dermatitis may also include oozing pustules and skin erosion.

Diagnosis

When the causative agent is known, the diagnosis of contact dermatitis is clinical. Patch testing is done if the allergens are unknown and is usually performed several weeks after the resolution of the original dermatitis.

Nonpharmacologic Therapy

In many cases, contact dermatitis may not require medical treatment at all. Nondrug therapy for contact dermatitis is aimed at relieving pruritus and maintaining skin hydration.[28] Effective agents used for this include the following:[26,28]

- Colloidal oatmeal baths
- Cool or tepid soapless showers
- Cool, moist compresses applied to the area for 30 minutes three times a day
- Emollients or lubricants applied to the area after bathing (mineral oil, petrolatum)

Pharmacologic Therapy

▶ Astringents

The drying effect of astringents will decrease oozing from lesions and relieve itching.[26,27] Due to their ability to cause blood vessel constriction, astringents can also decrease inflammation. Aluminum acetate (Burow's solution), calamine, and witch hazel are safe and effective.[26] Patients apply solutions as a compress for 15 to 30 minutes two to four times a day.

Adverse effects reported with these agents are minimal and include drying and tightening of the skin. Because of this, their use should be limited to no more than 7 days.[26,27,29]

▶ Topical Steroids

Erythema, inflammation, pain, and itching caused by contact dermatitis can be effectively treated with topically applied corticosteroids. With such a wide range of products and potencies, an appropriate steroid selection is based on severity and location of lesions (See Table 65–6 for a list of topical steroids and potencies.) Higher potency preparations are used in areas where penetration is poor, such as the elbows and knees. Lower potency products should be reserved for areas of higher penetration, such as the face, axillae, and groin. Low potency steroids are also recommended for the treatment of infants and children.[33,34]

Adverse effects from topical steroids are usually related to the potency of the steroid, frequency of application, duration of therapy and the site of application. Skin atrophy, hypopigmentation, striae and steroid-induced acne are all possible side effects associated with long-term use.[33,34]

Topical steroids are typically applied two to four times daily. As improvement begins, maintenance therapy should be limited to the lowest strength steroid that continues to control the condition. Once symptoms are completely resolved, use should be discontinued.

▶ Antihistamines

Whether due to their antihistaminic activity or their sedative side effects, pruritus caused by contact dermatitis can be relieved with the use of sedating oral antihistamines such as diphenhydramine or hydroxyzine. Topical antihistamines are available, but use is limited due to their high-sensitizing potential.[26,33]

In addition to sedation, many oral antihistamines can cause hypotension, dizziness, blurred vision, and confusion.[29]

Diphenhydramine and hydroxyzine can be safely administered to children older than 2 years and adults. Table 65–7 outlines the recommended doses for these medications.

OUTCOME EVALUATION

With adequate treatment, most cases of contact dermatitis should improve within 7 days. Complete resolution of symptoms may take up to 3 weeks.[26] If a patient experiences severe symptoms associated with fever or difficulty breathing, they should be instructed to seek medical attention immediately. Furthermore, patients should return to their health care provider if any of the following occur:

- Rash has not improved or has worsened after several days of treatment
- Rash has increased in size or has spread to other locations
- Patient is experiencing adverse effects from the treatment regimen

Table 65–6

Topical Steroids to Treat Contact Dermatitis

Corticosteroids	Dosage Forms	Strength (%)	USP Potency Ratings[a]	Vasoconstrictive Potency Rating[b]
Alclometasone dipropionate	Cream	0.05	Low	VI
	Ointment	0.05	Low	V
Amcinonide	Lotion, ointment	0.1	High	II
	Cream	0.1	High	III
Beclomethasone dipropionate	Cream, lotion, ointment	0.025	Medium	—
Betamethasone benzoate	Cream, gel	0.025	Medium	III
	Ointment	0.025	Medium	IV
Betamethasone dipropionate	Cream AF (optimized vehicle)	0.05	Very high	I
	Cream	0.05	High	III
	Gel, lotion, ointment (optimized vehicle)	0.05	Very high	I
	Lotion	0.05	High	V
	Ointment	0.05	High	II
	Topical aerosol	0.1	High	—
Betamethasone valerate	Cream	0.01, 0.05, 0.1	Medium	V
	Lotion, ointment	0.05, 0.1	Medium	III
	Foam	0.12	Medium	IV
Clobetasol propionate	Cream, ointment, solution, foam	0.05	Very high	I
Clobetasol butyrate	Cream, ointment	0.05	Medium	—
Clocortolone pivalate	Cream	0.1	Low	—
Desonide	Cream, lotion, ointment	0.05	Low	VI
Desoximetasone	Cream	0.05	Medium	II
	Cream, ointment	0.25	High	II
	Gel	0.05	High	II
Dexamethasone	Gel	0.1	Low	VII
	Topical aerosol	0.01, 0.04	Low	VII
Dexamethasone sodium phosphate	Cream	0.1	Low	VII
Diflorasone diacetate	Cream	0.05	High	III
	Ointment	0.05	High	II
	Ointment (optimized vehicle)	0.05	Very high	II
Diflucortolone valerate	Cream, ointment	0.1	Medium	—
Flumethasone pivalate	Cream, ointment	0.03	Low	—
Fluocinolone acetonide	Cream	0.01	Medium	VI
	Cream	0.025	Medium	V
	Cream	0.2	High	—
	Ointment	0.025	Medium	IV
	Solution	0.01	Medium	VI
Fluocinonide	Gel, cream, ointment	0.05	High	II
	Solution	0.05	High	II
Flurandrenolide	Cream, ointment	0.0125	Low	—
	Ointment	0.05	Medium	IV
	Cream, lotion	0.05	Medium	V
	Tape	4 mcg/cm^2	Medium	I
Fluticasone propionate	Cream	0.05	Medium	IV
	Ointment	0.05	Medium	III
Halcinonide	Cream	0.025, 0.1	High	II
	Ointment	0.1	High	III
	Solution	0.1	High	—
Halobetasol propionate	Cream, ointment	0.05	Very high	I
Hydrocortisone	Cream, lotion, ointment	All strengths	Low	VII
Hydrocortisone acetate	Cream, lotion, ointment	All strengths	Low	VII
Hydrocortisone butyrate	Cream	0.1	Medium	V
	Ointment	0.1	Medium	—
Hydrocortisone valerate	Cream	0.2	Medium	V
	Ointment	0.2	Medium	IV

(Continued)

Table 65–6

Topical Steroids to Treat Contact Dermatitis (*Continued*)

Corticosteroids	Dosage Forms	Strength (%)	USP Potency Ratings[a]	Vasoconstrictive Potency Rating[b]
Methylprednisolone acetate	Cream, ointment	0.25	Low	VII
	Ointment	1	Low	VII
Mometasone furoate	Cream	0.1	Medium	IV
	Lotion, ointment	0.1	Medium	II
Triamcinolone acetonide	Cream, ointment	0.1	Medium	IV
	Cream, lotion, ointment	0.025	Medium	—
	Cream (Aristocort)	0.1	Medium	VI
	Cream (Kenalog)	0.1	High	IV
	Lotion	0.1	Medium	V
	Ointment (Aristocort, Kenalog)	0.1	High	III
	Cream, ointment	0.5	High	III
	Topical aerosol	0.015	Medium	—

[a]USP ratings are low, medium, high, and very high.

[b]Vasoconstriction potency scale is I (highest) to VII (lowest);—denotes unknown vasoconstrictive properties.

From Ref. 32.

Table 65–7

Oral Antihistamines Used for Pruritus

Drug	Pediatric Dosage	Adult Dosage
Diphenhydramine (Benadryl)	Not recommended for use in infants or neonates Less than 6 years old: 6.25–12.5 mg every 4– 6 hours as needed 6–12 years old: 12.5–25 mg every 4–6 hours as needed	25–50 mg every 6–8 hours as needed
Hydroxyzine (Atarax)	0.6 mg/kg/dose every 6 hours as needed	25 mg every 6–8 hours as needed

From Ref. 15.

Patient Encounter 2

A 45-year-old female presents to a pharmacy with complaints of itching and wants a recommendation to treat it. Upon visual examination you see that she has erythematous papules on both legs. After further questioning, you learn that she has recently spent a great deal of time outside at a family picnic. She states that the picnic was in a wooded area near her home and that she and several others went on a short hike that day. She states that she was wearing shorts and "probably" came into contact with the grasses and weeds that lined the hiking trail. The rash appeared the same day as the picnic and she says that it seems to have spread since it first developed. From the information she has presented, you conclude that she has been exposed to poison ivy.

What information supports the possibility of poison ivy exposure?

Describe the symptoms that support this diagnosis.

Determine what the patient has tried to relieve her symptoms.

What are your treatment goals for this patient?

What nonpharmacologic and pharmacologic treatment options are available for this diagnosis?

Given the information presented, develop a treatment regimen for this patient including (a) a statement of the problem, (b) a patient-specific therapeutic plan, and (c) monitoring parameters to assess efficacy and safety.

Patient Care and Monitoring: Contact Dermatitis

1. Assess the patient's symptoms. Determine which form of contact dermatitis is present—irritant or allergic?

2. Obtain a thorough patient history. Has there been prior exposure to this agent? If so, what treatment regimens were used in the past to alleviate symptoms?

3. Obtain patient's allergy status.

4. Develop a treatment plan appropriate for contact dermatitis.

5. Discuss testing that may need to be performed to suggest or confirm the etiologic agent (patch testing).

6. Provide patient education on contact dermatitis and treatment:

    a. What is contact dermatitis and how does it develop?

    b. List various types of contact dermatitis.

    c. What drug therapies are available for treatment?

    d. What are the possible adverse effects of drug therapy?

    e. What are the symptoms that warrant physician referral.

    f. Explain the importance of treatment compliance.

    g. Educate on the recognition of agents that may cause contact dermatitis.

Clinical Presentation and Diagnosis of Diaper Dermatitis

Typical Symptoms

- Erythema is the most common symptom presented with a diaper rash. The rash may begin as light to medium pink with poorly defined edges, but when further developed may become dark red and raised lesions with distinct edges.

- Rashes generally appear in the folds of the skin around the diaper area, thighs, genitals, and buttocks.

- Other typical symptoms include irritation and pruritus.

Atypical symptoms

Patients presenting with the following symptoms may indicate the need for more aggressive antibiotic or antifungal therapy and should be referred to a primary care physician for further evaluation:

- Rashes not responding to typical creams and concurrent nonpharmacologic treatment

- Rashes extending beyond the diaper region (upper abdomen, back)

- Formation of papules, bullae, ulceration

- Excessive oozing

- Presence of genital discharge

- Concurrent fever

- Rashes appearing when diapers have not been used or rashes that fail to improve upon discontinuing diaper usage for extended periods of time (several days or more)

- Bleeding or open skin

Diagnosis

The diagnosis of diaper dermatitis is clinical. The presence of *Candida albicans* can be determined by KOH testing or culture, but is generally not necessary.

DIAPER DERMATITIS

EPIDEMIOLOGY AND ETIOLOGY

Diaper dermatitis, or more commonly known as diaper rash, is a form of irritant contact dermatitis that affects the buttocks, upper thighs, lower abdomen and genitalia of an estimated 7% to 35% of all infants.[35,36] Onset of occurrence is usually between 3 weeks and 2 years of age, with the most cases reported between 9 and 12 months of age.[37] The rise in the number of adults who use diapers for incontinence also increases the risk of developing diaper dermatitis.[35]

PATHOPHYSIOLOGY

6 *Although many factors contribute to the etiology of diaper rash, it is most likely the result of prolonged contact of the skin with urine and feces in the diaper.* If a diaper is not changed soon after urination or defecation, the protective layer of the skin can break down and make the area more susceptible to irritation and infection from the contents of the diaper.[38] While most mild cases of diaper rash present as erythema, moderate to severe cases can result

in the formation of papules, vesicles, and even ulceration. If these cases are not effectively treated, the likelihood of secondary fungal or bacterial infections developing is greatly increased.[35]

TREATMENT

Desired Outcomes and Goals

7 *The primary goal in the treatment of diaper rash is prevention and is most often accomplished through frequent diaper changes.* **8** *When a diaper rash is already present, repairing the damaged skin, relieving discomfort, and preventing secondary infections from occurring are important factors to consider when developing an effective treatment regimen.*[38]

Nonpharmacologic Therapy

Most mild cases of diaper rash can be resolved with the use of nonpharmacologic therapies. Keeping the diaper area clean and dry by changing diapers as soon as practically possible is highly effective for treatment and prevention.[35,36] Other nondrug options include[27,35]:

- Washing the area with lukewarm water and mild soap and allowing to completely dry before applying a new diaper
- Keeping diapers loose and well ventilated
- Avoiding plastic pants over diapers
- Allowing infants to take naps on an open diaper or absorbent pad to promote drying and healing

Pharmacologic Therapy

▶ Protectants

Protectants form an occlusive barrier between the skin and moisture from the diaper. Cream and ointment preparations are effective in providing a sufficient barrier in mild, irritant, and noninfected diaper rashes. For more severe cases, a paste is the topical agent of choice. Pastes are thicker and often contain additional ingredients (petrolatum, moisturizers) to help decrease discomfort and promote healing.[37] Zinc oxide is one of the most commonly used topical protectants. In addition to forming an effective barrier against moisture, it has astringent and antiseptic properties that provide added symptom relief.[35]

Protectants are generally applied to the affected area after every diaper change and can be discontinued when the rash resolves. Other available protectants that can be used alone or in combination for the safe and effective treatment of diaper rash include white petrolatum, Vitamins A & D, lanolin, and topical cornstarch. Many agents contain a combination of occlusive and protective agents such as Triple Paste and Calmoseptine.

▶ Topical Steroids

Because of the increased permeability of their skin, infants are at risk for excessive absorption and toxicity from the use of topical steroids. Although these agents are effective in decreasing inflammation and relieving pruritus, steroid use in infants for the treatment of diaper dermatitis should be limited to only the low potency preparations.[39]

A thin layer of hydrocortisone cream (0.25–1%) applied twice a day for no more than 2 weeks is an appropriate treatment regimen. The use of higher potency steroids or use extending beyond 2 weeks should be at the discretion of a physician only.

▶ Antifungals

Diaper rashes lasting longer than 48 to 72 hours are at increased risk for the development of fungal infections. These complications are most frequently caused by *Candida albicans* and will require treatment with a topical antifungal[36,37] (See Fig. 65–6.)

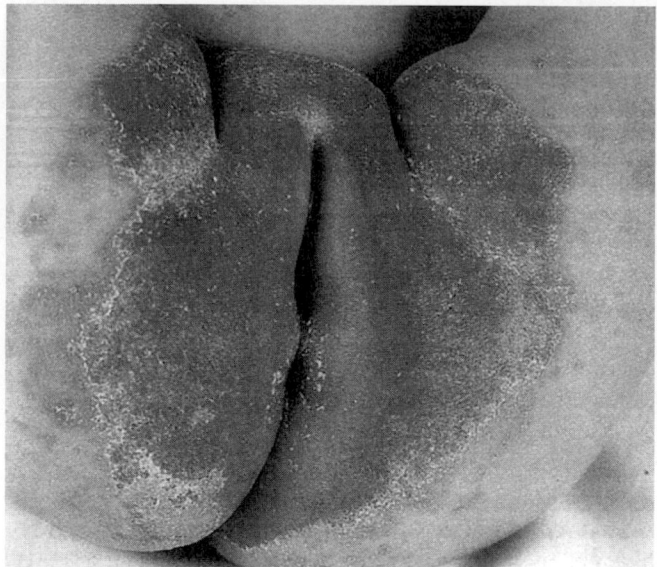

FIGURE 65–6. Candidiasis: diaper dermatitis. Confluent erosions, marginal scaling, and "satellite pustules" in the area covered by a diaper in an infant. (From Wolff K, Johnson RA. Cutaneous fungal infections. Fitzpatrick's Color Atlas & Synopsis of Clinical Dermatology. 5th ed. New York: McGraw-Hill, 2005: 721.)

Adverse events with the use of topical antifungals are generally limited to local irritation at the site of application.

Nystatin, clotrimazole, and miconazole creams or ointments applied two to four times daily with diaper changes have all shown to be effective in the treatment of candidal diaper rash. Although some of these products are available over-the-counter, parents and caregivers should be advised to initiate treatment with antifungal agents only after physician recommendation.

Antibacterials If conventional treatment fails, unresolved diaper rash can also lead to secondary bacterial infections. *Staphylococcus aureus* and *streptococcus* are the most likely pathogens responsible for these infections and require treatment with systemic antibiotics.[37,38] While topical protectants may be used as an adjunct in treatment, suspected bacterial infections should always be referred to a physician for accurate diagnosis and the selection of an appropriate antibacterial regimen.[35] Figure 65–7 shows a useful algorithm for the effective treatment of diaper dermatitis.

OUTCOME EVALUATION

Most diaper rashes can be effectively treated in less than 1 week. If symptoms do not resolve or begin to worsen, advise caregivers to seek medical attention to determine the presence of secondary fungal or bacterial infections. In addition, provide educational information on proper diaper hygiene techniques in order to prevent the development of future diaper rashes.

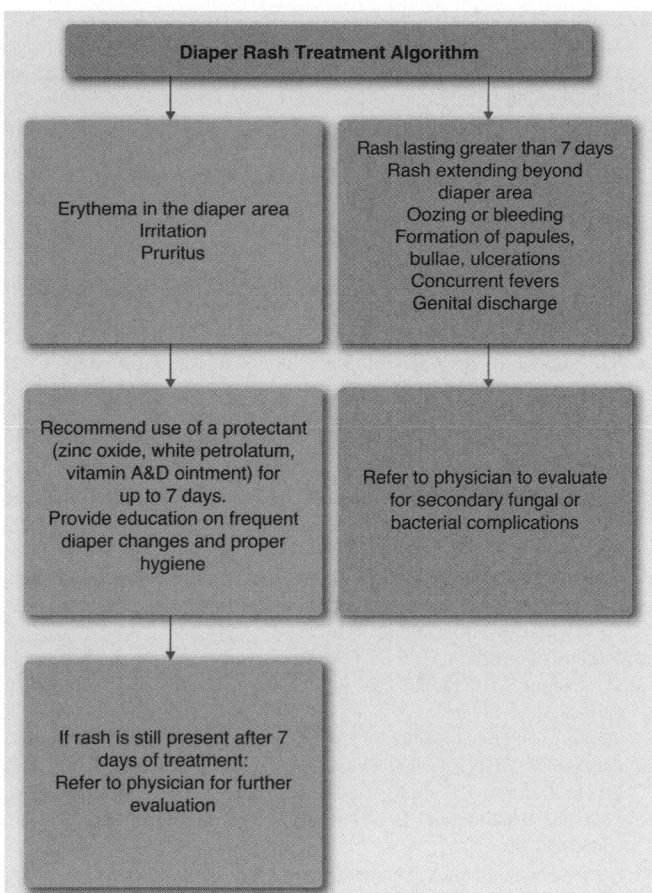

FIGURE 65–7. Diaper dermatitis treatment algorithm.

Patient Care and Monitoring: Diaper Dermatitis

1. Assess rash symptoms. Determine the level of severity—is there a possibility of a secondary fungal or bacterial infection?

2. Identify signs and symptoms which require immediate physician referral.

3. Inquire about the patient's history, including any similar rashes in the past.

4. Educate the caregiver on the importance of frequent diaper changes and proper hygiene.

5. Obtain patient allergy status.

6. Discuss labs that may be necessary if a secondary infection is suspected (cultures, biopsies).

7. Develop a treatment regimen for the patient, including a plan for assessing improvement of the condition.

8. Provide patient education about diaper rash etiology, treatment, and prevention:

   a. What is diaper rash and how does it develop? What exacerbates diaper rash?

   b. Symptoms to report to a physician (blistering, oozing, bleeding, changes in rash or no improvement in symptoms within 2–3 days).

   c. Available treatment options, including proper usage instructions and potential side effects.

   d. Importance of treatment compliance.

   e. Prevention measures.

Self-assessment questions and answers are available at *http://www.mhpharmacotherapy. com/pp.html*.

Patient Encounter 3

A gentleman presents to a community pharmacy with his 16-month-old daughter who recently developed a rash in her diaper area. He states that besides trying to keep the area clean and dry and changing her diapers more frequently than usual, he has tried to treat it with zinc oxide for the past 2 days. He says the rash is bright red, has persisted for 3 or 4 days and seems to be "spreading." Although there is no blistering or oozing, he thinks the rash must be painful because his daughter cries with every diaper change.

What reported symptoms support the diagnosis of diaper rash?

Elicit additional information to aid in your assessment of this patient.

What are your treatment goals for this patient?

What nonpharmacologic and pharmacologic treatment options are available for this diagnosis?

Given the information presented, develop a treatment regimen for this patient including (a) a statement of the problem, (b) a patient-specific therapeutic plan, and (c) monitoring parameters to assess efficacy and safety.

REFERENCES

1. Bello CE. Optimizing acne vulgaris treatment. US Pharmacist 2002;27(4):63–75.
2. Fitzpatrick TB, Johnson RA, Wolff C, Suurmond D. Color Atlas and Synopsis of Clinical Dermatology: Common and Serious Diseases. 5th ed. New York: McGraw-Hill, 2005:5, 20, 27, 721.
3. West DP, Loyd A, Bauer KA, West LE, Scuderi L, Micali G. Acne vulgaris. In: Dipiro JT, Talbert RL, Yee GC, et al., eds. Pharmacotherapy: A Pathophysiological Approach, 7th ed. New York: McGraw-Hill, 2008:1591–1602.
4. Berson DS, Chalker DK, Harper JC, et al. Current concepts in the treatment of acne: Report from a clinical roundtable. Cutis 2003;72:5–13.
5. Whitmore SE. Disorders of the pilosebaceous unit: Acne and related disorders and hair loss. In: Barker LB, Burton JR, Zieve PD, et al., eds. Principles of Ambulatory Medicine. 6th ed. Philadelphia: Lippincott Williams & Wilkins, 2003:1740–1746.
6. Taylor SC, Cook-Bolden F, Rahman Z, et al. Acne vulgaris in skin of color. J Am Acad Dermatol 2002;46(Suppl):S98–S106.

7. Harper JC, Fulton J. Acne Vulgaris. Emedicine. *http://www.emedicine. com/derm/topic2.htm.* Updated July 15, 2008.

8. Seaton TL. Acne. In: Koda-Kimble MA, Young LY, Kradjan WA, et al., eds. Applied Therapeutics: The Clinical Use of Drugs. 8th ed. New York: Lippincott Williams & Wilkins, 2005:39-1–39-11.

9. Hartsock M. Medical Illustrations. Cincinnati, OH: The Medical Art Company.

10. Baldwin HE. The interaction between acne vulgaris and the psyche. Cutis 2002;70(2):133–139.

11. Johnson BA, Nunley JR. Topical therapy for acne vulgaris: How do you choose the best drug for each patient? Postgrad Med 2000;107: 69–80.

12. Foster KT, Coffey CW. Acne. In: Berardi RR, Kroon LA, McDermott JH, et al., eds. The Handbook of Nonprescription Drugs, 15th ed. Washington, DC: American Pharmaceutical Association, 2006:803–816.

13. Del Rosso JQ. Fall clinical dermatology 2007: An update on advances in acne and excerpts from what's new in the medicine cabinet. Skin and Aging 2008:3(Suppl):1–11.

14. Ortho Dermalogical. Retin-A Micro Package Insert. Skillman, NJ: Ortho Dermalogical; May 2002.

15. Wickersham RM, ed. Drug Facts and Comparisons. St Louis, MO: Drug Facts and Comparisons, 2008.

16. Thiboutot D. New treatment and therapeutic strategies for acne. Arch Fam Med 2000;9(2):179–187.

17. Russell JJ. Topical therapy for acne. Am Fam Physician 2000;61: 357–368.

18. Hsu S, Quan LT. Topical antibacterial agents. In: Wolverton SE, ed. Comprehensive Dermatologic Drug Therapy. Philadelphia: WB Saunders, 2001:472–496.

19. Dermik Laboratories BenzaClin Topical Gel Package Insert. Berwyn, PA: Dermik Laboratories; 2005.

20. Kligman AM. Acne vulgaris: Tricks and treatments. Part II: The benzoyl peroxide saga. Cutis 1995;56:260–261.

21. Allergan Azelex package insert. Irvine, CA: Allergan; 2003(June).

22. White GM. Acne therapy. In: James WD, Cockerell CJ, Dzubow LM, et al., eds. Advances in Dermatology. St Louis: Mosby, 1999:29–59.

23. Sadick N. Systemic antibacterial agents. In: Wolverton SE, ed. Comprehensive Dermatologic Drug Therapy. Philadelphia: WB Saunders, 2001:(3):28–54.

24. DeSimone EM, Miller KM. Teratogenicity and dermatologic agents. US Pharmacist 2001;26(4):75–85.

25. Harper JC. Fall clinical dermatology 2007: Treating acne with oral contraceptives: A guide for safe, effective and efficient prescribing. Skin and Aging 2008:3(Suppl):12–14.

26. Keefner KR. Contact dermatitis. In: Berardi RR, Kroon LA, McDermott JH, et al., eds. Handbook of Nonprescription Drugs. 15th ed. Washington, DC: American Pharmaceutical Association, 2006:745–764.

27. Cheigh NH. Dermatologic drug reactions and self-treatable skin disorders. In: Dipiro JT, Talbert RL, Yee GC, et al., eds. Pharmacotherapy: A Pathophysiological Approach, 7th ed. New York: McGraw-Hill, 2008:1577–1590.

28. Nykamp D. Self-care of common dermatologic disorders. US Pharmacist 2001;26(4):31–48.

29. Shy BD, Schwartz DT. Dermatitis, Contact. Emedicine. *http://www. emedicine.com/emerg/topic131.htm.* Updated February 28, 2008.

30. Parker F. Skin diseases of general importance. In: Goldman L, Bennett JC, eds. Cecil Textbook of Medicine, 21st ed. Philadelphia: WB Saunders, 2000:2276–2298.

31. Whitmore, SE. Dermatitis and psoriasis. In: Barker LB, Burton JR, Zieve PD, et al., eds. Principles of Ambulatory Medicine, 6th ed. Philadelphia: Lippincott Williams & Wilkins, 2003:1746–1754.

32. West DP, West LE, Scuderi L, Micali G. Psoriasis. In: Dipiro JT, Talbert RL, Yee GC, et al., eds. Pharmacotherapy: A Pathophysiological Approach, 6th ed. New York: McGraw-Hill, 2005:1769–1783.

33. Cheigh NH. Atopic dermatitis. In: Dipiro JT, Talbert RL, Yee GC, et al., eds. Pharmacotherapy: A Pathophysiological Approach. 7th ed. New York: McGraw-Hill, 2008:1619–1626.

34. Marek-Thompson TA, Bond CA. Dermatotherapy. In: Koda-Kimble MA, Young LY, Kradjan WA, et al., eds. Applied Therapeutics: The Clinical Use of Drugs, 7th ed. New York: Lippincott Williams & Wilkins, 2001:36-1–36-22.

35. Padron VA. Diaper dermatitis and prickly heat. In: Berardi RR, Kroon LA, McDermott JH, et al., eds. Handbook of Nonprescription Drugs. 15th ed. Washington, DC: American Pharmaceutical Association, 2006:765–779.

36. Agrawal R, Sammeta V, Thomas I. Diaper Dermatitis. Emedicine. *http://www.emedicine.com/ped/TOPIC2755.HTM.* Updated June 28, 2006.

37. Borkowski S. Diaper rash care and management. Pediatr Nurs 2004;30(6):467–470.

38. Atherton JD. A review of the pathophysiology, prevention and treatment of irritant diaper dermatitis. Curr Med Res Opin 2004; 20(5):645–649.

39. Raimer SS. The safe use of topical corticosteroids in children. Pediatric Annals 2001;30(4):225–229.

66 Anemia

Edward C. Li and James M. Hoffman

LEARNING OBJECTIVES

● **Upon completion of the chapter, the reader will be able to:**

1. Identify common causes of anemia.

2. Describe common signs and symptoms of anemia.

3. Discuss the appropriate diagnostic evaluation to determine anemia type and guide therapeutic decisions.

4. State the desired therapeutic outcomes for patients with anemia.

5. Compare and contrast the various oral and parenteral iron preparations.

6. Explain the optimal use of folic acid and vitamin B_{12} in patients with macrocytic anemia.

7. Evaluate the proper use of epoetin and darbepoetin in anemia patients with cancer and kidney disease.

8. Recommend a specific treatment regimen for anemia considering the underlying cause of anemia and patient-specific variables.

9. Develop a plan to monitor the outcomes of anemia pharmacotherapy.

KEY CONCEPTS

❶ Anemia is a reduction below normal in the concentration of hemoglobin (Hgb) in the body that results in a reduction of the oxygen-carrying capacity of the blood.

❷ Common signs and symptoms of anemia include fatigue, lethargy, dizziness, shortness of breath, headache, edema, and tachycardia.

❸ A standard initial laboratory evaluation for anemia includes a CBC (evaluation of the serum Hgb and hematocrit [Hct] concentration, white blood cell count, platelets), measurement of the red blood cell (RBC) count and size, and review of peripheral smear.

❹ The goal of anemia therapy is to increase Hgb, which will improve red cell oxygen-carrying capacity, alleviate symptoms, and prevent anemia complications.

❺ The underlying cause of anemia (e.g., blood loss; iron, folic acid, or B_{12} deficiency; or chronic disease) must be determined and used to guide therapy.

❻ In patients with iron-deficiency anemia (IDA), appropriate oral iron therapy that delivers sufficient elemental iron should be attempted before giving parenteral iron.

❼ Anemia from vitamin B_{12} or folic acid deficiency is treated effectively by replacing the missing nutrient.

❽ In cancer and kidney disease patients with anemia, therapy with epoetin or darbepoetin can increase Hgb, decrease transfusion requirements, and improve quality of life, but this therapy has safety risks and must be carefully monitored.

❾ After treatment, patients should be monitored for symptom resolution, Hgb concentration, and adverse effects.

INTRODUCTION

❶ *Anemia is a reduction in the concentration of hemoglobin (Hgb) that results in a reduced oxygen-carrying capacity of the blood.* Some patients with anemia may be asymptomatic initially, but eventually, the lack of oxygen to the tissues could result in fatigue, lethargy, shortness of breath, headache, edema, and tachycardia. Common causes of anemia include blood loss, decreased production of red blood cells (RBCs), increased destruction of RBCs, or some combination of these factors. Determination of the underlying cause of anemia is essential for successful management. Appropriate treatment of anemia will result in an increase in Hgb, with a corresponding increase in oxygen-carrying capacity and reduction in symptoms.

EPIDEMIOLOGY AND ETIOLOGY

Anemia is a common condition, and the prevalence of anemia varies widely based on age, gender, race/ethnicity, and comorbid conditions. Studies have been done in the United States to describe differences in the prevalence of anemia in various populations.[1] The prevalence of anemia in children (ages 1–16 years) was 6% to 9%, but the prevalence of anemia increases to approximately 11% in adults over age 65 years and to at least 20% in adults 85 years of age and older. Anemia is generally more common in women, particularly during their reproductive years (ages 17–49) occurring in 12% of this group. However, in the same age range, only 2% of men are anemic. In the population over age 65, non-Hispanic whites and Mexican Americans had similar prevalence of anemia (9% and 10.4%, respectively), but anemia was significantly more common in non-Hispanic blacks with a prevalence of 27.8%.

Comorbid conditions can increase the risk of anemia substantially. Anemia is especially common in cancer patients receiving chemotherapy and patients with chronic kidney disease (CKD). The incidence of anemia in cancer patients varies based on tumor type and the level of myelosuppression of the chemotherapy regimen. For instance, severe anemia (Hgb 7.9 g/dL or less [79 g/L or 4.9 mmol/L]) occurs in at least 75% of patients who receive a common lymphoma chemotherapy regimen but severe anemia may occur in less than 10% of patients who receive common breast cancer chemotherapy regimen.[2] Overall, retrospective reviews demonstrate that chemotherapy-induced anemia is most common in patients with lymphomas, lung tumors, and ovarian tumors, with an incidence of 50% to 60%. In addition, up to 60% of patients with serious kidney disease have anemia, which demonstrates how common anemia is in patients with CKD.[3]

The causes of anemia can be divided into three main categories: decreased production, increased destruction, and blood loss. Drug therapy is the mainstay of treatment for anemias caused by reduced production of erythrocytes and will be the focus of this chapter, and anemias due to destruction of erythrocytes will not be discussed.

A decrease in erythrocyte production can be multifactorial. Nutritional deficiencies (such as iron, vitamin B$_{12}$, and folic acid) are common causes that are often easily treatable. In addition, patients with cancer and CKD are at risk for developing a hypoproductive anemia. Furthermore, patients with chronic immune-related diseases (such as rheumatoid arthritis and systemic lupus erythematosus) can develop anemia as a complication of their disease. Anemia related to chronic inflammatory conditions is typically termed *anemia of chronic disease.*

PATHOPHYSIOLOGY

Erythropoiesis

Erythropoiesis is a process that starts with a pluripotent stem cell in the bone marrow that differentiates into an erythroid colony-forming unit (CFU-E)[4] (Fig. 66–1). The development

Patient Encounter 1, Part 1

A 74-year-old Caucasian woman with a past medical history significant for hypertension and type II diabetes mellitus presents to her primary care physician complaining of shortness of breath and fatigue for the past few days. She denies any recent bleeding manifestations, including bright red blood per rectum, hemoptysis, melena, or epistaxis. She denies any fevers, chills, nausea, vomiting, or recent weight loss. A CBC was taken and revealed Hgb of 9.3 g/dL (93 g/L or 5.8 mmol/L). Recent colonoscopy and endoscopy were normal. The patient weighs 54 kg (119 lb).

Is this patient anemic? If so, what are possible causes of anemia?

What additional laboratory assessments are required to make an appropriate therapeutic plan?

How would the requested laboratory parameter(s) aid your decision making?

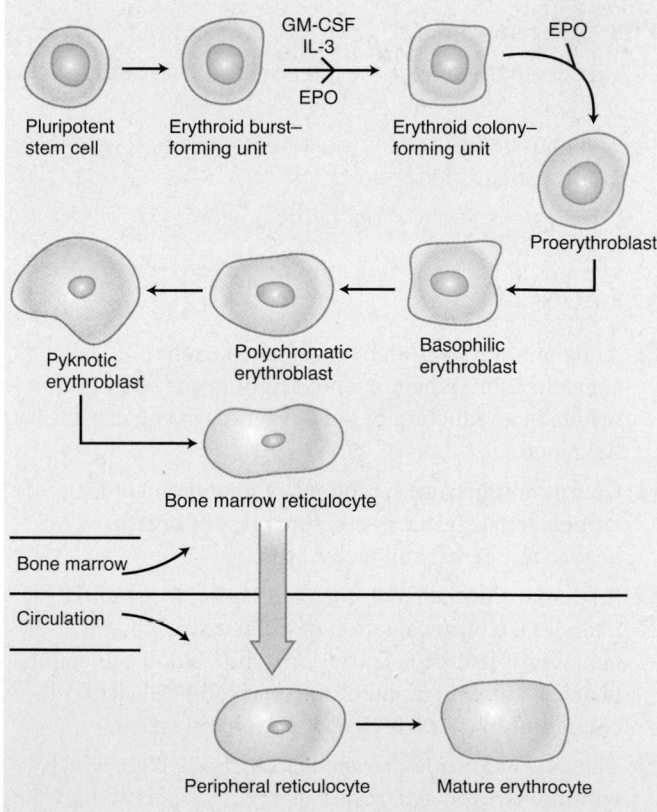

FIGURE 66–1. The process of erythropoiesis.

of these cells depends on stimulation from the appropriate growth factors, primarily the renally produced hormone erythropoietin (EPO). Other cytokines involved include granulocyte-monocyte colony-stimulating factor (GM-CSF) and interleukin 3 (IL-3). These CFU-Es then differentiate into reticulocytes and cross from the bone marrow into the peripheral blood. Throughout this process, the cells gradually accumulate more Hgb and lose their nuclei.[4] Finally, these reticulocytes mature into erythrocytes after 1 to 2 days in the bloodstream.

Hypoproliferative or Decreased-Production Anemias

▶ Nutritional

Deficiencies in nutrients such as folic acid and vitamin B_{12} may hinder the process of erythrocyte maturation.[4,5] Folic acid and vitamin B_{12} are required for the formation of DNA. When these nutrients are decreased, DNA synthesis is inhibited, and consequently, erythrocyte maturation also is inhibited.[4,5] Poor diet can be a contributor to the deficiencies in these nutrients. Similarly, patients with a condition called pernicious anemia are unable to absorb B_{12} via their GI tract due to a lack in a glycoprotein called intrinsic factor. This glycoprotein binds to vitamin B_{12} and facilitates its absorption in the ileum. This condition results in B_{12} deficiency despite adequate dietary B_{12} intake.[6]

Iron is also a vital nutrient in the development of functioning erythrocytes as it is essential for the formation of Hgb. Lack of iron leads to a decrease in Hgb synthesis and ultimately RBCs. Normal homeostasis of iron transport and metabolism is depicted in Figure 66–2.[7] Approximately 1 to 2 mg of iron is absorbed through the duodenum each day, and the same amount is lost via blood loss, desquamation of mucosal cells, or menstruation.

Since there is no true "excretion" of iron from the body, iron-deficiency anemia (IDA) typically occurs because of either inadequate absorption of iron or excess blood loss. Inadequate absorption may occur in patients who have congenital or acquired intestinal diseases, such as inflammatory bowel disease, celiac disease, or bowel resection. Achlorhydria and diets poor in iron also may contribute to iron deficiency states. In contrast, iron deficiency also may occur in patients who exhibit a higher rate of iron loss from the body. This is manifested in blood loss, either from the GI system, menstruation, cancer, or trauma.[7]

▶ Hypoproliferative Marrow

Patients with chronic diseases exhibit a different pathophysiologic mechanism of disease. For example, patients with cancer may suffer from anemia because of chemotherapy and/or the tumor effects on the marrow itself. Chemotherapy may cause destruction of highly proliferating stem cells, thereby decreasing the production of mature erythrocytes.[8] In addition, cancer can cause anemia via hemorrhage, replacing normal bone marrow with malignant cells, and releasing cytokines that lead to decreased EPO production. Both of these scenarios can lead to anemia from a hypoproliferative marrow.[8]

▶ Decreased EPO Production or Response

Patients with CKD suffer from a decrease in erythropoietin production because EPO is produced mainly in the kidneys.[4,5] In patients with anemia of chronic disease, there is a blunted EPO production as well as a diminished response to EPO.[9] Anemia of chronic disease also affects iron homeostasis, causing iron sequestration into storage sites and decreasing the amount available to the rest of the body.[9]

TREATMENT

Desired Outcomes

❹ *The goal of anemia therapy is to increase the Hgb level, which will improve red cell oxygen-carrying capacity, alleviate symptoms, and prevent complication from anemia.* Normal Hgb values are 14 to 17.5 g/dL (140–175 g/L or 8.69–10.9 mmol/L) for males and 12.3 to 15.3 g/dL (123–153 g/L or 7.63–9.5 mmol/L) for females. It is important to note that continuation of a patient's therapy should be assessed primarily by resolution of clinical signs and symptoms. Patients who experience a resolution in their symptoms such as shortness of breath, tachycardia, fatigue, dizziness, and edema may not require aggressive therapy to maintain their Hgb values within normal limits. Ultimately, prevention of complications owing to anemia such as hypoxia and cardiovascular sequelae can be avoided if Hgb levels are greater than 7 g/dL (70 g/L or 4.34 mmol/L).[10]

General Approach to the Anemic Patient

❺ *The underlying cause of anemia (e.g., blood loss; iron, folic acid, or vitamin B_{12} deficiency; or chronic disease) must*

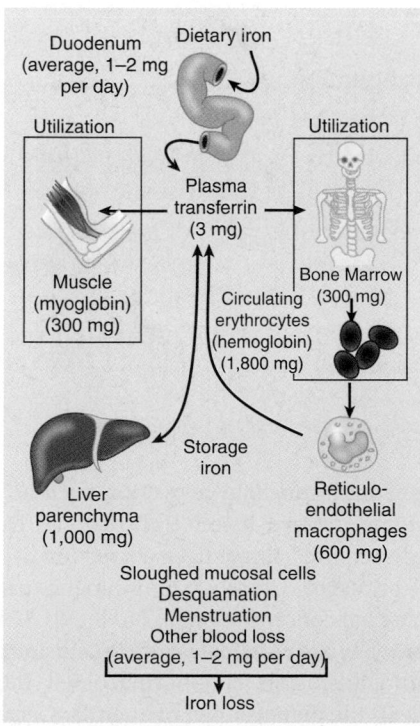

FIGURE 66–2. The distribution of iron use in adults. (From Ref. 7.)

Clinical Presentation and Diagnosis of Anemia

Signs and Symptoms

② *Generally, the signs and symptoms of anemia are nonspecific and may include:*

- Fatigue, lethargy, dizziness
- Shortness of breath
- Headache
- Edema
- Tachycardia

Other findings that may be present in some patients include:

- Dry skin, chapped lips
- Nail brittleness
- Hunger for ice, starch, or clay (termed *pica*)

Past Medical History

Inquire about the following conditions:

- History of blood loss, such as hemorrhoids, melena, or menorrhagia (IDA)
- Malnourished or recent weight loss (vitamin B_{12} or folate deficiency)
- Alcoholism (folate deficiency)
- Cancer or chronic kidney disease (CKD)
- Chronic autoimmune disorders or infections, such as HIV infection or rheumatoid arthritis (anemia of chronic disease)

Physical Examination

These findings aid the clinician in determining the severity of the anemia:

- Orthostatic hypotension and tachycardia secondary to volume depletion
- Mental status changes and confusion
- Cutaneous changes such as pallor, jaundice, and nail brittleness

Laboratory Evaluation

Table 66–1 describes common tests used to determine the etiology of anemia. A diagnostic and treatment algorithm for anemia is outlined in Figure 66–3.

1. **③** *A CBC is a necessary first step in evaluating a patient with anemia. If the Hgb and Hct are less than the normal range, the patient is anemic. Subsequent evaluations of RBC indices and the peripheral smear often are necessary to determine the etiology (and ultimately, the treatment) of the anemia.*

2. Evaluating the mean corpuscular volume (MCV) is the next step in an anemia workup. It is classified as microcytic, normocytic, or macrocytic if the MCV is below, within, or above the normal range of 80 to 96 fL/cell, respectively.

Microcytic Anemia and Iron Evaluation

Iron studies (see Table 66–1) should be evaluated in the setting of a low MCV. These include:

- Serum iron
- Serum ferritin—the best indirect determinant of body iron stores. It is commonly decreased in patients with IDA
- Total iron-binding capacity (TIBC)—quantifies the iron-binding capacity of transferrin and is increased in IDA
- Transferrin saturation (TSAT) (serum iron/TIBC)—indicates the amount of transferrin that is bound with iron; it is lower in IDA

Macrocytic Anemia

- Evaluate folic acid and vitamin B_{12} levels in the setting of an elevated MCV
- Further investigation by administering radiolabeled B_{12} (i.e., Schilling test) to determine if lack of intrinsic factor
- Consider obtaining homocysteine and methylmalonic acid levels

Normocytic Anemia

- Evaluate reticulocytes and CBC
- High reticulocyte counts may indicate RBCs loss via acute blood loss, hemolysis, or splenic sequestration
- Low reticulocyte counts may indicate a diseased bone marrow (e.g., aplastic anemia, myelodysplasia, or leukemia), especially if the WBC and platelets are low
- High WBC/platelets may be from anemia of chronic disease, malignancy, or CKD

be determined and used to guide therapy (see Fig. 66–3). Subsequently, the appropriate pharmacologic treatment should be initiated based on the cause of anemia.

Nonpharmacologic Therapy

The most important nonpharmacologic treatment of anemia is the transfusion of RBCs. However, because of the risk of infection, immunosuppression, and microcirculatory complications and the high cost of the procedure, the threshold for transfusion has been debated.[11] Generally, only patients requiring immediate correction such as those with acute symptoms, receive blood transfusions. Determining which patient requires immediate correction is left to the health care provider. Usually, symptomatic patients who present with a Hgb concentration of 7 to 8 g/dL (70–80 g/L or 4.34–4.96 mmol/L) are candidates for transfusion.[12]

Other than transfusion, nonpharmacologic therapy plays a limited role in the management of anemia. Certainly, some causes of anemia can be attributed to diets poor in iron, folic acid, or vitamin B_{12}. However, in the United States, nutrient-poor diets are rarely the sole cause of anemia in a patient.

Table 66–1

Pertinent Laboratory Tests in the Evaluation of Anemia

Test Name	Normal Range	Description/Significance
CBC		
Hgb	Males: 14–17.5 g/dL (140–175 g/L or 8.69–10.9 mmol/L) Females: 12.3–15.3 g/dL (123–153 g/L or 7.63–9.5 mmol/L)	Amount of Hgb in the blood; signifies oxygen-carrying capacity of the blood and determines if a patient is anemic
Hct	Males: 42–50% (0.42–0.50) Females: 36–45% (0.36–0.45)	The percent of blood that the erythrocytes encompass; also indicates anemia; the Hgb is measured, and the Hct is calculated
RBC	Males: 4.5–5.9 × 10⁶ cells/mL (4.5–5.9 × 10¹² cells/L) Females: 4.1–5.1 × 10⁶ cells/mL (4.1–5.1 × 10¹² cells/L)	The number of erythrocytes in a volume of blood; also indicates anemia, but seldom used
RBC Indices		
MCV	80–96 fL/cell	A widely used laboratory value to measure RBC "size"; higher values indicate macrocytosis and lower values indicate microcytosis
MCH	27–33 pg/cell	Amount of Hgb per RBC; may be decreased in IDA
MCHC	33.4–35.5 g/dL (334–355 g/L)	Hgb divided by the Hct; also low in IDA
Iron Studies		
Serum iron		
Males	45–160 mcg/dL (8.1–28.64 μmol/L)	Measures amount of iron bound to transferrin; low in IDA
Females	30–160 mcg/dL (5.4–28.64 μmol/L)	
Serum ferritin	12–300 mcg/L (26.4–660 pmol/L)	Ferritin is the protein–iron complex found in macrophages used for iron storage; low in IDA
TIBC	220–420 mcg/dL (39.4–75.2 μmol/L)	Measures the capacity of transferrin to bind iron; high in IDA
TSAT	30–50% (0.30–0.50)	TSAT = (serum iron/TIBC) × 100; a saturation of less than 15% is common in IDA
Other Tests		
RBC distribution width (RDW)	11.5–14.5% (0.115–0.145)	A higher value means the presence of many different sizes of RBCs; the MCV is therefore less reliable
Reticulocyte count		
Males	0.5–15% of RBCs (0.005–0.025)	Should be elevated in patients who are responding to treatment
Females	0.5–2.5% of RBCs (0.005–0.025)	
Folic acid (plasma)	3.1–12.4 ng/mL or mcg/L (7–28 nmol/L)	Used to determine folic acid deficiency
Folic acid (RBC)	125–600 ng/mL (283–1,360 nmol/L)	Used to determine folic acid deficiency
Vitamin B₁₂	180–600 pg/mL (133–738 pmol/L)	Used to determine vitamin B₁₂ deficiency
EPO level	2–25 mIU/mL (2–25 IU/L)	Patients may benefit from EPO therapy if they are anemic and EPO levels are normal or mildly elevated

EPO, erythropoietin; Hct, hematocrit; Hgb, hemoglobin; MCH, mean cell hemoglobin; MCHC, mean cell hemoglobin concentration; MCV, mean cell volume; RDW, RBC distribution width; TIBC, total iron-binding capacity; TSAT, transferrin saturation.

Therefore, ingesting a diet that is rich in iron, folic acid, or vitamin B_{12} should be encouraged but it is rarely the sole modality of treatment. Food sources of iron, folic acid, and vitamin B_{12} are listed in Table 66–2.[5]

Pharmacologic Therapy

▶ *Iron-Deficiency Anemia*

6 *The initial treatment of IDA is oral iron therapy with a goal of 200 mg of elemental iron daily for those who are able to tolerate the oral route.* Many different iron products and salt forms are available. Table 66–3 lists the various salt forms of oral iron available, the amount of elemental iron in each product, and the approximate daily dose of the salt to attain 200 mg of elemental iron daily.

Iron supplementation resolves anemia by replacing iron stores in the body that are necessary for RBC production and maturation. If treated properly, a response (via the presence of reticulocytosis) should be seen in 7 to 10 days, and Hgb values should rise by about 1 g/dL (10 g/L or 0.62 mmol/L) per week. Patients should be reassessed if Hgb does not increase by 2 g/dL (20 g/L or 1.24 mmol/L) in 3 weeks.

Dosing for iron should be divided equally into two to three doses daily. An empty stomach (1 hour before or

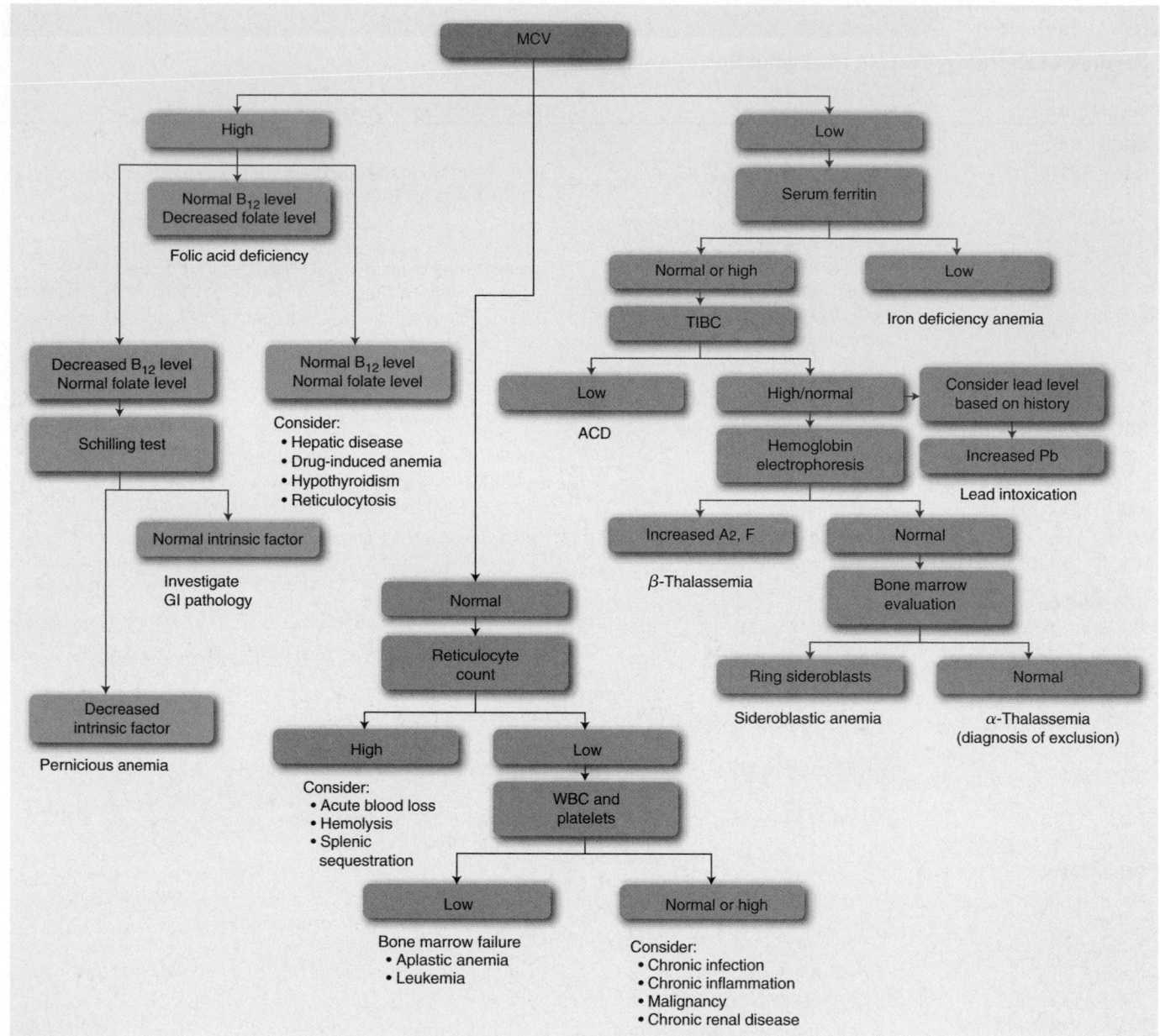

FIGURE 66-3. The anemia evaluation process. (ACD, anemia of chronic disease; MCV, mean corpuscular volume; Pb, lead; TIBC, total iron-binding capacity.)

2 hours after a meal) is preferred for maximal absorption. After absorption, iron binds to transferrin in the plasma and is transported to the muscles (for myoglobin), liver (for storage), or bone marrow (for red cell production). Iron is not actively excreted from the body but is "lost" through other measures already described.[7] Some studies suggest that iron absorption may be increased by adding ascorbic acid (vitamin C) to the drug regimen.[13] However, administration of iron on an empty stomach and with ascorbic acid may increase the incidence of GI side effects, such as abdominal pain, nausea, and heartburn. Patients who cannot tolerate iron on an empty stomach can take it with food, but iron absorption is reduced when it is taken with food.

Common toxicities associated with oral iron products include abdominal pain, nausea, heartburn, constipation, and dark stools. Drug interactions may occur with iron products, predominantly owing to iron-drug binding, resulting in decreased absorption of the interacting drug. Examples include fluoroquinolones, tetracyclines, and phenytoin. To avoid this interaction, doses of iron and the interacting drug should be separated by 2 to 4 hours.

Parenteral iron therapy may be appropriate in cases where patients are unable to tolerate the oral formulation because of toxicities or compliance. In addition, those who have IDA that has not responded to oral iron therapy (e.g., because of malabsorption) are also candidates for parenteral iron therapy.

Parenteral iron therapy currently is available in three different formulations, which are listed in Table 66-3. Iron dextran was the first parenteral iron formulation to be

Patient Encounter 1, Part 2

Additional laboratory parameters are ordered, and the following is observed:

CBC

- *WBC:* 5.50 × 10³/µL (5.50 × 10⁹/L)
- *Hgb:* 9.3 g/dL (93 g/L or 5.77 mmol/L)
- *Hct:* 27.8% (0.278)
- *Plt:* 170 × 10³/µL (170 × 10⁹/L)

RBC

- *MCV:* 78 fL/cell
- *MCH:* 26 pg/cell
- *MCHC:* 33.5 g/dL (335 g/L)

Others

- *RBC count:* 3 M/µL (3 × 10¹²/L)

- *RDW:* 15% (0.15)
- *Retic:* 3% (0.03)

Iron Studies

- *Serum iron:* 45 mcg/dL (8.1 µmol/L)
- *Serum ferritin:* 7 mcg/L (15.7 pmol/L)
- *TIBC:* 462 mcg/dL (82.7 µmol/L)
- *TSAT:* 10% (0.10)

B₁₂ and Folate

- *Serum folate:* 20 mcg/dL (45 nmol/L)
- Serum B_{12}: 675 pg/mL (498 pmol/L)

Is this a macrocytic or microcytic anemia?

Specifically, what is the etiology of the anemia?

What therapy should the patient receive?

Patient Encounter 1, Part 3

The patient is diagnosed with IDA and is started on ferrous sulfate 325 mg orally three times daily to be taken on an empty stomach. Follow-up CBC 1 month later reveals a Hgb of 10 g/dL (100 g/L or 6.2 mmol/L), previously 9.3 g/dL (93 g/L or 5.77 mmol/L). The patient complains of shortness of breath on exertion and constipation. She also admits to taking only one tablet a day because of nausea.

What Hgb level would constitute a therapeutic response in this patient?

How can nausea secondary to ferrous sulfate be reduced in this patient?

What changes to this patient's iron therapy do you recommend?

Table 66–2

Food Sources of Iron, Folic Acid, or Vitamin B₁₂

Nutrient	Food Sources
Iron	Red meat, organ meats, wheat germ, egg yolks, oysters
Folic acid	Green vegetables, liver, yeast, fruits
Vitamin B₁₂	Animal by-products, legumes

Table 66–3

Iron Products (IV and PO) and Elemental Iron Content

Salt Form	Brand Name(s)	Elemental Iron Content per Dose Form
Oral Formulations		
Ferrous sulfate	Feosol	65 mg/325-mg tablet 60 mg/300-mg tablet
Ferrous sulfate, anhydrous	N/A	65 mg/200-mg tablet
Ferrous gluconate	Fergon	39 mg/325-mg tablet 37 mg/300-mg tablet
Ferrous fumarate	Feostat	33 mg/100-mg tablet
Polysaccharide–iron complex	Niferex	150 mg/capsule 50 mg/tablet
Parenteral Formulations		
Iron dextran	InFED	50 mg/mL
Iron sucrose	Venofer	20 mg/mL
Sodium ferric gluconate	Ferrlecit	62.5 mg/5 mL

approved, followed by ferric gluconate, and then iron sucrose. Although these newer agents are only approved by the FDA to treat anemia associated with CKD in patients receiving EPO products, they are effective in treating IDA as well. Iron dextran is FDA approved for treating documented iron deficiency in patients who are unable to tolerate the oral formulation.

The dose of iron dextran can be calculated by the following equation: dose (mL) = 0.0442 (desired Hgb – observed Hgb) × body weight + (0.26 × body weight). The body weight that should be used is lean body weight for adults and children weighing more than 15 kg and actual body weight for children weighing 5 to 15 kg. The dose in milligrams can be calculated based on a standard concentration of 50 mg elemental iron per milliliter.[14] The prescribing information recommends administering iron dextran in 100-mg aliquots daily until the total dose is achieved. However, anecdotal evidence reports that the total calculated dose can be administered safely over 4 to 6 hours in 1 day. It is important to note that a test dose of iron dextran (0.5 mL over at least 30 seconds) must be administered to patients who are about to receive their

Patient Encounter 1, Part 4

Because the patient is not able to tolerate oral iron therapy (constipation and nausea), changing to IV iron therapy is appropriate.

What formulation of IV iron therapy should the patient receive?

What adverse effects are associated with parenteral iron?

first dose of iron dextran because of the risk of anaphylaxis. Patients should be monitored for signs of anaphylaxis for at least 1 hour after the test dose before administering the total dose. Other adverse effects include arthralgias, arrhythmias, hypotension, flushing, and pruritus.

The use of the newer parenteral iron products, iron sucrose and ferric gluconate, for the treatment of IDA is controversial; they are currently only FDA approved for the treatment of anemia associated with CKD. However, since the newer agents are relatively safe and have a lower risk of anaphylaxis, their use is attractive in other causes of anemia. However, the high cost and lack of reimbursement for these agents may preclude their routine use in IDA patients without kidney disorders.[12,13]

▶ Vitamin B₁₂ and Folic Acid Anemia

❼ *Anemia from vitamin B₁₂ or folic acid deficiency is treated effectively by replacing the missing nutrient.* Both folic acid and vitamin B₁₂ are essential for erythrocyte production and maturation. Replacing these factors allows for normal DNA synthesis and, consequently, normal erythropoiesis.

Vitamin B₁₂ (cyanocobalamin) administered both orally and parenterally is equally effective in treating anemia from vitamin B₁₂ deficiency. However, use of parenteral cyanocobalamin is the most common method of vitamin B₁₂ replacement because it may be more reliable and practical. Vitamin B₁₂ is absorbed completely following parenteral administration, whereas oral vitamin B₁₂ is absorbed poorly via the GI tract. Furthermore, use of parenteral vitamin B₁₂ to treat this type of anemia may circumvent the need to perform a testing to diagnose a deficiency of intrinsic factor.

A typical cyanocobalamin dosing regimen is 800 to 1,000 mcg/day for 1 to 2 weeks, followed by 100 to 1,000 mcg/day every week until the Hgb/Hct normalizes and with subsequent maintenance of 100 to 1,000 mcg monthly for life. A common oral dosing regimen is from 1,000 to 2,000 mcg/day. If parenteral cyanocobalamin is used initially, oral vitamin B₁₂ can be useful as maintenance therapy. Typically, the response to therapy is quick. Neurologic symptoms and megaloblastic cells disappear within a few days, and Hgb levels increase after a week of therapy.

Vitamin B₁₂ generally is well tolerated and exhibits minimal adverse effects. Injection-site pain, pruritus, rash, and diarrhea have been reported. Drug interactions have been observed with omeprazole and ascorbic acid that decrease oral absorption.

When treating folic acid deficiency, an initial daily dose of 1 mg/day by mouth typically is effective. Absorption of folic acid generally is rapid and complete. However, patients with malabsorption syndromes may require larger doses (up to 5 mg/day). Similar to vitamin B₁₂ deficiency, resolution of symptoms and reticulocytosis is prompt, occurring within days of commencing therapy. Hgb will start to rise after 2 weeks of therapy and may take from 2 to 4 months to resolve the deficiency completely. Afterwards, if the underlying deficiency is corrected, folic acid replacement can be discontinued. However, in cases where folic acid is consumed rapidly or absorbed poorly, chronic replacement may be required.

Folic acid is also well tolerated. Some nonspecific adverse effects include allergic reactions, flushing, malaise, and rash. Folic acid has been reported to decrease phenytoin levels by inducing its metabolism.

▶ Anemia of Chronic Disease

Anemia of chronic disease is a term given those with underlying conditions that contribute to or cause anemia in a patient. These chronic diseases can include cancer, CKD, and other inflammatory disorders. **❽** *In patients with anemia owing to cancer and CKD, therapy with epoetin or darbepoetin can increase Hgb, decrease transfusion requirements, and improve quality of life, but this therapy has safety risks and monitoring requirements that are discussed further below.*

Chemotherapy-Induced Anemia Studies have shown that in patients with chemotherapy-related anemia, therapy with the erythropoietin stimulating agents (ESA), epoetin-alfa and darbepoetin, can increase Hgb, and decrease transfusion requirements.[14] Epoetin is recombinant human EPO, and darbepoetin is structurally similar to endogenous EPO. Both bind to the same receptor to stimulate RBC production. Darbepoetin differs from epoetin in that it is a glycosylated form and exhibits a longer half-life in the body, allowing for a longer dosing interval. The half-lives of a single subcutaneous injection of epoetin or darbepoetin in patients are roughly 27 and 43 hours, respectively.

A number of clinical trials and a recent meta-analysis suggest that epoetin and darbepoetin may be detrimental to cancer patients.[15] This may be related to increased thrombotic events, increased tumor progression, or a combination of the two. In the meta-analysis, a total of 13,933 cancer patients from 53 trials were analyzed. ESAs increased on study mortality (combined hazard ratio [cHR] 1.17; 95% CI 1.06–1.30) and worsened overall survival (cHR 1.06; 95% CI 1.00–1.12). This corresponds to a 17% increased risk of mortality for patients treated with ESAs while on study and a 6% increase overall. Based on these findings, the use of ESAs is restricted to patients with chemotherapy-induced anemia without a curative intent. ESAs should only be used to prevent a transfusion, and should not be initiated unless the hemoglobin is less than or equal to 10 g/dL (10 g/L, 6.1 mmol/L).

Table 66–4		
EPO Products and Usual Doses for Anemia from Cancer/Chemotherapy and CKD		
	Epoetin-alfa (Epogen, Procrit)	**Darbepoetin-alfa (Aranesp)**
Cancer/chemotherapy dosing regimens	150 units/kg SC 3 × per week. 40,000 units SC once every week	2.25 mcg/kg SC once every week 3 mcg/kg SC once every 2 weeks; may increase to 5 mcg/kg 200 mcg SC fixed dose every 2 weeks, may increase to 300 mcg 300–500 mcg every 3 weeks
CKD dosing regimens[a]	50–100 units/kg SC 3 × per week	0.45 mcg/kg SC once every week 0.75 mcg/kg SC once every 2 weeks

[a]According to National Kidney Foundation guidelines for the use of epoetin in patients with anemia owing to kidney disease, the subcutaneous (SC) route is preferred. However, the IV route is used commonly in clinical practice.

Patients should be monitored every 4 to 6 weeks. If the Hg has not increased by 1 g/dL (1 g/L, 0.61 mmol/L) in this time period and remains less than 10 g/dL (10 g/L, 6.1 mmol/L), a one-time dose escalation of 25% may be performed. If the Hg increases by more than 1 g/dL (1 g/L, 0.61 mmol/L) or is more than 10 g/dL (10 g/L, 6.1 mmol/L), the ESA should be discontinued. ESAs should also be discontinued within 6 weeks of completing chemotherapy, whether the anemia has resolved or not.[14]

Cancer patients also may have concurrent iron deficiency secondary to EPO use ("functional" iron deficiency) or to cancer. Therefore, it is imperative that these patients have iron studies done to assess adequate iron stores needed to drive hematopoiesis. If the patient is determined to have suboptimal iron stores or is iron deficient, then replacement either orally or intravenously may be necessary, in addition to the use of EPO products. The use of iron in these patients is the same as discussed previously under iron-deficiency anemia (IDA).

Chronic Kidney Disease (CKD) Patients with CKD progress through five stages of disease based on the glomerular filtration rate (GFR).[16,17] Anemia is a common development in patients with CKD, and anemia evaluation and treatment should be initiated in patients with stage 3 CKD patients (GFR less than 60 mg/dL). Early treatment of anemia in patients with CKD has been associated with slower disease progression and a lower risk of death in dialysis patients.[18,19] Therefore, it is essential to evaluate and treat anemia in patients before they progress to stage 5 CKD, which is a GFR of less than 15 mg/dL or patients that require dialysis.

To rule out other causes of anemia, a thorough anemia evaluation should be completed in patients with CKD.[20] CKD anemia typically is a normocytic, normochromic anemia that is due to EPO deficiency. Therefore, therapy with epoetin and darbepoetin is effective in treating CKD anemia. The target Hgb value in patients with CKD is 11 to 12 g/dL (110–120 g/L or 6.82–7.44 mmol/L), but the epoetin and darbepoetin doses required for CKD anemia typically are lower than the doses for anemia from cancer/chemotherapy, and subcutaneous administration is the preferred route of administration (Table 66–4). According to the National Kidney Foundation Kidney Disease Outcomes Quality Initiative (NKFK/DOQI) guidelines, epoetin doses should be increased by 50% if patients do not have an adequate response (less than 2% increase in Hct) after 2 to 4 weeks of therapy and decreased by 25% if the absolute increase in Hgb is greater than 3 g/dL (30 g/L or 1.9 mmol/L) or the target Hgb is surpassed.

Although EPO deficiency is the primary cause of CKD anemia, iron deficiency is often present as well, and it is essential to assess and monitor the CKD patient's iron status (NKFK/DOQI guidelines). Iron stores in patients with CKD should be maintained so that TSAT is greater than 20% and serum ferritin is greater than 100 ng/mL (100 mcg/L or 225 pmol/L). If iron stores are not maintained appropriately, epoetin or darbepoetin will not be effective, and most CKD patients will require iron supplementation. Oral iron therapy can be used, but it is often ineffective, particularly in CKD patients on dialysis. Therefore, IV iron therapy is used extensively in these patients. Details of the pharmacology, pharmacokinetics, adverse effects, interactions, dose, and administration of EPO and iron products have been discussed previously.

Other Chronic Diseases Besides anemia associated with cancer and CKD, anemia of chronic disease can result from inflammatory processes and occurs commonly in autoimmune disorders such as rheumatoid arthritis and systemic lupus erythematosus. In treating these types of anemia of chronic disease, the most important principle is treating the underlying disease. These patients also may have iron deficiency and should be treated in the manner already discussed. EPO therapy such as epoetin-alfa therapy at a dose of 150 units/kg three times a week may also be used in these patients.

OUTCOME EVALUATION

❾ *After treatment, patients should be monitored for symptom and laboratory value resolution, Hgb concentration, and adverse effects.* The goal of anemia therapy is to correct the underlying source of the anemia, normalize the Hgb, and alleviate associated symptoms.

Patient Encounter 2

A 65-year-old male with a diagnosis of metastatic colon cancer being treated with irinotecan presents with chemotherapy-induced anemia, with a Hgb of 8.3 g/dL (83 g/L or 5.14 mmol/L).

What discussion must be presented to the patient before ESA therapy can be initiated?

What laboratory parameters and symptoms should be assessed prior to initiating ESA therapy?

If after 4 weeks of ESA therapy, the Hgb is 9.3 g/dL (93 g/L or 5.3 mmol/L), what action should be taken?

When should ESA therapy be stopped?

• Monitor the CBC to ensure the correct Hgb titration.

• A 1 g/dL (10 g/L or 0.62 mmol/L) per week titration is desirable in patients with IDA. Reevaluate patients with an increase of less than 2 g/dL (20 g/L or 1.24 mmol/L) in 3 weeks.

• In patients with folic acid deficiency, methylmalonic acid may be normal, and homocysteine may be high. Monitor Hgb periodically, and reevaluate patients who fail to normalize Hgb levels after 2 months of therapy.

• In patients with vitamin B_{12} deficiency, methylmalonic acid and homocysteine levels may be high. Monitor for resolution of neurologic symptoms (i.e., confusion and paresthesias), if applicable, and Hgb levels periodically until the levels normalize.

• Do not exceed more than 1 g/dL (10 g/L or 0.62 mmol/L) every 2 weeks when using ESAs to increase Hgb. Decrease the dose of the ESA if this occurs.

• When using ESAs, do not exceed Hgb of greater than 10 g/dL (10 g/L or 6.2 mmol/L) in cancer patients because of an increased risk of death and adverse effects.

• Monitor other laboratory tests, such as mean cell volume (MCV), iron studies, and presence of reticulocytosis.

Abbreviations Introduced in This Chapter

CFU-E	Erythroid colony-forming unit
CKD	Chronic kidney disease
EPO	Erythropoietin
ESA	Erythropoietin stimulating agent
GFR	Glomerular filtration rate
GM-CSF	Granulocyte-monocyte colony-stimulating factor
Hct	Hematocrit
Hgb	Hemoglobin
IDA	Iron-deficiency anemia
IL-3	Interleukin 3
MCV	Mean corpuscular volume
MCH	Mean corpuscular hemoglobin

Patient Care and Monitoring

1. Identify and treat the underlying cause of anemia.

2. Determine if immediate correction of anemia is required with a transfusion or if chronic therapy can be initiated.

3. Monitor symptoms such as fatigue, shortness of breath, lethargy, headache, edema, and tachycardia for resolution.

4. Monitor the CBC monthly.

5. When initiating ESAs, assess the patient's iron status.

6. Monitor side effects of therapy, such as

• *Oral iron:* nausea, vomiting, abdominal pain, heartburn, constipation, and dark stools

• *Parenteral iron:* anaphylaxis (test dose required for iron dextran and observe for 1 hour after), injection-site pain/irritation, arthralgias, myalgias, flushing, malaise, and fever

• *Folic acid:* bad taste and nausea, rash, and allergic reactions

• *Vitamin B_{12}:* hyperuricemia, hypokalemia, and sodium retention (rare)

• *ESAs:* hypertension (monitor blood pressure), thrombosis (e.g., DVT/PE, MI, CVA, and TIA), arthralgias, and headache

NCCN	National Comprehensive Cancer Network
NKF-K/DOQI	National Kidney Foundation Kidney Disease Outcomes Quality Initiative
TIBC	Total iron-binding capacity
TSAT	Transferrin saturation

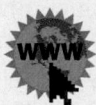 Self-assessment questions and answers are available at *http://www.mhpharmacotherapy. com/pp.html.*

REFERENCES

1. Guralnik JM, Eisenstaedt RS, Ferrucci L, Klein HG, Woodman RC. Prevalence of anemia in persons 65 years and older in the United States: Evidence for a high rate of unexplained anemia. Blood 2004;104(8):2263–2268.

2. Martin M, Pienkowski T, Mackey J, et al. Adjuvant docetaxel for node-positive breast cancer. N Engl J Med 2005;352:2302–2313.

3. Xue JL, St PW, Ebben JP, Everson SE, Collins AJ. Anemia treatment in the pre-ESRD period and associated mortality in elderly patients. Am J Kidney Dis 2002;40(6):1153–1161.

4. Guyton AC, Hall JE. Red blood cells, anemia, and polycythemia. In: Guyton AC, Hall JE, eds. Textbook of Medical Physiology, 11th ed. Philadelphia: WB Saunders, 2006:419–428.

5. Kaushansky K, Kipps TJ. Hemapoietic Agents: Growth Factors, Minerals, and Vitamins. In: Brunton LL, Laza LS, Parker KL, eds.

Goodman & Gilman's the Pharmacological Basis of Therapeutics, 11th ed. New York: McGraw-Hill, 2006:1433–1466.

6. Toh BH, van Driel IR, Gleeson PA. Pernicious anemia. N Engl J Med 1997;337(20):1441–1448.

7. Andrews NC. Disorders of iron metabolism. N Engl J Med 1999;341(26):1986–1995.

8. Spivak JL. The anaemia of cancer: Death by a thousand cuts. Nat Rev Cancer 2005;5(7):543–555.

9. Weiss G, Goodnough LT. Anemia of chronic disease. N Engl J Med 2005;352(10):1011–1023.

10. Aird William C. Anemia. In: Furie Bruce, Cassileth Peter A, Atkins Michael B, Mayer Robert J, eds. Clinical Hematology and Oncology, 1st ed. Philadelphia: Churchill Livingstone, 2003:232–240.

11. Petrides M. Red cell transfusion "trigger": A review. South Med J 2003;96(7):664–667.

12. Infed (Iron Dextran) Prescribing Information. Morristown, NJ: Watson Pharma, March 2006.

13. Silverstein SB, Rodgers GM. Parenteral iron therapy options. Am J Hematol 2004;76(1):74–78.

14. National Comprehensive Cancer Network Clinical Practice Guidelines in Oncology™—Cancer and Chemotherapy-Induced Anemia V.3. 2009. National Comprehensive Cancer Network 2009, URL: *http://www.nccn.org/professionals/physician_gls/PDF/anemia.pdf.*

15. Bohlius J, Schmidlin K, Brillant C, et al. Erythropoieten or darbepoieten for patients with cancer—meta-analysis based on individual patient data. Cochrane Database Syst Rev 2009;8:CD007303.

16. Levey AS, Coresh J, Balk E, et al. National Kidney Foundation practice guidelines for chronic kidney disease: Evaluation, classification, and stratification. Ann Intern Med 2003;139(2):137–147.

17. Fink J, Blahut S, Reddy M, Light P. Use of erythropoietin before the initiation of dialysis and its impact on mortality. Am J Kidney Dis 2001;37(2):348–355.

18. Jungers P, Choukroun G, Oualim Z, Robino C, Nguyen AT, Man NK. Beneficial influence of recombinant human erythropoietin therapy on the rate of progression of chronic renal failure in predialysis patients. Nephrol Dial Transplant 2001;16(2):307–312.

19. Eschbach J, DeOreo PB, Adamson J, et al. NKF-K/DOQI Clinical Practice Guidelines. National Kidney Foundation—Kidney Disease Outcomes Quality Initiative (NKF K/DOQI) 2000, Available from: URL: *http://www.kidney.org/professionals/kdoqi/guidelines_updates/doqi_uptoc.html#an.*

20. KDOQI; National Kidney Foundation. Am J Kid Dis 2006;47:S109–S116.

67 Coagulation and Platelet Disorders

Anastasia Rivkin

LEARNING OBJECTIVES

Upon completion of the chapter, the reader will be able to:

1. Describe the basics of the regulation of hemostasis and thrombosis.

2. Determine which factor replacement preparation is appropriate in a given clinical situation.

3. Calculate an appropriate factor-concentrate dose for a product, given the percentage correction desired.

4. List the complications from hemophilia bleeding episodes.

5. Devise a treatment plan for a patient with a specific variant of von Willebrand's disease (vWD).

6. Identify an appropriate treatment plan based on presentation of disseminated intravascular coagulation (DIC).

7. Recommend a treatment approach for the initial treatment of immune thrombocytopenic purpura (ITP).

8. Identify basic clinical features and causes of thrombotic thrombocytopenic purpura (TTP).

KEY CONCEPTS

❶ Intravenous factor replacement with recombinant or plasma-derived products to treat or prevent bleeding is the primary treatment of hemophilia.

❷ Type 1 patients unresponsive to desmopressin, patients with types 2 and 3 von Willebrand's disease (vWD), and major surgery patients require replacement therapy with plasma-derived intermediate- and high-purity factor VIII, virus-inactivated factor VIII concentrates containing von Willebrand's factor (vWF).

❸ The primary treatment of recessively inherited coagulation disorders (RICDs) is single-donor fresh-frozen plasma (FFP) that contains all coagulation factors.

❹ The cornerstone of the management of disseminated intravascular coagulation (DIC) is aggressive treatment of the underlying primary illness. Supportive measures may be used as necessary; however, owing to the heterogeneity of the DIC etiology, treatment should be guided by predominant symptoms (bleeding or clotting).

❺ The treatment of immune thrombocytopenic purpura (ITP) is determined by the symptom severity. In some cases, no therapy is needed.

❻ The present standard of treatment for thrombotic thrombocytopenic purpura (TTP) is urgent plasma exchange (PEX). If PEX is unavailable, treatment with plasma infusion and glucocorticoids is indicated until PEX is available.

INTRODUCTION

Components of the Hemostatic System

Following endothelial injury, vessel-wall response involves vasoconstriction, platelet plug formation, coagulation, and fibrinolysis regulation. In normal circumstances, platelets circulate in the blood in an inactive form. After injury, platelets undergo activation, which consists of (a) adhesion to the subendothelium, (b) secretion of granules containing chemical mediators (e.g., adenosine diphosphate, thromboxane A2, thrombin, etc.), and (c) aggregation. Chemical factors released from the injured tissue and platelets stimulate the coagulation cascade and thrombin formation. In turn, thrombin catalyzes the conversion of fibrinogen to fibrin and its subsequent incorporation into plug.

The coagulation system consists of intrinsic and extrinsic pathways. Both pathways are composed of a series of enzymatic reactions that ultimately produce thrombin, fibrin, and a stable clot. In parallel with the coagulation, the fibrinolytic system is activated locally. Plasminogen is converted to plasmin, which dissolves the fibrin mesh (Fig. 67–1).[1]

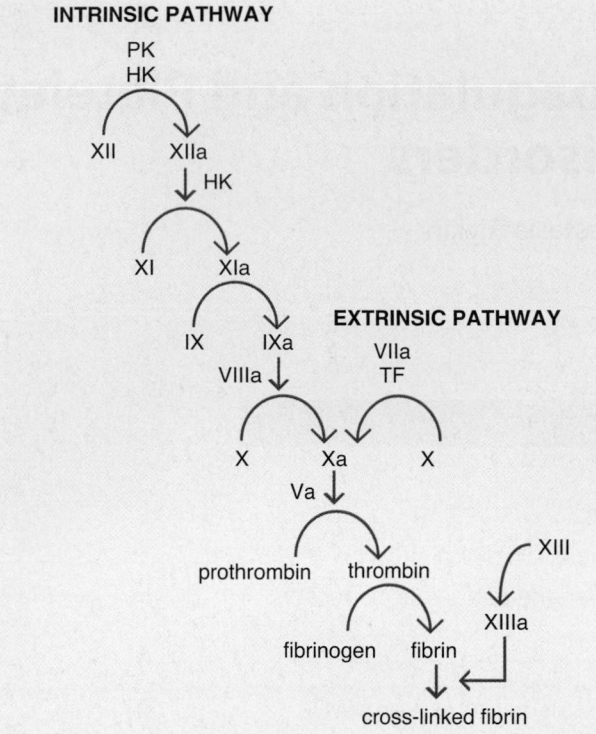

FIGURE 67–1. Cascade model of coagulation demonstrates activation via the intrinsic or extrinsic pathway. This model shows successive activation of coagulation factors proceeding from the top to the bottom where thrombin and fibrin are generated. (PK, prekallikrein; HK, high–molecular weight kininogen; TF, tissue factor.) (From Roberts HR et al. Molecular biology and biochemistry of the coagulation factors and pathways of hemostasis. In: Beutler et al., eds. Williams Hematology. 6th ed. New York: McGraw-Hill; 2001:1409–1434.)

INHERITED COAGULATION DISORDERS

HEMOPHILIA

Etiology and Epidemiology

Hemophilia A and B are coagulation disorders that result from defects in the genes encoding for plasma coagulation proteins. Hemophilia A (classic hemophilia) is caused by the deficiency of factor VIII, and hemophilia B (Christmas disease) is caused by the deficiency of factor IX. The incidences of hemophilia A and B are estimated at 1 in 5,000 and 1 in 30,000 male births, respectively. Both types of hemophilia are evenly distributed across all ethnic and racial groups.[1]

Pathophysiology

The pathophysiology of hemophilia is based on the deficiency of factor VIII or IX resulting in inadequate thrombin generation and an impaired intrinsic-pathway coagulation cascade (see Fig. 67–1). Factor VIII and IX genes are located on the X chromosome. Hemophilias are recessive X-linked diseases. Generally, affected males carrying either defective allele on their X chromosome do not transmit the gene to their sons. However, their daughters are obligate carriers. Over 2,100 mutations, deletions, and inversions have been identified throughout the factor VIII and IX genes.[2]

Consequently, hemophilia is not a result of a single genetic mutation. However, inversion at intron 22 of the factor VIII gene accounts for 45% of severe hemophilia A cases. Owing to the high incidence, this mutation is used for carrier and prenatal testing.[3]

Complications of Hemophilia

The severity of bleeding associated with hemophilia correlates with the degree of factor VIII or factor IX deficiency as measured against the normal plasma standard. Table 67–1 summarizes the age at onset and laboratory and clinical manifestations of hemophilia.[4]

Clinical Presentation and Diagnosis of Hemophilias A and B

Hemophilias A and B are clinically indistinguishable.

Symptoms

- Ecchymoses
- **Hemarthrosis**—bleeding into joint spaces* (especially knee, elbow, and ankle)
  - Joint pain, swelling and erythema
  - Cutaneous warmth
  - Decreased range of motion
- Muscle hemorrhage
  - Swelling
  - Pain with motion of affected muscle

- Signs of nerve compression
- Potential life-threatening blood loss, especially with thigh bleeding
- Mouth bleeding with dental extractions or trauma
- Genitourinary bleeding
- Hematuria
- Intracranial hemorrhage (spontaneous or following trauma), with headache, vomiting, change in mental status, and focal neurologic signs
- Excessive bleeding with surgery

---

*Hallmark of hemophilia; recurrent inadequately managed hemarthrosis leads to deformity and chronic pain.

Table 67–1			
Laboratory and Clinical Manifestations of Hemophilia			
	Severe (Less Than 0.01 IU/mL)[a]	**Moderate (0.01–0.05 IU/mL)[a]**	**Mild (More Than 0.05 IU/mL)[a]**
Age at onset	1 year or less	1–2 years	2 years–adult
Neonatal symptoms			
PCB	Usual	Usual	Rare
ICH	Occasional	Uncommon	Rare
Muscle/joint hemorrhage	Spontaneous	Minor trauma	Minor trauma
CNS hemorrhage	High risk	Moderate risk	Rare
Postsurgical hemorrhage (without prophylaxis)	Frank bleeding, severe	Wound bleeding, common	Wound bleeding, with factor less than 0.3 unit/mL
Oral hemorrhage following trauma, tooth extraction	Usual	Common	Common

CNS, central nervous system; ICH, intracranial hemorrhage; PCB, postcircumcisional bleeding.

Normal range of factor VIII/IX activity level is 0.5–1.5 IU/mL (50–150%). 1 IU/mL corresponds to 100% of the factor found in 1 mL of normal plasma.

[a]0.01 IU/mL = 0.00001 unit/L; 0.05 IU/mL = 0.00005 unit/L; 0.5 IU/mL = 0.0005 unit/L; 1 unit/mL = 1 IU/mL = 0.001 unit/L; 1.5 IU/mL = 0.0015 unit/L.

Treatment

▶ Desired Outcomes

Currently, there is no cure for hemophilia A or B. The life expectancy of hemophiliacs was only 8 to 11 years in the 1920s and 1930s. With the development of effective treatment strategies, life expectancy is currently about 65 years, or nearly that of the normal population.

The short-term goals of hemophilia treatment are to:
- Decrease the number of bleeding episodes per year or bleeding frequency
- Normalize or improve clotting factor concentrate levels

The long-term goals of hemophilia treatment are to:
- Maintain clinical joint function
- Normalize orthopedic joint score
- Normalize radiologic joint score
- Maintain quality-of-life measurements

▶ General Approach to Treatment

1 *Intravenous factor replacement with recombinant or plasma-derived products to treat or prevent bleeding is the primary treatment of hemophilia.* Primary prophylaxis is defined as the regular administration of factor concentrates with the intention of preventing joint bleeds.[5] The rationale for primary prophylaxis is that individuals with factor levels of greater than 0.02 IU/mL (0.00002 unit/L) rarely suffer from spontaneous bleeds and arthropathy. Therefore, to maintain a trough level above this might convert "severe" hemophilia to "moderate" disease, with the abolition of joint bleeds and the associated arthropathy.[6]

Although primary prophylaxis is expensive, historical cohorts show progressively better outcomes (joint function and radiologic appearances) with its use. The Medical and Scientific Advisory Council of the National Hemophilia Foundation of the United States recommends primary prophylaxis in patients with severe hemophilia A and B (factor VIII or factor IX less than 1%). The optimal duration of prophylactic therapy is unknown.[7,8] Vaccination against hepatitis A and B is recommended in all hemophiliacs.

▶ Nonpharmacologic Therapy

Surgery Surgical arthroscopic synovectomy reduces replacement-therapy-resistant disease and repetitive hemarthrosis of a single joint. This procedure removes inflamed joint tissue. Patients may have decreased range of motion after the surgery.

Orthotics Joint prostheses do not deal with the deformities directly. Orthotics in hemophilia serve as an important supportive measure before or after surgery.

▶ Pharmacologic Therapy

Hemophilia A

DDAVP. Primary therapy is based on disease severity and type of hemorrhage.[9] Most patients with mild to moderate disease and a minor bleeding episode can be treated with 1-desamino-8-D-arginine vasopressin (desmopressin acetate [DDAVP]), a synthetic analog of the antidiuretic hormone, vasopressin. DDAVP causes release of von Willebrand's factor (vWF) and factor VIII from endothelial storage sites. DDAVP increases plasma factor VIII levels by three- to five-fold within 30 minutes. The recommended dose is 0.3 mcg/kg IV (in 50 mL normal saline infused over 15–30 min) or subcutaneously or 150 to 300 mcg intranasally via concentrated nasal spray every 12 hours. Peak effect with intranasal administration occurs 60 to 90 minutes after administration, which is somewhat later than with IV administration. Desmopressin infusion may be administered daily for up to 2 to 3 days.

Facial flushing, hypertension or hypotension, GI upset, and headache are common side effects of desmopressin. Water retention and hyponatremia may occur; patients should be instructed to limit water intake while taking desmopressin. Serious side effects include seizures related to hyponatremia, most frequently seen in children younger than two years of age, and myocardial infarction in the elderly. Tachyphylaxis, an attenuated response with repeated administration, may occur after several doses.[10] Use of DDAVP is contraindicated in patients with creatinine clearance less than 50 mL/min.

Antifibrinolytic Therapy. Aminocaproic acid and tranexamic acid are antifibrinolytic agents that reduce plasminogen activity leading to inhibition of clot lysis and clot stabilization. These agents are usually used as adjuncts in dental procedures or in difficult-to-control epistaxis and menorrhagia episodes.

● ***Factor VIII Replacement.*** Patients with severe hemophilia may receive primary (before the first major bleed) or secondary (after the first major bleed) prophylaxis. All hemophiliacs with a major bleed require factor VIII replacement.[11] The therapy may include recombinant (produced via transfection of mammalian cells with the human factor VIII gene) or plasma-derived (concentrate from pooled plasma) factor VIII (Table 67–2). The choice of product and dose are based on the overall clinical scenario because the efficacy of various preparations does not differ. Newer-generation plasma-derived coagulation factor concentrates are considerably safer owing to advancements in viral testing and inactivation technology. While original recombinant factor VIII concentrates were stabilized with human serum albumin, potentially creating a source for viral contamination, new generation recombinant factor VIII concentrates are stabilized with sucrose, eliminating the concern for viral transmission.

● The severity of hemorrhage and its location are major determinants of percentage correction to target, as well as duration of therapy (Table 67–3). The normal range of factor VIII activity level is 1 IU/mL (0.001 IU/L), which corresponds to 100% of the factor found in 1 mL of normal plasma. Minor bleeding may be treated with a goal of 25% to 30% (0.25–0.30 IU/mL [0.00025–0.0003 IU/L]) of normal activity, whereas serious or life-threatening bleeding requires at least 50% of normal activity. Factor VIII is a large molecule that remains in the intravascular space and its estimated volume of distribution is approximately 50 mL/kg.

Table 67–2			
Factor Concentrates			
Brand Name	**Product Type**	**Viral Inactivation or Exclusion Method**	**Other Contents**
Factor VIII Concentrates			
Alphanate	Plasma	Solvent detergent, dry heat	Albumin, heparin, vWF
Hemophil M	Plasma	Solvent detergent, monoclonal antibody	Albumin
Humate-P	Plasma	Pasteurization	Albumin, vWF
Koāte-DVI	Plasma	Solvent detergent, dry heat	Albumin, heparin, vWF
Monarc-M	Plasma	Solvent detergent, monoclonal antibody	Albumin
Monoclate P	Plasma	Pasteurization, monoclonal antibody	Albumin
Advate	Recombinant	None	
Bioclate	Recombinant	None	Albumin
Helixate FS	Recombinant	Solvent detergent	Albumin (fermentation only); sucrose
Kogenate	Recombinant	Monoclonal antibody	Albumin
Kogenate FS	Recombinant	Solvent detergent, monoclonal antibody	Albumin (fermentation only); sucrose
Recombinate	Recombinant	Monoclonal antibody	Albumin
ReFacto	Recombinant B domain deleted	None	Albumin (fermentation only); sucrose
Factor IX Concentrates			
AlphaNine SD	Plasma	Solvent detergent, filtered	Heparin
Mononine	Plasma	Monoclonal antibody, ultrafiltration	Heparin
Benefix	Recombinant	None	
APCC			
Autoplex T	Plasma	Dry heat	Heparin, IIa, VIIa, trace VIIIa, IXa, Xa
Feiba VH Immuno	Plasma	Vapor heat	IIa, VIIa, VIIIa, IXa, Xa
PCC			
Bebulin VH	Plasma	Vapor heat	Heparin, II, IX, X
Profilnine SD	Plasma	Solvent detergent	Preservative free
Proplex T	Plasma	Dry heat	Heparin, II, VII, IX, X
Other			
NovoSeven	Recombinant VII	None	

APCC, activated prothrombin complex concentrate; PCC, prothrombin complex concentrate; vWF, von Willebrand's factor.

Table 67–3

Guidelines for Replacement Dosing With Factor VIII and Factor IX

Type of Hemorrhage	Desired Plasma Factor VIII Level (% of Normal)	Desired Plasma Factor XI Level (% of Normal)	Duration of Therapy (days)
CNS, intracranial, retropharyngeal, retroperitoneal, surgical prophylaxis	80–100	80–100	Factor VIII: q 8–12 h over 10–14 days Factor IX: q 12 h over 10–14 days
Mild hemarthrosis, mucosal (e.g., epistaxis), superficial hematoma	30	20–30	Factor VIII: q 8–12 h over 1–2 days Factor IX: q 12–24 h over 1–2 days

Generally, factor VIII levels increase by 2% (0.02 IU/mL [0.00002 unit/L]) for every 1 unit/kg of factor VIII concentrate infused. To calculate factor VIII replacement dose, the following equation can be used:

Dose of factor VIII (units)
    = weight (kg) × (desired percentage increase) × 0.5

Thus, to increase factor VIII levels by 50% (e.g., from 0 to 50%) in a 70 kg (154 lb) patient, an IV dose of 1,750 units is required. The half-life of factor VIII ranges from 8 to 15 hours. Half the initial dose is given every half-life (every 8–12 hours) to maintain the desired factor VIII level.[12] Although intermittent bolus infusions of factor VIII concentrates have been used successfully, continuous-infusion protocols are being instituted successfully in patients requiring prolonged treatment of acute hemorrhage to avoid dangerously low trough levels and decrease the overall cost of therapy.

▶ Hemophilia B

Factor IX Replacement Hemophilia B therapy may include recombinant (produced via transfection of mammalian cells with the human factor IX gene) or plasma-derived (concentrate from pooled plasma) factor IX (see Table 67–2). Guidelines for choosing the factor-concentrate formulation for hemophilia B are similar to the guidelines for hemophilia A. However, older-generation factor IX concentrates containing other vitamin K-dependent proteins (e.g., factors II, VII, and IX), called prothrombin complex concentrates (PCCs), have been associated with thrombogenic side effects. Consequently, these products are not first-line treatment for hemophilia B. Because it is a small protein, the factor IX molecule passes into both the intravascular and the extravascular spaces. Therefore, the volume of distribution of recombinant factor IX is twice that of factor VIII. Consequently, 1 unit of factor IX administered per kilogram of body weight yields a 1% rise in the plasma factor IX level (0.01 IU/mL [0.00001 units/L]). To calculate the factor IX replacement dose, the following equation can be used:

Dose of factor IX (units)
    = weight (kg) × (desired percentage increase) × F

Where F = 1 for human plasma-derived products and 1.2 for recombinant factor IX.

Thus, to increase factor IX levels by 50% (e.g., from 0 to 50%) in a 70 kg (154 lb) patient, the required dose of factor IX is 4,200 units IV (using the recombinant factor IX product). The half-life of factor IX ranges from 18 to 22 hours; therefore, doses are given every 12 to 24 hours.

▶ Treatment of Patients With Factor VIII or IX Inhibitors

Factor VIII and IX inhibitors are antibodies that develop in 20% and 5% of hemophilia A and hemophilia B patients, respectively, in response to replacement therapy. These antibodies bind to and neutralize the activity of infused factor concentrates. Although the inhibitors do not increase hemorrhage frequency, their existence challenges the treatment of bleeding episodes. Titers of inhibitors are measured and reported in Bethesda units (BU), and this measurement is used to guide therapy (Fig. 67–2). Management options for acute bleeding in patients with factor inhibitors include the administration of factor VIII concentrates, PCCs, recombinant factor VIIa (rFVIIa), and porcine factor VIII. Immune tolerance induction can be attempted to prevent future bleeding episodes.

Factor VIII concentrates can be used in patients with low inhibitor levels to control acute bleeding episodes. The dose of factor VIII is determined based on clinical response (see Fig. 67–2).

PCCs contain the vitamin K-dependent factors II, VII, IX, and X. These agents bypass factor VIII at which the antibody is directed (see Fig. 67–2). However, PCCs carry the risk of serious thrombotic complications.

Factor VIIa (rFVIIa) is a bypassing agent designed to generate thrombin only at tissue injury sites, where it binds tissue factor. Due to its local action, rFVIIa is associated with fewer systemic thrombotic events than PCC. rFVIIa is used effectively in surgeries and spontaneous bleeds.[13]

Plasma-derived porcine factor VIII participates in the coagulation cascade in place of human factor VIII. However, due to contamination with parvovirus, it is no longer

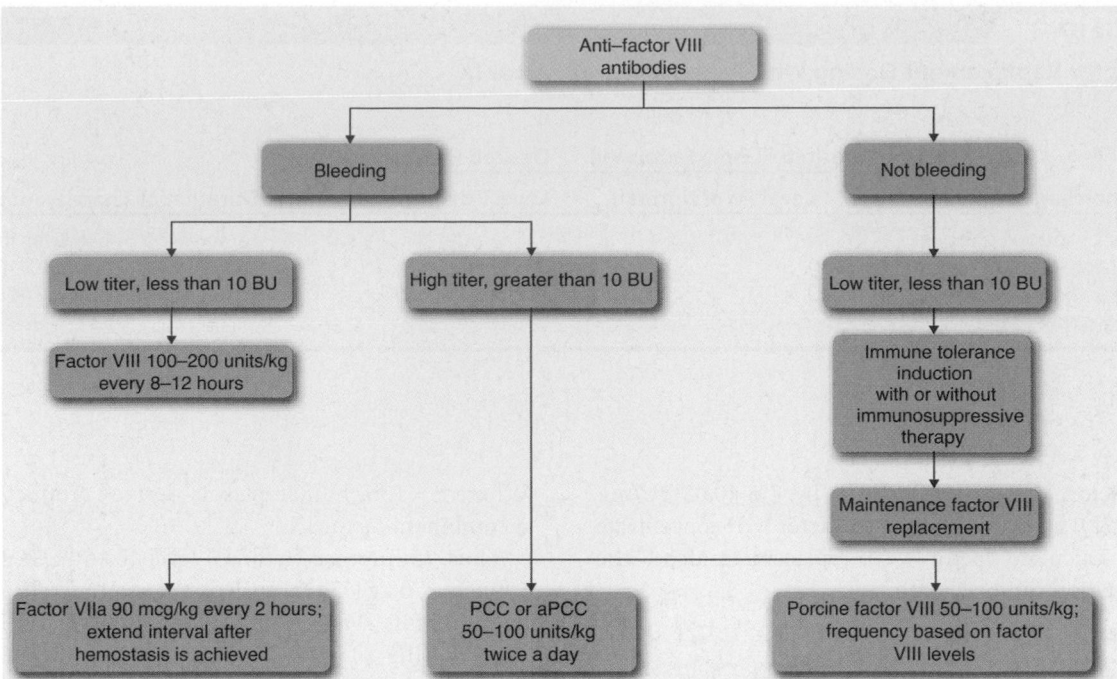

FIGURE 67–2. Treatment algorithm for the management of patients with hemophilia A and factor VIII antibodies. Porcine factor VIII is currently not available in the United States. (BU, Bethesda unit; PCC, prothrombin complex concentrate; aPCC, activated prothrombin complex concentrate.)

available. Recombinant porcine factor VIII is currently under review and could serve as a third-line agent (only after factor VIIa and a PCC have failed) owing to the relatively high incidence of cross-reactivity with factor VIII inhibitors.

Induction of immune tolerance is often performed with the goal of eliminating the inhibitor. Immune tolerance induction is accomplished by the administration of repetitive doses of factor VIII or IX with or without immunosuppressive therapy. It is effective in 70% of patients with hemophilia A and 30% of patients with hemophilia B.

Pain Associated With Hemophilia

Pain commonly occurs in patients with hemophilia. Acute bleeding episodes and long-term joint destruction are common sources of pain. Acetaminophen, cyclooxygenase-2 (COX-2) inhibitors, and opioid analgesics are recommended to control mild, moderate, and severe pain, respectively. Nonsteroidal anti-inflammatory drugs and aspirin should be avoided if possible, because these drugs bind to platelets and increase the risk of bleeding episodes.

Outcome Evaluation

The main goal of hemophilia treatment is to prevent bleeding episodes and their long-term complications. Clinicians should evaluate patients every 6 to 12 months for the following:

• Musculoskeletal status, including joint range of motion and radiologic assessment, as indicated.

• Number and type of bleeding episodes to assess adequacy of prophylactic treatment and home therapy.

• Use of clotting-factor concentrates to check for the development of inhibitors, especially in patients with severe disease and poor treatment responders.

von WILLEBRAND'S DISEASE

Epidemiology and Etiology

von Willebrand's disease (vWD) is the most common inherited bleeding disorder caused by a deficiency or dysfunction of vWF. It is classified based on the quantitative deficiency of vWF or qualitative abnormalities of vWF. The disease prevalence is estimated at 30 to 100 cases per million. In contrast to hemophilia, the majority of vWD cases are inherited as an autosomal dominant disorder, ensuing equal frequency in males and females.[14]

Pathophysiology

vWF is a large multimeric glycoprotein with two main functions in hemostasis: to aid platelet adhesion to injured blood vessel walls and to carry and stabilize factor VIII in plasma. Table 67–4 represents three main vWD phenotypes, their frequency, and genetic transmission.[15]

Treatment

▶ Desired Outcomes

Unlike hemophilia, the bleeding tendency in vWD is less frequent and generally less severe. Consequently, chronic

Table 67–4

Classification of vWD

Phenotype	Mechanism of Disease	Percentage of Cases	Genetic Transmission
Type 1 vWD	Partial (mild to moderate) quantitative deficiency of vWF and factor VIII	70–80	Autosomal dominant
Type 2 vWD	Qualitative abnormalities of vWF	10–30	
2A	Decreased platelet-dependent vWF function owing to lack of larger multimers	10–15	Autosomal dominant (or recessive)
2B	Increased platelet-dependent vWF function owing to lack of larger multimers	Uncommon	Autosomal dominant
2M	Defective platelet-dependent vWF functions not associated with multimer defects	Uncommon	Autosomal dominant (or recessive)
2N	Defective vWF binding to factor VIII	Uncommon	Autosomal recessive
Type 3 vWD	Severe quantitative deficiency of vWF	Rare	Autosomal recessive

Clinical Presentation and Diagnosis of vWD

Clinical manifestations vary depending on the subtype. Patients with mild disease may be asymptomatic into adulthood.

Symptoms

- Bruising
- Mucocutaneous bleeding
  - Epistaxis
  - Oral cavity bleeding
  - Menorrhagia
  - GI bleeding
- Joint and deep tissue bleeding
- Postoperative bleeding

Laboratory Testing

- Low or normal von Willebrand's factor antigen concentration in plasma (vWF:Ag)
- Low or normal factor VIII coagulation assay (FVIII:C)[a]
- Low ristocetin cofactor activity (vWF:RCo)[b]

---

[a]Factor VIII coagulation assay measures the ability of vWF to ind factor and maintain adequate levels of factor VIII.

[b]Ristocetin cofactor activity (vWF:RCo) assay measures the ability of vWF to interact with intact platelets (normal 50–200 IU/dL).

---

prophylaxis is usually unwarranted. The goal of two mainstay therapeutic options in vWD is:

- To stop spontaneous bleeding as necessary
- To prevent surgical and postpartum bleeding

▶ Nonpharmacologic Therapy

Local measures, including pressure and ice, may be used to control superficial bleeding.

▶ Pharmacologic Therapy

Systemic therapy is used to prevent bleeding associated with surgery, childbirth, and dental extractions and to treat bleeding that cannot be controlled with local measures. The two systemic approaches involve using desmopressin, which stimulates the release of endogenous vWF, or administering products that contain vWF. The general approach to the treatment of vWD is depicted in Figure 67–3. In 2008, The National Heart, Lung, and Blood Institute issued a comprehensive evidence-based guidelines for the diagnosis and management of vWD.[16]

DDAVP Most patients with type 1 vWD (functionally normal vWF) and a minor bleeding episode can be treated successfully with desmopressin, which induces release of factor VIII and vWF from endothelial cells through interaction with vasopressin V2 receptors. The recommended dose is the same as that used to treat mild factor VIII deficiency (0.3 mcg/kg IV in 50 mL of normal saline infused over 15–30 min). This therapy is generally ineffective in type 2A patients, who secrete abnormal vWF, and is controversial in type 2B patients because it may increase the risk of postinfusion thrombocytopenia. Type 3 vWD patients who lack releasable stores of vWF do not respond to DDAVP therapy.[17]

The individual responsiveness to desmopressin is consistent, and a test dose administered at the time of diagnosis or prior to therapy is the best predictor of response. Generally, DDAVP is more effective in vWD than in hemophilia patients, with an average two- to five-fold increase in vWF and factor VIII levels over baseline. In patients with an adequate response, desmopressin is first-line therapy because it allows for once-daily administration

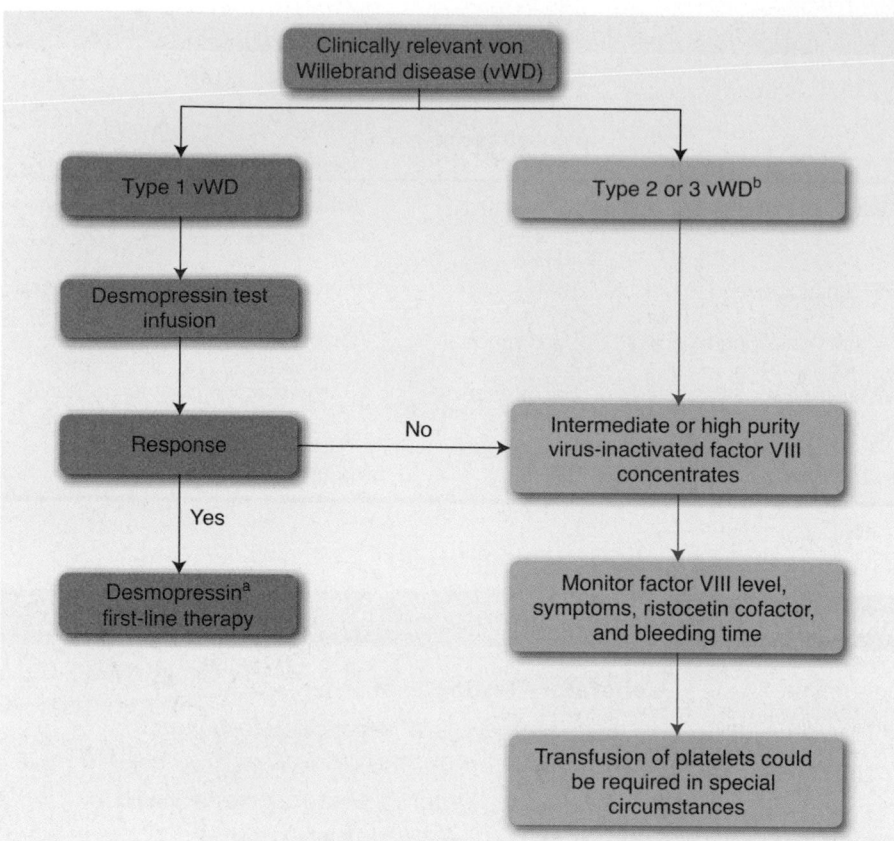

FIGURE 67–3. Guidelines for the treatment of vWD. [a]Use factor VIII concentrate for life-threatening bleeding. [b]Some patients with type 2 or 3 vWD may respond to desmopressin.

Table 67–5		
Replacement Therapy in vWD		
Condition	**Therapy**	**Recommended Dosage**
Major surgery	Maintain vWF:RCo and factor VIII levels at least 100 IU/dL followed by 50 IU/dL for 7–14 days To minimize risk of thrombosis: vWF:RCo levels should not exceed 200 IU/dL, and factor VIII levels should not exceed 250 IU/dL	40–60 units/kg[a] loading dose, followed by 20–40 units/kg every 8–24 hours DDAVP may be added after a few days
Minor surgery	Prophylaxis: maintain vWF:RCo and factor VIII levels at least 30 IU/dL (preferably >50 IU/dL) Minor surgery: maintain vWF:RCo and factor VIII levels at least 30 IU/dL (preferably >50 IU/dL) for 1–5 days	30–60 units/kg loading dose, followed by 20–40 units/kg every 12–48 hours DDAVP may be added after a few days

[a]vWF concentrates are dosed based on vWF:RCo units concentration in the preparation to achieve the desired vWF:RCo levels.

(elevates plasma levels for 8–10 hours), does not pose a threat in terms of viral transmission, and costs substantially less than that of the plasma-derived products.

Antifibrinolytic Therapy Fibrinolysis inhibitors and oral contraceptives are used successfully in the management of epistaxis and menorrhagia or as adjuvant treatments. Fibrinolysis inhibitors include aminocaproic acid (25–60 mg/kg orally or IV every 4–6 hours, to a maximum dose of 24 g/day) and tranexamic acid (10 mg/kg IV every 8 hours). Tranexaminic acid is not FDA-approved for oral administration;

however, IV form given as swish and swallow or spit every 6 to 8 hours has been used as bleeding prophylaxis in dental surgery. Both aminocaproic acid and tranexaminic acid are dose adjusted with renal insufficiency.

Replacement Therapy ❷ *Type 1 patients unresponsive to desmopressin, patients with types 2 and 3 vWD, and major surgery patients require replacement therapy with plasma-derived, intermediate- and high-purity factor VIII virus-inactivated factor VIII concentrates containing vWF.*[18] Table 67–5 provides typical dosing guidelines and target levels of replacement therapy–concentrates to control various types of hemorrhage. Ultra-high-purity (monoclonal) plasma-derived and recombinant factor VIII concentrates do not contain vWF and should not be used in the treatment of vWD. Cryoprecipitate contains considerable amounts of both factor VIII and vWF. However, this product is not a first-line treatment option because it does not undergo viral inactivation.

Outcome Evaluation

The main goal of vWF treatment is to prevent bleeding with surgery or dental procedures. Clinicians should evaluate patients every 6 to 12 months for the following:

- Number and type of bleeding episodes to assess the need for prophylactic treatment.
- Ensure adequate levels of vWF and factor VIII prior to minor and major surgical procedures and for the treatment of bleeding.
- Vaccination against hepatitis A and B is recommended in all patients with vWF deficiency.

OTHER CLOTTING FACTOR DEFICIENCIES

Etiology and Epidemiology

Recessively inherited coagulation disorders (RICDs) refer to relatively rare deficiencies in factor II, V, VII, and X to XIII resulting in either decreased clotting factor production or production of a dysfunctional molecule with reduced activity.[19] The clinical severity of bleeding varies and generally is poorly correlated with the factor blood levels. Table 67-6 illustrates these clotting factor deficiencies and some of their characteristics.

Pathophysiology

The RICDs are rare genetic disorders. Mutations in the genes responsible for the respective clotting factors results in impaired functionality or production of the factor.

Treatment

▶ Desired Outcomes

Therapeutic options for RICDs improve hemostasis via replacement of deficient blood coagulation factors while minimizing the development of immune tolerance.[20]

Hemostatic levels should be maintained for the following conditions:

- Spontaneous bleeding—until bleeding stops.
- Minor surgery—for two to three days.
- Major surgery—until incision site has healed.

▶ Nonpharmacologic Therapy

Transfusional Therapies ❸ *The primary treatment of RICDs is single-donor fresh-frozen plasma (FFP) that contains all coagulation factors.* Disadvantages of FFP treatment include the risk of becoming volume overloaded, especially when repeated infusions are administered in order to improve and maintain hemostasis, risk of infections, and risk of inhibitor development. PCCs licensed for the treatment of hemophilia B also contain significant levels of vitamin K-dependent factors and may be used off-label for treatment of RICD. Table 67–7 lists the recommended RICD treatment schedules in different clinical scenarios.

▶ Pharmacologic Therapy

Less severe hemorrhages may be treated successfully with antifibrinolytic amino acids alone or in combination

---

Table 67–6

Clotting Factor Deficiency Characteristics

Factor Deficient	Inheritance Pattern	Estimated Incidence	Laboratory Abnormalities	Severity and Site of Bleeding
II	Autosomal dominant or recessive	Extremely rare	Prolonged PT and aPTT	Mild to moderate umbilical cord, joint, and mucosal tract
V	Autosomal recessive	1:1,000,000	Prolonged PT and aPTT	Mild to moderate mucosal tract
VII	Autosomal recessive	1:500,000	Prolonged PT	Mild to severe mucosal tract and joint
X	Autosomal recessive	1:500,000	Prolonged PT and aPTT	Mild to severe umbilical cord, joint, and muscle
XI	Autosomal recessive	4% of Askenazi Jews: otherwise rare	Prolonged aPTT	Mild to moderate post-traumatic bleeding
XII	Unknown	Unknown	Prolonged aPTT	No bleeding
XIII	Autosomal recessive	Less than 1:2,000,000	Normal PT and aPTT	Moderate to severe umbilical cord, intracranial, and joint bleeding; recurrent miscarriages, impaired wound healing

aPTT, activated partial thromboplastin time; PT, prothrombin time.

Table 67–7			
Treatment of Factor Deficiencies			
Factor Deficient	**Major Surgery**	**Spontaneous Bleeding**	**Hemostatic Level^a (units/dL)**
II	1. PCC: 20–30 units/kg 2. FFP: 15–20 mL/kg	1. FFP: 15–20 mL/kg	20–40
V	1. FFP: 15–20 mL/kg	1. FFP: 15–20 mL/kg	15–25
VII	1. rFVIIa: 15–30 mcg/kg every 4–6 hours	1. rFVIIa: 15–30 mcg/kg every 12 hours	10–20
X	1. PCC: 20–30 units/kg 2. FFP: 15–20 mL/kg	1. PCC: 20–30 units/kg 2. FFP: 15–20 mL/kg	10–20
XI	1. FFP: 15–20 mL/kg	1. FFP: 15–20 mL/kg	10–20
XIII	1. Pasteurized plasma concentrate: 10–20 units/kg 2. FFP: 15–20 mL/kg 3. Cryoprecipitate (1 bag per 10 kg)	1. Pasteurized plasma concentrate: 10–20 units/kg 2. FFP: 15–20 mL/kg 3. Cryoprecipitate (1 bag per 10 kg)	3–5

^{a}The hemostatic level represents the lowest concentration of coagulation factor to sustain normal hemostasis. Patients undergoing major surgery or experiencing significant bleeding should achieve higher factor levels than are minimally required for normal hemostasis.

Numbers indicate lines of therapy. FFP, fresh-frozen plasma; PCC, prothrombin complex concentrates.

with factor replacement therapy. Tranexamic acid and aminocaproic acid may be administered IV or orally (for doses, see Pharmacologic Therapy for vWD).

ACQUIRED COAGULATION DISORDERS

DISSEMINATED INTRAVASCULAR COAGULATION

Etiology and Epidemiology

Disseminated intravascular coagulation (DIC) is a systemic thrombohemorrhagic disorder characterized by an increased propensity for clot formation secondary to a wide variety of clinical conditions (Table 67–8). Central to the etiology of DIC is excessive and unregulated generation of thrombin, leading to an aggressive compensatory fibrinolysis. Therefore, clinical manifestations of DIC result from a loss of balance between the clot-promoting (leading to thrombosis) and the clot-lysing (leading to hemorrhage) systems. Although this balance may tip in either direction, presenting as bleeding or clotting, bleeding is most common. Incidence of bleeding, end-organ dysfunction, and other manifestations depends on the etiology of DIC.[21]

Pathophysiology

Once injured or activated by a toxic substance (e.g., bacterial toxins, placenta chemicals, snake venom, etc.), endothelial cells and monocytes respond by generating tissue factor on the cell surface. Generation of tissue factor–factor VIIa complexes leads to extrinsic pathway activation, excessive generation of thrombin and fibrin, generation of systemic microthrombi, and consumption of coagulation factors and platelets. In addition, inhibition of naturally occurring endothelium-linked anticoagulant pathways (e.g., antithrombin, protein C, and tissue factor pathway inhibitor) and fibrinolytic system (due to a rise in plasminogen activator inhibitor, PAI-1 concentrations) leads to a vast procoagulant state. While bleeding into the subcutaneous tissues, skin, and mucous membranes takes place, microvascular thrombosis exacerbates tissue ischemia and organ damage.[22]

Treatment

▶ Desired Outcomes

❹ The cornerstone of the management of DIC is aggressive treatment of the underlying primary illness. Supportive measures may be used as necessary, but owing to the heterogeneity of DIC etiology, treatment should be guided by predominant symptoms (bleeding or clotting).[23]

Goals of DIC treatment include:

- Replace missing blood components
- Interrupt coagulation
- Treat underlying disease

▶ Pharmacologic Therapy

Anticoagulants While bleeding is the most frequently observed symptom of DIC, thrombotic events cause most of the mortality. Heparin is an effective anticoagulant which activates the antithrombin system and inhibits factors II (thrombin), IXa, and Xa; however, its use is limited by the potential for bleeding. Clinical trials of heparin in DIC have not shown a consistent improvement in organ function or

Table 67–8

Conditions Associated With DIC

Cardiovascular
Acute myocardial infarction
Angiopathy
Aortic aneurysm
Aortic balloon assist devices
Giant hemangiomas
Peripheral vascular disease
Postcardiac arrest
Prosthetic devices
Raynaud's syndrome

Infectious
Arbovirus
Aspergillus
Candida albicans
Cytomegalovirus
Ebola virus
Gram-negative bacteria
Gram-positive bacteria
Herpesvirus
Histoplasma
Human immunodeficiency virus
Influenza
Kala-azar
Malaria
Mycobacteria
Mycoplasma
Paramyxoviruses
Rocky Mountain spotted fever
Rubella
Typhoid
Varicella
Variola

Intravascular Hemolysis
Hemolytic transfusion reaction
Hemolytic uremic syndrome
Minor hemolysis
Massive transfusion

Newborn
Birth asphyxia
Hypothermia
Meconium or amniotic fluid aspiration
Necrotizing enterocolitis
Respiratory distress syndrome
Shock

Obstetrics
Abortion
Amniotic fluid embolism
Fatty liver of pregnancy
Placental abruption
Pre-eclampsia/eclampsia
Retained fetus syndrome

Pulmonary
Empyema
Hyaline membrane disease
Pulmonary embolism
Pulmonary infarction

Tissue injury
Burns
Crush injuries
Extensive surgery
Head trauma
Multiple trauma

Miscellaneous
Acid–base imbalance
Acute liver failure
Amphetamines
Anaphylaxis
Autoimmune diseases
Cholestasis
Chronic inflammatory diseases
Collagen vascular disease
Craniotomy
Extracorporeal circulation
Extracorporeal membrane oxygenation
Fat embolism
Heat stroke
Hemorrhagic telangiectasia
Hepatitis
Leukemia
Lightning strikes
Near drowning
Organic solvent poisoning
Paroxysmal nocturnal hemoglobinuria
Peritoneovenous or pleurovenous shunts
Polycythemia rubra vera
Renal vascular disorders
Severe anoxia
Snake bite
Solid tumors
Transplant rejection

Clinical Presentation of DIC

Clinical manifestations generally are associated with underlying primary illness, as described in Table 67–8.

Signs and Symptoms

- Thrombosis, hemorrhage, or both
- Hemorrhagic bullae
- Peripheral cyanosis
- Petechiae and purpura

Thrombus and End-Organ Dysfunction

- Skin
- Lungs
- Kidneys
- Liver
- Adrenal glands
- Heart

Laboratory Testing

- Increased D-dimer
- Thrombocytopenia
- Decreased fibrinogen
- Increased fibrin degradation products (FDP)
- Increased prothrombin time (PT)
- Evidence of end-organ dysfunction or failure

mortality benefit. DIC patients most likely to benefit from heparin are those with chronic symptomatic thromboemboli, extensive fibrin deposition, and solid tumors. Heparin is contraindicated in DIC patients with serious or life-threatening bleeding, such as intracranial bleeding.[24]

Heparin may be given IV or subcutaneously; there is no universally accepted dose. Heparin administered subcutaneously for venous thromboembolism prophylaxis (5,000 units every 8–12 hours) can be beneficial in DIC patients without serious or life-threatening bleeding. Full-dose

Patient Encounter 1, Part 1: DIC

A 48-year-old woman was admitted to the intensive care unit with sepsis and hemodynamic instability. Three days earlier, the patient had undergone an abdominal surgery. After the IV line was placed, the patient's nurse notified the medical team of blood oozing from the IV lines, abdominal drains, and nasogastric tube.

What information is suggestive of disseminated intravascular coagulation (DIC)?

What additional information do you need to create a treatment plan for this patient?

What is the most important intervention at this time?

Patient Encounter 1, Part 2: DIC

Meds
- Insulin via sliding scale SC
- Lorazepam 1 mg/h IV

Labs
- Platelet count: $30 \times 10^3/mm^3$ ($30 \times 10^9/L$) (normal $140–440 \times 10^3/mm^3$ [$140–440 \times 10^9/L$])
- aPTT: 46 seconds (normal 25–40 seconds)
- PT: 31 seconds (normal 10–12 seconds)
- D-dimer: 3 mcg/mL (3 mg/L) (normal 250 ng/mL)
- Fibrinogen: 0.8 g/L (normal 2–4 g/L)
- Hemoglobin: 7.8 g/dL (78 g/L or 4.8 mmol/L) (normal 12.1–15.1 g/dL or 121–151 g/L or 7.5–9.36 mmol/L)

Given this additional information, is this patient's presentation consistent with DIC?

Identify your treatment goals for this patient.

Patient Encounter 1, Part 3: DIC: Creating a Care Plan

Based on the information presented, create a care plan for this patient's DIC.

require an invasive procedure. In a bleeding patient, the platelet count should be maintained above $50 \times 10^3/mm^3$ ($50 \times 10^9/L$), and platelet concentrates should be given at a dose of 1 unit/10 kg of body weight. For patients who are not bleeding, a lower threshold of less than 10 to $20 \times 10^3/mm^3$ or less than 10 to $20 \times 10^9/L$ is used. FFP contains all the coagulant factors as well as fibrinogen. Adding fibrinogen to the blood system in a situation where the level of antithrombin is already low may predispose patients to widespread microvascular thrombosis and may aggravate end-organ damage. Therefore, FFP use is reserved for actively bleeding patients who have significantly elevated prothrombin time and a fibrinogen concentration less than 50 mg/dL (0.5 g/L). The recommended FFP dose is 10 to 15 mL/kg.

- **Cryoprecipitate** If FFP cannot maintain fibrinogen concentration above 100 mg/dL (1 g/L) in a symptomatic patient, 1 to 4 units/10 kg of cryoprecipitate may be administered.

Outcome Evaluation

- With each therapeutic option, postinfusion monitoring parameters (platelets, PT, aPTT, and fibrinogen) should be checked within 30 to 60 minutes and every 6 hours thereafter, and the dose should be adjusted accordingly.

- Monitor the patient for relief of symptoms and signs of hemorrhage.

PLATELET DISORDERS

IMMUNE THROMBOCYTOPENIC PURPURA

Etiology and Epidemiology

Immune (or idiopathic) thrombocytopenic purpura (ITP) is one of the most common causes of acquired thrombocytopenia. The estimated incidence is 100 cases per 1 million persons per year, about half of whom are children. ITP is an autoimmune disorder caused by the binding of antibodies (usually IgG) to platelet surface antigens resulting in shortened platelet life span. ITP can occur as an isolated condition or secondary to an underlying disorder. Childhood-onset and adult-onset ITP present very differently. Adult-onset ITP is generally chronic (greater than 6 months) and affects women two to three times more often than men. By contrast, childhood-onset ITP is acute in onset and usually follows an infectious illness, and both sexes

heparin therapy in adults is a bolus of 5,000 units, followed by a continuous infusion of 1,000 units/h. In general, full-dose heparin should be avoided in patients with DIC due to increased risk of bleeding, and a lower dose of 500 units/hour can be used. Since the aPTT is already elevated in individuals with DIC, monitoring heparin therapy may be difficult. Treatment with subcutaneous heparin and low–molecular weight heparins are other, less studied options.[25]

Antithrombin concentrate has been evaluated in clinical trials and has not been associated with reduced mortality in septic patients. Although activated protein C can normalize abnormal coagulation activation during severe sepsis, more data are necessary before its use can be recommended for patients with DIC.[26,27]

- **Platelets and FFP** Treatment with platelet concentrates and plasma is indicated in patients who are bleeding or who

Clinical Presentation and Diagnosis of ITP

General

The typical patient is well with the exception of bleeding.

Symptoms

- Petechiae
- Purpura
- Ecchymoses
- Cutaneous bleeding
- Mucosal site bleeding
- Epistaxis
- Gingival bleeding
- Hematuria
- Intracranial hemorrhage (rare)

Laboratory Testing

- Normal or slightly elevated thrombopoietin
- Decreased hemoglobin, hematocrit, platelets
- Prolonged bleeding time
- Peripheral blood smear for abnormal platelets
- *Helicobacter pylori* testing
- HIV, HCV testing

Patient Encounter 2, Part 1: ITP

GH is a 4-year-old boy who presents with gingival bleeding and hematuria for 1 day. His vital signs and physical exam are within normal limits, except for noticeable mucosal ecchymoses in the oral and nasal cavities.

What information is suggestive of immune thrombocytopenic purpura (ITP)?

What additional information do you need to create a treatment plan for this patient?

Patient Encounter 2, Part 2: ITP

Meds at Home

- Albuterol inhaler one to two inhalations as needed for asthma

PMH: Mild intermittent asthma, recent upper respiratory disease with rhinorrhea, fever, and vomiting (per mother's report)

Labs:

- Platelet count: $60 \times 10^3/mm^3$ ($60 \times 10^9/L$) (normal 140–$440 \times 10^3/ mm^3$ [140–$440 \times 10^9/L$])
- aPTT: 28 seconds (normal 25–40 seconds)
- PT: 12 seconds (normal 10–12 seconds)
- Hemoglobin 12.5 g/dL (125 g/L or 7.75 mmol/L) (normal 13.8–17.2 g/dL or 138–172 g/L or 8.6–10.7 mmol/L)
- Bleeding time 8 minutes (normal 3–7 minutes)

Given this additional information, is this patient's presentation consistent with ITP?

What is the likely etiology of this patient's ITP?

Identify your treatment goals for this patient.

are equally affected. Childhood ITP typically resolves on its own within 4 to 6 weeks without major sequelae. ITP occurs in 1 to 2 of every 1,000 pregnancies. In pregnant women with pre-existing ITP, both maternal and fetal complications may occur, requiring separate management.[28]

Pathophysiology

In ITP, IgG autoantibodies bind to platelet-antigen complex and are cleared from the blood via binding to mononuclear phagocytes by macrophage Fcγ receptor, leading to thrombocytopenia. Platelet survival time is significantly shorter in patients with ITP (from minutes to 2–3 days). Sequestration in spleen, liver, and bone marrow is partially responsible for decreased platelet survival. Megakaryopoiesis may be reduced due to antibody binding to megakaryocyte precursors in the bone marrow.

Treatment

▶ Desired Outcomes

The main goal of ITP treatment is to maintain the platelet count (greater than 20–$30 \times 10^3/mm^3$ [20–$30 \times 10^9/L$]) while awaiting spontaneous or treatment-induced remission.[29]

▶ General Approach to Treatment

⑤ *The treatment of ITP is determined by the symptom severity* (Table 67–9). *In some cases, no therapy is needed.* The initial treatment of children with ITP is controversial because 30% to 70% of cases resolve spontaneously irrespective of pharmacologic intervention. Currently, therapy is indicated in children with platelet counts less thaln 10 to 20×10^3 mm³ (10–$20 \times 10^9/L$) because most intracranial hemorrhages occur when platelets are in this range.[30] In adults, treatment is indicated when platelet counts are less than 20 to $30 \times 10^3/mm^3$ (20–$30 \times 10^9/L$) or less than $50 \times 10^3/mm^3$ ($50 \times 10^9/L$) with serious bleeding or risk factors for bleeding.[31]

Table 67–9

Guidelines for the Initial Management of ITP

Greater than 50×10^3 platelets/mm³ (50×10^9/L)	No treatment
$30–50 \times 10^3$ platelets/mm³ ($30–50 \times 10^9$/L)	Prednisone (1 mg/kg/day) or no treatment
Less than 30×10^3 platelets/mm³ (30×10^9/L)	Prednisone (1–1.5 mg/kg/day) Anti-D immune globulin (75 mcg/kg)
Hemorrhage	Platelet transfusion IVIg (1 g/kg/day for 2–3 days) Methylprednisolone (1 g/day for 3 days)

▶ Nonpharmacologic Therapy

In adults, splenectomy is generally considered after 3 to 6 months if the patient continues to require 10 to 20 mg/day of prednisone to maintain the platelet count greater than 30×10^3/mm³ 30×10^9/L) or within 6 weeks of diagnosis in nonbleeding patients with platelet counts of less than 10×10^3/mm³ (10×10^9/L) despite treatment. Splenectomy may also be considered for urgent treatment of neurologic symptoms or for managing relapse despite an adequate trial of corticosteroids, intravenous immunoglobulin (IVIg), or anti-Rh(D). Even though individual patient response cannot be predicted, approximately two-thirds of refractory adult patients have a favorable response to splenectomy within several days; however, 30% to 40% will have no response or will experience a relapse some time after splenectomy. In children, splenectomy is usually reserved due to the self-limited nature of ITP and fear of infectious complications of splenectomy. Splenectomy is recommended in children with ITP duration greater than one year with significant bleeding symptoms and platelet counts less than 10×10^3/mm³ (10×10^9/L), or platelet counts 10 to 30×10^3/mm³ ($10–30 \times 10^9$/L) with bleeding symptoms. Between 70% and 80% of children attain complete remission following splenectomy. Laproscopic splenectomy is preferable to open splenectomy because it speeds the recovery and shortens the duration of hospitalization. The major drawback of splenectomy is bacterial sepsis, occurring at incidence rates of approximately 1%. Immunization with *Haemophilus influenzae* type b, pneumococcal, and meningiococcal vaccines is indicated in all patients two weeks prior to splenectomy.[29]

▶ Pharmacologic Therapy

The general approach to initial management of ITP is summarized in Table 67–9.

Glucocorticoids Glucocorticoids may decrease splenic sequestration of antibody-coated platelets, diminish antibody generation by the spleen and the bone marrow, and increase platelet output by the bone marrow. In adults, the response rate to oral prednisone (1–1.5 mg/kg/day) is 50% to 75% with patients usually responding within the first three weeks. In children, severe life-threatening bleeding is treated with either high-dose oral (4–8 mg/kg/day prednisone) or parenteral (30 mg/kg/day methylprednisolone) glucocorticoids.

IV Immunoglobulin (IVIg) IVIg impairs the clearance of platelets coated with IgG by activating inhibitory receptor $FcR\gamma IIb$. It is generally indicated in emergencies, during pregnancy, and in chronic management of patients refractory to other treatment options. Roughly 80% of adults will respond to IVIg (1 g/kg/day for 2–3 days), but remission usually is not sustained. In adults, use of IVIg is reserved for severe life-threatening bleeding, platelet counts less than 5×10^3/mm³ (5×10^9/L), with extensive purpura. If treatment is indicated in children, a single dose of IVIg (0.8 g/kg) is usually effective, although other dosing regimens can also be used (1 g/kg × 1 day; 2 g/kg total dose over 2–5 days). IVIg use is complicated by many serious adverse effects and high cost.

Anti-Rh(D) Anti-Rh(D) can be used only in Rh(D)-positive patients. It is as efficacious as IVIg and is generally less expensive. The indications for use of anti-Rh(D) are identical to those for IVIg. Anti-Rh(D) is desirable form of treatment in chronic ITP when the goal is to circumvent long-term exposure to corticosteroids. At doses of 25 to 75 mcg/kg/day, anti-Rh(D) may increase the platelet count in about 70% to 80% of children with acute and chronic ITP. Response to anti-Rh(D) lasts about 3 to 5 weeks, and substantial numbers of patients treated repetitively with Rh(D) can postpone or avoid splenectomy.

Immunosuppressants Immunosuppressant therapy is generally utilized for patients with platelet counts below 20×10^3/mm³ (20×10^9/L) who are refractory to or intolerant of all other ITP treatments. Azathioprine and cyclophosphamide produce response rates of 20% to 40% in adult patients who are treated for 2 to 6 months. Other medications used in ITP include vincristine, vinblastine, cyclosporine, and rituximab; due to major toxicities, their use is reserved for refractory ITP.

Thrombopoietic Growth Factors New treatment options for ITP include a novel thrombopoiesis-stimulating protein and a small-molecule thrombopoietin (TPO) receptor agonist. These agents stimulate the bone marrow to make enough platelets to overcome the body's premature destruction of platelets. Romiplostim and eltrombopag are two new therapeutic agents that have been recently approved by the FDA for the treatment of thrombocytopenia in patients with chronic ITP who have had an insufficient response to corticosteroids, immunoglobulins, or splenectomy.

Romiplostim is a TPO peptide mimetic that binds to and activates the human TPO receptor. As a once weekly subcutaneous injection, romiplostim stimulates megakaryopoiesis resulting in enhanced platelet production. Initial dose of romiplostim is based on the actual body weight, adjusted weekly by increments of 1 mcg/kg until a maximum of 10 mcg/kg the patient achieves a platelet count greater than or equal to 50×10^3/mm³ (50×10^9/L) as necessary to reduce the risk for bleeding. In clinical studies, most patients

Patient Encounter 2, Part 3: ITP: Creating a Care Plan for ITP patient

Based on the information presented, create a care plan for this patient's ITP.

Table 67–10

Conditions Associated with TTP

- Infections
  Bacterial, fungal, viral, atypical
- Transplantation
  Solid organ or bone marrow
- Malignancy
- Pregnancy
- Collagen vascular diseases
- Medications
  Antineoplastic agents, ticlopidine, clopidogrel, antibiotics, immunosuppressants, others

---

who responded to romiplostim achieved and maintained platelet counts greater than or equal to $50 \times 10^3/mm^3$ ($50 \times 10^9/L$) with a median dose of 2 mcg/kg. Both agents need to be discontinued if platelet counts do not increase after 4 weeks at a maximum dose. Eltrombopag is a once-daily oral nonpeptide thrombopoietin receptor agonist with a low immunogenic potential that stimulates megakaryocyte proliferation and differentiation.

For most patients, the initial dose of eltrombopag is 50 mg once daily. The daily dose is subsequently adjusted to a maximum dose of 75 mg daily, in order to achieve and maintain a platelet count greater than or equal to $50 \times 10^3/mm^3$ ($50 \times 10^9/L$) in order to reduce the risk for bleeding.

Romiplostim and eltrombopag are effective in increasing platelet counts in patients with ITP and can be used in combination with therapies that inhibit platelet destruction. While usually well tolerated, a number of rare but serious risks have been reported, including; changes in the bone marrow, worsened thrombocytopenia and the risk of bleeding after cessation of the medication, thrombotic/thromboembolic complications, and worsening of blood cancers. Eltrombopag carries a black-box warning regarding hepatic toxicity. It is also associated with development of cataracts and has multiple drug–drug interactions. To enhance patient safety, both romiplostim and eltrombopag are available only through restricted access programs. For both programs, each institution must enroll in the program to receive drug and training kits and only prescribers, pharmacists, and patients registered with the program are able to prescribe, dispense, and receive the product, respectively.

Outcome Evaluation

- Monitor platelet counts as indicated clinically.
- Goal of therapy is to maintain platelet count greater than or equal to $30 \times 10^3/mm^3$ ($30 \times 10^9/L$).
- Monitor for signs and symptoms of bleeding.

THROMBOTIC THROMBOCYTOPENIC PUPURA

Etiology and Epidemiology

Thrombotic thrombocytopenic purpura (TTP) is a severe systemic disorder characterized by the thrombi formation within the circulation that results in the platelet consumption and subsequent thrombocytopenia. Acute idiopathic TTP is more common in women and African Americans, and most frequently occurs in people between 30- and 40-years-old. The estimated annual incidence of TTP is 3.8 cases per million.[32] Common conditions associated with TTP are summarized in Table 67–10.

Pathophysiology

Endothelial cells normally synthesize vWF in the form of a high–molecular weight multimer composed of smaller identical monomers. Each monomer is able to bind platelets, and the number of monomers on the vWF multimer is directly proportional to its platelet-binding capacity. Consequently, particularly adherent ultralarge molecules of the vWF (ULvWF) are broken down to smaller size by vWF-cleaving proteases such as ADAMTS13 (a disintegrin and metalloprotease with thrombospondin type 1 repeats) to avoid undesired clot formation. TTP results from genetic or acquired deficiency in the vWF-cleaving protease ADAMTS13 activity. This, in turn, elevates circulating levels of ultralarge molecules of the factor (ULvWF) leading to inappropriate platelet agglutination. Thrombocytopenia develops because the rate of aggregated platelet consumption is faster than megakaryocyte bone marrow production. Microangiopathic hemolytic anemia generally follows as a consequence of red blood cell damage by platelet clumps occluding the microcirculation. Occlusive ischemia of the brain or GI tract is common, and renal dysfunction may occur.

Treatment

▶ *Desired Outcomes*

The main goal of TTP treatment is to prevent end-organ damage.

▶ *Nonpharmacologic Therapy*

❻ *The present standard of treatment for TTP is urgent plasma exchange (PEX). If PEX is unavailable, treatment with plasma infusion and glucocorticoids is indicated until PEX is available.*[33]

Plasma Exchange The procedure involves removal of the patient's plasma and its substitution by donor plasma. In this manner, circulating antibody inhibitor of ADAMTS13 is

Clinical Presentation and Diagnosis of TTP

Typical Pentad of Symptoms (Rare That All Five Are Present)[a]

1. Thrombocytopenia
   - Thrombocytopenic purpura
   - Bleeding
2. Fever
3. Microangiopathic hemolytic anemia
4. Neurologic symptoms
   - Headache, confusion, difficulty speaking, transient paralysis, numbness
5. Renal abnormalities
   - Proteinuria, hematuria, mild renal insufficiency

Laboratory Testing

- Decreased hemoglobin, hematocrit, and platelets
- Peripheral blood smear for schistocytes
- Decreased serum haptoglobin
- Elevated lactate dehydrogenase (LDH)
- Elevated indirect bilirubin level
- Elevated reticulocyte count
- Normal PT and aPTT
- Elevated urine protein, red blood cells, and/or serum creatinine

[a]TTP diagnosis can be based on the presence of thrombocytopenia and microangiopathic hemolytic anemia in the absence of other possible causes

Patient Encounter 3, Part 1: TTP

A 58-year-old African American female presented to her primary care physician complaining of headache, weakness, fever, chills, chest pain, nausea, vomiting, and hematuria. She had a diagnostic cardiac catheterization performed 10 days ago and oral clopidogrel 75 mg daily was prescribed by her cardiologist after the test.

What information is suggestive of thrombotic thrombocytopenic purpura (TTP)?

What additional information do you need to create a treatment plan for this patient?

Patient Encounter 3, Part 2: TTP

Meds at Home: Clopidogrel 75 mg orally daily; metoprolol tartrate 25 mg orally twice a day; zolpidem 10 mg orally at bedtime as needed

PE: Wt 65 kg (143 lb)

Labs:

- Platelet count: $9 \times 10^3/mm^3$ ($9 \times 10^9/L$) (normal $140-440 \times 10^3/mm^3$ [$140-440 \times 10^9/L$])
- aPTT: 38 seconds (normal 25–40 seconds)
- PT: 10 seconds (normal 10–12 seconds)
- Haptoglobin 15 mg/dL (150 mg/L) (normal 30–200 mg/dL or 300–2,000 mg/L)
- LDH 1,950 units/L (32.5 μkat/L) (normal 100–250 units/L, or 1.67–4.17 μkat/L)
- Hemoglobin 6 g/dL (60 g/L or 3.72 mmol/L) (normal 12.1–15.1 g/dL or 121–151 g/L or 7.5–9.36 mmol/L)
- Blood peripheral smear: numerous schistocytes (11–12 per high power field)

Given this additional information, is this patient's presentation consistent with TTP?

What is the likely etiology of this patient's TTP?

Identify your treatment goals for this patient.

removed and enzyme is replenished. PEX involves placement of two IV lines (cannulae) into two separate veins. Blood removed through one cannula is centrifuged to separate the blood cells from the plasma. The blood cells are mixed subsequently with donor plasma and returned to the patient via the second cannula. The goal is to exchange 1 to 1.5 plasma volumes (40–60 mL/kg). The procedure generally is repeated daily until neurologic symptoms resolve and normal LDH and platelet counts are maintained for several days. After complete remission is achieved, PEX frequency can be reduced to every other day for an additional few days, with subsequent PEX discontinuation and close patient follow-up. When PEX is started immediately upon diagnosis, remission and survival rates at six months are approximately 80%. Although generally considered safe, complications from catheter insertion or catheter infection may occur and include hemorrhage, pneumothorax, sepsis, and thrombosis. Allergic reactions to plasma can cause severe hypotension and hypoxia.[33]

Splenectomy

Splenectomy is reserved for patients with frequently relapsing disease, refractory to PEX or immunosuppressive therapy.

▶ Pharmacologic Therapy

Corticosteroids Corticosteroids can be used for their immunosuppressive effect in combination with PEX; however, they are not efficacious as monotherapy in TTP.

Patient Encounter 3, Part 3: TTP: Creating a Care Plan

Based on the information presented, create a care plan for this patient's TTP.

Patient Care and Monitoring

1. Obtain a complete history.

2. In a patient presenting with a bleeding or clotting disorder, an initial evaluation should include bleeding time, prothrombin time (PT), activated partial thromboplastin time (aPTT), thrombin time, and platelet count.

   - Activated partial thromboplastin time: aPTT is performed by adding calcium phospholipids and kaolin to citrated blood and measures the time required for a fibrin clot to form. In this manner, aPTT measures the activity of intrinsic and common pathways. Prolongation of aPTT may be due to a deficiency or inhibitor for factors II, V, VIII, IX, X, XI, and XII. It also may be due to heparin, direct thrombin inhibitors, vitamin K deficiency, liver disease, or lupus anticoagulant.

   - Prothrombin time: PT is performed by adding thromboplastin (tissue) factor and calcium to citrate-anticoagulated plasma, recalcifying the plasma, and measuring the clotting time. The major utility of PT is to measure the activity of the vitamin K–dependent factors II, VII, and X. The PT is used in evaluation of liver disease, to monitor warfarin anticoagulant effect, and to assess vitamin K deficiency.

   - Thrombin time is an assessment of the time required for the appearance of the fibrin clot after thrombin is added to plasma. It may be affected by thrombin inhibitors or fibrinogen abnormalities. Most commonly, thrombin time is used to monitor fibrinolytic therapy.

   - Bleeding time indicates how well platelets interact with blood vessel walls to form blood clots by assessing the length of time to arrest the bleeding after a standardized skin cut. The bleeding time is prolonged in thrombocytopenia, fibrinogen disorders, and collagen defects.

3. After a diagnosis is made, institute specific therapy.

4. Monitor resolution of laboratory and clinical symptoms with treatment.

The most commonly used agents are methylprednisolone 1 g/day IV for 3 days and prednisone 1 to 2 mg/kg/day orally for the duration of PEX therapy.

Immunosuppressants TTP that fails to respond adequately to PEX can be treated with immunosuppressive agents. Cytotoxic immunosuppressive therapies with potential benefit in refractory TTP include vincristine, cyclophosphamide, azathioprine, rituximab, and the CHOP combination regimen (cyclophosphamide, doxorubicin, vincristine, and prednisone).[33]

Outcome Evaluation

Monitor platelet counts, hemoglobin, and LDH.

Abbreviations Introduced in This Chapter

ADAMTS13	A disintegrin and metalloprotease with thrombospondin type 1 repeats (vWF-cleaving metalloprotease)
BU	Bethesda units
DDAVP	1-Desamino-8-D-arginine vasopressin (desmopressin acetate)
DIC	Disseminated intravascular coagulation
FFP	Fresh-frozen plasma
HCV	Hepatitis C virus
ICH	Intracranial hemorrhage
ITP	Immune thrombocytopenic purpura
IVIg	Intravenous immunoglobulin
PCC	Prothrombin complex concentrate
PEX	Plasma exchange
rFVIIa	Recombinant factor VIIa
RICD	Recessively inherited coagulation disorders
TTP	Thrombotic thrombocytopenic purpura
ULvWF	Ultralarge molecules of vWF
vWD	von Willebrand's disease
vWF	von Willebrand's factor

 Self-assessment questions and answers are available at *http://www.mhpharmacotherapy.com/pp.html.*

REFERENCES

1. Soucie JM, Evatt B, Jackson D. Occurrence of hemophilia in the United States. The Hemophilia Surveillance System Project Investigators. Am J Hematol 1998;59:288–294.

2. Bolton-Maggs PH, Pasi KJ. Haemophilias A and B. Lancet 2003;361: 1801–1809.

3. Stobart K, Iorio A, Wu JK. Clotting factor concentrates given to prevent bleeding and bleeding-related complications in people with hemophilia A or B. Cochrane Database Syst Rev 2006:CD003429.

4. Astermark J, Petrini P, Tengborn L, et al. Primary prophylaxis in severe haemophilia should be started at an early age but can be individualized. Br J Haematol 1999;105:1109–1113.

5. Berntorp E. Prophylactic therapy for haemophilia: Early experience. Haemophilia 2003; 9(Suppl 1):5–9; discussion 9.

6. Blanchette VS, Manco-Johnson M, Santagostino E, et al. Optimizing factor prophylaxis for the haemophilia population: Where do we stand? Haemophilia 2004;10(Suppl 4):97–104.

7. MASAC Recommendation Concerning Prophylaxis (Regular Administration of Clotting factor Concentrate to Prevent Bleeding). MASAC Document #179. National Hemophilia Foundation 2007; 116 West 32nd Street, New York, NY 10001.

8. Manco-Johnson MJ, Abshire TC, Shapiro AD, et al. Prophylaxis versus episodic treatment to prevent joint disease in boys with severe hemophilia. N Engl J Med 2007;357:535–544.

9. Fiebig EW, Busch MP. Emerging infections in transfusion medicine. Clin Lab Med 2004;24:797–823.

10. Srivastava A. Optimizing clotting factor replacement therapy in hemophilia: A global need. Hematology 2005;10(Suppl 1):229–230.

11. MASAC Recommendations Concerning the Treatment of Hemophilia and Other Bleeding Disorders. MASAC Document #182. National Hemophilia Foundation 2008; 116 West 32nd Street, New York, NY 10001.

12. Mannucci PM, Tuddenham EG. The hemophilias-from royal genes to gene therapy. N Engl J Med 2001;344:1773–1779.

13. Shord SS, Lindley CM. Coagulation products and their uses. Am J Health Syst Pharm 2000;57:1403–1417; quiz 1418–1420.

14. Rodeghiero F, Castaman G, Dini E. Epidemiological investigation of the prevalence of von Willebrand's disease. Blood 1987;69:454–459.

15. Werner EJ, Broxson EH, Tucker EL, et al. Prevalence of von Willebrand disease in children: A multiethnic study. J Pediatr 1993;123:893–898.

16. Nichols WL, Hultin MB, James AH, et al. von Willebrand disease (vWD): Evidence-based diagnosis and management guidelines, the National Heart, Lung, and Blood Institute (NHLBI) Expert Panel report (USA). Haemophilia 2008;14:171–232.

17. Mannucci PM. Treatment of von Willebrand's disease. N Engl J Med 2004;351:683–694.

18. Friedman KD, Rodgers GM. Inherited coagulation disorders. In: Glader B, ed. Wintrobe's Clinical Hematology, Vol. 2. Philadelphia: Lippincott Williams and Wilkins, 2004:1619–1667.

19. Mannucci PM, Duga S, Peyvandi F. Recessively inherited coagulation disorders. Blood 2004;104:1243–1252.

20. Roberts HR, Escobar MA. Other clotting factor deficiencies. In: Hoffman R, Benz EJJ, Shattil SJ, eds. Hematology: Basic Principles and Practice. Philadelphia: Elsevier, 2005:2047–2069.

21. Okajima K, Sakamoto Y, Uchiba M. Heterogeneity in the incidence and clinical manifestations of disseminated intravascular coagulation: A study of 204 cases. Am J Hematol 2000;65:215–222.

22. Levi M. Disseminated intravascular coagulation. Crit Care Med 2007;35:2191–2195.

23. Rodgers GM. Acquired coagulation disorders. In: Greer JP, Foerster J, Lukens JN, et al., eds. Wintrobe's Clinical Hematology, Vol. 2. Philadelphia: Lippincott Williams and Wilkins, 2004:1669.

24. Levi M. Disseminated intravascular coagulation: What's new? Crit Care Clin 2005;21:449–467.

25. Bick RL. Disseminated intravascular coagulation: Pathophysiological mechanisms and manifestations. Semin Thromb Hemost 1998;24:3–18.

26. de Pont AC, Bakhtiari K, Hutten BA, et al. Recombinant human activated protein C resets thrombin generation in patients with severe sepsis—A case control study. Crit Care 2005;9:R490–R497.

27. Warren BL, Eid A, Singer P, et al. Caring for the critically ill patient. High-dose antithrombin III in severe sepsis: A randomized controlled trial. JAMA 2001;286:1869–1878.

28. Frederiksen H, Schmidt K. The incidence of idiopathic thrombocytopenic purpura in adults increases with age. Blood 1999;94:909–913.

29. George JN, Woolf SH, Raskob GE, et al. Idiopathic thrombocytopenic purpura: A practice guideline developed by explicit methods for the American Society of Hematology. Blood 1996;88:3–40.

30. Medeiros D, Buchanan GR. Major hemorrhage in children with idiopathic thrombocytopenic purpura: Immediate response to therapy and long-term outcome. J Pediatr 1998;133:334–339.

31. Cines DB, Blanchette VS. Immune thrombocytopenic purpura. N Engl J Med 2002;346:995–1008.

32. Furlan M, Robles R, Galbusera M, et al. von Willebrand factor-cleaving protease in thrombotic thrombocytopenic purpura and the hemolytic-uremic syndrome. N Engl J Med 1998;339:1578–1584.

33. Sadler J, Poncz M. Antibody-mediated thrombotic disorders: Idiopathic thrombotic thrombocytopenic purpura and heparin-induced thrombocytopenia. In: Lichtman M, ed. Williams Hematology. New York: McGraw-Hill, 2006:2031–2054.

68 Sickle Cell Anemia

Tracy M. Hagemann and Teresa V. Lewis

LEARNING OBJECTIVES

● **Upon completion of the chapter, the reader will be able to:**

1. Explain the underlying causes of sickle cell disease (SCD) and their relationship to patient signs and symptoms.

2. Identify the typical characteristics of SCD as well as symptoms that indicate complicated disease

3. Identify the desired therapeutic outcomes for patients with SCD.

4. Recommend appropriate pharmacotherapy and nonpharmacotherapy interventions for patients with SCD.

5. Recognize when chronic maintenance therapy is indicated for a patient with SCD.

6. Describe the components of a monitoring plan to assess effectiveness and adverse effects of pharmacotherapy for SCD.

7. Educate patients about the disease state, appropriate therapy, and drug therapy required for effective treatment and prevention of complications.

KEY CONCEPTS

❶ Sickle cell disease (SCD) is an inherited disorder caused by a defect in the gene for hemoglobin. Patients may have one defective gene (sickle cell trait [SCT]) or two defective genes (SCD).

❷ Although most often seen in persons of African ancestry, other ethnic groups can be affected.

❸ SCD involves multiple organ systems.

❹ Prophylaxis against pneumococcal infection reduces death during childhood.

❺ Hydroxyurea has been shown to decrease the incidence of painful crises. However, the patient population that receives hydroxyurea should be carefully monitored.

❻ Chronic transfusion therapy programs have been shown to be beneficial in decreasing the occurrence of stroke in children with SCD.

❼ Patients with fever greater than 38.5°C (101.3°F) should be evaluated and appropriate antibiotics should include coverage for encapsulated organisms, especially pneumococcal.

❽ Pain episodes can usually be managed at home. Hospitalized patients usually require parenteral analgesics. Analgesic options include opioids, nonsteroidal anti-inflammatory agents, and acetaminophen. The patient characteristics and the severity of the crisis should determine the choice of agent and regimen.

INTRODUCTION

❶ *"Sickle cell syndrome" refers to a collection of autosomal recessive genetic disorders that are characterized by the presence of at least one sickle hemoglobin gene (HbS).*[1,2]

Sickle cell disease (SCD) is a chronic illness that is associated with frequent crisis episodes. Acute complications are unpredictable and potentially fatal. Common symptoms include excruciating musculoskeletal pain, life-threatening pneumonia-like illness, cerebrovascular accidents, and splenic and renal dysfunction.[2] As the disease progresses, patients may develop organ damage from the combination of hemolysis and infarction. Because of the complexity and severity of SCD, it is imperative that patients have access to comprehensive care with providers who have a good understanding of the countless clinical presentations and the management options of this disorder.

EPIDEMIOLOGY AND ETIOLOGY

● Sickle cell trait (SCT) is the heterozygous form (HbAS) of SCD in which a person inherits one normal adult hemoglobin (HbA) gene and one sickle hemoglobin (HbS) gene. These individuals are carriers of the SCT and are usually asymptomatic.[2] Symptomatic disease is seen in homozygous and compound heterozygous genotypes of SCD. Sickle cell anemia (SCA) is the homozygous (HbSS) state of SCD.[2] It is the most common and severe form of SCD. Compound heterozygosity is seen when individuals inherit one copy of the mutation that causes HbS and one copy of another abnormal hemoglobin gene. Compound heterozygosity may also include the coinheritance of HbS and one of the many different mutations of β-thalasssemia (HbSβ^0-thalassemia and HbSβ^+-thalassemia).[1-3] SCA affects both males and females equally because it is not a sex-linked disease.

❷ *Nine percent of African Americans possess the SCT and 1 in 600 has HbSS.*[4] Two thousand infants are identified with SCD annually in the United States.[5] For every infant diagnosed with SCD, 50 are identified as carriers.[5] HbSS (approximately 45%) is the most common genotypic expression, followed by HbSC (approximately 25%), HbSβ^+-thalassemia (approximately 8%), and HbSβ^0-thalassemia (approximately 2%). Other variants account for less than 1% of patients.[2,5]

Having the sickle hemoglobin gene protects heterozygous carriers from succumbing to *Plasmodium falciparum* (malaria) infection.[1] The microorganism cannot parasitize abnormal red blood cells (RBCs) as easily as normal RBCs. Consequently, persons with heterozygous sickle gene (SCT) have a selective advantage in tropical regions where malaria is endemic.

The highest incidence of SCD is seen in those with African heritage, but SCD also affects persons of Indian, Saudi Arabian, Mediterranean, South and Central American, and Caribbean ancestry.[5,6]

Normal adult hemoglobin (HbA) is composed of two α-chains and two β-chains ($\alpha2\beta2$).[3] A single substitution of the amino acid valine for glutamic acid at position 6 of the β-polypeptide chain is responsible for the production of a defective form of hemoglobin called sickle hemoglobin (HbS).[1] Different genetic mutations encode for other hemoglobin variants such as hemoglobin C (HbC). HbC is produced by the substitution of lysine for glutamic acid at the sixth amino acid position in the β-globulin chain.[3] The α-chains of HbS, HbA, and HbC are structurally identical. The chemical differences in the β-chain are responsible for RBC sickling and its associated sequelae.

SCA is the homozygous (HbSS) state of SCD in which individuals inherit the mutant hemoglobin gene (HbS) from both parents. The progeny of two carriers will have a 25% probability of having SCD and a 50% risk of being a carrier (Fig. 68–1). β-Thalassemia can be found in conjunction with HbS. Patients with HbSS and HbSβ^0-thalassemia do not have normal β-globulin production and usually have a more severe course than those with HbSC and HbSβ^+-thalassemia. ❸ *SCD involves multiple organ systems, and its clinical manifestations vary greatly between and among genotypes.*

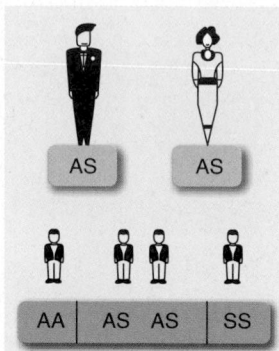

FIGURE 68–1. Sickle gene inheritance scheme for both parents with sickle cell trait (SCT). Possibilities with each pregnancy: 25% normal (AA); 50% SCT (AS); 25% sickle cell anemia (SS). (A, normal hemoglobin; S, sickle hemoglobin.) (From Chan CYJ, Moore R. Sickle cell disease. In: DiPiro JT, Talbert RL, Yee GC, et al., eds. Pharmacotherapy: A Pathophysiologic Approach, 7th ed. New York: McGraw-Hill, 2008.)

PATHOPHYSIOLOGY
Erythrocyte Physiology

A review of RBC physiology is important to understand the pathophysiology of SCD. Pediatric RBCs possess normal hemoglobin concentrations between 9 and 18.5 g/dL (90–185 g/L or 5.6–11.5 mmol/L), depending on the age of the child.[7] Adult RBCs contain 12 to 15.5 g/dL (120–155 g/L or 7.4–9.6 mmol/L) hemoglobin.[7] The predominant form of hemoglobin is adult hemoglobin or HbA (96%). Other forms of hemoglobin include HbA2 and fetal hemoglobin (HbF). HbA2 makes up less than 1% of hemoglobin in newborns. In adults, HbA2 constitutes approximately 1.6% to 3.5%.[7] Fetal hemoglobin (HbF) is present primarily in fetal RBCs (60–90%), whereas adult RBC's contain less than 1% HbF.[7] HbF is the primary oxygen transport protein in the fetus. After birth, only a small proportion of red cell clones remain to produce HbF. The elasticity of young erythroid cells enables them to deform and squeeze through capillaries (Fig. 68–2). As RBCs age, mean corpuscular hemoglobin concentration (MCHC) increases, deformability decreases, and the cells are removed by the reticuloendothelial system.

Impaired circulation, destruction of RBCs, and vascular stasis are three known problems that are primarily responsible for the clinical manifestations of SCD (Fig. 68–3).

Sickle Hemoglobin Polymerization

The primary event in the molecular pathogenesis of SCD involves polymerization of deoxygenated HbS. Since RBCs are packaged with such a high concentration of hemoglobin (32–34 g/dL, 320–340 g/L, or 19.9–21 mmol/L), it is important that the proteins be extremely soluble.[1] HbS carries oxygen normally, and when oxygenated, the solubility of HbS and HbA are the same. Once the oxygen is unloaded to the tissues HbS solubility decreases. This promotes hydrophobic interactions between the hemoglobin molecules and polymerization, which leads to the distortion of the RBC into the characteristic crescent or sickle shape.[1] Polymerization of deoxy-HbS is influenced by the degree of red cell deoxygenation, MCHC, temperature, intracellular pH, intraerythrocytic HbS concentration, and intracellular HbF concentration.[1]

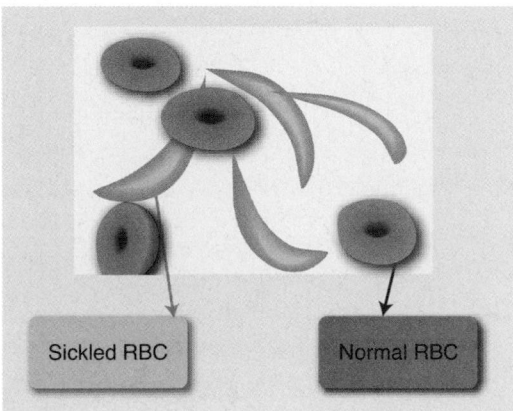

FIGURE 68–2. Elongated sickle-shaped and normal discoid-shaped red blood cells. (From Chan CYJ, Moore R. Sickle cell disease. In: DiPiro JT, Talbert RL, Yee GC, et al., eds. Pharmacotherapy: A Pathophysiologic Approach, 6th ed. New York: McGraw-Hill, 2005: 1856.)

Viscosity of Erythrocytes and Sickle Cell Adhesion

When HbS becomes reoxygenated, the polymers within the RBCs disappear, and the cells eventually return to normal shape. Vasoocclussion is caused by a combination of factors. Repeated assaults on RBCs from sickling and unsickling can lead to cell membrane damage, loss of membrane flexibility, and rearrangement of surface phospholipids. Damage to cell membranes can interfere with ion transport, leading to loss of potassium and water. This creates dehydrated, dense sickle cells, and irreversible sickle cells (ISCs). ISCs are the densest cells, and they tend to remain sickled even when oxygenated. Rigid ISCs can become trapped in microvasculature, leading to cell fragmentation and chronic hemolysis, thus contributing to short survival of RBCs. The life span of sickled RBCs is markedly shorter (10–20 days) than that of normal RBCs (100–120 days). As intracellular membrane viscosity of HbS-containing RBCs increases, blood viscosity increases, which further contributes to vasoocclussion.[8] There is also increasing evidence that suggest sickle cells adhere to vascular endothelium.[1,8] The combined effects of decreased RBC deformability, slow transit through microcirculation, and adhesion to vascular endothelium contribute to obstruction of small and sometimes large blood vessels. The resulting local tissue hypoxia can accentuate the pathologic process of SCD.

Protective Hemoglobin Types

Fetal hemoglobin binds oxygen more tightly than HbA, and it has a decreased propensity to sickling. HbA2 also possesses

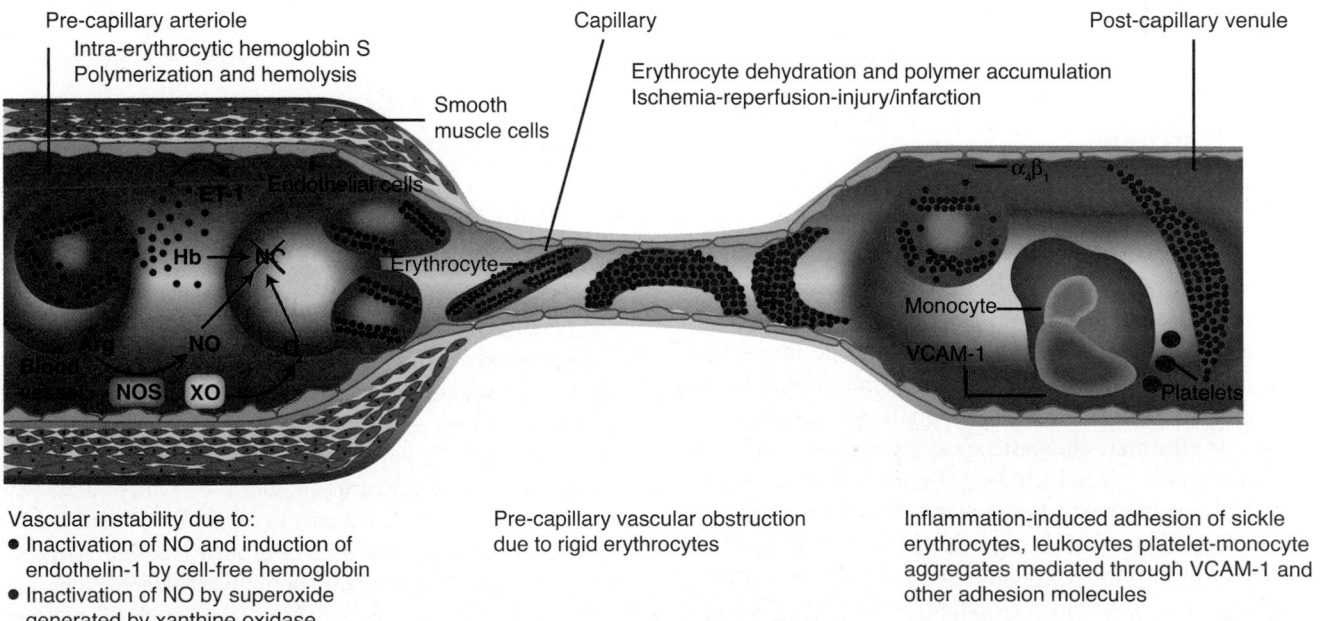

FIGURE 68–3. Pathophysiology of SCD. (Arg, arginine; ET-1, endothelin-1; Hb, hemoglobin; NO, nitric oxide; NOS, nitrous oxide synthase; VCAM-1, vascular cell adhesion molecule 1; XO, xanthine oxidase.) (From Kato GJ, Gladwin MT. Sickle cell disease. In: Hall JB, Schmidt GA, Wood LDH, (eds.). Principles of Critical Care, 3rd ed. New York: McGraw-Hill, 2005:1658.)

Clinical Presentation and Diagnosis of SCT

General
- Generally asymptomatic

Symptoms
- Females may have frequent urinary tract infections

Signs
- Microscopic hematuria occurs rarely
- Gross hematuria may occur spontaneously or with heavy intensity exercise

Laboratory Tests
- Normal Hgb values

Clinical Presentation and Diagnosis of SCD

General
- Indentified by neonatal screening before 2 months of age

Symptoms
- Painful vasoocclusive crises are the hallmark of SCD
- Dactylitis (hand–foot syndrome) before age 1 year
- May develop infarction of the spleen, liver, bone marrow, kidney, brain, and lungs
- Gallstones
- Priapism in males
- Slow healing lower extremity ulcers after trauma or infection
- Weakness, fatigue

Signs
- Chronic hemolytic anemia is common
- Enlargement of spleen, and heart
- Scleral icterus

Laboratory Tests
- Hgb 7 to 10 g/dL (70–100 g/L or 4.3–6.2 mmol/L)
- Low HgF and increased reticulocytes, platelets, and WBCs
- Presence of sickled cells on blood smear (see Fig. 68–2)
- Neonatal screening: hemoglobin electrophoresis, isoelectric focusing, or DNA analysis

---

this characteristic but to a lesser extent. RBCs that contain HbF sickle less readily than cells without. ISCs are found to have low HbF concentrations. In some patients, higher HbF may ameliorate the disease.

Other Pathophysiologic Effects

Other factors may be responsible for the pathogenesis of some of the clinical features of SCD. Sickle cells can obstruct blood flow to the spleen leading to functional asplenia. Impaired splenic function can increase the propensity to infection by encapsulated organisms, particularly *Streptococcus pneumoniae*.[1] Additionally, coagulation abnormalities are not uncommon since almost every component of hemostasis is altered in SCD.

TREATMENT
Desired Outcomes

Multidisciplinary, regularly scheduled care is required over the lifetime of the SCD patient with the goal of reduction of complications and hospitalizations. Comprehensive care should include medical, educational, and psychosocial aspects as well as genetic and medication counseling.

Therapeutic interventions for SCD should be targeted at preventing and/or minimizing the symptoms related to the disease and its complications. The goals of treatment are to reduce or eliminate the patient's symptoms; decrease the frequency of sickle crises, including vasoocclusive pain crises; prevent the development of complications; and maintain or improve the quality of life through decreased hospitalizations and decreased morbidity. Specific therapeutic options may:

- Maintain or increase the hemoglobin level to the patient's baseline
- Increase the HbF concentration
- Decrease the HbS concentration
- Prevent infectious complications
- Prevent or effectively manage pain
- Prevent CNS damage, including stroke

General Approach to Treatment

Patients should be educated to recognize the signs and symptoms of complications that would require urgent evaluation. Patients and parents of children with SCD should be educated to read a thermometer properly and to seek immediate medical care when a fever develops or signs of infection occur. With acute illnesses, prompt evaluation is important as deterioration may occur rapidly. Fluid status should be monitored to avoid dehydration or overhydration, both of which may worsen complications of SCD. Patients in acute distress should maintain oxygen saturation at 92% or at their baseline. Any supplemental oxygen requirements should be evaluated.[5,9]

Nonpharmacologic Therapy

Patients should avoid smoking and excessive alcohol intake. Patients with SCD should maintain adequate hydration in order to help decrease blood viscosity, and should be educated to avoid extreme temperature changes and to dress properly in hot and cold weather. Physical exertion that leads to complications should be avoided.[5] Regular exams, including ophthalmic, renal, pulmonary, and cardiac function, are required to monitor for organ damage. A treatment overview is shown in Table 68–1.

Pharmacologic Therapy

▶ *Health Maintenance*

Immunizations Children with SCD should receive the required immunizations as recommended by the American Academy of Pediatrics and the Advisory Committee on Immunization Practices.[10] Additionally, influenza vaccine should be administered yearly to SCD patients 6 months of age and older, including adult patients. Any SCD patient who is scheduled for splenectomy should receive the vaccine for meningococcal disease if over 2 years of age.[11]

Because patient with SCD have impaired splenic function they are less adequately protected against encapsulated organisms such as *Streptococcus pneumoniae*, *Haemophilus influenzae* and *Salmonella*. ❹ *The use of pneumococcal vaccine in SCD patients has dramatically decreased the rates of morbidity and mortality; however, there are still groups of SCD children who continue to have high rates of invasive pneumococcal infections.*[12] Infection is the leading

cause of death in children younger than 3 years of age.[13,14] Two pneumococcal vaccines are available. The 7-valent conjugate vaccine (PCV 7: Prevnar) is indicated for infants and children and provides good protection against the seven most common isolates seen in this age-range. Administer the first dose of PCV 7 between 6 weeks and 6 months of age, followed by two additional doses at 2 month intervals and a fourth dose at 12 to 15 months of age. The 23-valent polysaccharide vaccine (PPV 23: Pneumovax 23) is indicated for children over 2 years of age and adults. Because PPV 23 is a polysaccharide vaccine, children less than two years of age do not respond well. PPV 23 contains the 23 most common isolates of *S. pneumoniae* seen in older children and adults. Because of the difference serotypes seen in the two vaccines, it is recommended that SCD children receive both vaccines, with a dose of PPV 23 administered after the child turns 2 years of age. The dose of PPV 23 should be separated from the last dose of PCV 7 by at least 2 months. An additional dose of PPV 23 should be considered in children 3 to 5 years of age to ensure antibody response. All adults with SCD should be vaccinated once with PPV 23 also. Because some children fall behind on their childhood vaccinations, a catch-up schedule is presented in Table 68–2.[11]

Penicillin ❹ *Children with SCD should receive prophylactic penicillin until at least the age of 5 years, even if they have been appropriately immunized with PCV 7 against pneumococcal*

Table 68–1		
Management of SCD		
	Options and Comments	
Health maintenance		
Infection prophylaxis	• Pneumococcal vaccines (PCV 7 and PPV 23) • Penicillin prophylaxis for children less than 5 years of age • Annual influenza vaccine	
Induction of fetal hemoglobin	• Hydroxyurea is the primary agent • Other agents are butyrates (arginine butyrate and sodium phenylbutyrate), decitabine, clotrimazole, and erythropoietin • Combination HbF inducers have been proposed	
Chronic transfusion therapy	• Primary indication: stroke prevention in pediatric patients • May also reduce pain crisis and acute chest syndrome • Goal: maintain HbS less than 30%	
Future prospects		
Transplantation	• May potentially cure the disease • Most experience is with HLA-matched donors; umbilical cord blood transplantation is being evaluated	
Crises and complications		
Fever and infection	• Broad-spectrum antibiotic: cefotaxime or ceftriaxone (clindamycin for cephalosporin allergy); vancomycin for staphylococcal and resistant pneumococcal organisms	
Stroke	• Fluids • Acetaminophen or ibuprofen for fever • Exchange transfusion • Initiate chronic transfusion therapy to prevent recurrent strokes	
Acute chest syndrome	• Broad-spectrum antibiotics (include *Mycoplasma* coverage) • Bronchodilator if wheezing or history of reactive airway disease • Fluids • Pain management • Transfusion	
Pain crisis	• Hydration • Analgesics	

Table 68–2	
Pneumococcal Immunization for Children With SCD	
	Recommended Schedule
Previously unvaccinated	
Age 2–6 months	PCV 7 (Prevnar): three doses 6–8 weeks apart; then 1 dose at 12–15 months
Age 7–11 months	PCV 7 (Prevnar): two doses 6–8 weeks apart; then 1 dose at 12–15 months
Age greater than or equal to 12–23 months	PCV 7 (Prevnar): two doses 6–8 weeks apart
Age 24–59 months	PCV 7 (Prevnar): two doses 6–8 weeks apart
	PPV 23 (Pneumovax): two doses; first dose at least 6–8 weeks after last PCV 7 dose; second dose 3–5 years after the first PPV 23 dose
Age 5 years or older	PCV 7 (Prevnar): one dose
	PPV 23 (Pneumovax): two doses; first dose at least 6–8 weeks after last PCV 7 dose; second dose 3–5 years (for those age 10 years or younger) or more than 5 years (for those age 10 years or older) after the first PPV 23 dose
Previously vaccinated	
Age 12–23 months, incomplete PCV 7 series	PCV 7 (Prevnar): two doses 6–8 weeks apart
Age 24–59 months, received four doses	PPV 23 (Pneumovax): two doses; first dose at least 6–8 weeks after last PCV 7 dose; second dose 3–5 years after the first PPV23 dose of PCV 7
Age 24–59 months, three doses of PCV 7 given before 24 months of age	PCV 7 (Prevnar): one dose
	PPV 23 (Pneumovax): two doses; first dose at least 6–8 weeks after last PCV 7 dose; second dose 3–5 years after the first PPV 23 dose
Age 24–59 months, 1 dose PPV 23 given	PCV 7 (Prevnar): two doses 6–8 weeks apart; first dose at least 8 weeks after PPV 23 dose
	PPV 23 (Pneumovax): second dose 3–5 years after first PPV 23
Age 5 years or older, received PPV 23	PCV 7 (Prevnar): one dose 6–8 weeks after PPV 23
	If only received one dose of PPV 23 (Pneumovax): Second dose 6–8 weeks after PCV 7 *and* 3–5 years (for those age 10 years or less) or more than 5 years (for those age 10 years or older) after the first PPV 23 dose

Patient Encounter 1

An 18-month-old female is presenting for a routine check-up. She was diagnosed with sickle cell anemia at birth, identified through neonatal screening. Today, her hemoglobin is 8.6 g/dL (86 g/L or 5.3 mmol/L) and she is afebrile.

What acute complications is she at risk for developing?

What preventative treatment should she receive?

What additional information do you need to know before creating a plan for this patient?

infections. Penicillin V potassium is typically initiated at age 2 months with a dose of 125 mg orally twice daily until age 3 years, then 250 mg orally twice daily until 5 years of age. The intramuscular use of benzathine penicillin 600,000 units every 4 weeks from age 6 months to 6 years is also an option for noncompliant patients. Penicillin allergic patients may receive erythromycin 10 mg/kg twice daily. Penicillin prophylaxis usually is not continued in children over the age of 6 years, but may be considered in patients with a history of invasive pneumococcal infection or surgical splenectomy.[5,15–17]

Folic Acid Folic acid supplementation with 1 mg daily is generally recommended in adult SCD patients, women considering pregnancy, and any SCD patient with chronic hemolysis.[5] Because of accelerated erythropoiesis, these patients have an increased need for folic acid. There are conflicting studies in the SCD population, especially among infants and children, but if the child has chronic hemolysis, supplementation is recommended.[18]

Fetal Hemoglobin Inducers Fetal hemoglobin (HbF) induction in patients with SCD, especially those with frequent crises, has been shown to decrease RBC sickling and RBC adhesion. A direct relationship between HbF concentrations and the severity of disease have been demonstrated in studies.[2]

Hydroxyurea Hydroxyurea is a riboneucleotide reductase inhibitor that prevents DNA synthesis and traditionally has been used in chemotherapy regimens. Studies in the 1990s also found that hydroxyurea increases HbF levels as well as increasing the number of HbF-containing reticulocytes and intracellular HbF. Other beneficial effects of hydroxyurea include antioxidant properties, reduction of neutrophils and monocytes, increased intracellular water content leading to increased red cell deformability, decreased red cell adhesion to endothelium, and increased levels of nitric oxide, which is a regulator involved in physiologic disturbances.[19]

❺ *Hydroxyurea reduced the frequency of hospitalizations and the incidences of pain, acute chest syndrome, and blood transfusions by almost 50% in a landmark trial in adult SCD patients with moderate to severe disease.* Hemoglobin and HbF concentrations increased and hemolysis decreased.[19] A follow-up study demonstrated a 40% reduction in mortality over a 9-year period in patients continuing to receive hydroxyurea.[20] Not all patients responded equally therefore hydroxyurea may not be the best option for all patients.

The use of hydroxyurea in children and adolescents with SCD has been investigated and similar results were reported as in adult trials with no adverse effects on growth and development.[5,21,22] Hydroxyurea is recommended as an option for children with moderate to severe SCD.[23]

The most common adverse effect of hydroxyurea in reported studies is myelosuppression. Long-term adverse effects are unknown but myelodysplasia, acute leukemia, and chronic opportunistic infections have been reported.[24] Hydroxyurea is teratogenic in high doses in animal studies and this is a concern, which should be addressed with patients. Normal pregnancies with no birth defects have been reported in some women receiving hydroxyurea, but close monitoring and weighing risk versus benefit to the patient are vitally important. Hydroxyurea is excreted in breast milk and should be avoided in lactating mothers.[9]

Hydroxyurea should be considered in SCD with frequent vasoocclusive crises, severe symptomatic anemia, repeated history of acute chest syndrome (ACS), or other history of severe vasoocclusive crisis (VOC) complications.[5] The prevention of organ damage or reversal of previous damage has not been shown to occur with chronic use of hydroxyurea.[20] The goals of therapy with hydroxyurea are to decrease the acute complications of SCD, improve quality of life, and reduce the number and severity of pain crises.

Hydroxyurea is available in 200-, 300-, 400-, and 500-mg capsules. Extemporaneous liquid preparations can be prepared for children who cannot swallow capsules. Doses should start at 10 to 15 mg/kg daily in a single oral dose, which can be increased after 8 to 12 weeks if blood counts are stable and there are no side effects. Individualize the dosage based on the patient's response and the toxicity seen. With close monitoring, doses can be increased 5 mg/kg/day up to 35 mg/kg daily.[19] In patients with renal failure, dosing of hydroxyurea will need to be adjusted according to the creatinine clearance, as shown in Table 68-3.

Closely monitor patients for efficacy and toxicity while they are receiving hydroxyurea. Monitor mean corpuscular volume (MCV), since it increases as the level of HbF increases. If the MCV does not increase with hydroxyurea use, the marrow may be unable to respond, the dose may not be adequate, or the patient may be noncompliant.[9] HbF levels can also be monitored to assess response with a goal of increasing HbF to 15% to 20%. Assess blood counts every 2 weeks during dose titration and then every 4 to 6 weeks once the dose is stabilized. Temporary discontinuation of therapy is warranted if hemoglobin level is less than 5 g/dL (50 g/L or 3.1 mmol/L), absolute neutrophil count is less than $2 \times 10^3/\text{mm}^3$ ($2 \times 10^9/\text{L}$) platelets are less than $80 \times 10^3/\text{mm}^3$ ($80 \times 10^9/\text{L}$), or the reticulocytes are less than $80 \times 10^3/\text{mm}^3$ ($80 \times 10^9/\text{L}$) if the hemoglobin is less than 9 g/dL (90 g/L or 5.6 mmol/L). Monitor for increases in serum creatinine and transaminases. Once the patient's blood counts have returned to baseline, hydroxyurea may be restarted with a dose that is 2.5 to 5 mg/kg less than the dose associated with the patient's toxicity. Doses may then be increased by 2.5 to 5 mg/kg daily after 12 weeks with no toxicity.

Administer prophylactic folic acid supplementation to SCD patients receiving hydroxyurea, because folate deficiency may be masked by the use of hydroxyurea.

Table 68-3

Dosage Adjustments for Renal and Hepatic Dysfunction

Medication	Renal Adjustment	Hepatic Adjustment
Decitabine (Decagon)	For Scr greater than or equal to 2 mg/dL (177 μmol/L): hold therapy until values return to baseline	For serum alanine transaminase (ALT), serum glutamic pyruvic transaminase (SGPT), or total bilirubin values greater than 2 times the upper limit of normal: hold therapy until values return to baseline
Deferoxamine (Desferol)	Cl_{cr} less than 10 mL/min: decrease the dose by 50%	
Deferasirox (Exjade)		
Children	Greater than 33% increase in Scr (on two consecutive readings) and above the age-appropriate upper limits of normal: decrease daily dose by 10 mg/kg	Severe or persistent elevations in liver function tests: decrease the daily dose or discontinue therapy
Adults	Greater than 33% increase in Scr above pretreatment values on two consecutive readings: decrease daily dose by 10 mg/kg	Severe or persistent elevations in liver function tests: decrease the daily dose or discontinue therapy
Folic acid	No adjustment necessary	No adjustment necessary
Hydroxyurea	Cl_{cr} less than 60 mL/min: Initial dose of 7.5 mg/kg/day Cl_{cr} 10-50 mL/min: reduce the daily dose by 50% Cl_{cr} less than 10 mL/min: administer 20% of the usual dose Hemodialysis: 7.5 mg/kg/day given after dialysis	Monitor patient for bone marrow toxicity

From Refs. 25–30.

5-Aza-2′-Deoxycytine (Decitabine) For patients who do not respond to hydroxyurea, 5-azacytidine and 5-aza-2′-deoxycytidine (decitabine) may be useful. Both induce HbF by inhibiting methylation of DNA, preventing the switch from γ- to β-globin production. Decitabine appears to be safer and more potent than 5-azacytadine. In a small study in adults refractory to hydroxyurea, decitabine 0.2 mg/kg subcutaneously one to three times weekly was associated with an increase in HbF in all patients. Additionally, RBC adhesion was reduced. Neutropenia was the only significant toxicity reported.[31]

Combinations of HbF Inducers Very limited information is available on the use of combination therapy for potentiation of HbF production. Erythropoietin has shown inconsistent results in small numbers of patients. When used with hydroxyurea, erythropoietin has been shown to increase HbF to a greater extent than hydroxyurea alone; and although more studies are needed, this may provide an option for patients who do not respond to hydroxyurea alone.[9]

Chronic Transfusion Therapy Chronic transfusion therapy is warranted to prevent serious complications from SCD, including stroke prevention and recurrence. ❻ *Especially in children, chronic transfusions have been shown to decrease stroke recurrence from approximately 50% to 10% over 3 years.* Without chronic transfusions,

approximately 70% of ischemic stroke patients will have another stroke. Chronic transfusion therapy also may be used to prevent vasoocclusive pain and ACS, as well as prevent progression of organ damage. Patients receiving chronic transfusion therapy report increased energy levels, improved quality of life, and better exercise tolerance. Patients in whom chronic transfusion therapy should be considered, include those with severe or recurrent ACS, debilitating pain, splenic sequestration, recurrent priapism, chronic organ failure, transient ischemic attacks, abnormal transcranial Doppler studies, intractable leg ulcers, severe chronic anemia in the presence of cardiac failure, and complicated pregnancies.[5,9]

Several methods of transfusion may be used, including simple transfusion, exchange transfusion, or erythrocytapheresis. The goal of chronic transfusion therapy is to maintain the HbS level at less than 30% (0.30) of total hemoglobin concentration. Transfusions are usually administered every 3 to 4 weeks depending on the HbS concentration. For secondary stroke prevention, current studies have indicated that lifelong transfusion may be required, with increased incidence of recurrence once transfusions are stopped.[5]

The benefits of transfusion should be weighed with the risks. Risks associated with transfusions include alloimmunization (sensitization to the blood received), hyperviscosity, viral transmission, volume overload, iron overload, and transfusion reactions. Approximately 18% to 30% of SCD patients who receive transfusions will experience alloimmunization, which can be minimized by the use of leukocyte-reduced RBCs or HLA-matched units. Viral transmission is still a concern, despite increased screening of blood donors and units. While the risk of contraction of AIDS has decreased dramatically, hepatitis C remains a concern. All SCD patients should be vaccinated for hepatitis A and B, and should be serially monitored for hepatitis C and other infections. Parvovirus occurs in 1 of every 40,000 units of RBCs and can be associated with acute anemia and multiple sickle cell complications.[5] Iron overload remains a concern among those patients maintained on chronic transfusions for greater than 1 year. Counsel patients to avoid excessive dietary iron and monitor serum ferritin regularly. Chelation therapy with deferoxamine or deferasirox should be considered when the serum ferritin level is greater than 1,500 to 2,000 ng/mL (1,500–2,000 mcg/L). Deferoxamine should be initiated at 20 to 40 mg/kg daily (to a maximum of 1–2 g/day) over 8 to 12 hours subcutaneously, and has been associated with growth failure.[5] Monitor children receiving deferoxamine for adequate growth and development on a regular basis. Deferasirox should be initiated at 20 mg/kg daily, and is available in a tablet that should be dispersed in water, orange juice, or apple juice and taken orally 30 minutes before food.[32,33] Monitor all chelation patients for auditory and ocular changes on a yearly basis. Exchange transfusions may also be helpful in cases of iron overload.

Sickle cell hemolytic transfusion reaction syndrome is a unique problem in SCD patients. Due to alloimmunization, an acute or delayed transfusion reaction may occur. Delayed reactions typically occur 5 to 20 days post-transfusion. Alloantibodies and autoantibodies resulting from previous

---

Patient Encounter 2

LK is a 15-year-old female with a history of sickle cell disease (HbS).

PMH: Cholecystectomy at age 11 years; admitted for vasoocclusive crises five times over the past year; acute chest syndrome at age 13 and 14; immunizations up-to-date; multiple blood transfusions

FH: Father with SC trait; mother with SCD

SH: Student in the 9th grade; denies alcohol or drug use; is sexually active

Meds: Lortab 7.5 mg tablets orally every 4 to 6 hours as needed for pain; ibuprofen 600 mg orally three times a day as needed for pain; Folic acid 1 mg orally daily

The medical team wants to start LK on hydroxyurea.

Is she a candidate for hydroxyurea? Why or why not?

What initial laboratory work is required before initiating hydroxyurea?

Identify treatment goals for hydroxyurea in LK.

What is the initial dose and how will you monitor for efficacy?

What patient counseling is needed?

How will you monitor for toxicity?

transfusions can trigger the reaction, in which patients develop symptoms suggestive of a pain crisis or worsening symptoms if they are already in crisis. A severe anemia after transfusion also may occur due to a rapid decrease in hemoglobin and hematocrit, along with a suppression of erythropoiesis. Further transfusions may worsen the clinical picture due to autoimmune antibodies. Recovery may occur only after ceasing all transfusions, and is evidenced by a gradual increase in hemoglobin with reticulocytosis[5,9]

Allogeneic Hematopoietic Stem Cell Transplant

Allogeneic hematopoietic stem cell transplantation (HSCT) is the only potential cure for SCD. The best candidates are children with SCD who are younger than 16 years of age with severe complications, who have an identical HLA-matched donor, usually a sibling. The transplant related mortality rate is between 5% and 10% and graft rejection is approximately 10%. Other risks include secondary malignancies, development of seizures or intracranial bleeding, and infection in the immediate post-transplant period.[5,34,35]

Experience with HSCT in adult patients with SCD is very limited. Umbilical cord blood and hematopoietic cells from nonmatched donors are potential alternatives in some patients, but use is limited.[5,35]

▶ Acute Complications

Transfusions for Acute Complications Red cell transfusion is indicated in patients with acute exacerbations of baseline anemia; in cases of severe vasoocclusive episodes, including ACS, stroke, and acute multiorgan failure; and in preparation for procedures that will require the use of general anesthesia or ionic contrast products. Transfusions also may be useful in patients with complicated obstetric problems, refractory leg ulcers, refractory and prolonged pain crises, or severe priapism. Hyperviscosity may occur if the hemoglobin level is increased to greater than 10 to 11 g/dL (100–110 g/L or 6.2–6.8 mmol/L). Volume overload leading to congestive heart failure is more likely to occur if the anemia is corrected too rapidly in patients with severe anemia, and should be avoided.[5,9]

Infection and Fever ❼ *Any fever greater than 38.5°C (101.3°F) in a SCD patient should be immediately evaluated, and the patient should have a blood culture drawn and be started on antibiotics that provide empirical coverage for encapsulated organisms.*[9]

Patients who should be hospitalized include the following:

- Infants younger than 1 year of age
- Patients with a previous sepsis or bacteremia episode
- Patients with temperatures in excess of 40°C (104°F)
- Patients with WBC counts greater than 30×10^3/mm³ (30×10^9/L) or less than 0.5×10^3/mm³ (0.5×10^9/L) and/or platelets less than 100×10^3/mm³ (100×10^9/L) with evidence of other acute complications
- Acutely ill-appearing individuals

Broad IV antibiotic coverage for the encapsulated organisms can include ceftriaxone or cefotaxime. For patients

---

Clinical Presentation and Diagnosis of Infection in SCD

General

- Patients may become acutely distressed very rapidly
- A low threshold to begin empiric therapy is recommended

Symptoms

- Patients may complain of lethargy, nausea, cough, or a general "unwell" feeling

Signs

- Temperature greater than 38.5°C (101.3°F)

Laboratory Tests

- CBC with reticulocyte count
- Cultures (urine, blood, and throat)
- Lumbar puncture if toxic-looking or signs of meningitis
- Urinalysis
- Chest x-ray

Potential Pathogens

- *Streptococcus pneumoniae* (most common), *Haemophilus influenzae, Salmonella, Mycoplasma pneumoniae, Chlamydia,* and viruses (parvovirus B19)

---

with true cephalosporin allergy, clindamycin may be used. If staphylococcal infection is suspected due to previous history or the patient appears acutely ill, vancomycin should be initiated. Macrolide antibiotics, such as erythromycin or azithromycin, may be initiated if mycoplasma pneumonia is suspected. While the patient is receiving broad-spectrum antibiotics, their regular use of penicillin for prophylaxis can be suspended. Fever should be controlled with acetaminophen or ibuprofen. Because of the risk of dehydration during infection with fever, increased fluid requirements may be needed.[5,9]

Bone infarcts or sickling in the periosteum usually is indicated by pain and swelling over an extremity. Osteomyelitis also should also be considered. *Salmonella* species are the most common cause of osteomyelitis in SCD children, followed by *Staphylococcus aureus*.[9] Select an appropriate antibiotic to cover the suspected organisms empirically.

Cerebrovascular Accidents Acute neurologic events, such as stroke, will require hospitalization and close monitoring. Patients should have physical and neurologic examinations every 2 hours.[9] Acute treatment may include exchange transfusion or simple transfusion to maintain hemoglobin at around 10 g/dL (100 g/L or 6.2 mmol/L) and HbS concentration at less than 30%. Patients with a history of seizure may need anticonvulsants, and interventions for increased intracranial pressure should be initiated if necessary. Children with history of stroke should be initiated on chronic transfusion

Clinical Presentation and Diagnosis of Stroke in SCD

General

- Most common cause is cerebrovascular occlusion
- Initial episode most often occurs during first 10 years of life
- Silent infarcts seen on MRI have been reported in 22% of patients and may be associated with increased risk of stroke and decreased neurocognitive function

Symptoms

- Patients may present with headache, vomiting, stupor, hemiparesis, aphasia, visual disturbances and seizure

Evaluation

- CT scan and MRI for acute event
- Magnetic resonance angiography for asymptomatic infarction
- Transcranial Doppler to detect abnormal velocity and identify high-risk patients
- Electroencephalography if there is history of seizure
- Chest x-ray

Clinical Presentation and Diagnosis of ACS in SCD

General

- Occurs in 15% to 43% of patients and is responsible for 25% of deaths
- Risk factors include young age, low HbF level, high Hgb and WBCs, winter seasons, reactive airway disease
- Recurrences are up to 80% and can lead to chronic lung disease

Symptoms

- Patients may complain of cough, fever, dyspnea, chest pain

Signs

- Temperature greater than 38.5°C (101.3°F)
- Hypoxia
- New infiltrate on chest x-ray

Laboratory Tests

- Complete blood count with reticulocyte
- Blood gases
- Oxygen saturation
- Cultures (blood and sputum)

Other

- Closely monitor pulmonary status

therapy. Adults presenting with ischemic stroke should be considered for thrombolytic therapy if it has been less than 3 hours since the onset of symptoms.[5,9]

Early detection of ischemic stroke can be done with the use of transcranial Doppler ultrasonography. In the Stroke Prevention Trial in Sickle Cell Anemia (STOP) study, screening with this method followed by chronic transfusion therapy significantly reduced the incidence of stroke.[36] Screening is recommended in all patients over the age of two.

Acute Chest Syndrome ACS will require hospitalization for appropriate management of symptoms and to avoid complications. Patients should be encouraged to use incentive spirometry at least every 2 hours. Incentive spirometry helps the patient take long, slow breaths to increase lung expansion. Appropriate management of pain is important, but analgesic-induced hypoventilation should be avoided. Patients should maintain appropriate fluid balance because overhydration can lead to pulmonary edema and respiratory distress. Infection with gram-negative, gram-positive, or atypical bacterial is common in ACS and early use of broad-spectrum antibiotics, including a macrolide, quinolone, or cephalosporin is recommended. Fat emboli, from infarction of the long bones, may lead to ACS. Oxygen therapy should be utilized in any patient presenting with respiratory distress or hypoxia. Oxygen saturations, measured by pulse oximeter, should be maintained at 92% or above. Transfusions are often indicated and patients who present with wheezing may require inhaled bronchodilators.[5,37,38]

The use of corticosteroids is controversial. While they may decrease the inflammation and endothelial cell adhesion seen with ACS, their use has also been associated with higher readmission rates for other complications. Tapered corticosteroids, nitric oxide therapy, and L-arginine are being evaluated for use in ACS in studies.[37,39]

Priapism By age 18, approximately 90% of SCD males will have had at least one episode of priapism. Stuttering priapism, where erection episodes last anywhere from a few minutes to less than 2 hours, resolves spontaneously. Erections lasting more than 2 hours should be evaluated promptly. Goals of therapy are to provide pain relief, reduce anxiety, provide detumescense, and preserve testicular function and fertility. Initial treatment should include aggressive hydration and analgesia. Transfusion may or may not be helpful, but should be considered in anemic patients. Avoid the use of ice packs due to the risk of tissue damage.[5,9]

Both vasoconstrictors and vasodilators have been used in the treatment of priapism. Vasoconstrictors are thought to work by forcing blood out of the cavernosum and into the venous return. Aspiration of the penile blood followed by intracavenous irrigation with epinephrine (1:1,000,000 solution) has been effective with minimal complications.[40] In severe cases, surgical intervention to place penile shunts

Clinical Presentation and Diagnosis of Priapism in SCD

General

- Mean age of initial episode is 12 years of age
- Most males with SCD will have one episode by age 20
- Repeated episodes can lead to fibrosis and impotence

Symptoms

- Patients may complain of painful and unwanted erection lasting anywhere from less than 2 hours (stuttering type) to more than 2 hours (prolonged type)

Signs

- Urinary obstruction

Laboratory Tests

- CBC with reticulocyte

Other

- Monitor for duration of episode
- Prolonged episodes should be considered medical emergencies

Clinical Presentation and Diagnosis of Acute Aplastic Crisis in SCD

General

- Transient suppression of RBC production in response to bacterial or viral infection
- Most commonly due to infection with parvovirus B19

Symptoms

- Patients may complain of headache, fatigue, dyspnea, pallor, or fever
- Patients may also complain of upper respiratory or GI infection symptoms

Signs

- Temperature greater than 38.5°C (101.3°F) may occur
- Hypoxia
- Tachycardia
- Acute decrease in Hgb with decreased reticulocyte count

Laboratory Tests

- CBC with reticulocyte
- Chest x-ray
- Parvovirus titers
- Cultures (blood, urine, and throat)

has been used, but there is a high failure rate, and the risk of complications, from skin sloughing to fistulas, limits its use.

Pseudoephedrine dosed at 30 to 60 mg/day taken at bedtime, has been used to prevent or decrease the number of episodes of priapism.[5] Terbutaline 5 mg has been used orally to prevent priapism with mixed results.[41,42] Leuprolide, a gonadotropin-releasing hormone, also has been used for this indication. Hydroxyurea may be helpful in some patients. The use of antiandrogens is under investigation.[5,9]

▶ Treatment of Acute Complications

Aplastic Crisis Most patients in aplastic crisis will recover spontaneously and therefore treatment is supportive. If anemia is severe or symptomatic, transfusion may be indicated. Infection with human parvovirus B19 is the most common cause of aplastic crisis. Isolate infected patients, because parvovirus is highly contagious. Pregnant individuals should avoid contact with infected patients because midtrimester infection with parvovirus may cause hydrops fetalis and still birth.[5,9]

Sequestration Crisis RBC sequestration in the spleen in young children may lead to a rapid drop in hematocrit, resulting in hypovolemia, shock, and death. Treatment is RBC transfusion to correct the hypovolemia, as well as broad-spectrum antibiotics because infections may precipitate the crisis.[5,9]

Recurrent episodes are common and can be managed with chronic transfusion and splenectomy. Observation is used commonly in adults because their episodes are milder. Splenectomy is usually delayed until after 2 years

of age to lessen the risk of postsplenectomy septicemia. Patients with chronic hypersplenism should be considered for splenectomy.[5,43]

Vasoocclusive Pain Crisis The mainstay of treatment for vasoocclusive crisis includes hydration and analgesia (Table 68–4). Pain may involve the extremities, back, chest, and abdomen. ❽ *Patients with mild pain crisis may be treated as outpatients with rest, warm compresses to the affected (painful) area, increased fluid intake, and oral analgesia.* Moderate to severe crises should be hospitalized. Infection should be ruled out because it may trigger a pain crisis, and any patient presenting with fever or critical illness should be started on empirical broad-spectrum antibiotics. Patients who are anemic should be transfused to their baseline. IV or oral fluids at 1.5 times maintenance is recommended. Close monitoring of the patient's fluid status is important to avoid overhydration, which can lead to ACS, volume overload, or heart failure.[5,9]

Aggressive pain management is required in patients presenting in pain crisis. Assess pain on a regular basis (every 2–4 hours) and individualize management to the patient. The use of pain scales may help with quantifying the pain rating. Obtain a good medication history of what has worked well for the patient in the past. Use acetaminophen or a nonsteroidal anti-inflammatory drug (NSAID) for treatment of mild to moderate pain. Patients with bone or joint pain, who require IV medications may be helped by the use of

Clinical Presentation and Diagnosis of Sequestration Crisis in SCD

General
- Acute exacerbation of anemia due to sequestration of large blood volume by the spleen
- More common in patients with functioning spleens
- Onset often associated with viral or bacterial infections
- Recurrence is common and can be fatal

Symptoms
- Sudden onset of fatigue, dyspnea, and distended abdomen
- Patients may present with vomiting and abdominal pain

Signs
- Rapid decrease in Hgb and Hct with elevated reticulocyte count
- Splenomegaly
- May exhibit hypotension and shock

Evaluation
- Vital signs
- Spleen size changes
- Oxygen saturations
- CBC with reticulocyte count
- Cultures (blood, urine, throat)

Clinical Presentation and Diagnosis of Vasoocclusive Crisis in SCD

General
- Most often involves the bones, liver, spleen, brain, lungs, and penis
- Precipitating factors include: infection, extreme weather conditions, dehydration, and stresses
- Recurrent acute crises result in bone, joint, and organ damage and chronic pain

Symptoms
- Patients may complain of deep throbbing pain, local tenderness

Signs
- Erythema and swelling of painful area
- Dactylitis in young infants
- Temperature greater than 38.5°C (101.3°F)
- Leukocytosis

Laboratory tests
- CBC with reticulocyte
- Urinalysis
- Abdominal studies (if symptoms exist)
- Cultures (blood and urine)
- Liver function tests and bilirubin
- Chest x-ray

ketorolac, an injectable NSAID. Because of the concern for side effects, including GI bleeding, ketorolac should be used only for a maximum of 5 consecutive days. Monitor for the total amount of acetaminophen given daily, because many products contain acetaminophen. Maximum daily dose of acetaminophen for adults is 4 g/day, and for children, five doses over a 24-hour period.[44] Add an opioid if pain persists or if pain is moderate to severe in nature. Combining an opioid with an NSAID can enhance the analgesic effects without increasing adverse effects.[45–47]

Severe pain should be treated with an opioid such as morphine, hydromorphone, methadone or fentanyl. Moderate pain can be effectively treated in most cases with a weak opioid such as codeine or hydrocodone, usually in combination with acetaminophen. Meperidine should be avoided because of its relatively short analgesic effect and its toxic metabolite, normeperidine. Normeperidine may accumulate with repeated dosing and can lead to CNS side effects including seizures.

IV opioids are recommended for use in treatment of severe pain because of their rapid onset of action and ease in titration. Intramuscular injection should be avoided. Analgesia should be individualized and titrated to effect, either by scheduled doses or continuous infusion. The use of continuous infusion will avoid the fluctuations in blood levels between doses that

is seen with bolus dosing. As needed dosing of analgesia is only appropriate for breakthrough pain or uncontrolled pain. Patient-controlled analgesia (PCA) is commonly used and allows the patient to have control over his or her analgesic breakthrough dosing. As the pain crisis resolves, the pain medications can be tapered. Physical therapy and relaxation therapy can be helpful adjuvants to analgesia.[45–48]

Tolerance to opioids is seen when patients have had continuous long-term use of the medications and can be managed during acute crises by using a different potent opioid or using a larger dose of the same medication. Adverse effects associated with the use of opioids include respiratory depression, itching, nausea and vomiting, constipation, and drowsiness. Patients on continuous infusions of opioids should be on continuous pulse oximeter to assess oxygen saturations. Monitor the patient for oxygen saturations less than 92%. Oxygen should be administered as needed to keep the saturations above 92%. Itching can be managed with an antihistamine such as diphenhydramine. Nausea and vomiting can be treated and managed with the administration of antiemetics such as promethazine or the 5HT3 antagonists, but the use of promethazine is contraindicated in children younger than 2 years of age. Assess stool frequency in all patients on a continuous opioid,

Table 68–4

Management of Acute Pain of SCD

Principles

- Treat underlying precipitating factors
- Avoid delays in analgesia administration
- Use pain scale to assess severity
- Choice of initial analgesic should be based on previous pain crisis pattern, history of response, current status, and other medical conditions
- Schedule pain medication; avoid as-needed dosing
- Provide rescue dose for breakthrough pain
- If adequate pain relief can be achieved with one or two doses of morphine, consider outpatient management with a weak opioid; otherwise hospitalization is needed for parenteral analgesics
- Frequently assess to evaluate pain severity and side effects; titrate dose as needed
- Treating adverse effects of opioids is part of pain management
- Consider nonpharmacologic intervention
- Transition to oral analgesics as the patient improves; choose an oral agent based on previous history, anticipated duration, and ability to swallow tablets; if sustained-release products are used, a fast-release product is also needed for breakthrough pain

Analgesic Regimens

Mild to moderate pain:

Acetaminophen with codeine
- Dose based on codeine—children: 1 mg/kg per dose every 6 hours; adults: 30–60 mg/dose

Hydrocodone + acetaminophen:
- Dose based on hydrocodone—children: 0.2 mg/kg per dose every 6 hours; adults: 5–10 mg/dose

Anti-inflammatory agents
- Use with caution in patients with renal failure (dehydration) and bleeding
- Ibuprofen: children: 10 mg/kg every 6–8 hours; adults: 200–400 mg/dose
- Naproxen: 5 mg/kg every 12 hours; adults: 250–500 mg/dose
- Ibuprofen + hydrocodone: Each tablet contains 200 mg ibuprofen and 7.5 mg hydrocodone per tablet; only for older children who can swallow tablets

Moderate to severe pain:

Morphine—children: 0.1–0.15 mg/kg per dose every 3–4 hours; adults: 5–10 mg/dose
- Continuous infusion: 0.04–0.05 mg/kg/h; titrate to effect

Hydromorphone—children: 0.015 mg/kg per dose every 3–4 hours; adults: 1.5–2 mg/dose
- Continuous infusion: 0.004 mg/kg/h; titrate to effect

IV anti-inflammatory agents:
- Ketorolac: 0.5 mg/kg up to 30 mg/dose every 6 hours

Patient-controlled analgesics:
- Morphine: 0.01–0.03 mg/kg/h basal; demand 0.01–0.03 mg/kg every 6–10 minutes; 4 hours lockout 0.04–0.06 mg/kg
- Hydromorphone: 0.003–0.005 mg/kg/h basal; demand 0.003–0.05 mg/kg every 6–10 minutes; 4 hours lock out 0.4–0.6 mg/kg

Patient Encounter 3

CC: "My right leg and lower back hurt badly"

HPI: CD is a 21-year-old African American male diagnosed with sickle cell disease at birth. He has had repeated pain crises (average of about two per year) and presents today with another. He started feeling ill yesterday and this morning woke up with increased pain and a cough.

PMH: Frequent pain crises, acute chest syndrome last year, priapism

FH: Mother with sickle cell trait, Father with sickle cell disease. Father died at age 36 from stroke. Has an older brother with sickle cell disease and a younger sister with sickle cell trait.

SH: CD is a college student. He lives in the dorms. Enjoys basketball.

PE: Wt 64 kg (14 lb), ht 180 cm (6 ft), BP 130/80, HR 90, RR 30, temp 40°C (104°F)

Lungs: decreased breath sounds in bases

Skin: Warm, dry, tender, and increased warmth in right leg, nailbeds dusky, poor capillary refill

HEENT: Sclera slightly yellow

Meds: Tylenol #3, two tablets orally every 4 to 6 hours as needed for pain; pseudoephedrine 30 mg orally twice daily

Allergies: NKDA

Lab: All within normal limits except; Hemoglobin: 6.2 g/dL; hematocrit: 30 g/dL; WBC: 20,000/mm³; Total bilirubin: 2.2 mg/dL

Based on the information presented, create a care plan for this patient's vasoocclusive crisis. Your plan should include the following:

Statement of the drug-related needs and/or problems

Goals of therapy

Patient-specific, detailed therapeutic plan

Plan for follow-up and monitoring to determine whether the goals have been achieved and adverse effects avoided.

Table 68–5

Chronic Complications of SCD

System	Complications
Auditory	Sensorineural hearing loss due to sickling in cochlear vasculature with hair cell damage
Cardiovascular	Cardiomegaly, myocardial ischemia, murmurs, and abnormal ECG; patients with SCD have lower BP than the normal population; normal BP values for SCD should be used for diagnosis of hypertension ("relative" hypertension); heart failure usually is related to fluid overload
Dermatologic	Painful leg ulcers; failure to heal occurs in 50% of patients; recurrences are common
Genitourinary	Renal papillary necrosis, hematuria, hyposthenuria, proteinuria, nephrotic syndrome, tubular dysfunction, chronic renal failure, impotence
Growth and development	Delay in growth (weight and height) and sexual development; decreased fertility; increased complications during pregnancy; depression may be more prevalent than in general population, especially in patients with unstable disease
Hepatic and biliary	Cholelithiasis, biliary sludge, acute and chronic cholecystitis, and cholestasis (can be progressive and life-threatening)
Neurologic	"Silent" brain lesions on MRI are associated with poor cognitive and fine motor functions; pseudotumor cerebri (rare)
Ocular	Retinal or vitreous hemorrhage, retinal detachment, transient or permanent visual loss; central retinal veinocclusion
Pulmonary	Pulmonary fibrosis, pulmonary hypertension, cor pulmonale
Renal	Hematuria, hyposthenuria (inability to concentrate urine maximally), tubular dysfunction, enuresis duringearly childhood, acute renal failure can also occur
Skeletal	Aseptic necrosis of ball-and-socket joints (shoulder and hip); prostheses may be needed due to permanent damage; bone marrow hyperplasia resulting in growth disturbances of maxilla and vertebrae
Spleen	Asplenia (autosplenectomy or surgical splenectomy)

and start stool softeners or laxatives as needed. Excessive sedation is difficult to control and the concurrent use of an opioid with diphenhydramine or other sedative medications can exacerbate the drowsiness, leading to hypoxemia. A continuous very low dose of naloxone, an opioid antagonist, has been used in some cases where the adverse effects such as itching are unbearable.[49]

OUTCOME EVALUATION

SCD treatment and prevention are considered successful when complications are minimized. The major outcome

Patient Care and Monitoring

1. Assess the patient's symptoms to determine whether the patient should be evaluated by a physician and/or receive immediate care. Determine the type of symptoms, onset of symptoms, frequency and exacerbating factors. Does the patient have evidence of SCD-related complications?

2. Review any available diagnostic data to determine the severity and status of the patient's SCD. *When was the patient last hospitalized for SCD complications?*

3. Obtain a thorough history of prescription, nonprescription and natural drug product use. For pain control, determine which treatments have been helpful to the patient in the past. *Is the patient currently taking any medications on a chronic basis?*

4. Educate the patient on lifestyle modifications that may lessen complications. These include maintaining adequate hydration status, avoiding extreme temperature changes, dressing appropriately for hot or cold weather, and avoiding physical exertion, smoking, and excessive alcohol intake.

5. Is the patient up to date on immunizations? Have they received their annual influenza vaccine? If not, why?

6. Is the patient taking appropriate doses of their pain medication to achieve effect? If not, why?

7. Develop a plan to assess the effectiveness of pain medications.

8. Determine if the patient is a candidate for hydroxyurea therapy.

9. Assess improvement in quality of life measures, such as physical, psychological, and social functioning and well-being.

10. Evaluate the patient for the presence of adverse drug reactions, drug allergies, and drug interactions.

11. Stress the importance of adherence with the therapeutic regimen, including lifestyle modifications. Recommend a therapeutic regimen that is easy for the patient/parent to accomplish.

12. Provide patient education on disease state, lifestyle modifications, and drug therapy:
    - Possible complications of SCD, both long- and short-term.
    - When to take their medications.
    - What potential adverse effects may occur?
    - Which drugs may interact with their medication therapy
    - Warning signs to report to the physician (increased or new pain, sudden headache, bleeding or bruising, fever, loss of energy, loss of appetite)

parameters are a decrease in morbidity and mortality, measured by the number of hospitalizations, and the extent of end-organ damage seen over time. Today, with longer survival for SCD, chronic manifestations of the disease contribute to the morbidity later in life (Table 68–5). Thirty years ago, complications from SCD contributed to high mortality. It was estimated that approximately 50% of patients with SCD did not survive to reach adulthood.[4] Since that time data suggest improvement in mortality rates for patients with SCD. The survival age for individuals with HbSS has increased to at least the fifth decade of life. Recent reports suggest 85% survival by 18 years of age.[4] SCD is a chronic disease and cannot be cured, except in some patients with transplant.

Starting with birth, SCD patients should have regularly scheduled health assessments and interventions when necessary. Obtain a urine analysis, complete blood count, liver function tests, ferritin or serum iron level and total iron binding capacity, blood urea nitrogen (BUN), and creatinine on at least a yearly basis and more often for children younger than 5 years of age to monitor for complications. All SCD patients should have regular screening of their hearing and vision.

All patients and parents of children with SCD should have a plan for what to do in the event of symptoms of infection or pain. Obtain a medication history when patients are admitted to the hospital. Assess compliance with prophylactic penicillin and childhood immunization schedules in all pediatric SCD patients.

Abbreviations Introduced in This Chapter

ACS	Acute chest syndrome
HbA	Normal adult hemoglobin
HbAS	One normal and one sickle hemoglobin gene
HbC	Hemoglobin C
HbF	Fetal hemoglobin
HbS	Sickle hemoglobin
HbSβ^0-thalassemia	One sickle hemoglobin and one β^0-thalassemia gene
HbSβ^+-thalassemia	One sickle hemoglobin and one β^+-thalassemia gene
HbSC	One sickle hemoglobin and one hemoglobin C gene
HbSS	Homozygous sickle hemoglobin
Hgb	Hemoglobin
HSCT	Hematopoietic stem cell transplantation
ISC	Irreversibly sickled cell
MCHC	Mean corpuscular hemoglobin concentration
MCV	Mean corpuscular volume
NSAID	Nonsteroidal anti-inflammatory drug
PCA	Patient-controlled analgesia
PCV 7	7-Valent pneumococcal conjugate vaccine
PPV 23	23-Valent pneumococcal polysaccharide vaccine
SCA	Sickle cell anemia
SCD	Sickle cell disease
SCT	Sickle cell trait
STOP	Stroke Prevention Trial in Sickle Cell Anemia
VOC	Vasoocclusive crisis

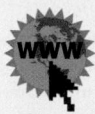

Self-assessment questions and answers are available at *http://www.mhpharmacotherapy.com/pp.html.*

REFERENCES

1. Stuart MJ, Nagel RL. Sickle-cell disease. Lancet 2004;364(9442):1343–1360. Review.
2. Ashley-Koch A, Yang Q, Olney RS. Sickle hemoglobin (HbS) allele and sickle cell disease: A huge review. Am J Epidemiol 2000;151:839–844.
3. Steinberg MH. Pathophysiologically based drug treatment of sickle cell disease. Trends Pharmacol Sci 2006;27(4):204–210.
4. Quinn CT, Rogers ZR, Buchanan GR. Survival of children with sickle cell disease. Blood 2004;103(11):4023–4027.
5. National Institutes of Health. The Management of Sickle Cell Disease. NIH Pub. No. 02–2117. Bethesda, MD, Division of Blood Diseases and Resources, Public Health Service, U.S. Department of Health and Human Services, June 2002:1–88.
6. World Health Organization Fifty-Ninth World Health Assembly 2006. Available at *http://www.who.int/gb/ebwha/pdf_files/WHA59/A59_9-en.pdf.*
7. Lanzkowsky P. Manual of Pediatric Hematology and Oncology, 4th ed. New York: Churchill Livingstone, 2005:160.
8. Rosse WF, Narla M, Petz LD, Steinberg MH. New views of sickle cell disease pathophysiology and treatment. Hematology Am Soc Hematol Educ Program 2000;2000:2–17.
9. Sickle Cell Disease Care Consortium. Sickle Cell Disease in Children and Adolescents: Diagnosis, Guidelines for Comprehensive Care, and Care Paths and Protocols for Management of Acute and Chronic Complications, November 2001. *http://www.scinfo.org/Protocol-2002.PDF.*
10. American Academy of Pediatrics Committee on Infectious Diseases. Recommended childhood and adolescent immunization schedule—United States, 2009. Pediatrics 2009;123:189–190.
11. Committee on Infectious Diseases, American Academy of Pediatrics. Policy Statement: Recommendations for the prevention of pneumococcal infections, including the use of pneumococcal conjugate vaccine (Prevnar), pneumococcal polysaccharide vaccine, and antibiotic prophylaxis. Pediatrics 2000;106:362–366.
12. Adamkiewicz TV, Sarnaik S, Buchanan GR, et al. Invasive pneumococcal infections in children with sickle cell disease in the era of penicillin prophylaxis, antibiotic resistance, and 23-valent pneumococcal polysaccharide vaccination. J Pediatr 2003;143:438–444.
13. Platt OS, Brambilla DJ, Rosse WF, et al. Mortality in sickle cell disease. Life expectancy and risk factors for early death. N Engl J Med 1994;330(23):1639–1644.
14. Miller ST, Sleeper LA, Pegelow CH, et al. Prediction of adverse outcomes in children with sickle cell disease. N Engl J Med 2000;342:83–89.
15. Advisory Committee on Immunization Practices, CDC. Preventing pneumococcal disease among infants and young children. Morb Mortal Wkly Rep 2000;49:1–38.
16. Falletta JM, Woods RM, Verter JI, et al. Discontinuing penicillin prophylaxis in children with sickle cell anemia. J Pediatr 1995;127:685–690.

17. Riddington C, Owusu-Ofori S. Prophylactic antibiotics for preventing pneumococcal infections in children with sickle cell disease. Cochrane Database 2002;(3):CD003427.

18. Kennedy TS, Fung EB, Kawchak DA, et al. Red blood cell folate and serum B12 status in children with sickle cell disease. J Pediatr Hematol Oncol 2001;23:165–169.

19. Charache S, Terrin ML, Moore RD, et al. Effect of hydroxyurea on the frequency of painful crises in sickle cell anemia. N Engl J Med 1995;332:1317–1322.

20. Steinberg MH, Bartin F, Castro O, et al. Effect of hydroxyurea on mortality and morbidity in adult sickle cell anemia. Risks and benefits up to 9 years of treatment. JAMA 2003;289:1645–1651.

21. Kinney TR, Helms RW, O'Branski EE, Ohene-Frempong K, et al. Safety of hydroxyurea in children with sickle cell anemia: Results of the HUG-KIDS study, a phase I/II trial. Pediatric Hydroxyurea Group. Blood 1999;94(5):1550–1554.

22. Zimmerman SA, Schultz WH, Davis JS, et al. Sustained long-term hematological efficacy of hydroxyurea at maximal tolerated dose in children with sickle cell disease. Blood 2004;103:2039–2045.

23. Hankins JS Ware RE, Rogers ZR, et al. Long-term hydroxyurea therapy for infants with sickle cell anemia: The HUSOFT extension study. Blood 2005;106:2269–2275.

24. Wilson S. Acute leukemia in a patient with sickle cell anemia treated with hydroxyurea (letter). Ann Intern Med 2000;133:925–926.

25. Hydroxyurea monograph. Lexi-Comp Online™, Pediatric Lexi-Drugs Online™, Hudson, Ohio: Lexi-Comp, inc.; 2008; September 29, 2008.

26. Deferoxamine monograph. Lexi-Comp Online™, Pediatric Lexi-Drugs Online™, Hudson, Ohio: Lexi-Comp, September 29, 2008.

27. Deferasirox monograph. Lexi-Comp Online™, Pediatric Lexi-Drugs Online™, Hudson, Ohio: Lexi-Comp, September 29, 2008.

28. Decitabine monograph. Lexi-Comp Online™, Lexi-Drugs Online™, Hudson, Ohio: Lexi-Comp, September 29, 2008.

29. Folic acid monograph. Lexi-Comp Online™, Lexi-Drugs Online™, Hudson, Ohio: Lexi-Comp, September 29, 2008.

30. Aronoff GR, Bennett WM, Berns JS, et al., eds. Drug Prescribing in Renal Failure, 15th ed. Philadelphia: American College of Physicians; 2007.

31. Koshy M, Dorn L, Bressler L, et al. 2-deoxy 5-azacytidine and fetal hemoglobin induction in sickle cell anemia. Blood 2000;248:378–381.

32. Porter J, Vinchinsky E, Rose C, et al. A Phase II study with ICL670 (Exjade), a once-daily oral iron chelator, in patients with various transfusion dependent anemias and iron overload (abstract). Blood 2004;104:3193.

33. Piga A, Galanello R, Foschini ML, et al. Once-daily treatment with the oral iron chelator ICL670 (Exjade): results of a Phase II study in pediatric patients with ß-thalassemia major (abstract). Blood 2004;104:3614.

34. Atkins RC, Walters MC. Haematopoietic cell transplantation in the treatment of sickle cell disease. Expert Opin Biol Ther 2003;3: 1215–1224.

35. Walters MC. Novel therapeutic approaches in sickle cell disease: Stem cell transplantation for sickle cell disease: How and when to intervene? Hematology Am Soc Hematol Educ Program 2002;22–29.

36. Adams RJ, Mckie VC, Bramilla D, Carl E, Gallagher D, Nichols FT, et al. Stroke prevention trial in sickle cell anemia. Control Clin Trials 1998;19:110–129.

37. Vichinsky E. Novel therapeutic approaches in sickle cell disease: Understanding the pathophysiology and treatment of pulmonary injury in sickle cell disease. Hematology Am Soc Hematol Edu Program 2002;16–22.

38. Knight-Madden J, Hambleton I. Inhaled bronchodilators for acute chest syndrome in people with sickle cell disease. Cochrane Database Syst Rev 2003;3:CD003733.

39. Sullivan KJ, Goodwin SR, Evangelist J, et al. Nitric oxide successfully used to treat acute chest syndrome of sickle cell disease in a young adolescent. Crit Care Med 1999;27:2563–2568.

40. Mantadakis E, Ewalt DH, Cavender JD et al. Outpatient penile aspiration and epinephrine irrigation for young patients with sickle cell anemia and prolonged priapism. Blood 2000;95:78–82.

41. Shantha TR, Finnerty DP, Rodriguez AP. Treatment of persistent penile erection and priapism using terbutaline. J Urol 1989;1427–1429.

42. Govier FE, Jonsson E, Kramer-Levien D. Oral terbutaline for the treatment of priapism. J Urol 1994:151:878–879.

43. Owusu-Ofori S, Riddington C. Splenectomy versus conservative management for acute sequestration crises in people with sickle cell disease. Cochrane Database of Systematic Reviews 2002;(4):CD003425.

44. AAP Committee on Drugs. APAP Toxicity in children. Peds 2001;108(1):1020–1024.

45. Jacob E, Miaskowski C, Savedra M, et al. Management of vaso-occlusive pain in children with sickle cell disease. J Pediatr Hematol Oncol 2003;25:307–311.

46. Berde CB, Sethna NF. Analgesics for the treatment of pain in children. N Engl J Med 2002;347(14):1094.

47. Stinson J, Naser B. Pain management in children with sickle cell disease. Paediatr Drugs 2003;5:229–238.

48. Yale SH. Approach to the vaso-occlusive crisis in adults with sickle cell disease. Am Fam Physician 2000;61:1349–1356, 1363–1364.

49. Maxwell LG, Kaufmann SC, Bitzer S, et al. The effects of a small-dose naloxone infusion on opioid-induced side effects and analgesia in children and adolescents treated with intravenous patient-controlled analgesia: A double-blind, prospective, randomized, controlled study. Anesth Analg 2005;100:953–958.

69 Antimicrobial Regimen Selection

Catherine M. Oliphant and Karl Madaras-Kelly

LEARNING OBJECTIVES

● **Upon completion of the chapter, the reader will be able to:**

1. Recognize that antimicrobial resistance is an inevitable consequence of antimicrobial therapy.

2. Describe how antimicrobials differ from other drug classes in terms of their effects on individual patients as well as on society as a whole.

3. Identify two guiding principles to consider when treating patients with antimicrobials, and apply these principles in patient care.

4. Differentiate between microbial colonization and infection based on patient history, physical examination, and laboratory and culture results.

5. Evaluate and apply at least six major drug-specific considerations when selecting antimicrobial therapy.

6. Evaluate and apply at least seven major patient-specific considerations when selecting antimicrobial therapy.

7. Select empirical antimicrobial therapy based on spectrum-of-activity considerations that provide a measured response proportional to the severity of illness. Provide a rationale for why a measured response in antimicrobial selection is appropriate.

8. Identify and apply five major principles of patient education and monitoring response to antimicrobial therapy.

9. Identify two common causes of patients failing to improve while on antimicrobials, and recognize other less common but potential reasons for antimicrobial failure.

KEY CONCEPTS

❶ An inevitable consequence of exposing microbes to antimicrobials is that some organisms will develop resistance to the antimicrobial.

❷ Antimicrobials are different from other classes of pharmaceuticals because they exert their action on bacteria infecting the host as opposed to acting directly on the host.

❸ Two guiding principles to consider when treating patients with antimicrobials are (a) make the diagnosis and (b) do no harm!

❹ Only bacteria that cause disease should be targeted with antimicrobial therapy, and colonizing flora should be left intact whenever possible.

❺ Bacterial cultures should be obtained prior to antimicrobial therapy in patients with a systemic inflammatory response, risk factors for antimicrobial resistance, or infections where diagnosis or antimicrobial susceptibility is uncertain.

❻ Drug-specific considerations in antimicrobial selection include the spectrum of activity, effects on nontargeted microbial flora, appropriate dose, pharmacokinetic and pharmacodynamic properties, adverse-effect and drug-interaction profile, and cost.

❼ Empirical therapy should be based on patient- and antimicrobial-specific factors such as the anatomic location of the infection, the likely pathogens associated with the presentation, the potential for adverse effects, and the antimicrobial spectrum of activity.

❽ Key patient-specific considerations in antimicrobial selection include recent previous antimicrobial exposures, identification of the anatomic location of infection through physical examination and diagnostic imaging, history of drug allergies, organ dysfunction that may affect drug clearance, immunosuppression, pregnancy, and compliance.

❾ Patient education, de-escalation of antimicrobial therapy based on culture results, monitoring for clinical response and adverse effects, and appropriate duration of therapy are important treatment components.

🔟 Inadequate diagnosis resulting in poor initial antimicrobial selection, poor source control, or the development of a new infection with a resistant organism are relatively common causes of antimicrobial failure.

The discovery of antimicrobials is among the greatest medical achievements of the 20th century. Prior to the antimicrobial era, patients who contracted common infectious diseases developed significant morbidity or perished. The discovery of penicillin in 1927, followed by the subsequent discovery of other antimicrobials, contributed to a significant decline in infectious disease–related mortality during the next five decades. However, since 1980, infectious diseases related mortality in the United States has begun to increase, in part owing to increases in antimicrobial resistance.

The discovery of virtually every new class of antimicrobials has occurred in response to the development of bacterial resistance and loss of clinical effectiveness to existing antimicrobials. ❶ *An inevitable consequence of exposing microbes to antimicrobials is that some organisms will develop resistance to the antimicrobial.* Today, there are dozens of antimicrobial classes and hundreds of antimicrobials available for clinical use. However, in many cases, differences in mechanisms of action between antimicrobials are minor, and the microbiologic properties of the agents are similar. ❷ *Antimicrobials are different from other classes of pharmaceuticals because they exert their action on bacteria infecting the host as opposed to acting directly on the host.* Because use of an antimicrobial in one patient affects not only that patient but also other patients if they become infected with resistant bacteria, correct selection, use, and monitoring of clinical response are paramount.

❸ *There are two guiding principles to consider when treating patients with antimicrobials: (a) make the correct diagnosis and (b) do no harm!* Patients with infections frequently present with signs and symptoms that are nonspecific for infection and may be confused with other noninfectious disease. Not only is it important to determine if a disease process is of infectious origin, but it is also important to determine the specific causative pathogen of the infection. Antimicrobials vary in their ability to inhibit or kill different species of bacteria, or their spectrum of activity. Antimicrobials that kill many different species of bacteria are called *broad-spectrum antimicrobials,* whereas antimicrobials that kill only a few different species of bacteria are called *narrow-spectrum antimicrobials.* One might argue that treating everybody with very broad antimicrobial coverage will increase the likelihood that a patient will get better without making a definitive diagnosis. However, counter to this argument is the principle of "Do no harm!" Very broad antimicrobial coverage does increase the likelihood of empirically targeting a causative pathogen; unfortunately, the development of

secondary infections caused by selection of antimicrobial-resistant nontargeted pathogens is a common problem. In addition, adverse events are thought to complicate up to 10% of all antimicrobial therapy, and for select agents, the adverse-event rates are similar to classical high-risk medications such as warfarin, digoxin, or insulin.[1] Therefore, the overall goal of antimicrobial therapy should be to cure the patient's infection; limit harm by minimizing patient risk for adverse effects, including secondary infections; and limit societal risk from antimicrobial-resistant bacteria.

EPIDEMIOLOGY AND ETIOLOGY

Infectious disease–related illnesses, particularly respiratory tract infections, are among the most common reasons patients seek medical care.[2] Approximately two-thirds of outpatient antimicrobial use is prescribed for respiratory tract infections, and the Centers for Disease Control and Prevention (CDC) estimate that one-third to one-half of all outpatient antimicrobials are used inappropriately to treat nonbacterial processes.[3] However, recent trends in prescribing suggest a modest reduction in antimicrobial use for these infections, suggesting an increased recognition of the negative consequences of antimicrobial use.[4] Prescription of antimicrobials in hospitalized patients is also common because up to one-half of all patients receive at least one antimicrobial during hospitalization. In addition, the CDC estimates that almost 2 million nosocomial or hospital-acquired infections and 90,000 related deaths occur annually.[5] Generally nosocomial infections tend be associated with more antimicrobial-resistant strains of bacteria. In recent years, there has been a shift in the etiology of some community-acquired infections. Increasingly, infections caused by antimicrobial-resistant pathogens, traditionally nosocomial in origin, are being identified in ambulatory care settings. Reasons for this change include an aging populace, improvement in the management of chronic comorbid conditions including immunosuppressive conditions, and increases in outpatient management of more debilitated patients. The majority of infections caused by antimicrobial-resistant pathogens in the ambulatory care setting have had recent exposure to some aspect of the health care system, therefore are defined as health care–associated infections. The converging bacterial etiologies and increasing resistance in all health care environments emphasize the need to "make the diagnosis."

PATHOPHYSIOLOGY

Normal Flora and Endogenous Infection

Many areas of the human body are colonized with bacteria—this is known as *normal flora.* Infections often arise from one's own normal flora (also called an *endogenous infection*). Endogenous infection may occur when there are alterations in the normal flora (e.g., recent antimicrobial use may allow for overgrowth of other normal flora) or disruption of host defenses (e.g., a break or entry in the skin). Knowing what organisms reside where can help to guide empirical antimicrobial therapy (Fig. 69–1). In addition, it is beneficial to know what anatomic sites are normally sterile. These include the cerebrospinal fluid, blood, and urine.

Determining Colonization Versus Infection

Infection refers to the presence of bacteria that are causing disease (e.g., the organisms are found in normally sterile anatomic sites or in nonsterile sites with signs/symptoms of infection). *Colonization* refers to the presence of bacteria that are not causing disease. ❹ *Only bacteria that cause disease should be targeted with antimicrobial therapy, and nondisease-producing colonizing flora should be left intact.* It is important to differentiate infection from colonization because antimicrobial therapy targeting bacterial colonization is inappropriate and may lead to the development of resistant bacteria.

Exogenously Acquired Bacterial Infections

Infections acquired from an external source are referred to as *exogenous infections*. These infections may occur as a result of human-to-human transmission, contact with exogenous bacterial populations in the environment, and animal contact. Resistant pathogens such as methicillin-resistant *Staphylococcus aureus* (MRSA) and vancomycin-resistant *Enterococcus* spp. (VRE) may colonize hospitalized patients or patients who access the health care system frequently. It is key to know which patients have acquired these organisms because patients generally become colonized prior to developing infection, and colonized patients should be placed in isolation (per infection-control policies) to minimize transmission to other patients.

Contrasting Bacterial Virulence and Resistance

Virulence refers to the pathogenicity or disease severity produced by an organism. Many bacteria may produce toxins or possess growth characteristics that contribute to their pathogenicity. Some virulence factors allow the organism to avoid the immune response of the host and cause significant disease. Virulence and resistance are different microbial characteristics. For example, *Streptococcus pyogenes*, a common cause of skin infections, produces toxins that can cause severe disease, yet it is very susceptible to penicillin. *Enterococcus faecium* is a highly resistant organism but is frequently a colonizing flora that causes disease primarily in the immunocompromised.

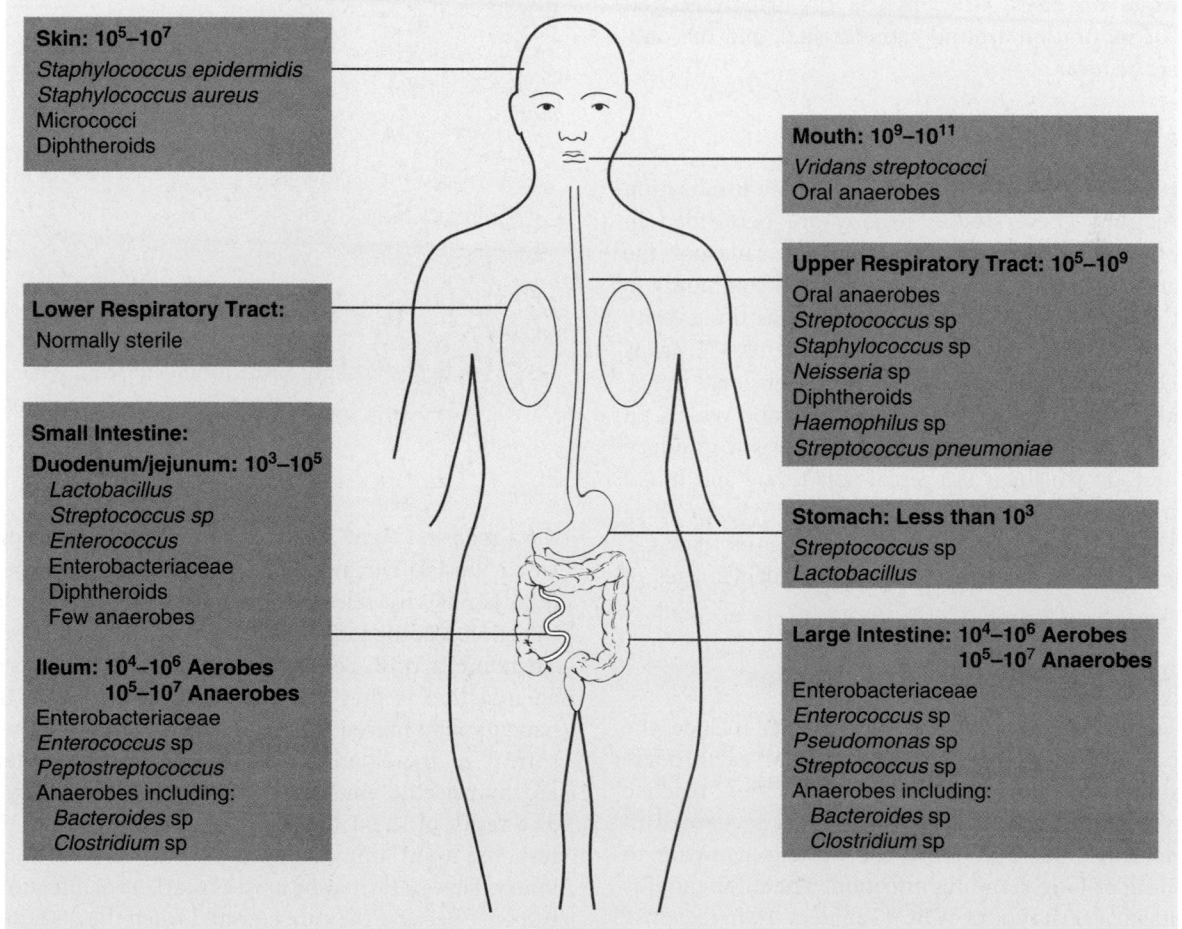

FIGURE 69–1. Normal flora and concentrations of bacteria (organisms per milliliter).

CLINICAL PRESENTATION AND DIAGNOSIS

Physical Examination

Findings on physical examination, along with the clinical presentation, can help to provide the anatomic location of the infection. Once the anatomic site is identified, the most probable pathogens associated with disease can be determined based on likely endogenous or exogenous flora.

Fever often accompanies infection and is defined as a rise in body temperature above the normal 37°C (98.6°F). Oral and axillary temperatures may underestimate core temperature by at least 0.6°C (1°F), whereas rectal temperatures best approximate core temperatures. Fever is a host response to bacterial toxins. However, bacterial infections are not the sole cause of fever. Fever also may be caused by other infections (e.g., fungal or viral), medications (e.g., penicillins, cephalosporins, salicylates, and phenytoin), trauma, or other medical conditions (e.g., autoimmune disease, malignancy, pulmonary embolism, and hyperthyroidism). Some patients with infections may present with hypothermia (e.g., patients with overwhelming infection). Elderly patients may be afebrile, as may those with localized infections (e.g., urinary tract infection).[6] For others, fever may be the only indication of infection. For example, neutropenic patients may not have the ability to mount normal immune responses to infection (e.g., infiltrate on chest x-ray, pyuria on urinalysis, and erythema or induration around catheter site), and the only finding may be fever.

Imaging Studies

Imaging studies also may help to identify anatomic localization of the infection. These studies usually are performed in conjunction with other tests to establish or rule out the presence of an infection. X-rays are performed commonly to establish the diagnosis of pneumonia, as well as the severity of disease (single versus multilobe involvement). CT scans are a type of x-ray that produces a three-dimensional image of the combination of soft tissue, bone, and blood vessels. In contrast, MRI use electromagnetic radio waves to produce two- or three-dimensional images of soft tissue and blood vessels with less detail of bony structures. MRI produce more detailed images of soft tissues and organs than CT scans, whereas CT scans produce more detailed images of bones.

Nonmicrobiologic Laboratory Studies

Common nonmicrobiological laboratory tests include the white blood cell count (WBC) and differential, erythrocyte sedimentation rate (ESR), and determination of the C-reactive protein level. In most cases, the WBC count is elevated in response to infection, but it may be decreased owing to overwhelming or long-standing infection. The differential is the percentage of each type of WBC (Table 69–1). In response to infection, neutrophils leave the bloodstream and enter

---

Patient Encounter 1

HPI: A 72-year-old man with a history of congestive heart failure, diabetes, hypertension, and hyperlipidemia presents to the local emergency room with complaints of increasing shortness of breath, cough productive of yellow-green sputum, chest pain, fever, and malaise. He was hospitalized 12 days ago for urosepsis, for which he received 10 days of levofloxacin.

PMH: Congestive heart failure, diabetes mellitus × 22 years, hypertension, hyperlipidemia

- Chronic renal insufficiency: baseline SCr 1.8 mg/dL (159 µmol/L)

FH: Father died of a myocardial infarction at age 75.

- Mother died of complications after cerebrovascular accident (CVA) at age 87.

SH:

- Retired accountant
- Alcohol: two to three drinks per day

Allergies: NKDA

Meds:

- Enalapril 10 mg twice daily
- Metoprolol XL 25 mg daily
- Furosemide 40 mg daily
- Insulin glargine (Lantus) 30 units SC at bedtime
- Glipizide 10 mg daily
- Atorvastatin 20 mg daily
- Aspirin 81 mg daily
- Home oxygen at 2 L/min

What information in the history supports an infectious etiology?

Is this patient at risk for resistant pathogens? Why?

---

the tissue to "fight" against the offending pathogens (i.e., leukocytosis). During an infection, immature neutrophils (e.g., bands) are released at an increased rate to help fight infection, leading to what is known as a bandemia or left shift. Therefore, a WBC count differential is key to determining if an infection is present. It is important to note that some patients may present with a normal total WBC with a left shift (e.g., the elderly). ESR and C-reactive protein (CRP) are nonspecific markers of inflammation. They increase as a result of the acute-phase reactant response, which is a response to inflammatory stimuli such as infection or tissue injury. These tests may be used as markers of infectious disease response because they are elevated when the disease is acutely active and usually fall in response to successful treatment.

Table 69-1

WBC and Differential

Type of Cell	Normal Value (%)	Function	Abnormalities
Neutrophil	Segs 40–60 Bands 3–5	Phagocytic	Leukocytosis • Bacterial infections • Fungal infections • Physiologic stress • Tissue injury (e.g., myocardial Infarction) • Medications (e.g., corticosteroids) Leukopenia • Long-standing infection • Cancer • Medications (e.g., chemotherapy)
Lymphocyte	20–40	T cells (cell-mediated immunity) B cells (humoral antibody response)	Lymphocytosis • Viral infections (e.g., mononucleosis) • Tuberculosis • Fungal infections Lymphopenia • HIV
Monocyte	2–8	Phagocytic Precursor to macrophage	Monocytosis • Tuberculosis • Protozoal infections • Leukemia
Eosinophil	1–4	Antigen-antibody reactions	Eosinophilia • Hypersensitivity reactions, including medications • Parasitic infections
Basophil	Less than 1		Hypersensitivity reactions

WBC, white blood cell count.

Clinicians may use these tests to monitor a patient's response to therapy in osteomyelitis and infective endocarditis. These tests should not be used to diagnose infection because they may be elevated in noninfectious inflammatory conditions (e.g., rheumatoid arthritis, polymyalgia rheumatica, and temporal arteritis).

Microbiologic Studies

Microbiologic studies that allow for direct examination of a specimen (e.g., sputum, blood, or urine) also may aid in a presumptive diagnosis and give an indication of the characteristics of the infecting organism. Generally, microbial cultures are obtained with a Gram stain of the cultured material.

A Gram stain of collected specimens can give rapid information that can be applied immediately to patient care.

Clinical Presentation of Antimicrobial Regimen Selection

- Review of symptoms consistent with an infectious etiology?
- Signs and symptoms may be nonspecific (e.g., fever) or specific.
- Specific signs and symptoms are beyond the scope of this chapter (see disease state-specific chapters for these findings).

Patient History

- History of present illness
- Comorbidities
- Current medications
- Allergies
- Previous antibiotic exposure (may provide clues as to colonization or infection with new specific pathogens or pathogens that may be resistant to certain antimicrobials)
- Previous hospitalization or health care utilization (also a key determinant in selecting therapy because the patient may be at risk for specific pathogens and/or resistant pathogens)
- Travel history
- Social history
- Pet/animal exposure
- Occupational exposure
- Environmental exposure

Physical Findings

- Findings consistent with an infectious etiology?
- Vital signs
- Body system abnormalities (e.g., rales, altered mental status, localized inflammation, erythema, warmth, edema, pain, and pus)

Diagnostic Imaging

- Radiographs (x-rays)
- CT scans
- MRI
- Labeled leukocyte scans

Nonmicrobiologic Laboratory Studies

- White blood cell count (WBC) with differential
- Erythrocyte sedimentation rate (ESR)
- C-reactive protein

Microbiologic Studies

- Gram stain
- Culture and susceptibility testing

A Gram stain is performed to identify if bacteria are present and to determine morphologic characteristics of bacteria (such as gram-positive or gram-negative or shape—cocci, bacilli). Certain specimens do not stain well or at all and must be identified by alternative staining techniques (*Mycoplasma* spp., *Legionella* spp., *Mycobacterium* spp.). Figure 69–2 identifies bacterial pathogens as classified by

Gram stain and morphologic characteristics. The presence of WBCs on a Gram stain indicates inflammation and suggests that the identified bacteria are pathogenic. The Gram stain may be useful in judging a sputum specimen's adequacy. For example, the presence of epithelial cells on sputum Gram stain suggests that the specimen is either poorly collected or contaminated. A poor specimen can give misleading

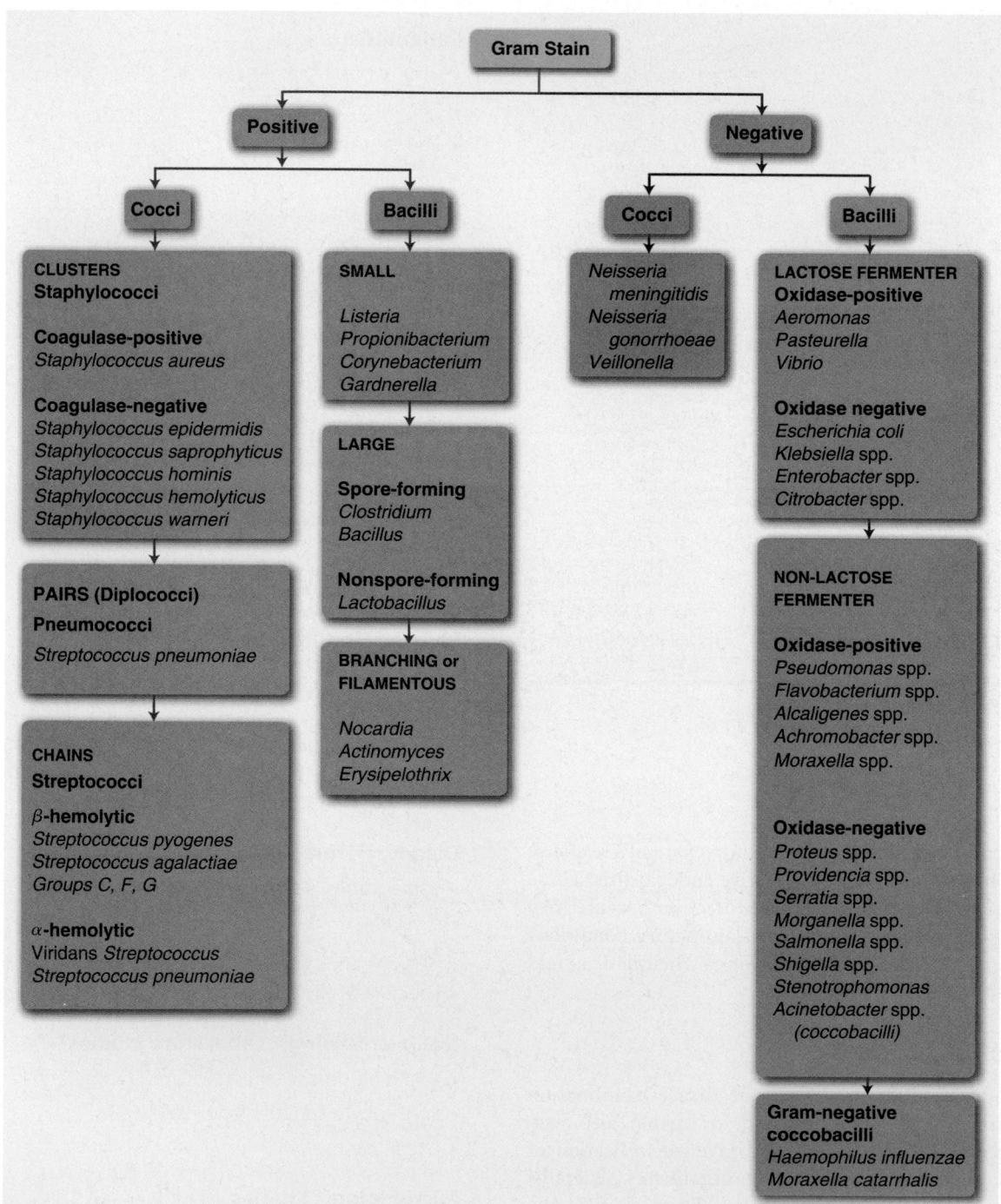

FIGURE 69–2. Important bacterial pathogens classified according to Gram stain and morphologic characteristics. (From Rybak MJ, Aeschlimann JR. Laboratory tests to direct antimicrobial pharmacotherapy. In: In DiPiro JT, Talbert RL, Yee GC, et al., eds. Pharmacotherapy: A Pathophysiologic Approach. 6th ed. New York: McGraw-Hill; 2005:1894.)

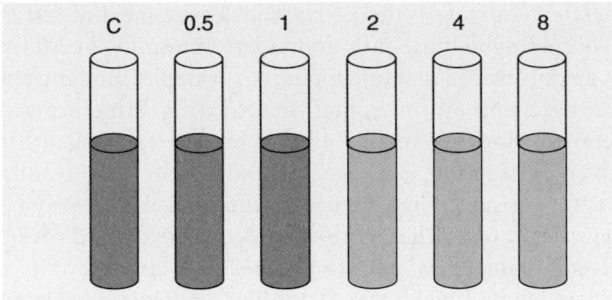

FIGURE 69-3. Macrotube minimal inhibitory concentration (MIC) determination. The growth control (C), 0.5 mg/dL, and 1 mg/dL tubes are visibly turgid, indicating bacterial growth. The MIC is read as the first clear test tube (2 mg/dL). (From Rybak MJ, Aeschlimann JR. Laboratory tests to direct antimicrobial pharmacotherapy. In: In DiPiro JT, Talbert RL, Yee GC, et al., eds. Pharmacotherapy: A Pathophysiologic Approach. 6th ed. New York: McGraw-Hill; 2005:1897.)

information regarding the underlying pathogen and is a waste of laboratory personnel time and patient cost.

Culture and susceptibility testing provides additional information to the clinician to guide appropriate therapy. Specimens are placed in or on culture media that provide the proper growth conditions. Once the bacteria grow on culture media, they can be identified through a variety of biochemical tests. Once a pathogen is identified, susceptibility tests can be performed to various antimicrobial agents. The *minimum inhibitory concentration* (MIC) is a standard susceptibility test. The MIC is the lowest concentration of antimicrobial that inhibits visible bacterial growth after approximately 24 hours (Fig. 69–3). Breakpoint and MIC values determine if the organism is susceptible (S), intermediate (I), or resistant (R) to an antimicrobial. The *breakpoint* is the concentration of the antimicrobial that can be achieved in the serum after a normal or standard dose of that antimicrobial. If the MIC is below the breakpoint, the organism is considered to be susceptible to that agent. If the MIC is above the breakpoint, the organism is said to be resistant. Reported culture and susceptibility results may not provide MIC values but report the S, I, and R results.

❺ *In general, bacterial cultures should be obtained prior to initiating antimicrobial therapy in patients with a systemic inflammatory response, risk factors for antimicrobial resistance, or infections where diagnosis or antimicrobial susceptibility is uncertain.* The decision to culture depends on the sensitivity and specificity of the physical findings, diagnostic examination findings, and whether or not the pathogens are readily predictable. Culture and susceptibility testing usually is not warranted in a young, otherwise healthy woman who presents with signs and symptoms consistent with a urinary tract infection (UTI) because the primary pathogen, *Escherichia coli*, is readily predictable. Cultures and susceptibility testing are routine for sterile-site specimens (e.g., blood and spinal fluid), as well as for material

presumed to be infected (e.g., material obtained from joints and abscesses). Cultures need to be interpreted with caution. Poor specimen collection technique and processing speed can result in misleading information and inappropriate use of antimicrobials.

TREATMENT

General Approach to Treatment, Including Nonantimicrobial Treatment

While selection of antimicrobial therapy may be a major consideration in treating infectious diseases, it may not be the only therapeutic intervention. Other important therapies may include adequate hydration, ventilatory support, and other supportive medications. In addition, antimicrobials are unlikely to be effective if the process or source that leads

---

Patient Encounter 2: Review of Symptoms, Physical Examination, and Laboratory Data

ROS: Patient with malaise, wheezing, dyspnea, cough, chest pain, and chills. No reports of emesis or diarrhea but with decreased appetite.

PE:

- **VS:** BP 160/88, P 84, RR 28, T 39.1°C (102.4°F), O$_2$ sat 86%, Ht 6 ft, 0 in. (183 cm), Wt 80 kg (176 lb)
- **HEENT:** Dry mucous membranes
- **Chest:** Rales and rhonchi R greater than L; diminished breath sounds RML and RLL
- **CV:** Tachycardic with regular rhythm; normal heart sounds

Labs:

- WBC 18.8 × 10³/mm³ (18.8 × 10⁹/L), segs 80%, bands 10%, lymphs 10%
- SCr 2.5 mg/dL (221 µmol/L)
- Glucose 322 mg/dL (17.9 mmol/L)
- Sputum Gram stain: less than 10 epithelial cells, greater than 25 WBCs, predominance of gram-negative bacilli

CXR: Pulmonary infiltrate right middle and lower lobes of right lung

What findings on physical examination are suggestive of an infectious process?

What laboratory findings and/or diagnostic studies have been performed to help establish the presence of an infection?

Are the findings of these laboratory and diagnostic studies suggestive of an infection?

What is your working diagnosis based on this patient encounter?

to the infection is not controlled. *Source control* refers to this process and may involve removal of prosthetic materials such as catheters and infected tissue or drainage of an abscess. Source control considerations should be a fundamental component of any infectious diseases treatment. It is also important to recognize that there may be many different antimicrobial regimens that may cure the patient. While the following therapy sections provide factors to consider when selecting antimicrobial regimens, an excellent and more in-depth resource for selecting antimicrobial regimens for a variety of infectious diseases is the *Infectious Diseases Society of America Guidelines.*[7]

Antimicrobial Considerations in Selecting Therapy

❻ *Drug-specific considerations in antimicrobial selection include spectrum of activity, effects on nontargeted microbial flora, appropriate dose, pharmacokinetic and pharmacodynamic properties, adverse-effect and drug-interaction profile, and cost* (Table 69–2).

▶ Spectrum of Activity and Effects on Nontargeted Flora

Most initial antimicrobial therapy is empirical because cultures usually have not had sufficient time to identify a pathogen. **❼** *Empirical therapy should be based on patient- and antimicrobial-specific factors such as the anatomic location of the infection, the likely pathogens associated with the presentation, the potential for adverse effects in a given patient, and the antimicrobial spectrum of activity.* Prompt initiation of appropriate therapy is paramount in hospitalized patients who are critically ill. Patients who receive initial antimicrobial therapy that provides coverage against the causative pathogen survive at twice the rate of patients who do not receive adequate therapy initially.[8] Empirical selection of antimicrobial spectrum of activity should be related to the severity of the illness. Generally, acutely ill patients may require broader-spectrum antimicrobial coverage, whereas less ill patients may be managed initially with narrow-spectrum therapy. While a detailed description of antimicrobial pathogen-specific spectrum of activity is beyond the scope of this chapter, this information can be obtained readily from a number of sources.[9,10]

TABLE 69–2

Considerations for Selecting Antimicrobial Regimens

Drug Specific	Patient Specific
Spectrum of activity and effects on nontargeted flora	Anatomic location of infection
Dosing	Antimicrobial history
Pharmacokinetic properties	Drug allergy history
Pharmacodynamic properties	Renal and hepatic function
Adverse-effect potential	Concomitant medications
Drug-interaction potential	Pregnancy or lactation
Cost	Compliance potential

Collateral damage is defined as the development of resistance occurring in a patient's nontargeted antimicrobial flora that can cause secondary infections. For example, clindamycin is an excellent antimicrobial for treating streptococcal infections. However, many antimicrobials can treat this relatively susceptible pathogen. Clindamycin also readily selects for resistance in a nontargeted organism that may be present in the intestinal tract, namely, *Clostridium difficile*. Collateral damage is manifested because clindamycin is considered to be a major risk factor for *C. difficile*–associated diarrhea.[11] If several different antimicrobials possess activity against a targeted pathogen, the antimicrobial that is least likely to be associated with collateral damage may be preferred.

▶ Single Versus Combination Therapy

A common subject of debate involves the need to provide similar bacterial coverage with two antimicrobials for serious infections. Proponents state that double coverage may be synergistic, prevent the emergence of resistance, and improve outcome. However, there are few clinical examples in the literature to support these assertions. Examples where double coverage is considered superior are limited to infections associated with large bacterial inocula and in species that are known to readily develop resistance such as active tuberculosis or enterococcal endocarditis.[12,13] A study of patients with *Pseudomonas aeruginosa* infections, an intrinsically resistant organism, demonstrated that empirical double coverage with two antipseudomonal antimicrobials improved survival.[14] The analysis found that combination therapy increased the likelihood of appropriate empirical coverage; however, once organism susceptibilities were known, there was no difference in outcome between double coverage and monotherapy. Double antimicrobial coverage with similar spectra of activity may be beneficial for selected infections associated with high bacterial loads or for initial empirical coverage of critically ill patients in whom antimicrobial-resistant organisms are suspected. Monotherapy usually is satisfactory once antimicrobial susceptibilities are established.

▶ Antimicrobial Dose

Clinicians should be aware that dosage regimens with the same drug maybe different depending on the infectious process. For example, ciprofloxacin, a fluoroquinolone, has various dosage regimens based on site of infection. The dosing for uncomplicated UTIs is 250 mg twice daily for 3 days. For complicated UTIs, the dose is 500 mg twice daily for 7 to 14 days. Severe complicated pneumonia requires a dosage regimen of 750 mg twice daily for 7 to 14 days. Clinicians are encouraged to use dosing regimens designed for treatment of the specific diagnosed infection because they have demonstrated proven efficacy and are most likely to minimize harm.

▶ Pharmacokinetic Properties

Pharmacokinetic properties of an antimicrobial may be important in antimicrobial regimens. *Pharmacokinetics* refers to a mathematical method of describing a patient's drug exposure in vivo in terms of absorption, distribution, metabolism, and elimination. *Bioavailability* refers to the amount of antimicrobial that is absorbed orally relative to an equivalent dose administered intravenously. Drug-related factors that may affect oral bioavailability include the salt formulation of the antimicrobial, the dosage form, and the stability of the drug in the gastrointestinal tract. Frequently, absorption may be affected by gastrointestinal tract blood flow. All patients that manifest systemic signs of infection such as hypotension or hypoperfusion should receive intravenous antimicrobials to ensure drug delivery. In almost all cases where patients have a functioning gastrointestinal tract and are not hypotensive, antimicrobials with almost complete bioavailability (greater than 80%) such as the fluoroquinolones, fluconazole, and linezolid may be given orally. With antimicrobials with modest bioavailability (e.g., many β-lactams), the decision to choose an oral product will depend more on the severity of the illness and the anatomic location of the infection. In sequestered infections, where higher systemic concentrations of antimicrobial may be necessary to reach the infected source (e.g., meningitis) or for antimicrobials with poor bioavailability, intravenous formulations should be used.

Several points regarding how the antimicrobial distributes into tissue are worth mentioning. First, only antimicrobials not bound to albumin are biologically active. Protein binding is likely clinically irrelevant in antimicrobials with low or intermediate protein binding. However, highly protein bound antimicrobials (greater than 50%) also may not be able to penetrate sequestered compartments, such as cerebral spinal fluid, resulting in insufficient concentration to inhibit bacteria. Second, some drugs may not achieve sufficient concentrations in specific compartments based on distribution characteristics. For example, *Legionella pneumophilia* is a nonenteric gram-negative organism that causes severe pneumonia. The organism is known to survive and reside inside pulmonary macrophages. Treatment with an antibiotic that works by inhibiting bacterial cell wall synthesis, such as a cephalosporin, will be ineffective because it only distributes into extracellular host tissues. However, macrolide or fluoroquinolone antimicrobials, which concentrate in human pulmonary macrophages, are highly effective against pneumonia caused by this organism.

Many antimicrobials undergo some degree of metabolism once ingested. Metabolism may occur via hepatic, renal, or nonorgan-specific enzymatic processes. The route of elimination of the metabolic pathway may be exploited for infections associated with tissues related to the metabolic pathways. For example, many fluoroquinolone antimicrobials are metabolized only in part and undergo renal elimination. Urinary concentrations of active drug are many times those achieved in the systemic circulation, making several of these agents good choices for UTIs.

▶ Pharmacodynamic Properties

Pharmacodynamics describes the relationship between drug exposure and pharmacologic effect of antibacterial activity or human toxicology. Antimicrobials generally are categorized based on their concentration-related effects on bacteria. Concentration-dependent pharmacodynamic activity occurs where higher drug concentrations are associated with greater rates and extents of bacterial killing. Concentration-dependent antimicrobial activity is maximized when peak antimicrobial concentrations are high. In contrast, *concentration-independent (or time-dependent) activity* refers to a minimal increase in the rate or extent of bacterial killing with an increase in antimicrobial dose. Concentration-independent antimicrobial activity is maximized when these antimicrobials are dosed to maintain blood and/or tissue concentrations above the MIC in a time-dependent manner. Fluoroquinolones, aminoglycosides, and metronidazole are examples of antimicrobials that exhibit concentration-dependent activity, whereas β-lactam and glycopeptide antimicrobials exhibit concentration-independent activity. Pharmacodynamic properties have been optimized to develop new dosing strategies for older antimicrobials. Examples include single-daily-dose aminoglycoside or β-lactam therapy administered by continuous infusion. The product labeling for many new antimicrobials takes pharmacodynamic properties into account.

Antimicrobials also can be classified as possessing bactericidal or bacteriostatic activity in vitro. Bactericidal antibiotics generally kill at least 99.9% (3 log reduction) of a bacterial population, whereas bacteriostatic antibiotics possess antimicrobial activity but reduce bacterial load by less than 3 logs. Clinically, bactericidal antibiotics may be necessary to achieve success in infections such as endocarditis or meningitis. A full discussion of the application of antimicrobial pharmacodynamics is beyond the scope of this chapter, but excellent sources of information are available.[15]

▶ Adverse-Effect and Drug-Interaction Properties

A major concern when selecting antimicrobial regimens should be the propensity for the regimen to cause adverse effects and the potential for interaction with other drugs. Patients may possess characteristics or risk factors that increase their likelihood of developing an adverse event, emphasizing the need to obtain a good patient medical history. In general, if several different antimicrobial options are available, antimicrobials with a low propensity to cause specific adverse events should be selected, particularly for patients with risk factors for a particular complication. Risk factors for adverse events may include the coadministration of other drugs that are associated with a similar type of adverse event. For example, coadministration of the known nephrotoxin gentamicin with vancomycin increases the risk for nephrotoxicity compared with administration of either drug alone.[16] Other drug interactions may predispose the patient to dose-related toxicity through inhibition of drug metabolism. For example, erythromycin has the potential to prolong cardiac QT intervals in a dose-dependent manner, potentially increasing the risk for sudden cardiac death. A cohort study of patients taking oral erythromycin found that patients with concomitantly prescribed medications that inhibited the metabolism of erythromycin exhibited a fivefold increase in cardiac death versus controls.[17]

▶ Antimicrobial Cost

A final consideration in selecting antimicrobial therapy relates to cost. It is important to remember that the most inexpensive antimicrobial is not necessarily the most cost-effective antimicrobial. Antimicrobial costs constitute a relatively small portion of the overall cost of care. Frequently, regulatory studies are not designed to identify differences in hospital length of stay, less common adverse events, monitoring costs, collateral damage, or antimicrobial-specific resistance issues, all of which may contribute to medical costs. Careful consideration of antimicrobial microbiologic, pharmacologic, and patient-related factors such as compliance and a variety of clinical outcomes is necessary to establish the cost versus benefit of an antimicrobial in a given patient. If there is no difference or a small difference in these factors, the least costly antimicrobial may be the best choice.

Patient Considerations in Antimicrobial Selection

8 *Key patient-specific considerations in antimicrobial selection include recent previous antimicrobial exposures, identification of the anatomic location of infection through physical examination and diagnostic imaging, history of drug allergies, pregnancy or breast-feeding status, organ dysfunction that may affect drug clearance, immunosuppression, compliance, and the severity of illness (see Table 69–2).*

▶ Host Factors

Host factors can help to ensure selection of the most appropriate antimicrobial agent. Age is an important factor in antimicrobial selection. With regard to dose and interval, renal and hepatic function varies with age. Populations with diminished renal function include neonates and the elderly. Hepatic function in the neonate is not fully developed, and drugs that are metabolized or eliminated by this route may produce adverse effects. For example, sulfonamides and ceftriaxone may compete with bilirubin for binding sites and may result in hyperbilirubinemia and kernicterus. Gastric acidity also depends on age; the elderly and children younger than 3 years of age tend to be achlorhydric. Drugs that need an acidic environment (e.g., ketoconazole) are not well absorbed, and those whose absorption is enhanced in an alkaline environment will have increased concentrations (e.g., penicillin G).

Disruption of host defenses owing to IV catheters, indwelling Foley catheters, burns, trauma, surgery, and increased gastric pH (secondary to antacids, H_2 blockers, and proton pump inhibitors) may place patients at higher risk for infection. Breaks in and entry into the skin provide a route for infection because the natural barrier of the skin is disrupted. Increased gastric pH can allow for bacterial overgrowth and has been associated with an increased risk of pneumonia.[18]

Recognizing the presumed site of infection and most common pathogens associated with the infectious source should guide antimicrobial choice, dose, and route of administration. For example, community-acquired pneumonia is caused most commonly by *S. pneumoniae*, *E. coli* is the primary cause of uncomplicated UTIs, and staphylococci and streptococci are implicated most frequently in skin and skin-structure infections (e.g., cellulitis).

Patients with a history of recent antimicrobial use may have altered normal flora or harbor resistant organisms. If a patient develops a new infection while on therapy, fails therapy, or has received antimicrobials recently, it is prudent to prescribe a different class of antimicrobial because resistance is likely. Previous hospitalization or health care utilization (e.g., residing in a nursing home, hemodialysis, and outpatient antimicrobial therapy) are risk factors for the acquisition of nosocomial pathogens, which are often resistant organisms.

Antimicrobial allergies are some of the most common drug-related allergies reported and have significant potential to cause adverse events. In particular, penicillin-related allergy is common and can be problematic because there is an approximately 4% cross-reactivity with cephalosporins as well as carbapenems.[19,20] In general, a patient's medical history should be reviewed to determine the offending β-lactam and nature of the allergic reaction. In some cases, patients with mild or nonimmunologic reactions may receive a β-lactam antimicrobial with low cross-reactive potential. However, patients with a history of physical findings consistent with IgE-mediated reactions such as anaphylaxis, urticaria, or bronchospasm should not be administered any type of β-lactam antimicrobial, including cephalosporins, unless there are no other alternatives. Administration of potentially cross-reactive agents in this situation should occur only under controlled conditions, and some patients may need to undergo desensitization. If the specific medical history relating to a reported allergy cannot be obtained, the patient should be assumed to have had an IgE-mediated reaction and should be managed in a similar manner.

Renal and/or hepatic function should be considered in every patient prior to initiation of antimicrobial therapy. In general, most antimicrobials undergo renal elimination and exhibit decreased clearance with diminished renal function, and dosing adjustments are found readily in the literature.[21] In contrast, dosing adjustments for antimicrobials that are not eliminated renally are less well documented. Failure to adjust the antimicrobial dose or interval may result in drug accumulation and an increase in adverse effects.

Concomitant administration of other medications may influence the selection of the antimicrobial, dose, and monitoring. Medications that are commonly associated with drug interactions include, but are not limited to, warfarin, rifampin, phenytoin, digoxin, theophylline, multivalent cations (e.g., calcium, magnesium, and zinc), and sucralfate. Drug interactions between antimicrobials and other medications may occur via the cytochrome P-450 system, protein-binding displacement, and alteration of vitamin K–producing bacteria. Interactions may result in increased concentrations of one or both agents, increasing the risk of adverse effects or additive toxicity. A key consideration in

Patient Encounter 3: Empirical Selection of Antibiotics

Based on the information presented, select an empirical antimicrobial regimen for this patient. Your plan should include

(a) a tentative infectious diagnosis or source, including likely pathogens or resistant organisms;
(b) a specific antimicrobial(s) regimen, including drug(s), dose, and route of administration;
(c) description of any ancillary treatments; and
(d) a rationale for your empirical antimicrobial selection based on drug- and patient-specific considerations.

selecting antimicrobial regimens starts with obtaining a good patient medical and drug history, recognizing drug-specific adverse-event characteristics, and anticipating potential problems proactively. If it is necessary to use an antimicrobial with a relatively high incidence of adverse effects, informing patients of the risks and benefits of therapy, as well as what to do if an adverse effect occurs, may improve patient compliance and may facilitate patient safety.

Antimicrobial agents must be used with caution in pregnant and nursing women. Some agents pose potential threats to the fetus or infant (e.g., quinolones, tetracyclines, and sulfonamides). For some agents, avoidance during a specific trimester of pregnancy is warranted (e.g., trimethoprim/sulfamethoxazole). Pharmacokinetic variables also are altered during pregnancy. Both the clearance and volume of distribution are increased during pregnancy. As a result, increased dosages and/or more frequent administration of certain drugs may be required to achieve adequate concentrations. This information can be obtained from a number of sources.[22,23]

Adherence is essential to ensure efficacy of a particular agent. Patients may stop taking their antibiotics once the symptoms subside and save them for a "future" infection. If the patient does not complete the course of therapy, the infection may not be eradicated, and resistance may emerge. Self-medication of saved antibiotics may be inappropriate and harmful and may select for resistant organisms. Poor patient adherence may be due to adverse effects, tolerability, cost, and lack of patient education.

OUTCOME EVALUATION

Figure 69–4 provides an overview of patient- and antimicrobial agent–specific factors to consider when selecting an antimicrobial regimen. It further delineates monitoring of therapy and actions to take depending on the patient's response to therapy. The duration of therapy depends on patient response and type of infection being treated.

Modifying Empirical Therapy Based on Cultures and Clinical Response

If a successful clinical response occurs and culture results are available, therapy should be de-escalated. *De-escalation* refers to decreasing antimicrobial regimen spectrum of activity to provide coverage against specific antimicrobial-sensitive pathogens recovered from culture. The purpose of de-escalation therapy is to minimize the likelihood of secondary infections owing to antimicrobial-resistant organisms. In cases where a specific organism is recovered that has a known preferred agent of choice, therapy might be changed to that specific agent. For example, antistaphylococcal penicillins are considered to be the agents of choice for methicillin-susceptible *S. aureus* owing to their bactericidal activity and narrow-spectrum activity and may be preferable to other antibiotic regimens. In other cases, empirical coverage might be discontinued if a specific suspected pathogen is excluded by culture or an alternative, noninfectious diagnosis is established. In addition, intravenous antimicrobials frequently are more expensive than oral therapy. Therefore, it is desirable to convert therapy to oral antimicrobials with a comparable antimicrobial spectrum or specific pathogen sensitivity as soon as the patient improves clinically.[24]

Failure of Antimicrobial Therapy

While many infections respond readily to antimicrobials, some infections do not. A relatively common question when a patient's condition fails to improve relates to whether the antimicrobial therapy has failed? Changing antimicrobials generally is one of the easiest interventions relative to other options. However, it is important to remember that antimicrobial therapy comprises only a portion of the overall disease treatment, and there may be many factors that contribute to a lack of improvement. ❿ *In general, inadequate diagnosis resulting in poor initial antimicrobial or other nonantibiotic drug selection, poor source control, or the development of a new infection with a resistant organism are relatively common causes of antimicrobial failure.* An infection-related diagnosis may be difficult to establish and generally has two components: (a) differentiating infection from noninfection-related disease and (b) providing adequate empirical spectrum of activity if the cause is infectious. Failure of improvement in a patient's condition should warrant broadening the differential diagnosis to include noninfection-related causes, as well as considering other potential infectious sources and/or pathogenic organisms. Another common cause of failure is poor source control. A diagnostic search for unknown sources of infection and removal of indwelling devices in the infected environment or surgical drainage of abscesses should be undertaken if the patient's condition is not improving. Less common but still frequent causes of therapeutic failure include the development of secondary infections. In this case, the patient generally improves, but then develops a new infection caused by an antimicrobial resistant pathogen and relapses. The emergence of resistance to a targeted pathogen while on antimicrobial therapy can be associated with clinical failure but usually is limited to tuberculosis, pseudomonads, or other gram-negative enterics. Drug- and patient-specific factors such as appropriate dosing, patient compliance, and drug interactions can be associated

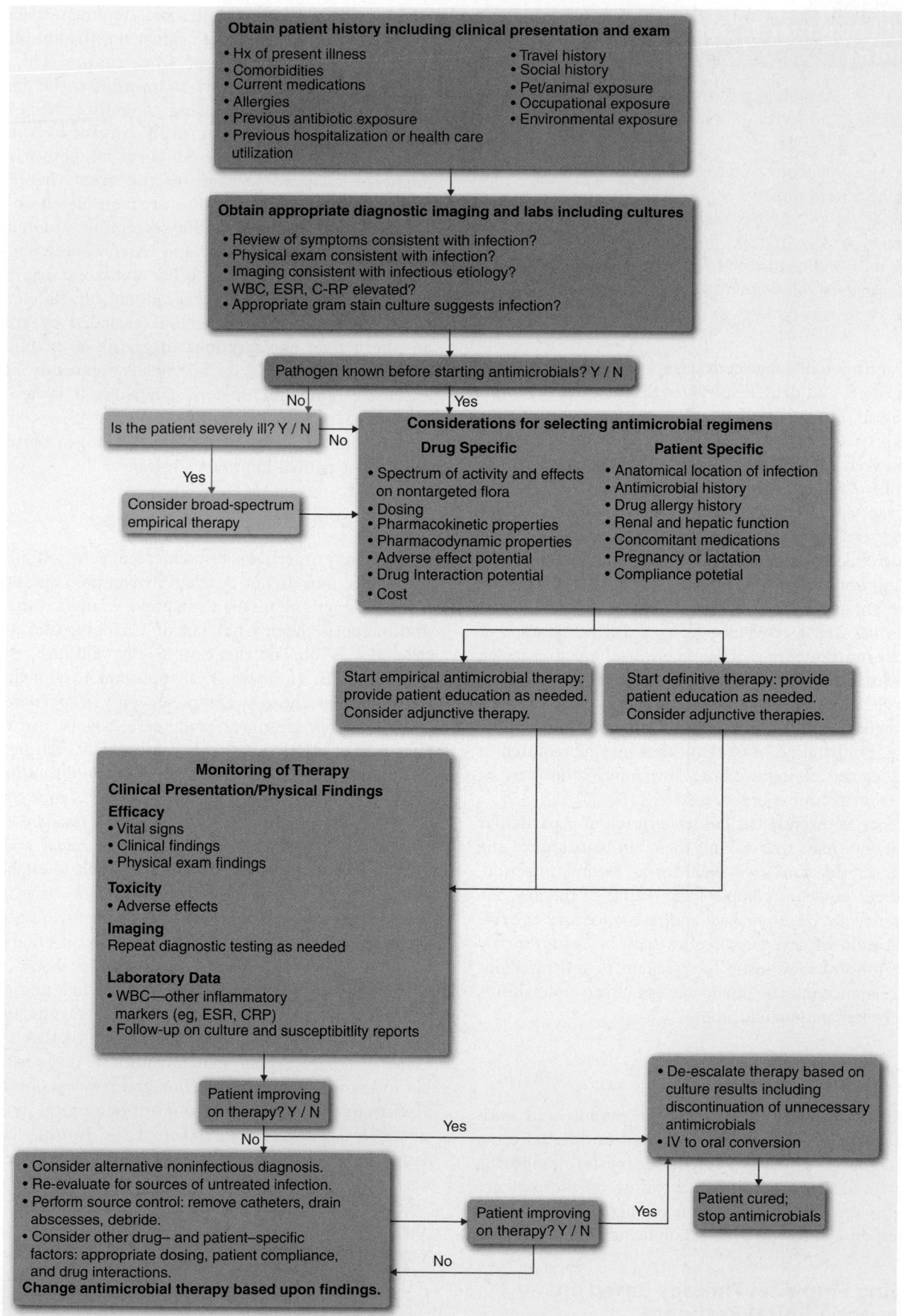

FIGURE 69–4. Approach to selection of antimicrobial therapy.

with therapeutic failure and also should be considered. A common assumption is that the correct diagnosis was made, but the patient was not treated long enough with antimicrobials. There are certain types of infections (e.g., endocarditis or osteomyelitis) where the standard of care is to treat for prolonged periods of time (i.e., weeks or months).

However, the optimal duration of therapy for many infectious diseases is somewhat subjective. Recently, studies of several infectious processes have suggested that shorter durations of therapy can result in similar clinical outcomes as longer durations of therapy, frequently with fewer complications or secondary infections.[25-27] The general trend has been to treat these disease processes with shortened courses of antibiotic therapy. In this period of extensive antimicrobial resistance, clinicians should keep abreast of changing recommendations emphasizing shorter durations of therapy.

Patient Encounter 4: Patient Care and Monitoring

Update: The patient was admitted to the hospital with a presumptive diagnosis of health care–associated pneumonia (based on the recent hospitalization). He received IV hydration with normal saline, 5 L oxygen via face mask, an insulin infusion to control his glucose, and empirical antimicrobial therapy with piperacillin-tazobactam 3.375 g IV every 6 hours and vancomycin 1 g IV every 48 hours. All other medications are continued with the exception of the diabetes medications.

After 48 hours of therapy, the following parameters are obtained:

PE

- **VS:** BP 145/82, P 77, RR 22, T 37.9°C (100.2°F), O_2 sat 92% on 4 L
- **Repeat CXR;** Increased fluid density in bases, infiltrate unchanged, rales and rhonchi unchanged

Labs:

- WBC $13.2 \times 10^3/mm^3$ ($13.2 \times 10^9/L$)
- SCr 1.9 mg/dL (168 μmol/L)
- Glucose 181 mg/dL (10.0 mmol/L)
- Urine and blood cultures × 2: Negative
- Sputum culture: 3+ *P. aeruginosa*

Sensitivity Report:

Cefepime sensitive (MIC = 1)

Ceftazidime sensitive (MIC = 1)

Piperacillin/taz sensitive (MIC = 4)

Imipenem resistant (MIC greater than 64)

Gentamicin sensitive (MIC = 1)

Amikacin sensitive (MIC = 0.5)

Ciprofloxacin resistant (MIC greater than 4)

What information suggests improvement in the patient's condition?

Do any of the antimicrobial doses need to be adjusted for changes in organ function?

Should antimicrobial therapy be modified based on the culture results?

Can the antimicrobial therapy be converted from IV to oral therapy?

Patient Care and Monitoring

After selection and initiation of antimicrobial regimen, there are a number of additional patient care and monitoring considerations that should be addressed to improve the likelihood of a successful outcome. ❾ *Patient education, de-escalation of antimicrobial therapy based on culture results, monitoring for clinical response and adverse effects, and appropriate duration of therapy are important.*

Patient Education

Provide patient education with regard to appropriate use of antimicrobials (e.g., dose, interval), adverse effects, and drug interactions (which may play a role in therapy failure and increased toxicity).

Therapeutic Monitoring

Monitor for therapeutic response by assessing efficacy and toxicity of the antimicrobial regimen.

- Clinical presentation/physical findings
- *Efficacy:* Assess vital signs (monitor for return to normal or lack of altered findings; e.g., fever), physical examination findings, patient's subjective impression
- *Toxicity:* Monitor and assess for adverse effects and evaluate antimicrobial serum concentrations when appropriate to minimize toxicity and improve outcomes
- *Diagnostic imaging*: Diagnostic testing is disease state-dependent
- Laboratory data
- Monitor and assess laboratory data: WBC with differential (goal is a reduction in WBC if elevated initially and resolution of left shift), renal and/or hepatic function (consider need for dosage adjustments), other labs as indicated (e.g., ESR, CRP)
- Follow-up on culture and susceptibility reports with subsequent de-escalation of therapy, if possible
- Reculture of specimens is not performed routinely except in few cases (e.g., endocarditis) or where a secondary infection is suspected because data may be misleading and lead to the addition of broader or more powerful antimicrobials

CONCLUSION

Antimicrobial regimen selection is a complex process involving the integration of a multitude of factors. The guiding principles to make the diagnosis and do no harm must be considered when choosing an antimicrobial for a given patient. In summary, when infection is suspected, rapid and accurate diagnosis should be followed by early intervention that includes administration of appropriately dosed antibiotics with appropriate empirical spectrums. De-escalation to suitable narrow-spectrum antibiotics if susceptibilities are known should occur as soon as possible, and therapy should be stopped as soon as the patient is cured. These fundamental actions improve infectious disease outcomes and minimize collateral damage and adverse effects.

Abbreviations Introded in This Chapter

CDC	Centers for Disease Control and Prevention
CRP	C-reactive protein
ESR	Erythrocyte sedimentation rate
HPI	History of present illness
MIC	Minimum inhibitory concentration
MRSA	Methicillin-resistant *Staphylococcus aureus*
PMH	Part medical history
UTI	Urinary tract infection
VRE	Vancomycin-resistant *Enterococcus*
WBC	White blood cell count

 Self-assessment questions and answers are available at *http://www.mhpharmacotherapy. com/pp.html.*

REFERENCES

1. Shehab N, Patel PR, Srinivasan A, Budnitz DS. Emergency department visits for antibiotic-associated adverse events. Clin Infect Dis 2008;47:735–743.
2. National Vital Statistics Reports 2005;(53)17.
3. Centers for Disease Control Antimicrobial Resistance. *http://www.cdc. gov/drugresistance/community/faqs.htm.*
4. Vanderweil SG, Pelletier AJ, Hamedani AG, Gonzales R, Metlay JP, Camargo CA Jr. Declining antibiotic prescriptions for upper respiratory infections, 1993–2004. Acad Emerg Med 2007;14:366–369.
5. Burke J. Infection control—A problem for patient safety. N Engl J Med 2003;348:651–655.
6. Mackowiak PA. Temperature regulation and the pathogenesis of fever. In: Mandell GL, Bennett JE, Dolin R. Mandell, Douglas, Bennett's, eds. Principles and Practice of Infectious Diseases. 5th ed. Philadelphia: Churchill Livingstone, 2000:604–620.
7. Practice Guidelines from the Infectious Diseases Society of America. *http://www.journals.uchicago.edu/IDSA/guidelines/.*
8. Kollef MH, Sherman G, Ward S, Fraser VJ. Inadequate antimicrobial treatment of infections: A risk factor for hospital mortality among critically ill patients. Chest 1999;115:462–474.
9. Antimicrobial spectra. In: Gilbert DN, Moellering RC, Eliopoulos GM, Sande MA, eds. The Sanford Guide to Antimicrobial Therapy 2008. 38th ed. Sperryville, VA: Antimicrobial Inc.
10. John Hopkins University Division of Infectious Diseases Antibiotic Guide. *http://www.hopkins-abxguide.org/.*
11. Johnson S, Samore MH, Farrow AF, et al. Epidemics of diarrhea caused by a clindamycin resistant strain of Clostridium difficile in four hospitals. N Engl J Med 1999;341:1645–1651.
12. Peloquin CA. Tuberculosis. In: DiPiro JT, Talbert RL, Yee GC, et al., eds. Pharmacotherapy: A Pathophysiological Approach. 6th ed. New York: McGraw-Hill, 2005:2015–2334.
13. Baddour LM, Wilson WR, Bayer AS, et al. Infective endocarditis: diagnosis, antimicrobial therapy, and management of complications: a statement for healthcare professionals from the Committee on Rheumatic Fever, Endocarditis, and Kawasaki Disease, Council on Cardiovascular Disease in the Young, and the Councils on Clinical Cardiology, Stroke, and Cardiovascular Surgery and Anesthesia, American Heart Association: endorsed by the Infectious Diseases Society of America. Circulation 2005;111:394–434.
14. Chamot E, Boffi E, Amari E, et al. Effectiveness of combination antimicrobial therapy for Pseudomonas aeruginosa bacteremia. Antimicrob Agents Chemother 2003;47:2756–2764.
15. Craig WA. Pharmacodynamics of antimicrobials. In: Nightingale CH, Murakawa T, Ambrose PG, eds. Antimicrobial Pharmacodynamics in Theory and Clinical Practice. 1st ed. New York: Marcel Dekker, 2002:1–22.
16. Rybak MJ. The pharmacokinetic and pharmacodynamic properties of vancomycin. Clin Infect Dis 2006;42(Suppl 1):S35–S39.
17. Ray WA, Murray KT, Meredith S, et al. Oral erythromycin and the risk of sudden death from cardiac causes. N Engl J Med 2004;351:1089–1096.
18. Laheij RJ, Sturkenboom MC, Hassing R, et al. Risk of community-acquired pneumonia and use of gastric acid-suppressing drugs. JAMA 2004;292:1955–1960.
19. Gruchalla RS, Pirmohamed M. Clinical practice. Antibiotic allergy. N Engl J Med 2006;354:601–609.
20. Weiss ME, Adkinson NF. B-lactam Allergy. In: Mandell GL, Bennett JE, Dolin R, eds. Principles and Practice of Infectious Diseases. 6th ed. Philadelphia, PA: Churchill Livingstone, 2005.
21. Frye RF, Matzke GR. Drug therapy individualization for patients with renal insufficiency. In: DiPiro JT, Talbert RL, Yee GC, et al., eds. Pharmacotherapy: A Pathophysiological Approach. 6th ed. New York: McGraw-Hill, 2005:919–933.
22. Briggs GG, Freeman RK, Yaffe SJ. Drugs in Pregnancy and Lactation. 7th ed. Philadelphia: Lippincott Williams & Wilkins, 2005.
23. Hale TW. Medications and Mothers' Milk. 11th ed. Amarillo, TX: Pharmasoft, 2004.
24. Press RA. The use of fluoroquinolones as antiinfective transition-therapy agents in community-acquired pneumonia. Pharmacotherapy 2001;21(7 pt 2):100S–104S.
25. Goff DA. Short-duration therapy for respiratory tract infections. Ann Pharmacother 2004;38(Suppl 9):S19–S23.
26. Chastre J, Wolff M, Fagon JY, et al. For the PneumA Trial Group. Comparison of 8 vs 15 days of antibiotic therapy for ventilator-associated pneumonia in adults: A randomized trial. JAMA 2003;290:2588–2598.
27. Kollef MH, Napolitano LM, Solomkin JS, Wunderink RG, Bae IG, Fowler VG, Balk RA, Stevens DL, Rahal JJ, Shorr AF, Linden PK, Micek ST. Healthcare-associated infection (HAI): A critical appraisal of the emerging threat-proceedings of the HAI Summit. Clin Infect Dis 2008 Oct 1;2 (Suppl 47):S55–S99.

70 Central Nervous System Infections

P. Brandon Bookstaver and April D. Miller

LEARNING OBJECTIVES

● **Upon completion of the chapter, the reader will be able to:**

1. Discuss the pathophysiology of CNS infections and the impact on antimicrobial treatment regimens (such as dosing and CNS penetration).

2. Describe the signs, symptoms, and clinical presentation of CNS infections.

3. List the most common pathogens causing CNS infections and identify risk factors for infection with each pathogen.

4. State the goals of therapy for CNS infections.

5. Design appropriate empirical antimicrobial regimens for patients suspected of having CNS infections caused by each of the following pathogens (taking age, vaccine history, and other patient-specific information into account), and analyze the impact of antimicrobial resistance on both empirical and definitive therapy: *Neisseria meningitidis* meningitis, meningitis, *Haemophilus influenzae* meningitis, *Listeria* meningitis, group B *Streptococcus* meningitis, gram-negative bacillary meningitis, postneurosurgical infection, CNS shunt infection, herpes simplex encephalitis.

6. Modify empirical antimicrobial regimens based on laboratory data and other diagnostic criteria.

7. Discuss the management of close contacts of patients diagnosed with CNS infections.

8. Identify candidates for vaccines and other prophylactic therapies to prevent CNS infections.

9. Describe the role of adjunctive agents (such as dexamethasone) in the management of CNS infections.

10. Formulate a monitoring plan to assess efficacy and adverse effects of therapy for CNS infections.

KEY CONCEPTS

❶ Meningitis is a neurologic emergency that requires prompt recognition, diagnosis, and management to prevent death and residual neurologic defects. Patients with fever, headache, and neck stiffness should be evaluated for meningitis.

❷ Ideally, lumbar puncture (LP) to obtain cerebrospinal fluid (CSF) for direct examination and laboratory analysis, as well as blood cultures and other relevant cultures, should be obtained before initiation of antimicrobial therapy. However, initiation of antimicrobial therapy should not be delayed if a pretreatment LP cannot be performed.

❸ The treatment goals for CNS infections are to prevent death and residual neurologic deficits, eradicate or control causative microorganisms, ameliorate clinical signs and symptoms, and identify measures (such as vaccination and suppressive therapy) to prevent future infections.

❹ Prompt initiation of IV high-dose bactericidal antimicrobial therapy directed at the most likely pathogen(s) is essential due to the high morbidity and mortality associated with CNS infections.

❺ IV therapy is administered for the full course of therapy for CNS infections to ensure adequate CSF penetration throughout the course of treatment.

❻ Empirical therapy should be directed at the most likely pathogen(s) for a specific patient, taking into account age, risk factors for infection (including underlying disease and immune dysfunction, vaccine history, and recent exposures), CSF Gram stain results, CSF antibiotic penetration, and local antimicrobial resistance patterns.

❼ Empirical antimicrobial therapy should be modified on the basis of laboratory data and clinical response.

❽ Close contacts of patients with CNS infections should be evaluated for possible antimicrobial prophylaxis.

⑨ Components of a monitoring plan to assess the efficacy and safety of antimicrobial therapy of CNS infections include clinical signs and symptoms and laboratory data (e.g., CSF findings, culture, and sensitivity data).

The term *CNS infections* describes a variety of infections involving the brain and spinal cord and associated tissues, fluids, and membranes, including meningitis, encephalitis, brain abscess, shunt infections, and postoperative infections (see Glossary). **❶** *CNS infections, such as meningitis, are considered neurologic emergencies that require prompt recognition, diagnosis, and management to prevent death and residual neurologic deficits.* Improperly treated, CNS infections are associated with high rates of morbidity and mortality. Despite advances in care, the overall mortality of bacterial meningitis remains greater than 20%, and at least 10% to 30% of survivors are afflicted with neurologic impairment, including hearing loss, hemiparesis, and learning disabilities.[1-3] Antimicrobial therapy and preventive vaccines have revolutionized management and improved outcomes of bacterial meningitis and other CNS infections dramatically.

EPIDEMIOLOGY AND ETIOLOGY

CNS infections are uncommon, with four to six cases of meningitis reported per 100,000 adults annually.[4] However, the severity of these infections demands prompt medical intervention and treatment. CNS infections can be caused by bacteria, fungi, mycobacteria, viruses, and spirochetes.

Bacterial meningitis is the most common cause of CNS infections. *Streptococcus pneumoniae* (pneumococcus) was the most common pathogen for bacterial meningitis (47%), followed by *Neisseria meningitidis* (meningococcus, 25%), group B *Streptococcus* (12%), *Listeria monocytogenes* (8%), and *Haemophilus influenzae* (7%).[5] Vaccines directed against bacteria causing meningitis and related infections (such as pneumonia and ear infections) have reduced the risk of infections due to *S. pneumoniae, N. meningitidis,* and *H. influenzae* type b (HIb) dramatically. Prior to the availability of Hib conjugate vaccines, Hib meningitis or other invasive disease was documented in one in 200 children by the age of 5 years.[5] Widespread use of the Hib vaccine has reduced the incidence of invasive Hib disease by 99% and has shifted the age distribution of bacterial meningitis to older age groups (from 15 months in 1986 to 25 years in 1995).[1,6] The routine use of the 7-valent conjugate pneumococcal vaccine (PCV7) in children has not only reduced the incidence of invasive pneumococcal disease in children but has also reduced invasive pneumococcal disease in adults 50 years of age and older by 28%.[7] Despite introduction of the PCV7, *S. pneumoniae* remains the most common pathogen for pediatric bacterial meningitis with nearly 50% of cases due to nonvaccine serotypes.[8]

Encephalitis may result from a number of viral, bacterial, parasitic, and other noninfectious causes. Herpes simplex virus (HSV) is the most common cause of encephalitis in the United States, accounting for 10% of all cases.[9] The annual incidence of viral encephalitis is estimated to be 3.5 to 7.4 infections per 100,000 persons.[9] Other pathogens include common bacterial meningitis causes, *Ricksettia* species, enteroviruses, arboviruses, varicella-zoster virus, rotavirus, coronavirus, influenza viruses A and B, West Nile virus, and Epstein-Barr virus may be associated with a meningo-encephalopathic presentation.[10] Approximately 20,000 hospitalizations each year are secondary to encephalitis accounting for $650 million in health care costs.[11] Over the past 10 to 20 years, mortality secondary to encephalitis has remained constant correlating well with the increased number of people living with HIV and AIDS. HIV infection is concurrent in nearly 20% of patients dying from encephalitis.[12]

Neurosurgical procedures may place patients at risk for meningitis due to bacteria (such as *Staphylococcus aureus,* coagulase-negative staphylococci, and gram-negative bacilli) acquired at the time of surgery or in the postoperative period. In addition to bacteria, other pathogens may cause meningitis in at-risk patients. Immunocompromised patients, such as solid-organ transplant patients and patients living with HIV infection, are at risk for fungal meningitis with *Cryptococcus neoformans* and encephalitis secondary to *Toxoplasma gondii* and JC virus (see Chap. 84). Tuberculosis can spread from pulmonary sites to cause clinical disease in the CNS. Life-threatening viral encephalitis and meningitis can occur in otherwise healthy, young individuals, as well as in patients immunocompromised by age or other factors. Because the treatments for different types of CNS infections are often different, it is important to pay close attention to patients' risk factors when choosing empirical antimicrobial therapy. Patients at extremes of age, those living in close contact with others, and those with immune defects are most susceptible to meningitis. Risk factors for CNS infections can be classified as follows:

- *Environmental*—recent exposures (such as close contact with meningitis or respiratory tract infection, contaminated foods), active or passive exposure to cigarette smoke, close living conditions

- *Recent infection in the patient*—respiratory infection, otitis media, sinusitis, mastoiditis

- *Immunosuppression*—anatomic or functional asplenia, sickle cell disease, alcoholism, cirrhosis, immunoglobulin or complement deficiency, cancer, HIV/AIDS, uncontrolled diabetes mellitus, debilitated state of health

- *Surgery, trauma*—neurosurgery, head trauma, CSF shunt, cochlear implant

- Noninfectious causes of meningitis include malignancy, medications (such as sulfonamides, nonsteroidal anti-inflammatory drugs [NSAIDs], IV Immunoglobulin), autoimmune disease (such as lupus), and trauma.[8,9]

- The most common pathogens causing bacterial meningitis, by age group and other risk factors, are found in Table 70–1.

PATHOPHYSIOLOGY

Meningitis is an inflammation of the membranes of the brain and spinal cord (meninges) and the CSF in contact with these

Table 70–1

Most Likely Pathogens and Recommended Empirical Therapy, by Risk Factor, for Bacterial Meningitis

Predisposing Factor	Most Likely Pathogens	Recommended Empirical Antibiotic Therapy
Age		
Less than 3 months	Group B *Streptococcus* *Escherichia coli* *Klebsiella pneumoniae* *Listeria monocytogenes*	Ampicillin *plus* cefotaxime or aminoglycoside
3 months to less than 18 years	*Neisseria meningitidis* *Streptococcus pneumoniae* *Haemophilus influenzae*	Cefotaxime or ceftriaxone *plus* vancomycin
18 years to less than 60 years	*Neisseria meningitidis* *S. pneumoniae*	Cefotaxime or ceftriaxone *plus* vancomycin
60 years or older	*S. pneumoniae* Gram-negative bacilli *L. monocytogenes*	Cefotaxime or ceftriaxone *plus* vancomycin *plus* ampicillin
Immunocompromised	*S. pneumoniae* *N. meningitidis* *L. monocytogenes* Gram-negative bacilli (including *Pseudomonas aeruginosa*)	Cefotaxime or ceftriaxone *plus* vancomycin *plus* ampicillin (double antibiotic coverage against *Pseudomonas* if suspected)
Surgery, Trauma		
Postneurosurgical infection	*S. aureus* (including MRSA) Coagulase-negative *Staphylococcus* (including MRSE) Gram-negative bacilli (including *P. aeruginosa*)	Vancomycin *or* linezolid *plus* ceftazidime or cefepime or meropenem
Penetrating head trauma	*S. aureus* (including MRSA) Coagulase-negative *Staphylococcus* Gram-negative bacilli (including *P. aeruginosa*)	Vancomycin *or* linezolid *plus* ceftazidime or cefepime or meropenem (double antibiotic coverage against *Pseudomonas* if suspected)
CSF shunt	Coagulase-negative *Staphylococcus (including MRSE)* *S. aureus (including MRSA)* Gram-negative bacilli (including *P. aeruginosa*)	Vancomycin *or* linezolid *plus* ceftazidime or cefepime or meropenem (double antibiotic coverage against *Pseudomonas* if suspected)

MRSA, methicillin-resistant *Staphylococcus aureus*; MRSE, methicillin-resistant *Staphylococcus epidermidis*.

From Refs. 14, 24.

Patient Encounter 1, Part 1

JD is a 17-year-old high school senior who visited her sister at her college dormitory for 1 week prior to her sister leaving for winter break. JD now presents to the emergency department with a 2-day history of headache and fever. Physical findings and laboratory values include temperature of 38.3°C (101°F) and WBC of 14.4 × 10³/mm³ (14.4 × 10⁹/L), with 90% polymorphonuclear cells. Examination reveals nuchal rigidity and a petechial truncal rash. JD reports light sensitivity and nausea with vomiting. She has tried nonprescription analgesics and antipyretics with no relief from her headache or fever.

What signs and symptoms consistent with meningitis are present in JD?

What clues to causative pathogen are present in JD?

What empiric antibiotics should be started?

---

membranes, whereas encephalitis is an inflammation of the brain tissue. CSF flows through the subarachnoid space, insulating and protecting delicate CNS tissue. CSF is produced within the ventricles of the brain and flows downward through the spinal cord, serving as a continuous flushing mechanism for the CNS.

The blood–brain barrier and blood–CSF barrier are made of specialized tissue capillaries that isolate the brain from substances circulating in the bloodstream or colonizing nearby tissues. To initiate a CNS infection, pathogens must gain entry into the CNS by **contiguous** spread, **hematogenous** seeding, direct inoculation, or reactivation of latent infection. **Contiguous** spread occurs when infections in adjacent structures (such as sinus cavities or the middle ear) invade directly through the blood–brain barrier (such as Hib). **Hematogenous** seeding occurs when a more remote infection causes bacteremia that seeds the CSF (such as pneumococcal pneumonia). Reactivation of latent infection results from dormant viral, fungal, or mycobacterial pathogens in the spine, brain, or nerve tracts. Direct inoculation of bacteria into the CNS is the result of trauma, congenital malformations, or complications of neurosurgery.

Once through the blood–brain barrier, pathogens thrive and replicate due to limited host defenses in the CNS. Figure 70–1 depicts the pathophysiologic changes associated

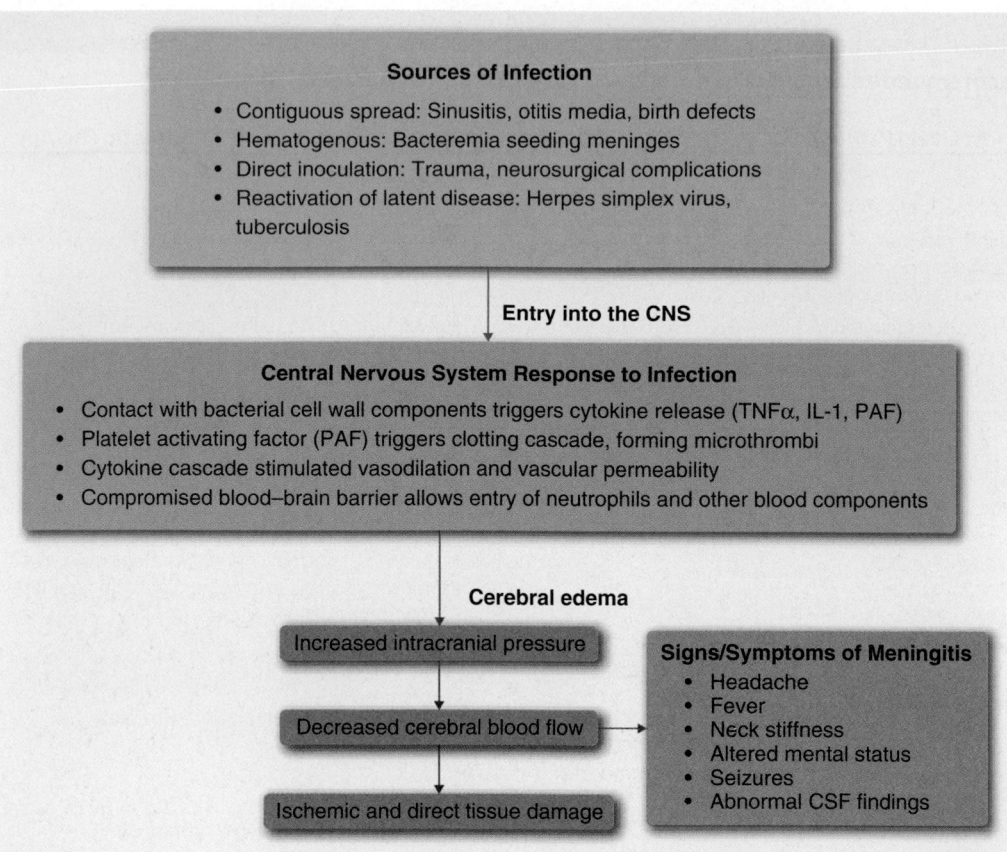

FIGURE 70–1.
Pathophysiology of bacterial meningitis.

Table 70–2

CNS Response to Infection (CSF Findings)

	Normal CSF	Bacterial Infection	Viral Infection	Fungal Infection	Tuberculosis
WBC ($\times 10^3$/mm³ or $\times 10^9$/L)	Less than 0.005	1.0–greater than 5.0	0.1–1	0.1–0.4	50–500 (0.05–0.5)
WBC differential (%, predominant cell type)	Greater than 85% monocytes	At least 80% PMNs	50% lymphocytes (PMN early)	Greater than 50% lymphocytes	Greater than 80% lymphocytes (PMNs early)
Protein (mg/dL, mg/L)	20–45 (200–450)	Greater than 100 (greater than 1,000)	50–100 (500–1,000)	100–200 (1,000–2,000)	40–150 (400–1,500)
Glucose (mg/dL, mmol/L)	45–80 (2.5–4.44)	5–40 (0.28–2.22)	30–70 (1.67–3.89)	Less than 30–70 (less than 1.67–3.89)	Less than 30–70 (less than 1.67–3.89)
CSF:serum glucose ratio	At least 0.6 serum glucose	Less than 0.4 serum glucose	At least 0.6 serum glucose	Less than 0.4 serum glucose	Less than 0.4 serum glucose
CSF stain	Negative	Positive Gram stain (60–90%)	Negative	Positive India ink stain (*Cryptococcus*)	Positive acid-fast bacilli stain

CSF, cerebrospinal fluid; PMNs, polymorphonuclear neutrophils.

From Refs. 4, 10, 19.

---

with meningitis. Neurologic tissue damage is the result of the host's immune reaction to bacterial cellular components (such as lipopolysaccharide, teichoic acid, and peptidoglycan) that triggers cytokine production, particularly tumor necrosis factor alpha (TNF-α) and interleukin 1 (IL-1), as well as other mediators of inflammation.[14] Bacteriolysis resulting from antibiotic therapy further contributes to the inflammatory process. Cytokines increase permeability of the blood–brain barrier, allowing influx of neutrophils and other host defense cells that contribute to the development of cerebral edema and increased intracranial pressure characteristic of meningitis.[15] The increase in intracranial pressure is responsible for the hallmark clinical signs and symptoms of meningitis: headache, neck stiffness, altered mental status, photophobia, and seizures. Unaltered, these pathophysiologic changes may result in cerebral ischemia and death.

The CNS response to infection is evident by demonstrable changes in the CSF. ❷ *Ideally, LP to obtain CSF for direct examination and laboratory analysis, as well as blood cultures and other relevant cultures, should be obtained before initiation of antimicrobial therapy. However, initiation of antimicrobial therapy should not be delayed if a pretreatment LP cannot be performed.*

Normal CSF has a characteristic composition in terms of protein and glucose content, as well as cell count. Table 70–2 lists CSF findings observed in the absence of infection, as well

as in patients with bacterial, viral, fungal, and tuberculous meningitis.

CLINICAL PRESENTATION AND DIAGNOSIS

A high index of suspicion should be maintained for patients at risk for CNS infections. Prompt recognition and diagnosis are essential so that antimicrobial therapy can be initiated as quickly as possible. A medical history (including risk factors for infection and history of possible recent exposures) and

---

Clinical Presentation and Diagnosis of CNS Infections

General

- Evaluate patient risk factors and recent exposures
- Evaluate other possible causes: space-occupying lesion (which may or may not be malignant), drug-induced CNS disease, autoimmune disease, and trauma[12,13]

Signs and Symptoms[2]

- 95% of patients with bacterial meningitis have two of the following: headache, fever, neck stiffness, and altered mental status
- Headache (87%)
- Nuchal rigidity (stiff neck) (83%)
- Fever (77%)
- Nausea (74%)
- Altered mental status (i.e., confusion, lethargy, and obtundation) (69%)
- Focal neurologic defects (including positive Brudzinski's sign and Kernig's sign) (33%)
- Seizures
- Malaise, restlessness
- Photophobia
- Skin lesions (diffuse petechial rash observed in 50% of patients with meningococcal meningitis)
- Signs and symptoms in neonates, infants, and young children: nonspecific findings, such as altered feeding and sleep patterns, vomiting, irritability, lethargy, bulging fontanel, seizures, respiratory distress, and petechial/purpuric rash[16]
- Predictors of an unfavorable outcome: seizures, focal neurologic findings, altered mental status, papilledema, hypotension, septic shock, and pneumococcal meningitis[3]

Laboratory Tests[4,17,18]

- CSF examination via lumbar puncture (LP, spinal tap); contraindicated in patients with cardiorespiratory compromise, increased intracranial pressure and papilledema, focal neurologic signs, seizures, bleeding

disorders, abnormal level of consciousness, and possible brain herniation (a CT scan should be performed before LP if there is a question of a CNS mass to avoid potential for brain herniation) (see Table 70–2 for specific CSF findings)
- Elevated opening pressure (may be decreased in neonates, infants, and children)
- Cloudy CSF
- Decreased glucose
- Elevated protein
- Elevated WBC (differential provides clues to offending pathogen)
- Gram stain (adequate for diagnosis in 60–90% of patients with bacterial meningitis)
- Culture and sensitivity (positive in 70–85% without prior antibiotic therapy, positive in less than 20% who have had prior therapy)
- If CSF Gram stain and/or culture is negative, rapid diagnostic tests (such as latex agglutination) may be useful; these tests are positive even if bacteria are dead
- Polymerase chain reaction (PCR; DNA amplification of the most common bacterial meningitis pathogens) may be useful to help exclude bacterial meningitis
- Elevated CSF lactate and C-reactive protein
- Blood cultures (at least two cultures, one "set"; positive in 66%)
- Scraping of skin lesions (such as rash) for direct microscopic examination and culture
- Other cultures should be obtained as clinically indicated (such as sputum)
- WBC with differential
- Fungal meningitis: CSF culture, CSF and serum cryptococcal antigen titers, microscopic examination of CSF specimens
- Tuberculous meningitis: CSF culture, PCR evaluation (preferred), and acid-fast stain

Patient Encounter 1, Part 2

The 17-year-old patient with signs and symptoms of meningitis underwent lumbar puncture. Initial results from CSF studies are WBC $2.2 \times 10^3/mm^3$ ($2.2 \times 10^9/L$) with 87% PMNs, protein 320 mg/dL (3,200 mg/L), glucose 10 mg/dL (0.56 mmol/L). Gram stain shows gram-negative diplococci and culture results confirm *N. meningitidis* infection. While in the ED, her clinical status deteriorated and her BP dropped to 85/60 mm Hg. She was transferred to the ICU for close monitoring.

Given this patient's clinical deterioration and identification of this pathogen, what complications should she be monitored for?

How can her antibiotic regimen be streamlined at this time?

How long should the antibiotics be continued?

Patient Encounter 1, Part 3

The parents and classmates at the high school of the 17-year-old patient with *N. meningitidis* call the hospital and are concerned about getting sick. They wonder about medications and vaccinations to prevent the disease.

Who should receive antimicrobial prophylaxis for N. meningitidis?

What antimicrobial regimens are effective for prophylaxis?

Who should receive vaccination against meningococcal disease?

physical examination yield important information to help guide the diagnosis and treatment of meningitis. Common signs and symptoms include fever, headache, nuchal rigidity (stiff neck), and photophobia. As common meningeal signs are not typically present in infants, nonspecific signs and symptoms including excessive irritability or crying, vomiting or diarrhea, tachypnea, altered sleep pattern, and poor eating should be noted. Depending on involved pathogens and disease severity, patients may also present with altered mental status, stupor, and seizures.

TREATMENT

Goals of Therapy

The introduction of antibiotic therapy and vaccines has reduced dramatically the mortality associated with bacterial meningitis.[19] Prior to these advances, bacterial meningitis was almost universally fatal, and those few patients who survived often suffered from debilitating residual neurologic deficits, such as permanent hearing loss. Although significant improvements have been made, the fatality rate of pneumococcal meningitis remains above 20% likely due to its occurrence in debilitated patient populations.

❸ *The treatment goals for CNS infections are to prevent death and residual neurologic deficits, eradicate or control causative micro-organisms, ameliorate clinical signs and symptoms, and identify measures to prevent future infections (such as vaccination and suppressive therapy).* These goals should be accomplished with minimal adverse drug reactions and interactions. Surgical debridement should be employed, if appropriate (as in postneurosurgical infections and brain abscess). Supportive care, consisting of hydration, electrolyte replacement, antipyretics, antiemetics, analgesics, antiepileptic drugs, and wound care (for surgical wounds), is an important adjunct to antimicrobial therapy, particularly early in the treatment course.

Treatment Principles

❹ *Prompt initiation of IV high-dose cidal antimicrobial therapy directed at the most likely pathogen(s) is essential due to the high morbidity and mortality associated with CNS infections.* Although there are no prospective studies that relate timing of antibiotic administration to clinical outcome in bacterial meningitis, a longer duration of symptoms and more advanced disease before treatment initiation increase the risk of a poor outcome.[3,17,20] Initiation of antibiotic therapy as soon as possible after bacterial meningitis is suspected or proven (even before hospitalization) reduces mortality and neurologic sequelae, as long as antibiotics were started before patients deteriorate to a score of 10 on the Glasgow Coma Scale.[21,22] Rapid sterilization of CSF is important; delayed CSF sterilization after approximately 24 hours of antibiotic therapy increases the risk of neurologic sequelae, including moderate to profound hearing loss.[23,24]

Meningitis occurs in a tissue with limited host defenses. Bacterial replication occurs rapidly in the absence of complement and specific antibodies directed toward common bacterial pathogens.[25] High-dose parenteral bactericidal antibiotic therapy is required to treat meningitis effectively. Data from animal studies and patients demonstrate better outcomes when bactericidal antibiotic therapy (versus bacteriostatic therapy) is used to sterilize the CSF.[26] However, successful treatment of meningitis has been reported with bacteriostatic agents. High doses of parenteral therapy are required to achieve CSF antibiotic concentrations adequate to rapidly sterilize the CSF and reduce the risk of complications. The presence of infection in the CSF reduces the activity of some classes of antibiotics. For example, the decreased pH of CSF associated with meningitis significantly reduces the activity of aminoglycoside antibiotics.[27]

Antimicrobial pharmacokinetics and pharmacodynamics must be considered when designing treatment regimens for CNS infections. Ability of antibiotics to reach and achieve effective concentrations at the infection site is the key to treatment success. In experimental models of meningitis, maximum bactericidal activity is achieved when CSF concentrations exceed the minimum bactericidal concentration (MBC) of the infecting pathogen by 10- to

30-fold.[16] In general, low-molecular-weight lipophilic antibiotics that are un-ionized at physiologic pH and not highly protein bound penetrate best into CSF and other body tissues and fluids.[25,27] In addition to drug characteristics, integrity of the blood–brain barrier determines antibiotic penetration into CSF. The CSF penetration of most, but not all, antibiotics is enhanced by the presence of infection and inflammation. Sulfonamides, trimethoprim, chloramphenicol, rifampin, and most antitubercular drugs achieve therapeutic CSF levels even without meningeal inflammation.[10] Most β-lactams and related antibiotics (i.e., carbapenems and monobactams),

vancomycin, quinolones, acyclovir, linezolid, daptomycin, and colistin achieve therapeutic CSF levels in the presence of meningeal inflammation.[10] Aminoglycosides, first-generation cephalosporins, second-generation cephalosporins (except cefuroxime), clindamycin, and amphotericin do not achieve therapeutic CSF levels, even with inflammation, but clindamycin does achieve therapeutic brain tissue levels.[10]

An adequate duration of therapy is required to treat meningitis successfully (Table 70–3). ❺ *Parenteral (IV) therapy is administered for the full course of therapy for CNS infections to ensure adequate CSF penetration*

Table 70–3

Pathogen-Based Definitive Treatment for CNS Infections

Pathogen	Recommended and Alternative Antimicrobial Therapy (Adult Doses; Pediatric Doses)	Renal and Hepatic Dose Adjustment	Adverse Effects/Safety Monitoring	Duration (Days)
Neisseria meningitidis Penicillin MIC 0.1 mg/L	*Standard Therapy* Penicillin G 4 million units IV every 4 hours *or*	*Renal*: CrCl less than 50 mL/min: 3 million units IV every 4 hours; CrCl less than 10 mL/min: 2 million units IV every 4 hours *Hepatic*: No dose adjustment	Hypersensitivity (rash, anaphylaxis), diarrhea	7
	Ampicillin 2 g IV every 4 hours	*Renal*: CrCl less than 50 mL/min: 2 g IV every 8 hours; CrCl less than 30 mL/min: 2 g IV every 12 hours; CrCl less than 10 mL/min: 2 g IV every 24 hours *Hepatic*: No dose adjustment	Hypersensitivity (rash, anaphylaxis), diarrhea	
	Alternative Therapies Ceftriaxone 2 g IV every 12 hours *or*	*Renal*: No dose adjustment *Hepatic*: Caution in severe hepatic impairment	Ceftriaxone: LFT elevation, cholecystitis	
	Cefotaxime 2 g IV every 4 hours	*Renal*: CrCl less than 80 mL/min: 2 g IV every 6–8 hours; CrCl less than 50 mL/min: 2 g IV every 8–12 hours; CrCl less than 30 mL/min: 2 g IV every 12 hours; CrCl less than 10 mL/min: 2 g IV every 24 hours *Hepatic*: No dose adjustment	Pseudocholelithiasis	
Penicillin MIC 0.1–1 mg/L	*Standard Therapy* Ceftriaxone *or* cefotaxime			
	Alternative Therapies Moxifloxacin 400 mg IV every 24 hours *or*	*Renal*: No dose adjustment *Hepatic*: Caution in severe hepatic impairment	Nausea/vomiting/diarrhea, dizziness, headache, QT prolongation	
	Meropenem 2 g IV every 8 hours *or*	*Renal*: CrCl less than 50 mL/min: 2 g IV every 12 hours; CrCl less than 30 mL/min: 500 mg to 1 g IV every 12 hours; CrCl less than 10 mL/min: 500 mg to 1 g IV every 24 hours *Hepatic*: No dose adjustment	Rash, hypersensitivity, diarrhea, decreased seizure threshold	
	Chloramphenicol 1–1.5 g IV every 6 hours	*Renal*: No dose adjustment *Hepatic*: Reduce dose in moderate to severe impairment; consider serum drug monitoring	Rash, diarrhea, seizures, anemia, gray baby syndrome, hypersensitivity, neurotoxicity (last choice due to toxicities)	

(Continued)

Table 70–3

Pathogen-Based Definitive Treatment for CNS Infections (*Continued*)

Pathogen	Recommended and Alternative Antimicrobial Therapy (Adult Doses; Pediatric Doses)	Renal and Hepatic Dose Adjustment	Adverse Effects/Safety Monitoring	Duration (Days)
Streptococcus pneumoniae Penicillin MIC 0.1 mg/L	**Standard Therapy** Penicillin G *or* ampicillin **Alternative Therapies** Ceftriaxone *or* cefotaxime *or* chloramphenicol			10–14
Penicillin MIC 0.1–1 mg/L (ceftriaxone/ cefotaxime-sensitive strains)	**Standard Therapy** Ceftriaxone *or* cefotaxime **Alternative Therapies** Cefepime 2 g IV every 8 hours *or* meropenem	*Renal*: CrCl less than 50 mL/min: 2 g IV every 12–24 hours; CrCl less than 30 mL/min: 1–2 g IV every 24 hours *Hepatic*: No dose adjustment	Hypersensitivity (rash, anaphylaxis) decreased seizure threshold	
Penicillin MIC 2 mg/L or greater	**Standard Therapy** Vancomycin 15 mg/kg IV every 8–12 hours (with dosing based on serum levels) *plus* ceftriaxone *or* cefotaxime **Alternative Therapies** Moxifloxacin	*Renal*: CrCl less than 50 mL/min: dosing every 24 hours; CrCl less than 20 mL/min: dosing based on serum levels; all dose adjustments should be made based on serum levels *Hepatic*: No dose adjustment	Vancomycin: rash, red man's syndrome (if infused too quickly) nephrotoxicity, neutropenia, thrombocytopenia	
Cefotaxime/ ceftriaxone MIC at least 1 mg/L	**Standard Therapy** Vancomycin *plus* ceftriaxone *or* cefotaxime **Alternative Therapies** Moxifloxacin			
H. influenzae β-Lactamase-negative	**Standard Therapy** Ampicillin **Alternative Therapies** Ceftriaxone *or* cefotaxime *or* cefepime *or* moxifloxacin *or* chloramphenicol			7
β-Lactamase-positive	**Standard Therapy** Ceftriaxone *or* cefotaxime **Alternative Therapies** Cefepime *or* moxifloxacin *or* chloramphenicol			
Listeria monocytogenes	**Standard Therapy** Ampicillin *or* penicillin G *plus* gentamicin (5 mg/kg/day, dosing based on serum levels)	*Renal*: CrCl less than 60 mL/min: Use of traditional pharmacokinetic dosing; dose adjustments per serum levels *Hepatic*: No dose adjustment	Gentamicin: nephrotoxicity, ototoxicity	At least 26
	Alternative Therapies Trimethoprim-sulfamethoxazole 10–20 mg/kg Trimethoprim IV per day in divided doses every 6–8 hours *or* meropenem	*Renal*: CrCl less than 50 mL/min: 10–15 mg/kg trimethoprim IV per day divided every 8 hours; CrCl less than 10 mL/min: 7–10 mg/kg trimethoprim IV per day divided every 8–12 hours *Hepatic*: No dose adjustment	Trimethoprim-sulfamethoxazole: Rash, Stevens-Johnson syndrome, bone marrow suppression, hepatotoxicity, elevated serum creatinine, hypertension	

(Continued)

Table 70–3

Pathogen-Based Definitive Treatment for CNS Infections (*Continued*)

Pathogen	Recommended and Alternative Antimicrobial Therapy (Adult Doses; Pediatric Doses)	Renal and Hepatic Dose Adjustment	Adverse Effects/Safety Monitoring	Duration (Days)
Streptococcus agalactiae (group B. *Streptococcus*)	*Standard Therapy* Ampicillin *or* penicillin G *Alternative Therapies* Ceftriaxone *or* cefotaxime			14–21
Enterobacteriaceae	*Standard Therapy* Ceftriaxone *or* cefotaxime			
	Alternative Therapies Aztreonam 2 g IV every 6–8 hours	*Renal*: CrCl less than 50 mL/min: 2 g IV every 8 hours; CrCl less than 30 mL/min: 2 g IV every 12 hours; CrCl less than 10 mL/min: 1 g IV every 12 hours *Hepatic*: No dose adjustment	Phlebitis, fever, rash, headache, confusion, seizures	21 (longer duration may be required for neonates)
	Moxifloxacin *or* meropenem *or* trimethoprim-sulfamethoxazole *or* ampicillin			
Pseudomonas aeruginosa	*Standard Therapy* cefepime *or* ceftazidime 2 g IV every 8 hours *or* meropenem (addition of aminoglycoside should be considered)	*Renal*: CrCl less than 50 mL/min: 1–2 g IV every 12 hours; CrCl less than 30 mL/min: 1–2 g IV every 24 hours; CrCl less than 10 mL/min: 1 g IV every 24 hours *Hepatic*: No dose adjustment	Hypersensitivity, rash, anemia, neutropenia, eosinophilia, LFT elevation	At least 21 days
	Alternative Therapies Aztreonam *or* ciprofloxacin 400 mg IV every 8–12 hours (addition of aminoglycoside should be considered)	Ciprofloxacin: *Renal*: CrCl less than 30 mL/min: 400 mg IV every 24 hours or 200 mg IV every 12 hours *Hepatic*: No dose adjustment	Nausea/vomiting/diarrhea, dizziness, headache, rash, confusion, seizures	
Staphylococcus aureus Methicillin-susceptible	*Standard Therapy* Nafcillin *or* oxacillin 1.5–3 g every 4 hours	*Renal*: No dose adjustment *Hepatic*: No dose adjustment (combined renal and hepatic impairment may require dose adjustment)	Rash, nausea/vomiting/diarrhea, acute interstitial nephritis	3–4 weeks (4–6 weeks if shunt involved)
Methicillin-resistant	*Alternative Therapies* Vancomycin *or* meropenem		Hepatotoxicity, red-orange discoloration of body fluids, skin rash, hepatic enzyme induction	
	Standard Therapy Vancomycin *plus* Rifampin 600 mg orally or IV daily if shunt involved	*Renal*: No dose adjustment *Hepatic*: Caution in moderate/severe hepatic impairment		
	Alternative Therapies Linezolid 600 mg IV every 12 hours *or* trimethoprim-sulfamethoxazole	*Renal*: No dose adjustment *Hepatic*: No dose adjustment	Pancytopenia, myalgias, arthralgias, neuropathy	
Staphylococcus epidermidis	*Standard Therapy* Vancomycin *plus* rifampin 600 mg orally or IV daily if shunt involved			3–4 weeks (4–6 weeks if shunt involved)

(Continued)

Table 70–3

Pathogen-Based Definitive Treatment for CNS Infections *(Continued)*

Pathogen	Recommended and Alternative Antimicrobial Therapy (Adult Doses; Pediatric Doses)	Renal and Hepatic Dose Adjustment	Adverse Effects/Safety Monitoring	Duration (Days)
	Alternative Therapies Linezolid			
Herpes simplex virus	*Standard Therapy* Acyclovir 10 mg/kg IV every 8 hours (adults); 20 mg/kg IV every 8 hours (neonates)	*Renal*: CrCl less than 50 mL/min: 10 mg/kg IV every 12 hours; CrCl less than 30 mL/min: 10 mg/kg IV every 24 hours; CrCl less than 10 mL/min: 5 mg/kg IV every 24 hours *Hepatic*: No dose adjustment	Nephrotoxicity, crystalluria, nausea/vomiting, neurotoxicity, phlebitis	14–21 (21 for neonates)
	Alternative Therapy Foscarnet 120–200 mg/kg IV per day in divided doses every 8–12 hours	*Renal*: CrCl: 1.0–1.4 mL/min/kg: 70 mg/kg IV every 12 hours; CrCl: 0.8–1.0 mL/min/kg: 50 mg/kg IV every 12 hours; CrCl: 0.6–0.8 mL/min/kg: 80 mg/kg IV every 24 hours; CrCl: 0.5–0.6 mL/min/kg: 60 mg/kg IV every 24 hours; CrCl: 0.4–0.5 mL/min/kg: 50 mg/kg IV every 24 hours; CrCl less than 0.4 mL/min/kg or less than 20 mL/min not recommended. *Hepatic*: No dose adjustment	Nephrotoxicity, electrolyte imbalances, nausea/vomiting, headache, penile ulceration, thrombophlebitis, seizures	

LFT, liver function tests; MIC, minimum inhibitory concentration.

Adapted, with permission, from Ref. 14.

throughout the course of treatment. Antibiotic treatment (and dexamethasone, if used as a treatment adjunct) reduces the inflammation associated with meningitis, which, in turn, reduces the penetration of some antibiotics into the CSF. To ensure adequate antibiotic concentrations throughout the treatment course, parenteral administration is continued for the full treatment course. Carefully selected patients who have close medical monitoring and follow-up may be able to receive a portion of their parenteral meningitis treatment on an outpatient basis.[17,28] A management algorithm for adults with suspected bacterial meningitis, as recommended by the Infectious Diseases Society of America (IDSA), is summarized in Figure 70–2.

Empirical Antimicrobial Therapy

After expeditious workup (i.e., evaluation of risk factors, clinical signs and symptoms, and laboratory data) and diagnosis, prompt and aggressive antimicrobial therapy is initiated. Appropriate empirical treatment is of the utmost importance in patients with suspected CNS infections. In most patients, a diagnostic LP will be performed before beginning antibiotics, but this never should delay initiation of antimicrobials. Antibiotic pretreatment may alter the CSF profile and complicate interpretation. ❻ *Empirical therapy should be directed at the most likely pathogen(s) for a specific patient, taking into account age, risk factors for infection (including underlying disease and immune*

dysfunction, vaccine history, and recent exposures), CSF Gram stain results, CSF antibiotic penetration, and local antimicrobial resistance patterns. Results of the CSF Gram stain may be used to help narrow empirical therapy for bacterial meningitis. In the absence of a positive Gram stain, empirical therapy should be continued for at least 48 to 72 hours, when meningitis may, in most cases, be ruled out by CSF findings inconsistent with bacterial meningitis, negative CSF culture, and negative PCR evaluations. A repeat LP may be useful in the absence of other findings. Table 70–1 outlines recommendations for empirical antibiotic therapy for bacterial meningitis by most likely pathogen(s) and patient risk factors.

Impact of Antimicrobial Resistance on Treatment Regimens for Meningitis

Development of resistance to β-lactam antibiotics, including penicillins and cephalosporins, has significantly impacted the management of bacterial meningitis. Approximately 17% of U.S. pneumococcal CSF isolates are resistant to penicillin, and 3.5% of CSF isolates are resistant to cephalosporins.[29] The Clinical and Laboratory Standards Institute (CLSI) has set a lower ceftriaxone susceptibility breakpoint for pneumococcal CSF isolates (1 mg/L) than for isolates from non-CNS sites (2 mg/L). Increasing pneumococcal resistance to penicillin G has changed empirical treatment regimens to the combination of a third-generation cephalosporin

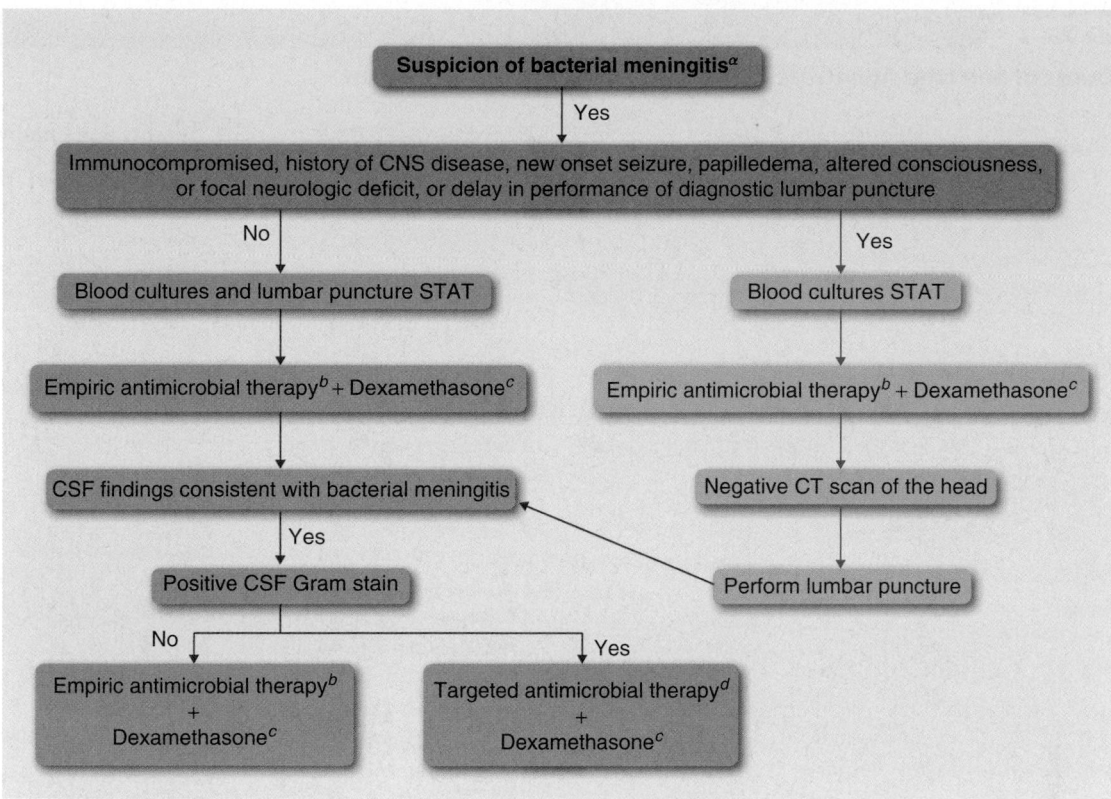

FIGURE 70–2. Management algorithm for adults with suspected bacterial meningitis. [a]Management algorithm is similar for infants and children with suspected bacterial meningitis. [b]See Table 70–1 for empirical treatment recommendations. [c]See text for specific recommendations for use of adjunctive dexamethasone in adults with bacterial meningitis. [d]See Table 70–3 for pathogen-based definitive treatment recommendations. (Adapted, with permission, from Ref. 14.)

plus vancomycin. Recognition of relative and high-level resistance to *N. meningitidis* in the laboratory, as well as in clinical treatment failures, has led to greater use of third-generation cephalosporins for empirical therapy of meningococcal meningitis.[20] Traditionally, ampicillin was the cornerstone of treatment for *H. influenzae* meningitis. Now, treatment of suspected or proven β-lactamase-mediated Hib meningitis requires a third-generation cephalosporin. Increasing rates of methicillin-resistant *S. aureus* (about one-third of staphylococcal CSF isolates) and coagulase-negative staphylococci require the use of vancomycin for empirical therapy when these pathogens are suspected.[29] As previously mentioned, hospitalized patients, especially those residing in an intensive care unit, are at risk for developing meningitis secondary to gram-negative pathogens. The emergence and continued rise of multidrug resistant strains of gram-negative organisms such as *Pseudomonas aeruginosa*, Acinetobacter species, AmpC and extended spectrum β-lactamase (ESBL)-producing strains of Enterobacteraciae have become a recognized threat nationally. Global and local resistance patterns should be taken into account and combined with optimized pharmacodynamic dosing strategies when designing empirical treatment regimens for bacterial meningitis.

Pathogen-Directed Antimicrobial Therapy

❼ *Empirical antimicrobial therapy should be modified on the basis of laboratory data and clinical response.* If cultures or other diagnostics, such as CSF Gram stain or bacterial antigen or antibody tests indicate a specific pathogen, therapy should be adjusted quickly as needed to ensure adequate coverage for the offending pathogen(s). Table 70–3 outlines recommended definitive pathogen-directed treatment regimens, recommended treatment duration, and key adverse effects that should be monitored during antibiotic therapy for meningitis. Treatment considerations for selected pathogens causing CNS infections are summarized below. Table 70–4 provides pediatric doses of selected agents used in bacterial meningitis treatment.

▶ *Neisseria meningitidis Meningitis*

N. meningiditis most commonly causes CNS infections in children and young adults. An estimated 1,400 to 2,800 cases of meningococcal meningitis occur annually in the United States, with a mortality of about 10%.[30] From 11% to 19% of survivors of meningococcal meningitis experience long-term sequelae, including hearing loss, limb loss, and neurologic deficits.[30] Nearly all meningococcal disease is caused by five serogroups: A, B, C, Y, and W-135. In the United States,

Table 70–4

Pediatric Doses of Selected Agents Used in Bacterial Meningitis Treatment

	Neonates, 0–7 Days	Neonates, 8–28 Days	Infants and Children
Ampicillin	150 mg/kg IV per day in divided doses every 8 hours	200 mg/kg IV per day in divided doses every 6–8 hours	300 mg/kg IV per day in divided doses every 8 hours
Cefepime	—	—	150 mg/kg per day in divided doses every 8 hours
Cefotaxime	100–150 mg/kg IV per day in divided doses every 8–12 hours	150–200 mg/kg IV per day in divided doses every 6–8 hours	225–300 mg/kg per day in divided doses every 6–8 hours
Ceftriaxone	—	—	80–100 mg/kg IV per day in divided doses every 12 hours
Gentamicin	5 mg/kg IV per day in divided doses every 12 hours (with dosing based on serum levels)	7.5 mg/kg IV per day in divided doses every 8 hours (with dosing based on serum levels	7.5 mg/kg IV per day in divided doses every 8 hours based on serum levels)
Meropenem	—	—	120 mg/kg IV per day in divided doses every 8 hours
Nafcillin/oxacillin	75 mg/kg IV per day in divided doses every 8–12 hours	Nafcillin: 100–150 mg/kg IV per day in divided doses every 6–8 hours Oxacillin: 150–200 mg/kg IV per day in divided doses every 6–8 hours	200 mg/kg IV per day in divided doses every 6 hours max, 2 g pediatrics greater than 3 months of age
Penicillin G	0.15 million units/kg IV per day in divided doses 8–12 hours	0.2 million units/kg IV per day in divided doses every 6–8 hours	0.3 million units/kg IV per day in divided doses every 4–6 hours
Vancomycin	20–30 mg/kg IV per day in divided doses every 8–12 hours	30–45 mg/kg IV per day in divided doses every 6–8 hours	60 mg/kg IV per day in divided doses every 6 hours

LFT, liver function tests; MIC, minimum inhibitory concentration.

Adapted, with permission, from Ref. 14.

serotypes B, C, and Y each are responsible for approximately 30% of cases.

Meningococcal meningitis is observed most commonly in individuals living in close quarters (such as college students and military personnel). Although infants younger than 1 year of age are at highest risk, nearly 60% of cases occur in patients over 11 years of age.[30,31] *N. meningitidis* colonizes the nasopharynx and usually is transmitted via inhaled respiratory droplets from patients or asymptomatic carriers. A subclinical bacteremia typically ensues, seeding the meninges. Meningococcal disease is often (approximately 50%) associated with a diffuse petechial rash, and patients may experience behavioral changes. Patients may develop fulminant meningococcal sepsis, characterized by shock, DIC, and multiorgan failure.[30,31] Meningococcal sepsis has a poor prognosis and carries a mortality rate of up to 80%.[20] Patients with suspected meningococcal infection should be kept on respiratory isolation for the first 24 hours of treatment.[4]

Traditionally, high-dose penicillin G was the treatment standard for meningococcal disease. However, increasing penicillin resistance requires that third-generation cephalosporins now be used for empirical treatment until in vitro susceptibilities are known.[27] Patients with a history of type I penicillin allergy or cephalosporin allergy may be treated with vancomycin. Treatment should be continued for seven days, after which no further treatment is necessary.

Prevention of meningococcal disease by vaccination is a key to reducing the incidence of meningococcal meningitis.

College freshmen living in dormitories, military recruits, patients undergoing splenectomy, HIV-infected patients and patients with complement deficiency should receive the meningococcal vaccine.[30] Both the older polysaccharide meningococcal vaccine and the quadrivalent conjugate meningococcal vaccine protect against four of the five serotypes causing invasive disease (A, C, Y, and W-135). Meningococcal vaccines do not protect against serotype B, which causes more than 50% of the cases of meningococcal meningitis in children younger than 2 years of age.[32] Either of the two available meningococcal vaccines can be used in outbreak situations, with protective antibodies measurable within 7 to 10 days. A possible advantage of the new conjugate vaccine is that it is believed to provide a longer duration of immunity than the older polysaccharide vaccine, although clinical studies to validate the duration of protection are not yet completed. The Centers for Disease Control and Prevention (CDC) Advisory Committee on Immunization Practices and the American Academy of Pediatrics recommend that all adolescents 11 to 12 years of age receive a dose of the new quadrivalent conjugate vaccine (currently approved by the FDA for patients 11–55 years of age). Until broader indications for the conjugate vaccine are licensed, the polysaccharide vaccine is available for patients 2 to 10 years of age, as well as patients over 55 years of age.

❽ *Close contacts of patients with meningococcal infections should be evaluated for antimicrobial prophylaxis.* Close contacts include members of the same household, individuals who share sleeping quarters, day-care contacts, and individuals exposed to oral secretions of meningitis patients. After consultation with the local health department, close contacts should receive prophylactic antibiotics to eradicate nasopharyngeal carriage of the organism. Household contacts of patients with meningococcal meningitis have a 400- to 800-fold increased risk of developing meningitis.[31] Prophylactic antibiotics should be started as soon as possible, preferably within 24 hours of exposure (and within 14 days, after which the benefit is significantly reduced). Recommended regimens, all of which are 90% to 95% effective, for adults include rifampin 600 mg orally every 12 hours for 2 days, ciprofloxacin 500 mg orally for one dose, or ceftriaxone 250 mg intramuscularly for one dose. Regimens for children include rifampin 5 mg/kg orally every 12 hours for 2 days (less than 1 month of age), rifampin 10 mg/kg orally every 12 hours for 2 days (greater than 1 month of age), or ceftriaxone 125 mg intramuscularly for one dose (less than 12 years of age).[30,31] It is not known if close contacts who have been vaccinated will benefit from prophylaxis. Patients with meningococcal meningitis who are treated with antibiotics other than third-generation cephalosporins also should be considered for prophylaxis to eradicate the nasopharyngeal carrier state.[32]

▶ Streptococcus pneumoniae *Meningitis*

S. pneumoniae is the most common cause of meningitis in adults and in children younger than 2 years of age. Pneumococcus is associated with the highest mortality observed with bacterial meningitis in adults (20–30%), and coma and seizures are more common in pneumococcal meningitis.[1–3] Patients at high risk for pneumococcal meningitis include the elderly, alcoholics, splenectomized patients, patients with sickle cell disease, and patients with cochlear implants. At least 50% of pneumococcal meningitis cases are due to a primary infection of the ears, sinuses, or lungs.

High-dose penicillin G traditionally has been the drug of choice for the treatment of pneumococcal meningitis. However, due to increases in pneumococcal resistance, the preferred empirical treatment now includes a third-generation cephalosporin in combination with vancomycin.[17] All CSF isolates should be tested for penicillin and cephalosporin resistance by methods endorsed by the CLSI. Once in vitro sensitivity results are known, therapy may be tailored (Table 70–3). Patients with a history of type I penicillin allergy or cephalosporin allergy may be treated with vancomycin. Treatment should be continued for 10 to 14 days, after which no further maintenance therapy is required. Antimicrobial prophylaxis is not indicated for close contacts.

Administration of vaccines to high-risk individuals is a key strategy to reduce the risk of invasive pneumococcal disease. The 23-valent pneumococcal vaccine targets serotypes that account for over 90% of invasive disease in high-risk patients. However, the 23-valent vaccine does not produce a reliable immunologic response in children younger than 2 years of age, nor does it reduce pneumococcal carriage. The 7-valent pneumococcal protein-polysaccharide conjugate vaccine introduced in 2,000 targets the seven most common serotypes in children and provides protection (94% reduction) against invasive pneumococcal disease (such as sepsis and meningitis) in children younger than 5 years of age.[33] Widespread administration of the 7-valent conjugate vaccine to children has also contributed to a 28% reduction in invasive pneumococcal disease in adults.[7] Unlike the 23-valent vaccine, the 7-valent vaccine reduces carriage and transmission. *S. pneumoniae* remains the most common cause of bacterial meningitis in children, with nearly 50% of strains due to nonvaccine serotypes.[8]

▶ Haemophilus influenzae *Meningitis*

Prior to the introduction of the Hib conjugate vaccine, *H. influenzae* type b was the most common cause of bacterial

---

Patient Encounter 2, Part 1

BB is a 4-month-old infant who is brought to the ED with a 3-day history of excessive crying, irritability, and poor eating. His parents report a tympanic temperature of 38.2°C (100.8°F) measured at home. Vital signs and laboratory values include a rectal temperature of 39°C (102.2°F), respirations 44 per minute, and peripheral WBC of 13.8 × 10³/mm³ (13.8 × 10⁹/L), with 65% PMNs. Physical examination reveals only that BB is more irritable while being held than when allowed to lie still. The child has not initiated routine vaccine schedule since receiving HBV initial dose at birth.

What signs and symptoms consistent with meningitis are present in BB?

What clues to causative pathogen are present in BB?

What empiric antimicrobial regimen should be started?

Patient Encounter 2, Part 2

BB underwent lumbar puncture. Initial results from CSF studies are WBC 1.76 × 10³/mm³ (1.76 × 10⁹/L) with 79% PMNs, protein 265 mg/dL (2,650 mg/L), glucose 30 mg/dL (1.67 mmol/L), with a concurrent serum glucose of 110 mg/dL (6.1 mmol/L). Gram stain shows gram-positive cocci and culture results confirm *S. pneumoniae* infection. The patient is admitted to an acute care unit and remains clinically stable.

What complications is he at risk for acutely? What potential long-term complications may result?

How can his antibiotic regimen be streamlined at this time?

How long should the antibiotics be continued?

meningitis in the United States.[5] Routine inoculation of pediatric patients against Hib since 1991 has reduced the incidence of invasive Hib disease (i.e., meningitis and sepsis) in children younger than 5 years of age by 99%,[6] with mortality from Hib meningitis now less than 5%.[2] The Hib vaccine is also recommended for patients undergoing splenectomy. Hib meningeal disease is often associated with a parameningeal focus such as a sinus or middle ear infection. Increases in β-lactamase-mediated resistance have changed the empirical treatment of choice from ampicillin to third-generation cephalosporins (e.g., ceftriaxone and cefotaxime). Treatment should be continued for 7 days, after which no further maintenance therapy is required.

❽ *Close contacts of patients with H. influenzae type B meningitis should be evaluated for antimicrobial prophylaxis.* The risk of Hib meningitis in close contacts may be up to 200- to 1,000-fold higher than in the general population.[10] Invasive Hib disease, including meningitis, should be reported to the local health department and the CDC. Prophylaxis to eliminate nasal and oropharyngeal carriage of Hib in exposed individuals should be initiated after consultation with local health officials. Rifampin (600 mg/day for adults; 20 mg/kg/day for children, maximum of 600 mg/day) is administered for 4 days.[16] Rifampin prophylaxis is not necessary for individuals who have received the full Hib vaccine series. Exposed, unvaccinated children between 12 and 48 months of age should receive one dose of vaccine, and unvaccinated children 2 to 11 months of age should receive three doses of vaccine, as well as rifampin prophylaxis.[16] Because of prior vaccine shortages, it cannot be assumed that all children have been vaccinated. Further, some children have not received all childhood vaccines because of parental fears regarding vaccine safety.

▶ Listeria monocytogenes *Meningitis*

L. monocytogenes is an intracellular gram-positive bacillus that has been reported to contaminate certain foods, such as soft cheese, unpasteurized milk, raw meats and fish, processed meats, and raw vegetables. Bacteria from contaminated foods colonize the GI tract, pass into the bloodstream, and overcome natural cellular immune responses to cause infection. *L. monocytogenes* meningitis, usually observed in patients at extremes of age and in immunocompromised patients with depressed cellular immunity (including patients with leukemia, solid-organ transplants, and HIV/AIDS), has an overall mortality rate of up to 30%.[34,35]

Only a limited number of antibiotics show bactericidal activity against *Listeria*. The combination of high-dose ampicillin or penicillin G and an aminoglycoside is synergistic and bactericidal against *Listeria*. A total treatment course of at least 3 weeks is required. Because of concerns about the risk of nephrotoxicity with an extended treatment course of aminoglycosides, patients are treated with combination therapy for 10 days and may finish out the remainder of their treatment with ampicillin or penicillin alone.[34] In penicillin-allergic patients, trimethoprim-sulfamethoxazole is the agent of choice due to documented in vitro bactericidal activity

against *Listeria*, as well as good CNS penetration. Vancomycin and cephalosporins are not effective treatments for *Listeria* meningitis. Prophylaxis is not needed for close contacts, nor is suppressive therapy indicated. Patients with severe depression of cell-mediated immunity should be advised to avoid foods that may be contaminated with *Listeria*.

▶ Group B Streptococcus *Meningitis*

Infection with group B *Streptococcus* (such as *S. agalactiae*) is the most common cause of neonatal sepsis and meningitis. One of every four to five pregnant women is a carrier of group B *Streptococcus* in the vagina or rectum. Group B streptococci can be acquired during childbirth after exposure to infected secretions from the mother's birth canal or rectum. Neonates born to women who are carriers are at very high risk (1 of every 100–200 babies) of developing invasive group B streptococcal disease, including sepsis and meningitis.[36] Neonatal meningitis is associated with significant morbidity and mortality. Synergistic treatment with penicillin or ampicillin, plus gentamicin, for 14 to 21 days is recommended for the treatment of group B streptococcal meningitis.[17]

To reduce the risk of clinical group B streptococcal disease in neonates, pregnant women should be screened at 35 to 37 weeks' gestation to determine if they are carriers of group B streptococci.[36] Intrapartum antibiotics (e.g., penicillin or ampicillin) are recommended for pregnant women with the following characteristics: group B streptococcal carrier state detected at screening, history of group B streptococcal bacteriuria at any time during pregnancy, and history of delivery of infant with invasive group B streptococcal disease.[36]

▶ Gram-Negative Bacillary Meningitis

Meningitis caused by enteric gram-negative bacilli is an important cause of morbidity and mortality in populations at risk, including those with diabetes, malignancy, cirrhosis, immunosuppression, advanced age, parameningeal infection, and/or a defect allowing communication from skin to CNS (such as neurosurgery, congenital defects, or cranial trauma).[10]

The optimal treatment for gram-negative bacillary meningitis is not well defined. The introduction of extended-spectrum cephalosporins has improved patient outcomes significantly. While the third-generation cephalosporins ceftriaxone and cefotaxime provide good coverage for most enterobacteriaceae, these antibiotics are not active against *P. aeruginosa*. Ceftazidime, cefepime, and carbapenems are effective in pseudomonal meningitis.[25,27] Addition of an aminoglycoside may improve treatment results; however, CNS penetration of aminoglycosides is extremely poor, even in the setting of inflamed meninges. Intrathecal or intraventricular administration of aminoglycosides may be useful, but intraventricular antibiotics have been associated with increased mortality in neonates.[25,37] Intrathecal therapy is accomplished by administering the antibiotic into the CSF via LP, whereas intraventricular therapy is usually administered into a reservoir implanted in the ventricles of the brain.

Initial therapy of suspected or documented pseudomonal meningitis should include an extended-spectrum β-lactam (e.g., ceftazidime, cefepime, or meropenem) plus an aminoglycoside (preferably tobramycin or amikacin). Although the carbapenem imipenem-cilastatin has similar activity to these β-lactams, its use is not recommended in meningitis because of the risk of seizures. Aztreonam, high-dose ciprofloxacin, and colistin are alternative treatments for pseudomonal meningitis. Local therapy (i.e., intrathecal or intraventricular therapy) may be indicated in patients with gram-negative bacillary meningitis (especially infections caused by multidrug-resistant *P. aeruginosa*) or in patients who fail to improve on IV antibiotics alone. In cases of multidrug-resistant pathogens, alternative pharmacodynamic dosing strategies such as continuous or extended infusion of β-lactam antimicrobials may be considered to optimize target attainment (time greater than minimum inhibitory concentration). Given the differences in local hospital resistance patterns, administration of pathogen-directed treatment is very important after microbiology results become available. Therapy for gram-negative bacillary meningitis should be continued for at least 21 days.

▶ Postoperative Infections in the Neurosurgical Patient and Shunt Infections

Patients who undergo neurosurgical procedures or have invasive or implanted foreign devices (such as CSF shunts, intraspinal pumps or catheters, or epidural catheters) are at risk for CNS infections. Key pathogens in postneurosurgical infections include coagulase-negative staphylococci, *S. aureus*, streptococci, propionobacteria, and gram-negative bacilli, including *P. aeruginosa*. Clinical signs and symptoms may be similar to those of other CNS infections, and there also may be evidence of malfunction of implanted hardware or visible signs of a postoperative wound infection.

Empirical therapy for postoperative infections in neurosurgical patients (including patients with CSF shunts) should include vancomycin in combination with either cefepime, ceftazidime, or meropenem. Linezolid reaches adequate CSF concentrations and resolves cases of meningitis refractory to vancomycin.[35,38] However, data with linezolid are limited. The addition of rifampin should be considered for treatment of shunt infections. When culture and sensitivity data are available, pathogen-directed antibiotic therapy should be administered. Removal of infected devices is desirable; aggressive antibiotic therapy (including high-dose IV antibiotic therapy plus intraventricular vancomycin and/or tobramycin) may be effective for patients in whom hardware removal is not possible.[39] If methicillin-resistant *S. aureus* is identified as the causative organism, daptomycin may be considered an alternative therapy.[40]

The use of prophylactic antibiotics against meningitis postcraniotomy remains controversial. A meta-analysis suggests that prophylaxis reduces rates of postoperative meningitis by nearly one-half.[42] Other studies have demonstrated no benefit and there is limited data on organism-specific reductions in infection rate.[43,44] Additionally, breakthrough meningitis that does occur may be a result of drug-resistant pathogens.[43]

Brain abscesses are localized collections of pus within the cranium. These infections are difficult to treat due to the presence of walled-off infections in the brain tissue that are hard for some antibiotics to reach. In addition to appropriate antimicrobial therapy (a discussion of which is beyond the scope of this chapter), surgical debridement is often required as an adjunctive measure. Surgical debridement may also be required in the management of neurosurgical postoperative infections.

▶ Viral Encephalitis and Meningitis

Viral encephalitis and meningitis may mimic bacterial meningitis on clinical presentation but often can be differentiated by CSF findings (Table 70–2). The most common viral pathogens are enteroviruses, which cause approximately 85% of cases of viral CNS infections.[10] Other viruses that may cause CNS infections include arboviruses, HSV, cytomegalovirus, varicella-zoster virus, rotavirus, coronavirus, influenza viruses A and B, West Nile virus, and Epstein-Barr virus. Viral CNS infections are acquired through hematogenous or neuronal spread.[10] Most cases of enteroviral meningitis or encephalitis are self-limiting with supportive treatment.[41] However, arbovirus, West Nile virus, and Eastern equine virus infections are associated with a less favorable prognosis.

In contrast to other viral encephalitides, HSV type 1 and 2 encephalitis are treatable. Although rare (1 case per 250,000 population per year in the United States), HSV encephalitis is a serious, life-threatening infection.[45] Over 90% of HSV encephalitis in adults is due to HSV type 1, whereas HSV type 2 predominates in neonatal HSV encephalitis (greater than 70%).[46] HSV encephalitis is the result of reactivation of a latent infection (two-thirds of cases) or a severe case of primary infection (one-third). Without effective treatment, the mortality rate may be as high as 85% and survivors often have significant residual neurologic deficits. In accordance with 2008 IDSA guidelines, high-dose IV acyclovir is the drug of choice, given for 2 to 3 weeks at a dose of 10 mg/kg intravenously every 8 hours in adults, based on ideal body weight, and for 3 weeks at a dose of 20 mg/kg intravenously every 8 hours in neonates.[47,48] Patients receiving acyclovir should maintain adequate hydration (consider continuous IV hydration in those receiving high-dose acyclovir) to help prevent acute kidney injury secondary to crystal nephropathy.[47,48] Foscarnet 120 to 200 mg/kg/day divided every 8 to 12 hours for 2 to 3 weeks is the treatment of choice for acyclovir-resistant HSV isolates.[47,48]

▶ Adjunctive Dexamethasone Therapy

The adjunctive agent dexamethasone improves outcomes in selected patient populations with meningitis. Dexamethasone inhibits the release of proinflammatory cytokines and limits the CNS inflammatory response stimulated by infection and antibiotic therapy.

Clinical benefit in reducing neurologic deficits (primarily by reducing hearing loss) has been observed in infants and children with *H. influenzae* meningitis, as well as other pathogens causing meningitis, if dexamethasone is initiated prior to antibiotic therapy.[1,13] The American Academy of Pediatrics recommends dexamethasone (0.15 mg/kg IV every 6 hours for 2–4 days) for infants and children at least 6 weeks of age with Hib meningitis and consideration of dexamethasone in pneumococcal meningitis.[17,49] In contrast to this recommendation, a large multicenter cohort study failed to show any mortality benefit of adjunctive dexamethasone therapy regardless of age or responsible pathogen (*S. pneumoniae* or *N. meningitidis*).[50] Dexamethasone should be initiated 10 to 20 minutes before or no later than the time of initiation of antibiotic therapy; it is not recommended for infants and children who have already received antibiotic therapy because it is unlikely to improve treatment outcome in these patients. There are insufficient data to make a recommendation regarding the use of adjunctive dexamethasone therapy in neonatal meningitis.

In adults, a significant benefit was observed with dexamethasone over placebo in reducing meningitis complications, including death, particularly in patients with pneumococcal meningitis.[51] The IDSA recommends dexamethasone 0.15 mg/kg intravenously every 6 hours for 2 to 4 days (with the first dose administered 10 to 20 minutes before or with the first dose of antibiotics) in adults with suspected or proven pneumococcal meningitis.[17] Dexamethasone is not recommended for adults who have already received antibiotic therapy. Some clinicians would administer dexamethasone to all adults with meningitis pending results of laboratory tests. Benefit of dexamethasone in bacterial meningitis in a HIV-positive population has not been clearly established.[52]

There is some controversy regarding the administration of dexamethasone to patients with pneumococcal meningitis caused by penicillin- or cephalosporin-resistant strains, for which vancomycin would be required. Animal models indicate that concurrent steroid use reduces vancomycin penetration into the CSF by 42% to 77% and delays CSF sterilization due to reduction in the inflammatory response.[27] A prospective evaluation in patients with pneumococcal meningitis receiving vancomycin and adjunctive dexamethasone demonstrated that adequate concentrations of vancomycin, nearly 30% of serum concentrations, were achievable in the CSF, provided appropriate vancomycin dosage was utilized.[53] Treatment failures have been reported in adults with resistant pneumococcal meningitis who were treated with dexamethasone, but the risk-benefit of using dexamethasone in these patients cannot be defined at this time. Animal models indicate a benefit of adding rifampin in patients with resistant pneumococcal meningitis whenever dexamethasone is used.[25,27]

OUTCOME EVALUATION

Monitor patients with CNS infections continuously throughout their treatment course to evaluate their progress toward achieving treatment goals, including relief of symptoms, eradication of infection, and reduction of inflammation to prevent death and the development of neurologic deficits.

Patient Encounter 2, Part 3

Further results reveal BB had confirmed bacterial meningitis secondary to *S. pneumoniae*, serotype 6B. It was noted that BB had not received any vaccinations since birth. The parents are concerned and inquire about the need for antibiotic prophylaxis for the family and vaccination for BB.

Who should receive antimicrobial prophylaxis for S. pneumoniae?

Who should receive vaccination against pneumococcal disease?

How is vaccination important in the prevention of invasive pneumococcal disease, specifically noting BB?

These treatment goals are best achieved by appropriate parenteral antimicrobial therapy, including empirical therapy to cover the most likely pathogens, followed by directed therapy after culture and sensitivity results are known. ❾ *Components of a monitoring plan to assess efficacy and safety of antimicrobial therapy of CNS infections include clinical signs and symptoms and laboratory data (such as CSF findings, culture, and sensitivity data).*

During the patient's treatment course, monitor clinical signs and symptoms at least three times daily. Trends are more important than one-time assessments. Expect fever, headache, nausea and vomiting, and malaise to begin to improve within 24 to 48 hours of initiation of antimicrobial therapy and supportive care. Evaluate the patient for resolution of neurologic signs and symptoms, such as altered mental status and nuchal rigidity, as the infection is eradicated and inflammation is reduced within the CNS. Expect improvement and subsequent resolution of signs and symptoms as the treatment course continues. At the time of hospital discharge, arrange outpatient follow-up for several weeks to months depending on the causative pathogen, clinical treatment course, and patient's underlying comorbidities. Specifically evaluate patients for the presence of residual neurologic deficits.

Monitoring of laboratory tests is important in patients receiving treatment for CNS infections. Monitor CSF and blood cultures so that antimicrobial therapy can be tailored to the etiologic organisms. Follow-up cultures may be obtained to prove eradication of the organism(s) or treatment failure. Although repeat LP generally is not performed, consider repeat LP for patients who do not respond clinically after 48 hours of appropriate antimicrobial therapy, especially those with resistant pneumococcus who receive dexamethasone.[13] Other candidates for repeat LP include the following: those with infection with gram-negative bacilli, prolonged fever, and recurrent meningitis. Repeat the LP in neonates to determine the duration of therapy. Repeat LP also may be performed to relieve elevated intracranial pressure. Expect repeat blood cultures to become negative quickly during

Patient Care and Monitoring

1. Assess the patient's signs, symptoms, and risk factors for meningitis. Do these offer any clues to the offending pathogen?

2. Determine if the patient can undergo an immediate LP or if the LP should be delayed until a CNS mass lesion can be ruled out. If the LP is delayed, blood cultures should be drawn and appropriate empirical antimicrobial therapy initiated immediately.

3. Based on patient-specific data, local resistance patterns, and other relevant data, design an appropriate empirical antimicrobial regimen directed at the most likely pathogens; empirical regimens should consist of high-dose IV cidal therapy.

4. Determine if adjunctive dexamethasone therapy is indicated; if so, start steroid therapy 15–20 minutes before the first dose of antimicrobial therapy.

5. Provide supportive care for patients with CNS infections, including hydration, electrolyte replacement, antipyretics, analgesics, and antiepileptic drugs.

6. Monitor culture and sensitivity data from the microbiology laboratory to determine whether any refinements are needed in the patient's treatment regimen. Design a therapeutic plan to finish out the patient's course of therapy for acute meningitis.

7. Monitor the patient's response to therapy (i.e., clinical signs/symptoms and laboratory data), as well as the development of complications, including seizures and hearing loss. Dexamethasone therapy may reduce antibiotic penetration, so antimicrobial drug dosing may have to be increased (especially vancomycin) to achieve dequate CSF levels. Serum levels of vancomycin should be measured and doses titrated to ensure adequate CNS concentrations. Evaluate whether intraventricular or intrathecal antibiotics are indicated.

8. Perform ongoing surveillance for adverse drug reactions, drug allergies, and drug interactions.

9. Determine whether prophylaxis is indicated for close contacts of patients with CNS infections. Close contacts should be located for patients with suspected meningococcal or Hib meningitis. After consultation with the local health department, antibiotic prophylaxis should be provided promptly to these individuals to avoid secondary disease.

10. Evaluate whether the patient is a candidate for finishing out his or her course of parenteral treatment on an outpatient basis. If so, the importance of close medical follow-up and medication compliance should be stressed to the patient and his or her family.

11. Consider how to minimize the patient's risk of contracting the current (and other) CNS infections in the future; administer appropriate vaccines after recovery from the acute infection.

12. Arrange for patient follow-up after discharge from the hospital. Continue to monitor for neurologic sequelae for several months after completion of treatment, and educate the patient and family in this regard. Serious complications that may occur include, among others, hearing loss, hemiparesis, quadriparesis, muscular hypertonia, ataxia, seizure disorders, mental retardation, learning disabilities, and obstructive hydrocephalus.

therapy and the serum WBC count to improve and normalize with appropriate antimicrobial therapy.

Evaluate antimicrobial dosing regimens to ensure efficacy of the treatment regimen. Trough vancomycin concentrations of 15 to 20 mg/L are recommended for the treatment of CNS infections.[17] Monitor patients for drug adverse effects, drug allergies, and drug interactions. The specific safety monitoring plan will depend on the antibiotic(s) used (Table 70–3). Pay close attention to concomitant medications in patients on rifampin for treatment or prophylaxis. Rifampin is a potent inducer of hepatic metabolism and may reduce the efficacy of other drugs metabolized by the cytochrome P-450 3A enzyme pathway.

Abbreviations Introduced in This Chapter

CDC	Centers for Disease Control and Prevention
CLSI	Clinical and Laboratory Standards Institute
DIC	Disseminated intravascular coagulation
GBS	Group B *Streptococcus*
Hib	*Haemophilus influenzae* type B
HSV	Herpes simplex virus
IDSA	Infectious Diseases Society of America
IL-1	Interleukin 1
LP	Lumbar puncture
MBC	Minimum bactericidal concentration
MIC	Minimum inhibitory concentration
MRSA	Methicillin-resistant *Staphylococcus aureus*
MRSE	Methicillin-resistant *Staphylococcus epidermidis*
PCR	Polymerase chain reaction
PMN	Polymorphonuclear cell
TNF-α	Tumor necrosis factor-alpha

 Self-assessment questions and answers are available at *http://www.mhpharmacotherapy. com/pp.html.*

REFERENCES

1. van de Beek D, de Gans J, McIntyre P, Prasad K. Corticosteroids for acute bacterial meningitis. Cochrane Database Syst Rev 2003;3:CD004405.

2. van de Beek D, de Gans J, Spanjaard L, et al. Clinical features and prognostic factors in adults with bacterial meningitis. N Engl J Med 2004;351(18):1849–1859.

3. Aronin SI, Peduzzi P, Quagliarello VJ. Common-acquired bacterial meningitis: Risk stratification for adverse clinical outcome and effect of antibiotic timing. Ann Intern Med 1998;129(11):862–869.

4. van de Beek D, de Gans J, Tunkel AR, Wijdicks EFM. Community-acquired bacterial meningitis in adults. N Engl J Med 2006;354:44–53.

5. Schuchat A, Robinson K, Wenger JD, et al. Bacterial meningitis in the United States in 1995. N Engl J Med 1997;337(14):970–976.

6. Centers for Disease Control and Prevention. Progress toward elimination of Haemophilus influenzae type b invasive disease among infants and children—United States, 1998–2000. MMWR Recomm Rep 2002; 51(RR11):234–237.

7. Lexau CA, Lynfield R, Danila R, et al. Changing epidemiology of invasive pneumococcal disease among older adults in the era of pediatric pneumococcal conjugate vaccine. JAMA 2005;294(16):2043–2051.

8. Nigrovic LE, Kuppermann N, Malley R, et al. Children with bacterial meningitis presenting to the emergency department during the pneumococcal conjugate vaccine era. Acad Emerg Med 2008;15:522–528.

9. Sejvar JJ. The evolving epidemiology of viral encephalitis. Curr Opin Neurol 2006;19:350–357.

10. Mitropoulous IF, Hermsen ED, Schafer JA, Rotschafer JC. Central nervous system infections. In: DiPiro JT, Talbert RL, Yee GC, et al., eds. Pharmacotherapy: A Pathophysiologic Approach, 7th ed. New York City: McGraw-Hill; 2008:1743–1760.

11. Khetsuriani N, Holman RC, Anderson LJ. Burden of encephalitis-associated hospitalizations in the United States, 1988–1997. Clin Infect Dis 2002;35:175–182.

12. Chamberlain MC. Neoplastic meningitis. J Clin Oncol 2005;23(15):3605–3613.

13. Moris G, Garcia-Monco JC. The challenge of drug-induced aseptic meningitis. Arch Intern Med 1999;159(11):1185–1194.

14. Scheld WM, Koedel U, Nathan B, Pfister HW. Pathophysiology of bacterial meningitis: mechanism(s) of neuronal injury. J Infect Dis 2002;186(Suppl 2):S225–S233.

15. Kim KS. Pathogenesis of bacterial meningitis: From bacteraemia to neuronal injury. Nat Rev Neurosci 2003;4:376–385.

16. Bashir HE, Laundy M, Booy R. Diagnosis and treatment of bacterial meningitis. Arch Dis Child 2003;88:615–620.

17. Tunkel AR, Hartman BJ, Kaplan SL, et al. Practice guidelines for the management of bacterial meningitis. Clin Infect Dis 2004;39:1267–1284.

18. Choi C. Bacterial meningitis in aging adults. Clin Infect Dis 2001;33:1380–1385.

19. Swartz MN. Bacterial meningitis—A view of the past 90 years. N Engl J Med 2004;351(18):1826–1828.

20. van Deuren M, Brandtzaeg P, van der Meer JWM. Update on meningococcal disease with emphasis on pathogenesis and clinical management. Clin Microbiol Rev 2000;13(1):144–166.

21. Lu CH, Huang CR, Chang, WN, et al. Community-acquired bacterial meningitis in adults: The epidemiology, timing of appropriate antimicrobial therapy, and prognostic factors. Clin Neurol Neurosurg 2002;104:352–358.

22. Miner JR, Heegaard W, Mapes A, Biros M. Presentation, time to antibiotics, and mortality of patients with bacterial meningitis at an urban county medical center. J Emerg Med 2001;21:387–392.

23. Radetsky M. Duration of symptoms and outcome in bacterial meningitis: An analysis of causation and the implications of a delay in diagnosis. Pediatr Infect Dis J 1992;11:694–698.

24. Schaad UB, Suter S, Gianella-Borradori A, et al. A comparison of ceftriaxone and cefuroxime for the treatment of bacterial meningitis in children. N Engl J Med 1990;322(3):141–147.

25. Quagliarello VJ, Scheld WM. Treatment of bacterial meningitis. N Engl J Med 1997;336(10):708–716.

26. Pankey GA, Sabath LR. Clinical relevance of bacterio-static versus bactericidal mechanisms of action in the treatment of gram-positive bacterial infections. Clin Infect Dis 2004;38:864–870.

27. Sinner SW, Tunkel AR. Antimicrobial agents in the treatment of bacterial meningitis. Infect Dis Clin N Am 2004;18:581–602.

28. Tice AD, Strait K, Ramey R, et al. Outpatient parenteral antimicrobial therapy for central nervous system infections. Clin Infect Dis 1999;29:1394–1399.

29. Jones ME, Draghi DC, Karlowsky JA, Sahm DF, Bradley JS. Prevalence of antimicrobial resistance in bacteria isolated from central nervous system specimens as reported by U.S. hospital laboratories from 2000 to 2002 (Online. Updated March 25, 2004). Ann Clin Microb 2004;3:3 (online journal published March 25, 2004).

30. Centers for Disease Control and Prevention. Prevention and control of meningococcal disease. MMWR Recomm Rep 2005;54(RR07): 1–21.

31. Rosenstein NE, Perkins BA, Stephens DS, Popovic T, Hughes JM. Meningococcal disease. N Engl J Med 2001;344(18):1378–1388.

32. Campos-Outcalt D. Meningococcal vaccine: New product, new recommendations. J Fam Pract 2005;54(4):324–326.

33. Centers for Disease Control and Prevention. Direct and indirect effects of routine vaccination of children with 7-valent pneumococcal conjugate vaccine on incidence of invasive pneumococcal disease—United States, 1998–2003. Morb Mortal Wkly Rep 2005;54(36):893–897.

34. Mylonakis D, Hohmann EL, Calderwood SB. Central nervous system infection with Listeria monocytogenes: 33 years' experience at a general hospital and review of 776 episodes from the literature. Medicine 1998;77(5):313–336.

35. Hof H. An update on the medical management of Listeriosis. Expert Opin Pharmacother 2004;5(8):1727–1735.

36. Centers for Disease Control and Prevention. Prevention of perinatal Group B streptococcal disease. MMWR Recomm Rep 2002;51(RR11): 1–22.

37. Shah S, Ohlsson A, Shah V. Intraventricular antibiotics for bacterial meningitis in neonates. Cochrane Database Syst Rev 2004;4:CD004496.

38. Villani P, Regazzi MB, Marubbi F, et al. Cerebrospinal fluid linezolid concentrations in postneurosurgical central nervous system infections. Antimicrob Agents Chemother 2002;46(3):936–937.

39. Anderson EJ, Yogev R. A rational approach to the management of ventricular shunt infections. Pediatr Infect Dis J 2005;24:557–558.

40. Lee DH, Palermo B, Chowdhury M. Successful treatment of methicillin-resistant Staphylococcus aureus meningitis with daptomycin. Clin Infect Dis 2008;47:588–589.

41. Sawyer MH. Enterovirus infections: Diagnosis and treatment. Pediatr Infect Dis J 1999;18(12):1033–1040.

42. Barker FG. Efficacy of prophylactic antibiotics against meningitis after craniotomy: A meta-analysis. Neurosurgery 2007;60:887–894.

43. Korinek AM, Golmard JL, Elcheick A, et al. Risk factors for neurosurgical site infections after craniotomy: A critical reappraisal of antibiotic prophylaxis on 4,578 patients. Br J Neurosurg 2005;19: 155–162.

44. Reichert MC, Medeiros EA, Ferraz FA. Hospital-acquired meningitis in patients undergoing craniotomy: Incidence, evolution, and risk factors. Am J Infect Control 2002;30:158–164.

45. Tyler KL. Herpes simplex virus infections of the central nervous system: Encephalitis and meningitis, including Mollaret's. Herpes 2004;11(Suppl 2):57A–64A.

46. Kimberlin D. Herpes simplex virus, meningitis and encephalitis in neonates. Herpes 2004;11(Suppl 2):65A–76A.

47. Tunkel AR, Glaser CA, Bloch KC, et al. The management of encephalitis: Clinical practice guidelines by the Infectious Diseases Society of America. Clin Infect Dis 2008;47:303–327.

48. Roos KL. Encephalitis. Neurol Clin 1999;17:813–833.

49. American Academy of Pediatrics. Pneumococcal infections. In: Pickering, LK, ed. Red Book: 2003 Report of the Committee on

Infectious Diseases, 26th ed. Elk Grove Village, IL: American Academy of Pediatrics; 2003:490–500.

50. Mongelluzzo J, Mohamad Z, Ten Have TR, Shah SS. Corticosteroids and mortality in children with bacterial meningitis. JAMA 2008;299(17):2048–2055.

51. de Gans J, van de Beek D, for the European Dexamethasone in Adulthood Bacterial Meningitis Study Investigators. N Engl J Med 2002;347(20):1549–1556.

52. Scarborough M, Gordon SB, Whitty CJM, et al. Corticosteroids for bacterial meningitis in adults in Sub-Saharan Africa. N Engl J Med 2007;357:2441–2450.

53. Ricard JD, Wolff M, Lacherade JC, et al. Levels of vancomycin in cerebrospinal fluid of adult patients receiving adjunctive corticosteroids to treat pneumo-coccal meningitis: A prospective multicenter observational study. Clin Infect Dis 2007;44:250–255.

71 Lower Respiratory Tract Infections

Diane M. Cappelletty

LEARNING OBJECTIVES

● **Upon completion of the chapter, the reader will be able to:**

1. List the common pathogens that cause community-acquired pneumonia (CAP), aspiration pneumonia, ventilator-associated pneumonia (VAP; early versus late onset), and health care–associated pneumonia.

2. Explain the host defenses that protect against infection.

3. Explain the pathophysiology of pneumonia.

4. Recognize the signs and symptoms associated with CAP and VAP.

5. Identify patient and organism factors required to guide the selection of a specific antimicrobial regimen for an individual patient.

6. Design an appropriate empirical antimicrobial regimen based on patient-specific data for an individual with CAP, aspiration pneumonia, and VAP or health care–associated pneumonia (early versus late onset).

7. Design an appropriate antimicrobial regimen based on both patient- and organism-specific data.

8. Develop a monitoring plan based on patient-specific information for a patient with CAP and health care–associated pneumonia or VAP.

9. Formulate appropriate educational information to be provided to a patient with pneumonia.

KEY CONCEPTS

❶ There are five classifications of pneumonia: community acquired, aspiration, hospital acquired, ventilator associated, and health care associated.

❷ The etiology of bacterial pneumonia varies in accordance with the type of pneumonia.

❸ *Streptococcus pneumoniae* is the most common bacterial pathogen associated with community-acquired pneumonia (CAP).

❹ The signs and symptoms and severity of pneumonia are needed not only to diagnose the patient but also to determine and assess response to therapy.

❺ The goal of therapy is to eliminate the patient's symptoms, minimize or prevent complications, and decrease mortality.

❻ Treatment of CAP is predominantly empirical.

❼ Empirical selection of antimicrobial therapy for ventilator-associated, health care–associated, and hospital-associated pneumonia is broad spectrum; however, once culture and susceptibility information are available the therapy should be narrowed (de-escalation) to cover the identified pathogen(s).

❽ Duration of therapy should be kept to the shortest duration possible.

❾ Monitoring response to therapy is essential for determining efficacy, identifying adverse reactions, and determining the duration of therapy.

❿ Prevention of pneumococcal disease by use of vaccination is a national goal.

Pneumonia is inflammation of the lung with consolidation. The cause of the inflammation is infection, which can be caused by a wide range of organisms. ❶ *There are five classifications of pneumonia: community-acquired, aspiration, hospital-acquired, ventilator-associated, and health care-associated.* Patients who develop pneumonia in the outpatient setting and have not been in any health care facilities including wound care and hemodialysis clinics have community-acquired pneumonia (CAP). Aspiration is of either oropharyngeal or GI contents. Hospital-acquired pneumonia (HAP) is defined as pneumonia that occurs 48 hours or more after admission.[1,2] Ventilator-associated pneumonia (VAP) requires endotracheal intubation for at least 48 to 72 hours before the onset of pneumonia.[2,3] The newest category is health care–associated pneumonia (HCAP), which is defined as pneumonia occurring in any patient hospitalized for at least 2 days within 90 days of the onset of the infection; residing in a nursing home or long-term care facility; received IV antibiotic therapy, wound care, or chemotherapy within the last 30 days of the onset of the infection; or having attended a hemodialysis clinic.[2,4,5]

EPIDEMIOLOGY AND ETIOLOGY

Etiology and Mortality Rates

❷ *The etiology of bacterial pneumonia varies in accordance with the type of pneumonia.* Table 71–1 lists the common pathogens associated with the various types or classifications of pneumonia. *S. pneumoniae* colonizes the nasopharyngeal flora in up to 50% of healthy adults and may colonize the lower airways in individuals with chronic bronchitis.[6,7] It possesses many virulence factors enhancing its ability to cause infection in the respiratory tract. ❸ *Therefore, it is not surprising that S. pneumoniae is the predominant bacterial pathogen associated with CAP.* The second most common pathogen is one of the atypical organisms, *Mycoplasma pneumoniae*. Nontypeable *Haemophilus influenzae* intermittently colonizes about 80% of the population and the incidence of permanent colonization increases in chronic obstructive pulmonary disease (COPD) patients and those with cystic fibrosis. Therefore the likelihood of nontypeable *H. influenzae* causing pneumonia increases in COPD patients. *Moraxella catarrhalis* is a more common cause of pneumonia in the young children and the elderly. *Chlamydia pneumoniae* and *Legionella*

Table 71–1

Common Pathogens by Type of Pneumonia

Type of Pneumonia	Common Pathogens
Community	Aerobic bacteria: *S. pneumoniae, H. influenzae, M. catarrhalis* Atypical: *M. pneumoniae, C. pneumoniae, L. pneumophila*, respiratory viruses
Aspiration	Oral contents: Anaerobes, *Viridans* streptococci GI contents with pH increase Enteric gram-negative bacilli
Hospital	(Early onset no risk factors for resistant pathogens)
Ventilator health care	*S. pneumoniae*, MSSA, *E. coli, K. pneumoniae*, (*M. pneumoniae, C. pneumoniae* are rare)
Hospital	(Late onset and/or risk factors for resistant pathogens)
Ventilator health care	MRSA, extended-spectrum β-lactamase-producing *K. pneumoniae, P. aeruginosa, Acinetobacter* spp.

MRSA, methicillin-resistant *Staphylococcus aureus*; MSSA, methicillin-susceptible *S. aureus*.

pneumophila are less frequent causes than the other bacterial and atypical organisms. Community-acquired methicillin-resistant *Staphylococcus aureus* (CA-MRSA) is associated with necrotizing and severe pneumonia in healthy children and young adults. Less than 2% of all CA-MRSA infections are pneumonia (most are skin and soft tissue); however, the number of reports of pneumonia are increasing.[8]

Viruses are a common cause of CAP in children (about 65%) and much less common in adults (about 15%).[9] Viruses often associated with pneumonia in adults include influenza A and B, adenoviruses while less common causes include rhinoviruses, enteroviruses, cytomegalovirus, varicella-zoster, herpes simplex, and others. In children, viral pneumonia is more commonly caused by respiratory syncytial virus, influenza A, and parainfluenza, and less commonly the viruses are similar to those listed above for adults.

Mortality associated with CAP is dependent upon the severity of the illness and the age of the patient. In elderly patients admitted to the hospital with severe pneumonia the mortality rate is up to 40%.[10–13] In the outpatient setting (mild to moderate disease) the mortality rate is less than 5%.[14] Mortality among case reports of CA-MRSA necrotizing pneumonia is 42%.[8] Pneumonia owing to aspiration of oral contents is caused by a variety of anaerobes (*Bacteroides* spp., *Fusobacterium* spp., *Prevotella* spp., and anaerobic gram-positive cocci) as well as *Streptococcus* spp. *M. catarrhalis* and *Eikenella corrodens* may be involved but much less frequently.[15,16] When gastric contents are aspirated enteric gram-negative bacilli and *S. aureus* are more commonly the pathogens.[16]

HAP, VAP, and HCAP may be caused by a wide spectrum of organisms. HCAP, early-onset HAP, and VAP commonly can be caused by enteric gram-negative bacilli in addition to the bacteria listed above for CAP. Late-onset HAP and VAP are more likely to be caused by more resistant enteric gram-negative bacilli or, *Pseudomonas aeruginosa*, or *Acinetobacter* spp., or *S. aureus*. Rarely are viruses or fungi a cause of HAP, VAP, or HCAP. The number of infections caused by multidrug-resistant (MDR) bacteria is increasing significantly in hospitalized patients.[17–22]

PATHOPHYSIOLOGY

Local Host Defenses

Local host defenses of both the upper and lower respiratory tract along with the anatomy of the airways are important in preventing infection. Upper respiratory defenses include the mucociliary apparatus of the nasopharynx, nasal hair, normal bacterial flora, IgA, and complement. Local host defenses of the lower respiratory tract include cough, mucociliary apparatus of the trachea and bronchi, antibodies (IgA, IgM, and IgG), complement, and alveolar macrophages. Mucous lines the cells of the respiratory tract forming a protective barrier for the cells that minimizes the ability of organisms to attach to the cells and initiating the infectious process. The squamous epithelial cells of the upper respiratory tract are not ciliated but those of the columnar epithelial cells of the lower tract are. The cilia beat in a uniform fashion upward, moving particles up and out of the lower respiratory tract.

Particles greater than 10 microns are efficiently trapped by mechanisms of the upper airway and are removed from the nasopharynx either by swallowing or by expulsion. The mucociliary apparatus of the trachea and bronchi along with the sharp angles of the bronchi, often are effective at trapping and eliminating particles that are 2 to 10 microns in size. Particles in the range of 0.5 to 1 micron may consistently reach the alveolar sacs of the lung. Microorganisms fall within this size range and if they reach the alveolar sacs, then infection may result if alveolar macrophages and other defenses cannot contain the organisms.

Aspiration

Aspiration of the oropharyngeal or gastric contents may lead to aspiration pneumonia or chemical (acid) pneumonitis. Risk factors for aspiration include:

- Dysphagia
- Change in oropharyngeal colonization
- Gastroesophageal reflux (GER)
- Decreased host defenses

Dysphagia can be caused by stroke or other neurologic disorders, seizures, alcoholism, and aging.[15] Oropharyngeal colonization may be altered by oral/dental disease, poor oral hygiene, tube feedings, or medications. This could result in a higher number of anaerobic organisms in the oral cavity or colonization with enteric gram-negative bacilli.[15] GER occurs in all individuals to a degree; however, those with GER disease (GERD) have it more frequently. Acid suppression is an important factor in the treatment of GERD, which may allow enteric gram-negative bacilli to colonize the gastric contents. Finally, impaired mucous production

or cilia function, decreased immunoglobulin in secretions, and altered cough reflex may increase the likelihood of infection following an aspiration. The infection can result in a necrotizing pneumonia or lung abscess.

HAP, VAP, HCAP

Risk factors for the development of HAP fall into four general categories:

- Intubation and mechanical ventilation
- Aspiration
- Oropharyngeal colonization
- Hyperglycemia

Intubation and mechanical ventilation increase the risk of HAP/VAP 6- to 21-fold.[2,23] VAP may also be related to colonization of the ventilator circuit.[24] Risk of aspiration is increased in these patients due to the supine positioning of the patient, the presence of the endotracheal tube preventing the closure of the epiglottis over the glottis, enteral feedings, GER, and medications.[24] Oropharyngeal colonization is affected by the use of antibiotics, oral antiseptics, and poor infection control measures, which may decrease normal commensal flora and allow pathogenic organisms to colonize the oral cavity. Hyperglycemia may directly or indirectly promote infection; two proposed mechanisms are inhibiting phagocytosis and providing additional nutrients for bacteria.

Once breakdown of the local host defenses occurs and organisms invade the lung tissue, an inflammatory response is generated either by the organisms causing tissue damage or by the immune response to the presence of the organisms. This inflammatory response either can remain localized in the infected tissue or can become systemic. The role of

---

Patient Encounter 1, Part 1

A 73-year-old woman presents to your clinic complaining of difficulty breathing and shortness of breath. Her physical examination reveals that she is alert and oriented ×3, has decreased breath sounds on the left side compared with the right, and has rales in the left lower lobe. Her temperature is 37.4°C (99.3°F), respiratory rate is 20 breaths per minute, and blood pressure is 110/76 mm Hg.

What are her signs and symptoms of pneumonia?

What are the top two organisms that could be causing the pneumonia?

What additional information do you need to know before creating a treatment plan for this patient?

Patient Encounter 2, Part 1

A 52-year-old man was admitted to the hospital for abdominal surgery. He developed complications postoperatively and was intubated 6 days ago. The nurses note an increase in the amount and purulence of his sputum. Attempts yesterday and today to wean the patient off the ventilator have failed. He is sedated but does respond to commands. His temperature is 38.4°C (101°F), his blood pressure is 120/84 mm Hg, and his WBC is $14.2 \times 10^3/mm^3$ ($14.2 \times 10^9/L$) with a cell differential of 76% neutrophils, 4% bands, 16% lymphocytes, and 4% monocytes.

What are his signs and symptoms of pneumonia?

What are the top three organisms that could be causing the pneumonia?

the alveolar macrophages is twofold. First, to engulf the organisms and to contain the infection and second to process the antigens for presentation in order to generate a specific immune response by either the cell-mediated or humoral system or both. The macrophages release cytokines in the area of the infection, which result in increased mucous production, constricting the local vasculature and lymphatic vessels, and attraction of other immune cells to the site. The increase in mucous is associated with symptoms such as cough, and sputum production. If tumor necrosis factor α (TNF-α), and interleukins 1 (IL-1) and (IL-6) are released systemically, then the symptoms become more severe and include hypotension, organ dysfunction and/or a septic or septic-shock clinical presentation.

CLINICAL PRESENTATION AND DIAGNOSIS

Several scoring systems are available for assessing the severity of the pneumonia: the Pneumonia Severity Index (PSI); Confusion, Uremia, Respiratory rate, Blood pressure (CURB); and CURB-65 (those 65 years and older).[10,25] Some of the characteristics evaluated with these models include but are not limited to age, comorbidities, blood pressure, mental status, respiratory rate, and organ function. These models are used by physicians to help determine the severity of illness, prognosis (mortality risk), the need for hospitalization, and then to help guide in the selection of antimicrobial therapy along with the use of published guidelines.[10,14,25]

Clinical Presentation of CAP or Aspiration Pneumonia

General

Patients may experience nonrespiratory symptoms in addition to respiratory symptoms. With increasing age, both respiratory and nonrespiratory symptoms decrease in frequency

❹ Symptoms

- Respiratory—cough (productive or nonproductive), shortness of breath, and difficulty breathing
- Nonrespiratory—fever, fatigue, sweats, headache, myalgias, mental status changes

Signs

- Temperature may increase or decrease from baseline, but most often it is elevated. The temperature may be sustained or intermittent
- Respiratory rate is often increased. Cyanosis, increased respiratory rate, and use of accessory muscles of respiration are suggestive of severe respiratory compromise
- Breath sounds may be diminished. Rales or rhonci may be heard
- Confusion, lethargy, and disorientation are relatively common in elderly patients

Diagnostic Tests

- Chest x-ray should reveal single or multiple infiltrates
- Oxygen saturation should be over 90%, as determined by pulse oximetry
- Arterial blood gases are beneficial primarily in patients with severe pneumonia

Laboratory Tests

- The WBC may or may not be elevated. In elderly patients, a drop in WBCs also can be a sign of infection. The differential should show a predominance of neutrophils if a bacterial infection is present. The presence of bands also could be an indicator of bacterial infection. Elevated lymphocytes are an indication of viral infection
- Blood urea nitrogen (BUN) and serum creatinine are needed to dose antibiotics appropriately and to minimize or prevent drug toxicity (especially in the elderly patient)

Microbiology Tests

- Sputum gram stain should demonstrate the presence of WBCs and the absence of squamous epithelial cells. It may or may not show a predominance of one type of organism
- Sputum culture and susceptibility are not obtained in the outpatient setting. The value of culturing is debated owing to the rapidity in which *S. pneumoniae* dies in transport media and the inability to reliably or routinely culture atypical organisms
- Bronchoscopy may be performed to improve the ability to diagnose pneumonia. Tracheal secretions often are better specimens than sputum owing to the lack of oral contamination
- Serology (IgM and IgG) is useful in determining the presence of atypical organisms such as *Mycoplasma* and *Chlamydia*
- Urinary direct fluorescence antigen (DFA) is used to diagnose *L. pneumophila*
- Polymerase chain reaction (PCR) is being used more frequently to detect the DNA of respiratory pathogens
- Blood cultures must be obtained in all patients hospitalized with pneumonia to comply with Joint Commission on Accreditation of Healthcare Organizations (JCAHO) pneumonia guidelines. Positive blood cultures are present in about 1% to 20% of patients with CAP

Clinical Presentation of Severe CAP or Aspiration Pneumonia

General

In approximately 10% of patients, CAP will be severe enough to require intensive care or mechanical ventilation

Symptoms ❹

- Respiratory—cough (productive or nonproductive), shortness of breath, difficulty breathing
- Nonrespiratory—fever, fatigue, sweats, headache, myalgias, mental status changes

Signs

- Temperature may increase or decrease from baseline, but most often it is elevated. The temperature may be sustained or intermittent
- Respiratory rate greater than 30 breaths per minute. Cyanosis and use of accessory muscles of respiration along with the increased respiratory rate are suggestive of severe respiratory compromise
- Hypotension (systolic blood pressure less than 90 mm Hg or diastolic blood pressure less than 60 mm Hg)

- Requirement for vasopressors
- Breath sounds may be diminished. Rales or rhonci may be heard
- Urine output less than 20 mL/h or less than 80 mL over 4 hours
- Confusion, lethargy, and disorientation are relatively common in elderly patients

Diagnostic Tests

As stated in the clinical presentation of community-acquired or aspiration pneumonia

Laboratory Tests

As stated in the clinical presentation of community-acquired or aspiration pneumonia

Microbiology Tests

As stated in the clinical presentation of community-acquired or aspiration pneumonia

TREATMENT

Desired Outcomes

❺ *The goal of antibiotic therapy is to eliminate the patient's symptoms, minimize or prevent complications, and decrease mortality.* Potential complications secondary to pneumonia include further decline in pulmonary function in patients with underlying pulmonary disease, prolonged mechanical ventilation, bacteremia/sepsis/septic shock, and death. Use of an antimicrobial agent with the narrowest spectrum of activity that covers the suspected pathogen(s) without having activity against organisms not involved in the infection is preferred to minimize the development of resistance.

General Approach to Treatment

Designing a therapeutic regimen for any patient with any type of pneumonia begins with three general categories of consideration:

1. Patient specific factors that will impact therapy
2. The top one to three organisms likely causing the infection, and resistance issues associated with each organism
3. The antimicrobials that will cover these organisms. The spectrum should not be too broad or narrow; they should penetrate into the site of infection and be the most cost effective.

Patient factors that need to be considered include age, renal function, drug allergies and/or drug intolerances, immune status (diabetes, neutropenia, or immunocompromised host), cardiopulmonary disease, pregnancy, medical insurance and prescription coverage, and prior antibiotic exposure(s) (what agents and when).

The most common pathogens vary with the type of pneumonia, and they are listed in Table 71–1. *M. pneumoniae* lack a cell wall; therefore, β-lactam antimicrobials have no activity against this organism. The atypical organisms have not changed in recent years with respect to antibiotic resistance. β-lactamase production in *H. influenzae* has remained relatively steady over the last 5 to 10 years and the rate is approximately 35%.[26] *S. pneumoniae* has developed resistance mechanisms against many classes of antimicrobials and the mechanisms include:

- Alteration of the penicillin binding proteins (PBPs) inactivating β-lactams
- Efflux or methylation of the ribosome inactivating macrolides
- Ribosome protection (*tetM* gene) inactivating tetracyclines
- Alteration of DNA gyrase or topoisomerase IV inactivating fluoroquinolones

Resistance to commonly prescribed antimicrobials such as the penicillins and macrolides/azalides dramatically increased in the late 1980s through the mid- to late 1990s. Table 71–2 provides resistance information collected nationally from 1999 to 2007 using the Tracking Resistance in the US Today (TRUST) surveillance database.[27] In 2007, the average national rate of resistance to penicillin and macrolides was approximately 13% and 32%, respectively. Susceptibility results alone do not account for clinical success or failures when treating pneumonia. Therefore, despite the 13% and 32% resistance to penicillin and macrolides,

Patient Encounter 1, Part 2: Medical History, Physical Examination, and Diagnostic Tests

The 73-year-old woman presents again to your clinic complaining of difficulty breathing and shortness of breath. Her daughter also states that she is easily confused and that this is not normal for her.

PMH: COPD for 15 years; hypertension for 4 years, currently controlled

FH: Father died of lung cancer at the age of 68 years; mother died of natural causes

SH: Smoked two packs per day for 23 years, quit 15 years ago; does not drink alcohol; lives with her daughter

Allergies: NKDA

Meds: Lisinopril 10 mg orally once daily; Ipratropium bromide four puffs four times per day; flunisolide three puffs two times per day; albuterol two puffs as needed

ROS: (+) difficulty breathing and shortness of breath; (−) chest pain, N/V/D, weight loss, change in appetite

PE:

VS: BP 110/76, P 82, RR 20, T 37.4°C (99.3°F)

CV: RRR, normal S_1, S_2; no murmurs, rubs, or gallops

Lungs: Decreased breath sounds on the left side compared with the right and rales in the left lower lobe

Abd: Soft, nontender, nondistended; (+) bowel sounds, no hepatosplenomegaly, heme (−) stool

Neuro: Oriented to name and place but not to date. She is easily confused by questions asked of her

Diagnostic Tests: Chest x-ray: left lower lobe infiltrates; oxygen saturation 92% on room air

Labs: Unavailable in the clinic

Given this additional information, what is your assessment of the patient's condition?

Identify your treatment goals for the patient

Table 71–2

Percentage of Resistance for Various Antimicrobials Against *S. pneumoniae*

Antimicrobial	1999	2001	2003	2005	2007
Penicillin	14.7	16.9	17.3	15.6	13.3
Azithromycin	22.7	27.5	27.5	28.2	32.3
Ceftriaxone[a]	3.4	3.0	1.5	0.7	1.4
Levofloxacin	0.6	0.8	0.9	0.8	0.7
Trimeth-sulfa	NA	NA	23.9	20.3	20.1
Tetracycline	NA	NA	NA	NA	18.8

NA, not available.

[a]Separation of ceftriaxone into nonmeningitis interpretation versus meningitis. Numbers presented are nonmeningitis.

one of those relates the timing of infection to the most likely pathogens. Early-onset infection is less likely to be caused by MDR pathogens than late-onset infection. In early-onset infection, community pathogens such as pneumococcus, *Legionella*, and *Mycoplasma* need to be considered as well as some of the hospital pathogens. Patients developing late-onset pneumonia are at increased risk of having a resistant pathogen or MDR pathogen such as MRSA, enteric gram-negative bacilli, *Pseudomonas*, and *Acinetobacter*. Another issue is how HCAP and HAP are studied compared to VAP. The majority of studies were performed using patients that were intubated. Therefore, the body of literature supporting the treatment recommendations is greatest for VAP and not for HCAP or HAP. The evidence-based guidelines generated by the American Thoracic Society (ATS) and Infectious Diseases Society of America (IDSA) were derived from VAP and applied to HCAP and HAP.

Risk factors for developing infection caused by a resistant pathogen are generally related to the prior use of antibiotics, insertion of catheters or other invasive devices, and hospitalization in a unit contaminated/colonized with resistant organisms. The following is a more complete list of factors influencing infection from a resistant organism:

- Antimicrobial therapy in preceding 90 days
- Current hospitalization of at least 5 days
- High occurrence of antibiotic resistance in the community or in the specific hospital unit
- Immunosuppressive disease and/or therapy
- Presence of the following risk factors for HCAP
  - Hospitalization for 2 days or more in the preceding 90 days
  - Residence in a nursing home or extended-care facility
  - Home infusion therapy (including antibiotics)
  - Peritoneal or hemodialysis within 30 days
  - Home wound care
  - Close contact family member with MDR pathogen

Once these issues are addressed, antimicrobial therapy can be selected and initiated. The patient- and drug-related

the clinical failure rate is less than this. Because CAP in the outpatient setting is treated empirically, establishing a meaningful clinical failure rate with any therapy is difficult to do. No studies have been performed that established a correlation between clinical failure rates with a particular antimicrobial agent and the percentage of resistant bacterial pathogens.

For HCAP, HAP, and VAP, the risk of infection from an MDR pathogen is relatively high. The number and type of organisms that are MDR vary from hospital to hospital making it more difficult to generate guidelines for treatment. Therefore, the treatment recommendations may be too broad or too narrow for any given institution. Treating patients with HCAP, HAP, or VAP is more complex than treating patients with CAP. There are many factors to consider and

Patient Encounter 2, Part 2: Medical History, Physical Examination, and Diagnostic Tests

The 52-year-old man who developed complications after abdominal surgery was intubated 6 days ago. The nurses note an increase in the amount and the purulence of his sputum. Attempts yesterday and today to wean the patient off the ventilator have failed. He is sedated, but he does respond to commands.

PMH: Small bowel obstruction, surgery 8 days ago; hypertension for 15 years, currently controlled

FH: Father died of acute MI at the age of 68 years; mother, age 72 years is alive, with hypertension and hypothyroid

SH: No tobacco use; drinks two beers per night. He lives with his wife; occupation—carpenter. He is 5'11" (180 cm) and weighs 85 kg (187 lb)

Allergies: Penicillin—hives

Meds: Lisinopril 40 mg orally once daily

PE:

VS: BP 120/84, P 78, T 38.4°C (101°F)

CV: RRR, normal S_1, S_2; no murmurs, rubs, or gallops

Abd: Soft, nontender, nondistended; (+) bowel sounds, no hepatosplenomegaly, incision looks good and is healing

Diagnostic Tests: Chest x-ray: left middle and lower lobe infiltrates; oxygen saturation 98% on ventilator

Labs: WBCs 18.2×10^3 /mm³ ($18.2 \times 109/L$) with a cell differential of 72% neutrophils, 8% bands, 16% lymphocytes, and 4% monocytes; BUN 10 mg/dL (3.57 mmol/L), SCr 0.9 mg/dL (80 μmol/L); sputum gram stain: many gram-negative bacilli, many WBCs; sputum culture is pending

Given this additional information, what is your assessment of the patient's condition?

Identify your treatment goals for the patient.

categories are common to all types of pneumonia, but the organisms vary with the type of pneumonia. Guidelines have been generated by experts in the field for all types of pneumonia. These guidelines were generated to provide practitioners with evidenced-based therapeutic options for the management of patients with pneumonia.

Pharmacologic Therapy for CAP

⑥ *Treatment of CAP is predominantly empiric, that is, treatment is started without knowing the causative pathogen.* As a way of incorporating an evidence-based approach to antibiotic selection, several different organizations have generated guidelines for the treatment of bacterial or atypical CAP in adults. The most recent guidelines are the result of a collaboration between the IDSA and the ATS.[28] The approach to patient care is based on the classification of patients into two broad categories, outpatient and inpatient, and then further divide the groups by comorbid conditions and location in the hospital, respectively. These guidelines use patient-specific data along with predominant pathogen information to design appropriate empirical antimicrobial regimens. Table 71–3 summarizes these therapeutic options. If influenza virus is the cause, supportive care is the best medical intervention available; antiviral agents against influenza are not very effective.

▶ Adult Outpatient Previously Healthy

First-line therapeutic options for treating previously healthy adults include use of a macrolide (erythromycin, clarithromycin) or an azalide (azithromycin) or doxycycline.[28] If a patient has failed therapy with a macrolide, azalide, or doxycycline, one has to consider why the patient failed. The most common reasons are either medication adherence issues or the presence of resistant organisms. If a resistant organism is suspected then use of one of the fluoroquinolones active against *S. pneumoniae* (gemifloxacin, levofloxacin, or moxifloxacin) is warranted.

▶ Adult Outpatient With Comorbid Conditions

The comorbid conditions that can impact therapy and outcomes in patients with CAP include diabetes mellitus, COPD, chronic heart, liver, or renal disease, alcoholism, malignancy, asplenia, and immunosuppressive condition or use of immunosuppressive drugs.[28] If the patient did not receive antibiotics in the last 3 months then either a respiratory fluoroquinolone alone or a combination of an oral β-lactam agent plus a macrolide or azalide is recommended. If the patient received an antibiotic in the last 3 months the recommendation is to use an agent from a different class. Doxycycline is an acceptable alternative to a macrolide or azalide. The β-lactam agents recommended are high-dose (3 g daily) amoxicillin or high-dose (4 g daily) amoxicillin-clavulanate. Alternative β-lactams are second- and third-generation cephalosporins such as cefuroxime, cefpodoxime, or ceftriaxone.

Telithromycin, a ketolide antibiotic approved for the treatment of mild to moderate CAP, is not included in the recommendations because of safety issues related to hepatotoxicity, loss of consciousness, and visual disturbances still pending resolution with the FDA. Telithromycin is similar in spectrum of activity to clarithromycin and azithromycin in that it covers primarily the respiratory pathogens and not gram-negative bacilli.

▶ Adult Inpatient Not in the ICU

For patients admitted to the hospital with CAP, the severity of illness is generally increased (caused either by the organism itself or underlying comorbidities in the patient) and the

Table 71–3

Summary of CAP Treatment

Adult outpatient otherwise healthy
Empirical coverage against *S. pneumoniae*, *M. pneumoniae*, *C. pneumoniae*, and *H. influenzae*

Monotherapy
Azithromycin, clarithromycin, erythromycin, doxycycline

Adult outpatient comorbidities
Empirical coverage against *S. pneumoniae*, *M. pneumoniae*, *C. pneumoniae*, and *H. influenzae*

Combination therapy
High-dose amoxicillin, high-dose amoxicillin-clavulanate (alternatives are cefpodoxime, or cefuroxime, or ceftriaxone) *plus* azithromycin, or clarithromycin or, doxycycline
Monotherapy
Gemifloxacin, levofloxacin, moxifloxacin

Adult inpatient (non-ICU)
Empirical coverage against *S. pneumoniae*, *H. influenzae*, *M. pneumoniae*, and *C. pneumoniae*

Combination therapy
Cefotaxime, or ceftriaxone, or ampicillin-sulbactam, or ertapenem *plus* azithromycin, or clarithromycin, or doxycycline
Monotherapy
Gemifloxacin, levofloxacin, moxifloxacin

Adult inpatient ICU (no Pseudomonas)
Empirical coverage against *S. pneumoniae*, *L. pneumophila*, *H. influenzae*, enteric GNB, and *S. aureus*

Combination therapy
Cefotaxime or ceftriaxone *plus* azithromycin, or levofloxacin, or moxifloxacin

Adult inpatient ICU (Pseudomonas is a concern)
Empirical coverage against *P. aeruginosa*, *S. pneumoniae*, *L. pneumophila*, *H. influenzae*, enteric GNB, and *S. aureus*

Combination therapy
Cefepime, or ceftazidime, or piperacillin-tazobactam, or imipenem, or meropenem *plus* or ciprofloxacin or levofloxacin or an aminoglycoside
If an aminoglycoside is chosen, then add azithromycin or levofloxacin or moxifloxacin.

Adult inpatient non-ICU or ICU (CA-MRSA is a concern)
Empirical coverage against *S. pneumoniae*, *L. pneumophila*, *H. influenzae*, enteric GNB, and *S. aureus* (*Pseudomonas* if ICU)

Add vancomycin or linezolid to the regimens listed above

Pediatric outpatient
Empirical coverage against *S. pneumoniae*, *M. pneumoniae*, and *C. pneumoniae*

Monotherapy
High-dose amoxicillin, or high-dose amoxicillin-clavulanate, or intramuscular ceftriaxone, or azithromycin, or clarithromycin

Pediatric inpatient (non-ICU)
Empirical coverage against *S. pneumoniae*, *H. influenzae*, *M. pneumoniae*, and *C. pneumoniae*

Combination therapy
IV cefuroxime, or cefotaxime, or ceftriaxone, or ampicillin-sulbactam plus azithromycin, or clarithromycin

Pediatric inpatient ICU
Empirical coverage against *S. pneumoniae*, *L. pneumophila*, *H. influenzae*, enteric GNB, and *S. aureus*

Combination therapy
Cefotaxime, or ceftriaxone plus azithromycin, or clarithromycin

---

pathogens are essentially the same as in the outpatient setting. Recommendations are to use either a respiratory fluoroquinolone alone or a combination of an IV β-lactam agent plus an advanced macrolide/azalide (clarithromycin/azithromycin) or doxycycline. The recommended β-lactams include cefotaxime, ceftriaxone, ampicillin-sulbactam, or ertapenem.[28] Therapy should be initiated in the emergency room; however, due to the controversy with a first antibiotic dose time of less than 4 or 8 hours, no recommendations were made regarding time to the first antibiotic dose. Conversion to oral therapy should occur when the patient is hemodynamically stable, improving clinically, and able to take oral medications, which often is within 48 to 72 hours for most patients. Discharge from the hospital should be as soon as the patient is stable and without other medical complications. The need to observe the patient in the hospital on their oral antibiotic is not necessary.[28]

Patient Encounter 1, Part 3: Creating a Care Plan

Based on the information presented, create a care plan for this patient's pneumonia. Your plan should include

(a) the goals of therapy,
(b) a patient-specific detailed therapeutic plan, and
(c) a plan for follow-up to determine whether the goals have been achieved and adverse effects avoided.

▶ Adult Inpatient in the ICU

Patients admitted to the ICU have severe pneumonia, and the likely etiology includes *S. pneumoniae*, *H. influenzae* as in the other categories; however, the incidence of *L. pneumophila* increases in this setting and should be included in the organism differential. In addition, enteric gram-negative bacilli and *S. aureus* are more frequently the cause of the pneumonia. The recommendations are to treat with an IV β-lactam plus either azithromycin or a respiratory fluoroquinolone. This combination therapy minimizes the risk of treatment failure due to a resistant pathogen as well as provides coverage against all of the potential pathogens.[28] The preferred β-lactams are ceftriaxone, cefotaxime, or ampicillin-sulbactam. If the patient is allergic to β-lactams then aztreonam plus a respiratory fluoroquinolone are preferred.

If *P. aeruginosa* is suspected (e.g., patient comes from a long-term care facility, or recent hospitalization) then the antimicrobial treatment must be broadened to cover *Pseudomonas* as well as the organisms listed above. Owing to the high resistance rates observed in *Pseudomonas*, the recommended regimens empirically double cover the *Pseudomonas* to ensure at least one of the antibiotics is active against *Pseudomonas*. The regimens include the use of an antipneumococcal, antipseudomonal β-lactam (cefepime, ceftazidime, piperacillin/tazobactam, imipenem, or meropenem) plus either ciprofloxacin or levofloxacin or an aminoglycoside. If the aminoglycoside is chosen, then either IV azithromycin or a respiratory fluoroquinolone should be added to cover *S. pneumoniae* and the atypical bacterial organisms.[28]

If CA-MRSA is suspected in the patient then the addition of vancomycin or linezolid to the above regimen should be considered. Daptomycin cannot be used because surfactant in the lung inactivates the drug thus rendering it ineffective for pneumonia. CA-MRSA can cause a necrotizing pneumonia, and the cause is believed to be due to the increased pathogenicity of this strain and its multiple toxins including the Panton-Valentine leukocidin toxin.[9] In these patients the use of an agent which decreases toxin production may be beneficial. Linezolid does decrease toxin production and the agents recommended to be added to vancomycin therapy are clindamycin or a respiratory fluoroquinolone.[28]

▶ Influenza

Influenza viruses A and B can cause pneumonia in pediatric and adult patients. Amantidine and rimantidine are available oral agents with activity against influenza virus type A. If started within 48 hours of the onset of the first symptoms, they reduce the duration of the illness by about 1.3 days. Oseltamivir and zanamivir also are oral agents that reduce the duration of the illness by about 1.3 days if initiated within 40 to 48 hours of the first symptoms.[29] For active infection beyond the first 48 hours, none of these agents is effective in treating infection, and supportive care is the best treatment for these patients.

▶ Aspiration

Anaerobes and *Streptococcus* spp. are the primary pathogens if a patient aspirates his or her oral contents and develops pneumonia. Antibiotics active against these organisms include penicillin G, ampicillin/sulbactam,

Patient Encounter 2, Part 3: Creating a Care Plan

Based on the information presented, create a care plan for this patient's pneumonia. Your plan should include

(a) the goals of therapy,
(b) a patient-specific detailed therapeutic plan, and
(c) a plan for follow-up to determine whether goals have been achieved and adverse effects avoided.

and clindamycin. If the patient aspirates oral and gastric contents then anaerobes and gram-negative bacilli are the primary pathogens. The preferred treatment regimen is a β-lactam/β-lactamase inhibitor combination (ampicillin/sulbactam, amoxicillin/clavulanate, piperacillin/tazobactam, or ticarcillin/clavulanate).[28]

▶ Pediatric Outpatient

If viral pneumonia is diagnosed, then treatment is often supportive (maintaining hydration, antipyretics) since we have very few effective antiviral agents. The bacterial pathogens are the same as for adults with *S. pneumoniae* as the predominant pathogen, then *M. pneumoniae*, and then the other organisms. Resistance issues with these organisms are similar to those seen in adult patients. Fluoroquinolones and tetracyclines should not be used in children younger than 5 years of age. High-dose amoxicillin (50 mg/kg/day), amoxicillin/clavulanate (70–90 mg/kg/day), intramuscular ceftriaxone (50 mg/kg/day), azithromycin (10 mg/kg/day), and clarithromycin (7.5 mg/kg/day) are all potential agents for use in children.[30] Dosing of antibiotics for pediatrics patients is presented in Table 71–4.

▶ Pediatric Inpatient

If the child is not admitted to the ICU, then the CDC recommends the use of IV cefuroxime, cefotaxime, ceftriaxone, or ampicillin/sulbactam plus a macrolide or azalide. If the child is admitted to the ICU, then only the third-generation cephalosporins (cefotaxime or ceftriaxone) plus a macrolide or azalide should be administered.[30]

Pharmacologic Therapy for HCAP/HAP/VAP

Nosocomial pneumonia was the term used to describe patients who develop pneumonia in an institutional setting but it has been replaced by the terms *health care–associated pneumonia*, *hospital-associated pneumonia*, and *VAP*. ❼ *Empirical selection of antimicrobial therapy for ventilator-, health care-, and hospital-associated pneumonia is broad spectrum; however, once culture and susceptibility information are available, the therapy should be narrowed (de-escalation) to cover the identified pathogen(s).* Two factors important to the empirical selection of antibiotics for these types of pneumonia are onset time after

Diagnosis of VAP

Clinical Strategy

- Chest x-ray should reveal a new infiltrate *plus* two of the following:
  - Temperature greater than 38°C (100.4°F)
  - Leukocytosis or leukopenia
  - Purulent secretions
  - Semiquantitative cultures are obtained to identify the pathogen(s)
- Tracheal aspirates grow more organisms than invasive quantitative cultures and often result in overuse of antibiotics
- The major limitation of the clinical strategy is the consistent overprescribing of antibiotics

Bacteriologic Strategy

- Uses quantitative culture of endotracheal aspirates, bronchoalveolar lavage (BAL), or protected specimen brush (PSB)
- Greater than or equal to 10^6 cfu/mL for endotracheal aspirates
- Greater than or equal to 10^4 to 10^5 cfu/mL for BAL
- Greater than or equal to 10^3 cfu/mL for PSB
- The advantage of this method is that it separates colonization from infection better than culturing tracheal aspirates

- The limitation is the potential misinterpretation of negative culture results. These samples should be obtained prior to antibiotics being started

Recommended Diagnostic Strategy

- Combination of the preceding two methods
- Obtain either a quantitative or semiquantitative culture of a lower respiratory sample. Initiate empirical broad-spectrum antibiotic therapy
- Days 2 and 3: Check culture results, and assess clinical response to therapy: temperature, WBCs, chest x-ray, oxygenation, purulent sputum, hemodynamic changes, and organ function
- Assess clinical improvement at 48 to 72 hours:
  - Improvement and culture negative—stop antibiotics
  - Improvement and culture positive—narrow antibiotic therapy
  - No improvement and culture negative—consider other pathogens, complications, or other diagnosis
  - No improvement and culture positive—change antibiotic therapy and consider other pathogens, complications, or other diagnosis

---

admission and risk factors for MDR organisms. If it is early onset (less than or equal to 5 days since admission) and there are no risk factors for MDR organisms then the most frequent pathogens include *S. pneumoniae, H. influenzae,* methicillin-susceptible *Staphylococcus aureus* (MSSA), and enteric gram-negative bacilli. Recommendations for therapy include third-generation cephalosporins such as ceftriaxone or cefotaxime, a respiratory fluoroquinolone such as gemifloxacin, levofloxacin, or moxifloxacin; or ampicillin/sulbactam or ertapenem.[31] If it is late-onset pneumonia and/or there are risk factors for MDR organisms, then the pathogen list includes *P. aeruginosa,* extended-spectrum *β*-lactamase producing *K. pneumoniae, Acinetobacter* spp., and MRSA. Empirical antibiotic selection must cover *P. aeruginosa,* which often then covers the other gram-negative pathogens. Available antibiotics include cefepime, ceftazidime, imipenem, meropenem, piperacillin/tazobactam, ticarcillin/clavulanate, levofloxacin, ciprofloxacin, gentamicin, tobramycin, and amikacin. Empirical therapy for late onset (listed in Table 71–5) could include any of the *β*-lactams, carbapenems, or fluoroquinolones alone or in combination with one of the aminoglycosides. If MRSA is suspected then either vancomycin or linezolid should be added to the regimen. Recommendations for vancomycin trough concentrations of 15 to 20 mcg/mL were based on expert opinion not evidence from clinical trials.[31]

Currently there is debate over whether or not double coverage for pseudomonas is required. In vitro studies have shown that aminoglycosides exhibit synergistic killing against gram-negative bacilli when combined with β-lactams. Dosing of the aminoglycosides is dependent upon the patient's renal function. A high-dose once-daily regimen (e.g., 4–7 mg/kg gentamicin or tobramycin or 15–20 mg/kg amikacin) can be utilized in patients with good renal function. Most of the studies enrolled patients with estimated creatinine clearances of at least 70 mL/min (1.17 mL/s). Meta-analyses have shown high-dose once-daily regimens to be as efficacious as and less toxic than divided daily dosing.[32–36]

In addition to obtaining a synergistic effect, another reason for double coverage when treating VAP, HAP, or HCAP is to broaden the coverage empirically to increase the likelihood of covering the majority of resistant pathogens. VAP is the most studied of these types of pneumonias and is often the most severe. Studies have demonstrated an increase in mortality when inadequate therapy is initiated for VAP. Crude mortality ranges from 35% to 92% with inadequate therapy compared to 25% to 47% with adequate therapy.[17]

❼ *Once a pathogen or pathogens have been identified, therapy should be narrowed to cover only those pathogens.* Use of broad-spectrum antibiotics for prolonged durations increases the risk of colonization with MDR pathogens.

Table 71–4

CAP Pediatric Dosing

Drug (Route)	Body Weight Less Than 2,000 g		Body Weight Greater Than 2,000 g		Greater Than 28 Days Old
	0–7 Days Old	7–28 Days Old	0–7 Days Old	7–28 Days Old	
Amoxicillin (orally)				15 mg/kg every 12 hours	17 mg/kg every 8 hours
Amoxicillin-clavulanate (orally)			15 mg/kg every 12 hours	15 mg/kg every 12 hours	45 mg/kg every 12 hours
Cefotaxime (IV)	50 mg/kg every 12 hours	50 mg/kg every 8 hours	50 mg/kg every 12 hours	50 mg/kg every 8 hours	50 mg/kg every 8 hours
Ceftriaxone (IM/IV)	25 mg/kg every 24 hours	50 mg/kg every 24 hours	25 mg/kg every 24 hours	50 mg/kg every 24 hours	50 mg/kg every 24 hours
Cefuroxime (orally)					15 mg/kg every 12 hours
Azithromycin (orally/IV)	5 mg/kg every 24 hours	10 mg/kg every 24 hours	5 mg/kg every 24 hours	10 mg/kg every 24 hours	10 mg/kg every 24 hours
Clarithromycin (orally)					7.5 mg/kg every 12 hours

Table 71–5

Empirical Therapy for Late-Onset HAP, HCAP, or VAP in Adults

Antibiotic (Route)	CrCl[a] Greater Than 50 mL/min	CrCl 30–50 mL/min	CrCl 10–30 mL/min	CrCl Less Than 10 mL/min
Cefepime (IV)	1–2 g every 12 hours	1–2 g every 24 hours	1 g every 24 hours	0.5–1 g every 24 hours
Ceftazidime (IV)	1–2 g every 8 hours	1–2 g every 12 hours	1–2 g every 12–24 hours	1–2 g every 24 hours
Imipenem (IV)	500 mg every 6 hours or 1 g every 8 hours	500 mg every 6–8 hours	500 mg every 8–12 hours	250 mg every 12 hours
Meropenem (IV)	1 g every 8 hours	1 g every 12 hours	500 mg every 12 hours	500 mg every 24 hours
Piperacillin-tazobactam (IV)	4.5 g every 6 hours or 3.375 g every 4 hours	4.5 g every 8 hours or 3.375 g every 6 hours	4.5 g every 8–12 hours or 3.375 g every 6–8 hours	4.5 g every 12 hours or 3.375 g every 8 hours or 2.25 g every 6 hours
Ticarcillin-clavulanate (IV)	3.1 g every 4–6 hours	2 g every 4–6 hours	2 g every 8 hours	2 g every 12 hours
Levofloxacin (IV/orally)	750 mg every 24 hours	750 mg every 48 hours	750 mg ×1 then 500 mg every 48 hours	750 mg ×1 then 500 mg every 48 hours
Ciprofloxacin (IV)	400 mg every 8 hours	400 mg every 8 hours	400 mg every 12 hours	400 mg every 24 hours
Ciprofloxacin (orally)	750 mg every 8 hours	750 mg every 8 hours	750 mg every 12 hours	750 mg every 24 hours
Gentamicin or Tobramcyin[b] (IV)	5–7 mg/kg every 24 hours	1.7–2 mg/kg every 12–24 hours	1.7–2 mg/kg every 36 hours	1.7–2 mg/kg every 48 hours
Amikacin[b] (IV)	20 mg/kg every 24 hours	7.5 mg/kg every 12–24 hours	7.5 mg/kg every 36 hours	7.5 mg/kg every 48 hours
Vancomycin[c] (IV)	15–20 mg/kg every 12 hours	15–20 mg/kg every 24 hours	15–20 mg/kg every 48 hours	15–20 mg/kg every 72 hours
Linezolid (IV/orally)	600 mg every 12 hours	600 mg every 12 hours	600 mg every 12 hours	600 mg every 12 hours

[a]CrCl, creatinine clearance.

[b]Trough concentrations ideally should be nondetectable; less than 1 mcg/mL for gentamicin (2.09 μmol/L) and tobramycin (2.14 μmol/L) and less than 4 to 5 mcg/mL (6.84–8.55 μmol/L) for amikacin are potentially acceptable.

[c]Trough concentrations should be between 15 and 20 mcg/mL (10–14 μmol/L).

▶ Duration of Therapy

❽ *The duration of therapy for pneumonia should be kept as short as possible* and depends upon several factors: type of pneumonia, inpatient or outpatient status, patient comorbidities, bacteremia/sepsis, and the antibiotic chosen.

If the duration of therapy is too prolonged, then it can have a negative impact on the patient's normal flora in the respiratory and GI tracts, vaginal tract of women, and on the skin. This can result in colonization with resistant pathogens, *Clostridium difficile* colitis, or overgrowth of yeast. In addition, the longer antibiotics are administered, the greater the chance for toxicity from the agent as well as an increase in cost.[17]

For treating outpatient CAP, two antibiotics are approved for a 5-day duration of therapy, levofloxacin (the 750-mg once daily dose) and azithromycin. The duration of therapy for all other agents used to treat CAP is 7 to 10 days. For treatment of CAP in patients admitted to the hospital, the duration is dependent upon whether or not blood cultures were positive. In the absence of positive blood cultures, the duration of therapy is 7 to 10 days. If blood cultures were positive, the duration of therapy should be 2 weeks from the day blood cultures first became negative.

The duration of therapy cited in the literature for HCAP, HAP, or VAP ranges from 10 to 21 days. Efforts should be made to shorten the duration of therapy from the traditional 14 to 21 days to periods as short as 7 days, provided that the etiologic pathogen is not *P. aeruginosa*, and that the patient has a good clinical response with resolution of clinical features of infection. Shortening the duration of therapy is acknowledged as beneficial because of the colonization, toxicity, and cost issues. The Clinical Pulmonary Infection Score (CPIS) has been used to determine when to end therapy for VAP. Luna and colleagues used the CPIS and found that patients who survived VAP and were treated with adequate therapy clinically improved within 3 to 5 days.[37] This study was instrumental in recommending a shortened duration of therapy of 6 days. Another study found that when the CPIS was six or less, those patients were at low risk of VAP or resistant pathogens and treatment only needed to be for 3 days.[38]

OUTCOME EVALUATION

For CAP, outcomes include preventing hospitalization, shortening the duration of hospitalization, and minimizing mortality. For patients admitted to the hospital, if antibiotics are initiated within 4 hours of presentation, the duration of hospitalization is decreased compared to when antibiotics are started after 4 hours.[39]

Improvement of symptoms should occur within 48 to 72 hours after initiation of therapy for most patients with CAP. Response to therapy could be slowed in patients with underlying pulmonary disease such as moderate to severe asthma, COPD, or emphysema. In patients not responding to therapy and when there are no underlying factors that would suggest a slowed response to therapy, then other infectious and noninfectious reasons must be considered. The infection could be caused by a pathogen not covered by the initial therapy, a drug-resistant isolate could be present, or more severe infection could be present (nonpulmonary) and the patient should be reevaluated. Noninfectious reasons to consider include pulmonary embolus, congestive heart failure, carcinoma, lymphoma, intrapulmonary hemorrhage, and certain inflammatory lung diseases.

Outcome parameters for VAP, HAP, and HCAP are similar to those with CAP. Clinical improvement should occur within 48 to 72 hours of the start of therapy. If a patient is not responding to therapy, then, again, consider infectious and

---

Patient Care and Monitoring

9 *Monitoring response to therapy is essential for determining efficacy, identifying adverse reactions, and determining the duration of therapy.*

1. Assess the patient's symptoms and status (i.e., inpatient, outpatient, or intubated) to determine the type of pneumonia and comorbid conditions. Does the patient have moderate to severe asthma, COPD, or emphysema or is a current smoker?

2. Review any available diagnostic data to determine severity of the disease.

3. Obtain a history of prescription and nonprescription medication use, as well as allergies and drug intolerances, noting the severity of the reaction.

4. What are the top two to three organisms associated with the type of pneumonia the patient has?

5. Select an appropriate empirical antibiotic regimen for the patient, ensuring that the doses are correct for renal function.

6. Develop a plan to assess the effectiveness of the antibiotic therapy after 24 to 72 hours. If the patient is not improving, then reevaluate the diagnosis and pathogen list, and make appropriate changes to therapy. Develop a plan to assess the effectiveness of the antibiotic therapy again at the end of therapy. When can conversion from IV to oral therapy occur?

7. Evaluate the patient for the presence of adverse drug reactions, drug allergies, and drug interactions.

8. For patients who meet the qualifications, discuss the value of vaccination against *S. pneumoniae* and/or influenza.

---

noninfectious reasons. Infectious explanations are the same as for CAP, but noninfectious are not. They include atelectasis, acute respiratory distress syndrome (ARDS), pulmonary embolism or hemorrhage, cancer, empyema or lung abscess.

PREVENTION

10 *Prevention of pneumococcal disease by use of vaccination is a national goal.* Vaccination is used to prevent or minimize the severity of pneumonia caused by *S. pneumoniae* or the influenza virus.

The influenza vaccine is available in two forms, injectable and nasal inhalation. The injectable product is an inactivated vaccine (containing killed virus) and is approved for use in people older than 6 months of age, including healthy people and people with chronic medical conditions. The nasal-spray influenza vaccine is made with live, weakened influenza viruses that do not cause influenza (live attenuated influenza vaccine). This formulation is approved for use in healthy people 5 to 49 years of age who are not pregnant. The ability of influenza vaccine to protect a person depends on two key factors: the age and health status of the person getting the vaccine, and the similarity or "match" between the virus strains in the vaccine and those in circulation. Given these factors, the vaccine has been effective. The influenza vaccine is recommended for the following groups of people[40]:

1. *People at high risk for complications from the flu*:
   - People 65 years and older
   - People who live in nursing homes and other long-term care facilities that house those with long-term illnesses
   - Adults and children 6 months and older with chronic heart or lung conditions, including asthma
   - Adults and children 6 months and older who needed regular medical care or were in a hospital during the previous year because of a metabolic disease (like diabetes), chronic kidney disease, or weakened immune system (including immune system problems caused by medicines or by infection with HIV)
   - Women who will be pregnant during the influenza season
   - Children 6 months to 18 years of age who are on long-term aspirin therapy
   - All children 5 to 18 years of age
   - People with any condition that can compromise respiratory function or the handling of respiratory secretions (i.e., a condition that makes it hard to breathe or swallow, such as brain injury or disease, spinal cord injuries, seizure disorders, or other nerve or muscle disorders)

2. *People 50 to 64 years of age*: Comorbid conditions are present in nearly one-third of people 50 to 64 years of age in the United States, and that places them at increased risk for serious flu complications. Therefore, vaccination is recommended for all persons aged 50 to 64 years.

3. *People who can transmit flu to others at high risk for complications*: Any person in close contact with someone in a high-risk group should get vaccinated. This includes all health care workers, household contacts, and out-of-home caregivers of children 0 to 23 months of age and adults 65 years and older.

There are two pneumococcal vaccines, a seven-valent conjugated vaccine for children younger than 6 years of age and a 23-purified-capsular polysaccharide antigen vaccine for adults. The 23 capsular types in the vaccine represent at least 85% to 90% of the serotypes that cause invasive pneumococcal infections among children and adults in the United States.[41] After vaccination, an antigen-specific antibody response, indicated by a twofold or greater rise in serotype-specific antibody, develops within 2 to 3 weeks in 80% or more of healthy young adults.[42] However, immune responses may not be consistent among all 23 serotypes in the vaccine.[42] Those who should receive the polysaccharide vaccine include[40]:

1. *All adults 65 years of age or older*

2. *Anyone over 6 years of age who has a long-term health problem* such as heart disease, lung disease, sickle cell disease, diabetes, alcoholism, cirrhosis, and leakage of cerebrospinal fluid.

3. *Anyone over 6 years of age who has a disease or condition or is taking any drug that lowers the body's resistance to infection,* such as Hodgkin's disease, lymphoma, leukemia, kidney failure, multiple myeloma, nephrotic syndrome, HIV infection or AIDS, damaged spleen or no spleen, organ transplant, long-term steroids, certain cancer drugs, or radiation therapy

4. *Alaskan Natives and certain Native American populations*: The conjugated pneumococcal vaccine is recommended for all children aged 2 to 23 months and for certain children aged 24 to 59 months. If there are underlying health issues such as diabetes mellitus, or cardiopulmonary disease then children 24 to 59 months should receive this vaccine as well. The seven capsular types in the vaccine represent at least 85% to 90% of the serotypes that cause invasive pneumococcal infections among children in the United States.[41]

Abbreviations Introduced in This Chapter

ARDS	Acute respiratory distress syndrome
ATS	American Thoracic Society
BUN	Blood urea nitrogen
CA-MRSA	Community-acquired methicillin-resistant *Staphylococcus aureus*
CAP	Community-acquired pneumonia
COPD	Chronic obstructive pulmonary disease
CPIS	Clinical Pulmonary Infection Score
DFA	Direct fluorescence antigen
GER(D)	Gastroesophageal reflux (disease)
HCAP	Health care–associated pneumonia
HAP	Hospital-acquired pneumonia
IDSA	Infectious Diseases Society of America
MDR	Multidrug resistant
MRSA	Methicillin-resistant *Staphylococcus aureus*
MSSA	Methicillin-susceptible *S. aureus*
PaO_2/FiO_2	Arterial oxygen pressure/fraction of inspired oxygen
PBP	Penicillin binding protein
PCR	Polymerase chain reaction
TNF-α	Tumor necrosis factor α
TRUST	Tracking Resistance in the United States Today
VAP	Ventilator-associated pneumonia

Self-assessment questions and answers are available at *http://www.mhpharmacotherapy.com/pp.html.*

REFERENCES

1. Masterton R. The place of guidelines in hospital-acquired pneumonia. J Hosp Infect 2007;66:116–122.

2. Tablan OC, Anderson LJ, Besser R, et al. Guidelines for preventing health-care–associated pneumonia, 2003: Recommendations of CDC and the Healthcare Infection Control Practices Advisory Committee. MMWR Recomm Rep 2004;53:1–36.

3. Hugonnet S, Eggimann P, Borst F, et al. Impact of ventilator-associated pneumonia on resource utilization and patient outcome. Infect Control Hosp Epidemiol 2004;25:1090–1096.

4. Hutt E, Kramer AM. Evidence-based guidelines for management of nursing home-acquired pneumonia. J Fam Pract 2002;51:709–716.

5. Mylotte JM. Nursing home-acquired pneumonia. Clin Infect Dis 2002;35:1205–1211.

6. Lees AW, McNaught W. Bacteriology of lower-respiratory-tract secretions, sputum, and upper-respiratory-tract secretions in "normals" and chronic bronchitis. Lancet 1959;2:1112–1115.

7. Hendley JO, Sande MA, Stewart PM, Gwaltney JMJ. Spread of *Streptococcus pneumoniae* in families. I. Carriage rates and distribution of types. J Infect Dis 1975;132:55–61.

8. Wallin CA, Hern HG, Frazee BW. Community-associated methicillin-resistant *Staphylococcus aureus*. Emerg Med Clin N Am 2008;26:431–455.

9. Howard LSGE, Sillis M, Pasteur MC, et al. Microbiological profile of community-acquired pneumonia in adults over the last 20 years. J Infect 2005;50:107–113.

10. Barlow GD, Lamping DL, Davey PG, et al. Evaluation of outcomes in community-acquired pneumonia: A guide for patients, physicians, and policymakers. Lancet Infect Dis 2003;3:476–488.

11. Lim WS, Macfarlane JT, Boswell TC, et al. Study of community acquired pneumonia aetiology (SCAPA) in adults admitted to hospital: Implications for management guidelines. Thorax 2001;56:296–301.

12. Lim WS, van der Eerden MM, Laing R, et al. Defining community acquired pneumonia severity on presentation to hospital: An international derivation and validation study. Thorax 2003;58:377–382.

13. Ewig S, de Roux A, Bauer T, et al. Validation of predictive rules and indices of severity for community acquired pneumonia. Thorax 2004;59:421–427.

14. Ayjesky D, Auble TE, Yealy DM, et al. Prospective comparison of three validated prediction rules for prognosis in community-acquired pneumonia. Am J Med 2005;118:384–392.

15. Kikawada M, Iwamoto T, Takasaki M. Aspiration and infection in the elderly: Epidemiology, diagnosis and management. Drugs Aging 2005;22:115–130.

16. Allewelt M, Schuler P, Bolcskei PL, et al. Ampicillin + sulbactam vs clindamycin +/– cephalosporin for the treatment of aspiration pneumonia and primary lung abscess. Clin Microbiol Infect 2004;10:163–170.

17. Chastre J, Fagon J-Y. Ventilator-associated pneumonia. Am J Respir Critical Care Med 2002;165:867–903.

18. Wunderink RG. Nosocomial pneumonia, including ventilator-associated pneumonia. Proc Am Thorac Soc 2005;2:440–444.

19. Edwards JR, Peterson KD, Andrus ML, et al. National Healthcare Safety Network (NHSN) Report, data summary for 2006, issued June 2007. Am J Infect Cont 2007;35:290–301.

20. El-Solh AA, Sikka P, Ramadan F, Davies J. Etiology of severe pneumonia in the very elderly. Am J Respir Critical Care Med 2001;163:645–651.

21. El-Solh AA, Aquilina AT, Dhillon RS, et al. Impact of invasive strategy on management of antimicrobial treatment failure in institutionalized older people with severe pneumonia. Am J Respir Crit Care Med 2002;166: 1038–1043.

22. Fridkin SK. Increasing prevalence of antimicrobial resistance in intensive care units. Crit Care Med 2001;29:N64–N68.

23. Kollef MH. Prevention of hospital-associated pneumonia and ventilator-associated pneumonia. Crit Care Med 2004;32:1396–1405.

24. Bonten MJM, Kollef MH, Hall JB. Risk factors for ventilator-associated pneumonia: From epidemiology to patient management. Clin Infect Dis 2004;38:1141–1149.

25. Society BT. BTS guidelines for the management of community acquired pneumonia in adults. Thorax 2001; 56(Suppl 4):IV1–IV64.

26. Gordon KA, Biedenbach DJ, Jones RN. Comparison of *Streptococcus pneumoniae* and *Haemophilus influenzae* susceptibilities from community-acquired respiratory tract infections and hospitalized patients with pneumonia: Five-year results for the SENTRY Antimicrobial Surveillance Program. Diagn Microbiol Infect Dis 2003;46:285–289.

27. Ortho-McNeil Pharmaceutical. TRUST Surveillance Database. Raritan, NJ: Ortho-McNeil Pharmaceutical, 1999–2007.

28. Mandell LA, Wunderink RG, Anzueto A, et al. Infectious Diseases Society of America/American Thoracic Society consensus guidelines on the management of community-acquired pneumonia in adults. Clin Infect Dis 2007;44:S27–S72.

29. Dreitlein WB, Maratos J, Brocavich J. Zanamivir and oseltamivir: Two new options for the treatment and prevention of influenza. Clin Ther 2001;23:327–355.

30. Esposito S, Principi N. Emerging resistance to antibiotics against respiratory bacteria: Impact on therapy of community-acquired pneumonia in children. Drug Resist Updat 2002;5:73–87.

31. Niederman MS, Craven DE. Guidelines for the management of adults with hospital–acquired, ventilator-associated, and healthcare-associated pneumonia. Am J Respir Crit Care Med 2005;171:388–416.

32. Contopoulos-Ioannidis DG, Giotis ND, Baliatsa DV, Ioannidis JPA. Extended-interval aminoglycoside administration for children: A meta-analysis. Pediatrics 2004;114:e111–e118.

33. Ferriols-Lisart R, Alos-Alminana M. Effectiveness and safety of once-daily aminoglycosides: A meta-analysis. Am J Health-Syst Pharm 1996;53:1141–1150.

34. Hatala R, Dinh T, Cook DJ. Once-daily aminoglycoside dosing in immunocompetent adults: A meta-analysis. Ann Intern Med 1996;124:717–725.

35. Munckhof WJ, Grayson ML, Turnidge JD. A meta-analysis of studies on the safety and efficacy of aminoglycosides given either once daily or as divided doses. J Antimicrob Chemother 1996;37:645–663.

36. Nestaas E, Bangstad H-J, Sandvik L, Wathne K-O. Aminoglycoside extended interval dosing in neonates is safe and effective: A meta-analysis. Arch Dis Child 2005;90:F294–F300.

37. Luna CM, Blanzaco D, Niederman MS, et al. Resolution of ventilator-associated pneumonia: Prospective evaluation of the clinical pulmonary infection score as an early clinical predictor of outcome. Crit Care Med 2003;31:676–682.

38. Singh N, Rogers P, Atwood CW, et al. Short-course empiric antibiotic therapy for patients with pulmonary infiltrates in the intensive care unit. A proposed solution for indiscriminate antibiotic prescription. Am J Respir Crit Care Med 2000;162:505–511.

39. Ziss DR, Stowers A, Feild C. Community-acquired pneumonia: Compliance with centers for Medicare and Medicaid services, national guidelines, and factors associated with outcome. S Med J 2003;96: 949–959.

40. Centers for Disease Control and Prevention. *www.cdc.gov/flu*.

41. Robinson KA, Baughman W, Rothrock G, et al. Epidemiology of invasive *Streptococcus pneumoniae* infections in the United States, 1995–1998: Opportunities for prevention in the conjugate vaccine era. JAMA 2001;285:1729–1735.

42. Musher DM, Luchi M, Watson DA, et al. Pneumococcal polysaccharide vaccine in young adults and older bronchitics: Determination of IgG responses by ELISA and the effect of adsorption of serum with non-type-specific cell wall polysaccharide. J Infect Dis 1990;161:728–735.

72 | Upper Respiratory Tract Infections

Heather VandenBussche

LEARNING OBJECTIVES

● **Upon completion of the chapter, the reader will be able to:**

1. List the most common bacterial pathogens that cause acute otitis media (AOM), acute bacterial rhinosinusitis (ABRS), and acute pharyngitis.

2. Explain the pathophysiologic causes of and risk factors for AOM, bacterial rhinosinusitis, and acute pharyngitis.

3. Identify clinical signs and symptoms associated with AOM, bacterial rhinosinusitis, streptococcal pharyngitis, and the common cold.

4. List treatment goals for AOM, bacterial rhinosinusitis, streptococcal pharyngitis, and the common cold.

5. Develop an appropriate antibiotic regimen for each infection based on patient-specific data.

6. Recommend appropriate adjunctive therapy for a patient with AOM or ABRS.

7. Recommend an appropriate treatment plan for a patient with the common cold.

8. Create a monitoring plan for a patient being treated for each infection using patient-specific information and prescribed therapy.

9. Educate patients about upper respiratory tract infections (URIs) and proper use of antibiotic therapy.

KEY CONCEPTS

❶ Most upper respiratory tract infections (URIs) have nonspecific symptoms, are viral in origin, and resolve spontaneously without significant morbidity.

❷ Antibiotic resistance patterns have greatly affected treatment options for bacterial URIs.

❸ Proper diagnosis of bacterial URIs is crucial to identify patients who require antibiotics to avoid unnecessary antibiotic use.

❹ Antibiotic therapy for acute otitis media (AOM) should be reserved for children who are most likely to benefit from therapy and is dependent upon patient age, illness severity, and diagnostic certainty.

❺ High dose amoxicillin (80–90 mg/kg/day) is the drug of choice for AOM. High dose amoxicillin-clavulanate is an alternative choice for severe illness or when a broader spectrum agent is desired.

❻ Antibiotic therapy for sinusitis should be reserved for patients with moderate persistent symptoms, clinical decompensation, or severe symptoms.

❼ Amoxicillin and amoxicillin-clavulanate are first-line antibiotics for acute bacterial rhinosinusitis (ABRS).

❽ The goals of therapy for streptococcal pharyngitis are to eradicate infection, reduce symptoms and infectivity, and prevent complications.

❾ Penicillin is the drug of choice for streptococcal pharyngitis, but cephalosporins may be appropriate alternative first-line agents owing to increasing failure rates after penicillin therapy.

❿ Treatment for the common cold is focused on symptom relief and is influenced by patient age, comorbid conditions, and balance of medication effectiveness and safety.

Upper respiratory tract infection (URI) is a term that refers to various upper airway infections, including otitis media, sinusitis, pharyngitis, laryngitis, and the common cold. Over 1 billion URIs occur annually in the United States, resulting in millions of physician office visits each year.[1] ❶ *Most URIs have nonspecific symptoms, are viral in origin, and resolve spontaneously without significant morbidity.*[2] Antibiotic use does not enhance resolution of most URIs, and excessive antibiotic use for these infections has contributed to the development of considerable bacterial resistance. Guidelines have been established to reduce inappropriate antibiotic use for viral URIs.[2] This chapter focuses on acute otitis media (AOM), sinusitis, and pharyngitis because bacteria frequently cause these infections and appropriate antibiotic therapy can minimize complications. Proper management of the common cold is also reviewed.

OTITIS MEDIA

Otitis media, or inflammation of the middle ear, is the most common reason for prescribing antibiotics in children. It usually results from a nasopharyngeal viral infection and can be subclassified as AOM or otitis media with effusion (OME). AOM is a rapidly developing symptomatic middle ear infection with effusion, or presence of fluid. OME is the presence of middle ear fluid without symptoms of acute illness. It is important to distinguish between AOM and OME because antibiotics are only useful for the treatment of AOM and effusions can be present for up to 6 months after an acute episode.

EPIDEMIOLOGY AND ETIOLOGY

Otitis media is most common in children between 6 months and 2 years of age but can occur in all age groups, including adults. By age 3 years, up to 85% of children have had at least one episode of otitis media, and up to 20% have recurrent infections by age 12 months.[3] At least 13 million antibiotic prescriptions are written annually in the United States for otitis media, resulting in $2 billion in direct costs.[4] Many risk factors (Table 72–1) predispose children to otitis media and can be associated with microbial resistance, such as daycare attendance, prior antibiotic exposure, and age younger than 2 years.[3,5,6]

Patient Encounter 1, Part 1

A 15-month-old girl presents to the pediatric clinic with 2 days of fever (38.9°C [102°F]), runny nose, and fussiness. Her mother states that she is more irritable than usual and cries many times throughout the night. She is not as interested in eating today. She attends daycare and has a 5-year-old brother who recently had a cold. Physical examination reveals erythema and bulging of the right tympanic membrane and the presence of middle ear fluid. The left tympanic membrane is obscured with cerumen.

What information is suggestive of acute otitis media (AOM)?

Does the child have risk factors for AOM?

Is there any additional information you need to know before recommending a treatment plan?

Table 72–1

Risk Factors for Otitis Media

Viral respiratory tract infection/ winter season	Native American or Inuit ethnicity
Daycare attendance[a]	Low socioeconomic status
Siblings	Pacifier use
Male sex	Lack of breast-feeding
Tobacco smoke exposure	Young age at first diagnosis[a]
Allergies	Immunodeficiency
Anatomic defects such as cleft palate	Gastroesophageal reflux
Positive family history/genetic predisposition	

[a]Risk factors for infection with a resistant pathogen (daycare attendee, age under 2 years, recent antibiotic use in previous 3 months).

From Refs. 3, 5, 6.

Bacteria are isolated from middle ear fluid in up to 70% of children with AOM, but viruses also play a predominant role.[5] *Streptococcus pneumoniae* traditionally has been the most common organism, responsible for up to half of bacterial cases.[4,7] *Haemophilus influenzae* and *Moraxella catarrhalis* cause 15% to 30% and 3% to 20% of cases, respectively. The microbiology of AOM has shifted toward a prevalence of *H. influenzae* because of routine childhood immunization with pneumococcal conjugate vaccine.[8,9] Bacteria that are less frequently associated with AOM include *Streptococcus pyogenes*, *Staphylococcus aureus*, and *Pseudomonas aeruginosa*. Viruses such as respiratory syncytial virus, influenza, parainfluenza, enteroviruses, rhinovirus, and adenoviruses are isolated from middle ear fluid with or without concomitant bacteria in about half of AOM cases.[5,10] Lack of improvement with antibiotic therapy is often a result of viral infection and subsequent inflammation rather than antibiotic resistance.

❷ *Bacterial resistance has significantly affected treatment options for AOM.* Penicillin-resistant *S. pneumoniae* (PRSP) encompasses both intermediate resistance (minimum inhibitory concentrations between 0.1 and 1.0 mcg/mL) and high-level resistance (minimum inhibitory concentration of 2.0 mcg/mL and higher). Altered penicillin-binding proteins cause resistance in approximately 35% of respiratory pneumococcal isolates, about half of which are highly penicillin-resistant.[11] Amoxicillin resistance occurs in less than 5% of pneumococcal isolates.[11] PRSP are also commonly resistant to other drug classes, including sulfonamides, macrolides, and clindamycin, and increasingly resistant to fluoroquinolones. Treatment for pneumococcal AOM is recommended because infection caused by *S. pneumoniae* is unlikely to resolve spontaneously and is the most common cause of recurrent infections.[5] β-Lactamase production occurs in 30% and nearly 100% of *H. influenzae* and *M. catarrhalis*, respectively.[12] Although infections caused by these organisms are more likely to resolve without treatment, they should be considered in cases of treatment failure.

PATHOPHYSIOLOGY

Multiple factors play a role in the development of AOM. Viral infection of the nasopharynx impairs eustachian tube function and causes mucosal inflammation, impairing mucociliary clearance and promoting bacterial proliferation and infection. Children are predisposed to AOM because their eustachian tubes are shorter, more flaccid, and more horizontal than adults, which make them less functional for drainage and protection of the middle ear from bacterial entry.[5] Clinical signs and symptoms of AOM are the result of host immune response and cellular damage caused by inflammatory mediators such as tumor necrosis factor and interleukins that are released from bacteria.[3]

Viscous middle ear effusions caused by allergy or irritant exposure may contribute to impaired mucociliary clearance and AOM in susceptible individuals.[3] OME occurs chronically in atopic children, and effusion can persist for months after an episode of AOM. Children with chronic OME usually require tympanostomy tube placement to reduce complications such as hearing and speech impairment and recurrent otitis media.

TREATMENT

Desired Outcomes

Therapy for AOM focuses on symptom relief and prevention of complications. The goals of treatment are to alleviate ear pain and fever, if present; eradicate infection; prevent complications; and minimize unnecessary antibiotic use.

General Approach to Treatment

1 *The majority of uncomplicated AOM cases resolve spontaneously without significant morbidity.* Untreated AOM improves in 80% of children between days 2 and 7 of illness without increasing the risk of complications.[13] Antibiotics improve ear pain in only 7% of children between days 2 and 7 of therapy and significantly improve recovery in children younger than 2 years of age and in those with severe AOM symptoms.[13] **3 4** *Therefore, antibiotics should be reserved for children most likely to benefit from therapy and is dependent upon patient age, illness severity, and diagnostic certainty.* Children younger than 2 years of age have a higher incidence of penicillin-resistant pneumococcal infections and have higher clinical and bacteriologic failure rates and complications when not treated initially with antibiotics as compared with older children.[4] Patients with severe illness, defined by degree of fever and pain severity, have lower spontaneous recovery rates than those with less severe disease.[13] Current guidelines recommend stratifying patients based on these criteria in order to identify those most likely to benefit from antibiotic therapy.[4]

Nonpharmacologic Therapy

Watchful waiting and safety-net antibiotic prescriptions (to be filled only if symptoms do not resolve after 48 hours'

Clinical Presentation and Diagnosis of AOM

It is important to differentiate AOM from OME because they are treated differently. Patients with AOM usually have cold symptoms, including rhinorrhea, cough, or nasal congestion before or at diagnosis.

Symptoms

- Young children: ear tugging, irritable, poor sleeping and eating habits
- Older patients: ear pain (mild, moderate, or severe), ear fullness, hearing impairment

Signs[4,7]

- Fever: present in less than 25% of patients; often in younger children
- Middle ear effusion
- Otorrhea (middle ear perforation with fluid drainage): uncommon
- Bulging tympanic membrane
- Limited or absent mobility of tympanic membrane
- Distinct erythema of tympanic membrane
- Opaque or cloudy tympanic membrane obscuring or reducing visibility of middle ear

Laboratory Tests

Gram stain, culture, and sensitivities of ear fluid if draining spontaneously or obtained via tympanocentesis (not performed routinely in practice)

Complications

- Infectious: mastoiditis, meningitis, osteomyelitis, intracranial abscess
- Structural: perforated eardrum, cholesteatoma
- Hearing and/or speech impairment

Diagnosis[4]

Certain AOM: Requires *all* the following:

- Rapid onset of signs and symptoms
- Middle ear effusion findings with pneumatic otoscopy
- Inflammation indicated by either otoscopic evidence (distinct erythema) or otalgia

Uncertain AOM: Not all three criteria are present

- Severe AOM: Moderate to severe ear pain or fever of 39°C (102.2°F) or greater
- Nonsevere AOM: Mild ear pain and fever of less than 39°C (102.2°F) in past 24 hours

observation) are approaches being used more frequently to attenuate microbial resistance and avoid unnecessary adverse events and costs of antibiotics. Delayed antibiotic therapy in older children and those with less severe disease does not result in more infectious complications, such as mastoiditis or meningitis, when compared with routine initial antibiotic treatment.[13,14] Use of an observation approach or use of a safety-net antibiotic prescription that can be filled 48 to 72 hours later if symptoms persist can reduce antibiotic use for AOM by 67% without increasing complications.[14] Observation or delayed antibiotic therapy should be considered only in otherwise healthy children without recurrent disease (Fig. 72–1) and only if proper follow-up and good communication exist between clinicians and the parent/caregiver.[3,4,14]

Other nondrug approaches include the use of external heat or cold to reduce postauricular pain and surgery. Tympanostomy tubes are most useful for patients with recurrent disease or chronic OME with impaired hearing or speech. Adenoidectomy may be necessary for children with chronic nasal obstruction, but tonsillectomy is rarely indicated.[3]

Pharmacologic Therapy

▶ Antimicrobial Therapy

When antimicrobial therapy is needed, many factors influence initial drug selection. Clinicians must consider drug

factors such as antimicrobial spectrum, likelihood of clinical response, middle ear fluid penetration, incidence of side effects, drug interactions, and cost, as well as patient factors, including risk factors for bacterial resistance, allergies, ease of dosing regimen, medication palatability, and presence of other medical conditions. Studies in uncomplicated AOM have not revealed significant differences between antibiotics in clinical response rates but most were confounded by spontaneous resolution in children likely to have had viral illnesses. Bacteriologic response varies among antibiotics and does not always correlate well with clinical response but is considered important when selecting an agent.[4,5]

Guidelines from the American Academy of Pediatrics and the American Academy of Family Physicians are available for children between 2 months and 12 years of age with uncomplicated AOM (Fig. 72–2) and are based on published trials and expert opinion.[4] ⑤ *Amoxicillin remains the drug of choice in most patients because of its proven effectiveness in AOM, high middle ear concentrations, excellent safety profile, low cost, good-tasting suspension, and relatively narrow spectrum of activity* (Table 72–2). High-dose amoxicillin (80–90 mg/kg/day) is preferred over conventional doses because higher middle ear fluid concentrations can overcome pneumococcal penicillin resistance without substantially increasing adverse effects.[15] ⑤ *In cases of severe illness or when coverage for β-lactamase-producing organisms is desired, high-dose amoxicillin-clavulanate is the preferred agent.* Pneumococcal resistance to trimethoprim-sulfamethoxazole

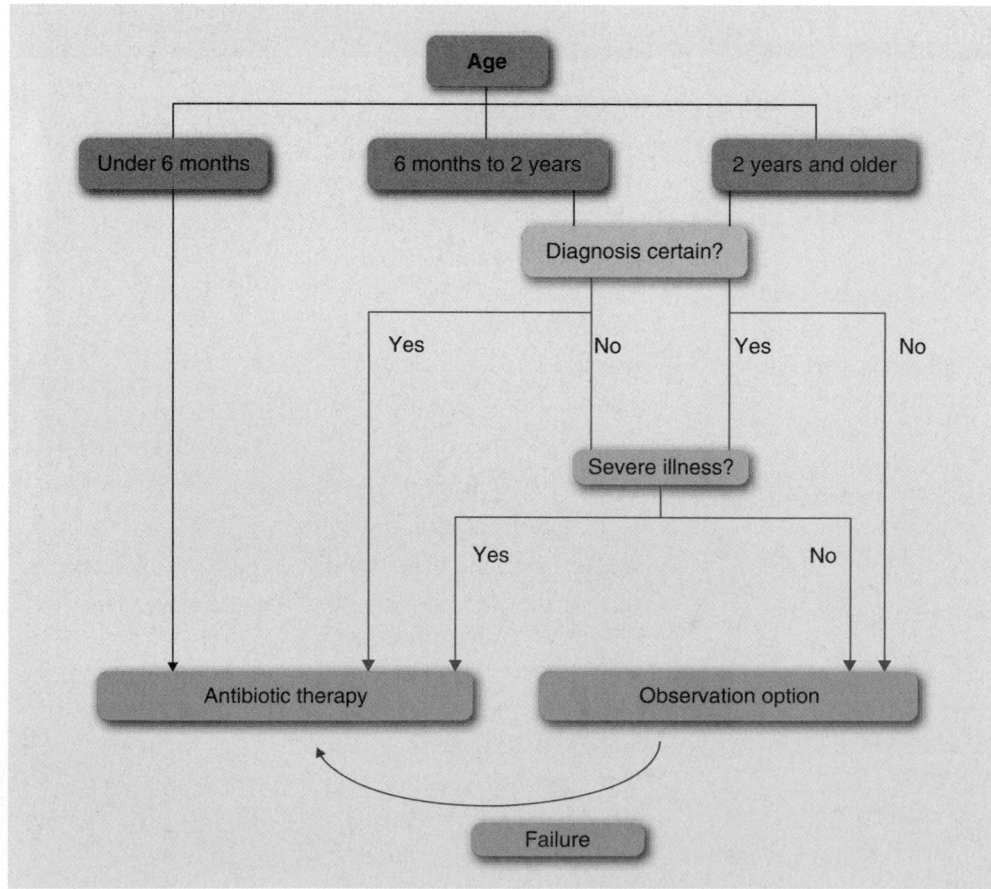

FIGURE 72–1. Treatment algorithm for initial antimicrobials or observation in children with suspected or certain uncomplicated AOM. (From Ref. 4.)

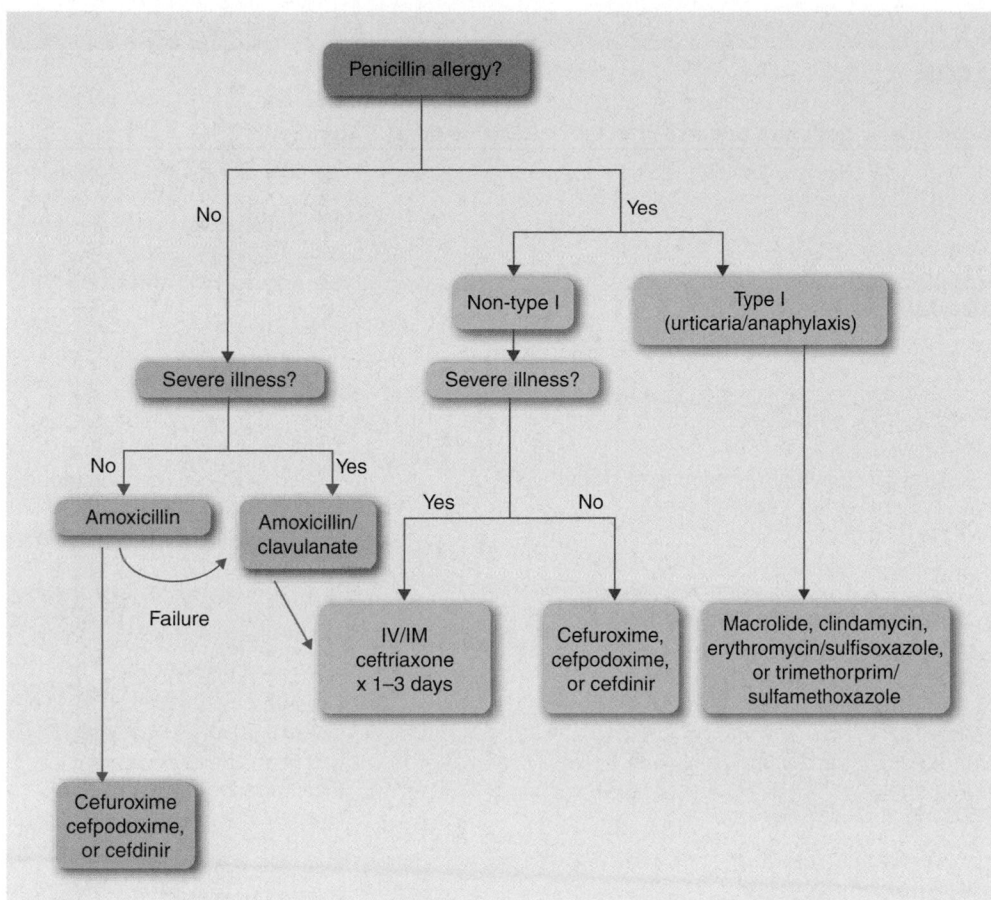

FIGURE 72–2. Treatment algorithm for uncomplicated AOM in children 2 months to 12 years of age. (From Refs. 4, 6.)

and macrolides is problematic and strikingly common in PRSP, making these agents less desirable for most patients.[6,11] Patients with penicillin allergies require alternative first-line therapy (see Fig. 72–2). Children who have received an antimicrobial in the previous month are more likely to harbor resistant organisms and should also receive alternative therapy.[6] A single dose of intramuscular ceftriaxone is effective for children who cannot tolerate oral medications, but a 3-day course may be preferred because of increasing pneumococcal resistance and failure of single doses.[16] Ototopic antibiotics are an alternative to systemic agents for AOM in patients with otorrhea or tympanostomy tubes.[17]

If there is a lack of improvement or worsening with initial therapy during the first 48 to 72 hours, antibiotic selection must be reassessed and other contributing diseases must be excluded.[4,6] Tympanocentesis can help to guide therapy in difficult cases.

Duration of therapy, like drug selection, depends on patient age and disease severity. Standard 10-day oral therapy is more effective than shorter courses for uncomplicated AOM in children younger than 2 years of age and those with recurrent infections, as well as in older patients with severe illness.[4,18] Exceptions to the 10-day regimen are for azithromycin and ceftriaxone. In older children with mild or moderate illness, antibiotic therapy is needed only for 5 to 7 days.

▶ Adjunctive Therapy

Pain is a central feature of AOM but is often overlooked in its management. Acetaminophen and ibuprofen are commonly used nonprescription agents for mild to moderate pain. Ibuprofen has a longer duration of effect than acetaminophen but is not used routinely in children younger than 6 months of age because of increased toxicity concerns. Alternating ibuprofen with acetaminophen is not recommended because of a lack of safety and efficacy data on combination therapy and the potential for dosing confusion and error. Topical anesthetic drops such as benzocaine (in Auralgan) provide pain relief within 30 minutes of administration and may be preferred over systemic analgesics when fever is absent. Myringotomy provides immediate relief but is performed rarely. Other medications such as decongestants, antihistamines, and corticosteroids have no role in the treatment of AOM and can, in some cases, prolong effusion duration.[4,19] Data are lacking on the safety and efficacy of complementary and alternative treatments.

▶ Prevention

Immunizations may prevent AOM in certain patients, such as those with recurrent infections. Influenza vaccine is more effective in preventing AOM in children older than 2 years of age than in younger patients possibly from

Table 72–2				
Antibiotics[a] for the Treatment of AOM				
Drug	**Usual Dose and Schedule**	**Common Adverse Effects**	**Relative Cost[b]**	**Comments**
Amoxicillin	80–90 mg/kg/day in 2 doses (adult: 875 mg twice daily)	Nausea, vomiting, diarrhea, rash	$	Drug of choice for AOM; experts recommended high-dose over conventional doses (40–45 mg/kg/day)
Amoxicillin-clavulanate	80–90 mg/kg/day in 2 doses (adult: 875 mg twice daily)	Nausea, vomiting, diarrhea, rash, diaper rash	$$$–$$$$	More diarrhea than amoxicillin, amoxicillin:clavulanate ratio of 14:1 preferred because of lower daily clavulanate component
Cefuroxime axetil	30 mg/kg/day in 2 doses (max 1 g/day with suspension; adult: 250 mg twice daily)	Nausea, vomiting, diarrhea, rash, diaper rash	$$$	Suspension gritty and bitter tasting, not interchangeable with tablets (less bioavailable)
Cefdinir	14 mg/kg/day in 1–2 doses (adult: 300 mg twice daily or 600 mg once daily)	Diarrhea, rash, vomiting, diaper rash, yeast infections	$$$	Preferred oral cephalosporin (good taste); separate from Al or Mg antacids and Fe supplements by 2 hours
Cefpodoxime proxetil	10 mg/kg/day in 2 doses (adult: 200 mg twice daily)	Diarrhea, diaper rash, vomiting, rash, yeast infections	$$$	Suspension is bitter tasting
Ceftriaxone	50 mg/kg IM or IV for 1–3 days (max 1 g/dose)	Injection site pain, swelling, or erythema, diarrhea, rash	$$$–$$$$	3-day regimen preferred for PRSP; avoid in children under 2 months
Azithromycin	10 mg/kg × 1 day, 5 mg/kg/day × 4 days; 10 mg/kg/day × 3 days; or 30 mg/kg single dose (adult dose 500 mg × 1 day, 250 mg × 4 days)	Nausea, vomiting, diarrhea, abdominal pain	$$	Separate from Al or Mg antacids by 2 hours; diarrhea/vomiting more common with single-dose regimen; 3- or 5-day courses preferred; increasing pneumococcal resistance; many failures with *H. influenzae* infection
Clarithromycin	15 mg/kg/day in 2 doses (adult: 250 mg twice daily)	Diarrhea, vomiting, rash, abnormal taste, abdominal pain	$$	Many drug interactions (inhibits cytochrome P-450 3A4); suspension cannot be refrigerated and has metallic taste; same microbiologic issues as azithromycin
Erythromycin-sulfisoxazole	50 mg/kg/day of erythromycin component in 3–4 doses	Nausea, vomiting, abdominal pain, diarrhea, rash	$$	Many drug interactions (like clarithromycin), contraindicated in children under 2 months; increasing pneumococcal resistance
Trimethoprim-sulfamethoxazole	8–10 mg/kg/day of trimethoprim component in 2 doses	Nausea, vomiting, anorexia, rash, urticaria	$	Increasing pneumococcal resistance; contraindicated in children under 2 months
Clindamycin	20–30 mg/kg/day in 3–4 doses (adult: 300 mg 4 times daily or 450 mg 3 times daily)	Nausea, diarrhea, *C. difficile* colitis, anorexia	$	Oral liquid has very poor taste; only for pneumococcal infection

[a]Other FDA-approved antibiotics for AOM not included in AAP/AAFP guidelines: cefaclor, cephalexin, cefprozil, cefixime, loracarbef, and ceftibuten.

[b]Approximate cost per course: $ (under $25), $$ ($25–$50), $$$ ($50–$100), $$$$ (over $100).

From Refs. 4, 7.

impaired immune responses and immature host defense in infants and toddlers.[20] Pneumococcal conjugate vaccine is protective against infection by vaccine serotypes only with a limited overall benefit for AOM.[21] Antibiotic prophylaxis is no longer recommended for otitis-prone children because of increasing resistance. Avoidance or minimization of risk factors associated with otitis media, such as tobacco smoke and bottle feeding, is advised, but the effects of these interventions remain unproven.

OUTCOME EVALUATION

Improvement of signs and symptoms (i.e., pain, fever, and tympanic membrane inflammation) should be evident by 72 hours of therapy. Children can appear clinically worse during the first 24 hours of treatment but often stabilize during the second day with defervescence and improved eating and sleeping patterns. If symptoms persist or worsen, reevaluation must occur to determine the proper diagnosis

Patient Encounter 1, Part 2

On further questioning, you discover that the child is allergic to penicillin. She developed a nonurticarial rash last year during treatment for pharyngitis. She has not received antibiotics since that time, and this is her first ear infection.

Immunizations: Up to date

Meds: Acetaminophen drops 120 mg orally every 4 to 6 hours as needed for fever or pain

ROS: (+) nasal congestion and rhinorrhea, (–) vomiting, diarrhea, or cough

PE:
- **Gen:** Irritable child but consolable
- **VS:** BP 100/60 mm Hg, P 120 bpm, RR 18 breaths per minute, T 38.6°C (101.5°F)
- **HEENT:** As noted before

Identify your treatment goals for this child.

Given this information, what nonpharmacologic and pharmacologic therapy do you recommend?

Patient Care and Monitoring of AOM

1. Assess the patient's signs and symptoms. Are they consistent with AOM?

2. Review diagnostic information to determine if acute infection is present. Are all three diagnostic criteria present? Was the proper method used for diagnosis (pneumatic otoscopy)?

3. Does the patient require antibiotic therapy, or is observation an appropriate option?

4. Obtain a complete medication history, including prescription drugs, nonprescription drugs, and natural product use, as well as allergies and adverse effects.

5. Determine what medication should be used for pain, if present.

6. If applicable, determine which antibiotic to use and the duration of therapy.

7. Develop a plan to assess effectiveness of the chosen therapy and course of action to take if the patient does not improve or worsens.

8. Provide patient education on:
   - What to expect from prescribed medication, including potential adverse effects
   - Avoidance of antihistamines and decongestants
   - Signs of treatment failure

9. Stress the importance of adherence to therapy, including antibiotic resistance concerns.

10. Determine the need for influenza and pneumococcal vaccinations.

11. Educate the family regarding risk factors for otitis media.

and treatment. Counsel patients and caregivers regarding common antibiotic adverse events such as rash, diarrhea, and vomiting that may prompt additional medical attention.

Presence of middle ear effusion in the absence of symptoms is not an indicator of treatment failure. Persistent effusion greater than 3 months in duration requires a hearing evaluation in children who are otherwise healthy.[22] Preschool-aged and younger children or those at risk for developmental difficulties may need reexamination earlier because speech and hearing impairment is more difficult to assess in these populations.

SINUSITIS

Sinusitis, or inflammation of the paranasal sinuses, is often described as **rhinosinusitis** that also involves inflammation of contiguous nasal mucosa, which occurs in nearly all cases of viral respiratory infections. Acute rhinosinusitis is characterized by symptoms that resolve completely in less than 4 weeks, whereas chronic rhinosinusitis typically persists as cough, rhinorrhea, or nasal obstruction for more than 90 days. Acute bacterial rhinosinusitis (ABRS) refers to an acute bacterial infection of the sinuses that can occur independently or be superimposed on chronic sinusitis. The focus of this section will be on ABRS and appropriate treatment.

EPIDEMIOLOGY AND ETIOLOGY

Rhinosinusitis is one of the most common medical conditions in the United States, affecting about 1 billion people annually.[1] It is caused mainly by respiratory viruses but also can be caused by allergies or environmental irritants. Viral rhinosinusitis is complicated by secondary bacterial infection in 0.5% to 2% of adults and 5% to 13% of children.[23,24] Upper respiratory infections of less than 7 days' duration are usually viral, whereas more prolonged disease or severe symptoms are often caused by bacteria. Risk factors for ABRS include prior viral respiratory infection, allergic rhinitis, anatomic defects, and certain medical conditions[23,25] (Table 72–3).

Bacterial pathogens that cause sinusitis are similar to those that cause AOM. *S. pneumoniae* and *H. influenzae* are responsible for over half of the cases in all patients, with an additional 20% of cases caused by *M. catarrhalis* in children.[23,25] Similar to AOM, an increased prevalence of *H. influenzae* has been reported in ABRS, and risk factors can predict the presence of drug-resistant pathogens.[1,26] Other pathogens that cause sinusitis include *S. pyogenes* (up to 5%), anaerobic bacteria such as *Bacteroides* and

Patient Encounter 2

A 36-year-old female presents to her primary care physician with purulent nasal/postnasal discharge, nasal congestion, headache, and fatigue. She reports that her symptoms began 7 days ago and have worsened over the past 2 days. She states that she has severe facial pressure when she bends forward and she has noticed that her upper molars ache when eating or brushing. She has taken ibuprofen and pseudoephedrine with little to no relief. She has a history of frequent sinus infections (1–2 per year). Her last course of antibiotics was 4 months ago for sinusitis when she received amoxicillin.

Immunizations: Up to date

Meds: Loratadine 10 mg orally daily, intranasal mometasone one spray each nostril daily, ibuprofen 400 mg orally as needed, pseudoephedrine 60 mg orally as needed

Allergies: Dust mites, cat dander, no medications

PE:

Gen: Tired-appearing, moderate distress, appears uncomfortable

VS: BP 102/60 mm Hg, P 88 bpm, RR 14 breaths per minute, T 38.2°C (100.8°F), wt 62 kg (136 lb)

HEENT: Thick, purulent green-brown postnasal discharge; nasal mucosal irritation and edema; facial pain (right maxillary) and upper molar hypersensitivity upon tapping; no oral lesions; erythematous pharynx with mild tonsillar hypertrophy

What information is suggestive of ABRS?

What risk factors are present?

What other diagnostic studies, if any, should be performed?

What are the treatment goals for this patient?

Create a care plan for this patient that includes nonpharmacologic and pharmacologic therapies and a monitoring plan.

Clinical Presentation and Diagnosis of ABRS

Sinusitis symptoms typically last 7 to 10 days after a viral infection and are caused by activation of the immune system and parasympathetic nervous system.

Acute Signs and Symptoms[23,24,28,29]

- *Adults:* Nasal congestion or obstruction, purulent nasal/postnasal discharge, facial pain or pressure or fullness (especially unilateral in a sinus area), diminished sense of smell, fever, cough, maxillary dental pain, fatigue, ear fullness or pain.

- *Children:* Purulent nasal/postnasal drainage, congestion and mouth breathing, persistent cough (particularly at night) or throat clearing, fever, pharyngitis, ear discomfort, halitosis, morning periorbital edema or facial swelling, fatigue, facial or tooth pain.

Complications

Orbital cellulitis or abscess, periorbital cellulitis, meningitis, cavernous sinus thrombosis, ethmoid or frontal sinus erosion, chronic sinusitis, and exacerbation of asthma or bronchitis.

③ Diagnosis[23,24,28]

- *Clinical diagnosis:* Most common method; acute rhinosinusitis signs and symptoms (as above) that have not resolved after 10 days or that worsen within 10 days after initial improvement. Sputum color is unreliable for diagnosis of bacterial infection because neutrophil presence causes color and can be found in viral sinusitis.

- *Radiographic studies:* Useful for assessing presence of abscess or intracranial complication.

- *Paranasal sinus puncture:* "Gold standard"; not performed routinely but can be useful in complicated or chronic cases.

- *Laboratory studies/nasopharyngeal cultures:* Not recommended for routine diagnosis.

Table 72–3

Risk Factors for ABRS

Viral respiratory tract infection/winter season	Anatomic defects (e.g., septal deviation)
Allergic or nonallergic rhinitis	Intranasal medications or illicit drugs
Tobacco smoke exposure	Immunodeficiency
Dental infections or procedures	Swimming/diving
Cystic fibrosis or ciliary dyskinesia	Mechanical ventilation
Nasogastric tubes	Traumatic head injury
Aspirin allergy, nasal polyps, and asthma	Female sex

ABRS, acute bacterial rhinosinusitis.

From Refs. 23, 25.

Peptostreptococcus spp. (up to 9% of adults), and *S. aureus* (up to 10% of adults).[23,27] Chronic infections are commonly polymicrobial with a higher incidence of anaerobes, gram-negative bacilli, and fungi.

PATHOPHYSIOLOGY

Rhinosinusitis is caused by mucosal inflammation and local damage to mucociliary clearance mechanisms from viral infection or allergy. Increased mucus production and reduced clearance of secretions can lead to blockage of the sinus ostia, or the opening of the sinuses to the upper airway. This environment is ideal for bacterial growth and promotes a cycle of local inflammatory response and mucosal injury characterized by increased concentrations of interleukins, histamine, and tumor necrosis factor.[23,25] Factors that contribute to bacterial invasion include nose blowing, reduced local immunity, viral virulence, and nasopharyngeal colonization with bacteria.[23,28] Damage to the host defense system perpetuates bacterial overgrowth and persistence of infection.

TREATMENT

Desired Outcomes

The goals of treatment for ABRS are to eradicate bacteria and prevent serious sequelae. Specific aims are to relieve symptoms, normalize the nasal environment, use antibiotics when appropriate, select effective antibiotics that minimize resistance, and prevent development of chronic disease or complications.

General Approach to Treatment

Initial management of rhinosinusitis focuses on symptom relief for patients with mild disease lasting less than 10 days. Clinicians often inappropriately prescribe antibiotics for clinically suspected rhinosinusitis that usually is viral, self-limiting, and infrequently complicated by bacterial infection. Studies comparing antimicrobials to placebo in ABRS report only modest symptom improvements but increased adverse events in patients treated with antibiotics and a high spontaneous improvement rate of over 70% at 7 to 12 days after diagnosis of nonsevere ABRS.[28,30] Therefore, watchful waiting is an option in nonsevere ABRS for up to 7 days after diagnosis if adequate follow-up can be assured.[28] ❻ *Antibiotic therapy should be reserved for persistent, worsening, or severe ABRS: patients with moderately severe symptoms that have persisted for greater than 10 days or worsened within 10 days after initial improvement and patients with severe disease regardless of duration.*[23,24,28] Empirical selection is often employed and should target likely pathogens because sinus cultures are rarely obtained.

Nonpharmacologic Therapy

Ancillary treatments such as humidifiers, vaporizers, and saline nasal spray or drops are used to moisturize the nasal canal and impair crusting of secretions along with promoting ciliary function. Although many patients report benefit from such therapies, there are no controlled studies that support their use.[24] Nasal irrigation with isotonic or hypertonic saline washes may improve quality of life, reduce medication usage, and improve symptoms especially in patients with recurrent or chronic sinusitis.[28]

Pharmacologic Therapy

▶ Adjunctive Therapy

Supportive medications that target symptoms of viral URIs are used widely in patients with rhinosinusitis, particularly in the early stage of infection. There is a lack of evidence supporting their use in ABRS, but they may provide temporary relief in certain patients.[24,28] Analgesics can be used to treat fever and pain from sinus pressure. Oral decongestants relieve congested nasal passages but should be avoided in children younger than 4 years of age and patients with ischemic heart disease or uncontrolled hypertension. Intranasal decongestants can be used for severe congestion in most patients 6 years of age or older, but use should be limited to 3 days or less to avoid rebound nasal congestion. Guaifenesin is often used as a mucolytic with no evidence to support its use in rhinosinusitis. Antihistamines should be avoided because they thicken mucus and impair its clearance, but they may be useful in patients with predisposing allergic rhinitis or chronic sinusitis. Similarly, intranasal corticosteroids usually are reserved for patients with allergies or chronic sinusitis, but they may be beneficial as monotherapy or with antibiotics in ABRS.[31]

▶ Antimicrobial Therapy

Although many clinical studies have been performed evaluating antibiotics for ABRS, no randomized, double-blind, placebo-controlled studies have used pre- and post-treatment sinus aspirate cultures as an outcome measure. In some studies, antimicrobials result in faster symptom resolution and lower failure rates and complications compared with no treatment, particularly in more severe disease.[24,28] Since diagnosis is based on clinical presentation and not sinus aspirate cultures, clinicians must attempt to differentiate ABRS from viral rhinosinusitis. ❻ *Therefore, it is important to limit antimicrobial use to cases where infection is unlikely to resolve without causing prolonged disease: patients with moderately severe symptoms that persist for greater than 10 days or worsen after initial improvement and patients with severe symptoms.*[23,24,28]

Treatment guidelines reflect antimicrobial choices that are likely to result in favorable clinical and bacteriologic outcomes based on pathogen distribution, spontaneous resolution rates, and nationwide resistance patterns.[23,24,28] ❷ *These guidelines (Figs. 72–3 and 72–4) stratify therapy based on severity of disease and risk of infection with resistant organisms, defined as prior antibiotic use within 4 to 6 weeks. Other risk factors for resistance include daycare attendance or frequent exposure to children in daycare and recurrent disease.* Severe disease requires evaluation and treatment in conjunction with specialized physicians such as otolaryngologists.

Antimicrobial therapy (Table 72–4) is targeted against *S. pneumoniae*, but consideration must be given to other pathogens such as *H. influenzae*, *M. catarrhalis*, *S. aureus*, and PRSP. ❼ *Patients with mild disease and no prior antimicrobial exposure should receive initial therapy with amoxicillin or amoxicillin-clavulanate.* Amoxicillin is effective for most mild infections and can be used in high doses to cover PRSP. It is less expensive and better tolerated than amoxicillin-clavulanate, which provides expanded coverage against β-lactamase-producing bacteria. Patients who are allergic to

Table 72–4

Antimicrobials[a] for the Treatment of ABRS

Drug	Adult Dose	Pediatric Dose[b]	Comments
Amoxicillin	1.5–4 g/day in 2–3 doses	90 mg/kg/day in 2 doses	Lacks coverage against β-lactamase producers
Amoxicillin-clavulanate	1.75–4 g/day in 2–3 doses	90 mg/kg/day in 2 doses	Broad coverage particularly with high doses; Augmentin XR (2 g every 12 hour) targeted toward PRSP
Cefdinir	600 mg/day in 1–2 doses	14 mg/kg/day in 1–2 doses	Preferred oral liquid cephalosporin owing to good palatability
Cefpodoxime proxetil	200 mg twice daily	10 mg/kg/day in 2 doses	
Cefuroxime axetil	250–500 mg twice daily	15–30 mg/kg/day in 2 doses	
Ceftriaxone	1 g IM/IV every 24 hour	50 mg/kg IM/IV every 24 hour	Experts recommend a 5-day treatment course
Trimethoprim-sulfamethoxazole	160/800 mg (1 DS tablet) twice daily	8–10 mg/kg/day of trimethoprim component in 2 doses	Considerable pneumococcal resistance limits use of this agent
Azithromycin	500 mg × 1 day, 250 mg/day × 4 days; 500 mg/day × 3 days; 2 g × 1 dose	10 mg/kg × 1 day, 5 mg/kg/day × 4 days; 10 mg/kg/day × 3 days	Increasing pneumococcal resistance and limited H. influenzae activity; single-dose regimen has high incidence of nausea, vomiting, and diarrhea
Clarithromycin	500 mg twice daily or 1 g once daily (XL only)	15 mg/kg/day in 2 doses	XL tablets reported to have fewer GI problems and taste disturbances than twice-daily preparation
Doxycycline	100 mg twice daily	Avoid in children under 8 years	Can cause photosensitivity, GI problems, tooth staining in young children; many drug–drug interactions (antacids, iron, calcium)
Levofloxacin	500–750 mg once daily (750 mg × 5 days)	Not available	Common fluoroquinolone side effects are nausea, vaginitis, diarrhea, dizziness; many drug–drug interactions (antacids, iron, calcium); tendon rupture, photosensitivity, QT prolongation possible; cost similar to amoxicillin/clavulanate
Moxifloxacin	400 mg once daily	Not available	
Clindamycin	150–450 mg 3–4 times daily	20–40 mg/kg/day in 3–4 doses	No gram-negative coverage; use in combination

[a]Refer to Table 72–2 for more information on antibiotics. Other FDA-approved antibiotics for ABRS not included in the Sinus and Allergy Health Partnership or American Academy of Pediatrics guidelines: cefaclor, cefprozil, cefixime, ciprofloxacin, erythromycin, loracarbef.

[b]Maximum dose not to exceed adult dose.

ABRS, acute bacterial rhinosinusitis.

From Refs. 23, 24.

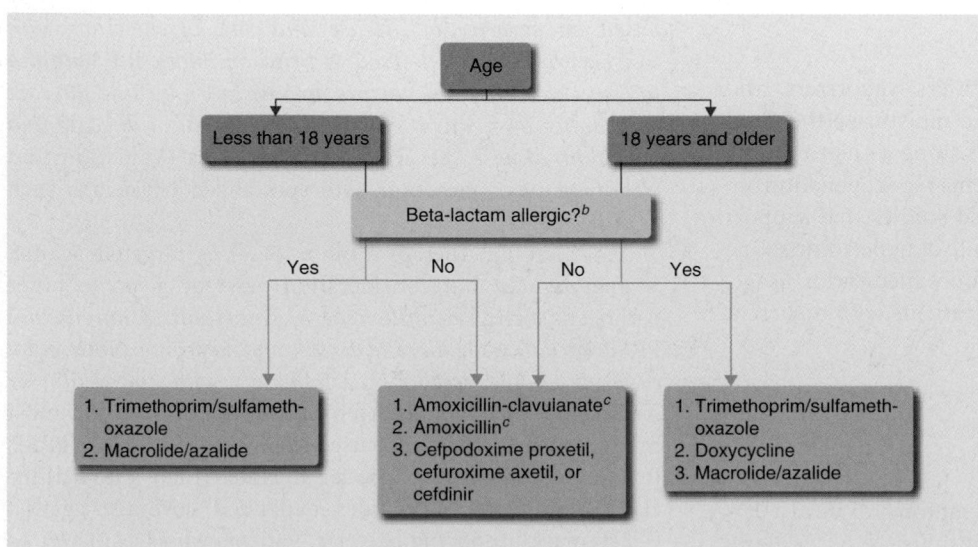

FIGURE 72–3. Treatment algorithm[a] for ABRS in patients with mild disease without recent antibiotic exposure. [a]Antimicrobials are listed in order of predicted efficacy based on predicted clinical and bacteriologic efficacy rates, clinical studies, safety, and tolerability. Doses can be found in Table 72–4. [b]Cephalosporins should be considered for patients with nontype I hypersensitivity to penicillins; they are more likely to be effective than the alternative agents. [c]High doses are recommended for adults with daycare contacts or frequent infections and most children. (From Refs. 23, 24.)

penicillins can be treated with an appropriate cephalosporin; severe penicillin allergies require treatment with alternative agents that may be less effective based solely on microbial resistance trends and not clinical data[11,23,24] (see Fig. 72–3).

Initial therapy for patients with moderate symptoms or those with recent antimicrobial exposure includes high-dose amoxicillin-clavulanate or a respiratory fluoroquinolone[23,24] (see Fig. 72–4).

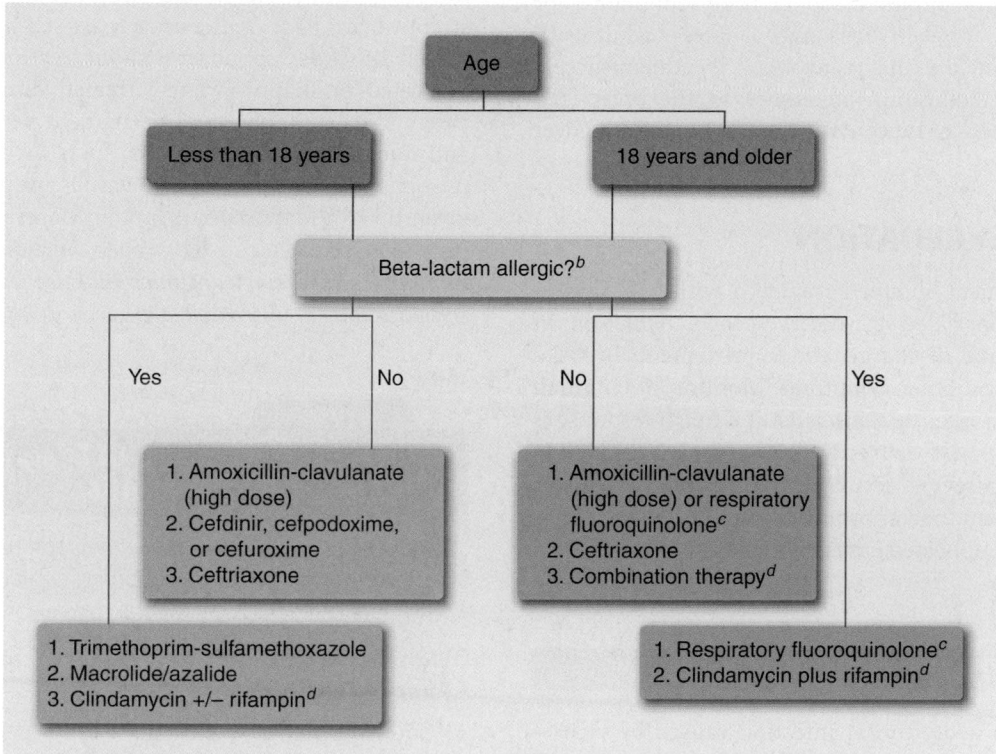

FIGURE 72–4. Treatment algorithm[a] for ABRS in patients with mild disease and recent antibiotic exposure or moderate disease. [a]Antimicrobials are listed in order of predicted efficacy based on predicted clinical and bacteriologic efficacy rates, clinical studies, safety, and tolerability. Doses can be found in Table 72–4. [b]Cephalosporins should be considered for patients with nontype I hypersensitivity to penicillins; they are more likely to be effective than the alternative agents. [c]Respiratory fluoroquinolone = levofloxacin, moxifloxacin. [d]Combination therapy should provide gram-positive and gram-negative coverage. Examples are high-dose amoxicillin or clindamycin plus rifampin or cefixime. There are no published clinical studies to support such combinations. (From Refs. 23, 24.)

Patient Care and Monitoring of ABRS

1. Assess the patient's signs and symptoms. Are they consistent with ABRS?

2. How long have the patient's symptoms been present? If symptoms are mild and present for fewer than 10 days, viral sinusitis is likely. Persistent moderate or acute severe symptoms are more indicative of bacterial infection.

3. Does the patient require antibiotic therapy? Avoid antibiotic use in viral disease.

4. Obtain a complete medication history, including prescription drugs, nonprescription drugs, and natural product use, as well as allergies and adverse effects.

5. Determine what adjunctive therapies should be used for symptoms, such as pain and congestion.

6. If applicable, determine which antibiotic to use and the duration of therapy.

7. Develop a plan to assess effectiveness of the chosen therapy and course of action to take if the patient does not improve or worsens.

8. Provide patient education on
   - What to expect from the antibiotic and other medications, including potential adverse effects
   - Avoidance of antihistamines, if appropriate
   - Signs of treatment failure
   - Role of viral infections in sinusitis and how to prevent disease transmission

9. Stress the importance of adherence to therapy, including antibiotic resistance concerns.

Failure to respond to initial therapy within 7 days requires reevaluation to consider changing therapy to cover resistant pathogens and to examine for complications.[28] Antimicrobials traditionally have been given for at least 10 to 14 days, with up to 21 days needed for resolution in some patients.[23] Five-day treatment courses of some fluoroquinolones or cephalosporins are as effective as longer courses in adults with uncomplicated acute maxillary sinusitis.[32] Treatment success is influenced by medication adherence to the prescribed regimen, where once- or twice-daily agents are preferred over multiple daily doses.

OUTCOME EVALUATION

Clinical improvement should be evident within 7 days of therapy, as demonstrated by defervescence, reduction in nasal congestion and discharge, and improvements in facial pain or pressure and other symptoms. Monitor for common adverse events and refer to a specialist if clinical response is not obtained with first- or second-line therapy. Referral is also important for severe, recurrent, or chronic sinusitis or acute disease in immunocompromised patients. Surgery may be indicated in complicated cases.

PHARYNGITIS

Pharyngitis is an acute throat infection caused by viruses or bacteria. Other conditions, such as gastroesophageal reflux, postnasal drip, or allergies, also can cause sore throat and must be distinguished from infectious causes. Acute pharyngitis is responsible for 1% to 2% of adult physician visits and 6% to 8% of pediatric visits but generally is self-limited without serious sequelae.[33,34] Antimicrobials are prescribed in 50% to 70% of cases in adults and children because of the inability to easily distinguish between viral and bacterial pathogens and fear of untreated streptococcal illness.[34,35]

EPIDEMIOLOGY AND ETIOLOGY

Pharyngitis is usually a component of upper respiratory infections caused by rhinovirus, coronavirus, adenovirus, influenza virus, parainfluenza virus, or Epstein-Barr virus. Group A *Streptococcus,* or *S. pyogenes*, is the most common bacterial cause of acute pharyngitis, responsible for 15% to 30% of cases in children and 5% to 10% of adult infections.[33,36] Infection is most common in late winter and early spring and is spread easily through direct contact with contaminated secretions. Clusters of infection are common within families, classrooms, and other crowded areas. Less common causes of bacterial pharyngitis are *Corynebacterium diphtheriae*, groups C and G streptococci, *Chlamydia pneumoniae*, *Mycoplasma pneumoniae*, and *Neisseria gonorrhoeae*. This section will focus on group A streptococcal disease in which antimicrobial therapy is indicated.

PATHOPHYSIOLOGY

Pharyngeal colonization with group A streptococci occurs in up to 20% of children and is a risk factor for developing streptococcal pharyngitis after a break in mucosal integrity.[37] Clinicians should recognize that the symptoms of streptococcal pharyngitis usually are self-limited and resolve within 2 to 4 days of onset without treatment.[36] Historically, untreated or inappropriately treated disease caused acute rheumatic fever, potential permanent heart valve damage, and infectious complications such as peritonsillar and retropharyngeal abscesses. Delayed antimicrobial therapy given up to 9 days after symptom onset can prevent these particular sequelae, so ❸ *proper diagnosis is important to minimize unnecessary antimicrobial use for viral disease and complications of untreated streptococcal infection.*[36,37]

Clinical Presentation and Diagnosis of Streptococcal Pharyngitis

Children between 5 and 15 years of age have the highest incidence of streptococcal pharyngitis. Parents and adults with significant pediatric contact are also at increased risk.

Signs and Symptoms of Streptococcal Pharyngitis[36,37]

- Sudden onset of sore throat with severe pain on swallowing
- Fever
- Headache, abdominal pain, nausea, or vomiting (especially in children)
- Pharyngeal and tonsillar erythema with possible patchy exudates
- Tender, enlarged anterior cervical lymph nodes
- Swollen and red uvula
- Soft palate petechiae
- Scarlatiniform Rash
- General absence of conjunctivitis, hoarseness, cough, rhinorrhea, discrete ulcerations, and diarrhea (suggestive of viral etiology)

Diagnosis[33,37]

- Rapid antigen detection test (RADT): 80% to 90% sensitivity; results available within minutes.
- Throat swab and culture: "Gold standard"; results available within 24 to 48 hours. Should be performed in all negative RADTs in children, adolescents, and adults with significant pediatric contact. Also recommended in outbreaks and to monitor for antibiotic resistance.
- These tests should be performed *only* if there is a clinical suspicion of streptococcal pharyngitis. Pharyngeal carriage of group A streptococci is 5% to 20% in children.

TREATMENT

Desired Outcomes

8 The goals of therapy for streptococcal pharyngitis are to eradicate infection in order to prevent complications, shorten the disease course, and reduce infectivity and spread to close contacts. Antimicrobial use only prevents peritonsillar or retropharyngeal abscesses, cervical lymphadenitis, and rheumatic fever. Immune-mediated, nonsuppurative complications of streptococcal infection that are not impacted by antimicrobial treatment include acute glomerulonephritis, reactive arthritis, and Pediatric Autoimmune Neuropsychiatric Disorders Associated with *Streptococcus* infection (PANDAS) that commonly presents with obsessive-compulsive or tic symptoms following streptococcal infection.[33,38]

Pharmacologic Therapy

3 Antimicrobials should be used only in cases of laboratory-documented streptococcal pharyngitis associated with clinical symptoms in order to avoid overtreatment[33,36,37] (Fig. 72–5). Effective therapy (Table 72–5) reduces the infectious period from approximately 10 days to 24 hours and shortens symptom duration by 1 to 2 days.[33] **9** Treatment guidelines recommend penicillin as the drug of choice because of its narrow antimicrobial spectrum, documented safety and history of nasopharyngeal streptococcal eradication, and low cost.[33,37] Studies proving that antimicrobials prevent rheumatic fever used intramuscular procaine penicillin, but other antimicrobials can also eradicate nasopharyngeal streptococci and presumably are effective for preventing rheumatic heart disease.[37]

Table 72–5

Antibiotics[a] for the Treatment of Streptococcal Pharyngitis

Drug	Adult Dose	Pediatric Dose	Duration	Comments
Penicillin V	250 mg 3–4 times daily or 500 mg twice daily	250 mg 2–3 times daily, 500 mg twice daily (over 12 years)	10 days	Drug of choice but increasing reports of treatment failures
Penicillin G benzathine	1.2 million units	600,000 units (if under 27 kg)	1 IM dose	Useful for nonadherence or emesis; painful injection
Amoxicillin	250 mg 3 times daily or 500 mg twice daily; 750–1,500 mg once daily being studied	40–50 mg/kg/day in 2–3 doses	10 days	Preferred over penicillin V for young children (more palatable)
Cephalexin	250–500 mg 4 times daily	25–50 mg/kg/day in 4 doses	10 days	Consider in penicillin allergy (if nontype I reaction)
Cefadroxil	500 mg twice daily	30 mg/kg/day in 2 doses	10 days	
Cefuroxime axetil	250 mg twice daily	20 mg/kg/day in 2 doses	10 days	
Cefdinir	300 mg twice daily or 600 mg once daily	14 mg/kg/day in 1–2 doses	5–10 days	Broad spectrum; expensive
Azithromycin	500 mg once daily	12 mg/kg once daily	5 days	Increasing resistance
Clindamycin	150 mg 4 times daily	20–30 mg/kg/day in 3 doses	10 days	Useful for recurrent infections

[a]Other FDA-approved agents include amoxicillin-clavulanate, cefixime, cefaclor, cefprozil, cefpodoxime, erythromycin, clarithromycin, and others.

From Refs. 36, 37.

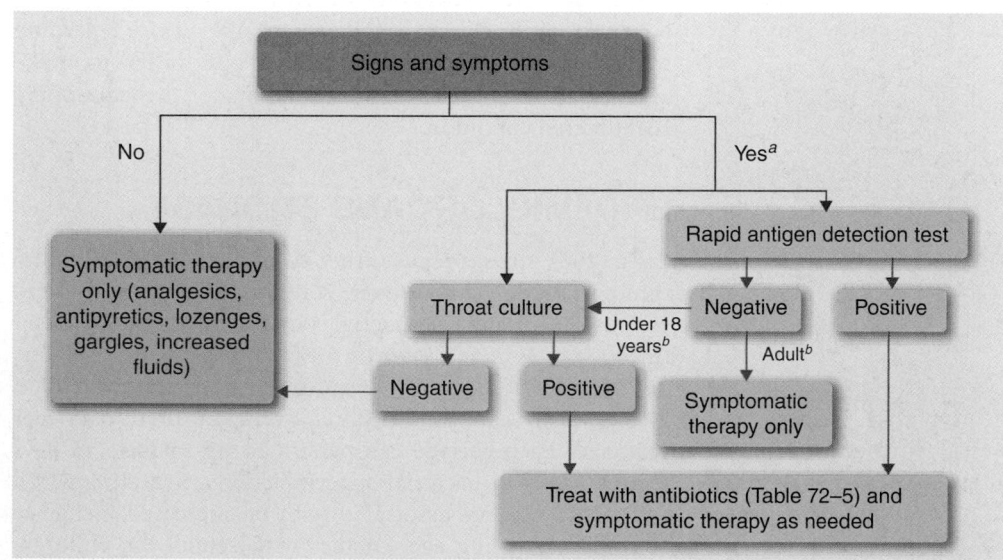

FIGURE 72–5. Treatment algorithm for management of pharyngitis in children and adults. [a]Rapid antigen detection tests (RADTs) are preferred if the test sensitivity exceeds 80%. [b]Parents, teachers, or other adults with significant pediatric contact should also be cultured if RADT is negative. (From Refs. 36, 37.)

Patient Encounter 3

A 7-year-old boy presents to the pediatrician with a sore throat and fever of 39.2°C (102.6°F) for 24 hours. His mother reports that other children in his class have had "strep throat" recently. He also complains of pain on swallowing and is not eating or drinking very much. He does not have any other symptoms and has no known drug allergies. Physical examination reveals pharyngeal and tonsillar erythema with exudates and painful cervical lymphadenopathy.

Does this child have streptococcal pharyngitis?

Is antibiotic therapy indicated? If so, what agent should be initiated and for how long?

What education should be provided to his mother regarding treatment?

Patient Care and Monitoring of Streptococcal Pharyngitis

1. Assess the patient's signs and symptoms. Are they consistent with streptococcal pharyngitis? Are symptoms of viral infection present?

2. Perform laboratory testing to confirm the presence of group A streptococci.

3. Does the patient require antibiotic therapy? Avoid antibiotic use in viral disease.

4. Obtain a complete medication history, including prescription drugs, nonprescription drugs, and natural product use, as well as allergies and adverse effects.

5. Recommend antipyretic or analgesic therapy, if needed.

6. If applicable, determine which antibiotic to use and the duration of therapy.

7. Develop a plan to assess effectiveness of chosen therapy and course of action to take if the patient does not improve or worsens.

8. Provide patient education on:
   - What to expect from the antibiotic, including potential adverse effects
   - Avoidance of close contacts for 24 hours
   - Signs of treatment failure

9. Stress the importance of adherence to therapy, including antibiotic resistance concerns.

❾ Cephalosporins are more effective than penicillin in producing bacteriologic and clinical cure and can be considered as first-line therapy alternatives in children and adults.[39] Possible reasons for improved cephalosporin efficacy include the copresence of β-lactamase-producing organisms that inactivate penicillin, improved eradication of commensal streptococci that are protective against group A streptococcal disease, and improved pharyngeal tissue penetration of cephalosporins. Usual duration of therapy is 10 days, but evidence is mounting that 5-day courses of certain cephalosporins are just as effective for bacterial eradication as 10 days of penicillin.[40]

Antimicrobial resistance plays a smaller role in pharyngitis therapy compared with other URIs. ❷ Penicillin resistance has not yet been documented in group A streptococci, but resistance and clinical failures occur more frequently with tetracyclines, trimethoprim-sulfamethoxazole, and to a lesser degree macrolides. As such, patients with penicillin allergies should be treated with a first-generation cephalosporin (if nontype I allergy), a macrolide/azalide, or clindamycin. Recurrent infections caused by reinfection, poor adherence to therapy, or true penicillin failure can be treated with amoxicillin-clavulanate, clindamycin, or penicillin G benzathine.[37]

OUTCOME EVALUATION

Antimicrobials relieve symptoms over 3 to 5 days, and patients can return to work or school if improved clinically after the first 24 hours of therapy. Follow-up cultures are not recommended to test for bacterial eradication. Lack of improvement or worsening of symptoms after 72 hours of therapy requires reevaluation. Recurrent symptoms following an appropriate treatment course should prompt reevaluation for possible retreatment.

COMMON COLD

The common cold is a self-limiting viral URI that occurs frequently throughout life. It is responsible for many missed days of school and work and is associated with significant health care resource utilization, including physician office and emergency department visits and nearly universal use of cough and cold medication for treatment or prevention.[41,42] It is important for clinicians to be aware of evidence regarding the use of cough and cold products in order to make appropriate treatment recommendations for this commonly encountered condition.

EPIDEMIOLOGY AND ETIOLOGY

Over 200 viruses cause the common cold, including rhinoviruses (most common), coronaviruses, parainfluenza viruses, respiratory syncytial virus, and adenoviruses.[43] Infection rates increase during the fall through spring seasons and are highest in the winter months. Adults experience 2 to 4 colds each year while children average 6 to 10 colds per year.[41,43,44] Each episode can persist for up to 10 to 14 days and can lead to bacterial superinfections, including AOM and ABRS. Factors associated with an increased incidence of colds are young age, contact with school-age children,

Clinical Presentation and Diagnosis of the Common Cold

Symptoms begin 24 to 72 hours after infectious contact. They usually peak around day 3 to 4 and begin to wane by day 7; colds typically last 10 to 14 days.

Signs and Symptoms[41,42,45]

- *Onset:* malaise, fatigue, headache, pharyngitis, low-grade fever (can be higher in infants and children); symptoms usually resolve over a few days.

- *Secondary:* Nasal/postnasal drainage (often clear at onset, but can become thick and purulent); nasal congestion; cough and/or throat clearing; sneezing; conjunctivitis; irritability; loss of smell or taste.

Complications

AOM, bacterial sinusitis, chronic bronchitis, bronchiolitis (in infants and children under 2 years of age), pneumonia, asthma exacerbation.

Diagnosis[45]

- *Clinical diagnosis:* Most common method; based on history, presence of symptoms, and physical examination.

- *Radiographic studies:* Not recommended routinely; useful for assessing complications such as pneumonia.

- *Laboratory studies:* Not recommended routinely; rapid viral antigen tests and nasopharyngeal cultures helpful for epidemiology and diagnosis in acutely ill young infants.

crowded conditions and poorly ventilated areas, and cigarette smoking. Children transmit viruses more rapidly than adults because of poorer hand hygiene, closer casual contacts, and sharing of toys.[42] Viral antigenic drifts and host immune system evasion contribute to the persistence of URIs in the community.

PATHOPHYSIOLOGY

Viruses enter the upper respiratory tract mucosa via inhalation of aerosols or infected droplets or direct contact with contaminated secretions. After cell entry, viral replication and shedding occur for several days to weeks. Clinical symptoms are a result of epithelial cell damage, inflammation, vasodilation, edema from increased vascular permeability, increased mucus production, and impaired mucociliary clearance from neutrophil migration, cytokine release, and cytotoxic immune responses.[42,45] Tracheobronchial inflammation and irritation induce cough via afferent nerve impulse transmission to the medulla.[42] Antibody production halts viral replication and inflammation as symptoms wane.

TREATMENT

Desired Outcomes

- The treatment goal for the common cold is to minimize discomfort from symptoms to allow patients to function as normally as possible. Antiviral use is not effective for cure. Preventative measures are also a focus to limit the spread to others.

General Approach to Treatment

Antimicrobials have no role in the treatment of the common cold. They are often prescribed inappropriately to patients with viral URIs and purulent secretions that has led to increased antimicrobial resistance.[2] Antimicrobials do not shorten symptom severity or duration and do not prevent bacterial complications from occurring in patients with the common cold.[2,41] Treatment measures should focus on symptomatic relief.

Nonpharmacologic Therapy

Supportive measures that assist with patient comfort include cool mist air humidification, use of intranasal saline drops or sprays with or without bulb suctioning, increased fluid intake, throat lozenges or saline gargles, and rest. Nasal strips have been advocated to relieve congestion by lifting the nares and opening the anterior nasal passages. These nondrug measures are particularly important for infants, children under 6 years of age, and pregnant women where medication safety is a significant concern. Although studies proving their benefits are lacking, these nondrug treatments are safe.

Pharmacologic Therapy

Nonprescription cough and cold preparations are used frequently to manage cold symptoms despite the lack of evidence to support their safety and efficacy. Over 10% of children per week receive nonprescription cough and cold remedies with highest use among children under 5 years of age.[46] Reports of serious adverse events and deaths have led to efforts to eliminate use of nonprescription cough and cold medications in young children.[47] Manufacturers have removed product labeling for children under 4 years of age while the FDA is reviewing their use in all children under 12 years.

Over 800 products are available to manage cold symptoms. ❿ *Choice of therapy is influenced by patient age, presence of comorbid conditions, and balance of effectiveness and safety.* Single ingredient agents are preferred over multi-ingredient products to target only active symptoms and to minimize the toxicity and overdose risk that can result from confusion and lack of knowledge on active components in marketed formulations. Cautious use of nonprescription preparations is warranted in certain patient populations: pregnant and/or lactating women, elderly, those with cardiovascular disease including hypertension, patients with diabetes, and glaucoma. Table 72–6 summarizes some of the available nonprescription

Table 72–6

Select Nonprescription Medications for the Common Cold for Patients 6 Years of Age and Above

Class/Drug	Adult Dose[a]	Pediatric Dose[b]	Comments
Analgesics/Antipyretics			
Acetaminophen[c,d]	325–1,000 mg every 4–6 hours (max 4 g/day)	10–15 mg/kg/dose every 4–6 hours (max 5 doses/day)	Use with caution in pre-existing liver disease
Ibuprofen[e]	200–400 mg every 6–8 hours (max 1,200 mg/day)	5–10 mg/kg/dose every 6–8 hours (max 4 doses/day)	Use with caution in cardiovascular disease; avoid use in elderly, renal impairment, and heart failure; avoid in third trimester of pregnancy
Decongestants			
intranasal:			
Oxymetazoline 0.05%[d]	2–3 sprays every 12 hours (max 2 doses/24 hours)	1–2 sprays every 12 hours (max 2 doses/24 hours)	Limit use of intranasal products to 3 to 5 days to minimize risk of rebound congestion; use with caution in patients with cardiovascular disease
Phenylephrine 0.25%, 0.5%, 1%	2–3 sprays no more than every 4 hours	2–3 sprays no more than every 4 hours (0.25% only)	
Systemic:			
Pseudoephedrine	60 mg every 4–6 hours (max 240 mg/day)	30 mg every 4–6 hours (max 120 mg/day)	Avoid use in patients with cardiovascular disease; children and elderly have increased risk of adverse effects (cardiovascular or CNS stimulation); use with caution in patients with diabetes, hyperthyroidism, prostatic hypertrophy; avoid in first trimester of pregnancy
Phenylephrine	10 mg every 4 hours (max 60 mg/day)	5 mg every 4 hours (max 30 mg/day)	
Cough Suppressants			
Dextromethorphan[d]	10–20 mg every 4 hours or 30 mg every 6–8 hours or 60 mg every 12 hours (max 120 mg/day)	5–10 mg every 4 hours or 15 mg every 6–8 hours or 30 mg every 12 hours (max 60 mg/day)	Increased adverse events in poor metabolizers (5–10% of Caucasians) and children; can cause dysphoria and serotonin syndrome; use caution in those taking psychotropic medications
Expectorants			
Guaifenesin	200–400 mg every 4 hours or 600–1,200 mg every 12 hours (max 2.4 g/day)	100–200 mg every 4 hours (max 1.2 g/day)	May cause nausea and abdominal pain, particularly in higher doses
Anticholinergics			
Intranasal ipratropium 0.06%[d]	2 sprays 3–4 times/day	2 sprays 3 times/day	Used for rhinorrhea only; does not improve congestion, postnasal drip, or sneezing

[a]Also for children greater than 12 years of age.

[b]For children 6 to 12 years of age.

[c]Preferred antipyretic/analgesic for children; can be used in newborns.

[d]Safe to use in pregnancy.

[e]Can be used in children older than 6 months of age.

From Refs. 41, 45, 48.

agents used for cold symptoms. Analgesics can be used for fever, pain, and discomfort from cold symptoms but only as single-ingredient formulations. Local anesthetics (e.g., benzocaine, dyclonine) relieve throat pain and are available in lozenges and sprays. Nasal decongestants cause vasoconstriction that can modestly improve nasal airway resistance and congestion, but use of intranasal products should be limited to 3 days to avoid rebound congestion.[41,49]

Antihistamines should be avoided when treating cold symptoms: first-generation antihistamines may help dry watery secretions via anticholinergic effects, but they impair mucociliary clearance of thick mucus which can worsen congestion and studies have not shown clear benefits for cough or cold symptoms.[41,49] Cough suppressant use is not supported by strong evidence showing benefit, and they can cause significant side effects and have been linked to abuse by teens for their euphoric effects in high doses.[41-43,49] Guaifenesin, an expectorant, may reduce cough frequency and sputum thickness in adults but has been poorly studied in children.[49] Routine high-dose vitamin C (more than 200 mg/day) treatment does not significantly impact cold severity or duration, but prevention in certain populations exposed to severe physical exercise or cold stress may be effective.[49] Use of *Echinacea purpurea* extracted from aerial parts may have benefit in adults when started early for treatment but its use is discouraged for prevention and in all children.[50] Other forms of echinacea have not shown consistent benefit for treatment of cold symptoms. Zinc lozenges are not effective for treating cold

Patient Encounter 4

A 25-year-old female presents to her family physician with a "sinus infection." Three days ago, she developed a sore throat, sneezing, and a "watery runny nose." Today, the nasal discharge is a thicker, yellow-green color and she has a mild headache. She also has some minor nasal congestion and a dry, nonproductive cough that started yesterday. She took acetaminophen 500 mg this morning which provided some headache relief. She has no medical conditions, but she does experience colds 4 to 5 times per year. She works in a daycare center and she has a 20-month-old son who developed a fever (38.0°C [100.4°F]) and clear rhinorrhea yesterday.

Immunizations: Up to date; needs influenza vaccine this season

Meds: Vitamin C 1,000 mg orally daily, Ortho Tri-Cyclen orally daily

Allergies: None

PE:

Gen: No apparent distress; pleasant

VS: BP 120/70 mm Hg, P 66 bpm, RR 16 breaths per minute, T 37.5°C (99.5°F), wt 80 kg (176 lb)

HEENT: Bilateral conjunctivitis with no discharge; green-yellow nasal discharge with mucosal hypertrophy and narrowed passages; erythematous pharynx with no exudates; no facial pain upon palpation; tympanic membranes normal appearing

Lungs: Clear to auscultation; occasional wheeze with cough; no crackles

What signs and symptoms are suggestive of the common cold? Which are suggestive of ABRS?

What other diagnostic studies, if any, should be performed?

Create a care plan that includes nonpharmacologic and pharmacologic therapies and a monitoring plan. Include preventative measures in your plan.

Patient Care and Monitoring of Common Cold

1. Assess the patient's signs and symptoms. Are they consistent with the common cold?

2. How long have the patient's symptoms been present? If symptoms have been present for fewer than 7 to 10 days, the common cold is likely. Persistent moderate or acute severe symptoms are more indicative of bacterial infections.

3. Has the patient tried any medications or nonpharmacologic methods to treat the symptoms? If yes, do they provide any relief?

4. Obtain a medication and medical history, including prescription and nonprescription drugs, natural product use, allergies, and current medical conditions.

5. Determine if nonprescription medications should be used to alleviate symptoms, such as pain and congestion.

6. Develop a treatment plan (including use of nonpharmacologic measures) to assess effectiveness of the chosen therapy and course of action to take if the patient does not improve or worsens.

7. Provide patient education on:
   - Role of viruses in colds, symptom resolution expectations, and how to prevent transmission to others
   - What to expect from the chosen therapy, including proper dosing and potential adverse effects
   - Avoidance of antibiotics to treat colds
   - When to seek additional medical care

8. Stress the importance of handwashing and limiting spread to others.

OUTCOME EVALUATION

Most colds will resolve within 7 to 10 days. Monitor patients for worsening symptoms and complications such as wheezing, difficulty breathing, moderate to severe facial or ear pain, and high fevers. If complications are suspected, referral to a physician is warranted.

Abbreviations Introduced in This Chapter

ABRS	Acute bacterial rhinosinusitis
AOM	Acute otitis media
OME	Otitis media with effusion
PANDAS	Pediatric Autoimmune Neuropsychiatric Disorders Associated with Streptococcus infection
PRSP	Penicillin-resistant *S. pneumoniae*
RADT	Rapid antigen detection test
URI	Upper respiratory tract infection

symptoms and concerns exist regarding the loss of smell with intranasal zinc preparations, so they should be avoided.[44]

Prevention

Minimizing contact with infected people and secretions is key to preventing the common cold. Frequent handwashing with soap and water or use of alcohol-based products is the cornerstone of prevention. Coughing and sneezing into the sleeve should be taught rather than using tissues or covering the mouth and nose with hands. Other methods that are often advocated include smoking cessation, maintenance of a healthy lifestyle through diet and exercise, and minimizing stress.

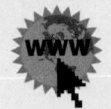

Self-assessment questions and answers are available at *http://www.mhpharmacotherapy. com/pp.html.*

REFERENCES

1. Poole MD. Acute bacterial rhinosinusitis: Clinical impact of resistance and susceptibility. Am J Med 2004;117:29S–38S.
2. Gonzales R, Bartlett JG, Besser RE, et al. Principles of appropriate antibiotic use for treatment of nonspecific upper respiratory tract infections in adults: Background. Ann Intern Med 2001;134:490–494.
3. Rovers MM, Schilder AGM, Zielhuis GA, Rosenfeld RM. Otitis media. Lancet 2004;363:465–473.
4. American Academy of Pediatrics and American Academy of Family Physicians. Diagnosis and management of acute otitis media. Pediatrics 2004;113(5):1451–1465.
5. Corbeel L. What is new in otitis media? Eur J Pediatr 2007;166:511–519.
6. Dowell SF, Butler JC, Giebink GS, et al. Acute otitis media: Management and surveillance in an era of pneumococcal resistance—a report from the Drug-Resistant *Streptococcus pneumoniae* Therapeutic Working Group. Pediatr Infect Dis J 1999;18:1–9.
7. McCracken GH. Diagnosis and management of acute otitis media in the urgent care setting. Ann Emerg Med 2004;39(4):413–421.
8. Casey JR, Pichichero ME. Changes in frequency and pathogens causing acute otitis media in 1995–2003. Pediatr Infect Dis J 2004;23:839–841.
9. Pichichero ME, Casey JR. Evolving microbiology and molecular epidemiology of acute otitis media in the pneumococcal conjugate vaccine era. Pediatr Infect Dis J 2007;26:S12–S16.
10. Nokso-Koivisto J, Räty R, Blomqvist S, et al. Presence of specific viruses in the middle ear fluids and respiratory secretions of young children with acute otitis media. J Med Virol 2004;72:241–248.
11. Jenkins SG, Brown SD, Farrell DJ. Trends in antibacterial resistance among *Streptococcus pneumoniae* isolated in the USA: Update from PROTEKT US Years 1–4. Ann Clin Microbiol Antimicrob. 2008;1;7:1.
12. Johnson DM, Stilwell MG, Fritsche TR, Jones RN. Emergence of multidrug resistant *Streptococcus pneumoniae*: Report from the SENTRY Antimicrobial Surveillance Program (1999–2003). Diagn Microbiol Infect Dis 2006;56:69–74.
13. Glasziou PP, Del Mar CB, Sanders SL, Hayem M. Antibiotics for acute otitis media in children. Cochrane Database Syst Rev 2004;CD000219.
14. Spiro DM, Arnold DH. The concept and practice of a wait-and-see approach to acute otitis media. Curr Opin Pediatr 2008;20:72–78.
15. Piglansky L, Leibovitz E, Raiz S, et al. Bacteriologic and clinical efficacy of high dose amoxicillin for therapy of acute otitis media in children. Pediatr Infect Dis J 2003;22:405–413.
16. Leibovitz E, Piglansky L, Raiz S, et al. Bacteriologic and clinical efficacy of one day vs. three day intramuscular ceftriaxone for treatment of nonresponsive acute otitis media in children. Pediatr Infect Dis J 2000;19:1040–1045.
17. Ototoxicity of ototopical drops—An update. Otolaryngol Clin N Am 2007;40:669–683.
18. Ovetchkine P, Cohen R. Shortened course of antibacterial therapy for acute otitis media. Paediatr Drugs 2003;5:133–140.
19. Flynn CA, Griffin GH, Schultz JK. Decongestants and antihistamines for acute otitis media in children. Cochrane Database Syst Rev 2004;CD001727.
20. Jenson HB, Baltimore RS. Impact of influenza and pneumococcal vaccines on otitis media. Curr Opin Pediatr 2004;16:58–60.
21. Straetemans M, Sanders EA, Veenhoven RH, et al. Pneumococcal vaccines for preventing otitis media. Cochrane Database Syst Rev 2004;(1):CD001480.
22. American Academy of Family Physicians; American Academy of Otolaryngology—Head and Neck Surgery; American Academy of Pediatrics Subcommittee on Otitis Media With Effusion. Otitis media with effusion. Pediatrics 2004;113:1412–1429.
23. Sinus and Allergy Health Partnership. Antimicrobial treatment guidelines for acute bacterial rhinosinusitis. Otolaryngol Head Neck Surg 2004;130:S1–S45.
24. American Academy of Pediatrics. Clinical practice guideline: Management of sinusitis. Pediatrics 2001;108:798–808.
25. Sande MA, Gwaltney JM. Acute community-acquired bacterial sinusitis: Continuing challenges and current management. Clin Infect Dis 2004;39:S151–S158.
26. Benninger MS. Acute bacterial rhinosinusitis and otitis media: Changes in pathogenicity following widespread use of pneumococcal conjugate vaccine. Otolaryngol Head Neck Surg 2008;138:274–278.
27. Payne SC, Benninger MS. *Staphylococcus aureus* is a major pathogen in acute bacterial rhinosinusitis: A meta-analysis. Clin Infect Dis 2007;45:e121–e127.
28. Rosenfeld RM, Andes D, Bhattacharyya N, et al. Clinical practice guideline: Adult sinusitis. Otolaryngol Head Neck Surg 2007;137:S1–S31.
29. Steele RW. Rhinosinusitis in children. Curr Allergy Asthma Rep 2006;6:508–512.
30. Rosenfeld RM, Singer M, Jones S. Systematic review of antimicrobial therapy in patients with acute rhinosinusitis. Otolaryngol Head Neck Surg 2007;137:S32–S45.
31. Meltzer EO, Teper A, Danzig M. Intranasal corticosteroids in the treatment of acute rhinosinusitis. Curr Allergy Asthma Rep 2008;8:133–138.
32. Elies W, Huber K. Short-course therapy for acute sinusitis: How long is enough? Treat Respir Med 2004;3:269–277.
33. Cooper RJ, Hoffman JR, Bartlett JG, et al. Principles of appropriate antibiotic use for acute pharyngitis in adults: Background. Ann Intern Med 2001;134:509–517.
34. Linder JA, Bates DW, Lee GM, Finkelstein JA. Antibiotic treatment of children with sore throat. JAMA 2005;294:2315–2322.
35. Linder JA, Stafford RS. Antibiotic treatment of adults with sore throat by community primary care physicians: A national survey, 1989–1999. JAMA 2001;286:1181–1186.
36. Shulman ST. Acute streptococcal pharyngitis in pediatric medicine. Pediatr Drugs 2003;5(Suppl 1):13–23.
37. Bisno AL, Gerber MA, Gwaltney JM, et al. Practice guidelines for the diagnosis and management of group A streptococcal pharyngitis. Clin Infect Dis 2002;35:113–125.
38. Moretti G, Pasquini M, Mandarelli G, et al. What every psychiatrist should know about PANDAS: A review. Clin Pract Epidemol Ment Health 2008;4:13.
39. Casey JR, Pichichero ME. The evidence base for cephalosporin superiority over penicillin in streptococcal pharyngitis. Diagn Microbiol Infect Dis 2007;57:39S–45S.
40. Casey JR, Pichichero ME. Metaanalysis of short course antibiotic treatment for group a streptococcal tonsillopharyngitis. Pediatr Infect Dis J 2005;24:909–917.
41. Simasek M, Blandino DA. Treatment of the common cold. Am Fam Physician 2007;75:515–520.
42. Kelley LK, Allen PJ. Managing acute cough in children: Evidence-based guidelines. Pediatr Nurs 2007;33:515–524.
43. Pratter MR. Cough and the common cold. ACCP evidence-based clinical practice guidelines. Chest 2006;129:72S–74S.
44. Caruso TJ, Prober CG, Gwaltney JM. Treatment of naturally acquired common colds with zinc: A structured review. Clin Infect Dis 2007;45:569–574.
45. Virk A, Henry NK. Upper respiratory tract infections. In: Wilson WR, Sande MA, eds. Current Diagnosis and Treatment of Infectious Diseases. New York: McGraw-Hill, 2002:98–117.
46. Vernacchio L, Kelly JP, Kaufman DW, Mitchell AA. Cough and cold medication use by US children, 1999–2006: Results from the Slone survey. Pediatrics 2008;122:e323–e329.
47. Ryan T, Brewer M, Small L. Over-the-counter cough and cold medication use in young children. Pediatr Nurs 2008;34:174–180.
48. Erebara A, Bozzo P, Einarson A, Koren G. Treating the common cold during pregnancy. Can Fam Physician 2008;54:687–689.
49. Arroll B. Non-antibiotic treatments for upper-respiratory tract infections (common cold). Respir Med 2005;99:1477–1484.
50. Linde K, Barrett B, Bauer R, et al. Echinacea for preventing and treating the common cold. Cochrane Database Syst Rev 2006;CD000530.

73 Skin and Soft Tissue Infections

Christie Nelson, Jaime R. Hornecker, and Randy Wesnitzer

LEARNING OBJECTIVES

Upon completion of the chapter, the reader will be able to:

1. Discuss characteristics of the skin that render it resistant to infection.

2. Describe the epidemiology, etiology, pathogenesis, clinical manifestations, diagnostic criteria, and complications associated with skin and soft tissue infections (SSTIs).

3. Identify the desired therapeutic outcomes for patients with SSTIs.

4. Recommend appropriate empirical and definitive antimicrobial regimens when given a diagnosis, patient history, physical examination, and laboratory findings.

5. Monitor chosen antimicrobial therapy for safety and efficacy.

KEY CONCEPTS

❶ Impetigo commonly afflicts young children, is usually caused by Group A streptococci or *Staphylococcus aureus*, and is characterized by numerous blisters that rupture and form crusts. Dicloxacillin, cephalexin, and topical mupirocin are considered the antibiotics of choice for treatment of impetigo.

❷ Folliculitis, furuncles, and carbuncles refer to the inflammation of one or more hair follicles, often attributed to infection with *S. aureus*. Treatment depends on severity and may involve local heat, incision and drainage, and/or oral or topical antibiotic therapy.

❸ Erysipelas is a superficial infection of the upper dermis and superficial lymphatics distinguished from cellulitis by its well-defined borders and slightly raised lesions. It is usually caused by *β*-hemolytic streptococci and treated with penicillin.

❹ Cellulitis, a bacterial infection of the dermis and subcutaneous tissue, is most commonly caused by *S. aureus* and *β*-hemolytic streptococci. Though *β*-lactams active against penicillinase-producing strains of *S. aureus* have historically been the drugs of choice, the increasing prevalence of infection with community-acquired methicillin-resistant *S. aureus* (CA-MRSA) is concerning. In areas with high rates of CA-MRSA, or in patients with risk factors for CA-MRSA infection, treatment with antibiotics active against this organism should be initiated.

❺ Persons who are immunocompromised, have diabetes or vascular insufficiency, or use injection drugs are at risk for polymicrobial cellulitis, often requiring broad-spectrum antibiotic coverage.

❻ Necrotizing fasciitis (NF) is an uncommon, rapidly progressive, life-threatening infection that causes necrosis of the subcutaneous tissue and fascia. Immediate surgical débridement is key to reducing its associated mortality.

❼ The pathogenesis of diabetic foot infection stems from three key factors: neuropathy, angiopathy, and immunopathy. Aerobic gram-positive cocci, such as *S. aureus* and *β*-hemolytic streptococci, are the predominant pathogens in acutely infected diabetic foot ulcers. However, chronically infected wounds are subject to polymicrobial infection and require treatment with broad-spectrum antibiotics.

❽ Prevention is key in the management of pressure sores. Mild superficial pressure sore infections may be treated with topical antimicrobial agents. Systemic antibiotics are indicated for serious pressure ulcer infections, including those associated with spreading cellulitis, osteomyelitis, or bacteremia.

❾ Bite wound infections generally are polymicrobial. Amoxicillin-clavulanate is the drug of choice for treating infected bite wounds and is also used as infection prophylaxis for human bites, deep punctures, and bites to the hand, or those requiring surgical repair.

❿ Every patient receiving antimicrobial therapy for skin and soft tissue infections (SSTIs) must be monitored for efficacy and safety. Efficacy typically is manifested by reductions in temperature, white blood cell count, erythema, edema, and pain that begin within 48 to 72 hours after treatment initiation. To ensure safety, adjust antibiotic dosages for renal and hepatic dysfunction as appropriate, and monitor for and minimize adverse drug reactions, allergic reactions, and drug interactions.

Skin and soft tissue infections (SSTIs) are frequently encountered in both acute and ambulatory care settings. They can range in severity from mild, superficial, and self-limiting, to life-threatening deep tissue infections that require intensive care, surgical intervention, and IV broad-spectrum antibiotics. *Staphylococcus aureus* and β-hemolytic streptococci are the most common causative bacteria.[1,2] Complicated infections in persons with immune suppression, diabetes, vascular insufficiency, burns, decubitus ulcers, or traumatic wounds are often polymicrobial.[2]

The role of MRSA, particularly Community-acquired methicillin-resistant *S. aureus* (CA-MRSA), is of increasing importance. In many U.S. cities, MRSA has become the most frequently isolated pathogen from patients presenting to emergency departments with SSTI.[3] MRSA infections were historically associated with exposures to health care settings (including hospitals, long-term care facilities, and dialysis centers), but have recently become problematic in previously healthy persons. Though risk factors for acquisition of CA-MRSA are not well established, outbreaks of CA-MRSA infection have occurred in prison inmates, homosexual males, athletes, military recruits, Native Americans, children, and injection drug users.[4] In these patients, or in areas with high rates of CA-MRSA, empiric therapy including antibiotics active against this pathogen must be considered.[2] This chapter will cover the epidemiology, pathogenesis, clinical manifestations, and pharmacologic management of the more common and severe bacterial SSTIs.

Intact skin generally is resistant to infection. In addition to providing a mechanical barrier, its relative dryness, slightly acidic pH, colonizing bacteria, frequent desquamation, and sweat (which contains IgG and IgA) prevent invasion by various microorganisms.[5] Conditions that predispose a patient to SSTIs include: (a) high bacterial load (greater than 10^5 microorganisms); (b) excessive skin moisture; (c) decreased skin perfusion; (d) availability of bacterial nutrients; and (e) damage to the corneal layer of the skin.[6]

IMPETIGO

EPIDEMIOLOGY AND ETIOLOGY

Impetigo, which stems from the Latin word for "attack," is a common skin infection worldwide.[7] ❶ *It predominately afflicts children between 2 and 5 years of age but may occur in any age group.*[1] β-hemolytic streptococci and *S. aureus* are the most common causative pathogens[1,7] Impetigo is a superficial infection and is spread easily, especially in settings of poor hygiene and crowding, and particularly during the summer months. The offending microorganisms colonize the skin surface and invade through abrasions, insect bites, or other small traumas. The scabby, crusty eruption of impetigo ensues. These lesions may occur anywhere on the body, but are most common on the face and extremities.[1]

CLINICAL PRESENTATION AND DIAGNOSIS

Impetigo lesions are numerous, well-localized, and erythematous. ❶ *They develop either as small, thin-walled blisters (impetigo contagiosum), or as larger blisters (bullous impetigo) which may be associated with mild systemic symptoms.*[1,7-9] *S. aureus* is most often implicated in bullous impetigo. The blisters rupture easily, leaving behind a friable crust reminiscent of cornflakes. The lesions of impetigo are rarely painful, but are pruritic. Scratching the lesions can spread the infection to other areas of the body.[7]

In order to avoid further spread and complications, antibiotic therapy is usually indicated. If left untreated, mild, localized cases of impetigo typically resolve within two to three weeks.[7,10] Sequelae of impetigo are uncommon, and when complications do occur, they seem to be more frequent in adults. Rarely, glomerulonephritis secondary to Group A streptococcus (GAS) may occur in nonbullous impetigo. Development of impetigo into more serious infections such as cellulitis or sepsis is another rare, but serious consequence.[9]

TREATMENT

Desired Outcomes

The primary goals of therapy for impetigo include preventing the spread of infection within the patient and to others, resolution of infection, and preventing recurrence. Secondarily, relief of symptoms associated with impetigo, such as itching, and improving cosmetic appearance are also important. Prevention of the rare, but serious complications of impetigo is an alternative goal.[10]

Nonpharmacologic Treatment

Because impetigo is rarely painful, there is often a delay in seeking medical attention. However, the lesions will resolve with time and increased hygiene. Soaking and cleansing the lesions with mild soap and water and the use of skin emollients to dry skin areas may reduce spread.[7]

Pharmacologic Treatment

Antibiotic therapy is recommended to achieve the desired outcomes of preventing the spread of infection and complications. Because GAS historically has been the primary causative organism, penicillin has been the mainstay of therapy. ❶ *However, the incidence of S. aureus impetigo is increasing, so oral penicillinase-stable penicillins or first-generation cephalosporins are now preferred.* Clindamycin or a macrolide are alternative choices when penicillin allergy is a concern; however, the clinician should be aware that some strains of GAS and *S. aureus* may be resistant to macrolides. ❶ *Topical mupirocin may be used alone when there are few lesions.*[1]

Table 73–1			
Folliculitis, Furuncles, and Carbuncles			
	Folliculitis	**Furuncles**	**Carbuncles**
Epidemiology/ etiology	❷ *Folliculitis is a superficial inflammatory reaction involving the hair follicle. The most familiar form of folliculitis is acne.* It can be infectious, caused by microorganisms such as *Staphylococcus aureus, Pseudomonas,* and *Candida.* Folliculitis can also be chemically-induced	Also known as boils, furuncles might be described as a deep form of folliculitis. A furuncle is a bacterial infection that has spread into the subcutaneous skin layers but still only involves individual follicles. Furuncles occur primarily in young men. Diabetes and obesity are other predisposing factors. Staphylococci are the most common cause	Carbuncles share all the characteristics of furuncles. However, a carbuncle is larger and involves several adjacent follicles and may extend into the subcutaneous fat. Carbuncles are more likely to occur in patients with diabetes, and tend to form on the back of the neck
Presentation and diagnosis	Folliculitis presents as small, pruritic, erythematous papules. Location of the lesions and a good patient history are often all that are required in the diagnosis of folliculitis. While Gram stain and culture of the papules may be considered to help determine the causative agent, they are not generally required as folliculitis typically resolves spontaneously	Furuncles most commonly develop on the face, neck, axilla, and buttock. A furuncle typically starts as a small, red, tender nodule. Within a few days, the nodule becomes painful and pustular. Typically, a furuncle will spontaneously discharge pus, heal, and leave a small scar	Carbuncles are similar to furuncles, only they are larger and exquisitely painful
Desired outcomes	The goals of therapy for folliculitis, furuncles, and carbuncles are resolution of infection with no or minimal scarring. A secondary goal of therapy for larger furuncles and all carbuncles is to minimize the risk of endocarditis or osteomyelitis by reducing bloodstream invasion		
Nonpharmacologic treatment	❷ *Warm compresses are generally sufficient*	*Moist heat is indicated to facilitate drainage. Large furuncles require incision and drainage*	*Incision and drainage are indicated*
Pharmacologic treatment	❷ *Often resolves spontaneously. A topical antibiotic or antifungal may be used to control the spread of infection but generally is unnecessary.* For staphylococcal or streptococcal folliculitis, antibiotic ointments such as mupirocin might be administered three times daily. Antifungal shampoo can be used for dermatophytes	*Carbuncles and furuncles that have surrounding cellulitis and fever or are located midline on the face must be treated systemically with an antibiotic that will cover* Staphylococcus aureus, *such as dicloxacillin or cephalexin. Trimethoprim-sulfamethoxazole DS, doxycycline, or clindamycin are preferred if CA-MRSA is suspected or if the patient has a severe allergy to penicillin.* Treatment should continue until acute inflammation has resolved, usually a 5- to 10-day course	

From Refs. 1, 8, 11.

FOLLICULITIS, FURUNCLES, AND CARBUNCLES

See Table 73–1.

CELLULITIS AND ERYSIPELAS

EPIDEMIOLOGY AND ETIOLOGY

Cellulitis and erysipelas are bacterial infections involving the skin. ❸ ❹ *Cellulitis is an infection of the dermis and subcutaneous tissue, whereas erysipelas is a more superficial infection of the upper dermis and superficial lymphatics. Although both can occur on any part of the body, about 90% of infections involve the leg.*[12,13] These infections develop after a break in skin integrity, resulting from trauma, surgery, ulceration, burns, tinea infection, or other skin disorder. However, they may occur after an inapparent break in the skin, and the skin may appear previously intact. In rare cases, cellulitis develops from blood-borne or contiguous spread of pathogens.[1,14]

Etiologic microorganisms vary according to the area involved, host factors, and exposures. ❸ *Erysipelas is generally caused by β-hemolytic streptococci, mainly GAS, and rarely by S. aureus.* ❹ *The predominant pathogens associated with cellulitis are S. aureus, including methicillin-resistant strains, and β-hemolytic streptococci.* ❺ *Persons who are immunocompromised, have diabetes or vascular insufficiency, or use injection drugs are at risk for polymicrobial cellulitis.*[1,2]

CLINICAL PRESENTATION AND DIAGNOSIS

The manifestations of and diagnostic criteria for erysipelas and cellulitis are presented in Table 73–2. Once diagnosed, cellulitis may be characterized as complicated or uncomplicated. Complicated infections are those that involve abnormal skin or wounds, occur in immunocompromised hosts, require substantial surgical intervention, or are polymicrobial in origin.[15]

Table 73–2

Presentation of Erysipelas and Cellulitis

Symptoms
- The infected area is described as painful or tender. In the case of erysipelas, the patient may complain of "burning pain" at the lesion site

Signs
- Both erysipelas and cellulitis are manifested by rapidly spreading areas of redness, edema, and heat. Lymphangitis and regional lymphadenopathy may be observed
- Important clinical differences between erysipelas and cellulitis exist:
  - In erysipelas, low-grade fever and flu-like illness are common prior to development of the lesion. The lesion is fiery red, raised above the level of surrounding skin, and has well-defined borders
  - In cellulitis, the lesion is not raised and has poorly defined margins

Laboratory Tests
- Leukocytosis may be present
- Cultures and sensitivities:
  - Blood cultures are only positive about 4% of the time but should be obtained for complicated or severe cases. Cultures aspirated from the lesion have an organism isolation rate of less than 20%, but also may be considered
  - Abscess drainage and débrided tissue, if obtainable, should be cultured and will yield the causative organism(s) up to 90% of the time

Imaging Studies
- Imaging studies may identify abscess formation, gas in the soft tissues, or osteomyelitis

From Refs. 1, 13, 14.

With early diagnosis and appropriate therapy, the prognoses for cellulitis and erysipelas are excellent. Severe or repeated episodes can cause lymphedema. Rare complications include the spread of infection to deeper skin and soft tissue layers, bacteremia and sepsis.[1] If the circumference of an extremity is cellulitic, compartment syndrome becomes a concern, and a surgical consult may be required. Recurrent cellulitis can be problematic. About 30% of patients hospitalized with cellulitis will develop a recurrent episode within 3 years. Vascular and lymphatic insufficiencies increase the risk of recurrences.[14,16]

TREATMENT

Desired Outcomes

The goals of therapy for cellulitis and erysipelas are rapid and successful eradication of the infection and prevention of related complications.

Nonpharmacologic Treatment

Nonpharmacologic treatment includes elevating and immobilizing the involved limb to decrease swelling. Sterile saline dressings should be placed on any open lesions to cleanse them of purulent materials. Surgical débridement

Patient Encounter 1, Part 1: Cellulitis

A 56-year-old male presents to the emergency department with complaints of right lower leg pain and redness. Examining his leg, you notice that he has erythema and edema extending from his ankle to proximal tibia. The area feels warm. The patient states that the redness started approximately 2 days ago. He has felt feverish over the previous 48 hours but did not check his temperature. He has had no other symptoms. He states that he bumped his shin on the bed frame last week and sustained a bruise but no apparent breaks in the skin. His vital signs at the clinic reveal a temperature of 38.3°C (100.9°F), pulse 110 bpm, blood pressure 110/72 mm Hg, and respiratory rate 25 breaths per minute. The physician diagnoses this patient with cellulitis.

What clinical manifestations are suggestive of cellulitis?

What additional information do you need before developing a therapeutic plan for this patient?

is indicated occasionally for severe infection. Drainage of abscesses are imperative to achieving clinical cure.[14]

Pharmacologic Treatment

Most patients with erysipelas or cellulitis are not hospitalized. Hospitalization and treatment with IV antibiotics should be considered if there are systemic signs and symptoms of infection (such as fever, chills, or hypotension), the patient has significant comorbid conditions (such as immunocompromise, diabetes, cirrhosis, cardiac failure, or renal insufficiency), or the cellulitis is spreading rapidly, involves a large area of the body, or is chronic.[14]

❸ *Penicillin is the treatment of choice for erysipelas.* In uncomplicated cases, a 5-day course is as effective as a 10-day course.[1] Other agents that are acceptable for treatment include clindamycin, cephalexin, and dicloxacillin.

❹ Though β-lactams, such as dicloxacillin, active against penicillinase-producing strains of *S. aureus* (commonly known as methicillin-sensitive *S. aureus*, or MSSA) have historically been the drugs of choice for acute bacterial cellulitis in otherwise healthy individuals, the increasing prevalence of infection with CA-MRSA is concerning, particularly in patients presenting with abscess.[1,17,18] In areas with high rates of CA-MRSA (e.g., greater than 15% of community *S. aureus* isolates show methicillin resistance), or in patients with risk factors for CA-MRSA infection, treatment with antibiotics active against this organism should be initiated.[2,17] Vancomycin continues to be the drug of choice for severe cellulitis due to MRSA because of its efficacy, safety, and low cost. Daptomycin or linezolid are also acceptable. Tigecycline is an alternative, however, due to its broad spectrum of activity, it is best reserved for patients with intolerances to the aforementioned drugs or in those with polymicrobial infections. For less severe, uncomplicated infections, many CA-MRSA strains can be treated with clindamycin, doxycycline, or trimethoprim-sulfamethoxazole.[1,2,17–20] However, it should be mentioned that though these agents are widely used for uncomplicated SSTI, this is an off-label use supported predominantly by data from observational and small interventional trials.[21] Also, trimethoprim-sulfamethoxazole and doxycycline have less than optimal activity against GAS and should be empirically combined with an agent with such activity (e.g., cephalexin) if GAS is also a suspected causative organism.[17,18]

⑤ In addition to being at risk for staphylococcal and streptococcal cellulitis, patients with immune suppression, diabetes, vascular insufficiency, or wounds are also at risk for disease caused by gram-negative bacilli such as *Escherichia coli* and *Pseudomonas aeruginosa*, with or without anaero-

bes.[2] Empirical broad-spectrum antimicrobial coverage, including coverage for resistant organisms such as health care–associated MRSA (HA-MRSA) and *P. aeruginosa*, is appropriate for severe cellulitis and/or severe systemic illness. The clinician should be diligent in attempting to isolate a causative pathogen in these individuals.[1]

Injection drug use also predisposes individuals to polymicrobial cellulitis. The antecubital region of the arm is usually the site of infection. *S. aureus*, the most common isolate, is frequently associated with abscess formation. Because some injection drug users lick their needles to "clean" them, antibiotics that cover oropharyngeal anaerobes should be included. Occasionally, *Candida* spp. are isolated, and the patient may require antifungal therapy.[22]

Table 73–3

Empirical Antimicrobial Therapy for Cellulitis

Host Factors	Probable Etiologic Bacteria	Mild Infection or Step-Down Therapy[a] (Oral Antibiotic Therapy)	Moderate–Severe Infection[a] (IV Antibiotic Therapy)
Previously healthy	MSSA GAS CA-MRSA	Dicloxacillin 500 mg every 6 hours Cephalexin 500 mg every 6 hours Clindamycin 300–600 mg every 6–8 hours CA-MRSA suspected or allergy to PCNs: Clindamycin[b] 300–600 mg every 6–8 hours Trimethoprim-sulfamethoxazole DS[c] 1–2 tabs every 12 hours Doxycycline[c] 100 mg every 12 hours	Nafcillin 1–2 g every 4 hours Cefazolin 1–2 g every 8 hours Clindamycin 600–900 mg every 8 hours CA-MRSA suspected or allergy to PCNs: Vancomycin 15 mg/kg every 12 hours (max: 2g/day) Linezolid 600 mg every 12 hours Daptomycin 4 mg/kg every 24 hours
Immunocompromise, diabetes mellitus, vascular insufficiency, pressure ulcer infection, or other polymicrobial infection suspected	MSSA HA-MRSA CA-MRSA Enterobactericiae *Pseudomonas aeruginosa* Anaerobes	Amoxicillin-clavulanate[d] 875 mg every 12 hours Levofloxacin[e] 750 mg every 24 hours + clindamycin 300–600 mg every 6 hours Moxifloxacin[d] 400 mg every 24 hours	Vancomycin, daptomycin, or linezolid[f] in combination with one of the following choices: Piperacillin-tazobactam[e] 3.375 g every 6 hours Ampicillin/sulbactam 3 g every 6 hours Imipenem-cilastatin[e] 500 mg every 6 hours Ertapenem 1 g every 24 hours Cefepime[e] 2 g every 12 hours ± metronidazole 500 mg every 8 hours Ceftazidime[e] 2 g every 8 hours + clindamycin 600–900 mg every 8 hours Levofloxacin[e] 750 mg every 24 hours ± clindamycin 600 mg every 8 hours OR Tigecycline 100 mg load, then 50 mg every 12 hours

[a]Doses given are for adults with normal renal function. IV therapy can be switched to oral therapy (as for mild infection) when the patient is afebrile and signs of infection are resolving.

[b]CA-MRSA isolates resistant to erythromycin should be evaluated for inducible clindamycin resistance via a D-test.

[c]Limited clinical data exist for the treatment of MRSA infections. Poor activity against GAS; consider using in combination with clindamycin or cephalexin if empirical coverage for GAS is desired.

[d]If CA-MRSA suspected, clindamycin, TMP-SMX, or doxycycline must be added to this regimen.

[e]*Pseudomonas aeruginosa* generally is susceptible to this agent.

[f]MRSA coverage indicated for patients with severe cellulitis or systemic illness, whom have risk factors for HA-MRSA or CA-MRSA infection, or reside in areas with high CA-MRSA prevalence. Otherwise, the broad-spectrum regimens listed below, without MRSA coverage, are appropriate.

From Refs. 1, 2, 8, 14, 17–20.

Patient Encounter 1, Part 2: Cellulitis: Medical History, Physical Examination, and Diagnostic Tests

PMH: Hypertension. He is not aware of any other illnesses.

FH: Father died of stroke at age 72. Mother, age 79, is alive with diabetes and a history of breast cancer. One brother, age 59, is alive and healthy.

SH: Works as a college professor; married; three grown children. Denies tobacco use; drinks approximately four glasses of wine on weekends; denies illicit drug use.

Meds: Atenolol 100 mg by mouth daily, multiple vitamin 1 tablet by mouth daily.

Allergies: No known drug allergies.

ROS: (+) pain and swelling in the right lower extremity; (−) headache, chest pain, shortness of breath, cough, nausea, vomiting, diarrhea, and weight loss.

PE:

Gen: Patient is in no acute distress. Wt 95 kg (209 lb); ht 5 ft, 11 in. (180 cm).

Chest: Lungs bilaterally clear to auscultation.

CV: Regular rate, rhythm. No murmurs/rubs/gallops.

Ext: Right lower extremity with erythema and edema from the ankle to just below the knee. Warm to the touch. LLE within normal limits.

Labs: WBC $17.3 \times 10^3/mm^3$ ($17.3 \times 10^9/L$), serum creatinine 0.8 mg/dL (70.7 μmol/L) The patient is diagnosed with cellulitis and admitted to the medical floor.

What are the most likely causative organisms in this case of cellulitis?

What are the goals of therapy for this patient?

What nonpharmacologic interventions would you recommend for him?

What antimicrobial therapy would you recommend? Include drug, dosage, route, interval, and duration of therapy.

How would you monitor your selected regimen for safety and efficacy?

If CA-MRSA represents 35% of all S. aureus *isolates at your hospital, would you change your pharmacologic recommendation? If so, how?*

Table 73–3 lists some recommended antibiotic regimens for the treatment of cellulitis. Because antimicrobial susceptibilities vary considerably between geographic locations, clinicians should select empirical treatment based on the antibiograms at their respective institutions. To decrease the spread of resistance, antibiotic therapy should be narrowed based on culture and sensitivity results whenever possible. The duration of therapy for uncomplicated cellulitis typically ranges from 7 to 10 days. For complicated cellulitis,

therapy with IV antibiotics is generally initiated and a switch to oral therapy can be made once the patient is afebrile and skin findings begin to resolve. Typically, this is done after 3 to 5 days. The complete duration of therapy can range from 10 to 14 days and longer in cases where abscess, tissue necrosis, underlying skin wounds, or delayed response to therapy are involved.[1,14]

NECROTIZING FASCIITIS

EPIDEMIOLOGY AND ETIOLOGY

Necrotizing fasciitis (NF) is an uncommon, rapidly progressive, life-threatening infection that causes necrosis of the subcutaneous tissue and fascia. When due to GAS infection, its associated mortality rate approaches 25%.[23] NF can affect any age group. Although the risk of NF is higher in injection drug users and in patients with diabetes, immune suppression, or obesity, healthy hosts can become infected as well.[24]

NF typically erupts after an initial trauma, which can range from a small abrasion to a deep penetrating wound. The infection begins in the fascia, where bacteria replicate and release toxins that facilitate their spread.[25]

In approximately 70% of cases, NF is polymicrobial and typically involves anaerobes (i.e., *Bacteroides* or *Peptostreptococcus*), facultative anaerobes (i.e., β-hemolytic streptococci), and Enterobacteriaceae (e.g., *Escherichia coli, Enterobacter, Klebsiella*). *P. aeruginosa* is occasionally implicated as well.[24] Polymicrobial NF develops in the following clinical settings: after surgery or deep penetrating wounds involving the bowel; from decubitous ulcer, perianal, or vulvovaginal infection; or from the injection site in an IV drug user.[1,8]

The remaining 30% are monomicrobial, caused by invasive GAS, or less frequently, *Clostridium perfringens*. CA-MRSA is more recently being implicated in these infections as well.[24] Monomicrobial NF is generally more severe than polymicrobial NF. GAS NF often occurs after minor trauma, such as an insect bite or abrasion, whereas infection with *C. perfringens* typically develops from surgical or traumatic wounds.[1,26] Once introduced, these organisms produce toxins that induce systemic toxicity, multiorgan failure, and shock.[26,27] Clostridial myonecrosis is more commonly known as gas gangrene.[1,26]

CLINICAL PRESENTATION AND DIAGNOSIS

Patient outcomes rely on the clinician's ability to recognize NF early in the course of disease. This is often difficult because early disease tends to be indistinguishable from cellulitis. The clinical presentation of NF is presented in Table 73–4.

NF is perhaps the most devastating SSTI. Left untreated, it can invade the muscles and circulation, resulting in myonecrosis and septic shock, respectively. Half of the cases

Table 73–4
Presentation of NF

Symptoms

- Early: Severe pain that is disproportionate to clinical signs and extends beyond the margins of the infected area
- Late: Area may become numb secondary to muscle and nerve involvement

Signs

- Early: Skin is erythematous, edematous, and warm; the clinical presentation is similar to that of cellulitis
- Intermediate (within 24–48 hours): Blisters and bullae indicate severe skin and tissue ischemia
- Late: The skin becomes violaceous and progressively gangrenous; hemorrhagic bullae may be present. Systemic signs may include fever, tachycardia, hypotension, and shock

Laboratory Tests

- White blood count, serum creatinine, and C-reactive protein may be elevated
- Deep tissue specimens obtained during surgical irrigation and débridement should be sent for Gram stain, culture, and sensitivity

Imaging Studies

- MRI and CT scans may reveal fluid and gas along fascial planes
- Typically, imaging studies are avoided when making a diagnosis because they may delay surgical intervention and increase mortality

NF, Necrotizing fasciitis.

From Refs. 1, 24, 25.

caused by GAS are accompanied by GAS toxic shock-like syndrome. The syndrome is endotoxin-mediated, manifested by hypotension and multiorgan dysfunction, and highly lethal.[8,24] Amputation is required in up to 50% of patients with extremity infections.[28] Once the patient recovers from acute NF, he or she often requires skin and/or muscle grafting and consequent physical rehabilitation depending on the amount and types of tissues removed during surgical intervention and the duration of hospital stay.[29]

TREATMENT

Desired Outcomes

The goals of therapy for NF include eradication of infection and reduction of related morbidity and mortality.

Nonpharmacologic Treatment

6 After resuscitation and hemodynamic stabilization, *prompt surgical intervention is key in the treatment of NF. Delayed operative débridement increases mortality.*[1,25] Some clinicians recommend hyperbaric oxygen (HBO) as an adjunct treatment for NF, although its use is controversial. Clinical data supporting the use of HBO in NF are inconsistent, with some trials showing reduced mortality rates and others showing no benefit.[30]

Pharmacologic Treatment

As an adjunct to surgery, broad-spectrum IV antibiotic therapy should be initiated immediately in patients with NF. Piperacillin/tazobactam or a carbapenem is appropriate for empiric therapy. These agents should be used in combination with vancomycin, daptomycin, or linezolid until MRSA infection is ruled out. The protein synthesis inhibitors clindamycin or linezolid are often utilized to decrease bacterial toxin production, thereby limiting tissue damage. This is particularly beneficial in streptococcal or clostridial infection.[24]

If GAS or *C. perfringens* is identified as the sole causative organism from deep tissue culture, antimicrobial therapy can be narrowed to high-dose IV penicillin G plus clindamycin. Antibiotic therapy should be continued until further operative débridements are unnecessary, the patient displays substantial clinical improvement, and fevers have abated for at least 48 to 72 hours.[1]

IV immune globulin (IVIG) may also be a useful adjunctive treatment in patients with GAS NF who present with shock. In one small randomized study, IVIG was associated with a reduction in mortality in such patients, however the finding was not statistically significant.[31]

DIABETIC FOOT INFECTIONS

EPIDEMIOLOGY AND ETIOLOGY

Foot ulcers and related infections are among the most common, severe, and costly complications of diabetes mellitus. Fifteen percent of all patients with diabetes develop at least one foot ulcer, resulting in direct health care expenditures of approximately $9 billion annually in the United States.[32,33]

Infected diabetic foot ulcers typically contain a multitude of microorganisms. **2** *Aerobic gram-positive cocci, such as S. aureus and β-hemolytic streptococci, are the predominant pathogens in acutely infected diabetic foot ulcers. However, chronically infected wounds are subject to polymicrobial infection.* The clinician should suspect the involvement of gram-negative (Enterobacteriaceae and *P. aeruginosa*) and possibly low-virulence pathogens (including enterococci and *S. epidermidis*) in chronic or necrotic wounds. Foul-smelling, necrotic or gangrenous wounds are also commonly infected with anaerobic bacteria. Patients recently hospitalized or treated with broad-spectrum antibiotics are at risk for infection with antibiotic-resistant organisms, including MRSA and vancomycin-resistant enterococci (VRE).[34]

PATHOPHYSIOLOGY

7 *The pathogenesis of diabetic foot infection stems from three key factors:* **neuropathy**, *angiopathy, and immunopathy.*[35,36] Neuropathy, the most prominent risk factor for diabetic foot ulcers, develops when continuously high blood glucose levels damage motor, autonomic, and sensory nerves. Damage to motor neurons that supply the small intrinsic muscles of the foot causes deformation, resulting in altered muscular balance, abnormal areas of pressure on tissues and bone, and repetitive injuries. Damage to autonomic neurons results in the shunting of blood through direct arteriole-venous communications, thereby decreasing capillary flow. The secretion of sweat and oil is also diminished, producing dry, cracked skin that is more prone to infection. Finally, damage to sensory neurons produces a loss of protective sensation so that the patient becomes unaware of injury or ulceration.[35,36]

Angiopathy of large (macroangiopathy) and small (microangiopathy) vessels is also the result of high blood glucose concentrations. Angiopathy results in ischemia and skin breakdown.[35,36]

Finally, persons with diabetes have altered immune function that predisposes them to infection. Although their humoral immune responses remain intact, leukocyte function and cell-mediated immunity are compromised in poorly-controlled disease. Achieving and maintaining tightly controlled blood glucose levels can wholly or partially reverse diabetic immunopathy.[35,36]

CLINICAL PRESENTATION AND DIAGNOSIS

Not all diabetic foot ulcers are infected. However, infection is often difficult to detect when perfusion and the inflammatory response are limited in the patient with diabetes. The common signs and symptoms (i.e., pain, erythema, and edema) of infection may be absent.[37] Still, the diagnosis of diabetic foot infection depends mostly on clinical evaluation.

Purulent drainage from the ulcer is indicative of infection. When pus and inflammatory symptoms are not present, the clinician must be astute to more subtle findings. These include delayed healing, increase in lesion size, prolonged exudate production, malodor, and tissue friability. Abnormal granulation tissue also may be present, as evidenced by color change (from bright red to dark red, brown, or gray) and increased bleeding. The ability to probe the ulcer to the underlying bone is highly indicative of osteomyelitis.[37]

Diabetic foot infections are classified into four categories based on clinical presentation using the PEDIS scale (perfusion, extent/size, depth/tissue loss, infection, sensation). Grade 1 signifies no infection; grade 2, involvement of skin and subcutaneous tissue only; grade 3, extensive cellulitis or deeper infection; and grade 4, systemic inflammatory response syndrome.[34] Grade 2 infections are classified as nonlimb-threatening infections, whereas grades 3 and 4 infections are limb-threatening.[34,36] Table 73–5 provides detailed information regarding these grades.

Imaging studies, such as x-ray and MRI, can identify osteomyelitis. Blood cultures should be obtained from all patients with signs and symptoms of systemic illness. Deep tissue cultures may help to direct therapy. Bone also may be sent for culture in cases of osteomyelitis. Superficial cultures of ulcers are unreliable and should be avoided.[34]

Spreading soft tissue infection and osteomyelitis are often the first complications that develop from diabetic foot infection. Some patients develop bacteremia and sepsis.

Table 73–5

Clinical Classification of a Diabetic Foot Infection

Infection Severity	PEDIS Grade	Clinical Manifestations of Infection
Uninfected	1	Wound lacking purulence or any manifestations of inflammation
Mild	2	Presence of at least two manifestations of inflammation (purulence or erythema, pain, tenderness, warmth, or induration), but any cellulitis/erythema extends no more than 2 cm around the ulcer, and infection is limited to the skin or superficial subcutaneous tissues; no other local complications or systemic illness
Moderate	3	Infection (as above) in a patient who is systemically well and metabolically stable but who has at least one of the following characteristics: cellulitis extending greater than 2 cm, lymphangitic streaking, spread beneath the superficial fascia, deep tissue abscess, gangrene, and involvement of muscle, tendon, joint, or bone
Severe	4	Infection in a patient with systemic toxicity or metabolic instability (e.g., fever, chills, tachycardia, hypotension, confusion, vomiting, leukocytosis, acidosis, severe hyperglycemia, or azotemia)

From Ref. 34.

Patient Encounter 2, Part 1: Diabetic Foot Infection

A 47-year-old man with a long-standing history of type 1 diabetes presents to the primary care clinic with complaints of a nonhealing sore on his left foot. He has also noticed more pain and swelling than usual in his left lower extremity. While examining his foot, you see a mildly purulent lesion with induration 4 cm (1.6 in.) in diameter, and the presence of lymphangitic streaking. His foot is erythematous, warm, and tender to touch, and slightly malodorous, despite good foot hygiene. The patient indicates that the sore has been present for about 3 months, and he first noticed it after a day at the beach, where he spent most of the day barefoot. The patient's vital signs are within normal limits with the exception of a blood pressure of 135/88 mm Hg. He is afebrile.

What signs and symptoms present in this patient are indicative of a diabetic foot infection?

Based on presentation, classify this patient's diabetic foot infection using the PEDIS grading scale.

What additional information do you need before developing a therapeutic plan for this patient?

The most feared complication of infected diabetic foot ulcers is lower extremity amputation. More than 60% of all nontraumatic lower extremity amputations performed each year in Western nations are linked to diabetic foot infection; nearly 71,000 were performed in the United States in 2004.[38]

TREATMENT

Desired Outcomes

● The goals of therapy for diabetic foot infection are eradication of the infection and avoidance of soft tissue loss and amputation.

Prevention

● Comprehensive foot care programs can reduce the rate of diabetic foot ulcers and associated amputations by 45% to 85%.[35] Periodic foot examinations with monofilament testing and patient education regarding proper foot care, optimal

glycemic control, and smoking cessation are key preventative strategies. Custom orthotic footwear and prophylactic reconstructive foot surgeries also may be effective in reducing the incidence of foot ulcers.[32]

Nonpharmacologic Treatment

The nonpharmacologic treatment of diabetic foot ulcers may include off-loading, chemical or surgical débridement of necrotic tissue, wound dressings, HBO, vascular or orthopedic surgery, and the use of human skin equivalents.[36]

Pharmacologic Treatment

The severity of a patient's infection, based on the PEDIS scale, guides the selection of empirical antimicrobial therapy. While most patients with grade 2 diabetic foot infections can be treated as outpatients with oral antimicrobial agents, all

Table 73–6

Empirical Pharmacologic Treatment of Diabetic Foot Infection

Infection Severity	PEDIS Grade	General Approach to Empirical Pharmacologic Treatment	Examples of Appropriate Empirical Antibiotics[a]
Uninfected	1	None. Avoid treating uninfected diabetic foot ulcers	Not applicable
Mild	2	Oral, narrow-spectrum antibiotic therapy with activity against *Staphylococcus aureus* and streptococcal species. Include coverage for MRSA (HA- or CA-MRSA) according to patient history and resistance patterns in the area	MRSA not suspected: cephalexin, dicloxacillin, or clindamycin HA-MRSA suspected: vancomycin (IV), linezolid, or daptomycin (IV) CA-MRSA suspected: clindamycin[b], trimethoprim-sulfamethoxazole[c], or doxycycline[c]
Moderate	3	Difficult to define a general approach. In many patients, highly bioavailable oral therapy is appropriate. IV therapy should be initiated in patients with more extensive or chronic infections, or those with abscess, deep tissue or bone involvement or gangrene	Oral options for Grade 3 infections: Amoxicillin-clavulanate, levofloxacin[d] + clindamycin, or moxifloxacin CA-MRSA suspected: Include clindamycin[b], trimethoprim-sulfamethoxazole or doxycycline
Severe	4	Parenteral, broad-spectrum antibiotic therapy should be initiated. Ideally drugs with activity against gram-positive, gram-negative, and anaerobic bacteria (especially if wound is malodorous) should be selected. Include coverage for MRSA	IV options for Grade 3–4 infection: Vancomycin, daptomycin, or linezolid[e] In combination with one of the following choices: Piperacillin-tazobactam[d], ampicillin-sulbactam, imipenem-cilastatin[d], ertapenem, moxifloxacin, levofloxacin[d] + clindamycin, cefepime[d] + metronidazole, ceftazidime[d] + clindamycin *OR* Tigecycline[f] monotherapy

[a]Please refer to Table 73–3 for dosing in adults with normal renal function.

[b]CA-MRSA isolates resistant to erythromycin should be evaluated for inducible clindamycin resistance via a D-test.

[c]Limited clinical data exist for the treatment of MRSA infections. Poor activity against GAS; consider using in combination with clindamycin or cephalexin if empirical coverage for GAS is desired.

[d]*Pseudomonas aeruginosa* generally is susceptible to this agent.

[e]MRSA coverage indicated for patients with severe cellulitis or systemic illness, whom have risk factors for HA-MRSA or CA-MRSA infection, or reside in areas with high CA-MRSA prevalence. Otherwise, the broad-spectrum regimens listed below, without MRSA coverage, are appropriate.

[f]Tigecycline is not currently approved for the treatment of diabetic foot infections.

From Refs. 34, 38–40.

Patient Encounter 2, Part 2: Diabetic Foot Infection: Medical History, Physical Examination, and Diagnostic Tests

PMH: Type 1 diabetes mellitus × 37 years, hypertension, dyslipidemia, peripheral neuropathy, and GERD

FH: Father died of an MI at age 77; mother died at age 56 of esophageal cancer. Two siblings alive with no significant PMH.

SH: Divorced, with two teenage children who live with their mother. Works in the computer tech industry. Smoked 1 PPD for 20 years, quit at age 39. Denies alcohol use.

Meds: Lantus 55 units at bedtime, Humalog Sliding Scale with meals, lisinopril 20 mg daily, hydrochlorothiazide 25 mg daily, Lipitor 40 mg at bedtime, gabapentin 600 mg three times daily, Prilosec OTC 20 mg daily, and aspirin 81 mg daily

Allergies: Sulfa (rash)

ROS: (+) left foot findings per HPI; (−) headache, chest pain, shortness of breath, cough, nausea, vomiting, diarrhea, and weight loss

PE:

Gen: Patient is in no acute distress. Wt 84 kg (185 lb); ht 5 ft 11 in. (180 cm)

Chest: CTAB

CV: RRR. No murmurs/rubs/gallops

Ext: 4-cm purulent, erythematous lesion present on the plantar aspect of the left foot proximal to the great toe. 1+ edema in the left foot; diminished sensation bilaterally

Labs: At previous visit 4 months ago: BUN 14 mg/dL (5.0 mmol/L), SCr 1.0 mg/dL (88.4 μmol/L), Glu 154 mg/dL (8.5 mmol/L), A1C 7.7%

The patient is diagnosed with a diabetic foot infection.

Explain the role of neuropathy, angiopathy, and immunopathy in the development of this patient's diabetic foot infection.

What are the best preventative strategies for diabetic foot infections, and complications such as LEA?

Antimicrobial therapy for this patient's infection should provide coverage for which microorganisms?

What antimicrobial therapy would you recommend? Include drug, dosage, route, interval, and duration of therapy.

How would you monitor your selected regimen for safety and efficacy?

How would your antimicrobial therapy change if this patient was experiencing fever, chills, blood glucose values in the 400s, and obvious deep tissue involvement?

---

grade 4 and many grade 3 infections require hospitalization, stabilization of the patient, and broad-spectrum IV antibiotic therapy.[34]

Multiple antibiotic options exist for the treatment of diabetic wound infections. Table 73–6 provides both general treatment strategies and specific, though not all-inclusive, antibiotic recommendations. The duration of therapy correlates with infection severity. Antibiotics should be continued until the infection has resolved, but not necessarily until the ulcer has healed. Grade 2 infections generally require 7 to 14 days of therapy, whereas grade 3 to 4 necessitate treatment durations of 14 to 28 days. If osteomyelitis is present, treatment duration depends on whether infected and necrotic bone is surgically debrided. In the case of amputation, where all infected bone and tissue is removed, 2 to 5 days of therapy is sufficient. Residual infection, status-post surgical debridement, requires 2 to 6 weeks of antibiotic therapy. Without surgery, antibiotic therapy should continue for at least 12 weeks.[34]

INFECTED PRESSURE SORES

EPIDEMIOLOGY AND ETIOLOGY

Pressures sores, also known as *decubitus ulcers* or *bedsores*, affect approximately 7% to 24% of long-term care and 10% to 18% of hospitalized patients. Patients of advanced age and those with spinal cord or orthopedic injuries are highest risk.[41]

A pressure sore is a chronic wound that results from continuous pressure on the tissue overlying a bony prominence. This pressure impedes blood flow to the dermis and subcutaneous fat, resulting in tissue damage and necrosis.[42,43]

Pressure sore infections develop from breaks in skin integrity and contamination from dirty areas of close proximity. Pressure sore infections generally are polymicrobial.[44]

CLINICAL PRESENTATION AND DIAGNOSIS

Approximately two-thirds of all pressure sores occur on the sacrum and heels. The remaining third occur predominately on the elbows, ankles, trochanters, ischia, knees, scapulas, shoulders, or occiput.[45] Pressure sores are classified according to the extent of tissue destruction.[46] The most commonly used system for staging of pressure sores is presented in Table 73–7.

Bacterial colonization of pressure sores is common. Because infection impairs wound healing and may require systemic antimicrobial therapy, the clinician must be able to distinguish it from colonization. Table 73–8 describes the clinical presentation of infected pressure sores.

Most complications are infectious. The most common is osteomyelitis, which is present in approximately 38% of

---

Table 73–7

Staging of Pressure Ulcers

Suspected Deep Tissue Injury

- Intact skin with localized area of purple or maroon discoloration or presence of a blood-filled blister
- The area may be preceded by tissue that is painful, firm, mushy, boggy, warmer or cooler as compared to adjacent tissue

Stage I

- Intact skin with localized area of nonblanchable redness, usually over a bony prominence
- May be difficult to detect in darkly pigmented skin; its color may differ from the surrounding area

Stage II

- Partial-thickness loss of dermis presenting as a shallow open ulcer with a red pink wound bed or an intact or ruptured serum-filled blister
- This stage should not be used to describe skin tears, tape burns, perineal dermatitis, maceration, or excoriation

Stage III

- Full thickness tissue loss. Subcutaneous fat may be visible but bone, tendon, or muscle are not exposed. Slough may be present but does not obscure the depth of tissue loss. May include undermining and tunneling

Stage IV

- Full thickness tissue loss with exposed bone, tendon or muscle. Slough or eschar may be present on some parts of the wound bed. Often include undermining and tunneling

Unstageable

- Full thickness tissue loss in which the base of the ulcer is covered by slough (yellow, tan, gray, green, or brown) and/or eschar (tan, brown, or black) in the wound bed
- Until enough slough and/or eschar is removed to expose the base of the wound, the true depth, and therefore stage, cannot be determined. Stable (dry, adherent, intact without erythema or fluctuance) eschar on the heels serves as "the body's natural (biological) cover" and should not be removed

From Ref. 46.

Table 73–8

Presentation of Infected Pressure Sores

Symptoms

- Because many high-risk patients lack sensation, pain may not be a primary symptom

Signs

- Infection generally is diagnosed when erythema and edema of the surrounding skin, purulent drainage, malodor, or delayed wound healing are present
- Patients with bacteremia often develop fever, chills, confusion, and/or hypotension

Laboratory Tests

- Deep tissue cultures may help to direct therapy. Bone also may be sent for culture in cases of osteomyelitis. Superficial cultures are unreliable and should be avoided

Imaging Studies

- Imaging studies, such as CT, MRI, or bone scan, can be used to detect osteomyelitis and to determine the depth and extent of tissue destruction

From Refs. 43, 45.

Careful monitoring and preventative care of high-risk patients can begin once these patients are identified. Intrinsic, or host-related risk factors for the development of pressure sores include age greater than 75 years, limited mobility, loss of sensation, unconsciousness or altered sense of awareness, and malnutrition. Extrinsic, or environmental risk factors include pressure, friction, shear stress, and moisture.[42,47]

Turning and repositioning the patient at least every 2 hours can reduce skin pressure and prevent pressure sores. However, because this level of care is difficult to achieve in most hospital and nursing home environments, multitudes of pressure-reducing mattresses have been manufactured. Although these can help to decrease pressure on susceptible areas, they do not negate the need for position changes.[42,47]

Maintaining a clean, dry environment can prevent skin maceration and subsequent tissue damage. This can be accomplished with frequent changes of bed sheets and clothing, thorough drying of skin after bathing, and prompt disposal of incontinent stool or urine.

Malnutrition is a significant but reversible risk factor. High-protein diets have been shown in multiple studies to improve wound healing in patients with pressure sores.[42]

Nonpharmacologic Treatment

Pressure relief, adequate nutrition (high-protein diet), and surgical débridement or abscess drainage are the mainstays of nonpharmacologic treatment.[43]

Pharmacologic Treatment

❽ *Systemic antibiotics are indicated for serious pressure ulcer infections, including those associated with spreading cellulitis, osteomyelitis, or bacteremia.*[43] Pressure ulcer infections are

---

infected pressure sores.[42] Less frequently, NF, clostridial myonecrosis, and sepsis can occur.

TREATMENT

Desired Outcomes

The goals of therapy for infected pressure sores include resolution of infection, promotion of wound healing, and establishment of effective infection control.[43]

Prevention

❽ *Prevention is the most humane and cost-effective component in the management of pressure sores.* Key prevention strategies include monitoring of high-risk patients, reducing skin exposure to pressure and moisture, and promoting good nutritional status.

generally polymicrobial. Thus, antimicrobial agents with a broad spectrum of activity should be initiated and narrowed according to the results of cultures obtained surgically. The duration of treatment is generally 10 to 14 days, unless osteomyelitis is present.[43]

Mild superficial infections, such as those that present clinically with delayed wound healing or minimal cellulitis, may be treated with topical antimicrobial agents such as silver sulfadiazine 1% cream or combination antibiotic ointments.[42] Systemic options for more extensive cellulitis are available in Table 73–3.

INFECTED BITE WOUNDS

EPIDEMIOLOGY AND ETIOLOGY

Fifty percent of Americans will be bitten by an animal at least once during their lifetimes. Although most of these injuries are minor, approximately 20% will require medical treatment.[1]

Dogs cause approximately 80% of all bites. These bites most commonly involve the extremities, and young children are particularly at risk.[48,49] Approximately 15% to 25% of dog bites become infected.[49]

Cat bites are the second most common animal bite, most often occurring in women and elderly individuals. Most involve the hand. Because cats have long, thin teeth that cause puncture wounds, their bites are more likely to become infected than a dog bite. Approximately 50% of cat bites become infected.[48,49]

Human bites are third most common and the most serious.[49] Before the availability of antibiotics, up to 20% resulted in amputation. Currently, human bite–associated amputation rates remain at 5%, secondary to vascular compromise and infectious complications.[49]

There are two types of human bite injuries. Occlusal injuries are inflicted by actual biting, whereas clenched-fist injuries are sustained when a person's closed fist hits another's teeth. Of the two, clenched-fist injuries typically are more prone to infectious complications.[48,49]

❾ *Bite wound infections generally are polymicrobial.* On average, five different bacterial species can be isolated from an infected animal bite wound.[1] Both the normal flora of the biter's mouth and that of the bite recipient's skin can be implicated. The bacteriology of the cat and dog mouth is quite similar. *Pasteurella multocida*, a gram-negative aerobe, is one of the predominant pathogens, isolated in up to 50% of dog and 75% of cat bites. Viridans streptococci are the most frequently cultured bacteria from human bite wounds.[1,48] Table 73–9 provides a comprehensive list of cat, dog, and human bite-wound pathogens.

CLINICAL PRESENTATION AND DIAGNOSIS

The clinical presentation of infected bite wounds is presented in Table 73–9.

Complications of infected bite wounds include lymphangitis, abscess, septic arthritis, tenosynovitis, and osteomyelitis. Bites to the hand are particularly complication-prone.[48,49]

Table 73–9
Etiology and Presentation of Infected Bite Wounds

Bacterial Pathogens

- *Dog and cat:* *Pasteurella multocida*, staphylococci, streptococci *Moraxella* spp., *Eikenella corrodens*, *Capnocytophaga canimorsus*, *Actinomyces*, *Fusobacterium*, *Prevotella*, and *Porphyromonas* spp.
- *Human:* Viridans streptococci, *Staphylococcus aureus*, *E. corrodens*, *Haemophilus influenzae*, and β-lactamase-producing anaerobic bacteria

Signs and Symptoms

- The onset of infectious symptomatology is typically 12–24 hours after the bite
- Pain at the wound site is common
- Erythema, edema, and purulent or malodorous drainage at the wound site are manifestations of infected wounds. The patient may be febrile
- Limited range of motion may be present, especially if the hand is bitten

Laboratory Tests

- Leukocytosis may be present
- The clinician should obtain anaerobic and aerobic wound cultures only if the wound appears clinically infected

Imaging Studies

- X-rays should be obtained if the bite is on the hand, could have damaged bone or joints, or if an embedded object or tooth fragment is suspected

From Refs. 48, 49.

TREATMENT

Desired Outcomes

The goals of therapy for an infected bite wound are rapid and successful eradication of infection and prevention of related complications.

Nonpharmacologic Treatment

Thorough irrigation with normal saline is the first step in the care of an infected bite wound. The wound should be elevated and immobilized. Surgical closure may be advocated, especially for facial wounds. Wounds that are infected, at higher risk for infection, or older than 24 hours should be left open because premature closure can lead to disastrous infectious complications. ❾ *Wounds at higher risk for infection include human bites, deep punctures, and bites to the hand.*[48]

Pharmacologic Treatment

Most bite wounds require antibiotic therapy only when clinical infection is present. ❾ *However, prophylactic therapy is recommended for wounds at higher risk for infection and bites requiring surgical repair.*[48]

❾ *The most effective agent for the treatment (and prophylaxis) of human and animal bite-wound infections is amoxicillin-clavulanate.* Alternatives for patients with significant penicillin

Patient Care and Monitoring

Choosing antibiotic therapy for SSTIs:

1. To select the most effective *empirical* antibiotic agent(s) for SSTIs, review the following:
   - The diagnosis
   - Clinical manifestations and severity of illness (to assess the need for IV versus oral therapy).
   - Past medical history, chronic disease states (to determine suspected pathogens).
   - Patient's ability to adhere to the regimen (if outpatient treatment indicated).

   In pediatric patients especially, consider duration of therapy, frequency of dosing, method and ease of administration, and palatability and tolerability of oral formulations.

2. To ensure the safety of your selected antibiotic agent(s), review the following:
   - Current medications (over-the-counter, prescription, and alternative) for potential drug interactions.
   - History of medication allergies and adverse effects.
   - Current laboratory analyses to determine renal and hepatic function.
   - Chronic disease states or acute conditions that could be worsened by certain antimicrobial agents (e.g., QT prolongation or acute renal failure).
   - Other disease modifiers that may preclude use (e.g., pregnancy, age).

Monitoring antibiotic therapy for SSTIs:

1. Ensure that antimicrobial therapy is effective by monitoring for:
   - Resolution of local and systemic signs and symptoms of infection.
   - Resolution of laboratory evidence of infection.
2. Narrow antibiotic coverage when possible with the use of culture and sensitivity data.
3. Assess patient adherence.
4. Ensure that antimicrobial therapy is safe by monitoring for and treating (as appropriate):
   - Common and severe adverse effects.
   - Drug interactions.

Patient education regarding antibiotic therapy for SSTIs:

1. It is imperative to take the antibiotic as prescribed and to finish the therapy.
2. If no symptomatic improvement is noted within 3 days, contact your health care provider.
3. Many antibiotics cause diarrhea. If it is severe, contact your health care provider.
4. Consider health initiatives to improve wound healing, such as smoking cessation and glycemic control.

allergies include either a fluoroquinolone (such as ciprofloxacin) or trimethoprim-sulfamethoxazole in combination with clindamycin. The durations of prophylaxis and treatment generally are 3 to 5 and 10 to 14 days, respectively.[1]

If the wound is associated with significant cellulitis and edema, systemic signs of infection, or possible joint or bone involvement, hospitalization and IV antibiotics (typically ampicillin-sulbactam 3 g IV every 6 hours) should be initiated. Bone and joint infections will require longer durations of therapy of up to 6 weeks.[49]

RABIES AND TETANUS

Patients with animal bite wounds may require rabies prophylaxis.[48,49] If the bite is from a bat, a wild animal, a domestic animal that has or is suspected to have rabies, or an unavailable animal, the patient should receive rabies immune globulin and vaccine immediately.[50]

Crush injuries and those greater than 1 cm (0.4") in depth are at risk for tetanus. A tetanus and diphtheria toxoid booster (Td) should be administered to any patient who has not received one in 5 or more years. A Td and tetanus immune globulin are indicated in those patients who have not previously received at least three Td boosters or whose immunization history is unknown.[48,49]

OUTCOME EVALUATION

❿ *Patients receiving antibiotic therapy for SSTIs require monitoring for efficacy and safety. Efficacy typically is manifested by reductions in temperature, white blood cell count, erythema, edema, and pain.* Initially, signs and symptoms of infection may worsen owing to toxin release from certain organisms (i.e., GAS); however, they should begin to resolve within 48 to 72 hours of treatment initiation. If no response, or worsening infection is noted after the first 3 days of antibiotics, reevaluate the patient.[1] Lack of response may be due to a noninfectious or nonbacterial diagnosis, a pathogen not covered by or resistant to current antibiotic therapy, poor patient adherence, drug or disease interactions causing decreased antibiotic absorption or increased clearance, immunodeficiency, or the need for surgical intervention. **❿** *To ensure the safety of the regimen, dose antibiotics according to renal and hepatic function as appropriate, and monitor for or minimize adverse drug reactions, allergic reactions, and drug interactions.*

Abbreviations Introduced in This Chapter

CA-MRSA	Community-acquired methicillin-resistant *S. aureus*
GAS	Group A *Streptococcus* (also known as *Streptococcus pyogenes*, one of the β-hemolytic streptococci)
HA-MRSA	Health care-associated methicillin-resistant *S. aureus*

HBO	Hyperbaric oxygen
MSSA	Methicillin-sensitive *S. aureus*
NF	Necrotizing fasciitis
SSTI	Skin and soft tissue infection

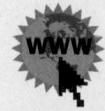 Self-assessment questions and answers are available at *http://www.mhpharmacotherapy.com/pp.html.*

REFERENCES

1. Stevens DL, Bisno AL, Chambers HF, et al. Practice guidelines for the diagnosis and management of skin and soft tissue infections. Clin Infect Dis 2005;41:1373–1406.
2. Choice of antibacterial drugs. Treatment Guidelines from The Medical Letter 2007 May;5(57):33–50.
3. Moran GJ, Krishnadasan A, Gorwitz RJ, et al. Methicillin-resistant *S. aureus* infection among patients in the emergency department. N Engl J Med 2006;355(7):666–674.
4. Boucher HW, Corey GR. Epidemiology of methicillin-resistant *Staphylococcus aureus.* Clin Infect Dis 2008;46(Suppl 5):S344–S349.
5. Dieffenbach CW, Tramont EC. Innate (general or nonspecific) host defense mechanisms. In: Mandell GL, Bennett JE, Dolin R, eds. Principles and Practice of Infectious Diseases. 6th ed. Philadelphia: Elsevier, 2005; 34–41.
6. Yagupski P. Bacteriologic aspects of skin and soft tissue infections. Pediatr Ann 1993;22:217–224.
7. Watkins P. Impetigo: Aetiology, complications, and treatment options. Nurs Stand 2005;19(36):50–54.
8. Swartz MN, Pasternack MS. Cellulitis and subcutaneous tissue infections. In: Mandell GL, Bennett JE, Dolin R, eds. Principles and Practice of Infectious Diseases. 6th ed. Philadelphia: Elsevier, 2005:1172–1193.
9. Stanley JR, Amagai M. Pemphigus, bullous impetigo, and staphylococcal scalded-skin syndrome. N Engl J Med 2006;355:1800–1810.
10. Cole C, Gazewood J. Diagnosis and treatment of impetigo. Am Fam Physician 2007;75:859–864, 868.
11. Luelmo-Aguilar J, Santandreu MS. Folliculitis: Recognition and management. Am J Clin Dermatol 2004;5(5):301–310.
12. Stulberg DL, Penrod MA, Blatny RA. Common bacterial skin infections. Am Fam Physician 2002;66:119–124.
13. Bonnetlanc JM, Bedane C. Erysipelas: Recognition and management. Am J Clin Dermatol 2003;4(3):157–163.
14. Swartz MN. Clinical practice. Cellulitis. N Engl J Med 2004;350(9):904–912.
15. DiNubile MJ, Lipsky BA. Complicated infections of skin and skin structures: When the infection is more than skin deep. J Antimicrob Chemother 2004;53(Suppl S2):ii37–ii50.
16. Morris A. Cellulitis and erysipelas. Clin Evid 2004 June;(1):2133–2139.
17. Stryjewski ME, Chambers HF. Skin and soft-tissue infections caused by community-acquired methicillin-resistant *Staphylococcus aureus.* Clin Infect Dis 2008;46(Suppl 5):S368–S377.
18. Cohen P. Community-acquired methicillin-resistant *Staphylococcus aureus* skin infections: Implications for patients and practitioners. J Clin Dermatol 2007;8(5):259–270.
19. Grim SA, Rapp RP, Martin CA, et al. Trimethoprim-Sulfamethoxazole as a viable treatment option for infections caused by methicillin-resistant *Staphylococcus aureus.* Pharmacotherapy 2005;25(2):253–264.
20. Ruhe JJ, Monson T, Bradsher RW, et al. Use of long-acting tetracyclines for methicillin-resistant *Staphylococcus aureus* infections: Case series and review of the literature. Clin Infect Dis 2005;40(10):1429–1434.
21. Cenizal MJ, Skiest D, Luber S, et al. Prospective randomized trial of empiric therapy with trimethoprim-sulfamethoxazole or doxycycline for outpatient skin and soft tissue infections in an area of high prevalence of methicillin-resistant *Staphylococcus aureus.* Antimicrob Agents Chemother 2007;51(7):2628–2630.
22. Bisbe J, Miro J, Latorre, et al. Disseminated candidiasis in addicts who use brown heroin: Report of 83 cases and review. Clin Infect Dis 1992;15:910–923.
23. Group A Streptococcal (GAS) Disease. Department of Health and Human Services. Centers for Disease Control and Prevention. April 3, 2008, *http://www.cdc.gov/ncidod/dbmd/diseaseinfo/groupastreptococcal_t.htm.*
24. Anaya DA, Dellinger EP. Necrotizing soft-tissue infection: Diagnosis and management. Clin Infect Dis 2007;44:705–710.
25. Wong C, Wang Y. The diagnosis of necrotizing fasciitis. Curr Opin Infect Dis 2005;18:101–106.
26. Finsterer J, Hess B. Neuromuscular and CNS manifestations of *Clostridium perfringens* infections. Infection 2007;35(6):396–405.
27. Wolf JE, Rabinowitz LG. Streptococcal toxic shock-like syndrome. Arch Dermatol 1995;131:73–77.
28. Jallali N. Necrotising fasciitis: Its aetiology, diagnosis and management. J Wound Care 2003;12(8):297–300.
29. Cunningham JD, Silver L, Rudikoff D. Necrotizing fasciitis: A plea for early diagnosis and treatment. Mt Sinai J Med 2001;68(4–5):253–261.
30. Jallali N, Withey S Butler PE. Hyperbaric oxygen as adjuvant therapy in the management of necrotizing fasciitis. Am J Surg 2005;189:462–466.
31. Darenberg J, Ihendyane N, Sjolin J, et al. IV immunoglobulin G therapy in streptococcal toxic shock syndrome: A European randomized, double-blind, placebo-controlled trial. Clin Infect Dis 2003;37(3):333–340.
32. Singh N, Armstrong DG, Lipsky BA. Preventing foot ulcers in patients with diabetes. JAMA 2005;293(2):217–228.
33. Ulbrecht JS, Cavanagh PR, Caputo GM. Foot problems in diabetes: An overview. Clin Infect Dis 2004;39(Suppl 2):S73–S82.
34. Lipsky BA, Berendt AR, Deery G, et al. Diagnosis and treatment of diabetic foot infections. Clin Infect Dis. 2004;39:885–910.
35. National Diabetes Fact Sheet, United States. Department of Health and Human Services. Centers for Disease Control and Prevention. 2007, *http://www.cdc.gov/diabetes/pubs/pdf/ndfs_2007.pdf.*
36. Calhoun JH, Overgaard KA, Stevens CM, et al. Diabetic foot ulcers and infections: Current concepts. Adv Skin Wound Care 2002;15:31–45.
37. Williams DT, Hilton JR, Harding KG. Diagnosing foot infection in diabetes. Clin Infect Dis 2004;39(2):S83–S86.
38. Bader MS. Diabetic foot infection. Am Fam Physician 2008;78(1):71–79,81–82.
39. Matthews PC, Berendt AR, Lipsky BA. Clinical management of diabetic foot infection: Diagnostics, therapeutics and the future. Expert Rev Anti Infect Ther 2007;5(1):117–127.
40. Lipsky BA, Giordano P, Shurjeel C, et al. Treating diabetic foot infections with sequential IV moxifloxacin compared with piperacillin-tazobactam/amoxicillin-clavulanate. J Antimicrob Chemother 2007;60:370–376.
41. National Pressure Ulcer Advisory Panel Board of Directors. Pressure ulcers in America: Prevalence, incidence, and implications for the future. Adv Skin Wound Care 2001;14:208–215.
42. Thomas DR. Prevention and treatment of pressure ulcers: What works? What doesn't? Cleve Clin J Med 2001;68(8):704–707.
43. Livesley NJ, Chow AW. Pressure ulcers in elderly individuals. Clin Infect Dis 2002;35:1390–1396.
44. Darouiche R. Infections in patients with spinal cord injury. In: Mandell GL, Bennett JE, Dolin R, eds. Principles and Practice of Infectious Diseases, 6th ed. Philadelphia: Elsevier Inc., 2005; 3512–3517.
45. Cannon BC, Cannon JP. Management of pressure ulcers. Am J Health Syst Pharm 2004;61:1895–1907.
46. National Pressure Ulcer Advisory Panel. Updated staging system. 2007, *http://www.npuap.org/pr2.htm.*
47. Pressure Sores. The Merck Manual. November 2005, *http://www.merck.com/mmpe/sec10/ch126/ch126a.html.*
48. Bower MG. Managing dog, cat, and human bite wounds. Nurs Pract 2001;26(4):36–38, 41, 42, 45.
49. Taplitz RA. Managing bite wounds. Postgrad Med 2004;116(2):49–55.
50. CDC. Human rabies prevention-United States, 1999 recommendations of the Advisory Committee on Immunization Practices (ACIP). MMWR 1999;48(RR-1):1–21.

74 Infective Endocarditis

Ronda L. Akins

LEARNING OBJECTIVES

Upon completion of the chapter, the reader will be able to:

1. Differentiate the causes and development of infective endocarditis (IE).

2. Identify the clinical presentation and laboratory evaluation for IE.

3. Assess diagnostic criteria used to evaluate a patient suspected of having IE.

4. Describe the most likely causative organisms of IE, particularly in specific patient populations.

5. Develop appropriate pharmacologic treatment recommendations for patients with IE.

6. Define appropriate patient populations requiring prophylactic treatment, and differentiate appropriate drug regimens.

7. Devise a monitoring plan for patients with IE to determine treatment efficacy and discern any adverse effects.

KEY CONCEPTS

❶ For infective endocarditis (IE) to develop, the occurrence of several factors is required. These factors involve alterations to the endocardial surface which allow bacterial adherence and eventual infection.

❷ Persistent fever is the most common symptom present in patients with IE.

❸ Blood cultures are the essential laboratory test for the diagnosis and treatment of IE. Typically, patients with IE have a low-grade consistent bacteremia. Blood culture results are critical for determining the most appropriate therapy.

❹ Echocardiograms are used for detecting the presence of a vegetation. Either a transthoracic echocardiogram (TTE) or a transesophageal echocardiogram (TEE) may be used depending on certain patient characteristics.

❺ Choosing the appropriate antimicrobial therapy is crucial to achieve adequate organism kill.

❻ An extended treatment course of 4 to 6 weeks (in most cases) is required to achieve an adequate cure.

❼ The overall goal of therapy is to eradicate the infection and minimize/prevent any complications.

❽ In an effort to prevent the development of IE, prophylactic treatment generally is considered appropriate for patients with high-risk factors.

❾ Monitoring the patient's clinical course is necessary to assess the effectiveness of therapy, detect the potential development of bacterial resistance, and determine outcome.

Infective endocarditis (IE) is a serious infection affecting the lining and valves of the heart. While this disease is mostly associated with infection of the heart valves, the septal defects may become involved as well. Infections also occur in patients with prosthetic or mechanical devices, such as mechanical heart valves or who are IV drug users (IVDUs). Bacteria is the primary cause of IE; however, fungi and atypical organisms may also be responsible pathogens.

Typically IE is classified into two categories: acute or subacute. The difference between the two categories is based on the progression and severity of the disease. Acute disease is more aggressive, characterized by high fevers, elevated WBC counts, and systemic toxicity, with death occurring within a few days to weeks. This type of IE is often caused by more virulent organisms, particularly *Staphylococcus aureus*. Subacute disease is typically caused by less virulent organisms, such as *viridans* streptococci, producing a slower and more subtle presentation. It is characterized by weakness, fatigue, low-grade fever, night sweats, weight loss, and other nonspecific symptoms, with death occurring in several months.

Successful management of patients with IE is based on proper diagnosis, treatment with adequate therapy, and monitoring for complications, adverse events, or development of resistance. The treatment and management of IE are best determined through identification of the causative organism.

IE has varied clinical presentations; therefore, patients with this infection may be found in any medical subspecialty (i.e., medicine, surgery, critical care, etc.).

EPIDEMIOLOGY AND ETIOLOGY

Despite IE being a fairly uncommon infection, in the United States, there are about 10,000 to 20,000 new cases annually, and IE accounts for approximately 1 case per 1,000 hospital admissions.[1] Although the exact number of cases is often difficult to determine owing to the diagnostic criteria and reporting methods for this disease, it continues to rise. IE is now considered the fourth leading cause of serious infectious disease syndromes following urosepsis, pneumonia, and intra-abdominal sepsis.[2] Men are affected more commonly than women at a ratio of 1.7:1. Although IE occurs at any age, more than 50% of cases occur in patients older than 50 years.[1] IE in children continues to be uncommon and is mainly associated with underlying structural defects, surgical repair of the defects, or nosocomial catheter-related bacteremia.[1] With the increased use of mechanical valves, prosthetic-valve endocarditis (PVE) now accounts for approximately 7% to 25%.[3] Patients who are IVDUs are also at an increased risk for IE, with 150 to 2,000 cases per 100,000 persons per year, most being younger adults.[3] Additionally, other patients at high risk for IE include patients with any congenital or structural cardiac defects, including valvular disease; long-term hemodialysis; diabetes mellitus; poor oral hygiene; major dental treatment; previous endocarditis; hypertrophic cardiomyopathy; and mitral valve prolapse with regurgitation.[4–8]

Although almost any type of organism is capable of causing IE, the majority of cases are caused by gram-positive organisms. These consist primarily of streptococci, staphylococci, and enterococci. Consideration of gram-negative, fungal, and other atypical organisms must be taken into account, particularly in certain patient populations. In Table 74–1, approximate percentages are given for each organism based on the type of IE, including native valve (community acquired versus health care–associated), prosthetic valve (grouped by months postsurgery) and IVDUs.

Patient Encounter, Part 1

A 56-year-old man with a history of diabetes and coronary artery disease presents to the emergency department with complaints of weakness, fever, and chills. On interviewing the patient, you determine that he went to the dentist about 3 weeks ago and since that time has lost about 2.3 kg (5 lb). His current weight is 63.6 kg (140 lb). The patient reports that the symptoms began about 1 to 2 weeks ago. He denies any use of alcohol or illicit drugs but admits to smoking about half a pack of cigarettes per day.

What information would make you suspect infective endocarditis (IE)?

Does he have any risk factors for IE?

What additional information would you like to know before deciding on an empirical treatment for this patient?

Table 74–1

Etiologic Organisms of IE

| Organism | Percent of Cases | | | | | |
| | Native-Valve IE | | PVE (Indicated in Months After Valve Surgery) | | | IVDU (Right- and Left-Sided) |
	Community Acquired	Health care–Associated	Less Than 2	2–12	Greater Than 12	Total
Streptococci[a]	32	8	1	9	31	12
Enterococci	8	16	8	12	11	9
Staphylococcus aureus	35	44b	22	12	18	57
CNS	4	15	33	32	11	—
HACEK group	3	—	—	—	6	—
Gram-negative bacilli	3	5	13	3	6	7
Fungi (*Candida* spp.)	1	6	8	12	1	4
Polymicrobial/miscellaneous	6	1	3	6	5	7
Culture-negative	5	5	5	6	8	3

CNS, coagulase-negative staphylococci; HACEK, *Haemophilus* spp. (primarily *H. paraphrophilus*, *H. parainfluenzae*, and *H. aphrophilus*), *Actinobacillus actinomycetemcomitans*, *Cardiobacterium hominis*, *Eikenella corrodens*, and *Kingella kingae*.

[a]Includes viridans group streptococci; *S. bovis*; other nongroup A, groupable streptococci; and nutritionally variant streptococci.

[b]Methicillin resistance is common among these *S. aureus* strains.

Modified from Karchmer AW. Infective endocarditis. In: Fauci AS, Braunwald E, Kasper DL, Hauser SL, Longo DL, Jameson JL, Loscalzo J, eds. Harrison's Principles of Internal Medicine, 17th ed. New York: McGraw Hill, 2008: Chap. 118.

PATHOGENESIS AND PATHOPHYSIOLOGY

❶ *For IE to develop, the occurrence of several factors is required. Typically, there must be an alteration of the endothelial surfaces of the heart valves to allow for organism attachment and colonization.* These alterations may be produced by an inflammatory process such as rheumatic heart disease or by injury from turbulent blood flow. Platelets and fibrin now deposit on the damaged valves, forming a nonbacterial thrombotic endocarditis (NBTE). At this point, bacteria through hematogenous spread (i.e., bacteremia) adhere to and colonize the nidus, forming a vegetation.[8] Further deposits of platelets and fibrin cover the bacteria, providing a protective coating that allows for the development of a suitable environment for continued organism and vegetation progression, often producing an organism density of 10^9 to 10^{10} colony-forming units (CFU) per gram. This sequence of events is summarized in Figure 74–1.

Acquisition of PVE differs in early stages, where direct inoculation may occur during surgery instead of through hematogenous seeding. The prosthetic valve also has a greater propensity for organism colonization than native valves. However, in late PVE, the process of colonization and vegetation formation is similar to native-valve IE, as described earlier.[9]

Classically, vegetations are located on the line along valve closure on the atrial surface of the atrioventricular valves (tricuspid and mitral) or on the ventricular surface of the semilunar valves (pulmonary and aortic) (Fig. 74–2). The vegetations can vary significantly in size ranging from millimeters to several centimeters and may be single or multiple masses. Often, destruction of underlying tissue occurs and may cause perforation of the valve leaflet or rupture of the chordae tendinae, interventricular septum, or papillary muscle. Valve ring abscesses may occur, resulting in fistulas penetrating into the myocardium or pericardial sac, particularly with staphylococcal endocarditis.

Embolic events are also common. Embolization occurs as portions of the friable vegetation break lose and enter the bloodstream. These infected pieces are called *septic emboli*. Pulmonary abscesses are commonly formed as a result of septic emboli from right-sided IE (tricuspid and pulmonary valves). However, left-sided IE (mitral and aortic valves) is more likely to have an embolus travel to any organ system, especially the kidneys, spleen, and brain. Along with emboli, immune complex deposition may occur in organ systems, causing extracardiac manifestations of the disease. This commonly occurs in the kidneys, producing abscesses, infarction, or glomerulonephritis. Immune complexes or emboli also may produce skin manifestations of the disease, as seen with petechiae, Osler's nodes, and Janeway's lesions, or within the eye (e.g., Roth's spots).

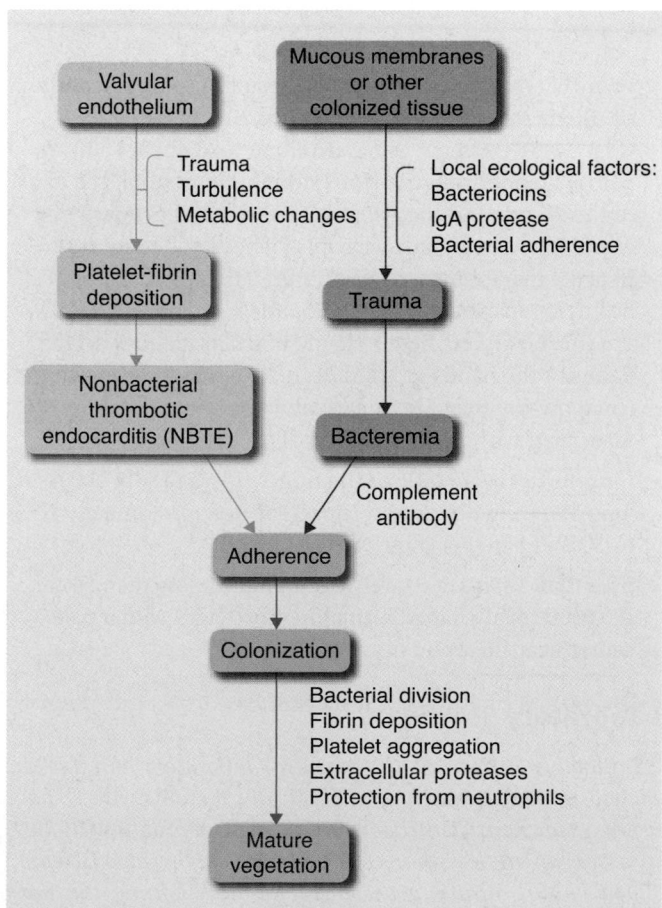

FIGURE 74–1. Pathogenesis of infective endocarditis. (From Ref. 1, Copyright 2005, with permission from Elsevier.)

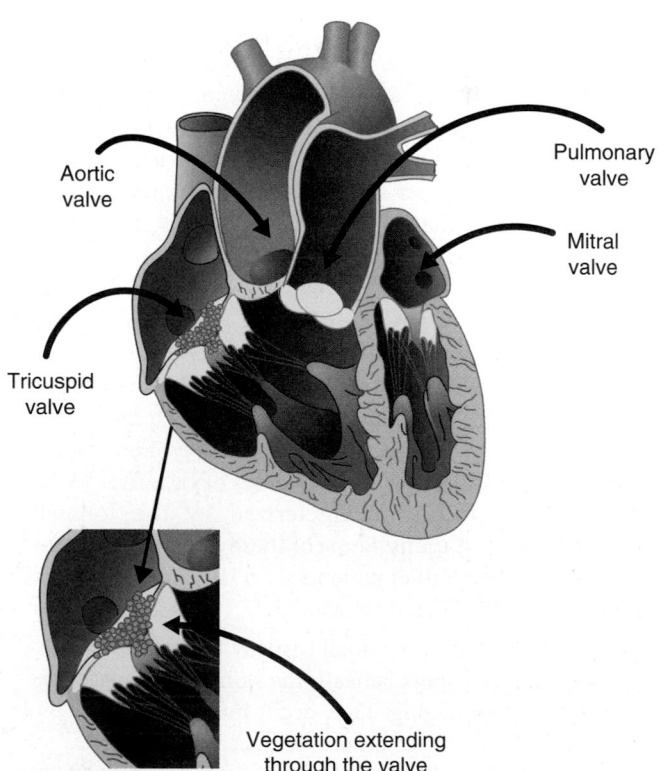

FIGURE 74–2. Diagram of the heart indicating common sites of infection.

Clinical Presentation of IE

General

Patients typically present with nonspecific and variable signs or symptoms.

Symptoms

Complaints from patients may include:
- Fever
- Chills
- Night sweats
- Weakness
- Dyspnea
- Weight loss
- Myalgia or arthralgias

Signs

- Fever is the most common sign of IE
- New or changing heart murmur
- Embolic phenomena (emboli affect the heart, lungs, abdomen, or extremities)
- Skin manifestations (e.g., petechiae, splinter hemorrhages, Osler's nodes, Janeway's lesions)

- Splenomegaly
- Clubbing of extremities

Laboratory Tests

- Blood cultures are the most important laboratory assessment for persistent bacteremia, which occurs commonly in IE. A minimum of three blood culture sets should be collected during the initial 24 hours
- Hematologic tests for anemia (normochromic, normocytic)
- WBC count may be elevated in acute disease but could be normal in subacute IE
- Nonspecific findings such as thrombocytopenia, elevated erythrocyte sedimentation rate or C-reactive protein, and abnormal urinalysis (i.e., proteinuria or microscopic hematuria)

Other Diagnostic Tests

An echocardiogram (TTE or TEE) should be performed on any patient with suspected IE to detect the presence of vegetations.

CLINICAL PRESENTATION AND DIAGNOSIS

The clinical presentation for IE is quite variable and often nonspecific. ❷ *A fever is the most frequent and persistent symptom in patients but may be blunted with previous antibiotic use, congestive heart failure, chronic liver or renal failure, or infection caused by a less virulent organism (i.e., subacute disease).*[3] Other signs and symptoms that also may occur are listed in the Clinical Presentation box with some discussed further in detail below.

Heart murmurs are heard frequently on auscultation (over 85% of cases), but a new murmur or change in murmurs is only found in 5% to 10% or 3% to 5%, respectively.[1] Additionally, over 90% of patients who have a new murmur will develop congestive heart failure, which is a major cause of morbidity and mortality. Splenomegaly and mycotic aneurysms are also noted in many cases of IE.

This disease is also characterized by the following peripheral manifestations. Some of these clinical findings are found in up to one-half of patients with IE, although recently the prevalence has been decreasing.[10]

- Skin: *Petechiae* are very small (usually less than 3 mm) pinpoint flat red spots beneath the skin surface caused by microhemorrhaging. They occur in 20% to 40% of chronic IE, often found on the buccal mucosa, conjunctivae (Fig. 74–3A), and extremities.[1] *Splinter hemorrhages* appear as small dark streaks beneath the finger- or toenails and occur most commonly proximally

with IE, typically occurring as a result of local vasculitis or microemboli occurring in about 20% of patients (Fig. 74–3B). *Osler's nodes* are small (usually 2–15 mm), painful, tender subcutaneous nodules located on the pads of the fingers and toes (Fig. 74–3D) caused primarily by either septic emboli or vasculitis. These nodes are rare in acute disease but are also nonspecific for IE despite occurring in 10% to 25% of all patients.[1] *Janeway's lesions* are small, painless hemorrhagic macular plaques on the palms of the hands or soles of the feet due to septic emboli (in approximately 5% of patients) and more commonly associated with acute *S. aureus* IE (Fig. 74–3E).
- Extremities: *Clubbing* of the finger tips typically occurs in long-standing illness and is present in approximately 10% to 20% of patients (Fig. 74–3C).[1]
- Eye: *Roth's spots* are rarely occurring (in less than 5% of IE cases), oval-shaped retinal hemorrhages with a pale center near the optic disc (Fig. 74–3F).

Laboratory Studies

❸ *Blood cultures are the essential laboratory test for the diagnosis and treatment of IE. Typically, patients with IE have a low-grade consistent bacteremia, with approximately 80% of cases having less than 100 CFU/mL in the bloodstream.*[1] *Blood culture results are critical for determining the most appropriate therapy.* Three blood culture sets should be drawn within the initial 24 hours to determine the etiologic agent. Approximately 90% of the first two cultures will yield

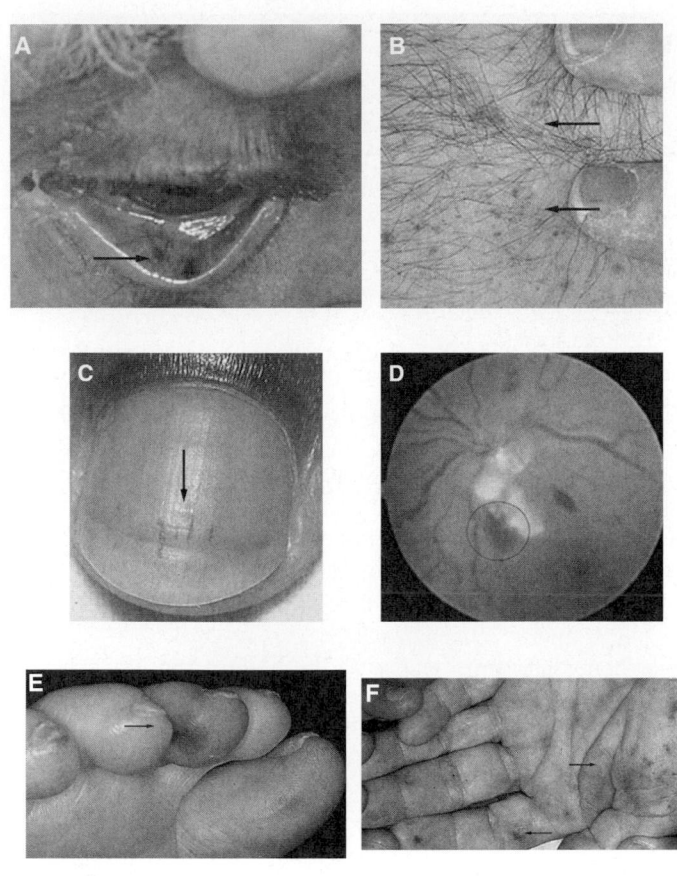

FIGURE 74–3. **A.** Conjunctival petechiae. (From Wolff K, Johnson RA, Suurmond D. In: Fitzpatrick's Color Atlas & Synopsis of Clinical Dermatology, 5th ed. New York: McGraw Hill. Copyright 2005.) **B.** Splinter hemorrhage. (From Collins SP. In: Atlas of Emergency Medicine, 2nd ed. New York: McGraw Hill. Copyright 2002.) **C.** Clubbing of finger. (From Tosti A, Piraccini BM. In: Fitzpatrick's Dermatology in General Medicine, 7th ed. New York: McGraw Hill. Copyright 2007.) **D.** Osler's nodes. (From Collins SP. In: Atlas of Emergency Medicine, 2nd ed. New York: McGraw Hill. Copyright 2002.) **E.** Janeway's lesions. (From Wolff K, Johnson RA, Suurmond D. In: Fitzpatrick's Color Atlas & Synopsis of Clinical Dermatology, 5th ed. New York: McGraw Hill. Copyright 2005.) **F.** Roth's spots (From Effron D, Forcier BC, Wyszynski RE. In: Atlas of Emergency Medicine, 2nd ed. New York: McGraw Hill. Copyright 2002.)

a positive result. If a positive blood culture is not obtained from a patient with suspected IE, the microbiology laboratory should be notified and cultures requested to be monitored for growth of fastidious organisms for up to 1 month.

❹ *Another important tool aiding in the diagnosis of IE is the echocardiogram. This imaging tool is used to visualize vegetations. Two methods of the echocardiogram are used: the transthoracic echocardiogram (TTE) and the transesophageal echocardiogram (TEE).* The TTE has been used since the 1970s; however, it is less sensitive (58–63%) than the TEE (90–100%).[10] Despite the TEE being more sensitive, use of the TTE for patients with suspected native-valve IE is usually

sufficient.[11,12] The TEE may be used as a secondary test for patients whose TTE was negative and in whom a high clinical suspicion of IE exists. Additionally, a TEE is often preferred in patients who have complicated disease, including left-sided IE, prosthetic valves, or perivalvular extension of the vegetation.[2,12] Echocardiograms also may be employed to assess the need for surgical intervention or to determine the possible source of emboli.[11,13]

Additional nonspecific tests for IE may be performed. These include hematologic parameters to determine whether the patient is anemic, which occurs in a majority of patients. The WBCs may be elevated, particularly in acute disease. However, in a subacute infection, the WBCs may be normal. An erythrocyte sedimentation rate (ESR) may also be obtained to determine the presence of inflammation, although this test is highly nonspecific and almost always elevated in IE.

DIAGNOSTIC CRITERIA

● A definitive diagnosis of IE would consist of a biopsy or culture directly from pathologic specimens from the endocardium. However, this would be a highly invasive test. Therefore, diagnosis of IE relies on clinical presentation as well as laboratory and echocardiogram results. To guide this clinical diagnosis, criteria have been established to assess major and minor criteria for IE[14,15] (Table 74–2A). Depending on the number of major or minor criteria a patient demonstrates, he or she will be classified as having a definite, possible, or rejected diagnosis of IE (Table 74–2B).

CAUSATIVE ORGANISMS

● Gram-positive bacteria are the most common organisms that produce IE. Streptococci and staphylococci species account for the majority of cases at more than 80%.[16] *Viridans* group streptococci have been considered the primary pathogens in IE. However, staphylococci have been increasing in prevalence as causative organisms and are the dominant causative organisms in some reports (Table 74–1).[5,17,18] Other gram-positive, gram-negative, atypical, and fungal organisms are less common but still must be considered in certain patient populations.

Streptococci

Streptococci causing IE are most commonly a group of species called *viridans* group streptococci. The most common of this group are *Streptococcus salivarius, Streptococcus mutans, Streptococcus mitus,* and *Streptococcus sanguis.* This group of bacteria, considered normal flora in the human mouth, is α-hemolytic, and typically, most clinical microbiology laboratories do not differentiate the exact species. These organisms may cause bacteremia after dental procedures, which can lead to the development of IE in at-risk patients. *Viridans* group streptococci are also the predominant pathogen of IE associated with mitral valve

---

Table 74–2

Modified Duke's Criteria for IE

2A. Definitions of Modified Duke's Criteria

Major Criteria

Blood culture positive for IE:

Typical microorganisms consistent with IE from two separate blood cultures:

Viridans streptococci, *S. bovis*, HACEK group, *S. aureus*, or community-acquired enterococci in the absence of a primary focus, or

Microorganisms consistent with IE from persistently positive blood cultures, defined as follows:

At least two positive cultures of blood samples drawn greater than 12 hours apart, or

All of three or a majority of four separate cultures of blood (with first and last sample drawn at least 1 hour apart)

Single positive blood culture for *C. burnetii* or antiphase I IgG antibody titer greater than 1:800

Evidence of endocardial involvement:

Echocardiogram positive for IE (TEE recommended in patients with prosthetic valves, rated at least "possible IE" by clinical criteria, or complicated IE [paravalvular abscess] TTE as first test in other patients), defined as follows:

Oscillating intracardiac mass on valve or supporting structures, in the path of regurgitant, or on implanted material in the absence of an alternative anatomic explanation, or

Abscess, or

New partial dehiscence of prosthetic valve

New valvular regurgitation (worsening or changing of pre-existing murmur not sufficient)

Minor Criteria

Predisposition, predisposing heart condition or injection drug use

Fever, temperature greater than 38°C (100.4°F)

Vascular phenomena, major arterial emboli, septic pulmonary infarcts, mycotic aneurysm, intracranial hemorrhage, conjunctival hemorrhages, and Janeway's lesions

Immunologic phenomena: glomerulonephritis, Osler's nodes, Roth's spots, and rheumatoid factor

Microbiological evidence: positive blood culture but does not meet a major criterion as noted above[a] or serological evidence of active infection with organism consistent with IE

2B. Modified Duke's Criteria for the Diagnosis of IE

Definite IE

Pathologic criteria:

(1) Microorganisms demonstrated by culture or histologic examination of a vegetation that has embolized, or an intracardiac abscess specimen, or

(2) Pathologic lesions; vegetation or intracardiac abscess confirmed by histologic examination showing active endocarditis

Clinical criteria[b]:

(1) Two major criteria, or

(2) One major criterion and three minor criteria, or

(3) Five minor criteria

Possible IE

(1) One major criterion and one minor criterion, or

(2) Three minor criteria

Rejected

(1) Firm alternate diagnosis explaining evidence of IE, or

(2) Resolution of IE syndrome with antibiotic therapy for less than or equal to 4 days, or

(3) No pathologic evidence of IE at surgery or autopsy, with antibiotic therapy for less than or equal to 4 days, or

(4) Does not meet criteria for possible IE, as above

CNS, coagulase-negative staphylococci; TEE, transesophageal echocardiography; TTE, transthoracic echocardiography.

[a]Excludes single positive cultures for CNS and organisms that do not cause endocarditis.

[b]See above for definitions of major and minor criteria.

From Ref. 15, with permission. University of Chicago Press, 2000 by the Infectious Diseases Society of America. All rights reserved.

prolapse and native valves and in children.[19,20] Another streptococci species that is commonly associated with IE is *Streptococcus bovis*, classified as group D streptococci, found in the GI tract. However, owing to the similarities of these streptococci, including microbiologic susceptibility, treatment is similar regardless of the species.

IE caused by these streptococci typically has a subacute clinical course. The current cure rate is often over 90% unless complications occur, and they do occur in more than 30% of patients.[20,21] The majority of *viridans* streptococci remain very susceptible to penicillin, with most strains having a minimum inhibitory concentration (MIC) of less than 0.125 mcg/mL.[19,22] Organisms with decreased susceptibilities are increasing. Therefore, antibiotic susceptibilities need to be assessed in order to determine the most appropriate treatment regimen.

Staphylococci

Staphylococcal endocarditis is increasing in prevalence, causing a minimum 30% of all cases of IE, with the majority (80–90%) being due to *S. aureus* (a coagulase-positive staphylococci).[18,23] This increase in staphylococci has been primarily attributed to expanded use of venous catheters, more frequent valve replacement, and increased IVDU.[24] Coagulase-negative staphylococci (CNS) also cause IE; however, these organisms typically infect prosthetic valves or indwelling catheters.[25]

Historically, *S. aureus* was considered community acquired[23]; however, now almost half the cases are nosocomial in origin.[18] Any patient who is bacteremic with *S. aureus* is at an increased risk of developing IE. *S. aureus* also may infect "normal" heart valves (no prior detected valvular disease) in a third of cases.[23,24] Therefore, it is imperative to assess these patients adequately for the presence of vegetations. Any heart valve may be affected; however, when the mitral or aortic valve is involved, it often results in extensive systemic infection with a mortality rate of approximately 20% to 65%.[16,23] When treating *S. aureus* IE, one must consider whether the isolate displays methicillin resistance, the location of the infection (right or left side), presence of prosthetic valves, and history of IVDU. Despite significant resistance to penicillinase-resistant penicillins (e.g., methicillin and nafcillin), most isolates remain susceptible to vancomycin. However, there is an increasing incidence of *S. aureus* intermediately resistant or fully resistant to vancomycin.[26,27] Fortunately, at this point they are not widespread enough to affect empirical antibiotic selection. Susceptibility reports should be assessed to ensure antibiotic activity.

Over the past decade there has been an increasing emergence of community-acquired methicillin-resistant *S. aureus* (CA-MRSA) that differs from health care–associated MRSA. This organism tends to be less resistant to many antibiotics with sensitivity to clindamycin, trimethoprim-sulfamethoxazole (TMP-SMX), and minocycline, as well as vancomycin, linezolid, and daptomycin. However, this organism has a virulence gene (Panton-Valentine leukocidin), which produces a toxin causing necrosis. To date this organism primarily causes skin/skin-structure infections or pneumonias (see skin and soft-tissue infections chapter). There have been a limited number of cases of IE caused by CA-MRSA.[28] If CA-MRSA is suspected, treatment with vancomycin with or without gentamicin and/or rifampin remains the standard of care.

The predominant coagulase-negative organism causing IE has been *S. epidermidis*. However, in the past few years, an increase in isolation of another coagulase-negative species (*S. lugdunensis*) has been noted.[29-31] Typically, coagulase-negative staphylococcal IE has a subacute course with numerous complications. Treatment (with or without surgical intervention) is usually successful. On the other hand, *S. lugdunensis* produces a more virulent infection and, despite similar antibiotic susceptibilities, has a much higher mortality rate.[30-32]

Enterococci

Enterococci are normal flora of the human GI tract and sometimes found in the anterior urethra. Historically, enterococci were considered part of the streptococci genus but now are separated despite similarities, such as group D classification and causing subacute disease. Frequently affected patients are older males who have undergone genitourinary manipulations or younger females who have had obstetric procedures. Although enterococci are a less common cause of IE, there are two predominant species: *Enterococcus faecium* and *Enterococcus faecalis*. *E. faecalis* is the most common and the more susceptible of the strains. However, enterococci overall are more intrinsically resistant, with enterococcal IE representing one of the most problematic gram-positive infections to treat and cure. Frequently, enterococci display resistance to multiple antibiotics, including penicillins, vancomycin, aminoglycosides, and some of the newer agents (e.g., linezolid or quinupristin/dalfopristin).[33]

Gram-Negative Organisms

Gram-negative IE is much less common (approximately 2–5%) but is typically much more difficult to treat than gram-positive infections. Fastidious organisms, such as the HACEK group, tend to be seen most commonly, causing 3% of all IE.[34] This group consists of *Haemophilus* spp. (primarily *H. paraphrophilus*, *H. parainfluenzae*, and *H. aphrophilus*), *Actinobacillus actinomycetemcomitans*, *Cardiobacterium hominis*, *Eikenella corrodens*, and *Kingella kingae*. The clinical presentation of IE by these organisms is subacute, with approximately 50% of patients developing complications. These complications are primarily due to the presence of large, friable vegetations and numerous emboli along with the development of acute congestive heart failure often requiring valve replacement.[35,36] It is important to allow cultures sufficient incubation time (often 2–3 weeks) in order to isolate these organisms. Often these organisms may not be isolated on culture and thus present as culture-negative IE.

Other gram-negative organisms, such as *Pseudomonas* spp., cause IE, especially in IVDUs and patients with prosthetic valves. Additionally, IE may be caused by *Salmonella* spp., *Escherichia coli*, *Citrobacter* spp., *Klebsiella* spp., *Enterobacter* spp., *Serratia marcescens*, *Proteus* spp. and *Providencia* spp.[1,37]

Gram-negative IE typically has a poor prognosis with high mortality rates (as high as 83%).[1] Treatment usually consists of high-dose combination therapy, with valve replacement often a necessity in many patients.

Culture Negative

Negative blood cultures are reported in approximately 5% of confirmed IE cases, often delaying diagnosis and treatment.[3,36,38] Sterile cultures may be the result of previous antibiotic use, subacute right-sided disease, slow growth of fastidious organisms, nonbacterial endocarditis (e.g., fungal or intracellular parasitic infections), noninfective endocarditis, or improper collection of blood cultures. If nonbacterial or fastidious organisms are suspected, additional testing is essential. The choice of treatment regimen depends on patient history and risk factors.

Other Organisms

Numerous bacteria, including gram-positive bacilli, unusual gram-negative bacteria, atypical bacteria, and anaerobes, as well as spirochetes, may cause IE, but these infections are rare.[34] Some of the more common organisms include *Legionella*, *Coxiella burnetii* (Q fever), and *Brucella*. These rare organisms occur primarily in at-risk patients such as those who have a prosthetic valve or are IVDUs. A comprehensive discussion of these organisms is not feasible for this chapter; for further information, other references sources (particularly references 1–5) should be examined. Treatment of these organisms is difficult, and cure rates are low. Therefore, consulting an infectious diseases specialist is warranted.

Fungi

Fungal endocarditis is quite uncommon but has significant mortality, typically affecting patients who have had cardiovascular surgery, received a prolonged course of broad-spectrum antibiotics, have long-term catheter placement, are immunocompromised, or are IVDUs.[10,39] Survival rates have remained poor, at approximately 15%, but improvements (approximately 30%) have been reported owing to advances in diagnosis and treatment.[39] The poor prognosis has been attributed to large vegetations, propensity for organism invasion into the myocardium, extensive septic emboli, poor antifungal penetration into the vegetation, and low toxic-to-therapeutic ratio and lack of cidal activity of certain antifungals.[39,40] The two most commonly associated organisms are *Candida* spp. and *Aspergillus* spp. Lack of clinical studies makes treatment decisions difficult. Typically, combination and/or high-dose therapy in conjunction with surgery is required.

TREATMENT

Therapeutic Considerations

● Treatment of IE often is complicated and difficult. Numerous factors involving the vegetation influence the effectiveness of the antimicrobial agents. The vegetation consists of a fibrin matrix (as discussed earlier) that provides an environment where organisms are relatively free to replicate unimpeded, allowing the microbial density to reach very high concentrations (10^9–10^{10} CFU/g). Once the organism density has reached this level, the organisms are virtually in a static growth phase. These factors hinder host defenses, as well as the ability of antimicrobials to produce sufficient kill. This is seen often with β-lactams and glycopeptides because their effectiveness can be significantly affected by the bacterial inoculum.

❺ *Selection of an appropriate antimicrobial agent must combine characteristics such as the ability to penetrate into the vegetation, the ability to achieve adequate drug concentrations, and the ability to be minimally affected by high bacterial inoculum in order to achieve adequate kill rates.* **❻** *To accomplish this, antimicrobials typically have to be given parenterally at high doses with an extended treatment course of 4 to 6 weeks (in most cases).* Other desirable drug characteristics include bactericidal and synergistic activity.

Empirical Therapy

● **❼** *The overall goal of therapy is to eradicate the infection and minimize/prevent any complications.* Patients with suspected IE should be evaluated for risk factors that may provide some indication as to the most likely organism causing the infection. If no risk factors can be determined, empirical therapy should primarily cover gram-positive organisms. Generally, if streptococci are suspected, empirical treatment should consist of penicillin plus gentamicin. However, if staphylococci or enterococci are suspected, empirical treatment should consist of vancomycin plus gentamicin. It is important to monitor the patient's response to therapy closely until cultures and susceptibilities are determined to ensure adequate treatment.

Specific Therapy

● The American Heart Association (AHA) has published guidelines for the management of IE, including specific treatment recommendations.[5] A summary of these treatments for the most common organisms (streptococci, staphylococci, and enterococci) is provided in Tables 74–3 through 74–6. However, for more detailed information (including dosing, length of treatment, etc.) for these organisms or less common organisms, refer to the complete guidelines.[5] These guidelines include primary and alternative regimens, as indicated in the treatment tables under strength of recommendation.

▶ *Streptococci*

Most isolates are highly susceptible to penicillin; therefore, penicillin G remains the regimen of choice. However, ceftriaxone

Patient Encounter, Part 2: Medical History, Physical Examination, and Diagnostic Tests

PMH: Type II diabetes mellitus since age 48; admits that his diet prevents his diabetes from being well controlled; coronary artery disease; cardiac pacemaker since 1998

FH: Father had a history of diabetes and died at age 72 with end-stage renal disease; mother died at age 75 from complications of a broken hip

SH: Smokes about half a pack of cigarettes per day. Initially denied use of alcohol of illicit drugs—now states that he has used illicit IV drugs in the past

Meds: Metformin 850 mg orally three times daily; sotalol 80 mg orally twice daily

Allergies: NKDA

ROS: Recent weight loss of 2.3 kg (5 lb), decreased appetite, significant fatigue × 2 weeks

PE:

VS: BP 168/89 mm Hg, P 88 bpm, RR 19 breaths per minute, T 38.5°C (101.3°F)

CV: Slight tachycardia, positive murmur

Abd: Obese, soft, nontender, nondistended; (+) bowel sounds

Labs: Within normal limits, except WBC = $16.4 \times 10^3/mm^3$ $(16.4 \times 10^9/L)$

Four sets of blood cultures were drawn. Two sets were drawn on admission and two sets were drawn about 12 hours later when the patient spiked a fever. Results are pending.

Diagnostic Tests

A transthoracic echocardiogram (TTE) has been ordered. Results are pending.

Given this additional information, what is your assessment of the patient's condition?

Identify your empirical treatment recommendations for this patient.

What other information would be beneficial to obtain?

Patient Encounter, Part 3: Additional Laboratory and Diagnostic Tests

Blood Cultures: All cultures are positive for viridans group streptococci.

Labs: Within normal limits

Echo: 3-mm vegetation on the tricuspid valve

Given this additional information, are there any changes in your assessment of the patient?

How would you tailor your treatment based on these new data?

What would be your treatment goals, including length of treatment?

What other information would be beneficial to have?

may be used as an alternative agent if the patient is allergic or resistance is suspected to penicillin. Typically, the length of treatment is 4 weeks and remains the most common regimen. However, a shorter course (i.e., 2 weeks) may be employed for a patient with uncomplicated IE due to highly penicillin-susceptible strains with no extracardiac infection or whose creatinine clearance is greater than 20 mL/min. If the shorter length of therapy is chosen, gentamicin should be added to the previous regimens for the entire course (i.e., 2 weeks). Recommended therapies for highly penicillin-susceptible *viridans* streptococci are summarized in Table 74–3.

As penicillin MICs increase (greater than 0.12 mcg/mL but less than or equal to 0.5 mcg/mL) for *viridans* group streptococci, treatment doses are increased, and 4 weeks of treatment is suggested. In addition, combination therapy with gentamicin is recommended during the first 2 weeks.

In patients who are allergic or intolerant to either of the β-lactams, vancomycin is an alternative treatment option. Additionally, in patients with resistant strains of *viridans* group streptococci (MIC greater than 0.5 mcg/mL), treatment should employ antimicrobial agents for enterococcal IE (precise agents determined by the susceptibility report).

Patients with PVE caused by penicillin-susceptible strains of *viridans* streptococci require treatment for 6 weeks with penicillin G or ceftriaxone with or without gentamicin during the initial 2 weeks of therapy. However, if the organism demonstrates less susceptibility to penicillin (MIC greater than 0.12 mcg/mL), a combination therapy with penicillin G or ceftriaxone plus gentamicin should be given for the entire 6 weeks. Vancomycin remains the primary alternative if the patient is allergic to β-lactams (e.g., penicillins, cephalosporins, etc.).

▶ *Staphylococci*

It is important to determine (a) whether the isolate is methicillin-susceptible or methicillin-resistant and (b) whether the patient has a prosthetic valve. For patients with no prosthetic material, methicillin-susceptible staphylococci treatment should consist of a penicillinase-resistant penicillin (e.g., nafcillin or oxacillin) with or without gentamicin, and for methicillin-resistant strains, therapy should consist of vancomycin (see Table 74–4). Combination therapy with aminoglycosides, when used in these patients, typically is given only during the first 3 to 5 days of therapy. In the absence of prosthetic material, some treatment guidelines do not recommend combination therapy against MRSA. However, many clinicians may combine either gentamicin or rifampin with vancomycin if the patient is unresponsive to monotherapy.

Increasing resistance of staphylococci necessitates the expanded use of alternative therapies. A recent clinical study demonstrated similar activity for daptomycin compared to standard therapy (i.e., penicillinase-resistant penicillin for *methicillin*-sensitive *S. aureus* (MSSA) or vancomycin for MRSA) in staphylococcal IE.[41] The FDA, based on this study, has approved an indication of daptomycin for the treatment of right-sided IE or bacteremia caused by *S. aureus*.

Table 74–3

Therapy of Native-Valve Endocarditis Caused by Highly Penicillin-Susceptible Viridans Group Streptococci and *S. bovis*

Regimen	Dosage[a] and Route	Duration (weeks)	Strength of Recommendation[b]	Comments
Aqueous crystalline penicillin G sodium *OR*	12–18 million units/24 hours (IV either continuously or in 4 or 6 equally divided doses	4	IA	Preferred in most patients 65 years of age or older or patients with impairment of eighth cranial nerve function or renal function
ceftriaxone sodium	2 g/24 hours IV/IM in 1 dose *Pediatric dose[c]*: penicillin 200,000 units/kg per 24 hours IV in 4–6 equally divided doses; ceftriaxone 100 mg/kg per 24 hours IV/IM in 1 dose	4	IA	
Aqueous crystalline penicillin G sodium *OR* ceftriaxone plus gentamicin sulfate[d]	12–18 million units/24 hours IV either continuously or in 6 equally divided doses 2 g/24 hours IV/IM in 1 dose 3 mg/kg per 24 hours IV/IM in 1 dose *Pediatric dose*: penicillin 200,000 units/kg per 24 hours IV in 4–6 equally divided doses; ceftriaxone 100 mg/kg per 24 hours IV/IM in 1 dose; gentamicin 3 mg/kg per 24 hours IV/IM in 1 dose or 3 equally divided doses[f]	2	IB	2-week regimen not intended for patients with cardiac or extracardiac abscess or for those with creatinine clearance of less than 20 mL/min, impaired eighth cranial nerve function, or *Abiotrophia*, *Granulicatella*, or *Gemella* spp. infection; gentamicin dosage should be adjusted to achieve peak serum concentration of 3–4 mcg/mL (6.3–8.4 µmol/L) and trough serum concentration of less than 1 mcg/mL (2.1 µmol/L) when 3 divided doses are used; nomogram used for single daily dosing[e]
Vancomycin hydrochloride[g]	30 mg/kg per 24 hours IV in 2 equally divided doses not to exceed 2 g/24 hours unless concentrations in serum are inappropriately low *Pediatric dose*: 40 mg/kg per 24 hours IV in 2–3 equally divided doses MIC less than or equal to 0.12 mcg/mL	4	IB	Vancomycin therapy recommended only for patients unable to tolerate penicillin or ceftriaxone; vancomycin dosage should be adjusted to obtain peak (1 hour after infusion completed) serum concentration of 30–35 mcg/mL (21–24 µmol/L) and a trough concentration range of 10–15 mcg/mL (6.9–10 µmol/L)

IV, intravenously; IM, intramuscularly; MIC, minimum inhibitory concentration.

[a]Dosage recommended are for patients with normal renal function.

[b]IA, condition with evidence and/or general agreement that a procedure or treatment is useful and effective, based on data from multiple randomized clinical trials; IB, condition with evidence and/or general agreement that a procedure or treatment is useful and effective-based on data from a single randomized trial or nonrandomized studies.

[c]Pediatric dose should not exceed that of a normal adult.

[d]Other potentially nephrotoxic drugs (e.g., nonsteroidal anti-inflammatory drugs) should be used with caution in patients receiving gentamicin therapy.

[e]See Nicolau DP, Freeman CD, Belliveau PB, et al. Experience with a once-daily aminoglycoside program administered to 2184 adult patients. Antimicrob Agents Chemother 1995;39:650–655.

[f]Data for once-daily dosing of aminoglycosides for children exist, but no data for treatment of IE exist.

[g]Vancomycin dosages should be infused during course of at least 1 hour to reduce risk of histamine-release "red man" syndrome.

From Ref. 5.

Table 74–4

Therapy for Endocarditis Caused by Staphylococci in the Absence of Prosthetic Materials

Regimen	Dosage[a] and Route	Duration (weeks)	Strength of Recommendation[b]	Comments
Oxacillin-Susceptible Strains				
Nafcillin or oxacillin[c]	12 g/24 hours IV in 4–6 equally divided doses	6	IA	For complicated right-sided IE and for left-sided IE, 6-week treatment; for uncomplicated right-sided IE, 2-week treatment
with optional addition of gentamicin sulfate[d]	3 mg/kg per 24 hours IV/IM in 2 or 3 equally divided doses *Pediatric dose[e]*: nafcillin or oxacillin 200 mg/kg per 24 hours IV in 4–6 equally divided doses; gentamicin 3 mg/kg per 24 hours IV/IM in 3 equally divided doses	3–5 days		Clinical benefit of aminoglycosides has not been established
For penicillin-allergic (nonanaphylactoid type) patients: cefazolin	6 g/24 hours IV in 3 equally divided doses	6	IB	Consider skin testing for oxacillin-susceptible staphylococci and questionable history of immediate-type hypersensitivity to penicillin; cephalosporins should be avoided in patients with anaphylactoid-type hypersensitivity to β-lactams; vancomycin should be used in these cases[e]
with optional addition of gentamicin sulfate	3 mg/kg per 24 hours IV/IM in 2 or 3 equally divided doses *Pediatric dose*: cefazolin 100 mg/kg per 24 hours IV in 3 equally divided doses; gentamicin 3 mg/kg per 24 hours IV/IM in 3 equally divided doses	3–5 days		Clinical benefit of aminoglycosides has not been established
Oxacillin-Resistant Strains				
Vancomycin hydrochloride[f]	30 mg/kg per 24 hours IV in 2 equally divided doses *Pediatric dose*: 40 mg/kg per 24 hours IV in 2–3 equally divided doses	6	IB	Adjust vancomycin dosage to achieve 1 hour (peak) serum concentration of 30–45 mcg/mL (21–31 μmol/L) and trough concentration of 10–15 mcg/mL (6.9–10 μmol/L) (see text for vancomycin alternatives)

MIC, minimum inhibitory concentration.

[a]Dosages recommended are for patients with normal renal function.

[b]IA, condition with evidence and/or general agreement that a procedure or treatment is useful and effective, based on data from multiple randomized clinical trails; IB, condition with evidence and/or general agreement that a procedure or treatment is useful and effective, based on data from a single randomized trial or nonrandomized studies.

[c]Penicillin G 24 million units/24 hours IV in 4 to 6 equally divided doses may be used in place of nafcillin or oxacillin if strain is penicillin-susceptible (MIC less than or equal to 0.1 mcg/mL) and does not produce β-lactamase.

[d]Gentamicin should be administered in close temporal proximity to vancomycin, nafcillin, or oxacillin dosing.

[e]Pediatric dose should not exceed that of a normal adult.

[f]For specific dosing adjustment and issues concerning vancomycin, see Table 74–3 footnotes.

From Ref. 5.

Table 74–5

Therapy for PVE Caused by Staphylococci

Regimen	Dosage[a] and Route	Duration (weeks)	Strength of Recommendation[b]	Comments
Oxacillin-Susceptible Strains				
Nafcillin or oxacillin	12 g/24 hours IV in 4–6 equally divided doses	6 weeks or longer	IB	Penicillin G 24 million units/24 hours IV in 4 to 6 equally divided doses may be used in place of nafcillin or oxacillin if strain is penicillin-susceptible (MIC less than or equal to 0.1 mcg/mL) and does not produce β-lactamase; vancomycin should be used in patients with immediate-type hypersensitivity reactions to β-lactam antibiotics (see Table 74–3 for dosing guidelines); cefazolin may be substituted for nafcillin or oxacillin in patients with nonimmediate-type hypersensitivity reactions to penicillins
plus rifampin	900 mg per 24 hours IV/orally in 3 equally divided doses	6 weeks or longer		
plus gentamicin sulfate[c]	3 mg/kg per 24 hours IV/IM in 2 or 3 equally divided doses	2		
	Pediatric dose[d]: nafcillin or oxacillin 200 mg/kg per 24 hours IV in 4–6 equally divided doses; rifampin 20 mg/kg per 24 hours IV/oral doses; in 3 equally divided doses; gentamicin 3 mg/kg per 24 hours in 3 equally divided doses			
Oxacillin-Resistant Strains				
Vancomycin hydrochloride	30 mg/kg per 24 hours IV in 2 equally divided doses	6 weeks or longer	IB	Adjust vancomycin to achieve 1 hour (peak) serum concentration of 30–45 mcg/mL (21–31 µmol/L) and trough concentration of 10–15 mcg/mL (6.9–10 µmol/L)
plus rifampin	900 mg/24 hours IV/oral in 3 equally divided doses	6 weeks or longer		
plus gentamicin sulfate	3 mg/kg per 24 hours IV/IM in 2 or 3 equally divided doses	2		
	Pediatric dose: vancomycin 40 mg/kg per 24 hours IV in 2 or 3 equally divided doses; rifampin 20 mg/kg per 24 hours IV/oral in 3 equally divided doses (up to adult dose); gentamicin 3 mg/kg per 24 hours IV/IM in 3 equally divided doses			

[a]Dosages recommended are for patients with normal renal function.

[b]IB, condition with evidence and/or general agreement that a procedure or treatment is useful and effective, based on data from a single randomized trial or nonrandomized studies.

[c]Gentamicin should be administered in close proximity to vancomycin, nafcillin, or oxacillin dosing.

[d]Pediatric dose should not exceed that of a normal adult.

Reproduced, with permission, from Ref. 5.

Recommended dosing for these indications are 6 mg/kg/day (unless renal adjustments are necessary).[41] This study along with another retrospective study reported daptomycin safe and well tolerated.[41,42] Additionally, other antibiotics, such as linezolid and quinupristin/dalfopristin, have been used in patients who were unresponsive to standard therapy, although they have had variable response rates.[43–45] These therapies often are reserved for patients who have been unresponsive

to traditional therapy (e.g., β-lactams or vancomycin) or for organisms that remain susceptible to these agents when resistant to traditional therapy.

For staphylococcal PVE, treatment length increases significantly, typically requiring a minimum of 6 weeks (see Table 74–5). For MSSA, a penicillinase-resistant penicillin is still employed, as well as vancomycin for MRSA. However, with either regimen, the addition of both gentamicin for first

Table 74-6

Therapy for Native-Valve or Prosthetic-Valve Enterococcal Endocarditis Caused by Strains Susceptible to Penicillin, Gentamicin, and Vancomycin

Regimen	Dosage[a] and Route	Duration (weeks)	Strength of Recommendation[b]	Comments
Ampicillin sodium *or*	12 g/24 hours IV in 6 divided doses	4–6	IA	Native valve: 4-week therapy recommended for patients with symptoms of illness less than or equal to 3 months; 6-week therapy recommended for patients with symptoms greater than 3 months
Aqueous crystalline penicillin G sodium	18–30 million units/24 hours IV either continuously or in 6 equally divided doses	4–6	IA	Prosthetic valve or other prosthetic cardiac material: minimum of 6 weeks of therapy recommended
plus gentamicin sulfate[c]	3 mg/kg per 24 hours IV/IM in 3 equally divided doses	4–6		
	Pediatric dose[d]: ampicillin 300 mg/kg per 24 hours IV in 4–6 equally divided doses; penicillin 300,000 units/kg per 24 hours IV in 4–6 equally divided doses; gentamicin 3 mg/kg per 24 hours IV/IM in 3 equally divided doses			
Vancomycin hydrochloride[e]	30 mg/kg per 24 hours IV in 2 equally divided doses	6	IB	Vancomycin therapy recommended only for patients unable to tolerate penicillin or ampicillin
plus gentamicin sulfate	3 mg/kg per 24 hours IV/IM in 3 equally divided doses	6		6 weeks of vancomycin therapy recommended because of decreased activity against enterococci
	Pediatric dose: vancomycin 40 mg/kg per 24 hours IV in 2 or 3 equally divided doses; gentamicin 3 mg/kg per 24 hours IV/IM in 3 equally divided doses			

[a]Dosages recommended are for patients with normal renal function.

[b]IA, condition with evidence and/or general agreement that a procedure or treatment is useful and effective, based on data from multiple randomized clinical trials; IB, condition with evidence and/or general agreement that a procedure or treatment is useful and effective, based on data from a single randomized trial or nonrandomized studies.

[c]Dosage of gentamicin should be adjusted to achieve peak serum concentration of 3 to 4 mcg/mL (6.3–8.4 μmol/L) and a trough concentration of less than 1 mcg/mL (2.1 μmol/L). Patients with a creatinine clearance of less than 50 mL/min should be treated in consultation with an infectious diseases specialist.

[d]Pediatric dose should not exceed that of a normal adult.

[e]See Table 74–3 for appropriate dosage of vancomycin.

From Ref. 5.

2 weeks and rifampin for the entire length of treatment is recommended.

▶ *Enterococci*

For enterococci, it is imperative to determine species and antibiotic susceptibilities. If the organism is susceptible to penicillin and vancomycin, treatment may consist of high-dose penicillin G, ampicillin, or vancomycin plus gentamicin

(see Table 74–6). Treatment length is usually 4 to 6 weeks, with the aminoglycoside used over the entire course. As resistance develops to penicillin, ampicillin and vancomycin remain treatment options. Once the isolate becomes resistant to ampicillin, vancomycin is considered the treatment of choice.

If the isolate is determined to be vancomycin-resistant, it is most important to know the exact species because some of the treatment options, such as quinupristin/dalfopristin, are not active against *E. faecalis*. Currently, the treatment options for vancomycin-resistant enterococci (VRE) are not well established by clinical studies or patient experience. The treatment recommendations for vancomycin-resistant *E. faecium* include linezolid or quinupristin/dalfopristin for a minimum of 8 weeks. However, newer agents, such as daptomycin, may provide another option for treatment for either enterococci species (*E. faecium* and *E. faecalis*). Additionally, guidelines suggest the use of imipenem-cilastatin plus ampicillin or ceftriaxone plus ampicillin for the treatment of *E. faecalis* with a minimum of 8 weeks of therapy. Consultation with an infectious diseases specialist is recommended.

▶ Gram-Negative Organisms

Identification of the exact isolate is crucial in gram-negative IE because treatment decisions depend on which organism is isolated. Therapy is usually targeted to the most susceptible antibiotics. Combination therapy (usually the addition of an aminoglycoside) is commonly used. For example, *Pseudomonas* spp. are treated with an antipseudomonal (e.g., piperacillin, cefepime, imipenem, etc.) plus high-dose aminoglycoside (typically tobramycin 8 mg/kg/day). However, exact dosing of antibiotics depends on the organism isolated. Length of treatment is usually a minimum of 6 weeks.

▶ HACEK Group

The HACEK group is difficult to isolate, often taking weeks for identification. If one of these organisms is suspected (e.g., subacute disease, embolism, large vegetations, etc.), it is important to initiate appropriate empirical treatment. The preferred regimen is ceftriaxone (or another third- or fourth-generation cephalosporin), followed by ampicillin-sulbactam. However, for patients who are intolerant of these treatments, ciprofloxacin may be used. The length of treatment typically is 4 weeks for these organisms.

▶ Culture-Negative

Treatment for culture-negative IE presents a significant dilemma. Therapeutic regimens are guided by specific isolated organisms. When cultures fail to identify a specific organism, decisions regarding treatment should cover the most common causative organisms. If the patient is unresponsive to this initial treatment, then additional coverage for less common organisms is warranted. An infectious diseases specialist should be consulted for managing a patient with this type of infection.

▶ Fungi

Treatment of fungal IE is exceptionally difficult. There is a significant lack of studies to identify and recommend the most appropriate therapy. Currently, amphotericin B is the most common treatment. However, valve replacement surgery is often considered an adjunct therapy. IV antifungal therapy requires high doses for a minimum of 8 weeks of treatment. Oral azoles (e.g., fluconazole) are used as long-term suppressive therapy to prevent relapse. The exact role of some of the newer antifungals (e.g., voriconazole and caspofungin) is unknown, but they should provide a viable option.[46,47]

Surgery

Surgical intervention has become an integral therapy in combination with pharmacologic management of IE. Valve replacement is the predominant intervention, and it is used in a minimum of 25% for all cases of IE.[1] Surgery may be indicated if the patient has unresolved infection, ineffective antimicrobial therapy (often associated with fungal IE), more than one episode of serious emboli, refractory congestive heart failure, significant valvular dysfunction, a mycotic aneurysm requiring resection, local complications (perivalvular or myocardial abscesses), or a prosthetic-valve infection associated with a pathogen that demonstrates higher antimicrobial resistance (e.g., staphylococci, gram-negative organisms, and fungi).[40,48,49] Often a patient's hemodynamic status (i.e., blood pressure, heart rate, pulmonary artery pressure, etc.) is used to determine when surgical intervention is warranted.[50] Despite appropriate medical management and cure, a significant number of people who develop native-valve endocarditis require valve replacement surgery. Involvement of the aorta is considered an indication for surgery in over 70% of patients with PVE.[50]

Dosing Considerations

The majority of antibiotic and antifungal agents used for the treatment of IE require dosing modifications based on renal or hepatic function. However, the most closely monitored is vancomycin and aminoglycosides. This is due in part because (a) therapeutic levels are normally monitored, and (b) the increased likelihood of developing toxicities (i.e., nephrotoxicity) if the level is too high or adverse outcomes (i.e., clinical failure or resistance development) if level is too low. General dosing considerations are included in Table 74–7 for the most commonly used drugs for treating IE. However, specific dosing adjustments for individual patients should be determined by referring to an appropriate drug dosing reference.

Patient Encounter, Part 4: Additional Laboratory

Susceptibility Report

Drug:	Penicillin	Ceftriaxone	Vancomycin
MIC (mcg/mL):	0.25	0.125	Less than 1

Given this additional information, are there any changes in your assessment of the patient?

Do you need to adjust your treatment regimen based on these data?

Would your treatment goals, particularly length of treatment, change?

Prophylaxis

8 *Certain conditions have been associated more commonly with IE due to pre-existing cardiac disease in the presence of a transient bacteremia. In an effort to prevent the development of IE, prophylactic treatment generally is considered*

Patient Encounter, Part 5: Create a Care Plan

Based on this patient's information, create a care plan for the management of his IE. Be sure to include

(a) a statement regarding treatment requirements and/ or possible problems, (b) goals of therapy, (c) a patient-specific plan, including preventive plans, and (d) a follow-up plan to assess whether the goals have been met and to determine whether the patient experienced any adverse effects.

appropriate for these at-risk patients. Although there are no well-controlled clinical studies of these recommendations, it is thought that if antibiotics are given just prior to a procedure, the number of bacteria may be decreased in the bloodstream and prevent the bacteria from adhering to the valves.

Cardiac conditions in which prophylaxis is reasonable include presence of prosthetic valves or material, prior IE, congenital cardiac disease (specific forms only), cardiac transplant patients with cardiac valvulopathy (Table 74–8).[7] While many patients have other cardiac dysfunction, only patients with these conditions are considered to be at a high risk of developing IE. No prophylaxis is advised in other patients.

Transient bacteria may occur due to many types of dental and surgical procedures. However, the AHA has recently published new guidelines significantly limiting the types of procedures where prophylaxis is appropriate. Only dental procedures involving manipulation of gingival tissue or the periapical region of teeth or perforation of the oral mucosa are considered to increase the likelihood that high-risk patients

Table 74–7

Dosage Considerations for Standard Antibiotics for Treatment of IE[a]

Drug	Renal Adjustments	Hepatic Adjustments	Comments
Penicillin G	Required	None	Extension of dosing interval primarily used for adjustment
Ampicillin	Required	None	Seizures most common AE if dosing not adjusted
Nafcillin	None	Severe (see comment)	Adjustments necessary ONLY if in patients with severe hepatic AND renal impairment
Oxacillin	Severe (see comment)	None	Adjustments for CrCl less than 10 mL/min to lower range of normal dose
Cefazolin	Required	None	Dose and/or dosing interval require adjustment. Based on patient's CrCl
Ceftriaxone	Severe (see comment)	None	Do not exceed 2 g/day if patient has BOTH severe renal AND hepatic impairment
Vancomycin	Required	None	Monitor therapeutic levels to guide dosage adjustments (see treatment guidelines for target ranges)
Gentamicin	Required	None	Used for synergy only with gram-positives. Therapeutic levels vary for gram-negative organisms
			Monitor therapeutic levels to guide dosage adjustments
			(synergy target levels: peak 3 mcg/mL [6.3 μmol/L] and trough less than 1 mcg/mL [2.1 μmol/L])
Rifampin	None	Required	Adjustment based on hepatic dysfunction
Newer and Salvage Drugs			
Daptomycin	Required	None	Adjustment in dosing interval CrCl less than 30 mL/min
			CPK should be monitored prior to and during therapy
Linezolid	None	None	Metabolites may accumulate in severe renal impairment
			Monitor for hematologic AE
			Use in severe hepatic impairment not established
Quinupristin/dalfopristin	None	Possibly	Adjustments suggested based on pharmacokinetic data. However, no specific recommendations are described

AE, adverse event; CPK, creatinine phosphokinase; CrCl, creatinine clearance.

[a]Gram-negative bacteria, fungal or atypical treatments are not listed. It is suggested that an Infectious Diseases Consult be obtained if a patient has IE caused by one of these organisms due to the complexity and difficulty in managing these patients.

Table 74–8

Cardiac Conditions Associated With the Highest Risk of Adverse Outcome From Endocarditis for Which Prophylaxis With Dental Procedures Is Reasonable[a]

Prosthetic cardiac valve or prosthetic material used for cardiac-valve repair

Previous IE

CHD[b]

Unrepaired cyanotic CHD, including palliative shunts and conduits

Completely repaired congenital heart defect with prosthetic material or device, whether placed by surgery or by catheter intervention, during the first 6 months after the procedure[c]

Repaired CHD with residual defects at the site or adjacent to the site of a prosthetic patch or prosthetic device (which inhibit endothelialization)

Cardiac transplantation recipients who develop cardiac valvulopathy

CHD, congenital heart disease.

[a]*All dental procedures* that involve manipulation of gingival tissue or the periapical region of teeth or perforation of the oral mucosa is reasonable to give prophylaxis in the patient conditions listed above.

[b]Except for the conditions listed above, antibiotic prophylaxis is no longer recommended for any other form of CHD.

[c]Prophylaxis is reasonable because endothelialization of prosthetic material occurs within 6 months after the procedure.

From Ref. 7. Copyright 2007, American Heart Association. All rights reserved.

Table 74–9

Prophylactic Regimens for Dental Procedure

Situation	Agent	Regimen: Single Dose 30–60 minutes Before Procedure	
		Adults	Children
Oral	Amoxicillin	2 g	50 mg/kg
Unable to take oral medications	Ampicillin **or** Cefazolin or Ceftriaxone	2 g IM or IV	50 mg/kg IM or IV
Allergic to penicillins or ampicillin—oral	Cephalexin[a,b] **or** Clindamycin **or** Azithromycin **or** Clarithromycin	2 g 600 mg 500 mg	50 mg/kg 20 mg/kg 15 mg/kg
Allergic to penicillins or ampicillin and unable take oral medications	Cefazolin or Ceftriaxone[b] **or** Clindamycin	1g IM or IV 600 mg IM or IV	50 mg/kg IM or IV 20 mg/kg IM or IV

IM, intramuscular; IV, intravenous.

[a]Or other first- or second-generation oral cephalosporin in equivalent adult or pediatric dosage.

[b]Cephalosporins should not be used in an individual with a history of anaphylaxis, angioedema, or urticaria with penicillins or ampicillin.

With permission from Ref. 7. Copyright 2007, American Heart Association. All rights reserved.

---

will develop IE.[7] *Viridans* group streptococci are the primary bacteria targeted for prophylaxis in this circumstance. On the other hand, prophylaxis for GI or genitourinary surgeries primarily targets enterococci.

The AHA guidelines include suggested antibiotic regimens for dental procedures where prophylaxis is warranted.[7] Recommended regimens for dental procedures are listed in Table 74–9. These guidelines recommend a single oral or intramuscular/IV dose initiated shortly before the procedure. The regimen for dental procedures consists primarily of a penicillin as first choice, with a cephalosporin for nonanaphylactic penicillin-allergic patients and clindamycin or a macrolide for penicillin-allergic patients. A second prophylactic dose is not recommended. However, if an infection develops at the procedure site, additional antibiotics (i.e., a therapeutic course) may be required.

OUTCOME EVALUATION

Monitoring for successful therapy is critical in this serious infection to prevent complications, prevent resistance development, and decrease mortality. Routine assessment of clinical signs and symptoms, as well as laboratory tests (i.e., repeat blood cultures), microbiologic testing, and serum drug concentrations (if appropriate), must be performed.

Resolution of signs and symptoms typically occurs within a few days to a week in most cases. Monitor the patient daily for febrile episodes, as well as other vital signs, with expected normal values within 2 to 3 days of initiating antimicrobial therapy.[3] Persistent signs or symptoms could be indicative of inadequate treatment or development of resistance.

Blood cultures are the primary laboratory evaluation to assess response to therapy. Typically, with appropriate treatment, they should become negative within 3 to 7 days. Use subsequent blood cultures if the patient appears not to be responding to therapy or on completing treatment to confirm eradication of infection. Evaluate all susceptibility reports to assess antimicrobial therapy.

Additionally, the patient needs to be counseled on the necessity of prophylactic antibiotics prior to major dental treatments (in appropriate patients) in order to prevent recurrent infections. This is critical in patients with risk factors that predispose them to developing IE, such as prosthetic heart valves, other valvular defects, or previous IE.

Develop a follow-up plan to determine whether the patient has achieved a cure, which includes a clinical evaluation of signs/symptoms, repeat blood cultures, and possibly a repeat echocardiogram. The patient should also be assessed for any adverse events. This should be performed usually within a few weeks after the completion of therapy.

Patient Care and Monitoring

1. Assess the patient's symptoms and/or laboratory results to determine if the empirical therapy is effective. Is the patient's fever resolving? Is the patient's WBC decreasing?

2. Review available microbiologic cultures and sensitivity to assess whether the initial antimicrobial regimen needs to be tailored?

3. Review any additional diagnostic tests to determine if treatment may be needed to prevent/minimize complications (e.g., emboli, congestive heart failure).

4. Evaluate therapeutic serum drug concentrations as appropriate (e.g., vancomycin and gentamicin).

5. Monitor serum creatinine in order to make appropriate renal adjustments of the antimicrobials as necessary.

6. Assess any repeat blood cultures and vital signs to determine continued treatment effectiveness.

7. Evaluate the patient for occurrence of any adverse drug reactions and possible drug allergies and/or drug interactions.

8. Develop a plan if the patient is going to continue therapy at home. Once defervescence has occurred, the patient may complete therapy outside the hospital by receiving the antimicrobials from an outpatient infusion center or through a home health agency.

9. Develop a follow-up plan to assess the resolution of infection once the patient has completed therapy. Assessment of any adverse events also should be conducted at this time.

10. Educate high-risk patients on the importance of taking prophylactic antibiotics prior to having certain dental procedures in an effort to prevent the future development of another infection. Stress the potential complications as well as the morbidity and mortality that are associated with IE and that taking precautions can minimize or prevent them.

Abbreviations Introduced in This Chapter

AHA	American Heart Association
CFU	Colony-forming units
ESR	Erythrocyte sedimentation rate
HACEK	Group of bacteria consisting of *Haemophilus* spp., *Actinobacillus actinomycetemcomitans*, *Cardiobacterium hominis*, *Eikenella corrodens*, and *Kingella kingae*
IE	Infective endocarditis
IVDUs	IV drug users
MIC	Minimum inhibitory concentration

MRSA	Methicillin-resistant *S. aureus*
MSSA	Methicillin-sensitive *S. aureus*
NBTE	Nonbacterial thrombotic endocarditis
PVE	Prosthetic-valve endocarditis
TEE	Transesophageal echocardiogram
TMP-SMX	Trimethoprim-sulfamethoxazole
TTE	Transthoracic echocardiogram
VRE	Vancomycin-resistant enterococci

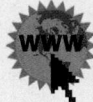 Self-assessment questions and answers are available at *http://www.mhpharmacotherapy.com/pp.html*.

REFERENCES

1. Fowler VG Jr, Scheld WM, Bayer AS. Endocarditis and intravascular infections. In: Mandell GL, Bennett JE, Dolin R, eds. Principles and Practice of Infectious Diseases, 6th ed. Philadelphia: Elsevier, 2005:975–1022.

2. Bayer AS, Bolger AF, Taubert KA, et al. Diagnosis and management of infective endocarditis and its complications. Circulation 1998;98: 2936–2948.

3. Mylonakis E, Calderwood SB. Infective endocarditis in adults. N Engl J Med 2001;345:1318–1320.

4. Habib B. Management of infective endocarditis. Heart 2006;92: 124–130.

5. Baddour LM, Wilson WR, Bayer AS, et al. American Heart Association Scientific Statement. Infective endocarditis: Diagnosis, antimicrobial therapy, and management of complications. Circulation 2005;111: e394–e433.

6. Millar BC, Moore JE. Emerging issues in infective endocarditis. Emerg Infect Dis 2004;10:110–116.

7. Wilson W, Taubert KA, Gewitz M, et al. Prevention of infective endocarditis: Guidelines from the American Heart Association. Circulation 2007;116:1736–1754.

8. Moreillon P, Que Y. Infective endocarditis. Lancet 2004;363:139–149.

9. Baddour LM, Wilson WR. Infections of prosthetic valves and other cardiovascular devices. In: Mandell GL, Bennett JE, Dolin R, eds. Principles and Practice of Infectious Diseases, 6th ed. Philadelphia: Elsevier, 2005:1022–1044.

10. Karchmer AW. Infective endocarditis. In: Braunwald E, ed. Heart Disease: A Textbook of Cardiovascular Medicine, 6th ed. Philadelphia: Saunders, 2001:1723–1748.

11. Cecchi E, Imazio M, Trinchero R. Infective endocarditis: Diagnostic issues and practical clinical approach based on echocardiography. J Cardiovasc Med 2008;9:414–418.

12. Sachdev M, Peterson GE, Jollis JG. Imaging techniques for diagnosis of infective endocarditis. Cardiol Clin 2003;21:185–195.

13. Di Salvo G, Habib G, Pergola V, et al. Echocardiography predicts embolic events in infective endocarditis. J Am Coll Cardiol 2001;37:1069–1076.

14. Durack DT, Lukes AS, Bright DK Duke Endocarditis Service. New criteria for diagnosis of infective endocarditis: Utilization of specific echocardiographic findings. Am J Med 1994;96:200–209.

15. Li JS, Sexton DJ, Mick N, et al. Proposed modifications to the Duke criteria for the diagnosis of infective endocarditis. Clin Infect Dis 2000;30:633–638.

16. Bridger A. Infective endocarditis: New strategies for diagnosis and prophylaxis. JAAPA 2001;14:35–47.

17. Cabell CH, Jollis JG, Peterson GE, et al. Changing patient characteristics and the effect on mortality in endocarditis. Arch Intern Med 2002;162:90–94.

18. Fowler VG Jr., Miro JM, Hoen B, et al. Staphylococcus aureus endocarditis: A consequence of medical progress. JAMA 2005;293:3012–3021.

19. Hoen B. Special issues in the management of infective endocarditis caused by gram-positive cocci. Infect Dis Clin North Am 2002;16:437–452.

20. Ferrieri P, Gewitz MH, Gerber MA, et al. Unique features of infective endocarditis in childhood. Circulation 2002;105:2115–2127.

21. Knoll B, Tleyjeh IM, Steckelberg JM, et al. Infective endocarditis due to penicillin-resistant viridans group streptococci. Clin Infect Dis 2007;44:1585–1592.

22. Upton A, Drinkovic D, Pottumarthy S, et al. Culture results of heart valves resected because of streptococcal endocarditis: Insights into duration of treatment to achieve valve sterilization. J Antimicrob Chemother 2005;55:234–239.

23. Murray RJ. Staphylococcus aureus infective endocarditis: Diagnosis and management guidelines. Intern Med J 2005;35:S25–S44.

24. Petti CA, Fowler VG Jr. Staphylococcus aureus bacteremia and endocarditis. Cardiol Clin 2003;21:219–233.

25. Miele PS, Kogulan PK, Levy CS, et al. Seven cases of surgical native valve endocarditis caused by coagulase-negative staphylococci: An underappreciated disease. Am Heart J 2001;142:571–576.

26. Woods CW, Cheng AC, Fowler VG Jr, et al. Endocarditis caused by Staphylococcus aureus with reduced susceptibility to vancomycin. Clin Infect Dis 2004;38:1188–1191.

27. Centers for Disease Control. Staphylococcus aureus resistant to vancomycin—United States, 2002. MMWR 2002;51:565–567.

28. Millar BC, Prendergast BD, Moore JE. Community-associated MRSA (CA-MRSA): An emerging pathogen in infective endocarditis. J Antimicrob Chemother 2008;61:1–7.

29. Anguera I, Del Rio A, Miro JM, et al. Staphylococcus lugdunensis infective endocarditis: Description of 10 cases and analysis of native valve, prosthetic valve, and pacemaker lead endocarditis clinical profiles. Heart 2005;91:e10.

30. Van Hoovels L, De Munter P, Colaert J, et al. Three cases of destructive native valve endocarditis caused by Staphylococcus lugdunensis. Eur J Clin Microbiol Infect Dis 2005;24:149–152.

31. Frank KL, Luiz del Pozo J, Patel R. From clinical microbiology to infection pathogenesis: How daring to be different works for Staphylococcus lugdunensis. Clin Microbiol Rev 2008;21:111–133.

32. Burgert SJ. Destructive native valve endocarditis caused by Staphylococcus lugdunensis. South Med J 1999;92:812–814.

33. Linden PK. Optimizing therapy for vancomycin-resistant enterococci (VRE). Semin Respir Crit Care Med 2007;28:632–645.

34. Brouqui P, Raoult D. Endocarditis due to rare and fastidious bacteria. Clin Microbiol Rev 2001;14:177–207.

35. Feder HM Jr., Roberts JC, Salazar JC, et al. HACEK endocarditis in infants and children: Two cases and a literature review. Pediatr Infect Dis J 2003;22:557–562.

36. Naber CK, Erbel R. Diagnosis of culture negative endocarditis: Novel strategies to prove the suspect guilty. Heart 2003;89:241–243.

37. Morpeth S, Murdoch D, Cabell CH, et al. Non-HACEK gram-negative bacillus endocarditis. Ann Intern Med 2007;147:829–835.

38. Houpikian P, Raoult D. Blood culture-negative endocarditis in a reference center: Etiologic diagnosis of 348 cases. Medicine 2005;84:162–173.

39. Ellis ME, Al-Abdely H, Sandridge A, et al. Fungal endocarditis: Evidence in the world literature, 1965–1995. Clin Infect Dis 2001;32:50–62.

40. Pierrotti LC, Baddour LM. Fungal endocarditis, 1995–2000. Chest 2002;122:302–310.

41. Fowler V, Boucher HW, Corey GR, et al. Daptomycin versus standard therapy for bacteremia and infective endocarditis caused by Staphylococcus aureus. N Engl J Med 2006;355:653–665.

42. Segreti JA, Crank CW, Finney MS. Daptomycin for the treatment of gram-positive bacteremia and infective endocarditis: A retrospective case series of 31 patients. Pharmacotherapy 2006;26:347–352.

43. Nathani N, Iles P, Elliott TSJ. Successful treatment of MRSA native valve endocarditis with oral linezolid therapy: A case report. J Infect 2005;51:e213–e215.

44. Corne P, Marchandin H, Macia J-C, Jonquet O. Treatment failure of methicillin-resistant Staphylococcus aureus endocarditis with linezolid. Scand J Infect Dis 2005;37:946–949.

45. Drew RH, Perfect JR, Srinath L, et al. Treatment of methicillin-resistant Staphylococcus aureus infections with quinupristin/dalfopristin in patients intolerant of/or failing prior therapy: For the Synercid Emergency-Use Study Group. J Antimicrob Chemother 2000;46:775–784.

46. Rajendram R, Alp NJ, Mitchell AR, et al. Candida prosthetic valve endocarditis cured by caspofungin therapy without valve replacement. Clin Infect Dis 2005;40:e72–e74.

47. Reis LJ, Barton TD, Pochettino A, et al. Successful treatment of Aspergillus prosthetic valve endocarditis with oral voriconazole. Clin Infect Dis 2005;41:752–753.

48. Sohail MR, Martin KR, Wilson WR, et al. Medical versus surgical management of Staphylococcus aureus prosthetic valve endocarditis. Am J Med 2006;119:147–154.

49. Rivas P, Alonso J, Moya J, et al. The impact of hospital-acquired infections on the microbial etiology and prognosis of late-onset prosthetic valve endocarditis. Chest 2005;128:764–771.

50. Akowuah EF, Davies W, Oliver S. Prosthetic valve endocarditis: Early and late outcome following medical or surgical treatment. Heart 2003;89:269–272.

75 Tuberculosis

Charles A. Peloquin and Rocsanna Namdar

LEARNING OBJECTIVES

● **Upon completion of the chapter, the reader will be able to:**

1. Compare the risk for active tuberculosis (TB) disease among patients based on their age, immune status, place of birth, and time since exposure to an active case.

2. Design, evaluate, and assess an appropriate therapeutic plan for an immunocompetent, immunocompromised, pregnant, and pediatric patient with pulmonary TB.

3. Assess the effectiveness of therapy in TB patients.

4. Describe the common and important adverse drug effects caused by TB drugs.

5. Select patients for whom therapeutic drug monitoring (TDM) may be valuable and identify the necessary laboratory monitoring parameters for patients on antituberculosis medications.

6. Design, evaluate, and assess appropriate regimens for the treatment of latent TB infection (LTBI) in all patient populations.

7. Design a therapeutic plan for a patient with TB meningitis or TB osteomyelitis.

KEY CONCEPTS

❶ Tuberculosis (TB) is the most prevalent communicable infectious disease on earth and remains out of control in many developing nations. These nations require medical and financial assistance from developed nations in order to control the spread of TB globally.

❷ In the United States, TB disproportionately affects ethnic minorities as compared with whites, reflecting greater ongoing transmission in ethnic minority communities. Additional TB surveillance and preventive treatment are required within these communities.

❸ Coinfection with HIV and TB accelerates the progression of both diseases, thus requiring rapid diagnosis and treatment of both diseases.

❹ Mycobacteria are slow-growing organisms; in the laboratory, they require special stains, special growth media, and long periods of incubation to isolate and identify.

❺ TB can produce atypical signs and symptoms in infants, the elderly, and immunocompromised hosts, and it can progress rapidly in these patients.

❻ Latent tuberculosis infection (LTBI) can lead to reactivation disease years after the primary infection occurred.

❼ The patient suspected of having active TB disease must be isolated until the diagnosis is confirmed and he or she is no longer contagious. Often, isolation takes place in specialized "negative pressure" hospital rooms to prevent the spread of TB.

❽ Isoniazid and rifampin are the two most important TB drugs; organisms resistant to both these drugs (multidrug resistant tuberculosis [MDR-TB]) are much more difficult to treat.

❾ Never add only a single antituberculosis drug to a failing regimen for active TB!

❿ Directly observed therapy (DOT) should be used whenever possible to reduce treatment failures and the selection of drug-resistant isolates.

Worldwide, tuberculosis (TB) kills about 1.5 million people each year, more than any other infectious organism. TB is caused by *Mycobacterium tuberculosis*, it presents either as latent TB infection (LTBI) or as progressive active disease.[1] The latter typically causes progressive destruction of the lungs, leading to death in most patients who do not receive treatment. Currently, one-third of the world's population is infected, and drug resistance is increasing in many areas.[1]

EPIDEMIOLOGY

❶ *Roughly one of every three people on earth is infected by Mycobacterium tuberculosis.[1-3] The distribution is uneven, with the highest incidences found in southern Asia and sub-Saharan Africa. In the United States, about 13 million people have LTBI, evidenced by a positive skin test (purified protein derivative ([PPD]) but no signs or symptoms of disease.* Such patients have roughly a 1 in 10 chance of active disease during their lives, with the greatest risk in the first 2 years after infection. Active disease occurs in over 13,000 Americans each year, resulting in about 1,500 deaths.[4] (For detailed data analysis, visit the Centers for Disease Control and Prevention [CDC] website at *www.cdc.gov/nchstp/tb.*)

M. tuberculosis is transmitted from person to person by coughing or sneezing.[2,6,18] This produces small particles known as droplet nuclei that float in the air for long periods of time. Each droplet contains one to three organisms. Thirty percent of individuals with prolonged contact with an infectious TB patient become infected.

Risk Factors for Infection

▶ Location and Place of Birth

- California, New York, Florida, and Texas accounted for 48% of all TB cases in 2006, reflecting the high immigration rates into these states.[4] TB is most prevalent in large urban areas, exacerbated by crowding in poor immigrant neighborhoods,
- where 57% of all U.S. cases were found in 2006.[3,4] Mexico, the Philippines, Vietnam, India, China, Haiti, Guatemala, and South Korea account for the largest numbers of these immigrants.[4] Those in close contact with patients with active pulmonary TB are most likely to become infected.[2,3] These include family members, coworkers, or coresidents in places such as prisons, shelters, and nursing homes.

▶ Race, Ethnicity, Age, and Gender

❷ *In the United States, the incidence of TB is more concentrated in nonwhite individuals. In 2007, non-Hispanic blacks accounted for 26% of all TB cases, followed by Hispanics at 29%.[5] Asians and Pacific Islanders accounted for 26%, whereas non-Hispanic whites accounted for only 17% of the new TB cases.[5] TB is most common among people 25 to 44 years of age (32% of all cases), followed by those 45 to 64 years of age (30%) and 65 or more years of age (19%).*

▶ Coinfection With HIV

❸ HIV is the most important risk factor for active TB because the immune deficit prevents patients from containing the initial infection.[2,3,5,6] *Roughly 10% of TB patients in the United States are coinfected with HIV, and roughly 20% of TB patients ages 25 to 44 years are coinfected with HIV.[4,5] Consistent with HIV in general, HIV-associated TB is most common among 25 to 44 year olds. Substance abuse and other risk factors are shared among some TB and HIV-infected individuals, promoting the spread of both diseases.[2,7,8]*

Patient Encounter 1

HPI: AF is a 56-year-old man who presents to the medical clinic complaining of a 1-month history of a persistent cough that has become productive over the past 2 weeks. He also complains of malaise, fever, night sweats, and a 6-kg (13-lb) weight loss over the past 2 months.

PMH: Type II diabetes mellitus (NIDDM)—well controlled; hypertension (HTN) × 5 years—well controlled

FH: Mother and father died in an MVA 10 years ago; one brother, age 54, is HIV positive and lives with the patient; one sister, age 50, is alive and has had breast cancer

SH: Single, one daughter. He works as an undercover agent and just returned from an operation in Cambodia. He denies smoking or IV drug use. He had a 20-year history of alcohol abuse but has been sober for 10 years.

Meds: Lisinopril 20 mg daily; amlodipine 5 mg daily; metformin 500 mg twice daily. Patient reports that he tries to be compliant with his therapies and takes them regularly except when he is unable to get his refills; over the past 2 months, he has gone 3 to 4 days without medication.

Allergies: NKDA

What information is suggestive of TB?

What factors place this patient at increased risk for acquiring TB?

Risk Factors for Disease

- Once infected with *M. tuberculosis*, a person's lifetime risk of active TB is about 10%, with about half this risk evident during the first 2 years after infection.[2,3,6] Young children, the elderly, and immunocompromised patients have greater risks. HIV-infected patients with *M. tuberculosis* infection are roughly 100 times more likely to develop active TB than normal hosts owing to the lack of normal cellular immunity.[3,9]

ETIOLOGY

❹ *Microscopic examination of infected material ("smear") detects about 8 to 10 × 10³ mm³/ organisms of specimen using the older AFB (acid-fast bacillus) stain. The newer auramine-rhodamine fluorsecent technique is one-third more sensitive. A smear-negative patient still can grow M tuberculosis on culture, which is more sensitive than either staining technique. Unfortunately, culture is much slower than staining due to the doubling time of the bacilli of about 20 hours. Further, microscopic examination cannot determine which of over 90 mycobacterial species is present. The usual practice is to assume the worst (TB) until confirmed by genetic probe or positive culture.*

Culture and Susceptibility Testing

Susceptibility testing is essential for directing proper treatment. The most common agar method, known as the *proportion method,* takes many weeks to produce results. The Bactec and newer mycobacterial growth indicator tube (MGIT) systems use liquid media and detect live mycobacteria in about 2 weeks.[1,10,11] Rapid-identification tests include nucleic acid probes and DNA fingerprinting using restriction fragment length polymorphism (RFLP) analysis, and polymerase chain reaction (PCR).[1,6,10,12–14] These tests differentiate among mycobacterial species but currently cannot provide susceptibility data. New tests looking for specific mutations associated with drug resistance may facilitate rapid drug therapy decisions in the future. Nitrate reductase assays and porous ceramic support systems are among other rapid drug susceptibility testing techniques currently being investigated.[15, 16]

PATHOPHYSIOLOGY

Primary Infection

Primary infection usually results from inhaling droplet nuclei that contain *M. tuberculosis.*[2,6,17] The progression to clinical disease depends on three factors: (a) the number of *M. tuberculosis* organisms inhaled (infecting dose), (b) the virulence of these organisms, and (c) the host's cell-mediated immune response.[2,4,6,12,18,19] If pulmonary macrophages inhibit or kill the bacilli, the infection is aborted.[18] If not, *M. tuberculosis* eventually spreads throughout the body through the bloodstream.[2,6,18] *M. tuberculosis* most commonly infects the posterior apical region of the lungs, where conditions are most favorable for its survival.

T lymphocytes become activated over the course of 3 to 4 weeks, producing interferon-γ (IFN-γ) and other cytokines. These stimulate microbicidal macrophages to surround the tuberculous foci and form granulomas to prevent further extension.[18] At this point, the infection is largely under control, and bacillary replication falls off dramatically. Any remaining mycobacteria are believed to reside primarily within granulomas or within macrophages that have avoided detection and lysis. Over 1 to 3 months, tissue hypersensitivity occurs, resulting in a positive tuberculin skin test.[2,6,17] ⑤ *Progressive primary disease occurs in roughly 5% of patients, especially children, the elderly, and immunocompromised patients.*[20,21] *This presents as a progressive pneumonia and frequently spreads, leading to meningitis and other severe forms of TB, even before their skin tests become positive.*[20]

Reactivation Disease

⑥ *About 10% of infected patients develop reactivation TB, with half occurring in the first 2 years after infection.*[2,6,12] Upper lobe pulmonary disease is the most common (85% of cases).[2] Caseating granulomas result from the vigorous immune response, and liquefaction leads to local spread. Eventually, a pulmonary cavity results, and this provides a portal to the outside that allows for person-to-person spread. Bacterial counts in the cavities can be as high as 10^{11}/L of cavitary fluid (10^8/mL).[2,18] Prior to the chemotherapy era, pulmonary TB usually was associated with hypoxia, respiratory acidosis, and eventually death.

Extrapulmonary and Miliary Tuberculosis

Caseating granulomas, regardless of location, can undergo liquefaction, spread tubercle bacilli and cause symptoms.[2,6] Because of muted or altered symptoms, the diagnosis of TB is difficult and often delayed in immunocompromised hosts.[2,3,6] HIV-infected patients may present with only extrapulmonary TB, which is uncommon in HIV-negative persons. A widely disseminated form of the disease called *miliary TB* can occur, particularly in children and immunocompromised hosts, and it can be rapidly fatal.[17] Immediate treatment is required.

Influence of HIV Infection on Pathogenesis

HIV infection is the most important risk factor for active TB.[2,6,17] As CD4+ lymphocytes multiply in response to the mycobacterial infection, HIV multiplies within these cells and selectively destroys them, gradually eliminating the TB-fighting lymphocytes.[17] HIV-infected patients coinfected with TB are at a substantially higher risk of early mortality compared with HIV-negative TB patients.[22,23] Because of the large pill burden, overlapping toxicities, and paradoxical worsening of the TB when TB and HIV treatments are initiated simultaneously, most clinicians elect to begin TB treatment first.[12,24] A reasonable time to begin HIV treatment is after 2 months of TB treatment, although individual circumstances often dictate the exact timing.

CLINICAL PRESENTATION

Fever, night sweats, weight loss, fatigue, and a productive cough are the classic symptoms of TB.[1,2,6,19] Onset may be gradual, and the diagnosis is easily missed if the symptoms are muted, such as in the elderly.[2,6,19] Progressive pulmonary disease leads to cavitation visible on x-ray. Physical examination is nonspecific but may be consistent with pneumonia. Dullness to chest percussion, rales, and increased vocal fremitus may be observed on examination. Laboratory data often are uninformative, but a modest increase in the white blood cell (WBC) count with a lymphocyte predominance can be seen.

Atypical presentations are common in patients coinfected with HIV.[1,2,6,19,25] HIV-positive patients often have negative skin tests and fail to produce cavitary lesions, and fever may be absent. Symptoms for these patients range from classic pulmonary to muted and nonspecific. Extrapulmonary TB typically presents as a slowly progressive decline in organ function, and lymphadenopathy is relatively common.[26,18,19] Abnormal behavior, headaches, or convulsions suggest tuberculous meningitis, although other acute CNS infections must be exlcuded.[6,19]

The Elderly

❺ *Many clinical findings are muted in the elderly or absent altogether, so there can be considerable diagnostic uncertainty. Positive skin tests, fevers, night sweats, sputum production, or hemoptysis may be absent, making TB hard to distinguish from other bacterial or viral infections or chronic lung diseases.*[2,19,26,27] In contrast, mental status changes are twice as common in the elderly, and CNS disease must be considered when TB is entertained. Mortality is six times higher in the elderly in part owing to delays in diagnosis.[2,19,26] Ethnic distributions of disease are different in the elderly and include more white patients because these patients often were infected decades ago, when TB was more prevalent in the United States.

Children

❺ *Because very young children (less than 5 years old) have immature cellular immunity, TB can be particularly dangerous in this population. TB in children may present as a typical bacterial pneumonia, called progressive primary TB, and often involves the lower and middle lobes.*[17,19–21] Dissemination to the lymph nodes, GI and genitourinary tracts, bone marrow, and meninges is fairly common. For these reasons, bacille Calmette-Guérin (BCG) vaccinations are administered in countries where TB remains common. BCG appears to stimulate the children's immune systems just enough to ward off the most serious forms of the disease. However, BCG does not block infection, and these same children often experience reactivation TB as young adults. Because cavitary lung lesions are uncommon, children do not spread TB readily. From the public health perspective, pediatric TB is the clearest indication of recent spread of TB.

DIAGNOSIS

Skin Testing

TB skin testing with the 5-TU strength of Tubersol PPD, also known as the *Mantoux test,* is the preferred method for skin testing.[2,19,22] The product is injected into the skin (not subcutaneously) with a fine (27-gauge) needle and produces a small, raised, blanched wheal to be read by an experienced professional in 48 to 72 hours. Criteria for interpretation are listed in Table 75–1.[1,2,6,19,22] The CDC does not recommend the routine use of anergy panels.[22,28] The "booster effect" occurs in patients who do not respond to an initial skin test but show a positive reaction if retested about a week later.[19,28]

Additional Tests

Morning sputum collections have the highest yield of organisms.[2,10,19] Daily sputum collections over three

---

Table 75–1		
Criteria for Tuberculin Positivity by Risk Group		
Reaction Greater Than or Equal to 5 mm of Induration	**Reaction Greater Than or Equal to 10 mm of Induration**	**Reaction Greater Than or Equal to 15 mm of Induration**
HIV-positive persons	Recent immigrants (i.e., within the last 5 years) from high-prevalence countries	Persons with no risk factors for TB
Recent contacts of TB case patients	Injection drug users	
Fibrotic changes on chest radiograph consistent with prior TB	Residents and employees[b] of the following high-risk congregate settings: prisons and jails, nursing homes and other long-term facilities for the elderly, hospitals and other healthcare facilities, residential facilities for patients with AIDS, and homeless shelters	
Patients with organ transplants and other immunosuppressed patients (receiving the equivalent of greater than or equal to 15 mg/day of prednisone for 1 month or more)[a]	Mycobacteriology laboratory personnel	
	Persons with the following clinical conditions that place them at high risk: silicosis, diabetes mellitus, chronic renal failure, some hematologic disorders (e.g., leukemias and lymphomas), other specific malignancies (e.g., carcinoma of the head or neck and lung), weight loss of greater than or equal to 10% of ideal body weight, gastrectomy, and jejunoileal bypass	
	Children younger than 4 years of age or infants, children, and adolescents exposed to adults at high risk	

[a]Risk of TB in patients treated with corticosteroids increases with higher dose and longer duration.

[b]For persons who are otherwise at low risk and are tested at the start of employment, a reaction of greater than or equal to 15 mm of induration is considered positive.

From Ref. 22.

Patient Encounter 2

PE:

Gen: Thin, emaciated man.

VS: BP 126/78, P 90 bpm, RR 18, T 39.3°C (102.7°F), O_2 sat 82% on room air, wt 51 kg (112 lb)

HEENT: PERRLA; EOMI

Neck: Supple; no lymphadenopathy, bruits, or JVD; no thyromegaly

Chest: Diffuse rhonchi, decreased breath sounds on left

CV: RRR; no murmurs, rubs, gallops

Abd: (+) BS; nontender, nondistended

Neuro: A&O × 3

Laboratory Values (U.S. Units):

Lab	Normal	Lab	Normal
Na 139 mEq/L	135–145 mEq/L	Hgb 13.5 g/dL	13.5–17.5 g/dL
K 3.9 mEq/L	3.5–5 mEq/L	Hct 40%	40–54%
Cl 98 mEq/L	95–105 mEq/L	RBC $4.6 \times 10^6/mm^3$	$4.6–6 \times 10^6/mm^3$
CO_2 38 mEq/L	22–30 mEq/L	WBC $4.5 \times 10^3/mm^3$	$4–10 \times 10^3/mm^3$
BUN 20 mg/dL	5–25 mg/dL	PMN 62%	50–65%
SCr 1.3 mg/dL	0.8–1.3 mg/dL	Lymph 34%	25–35%
Gluc 123 mg/dL	Less than 140 mg/dL	Mono 6%	2–6%
AST 36 IU/L	5–40 international units/L	Other: HIV negative	
ALT 28 IU/L	5–35 international units/L		
Tbili 1 mg/dL	0.1–1.2 mg/dL		
PT 10 second	10–12 second		

Laboratory Values (SI Units)

Lab	Normal	Lab	Normal
Na 139 mmol/L	135–145 mmol/L	Hgb 135 g/L or 0.84 mmol/L	135 – 175 g/L or 0.84–1.08 mmol/L
K 3.9 mmol/L	3.5–5 mmol/L	Hct 0.4 vol fraction	0.4–0.54 vol fraction
Cl 98 mmol/L	95–105 mmol/L	RBC $4.6 \times 10^{12}/L$	$4.6–6.0 \times 10^{12}/L$
CO_2 38 mmol/L	22–30 mmol/L	WBC $4.5 \times 10^9/L$	$4.0–10 \times 10^9/L$
BUN 7.1 mmol/L	1.8–8.9 mmol/L	PMN 62%	50–65%
SCr 115 μmol/L	71–115 μmol/L	Lymph 34%	25–35%
Gluc 6.8 mmol/L	Less than 7.8 mmol/L	Mono 6%	2–6%
AST 0.60 μKat/L	0.08–0.67 μKat/L	Other: HIV negative	
ALT 0.47 μKat/L	0.08–0.58 μKat/L		
Tbili 17 μmol/L	1.7–20.5 μmol/L		
PT 10 second	10–12 second		

CXR: Profound bilateral upper lobe infiltrates with cavitation on left; small left pneumothorax

Clinical Course: The patient was admitted and placed on respiratory isolation. Three separate sputum AFB stain specimens were reported to contain 3+ AFB. A PPD tuberculin skin test was placed. Sputum samples were sent for AFB, fungi, and bacterial cultures and sensitivities. After 48 hours, the PPD skin test was read as a 12-mm area of induration.

Assessment: Active pulmonary TB; pneumothorax; HTN; type II diabetes mellitus

Which signs, symptoms, and other findings are consistent with active TB infection?

consecutive days improve the yield of positive results. Sputum induction with aerosolized hypertonic saline may produce a diagnostic sample in patients unable to produce sputum. Bronchoscopy or aspiration of gastric fluid via a nasogastric tube may be attempted in selected patients, the latter being used more often in children.[19] For patients with suspected extrapulmonary TB, samples of draining fluid, biopsies of the infected site, or both may be attempted. Blood cultures are positive occasionally, especially in AIDS patients who have low CD4 counts.[19,25,29]

Advances in TB diagnosis include methods for rapid identification of patients with suspected TB. Improved smear microscopy, automated liquid cultures, nucleic acid amplification tests, antibody detection tests, antigen detection tests are under development.[30]

Interferon-gamma release assay (IGRA) is a new method for the diagnosis of LTBIs. The main advantage of this assay with respect to tuberculin skin test is the lack of cross-reaction with BCG and most nontuberculous mycobacteria. It also eliminates the need for the patient to return for test reading in 48 to 72 hours. The IGRAs cannot distinguish between latent and active TB and data are lacking in children and HIV-infected individuals.[31–33]

TREATMENT

General Approaches to Treatment

Monotherapy can be used only for infected patients who do not have active TB (LTBI, as shown by a positive skin test in the absence of signs or symptoms of disease). Once active disease is present, a minimum of two drugs and typically *three or four drugs* must be used simultaneously from the outset of treatment.[2,6,12,34] For most patients, the shortest duration of treatment is 6 months, and 2 to 3 years of treatment may be necessary for advanced cases of MDR-TB.[2,6,12,35] DOT is a method used to insure compliance. Patients are directly observed by a health care worker while taking their antituberculosis medication. This is also a cost-effective way to ensure completion of treatment.[2,6,12,34–36]

Nonpharmacologic Therapy

7 *Steps should be taken to: (a) prevent the spread of TB (respiratory isolation); (b) find where TB has already spread (contact investigation); and (c) return the patient to a state of normal weight and well-being.* The older term for TB is *consumption* because wasting was a primary symptom of disease progression in the prechemotherapy era and remains descriptive today. Items 1 and 2 are performed by public health departments. Clinicians involved in the treatment of TB should verify that the local health department has been notified of all new cases of TB. Surgery may be needed to remove destroyed lung tissue, space-occupying infected lesions (tuberculomas), and certain extrapulmonary lesions.[2,12,34]

Pharmacologic Therapy

▶ Treating Latent Tuberculosis Infection (LTBI)

Isoniazid is used for treating LTBI.[2,6,12,34] Typically, isoniazid 300 mg daily (5–10 mg/kg of body weight) is given alone for 9 months. Lower doses usually are less effective.[2,37] The treatment of LTBI reduces a person's lifetime risk of active TB from about 10% to about 1%[22] (Table 75–2). Rifampin 600 mg daily for 4 months can be used when isoniazid resistance is suspected or when the patient cannot tolerate

isoniazid.[2,21,37,38] Rifabutin 300 mg daily might be substituted for rifampin in patients at high risk of drug interactions. A 12-dose, once weekly regimen of isoniazid and rifapentine, a long half-life cyclopentyl-rifampin derivative, is under study. The combination of pyrazinamide and rifampin is no longer recommended because of unacceptable rates of hepatotoxicity.[39] When resistance to isoniazid and rifampin is suspected in the isolate causing infection, there is no regimen proven to be effective.[2,34]

▶ Treating Active Disease

In the United States, all patients diagnosed with TB can receive treatment free of charge through the local health department, and this is encouraged because local health departments generally have the greatest expertise. Treating active TB disease requires combination chemotherapy. Generally, *four drugs* are given at the onset of treatment. **8** *Isoniazid and rifampin should be used together for most cases because they are the best drugs for preventing drug resistance.*[2,6,34,40,41] Drug susceptibility testing should be done on the initial isolate for all patients with active TB and should be used to guide the selection of drugs over the course of treatment.[2,6,12,34] Susceptibility testing may be repeated in cases where the patient remains culture-positive 8 weeks or more into therapy.

8 *The standard TB treatment regimen is isoniazid, rifampin, pyrazinamide, and ethambutol for 2 months, followed by isoniazid and rifampin for 4 months, for a total of 6 months of treatment.*[2,12,34] *Extending treatment to 9 months of isoniazid and rifampin treatment is recommended for patients at greater risk of failure and relapse, including those with cavitation on initial chest radiograph or positive cultures at the completion of the initial 2-month phase of treatment, as well as for patients treated initially without pyrazinamide. Treatment should be continued for at least 6 months from the time that patients convert to a negative smear and culture.*[2,6,12,34] Some authors recommend TDM for such patients because one of the proven reasons for treatment failure is malabsorption of orally administered drugs.[2,34,41,42] Table 75–3 shows the recommmended treatment regimens for TB. When intermittent therapy is used, DOT is essential. Doses missed during an intermittent TB regimen decrease the efficacy of the regimen and increase the relapse rate. Further, outcomes appear to be worse for immunocompromised patients when intermittent treatment, especially twice-weekly treatment, is used. Therefore, HIV-positive TB patients should receive TB drugs at least three times weekly. When the patients' sputum smears convert to negative, the risk of them infecting others is greatly reduced, but it is not zero.[2,15,34] Such patients can be removed from respiratory isolation, but they must be careful not to cough on others and should meet only in well-ventilated places.

Adjustments to the regimen should be made once the susceptibility data are available.[2,12,34] Drug resistance should be expected in patients who have been treated previously for TB. Two or more drugs with in vitro activity against

Table 75–2

Recommended Drug Regimens for Treatment of LTBI in Adults

Drug	Interval and Duration	Comments	Rating[a] HIV–	Evidence HIV+
Isoniazid	Daily for 9 months[c,d]	In HIV infected patients, isoniazid may be administered concurrently with nucleoside reverse transcriptase inhibitors (NRTIs), protease inhibitors, or NNRTIs	A (II)	A (II)
	Twice weekly for 9 months[c,d]	DOT must be used with twice-weekly dosing	B (II)	B (II)
Isoniazid	Daily for 6 months[d]	Not indicated for HIV-infected persons, those with fibrotic lesions on chest radiographs, or children	B (I)	C (I)
	Twice weekly for 6 months[d]	DOT must be used with twice-weekly dosing	B (II)	C (I)
Rifampin	Daily for 4 months	For persons who are contacts of patients with isoniazid-resistant rifampin susceptible TB In HIV infected patients, protease inhibitors or NNRTIs generally should not be administered concurrently with rifampin; rifabutin can be used as an alternative for patients treated with indinavir, nelfinavir, amprenivir, ritonavir, or efavirenz, and possibly with nevirapine or soft-gel saquinavir[e]	B (II)	B (III)

[a]*Strength of recommendation*: A = preferred; B = acceptable alternative; C = offer when A and B cannot be given.

[b]*Quality of evidence*: I = randomized clinical trial data; II = data from clinical trials that are not randomized or were conducted in other populations; III = expert opinion.

[c]Recommended regimen for children younger than 18 years of age.

[d]Recommended regimens for pregnant women. Some experts would use rifampin and pyrazinamide for 2 months as an alternative regimen in HIV-infected pregnant women, although pyrazinamide should be avoided during the first trimester.

[e]Rifabutin should not be used with hard-gel saquinavir or delavirdine. When used with other protease inhibitorsor NNRTIs, dose adjustment of rifabutin may be required.

From Ref. 35.

the patient's isolate that were not used before should be added to the regimen as needed.[2,12,34] When isoniazid and rifampin cannot be used, treatment durations typically become 2 years or more, regardless of immune status.[2,12,34,41] TB specialists should be consulted regarding cases of drug-resistant TB or in any setting where there is uncertainty regarding appropriate treatment.[2,12,34] ❾ *It is critical to avoid monotherapy, and it is critical to avoid adding only a single drug to a failing regimen.*[2,12,34]

Special Populations

Patients with CNS TB usually are treated for longer periods (9–12 months instead of 6 months) because the consequences of undertreatment are severe.[2,12,34] TB of the bone typically is treated for 6 to 9 months, occasionally with surgical débridement.[2,12,34] Drug selection is the same as for pulmonary disease. Extrapulmonary TB of the soft tissues can be treated with conventional regimens.[2,12,34] TB in children may be treated with regimens similar to those used in adults, although some physicians extend treatment to 9 months.[2,12,19,20,34,38,43] Pediatric doses of isoniazid and rifampin on a milligram per kilogram basis are higher than those used in adults[34] (Table 75–4).

Pregnant women receive the usual treatment of isoniazid, rifampin, and ethambutol for 9 months.[2,34,38,41,43] Pyrazinamide

has not been studied in large numbers of pregnant women, but anecdotal data suggest that it may be safe.[34] B vitamins should be provided. Streptomycin, other aminoglycosides, capreomycin, and ethionamide generally are avoided because they have been associated with toxic effects on the fetus.[34,44] *Para*-aminosalicylic acid and cycloserine are used sparingly.[44] Quinolones generally are avoided in pregnancy because of concern about adverse effects on cartilage development.[34,44] Although most antituberculosis drugs are excreted in breast milk, the amount of drug received by the infant through

Patient Encounter 3: Creating a Care Plan

Based on the information provided, what are the goals of therapy for this patient? Select and recommend a therapeutic plan for treatment of this patient's TB infection. What drugs, dose, schedule, and duration of therapy are best for this patient? How should any contacts infected by this patient be evaluated and treated? What drugs, dose, and schedule of therapy are best for his close contacts?

Table 75–3

Drug Regimens for Culture-Positive Pulmonary Tuberculosis Caused by Drug-Susceptible Organisms

Initial Phase			Continuation Phase			
Regimen	Drugs	Interval and Doses[a] (Minimal Duration)	Regimen	Drugs	Interval and Doses[a,b] (Minimal Duration)	Range of Minimal Doses (mg)
1	Isoniazid Rifampin Pyrazinamide Ethambutol	7 days/week for 56 doses (8 weeks) or 5 days/ week for 40 doses (8 weeks)[c]	1a	Isoniazid/ Rifampin	7 days/week for 126 doses (18 weeks) or 5 days/week for 90 doses (18 weeks)[c]	182–130 (26 weeks)
			1b	Isoniazid/ Rifampin	Twice weekly for 36 doses (18 weeks)	92–76 (26 weeks)[d]
			1c[e]	Isoniazid/ Rifapentine	Once weekly for 18 doses (18 weeks)	74–58 (26 weeks)
2	Isoniazid Rifampin Pyrazinamide Ethambutol	7 days/wk for 14 doses (2 weeks)[c], *then* twice weekly for 12 doses (6 weeks) or 5 days/week for 10 doses (2 weeks), *then* twice weekly for 12 doses (6 weeks)	2a	Isoniazid/ Rifampin	Twice weekly for 36 doses (18 weeks)	62–58 (26 weeks)[d]
			2b[e]	Isoniazid/ Rifapentine	Once weekly for 18 doses (18 weeks)	44–40 (26 weeks)
3	Isoniazid Rifampin Pyrazinamide Ethambutol	3× weekly for 24 doses (8 weeks)	3a	Isoniazid/ Rifampin	3× weekly for 54 doses (18 weeks)	78 (26 weeks)
4	Isoniazid Rifampin Ethambutol	7 days/week for 56 doses (8 weeks) or 5 days/ week for 40 doses (8 weeks)[c]	4a	Isoniazid/ Rifampin	7 days/week for 217 doses (31 weeks) or 5 days/week for 155 doses (31 weeks)[c]	273–195 (39 weeks)
			4b	Isoniazid/ Rifampin	Twice weekly for 62 doses (31 weeks)	118–102 (39 weeks)

[a]When DOT is used, drugs may be given 5 days/week and the necessary number of doses adjusted accordingly. Although there are no studies that compare five with seven daily doses, extensive experience indicates this would be an effective practice.

[b]Patients with cavitation on initial chest radiograph and positive cultures at completion of 2 months of therapy should receive a 7-month (31-week; either 217 doses [daily] or 62 doses [twice weekly]) continuation phase.

[c]Five-day-a-week administration is always given by DOT. Rating for 5 day/week regimens is A(III).

[d]Not recommended for HIV-infected patients with CD4+ cell counts less than 100 cells/mL.

[e]Options 1c and 2b should be used only in HIV-negative patients who have negative sputum smears at the time of completion of 2 months of therapy and who do not have cavitation on the initial chest radiograph. For patients started on this regimen and found to have a positive culture from the 2-month specimen, treatment should be extended an extra 3 months.

From Ref. 35.

nursing is insufficient to cause toxicity. Quinolones should be avoided in nursing mothers, if possible, for the same reason as above.

▶ Human Immunodeficiency Virus

Patients with AIDS and other immunocompromised hosts may be managed with chemotherapeutic regimens similar to those used in immunocompetent individuals, although treatment is often extended to 9 months[2,12,34] (Table 75–3). The precise duration to recommend remains a matter of debate. Highly intermittent regimens (twice or once weekly) are not recommended for HIV-positive TB patients.[34] Prognosis has been particularly poor for HIV-infected patients infected

with MDR-TB. Some patients with AIDS malabsorb their oral medications, and drug interactions are common.[2,34,41,42] It is advisable that such patients are managed by TB-HIV experts because the challenges are many.

▶ Renal Failure

Because they are primarily hepatically cleared, isoniazid and rifampin usually do not require dose modification in renal failure.[41,44,45] Pyrazinamide and ethambutol typically are reduced to three times weekly to avoid accumulation of the parent drug (ethambutol) or metabolites (pyrazinamide).[34,45] Renally cleared TB drugs include the aminoglycosides (e.g., amikacin, kanamycin, and streptomycin), capreomycin,

Table 75–4

Antituberculosis Drugs for Adults and Children[a]

Drug	Daily Doses[b]	Adverse Effects	Monitoring
Isoniazid	*Adults*: 5 mg/kg (300 mg) *Children*: 10–15 mg/kg (300 mg)	Asymptomatic elevation of aminotransferases, clinical hepatitis, fatal hepatitis, peripheral neurotoxicity, CNS system effects, lupus-like syndrome, hypersensitivity, monoamine poisoning, diarrhea	LFT monthly in patients who have preexisting liver disease or who develop abnormal liver function that does not require discontinuation of drug. Dosage adjustments may be necessary in patients receiving anticonvulsants or warfarin
Rifampin	*Adults*[c]: 10 mg/kg (600 mg) *Children*: 10–20 mg/kg (600 mg)	Cutaneous reactions, GI reactions (nausea, anorexia, abdominal pain), flu-like syndrome, hepatotoxicity, severe immunologic reactions, orange discoloration of bodily fluids (sputum, urine, sweat, tears), drug interactions owing to induction of hepatic microsomal enzymes	Rifampin causes many drug interactions. For a complete list of drug interactions and effects refer to CDC website: *www. cdc.gov/nchstp/tb/tb*
Rifabutin	*Adults*[c]: 5 mg/kg (300 mg) *Children*: Appropriate dosing unknown	Hematologic toxicity, uveitis, GI symptoms, polyarthralgias, hepatotoxicity, pseudojaundice (skin discoloration with normal bilirubin), rash, flu-like syndrome, orange discoloration of bodily fluids (sputum, urine, sweat, tears)	Drug interactions are less problematic than rifampin
Rifapentine	*Adults*: 10 mg/kg (continuation phase) (600 mg) Dosed weekly. *Children*: The drug is not approved for use in children	Similar to those associated with rifampin	Drug interactions are being investigated and are likely similar to RIFAMPIN
Pyrazinamide	*Adults*: Based on IBW: 40–55 kg: 1,000 mg; 56–75 kg: 1,500 mg; 76–90 kg: 2,000 mg *Children*: 15–30 mg/kg	Hepatotoxicity, GI symptoms (nausea, vomiting), nongouty polyarthralgia, asymptomatic hyperuricemia, acute gouty arthritis, transient morbilliform rash, dermatitis	Serum uric acid can serve as a surrogate marker for compliance. LFTs in patients with underlying liver disease
Ethambutol[d]	*Adults*: Based on IBW: 40–55 kg: 800 mg; 56–75 kg: 1,200 mg; 76–90 kg: 1,600 mg *Children*[c]: 15–20 mg/kg daily	Retrobulbar neuritis, peripheral neuritis, cutaneous reactions	Baseline visual acuity testing and testing of color discrimination. Monthly testing of visual acuity and color discrimination in patients taking greater than 15–20 mg/kg, renal insufficiency, or receiving the drug for greater than 2 months
Cycloserine	*Adults*[e]: 10–15 mg/kg/day, usually 500–750 mg/day in 2 doses *Children*: 10–15 mg/kg/day	CNS effects	Monthly assessments of neuropsychiatric status. Serum concentration may be necessary until appropriate dose is established
Ethionamide	*Adults*[f]: 15–20 mg/kg/day, usually 500–750 mg/day in a single daily dose or 2 divided doses *Children*: 15–20 mg/kg/day	GI effects, hepatotoxicity, neurotoxicity, endocrine effects	Baseline LFTs. Monthly LFTs if underlying liver disease is present. TSH at baseline and monthly intervals
Streptomycin	*Adults*[g] *Children*: 20–40 mg/kg/day	Ototoxicity, neurotoxicity, nephrotoxicity	Baseline audiogram, vestibular testing, Romber testing and SCr. Monthly assessments of renal function and auditory or vestibular symptoms
Amikacin/ kanamycin	*Adults*[g] *Children*: 15–30 mg/kg/day IV or intramuscular as a single daily dose	Ototoxicity, nephrotoxicity	Baseline audiogram, vestibular testing, Romberg testing and SCr. Monthly assessments of renal function and auditory or vestibular symptoms
Capreomycin	*Adults*[g] *Children*: 15–30 mg/kg/day as a single daily dose	Nephrotoxicity, ototoxicity	Baseline audiogram, vestibular testing, Romber testing and SCr. Monthly assessments of renal function and auditory or vestibular symptoms. Baseline and monthly serum K[+] and Mg[2+]
p-Aminosalicylic acid (PAS)	*Adults*: 8–12 g/day in 2 or 3 doses *Children*: 200–300 mg/kg/ day in 2–4 divided doses	Hepatotoxicity, GI distress, malabsorption syndrome, hypothyroidism, coagulopathy	Baseline LFTs and TSH. TSH every 3 months

(Continued)

Table 75–4			
Antituberculosis Drugs for Adults and Children*^a* (Continued)			
Drug	**Daily Doses^b**	**Adverse Effects**	**Monitoring**
Levofloxacin	*Adults*: 500–1,000 mg daily Children^h	GI disturbance, neurologic effects, cutaneous reactions	No specific monitoring recommended
Moxifloxacin	*Adults*: 400 mg daily Childrenⁱ		
Gatifloxacin	*Adults*: 400 mg daily Children		

LFT, liver function test; SCr, serum creatinine; TSH, thyroid-stimulating hormone.

*^a*For purposes of this document, adult dosing begins at age 15 years.

*^b*Dose per weight is based on ideal body weight. Children weighing more than 40 kg should be dosed as adults.

*^c*Dose may need to be adjusted when there is concomitant use of protease inhibitors or nonnucleoside reverse transcriptase inhibitors.

*^d*The drug likely can be used safely in older children but should be used with caution in children younger than 5 years of age, in whom visual acuity cannot be monitored. In younger children, ethambutol at the dose of 15 mg/kg/day can be used if there is suspected or proven resistance to isoniazid or rifampin.

*^e*It should be noted that although this is the dose recommended generally, most clinicians with experience using cycloserine indicate that it is unusual for patients to be able to tolerate this amount. Serum concentration measurements are often useful in determining the optimal dose for a given patient.

*^f*The single daily dose can be given at bedtime or with the main meal.

*^g*Dose: 15 mg/kg /day (1 g) and 10 mg/kg in persons older than 50 years of age (750 mg). Usual dose: 750–1,000 mg administered intramuscularly or IV, given as a single dose 5–7 days/week, and reduced to 2–3× per week after the first 2–4 months or after culture conversion, depending on the efficacy of the other drugs in the regimen.

*^h*The long-term (more than several weeks) use of levofloxacin in children and adolescents has not be approved because of concerns about effects on bone and cartilage growth. However, most experts agree that the drug should be considered for children with TB caused by organisms resistant to both isoniazid and rifampin. The optimal dose is not known.

*ⁱ*The long-term (more than several weeks) use of moxifloxacin in children and adolescents has not been approved because of concerns about effects on bone and cartilage growth. The optimal dose is not known.

From Ref. 34.

ethambutol, cycloserine, and levofloxacin.[34,35,44,45] Dosing intervals need to be extended for these drugs. Serum concentration monitoring must be performed for cycloserine to avoid dose-related toxicities in renal failure patients.[37,41,42]

▶ Hepatic Failure

Elevations of serum transaminase concentrations generally are not correlated with the residual capacity of the liver to metabolize drugs, so these markers cannot be used directly as guides for residual metabolic capacity. Hepatically cleared TB drugs include isoniazid, rifampin, pyrazinamide, ethionamide, and p-aminosalicylic acid.[44] Ciprofloxacin and moxifloxacin are about 50% cleared by the liver. Further, isoniazid, rifampin, pyrazinamide, and to a lesser degree ethionamide, p-aminosalicylic acid, and rarely ethambutol may cause hepatotoxicity.[34,41,44] These patients require close monitoring, and serum concentration monitoring may be the most accurate way to dose them.

▶ The TB Drugs

The interested reader is referred to several other publications for more detailed information regarding these drugs.[2,11,34,39–42,44–47]

A summary of daily doses, adverse effects, and monitoring parameters of first- and second-line antituberculosis drugs is provided in Table 75–4.[34] Isoniazid and rifampin are considered the two key drugs for the treatment of active TB, followed by pyrazinamide, which has a special role in the first 2 months of treatment. Other drugs are used to suppress the emergence of drug resistance in conjunction with the first-line drugs or for pre-existing drug-resistant TB. In general, the most important toxicity with first-line drugs is hepatotoxicity, whereas various organs may be affected by each of the second-line drugs. Recent research is placing emphasis on the potential role of quinolones such as moxifloxacin in the treatment of TB. The role of these agents in the first 2-month intensive phase of therapy is currently being evaluated. It is possible that future regimens may consider these agents part of the first-line drugs.[48] Other new therapies include investigational vaccines, and investigational drugs such as PA-824, OPC67683, TMC207, and SQ109 which are in clinical trials.[49,50]

EVALUATION OF OUTCOMES

● Effectiveness of TB therapy is determined by AFB smears and cultures. Sputum samples should be sent for AFB staining and microscopic examination (smears) every 1 to 2 weeks until two consecutive smears are negative. This provides early evidence of a response to treatment.[34] Once on maintenance therapy, sputum cultures can be performed monthly until two consecutive cultures are negative, which generally occurs over 2 to 3 months. If sputum cultures continue to be positive after 2 months, drug susceptibility testing should be repeated, and serum concentrations of the drugs should be checked.

⑩ The most serious problem with TB therapy is patient nonadherence to the prescribed regimen.[51,52] Unfortunately, there is no reliable way to identify such patients a priori. The most effective way to achieve this end is with DOT.[2,11,34] The use of DOT in noncompliant patients will be of benefit.[53] DOT also provides increased opportunities to observe the patient for any apparent toxicities, thus improving overall care.

Serum chemistries, including blood urea nitrogen (BUN), creatinine, aspartate transaminase (AST), and alanine transaminase (ALT), and a complete blood count with platelets should be performed at baseline and periodically thereafter depending on the presence of other factors that may increase the likelihood of toxicity (e.g., advanced age, alcohol abuse, and pregnancy).[2,34] Hepatotoxicity should be suspected in patients whose transaminases exceed five times the upper limit of normal or whose total bilirubin exceeds 3 mg/dL (51 μmol/L) and in patients with symptoms such as nausea, vomiting, and jaundice. At this point, the offending agent(s) should be discontinued. Sequential reintroduction of the drugs with frequent testing of liver enzymes is often successful in identifying the offending agent; other agents may be continued[34] (Table 75–4).

Therapeutic Drug Monitoring

TDM or applied pharmacokinetics is the use of serum drug concentrations to optimize therapy.[34,41,42] Non-AIDS patients with drug-susceptible TB generally do well. TDM may be used if patients are failing appropriate DOT (no clinical improvement after 2–4 weeks or smear-positive after 4–6 weeks). On the other hand, patients with AIDS, diabetes, and various GI disorders often fail to absorb these drugs properly and are candidates for TDM. Also, patients with hepatic or renal disease should be monitored, given their potential for overdoses. In the treatment of MDR-TB, TDM may be particularly useful.[44,46] Finally, TDM of the TB and HIV drugs is perhaps the most logical way to untangle the

Patient Encounter 4: Creating a Care Plan

Based on the information provided, which clinical and laboratory parameters should be monitored in this patient to determine efficacy and avoid toxicity?

Is this patient a candidate for therapeutic drug monitoring? Why or why not?

Patient Care and Monitoring

1. Rapidly identify a new TB case.

2. Assess the patient's risk factors and signs and symptoms to determine if the patient might be infected with TB.

3. Isolate the patient with active disease to prevent the spread of the disease.

4. Collect appropriate samples for smears and cultures.

5. Obtain a thorough medication history.

6. Select and recommend appropriate antituberculosis treatment. Consider HIV status, pregnancy, type of TB infection, renal function, liver function etc.

7. Ensure adherence to the treatment regimen by the patient.

8. Obtain AFB stains to evaluate the effectiveness of treatment.

9. Consider TDM if no clinical improvement.

10. Secondary goals are identification of the index case that infected the patient, identification of all persons infected by both the index case and the new case of TB, and the completion of appropriate treatments for those individuals.

complex drug interactions that take place. For a complete list of drug interactions visit the CDC website at *www.cdc.gov/nchstp/tb/tb_hiv_drugs/toc.htm*.[54] In particular, interactions between the rifamycins (e.g., rifampin, rifapentine, and rifabutin) and the HIV protease inhibitors and NRTIs are common and require dose and frequency modifications in many cases. Since these are constantly being updated, the preceding link is an excellent way to keep current.

Abbreviations Introduced in This Chapter

AFB	Acid fast bacillus
ALT	Alanine transaminase
AST	Aspartate transaminase
BCG	Bacille Calmette-Guérin
DOT	Directly observed therapy
HTN	Hypertension
IFN-γ	Interferon-γ
IGRA	Interferon-gamma release assay
LTBI	Latent tuberculosis infection
MGIT	Mycobacterial growth indicator tube
NIDDM	Noninsulin dependent diabetes mellitus
NRTI	Nucleoside reverse transcriptase inhibitors
PCR	Polymerase chain reaction
PPD	Purified protein derivative
RFLP	Restriction fragment length polymorphism
TB	Tuberculosis
TDM	Therapeutic drug monitoring

Self-assessment questions and answers are available at *http://www.mhpharmacotherapy. com/pp.html.*

REFERENCES

1. World Health Organization Report on the Global Tuberculosis Epidemic 1998.
2. Iseman MD. A Clinician's Guide to Tuberculosis. Philadelphia, Lippincott Williams & Wilkins, 2000.
3. McCray E, Weinbaum CM, Braden CR, et al. The epidemiology of tuberculosis in the United States. Clin Chest Med 1997;18:99–113.
4. Centers for Disease Control and Prevention. Trends in Tuberculosis Morbidity–United States, 1992–2002. MMWR 2003;52:222-224.
5. CDC. Reported tuberculosis in the United States, 2007. Atlanta, GA: U.S. Department of Health and Human Services, CDC, September, 2008.
6. Haas DW. Mycobacterium tuberculosis. In: Mandell GL, Bennett JE, Dolin R, eds. Principles and Practice of Infectious Diseases, 5th ed. New York, Churchill Livingstone, 2000:2576–2607.
7. Small PM, Shafer RW, Hopewell PC, et al. Exogenous reinfection with multidrug-resistant Mycobacterium tuberculosis in patients with advanced HIV infection. N Engl J Med 1993;328;1137–1144.
8. Beck-Sague C, Dooley SW, Hutton MD, et al. Hospital outbreak of multidrug-resistant Mycobacterium tuberculosis infections: Factors in transmission to staff and HIV-infected patients. JAMA 1992:268;1280–1286.
9. Centers for Disease Control and Prevention. Meeting the challenge of multidrug-resistant tuberculosis: Summary of a conference. MMWR 1992;41(RR-11):51-57.
10. Heifets L. Mycobacteriology laboratory. Clin Chest Med 1997;18: 35–53.
11. Heifets LB. Drug susceptibility tests in the management of chemotherapy of tuberculosis. In: Heifets LB, ed. Drug Susceptibility in the Chemotherapy of Mycobacterial Infections. Boca Raton, FL: CRC Press, 1991:89–122.
12. Daley CL, Chambers HF. Mycobacterium tuberculosis complex. In: Yu VL, Weber R, Raoult D, eds. Antimicrobial therapy and vaccines, Volume I: Microbes, 2nd ed. New York, Apple Trees Productions, LLC, 2002:841–865.
13. Roberts GD, Böttger EC, Stockman L. Methods for the rapid identification of mycobacterial species. Clin Lab Med 1996;16: 603–615.
14. Sandin RL. Polymerase chain reaction and other amplification techniques in mycobacteriology. Clin Lab Med 1996;16:617–639.
15. Ingham CJ, Ayad AB, Nolsen K, Mulder B. Rapid drug susceptibility testing of mycobacteria by culture on a highly porous ceramic support. Int J Tuberc Lung Dis 2008;12(6):645–650.
16. Martin A, Panaiotov S, Portaels F, Hoffner S, Palomino JC, Angeby K. The nitrate reductase assay for the rapid detection of isoniazid and rifampicin resistance in Mycobacterium tuberculosis: A systematic review and meta-analysis. Journal of Antimicrobial Chemotherapy 2008;62(1):56–64.
17. Daniel TM, Boom WH, Ellner JJ. Immunology of Tuberculosis. In: Reichman LB, Hershfield ES. Tuberculosis. A Comprehensive International Approach, 2nd ed. New York, Marcel Dekker, 2000:157–185.
18. Piessens WF, Nardell EA. Pathogenesis of Tuberculosis. In: Reichman LB, Hershfield ES. Tuberculosis. A Comprehensive International Approach, 2nd ed. New York, Marcel Dekker, 2000:241–260.
19. American Thoracic Society / Centers for Disease Control and Prevention. Diagnostic standards and classification of tuberculosis in adults and children. Am J Respir Crit Care Med 2000;161:1376–1395.
20. Peloquin CA, Berning SE. Tuberculosis and multi-drug resistant tuberculosis in children. Pediatr Nurs 1995;21:566–572.
21. Correa AG. Unique aspects of tuberculosis in the pediatric population. Clin Chest Med 1997;18:89–98.
22. American Thoracic Society / Centers for Disease Control and Prevention. Targeted tuberculin skin testing and treatment of latent tuberculosis infection. Am J Respir Crit Care Med 2000;161: S221–S247.
23. Pape JW, Jean SS, Ho JL, et al. Effect of isoniazid prophylaxis on incidence of active tuberculosis and progression of HIV infection. Lancet 1992;342:268–272.
24. Narita M, Ashkin D, Hollender ES, Pitchenik AE. Paradoxical worsening of tuberculosis following antiretroviral therapy in patients with AIDS. Am J Respir Crit Care Med 1998;158:157–161.
25. Barnes PF, Bloch AB, Davidson PT, Snider DE. Tuberculosis in patients with human immunodeficiency virus infection. N Engl J Med 1991;324:1644–1650.
26. Alvarez S, Shell C, Berk SL. Pulmonary tuberculosis in elderly men. Am J Med 1987;82:602–606.
27. Umeki S. Comparison of younger and elderly patients with pulmonary tuberculosis. Respiration 1989;55:75–83.
28. Centers for Disease Control and Prevention. Anergy skin testing and preventive therapy for HIV-infected persons: revised recommendations. MMWR 1997; 46 (RR-15):1–10.
29. Bouza E, Diaz-Lopez MD, Moreno S, et al. Mycobacterium tuberculosis bacteremia in patients with and without human immunodeficiency virus infection. Arch Intern Med 1993;153:496–500.
30. Pai M, O'Brien R. New Diagnostics for latent and active tuberculosis: State of the art and future prospects. Semin Respir Crit Care Med 2008;29:560–568.
31. Nienhaus A, Schablon A, Diel R. Interferon-gamma release assay for the diagnosis of latent TB infection—Analysis of discordant results, when compared to the tuberculin skin test. PLoS ONE 2008;3(7):e2665.
32. Pai M, Zwerling A, Menzies D. Systematic review: T-cell based assays for the diagnosis for latent tuberculosis infection. Ann Intern Med 2008;149:177–184.
33. Pai M, Dheda K, Cunningham J, Scano F, O'Brien R. T-cell assays for the diagnosis of latent tuberculosis infection: moving the research agenda forward. Lance Infect Dis 2007;7:428–438.
34. American Thoracic Society / Centers for Disease Control / Infectious Disease Society of America. Treatment of tuberculosis. Am J Respir Crit Care Med 2003;167:603-662.
35. Fujiwara PI, Larkin C, Frieden TR. Directly observed therapy in New York City. Clin Chest Med 1997;18:135–148.
36. Weis SE. Universal directly observed therapy. Clin Chest Med 1997;18:155–163.
37. Malone RS, Fish DN, Spiegel DM, Childs JM, Peloquin CA. The effect of hemodialysis on cycloserine, ethionamide, para-aminosalicylate, and clofazimine. Chest 1999;116:984–990.
38. Vallejo JG, Starke JR. Tuberculosis and pregnancy. Clin Chest Med 1992;13:693–707.
39. Centers for Disease Control and Prevention. Update: Fatal and severe liver injuries associated with rifampin and pyrazinamide for latent tuberculosis infection, and revisions in the American Thoracic Society/CDC recommendations. MMWR 2001;50(34):733–735.
40. Mitchison DA. Basic mechanisms of chemotherapy. Chest 1979;76 (Suppl):771–781.
41. Peloquin CA. Pharmacological Issues in the Treatment of Tuberculosis. Ann NY Acad Sci 2001;953:157–164.
42. Peloquin CA. Therapeutic Drug Monitoring in the Treatment of Tuberculosis. Drugs 2002;62:2169–2183.
43. Hamadeh MA, Glassroth J. Tuberculosis and pregnancy. Chest 1992; 101:1114–1120.
44. Peloquin CA. Antituberculosis drugs: Pharmacokinetics. In: Heifets LB, ed. Drug Susceptibility in the Chemotherapy of Mycobacterial Infections. Boca Raton, FL: CRC Press, 1991:59–88.
45. Malone RS, Fish DN, Spiegel DM, Childs JM, Peloquin CA. The effect of hemodialysis on isoniazid, rifampin, pyrazinamide, and ethambutol. Am J Respir Crit Care Med 1999;159:1580–1584.
46. Holdiness MR. Clinical pharmacokinetics of the antituberculosis drugs. Clin Pharmacokinet 1984;9:511–544.
47. Girling DJ. Adverse effects of antituberculous drugs. Drugs 1982;23: 56–74.

48. Burman WJ. Moxifloxacin versus ethambutol in the first 2 months of treatment for pulmonary tuberculosis. Am J Respir Crit Care Med 2006;174:331–338.

49. Johnson JL. Early and extended early bactericidal activity of levofloxacin, gatifloxacin and moxifloxacin in pulmonary tuberculosis. Int J. Tuberc Lund Dis 2006;10:605–612.

50. Zhang Y. Advances in the treatment of tuberculosis. Clinical Pharmacology and Therapeutics 2007;82:595–600.

51. Brudney K, Dobkin J. Resurgent tuberculosis in New York City: Human immunodeficiency virus, homelessness, and the decline of tuberculosis control programs. Am Rev Resp Dis 1991;144:745–749.

52. Mahmoudi A, Iseman MD. Pitfalls in the care of patients with tuberculosis: Common errors and their association with the acquisition of drug resistance. JAMA 1993;270:65–68.

53. Chaulk CP, Bartlett JG, Chaisson RE. 15 years of directly observed therapy for TB. Program and Abstracts, 32nd Annual Meeting, Infectious Diseases Society of America, Orlando, FL, October 7–9, 1994. Abstract 181.

54. Namdar R, Ebert S, Peloquin CA. Drugs for Tuberculosis. In: Piscitelli SC, Rodvold KA, eds. Drug Interactions in Infectious Diseases, 2d., Totowa, NJ, Humana Press, 2000,191–214.

76 Gastrointestinal Infections

Elizabeth D. Hermsen and Ziba Jalali

LEARNING OBJECTIVES

● **Upon completion of the chapter, the reader will be able to:**

1. Describe the epidemiology and clinical presentation of the various GI infections.
2. Develop an individualized treatment plan given a patient with each of the GI infections.
3. Understand the impact of resistance on the treatment of the various GI infections.
4. Recognize the effect of immunosuppression on GI infections.
5. Educate patients on appropriate prevention measures.
6. Describe the role of antimicrobial prophylaxis and/or vaccination for GI infections.

KEY CONCEPTS

❶ Rehydration is the foundation of therapy for GI infections.

❷ Blood in the stool indicates the possibility of inflammatory mucosal disease of the colon such as enterohemorrhagic *Escherichia coli* (EHEC), which is an important cause of bloody diarrhea in the United States.

❸ Traveler's diarrhea is most commonly caused by bacteria such as *Shigella, Salmonella, Campylobacter,* and *E. coli,* although viruses are being recognized increasingly as a significant cause of traveler's diarrhea as well.

❹ Education of travelers about high-risk food items is the key to the prevention of traveler's diarrhea.

❺ Nosocomial *Clostridium difficile*–associated diarrhea (CDAD) is almost always associated with antimicrobial use; therefore, unnecessary and inappropriate antibiotic therapy should be avoided. Almost all antibiotics except aminoglycosides have been associated with CDAD.

❻ Viruses are the most common cause of diarrheal illness in the world. A live, oral vaccine is licensed and recommended for use in infants for the prevention of rotavirus infection.

INTRODUCTION

One of the primary concerns related to GI infection, regardless of the cause, is dehydration, which is the second leading cause of worldwide morbidity and mortality.[1] Worldwide, dehydration is especially problematic for children younger than age 5. However, the highest rate of death in the United States occurs among the elderly.[1] ❶ *Rehydration is the* *foundation of therapy for GI infections, and oral rehydration therapy (ORT) is usually preferred* (Table 76–1).

BACTERIAL INFECTIONS

SHIGELLOSIS

Epidemiology

Shigella causes bacillary dysentery, which refers to diarrheal stool containing pus and blood. Worldwide, there are an estimated 165 million cases of shigellosis annually with 1 million associated deaths.[2] Shigellosis mostly affects children 6 months to 10 years of age. In the United States, shigellosis is a serious problem in daycare centers and areas with crowded living conditions such as urban centers. Most cases of shigellosis are a result of person-to-person transmission. *Shigella* transmission from contaminated food and water, although less common, is associated with large outbreaks.

Pathogenesis

*Shigella*s are nonmotile, gram-negative, nonlactose-fermenting rods and are members of the family Enterobacteriaceae. There are four species of *Shigella*: *S. dysenteriae* (serogroup A), *S. flexneri* (serogroup B), *S. boydii* (serogroup C), and *S. sonnei* (serogroup D). Infection with *Shigella* occurs after ingestion of as few as 10 to 100 organisms.[3] This low dose of organisms probably explains the person-to-person spread and the high secondary attack rate when an index case is introduced into a family.

Shigella strains invade intestinal epithelial cells with subsequent multiplication, inflammation, and destruction.[4]

Table 76–1

Clinical Assessment of Degree of Dehydration in Children Based on Percentage of Body Weight Loss

Variable	Mild (3–5%)	Moderate (6–9%)	Severe (10% or More)
Blood pressure	Normal	Normal	Normal to reduced
Quality of pulses	Normal	Normal to slightly decreased	Moderately decreased
Heart rate	Normal	Increased	Increased (bradycardia in severe cases)
Skin turgor	Normal	Decreased	Decreased
Fontanelle	Normal	Sunken	Sunken
Mucous membranes	Slightly dry	Dry	Dry
Eyes	Normal	Sunken orbits/ decreased tears	Deeply sunken orbits/ decreased tears
Extremities	Warm, normal capillary refill	Delayed capillary refill	Cool, mottled
Mental status	Normal	Normal to listless	Normal to lethargic to comatose
Urine output	Slightly decreased	Less than 1 mL/kg/h	Less than 1 mL/kg/h
Thirst	Slightly increased	Moderately increased	Very thirsty
Fluid replacement	ORT 50 mL/kg over 2–4 hours	ORT 100 mL/kg over 2–4 hours	Lactated Ringer's 40 mL/kg in 15–30 minutes, then 20–40 mL/kg if skin turgor, alertness, and pulse have not returned to normal *or* Lactated Ringer's or normal saline 20 mL/kg, repeat if necessary, and then replace water and electrolyte deficits over 1–2 days, followed by ORT 100 mL/kg over 4 hours

From Ref. 1.

Clinical Presentation and Diagnosis of Shigellosis

- Biphasic illness
  - Early—high fever, watery diarrhea without blood
  - Later—after approximately 48 hours, colitis develops with urgency, tenesmus, and dysentery.
  - Low-grade fever
  - More frequent small-volume stools ("fractional stools")
  - Abdominal cramping
- Major complications of shigellosis include
  - Proctitis or rectal prolapse (infants and young children)
  - Toxic megacolon (primarily in the setting of *S. dysenteriae* 1 infection)
  - Intestinal obstruction
  - Colonic perforation
  - Bacteremia (more common in children)
  - Metabolic disturbances
  - **Leukemoid reaction**
  - Neurologic disease
  - Reactive arthritis or Reiter's syndrome
  - **Hemolytic-uremic syndrome (HUS)**
- Microscopic examination of stool is extremely useful and reveals multiple polymorphonuclear leukocytes and red blood cells (RBCs). Diagnosis is usually confirmed by stool culture

The organism infects the superficial layer of the gut, rarely penetrates beyond the mucosa, and seldom invades the bloodstream. However, bacteremia can occur in malnourished children and immunocompromised patients.

Treatment and Monitoring

Although infection with *Shigella* generally is self-limited and responds to supportive care, antibiotic therapy is indicated because it shortens the duration of illness and shedding and consequently reduces the risk of transmission. Antibiotic resistance is a worldwide concern and growing problem for enteric bacterial pathogens. The treatment of choice is a fluoroquinolone when the antibiotic susceptibility of the organism is unknown[5] (Table 76–2). Cephalosporins or azithromycin can be used in the management of pediatric shigellosis. Rifaximin is likely to be effective in the treatment of milder forms of shigellosis and is effective at preventing infection with *S. flexneri*.[6] Antimotility agents are not recommended because they can worsen dysentery and may

Patient Encounter 1

A 55-year-old man presents with headache, fever, abdominal pain, and bloody diarrhea for 48 hours. He states that his wife had similar symptoms several days ago. His stool Gram stain reveals the presence of leukocytes, and his WBC is $52 \times 10^3/mm^3$ ($52 \times 10^9/L$).

What test should you send?

Stool culture showed many Shigella sonnei.

What treatment do you recommend?

Table 76–2

Antibacterial Therapy for Shigellosis

Agent	Adult Dosage	Pediatric Dosage	Renal/Hepatic Dosing Considerations
Levofloxacin	500 mg daily × 3 days	Not approved for use in patients less than 18-year-old.	CrCl 20–49: 500 mg once, then 250 mg daily CrCl 10–19/dialysis: 500 mg once, then 250 mg every other day
Ciprofloxacin	500 mg twice daily × 3 days	10 mg/kg twice daily × 5 days	CrCl less than 30/dialysis: same dose given daily
Norfloxacin	400 mg twice daily × 3 days	Not approved for use in patients less than 18-year-old.	CrCl 10–30: 400 mg daily CrCl less than 10: 200 mg daily
Azithromycin	500 mg daily × 3 days	10 mg/kg daily × 3 days	No dosage adjustment necessary
Rifaximin	200 mg three times daily × 3 days	Not approved for use in patients less than 12-year-old.	Lack of information regarding renal insufficiency No dosage adjustment necessary for hepatic impairment

CrCl, Creatinine clearance (mL/min).

be related to the development of toxic megacolon. No vaccines are licensed currently for the prevention of shigellosis.

SALMONELLOSIS

Epidemiology

Salmonella typhi and *Salmonella paratyphi,* which cause typhoid fever, have high host specificity for humans. In the United States, typhoid fever has become less prevalent and is associated primarily with international travel, especially to developing countries. Nontyphoidal *Salmonella* are important causes of reportable food-borne infection. There are an estimated 1.4 million cases of nontyphoid *Salmonella* illness annually in the United States.[7] The highest incidence is in those younger than 1 year of age and older than 65 years of age or in those with HIV/AIDS. Outbreaks of intestinal salmonellosis have been associated with unpasteurized orange juice, tomatoes, cantaloupe, alfalfa sprouts, and cilantro, among others. Exotic pets, especially reptiles (e.g., snakes, turtles, and iguanas), are an increasing source of human salmonellosis, accounting for 3% to 5% of all cases.

Risk factors for salmonellosis include extremes of age, alteration of the endogenous bowel flora of the intestine (e.g., as a result of antimicrobial therapy or surgery), diabetes, malignancy, rheumatologic disorders, HIV infection, and therapeutic immunosuppression of all types.

Pathogenesis

Salmonella are motile, nonlactose-fermenting, gram-negative bacilli. In salmonellosis, the organisms penetrate the epithelial lining to the lamina propia with production of diffuse inflammation. The distal ileum and colon are sites of infection.

Treatment and Monitoring

Gastroenteritis *Salmonella* gastroenteritis is usually self-limited, and antibiotics have no proven value. Patients respond well to ORT. Symptoms typically diminish in 3 to 7 days without sequelae. Antibiotic use may result in a higher rate of chronic carriage and relapse. Antimicrobial use should be limited to pre-emptive therapy among patients at higher risk for extraintestinal spread or invasive disease (Table 76–3). Antimotility agents should not be used.

Enteric Fever

The current drug of choice for typhoid fever is a fluoroquinolone, such as ciprofloxacin. The recommended adult dose of ciprofloxacin for uncomplicated typhoid is 500 mg orally twice daily for 5 to 7 days. Drug resistance is a recognized problem in the Indian subcontinent, Southeast Asia, Mexico, the Arabian Gulf, and Africa. All *S. typhi* isolates should be screened for nalidixic acid and fluoroquinolone resistance. If nalidixic acid resistance is present, the patient should be given higher doses of ciprofloxacin or ofloxacin (10 mg/kg twice daily) for 10 to 14 days. A third-generation cephalosporin and azithromycin (1,000 mg once on day 1 followed by 5 days of 500 mg daily) are alternative agents for *S. typhi* strains, with minimum inhibitory concentration (MIC) values for ciprofloxacin of 2 mcg/mL or greater.[8] Children may receive intravenous ceftriaxone 75 mg/kg daily

---

Table 76–3

Antimicrobial Indications for Nontyphoidal Salmonellosis

Age 3 months or less; 65 years or more
Fever and systemic toxicity
AIDS and other immunodeficiencies (including steroid use or organ transplantation)
Uremia or hemodialysis or renal transplant
Malignancy
Sickle cell anemia or hemoglobinopathy
Inflammatory bowel disease
Aortic aneurysm, prosthetic heart valve, vascular or orthopedic prosthesis

Clinical Presentation and Diagnosis of Salmonellosis

Gastroenteritis

- Onset 8 to 48 hours after ingestion of contaminated food.
- Fever, diarrhea, and cramping
- Stools are loose, of moderate volume, and without blood.
- Headache, myalgias, and other systemic symptoms can occur.
- Diagnosis relies on isolation of the organism from stool or ingested food.
- Certain underlying conditions (e.g., AIDS, inflammatory bowel disease, and prior gastric surgery) predispose the patient to more severe disease.

Enteric Fever

- Febrile illness 5 to 21 days after ingestion of contaminated food or water
- Chills, diaphoresis, headache, anorexia, cough, weakness, sore throat, dizziness, and muscle pains are frequently present before the onset of fever.
- Diarrhea is an early symptom and occurs only in 50% of cases. Intestinal hemorrhage or perforation, leukopenia, anemia, and subclinical disseminated intravascular coagulopathy may be seen.
- Culture of stool, blood, or bone marrow for *Salmonella* species is helpful.

Vascular Infection and Bacteremia

S. choleraesuis and *S. dublin* are the most common causative organisms. The risk of bacteremia is greater for infants, the elderly, and the immunocompromised.

Localized Infections

Localized infections occur in 5% to 10% of cases with *Salmonella* bacteremia. Sites for extraintestinal complications of salmonellosis include endocarditis, arteritis, central nervous system, lung, bone, joints, muscle/soft tissue, splenic, and genitourinary.

Chronic Carriers

The chronic carrier state, defined as positive stool or urine cultures for more than 12 months, develops in 1% to 4% of adults with typhoid fever. Persistence of the organism, in many cases, is due to billiary tract carriage, and the frequency of chronic carriage is higher in persons with biliary abnormalities.

Salmonella and HIV Infection

Salmonella is more likely to cause severe invasive infection in the HIV-infected population. Recurrent nontyphoidal *Salmonella* bacteremia is an AIDS-defining illness.

---

or oral azithromycin 20 mg/kg (up to 1 g) daily, although relapse rates are higher with ceftriaxone.

Patients with complicated typhoid fever (i.e., metastatic foci, ileal perforation, etc.) should receive parenteral therapy with ciprofloxacin 400 mg twice daily or ceftriaxone 2,000 mg once daily. Antimicrobial therapy can be completed with an oral agent after initial control of the symptoms of typhoid fever. In persons with AIDS and a first episode of *Salmonella* bacteremia, a longer duration of antibiotic therapy (1–2 weeks of parenteral therapy followed by 4 weeks of oral fluoroquinolone) is recommended to prevent relapse of bacteremia.

Three typhoid vaccines are available currently for use in the United States: (a) an oral live-attenuated vaccine (Vivotif Berna-TM vaccine, Swiss Serum and Vaccine Institute), (b) a parenteral heat-phenol-inactivated vaccine (Typhoid Vaccine, Wyeth-Ayerst), and (c) a parenteral capsular polysaccharide vaccine (Typhim Vi, Pasteur Merieux). Immunization is recommended only for travelers going to endemic areas such as Latin America, Asia, and Africa; household contacts of a chronic carrier; and laboratory personnel who frequently work with *S. typhi*.[9]

▶ *Chronic Carriers*

In patients with normal gallbladder function, effective agents for eradication of chronic carriage include amoxicillin (3 g divided three times a day in adults for 3 months), trimethoprim-sulfamethoxazole (one double-strength tablet twice a day for 3 months), and ciprofloxacin (750 mg twice

Patient Encounter 2

A 45-year-old Hispanic man with AIDS presents to the emergency department (ED) with fever, nausea, two episodes of vomiting, abdominal pain, and nonbloody diarrhea for 2 days. He reports that his diarrhea is improving, but he developed fever and chills a few hours before he came to the ED. Other history is noncontributory. His physical examination is positive for fever and diffuse abdominal pain. An abdominal ultrasound did not show any abnormal findings. Two sets of blood cultures were sent. He was admitted to the hospital.

What GI pathogen(s) do you suspect in this patient given that his blood cultures came back positive for nontyphoidal Salmonella?

What treatment do you recommend? Do any further tests need to be performed before you can decide on treatment recommendation? Are there any special considerations owing to this patient's HIV infection?

daily for 4 weeks). In patients with anatomic abnormalities, such as biliary or kidney stones, surgery combined with antibiotic therapy is indicated.

CAMPYLOBACTERIOSIS

Epidemiology

Campylobacter jejuni is the most commonly identified bacterial cause of diarrhea worldwide. The organism accounts for 2.1 to 2.4 million cases of illness in the United States each year. Risk factors for *Campylobacter* infection include consumption of chicken, sausage, red meat, and contaminated water; foreign travel; receipt of an antimicrobial agent; household exposure to chickens; and contact with pets (especially birds and cats). Between 25% and 50% of *C. jejuni* infections in the United States appear to be related to chicken exposure or consumption.

The age and sex distributions of *Campylobacter* infections are unique among bacterial enteric pathogens. In developed countries, there are two age peaks: younger than 1 year of age and 15 to 44 years of age. There is a mild male predominance among infected persons. The reason for this distinct age and sex distribution remains unknown. The epidemiology of *Campylobacter* infections is quite different in developing countries; *Campylobacter* diarrhea is primarily a pediatric disease in developing countries.

Pathogenesis

Campylobacter spp. are gram-negative bacilli that have a curved or spiral shape. *Campylobacter* are sensitive to stomach acidity; as a result, diseases or medications that buffer gastric acidity may increase the risk of infection. The infectious dose for *C. jejuni* is low, similar to that for *Salmonella* spp. After an incubation period, infection is established in the jejunum, ileum, colon, and rectum.

Treatment and Monitoring

Hydration and electrolyte balance, often with ORT, are the cornerstone of treatment. The specific circumstances for which antibiotics should be considered include high fevers, bloody stools, symptoms longer than 1 week, pregnancy, infection with HIV, and other immunocompromised hosts.

Until a few years ago, fluoroquinolones were the drug of choice for campylobacteriosis. However, a major problem among *Campylobacter* strains is growing resistance, occurring worldwide. Fluoroquinolone resistance in human isolates of *C. jejuni* in the United States occurs at a rate of 18%, and resistance levels in Barcelona and Thailand are over 80%. Fluoroquinolones should not be used unless susceptibility is confirmed.

Macrolides are considered the optimal drug class for treatment of *Campylobacter* infections. The rate of resistance of *Campylobacter* to macrolides remains low. Other advantages include ease of administration, low cost, lack of major toxicity, and narrow spectrum of activity.[10]

Clinical Presentation and Diagnosis of Campylobacteriosis

- Incubation period of 1 to 7 days
- Abdominal cramps, fever, and diarrhea
- Dysentery is seen in approximately 50% of cases.
- Diarrhea is either loose and watery or grossly bloody.
- Some patients present mainly with abdominal cramps and pain and minimal diarrhea.
- Fecal leukocytes and red blood cells (RBCs) are detected in the stools of 75% of infected individuals. Diagnosis of *Campylobacter* is established by stool culture.
- Extraintestinal *C. jejuni* infection, including septic arthritis, cholecystitis, pancreatitis, meningitis, endocarditis, osteomyelitis, and neonatal sepsis, can present in three different ways:
  - Transient bacteremia with acute campylobacter enteritis in a normal host with benign course
  - Sustained bacteremia or deep focus of infection in a previously normal host that responds to antimicrobial therapy
  - Sustained bacteremia or deep infection in a compromised host
- The most important postinfectious complication of *C. jejuni* is Guillain-Barré syndrome (GBS). The risk of developing GBS is very small (less than one case of GBS per 1,000 *C. jejuni*). GBS typically occurs 1 to 3 weeks after diarrhea.

The recommended dosage of azithromycin for adults is 500 mg orally daily for 3 days and for erythromycin is 500 mg orally four times daily for 5 days. The recommended regimen for children is azithromycin 20 mg/kg (up to 1 g) orally daily. For very ill patients, treatment with gentamicin,

---

Patient Encounter 3

A 55-year-old woman presents with a 3-day history of high fevers, headaches, and diarrhea. She reports having 7 to 10 loose watery stools per day. She had chicken for lunch in a local restaurant last week, which she really liked. Otherwise, she denies any unusual foods, any recent travel, or any sick contacts. She doesn't have any pets at home. She is able to keep food down. The only positive physical findings are diffuse abdominal tenderness, fever, and high blood pressure. Fecal leukocytes were negative. A stool culture was sent, which showed moderate *Campylobacter jejuni*.

How would you treat this patient?

imipenem, cefotaxime, or chloramphenicol is indicated, but susceptibility tests should be performed.

ENTEROHEMORRHAGIC *ESCHERICHIA COLI*

Epidemiology

● Enterohemorrhagic *E. coli* (EHEC) are the pathogenic subgroup of shiga toxin-producing *E. coli* (STEC). Acute hemorrhagic colitis has been associated mainly with the O157:H7 serotype. This serotype has been responsible for larger outbreaks of infection, has higher rates of complications, and appears to be more pathogenic than non-EHEC STEC strains. ❷ *The spectrum of disease associated with E. coli O157:H7 includes bloody diarrhea, which is seen in as many as 95% of patients, nonbloody diarrhea, HUS, and thrombotic thrombocytopenic purpura.*

Approximately 70,000 cases of EHEC illness occur every year in the United States. The highest incidence is in patients aged 5 to 9 years and 50 to 59 years. Outbreaks of diarrhea due to *E. coli* O157:H7 and other STECs have occurred from contaminated beef, classically hamburgers served at fast-food chains, unpasteurized milk and other dairy products, vegetables (e.g., alfalfa sprouts, coleslaw, and lettuce), and apple juice. The most important reservoir for *E. coli* O157:H7 is the GI tract of cattle. Person-to-person transmission is also possible because of the low infectious dose required. Swimming in infant pools or contaminated lakes or drinking municipal water also appears to be a risk factor. The incidence of diagnosed *E. coli* O157:H7 infections in the United States are greater among rural than urban populations, and *E. coli* O157:H7 infections occur in summer and autumn.

Clinical Presentation and Diagnosis of EHEC

- Incubation period of 3 to 5 days
- Bloody stools
- Fever usually absent
- Leukocytosis
- Abdominal tenderness
- HUS in 2% to 10% of patients (especially children 1–5 years of age and the elderly in nursing homes); develops on average 1 week after the onset of diarrhea.
- EHEC belonging to serotype 0157:H7 characteristically do not ferment sorbitol, whereas more than 70% of intestinal floral *E. coli* do. To properly screen EHEC strains in cases of diarrhea, stool should be placed on special sorbitol-MacConkey agar. Colonies of *E. coli* 0157:H7, which do not ferment the sorbitol, can be identified readily and confirmed by serotyping with specific antisera. In addition, stool should be tested directly for the presence of Stx I and II by enzyme immunoassay (EIA).

Patient Encounter 4

A very pleasant 73-year-old white female with a 48-hour history of hematochezia and hemoptysis presents to the ED. She denies any recent travel, exotic foods, raw foods, or sick contacts. She does note that she ate cold-cut sandwiches at a fundraiser approximately 3 days before her symptoms started. She also noticed that she has three friends who developed bloody diarrhea who also ate at this same fundraiser. She denies any fevers, shakes, chills, cough, sore throat, shortness of breath, chest pain, nausea or vomiting, dysuria, hematuria, edema, or night sweats. On her initial presentation, she had a CT that showed pan-colitis and terminal ileitis. She was started on antibiotic therapy including ciprofloxacin and metronidazole. Fecal leukocytes were negative. A stool culture was sent and was positive for Stx. The final culture result was positive for *Escherichia coli* O157:H7.

What would be your next step for this patient?

Two days later, she develops acute kidney injury and thrombocytopenia. What is the most likely diagnosis?

Pathogenesis

The infectious dose of EHEC is very low, between 1 and 100 colony-forming units (CFUs).[11] The two major virulence factors for EHEC are the production of two Shiga-like cytotoxins (Shiga toxin [Stx] I and II) and adhesion-causing attachment-effacement (A/E) lesions. These Stx cytotoxins are responsible for vascular damage and systemic effects such as HUS. Adhesion mediates initial attachment of EHEC to intestinal epithelial cells. Following attachment, these organisms produce A/E lesions on individual intestinal epithelial cells. A/E lesions infect the small or large intestine and cause diarrhea.

Treatment and Monitoring

● The only recommended treatment of EHEC infection is supportive, including fluid and electrolyte replacement, often in the form of ORT. Most illnesses resolve in 5 to 7 days. Patients should be monitored for the development of HUS. Antibiotics are currently contraindicated because they can induce the expression and release of toxin. Antimotility agents should be avoided because they may delay clearance of the pathogen and toxin. This, in turn, may increase the risk of systemic complications.

Proper cooking of foods is essential. Supervision of hand washing by children in daycare centers and exclusion of symptomatic children may reduce person-to-person spread.

CHOLERA

Epidemiology

● Cholera, the first reportable disease, is endemic in South Asia, particularly in the Ganges delta region.[12] The biotypes of *Vibrio cholerae* responsible for pandemics are serogroup

O1 (El Tor) and serogroup O139.[13,14] Although not associated with pandemics, serogroups O75 and O141 have caused small outbreaks of severe diarrhea in the United States. Cholera can be transmitted by water or by food contaminated with contaminated water, particularly undercooked seafood. *V. cholerae* grows well in warm temperatures, causing marked seasonality in the incidence of cholera.[12]

People of blood type O are more susceptible to El Tor vibrios than people of other blood types.[15] Inoculum size affects the likelihood and severity of cholera infection. The infectious dose is lower in patients who are taking antacids owing to the neutralization of gastric acid.[16]

Pathogenesis

V. cholerae is a gram-negative bacillus. Vibrios pass through the stomach to colonize the upper small intestine. Vibrios have filamentous protein extensions that attach to receptors on the intestinal mucosa, and their motility assists with penetration of the mucus layer.[12] The cholera enterotoxin consists of two subunits, one of which (subunit A) is transported into the cells and causes an increase in cyclic adenosine monophosphate (cAMP), which leads to a deluge of fluid into the small intestine.[17] This large volume of fluid results in the watery diarrhea that is characteristic of cholera. The stools are an electrolyte-rich isotonic fluid, the loss of which results in blood volume depletion followed by low blood pressure and shock.[12] Of note, the diarrheal fluid is highly infectious.

Treatment and Monitoring

- The cornerstone of cholera treatment is fluid replacement. Without treatment, the case-fatality rate for severe cholera is approximately 50%. For cholera, rice-based ORT is better than glucose-based ORT because it reduces the number of stools.[18] Patients with significant disease should receive a short antibiotic course to shorten the duration of illness and decrease the number of stools. Azithromycin 1 g (20 mg/kg for children) orally given once is the regimen of choice. Ciprofloxacin 1 g (20 mg/kg for children) orally given once is an alternative but is associated with higher failure rates.

Clinical Presentation and Diagnosis of Cholera[12]

- Incubation period of 18 hours to 5 days
- Abrupt onset of watery diarrhea and vomiting
- Large volumes of rice-water stools
- Dehydration, may be severe. Patients suffering from severe dehydration owing to rapid fluid loss are at risk for death within several hours of disease onset.
- Severe muscle cramps in extremities owing to the electrolyte imbalance are caused by the fluid loss. These cramps should resolve with treatment.
- Metabolic acidosis

Ciprofloxacin is associated with joint damage in children and should not be given to children under 18 years of age unless they cannot be treated with other antibiotics. Antibiotic resistance has been documented in *V. cholerae* since 1977.[12] Antibiotic prophylaxis is not warranted.

The main prevention strategies include ensuring a safe water supply and safe food preparation, improving sanitation, and patient education. Several oral vaccines are in development, and two are available in countries outside the United States.[19–24] However, these vaccines do not provide protection against all cases of cholera because the immunity may be overcome by high inocula.[12]

TRAVELER'S DIARRHEA
Epidemiology

- Traveler's diarrhea occurs commonly when visitors from developed countries travel to developing countries. Over 50 million people are at risk for traveler's diarrhea each year.[25] Traveler's diarrhea can occur following the consumption of food or water contaminated with bacteria, viruses, or parasites. ❸ *Bacteria such as Shigella, Salmonella, Campylobacter, and E. coli are responsible for 60% to 85% of the traveler's diarrhea cases.[25] Noroviruses are being recognized increasingly as a significant cause of traveler's diarrhea as well.[26]*

Risky foods include tap water; uncooked foods, including seafood, fruits, and vegetables; and foods that are stored inadequately, particularly buffet-style meals. Additionally, alcohol consumption of more than five drinks per day has been demonstrated to be a risk factor, especially in males.[27] Education about the types of foods to avoid during travel can be an effective method of prevention.

Pathogenesis

Refer to the specific microorganism sections of this chapter for pathogenesis information.

Treatment and Monitoring

- The goal of treatment is to maintain hydration and functional status to prevent disruption of travel plans. For travelers with mild cases of diarrhea, ORT is often all that is needed. However, antibiotics are effective at reducing the duration

---

Clinical Presentation and Diagnosis of Traveler Diarrhea

- Frequent, loose stools
- Associated with nausea and vomiting
- Abdominal pain
- Fecal urgency
- Dysentery
- Signs and symptoms related to specific causative pathogen

of illness. The use of trimethoprim-sulfamethoxazole has fallen out of favor because of the development of resistance in many regions. In general, fluoroquinolones, specifically levofloxacin (500 mg once daily for adults) and ciprofloxacin (500 mg twice daily for adults), are the drugs of choice for traveler's diarrhea. A 24-hour regimen can be used unless the traveler has a fever or bloody stools, in which case a 3-day regimen is necessary.[25] Alternatives to fluoroquinolones should be used in Asia, where resistance is high among *Campylobacter*. Azithromycin, as a single adult dose of 1,000 mg, represents an alternative to the fluoroquinolone class.[25] The recommended regimen for children is azithromycin 5 to 10 mg/kg orally as a single dose. Additionally, the FDA recently approved rifaximin for the treatment of traveler's diarrhea at an adult dose of 200 mg three times daily for 3 days; rifaximin is not indicated for use in children under the age of 12 years. Rifaximin is not effective against *C. jejuni*, and efficacy has not been documented against *Salmonella*.

Although antimotility agents are effective at shortening the duration of illness, they do not eradicate microorganisms and should not be used in moderate to severe cases with systemic symptoms unless in combination with an antibiotic. The combination of an antimotility agent and an antibiotic can reduce the duration of illness to a few hours.[25]

❹ *Education of travelers about high-risk food items is the key to the prevention of traveler's diarrhea.* Slogans such as "Peel it, boil it, cook it, or forget it" can help to remind travelers of the foods that may be contaminated. Prophylaxis of traveler's diarrhea with antibiotics is effective but should be restricted to individuals who have a repeated history of traveler's diarrhea; cannot afford to make travel alterations (e.g., business trip, competitors, or politicians); have a predisposing factor for traveler's diarrhea, such as achlorhydria, gastrectomy, or inflammatory bowel disease; or are immunosuppressed.[25] The use of antibiotics for prophylaxis is not widely recommended because of the selective pressure for the development of resistance, adverse effects, effect on the normal flora of the GI tract, and cost. The fluoroquinolones are used when prophylaxis is necessary. However, rifaximin may represent an ideal option for prophylaxis of traveler's diarrhea, with virtually no systemic absorption and an excellent safety profile, although it is not approved by the FDA for this indication. Bismuth subsalicylate 525 mg one to four times daily is also effective for traveler's diarrhea prophylaxis. No effective vaccines exist for traveler's diarrhea.

CLOSTRIDIUM DIFFICILE–ASSOCIATED DIARRHEA

Epidemiology

C. difficile is the leading cause of nosocomial enteric infection. Notably, the incidence and severity of illness associated with *C. difficile* has been increasing. *C. difficile* toxins can be found in the stool of 15% to 25% of patients with antibiotic-associated diarrhea (AAD) and more than 95% of patients with pseudomembranous colitis.[28] More than 90% of health care–associated *clostridium difficile*–associated diarrhea (CDAD) occur after or during antimicrobial therapy. **❺** *Clindamycin, cephalosporins, and penicillins are the antibiotics most associated with CDAD, but almost all antimicrobial agents except aminoglycosides have been associated with CDAD.*[29] Fluoroquinolones are strongly associated with CDAD.[30,31] Other risk factors for CDAD include increasing age, severe underlying disease, nonsurgical GI procedures, presence of a nasogastric tube, receipt of antiulcer medications, hospitalization in an intensive care unit (ICU), long duration of hospital stay, long duration of antibiotic, and receiving multiple antibiotics.[32]

The incidence of community-associated *C. difficile* infection (defined as occurring in patients not hospitalized in the year prior to diagnosis) is increasing.[33] In addition to antibiotic use, community-associated *C. difficile* cases are associated with the use of gastric acid-suppressive agents (e.g., proton pump inhibitors and H_2-receptor antagonists).

Pathogenesis

C. difficile is spread by the fecal-oral route, and patient-to-patient transmission has been documented. *C. difficile* is a gram-positive, spore-forming anaerobe. The organism is ingested either as the vegetative form or spores, which can survive for long periods in the environment and can traverse the acidic stomach. In the small intestine, spores germinate into the vegetative form. In the large intestine, CDAD can develop if the normal flora is disrupted by antibiotic therapy. Toxin production is essential for disease to occur. The main virulence factor for disease related to *C. difficile* is the production of toxins A and B. These toxins are responsible for inflammation, fluid and mucus secretion, and mucosal damage, which lead to diarrhea or colitis.

Treatment and Monitoring

Stopping the inciting antibiotic is the most important step in the initial treatment of CDAD. If stopping antibiotic therapy is not effective or not practical, antimicrobial therapy directed specifically against *C. difficile* should be given for 10 days. Oral metronidazole (adult dosing: 500 mg three times daily or 250 mg four times daily; pediatric dosing: 30 mg/kg/day divided four times daily, not to exceed 4 g/day) and oral vancomycin (adult dosing: 125 mg four times daily; pediatric dosing: 40 mg/kg/day divided four times daily, not to exceed 2 g/day) have similar rates of efficacy, but metronidazole is considered the drug of choice for most cases because of cost and concerns regarding the emergence of vancomycin-resistant enterococcus (VRE). Rifaximin and nitazoxanide have demonstrated the potential for treatment of CDAD, although further study is recommended.

Severe disease occurs when patients with CDAD also have marked leukocytosis and/or new onset renal insufficiency. Severe complicated disease is defined as severe disease plus the presence of colitis complications, such as sepsis, volume depletion, electrolyte imbalance, hypotension, paralytic ileus, and toxic megacolon. Patients with signs of severe disease should receive oral vancomycin as initial therapy. Severe

Clinical Presentation and Diagnosis of CDAD

- Symptoms can start as early as the first day of antimicrobial therapy or several weeks after antibiotic therapy is completed.
- Asymptomatic carriage
- Diarrhea
  - Acute watery diarrhea with lower abdominal pain, low-grade fever, and mild or absent leukocytosis
  - Mild, with only three or four loose watery stools per day
  - *C. difficile* toxins are present in stool, but sigmoidoscopic examination is normal.
- Colitis
  - Profuse, watery diarrhea with 5 to 15 bowel movements per day, abdominal pain, abdominal distention, nausea, and anorexia
  - Left or right lower quadrant abdominal pain and cramps that are relieved by passage of diarrhea.
  - Dehydration and low-grade fever
  - Sigmoidoscopic examination may reveal a nonspecific diffuse or patchy erythematous colitis without pseudomembranes.
- Pseudomembranous colitis: Same symptoms as colitis, but sigmoidoscopic examination reveals a characteristic membrane with adherent yellow or off-white plaques, usually in distal colon.
- Toxic megacolon: Suggested by acute dilation of the colon to a diameter greater than 6 cm, associated systemic toxicity, and the absence of mechanical obstruction. It carries a high mortality rate.
- Fulminant colitis: Acute abdomen and systemic symptoms such as fever, tachycardia, dehydration, and hypotension. Some patients have marked leukocytosis (up to 40×10^3 white blood cells/mm^3 [40×10^9/l]). Diarrhea is usually prominent but may not occur in patients with paralytic ileus and toxic megacolon.
- Relapsing colitis
  - Risk factors include increased age, recent abdominal surgery, increased number of *C. difficile* diarrheal episodes, and leukocytosis.
  - 12% to 24% of patients develop a second episode of CDAD within 2 months of the initial diagnosis.
- In most instances, *C. difficile* toxin testing of a single stool specimen effectively establishes the diagnosis. Various enzyme-linked immunosorbent assay (ELISA) kits are available to detect toxin A or toxin B or both. Those that detect both toxin A and B are preferred. Repeated testing can boost sensitivity.
- Leukocytosis, hypoalbuminemia, and fecal leukocytes are nonspecific but suggestive of *C. difficile* infection.
- In selected patients, sigmoidoscopy, colonoscopy, or abdominal CT scan can provide useful diagnostic information.

Patient Encounter 5

A 70-year-old man presents to the ED because of diffuse abdominal pain and nonbloody diarrhea. One day earlier he had been discharged from the hospital, where he had received ceftriaxone and levofloxacin for 7 days for an upper respiratory infection. Soon after going home, he passed numerous liquid brown stools. A few hours later, the patient became disoriented, and an ambulance was called. His medical history is unremarkable. Laboratory values: WBC count 50×10^3/mm^3 (50×10^9/L)/mm^3, hematocrit 43%, sodium 125 mEq/L (125 mmol/L), potassium 5.6 mEq/L (5.6 mmol/L), CO$_2$ 14 mEq/L (14 mmol/L), and metabolic acidosis. An abdominal radiograph series show no evidence of obstruction. The patient was admitted to the hospital.

What GI disease do you suspect based on this information? From your suspicion, what diagnostic tests and treatment would you recommend for this patient?

In the hospital, he receives fluids and vancomycin 125 mg orally four times daily. Stool was sent for *C. difficile* toxin assay, which came back positive. The patient continues to have abdominal pain but no bowel movement. On day 3 of hospitalization, his abdomen is distended with diffuse pain. His WBC count remains elevated. A CT scan of the abdomen showed colonic dilation to greater than 6 cm. The patient became febrile and hypotensive, requiring multiple pharmacologic support for hypotension.

What are this patient's risk factors for Clostridium difficile–associated diarrhea (CDAD)?

What do these new findings suggest?

How does this progression change your treatment recommendations?

complicated disease should be treated with a combination of oral vancomycin and intravenous metronidazole. Surgical intervention may be indicated and lifesaving, particularly in cases complicated by toxic megacolon or colonic perforation.

In circumstances where oral therapy cannot be given, intravenous metronidazole (500 mg every 6–8 hours in adults), vancomycin retention enemas (500 mg every 4–8 hours in adults), or vancomycin via colonic catheter should be considered.[34] Antiperistaltic agents should not be given because the use of these agents is associated with the development of toxic megacolon.

Therapeutic response should be based on clinical signs and symptoms. A repeat toxin assay as a "test of cure" is not recommended because some patients may remain colonized with this organism following recovery. Treatment of asymptomatic colonized patients is not recommended as an infection-control measurement.

Relapse is suggested by the returning of symptoms 3 to 21 days after stopping metronidazole or vancomycin. Since antibiotic resistance is not a factor in relapse, most relapses usually respond to another course of either metronidazole or vancomycin. Currently, metronidazole is recommended for treatment of the first recurrence, while vancomycin pulse dosing (125 mg orally every 3 days for 3 weeks) or tapered dosing (125 mg orally four times daily for 10–14 days, then 125 mg orally twice daily for 7 days, then 125 mg orally daily for 7 days) is recommended for treatment of subsequent recurrences.

Vigilant hand washing and isolation precautions are keys to controlling *C. difficile*. Use of antimicrobial hand gel instead of soap and water is not a recommended alternative for patients infected with *C. difficile*.

PARASITIC INFECTIONS

Please refer to Chapter 75 for information regarding giardiasis.

CRYPTOSPORIDIOSIS

Epidemiology

Cryptosporidiosis has been recognized as a human disease since the 1970s, with increasing importance in the 1980s and 1990s because of its relationship with HIV/AIDS. *Cryptosporidium* accounts for 2.2% and 6.1% of diarrhea cases in immunocompetent people in developed and developing countries, respectively.[35] These percentages increase to 7% and 12% in children in developed and developing countries, respectively, and to 14% and 24% in immunocompromised persons in developed and developing countries, respectively.[35]

Infection is spread person-to-person, usually via the fecal-oral route; by animals, particularly cattle and sheep; and through the environment, especially water. People at increased risk of contracting cryptosporidiosis include household and family contacts and sexual partners of someone with the disease,

---

Clinical Presentation and Diagnosis of Cryptosporidiosis[35,36]

General

- 7- to 10-day incubation period
- Profuse, watery diarrhea with mucus but not blood or leukocytes that lasts for approximately 2 weeks
- Nausea, vomiting, and abdominal cramps often accompany the diarrhea.
- Fever may be present.
- Simplest method of diagnosis is detection of oocysts by modified acid-fast staining of a stool specimen. Standard ova and parasite test does not include *Cryptosporidium*.

Immunocompetent

- May manifest as asymptomatic disease, acute diarrhea, or persistent diarrhea lasting for several weeks
- Usually self-limiting

Immunocompromised

- May manifest as asymptomatic disease; transient infection for less than 2 months; chronic diarrhea lasting at least 2 months, or fulminant infection, with at least 2 L of watery stool per day
- Asymptomatic disease more common in those with a CD4+ cell count greater than 200 cells/mm³, and fulminant infection more common in those with a CD4+ cell count of less than 50 cells/mm³

---

health care workers, daycare workers, users of public swimming areas, and people traveling to regions of high endemicity.[35]

Pathogenesis

Cryptosporidium is an intracellular protozoan parasite that is capable of completing its entire life cycle within one host. Humans become infected on ingestion of the oocysts, and autoinfection and persistent infections are possible owing to repeated life cycles within the GI tract.[35] As few as 10 to 100 oocysts can cause infection.[35]

Treatment and Monitoring

There is no antimicrobial available that is effective at consistently eradicating *Cryptosporidium*, particularly in immunocompromised hosts. In general, immunocompetent persons and those with asymptomatic infection do not require antimicrobial therapy. In patients with HIV/AIDS, the optimal therapy is restoration of immune function through the use of antiretroviral therapy (ART). In persons in whom antimicrobial therapy is deemed necessary or in HIV/AIDS patients in whom ART is ineffective, a combination of an antimicrobial and an antidiarrheal agent is recommended.[35]

Azithromycin and clarithromycin have shown some treatment success for cryptosporidiosis, even in HIV-positive

Patient Encounter 6

A 35-year-old man with a past medical history significant for recent kidney transplant presents with diarrhea for one month. He reports 4 to 5 watery stools per day. He also complains of abdominal pain and weight loss. He denies any fever, nausea, and vomiting. Stool studies including fecal leukocytes, culture, and ova and parasites were all negative.

What additional diagnostic test should you order and why?

An acid-fast staining of stool was positive for Cryptosporidium parvum. What treatment would you recommend for this patient?

patients.[36] However, the most promising agent is nitazoxanide, which is approved by the FDA for the treatment of cryptosporidiosis in adults and children. In randomized, placebo-controlled trials, nitazoxanide has demonstrated efficacy in cryptosporidiosis in immunocompetent persons, malnourished children, and HIV/AIDS patients with CD4+ cell counts above 50 cells/mm³.[37] Limited evidence suggests that patients with CD4+ cell counts of less than 50 cells/mm³ may benefit from higher doses, longer durations, or both.[37]

Prevention of cryptosporidiosis can prove difficult because the oocysts are resilient to many disinfectants and antiseptics, including ammonia, alcohol, and chlorine.[35] Therefore, most traditional water-treatment methods, including filtration, do not eradicate all oocysts, which is problematic in the face of the small infective dose of *Cryptosporidium*. Routine screening of drinking water should be considered for water-treatment plants, and severely immunocompromised individuals should be advised to avoid water in lakes and streams and contact with young animals.[35] For these persons, drinking water should be brought to a boil and cooled before ingestion.

VIRAL GASTROENTERITIS

6 Viruses are the most common cause of diarrheal illness in the world, resulting in about 450,000 and 160,000 hospitalizations for adults and children, respectively, and over 4,000 deaths.[38,39] Many viruses may cause gastroenteritis, including rotaviruses, noroviruses, astroviruses, enteric adenoviruses, and coronaviruses (Table 76–4). This chapter will focus on rotaviruses.

ROTAVIRUS

Epidemiology

Rotavirus causes between 600,000 and 875,000 deaths each year, with the highest rates in the very young and in developing countries.[40] Rotavirus is the leading cause of childhood gastroenteritis and death worldwide. Most infections occur in children between 6 months and 2 years old, typically during the winter season, but adults may be infected as well. Rotavirus causes over 2 million hospitalizations and 600,000 deaths per year in children younger than 5 years of age.[41] Person-to-person transmission occurs through the fecal–oral route.

Pathogenesis

The mechanism of diarrhea has not been clearly elucidated, but theories include a reduction in the absorptive surface along with impaired absorption owing to cellular damage, enterotoxigenic effects of a rotavirus protein, and stimulation of the enteric nervous system.[42]

Clinical Presentation and Diagnosis of Rotavirus Infection[40]

- Incubation period of 2 days
- 2- to 3-day prodrome of fever and vomiting
- Profuse diarrhea without blood or leukocytes (up to 10–20 stools per day)
- Severe dehydration
- Anorexia
- Fever may be present.
- Presentation in adults may vary from asymptomatic to nonspecific symptoms of headache, malaise, and chills to severe diarrhea, nausea, and vomiting.
- Diagnosis can be made by polymerase chain reaction (PCR) of the stool.

Table 76–4

Agents Responsible for Acute Viral Gastroenteritis and Diarrhea

Virus	Peak Age	Peak Time	Duration	Transmission	Symptoms
Rotavirus	6 months–2 years	Winter	3–8 days	Fecal-oral, water, food	Diarrhea, vomiting, fever, abdominal pain
Enteric adenovirus	Less than 2 years	Year-round	7–9 days	Fecal-oral	Diarrhea, respiratory symptoms, vomiting, fever
Astrovirus	Less than 7 years	Winter	1–4 days	Fecal-oral, water, shellfish	Vomiting, diarrhea, fever, abdominal pain
Noroviruses	Greater than 5 years	Variable	12–24 hours	Fecal-oral, food, aerosol	Nausea, vomiting, diarrhea, abdominal cramps, headache, fever, chills, myalgia

Modified from Ref. 1.

Patient Encounter 7

A 12-month-old female was brought to the ED for 10 watery stools in the last 36 hours. She attends a home daycare. Her mom reports that three other kids at the same daycare developed the same symptoms. She also vomited four times today. Positive physical findings include low-grade fever plus hyperactive bowel sounds.

What diagnostic test would you recommend?

What treatment would you recommend for this patient?

How can you prevent this infection?

Patient Care and Monitoring

1. Observe the patient for signs and symptoms of dehydration, and rehydrate as necessary (see Tables 76–1 and 76–2).

2. Monitor for increase in stool consistency and decrease in stool frequency.

3. If pharmacologic agents are used, monitor for any adverse effects.

4. Evaluate the patient for any complications or effects specific to the afflicting pathogen.

Treatment and Monitoring

● The cornerstone of rotavirus treatment is supportive care and rehydration with ORT or intravenous fluids if necessary. Antimotility and antisecretory agents should not be used owing to their potential side effects in children and the self-limited nature of the disease. ❻ *A live oral rotavirus vaccine is approved by the FDA for use in infants aged 6 weeks to 32 weeks and provides protection against rotavirus infection for at least 24 months.*[43] The Centers for Disease Control and Prevention (CDC) Advisory Committee on Immunization Practices recommends vaccination at 2, 4, and 6 months.

FOOD POISONING

Each year in the United States, approximately 76 million food-borne illnesses occur, leading to 325,000 hospitalizations and over 5,000 deaths.[38] Many bacterial and viral pathogens that have been discussed previously in this chapter (e.g., *Salmonella*, *Shigella*, *Campylobacter*, *E. coli*, and noroviruses) can cause food poisoning. Other bacteria that can cause food-borne illness include *Staphylococcus aureus*, *C. perfringens*, *C. botulinum*, and *Bacillus cereus* (Table 76–5). Food poisoning should be suspected if at least two individuals present with similar symptoms after the ingestion of a common food in the prior 72 hours.

OUTCOME EVALUATION

Patients with GI infections should be evaluated for resolution of GI symptoms, as well as any related systemic signs and symptoms. If antimicrobial therapy was used, completion of the course of therapy should be assessed. Documented clearance of the offending microorganism is not necessary.

Abbreviations Introduced in This Chapter

A/E	Attachment-effacement
AAD	Antibiotic-associated diarrhea
ART	Antiretroviral therapy
cAMP	Cyclic adenosine monophosphate
CDAD	*Clostridium difficile*–associated diarrhea

Table 76–5

Food Poisonings

Organism	Onset (Hours)	Associated Foods	Duration	Symptoms	Treatment
Staphylococcus aureus	1–6	Salad, pastries, ham, poultry	12 hours	Nausea, vomiting	Supportive
Bacillus cereus—emetic	0.5–6	Rice, noodles, pasta, pastries	24 hours	Vomiting	Supportive
Bacillus cereus—diarrheal	8–16	Meats, vegetables, soups, sauces, milk products	24 hours	Diarrhea, abdominal pain	Supportive
Clostridium perfringens (type A)	8–12	Meats, poultry	24 hours	Nausea, abdominal cramps, profuse, watery diarrhea	Supportive
Clostridium botulinum	18–24	Canned fruits, vegetables, meats, honey, salsa, relish	Weeks	Acute GI symptoms followed by symmetric, descending, flaccid paralysis; death is possible	Supportive (including mechanical ventilation); trivalent antitoxin

CFUs	Colony-forming units
EHEC	Enterohemorrhagic *Escherichia coli*
EIA	Enzyme immunoassay
ELISA	Enzyme-linked immunosorbent assay
GBS	Guillain-Barré syndrome
HUS	Hemolytic-uremic syndrome
ORT	Oral rehydration therapy
MIC	Minimum inhibitory concentration
PCR	Polymerase chain reaction
STEC	Shiga toxin-producing *E. coli*
Stx	Shiga toxin
VRE	Vancomycin-resistant enterococcus

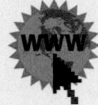 Self-assessment questions and answers are available at *http://www.mhpharmacotherapy.com/pp.html.*

REFERENCES

1. Martin S, Jung R. Gastrointestinal infections and enterotoxigenic poisonings. In: DiPiro JT, Talbert RL, Yee GC, et al., eds. Pharmacotherapy: A Pathophysiologic Approach, 6th ed. New York: McGraw-Hill, 2005:2035–2053.
2. Kotloff KL, Winickoff JP, Ivanoff B, et al. Global burden of Shigella infections: Implications for vaccine development and implementation of control strategies. Bull World Health Organ 1999;77:651–666.
3. DuPont HL, Levine MM, Hornick RB, Formal SB. Inoculum size in shigellosis and implications for expected mode of transmission. J Infect Dis 1989;159:1126–1128.
4. Sansonetti PJ. Rupture, invasion and inflammatory destruction of the intestinal barrier by Shigella, making sense of prokaryote-eukaryote cross-talks. FEMS Microbiol Rev 2001;25:3–14.
5. The choice of antibacterial drugs. Med Lett Drugs Ther 2001;43:69–78.
6. Taylor DN, McKenzie R, Durbin A, et al. Rifaximin, a nonabsorbed oral antibiotic, prevents shigellosis after experimental challenge. Clin Infect Dis 2006;42:1283–1288.
7. Ackers ML, Puhr ND, Tauxe RV, Mintz ED. Laboratory-based surveillance of Salmonella serotype Typhi infections in the United States: Antimicrobial resistance on the rise. JAMA 2000;283:2668–2673.
8. Butler T, Frenck RW, Johnson RB, Khakhria R. In vitro effects of azithromycin on Salmonella typhi: Early inhibition by concentrations less than the MIC and reduction of MIC by alkaline pH and small inocula. J Antimicrob Chemother 2001;47:455–458.
9. ACIP revises typhoid immunization recommendations. Am Fam Physician 1995;51:969–970.
10. Skirrow MB. In: Blaser MJ, Smith PD, Ravdin J, eds. Infections of the Gastrointestinal Tract, 2nd ed. Philadelphia: Lippincott-Raven, 2002:825–848.
11. Paton JC, Paton AW. Pathogenesis and diagnosis of Shiga toxin-producing Escherichia coli infections. Clin Microbiol Rev 1998;11:450–479.
12. Sack DA, Sack RB, Nair GB, Siddique AK. Cholera. Lancet 2004;363:223–233.
13. Blake PA, Allegra DT, Snyder JD, et al. Cholera—a possible endemic focus in the United States. N Engl J Med 1980;302:305–309.
14. Faruque SM, Chowdhury N, Kamruzzaman M, et al. Reemergence of epidemic Vibrio cholerae O139, Bangladesh. Emerg Infect Dis 2003;9:1116–1122.
15. Glass RI, Holmgren J, Haley CE, et al. Predisposition for cholera of individuals with O blood group. Possible evolutionary significance. Am J Epidemiol 1985;121:791–796.
16. Sack DA, Tacket CO, Cohen MB, et al. Validation of a volunteer model of cholera with frozen bacteria as the challenge. Infect Immun 1998;66:1968–1972.
17. Field M, Fromm D, al-Awqati Q, Greenough WB 3rd. Effect of cholera enterotoxin on ion transport across isolated ileal mucosa. J Clin Invest 1972;51:796–804.
18. Zaman K, Yunus M, Rahman A, et al. Efficacy of a packaged rice oral rehydration solution among children with cholera and cholera-like illness. Acta Paediatr 2001;90:505–510.
19. Cohen MB, Giannella RA, Bean J, et al. Randomized, controlled human challenge study of the safety, immunogenicity, and protective efficacy of a single dose of Peru-15, a live attenuated oral cholera vaccine. Infect Immun 2002;70:1965–1970.
20. Holmgren J, Clemens J, Sack DA, Svennerholm AM. New cholera vaccines. Vaccine 1989;7:94–96.
21. Tacket CO, Cohen MB, Wasserman SS, et al. Randomized, double-blind, placebo-controlled, multicentered trial of the efficacy of a single dose of live oral cholera vaccine CVD 103-HgR in preventing cholera following challenge with Vibrio cholerae O1 El Tor Inaba three months after vaccination. Infect Immun 1999;67:6341–6345.
22. Tacket CO, Kotloff KL, Losonsky G, et al. Volunteer studies investigating the safety and efficacy of live oral El Tor Vibrio cholerae O1 vaccine strain CVD 111. Am J Trop Med Hyg 1997;56:533–537.
23. Tacket CO, Losonsky G, Nataro JP, et al. Initial clinical studies of CVD 112 Vibrio cholerae O139 live oral vaccine: Safety and efficacy against experimental challenge. J Infect Dis 1995;172:883–886.
24. Trach DD, Clemens JD, Ke NT, et al. Field trial of a locally produced, killed, oral cholera vaccine in Vietnam. Lancet 1997;349:231–235.
25. Okhuysen PC. Current concepts in travelers' diarrhea: Epidemiology, antimicrobial resistance and treatment. Curr Opin Infect Dis 2005;18:522–526.
26. Chapin AR, Carpenter CM, Dudley WC, et al. Prevalence of norovirus among visitors from the United States to Mexico and Guatemala who experience traveler's diarrhea. J Clin Microbiol 2005;43:1112–1117.
27. Huang DB, Sanchez AP, Triana E, et al. United States male students who heavily consume alcohol in Mexico are at greater risk of travelers' diarrhea than their female counterparts. J Travel Med 2004;11:143–145.
28. Bartlett JG. Clostridium difficile: History of its role as an enteric pathogen and the current state of knowledge about the organism. Clin Infect Dis 1994;18(Suppl 4):S265–S272.
29. Wistrom J, Norrby SR, Myhre EB, et al. Frequency of antibiotic-associated diarrhoea in 2462 antibiotic-treated hospitalized patients: A prospective study. J Antimicrob Chemother 2001;47:43–50.
30. Gaynes R, Rimland D, Killum E, et al. Outbreak of Clostridium difficile infection in a long-term care facility: Association with gatifloxacin use. Clin Infect Dis 2004;38:640–645.
31. Pepin J, Saheb N, Coulombe MA, et al. Emergence of fluoroquinolones as the predominant risk factor for Clostridium difficile-associated diarrhea: A cohort study during an epidemic in Quebec. Clin Infect Dis 2005;41:1254–1260.
32. Bignardi GE. Risk factors for Clostridium difficile infection. J Hosp Infect 1998;40:1–15.
33. Dial S, Delaney JA, Barkun AN, Suissa S. Use of gastric acid-suppressive agents and the risk of community-acquired Clostridium difficile-associated disease. JAMA 2005;294:2989–2995.
34. Apisarnthanarak A, Razavi B, Mundy LM. Adjunctive intracolonic vancomycin for severe Clostridium difficile colitis: Case series and review of the literature. Clin Infect Dis 2002;35:690–696.
35. Chen XM, Keithly JS, Paya CV, LaRusso NF. Cryptosporidiosis. N Engl J Med 2002;346:1723–1731.
36. Smith HV, Corcoran GD. New drugs and treatment for cryptosporidiosis. Curr Opin Infect Dis 2004;17:557–564.

37. White AC. Nitazoxanide: A new broad spectrum antiparasitic agent. Expert Rev Anti Infect Ther 2004;2:43–50.

38. Mead PS, Slutsker L, Dietz V, et al. Food-related illness and death in the United States. Emerg Infect Dis 1999;5:607–625.

39. Mounts AW, Holman RC, Clarke MJ, et al. Trends in hospitalizations associated with gastroenteritis among adults in the United States, 1979–1995. Epidemiol Infect 1999;123:1–8.

40. Clark B, McKendrick M. A review of viral gastroenteritis. Curr Opin Infect Dis 2004;17:461–469.

41. Parashar UD, Hummelman EG, Bresee JS, et al. Global illness and deaths caused by rotavirus disease in children. Emerg Infect Dis 2003;9:565–572.

42. Wilhelmi I, Roman E, Sanchez-Fauquier A. Viruses causing gastroenteritis. Clin Microbiol Infect 2003;9:247–262.

43. Vesikari T, Matson DO, Dennehy P, et al. Safety and efficacy of a pentavalent human-bovine (WC3) reassortant rotavirus vaccine. N Engl J Med 2006;354:23–33.

77 Intra-Abdominal Infections

Joseph T. DiPiro and Thomas R. Howdieshell

LEARNING OBJECTIVES

● **Upon completion of the chapter, the reader will be able to:**

1. Define and differentiate between primary and secondary intra-abdominal infections.

2. Describe the microbiology typically seen with primary and secondary intra-abdominal infections.

3. Describe the clinical presentation typically seen with primary and secondary intra-abdominal infections.

4. Describe the role of culture and susceptibility information for diagnosis and treatment of intra-abdominal infections.

5. Recommend the most appropriate drug and nondrug measures to treat intra-abdominal infections.

6. Recommend an appropriate antimicrobial regimen for treatment of a primary and a secondary intra-abdominal infection.

7. Describe the patient-assessment process during the treatment of intra-abdominal infections.

KEY CONCEPTS

❶ Most intra-abdominal infections are "secondary" infections that are caused by a defect in the GI tract that must be treated by surgical drainage, resection, and/or repair.

❷ Primary peritonitis generally is caused by a single organism (*Staphylococcus aureus* in patients undergoing continuous ambulatory peritoneal dialysis [CAPD] and *Escherichia coli* in patients with cirrhosis).

❸ Secondary intra-abdominal infections usually are caused by a mixture of enteric gram-negative bacilli and anaerobes. This mix of organisms enhances the pathogenic potential of the bacteria.

❹ For peritonitis, early and aggressive IV fluid resuscitation and electrolyte replacement therapy are essential. A common cause of early death is hypovolemic shock caused by inadequate intravascular volume expansion and tissue perfusion.

❺ Cultures of secondary intra-abdominal infection sites generally are not useful for directing antimicrobial therapy. Treatment generally is initiated on a "presumptive" or empirical basis.

❻ Antimicrobial regimens for secondary intra-abdominal infections should include coverage for enteric gram-negative bacilli and anaerobes. Antimicrobial agents that may be used for treatment of secondary intra-abdominal infections include the following: (a) a β-lactam–β-lactamase-inhibitor combination, (b) a carbapenem, and (c) a quinolone plus metronidazole or an aminoglycoside plus clindamycin (or metronidazole).

❼ Treatment of primary peritonitis for CAPD patients should include an antistaphylococcal antimicrobial such as a first-generation cephalosporin (cefazolin) or vancomycin, usually given by the intraperitoneal (IP) route.

❽ The duration of antimicrobial treatment should be for a total of 5 to 7 days for most intra-abdominal infections.

Intra-abdominal infections are those contained within the peritoneal cavity or retroperitoneal space. The peritoneal cavity extends from the undersurface of the diaphragm to the floor of the pelvis and contains the stomach, small bowel, large bowel, liver, gallbladder, and spleen. The duodenum, pancreas, kidneys, adrenal glands, great vessels (aorta and vena cava), and most mesenteric vascular structures reside in the retroperitoneum. Intra-abdominal infections may be generalized or localized. They may be contained within visceral structures, such as the liver, gallbladder, spleen, pancreas, kidney, or female reproductive organs. Two general types of intra-abdominal infection are discussed throughout this chapter: peritonitis and abscess.

Peritonitis is defined as the acute inflammatory response of the peritoneal lining to microorganisms, chemicals,

Patient Encounter 1, Part 1

A 67-year-old man presents to the emergency room in acute distress with abdominal pain, nausea, and vomiting. The patient was in a reasonably good state of health until yesterday evening when he had a sudden onset of excruciating abdominal pain. During the night, he had a few episodes of vomiting, and the pain did not diminish. His physical exam is completely normal and no focal neurologic deficits were observed.

The patient is taking glyburide for noninsulin-dependent diabetes mellitus and has been treated in the past for peptic ulcer disease with ranitidine and omeprazole. He has a history of allergy to various types of pollen but reports no allergies to drugs. He reports moderate consumption of alcohol and smoking two packs of cigarettes per day.

What other information would you like to have about this patient before beginning treatment?

What are the goals of treatment?

Patient Encounter 2, Part 1

A 28-year-old woman, who has been undergoing peritoneal dialysis for chronic renal failure and reports to her doctor's clinic with cloudy dialysate and generalized abdominal pain and cramping.

HPI: The abdominal pain began about two days ago.

PMH: The patient has had renal failure since 22 years of age as a result of diabetes. She has been on peritoneal dialysis for the past three years. She also has hyperlipidemia. She reports two prior episodes in the past year similar to the present one.

Meds: She usually takes a combination of NPH and regular human insulin which controls her blood sugar. She takes simvastatin for dyslipidemia.

SOC: The patient is married with no children. She does not smoke or drink alcohol. There is no history of renal disease in her family.

PE: The abdomen is found to be tender. Bowel sounds are hypoactive. The remainder of the physical exam in not contributory.

VS: T 99°F (37.2°C), BP 128/82 mm Hg, P 96 bpm, wt 76 kg (167 lb), ht 5'7" (170 cm), RR 20 per minute.

Labs: Hct 40%, Hgb 13.4 g/dL (134 g/L or 8.3 mmol/L), WBC $9.2 \times 10^3/mm^3$ ($9.2 \times 10^9/L$), serum: glucose 256 mg/dL (14.2 mmol/L), serum creatinine 3.2 mg/dL (283 μmol/L), BUN 43 g/dL (15.4 mmol/L), Na 138 mEq/L (138 mmol/L), K 4.2 mEq/L 4.2 mmol/L), Cl 103 mEq/L (103 mmol/L), CO_2 23 mEq/L (23 mmol/L), total bilirubin 0.3 mg/dL (5.13 μmol/L), albumin 3.9 g/dL (39 g/L).

What is the likely diagnosis?

How does this type of infection differ from secondary peritonitis?

What are the likely pathogens? Should a culture be performed in this patient? If so, what sites?

What else would you want to know about this patient?

---

irradiation, or foreign-body injury. This chapter deals only with peritonitis of infectious origin.

An abscess is a purulent collection of fluid separated from surrounding tissue by a wall consisting of inflammatory cells and adjacent organs. It usually contains necrotic debris, bacteria, and inflammatory cells. Peritonitis and abscess differ considerably in presentation and approach to treatment.

EPIDEMIOLOGY AND ETIOLOGY

Peritonitis may be classified as primary, secondary, or tertiary. Primary peritonitis, also called *spontaneous bacterial peritonitis*, is an infection of the peritoneal cavity without an evident source of bacteria from the abdomen.[1,2] In secondary peritonitis, a focal disease process is evident within the abdomen. Secondary peritonitis may involve perforation of the GI tract (possibly because of ulceration, ischemia, or obstruction), postoperative peritonitis, or post-traumatic peritonitis (e.g., blunt or penetrating trauma). Tertiary peritonitis occurs in critically ill patients; and it is an infection that persists or recurs at least 48 hours after apparently adequate management of primary or secondary peritonitis.

① *Primary peritonitis develops in 10% to 30% of patients with alcoholic cirrhosis.*[3] Patients undergoing continuous ambulatory peritoneal dialysis (CAPD) average one episode of peritonitis every 2 years.[4] Secondary peritonitis may be caused by perforation of a peptic ulcer; traumatic perforation of the stomach, small or large bowel, uterus, or urinary bladder, appendicitis, pancreatitis, diverticulitis,

bowel infarction, inflammatory bowel disease, cholecystitis, operative contamination of the peritoneum, or diseases of the female genital tract such as septic abortion, postoperative uterine infection, endometritis, or salpingitis. Appendicitis is one of the most common causes of intra-abdominal infection. In 2006, 341,000 appendectomies were performed in the United States for suspected appendicitis.[5]

Primary peritonitis in adults occurs most commonly in association with alcoholic cirrhosis, especially in its end stage, or with ascites caused by postnecrotic cirrhosis, chronic active hepatitis, acute viral hepatitis, congestive heart failure, malignancy, systemic lupus erythematosus, and nephrotic syndrome. It also may result from the use of a peritoneal catheter for dialysis with renal failure or CNS ventriculoperitoneal shunting for hydrocephalus. Abscesses are the result of chronic inflammation and may occur without preceding generalized peritonitis. They may be located within the peritoneal cavity or in a visceral organ and may vary in size, taking a few weeks to years to form.

The causes of intra-abdominal abscess overlap those of peritonitis and, in fact, may occur sequentially or simultaneously. Appendicitis is the most frequent cause of abscess.

PATHOPHYSIOLOGY

Intra-abdominal infection results from bacterial entry into the peritoneal or retroperitoneal spaces or from bacterial collections within intra-abdominal organs. In primary peritonitis, bacteria may enter the abdomen via the bloodstream or the lymphatic system by transmigration through the bowel wall, through an indwelling peritoneal dialysis (PD) catheter, or via the fallopian tubes in females. Hematogenous bacterial spread (through the bloodstream) occurs more frequently with tuberculosis peritonitis or peritonitis associated with cirrhotic ascites. When peritonitis results from PD, skin-surface flora are introduced via the peritoneal catheter. In secondary peritonitis, bacteria most often enter the peritoneum or retroperitoneum as a result of perforation of the GI or female genital tracts caused by diseases or traumatic injuries.

If bacteria that enter the abdomen are not handled by cellular and humoral defense mechanisms, bacterial dissemination occurs throughout the peritoneal cavity, resulting in peritonitis. This is more likely to occur in the presence of a foreign body, hematoma, necrotic tissue, large bacterial inoculum, continuing bacterial contamination, and contamination involving a mixture of synergistic organisms.

The fluid and protein shift into the abdomen (called *third spacing*) may be so dramatic that circulating blood volume is decreased, which causes decreased cardiac output and hypovolemic shock. Accompanying fever, vomiting, or diarrhea may worsen the fluid imbalance. A reflex sympathetic response, manifested by sweating, tachycardia, and vasoconstriction, may be evident. With an inflamed peritoneum, bacteria and endotoxins are absorbed easily into the bloodstream (translocation), and this may result in septic shock.[1] Other foreign substances present in the peritoneal cavity potentiate peritonitis, notably feces, dead tissues, barium, mucus, bile, and blood.

Many of the manifestations of intra-abdominal infections, particularly peritonitis, result from cytokine activity. Inflammatory cytokines are produced by macrophages and neutrophils in response to bacteria and bacterial products or to tissue injury, resulting from the surgical incision.[1] These cytokines produce wide-ranging effects on the endothelium of organs, particularly the liver, lungs, kidneys, and heart. With uncontrolled activation of these mediators, sepsis may

result.[6] Peritonitis may result in death because of the effects on major organ systems.

An abscess occurs if peritoneal contamination is localized but bacterial elimination is incomplete. The location of the abscess often is related to the site of primary disease. For example, abscesses resulting from appendicitis tend to appear in the right lower quadrant or the pelvis; those resulting from diverticulitis tend to appear in the left lower quadrant or pelvis. A mature abscess may have a fibrinous capsule that isolates bacteria and the liquid core from antimicrobials and immunologic defenses.

Microbiology of Intra-Abdominal Infection

❷ *Primary bacterial peritonitis is often caused by a single organism.* In children, the pathogen is usually *Streptococcus pneumoniae* or a group A *Streptococcus*, *E. coli*, *S. pneumoniae*, or Bacteroides species.[4,7] When peritonitis occurs in association with cirrhotic ascites, *E. coli* and *Klebsiella* are isolated most frequently.[8] Other potential pathogens are *Haemophilus pneumoniae*, *Klebsiella*, *Pseudomonas*, *anaerobes*, and *S. pneumoniae*.[9] Occasionally, primary peritonitis may be caused by *Mycobacterium* tuberculosis. Peritonitis in patients undergoing PD is caused most often by common skin organisms such as *S. epidermidis*, *S. aureus*, *Streptococci*, and diphtheroids. Occasionally, aerobic gram-negative bacilli may cause infections, particularly in patients undergoing dialysis during hospitalization. Death from primary peritonitis caused by gram-negative bacteria occurs much more frequently than from gram-positive bacteria.[10]

❸ *Because of the diverse bacteria present in the GI tract, secondary intra-abdominal infections are often polymicrobial.*[2,11] The mean number of different bacterial species isolated from infected intra-abdominal sites ranged from 3 when infection involves the small intestine to 26 with the colon.[11]

Bacterial Synergism

A combination of aerobic and anaerobic organisms appears to increase the severity of infection. Facultative bacteria (such as *E. coli*) may provide an environment conducive to the growth of anaerobic bacteria.[2] Although many bacteria isolated in mixed infections are nonpathogenic by themselves, their presence may be essential for the pathogenicity of the bacterial mixture.[3] Facultative bacteria in mixed infections have the ability to:

- Promote an appropriate environment for anaerobic growth through oxygen consumption
- Produce nutrients necessary for anaerobes
- Produce extracellular enzymes that promote tissue invasion by anaerobes.

Bacteria such as *E. coli* appear responsible for the early mortality from peritonitis, whereas anaerobic bacteria are major pathogens in abscesses, with *B. fragilis* predominating.[12] *Enterococcus* can be isolated from many intra-abdominal infections in humans, but its role as a pathogen is not clear.[13]

Clinical Presentation of Primary Peritonitis

General

Patients may not be in acute distress, particularly with peritoneal dialysis.

Symptoms

Patient may complain of nausea, vomiting (sometimes with diarrhea), and abdominal tenderness.

Signs

- Temperature may be only mildly elevated or not elevated in patients undergoing peritoneal dialysis.
- Bowel sounds are hypoactive
- Cirrhotic patients may have worsening encephalopathy.
- There may be cloudy dialysate fluid with peritoneal dialysis.

Laboratory Tests

- The WBC may be only mildly elevated.
- Ascitic fluid usually contains more than $0.3 \times 10^3/mm^3$ $(0.3 \times 10^9/L)$ leukocytes, and bacteria may be evident on gram stain of a centrifuged specimen.

Other Diagnostic Tests

Culture of peritoneal dialysate or ascitic fluid should be positive.

Clinical Presentation of Secondary Peritonitis

General

Patients may be in acute distress.

Symptoms

- Patients may complain of nausea, vomiting, and generalized abdominal pain.
- Patients may demonstrate abdominal guarding and a "boardlike abdomen."

Signs

- Tachypnea and tachycardia are present.
- Temperature is normal initially, then may increase to 100°F to 102°F (37.7–38.9°C) within the first few hours, and may continue to rise for the next several hours.
- Hypotension and shock may develop if intravascular volume is not restored.
- Decreased urine output may develop owing to dehydration.
- Bowel sounds are faint initially and eventually cease.

Laboratory Tests

- The WBC is high (WBCs $15–20 \times 10^3/mm^3$ $[15–20 \times 10^9/L]$), with neutrophils predominating and an elevated percentage of immature neutrophils (bands).
- The hematocrit and blood urea nitrogen increase because of dehydration.
- Hyperventilation and vomiting result in early alkalosis, which changes to acidosis and lactic academia to reduced intravascular volume and diminished tissue perfusion.

Other Diagnostic Tests

Abdominal radiographs may be useful because free air in the abdomen (indicating intestinal perforation) or distension of the small or large bowel is often evident.

CLINICAL PRESENTATION AND DIAGNOSIS

Intra-abdominal infections have a wide spectrum of clinical features. Peritonitis usually is easily recognized, but intra-abdominal abscess often may continue unrecognized for long periods of time. Patients with primary and secondary peritonitis present quite differently.

TREATMENT

Desired Outcomes

The primary goals of treatment are correction of the intra-abdominal disease processes or injuries that have caused infection and drainage of collections of purulent material (abscess). A secondary objective is to resolve the infection without major organ system complications (e.g., pulmonary, hepatic, cardiovascular, or renal failure) or adverse drug effects. Ideally, the patient should be discharged from the hospital with full function for self-care and routine daily activities.

General Approach to Treatment

The treatment of intra-abdominal infection most often requires the coordinated use of three major modalities: (a) prompt drainage; (b) support of vital functions; and (c) appropriate antimicrobial therapy to treat infection not eradicated by surgery.[14] Antimicrobials are an important adjunct to drainage procedures in the treatment of secondary intra-abdominal infections; however, the use of antimicrobial agents without surgical intervention usually is inadequate. For most cases of primary peritonitis, drainage procedures may not be required, and antimicrobial agents become the mainstay of therapy.

Patient Encounter 1, Part 2: Physical Examination and Diagnostic Tests

PE:

The patient is found responsive but in acute distress. He is lying on the examination table with knees drawn up to his chest. There is involuntary abdominal guarding with a rigid abdomen. There are no audible bowel sounds. He is alert and oriented times 3. Neurologic function is intact. Mucous membranes are dry. Stool is heme-negative.

VS: T 101°F (38.3°C), BP 105/70 mm Hg, P 132 bpm, wt 82 kg (180 lb), ht 5'7" (170 cm), RR 24 per minute.

Labs: Hct 46% (0.46 volume fraction), Hgb 15.4 g/dL (154 g/L or 9.5 mmol/L), WBC count 15.2 × 10³/mm³ (15.2 × 10⁹/L) (45% neutrophils, 20% bands)

Serum: Glucose 213 mg/dL (11.8 mmol/L), serum creatinine 1.9 mg/dL (168 μmol/L), BUN 42 g/dL (15 mmol/L), Na 138 mEq/L (138 mmol/L), K 3.7 mEq/L (3.7 mmol/L), Cl 101 mEq/L (101 mmol/L), CO₂ 21 mEq/L (21 mmol/L), calcium 9.8 mg/dL (2.45 mmol/L), magnesium 2.0 mEq/L (1.0 mmol/L), total bilirubin 0.4 mg/dL (6.84 μmol/L), albumin 4.2 g/dL (42 g/L), lactic acid 3.2 mEq/L (3.2 mmol/L)

KUB: An upright abdominal x-ray shows dilated loops of small bowel and free air under the diaphragm.

DPL (diagnostic peritoneal lavage: examination of fluid in peritoneal cavity): No blood is found, but WBCs are evident.

Develop a care plan for this patient for the first 7 days of his hospitalization. This plan should include specific drug recommendations, and monitoring parameters to evaluate outcome.

Patient Encounter 2, Part 2

A sample of dialysate fluid was found to be cloudy. A spun specimen had numerous white cells and gram-positive cocci on gram stain.

Suggest an initial regimen for this patient (agent, dose, and route of administration).

What are some factors that would be considered when deciding the route of antimicrobial administration for this patient?

How long should the antimicrobial be continued?

What can be done to prevent future infections like this?

Nonpharmacologic Therapy

▶ Drainage Procedures

Primary peritonitis is treated with antimicrobials and rarely requires drainage. Secondary peritonitis requires surgical removal of the inflamed or gangrenous tissue to prevent further bacterial contamination. If the surgical procedure is suboptimal, attempts are made to provide drainage of the infected or gangrenous structures.

The drainage of purulent material is the critical component of management of an intra-abdominal abscess. This may be performed surgically or with percutaneous image-guided techniques.[15] Without adequate drainage of the abscess, antimicrobial therapy and fluid resuscitation can be expected to fail. The most valuable microbiologic information may be obtained at the time of percutaneous or operative abscess drainage.

▶ Fluid Therapy

In patients with peritonitis, hypovolemia is often accompanied by acidosis and large volumes of a solution such as lactated Ringer's may be required initially to restore intravascular volume. Maintenance fluids should be instituted (after intravascular volume is restored) with 0.9% sodium chloride and potassium chloride (20 mEq/L [20 mmol/L]) or 5% dextrose and 0.45% sodium chloride with potassium chloride (20 mEq/L [20 mmol/L]). The administration rate should be based on estimated daily fluid loss through urine and nasogastric suction, including 0.5 to 1.0 L for insensible fluid loss. Potassium would not be included routinely if the patient is hyperkalemic or has renal insufficiency. Aggressive fluid therapy often must be continued in the postoperative period because fluid will continue to sequester in the peritoneal cavity, bowel wall, and lumen.

Pharmacologic Therapy

▶ Antimicrobial Therapy

The goals of antimicrobial therapy are as follows:

- To control bacteremia and prevent the establishment of metastatic foci of infection

❹ *In the early phase of serious intra-abdominal infections, attention should be given to preserving major organ system function.* With generalized peritonitis, large volumes of IV fluids are required to maintain intravascular volume, to improve cardiovascular function, and to ensure adequate tissue perfusion and oxygenation. Adequate urine output should be maintained to ensure appropriate fluid resuscitation and to preserve renal function. A common cause of early death is hypovolemic shock caused by inadequate intravascular volume expansion and tissue perfusion.

An additional important component of therapy is nutrition. Intra-abdominal infections often involve the GI tract directly or disrupt its function (paralytic ileus). The return of GI motility may take days, weeks, and occasionally, months. In the interim, enteral or parenteral nutrition as indicated facilitates improved immune function and wound healing to ensure recovery.

- To reduce suppurative complications after bacterial contamination
- To prevent local spread of existing infection

After suppuration has occurred (e.g., an abscess has formed), a cure by antibiotic therapy alone is difficult to achieve; antimicrobials may serve to improve the results with surgery.

5 *An empirical antimicrobial regimen should be started as soon as the presence of intra-abdominal infection is suspected and before identification of the infecting organisms is complete.* Therapy must be initiated based on the likely pathogens, which vary depending on the site of intra-abdominal infection and the underlying disease process. Cultures of secondary intra-abdominal infection sites generally are not useful for directing antimicrobial therapy. Table 77–1 lists the likely pathogens against which antimicrobial agents should be directed.

▶ Antimicrobial Experience

Many studies have been conducted evaluating or comparing the effectiveness of antimicrobials for treatment of intra-abdominal infections. Substantial differences in patient outcomes from treatment with a variety of agents generally have not been demonstrated.[16]

Important findings from the last 25 years of clinical trials regarding selection of antimicrobials for intra-abdominal infections are as follows:

- Antimicrobial regimens for secondary intra-abdominal infections should cover a broad spectrum of aerobic and anaerobic bacteria from the GI tract.

- Single-agent regimens (such as antianaerobic cephalosporins, extended-spectrum penicillins with β-lactamase inhibitors, or carbapenems) are as effective as combinations of aminoglycosides or fluoroquinolones with antianaerobic agents. This is also true for antimicrobial treatment of acute bacterial contamination from penetrating abdominal trauma.

- Clindamycin and metronidazole appear to be equivalent in efficacy when combined with agents effective against aerobic gram-negative bacilli (e.g., gentamicin or aztreonam).

- For most patients, antimicrobial treatment can be completed orally with amoxicillin–clavulanate or the combination of ciprofloxacin and metronidazole.

- Five to seven days of antimicrobial treatment are sufficient for most intra-abdominal infections of mild to moderate severity.

Intra-abdominal infection presents in many different ways and with a wide spectrum of severity. The antibiotic regimen employed and duration of treatment depend on the specific clinical circumstances (i.e., the nature of the underlying disease process and the condition of the patient).

▶ Recommendations

6 *For most intra-abdominal infections, the antimicrobial regimen should be effective against both aerobic and anaerobic bacteria.*[17] Although it is impossible to provide antimicrobial activity against every possible pathogen, agents with activity against enteric gram-negative bacilli, such as *E. coli* and *Klebsiella*, and anaerobes, such as *B. fragilis* and *Clostridia* spp., should be administered.

Table 77–2 presents the recommended agents for treatment of community-acquired and complicated intra-abdominal infections from the Infectious Diseases Society of America and the Surgical Infection Society.[18,19] These recommendations were formulated using an evidence-based approach. Most community-acquired infections are "mild to moderate," whereas health care–associated infections tend to be more severe and difficult to treat. Table 77–3

Table 77–1

Likely Intra-Abdominal Pathogens

Type of Infection	Aerobes	Anaerobes
Primary Bacterial Peritonitis		
Children (spontaneous)	Group A *Streptococcus, Escherichia coli,* pneumococci	
Cirrhosis	*E. coli, Klebsiella,* pneumococci (many others)	–
Peritoneal dialysis	*Staphylococcus, Streptococcus*	–
Secondary Bacterial Peritonitis		
Gastroduodenal	*Streptococcus, E. coli*	–
Biliary tract	*E. coli, Klebsiella,* enterococci	Clostridium or Bacteroides (infrequent)
Small or large bowel	*E. coli, Klebsiella* spp., *Proteus* spp.	Bacteroides fragilis and other Bacteroides; Clostridium
Appendicitis	*E. coli, Pseudomonas*	*Bacteroides spp.*
Abscesses	*E. coli, Klebsiella,* enterococci	*B. fragilis* and other Bacteroides, Clostridium, anaerobic cocci
Liver	*E. coli, Klebsiella,* enterococci, staphylococci, amoeba	Bacteroides (infrequent)
Spleen	*Staphylococcus, Streptococcus*	

From DiPiro JT, Talbert RL, Yee GC, et al., (eds.) Pharmacotherapy: A Pathophysiologic Approach. 7th ed. New York: McGraw-Hill; 2008.

Table 77–2

Recommended Agents for the Treatment of Community-Acquired Complicated Intra-Abdominal Infections

Agents Recommended for Mild to Moderate Infections	Agents Recommended for High-Severity Infections

β-Lactam/β-Lactamase Inhibitor Combinations
  Ampicillin-sulbactam
  Ticarcillin-clavulanate
	Piperacillin-tazobactam

Carbapenems Ertapenem	Imipenem/cilistatin Meropenem
Combination Regimens Cefazolin or cefuroxime plus metronidazole Ciprofloxacin, levofloxacin moxifloxacin, or gatifloxacin, in combination with metronidazole	Third- or fourth-generation cephalosporins (cefotaxime, ceftriaxone, ceftizoxime, ceftazidime, cefepime) plus metronidazole Ciprofloxacin, in combination with metronidazole Aztreonam plus metronidazole

From Refs. 17 and 18.

Table 77–3

Guidelines for Initial Antimicrobial Agents for Intra-Abdominal Infections

Primary Agents		Alternatives
Primary Bacterial Peritonitis		
Cirrhosis	Cefotaxime	1. Add clindamycin or metronidazole if anaerobes are suspected 2. Other third-generation cephalosporins, extended-spectrum penicillins, aztreonam, and imipenem as alternatives 3. Aminoglycoside with antipseudomonal penicillin
Peritoneal dialysis	Initial empiric regimens	
	Cefazolin or cephalothin plus ceftazidime or cefepime	1. An aminoglycoside may be used in place of ceftazidime or cefepime 2. Imipenem/cilsaatin or cefepime may be used alone 3. Quinolones may be used in place of ceftazidime or cefepime if local susceptibilities allow
	Staphylococcus: penicillinase-resistant penicillin or first-generation cephalosporin	1. Alternative for methicillin resistant staphylococci is vancomycin 2. For vancomycin-resistant Staphylococcus aureus, linezolid, daptomycin, or quinupristin-dalfopristin must be used
	Sterptococcus or Enterococcus: ampicillin	1. An aminoglycoside may be added for enterococcal peritonitis 2. Linezolid or quinupristin-dalfopristin should be used to treat vancomycin-resistant enterococcus not susceptible to ampicillin
	Aerobic gram-negative bacillic ceftazidime or cefepime	1. The regimen should be based on in vitro sensitivity tests
	Pseudomonas aeruginosa: two agents with differing mechanisms of actions, such as an oral quinolone plus ceftazidime, cefepime, tobramycin, or piperacillin	
Secondary Bacterial Peritonitis		
Perforated peptic ulcer	First-generation cephalosporins	1. Antianaerobic cephalosporins[a] 2. Possibly add aminoglycoside if patient condition is poor 3. Aminoglycoside with clindamycin or metronidazole; add ampicillin if patient is immunocompromised or if biliary tract origin of infection
Other	Imipenem-cilistatin, meropenem, ertapenem, or extended-spectrum penicillins with β-lactamase inhibitor	1. Ciprofloxacin with metronidazole 2. Aztreonam with clindamycin or metronidazole 3. Antianaerobic cephalosporins[a]

(Continued)

Table 77–3

Guidelines for Initial Antimicrobial Agents for Intra-Abdominal Infections (*Continued*)

Primary Agents		Alternatives
Abscess		
General	Imipenem-cilastatin, meropenem, ertapenem, or extended-spectrum penicillins with β-lactamase inhibitor	1. Aztreonam with clindamycin or metronidazole 2. Ciprofloxacin with metronidazole 3. Aminoglycoside with clindamycin or metronidazole
Liver	As above but add a first-generation cephalosporin	1. Use metronidazole if amoebic liver abscess is suspected
Spleen	Aminoglycoside plus penicillinase-resistant penicillin	1. Alternatives for penicillinase-resistant penicillin are first-generation cephalosporins or vancomycin
Appendicitis		
Normal or inflamed	Antianaerobic cephalosporins[a] (discontinued immediately postoperation)	1. Ampicillin-sulbactam
Gangrenous or perforated	Imipenem-cilastatin, meropenem, ertapenem, antianaerobic cephalosporins or extended-spectrum penicillins with β-lactamase inhibitor	1. Aztreonam with clindamycin or metronidazole 2. Ciprofloxacin with metronidazole 3. Aminoglycoside with clindamycin or metronidazole
Acute cholecystitis	First-generation cephalosporin	1. Aminoglycoside plus ampicillin if severe infection
Cholangitis	Aminoglycoside with ampicillin with or without clindamycin or metronidazole	1. Use vancomycin instead of ampicillin if patient is allergic to penicillin
Acute Contamination from abdominal trauma	Antianaerobic cephalosporins[a] or ampicillin-sulbactam	1. A carbapenem 2. Ciprofloxacin plus metronidazole
Pelvic inflammatory disease	Cefotetan or cefoxitin with doxycycline	1. Clindamycin with gentamicin 2. Ampicillin-sulbactam with doxycycline 3. Ciprofloxacin with doxycycline and metronidazole

[a]Cefoxitin, cefotetan, and ceftizoxime.

From DiPiro JT, Talbert RL, Yee GC, et al., (eds.) Pharmacotherapy: A Pathophysiologic Approach. 7th ed. New York: McGraw-Hill; 2008.

presents guidelines for treatment and alternative regimens for specific situations. These are general guidelines; there are many factors that cannot be incorporated into such a table.

When used for intra-abdominal infection, aminoglycosides should be combined with agents that are effective against the majority of *B. fragilis*. Clindamycin or metronidazole is the agent of first choice, but others, such as antianaerobic cephalosporins (e.g., cefoxitin, cefotetan, or ceftizoxime), piperacillin, mezlocillin, and combinations of extended-spectrum penicillins with β-lactamase inhibitors, would be suitable alternatives. Patients receiving multiple broad-spectrum antimicrobial agents who are immunocompromised should receive an oral antifungal agent (nystatin) for prevention of fungal overgrowth in the mouth and GI tract. The benefits of systemic antifungal prophylaxis (with fluconazole) have not been established for intra-abdominal infection and should not be used routinely.

In immunocompromised patients or patients with valvular heart disease or a prosthetic heart valve, there is justification to provide specific antimicrobial activity against *enterococci*. Ampicillin or other penicillins that are active against *enterococci* (e.g., penicillin, piperacillin, and mezlocillin) should be used in patients at high-risk, patients with persistent or recurrent intra-abdominal infection, or patients who are immunosuppressed, such as after organ transplantation. Ampicillin remains the drug of choice for this indication because it is most active in vitro against *enterococci* and is relatively inexpensive. Vancomycin is active against most *enterococci*; however, resistance is increasing, and this agent should be reserved for established infections when first-line therapies cannot be used.

IP administration of antibiotics is preferred over IV therapy in the treatment of peritonitis that occurs in patients undergoing CAPD.[20] The International Society of Peritoneal Dialysis (ISPD) revised its guidelines for the diagnosis and pharmacotherapy of PD-associated infections.[21] The guidelines provide dosing recommendations for intermittent and continuous therapy based on the modality of dialysis (CAPD or automated peritoneal dialysis [APD]) and the extent of the patient's residual renal function.

❼ *Antimicrobial agents effective against both gram-positive and gram-negative organisms should be used for initial IP empirical therapy for peritonitis in PD patients.* The most important factors to take into consideration for initial antimicrobial selection are the dialysis center's and the patient's history of infecting organisms and their sensitivities. The use of cefazolin (loading dose [LD] 500 mg/L, maintenance dose [MD] 125 mg/L) plus ceftazidime (LD 500 mg/L, MD 125 mg/L) or cefepime (LD 500 mg/L, MD 125 mg/L) or an aminoglycoside (gentamicin-tobramycin LD 8 mg/L, MD 4 mg/L) is suitable for initial empirical therapy; if patients are allergic to cephalosporin antibiotics, vancomycin (LD 1,000 mg/L, MD 25 mg/L) or an aminoglycoside should be substituted. Another option is monotherapy with imipenem-cilastin (LD 500 mg/L, MD 200 mg/L) or cefepime. Antimicrobial doses should be increased empirically by 25% in patients with residual renal function (more than 100 mL/day urine output).[21] Antimicrobial therapy should be continued for at least 1 week after the dialysate fluid is clear and for a total of at least 14 days. The reader is referred to these guidelines for additional information.[21]

After acute bacterial contamination, such as with abdominal trauma where GI contents spill into the peritoneum, combination antimicrobial regimens are not required. If the patient is seen soon after injury (within 2 hours) and surgical measures are instituted promptly, antianaerobic cephalosporins (such as cefoxitin or cefotetan) or extended-spectrum penicillins are effective in preventing most infectious complications. Antimicrobials should be administered as soon as possible after injury.[22]

For appendicitis, the antimicrobial regimen used should depend on the appearance of the appendix at the time of operation, which may be normal, inflamed, gangrenous, or perforated. Because the condition of the appendix is unknown preoperatively, it is advisable to begin antimicrobial agents before the appendectomy is performed. Reasonable regimens would be antianaerobic cephalosporins or, if the patient is seriously ill, a carbapenem or β-lactam–β-lactamase-inhibitor combination. If, at operation, the appendix were normal or inflamed, postoperative antimicrobials would not be required. If the appendix is gangrenous or perforated, a treatment course of 5 to 7 days with the agents listed in Table 77–2 is appropriate.

⑧ *Acute intra-abdominal contamination, such as after a traumatic injury, may be treated with a short course (24 hours) of antimicrobials.*[22] *For established infections (i.e., peritonitis or intra-abdominal abscess), an antimicrobial course limited to 5 to 7 days is justified.* Under certain conditions, therapy for longer than 7 days would be justified, for example, if the patient remains febrile or is in poor general condition, when relatively resistant bacteria are isolated, or when a focus of infection in the abdomen still may be present. For some abscesses, such as pyogenic liver abscess, antimicrobials may be required for a month or longer.

OUTCOME EVALUATION

• Whether diagnosed with primary or secondary peritonitis, monitor the patient for relief of symptoms. Once antimicrobials are initiated and the other important therapies described earlier are used, most patients should show improvement within 2 to 3 days. Successful antimicrobial therapy with

resolution of infection will result in decreased pain, manifested as resolution of abdominal guarding and decreased use of pain medications over time. The patient should not appear in distress, with the exception of recognized discomfort and pain from incisions, drains, and a nasogastric tube.

Monitor vital signs and WBC count with differential; each should normalize as the infection resolves. At 24 to 48 hours, aerobic bacterial culture results should be available. If a suspected pathogen is not sensitive to the antimicrobial agents being given, the regimen should be changed if the patient has not shown sufficient improvement. If the isolated pathogen is extremely sensitive to one antimicrobial and the patient is progressing well, concurrent antimicrobial therapy often may be discontinued.

With anaerobic culturing techniques and the slow growth of these organisms, anaerobes often are not identified until 4 to 7 days after culture, and sensitivity information is difficult to obtain. For this reason, anaerobic culture information generally is not helpful for selection of the antianaerobic component of the antimicrobial regimen. A report indicating that anaerobes were not isolated should not be the sole justification for discontinuing antianaerobic drugs because anaerobic bacteria that were present in the infectious process may not have been transported properly to the microbiology laboratory, or other problems may have led to bacterial death in vitro.

Once the patient's temperature is normal for 48 to 72 hours and the patient is eating, consider changing the IV antibiotic to an oral regimen for the duration of antibiotic treatment. Monitor the serum creatinine level to evaluate for renal complications as well as potential drug toxicity, especially if an aminoglycoside is a component of the antibiotic regimen. Bowel sounds should return to normal. Evaluate the patient daily for development of rash or other drug-related adverse effects.

For patients with primary peritonitis, if peritoneal dialysate cultures were positive initially, repeat cultures should be negative. For patients with secondary peritonitis, monitor the amount of fluid draining if a drain was placed. The volume of drainage should lessen as the infection resolves. Repeat abdominal radiographs should return to normal.

If symptoms do not improve, the patient should be evaluated for persistent infection. There are many reasons for poor patient outcome with intra-abdominal infection; improper antimicrobial selection is only one. The patient may be immunocompromised, which decreases the likelihood of successful outcome with any regimen. It is impossible for antimicrobials to compensate for a nonfunctioning immune system. There may be surgical reasons for poor patient outcome. Failure to identify all intra-abdominal foci of infection or leaks from a GI anastomosis may cause continued intra-abdominal infection. Even when intra-abdominal infection is controlled, accompanying organ system failure, most often renal or respiratory, may lead to patient demise.

The outcome from intra-abdominal infection is not determined solely by what transpires in the abdomen. Unsatisfactory outcomes in patients with intra-abdominal

Patient Care and Monitoring

1. A thorough patient medication history should be taken at the time of admission to document all recent medication use, including nonprescription medications and use of complementary or alternative medicines. Any drug allergies or intolerances also should be documented.

2. The initial antimicrobial regimen should conform to standard guidelines unless an appropriate justification for an alternative regimen is evident. With the first few doses of antimicrobial, assess the patient for hypersensitivity reactions or other acute intolerances.

3. Review the dosages of all medications to be sure that they are appropriate for age, weight, and major organ function Verify that the drugs selected are not contraindicated in the patient with allergies or other intolerances.

4. Confirm that all necessary acute and chronic medications are continued postoperatively.

5. Monitor vital signs (i.e., temperature and heart rate) and laboratory assessments (i.e., WBC count) daily to assess resolution of infection and efficacy of pain medications. When possible, interview the patient to obtain additional information about pain control.

6. Evaluate fluid status to ensure that the patient is not hypovolemic. In a seriously ill patient, assess intravascular volume by monitoring blood pressure and heart rate, but do so more accurately by measuring central venous pressure or urinary output via a urinary bladder catheter. Urine output should equal or exceed 0.5 mL/kg of body weight per hour.

7. Review results of cultures obtained preoperatively or during the surgical procedure. Evaluate the appropriateness of antibiotic therapy based on susceptibility information. Although some investigators suggest that routine culturing of patients with community-acquired intra-abdominal infections contributes little to their management other investigators suggest that antimicrobial therapy should be based on susceptibility of the bacteria collected from the operative site because this has been shown to correlate with clinical outcome.[24]

8. Assess serum creatinine and aminoglycoside serum concentrations if the patient is being treated with an aminoglycoside. Adjust aminoglycoside dose based on serum concentrations; target peak concentration with multiple doses per day = 6 mcg/mL (12.5 μmol/L gentamicin or 12.8 μmol/L tobramycin).

9. On the fifth day of antimicrobial treatment or when GI function returns, determine if parenteral antimicrobial agents can be switched to oral agents to complete therapy.

10. Assess nutritional needs and recommend appropriate supplementation. When the patient is tolerating an oral diet, determine if any parenteral medications can be switched to the oral route.

11. Monitor the patient for the development of potential complications of treatment such as delayed hypersensitivity reactions, antibiotic-induced diarrhea, pseudomembraneous colitis, or fungal superinfections (manifested as oral thrush).

12. Provide information to the patient concerning the medications administered in the hospital as well as any new medications prescribed for use at home. Advise the patient to contact his or her doctor or pharmacist if he or she experience any adverse effects from medications.

---

infections may result from complications that arise in other organ systems. Infectious complications commonly associated with mortality after intra-abdominal infection are urinary tract infections and pneumonia.[23] Reasons for antimicrobial failure may not always be apparent. Even when antimicrobial susceptibility tests indicate that an organism is susceptible in vitro to the antimicrobial agent, therapeutic failures may occur. Possibly there is poor penetration of the antimicrobial agent into the focus of infection, or bacterial resistance may develop after initiation of antimicrobial therapy. Also, it is possible that an antimicrobial regimen may encourage the development of infection by organisms not susceptible to the regimen being used. Superinfection in patients being treated for intra-abdominal infection can be caused by *Candida*; however, *Enterococci* or opportunistic gram-negative bacilli such as *Pseudomonas* and *Serratia* may be involved.

Treatment regimens for intra-abdominal infection can be judged as successful if the patient recovers from the infection without recurrent peritonitis or intra-abdominal abscess and without the need for additional antimicrobials. A regimen can be considered unsuccessful if a significant adverse drug reaction occurs, reoperation or percutaneous drainage is necessary, or patient improvement is delayed beyond 1 or 2 weeks.

Abbreviations Introduced in This Chapter

APD	Automated peritoneal dialysis
CAPD	Continuous ambulatory peritoneal dialysis
DPL	Diagnostic peritoneal lavage
IP	Intraperitoneal
ISPD	International Society of Peritoneal Dialysis

LD   Loading dose
MD   Maintenance dose
PD   Peritoneal dialysis
TNF   Tumor necrosis factor

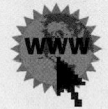 Self-assessment questions and answers are available at *http://www.mhpharmacotherapy.com/pp.html.*

REFERENCES

1. Ordonez CA, Puyana JC. Management of peritonitis in the critically ill patient. Surg Clin North Am 2006;86:1323–1349.
2. Marshall JC. Intra-abdominal infections. Microbes Infect 2004;6:1015–1025.
3. Mowat C, Stanley AJ. Spontaneous bacterial peritonitis—Diagnosis, treatment, and prevention. Aliment Pharmacol Therap 2001;15:1851–1859.
4. Vas S, Oreopoulos DG. Infections in patients undergoing peritoneal dialysis. Infect Dis Clin North Am 2001;15:743–774.
5. DeFrances CJ, Lucas CA, Buie VC, Golosinskiy A. 2006 National Hospital Discharge Survey, National Center for Health Statistics.
6. Riche FC, Cholley BP, Panis YH, et al. Inflammatory cytokine response in patients with septic shock secondary to generalized peritonitis. Crit Care Med 2000;28:433–437.
7. Thompson AE, Marshall JC, Opal SM. Intraabdominal infections in infants and children: Descriptions and definitions. Pediatr Crit Care Med 2005;6:S30–S35.
8. Căruntu FA, Benea L. Spontaneous bacterial peritonitis: Pathogenesis, diagnosis, treatment. J Gastroint Liver Dis 2006;15:51–56.
9. Johnson DH, Cuhna BA. Infections in cirrhosis. Infect Dis Clin North Am 2001;15:363–371.
10. Troidle L, Gordon-Brennan N, Kliger A, Finkelstein F. Differing outcomes of gram-positive and gram-negative peritonitis. Am J Kidney Dis 1998;32:623–628.
11. Brook I. Microbiology and management of abdominal infections. Dig Dis Sci 2008;53:2585–2591.
12. Onderdonk AB, Bartlett JG, Louie T, et al. Microbial synergy in experimental intraabdominal abscess. Infect Immun 1997;13:22–26.
13. Sitges-Serra A, Lopez MJ, Girvent M, et al. Postoperative enterococcal infection after treatment of complicated intraabdominal sepsis. Br J Surg 2002;89:361–367.
14. Gauzit R, Pean Y, Barth X, et al. Epidemiology, management, and prognosis of secondary non-postoperative peritonitis: A French prospective observational multicenter study. Surg Infect 2009;10(2):119–127.
15. Jaffe TA, Nelson RC, Delong DM, Paulson EK. Practice patterns in percutaneous image-guided intraabdominal abscess drainage: Survey of academic and private practice centers. Radiology 2004;233:750–756.
16. Wong PF, Gilliam AD, Kumar S, Shenfine J, O'Dair GN, Leaper DJ. Antibiotic regimens for secondary peritonitis of gastrointestinal origin in adults. Cochrane Database Syst Rev 2005;(2):CD004539.
17. Solomkin JS, Mazuski JE, Baron EJ, et al. Guidelines for the selection of antiinfective agents for complicated intraabdominal infections. Clin Infect Dis 2003;37:997–1005.
18. Mazuski JE, Sawyer RG, Nathens AB, et al. The Surgical Infection Society guidelines on antimicrobial therapy for intraabdominal infections: An executive summary. Surg Infect (Larchmt) 2002;3:161–174.
19. Mazuski JE, Sawyer RG, Nathens AB, et al. The Surgical Infection Society guidelines on antimicrobial therapy for intraabdominal infections: Evidence for recommendations. Surg Infect (Larchmt) 2002;3:175–234.
20. Wiggins KJ. Craig JC. Johnson DW. Strippoli GF. Treatment for peritoneal dialysis-associated peritonitis. Cochrane Database Syst Rev 2008;(1):CD005284.
21. Piraino B, Bailie GR, Bernardini J, et al. Peritoneal dialysis related infections: 2005 update. Perit Dial Int 2005;25:107–131.
22. Bozorgzadeh A, Pizzi WF, Barie PS, et al. The duration of antibiotic administration in penetrating abdominal trauma. Am J Surg 1999;172:125–135.
23. Merlino JI, Yowler CJ, Malangoni MA. Nosocomial infections adversely affect the outcomes of patients with serious intraabdominal infections. Surg Infect (Larchmt) 2004;5:21–27.
24. Nathens AB. Relevance and utility of peritoneal cultures in patients with peritonitis. Surg Infect (Larchmt) 2001;2:153–160.

78 Parasitic Diseases

J.V. Anandan

LEARNING OBJECTIVES

● **Upon completion of the chapter, the reader will be able to:**

1. Identify the primary reasons why some parasitic diseases may be more prevalent in the U.S. population.

2. Describe the treatment algorithm for giardiasis and amebiasis.

3. List one effective therapy for nematodes and select the drugs of choice for strongyloidiasis and tapeworms.

4. List three major reasons why travelers are infected with malaria.

5. Describe the presenting signs and symptoms of malaria.

6. List some specific toxicities of mefloquine.

7. Identify the monitoring parameters for quinidine gluconate in severe malaria.

8. Define the major complications of falciparum malaria.

9. Discuss the cardiovascular complications of chronic South American trypanosomiasis.

10. Describe the steps to take to eradicate lice infestation and scabies.

KEY CONCEPTS

❶ For treatment of giardiasis (or as empirical treatment), metronidazole 250 mg three times daily for 7 days or tinidazole 2 g as a single dose is recommended.

❷ Diagnostic tests for amebiasis include stool for ova, antigen detection, or polymerase chain reaction (PCR) testing.

❸ The drug of choice for nematode infestations (hookworm, enterobiasis, and ascariasis) is mebendazole, while ivermectin is indicated for strongyloidiasis and praziquantel is indicated for tapeworms.

❹ The primary reasons why travelers are infected with malaria are failure to take chemotherapy, inappropriate chemotherapy, and delay in seeking medical care.

❺ Falciparum malaria must be considered a life-threatening medical emergency.

❻ Treatment of serious malarial infection requires admission to an acute care service, IV administration of quinidine gluconate, and symptomatic support.

❼ Complications of falciparum malaria include hypoglycemia, acute renal failure, pulmonary edema, seizure, and coma.

❽ The chronic presentation of American trypanosomiasis includes cardiovascular, GI, and CNS manifestations.

❾ Lice infestation should be treated with 1% permethrin followed by treatment of immediate family members and sexual partners. Bedding and clothes should be sterilized by washing in the hot cycle of the washing machine.

❿ The diagnosis of scabies is made by obtaining skin scrapings and detecting the mite in a wet mount. Topical therapy is 5% permethrin.

Parasitic medicine is an ever changing field. The increased desire of large segments of the U.S. population to travel to Asia, Africa, and other parts of the world can expose them to parasitic infections that are endemic in those areas. The influx of refugees and new immigrant populations from Asia and other parts of the world have brought new parasitic infections to our shores. Migrant farm workers who work and live in substandard hygienic conditions, the large and growing Central and South American immigrant population, and the presence of immunosuppressed populations (e.g., those with the AIDS and transplant patients) represent other significant sources of parasitic infections in the United States.[1–10] Clearly, there is a need for health professionals in the United States to be familiar with the pathophysiology and treatment of parasitic diseases.

Defined below are some terms that are frequently used when discussing parasitic diseases.[9] *Symbiosis* is defined as "living together," when two species are dependent on each other for food and protection. The term *commensalism*, from the Latin translation of "eating at the same table," implies a mutual association in which both organisms may benefit, or at least one benefits but does no harm to the other. In contrast, *parasitism*, although resembling symbiosis in one aspect (i.e., it is also an intimate relationship between two species), does not represent a mutually beneficial association. One species (the host) does not benefit from the relationship, and in fact the relationship may be detrimental to its very survival. Parasites have made morphologic, biochemical, reproductive, and defensive adaptations over time. These adaptations have increased the ability of parasites to survive host defenses and have allowed them to utilize the host's biochemical systems to synthesize necessary cellular components. Beef and pork tapeworms (cestodes) possess highly developed reproductive systems which allow them to transfer easily to new hosts. Because of the lack of digestive systems cestodes are completely host-dependent for all nutrients. Cestodes (tapeworms) (*Taenia saginata* and *T. solium*) use specialized suckers which enable them to obtain blood and vital nutrients from their host. *Entamoeba histolytica*, the causative agent for amebiasis, once it has gained access to the human colon or large intestine is able to invade and utilize its specialized proteolytic enzyme to penetrate and erode the GI mucosa. *E. histolytica* is also able to survive in adverse conditions when it leaves the host by walling itself off and forming cysts; this protects the parasite from environmental conditions until it is ready to infect the next host.

Although acquired immunity to some parasitic diseases may lower the level of infection, absolute immunity as seen in bacterial and viral infections is seldom seen in parasitic diseases. Since parasitic infections produce a wide variety of antigens because of the many life cycle phases, it is more difficult to identify a constant antigenic protein against which specific antibodies are protective. However, malaria remains a likely candidate for a vaccine and there are ongoing studies to develop one.

Space constraints do not allow detailed discussions of the world of parasites, and clinicians and students are directed to some excellent resources for further details on parasites and parasitic diseases.[9,11] Discussion in this chapter will include those parasitic diseases that are more likely to be seen in the United States and will include GI parasites (primarily giardiasis and amebiasis), protozoan infections (malaria and South American trypanosomiasis), some common helminthic diseases (specifically those caused by nematodes and cestodes), and ectoparasites (lice and scabies).

GIARDIASIS

EPIDEMIOLOGY AND ETIOLOGY

Giardia lamblia (also known as *G. intestinalis* or *G. duodenalis*), an enteric protozoan, is the most common intestinal parasite

---

Patient Encounter 1: Giardiasis

MK is a 15-year-old high school student who had traveled to Mexico as part of a school group to practice his Spanish language skills. While in Mexico, he was careful not to drink any local water and only consumed warm or heated food and soda. He is seen in the travel clinic with complaints of some "explosive" crampy diarrhea and has had constipation alternating with diarrhea for the last 2 weeks. MK indicates that his stools have been foul smelling.

Are his symptoms characteristic of giardiasis?

How would you differentiate giardiasis from possible Escherichia coli–*induced diarrhea?*

---

responsible for diarrheal syndromes throughout the world. Giardia is the most frequently identified intestinal parasites in the United States, with a prevalence rate of 5% to 15% in some areas. *G. lamblia* has been identified as the first enteric pathogen seen in children in developing countries, with prevalence rates between 15% and 30%.

There are two stages in the life cycle of *G. lamblia*: the trophozoite and the cyst. *G. lamblia* is found in the small intestine, the gallbladder, and in biliary drainage. The distribution of giardiasis is worldwide with children being more susceptible than adults.

PATHOPHYSIOLOGY

Giardiasis is caused by ingestion of *G. lamblia* cysts in fecally-contaminated water or food.[9–15] The protozoan excysts in the low gastric pH to release the trophozoite. Colonization and multiplication of the trophozoite lead to mucosal invasion, localized edema, and flattening of the villi, resulting in malabsorption states in the host. Achlorhydria, hypogammaglobulinemia, or deficiency in secretory immunoglobulin A (IgA) predispose to giardiasis. Individuals with HIV infection and AIDS may have higher carriage rates than the general population. Some patients may develop lactose intolerance after chronic giardiasis.

CLINICAL PRESENTATION AND DIAGNOSIS

Pharmacologic Therapy

❶ *All symptomatic adults and children over the age of 8 years with giardiasis should be treated with metronidazole 250 mg three times daily for 7 days, or tinidazole 2 g as a single dose, or nitazoxanide (Alinia) 500 mg twice daily for 3 days.*[12,16] The pediatric dose of metronidazole is 15 mg/kg/day three times daily for 7 days. Alternative drugs include furazolidone 100 mg four times daily or paromomycin 25 to 35 mg/kg/day in divided doses daily for 7 days. Paromomycin may be used in pregnancy instead of metronidazole. Pediatric patients

Clinical Presentation and Diagnosis of Giardiasis

Acute Onset

- Diarrhea, cramp-like abdominal pain, bloating, and flatulence
- Malaise, anorexia, nausea, and belching

Chronic Symptoms

- Diarrhea: Foul-smelling, copious, light-colored and greasy stools
- Weight loss, steatorrhea, and vitamin B_{12} and fat-soluble vitamin deficiencies
- Constipation alternating with diarrhea

Diagnosis

- Diagnosis is made by examination of fresh stool or a preserved specimen during acute diarrheal phase
- Fresh stool may show trophozoites while preserved specimens yield cysts. (*Note*: stool for ova may show the presence of other parasites [e.g., *Cryptosporidium parvum*, *E. histolytica*, or *E. hartmanni*]; multiple stool samples may be needed.)
- Even though stool examination for ova and parasites has remained the major means of diagnosis, other diagnostic tests include enzyme-linked immunosorbent assay (ELISA), which is considered to be between 85% and 98% sensitive and almost 100% specific (ProSpec T, Giardia Microplate Assay, Remel, Lenexa, KS).

can also be treated with suspensions of either furazolidone 6 mg/kg/day in four divided doses for 7 days.

Quinacrine 100 mg three times in adults or 5 mg/kg/day in pediatric patients for 5 to 7 days, is available from a specialized pharmacy (e.g., Ponorama Compounding Pharmacy).[12]

Patient Care and Monitoring: Giardiasis

- Metronidazole produces cure rates between 85% and 95%.
- Diarrhea will cease within a few days, although in some patients it may take 1 to 2 weeks.
- Cyst excretion will cease within days.
- Intestinal dysfunction (manifested as increased transit time) and radiologic changes primarily due to chronic infection may take months to resolve.
- Patients who fail therapy with metronidazole should receive a second course with either metronidazole or an alternative agent; nitazoxanide has been shown to be effective in resistant giardiasis.

OUTCOME EVALUATION

Patients with symptomatic giardiasis and positive stool samples or positive enzyme-linked immunosorbent assay (ELISA) tests should be treated with metronidazole for 7 days. Patients who fail initial therapy with metronidazole should receive a second course of therapy. Pregnant patients can receive paromomycin 25 to 35 mg/kg/day in divided doses for 7 days. Giardiasis can be prevented by good hygiene and by using caution in food and drink consumption.

AMEBIASIS

EPIDEMIOLOGY AND ETIOLOGY

Amebiasis remains one of the most important parasitic diseases because of its worldwide distribution and serious GI manifestations. The major causative agent in amebiasis is *E. histolytica*, which invades the colon and must be differentiated from *E. dispar*, which is associated with an asymptomatic carrier state and is considered nonpathogenic.[17–20] Invasive amebiasis is almost exclusively the result of ingesting *E. histolytica* cysts found in fecally-contaminated food or water. Approximately 50 million cases of invasive disease result each year worldwide, leading to an excess of 100,000 deaths. In the general population, the highest incidence is found in institutionalized mentally retarded patients, sexually active homosexuals, AIDS patients, the Native American population, and new immigrants from endemic areas (e.g., Mexico, South and Southeast Asia, West and South Africa, and portions of Central and South America).

PATHOPHYSIOLOGY

E. histolytica invades mucosal cells of colonic epithelium, producing the classic flask-shaped ulcer in the submucosa. The trophozoite toxin has a cytocidal effect on cells. If the trophozoite gets into the portal circulation, it will be carried to the liver, where it produces abscess and periportal fibrosis. Liver abscesses are more common in men than women and are rarely seen in children. Amebic ulcerations can affect the perineum and genitalia, and abscesses may occur in the lung and brain.

Erosion of liver abscesses can result in peritonitis. Liver abscesses that are located in the right lobe can spread to the lungs and pleura. Pericardial infection, although rare, may be associated with extension of the amebic abscesses from the liver.[21–23]

CLINICAL PRESENTATION AND DIAGNOSIS

Pharmacologic Therapy

Metronidazole (Flagyl), dehydroemetine, and chloroquine (Aralen) are tissue-acting agents, and iodoquinol (Yodoxin),

Clinical Presentation and Diagnosis of Amebiasis

Review of the patient's history should include: recent travel, type of foods ingested (e.g., salads or unpeeled fruit), the nature of water and fluid consumed, and description of any symptoms of friends or relatives who ate the same food.

Intestinal Disease

- Vague abdominal discomfort
- Symptoms may range from malaise to severe abdominal cramps, flatulence, and nonbloody or bloody diarrhea (heme-positive in 100% of cases) with mucus
- May have low-grade fever, but this may be absent in many patients
- Eosinophilia is usually absent, although mild leukocytosis is not unusual

Note: Fecal screening may show other intestinal parasites, including *Cryptosporidium* spp., *Balantidium coli*, *Dientamoeba fragilis*, *Isospora belli*, *G. lamblia*, or *Blastocystis hominis*.

Amebic Liver Abscess

- May present with high fever with significant leukocytosis with left shift, anemia, elevated alanine aminotransferase, and dull abdominal pain on palpation
- Physical findings: Right upper quadrant pain, hepatomegaly, and liver tenderness, with referred pain to the left or right shoulder (*Note:* Erosion of liver abscesses may present as peritonitis.)

❷ Diagnosis

- *Intestinal amebiasis is diagnosed by demonstrating* E. histolytica *cysts or trophozoites (may contain ingested erythrocytes) in fresh stool or from a specimen obtained by sigmoidoscopy.*
- *Microscopy may not differentiate between the pathogenic* E. histolytica *and the nonpathogenic* E. dispar *or* E. moshkovskii *in stools.*
- *Sensitive techniques are available to detect* E. histolytica *in stool: antigen detection, antibody test (ELISA) and PCR.*
- Endoscopy with scrapings or biopsy and stained slides (iron hematoxylin or trichrome) may provide more definitive diagnosis of amebiasis.
- Diagnosis for liver abscess includes serology and liver scans (using isotopes by ultrasound or CT) or MRI; however, none of these are specific for liver abscess. In rare instances, needle aspiration of hepatic abscess may be attempted using ultrasound guidance.

---

diloxanide furoate (Furamide), and paromomycin (Humatin) are luminal amebicides. A systemic or tissue-acting agent may be so well absorbed that the amounts of the drug remaining in the bowel may be insufficient to have luminal or local effects. A luminally-active agent, on the other hand, may not attain effective enough levels in the tissue to be efficacious. Asymptomatic cyst passers (identified by stool examinations, and who may develop invasive disease) and patients with mild intestinal amebiasis should receive a luminal agent: paromomycin 25 to 35 mg/kg/day three times daily for 7 days, or iodoquinol 650 mg three times daily for 20 days, or diloxanide furoate 500 mg three times daily for 10 days. These regimens have cure rates of between 84% and 96%. Diloxanide furoate is available from Ponorama Compounding Pharmacy (6744 Balboa Blvd., Lake Balboa, CA 91406; [800] 247-9767).[12] The pediatric dose of paromomycin is the same as that used in adults, whereas the pediatric dose of iodoquinol is 30 to 40 mg/kg (maximum: 2 g) per day in three doses for 20 days, and the pediatric dose of diloxanide furoate is 20 mg/kg/day in three doses for 10 days. Paromomycin is the preferred agent in pregnant patients.[12]

Patients with severe intestinal disease or liver abscess should receive metronidazole 750 mg three times daily for 10 days, followed by the luminal agents indicated above. The pediatric dose of metronidazole is 50 mg/kg/day in divided doses, which should be followed by a luminal agent. An alternative regimen of metronidazole is 2.4 g/day for 2 days in combination with the luminal agent.[20,21] Tinidazole (Tindamax, recently introduced in the U.S. market) administered in a dose of 2 g daily for 3 days (pediatric dose: 50 mg/kg for 3 days) is an alternative to metronidazole. If there is no prompt response to metronidazole or aspiration of the abscess, an antibiotic regimen should be added. Patients who cannot tolerate oral doses of metronidazole should receive an equivalent dose IV.

Patient Encounter 2: Amebiasis

WR is a 37-year-old native of India and a permanent resident in the United States who has recently returned from a trip to Calcutta where he was visiting a relative. He presents in the emergency department with complaints of a 3-week history of sharp, crampy, and postprandial abdominal pain. The pain is more intense over the right lower quadrant and associated with watery nonbloody diarrhea and tenesmus.

What specific findings in this patient suggest that he may have giardiasis or amebiasis?

What other information do you need to confirm a diagnosis of amebiasis?

What is the major complication of amebiasis?

Patient Care and Monitoring: Amebiasis

1. Follow-up in patients with amebiasis should include repeat stools (1–3), colonoscopy (in colitis) or CT (in liver abscess) between days 5 and 7, at the end of the course of therapy, and a month after the end of therapy.

2. Most patients with either intestinal amebiasis or colitis will respond in 3 to 5 days with amelioration of symptoms.

3. Those with liver abscess may take up to 7 days before there will be decreases in pain and fever. In liver abscess, patients not responding by the fifth day may require aspiration of the abscesses or exploratory laparotomy.

4. Serial liver scans have demonstrated that healing of liver abscesses take from 4 to 8 months following adequate therapy.

Preventive Measures

- Travelers and tourists visiting endemic areas should avoid local tap water, ice, salads, and unpeeled fruits. Boiled water is safe.

- Water can be disinfected by the use of iodine 2% (5 drops/L) or chlorine 6% (laundry bleach: 4 drops/L) or use of a commercial water purifier, such as Portable Aqua tablets (Wisconsin Pharmaceutical).

OUTCOME EVALUATION

Follow-up in patients with amebiasis should include repeat stool examinations, serology, colonoscopy (in colitis) or CT on day 7, at the end of therapy, and a month after the end of therapy. Serial liver scans have demonstrated healing of liver abscesses over 4 to 8 months after adequate therapy.[20,21]

HELMINTHIC DISEASES

Helminthic infections include three groups of organisms: roundworms or nematodes, flukes (trematodes), and tapeworms (cestodes). Because of space constraints, only brief descriptions of some of the helminthic infections most commonly seen in North America and their treatments will be provided here. Although helminthic infections may not produce clinical manifestations, they can cause significant pathology. One factor that determines the pathogenicity of helminthic infections is their population density; a high-density population ("worm burden") results in predictable disease presentation. In the United States, these infections are reported most frequently in recent immigrants from Southeast Asia, the Caribbean, Mexico, and Central America.[5,6] Populations at risk include institutionalized patients (both young and elderly), preschool children in daycare centers, residents of Native American reservations, and homosexuals.[17,24] Certain conditions and drugs (anesthesia and corticosteroids) can cause atypical localization of worms. Immunocompromised hosts can be overwhelmed by some helminthic infections, such as *Strongyloides stercoralis*.

NEMATODES

Hookworm Disease

Hookworm infection is caused by *Ancylostoma duodenale* or *Necator americanus*. *N. americanus* is found in the southeastern United States.[24–26] Infective larvae enter the host in contaminated food or water, or penetrate the skin and migrate to the small intestine. The adult worm attaches to GI mucosa and causes injury by lytic destruction of the tissue. Over a period of time, the adult worm can cause anemia and hypoproteinemia in the host.[27,28]

Treatment

❸ *The drug of choice is mebendazole (Vermox), which is also active against ascariasis, enterobiasis, trichuriasis, and hookworm.*[12] The adult and pediatric (age greater than 2 years) oral dose of mebendazole for hookworm is 100 mg twice daily for 3 days. An alternative agent that can be used in both pediatric and adult patients is albendazole (Zentel), 400 mg as a single oral dose. Diagnosis is by detection of eggs or larvae in stool. Stool examination for eggs and the larvae should be repeated in 2 weeks and the patient retreated if necessary.

ASCARIASIS

The causative agent in ascariasis is the giant roundworm *Ascaris lumbricoides,* which is found worldwide and is responsible about 4 million infections in the United States (it primarily affects residents of the Appalachian mountain range and the Gulf Coast states).[29–31] Migration of the worm into the lungs usually produces pneumonitis, fever, cough, eosinophilia, and pulmonary infiltrates. *Ascaris* infection can also cause abdominal discomfort, intestinal obstruction, and appendicitis. Diagnosis is made by detection of the characteristic eggs in the stool or passed worms.

Treatment

In both adults and pediatric patients older than 2 years of age, mebendazole 100 mg orally twice daily for 3 days is the treatment to use. An alternative agent is pyrantel pamoate (Antiminth).[12] The stool should be checked within 2 weeks and the patient retreated when warranted.

ENTEROBIASIS

Enterobiasis, or pinworm infection, is caused by *Enterobius vermicularis*. It is the most widely distributed helminthic infection in the world.[24,32] There are approximately 42 million cases in the United States, primarily affecting children. The most common manifestation of the infection is cutaneous irritation in the perianal region, resulting from the migrating female or the presence of eggs. The intense pruritus may lead to dermatitis and secondary bacterial infections. Diagnosis is made by the use of a perianal swab and cellophane tape sampling, which will aid in egg identification.

Treatment

The three agents that are administered for enterobiasis include pyrantel pamoate, mebendazole, and albendazole. The oral dose of pyrantel pamoate is 11 mg/kg (maximum: 1 g) as a single dose that can be repeated in 2 weeks. The oral dose of mebendazole for both adults and children older than 2 years of age is 100 mg as a single dose. This may be repeated in 2 weeks.[12] Following treatment, to eradicate the eggs, all bedding and underclothing should be sterilized by steaming or washing in the hot cycle of the washing machine.

STRONGYLOIDIASIS

Strongyloidiasis is caused by *Strongyloides stercoralis*, which has a worldwide distribution and is predominantly prevalent in South America (Brazil and Columbia) and in Southeast Asia.[33–38] Strongyloidiasis is primarily seen among institutionalized populations (those in mental hospitals and children's hospitals) and immunocompromised individuals (those with HIV infection, AIDS, and patients with hematologic malignancies).[33,35] The worm is usually found in the upper intestine where the eggs are deposited and hatch to form the rhabditiform larvae. The rhabditiform larva (male and female) migrate to the bowel where they may be excreted in the feces. If excreted in the feces, the larva can evolve into either one of two forms after copulation: a free-living noninfectious rhabditiform larvae, or an infectious filariform larvae. The filariform larva can penetrate host skin and migrate to the lungs and produce progeny, a process called autoinfection. This can result in hyperinfection (i.e., an increased number of larva in the intestine, lungs, and other internal organs), especially in an immunocompromised host.

Patients with acute infection may develop a localized pruritic rash, but heavy infestations can produce eosinophilia (10–15%), diarrhea, abdominal pain, and intestinal obstruction. Administration of corticosteroids or other immunosuppressive drugs to an infected individual can result in hyperinfections and disseminated strongyloidiasis.[33,35] Diagnosis of strongyloidiasis is made by identification of the rhabditiform larva in stool, sputum, or duodenal fluid, or from small bowel biopsy specimens or via antigen testing (ELISA essay). Multiple stool and other samples may need to be checked, both for diagnosis and to ensure eradication of the larva in patients after treatment.

Treatment

❸ *The drug of choice for strongyloidiasis is oral ivermectin 200 mcg/kg/day for 2 days, while albendazole 400 mg twice daily is given for 7 days as an alternative.*[12,39] With hyperinfe-

ction or disseminated strongyloidiasis, immunosuppressive drugs should be discontinued and treatment should be initiated with ivermectin 200 mcg/kg/day until all symptoms are resolved. Patients should be tested periodically to ensure the elimination of the larva. Individuals from an endemic area who are candidates for organ transplantation should be screened for *S. stercoralis*.

CESTODIASIS

Cestodiasis (tapeworm infection) is caused by species of the phylum Platyhelminthes (flatworms), and include among others the pork tapeworm (*Taenia solium*) and the beef tapeworm (*T. saginata*).[9,40] The tapeworm attaches itself to the mucosal wall of the upper jejunum by the scolex (mouth parts), and by two to four cup-shaped suckers and a structure called a rostellum, which may have hooks in some species. Since the parasite lacks a digestive system it obtains all nutrients directly from the host. The scolex, proglottids (segments), and eggs are specific for each species and used for identification of tapeworms. Tapeworm infections are caused by ingestion of poorly cooked meat which contains the larva or cysticerci. Cysticerci, when released from the contaminated meat by host digestive juices, mature in the host jejunum. Cystericercosis is a systemic disease caused by the larva of *T. solium* (oncosphere or hexacanth), and is usually acquired by ingestion of eggs in contaminated food or by autoinfection.[41–45] The larvae can penetrate the bowel and migrate through the bloodstream to infect different organs including the CNS (neurocysticercosis). Diagnosis of both *T. saginata* and *T. solium* is accomplished by recovery of the gravid proglottids and the scolex in the stool.

Treatment

❸ *Tapeworm infections (*T. saginata *and* T. solium*) are treated with praziquantel 5 to 10 mg/kg as a single dose (use the same dose for adults and pediatric patients).*[12] The treatment for cysticercosis and neurocysticercosis may include surgery, anticonvulsants (neurocysticercosis can cause seizures), and anthelmintic therapy. The anthelmintic therapy of choice is albendazole 400 mg twice daily for 8 to 30 days.[45,46] The pediatric dose of albendazole is 15 mg/kg (maximum: 800 mg) in two divided doses for 8 to 30 days. The doses for both adults and pediatric subjects can be repeated if necessary. Praziquantel is an alternative therapy.[12]

OUTCOME EVALUATION

Morbidity and disease due to helminthic infections is related to the intensity of infection. The major adverse effects of helminthic infections are malnutrition, fatigue, and diminished work capacity. Unlike other helminthic infections, strongyloidiasis can cause autoinfection, and in the presence of immunosuppression, it can cause CNS and disseminated infections which have high mortality.[33]

The most serious complication of cysticercosis is neurocysticercosis that can cause strokes and seizures.[45] Treatment of neurocysticercosis with anthelmintic treatment remains controversial.

MALARIA

Malaria is one of the most devastating parasitic diseases, affecting a population in excess of 500 million and causing between 700,000 and 2.7 million deaths a year worldwide.[3,5,7] In the year 2000, approximately 27 million U.S. travelers visited countries where malaria is endemic. In 2002, the Centers for Disease Control and Prevention indicated that there were 1,337 cases of malaria, of which 849 were in U.S. civilians, 33 in U.S. military personnel, and the rest in foreign civilians.[5] There were eight fatalities, all due to *Plasmodium falciparum*. ❹ *The primary reasons for morbidity and death in malaria are failure to take recommended chemoprophylaxis, inappropriate chemoprophylaxis, delay in seeking medical care or in initiating therapy promptly, and misdiagnosis.* Evaluation of a patient should include specific travel history, details of chemoprophylaxis, and physical findings (e.g., splenomegaly).

Malaria is transmitted by the bites of the *Anopheles* mosquitoes which introduce into the bloodstream one of four species of sporozoites of the plasmodia (*Plasmodium falciparum, P. ovale, P. vivax,* or *P. malariae*).[47–56] Initial symptoms of malaria are nonspecific and may resemble influenza and include: chills, headache, fatigue, muscle pain, rigors, and nausea. The onset of the symptoms is between 1 and 3 weeks following exposure. Fever may appear 2 to 3 days after initial symptoms and may follow a pattern and occur every 2 or 3 days (*P. vivax, P. ovale,* and *P. malariae*). Fever with *P. falciparum* can be erratic and may not follow specific patterns. It is not unusual for patients to have concomitant infections with *P. vivax* and *P. falciparum*. Falciparum malaria must always be regarded as a life-threatening medical emergency.

EPIDEMIOLOGY AND ETIOLOGY

The distribution of the various species of malaria is not well defined but *P. vivax* is reported to be prevalent in the Indian subcontinent, Central America, North Africa, and the Middle East, whereas *P. falciparum* is predominantly in Africa (including sub-Saharan Africa), both East and West Africa, Haiti, the Dominican Republic, the Amazon region of South America, Southeast Asia, and New Guinea.[5,48,51] Most *P. ovale* infections occur in Africa, while the distribution of *P. malariae* is worldwide.[7] Most infections in the United States are reported in American travelers, recent immigrants, or immigrants who have visited friends and family in an endemic area.[4,7] Placental transmission and blood transfusions are also sources of malaria.

Within minutes after the bite of the *Anopheles* mosquito, the sporozoites invade hepatocytes in the liver and begin

Patient Encounter 3, Part 1: Malaria

TW is a 27-year-old male who had returned from Bamako, Mali in West Africa, after visiting his college classmate who was in the Peace Corps. While there, he accompanied his friend on a river trip to visit a number of villages. He indicates that he took steps to minimize mosquito bites and had slept under a mosquito net. He was well since returning from Africa until the previous day, when he had a temperature as high as 39°C (102.2°F), with anorexia, headache, chills, sweats, myalgias, and abdominal pain. He took a few doses of ibuprofen but his fever came back after a few hours and he now presents in the emergency department with chills, high fever (greater than 39.8°C) (greater than 103.6°F), headache, abdominal pain, nausea, stiffness of the neck, and back pain.

Are the symptoms in this patient consistent with malaria?

What places this patient at risk for malaria?

What additional information do you need to develop a therapeutic plan for this patient?

an asexual phase called schizonts (exoerythrocytic stage or schizogony). The patient may be asymptomatic during this period. After a lapse of between 5 and 15 days (depending on the species), schizonts rupture to release daughter cells (merozoites) into the blood, which then invade erythrocytes. In erythrocytes the merozoites undergo a number of sequential forms: a ring form, trophozoite, schizont, and merozoite, which then invade new erythrocytes. This asexual phase is about 48 hours for *P. falciparum, P. vivax,* and *P. ovale,* and 72 hours for *P. malariae*. Subsequently, the merozoites develop into gametocytes and undergo a sexual phase (sporogony) in the *Anopheles* mosquito. In the mosquito, the gametocytes undergo a number of stages: zygote, ookinete, and oocyst, and finally transform into sporozoites in the salivary glands where it is again able to infect the next host. Unlike *P. falciparum* and *P. malariae,* which only remain in the liver for about 3 weeks before invading erythrocytes, *P. ovale* and *P. vivax* can remain in the liver for extended periods in a latent stage (as hypnozoites); this can result in the recurrence of the infection after weeks or months. Primaquine therapy is necessary to eradicate this stage of the infection.

PATHOPHYSIOLOGY

The clinical presentation of malaria can be quite variable. Normally, the appearance of a prodrome with headache, abdominal pain, fatigue, fever, and chills, which coincides with the erythrocytic phase of malaria occurs frequently between 10 and 21 days after being exposed.[48,51] This phase causes extensive hemolysis, which results in anemia and splenomegaly. The most serious complications are caused by *P. falciparum* infections. Infants and children under the age of 5 years and nonimmune pregnant women are at high risk for severe complications with falciparum infections.[52–58]

The complications associated with falciparum malaria are related to two unique features of *P. falciparum*: (a) its ability to produce high parasitism (up to 80%) of red cells of all ages; and (b) the propensity to be sequestered in postcapillary venules of critical organs such as brain, liver, heart, lungs, and kidneys.[53,54] It has been postulated that tissue hypoxia from anemia, together with *P. falciparum*–parasitized red blood cell adherence to endothelial cells in capillaries, contribute to severe ischemia and metabolic derangements. *P. malariae* is implicated in immune-mediated glomerulonephritis and nephrotic syndrome.

CLINICAL PRESENTATION AND DIAGNOSIS

Recent innovations for detecting malaria include DNA or RNA probes by polymerase chain reaction (PCR).[59] These,

Clinical Presentation and Diagnosis of Malaria

Initial Presentation

Include a careful travel history of patient and physical findings (e.g., splenomegaly) and details of antimalarial chemoprophylaxis, when obtainable.

Erythrocytic Phase

1. Prodrome: Headache, anorexia, malaise, fatigue, and myalgia
2. Nonspecific complaints include: abdominal pain, diarrhea, chest pain, and arthralgia
3. Paroxysm: High fever, chills, and rigor
4. Cold phase: Severe pallor, cyanosis of the lips and nail beds
5. Hot phase: Fever between 40.5°C (104.9°F) and 41°C (105.8°F) (seen more frequently with *P. falciparum*)
6. Sweating phase: Follows the hot phase by 2 to 6 hours
7. When fever resolves, it is followed by marked fatigue and drowsiness, warm dry skin, tachycardia, cough, headache, nausea, vomiting, abdominal pain, diarrhea and delirium, anemia, and splenomegaly

⑤ *P. falciparum malaria is a life-threatening emergency. Complications include hypoglycemia, acute renal failure, pulmonary edema, severe anemia (high parasitism), thrombocytopenia, heart failure, cerebral congestion, seizures, coma, and adult respiratory distress syndrome.*

Diagnostic Procedures for Malaria

1. To ensure a positive diagnosis, blood smears (both thick and thin films) should be obtained every 12 to 24 hours for three consecutive days.
2. The presence of parasites in the blood 3 to 5 days after initiation of therapy suggests resistance to the drug regimen.

however, are not widely available for clinical use. A rapid dip-stick test (ParaSight F, Becton-Dickinson, Cockeyville, MD) reportedly has a sensitivity of 88% and a specificity of 97%, which is comparable to microscopy. However, ParaSight F can give false-positive results with rheumatoid factor; thus microscopy remains the optimal test.

TREATMENT

The primary goal in the management of malaria is the rapid identification of the *Plasmodium* species by blood smears (both thick and thin smears repeated every 12 hours for 3 days). Antimalarial therapy should be initiated promptly to eradicate the infection within 48 to 72 hours and avoid complications such as hypoglycemia, pulmonary edema, and renal failure.[53,54]

PHARMACOLOGIC THERAPY

The chemoprophylaxis regimen for malaria is outlined in Table 78–1.[12]

Chemotherapy for Malarial Infection

In an uncomplicated attack of malaria (for all plasmodia except chloroquine-resistant *P. falciparum* and *P. vivax*), the recommended oral regimen is chloroquine 600 mg (base) initially, followed by 300 mg (base) 6 hours later, and then 300 mg (base) daily for 2 days.[12] **⑥** *In severe illness or falciparum malaria, patients should be admitted to an acute care unit and quinidine gluconate 10 mg salt/kg as a loading dose (maximum 600 mg) in 250 mL normal saline should be administered IV slowly over 1 to 2 hours. This should be followed by continuous infusion of 0.02 mg/kg/min of quinidine for at least 24 hours until oral therapy can be started. In patients who have received either quinine or mefloquine, the loading dose of quinidine should be omitted. Oral quinine salt (650 mg every 8 hours) plus doxycycline 100 mg twice daily should follow the IV dose of quinidine to complete 7 days of therapy.*[53,54] The pediatric dose of IV quinidine gluconate is the same as the dose for adults. The pediatric dose of oral quinine is 25 mg/kg/day in three divided doses, while the dose of doxycycline (children greater than 8-year-old) is 4 mg/kg in two divided doses for 7 days. An alternative to doxycycline is clindamycin 900 mg (20 mg/kg/day) three times daily for 3 days. The pediatric dose of clindamycin is the same as in adults. *(In patients who cannot tolerate quinidine or quinidine is not readily available, IV artesunate 2.4 mg/kg/dose × 3 days, at 0,12, 24, 48, and 72 hours may be used, followed by oral therapy. Artesunate is available from CDC under an investigational new drug application. Pediatric dose of artesunate is same as in adults. Oral therapy may include atovaquone/proguanil, doxycycline,mefloquine or clindamycin.)*[12]

In *P. falciparum, P. vivax, P. ovale,* or *P. malariae* (chloroquine-resistant) infections, a dose of 750 mg mefloquine followed by 500 mg 12 hours later is recommended. The pediatric dose of mefloquine is 15 mg/kg (less than 45 kg)

Table 78–1

Chemoprophylaxis for Malaria

Plasmodia-Sensitive	Drug	Dose	Pediatric Dose	Comments
Chloroquine-sensitive	Chloroquine phosphate (oral)[a]	300 mg (base) once weekly beginning 1 week prior to departure and continued for 4 weeks after leaving endemic area	5 mg (base) per kg of body weight once weekly (maximum 300 mg)	Hydroxychloroquine sulfate 310 (base) or 400 mg salt once a week may be used instead of chloroquine; regimen will be similar to chloroquine
When leaving an area endemic for *P. vivax* or *P. ovale*	Primaquine (oral)	30 mg base (52.6 mg salt) daily for 14 days after departure, in addition to the above	0.6 mg/kg base (1 mg/kg salt) daily for 14 days after departure	*Contraindicated* in those with G6PD deficiency and in pregnancy and lactation
Chloroquine-resistant *P. falciparum*	Atovaquone-proguanil (oral)	250 mg atovaquone and 100 mg proguanil (1 tablet) once daily	62.5 mg atovaquone and 25 mg proguanil once daily 11–20 kg: 1 tablet 21–30 kg: 2 tablets 31–40 kg: 3 tablets Greater than or equal to 40 kg: 1 adult tablet daily	Begin 1–2 days before departure and continue for 1 week after leaving high-risk area Recommended also for primary prophylaxis in mefloquine-resistant *P. falciparum*
	Alternatives Doxycycline (oral)	100 mg daily	Greater than or equal to 8 years of age 2 mg/kg (maximum 100 mg)	Effective for mefloquine-resistant *P. falciparum* Start 1–2 days before departure, continue through stay in endemic area, and continue regimen for 4 weeks after returning
	Mefloquine (oral)	228 mg (base) (250 mg salt) weekly	Less than or equal to 15 kg: 4.6 mg/kg base (5 mg/kg salt) once weekly 15–19 kg: 1/4 tablet 20–30 kg: 1/2 tablet 31–45 kg: 3/4 tablet Greater than or equal to 45 kg: 1 tablet	Start 1–2 week before departure and continue for 4 week after leaving endemic area; may start 3–4 week earlier to assess tolerance *Contraindications*: History of seizure, psychiatric disorders (including depression and anxiety), or arrhythmias
	Primaquine (oral)	30 mg base (1 mg/kg salt for adult) daily	0.6 mg/kg base (1 mg/kg salt up to adult dose)	Alternative or second-line regimen; see above for contraindications

G6PD, glucose-6-phosphate dehydrogenase deficiency.

[a]Pediatric dose can be calculated and tablet pulverized and placed in gelatin capsules. Parents can be instructed to suspend dose in food, simple syrup, or drink.

For further information, see Ref. 68 (see table on p. 2858: Pretravel Resources).

followed by 10 mg/kg 8 to 12 hours later. Mefloquine is associated with sinus bradycardia, confusion, hallucinations, and psychosis and should be avoided in patients with a history of cardiovascular problems or depression. IV quinidine gluconate followed by quinine plus doxycycline or clindamycin should be administered for severe illness as indicated above. The IV quinidine regimen requires close monitoring of the ECG (QT-segment) and other vital signs (hypotension and hypoglycemia). An alternative oral treatment for *P. falciparum* infections in adults, especially those with history of seizures,

psychiatric disorders, or cardiovascular problems, is the combination of atovaquone 250 mg and proguanil 100 mg (Malarone) (two tablets twice daily for 3 days).[12] The pediatric dose of Malarone is as follows: child less than 5 kg: not indicated; 9 to 10 kg: 3 pediatric tablets/day × 3 days; 11 to 20 kg: one adult tablet/day × 3 days; 21 to 30 kg: 2 adult tablets/day 3 days; 31 to 40 kg: 3 adult tablets/day 3 days; greater than 40 kg: 2 adults tablets twice daily × 3 days. ❼ *Since falciparum malaria is associated with serious complications, including pulmonary edema, hypoglycemia, jaundice, renal*

Patient Encounter 3, Part 2: Falciparum Malaria

TW presents with fever, nausea, headache, myalgias, chills, and body aches including back pain. When questioned about his travels, he indicates that he had not taken any antimalarial prophylaxis.

PMH: Healthy 27-year-old male

FH: Father died of stroke at age 87 years; mother, who is 82-year-old, has rheumatoid arthritis and lives with an unmarried daughter

SH: Systems analyst, works for local school district; occasionally drinks wine with meals

Meds: Ibuprofen 200 mg

ROS: In addition to the complaints noted above, he complains of severe nausea and fatigue

PE:

Gen: Patient is lucid but slightly agitated and febrile

VS: BP 105/70 mm Hg; P 120 bpm, RR 32 per minute, T 40.1°C (104.2°F)

Skin: Warm and dry to touch

HEENT: Slightly icteric sclerae and dry oral mucosa

ABD: Soft with diffuse tenderness with hepatomegaly and splenomegaly

Rest of the systems were WNL

Labs: Sodium 131 mEq/L (131 mmol/L); hemoglobin 10.2 g/dL (102 g/L or 6.3 mmol/L); potassium 4.9 mEq/L (4.9 mmol/L); hematocrit 31% (0.31); chloride 96 mEq/L (96 mmol/L); WBC 14.8 × 10³/mm³ (14.8 × 10⁹/L); BUN 28 mg/dL (10 mmol/L); total bilirubin 1.8 mg/dL (30.8 μmol/L); Scr 1.4 mg/dL (124 μmol/L); platelets 110 × 10³/mm³ (110 × 10⁹/L); glucose 77 mg/dL (4.27 mmol/L); aspartate aminotransferase 87 units/L (1.45 μkat/L); albumin 3.2 g/dL (32 g/L); alanine aminotransferase 94 units/L (1.57 μkat/L); blood smear (Giemsa stain): *P. falciparum*

In view of the above information, what is your assessment of this patient?

Identify your treatment goals and monitoring parameters.

Patient Encounter 3, Part 3: Malaria

Following treatment of falciparum malaria, TW has remained well for 2 months. However, 2 days ago, he started developing fever and chills, nausea, and abdominal pain. When seen in the emergency department he has a fever of 38.4°C (101.1°F) and complains of severe headache. Examinations of a thick and thin blood smear of the patient's blood identified *P. vivax* infection. TW received a course of chloroquine and primaquine. In a follow-up 2 weeks later, a repeat blood smear was negative for parasites and the patient was asymptomatic.

Patient Care and Monitoring: Malaria

- Acute *P. falciparum* malaria resistant to chloroquine should be treated with IV quinidine via central venous catheter and fluid status and the electrocardiogram (ECG) should be monitored closely.

- The loading dose of quinidine should be omitted in those patients who have received quinine or mefloquine.

- Hypoglycemia that is associated with both *P. falciparum* and quinidine administration, should be checked every 4 to 6 hours and corrected with dextrose infusions (5–10%).

- Quinidine infusions should be slowed temporarily or stopped if the QT interval is greater than 0.6 second, the increase in the QRS complex is greater than 25%, or hypotension unresponsive to fluid challenge results.

- The suggested quinidine levels should be maintained at 3 to 7 mg/dL (9.2–21.6 μmol/L).

- Blood smears should be checked every 12 hours until parasitemia is less than 1%.

- Resolution of fever should take place between 36 and 48 hours after initiation of the IV quinidine therapy, and the blood should be clear of parasites in 5 days.

- When parenteral therapy is required for more than 48 hours or the patient's renal function deteriorates, the dose of quinidine should be lowered by half.

Advice to Travelers

All travelers to endemic areas should be advised to remain in well-screened areas, to wear clothes that cover most of the body, and sleep in mosquito nets. Travelers should adhere to malaria chemoprophylaxis regimens and carry the insect repellant DEET (*N, N*-diethylmetatoluamide) or other insect sprays containing DEET for use in mosquito-infested areas.

failure, confusion, delirium, seizures, coma, and death; careful monitoring of fluid status and hemodynamic parameters is mandatory. Exchange transfusion that may be required in patients with *P. falciparum* malaria in whom parasitemia may be between 5% and 15% remains a questionable modality.[57] Either peritoneal or hemodialysis may be indicated in renal failure.

OUTCOME EVALUATION

When advising potential travelers on prophylaxis for malaria, be aware of the incidence of chloroquine-resistant *P. falciparum* malaria and the countries where it is prevalent.[60–74] In patients who have *P. vivax* or *P. ovale* malaria (note that some patients can have *P. falciparum* and one of these species), following the treatment of the acute phase of malaria and screening for glucose-6-phosphate dehydrogenase deficiency, patients should receive a regimen of primaquine for 14 days to ensure eradication of the hypnozoite stage of *P. vivax* or *P. ovale*.[63] For detailed recommendations for prevention of malaria go to *www.cdc.gov/travel/*.

AMERICAN TRYPANOSOMIASIS

ETIOLOGY

Two distinct forms of the genus *Trypanosoma* occur in humans. One is associated with African trypanosomiasis (sleeping sickness) and the other with American trypanosomiasis (Chagas' disease). *T. brucei gambiense* and *T. brucei rhodesiense* are the causative organisms for the East African and West African trypanosomiasis, respectively. *T. brucei rhodesiense* causes the acute disease and is the more virulent of the two species. Both East and West African trypanosomiasis are transmitted by various species of tsetse fly belonging to the genus *Glossina*. Further discussion of this subject will focus on American trypanosomiasis.

T. cruzi is the agent that causes American trypanosomiasis. American trypanosomiasis is transmitted by a number of species of reduviid bugs (*Triatoma infestans* and *Rhodrium prolixus*) that live in wall cracks of houses in rural areas of

---

Clinical Presentation and Diagnosis of Trypanosomiasis

Acute
- Unilateral orbital edema (Romana's sign)
- Granuloma (chagoma)
- Fever, hepatosplenomegaly, and lymphadenopathy

Chronic ❽
- *Cardiac: cardiomyopathy and heart failure*
- *ECG: first-degree heart block, right bundle-branch block, and arrhythmias*
- *GI: enlargement of the esophagus and colon ("mega" syndrome)*
- *CNS: meningoencephalitis, strokes, seizures, and focal paralysis*

Diagnosis
Positive history of exposure and use of serology: indirect hemagglutination test, ELISA (Chagas EIA, Abbott Labs, Abbott Park, IL), and complement fixation (CF) test. (*Note:* CF may produce false-positive reactions in those exposed to leishmaniasis, syphilis, and malaria. PCR may be more definitive for diagnosis.)

Patient Care and Monitoring

- It is essential to identify *T. cruzi*–infected patients by serology and to monitor the cardiovascular status of these patients by ECG periodically.
- Some patients will benefit from implantation of pacemakers.
- All transplant candidates from areas endemic for Chagas' disease need to be screened for *T. cruzi*. Immunosuppression in these patients can lead to overwhelming infections.

North, Central, and South America.[75-79] The reduviid bug is infected by sucking blood from animals (e.g., opossums, dogs, and cats) or humans infected with circulating trypomastigotes. American trypanosomiasis is endemic in all Latin American countries and can be transmitted congenitally, by blood transfusion, and by organ transplantation.

CLINICAL PRESENTATION AND DIAGNOSIS

Pharmacologic Therapy

The drugs used for *T. cruzi* include nifurtimox (Lampit) and benznidazole (Rochagan). Oral nifurtimox is available from the CDC, while benznidazole is only available in Brazil.[12,80-83] The adult dose of nifurtimox is 8 to 10 mg/kg/day in divided doses for 120 days. Since children seem to tolerate the dose better than adults, the pediatric dose of nifurtimox in children 1- to 10-year-old is 15 to 20 mg/kg/day, and the dose for children 11- to 16-year-old is 12.5 to 15 mg/kg/day in divided doses. Symptomatic treatment for heart failure associated with Chagas' disease should be initiated. The GI complications may require surgical revisions and reconstruction.

OUTCOME EVALUATION

Treatment of the acute phase of the disease (i.e., fever, malaise, edema of the face, and hepatosplenomegaly) is nifurtimox. The congestive heart failure associated with cardiomyopathy of Chagas' disease is treated the same way as cardiomyopathy from other causes.[76,80]

ECTOPARASITES

A parasite that lives outside the body of the host is called an ectoparasite. Approximately 6 to 12 million subjects become infested with pediculosis (lice infestation) yearly in the United States. Pediculosis is usually associated with poor hygiene, and infections are passed from person to person through social and sexual contact.

LICE

The two species that belong to this group include *Pediculus humanus capitis* (head louse) and *P. humanus corporis* (body louse).[84-88] The eggs (or nits) remain firmly attached to the hair, and in about 10 days the lice hatch to form nymphs, which mature in 2 weeks. The lice become attached to the base of the hair follicle and feed on the blood of the host.[10] Pubic or crab lice is found on the hairs around the genitals but may occur in other parts of the body (e.g., eyelashes or axillae). Hypersensitivity to the secretions from lice can produce macular swellings and lead to secondary bacterial infections.

Treatment

9 *The agent of choice for all three infections (body, head, and crab lice) is 1% permethrin (Nix).* Permethrin has both pediculicidal and ovicidal activity against *P. humanus capitis*. The cure rate is reported to be between 90% and 97%. A cream rinse of permethrin 1% (Nix-Crème Rinse) is also available. Individuals with a history of hypersensitivity to ragweed or chrysanthemum may react to permethrin and should avoid this preparation. An alternative agent is oral ivermectin 100 mcg/kg for 3 days (days 1, 2, and 10). Permethrin can cause itching, burning, stinging, and tingling with application. Permethrin 1% should be applied to the dry scalp after shampooing and be left on the scalp for 10 minutes. The application may need to be repeated. Because of the reports of resistance to permethrin, an alternative agent is 0.5% malathion (Ovide), which has to be left on the scalp for 90 minutes and has also been found to be effective. For the relief of pruritus, calamine lotion with 0.1% menthol or an equivalent agent may be used. *All individuals, including immediate family members and sexual partners of the primary host, should be treated. All bedding and clothes should be sterilized as previously indicated for enterobiasis.*

SCABIES

10 *Scabies is caused by the itch mite* Sarcoptes scabiei hominis, *which affects both humans and animals. Infection usually affects the interdigital and popliteal folds, axillary folds, the umbilicus, and the scrotum.* The infection causes severe itching and excoriations in the interdigital web spaces, buttocks, groin, and scalp.[89,90] *Diagnosis is made by identifying the mite from skin scrapings on a wet mount.*

Treatment

10 *The agent of choice for scabies is permethrin 5% (Elimite) cream.* Alternative agents in subjects who cannot use permethrin are crotamiton 10% (Eurax) and oral ivermectin (Stromectal) 200 mcg/kg as a single dose. To initiate the treatment with permethrin, the skin should be scrubbed in a warm soapy bath to remove the scabs. The permethrin lotion should then be applied to the whole body, avoiding the face, mucous membranes, and eyes, and left on for 8 to 14 hours. A single application eradicates 97% of scabies. All

close contacts should be treated appropriately. The pruritus associated with scabies may persist for 2 to 4 weeks because of the remnants of mite parts in the skin.

OUTCOME EVALUATION

Infections due to arthropods can be controlled by preventing their access to the host. Improving living conditions and avoiding sharing common personal items like hats and hair brushes may minimize these infections due to arthropods. Permethrin (1–5%) is an effective agent for all these infections.

Abbreviations Introduced in This Chapter

CF	Complement fixation
DEET	*N, N*-Diethylmetatoluamide
ELISA	Enzyme-linked immunosorbent assay
IgA	Immunoglobulin A
PCR	Polymerase chain reaction

 Self-assessment questions and answers are available at *http://www.mhpharmacotherapy. com/pp.html.*

REFERENCES

1. Garg PK, Perry S, Dorn M, et al. Risk of intestinal helminth and protozoan infection in a refugee population. Am J Trop Med Hyg 2005;73:386–391.
2. White AC, Atmar RL. Infections in Hispanic immigrants. Clin Infect Dis 2002;34:1627–1632.
3. Bledsoe GH. Malaria primer for clinicians in the United States. South Med J 2005;98:1197–1204.
4. Chen LH, Wilson ME, Schlagenhauf P. Controversies and misconceptions in malaria chemoprophylaxis for travelers. JAMA 2007;297:2251–2263.
5. Malaria Surveillance—United States, 2007. MMWR Surveill Summ 2009;58(SS-02):1–16.
6. Vicas AE, Albrecht H, Lennox JL, del Rio C. Imported malaria at an inner-city hospital in the United States. Am J Med 2005;329:6–12.
7. Franco-Paredes C, Santos-Preciado JI. Problem pathogens: Prevention of malaria in travelers. Lancet Infect Dis 2006;6:139–149.
8. Nuesch R, Zimmerli L, Stockli R, et al. Imported Strongyloidosis: A longitudinal analysis of 31 cases. J Travel Med 2005;29:80–84.
9. John DT, Petri WA Jr. Markell and Voge's Medical Parasitology, 9th ed. Philadelphia: Saunders, 2006.
10. Escobedo AA, Cimerman S. Giardiasis: A pharmacotherapy review. Expert Opin Pharmacother 2007;8(12):1885–1902.
11. Hill DR. Giardia lamblia. In: Mandell GL, Bennett JE, Dolin R, eds. Principles and Practice of Infectious Diseases, 7th ed. New York: Elsevier Churchill-Livingstone, 2009:3527–3534.
12. Drugs for parasitic infections. In: Handbook of Antimicrobial Therapy, 18th ed. New Rochelle, NY: Medical Letter, 2008:225–280.
13. Lebwohl B, Deckelbaum RJ, Green PHR. Giardiasis. Gastrointest Endosc 2003;57:906–913.
14. Huang DB, White AC. An updated review on Cryptosporium and Giardia. Gastroenterol Clin North Am 2006;35:291–314.
15. Sorell L, Garrote JA, Galvan JA, et al. Celiac disease diagnosis in patients with giardiasis: High value of antitransglutaminase antibodies. Am J Gastroenterol 2004;99:1330–1332.

16. Nitazoxanide (alina): A new antiprotozoal agent. Med Lett Drugs Ther 2003;45:29–31.

17. Hung C-C, Deng H-Y, Hsiao W-H, et al. Invasive amebiasis as an emerging parasite disease in patients with human immunodeficiency virus type 1 infection in Taiwan. JAMA 2005;165:409–415.

18. Farthing MJG. Intestinal protozoa. Entamoeba histolytica. In: Manson's Tropical Diseases, 22nd ed. London: WB Saunders, 2009: 1375–1386.

19. Haque R, Huston CD, Hughes M, et al. Amebiasis. N Engl J Med 2003;348:1565–1573.

20. Petri Jr WA, Haque R. Entamoeba histolytica (amebiasis). In: Mandell GL, Bennett JA, Dolin R, eds. Principles and Practice of Infectious Diseases, 7th ed. New York: Elsevier Churchill-Livingstone, 2009:3411–3425.

21. Salles JM, Morales LA, Salles MC. Hepatic Amebiasis. Braz J Infect Dis 2003;7:96–110.

22. Bercu TE, Petri Jr WA, Behm BW. Amebic colitis: New insights into pathogenesis and treatment. Curr Gastroenterol Rep 2007;9:429–433.

23. Ozdogan M, Baykal A, Aran O. Amebic perforation of the colon: Rare and frequently fatal complication. World J Surg 2004;28:926–929.

24. Maguire JH. Intestinal nematodes (roundworms). In: Mandell GL, Bennett JE, Dolin R, eds. Principles and Practice of Infectious Diseases, 7th ed. New York: Elsevier Churchill-Livingstone, 2009:3577–3586.

25. Bethony J, Brooker S, Albonico M, et al. Soil-transmitted helminth infection: Ascariasis, trichuriasis, and hookworm. Lancet 2006;367: 1521–1532.

26. Hotez PJ, Brooker S, Bethony JM, et al. Hookworm infection. N Engl J Med 2004;357:799–807.

27. Gabriella AF, Ramsan M, Naumann C, et al. Soil-transmitted helminthes and haemoglobin status among Afghan children in World Food Programme Assisted Schools. J Helminthol 2005;79:381–384.

28. Larocque R, Casapia M, Gotuzzo E, Gyorkos TW. Relationship between intensity of soil-transmitted helminth infections and anemia in pregnancy. Am J Trop Med Hyg 2005;73:783–789.

29. Sahoo PK, Satapathy AK, Michael E, Ravindran B. Concomitant parasitism: Bancroftian filariasis and intestinal helminthes and response to albendazole. Am J Trop Med Hyg 2005;73:877–880.

30. Malik AH, Saima BD, Wani MY. Management of hepatobiliary and pancreatic ascariasis in children of endemic area. Pediatr Surg Int 2006;22:164–168.

31. Huratado RM, Sahani DV, Kradin RL. Case records of the Massachusetts General Hospital. Case 9-2006. A 35-year-old woman with recurrent-upper-quadrant pain. N Engl J Med 2006;354:1295–1303.

32. Petro M, Iavu K, Minocha A. Unusual endoscopic and microscopic view of Enterobius vermicularis: A case report with review of the literature. South Med J 2005;98:927–929.

33. Keiser PB, Nutman TB. Strongyloides stercoralis in the immuno-compromised population. Clin Microbiol Rev 2004;17:208–217.

34. Lim S, Katz K, Krajden S, et al. Complicated and fatal Strongyloides infection in Canadians: Risk factors, diagnosis and management. Can Med Assoc J 2004;171:479–484.

35. Schaeffer MW, Buell JF, Gupta M, et al. Strongyloides hyperinfection syndrome after heart transplantation: Case report and review of literature. J Heart Lung Transplant 2004;23:905–911.

36. Concho R, Harrington W, Rogers AI. Intestinal Strongyloidiasis: Recognition, management, and determinants of outcome. Clin Gastroenterol 2005;39:203–211.

37. Newberry AM, Williams DN, Stauffer WM, et al. Strongyloides hyperinfection presenting as acute respiratory failure and gram-negative sepsis. Chest 2005;128:3681–3684.

38. Satoh M, Kokaze A. Treatment strategies in controlling strongyloidiasis. Expert Opin Pharmacother 2004;5:2293–2301.

39. Muennig P, Pallin D, Challah C, Khan K. The cost-effectiveness of ivermectin vs albendazole in the presumptive treatment of strongyloidiasis in immigrants to the United States. Epidemiol Infect 2004;132:1055–1063.

40. King CH. Cestodes (tapeworms). In: Mandell GL, Dolin R, Bennett JE, eds. Principles and Practice of Infectious Diseases, 7th ed. New York: Elsevier Churchill-Livingstone, 2009:3607–3616.

41. Garcia HH, Gonzalez AE, Evans CAW, Gilman RH. Taenia solium cysticercosis. Lancet 2003;361:547–556.

42. Del La Garza Y, Graviss EA, Daver NG, et al. Epidemiology of neurocysticercosis in Houston, Texas. Am J Trop Med Hyg 2005;73:766–770.

43. Townes JM, Hoffmann CJ, Kohn MA. Neurocysticercosis in Oregon, 1995-2000. Emerging Infect Dis 2004;10:508–510.

44. Dua T, Aneja S. Neurocysticercosis: Management issues. Indian Pediatr 2006;43:227–235.

45. Garcia HH, Del Brutto OH, Nash TE, et al. New concepts in the diagnosis and management of neurocysticercosis (Taenia solium). Am J Trop Med Hyg 2005;72:3–9.

46. Gongora-Rivera F, Soto-Hernandez JL, Esquivel DG, et al. Albendazole trial at 15 or 30 mg/kg/day for subarachnoid and intraventricular cysticercosis. Neurology 2006;66:436–438.

47. Fairhurst RM, Wellems TE. Plasmodium species (malaria). In: Mandell GL, Dolin R, Bennett JE, eds. Principles and Practice of Infectious Diseases, 7th ed. New York: Elsevier Churchill-Livingstone, 2009:3437–3462.

48. White NJ, Breman JG. Malaria and babesiosis: Diseases caused by red blood cell parasites. In: Harrison's Principles of Internal Medicine, 18th ed. New York: McGraw-Hill, 2008:1280–1294.

49. Newman RD, Parise ME, Barber AM, Steketee RW. Malaria-related deaths among travelers, 1963-2001. Ann Intern Med 2004;141:547–555.

50. Kitchen AD, Chiodini PL. Malaria and blood transfusion. Vox Sang 2006;90:77–84.

51. White NJ. Malaria. In: Cook GC and Zumla A, eds. Manson's Tropical Diseases, 21st ed. London: WB Saunders, 2003:1205–1295.

52. Idro R, Carter JA, Fegan G, et al. Risk factors for persisting neurological and cognitive impairment following cerebral malaria. Arch Dis Child 2006;91:142–148.

53. Idro R, Jenkins NE, Newton CRJC. Pathogenesis, clinical features, and neurological outcome of cerebral malaria. Lancet Neurol 2005;4:827–840.

54. Pasvol G. Management of severe malaria: Interventions and controversies. Infect Dis Clin North Am 2005;19:211–240.

55. Eiam-Ong S. Malarial nephropathy. Semin Nephrol 2003;23:21–33.

56. Trampuz A, Jereb M, Muzlovic I, Prabhu RM. Clinical Review: Severe Malaria. Crit Care 2003;7:315–323.

57. Riddle MS, Jackson JL, Sanders JW, Blazes DL. Exchange transfusion as an adjunct therapy in severe Plasmodium falciparum malaria: A meta-analysis. Clin Infect Dis 2002;34:1192–1198.

58. Taylor WRJ, White NJ. Malaria and the lung. Clin Chest Med 2002;23:457–468.

59. Singh N, Saxena A. Usefulness of a rapid on-site plasmodium falciparum diagnosis (PARACHECK® PF) in forest migrants and among the indigenous population at the site of their occupational activities in central India. Am J Trop Med Hyg 2005;72:26–29.

60. Magill AJ. The prevention of malaria. Prim Care 2002;29:815–842.

61. Chen LH, Wilson ME, Schlagenhauf P. Prevention of malaria in long-term travelers. JAMA 2006;296:2234–2244.

62. Shanks GD, Edstein MD. Modern malaria chemoprophylaxis. Drugs 2005;65:2091–2110.

63. Taylor WRJ, White NJ. Antimalarial drug toxicity. Drug Saf 2004;27:25–61.

64. Tako EA, Zhou A, Lohoue J, et al. Risk factors for placental malaria and its effect on pregnancy outcome in Yaounde, Cameroon. Am J Trop Med Hyg 2005;72:236–242.

65. Sharma S, Pathak S. Malaria vaccine: A current perspective. J Vector Borne Dis 2008;45:1–20.

66. Ballou WR, Arevalo-Herrera M, Carucci D, et al. Update on the clinical development of candidate malaria vaccines. Am J Trop Med Hyg 2004;71:239–247.

67. Alonso P, Sacarlal J, Aponte JJ, et al. Efficacy of the RTS, S/ASO2A vaccine against Plasmodium infection and disease in young African children: Randomized controlled trial. Lancet 2004;364:1411–1420.

68. Bacaner N, Stauffer B, Boulware DR, Walker PF, Keystone JS. Travel medicine considerations for North American immigrants visiting friends and relatives. JAMA 2004;291:2856–2864.

69. Rathore D, McCutchan TF, Sullivan M, Kumar S. Antimalarial drugs: Current status and new developments. Expert Opin Investig Drugs 2006;14:871–883.

70. Chen LH, Keystone JS. New strategies for the prevention of malaria in travelers. Infect Dis Clin North Am 2005;19:185–210.

71. Rosenthal PJ. Artesunate for the treatment of severe Falciparum malaria. N Engl J Med 2008;358:1829–1836.

72. Price RN, Uhlemann A-C, van Vugt M, et al. Molecular and pharmacological determinants of the therapeutic response to artemether-lumefantrine in multi-resistant Plasmodium falciparum malaria. Clin Infect Dis 2006;42:1570–1577.

73. Fradin MS, Day JF. Comparative efficacy of insect repellents against mosquito bites. N Engl J Med 2002;347:13–18.

74. Rosenthal PJ. Antiprotozoal drugs. In: Katzung BG, ed. Basic and Clinical Pharmacology, 11th ed. New York: Lange Medical Books/McGraw-Hill, 2009:899–921.

75. Barrett MP, Burchmore RJS, Stich A, et al. The trypanosomiasis. Lancet 2003;362:1469–1480.

76. Marin-Neto JA, Cunha-Neto E, Maciel BC, Simoes MV. Pathogenesis of chronic Chagas heart disease. Circulation 2007;115:1109–1123.

77. Kirchhoff LV. Trypanosoma species (American trypanosomiasis, Chagas' disease): Biology of trypanosomes. In: Mandell GL, Bennett JE, Dolin R, eds. Principles and Practice of Infectious Diseases, 7th ed. New York: Elsevier Churchill-Livingstone, 2009:3481–3488.

78. Kirchhoff LV. American trypanosomiasis (Chagas disease). In: Guerrant RL, Walker H, Weller PF, eds. Tropical Infectious Diseases: Principles, Pathogens, and Practice, 2nd ed. 2006:1082–1094.

79. Carod-Artal FJ, Vargas AP, Melo M, Horan TA. American trypanosomiasis (Chagas' disease): An unrecognized cause of stroke. J Neurol Neurosurg Psychiatry 2003;74:516–518.

80. Schijman AG, Vigliano CA, Viotti RJ, et al. Trypanosoma cruzi DNA in cardiac lesions of Argentine patients with end-stage chronic Chagas heart disease. Am J Trop Med Hyg 2004;70:210–220.

81. Chagas disease after organ transplantation – Los Angeles, California, 2006. MMWR Morb Mortal Wkly Rep 2006;55:798–800.

82. Viotti R, Vigliano C, Lococo B, et al. Long-term cardiac outcomes of treating chronic Chagas disease with benznidazole versus no treatment. A nonrandomized trial. Ann Intern Med 2006;144:724–734.

83. Rosenthal PJ. Clinical pharmacology of the anthelmintic drugs. In: Katzung BG, ed. Basic and Clinical Pharmacology, 11th ed. New York: Lange Medical Books/McGraw-Hill, 2009:923–934.

84. Diaz SH. Lice (pediculosis). In: Mandell GL, Bennett JR, Dolin R, eds. Principles and Practice of Infectious Diseases, 7th ed. New York: Elsevier Churchill-Livingstone, 2009:3629–3632.

85. Roberts RJ. Head lice. N Engl J Med 2002;346:1645–1650.

86. Yoon KS, Gao J-R, Taplin D, et al. Permethrin-resistant human head lice, pediculus capitis, and their treatment. Arch Dermatol 2003;139:994–1000.

87. Burkhart CG. Relationship of treatment-resistant head lice to the safety and efficacy of pediculicides. Mayo Clin Proc 2004;79:661–666.

88. Jones KN, English III JC. Review of common therapeutic options in the United States for the treatment of pediculosis capitis. Clin Infect Dis 2003;36:1355–1361.

89. Johnson G, Sladden M. Scabies: Diagnosis and treatment. Br Med J 2005;331:619–622.

90. Chosidow O. Scabies. N Engl J Med 2006;354:1718–1727.

79 Urinary Tract Infections

Kathryn R. Matthias and Brian A. Potoski

LEARNING OBJECTIVES

● **Upon completion of the chapter, the reader will be able to:**

1. Explain the diagnostic criteria for significant bacteriuria.

2. Recognize the signs and symptoms of urinary tract infections (UTIs) and how they differ in upper versus lower urinary tract disease.

3. Identify the organism responsible for the majority of uncomplicated UTIs.

4. Assess the laboratory tests that help in diagnosing patients with UTI.

5. Determine appropriate drug, dose, and duration for uncomplicated and complicated UTI prophylaxis and empiric treatment.

6. Evaluate and select therapy for uncomplicated and complicated UTIs based on specific urine culture results and patient characteristics.

7. Formulate appropriate monitoring and education information for patients with UTIs.

KEY CONCEPTS

❶ Urinary tract infections (UTIs) are thought of as either uncomplicated or complicated. Generally this refers to absence or presence, respectively, of functional or structural abnormalities within the urinary tract.

❷ The majority (85%) of uncomplicated UTIs are caused by *Escherichia coli*. The majority of the remaining 15% are caused by *Staphylococcus saprophyticus* along with *Klebsiella* spp., *Proteus* spp., *Pseudomonas* spp., *Enterobacter* spp., and *Enterococcus* spp.

❸ Symptoms of lower UTIs include dysuria, gross hematuria, suprapubic heaviness, nocturia, increased urinary frequency, and urgency.

❹ Symptoms of upper UTIs include fever, nausea, vomiting, malaise, and often severe flank pain.

❺ The goals of treatment of UTIs are to eradicate the offending organism, to prevent or treat consequences of infection, and to prevent recurrence of infection.

❻ Uncomplicated UTIs may be managed with 3-day or even 1-day regimens, while complicated UTIs should be treated for at least 7 days and sometimes 2 weeks or longer.

Urinary tract infections (UTIs) are comprised of a diverse array of syndromes depending on the location of the infection within the urinary tract. UTIs occur frequently and are responsible for approximately 8.3 million physician office and hospital outpatient visits annually.[1-3] In simplest of terms, a UTI is bacteria in the urinary tract, that does not represent contamination.

● Bacteriuria, or bacteria in the urine, does not always represent infection. For this reason a number of quantitative diagnostic criteria have been created to identify the amount of bacteria in the urine that most likely represents true infection (hence the term "significant bacteriuria").[4] These criteria are shown in Table 79–1. Furthermore, UTIs are classified as lower tract or upper tract disease. Patients can present differently with upper versus lower tract disease, and upper tract disease is thought of as a much more severe infection since patients are more likely to be admitted to the hospital with upper urinary tract disease than lower tract disease. An example of lower tract syndrome is cystitis which involves inflammation of the bladder and commonly causes symptoms such as dysuria, nocturia, gross hematuria, and occasional suprapubic tenderness. An example of upper urinary tract disease is pyelonephritis. Pyelonephritis is an inflammation of the kidney usually due to infection. Patients with uncomplicated UTI are more frequently treated as outpatients compared to those patients with complicated UTIs.

EPIDEMIOLOGY AND ETIOLOGY

The prevalence and type of UTIs generally varies by age and gender.[5,6] UTIs may occur at any age, even in the very young. Premature infants, for example, have a higher rate than

Table 79–1
Diagnostic Criteria for Significant Bacteriuria
• Greater than or equal to 10^2 CFU coliforms/mL or greater than or equal to 10^5 CFU noncoliforms/mL in a symptomatic female
• Greater than or equal to 10^3 CFU organisms/mL in a symptomatic male
• Greater than or equal to 10^5 CFU same organisms/mL in asymptomatic individuals on two consecutive specimens
• Any growth of bacteria on suprapubic catheterization in a symptomatic patient
• Greater than or equal to 10^2 CFU organisms/mL in a catheterized patient

CFU, colony-forming unit.

full-term infants, and neonatal boys are five to eight times more likely to have UTIs than neonatal girls. In young children 1 to 5 years of age, significant bacteriuria occurs more in girls than boys, 4.5% compared to 0.5%, respectively.[7] Once adulthood is reached, bacteriuria increases in young, nonpregnant women (range, 1–3%), yet remains low in men (up to 0.1%).[8] Symptomatic UTI affects 30% of women between 20 and 40 years of age, which represents a prevalence that is 30 times greater than men of the same age group. Upwards of 40% to 50% of the female population will experience a symptomatic UTI at sometime during their life.[1]

The etiology of UTIs has remained relatively unchanged over the past several decades. ❶ *UTIs are either uncomplicated or complicated.* There is a lack of consensus regarding the definition of what makes a UTI complicated, but in general a complicated UTI refers to a structural or functional abnormality of the urinary tract. Patients with complicated UTIs are typically given longer treatment durations than those patients with uncomplicated infections. Those with complicated UTIs by definition are also prone to more frequent infections. It is important to note that an upper UTI does not necessarily imply complicated UTI, nor does lower UTI imply uncomplicated UTI.

While the frequency of causative organisms changes depending on the location of infection and patient characteristics, over 95% of uncomplicated UTIs are the result of a single causative organism. ❷ *In 85% of the uncomplicated UTI cases, the causative organism is* E. coli.[9] A variety of other organisms may cause uncomplicated UTIs, but represent the minority of pathogens. Other organisms include gram-positives such as *Staphylococcus saprophyticus* and *Enterococcus* spp. and gram-negative bacteria such as *Pseudomonas aeruginosa*, *Klebsiella pneumoniae*, *Proteus* spp., and *Enterobacter* spp.[10–12] The chances of isolating an organism other than *E. coli* are higher in patients that have recurrent UTIs, particularly those patients whose UTI is considered complicated. It is also more common for organisms other than *E. coli* to cause UTIs in the hospitalized population than in the general population.[13,14]

Patient Encounter, Part 1

VN is a 23-year-old female who presents to a local urgent care center with complaints of painful urination and frequent need to urinate especially at night which began 3 days ago. She denies vomiting, fever, nausea, or flank pain. Upon questioning she does admit that she is sexually active with only one partner and uses a diaphragm.

What symptoms are suggestive of urinary tract infection (UTI)?

Does she have risk factors for UTI?

What additional information do you need to know before creating a treatment plan for this patient?

PATHOPHYSIOLOGY

There are three potential ways for bacteria to enter into the urinary tract and cause infection: the ascending, hematogenous, and lymphatic pathways.

Ascending Pathway

The ascending pathway occurs when bacteria colonizing the urethra subsequently travel upwards, or ascend, the urethra to the bladder and cause cystitis (Fig. 79–1). The ascending route may help to explain why UTIs occur more commonly in women than in men. Women have a shorter urethra than men, and colonization of the female urethra is likely due to its proximity to the perirectal area. The use of spermicidal agents increases the colonization of the vagina with uropathogens.[15] Additionally, massage of the urethra in women as well as sexual intercourse may lead to bacteria gaining entrance into the bladder.[16,17] Once in the bladder, bacteria are not limited to causing cystitis. These bacteria may continue to ascend the urinary tract via the ureters and cause more complicated infections, such as pyelonephritis.

Hematogenous Pathway

The hematogenous route occurs through the seeding of the urinary tract with pathogens carried by the blood supply. These pathogens represent an infection at some other primary site in the body. *Staphylococcus aureus* bacteremia, for example, can cause renal abscesses via the hematogenous route, and pyelonephritis can be experimentally produced by IV injection of *Salmonella* spp., *Mycobacterium tuberculosis*, or even yeast (*Candida* spp.) into rabbits.[18] However, experimentally creating this pathway has not been successful with all organisms. Experimental hematogenous seeding of the kidneys could not be created with the IV injection of large innocula of *E. coli* or *P. aeruginosa* in a mouse model.[19]

Lymphatic Pathway

The lymphatic system, also known as the secondary circulatory system, connects the bladder to the kidney and

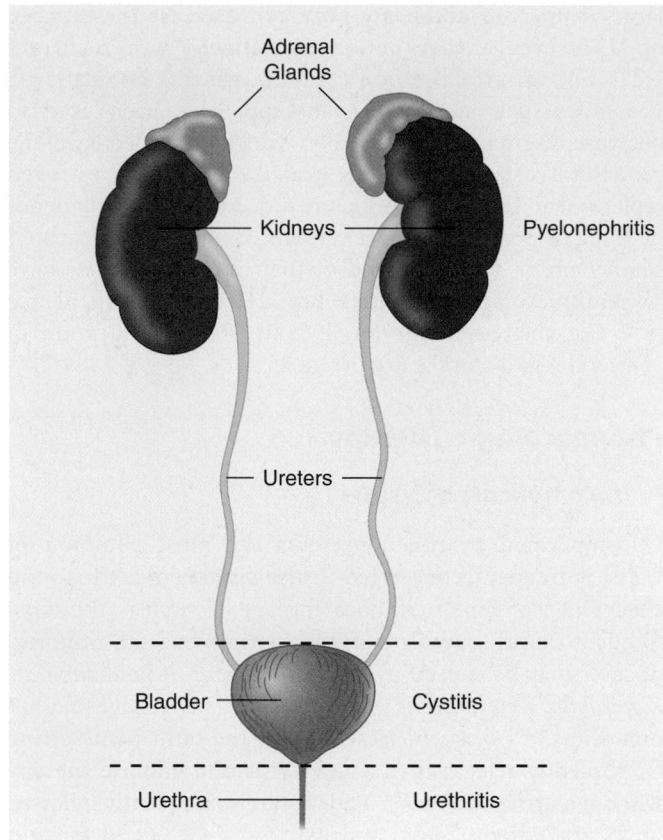

FIGURE 79–1. Anatomy and associated infections of the urinary tract. (From Sprandel KA, Lesch CA, Rodvold KA. Lower urinary tract infection. In: Schwinghammer TL (ed.) Pharmacotherapy Casebook: A Patient-Focused Approach, 6th ed. New York City: McGraw-Hill; 2005:315, with permission).

Clinical Presentation and Diagnosis of UTIs

General

- Most women present with hematuria; however, this is not a presentation restricted only to UTIs.
- Elderly patients frequently will not present with common signs and symptoms of UTI, but may present with altered mental status.
- More than 95% of UTIs are caused by a single organism.
- Patients may present with urosepsis.
- ❸ *Signs and Symptoms of Lower UTI*
- *Dysuria, gross hematuria, suprapubic heaviness, nocturia, increased urinary frequency and urgency*
- ❹ *Signs and Symptoms of Upper UTI*
- *Fever, nausea, vomiting, malaise, and often severe flank pain*

Laboratory Tests

Urinalysis should show:

- **Pyuria** typically greater than 10 white blood cells/mm^3 urine
- Bacteriuria, usually greater than 10^5 CFU organisms/mL
- Nitrites present
- Leukocyte esterase present

Other Diagnostic Tests

- Bacterial urine culture
- Upper UTI: presence of costovertebral tenderness

may represent a way for bacteria to be transported and subsequently cause infection. Although this pathway is classically included as a route of infection, there is a lack of data showing the lymphatic pathway as a significant mechanism for development of infection. As a result this pathway is not believed to be a significant host mechanism.

Host Defense Mechanisms

Urine, although not an antimicrobial itself, possesses characteristics that are less than ideal for bacterial growth. Some of these characteristics include low pH, significant urea concentration, and high osmolality. Also, bacteria in the bladder can stimulate an urge to urinate. Additionally, prostatic fluid secretions in men can inhibit bacterial growth while normal vaginal flora in women such as *Lactobacillus* spp. can secrete lactic acid which can decrease the pH of the enviroment.[20–22]

There are several other host factors that inhibit what are known as bacterial virulence factors. These virulence factors are mechanisms that bacteria utilize to cause infection and/or ensure their survival. The first is glycosaminoglycan, a compound produced by the body that coats the epithelial cells of the bladder. This compound essentially separates the bladder from the urine by forming a protective layer against bacterial adhesion.[23] A second compound known as Tamm-Horsfall protein is secreted into the urine, and prevents *E. coli* from binding to receptors present on the surface of the bladder. Other factors implicated in contributing to host defense mechanisms against UTIs include immunoglobulins, specifically IgA.

Risk Factors

There are several risk factors for development of UTIs.[8] Common risk factors for UTIs in women include sexual intercourse, use of a diaphragm, use of spermicidal jellies, diabetes, and pregnancy.[24–26] In men, the risks primarily relate to lack of circumcision and at an older age include prostatic hyperplasia. Common risk factors for both men and women include urologic instrumentation, renal transplantation, neurogenic bladder, and urinary tract obstruction.[27,28]

TREATMENT

Desired Outcomes

❺ *The goals of treatment are to eradicate the invading organism, to prevent or treat consequences of infection,*

Patient Encounter, Part 2: Medical History, Physical Exam, and Diagnostic Tests

PMH: Asthma (controlled)

FH: Father living with diabetes mellitus, type 2 (controlled) and chronic obstructive pulmonary disease; mother living with hypertension (controlled)

SH: Second year pharmacy student. Works as a pharmacy intern at a local hospital

Allergies: Penicillin (patient states she was admitted to a hospital at the age of 7 years with hives and throat swelling after receiving amoxicillin)

Meds: Albuterol (salbutamol) inhaler as needed

ROS: (+) dysuria, urinary frequency; (–) fever, nausea, vomiting, flank pain

PE:

VS: BP 122/64 mm Hg, P 62 bpm, RR 16 per minute, afebrile

CV: RRR, normal S1, S2; normal findings

Abd: Soft, nontender, nondistended; (+) bowel sounds, no hepatosplenomegaly, heme (–) stool

Labs: Within normal limits; (–) pregnancy test

Given this additional information, what is your assessment of the patient's condition?

Identify your treatment goals for the patient.

What nonpharmacologic pharmacologic alternatives are available for the patient?

and to prevent, if possible, recurrence of infection. Therapy is directed at microbiologic eradication of the offending organism through antibiotics.

General Approach to Treatment

Antimicrobial therapy is the cornerstone of treatment in UTIs. Antimicrobials should ideally be well tolerated, narrow in antimicrobial spectrum, lend itself to patient compliance (low total number of doses), have adequate concentrations at the site of the infection, and have good oral bioavailability. Table 79–2 reviews oral and IV antibiotics frequently used to treat UTIs with comments on their use, and Table 79–3 reviews frequency, duration, and doses of oral antibiotics used commonly for outpatient treatment of UTIs.

Nonpharmacologic Therapy

Although there is limited data in the literature and sometimes conflicting results, several nonpharmacologic therapies have been proposed for prevention of UTIs. The intake of large volumes of cranberry juice can decrease the number of UTIs over a year period in patients with recurrent UTIs but uncertain efficacy in the general population.[29] Probiotics such as *Lactobacillus* spp. have been used to decrease vaginal pH in women which may decrease the growth of certain pathogenic bacteria.[21–22] Topical estrogen replacement therapy significantly decreases the incidence of UTIs in postmenopausal women compared to placebo.[30] Methenamine hippurate and methenamine mandalate have no antimicrobial properties but decrease the incidence of UTIs when used for prophylaxis. Patient education of common risk factors is important.

Pharmacologic Therapy

▶ Uncomplicated Cystitis

Uncomplicated cystitis represents the most common of UTIs, is frequently managed in the outpatient setting, and occurs in women of childbearing age.[3] *E. coli* is the most frequent causal organisms in this setting, but in a minority of cases may be caused by *S. saprophyticus*, *K. pneumoniae*, *P. mirabilis*, *Enterococcus* spp., and a small percentage of other organsims.[9–12] As such, treatment in the outpatient setting is frequently relegated to a urinalysis and empiric therapy without a urine culture.[31,32] Patients are subsequently followed up for resolution of signs and symptoms. ❻ *One significant benefit of treatment in the setting of uncomplicated cystitis is that treatment duration can be less than 7 days, and often may be 3 days or even 1 day.*

Although treatment duration of 1 day is advantageous because it strictly limits adverse events and drug interactions, and increases compliance, health care providers should know that 3-day courses of fluoroquinolones and trimethoprim-sulfamethoxazole are superior to single-doses in terms of cure rates in uncomplicated UTIs.[10,33] For acute uncomplicated UTIs, it is reasonable to pursue a 1-day course of therapy. Which agent to choose empirically partly hinges on known resistance rates in the geographic region, particularly *E. coli* resistance to trimethoprim-sulfamethoxazole.[9,34,35] No consensus has been reached on what percentage of *E. coli* isolates resistant to trimethoprim-sulfamethoxazole should preclude its use; however, a model has been created that suggests that this threshold resistant rate is between 19% and 21% in the empiric setting.[36]

▶ Acute Pyelonephritis

In contrast to patients that present with lower UTIs, those that present with pyelonephritis usually have high-grade fever (greater than 38.3°C [100.9°F]) and severe flank pain. Select patients with pyelonephritis may be treated in the outpatient setting; however, patients whose infection is severe enough to cause vomiting, decreased food intake, and dehydration may need to be treated in an inpatient hospitalized setting. These patients will usually receive IV antibiotics at first before being switched to oral therapy depending on susceptibility testing.

Table 79–2

Commonly Used Antimicrobial Agents for the Treatment of UTIs

Agent	Comments
Oral Therapy	
Penicillins Amoxicillin Amoxicillin- clavulanic acid	Increasing *E. coli* resistance has limited amoxicillin use in acute cystitis despite broad-spectrum activity. Amoxicillin-clavulanic acid is empirically preferred due to resistance. Ampicillin is the drug of choice for enterococci sensitive to penicillin but oral bioavailability approximately 50%
Cephalosporins Cefaclor Cefadroxil Cefixime Cefpodoxime Cefuroxime Cephalexin Cephradine	There are no major advantages of these agents over other oral agents in the treatment of UTIs, and they are usually more expensive. They may be useful in cases of resistance to amoxicillin and trimethoprim-sulfamethoxazole. These agents are not active against enterococci
Tetracyclines Doxycycline Minocycline Tetracycline	These agents have been effective for initial episodes of UTI; however, resistance can develop rapidly. Avoid during pregnancy
Fluoroquinolones Ciprofloxacin Levofloxacin Norfloxacin Ofloxacin	The newer quinolones have a greater spectrum of activity. These agents are effective for pyelonephritis. Avoid in pregnancy and children. Moxifloxacin is not listed due to limited urinary excretion
Miscellaneous Trimethoprim- sulfamethoxazole	This combination is highly effective against most aerobic enteric bacteria except *P. aeruginosa*. High urinary tract tissue levels and urine levels are achieved, which may be important in complicated UTI treatment. Also effective as prophylaxis for recurrent infections. Generally well tolerated and low cost. Its use may be precluded in patients with sulfa allergies
Nitrofurantoin	This agent is effective in treatment and prophylaxis in patients with recurrent lower tract UTIs. Should not be used in patients with low estimated CrCl (less than 40 to 60 mL/min) due to limited urine concentrations and potential increased risk of neuropathy
Azithromycin	Commonly used for sexually transmitted diseases (i.e., Chlamydia infections) rather than for UTIs
Fosfomycin	Single-dose therapy for uncomplicated UTI
Parenteral Therapy	
Aminoglycosides Amikacin Gentamicin Tobramycin	Gentamicin and tobramycin are generally equally effective while tobramycin has slightly better coverage of certain *Pseudomonas* spp. Amikacin generally is reserved for multidrug resistant bacteria. Typically used as a short course of therapy followed by a switch to an oral agent. Concern for neurotoxicity and ototoxicity generally limit use especially in patients with impaired renal function
Penicillins Ampicillin Ampicillin-sulbactam Ticarcillin-clavulanate Piperacillin Piperacillin- tazobactam	These agents are generally effective for susceptible bacteria. The extended-spectrum penicillins are active against certain strains of *Pseudomonas* spp. They are very useful in renally impaired patients since urine concentration can remain adequate or when an aminoglycoside is avoided

Cephalosporins
First-, second-,
    third-, and fourth-
    generation
	Second- and third-generation cephalosporins have a broad spectrum of activity against gram-negative bacteria, but are not active against enterococci. Only ceftazidime and cefepime have activity against certain strains of *Pseudomonas* spp. They are useful for nosocomial infections and urosepsis due to susceptible pathogens

Carbapenems Doripenem Ertapenem Imipenem-cilastatin Meropenem	These agents have broad-spectrum activity, including gram-positive, gram-negative, and anaerobic bacteria. Ertapenem is not active against *Pseudomonas* spp. All may be associated with *Candida* spp. superinfections. Rarely used for UTIs

(Continued)

Table 79–2

Commonly Used Antimicrobial Agents for the Treatment of UTIs (*Continued*)

Agent	Comments
Fluoroquinolones Ciprofloxacin Levofloxacin	These agents have broad-spectrum activity against both gram-negative and gram-positive bacteria. They provide high urine and tissue concentrations and are actively secreted in reduced renal function. Switch to oral therapy when possible due to excellent bioavailability
Monobactam Aztreonam	Only active against gram-negative bacteria including some strains of *P. aeruginosa*. Generally useful for nosocomial infections when aminoglycosides are to be avoided and in patients with Type 1/immediate hypersensitivity to penicillins
Glycopeptide Vancomycin	May be considered in combination for empiric therapy based on patient risk factors for multidrug resistant organisms and gram-positive cocci shown in urinalysis

CrCl, creatinine clearance.

Table 79–3

Overview of Outpatient, Oral Antimicrobial Therapy for Lower and Upper Tract UTIs

Indications	Antibiotic	Adult Dose[a]	Frequency	Duration
Lower Tract UTIs				
Uncomplicated	Trimethoprim-sulfamethoxazole	2 DS[b] tablets	Single dose	1 day
		or 1 DS[b] tablet	Every 12 hours	3 days
	Trimethoprim	100 mg	Every 12 hours	3 days
	Ciprofloxacin	250 mg	Every 12 hours	3 days
	Levofloxacin	250 mg	Every 24 hours	3 days
	Norfloxacin	400 mg	Every 12 hours	3 days
	Nitrofurantoin macrocrystals	50 *or* 100 mg	Every 6 hours	3–7 days
	Nitrofurantoin monohydrate	100 mg	Every 12 hours	7 days
	Amoxicillin	6 × 500 mg	Single dose	1 day
		or 500 mg	Every 12 hours	3 days
	Amoxicillin-clavulanic acid	500 mg	Every 8 hours	3 days
	Fosfomycin	3,000 mg	Single dose	1 day
Complicated	Trimethoprim-sulfamethoxazole	1 DS[b] tablet	Every 12 hours	7–10 days
	Trimethoprim	100 mg	Every 12 hours	7–10 days
	Ciprofloxacin	500 mg	Every 12 hours	7–10 days
	Norfloxacin	400 mg	Every 12 hours	7–10 days
	Levofloxacin	250 mg	Every 24 hours	7–10 days
	Amoxicillin-clavulanic acid	500 mg	Every 8 hours	7–10 days
Recurrent infections—continuous prophylaxis	Trimethoprim-sulfamethoxazole	½ SS[c] tablet	Every 24 hours	6 months
	Trimethoprim	100 mg	Every 24 hours	6 months
	Ciprofloxacin	125 mg	Every 24 hours	6 months
	Nitrofurantoin	50 *or* 100 mg	Every 24 hours	6 months
	Cefaclor	250 mg	Every 24 hours	6 months
	Cephalexin	125 mg	Every 24 hours	6 months
Upper Tract UTIs				
Acute pyelonephritis[d]	Amoxicillin-clavulanic acid	875 mg	Every 12 hours	14 days
		or 500 mg	Every 8 hours	14 days
	Ciprofloxacin	500 mg	Every 12 hours	7 days
	Levofloxacin	250 *or* 500 mg	Every 24 hours	14 days
	Trimethoprim-sulfamethoxazole	1 DS[b] tablet	Every 12 hours	14 days

[a]Majority of listed antimicrobial agents require dosage adjustment in patients with significant renal dysfunction.

[b]DS, double strength (160 mg trimethoprim/800 mg sulfamethoxazole).

[c]SS, single strength (80 mg trimethoprim/400 mg sulfamethoxazole).

[d]Doses listed for acute pyelonephritis are for oral regimens.

Patients with pyelonephritis are traditionally given 14 days of therapy; however, there are limited data showing success in treating acute uncomplicated pyelonephritis for 7 to 10 days. More studies need to be conducted on treating for these shorter durations.[3] Gram stain and culture are important in ensuring that appropriate antimicrobial coverage is selected. Stratification is used to manage patients with acute pyelonephritis. Women who present with mild cases of pyelonephritis (defined as low-grade fever and a normal to slightly elevated peripheral white blood count, without nausea or vomiting) may be treated as outpatients.[3] Those women who exhibit more severe signs and symptoms will need to be admitted to an acute care setting for appropriate treatment. The same holds true for antibiotic selection in these patients. Those who are treated in an outpatient setting can be treated with trimethoprim-sulfamethoxazole, fluoroquinolones, or even β-lactam/β-lactamase inhibitors, such as amoxicillin-clavulanic acid. In those patients that are admitted to the hospital, antibiotic therapy is usually broader in nature, especially in patients suspected of having bacteremia or urosepsis. These patients will typically receive IV therapy such as a fluoroquinolone, or a β-lactam plus an aminoglycoside.[3,37,38]

Special Populations

▶ Pregnant Women

Changes to the urinary tract in pregnant women predispose them to an increased incidence of bacteriuria, and subsequent UTIs that may follow. These changes include alterations in amino acid and other nutrient concentrations in the urine along with physiologic changes such as reduced bladder tone and dilation of the renal pelvis and ureters.[39,40]

An association exists between maternal UTI during pregnancy and fetal death, mental retardation, and developmental delay.[41] Due to this known association and since up to 7% of pregnant women will develop an asymptomatic bacteriuria that may progress to pyelonephritis, screening for UTI is necessary.[24,42] In pregnant patients with significant bacteriuria, whether symptomatic or asymptomatic, treatment is recommended to avoid the complications discussed previously. In the majority of patients, a sulfonamide (not in the third trimester due to concerns for hyperbilirubinemia), amoxicillin-clavulanic

acid, cephalexin, or nitrofurantoin are effective treatment options. Tetracyclines and fluoroquinolones should be avoided due to risk of teratogenicity and ability to inhibit cartilage and bone development, respectively. Follow-up usually consists of a urine culture 1 to 2 weeks after completion of therapy, and afterwards monthly until birth.

▶ Catheterized Patients

An indwelling catheter is commonly used in various health care settings and is associated with UTIs.[27] Bacteria may be introduced into the bladder via the catheter in several ways including direct infection introduction during catheterization (via colonization and subsequently traveling the length of the catheter through bacterial motility or capillary action). UTIs as a result of an indwelling catheter are common and occur at a rate of 5% per day of catheter presence.[43]

The approach in the setting of a patient with bacteriuria and an indwelling urinary catheter follows two paths. The first, in asymptomatic patients with catheterization, is to hold antibiotics and remove the catheter if possible. The second, in symptomatic patients with catheterization, is to initiate antibiotic therapy and removal of the catheter if possible. In both of the above situations, if discontinuation of the catheter is not possible, the patient should be recatheterized with a new urinary catheter if the previous catheter is greater than 2 weeks old.

▶ UTIs in Men

Although UTIs in men are not always complicated by definition, due to the relative infrequency of UTIs in men compared to women, an abnormality (structural or functional) should be suspected and therefore treated as a probable complicated infection until proven otherwise.[44] For this reason, men should not be treated with a single dose or short course of therapy if diagnosed with a UTI. Typically these patients will receive 2 weeks of therapy, and in situations of failure may be treated up to 6 weeks, particularly if a prostatic source of infection is suspected. Prostatic enlargement, as previously mentioned, is a risk factor in men, and the prevalence of benign prostatic hyperplasia in the elderly population may predispose this population to UTIs.

OUTCOME EVALUATION

- Monitor the patient for resolution of symptoms with a goal of 48 to 72 hours to resolution after start of antimicrobial therapy
- If possible, follow-up on susceptibilities of the infecting organism (urine culture)
- Repeat culture is necessary only if symptoms do not acutely abate or reinfection or recurrence occurs
- Depending on chosen antibiotic therapy, evaluate patient based on drug therapy monitoring parameters including those presented in Table 79–4 to optimize therapy and decrease incidence of adverse drug events.

Patient Encounter, Part 3: Creating a Care Plan

Based on the information presented, create a care plan for this patient's UTI. Your plan should include:

(a) a statement of the drug-related needs and/or problems, (b) a patient-specific detailed therapeutic plan, and (c) monitoring parameters to assess efficacy and safety.

Table 79–4

Monitoring Parameters for Select Antibiotics Used in the Treatment of UTIs

Drug Class or Drug	What to Monitor	Frequency	Endpoint
Aminoglycosides	SCr, urine output	Every 24 hours	Prevention of nephrotoxicity manifested by a rise in SCr
	Aminoglycoside serum concentrations	Depends on duration of therapy. At least once weekly; more frequently if evidence of changing renal function	Trough serum concentrations less than 2 mg/L (less than 4.2 µmol/L for gentamicin and less than 4.3 µmol/L for tobramycin) or (less than 8 mg/L or 13.7 µmol/L for amikacin)[a] to decrease risk of nephrotoxicity and ototoxicity
Nitrofurantoin	SCr	Only if renal function changing or unstable	Nitrofurantoin metabolites may accumulate in renal insufficiency and lead to neuropathy; avoid if CrCl less than 40 mL/min
	Liver profile	Periodic monitoring	Prevention of cholestasis
Aminoglycosides Nitrofurantoin Tetracyclines Sulfonamides	SCr	Only if renal function changing or unstable	Decreases in glomerular filtrate rate can significant decrease the urine concentration of these agents

CrCl, creatinine clearance; SCr, serum creatinine

[a]Streptomycin concentrations are different than those listed here; because streptomycin is not used to treat UTIs, monitoring for this agent is not included.

Patient Care and Monitoring

1. Assess the patient's symptoms to determine response to the antimicrobial regimen you have chosen.

2. Review any microbiologic data:

   - Based on urinalysis and gram stain (if available), is your empiric selection reasonable?

   - Based on culture and susceptibility data (if available), are there any changes that need to be made from your initial empiric antimicrobial selection (i.e., resistance to the regimen initially selected)?

3. Determine if the patient may benefit from prophylactic therapy (i.e., recurrent UTIs secondary to chronic urinary catheterization due to paraplegia).

4. Evaluate the patient for the presence of adverse drug reactions, drug allergies, and potential drug interactions.

5. Stress the importance of complying with the prescribed antimicrobial regimen and to follow-up with the health care provider if signs and symptoms recur.

Abbreviations Introduced in This Chapter

CFU	Colony-forming units
CrCl	Creatinine clearance
SCr	Serum creatinine
UTI	Urinary tract infection

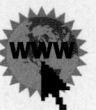

Self-assessment questions and answers are available at *http://www.mhpharmacotherapy. com/pp.html.*

REFERENCES

1. Foxman B. Epidemiology of urinary tract infections: Incidence, morbidity, and economic costs. Am J Med 2002;113(Suppl 1A): 5S–13S.
2. Fihn SD. Clinical practice. Acute uncomplicated urinary tract infection in women. N Engl J Med 2003;349:259–266.
3. Warren JW, Abrutyn E, Hebel JR, et al. Guidelines for antimicrobial treatment of uncomplicated acute bacterial cystitis and acute pyelonephritis. Clin Infect Dis 1999;29:745–758.
4. Bent S, Nallamothu BK, Simel DL, et al. Does this woman have an acute, uncomplicated urinary tract infection? JAMA 2002;287: 2701–2710.
5. Alper BS, Curry SH. Urinary tract infection in children. Am Fam Physician 2005;72:2483–2488.
6. Shortliffe LM, McCue JD. Urinary tract infections at the age extremes: Pediatrics and geriatrics. Am J Med 2002;113(Suppl 1A):55S–66S.
7. Smellie JM, Prescod NP, Shaw PJ, et al. Childhood reflux and urinary infection: A follow-up of 10–41 years in 225 adults. Pediatr Nephrol 1998;12:727–736.
8. Ronald AR, Pattullo AL. The natural history of urinary tract infection in adults. Med Clin North Am 1991;75:299–312.
9. Zhanel GG, Hisanaga TL, Laing NM, et al. Antibiotic resistance in *Escherichia coli* outpatient urinary isolates: Final results from the North American Urinary Tract Infection Collaborative Alliance (NAUTICA). Int J Antimicrob Agents 2006;27:468–475.
10. Stamm WE, Hooton TM. Management of urinary tract infections in adults. N Engl J Med 1993;329:1328–1334.

11. Ronald A. The etiology of urinary tract infection: Traditional and emerging pathogens. Am J Med 2002;113(Suppl 1A):14S–19S.

12. Raz R, Colodner R, Kunin CM. Who are you – *Staphylococcus saprophyticus*? Clin Infect Dis 2005;40:896–898.

13. Wagenlehner FM, Naber KG. Hospital-acquired urinary tract infections. J Hosp Infect 2000;46:171–181.

14. Lundstrom T, Sobel J. Nosocomial candiduria: A review. Clin Infect Dis 2001;32:1602–1607.

15. Hooten TM, Hillier S, Johnson C, et al. *Escherichia coli* bacteriuria and contraceptive method. JAMA 1991;265:64–69.

16. Stamatiou C, Bovis C, Panaguopoulos P, et al. Sex-induced cystitis – patient burden and other epidemiological features. Clin Exp Obstet Gynecol 2005;32:180–182.

17. Bran JL, Levison ME, Kaye D. Entrance of bacteria into the female urinary bladder. N Engl J Med 1972;286:626–629.

18. Freedman LR. Experimental pyelonephritis. VI. Observation on susceptibility of the rabbit kidney to infection by a virulent strain of *Staphylococcus aureus*. Yale J Biol Med 1960;32:272–279.

19. Gorrill RH, DeNavasquez SJ. Experimental pyelonephritis in the mouse produced by *Escherichia coli, Pseudomonas aeruginosa*, and *Proteus mirabilis*. J Pathol Bacteriol 1964;87:79–87.

20. Stamey TA, Fair WR, Timothy MM, et al. Antibacterial nature of prostatic fluid. Nature 1968;218:444–447.

21. Kwok L, Staphleton AE, Stamm WE, et al. Adherence of *Lactobacillus crispatus* to vaginal epithelial cells from women with or without a history of recurrent urinary tract infection. J Urol 2006;176; 2050–2054.

22. Gupta K, Stapleton AE, Hooton TM, et al. Inverse association of H_2O_2-producing lactobacilli and vaginal *Escherichia coli* colonization in women with recurrent urinary tract infections. J Infect Dis 1998;178:446–450.

23. Parsons CL, Schrom SH, Hanno P, et al. Bladder surface mucin: Examination of possible mechanisms for its antibacterial effect. Invest Urol 1978;6:196–200.

24. U.S. Preventive Services Task Force. Screening for asymptomatic bacteriuria in adults: U.S. Preventive Services Task Force reaffirmation recommendation statement. Ann Intern Med 2008;149:43–47.

25. Nicolle LE. Urinary tract infection in diabetes. Curr Opin Infect Dis 2005;18:49–53.

26. Harding GK, Zhanel GG, Nicolle LE, et al. Antimicrobial treatment in diabetic women with asymptomatic bacteriuria. N Engl J Med 2002;347:1576–1583.

27. Niël-Weise BS, van den Broek PJ. Urinary catheter policies for long-term bladder drainage. Cochrane Database Syst Rev 2005;1:CD004201.

28. Sobel JD, Kaye D. Urinary tract infection. In: Mandell GL, Bennett JE, Dolin R, eds. Principles and Practice of Infectious Diseases, 6th ed. Philadelphia: Elsevier, 2005:875.

29. Jepson RG, Craig JC. Cranberries for preventing urinary tract infection. Cochrane Database Syst Rev 2008;1:CD001321.

30. Raz R, Stamm WE. A controlled trial of intravaginal estriol in post-menopausal women with recurrent urinary tract infections. N Engl J Med 1993;329:753–756.

31. Carson C, Naber KG. Role of fluoroquinolones in the treatment of serious bacterial urinary tract infections. Drugs 2004;64:1359–1373.

32. Miller LG, Tang AW. Treatment of uncomplicated urinary tract infections in an era of increasing antimicrobial resistance. Mayo Clin Proc 2004;79:1048–1054.

33. Wong ES, McKevitt M, Running K, et al. Management of recurrent urinary tract infections with patients-administered single-dose therapy. Ann Intern Med 1985;102:302–307.

34. Wagenlehner FME, Naber KG. Treatment of bacterial urinary tract infections: Presence and future. Eur Urol 2006;49:235–244.

35. Gupta K, Sahm DF, Mayfield D, et al. Antimicrobial resistance among uropathogens that cause community-acquired urinary tract infections in women: A nationwide analysis. Clin Infect Dis 2001;33:89–94.

36. Perfetto EM, Gondek EK. *Escherichia coli* resistance in uncomplicated urinary tract infection: A model for determining when to change first-line empirical antibiotic choice. Manag Care Interface 2002;6: 35–42.

37. Wagenlehner FM, Pilatz A, Naber KG, et al. Anti-infective treatment of bacterial urinary tract infections. Curr Med Chem 2008;15: 1412–1427.

38. Rubenstein JN, Schaeffer AJ. Managing complicated urinary tract infections: The urologic view. Infect Dis Clin North Am 2003;17: 333–351.

39. Ovalle A, Levancini M. Urinary tract infections in pregnancy. Curr Opin Urol 2001;11:55–59.

40. Christensen B. Which antibiotics are appropriate for treating bacteriuria in pregnancy? J Antimicrob Chemother 2000;46(suppl S1): 29–34.

41. McDermott S, Daguise V, Mann H, et al. Perinatal risk for mortality and mental retardation associated with maternal urinary tract infections. J Fam Pract 2001;50:433–437.

42. Nicolle LE, Bradley S, Colgan R, et al. Infectious Diseases Society of America guidelines for the diagnosis and treatment of asymptomatic bacteriuria in adults. Clin Infect Dis 2005;40:643–654.

43. Warren JW. The catheter and urinary tract infection. Med Clin North Am 1991;75:481–493.

44. Naber KG, Bergman B, Bishop MC, et al. EAU guidelines for management of urinary and male genital tract infections. Urinary Tract Infection Working Group of the Health Care Office of the European Associated of Urology. Eur Urol 2001;40:576–588.

80 Sexually Transmitted Infections

Marlon S. Honeywell and Michael D. Thompson

LEARNING OBJECTIVES

● **Upon completion of the chapter, the reader will be able to:**

1. Analyze the behavioral considerations and assess the importance of contraception with regard to the contributing factors of sexually transmitted infections (STIs).

2. Apply the "expedited partner treatment" method when recommending treatment.

3. Identify the patient populations that are epidemiologically affected.

4. Identify causative organisms.

5. Devise a list of the clinical signs and symptoms corresponding to each disease state and classify patients based on recommended criteria.

6. Select appropriate diagnostic procedures.

7. Identify treatment regimens and recommend therapy when appropriate.

8. Design a patient care plan based on the monitoring parameters.

KEY CONCEPTS

❶ Optimal detection and treatment of sexually transmitted diseases depends on counseling by a patient-friendly and knowledgeable clinician who can establish open communication with the patient. Patients, especially adolescents, should be counseled on the importance of using condoms, spermicides, and diaphragms properly.

❷ Generally, when treating a sexually transmitted infection (STI), the patient being treated should be provided with a sufficient quantity of medication for his/her partner also, increasing the probability that the initial infection will be cured in both individuals.

❸ Patients treated for gonorrhea should be assumed to be coinfected with *Chlamydia trachomatis*; treatment recommendations should cover both organisms. Treatment of *Neisseria gonorrhoeae* with fluoroquinolones is inadvisable in those with a history of recent foreign travel, infections acquired in California or Hawaii, infections in other areas with increased gonococcal resistance, or in men who have sex with men (MSM).

❹ Parenteral penicillin is the drug of choice for treatment of all stages of syphilis. Though the dose may vary with the stages of syphilis, benzathine penicillin is the drug of choice.

❺ Metronidazole and tinidazole are the standard agents for trichomoniasis; advise patients to avoid the consumption of alcohol during treatment.

❻ Due to the variable appearance of genital warts, treatment may be based on the size, site, and morphology of the lesions. Treatment options include podofilox, imiquimod, podophyllin resin, and bichloro- and trichloroacetic acid.

❼ Acyclovir, valacyclovir, and famciclovir may be prescribed to treat first and intermittent episodes of genital herpes and to suppress active herpetic infections.

❽ Bacterial vaginosis (BV) is caused by overgrowth of anaerobic organisms and may be treated with oral or intravaginal metronidazole or intravaginal clindamycin.

❾ In patients with pelvic inflammatory disease (PID), resolution of infection (i.e., *N. gonorrhoeae, C. trachomatis, Streptococcus* spp., and gram-negative facultative bacteria) and mitigation of sequelae should be the main goal of pharmacologic therapy.

❿ Approximately 10% of persons who have chancroid acquired in the United States are coinfected with *Treponema pallidum* or herpes simplex virus.

Though we have made progress in medicine, age-old problems of infectious disease continue to plague us.[1] Even with the discovery of newly improved antibiotics, few sexually transmitted infections (STIs) have been completely eradicated. Many have reemerged secondary to modern social trends of sexual activity, and some as a result of the HIV epidemic, socioeconomic concerns, and the global lack of preventive education. Educating the public decreases the probability of infection in some individuals; however, this tactic alone may not be sufficient. ❶ *Optimal detection and treatment of sexually transmitted diseases depends on counseling by a patient-friendly and knowledgeable clinician who can establish open communication with the patient.*

BEHAVIORAL CONSIDERATIONS

● The correlation between risky sexual behavior and STIs is well documented.[2] Inconsistent and incorrect condom use has been recognized to increase the incidence of new STIs. ❶ *Assuming that patients, especially adolescents, consistently use and understand how to use condoms, spermicides, or diaphragms can be detrimental and may contribute to nonpharmacologic mismanagement.*[3] Health care providers who manage persons at risk for STIs should counsel women concerning the option for emergency contraception, if indicated, and provide it in a timely fashion if desired by the woman. Plan B (two 750 mcg levonorgestrol) has been approved in the United States for the prevention of unintended pregnancy.[4]

In addition to the increasing number of adolescents engaging in unsafe sexual practices is a high incidence of men who have sex with men (MSM) and women who have sex with women (WSW). Many MSM do not disclose their HIV status. This "don't ask, don't tell" practice has been linked to an upsurge in newly diagnosed HIV infections and STIs among previously noninfected people.[5] Although limited data are available with regard to STIs in WSW, risk of transmission probably varies by the specific STI and sexual techniques. Sharing penetrative items or employing practices involving digital vaginal or digital anal contact most likely represent common modes of transmission. This possibility is supported by reports of metronidazole-resistant trichomoniasis and genotype-specific HIV transmitted sexually between women who reported such behaviors and an increased prevalence of bacterial vaginosis (BV) among monogamous WSW.[6]

❷ *Optimally, both sex partners should be treated simultaneously for a STI; however, this is difficult to accomplish. Clinics and health departments often proactively attempt dual treatment by providing a prescription for the partner to the* index patient (the patient who is evaluated by a clinician), *a practice commonly known as expedited partner treatment.*

GONORRHEA

● Gonorrhea is a curable STI caused by the gram-negative diplococcus *Neisseria gonorrhoeae*. Proper therapeutic management with antimicrobial agents is essential to eradicate this infection and prevent the development of associated sequelae such as a urethritis, cervicitis, or dysuria.

In the United States, the highest rate of gonococcal infection is seen within the 15- to 24-year-old age groups for both sexes; although more cases are reported in men. Approximately 600,000 new cases occur annually in the United States.[7] Factors associated with an increased risk of infection include ethnicity, low socioeconomic status, and illicit drug use. The risk of a cervical infection after a single episode of vaginal intercourse is approximately 50% and increases with multiple exposures. Furthermore, rates of reinfection are significantly higher among ethnic minorities.

PATHOPHYSIOLOGY

Attachment to mucosal epithelium, mediated in part by pili and Opa (outer membrane opacity proteins), is followed by penetration of *N. gonorrhoeae* through epithelial cells to the submucosal tissue within 24 to 48 hours. A vigorous response by neutrophils begins with sloughing of the epithelium, development of submucosal microabscesses, and exudation of pus. Stained smears usually reveal large numbers of gonococci within a few neutrophils, whereas most cells contain no organisms.[8]

DIAGNOSIS

● Several laboratory tests are available to aid in the diagnosis of gonorrhea and include gram-stained smears, culture,

---

Clinical Presentation of Gonorrhea[7,9]

General
- Purulent discharge

Signs
- Painful or swollen testicles
- Tubal scarring

Symptoms

Men:
- May be asymptomatic, though acute urethritis is the predominant manifestation
- Urethral discharge and dysuria, usually without urinary frequency or urgency
- When compared with nongonococcal urethritis, the discharge in gonococcal urethritis is generally more profuse and purulent
- Pain during urination

Women:
- Cervicitis, urethritis, increased vaginal discharge, dysuria and intermenstrual bleeding
- Pain during urination
- Abdominal pain

Patient Encounter 1, Part 1

KL is a 27-year-old African American female who visits a clinic complaining of profuse urethral discharge for the past several days. She also informs the nurse that she did not have a menstrual cycle last month and that a home pregnancy test taken this morning revealed that she was indeed pregnant. The patient admits to having sexual intercourse without barrier contraception (condoms) with her boyfriend within the past week or two and is not sure of other sexual encounter(s) in which he may have been involved.

What information is suggestive of gonorrhea?

What potential risk factors for STIs are present?

What impact will pregnancy have on diagnostic and treatment plans for STI management?

Patient Encounter 1, Part 2

PMH: Currently receiving no medications; no prior history of STIs; no drug allergies noted

FH: Noncontributory

SH: Admits to having unprotected sex with boyfriend. Does not smoke or drink alcohol

ROS: C/o vaginal discharge, recent nonpruritic rash development across abdominal area noted over past 3 to 5 days

PE:

VS: BP 130/80 mm Hg, P 70 bpm, T 37°C (98.6°F)

Lab: Urethral discharge swab revealed *N. gonorrhoeae*; rapid plasma reagin (RPR) test was positive.

Given this additional information, what is your assessment of the patient's condition?

What consideration should be given to other STIs?

Identify your treatment goals for this patient.

What pharmacologic alternatives are available for this patient?

or the DNA hybridization probe. A gram stain of a male urethral specimen that demonstrates polymorphonuclear leukocytes with intracellular gram-negative diplococci may be considered diagnostic in symptomatic men. A gram-negative stain should not be considered sufficient for ruling out infection in asymptomatic men.[4] All patients who test positive for gonorrhea should be tested for other STIs, including chlamydia, syphilis, and HIV.

TREATMENT

Desired Outcome

The desired outcome is complete eradication of *N. gonorrhoeae* and avoidance of sequelae.

Pharmacologic Therapy [4,9,10]

❸ *Patients infected with gonorrhea often are coinfected with Chlamydia trachomatis and should receive therapy to eradicate both organisms concurrently.* While fluoroquinolones and broad-spectrum cephalosporins have been effective in the treatment of gonorrhea, resistant strains of *N. gonorrhoeae* have still emerged. In the far-eastern countries, as many as 50% of gonococcal strains exhibit decreased susceptibility to fluoroquinolones. Though ciprofloxacin is still an option for treatment, gonococcal resistance to ciprofloxacin is usually indicative of its resistance to other fluoroquinolones. As a result, monitoring for fluoroquinolone resistance is now essential to ensure proper treatment and to ascertain the maximum time that this class may be employed as a treatment option.

Fluoroquinolones should not be prescribed for infections in MSM, or in those with a history of recent foreign travel or partners' travel, infections acquired in California or Hawaii, or infections in other areas with increased gonococcal resistance.[11]

Treatment of gonorrhea may vary according to clinical presentation and is indicated as follows:

Uncomplicated Gonococcal Infection of the Cervix, Urethra, and Rectum*: Ceftriaxone 125 mg intramuscularly *or* ciprofloxacin 500 mg orally *or* cefixime 400 mg orally *or* levofloxacin 250 mg orally *plus* treatment for chlamydial infection if it has not been ruled out.

MSM or Heterosexuals With a History of Recent Travel*: Ceftriaxone 125 mg intramuscularly *or* cefixime 400 mg orally *plus* treatment for chlamydial infection if it has not been ruled out.

Uncomplicated Gonococcal Infection of the Pharynx*: Ceftriaxone 125 mg intramuscularly *or* ciprofloxacin 500 mg orally *plus* treatment for chlamydial infection if it has not been ruled out.

MSM or Heterosexuals With a History of Recent Travel*: Ceftriaxone 125 mg intramuscularly *plus* treatment for chlamydial infection if it has not been ruled out.

Coverage for Coinfection With *Chlamydia trachomatis*: Azithromycin 1 g orally as a single dose *or* doxycycline 100 mg orally twice daily for 7 days.

---

*Regimens are given for one dose only.

Patient Encounter 1, Part 3

Unprotected sex is a major risk factor for contracting STIs. Although the purulent discharge is consistent with gonorrhea infection, a positive urethral swab coupled with an incubation period consistent with gonorrhea confirms the diagnosis. A serologic test for syphilis should be performed on all pregnant women at the first prenatal visit and a RPR should be performed at the time pregnancy is confirmed and treatment provided. Although the patient has confirmed gonorrhea, infection with *Chlamydia trachomatis* occurs commonly in this setting. Additionally, pregnant patients should be tested for this infection during the first prenatal visit and treated appropriately. Further, the presence of a rash could possibly suggest that the patient may have contracted syphilis previously, potentially indicative of secondary syphilis.

If this patient had an allergy to penicillin, how would the therapeutic management of the identified problems change?

▶ Treatment of Gonorrhea in Special Situations

Uncomplicated infections of the cervix, urethra, and rectum can be treated with one of the following regimens in adults:

Recommendations During Pregnancy:

- Ceftriaxone 125 mg intramuscularly as a single dose *plus* therapy recommended for coinfection with *Chlamydia*
- Spectinomycin 2 g intramuscularly as a single dose *plus* therapy recommended for coinfection with *Chlamydia*
- Doxycycline and fluoroquinolones are contraindicated

Recommendations for Disseminated Gonococcal Infection (Regimens Should Be Continued for 24 to 48 Hours): Ceftriaxone 1 g intramuscularly or IV every 24 hours *or* cefotaxime 1 g IV every 8 hours *or* ceftizoxime 1 g IV every 8 hours *or* levofloxacin 250 mg IV every 24 hours *or* spectinomycin 2 g intramuscularly every 12 hours

After improvement begins, therapy is then switched to *one* of the following 7-day oral regimens: Cefixime 400 mg orally twice daily *or* ciprofloxacin 500 mg orally twice daily *or* levofloxacin 500 mg orally once daily.

Uncomplicated Infections of the Cervix, Urethra, and Rectum in Children Less Than 45 kg: Ceftriaxone 125 mg intramuscularly as a single dose *or* spectinomycin 40mg/kg intramuscularly as a single dose *or* ceftriaxone 50 mg/kg intramuscularly or IV once daily for 7 days in children with bacteremia or arthritis.

Gonococcal Conjunctivitis: Ceftriaxone 1 g intramuscularly once for adults *or* ceftriaxone 25 to 50 mg/kg IV or intramuscularly as a single dose for ophthalmia neonatorum or infants born to mothers with gonococcal infection as prophylaxis.

Ophthalmic Neonatorum or Prophylactic Treatment for Infants Whose Mothers Have Gonococcal Infection:
- Ceftriaxone 25 to 50 mg/kg IV or intramuscularly in a single dose, not to exceed 125 mg.
- **Ophthalmic Neonatorum Prophylaxis:** Erythromycin (0.5%) ophthalmic ointment in a single application to the eyes *or* tetracycline (1%) ophthalmic ointment in a single application to the eyes.

PATIENT CARE AND MONITORING

Monitoring is generally not required.

CHLAMYDIA

EPIDEMIOLOGY

Infection with *C. trachomatis* has increased dramatically in recent years. This bacterium is the most common cause of nongonococcal urethritis, accounting for as many as 50% of cases. The prevalence is highest in individuals lesser than or equal to 25 years. Associated sequelae include pelvic inflammatory disease (PID), ectopic pregnancy, and infertility.

PATHOPHYSIOLOGY

C. trachomatis possesses characteristics resembling both bacteria and viruses. Its major membrane is comparable to that of gram-negative bacteria, although it lacks a peptidoglycan cell wall and requires cellular components from the host for replication. Chlamydia transmission risk is thought to be less than that of gonorrhea.

DIAGNOSIS

Common tests used to diagnose *C. trachomatis* include culture, the enzyme immunoassay, the DNA hybridization probe, or the direct fluorescent monoclonal antibody test. Diagnosis has been confirmed in women through urine or swab specimen collected from the endocervix and in men using a urethral swab or urine specimen. Most women are asymptomatic; therefore, an annual screening or physical is necessary, as early detection may reduce rates of transmission.

TREATMENT[12]

Uncomplicated Urethral, Endocervical, or Rectal Infection in Adults: The recommended adult regimen is azithromycin 1 g orally in a single dose *or* doxycycline

Clinical Presentation of Chlamydia[10]

General

- Asymptomatic

Signs

- Beefy red cervix that bleeds easily (women)

Symptoms

- When present, the urethral discharge is watery and less purulent than that seen with acute gonococcal urethritis. Complications resulting from lack of treatment or inadequate treatment include: epididymitis (in males), and PID including associated complications in women.

Other Diagnostic Tests

- Culture is usually positive for both chlamydia and gonorrhea.

---

100 mg orally twice daily for 7 days. An *alternate regimen is* erythromycin ethylsuccinate 800 mg orally four times daily for 7 days *or* erythromycin base 500 mg orally four times daily for 7 days *or* levofloxacin 500 mg orally once daily for 7 days.

The recommended regimen for pregnancy is azithromycin 1 g orally in a single dose *or* amoxicillin 1 g orally in a single dose *or* amoxicillin 500 mg orally three times daily for 7 days.

Alternate regimens include erythromycin base 500 mg orally four times daily for 7 days *or* 250 mg orally four times daily for 14 days *or* erythromycin ethylsuccinate 800 mg orally four times daily for 7 days *or* 400 mg orally four times daily for 14 days.

C. trachomatis Infection in Infants: Treatment of ophthalmia neonatorum or infant pneumonia should be with erythromycin base or ethylsuccinate 50 mg/kg/day orally divided into four doses daily for 14 days.

PATIENT CARE AND MONITORING

Monitoring is generally not required.

SYPHILIS

Syphilis, attributed to the spirochete *Treponema pallidum*, can have numerous and complex manifestations. Clinician familiarity, stage-specific diagnosis, and effective treatment are vital. Missed or inappropriately treated syphilis may result in cardiovascular complications, neurologic disease, or congenital syphilis.

EPIDEMIOLOGY

Since the 1940s, the incidence of syphilis declined drastically following the introduction of penicillin, but rose when

HIV arrived from obscurity in the 1980s. In 2000, the rate of primary and secondary syphilis in the United States was 2.1 cases per 100,000 population. From 2001 to 2004, the rate increased to 2.7, primarily as a result of increases in cases among MSM. The 2006 morbidity and mortality report also reflects a substantial increase of syphilis among black men, emphasizing the need for enhanced preventive measures among blacks and MSM. The disparity among men and women has been observed across racial and ethnic groups and is highest in the South and among non-Hispanic blacks.[13]

PATHOPHYSIOLOGY

T. pallidum rapidly penetrates intact mucous membranes or microscopic dermal abrasions, and within a few hours, enters the lymphatics and blood to produce systemic illness. During the secondary stage, examinations commonly demonstrate abnormal findings in the cerebrospinal fluid (CSF). As the infection progresses, the parenchyma of the brain and spinal cord may subsequently be damaged.

Stages of Syphilis

Primary Syphilis Usually manifests as a solitary, painless chancre. Primary syphilis develops at the site of infection approximately 3 weeks after exposure to *T. pallidum*; the chancre is highly infectious.[14]

Secondary Syphilis Without appropriate treatment, primary syphilis will advance to secondary syphilis, a stage usually apparent from its clinical symptomatology. Symptoms include fatigue, diffuse rash, fever, lymphadenopathy, and genital or perineal condyloma latum. Also, the skin is most often affected and a rash may present as macular, macropapular, or pustular lesions, or involve skin surfaces including the palms of the hands and soles of the feet.

Patient Encounter 2

KG is an HIV-positive male who complains of the appearance of a "sore" on his penis. He reports having unprotected sexual intercourse with another male approximately 5 to 7 days prior to the appearance of the lesion. He denies pain or itching at the site of the lesion, dysuria, or frequent urination. Additionally, there appears to be no vesicles in the genital area.

What information is suggestive of syphilis?

What potential risk factors for STIs are present?

How should the diagnosis of syphilis be confirmed in this patient?

If the diagnosis of syphilis is confirmed, what therapeutic options exist for this patient?

Latent Syphilis

Early Latent. Involves the first year after infection and may be established in patients who have seroconverted in the past year, who have had symptoms of primary or secondary syphilis in the past year, or who have had sex with a partner with primary, secondary, or latent syphilis in the past year.

Late Latent. Patients should be considered to have late latent syphilis if the aforementioned criteria (early latent) are not met. In both stages, patients are usually asymptomatic and the lesions noted in the primary and secondary phase usually resolve; however, individuals are still seropositive for *T. pallidum*.

Tertiary Syphilis. Develops years after the initial infection and may involve any organ in the body.

Congenital Syphilis

Congenital syphilis is a condition in which the fetus is infected with *T. pallidum* as a result of the hematogenous spread from an infected mother, although transmission may also occur from direct contact with the infectious genitalia of the mother. Since the primary stage of syphilis is characterized by spirochetemia, infectious rates of the fetus are nearly 100% if the mother has primary syphilis.[15]

DIAGNOSIS

Diagnostic procedures include dark-field microscopy,[16] nontreponemal exams[14] (i.e., the Venereal Disease Laboratory and the rapid plasma reagin [RPR] test), and treponemal exams (i.e., enzyme immunoassay, the *T. pallidum* hemagglutination test, the fluorescent treponemal antibody test, and the enzyme-linked immunosorbent assay).

TREATMENT

Desired Outcome

After confirming the diagnosis of syphilis, the desired outcome is a fourfold decrease in quantitative nontreponemal titers over a 6-month period and within 12 to 24 months after treatment of latent or late syphilis. An algorithm for the treatment of syphilis is shown in Figure 80–1.

With regard to neurosyphilis, a reduction in neurologic manifestations is desired, which may include seizures, paresis, hyperreflexia, visual disturbances, hearing loss, neuropathy, or loss of bowel and bladder function. In late neurosyphilis, vascular lesions (meningovascular neurosyphilis) may also be observed; thus, a reduction in the number of observed lesions is warranted. A diminution in CSF WBC (less than $10 \times 10^3/mm^3$ [$10 \times 10^9/L$]) or protein levels (0.05 g/dL [0.5 g/L]) is also preferred.

Pharmacologic Therapy

❹ *Parenterally administered penicillin is recommended for all stages of syphilis* (Table 80–1). Although penicillin is the drug of choice, combinations of benzathine penicillin with procaine penicillin or oral penicillin preparations are not considered appropriate treatment regimens. Several reports have demonstrated the misuse of the benzathine–procaine combination (Bicillin C-R) instead of the standard benzathine penicillin (Bicillin L-A).[17] Pertinent information related to benzathine penicillin G is found in Table 80–1.

Alternative agents may be used in allergic individuals and include doxycycline, minocycline, tetracycline, or erythromycin base or stearate. Some patients (such as young children or pregnant women) may not respond favorably to alternative modalities or should not receive tetracyclines. Therefore, in patients who must be administered penicillin (i.e., patients who are pregnant or have CNS involvement) or are allergic, desensitization must be performed before the drug is initiated.

Patients may experience fever, chills, tachycardia, and tachypnea, a condition commonly known as the Jarisch-Herxheimer reaction. This reaction is postulated to occur secondary to spirochete lysis and proinflammatory cytokine cascades. It may transpire as early as 2 hours after penicillin administration and usually resolves within 24 hours. Treatment is supportive and may include antipyretic and anti-inflammatory agents, as well as fluid resuscitation and bed rest.

▶ *Primary Syphilis*

Drug of Choice

Adults. Benzathine penicillin, 2.4 million units intramuscularly as a single dose.

Children. Benzathine penicillin 50,000 units/kg intramuscularly, up to the adult dose of 2.4 million units in a single dose.

Alternatives Oral doxycycline 100 mg twice daily for 2 weeks *or* tetracycline 500 mg by mouth four times daily for 2 weeks. Limited literature also supports the use of ceftriaxone 1 g intramuscularly or IV once daily for 10 days *or* oral azithromycin as a single 2-g dose.[13]

▶ *Secondary and Early Latent Syphilis*

Treatment modalities administered in primary syphilis are also effective in secondary syphilis and early latent syphilis (less than 1 year duration).

▶ *Late Latent Syphilis*

Benzathine penicillin, 7.2 million units total, administered as three doses of 2.4 million units intramuscularly each at 1-week intervals.

▶ *Tertiary Syphilis*

Drug of Choice Benzathine penicillin 2.4 million units administered intramuscularly once weekly for 3 weeks.

Alternatives In nonpregnant patients with a penicillin allergy, alternative regimens include doxycycline 100 mg orally two times daily for 4 weeks *or* tetracycline 500 mg orally four times daily for 4 weeks.

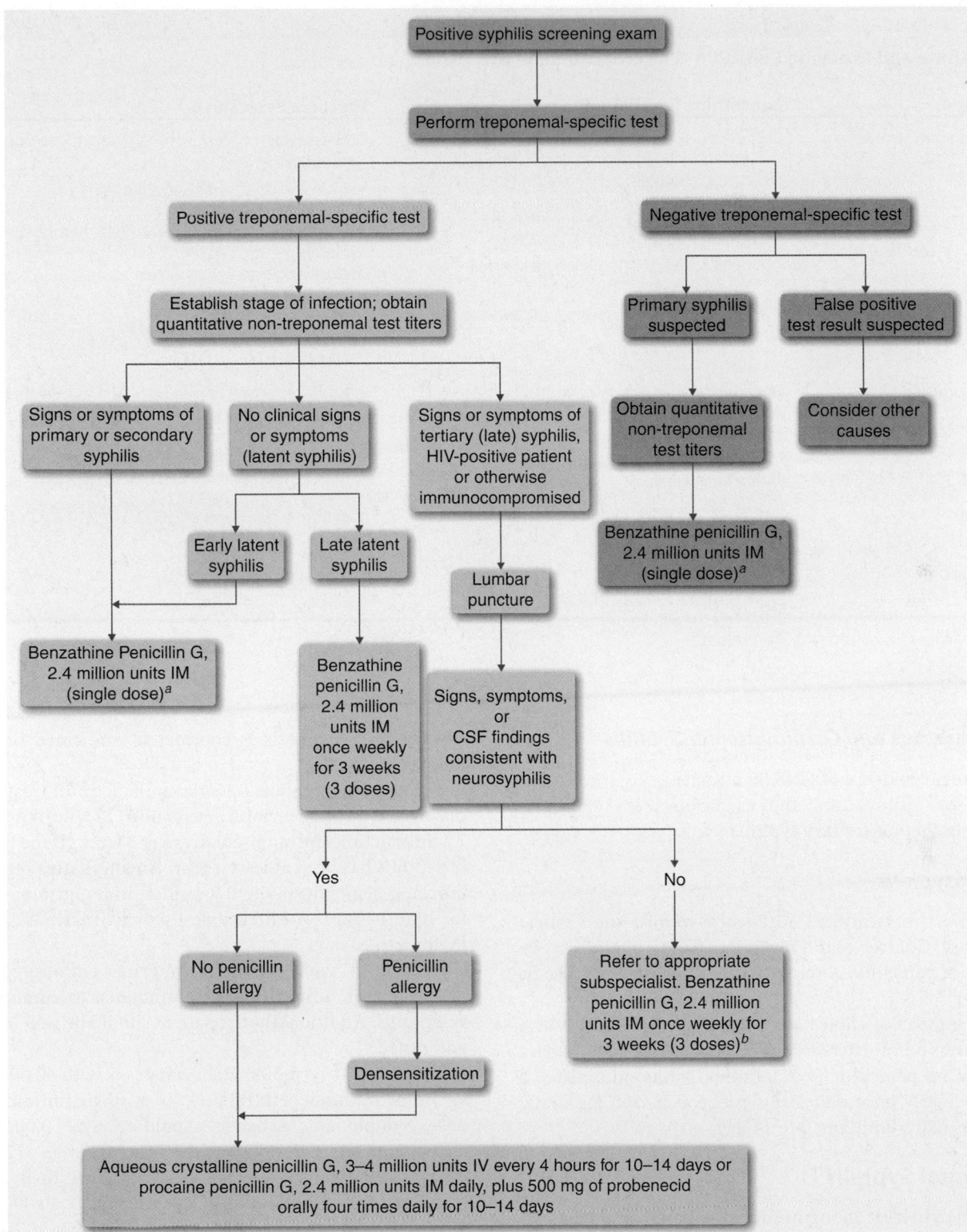

FIGURE 80–1. Treatment of syphilis. (CSF, cerebrospinal fluid; IM, intramuscularly.) (From Brown D, Frank J. Diagnosis and Management of Syphilis. Am Fam Physician. 2003;68(2):283–290.) [a]Alternative treatments for nonpregnant penicillin-allergic patients: doxycycline 100 mg orally twice daily for 2 weeks, or tetracycline 500 mg four times daily for 2 weeks; limited data support ceftriaxone 1 g once daily IM or IV for 8 to 10 days; or azithromycin, 2 g orally (single dose). [b]Alternative treatments for nonpregnant penicillin-allergic patients: doxycycline, 100 mg orally twice daily for 4 weeks, or tetracycline 500 mg orally four times daily for 4 weeks.

Table 80–1		
Benzathine and Procaine Penicillin G Informational Chart		
Categories	**Benzathine Penicillin G**	**Procaine Penicillin G**
Potential adverse reactions	CNS: convulsions, confusion, drowsiness, myoclonus, fever; dermatologic: rash; metabolic: electrolyte imbalance; Hematologic: positive Coombs test, hemolytic anemia; local: pain, thrombophlebitis; renal: acute interstitial nephritis; miscellaneous: anaphylaxis, hypersensitivity, Jarisch-Herxheimer reaction	CNS: seizures, confusion, drowsiness, myoclonus, CNS stimulation Cardiovascular: myocardial depression, vasodilation, conduction disturbances Hematologic: positive Coombs test, hemolytic anemia, neutropenia Local: thrombophlebitis, sterile abscess at injection site Renal: interstitial nephritis Miscellaneous: pseudoanaphylactic reactions, hypersensitivity, Jarisch-Herxheimer reaction, serum sickness
Monitoring parameters	Observe for anaphylaxis during first dose	Periodic renal and hematologic function tests with prolonged therapy; fever, mental status, WBC
Pregnancy category	B	B
Lactation	Enters breast milk	Enters breast milk
Availability	Bicillin L-A: 600,000 units/mL (1, 2, and 4 mL); Permapen Isoject: 600,000 units/mL (2 mL)	Injection, suspension: 600,000 units/mL (1, 2 mL)
Combination	Bicillin C-R: (1, 2, 4 mL) Bicillin C-R: 900/300: (2 mL)	Same

CNS, central nervous system; IM, intramuscular.

From Ref. 32.

► *Gummatous and Cardiovascular Syphilis*

As long as no evidence of CNS involvement exists, antibiotic therapy for gummatous and cardiovascular syphilis is identical to that for tertiary syphilis.

► *Neurosyphilis*

As an effective treatment for neurosyphilis, the Centers for Disease Control and Prevention (CDC) endorses two regimens of penicillin. Alternatively, ceftriaxone may also be prescribed.[18]

The regimens of choice are aqueous penicillin G 3 to 4 million units administered IV every 4 hours for 10 to 14 days OR procaine penicillin G 2.4 million units administered intramuscularly once daily, plus probenecid 500 mg orally four times daily, both for 10 to 14 days.

Congenital Syphilis[19]

The decision to treat an infant should be based on a diagnosis of syphilis in the mother and confirmation of adequacy of maternal treatment. Clinical, laboratory, or radiographic evidence of syphilis in the infant should be documented. Maternal nontreponemal titers (at delivery) should be compared with the infant's nontreponemal titers. Since diagnosis based on neonatal serologic testing is complicated by the transplacental transfer of maternal IgG antibodies, which can cause a positive test in the absence of infection, neonatal titers are assessed. A titer greater than four times the maternal titer would not generally result from passive transfer and diagnosis is considered confirmed or highly probable.

The following regimens are recommended for treatment of maternal syphilis: benzathine penicillin G 2.4 million units or 7.2 million units intramuscularly over 3 weeks if the duration of syphilis has been at least a year. An alternative regimen is procaine penicillin 0.6 to 0.9 million units intramuscularly for 10 to 14 days, or ceftriaxone 1 g daily intramuscularly or IV for 8 to 10 days.

In women who experience uterine cramping, pelvic pain, or fever, administer acetaminophen to combat these symptoms. Additionally, the patient should be well hydrated and rested.

Treatment of asymptomatic neonates is with 50,000 units/kg of benzathine penicillin G in a single intramuscular dose. Symptomatic neonates should receive 50,000 units/kg of aqueous crystalline penicillin G every 12 hours intramuscularly for the first 7 days of life, then every 8 hours for 3 days, OR procaine penicillin G 50,000 IU/kg intramuscularly as a single dose daily for 10 days.

PATIENT CARE AND MONITORING

The CDC has provided patient care monitoring guidelines for syphilis (Fig. 80–2).[4,14,20]

Primary and Secondary Syphilis

- After 6, 12, and 24 months of treatment, reexamine the patient and recommend a follow-up quantitative

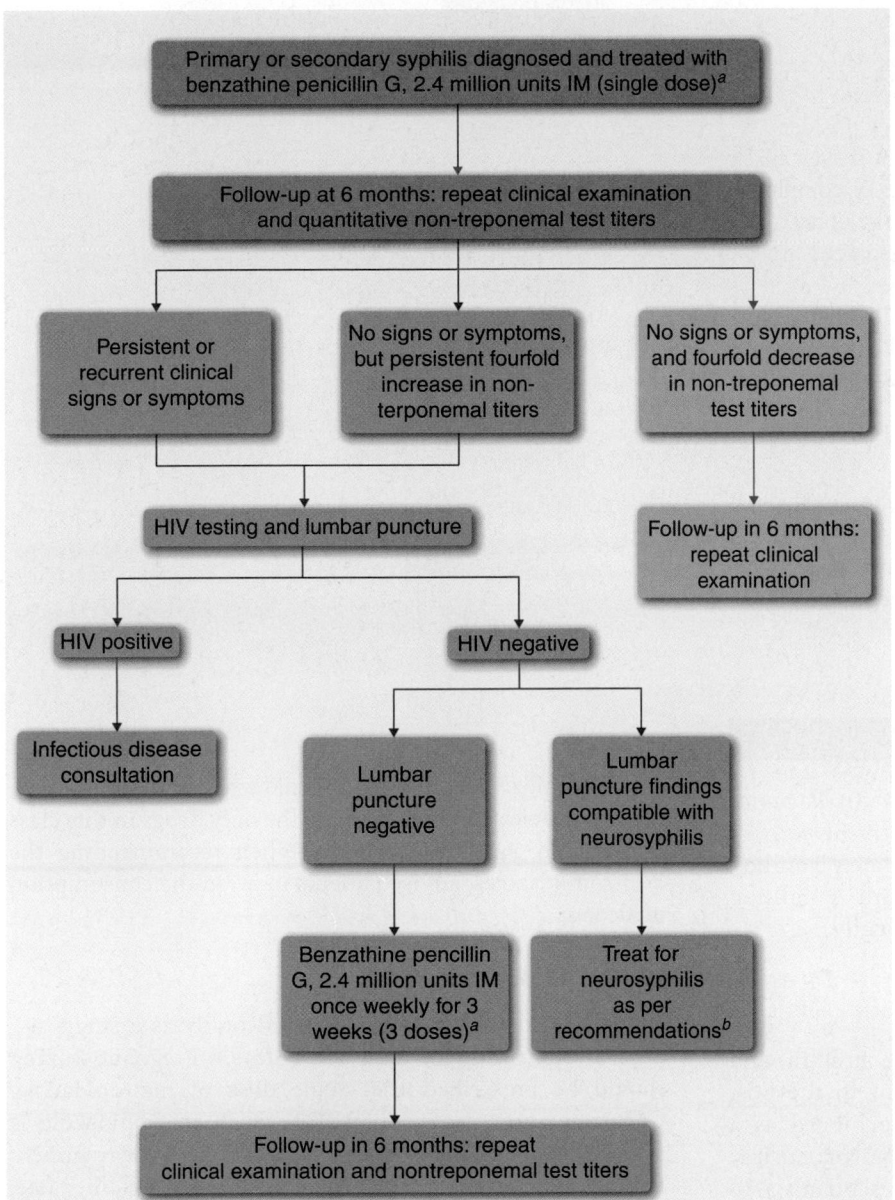

FIGURE 80–2. Patient care monitoring for syphilis. (From Brown D, Frank J. Diagnosis and Management of Syphilis. Am Fam Physician. 2003;68(2):283–290.) ([a]See text for alternative treatment recommendations for nonpregnant penicillin-allergic patients. [b]See text for treatment recommendations for neurosyphilis.)

nontreponemal titer. If the patient is asymptomatic, yet has a fourfold increase in nontreponemal titer or persistent or recurrent symptoms are observed, order an HIV test and a lumbar puncture; if the patient is HIV-positive, suggest an infectious disease consult.

• In patients who are both negative for HIV and the lumbar puncture, administer benzathine penicillin G 2.4 million units intramuscularly once weekly for three additional weeks. Perform a patient follow-up in 6 months including a clinical examination and another nontreponemal titer. In HIV-negative patients with lumbar puncture findings compatible with neurosyphilis, treat the patient accordingly for neurosyphilis.

• Six months after the original diagnosis, institute a standard clinical follow-up exam in patients who show no symptomatology and a fourfold decrease in nontreponemal titers. By testing and observing the patient for signs of remission, you may be able to initiate proper treatment or recommend a consult in a timely fashion, thereby decreasing the propensity of the patient's condition to advance to a higher stage.

Early and Late Latent Syphilis

• Order nontreponemal titers 6, 12, and 24 months after instituting treatment for early or late latent syphilis. Neurosyphilis should be strongly considered in patients who show a fourfold increase in titers, patients who have an initially high titer (1:32 or greater) that fails to decline at least fourfold, HIV-infected patients, and patients who develop signs or symptoms associated with neurosyphilis.

Neurosyphilis

- Follow-up is dependent on the CSF findings. If pleocytosis is present, reexamine the CSF every 6 months until the WBC count normalizes. Consider recommending a second course of treatment if the CSF white count does not decline after 6 months or completely normalize after 2 years.[4,14] Failure to normalize may require retreatment; most treatment failures occur in immunocompromised patients.

Congenital Syphilis

- Observe the patient for changes in clinical features; hepatomegaly, jaundice, and bone changes will usually resolve in 3 months.

- Monitor elevated serologic markers (nontreponemal tests) for reduction in titer levels. Given effective treatment, clinical features will usually disappear after 6 months. On this basis, evaluate seropositive infants periodically for at least 6 months.[19]

TRICHOMONIASIS

Trichomoniasis is caused by the protozoan *Trichomonas vaginalis* and is far more prevalent than *C. trachomatis* or *N. gonorrhoeae*. In the United States, approximately 5 million new cases appear annually, compared with 3 million chlamydial and 650,000 gonococcal cases annually.[21]

PATHOPHYSIOLOGY

T. vaginalis may be isolated from the vagina, urethra, and Bartholin or Skene glands. After attachment to the host cells, it ignites an inflammatory response exhibited as a discharge containing elevated levels of polymorphonuclear leukocytes. The protozoal pathogen causes direct damage to the epithelium, leading to microulcerations.

DIAGNOSIS

Diagnosis is usually performed with a wet mount or Papanicolaou smear. In women, symptoms are characterized by diffuse, malodorous, yellow-green vaginal discharge with vulvar irritation. Some women may be asymptomatic.

TREATMENT

Desired Outcome

The desired outcome is the complete eradication of *T. vaginalis* in both partners and elimination of the signs and symptoms observed.

Pharmacologic Therapy

❺ *The 5-nitroimidazoles have been the standard therapy for trichomoniasis for over 40 years.* Drugs included in this class

---

Clinical Presentation of Trichomoniasis[21]

General
- Asymptomatic

Signs
- Strawberry cervix (women)
- Colpitis macularis (women)
- Prostatitis or epididymitis (men)

Symptoms
- Vaginal/vulvar erythema
- Excessive yellow-green discharge
- Vulvar itching
- Vaginal odor
- Urethral discharge or irritation
- Dysuria
- Vaginal pH greater than 4.5

---

are metronidazole, tinidazole, ornidazole, and secnidazole; metronidazole and tinidazole are the only drugs in this class available in the United States. When recommending the 5-nitroimidazoles, advise patients to avoid the consumption of alcohol.

▶ Metronidazole

Metronidazole may be administered orally as a single 2-g dose or 500 mg twice daily for 7 days.[22] Pregnant women should be prescribed the single dose of metronidazole. Cure rates are greater than 90% when metronidazole is administered as either a single 2-g dose or a 7-day regimen. Possible adverse effects include an unpleasant metallic taste, reversible neutropenia, urticaria, rash, flushing, dry mouth, darkened urine, and a disulfiram-like reaction.

▶ Tinidazole

Tinidazole, a second-generation nitroimidazole with protozoal and anaerobic activity, has been available outside the United States for over 30 years.[23] As a single 2-g dose, tinidazole has an efficacy equivalent to a 2-g dose of metronidazole. Tindazole also has a longer half-life than metronidazole, 14 and 7 hours respectively, and penetrates into male reproductive tissue better than metronidazole.

Tinidazole is effective for metronidazole-resistant trichomoniasis.[24] Possible side effects include a metallic taste, dizziness, loss of coordination, seizures, severe diarrhea, darkened urine, nausea, vomiting, and a swollen or discolored tongue.

PATIENT CARE AND MONITORING

Monitoring for *T. vaginalis* is generally not required.

GENITAL WARTS

Genital warts, caused by the human papillomavirus (HPV), are regularly encountered in primary care. Responsible for various visible, keratotic, and nonkeratotic manifestations, HPV has nearly 120 noted strains, some of which have been linked to squamous cell carcinoma.[25] More than 30 strains have been linked to the genital area.

EPIDEMIOLOGY

Affecting over 20 million Americans, HPV is one of the most common STIs in the United States, with a prevalence of approximately 15%. Furthermore, among adolescent and college-aged women, HPV may be the most common STI.[4,20] The frequency of cervicovaginal HPV infection among sexually-active women has been observed at 43%, with the greatest incidence noticed in men with three or more sex partners and women whose most recent regular sexual partner had two or more lifetime partners.

PATHOPHYSIOLOGY

HPV replicates in terminally differentiated squamous cells in the intermediate layers of the genital mucosa. Hence, these effects of the viral early region genes on DNA synthesis are critical for viral survival. Genital warts are the clinical manifestation of active viral replication and virion production at the infection site.

DIAGNOSIS

- A definitive diagnosis of HPV is based on DNA or RNA or capsid protein detection.
- Diagnosis is generally made from the clinical presentation and may be classified into several categories: classic condyloma acuminata, which are pointed or cauliform; keratotic warts with a thick, horny surface resembling common skin warts; and flat warts, frequently observed on the surface.

Clinical Presentation of Genital Warts[27,28]

General
- Appear as rough, thick, cauliflower-like lesions

Signs
- Black dots within warts
- Disrupted surface

Symptoms
- Anogenital pruritus
- Burning
- Vaginal discharge or bleeding
- Although rare, **dyspareunia** may occur with vulvovaginal condyloma

- Tissue **biopsy** or viral typing is only indicated if diagnosis is uncertain and is not recommended for patients with routine or typical lesions.
- Since HPV is highly associated with cervical cancer and since there are more than 20 different cancer-associated HPV types, patients who are diagnosed with HPV should be tested for cervical cancer.

TREATMENT

Desired Outcome

Removal of visible warts and reduction of infectivity are the goals of treatment.

Pharmacologic Therapy[4,26]

6 *Currently, the choice of therapy is based on the size, site, and morphology of lesions, as well as patient preference, treatment costs, convenience, adverse effects, and clinician experience. Factors that might affect response include the presence of immunosuppression and patient compliance. Assuming that the diagnosis is correct, switching to alternate therapy is appropriate if there has been no response observed after three treatment cycles. A comparison of adverse effects related to treatment options may be found in Table 80–2.*

Table 80–2	
Comparison of Adverse Effects Seen With Treatments for Genital Warts	
Treatment	**Adverse Effects**
Podofilox	Burning at site of application, pain, inflammation
Imiquimod	Erythema, irritation, ulceration, pain, burning, edema, pigmentary changes
Podophyllin resin	Local irritation, erythema, burning, soreness at application site; possibly oncogenic
Bichloroacetic and trichloroacetic acid	Local irritation and pain, minimal systemic effects
Cryotherapy	Pain or blisters at application site
Surgical excision	Pain, bleeding, scarring; possible burning or allergic reaction to local anesthetic
Vaporization	Pain, bleeding, scarring; risk of HPV spreading via smoke plumes
Intralesional interferon	Burning, itching, irritation at injection site, systemic myalgia, headache, fever, chills, leukopenia, elevated liver enzymes, and thrombocytopenia

HPV, human papillomavirus.

From Refs. 25, 41.

▶ *Patient-Applied Treatment*

● **Podofilox** Available as a 0.5% gel or solution containing purified extract of the most active compound of podophyllin, podofilox arrests the formation of the mitotic spindle, prevents cell division, and may also induce damage in blood vessels within the warts. The surface area treated must not exceed 10 cm², and a maximum of 0.5 mL should be used on a daily basis.

Apply twice daily for three consecutive days followed by four consecutive days without treatment. This cycle may be repeated until there are no visible warts or for a maximum of 4 weeks. Side effects are generally local and may include erythema, swelling, and erosions. Podofilox is not recommended for use in the vagina, anus, or during pregnancy.

● **Imiquimod** Imiquimod is a cell-mediated immune-response modifier, available as a topical 5% cream in single-dose application packets. There are two recommended dosage regimens:

1. Apply at bedtime, three times a week for up to 16 weeks.

2. Apply every other day for three applications.

The treatment area should be washed with soap and water 6 to 10 hours after application. Mild to moderate erythema has been noted with imiquimod use; however, this generally suggests that the drug is reaching a therapeutic range and may be clearing the lesion.[27]

▶ *Physician-Applied Treatments*

● **Podophyllin Resin**[28] A 10% to 25% solution of podophyllin resin has been the standard in-office treatment for genital warts. It is neurotoxic and due to its systemic absorption, a small amount (no more than 0.5 mL) should be applied. Application should be limited to less than 0.5 mL of podophyllin on an area of less than 10 cm² of warts per session and no open lesions or wounds should exist in the area to which treatment is administered. The affected area will likely become erythematous and painful within 48 hours of application.

Topical podophyllin is applied once weekly and the area should be allowed to dry. Immediately following treatment, the dried drug should be removed using alcohol or soap and water. It is contraindicated in pregnant patients.

● **Bichloroacetic and Trichloroacetic Acids** These products are available in 80% to 90% concentrations and are not systemically absorbed. The products are effective when used to treat a few, small, moist lesions. They may be applied to both keratinized epithelial and mucosal surfaces and may be used in pregnancy.

A noted reaction to these medications is transient burning, and contact with surrounding epithelium may prove to be painful, producing significant local erythema and swelling. To avoid these effects, place petroleum jelly around the external lesion, including unaffected skin, and carefully apply the agent with a small applicator. If an excess amount of acid is used, talc or sodium bicarbonate (baking soda) may be used to neutralize unreacted acid.

Other Treatments[26] Other treatments may include fluoro-uracil/epinephrine/bovine collagen gel, an intralesional injection that has been proven effective in clinical trials for refractory patients, or an intralesional injection of interferon.

▶ *Ablative Therapy*

Several ablative options have been employed in the treatment of genital warts and include cryotherapy, surgical removal, and vaporization.

▶ *Special Therapeutic Issues*[26,28]

Large Warts Treat warts greater than 10 mm in diameter with surgical excision. Use imiquimod for three to four treatment cycles to reduce the number of warts and improve surgical outcomes. Fifty percent reduction in wart size after four treatment cycles warrants continued use of imiquimod until warts clear or eight cycles have been completed; less than 50% reduction warrants surgical excision or other ablative therapy.

Subclinical Warts Subclinical warts may be identified through colonoscopy, biopsy, acetic acid application, or laboratory serology. However, early treatment has not been linked to a favorable effect during the course of therapy in the index patient or the partner with regard to reduction of the transmission rate.

Pregnancy Agents contraindicated in pregnancy include podofilox, fluorouracil, and podophyllin. Imiquimod is not approved for use in pregnancy, although it has been considered after signed consent has been obtained. Bichloroacetic and trichloroacetic acids have been used without problems. Ablative therapy is also a viable option.

PATIENT CARE AND MONITORING

Monitor patients every 3 to 6 months for a reduction in lesions or disease remission. Monitoring parameters include patient compliance, disease remission, and benign or cancerous tumors.

GENITAL HERPES

● Genital herpes, caused by herpes simplex virus (HSV) types 1 and 2, is a common STI for which there is no cure. Once latency is established, neither competent host immunity nor therapeutic agents can eradicate the virus. Currently, there is no vaccine available for HSV, and it seems that the development of one is unlikely in the near future.

EPIDEMIOLOGY

● Despite a decline in the number of bacterial STIs, HSV-2 in adults has increased from approximately 20% to 32%.[29] Prevalence of HSV-2 infection has grown by approximately 30% since the late 1970s, and currently over 500,000 new cases of HSV-2 occur annually.

Clinical Presentation of Genital Herpes[30]

General
- Asymptomatic

Classic Sign
- A cluster of painful vesicles on an erythematous base

Symptoms
- Itching
- Burning
- Tingling
- Groin lump
- Dysuria
- Dyspareunia
- Increased urinary frequency

Other Symptoms
- Ulcerative lesions, fissures, cervicitis

Patient Encounter 3

MR is a 19-year-old Caucasian female who visits a clinic complaining of intense itching and burning in the genital area for the past few days. She informed the clinician that she engaged in sexual intercourse within the past month and has also noticed an eruption of painful vesicles in the genital area. She is not sure of her partner's sexual contacts.

What information is suggestive of genital herpes?

What potential risk factors for STIs are present?

What therapy should be recommended for this patient initially and how will this differ if episodic infection recurs?

PATHOPHYSIOLOGY

Since HSV is only found in humans, infection may only be transmitted from infectious secretions onto mucosal surfaces (i.e., cervix or urethra) or abraded skin. The virus may survive for a limited amount of time on environmental surfaces.

DIAGNOSIS

Laboratory confirmation is vital to effective treatment of HSV, especially in individuals in whom a clinical diagnosis cannot be obtained. There are several methods by which a definitive diagnosis may be acquired, and these include virologic typing, serologic diagnosis, rapid point-of-care antigen detection, enzyme-linked immunosorbent assay (ELISA), immunoblot, and DNA polymerase chain reaction.[30] Additionally, the FDA recently approved glycoprotein G-based assays to aid in the diagnosis of HSV.

TREATMENT

Desired Outcome

The desired outcome is to curtail the number of episodic prodromes and to minimize any side effects experienced due to the antivirals. Counseling of infected persons and their partners is vital to the management of HSV.

Pharmacologic Therapy

❼ *Treatment is based on several factors including likelihood of patient compliance, whether it is the first or a recurrent episode, host immunity, and pregnancy. However, patient response has been linked to the time it takes to initiate treatment after symptom onset.*

▶ First Episode

The first episode is a systemic illness associated with the vesicular lesions, may last up to 21 days, usually has an uncomplicated course of infection, and in severe cases may require hospitalization. Several agents are effective during this period (Table 80–3).[31,32] At the cited dosages, these agents have had excellent outcomes with regard to lesion healing time, viral shedding, and loss of pain. Common adverse effects are nausea, headache, and diarrhea.

▶ Episodic Therapy

In a patient with a previous diagnosis of genital herpes, the appearance of new vesicular lesions is synonymous with HSV reactivation. For most patients, genital herpes recurrence is self-limiting and shortlived, lasting approximately 6 to 7 days.

▶ Suppressive Therapy

Suppressive therapy is effective for controlling all symptoms related to the disease and may impact troublesome complications of infection. Before beginning suppressive therapy, discuss patient expectations. Encourage patients to record any breakthrough episodes, as this may require treatment reevaluation and adjustment.

▶ Preventive Therapy

Valacyclovir 500 mg orally once daily has been implicated to prevent the sexual transmission of HSV to an uninfected partner. In addition to pharmacologic therapy, counsel patients regarding safe sex practices.

▶ Drug Resistance

Foscarnet, cidofovir, and trifuridine have been administered in acyclovir-resistant patients.[33] These agents are usually reserved for use after other agents have failed because of their associated toxicities.

▶ Pregnancy

Women who are pregnant may transmit the virus to the neonate during delivery. There are two management

Table 80–3

Comparison of Antivirals Used for Herpes Simplex Infection

Agent	Dose	Side Effects
First Episode		
Acyclovir	*200 mg orally every 4 hours × 7–10 days* 400 mg orally 3 times daily × 7–10 days[a] 200 mg orally every 12 hours × 7–10 days[b]	Headache, confusion, nausea, vomiting, thrombocytopenia, renal insufficiency, rash, pruritus, fever, arthralgias, myalgia, thrombotic thrombocytopenic purpura, hallucinations, somnolence, depression
Valacyclovir	*1 g orally 2 times daily × 7–10 days* 1 g orally daily × 7–10 days[c] or 500 mg orally daily × 7–10 days[c]	Refer to acyclovir
Famciclovir	250 mg orally 3 times daily × 7–10 days	Refer to acyclovir
Episodic		
Acyclovir	*200 mg orally every 4 hours × 5 days* or 400 mg orally every 8 hours × 5 days or 800 mg orally 2 times daily × 5 days or 800mg orally 3 times daily × 2 days	Refer to acyclovir
Valacyclovir	*500 mg orally 2 times daily × 3 days* 500 mg orally once daily × 5 days[c] 1 g orally once daily × 5 days	Refer to acyclovir
Famciclovir[d]	*125 mg orally 2 times daily × 5 days* 125 mg orally once daily × 5 days[c]	Refer to acyclovir
Suppressive		
Acyclovir	*400 mg orally 2 times daily up to 1 year* or 200 mg orally 3–5 × daily up to 1 year	Refer to acyclovir
Valacyclovir[e]	*250 mg orally 2 times daily up to 1 year* or 500 mg orally once daily up to 1 year or 1 g orally once daily up to 1 year	Refer to acyclovir
Famciclovir	250 mg orally 2 times daily up to 1 year	Refer to acyclovir
Reserved Agents		
Foscarnet	40 mg/kg IV every 8–12 hours × 2–3 weeks or until clinical resolution is attained	Renal insufficiency, metabolic disturbances, hypophosphatemia
Cidofovir	0.3%, 1%, and 3% topical agent used on a compassionate basis for acyclovir-resistant herpes lesions (3–7 days)	Application site reactions, lesion recrudescence
Trifluridine	1% topical agent used for acyclovir-resistant herpes infections for 7–14 days	Transient burning or stinging, palpebral edema, superficial punctuate, keratopathy, changes in intraocular pressure

Italicized data indicate recommended dosages. CrCl, creatinine clearance.

[a]The Centers for Disease Control and Prevention states that this dosage may be useful for immunocompromised patients.

[b]Dose for administration in renal impairment (CrCl 10 mL/min or less).

[c]Dose for administration in renal impairment (CrCl 30 mL/min or less).

[d]If administered at the same frequency, there is no evidence that 250 mg or 500 mg will provide greater benefit than 125 mg.

[e]Dose is based on the number of symptomatic recurrences.

From Ref. 41.

strategies: cesarean section and antiviral therapy. A few studies indicate that acyclovir 200 to 400 mg every 8 hours has been administered from 38 weeks gestation until delivery. The goal of therapy is to reduce the number of lesions and asymptomatic shedding at delivery.

▶ Neonates

Herpes simplex virus infections should be considered in all neonates who present with nonspecific symptoms such as fever, poor feeding, lethargy, or seizures in the first month of life. Infants suspected to have or who are diagnosed with an

HSV infection should be treated parenterally. Acyclovir 60 mg/kg/day in three divided doses IV for 14 days for disease limited to skin, eyes, and mucous membranes, and 21 days for CNS or disseminated disease is suggested.

PATIENT CARE AND MONITORING

Reevaluation of the patient's condition and therapy adjustment are key elements in effective monitoring. Parameters may include:

- The patient's psychosocial and psychosexual status
- Frequent reassessment of recurrent episodes and therapy adjustment
- Ordering tests for malignancy
- Yearly testing of HIV status
- Side effects of drugs

VACCINATIONS

Several HPV genotypes have been linked to the development of cervical cancer. HPV vaccine (Gardasil), developed to protect against HPV genotypes 6, 11, 16, and 18, is the first employed to prevent cervical cancer, precancerous genital lesions, and genital warts due to HPV. The CDC recommends the HPV vaccine for all 11- and 12- year-old females. Vaccination is also recommended for females aged 13 through 26 years who have not been previously vaccinated or who have not completed the full series of shots.[34]

The vaccine is given in a series of three injections over a 6-month period. The second and third doses should be given at 2 and 6 months (respectively) after the first dose. HPV vaccine may be given at the same time as other vaccines.

BACTERIAL VAGINOSIS

BV is a common infection and a recurrent cause of abnormal vaginal discharge in women of childbearing age. BV is categorized by an overgrowth of anaerobic organisms such as *Gardenella vaginalis*, *Prevotella* species, *Mycoplasma hominis*, and *Mobiluncus* species, leading to the replacement of lactobacillus and an increase in vaginal pH from 4.5 to 7.[35] BV is the most prevalent cause of vaginal discharge and malodor.

EPIDEMIOLOGY

BV has been found in 12% to 25% of women in routine clinic populations, 10% to 26% of women in obstetrics clinics, and 32% to 64% of women in clinics for STIs. BV infection usually results from sexual activity, although some cases have been reported in women who are not sexually active.

PATHOPHYSIOLOGY

A complex and intricate balance of microorganisms maintains the normal vaginal flora (i.e., lactobacilli, corynebacteria,

Clinical Presentation of Bacterial Vaginosis[36]

General
- Offensive fishy-smelling vaginal discharge

Signs
- Thin, white, homogenous discharge, coating the walls of the vagina

Symptoms
- Many women are asymptomatic; usually not associated with soreness, itching, or irritation

and yeast). The normal postmenarchal and premenopausal vaginal pH is 3.8 to 4.2. At this pH, growth of pathogenic organisms is usually inhibited; however, disturbance of the normal vaginal pH can alter the vaginal flora, leading to overgrowth of pathogens.

DIAGNOSIS

❽ BV is diagnosed according to the Amsel criteria. In order for diagnosis to be confirmed, three of the four criteria must be present:

1. Thin, white, homogenous discharge
2. Clue cells on microscopy (clue cells are epithelial cells of the vagina that get their distinctive stippled appearance by being covered with bacteria)
3. pH of vaginal fluid greater than 4.5
4. Release of a fishy odor upon the addition of an alkali (10% potassium hydroxide) to a vaginal sample.

❾ *Alternatively, a gram-stain vaginal smear may be used to diagnose BV using the Nugent criteria.* This relies on estimating the proportions of bacteria morphotypes to provide a score between 0 and 10. A score of less than 4 is normal, 4 to 6 is intermediate, and greater than 6 is consistent with BV. Isolation of *G. vaginalis* may not be diagnostic because it can be cultured from the vagina in some normal women, although a high concentration may be indicative of infection.[36]

TREATMENT

Desired Outcome

Reduction in the number of causative bacteria, cessation of vaginal discharge, and decrease in vaginal pH are the desired outcomes.

Pharmacologic Therapy[4,37]

Adults Recommended adult regimens include: Metronidazole 500 mg orally twice daily for 7 days *or* metronidazole gel (0.75%), one full applicator (5 g) intravaginally once daily for 5 days *or* clindamycin cream (2%), one full applicator (5 g) intravaginally at bedtime for 7 days.

Alternative regimens include: Clindamycin ovules 100 mg intravaginally once at bedtime for 3 days *or* clindamycin 300 mg orally twice daily for 7 days.

Pregnancy Pregnant symptomatic women should receive treatment. Treatment of BV in asymptomatic women at high-risk for preterm delivery with a recommended oral regimen mitigates preterm delivery. Screening should be performed during the first prenatal visit. Recommended regimens for pregnant women include: metronidazole 500 mg orally twice daily for 7 days *or* metronidazole 250 mg orally three times daily for 7 days *or* clindamycin 300 mg orally twice daily for 7 days.

PATIENT CARE AND MONITORING

A test to determine if the patient has been cured is generally not recommended. However, in patients with recurrent BV, a follow-up after the course of therapy may be warranted. If treatment has been prescribed during pregnancy to reduce preterm birth, perform a repeat exam in 1 month and advise further treatment for recurrent BV.

PELVIC INFLAMMATORY DISEASE

PID usually affects young, sexually-active, reproductive-age women. In the majority of cases, the pathogens responsible are *C. trachomatis* and *N. gonorrhoeae;* although anaerobes, enteric gram-negative rods, and cytomegalovirus have also been implicated in the pathogenesis.[38] PID has been correlated with ectopic pregnancy, infertility, tubo-ovarian abscess, and chronic pelvic pain.

PATHOPHYSIOLOGY

Chlamydia may produce a heat-shock protein that causes tissue damage through a delayed hypersensitivity reaction. *C. trachomatis* may also possess DNA evidence of toxin-like genes that code for high-molecular-weight proteins with structures similar to *Clostridium difficile* cytotoxins, enabling inhibition of immune activation. This may explain the observation of a chronic *C. trachomatis* infection in subclinical PID.

DIAGNOSIS[38,39]

To be diagnosed with PID, patients must have uterine tenderness, cervical motion tenderness, and adnexal tenderness with no other cause of these signs. Additional criteria include:

- Oral temperature greater than 38.3°C (101°F)
- Abnormal cervical or vaginal discharge
- WBC presence on saline microscopy of vaginal secretions
- Elevated erythrocyte sedimentation rate
- Elevated C-reactive protein

Clinical Presentation of Pelvic Inflammatory Disease[39]

General
- Signs and symptoms may vary from mild to severe

Signs
- Vague

Symptoms
- Lower abdominal or pelvic pain
- Malodorous vaginal discharge
- Abnormal uterine bleeding
- Dyspareunia
- Dysuria
- Nausea and/or vomiting
- Fever

- Laboratory documentation of cervical infection with *N. gonorrhoeae* or *C. trachomatis*

TREATMENT

Desired Outcome

The removal of causative bacteria and reduction of any related sequelae are the desired goals of treatment.

Pharmacologic Treatment

❾ *Resolution of infection (i.e., N. gonorrhoeae, C. trachomatis, Streptococcus spp., and gram-negative facultative bacteria) and mitigation of sequelae should be the main goal of pharmacologic therapy.* CDC-approved treatment regimens are shown in Table 80–4.[4,38,43] Optimal management of PID should be individualized based on clinical setting and patient characteristics. For some patients, hospitalizations, IV antibiotics, and surgical treatment of complications may be needed. Though outpatient management remains contentious, many feel that outpatient management should be limited to individuals who: remain afebrile, have a WBC counts less than $11 \times 10^3/mm^3$ (11×10^9L), have minimal evidence of peritonitis, have active bowel sounds, and can tolerate oral nourishment. Nonetheless, outpatient therapy with a parenteral cephalosporin or levofloxacin followed by doxycycline and metronidazole is recommended.

PATIENT CARE AND MONITORING

The goals of monitoring patients with PID are related to reducing long-term complications. To this end, the primary approach should be prevention and education of at-risk women. Secondary prevention may include screening by conducting a pelvic exam during a routine check-up.

Table 80–4

Treatment Regimens for PID

Parenteral

Cefotetan 2 g IV every 12 hours or cefoxitin 2 g IV every 6 hours and doxycycline 100 mg orally or IV every 12 hours

Clindamycin 900 mg IV every 8 hours and gentamicin, loading dose IV or IM (2 mg/kg) followed by maintenance dose (1.5 mg/kg) every 8 hours (a single daily dose may be used)

Levofloxacin 500 mg IV every 24 hours with or without metronidazole 500 mg IV every 8 hours

Ampicillin-sulbactam, 3 g IV every 6 hours and doxycycline 100 mg orally or IV every 12 hours

Ofloxacin 400 mg IV every 12 hours with or without metronidazole 500 mg IV every 8 hours

Oral

Levofloxacin 500 mg orally daily for 14 days with or without metronidazole, 500 mg orally twice daily for 14 days

Ceftriaxone 250 mg IM single dose and probenecid 1 g single dose, plus doxycycline 100 mg orally twice daily for 14 days with or without metronidazole, 500 mg orally twice daily for 14 days

Cefoxitin 2 g IM single dose and probenecid 1 g single dose, plus doxycycline 100 mg orally twice daily for 14 days with or without metronidazole, 500 mg orally twice daily for 14 days

Third-generation cephalosporin plus doxycycline 100 mg orally twice daily for 14 days with or without metronidazole, 500 mg orally twice daily for 14 days

From Refs. 40–42.

CHANCROID

Haemophilus ducreyi, a gram-negative bacterium, has been isolated as the causative organism of chancroid, a genital ulcerative disease usually accompanied by inguinal lymphadenitis and bubo formation. Chancroid may possibly spread to other anatomic sites, a clinical feature first discovered by Ducrey in 1889.[44]

Clinical Presentation of Chancroid[43]

General

- The ulcer edge is commonly ragged and poorly defined.

Signs

- Four to seven days after infection, a tender, erythematous papule usually develops and subsequently progresses to the pustular stage.[37] The pustules often rupture after 2 to 3 days.

- Lesions typically occur on the prepuce and frenulum in men and on the vulva, cervix, and perianal area in women. Some extragenital cases have been noted on the inner thighs, breasts, and fingers, though rarely seen in practice.

Symptoms

- Painful and tender lesions
- Painful shallow ulcers with granulomatous bases and purulent exudates.

EPIDEMIOLOGY

In 2003, more than 50,000 patients were diagnosed with chancroid in the United States. The majority of cases were diagnosed in the South Atlantic region, which included Delaware, North and South Carolina, Georgia, and Florida.[45] ❿ *Approximately 10% of persons who have chancroid that was acquired in the United States are coinfected with* T. pallidum *or HSV*[a]; *this percentage is higher in individuals who acquired chancroid outside of the United States.*

PATHOPHYSIOLOGY

Transmission commences through direct contact with the skin, presumably through minor abrasions. The ulcer may be quite deep, and more than half of patients have multiple ulcers.

DIAGNOSIS

The multiplex polymerase chain reaction has been used successfully in diagnosis, demonstrating approximately 75% specificity in studies employing genital ulcer swabs. It offers an acceptable sensitivity in the detection of the three most common organisms involved in the etiology of genital ulcer disease: HSV, *T. pallidum*, and *H. ducreyi*.[44,46] Additionally, several amplification techniques have been created in hopes of improving the sensitivity of laboratory diagnosis.

TREATMENT

Management of the syndrome has been the accepted approach of the WHO in lieu of the limitations seen with most diagnostic procedures. The prevailing thought is that patients

Table 80–5

Recommended Treatment Regimens for Chancroid from WHO and CDC

Antimicrobial	Regimen	Recommending Body
Erythromycin	500 mg orally 3 times daily for 7 days *or* 500 mg orally 4 times daily for 7 days	WHO, CDC
Azithromycin	1 g orally as a single dose	CDC
Ceftriaxone	250 mg IM as a single dose	WHO, CDC
Ciprofloxacin	500 mg orally as a single dose *or* 500 mg orally 2 times daily for 3 days	WHO, CDC
Spectinomycin	2 g IM as a single dose	WHO

IM, intramuscularly.

From Ref. 44.

should be treated during the first visit with a combination of antibiotics to cover for probable etiologic organisms.[46]

Desired Outcome

The desired outcome is to treat the ulceration, resolve the symptoms, and reduce the spread of infection to others.

Pharmacologic Therapy

The WHO- and CDC-recommended treatment regimens are shown in Table 80–5.[4,44] There has been some debate about a suitable dosage of ciprofloxacin in the treatment of chancroid. Though the CDC recommends 500 mg orally three times daily, the WHO supports a single 500-mg oral dose. Ciprofloxacin has demonstrated an acceptable cure rate for a single dose (92%) when compared to erythromycin (91%). Ciprofloxacin is contraindicated for pregnant and lactating women.

PATIENT CARE AND MONITORING

Follow-up should include patient education, counseling, and repeated inspections of the ulceration to ensure healing. Examine patients 3 to 7 days after commencing with treatment. Ulcers usually improve symptomatically within 3 days and objectively within 7 days. If improvement is not evident, consider the following: (a) the diagnosis is incorrect; (b) the patient is coinfected with another STI; (c) the patient is infected with HIV; (d) the patient was noncompliant; or (e) the *H. ducreyi* strain may be resistant to therapy.

PREVENTION STRATEGIES

A combination of prevention efforts is advised. Alteration in sexual behavior should undoubtedly be the first counseling concern, as promiscuous sexual activity has been shown to augment the probability of infection.

Abstinence is the best course of action, especially in patients with herpes during lesional episodes. However, compliance in some may be minimal, in which case, appropriate condom use should always be recommended.

To alleviate any possible misconceptions about condom application, either demonstrate how to apply a condom or ask the patient to demonstrate. During the demonstration, explicitly educate the patient with regard to application, storage, and the use of lubricants.[47]

Abbreviations Introduced in This Chapter

BV	Bacterial vaginosis
CSF	Cerebrospinal fluid
ELISA	Enzyme-linked immunosorbent assay
HPV	Human papillomavirus
HSV	Herpes simplex virus
MSM	Men who have sex with men
PID	Pelvic inflammatory disease
RPR	Rapid plasma reagin
STI	Sexually transmitted infection
WSW	Women who have sex with women

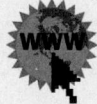 Self-assessment questions and answers are available at *http://www.mhpharmacotherapy.com/pp.html*.

REFERENCES

1. Birley H, Duerden B, Hart C. Sexually transmitted diseases: Microbiology and management. J Med Microbiol 2002;51:793–807.
2. Aral S. Sexually risky behaviour and infection: Epidemiological considerations. Sex Transm Infect 2004;80(Suppl II):ii8–ii12.
3. Biddlecom A. Trends in sexual behaviours and infections among young people in the United States. Sex Transm Infect 2004;80(Suppl II):ii74–ii79.
4. Sexually Transmitted Diseases. MMWR Recommendations and Reports. 2006;55 RR-11:1–92.
5. Gorbach P, Galea J, Amani A, et al. Don't ask, don't tell: Patterns of HIV disclosure among HIV positive men who have sex with men with recent STI practicing high risk behaviour in Los Angeles and Seattle. Sex Transm Infect 2004;80:512–517.
6. Fethers K, Marks C, Mindel A, et al. Sexually Transmitted Infections and risk behaviors in women who have sex with women. Sex Transmit Infect. 2000;76:345–349.

7. Kodner C. Sexually transmitted infections in men: Primary care. Clin Office Pract 2003;30:173–191.
8. Mandell. Principles and Practice of Infectious Diseases, 5th ed. Church Livingstone; 2002.
9. Moran J. Gonorrhea. Clin Evid 2004(Jun);(11):2104–2112.
10. Lyss S, Kamb M, Peterman T, et al. *Chlamydia trachomatis* among patients infected with and treated for *Neisseria gonorrhea* in sexually transmitted disease clinics in the United States. Ann Intern Med. 2003;139:178–185.
11. Tapsall JW. What management is there for gonorrhea in the postquinolone era? Sex Transm Dis. 2006;33:8–10.
12. Young F. Sexually transmitted infections. Genital chlamydia: Practical management in primary care. J Fam Health Care 2005;15:19–21.
13. Summary of Notifiable Diseases in the United States 2006. Morbidity and Mortality Weekly Report. March 21, 2008;55(53):1–94.
14. Brown D, Frank J. Diagnosis and management of syphilis. Am Fam Physician 2003;68:283–290.
15. Berman S. Maternal syphilis: Pathophysiology and treatment. Bull World Health Organ 2004(Jun);82(6):433–438.
16. Peeling R, Ye H. Diagnostic tools for preventing and managing maternal and congenital syphilis: An overview. Bull World Health Organ 2004(Jun);82(6):439–446.
17. CDC. Inadvertent use of Bicillin® C-R to treat syphilis infection. MMWR. 2005;54:217–219.
18. Med Let. 2004(Oct);26(2):2.
19. Saloojee H, Sithembiso V, Goga Y, et al. The prevention and management of congenital syphilis: An overview and recommendations. Bull World Health Organ 2004(Jun);82(6):424–430.
20. Centers for Disease Control and Prevention. Sexually transmitted diseases treatment guidelines, 2002. MMWR Recomm Rep 2002;51(RR-6):18–25, 28–30.
21. Soper D. Trichomoniasis: Under control or undercontrolled? Am J Obstet Gynecol 2004;190:281–290.
22. National guidelines for the management of trichomonas vaginalis. Sex Transm Inf 1999;75(Suppl 1):S21–S23.
23. Tindamax. *www.tindamax.com.* 24. Sobel J, Nyirjesy P, Brown W. Tinidazole therapy for metronidazole resistant vaginal trichomoniasis. Clin Infect Dis 2001;33:1341–1346.
25. Kodner C, Nasraty S. Management of genital warts. Am Fam Physician 2004;70:2335–2342, 2345–2346.
26. Gunter J. Genital and perianal warts: New treatment opportunities for human papillomavirus infection. Am J Obstet Gynecol 2003;189:S3–S11.
27. Bowden F, Tabrizi S, Garland S, et al. Sexually transmitted infections: New diagnostic approaches and treatments. MJA 2002;176:551–557.
28. Woodward C, Fisher M. Drug treatment of common STDs: Part II. Vaginal infections, pelvic inflammatory disease and genital warts. Am Fam Physician 1999;60:1716–1722.
29. Solomon L, Cannon M, Reyes M, et al. Epidemiology of recurrent herpes simplex virus types 1 and 2. Sex Transm Infect 2003(Dec);79(6):456–459.
30. Patel R. Progress in meeting today's demands in genital herpes: An overview of current management. J Infect Dis 2002;186(Suppl I):S47–S56.
31. Alexander L, Naisbett B. Patient and physician partnerships in managing genital herpes. J Infect Dis 2002;186(Suppl I):S57–S65.
32. Lacy C, Armstrong L, Goldman M, Lance L. Lexi-Comp's Drug Information Handbook, 12th ed. 2004:1128–1132.
33. Wald A. New therapies and prevention strategies for genital herpes. Clin Inf Dis 1999;28(Suppl 1):S4–S13.
34. Gardasil. *http://www.cdc.gov/vaccines/vpd-vac/hpv/vac-faqs.html.*
35. Klebanoff M, Hauth J, MacPherson C, et al. Time course of the regression of asymptomatic bacterial vaginosis in pregnancy with and without treatment. Am J Obstet Gynecol 2004;190:363–370.
36. Sobel J. What's new in bacterial vaginosis and trichomoniasis? Infect Dis Clin North Am 2005;19:387–406.
37. Clinical Effectiveness Group. National guidelines for the management of bacterial vaginosis. Sex Transm Inf 1999;75(Suppl I):S16–S18.
38. Miller K, Ruiz D, Graves J. Update on the prevention and treatment of sexually transmitted diseases. Am Fam Physician 2003;67(9):1915–1922.
39. Beigi R, Wiesenfeld H. Pelvic inflammatory disease: New diagnostic criteria and treatment. Obstet Gynecol Clin North Am 2003(Dec);30(4):777–793.
40. Teva Pharmaceuticals USA. Metronidazole package insert. North Wales, PA: Teva Pharmaceuticals USA, 2005.
41. McEvoy G, ed. AHFS Drug Information. Bethesda, MD: ASHP, 2005.
42. Epperly AT, Viera AJ. Pelvic inflammatory disease. Clin Fam Pract 2005;7:67–78.
43. Lagley C. Update on chancroid: An important cause of genital ulcer disease. AIDS Patient Care STDS 1996(Aug);10(4):221–226.
44. Lewis D. Diagnostic tests for chancroid. Sex Transm Infect 2000;76:137–141.
45. Morbidity and Mortality Weekly Report. Notifiable diseases. *http://www.cdc.gov/ncphi/disss/nndss/casedef/chancroid_current.htm.*
46. Htun Y, Morse S, Dangor Y, et al. Comparison of clinically directed, disease specific, and syndromic protocols for the management of genital ulcer disease in Lesotho. Sex Transm Infect 1998;74(Suppl 1):S23–S28.
47. FDA. Condoms and Sexually Transmitted diseases. *http://www.fda.gov/oashi/aids/condom.html.*

81 Osteomyelitis

Melinda M. Neuhauser and Susan L. Pendland

LEARNING OBJECTIVES

● **Upon completion of the chapter, the reader will be able to:**

1. Discuss the pathophysiology of osteomyelitis.
2. List common risk factors for osteomyelitis.
3. Compare and contrast the classic signs and symptoms of acute and chronic osteomyelitis.
4. Evaluate microbiology culture data and other laboratory tests utilized for the diagnosis and treatment of bone infections.
5. List the most common pathogens isolated in acute and chronic osteomyelitis.
6. Develop a treatment plan for osteomyelitis.
7. Recommend parameters to monitor antimicrobial therapy for effectiveness and toxicity.
8. Educate patients regarding disease state and drug therapy.

KEY CONCEPTS

❶ Osteomyelitis, an infection of the bone, can be an acute or chronic process.

❷ Osteomyelitis is most often classified by route of infection and duration of disease.

❸ *Staphylococcus aureus* is the predominant pathogen seen in all types of osteomyelitis. However, the spectrum of potential causative pathogens varies with patient-specific risk factors and route of infection.

❹ Typical signs and symptoms of osteomyelitis include local pain and tenderness over the affected bone, as well as inflammation, erythema, edema, and decreased range of motion. Patients with acute hematogenous osteomyelitis may also present with fever, chills, and malaise.

❺ The gold standard for diagnosis of osteomyelitis is a bone biopsy with isolation of microorganism(s) from culture and the presence of inflammatory cells and osteonecrosis on histological exam.[1-3] Due to the invasive nature of the bone biopsy, the diagnosis of osteomyelitis is often based upon on clinical findings, laboratory tests, and imaging studies rather than bone biopsy.[4] A thorough history and physical examination are especially important for diagnosis in patients with limited or atypical symptoms.

❻ The treatment goals for acute and chronic osteomyelitis are to eradicate the infection and prevent recurrence.

Higher cure rates are seen with acute compared to chronic osteomyelitis. Therefore, in chronic osteomyelitis, a common treatment goal for many patients is to prevent complications such as amputation.

❼ Treatment of osteomyelitis is dependent on the extent of bone necrosis. For acute osteomyelitis with minimal bone destruction, an extended course of antimicrobial therapy should effectively treat the infection; however, in chronic osteomyelitis surgical intervention is also typically required.

❽ Empiric antimicrobial therapy should target likely causative pathogen(s) based on patient-specific risk factors and route of infection. However, therapy should be modified based on culture and sensitivity data.

❾ The total duration of antimicrobial therapy is typically 4 to 6 weeks. Therapy is often administered IV for 1 or 2 weeks and then switched to the oral route.

❿ Patients should be monitored for clinical and laboratory response, development of adverse drug reactions, and potential drug–drug interactions. Patients should also be closely monitored for compliance in the outpatient setting.

INTRODUCTION

❶ *Osteomyelitis is an infection of the bone that is associated with high morbidity and increased health care costs. The inflammatory response associated with acute osteomyelitis*

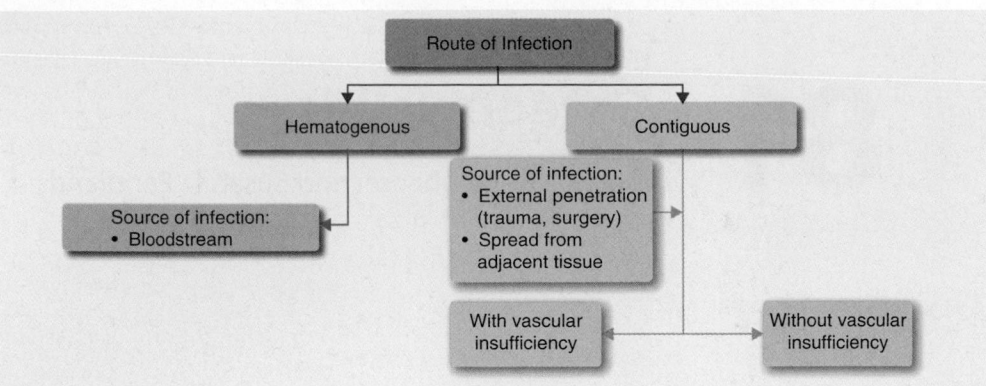

FIGURE 81–1. Classification by route of infection.

can lead to bone necrosis and subsequently chronic infections. Bacterial pathogens, particularly *Staphylococcus aureus*, are the most common microorganisms implicated in these infections. Diagnosis and treatment are often difficult due to the heterogeneous nature of osteomyelitis. Medical management is the mainstay of treatment for acute infections; however, surgical intervention is necessary for chronic cases that involve bone necrosis. Outcomes may vary based on patient-specific risk factors, duration of disease, and site of infection.

EPIDEMIOLOGY AND ETIOLOGY

❷ *There are multiple classification schemes for osteomyelitis.*[5] *Due to the heterogeneity of bone infections, no single classification system has been universally accepted.*[1] *Two of the most common classification schemes are based on* route of infection *and* duration of disease.[1,4–6] In the classification scheme developed by Waldvogel and colleagues,[6] the route of infection is categorized as either hematogenous or contiguous (Fig. 81–1). Osteomyelitis secondary to a contiguous focus was further subdivided into infections with or without vascular insufficiency.

Historically, osteomyelitis has been classified as acute or chronic based on duration of disease (Fig. 81–2).[1] However, there are no established definitions for acute and chronic infections.[1,4] Acute infection has been defined as first episode or recent onset of symptoms (less than 1 week).[4] Chronic osteomyelitis is generally defined as relapse of the disease or symptoms persisting beyond 4 weeks.[4] Others describe chronic osteomyelitis as the presence of necrotic bone.[4]

An alternative classification, the Cierny-Mader staging system, is based on anatomic site and physiologic status of the patient.[5] This classification scheme was developed for chronic osteomyelitis involving long bones, but has limited application for small bones and digits. The detailed stratification has the greatest utility in clinical trials since it permits comparison of treatment regimens in patients with diverse comorbidities and infection sites.

The epidemiology of osteomyelitis in adults has been changing over the past several decades.[5] The frequency of contiguous osteomyelitis has been increasing. This trend may be related to the rising rates of diabetes and peripheral vascular disease (PVD), as well as the increased presence of prosthetic implants and surgical interventions.[4,7,8] In contrast, the incidence of acute hematogenous osteomyelitis, which is most often seen in children, has been declining.[7,9]

❸ The etiology of osteomyelitis has remained relatively unchanged, with *S. aureus being the predominant pathogen seen in all types of osteomyelitis.*[1,10] However, the susceptibility of *S. aureus* has been shifting from methicillin-sensitive to methicillin-resistant in both the health care and community settings.[11–16] Risk factors for health care–associated methicillin-resistant *S. aureus* (MRSA) include previous antimicrobial therapy, prolonged hospitalization, hemodialysis, or presence of an indwelling catheter.[17] In contrast, community-associated MRSA has emerged in patients with no prior health care exposure or apparent risk factors.[14–17] While more

FIGURE 81–2. Classification by duration of disease.

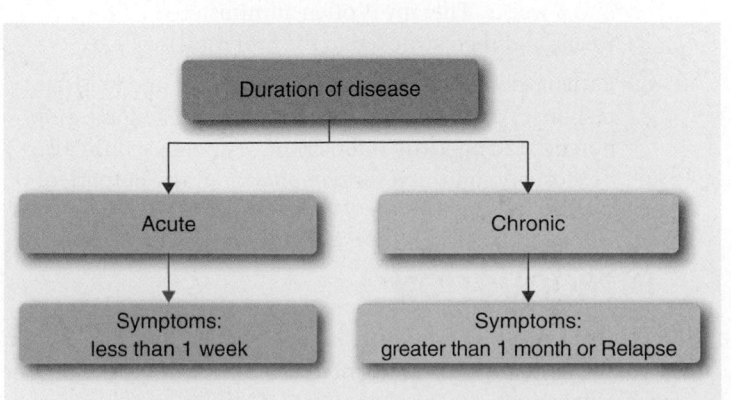

common in skin and soft tissue infections, both health care- and community-associated MRSA have been increasingly reported in osteomyelitis.[18,19]

Host factors such as age, comorbidities, medication, and presence of foreign devices can influence the spectrum of infection (i.e., bone and pathogen involvement) (Table 81–1).[1]

For example, patients with diabetes and PVD have poor wound healing and often present with nonhealing skin ulcers. These wounds are typically colonized with a mixture of aerobic and anaerobic microorganisms, which can lead to polymicrobial osteomyelitis. Therefore, if a wound is deep or extensive, these patients should be evaluated for

Acute Hematogenous Osteomyelitis

- Single pathogen most often isolated
- *Staphylococcus aureus* is the predominant pathogen
- Other pathogens based on risk factors:
  - Neonates: *Eschericia coli* or group B streptococci
  - Elderly: *E. coli* (secondary to urinary tract infections)

Contiguous Focus Osteomyelitis With Vascular Insufficiency

- Multiple pathogens often isolated
- Mixture of aerobic and anaerobic organisms
  - *Staphylococcus aureus, Enterococcus* spp., Enterobacteriaceae, *Pseudomonas aeruginosa*, anaerobes

Table 81–1

Empiric Antimicrobial Therapy for Osteomyelitis

Classification	Age of Onset	Infection Site	Risk Factors	Typical Pathogens	Antimicrobial Therapy
Hematogenous	Neonates	Long bones (femur, tibia)		*S. aureus* *E. coli* Group B streptococci	Antistaphylococcal agent[a] (e.g., nafcillin or vancomycin) *and* 3rd/4th generation cephalosporin with exception of ceftriaxone
	Prepubertal children	Long bones (femur, tibia)		*S. aureus*	Antistaphylococcal agent[a] *or* Clindamycin[b]
	Elderly	Vertebra	UTI	*S. aureus* *E. coli*	Antistaphylococcal agent[a] *and* 3rd/4th generation cephalosporin
Contiguous With vascular insufficiency	Adult (older than 50 years)	Feet, fingers	Diabetes, PVD, peripheral neuropathy	*S. aureus* (MRSA) Enterobacteriaceae *P. aeruginosa* *Enterococcus* spp. Anaerobes	Several therapeutic options: Vancomycin[c] *and* (1) Piperacillin/tazobactam *or* (2) Imipenem/cilastatin, meropenem or doripenem *or* (3) Cefepime or ceftazidime and clindamycin or metronidazole *or* (4) Ciprofloxacin or levofloxacin and clindamycin or metronidazole
Without vascular insufficiency	Adult (older than 50 years)	Postoperative (e.g., hip fractures), Soft-tissue infections		*S. aureus*	Antistaphylococcal agent[a]

MRSA, methicillin-resistant *Staphylococcus aureus*; PVD, peripheral vascular disease; UTI, urinary tract infection.

[a]If the patient has risk factors for MRSA or prevalence of community-associated MRSA is high, vancomycin should be substituted for nafcillin, oxacillin, and cefazolin.

[b]The isolated must be fully susceptible (D-disk) to clindamycin.

[c]If vancomycin minimum inhibitory concentration (MIC) is greater than or equal to 2.0 mcg/mL (1.4 μmol/L) against MRSA, consider an alternative agent such as linezolid or daptomycin.

From Refs. 2, 3, 9–17, 22, 23, 30–32, 34–36, 38.

> ## Contiguous Focus Osteomyelitis Without Vascular Insufficiency
>
> - Single or multiple pathogens isolated
> - *S. aureus* is predominant pathogen
> - Other pathogens based on source of infection:
>   - Mandibular osteomyelitis (mixture of aerobic and anaerobic oral flora)

underlying osteomyelitis.[2] Other special populations that have a varied pathogen spectrum include intravenous drug abusers (IVDA) (*Pseudomonas aeruginosa* and MRSA), sickle cell patients (*Salmonella*), and individuals with prosthetic implants (coagulase-negative staphylococci).[4] Recently, rare cases of osteomyelitis of the jaw have been reported in patients receiving bisphosphonate therapy.[20,21] Risk factors include cancer, chemotherapy, corticosteroids, tooth extraction and poor oral hygiene. Bisphosphates may induce osteoclast apoptosis and slow wound healing, leaving oral lesions susceptible to infection from oral microflora.[21]

PATHOPHYSIOLOGY

Both microbial and host factors are important determinants in the development of osteomyelitis.[1,3,4] Healthy bone tissue is normally resistant to infection but may become susceptible under certain conditions.[1,3] Bone can become infected: (a) via the presence of bacteria in the bloodstream, (b) by direct inoculation from trauma or surgery, and (c) by spread from an adjacent site (e.g., soft-tissue infection).[1,3] The latter is particularly problematic in patients with foreign body implants (e.g., hip replacement) and chronic skin ulcers.[2,4] *Staphylococcus* species possess bacterial adhesins, which promote their attachment to tissues and foreign devices.[3] Microbial adherence to bone elicits an inflammatory response.[4] The subsequent release of leukocytes and cytokines leads to edema and ischemia. In some cases, these processes can lead to bone necrosis.[3] Pieces of dead bone may become separated forming sequestra.[3,4] These areas typically cannot be penetrated by antimicrobials and phagocytic cells and thus require surgical intervention to eradicate the bacterial nidus (Fig. 81–3).[4]

CLINICAL PRESENTATION AND DIAGNOSIS

The clinical presentation of osteomyelitis may vary depending on route and duration of infection, as well as patient-specific factors such as infection site, age, and comorbidities.

❹ *In hematogenous osteomyelitis, the patient typically experiences systemic and localized signs and symptoms.*[4,9,22,23] *In comparison, patients with chronic infection typically present with only localized signs and symptoms.*[7] A cardinal sign of chronic osteomyelitis is the formation of sinus tracts with purulent drainage.[4,7]

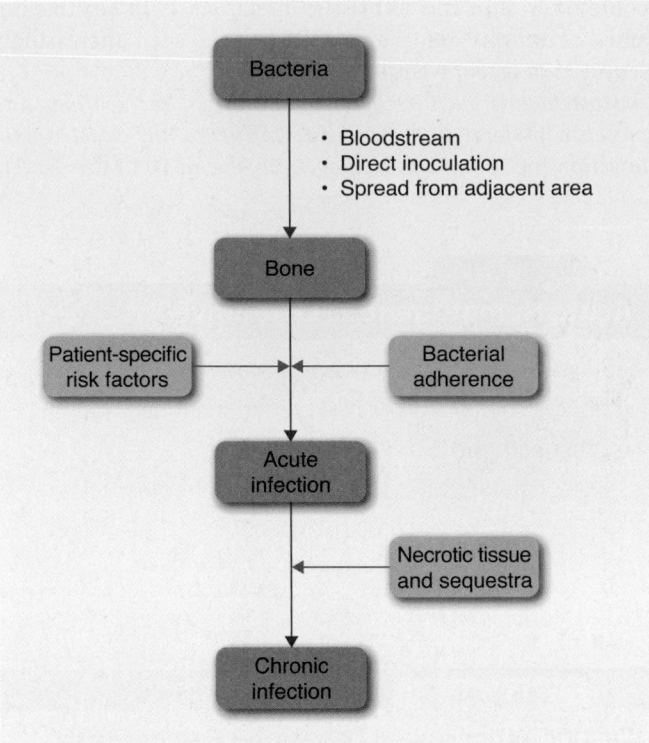

FIGURE 81–3. Pathogenesis of osteomyelitis.

> ## Patient Encounter, Part 1
>
> A 62-year-old male with history of diabetes, hypertension, and PVD comes to the emergency department complaining of a "painful sore" on his left lower leg. After questioning him, you determine that the wound has been present for months and has not responded to oral antibiotic therapy. On physical examination, a large, deep wound with purulent drainage is seen.
>
> *What information is suggestive of osteomyelitis?*
>
> *What risk factors, if any, does he have for osteomyelitis?*

Common signs and symptoms of osteomyelitis include:

Systemic: Fever, chills, malaise

Localized: Pain or tenderness, edema, erythema, inflammation, decreased range of motion of infected area

❺ *The gold standard for diagnosis of osteomyelitis is a bone biopsy with isolation of microorganism(s) from culture and the presence of inflammatory cells and osteonecrosis on histological exam.*[1–3] Due to the invasive nature of the bone biopsy, the diagnosis of osteomyelitis is often based upon clinical findings, laboratory tests, and imaging studies rather than bone biopsy.[4] A thorough history and physical examination are especially important for diagnosis in patients with limited or atypical symptoms.

No single noninvasive laboratory test is currently available for the diagnosis of osteomyelitis. However, despite their low specificity, several tests are commonly used to aid in the diagnosis and to monitor response to therapy. Nonspecific inflammatory markers for infection include white blood cell count (WBC), erythrocyte sedimentation rate (ESR), and C-reactive protein (CRP):[4,7,22]

- WBC, ESR and CRP are often elevated, but may also be within normal limits. An elevated WBC is mostly seen in patients with acute osteomyelitis.

- CRP rises faster than ESR during early stages of infection and also returns to normal levels more quickly than ESR. This makes CRP a more useful tool for both diagnosis and monitoring of therapeutic response.

A number of different imaging tests are used to assist in the diagnosis of osteomyelitis. These include plain film radiographs, MRI, CT scans and nuclear medicine scans.[1–4,7,8]

- *Plain film radiographs.* Most commonly used for initial screening. Bone abnormalities are not apparent for 10 to 21 days, so early infection may be missed.

- *MRI.* Most accurate for diagnosing bone infection and can detect early infection. However, it is more expensive than radiographs.

- *CT scan.* Less specific than MRI, but superior to MRI in detection of sequestra. CT is useful for monitoring clinical improvement. It cannot be used to diagnose infections with metallic implants.

- *Nuclear medicine scans.* Useful for early detection (24–48 hours after onset of symptoms). Radionuclide scans are more sensitive than radiographs, but lack specificity and are expensive. Bone scans demonstrate low specificity in diagnoses involving trauma, surgery, orthopedic implants and diabetes. Leukocyte scans have increased specificity compared to bone scans, but have limited resolution in some anatomical sites.

Microbiologic evaluation.[2,4,7,22]

- Isolation of causative pathogen is essential for targeted antimicrobial therapy

- Bone biopsy can provide definitive diagnosis: Samples should be submitted for culture and histology (rarely performed due to invasive nature)

- Blood cultures may be positive in patients with hematogenous osteomyelitis

- Superficial swabs should have a limited role in directing therapy as they may represent colonization rather than infecting organism(s)

TREATMENT

Desired Outcomes

6 *The treatment goals for osteomyelitis are to eradicate the infection and prevent recurrence. Cure rates of greater than 85% have been reported for acute hematogenous osteomyelitis.*[9,23] *In contrast, chronic osteomyelitis is associated with higher failure rates largely due to the presence of necrotic bone.*[1] These patients typically require surgical intervention to remove the necrotic bone and tissue, and if applicable, to replace infected hardware.[4,24] Comorbidities such as vascular insufficiency can further contribute to the poor outcomes seen with chronic osteomyelitis. Due to the high failure rates, treatment in this patient population may require prolonged therapy with the primary goal of preventing amputation of infected areas.[2,4,7,25]

General Approach to Treatment

7 *Antimicrobial therapy alone is the mainstay of treatment for acute osteomyelitis.*[9,22] *In comparison, treatment for chronic osteomyelitis typically requires a combination of antimicrobial therapy and surgical intervention.*[2–4,7,24,25] If the patient is not a candidate for surgical intervention, prolonged antimicrobial therapy is generally necessary.[2,7,26]

▶ *Pharmacologic Therapy*

8 *Empiric antimicrobial therapy should target likely causative pathogen(s) based on patient-specific risk factors and route of infection (Table 81–1). Empiric antimicrobial coverage against* S. aureus *should be considered for all classifications of osteomyelitis. Specific recommendations may vary based on factors such as patient allergies, potential for harboring a resistant organism, institution formulary, and cost considerations. Antimicrobial therapy should be modified based on culture and sensitivity data of appropriately collected specimens (Table 81–2).*[27]

9 *Typically, treatment is initiated with IV antimicrobials to ensure that therapeutic drug concentrations will be achieved in the bone.*[26] *IV therapy can be administered in the inpatient or outpatient setting.*[25,28] *Following 1 to 2 weeks of IV therapy, a switch to oral antibiotics may be considered in patients with good adherence and outpatient follow-up.*[22,25,29] Oral agents should possess such characteristics as high bioavailability, good bone penetration, and long half-life (i.e., extended dosing interval).[26,29] Antimicrobials commonly used as oral therapy for osteomyelitis include fluoroquinolones, clindamycin,

---

Patient Encounter, Part 2

The medical resident suspected osteomyelitis and ordered plain film radiographs. He also swabbed the open wound and sent the swab to the microbiology laboratory for culture and sensitivity. The following result was reported:

Radiograph: Lytic changes consistent with bone destruction

How would you classify the infection in this patient?

How should the results of the wound swab culture be utilized to target the patient's antimicrobial therapy?

Table 81–2

Pathogen-Targeted Antimicrobial Therapy and Dosing Recommendations in Pediatric and Adult Patients

Microorganism	Recommended Therapy	Alternatives
Staphylococcus aureus		

MSSA	Antistaphylococcal penicillin:
	Nafcillin^a/oxacillin^c:
	    Adult: 2 g IV every 4–6 hours
	    Pediatric^b: 100–200 mg/kg/day IV in divided doses every
	      4–6 hours
	First-generation cephalosporin:
	Cefazolin^c:
	    Adult: 1–2 g IV every 8 hours
	    Pediatric^b: 50–100 mg/kg/day IV in divided doses every
	      6–8 hours
		β-Lactam allergy:
		  Vancomycin or clindamycin

MRSA	*Clindamycin* (often used in pediatric patients for serious MRSA
	  infections; perform D-test to confirm susceptibility)
	Pediatric^b: 25–40 mg/kg/day IV in divided doses every
	  6–8 hours; 10–30 mg/kg/day orally in divided doses every
	  6–8 hours	

Vancomycin MIC less than
  or equal to 1 mcg/mL
  (0.7 μmol/L)
	Vancomycin^c:
	  Goal steady state trough: 15–20 mcg/mL (10–14 μmol/L)
	  Adult: 15–20 mg/kg per dose IV every 8–12 hours
	  Pediatric^b: 10–15 mg/kg per dose IV every 6 hours
	  Dosage should be based upon actual body weight	

Vancomycin MIC greater than
  1 mcg/mL (0.7 μmol/L)
	Consider alternative agent:
	Linezolid:
	    Adult: 600 mg IV/oral every 12 hours
	    Pediatric^b: 10 mg/kg per dose IV/oral every 8 hours
	Daptomycin^c
	    Adult: 6 mg/kg IV every 24 hours	

***Enterococcus* spp.**		

Ampicillin-sensitive	*Ampicillin^c*:
	  Adult: 2 g IV every 4–6 hours
	  Pediatric^b: 100–200 mg/kg/day IV in divided doses
	    every 4–6 hours
		β-Lactam allergy:
		  Vancomycin

Ampicillin-resistant	*Vancomycin*	
Vancomycin-resistant	*Linezolid or daptomycin*	

***Streptococcus* spp.**	*Penicillin G^c*:
	  Adult: 2–4 million units IV every 4–6 hours
	  Pediatric^b: 250,000–400,000 units/kg/day IV in divided
	    doses every 4–6 hours
		β-Lactam allergy:
		  Vancomycin

Enterobacteriaceae	Third- or fourth-generation cephalosporin:
	Ceftriaxone^a
	    Adult: 1–2 g IV every 24 hours
	    Pediatric^b: 50–75 mg/kg per dose IV every 24 hours
	Cefotaxime^{a,c}:
	    Adult: 1–2 g IV every 8 hours
	    Pediatric^b: 50–200 mg/kg/day IV in divided doses
	      every 8 hours
	Ceftazidime^c:
	    Adult: 1–2 g IV every 8 hours
	    Pediatric^b: 100–150 mg/kg/day IV in divided doses
	      every 8 hours
	Cefepime^c:
	    Adult: 1–2 g IV every 8–12 hours
	    Pediatric^b: 50 mg/kg per dose IV every 8–12 hours
	Piperacillin/tazobactam^c:
	    Adult: 3.375 g IV every 4–6 hours *or* 4.5 g IV every
	      6–8 hours
	Fluoroquinolones^e:
	Ciprofloxacin^c
	    Adult: 400 mg IV every 12 hours; 500–750 mg oral twice daily
		Carbapenems:
		Imipenem/cilastatin^c:
		    Adult: 500 mg IV every 6–8 hours
		    Pediatric^b: 60–100 mg/kg/day
		      in divided doses every 6 hours
		Meropenem^c:
		    Adult: 1 g IV every 8 hours
		    Pediatric^b: 60–120 mg/kg/day
		      in divided doses every 8 hours:
		Doripenem^c
		    Adult: 500mg IV every 8 hours
		Ertapenem^c
		    Adult: 1 g IV every 24 hours

(Continued)

Table 81-2

Pathogen-Targeted Antimicrobial Therapy and Dosing Recommendations in Pediatric and Adult Patients *(Continued)*

Microorganism	Recommended Therapy	Alternatives
Enterobacteriaceae *(continued)*	*Levofloxacin[c]*: Adult: 500–750 mg IV/oral once daily *Moxifloxacin[d]*: Adult: 400 mg IV/oral once daily	
Pseudomonas aeruginosa	Antipseudomonal cephalosporin: Ceftazidime Cefepime Antipseudomonal fluoroquinolone[e] Ciprofloxacin Levofloxacin	Piperacillin/tazobactam Carbapenems (only imipenem/ cilastatin, meropenem, or doripenem)
Anaerobes	*Clindamycin[d]*: Adult: 600–900 mg IV every 8 hours; 300–450 mg oral every 6–8 hours Pediatric[b]: Refer to MRSA dosage recommendations *Metronidazole[c,d]*: Adult: 500 mg IV/oral every 8 hours Pediatric[b]: 30 mg/kg/day IV/oral in divided doses every 6–8 hours	

D-test, disk diffusion test; MIC, minimum inhibitory concentration; MRSA, methicillin-resistant *S. aureus*; MSSA, methicillin-sensitive *S. aureus*.

[a]Dosage adjustment necessary in patients with concomitant renal and hepatic dysfunction.

[b]Refer to specialized pediatric reference for maximum pediatric dose and neonatal recommendations and dosing.

[c]Dosage adjustment necessary in renal dysfunction.

[d]Dosage adjustment necessary in severe hepatic dysfunction.

[e]Fluoroquinolones: Not approved by the U.S. FDA for use in children except for anthrax (ciprofloxacin, levofloxacin) and complicated UTI and pyelonephritis (ciprofloxacin).

From Refs. 2, 3, 7, 8, 10–17, 23, 27, 30–32, 34–36, 38–41, 45.

linezolid, and trimethoprim-sulfamethoxazole.[1,7,10,23,27,29,30] Additionally, oral rifampin may be used in combination with another antibiotic in the treatment of chronic osteomyelitis, particularly in patients with foreign devices.[25,29]

With increasing methicillin resistance, clinicians will need to be aware of changing treatment strategies for infections that are often staphylococcal in origin. Historically, IV vancomycin has been first-line therapy for serious MRSA infections. Based upon pharmacokinetic/ pharmacodynamic principles, higher vancomycin trough levels (15–20 mcg/mL; 10–14 µmol/L) have been recommended for serious infections including osteomyelitis.[31,32] Although susceptibility of MRSA to vancomycin remains almost 100%,[32] vancomycin displays reduced activity against MRSA with minimum inhibitory concentrations (MICs) at the high end of the susceptible range (MIC 1–2 mcg/mL [0.7–1.4 µmol/L]).[32–37] As a result, clinicians should know the specific MIC of vancomycin for MRSA. If the MIC is greater than or equal to 2 mcg/mL (1.4 µmol/L), switching to another anti-MRSA agent may be advisable, despite lack of FDA approval.[38] Clinical effectiveness has been reported with linezolid and daptomycin in several small, nonrandomized studies against MRSA osteomyelitis (Table 81–3).[39–41]

However, some in vitro studies have shown reduced susceptibility to daptomycin in vancomycin-intermediate or -resistant *S. aureus* strains;[42–44] therefore, daptomycin susceptibility should be established prior to switching from vancomycin to daptomycin. Clinical trials being conducted with newer agents include daptomycin versus vancomycin for treatment of osteomyelitis related to prosthetic infections, and tigecycline versus ertapenem for treatment of diabetic foot infections.[45] In children, clindamycin is an effective antibiotic against susceptible strains of MRSA.[10,30] However, microbiology laboratories must screen with a disk diffusion test (D-test) for inducible resistance via the macrolide-lincosamide-streptogramin (MLS) gene as clindamycin failures have been associated with infections caused by these isolates.[10,30] Oral anti-MRSA agents often utilized for treatment of osteomyelitis include linezolid, trimethoprim-sulfamethoxazole and clindamycin (mostly in pediatrics).[27,29,30]

❾ *The duration of treatment is typically 4 to 6 weeks for acute osteomyelitis.[25] Chronic osteomyelitis also requires 4 to 6 weeks of therapy. In patients who have undergone surgical intervention, the total length of therapy should be counted after the last major surgical intervention.[25] Therapy should be continued until the infection has resolved. Prolonged therapy*

Patient Encounter, Part 3: The Medical History, Physical Exam, and Diagnostic Tests

PMH: Diabetes mellitus, PVD, hypertension

SH: Tobacco smoker (2 packs per day for the past 30 years), social drinker ("3 cans of beer per day"), nonemployed with medical disability

Allergies: NKDA

Meds: Aspirin 81 mg orally once daily; atorvastatin 40 mg orally once daily; clopidogrel 75 mg orally once daily; lisinopril 10 mg orally once daily; insulin glargine 20 units every day at bedtime; insulin lispro 7 units before breakfast and lunch; insulin lispro 9 units before dinner

PE:

Gen: His general appearance is that of an obese male with tenderness and pain in the region of the nonhealing skin ulcer

Skin: Large, deep ulcer with purulent drainage on his left lower leg

VS: BP 145/87 mm Hg, P 80 bpm, RR 18/min, T 36.0°C (96.8°F), ht 5'6"(168 cm), wt 93 kg (205 lb)

Labs: WBC 13 x 10³/mm³ (13 × 10⁹/L), BUN 19 mg/dL (6.8 mmol/L), serum creatinine (Scr) 1.6 mg/dL (141 μmol/L), fasting blood glucose 156 mg/dL (8.7 mmol/L), ESR 80 mm/h, CRP 49 mg /dL (490 mg/L or 0.49 g/L)

Microbiology: Culture from wound swab: *Enterococcus*, coagulase-negative staphylococci, and *P. aeruginosa*; culture from bone biopsy during débridement: MRSA and *Bacteroides fragilis*

Against which organisms should the antimicrobial therapy be targeted?

Based on the information presented, create a care plan for this patient's osteomyelitis. Your plan should include: (a) goals of therapy, (b) patient-specific detailed therapeutic plan, (c) nonpharmacologic interventions, and (d) follow-up plan to determine if outcomes have been achieved.

Table 81–3

Monitoring Considerations for Select Parenteral Antistaphylococcal Agents

Antimicrobial	Monitoring Considerations
Daptomycin	Muscle pain or weakness particularly of the distal extremities; monitor CPK weekly with more frequent monitoring in patients with renal insufficiency or receiving (or recent discontinuation) of HMG-CoA reductase inhibitors Consider temporarily discontinuing HMG-CoA reductase inhibitors while patient receiving daptomycin
Linezolid	Myelosuppression: monitor CBC once weekly if more than 2 weeks of therapy Mild MAO inhibitor; evaluate for potential drug-drug or drug-food interactions Peripheral and/or optic neuropathy has been reported with long-term therapy; perform routine neurologic and ophthalmic evaluations in these patients
Vancomycin	Renal dysfunction: Monitor weekly renal function (BUN/SCr) and troughs in stable patients Potential for additive renal toxicity if being coadministered with a nephrotoxic agent (e.g., aminoglycoside)

BUN, blood urea nitrogen; CPK, creatinine phosphate; HMG-CoA, hydroxymethylglutaryl coenzyme-A; MAO, monoamine oxidase; SCr, serum creatinine.

From Refs. 27, 32, 45.

Patient Encounter, Part 4

The patient received 4 weeks of IV antimicrobial therapy following débridement. Due to clinical improvement, the physician contacts you for a recommendation for an oral antibiotic to complete a total of 6 weeks of therapy.

What antimicrobial therapy would you recommend for this patient?

Evaluate the patient's medication profile for drug-drug interactions.

Counsel the patient regarding this drug therapy.

may be necessary for certain populations such as patients with vascular insufficiency or patients with recalcitrant infections that do not respond to 4 to 6 weeks of therapy.[2,4,7,26]

In addition to medical and surgical management, nonpharmacologic interventions that reduce risk factors for developing osteomyelitis should be communicated to the patient. Examples include smoking cessation, weight-control, exercise, and good nutrition. Additionally, a diabetic patient should be counseled regarding the necessity of controlled blood glucose, routine care and self-examination of lower extremities, and aggressive wound care.[2]

OUTCOME EVALUATION

Therapeutic success is measured by the extent to which the care plan (a) resolves signs and symptoms, (b) eradicates the microorganism(s), (c) prevents relapses, and (d) prevents complications such as amputation. Patients should be evaluated for resolution of clinical signs and symptoms and normalization of laboratory tests (WBC, CRP, ESR, and cultures). Hospitalized patients should be examined daily. Improvement in clinical manifestations should be seen within 48 to 72 hours of initiation of IV antimicrobial therapy.[2] In the outpatient setting, patients should be evaluated weekly during the initial 4 to 6 weeks of therapy. A reduction in CRP should be seen within 1 week of therapy and should be monitored weekly throughout therapy for a continued downward trend. ESR can also be monitored weekly although normalization will be slower than for CRP. Patients should also be monitored for antimicrobial tolerability and toxicity (see Table 81–3). If poor response is noted, the following should be evaluated: (a) patient compliance, (b) significant drug–drug or drug–food interactions, (c) appropriate dosage to achieve therapeutic concentrations, (d) development of antimicrobial resistance necessitating a change in the treatment regimen, (e) need for additional imaging studies, and (f) diagnostic reevaluation.[2] Treatment is considered successful if all clinical signs and symptoms are resolved and all laboratory tests have returned to normal following 4 to 6 weeks of appropriate treatment. Due to high rates of relapse, patients should have medical follow-up for at least 1 year following resolution of symptoms.[2] Patients should be evaluated at 3- to 6-month intervals for any clinical manifestations of recurring infection and continued normalization of laboratory tests. Follow-up imaging studies at 1 to 2 years may be useful in some patients to confirm therapeutic success.

Abbreviations Introduced in This Chapter

BUN	Blood urea nitrogen
CRP	C-reactive protein
CPK	Creatine phosphokinase
CYP	Cytochrome P-450 isoenzyme
D-test	Disk diffusion test
ESR	Erythrocyte sedimentation rate
IVDA	Intravenous drug abuser
LFT	Liver function test
MAO	Monoamine oxidase
MIC	Minimum inhibitory concentration
MLS	Macrolide-lincosamide-streptogramin
MRSA	Methicillin-resistant *Staphylococcus aureus*
MSSA	Methicillin-sensitive *S. aureus*
PVD	Peripheral vascular disease
Scr	Serum creatinine
TMP-SMX	Trimethoprim-sulfamethoxazole
UTI	Urinary tract infection

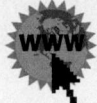 Self-assessment questions and answers are available at *http://www.mhpharmacotherapy.com/pp.html*.

Patient Care and Monitoring

1. ⑩ *Assess the patient's symptoms and laboratory test results to determine if patient-directed therapy is appropriate.*

2. *Obtain a thorough history of prescription, nonprescription, and natural drug product use.*

3. *Educate the patient on lifestyle modifications that will reduce the risk of recurrent infections.*

4. *Develop a plan to assess the effectiveness of antimicrobial therapy.*

5. *Evaluate the patient for the presence of adverse drug reactions, drug allergies, and drug interactions (Table 81–3).*

6. *Stress the importance of adherence to the therapeutic regimen.*

7. *Provide patient education with regard to disease state and drug therapy. Explain the following:*

   - *Causes of osteomyelitis*
   - *Complications associated with osteomyelitis*
   - *The drug, dose, duration, and route of administration of the patient's antimicrobial regimen*
   - *Optimal medication administration time for the patient's lifestyle and other concurrent medications*
   - *Available options for missed dose(s)*
   - *Adverse effects that may occur*
   - *Provide patient education monographs for antibiotic(s)*

REFERENCES

1. Calhoun JH, Manring MM. Adult osteomyelitis. Infect Dis Clin N Am 2005;19:765–786.
2. Lipsky BA, Berendt AR, Deery HG, et al. Diagnosis and treatment of diabetic foot infections. Clin Infect Dis 2004;39:885–910.
3. Hartemann-Heurtier A, Senneville E. Diabetic foot osteomyelitis. Diabetes Metab 2008;34:87–95.
4. Lew DP, Waldvogel FA. Osteomyelitis. Lancet 2004;364:369–378.
5. Mader JT, Shirtliff M, Calhoun JH. Staging and staging application in osteomyelitis. Clin Infect Dis 1997;25:1303–1309.
6. Waldvogel FA, Medoff G, Swartz MN. Osteomyelitis: A review of clinical features, therapeutic considerations and unusual aspects. N Engl J Med 1970;282:198–206.
7. Lazzarini L, Mader JT, Calhoun JH. Osteomyelitis in long bones. J Bone Joint Surg Am 2004;86:2305–2318.
8. Mandracchia VJ, Sanders SM, Jaeger AJ, Nickles WA. Management of osteomyelitis. Clin Podiatr Med Surg 2004;21:335–351.
9. Vazquez M. Osteomyelitis in children. Curr Opin Pediatr 2002;14:112–115.
10. Kaplan SL. Osteomyelitis in children. Infect Dis Clin N Am 2005;19:787–797.
11. Gafur OA, Copley LA, Hollmig ST, et al. The impact of the current epidemiology of pediatric musculoskeletal infection on evaluation and treatment guidelines. J Pediatr Orthop 2008;28:777–785.
12. Saavedra-Lozano J, Mejías A, Ahmad N, et al. Changing trends in acute osteomyelitis in children: Impact of methicillin-resistant Staphylococcus aureus infections. J Pediatr Orthop 2008;28:569–575.
13. Klevens RM, Edwards JR, Tenover FC, et al. Changes in the epidemiology of methicillin-resistant Staphylococcus aureus in intensive care units in US hospitals, 1992–2003. Clin Infect Dis 2006 Feb 1;42:389–391.
14. Boucher HW, Corey GR. Epidemiology of methicillin-resistant Staphylococcus aureus. Clin Infect Dis 2008;46(suppl 5):S344–S349.
15. King MD, Humphrey BJ, Wang YF, Kourbatova EV, Ray SM, Blumberg HM. Emergence of community-acquired methicillin-resistant Staphylococcus aureus USA 300 clone as the predominant cause of skin and soft-tissue infections. Ann Intern Med 2006;144:309–317.

16. Moran GJ, Krishnadasan A, Gorwitz RJ, et al. Methicillin-resistant S. aureus infections among patients in the emergency department. N Eng J Med 2006;355:666–674.

17. Klevens RM, Morrison MA, Nadle J, et al. Invasive methicillin-resistant Staphylococcus aureus infection in the United States. JAMA 2007;298:1763–1771.

18. Game F, Jeffcoate W. MRSA and osteomyelitis of the foot in diabetes. Diabet Med 2004;21(suppl 4):16–19.

19. Naimi TS, LeDell KH, Como-Sabetti K, et al. Comparison of community- and health care-associated methicillin-resistant Staphylococcus aureus infection. JAMA 2003;290:2976–2984.

20. Hess LM, Jeter JM, Benham-Hutchins M, Alberts DS. Factors associated with osteonecrosis of the jaw among bisphosphonate users. Am J Med 2008;121:475–483.

21. Bertoldo F, Santini D, Lo Cascio V. Bisphosphates and osteomyelitis of the jaw: A pathogenic puzzle. Nat Clin Pract Oncol 2007;4(12):711–721.

22. Steer AC, Carapetis JR. Acute hematogenous osteomyelitis in children: Recognition and management. Pediatric Drugs 2004;6:333–346.

23. Gutierrez K. Bone and joint infections in children. Pediatr Clin North Am 2005;52:779–794.

24. Parsons B, Strauss E. Surgical management of chronic osteomyelitis. Am J Surg 2005;188:S57–S66.

25. Darley ES, MacGowan AP. Antibiotic treatment of gram-positive bone and joint infections. J Antimicrob Chemother 2004;53:928–935.

26. Lazzarini L, Lipsly BA, Mader JT. Antibiotic treatment of osteomyelitis; what have we learned from 30 years of clinical trials? Int J Infect Dis 2005;9:127–138.

27. Rayner CR, Baddour LM, Birmingham MC, et al. Linezolid in the treatment of osteomyelitis: Results of compassionate use experience. Infection 2004;32:8–14.

28. Tice AD, Hoaglund PA, Shoultz DA. Outcomes of osteomyelitis among patients treated with outpatient parenteral antimicrobial therapy. Am J Med 2003;114:723–728.

29. Shuford JA, Steckelberg JM. Role of oral antimicrobial therapy in the management of osteomyelitis. Curr Opin Infect Dis 2003;16:515–519.

30. Moellering Jr RC. Current treatment options for community-acquired methicillin-resistant Staphylococcus aureus infection. Clin Infect Dis 2008;46:1032–1037.

31. Toma MB, Smith KM, Martin CA, Rapp RP. Pharmacokinetic considerations in the treatment of methicillin-resistant Staphylococcus aureus osteomyelitis. Orthopedics 2006;29(6):497–501.

32. Rybak M, Lomaestro B, Rotschafer JC, et al. Therapeutic monitoring of vancomycin in adult patients: A consensus review of the American Society of Health-System Pharmacists, the Infectious Diseases Society of America, and the Society of Infectious Diseases Pharmacists. Am J Health-Syst Pharm 2009;66:82–98.

33. Jones RN. Microbiological features of vancomycin in the 21st century: Minimum inhibitory concentration creep, bactericidal/static activity, and applied breakpoints to predict clinical outcomes or detect resistant strains. Clin Infect Dis 2006;42(Suppl 1):S13–S24.

34. Sakoulas G, Moise Broder PA, Schentag J, et al. Relationship of MIC and bactericidal activity to efficacy of vancomycin for treatment of methicillin-resistant Staphylococcus aureus bacteremia. J Clin Microbiol 2004;42:2398–2402.

35. Moise PA, Sakoulas G, Forrest A et al. Vancomycin in vitro bactericidal activity and its relationship to efficacy in clearance of methicillin-resistant Staphylococcus aureus bacteremia. Antimicrob Agents Chemother 2007;51:2582–2588.

36. Hidayat LK, Hsu DI, Quist R, et al. High-dose vancomycin therapy for methicillin-resistant Staphylococcus aureus infections: Efficacy and toxicity. Arch Intern Med 2006;166:2138–2144.

37. Steinkraus G, White R, Friedrich L. Vancomycin MIC creep in non-vancomycin-intermediate Staphylococcus aureus (VISA), vancomycin-susceptible clinical methicillin-resistant S. aureus (MRSA) blood isolates from 2001–2005. J Antimicrob Chemother 2007;60:788–794.

38. Awad SS, Elhabash SI, Lee L, Farrow B, Berger DH. Increasing incidence of methicillin-resistant Staphylococcus skin and soft-tissue infections: Reconsideration of empiric antimicrobial therapy. Am J Surg 2007;194:606–610.

39. Lamp KC, Friedrich LV, Mendez-Vigo L, Russo R. Clinical experience with daptomycin for the treatment of osteomyelitis. Am J Med 2007;120: S13–S20.

40. Falagas ME, Giannopoulou KP, Ntziora F, Papagelopoulous PJ. Daptomycin for treatment of patients with bone and joint infections: A systemic review of the clinical evidence. Int J Antimicrob Agents 2007;30:202–209.

41. Falagas ME, Siempos II, Papagelopoulos P, Vardakas KZ. Linezolid for the treatment of adults with bone and joint infections. Int J Antimicrob Agents 2007;29:233–239.

42. Sakoulas G, Alder J, Thauvin-Eliopoulos C, et al. Induction of daptomycin heterogeneous susceptibility in Staphylococcus aureus by exposure to vancomycin. Antimicrob Agents Chemother 2006;50:1581–1585.

43. Pfaller MA, Sader HS, Jones RN. Evaluation of the in vitro activity of daptomycin against 19,615 clincial isolates of Gram-positive cocci collected in North American hospitals (2002–2005). Diagn Microbiol Infect 2007;57:459–465.

44. Clinicaltrials.gov. A Service of National Institutes of Health. Osteomyelitis.*www.clinicaltrials.gov/ct2/results?term=osteomyelitis*.

44. Graber CJ, Wong MK, Carleton HA, Perdreau-Remington F, Haller BL, Chamber HF. Intermediate vancomycin susceptibility in a community-associated MRSA clone. Emerg Infect Dis 2007;13:491–493.

45. Lexi-Drugs Online. *www.crlonline.com*.

82 Sepsis and Septic Shock

S. Scott Sutton

LEARNING OBJECTIVES

● **Upon completion of the chapter, the reader will be able to:**

1. Compare and contrast the definitions of syndromes related to sepsis.

2. Identify the pathogens associated with sepsis.

3. Discuss the pathophysiology of sepsis as it relates to pro- and anti-inflammatory mediators.

4. Identify patient symptoms as early or late sepsis and evaluate diagnostic and laboratory tests for patient treatment and monitoring.

5. Assess complications of sepsis and discuss their impact on patient outcomes.

6. Design desired treatment outcomes for septic patients.

7. Formulate a treatment and monitoring plan (pharmacologic and nonpharmacologic) for septic patients.

8. Evaluate patient response and devise alternative treatment regimens for nonresponding septic patients.

KEY CONCEPTS

❶ Sepsis is a continuum of physiologic stages defined by physiologic measures and signs and symptoms of sepsis process.

❷ Gram-positive and gram-negative bacteria, fungal species, and viruses may cause sepsis.

❸ Inflammation is the key factor in the development of sepsis. Patients with severe infections, trauma, debilitating conditions, or an immunocompromised status may experience an imbalance between inflammatory mediators that progresses to sepsis.

❹ The cumulative burden of sepsis complications is the leading factor of mortality. The risk of death increases 20% with failure of each additional organ. Severe sepsis averages two failed organs, with a mortality rate of 40%.

❺ Treatment is aimed at early goal-directed resuscitation; reducing or eliminating organ failures; treating and eliminating the source of infection; avoiding adverse reactions of treatment; and providing cost-effective therapy.

❻ Appropriate empiric anti-infective therapy administered within 1 hour of the recognition of sepsis decreases complications and 28-day mortality.

❼ Drotrecogin alfa may be utilized for patients at a high risk of mortality (as defined by Acute Physiology, Age, and Chronic Health Evaluation II [APACHE II] scores).

Sepsis is a continuum of physiologic stages characterized by infection, systemic inflammation, and hypoperfusion with widespread tissue injury.[1] ❶ *The American College of Chest Physicians and the Society of Critical Care Medicine developed definitions to utilize for sepsis (Table 82–1).*[2] Physiologic parameters categorize patients as having: bacteremia, infection, systemic inflammatory response syndrome (SIRS), sepsis, severe sepsis, septic shock, or multiple-organ dysfunction syndrome (MODS).[2] Standardized definitions have been developed for infections in critically ill patients.[3]

EPIDEMIOLOGY AND ETIOLOGY

Sepsis is the leading cause of morbidity and mortality for critically ill patients, and the tenth leading cause of death overall.[1,4] Sepsis causes 660,000 to 750,000 cases annually, a fourfold increase from 1979.[1,4,5] Care of septic patients costs $17 billion in the United States annually ($22,000–$50,000 per patient).[4,6]

Table 82–1

Definitions Related to Sepsis

Bacteremia (fungemia): Presence of viable bacteria or fungi in the bloodstream

Infection: Inflammatory response to invasion of normally sterile host tissue by microorganisms

SIRS: A systemic inflammatory response to a variety of clinical insults which can be infectious, but can have a noninfectious etiology. The response is manifested by two or more of the following conditions: temperature greater than 38°C (100.4°F) or less than 36°C (96.8°F); pulse greater than 90 bpm; respiratory rate greater than 20 breaths/min or $PaCO_2$ less than 32 torr; WBC count greater than $12 \times 10^3/mm^3$ ($12 \times 10^9/L$), less than $4 \times 10^3/mm^3$ ($4 \times 10^9/L$), or greater than 10% immature (band) forms

Sepsis: The SIRS and documented infection (culture or Gram stain of blood, sputum, urine, or normally sterile body fluid positive for pathogenic microorganisms

Severe sepsis: Sepsis associated with organ dysfunction, hypoperfusion, or hypotension (systolic blood pressure less than 90 mm Hg). Hypoperfusion and perfusion abnormalities may include, but are not limited to, lactic acidosis, oliguria, or acute alteration in mental status

Septic shock: Sepsis with hypotension, despite fluid resuscitation, along with the presence of perfusion abnormalities. Patients who are on inotropic or vasopressor agents may not be hypotensive at the time perfusion abnormalities are measured

MODS: Presence of altered organ function requiring intervention to maintain homeostasis

MODS, multiple-organ dysfunction syndrome; $PaCO_2$, partial pressure of carbon dioxide; SIRS, systemic inflammatory response syndrome.

From Ref. 2.

Table 82–2

Pathogens in Sepsis

Organism	Frequency (%)
Gram-positive bacteria	30–50
Methicillin-susceptible *Staphylococcus aureus*	14–24
Methicillin-resistant *Staphylococcus aureus*	5–11
Other *Staphylococcus* species	1–3
Streptococcus pneumoniae	9–12
Other *Streptococcus* species	6–11
Enterococcus species	3–13
Anaerobes	1–2
Other gram-positive bacteria	1–5
Gram-negative bacteria	25–30
Escherichia coli	9–27
Pseudomonas aeruginosa	8–15
Klebsiella pneumoniae	2–7
Enterobacter species	6–16
Haemophilus influenzae	2–10
Anaerobes	3–7
Other gram-negative bacteria	3–12
Fungi	
Candida albicans	1–3
Other *Candida* species	1–2
Parasites	1–3
Viruses	2–4

From Refs. 4–7.

PATHOPHYSIOLOGY

The development of sepsis is complex and multifactorial. The normal host response to infection is designed to localize and control bacterial invasion and initiate repair of injured tissue through phagocytic cells and inflammatory mediators.[1] Sepsis results when the inflammatory response becomes exaggerated and extends to normal tissue distant from the initial tissue site.

Pro- and Anti-inflammatory Mediators

❸ *The key factor in the development of sepsis is inflammation, which is intended to be a local and contained response to infection or injury. Infection or injury is controlled through pro- and anti-inflammatory mediators.* Proinflammatory mediators facilitate clearance of the injuring stimulus, promote resolution of injury, and are involved in processing of damaged tissue.[1,13–16] In order to control the intensity and duration of the inflammatory response, anti-inflammatory mediators are released that act to regulate proinflammatory mediators.[15–16] The balance between pro- and anti-inflammatory mediators localizes infection/injury of host tissue.[13–16] However, systemic responses ensue when equilibrium in the inflammatory process is lost.

The inflammatory process in sepsis is linked to the coagulation system. Proinflammatory mediators may be procoagulant and antifibrinolytic, whereas anti-inflammatory mediators may be fibrinolytic. A key factor in the inflammation of sepsis is activated protein C, which

Risk factors for sepsis include: age, cancer, immunodeficiency, chronic organ failure, genetic factors (male, and nonwhite ethnic origin in North America), bacteremic patients, and polymorphisms in genes that regulate immunity.[4,7–10] Pulmonary, GI, genitourinary, and bloodstream infections account for the majority of sepsis cases.[4,7,8]

❷ *Gram-positive and gram-negative bacteria, fungal species, and viruses cause sepsis (Table 82–2).* Gram-positive infections account for 30% to 50% of sepsis and septic shock cases.[4,7,8] The percentages of gram-negative, polymicrobial, and viral sepsis cases are 25%, 25%, and 4%, respectively.[4,7,8,11] Multidrug resistant (MDR) bacteria are responsible for approximately 25% of sepsis cases, are difficult to treat, and increase mortality.[7,8] The rate of fungal infections increased 200% from 1979 to 2000.[4] *Candida albicans* is the most common fungal species; however, nonalbicans species (*C. glabrata*, *C. krusei*, and *C. tropicalis*) have increased from 24% to 46%.[4,11,12] Other fungi identified as causes of sepsis include *Cryptococcus*, *Coccidioides*, *Fusarium*, and *Aspergillus*.

enhances fibrinolysis and inhibits inflammation. Protein C levels are decreased in septic patients.

CLINICAL PRESENTATION AND DIAGNOSIS

The clinical presentation of sepsis varies and the rate of development of clinical manifestations may differ from patient to patient. Immunosuppressed patients, those with meningococcemia or *Pseudomonas aeruginosa* infections may progress to late sepsis more rapidly.

A physical examination should be performed rapidly and efficiently, with efforts directed toward uncovering the most likely cause of sepsis. The patient may not provide any medical history; therefore historical data may be obtained from medical records and/or family. The patient's medical condition, recent illnesses, infections, or activities may provide valuable information about the cause of sepsis.

Diagnostic and Laboratory Tests

Microbiologic cultures should be obtained before anti-infective therapy is initiated. However, cultures take 6 to 48 hours for results to be returned and may be negative (no growth of bacterial organisms). Negative cultures do not rule out infection. Administering anti-infectives prior to obtaining cultures may lead to a false negative culture.

Two sets of blood cultures should be obtained to rule out contamination. At least one set should be drawn percutaneously and one drawn through each vascular access device, unless the device was recently (less than 48 hours) inserted.

Physical Examination Results in Sepsis

HEENT: Scleral icterus, dry mucous membranes, pinpoint pupils, dilated and fixed pupils, nystagmus

Neck: Jugular venous distention, carotid bruits

Lungs: Crackles (rales), consolidation, egophony, absent breath sounds

CV: Irregular rhythm, S_3 gallop, murmurs

Abd: Tense, distended, tender, rebound, guarding, hepatosplenomegaly

Rectal: Decreased tone, bright red blood

Exts: Swollen calf, disparity of blood pressure between upper extremities

Neurologic: Agitation, confusion, delirium, obtundation, coma

Skin: Cold, clammy, or warm; hyperemic skin; rashes

Clinical Presentation and Diagnosis of Sepsis

The signs and symptoms of septic patients are referred to as early and late sepsis.

Signs and Symptoms

The initial clinical signs and symptoms represent early sepsis, and they include: fever, chills, and change in mental status. Other signs and symptoms include:

- Tachycardia
- Tachypnea
- Nausea and vomiting
- Hyperglycemia
- Myalgias
- Lethargy and malaise
- Proteinuria
- Leukocytosis
- Hypoxia
- Hyperbilirubinemia

Septic patients may have an elevated, low, or normal temperature. The absence of fever is common in neonates and elderly patients. Hypothermia is associated with a poor prognosis. Hyperventilation may occur before fever and chills and may lead to respiratory alkalosis. Disorientation and confusion may develop early in septic patients, particularly in the elderly and patients with pre-existing neurologic impairment. Disorientation and confusion may be related to the infection or due to sepsis signs and symptoms (e.g., hypoxia).

Late sepsis represents a slow process that develops over several hours of hemodynamic instability. Signs and symptoms of late sepsis include:

- Lactic acidosis
- Oliguria
- Leukopenia
- Thrombocytopenia
- Myocardial depression
- Pulmonary edema
- Hypotension
- Hypoglycemia
- GI hemorrhage

Oliguria often follows hypotension because of decreased perfusion. Metabolic acidosis ensues because of diminished clearance by the kidneys and liver of lactic acid.

Patient Encounter, Part 1

A 67-year-old man with a history of chronic obstructive pulmonary disease presents to the emergency department with high fevers, shaking chills, severe chest pain, and shortness of breath. His family members state that he has been confused all day. He started having a severe cough 2 days ago, with excessive sputum production. He received doxycycline 100 mg twice daily for an upper respiratory tract infection 7 days ago.

What information is suggestive of infection and/or sepsis?

Does this patient have factors that could lead to the development of sepsis?

What information do we need in order to confirm or diagnose sepsis in this patient?

Cultures to obtain if clinical situation suggests infection of specific fluids, tissues, or organs include:

- Urine culture and urinalysis, respiratory secretions, cerebrospinal fluid, wounds
- Laboratory tests to evaluate infection or complications of sepsis include: CBC with differential; coagulation parameters; basic metabolic panel; serum lactate concentration; arterial blood gas.

The use of biomarkers of sepsis have been controversial. Measurement of endotoxin, procalcitonin, or other markers in blood or serum is not routinely recommended. Concentrations of procalcitonin in serum are usually increased in sepsis, but fail to differentiate between infection and inflammation. However, procalcitonin has a high negative predictive value and could allow for the discontinuation of antibiotics.

Complications of Sepsis

❹ Recognition and treatment of sepsis complications, particularly organ failure is essential to improve outcomes. The cumulative burden of sepsis complications is the leading factor of mortality. The risk of death increases 20% with failure of each additional organ. Severe sepsis averages two failed organs, with a mortality rate of 40%. The most common complications are: disseminated intravascular coagulation, acute respiratory distress syndrome (ARDS), acute renal failure (ARF), and hemodynamic compromise.

Disseminated Intravascular Coagulation

Disseminated intravascular coagulation (DIC) complicates 25% to 50% of septic patients, and is an independent predictor of mortality.[17] DIC is a syndrome characterized by coagulation and activation and production of proinflammatory **cytokines**, culminating in intravascular fibrin formation and deposition in the microvasculature. Bleeding results from consumption and exhaustion of coagulation proteins and platelets, because of continued activation of the coagulation system.[17] DIC may produce ARF, hemorrhagic necrosis of the GI mucosa, liver failure, acute pancreatitis, ARDS, and pulmonary failure.[17]

Acute Respiratory Distress Syndrome

ARDS is an acute and persistent lung inflammatory process with increased vascular permeability leading to severe hypoxia that can affect 20% of septic shock patients.[18,19] Lung deterioration is a multiphase process that begins after infection, injury, or exacerbation of the medical condition. The patient appears stable; however, the chest radiograph reveals parenchymal infiltrates. At this time the patient has pulmonary edema and may be hyperventilating.[18,19] During the next phase the patient develops respiratory insufficiency and pulmonary edema can be seen on chest radiographs. Severe hypoxia may ensue, leading to mechanical ventilation.

Acute Renal Failure

ARF occurs in 19% of septic patients, 25% of severe septic patients, and 51% of septic shock patients.[20] Sepsis and ARF together have a 70% mortality, compared to 45% among patients with ARF alone.[20] ARF leads to fluid in the extravascular space, including the lungs, followed by impairment in gas exchange and severe hypoxemia. The hypoxemia will exacerbate ischemia and organ damage. Renal replacement therapy with the use of continuous venovenous hemofiltration and intermittent hemodialysis can be used to facilitate volume and electrolytes.[20]

Hemodynamic Compromise

Arterial vasodilatation is the hallmark of hemodynamic effects related to sepsis. High cardiac output and low systemic vascular resistance characterize arterial vasodilation. Inflammatory cytokines (i.e., tumor necrosis factor-α [TNF-α]) and endotoxin directly depress cardiovascular function. Persistent hypotension offsets the delivery of oxygen to tissues (DO_2) and oxygen consumption by tissues (VO_2).[21] Certain tissues may receive adequate oxygen during sepsis; however, in other tissues oxygen demands may not be met because of decreased perfusion. This perfusion defect is accentuated by increased precapillary atrioventricular shunt. If perfusion decreases, oxygen extraction increases, and the atrioventricular oxygen gradient widens. Cellular DO_2 is decreased, but VO_2 remains unchanged. If perfusion decreases significantly, reserve DO_2 will be exceeded, and tissue ischemia results. Tissue ischemia leads to organ failure. Therefore, increasing oxygen delivery or decreasing oxygen consumption in a hypermetabolic patient should optimize systemic DO_2 relative to VO_2.[21]

TREATMENT AND OUTCOME EVALUATION

Desired Outcomes

⑤ The primary treatment goal of sepsis is to prevent morbidity and mortality. Treatment is aimed at early goal-directed resuscitation; reducing or eliminating organ failures; treating and eliminating the source of infection; avoiding adverse reactions of treatment; and providing cost-effective therapy.[22-28]

General Approach to Treatment

The speed and appropriateness of therapy administered in the initial hours after sepsis develops influences outcome, as is the case for acute myocardial infarction and cerebrovascular accidents.[22]

Pertinent issues in the management of septic patients are (Fig. 82–1):[24]

1. Early goal-directed resuscitation of septic patients during the first 6 hours after recognition.

2. Early administration of broad-spectrum anti-infective therapy.

3. Activated protein C in patients with severe sepsis and high risk of death (Acute Physiology, Age, and Chronic Health Evaluation II [APACHE II] score greater than 25).

4. Hydrocortisone for septic shock patients refractory to resuscitation and vasopressors.

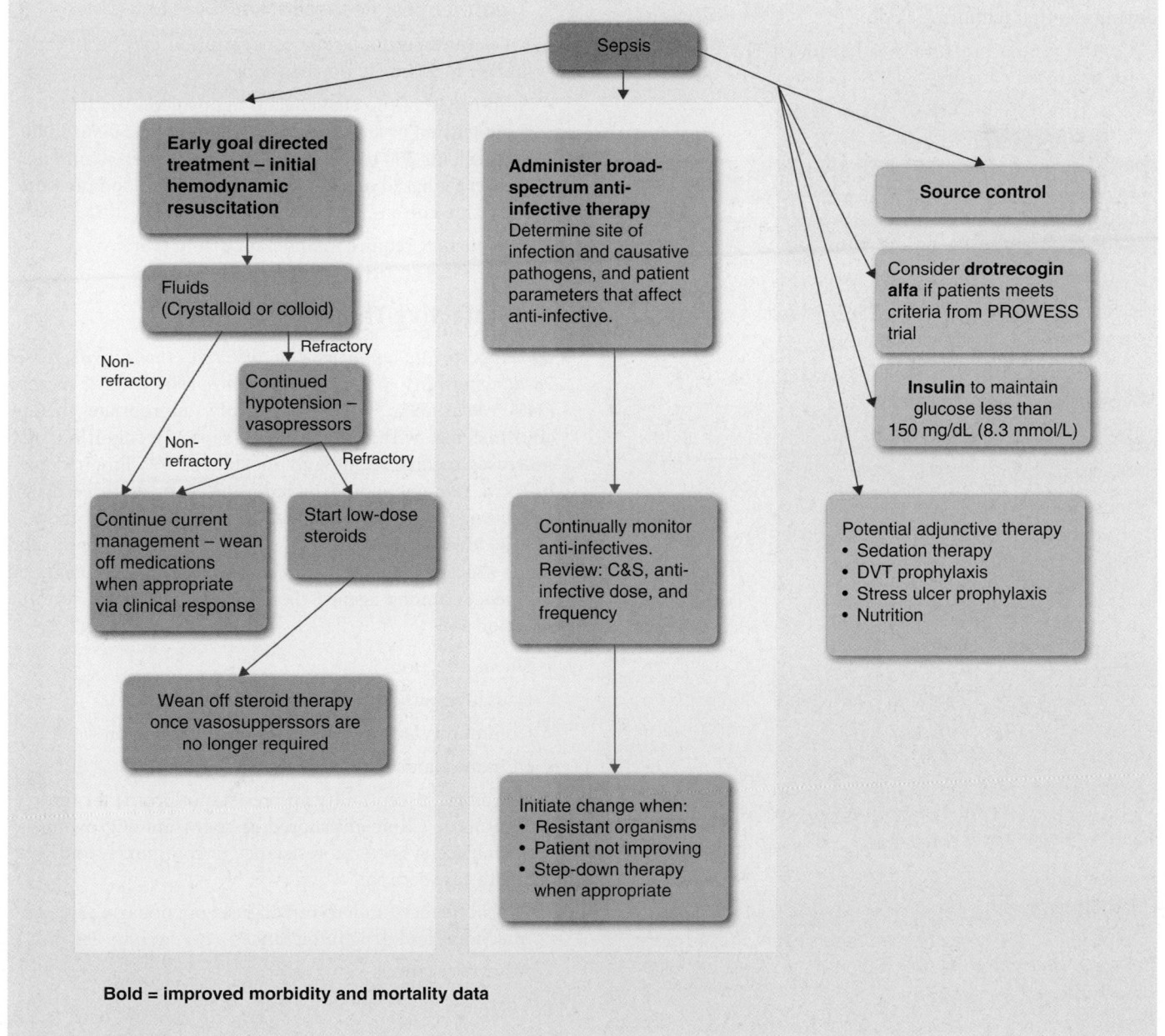

Bold = improved morbidity and mortality data

FIGURE 82–1. Therapeutic approach to sepsis. (C&S, culture and sensitivity.)

5. Glycemic control via infusion of insulin and glucose, to maintain a glucose level less than 150 mg/dL (8.3 mmol/L).

6. Adjunctive therapies: nutrition, deep vein thrombosis (DVT) prophylaxis, stress ulcer prophylaxis, and sedation for mechanically ventilated patients.

Pharmacologic Therapy

Treatment for sepsis focuses on infection, inflammation, hypoperfusion, and widespread tissue injury. Septic patients may require multiple simultaneous treatment regimens to achieve desired outcomes of decreased morbidity and mortality.

Initial Resuscitation

❺ *Early goal-directed resuscitation decreases 28-day mortality in septic patients.* The treatment goals of sepsis-induced hypoperfusion (hypotension or lactic acidosis) during the first 6 hours include[24,27–29]:

- Central venous pressure: 8 to 12 mm Hg (12–15 mm Hg for intubated patients)

Patient Encounter, Part 2: Medical History, Physical Exam, and Diagnostic Tests

PMH: Chronic obstructive pulmonary disease; hypertension; diabetes mellitus; chronic renal insufficiency (baseline serum creatinine 1.6 mg/dL [141 μmol/L])

FH: Father had stroke at age 59; mother has history of hypertension and diabetes mellitus

SH: Construction worker; smoker with a 35 pack-year history

Allergies: NKDA

Meds: No know drug allergies; albuterol/ipratropium inhaler two puffs every 6 hours; glipizide 10 mg once daily; hydrochlorothiazide 25 mg once daily; lisinopril 20 mg once daily

ROS: Unable to obtain; patient has become more confused

PE:

VS: BP 87/53 mm Hg, P 97 bpm, RR 34/min, T 39.3°C (102.7°F)

Lungs: Decreased breath sounds

Labs: Serum creatinine 2.7 mg/dL (239 μmol/L); glucose 298 mg/dL (16.5 mmol/L); white blood cells: leukocytosis with left shift. APACHE II score 27

Cultures: Blood, urine, and respiratory cultures pending.

Radiology: Chest x-ray shows infiltrates in left lower lobe

According to the patient's parameters what does he have (i.e., systemic inflammatory response syndrome, sepsis, or septic shock)?

Identify treatment goals (nonpharmacologic and pharmacologic).

- Mean arterial pressure greater than or equal to 65 mm Hg
- Urine output greater than or equal to 0.5 mL/kg/h
- Central venous or mixed venous oxygen saturation greater than or equal to 70% or 65%, respectively.

Crystalloid (such as 0.9% sodium chloride or lactated Ringer's solutions) or colloid fluids (5% albumin or 6% hetastarch) are used for resuscitation and clinical studies comparing the fluids found them to be equivalent.[29] Crystalloids require more fluids, which may lead to more edema (utilize caution in patients at risk for fluid overload, e.g., congestive heart failure and ARDS); however, colloids are significantly more expensive. Most patients require aggressive fluid resuscitation during the first 24 hours because of persistent venodilation and capillary leak.[24]

▶ *Monitoring Parameters and Alternative Treatment for Resuscitation*[24,27–29]

- An elevated serum lactate concentration may be an early marker for tissue hypoperfusion.
- Administer a fluid challenge to hypovolemic patients (hypotension or lactic acidosis): crystalloids 500 to 1,000 mL; colloids 300 to 500 mL. Administer over 30 minutes and repeat based on response (increase in blood pressure and urine output).
- Patients may require maintenance fluid therapy.

Anti-infective Therapy

❻ *Appropriate empiric anti-infective therapy decreases 28-day mortality compared to inappropriate empiric therapy (24% versus 39%).*[22,23,30] Additionally, appropriate therapy administered within 1 hour of sepsis recognition also decreases complications and mortality.[22,23,30] Empiric anti-infective therapy should include one, two, or three drugs, depending on the site of infection and causative pathogens (Table 82–3). Anti-infective clinical trials in sepsis and septic shock patients are scarce and have not demonstrated differences among agents; therefore, factors that determine selection are:

- Site of infection
- Causative pathogens
- Community- or nosocomial-acquired infection
- Immune status of patient
- Antibiotic susceptibility and resistance profile for the institution. Clinicians should be cognizant of growing prevalence of bacterial resistance in community and health care setting.
- Patient history (underlying disease, previous cultures or infections, and drug intolerance)
- Adverse reactions
- Cost

Anti-infective regimens should be broad-spectrum since there is little margin for error in critically ill patients.

Table 82–3		
Empirical IV Antimicrobial Regimens in Sepsis		
Infection (Site or Type)	**Community Acquired**	**Hospital Acquired**
Urinary tract	Third-generation cephalosporin (ceftriaxone) *or* fluoroquinolone (levofloxacin or ciprofloxacin)	Antipseudomonal penicillin *or* antipseudomonal cephalosporin *or* antipseudomonal carbapenem *plus* aminoglycoside
Community-acquired pneumonia	Third-generation cephalosporin *plus* a macrolide or doxycycline	
Health care–associated, ventilator-associated, or nosocomial pneumonia (early onset; no risk factors for MDR pathogens)		Third-generation cephalosporin *or* fluoroquinolone *or* ampicillin-sulbactam *or* ertapenem
Health care–associated, ventilator-associated, or nosocomial pneumonia (late onset and/or MDR pathogen risk factors)		Antipseudomonal penicillin *or* antipseudomonal cephalosporin *or* antipseudomonal carbapenem *plus* aminoglycoside *or* antipseudomonal fluoroquinolone *plus* vancomycin or linezolid
Intra-abdominal	Ampicillin-sulbactam *or* fluoroquinolone + metronidazole	Piperacillin-tazobactam *or* imipenem or meropenem *or* cefepime *plus* metronidazole *or* ciprofloxacin or levofloxacin *plus* metronidazole
Skin and soft-tissue: Catheter-related Unknown source of infection	Nafcillin or cefazolin	Ceftriaxone ± vancomycin Vancomycin Antipseudomonal penicillin ± antipseudomonal cephalosporin *or* antipseudomonal carbapenem *plus* aminoglycoside *plus* vancomycin

MDR, multidrug resistant.

From Refs. 31–37.

▶ Monitoring and Treatment Strategies to Maximize Efficacy and Minimize Toxicity for Anti-infectives

- Administer broad-spectrum anti-infectives for initial therapy, as early as possible and within first hour of recognition of sepsis.
- Appropriate cultures should be obtained before initiating antibiotic therapy, but should not prevent prompt administration of treatment.
- Administer antibiotics that concentrate at the site of infection.
- Monitor patient parameters to ensure adequate dosing.
- Abnormal renal and hepatic function will increase drug concentration and predispose the patient to toxicity.
- Septic patients may have altered volume of distribution due to initial resuscitation.
- Reevaluate the initial regimen daily to optimize activity, prevent development of resistance, reduce toxicity, and decrease costs.
- Initiate step-down therapy based on microbiologic cultures to: prevent resistance, reduce toxicity, and cost.
- Monotherapy is equivalent to combination therapy once a causative pathogen has been identified. Empiric therapy should include combination regimens to ensure coverage of causative organisms.

Clinical Parameters for Aminoglycosides

Tobramycin is more active against *Pseudomonas aeruginosa* than gentamicin, whereas gentamicin is more active against *Serratia* species. Amikacin is the most potent aminoglycoside against the Enterobacteriaceae; however, it should be reserved for bacterial organisms resistant to gentamicin and tobramycin. Select an aminoglycoside based on:

- Local susceptibility patterns
- Patient parameters (infection and microbiologic culture history)
- Cost

Aminoglycosides may be administered by traditional methods (1.5–2 mg/kg every 8 hours) or by an extended dosing interval method (4–7 mg/kg every 24 hours). The extended dosing method maximizes the pharmacodynamic properties of aminoglycosides (concentration-dependent killing and postantibiotic effect) and reduces the incidence of nephrotoxicity. Extended dosing interval aminoglycosides have prolonged drug-free periods, during which the saturable uptake of aminoglycosides into the proximal renal tubular cells can be completed. Extended dosing interval aminoglycosides should not be used in pediatric patients, burn victims, pregnant patients, patients with pre-existing or progressive renal insufficiency, or for synergy with gram-positive organisms.[38]

Selection of Antimicrobial Agents

▶ *Urinary Tract Infections*

● Septic patients with a community-acquired urinary tract infection should be treated with a third-generation cephalosporin (ceftriaxone or cefotaxime) or a fluoroquinolone (ciprofloxacin or levofloxacin). ❷ The causative pathogen is commonly an enteric gram-negative bacilli (i.e., *Escherichia coli*). ❷ Nosocomially-acquired urinary tract infections are often related to catheters and are caused by fermenting and nonfermenting (*Pseudomonas*) gram-negatives, and *enterococci* (see Table 82–3). β-Lactam/β-lactamase inhibitors (i.e., piperacillin-tazobactam), an antipseudomonal cephalosporin (i.e., cefepime or ceftazidime), or an antipseudomonal carbapenem (imipenem, meropenem, or doripenem), plus an aminoglycoside are recommended treatment options until susceptibilities are known (see Table 82–3).[31]

▶ *Community-Acquired Pneumonia*

● Septic patients with community-acquired pneumonia (CAP) are treated with a third-generation cephalosporin (ceftriaxone or cefotaxime) plus a macrolide (azithromycin or clarithromycin) or doxycycline, or a respiratory fluoroquinolone (levofloxacin, moxifloxacin, gemifloxacin) (see Table 82–3).[32] ❷ *The causative organisms for CAP are Streptococcus pneumoniae, Haemophilus influenzae, Moraxella catarrhalis, and atypical organisms (Mycoplasma pneumoniae, Chlamydia pneumoniae, and Legionella pneumophila).* S. pneumoniae accounts for 60% of the deaths associated with CAP, and is resistant to penicillin and macrolides (multidrug resistant *S. pneumoniae*; MDRSP) 30% to 40% of the time.[32,33] Controversy exists relating to the clinical significance of this resistance for nonmeningitis infections. Respiratory fluoroquinolones (levofloxacin, moxifloxacin, and gemifloxacin) may be utilized for MDRSP; however, clinical data have not shown them to be superior to cephalosporins plus a macrolide or doxycycline. The Centers for Disease Control and Prevention recommends reserving fluoroquinolones as last-line options in order to maintain their broad-spectrum antibacterial activity.[33] Treatment of methicillin-resistant *Staphylococcus aureus* (MRSA) or *Pseudomonas aeruginosa* is a potential reason to modify the standard empirical regimen for CAP. Risk factors for the development of these pathogens are listed in Table 82–4.

▶ *Hospital-, Ventilator-, and Health Care–Associated Pneumonia*

● Treatment for septic patients with hospital-acquired, ventilator-acquired, and health care–associated pneumonia is dependent on risk factors for MDR organisms (Fig. 82–2). Recommended treatment for patients with no MDR risk factors are: third-generation cephalosporins (ceftriaxone or cefotaxime), fluoroquinolones (levofloxacin and moxifloxacin),

Table 82–4
Risk Factors for MRSA, *Pseudomonas*, and Gram-Negatives in CAP
Methicillin-Resistant *Staphylococcus aureus*
End stage renal disease
Injection drug abuse
Prior influenza
Prior antibiotic therapy (especially fluoroquinolones)
Pseudomonas aeruginosa
Structural lung disease
Exacerbations of severe chronic obstructive pulmonary diseases leading to frequent steroid and/or antibiotic use, as well as prior antibiotic therapy
Other Gram-negatives (*Klebsiella pneumoniae* or *Acinetobacter* species)
Chronic alcoholism

From Ref. 33.

ampicillin-sulbactam, or ertapenem (see Table 82–3).[34] Recommended treatment for patients with MDR risk factors are: β-lactam/β-lactamase inhibitors (piperacillin/tazobactam), antipseudomonal cephalosporin (cefepime or ceftazidime), or an antipseudomonal carbapenem (imipenem, meropenem, or doripenem), plus an aminoglycoside, plus vancomycin or linezolid (see Table 82–3).[34] If an aminoglycoside is undesirable, a antipseudomonal fluoroquinolone (ciprofloxacin or levofloxacin) may be utilized with a antipseudomonal β-lactam (piperacillin/tazobactam, cefepime, ceftazidime, imipenem, meropenem, or doripenem).

▶ *Skin and Soft-Tissue Infections*

● ❷ *Community-acquired skin and soft-tissue infections are caused by Streptococcus pyogenes and S. aureus.* Treatment with nafcillin or cefazolin is recommended (see Table 82–3).[35] Soft-tissue infections caused by S. pyogenes can lead to streptococcal toxic shock syndrome. Although penicillins and cephalosporins are efficacious, experimental models show clindamycin to be more effective than penicillin.[31] Hospital-acquired skin and soft-tissue infections are caused by S. pyogenes, S. aureus, ● and enteric gram-negatives. Recommended treatment is a third-generation cephalosporin (cefotaxime or ceftriaxone), ampicillin-sulbactam, or ertapenem, plus vancomycin (see Table 82–3).[35]

▶ *Intra-abdominal Infections*

● ❷ *Intra-abdominal infections are polymicrobial, including enteric aerobes and anaerobes.* Patients with community-acquired intra-abdominal infections of mild to moderate severity should be administered antibiotics with activity against enteric ● gram-negative bacilli, gram-negative anaerobes, and gram-positive cocci. Recommended treatment for mild to moderate community-acquired intra-abdominal infections are: ampicillin/sulbactam; cephalosporins (ceftriaxone or cefotaxime) plus metronidazole; fluoroquinolones (levofloxacin, ciprofloxacin, or moxifloxacin) plus metronidazole; and ertapenem (see

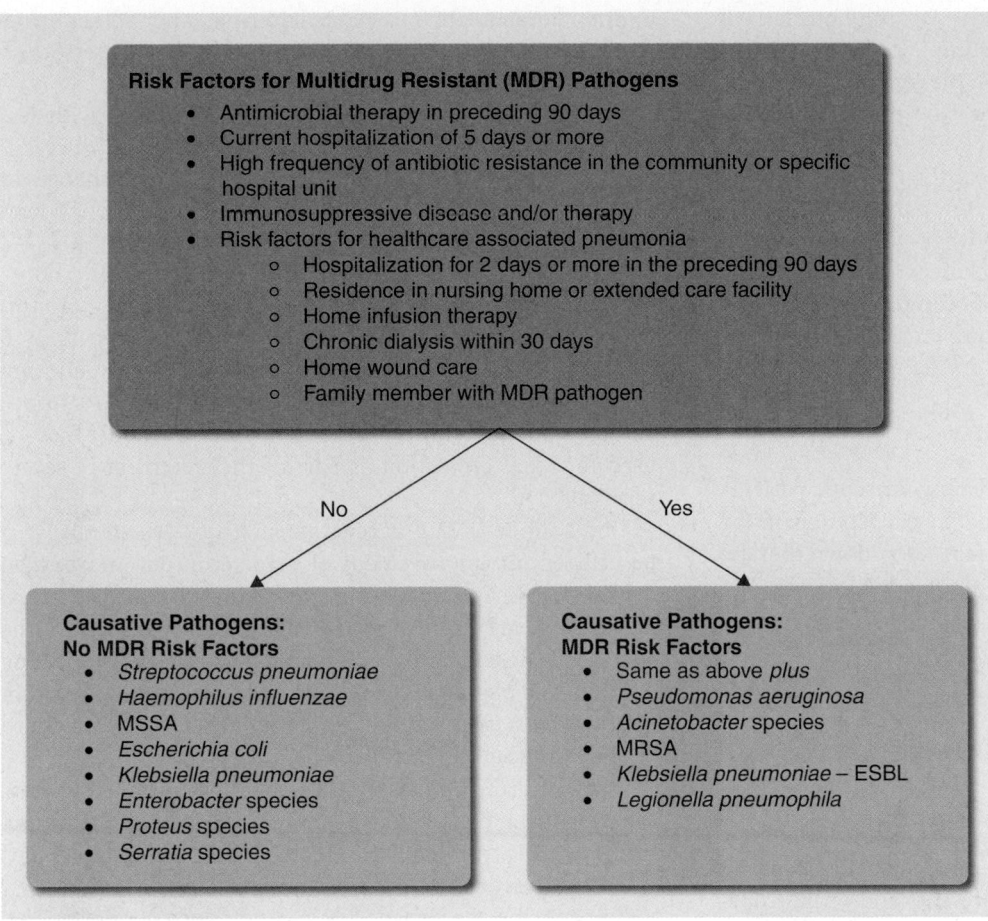

Risk Factors for Multidrug Resistant (MDR) Pathogens
- Antimicrobial therapy in preceding 90 days
- Current hospitalization of 5 days or more
- High frequency of antibiotic resistance in the community or specific hospital unit
- Immunosuppressive disease and/or therapy
- Risk factors for healthcare associated pneumonia
  - Hospitalization for 2 days or more in the preceding 90 days
  - Residence in nursing home or extended care facility
  - Home infusion therapy
  - Chronic dialysis within 30 days
  - Home wound care
  - Family member with MDR pathogen

No   Yes

Causative Pathogens: No MDR Risk Factors
- *Streptococcus pneumoniae*
- *Haemophilus influenzae*
- MSSA
- *Escherichia coli*
- *Klebsiella pneumoniae*
- *Enterobacter* species
- *Proteus* species
- *Serratia* species

Causative Pathogens: MDR Risk Factors
- Same as above *plus*
- *Pseudomonas aeruginosa*
- *Acinetobacter* species
- MRSA
- *Klebsiella pneumoniae* – ESBL
- *Legionella pneumophila*

FIGURE 82–2. Risk factors for multidrug resistant pathogens and causative pathogens for hospital, ventilator, and health care–associated pneumonia.[34] (ESBL, extended spectrum β-lactamase; MDR, multidrug resistant; MRSA, methicillin-resistant *Staphylococcus aureus*; MSSA, methicillin-sensitive *Staphylococcus aureus*.)

Clinical Dilemma About MRSA

MRSA is a common hospital-acquired pathogen and is also increasing in the community. MRSA has presented a problem in the past because it required treatment with vancomycin. Community-acquired MRSA presents a major therapeutic challenge. MRSA can cause pneumonia, cellulitis, and other infections. Clinicians should be aware of the rate of hospital and community MRSA in your geographic area. New treatment options are available for MRSA. They include linezolid, tigecycline, and daptomycin. Prospective clinical trials have not demonstrated benefits of these agents over vancomycin.[39,40]

Patient Encounter, Part 3

Treatment and Outcome Evaluation

The patient has continued hypotension despite previous intervention. Continued hypoxia has led to mechanical ventilation. The patient's serum creatinine has risen to 6.8 mg/dL (601 μmol/L). Blood cultures reveal gram-positive cocci and lactose-negative oxidase-positive gram-negative rods.

Design a therapeutic regimen for this patient. Include all necessary medications.

Table 82–3).[36] Patients with nosocomial-acquired, high-severity intra-abdominal infections or immunosuppression should receive empiric treatment with broad-spectrum antibiotics. Broad-spectrum antibiotics such as antipseudomonal β-lactam/β-lactamase inhibitors (piperacillin/tazobactam), carbapenems (imipenem, meropenem, or doripenem), antipseudomonal cephalosporins (cefepime or ceftazidime) plus metronidazole, or antipseudomonal fluoroquinolones (ciprofloxacin or levofloxacin) plus metronidazole are recommended (see Table 82–3).[36]

Antifungal Therapy

❷ *Septic patients not responding to conventional antibiotics should be evaluated for fungal infections. Candida albicans is the most common fungal species; however, the prevalence of nonalbicans species is increasing. Amphotericin B is utilized in septic patients with fungal or suspected fungal infections because of greater activity against nonalbicans Candida compared to fluconazole.*[37] However, amphotericin B has a significantly higher rate of adverse reactions.

Lipid formulations of amphotericin B (amphotericin B cholesteryl sulfate complex, lipid complex, and liposomal amphotericin B) are available that are less nephrotoxic and have decreased infusion-associated side effects. Efficacy among the amphotericin products is equivalent, but the lipid formulations are significantly more expensive. Lipid products are recommended for patients intolerant of conventional amphotericin. Other alternatives for treatment of fungal infections include voriconazole and echinocandins (anidulafungin, caspofungin, micafungin). Data are lacking that demonstrate clinical superiority between agents.

Duration of Therapy

Average duration of anti-infective therapy for septic patients is 7 to 10 days. However, the durations vary depending on the site of infection and response to therapy. Step-down therapy from IV to oral anti-infectives is recommended for:

- Hemodynamically stable patients
- Patients afebrile for 48 to 72 hours
- Patients with normalized WBC
- Patients able to take oral medications

Vasopressors and Inotropic Therapy

When fluid resuscitation does not provide adequate arterial pressure and organ perfusion, vasopressors and/or inotropic agents should be initiated. Vasopressors are recommended in patients with a systolic blood pressure less than 90 mm Hg or mean arterial pressure (MAP) lower than 60 to 65 mm Hg, after failed treatment with crystalloids.[24,27,28] Vasopressors and inotropes are effective in treating life-threatening hypotension and improving cardiac index, but complications such as tachycardia and myocardial ischemia require slow titration of the adrenergic agents to restore MAP without impairing stroke volume. Vasopressor therapy may also be required transiently to sustain life and maintain perfusion in the face of life-threatening hypotension, even when fluid resuscitation is in progress and hypovolemia has not yet been corrected. Agents commonly considered for vasopressor or inotropic support include dopamine, dobutamine, norepinephrine, phenylephrine, and epinephrine. Norepinephrine or dopamine are first-line vasopressors to correct hypotension in septic shock.[24,27,28]

Norepinephrine is a potent α-adrenergic agent with less pronounced β-adrenergic activity. Doses of 0.01 to 3 mcg/kg/min can reliably increase blood pressure with small changes in heart rate or cardiac index. Norepinephrine is a more potent agent than dopamine in refractory septic shock.[24,27,28]

Dopamine is a α- and β-adrenergic agent with dopaminergic activity. Low doses of dopamine (1–5 mcg/kg/min) maintain renal perfusion, higher doses (greater than 5 mcg/kg/min) exhibit α- and β-adrenergic activity and are frequently utilized to support blood pressure and to improve cardiac function. Low doses of dopamine should not be used for renal protection as part of the treatment of severe sepsis.[24,27,28]

Dobutamine is a β-adrenergic inotropic agent that can be utilized for improvement of cardiac output and oxygen delivery. Doses of 2 to 20 mcg/kg/min increase cardiac index; however, heart rate increases significantly. Dobutamine should be considered in septic patients with adequate filling pressure and blood pressure, but low cardiac index. If used in hypotensive patients, dobutamine should be combined with vasopressor therapy.[24,27,28]

Phenylephrine is a fast-acting, short-duration $\alpha1$ agonist. Phenylephrine has primarily vascular effects, and does not impair cardiac or renal function. Phenylephrine is useful when tachycardia limits the use of other vasopressors.[24,27-28]

Epinephrine is a nonspecific α- and β-adrenergic agonist. Epinephrine can increase cardiac index and produce significant peripheral vasoconstriction. However, it can also increase lactate levels and impair blood flow to the splanchnic system. Because of these undesirable effects, epinephrine should be reserved for patients who fail to respond to traditional therapies.[24,27,28]

Vasopressin levels are increased during hypotension to maintain blood pressure by vasoconstriction. However, there is a vasopressin deficiency in septic shock. Low doses of vasopressin increase MAP, leading to the discontinuation of vasopressors. However, routine use of vasopressin is not recommended because of lack of evidence of efficacy. Vasopressin is a direct vasoconstrictor without inotropic or chronotropic effects and may result in decreased cardiac output and hepatosplanchnic flow. Vasopressin use may be considered in patients with refractory shock despite adequate fluid resuscitation and high-dose vasopressors.[24,27,28]

Recombinant Human Activated Protein C

⑦ Recombinant human activated protein C (drotrecogin alfa) is recommended for patients at a high risk of death (APACHE II score greater than or equal to 25, multiple-organ failure, septic shock, or ARDS) and no absolute contraindications related to bleeding.[41] Drotrecogin alfa has antithrombotic, anti-inflammatory, and profibrinolytic properties. The Recombinant Human Activated Protein C Worldwide Evaluation in Severe Sepsis (PROWESS) trial

---

Clinical Controversy

Enterococcus species are normal inhabitants of the GI tract, but should empiric treatment of intra-abdominal infections have activity against *Enterococcus* species? Empiric treatment that covered *Enterococcus* species in intra-abdominal infections was equivalent to empiric treatment that lacked enterococcal coverage. Routine coverage for *Enterococcus* is not necessary for patients with community-acquired intra-abdominal infections. However, in patients with nosocomial or high-severity infections, enterococcal coverage may be warranted.[36]

evaluated the effects of a 96-hour continuous infusion of drotrecogin alfa. Drotrecogin alfa decreased 28-day mortality compared to placebo (30.8% versus 24.7%). A higher incidence of serious bleeding occurred during the 28-day period in the drotrecogin alfa group (3.5%) than in the placebo group (2.0%). An analysis of secondary endpoints suggested that the incidence of multiple-organ dysfunction was lower in patients treated with drotrecogin alfa, and that therapy was associated with more rapid recovery of cardiac and pulmonary function. A second study of patients with severe sepsis, Extended Evaluation of Recombinant Human Activated Protein C (ENHANCE) trial noted that 28-day all cause mortality for patients treated with drotrecogin alfa was similar to that observed in PROWESS. ENHANCE also found that patients treated within the first 24 hours of their first sepsis-induced organ dysfunction had significantly lower mortality than those treated after 24 hours (22.9–27.4%). Cost-effectiveness models have found that for septic patients with a APACHE II score greater than or equal to 25, the cost per year of life saved with drotrecogin alfa is $24,000 to $27,000, suggesting that this is a cost-effective therapy in patients with severe sepsis and septic shock. The effect of drotrecogin alfa on long-term survival was evaluated in a retrospective analysis of patients in PROWESS. The mortality benefit of drotrecogin alfa persisted up to hospital discharge; however, there were no mortality differences between drotrecogin alfa and placebo thereafter.[42]

❼ Drotrecogin alfa is not recommended for severe sepsis patients at low risk for death. The Administration of Drotrecogin Alpha in Early Stage Severe Sepsis (ADDRESS) trial evaluated the effects of a 96-hour continuous infusion of drotrecogin alfa. There were no statistically significant differences between drotrecogin alfa and placebo in 28-day mortality (18.5% versus 17.0%).[43] The rate of serious bleeding was higher for drotrecogin alfa during the 96-hour infusion and the 28-day study period.

Steroids

Stress-induced adrenal insufficiency complicates 9% to 24% of septic patients and is associated with increased mortality. Septic shock patients refractory to resuscitation and vasopressors should be administered IV hydrocortisone 200 to 300 mg/day in three divided doses.[24,44] Patients should be weaned from steroid therapy when vasopressors are no longer required.

Patient Encounter, Part 4

During medical rounds, you are asked to discuss clinical trials.

What antibiotics are found to be superior in septic patients?

What are the results of the PROWESS and ADDRESS trials?

Is this patient a candidate for drotrecogin alfa?

Sedation and Neuromuscular Blockade

Patients with ARDS and progressive hypoxia require mechanical ventilation. Critically ill patients may require sedation when high ventilator settings are used or when patients fight the ventilator. Mechanically ventilated patients should receive sedation by a protocol that includes a daily interruption or lightening of a sedative infusion until the patient is awake.[24] The utilization of sedation protocols decreases the duration of mechanical ventilation, length of hospitalization, and tracheostomy rates.

Paralysis usually is reserved for patients in whom sedation alone does not improve the effectiveness of mechanical ventilation. Neuromuscular blockers may lead to prolonged skeletal muscle weakness and should be avoided if possible. Patients requiring neuromuscular blockade should be monitored and intermittent boluses or continuous infusion should be utilized. Monitor depth of neuromuscular blockade with train-of-four stimulation when using continuous infusion.

Glucose Control

Glycemic control improves survival in postoperative surgical patients and is recommended in septic patients. Following initial stabilization of septic patients, maintain blood glucose concentrations less than 150 mg/dL (8.3 mmol/L).[24,45] Septic patients with high glucose concentrations should receive insulin and glucose with frequent blood glucose monitoring (every 1 to 2 hours until glucose values and insulin infusion rates are stable, then every 4 hours).

Adjunctive Therapies

Enteral nutrition is recommended in septic patients to meet the increased energy and protein requirements. Protein requirements are increased to 1.5 to 2.5 g/kg/day. Nonprotein caloric requirements range from 25 to 40 kcal/kg/day (105–168 kJ/kg/day).[24]

DVT prophylaxis is recommended for septic patients. Low-dose unfractionated heparin or low-molecular-weight heparin (such as enoxaparin or dalteparin) may be utilized. Graduated compression stockings or an intermittent compression device is recommended for patients with a contraindication to heparin products (thrombocytopenia, severe coagulopathy, active bleeding, or recent intracerebral hemorrhage).[24] Patients with severe sepsis and history of DVT, trauma, or orthopedic surgery should receive a combination of pharmacologic and mechanical therapy unless contraindicated or not practical.

Stress ulcer prophylaxis is recommended in septic patients. Patients at greatest risk for stress ulcers are: coagulopathic, mechanically ventilated, and hypotensive. Histamine-receptor antagonists (such as ranitidine) are more efficacious than sucralfate, and proton pump inhibitors (such as omeprazole) have not been compared to histamine-receptor antagonists. However, they do demonstrate equivalence in the ability to increase gastric pH.[24] The benefit of prophylaxis must be weighed against the potential effect of an increased stomach pH and development of hospital-acquired pneumonia.

Nonpharmacologic Therapy

❺ *Evaluate septic patients for the presence of a localized infection amenable to source control measures.* Common source control measures include drainage and debridement, device removal, and prevention.[24-26] Implementation of source control methods should be instituted as soon as possible following initial fluid resuscitation. The selection of optimal source control methods must weigh benefits and risks of the intervention. Source control measures may cause complications (bleeding, fistulas, and organ injury), therefore the method with the least risk should be employed.[24]

Prognosis

There are various factors that influence outcome. Gram-negative bacteria are more likely to produce septic shock than gram-positive bacteria (50% versus 25%) and have a higher mortality than other pathogens. This may be related to the severity of the underlying condition. Patients with rapidly fatal conditions, such as leukemia, aplastic anemia, and burn patients have a worse prognosis than patients with nonfatal underlying conditions, such as diabetes mellitus or chronic renal insufficiency. Other factors that worsen the prognosis of septic patients are: advanced age, malnutrition, resistant bacteria, utilization of medical devices, and immunosuppression. Data for long-term mortality are lacking (it is estimated that the mortality for sepsis survivors within the first year is 20%).[5] Patients may have prolonged physical disability related to muscle weakness and posttraumatic stress.

Abbreviations Introduced in This Chapter

ADDRESS	Administration of Drotrecogin Alpha in Early Stage Severe Sepsis
APACHE II	Acute Physiology, Age, and Chronic Health Evaluation II
ARDS	Acute respiratory distress syndrome
ARF	Acute renal failure
CAP	Community-acquired pneumonia
DIC	Disseminated intravascular coagulation
DO_2	Delivery of oxygen to tissues
DVT	Deep vein thrombosis
ENHANCE	Extended Evaluation of Recombinant Human Activated Protein C
MAP	Mean arterial pressure
MDR	Multidrug resistant
MDRSP	Multidrug resistant *Streptococcus pneumoniae*
MODS	Multiple-organ dysfunction syndrome
MRSA	Methicillin-resistant *Staphylococcus aureus*
MSSA	Methicillin-sensitive *S. aureus*
$PaCO_2$	Partial pressure of carbon dioxide
PROWESS	Recombinant Human Activated Protein C Worldwide Evaluation in Severe Sepsis (study) systemic inflammatory response syndrome
SIRS	Systemic inflammatory response syndrome
TNF-α	Tumor necrosis factor-α
VO_2	Oxygen consumption by tissues

Patient Care and Monitoring

1. Evaluate patient parameters and classify as infection, SIRS, sepsis, severe sepsis, septic shock, or MODS.

2. Review available diagnostic and laboratory data.

3. Evaluate early goal-directed resuscitation therapy. Understand what parameters define efficacy and failure of initial therapy. Recommend alternative resuscitation therapy if the patient does not respond to initial fluid challenge.

4. Evaluate the source of infection and make recommendations to remove potential source(s).

5. Analyze anti-infective therapy (dose, frequency, and duration) and revise as necessary based on clinical response and culture and sensitivity reports. Prepare an appropriate step-down therapy for the patient.

6. Determine the risk of sepsis complications and construct recommendations for treatment and monitoring.

7. Formulate appropriate doses of medications involved in patient therapy and revise as needed. Patient parameters may change frequently, thus requiring different doses and/or medications. Examples include: antibiotic therapy, sedatives, insulin, fluids, or vasopressors.

8. Continually monitor patient parameters to ensure optimal therapy to maximize outcomes.

 Self-assessment questions and answers are available at *http://www.mhpharmacotherapy.com/pp.html.*

REFERENCES

1. Hotchkiss RS, Karl IE. The pathophysiology and treatment of sepsis. N Engl J Med 2003;348:138–150.
2. American College of Chest Physicians, Society of Critical Care Medicine Consensus Conference. Definitions for sepsis and organ failure and guidelines for the use of innovative therapies in sepsis. Crit Care Med 1992;20:864–874.
3. Calandra T, Cohen J. The international sepsis forum consensus conference on definitions of infection in the intensive care unit. Crit Care Med 2005;33:1538–1548.
4. Martin GS, Mannino DM, Eaton S, Moss M. The epidemiology of sepsis in the United States from 1979 through 2000. N Engl J Med 2003;348:1546–1554.
5. Annane D, Bellissant E, Cavaillon JM. Septic shock. Lancet 2005;365: 63–78.

6. Angus DC, Linde-Zwirble WT, Lidicker J, et al. Epidemiology of severe sepsis in the United States: Analysis of incidence, outcome, and associated costs of care. Crit Care Med 2001;29:1303–1310.

7. Annane D, Aegerter P, Jars-Guincestre MC, Guidet B. Current epidemiology of septic shock: The CUB-Rea Network. Am J Respir Crit Care Med 2003;1687:165–172.

8. Alberti C, Brun-Buisson C, Burchardi H, et al. Epidemiology of sepsis and infection in ICU patients from an international multicentre cohort study. Intensive Care Med 2002;28:108–121.

9. Hubacek JA, Stuber F, Frohlich D, et al. Gene variants of the bactericidal/permeability increasing protein and lipopolysaccharide binding protein in sepsis patients: Gender-specific genetic predisposition to sepsis. Crit Care Med 2001;29:557–561.

10. Lin MT, Albertson TE. Genomic polymorphisms in sepsis. Crit Care Med 2004;32:569–579.

11. Bodey GP, Mardani M, Hanna HA, et al. The epidemiology of Candida glabrata and Candida albicans fungemia in immunocompromised patients with cancer. Am J Med 2002;112:380–385.

12. Costa SF, Marino I, Araujo EA, et al. Nosocomial fungemia: A 2-year prospective study. J Hosp Infect 2000:45:69–72.

13. Marie C, Muret J, Fitting C, et al. Interleukin-1 receptor antagonist production during infectious and noninfectious systemic inflammatory response syndrome. Crit Care Med 2000;28:2277–2282.

14. Opal SM, Girard TD, Ely EW. The immunopathogenesis of sepsis in elderly patients. Clin Infect Dis 2005;41:S504–S512.

15. Kim PK, Deutschman CS. Inflammatory responses and mediators. Surg Clin North Am 2000;80:885–894.

16. van der Poll T, van Deventer SJH. Cytokines and anticytokines in the pathogenesis of sepsis. Infect Dis Clinic North Am 1999;13:413–426.

17. Zeerleder S, Hack CE, Wuillemin WA. Disseminated intravascular coagulation in sepsis. Chest 2005;128:2864–2875.

18. Wheeler AP, Bernard GR. Treating patients with severe sepsis. N Engl J Med 1999;340:207–214.

19. Hirrela E. Advances in the management of acute respiratory distress syndrome. Arch Surg 2000;135:126–134.

20. Schrier RW, Wang W. Acute renal failure and sepsis. N Engl J Med 2004;351:159–169.

21. Awad SS. State-of-the-art therapy for sepsis and multisystem organ failure. Am J Surg 2003;186:23S–30S.

22. Harbarth S, Garbino J, Pugin J, et al. Inappropriate initial antimicrobial therapy and its effects on survival in a clinical trial of immunomodulating therapy for severe sepsis. Am J Med 2003;115:529–535.

23. Garnacho-Montero J, Garcia-Garmendia JL, Barrero-Almodovar A, et al. Impact of adequate empirical antibiotic therapy on the outcome of patients admitted to the intensive care unit with sepsis. Crit Care Med 2003;31:2742–2751.

24. Dellinger RP, Levy MM, Carlet JM, et al. Surviving Sepsis Campaign: International guidelines for the management of severe sepsis and septic shock:2008. Crit Care Med 2008;36:296–327.

25. Jimenez MF, Marshall JC. Source control in the management of sepsis. Intensive Care Med 2001;27:S49–S62.

26. Centers for Disease Control and Prevention. Guidelines for the prevention of catheter-related infections. MMWR 2002;51:1–29.

27. Rivers E, Nguyen B, Havstad S, et al., for the Early Goal-directed Therapy Collaborative Group. Early goal-directed therapy in the treatment of severe sepsis and septic shock. N Engl J Med 2001;345:1368–1377.

28. Hollenberg SM, Ahrens TS, Annane D, et al. Practice parameters for hemodynamic support of sepsis in adult patients: 2004 update. Crit Care Med 2004;32:1928–1948.

29. Finfer S, Bellomo R, Boyce N, et al. A comparison of albumin and saline for fluid resuscitation in the intensive care unit. N Engl J Med 2004;350:2247–2256.

30. MacArthur RD, Miller M, Albertson T, et al. Adequacy of early empiric antibiotic treatment and survival in severe sepsis: Experience from the MONARCS trial. Clin Infect Dis 2004;38:284–288.

31. Simon D, Trenholme G. Antibiotic selection for patients with septic shock. Crit Care Clin 2000;16:215–231.

32. Mandell LA, Wunderink RG, Anzueto A, et al. Infectious Diseases Society of America / American Thoracic Society Consensus Guidelines on the Management of Community-Acquired Pneumonia in Adults. Clin Infect Dis 2007;44:S27–S72.

33. Heffelfinger JD, Dowell SF, Jorgensen JH, et al. Management of community-acquired pneumonia in the era of pneumococcal resistance: A report from the Drug-Resistant Streptococcus pneumoniae Therapeutic Working Group. Arch Intern Med 2000;160:1399–1408.

34. American Thoracic Society and the Infectious Diseases Society of America. Guidelines for the management of adults with hospital-acquired, ventilator-associated, and healthcare-associated pneumonia. Am J Respir Crit Care Med 2005;171:388–416.

35. Stevens DL, Bisno AL, Chambers HF, et al. Practice guidelines for the diagnosis and management of skin and soft-tissue infections. Clin Infect Dis 2005;41:1373–1406.

36. Solomkin JS, Mazuski JE, Baron EL, et al. Guidelines for the selection of anti-infective agents for complicated intra-abdominal infections. Clin Infect Dis 2003;37:997–1005.

37. Pappas PG, Rex JH, Sobel JD, et al. Guidelines for treatment of candidiasis. Clin Infect Dis 2004;38:161–189.

38. Wallace AW, Jones M, Bertino JS. Evaluation of four once-daily aminoglycoside dosing nomograms. Pharmacotherapy 2002;22:1077–1083.

39. Zetola N, Francis JS, Nuermberger EL, Bishai WR. Community-acquired methicillin-resistant Staphylococcus aureus: An emerging threat. Lancet Infect Dis 2005;5:275–286.

40. Crum NF. The emergence of severe, community-acquired methicillin-resistant Staphylococcus aureus infections. Scand J Infect Dis 2005;39:651–656.

41. Bernard GR, Vincent JL, Laterre PF, et al., for the Recombinant Human Protein C Worldwide Evaluation in Severe Sepsis (PROWESS) study group. Efficacy and safety of recombinant human activated protein C for severe sepsis. N Engl J Med 2001;344:699–709.

42. Angus DC, Laterre PF, Helterbrand J, et al. The effect of drotrecogin alfa (activated) on long-term survival after severe sepsis. Crit Care Med 2004;32:2199–2206.

43. Abraham E, Laterre PF, Garg R, et al., for the Administration of Drotrecogin Alfa (Activated) in Early Stage Severe Sepsis (ADDRESS) Study Group. Drotrecogin alfa (activated) for adults with severe sepsis and a low risk of death. N Engl J Med 2005;353:1322–1341.

44. Annane D, Sebille V, Charpentier C, et al. Effect of treatment with low doses of hydrocortisone and fludrocortisone on mortality in patients with septic shock. JAMA 2002;288:862–871.

45. van den Berghe G, Wouters P, Weekers F, et al. Intensive insulin therapy in the critically ill patient. N Engl J Med 2001;345:1359–1367.

83 Superficial Fungal Infections

Lauren S. Schlesselman

LEARNING OBJECTIVES

● **Upon completion of the chapter, the reader will be able to:**

1. Explain the underlying pathophysiology of vulvovaginal candidiasis (VVC), oropharyngeal candidiasis (OPC), esophageal candidiasis, and fungal skin infections.

2. Identify symptoms of VVC, OPC, esophageal candidiasis, and fungal skin infections.

3. Identify the desired therapeutic outcomes for patients with uncomplicated and complicated VVC, OPC, esophageal candidiasis, and fungal skin infections.

4. Recommend appropriate lifestyle modifications and pharmacotherapy interventions for patients with VVC, OPC, esophageal candidiasis, and fungal skin infections.

5. Recognize when long-term suppressive therapy is indicated for a patient with VVC.

6. Recognize when topical versus oral treatment is indicated for a patient with OPC, esophageal candidiasis, VVC, and fungal skin infections.

7. Educate patients about the disease state, appropriate lifestyle modifications, and medication therapy required for effective treatment of VVC, OPC, esophageal candidiasis, and fungal skin infections.

KEY CONCEPTS

❶ The predominant pathogen associated with vulvovaginal candidiasis (VVC) is *Candida albicans*, although a small percentage of cases are caused by *C. glabrata*, *C. tropicalis*, *C. krusei*, and *C. parapsilosis*.

❷ A variety of factors including antibiotic use, diabetes, and immunosuppression may increase the risk of developing symptomatic VVC. No risk factors are consistently associated with any case of VVC.

❸ Asymptomatic vaginal colonization of *C. albicans* is not diagnostic of VVC since 10% to 20% of women are asymptomatic carriers of *Candida* species. Asymptomatic vaginal colonization does not require treatment.

❹ Selection of antifungal agents to treat uncomplicated VVC is influenced by patient preference, including route of administration, duration of therapy, cost, risk of adverse effects, and potential for medication interactions.

❺ Recurrent VVC, defined as four or more infections per year, requires long-term suppressive therapy for 6 months.

❻ The occurrence of oropharyngeal candidiasis (OPC) and esophageal candidiasis is an indicator of immune suppression, often developing in infants, the elderly, and the immunocompromised.

❼ Topical antifungal agents are first-line therapy for OPC, although oral agents may be used for severe or unresponsive cases.

❽ Esophageal candidiasis is a severe extension of OPC that requires oral antifungal therapy.

❾ Since dermatophyte hyphae seldom penetrate into the living layers of the skin, instead remaining in the stratum corneum, most mycotic infections of the skin can be treated with topical antifungals. Infections covering large areas of the body or infections involving nails or hair may require oral therapy.

❿ Onychomycosis, fungal infections involving the nails, requires oral antifungal therapy. Topical agents do not adequately penetrate the nail.

VULVOVAGINAL CANDIDIASIS

Vulvovaginal candidiasis (VVC), whether symptomatic or asymptomatic, refers to infections in women whose vaginal cultures are positive for *Candida* species.

EPIDEMIOLOGY AND ETIOLOGY

VVC, also known as moniliasis, is a common form of vaginitis, accounting for 20% to 25% of vaginitis cases. Although VVC is uncommon prior to menarche, nearly 50% of women will experience one or more episodes by the age of 25 years.[1] A survey of women in the United States found that 6.5% of women over the age of 18 years reported experiencing at least one episode of vaginitis during the previous 2 months.[2]

According to the treatment guidelines of the Centers for Disease Control and Prevention (CDC),[3] VVC can be classified as uncomplicated or complicated. Uncomplicated infections are typically infrequent and cause mild to moderate symptoms. Complicated infections, including recurrent or severe infections, may be caused by azole-resistant fungal organisms. Immunocompromise, including immunosuppression, uncontrolled diabetes, pregnancy, or debilitation, is a risk factor for developing recurrent infection. Recurrent VVC, defined as four or more infections per year, occurs in less than 5% of women.[4] Recurrent infection is distinguishable from a persistent infection by the presence of a symptom-free interval between infections.

❶ *Candida albicans is the primary pathogen responsible for VVC, accounting for more than 90% of cases.*[5] A small percentage of cases are caused by nonalbicans species including *C. glabrata, C. tropicalis, C. krusei,* and *C. parapsilosis.* In patients with recurrent vaginitis, the causative *Candida* is twice as likely to be nonalbicans.[6] The incidence of nonalbicans VVC is increasing, possibly due to overuse of nonprescription vaginal antifungal products, short-course antifungal treatments, and long-term suppressive therapy with antifungals.[7]

PATHOPHYSIOLOGY

The normal vaginal environment protects women against vaginal infections. Under the influence of estrogen, vaginal epithelium cornifies to reduce the risk of infection. Vaginal discharge, comprised of exfoliated cells, cervical mucus, and colonized bacteria, cleans the vagina. The volume of discharge varies during pregnancy, during oral contraceptive use, with age, and at mid-menstrual cycle near ovulation. The normal pH of vaginal secretions, near 4, is maintained by *Lactobacillus acidophius,* diphtheroids, and *Staphylococcus epidermidis.* The low pH is toxic to many pathogens.

Any alteration in the vaginal environment allows for overgrowth of organisms that are normally suppressed. Increases in the vaginal pH are associated with increased vulvovaginitis. pH changes are caused by stress, changes in hormone level, sexual activity, pregnancy, phases of the menstrual cycle, contraceptive use, presence of foreign bodies or necrotic tissue, use of douches, or the use of antibiotics. An increase in glycogen production, associated with altered estrogen and progesterone levels, can also increase the risk of infection through increased adherence of *C. albicans* to epithelial cells.

RISK FACTORS

❷ *Although no risk factors are consistently associated with conversion to symptomatic infection, a variety of factors may increase the risk of developing symptomatic VVC in certain women* (Table 83–1).

TREATMENT

The goals of treatment of VVC are as follows:

- Relief of symptoms
- Eradication of infection
- Re-establishment of normal vaginal flora
- Prevention of recurrence in complicated infections

Clinical Presentation and Diagnosis of VVC

Patients with VVC may present with vulvar and/or vaginal symptoms. Symptoms often develop the week before menses and resolve with the onset of menses.

Symptoms include:

- Itching
- Soreness
- Burning
- Irritation
- External dysuria
- Dyspareunia

Signs include:

- Nonodorous discharge (may vary from watery to curd-like)
- Yellow or yellowish-green discharge
- Erythema and edema of the labia and vulva
- Fissures
- Pustulopapular lesions
- Normal cervix

Diagnostic Testing

- Microscopic investigation for the presence of blastospores or pseudohyphae; saline wet mount has a sensitivity of 40% to 50%, while a KOH preparation has a sensitivity of 50% to 70%.[7] ❸ *Asymptomatic vaginal colonization of Candida albicans is not diagnostic of VVC since 10% to 20% of women are asymptomatic carriers of* Candida *species. Asymptomatic vaginal colonization does not require treatment; therefore the presence alone of* Candida *should not determine care.*

- Vaginal pH less than or equal to 4.5; pH should remain normal in cases of fungal infection, while an elevated pH suggests bacterial infection.

- *Candida* cultures should be obtained only if signs and microscopy are inconclusive or in cases of recurrent VVC.

Table 83–1

Possible Risk Factors Associated With VVC

Risk Factor	Proposed Mechanism
Broad-spectrum antibiotic use	Altered vaginal flora allowing overgrowth of *Candida* organisms; risk increases with duration of antibiotic use
Systemic cortico-steroid or immuno-suppressant use	Reduced vaginal protection by immunoglobulins
Sexual activity	A small percentage of male partners have penile or oral colonization of identical strains; VVC is often associated with the onset of sexual activity
Tight-fitting and nonabsorbent clothing	Promotes warm, moist environment for fungus growth
Elevated estrogen levels, hormonal contraceptives, and pregnancy	Estrogen enhances *Candida* adherence to vaginal epithelial cells and yeast-mycelial transformation; this is supported by the fact that infection rates are lower before menarche and after menopause (except in women taking hormone replacement therapy), while rates are higher during pregnancy
Vaginal pH	Changes in glycogen and lactic acid levels
GI reservoir of *Candida* organisms	Transfer of organism from rectum to vagina; irritation of the vulvovaginal area during sexual intercourse may enhance invasion of organisms
Diabetes	Enhanced binding of *Candida* to epithelial cells due to hyperglycemia; asymptomatic colonization is more common in patients with diabetes; elevated sugar levels may cause conversion to symptomatic infection

Patient Encounter 1

A 28-year-old woman with a history of diabetes presents to your clinic complaining of what she calls "itching in my private areas." After questioning her, you determine that she has vaginal burning and itching, accompanied by a curd-like discharge. On examination, she has erythema of the labia and a nonodorous discharge.

What information is suggestive of vulvovaginal candidiasis (VVC)?

What additional information do you need to know before creating a treatment plan for this patient?

Nonpharmacologic Treatments

In combination with pharmacologic treatment, the practitioner should recommend basic nonpharmacologic

approaches to treatment and prevention of VVC:

- Keep the genital area clean and dry.
- Avoid prolonged use of hot tubs.
- Avoid constrictive clothing.
- Wear underwear made of breathable materials, such as cotton.
- To reduce vulvar irritation, avoid soaps and perfumes in the genital area.
- Although study results are conflicting, the daily consumption of active *L. acidophilus* may reduce recurrence. One study found that the daily ingestion of 8 ounces of yogurt produced a threefold reduction in the incidence of infection,[8] while other studies found no difference in infection rates in women who ingested yogurt.[9,10]

Pharmacologic Treatment of Uncomplicated VVC

Most cases of uncomplicated VVC will resolve with a single course of antifungal therapy. Treatment with an oral or vaginal antifungal agent, either prescription or nonprescription, is appropriate for most uncomplicated cases. Nonprescription azole antifungal products are available as one-night, three-night, and seven-night regimens in a variety of formulations, including cream, suppository, and vaginal tablets (Table 83–2). Oral fluconazole offers the option of treatment with one dose administered without regard to time of day. Some practitioners opt to retreat with a second dose of fluconazole 3 days later. Due to the risk of severe hepatotoxicity, the use

Table 83–2

Treatment Options for Uncomplicated VVC

1-Day Therapies

Butoconazole 2% sustained-release cream, 5 g intravaginally as a single application
Fluconazole 150 mg, one tablet orally as a single dose
Tioconazole 6.5% ointment, 5 g intravaginally as a single application

3-Day Therapies

Butoconazole 2% cream, 5 g intravaginally daily for 3 nights
Clotrimazole 100-mg vaginal tablet, two tablets daily for 3 nights
Miconazole 200-mg vaginal suppository, one suppository daily for 3 nights
Terconazole 0.8% cream, 5 g intravaginally daily for 3 nights
Terconazole 80-mg vaginal suppository, one suppository daily for 3 nights

7- to 14-Day Therapies

Boric acid 600-mg vaginal suppository, one suppository intravaginally twice daily for 14 days
Clotrimazole 1% cream, 5 g intravaginally daily for 7–14 nights
Clotrimazole 100-mg vaginal tablet, one tablet daily for 7 nights
Miconazole 2% cream, 5 g intravaginally daily for 7 nights
Miconazole 100-mg vaginal suppository, one suppository daily for 7 nights
Nystatin 100,000-unit vaginal tablet, one tablet daily for 14 nights
Terconazole 0.4% cream, 5 g intravaginally daily for 7 nights

of oral ketoconazole should be reserved for severe fungal infections resistant to other antifungal options.

To avoid inappropriate use of nonprescription products, the practitioner should only recommend them to women who have previously been diagnosed with VVC. Estimates of how accurately women self-diagnose VVC are difficult to assess. One study found that only one-third of women accurately diagnosed an episode of vaginitis.[11] Women with a previous clinically based diagnosis of VVC are no more accurate at self-diagnosing than women without prior clinical diagnosis.[11]

Inability to resolve an infection may indicate a mixed infection, infection due to a nonalbicans strain, or an infection that is not fungal. Difficulty treating VVC can also be indicative of serious underlying conditions, such as diabetes or HIV infection. For these reasons, if infection does not resolve easily with a single course of antifungal therapy or if symptoms return within 2 months, practitioners should check cultures and further evaluate the patient's health status or refer the patient to a physician.

❹ *Due to the numerous treatment options available, a variety of factors can influence product selection, with patient preference playing a significant role.* To improve adherence with therapy, the practitioner should discuss with the patient what options are available and what her preferences are.

Adherence rates are greater with oral treatment than with vaginal therapy. This may be due to the ease of administration, short duration, and flexibility on time of administration. Vaginal creams provide rapid relief of itching and burning. The practitioner may wish to advise a patient to apply a vaginal cream externally to reduce itching and burning if using an oral agent. The need to clean the vaginal applicator for reuse is unappealing for some women. Many nonprescription vaginal products are now packaged with sufficient disposable applicators to prevent the need for reuse with subsequent doses. Available regimens range from 1 to 7 days for topical preparations and fluconazole. Cure rates are similar among different durations of therapy.[12] Most OTC products cost $10 to $20 per course of therapy. The cost of prescription products can vary based on whether or not the patient has insurance coverage as well as the type of coverage the patient has. If the patient does not have prescription coverage, nonprescription products may prove less expensive than even one or two fluconazole tablets.

▶ Risk of Adverse Effects and Interactions

Systemic adverse effects associated with vaginal azoles are less frequent than with oral products. Common adverse effects associated with fluconazole include headache, diarrhea, nausea, dizziness, abdominal pain, and taste alterations. With topical products, local discomfort such as burning, itching, stinging, and redness may occur, particularly with the first application. Fifteen percent of patients experience GI side effects with orally administered antifungal agents.[13] Oral ketoconazole is associated with hepatic toxicity at a rate of 1 in 15,000.[14]

Oral azoles are associated with significant interactions, particularly due to cytochrome P450 isoenzymes. Medications that interact with azoles include warfarin, phenytoin, theophylline, rifampin, cyclosporine, and zidovudine. For patients receiving only a few doses, these interactions do not pose a significant risk. These interactions may pose a risk for patients receiving long-term suppressive therapy for recurrent infections.

TREATMENT OF RECURRENT VVC

The goal of treating recurrent VVC is control of the infection, rather than cure. First, any acute episodes are treated, followed by maintenance therapy. For the treatment of acute episodes, intravaginal or oral azoles can be utilized. Although acute episodes of recurrent VVC will respond to azole therapy, some patients may require prolonged therapy in order to achieve remission. To achieve remission, a second dose of oral fluconazole 150 mg repeated 3 days after the first dose or 14 days of topical azole therapy can be used. The practitioner should consider that nonalbicans infections are more common in recurrent VVC; therefore, fluconazole and itraconazole resistance may make these agents less effective.

❺ *After achieving remission, recurrent VVC requires long-term suppressive therapy for 6 months (Table 83–3).* To improve adherence to long-term suppressive therapy, oral therapy, typically with fluconazole, is preferred. Fluconazole 150 mg weekly for 6 months will prevent recurrence of infection in 90% of women.[15] Cessation of suppressive therapy is associated with resurgence of symptomatic infection in 50% of women.[16]

TREATMENT OF NONALBICANS INFECTIONS

Treatment response rates are lower for nonalbicans infections. Although an optimal regimen is unknown, use of intravaginal azole therapy for 7 to 14 days is recommended. Terconazole may prove more effective than other azoles in the treatment of nonalbicans infections since *C. glabrata* and *C. tropicalis* are more susceptible to terconazole.[17] For second-line therapy, boric acid 600 mg in a gelatin capsule administered vaginally twice daily for 2 weeks followed by once daily during menstruation is effective.[18] Local irritation

Table 83–3
Treatment Options for Maintenance Therapy

Daily
Boric acid 600 mg in gelatin capsule vaginally daily during menses (5 days)
Itraconazole 100 mg orally once daily
Ketoconazole 100 mg orally once daily

Weekly
Clotrimazole 500 mg vaginal suppository once weekly
Fluconazole 100 or 150 mg orally once weekly
Terconazole 0.8% cream 5 g vaginally once weekly

Monthly
Fluconazole 150 mg orally once monthly
Itraconazole 400 mg orally once monthly

often limits the use of boric acid. Topical 4% flucytosine is also effective but use should be limited due to the potential for resistance.

VVC DURING PREGNANCY

During pregnancy, VVC may prove difficult to treat due to elevated estrogen levels, accompanied by concern about harm to the fetus. Response rates are lower and recurrences are frequent during pregnancy. Vaginal antifungals remain the preferred treatment during pregnancy, although therapy should continue for 1 to 2 weeks to ensure effectiveness.[16] Most topical antifungals are classified as risk category C, while clotrimazole is classified as risk category B. The primary reason for the risk category C classification is the lack of studies, rather than increased risk. Fluconazole is also classified as risk category C. Despite oral fluconazole's classification, studies have not demonstrated an increased risk to the fetus when the pregnant mother was exposed to fluconazole,[19,20] although case studies have reported congenital limb deformities.[21]

Cultural Awareness During Treatment of VVC

As with all gynecological issues, the practitioner is faced with cultural perceptions of female genitalia. In particular, practitioners are treating an increased number of patients who have undergone female genital mutilation. More than 100 million women and girls worldwide have undergone such procedures for cultural and religious reasons.[22] Female genital mutilation, formerly known as female circumcision, describes the intentional alteration or injury of female genitalia. Some authorities suggest using the term "genital cutting" when dealing with patients to avoid appearing judgmental.[23] Regardless of the terminology used, many immigrants are aware of common cultural views in the United States pertaining to female genital mutilation. Women who have undergone this procedure suffer acute and chronic complications. Within the scope of this chapter, the practitioner may find patients with female genital mutilation suffer from recurrent VVC due to inadequate drainage of vaginal fluids. Regardless of what the practitioner's opinion is about female genital mutilation, the practitioner must be sensitive to the patient's feeling and cultural values.

OUTCOME EVALUATION

Patients should notice relief of itching and discomfort within 1 to 2 days. The volume of discharge should also begin to decrease within a few days. The entire course of therapy should be continued even if symptoms have resolved. If the condition does not resolve or worsens, the patient should be referred to a physician for aggressive therapy. If the condition recurs within 4 weeks or more than four times per year, the patient should be further evaluated or referred to a physician for evaluation of

---

Patient Care and Monitoring of VVC

1. Assess the patient's symptoms to determine if self-treatment with OTC antifungal therapy is appropriate or whether the patient should be evaluated by a practitioner or physician. OTC preparations should only be recommended for patients who have previously been diagnosed with VVC. Patients who experience more than four episodes per year should be referred to a physician for culturing and initiation of maintenance therapy.

2. Review any available diagnostic data, including cultures and potassium hydroxide (KOH) preps.

3. Obtain a thorough history of prescription, nonprescription, and natural drug product use. Is the patient taking any medications, such as steroids, antibiotics, or immunosuppressants, that may contribute to VVC? Is the patient taking any medications that may interfere with treatment?

4. If the patient has had VVC previously, determine what treatments were helpful to the patient in the past.

5. Educate the patient on lifestyle modifications that may prevent recurrence, including decreased consumption of sucrose and refined carbohydrates, increased consumption of yogurt containing live cultures, and wearing cotton underwear.

6. Develop a plan to assess effectiveness of antifungal therapy.

7. Determine if long-term suppressive therapy is necessary.

8. Evaluate the patient for the presence of adverse drug reactions, drug allergies, and drug interactions.

9. Stress the importance of adherence with the antifungal regimen, including lifestyle modifications.

10. Provide patient education pertaining to VVC and antifungal therapy.

   - Causes of VVC
   - How to administer vaginal antifungal creams
   - Adverse effects of vaginal antifungal creams and suppositories on latex condoms and diaphragms
   - Potential adverse effects that may occur with antifungal therapy
   - Medications that may interact with antifungal therapy
   - Preventing the spread of infection
   - Warning signs to report to a physician (recurrent or difficult-to-cure infections, infections with malodorous discharge)

---

possible non-*Candida* infections, resistant organism, or other complicating factors, along with assessment of need for long-term suppressive therapy.

OROPHARYNGEAL AND ESOPHAGEAL CANDIDIASIS

Oropharyngeal candidiasis (OPC) is a common fungal infection, usually associated with immune suppression. If left untreated, it will progress to more serious oral disease. Esophageal candidiasis, representing a serious progression of OPC, is associated with increased morbidity.

EPIDEMIOLOGY AND ETIOLOGY

❻ *The occurrence of oropharyngeal and esophageal candidiasis is an indicator of immune suppression, often developing in infants, the elderly, and the immunocompromised.* One-third to one-half of geriatric inpatients develop OPC. Denture stomatitis is present in 24% to 60% of denture wearers,[24] more commonly in women than men. Oral candidiasis is the most commonly reported adverse drug event among patients receiving inhaled corticosteroids.[25] The prevalence of esophageal candidiasis is 37% among patients treated with inhaled corticosteroids.[26] The incidence is highest among patients receiving high doses of corticosteroids or those with diabetes.

The prevalence of HIV infection plays a significant role in the incidence of OPC and esophageal candidiasis. In the 1980s, the incidence of OPC increased fivefold, in association with the spread of HIV infections.[27] Although HIV infection remains a risk factor for candidiasis, the introduction of highly active antiretroviral therapy precipitated a decline in the incidence of both infections by 50% to 60%.[28]

OPC remains the most common opportunistic infection in patients with HIV. Eighty to ninety percent of HIV-positive patients develop OPC.[29] For 70% of these patients, it is the first manifestation of HIV infection.[30] The incidence of oropharyngeal infection increases with decreasing CD4 lymphocyte counts, with an incidence of 60% in patients with a CD4 count less than 200 cells/mm³.

Although esophageal candidiasis represents the first manifestation of HIV infection in less than 10% of cases, it is the second most common AIDS-defining disease.[31] As with OPC, the incidence of esophageal candidiasis increases with decreasing CD4 counts.

C. albicans accounts for 80% of cases of OPC and esophageal candidiasis. Over the last 20 years, an increasing incidence of *C. albicans* resistance has been accompanied by an increased incidence of nonalbicans species infections, including *C. glabrata*, *C. tropicalis*, *C. krusei*, and *C. parapsilosis*. In patients with cancer, nonalbicans *Candida* species account for almost half of all cases.[29]

PATHOPHYSIOLOGY

Similar to VVC, the development of OPC occurs when the normal environment is altered. *Candida* organisms frequently colonize the oropharynx and mucous membranes. These organisms do not become pathogenic until the environmental balance is disturbed. This occurs in the setting of broad-spectrum antibiotic use, tissue damage (due to chemotherapy, catheter tubing, trauma), or immune deficiency.

Table 83–4	
Risk Factors for OPC and Esophageal Candidiasis	
Factor	**Proposed Mechanism**
Extremes of age	Immature immunity in infants and reduced immunity in the elderly
Impaired mucosal integrity	Breaks in the protective barrier allows fungal invasion; often due to radiation, surgery, or mucositis
Dentures	Adherence of fungus to dentures, along with reduced salivary flow under dentures; ill-fitting dentures may impair mucosal integrity
Xerostomia	Reduced cleansing and defense factors of saliva
Use of antibiotics	Altered flora of mucosa allowing fungal overgrowth
Use of steroids	Suppression of immunity
Use of immunosuppressants	Suppression of immunity
HIV infection	Decreased CD4 T lymphocytes
Diabetes mellitus	Elevated glucose levels and defense factors in saliva
Nutritional deficiencies	Altered defense mechanisms, impaired mucosal integrity, or enhanced pathogenic potential of fungus

RISK FACTORS

Risk factors for OPC can be found in Table 83–4.

CLINICAL PRESENTATION AND DIAGNOSIS

See text boxes for clinical presentations and diagnosis of OPC and esophageal candidiasis.

TREATMENT

Along with selecting an effective treatment, selection of an appropriate antifungal agent requires consideration of location and severity of infection, medication adherence, potential drug interactions, concomitant medical conditions, and presence of sucrose or dextrose. Topical agents require frequent dosing and prolonged contact time with oral mucosa. Rough surfaces of tablets and troches may irritate sensitive mucosa. Patients with xerostomia may have inadequate saliva to dissolve troches. Topical agents containing sucrose or dextrose may increase the risk of caries or cause elevated blood sugar in patients with diabetes. Along with being expensive, oral azoles exhibit an increased risk of toxicity and drug interactions due to cytochrome P450.

Since oropharyngeal and esophageal candidiasis are signs of immunocompromise, the immune status of the patient

Clinical Presentation and Diagnosis of OPC

OPC is often a presumptive diagnosis based on signs and symptoms, along with the resolution of them after treatment with antifungal agents.

Symptoms

- Sore, painful mouth and tongue
- Burning tongue
- Dysphagia
- Metallic taste

Signs

Signs vary depending on the type of OPC:

- Diffuse erythema on the surface of buccal mucosa, throat, tongue, and gums.
- White patches on tongue, gums, or buccal mucosa; removal of patches reveals erythematous and bloody tissue; ability to remove patches distinguishes OPC from oral hairy leukoplakia.
- Angular cheilitis presents with small cracking lesions, erythema, and soreness at the corners of the mouth; associated with vitamin and iron deficiency.
- Denture stomatitis presents with flat, red lesions on mucosa beneath dentures; signs of chronic erythema and edema on mucosa.
- Hyperplastic OPC presents with discrete, transparent raised lesions on the inner mucosa of the cheek; typically found in men who smoke.
- Pseudomembranous OPC presents with yellow–white plaques that may be small and discrete or confluent; most common form found in HIV patients.

Diagnostic Testing

Diagnosis is primarily based on identification of characteristic lesions. Although rarely necessary, diagnostic testing is possible if a definitive diagnosis is required.

- Cytology, although presence of *Candida* is not diagnostic since colonization is common.
- Culture to identify species of yeast or presence of resistance.
- Biopsy.

Clinical Presentation and Diagnosis of Esophageal Candidiasis

Symptoms

- Fever
- Odynophagia
- Dysphagia
- Retrosternal pain

Signs

- Fever
- Hyperemic or edematous white plaques
- Ulceration of esophagus
- Increased mucosal friability
- Narrowing of lumen

Diagnostic Testing

Unlike OPC, diagnosis of esophageal candidiasis is not based solely on clinical presentation, instead requiring endoscopic visualization of lesions and culture confirmation. Due to the invasive nature of these procedures, most practitioners opt to treat the infection presumptively, reserving endoscopic evaluation for patients who fail therapy.

- Cytology and culture to identify species of yeast or presence of resistance
- Barium esophagogram
- Endoscopy revealing whitish plaques with progression to superficial ulceration of the esophageal mucosa
- Mucosal biopsy

Patient Encounter 2

A 35-year-old woman presents to your clinic complaining of "burning and soreness in my mouth" along with a metallic taste and "this funny white stuff." On initial examination, she has white patches on her tongue, gums, and buccal mucosa. These patches are easily removed, revealing erythematous tissue underneath.

This is the woman's first visit to your clinic, therefore no medical history is available in her chart.

What additional information do you need to know before creating a treatment plan for this patient?

What underlying medical conditions might make her susceptible to fungal infections?

How is the treatment care plan altered if the patient has a history of frequent and severe OPC? If the patient is HIV-positive? If the patient is neutropenic?

should be considered in the therapeutic care plan. For HIV-infected patients, this should also include an evaluation of the patient's antiretroviral therapy since fungal infections may represent deterioration in immune status.

❼ *For low-risk patients, topical agents are first-line therapy for OPC, although systemic agents may be used for severe or unresponsive cases.* For patients with severe OPC, oral fluconazole remains the agent of choice. Oral fluconazole administered for 2 weeks exhibits a mycological cure rate of 48% and a clinical cure rate of 84% in HIV patients.[32] Response occurs within 5 days in patients receiving 100 to 200 mg daily.[16] Doses as low as 50 mg are effective, but clinical response is slow and potentially leads to resistance. Two weeks of oral itraconazole solution is as effective as fluconazole but is less well tolerated. Due to variable absorption, risk of toxicity, and potential for drug interactions, ketoconazole and itraconazole capsules are considered second-line alternatives to fluconazole.

For non–HIV-infected patients who have suppressed immune systems, the practitioner must consider the patient's risk of dissemination. Patients with cell-mediated immune deficiency but near-normal granulocyte function, such as patients with diabetes, solid organ transplant, or solid tumors, are at low-risk for dissemination. The risk of dissemination is higher for patients who develop neutropenia, including patients with leukemia or bone marrow transplant. These patients should be treated aggressively to prevent invasive fungal infection.

For the treatment of OPC in HIV-infected individuals, initial episodes can be adequately controlled with topical agents, such as clotrimazole troches, so long as symptoms are not severe and no esophageal involvement is suspected.[28] Topical nystatin is the least effective agent, especially in severely immunocompromised patients.[33] Topical clotrimazole appears to be the most effective topical antifungal, exhibiting clinical responses equivalent to oral fluconazole and itraconazole solution, but mycological cure rates are lower and relapse rates higher with clotrimazole.[31]

❽ *Representing a severe extension of OPC, esophageal candidiasis requires systemic antifungal therapy.* The significant morbidity associated with esophageal candidiasis warrants aggressive treatment. The diagnosis of esophageal candidiasis requires endoscopic evaluation, but rather than employing invasive procedures, patients can be treated with an appropriate course of antifungal based on clinical presentation. If patients do not respond, endoscopy should be considered.

Two to three weeks of fluconazole or itraconazole solution are highly effective and demonstrate similar clinical response rates.[34] Oral doses of 100 to 200 mg are effective in immunocompetent patients but doses up to 400 mg are recommended for immunocompromised patients. Due to variable absorption, ketoconazole and itraconazole capsules should be considered second-line therapy. In severe cases, oral azoles may prove ineffective, warranting the use of IV amphotericin B for 10 days. Although echinocandins and voriconazole are effective in treatment of esophageal candidiasis, experience remains limited.

Fluconazole-Resistant Infections

Twenty percent of HIV-infected patients develop fluconazole resistant *C. albicans* isolates after repeated exposure to fluconazole.[35] To treat fluconazole-resistant OPC, daily itraconazole for 2 to 4 weeks may be used. Oral itraconazole solution exhibits a mycological cure rate of 88% and a clinical cure rate of 97% in immunocompromised patients.[36] Fluconazole-resistant esophageal candidiasis should be treated with IV amphotericin B or caspofungin.

Recurrent Infections

If immunocompromised patients experience frequent or severe recurrences, particularly of esophageal candidiasis, chronic maintenance therapy with fluconazole 100 to 200 mg daily should be considered. In patients with infrequent or mild cases, secondary prophylaxis is not recommended. The rationale for not giving prophylaxis includes availability of effective treatments for acute episodes, risk of developing

---

Patient Care and Monitoring of OPC

1. Assess the patient's symptoms to determine if symptoms are consistent with OPC or esophageal candidiasis. All patients with suspected OPC or esophageal candidiasis should be referred to a practitioner or physician since no antifungal products appropriate for oral use are available without a prescription.

2. Review any available diagnostic data, including cultures.

3. Obtain a thorough history of prescription, nonprescription, and natural drug product use. Is the patient taking any medications that may contribute to candidiasis? Is the patient taking any medications that may interfere with treatment?

4. If the patient has had OPC or esophageal candidiasis previously, determine what treatments were helpful to the patient in the past.

5. If the patient has had OPC or esophageal candidiasis previously, determine if the patient has risk factors for recurrent infection.

6. Develop a plan to assess effectiveness of antifungal therapy.

7. Determine if long-term suppressive therapy is necessary.

8. Evaluate the patient for the presence of adverse drug reactions, drug allergies, or drug interactions.

9. Stress the importance of adherence with the antifungal regimen.

10. Provide patient education pertaining to OPC or esophageal candidiasis and antifungal therapy.

   - Causes of OPC or esophageal candidiasis
   - Risk factors for developing candidiasis
   - How to administer topical antifungal agents, including cleaning the oral cavity prior to administration, shaking suspensions prior to use, administering after meals, how to dissolve troches, and how to swish suspensions
   - Importance of completing the course of therapy
   - Potential adverse effects that may occur with antifungal therapy
   - Medications that may interact with antifungal therapy
   - Warning signs to report to a physician (recurrent or difficult-to-cure infections, or worsening symptoms)

resistant organisms, potential for drug interactions, and the cost of therapy.

OUTCOME EVALUATION

- Patients should notice symptomatic relief within 2 to 3 days of initiating therapy. Complete resolution typically occurs within 7 to 10 days. The entire course of therapy should be continued even if symptoms have resolved. If the condition does not resolve or worsens, the patient should be referred to a specialist for aggressive therapy.

- Short courses of oral azoles are associated with GI upset, while courses lasting longer than 7 to 10 days are associated with increased risk of hepatotoxicity. In patients receiving prolonged therapy lasting more than 3 weeks, periodic monitoring of liver function tests should be considered.

- Immunocompetent patients generally do not require reassessment after treatment. Patients with neutropenia exhibit an increased risk of dissemination of infection, and therefore should be monitored for signs of systemic fungal infection. Due to an increased risk of recurrence, HIV-positive patients should routinely be evaluated for recurrence at each visit.

MYCOTIC INFECTIONS OF THE SKIN, HAIR, AND NAILS

Tinea infections are superficial fungal infections in which the pathogen remains within the keratinous layers of the skin or nails (Table 83–5). Typically these infections are

Clinical Presentation and Diagnosis of Mycotic Infections

Symptoms and Signs
- See Table 83–5

Diagnostic Testing
- KOH prep
- Wood's ultraviolet lamp
- Microscopic examination
- Fungal cultures
- Periodic acid-Schiff (PAS) staining of nail

Treatment of Skin and Hair Infections
The goals of treatment include:
- Providing symptomatic relief
- Resolution of infection
- Preventing spread of infection

named for the affected body part, such as tinea pedis (feet), tinea cruris (groin), and tinea corporis (body). Tinea infections are commonly referred to as ringworm due to the characteristic circular lesions. In actuality, tinea lesions can vary from rings to scales and single or multiple lesions.

EPIDEMIOLOGY AND ETIOLOGY

Tinea infections are second only to acne in frequency of reported skin disease.[37] The common tinea infections are tinea pedis, tinea corporis, and tinea cruris. Tinea pedis, the most prevalent cutaneous fungal infection, afflicts more than 25 million people annually in the United States.

Fungal skin infections are primarily caused by dermatophytes such as *Trichophyton*, *Microsporum*, and *Epidermophyton*. *T. rubrum* accounts for more than 75% of all cases in the United States.[38] To a lesser extent, *Candida* and other fungal species cause skin infections. With tinea infections, the causative dermatophyte typically invades the stratum corneum without penetration into the living tissues, leading to a localized infection.

PATHOPHYSIOLOGY

- The primary mode of transmission of tinea infections is direct contact with other persons or surface reservoirs. Upon contact, the dermatophytes attach to the keratinized cells, leading to thickening of the cells. Although infection remains localized, bacterial superinfections may develop.

The pathophysiology of onychomycosis depends on the clinical type. With the most common form of onychomycosis, distal lateral subungual, the fungus spreads from the plantar skin. The fungus invades the underside of the nail through the distal lateral nail bed, leading to inflammation of the area. In cases of white superficial onychomycosis, the fungus invades the surface of the nail plate directly and the nail bed and hyponychium are infected secondarily. Proximal subungual onychomycosis infections begin in the cuticle and the proximal nail fold, then penetrate the dorsum of the nail plate.

RISK FACTORS

- Prolonged exposure to sweaty clothing
- Excessive skin folds
- Sedentary lifestyle
- Warm, humid climate
- Use of public pools
- Walking barefoot in public areas
- Skin trauma
- Poor nutrition
- Diabetes mellitus
- Immunocompromise
- Impaired circulation

Table 83–5

Signs, Symptoms, and Risk Factors of Superficial Fungal Infections

Infection	Symptoms, Signs, and Risk Factors
Tinea pedis	• Involves plantar surface and interdigital spaces of foot • Interdigital infections produce itching; presents as fissures, scaling, or macerated skin; can occur between any toes but most often between fourth and fifth toes; may cause foul smell due to superinfection with *Pseudomonas* or diphtheroids • Hyperkeratotic infections present with silvery-white scales on a thickened, red base; usually covers entire foot; occasionally may also affect hand • Vesiculobullous tinea pedis presents as pustules or vesicles on soles of feet; associated with maceration, itching, and thickening of sole; may cause lymphangitis and cellulitis; most common during summer months • Ulcerative tinea pedis presents as macerated, denuded, and weeping ulcers on soles; may produce extreme pain and erosion of interdigital spaces; typically complicated by opportunistic gram-negative infections • Risk factors include occlusive footwear, foot trauma, and use of public showers
Tinea manuum	• Infection of the interdigital and palmar surfaces • Presents as white scales in palmar folds; may also develop scales on remainder of palm; may present as singular plaque • More commonly affecting only one hand • Presents with hyperkeratotic skin
Tinea cruris	• Presents with follicular papules and pustules on the medial thigh and inguinal folds • Ringed lesions may extend from inguinal fold over adjacent inner thigh • Lesions usually spare the penis and scrotum, in contrast to candidiasis • Frequency increases during summer • Primarily develops in young men • Risk factors include tight-fitting clothing, excessive sweating, poor hygiene, increased humidity and temperatures • Commonly referred to as jock itch
Tinea corporis	• Presents with circular, scaly patch with enlarged border • Lesions may have red papules or plaque in center that clears, leaving hypopigmentation or hyperpigmentation • Itching may be present • Commonly referred to as ringworm of the body • Risk factors include animal to human contact
Tinea versicolor	• Characterized by skin depigmentation but can present as hyperpigmentation, particularly in dark-skinned patients • Typically occurs in areas with sebaceous glands, including neck, trunk, and arms • Depigmentation may persist for years • Primarily develops in young and middle-aged adults • Risk factors include application of oil, greasy skin, high ambient temperature, high relative humidity, tight-fitting clothing, immunodeficiency, malnutrition, hereditary predisposition
Tinea barbae	• Infection of beard area
Tinea capitis	• Infection of the head and scalp • May be asymptomatic initially, then progresses to inflammatory alopecia • "Black dot" alopecia may develop due to breakage of hair at the root • May form kerions (nodular swellings) • Scaling or favus may develop on scalp • Cervical lymphadenopathy is common • Primarily found in infants, children, and young adolescents, often in African American and Hispanic populations • Can be spread from person to person or animal to person
Onychomycosis (tinea unguium)	• Infection of nail plate and bed • Nail becomes opaque, thick, rough, yellow, and friable; nail may separate from bed • Toenails affected more frequently than fingernails • Prevalence increases with advanced age

Nonpharmacologic Therapy

• Since fungi thrive in warm, moist environments, the practitioner should encourage patients to wear loose-fitting clothing and socks, preferably garments made of cotton or other fabrics that wick moisture away from the body. Avoid clothing made with synthetic fibers or wool.

• Clean the infected area daily with soap and water.

• The infected area should be dried completely prior to dressing, paying particular attention to skin folds.

• To allow circulation of air, the infected area should not be bandaged.

• For foot infections, cotton socks are recommended, although these should be changed two to three times a day to reduce moisture.

• To prevent spreading of the infection towels, clothing, and footwear should not be shared with other persons.

• Wear protective footwear in public showers and pool areas.

Table 83–6
Available Topical Antifungal Agents

Medication	Rx/OTC	Cream/Ointment	Gel	Lotion	Spray/Solution	Powder
Butenafine	Rx	x				
Ciclopirox	Rx	x		x	Lacquer and shampoo	
Clotrimazole	OTC	x		x	x	x
Econazole	Rx	x				
Haloprogin	Rx	x			x	
Ketoconazole	Rx/OTC	x			Shampoo	
Miconazole	OTC	x		x	x	x
Naftifine	Rx	x	x			
Nystatin	Rx	x		x		x
Oxiconazole	Rx	x		x		
Sertaconazole	Rx	x				
Sulconazole	Rx	x				
Terbinafine	OTC	x	x		x	
Tolnaftate	OTC	x		x	x	

Table 83–7
Dosing of Systemic Therapy for Tinea Infections

Medication	Adult Dosing	Pediatric Dosing
Fluconazole	150 mg/week	6 mg/kg/week
Griseofulvin	0.5–1 g/day	10–25 mg/kg/day
Itraconazole	200 mg twice daily	Not studied
Ketoconazole	200–400 mg/day	3.3–6.6 mg/kg/day
Terbinafine	250 mg/day	Less than 20 kg: 67.5–125 mg/day 20–40 kg: 125–200 mg/day

Pharmacologic Therapy of Tinea Infections

9 *Since dermatophyte hyphae seldom penetrate into the living layers of the skin, instead remaining in the stratum corneum, most infections can be treated with topical antifungals.* Infections covering large areas of the body or infections involving nails or hair may require systemic therapy. Treatment is typically initiated based on symptoms, rather than on microscopic evaluation. For infections accompanied by inflammation, combination therapy with a topical steroid can be considered (Tables 83–6 and 83–7). Patients with chronic infections or infections that do not respond to topical therapy are also candidates for systemic therapy.

For the treatment of tinea pedia, corporis, and cruris, topical agents can be utilized unless the infection is refractory. Typically, tinea pedis requires treatment one to two times daily for 4 weeks, while tinea corporis and tinea cruris require treatment one to two times daily for 2 weeks. When applying treatment, the medication should be applied at least 1 inch beyond the affected area. Treatment of any infection should continue at least 1 week after resolution of symptoms. Many practitioners opt to initiate therapy with nonprescription clotrimazole or terbinafine, reserving prescription topical agents, such as naftifine, ciclopirox, and butenafine, for second-line therapy or refractory cases. For refractory cases or widespread lesions, systemic therapy can be prescribed.

When recommending topical therapy, the selection of vehicle is based on the type of lesion and location of the infection. Solutions are recommended for hairy areas and oozing lesions, while creams are better for moderately scaling and nonoozing lesions. For hyperkeratotic lesions, ointments can be considered. The selected formulation should be applied to the affected area that is cleaned and dried. The medication should be rubbed into the infected area for improved penetration. Since most patients do not rub in sprays and powders, penetration of the epidermis is minimal, making them less effective than other formulations. Sprays and powders should be considered as adjuvant therapy with a cream or lotion or as prophylactic therapy to prevent recurrence.

Due to the severity of infection and inflammation, tinea capitis does not adequately respond to topical agents. Oral agents for 6 to 8 weeks are recommended for eradication of tinea capitis. Griseofulvin has long been considered the treatment of choice due to its ability to achieve high levels within the stratum corneum. Itraconazole has also demonstrated effectiveness. Due to its lipophilicity, itraconazole achieves high levels in the skin. These levels are maintained for 4 weeks after medication is discontinued. Some practitioners recommend adjunct therapy with the oral agent to decrease dissemination, including ketoconazole or selenium sulfide shampoos.

TREATMENT OF ONYCHOMYCOSIS

Onychomycosis is a chronic infection that rarely remits spontaneously. Adequate treatment is essential to prevent spread to other sites, secondary bacterial infections, cellulitis, or gangrene. **10** *Due to the chronic nature and impenetrability of nails, topical agents have low efficacy rates for treating onychomycosis.* Oral agents that can penetrate the nail matrix and nail base, such as itraconazole and terbinafine, are more effective than ciclopirox lacquer. Itraconazole and terbinafine demonstrate mycological cure rates of 62%[39] and 76%,[40] respectively, while ciclopirox has a cure rate of 29% to 36%.[41]

Itraconazole can be administered continuously (200 mg orally daily) or as pulse therapy (200 mg orally twice daily for 1 week per month). Terbinafine is administered orally 250 mg per day as continuous therapy. Whether administered continuously or as pulse therapy, oral treatment for toenail infections should continue for at least 3 months, while treatment for fingernail infections should continue for at least 2 months. Terbinafine is an inhibitor of CYP450 2D6 isozyme. When administered with other medications metabolized via this isozyme, the other medication should be started at a low dose if it has a narrow therapeutic range. Griseofulvin is also effective for the treatment of onychomycosis, but therapy must be continued for 4 months for fingernail infections or 6 months for toenail infections. For patients with liver disease or who are unable to use oral agents, ciclopirox nail lacquer remains a reasonable alternative, although it requires 48 weeks of therapy.

The FDA has released warnings pertaining to itraconazole and terbinafine as there is a small but real risk of developing congestive heart failure with itraconazole therapy due to its negative inotropic effects. Itraconazole should not be administered to patients with ventricular dysfunction such as congestive heart failure. The FDA also released warnings that itraconazole and terbinafine are associated with serious hepatic toxicity, including liver failure and death. Liver failure associated with these medications has occurred in patients with no pre-existing living disease or serious underlying medical conditions. Treatment with itraconazole or terbinafine for prolonged periods requires laboratory monitoring of liver function tests before initiation of therapy and at monthly intervals thereafter.

Cultural Awareness When Treating Mycotic Infections

Awareness of cultural beliefs related to feet and hands is essential when treating patients with fungal infections. In Arab countries, showing the bottom of the foot is a grave insult. The foot is considered the dirtiest part of the body. As such, patients from these countries may be hesitant to show their feet to the practitioner. In other countries, the open palm "high five" gesture is considered insulting. When treating patients with infections on the hand, the practitioner should refrain from making this gesture while discussing the patient's hand infection.

OUTCOME EVALUATION

For infections of the skin, patients should notice relief of symptoms, including pruritus, scales, and inflammation, within 1 to 2 weeks. Therapy should be continued at least 1 week after complete resolution of symptoms. If the condition worsens or does not resolve within 4 weeks, the patient should be treated with oral therapy.

For onychomycosis, relief of symptoms is slow. The infected nail will need months to grow out. The practitioner should

---

Patient Care and Monitoring of Mycotic Infections

1. Assess the patient's symptoms to determine if self-treatment with OTC antifungal therapy is appropriate or whether the patient should be evaluated by a practitioner. Exclusions for self-treatment include infection of nails or hair, unsuccessful initial treatment, worsening condition, signs of secondary bacterial or systemic infection, large infected areas, or chronic medical conditions such as diabetes, immunosuppression, or impaired circulation.

2. Review any available diagnostic data, including cultures and KOH preps.

3. Obtain a thorough history of prescription, nonprescription, and natural drug product use.

4. If the patient has had a mycotic infection previously, determine what treatments were helpful to the patient in the past.

5. Educate the patient on lifestyle modifications that will prevent recurrence, which includes keeping the area dry, wearing shower shoes, washing clothing in hot water, using drying powders, avoiding sharing of towels or clothing, and wearing loose-fitting clothing.

6. Develop a plan to assess effectiveness of antifungal therapy.

7. Determine if long-term prophylactic therapy is necessary to prevent recurrence.

8. Evaluate the patient for the presence of adverse drug reactions, drug allergies, and drug interactions.

9. Stress the importance of adherence with the antifungal regimen.

10. Provide the patient education pertaining to mycotic infections and antifungal therapy.

   - Causes of mycotic infections of the skin, hair, or nails
   - Different types of OTC antifungal products, such as creams, sprays, shampoos, ointments, gel, lotions, solutions, and powders
   - How to apply various OTC antifungal products
   - How long therapy should be continued
   - How to avoid spread of infection
   - How to avoid recurrent infection
   - Potential adverse effects that may occur with antifungal therapy
   - Dietary modifications that are necessary with oral agents
   - Medications that may interact with antifungal therapy, particularly with oral agents used for nail infections
   - Warning signs to report to a physician (recurrent or difficult-to-cure infections, infections with malodorous discharge or bleeding)

advise the patient not to become frustrated by the slow resolution. Despite the slow progress, the antifungal agent is curing the infection. The practitioner should also advise the patient that even after the infection is cured, the nail may not look "normal."

Abbreviations Introduced in This Chapter

CDC   Centers for Disease Control and Prevention
KOH   Potassium hydroxide
OPC   Oropharyngeal candidiasis
OTC   Over-the-counter
PAS   Periodic acid-Schiff test
VVC   Vulvovaginal candidiasis

 Self-assessment questions and answers are available at *http://www.mhpharmacotherapy. com/pp.html.*

REFERENCES

1. Cleveland A. Vaginitis: Finding the cause prevents treatment failure. Cleve Clin J Med 2000;67(9):634–646.
2. Foxman B, Barlow R, D'Arcy H, et al. Candida vaginitis: Self-reported incidence and associated costs. Sex Transm Dis 2000;27:230–235.
3. Center for Disease Control and Prevention. Sexually transmitted diseases treatment guidelines, 2002. *www.cdc.gov/STD/treatment/5-2002TG.htm.*
4. Sobel JD. Vaginitis. N Engl J Med 1997;337(26):1896–1903.
5. Clinical Effectiveness Group. National guideline for the management of vulvovaginal candidiasis. Sex Transm Infect 1999;75(Suppl 1):S19–S20.
6. Richter SS, Galask RP, Messer SA, et al. Antifungal susceptibilities of Candida species causing vulvovaginitis and epidemiology of recurrent cases. J Clin Microbiol 2005;43(5):2155–2162.
7. Sobel JD, Faro S, Force R, et al. Vulvovaginal candidiasis: Epidemiologic, diagnostic, and therapeutic considerations. Am J Obstet Gynecol 1998;178:203–211.
8. Hilton E, Isenberg HD, Alperstein P, et al. Ingestion of yogurt containing Lactobacillus acidophilus as prophylaxis for candidal vaginitis. Ann Intern Med 1992;116:353–357.
9. Shalev E, Battino S. Weiner E, et al. Ingestion of yogurt containing Lactobacillus acidophilus compared with pasteurized yogurt as prophylaxis for recurrent candidal vaginitis and bacterial vaginosis. Arch Fam Med 1996;5:593–596.
10. Pirotta M, Chondros, P, Grover S, et al. Effect of lactobacillus in preventing postantibiotic vulvovaginal candidiasis: A randomized controlled trial. BMJ doi:10.1136/bmj.38210.494977.DE.
11. Ferris DG, Nyirjesy P, Sobel JD, et al. Over-the-counter antifungal drug misuse associated with patient-diagnosed vulvovaginal candidiasis. Obstet Gynecol 2002;99:419–425.
12. Edelman DA, Grant S. One-day therapy for vaginal candidiasis. A review. J Reprod Med 1999;44:543–547.
13. Fluconazole. In AHFS drug information. Am Soc of Health-Sys Pharm, 2008:500–511.
14. Janssen Pharmaceutical. Nizoral package insert. Titusville, NJ: Janssen Pharmaceutical; 1997.
15. Sobel JD, Wiesenfeld HC, Martens M, et al. Maintenance fluconazole therapy for recurrent vulvovaginal candidiasis. N Engl J Med 2004;351:876–883.
16. Vazquez JA, Sobel JD. Mucosal candidiasis. Infect Dis Clin N Am 2002;16:793–820.
17. Ringdahl EN. Treatment of recurrent vulvovaginal candidiasis. Am Fam Physician 2000;61:3306–3312, 3317.
18. Jovanovic R, Congema E, Nguyen HT. Antifungal agents vs boric acid for treating chronic mycotic vulvovaginitis. J Reprod Med 1991;36:593–597.
19. Mastroiacovo P, Mazzone T, Botto L, et al. Prospective assessment of pregnancy outcomes after first-trimester exposure to fluconazole. Am J Obstet Gynecol 1996;175:1645–1650.
20. Jick SS. Pregnancy outcomes after maternal exposure to fluconazole. Pharmacotherapy 1999;19:221–222.
21. Pursley TJ, Blomquist IK, Abraham J, et al. Fluconazole-induced congenital anomalies in three infants. Clin Infect Dis 1996;22:336–340.
22. World Health Organization Website. Female genital mutilation. *http://www.who/int/mediacentre/factsheets/fs241/en/print.html.*
23. Braddy CM, Files JA. Female genital mutiliation: Cultural awareness and clinical considerations. J Midwifery Womens Health 2007;52:159–163.
24. Budtz-Jorgensen E, Stenderup A, Grabowski M. An epidemiological study of yeasts in elderly denture wearers. Community Dent Oral Epidemiol 1975;3:115–119.
25. Kaliner M, Amin A, Gehling R, et al. Impact of inhaled corticosteroid-induced oropharyngeal adverse effects on treatment patterns and costs in asthmatic patients: Results from a Delphi panel. P&T 2005;30(10):573–589.
26. Kanda N, Yasuba H, Takahashi T, et al. Prevalence of esophageal candidiasis among patients treated with inhaled fluticasone propionate. Am J Gastroenterol 2003;98:2146–2148.
27. Fotos PG, Lilly JP. Clinical management of oral and perioral candidosis. Dermatol Clin 1996;14(2):273–280.
28. Powderly WG, Mayer KH, Perfect JR. Diagnosis and treatment of oropharyngeal candidiasis in patients infected with HIV: A critical reassessment. AIDS Res Hum Retroviruses 1999;15:1405–1412.
29. Vazquez JA. Options for the management of mucosal candidiasis in patients with AIDS and HIV infection. Pharmacotherapy 1999;19(1):76–87.
30. Minamoto GY, Rosenberg AS. Fungal infection in patients with acquired immunodeficiency syndrome. Med Clin North Am 1997;81(2):381–409.
31. Darouiche RO. Oropharyngeal and esophageal candidiasis in immunocompromised patients: Treatment issues. Clin Infect Dis 1998;26:259–274.
32. Hay RJ. Overview of studies of fluconazole in oropharyngeal candidiasis. Rev Infect Dis 1990;12:S334–S337.
33. Epstein JB, Polsky B. Oropharyngeal candidiasis: A review of its clinical spectrum and clinical therapies. Clin Ther 1998;20(1):40–57.
34. Dewit S, Urbain D, Rahir F, et al. Efficacy of oral fluconazole in the treatment of AIDS-associated esophageal candidiasis. Eur J Clin Microbiol Infect Dis 1991;10:503–505.
35. Ruhnke M, Eigler A, Tennagen I, et al. Emergence of fluconazole-resistant strains of candida albicans in patients with recurrent oropharyngeal candidosis and human immunodeficiency virus infection. J Clin Microbiol 1994;32:2092–2098.
36. Saag MS, Fessel WJ, Kaufman CA, et al. Treatment of fluconazole-refractory oropharyngeal candidiasis with itraconazole oral solution in HIV-positive patients. AIDS Res Hum Retroviruses 1999;15:1413–1417.
37. Stern RS. The epidemiology of dermatophyte infections. In: Freedberg IM, Fitzpatrick TB, eds. Fitzpatrick's Dermatology in General Medicine. 5th ed. New York: McGraw-Hill; 1999:7–12.
38. Kemna ME, Elewski BE. A U.S. epidemiologic survey of superficial fungal diseases. J Am Acad Dermatol 1996;35:539–542.
39. Gupta AK, Maddin S, Arlette J, et al. Itraconazole pulse therapy is effective in dermatophyte onychomycosis of the toenail: A double-blind placebo-controlled study. J Dermatolog Treat 2000;11:33–37.
40. Evans EG, Sigurgeirsson B. Double-blind, randomized study of continuous terbinafine compared with intermittent itraconazole in treatment of toenail onychomycosis. The LION study group. BMJ 1999;318:1031–1035.
41. Dermik Laboratories. Penlac nail lacquer topical solution prescribing information. Dermik Laboratories; 2000.

84 Invasive Fungal Infections

Russell E. Lewis and P. David Rogers

LEARNING OBJECTIVES

● **Upon completion of the chapter, the reader will be able to:**

1. Differentiate epidemiologic differences and host risk factors for acquisition of primary and opportunistic invasive fungal pathogens.

2. Recommend appropriate empiric or targeted antifungal therapy for the treatment of invasive fungal infections.

3. Describe the components of a monitoring plan to assess effectiveness and adverse effects of pharmacotherapy for invasive fungal infections.

4. Evaluate the role of antifungal prophylaxis in the prevention of opportunistic fungal pathogens.

KEY CONCEPTS

❶ The diagnosis of endemic fungal infections is often prompted by a patient history of prolonged infectious symptoms, travel or residence in an endemic area, and/or participation in activities that result in exposures to soil contaminated by endemic fungi.

❷ The approach to antifungal therapy in patients with endemic fungal infections is determined by the severity of clinical presentation, the patient's underlying immunosuppression, and potential toxicities and drug interactions associated with antifungal treatment.

❸ Secondary prophylaxis or suppressive therapy is recommended for endemic mycoses in immunocompromised patients, especially in hosts with pronounced defects in T-cell–mediated immunity (i.e., AIDS).

❹ Commensal or environmental fungi that are typically harmless can become invasive mycoses when the host immune defenses are impaired. Host immune suppression and risk for opportunistic mycoses can be broadly classified into three categories: (a) quantitative or qualitative deficits in neutrophil function, (b) deficits in cell-mediated immunity, and (c) disruption of integument and/or microbiologic barriers.

❺ Familiarity with the epidemiology and frequency of nonalbicans Candida species in the institution is essential before selecting empiric antifungal therapy for invasive candidiasis.

❻ Laboratory identification of *Candida* in clinical samples must be performed to the species level whenever possible, as Candida species differ considerably in their susceptibility to antifungal agents.

❼ If a patient is non-neutropenic, clinically stable, and has never received prior azole therapy, fluconazole 800 mg/day (12 mg/kg/day) is an appropriate first-line therapy for invasive candidiasis until identification of the *Candida* isolate. Liposomal amphotericin B 3 mg/kg, an echinocandin (i.e., caspofungin 70 mg on day 1, then 50 mg/day), or voriconazole, are suitable options for empiric therapy in patients with neutropenic fever.

❽ Clinical trials performed by the National Institute of Allergy and Infectious Diseases (NIAID) Mycoses Study Group showed that 2 weeks of induction antifungal therapy with combination amphotericin B (0.7 mg/kg/day) plus flucytosine (100 mg/kg/day) for cryptococcal meningitis, followed by consolidation therapy with fluconazole (400 mg daily) for 8 weeks was as effective as 4 weeks of combination therapy, and had fewer toxicities.

❾ Nodular or halo-like lesions detected by high-resolution computed tomography (HRCT) scans are often the first indication of invasive pulmonary aspergillosis.

❿ Immunocompromised patients on fluconazole with progressive sinus or pulmonary disease by radiography should be evaluated for possible mold infection.

⓫ Many experts now consider voriconazole as the first-line treatment for invasive aspergillosis (IA) in patients without significant contraindications (e.g., drug interactions or pre-existing liver dysfunction) to azole therapy.

Invasive fungal infection or invasive mycoses are general terms for diseases caused by invasion of living tissue by fungi. Unlike superficial mycoses (see Chap. 80), invasive mycoses invade internal organs, can disseminate throughout the body, and are associated with high rates of morbidity and mortality, particularly in the immunocompromised host. Invasive fungal infections are broadly categorized as either primary or opportunistic invasive mycoses. Primary invasive fungal infections are caused by fungal spores or conidia in the soil that, when disturbed, can become aerosolized and inhaled leading to infection, even in an immunocompetent patient. Because these fungi are often endemic to certain soil types and hence geographically restricted, primary invasive fungal pathogens are also known as endemic fungi. In the United States, three species (*Histoplasma capsulatum*, *Blastomyces dermatitidis,* and *Coccidioides immitis*) account for most of these infections (Table 84–1). In contrast, opportunistic fungal infections occur only in the setting of compromised host immune defenses and are caused by a wider spectrum of less virulent fungal species that are generally incapable of causing infection in healthy patients (see Table 84–1). Hence, the spectrum, severity, and outcome of opportunistic fungal infections are heavily influenced by the degree, type, and severity of host immunosuppression. As a general rule, opportunistic fungal infections are difficult to diagnose, uniformly fatal if not treated early and aggressively, and associated with high rates of morbidity and mortality.

Table 84–1

Invasive Mycoses

Primary (Endemic) Invasive Fungi
Histoplasma capsulatum[a]
Coccidioides immitis[a]
Blastomyces dermatitidis[a]

Opportunistic Invasive Fungi

Yeast
Candida species (*C. albicans, C. glabrata, C. parapsilosis, C. tropicalis, C. krusei,* and others)
Cryptococcus neoformans[a]
Trichosporon spp. and others

Mold
Hyalohyphomycetes
   Aspergillus fumigatus and other species[a]
   Fusarium solani and *Fusarium oxysporum*
   Zygomycoses (*Mucor, Absidia, Rhizopus, Cunninghamella,* and *Rhizomucor*)
   Penicillium
Phaeohyphomycetes
   Pseudallescheria boydii (*Scedosporium* spp.)
   Bipolaris
   Alternaria

Other
Pneumocystis jiroveci (formerly *P. carinii*)[a,b]

[a]Most common.

[b]Recently reclassified as a fungus.

ENDEMIC MYCOSES

EPIDEMIOLOGY

Endemic mycoses are true primary fungal pathogens capable of causing infection in otherwise healthy individuals. In immunocompromised patients, endemic fungal infections often present with a more fulminant course (in the case of primary infections) or reactivate to cause life-threatening infection. Because initial symptoms of an endemic fungal infection are often nonspecific and overlap with other slowly-progressing infections (e.g., tuberculosis), a careful patient history concerning travel and activities associated with potential exposure to soil contaminated with endemic fungi is essential for the diagnosis and early treatment of infection.

Two of the most common endemic fungal infections (histoplasmosis and North American blastomycosis) are found in overlapping regions in the eastern and central river basins of the United States (Fig. 84–1).[1] *Histoplasma capsulatum* var. *capsulatum*, the causative fungus of histoplasmosis, grows heavily in soil contaminated with bird or bat excreta, which serve to enhance sporulation of the fungus.[2] Activities in endemic regions that are classically associated with high exposures to *Histoplasma capsulatum* include cave exploration (spelunking), working in or demolishing chicken coops, demolition of older buildings, woodcutting in forests with large bird roosts, or spreading avian excreta as fertilizer. For blastomycosis, decaying organic matter, warm humid conditions, and proximity to water or frequent rainfall seems to support growth of this fungus.[3] Occupational or recreational activities that disturb soil heavily contaminated with *Blastomyces dermatitidis* are common risk factors for development of blastomycosis. Coccidioidomycosis differs from histoplasmosis and blastomycosis, as the fungus is associated with arid to semiarid climates, hot summers, low altitude, alkaline soil, and sparse flora. Hence the fungus is found in the southwestern regions of the United States stretching from western Texas to southern California (see Fig. 84–1).[4] Epidemics of coccidioidomycosis have been reported in California following dust storms and earthquakes, including cycles of intense drought and rain, which favor the growth cycle of the fungus and enhance dispersion of its specialized spore forms called arthroconidia.

PATHOPHYSIOLOGY

Endemic fungi share several key biologic and ecological characteristics that contribute to their pathogenicity in humans. All endemic fungi exhibit temperature-dependent dimorphism, meaning they can propagate as either yeast (single cells that reproduce by budding into daughter cells) or molds (multicellular filamentous fungi that reproduce through production of conidia or spores). At environmental temperatures (25–30°C [77–86°F]), *H. capsulatum*, *B. dermatitidis*, and *C. immitis* grow in the mold form producing 2- to 10-μm round to oval shaped (*Histoplasma* and *Blastomyces*) or barrel-shaped (*Coccidioides*) conidia that are dispersed throughout the environment and in air

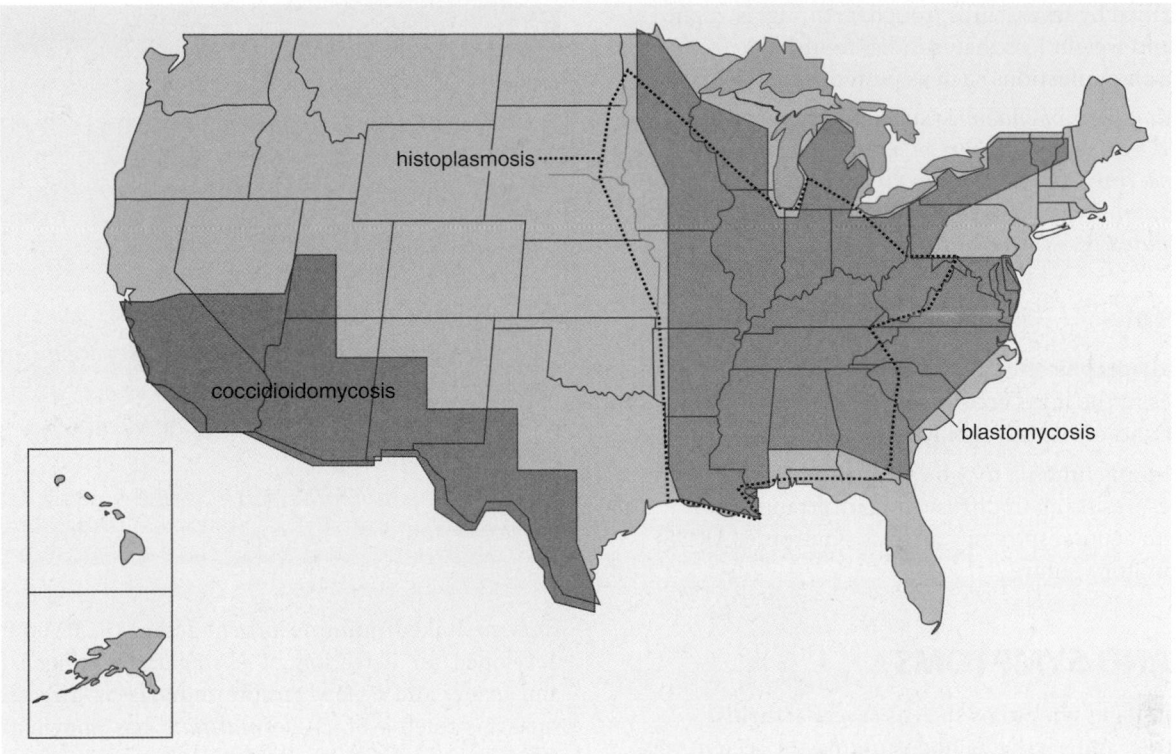

FIGURE 84–1. Geographic localization of primary (endemic) fungi in the United States.

currents. At physiologic temperatures, the conidia germinate into yeast (*Histoplasma* and *Blastomyces*) or in specialized cell forms called spherules (*Coccidioides*) that are resistant to killing by resident alveolar macrophages and neutrophils in the lung. Control of infection is mediated by the development of antigen-specific T-lymphocyte response that enhances macrophage fungicidal activity, and formation of a granuloma to contain the fungus.[5] Not surprisingly, patients with T-cell–mediated immune deficiency (e.g., AIDS patients and transplant recipients) or suppressed cellular immunity due to drug therapy (e.g., chemotherapy, high-dose corticosteroids, or tumor necrosis-α-blockers) are especially prone to severe reactivation of fungal disease.

The most common route of infection for endemic fungi is the respiratory tract, where conidia aerosolized from contaminated soil are inhaled into the lung. Once in the lung, conidia are phagocytosed but not destroyed by resident macrophages and neutrophils in the alveoli and bronchioles. Within 2 to 3 days, conidia germinate into facultative yeast resistant to phagocytosis and killing by macrophages and neutrophils (Fig. 84–2A and B). For *C. immitis,* germination of the arthroconidia results in the formation of a sac-like structure called a spherule filled with endospores (Fig. 84–2C). Spherules then rupture to release large numbers of endospores, which are the propagating form of the infection. Control of infection in the lungs is typically accomplished through formation of granulomas. However, in patients exposed to an overwhelming inoculum, or lower inocula in the setting of suppressed T-cell–mediated immunity, dissemination outside the lung to the skin and oral mucosa (especially blastomycoses), adrenal glands, bone, spleen, thyroid, GI tract, heart, and CNS is possible and uniformly fatal if left untreated.

CLINICAL PRESENTATION AND DIAGNOSIS

Histoplasmosis and coccidioidomycosis are frequently asymptomatic infections in immunocompetent patients or present as a self-limiting, influenza-like illness 1 to 3 weeks after inhalation of conidia. The clinical presentation of blastomycosis can range from asymptomatic infection, to acute or chronic pneumonia that develops 30 to 40 days after exposure, to full-blown disseminated disease.

General

- Symptomatic endemic fungal infections generally present as persistent and sometimes progressive pneumonia

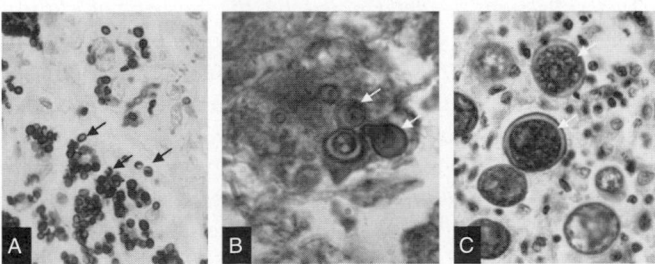

FIGURE 84–2. Histopathology of endemic mycoses in tissue. A. Histoplasmosis (yeast). B. Blastomycoses (broad-based budding yeast). C. Coccidioidomycoses (spherules with endospores).

accompanied by fever, chills, cough, arthralgias, night sweats, and weight loss that is indistinguishable from other chronic infections such as pulmonary tuberculosis.

- ❶ *The diagnosis of endemic fungal infection is often prompted by a patient history of a prolonged infectious symptoms, travel or residence in an endemic area, and/or participation in activities that result in exposures to soil contaminated by endemic fungi.*

Radiographs

- Chest radiographs often reveal either diffuse or nodular infiltrates in the lung, accompanied by enlargement of the hilar and/or mediastinal lymph nodes.

- Fulminant pneumonia may be seen with high inoculum exposures, resulting in diffuse lung infiltrates that proceed to acute respiratory distress syndrome (ARDS) and respiratory failure.

SIGNS AND SYMPTOMS

- Rheumatologic symptoms such as severe arthritis, pericarditis, and erythema nodosum may be seen in 10% to 30% of patients with endemic fungi.[2,6]

- Dissemination outside the lung is common in patients with suppressed cellular immunity and frequently produces signs of progressing infection.

- Ulcerative oral and cutaneous lesions may also arise with any endemic fungal infections.

- Verrucose skin lesions on sun-exposed areas on the face are particularly suggestive of progressing blastomycosis and are frequently mistaken for cutaneous malignancy.[6]

- Dissemination of the fungi to bone marrow may result in anemia or thrombocytopenia.

- Hepatomegaly, splenomegaly, and adrenal insufficiency can also occur with dissemination of the endemic fungi to these internal organs.

- Seizures, meningeal signs, and hydrocephalus are common findings with dissemination to the CNS and portend an especially poor prognosis in the setting of disseminated coccidioidomycosis.

Definitive diagnosis of an endemic fungal infection requires growth of the fungus from body fluids or tissue, or evidence of cellular or tissue invasion in clinical samples by histopathologic staining. However, cultures may only be positive in the setting of high inoculum exposures, pneumonia, or disseminated disease.[7] Serologic testing is helpful in the diagnosis and management of patients with histoplasmosis or coccidioidomycosis but lacks sufficient specificity for diagnoses of *B. dermatitidis*.[6] In general, a fourfold rise in antibody titers of *Histoplasma* or *Coccidioides*, or any titer greater than 1:16 suggests active infection. However, many clinicians still consider titers as low as 1:8 as evidence of active disease because undetectable titers may be present in one-third of all active infections.[4]

Patient Encounter 1, Part 1

A 39-year-old male with chronic steroid-dependent asthma who recently relocated to Phoenix, Arizona presents with a 4-week history of increasing fever, dry cough, and pain upon deep inspiration. He also reports arthralgias and night sweats over the last 3 weeks. A chest radiograph reveals a small area of consolidation in the left lower lobe and some hilar adenopathy. Otherwise, all other routine tests and cultures appear negative.

What are this patient's risk factors for developing an endemic fungal infection?

What is the most likely endemic fungal pathogen based on this patient's history?

What additional information is needed to select antifungal therapy?

Enzyme-linked immunosorbent assays (ELISAs) have been developed for detection of *Histoplasma* antigen in serum and urine, and a new radioimmunoassay directed against surface proteins of *B. dermatitidis* has shown promising sensitivity and specificity. Serial antigen testing can also provide a means for assessing response to antifungal therapy and early detection of relapse in patients with histoplasmosis or coccidioidomycosis.

The clinical presentation of blastomycosis covers a wide spectrum ranging from asymptomatic infections to flu-like illness resembling other upper respiratory tract illnesses; to infections resembling bacterial pneumonia with acute onset, high fever, lobar infiltrates, and cough; to subacute or chronic respiratory illness with complex symptoms resembling tuberculosis or lung cancer or fulminant lung infections with high fever, diffuse infiltrates, and an ARDS-like presentation.[6] As mentioned previously, the skin is the most common site of dissemination typically involving sunlight exposed body areas (i.e., nose, face, and arms) and mucous membranes.

TREATMENT
General Approach

❷ *The approach to antifungal therapy in patients with endemic fungal infections is determined by the severity of clinical presentation, the patient's underlying immunosuppression, and potential toxicities and drug interactions associated with antifungal treatment.* Immunocompetent patients with mild disease following exposure to *H. capsulatum* or *C. immitis* often experience a benign course of infection and rarely require antifungal therapy. Typically, these patients are followed in the outpatient setting with serial antigen testing to confirm resolving infection. Patients without clinical improvement within the first month are typically treated with oral itraconazole for 6 to 12 weeks (Table 84–2).[1,4,6] Other newer azoles such as voriconazole and posaconazole appear to have good activity against endemic fungi; however,

Table 84–2

Therapeutic Approach to Endemic Fungal Infections

Mycosis	Recommended Treatment Regimens	Comments
Histoplasmosis		
Mild to moderate acute pulmonary disease	Observation *or* If symptoms persist greater than 1 month, Itraconazole 200 mg orally 3 × daily for 3 days and then 200 mg once or twice daily for 6–12 weeks	Itraconazole is less effective for CNS infections
Moderately severe to severe acute pulmonary disease	Lipid formulation of Amphotericin B (3–5 mg/kg/day IV for 1–2 weeks) followed by itraconazole (200 mg 3 × daily for 3 days and then 200 mg twice daily, for a total for 12 weeks)	Amphotericin B deoxycholate (0.7–1 mg/kg daily IV) is an alternative in patients with low risk of nephrotoxicity Methylprednisolone (0.5–1 mg/kg daily IV) during the first 1–2 weeks for patients who develop respiratory complications (hypoxemia, significant respiratory distress, etc.)
Chronic cavitary pulmonary disease	Itraconazole (200 mg 3 × daily for 3 days and then once or twice daily for 1–2 years	Blood levels of itraconazole should be obtained after 2 weeks of therapy to ensure adequate exposure
Mild to moderate progressive disseminated disease	Itraconazole 200 mg 3 × daily for 3 days and then twice daily for at least 12 months	
Moderately severe to severe progressive disseminated disease	Liposomal Amphotericin B (3 mg/kg daily) for 1–2 weeks, followed by oral itraconazole (200 mg 3 × daily for 3 days and then 200 mg twice daily for a total of at least 12 months)	Substitution of another lipid formulation at a dosage of 5 mg/kg daily may be preferred in some patients due to cost or tolerability Amphotericin B deoxycholate (0.7–1 mg/kg daily IV) is an alternative in patients with low risk of nephrotoxicity Lifelong suppressive therapy with itraconazole (200 mg daily) may be required in immunosuppressed patients if immunosuppression cannot be reversed and in patients who relapse despite receipt of appropriate therapy Blood levels of itraconazole should be obtained to ensure adequate drug exposure Antigen levels should be measured during therapy and for 12 months after therapy is ended to monitor for relapse
CNS disease	Liposomal amphotericin B (5 mg/kg daily for a total of 175 mg/kg given over 4–6 weeks) followed by itraconazole (200 mg 2 × or 3 × daily) for at least 1 year and until resolution of CSF abnormalities, including Histoplasma antigen levels, is recommended	Blood levels of itraconazole should be obtained to ensure adequate drug exposure
Blastomycosis		
Mild to moderate pulmonary disease	Itraconazole, 200 mg 3 × per day for 3 days and then once or twice per day for 6–12 months	Serum levels of itraconazole should be determined after the patient has received this agent for at least 2 weeks, to ensure adequate drug exposure
Moderately severe to severe pulmonary disease	Lipid formulation of Amphotericin B at a dosage of 3–5 mg/kg/day or Amphotericin B deoxycholate at a dosage of 0.7–1 mg/kg/day for 1–2 weeks or until improvement is noted, followed by oral itraconazole, 200 mg 3 × per day for 3 days and then 200 mg twice per day, for a total of 6–12 months	
Mild to moderate disseminated extrapulmonary disease	Itraconazole, 200 mg 3 × per day for 3 days and then once or twice per day for 6–12 months	Patients with osteoarticular blastomycosis should receive a total of at least 12 months of antifungal therapy Serum levels of itraconazole should be determined after the patient has received this agent for at least 2 weeks, to ensure adequate drug exposure

(Continued)

Table 84–2

Therapeutic Approach to Endemic Fungal Infections *(Continued)*

Mycosis	Recommended Treatment Regimens	Comments
Moderately severe to severe disseminated extrapulmonary disease	Lipid formulation of Amphotericin B, 3–5 mg/kg/day, or Amphotericin B deoxycholate, 0.7–1 mg/kg/day, for 1–2 weeks or until improvement is noted, followed by oral itraconazole, 200 mg 3 × per day for 3 days and then 200 mg twice per day for a total of at least 12 months	
CNS disease	Lipid formulation of Amphotericin B, 5 mg/kg/day over 4–6 weeks followed by an oral azole	Options for azole therapy include fluconazole, 800 mg/day, itraconazole, 200 mg 2 or 3 × per day, or voriconazole, 200–400 mg twice per day, for at least 12 months and until resolution of CSF abnormalities
Coccidioidomycosis		
Mild to moderate	Observation or itraconazole 200 mg orally twice daily for 6–8 months *or* Fluconazole 6–12 mg/kg/day orally daily	Itraconazole demonstrated trend toward superiority over fluconazole in a randomized controlled trial for progressive, nonmeningeal coccidioidomycosis; however, fluconazole is better tolerated than itraconazole
Diffuse pneumonia or disseminated infection	Amphotericin B 1–1.5 mg/kg/day with dose and frequency decreased as improvement occurs *or* Lipid Amphotericin B formulations	Fluconazole 800–1,000 mg/day is sometimes recommended after initial Amphotericin B therapy for meningitis

there are currently insufficient data to recommend their routine first-line use. Fluconazole (400–800 mg/day) is somewhat less effective than itraconazole but may have fewer GI adverse effects and drug interactions than itraconazole in patients who require prolonged therapy.[1,4,6] Patients with progressive symptoms longer than 2 weeks or titers greater than 1:8 of histoplasmosis or coccidioidomycosis antigen are candidates for immediate antifungal therapy.[1,4] Any patient with underlying immunosuppression should also receive immediate antifungal therapy. The following signs and symptoms are considered to be indicators of severe disease that requires hospitalization and initial treatment with systemic amphotericin B (see Table 84–2).[1,4,6]

- Hypoxia indicated by a partial pressure of oxygen less than 80 mm Hg
- Hypotension (systolic blood pressure less than 90 mm Hg)
- Impaired mental status
- Anemia (hemoglobin less than 10 g/dL [100 g/L or 6.2 mmol/L])
- Leukopenia (less than $1 \times 10^3/mm^3$ [$1 \times 10^9/L$])
- Elevated hepatic transaminases (greater than five times upper limit of normal) or bilirubin (greater than 2.5 times upper limit of normal)

- Coagulopathy
- More than 10% loss in body weight
- Evidence of dissemination including cutaneous manifestations
- Meningitis

The treatment of blastomycoses is heavily dependent on the severity of clinical manifestations. Generally, patients with mild disease can be managed as outpatients with oral

Patient Encounter 1, Part 2

Selecting Antifungal Therapy

The patient's serum titer for coccidioidomycosis returns as greater than 1:32. Based on the information presented, select an appropriate treatment plan for the patient's coccidioidomycosis.

Does the patient require antifungal treatment at this time?

If the patient is considered to have moderately severe disease, what are the recommended treatment options?

itraconazole.[6] Patients with evidence of severe pulmonary disease or dissemination require initial treatment as inpatients with amphotericin B–based regimens until they are clinically stable, whereupon they can complete a 6- to 12-month treatment course as outpatients with oral azoles.[6] Methylprednisolone (0.5–1 mg/kg daily IV) during the first 1 to 2 weeks of antifungal therapy is often considered for patients who develop respiratory complications during initial treatment, including hypoxemia or significant respiratory distress.

PATIENT MONITORING AND SIDE EFFECTS

Response to antifungal therapy may be slow in patients with a prolonged history of infection or severe manifestations. However, gradual improvements in symptoms and reduction in fever are indicators of response to antifungal therapy. For histoplasmosis and coccidioidomycosis, decreasing antigen titers are also indicative of response to antifungal therapy.[1,4]

Antifungals used for the treatment of endemic mycoses can be associated with clinically-significant drug interactions and toxicities, especially with the prolonged treatment courses that are often required in the management of endemic mycoses. Itraconazole is available as a capsule formulation and as a liquid. The liquid formulation of itraconazole has several advantages over the capsule: it has a better oral bioavailability and does not require the low gastric pH that is required for dissolution and absorption of the capsule. However, the oral solution is somewhat dilute, has an unpalatable aftertaste (an issue when taking months of therapy), and has a much higher rate of GI side effects. Therefore, the capsule formulation is often preferred provided patients are not on acid-suppression therapy (i.e., proton pump inhibitors, histamine antagonists, or antacids).

Drug interactions are an important concern in patients taking long-term azole therapy. Itraconazole is a substrate and inhibitor of the cytochrome P450 (CYP)3A4 enzyme and the drug transporter, P-glycoprotein. Coadministration of itraconazole with inducers of this enzyme system (e.g., rifampin, phenytoin, and phenobarbital) can dramatically increase the clearance of itraconazole (and to a lesser extent fluconazole), resulting in ineffective plasma and tissue concentrations of the drug.[8–11] In general, coadministration of itraconazole with these inducers should be avoided. In some cases, plasma trough levels can be drawn once the patient reaches steady state (greater than 7 days of therapy) to ensure adequate drug absorption. Concentrations less than 0.25 mcg/mL (0.25 mg/L) should be considered evidence of insufficient itraconazole absorption[11] as trough concentrations should ideally approach 1 mcg/mL (1 mg/L) by the time the patient is in steady state.[12]

As a potent inhibitor of CYP450 enzymes including CYP3A4, itraconazole can dramatically decrease the clearance of many important medications metabolized through this enzyme, leading to potentially dangerous drug interactions. Patients receiving anticoagulation therapy with warfarin, immunosuppressive therapy with cyclosporine or tacrolimus, those taking midazolam, HMG-CoA reductase inhibitors

(statins), rifabutin, chemotherapy agents (e.g., vinca alkaloids, busulfan, and cyclophosphamide), and digoxin will require dosage adjustment and careful monitoring while receiving itraconazole therapy.[13] Although fluconazole is not as potent an inhibitor of CYP3A4 as itraconazole, drug interactions can still be severe, especially at higher fluconazole dosages (i.e., 800 mg/day).[13]

All azole antifungals carry the potential for rash, photosensitivity, and hepatotoxicity. In general, hepatotoxicity is mild and reversible, presenting as asymptomatic increases in liver transaminases or less commonly, an increase in total bilirubin. Fulminant hepatic failure has been reported with itraconazole. Therefore, serial monitoring of liver function is recommended in all patients on long-term azole therapy. Long-term therapy with itraconazole has also been associated with reversible adrenal suppression and cardiomyopathy associated with the drug's negative inotropic effects. These adverse effects can be prevented or managed with close monitoring and follow-up of patients on long-term therapy.

Amphotericin B is the mainstay of treatment of patients with severe endemic fungal infections. The conventional deoxycholate formulation of the drug can be associated with substantial infusion-related adverse effects (e.g., chills, fever, nausea, rigors, and in rare cases hypotension, flushing, respiratory difficulty, and arrhythmias). Premedication with low doses of hydrocortisone, acetaminophen, nonsteroidal anti-inflammatory agents, and meperidine is common to reduce acute infusion-related reactions. Venous irritation associated with the drug can also lead to thrombophlebitis; hence, central venous catheters are the preferred route of administration in patients receiving more than a week of therapy.

The most severe adverse effect associated with amphotericin B therapy is nephrotoxicity, which occurs through the renal vascular effects of the drug (constriction of the afferent arterioles in the kidney tubule), and direct toxicity to the kidney tubular membrane. Generally, nephrotoxicity with amphotericin B is reversible provided the drug is stopped. However, treatment interruptions can be problematic in patients with severe infections. Precipitous decreases in glomerular filtration occasionally are seen with the initiation of amphotericin B therapy, especially in patients with marked dehydration. Infusion of normal saline before and after amphotericin B, a practice known as "sodium loading" can blunt precipitous decreases in renal perfusion pressure and slow that rate of decline in the glomerular filtration rate. Tubular toxicity can be delayed by avoiding the use of other drugs with known tubular toxicity such as aminoglycosides, cyclosporine, cisplatin, or foscarnet. Generally, tubular toxicity manifests in patients with severe wasting of potassium and magnesium in the urine. Therefore, patient electrolytes must be carefully monitored and potassium and magnesium supplementation is often required. Hypokalemia and hypomagnesemia frequently precede decreases in glomerular filtration (increased serum creatinine) especially in patients who are adequately hydrated.[14] Continued tubular damage, however, eventually results in decreases in renal blood flow and glomerular filtration through tubuloglomerular feedback mechanisms that further constrict the afferent arteriole.

During the 1990s, amphotericin B was reformulated into three different lipid-based formulations (Abelcet, Ambisome, and Amphotec) that have reduced rates of nephrotoxicity compared to the conventional deoxycholate formulation (Fungizone). Two of the formulations (Abelcet and Ambisome) have also shown reductions in the rates of infusion-related reactions. Although these lipid formulations are generally considered to be as effective as conventional amphotericin B deoxycholate, they are not dosed equivalently to the standard formulation. Unlike conventional amphotericin B, which is administered at dosages ranging from 0.6 to 1.5 mg/kg/day, lipid formulation doses are threefold to fivefold higher on a milligram-per-milligram basis, ranging from 3 to 5 mg/kg/day. Only one prospective study has directly compared the efficacy of a lipid amphotericin formulation to the conventional formulation.[15] In a small study of AIDS patients with moderate to severe histoplasmosis, liposomal amphotericin B (Ambisome) was more effective than amphotericin B, with response rates of 84% and 64%, respectively. Ambisome may also be the preferred agent in patients with CNS infections over other lipid formulations, due to its improved CNS penetration.[16]

PROPHYLAXIS

Primary prophylaxis, before development of infection, is generally not recommended for endemic fungi but may be considered for patients who are severely immunocompromised. Patients with HIV infection with CD4 cell counts less than 150 cells/mm³ (histoplasmosis) or less than 250 cells/mm³ (coccidioidomycosis) living in endemic areas with high endemic case rates (greater than 10 cases per 100 patient-years) or with positive IgM or IgG antibodies to the fungal pathogen serology should receive itraconazole 200 mg daily.[12] ❸ *Secondary prophylaxis or suppressive therapy with itraconazole 200 mg daily, to prevent*

recurrence of infection is recommended for blastomycosis in immunosuppressed patients if immunosuppression cannot be reversed.[6,12] In patients with prior CNS disease, fluconazole or voriconazole are the preferred drug due to the limited penetration of itraconazole into the CNS.

OPPORTUNISTIC MYCOSES

❹ *Commensal or environmental fungi that are typically harmless can become invasive mycoses when the host immune defenses are impaired. Host immune suppression and risk for opportunistic mycoses can be broadly classified into three categories:*

- *Quantitative or qualitative deficits in neutrophil function*
- *Deficits in cell-mediated immunity*
- *Disruption of the integument and/or microbiologic barriers*

Quantitative defects in neutrophils (neutropenia) resulting from neoplastic diseases, cytotoxic chemotherapy, marrow transplantation, or aplastic anemia are among the most common risk factors for opportunistic mycoses. Qualitative defects may be seen in certain disease states (e.g., advanced diabetes mellitus and chronic granulomatous disease) or with high-dose corticosteroid therapy. Deficits in T-cell–mediated immunity secondary to AIDS, high-dose corticosteroid therapy, cyclosporine or other immunosuppressive drugs, chemotherapy, transplantation, bone marrow failure, and various other disorders have become increasingly common with the prolonged survival of transplant patients on chronic immunosuppressive therapy.

Immune deficits arising from disruption of the integument or GI/genitourinary barriers can also predispose patients to fungal infections. The most common types of integument/barrier disruptions are surgery, use of central venous and urinary catheters, hyperalimentation, and mucositis secondary to cytotoxic chemotherapy. Broad-spectrum antibacterial therapy can also predispose patients to fungal infections through disruption of the microbiologic flora in the gut, which allows overgrowth of Candida species. Successful management of opportunistic fungal pathogens, therefore, requires the reversal or reduction of underlying deficits in the host immune system.

All of the opportunistic mycoses are difficult to diagnose and often must be treated empirically before diagnosis is proven. Deciding when to initiate antifungal therapy and what opportunistic pathogens to cover is a decision governed largely by the *cumulative* immune deficits and clinical status of the host.

Patient Encounter 2, Part 1

A 43-year-old male in the surgical ICU after exploratory laparotomy following a motor vehicle accident develops fever that is unresponsive to broad-spectrum antibacterial therapy (piperacillin-tazobactam 3.75 g every 6 hours, gentamicin 120 mg every 8 hours, and vancomycin 1 g every 12 hours). The patient has a central venous catheter and a Foley catheter. Blood cultures are negative at the time, but the patient has yeast growing in the sputum and urine. Laboratory studies reveal a white blood cell count of $11.3 \times 10^3/mm^3$ $(11.3 \times 10^9/L)$

What are this patient's risk factors for developing an invasive fungal infection?

What current evidence suggests that this patient has an invasive fungal infection?

If antifungal therapy is empirically started in this patient, which species need to be treated?

INVASIVE CANDIDIASIS

EPIDEMIOLOGY

Candida species are the most common opportunistic fungal pathogens encountered in hospitals, ranking as the third to fourth most common cause of nosocomial bloodstream infections in United States.[17] The incidence of nosocomial candidiasis has increased steadily since the early 1980s, with the widespread use of central venous catheters, broad-spectrum antimicrobials, and other advancements in the supportive care of critically ill patients. In the 1980s, *C. albicans* accounted for over 80% of all bloodstream yeast isolates cultured from patients. By the late 1990s, this relative frequency of *C. albicans* had decreased to 50% in national surveys of bloodstream infections without a corresponding decrease in infections caused by nonalbicans species. Because of the inherent resistance (e.g., *C. krusei*) or diminished susceptibility (e.g., *C. glabrata*) of many of the nonalbicans species, the introduction of fluconazole in the early 1990s is often cited as the key element driving the shift in the microbiology of invasive candidiasis. However, it is likely that other institution-specific factors (e.g., increasing use of central venous catheters and increasing intensity of cytotoxic/mucotoxic chemotherapy) and use of broad-spectrum antibiotic therapy have contributed equally to this trend.[18,19] ❺ *It is important to be familiar with the relative epidemiology and frequency of nonalbicans Candida species in the institution or intensive care unit (ICU) before selecting empiric antifungal therapy for invasive candidiasis.*

PATHOGENESIS AND CLINICAL PRESENTATION

Invasive candidiasis is not a single syndrome, rather a spectrum of infections that differ in terms of clinical presentation and course depending on the type of host immune immunosuppression. Many forms of invasive candidiasis are potentially severe, however, with high (30–60%) rates of crude morbidity and mortality.[19] The most common form of invasive candidiasis is seen in non-neutropenic patients with disruption of the GI, skin or microbiologic barriers giving rise to a bloodstream infection (fungemia) from, or seeding to, a central venous catheter. Catheter-related candidemia carries a good prognosis if appropriate antifungal therapy is instituted early with catheter removal.[19] Fungemia can be of high density, however, leading to metastatic sites of infection and invasion of deep organs with increased morbidity. Therefore, the infection must be taken seriously, especially in patients with poor performance status (i.e., a high Acute Physiology, Age, and Chronic Health Evaluation II score) in the ICU.

Patients with acute disseminated candidiasis share many similar features as patients with catheter-related candidemia, except infection generally arises from the gut following mucotoxic chemotherapy and the patients are often profoundly ill. Hematogenous spread to noncontiguous organs is common in patients with acute disseminated candidiasis, and outcome is heavily dependent upon recovery from neutropenia.[19] Fluconazole prophylaxis has markedly decreased the incidence of acute disseminated candidiasis among high-risk patient groups such as bone marrow transplant and acute leukemia patients.[19] However, breakthrough infections

with fluconazole-resistant *C. glabrata* and *C. krusei* are still a concern.

Some forms of invasive candidiasis are dominated by deep-organ infection and may never be detected by blood cultures. Chronic disseminated candidiasis or hepatosplenic candidiasis is a unique presentation of candidemia seen after recovery from neutropenia. Candidemia during the period of neutropenia may be initially localized to the portal circulation with dissemination to contiguous organs. After recovery of neutrophils, an inflammatory response is seen against areas of focal infection in the liver and spleen. This inflammatory response produces abdominal pain that is associated with increases in alkaline phosphatase levels and hepatocellular enzymes.[19] Diagnosis is typically confirmed by patient history (recent neutropenia), and multiple areas of lucency in the liver and spleen on CT.

Focal invasive candidiasis has been reported for virtually every organ, even following apparently uncomplicated catheter-related fungemia. The most common sites of infection are the kidney, eye, and bone. *Candida* in the urine can be an indication of renal candidiasis or an obstructing fungus ball; however, it must be distinguished from more benign colonization of the urinary tract, especially in patients with chronic indwelling urinary catheters.[19] All patients with candidemia should undergo an eye exam to rule out *Candida* endophthlamitis, which can be sight-threatening if not recognized early.[19]

Laboratory diagnosis of invasive candidiasis is established by detection of the yeast in blood cultures or another sterile site (Fig. 84–3A).[19] Growth of Candida from urine, sputum, or respiratory secretions (including bronchoalveolar lavage) is not considered to be evidence of invasive infection, as these areas frequently become colonized with Candida species in patients receiving broad-spectrum antibiotics.[19] Colonization at multiple distinct body sites or with high

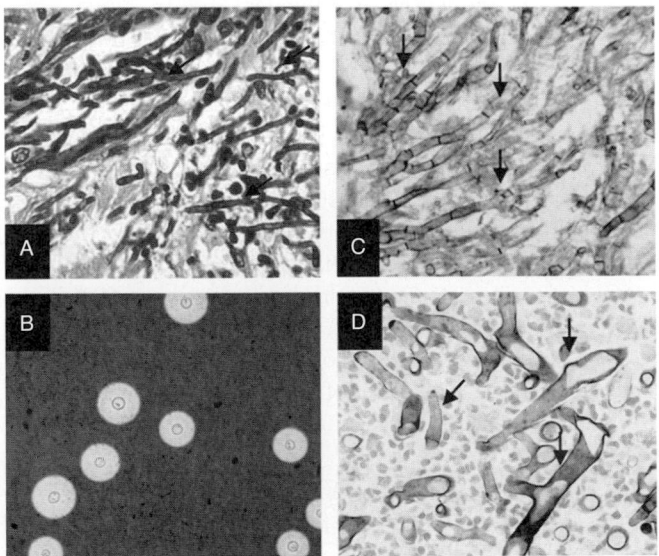

FIGURE 84–3. Opportunistic mycoses in clinical samples. *A.* Candidiasis (tissue). *B.* Cryptococcosis (India ink stain of CSF). *C.* Aspergillosis (tissue). *D.* Zygomycosis (tissue).

density of Candida species, however, may precede invasive infection. Therefore, preemptive antifungal therapy may be indicated in colonized high-risk populations such as those with neutropenic fever, transplant recipients, or following major abdominal surgery.[19] Although *Candida* are not particularly fastidious organisms, the sensitivity of blood cultures is relatively poor (less than 60%) and a negative culture does not rule out infection.[19] The poor sensitivity of blood cultures for detecting invasive disease has led to the study of novel serodiagnostic tests to detect antibodies, fungal metabolites, fungal cell wall antigens, or nucleic acids of Candida species. Of the four approaches, antigen testing based on the detection of β-glucan polymers in the cell wall of *Candida* have appeared most promising; however, none of these diagnostic tests have achieved routine clinical use.

6 *Laboratory identification of Candida in clinical samples must be performed to the species level whenever possible, as Candida species differ considerably in their susceptibility to antifungal agents.*[19,20] Rapid discrimination of *C. albicans* from common nonalbicans Candida species can be accomplished by the germ-tube test, which presumptively identifies *C. albicans* by the early formation (less than 4 hours) of a hyphae-like structure when the yeast in incubated in serum at 37°C (98.6°F). Definitive species identification, however, may require an additional 48 to 72 hours after the organism is isolated on agar. Fluorescent in situ hybridization (FISH) of Candida species-specific DNA sequences can reduce the time needed for definitive species identification, but is not available at most hospitals.

C. albicans remains the most common cause of invasive candidiasis, is the most virulent of Candida species, but is the most susceptible to commonly used antifungals including fluconazole.[19,20] Like *C. albicans*, *C. tropicalis* is a relatively virulent species that has a tropism for causing deep tissue invasion. *C. tropicalis* is generally sensitive to antifungals including fluconazole.[19,20] *C. parapsilosis* is a less virulent species seen frequently in neonates and in adults with central venous catheters. Although *C. parapsilosis* is less virulent, many isolates form thick biofilms on prosthetic materials and catheters that make the organism difficult to eradicate.[19,20] *C. parapsilosis* is generally susceptible to most antifungals including fluconazole. However, higher dosages of echinocandins (e.g., 70–100 mg/day of caspofungin) have been suggested due to the decreased potency of the echinocandin class against this species. *C. krusei* is a less-common species associated with breakthrough infections in heavily immunocompromised patients and should always be considered resistant to fluconazole.[19,20] Interestingly, most fluconazole-resistant isolates of *C. krusei* retain susceptibility to itraconazole and voriconazole, based on laboratory analysis.

C. glabrata has become a common cause of both de novo candidemia in heavily immunocompromised hosts and breakthrough infection in patients on fluconazole prophylaxis. Although *C. glabrata* is less virulent than other Candida species, infections with this organism are typically seen in patients with poor performance status, therefore mortality remains high. The marginal susceptibility of *C. glabrata* to fluconazole dictates that other agents such as amphotericin B or the echinocandins be considered as first-line therapy until susceptibility to fluconazole can be documented.[19,20] The effectiveness of voriconazole or posaconazole for fully fluconazole-resistant *C. glabrata fungemia* is not well established, and cross-resistance among these triazole antifungals has been documented in laboratory studies.[21,22]

TREATMENT

Six antifungals (amphotericin B, fluconazole, voriconazole, caspofungin, micafungin, and anidulafungin) have been studied as montherapy in prospective, randomized comparative clinical trials for the treatment of invasive candidiasis.[19,23–27] While these treatment options are considered to have relatively equivalent efficacy, they differ somewhat in toxicity and associated drug-drug interaction profiles. Lipid amphotericin B formulations are probably as effective as the aforementioned agents; however, evidence supporting their use is derived principally from open-label observational studies and empiric therapy trials of febrile neutropenia.[19] Moreover, the acquisition cost of lipid amphotericin B formulations is relatively higher compared to fluconazole and the echinocandins. As a result, their first-line use is not prominently recommended in evidence-based guidelines for proven infection.[20] No prospective randomized, controlled clinical trials have been published comparing antifungal therapies for proven acute disseminated candidiasis in neutropenic patients, chronic disseminated candidiasis, or other forms of deep-organ candidiasis.[19]

A majority of patients are treated empirically for invasive candidiasis before conclusive evidence of infection is available to direct therapy. Empiric therapy for invasive candidiasis

---

Patient Encounter 2, Part 2

Selecting Antifungal Therapy

The patient is started on fluconazole 400 mg/day, but 3 days later has persistent fever and develops hypotension and decreased urine output. Blood cultures reveal a germ tube–negative yeast growing in the blood. Laboratory studies revealed a WBC of $12.3 \times 10^3/mm^3$ ($12.3 \times 10^9/L$), aspartate aminotransferase 68 IU/L (1.13 μKat/L), alanine aminotransferase 75 IU/L (1.25 μKat/L), alkaline phosphatase 168 IU/L (2.8 μKat/L), and normal bilirubin. Serum creatinine is 1.8 mg/dL (159 μmol/L).

What factors suggest empiric antifungal therapy should be changed in this patient?

What are the most likely fungal species growing from the blood?

What other procedures should be recommended in this patient to improve response to antifungal therapy?

should be considered in any patient with persistent, unexplained fever and host deficits that predispose patients to candidemia, including broad-spectrum antibacterial therapy, presence of a central venous catheter, patients with severe organ dysfunction or on dialysis, patients with neutropenia or qualitative deficiencies in host immunity (e.g., due to high-dose corticosteroid therapy), or colonization with *Candida* at one or more body sites. ❼ *If a patient is non-neutropenic, clinically stable (i.e., normotensive with relatively normal organ function), and has never received prior azole therapy, fluconazole 800 mg/day (12 mg/kg/day) is an appropriate first-line therapy for invasive candidiasis until speciation of the Candida isolate is confirmed.*[19] Echinocandins (caspofungin, micafungin, anidulafungin) are preferred as first-line agents in more critically ill patients with compromised renal function, hypotension/sepsis, or in institutions/ICUs with relatively high rates (greater than 10%) of *C. glabrata* or *C. krusei* (Table 84–3).[19] Treatment is continued for at least 2 weeks or longer for complicated infections (endovascular source, metastatic seeding).

One caveat is that cryptococcoisis or endemic fungi occasionally produce fungemia in lymphopenic patients that initially misidentified as *Candida*. Therefore, initial treatment with a lipid amphotericin B formulation may be judicious in profoundly lymphopenic patients (i.e., CD4+ less than 250/mm³) with yeast in blood cultures until fungal identification is confirmed, as echinocandins have poor activity against non-*Candida* yeast. Timely initiation of appropriate antifungal therapy is critical as any delay in the initiation of antifungal therapy once a patient has a positive blood culture significantly increases mortality and the potential for metastatic infections.[28]

Amphotericin B deoxycholate 0.7 mg/kg/day or an echinocandin (i.e., caspofungin, micafungin, or anidula-fungin); voriconazole; or a lipid amphotericin B formulation are recommended as empiric therapy in patients with neutropenic (i.e., absolute neutrophil count less than 500 PMN/mm³) fever. Other newer echinocandins (micafungin and anidulafungin) are effective alternatives to caspofungin. If the neutropenia is of shorter duration and the patient is at lower risk for mold infections (e.g., solid tumor patients with 2 weeks or less of neutropenia), higher-dose fluconazole (i.e., 800 mg/day or 12 mg/kg) could be considered.[19] Lipid amphotericin B formulations, an echinocandin, or voriconazole are often the preferred agents in febrile patients with 3 weeks or more of neutropenia to expand coverage against molds.[19,29] If the yeast is identified as *C. glabrata*, published treatment guidelines recommend the use of either caspofungin or possibly amphotericin B formulations.[19] Voriconazole is not recommended until further clinical data support its use for *C. glabrata*, as laboratory studies have suggested potential cross-resistance with fluconazole-resistant isolates of this species. Fluconazole can also be considered for *C. glabrata* infections if the isolate is documented to be susceptible or susceptible-dose-dependent to fluconazole.[19] *C. krusei* infections can be treated with an echinocandin, amphotericin B, or voriconazole. Patients who

respond to therapy are medically stable, are not neutropenic, and are taking oral medications can be transitioned to oral fluconazole provided isolate susceptibility is documented by minimum inhibitory concentration testing.

For uncomplicated catheter-related candidemia (no evidence of organ involvement), therapy should be continued for at least 2 weeks from the last positive blood culture.[19] In neutropenic patients, therapy should be continued until resolution of neutropenia.[19] Whenever possible, central venous catheters should be removed to decrease the duration of fungemia and risk of recurrent infections.[19]

Treatment recommendations for other forms of invasive candidiasis are based primarily on anecdotal evidence and expert opinion. Deep-organ candidiasis requires prolonged therapy to achieve a cure; therefore, importance is placed on the use of convenient and nontoxic long-term treatment regimens. Fluconazole (400 mg/day or 6 mg/kg/day) is the preferred regimen in clinically-stable patients. Amphotericin B, lipid amphotericin B formulations, and possibly caspofungin can be considered for refractory cases or clinically unstable patients. Infections of the eye, bone, pancreas, or gallbladder are typically treated with either amphotericin B or fluconazole; however, there are few data to support the use of echinocandins. Urinary candidiasis is an ill-defined group of syndromes that can range from benign colonization (candiduria) to invasive disease of the renal parenchyma. Asymptomatic non-neutropenic patients with candiduria do not require antifungal therapy, as no study has demonstrated the value of transiently clearing *Candida* from the urine. Patients should receive 7 to 14 days of antifungal therapy for urinary candidiasis if they are: (a) symptomatic; (b) have clinical or laboratory evidence of infection; (c) are neutropenic; (d) are low-birth-weight infants; (e) will undergo urologic manipulations; or (f) have renal allografts. Removal of urinary tract instruments, including Foley catheters and stents, is recommended whenever possible. The preferred therapy is fluconazole 200 mg daily, although IV amphotericin B deoxycholate 0.3 to 1 mg/kg/day is also effective. Other antifungal agents do not achieve appreciable concentrations in the urine and therefore should not be considered for urinary candidiasis. Irrigation with amphotericin B is not effective for infections above the bladder and should not be used in higher-risk patients with the exception of its use as a diagnostic tool for confirming a localized infection of the bladder. *Candida* infections of the renal parenchyma secondary to metastatic seeding from the bloodstream are treated in a similar fashion to candidemia.

Mucocutaneous candidiasis is generally not life threatening nor invasive and can be treated with topical azoles (clotrimazole troches), oral azoles (fluconazole, ketoconazole, or itraconazole), or oral polyenes (such as nystatin or oral amphotericin B). Orally administered and absorbed azoles (ketoconazole, fluconazole, or itraconazole solution), amphotericin B suspension, IV echinocandins, or IV amphotericin B are recommended for refractory or recurrent infections.[19]

Table 84–3

Therapeutic Approach to Opportunistic Fungal Infections in Adults

Mycoses	Recommended Treatment Regimens	Comments
Candidiasis Catheter-related and acute hematogenous	Fluconazole 6–12 mg/kg/day IV every 24 hours *or* caspofungin[a] 70 mg IV on day 1, then 50 mg every 24 hours[a] *or* amphotericin B + fluconazole *Second line:* Lipid amphotericin B formulation 3–5 mg/kg/day[b] *or* amphotericin B 0.5–7 mg/kg/day or voriconazole 6 mg/kg every 12 hours for 1 day, then 3 mg/kg every 12 hours	Treat for 14 days after the last positive blood culture and resolution of signs and symptoms catheter should be removed whenever possible Patients can be switched to oral fluconazole when clinically stable if isolate is susceptible An echinocandin or amphotericin B are preferred agents for fluconazole-resistant species Voriconazole appears to be effective against fluconazole-resistant *C. krusei*
Empirical therapy in neutropenic patient	Fluconazole 6–12 mg/kg/day (low risk) *or* amphotericin B 0.7 mg/kg/day IV *or* liposomal amphotericin B 3 mg/kg every 24 hours	Antifungals with coverage of *Aspergillus* should be used in higher-risk patients or prolonged neutropenia (i.e., longer than 2 weeks) Asymptomatic candiduria does not required therapy However, treatment is recommended in neutropenic, low-birth-weight infants, and patients undergoing urologic manipulations or those with renal allografts Amphotericin B bladder irrigation no longer recommended
Urinary candidiasis	Fluconazole 200 mg IV or orally for 7–14 days *or* amphotericin B 0.3 mg/kg/day IV for 1–7 days	
Cryptococcosis Pulmonary-isolated severe pulmonary and meningitis	Fluconazole 6 mg/kg/day IV or orally for 6–12 months *Induction:* Amphotericin B 0.7–1 mg/kg/day + flucytosine 100 mg/kg/day orally divided every 6 hours for 2 weeks *Consolidation:* Fluconazole 6–12 mg/kg/day for 10 weeks *Second line:* Fluconazole + flucytosine for 2 weeks then fluconazole for 10 weeks *or* amphotericin + fluconazole for 2 weeks then fluconazole for 10 weeks *or* liposomal amphotericin B 5 mg/kg/day × 2 weeks then fluconazole for 10 weeks	Regimens reported to produce faster sterilization of CSF compared to amphotericin B deoxycholate alone during the first 2 weeks: Amphotericin B + 5-flucytosine Amphotericin B + Liposomal amphotericin B Fluconazole Echinocandins have no activity against cryptococci
Aspergillosis	Voriconazole 6 mg/kg every 12 hours for 1 day, then 4 mg/kg every 12 hours *or* lipid formulations of amphotericin B *or* caspofungin 70 mg IV for 1 dose, then 50 mg IV every 24 hours[a] *or* posaconazole 200 mg orally 4 × daily × 14 days, then 200 mg orally twice daily *or* combination therapy	Voriconazole can be administered as oral therapy in patients taking oral medications Voriconazole can cause reversible visual disturbances and occasionally hallucinations Because of the high dosages and prolonged treatment courses, lipid formulations are preferred for amphotericin B–based therapy Preclinical studies suggest mold-active azoles plus echinocandins have enhanced activity against *Aspergillus* *A. terreus* should be considered resistant to amphotericin B Activity of amphotericin B and voriconazole is decreased versus *Aspergillus* species; higher doses or combination therapy may be indicated in more refractory cases
Fusariosis	Lipid formulations of amphotericin B *or* voriconazole 6 mg/kg every 12 hours for 1 day, then 4 mg/kg every 12 hours *or* posaconazole 200 mg orally 4 × daily for 14 days, then 200 mg orally every 12 hours *or* combination therapy	
Zygomycoses	High-dose lipid amphotericin B (e.g., 7.5–10 mg/kg/day) *or* posaconazole 200 mg orally 4 × daily for 14 days, then 200 mg orally every 12 hours *or* combination therapy +/– echinocandin	Prompt diagnosis and surgical debridement are essential for successful outcome; high dosages of lipid amphotericin B are required; posaconazole is the only azole with activity against zygomycoses

CSF, cerebrospinal fluid.

[a]Or equivalent echinocandin (micafungin 100 mg/day, anidulafungin 200 mg/day 1, then 100 mg/day).

[b]Ambisome 3 to 5 mg/kg/day; 7.5 to 10 mg/kg for zygomycosis; Abelcet 5 mg/kg/day; Amphotec 4 mg/kg/day.

Although more invasive, esophageal candidiasis does not typically evolve into a life-threatening infection. However, topical therapy is ineffective. Azoles (fluconazole, itraconazole solution, or voriconazole), echinocandins, or IV amphotericin B (in cases of unresponsive infections) are effective treatment options. Parenteral therapy should be used in patients who are unable to take oral medications.[19]

PATIENT MONITORING AND SIDE EFFECTS

Response to antifungal therapy in invasive candidiasis is often more rapid than for endemic fungal infections. Resolution of fever and sterilization of blood cultures are indications of response to antifungal therapy. Toxicity associated with antifungal therapy is similar in these patients as described earlier with the caveat that some toxicities may be more pronounced in critically-ill patients with invasive candidiasis. Nephrotoxicity and electrolyte disturbances, with amphotericin B in particular, are problematic and may not be avoidable even with lipid amphotericin B formulations. Therefore, there is a growing emphasis on the first-line use of fluconazole in lower-risk patients and echinocandins in higher-risk patients to reduce the potential for patient adverse effects. Decisions to use one class of antifungal agents over the other are principally driven by concerns of nonalbicans species, patient tolerability, or history of prior fluconazole exposure (risk factor for nonalbicans species.).

PROPHYLAXIS

Fluconazole (400 mg/day) has been extensively studied as a prophylactic regimen to prevent invasive candidiasis in patients with prolonged (greater than 2 weeks) neutropenia.[29-34] Placebo-controlled, prospective randomized trials performed in the 1990s demonstrated that fluconazole was effective in reducing the frequency, morbidity, and in some trials mortality, due to invasive candidiasis when administered until marrow recovery. However, the major limitation with fluconazole is its lack of mold coverage needed for high-risk patients with persistent neutropenia. Studies have examined the use of itraconazole, voriconazole, posaconazole, or the echinocandin micafungin as prophylaxis in hematopoietic cell transplant recipients until engraftment to provide protection against both *Candida* and *Aspergillus* species.[34-37] Although all antifungals studies have demonstrated a benefit in reducing fungal infections, all of the drugs have limitations with respect to prolonged administration in high-risk patients. Therefore, the approach toward antifungal prophylaxis is highly institution-specific depending on the patient population, epidemiology of invasive fungal infections, and options for outpatient IV drug therapy.

Use of antifungal prophylaxis for invasive candidiasis in the non-neutropenic patients remains an area of controversy.

Prophylaxis should be targeted toward clearly-defined high-risk transplant populations (e.g., liver, pancreatic, or small-bowel transplantation) or ICU patients (i.e., neonatal intensive care) with rates of invasive candidiasis exceeding 10%, despite aggressive infection-control procedures.[38,39] Fluconazole prophylaxis (400 mg/day) reduces the rate of *Candida* peritonitis in patients with refractory GI perforation and trended toward decreased rates of invasive candidiasis in select adult patients admitted to a surgical ICU for more than 3 days.[38,39] Fluconazole is also effective in reducing the rate of invasive candidiasis in neonates.[36] However, prophylaxis can result in excessive antifungal use in lower-risk patients; therefore, many experts have advocated preemptive (i.e., starting therapy based on biomarkers of infection) or empirical (symptoms of infection) treatment approaches in this population in lieu of prophylaxis. A recently completed multi-institutional prospective randomized trial of administering empirical fluconazole (800 mg/day vs. placebo) in ICU patients with persistent fever, however, did not demonstrate a benefit for in the non-neutropenic population.[40] It is hoped that ongoing studies will better define the risks versus benefits of routine antifungal prophylaxis or preemptive treatment approaches in the ICU setting.

CRYPTOCOCCOSIS

EPIDEMIOLOGY

Cryptococcus neoformans is an encapsulated yeast that can infect apparently normal hosts but is more frequently associated with severe infections in immunocompromised patients. *C. neoformans* is divided into two varieties based on serotype: *C. neoformans* var. *neoformans* (serotypes a and d) and *C. neoformans* var. *gatti* (serotypes b and c). *C. neoformans* var. *gatti* is found predominantly in tropical and subtropical climates associated with eucalyptus trees, whereas *C. neoformans* var. *neoformans* is found worldwide and is associated with pigeon droppings and other avian excreta. Before the AIDS pandemic, cryptococcosis was a relatively uncommon disease but became a leading cause of meningitis among HIV-infected patients. Although the incidence of this infection has declined somewhat with the widespread use of highly active antiretroviral therapy (HAART), *C. neoformans* remains an important pathogen in immunocompromised patients, including cancer patients who often present with the pulmonary form of the infection.

PATHOGENESIS AND CLINICAL PRESENTATION

C. neoformans is acquired primarily through inhalation of the desiccated yeast particles found in the environment. Inhaled cells reach distal alveolar spaces where they gradually rehydrate and form their characteristic polysaccharide

Patient Encounter 3

Invasive Mold Infection

A 40-year-old female with acute myelogenous leukemia at day 115 post matched-allogeneic donor hematopoietic stem cell transplantation presents to the clinic with increasing complaints of nausea, stomach cramping, and rash on the hands spreading up her arms. She also complains of pain upon deep inspiration. By laboratory examination, she is noted to have an alanine aminotransferase of 85 IU/L (1.42 μKat/L), aspartate aminotransferase 75 IU/L (1.25 μKat/L) and total bilirubin of 2.1 mg/dL (36 μmol/L). Her current medications include tacrolimus 5 mg twice daily (most recent level: 8 ng/mL [8 mcg/L]), levofloxacin 500 mg daily, fluconazole 200 mg/day, valacyclovir 500 mg twice daily, metoprolol 25 mg twice daily, and benzonatate (tessalon) pearls. She is admitted to the hospital for suspected graft-versus-host disease exacerbation. CT scan of the chest reveals three to four dense pleural base nodules in both lung fields. The primary service wishes to start voriconazole.

What are the patient's risk factors for developing an invasive mold infection?

Is voriconazole an acceptable option in this patient? Are there any drug interaction concerns?

capsules that enable resistance to phagocytosis. Defects in cellular immunity allow reconstitution of the protective capsule and multiplication of yeast in the lungs. Although alveolar macrophages phagocytose the yeast, containment and killing requires a coordinated response between innate and adaptive humoral (complement and anticryptococcal antibodies) and T-cell–mediated host responses.[5] Deficiencies in cell-mediated immunity allow the yeast to survive as a facultative intracellular pathogen in macrophages as they migrate from the lung to draining lymph nodes, leading to dissemination via the bloodstream to the meninges.

Unlike most opportunistic fungi, true virulence factors have been identified for *C. neoformans*. The capsules, including the soluble polysaccharides released from the yeast cells during infection, impair phagocytosis and binding of anticryptococcal antibodies. Primary cryptococcal infection begins in the lung, presenting as a mildly symptomatic or asymptomatic infection that resolves spontaneously or results in an encapsulated, usually noncalcified lung nodule. It is common for these isolated nodules to be detected on chest x-rays during routine workup. Diagnosis of primary cryptococcosis is only made if the nodule is aspirated or removed because of concerns of primary lung cancer.

In the immunocompromised host, infection of the lung may present with more diffuse, bilateral, and interstitial disease that mimics the presentation of *Pneumocystis jiroveci (carinii)* pneumonia (PCP). Dissemination to other organs, particularly the CNS, eye, and possibly the skin, is more likely to occur in patients with severe deficits in cell-mediated immunity. Fever, cough, dyspnea, and pleural pain are common at presentation with accompanying hypoxemia that can rapidly evolve to acute respiratory failure. Because of the features of diffuse pulmonary cryptococcosis overlap with other opportunistic pathogens, early diagnosis requires bronchoalveolar lavage or transbronchial biopsy, which can effectively diagnose 80% to 100% of cases.[41] The clinical course of diffuse cryptococcal pneumonia can be as severe as PCP, with mortality rates approaching 100% in untreated patients by 48 hours.

C. neoformans is strongly neurotropic and readily disseminates from the lung to the CNS, specifically the leptomeninges, and occasionally the parenchyma of the brain. The clinical characteristics of cryptococcal meningitis differ somewhat, however, between patients with and without underlying AIDS. In patients without AIDS, disease presentation is more insidious and symptoms such as dizziness, irritability, decreased comprehension, and unstable gait may present many weeks to months before the diagnosis is established.[41] Patients with AIDS generally present much later in the course of disease with severe meningoencephalitis.[37] The most common signs and symptoms on presentation are fever, headache, meningismus, photophobia, mental status changes, and seizures. CT or more sensitive MRI may reveal cerebral edema, multiple areas of enhanced nodules, or a single mass lesion (cryptococcoma). Examination of the cerebrospinal fluid (CSF) often reveals increased opening pressure upon lumbar puncture, but glucose, protein, and leukocyte levels can be normal.[41]

LABORATORY DIAGNOSIS

Clinical diagnosis is confirmed by cultures from the blood, CSF, or other clinically relevant fluids or tissue. However, early diagnosis is suggested by direct observation of *C. neoformans* in the CSF by India ink staining (Fig. 84–3B).[41] Similarly, detection of cryptococcal antigen in either serum or CSF can provide a rapid diagnosis with greater than 95% sensitivity and specificity and appears to correlate with fungal burden.[41] A positive serum antigen test of greater than 1:4 strongly suggests cryptococcal infection, and greater than or equal to 1:8 is indicative of active disease. Antigen titers in serum are positive in 99% of patients with cryptococcal meningitis and typically exceed titers of 1:2,048 in patients with AIDS.[41] However, the time course of cryptococcal antigen elimination is unknown, and a positive test result can persist for many years. Changes in the CSF cryptococcal antigen titers have limited value in the monitoring of drug therapy for cryptococcal meningitis, although it is expected that a decrease should be seen after two or more weeks of antifungal therapy.[41]

TREATMENT

Cryptococcal meningitis is fatal if left untreated. Because pneumonia frequently precedes dissemination of disease and subsequent meningitis, all patients with culture-, histopathology-, or serology-proven disease should receive antifungal therapy. In patients with isolated pulmonary cryptococcosis, fluconazole is generally considered to be the therapy of choice (see Table 84–2).[41] Alternatively, itraconazole, voriconazole, or combination therapy (fluconazole plus flucytosine) has also been used with some success but these regimens are generally considered inferior to amphotericin B and are recommended only for persons unable to tolerate or unresponsive to standard treatment. Echinocandins do not have clinically useful activity against *C. neoformans*.

Disseminated or CNS cryptococcosis requires a more aggressive treatment approach. Pretreatment predictors of poor outcome with antifungal therapy include:

- Progressive underlying disease or immunodysfunction
- Abnormal mental status at the time of presentation
- Increased opening pressure on lumbar puncture (greater than 260 mm H_2O)
- High fungal burden as reflected by a CSF antigen titer (in AIDS patients) of greater than 1:2,048

Prospective randomized trials completed prior to the recognition of AIDS demonstrated high response rates (approximately 80%) with the combined use of amphotericin B and flucytosine for 4 to 6 weeks. Although sterilization of the CSF could be achieved in most patients within 2 weeks with this regimen, a substantial number of patients (30–40%) developed dose-limiting toxicities and relapse was seen in roughly 50% of patients. Therefore, a treatment approach was devised that consisting of distinct treatment phases to minimize toxicity and reduce the risk of relapse. ❽ *Clinical trials performed by the National Institute of Allergy and Infectious Diseases (NIAID) Mycoses Study Group after the recognition of AIDS showed that 2 weeks of induction antifungal therapy with combination amphotericin B (0.7 mg/kg/day) plus flucytosine (100 mg/kg/day) for cryptococcal meningitis, followed by consolidation therapy with fluconazole (400 mg daily) for 8 weeks was as effective as 4 weeks of combination therapy, with fewer toxicities (see Table 84–2).[12,41]* Other studies have suggested fluconazole plus amphotericin may be an acceptable option in patients who cannot tolerate therapy with flucytosine (see Table 84–2).[12]

PROPHYLAXIS

Fluconazole (200 mg/day) is recommended as maintenance therapy for life in patients with persistent underlying immune dysfunction to prevent recurrent cryptococcal meningitis.[12] Available data have demonstrated that it is safe to discontinue maintenance therapy in AIDS patients who have had a sustained immunologic response on effective antiretroviral therapy.[12] Occasionally, initiation of HAART can result in the reactivation of a subclinical, immunologic manifestation of cryptococcal infection (or other opportunistic infections). Manifestations of this so-called *immune reconstitution syndrome* (IRIS) may include exacerbations of meningitis or necrotizing pneumonia. Antifungal therapy plus a nonsteroidal anti-inflammatory agent or prednisone have been used successfully in patients with cryptococcal-associated immune reconstitution syndrome.[12] However, the optimal management of this recently defined clinical entity remains unknown.

INVASIVE ASPERGILLOSIS

EPIDEMIOLOGY

Invasive molds, particularly *Aspergillus*, have become an increasingly important complication of cancer therapy and organ transplantation. Patients with acute leukemia and recipients of allogeneic hematopoietic cell transplants are at especially high risk for invasive aspergillosis (IA) due to prolonged neutropenia and deficiencies in cell-mediated immunity associated with graft-versus-host disease and its treatment. More than 180 species within the genus *Aspergillus* have been described, but only four species are commonly associated with invasive infection: *Aspergillus fumigatus*, *Aspergillus flavus*, *Aspergillus terreus*, and *Aspergillus niger*. Of these four species, *A. fumigatus* accounts for most of human infections. However, identification of *Aspergillus* mold in culture to the species level is still essential because the incidence of amphotericin B–resistant *Aspergillus terreus* and *Aspergillus flavus* have increased over the last 10 years among high-risk patients. Early and accurate diagnosis of IA remains the most important barrier to the effective management of this infection, which is associated with crude mortality rates ranging from 60% to 100%.[42]

PATHOGENESIS AND CLINICAL PRESENTATION

The pathogenesis of IA is defined largely by the underlying immune dysfunction of the host. The most common route of acquisition for *Aspergillus* is through the respiratory tract. Conidia dispersed in air currents are continuously inhaled through the sinuses and mouth and penetrate down to distal alveolar spaces (see Fig. 84–3C). Most conidia are rapidly phagocytosed and removed by resident macrophages and neutrophils in the upper and lower respiratory tract.[5] However, macrophage function may be suppressed following transplantation, cytotoxic chemotherapy, or in patients who have received high-dose corticosteroid therapy. Conidia that escaped phagocytosis begin to germinate into hyphal forms that are too large for ingestion by macrophages. Hyphal forms of *Aspergillus* then invade blood vessels or contiguous tissues or bone (in sinuses) resulting in hemorrhage and/or infarction, and coagulative necrosis. Once in the bloodstream, viable hyphal fragments can break off and disseminate to distal organs including the brain. Control of the infection at this stage requires development of an adaptive Th-1 type response to enhance the fungicidal activity of professional effector cells (i.e., neutrophils) against hyphal elements.[5] Patients with dysregulated, suppressed T-cell–mediated immunity, or prolonged neutropenia are unable to control the infection and are at high risk for dissemination of the infection. Without antifungal therapy, IA in immunosuppressed patients is uniformly fatal.

Signs and symptoms of IA are predictably muted in the immunocompromised host. Fever is common but nonspecific for infection and may be accompanied by pleuritic chest pain, cough, hemoptysis, and/or friction rub.[40] Neurologic signs including seizures, hemiparesis, and stupor may be present in patients with dissemination to the brain. Cutaneous plaques or papules characterized by a central necrotic ulcer or eschar occur in up to 10% of patients with disseminated disease; however, concomitant blood cultures are often negative. Chest radiographs cannot detect early forms of disease and may remain negative in up to 10% of patients within 1 week of death.[43,44] ❾ *Nodular lesions detected by high-resolution computed tomography (HRCT) scans are often the first indication of invasive pulmonary aspergillosis* along with fever, and reveal small wedge-shaped or nodular lesions, typically surrounded by intermediate attenuation called the "halo sign."[43,44] These early lesions on CT scans represent hemorrhage and edema surrounding an infarcted blood vessel. Despite "effective" antifungal therapy, lesions on CT scan may continue to increase in size in neutropenic patients until neutrophil counts recover, at which time they begin to cavitate, forming the "air-crescent sign" on chest radiographs, indicative of resolving infection. ❿ *Immunocompromised patients on fluconazole with progressive sinus or pulmonary disease by radiography should be considered to have a possible mold infection* and receive empiric antifungal therapy directed (at minimum) against *Aspergillus* species.[42]

LABORATORY DIAGNOSIS

Like other invasive mycoses, definitive diagnosis of aspergillosis requires histopathologic evidence of hyphal invasion in tissue (Fig. 84–4). However, procedures needed to establish a definitive diagnosis by sampling of suspicious lesions (e.g., fine-needle aspiration or thoracoscopic lung biopsy) are not feasible in many patients with underlying thrombocytopenia secondary to hematologic malignancies or chemotherapy. Even if hyphae are observed in tissue, histopathology alone cannot distinguish *Aspergillus* from other angioinvasive septate molds such as *Fusarium*, which have different patterns of antifungal susceptibility.[42] Therefore, respiratory and/or wound cultures (if cutaneous

or sinus/hard palate lesions are present) are important factors in the modification of empiric antifungal therapy.

Respiratory cultures including sputum, bronchial washings, or bronchoalveolar lavage have a low sensitivity for diagnosis of IA but a high positive predictive value in immunocompromised patients.[42] Therefore, a negative bronchoalveolar lavage culture does not rule out invasive pulmonary aspergillosis, but a positive culture in a high-risk patient (e.g., allogeneic hematopoietic cell transplant patients) indicates pulmonary aspergillosis in at least 60% of such patients. Blood cultures have little diagnostic value for IA but may reflect true disease with *A. terreus*. Patients with limited lung involvement or on prophylactic or empiric antifungal therapy may continue to be culture-negative for *Aspergillus* species, despite the appearance of progressing disease.[42] Therefore, clinical specialists should never consider negative cultures as an indication for stopping antifungal therapy in patients with suspected or proven aspergillosis.

Considerable effort has been focused in the last decade to develop nonculture based laboratory methods (antigen detection, polymerase chain reaction [PCR], and metabolite detection) for the diagnosis of IA. The hope is that these surrogate tests could detect early evidence of *Aspergillus* infection before significant target organ damage eventually detected by CT scans occurs. The FDA has approved an ELISA-based assay for the detection of a polysaccharide component of the *Aspergillus* cell wall called galactomannan. Although several large prospective studies have found that the sensitivity and specificity of the assay exceeded 90% in neutropenic patients with hematologic malignancies, the median time span between galactomannan detection and clinical signs and symptoms of IA averages less than 6 days.[42] Other factors such as patient immune status (neutropenia versus graft-versus-host disease), antifungal therapy, and diet may affect the interpretation of the galactomannan test.[42] For example, false-positive results have been reported in pediatric patients, patients receiving piperacillin-tazobactam for neutropenic fever, and following the ingestion of certain cereals, pastas, nutritional supplements, or soy sauce.[42] Hence, there are numerous opportunities for false-positive tests. Although some animal studies and clinical data suggest that rising galactomannan levels are a harbinger of breakthrough infection, there are still limited data supporting the use of this test to guide and monitor antifungal therapy. At this time it appears that the galactomannan test (and other nonculture based strategies) will serve as complementary methods to confirm results from microbiologic, histopathologic, and radiographic investigations directed toward diagnosing IA.

TREATMENT

To date, only two comparative randomized controlled clinical trials have evaluated antifungal therapies for the treatment of diagnosis-proven IA and only one study was sufficiently powered to measure differences in response to antifungal therapy.[45] In that study, unblinded investigators

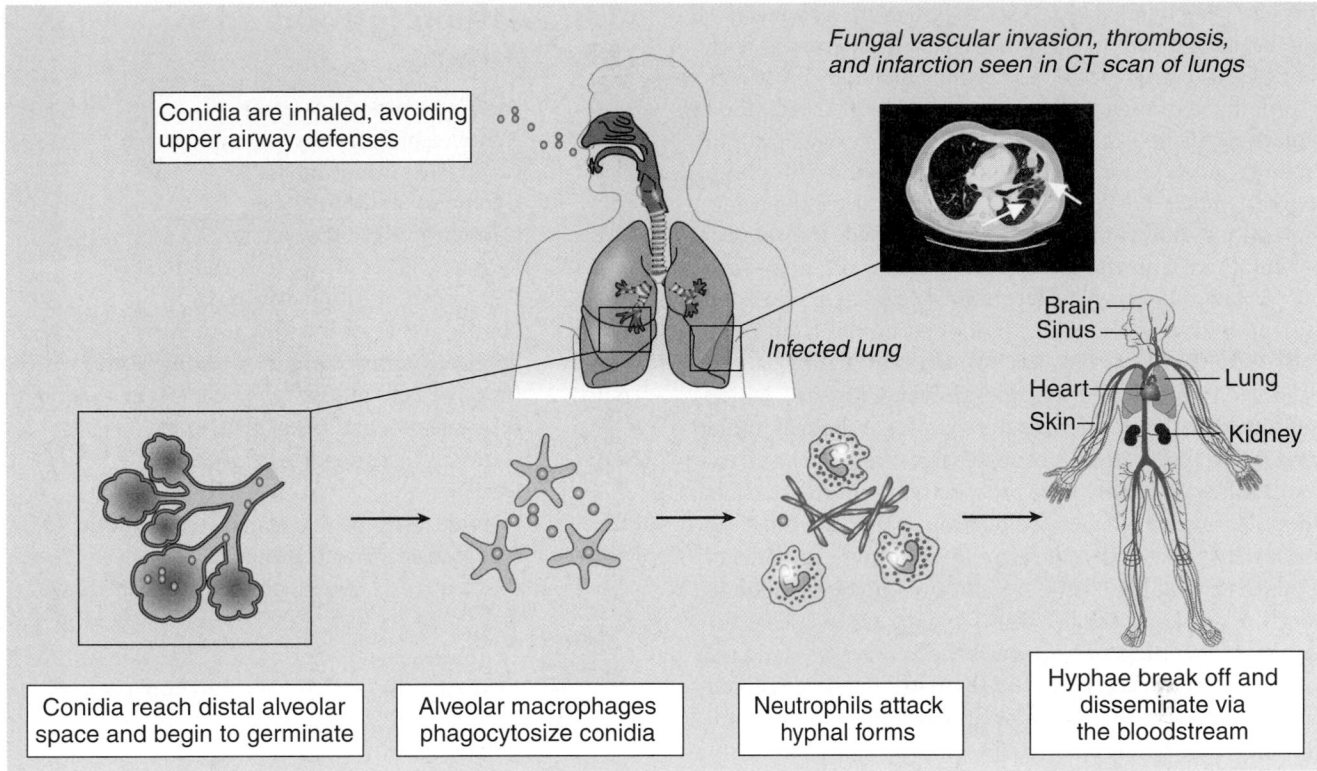

Fungal vascular invasion, thrombosis, and infarction seen in CT scan of lungs

Conidia are inhaled, avoiding upper airway defenses

Infected lung

Brain
Sinus
Heart
Skin
Lung
Kidney

Conidia reach distal alveolar space and begin to germinate

Alveolar macrophages phagocytosize conidia

Neutrophils attack hyphal forms

Hyphae break off and disseminate via the bloodstream

FIGURE 84–4. Pathogenesis of invasive aspergillosis (IA).

compared patients initially randomized to the newer triazole, voriconazole, to patients initially treated with amphotericin B deoxycholate.[45] The study design was unique in that it allowed a change from the randomized drug to any other licensed antifungal therapy, without requiring that the patient be classified as a treatment failure on randomized therapy. Nearly 80% of patients randomized to receive amphotericin B deoxycholate were switched to other licensed antifungal therapies (mean duration 10 days) versus 36% of patients in the voriconazole arm (mean duration 77 days). The poor tolerability of amphotericin B deoxycholate was not surprising given the relatively higher dosages (1 mg/kg/day IV) and prolonged treatment courses required in the treatment of IA. At the end of the study (12 weeks), a higher proportion of patients in the voriconazole arm remained alive (70.8%) compared to amphotericin B deoxycholate–treated patients (57.9%). ⓫ *On the basis of these results, many experts now consider voriconazole as the initial drug of choice for IA in patients without significant contraindications (e.g., drug interactions or pre-existing liver dysfunction) to azole therapy* (see Table 84–2).[42] Voriconazole also appears to have some efficacy in CNS aspergillosis, a form of IA with historical mortality rates approaching 100%. Itraconazole has activity against *Aspergillus* and is frequently used as prophylaxis, but is not considered a particularly effective treatment option for invasive disease.[42]

Lipid formulations of amphotericin B, echinocandins, or posaconazole can be considered as possible alternatives to voriconazole therapy and may be preferred agents in patients with breakthrough infection on azole antifungals (including itraconazole or fluconazole). Several recent open-label case series have suggested that combination therapy, with an echinocandin and mold-active triazole such as voriconazole, may be more effective than voriconazole alone for IA that has failed amphotericin B–based therapy.[42] Once antifungal therapy has begun, the duration and intensity of antifungal therapy is directed by host-specific factors including clinical response, underlying immunosuppression, tolerability, and plans for future chemotherapy/immunosuppression. In the heavily immunocompromised patient, complete eradication of the fungus is unlikely and suppressive therapy may be required until well after recovery of cellular immune function. Reactivation from residual infarcts or devitalized tissue in the sinus or lung harboring aspergillosis is a concern if the patient will receive further immunosuppressive therapy. Therefore, surgical débridement of the sinus or excision of large lung lesions is often pursued if the patient is not profoundly thrombocytopenic. Relapsing or breakthrough *Aspergillus* infections respond less favorably to antifungal therapy than de novo IA and may require more aggressive measures (combination therapy, immunotherapy, or surgery) to stabilize the infection.

PROPHYLAXIS

Although recently published guidelines for preventing opportunistic infections in hematopoietic cell transplant recipients do not provide concrete recommendations for antifungal prophylaxis against *Aspergillus*, prophylaxis should be considered in certain high-risk subgroups with rates of IA exceeding 10%. These groups include: (a) patients with prolonged pre-engraftment periods (e.g., cord-blood transplant recipients), (b) patients with a history of IA prior to transplantation, (c) patients receiving transplants with a high risk of graft-versus-host disease (e.g., haploidentical allogeneic transplant) or infection (e.g., T-cell–depleted transplant), any patient with graft-versus-host disease on high-dose corticosteroid therapy (greater than 1 mg/kg prednisone equivalent) with or without antithymocyte globulin or tumor necrosis factor blockade (i.e., infliximab), and (d) any patient transplanted with active cytomegalovirus disease, which is associated with an increased risk of subsequent mold infections due to the immunosuppressive effect of the virus. Posaconazole was shown in two prospective randomized trials to reduce *Aspergillus*-associated death in patients with acute high-risk leukemia and reduce mold infections in patients with graft-versus-host disease following hematopoetic stem cell transplantation.[35,36] Similar data are available for voriconazole,[37] but less benefit was observed versus standard fluconazole prophylaxis in the hematopoetic stem cell transplant patients. Prophylactic approaches, however, are often highly institution and patient specific.

PATIENT MONITORING AND SIDE EFFECTS

Response to antifungal therapy in invasive molds is slow and difficult to judge by clinical signs alone. Resolution of fever and eventual clearing of CT scans (in the case of lung infections) are indications of response to antifungal therapy. Toxicity associated with antifungal therapy is similar in these patients as in those described earlier. In addition to the adverse effects mentioned earlier, voriconazole may cause transient visual changes (photopsia) in approximately one-third of patients with the first few doses of therapy. Occasionally, these visual disturbances are accompanied by hallucinations and may require discontinuation of therapy. Voriconazole and posaconazole exhibit wide intrapatient and interpatient pharmacokinetic variability due to variable absorption and metabolism, respectively.[42] Therefore, many experts advocate therapeutic drug monitoring in patients with documented disease receiving the drugs as monotherapy, or in patients with suspected progression (voriconazole, posaconazole) or toxicities (voriconazole) while on therapy. Although the therapeutic ranges are not well established, improved responses in patients receiving posaconazole as salvage therapy have been noted when plasma concentrations 3 to 4 hours after the oral dose approached 1 mcg/mL (1 mg/L).[46] For voriconazole, patient response rates are improve if steady-state trough concentrations surpass 1 mcg/mL (1 mg/L); however, the risk of CNS toxicity increases as plasma concentrations increase above 5.5 mcg/mL (5.5 mg/L).[47] Patients often require prolonged therapy, particularly if they remain immunosuppressed. In many cases, antifungal therapy may be continued indefinitely until complete resolution of underlying immunosuppression.

Abbreviations Introduced in This Chapter

ALT	Alanine aminotransferase
ARDS	Acute respiratory distress syndrome
AST	Aspartate aminotransferase
CSF	Cerebrospinal fluid
CYP	Cytochrome P450 isoenzyme
ELISA	Enzyme-linked immunosorbent assay
FISH	Fluorescent *in situ* hybridization
HAART	Highly active antiretroviral therapy
HRCT	High-resolution computed tomography
IA	Invasive aspergillosis
IRIS	Immune reconstitution syndrome
NIAID	National Institute of Allergy and Infectious Diseases
PCP	*Pneumocystis jiroveci (carinii)* pneumonia
PCR	Polymerase chain reaction

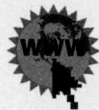 Self-assessment questions and answers are available at *http://www.mhpharmacotherapy.com/pp.html.*

REFERENCES

1. Wheat LJ, Freifeld AG, Kleiman MB, et al. Clinical practice guidelines for the management of patients with histoplasmosis: 2007 update by the Infectious Diseases Society of America. Clin Infect Dis 2007;45:807–825.
2. Wheat LJ, Kauffman CA. Histoplasmosis. Infect Dis Clin North Am 2003;17:1–19.
3. Pappas PG. Blastomycosis. Semin Respir Crit Care Med 2004;25:113–121.
4. Galgiani JN, Ampel NM, Blair JE, et al. Coccidioidomycosis. Clin Infect Dis 2005;41:1217–1223.
5. Romani L. Immunity to fungal infections. Nat Rev Immunol 2004;4:11–23.
6. Chapman SW, Dismukes WE, Proia LA, et al. Clinical practice guidelines for the management of blastomycosis: 2008 update by the Infectious Diseases Society of America. Clin Infect Dis 2008;46:1801–1812.
7. Lortholary O, Denning DW, Dupont B. Endemic mycoses: A treatment update. J Antimicrob Chemother 1999;43:321–331.
8. Albengres E, Le Louet H, Tillement JP. Systemic antifungal agents. Drug interactions of clinical significance. Drug Saf 1998;18:83–97.
9. Todd JR, Arigala MR, Penn RL, King JW. Possible clinically significant interaction of itraconazole plus rifampin. AIDS Patient Care STDS 2001;15:505–510.
10. Nicolau DP, Crowe HM, Nightingale CH, Quintiliani R. Rifampin-fluconazole interaction in critically ill patients. Ann Pharmacother 1995;29:994–996.
   • Glasmacher A, Hahn C, Leutner C, et al. Breakthrough invasive fungal infections in neutropenic patients after prophylaxis with itraconazole. Mycoses 1999;42:443–451.
   • Guidelines for Prevention and Treatment of Opportunistic Infections in HIV-Infected Adults and Adolescents - June 18, 2008. AIDSinfo June 18, 2008.
11. Gubbins PO, McConnell SA, Penzak SR. Antifungal agents. In: Piscitelli SC, Rodvold KA, eds. Drug Interactions in Infectious Diseases. Totowa, NJ: Humana Press, 2001.
12. Groll AH, Piscitelli SC, Walsh TJ. Clinical pharmacology of systemic antifungal agents: A comprehensive review of agents in clinical use,

current investigational compounds, and putative targets for antifungal drug development. Adv Pharmacol 1998;44:343–499.

13. Johnson PC, Wheat LJ, Cloud GA, et al. Safety and efficacy of liposomal amphotericin B compared with conventional amphotericin B for induction therapy of histoplasmosis in patients with AIDS. Ann Intern Med 2002;137:105–109.

14. Groll AH, Giri N, Petraitis V, et al. Comparative efficacy and distribution of lipid formulations of amphotericin B in experimental Candida albicans infection of the central nervous system. J Infect Dis 2000;182:274–282.

15. Wisplinghoff H, Seifert H, Wenzel RP, Edmond MB. Current trends in the epidemiology of nosocomial bloodstream infections in patients with hematological malignancies and solid neoplasms in hospitals in the United States. Clin Infect Dis 2003;36:1103–1110.

16. Rex JH, Bennett JE, Sugar AM, et al. A randomized trial comparing fluconazole with amphotericin B for the treatment of candidemia in patients without neutropenia. N Engl J Med 1994;331:1325–1330.

17. Pappas PG, Rex JH, Sobel JD, et al. Guidelines for treatment of candidiasis. Clin Infect Dis 2004;38:161–189.

18. Rex JH, Pfaller MA, Walsh TJ, et al. Antifungal susceptibility testing: Practical aspects and current challenges. Clin Microbiol Rev 2001;14:643–658.

19. Pfaller MA, Diekema DJ, Messer SA, et al. Activities of fluconazole and voriconazole against 1,586 recent clinical isolates of Candida species determined by broth microdilution, disk diffusion, and Etest methods: Report from the ARTEMIS global antifungal susceptibility program, 2001. J Clin Microbiol 2003;41:1440–1446.

20. Pfaller MA, Messer SA, Boyken L, et al. In vitro activities of voriconazole, posaconazole, and fluconazole against 4,169 clinical isolates of Candida spp. and Cryptococcus neoformans collected during 2001 and 2002 in the ARTEMIS global antifungal surveillance program. Diagn Microbiol Infect Dis 2004;48:201–205.

21. Mora-Duarte J, Betts R, Rotstein R, et al. Comparison of caspofungin and amphotericin B for invasive candidiasis. N Engl J Med 2002;347:2020–2029.

22. Kullberg BJ, Sobel JD, Ruhnke M, et al. Voriconazole versus a regimen of amphotericin B followed by fluconazole for candidaemia in non-neutropenic patients: A randomised non-inferiority trial. Lancet 2005;366:1435–1442.

23. Kuse E, Chetchotisakd P, da Cunha C, et al. Micafungin versus liposomal amphotericin B for candidemia and invasive candidiasis: A phase III randomized double-blind trial. Lancet 2007;369:1519–1527.

24. Pappas P, Rotstein C, Betts R, et al. Micafungin versus caspofungin for the treatment of candidemia and other forms of invasive candidiasis. Clin Infect Dis 2007;45:883–893.

25. Reboli A, Rotstein C, Pappas P, et al. Anidulafungin versus fluconazole for invasive candidiasis. New Eng J Med 2007;356:2472–2482.

26. Morrell M, Fraser V, Kollef M. Delaying the empiric treatment of Candida bloodstrem infection until positive blood culture results are obtained: A potential risk factor for hospital mortality. Antimicrob Agent Chemother 2005;49:3640–3645.

27. Hughes WT, Armstrong D, Bodey GP, et al. 2002 guidelines for the use of antimicrobial agents in neutropenic patients with cancer. Clin Infect Dis 2002;34:730–751.

28. Goodman JL, Winston DJ, Greenfield RA, et al. A controlled trial of fluconazole to prevent fungal infections in patients undergoing bone marrow transplantation. N Engl J Med 1992;326:845–851.

29. Winston DJ, Chandrasekar PH, Lazarus HM, et al. Fluconazole prophylaxis of fungal infections in patients with acute leukemia. Results of a randomized placebo-controlled, double-blind, multicenter trial. Ann Intern Med 1993;118:495–503.

30. Slavin MA, Osborne B, Adams R, et al. Efficacy and safety of fluconazole prophylaxis for fungal infections after bone marrow transplantation—a prospective, randomized, double-blind study. J Infect Dis 1995;171:1545–1552.

31. Winston DJ, Maziarz RT, Chandrasekar PH, et al. Intravenous and oral itraconazole versus intravenous and oral fluconazole for long-term antifungal prophylaxis in allogeneic hematopoietic stem-cell transplant recipients—a multicenter, randomized trial. Ann Intern Med 2003;138:705–713.

32. Van Burik J, Ratanatharathorn V, Lipton J, et al. Randomized, double-blind trial of micafungin versus fluconazole for prophylaxis of invasive fungal infections in patients undergoing hematopoietic stem cell transplant. Clin Infect Dis 2004;39:1407–1416.

33. Cornely O, Maertens J, Winston D, et al. Posaconazole versus fluyconazole or itraconazole prophylaxis in patients with neutropenia. N Eng J Med 1007;356:348–359.

34. Ullman A, Lipton J, Vesole D, et al. Posaconazole or fluconazole for prophylaxis in severe graft versus host disease. N Eng J Med 2007;356:335–347.

35. Wingard J, Carter S, Walsh T, et al. Results of a randomized, double-blind trial of Fluconazole (FLU) vs. Voriconazole (VORI) for the prevention of invasive fungal infections (IFI) in 600 allogeneic blood and marrow transplant (BMT) patients. Blood 2007;110: Abstract #163.

36. Pelz RK, Hendrix CW, Swoboda SM, et al. Double-blind placebo-controlled trial of fluconazole to prevent candidal infections in critically ill surgical patients. Ann Surg 2001;233:542–548.

37. Rex JH, Sobel JD. Prophylactic antifungal therapy in the intensive care unit. Clin Infect Dis 2001;32:1191–1200.

38. Shuster M, Edward J, Sobel J, et al. Empirical fluconazole versus placebo for intensive care unit patients: A randomized trial. Ann Intern Med 2008;149:83–90.

39. Saag MS, Graybill RJ, Larsen RA, et al. Practice guidelines for the management of cryptococcal disease. Infectious Diseases Society of America. Clin Infect Dis 2000;30:710–718.

40. Walsh TJ, Anaissie EJ, Denning DW, et al. Treatment of aspergillosis: Clinical Practice Gudelines of the Infectious Diseases Society of America. Clin Infect Dis 2008;46:327–360.

41. Caillot D, Mannone L, Cuisenier B, Couaillier JF. Role of early diagnosis and aggressive surgery in the management of invasive pulmonary aspergillosis in neutropenic patients. Clin Microbiol Infect 2001;7:54–61.

42. Caillot D, Casasnovas O, Bernard A, et al. Improved management of invasive pulmonary aspergillosis in neutropenic patients using early thoracic computed tomographic scan and surgery. J Clin Oncol 1997;15:139–147.

43. Herbrecht R, Denning DW, Patterson TF, et al. Voriconazole versus amphotericin B for the primary treatment of aspergillosis. New Eng J Med 2002;347:408–415.

44. Walsh T, Raad I, Patterson T, et al. Treatment of invasive aspergillosis with posaconazole in patients who are refractory to or intolerant of conventional therapy: An externally controlled trial. Clin Infect Dis 2007;44:2–12.

45. Pascual A, Calandra T, Bolay S. Voriconazole therapeutic drug monitoring in patients with invasive mycoses improves safety and efficayc outcomes. Clin Infect Dis 2007;46:201–211.

46. Lionakis MS, Kontoyiannis DP. Fusarium infections in critically ill patients. Semin Respir Crit Care Med 2004;25:159–169.49.

47. Kontoyiannis DP, Lionakis MS, Lewis RE, et al. Zygomycosis in a tertiary-care cancer center in the era of Aspergillus-active antifungal therapy: A case-control observational study of 27 recent cases. J Infect Dis 2005;191:1350–1360.

85 Antimicrobial Prophylaxis in Surgery

Mary A. Ullman, Jeremy A. Schafer, and
John C. Rotschafer

LEARNING OBJECTIVES

● **Upon completion of the chapter, the reader will be able to:**

1. Discuss the epidemiology and impact of surgical wound infections on patient outcomes and health care costs.

2. Name and differentiate the four different types of wound classifications.

3. Recognize at least three risk factors for postoperative surgical site infections (SSIs).

4. Identify likely pathogens associated with different surgical operations.

5. Compare and contrast antimicrobials used for surgical prophylaxis and identify potential advantages and disadvantages for each antibiotic.

6. Discuss the importance of β-lactam allergy screening and how this could impact resistance and health care costs.

7. Identify nonantimicrobial methods that can reduce the risk of postoperative infection.

8. Discuss the possible impact of antimicrobial-impregnated bone cement and how this affects the use of antimicrobial prophylaxis in surgery.

9. Discuss the importance of timing, duration, and redosing in relation to antimicrobial prophylaxis in surgery.

10. Recommend appropriate prophylactic antimicrobial(s) given a surgical operation.

KEY CONCEPTS

❶ Surgical site infections (SSIs) are a significant cause of morbidity and mortality.

❷ The distinction between prophylaxis and treatment influences the choice of antimicrobial and duration of therapy.

❸ Surgical operations are classified as clean, clean-contaminated, contaminated, or dirty.

❹ Choosing the appropriate prophylactic antimicrobial relies on anticipating which organisms are likely to be encountered during the operation.

❺ A thorough drug allergy history should be taken to discern true allergy (anaphylaxis) from other adverse events (stomach upset).

❻ Further study is needed before antibiotic-impregnated bone cements can be recommended as an alternative to preoperative prophylaxis with traditional antimicrobials for orthopedic operations.

❼ For prevention of SSIs, correct timing of antimicrobial administration is imperative so as to allow the persistence of therapeutic concentrations in the blood and wound tissues during the entire course of the operation.

❽ The goal of antimicrobial dosing for surgical prophylaxis is to optimize the pharmacodynamic parameter of the selected agent against the suspected organism for the duration of the operation.

❾ The duration of antimicrobial prophylaxis should not exceed 24 hours (48 hours for cardiac surgery); additional doses of antimicrobial past this time point do not demonstrate added benefits.

❿ According to Centers for Disease Control and Prevention criteria, SSI may appear up to 30 days after an operation and up to 1 year if a prosthesis is implanted.

❶ *Surgical site infections (SSIs) are a significant cause of morbidity and mortality.* Approximately 2% to 5% of patients undergoing clean extra-abdominal operations and 20% undergoing intra-abdominal operations will develop an SSI.[1] SSIs have become the second most common cause of nosocomial infection and these data are likely underestimated.[1] More than 70% of surgical procedures are now performed on an outpatient basis, creating a significant potential for under-reporting.[2]

SSIs negatively affect patient outcomes and increase health care costs. Patients who develop SSIs are five times more likely to be readmitted to the hospital and have twice the mortality of patients who do not develop an SSI.[1] A patient with an SSI is also 60% more likely to be admitted to an ICU.[1] SSIs increase lengths of hospital stay and costs.[1,3,4] The type of SSI can also affect the severity of a patient's negative outcome due to surgery. Deep SSIs, involving organs or spaces, result in longer durations of hospital stay and higher costs compared to SSIs that are limited to the incision.[5] Additionally, beginning in 2008, Medicare and Medicaid Services will no longer reimburse the hospitals for any cost incurred from treating certain hospital-acquired infections, including SSIs.[6] Thus, even greater importance is placed on preventing infection, and, if infection should occur, treatment of the infection should be for the shortest duration possible and in the most cost effective manner.

SSIs are defined and reported according to Centers for Disease Control and Prevention (CDC) criteria.[5] SSIs are classified as either incisional or organ/space. Incisional SSIs are further divided into superficial incisional SSI (skin or subcutaneous tissue) and deep incisional SSI (deeper soft tissues of the incision). Organ/space SSIs involve any anatomic site other than the incised areas. For example, a patient who develops meningitis after removal of a brain tumor could be classified as having an organ/space SSI. An infection is considered as SSI if any of the above criteria is met and the infection occurs within 30 days of the operation. If a prosthetic is implanted, the timeline extends out to 1 year.

EPIDEMIOLOGY AND ETIOLOGY

Numerous risk factors for SSI have been identified in the literature.[5,7,8] These factors can be divided into two categories: patient and operative characteristics. Patient risk factors for SSI include: age, comorbid disease states (especially chronic lung disease and diabetes), malnutrition, immunosuppression, nicotine or steroid use, and colonization of the nares with *Staphylococcus aureus*. Many patients developing postoperative wound infections bring the organism with them into the hospital. Modifying risk factors may decrease the threat of SSI. Malnutrition can be corrected using enteral or parenteral feedings. Additional nonantimicrobial strategies to reduce SSI will be discussed later.

Operative characteristics are based on the actions of both the patient and the operating staff. Shaving of the surgical site prior to operating can produce microscopic lacerations and increase the chance of SSI and is, therefore, not accepted as a method of hair removal.[5] Maintaining aseptic technique and proper sterilization of medical equipment is effective in preventing SSI. Surgical staff should wash their hands thoroughly. In clean surgeries, most bacterial inoculums introduced postoperatively are generally small. However,

subsequent patient contact between contaminated areas (nares or rectum) and the surgical site can lead to SSI. Finally, the appropriate use of antimicrobial prophylaxis can have a significant impact on decreasing SSIs.

PATHOPHYSIOLOGY

Prophylaxis Versus Treatment

Properly identifying the state of an infection is important when using antimicrobial prophylaxis in surgery. Antibiotic prophylaxis begins with the premise that no infection exists but that during surgery there can be a low level inoculum of bacteria introduced into the body. However, if sufficient antimicrobial concentrations are present, the situation can be controlled without infection developing. This is the case when surgery is done under controlled conditions, there are no major breaks in sterile technique or spillage of GI contents, and perforation or damage to the surgical site is absent. An example would be an elective hysterectomy done with optimal surgical technique.

If an infection is already present, or presumed to be present, then antimicrobial use is for treatment, not prophylaxis, and the goal is to eliminate the infection. This is the case when there is spillage of GI contents, gross damage or perforation is already present, or the tissue being operated on is actively infected (pus is present and cultures are positive). An example would be a patient undergoing surgery for a ruptured appendix with diffuse peritonitis.

❷ *The distinction between prophylaxis and treatment influences the choice of antimicrobial and duration of therapy.* Appropriate antimicrobial selection, dosing, and duration of therapy differ significantly between these two situations. A regimen for antimicrobial prophylaxis ideally involves one agent and lasts less than 24 hours. Treatment regimens can involve multiple antimicrobials with durations lasting weeks to months depending on desired antimicrobial coverage and the surgical site.

Types of Surgical Operations

❸ *Surgical operations are classified at the time of operation as clean, clean-contaminated, contaminated, or dirty.* Antimicrobial prophylaxis is appropriate for clean, clean-contaminated, and contaminated operations. Dirty operations take place in situations of existing infection and antimicrobials are used for treatment, not prophylaxis (Table 85–1).

Microbiology

❹ *Choosing the appropriate prophylactic antimicrobial relies on anticipating which organisms will be encountered during the operation.* SSIs associated with extra-abdominal operations are the result of skin flora organisms in nearly all cases. These organisms include gram-positive cocci, with *S. aureus* and *Staphylococcus epidermidis* being among the most frequently isolated SSI pathogens according to the National Nosocomial Infections Surveillance System

Table 85–1

National Red Cross Wound Classification, Risk of SSI, and Antibiotic Indication

Classification	Description	SSI Risk	Antibiotic Prophylaxis
Clean	No acute inflammation or transection of GI, oropharyngeal, GU, biliary, or respiratory tracts; elective case, no technique break	Low	Indicated
Clean-contaminated	Controlled opening of aforementioned tracts with minimal spillage or minor technique break; clean procedures performed emergently or with major technique breaks	Medium	Indicated
Contaminated	Acute, nonpurulent inflammation present; major spillage or technique break during clean-contaminated procedures	High	Indicated
Dirty	Obvious pre-existing infection present (abscess, pus, or necrotic tissue present)	—	Not indicated; antibiotics used for treatment

GU, genitourinary.

From Refs. 7, 9.

Table 85–2

Major Pathogens in Surgical Wound Infections

Pathogen	Percentage of Infections[a]
Staphylococcus aureus	20
Coagulase-negative staphylococci	14
Enterococci	12
Escherichia coli	8
Pseudomonas aeruginosa	8
Enterobacter spp.	7
Proteus mirabilis	3
Klebsiella pneumoniae	3
Other *Streptococcus* spp.	3
Candida albicans	3
Group D streptococci	2
Other gram-positive aerobes	2
Bacteroides fragilis	2

[a]Data reported by the NNIS from 1990 to 1996, adapted from National Academy of the Sciences National Research Council. Postoperative wound infections: The influence of ultraviolet irradiation of the operating room and of various other factors. Ann Surg 1984; 160:32–135.

From Kanji S, Devlin JW. Antimicrobial prophylaxis in surgery. In: DiPiro JT, Talbert RL, Yee GC, et al., (eds.) Pharmacotherapy: A Pathophysiologic Approach. 6th ed. New York: McGraw-Hill; 2005: 2219, with permission.

(NNIS)[5] (Table 85–2). *Streptococcus* spp. and other gram-positive aerobes may also be implicated.

Intra-abdominal operations involve a diverse flora with the potential for polymicrobial SSIs. *Escherichia coli* make up a large portion of bowel flora and are frequently isolated as pathogens according to the NNIS.[5] Other enteric gram-negative bacteria, as well as anaerobes (especially *Bacteroides* spp.), may be encountered during intra-abdominal operations.

Candida albicans is being implicated as the cause of a growing number of SSIs. According to the NNIS, from 1991 to 1995, the incidence of fungal SSIs rose from 0.1 to 0.3 per 1,000 discharges.[5] Increased use of broad-spectrum antimicrobials and rising prevalence of immunocompromised and human immunodeficiency virus-infected individuals are factors in fungal SSIs. Despite this increase, antifungal prophylaxis for surgery is not currently recommended.

Choosing an Antibiotic

An antimicrobial used in surgical prophylaxis should meet certain criteria. Selecting an antimicrobial with a spectrum that covers expected pathogens is crucial. The antimicrobial should be inexpensive, available in a parenteral formulation, and easy to use. Adverse-event potential should be minimal. Choosing an agent with a longer half-life reduces the likely need to redose unless the surgical procedure is prolonged.

Operations can be separated into two basic categories: extra-abdominal and intra-abdominal. SSIs resulting from extra-abdominal operations are frequently caused by gram-positive aerobes. Thus, an antimicrobial with strong gram-positive coverage is useful. Cefazolin benefits from a benign adverse-event profile, simple dosing, and low cost. These aspects have made cefazolin the mainstay for surgical prophylaxis of extra-abdominal procedures. For patients with a β-lactam allergy, clindamycin or vancomycin can be used as an alternative.

Intra-abdominal operations necessitate broad-spectrum coverage of gram-negative organisms and anaerobes. Antianaerobic cephalosporins, cefoxitin and cefotetan, are widely used. Fluoroquinolones or aminoglycosides, paired with clindamycin or metronidazole, should provide adequate coverage for intra-abdominal operations; these regimens are recommended as appropriate regimens for use in patients with β-lactam allergies.

The Hospital Infection Control Practices Advisory Committee allows for the use of vancomycin for surgical prophylaxis when methicillin-resistant *Staphylococcus aureus* (MRSA) rates at an institution are "high."[1] Unfortunately, a "high" rate of MRSA has not been standardized. Additionally, vancomycin use in institutions where MRSA rates are "high" may not translate into a lower incidence of SSI. Finkelstein and associates found that the incidence of

SSI for patients on cefazolin or vancomycin did not differ despite a high MRSA rate at the study institution. However, patients who received cefazolin were more likely to develop an SSI due to MRSA.[10] The increasing prevalence of community-associated methicillin-resistant *Staphylococcus aureus* (CA-MRSA) in patients admitted to the hospital creates an added concern, although this pathogen is often sensitive to clindamycin. Vancomycin should be considered appropriate surgical prophylaxis for those patients identified as being colonized with MRSA (prior to or at admission).[1]

Due to antimicrobial shortages of the recommended antimicrobials and development of newer antimicrobials (e.g., carbapenems, third and fourth generation cephalosporins, and antipseudomonal penicillins), some interest has been generated in the use of these newer antimicrobials for surgical prophylaxis. Recently, ertapenem was determined to be superior to standard cefotetan in the prevention of SSIs after elective colorectal surgery.[11] However, the ertapenem treatment group had a larger proportion of *Clostridium difficile* infections than those in the cefotetan treatment group. Ertapenem has been included as an approved antibiotic for colon surgery by some agencies.[12] At this time, it is not considered appropriate to use these newer antimicrobials for surgical prophylaxis; overuse of these antimicrobials may contribute to collateral damage and the development of bacterial resistance. Further research is needed before any of these newer agents are routinely used for surgical prophylaxis. New guidelines are likely to be published soon and may offer guidance on the use of newer antimicrobials.

β-Lactam Allergy

Penicillin allergy is one of the most common reported drug allergies. Concerns over cross-reactivity may limit the use of β-lactams for surgical prophylaxis. ❺ *A thorough drug allergy history should be taken to discern true allergy (e.g., anaphylaxis) from adverse event (e.g., stomach upset).* Allergy testing may be helpful in confirming a patient's penicillin allergy and could spare vancomycin. However, practitioners should be aware allergy testing may be difficult to perform due to the removal of a major component (penicilloyl-polylisine) of the testing from the commercial market.[13] If a practitioner desires to perform allergy testing, the individual reagents required for penicillin allergy testing must be prepared at the health care facility, on a case-by-case basis. Cross-allergenicity between penicillin and cephalosporins is low. The increased risk of cephalosporin allergy in patients with a history of penicillin allergy may be as low as 0.4% for first-generation cephalosporins and nearly zero for second- and third-generation agents.[14] Other studies also found the risk of cross-reactivity to be very low.[15] However, in the case of severe penicillin allergy (anaphylaxis), cephalosporins should be avoided.

Alternative Methods to Decrease SSI

Several nonantimicrobial methods have been studied for reducing the risk of SSI.[16] Providing supplemental warming to patients (36.6°C [98°F]) during the intraoperative period reduced infection rates compared to control patients (34.7°C [94.5°F]).[17] Intensive glucose control (maintaining blood glucose to 80 to 110 mg/dL [4.4–6.1 mmol/L]) versus conventional control (blood glucose less than 220 mg/dL [less than 12.2 mmol/L]) reduced infections and improved outcomes in cardiac patients who received intensive insulin control in the ICU after surgery.[18] Also, patients randomized to 80% inspired oxygen had lower SSI rates compared to patients on 30% oxygen after colorectal resection.[19] Despite these findings, there are insufficient data to make definitive recommendations on the use of these therapies.

Antimicrobial-impregnated bone cement is being used as an adjunct or alternative to traditional antimicrobial prophylaxis for orthopedic operations. Cefuroxime-impregnated cement lowered the risk of deep infection after primary total knee arthoplasty.[20] Other studies have been inconclusive regarding superiority of antimicrobial-impregnated bone cement versus conventional therapies.[21] Confounding this issue is the lack of standards regarding antimicrobial-impregnated cements. An array of drugs, from aminoglycosides to macrolides, is used in these preparations. Some cements are produced commercially whereas others are made in the operating room. The long-term durability of impregnated cements is also unknown, as the addition of antimicrobials may reduce the tensile strength of bone cement. ❻ *Further study is needed before antimicrobial-impregnated bone cements can be recommended as an alternative to preoperative prophylaxis with traditional antimicrobials.*

Antimicrobial irrigation may also be encountered in the surgical arena as an adjunct or alternative to traditional parenteral antimicrobial prophylaxis. Irrigation of wounds allows debris removal as well as an additional way to lessen bacterial contamination. However, as with the antimicrobial bone cement, evidence is mixed on the advantages of using this approach. Irrigation with detergent solutions, rather than antimicrobials, appears to provide the same results but with less wound-healing problems encountered with antimicrobial irrigation.[22] Additionally, because antimicrobial irrigation solutions are not commercially available, irrigants are often made in the operation rooms, allowing for the possibility of higher than or lower than desired concentrations. If concentrations are higher than desired, local chemical irritation may occur as well as systemic absorption and toxicity. If concentrations fall below desired targets, development of resistant organisms may occur. Further study is required before antimicrobial irrigation is recommended for use in surgical prophylaxis.

With the increase of CA-MRSA, increased importance has been placed on screening for *S. aureus*, especially MRSA and decolonization. Surgical patients with nasal colonization of *S. aureus* have a higher risk of an SSI due to *S. aureus*, and decolonization leads to a lower incidence of SSIs.[23–25] However, while this evidence may imply the opportunity for some real benefits in the surgical population, a clear consensus on how the nasal colonization should be approached has not been reached. British guidelines recommend an attempt at decolonization for patients undergoing planned surgical procedures to minimize the risk of infection.[26] Harbarth and colleagues suggest MRSA screening be targeted to patients undergoing elective surgical procedures that have a high risk of MRSA infection. In addition, each hospital's infection control team, along with the surgical team, should analyze their patient population and MRSA epidemiology to appropriately select screening guidelines,[27] keeping in mind state and federal statutes regarding the use of active surveillance cultures. Screening methods that utilize rapid, PCR-based testing may provide an advantage in quickly identifying colonized patients and allowing decolonization to occur prior to surgery.

The most studied approach to eradication of methicillin-sensitive *S. aureus* (MSSA) and/or MRSA has been mupirocin applied to the anterior nares for 5 days prior to surgery.[28] Additionally, skin decolonization with 4% chlorhexidine for 5 days prior to surgery has also been recommended. While decolonization of the anterior nares is the most common and most studied, some controversy exists because patients may be colonized elsewhere (rectum, throat, vagina, etc.) and often do not receive complete decolonization.[28] Furthermore, decolonization usually does not lead to life-long eradication. Other drugs, both topical and systemic, have been studied for decolonization/eradication of MRSA, but a review of randomized controlled trials for the eradication of MRSA found insufficient evidence for the use of any agent for eradication of MRSA.[29] Further studies are needed to elucidate this area of surgical prophylaxis.

Principles of Antimicrobial Prophylaxis

▶ Route of Administration

IV antimicrobial administration is the most common delivery method for surgical prophylaxis. IV administration ensures complete bioavailability while minimizing the impact of patient-specific variables. Oral administration is also used in some bowel operations. Nonabsorbable compounds like erythromycin base and neomycin are given up to 24 hours prior to surgery to cleanse the bowel. Note that oral agents are used adjunctively and do not replace IV agents.

▶ Timing of First Dose

7 *For prevention of SSIs, correct timing of antimicrobial administration is imperative so as to allow the persistence of therapeutic concentrations in the blood and wound tissues during the entire course of the operation.* The National Surgical Infection Prevention Project recommends infusing antimicrobials for surgical prophylaxis within 60 minutes of the first incision. Exceptions to this rule are fluoroquinolones and vancomycin, which can be infused 120 minutes prior to avoid infusion-related reactions.[1] No consensus has been reached on whether the infusion should be complete prior to the first incision. However, if a proximal tourniquet is used, antimicrobial administration should be complete prior to inflation.

Administration of the antimicrobial should begin as close to the first incision as possible. This is important for antimicrobials with short half-lives so that therapeutic concentrations are maintained during the operation and reduce the need for redosing. Beginning the antimicrobial infusion after the first incision is of little value in preventing SSI. Administration of the antimicrobial after the first incision had SSI rates similar to patients who did not receive prophylaxis.[30]

▶ Dosing and Redosing

8 *The goal of antimicrobial dosing for surgical prophylaxis is to optimize the pharmacodynamic parameter of the selected agent against the suspected organism for the duration of the operation.* Dosing recommendations can vary between institutions and guidelines. Clinical judgment should be exercised regarding dose modifications for renal function, age, and especially weight. Obese patients often require higher doses than do nonobese patients.[1] Morbidly obese patients (body mass index greater than 40) who received 2 g of cefazolin had a lower incidence of SSI compared to patients receiving 1 g.[31] An advisory statement from the National Surgical Infection Prevention Project suggested that for patients less than 80 kg, cefazolin should be dosed at 1 g; patients that are 80 kg or greater should receive 2 g of cefazolin for adequate prophylaxis.[1]

If an operation exceeds two half-lives of the selected antimicrobial, then another dose should be administered.[1] Repeat dosing reduces rates of SSI. For example, cefazolin has a half-life of about 2 hours, thus another dose should be given if the operation exceeds 4 hours. The clinician should have extra doses of antimicrobial ready in case an operation lasts longer than planned.

▶ Duration

The National Surgical Infection Prevention Project and published evidence suggest that the continuation of antimicrobial prophylaxis beyond wound closure is unnecessary.[1] **9** *The duration of antimicrobial prophylaxis should not exceed 24 hours (48 hours for cardiac surgery); additional doses of antimicrobial past this time point do not demonstrate added benefits. Longer durations of antimicrobial prophylaxis are advocated by some guidelines and will be discussed later.*

TREATMENT

Antimicrobial Prophylaxis in Specific Surgical Procedures

▶ Gynecologic and Obstetric

Enteric gram-negative bacilli, anaerobes, group B streptococci, and enterococci are all possible pathogens that may be encountered in gynecologic or obstetric surgeries. For patients undergoing hysterectomy, cefoxitin or cefotetan are appropriate therapies (Table 85–3). Cefazolin or ampicillin/ sulbactam may be used.

Table 85–3

Recommended Regimens for Antimicrobial Prophylaxis of Specific Surgical Procedures[a]

Type of Operation	Recommended Prophylaxis Regimen	Alternative Regimen
Vascular	Cefazolin 1–2 g IV every 8 hours for a total of 24 hours or cefuroxime 1.5 g IV × 1, then 750 mg every 8 hours for a total of 24 hours	Clindamycin 600–900 mg IV every 6 hours for a total of 24 hours or vancomycin 1 g IV every 8–12 hours for a total of 24 hours
Neurosurgery	Cefazolin 1–2 g IV every 8 hours for a total of 24 hours	Vancomycin 1 g IV every 8–12 hours for a total of 24 hours
Head and neck	Cefazolin 1–2 g IV every 8 hours for a total of 24 hours	Clindamycin 600–900 mg IV every 6 hours for a total of 24 hours
Urologic	Cefazolin 1–2 g IV × 1	Ciprofloxacin 400 mg IV × 1
Cesarean section	Cefazolin 1–2 g IV × 1	See hysterectomy
Hysterectomy	Cefotetan 1 g IV × 1, cefazolin 1–2 g IV × 1, cefoxitin 1–2 g IV × 1	Antianaerobic agent (metronidazole 0.5–1 g IV × 1 or clindamycin 600–900 mg IV × 1 combined with gentamicin 1.5 mg/kg IV × 1, aztreonam 1–2 g IV × 1, or ciprofloxacin 400 mg IV × 1) Ampicillin/sulbactam 3 g IV × 1
Gastroduodenal (high-risk only: obstruction, acid suppression, morbid obesity, hemorrhage, malignancy)	Cefazolin 1–2 g IV × 1	Ciprofloxacin 400 mg IV × 1
Biliary tract (high-risk only: age greater than 70, acute cholecystitis, obstructive jaundice, duct stones, nonfunctioning gallbladder)	Cefazolin 1–2 g IV × 1 or cefoxitin 1–2 g IV × 1	Ciprofloxacin 400 mg IV × 1
Colorectal	[b]Oral: neomycin 1 g plus erythromycin base 1 g (give 19, 18, and 9 hours prior to procedure) IV: cefoxitin 1–2 g × 1	Cefazolin 1–2 g IV plus metronidazole 0.5–1 g IV × 1 or hysterectomy regimens Ertapenem 1 g × 1
Appendectomy	Cefoxitin 1–2 g IV × 1; cefotetan 1 g IV × 1	Metronidazole 0.5–1 g IV plus gentamicin 1.5 mg/kg IV × 1
Orthopedic	Cefazolin 1–2 g IV every 8 hours for a total of 24 hours	Vancomycin 1 g IV every 12 hours or clindamycin 600–900 mg IV q 6 h
Cardiothoracic	Cefazolin 1–2 g IV every 8 hours for a total of 48 hours or cefuroxime 1.5 g IV every 12 hours for a total of 48 hours	Vancomycin 1 g IV every 12 hours for a total of 48 hours or clindamycin 600–900 mg IV every 6 hours

[a]Dosing recommendations are based on common clinical doses for adult patients with normal renal function*; dosing for individual patients and institutions may vary.

[b]Oral regimens should be used in conjunction with IV prophylaxis.

From Refs. 1, 9, 15.

In the case of β-lactam allergy, the following regimens are appropriate: clindamycin combined with gentamicin, aztreonam, or ciprofloxacin; metronidazole combined with gentamicin or ciprofloxacin, or clindamycin monotherapy. Metronidazole monotherapy is also indicated but is less effective than other regimens.[1]

Cesarean sections are stratified into low- and high-risk groups. Patients who undergo emergency operations or have cesarean sections after the rupture of membranes and/or onset of labor are considered high risk. Prophylactic antimicrobials are most beneficial for high-risk patients but are used in both groups. Antimicrobial regimens similar to those for hysterectomy are appropriate. Antimicrobials should not be administered until after the first incision and the umbilical cord has been clamped. This practice prevents potentially harmful antimicrobial concentrations from reaching the newborn.

▶ Orthopedic Surgery

Orthopedic operations are generally clean and are done under controlled conditions. Likely pathogens include gram-positive cocci, mostly staphylococci. In the case of total joint (knee and hip) arthroplasty, cefazolin is the antimicrobial of choice. Patients with a β-lactam allergy should receive either clindamycin or vancomycin. Antimicrobial prophylaxis should not exceed 24 hours and does not need to be continued until all drains and catheters have been removed. Antimicrobial-impregnated bone cement can be useful in lowering infection rates in orthopedic surgery but has not been approved for prophylaxis.

▶ Cardiothoracic and Vascular Surgery

Cefazolin or cefuroxime are appropriate for prophylaxis in cardiothoracic and vascular surgeries. In the case of β-lactam

Patient Encounter 1, Part 1

AD is a 60-year-old woman with a history of poorly controlled diabetes mellitus and MSSA nasal colonization. She weighs 54 kg (119 lb) and is 5′ 1″ (155 cm) tall. She presents today for a hysterectomy. She has no allergies to any medications. The surgeon approaches you for recommendations on prophylactic antibiotic use.

PE:

VS: BP 128/76 mm Hg, P 76 bpm, RR 15 per minute, T 36.4°C (97.5°F)

Labs: WBC 5 × 10³/mm³ (5 × 10⁹/L), serum creatinine 80 μmol/L (0.9 mg/dL), glucose 5.3 mmol/L (95 mg/dL)

What drug would you choose for this operation and why?

What organisms are likely to be encountered in this operation?

The surgeon asks about using metronidazole as a solo agent; what is your opinion on this?

The surgeon agrees with your decision and wants to begin infusing the antibiotic 1 hour after *the first incision. Comment on this.*

What other interventions besides antibiotic use could prove useful in lowering AD's risk of SSI?

Patient Encounter 1, Part 2

AD has been admitted to the ward after completion of her hysterectomy. A physical examination is performed and laboratory data are collected in the immediate postoperative period. AD complains of tenderness around the incision site but no erythema is noted.

PE:

VS: BP 132/80 mm Hg, P 82 bpm, RR 20 per minute, T 37.8°C (100°F)

Labs: WBC 11 × 10³/mm³ (11 × 10⁹/L), serum creatinine 88 μmol/L (1 mg/dL), glucose 5.55 mmol/L (100 mg/dL)

Based on the available data, does AD have an SSI?

What interventions may increase AD's comfort?

How should AD be screened for SSI?

How long should AD be followed in order to identify a possible SSI?

Patient Encounter 2

GL is a 56-year-old male who presents to the emergency department with crushing chest pain described as a "10/10" and shortness of breath. He weighs 82 kg (180 lb) and is 5′ 9″ (175 cm) tall. An ECG reveals an elevated ST segment and lab data are significant for elevated troponins. GL is diagnosed with acute myocardial infarction. After GL is stabilized, the decision is made to place multiple stents. The surgeon consults with you on recommendations for antibiotic prophylaxis. Significant history for GL: allergy to amoxicillin (anaphylaxis), smokes two packs of cigarettes per day, and lives with his wife and two children.

PE:

VS: BP 162/95 mm Hg, P 120 bpm, RR 28 per minute, T 35.8°C (96.4°F)

Labs: Serum creati nine 0.9 mg/dL (80 μmol/L), troponins 0.8 ng/mL (0.8 mcg/L)

The surgeon wants to use vancomycin for this case; what is your opinion on this?

The surgeon decides to use vancomycin at a dose of 1 g over 30 minutes. During the infusion, GL experiences a rash and a call is made for an epinephrine pen. What is happening to GL and how would you alter the therapy?

What is the risk of overuse of vancomycin in hospitals and what pathogens are becoming problematic?

allergy, vancomycin or clindamycin are advised. Debate exists on the duration of antimicrobial prophylaxis. SSIs are rare after cardiothoracic operations, but the potentially devastating consequences lead some clinicians to support longer periods of prophylaxis. The National Surgical Infection Prevention Project cites data that extending prophylaxis beyond 24 hours does not decrease SSI rates and may increase bacterial resistance.[1] However, the Society of Thoracic Surgeons issued practice guidelines in 2006 to extend the duration of antibiotics to 48 hours following cardiac surgeries.[32] Duration of therapy should be based on patient factors and risk of development of an SSI.

▶ Colorectal Surgery

Antimicrobial prophylaxis for colorectal operations must cover a broad range of gram-positive, gram-negative, and anaerobic organisms. Strategies include oral antimicrobial bowel preparations, parenteral antimicrobials, or both. Oral prophylaxis combinations of neomycin and erythromycin or neomycin and metronidazole are common. Oral antimicrobials should be administered at 19, 18, and 9 hours prior to surgery. A delay in surgery may require a redose, depending on the length of postponement. For parenteral prophylaxis, cefoxitin or cefotetan is appropriate. Cefazolin combined with metronidazole or ampicillin/sulbactam is an effective alternative if antianaerobic cephalosporins are not available. For patients with β-lactam allergies, use clindamycin combined with gentamicin, aztreonam, or ciprofloxacin; metronidazole combined with gentamicin or ciprofloxacin is also appropriate.

Appendectomy is one of the most common intra-abdominal operations. Antimicrobial prophylaxis used for appendectomy is similar to that used for colorectal regimens. In the case of ruptured appendix, antimicrobials are used for treatment, not prophylaxis.

OUTCOME EVALUATION

The clinician should consistently follow-up postoperative patients and screen for any sign of SSI. ❿ *According to CDC criteria, SSI may appear up to 30 days after an operation and up to 1 year if a prosthesis is implanted.*[5] This period often extends beyond hospitalization so patients should be educated on warning signs of SSI and be encouraged to contact a clinician immediately if necessary. The presence of fever or leukocytosis in the immediate postoperative period does not constitute SSI and should resolve with proper patient care. Distal infections, such as pneumonia, are not considered SSIs even if these infections occur in the 30-day period. The appearance of the surgical site should be checked regularly and changes should be documented (e.g., erythema, drainage, or pus). The presence of pus or other signs suggestive of SSI must be treated accordingly. Any wound requiring incision and drainage is considered an SSI regardless of appearance. Prompt cultures should be collected and appropriate antimicrobial therapy initiated to reduce any chance of morbidity and mortality.

Abbreviations Introduced in This Chapter

ASHP	American Society of Health-System Pharmacists
CA-MRSA	Community-associated methicillin-resistant *Staphylococcus aureus*
MIC	Minimum inhibitory concentration
MRSA	Methicillin-resistant *Staphylococcus aureus*
MSSA	Methicillin-sensitive *S. aureus*
NNIS	National Nosocomial Infections Surveillance System
SSI	Surgical site infection

Self-assessment questions and answers are available at *http://www.mhpharmacotherapy. com/pp.html.*

Patient Care and Monitoring

- Conduct a thorough medication history including prescription and nonprescription medications, as well as herbals and vitamins.

- Verify the patient's allergy history and the type of reaction experienced. Attempt to discern between true allergy and adverse event. β-Lactam–allergic patients may receive clindamycin, vancomycin, or other antimicrobials. Cross-reactivity between penicillin allergy and cephalosporins is low but cephalosporins should be avoided in patients with a history of anaphylaxis to penicillins.

- Document the type of operation the patient is undergoing. Verify the surgical procedure with the patient.

- Prophylactic antimicrobials should be started within an hour of the first incision to optimize patient outcomes. Exceptions to this include vancomycin and fluoroquinolones.

- The patient should be monitored for signs of an allergic reaction during the operation. These include rash, hives, difficulty breathing, or substantial drops in blood pressure.

- Major breaks in surgical technique may cause the classification of the operation to change and require adjustments in antimicrobial prophylaxis.

- The patient should be monitored for signs and symptoms of infection postoperatively. These could include pus, erythema, and fever. If signs consistent with SSI appear, cultures should be taken and additional antimicrobial therapy should be considered.

- Patients being discharged should be counseled on recognizing signs and symptoms of SSI. An SSI can appear up to 30 days after an operation is completed.

REFERENCES

1. Bratzler DW, Houck PM, for the Surgical Infection Prevention Guideline Writers Workgroup. Antimicrobial prophylaxis for surgery: An advisory statement from the National Surgical Infection Prevention Project. Am J Surg 2005;189:395–404.
2. Barie PS, Eachempati SR. Surgical site infections. Surg Clin North Am 2005;85:1115–1135.
3. Kirkland KB, Briggs JP, Trivette SL, et al. The impact of surgical site infections in the 1990s: Attributable mortality, excess length of hospitalization, and extra costs. Infect Control Hosp Epidemiol 1999;20:725–730.
4. Hollenbeak CS, Murphy D, Dunagan WC, et al. Nonrandom selection and the attributable cost of surgical-site infections. Infect Control Hosp Epidemiol 2002;23:174–176.
5. Mangram AJ, Horan TC, Pearson ML, et al. Guideline for prevention of surgical site infection, 1999. Infect Control Hosp Epidemiol 1999;20:247–266.
6. Department of Health and Human Services: Centers for Medicare & Medicaid Services. Medicare Program; Changes to the Hospital Inpatient Prospective Payment Systems and Fiscal Year 2008; Final Rule. Federal Register 2007;72:47200–47206.
7. Dionigi R, Rovera F, Dionigi G, et al. Risk factors in surgery. J Chemother 2001;13:6–11.
8. Pessaux P, Atallah D, Lermite E, et al. Risk factors for prediction of surgical site infections in "clean surgery." Am J Infect Control 2005;33:292–298.

9. Devlin JW, Kanji S, Janning SW, et al. Antimicrobial prophylaxis in surgery. In: Dipiro JT, Talbert RL, Yee GC, et al. Pharmacotherapy: A Pathophysiologic Approach, 5th ed. New York: McGraw-Hill, 2002:2111–2122.

10. Finkelstein R, Rabino G, Mashiah T, et al. Vancomycin versus cefazolin prophylaxis for cardiac surgery in the setting of a high prevalence of methicillin-resistant staphylococcal infections. J Thorac Cardiovasc Surg 2002;123:326–332.

11. Itanu KMF, Wilson SE, Awad SS, et al. Ertapenem versus cefotetan prophylaxis in elective colorectal surgery. N Engl J Med 2006;355:2640–2651.

12. Centers for Medicare & Medicaid Services and The Joint Commission. *The Specifications Manual for National Hospital Inpatient Quality Measures (Specifications Manual)* Version 3.0b. Available at http://www.qualitynet.org/dcs/contentserver?cid=1141662756099&pagename=Qnetpublic%2Fpage%2FQnetTier2&c=page. Last accessed 29 September 2009.

13. Schafer JA, Mateo N, Parlier GL, Rotschater JC. Penicillin allergy skin testing: What do we do know? Pharmacotherapy 2007;27:542–545.

14. Pichichero ME. A review of evidence supporting the American Academy of Pediatrics recommendation for prescribing cephalosporin antibiotics for penicillin-allergic patients. Pediatrics 2005;115:1048–1057.

15. Apter AJ, Kinman JL, Bilker WB, et al. Is there cross-reactivity between penicillins and cephalosporins? Am J Med 2006;119:354.e11–e20.

16. Weed HG. Antimicrobial prophylaxis in the surgical patient. Med Clin North Am 2003;87:59–75.

17. Kurz A, Sessler D, Lenhardt R. Perioperative normothermia to reduce the incidence of surgical-wound infection and shorten hospitalization. Study of Wound Infection and Temperature Group. N Engl J Med 1996;334:1209–1215.

18. Ingels C, Debaveye Y, Milants I, Buelens E, et al. Strict blood glucose control with insulin during intensive care after cardiac surgery: Impact on 4-years survival, dependency on medical care, and quality of life. Eur Heart J 2006;27(22):2716–2724.

19. Greif R, Akca O, Horn E, et al., for the Outcomes Research Group. Supplemental perioperative oxygen to reduce the incidence of surgical-wound infection. N Engl J Med 2000;342:161–167.

20. Chiu FY, Chen CM, Lin CF, et al. Cefuroxime-impregnated cement in primary total knee arthroplasty. J Bone Joint Surg 2002;84:759–762.

21. Joseph TN, Chen AL, Di Cesare PE. Use of antibiotic-impregnated cement in total joint arthroplasty. J Am Acad Orthop Surg 2003;11:38–47.

22. Fletcher N, Sofianos D, Berkes MB, Obremskey WT. Prevention of perioperative infection. J Bone Joint Surg Am 2007;89:1605–1618.

23. Wilcox MH, Hall J, Pike H, et al. Use of perioperative mupirocin to prevent methicillin-resistant staphylococcus aureus (MRSA) orthopaedic surgical site infections. J Hosp Infect 2003;54:196–201.

24. Perl TM, Cullen JJ, Wenzel RP, et al. Intranasal mupirocin to prevent postoperative *Staphylococcus aureus* infections. N Engl J Med 2002;346:1871–1877.

25. Munoz P, Hortal J, Giannella M, et al. Nasal carriage of *S. aureus* increases the risk of surgical site infection after major heart surgery. J Hosp Infect 2008;68:25–31.

26. Coia JE, Duckworth GJ, Edwards DI, et al. Guidelines for the control and prevention of meticillin-resistant *Staphylococcus aureus* (MRSA) in healthcare facilities. J Hosp Infect 2006;63:S1–S44

27. Harbath S, Fankhauser C, Schrenzel J, et al. Universal screening for methicillin-resistant Staphylococcus aureus at hospital admission and noscomial infection in surgical patients. JAMA 2008;299:1149–1157.

28. Loveday HP, Pellowe CM, Jones SRLJ, Pratt RJ. A systematic review of the evidence for interventions for the prevention and control of meticillin-resistant *Staphylococcus aureus* (1996 – 2004): Report to the Joint MRSA Working Party (Subgroup A). J Hosp Infect. 2006;63:S45–S70.

29. Loeb M, Main C, Walker-Dilks C, Eady A. Antimicrobial drugs for treating methicillin-resistant Staphylococcus aureus colonization. Cochrane Database of Systemic Reviews 2003,Issue 4.

30. Stone HH, Hooper CA, Kolb LD, et al. Antibiotic prophylaxis in gastric, biliary and colonic surgery. Ann Surg 1976;184:443–452.

31. Forse RA, Karam B, MacLean LD, et al. Antibiotic prophylaxis for surgery in morbidly obese patients. Surgery 1989;106:750–756.

32. Edwards FH, Engelman RM, Houck P, et al. The Soceity of Thoracic Surgeons Practice Guideline Series: Antibiotic Prophylaxis in Cardiac Surgery, Part I: Duration. Ann Thorac Surg 2006;81:397–404.

86 Vaccines and Toxoids

Marianne Billeter

LEARNING OBJECTIVES

● **Upon completion of the chapter, the reader will be able to:**

1. Define vaccination and immunization.

2. Classify each of the routine vaccines as an inactivated, polysaccharide, conjugate, toxoid, or subunit vaccine.

3. Describe the effect of each routine vaccine on preventing infection.

4. Recommend an immunization schedule for a child, including immunocompromised children.

5. Recommend an immunization schedule for an adult based on comorbid conditions and lifestyle issues.

6. Evaluate an adverse reaction and its probable association with a vaccine.

KEY CONCEPTS

❶ Vaccines provide active immunity against viral and bacterial pathogens.

❷ Polysaccharide vaccines are poorly immunogenic in children younger than 2 years of age.

❸ Combination vaccines decrease the number of injections and increase the likelihood of completing the immunization schedule.

❹ Health care professionals should report vaccine-adverse events.

❺ Live virus vaccines should not be given to an immunocompromised host.

❻ Vaccines are cost effective in preventing disease.

The development and widespread use of vaccines is one of the greatest public health achievements of the 20th century. Other than safe drinking water, no other modality has had a greater impact on reducing mortality from infectious diseases. The first accounts of deliberate inoculation to prevent disease date back as far as the tenth century. However it wasn't until 1798 that Edward Jenner published his work on inoculation of natural cowpox as a means to prevent infection with smallpox. This was the first scientific attempt to prevent infection by inoculation. Since 1900, vaccines have been developed against more than 20 diseases, with half of these recommended for routine use. The widespread use of vaccines has resulted in the eradication of smallpox worldwide and wild-type poliovirus from the Western hemisphere. There have also been dramatic declines in the incidence of diphtheria, pertussis, tetanus, measles, mumps, rubella, and *Haemophilus influenzae* type b.

❶ *Vaccines have traditionally been preparations of killed or attenuated microorganisms that provide active immunity against a variety of viral and bacterial infections.* Most vaccines are designed to prevent acute infections that can be rapidly controlled and cleared by the immune system. Successful immunization involves activation of antigen-presenting cells with processing of the antigen by lysosomal or cytoplasmic pathways. T and B lymphocytes will be activated to replicate and differentiate to form large pools of memory cells for protection against subsequent exposure to the antigen.[1]

Vaccines against viral infections may be **attenuated** live viruses or inactivated viral particles. Attenuation may be accomplished by several methods to decrease the viruses' virulence while retaining their **immunogenicity**. Bacterial vaccines utilize antigenic particles of the outer membrane to elicit an immune response. ❷ *Outer membrane polysaccharides are poorly immunogenic in children less than 2 years of age* unless conjugated with a carrier protein. Also, bacterial toxins may undergo chemical treatment to render them nontoxic to form **toxoids** against infectious agents.

COMMON TERMINOLOGY

Often the terms vaccination and immunization are used interchangeably even though they are distinct concepts. ● Vaccination refers to the act of administering a vaccine, while immunization refers to the development of immunity to a pathogen. The delivery of a vaccine does not imply that

Patient Encounter 1

A 1-year-old child is brought to the pediatrician's office for a routine 1-year checkup. The child is healthy and meeting all growth and developmental targets. The child has received all vaccinations to date. The pediatrician discusses with the mother the need for more vaccinations during this visit.

Which vaccine should the child receive during this visit?

Is there a way to minimize the number of shots the child receives?

What risks are involved with vaccinating this child?

the individual mounted an adequate immune response to the vaccine to elicit protection. However, immunization implies that the act of vaccination resulted in the development of protective immunity.

Herd immunity refers to high levels of immunization in one population resulting in protection of another unvaccinated population. For example, concentrated vaccination of children with the 7-valent pneumococcal conjugate vaccine resulted in decreased invasive *Streptococcus pneumoniae* infection not only in the vaccinated children, but also in elderly persons within the same community.

Cocoon immunization is a strategy used to immunize all persons surrounding another high-risk individual, such as vaccinating parents, siblings, and grandparents of a new infant who is too young to be vaccinated. This strategy is used to protect individuals who are not able to be vaccinated themselves.

THE ROUTINE VACCINES

Diphtheria, Tetanus, and Pertussis Vaccines

▶ Diphtheria Toxoid

Diphtheria is a bacterial respiratory infection characterized by membranous pharyngitis. The membrane may cover the pharynx, tonsillar areas, soft palate, and uvula. Diphtheria may also cause anal, cutaneous, vaginal, and conjunctival infections. The impact of diphtheria is not from the causative bacteria, *Corynebacterium diphtheriae*, but rather from complications attributed to its exotoxin, such as myocarditis and peripheral neuritis. In the late 1800s, annual death rate from diphtheria ranged from 46 to 196 cases per 100,000. Mortality from diphtheria dropped in the 1900s mostly due to the availability of diphtheria antitoxin, which elicited passive immunity. Diphtheria is rarely reported in the United States since the introduction of vaccination with diphtheria toxoid; however, diphtheria continues to be a major problem in developing countries.

In the early 1900s, a balanced mixture of diphtheria toxin and antitoxin was found to produce active immunity in both animals and humans. This preparation gained widespread acceptance and protected approximately 85% of recipients. Several years later, diphtheria toxoid was developed by treating the toxin with small amounts of formalin. This process caused the toxin to lose its toxic properties while maintaining its immunogenic properties. In the mid-1920s, the addition of an alum precipitate enhanced the immunogenic properties of the toxoid.

In the 1940s, diphtheria toxoid was combined with tetanus toxoid and whole cell pertussis vaccines, and later with the acellular pertussis vaccine. The diphtheria toxoid, tetanus toxoid, and acellular pertussis vaccine are part of the routine childhood immunization schedule. Diphtheria toxoid is also combined with tetanus toxoid and is commonly used as a booster vaccine. The pediatric product (DT) has a higher amount of diphtheria toxoid than does the adult product (Td). Diphtheria toxoid is not available as an individual vaccine.

Recent outbreaks of diphtheria have demonstrated that immunity wanes in adulthood. Approximately 50% of all adults no longer have immunity to diphtheria. Regular boosters with tetanus and diphtheria toxoids every 10 years will provide adequate recall immunity to diphtheria provided the adult was previously immunized.[2]

▶ Tetanus Toxoid

The tetanus vaccine differs from others in that it does not protect against a contagious disease such as diphtheria, but rather against an environmental pathogen. *Clostridium tetani* is widely found in the environment, especially in dirt and soils. Additionally, animals and humans may harbor and excrete the organism. *C tetani* produces two neurotoxins, tetanospasmin and tetanolysin, which are responsible for producing the painful muscular contractions associated with tetanus. Tetanus continues to be a major problem in the developing world, causing approximately 1 million deaths each year.[3] Approximately 40% of the cases are neonatal tetanus most likely associated with the use of nonsterile instruments or poultices on the umbilical cord. Tetanus is rarely seen in developed countries.

Immunity to tetanus decreases with increasing age; therefore, a regular booster every 10 years with tetanus toxoid is recommended. The preferred agent to use in adults is tetanus and diphtheria toxoid (Td) in order to give a booster for diphtheria. Tetanus immunization status should be assessed in the management of wounds in individuals seeking medical care. A tetanus booster should be administered if a tetanus-containing vaccine has not been given in the preceding 5 years for moderate and severe wounds or contaminated wounds. If the wound is minor and uncontaminated, then a tetanus booster is needed if the previous tetanus vaccination was more than 10 years ago.

▶ Pertussis

Pertussis is a highly contagious respiratory tract infection caused by the bacteria *Bordetella pertussis*. Pertussis is characterized by a protracted severe cough with or without posttussive vomiting, whoop, difficulty breathing, difficulty sleeping, and rib fractures. It is often referred to as "whooping cough" or the 100-day cough. In the prevaccinc cra, pertussis accounted for more than 250,000 cases of severe illness and 10,000 deaths per year in the United States. Pertussis has always been thought of as a pediatric disease since most cases occurred in preschool-aged children with relatively no cases seen in adolescents and adults. The first pertussis vaccine was introduced in the 1940s and within 30 years resulted in a 99% reduction in disease. However, during the past two decades there has been a steady increase in reported cases of pertussis among adolescents and adults, indicating a waning immunity after primary immunization.[4]

The first pertussis whole cell vaccine was a mixture of killed organisms that was associated with frequent local and systemic reactions. In the late 1980s, an acellular pertussis vaccine was introduced that contains purified pertussis components that are immunogenic but associated with fewer adverse reactions. Acellular pertussis vaccine is available in combination with tetanus and diphtheria toxoids. Pertussis is not available as a separate vaccine component. In the spring of 2005, the FDA-approved tetanus toxoid, reduced diphtheria toxoid, and acellular pertussis vaccines for use in adolescents and adults.

▶ Use of Diphtheria, Tetanus, and Acellular Pertussis Vaccine

Diphtheria and tetanus toxoids and acellular pertussis (Dtap) vaccine should be administered in a five-shot series to all children beginning at 2 months of age (Table 86–1). The shots are given at 2, 4, 6, and 15 to 18 months, and 4 to 6 years. Complete immunity to diphtheria and tetanus is achieved after the third vaccination.

Tetanus toxoid, reduced diphtheria toxoid, and acellular pertussis vaccine (Tdap) is recommended as a single booster for the following groups in place of a tetanus booster.[5]

- *Adolescents 11 to 18 years of age*: An interval of 5 years, with a minimum of 2 years, between the last tetanus-containing vaccine is recommended to minimize local and systemic adverse events; however, shorter intervals may be used.
- *Adults 19 to 64 years of age*: Tdap should replace the next routine tetanus booster. Intervals as short as 2 years between Tdap and Td may be used.
- *Tetanus prophylaxis in wound management*: Adolescents and adults 11 to 64 years of age, who have completed a primary series and require a tetanus-containing product should receive Tdap instead of Td if they have not already received Tdap.
- *Prevention of pertussis among infants less than 12 months of age*: Adults who have close contact with infants less than 12 months of age, especially parents, grandparents less than 65 years of age, and child care providers, should receive a single dose of Tdap. An interval of at least 2 years since the last tetanus-containing vaccine was given is suggested, but shorter intervals may be used. Ideally, Tdap should be given 2 weeks prior to contact with the infant.

- *Postpartum women*: Women should receive a single dose of Tdap in the immediate postpartum period if Tdap has not been previously received. Ideally this should be administered prior to discharge from the hospital or birthing center.
- *Health care workers with direct patient contact*: Such workers should receive a single dose of Tdap.

Haemophilus influenzae Type b Vaccine

Haemophilus influenzae is a bacterial respiratory pathogen that causes a wide spectrum of disease ranging from colonization of the airways to bacterial meningitis. It causes considerable morbidity and mortality, especially in children less than 5 years of age. *H influenzae* is either encapsulated or unencapsulated. The encapsulated strains can be further differentiated into six antigenically distinct serotypes, a through f. *H influenzae* type b was primarily found in cerebrospinal fluid and blood of children with meningitis, while the unencapsulated strains were found in the upper respiratory tract of adults. Before the introduction of the vaccine, *H influenzae* was responsible for 20,000 to 25,000 cases of invasive disease annually and was the most common cause of bacterial meningitis. Since the introduction of the vaccine, invasive disease due to *H influenzae* type b has been nearly eliminated.

The *H influenzae* type b vaccine is a protein conjugate that utilizes a carrier-hapten for antigen presentation. The polysaccharide is conjugated to an immunogenic protein carrier, which is recognized by T cells and macrophages that stimulates T-dependent immunity. The conjugated vaccine elicits an immune response characterized by T-helper cell activation. The T-dependent antigens induce an enhanced immune response in younger children. Within 10 years of its introduction, the *H influenzae* type b vaccine use has resulted in widespread herd immunity.

H influenzae type b conjugate vaccine is a recommended routine childhood vaccine given at 2, 4, 6, and 12 to 15 months of age. Adolescents and adults with functional or anatomic asplenia should also receive a booster dose of *H influenzae* type b vaccine. The currently available vaccines are labeled for pediatric use, but can be used in adults when vaccination is indicated. There are several *H influenzae* type b vaccines on the market that differ in the size of the polysaccharide and type of carrier protein; however, the immune response to *H influenzae* type b is similar among the different vaccines. The different brands are interchangeable without affecting the primary immune response or booster response.

II *influenzae* type b and influenza vaccines have the potential for confusion and medication errors because of the similarity of the names. Care should be taken when ordering, dispensing, and administering these vaccines.

Hepatitis A Vaccine

Hepatitis A virus continues to be a frequent cause of illness despite the availability of a highly effective vaccine.

Table 86–1

Vaccine Dosing

Vaccine	Common Abbreviation	Dose	Route	Cautions
Diphtheria and tetanus toxoid	DT	0.5 mL	Intramuscular	
Diphtheria, tetanus, acellular pertussis	Dtap	0.5 mL	Intramuscular	Systemic neurologic reaction from previous vaccine Brachial neuritis Cries for 3 hours nonstop after previous dose Temperature greater than 40.5°C (105°F)
Haemophilus influenzae type b	HIB	0.5 mL	Intramuscular	
Hepatitis A	HAV	C: 0.5 mL A: 1 mL	Intramuscular	
Hepatitis B	HBV	C: 0.5 mL A: 1 mL	Intramuscular	Allergic reaction to yeast (baking yeast)
Human papillomavirus	HPV	0.5 mL	Intramuscular	Pregnant women
Inactivated influenza	TIV	0.5 mL	Intramuscular	Severe egg allergy History of Guillain-Barré syndrome
Live attenuated influenza	LAIV	0.5 mL	Intranasal	Severe egg allergy Asthma Chronic health problems Immunocompromised host Pregnant women History of Guillain-Barré syndrome
Measles, mumps, rubella	MMR	0.5 mL	Subcutaneous	Allergic reaction to gelatin or neomycin Pregnant women Immunocompromised host Recently received a blood transfusion Severe egg allergy
Meningococcal polysaccharide	MPSV4	0.5 mL	Subcutaneous	History of Guillain-Barré syndrome
Meningococcal conjugate	MCV4	0.5 mL	Intramuscular	History of Guillain-Barré syndrome
Pneumococcal 7-valent conjugate	PCV7	0.5 mL	Intramuscular	
Pneumococcal polysaccharide	PPV23	0.5 mL	Intramuscular route preferred; subcutaneous	Children less than 2 years of age
Poliovirus, inactivated	IPV	0.5 mL	Intramuscular, subcutaneous	Allergic reaction to neomycin, streptomycin, polymyxin B
Rotavirus vaccine	RV	2 mL	Oral	Immunocompromised host
Tetanus and diphtheria toxoid	Td	0.5 mL	Intramuscular	
Tetanus, reduced diphtheria, acellular pertussis	Tdap	0.5 mL	Intramuscular	History of Guillain-Barré syndrome Systemic neurologic reaction from previous vaccine
Varicella	VAR	0.5 mL	Subcutaneous	Allergic reaction to gelatin or neomycin Pregnant women Immunocompromised host Recently received a blood transfusion Hematopoietic stem cell transplant
Zoster	ZOS	0.65 mL	Subcutaneous	Allergic reaction to gelatin or neomycin Immunocompromised host Recently received a blood transfusion Hematopoietic stem cell transplant

C, children; A, adult.

Hepatitis A typically has an abrupt onset of symptoms including fever, malaise, nausea, abdominal discomfort, and jaundice. Frequently children less than 6 years of age are asymptomatic while adults typically have symptomatic disease. Symptoms may persist for 2 months or longer. There is wide geographic variation in the incidence of hepatitis A infection, with the number of cases ranging from 50 to more than 700 cases per 100,000 persons annually. The economic burden of hepatitis A is greater than $300 million annually in combined direct and indirect costs. Widespread use of the vaccine offers the opportunity to substantially decrease the disease burden caused by hepatitis A infection.[6]

Hepatitis A vaccine was licensed in the United States in 1995. It is an inactivated whole virus vaccine that is administered in a two-dose series. More than 94% of children, adolescents, and adults will have protective antibodies 1 month after receiving the first dose and 100% following the second dose.[6] Recommended use of the hepatitis A vaccine utilizes an incremental implementation schedule beginning with high-risk populations or those at increased risk for serious complications from the disease. Currently hepatitis A vaccine is recommended for all children following the first birthday, with the second dose administered 6 months later. Adults who are at high-risk for hepatitis A should receive two doses at least 6 months apart. High-risk adults include persons with clotting disorders or chronic liver disease, men who have sex with men, illicit drug users, international travelers going to areas with high to intermediate endemicity of hepatitis A, or any other person who wishes to become immune.

Hepatitis B Vaccine

Hepatitis B virus is a blood-borne or sexually transmitted virus. Most acute infections occur in adults, while chronic infections usually occur in individuals infected as infants or children. However, about 10% of adults who contract hepatitis B virus will fail to clear their infection and develop chronic hepatitis B infection. Individuals with chronic hepatitis B infection are at risk for cirrhosis or hepatocellular carcinoma. Vaccination with hepatitis B vaccine is the most effective way to prevent hepatitis B infection.[7]

Hepatitis B vaccine is manufactured using recombinant DNA technology to express hepatitis B surface antigen (HBsAg) in yeast. This is further purified with biochemical separation techniques to produce the vaccine. The vaccines are formulated to contain 10 to 40 mcg of HBsAg protein/mL. Hepatitis B vaccine is available as a single component or in combination vaccines.

Hepatitis B vaccine is recommended for routine use in children. The first dose should be given within 12 hours of birth. The second and third doses are given at 2 months and 6 months after the first dose if using the single component vaccine, or at 2, 4, and 6 months if using a hepatitis B containing combination vaccine. If the infant weighs less than 2,000 g at birth, the birth dose is not counted in the three-dose series. Infants less than 2,000 g do not produce an adequate immune response to the birth dose of hepatitis B vaccine. Adolescents should receive the three-dose series if not previously vaccinated.[7]

Adults at high-risk for hepatitis B because of occupation or lifestyle should receive the hepatitis B vaccine series. The typical series has the second and third doses given 1 month and 6 months after the first dose. Accelerated schedules may also be used. Frequently, individuals do not follow through with the complete three-dose series and questions arise about restarting the series. Hepatitis B vaccine produces an amnesic response; therefore the series may be continued at any time in order to complete the three doses.

Following vaccination with hepatitis B vaccine, hepatitis B virus serologic markers will remain negative with the exception of anti-HBs (antibody to hepatitis B surface antigen), which will be positive indicating immunity. Persons with anti-HBs concentration greater than 10 mIU/mL after vaccination will have complete protection against acute and chronic infection.[7] It is unclear if a booster dose of hepatitis B vaccine should be administered when anti-HBs concentrations fall below 10 mIU/mL, since a good memory response will occur following exposure to hepatitis B virus.

Human Papillomavirus Vaccine

Human papillomavirus (HPV) is the most common sexually transmitted virus and is associated with a wide range of diseases, including genital warts and cervical cancer. More than 100 HPVs have been sequenced and classified as low-risk, nononcogenic or high-risk oncogenic types based on their ability to cause malignant disease. The predominant low-risk types HPV 6 and 11 are associated with 90% of genital warts. High-risk types HPV 16 and 18 are associated with 70% of cervical cancer cases and cervical intra-epithelial neoplasia.[8] HPV is also associated with other gynecologic cancers, such as vaginal and vulvovaginal tumors.

Two HPV L-1 virus-like particle vaccines have been developed. The quadrivalent vaccine contains HPV types 6, 11, 16, and 18, and has been approved for use in the United States for the prevention of cervical cancer, precancerous or dysplastic lesions and genital warts in girls and women 9 through 26 years of age. The bivalent vaccine contains HPV types 16 and 18; this vaccine is under review by the FDA, but not yet approved. Both vaccines have shown greater than 95% efficacy in preventing precancerous lesions of the cervix, vulva, and vagina. Additionally, the quadrivalent vaccine is also effective against genital warts. Both HPV vaccines are safe with no unexpected adverse events.

These vaccines are unique in that preventing infection by HPV will translate into prevention of cancer, making these the first cancer prevention vaccines. Clinical trials are utilizing surrogate markers, prevention of precancerous lesions, to determine efficacy of the vaccines. However, the true impact on preventing cancerous tumors will not be known for years. The HPV vaccine is recommended for use in girls and women 9 through 26 years of age.[9] Ideally it should be administered to girls before they become sexually active. However, sexually active girls and women should still receive the vaccine. Additionally, girls and women who have been infected with HPV should still receive the vaccine since the vaccine provides protection against more than one type of HPV. Use of the HPV in boys and men is not recommended at this time.

Influenza Vaccine

Influenza is a contagious viral respiratory infection that usually occurs during the winter months in the Northern Hemisphere and all year round in the Southern Hemisphere. All age groups are affected by influenza; however, children have the highest rate of infection. Serious illness and death due to influenza usually occurs in extremes of age, those over 65 years or under 2 years. Influenza is responsible for approximately 36,000 deaths annually in the United States.[10]

Influenza A and B viruses are responsible for causing human disease. Influenza A is further categorized into subgroups by its surface antigens, hemagglutinin and neuraminidase (e.g., influenza A H1N1 virus). Influenza B virus is not subtyped. Both influenza A and B undergo frequent antigenic drift, creating new influenza variants. Immunity to the surface antigens decreases the likelihood of infection. Unfortunately, antibody to one influenza subgroup does not give complete protection against other influenza subtypes. Therefore, annual influenza vaccination is recommended during October and November, and continuing until the vaccine supply is exhausted.

The best way to protect against influenza is through vaccination. The influenza vaccine is composed of two influenza A subtypes and one influenza B subtype. The viral subtypes contained in the vaccine usually changes each year. The exact composition is selected by a panel of experts and announced by the Centers for Disease Control and Prevention (CDC) in March or April each year. The vaccine becomes available for use in late August and September. Two types of influenza vaccine are licensed for use in the United States; both vaccines contain the same viral subunits. The influenza viruses for both vaccine preparations are grown in eggs. Therefore, the vaccines are contraindicated in individuals with severe allergy to eggs.

The influenza vaccine should be administered to any person wanting to reduce the risk of infection with the influenza virus. Target groups for annual influenza vaccination are all children age 6 months through 18 years, all adults 50 years and older and younger adults at high-risk of complications from influenza. The trivalent inactivated influenza vaccine can be administered to all age groups and risk populations. The live attenuated influenza vaccine may be administered to healthy individuals between the age of 2 and 49 years. If the child is less than 8 years old and is receiving influenza vaccine for the first time, two doses separated by 4 to 6 weeks should be given.[10]

Measles, Mumps, and Rubella Vaccine

▶ *Measles*

Measles, also known as rubeola, is characterized by a rash that is often complicated by diarrhea, middle ear infection, or pneumonia. Encephalitis occurs in 1 of every 1,000 reported cases. Individuals who recover from encephalitis usually have permanent brain damage. Death occurs in 1 to 2 of every 1,000 reported measles cases.[11]

Prior to measles vaccine availability the number of cases of measles approached the birth rate of approximately 3 to 4 million annually. The first measles vaccine was licensed in 1963. Since that time there has been a 99% reduction in reported measles cases. Currently, there is a goal to eliminate measles transmission in the United States through aggressive immunization programs.

There have been several types of measles vaccines used since its introduction. There have been inactive and live attenuated vaccines using different strains of the virus. The current vaccine uses a live attenuated preparation of the Enders-Edmonston virus strain. Following vaccination with measles containing vaccine, a mild noncommunicable infection develops. Approximately 95% of individuals will develop antibodies following a single dose if administered after 12 months of age. More than 99% of individuals who receive two inoculations will develop long-term, probably lifelong, immunity to measles.[11]

▶ *Mumps*

Mumps is usually thought of as a disease of children, but it has also gained notoriety as a prominent illness affecting military units. Mumps produces a typical acute parotitis, but may also cause nonspecific respiratory symptoms. In postpubertal males, mumps may also cause orchitis in 38% of those infected, which may result in infertility.[11]

Since the introduction of the mumps vaccine in 1967 there has been a 99% reduction in reported cases. The mumps vaccine is a live virus preparation of the Jeryl-Lynn strain. It produces a subclinical, noncommunicable infection following vaccination. Single doses of mumps vaccine will elicit immunity in 75% to 95% of individuals. Vaccine-induced immunity lasts for more than 30 years.

▶ *Rubella*

German measles, also known as rubella, is a mild exanthematous illness in children and young adults; however, rubella infection in pregnant women can cause a variety of congenital malformations in the infant. Congenital rubella syndrome occurs in approximately 25% of infants whose mother acquires rubella during the first trimester. Congenital rubella syndrome is characterized by congenital cataracts, heart disease, deafness, thrombocytopenia, mental retardation, and numerous other abnormalities.[11]

The first rubella vaccine was licensed in 1969. Initial vaccination campaigns were targeting young children, as this age group had the highest rate of rubella infection. This strategy significantly decreased rubella cases in children, but did not have the desired effect on infection in adolescents and adults or on congenital rubella syndrome. Adolescents, especially young girls, were then targeted for vaccination. This has resulted in a significant reduction in the number of cases of congenital rubella syndrome.

The live rubella vaccine available in the United States contains the RA 27/3 strain of the virus. Following a single dose of rubella vaccine after the first birthday, more than 90% of individuals will develop long-term immunity. Rarely has congenital rubella syndrome been reported in infants born to mothers with adequate rubella immunization.

▶ Use of Measles, Mumps, and Rubella Vaccine

Measles, mumps, and rubella vaccines are available as single component vaccines or as combinations. Most authorities recommend use of the measles, mumps, and rubella combination vaccine and discourage use of the single- or double-component vaccines. Two doses of the measles, mumps, and rubella vaccine are recommended for all individuals born after 1957. The first dose should be administered soon after the first birthday and the second prior to entering school. For high-risk adolescents and adults who do not have adequate immunity, two doses of the vaccine should be separated by a minimum of 28 days.[11]

Measles, mumps, and rubella vaccine is a live virus vaccine that should be used with caution in immunosuppressed children, such as those with cancer receiving chemotherapy, solid organ or bone marrow transplantation, or receiving other immunosuppressive drugs, such as steroids in a dose equivalent to prednisone 1 mg/kg/day or higher or 20 mg/day for 2 weeks or longer. If possible, vaccines should be given prior to becoming immunosuppressed. Otherwise, it may be prudent to defer the vaccine until after the immuno-suppression resolves.

Meningococcal Vaccines

Neisseria meningitidis is a significant cause of meningitis and severe sepsis. Meningococcus causes an estimated 2,500 cases of invasive disease each year in the United States. Invasive meningococcal disease is associated with an estimated 15% mortality rate. Morbidity in survivors is substantial, with approximately 20% having loss of limb or neurologic sequelae. The highest rates of meningococcal disease are among young children; however, rates have been increasing in adolescents and young adults. Thirteen meningococcal serogroups have been identified; however, five serogroups, A, B, C, Y, and W-135, are responsible for epidemic and endemic disease worldwide. Despite the availability of highly active antibacterial agents against *N meningitidis,* there has been little impact on decreasing the morbidity and mortality due to invasive meningococcal disease.[12]

A meningococcal polysaccharide vaccine containing serogroups A, C, Y, and W-135 has been available in the United States for a number of years. Meningococcal polysaccharide vaccine is similar to other polysaccharide vaccines, in that it is poorly immunogenic in infants and children less than 2 years of age, and does not produce lasting immunity. Meningococcal polysaccharide vaccine produces a T-cell–independent response and fails to induce a memory response. Repeated vaccination results in hyporesponsiveness to serogroups A and C; the clinical implication of this finding is unknown.

In January 2005, a new meningococcal polysaccharide diphtheria toxoid conjugate vaccine was approved by the FDA. This vaccine also contains meningococcal serogroups A, C, Y, and W-135. Polysaccharide-protein conjugate vaccines are known to produce improved immunogenicity and memory responses. Meningococcal conjugate vaccine has shown similar immunologic response for all four serogroups when compared to meningococcal polysaccharide vaccine. However, this vaccine does not offer protection against diphtheria.

Meningococcal conjugate vaccine is recommended for routine vaccination in individuals 11 to 18 years of age. Ideally, this should be done at the routine preadolescent health care visit. Routine meningococcal vaccination is also recommended for persons aged 19 to 55 years at increased risk for meningococcal disease, such as college freshman living in dormitories, microbiologists who are routinely exposed to isolates of *N meningitidis*, military recruits, persons who travel to or reside in countries in which *N meningitidis* is hyperendemic or epidemic, persons who have terminal complement component deficiencies, and persons who have anatomic or functional asplenia.[13] Additionally, meningococcal conjugate vaccine should be administered to children 2 to 10 years of age who are high-risk of meningococcal disease.[14] Routine revaccination is not recommended at this time.[12] A history of Guillain-Barré syndrome is a relative contraindication to receiving meningococcal conjugate vaccine, and the risk versus benefit should be carefully considered. Individuals may be given the meningococcal polysaccharide vaccine in lieu of the conjugate vaccine.

Pneumococcal Vaccines

Streptococcus pneumoniae is the most common bacterial cause of community-acquired respiratory tract infections. *S pneumoniae* causes approximately 3,000 cases of meningitis, 50,000 cases of bacteremia, 500,000 cases of pneumonia, and over 1 million cases of otitis media each year. The increasing

---

Patient Encounter 2

An 18-year-old male is having a routine physical before leaving for college. He will be a freshman and is looking forward to dormitory life. The health care provider recommends some vaccinations be given at this visit.

Which vaccines should be administered?

What is the risk of not receiving the vaccines?

prevalence of drug-resistant *S pneumoniae* has highlighted the need to prevent infection through vaccination. Both licensed pneumococcal vaccines are highly effective in preventing disease from the common *S pneumoniae* serotypes that cause human disease.

The 23-valent pneumococcal polysaccharide vaccine contains 23 serotypes that are responsible for causing more than 80% of invasive *S pneumoniae* infections in adults. The vaccine includes those serotypes that are associated with drug resistance. Use of the vaccine will not prevent the development of antibiotic-resistant *S pneumoniae*, but is likely to prevent infection from drug-resistant strains. The 23-valent pneumococcal polysaccharide vaccine has demonstrated good immunogenicity in adults, but an individual will not develop immunity to all 23 serotypes following vaccination.[15]

The 23-valent pneumococcal polysaccharide vaccine is recommended for use in all adults 65 years of age or older and adults less than 65 years who have medical comorbidities that increase the risk for serious complications from *S pneumoniae* infection, such as chronic pulmonary disorders, cardiovascular disease, diabetes mellitus, chronic liver disease, chronic renal failure, functional or anatomic asplenia, and immunosuppressive disorders. Alaskan natives and certain Native American populations are also at increased risk. Children over the age of 2 years may be vaccinated with the 23-valent pneumococcal polysaccharide vaccine if they are at increased risk for invasive *S pneumoniae* infections, such as children with sickle cell anemia or those receiving cochlear implants.

Revaccination with the 23-valent pneumococcal polysaccharide vaccine is recommended for adults over the age of 65 years if the first dose was administered when they were less than 65 years of age and at least 5 years have passed. Revaccination results in a blunted immune response and increased local adverse reactions, therefore routine revaccination is not recommended.[15] Adults vaccinated at age 65 or greater do not require revaccination.

The 7-valent pneumococcal conjugate vaccine was licensed in February 2000 for use in children. It induces good immunogenicity in children under the age of 2 years. It is now part of the routine childhood immunization schedule beginning at 2 months of age. It is given at 2, 4, 6, and 12 to 18 months of age. The 7-valent pneumococcal conjugate vaccine decreases the carriage rate of *S pneumoniae* and the incidence of invasive disease in vaccinated populations. Widespread use of the 7-valent pneumococcal conjugate vaccine has resulted in herd immunity and decreased the incidence of invasive *S pneumoniae* disease among unvaccinated adults over 20 years of age.[15]

Poliovirus Vaccine

Poliomyelitis is a highly contagious disease that is often asymptomatic; however, approximately 1 in every 100 to 1,000 cases will develop a rapidly progressive paralytic disease. Polio is caused by poliovirus which has three serotypes; type 1 is most frequently associated with paralytic disease. Poliovirus replicates in the oropharynx and intestinal tract and is excreted in oral secretions and feces, which can infect others. As a result, more than 90% of unvaccinated individuals will become infected with poliovirus following household exposure to wild-type poliovirus. Since the introduction of the first poliovirus vaccine, there has been a significant reduction in the number of polio cases. Today, polio caused by wild-type poliovirus has been eradicated from the Western Hemisphere with the goal of eradicating it from the world.[16]

The first inactivated poliovirus vaccine was introduced in the 1950s in an injectable formulation, and replaced in the 1960s by a live oral poliovirus vaccine. The oral poliovirus vaccine not only elicits systemic immunogenicity but also a localized immune response in the intestinal tract. Unfortunately, the oral poliovirus vaccine has the risk of vaccine-associated paralytic poliomyelitis occurring in approximately 1 case of every 2.4 million doses distributed. The risk with the first dose of oral poliovirus vaccine is 1 case in 750,000 doses.[16]

The last reported case of indigenous wild-type poliovirus in the United States was in 1979; subsequent cases were all vaccine-associated. In 1997, a transition period to the inactivated poliovirus vaccine was begun to reduce the risk of vaccine-associated paralytic poliomyelitis. By January 2000, the oral vaccine was no longer recommended for routine use. Currently, the inactivated poliovirus vaccine is recommended for routine use in the United States. The oral poliovirus vaccine is still widely used in some countries where poliovirus eradication has been more difficult.

The enhanced potency inactivated poliovirus vaccine contains all three serotypes. After two doses, more than 90% of those vaccinated will have immunity to the three serotypes and 99% after three doses. Inactivated poliovirus vaccine is recommended to be given at 2, 4, 6 to 18 months, and 4 to 6 years of age.

Rotavirus Vaccine

Rotavirus is the most common cause of diarrhea worldwide. Most children will become infected by the age of 5 years. In the United States, rotavirus is responsible for approximately 50,000 hospitalizations for severe diarrhea and dehydration, and 20 to 40 deaths annually. Most hospitalizations occur in children less than 3 years of age. Rotavirus infections follow a winter–spring seasonal pattern. Rotavirus G1 is the most prevalent strain found in the United States. However, in any given year other strains G2, G3, G4, and G9 may predominate.

The first rotavirus vaccine was a tetravalent rhesus-based rotavirus strain. It was licensed in the United States in 1998 and subsequently withdrawn from the market within the first year due to an association with intussusception. A pentavalent human-bovine reassortant rotavirus vaccine was approved by the FDA in February 2006. This vaccine contains outer capsid proteins for G1, G2, G3, G4 and P1. A monovalent, G1 vaccine has been approved for use in the United States.[17] The exact mechanism by which these vaccines produce an immune response is unknown; however, these live virus vaccines replicate in the small intestine and induce immunity.

The rotavirus vaccine is administered in either a two-dose or three-dose series that is orally administered. The first dose is given to infants between 6 and 12 weeks of age.[17] One year after the introduction of the rotavirus vaccine the CDC reported a 50% reduction in reported cases of rotavirus in the United States.

Varicella Vaccine

Varicella zoster virus is a herpes virus that infects nearly all humans. Primary infection with Varicella zoster causes chickenpox (varicella), which is one of the most common childhood diseases. Chickenpox has always been thought to be a benign disease causing few serious complications in children. The rate of chickenpox prior to the vaccine becoming available was thought to approximate the birth rate with 3 to 4 million cases annually resulting in 11,000 hospitalizations and 100 deaths. Adults who develop chickenpox have a 25% greater risk for developing serious complications from varicella compared to children. Chickenpox is highly contagious and has a secondary household transmission rate of 87%. Following resolution of the primary infection, varicella becomes latent in cranial nerve, dorsal routs, and autonomic ganglia.

The varicella vaccine is made up of an attenuated Oka strain of varicella zoster virus. This is a live attenuated vaccine. Attenuation was achieved by performing serial passages through human embryonic lung cells, embryonic guinea pig cells, and human diploid cells.

Children less than 12 years of age will have a 97% seroconversion rate following a single vaccination. Adolescents and adults more than 13 years old will only have 78% seroconversion after a single inoculation, but will have 99% conversion after the second vaccination administered 4 to 8 weeks after the first. Antibody titers appear to persist for at least 20 years following immunization. Despite excellent seroconversion rates, breakthrough chickenpox is reported at a rate of 1 case per 10,000 doses distributed. Most cases occurred within the first year following vaccination, and were due to wild-type varicella zoster virus. The majority of breakthrough cases were mild and of short duration.[18]

Secondary transmission to household contacts is always a concern with administration of a live vaccine. There are a few cases of possible secondary transmission of varicella following vaccination. Of the cases that varicella typing was done, 62% were wild-type virus, indicating exposure to an unvaccinated person. There are less than 10 confirmed cases of secondary transmission of the Oka vaccine strain following vaccination. A mild rash occurring in less than 5% of persons has been reported following vaccination. The varicella virus may be shed from the rash. Rashes due to the Oka vaccine strain typically occur more than 20 days following vaccination.[18]

Varicella vaccine should be administered after 12 months of age and a second dose at 4 years of age. Adolescents and adults without evidence of immunity to varicella zoster should receive two doses of varicella vaccine given 4 to 8 weeks apart. Varicella vaccine is available as a single-component vaccine or in combination with measles, mumps, and rubella vaccine.

Zoster Vaccine

Later in life, approximately 15% of the population will develop herpes zoster (shingles). Zoster is the reactivation of latent varicella zoster virus in the sensory ganglia. It produces a classic rash along a single nerve track. Approximately 20% of persons with herpes zoster will develop postherpetic neuralgia, which is a painful debilitating condition that can persist for months after resolution of the herpes zoster rash. Adults get a boost in immunity with repeated exposure to children with the chickenpox. Zoster most frequently occurs in the elderly and immunocompromised individuals who have decreased circulating antibodies to varicella zoster virus.[19]

Zoster vaccine is a more concentrated form of the varicella vaccine. It is recommended for use in individuals 60 years of age and older. Use of the zoster vaccine has shown a 60% reduction in the incidence of zoster and postherpetic neuralgia. There is decreased effectiveness of the vaccine with increasing age.

The varicella vaccine is relatively new and has only been recommended for use since 1996, therefore its true impact on chickenpox and zoster is not yet known. Continued use of the varicella vaccine will undoubtedly change the epidemiology of both of these diseases. As the prevalence of chickenpox declines, the rate of zoster will likely increase in the elderly making vaccination with the zoster vaccine more prudent.[19]

COMBINATION VACCINES

The childhood immunization schedule is complex and requires a large number of injections. In small infants the large number of injections can be intolerable to the infant, parent, and health care provider. Limiting the number of injections at each visit can lead to missed vaccinations and increased expense for return visits. ❸ *Use of combination vaccines decreases the number of injections and increases the likelihood that the immunization schedule would be completed.*

Many factors have to be considered when developing combination vaccines. First the selected components need to be given on a similar schedule and all components should already be licensed in the United States. The excipients contained in the individual vaccines may interfere with another component when combined, altering a component's immunogenicity. Finally, the immunogenicity of the combination must be similar (within 10%) to the immune response when the components are administered separately.[20]

There are several combination vaccines available in the United States. One of the most popular pediatric combinations is Pediarix, a combination of diphtheria and tetanus toxoids, acellular pertussis, inactivated poliovirus, and hepatitis B vaccines. Pentacel was recently approved and is a combination of diphtheria and tetanus toxoids, acellular pertussis, inactivated poliovirus, and *H influenza* type b vaccines. ComVax is a combination of *H influenzae* type b and hepatitis B vaccines. ProQuad contains measles, mumps, rubella, and varicella vaccines. The only combination available for adults is Twinrix, which has hepatitis A and hepatitis B vaccines.

VACCINE ADMINISTRATION SCHEDULES

Most vaccines are administered in two- to four-shot series in order to elicit the best protection. Childhood and adult immunization schedules are revised frequently and published annually by the CDC Advisory Committee on Immunization Practices. Current immunization schedules can be found at *www.cdc.gov*. The childhood schedule is published in January and the adult schedule in October of each year. Recommendations will be published throughout the year in the *Morbidity and Mortality Weekly Report* (*MMWR*) as new vaccines are licensed or new information necessitates a change in previous recommendations.

VACCINE SAFETY

Vaccination is one of the most powerful tools used to prevent disease. As with all drugs, most vaccines have been reported to cause adverse reactions. The reactions are either acute, such as local reactions, or are related to the risk of developing another disease. Health care professionals are to give vaccine information sheets to individuals or caregivers prior to vaccination; these provide information about the risks and benefits of each vaccine.

Vaccine safety is monitored by the FDA and CDC through a passive reporting system that allows anyone, health professionals or lay public, to report any event. ❹ *Health care professionals are bound by federal regulation to report certain adverse events* (*Table 86–2*). Additionally, any serious, life-threatening or unusual reactions should also be reported. The Vaccine Adverse Event Reporting System (VAERS) can be found at *http://vaers.hhs.gov*.

The VAERS database is continually monitored to determine if the prevalence of reactions is changing and to identify previously unreported reactions to a particular vaccine. One of the limitations of the VAERS data is that it does not contain denominator data. Therefore it is not possible to calculate a true rate of reaction occurrence: the number of cases of reaction per dose of vaccine administered. Rates

Table 86–2

Vaccine Reportable Events

Vaccine/Toxoid	Event	Interval From Vaccination
Tetanus in any combination (DTaP, DTP, DTP-Hib, DT, Tdap, Td, or TT)	Anaphylaxis or anaphylactic shock	7 days
	Brachial neuritis	28 days
	Systemic allergic reaction	7 days
	Systemic neurologic reaction	
Pertussis in any combination (DTaP, DTP, DTP-Hib, or Tdap)	Anaphylaxis or anaphylactic shock	7 days
	Encephalopathy or encephalitis	7 days
	Progressive neurologic disorders, such as infantile spasms or uncontrolled epilepsy	7 days
Measles, mumps, and rubella in any combination (MMR, MR, M, or R)	Anaphylaxis or anaphylactic shock	7 days
	Encephalopathy or encephalitis	15 days
Rubella in any combination (MMR, MR, or R)	Chronic arthritis	42 days
Measles in any combination (MMR, MR, or M)	Thrombocytopenic purpura	7–30 days
	Vaccine strain measles in immunodeficient recipient	6 months
Oral polio (OPV)	Paralytic polio	30 days to 6 months
	Vaccine strain polio infection	30 days to 6 months
Inactivated polio (IPV)	Anaphylaxis or anaphylactic shock	7 days
	Systemic allergic reaction	7 days
Hepatitis B	Anaphylaxis or anaphylactic shock	7 days
	Systemic allergic reaction	7 days
Haemophilus influenzae type b (conjugate)	Anaphylaxis or anaphylactic shock	7 days
	Systemic allergic reaction	7 days
Varicella (chickenpox)	Anaphylaxis or anaphylactic shock	7 days
	Systemic allergic reaction	7 days
Rotavirus	Intussusception	30 days
Pneumococcal conjugate	Anaphylaxis or anaphylactic shock	7 days
	Systemic allergic reaction	7 days

are usually calculated using the number of doses distributed from the manufacture as the denominator. This makes the assumption that each dose distributed is administered.

Local Reactions

Pain at the injection site is one of the most commonly reported adverse effects of vaccination. The reaction is usually mild with complaints of pain and tenderness at the injection site that may or may not be accompanied by erythema. Local reactions tend to be more frequent with repeated doses or booster doses of vaccine. The frequency and degree of the reactions appear to be related to the amount of preformed antibodies and rapid immunologic responses reflective of priming from previous doses. More serious Arthus reactions are infrequently reported. Arthus reactions are classified as type III hypersensitivity reactions, and are characterized by a massive local response involving the entire thigh or deltoid. Arthus reactions are also related to preformed antibody complexes that induce an inflammatory lesion.[21]

Tetanus-containing vaccines are well known for causing localized reactions; however, all vaccines can cause local reactions.

Fever

Fever is the most frequently reported adverse effect in children and adolescents. Fever associated with vaccination is defined as a temperature of greater than or equal to 38°C (100.4°F) measured at any site using a validated device. Fever is caused by a complex reaction induced by the production of cytokines that affect the hypothalamic neurons. This results in raising the hypothalamic set point. Temperature elevations above 40°C (104°F) can result in cellular and multi-organ dysfunction. Excessive temperature elevations rarely result from fever alone, but are usually coupled with other thermoregulatory dysfunction.[22]

The whole cell pertussis vaccine has been highly associated with temperature elevations; however, the prevalence has significantly decreased since the introduction of the acellular pertussis vaccine. Live virus vaccines are also associated with fever.

Guillain-Barré Syndrome

Guillain-Barré syndrome is a transient neurologic disorder involving inflammatory demyelination of the peripheral nerves. The syndrome is characterized by progressive symmetric weakness of the legs and arms with loss of reflexes. Occasionally sensory abnormalities and paralysis of respiratory muscles will occur.[23]

The etiology of Guillain-Barré syndrome is unknown, but increasing evidence suggests it is probably a humoral and cellular autoimmune disease induced by infection with a variety of microorganisms. The background rate of Guillain-Barré syndrome is one to two cases per 100,000 persons annually. Guillain-Barré syndrome has been associated with several vaccines. An influenza vaccine used in the mid-1970s (swine flu vaccine) increased the incidence of Guillain-Barré syndrome by a factor of eight.[23] Warnings about Guillain-Barré syndrome continue to be given with annual influenza vaccinations. The hepatitis B vaccine derived from pooled plasma was also associated with Guillain-Barré syndrome; however, Guillain-Barré has not been reported with use of the currently available hepatitis B vaccines produced through recombinant DNA technology. Most recently, Guillain-Barré syndrome has been reported to occur with the meningococcal conjugate vaccine.

Other Safety Concerns

A clear cause-and-effect relationship between vaccine administration and chronic diseases, such as diabetes mellitus, multiple sclerosis, and chronic arthritis, has never been scientifically proven.

Thimerosal is a preservative used in vaccines that has been purported to cause autism in children. The assumption is that thimerosal, also known as ethyl mercury, causes similar effects as methyl mercury, which has neurotoxic and nephrotoxic effects at high-doses. Several epidemiologic studies have not shown a higher rate of autism among children receiving thimerosal-containing vaccines when compared to the normal background rate of autism. Additionally, the mercury exposure with vaccination is much lower than through many other environmental exposures. Despite the lack of evidence of thimerosal causing neurologic disorders, vaccine manufacturers are producing vaccines that are thimerosal-free or only contain trace amounts of thimerosal.[21]

SPECIAL POPULATIONS
Immunocompromised Host

The number of immunocompromised persons is continually increasing as advances are made in medicine. The life expectancy for persons with cancer, HIV infection, and solid organ or bone marrow transplantation is increasing.

Patient Encounter 3

A 7-year-old child with acute leukemia is 1-year post bone marrow transplantation. The child's clinical course has been uneventful since transplantation and everything is going as expected. The physician discusses with the child's parents the continued need for protection against infections and suggests that the child should receive some vaccinations.

When should the child begin receiving vaccinations?

Which vaccines should be administered and on what schedule?

Should any vaccines be avoided?

Which vaccines should household contacts receive?

Vaccination provides one tool to prevent infection in the immunocompromised host; however, the individual's immunosuppressed state will alter the response to the vaccine. In general all vaccinations should be updated prior to the person becoming immunosuppressed, if possible. ❺ *Once a person becomes significantly immunosuppressed, live virus vaccines should be avoided.*

Adults with HIV infection should be vaccinated with the 23-valent pneumococcal polysaccharide and hepatitis B vaccines as early in the course of the disease as possible. Inactivated influenza vaccine should be given yearly. Children should continue to receive vaccinations on the standard childhood immunization schedule. The individual may experience a transient elevation in HIV viral load following vaccination.[24]

Following hematopoietic stem cell transplantation the patient will need virtually all routine vaccines to be administered again; however, the patient will not be able to mount an adequate response for 6 to 12 months posttransplant. Diphtheria, tetanus, acellular pertussis, *H influenzae* type b, hepatitis B, pneumococcal, and inactivated poliovirus should be given at 12, 14, and 24 months posthematopoietic stem cell transplantation. Inactivated influenza vaccine should be given yearly, starting 6 months after transplant. Measles, mumps, and rubella can be given 2 years after transplant and varicella vaccine is contraindicated.[24]

Solid organ transplant recipients have a blunted immune response to vaccines because the immunosuppressive regimens used to prevent organ rejection inhibit both T- and B-cell proliferation. Many of these patients will also have secondary hypogammaglobulinemia posttransplantation. Prior to transplant, children should complete primary immunization schedules if possible; accelerated schedules may be used. Adults should have all vaccinations updated prior to transplantation.[24]

Household contacts of immunocompromised persons should have all routine vaccines as scheduled, including yearly influenza vaccination. Children in the household may receive live virus vaccines without special precautions; however, if a rash develops following varicella vaccination, contact should be avoided with the immunocompromised host until the rash resolves.

Pregnancy

Immunization during pregnancy is done to ensure that the infant has sufficient antibodies during the period the infant is most vulnerable to disease. Maternal antibodies are actively transported to the fetus throughout the pregnancy. However, in the last 4 to 6 weeks of gestation the active transport of immunoglobulins substantially increases. Vaccines administered during pregnancy should produce high antibody concentrations following a single vaccination and are administered in the second and third trimester, but no later than 2 weeks prior to delivery. Maternal vaccination has not shown any harmful effects to the developing fetus. However, live virus vaccines are avoided due to theoretical concerns of the virus being transported across the placenta and infecting the fetus. It is recommended that pregnant women be up to date on tetanus vaccine and receive the influenza vaccine if the second and third trimester will occur during the winter months.[25]

Health Care Workers

Most health care workers are at risk for exposure to many diseases in the normal course of their work. Additionally, health care workers may transmit vaccine-preventable diseases to their patients. At the time of employment and on a regular basis, health care workers should be screened for immunity to measles, mumps, rubella, and varicella; if found to be nonimmune, the measles, mumps, and rubella, and varicella vaccines should be administered. The hepatitis B series should be given if not already completed. Tetanus should be updated and given every 10 years. Health care personnel in hospitals and ambulatory settings with direct patient contact should receive Tdap if not already received; an interval as short as 2 years from the last tetanus-containing vaccine should be used.

All health care personnel should be strongly encouraged to receive the influenza vaccine yearly in order to prevent transmission of influenza within the health care facility and to decrease employee absenteeism for influenza-related reasons. The vaccine should be made available to employees at the workplace free of charge. Employees should be asked to sign a declination if refusing to receive the influenza vaccine. Additionally, health care facilities should report the number of health care personnel receiving influenza vaccine as a patient safety measure.[26]

OUTCOME MEASURES

❻ *Vaccines are a cost-effective means for disease prevention.* For every dollar spent on routine childhood vaccines there will be a savings of $0.90 to $24.00 in direct medical expense. The rates of vaccination for children are well over 90%. This has been attributed to the requirements for proof of vaccination by states for enrollment into day care centers and school. Additionally, children (18 years of age or younger) may receive routine vaccinations free of charge through state health departments or other assistance programs, such as the national Vaccines for Children program. Many states have developed universal immunization databases to document pediatric and adult vaccination status. This eliminates the problems of lost immunization records if a child changes health care providers.

The vaccination rate in adults is much lower than that in children. Only 50% to 60% of adults who meet criteria have received pneumococcal or influenza vaccination. Comprehensive initiatives need to be implemented to increase the adult vaccination rate. Some proven concepts are providing reminders to patients that vaccines are due and implementation of standing orders for vaccines. This latter concept allows nurses and pharmacists to screen patients to see if pneumococcal, influenza, or other vaccines are needed and to vaccinate without a physician's order.

The Centers for Medicare and Medicaid Services has incorporated pneumococcal and influenza immunization rates into some of their quality standards. Patients admitted to a hospital for community-acquired pneumonia should be screened for, offered, and vaccinated with pneumococcal and influenza vaccines prior to discharge if not previously administered. In physicians' office practice, all persons over 65 years of age who have been hospitalized in the past year should be screened for, offered, and vaccinated with pneumococcal and influenza vaccines if not previously administered. Both of these standards will affect payment if the standard is not met. The Joint Commission has also incorporated these standards into their accreditation reviews of health care facilities.

Abbreviations Introduced in This Chapter

anti-HBs	Antibody to hepatitis B surface antigen
DT	Diphtheria and tetanus toxoid vaccine (pediatric)
Dtap	Diphtheria and tetanus toxoids and acellular pertussis vaccine
HBsAg	Hepatitis B surface antigen
Td	Tetanus and diphtheria toxoid vaccine (adult)
Tdap	Tetanus toxoid, reduced diphtheria toxoid, and acellular pertussis vaccine
VAERS	Vaccine Adverse Event Reporting System

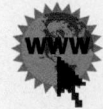 Self-assessment questions and answers are available at *http://www.mhpharmacotherapy. com/pp.html.*

REFERENCES

1. MacKay IR, Rosen FS. Vaccines and vaccination. N Engl J Med 2001;345:1042–1053.
2. Mattos-Guaraldi AL, Moreira LO, Damasco PV, Junior RH. Diphtheria remains a threat to health in the developing world—An overview. Mern Inst Oswaldo Cruz 2003;98:987–993.
3. Rhee P, Nunley MK, Demetriades D, Velmahos G, Doucet JJ. Tetanus and trauma: A review and recommendations. J Trauma 2005;58:1082–1088.
4. Hewlett El, Edwards KM. Pertussis—Not just for kids. N Engl J Med 2005;352:1215–1222.
5. Centers for Disease Control and Prevention. Preventing tetanus, diphtheria, and pertussis among adults: Use of the tetanus toxoid, reduced diphtheria toxoid and acellular pertussis vaccine. MMWR 2006;55 (No. RR-17):1–34.
6. Centers for Disease Control and Prevention. Prevention of hepatitis A through active and passive immunization: Recommendations of the Advisory Committee on Immunization Practices (ACIP). MMWR 1999; 48(No. RR-12):1–37.
7. Centers for Disease Control and Prevention. A comprehensive immunization strategy to eliminate transmission of hepatitis B virus infection in the United States: Recommendations of the Advisory Committee on Immunization Practices (ACIP); Part 1 immunization of infants, children, and adolescents. MMWR 2005; 55(No. RR-16):1–32.
8. Govan VA. A novel vaccine for cervical cancer: Quadrivalent human papillomavirus (types 6, 11, 16 and 18) recombinant vaccine (Gardasil®). Ther Clin Risk Manag 2008;4:65–70.
9. Centers for Disease Control and Prevention: Quadrivalent human papillomavirus vaccine: Recommendations of the Advisory Committee on Immunization Practices (ACIP). MMWR 2007;57 (No. RR-2):1–23.
10. Centers for Disease Control and Prevention. Prevention and control of influenza: Recommendations of the Advisory Committee on Immunization Practices (ACIP), 2008. MMWR 2008;57(No. RR-7): 1–59.
11. Centers for Disease Control and Prevention. Measles, mumps, and rubella—Vaccine use and strategies for elimination of measles, rubella, and congenital rubella syndrome and control of mumps: recommendations of the Advisory Committee on Immunization Practices (ACIP). MMWR 1998;47(No. RR-8):1–57.
12. Centers for Disease Control and Prevention. Prevention and control of meningococcal disease recommendations of the Advisory Committee on Immunization Practices (ACIP). MMWR 2005;54(No. RR-7):1–21.
13. Centers for Disease Control and Prevention. Revised recommendations of the Committee on Immunization Practices to vaccinate all persons aged 11–18 years with meningococcal conjugate vaccine. MMWR 2007;56: 794–795.
14. Centers for Disease Control and Prevention. Recommendation from the Committee on Immunization Practices (ACIP) for use of the quadrivalent meningococcal conjugate vaccine (MCV4) in children aged 2–10 years at increased risk for invasive meningococcal disease. MMWR 2007;56:1265–1266.
15. American Society of Health-Systems Pharmacists. ASHP therapeutic position statement on strategies for identifying and preventing pneumococcal resistance. Am J Health-Syst Pharm 2004;61: 2430–2435.
16. Centers for Disease Control and Prevention. Poliomyelitis in the United States: Updated recommendations of the Advisory Committee on Immunization Practices (ACIP). MMWR 2000;49(No. RR-5):1–22.
17. Centers for Disease Control and Prevention. Prevention of rotavirus gastroenteritis among infants and children: Recommendations of the Advisory Committee on Immunization Practices (ACIP). MMWR 2006; 55 (No. RR-12):1–13.
18. Sharrar RG, LaRussa P, Galea SA, et al. The postmarketing safety profile of varicella vaccine. Vaccine 2001;19:916–923.
19. Quan D, Cohrs RJ, Mahalingam R, Gilden DH. Prevention of shingles: Safety and efficacy of live zoster vaccine. Ther Clin Risk Manag 2007; 3:633–639.
20. Edwards KM, Decker MD. Combination vaccines. Infect Dis Clin N Am 2001;15:209–230.
21. Moylett EH, Hanson IC. Mechanistic actions of the risks and adverse events associated with vaccine administration. J Allerg Clin Immunol 2004;114: 1010–1020.
22. Kohl KS, Marcy SM, Blum M, et al. Fever after immunization: Current concepts and improved future scientific understanding. Clin Infect Dis 2004;39:389–394.
23. Shoenfeld Y, Aron-Maor A. Vaccination and autoimmunity – 'vaccinosis': A dangerous liaison? J Autoimmune 2000;14:1–10.
24. Weber DJ, rutala WA. Immunization of immunocompromised persons. Immunol Allergy Clin North Am 2003;23:605–634.
25. Munoz FM, Englund JA. Vaccines in pregnancy. Infect Dis Clin North Am 2001;15:253–271.
26. Centers for Disease Control and Prevention. Influenza vaccination of health-care personnel: Recommendations of the Healthcare Infection Control Practices Advisory Committee (HICPAC) and the Advisory Committee on Immunization Practices (ACIP). MMWR Recomm Rep 2006:55 (RR-2):1–16.

87 Human Immunodeficiency Virus Infection

Amanda Corbett, Rosa Yeh, Julie Dumond, and Angela D.M. Kashuba

LEARNING OBJECTIVES

Upon completion of the chapter, the reader will be able to:

1. Explain the routes of transmission for HIV, and its natural disease progression.

2. Identify typical and atypical signs and symptoms of acute and chronic HIV infection.

3. Identify the desired therapeutic outcomes for patients with HIV infection.

4. Recommend appropriate first-line pharmacotherapy interventions for patients with HIV infection.

5. Recommend appropriate second-line pharmacotherapy interventions for patients with HIV infection.

6. Describe the components of a monitoring plan to assess effectiveness and adverse effects of pharmacotherapy for HIV infection.

7. Educate patients about the disease state, appropriate lifestyle modifications, and drug therapy required for effective treatment.

KEY CONCEPTS

❶ The treatment goals for HIV infection are to maximally and durably suppress HIV replication, avoid the development of drug resistance, restore and preserve immune function, prevent opportunistic infections, and minimize adverse effects.

❷ HIV RNA plasma concentrations and CD4+ T-cell counts are used to assess risk of progression to AIDS (or risk for opportunistic infection) and to monitor efficacy and durability of treatment.

❸ Effective and complete treatment of HIV infection involves a multidisciplinary approach, which includes pharmacists, clinicians, social workers, and others.

❹ Treatment with two nucleoside reverse transcriptase inhibitors (NRTIs) *and* either a nonnucleoside reverse transcriptase inhibitor (NNRTI) or a ritonavir-boosted protease inhibitor (PI) is the mainstay of initial treatment for HIV infection.

❺ All patients with HIV infection relapse if medication is withdrawn. Therefore, long-term maintenance treatment is required.

❻ Eventually, HIV becomes resistant to current medication therapy. To prolong this time to resistance, both strict adherence to the drug regimen and avoidance of deleterious drug interactions is critical.

❼ The majority of antiretroviral medications are metabolized by the cytochrome P-450 enzyme system (CYP). Therefore, it is important to review patient medication profiles for drugs that may interact with antiretroviral drugs.

❽ Most antiretroviral medications cause acute and chronic adverse effects. Patients should be closely monitored for these toxicities so that interventions can occur quickly.

The acquired immune deficiency syndrome (AIDS) was first recognized in 1981, and described in a cohort of young homosexual men with significant immune deficiency. Since then, human immunodeficiency virus type 1 (HIV-1) has been clearly identified as the major cause of AIDS.[1] HIV-2 is much less prevalent than HIV-1, but also causes AIDS. HIV primarily targets CD4+ lymphocytes, which are critical to proper immune system function. If left untreated, patients experience a prolonged asymptomatic period followed by rapid, progressive immunodeficiency. Therefore, most complications experienced by patients with AIDS involve opportunistic infections and cancers.

HIV is primarily transmitted by sexual contact, by contact with blood or blood products, and from mother to child during gestation, delivery, or breast-feeding. The prevalence and incidence of HIV is rising globally, and to date there are no treatments which eradicate HIV from the body. Combinations of potent antiretroviral agents (called highly active antiretroviral therapy, or HAART) can suppress HIV replication to undetectable levels, delay the onset of AIDS, and prolong survival. However, there are a number of drug-induced, long-term toxicities that challenge effective patient management. This chapter will address HIV treatment options and challenges, and give practical suggestions for patient management.

EPIDEMIOLOGY

Since the first cases of AIDS were identified in 1981, over 25 million people have died as a result of HIV infection.[1] This makes AIDS one of the most destructive epidemics in recorded history. The epidemic remains extremely dynamic, and no country in the world is unaffected. It is estimated that HIV currently infects approximately 35 million people worldwide. Approximately 68% of these cases are in subsaharan Africa, with a prevalence of approximately 5%. East Asia, Central Asia, and Eastern Europe are also seeing rapidly rising infection rates.

In 2007 alone, approximately 2.1 million people died from AIDS and 2.5 million people were newly infected with HIV. Most of these infections were acquired through heterosexual transmission. As of December 2007, women accounted for 47% of all people living with HIV worldwide; in subsaharan Africa, women account for 61%. Persons aged 15 to 24 years accounted for nearly one-half of new HIV infections worldwide.

In the United States, at the end of 2006, an estimated 1,039,000 to 1,185,000 persons were living with HIV/AIDS. Approximately 30% of these are undiagnosed and unaware of their HIV infection, and could be unknowingly transmitting the virus to others. In 2006, of the total number of HIV-infected patients, approximately 509,681 were living with AIDS, while 14,627 died with AIDS. The cumulative estimated number of diagnoses of AIDS through 2006 was 1,014,797, one-half of whom (565,927) had died. Approximately 56,300 people were newly infected with HIV in 2006.

Compared with their distribution in the U.S. population, African American and Hispanic populations are disproportionately affected by HIV/AIDS, representing 48% and 19% of cases, respectively. HIV/AIDS is among the top four causes of death for African American men aged 25 to 44 years and is among the top three causes of death for African American women of the same age. In 2006, HIV/AIDS rates for African American males were seven times those for white males and two times those for Hispanic males. HIV/AIDS rates for African American females were 19 times the rates for white females and four times the rates for Hispanic females.

ETIOLOGY AND PATHOGENESIS

HIV-1 is a retrovirus and member of the genus *Lentivirus*. These viruses have a characteristically prolonged latency period. There are two molecularly and serologically distinct but related types of HIV: HIV-1 and HIV-2. HIV-2 is a less common cause of the epidemic and is found primarily in West Africa. HIV-1 is categorized by phylogenetic lineages into three groups (M [main], N [new], and O [outlier]). HIV-1 group M can be further categorized into nine subtypes: A

through D, F through H, and J and K. HIV-1 subtype B is primarily responsible for the North American and Western European epidemic.

HIV in humans is believed to result from cross-species transmission from primates infected with simian immunodeficiency virus (SIV). HIV-2 is closely related to the SIV found in sooty mangabeys in West Africa, and HIV-1 is similar to the SIV found in chimpanzees. The earliest known human HIV infection was in central Africa in 1959. Cultural practices such as the preparation and eating of bush-meat, or keeping primates as pets, may have allowed the virus to transmit from animal to human. The rapid spread of the virus throughout the world can be primarily attributed to sexual promiscuity, drug abuse, and high mobility due to modern transportation.

HIV infection occurs through three primary modes of transmission: sexual, parenteral, and perinatal. The most common method for transmission is receptive anal and vaginal intercourse, with the probability of transmission up to 30% per sexual contact. The probability of transmission increases when the index partner has a high level of viral replication (which occurs at the beginning of infection or late in disease), or when the uninfected partner has ulcerative disease, compromised mucosal surfaces, or (in the case of men) has not been circumcised.

Parenteral transmission of HIV primarily occurs through injection drug use by sharing contaminated needles or injection-related supplies. As a result of a comprehensive North American screening program, less than 1% of all cases of HIV infection occurs as a result of transfusions of contaminated blood or blood products, or infected transplant organs. Health care workers have a 0.3% estimated risk of acquiring HIV infection through percutaneous needlestick injury.

Perinatal infection (also known as vertical transmission or mother-to-child transmission [MTCT]) can occur during gestation, at or near delivery, and during breast-feeding. The risk of MTCT up to and including delivery is approximately 25%, while the risk of transmission during breast-feeding is approximately 15% to 20% within the first 6 months of life. Because a high rate of HIV replication in the blood is a significant risk factor for transmission of HIV, it is important to treat women for their HIV infection during pregnancy. After delivery, mothers are strongly recommended not to breast-feed if safe alternatives are available.

Understanding the life cycle of the virus is important to know how antiretroviral drugs are combined for optimal therapy (Fig. 87–1). Once HIV enters the body, an outer glycoprotein called gp120 binds to CD4 receptors found on the surface of dendritic cells, T lymphocytes, monocytes, and macrophages. This allows further binding to other chemokine receptors on the cell surface called CCR5 and CXCR4. Greater than 95% of newly infected patients have viruses that preferentially use CCR5 to enter the cell, and most patients with advanced disease have viruses that preferentially use CXCR4 to enter the cell. This becomes important in understanding the place in therapy for some of the new drugs in development.

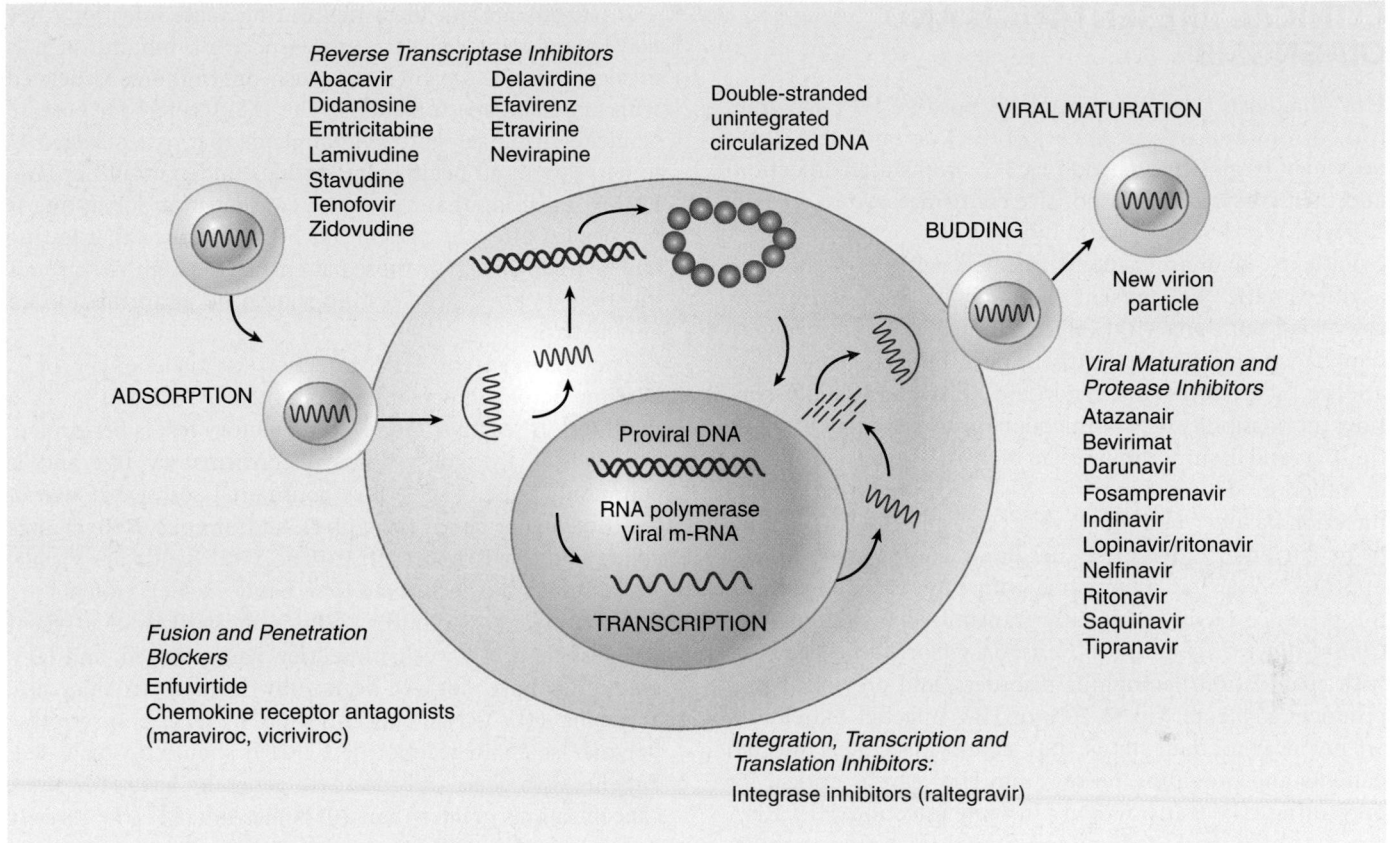

FIGURE 87–1. Life cycle of HIV and targets for antiretroviral drugs. (From Fletcher CV, Kakuda TN. Human immunodeficiency virus infection. In: DiPiro JT, Talbert RL, Yee GC, et al., eds. Pharmacotherapy: A Pathophysiologic Approach. 6th ed. New York: McGraw-Hill; 2005: 2258, with permission.)

After the virus has attached to CD4 and chemokine receptors, another viral glycoprotein (gp41) assists with viral fusion to the cell and internalization of the viral contents. The viral contents include single-stranded RNA, an RNA-dependent DNA polymerase (also known as reverse transcriptase), and other enzymes. Using the single-stranded viral RNA as a template, reverse transcriptase synthesizes a complementary strand of DNA. The single-stranded viral RNA is removed from the newly formed DNA strand by ribonuclease H, and reverse transcriptase completes the synthesis of double-stranded DNA. The viral reverse transcriptase enzyme is highly error-prone, and many mutations occur in the conversion of RNA to DNA. This inefficient reverse transcription activity is responsible for HIV's ability to rapidly mutate and develop drug resistance.

A chronic infection is established when the double-stranded DNA migrates to the host cell nucleus and is integrated into the host cell chromosome by an HIV enzyme called integrase. Once the cell becomes activated by antigens or cytokines, HIV replication starts: host DNA polymerase transcribes viral DNA into messenger RNA, and messenger RNA is translated into viral proteins. These proteins assemble beneath the bilayer of the host cell, a nucleocapsid forms containing these proteins, and the virus buds from the cell.

After budding, the virus matures when an HIV protease enzyme cleaves large polypeptides into smaller functional proteins. Without this process, the virus is unable to infect other cells.

During the early stages of infection, approximately 10 billion virions can be produced each day. Most of the cells containing these viruses will be lysed as a result of budding virions, killed by cytotoxic T-lymphocytes, or undergo apoptosis. However, virus will be protected within some cells (macrophages, T cells in lymph nodes), which can stay dormant for years. The initial immune response against HIV is relatively effective, but it is unable to completely clear the infection, and the patient enters a latent, asymptomatic or mildly symptomatic stage lasting 5 to 15 years. During this time, a high rate of viral replication can be seen in the lymph nodes. Eventually immune deficiency occurs when the body is no longer able to replenish helper T cells at a rate equal to that at which HIV is destroying them.

❶ *The goal of therapy is to maximally and durably suppress HIV replication in order to restore and preserve immune system function and minimize morbidity and mortality.* Because HIV replication has been found in all areas of the body, it is important to use potent drug therapy that can achieve adequate concentrations in all tissues, including protected sites such as the brain and genital tract.

CLINICAL PRESENTATION AND DIAGNOSIS

HIV diagnosis is made either by a positive **HIV enzyme-linked immunosorbent assay** (**ELISA**) or rapid test (these tests may be positive as soon as 3–6 weeks after infection) and then confirmed by a positive confirmatory test, usually the HIV Western blot (WB) (Table 87–1).

Patients who are acutely infected with HIV may be asymptomatic or present with signs and symptoms associated with any viral infection, such as fever, myalgias, lymphadenopathy, pharyngitis, or rash. Taken together, these are the "acute retroviral syndrome." Providers should consider the possibility of HIV infection in any patients with these findings and inquire about recent high-risk sexual encounters or other modes of exposure. Risk factors for HIV/AIDS infection include: men who have sex with men (MSM); history of or current IV drug use (needle or equipment sharing); unprotected sexual intercourse with high-risk individuals; the presence of other sexually transmitted infections (e.g., *Chlamydia trachomatis* or *Neisseria gonorrhoeae*); persons with coagulation/hemophilia disorders; and previous blood product recipients. Up to 50% of HIV-infected individuals are not aware of their status, thus identifying acutely infected patients and providing referral into HIV care is critical for preventing HIV transmission.[2] In acute infection, HIV RNA concentrations in blood and the genital tract are very high, increasing the risk of transmission to others.[3] Increased infectiousness coupled with undiagnosed HIV infection in these patients may account for a substantial proportion of sexual HIV transmission.

If patients are not identified during acute infection, they may later present with various nonspecific symptoms such as myalgias, fatigue, weight loss, thrush, or symptoms associated with opportunistic infections. The U.S. Centers for Disease Control (CDC) currently recommends that patients aged 13 to 64 years in all health care settings undergo opt-out HIV testing, meaning that a separate consent form for testing is not needed after the patient has been informed that testing will be performed. For those patients in the high-risk groups mentioned above, HIV testing should be performed on an annual basis.[4]

The diagnosis of HIV infection is made either by a baseline serologic screening test such as the ELISA or a rapid test. If reactive, then a confirmatory test is performed. The **WB** is the gold standard confirmatory test and is commonly used. The WB is considered reactive if two of the three major bands (p24, gp41, and/or gp120/160) change color. The test is nonreactive if no viral bands are visible. If the test is indeterminate (one band visible), patients are retested in 2 to 3 months. This is most likely if a recent (i.e., less than 3–6 weeks) infection has occurred, and HIV antibodies have not yet been fully formed. In this case, a plasma HIV RNA concentration (reverse transcriptase polymerase chain reaction [RT-PCR]) should be evaluated. Patients with acute infection will generally have HIV RNA concentrations greater than 10^6 copies/mL. ❷ *HIV severity is determined by following: (a) the CD4+ lymphocyte count (CD4 count) and percentage and (b) HIV RNA (viral load).* The CD4 percentage is followed because the absolute count may fluctuate and does not necessarily indicate a change in the patient's condition.

Table 87–1			
HIV Diagnostic Tests			
Test	**Minimum Time to Detection After Exposure**	**Sample(s) Tested**	**Comments**
Initial Screening Tests			
ELISA	3–6 weeks	Plasma	If nonreactive, no further testing is required, unless acute infection suspected
HIV RNA assay	Up to 14 days	Plasma	Obtain if recent high-risk exposure; if initially negative, repeat at months 1, 3, and 6
Rapid tests (currently FDA-approved products):	Detects HIV antibodies within minutes of sample application		
OraQuick ADVANCE	3–6 weeks	Whole blood, plasma, or oral fluid	Detects HIV-1 and HIV-2
Reveal Rapid HIV-1 Antibody Test	3–6 weeks	Plasma or serum	Detects HIV-1
Uni-Gold Recombigen HIV Test	3–6 weeks	Whole blood, plasma, or serum	Detects HIV-1
Confirmatory Tests			
Western blot (WB)	3–6 weeks	Plasma	Gold standard confirmatory test
Indirect immunofluorescence assay (IFA)	3–6 weeks	Plasma	Simple to perform, but requires expertise to interpret results

ELISA, enzyme-linked immunosorbent assay.

Clinical Presentation and Diagnosis of HIV

Patients with acute HIV infection may display symptoms described as "acute retroviral syndrome." Patients with chronic HIV infection may present with these same nonspecific symptoms and/or opportunistic infections.

Acute Retroviral Syndrome

The majority of patients may present with fever, lymphadenopathy, pharyngitis, and/or rash. Other symptoms include:

- Myalgia or arthralgia
- Diarrhea
- Headache
- Nausea and vomiting
- Hepatosplenomegaly
- Weight loss
- Thrush
- Neurologic symptoms (meningoencephalitis, aseptic meningitis, peripheral neuropathy, facial palsy, or cognitive impairment or psychosis)

Opportunistic Infections

Depending on the severity of immunosuppression (the CD4+ T lymphocyte count), patients may present with the following opportunistic infections (grouped by CD4+ count):

Any CD4+ count

- *Mycobacterium tuberculosis* disease

- Bacterial pneumonia (commonly *Streptococcus pneumoniae*, *Haemophilus influenzae*, *Pseudomonas aeruginosa*, and *Staphylococcus aureus*)
- Herpes simplex virus disease
- Varicella zoster virus disease
- Bacterial enteric disease (most commonly *Salmonella*, *Campylobacter*, and *Shigella*)
- Syphilis
- Bartonellosis

Less than 250 cells/mm³

- Coccidioidomycosis
- *Pneumocystis jiroveci* (formerly *carinii*) pneumonia (PCP)
- Oropharyngeal and esophageal candidiasis
- Kaposi's sarcoma or human herpesvirus-8 disease

Less than 150 cells/mm³

- Disseminated histoplasmosis

Less than 100 cells/mm³

- Cryptosporidiosis
- Microsporidiosis

Less than 50 cells/mm³

- Disseminated *Mycobacterium avium* complex disease
- Cytomegalovirus disease
- Cryptococcosis, aspergillosis, and *Toxoplasma gondii* encephalitis

Patient Encounter, Part 1

A 46-year-old Caucasian man with a history of hypertension and gastroesophageal reflux disease (GERD) comes to your clinic complaining of increased fatigue, shortness of breath, and cough. He has noticed feeling tired more easily for the past 3 months, but the difficulty breathing and cough appeared 2 weeks ago. After questioning him further, he says he has sex with men, but he has had the same sexual partner for the past 8 years. They do not use condoms. He also says that he smokes about one pack of cigarettes per day.

What information is suggestive of HIV/AIDS?

What risk factors are present for having HIV/AIDS?

What additional information do you need to know before creating a treatment plan for this patient?

TREATMENT

❶ *The goals of treatment are to maximally and durably suppress viral replication, avoid the development of drug* resistance, restore and preserve immune function, prevent opportunistic infections, and minimize drug adverse effects. Elimination of HIV is not possible with currently available therapies. Instead, maximal suppression of viral replication (defined as HIV RNA concentrations undetectable by the most sensitive assay available) is desired. After the initiation of antiretroviral therapy, a rapid decline to undetectable HIV RNA in 16 to 24 weeks is a predictor of improved clinical outcomes.[5]

❷ *Degree of immune function preservation also correlates with decreased viral replication, and is measured by CD4+ T-cell counts. CD4 measures are the best predictor of progression to AIDS, and help decide when to initiate treatment.* At CD4+ T-cell counts of 200 cells/mm³ and lower, patients require drug prophylaxis for opportunistic infections. Table 87–2 details the monitoring end points of HIV treatment for HIV RNA and CD4+ T-cell counts.

Six classes of drugs are available to treat HIV infection: **nucleoside (NRTI)/nucleotide (NtRTI) reverse transcriptase inhibitor, protease inhibitor (PI), nonnucleoside reverse transcriptase inhibitor (NNRTI), fusion inhibitors, CCR5 inhibitors, and integrase inhibitors.** ❸ *Currently, combination antiretroviral drug therapy with three or more active*

Table 87–2

Monitoring End Points for CD4+ T-Cell Counts and HIV RNA

CD4+ T Cell Counts			HIV RNA Concentration		
When to Monitor?	**Why?**	**Goal**	**When to Monitor?**	**Why?**	**Goal**
Initial diagnosis	Assess need for ART	Start therapy in appropriate patients	Initial diagnosis/ evaluation	Establish baseline and assess need for ART	Start ART in appropriate patients
	Assess need for OI chemoprophylaxis	Start therapy when counts less than 200 cells/mm³	2–8 weeks after starting or changing ART	Early assessment of regimen efficacy	Decrease of at least a 1 log$_{10}$ copies/mL
Every 3–6 months	Receiving ART: monitor success of treatment	Average increase of 100–150 cells/ mm³/year	3–4 months after starting ART	Assess virologic efficacy of regimen	Undetectable levels
	Not receiving ART: assess need to begin therapy	Start ART in appropriate patients	Every 3–4 months	Receiving ART: assess durability of virologic suppression with current regimen	Steadily decreasing levels and/or consistently low levels
	Assess need for OI chemoprophylaxis	Start therapy when counts less than 200 cells/mm³		Not receiving ART: monitor changes in viral load	Start therapy in appropriate patients

ART, antiretroviral therapy; OI, opportunistic infection.

Adapted from Ref. 5.

---

drugs is the standard of care, which increases the durability of viral suppression and decreases the potential for the development of resistance. ❹ *Two nucleoside (nucleotide) reverse transcriptase inhibitors and either a NNRTI or a ritonavir-boosted PI are the mainstay regimens of combination therapy in initial treatment.* In the late 1980s, when only zidovudine was available, achieving and maintaining viral suppression for more than 4 months was rarely possible. As more agents became available in the mid-1990s (most notably the PIs), HIV RNA was suppressed to undetectable concentrations and maintained there for long periods of time. Currently recommended combination regimens decrease HIV RNA to less than 50 copies/mL in 80% to 90% of patients in clinical trials. Therefore, monotherapy with any agent or the use of NRTIs without a PI or NNRTI are not routine treatment options. Fusion inhibitors, CCR5 inhibitors, and integrase inhibitors are only FDA-approved for use in treatment experienced patients with drug resistance to NRTIs, NNRTIs, and/or PIs, although clinical trials are ongoing to determine their role in the initial treatment of HIV infection. Figure 87–1 details the mechanisms of action of the drug classes within the life cycle of HIV.

Nonpharmacologic Interventions

❻ *Patient adherence is a key component in treatment success.* Drug therapy is required for a lifetime, as the virus begins to replicate at high levels when medications are stopped. Early HIV combination therapy was exceedingly complicated for patients, with multiple daily doses, varying food restrictions, and large pill burdens. Advances in delivery and formulations now make possible once- or twice-daily dosing with fewer than six pills per day. Currently, a combination tablet of tenofovir + emtricitabine + efavirenz (Atripla) supplies a one pill, once-daily regimen. The use of low-dose ritonavir to enhance the concentrations of other PIs (known as pharmacokinetic enhancement or "boosting") allows for significantly fewer doses and lower pill burdens. Atazanavir with ritonavir boosting is a potent, once-daily PI option. These advances, however, do not replace the need for patient counseling by a trained pharmacist and a multidisciplinary approach to promoting adherence.

Counsel all patients initially and repeatedly on ways to prevent viral transmission. Preventing the spread of resistant virus is particularly important. Patients receiving antiretroviral therapy can still transmit virus to sexual partners, and to those with whom they share needles or other drug equipment. Where both partners are HIV-positive, safe sex and needle practices reduce the risk of superinfection with differing strains of HIV and the transmission of other sexually transmitted diseases. General guidelines for preventing viral transmission include using condoms with a water-based lubricant for vaginal or anal intercourse, using condoms without lubricant or dental dams for oral sex, and not sharing equipment used to prepare, inject, or inhale drugs. Treating other sexually transmitted infections (STIs), particularly genital herpes, in HIV-infected patients may help to prevent HIV transmission. The presence of STIs increases genital tract HIV viral load, and correspondingly the risk of HIV transmission to sexual partners.

❸ *Nutrition and dietary counseling should also be included in the care of the HIV patient, as poor nutrition leads to poorer outcomes and complicates treatment.* Antiretroviral therapy itself introduces a host of nutritional issues, including drug-food interactions, GI adverse effects that may affect appetite and limit dietary intake, lipid abnormalities, and fat redistribution. The American Dietetics Association currently recommends assessing HIV-infected patients for their level of nutritional risk and involving a registered dietician as part of the clinical team for optimal nutrition care.[6]

Pharmacologic Therapy for Antiretroviral-Naïve Patients

Two major panels of experts publish guidelines for the treatment of HIV-infected individuals. Although the recommendations are quite similar, slight differences do exist between the Department of Health and Human Services (DHHS) Guidelines[5] and the International AIDS Society-USA (IAS-USA) Panel Recommendations.[7] The DHHS Guidelines are updated every 6 months and current and archived versions are available online at *www.aidsinfo.nih. gov*. The IAS-USA Guidelines were last updated in 2008, and in 2006 prior to that revision. Due to the intense research and constant modifications to therapeutic approaches in the treatment of HIV, the majority of the treatment algorithms and recommendations presented herein follow the most up-to-date information found in the DHHS recommendations.

❷ *The decision of when to begin antiretroviral therapy is complex. Recommendations are based on the CD4+ T-cell count, which predicts disease-free survival* (Table 87–3). Other factors to consider include the patient's viral load, willingness to begin therapy and maintain medication adherence, and the risk versus benefit of treating an asymptomatic patient. The clinical evidence is strongest for beginning treatment at CD4+ counts less than 200 cells/mm³, but more recent evidence from long-term studies and the availability of potent drugs with improved tolerability support earlier treatment at higher CD4+ counts. Once the decision is made to initiate treatment, the regimen is selected based on patient-specific factors. ❹ *All recommended regimens for initial treatment contain either an NNRTI or a ritonavir-boosted PI in combination with two NRTIs (or NtRTI). The preferred agents are:*

1. NRTI/NtRTI combinations:
   a. Tenofovir *and* emtricitabine
2. PIs:
   b. Lopinavir/ritonavir (dosed once or twice daily)
   c. Atazanavir/ritonavir (dosed once daily)
   d. Fosamprenavir/ ritonavir (dosed twice daily)
   e. Darunavir/ritonavir (dosed once daily)
3. NNRTI:
   a. Efavirenz

The decision to choose a NNRTI- or PI-based regimen as initial therapy is based on many patient- and clinician-specific factors. Drug resistance testing should be performed at diagnosis, and again prior to initiating treatment, if time has elapsed between diagnosis and treatment (see Pharmacologic Treatment for Antiretroviral-Experienced Patients for further discussion of drug resistance testing). The results of resistance testing may dictate which drug class is preferred; 6% to 16% of newly diagnosed patients will have drug-resistant virus. This initial resistance pattern often involves the NNRTIs, but may involve other drug classes. NNRTI-based regimens have low pill burdens and may have decreased incidences of long-term adverse effects (e.g., dyslipidemia) in comparison to some PI-based regimens. However, this class also has a low threshold for drug resistance (the K103N mutation causes high level cross-class resistance), and patient adherence is a critical consideration. In pregnant women, or women with the potential to become pregnant, a PI-based regimen is preferred due to the potential teratogenicity of efavirenz (pregnancy category D).

In patients who cannot tolerate the above preferred first-line therapies, or have a compelling reason to choose a different agent, the following alternatives are recommended.

1. NRTI:
   a. Zidovudine and lamivudine
   b. Didanosine and (emtricitabine *or* lamivudine)
   c. Abacavir and lamivudine
2. PIs:
   a. Atazanavir (if tenofovir is included in the regimen, ritonavir must be used)
   b. Fosamprenavir (dosed twice daily)
   c. Fosamprenavir/ritonavir (dosed once daily)
   d. Saquinavir/ritonavir
3. NNRTI:
   a. Nevirapine in selected populations (due to a more frequent incidence of hepatotoxicity, nevirapine should only be used in patients with low to moderate CD4+ T-cell counts: less than or equal to 250 cells/mm³ for females, less than or equal to 400 cells/mm³ for males)

If abacavir is included in a regimen, patients should undergo HLA-B*5701 testing prior to initiation to reduce the

---

Table 87–3

Summary of Recommendations for Initiating Antiretroviral Therapy

Clinical Indicator/CD4 Count	Recommended Action
History of AIDS-defining illness CD4 count less than 200 cells/mm³	
CD4 count 200–350 cells/mm³ Pregnant women HIV-associated nephropathy HBV coinfection, where HBV treatment is indicated	Start ART
CD4 count greater than 350 mm³	Currently not well-defined; depends on the patient characteristics and individual risk-benefit assessment

ART: antiretroviral therapy; HBV, hepatitis B virus.

Adapted from Ref. 5.

risk of abacavir hypersensitivity. Patients who test positive for the allele are at high risk (approximately 70%) of developing this reaction, and should not be given abacavir. An abacavir allergy should also be documented in the patient's medical record to prevent future administration. Those patients with a negative test may receive abacavir, but should still be monitored for the development of hypersensitivity.

Therapies *not recommended* for initial treatment due to poor potency or significant toxicity include triple-NRTI regimens, delavirdine, nevirapine in patients with moderate to high CD4+ T-cell counts, indinavir ± ritonavir, saquinavir used without ritonavir ("unboosted"), ritonavir used without another PI, nelfinavir, tipranvir/ritonavir, and tenofovir with didanosine. Due to lack of data in antiretroviral naïve patients, maraviroc, etravirine, enfuvirtide, and raltegravir are not recommended in the DHHS guidelines.

Drugs that should *not be combined* due to overlapping toxicities include: atazanavir plus indinavir (due to enhanced hyperbilirubinemia), two NNRTIs, and didanosine plus stavudine. Emtricitabine and lamivudine should not be combined because of their similar chemical structures, and antagonism can result when stavudine is combined with zidovudine.

Pharmacologic Therapy for Antiretroviral-Experienced Patients

6 *Ongoing viral replication, whether at low levels in the face of adequate drug concentrations or at higher levels due to inconsistent systemic concentrations (or low concentrations in sanctuary sites; e.g., male and female genital fluids, cerebrospinal fluid, or lymph nodes), will eventually lead to resistance to the prescribed medications.* There is no consensus on the optimal time to change therapy based on virologic or immunologic failure (Table 87–4). **2** *Virologic failure is defined as HIV RNA greater than 400 copies/mL after 24 weeks, greater than 50 copies/mL after 48 weeks, or a repeated HIV RNA greater than 400 copies/mL after prior suppression to less than 400 copies/mL.*[5] Some clinicians may change therapy with any repeated, detectable viremia (HIV RNA greater than 50–400 copies/mL), while others will set arbitrary thresholds of 1,000 to 1,500 copies/mL. Immunologic failure is defined as having an increase of less than 25 to 50 cells/mm³ in CD4+ T lymphocyte count above baseline after 1 year of therapy, or a decline in CD4+ cell count below baseline while taking antiretroviral therapy.

Treatment considerations for antiretroviral-experienced patients are much more complex than for patients who are naïve to therapy. Prior to changing therapy, the reasons for treatment failure should be identified. A comprehensive review of the patient's severity of disease, antiretroviral treatment history, adherence to therapy, intolerance or toxicity, concomitant drug therapies, comorbidities, and results of current and past HIV resistance testing should be performed. If patients fail therapy due to poor adherence, the underlying reasons must be determined and addressed prior to initiation of new therapy. Reasons for poor adherence

---

Table 87–4

Treatment Options Following Virologic Failure With the Initial Regimen

Initial Regimen	Recommended Change
2 NRTIs + NNRTI	2 NRTIs (based on resistance testing) + PI (with or without low-dose ritonavir)
2 NRTIs + PI (with or without low-dose ritonavir)	2 NRTIs (based on resistance testing) + NNRTI
3 NRTIs	2 NRTIs (based on resistance testing) + NNRTI *or* PI (with or without low-dose ritonavir)
	NNRTI + PI (with or without low-dose ritonavir)
	NRTI (based on resistance testing) + NNRTI + PI (with or without low-dose ritonavir)

NRTI, nucleoside reverse transcriptase inhibitor; NNRTI, nonnucleoside reverse transcriptase inhibitor; PI, protease inhibitor.

Adapted from Ref. 5.

---

include: problems with medication access, active substance abuse, depression and/or denial of the disease, and a lack of education on the importance of 100% adherence to therapy. Medication intolerance or toxicity can be remedied with therapy for the adverse event, exchanging the drug causing the toxicity with another in the same class, or changing the entire regimen. Pharmacokinetics or systemic drug exposure can be optimized by ensuring maximal drug absorption (taking the drug with or without food can alter exposure by up to 30%), and avoiding interactions with concomitant prescription or nonprescription medications and dietary supplements or natural products (e.g., antacids, St. John's wort, and garlic). When causes for treatment failure are identified, appropriate strategies for therapy can be determined.

An additional consideration when stopping or changing therapy is a staggered discontinuation of antiretrovirals with different half-lives. For example, in patients taking Atripla (tenofovir, emtricitabine, and efavirenz) tenofovir and emtricitabine should be continued for at least 4 days after discontinuation of efavirenz due to the much prolonged half-life of efavirenz as compared to tenofovir and emtricitabine. Otherwise, the potential for monotherapy with efavirenz exists. If new antiretroviral therapy is to be initiated immediately, no overlap is necessary; however, it should be noted that efavirenz concentrations will persist for some period of time.

Drug interactions between antiretrovirals and between antiretrovirals and concomitant medications should be evaluated for each patient to avoid under- and/or overexposure of either therapy. **7** *NNRTIs and PIs are metabolized by CYP450 enzymes and are inducers and/or inhibitors of this enzyme system.* In addition, some of the antiretrovirals are substrates, inhibitors, and/or inducers of transporters such as P-glycoprotein, and therefore may lead to drug interactions. Information provided in Table 87–5 describes

Table 87-5

Summary of Currently Available Antiretroviral Agents

Generic Name [Abbreviation] (Trade Name)	Dosage Forms	Commonly Prescribed Doses	Dose Adjustments	Food Restrictions	Significant Adverse Events	Drug Interaction Potential
Nucleoside(tide) Reverse Transcriptase Inhibitors						
Abacavir (Ziagen)	300-mg tablet; 20 mg/mL oral solution	300 mg twice daily or 600 mg once daily	None	None (alcohol increases abacavir conc. by 41%)	Potentially fatal hyper-sensitivity reaction (rash, fever, malaise, nausea, vomiting, shortness of breath, sore throat, loss of appetite)	Alcohol dehydrogenase and glucuronyl transferase, 82% renal excretion of metabolites
Didanosine (Videx EC) Generic didanosine EC	125-, 200-, 250-, 400-mg capsules; 125-, 200-, 250-, 400-mg capsules	Greater than 60 kg: 400 mg daily; Less than 60 kg: 250 mg daily	CrCl (mL/min): / 30–59 / 10–29 / Less than 10 → Greater than 60 kg: 200-mg / 125-mg / 125 mg; Less than 60 kg: 125 mg / 100 mg / 75 mg	Take 30 minutes prior or 2 hours after meal (conc. decreases 55% with food)	Pancreatitis; peripheral neuropathy; nausea; diarrhea	Renal excretion
Emtricitabine (Emtriva)	200-mg capsule; 10 mg/mL oral solution	200 mg daily; 240 mg (24 mL) oral solution daily	CrCl (mL/min): / 30–49 / 15–29 / Less than 15/HD (Dose after dialysis on dialysis days) → Capsule: 200 mg every 48 hours / 200 mg every 72 hours / 200 mg every 96 hours; Solution: 120 mg every 24 hours / 80 mg every 24 hours / 60 mg every 24 hours	None	Minimal	Renal excretion
Lamivudine (Epivir)	150-mg and 300-mg tabs or 10 mg/mL oral solution	150 mg twice daily or 300 mg once daily	CrCl (mL/min): / 30–49 / 15–29 / 5–14 / Less than 5/HD (Dose after dialysis on dialysis days) → Dose: 150 mg qday / 150 mg, then 100 mg every day / 150 mg, then 50 mg every day / 50 mg, then 25 mg every day	None	Minimal	Renal excretion
Stavudine (Zerit)	15-, 20-, 30-, 40-mg capsules or 1 mg/mL for oral solution	Greater than 60 kg: 40 mg twice daily; Less than 60 kg: 30 mg twice daily	CrCl (mL/min): / 26–50 / 10–25/HD → Greater than 60 kg: 20 mg every 12 hours / 20 mg every 24 hours; Less than 60 kg: 15 mg every 12 hours / 15 mg every 24 hours	None	Peripheral neuropathy; lipodystrophy; rapidly progressive ascending neuromuscular weakness (rare); pancreatitis; lactic acidosis with hepatic steatosis (higher incidence with stavudine than with other NRTIs); hyperlipidemia	Renal excretion

(Continued)

Table 87–5

Summary of Currently Available Antiretroviral Agents (Continued)

Generic Name [Abbreviation] (Trade Name)	Dosage Forms	Commonly Prescribed Doses	Dose Adjustments		Food Restrictions	Significant Adverse Events	Drug Interaction Potential
Tenofovir disoproxil fumarate (Viread)	300-mg tablet	300 mg daily	CrCl (mL/min): 30–49, 10–29, ESRD/HD (Dose after dialysis on dialysis days)	Dose: 300 mg every 48 hours, 300 mg twice weekly, 300 mg every 7 days	None	Asthenia, headache, diarrhea, nausea, vomiting, and flatulence; renal insufficiency	Renal excretion
Zidovudine (Retrovir)	100-mg capsule, 300-mg tablet, 10 mg/mL IV solution, 10 mg/mL oral solution	300 mg twice daily	100 mg 3 times daily or 300 mg once daily in severe renal impairment or HD		None	Bone marrow suppression: macrocytic anemia or neutropenia; GI intolerance, headache, insomnia, asthenia	Glucuronyl transferase and renal
Zidovudine + lamivudine (Combivir)	Zidovudine 300 mg + Lamivudine 150-mg tablet	1 tablet twice daily	Do not use with CrCl less than 50 mL/min		None	See adverse events for zidovudine and lamivudine	See zidovudine and lamivudine
Abacavir + lamivudine + zidovudine [abacavir/lamivudine/zidovudine] (Trizivir)	Abacavir 300 mg + lamivudine 150 mg + zidovudine 300-mg tablet	1 tablet twice daily	Do not use with CrCl less than 50 mL/min		None	See adverse events for zidovudine, lamivudine, and abacavir	See zidovudine, lamivudine, and abacavir
Abacavir + lamivudine [abacavir/lamivudine] (Epzicom)	Abacavir 600 mg + lamivudine 300-mg tablet	1 tablet daily	Do not use with CrCl less than 50 mL/min		None	See adverse events for abacavir and lamivudine	See abacavir and lamivudine
Tenofovir + emtricitabine [Tenofovir/emtricitabine] (Truvada)	Tenofovir 300 mg + emtricitabine 200-mg tablet	1 tablet daily	CrCl (mL/min): 30–49, Less than 30	Dose: 1 tablet every 48 hours, Not recommended	None	See adverse events for tenofovir and emtricitabine	See tenofovir and emtricitabine
Nonnucleoside Reverse Transcriptase Inhibitors							
Delavirdine (Rescriptor)	100-, 200-mg tablets	400 mg 3 times daily (100-mg tablet can be dispersed in 3 oz or more of water to produce slurry); 200-mg tablet should be administered whole; separate dosing from buffered didanosine or antacids by 1 hour	Use with caution in patients with hepatic impairment		None	Rash; increased LFTs, headaches	Metabolized by cytochrome P-450 (CYP); CYP3A inhibitor; 51% excreted in urine (less than 5% unchanged); 44% in feces

Drug	Available Formulation	Usual Dose	Dosage Adjustment	Food/Administration	Adverse Effects	Metabolism/Elimination
Efavirenz (Sustiva)	50-, 100-, 200-mg capsules or 600-mg tablet	600 mg daily at or before bedtime	Use with caution in patients with hepatic impairment	Take on an empty stomach (high-fat/calorie meals increases C_{max} of capsule 39% and C_{max} of tablet 79%)	Rash; CNS symptoms (insomnia, irritability, lethargy, dizziness, vivid dreams) usually resolve in 2 weeks; increased LFTs; false-positive cannabinoid test; teratogenic in monkeys	Metabolized by CYP2B6 and CYP3A (3A mixed inducer/inhibitor); 14–34% excreted in urine (glucuronidated metabolites, less than 1% unchanged); 16–61% in feces
Etravirine (Intelence)	100-mg tablet	200 mg twice daily following a meal	No dosage adjustment for Child-Pugh Class A or B. Has not been evaluated for Class C	Take following a meal. Fasting decreases by 50%	Rash, nausea	Metabolized by CYP3A, 2C9, and 2C19; Induces 3A4 and inhibits 2C9 and 2C19
Nevirapine (Viramune)	200-mg tablet or 50 mg/5 mL oral suspension	200 mg once daily for 14 days; then 200 mg twice daily	Use with caution in patients with hepatic impairment; avoid use with moderate to severe hepatic impairment	No food restrictions	Rash including Stevens-Johnson syndrome; symptomatic hepatitis, including fatal hepatic necrosis	Metabolized by CYP2B6 and CYP3A (3A inducer); 80% excreted in urine (glucuronidated metabolites; less than 5% unchanged); 10% in feces
Tenofovir + emtricitabine + efavirenz [tenofovir/emtricitabine/efavirenz] (Atripla)	Tenofovir 300 mg Emtricitabine 200 mg Efavirenz 600 mg	1 tablet daily	Do not use in patients with CrCl less than 50 mL/min	High-fat/high-caloric meals increase peak plasma concentrations of efavirenz capsules by 39% and efavirenz tablets by 79%; take on empty stomach	See adverse events of tenofovir, emtricitabine, and efavirenz	See tenofovir, emtricitabine, and efavirenz
Protease Inhibitors						
Atazanavir (Reyataz)	100-, 150-, 200-, 300-mg capsules	400 mg daily If taken with tenofovir use the following: atazanavir 300 mg daily + ritonavir 100 mg daily If taken with efavirenz in treatment naïve patients only: atazanavir 400 mg daily + ritonavir 100 mg daily (do not use with efavirenz in treatment-experienced patients)	Child-Pugh Class: 7–9 / Greater than 9 Dose: 300 mg daily / Not recommended; Treatment-naïve patients on hemodialysis: atazanavir 300 mg + ritonavir 100 mg daily; treatment-experienced patients on hemodialysis: Not recommended	Take with food (AUC increases 30%); pH-sensitive dissolution—special considerations needed when coadministered with antacids	Indirect hyperbilirubinemia; prolonged PR interval (asymptomatic first-degree AV block); use with caution in patients with underlying conduction defects or on concomitant medications that can cause PR prolongation; hyperglycemia; fat maldistribution; increased bleeding episodes in patients with hemophilia	CYP3A4 inhibitor and substrate; UGT1A1 inhibitor

(Continued)

Table 87–5

Summary of Currently Available Antiretroviral Agents (*Continued*)

Generic Name [Abbreviation] (Trade Name)	Dosage Forms	Commonly Prescribed Doses	Dose Adjustments	Food Restrictions	Significant Adverse Events	Drug Interaction Potential
Darunavir (Prezista)	400-, 600-mg tablets	Darunavir 600 mg + ritonavir 100 mg twice daily	Use with caution in patients with hepatic impairment	Should be given with food	Skin rash (has a sulfonamide moiety, Stevens Johnson and erythema multiforme have been reported); diarrhea, nausea; headache; hyperlipidemia; transaminase elevation; hyperglycemia; fat maldistribution; possible increased bleeding episodes in patients with hemophilia	CYP3A4 inhibitor and substrate
Fosamprenavir (Lexiva)	700-mg tablet; 50 mg/mL oral suspension	ARV-naïve patients: fosamprenavir 1,400 mg twice daily, Fosamprenavir 700 mg + ritonavir 100 mg twice daily, or fosamprenavir 1,400 mg + ritonavir 200 mg once daily; PI-experienced patients: fosamprenavir 700 mg + ritonavir 100 mg twice daily Coadministration with efavirenz: fosamprenavir 700 mg + ritonavir 100 mg twice daily or fosamprenavir 1,400 mg + ritonavir 300 mg once daily	**Child-Pugh Class:** **Dose:** 5–8 — 700 mg twice daily 9–12 — Not recommended Ritonavir should not be used in patients with hepatic impairment	None	Skin rash; diarrhea, nausea and vomiting; headache; hyperlipidemia; LFT elevation; hyperglycemia; fat maldistribution; increased bleeding episodes in patients with hemophilia	CYP3A4 inhibitor, inducer, and substrate
Indinavir (Crixivan)	200-, 333-, 400-mg capsules	800 mg every 8 hours; indinavir 800 mg + ritonavir 100 twice daily; indinavir 800 mg + ritonavir 200 mg twice daily	Mild to moderate hepatic insufficiency due to cirrhosis: 600 mg every 8 hours	*For unboosted indinavir:* Take 1 hour before or 2 hours after heavy meals, or concomitantly with low-fat meal. No restrictions when used with ritonavir	Nephrolithiasis; GI intolerance, nausea; indirect hyperbilirubinemia; hyperlipidemia; headache, asthenia, blurred vision, dizziness, rash, metallic taste, thrombocytopenia, alopecia, hemolytic anemia; hyperglycemia; fat maldistribution; increased bleeding episodes in patients with hemophilia	CYP3A4 inhibitor (less than ritonavir)

Drug	Dosage Forms	Dosage	Hepatic Impairment	Administration	Adverse Effects	Metabolism
Lopinavir + ritonavir (Kaletra)	Lopinavir 200 mg + ritonavir 50-mg tablet, lopinavir 400 mg + ritonavir 100 mg/5 mL oral solution (contains 42% alcohol)	2 tablets or 5 mL twice daily 4 tablets once daily; with efavirenz or nevirapine: 3 tablets or 6.7 mL twice daily	Use with caution in patients with hepatic impairment	Take with food (AUC increases 48–80%)	Nausea, vomiting, diarrhea; asthenia; hyperlipidemia; LFT elevation; hyperglycemia; fat maldistribution; increased bleeding episodes in hemophiliacs	CYP3A4 inhibitor and susbstrate CYP2C9, 2C19, 1A2 inducer
Nelfinavir (Viracept)	250–625-mg tablets, 50 mg/g oral powder	1,250 mg twice daily or 750 mg 3 times daily	Use with caution in patients with hepatic impairment	Take with meal or snack	Diarrhea; hyperlipidemia; hyperglycemia; fat maldistribution; increased bleeding in hemophiliacs; LFT elevation	CYP3A4 inhibitor and substrate
Ritonavir (Norvir)	100-mg capsule, 600 mg/7.5 mL solution	600 mg twice daily (when ritonavir is used as sole PI); 100–200 mg/dose when used as pharmacokinetic enhancer	No dosage adjustment in mild hepatic impairment. No data for moderate to severe impairment; use with caution	Take with food to improve tolerability	GI intolerance, nausea, diarrhea; paresthesias; hyperlipidemia; hepatitis; asthenia; taste perversion; hyperglycemia; fat maldistribution; increased bleeding in hemophiliacs	CYP3A4 inhibitor (potent) and substrate; CYP2D6 substrate; mixed dose-dependent induction and inhibition of other Phase I and II enzymes
Saquinavir tablets and hard gel capsules (Invirase)	200-mg capsule, 500-mg tablet	Unboosted saquinavir not recommended *With ritonavir:* (ritonavir 100 mg + saquinavir 1,000 mg) twice daily	Use with caution in patients with hepatic impairment	Take within 2 hours of a meal when taken with ritonavir	Nausea, diarrhea; headache; LFT elevation; hyperlipidemia; hyperglycemia; fat maldistribution; increased bleeding in hemophiliacs	CYP3A4 inhibitor and substrate
Tipranavir (Aptivus)	250-mg capsules	500 mg twice daily with ritonavir 200 mg twice daily	Contraindicated in patients with moderate to severe hepatic insufficiency	Take with food	Hepatotoxicity; skin rash; hyperlipidemia; hyperglycemia; fat maldistribution; possible increased bleeding in hemophiliacs	Tipranavir/ritonavir mixed CYP inhibitor/ inducer; Tipranavir is CYP3A4 substrate
Fusion Inhibitors						
Enfuvirtide (Fuzeon)	Injectable, in lyophilized powder Each single-use vial contains 108 mg of enfuvirtide to be reconstituted with 1.1 mL of sterile water for injection for delivery of approximately 90 mg/1 mL	90 mg (1 mL) subcutaneously 2 times per day	No dosage recommendation	N/A	Local injection site reaction (pain, erythema, induration, nodules and cysts, pruritus, eachymosis) in most patients; increased rate of bacterial pneumonia; less than 1% hypersensitivity reaction (rash, fever, nausea, vomiting, chills, rigors, hypotension, or elevated serum transaminases); do not rechallenge	Catabolism to amino acids, with subsequent recycling in the body pool

(Continued)

Table 87-5

Summary of Currently Available Antiretroviral Agents (Continued)

Generic Name [Abbreviation] (Trade Name)	Dosage Forms	Commonly Prescribed Doses	Dose Adjustments	Food Restrictions	Significant Adverse Events	Drug Interaction Potential
Chemokine Receptor Antagonists (CCR5 Antagonists)						
Maraviroc (Selzentry)	150-mg and 300-mg tablets	150 mg twice daily when given with strong CYP3A inhibitors (with or without CYP3A inducers) including PIs (except tipranavir/ritonavir) 300 mg twice daily when given with NRTIs, Enfuvirtide, tipranavir/ritonavir, nevirapine and other drugs that are not potent P450 inhibitors 600 mg twice daily when given with CYP3A inducers, including efavirenz, rifampin, etc. (without a CYP3A inhibitor)	Patients with CrCl less than 50 mL/min should receive maraviroc with a CYP3A inhibitor only if benefit outweighs the risk	No food restrictions	Abdominal pain; cough; dizziness; musculoskeletal symptoms; pyrexia; rash; upper RTI; hepatotoxicity; orthostatic hypotension	CYP3A substrate
Integrase Inhibitors						
Raltegravir (Isentress)	400-mg tablet	400 mg twice daily	No dosage adjustment	No food restrictions	Nausea; headache; diarrhea; pyrexia; CPK elevation	UGT1A1 substrate (glucuronidation)

AUC, area under the time-concentration curve; ARV, antiretroviral; AV, atrioventricular; C_{max}, maximum concentration; CrCl, creatinine clearance; ESRD, end-stage renal disease; HD, hemodialysis; LFT, liver function test; NRTI, nucleoside reverse transcriptase inhibitor; UGT, uridine diphosphate-glucuronosyltransferase.

Adapted from the DHHS Guidelines for the Use of Antiretroviral Agents in HIV-1-Infected Adults and Adolescents, January 29, 2008.

the drug interaction potential of each antiretroviral. Due to the ever-changing drug interactions with this class of medications, the regularly updated DHHS Guidelines for the Use of Antiretroviral Agents in HIV-1–Infected Adults and Adolescents are a recommended source of specific drug interactions.[5]

The goals of therapy differ for antiretroviral-experienced patients that have limited drug exposure (i.e., developing resistance to their first antiretroviral regimen) versus those with extensive exposure (i.e., developing resistance to their third or fourth antiretroviral regimen). It is reasonable to expect maximal viral suppression in those with limited drug exposure. However, this may not be feasible for patients with prior exposure to multiple medications. **❶** *In antiretroviral-experienced patients, a reasonable goal is to simply preserve immune function and prevent clinical progression.*

Several issues need to be considered in choosing a salvage regimen for HIV infection. Knowing prior medication exposure can assist in identifying which drugs to avoid. However, direct HIV resistance testing can better identify the resistance and susceptibility patterns of the major viral strains. Because HIV may be susceptible to certain components of the failing antiretroviral regimen, these drugs can be recycled into future regimens. Resistance testing should be used when all patients enter into care, in patients with virologic failure on a current ARV regimen, or with suboptimal suppression after initiation of ARV therapy. Testing is generally preferred for antiretroviral naïve patients. For resistance testing to be useful, the patient should have a plasma HIV RNA of at least 1,000 copies/mL, and should be currently taking their antiretroviral medications (or be within 4 weeks of discontinuing antiretroviral therapy). This viral concentration is necessary to yield reliable amplification of the virus, and the antiretroviral medications are needed because the dominant viral species reverts to wild-type within 4 to 6 weeks after medications are stopped.

Two types of HIV resistance testing are available, genotyping and phenotyping. Genotyping involves detecting mutations by genetically sequencing the virus, while phenotyping determines the ability of the virus to replicate in the presence of varying ARV concentrations. Genotyping is more rapid and less costly than phenotyping, but results in a list of mutations that may be more difficult to interpret than phenotyping. A *virtual phenotype* report may also be obtained when genotypes are ordered.[8–15] This compares the patient's viral sequence to a database of matched genotypes and drug susceptibilities. Because the predictability of *virtual phenotypes* are dependent on the robustness of the database from which they are derived, some clinicians believe their utility is limited. Web-based tools are available to assist with interpretation of resistance mutations (e.g., Stanford University's HIV Drug Resistance Database; *http://hivdb.stanford.edu/index.html*). However, expert interpretation of genotype and phenotype reports is recommended.

Certain guiding principles should be considered when treating ARV-experienced patients, and expert opinion is advised before selecting therapy. **❹** *As with ARV-naïve patients, three or more active drugs should be prescribed.*[11,16–18] Because considerable cross-resistance can occur between medications within an antiretroviral class, simply using drugs to which the patient has not been exposed may be insufficient. Complete cross-resistance occurs within the NNRTI class, whereas the NRTIs and PIs have variable overlapping resistance patterns. For this reason, HIV resistance assays are important tools for choosing subsequent effective therapies. The following factors are associated with superior virologic response: lower viral load at the time therapy is changed, using a new class of antiretroviral agent, and using ritonavir enhanced PIs in patients previously exposed to PIs.[19,20]

Table 87–4 provides general treatment options based on previous drug use. If patients fail therapy with resistance to only one drug, one or two active agents may be substituted for this drug while retaining the remaining drugs in the regimen. If patients fail therapy with resistance to more than one drug, changing classes of antiretrovirals and/or adding new active drugs is warranted. New NRTIs should be selected from resistance testing. If this is not available, the assumption should be made that resistance has developed to all NRTIs used in the failing regimen. In general, HIV that is resistant solely to lamivudine and/or emtricitabine will be susceptible to other NRTIs. If HIV develops resistance solely to tenofovir, then it may have reduced susceptibility to didanosine, but should remain susceptible to zidovudine, stavudine, lamivudine, emtricitabine, and abacavir. Cross-resistance occurs between zidovudine and stavudine.

Three new antiretrovirals have been FDA-approved for use in antiretroviral experienced patients. Two of these agents, Isentress (raltegravir) and Selzentry (maraviroc) have unique mechanisms of action compared to previous agents lending to their advantage in treating antiretroviral experienced patients with limited treatment options and resistance. The final agent, Intelence (etravirine), a member of the NNRTI class, is known as a second-generation NNRTI which is effective at reducing viral load in patients with first generation NNRTI resistance virus. These agents add to the antiretroviral armamentarium in HIV infected treatment experienced patients.

If a patient appears to fail an antiretroviral regimen without detectable HIV resistance, adherence should be investigated, and the adequacy of the plasma HIV RNA concentration in the resistance sample confirmed. Options include continuing the current regimen or starting a new regimen and repeating the resistance test 2 to 4 weeks after adherence is verified. An increasing number of patients have extensive HIV resistance, such that antiretroviral regimens cannot be designed to which the virus is fully susceptible. For these patients, continuing the current regimen may be beneficial because drug-resistant virus may have a compromised replication capacity. Other strategies may be considered for this type of patient, including pharmacokinetic enhancement with ritonavir, retreatment with prior antiretroviral agents, treatment with multidrug regimens (four or more antiretroviral drugs), and the use of new agents through expanded access programs or clinical trials.

Treatment Considerations in Special Populations

▶ Acute HIV Infection

Diagnosis of acute HIV infection is difficult, since many patients are asymptomatic, or have nonspecific clinical symptoms similar to other common respiratory infections. If acute HIV infection is suspected, HIV antibody tests and a plasma HIV RNA concentration should be obtained. A clear diagnosis is made when an HIV antibody test is negative and the plasma HIV RNA concentration is high. There are limited outcomes data for treating acutely infected patients. Treatment of acute infection can decrease the severity of acute disease and decrease the viral set point; this may decrease progression rates and reduce the rate of viral transmission.[21–25] Limitations include an increased risk of chronic drug-induced toxicities and the development of viral resistance. Resistance testing should be performed prior to initiation of therapy due to an increase in resistance of antiretroviral naïve patients.[5]

▶ Adolescent Patients

As a result of similar modes of HIV transmission, adolescents infected after puberty are treated with similar considerations as adults. In this population, dosing of antiretroviral drugs should not be based on age, but on the Tanner stage (which considers external primary and secondary sexual characteristics). Adolescents in early puberty should be dosed according to pediatric guidelines, while those in late puberty should be dosed as adults. During growth spurts, adolescents should be monitored closely for drug efficacy and toxicity, since rapid changes in weight can lead to altered drug concentrations. Adherence is of concern in this population due to denial of the disease, misinformation, distrust of health care professionals, low self-esteem, and lack of family and/or social support. Additionally, asymptomatic patients this age find it more difficult to adhere to therapy while feeling well.

▶ Pediatric Patients

There are unique considerations in the treatment of HIV-infected children. Specific treatment guidelines exist,[26] but a thorough review is outside the scope of this chapter. Most children acquire HIV infection through perinatal transmission either in utero, intrapartum, or postpartum through breast-feeding, although antiretroviral interventions have dramatically reduced transmission rates.[5]

Antiretroviral therapy is limited in pediatric patients, as some drugs have no dosing recommendations for this population, or are not available in a formulation that can be easily administered to children. Additionally, drug exposures can change dramatically during ontogeny due to altered drug-metabolizing enzyme and drug transporter activities.

▶ Drugs of Abuse

Treatment challenges in illicit drug users include comorbidities (such as hepatitis infection), limited access to care, inadequate adherence to therapy, side effects and toxicities, and the need for treatment of substance abuse which can lead to drug interactions. *Many drugs of abuse have the potential to interact with antiretroviral medications, and a number of case reports have documented drug overdose when combined with PI therapy.*[27] In these populations, without addiction control, adherence is suboptimal and treatment failure is common.[2] Most PIs and NNRTIs decrease methadone concentrations up to 50%. As this can result in the development of withdrawal symptoms, patients should be closely monitored for 4 to 8 weeks after initiation of antiretroviral therapy. Withdrawal symptoms can be alleviated with a methadone dose increase of 5 to 10 mg. Although there are fewer data, buprenorphine concentrations may be similarly affected, and therefore this drug requires close monitoring.

▶ Pregnancy and Women of Reproductive Potential

The goals of antiretroviral therapy for women of reproductive age and pregnant women are the same as for other adult patients. Specific guidelines for HIV-infected pregnant women are available.[28] Recommended therapies in pregnancy include zidovudine, lamivudine, lopinavir/ritonavir, and if the CD4+ count is less than 250 cells/mm^3, nevirapine. Drugs to be avoided include efavirenz (due to potential teratogenicity), the combination of didanosine and stavudine (due to a high incidence of lactic acidosis), nevirapine in patients with a CD4 count greater than 250 cells/mm^3 (due to an increased risk of hepatotoxicity), and the liquid formulation of amprenavir (due to high concentrations of propylene glycol). The goal of therapy is to reduce plasma HIV RNA below 1,000 copies/mL and prevent MTCT of HIV. Limited data are available on antiretroviral pharmacokinetics in pregnancy, and standard doses of antiretroviral drugs are currently recommended with close HIV RNA and CD4 monitoring in the third trimester of pregnancy. Some experts will consider increasing lopinavir/ritonavir dosing in the third trimester from 2 to 3 tablets twice daily; however, studies are underway to better assess this approach.[28]

Women of reproductive potential prescribed efavirenz should be counseled on its potentially teratogenic effects and the importance of birth control. ❼ *Additionally, nevirapine, nelfinavir, ritonavir, lopinavir/ritonavir, and tipranavir/ritonavir decrease the concentrations of estrogens and/or progestins in oral contraceptives, which could lead to failure.*[5] For patients prescribed these drugs, barrier forms of contraception are preferred to prevent pregnancy. Atazanavir may be taken with oral contraceptives with caution, as it can increase or decrease the exposure to estrogen and progesterone, depending on whether it is used in combination with ritonavir. DepoProvera may be a safe alternative, as it does not affect nelfinavir, efavirenz, or nevirapine concentrations; although the effect of antiretrovirals on medroxyprogesterone concentrations has not been examined, no evidence of ovulation has been seen in women on these combinations.[29]

▶ Hepatitis B Coinfection

HIV-infected patients coinfected with hepatitis B virus (HBV) have higher concentrations of DNA and hepatitis B early antigen (HBeAg), and higher rates of HBV-associated liver disease. Therapy for HBV should be offered to patients who are HBeAg-positive, or have HBV DNA greater than 10^5 copies/mL and have either liver serologies (alanine aminotransferase) greater than two times the upper limit of normal or histologic evidence of moderate disease or fibrosis. Options include interferon alfa 2a or 2b and nucleoside/tide analogs. Nucleoside/tide analogs that treat HBV but not HIV are adefovir and entecavir. Nucleoside/tide analogs that treat HBV and HIV are lamivudine, emtricitabine, and tenofovir. These latter agents should be considered when treating HIV infection in HBV coinfected patients.

▶ Hepatitis C Coinfection

Patients coinfected with hepatitis C virus (HCV) and HIV have a threefold increase in rate of progression to cirrhosis compared to those with HCV alone. Therapy for HCV is considered in patients with detectable plasma HCV RNA and a liver biopsy showing bridging or portal fibrosis. Patients with HCV genotype 2 and 3 (and a CD4 count greater than 200 cells/mm³) treated with pegylated interferon plus ribavirin have a better sustained viral response at 48 weeks (60%–70%) compared to those with HCV genotype 1 (15%–28%). Comprehensive treatment guidelines for HIV/HCV coinfected patients are available.[30-32] Important considerations addressed in these guidelines include avoiding the combination of ribavirin with didanosine,and stavudine (due to increased risk of pancreatitis and/or lactic acidosis) and ribavirin with zidovudine (due to increased risk of anemia). Growth factors and erythropoietin may be needed to treat neutropenia from interferon and anemia from ribavirin. Antiretrovirals such as nevirapine, efavirenz, and tipranavir are hepatotoxic and in most cases should be avoided in HCV/HIV-infected patients.

Patient Encounter, Part 2: Medical History, Physical Exam, and Diagnostic Tests

PMH: Hypertension for 5 years; it is often not well controlled because of poor patient adherence; GERD, currently controlled on histamine antagonists; history of hepatitis B

FH: Father died of myocardial infarction at the age of 68 years; mother is still alive with history of diabetes

SH: Works as a truck driver; reports distant history of IV drug use in his 20s; drinks alcohol occasionally

Meds: Hydrochlorothiazide 25 mg by mouth once daily; famotidine 20 mg by mouth twice daily

ROS: (+) weight loss, decreased appetite, shortness of breath, and cough; (–) chest pain, nausea, vomiting, diarrhea

PE:

VS: BP 144/84 mm Hg, P 100 bpm, RR 22 per minute, T 38.3°C (100.9°F)

HEENT: Mild thrush on tongue

CV: RRR, normal S_1, S_2; no murmurs, rubs, gallops

Abd: Soft, nontender, nondistended; (+) bowel sounds, no hepatosplenomegaly

Rectal: Deferred

Labs: Sodium 135 mEq/L (135 mmol/L), potassium 3.6 mEq/L (3.6 mmol/L), chloride 100 mEq/L (100 mmol/L), bicarbonate 24 mEq/L (24 mmol/L), blood urea nitrogen 14 mg/dL (5 mmol/L), creatinine 1.0 mg/dL (88 μmol/L), WBC 5.2 × 10³/mm³ (5.2 × 10⁹/L), hemoglobin 11.5 g/dL (115 g/L or 7.1 mmol/L), hematocrit 34.1%, platelets 151 × 10³/mm³ (151 × 10⁹/L), neutrophils 58%, bands 9%, lymphocytes 32%, monocytes 1%, eosinophils 0%, basophils 0%, CD4 150 cells/mm³

HIV ELISA: Pending

CXR: Diffuse interstitial infiltrates bilaterally

Given this additional information, what is your assessment of the patient's condition?

What other laboratory tests would you recommend?

Identify your treatment goals for the patient.

What nonpharmacologic and pharmacologic alternatives are available for the patient?

OUTCOME EVALUATION

❶ *The success of antiretroviral therapy is measured by the degree to which the therapy: (a) restores and preserves immunologic function, (b) maximally and durably suppresses HIV RNA, (c) improves quality of life, (d) reduces HIV-related morbidity and mortality, and (e) prevents opportunistic infections.* **❷** *The major outcome parameters are CD4+ lymphocyte absolute count and percentage, and plasma HIV RNA.* Adequate immunologic response in antiretroviral-naïve patients consists of an increase in CD4+ cell count that averages 50 to 150 cells/mm³ (with a faster response in the first 3 months), and a 1 log decrease in HIV RNA by 2 to 8 weeks after starting medications, followed by concentrations less than 50 copies/mL by 12 to 16 weeks (if HIV RNA less than 100,000/mL or by 16–24 weeks if HIV RNA greater than 100,000/mL). Upon initiating or changing antiretroviral therapy, HIV RNA should be measured after 2 to 8 weeks and every 4 to 8 weeks until undetectable. Once stable, HIV RNA and CD4 count are monitored generally every 3 to 6 months. In highly treatment-experienced patients, adequate immunologic response may be only a stable, or slightly increased, CD4 T-cell count, and a stable HIV RNA. This may be enough to prevent clinical progression. However, with the recent new agents and new therapeutic classes of antiretrovirals available for treatment-experienced patients, the goal of treatment should be to reestablish maximal viral suppression to less than 50 HIV RNA copies/mL.

Each patient should have a plan to assess the effectiveness of antiretroviral therapy after initiation. At each clinic visit, patients should be evaluated for the presence of adverse drug reactions, drug allergies, medication adherence, and potential drug interactions. **❽** *Antiretrovirals have both class-associated and drug-specific adverse effects* (see Table 87–5). If the patient experiences any of the serious, life-threatening effects (Table 87–6), the offending agent should be discontinued promptly, and in most cases the patient cannot be rechallenged. Potential long-term complications that may reduce the quality of life are listed in Table 87–7. For drugs with a high likelihood of intolerability (such as nelfinavir-associated diarrhea), patients should be counseled to anticipate these effects and have concomitant prescriptions available for preemptive management (such as an antidiarrheal agent). Patients should have follow-up within the 1st week after initiating a new drug regimen. If the patient does not tolerate a medication despite all efforts to the contrary, consider changing the drug.

❺ *Currently, treatment of HIV infection is lifelong.* Unplanned short-term treatment interruptions may be necessary due to drug toxicity or illness that precludes administration of oral therapy. If a patient must interrupt therapy due to toxicity, all drugs of the regimen should be stopped at the same time, regardless of half-life. The strategy of scheduling elective treatment interruptions (where patients stop and start antiretroviral therapy based on CD4 T-cell count criteria) has been evaluated in several clinical trials.

Viral rebound occurs quickly after stopping therapy, and worsens immune function, clinical progression, and may even result in death. If either short-term (less than 7 days) or long-term treatment interruption is needed, drug half-life must be taken into consideration. For regimens where all components have similar half-lives, all drugs can be stopped simultaneously. If the regimen contains components with significantly different half-lives (e.g., Atripla), stopping all drugs at the same time could result in the drug with the longest half-life (usually NNRTIs) lingering in the body and functioning as monotherapy. The ideal time to stop the NNRTIs (efavirenz, etravirine, or nevirapine) is unknown as these drugs can continue to be detectable 1 to 3+ weeks in patients. Options include either: (a) stopping the NNRTI first and continuing the other drugs in the regimen for up to 4 weeks or (b) substituting the NNRTI with a PI and continuing the PI with dual NRTIs for up to 4 weeks. In this situation, therapeutic drug monitoring of the long half-life drug can be useful in determining when to stop the NRTI ± PI coverage.

Patient Encounter, Part 3

Based on the information presented, create a care plan for this patient's HIV/AIDS. Your plan should include:

(a) A statement of the best drug combinations and reasons supporting each drug recommended, as well as any adverse effects or potential drug-related problems.
(b) Goals of therapy.
(c) A patient-specific, detailed therapeutic plan.
(d) A plan for follow-up to determine whether the goals have been achieved and adverse effects avoided.

Patient Encounter, Part 4

Your patient begins treatment with atazanavir 300 mg by mouth once daily, ritonavir 100 mg by mouth once daily, tenofovir 300 mg by mouth once daily, and lamivudine 300 mg by mouth once daily. He initially does well on this regimen, but after about 3 months, he has difficulty taking his medications at the same time every day due to his busy schedule. Because of his job, he relocated to Alabama, and has not been seen in your clinic for 2 years. He returns today to see you in clinic and complains of feeling tired, but otherwise no specific complaints.

What laboratory tests do you recommend?

What additional information do you need to know before creating a treatment plan for this patient?

Table 87-6

Serious Adverse Effects and Management

Adverse Effects	Drug	Signs and Symptoms	Risk Factors	Prevention/ Monitoring	Management
Hepatotoxicity	Nevirapine	**Onset** Up to 18 weeks postinitiation **Symptoms** Abrupt onset of flu-like symptoms, abdominal pain, jaundice, fever ± rash	Increased CD4 + count at initiation Female Elevated baseline AST/ALT Any liver disease High nevirapine concentration	2-week dose escalation Avoid starting nevirapine in women with CD4 greater than 250 cells/ mm^3, men with CD4 greater than 400 cells/mm^3 AST/ALT every 2 weeks for 1st month, monthly for 3 months, then every 3 months	D/C antiretrovirals; D/C all hepatotoxic agents; rule out other causes; do not rechallenge with nevirapine
	Other NNRTIs, PIs, most NRTIs, and MVC	**Onset:** NNRTI—60% within first 12 weeks PI—weeks to months NRTI—months to years **Symptoms:** NNRTI—asymptomatic to nonspecific symptoms, such as anorexia, weight loss, or fatigue PI—generally asymptomatic, some with anorexia, weight loss, jaundice Didanosine NRTI—zidovudine, didanosine, stavudine may cause hepatotoxicity associated with lactic acidosis; lamivudine, emtricitabine, or tenofovir may cause HBV flare when these drugs are withdrawn	HBV or HCV coinfection Alcoholism Concomitant hepatotoxic drugs	Monitor LFTs at least every 3–4 months	Rule out other causes. For symptomatic patients: D/C all antiretrovirals and other potential hepatotoxic agents; after symptoms and LFTs normalize, begin new antiretroviral regimen (without the potential offending agents). For asymptomatic patients: If ALT greater than 5–10 × ULN, may consider D/C antiretrovirals or continue with close monitoring; after symptoms and LFTs normalize, begin new antiretroviral regimen (without the potential offending agents)
Lactic acidosis/ hepatic steatosis +/− pancreatitis	NRTIs (esp. stavudine, didanosine, zidovudine)	**Onset:** Months after initiation **Symptoms:** Nonspecific GI (nausea, anorexia, abdominal pain, vomiting, weight loss, fatigue) Laboratory values: ↑ lactate, ↓ arterial pH, ↓ serum bicarbonate, ↑ AST/ALT, ↑ PT, ↑ T.bili, ↓ serum albumin, ↑ amylase/ lipase (with pancreatitis)	Stavudine + didanosine Female Obesity Pregnancy Didanosine + hydroxyurea or ribavirin ↑ Duration of NRTI use	None unless symptoms present Consider lactate concentrations in patients with ↓ serum bicarbonate or ↑ anion gap	D/C all antiretrovirals; symptomatic support with fluids; some patients require IV bicarbonate, hemodialysis, parenteral nutrition, or mechanical ventilation; once syndrome resolves, consider using NRTIs with ↓ mitochondrial toxicity (abacavir, tenofovir, lamivudine, or emtricitabine); monitor lactate after restarting NRTIs; some clinicians use NRTI-sparing regimens

(Continued)

Table 87–6

Serious Adverse Effects and Management (Continued)

Adverse Effects	Drug	Signs and Symptoms	Risk Factors	Prevention/ Monitoring	Management
Stevens-Johnson syndrome/ toxic epidermal necrosis	Nevirapine greater than efavirenz, delavirdine, etravirine; Also, amprenavir, abacavir, zidovudine, didanosine, indinavir lopinavir/r, atazanavir	**Onset:** 1st day–weeks after therapy start **Symptoms:** Skin eruption with mucosal ulcerations; fever, tachycardia, malaise, myalgia, arthralgia; for nevirapine may also have hepatic toxicity	Nevirapine—female, black, Asian, Hispanic	Nevirapine: use 2-week lead in 200 mg daily, then 200 mg twice a day Avoid corticosteroid use during dose escalation—may increase rash incidence Educate patients to report symptoms as soon as they appear	D/C all antiretrovirals as well as any other possible cause; aggressive symptom support; do not rechallenge patient with offending agent; if caused by nevirapine, avoid NNRTI class, if possible
Hypersensitivity reaction (HSR)	Abacavir	**Onset:** Median = 9 days; 90% within first 6 weeks **Symptoms:** Acute onset of symptoms (most frequent to least): high fever, diffuse skin rash, malaise, nausea, headache, myalgia, chills, diarrhea, vomiting, abdominal pain, dyspnea, arthralgia, respiratory symptoms	HLA-B*5701, HLA-DR7, HLA-DQ3 Antiretroviral-naïve patients Higher incidence with 600 mg every day compared to twice a day dosing	HLA-B*5701 screening prior to abacavir if (+), label as abacavir allergic in medical chart Educate patients about signs and symptoms of HSR and the need of prompt report	D/C abacavir and other antiretrovirals; rule out other causes of symptoms, most signs and symptoms resolve 48 hours after abacavir/DC; do not rechallenge with abacavir after suspected HSR
Lactic acidosis/ rapidly progressive ascending neuromuscular weakness	Stavudine	**Onset:** Months, then striking motor weakness within days to weeks **Symptoms:** Rapidly progressive ascending demylenating polyneuropathy (similar to Guillain-Barré); respiratory paralysis	Prolonged stavudine use	Early recognition and D/C of offending agent to avoid progression	D/C antiretrovirals; supportive care; recovery may take months, sometimes irreversible; do not rechallenge with offending agent
Bleeding events	Tipranavir/ritonavir: intracranial hemorrhage (ICH); other PIs: ↑ bleeding in hemophiliacs	**Onset:** ICH: median = 525 days on tipranavir/ritonavir Hemophiliacs: Few weeks **Symptoms:** ↑ Spontaneous bleeding tendency (in joints, muscles, soft tissues, and hematuria)	ICH: CNS lesions, head trauma, recent neurosurgery, coagulopathy, alcohol abuse, or on anticoagulant or antiplatelet agents Hemophiliac patients: PI use	ICH: Avoid tipranavir/ ritonavir use in high risk patients Hemophiliacs: Consider using a NNRTI-based regimen; monitor for spontaneous bleeding	ICH: D/C tipranavir/ritonavir; supportive care Hemophiliacs: May require increased use of factor VIII products

	Drug	Onset/Symptoms	Predisposing/Risk Factors	Prevention/Monitoring	Management
Bone marrow suppression	Zidovudine	**Onset:** Few weeks–months **Symptoms:** Fatigue, risk of ↑ bacterial infections due to neutropenia; anemia, neutropenia	Advanced HIV High dose zidovudine Preexisting anemia or neutropenia Concomitant use of bone marrow suppressants	Avoid in patients at high risk for bone marrow suppression; avoid other suppressing agents; monitor CBC with differential at least every 3 months	Switch to another NRTI; D/C concomitant bone marrow suppressant, if possible; for anemia: Identify and treat other causes; consider erythropoietin treatment or blood transfusion, if indicated; for neutropenia: Identify and treat other causes; consider filgrastim treatment, if indicated
Nephrolithiasis/ urolithiasis/ crystalluria	Indinavir	**Onset:** Any time after initiation of therapy, especially if ↓ fluid intake **Symptoms:** Flank pain and/or abdominal pain, dysuria, frequency; pyuria, hematuria, crystalluria; rarely, ↑ serum creatinine and acute renal failure	History of nephrolithiasis Patients unable to maintain adequate fluid intake High peak indinavir concentration ↑ duration of exposure	Drink at least 1.5–2 L of noncaffeinated fluid per day; ↑ fluid intake at first sign of darkened urine; monitor urinalysis and serum creatinine every 3–6 months	Increased hydration; pain control; may consider switching to alternative agent; stent placement may be required
Nephrotoxicity	Indinavir, tenofovir	**Onset:** Indinavir—months after therapy Tenofovir—weeks to months after therapy **Symptoms:** Indinavir—asymptomatic; rarely develop end-stage renal disease; ↑ serum creatinine, pyuria; hydronephrosis, renal atrophy Tenofovir—asymptomatic to symptoms of nephrogenic diabetes insipidus, Fanconi syndrome; ↑ serum creatinine, proteinuria, hypophosphatemia, glycosuria, hypokalemia, non–anion gap metabolic acidosis	History of renal disease Concomitant use of nephrotoxic drugs	Avoid use of other nephrotoxic drugs; adequate hydration if on indinavir; monitor creatinine, urinalysis, serum potassium and phosphorus in patients at risk	D/C offending agent, generally reversible; supportive care; electrolyte replacement as indicated
Pancreatitis	Didanosine; didanosine + stavudine;	**Onset:** Usually weeks–months	High intracellular and/or serum Didanosine concentrations	Didanosine should not be used in patients with history of	D/C offending agents; symptomatic management of pancreatitis—bowel rest, IV hydration, pain

(Continued)

Table 87–6

Serious Adverse Effects and Management (*Continued*)

Adverse Effects	Drug	Signs and Symptoms	Risk Factors	Prevention/ Monitoring	Management
	didanosine + hydroxyurea or ribavirin; tenofovir	**Symptoms:** Postprandial abdominal pain, nausea, vomiting; ↑ serum amylase and lipase	History of pancreatitis Alcoholism Hypertriglyceridemia Concomitant use of didanosine with stavudine, hydroxyurea, or ribavirin Use of didanosine + tenofovir without didanosine dose reduction	pancreatitis; avoid concomitant use of ddI with stavudine, hydroxyurea, or ribavirin; ↓ ddI dose when used with tenofovir	control, gradual resumption of oral intake

AST, aspartate aminotransferase; ALT, alanine aminotransferase; CBC, complete blood cell count; CPK, creatine phosphokinase; D/C, discontinue; HBV, hepatitis B virus; HCV, hepatitis C virus; LFT, liver function tests; NNRTI, nonnucleoside reverse transcriptase inhibitor; NRTI, nucleoside reverse transcriptase inhibitor; PI, protease inhibitor; PT, prothrombin time; T.bili, total bilirubin; ULN, upper limit of normal.

Table 87-7

Other Adverse Effects and Management

Adverse Effects	Drug	Signs and Symptoms	Risk Factors	Prevention/ Monitoring	Management
Potential Long-Term Complications					
Cardiovascular	Potentially all PIs and other antiretrovirals (efavirenz, stavudine—unfavorable lipid effect; abacavir, didanosine—unknown)	Onset: months–years after therapy initiation; symptoms: premature CVD	Other risk factors for CVD	Consider non-PI based regimen; lifestyle modification counseling	Early diagnosis, prevention, and pharmacologic therapy for hyperlipidemia, HTN, insulin-resistance/diabetes mellitus; assess cardiac risk factors; switch to NNRTI- or atazanavir-based regimen; avoid stavudine
Hyperlipidemia	All PIs (except atazanavir); stavudine; efavirenz (to a lesser extent)	Onset: weeks–months after therapy initiation; symptoms: All PIs except atazanavir—↑ LDL and total cholesterol (TC), ↓↑ HDL; lopinavir/r and ritonavir—disproportionate ↑ TG; stavudine—↑ TG; may also ↑ LDL and TC; efavirenz or nevirapine—↑ HDL, slight ↑ TG	Underlying hyperlipidemia PI: Tipranavir/r greater than lopinavir/r and ritonavir greater than nelfinavir and amprenavir greater than indinavir and saquinavir greater than atazanavir NNRTI: less than PIs; efavirenz greater than nevirapine NRTI: stavudine greater than zidovudine and tenofovir most common	Use non-PI, non-stavudine-based regimens; use atazanavir-based regimen; monitor fasting lipid profile at baseline, 3–6 months after new regimen, then at least annually	Assess cardiac risk factor; lifestyle modification; switch to antiretrovirals with fewer lipid effects; total cholesterol greater than 200 mg/dL, LDL, TG 200–500 mg/dL => pravastatin or atorvastatin; TG greater than 500 mg/dL gemfibrozil or micronized fenofibrate
Insulin resistance/ diabetes mellitus	All PIs	Onset: weeks–months after therapy initiation; symptoms: polyuria, polydipsia, polyphagia, fatigue, weakness; exacerbation of hyperglycemia in patients with underlying diabetes	Underlying hyperglycemia, family history of diabetes mellitus	Use PI-sparing regimens; monitor fasting blood glucose 1–3 months after starting new regimen, then at least every 3–6 months	Diet and exercise; consider switching to an NNRTI-based regimen; if need for pharmacologic therapy, consider metformin, sulfonylurea, "glitazones," or insulin, where indicated
Osteonecrosis	All PIs	Onset: insidious; symptoms: mild to moderate periarticular pain; 85% of cases involve one or both femoral heads	Diabetes Prior steroid use Advanced age Alcohol use Hyperlipidemia	Risk reduction (limit steroid and alcohol use): for asymptomatic cases with less than 15% bony head involvement, monitor with MRI every 3–6 months × 1 year, then every 6 months × 1 year, then annually	Conservative: reduce weight-bearing activity on affected joint; reduce risk factors; analgesics as needed; Surgical: core decompression +/− bone grafting (early disease); total joint arthroplasty (severe disease)
Quality of Life Complications					
CNS effects	Efavirenz	Onset: first few doses; symptoms: one or more of the following: drowsiness, insomnia,	Pre-existing or unstable psychiatric illness Use of other drugs with CNS effects	Take no earlier than 2–3 hours before bedtime; take on an empty stomach; counsel patients	Symptoms usually diminish or resolve after 2–4 weeks; may consider discontinuing therapy if symptoms persist and significantly

(Continued)

Table 87-7

Other Adverse Effects and Management (Continued)

Adverse Effects	Drug	Signs and Symptoms	Risk Factors	Prevention/Monitoring	Management
		abnormal dreams, dizziness, impaired concentration, depression, hallucination; exacerbation of psychiatric disorders; psychosis; suicidal ideation	May be more common in African Americans due to genetic predisposition of ↓ clearance	to avoid operating machinery during first 2–4 weeks of therapy	impair daily function or exacerbate psychiatric illness
Fat maldistribution	PIs, thymidine analogs (stavudine more common than zidovudine)	Onset: gradually, months after therapy initiation; symptoms: lipoatrophy—peripheral fat loss (facial thinning, thinning of extremities and buttocks); lipohypertrophy—increase in abdominal girth, breast size, and dorsocervical fat pad (buffalo hump)	Lipoatrophy—low baseline body mass index	DEXA scan; lipoatrophy: avoid thymidine analogs or switch from ZDV or stavudine to abacavir or tenofovir	Switching to other agents may slow or stop progression, but may not reverse effects; injectable poly-L-lactic acid for facial lipoatrophy
GI intolerance	All PIs, zidovudine, didanosine	Onset: first few doses; symptoms: nausea, vomiting, abdominal pain; diarrhea commonly seen with nelfinavir, lopinavir/ritonavir, and didanosine -buffered formulations	All patients	Taking with food may reduce symptoms (not for didanosine or unboosted indinavir); may preemptively need antiemetics or antidiarrheals	May spontaneously resolve or become tolerable with time; nausea and vomiting: consider antiemetic prior to dosing; switch to less emetogenic agent; diarrhea: consider antimotility agents, calcium tablets, bulk-forming agents, and/or pancreatic enzymes
Injection site reactions	Enfuvirtide	Onset: first new doses; symptoms: pain, pruritus, erythema, ecchymosis, warmth, nodules, rarely injection site infection	All patients	Educate regarding use of sterile technique, solution at room temperature, rotation of injection sites, avoidance of sites with little subcutaneous fat or existing reactions	Massaging the area vigorously before and after injection may reduce pain; wear loose clothing around injection site areas; take warm shower or bath prior to injection; rarely, warm compact or analgesics may be necessary
Peripheral neuropathy	Didanosine, stavudine, zalcitabine	Onset: weeks–months after therapy initiation; symptoms: begins with numbness and paresthesias of toes and feet; may progress to painful neuropathy; upper extremities less frequently involved; may be irreversible despite drug discontinuation	Preexisting peripheral neuropathy Combined use of these NRTIs or other drugs which may cause neuropathy Advanced HIV High dose of offending drugs or drugs that may increase Didanosine intracellular activities (hydroxyurea, ribavirin)	Avoid using these agents in patients at risk; if possible, avoid combined use of these agents; ask patient at each encounter	Consider D/C offending agent prior to onset of disabling pain; pharmacologic treatment (variable effectiveness): gabapentin, tricyclic antidepressants, lamotrigine, oxcarbamazepine, topiramate, tramadol, narcotic analgesics, capsaicin cream, topical lidocaine

CVD, cardiovascular disease; D/C, discontinue; DEXA, dual-energy x-ray absorptiometry; HDL, high-density lipoprotein; HTN, hypertension; LDL, low-density lipoprotein; NNRTI, nonnucleoside reverse transcriptase inhibitor; NRTI, nucleoside reverse transcriptase inhibitor; PI, protease inhibitor; TG, triglyceride.

Patient Care and Monitoring

Patient Assessment

1. Medication history

   - Get a thorough history of prescription, nonprescription, and natural drug product use. Determine what prior antiretroviral regimens, if any, were used in the past.

   - *Is the patient taking the appropriate dose of each medication? Are the doses adjusted for renal or hepatic failure? Are the doses adjusted for drug interactions with concomitant medications?*

   - Evaluate the patient for the presence of adverse drug reactions, drug allergies, and drug interactions.

   - Assess improvement in quality-of-life measures such as physical, psychological, and social functioning and well-being. *Is the patient experiencing any drug-induced adverse effects? What can you do to help manage these adverse effects?*

2. Review any available diagnostic data to determine status of his HIV/AIDS.

3. Determine if initiation of antiretroviral therapy is indicated. Evaluate the patient's ability to adhere to medications, daily routine, social support, and financial stability. *Is the patient taking any medications that may interfere with the individual components of potential regimens? Does the patient have medical insurance and prescription coverage?*

4. Develop a plan to assess the effectiveness and tolerability of antiretroviral therapy.

Patient Education

1. Educate the patient on HIV/AIDS disease and the importance of strict adherence to medication (the patient must ideally take his or her medications at the same time every day). Recommend a therapeutic regimen that is as easy as possible for the patient to take. Talk to the patient specifically about when and how the patient will be taking the medications. *What time do they eat meals? When do they wake up? What other medications are they taking at the same time?* Educate patients whether to take their medications with or without food.

2. Educate the patient on common adverse drug effects and a few of the key signs and symptoms of severe toxicity (i.e., jaundice and abacavir hypersensitivity reaction). Tell them to call their provider immediately if any of those symptoms occur. Make sure they have the correct telephone number for the clinic.

Abbreviations Introduced in This Chapter

ALT	Alanine aminotransferase
ARV	Antiretroviral
AST	Aspartate aminotransferase
CPK	Creatine phosphokinase
CVD	Cardiovascular disease
CYP	Cytochrome P-450 isoenzyme
D/C	Discontinue
DEXA	Dual-energy x-ray absorptiometry
DHHS	Department of Health and Human Services
ELISA	Enzyme-linked immunosorbent assay
GERD	Gastroesophageal reflux disease
HAART	Highly active antiretroviral therapy
HBeAg	Hepatitis B early antigen
HBV	Hepatitis B virus
HCV	Hepatitis C virus
HDL	High-density lipoprotein
HTN	Hypertension
IAS-USA	International AIDS Society-USA
IFA	Indirect immunofluorescence assay
LDL	Low-density lipoprotein
LFT	Liver function tests
MSM	Men who have sex with men
MTCT	Mother-to-child transmission
NNRTI	Nonnucleoside reverse transcriptase inhibitor
NRTI	Nucleoside reverse transcriptase inhibitor
NtRTI	Nucleotide reverse transcriptase inhibitor
PCP	Pneumocystis jiroveci (formerly carinii) pneumonia
PI	Protease inhibitor
PT	Prothrombin time
RT-PCR	Reverse transcriptase polymerase chain reaction
SIV	Simian immunodeficiency virus
T.bili	Total bilirubin
TDF	Tenofovir disoproxil fumarate
TG	Triglyceride
ULN	Upper limit of normal
WB	Western blot

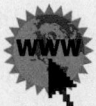 Self-assessment questions and answers are available at *http://www.mhpharmacotherapy.com/pp.html.*

REFERENCES

1. Gallo RC, Salahuddin SZ, Popovic M, et al. Frequent detection and isolation of cytopathic retroviruses (HTLV-III) from patients with AIDS and at risk for AIDS. Science 1984;224:500–503.

2. Centers for Disease Control and Prevention. HIV prevalence, unrecognized infection, and HIV testing among men who have sex with men—Five U.S. cities, June 2004-April 2005. MMWR 2005;54: 597–601.

3. Wawer MJ, Gray RH, Sewankambo NK, et al. Rates of HIV-1 transmission per coital act, by stage of HIV-1 infection, in Rakai, Uganda. J Infect Dis 2005;191:1403–1409.

4. Branson BM, Handsfield HH, Lampe MA, et al. Revised recommendations for HIV testing of adults, adolescents, and pregnant women in health-care settings. MMWR Recomm Rep 2006;55:1–17.

5. Panel on Antiretroviral Guidelines for Adults and Adolescents. Guidelines for the Use of Antiretroviral Agents in HIV-1 Infected Adults and Adolescents. Department of Health and Human Services. November 3, 2008:1–139. *http://www.aidsinfo.nih.gov/ContentFiles/AdultandAdolescentGL.pdf.*

6. Nerad J, Romeyn M, Silverman E, et al. General nutrition management in patients infected with human immunodeficiency virus. Clin Infect Dis 2003;36:S52–S62.

7. Hammer SM, Eron JJ, Reiss P, et al. Antiretroviral treatment of adult HIV infection: 2008 recommendations of the International AIDS Society-USA panel. JAMA 2008;300(5):555–570.

8. Baxter JD, Mayers DL, Wentworth DN, et al., for the CPCRA 046 Study Team for the Terry Beirn Community Programs for Clinical Research on AIDS. A randomized study of antiretroviral management based on plasma genotypic antiretroviral resistance testing in patients failing therapy. AIDS 2000;14:F83–F93.

9. Cohen CJ, Hunt S, Sension M, et al. A randomized trial assessing the impact of phenotypic resistance testing on antiretroviral therapy. AIDS 2002;16:579–588.

10. Durant J, Clevenbergh P, Halfon P, et al. Drug-resistance genotyping in HIV-1 therapy: The VIRADAPT randomised controlled trial. Lancet 1999;353:2195–2199.

11. Cingolani A, Antinori A, Rizzo MG, et al. Usefulness of monitoring HIV drug resistance and adherence in individuals failing highly active antiretroviral therapy: A randomized study (ARGENTA). AIDS 2002;16:369–379.

12. Meynard JL, Vray M, Morand-Joubert L, et al. Phenotypic or genotypic resistance testing for choosing antiretroviral therapy after treatment failure: A randomized trial. AIDS 2002;16:727–736.

13. Vray M, Meynard JL, Dalban C, et al. Predictors of the virological response to a change in the antiretroviral treatment regimen in HIV-1-infected patients enrolled in a randomized trial comparing genotyping, phenotyping and standard of care (Narval trial, ANRS 088). Antivir Ther 2003;8:427–434.

14. Wegner SA, Wallace MR, Aronson NE, et al. Long-term efficacy of routine access to antiretroviral-resistance testing in HIV type 1-infected patients: Results of the clinical efficacy of resistance testing trial. Clin Infect Dis 2004;38:723–730.

15. Tural C, Ruiz L, Holtzer C, et al. Clinical utility of HIV-1 genotyping and expert advice: The Havana trial. AIDS 2002;16:209–218.

16. Gallego O, Martin-Carbonero L, Aguero J, et al. Correlation between rules-based interpretation and virtual phenotype interpretation of HIV-1 genotypes for predicting drug resistance in HIV-infected individuals. J Virol Methods 2004;121:115–118.

17. Ravela J, Betts BJ, Brun-Vezinet F, et al. HIV-1 protease and reverse transcriptase mutation patterns responsible for discordances between genotypic drug resistance interpretation algorithms. J Acquir Immune Defic Syndr 2003;33:8–14.

18. Wensing A, Keulen W, Buimer M, et al. Analysis of the world-wide evaluation study on HIV-1 genotype interpretation: ENVA-3. Antivir Ther 2001;6:101.

19. Gulick RM, Hu XJ, Fiscus SA, et al. Randomized study of saquinavir with ritonavir or nelfinavir together with delavirdine, adefovir, or both in human immunodeficiency virus-infected adults with virologic failure on indinavir: AIDS Clinical Trials Group Study 359. J Infect Dis 2000;182:1375–1384.

20. Hammer SM, Vaida F, Bennett KK, et al. Dual vs single protease inhibitor therapy following antiretroviral treatment failure: A randomized trial. JAMA 2002;288:169–180.

21. Hoen B, Dumon B, Harzic M, et al. Highly active antiretroviral treatment initiated early in the course of symptomatic primary HIV-1 infection: Results of the ANRS 053 trial. J Infect Dis 1999;180:1342–1346.

22. Lafeuillade A, Poggi C, Tamalet C, et al. Effects of a combination of zidovudine, didanosine, and lamivudine on primary human immunodeficiency virus type 1 infection. J Infect Dis 1997;175:1051–1055.

23. Lillo FB, Ciuffreda D, Veglia F, et al. Viral load and burden modification following early antiretroviral therapy of primary HIV-1 infection. AIDS 1999;13:791–796.

24. Malhotra U, Berrey MM, Huang Y, et al. Effect of combination antiretroviral therapy on T-cell immunity in acute human immunodeficiency virus type 1 infection. J Infect Dis 2000;181:121–131.

25. Smith DE, Walker BD, Cooper DA, et al. Is antiretroviral treatment of primary HIV infection clinically justified on the basis of current evidence? AIDS 2004;18:709–718.

26. Working Group on Antiretroviral Therapy and Medical Management of HIV-Infected Children. Guidelines for the Use of Antiretroviral Agents in Pediatric HIV Infection. July 29, 2008. *http://aidsinfo.nih.gov/contentfiles/PediatricGuidelines.pdf*

27. Institute NYSDoHA. Drug-Drug Interactions Between HAART, Medications Used in Substance Use Treatment, and Recreational Drugs, 2008. *http://www.hivguidelines.org.*

28. Public Health Service Task Force. Recommendations for Use of Antiretroviral Drugs in Pregnant HIV-Infected Women for Maternal Health and Interventions to Reduce Perinatal HIV-1 Transmission in the United States. July 8, 2008. *http://aidsinfo.nih.gov/contentfiles/PerinatalGL.pdf*

29. Cohn SE, Watts D, Lertora J, Park JG, Yu S. Depo-medroxyprogesterone in women on antiretroviral thearpy: Effective contraception and lack of clinically significant interactions. Clin Pharmacol Ther 2007;81:222–227.

30. Koziel MJ and Peters MG. Viral hepatitis in HIV infection. N Engl J Med 2007;356:1445–1454.

31. Tien PC. Management and treatment of hepatitis C virus infection in HIV-infected adults: Recommendations from the Veterans Affairs Hepatitis C Resource Center Program and National Hepatitis C Program Office. Am J Gastroenterol 2005;100:2338–2354.

32. Rockstroh JK, Bhagani S, Benhamou Y, et al. European AIDS Clinical Society (EACS) guidelines for the clinical management and treatment of chronic hepatitis B and C coinfection in HIV-infected adults. HIV Med 2008;9:82–88.

88 Cancer Chemotherapy and Treatment

Dianne Brundage

LEARNING OBJECTIVES

● **Upon completion of the chapter, the reader will be able to:**

1. Describe the etiology of cancer.

2. Define the tumor, nodes, metastases (TNM) system of cancer staging.

3. Classify each drug used in the treatment of cancer, and compare and contrast the mechanisms of action, uses, and side effects.

4. Outline actions for all health care providers to prevent medication errors with cancer treatments.

5. Describe the role of the health care practitioner in the care of cancer patients.

KEY CONCEPTS

❶ The word cancer covers a diverse array of tumor types that affect a significant number of Americans and are a significant cause of mortality.

❷ Numerous cellular changes occur in the genetic material of the cancer cell so that programmed cell death, or **apoptosis,** does not occur. Proliferation of cancer cells goes unregulated.

❸ Many tumors are staged according to the tumor, nodes, metastases (TNM) system. Metastases are cancer cells that have spread to sites distant from the primary tumor site and have started to grow. The most frequently-occurring sites of metastases of solid tumors are the brain, bone, liver, and lungs.

❹ Each category of chemotherapy drugs has some similar side effects, usually on the most rapidly-growing cells of the body. However, there are unique toxicities of various pharmacologic categories of antineoplastic agents. Anthracyclines cause cardiac toxicity, which is related to the cumulative dose. Tubulin-interactive agents are associated with neuropathy and ileus. Alkylating agents are associated with secondary malignancies.

❺ Because of the severe toxicities associated with many of the chemotherapy agents, safety precautions must be in place to prevent chemotherapy errors, accidental chemotherapy exposures, and overdosages.

❻ Clinicians should play a role in chemotherapy safety, patient education, and monitoring patient response to therapy. For example, cumulative doses of anthracyclines should be monitored along with signs and symptoms of heart failure. Clinicians also should monitor for drug interactions between other current medications and chemotherapy agents.

EPIDEMIOLOGY

❶ *The word cancer covers a diverse array of tumors types that affect a significant number of Americans and are a significant cause of mortality.* The term *cancer* actually refers to more than 100 diseases. What is common to all cancers is that the cancerous cell has uncontrolled growth so that it invades tissues and spreads to other parts of the body, called **metastases.** In 2008, it was projected that over 1.4 million Americans will be diagnosed with cancer, and more than 565,000 Americans will die from the cancer.[1] Figure 88–1 describes cancers by gender, new cases, and deaths.

A cancer patient may encounter many different health care professionals: phlebotomists, pathologists, surgeons, medical and radiation oncologists, physician assistants, pharmacists, nurses, counselors, dieticians, social workers, and chaplains all may be involved with a single patient. The pharmacist's role may include recommendations of various pharmacologic agents, education of patients and family members, education of staff about new agents and safety issues, preparation of therapies, resolution of reimbursement issues, development of order sets, and participation in clinical trials. Each patient should have access to an interdisciplinary team to assist him or her during treatment.

Cancer treatments have exploded due to advances in technology in the last couple of decades. The fields of radiation therapy, surgery, and pharmaceuticals have had numerous developments, so patients are receiving not only less toxic treatments but also treatments that have improved outcomes over those of 15 years ago. Supportive-care therapies have

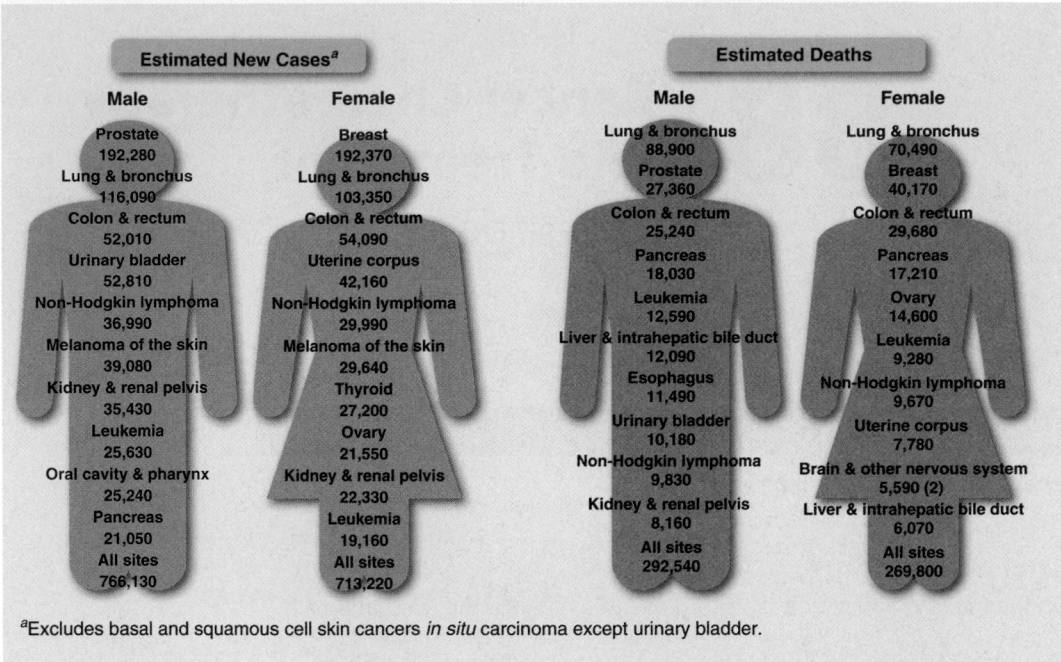

FIGURE 88–1. Cancer incidences (*left*) and deaths (*right*) in the United States for males and females estimated for 2009. (Reprinted with permission from American Cancer Society. Cancer facts and figures—2009. Atlanta: American Cancer Society; 2009.)

improved, so patients may be at less risk for toxicity and have a better **quality of life** than patients 10 to 15 years ago. In the early 1990s, most patients received chemotherapy in the hospital because of side effects. Today, most patients receive chemotherapy in the clinic and/or are taking oral agents at home.

Cancer Prevention

Because most cancers are not curable in advanced stages, cancer prevention is an important avenue of exploration. Both lifestyle modifications and chemoprevention agents ultimately may reduce the risk of developing cancer.

Tobacco

Tobacco smoking increases the risk of developing not only lung cancer but also many other types of cancer, including cancer of the bladder, mouth, pharynx, larynx, and esophagus. While the immediate benefit of smoking cessation is minimal for lung cancer, documented benefit has been observed 6 or more years after stopping.

Sun Exposure

Ultraviolet light and increased skin exposure may increase the risk of skin malignancies, especially in individuals who are fair-skinned. Practitioners can counsel patients to minimize skin exposure to the sun and to use strong sunscreens on exposed areas.

CARCINOGENESIS

The exact cause of cancer remains unknown and probably is very diverse given the vast array of diseases called cancer. It

is thought that cancer develops from a single cell in which the normal mechanisms for control of growth and proliferation are altered. Initiation occurs when a carcinogenic substance encounters a normal cell to produce genetic damage, or a mutated cell. Environmental or other factors that favor the growth of the mutated cell refer to promotion. Transformation occurs when the mutated cell becomes malignant, and progression occurs when cell proliferation takes over and the tumor spreads or develops metastases. Depending upon the type of cancer, many years may go by between the carcinogenic phases and the development of a clinically detectable tumor.

Carcinogenic agents include chemicals in the environment, such as aniline and benzene, which are associated with the development of bladder cancer and leukemia, respectively. Environmental factors, such as excessive sun exposure, also may result in cancer. Viruses, including the human papilloma virus and hepatitis B, may be associated with the development of cancer. Some of the chemotherapy agents cause secondary cancers after therapy has been completed. Numerous factors may contribute to the development of cancer. In addition to the carcinogenic agents mentioned, factors such as the patient's age, gender, diet, and chronic irritation or inflammation may be considered to be promoters of carcinogenesis.

Cancer Genetics

Because the human genome has been sequenced, and with the great improvements in genetic technology, there is an ever-increasing body of knowledge regarding the genetic changes of cancer. Currently, there are two major classes of genes involved in cancer: oncogenes and tumor-suppressor genes. Protooncogenes are normal genes that, through some genetic alteration caused by carcinogens, change into oncogenes. Protooncogenes are present in all normal cells and regulate cell function and replication. Genetic damage of the protooncogene may occur through point mutation, chromosomal rearrangement, or an increase in gene function, resulting in the oncogene. The oncogene produces abnormal or excessive gene product that disrupts normal cell growth and proliferation.[2] This may cause the cell to have a distinct growth advantage, increasing its likelihood of becoming cancerous. Table 88–1 provides examples of oncogenes.

Tumor-suppressor genes inhibit inappropriate cellular growth and proliferation by gene loss or mutation. This results in loss of control over normal cell growth. The *p53* gene is one of the most common tumor-suppressor genes, and mutations of *p53* may occur in up to 50% of all malignancies. This gene stops the cell cycle to enable "repairs" of the cell. If

p53 is inactivated, then the cell allows the mutations to occur. While mutations of the *p53* gene are found in many tumors, such as breast, colon, and lung cancer, it is also associated with drug resistance of cancer cells. DNA-repair genes fix errors in DNA that occur because of environmental factors or errors in replication and sometimes are referred to as *tumor-suppressor genes*. Mutations in DNA-repair genes have been reported in hereditary nonpolyposis colon cancer and in some breast cancer syndromes.

❷ *Numerous cellular changes occur in the genetic material of the cancer cell so that programmed cell death, or apoptosis, does not occur. Proliferation of cancer cells goes unregulated.* If mutations persist and cells aren't repaired or suppressed, cancer may develop. **Apoptosis,** or programmed cell death, may prevent the mutated cell from becoming cancerous.

Table 88–1

Examples of Oncogenes and Tumor-Suppressor Genes

Gene	Function	Associated Human Cancer
Oncogenes		
Genes for growth factors or their receptors		
EGFR or ERB-B1	Codes for EGFR	Glioblastoma, breast cancer, squamous carcinoma
HER-2/neu or ERB-B2	Codes for a growth factor receptor	Breast, salivary gland, prostate, bladder and ovarian cancers
RET	Codes for a growth factor receptor	Thyroid cancer
Genes for cytoplasmic relays in stimulatory signaling pathways		
KRAS	Codes for guanine nucleotide-proteins with GTPase activity	Lung, ovarian, colon, pancreatic binding cancers
NRAS		Neuroblastoma, acute leukemia
Genes for transcription factors that activate growth-promoting genes		
c-MYC		Leukemia and breast, colon, gastric, and lung cancers
N-MYC		Neuroblastoma, small cell lung cancer, and glioblastoma
Genes for cytoplasmic kinases		
BCR-ABL	Codes for a nonreceptor tyrosine kinase	Chronic myelogenous leukemia
Genes for other molecules		
BCL-2	Codes for a protein that blocks apoptosis	Indolent B-cell lymphomas
BCL-1 or PRAD1	Codes for cyclin D1, a cell cycle clock stimulator	Breast, head, and neck cancers
MDM2	Protein antagonist of *p53* tumor suppressor protein	Sarcomas
Tumor Suppressor Genes		
Genes for proteins in the cytoplasm		
APC	Step in a signaling pathway	Colon and gastric cancer
NF-1	Codes for a protein that inhibits the stimulatory *Ras* protein	Neurofibroma, leukemia, and pheochromocytoma
NF-2	Codes for a protein that inhibits the stimulatory *Ras* protein	Meningioma, ependymoma, and schwannoma
Genes for proteins in the nucleus		
MTS1	Codes for *p16* protein, a cyclin-dependent kinase inhibitor	Involved in a wide range of cancers
RB1	Codes for the *pRB* protein, a master brake of the cell cycle	Retinoblastoma, osteosarcoma, bladder, small cell lung, prostate, and breast cancers
p53	Codes for the *p53* protein, which can halt cell division and induce apoptosis	Involved in a wide range of cancers
Genes for protein whose cellular location is unclear		
BRCA1	DNA repair, transcriptional regulation	Breast and ovarian cancers
BRCA2	DNA repair	Breast cancer
VHL	Regulator of protein stability	Renal cell cancer
MSH2, MLH1, PMS1, PMS2, MSH6	DNA mismatch repair enzymes	Hereditary nonpolyposis colorectal cancer

EGFR, epidermal growth factor receptor.

From DiPiro JT, Talbert RL, Yee GC, et al. (eds.) Pharmacotherapy: A Pathophysiologic Approach. 6th ed. New York: McGraw-Hill; 2005: Table 124–2.

● Loss of *p53* and overexpression of *bcl-2* are two examples of changes within the cell that occur to result in enhanced cell survival. Cellular senescence refers to cell death that occurs after a preset number of cell doublings. Telomeres are DNA segments at the ends of chromosomes that shorten with each replication to the point where senescence is triggered.

Cancer genetics may be done on the tumor itself to determine if a particular drug will be effective, or if the patient will suffer toxicity. Table 88–2 presents the genetic tests currently recommended for either tumor or patient.

Principles of Tumor Growth

It takes about 10^9 cancer cells to be clinically detectable by palpation. Figure 88–2 demonstrates the classic Gompertzian

kinetics tumor-growth cycle. From the diagram, one can see that malignant cell growth occurs many times before a mass may be palpated. The number of malignant cells may plummet drastically because of surgery or in decreasing steps by each administration of chemotherapy. One dosing round, or cycle, of chemotherapy does not eliminate all malignant cells, and therefore, repeated cycles of chemotherapy are administered to eliminate tumor-cell burden. The cell kill hypothesis states that a fixed percentage of tumor cells will be killed with each cycle of chemotherapy. According to this hypothesis, the number of tumor cells will never reach zero. There are three assumptions to this theory: all cancers are equally responsive and drug resistance and metastases do not occur.

Metastases

A **metastasis** is a growth of the same cancer found at some distance from the primary tumor site.[3] The metastasis may be large, or it may be just a few cells that may be detected through polymerase chain reaction (PCR); however, the presence of metastasis at staging usually is associated with a poorer prognosis than the patient with no known metastatic disease. As the technology to find malignant cells evolves, the dilemma exists on how to treat patients based on current guidelines that were not based on cellular detection technology.

Cancers spread usually by two pathways: hematogenous (through the bloodstream) or through the lymphatics (drainage through adjacent lymph nodes). The malignant cells that split from the primary tumor find a suitable environment for growth. It is believed that malignant cells secrete mediators that stimulate the formation of blood vessels for growth and oxygen, the process of angiogenesis.

Table 88–2	
RECIST Criteria	
Term	**Description**
Complete response (CR)	Disappearance of all targeted lesions
Partial response (PR)	At least a 30% decrease in the sum of the longest diameter of target lesions from baseline
Progressive disease (PD)	At least a 20% increase in the sum of the longest diameter of target lesions from baseline, including new lesions discovered during treatment
Stable disease (SD)	Neither sufficient shrinkage to qualify for PR nor sufficient increase to qualify for PD

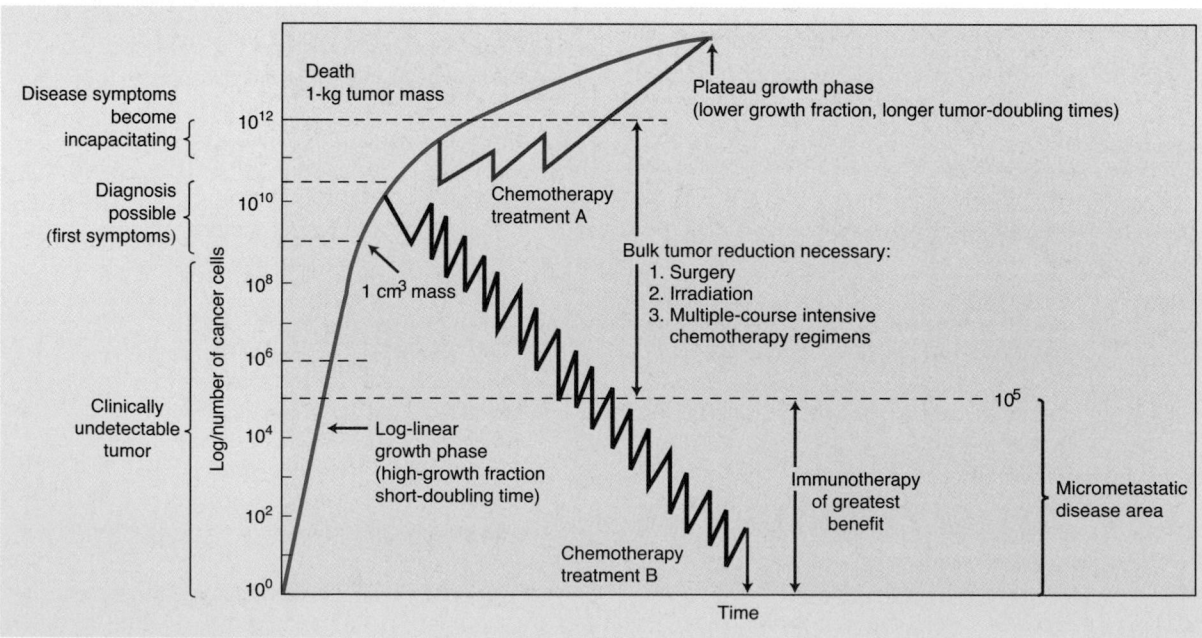

FIGURE 88–2. The Gompertzian growth curve demonstrating symptoms and treatments versus tumor volume. (From Buick RN. Cellular basis of chemotherapy. In: Dorr RT, Von Hoff DD, eds. Cancer Chemotherapy Handbook. 2nd ed. New York: Elsevier; 1994: 3–14.)

The usual metastatic sites for solid tumors are the brain, the bone, the lung, and the liver. It is important to realize and educate patients that breast cancer cells may metastasize to the brain, so the individual does not have brain and breast cancer but breast cancer with metastases to the brain.

PATHOPHYSIOLOGY

Tumor Characteristics

Tumors are either benign or malignant.[4] Benign tumors often are encapsulated, localized, and indolent; they seldom metastasize; and they recur rarely once removed. Histologically, the cells resemble the cells from which they developed. Malignant tumors are invasive and spread to other locations, even if the primary tumor is removed. The cells no longer perform their usual functions, and their cellular architecture changes. This loss of structure and function is called *anaplasia*. Despite improvements in screening procedures, many patients have metastatic disease at the time of diagnosis. Usually, once distant metastases have occurred, the cancer is deemed to be incurable.

Tumor Origin

Tumors may arise from epithelial, connective (i.e., muscle, bone, and cartilage), lymphoid, or nerve tissue. The suffix *-oma* is added to the name of the cell type if the tumor cells are benign. A *lipoma* is a benign growth that resembles fat tissue.

Precancerous cells have cellular changes that are abnormal but not yet malignant and may be described as *hyperplastic* or *dysplastic*. Hyperplasia occurs when a stimulus is introduced and reverses when the stimulus is removed. Dysplasia is an abnormal change in the size, shape, or organization of cells or tissues.

Malignant cells are divided into categories based on the cells of origin. Carcinomas arise from epithelial cells, whereas sarcomas arise from muscle or connective tissue. Adenocarcinomas arise from glandular tissue. *Carcinoma in situ* refers to cells limited to epithelial origin that have not yet invaded the basement membrane. Malignancies of the bone marrow or lymphoid tissue, such as leukemias or lymphomas, are named differently.

DIAGNOSIS OF CANCER

Cancer can present as a number of different signs and symptoms as well as pain and loss of appetite. Unfortunately, many people fear a diagnosis of cancer, and may not seek medical attention at the first warning signs, when the disease is at its most treatable stage. After the initial visit with the physician, a variety of tests will be performed, which are somewhat dependent on the initial differential diagnosis. Appropriate blood work, radiologic scans, and tissue sample are necessary. The sample of tissue may be obtained by a biopsy, fine-needle aspiration, or exfoliative cytology. No treatment of cancer should be initiated without a pathologic diagnosis of cancer. During the pathologic workup, cytogenetics may be done. Depending on the type of cancer, the cytogenetics can provide the additional information on prognosis of the malignancy, and whether certain therapies may be appropriate.

Once the pathology of cancer is established, then the staging of the disease is done before treatment is initiated. Each cancer disease chapter will discuss the specifics of staging of the disease. Cancer staging will be done according to the primary tumor size, extent of lymph node involvement, and the presence, or absence of metastases, or sometimes referred to the tumor, nodes, metastases (TNM) system (Table 88–3). The stage of the disease is a compilation of the primary tumor size, the nodal involvement, and metastases, and is usually referred to as stages I through IV. Not all cancers can be staged according to this system, but many of the solid tumors are classified this way.

Why are tumors staged? First, the stage of the disease is an important part of determining prognosis of the cancer. Second, staging of the cancers allows comparison of patient groups when examining data from clinical trials; staging reflects the extent of disease. Third, the clinician uses it as a guide to treatment, and may use restaging after treatment to guide further treatment.

Some cancers produce substances that are detected by a blood test, that may be useful in following response to therapy or detecting a recurrence; these are referred to as tumor markers. Unfortunately, some tumor markers are nonspecific and may be elevated from nonmalignant causes. Some tumors may express a marker in some patients, and not in others. The full role of tumor markers has not been fully elucidated.

TREATMENT

Desired Outcome

While at the time of surgery the surgeon may be able to remove all macroscopic disease, microscopic cells may be present near the surgical site or may have traveled to other parts of the body. When malignant cells have traveled to other parts of the body and become established there and are able to grow in this new environment, they are called metastatic cancer cells. Thus, for chemotherapy-sensitive diseases, systemic therapies may be administered after surgery to destroy these microscopic malignant cells; this is called *adjuvant therapy*. The goals of adjuvant therapy are to decrease recurrence of the cancer and to prolong survival. Chemotherapy may also be given prior to surgical resection of the tumor; this is referred to as neoadjuvant therapy. Chemotherapy given prior to surgery should decrease the tumor burden to be removed (which may result in a shorter surgical procedure) and make the surgery easier to perform because the tumor has shrunk away from vital organs or vessels. Neoadjuvant chemotherapy also gives the clinician an idea of the responsiveness of the tumor to that particular chemotherapy.

Chemotherapy may be given to cure cancers that are curable, or it may be given to help control the symptoms of an incurable cancer, which is referred to as palliative therapy.

Table 88–3

TNM Staging Classification System for Colorectal Cancer

Primary tumor (T)
T_x Primary tumor cannot be assessed
T_0 No evidence of primary tumor
T_{is} Carcinoma *in situ*: intraepithelial or invasion of lamina propria
T_1 Tumor invades submucosa
T_2 Tumor invades muscularis propria
T_3 Tumor invades through the muscularis propria into the subserosa, or into nonperitonealized pericolic or perirectal tissues
T_4 Tumor perforates the visceral peritoneum, and/or directly invades other organs or structures

Regional lymph nodes (N)
N_x Regional lymph nodes cannot be assessed
N_0 No regional lymph node metastasis
N_1 Metastasis in one to three pericolic or perirectal lymph nodes
N_2 Metastasis in four or more pericolic or perirectal lymph nodes

Distant metastasis (M)
M_x Presence of distant metastasis cannot be assessed
M_0 No distant metastasis
M_1 Distant metastasis

Stage	Grouping			Dukes	Modified Astler-Collier
Stage 0	T_{is}	N_0	M_0		
Stage 1	T_1	N_0	M_0	A	A
	T_2	N_0	M_0	A	B1
Stage IIA	T_3	N_0	M_0	B	B2
Stage IIB	T_4	N_0	M_0	B	B2, B3
Stage IIIA	T_{1-2}	N_1	M_0	C	C1–3
Stage IIIB	T_{3-4}	N_1	M_0	C	C1–3
Stage IIIC	Any T	N_2	M_0	C	C1–3
Stage IV	Any T	Any N	M_1	"D"	D

From DiPiro JT, Talbert RL, Yee GC, et al. (eds.) Pharmacotherapy: A Pathophysiologic Approach. 6th ed. New York: McGraw-Hill; 2005: Table 124–7.

Clinical Presentation and Diagnosis Cancer Chemotherapy and Treatment

Signs and Symptoms

The seven warning signs of cancer are:

- Change in bowel or bladder habits
- A sore that does not heal
- Unusual bleeding or discharge
- Thickening or lump in breast or elsewhere
- Indigestion or difficulty in swallowing
- Obvious change in wart or mole
- Nagging cough or hoarseness

The eight warning signs of cancer in children are:

- Continued, unexplained weight loss
- Headaches with vomiting in the morning
- Increased swelling or persistent pain in bones or joints
- Lump or mass in abdomen, neck, or elsewhere
- Development of a whitish appearance in the pupil of the eye
- Recurrent fevers not caused by infections
- Excessive bruising or bleeding
- Noticeable paleness or prolonged tiredness

Diagnostic Procedures

- Laboratory tests: CBC, lactate dehydrogenase (LDH), renal function, and liver function tests
- Radiologic scans: x-rays, CT scans, MRI, position-emission tomography (PET)
- Biopsy of tissue or bone marrow with pathologic evaluation
- Cytogenetics
- Tumor markers
- Staging determination of the primary tumor size, extent of lymph node involvement, and the presence or absence of metastases, or sometimes referred to the TNM system (Table 88–2). ❸ *Many tumors are staged according to the TNM system. Metastases are cancer cells that have spread to sites distant from the primary tumor site and have started to grow. The most frequently-occurring sites of metastasis are the brain, bone, liver, and lungs.*

Response

The responses to chemotherapy may be referred to as complete response (CR), partial response (PR), stable disease (SD), or disease progression. A cure in oncology implies that the cancer is completely gone, and the patient will have the same life expectancy as a patient without cancer. The World Health Organization response criteria were updated in 2000. The Response Evaluation Criteria in Solid Tumors (RECIST) is considered to be the standard criteria to evaluate a response to therapy (see Table 88–2). A CR refers to complete disappearance of all cancer for 1 month after treatment. A PR is defined as a 30% or greater decrease in tumor diameter along with no new disease for 1 month. The term overall objective response rate refers to the combination of PR and CR. SD occurs in a patient whose tumor size neither grows nor shrinks by the above criteria. Disease progression refers to tumor that has spread or the primary tumor that has increased in size by 20% while receiving treatment. Some cancers, such as leukemia, cannot be measured by size, so biopsy of the bone marrow provides a cellular indication of absence or presence of disease.

Cancer chemotherapy and the treatment of cancers are analogous to anti-infectives and the treatment of infections. Cancer cells may be sensitive to certain chemotherapy agents, but then with repeated exposure, the cells become resistant to treatment. The resistant cells then may grow and multiply. While tumors may be tested for chemotherapy sensitivity, this area is still developing. Today, tumor sensitivity can demonstrate tumor resistance so that needless exposure to an inadequate therapy and its toxicity can be avoided.

Tumor cells may become resistant when genetic changes occur during cell proliferation. Resistant cancer cells with the mdr-1 gene may possess a membrane-associated protein, p-glycoprotein, that facilitates efflux of chemotherapy agents out of the cells. Numerous attempts at blocking this efflux pump have been unsuccessful.

Nonpharmacologic Therapy

The three primary treatment modalities of cancer are surgery, radiation, and pharmacologic therapy. Surgery is useful to gain tissue for diagnosis of cancer and for treatment, especially those cancers with limited disease. Radiation plays a key role not only in the treatment and possible cure of cancer but also in palliative therapy. Together, surgery and radiation therapy may provide local control of symptoms of the disease. However, when cancer is widespread, surgery may play little or no role, whereas radiation therapy localized to specific areas may palliate symptoms.

Pharmacologic Therapy

Chemotherapy of cancer started in the early 1940s when nitrogen mustard was administered to patients with lymphoma. Since then, numerous agents have been developed for the treatment of different cancers.

Dosing of Chemotherapy

Chemotherapeutic agents typically have a narrow therapeutic index. Many chemotherapy agents have significant organ toxicities that preclude using larger and larger doses to treat the cancer. The doses of chemotherapy must be spaced out to allow the patient to recover from the toxicity of the chemotherapy; each period of chemotherapy dosing is referred to as a cycle. Each cycle of chemotherapy may have the same dosages, or the dosages may be modified based on toxicity, or a chemotherapy regimen may alternate from one set of drugs given during the first, third, and fifth cycles to another set of different drugs given during the second, fourth, and sixth cycles. Dose density of chemotherapy refers to shortening of the period between doses of chemotherapy. This can accomplish two things: First, the tumor has less time between doses of chemotherapy to grow, and second, patients receive chemotherapy over a shorter period of time and hopefully can get back to a normal life sooner. Usually dose-dense chemotherapy regimens require colony-stimulating factors to be administered to shorten the time of neutropenia. The chemotherapy regimens that are dose-dense tend to be adjuvant regimens, where the tumor burden is not measurable, and the cancer outcome is a cure. When a chemotherapy regimen is used as palliative therapy (to control symptoms), the dosages of chemotherapy should be decreased based on toxicity, or the interval between dosages should be lengthened to maintain quality of life.

Patient and tumor biology also affect how cancer therapy is dosed. Patients with a uridine diphosphate–glucuronosyltransferease 1A1 enzyme deficiency can have life-threatening diarrhea and complications from irinotecan. The patient may have a blood test prior to therapy to determine if there is a genetic problem prior to receiving irinotecan (see Table 88–4). In the case of the some of the monoclonal antibodies, flow cytometry results will reveal whether the tumor has the receptor where the drug will bind and exert the pharmacologic effect.

Another consideration of chemotherapy administration is the patient. Factors that affect chemotherapy selection and dosing are age, concurrent disease states, and performance status. Performance status can be assessed through either the Eastern Cooperative Oncology Group Scale or the Karnofsky Scale (Table 88–5). The patient is evaluated on whether he or she is active to bedridden most of the day; performance status is a very important prognostic factor for many types of cancer. If a patient has kidney dysfunction, and the chemotherapy is eliminated primarily by the kidney, dosing adjustments will need to be made. If a patient has had a myocardial infarction recently, the clinician will weigh the risks of anthracycline therapy against the benefit of the treatment of the cancer.

Another important consideration for treatment of cancers is reimbursement by third-party payors for off-label use of chemotherapy agents because of the high expense. The American Association of Cancer Centers (*www.accc-cancer.org*) provides a drug compendium quarterly to which clinicians may refer to verify coverage by Medicare based on

Table 88–4

Oncology Drugs With Valid Genomic Biomarkers

Biomarker	Drug	Approved Label Content
Biomarkers for selection of therapy		
c-kit	Imatinib	Imatinib is indicated for the treatment of patients with kit (CD117)-positive unresectable and/or metastatic malignant GIST
Chromosome 5 deletion	Lenalidomide	Lenalidomide is indicated for the treatment of patients with transfusion dependent anemia due to Low- or Intermediate-1-risk myelodysplastic syndromes associated with a deletion 5q cytogenetic abnormality with or without additional cytogenetic abnormalities
EGFR expression	Erlotinib, Panitumumab, Gefitinib Cetuximab	Erlotinib *EGFR* expression was determined using the *EGFR* pharmDx kit. In contrast to the 1% cut-off specified in the pharmDx kit instructions, a positive EGFR expression status was defined as having at least 10% of cells staining for EGFR. The pharmDx kit has not been validated for use in pancreatic cancer. An apparently larger effect, however, was observed in two subsets: patients with EGFR positive tumors (HR 0.68) and patients who never smoked (HR 0.42). Cetuximab (colon cancer) Patients enrolled in the clinical studies were required to have immunohisto-chemical evidence of positive EGFR expression using the DakoCytomation EGFR pharmDx test kit
HER-2/neu	Trastuzumab, Lapatinib	Detection of *HER-2* protein overexpression is necessary for selection of patients appropriate for trastuzumab and lapatinib therapy
Philadelphia chromosome	Busulfan, Dasatinib	Busulfan is clearly less effective in patients with chronic myelogenous leukemia who lack the Philadelphia (Ph1) chromosome Dasatinib is indicated for the treatment of adults with Philadelphia-chromosome-positive acute lymphoblastic leukemia (Ph+ ALL) with resistance or intolerance to prior therapy
PML/RAR fusion gene	Tretinoin	Initiation of therapy with tretinoin may be based on the morphological diagnosis of acute promyelocytic leukemia (APL). Confirmation of the diagnosis of APL should be sought by detection of the t (15; 17) genetic marker by cytogenetic studies. If these are negative, PML/ RAR (alpha) fusion should be sought using molecular diagnostic techniques. The response rate of other AML subtypes to tretinoin has not been demonstrated; therefore, patients who lack the genetic marker should be considered for alternative treatment
Biomarkers for preventing toxicity		
TPMT	Azathioprine, Mercaptopurine	Thiopurine methyltransferase deficiency or lower activity due to mutation at increased risk of myelotoxicity. TPMT testing is recommended and consideration be given to either genotype or phenotype patients for TPMT
UGT1A1	Irinotecan	Individuals who are homozygous for the UGT1A*28 allele are at increased risk for neutropenia following initiation of irinotecan treatment. A reduced initial dose should be considered for patients known to be homozygous for the UGT1A*28 allele. Heterozygous patients may be at increased risk of neutropenia; however clinical results have been variable that patients have been shown to tolerate normal starting doses
DPD deficiency	5-FU, Capecitabine	Rarely, unexpected, severe toxicity (e.g., stomatitis, diarrhea, neutropenia and neurotoxicity) associated with 5-fluorouracil has been attributed to a deficiency of dihydropyrimidine dehydrogenase (DPD) activity. A link between decreased levels of DPD and increased, potentially fatal toxic effects of 5-fluorouracil therefore cannot be excluded

ICD-9 codes. The drugs used according to FDA-approved indications are almost always reimbursed. If sufficient literature exists, an insurer may pay for an off-label use.

During the time of chemotherapy, patients will experience toxicity from it. The National Cancer Institute (NCI) has provided a standardized system for evaluating and grading the toxicity from chemotherapy to provide uniform grading of toxicity and evaluation of new agents and new regimens (see Table 88–6).

Combination Chemotherapy

Again, the analogy to antibiotic therapy can be made when deciding on monotherapy versus combination therapy for the treatment of cancer. The underlying principles of using combination therapy are to use (a) agents with different pharmacologic actions, (b) drugs with different organ toxicities, (c) agents that are active against the tumor and ideally synergistic when used together, and (d) agents that

Table 88–5

Performance Status Scales

Description: Karnofsky Scale	Karnofsky Scale (%)	Zubrod Scale (ECOG)	Description: ECOG Scale
No complaints; no evidence of disease	100	0	Fully active, able to carry on all predisease activity
Able to carry on normal activity; minor signs or symptoms of disease	90		
Normal activity with effort, some signs or symptoms of disease	80	1	Restricted in strenuous activity, but ambulatory and able to carry out work of a light or sedentary nature
Cares for self; unable to carry on normal activity or to do active work	70		
Requires occasional assistance but is able to care for most personal needs	60	2	Out of bed more than 50% of time; ambulatory and capable of self-care, but unable to carry out any work activities
Requires considerable assistance and frequent medical care	50		
Disabled; requires special care and assistance	40	3	In bed more than 50% of time; capable of only limited self-care
Severely disabled; hospitalization indicated, although death not imminent	30		
Very sick; hospitalization necessary; requires active supportive treatment	20	4	Bedridden; cannot carry out any self-care; completely disabled
Moribund; fatal processes progressing rapidly	10		
Dead	0		

ECOG, Eastern Cooperative Oncology Group.

Table 88–6

Selected NCI Common Toxicity Criteria

Toxicity	Grade 1	Grade 2	Grade 3	Grade 4	Grade 5
General	Mild	Moderate	Severe	Life-threatening	Death
Neutropenia	Lowest baseline: 1,500/mm^3 (1.5 × 10^9/L)	Less than 1,500–1,000/mm^3 (1.5–1 × 10^9/L)	Less than 1,000–500/mm^3 (1–0.5 × 10^9/L)	Less than 500/mm^3 (5 × 10^9/L)	
Thrombo-cytopenia	Lowest baseline: 75,000/mm^3 (75 × 10^9/L)	Less than 75,000–50,000/mm^3 (75–50 × 10^9/L)	Less than 50,000–25,000/mm^3 (50–25 × 10^9/L)	Less than 25,000 mm^3 (25 × 10^9/L)	Death
Diarrhea	Increase of less than 4 stools per day over baseline or mild increase in ostomy output	Increase of 4–6 stools per day over baseline, IV fluids indicated less than 24 hours moderate increase in ostomy output compared with baseline, not interfering with ADL	Increase of greater than or equal to 7 stools per day over baseline, incontinence, IV fluids greater than or equal to 24 hours; hospitalization; severe increase in ostomy output compared to baseline; interfering with ADL	Life-threatening consequences (e.g., hemo-dynamic collapse)	Death
Esophagitis	Asymptomatic pathologic, radiographic, or endoscopic findings only	Symptomatic altered eating/swallowing IV fluids indicated less than 24 hours	Symptomatic and severely altered eating/swallowing; IV fluids, tube feedings, or TPN indicated 24 hours or more	Life-threatening consequences	Death
Nausea	Loss of appetite without alteration in eating habits	Oral intake decreased without significant weight loss, dehydration or malnutrition; IV fluids indicated less than 24 hours	Inadequate oral caloric or fluid intake; IV fluids, tube feedings, or TPN indicated greater than 24 hours	Life-threatening consequences	Death
Vomiting	1 episode in 24 hours	2–5 episodes in 24 hours; IV fluids indicated less than 24 hours	6 episodes or more in 24 hours; IV fluids or TPN indicated greater than or equal to 24 hours	Life-threatening consequences	Death

NCI, National Cancer Institute.

From *http://ctep.cancer.gov.*

do not result in significant drug interactions (although these can be studied carefully and the interactions addressed). When two or more agents are used together, the development of resistance may be slowed, but increased toxicity may result. ❹ *Each category of chemotherapy drugs has similar side effects. Anthracyclines cause cardiac toxicity, which is related to the cumulative dose. Tubulin-interactive agents are associated with neuropathy and ileus. Alkylating agents are associated with secondary malignancies.*

Currently, anticancer agents are categorized by the mechanism of action. As depicted in Figure 88–3, different agents work in different parts of the cell.

Antimetabolites

▶ *Fluorouracil*

5-Fluorouracil, commonly referred to as 5-FU, is an analog of the pyrimidine uracil. It is metabolized by dihydropyrimidine dehydrogenase. 5-FU ultimately is metabolized to fluorodeoxyuridine monophosphate (FdUMP), which interferes with the function of thymidylate synthase, which is required for synthesis of thymidine. The triphosphate metabolite of 5-FU is incorporated into RNA to produce the second cytotoxic effect of 5-FU. It appears that inhibition of

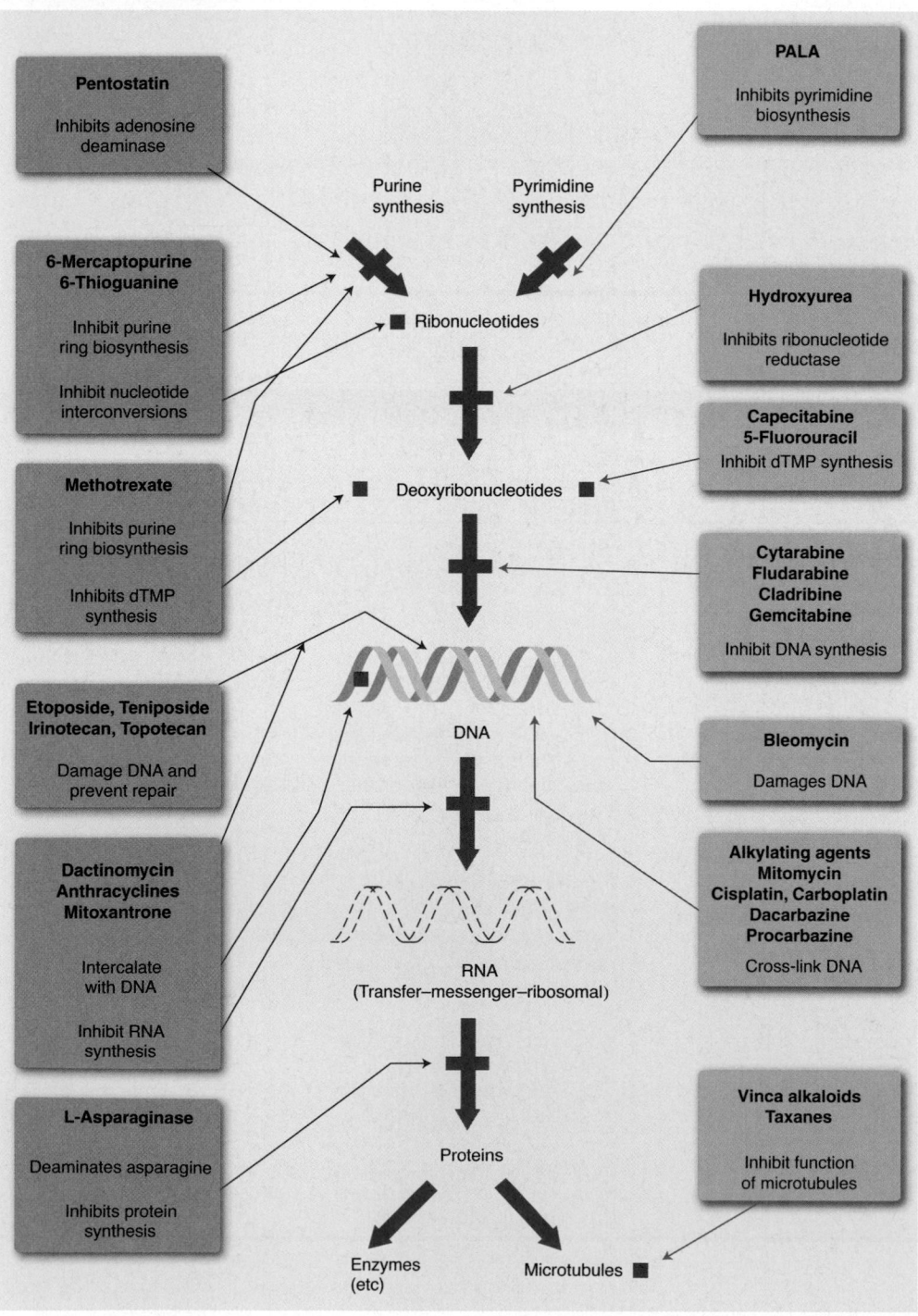

FIGURE 88–3. The mechanisms of action of antineoplastic agents. (From Chabner BA, Ryan DP, Paz-Ares L, et al. Antineoplastic agents. In: Hardman JG, Limbird LE, Gilman AG, eds. Goodman & Gilman's The Pharmacologic Basis of Therapeutics. 10th ed. New York: McGraw-Hill; 2001: 1381.)

thymidylate synthesis occurs with the continuous infusion regimens, whereas the triphosphate form is associated with bolus administration. Patients with low activity of dihydropyrimidine dehydrogenase appear to be at risk for life-threatening toxicities.[5] Folates appear to increase the stability of the FdUMP-thymidylate synthase inhibition, which enhances the activity of the drug in certain cancers. 5-FU has shown to be useful in the treatment of cancers of the colon, rectum, gastric, head and neck, and breast. 5-FU is metabolized extensively by the liver, whereas up to 15% of a dose may be found unchanged in the urine. The clearance of 5-FU ranges from 155 L/m²/h (range 56–466 L/m²/h) in women to 179 L/m²/h (range 29–739 L/m²/hr) in men. Age does not appear to alter the pharmacokinetics of 5-FU. 5-FU has shown clinical activity in the treatment of colorectal, breast, esophageal, pancreas, stomach, anal, and head and neck cancers. Side effects of 5-FU include stomatitis, diarrhea, cardiac abnormalities, and rarely reported cerebellar toxicities. Esophagitis and gastric ulcerations also may occur. Some alopecia may occur, but hair regrowth may occur with subsequent doses. A recent study demonstrated that if the patient uses ice chips in the mouth for 30 minutes while receiving bolus 5-FU, mucositis may be decreased significantly. Neurotoxicity may consist of headaches, visual disturbances and cerebellar ataxia. Cardiac toxicity may consist of ST-segment elevation, which appears to be more common in patients with a prior history of coronary artery disease.

▶ Capecitabine

Capecitabine is the prodrug of 5-FU and comes as oral tablets that are administered with food twice a day. Capecitabine has shown to be active in tumors of the colon, rectum, and breast. The toxicity profile of capecitabine is similar to that of 5-FU and includes diarrhea, mucositis, palmar-plantar erythrodyesthesia, nausea, and myelosuppression. Palmar-plantar erythrodyesthesia refers to redness, itching, and blistering of the palms of the hands and soles of the feet. Patients should be educated to notify the prescriber when palmar-plantar erythrodyesthesia occurs. Significant increases in International Normalization Ratio (INR) and prothrombin time may occur within several days when capecitabine is started in patients who are on warfarin, and the INR should be monitored closely, or the patient may be switched to a low–molecular weight heparin. Phenytoin levels may become elevated related to possible CYP2C9 inhibition by capecitabine. Patients should be instructed to take capecitabine within 30 minutes of a meal.

▶ Cytarabine

Cytarabine, often referred to as Ara-C, is an analog of cytosine and is phosphorylated intracellularly to the active triphosphate form, which inhibits DNA polymerase. The triphosphate form also may be incorporated into DNA to result in chain termination to prevent DNA elongation. The drug may be administered as a low-dose continuous infusion, high-dose intermittent infusion, and into the subdural space via intrathecal or intraventricular administration. There is also a liposomal formulation available for less-frequent administration into the CNS. Cytarabine pharmacokinetics are best described by a two-compartment model, with an α-half-life of 15 minutes and a β-half-life of 2 hours. Cytarabine is eliminated by the kidney with a renal clearance of 90 mL/min. Cytarabine has shown efficacy in the treatment of acute leukemias and some lymphomas. The toxicities of cytarabine in high doses include myelosuppression, cerebellar syndrome (i.e., nystagmus, dysarthria, and ataxia), and eye irritation that requires round-the-clock steroid eye drop administration. The risk of CNS toxicity is increased with the high-dose cytarabine regimen with renal dysfunction; dosage modification is necessary with the high-dose regimen with renal dysfunction.

▶ Gemcitabine

Gemcitabine is a deoxycytidine analog that is structurally related to cytarabine. Gemcitabine inhibits DNA polymerase activity and ribonucleotide reductase to result in DNA chain elongation. The pharmacokinetics of gemcitabine are best described by a two-compartment model, with a terminal half-life of 6 to 20 minutes. Approximately 5% of the dose is excreted unchanged by the kidney.[6] Gemcitabine has shown activity in cancers of the pancreas, breast, lung, ovary, and lung (nonsmall cell), along with some lymphomas. The toxicities include myelosuppression, flu-like syndrome with fevers during the first 24 hours after administration, rash that appears 48 to 72 hours after administration, and hemolytic uremic syndrome. While hemolytic uremic syndrome is uncommon, it is a life-threatening side effect. Patients should be counseled about using acetaminophen to treat the fevers during the first 24 hours; however, fevers occurring 7 to 10 days after gemcitabine are likely to be febrile neutropenias and need prompt treatment with broad-spectrum antibiotics.

▶ Azacitidine

Azacitidine, a cytidine analog, causes hypomethylation of DNA, which normalizes the function of genes that control cell differentiation to promote normal-cell maturation. The suspension is administered as a subcutaneous injection daily for 7 days for the treatment of myelodysplastic syndrome, a preleukemia disease. The pharmacokinetics of azacitidine are best described by a two-compartment model, with a terminal half-life of 3.4 to 6.2 hours, whereas peak concentrations are achieved 30 minutes after a subcutaneous injection.[7] Azacitidine has been shown to be clinically active in the treatment of myelodysplastic syndromes. The side effects include myelosuppression, renal tubular acidosis, renal dysfunction, and injection-site reactions.

▶ Decitabine

Decitabine, approved by the FDA in 2006 for the treatment of myelodysplastic syndrome, is incorporated into DNA and directly inhibits DNA methyltransferase which causes hypomethylation of DNA. The pharmacokinetics of decitabine are best described by a two-compartment model, with a terminal half-life of 0.5 hours. Side effects include myelosuppression, constipation, edema, headache, and nausea.

▶ *Nelarabine*

Nelarabine is indicated for the treatment of patients with T-cell acute lymphoblastic leukemia and T-cell lymphoblastic lymphoma, whose disease has been already treated with at least two other chemotherapy regimens. Nelarabine is a prodrug, which accumulates as the active 5′-triphosphate form in leukemic blasts to result in inhibition of DNA synthesis and cell death. The plasma half-life of nelarabine is approximately 30 minutes. Nelarabine is primarily metabolized by demethylation, with only 5% to 10% excreted unchanged by the kidney.

Purines and Purine Antimetabolites

▶ *6-Mercaptopurine*

6-Mercaptopurine (6-MP) is an oral purine analog that is converted to a ribonucleotide to inhibit purine synthesis. Mercaptopurine is converted into thiopurine nucleotides, which are catabolized by thiopurine *S*-methyltransferase (TPMT), which is subject to genetic polymorphisms and may cause severe myelosuppression. TPMT status may be assessed prior to therapy to reduce drug-induced morbidity and the costs of hospitalizations for neutropenic events. Mercaptopurine is poorly absorbed, with a time to peak concentration of 1 to 2 hours after an oral dose. The half-life is 21 minutes in pediatric patients and 47 minutes in adults. Mercaptopurine is used in the treatment of acute lymphocytic leukemia and chronic myelogenous leukemia. Significant side effects include myelosuppression, mild nausea, skin rash, and cholestasis. When allopurinol is used in combination with 6-MP, the dose of 6-MP must be reduced by 66% to 75% of the usual dose because allopurinol blocks the metabolism of 6-MP.

▶ *6-Thiogaunine*

6-Thioguanine (6-TG) is another oral purine analog that works similarly to 6-MP, and because of this, cross-resistance is observed. While little is known about the pharmacokinetics of thioguanine, it appears that absorption is incomplete and approximates 30% of the dose. Thioguanine may be used in the treatment of acute and chronic myelogenous leukemia. Side effects include myelosuppression, mild nausea, cholestasis, and rarely, veno-occlusive disease.

▶ *Fludarabine*

Fludarabine is an analog of the purine adenine. It interferes with DNA polymerase to cause chain termination and inhibits transcription by its incorporation into RNA. Fludarabine is dephosphorylated rapidly and converted to 2-fluoro-Ara-AMP (2-FLAA), which enters the cells and is phosphorylated to 2-fluoro-Ara-ATP, which is cytotoxic. Fludarabine is converted rapidly to 2-FLAA. The pharmacokinetics of 2-FLAA are best described by a two-compartment model, with an α-half-life of 0.6 hours and a terminal half-life of 9.3 hours.[8] Fludarabine is used in the treatment of chronic lymphocytic leukemia, some lymphomas, and refractory acute myelogenous leukemia. This drug is given IV usually daily for 5 days every 4 weeks. Significant myelosuppression may occur, along with immunosuppression, so patients are susceptible to opportunistic infections. Mild nausea and vomiting and diarrhea have been observed. Rarely, interstitial pneumonitis has occurred.

▶ *Cladribine*

Cladribine (2-chlorodeoxyadenosine, or 2-CDA) is a purine nucleoside that once it is in the triphosphate form is incorporated into DNA, which results in inhibition of DNA synthesis and chain termination. The pharmacokinetics of cladribine are best described by a two-compartment model, with an α-half-life of 35 minutes and a terminal half-life of 6.7 hours.[9] It may be administered as a continuous 7-day IV infusion or as a 2-hour infusion daily for 5 days; both regimens deliver the same total dose of drug. Cladribine is used to treat hairy cell leukemia and, therefore, is myelosuppressive. Unfortunately, one of the other side effects of the drug is fever, so the clinician struggles with the dilemma of whether the fever is due to the drug or an infection. Rash occurs in approximately 50% of patients with hairy cell leukemia. Cladribine also may be used to treat chronic lymphocytic leukemia, refractory low-grade non-Hodgkin's lymphoma, and Waldenström's macroglobulinemia.

▶ *Clofarabine*

Clofarabine was developed based on the structures of fludarabine and cladribine, with the hope it would be resistant to deamination by adenosine deaminase. Clofarabine has shown activity in myeloid leukemia and myelodysplastic syndrome.[10] The pharmacokinetics are best described by a two-compartment model with a terminal half-life of approximately 5.2 hours. Clofarabine is 47% bound to plasma proteins, primarily albumin. In children, 49% to 60% of the dose is excreted unchanged in the urine. No dosing adjustments are available for renal dysfunction. Side effects include bone marrow suppression, severe but transient liver dysfunction in 15% to 25% of patients, skin rashes, and hand-foot syndrome.

▶ *Pentostatin*

Pentostatin is an inhibitor of adenosine deaminase, an enzyme important in purine base metabolism. Pentostatin irreversibly inhibits adenosine deaminase, which ultimately is believed to block DNA synthesis through inhibition of RNA ribonucleotide reductase. The pharmacokinetics of pentostatin are best described by a two-compartment model with a half-life of 2.6 to 6 hours. While the drug is primarily eliminated unchanged by the kidney, preliminary data suggest no dosage adjustments are necessary for renal dysfunction. Side effects include bone marrow suppression, myalgias, conjunctivitis, and rash.

▶ Antifolates

Folates carry one-carbon groups in transfer reactions required for purine and thymidylic acid synthesis. Dihydrofolate reductase is the enzyme responsible for supplying reduced folates intracellularly for thymidylate and purine synthesis.

▶ Methotrexate

Methotrexate inhibits dihydrofolate reductase of both malignant and nonmalignant cells. When high doses of methotrexate are given, leucovorin, a reduced folate, is administered to bypass the methotrexate inhibition of dihydrofolate reductase of normal cells and is usually initiated 24 hours after methotrexate administration. For safety purposes, the term folinic acid, another term used for leucovorin, should not be used because of medication errors where folic acid was given instead. Methotrexate concentrations should be monitored to determine when to stop leucovorin administration. Generally, leucovorin administration may be stopped when methotrexate concentrations decrease to 5×10^{-8} M, although this may vary by the chemotherapy regimen. High dosages of methotrexate may cause methotrexate to crystallize out in the kidney, which may result in renal dysfunction and decreased methotrexate clearance. IV hydration with sodium bicarbonate to maintain urinary pH greater than or equal to 7 helps to prevent methotrexate-induced renal dysfunction. The pharmacokinetics of methotrexate are best described by either a two- or three-compartment model. The α-half-life is less than 1 hour, whereas the β-half-life is 3 to 4 hours, and the γ-half-life is 8 to 10 hours or longer with impaired kidney function. Approximately 60% to 100% of methotrexate is eliminated primarily as unchanged drug by the kidney. Since methotrexate is eliminated by tubular secretion, concomitant drugs that may inhibit or compete for tubular secretion should be avoided. Methotrexate doses must be adjusted for renal dysfunction. A recommended dosing adjustment is to divide the creatinine clearance of the patient by 70 mL/minute, which is the average creatinine clearance of patients who received methotrexate during clinical trials, and then to multiple this fraction by the dosage recommended for that disease state. Again, close monitoring of methotrexate concentrations in patients with renal impairment is advised. Methotrexate has shown activity in lymphoma, gastric, esophageal, bladder, and breast cancer and acute lymphocytic leukemia. Side effects of methotrexate include myelosuppression, nausea and vomiting, and mucositis. Methotrexate also may be administered via the intrathecal route in very low doses as small as 12 mg to doses of 20 g IV, so it is crucial for the clinician to know the correct dose by the correct route in order to avoid substantial toxicity. Methotrexate is also administered as an intrathecal injection into the cerebrospinal fluid or directly into the ventricle via an Ommaya reservoir. The methotrexate used for intrathecal and intraventricular injection must be preservative free. Drugs that may block the tubular secretion of methotrexate include probenecid, salicylates, penicillin G, and ketoprofen.

▶ Pemetrexed

Pemetrexed inhibits at least three pathways in thymidine and purine synthesis. Pemetrexed is excreted primarily as unchanged drug by the kidney, with 70% to 90% of a dose recovered in 24 hours as unchanged drug in the urine. Patients with normal kidney function have a half-life of 3.5 hours.[11] Pemetrexed has shown activity in the treatment of mesothelioma and nonsmall cell lung cancer. Side effects include myelosuppression, rash, diarrhea, and nausea and vomiting. Patients should receive folic acid and cyanocobalamin to reduce bone marrow toxicity and diarrhea. Doses of folic acid of at least 400 mcg/day starting 5 days before treatment and continuing throughout therapy, as well as for 21 days after the last pemetrexed dose, have been used. Cyanocobalamin 1,000 mcg is given intramuscularly the week prior to pemetrexed and then every three cycles thereafter. Dexamethasone 4 mg twice daily the day before, the day of, and the day after pemetrexed administration helps to decrease the incidence and severity of rash.

Tubulin Active Agents

The periwinkle, or vinca plant, served as a source for the drugs vincristine and vinblastine, which are commonly referred to as the vinca alkaloids. The vinca alkaloids inhibit the assembly of microtubules, which interferes in the formation of the mitotic spindle. Care must be taken not to confuse the names and doses of vincristine and vinblastine.

▶ Vincristine

Vincristine causes mitotic inhibition to arrest cells in metaphase. The pharmacokinetics of vincristine have been described by a three-compartment model, with an α-half-life of 0.8 minutes, a β-half-life of 7 minutes, and an α-half-life of 164 minutes.[12] Biliary excretion accounts for a significant portion of elimination of vincristine and its metabolites, so doses need to be adjusted for obstructive liver disease. Vincristine has been useful in the treatment of sarcomas, Wilms' tumor, many kinds of lymphoma, multiple myeloma, and acute lymphocytic leukemia. Vincristine is a vesicant that may cause significant neuropathy. Patients should be counseled regarding prevention of constipation and ileus caused by vincristine. Many clinicians cap IV vincristine doses at 2 mg to prevent severe neuropathic side effects, however, if the intent of chemotherapy is curative, the vincristine dose is often not capped at 2 mg. Several patients have died as a result of vincristine being administered intrathecally; it should only be administered IV and appropriate labeling should be placed on all doses. Itraconazole has been reported to cause severe neurotoxicity when administered to patients receiving vincristine. Patients have been reported to experience paralytic ileus, neurogenic bladder, absence of deep reflexes, and severe paralysis of the lower extremities within 10 days of starting itraconazole. Clinicians need to be aware of the potential interactions of the newer azoles with vincristine and the agents should only be used in combination when the benefit clearly outweighs the risk In most cases, alternative antifungals can be administered.

▶ Vinblastine

Vinblastine is another vesicant vinca alkaloid that causes myelosuppression and less neurotoxicity than vincristine. The pharmacokinetics of vinblastine are best described by a three-compartment model, with an α-half-life of 25 minutes, a β-half-life of 53 minutes, and a terminal half-life of 19 to 25 hours.[13] Vinblastine has shown activity in the treatment of bladder, breast, and kidney cancer, as well as some lymphomas. The doses of vinblastine tend to be higher on a milligram per meter squared basis than vincristine. Nausea and vomiting are minimal with vinblastine. Other side effects include mild alopecia, rash, photosensitivity, and stomatitis.

▶ Vinorelbine

The vesicant vinorelbine is structurally similar to vincristine and may cause many of the same side effects as vincristine. Vinorelbine is administered IV over 6 to 10 minutes, and patients should be counseled about neuropathy, ileus, and myelosuppression. The pharmacokinetics of vinorelbine are best described by a three-compartment model, with an α-half-life of 2 to 6 minutes, a β-half-life of 1.9 hours, and a γ-half-life of 40 hours. Vinorelbine has shown efficacy in the treatment of breast cancer and non–small cell lung cancer. Additional side effects include myelosuppression, paresthesias, and mild nausea and vomiting.

▶ Paclitaxel

Paclitaxel, a taxane, binds to tubulin to promote microtubule assembly and to prevent microtubule disassembly. The pharmacokinetics of paclitaxel can be described by a two-compartment model, with an α-half-life of 30 to 45 minutes and a β-half-life of 4 to 8 hours. Hepatic metabolism and biliary excretion account for the majority of paclitaxel's elimination. Paclitaxel has demonstrated activity in ovarian, breast, nonsmall cell lung, prostate, esophageal, gastric, and head and neck cancers. Considerable variability exists in paclitaxel dosing, from weekly 1-hour infusions to 24-hour infusions administered every 3 weeks. The diluent for paclitaxel, Cremophor EL, is composed of ethanol and castor oil. Infusions must be prepared and administered in non-PVC–containing bags and tubings, and solutions must be filtered. Patients receive dexamethasone, diphenhydramine, and an H_2 blocker to prevent hypersensitivity reactions from paclitaxel/Cremophor EL. Patients also may have asymptomatic bradycardia (i.e., heart rates around 45 bpm) during the infusion. Approximately 3 to 5 days after administration, patients may complain of myalgias and arthralgias that may last several days. Myelosuppression, flushing, neuropathy, ileus, and total-body alopecia are

other common side effects. Because paclitaxel is a substrate for CYP 3A4, steady-state concentrations of paclitaxel were 30% lower in patients receiving phenytoin than in patients not receiving phenytoin. Paclitaxel clearance was decreased by 33% when it was administered following cisplatin, so paclitaxel is administered before cisplatin.

Recently, a nanoparticle albumin-bound paclitaxel product became available commercially for the treatment of metastatic breast cancer. This product does not have the serious allergic reactions encountered with paclitaxel in Cremophor EL, so premedication with H_1 and H_2 blockers and steroids is not necessary. The dose is infused over 30 minutes and does not require a special IV bag, tubing, or filter. The dosing of this product is different from that of the original paclitaxel, so practitioners need to be aware of which product is being prescribed. The pharmacokinetics of the albumin-bound paclitaxel display a higher clearance and larger volume of distribution than paclitaxel. The drug is eliminated primarily via fecal excretion.[14] The side effects of bone marrow suppression, neuropathy, ileus, arthralgias, and myalgias still occur.

▶ Docetaxel

Docetaxel, a semi-synthetic taxane, binds to tubulin to promote microtubule assembly. The pharmacokinetics of docetaxel are best described by a three-compartment model, with an α-half-life of 0.08 hours, a β-half-life of 1.6 to 1.8 hours, and a terminal half-life of 65 to 73 hours.[15] Docetaxel has activity in the treatment of breast, nonsmall cell lung, prostate, bladder, esophageal, stomach, ovarian, and head and neck cancers. Dexamethasone, 8 mg twice daily for 3 days starting the day before treatment, is used to prevent the fluid-retention syndrome associated with docetaxel and possible hypersensitivity reactions. The fluid-retention syndrome is characterized by edema and weight gain that is unresponsive to diuretic therapy and is associated with cumulative doses greater than 800 mg/m². Myelosuppression, alopecia, and neuropathy are other side effects associated with docetaxel treatment.

▶ Estramustine

Estramustine, an oral drug, also inhibits microtubule assembly and has weak estrogenic activity at the estradiol hormone receptors of the cell. Approximately 75% of a dose of estramustine is absorbed.[16] The terminal half-life ranges between 20 and 24 hours, with nonrenal excretion as the major route of elimination. This drug is used primarily for the treatment of prostate cancer, but its use is limited by the side effects, which include nausea and vomiting, diarrhea, thromboembolic events, and gynecomastia.

▶ Ixabepilone

Ixabepilone, an epothilone analog, bind to β-tubulin sub-units on microtubules which leads to suppression of microtubule dynamics. Ixabepilone is primarily eliminated by the liver by oxidation through the CYP3A4 system, with a terminal half-life of 52 hours. Approximately 5% of the drug is excreted unchanged by the kidney. Ixabepilone is indicated for the treatment of metastatic or locally advanced breast cancer after failures of anthracyclines and a taxane. Side effects include hypersensitivity reactions, myelosuppression, and peripheral neuropathy. To minimize the occurrence of hypersensitivity reactions, patients must receive both H1 and H2 antagonists prior to therapy. If a reaction still occurs, corticosteroids should be added to the premedications.

Topoisomerase Inhibitors

Topoisomerase is responsible for relieving the pressure on the DNA structure during unwinding by producing strand breaks. Topoisomerase I produces single-strand breaks, whereas topoisomerase II produces double-strand breaks.

▶ Etoposide

Etoposide causes multiple DNA double-strand breaks by inhibiting topoisomerase II. The pharmacokinetics of etoposide are described by a two-compartment model, with an α-half-life of 0.5 to 1 hour and a β-half-life of 3.4 to 8.3 hours. Approximately 30% of the dose is excreted unchanged by the kidney.[17] Etoposide has shown activity in the treatment of several types of lymphoma, testicular and lung cancer, retinoblastoma, and carcinoma of unknown primary. The IV preparation has limited stability, so final concentrations should be 0.4 mg/mL. IV administration needs to be slow to prevent hypotension. Oral bioavailability is approximately 50%, so oral dosages are approximate two times those of IV doses; however, relatively low oral daily dosages are used for 1 to 2 weeks. Side effects include mucositis, myelosuppression, alopecia, phlebitis, hypersensitivity reactions, and secondary leukemias.

▶ Teniposide

Teniposide, a topoisomerase-II inhibitor, is administered as an infusion over 30 to 60 minutes to prevent hypotension. The pharmacokinetics are described by a three-compartment model, with an α-half-life of 0.75 hours, a β-half-life of 4 hours, and a terminal half-life of 20 hours. Considerable variability in clearance of teniposide in children has been reported.[18] Teniposide has shown activity in the treatment of acute lymphocytic leukemia, neuroblastoma, and non-Hodgkin's lymphoma. Side effects include myelosuppression, nausea, vomiting, mucositis, and venous irritation. Hypersensitivity reactions may be life-threatening.

▶ Irinotecan

Irinotecan, a camptothecin analog, inhibits topoisomerase I to interfere with DNA synthesis through the active metabolite SN38, which is 100-fold more potent in vitro. The pharmacokinetics of irinotecan are best described by a three-compartment model, with an α-half-life of 0.07 hours, a β-half-life of 2.2 hours, and a terminal half-life of about 18 hours.[19] Irinotecan has shown activity in the treatment of cancers of the colon, rectum, cervix, and lung. Irinotecan induced diarrhea may be life-threatening. IV atropine should be used to treat diarrhea that occurs during the first 24 hours of administration. Loperamide, 2 mg every 2 hours or 4 mg every 4 hours until diarrhea has stopped for 12 hours, should be used for diarrhea occurring for more than 24 hours after administration. Other side effects include myelosuppression, fatigue, and alopecia. Individuals homozygous for *UGT1A1*28* have an increased risk of febrile neutropenia and diarrhea and should be considered for an upfront dose reduction of one level; and heterozygotes should receive closer monitoring, including more frequent CBC.

▶ Topotecan

Topotecan inhibits topoisomerase I to cause single-strand breaks in DNA. The pharmacokinetics of topotecan can be described by a two-compartment model, with a terminal half-life of 80 to 180 minutes, with renal clearance accounting for approximately 70% of the clearance.[20] Topotecan has shown clinical activity in the treatment of ovarian and lung cancer, myelodysplastic syndromes, and acute myelogenous leukemia. The IV infusion may be daily for 5 days or once weekly. Side effects include myelosuppression, mucositis, and diarrhea.

Anthracyclines

All the anthracyclines contain a four-membered anthracene ring, a chromophore, with an attached sugar portion. Free radicals formed from the anthracyclines combine with oxygen to form superoxide, which can make hydrogen peroxide. Oxygen-free-radical formation is a cause of cardiac damage and extravasation injury, which is common to these drugs. Daunorubicin, doxorubicin, epirubicin, and idarubicin cause cardiac toxicity, as manifested by a congestive heart failure/cardiomyopathy symptomotology, mucositis, and myelosuppression. These drugs are vesicants; significant tissue damage may occur with extravasation.

▶ Daunorubicin

Daunorubicin is an anthracycline that is sometimes referred to as an antitumor antibiotic. Daunorubicin inserts between base pairs of DNA to cause structural changes in DNA; however, the primary mechanism of cytotoxicity is the inhibition of topoisomerase II. The pharmacokinetics are best described by a two-compartment model, with a terminal half-life of about 20 hours. The predominant route of elimination of daunorubicin and hydroxylated metabolites is hepatobiliary secretion. Daunorubicin has shown clinical activity in the treatment of acute lymphocytic leukemia, non-Hodgkin's lymphoma, neuroblastoma, and Ewing's and Kaposi's sarcomas. Myelosuppression is the major toxicity, along with alopecia, stomatitis, and mild to moderate nausea and vomiting, and it imparts a red to color to the urine so that patients need to be educated on side effects. Cardiac toxicity is dose related and manifested as congestive heart failure. To reduce the risk of cardiotoxicity, the maximum cumulative dose in children older than 2 years of age is 300 mg/m^2, and the cumulative dose is 400 to 600 mg/m^2 in adults. Ventricular ejection fractions should be measured before therapy, and periodically if therapy is continued. Therapy should be halted if there is a 10% to 20% decrease from baseline in ejection fraction. Daunorubicin is a vesicant also.

▶ Doxorubicin

The addition of a hydroxyl group to daunorubicin, resulted in the drug hydroxydaunorubicin (the H in CHOP therapy), or doxorubicin, which inhibits topoisomerase II. The pharmacokinetics of doxorubicin may be described by either a two- or three-compartment model, with a terminal half-life of 30 to 40 hours. Doxorubicin is metabolized extensively, and doxorubicinol, a major metabolite, is also a cardiotoxin. Biliary excretion accounts for about 40% of a dose; patients with cholestasis experience greater toxicity from standard doses. Doxorubicin has shown clinical activity in breast, esophageal, bladder, lung, ovarian, and head and neck cancers, along with lymphomas and multiple myeloma. This red drug causes a red-orange discoloration of the urine. Cumulative doses greater than 550 mg/m^2 are associated with cardiomyopathy. Doxorubicin is a vesicant and may cause significant pain when administered into the peritoneal cavity. Other side effects include myelosuppression, alopecia, mucositis, and nausea and vomiting.

▶ Doxorubicin, Liposomal

Liposomal doxorubicin is an irritant, not a vesicant, and is dosed differently from doxorubicin, so clinicians need to be very careful when prescribing these two drugs. The pharmacokinetics of liposomal doxorubicin are best described by a two-compartment model, with a terminal half-life of 30 to 90 hours.[21] Liposomal doxorubicin has shown significant activity in the treatment of breast and ovarian cancer, along with multiple myeloma and Kaposi's sarcoma. Side effects include mucositis, myelosuppression, alopecia, and palmar-plantar erythrodysesthesia. The liposomal doxorubicin may be less cardiotoxic than doxorubicin.

▶ Epirubicin

Epirubicin inhibits both DNA and RNA polymerases and thus inhibits nucleic-acid synthesis and topoisomerase-II enzymes. Epirubicin pharmacokinetics are best described by a three-compartment model, with an α-half-life of 4 to 5 minutes, a β-half-life of 2.4 hours, and a terminal half-life of 30 hours. Dosage alterations should be made in the presence of cholestasis because approximately 35% of a dose undergoes biliary excretion.[22] Epirubicin has shown clinical activity in the treatment of breast, esophageal, lung, ovarian, and stomach cancers. Epirubicin also has been used in the treatment of lymphomas and soft-tissue sarcomas. Cumulative doses of epirubicin greater than 900 mg/m^2

are associated with cardiomyopathy, so this drug may be less cardiotoxic on a milligram-per-milligram basis than doxorubicin. This topoisomerase-II inhibitor may cause red-orange urine, myelosuppression, alopecia, and significant nausea and vomiting.

▶ Idarubicin

Idarubicin inhibits both DNA and RNA polymerase, as well as topoisomerase II. The pharmacokinetics of idarubicin can best be described by a three-compartment model, with an α-half-life of 13 minutes, a β-half-life of 2.4 hours, and a terminal half-life of 16 hours.[23] Idarubicin is metabolized to an active metabolite, idarubicinol, which has a half-life of 41 to 69 hours. Idarubicin and idarubicinol are eliminated by the liver and through the bile. Idarubicin has shown clinical activity in the treatment of acute leukemias, chronic myelogenous leukemia, and myelodysplastic syndromes. Idarubicin causes cardiomyopathy at cumulative doses of greater than 150 mg/m^2 and produces cumulative cardiotoxic effects with other anthracyclines. Idarubicin is a vesicant and causes red-orange urine, mucositis, mild to moderate nausea and vomiting, and bone marrow suppression.

▶ Mitoxantrone

This royal-blue-colored drug is an anthracenedione that inhibits DNA topoisomerase II. The pharmacokinetics of mitoxantrone may best be described by a three-compartment model, with an α-half-life of 3 to 10 minutes, a β-half-life of 0.3 to 3 hours, and a median terminal half-life of 12 days. Biliary elimination appears to be the primary route of elimination, with less than 10% of the drug eliminated by the kidney.[24] Mitoxantrone has shown clinical activity in the treatment of acute leukemias, breast and prostate cancer, and

---

Patient Encounter 1

AB is a 40-year-old white woman who went to urgent care because she has not been feeling well for a couple of days and has a fever. Her WBC results are greater than 100×10^9/L (100×10^3/μL) with greater than 85% blast cells, which is indicative of acute leukemia. AB is admitted directly to the hospital to start chemotherapy.

The oncologist prescribes the normal doses of idarubicin 12 mg/m^2 IV daily for 3 days and cytarabine 100 mg/m^2/day by continuous infusion for 7 days to treat her acute myelogenous leukemia. Her baseline laboratory measurements are significant for an elevated WBC, a creatinine concentration of 2.5 mg/dL (221 μmol/L), and a bilirubin level of 1.6 mg/dL (27 μmol/L).

Should her chemotherapy dosages be adjusted? If so, how would you adjust the dosages?

What should be monitored while she is receiving her chemotherapy?

non-Hodgkin's lymphomas. Myelosuppression, mucositis, nausea and vomiting, and cardiac toxicity are side effects of this drug. The total cumulative dose limit is 160 mg/m² for patients who have not received prior anthracycline or mediastinal radiation. Patients who have received prior doxorubicin or daunorubicin therapy should not receive a cumulative dose greater than 120 mg/m² of mitoxantrone. Patients should be counseled that their urine will turn a blue-green color.

Alkylating Agents

The alkylating drugs are the oldest category of chemotherapy agents. Alkylating agents add a alkyl group to the DNA, which , inhibits DNA replication because interlinked strands do not separate.

▶ Busulfan

Busulfan is an alkylating agent that forms DNA-DNA and DNA-protein cross-links to inhibit DNA replication. Oral busulfan is well absorbed, has a terminal half-life of 2 to 2.5 hours, and is eliminated primarily by metabolism. Busulfan has shown significant clinical activity in the treatment of acute myelogenous leukemia and chronic myelocytic leukemia. Side effects include bone marrow suppression, hyperpigmentation of skin creases, and rarely, pulmonary fibrosis. High doses used for bone marrow transplant preparatory regimens result in severe nausea and vomiting, tonic-clonic seizures, and sinusoidal obstruction syndrome (formerly known as *veno-occlusive disease*). Patients receiving high-dose busulfan should receive anticonvulsant prophylaxis.

▶ Cyclophosphamide

Cyclophosphamide prevents cell division by cross-linking DNA strands. Cyclophosphamide is activated to phosphoramide mustard and acrolein. Acrolein, which has no tumor activity, causes hemorrhagic cystitis of the bladder. The pharmacokinetics of cyclophosphamide are best described by a two-compartment model, with a terminal half-life that ranges from 4 to 10 hours. Approximately 15% of the dose is excreted unchanged by the kidney. Cyclophosphamide has shown clinical activity in numerous types of cancer, ranging from leukemias to lymphomas to breast and ovarian cancer. Whether the drug is administered orally or IV, patients need to be counseled on the importance of good hydration and frequent voiding to prevent hemorrhagic cystitis. Nausea and vomiting may occur 12 hours after administration, so patients need to have antiemetics available after the acute treatment period. Other side effects include myelosuppression, alopecia, SIADH (usually with doses greater than 50 mg/kg), secondary malignancies (e.g., bladder cancers and acute leukemias), and infertility issues.

▶ Ifosfamide

Hemorrhagic cystitis is such a predominant side effect of the alkylator ifosfamide that mesna always must be given with ifosfamide, along with hydration. Dosing regimens of mesna

Patient Encounter 2

JP is receiving a highly myelosuppressive chemotherapy regimen for the next 3 days for his lymphoma. The chemotherapy orders specify ifosfamide, carboplatin, and etoposide. The goal of this cycle of chemotherapy is to put the cancer into remission so that his lymphoma can be cured with a bone marrow transplant.

What drug is missing from his ifosfamide orders?

What instructions should the patient receive about ifosfamide?

range from an equal milligram dose to the ifosfamide mixed in the same IV bag to 20% of the dose prior to ifosfamide and 20% of the dose repeated at 4 and 8 hours after the dose. The pharmacokinetics of ifosfamide are best described by a one-compartment model, with a terminal half-life of 7 to 15 hours. Approximately 50% of a dose is excreted unchanged by the kidney. Ifosfamide has shown clinical activity in the treatment of acute lymphocytic leukemia, lymphomas, and breast, ovarian, lung, and head and neck cancers. CNS side effects of confusion, delirium, and somnolence are associated with high doses infused quickly.

▶ Carmustine

Carmustine, a nitrosurea, cross-links DNA strands to inhibit DNA replication. Carmustine, which is reconstituted with ethanol, crosses the blood–brain barrier when given IV. It also comes as a wafer formulation that may be implanted surgically for brain tumors. The pharmacokinetics are best described by a two-compartment model, with an α-half-life of 6 minutes and a terminal half-life of 21 minutes.[25] Carmustine has shown clinical activity in the treatment of lymphoma, melanoma, and brain tumors. Side effects include myelosuppression, severe nausea and vomiting, and pulmonary fibrosis with long-term therapy.

▶ Lomustine

Lomustine is an orally available nitrosurea alkylating agent. Lomustine is converted rapidly to the *cis*- and *trans*-4-hydroxy metabolites; the range of half-lives of these two metabolites is 2 to 4 hours.[26] Lomustine has shown clinical activity in the treatment of non-Hodgkin's lymphoma and melanoma. Side effects are similar to those of carmustine. Patients should receive only enough drug for one cycle at a time to prevent confusion and accidental overdose.

▶ Dacarbazine

While the exact mechanism of action remains unclear, dacarbazine appears to inhibit DNA, RNA, and protein synthesis. Dacarbazine disappears rapidly from the plasma, with a terminal half-life of about 40 minutes. Dacarbazine has shown clinical benefit in the treatment of melanoma,

Hodgkin's lymphoma, and soft-tissue sarcomas. Side effects include myelosuppression, severe nausea and vomiting, and a flu-like syndrome that starts about 7 days after treatment and lasts 1 to 3 weeks.

▶ Temozolomide

Temozolomide is an orally active agent with the same mechanism of action as dacarbazine. It is well absorbed and crosses the blood–brain barrier. Temozolomide is converted enzymatically to the active metabolite 5-(3-methyltriazeno)-imidazole-4-carboxamide. Temozolomide has a terminal half-life of 1.8 hours, with a mean time to peak concentrations of 1.4 hours, and a small amount of the drug is excreted unchanged by the kidney.[27] The active metabolite has a terminal half-life of 1.5 hours and is metabolized primarily. Temozolomide may be used in the treatment of melanoma, refractory anaplastic astrocytoma, and glioblastoma multiforme. Nausea may be minimized by administering the drug at bedtime. Because patients receiving temozolomide may have confusion secondary to their brain tumor, and because dosing can consist of multiple capsule sizes, care must be taken by all providers to simplify regimens to prevent chemotherapy overdose.

▶ Procarbazine

While the exact mechanism of action of procarbazine is unknown, it does inhibit DNA, RNA, and protein synthesis. The pharmacokinetics have never been fully characterized, but it is known that the drug is metabolized extensively. Procarbazine is used most often in the treatment of lymphoma. Myelosuppression is the major side effect. Nausea, vomiting, and a flu-like syndrome occur initially with therapy. Patients must be counseled to avoid tyramine-rich foods because procarbazine is a monoamine oxidase inhibitor. Patients should be provided a list of foods and beverages to avoid to prevent a hypertensive crisis. A disulfiram-like reaction can occur with the ingestion of alcohol.

▶ Bendamustine

Bendamustine has three chemically active groups: a 2-chlorethyl group, a butyric acid side chain, and a benzimidazole ring. The 2-chloroethyl group, which confers alkylating properties, is shared with chlorambucil and other agents from the nitrogen mustard class. The butyric acid side chain, also common to chlorambucil, confers water solubility. The benzimidazole ring, structurally similar to a purine ring, occupies the position of the benzene ring in chlorambucil. Bendamustine has shown activity in chronic lymphocytic leukemia and non-Hodgkin's lymphoma. The recommended dose of bendamustine is 100 mg/m^2 given IV over 30 minutes on days 1 and 2 of a 28-day cycle. Bendamustine is oxidized by the liver to two weakly active metabolites with 45% of the dose excreted unchanged by the kidney. The terminal half-life of bendamustine is about 40 minutes. Side effects include nausea, vomiting, bone marrow suppression, headache and dyspnea.

▶ Thiotepa

Thiotepa is an alkylating agent that reacts with DNA phosphate groups to produce chromosomal cross-linkage. The pharmacokinetics of thiotepa are best described by a two-compartment model, with an α-half-life of 6 to 24 minutes and a terminal half-life of 78 to 160 minutes. Thiotepa has shown clinical activity in the treatment of breast, bladder, and ovarian cancer, along with carcinomatous meningitis and malignant effusions, and usually is administered IV or as an intravesicular infusion. It also may be used intrathecally. Side effects include myelosuppression, nausea and vomiting, and venous irritation.

Heavy-Metal Compounds

Platinum drugs form reactive platinum complexes that bind to cells, so the pharmacokinetics of the individual drug may be of the platinum, both free and bound, rather than of the parent drug.

▶ Cisplatin

Cisplatin forms inter- and intrastrand DNA cross-links to inhibit DNA synthesis. The pharmacokinetics are best described by a three-compartment model, with an α-half-life of 20 minutes, a β-half-life of 48 to 70 minutes, and a terminal half-life of 24 hours. Ninety percent of the drug is removed by the kidney by glomerular filtration and tubular secretion. Cisplatin has shown clinical activity in the treatment of numerous tumor types, from head and neck cancers to anal cancer, including many types of lymphoma and carcinoma of unknown primary. Cisplatin is highly emetogenic, even when low doses are given daily for 5 days, and causes delayed nausea and vomiting as well; patients require aggressive antiemetic regimens for both delayed and acute emesis. Significant nephrotoxicity and electrolyte abnormalities can occur if inadequate hydration occurs. Ototoxicity, which manifests as a high-frequency hearing loss, and a glove-and-stocking neuropathy may limit therapy.

▶ Carboplatin

While carboplatin has the same mechanism of action as cisplatin, it has a much less toxic side-effect profile than cisplatin. The pharmacokinetics of carboplatin are best described by a two-compartment model, with an α-half-life of 90 minutes and a terminal half-life of 180 minutes. Carboplatin is eliminated almost entirely by the kidney by glomerular filtration and tubular secretion. Many chemotherapy regimens dose carboplatin based on an area under the curve (AUC), which is referred to as the *Calvert equation*. According to the Calvert equation, the dose in milligrams = (CrCl + 25) × AUC desired.[28] Carboplatin has shown clinical activity in the treatment of ovarian, lung, breast, testicular, esophageal, and head and neck cancers, as well as lymphomas. Thrombocytopenia, nausea and vomiting, and hypersensitivity reactions are side effects.

► *Oxaliplatin*

The pharmacokinetics of oxaliplatin are best described by a three-compartment model, with an α-half-life of 0.28 hours, a β-half-life of 16.3 hours, and a terminal half-life of 273 hours.[29] Oxaliplatin has shown clinical activity in the treatment of colorectal cancer. Oxaliplatin, while similar in action to cisplatin and carboplatin, causes a cold-induced neuropathy. Patients should be counseled to avoid cold beverages, to use gloves to remove items from the freezer, and to wear protective clothing in cold climates for the first week after treatment. A glove-and-stocking neuropathy also occurs with long-term dosing. Hypersensitivity reactions and moderate nausea and vomiting are also side effects.

mTOR Inhibitors

The mammalian target of rapamycin (mTOR) is a downstream mediator in the phosphatidylinositol 3-kinase/Akt signaling pathway which controls translation of proteins that regulate cell growth and proliferation, but also angiogenesis and cell survival.

► *Temsirolimus*

The mTOR is an intracellular component which stimulates protein synthesis by phosphorylating translation regulators, and contributes to protein degradation and angiogenesis. Temsirolimus is approved for the treatment advanced renal cell carcinoma. The pharmacokinetics of temsirolimus are best described by a two-compartment model, with a terminal half-life of 13 to 25 hours. Elimination is primarily via the feces. Temsirolimus, and its metabolite sirolimus, are substrates of the cytochrome P4503A4/5 isoenzyme system. The primary side effects of temsirolimus include mucositis, diarrhea, maculopapular rash, nausea, leucopenia, thrombocytopenia, and hyperglycemia.

Miscellaneous Agents

► *Altretamine*

Altretamine, formerly known as hexamethylmelamine, is similar in structure to alkylating agents but is known to have anticancer activity in cancer cells resistant to alkylating agents. Altretamine is well absorbed after oral administration and undergoes rapid and extensive demethylation in the liver. Peak plasma concentrations were observed 0.5 to 3 hours after administration. The terminal half-life is 4.7 to 10.2 hours. Altretamine has shown activity in the treatment of ovarian and lung cancer. This orally administered drug has the dose-limiting side effects of anorexia, nausea, vomiting, diarrhea, and abdominal cramping. Other side effects include neuropathy, agitation, confusion, and depression.

► *Bleomycin*

Bleomycin is a mixture of peptides with drug activity expressed in units, where 1 unit equals 1 mg. Bleomcyin causes DNA strand breakage. The pharmacokinetics of bleomycin are best described by a two-compartment model, where the α-half-life is 10 to 20 minutes and a terminal elimination half-life of 2 to 3 hours, which can be prolonged to 21 hours in patients with renal impairment.[30] Bleomycin has shown clinical activity in the treatment of testicular cancer and malignant effusions, squamous cell carcinomas of the skin, and Kaposi's sarcoma. Hypersensitivity reactions and fever may occur, so premedication with acetaminophen may be required. The most serious side effect is the pulmonary toxicity that presents as a pneumonitis with a dry cough, dyspnea, rales, and infiltrates. Pulmonary function studies will show decreased carbon monoxide diffusing capacity and restrictive ventilatory changes. "Bleomycin lung" is associated with cumulative dosing greater than 400 units and occurs rarely with a total dose of 150 units. The pulmonary toxicity is potentiated by thoracic radiation and by hyperoxia. Additional side effects include fever with or without chills, mild to moderate alopecia, and nausea and vomiting. Bleomycin has been used to manage malignant effusions at doses of 15 to 60 units through installation into the affected area. The drainage tube of the effusion is clamped off for some period of time after administration of the bleomycin (time varies based on the location of the effusion), and then the amount of drainage is monitored to determine efficacy of the bleomycin treatment.

► *Hydroxyurea*

Hydroxyurea is an oral drug that inhibits ribonucleotide reductase, which converts ribonucleotides into the deoxyribuoncleotides used in DNA synthesis and repair. The time to peak concentrations of hydroxyurea is 1 to 2 hours after oral administration. Approximately 50% is degraded by the liver to form urea and respiratory carbon dioxide. The remainder is excreted by the kidney. The half-life ranges from 3.5 to 4.5 hours. Hydroxyurea has shown clinical activity in the treatment of chronic myelocytic leukemia, polycythemia vera, and thrombocytosis. The major side effects are myelosuppression, nausea and vomiting, diarrhea, and constipation. Rash, mucositis, and renal tubular dysfunction occur rarely.

► *L-Asparaginase*

L-Asparaginase is an enzyme that may be produced by *Escherichia coli*. Asparaginase hydrolyzes the reaction of asparagines to aspartic acid and ammonia to deplete lymphoid cells of asparagine, which inhibits protein synthesis. The pharmacokinetics of L-asparaginase are best described by a two-compartment model, with an initial half-life of 4 to 9 hours and a terminal half-life of 1.4 to 1.8 days. L-Asparaginase has shown clinical activity in the treatment of acute lymphocytic leukemia and childhood acute myeloid leukemia. Severe allergic reactions may occur when the interval between doses is 7 days or greater, so while a skin test may be negative, patients should be observed closely after asparaginase administration. Pancreatitis and fibrinogen depletion also may occur during therapy. Repletion of fibrinogen should be done to prevent disseminated intravascular coagulation and fatal bleeding. If the patient suffers an allergic reaction to L-asparaginase, pegaspargase, which is L-asparaginase modified through a linkage with polyethylene glycol, which extends the half-life and allows for lower doses and less frequent administration, may be given. Cost and limited availability are the reasons why pegaspargase is not used first.

▶ Arsenic Trioxide

Arsenic trioxide, which was approved recently for the treatment of acute promyelocytic leukemia, induces the growth of cancer cells into mature, more normal cells, as well as induces programmed cell death, or apoptosis. The pharmacokinetics of arsenic trioxide are best described by a two-compartment model, with an α-half-life of 0.89 hours and a β-half-life of 12.1 hours. Less than 10% of a dose is excreted by the kidney.[31] Arsenic trioxide causes QT-interval prolongation, so frequent ECGs need to be done prior to each dose, and other drugs that may prolong the QT interval need to be avoided during therapy. Monitoring of potassium and magnesium should be done, and active replacement undertaken to prevent QT prolongation. Other side effects include dry skin with itching, nausea and vomiting, loss of appetite, and elevations of serum hepatic enzymes. An uncommon but serious side effect is a syndrome similar to the retinoic acid syndrome, which appears similar to pneumonia but is related to the arsenic therapy.

▶ Mitomycin C

Mitomycin C is an alkylating agent that forms cross-links with DNA to inhibit DNA and RNA synthesis. The pharmacokinetics of mitomycin C are best described by a two-compartment model, with an α-half-life of 8 minutes and a terminal half-life of 48 minutes.[32] Liver metabolism is the primary route of elimination. Mitomycin C has shown clinical activity in the treatment of anal, bladder, cervix, gallbladder, esophageal, and stomach cancer. Side effects consist of myelosuppression and mucositis, and it is a vesicant.

▶ Tretinoin

Tretinoin, also referred to *ATRA*, which stands for all transretinoic acid, is a retinoic acid that is not cytotoxic but promotes the maturation of early promyelocytic cells and is specific to the t(15;17) cytogenetic marker. The time to peak concentrations is 1 to 2 hours after an oral dose. The elimination half-life is 21 to 51 minutes.[33] These maroon-and-gold capsules are dosed at 45 mg/m²/day divided into two doses. The most significant side effect is the retinoic acid syndrome, which may occur anywhere from the first couple of days of therapy until the end of therapy and consists of symptoms of fever, respiratory distress, and hypotension. Chest radiographs are consistent with a pneumonia-like process. The syndrome can be confused easily with

pneumonia in a patient with possible neutropenia. The treatment for retinoic acid syndrome is dexamethasone 10 mg IV every 12 hours; the syndrome may resolve within 24 hours of the start of dexamethasone therapy. However, the use of steroids in a febrile neutropenic patient may further compromise the treatment of infection.

▶ Thalidomide

Thalidomide was introduced into the market on October 1, 1957, as a sedative-hypnotic, and when it was taken by pregnant women, it resulted in severe limb deformities (phocomelia). Thalidomide is used for the treatment of leprosy but now is part of the treatment of multiple myeloma. While thalidomide is believed to be an angiogenesis inhibitor, the mechanism of action is still unknown. Possible mechanisms of action include free-radical oxidative damage to DNA, inhibiting tumor necrosis factor α production, altering the adhesion of cancer cells, and altering cytokines that affect the growth of cancer cells. The pharmacokinetics of thalidomide demonstrate a time to peak concentration of 2 to 3 hours and a terminal half-life of 4 to 7 hours.[34] Thalidomide has shown clinical activity in the treatment of multiple myeloma and is still being studied for the treatment of several other cancers. Because of thalidomide's potential to cause phocomelia, each patient must be counseled on the risks of thalidomide not only for the patient but also the patient's reproductive partner. Physicians must be registered to prescribe thalidomide. Pharmacists can fill prescriptions only where both the patient and the physician have completed surveys on a monthly basis.

▶ Lenalidomide

Lenalidomide is approved for the treatment of myelodysplastic syndrome where the 5q deletion is present and multiple myeloma. Since lenalidomide is an analog of thalidomide, all the same precautions must be taken to prevent phocomelia. The time to maximum lenalidomide concentrations occurs 0.5 to 4 hours after the dose. The terminal half-life ranges from 3 to 9 hours. Approximately 65% of lenalidomide is eliminated unchanged in the urine, with clearance exceeding the glomerular filtration rate. Dosing adjustments are necessary for renal dysfunction.[35] Lenalidomide is used in the treatment of myelodysplastic syndrome and multiple myeloma. Other side effects are neutropenia, thrombocytopenia, deep vein thrombosis, and pulmonary embolus.

▶ Bexarotene

Bexarotene is a retinoid that selectively activates retinoid X receptors which affects cellular differentiation and proliferation. The time of maximum concentration after an oral dose of bexarotene is about 2 hours, while the terminal half-life is about 7 hours. Bexarotene is eliminated primarily by the hepatobilliary system. Bexarotene is indicated for the treatment of cutaneous manifestations of cutaneous T-cell lymphoma in patients who are refractory to other therapy. Side effects include hypercholesterolemia, elevations in triglycerides, pancreatitis, hypothyroidism, and leukopenia, headache, and dry skin.

▶ *Vorinostat*

Vorinostat is indicated for the treatment for cutaneous T-cell lymphoma in patients with progressive, persistent, or recurrent disease after treatment with other drugs. Vorinostat inhibits the activity of histone deacetylases which results in repression of gene transcription. Vorinostat is eliminated primarily by glucuronidation and hydrolysis to pharmacologically inactive metabolites, with a terminal half-life of 2 hours. Side effects include diarrhea, fatigue, nausea and anorexia, hypercholesterolemia, hypertriglyceridemia, and hyperglycemia. Despite anemia, thrombocytopenia and neutropenia, patients have developed pulmonary embolism and deep vein thromboses while on therapy.

Immune Therapies

▶ *Interferons*

The categories of α, β, and γ interferons exist; the α interferons are used in the treatment of cancer. Interferon enhances the immune system's attack on cancer cells, can decrease new blood vessel formation, and can augment expression of antigen on tumor cell surfaces. Interferon has an elimination half-life of 3.7 to 8.5 hours. Interferon is filtered through the glomeruli and then degraded during tubular reabsorption. Interferon has shown clinical activity in the treatment of melanoma, kidney cancer, Kaposi's sarcoma, and chronic myelocytic and lymphocytic leukemia. Unfortunately, interferon is not well tolerated by patients because it causes a flu-like syndrome that consists of fevers and chills; depression, malaise, and fatigue are other side effects. Premedication with acetaminophen will help alleviate the flu-like symptoms, which will decrease with chronic administration.

▶ *Aldesleukin*

Aldesleukin, commonly referred to as *interleukin 2*, is a lymphokine that promotes B- and T-cell proliferation and triggers a cytokine cascade to attack the tumor. The pharmacokinetics are best described by a two-compartment model, with an α-half-life of 13 minutes and a terminal half-life of 85 minutes. Aldesleukin is eliminated by both glomerular filatration and peritubular extraction in the kidney. Aldesleukin has shown clinical activity in the treatment of kidney cancer and melanoma. Side effects of interleukin 2 vary by dose and route. IV high-dose interleukin 2 causes a drug-induced shock-like picture. Patients may develop hypotension despite aggressive IV hydration. Patients develop a red, itching skin; liver and kidney function tests change; fluid and electrolyte imbalances occur; and high fevers occur while receiving scheduled acetaminophen and nonsteroidal anti-inflammatory agents. Severe rigors and chills may require IV meperidine for symptom control. All the side effects reverse within 24 hours of stopping the drug. The toxicity profile is much less with

subcutaneous administration. However, with subcutaneous administration, little nodules form at the injection site and may take months to resolve. Corticosteroids should not be administered to patients while receiving aldesleukin unless a life-threatening emergency should occur. Steroids will reverse all the symptoms and the antitumor effect, even with topical administration. The itching, red skin may be treated with topical creams and antihistamines.

▶ *Denileukin Diftitox*

Denileukin diftitox is a combination of the active sections of interleukin 2 and diphtheria toxin. It binds to high-affinity interleukin 2 receptors on the cancer cell (and other cells), and the toxin portion of the molecule inhibits protein synthesis to result in cell death. The pharmacokinetics of denileukin diftitox are best described by a two-compartment model, with an α-half-life of 2 to 5 minutes and a terminal half-life of 70 to 80 minutes. Denileukin diftitox is used for the treatment of persistent or recurrent cutaneous T-cell lymphoma whose cells express the CD25 receptor. Side effects include vascular leak syndrome, fevers/chills, hypersensitivity reactions, hypotension, anorexia, diarrhea, and nausea and vomiting.

Monoclonal Antibodies

The cell surface contains antigens, which are referred to as CD, which stands for "cluster of differentiation." The antibodies are produced against a specific antigen. When administered, usually by an IV injection, the antibody binds to the antigen, which may trigger the immune system to result in cell death through complement-mediated cellular toxicity, or the antigen–antibody cell complex may be internalized to the cancer cell, which results in cell death. Monoclonal antibodies also may carry radioactivity, sometimes referred to as *hot antibodies*, and may be referred to as *radioimmunotherapy*, so the radioactivity is delivered to the cancer cell. Antibodies that contain no radioactivity are referred to as *cold antibodies*.

All monoclonal antibodies end in the suffix -*mab*. The syllable before -*mab* indicates the source of the monoclonal antibody (see Table 88–7). When administering an antibody for the first time, one should consider the source. The less humanized an antibody, the greater is the chance for the patient to have an allergic-type reaction to the antibody. The more humanized the antibody, the lower is the risk of a reaction. The severity of the reactions may range from fever and chills to life-threatening allergic reactions (which have resulted in death). Premedication with acetaminophen and diphenhydramine is common before the first dose of any antibody. If a severe reaction occurs, the infusion should be stopped and the patient treated with antihistamines, corticosteroids, or other supportive measures.

▶ *Alemtuzumab*

Alemtuzumab is the antibody to the CD52 receptor present on B and T lymphocytes. The pharmacokinetics of

Table 88–7

Syllable Source Indicators for Monoclonal Antibodies

U	Human
O	Mouse
A	Rat
E	Hamster
I	Primate
Xi	A cross between humanized and animal source

These letters appear before mab, which stands for monoclonal antibody.

From Programme on International Nonproprietary Names (INN) Division of Drug Management and Policies, World Health Organization, Geneva. 1997.

alemtuzumab demonstrate a terminal half-life of 7 days. Alemtuzumab has shown clinical activity in the treatment of chronic lymphocytic leukemia. Severe and prolonged (6 months) immunosuppression may result, which necessitates prophylaxis with cotrimoxazole and antivirals to prevent opportunistic infections.

▶ Bevacizumab

Bevacizumab is a humanized monoclonal antibody that binds to vascular endothelial growth factor, which prevents it from binding to its receptors, ultimately resulting in inhibition of angiogenesis. The pharmacokinetics of bevacizumab demonstrate a terminal half-life of 21 days, with a volume of distribution consistent with limited extravascular distribution.[36] Bevacizumab has shown clinical activity in the treatment of colorectal, kidney, lung, breast, and head and neck cancer. Patients may develop hypertension requiring chronic medication during therapy. Impaired wound healing, thromboembolic events, proteinuria, bleeding, and perforation are serious side effects.

▶ Cetuximab

Cetuximab is a chimeric antibody that binds to the epidermal growth factor receptor (EGFR) to block its stimulation. Recently investigators found that colorectal tumors that have *KRAS* mutations do not respond to treatment with cetuximab; therefore tumors should be tested for *KRAS* mutations prior to initiating therapy. The pharmacokinetics of cetuximab demonstrate a volume of distribution that approximates the vascular space and a terminal half-life of 70 to 100 hours. Cetuximab has shown clinical activity in the treatment of colorectal and head and neck cancers. An acne-like rash may appear on the face and upper torso 1 to 3 weeks after the start of therapy. Other side effects include hypersensitivity reactions, interstitial lung disease, fever, malaise, diarrhea, abdominal pain, and nausea and vomiting.

▶ Gemtuzumab Ozogamicin

Gemtuzumab ozogamicin is a humanized antibody to the CD33 receptor present on about 80% of acute myelogenous leukemia cells. The antibody is linked to calicheamicin, a cellular toxin that is released intracellularly after the antigen-antibody complex is internalized. The pharmacokinetics of gemtuzumab ozogamicin show a terminal half-life of 67 to 78 hours of the antibody portion of the drug and a terminal half-life of about 45 hours of the calicheamicin.[37] Gemtuzumab ozogamicin has shown clinical activity in the treatment of acute myeloid leukemia. Severe rigors and chills, which may occur after the infusion is completed, respond to meperidine IV. Premedications should include acetaminophen, diphenhydramine, and methylprednisolone to prevent rigors and chills.

▶ Ibrotumomab Tiuxetan

This "hot antibody" is linked to yttrium and binds to the CD20 receptor of B lymphocytes (see Rituximab below). Hematologic toxicity may occur several weeks after administration and may take weeks to resolve.

▶ Panitumumab

Panitumumab binds to the EGFR to prevent receptor auto-phosphorylation and activation of receptor-associated kinases, which results in inhibition of inhibition of cell growth and induction of apoptosis. Recently data were presented that demonstrated that colorectal tumors without KRAS mutations responded to panitumumab therapy, and had a longer median time to progression. Panitumumab demonstrates nonlinear pharmacokinetics with a terminal half-life of 7.5 days. Panitumumab has demonstrated activity against tumors of the colon and rectum. Side effects include dermatitis, pruritus, exfoliative rash, infusion reactions, pulmonary fibrosis, diarrhea, hypomagnesemia, hypocalcemia, and photosensitivity.

▶ Rituximab

Rituximab is a monoclonal antibody to the CD20 receptor expressed on the surface of B lymphocytes; the presence of the antibody is determined during flow cytometry of the tumor cells. Cell death results from antibody-dependent cellular cytotoxicity. The pharmacokinetics of rituximab are best described by a two-compartment model, with a terminal half-life of 76 hours after the first infusion and a terminal half-life of 205 hours after the fourth dose.[38] Rituximab has shown clinical activity in the treatment of B-cell lymphomas that are CD20 positive . Side effects include hypersensitivity reactions, hypotension, fevers, chills, rash, headache, and mild nausea and vomiting.

▶ Tositumomab

This "hot antibody" is linked to radioactive iodine and binds to the CD20 receptor present on B lymphocytes (see Rituximab above). Tositumomab has shown activity in non-Hodgkin's lymphoma. Hematologic toxicity occurs several weeks after administration and may persist for months. Because radioactive iodine may have adverse effects on the thyroid, all patients must receive thyroid-blocking agents.

▶ *Trastuzumab*

Trastuzumab is the antibody directed against human epidermal receptor 2 (*HER-2*), which is overexpressed by 25% to 30% of breast cancers and is associated with aggressive disease and decreased survival. Breast cancer tissue must be tested for the presence of *HER-2*, as patients that do not expresses *HER-2* do not respond to trastuzumab. The pharmacokinetics of trastuzumab are best described by a two-compartment model, with a terminal half-life of 19 to 28 days.[39] Severe congestive heart failure may occur with concurrent anthracycline administration. Cardiac toxicity may be seen when the drug is administered months after anthracycline administration, so patients must be counseled on the signs and symptoms of heart failure. Other side effects include hypersensitivity reactions, fever, diarrhea, infections, chills, cough, headache, rash, and insomnia.

Tyrosine-Kinase Inhibitors

There are more than 100 different types of tyrosine-kinases present in the body. Sometimes tyrosine-kinase inhibitors are referred to as small-molecule inhibitors. Each of the following drugs was developed to block either several or a specific tyrosine kinase.

▶ *Imatinib*

Imatinib was the first FDA-approved tyrosine-kinase inhibitor. The drug was designed to block the breakpoint cluster region tyrosine kinase (BCR:ABL) produced by the Philadelphia chromosome associated with chronic myelogenous leukemia and acute lymphocytic leukemia. The pharmacokinetics of imatinib demonstrate a mean time to maximum concentration of 2 to 4 hours, with a terminal half-life of 15 hours.[40] Imatinib also has shown activity against GI stroma tumors (GIST) that are positive for c-kit (CD117). Numerous drug interactions have been reported for imatinib. CYP450 3A4 inducers, such as rifampicin and St. John's wort, increase the clearance of imatinib.[41,42] Ketoconazole, a CYP450 3A4 inhibitor, has been shown to decrease imatinib clearance by almost 30%.[43] Imatinib also may increase the exposure of simvastatin, a CYP450 3A4 substrate.[44]

▶ *Dasatinib*

Dasatinib is a second generation tyrosine kinase inhibitor that shares the same binding site on the BCR:ABL cluster region as imatinib, but maintains activity despite imatinib resistance, with more higher potency than imatinib. Dasatinib also inhibits SRC kinases, which are tyrosine kinases that mediate cellular differentiation, proliferation and survival. The terminal half-life of dasatinib is 3 to 5 hours, with elimination primarily via the liver and feces. Dasatinib is used in the treatment of chronic myeloid leukemia with resistance or intolerance to imatinib, and for the treatment of Philadelphia chromosome-positive acute lymphoblastic leukemia. Side effects of dasatinib include myelosuppression, nausea and vomiting, headache, fluid retention, hypocalcemia and pleural effusions.

▶ *Nilotinib*

Nilotinib also blocks the breakpoint cluster region tyrosine kinase (BCR:ABL) produced by the Philadelphia chromosome associated with chronic myelogenous leukemia and acute lymphocytic leukemia. Nilotinib is primarily eliminated by oxidation and hydroxylation, with a terminal half-life of 17 hours. Nilotinib should be administered on an empty stomach, or 2 hours after a meal. Nilotinib is indicated for the treatment of Philadelphia-chromosome-positive chronic myelogenous leukemia also. Side effects include QT prolongation, bone marrow suppression, elevations in lipase, and hepatotoxicity.

▶ *Erlotinib*

Erlotinib, whose pharmacology is not entirely understood, is believed to inhibit the intracellular phosphorylation of the EGFR. Erlotinib is about 60% absorbed after oral administration; food increases bioavailability to almost 100%, however this is variable and experts recommend administering erlotinib on an empty stomach. The time to peak concentrations is approximately 4 hours after a dose. The half-life of erlotinib is about 36 hours, and it is eliminated predominately by CYP450 3A4. Smoking increases the clearance of erlotinib by 24%, which may result in treatment failure.[45] Erlotinib is used in the treatment of nonsmall cell lung cancer and cancer of the pancreas. Side effects include interstitial lung disease, rash, diarrhea, anorexia, pruritus, conjunctivitis, and drug skin. Again, significant drug interactions have been documented with CYP450 3A4 inducers and inhibitors.

▶ *Lapatinib*

Lapatinib inhibits the intracellular kinase domains of both EGFR and *HER-2*, and has been shown to retain activity against breast cancer cells that have become resistant to trastuzumab. The pharmacokinetics of lapatinib with repeated dosing display a time-dependent increase in systemic exposure. Absorption is enhanced when administered with food. A single-dose study demonstrated a terminal half-life of 14 hours, while repeated dosing studies indicated an effective half of 24 hours. Patients with Child-Pugh class C liver disease should have a dosage reduction to 750 mg daily to adjust the AUC to the normal range. Lapatinib is indicated for the treatment of patients with breast cancer whose tumors overexpress *HER-2*. Side effects of lapatinib include decreased left-ventricular ejection fraction, diarrhea, hepatotoxicity, rash, and QT prolongation.

▶ *Sorafenib*

Sorafenib is a multikinase inhibitor that inhibits both intracellular and extracellular kinases to decrease renal cell cancer proliferation. The half-life of sorafenib is 25 to 48 hours, with a bioavailability of 38% to 49% and a time to peak concentration of 3 hours. Sorafenib is metabolized primarily by the liver by CYP450 3A4. Sorafenib is used for the treatment of renal cell cancer. The primary side effects of sorafenib include rash, hand-foot skin reaction, diarrhea, pruritus, and elevations in serum lipase.

▶ Sunitinib

Sunitinib blocks several tyrosine kinases, so it inhibits platelet-derived growth factor, vascular endothelial growth factor receptor, stem cell factor receptor, fms-like receptor growth factor, colony-stimulating growth factor receptor type 1, and glial-cell-line-derived neurotrophic factor receptor. The active metabolite of sunitinib blocks these same enzymes with similar potency. The pharmacokinetics of sunitinib demonstrate a time of peak concentration of about 5 hours, with a half-life of 41 to 86 hours.[46] It is indicated for the treatment of GISTs after disease progression or intolerance to imatinib. It is also indicated for the treatment of advanced renal cell cancer. Significant side effects include left ventricular dysfunction, hemorrhage, asthenia, hypertension, nausea and vomiting, and diarrhea. Approximately one-third of patients may develop a yellow color of the skin, along with dryness and cracking of the skin. Also, hair may become depigmented with doses of 50 mg/day or more, and the depigmentation is reversible when therapy is stopped. Clinically significant drug interactions exist with drugs metabolized via the CYP450 3A4 system; ketoconazole has been shown to increase concentrations of sunitinib, whereas rifampin has been shown to decrease concentrations of sunitinib.

Hormonal Therapies

Hormonal therapies have shown activity in the treatment of cancers whose growth is affected by gonadal hormonal control. Hormonal treatments either block or decrease the production of endogenous hormones.

▶ Antiandrogens: Bicalutamide, Flutamide, and Nilutamide

The antiandrogens block androgen receptors to inhibit the action of testosterone and dihydrotestosterone in prostate cancer cells. Unfortunately, prostate cancer cells may become hormone refractory.

Flutamide is an androgen receptor antagonist that achieves peak concentrations approximatley 2 to 4 hours after an oral dose. Flutamide is metabolized extensively, with a terminal half-life of about 8 hours. Bicalutamide achieves peak concentrations approximately 6 hours after the dose, with a terminal half-life of 6 to 10 days. Bicalutamide undergoes stereospecific metabolism, where the *S*-enantiomer is cleared more rapidly by the liver than the *R*-enantiomer. Nilutamide achieves peak serum concentrations between 1 and 4 hours after an oral dose and has a terminal half-life of 38 to 60 hours. Nilutamide is metabolized extensively, with less than 2% excreted as unchanged drug by the kidney. Side effects common to these agents are hot flashes, gynecomastia, and decreased libido. Flutamide tends to be associated with more diarrhea and requires three-times-daily administration, whereas bicalutamide is dosed once daily. Nilutamide may cause

interstitial pneumonia and is associated with the visual disturbance of delayed adaptation to darkness.

▶ Luteinizing Hormone–Releasing Hormone Agonists: Goserelin and Leuprolide

Initially, luteinizing hormone–releasing hormone (LHRH) agonists increase levels of leutinizing hormone and follicle-stimulating hormone, but testosterone and estrogen levels are decreased because of continuous negative-feedback inhibition. Major side effects are testicular atrophy, decreased libido, gynecomastia, and hot flashes. Leuprolide is well absorbed, with a terminal half-life of 2.9 hours, whereas goserelin has a terminal half-life of 4.9 hours. Goserelin is injected as a pellet under the skin, so subcutaneous injection of lidocaine prior to administration helps to decrease the pain associated with goserelin administration. Numerous dosage forms are available for leuprolide with varying strengths and dosing intervals. Antiandrogens may be administered during initial therapy to decrease symptoms of tumor flare (e.g., bone pain and urinary tract obstruction).

▶ Ketoconazole

While ketoconazole is an antifungal agent, it has been used for treatment of prostate cancer. In high doses of 400 mg three times daily, ketoconazole blocks the production of testosterone.

▶ LHRH Antagonist: Abarelix

Abarelix is a gonadotropin-releasing hormone antagonist that is associated with life-threatening hypersensitivity reactions. Patients must be observed for 30 minutes after administration. The drug is limited to men who cannot risk tumor flare and refuse orchiectomy.

▶ Aminoglutethimide

Aminoglutethimide blocks the conversion of androgens to estrogens and decreases the synthesis of glucocorticoids. Adrenocorticoid suppression may occur, so replacement therapy with hydrocortisone may be required. Other side effects include rash (which usually resolves in 5–8 days), lethargy, and anorexia.

▶ Anastrozole

Anastrozole is a selective nonsteroidal aromatase inhibitor that lowers estrogen levels. The pharmacokinetics of anastrozole demonstrate good absorption, with hepatic metabolism the primary route of elimination and only 10% excreted unchanged by the kidney. The elimination half-life is approximately 50 hours. Anastrozole is used for the adjuvant treatment of postmenopausal women with hormone-positive breast cancer and in breast cancer patients who have had disease progression following tamoxifen. Side effects include hot flashes, arthralgias, osteoporosis/bone fractures, and thrombophlebitis.

▶ Exemestane

Exemestane is an irreversible aromatase inactivator that binds to the aromatase enzyme to block the production of estrogen from androgens. Exemestane is absorbed rapidly after oral administration, with a terminal half-life of 24 hours. The drug is eliminated primarily by the liver and feces, with less than 1% of the dose excreted unchanged in the urine. Exemestane is indicated for the treatment of advanced breast cancer in postmenopausal women who have had disease progression following tamoxifen therapy. Side effects include hot flashes, fatigue, osteoporosis/bone fractures, and flu-like symptoms.

▶ Fulvestrant

Fulvestrant is an estrogen receptor antagonist that binds to the estrogen receptor and is given as a monthly intramuscular injection. Fulvestrant has a terminal half-life of 40 days and a large volume of distribution of 3 to 5 L/kg. Fulvestrant is metabolized primarily, with excretion primarily via feces. Fulvestrant is used for the treatment of hormone-receptor-positive metastatic breast cancer in postmenopausal women with disease progression following antiestrogen therapy. Side effects are hot flashes, abdominal pain, depression, and myalgias.

▶ Letrozole

Letrozole is another selective aromatase that inhibits the conversion of androgens to estrogen. Maximum plasma concentrations occur 1 hour after oral dosing; concomitant food has not been shown to have an effect on the extent of absorption of letrozole. The terminal half-life is approximately 2 days. Letrozole is used in the treatment of postmenopausal women with hormone-receptor-positive or unknown advanced breast cancer. Side effects include bone pain, hot flushes, back pain, nausea, arthralgia, osteoporosis/bone fractures, and dyspnea.

▶ Megestrol Acetate

Megestrol is a synthetic progestin with antiestrogen properties that is used for breast cancer and in higher doses for weight gain. Side effects include fluid retention, hot flashes, vaginal bleeding and spotting, breast tenderness, and thrombosis.

▶ Tamoxifen

Tamoxifen is an estrogen receptor antagonist. Most of a dose of tamoxifen is eliminated primarily by metabolism, with significant enterohepatic recirculation. The time to a peak concentration is 6 hours after an oral dose, and the terminal half-life is 7 days. Tamoxifen is used primarily for the treatment of postmenopausal hormone-receptor-positive breast cancer patients and the prevention of breast cancer in postmenopausal women. Side effects include hot flashes, fluid retention, mood swings, thrombosis, endometrial and uterine cancer, and corneal changes and cataracts. Since tamoxifen is a substrate of CYP450 3A4, decreased tamoxifen levels have occurred with use of St. John's wort, and decreased tamoxifen levels have been observed with use of rifampin. Tamoxifen is also a substrate for CYP450 2D6, and recent evidence suggests that those who are CYP2D6*4/*4 may have a poorer response and more toxicity with tamoxifen.[47] Significant drug interactions exist with antidepressants which may be used to treat depression or help relieve hot flashes.

▶ Toremifene

Toremifene is an estrogen receptor antagonist. The pharmacokinetics of toremifene are best described by a two-compartment model, with an α-half-life of 4 hours and an elimination half-life of 5 days. Peak plasma concentrations are achieved approximately 3 hours after an oral dose. Toremifene is metabolized extensively, with metabolites found primarily in the feces. Toremifene is used for the treatment of metastatic breast cancer in postmenopausal women with estrogen-receptor-positive or unknown tumors. Toremifene causes hot flashes, vaginal bleeding, thromboembolism, and visual acuity changes.

ADMINISTRATION ISSUES

Extravasation

Another issue of chemotherapy safety is extravasation. Antineoplastic agents that cause severe tissue damage when they escape from the vasculature are called *vesicants*. Some examples of vesicants are the anthracyclines and the vinca alkaloids. The tissue damage may be severe, with tissue sloughing and loss of mobility, depending on the area of extravasation. Patients need to be educated to notify the nurse immediately if there is any pain on administration. If extravasation of a vesicant occurs, the injection should be stopped, and any fluid aspirated out of the injection site. If an antidote should be administered, such as with nitrogen mustard extravasation, the pharmacy should be notified immediately so that the sodium thiosulfate can be prepared and delivered quickly. Cold compresses should be applied (heat should be used for vincas) to the affected area. The area of extravasation should be recorded and inked and followed closely to detect early signs of infection and to treat pain. Obviously, prevention of extravasation is very important. Good IV access is key, which may include the placement of a central venous catheter, along with free-flowing IV fluids. During administration of a vesicant, blood return should be checked to be sure that the drug is going into the vein. Central venous catheters can be placed for patients needing infusions of vesicants or for patients with small, friable veins to prevent extravasation.

Hypersensitivity Reactions

Recently more attention has been focused on hypersensitivity reactions of cancer treatments because of cross-reactivity between agents, and the desire to continue active therapies against the cancer.[48] Bleomycin and asparaginase have skin tests suggested to be administered prior to administration.

However, a negative skin test does not preclude an allergic reaction. For documented immediate hypersensitivity reactions to a particular agent, further administration of the agent may be achieved through extensive premedication with H1 and H2 antihistamines and corticosteroids, and through use of escalating doses of the offending agent given at doses of one-hundredth, one-tenth, and the balance of the dose (so the total dose administered is equivalent to the normally prescribed dose) administered over a much longer period of time. These treatments must be given in an environment where resuscitation is readily available in case of medical emergency.

Secondary Malignancies

Chemotherapy and radiation therapy treatments may cause cancers later in life; these are referred to as secondary cancers. The most common type of secondary cancer is myelodysplastic syndrome, or acute myeloid leukemia. The antineoplastic agents most commonly associated with secondary malignancies are alkylating agents, etoposide, teniposide, and anthracyclines. While the risk for secondary cancers is extremely low, it must outweigh the risk of survival produced by treatment of the primary malignancy. Because secondary malignancies may not occur for several years after treatment, patients with relatively short-term survival owing to the primary malignancy should consider the more immediate benefits of chemotherapy. Radiation therapy rarely may cause solid tumors as secondary cancers decades after treatment. The most common example of radiation therapy–induced secondary malignancy is breast cancer, which rarely occurs after mantle field radiation therapy for Hodgkin's disease.

CHEMOTHERAPY SAFETY

One of the first Institute of Medicine reports starts out with a patient who died from an overdose of chemotherapy; the patient did not have an immediately life-threatening cancer, so her death was hastened by a medication error. Chemotherapy agents may cause harm to patients, health care workers, and the environment if not handled correctly. ❺ *Because of the severe toxicities associated with many of the chemotherapy agents, safety precautions must be in place to prevent chemotherapy errors, accidental chemotherapy exposures, and overdosages.* The Oncology Nursing Society and the American Society of Health-System Pharmacists have

---

Table 88–8

Dosing Adjustment Guidelines for Chemotherapy for Renal Dysfunction

Drug	Dosing Adjustment
Bleomycin	Creatinine 1.5–2.0 mg/dL (133–177 µmol/L): decrease dose by 50% CrCl less than 20 mL/min (0.19 mL/s × m²): decrease dose by 60%
Capecitabine	CrCl 30–50 mL/min (0.29–0.48 mL/s × m²): decrease dose by 75% CrCl less than 30 mL/min (0.29 mL/s × m²)
Cladribine	No dosing guidelines
Cytarabine	High dose (greater than 2 g/m²) Creatinine 1.5–1.9 mg/dL (133–177 µmol/L) or increase of 0.5–1.2 mg/dL (44–106 µmol/L): decrease dose to 1 g/m² Creatinine greater than 1.9 mg/dL (168 µmol/L) or an increase greater than 1.2 mg/dL (106 µmol/L): decrease dose to 0.1 g/m²/day continuous infusion
Etoposide	CrCl 15–50 mL/min (0.001–0.48 mL/s × m²): decrease dose by 25%
Carboplatin	Dosing adjustment based on Calvert equation
Cisplatin	Proportional to lower creatinine clearance, where normal equal to 70 mL/min (0.67 mL/s × m²)
Ifosfamide	CrCl 46–60 mL/min (0.44–0.57 mL/s × m²): reduce by 20% CrCl 31–45 mL/min (0.3–0.43 mL/s × m²): reduce by 25% CrCl less than 31 mL/min (0.3 mL/s × m²): reduce by 30%
Lenalidomide	Multiple myeloma: greater than 50 mL/min (0.48 mL/s × m²): 25 mg daily 30–49 mL/min (0.29–0.47 mL/s × m²): 10 mg daily less than 30 mL/min (0.29 mL/s × m²); no dialysis: 15 mg every 48 hours; dialysis: 15 mg three times weekly after dialysis Myelodysplastic syndromes: greater than 50 mL/min (0.48 mL/s × m²): 25 mg daily 30–49 mL/min (0.29–0.47 mL/s × m²): 5 mg daily less than 30 mL/min (0.29 mL/s × m²); no dialysis: 15 mg every 48 hours; dialysis: 5 mg three times weekly after dialysis
Methotrexate	Proportional to lowered creatinine clearance, where normal equal to 70 mL/min (0.67 mL/s × m²)
Melphalan	If BUN greater than 30 mg/dL (10.7 mmol/L) and creatinine greater than 1.5 mg/dL (132 µmol/L): decrease dose by 50%
Pemetrexed	Greater than or equal to 80 mL/min (0.77 mL/s × m²): 600 mg/m² 40–79 mL/min (0.38–0.76 mL/s ×m²): 500 mg/m²
Topotecan	20–39 mL/min (0.2–0.37 mL/s × m²): decrease dose by 50% less than 20 mL/min (0.2 mL/s × m²): not established

Adapted from DiPiro JT, Talbert RL, Yee GC, et al. (eds.) Pharmacotherapy a Pathophysiologic Approach. 7th ed. New York: McGraw-Hill; 2008: Table 130–8.

information to assist in the safe handling of chemotherapy agents.[49] National, state, and local regulations regarding the safe disposal of chemotherapy agents and the equipment used to administer them need to be followed to protect the environment.

Each organization should have chemotherapy safety checks built into the prescribing, preparation, and administration of chemotherapy.[50] Dosing based on patient-specific body information should be included on every order for chemotherapy, whether it is oral or parenteral. Many chemotherapy regimens are acronyms; these should not be allowed in the prescribing of chemotherapy. Also, abbreviations for the names of chemotherapy agents should be avoided because one abbreviation may stand for two different drug entities. For drugs such as doxorubicin and liposomal doxorubicin, the names should be written out fully, and in this case, the addition of the brand name may help to prevent a mistake.

The measured height and weight, along with the body surface area, if applicable, should be readily available, along with the dosage in milligrams per meter squared or kilogram, so that the dosage may be checked. If a chemotherapy regimen is a continuous infusion of 800 mg/m^2/day for 4 days, an added safety feature would be to include the total dosage of 3,200 mg in order to prevent any ambiguity. In cases where the clinician wants to decrease the dosage based on a laboratory value or side effect, it is recommended that the clinician include that information with the order so that everyone understands what the correct

dosage is for that patient. Chemotherapy dosages should be checked for route and dose to determine that the dosages prescribed are correct according to the regimen and do not exceed dosing guidelines. Appropriate laboratory values should be checked to verify that dosages are correct for any organ dysfunction present, and drug interactions should be scrutinized closely (Tables 88–8 and 88–9). Health care practitioners administering chemotherapy should check the dosage calculation for the body size, along with the five Rs of administering medication (i.e., right patient, right medication, right dose, right route, at the right time). If there is any question about the safe dosage or safe administration of a chemotherapy agent, the chemotherapy should not be administered until the question is resolved.

An area of controversy with chemotherapy dosing: What weight should be used for patients who are morbidly obese? Currently, there is no consensus. Some clinicians will cap BSA at some value; some clinicians will use an adjusted weight for the BSA calculation even though there is no recommendation on what adjust weight to use. This is an area for future research.

Many of the newer agents used to treat cancer are orally administered agents. The clinician needs to be aware of drug-herbal interactions, timing of agents with respect to meals, patient education on correct dosing when multiple dosage forms are used, and reimbursement issues. Table 88–10 presents a summary of timing of oral chemotherapy with respect to food. Information should be provided to the patient

---

Table 88–9

Dosing Adjustment Guidelines for Chemotherapy for Hepatic Impairment

Drug	Dosing Adjustment
Doxorubicin	Bilirubin greater than 1.5 mg/dL (26 μmol/L), reduce dose by 50%
Daunorubicin Vincristine Vinblastine	Bilirubin greater than 3.0 mg/dL (51 μmol/L), reduce dose by 75%
Vinorelbine	Bilirubin greater than 2.0 mg/dL (34 μmol/L), reduce dose by 50% Bilirubin greater than 3.0 mg/dL (51 μmol/L), reduce dose by 75%
Gemcitabine	Bilirubin greater than 1.6 mg/dL (27 μmol/L), reduce dose by 20% Bilirubin greater than 7.5 mg/dL (128 μmol/L), should be avoided
Idarubicin	Bilirubin greater than 5 mg/dL (86 μmol/L): avoid use
Docetaxel	Contraindicated with bilirubin greater than 1.5 × ULN or greater than 1.5 × ULN or transaminases greater than 1.5 × ULN or alkaline phosphatases greater than 2.5 × ULN
Imatinib	Bilirubin greater than 3 × ULN or AST/ALT greater than 5 × ULN: hold until bilirubin less than 1.5 × ULN and AST/ALT less than 2.5 × ULN and resume at reduced dose
Irinotecan	Contraindicated with bilirubin greater than 2 mg/dL (34 μmol/L) or transaminases greater than 3 × ULN (without liver metastases), greater than 5 × ULN (with liver metastases)
Ixabepilone	AST or ALT less than 10 × ULN and bilirubin less than 1.5 × ULN: 32mg/m^2 AST and AKT less than 10 × ULN and bilirubin greater than 1.6–3 × ULN: 20–30 mg/m^2
Paclitaxel	If transaminase levels less than 10 × ULN and bilirubin 1.5–2.4 mg/dL (26–41 μmol/L): reduce dose by 25% Bilirubin 2.5–7.5 mg/dL (43–128 μmol/L): reduce dose by 50% Bilirubin greater than 7.5 mg/dL (128 μmol/L): not recommended

ULN, upper limit of normal.

Adapted from DiPiro JT, Talbert RL, Yee GC, et al. (eds.) Pharmacotherapy a Pathophysiologic Approach. 7th ed. New York: McGraw-Hill; 2008: Table 130–8.

Table 88–10

Oral Chemotherapy Administration with Respect to Food

	With Food	Empty Stomach	With or Without Food
Anastrozole			X
Bexarotene	X		
Bicalutamide			X
Capecitabine	X		
Dasatinib			X
Erlotinib		X	
Estramustine			X
Etoposide			X
Exemestane	X		
Imatinib	X		
Lapatinib		X	
Lenalidomide			X
Letrozole			X
Nilutamide			X
Sorafenib		X	
Sunitinib			X
Tamoxifen			X
Temozolomide		X	
Thalidomide			X
Toremifene			X
Vorinostat	X		

both in writing and verbally, and to family caregivers if brain metastases are present in order to avoid mistakes. Particular attention should be paid to educating patients on regimens given Monday through Friday only, daily times 4 weeks and then off 2 weeks. Patients should be encouraged to bring in oral medications with visits so adherence can be checked.

OUTCOME EVALUATION

Once a pathologic diagnosis of cancer is made, the patient may be evaluated by a radiation oncologist, a surgical oncologist, and a medical oncologist. Options for treatment are presented that may include surgery, radiation, chemotherapy, or some combination of these modalities. The goals of treatment will vary by the cancer and the stage of disease. For example, the patient who has metastatic kidney cancer could be cured by high-dose aldesleukin or receive palliative therapy with sorafenib or sunitinib or may decline any therapy because of fears of significant toxicity that would decrease quality of life. In this case, if the patient's performance status is poor, such as an Eastern Cooperative Oncology Group (ECOG) performance status 3, then the patient would not be a candidate for aldesleukin therapy because of significant toxicity or even death from treatment for a patient who has a performance status of 3. The patient with the poor performance status will receive palliative therapy to control symptoms of the disease to improve the quality of life at the end of life. For the patient

Patient Encounter 3

DQ is a 57-year-old man who came to the emergency department because of shortness of breath. A radiographic examination demonstrates a large mass pressing on the bifurcation of the main stem bronchus. A biopsy demonstrates an aggressive lymphoma; a five-drug chemotherapy regimen with both IV and intrathecal chemotherapy will start today.

What steps should be taken to make sure that DQ gets the correct dosages of chemotherapy?

Patient Care and Monitoring

❻ *Clinicians should play a role in chemotherapy safety, patient education, and monitoring patient response to therapy.*

Chemotherapy Administration

1. Evaluate the chemotherapy regimen to ensure the correct dose and route of administration.

2. Check patient laboratory values to ensure that the CBC and organ function studies are normal prior to administering chemotherapy.

3. If a patient has renal or hepatic impairment or a poor metabolizer genotype, adjust chemotherapy doses if necessary.

4. Ensure appropriate antiemetic therapy for the degree of emetogenicity.

5. Assess the regimen to determine if primary prophylaxis with colony-stimulating factors is needed.

6. Assess the patient's concurrent medications for the possibility of drug interactions, and discontinue potentially interacting medications, if possible.

7. Employ safe handling and disposal methods.

Monitoring

1. *Efficacy:* Monitor CT scans or other imaging studies, and categorize patient with a complete response (CR), partial response (PR), stable disease (SD), or progressive disease.

2. *Toxicity:*

   • Monitor CBC and other lab tests

   • Monitor patient for other known toxicities of the chemotherapy regimen, and decrease the dose or discontinue the regimen if necessary

with a poor performance status and extensive metastatic disease, no treatment of the cancer may be appropriate, and the patient may be enrolled in a hospice program or provided comfort care.

Abbreviations Introduced in This Chapter

2-CDA	2-Chlorodeoxyadenosine
2-FLAA	2-Fluoro-Ara-AMP
5-FU	Fluorouracil
6-MP	6-Mercaptopurine
6-TG	6-Thioguanine
Ara-C	Cytarabine
ATRA	All-transretinoic acid
CD	Cluster of differentiation
CTC	Common toxicity criteria
FdUMP	Fluorodeoxyuridine monophosphate
IL	Interleukin
NCI	National Cancer Institute
PCR	Polymerase chain reaction
TNM	Tumor, nodes, metastases
TPMT	Thiopurine S-methyltransferase

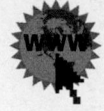 Self-assessment questions and answers are available at *http://www.mhpharmacotherapy. com/pp.html.*

REFERENCES

1. Jemal A, Siegel R, Ward E, et al. Cancer statistics, 2008. CA Cancer J Clin 2008;58:71–96.
2. Blagosklonny MV. Molecular theory of cancer. Cancer Biol Ther 2005 Jun;4(6):621–627.
3. Folkman J. Angiogenesis. Annu Rev Med 2006;57:1–18.
4. Mountford CE, Doran S, Lean CL, Russell P. Cancer pathology in the year 2000. Biophys Chem 1997 Oct;68(1–3):127.
5. Paolo A, Danesi R, Vannozzi F, et al. Limited sampling model for the analysis of 5-fluorouracil pharmacokinetics in adjuvant chemotherapy for colorectal cancer. Clin Pharmacol Ther 2002;72: 627–637.
6. Abbruzzese JL, Grunewald R, Weeks, EA, et al. A phase I clinical, plasma, and cellular pharmacology study of gemcitabine. J Clin Oncol 1991;9(3):491–498.
7. Israili ZH, Vogler WR, Mingioli ES, et al. The disposition and pharmacokinetics in humans of 5-azacytidine administered intravenously as a bolus or by continuous infusion. Cancer Res 1976;36:1453–1461.
8. Hersh MR, Kuhn JG, Phillips JL, et al. Pharmacokinetic study of fludarabine phosphate. Cancer Chemother Pharmacol 1986;17: 277–280.
9. Lilliemark J, Juliusson G. On the pharmacokinetics of 2-chloro-2'-deoxyadenosine in humans. Cancer Res 1991;51:5570–5572.
10. Kantarjian H, Gandhi V, Cortes J, et al. Phase 2 clinical and pharmacologic study of clofarabine in patients with refractory or relapsed acute leukemia. Blood 2003;1202:2379–2386.
11. Villela LR, Stanford BL, Shah SR. Pemetrexed, a novel antifolate therapeutic alternative for cancer chemotherapy. Pharmacotherapy 2006;26(5):641–654.
12. Bender R, Castle M, Margileth D, et al. The pharmacokinetics of [3H] vincristine in man. Clin Pharmacol Ther 1977;22(4):430–438.
13. Owellen RJ, Hartke CA, Hains FO. Pharmacokinetics and metabolism of vinblastine in humans. Cancer Res 1977;37:2597–2602.
14. Sparreboom A, Scripture CD, Trieu V, et al. Comparative preclinical and clinical pharmacokinetics of a Cremophor-free, nanoparticle
albumin-bound paclitaxel (ABI-007) and paclitaxel formulated in Cremophor (Taxol). Clin Cancer Res 2005;11(11):4136–4143.
15. Tije AJ, Verweij J, Carducci MA, et al. Prospective evaluation of the pharmacokinetics and toxicity profile of docetaxel in the elderly. J Clin Oncol 2005;23:1070–1077.
16. Nilsson T, Jonsson G. Clinical results with estramustine phosphate: A comparison of the intravenous and oral preparations. Cancer Chemother Rep 1975;59:229–232.
17. Dorr RT, Von Hoff DD, eds. Cancer Chemotherapy Handbook. 2nd ed. New York: Elsevier; 1994:464.
18. Rodman JH, Abromowitch M, Sinkule JA, et al. Clinical pharmacodynamics of continuous infusion teniposide: Systemic exposure as a determinant of response in a phase I trial. J Clin Oncol 1987;5(7):1007–1014.
19. Chabot GG, Bariler I, Armand JP, et al. Pharmacokinetics of the camptothecin analog CPT-11 and its active metabolite SN-38 in cancer patients. Proc Am Assoc Cancer Res 1991;32:175.
20. Rowinsky E, Grochow L, Hendricks C, et al. Phase I and pharmacologic study of topotecan: A novel topoisomerase I inhibitor. Proc Am Soc Clin Oncol 1991;10:93.
21. Gabizon A, Shmeeda H, Barenholz Y. Pharmacokinetics of pegylated liposomal doxorubicin: Review of animal and human studies. Clin Pharmacokinet 2003;42(5):419–436.
22. Ormrod D, Holm K, Goa K, Spencer C. Epirubicin: A review of its efficacy as adjuvant therapy and in the treatment of metastatic disease in breast cancer. Drugs Aging 1999;5:389–416.
23. Robert J. Clinical pharmacokinetics of idarubicin. Clin Pharmacokinet 1993;24(4):275–288.
24. Faulds D, Balfour JA, Chrisp P, Langtry HD. Mitoxantrone: A review of its pharmacodynamic and pharmacokinetic properties, and therapeutic potential in the chemotherapy of cancer. Drugs 1991; 41(3):400–449.
25. Levin VA, Hoffman W, Weinkam RJ. Pharmacokinetics of BCNU in man: A preliminary study of 20 patients. Cancer Treat Rep 1978;62:1305–1312.
26. Lee FYF, Workman P, Roberts JT, Bleechen NM. Clinical pharmacokinetics of oral CCNU. Cancer Chemother Pharmacol 1985; 14:125–131.
27. Rudek MA, Donehower RC, Statkevich P, et al. Temozolomide in patients with advanced cancer: Phase I and pharmacokinetic study. Pharmacotherapy 2004;24(1):16–25.
28. Calvert AH, Newell DR, Gumbrell LA, et al. Carboplatin dosage: Prospective evaluation of a simple formula based on renal function. J Clin Oncol 1989;7(11):1748–1756.
29. Graham MA, Lockwood GF, Greenshade D, et al. Clinical pharmacokinetics of oxaliplatin: A critical review. Clin Cancer Res 2000;6:1205–1218.
30. Dorr RT. Bleomycin pharmacology: Mechanism of action and resistance, and clinical pharmacokinetics. Semin Oncol 1992;19(2 suppl 5):3–8.
31. Zhi-Xiang S, Chen, G, Ni J, et al. Use of arsenic trioxide in the treatment of acute promyelocytic leukemia: II. Clinical efficacy and pharmacokinetics in relapsed patients. Blood 1997;89(9): 3354–3360.
32. Van Hazel GA, Scott M, Rubin J, et al. Pharmacokinetics of mitomycin C in patients receiving the drug alone or in combination. Cancer Treat Rep 1983;67(9):805–810.
33. Avvisati G, Tallman MS. All-trans retinoic acid in acute promyelocytic leukaemia. Best Pract Res Clin Haematol 2003;16(3):419–432.
34. Wohl DA, Aweeka FT, Schmitz J, et al. Safety, tolerability, and pharmacokinetic effects of thalidomide in patients infected with human immunodeficiency virus: AIDS clinical trials group 267. J Infect Dis 2002;185:1359–1363.
35. Chen N, Lau H, Kong L, et al. Pharmacokinetics of lenalidomide in subjects with various degrees of renal impairment and in subjects on hemodialysis. J Clin Pharmacol 2007;47:1466–1475.
36. Gordon MS, Margolin K, Talpaz M, et al. Phase I safety and pharmacokinetic study of recombinant human anti-vascular endothelial growth factor in patients with advanced cancer. J Clin Oncol 2001;19(3):843–850.

37. Korth-Bradley JM, Dowell JA, King SP, et al. Impact of age and gender on the pharmacokinetics of gemtuzumab ozogamicin. Pharmacotherapy 2001;21(10):1175–1180.

38. Wood AM. Rituximab: An innovative therapy for non-Hodgkin lymphoma. Am J Health Syst Pharm 2001;58(3):215–232.

39. Leyland-Jones B, Gelman K, Ayoub J, et al. Pharmacokinetics, safety, and efficacy of trastuzumab administered every three weeks in combination with paclitaxel. J Clin Oncol 2003;21:3965–3971.

40. Peng B, Hayes M, Resta D, et al. Pharmacokinetics and pharmacodynamics of imatinib in a phase I trial with chronic myeloid leukemia patients. J Clin Oncol 2004;22:935–942.

41. Bolton AE, Peng B, Hubert M, et al. Effect of rifampicin on the pharmacokinetics of imatinib mesylate in healthy subjects. Cancer Chemother Pharmacol 2004;53(2):102–106.

42. Frye RF, Fitzgerald SM, Lagattuta TF, et al. Effect of St. John's Wort on imatinib mesylate pharmacokinetics. Clin Pharmacol Ther 2004;76(4):323–329.

43. Dutreix C, Peng B, Mehring G, et al. Pharmacokinetic interaction between ketoconazole and imatinib mesylate in healthy subjects. Cancer Chemother Pharmacol 2004;54(4):290–294.

44. O'Brien SG, Meinhardt P, Bond E, et al. Effects of imatinib mesylate on the pharmacokinetics of simvastatin, a cytochrome p450 3A4 substrate, in patients with chronic myeloid leukaemia. Br J Cancer 2003;89(3):1855–1859.

45. Hamilton M, Wolf JL, Rusk J, et al. Effects of smoking on the pharmacokinetics of erlotinib. Clin Cancer Res 2006;12:2166–2171.

46. Faivre S, Delbaldo C, Vera K, et al. Safety, pharmacokinetic, and antitumor activity of SU11248, a novel oral multitarget tyrosine kinase inhibitor, in patients with cancer. J Clin Oncol 2006;24:25–35.

47. Goetz MP, Knox SK, Suman VJ, et al. The impact of cytochrome P450 2D6 metabolism in women receiving adjuvant tamoxifen. Breast Cancer Res Treat 2007;101:113–121.

48. Gonzalez ID, Saez RS, Rodilla EM, Yges EL, Toledano FL. Hypersensitivity reactions to chemotherapy drugs. Alergo Immunol Clin 2000;15:151–181.

49. Cohen MR, Anderson RW, Attilio RM, et al. Preventing medication errors in cancer chemotherapy. Am J Health Syst Pharm 1996;53:737–746.

50. ASHP technical assistance bulletin on handling cytotoxic and hazardous drugs. Am J Hosp Pharm 1990;47:1033–1049.

89 Breast Cancer

Gerald Higa

LEARNING OBJECTIVES

● **Upon completion of the chapter, the reader will be able to:**

1. List factors associated with an increased risk of breast cancer in the United States.

2. Assess patients for signs and symptoms related to breast cancer in early and late stages of the disease.

3. List all modalities that are appropriate screening tools for breast cancer and determine how they should best be used in the public domain.

4. Discuss available options for breast cancer prevention.

5. Critique available prognostic variables for clinical utility.

6. Determine which patient populations may benefit from systemic adjuvant therapy for breast cancer.

7. Determine the treatment goals for early stage, locally advanced and metastatic breast cancer.

8. Determine appropriate indications for endocrine therapy, chemotherapy and biologic therapy for patients with metastatic breast cancer.

9. Evaluate available chemotherapy options for patients with metastatic breast cancer based on pertinent patient and disease state characteristics.

10. Discuss the role of trastuzumab in the management of early and advanced stage breast cancer.

KEY CONCEPTS

❶ Nearly 75% of breast cancers are diagnosed in women older than 50 years. Regular use of screening in this age group decreases the mortality from breast cancer by 20 to 40%.

❷ Breast cancer is diagnosed most commonly in early stages, when it is highly curable.

❸ Local therapy of early-stage breast cancer consists of modified radical mastectomy or lumpectomy plus external-beam radiation therapy. The surgical approach to the ipsilateral axilla may consist of a full level I/II axillary lymph node dissection or a lymph node mapping procedure with sentinel lymph node biopsy.

❹ Adjuvant endocrine therapy reduces the rates of relapse and death in patients with hormone receptor-positive early breast cancer. Adjuvant chemotherapy reduces the rates of relapse and death in all patients with early-stage disease.

❺ The choice of chemotherapy regimen, dose, schedule, and duration of therapy, as well as endocrine therapy, are controversial and changing as results from ongoing clinical trials are reported.

❻ Neoadjuvant chemotherapy is appropriate for patients with locally advanced or inflammatory breast cancer, followed by local therapy and further systemic adjuvant therapy.

❼ The goal of adjuvant chemotherapy is cure, whereas the goal of chemotherapy in the metastatic setting is improving or preserving quality of life.

❽ Initial therapy of metastatic breast cancer in women with hormone receptor-positive tumors usually consists of hormonal therapy.

❾ Women with metastatic breast cancer who have hormone receptor-positive tumors and respond to initial hormonal manipulation usually will respond to a second-hormonal therapy.

❿ Approximately 50% to 60% of women who have not received prior chemotherapy for metastatic disease will respond to chemotherapy regimens; anthracycline- and taxane-containing regimens are the most active.

Although the incidence of breast cancer has been increasing in the United States, the mortality rate has been decreasing over the past two decades. This trend reflects the success of early detection and the development of effective treatment regimens. Treatment for most breast cancer patients includes a combination of pharmacologic and nonpharmacologic therapy.

EPIDEMIOLOGY AND ETIOLOGY

Breast cancer is the most common type of cancer and is second only to lung cancer as a cause of cancer death in American women. It is estimated that 194,280 new cases of breast cancer were diagnosed and that 40,610 women died of breast cancer in 2009.[1] Whites account for the largest portion of estimated cases (82%) and deaths (80%). In addition to invasive breast cancers, it is estimated that 62,000 cases of in situ cancer were diagnosed among women in the United States in 2007. The median age for the diagnosis of breast cancer is between the ages of 60 and 65 years.[2]

Most breast cancers diagnosed are small tumors (less than or equal to 2 cm), and disease is localized in all racial and ethnic groups. However, blacks and other minority women have proportionally more cases of disease diagnosed at more advanced stages compared with white women. This is thought to reflect access to and use of screening mammography and timely treatment.

The etiology of breast cancer is unknown, but a number of factors that increase a woman's chances of developing the disease have been identified. These risk factors, as well as information regarding the biology of the disease, suggest that a complex interplay between hormones, genetic factors, and environmental and lifestyle influences contributes to the etiology of this disease.

The two variables most strongly associated with the occurrence of breast cancer are gender and age. Although one commonly thinks of breast cancer as a disease confined to women, about 2,000 cases of male breast cancer were diagnosed in the United States in 2006.[1] When stage and other known prognostic factors are controlled for, men do not fare any differently from their female counterparts and receive similar treatment regimens.

The incidence of breast cancer increases with advancing age. Perhaps the most frequently quoted breast cancer statistic is that one in seven women will develop breast cancer during their lifetime. It should be emphasized that this is a cumulative lifetime risk of developing the disease from birth to age 110 and that the estimates are weighted by the probability of surviving through each decade of life.[3] The one in seven women figure is often misinterpreted by women who assume that it translates into one in seven women being diagnosed with breast cancer each year. Feuer and colleagues developed a more useful method of presenting the risk data based on age intervals.[3] As Table 89–1 demonstrates, the risk of a woman developing breast cancer before the age of 40 years is about 1 in 250. It is apparent from this table that although the cumulative probability of developing breast

Table 89–1	
Risk of Developing Breast Cancer: SEER Areas, Women, All Races, 1998 to 2000	
Age Interval (years)	**Probability (%) of Developing Invasive Breast Cancer During the Interval**
30–40	0.40 or 1 in 250
40–50	1.45 or 1 in 69
50–60	2.78 or 1 in 36
60–70	3.81 or 1 in 26
From birth to death	13.51 or 1 in 7

From Ref. 2.

cancer increases with increasing age, more than half the risk occurs after the age of 60.

As many as 85% of American women have "lumpy breasts" and may have a clinical diagnosis of fibrocystic breast disease or benign breast disease. Data suggest that benign breast disease or fibrocystic disease is most often not associated with proliferation and that these women are not at an increased risk for developing breast cancer.[4] However, it must be noted that "lumpy breasts" may lead to a delay in diagnosis of breast cancer because of an inability of the patient or physician to detect a true malignant lesion.

Endocrine Factors

A number of endocrine factors have been linked to the incidence of breast cancer.[5,6] Many of these relate to the total duration of menstrual life. Early menarche (prior to age 12) and late menopause (after age 55) increase a women's breast cancer risk. Similarly, investigators have reported that bilateral oophorectomy prior to age 35 reduces the relative risk of developing breast cancer. Nulliparity and a late age at first birth (greater than or equal to 30 years) have been reported to increase the lifetime risk of developing breast cancer twofold.

Long-term use of hormone-replacement therapy and concurrent use of progestins appear to contribute to breast cancer risk.[7] The use of postmenopausal estrogen-replacement therapy in women with a history of breast cancer generally is considered contraindicated. However, most experts believe that the safety and benefits of low-dose oral contraceptives currently outweigh the potential risks and that changes in the prescribing practice for the use of oral contraceptives are not warranted. Oral contraceptives are known to reduce the risk of ovarian cancer by about 40% and the risk of endometrial cancer by about 60%.

Genetic Factors

Both personal and family histories influence a woman's risk of developing breast cancer. A past medical history for breast cancer is associated with about a fivefold increased risk of contralateral breast cancer. Cancer of the uterus and ovary also has been associated with an increased risk of the development of breast cancer.

It has been recognized for some time that a family history of breast cancer is associated rather strongly with a woman's own risk for developing the disease. The percentage of all breast cancers in the population that can be attributed to family history range between 6% and 12%.[8] Empirical estimates of the risks associated with particular patterns of family history of breast cancer indicate the following:[8]

1. Having any first-degree relative with breast cancer increases a woman's risk of breast cancer 1.5- to 3-fold, depending on age.

2. The higher relative risk is associated with breast cancer with onset younger than age 45 years in one or more first-degree relatives.

3. Having multiple first-degree relatives affected has been inconsistently associated with elevated risks.

4. Having a second-degree relative affected increases a woman's risk of developing breast cancer by approximately 50% (relative risk [RR] 1.5).

5. Affected family members on the maternal side and the paternal side contribute similarly to the risk.

In the early 1990s, the *BRCA1* gene on the long arm of chromosome 17 (17q21) was identified as abnormal in a large percentage of hereditary breast and ovarian cancer patients.[9,10] A second breast cancer gene, called *BRCA2*, has been mapped to chromosome 13. Both genes are tumor suppressors. A woman with a strong family history of breast or ovarian cancer, or both, who carries a germ-line mutation of *BRCA1* faces roughly an 85% lifetime risk of breast cancer and a 60% risk of ovarian cancer.[11] Carriers of the *BRCA2* mutation have similar risks for breast cancer but much lower risks for ovarian cancer. Jewish people of Eastern European decent (Ashkenazi Jews) have an unusually high (2.5%) carrier rate of germ-line mutations in *BRCA1* and *BRCA2* compared with the rest of the U.S. population.

There is a commercially available test for screening that should be done under the guidance of a genetic counselor. Oophorectomy at completion of childbearing is recommended for carriers of *BRCA1* and *BRCA2* from high-risk families. Bilateral total mastectomy does reduce the risk of breast cancer occurrence; however, both breast and ovarian cancer have been reported in patients who have had prophylactic removal of these organs. In *BRCA* carriers who do not opt for surgical prophylaxis, mammography every 6 months is recommended and tamoxifen therapy can be considered.

Environmental and Lifestyle Factors

Experimental and epidemiologic evidence suggests an association between breast cancer and the Western diet (high in calories, fat, and cooked meats). Obesity in postmenopausal women and distribution of body fat around the abdominal region also appear to increase the risk of breast cancer. A recent meta-analysis[12] indicates both a modest positive association between alcohol ingestion and breast cancer and a dose-response relationship. Cigarette smoking and augmentation mammoplasty do not appear to increase

---

Patient Encounter, Part 1

BB is a 65-year-old woman who presents with a history of a small, hard lump in the upper outer quadrant of her right breast. This lump has been there for at least 3 months. She reports having mammograms in the past that were normal, but she has not had one in about 3 years. The lump in her breast is not painful. She has no nipple discharge or drainage from that breast and the skin appears normal. The left breast is normal. She has a history of hypertension and has been postmenopausal for approximately 10 years. She does not smoke and drinks an occasional glass of wine. She has no family history of breast cancer, but does have a sister with ovarian cancer at age 58 and her father had prostate cancer at age 85. She began menses at age 10, had two pregnancies (first at age 25) with two healthy daughters, and has taken Prempro since menopause at age 55 (for 10 years).

What risk factors for breast cancer does this patient have?

---

the risk of breast cancer. Exercise may provide a modest protection against breast cancer.

Radiation is associated with an increased risk of breast cancer in survivors of the atomic bomb, in patients given radiation for postpartum mastitis, in women receiving multiple fluoroscopic examinations during therapy for tuberculosis, and in patients who receive mediastinal radiation for malignancies. Interestingly, this risk appears to be confined to exposure to radiation prior to age 40, which suggests that a "window of initiation" for breast cancer occurs at a relatively early age. Exposure to diagnostic x-rays, including annual screening mammography, does not impart a sufficient dose of radiation for clinical concern.

It should be emphasized that more than 60% of women with breast cancer have no identifiable major risk factor, indicating that the search for the etiology of this disease is largely incomplete.

A number of calculators are available on the Internet to estimate a patient's risk of developing breast cancer. The National Cancer Institute (NCI) has an online version of the Breast Cancer Risk Assessment Tool that is considered to be the most authoritative and accurate standard (*www.cancer. gov/bcrisk-tool*). The Breast Cancer Risk Assessment Tool was designed for health professionals to project a women's individualized risk for invasive breast cancer over a 5-year period and over her lifetime.

PATHOPHYSIOLOGY

The pathologic evaluation of breast lesions serves to establish the histologic diagnosis and to confirm the presence or absence of other factors believed to influence prognosis. These prognostic factors include the presence of necrosis, lymphatic or vascular invasion, nuclear grade, hormone-receptor status, proliferative index, amount of aneuploidy, and *HER-2/neu* expression.

Invasive Carcinoma

Invasive breast cancers are a histologically heterogeneous group of lesions. Most breast carcinomas are adenocarcinomas and are classified on the basis of their microscopic appearance as either ductal or lobular, corresponding to the ducts and lobules of the normal breast. The various histologic types of breast cancer have different prognoses, but it is unknown whether their response to therapy differs because patients in therapeutic trials typically are not stratified according to histologic type. *Infiltrating lobular carcinoma* commonly metastasizes to meningeal and serosal surfaces and other unusual sites, whereas other types usually metastasize to the bone, brain, or liver.

Noninvasive Carcinoma

As with invasive carcinoma, the noninvasive lesions may be divided broadly into ductal and lobular categories. The widespread use of screening mammography and subsequent biopsy, coupled with recognition of noninvasive breast carcinoma by pathologists, has resulted in a significant increase in the diagnosis of in situ breast cancer during the past decade. A detailed discussion of the biology and appropriate management of noninvasive breast cancer is beyond the scope of this chapter, but some of the more salient characteristics of ductal carcinoma in situ (DCIS) and lobular carcinoma in situ (LCIS) are described below, and the reader is referred to a number of excellent reviews for a more comprehensive discussion.[13,14]

DCIS is seen more frequently than LCIS. It is important to note that carcinoma in situ is treated as cancer. *Simple* or *total mastectomy* (without lymph node dissection) has been the standard treatment of DCIS for several decades. Breast conservation, i.e., wide local excision followed by irradiation of breast tissue, may be an effective alternative to mastectomy. Although radiation following lumpectomy does not appear to change the survival of patients with DCIS, it significantly reduces the incidence of local recurrences and enhances the breast preservation rate in these women. Axillary dissection generally is not indicated because there is only a 1% incidence of axillary node involvement. There is currently no proven benefit for the use of cytotoxic chemotherapy in patients who receive local therapy for DCIS. However, there are subgroups of patients with DCIS, such as hormone receptor-positive patients, who may benefit from the addition of tamoxifen to lumpectomy plus radiation.[15]

CLINICAL PRESENTATION AND DIAGNOSIS

Prevention and Early Detection

Current efforts at breast cancer prevention are directed toward the identification and removal of risk factors. Unfortunately, a number of risk factors associated with the development of breast cancer, such as family history of breast cancer or personal history of breast or other gynecologic malignancies, cannot be modified. Isolation and cloning of breast cancer susceptibility genes now allows screening of women with histories suggestive of "breast cancer families" and identification of appropriate candidates for prophylactic bilateral mastectomy. There are currently no absolute indications for prophylactic bilateral mastectomy. This surgery is considered for women at very high risk for the development of breast cancer, particularly if the women's breasts are difficult to evaluate by both physical examination and mammography, and the women have persistent disabling fears that they will be diagnosed with the disease.

Clinical Presentation and Diagnosis of Breast Cancer

Common early symptoms include:
- Painless lump (90% of cases) that is:
  - Solitary
  - Unilateral
  - Solid
  - Hard
  - Irregular
  - Nontender
- Stabbing or aching pain (10% of cases) as the first symptom

Uncommon early symptoms include:
- Nipple discharge (3% of women and 20% of men), retraction, or dimpling

- Eczema appearance of the nipple (Paget's carcinoma)
- Prominent skin edema, redness, warmth, and induration of the underlying tissue (inflammatory carcinoma)

Metastatic symptoms—tissues most commonly involved with metastases are lymph nodes (other than axillary or internal mammary), skin, bone, liver, lungs, and brain. The following symptoms of metastases will be present in about 10% of patients when they first seek treatment:

- Bone pain
- Difficulty breathing
- Abdominal enlargement
- Jaundice
- Mental status changes

The idea that prevention could also be achieved pharmacologically was based on results from clinical trials of tamoxifen, an antiestrogen used as adjuvant therapy for early breast cancer. Not only was the development of contralateral breast cancer lower, but a survival advantage was also clearly demonstrated in women who received tamoxifen for 2 to 5 years following mastectomy.[16–18] Provided with an appropriate scientific rationale, several clinical trials were conducted with tamoxifen, which provided proof of principle that breast cancer risk reduction could be achieved through chemoprevention.[19–21] A recent meta-analysis of these trials indicates a consistent benefit in reducing the risk of developing estrogen receptor (ER)-positive breast cancers in premenopausal and postmenopausal women.[22]

However, results of the prevention trials also confirmed the increased incidence of tamoxifen-induced endometrial cancer. That this concern could have a direct impact on patient acceptance of chemoprevention, a search was begun for an agent with a better safety profile. A compound related to tamoxifen known as raloxifene was found to reduce the incidence of spinal fractures in postmenopausal women at high-risk for osteoporosis.[23] Because raloxifene was also an antiestrogen, the effects on breast and endometrium were also closely monitored. After 3 years of raloxifene therapy, investigators found a significant decrease in the incidence of breast cancer without the carcinogenic effect on the endometrium.[24]

The Study of Tamoxifen and Raloxifene (STAR) trial compared the two agents in postmenopausal women who were considered to be at increased risk (as determined by the Gail model)[25] for developing invasive breast cancer.[26] Although there was a similar reduction in the incidence of breast cancer, raloxifene had a superior safety profile with regards to uterine cancer and thromboembolic events. Thus, raloxifene is the chemopreventive agent of choice for postmenopausal women at high-risk for breast cancer. Since premenopausal women were not included in the STAR trial, tamoxifen is the only agent approved for reducing the risk of breast cancer in younger patients.

The impressive data of the aromatase inhibitors in the adjuvant setting have provided the rationale and impetus for studying their potential as breast cancer chemoprevention agents also. Clinical trials have begun to investigate the use of third-generation aromatase inhibitors.[27]

The rationale for early detection of breast cancer is based on the clear relationship between stage of breast cancer at diagnosis and the probability of cure. Thus, if all breast cancers could be detected at a very early stage of the disease (i.e., small primary tumor and negative lymph nodes), then more patients with the disease could be cured. Screening guidelines for early detection of breast cancer have been put forward by the American Cancer Society, the United States Preventive Services Task Force, and the National Cancer Institute[28–30] (Table 89–2). These all include recommendations for women at average risk, with some general statements regarding screening for high-risk women as well. ❶ *Nearly 75% of all breast cancer occurs in women 50 years of age or older, and regular use of screening mammography can reduce mortality from breast cancer by 20% to 40% in this age group. Controversy regarding the use of screening mammography is largely confined to women younger than 50 years of age. After many years of debate, the three available guidelines discussed here recommend mammograms in this age group of women every 1 to 2 years.*[28–30]

Diagnosis

Initial workup for a woman presenting with a lesion or symptoms suggestive of breast cancer should include a careful history, physical examination of the breast, three-dimensional mammography, and possibly other breast imaging techniques such as ultrasound. Most (80–85%) breast cancers can be visualized on a mammogram as a mass, a cluster of calcifications, or a combination of both. Breast biopsy is indicated for a mammographic abnormality that suggests malignancy or for a palpable mass on physical examination.

Clinical Staging

Stage (anatomic extent of disease) is defined on the basis of the primary tumor size (T_{1-4}), presence and extent of lymph node involvement (N_{1-3} or pN_{1-3} if pathologic examination of lymph nodes is conducted), and presence or absence of

---

Table 89–2

Guidelines for Early Detection of Breast Cancer

	American Cancer Society[18]	U.S. Preventive Services Task Force[19]	National Cancer Institute[20]
BSE	Age 20 years and older: Risk/benefit discussion	All ages: ±	NR
CBE	Age 20 to 30: Every 3 years Age 40 years and older: Every year	All ages: ± (recommended with mammogram)	All ages: Every year
Mammogram	Age 40 years and older: Interval not designated	Age greater than or equal to 40: Every 1–2 years (with or without CBE)	Age 40–49: Every 1–2 years Age 50 years and older: Every 1–2 years

BSE, breast self-examination; CBE, clinical breast examination; NR, not recommended; ±, insufficient data to recommend for or against.

Table 89–3

TNM Stage Grouping for Breast Cancer

Stage Grouping

Stage	T	N	M
0	T_{is}	N_0	M_0
I	T_1 [a]	N_0	M_0
IIA	T_0	N_1	M_0
	T_1 [a]	N_1	M_0
	T_2	N_0	M_0
IIB	T_2	N_1	M_0
	T_3	N_0	M_0
IIIA	T_0	N_2	M_0
	T_1 [a]	N_2	M_0
	T_2	N_2	M_0
	T_3	N_1	M_0
	T_3	N_2	M_0
IIIB	T_2	N_0	M_0
	T_2	N_1	M_0
	T_2	N_2	M_0
IIIC	Any T	N_3	M_0
IV	Any T	Any N	M_1

T_0, no evidence of tumor; T_{is}, carcinoma in situ or Paget's disease of the nipple with no tumor; T_1, less than or equal to 2 cm; T_2, greater than 2 to 5 cm; T_3, greater than 5 cm; T_4, any size; direct extension to chest wall (excluding pectoral muscle) or skin infiltration; regional lymph nodes (N); N_x, regional lymph nodes cannot be assessed (e.g., previously removed); N_0, no regional lymph node metastasis; pN, metastasis in one to three lymph nodes; N_2, metastasis in four to nine lymph nodes; N_3, metastasis in 10 or more lymph nodes; metastasis (M); M_0, no distant metastases; M_1, distant metastasis.

[a] T_1 includes T_1mic tumor (T).

Adapted with permission of the American Joint Committee on Cancer (AJCC), Chicago, IL. The original source for this material is the AJCC Cancer Staging Manual, 6th ed (2002). Published by Springer-Verlag New York. *www.springer-ny.com.*

distant metastases (M_{0-1}) (Table 89–3). For a more complete description of the staging system, the reader is referred to the guidelines.[31] Although many possible combinations of T and N are possible within a given stage, simplistically, stage 0 represents carcinoma in situ (T_{is}) or disease that has not invaded the basement membrane. Stage I represents small primary tumor without lymph node involvement, and the majority of stage II disease involves regional lymph nodes. Stages I and II are often referred to as *early breast cancer*. It is in these early stages that the disease is curable. Stage III, also referred to as *locally advanced disease*, usually represents a large tumor with extensive nodal involvement in which either node or tumor is fixed to the chest wall. Stage IV disease is characterized by the presence of metastases to organs distant from the primary tumor and is often referred to as *advanced* or *metastatic disease*, as described earlier. Most cancer today presents in early stages, where the prognosis is favorable (Table 89–4).

Prognostic Factors

A number of potential prognostic factors have been identified for breast cancer. *Prognostic factors* are measurements

Table 89–4

Estimated Stage at Presentation and 5-Year Disease-Free Survival (DFS): Breast Cancer

	Percentage of Total Cases	5-Year DFS[a] (%)
Stage I	40	70–90
Stage II	40	50–70
Stage III	15	20–30
Stage IV	5	0–10[b]

[a] With current conventional local and systemic therapy.

[b] Patients in stage IV are rarely free of disease; however, 10% to 20% of these patients may survive with minimal disease for 5 to 10 years.

available at diagnosis or time of surgery that in the absence of adjuvant therapy are associated with recurrence rate, death rate, or other clinical outcome.

- *Patient age.* Patients diagnosed at age younger than 35 years have a worse prognosis.
- *Tumor size.* In general, patients with a larger tumor have a worse prognosis.
- *Nuclear grade* describes the size and shape of the nucleus in tumor cells and the percentage of tumor cells that are dividing. A high nuclear grade signifies that a tumor is growing quickly and indicates a worse prognosis.
- *Lymph node involvement.* Patients with node-positive disease have a worse prognosis.
- *Hormone-receptor status.* Patients with negative-ER and negative-progesterone-receptor (PR) tumors have a worse prognosis.
- *HER-2/neu protein expression.* Patients with *HER-2/neu* overexpression have a worse prognosis.

EARLY BREAST CANCER

TREATMENT

Desired Outcome

❷ *Most patients presenting with breast cancer today have either an in situ tumor, a small tumor with negative lymph nodes (stage I), or a small stage II cancer. The goal of therapy in early breast cancer is curative.* Surgery alone can cure most, if not all, patients with in situ cancers and approximately half of all patients with stage II cancers.

Nonpharmacologic Local-Regional Therapy

The choice of surgical procedures has changed drastically over the past 50 years. ❸ *Current surgical management options for early invasive breast cancer include the modified radical mastectomy (also termed total mastectomy with ipsilateral axillary lymph node dissection) and breast conservation.* In the modified radical mastectomy, the pectoralis minor muscle may be excised, divided, or left intact, and more important,

Patient Encounter, Part 2: Medical History and Physical Exam

PMH: Hypertension for 15 years, currently controlled.

Endocrine History: Menarche age 10; menopause age 55 (natural); first child age 25; $G_2P_2A_0$. Last Pap smear 10 years ago. HRT with Prempro since age 55 (10 years). No other exogenous hormone exposure

Meds: Valsartan 160 mg by mouth daily; prempro one tablet by mouth daily.

ROS: (+) lump in right breast; otherwise (−).

PE:

Gen: Obese 65-year-old Caucasian woman who appears her stated age, in NAD

VS: BP 135/76, P 78, RR 18, T 38.1°C (100.6°F); ht 5′4″, wt 100 kg (220 lbs).

Breast: Right: Hard 2.4 x 3 cm mass in upper outer quadrant without associated erythema, dimpling or skin changes, not fixed to skin, no ulceration. No palpable lymph nodes in axilla. Left: Without masses or lymphadenopathy

Labs: All within normal limits

CXR: Lungs are clear

What information is suggestive of breast cancer?

What other tests do you need to make a diagnosis and develop a treatment plan?

there may be variation in the extent of axillary lymph node dissection, ranging from sampling to full dissection. It is important to note that in the elderly, patients with comorbid conditions, patients with particularly favorable tumors, or patients whose adjuvant therapy likely would not be affected by node status, axillary dissection can be considered optional. Breast conservation consists of lumpectomy, also referred to as segmental mastectomy, or partial mastectomy, and is defined as excision of the primary tumor and adjacent breast tissue, followed by radiation therapy to reduce the risk of local recurrence. Removal of level I/II axillary lymph nodes is recommended for completeness of staging and prognostic information. The National Institutes of Health (NIH) Consensus Conference on the Treatment of Early-Stage Breast Cancer addressed the roles of modified radical mastectomy versus breast conservation and concluded that primary therapy for breast cancer stages I and II should be breast conservation.[32] The reason given for favoring breast conservation therapy is that it achieved similar results to more extensive surgical procedures and had superior results cosmetically.

In most instances, external-beam radiation therapy used in conjunction with breast-conserving procedures involves 4 to 6 weeks of radiation therapy directed to the breast tissue to eradicate residual disease. Complications associated with radiation therapy to the breast are minor and include reddening and erythema of the breast tissue and subsequent shrinkage of total breast mass beyond that predicted on the basis of breast tissue removal. Some clinical situations also require postmastectomy radiation therapy as well (see section on locally advanced breast cancer).

There are several contraindications to breast conservation that must be considered when selecting patients:

- Multiple sites of cancer within the breast
- Pregnancy (patient cannot receive radiation)
- Inability to attain negative pathologic margins on the excised breast specimen
- Pre-existing collagen-vascular diseases (e.g., scleroderma and systemic lupus erythematosus)
- Diffuse malignant-appearing microcalcifications on mammogram
- Prior radiation treatment to the breast or chest wall
- Large tumor volume in a woman with small breasts (better cosmetic results often can be obtained with mastectomy and reconstruction).

The importance of stage I/II axillary dissection is being challenged. Although highly accurate, its morbidity is significant, with an acute complication rate as high as 20% to 30% and rates of chronic lymphedema also on the order of 20% to 30%.[33,34] A new procedure involving lymphatic mapping and sentinel lymph node biopsy is becoming more acceptable at many academic centers across the United States.[35] The sentinel lymph node is the first lymph node that drains a cancer. Injection of a dye around the primary breast tumor results in identification of the sentinel lymph node in the majority of patients, and the status of this lymph node may predict the status of the remaining nodes in the nodal basin. A sentinel lymph node can be identified in 90% of patients and can accurately predict the status of the remaining axillary nodes in 95% of patients.[36]

Pharmacologic Systemic Adjuvant Therapy

Unfortunately, breast cancer cells often spread by contiguity, lymph channels, and through the blood to distant sites. This often occurs early in the breast cancer growth, and deposits of tumor cells form in distant sites that cannot be detected with current diagnostic methods and equipment (micrometastases). *Systemic adjuvant therapy* is defined as the administration of systemic therapy following definitive local therapy (i.e., surgery, radiation, or a combination of these) when there is no evidence of metastatic disease but a high likelihood of disease recurrence. ❹ *Most published results confirm that chemotherapy (in all patients), hormonal therapy (in patients with hormone-receptor-positive disease), or both result in improved DFS and/or overall survival (OS) for patients with early-stage breast cancer.*

A standard approach was formalized at the National Institute of Health's 2000 Consensus Development Conference on adjuvant therapy for breast cancer.[32] The conference panel recommended consideration of adjuvant hormonal therapy for women whose tumors contain hormone-receptor protein regardless of age, menopausal status, involvement of axillary lymph nodes, or tumor size. They also recommended that adjuvant chemotherapy be given for essentially all patients with lymph node metastases or breast tumors 1 cm or larger in size.[32]

Another group, the St. Gallen expert panel, is convened every 2 years to review new information and establish evidence-based recommendations regarding the treatment of early breast cancer.[37] In 2007, the panel endorsed the concept and definition of "endocrine-responsive" tumors, as well as the classification of patients into three risk groups, which were established in 2005. Briefly, tumors were categorized as endocrine responsive (10% or greater number of ER-positive tumor cells), endocrine nonresponsive (0% ER-positive tumor cells), and endocrine responsive uncertain (1–9% ER-positive tumor cells). Risk classification was based on a number of tumor and patient characteristics with the regional lymph node status being the major criterion. The most prominent new recommendation in 2007 was the addition of adjuvant trastuzumab for all patients with *HER-2/neu* overexpressing tumors. A summary of the risk classification and therapy recommendations is provided in Table 89–5.

The National Comprehensive Cancer Network (NCCN) also has developed practice guidelines for the treatment of early breast cancer.[38] Whereas the 2008 guidelines already included the use of trastuzumab, the 2009 version added further recommendations related to *HER-2/neu* overexpressing tumors. First, although the prognosis of patients with tumors 1 cm or smaller and negative or micro tumor-involved nodes is generally good, the decision to use trastuzumab must consider the relative clinical benefits and drug-associated toxicities. Second, adjuvant trastuzumab should be given for at least 1 year in the absence of treatment-limiting toxicity. Third, the use of preoperative (*neoadjuvant*)

systemic therapy is gaining favor in both early-stage and locally advanced breast cancers. When used prior to surgery, treatments incorporating trastuzumab should be given for at least 9 weeks before the operation is performed.

Although neoadjuvant therapy most often consists of cytotoxic chemotherapy, hormonal agents may be preferable in patients with significant comorbidities. Nonetheless, this strategy can be used to determine tumor response in vivo (an important prognostic indicator) as well as minimize the amount of breast tissue resected. While this approach to therapy generally is reserved for patients with inoperable tumors (locally advanced), early-stage breast cancer patients who meet the criteria for breast-conserving therapy except for the size of the tumor may be considered for preoperative systemic therapy.

▶ Adjuvant Chemotherapy

5 *Cytotoxic drugs that have been used alone and in combination as adjuvant therapy in breast cancer include doxorubicin, epirubicin, cyclophosphamide, methotrexate, fluorouracil, paclitaxel, docetaxel, melphalan, prednisone, vinorelbine, and vincristine.* The most common combination chemotherapy regimens employed in the adjuvant and metastatic setting are listed in Table 89–6. The dose-limiting toxicities and other significant toxicities are listed for each chemotherapeutic agent in Table 89–7.

The basic principle of adjuvant therapy for any cancer type is that the regimen with the highest response rate in advanced disease should be the optimal regimen for use in the adjuvant setting. Early administration of effective combination chemotherapy at a time when the tumor burden is low should increase the likelihood of cure and minimize the emergence of drug-resistant tumor cell clones. Anthracyclines (e.g., doxorubicin and epirubicin) historically have been

---

Table 89–5

St. Gallen Risk Classification and Therapy Recommendations, 2007

Risk Classification	Low Risk	Intermediate Risk	High Risk
Tumor and patient criteria	Node-negative (and all of the following): ER/PR positive; *HER-2* negative; 2 cm or smaller in size; grade 1; no vascular invasion; 35 years of age or older	1–3 nodes involved with tumor and HER-2 negative *or* Node-negative (and at least one of the following): *HER-2* over-expressed greater than 2 cm in size; grade greater than 1; presence of vascular invasion; less than 35 years of age	Greater than 4 nodes involved with tumor *or* 1–3 nodes involved with tumor and *HER-2* positive
Adjuvant therapy	Endocrine or no therapy	Endocrine responsive: Endocrine therapy or chemotherapy followed by endocrine therapy; add trastuzumab if *HER-2* positive Endocrine uncertain: Chemotherapy followed by endocrine therapy; add trastuzumab if *HER-2* positive Endocrine nonresponsive: Chemotherapy; add trastuzumab if *HER-2* positive	Endocrine responsive or uncertain: Chemotherapy followed by endocrine therapy; add trastuzumab if *HER-2* positive Endocrine nonresponsive: Chemotherapy; add trastuzumab if *HER-2* positive

From Ref. 37.

Table 89–6

Common Chemotherapy Regimens for Breast Cancer

Adjuvant Chemotherapy Regimens

AC
Doxorubicin 60 mg/m² IV, day 1
Cyclophosphamide 600 mg/m² IV, day 1
Repeat cycles every 21 days for 4 cycles[a]

FAC[w]
Fluorouracil 500 mg/m² IV, days 1 and 4
Doxorubicin 50 mg/m² IV continuous infusion over
 72 hours[w]
Cyclophosphamide 500 mg/m² IV, day 1
Repeat cycles every 21–28 days for
 6 cycles[c]

CAF
Cyclophosphamide 600 mg/m² IV, day 1
Doxorubicin 60 mg/m² IV bolus, day 1
Fluorouracil 600 mg/m² IV, day 1
Repeat cycles every 21–28 days for 6 cycles[e]

FEC
Fluorouracil 500 mg/m² IV, day 1
Epirubicin 100 mg/m² IV bolus, day 1
Cyclophosphamide 500 mg/m² IV, day 1
Repeat cycle every 21 days for 6 cycles[g]

CEF
Cyclophosphamide 75 mg/m² orally on days 1–14
Epirubicin 60 mg/m² IV, days 1 and 8
Fluorouracil 500 mg/m² IV, days 1 and 8
Repeat cycles every 28 days for 6 cycles (requires
 prophylactic antibiotics or growth factor support)[i and j]

AC → Paclitaxel (CALGB 9344)
Doxorubicin 60 mg/m² IV, day 1
Cyclophosphamide 600 mg/m² IV, day 1
Repeat cycles every 21 days for 4 cycles

TAC (BCIRG 001)
Docetaxel 75 mg/m² IV, day 1
Doxorubicin 50 mg/m² IV bolus, day 1
Cyclophosphamide 500 mg/m² IV, day 1
(Doxorubicin should be given first)
Repeat cycles every 21–28 days for 6 cycles[d]

Paclitaxel → FAC[f, w]
Paclitaxel 80 mg/m²/weak IV over 1 hour every week for 12 weeks
Followed by:
 Fluorouracil 500 mg/m² IV, days 1 and 4
 Doxorubicin 50 mg/m² IV continuous infusion over 72 hours
 Cyclophosphamide 500 mg/m² IV, day 1
Repeat cycles every 21–28 days for 4 cycles[n]

CMF
Cyclophosphamide 100 mg/m²/day orally, days 1–14
Methotrexate 40 mg/m² IV, days 1 and 8
Fluorouracil 600 mg/m² IV, days 1 and 8
Repeat cycles every 28 days for 6 cycles[h, j]
or
Cyclophosphamide 600 mg/m² IV, day 1
Methotrexate 40 mg/m² IV, day 1
Fluorouracil 600 mg/m² IV, days 1 and 8
Repeat cycles every 28 days for 6 cycles[j]

Dose-Dense AC → Paclitaxel
Doxorubicin 60 mg/m² IV bolus, day 1
Cyclophosphamide 600 mg/m² IV, day 1
Repeat cycles every 14 days for 4 cycles (must be given with growth factor support)
Followed by:
 Paclitaxel 175 mg/m² IV over 3 hours
 Repeat cycles every 14 days for 4 cycles (must be given with growth factor
  support)[k]
Followed by:
 Paclitaxel 175 mg/m² IV over 3 hours
 Repeat cycles every 21 days for 4 cycles[b]

Metastatic Single-Agent Chemotherapy

Paclitaxel
Paclitaxel 175 mg/m² IV over 3 hours
Repeat cycles every 21 days[l]
or
Paclitaxel 80 mg/m²/weak IV over 1 hour
Repeat dose every 7 days[m]

Docetaxel
Docetaxel 60–100 mg/m² IV over 1 hour
Repeat cycles every 21 days[o]
or
Docetaxel 30–35 mg/m²/weak IV over 30 minutes
Repeat dose every 7 days[p]

Capecitabine
Capecitabine 2,000–2,500 mg/m²/day orally, divided
 twice daily for 14 days
Repeat cycles every 21 days[q,r]

Vinorelbine
Vinorelbine 30 mg/m² IV, days 1 and 8
Repeat cycles every 21 days
or
Vinorelbine 25–30 mg/m²/weak IV
Repeat cycles every 7 days (adjust dose based on absolute neutrophil count; see
 product information)[n]

Gemcitabine
Gemcitabine 600–1,000 mg/m²/weak IV, days 1, 8, and 15
Repeat cycles every 28 days (may need to hold day-15 dose based on
 blood counts)[q]

Liposomal doxorubicin
Liposomal doxorubicin 30–50 mg/m² IV over 90 minutes
Repeat cycles every 21–28 days[s]

(Continued)

Table 89–6

Common Chemotherapy Regimens for Breast Cancer (*Continued*)

Metastatic Combination Chemotherapy Regimens

Docetaxel + capecitabine
Docetaxel 75 mg/m² IV over 1 hour, day 1
Capecitabine 2,000–2,500 mg/m²/day orally divided
  twice daily for 14 days
Repeat cycles every 21 days[t]

Doxorubicin + docetaxel[x]
Doxorubicin 50 mg/m² IV bolus, day 1
Followed by:
  Docetaxel 75 mg/m² IV over 1 hour, day 1
  Repeat cycles every 21 days[u]

Epirubicin + docetaxel[x]
Epirubicin 70–90 mg/m² IV bolus
Followed by:
Docetaxel 70–90 mg/m² IV over 1 hour
Repeat cycles every 21 days[v]

---

[a]From Fisher B, et al. J Clin Oncol 1990;8:1483. [b]From Henderson CI, et al. J Clin Oncol 2003;21:976. [c]From Buzdar AU, et al. In: Salmon S, ed. Adjuvant Therapy of Cancer, VIII. Philadelphia, Lippincott-Raven, 1997:93–100. [d]From Martin et al. San Antonio Breast Cancer Symposium 2003;A43. [e]From Wood WC, et al. N Engl J Med 1994;330:1253. [f]From Green et al. Proc Am Soc Clin Oncol 2002;A135. [g]French Adjuvant Study Group. J Clin Oncol 2001;19:602. [h]From Bonadonna G, et al. N Engl J Med 1976;294:405. [i]From Fisher B, et al. N Engl J Med 1989;32:473. [j]From Levine MN, et al. J Clin Oncol 1998;16:2651. [k]From Citron et al. J Clin Oncol 2003;21;1431. [l]From Taxol (paclitaxel) product information. Bristol-Myers Squibb, April 2003. [m]From Perez EA, et al. Clin Oncol 2001;19:4216. [n]From Zelek L. Cancer 2001;92:2267. [o]From Taxotere (docetaxel) product information. Aventis Pharmaceuticals Inc., April 2003. [p]From Hainsworth JD, et al. J Clin Oncol 1998;16:2164. [q]From Carmichael J, et al. J Clin Oncol 1995;13:2731. [r]From Michaud et al. Proc Am Soc Clin Oncol 2000;A402, and Xeloda product information. [s]From Ranson MR, et al. J Clin Oncol 1997;15:3185. [t]From O'Shaughnessy et al. J Clin Oncol 2002;20:2812. [u]From Nabholtz JM, et al. J Clin Oncol 2003;21:968. [v]From Levin MN, et al. J Clin Oncol 1998;16:2651. [w]FAC may also be given with bolus doxorubicin administration, and the fluorouracil dose is then given on days 1 and 8. [x]Paclitaxel may also be given concurrently with doxorubicin or epirubicin as a combination regimen. Pharmacokinetic interactions make these regimens more difficult to give.

Table 89–7

Toxicities of Common Chemotherapies Used for Breast Cancer

Class	Drug	Dose-Limiting Toxicities	Other Toxicities
Anthracyclines	Doxorubicin, epirubicin	Myelosuppression, cardiomyopathy	Alopecia, nausea, vomiting, stomatitis, ulceration, and necrosis with extravasation, red-colored urine, radiation-recall effect
	Liposomal doxorubicin	Myelosuppression, palmar-plantar erythrodysesthesia (hand-foot syndrome)	Alopecia, infusion reactions, stomatitis, fatigue, nausea, vomiting
Taxanes	Paclitaxel	Neutropenia, peripheral neuropathy, hypersensitivity reactions	Alopecia, fluid retention, myalgia, skin reactions, ulceration, and necrosis with extravasation, bradycardia, stomatitis
	Docetaxel	Myelosuppression, severe fluid retention	Alopecia, fatigue, stomatitis, nausea, vomiting, diarrhea, peripheral neuropathy, nail disorder, skin reactions, hypersensitivity reactions
Antimetabolites	Capecitabine	Diarrhea, palmar-plantar erythrodysesthesias (hand-foot syndrome)	Myelosuppression, stomatitis, nausea, vomiting
	Gemcitabine	Myelosuppression (especially thrombocytopenia)	Flu-like syndrome (fever, chills, myalgias, and arthralgias), nausea
	Fluorouracil	Myelosuppression	Stomatitis, diarrhea, alopecia
	Methotrexate	Myelosuppression, stomatitis	Diarrhea, nausea, vomiting, renal toxicity
Vinca alkaloids	Vinorelbine	Neutropenia	Fatigue, nausea, vomiting, ulceration, and necrosis with extravasation
Alkylating agents	Cyclophosphamide	Myelosuppression, hemorrhagic cystitis	Alopecia, stomatitis, amenorrhea, aspermia

---

referred to as the most active class of chemotherapy agents in the treatment of metastatic breast cancer. This has led to the assumption that anthracycline-containing regimens are associated with a higher cure rate than nonanthracycline-containing regimens when used in the adjuvant setting.

The taxanes (e.g., paclitaxel and docetaxel) are a newer class of agents that rival the anthracyclines in their activity in metastatic breast cancer, becoming (arguably) the most active class of chemotherapy for this disease.

Although the optimal duration of adjuvant chemotherapy administration is unknown, it appears to be on the order of 12 to 24 weeks and may depend on the regimen being used. Chemotherapy is usually initiated within 3 weeks of surgical removal of the primary tumor. Dose intensity and dose density appear to be critical factors in achieving optimal outcomes in adjuvant breast cancer therapy. *Dose intensity* is defined as the amount of drug administered per unit of time and typically is reported in milligrams per square meter of body surface area per week (mg/m^2/weak). Increasing dose, decreasing time, or both can increase dose intensity. *Dose density* is equivalent to the concept of increasing dose intensity but not by increasing the amount of drug given, as occurs with dose escalation, but instead by decreasing the time between treatment cycles. Reducing the dose for standard treatment regimens should be avoided unless necessitated by severe toxicity. On the other hand, increasing doses beyond those contained in standard treatment regimens does not appear to add benefit because there is a threshold for dosing adjuvant chemotherapy above which only additional toxicity is seen without any improvement in patient outcomes.

The short-term toxic effects of chemotherapy used in the adjuvant setting generally are well tolerated. Although a number of investigators have demonstrated a reduction in quality of life, most patients are able to maintain a reasonable level of function and emotional and social well-being during treatment.[39] In general, supportive therapy of the patient receiving systemic adjuvant chemotherapy has improved in the past decade. Increased attention to the impact of symptoms on quality of life may account for some of this improvement. In addition, antiemetics that block serotonin and substance P have become available to assist in managing chemotherapy-induced nausea and vomiting, and colony-stimulating factors often are helpful in preventing febrile neutropenia, particularly in elderly patients or patients receiving high-dose and dose-dense chemotherapy regimens. A number of side effects are common with the regimens employed, and patients should be counseled appropriately regarding the likelihood of alopecia, weight gain, and fatigue. Patients who are menstruating usually experience a cessation of menses that may or may not return. Along with cessation of menses are accompanying signs and symptoms of menopause. Deep vein thrombosis has been reported in women receiving combination chemotherapy regimens.[40] A recent study estimated that 1 to 10 of 10,000 patients treated for 6 months with cyclophosphamide-based regimens might be expected to have leukemia within 10 years of diagnosis of breast cancer.[41] Cardiomyopathy induced by doxorubicin occurs less than 1% of the time in women whose total dose of doxorubicin is less than 320 mg/m^2.[42] It should be noted that epirubicin in the adjuvant setting is given at a dose of 100 to 120 mg/m^2.[43] At this dose, epirubicin has an equal chance of causing cardiomyopathy as standard doxorubicin doses when both agents are given as bolus or short infusions. Taxanes often are associated with hypersensitivity reactions, peripheral neuropathy, and/or myalgias and arthralgias for a few days following the infusion.

It is important to note that the magnitude of survival benefit for chemotherapy appears to be small, with an absolute reduction in mortality of only 5% at 10 years for patients with negative axillary lymph nodes and 10% for patients with positive axillary lymph nodes. Regardless, it has been reported that most patients with early breast cancer would accept drug-related toxicities in order to achieve the modest overall benefits.[44,45] Because the risks are not insignificant, investigators have been searching for ways to identify patients who could avoid chemotherapy without altering the disease prognosis. Recently, three gene expression assays (e.g., Oncotype DX, MammaPrint, and H/I) with the potential to do this have become commercially available. Of the three, Oncotype DX provides the strongest evidence that a subset of patients, especially those with ER-positive, lymph node-negative tumors derive little or no benefit from adjuvant chemotherapy when compared to the use of hormonal therapy alone.[46] Some newer data also suggest this is true for patients with lymph node-positive disease.[47] In essence, genomic analyses may play an important role in improving risk stratification and determining chemotherapy benefit.[48]

▶ Adjuvant Biologic Therapy

Trastuzumab is a monoclonal antibody directed against the *HER-2/neu* receptor. *HER-2/neu* is a member of the erbB (or HER) growth factor receptor family and is expressed at low levels in the epithelial cells of normal breast tissue. The overexpression of *HER-2/neu* is associated with increased transmission of growth signals that control aspects of cell growth and division. Most experts would agree that women whose tumors overexpress *HER-2/neu* appear to be relatively resistant to alkylating agent-based adjuvant therapy, and they might derive greater benefit from an anthracycline-based adjuvant therapy regimen.[49-51]

While *HER-2/neu* positively (but not absolutely) predicts response to trastuzumab therapy, receptor over expression is also considered a negative prognostic factor. Currently, the use of trastuzumab is indicated for treatment of adjuvant and metastatic breast cancer in patients who have tumors that overexpress *HER-2/neu*.[38] It is important to note that trastuzumab therapy should not be given concurrently with the anthracyclines because of an increased risk of cardiotoxicity (see section on metastatic breast cancer). Doses and common toxicities for trastuzumab are listed in Table 89–8.

▶ Adjuvant Endocrine Therapy

❺ *Hormonal therapies that have been studied in the treatment of primary or early breast cancer include antiestrogens, oophorectomy, ovarian irradiation, luteinizing hormone-releasing hormone (LHRH) agonists, and aromatase inhibitors.*

Hormone receptors are used clinically as indicators of prognosis and to predict response to hormone therapy. Hormone receptors are cytoplasmic proteins that transmit signals to the nucleus of the cell for growth and proliferation.

The hormone receptors clinically useful in discussions of breast cancer include the ER and the PR. The presence of these proteins in the primary tumor (or less often in metastases) is measured routinely by enzyme-linked immunochemical assays and radio assays (enzyme-linked immunosorbent assay). About 50% to 70% of patients with primary or metastatic breast cancer have hormone-receptor-positive tumors. Hormone-receptor positivity is associated with a superior response to hormone therapy and a longer disease-free interval between primary and subsequent metastatic disease and overall a more favorable prognosis. Hormone-receptor-positive tumors are more common in postmenopausal patients than in premenopausal patients. Many experts suggest that breast cancer in postmenopausal women is substantively different from that occurring in premenopausal women.

Tamoxifen traditionally was the "gold standard" adjuvant hormonal therapy and has been used in the adjuvant setting for three decades. Tamoxifen is antiestrogenic in breast cancer cells, but it appears to have estrogenic properties in other tissues and organs.[52,53] Newer information confirms that tamoxifen and other similar drugs have many estrogenic and antiestrogenic effects that depend on the tissue and the gene in question, and they are more appropriately called *selective estrogen-receptor modulators* (SERMs). Women receiving adjuvant tamoxifen therapy have a reduction in recurrence and mortality compared with women not receiving adjuvant tamoxifen therapy.[54] This observation, coupled with evidence of tamoxifen's tolerability, including beneficial estrogenic effects on the lipid profile and bone density, led to tamoxifen being the hormonal agent of choice.

Adjuvant tamoxifen therapy generally is initiated shortly after surgery or as soon as pathology results are known and the decision to administer tamoxifen as adjuvant therapy is made. The administration of tamoxifen should be limited to administration after completion of chemotherapy based on results from a study that randomized patients to receive chemotherapy for six cycles with concurrent tamoxifen, followed by continued tamoxifen for a total of 5 years, or chemotherapy with sequential tamoxifen for 5 years.[55] After a median follow-up of 8.5 years, the administration of sequential tamoxifen resulted in an estimated DFS advantage of 18% (hazard ratio [HR] 1.18) compared with the concurrent use of tamoxifen with chemotherapy.[55] It is believed the growth-inhibitory effect of tamoxifen therefore may diminish the cytotoxic effect of chemotherapy, resulting in subsequent recurrence of disease in women who received the two agents concurrently.

The optimal duration of tamoxifen therapy (20 mg/day) in the adjuvant setting is currently defined as 5 years. Studies examining prolonged administration (e.g., 10 years) have failed to demonstrate any advantage and may, in fact, be associated with a slightly worse survival.[56] Owing to the potential serious side effects of tamoxifen, all patients must be counseled properly about warning signs of endometrial cancer (i.e., vaginal bleeding or groin pain/pressure) and thromboembolism (i.e., chest pain, trouble breathing, changes in vision, one-sided weakness, or pain/swelling in the legs).

One of the most intriguing observations associated with the adjuvant tamoxifen trials relates to the role of pharmacogenomics in terms of tailoring therapy to individual patients (Table 89–9). For example, compelling evidence

---

Table 89–8

Breast Cancer Pharmacogenomics

Gene/Gene Product	Drug	Effect on Drug	Comment
CYP2D6	Tamoxifen	Enzyme responsible for metabolic activation of tamoxifen	Genetic variants of CYP2D6 with low metabolizing activity or coprescribed drugs that inhibit CYP2D6 (e.g., fluoxetine and paroxetine) associated with increased risk of disease recurrence and shorter DFS
HER2/neu	Anthracycline-containing chemotherapy regimens	Precise mechanistic effect on drug therapy not known	Clinical trial data indicate a differential benefit of the anthracyclines. These data also support the belief that the anthracyclines are one of the most active class of drugs for breast cancer
	Trastuzumab	Gene amplification and protein overexpression has predictive value	Predictive value relates to the likelihood of response to trastuzumab (conversely the agent is of no benefit in patients with HER-2 negative disease)
	Lapatinib	Gene amplification and protein overexpression has predictive value	Beneficial in patients with trastuzumab resistant disease; may be beneficial in brain metastasis
Dihydropyrimidine dehydrogenase (DPD)	5-Fluorouracil (5-FU)	Inactivates 5-FU	Low DPD activity associated with increased normal tissue toxicity
Thymidine phosphorylase (TP)	Capecitabine	Converts drug to 5-FU	Oral TP/DPD ratio appears to determine tumor 5-FU levels.

From Refs. 50, 51, 57–61, 83, 89.

from a number of studies indicate that women with germ-line variants of CYP2D6 is associated with substantially lower concentrations of the active tamoxifen metabolite endoxifen and significantly more disease recurrence and shorter DFS.[57,58] Consistent with this finding are additional data that concomitant administration of drugs that inhibit CYP2D6 resulted in reduced plasma levels of endoxifen and was an independent predictor of breast cancer outcomes in patients receiving tamoxifen.[59-61]

Toremifene is a recently marketed antiestrogen whose primary advantage is a lower estrogenic: antiestrogenic ratio than tamoxifen (based on laboratory data).[62] Toremifene (60 mg orally daily) has been found to have efficacy similar to that of tamoxifen in metastatic disease and a generally similar side-effect profile.[63] Currently, toremifene is indicated as an alternative to tamoxifen in patients with metastatic breast cancer, but studies are ongoing that evaluate its safety and efficacy in the adjuvant setting.

In premenopausal women, the use of LHRH agonists or other means of ovarian ablation have been shown to provide benefit in the adjuvant setting.[64] The use of goserelin (an LHRH agonist), alone or with tamoxifen, has been compared with standard chemotherapy (CMF) for six cycles. As a single agent, goserelin appears to provide similar benefit to CMF for six cycles for node-positive, ER-positive premenopausal breast cancer patients.[65] In another trial, the combination of goserelin and tamoxifen was compared with CMF for six cycles.[66] After a median follow-up of 6 years, this trial demonstrated a significant advantage of endocrine therapy in terms of DFS over chemotherapy alone. Retrospective reviews have found that premenopausal women who cease to menstruate with chemotherapy may have a better survival than women who continue to menstruate.[67] Therefore, the role of an LHRH agonist after chemotherapy in women who continue to menstruate is being investigated.

In postmenopausal women, recently reported evidence supporting the use of aromatase inhibitors in the adjuvant setting is intriguing and may usurp the role of tamoxifen. Three different approaches to therapy have been undertaken with these new agents: (a) direct comparison with tamoxifen for adjuvant hormonal therapy; (b) sequential use after 5 years of adjuvant tamoxifen therapy; and (c) sequential use after 2 to 3 years of adjuvant tamoxifen. Based on results of several studies, it has been concluded that therapy for postmenopausal women with ER-positive breast cancer should include an aromatase inhibitor.[37,68] It is still unclear if the aromatase inhibitor should be used instead of tamoxifen or sequentially after receiving tamoxifen for 2 to 5 years.[37] Nonetheless, the 2009 NCCN Practice Guidelines recommend "bone mineral density determination at initiation of aromatase inhibitor therapy and periodically thereafter."[38] Other concerns related to changes in blood lipids and cardiovascular disease require further study. Successful coadministration of bisphosphonates with the aromatase inhibitors has been accomplished in many patients in the metastatic setting. The three available aromatase inhibitors are exemestane, anastrozole, and letrozole.

Table 89–9			
Endocrine Therapies Used for Metastatic Breast Cancer			
Class	**Drug**	**Dose**	**Side Effects**
Aromatase inhibitors			
Nonsteroidal	Anastrozole	1 mg orally daily	Hot flashes, arthralgias, myalgias, headaches, diarrhea, mild nausea
	Letrozole	2.5 mg orally daily	
Steroidal	Exemestane	25 mg orally daily	
Antiestrogens			
SERMs	Tamoxifen	20 mg orally daily	Hot flashes, vaginal discharge, mild nausea, thromboembolism, endometrial cancer
	Toremifene	60 mg orally daily	
SERDs	Fulvestrant	250 mg IM every 28 days	Hot flashes, injection-site reactions, possibly thromboembolism.
LHRH analogs	Goserelin	3.6 mg SC every 28 days	Hot flashes, amenorrhea, menopausal symptoms, injection-site reactions
	Leuprolide	7.5 mg IM every 28 days	
	Triptorelin	3.75 mg IM every 28 days	
Progestins	Megestrol acetate	40 mg orally 4 for a day	Weight gain, hot flashes, vaginal bleeding, edema, thromboembolism
	Medroxyprogesterone	400–1,000 mg IM every week	
Androgens	Fluoxymesterone	10 mg orally twice a day	Deepening voice, alopecia, hirsutism, facial/truncal acne, fluid retention, menstrual irregularities, cholestatic jaundice
Estrogens	Diethylstilbestrol	5 mg orally 3 for a day	Nausea/vomiting, fluid retention, anorexa, thromboembolism, hepatic dysfunction
	Ethinyl estradiol	1 mg orally 3 for a day	
	Conjugated estrogens	2.5 mg orally 3 for a day	

IM, intra muscular; LHRH, luteinizing hormone-releasing hormone; SERD, selective estrogen-receptor downregulator; SERM, selective estrogen-receptor modulator.

LOCALLY ADVANCED BREAST CANCER (STAGE III)

TREATMENT

Desired Outcome

Locally advanced breast cancer generally refers to breast carcinomas with significant primary tumor and nodal disease but in which distant metastases cannot be documented. A wide variety of clinical scenarios can be seen within this group of patients, including neglected tumors that have spread locally and inflammatory breast cancers that are a unique clinical entity. Many locally advanced breast cancers are diagnosed in patients who have had symptoms for months to years and have neglected to seek medical attention. Patients with inflammatory breast cancer often are treated inappropriately for cellulitis with antibiotics for several weeks to months.

Treatment of stage III breast cancer generally consists of a combination of surgery, radiation, and chemotherapy administered in an aggressive approach. The natural history of locally advanced breast cancer suggested that even when local-regional control was accomplished, systemic relapse and death from breast cancer occurred eventually in most patients.[69] This led to interest in the use of neoadjuvant or primary chemotherapy in locally advanced breast cancer, as discussed previously. This approach to therapy renders inoperable tumors resectable and can increase rates of breast-conserving therapy. Theoretical advantages also include potential benefits related to early initiation of systemic therapy, delivery of drugs through an intact vasculature, in vivo assessment of response to therapy, and the opportunity to study the biologic effects of the systemic treatment. However, this approach to therapy also results in a loss of standard, well-validated pathologic prognostic markers, such as initial tumor size and the number of axillary lymph nodes involved. Also, as discussed earlier, OS with adjuvant compared with neoadjuvant chemotherapy is similar, making either approach reasonable for a patient with operable breast cancer.

Pharmacologic Therapy

❻ *For patients with inoperable breast cancer, including inflammatory breast cancer, the initial approach to therapy should be chemotherapy with the goal of achieving resectability.* After neoadjuvant chemotherapy, most tumors respond with more than a 50% decrease in tumor size; about 70% of patients experience downstaging. Chemotherapy regimens used in this setting are similar to those used in the adjuvant setting. Supporting evidence for each individual regimen differs, but most of the available data support the use of anthracycline-containing regimens, incorporation of the taxanes in some manner, and other approaches to improve dose density or dose intensity. For more details regarding the specific regimens, the reader is referred to a recently published review.[69] Neoadjuvant endocrine therapy may be an option for patients who have unresectable hormone-receptor-positive tumors who are unable to receive chemotherapy (e.g., multiple comorbid conditions). In terms of local therapy, this usually follows chemotherapy, and the extent of surgery will be determined by response to chemotherapy, the wishes of the patient, and the cosmetic results likely to be achieved. Many patients may be able to have breast-conserving surgery if an acceptable response to chemotherapy is achieved. Adjuvant radiation therapy should be administered to all locally advanced breast cancer patients to minimize local recurrences regardless of the type of surgery used for that individual patient (e.g., mastectomy or segmental mastectomy). Inoperable tumors that are unresponsive to systemic chemotherapy may require radiation therapy for local management and may or may not be eligible for surgical resection after that radiation. Such patients are not seen commonly, but they have a very poor prognosis. For most patients in this category, cure is still the primary goal of therapy and can be achieved in a large number of patients when all treatment modalities are employed.

METASTATIC BREAST CANCER (STAGE IV)

TREATMENT

Desired Outcome

The goal of therapy with early and locally advanced breast cancer is to cure the disease. **❼** *Breast cancer is currently incurable after it has advanced beyond local-regional disease.* The goal of treatment of metastatic breast cancer is to improve symptoms, maintain quality of life, and extend survival. Thus, it is important to choose therapy with good activity while minimizing toxicities. Treatment of metastatic breast cancer with either cytotoxic or endocrine therapy often results in regression of disease and improvements in quality of life.

General Approach to Treatment

The choice of therapy for metastatic disease is based on the site of disease involvement and presence or absence of certain characteristics (i.e., hormone and HER-2 receptor status of the primary tumor). For example, patients who experience a long DFS following local-regional therapy or have disease that is located primarily in the bone or soft tissue likely will respond to endocrine therapy. Patients with asymptomatic visceral involvement (e.g., liver or lung) may be candidates for hormonal therapy depending on the clinical circumstance (generally, hormones work more slowly than chemotherapy). **❽** *Patients who are hormone-receptor-positive generally will receive initial endocrine therapy followed by combination chemotherapy when endocrine therapy fails.* **❾** *Patients who respond to initial endocrine therapy often respond to a second (or even third) hormonal manipulation.* Response rate is lower and duration of response is shorter with second (and third) hormonal manipulations. Patients are treated sequentially with endocrine therapy until their tumors cease to respond, at which time cytotoxic chemotherapy can be given. Between 50% and 60% of ER-positive patients and 75% and 80% of ER- and PR-positive patients will respond to hormonal therapy, whereas those with ER- and PR-negative tumors have a less than 10% response rate. Thus, the largest factor determining choice of endocrine versus cytotoxic chemotherapy is the presence of hormone receptors in the primary breast tumor.

Patients who are hormone-receptor-negative with rapidly progressive or symptomatic disease involving the liver, lung, or CNS or those having progressed on initial endocrine therapy usually are treated with cytotoxic chemotherapy initially. ❿ *Chemotherapy will result in an objective response in about 50% to 60% of patients previously unexposed to chemotherapy.* Most patients have partial response, and complete disappearance of disease occurs in fewer than 20% of patients treated. Median duration of response is 5 to 12 months, although some patients will have an excellent response to an initial course of chemotherapy and may live 5 to 10 years without evidence of disease. In general, survival of patients after treatment with commonly used drug combinations for metastatic breast cancer is a median of 14 to 33 months. The response rate to second- and third-line combination chemotherapy varies from 20% to 40% depending on the previous chemotherapy regimens the patient has received. Combinations of different hormonal therapies or chemotherapy plus hormones are not employed in the setting of metastatic breast cancer owing to the lack of increased efficacy and evidence of increased toxicity. Patients with tumors that have *HER-2/neu* overexpression should be considered for treatment with trastuzumab, alone or with chemotherapy.

Pharmacologic Systemic Therapy

▶ *Endocrine Therapy*

The pharmacologic goals of endocrine therapy for breast cancer are either to decrease circulating levels of estrogen and/or to prevent the effects of estrogen on the breast cancer cell (targeted therapy) through blocking the hormone receptors or downregulating the presence of those receptors. Achievement of the first goal depends on the menopausal status of the patient, but achievement of the second goal is independent of menopausal status. Many endocrine therapies are available to target either goal of therapy, and combination studies also have been conducted in an attempt to combine differing mechanisms of action and improve outcomes. Unfortunately, combinations have not demonstrated any efficacy benefits but have increased toxicity. Therefore, combinations of endocrine agents for breast cancer are not recommended outside the context of a clinical trial. Patients often are treated with a series of endocrine agents, frequently over several years, before chemotherapy is considered.

Until recently, there was little evidence that the response or survival benefit from one endocrine therapy was clearly superior to that achieved with other therapies. Given this equality in efficacy, the choice of a particular endocrine therapy was based primarily on toxicity (Table 89–9). Based on these criteria, tamoxifen has been the preferred initial agent when metastases are present. An exception to this occurs when the patient is receiving adjuvant tamoxifen at the time or within 1 year of occurrence of metastatic disease.

Over the past decade, new information has been published regarding the use of a new generation of aromatase inhibitors. These data have changed the way we treat metastatic breast cancer, as well as early-stage breast cancer (as noted previously). In postmenopausal and castrated women, the main source of estrogen is derived from the peripheral conversion of androstenedione, produced by the adrenal gland, to estrone and estradiol. This conversion requires the enzyme aromatase. Aromatase also catalyzes the conversion of androgens to estrogens in the ovary in premenopausal women and in extraglandular tissue, including the breast itself, in postmenopausal women. Therefore, aromatase inhibitors (e.g., anastrozole, letrozole, and exemestane) effectively reduce the level of circulating estrogens, as well as estrogens in the target organ. Their toxicity profile consists mainly of nausea, hot flashes, arthralgias/myalgias, and mild fatigue. Anastrozole and letrozole are nonsteroidal compounds that exhibit reversible, competitive inhibition of aromatase. Exemestane is a steroidal compound that binds irreversibly to aromatase, forming a covalent bond. There is no clinical evidence that exemestane produces superior results over the other agents in this class.

Aromatase inhibitors are used for first-line therapy for advanced breast cancer in postmenopausal women. Large trials have compared these agents with tamoxifen and have found similar response rates and a longer median time to progression for patients receiving the selective aromatase inhibitor.[49] A consistent finding in these trials was a lower incidence of thromboembolic events and vaginal bleeding in patients who received selective aromatase inhibitors, which, together with the advantage in terms of time to progression, led to the conclusion that the new aromatase inhibitors are superior to tamoxifen as first-line therapy for advanced breast cancer in postmenopausal women. Use of a steroidal aromatase inhibitor (exemestane) after a patient progresses on a nonsteroidal inhibitor (anastrozole or letrozole) may provide some benefit and is a common practice based on small clinical trials investigating this sequential approach to therapy.[70] The opposite sequence also has shown some benefit. Therefore, patients may receive two aromatase inhibitors (first and second line sequentially), especially patients who progress while on adjuvant tamoxifen therapy.

As mentioned several times so far, the aromatase inhibitors are only used appropriately in women who are postmenopausal. Premenopausal or perimenopausal women, whose ovaries are functioning, are not appropriate candidates for these therapies, at least based on the available evidence. Use of the aromatase inhibitors in addition to ovarian ablation (e.g., oophorectomy or LHRH agonists) is currently being investigated. Also, the use of aromatase inhibitors in men with advanced breast cancer should be avoided. Available evidence suggests that use of these agents in men increases circulating levels of testosterone, which may negate the therapeutic effects of the drug.[71]

Antiestrogens bind to estrogen receptors, preventing receptor-mediated gene transcription, and therefore are used to block the effect of estrogen on the end target. This class of agents now is subdivided into two pharmacologic categories, SERMs and pure antiestrogens. SERMs include tamoxifen and toremifene and demonstrate tissue-specific activity, both estrogenic and antiestrogenic, as described previously. The agonistic activity is thought to be responsible for many of the adverse reactions seen with these agents, including the increased risk of endometrial cancer. Research into how to minimize this agonistic activity has led to the production of pure estrogen-receptor antagonists that lack estrogen agonist activity. Pure antiestrogens are a new class of agents that are also referred to as *selective estrogen-receptor downregulators* (SERDs). These molecules bind to the ER, inhibiting estrogen binding, and cause a degradation of the drug-ER complex, decreasing the amount of ER on the tumor cell surface. There is currently only one pure antiestrogen available commercially in the United States, namely, fulvestrant.

Tamoxifen can be used in both premenopausal and postmenopausal women with metastatic breast cancer who have tumors that are hormone-receptor-positive. The toxicities of tamoxifen are described in the section on adjuvant endocrine therapy. The only additional toxicity that one might expect to find in the setting of metastatic breast cancer (specifically bone metastases) is a tumor flare or hypercalcemia, which occurs in approximately 5% of patients following the initiation of any SERM therapy and is not an indication to discontinue SERM therapy. It is generally accepted that this is a positive indication that the patient will respond to endocrine therapy.

Toremifene is another commercially available SERM for the treatment of breast cancer. It exhibits similar efficacy and tolerability to tamoxifen in the metastatic setting. Cross-resistance to toremifene has been demonstrated in patients with tamoxifen-refractory disease.[72] Therefore, toremifene appears to be an alternative to tamoxifen in postmenopausal patients with positive or unknown hormone-receptor status with metastatic breast cancer.

Fulvestrant is a new agent approved for the second-line therapy of postmenopausal metastatic breast cancer patients who have tumors that are hormone-receptor-positive. Studies examining the role of fulvestrant in the treatment of metastatic breast cancer have compared this agent with anastrozole. Given anastrozole's mechanism of action, only postmenopausal women were eligible for these trials. There is no biologic reason why fulvestrant should not produce similar outcomes in premenopausal women, but no data exist to confirm the safety or efficacy in premenopausal women. In the comparative trials with fulvestrant and anastrozole, similar efficacy and safety were demonstrated with both agents when given after patients progressed on tamoxifen therapy.[73,74] Adverse events related to fulvestrant include injection-site reactions, hot flashes, asthenia, and headaches. This agent is a good option for patients who are unable to take an oral medication because it is given as an intramuscular injection over 28 days.

Another goal of antitumor treatment is to reduce estrogen production in premenopausal women with surgery, irradiation, or medication. No difference has been found in two randomized trials of the overall response rate between tamoxifen and oophorectomy in premenopausal women. However, the secondary response rate to oophorectomy after tamoxifen treatment was somewhat higher than the response to tamoxifen after primary oophorectomy (33% versus 11%).[75] Some experts interpret this as suggesting that tamoxifen does not completely antagonize available estrogen, particularly in premenopausal women. Ovarian ablation (surgically or chemically) is still used commonly in some parts of the United States and is considered by many specialists to be the endocrine therapy of choice in premenopausal women. The mortality rate with surgical oophorectomy is low, usually less than 2% to 3% in appropriately selected patients. Irradiation of the ovaries was a means of castration many years ago but was associated with multiple complications and is no longer performed for these purposes. Medical castration with LHRH analogs is used increasingly in lieu of oophorectomy in premenopausal women.

Medical castration with LHRH analogs has been used in premenopausal metastatic breast cancer patients and induces remission in about one-third of unselected patients. The mechanism of action of LHRH analogs in breast cancer is thought to result from down-regulation of LHRH receptors in the pituitary. Decreased levels of luteinizing hormone (LH) subsequently lead to a decrease in estrogen to castrated levels. The three agents available in the United States are leuprolide, goserelin, and triptorelin, but only goserelin is approved for the treatment of metastatic breast cancer. These agents are administered as an injection and are associated with minimal side effects, including amenorrhea, hot flashes, and occasionally nausea. A recent metaanalysis was reported on combined tamoxifen and LHRH agonists versus LHRH agonists alone in premenopausal patients with metastatic breast cancer.[76] With a median follow-up of 6.8 years, there was a significant survival benefit and progression-free survival (PFS) benefit in favor of the combined treatment. The overall response rate was significantly higher on combined endocrine treatment. However, this analysis did not compare tamoxifen alone against the combination of an LHRH agonist with tamoxifen. LHRH agonists also may produce a flare response owing to an initial surge in LH and estrogen production for the first 2 to 4 weeks. This flare response is similar to that seen with tamoxifen, and patients should be monitored for increasing pain and/or hypercalcemia during the initiation period.

Progestins such as megestrol acetate and medroxyprogesterone acetate have been compared with tamoxifen in randomized trials and have been found to yield equal response rates. Although there were no direct comparisons of these two forms of progestational therapy, they appear to be equally effective. Medroxyprogesterone acetate is used more frequently in Europe, and megestrol acetate is used more frequently in the United States. Based on efficacy and tolerability, these agents generally are reserved as third-line therapy after patients have received an aromatase inhibitor and a SERM (i.e., tamoxifen or toremifene). The most common side effect is weight gain, occurring in 20% to 50% of patients. Patients experiencing weight gain may have fluid retention, but fluid retention is not totally responsible for the weight gain. In cachectic cancer patients, the weight gain may be desirable, but this is not uniformly true of all patients with metastatic breast cancer. Additional side effects associated with progestins include vaginal bleeding in 5% to 10% of patients, either while patients are taking the progestational agent or when it is discontinued, and somewhat less than a 10% incidence of hot flashes. Thromboembolic complications are also significant with these agents.

High-dose estrogens and androgens are used rarely today because these agents are more toxic than the other hormonal agents discussed thus far. About one-third of patients placed on high-dose estrogens will discontinue them because of side effects, the most important of which are thromboembolic events, vomiting, and fluid retention. Given the recent availability of the aromatase inhibitors, use of androgens and estrogens has become rare.

▶ Cytotoxic Chemotherapy

Cytotoxic chemotherapy is eventually required in most patients with metastatic breast cancer. Patients with hormone-receptor-negative tumors r-equire chemotherapy as initial therapy of symptomatic metastases. Patients who respond initially to hormonal manipulations eventually cease to respond and go on to require chemotherapy. The median duration of response is 5 to 12 months, but some patients will have an excellent response to an initial course of chemotherapy and may live 5 to 10 years or longer without evidence of disease. In general, median survival of patients after treatment with commonly used drug combinations for metastatic breast cancer is 14 to 33 months. The median time to response has ranged from 2 to 3 months in most studies, but this period depends in large part on the site of measurable disease. The median time to appearance of response is between 3 and 6 weeks in patients whose disease is primarily in the skin and lymph nodes, 6 to 9 weeks in patients with metastatic lung involvement, 15 weeks in patients with hepatic involvement, and nearly 18 weeks in patients with bone involvement. Thus it is often the case that an immediate response to therapy is not apparent, and in general, once a chemotherapy regimen has been initiated, it is continued until there is unequivocal evidence of progressive disease.

There are no well-defined clinical characteristics or established tests to identify patients likely to benefit from chemotherapy. Factors associated with an increased probability of response that have been identified include a good performance status, a limited number (one–two) of disease sites, and patients who respond to chemotherapy or hormonal therapy with a long disease-free interval. Patients who have progressive disease during chemotherapy have a lower probability of response to a different type of chemotherapy. However, this is not necessarily true for patients who are given chemotherapy after some interval during which they have received no chemotherapy. Patients who do not respond to endocrine therapy are as likely to respond to chemotherapy as patients who are treated with chemotherapy as their initial treatment modality. Age, menopausal status, and receptor status have not been associated with favorable or unfavorable response to chemotherapy.

A number of chemotherapeutic agents have demonstrated activity in the treatment of breast cancer, including doxorubicin, epirubicin, paclitaxel, nab-paclitaxel, docetaxel, capecitabine, fluorouracil, cyclophosphamide, methotrexate, vinblastine, vinorelbine, ixabepilone, gemcitabine, mitoxantrone, mitomycin-C, thiotepa, and melphalan. ❿ *The most active classes of chemotherapy in metastatic breast cancer are the anthracyclines and the taxanes, producing response rates as high as 50% to 60% in patients who have not received prior chemotherapy for metastatic disease.*[77] The most useful weekly dose of paclitaxel in the metastatic setting appears to be 80 mg/m^2/weak with no breaks in therapy. With this approach, the toxicity profile of paclitaxel changes with less myelosuppression and delayed onset of peripheral neuropathy but slightly more fluid retention and skin and nail changes. Patients should be premedicated with a steroid (dexamethasone), H$_1$ antagonist (diphenhydramine), and H$_2$ antagonist (ranitidine or famotidine) prior to treatment to minimize hypersensitivity reactions. A randomized study comparing doses of 60, 75, and 100 mg/m^2 docetaxel was published recently and demonstrates a dose-response relationship with regard to response rates only.[78] Time to progression and os were similar among all three dose levels. Therefore, dose remains important for symptomatic patients who require a rapid response to therapy. In asymptomatic patients requiring docetaxel chemotherapy, lower doses may be appropriate. Results from a single randomized trial appear to indicate that docetaxel is associated with less neuropathy, myalgia, and hypersensitivity than paclitaxel given every 3 weeks, but febrile neutropenia, fluid retention, and skin reactions appear to occur more frequently with the newer taxane.[79] The median cumulative docetaxel dose to the onset of fluid retention is 400 mg/m^2 in nonpremedicated patients. Premedication with a steroid (dexamethasone) prior to beginning docetaxel and continued for 3 days helps to prevent hypersensitivity reactions and fluid retention.

Regardless of the minor controversy regarding whether a new formulation of an old drug can be considered a "new" drug, nanoparticle albumin-bound paclitaxel or nab-paclitaxel exhibits some distinct advantages over conventional paclitaxel. In a pivotal clinical study designed to compare the efficacy and safety of nab-paclitaxel with the older formulation, patients with metastatic breast cancer were enrolled into a randomized trial.[80] Patients received either 260 mg/m^2 nab-paclitaxel or 175 mg/m^2 conventional paclitaxel. Because the albumin-bound drug does not require solvents, standard premedications to prevent acute drug reactions were not given to those randomized to the newly formulated product. Results of the trial indicated significantly better outcomes in patients treated with nab-paclitaxel compared to those receiving standard paclitaxel. The overall response rates of 33% and 19% favored patients in the nab-paclitaxel arm; $P = 0.001$; and median time to progression for the nab-paclitaxel group and conventional paclitaxel group was 23 weeks versus 16.9 weeks, respectively, $P = 0.006$. Despite the higher dosage, the incidence of severe neutropenia was significantly lower with nab-paclitaxel compared to conventional paclitaxel, 9% versus 22%, respectively; $P < 0.001$. In addition, even in the absence of premedication, no acute hypersensitivity reactions were observed with nab-paclitaxel administration. Nab-paclitaxel is currently indicated for patients with metastatic breast cancer resistant to conventional chemotherapy or progressing within 6 months of receiving an adjuvant anthracycline-containing chemotherapy regimen.

Ixabepilone is a member of a distinct class of microtubule-targeted agents known as the epothilones. In vitro studies show that the antitumor activity of ixabepilone, like the taxanes, occurs primarily by blocking disassembly, thus kinetically "stabilizing" the microtubule structure. The results of an international phase III clinical trial demonstrated that the combination of ixabepilone plus capecitabine significantly prolonged PFS by approximately 1.6 months compared to capecbine alone (median 5.8 months versus 4.2 months, respectively; $P = 0.0003$).[81] This relatively modest improvement represented a 38% overall increase in PFS. The objective response rate (ORR) was more than twice as high with the combination compared to capecitabine alone, 35% versus 14%, respectively. Notably, the response rates were nearly identical to the ORRs (33% versus 14%) in patients who had disease which was intrinsically resistant to previous taxane therapy. The findings from this study support preclinical data that the antitumor activity between ixabepilone and capecitabine are at least additive, and may in fact, be synergistic.[82]

However, a much higher incidence of adverse effects involving the bone marrow and peripheral nervous system was apparent in those receiving ixabepilone plus capecitabine. Five infection-related deaths were associated with abnormal liver function at the time of enrollment. In addition, two-thirds of the patients developed variable grades of sensory neuropathy; 21% of the all patients discontinued treatment due to this adverse effect.

Ixabepilone is approved for use in combination with capecitabine for patients with advanced breast cancer resistant to or progressing on previous anthracycline and taxane therapy or for patients in whom anthracyclines are contraindicated. The use of single-agent ixabepilone is approved for use in patients with disease resistant capecitabine as well as any drugs in the two classes mentioned above.

Capecitabine is a novel oral agent approved in the mid-1990s with significant activity in metastatic breast cancer patients who have progressed on an anthracycline-containing regimen as well as a taxane regimen. This agent is a prodrug for fluorouracil with somewhat targeted activity toward malignant cells. The parent compound undergoes a three-step enzymatic conversion to become fluorouracil at the target cell (Table 89–9).[83] The third and final step in this conversion is more likely to occur in malignant cells than normal cells owing to the presence of higher levels of the responsible enzyme in malignant tissues. Approximately 85% of fluorouracil is degraded by dihydropyrimidine dehydrogenase (Table 89–9). In patients who have been exposed to an anthracycline and a taxane, capecitabine produces response rates of about 25%, which is impressive compared with other tested chemotherapy agents.[84]

Vinorelbine, a microtubule interactive agent, also has shown impressive response rates in metastatic breast cancer.[85] Vinorelbine was approved by the FDA in 1994 for the treatment of nonsmall cell lung cancer. It is not approved for breast cancer, but response rates to vinorelbine range from 30% to 50%, with an overall 5% complete response rate in phase I and phase II studies in patients with advanced breast cancer. Importantly, paclitaxel, docetaxel, and vinorelbine do not appear to be cross-resistant with anthracyclines, which are arguably considered first-line treatment of metastatic breast cancer.

Gemcitabine is another agent that is used quite frequently in patients who have received the aforementioned chemotherapy regimens, who still have a good performance status, and who may benefit from additional chemotherapy. This is a nucleotide analog that inhibits DNA synthesis. Response rates ranging from 13% to 42% have been reported in a number of phase II trials.[85] In patients who have been exposed to an anthracycline and a taxane, gemcitabine appears to provide similar benefit to capecitabine. This agent appears to affect platelets more frequently than other chemotherapy previously mentioned, and close monitoring is required for patients receiving this agent.

Combination chemotherapy regimens are associated with higher response rates than are single-agent therapies in the treatment of metastatic breast cancer, but the higher response rates usually have not translated into significant differences in time to progression and OS. The use of sequential single-agent chemotherapies versus the combination regimens has been debated widely for metastatic breast cancer. Current consensus is that first-line chemotherapy includes sequential single agents or combination chemotherapy.[38] In the palliative metastatic setting, using the least toxic approach is preferred when efficacy is considered equal. In clinical practice, patients who require a rapid response to chemotherapy (e.g., those with symptomatic bulky metastases) often receive combination therapy despite the added toxicity. This decision is complex and should be made on an individual patient basis.

Because most patients are given adjuvant chemotherapy, regimens chosen for first-line use in the metastatic setting often are different from those used in the adjuvant setting. If a patient's cancer recurs within 1 year of finishing adjuvant chemotherapy, those chemotherapy agents are not considered effective for treatment of the metastatic disease. However, if the patient recurs more than 1 year after the end of her adjuvant chemotherapy, the same agents also may be helpful in the metastatic setting.

► *Biologic Therapy*

Trastuzumab is a humanized monoclonal antibody that binds with a specific epitope of the *HER-2/neu* protein. Single-agent treatment with trastuzumab has a response rate of 15% to 20% and a clinical benefit rate of nearly 40% in patients with *HER-2/neu*-overexpressing cancers.[86] Trastuzumab has additive and perhaps synergistic activity with other chemotherapeutic agents.[87] In the pivotal trial, patients who received the doxorubicin-trastuzumab combination had a very high incidence of cardiotoxicity (27%), leading to a black-box warning regarding this combination in the product information for trastuzumab. Many investigators are attempting to circumvent this toxicity while giving these two classes of agents together (e.g., liposomal doxorubicin or continuous-infusion doxorubicin). Until further information regarding the safety of these approaches becomes available, this combination should not be given outside the context of a clinical trial. Other chemotherapy agents that are being evaluated in combination with trastuzumab include docetaxel, vinorelbine, gemcitabine, capecitabine, and the platinum agents (e.g., cisplatin and carboplatin).[88]

Trastuzumab is reasonably well tolerated. The most common adverse effects are infusion-related, primarily fever and chills, and occur in about 40% of patients during the initial infusion. Acetaminophen and diphenhydramine may be given and/or the infusion rate reduced to help alleviate the symptoms related to these reactions. A more severe adverse effect consisting of severe hypersensitivity and/or pulmonary reactions has been reported but is rare. It is important to educate patients regarding the pulmonary reactions because these may occur up to 24 hours after the infusion and can be fatal if not treated promptly. Trastuzumab may increase the incidence of infection, diarrhea, and/or other adverse events when given with chemotherapy. As mentioned previously, when given with an anthracycline, the rates of heart failure are unacceptably high, but even when given as a single agent, there is about a 5% incidence of heart failure. Fortunately, the heart failure seen with trastuzumab is somewhat reversible with pharmacologic management, and some patients have continued therapy with trastuzumab after their left ventricular ejection fraction has returned to normal. Close monitoring for clinical signs and symptoms of heart failure is important in order to intervene with appropriate cardiac treatments.

It should be noted that only 20% to 30% of patients with metastatic breast cancer overexpress *HER-2/neu*, and commercially available immunohistochemistry (IHC) tests that are reported back as 2+ for *HER-2/neu* are often negative by the more sensitive and specific fluorescence in situ hybridization (FISH) technique. To date, there is no benefit associated with the administration of trastuzumab to the subset of patients who are *HER-2/neu*-negative and a very questionable benefit associated with administration of trastuzumab to women who are 2+ for *HER-2/neu* by IHC staining alone. The patients who benefit most from trastuzumab therapy include those whose tumors express *HER-2* protein at the 3+ level and/or demonstrate gene amplification by FISH testing.[89]

Lapatinib is a dual inhibitor of *HER-2/neu* and the epidermal growth factor receptor (EGFR). In contrast to the extracellular recognition site of trastuzumab, the specific targets of lapatinib are the receptors' intracellular kinase domain. A critical phase III trial was conducted to assess the efficacy and safety of lapatinib plus capecitabine versus capecitabine alone in patients with trastuzumab-refractory advanced breast cancer.[90] Of note, the trial was terminated early when a preplanned interim analysis indicated a significant reduction in risk of disease progression (time to progression [TTP], $P < 0.001$) which favored the group receiving the combination to capecitabine alone. Efficacy data of the entire patient cohort were reanalyzed 4 months later. Based on an independent review, the median TTP was 27.1 weeks and 18.6 weeks ($P = 0.00013$, HR 0.57) and response rates were 23.7% and 13.9% for the lapatinib combination arm and capecitabine monotherapy arm, respectively. Interestingly, tumor cell expression of EGFR was not an eligibility criterion. This is especially notable because results from an earlier study of lapatinib suggested that clinical response may be higher in breast tumors that coexpressed EGFR and HER2.[91] Another relevant outcome was the significantly lower incidence of brain metastasis in the lapatinib-treated group compared to capecitabine alone, 2% versus 11%, respectively, $P = 0.0445$.[92]

Clinical trials of lapatinib have revealed a remarkably similar side-effect profile which included nontreatment-limiting diarrhea, rash, nausea and fatigue among the most frequently reported side effects. The incidence of diarrhea, dyspepsia, and rash was higher when lapatinib was combined with capecitabine.[81] Cardiac events were also monitored because severe toxicity related to blockade of the *HER-2/neu* signaling pathway has been previously reported.[93,94] Although addition of lapatinib was not associated with any cardiac event resulting in subject withdrawal, the answer related to this issue is not final as the possibility of selection bias and the relatively short observation period.

Based on these data, lapatinib in combination with capecitabine was approved in March 2007 for patients with *HER-2/neu*-overexpressing metastatic breast cancer progressing on prior anthracycline, taxane, and trastuzumab therapy.

Another monoclonal antibody, bevacizumab, was combined with paclitaxel in a clinical trial for first-line chemotherapy in women with metastatic breast cancer. The PFS was improved for the combination regimen over paclitaxel alone.[38] Bevacizumab targets vascular endothelial growth factor (VEGF), thereby preventing angiogenesis, which is a necessary process to support tumor growth and metastasis. Bevacizumab was first approved by the FDA for the treatment of colorectal cancer and in February 2008, received FDA approval as first-line therapy in combination with paclitaxel for metastatic *HER-2*-negative breast cancer. Additional studies are being conducted to elucidate bevacizumab's role in the treatment of breast cancer, including combination with trastuzumab.

Patient Encounter 1, Part 3: Creating a Care Plan

BB is diagnosed with stage IV metastatic, ER+ *HER-2/neu+* breast cancer that is metastatic to the bone.

What are the goals of therapy?

What patient-specific therapeutic plan do you recommend?

How should the patient be monitored for efficacy and toxicity?

▶ *Bisphosphonates*

For women whose breast cancer has metastasized to bone, bisphosphonates are recommended, in addition to chemotherapy or endocrine therapy, to reduce bone pain and fractures.[38,95] Pamidronate (90 mg) and zoledronate (4 mg) can be given IV once each month. These bisphosphonates are given in combination with calcium and vitamin D.

Local-Regional Control

▶ *Radiation Therapy*

Radiation is an important modality in the treatment of symptomatic metastatic disease. The most common indication for treatment with radiation therapy is painful bone metastases or other localized sites of disease refractory to systemic therapy. Radiation therapy gives significant pain relief to approximately 90% of patients who are treated for painful bone metastases. Radiation is also an important modality in the palliative treatment of metastatic brain lesions and spinal cord lesions, which respond poorly to systemic therapy, as well as eye or orbit lesions and other sites where significant accumulation of tumor cells occurs. Skin and/or lymph node metastases confined to the chest wall area also may be treated with radiation therapy for palliation (e.g., open wounds or painful lesions).

OUTCOME EVALUATION

Early breast cancer is resected completely with curative intent, and adjuvant chemotherapy and hormonal therapy are initiated to prevent recurrence. During adjuvant chemotherapy, laboratory values to monitor chemotherapy toxicity are obtained prior to each cycle of chemotherapy. After completion of adjuvant therapy, patients are monitored every 3 months for the first few years after diagnosis, with intervals between exams extended as time from diagnosis lengthens.

- Physical examination to detect breast cancer recurrence
- Annual mammography
- Symptom-directed workup

Locally advanced breast cancer often is treated with neoadjuvant therapy to make the tumor surgically resectable.

During neoadjuvant chemotherapy, laboratory values to monitor chemotherapy toxicity are obtained prior to each cycle of chemotherapy, and a physical and ultrasound examinations to detect size of tumor are performed after the cycles of neoadjuvant therapy are completed. After a complete surgical resection, monitoring proceeds as described earlier for early breast cancer.

Patient Care and Monitoring

1. Review the patient's diagnostic information to determine the stage of disease, overall prognosis and goals of therapy.

2. Obtain a thorough history of prescription, nonprescription, and natural drug product use. Is the patient taking any medications that may contribute to breast cancer and require discontinuation?

3. Review the patient's past medical history to determine the risks associated with any potential therapies and/or surgery and/or radiation therapy.

4. Educate the patient on the chemotherapy or endocrine therapy regimen chosen for the patient, focusing on what adverse events to expect, when to expect them, and how to manage them if they do occur. Also, include in the initial education an overall plan of care, including the duration of therapy, other treatment modalities that will follow (e.g., radiation therapy, surgery, endocrine therapy) and when they will receive them.

5. Develop a premedication and postmedication plan for the chemotherapy or endocrine therapy regimen chosen based on the patient's risk factors for adverse events, chemotherapy/endocrine therapy drugs chosen, and dose, route, and timing of administration chosen.

6. Develop a plan to assess effectiveness of the overall treatment plan, focusing on educating the patient on ways to monitor and track adverse events and/or disease-related symptoms throughout therapy.

7. Determine success of the overall treatment plan by obtaining a thorough history of adverse events experienced with the previous chemotherapy/endocrine therapy treatment and objective measures of response to therapy. Assess effects on quality of life measures such as physical, psychological, and social function and well-being.

8. Address any adverse events the patient experienced and alter the premedication and postmedication plan for the next treatment accordingly.

9. Provide follow-up patient education regarding the new plan for side effect management.

10. Stress importance of reporting adverse events and adherence with the prescribed medication regimen. Attempt to develop a therapeutic regimen that is easy for the patient to accomplish.

Metastatic breast cancer is not curable, and therapy is intended to palliate symptoms. In most cases, hormonal therapy is the mainstay. While on therapy, patients are monitored monthly for signs of disease progression or metastasis to common sites, such as the bones, brain, or liver:

- Pain
- Mental status or other neurologic findings
- Laboratory tests
- Liver function tests
- CBC
- Calcium, electrolytes

Abbreviations Introduced in This Chapter

BSE	Breast self-examination
CBE	Clinical breast examination
CMF	Cyclophosphamide, methotrexate, fluorouracil (regimen)
DCIS	Ductal carcinoma in situ
ER	Estrogen receptor
FISH	Fluorescence in situ hybridization
IHC	Immunohistochemistry
IM	Intramuscular
LCIS	Lobular carcinoma in situ
LHRH	Luteinizing hormone-releasing hormone
NCI	National Cancer Institute
NIH	National Institutes of Health
NCCN	National Comprehensive Cancer Network
OS	Overall survival
PFS	Progression-free survival
PR	Progesterone receptor
SERD	Selective estrogen-receptor downregulator
SERM	Selective estrogen-receptor modulators
TNM	Tumor-node-metastasis staging system
VEGF	Vascular endothelial-derived growth factor

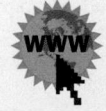 Self-assessment questions and answers are available at *http://www.mhpharmacotherapy.com/pp.html.*

REFERENCES

1. Jemal A, Siegel R, Ward E, et al. Cancer statistics, 2008. CA Cancer J Clin 2008;58:71–96.
2. Ries LAG, Eisner MP, Kosary CL, et al. SEER Cancer Statistics Review, 1975–2001. Bethesda, MD, National Cancer Institute. 2004, *http://seer.cancer.gov/csr/1975–2001/*
3. Feuer EJ, Wun LM, Boring CC, et al. The lifetime risk of developing breast cancer. J Natl Cancer Inst 1993;85:892–897.
4. Dupont WD. Risk factors for breast cancer in women with proliferative breast disease. N Engl J Med 1985;312:146–151.
5. Clemons M, Goss P. Estrogen and the risk of breast cancer. N Engl J Med 2001;344:276–285.
6. Kelsey JL, Gammon MD, John EM. Reproductive factors and breast cancer. Epidemiol Rev 1993;15:36.
7. Risks and benefits of estrogen and progestin in healthy postmenopausal women: Principal results from the Women's Health Initiative randomized controlled trial. JAMA 2002;288:321.
8. Familial breast cancer: Collaborative reanalysis of individual data from 52 epidemiological studies including 58,209 women with breast cancer and 101,986 women without the disease. Lancet 2001;358:1389.
9. Weber BL, Abel JK, Brody LC, et al. Familial breast cancer. Cancer 1994;74:1013–1020.
10. Wooster R, Weber BL. Genomic medicine: Breast and ovarian cancer. N Engl J Med 2003;348:2339–2347.
11. King MC, Marks JH, Mandell JB. Breast and ovarian cancer risks due to inherited mutations in BRCA1 and BRCA2. Science 2003;302:643–646.
12. Longnecker MP. Alcohol consumption in relation to risk of breast cancer. Cancer Causes Control 1994;5:73–82.
13. Frykberg ER, Bland KI. Overview of the biology and management of ductal carcinoma in situ of the breast. Cancer 1994;74:350–361.
14. Frykberg ER, Ames FC, Bland KI. Current concepts for management of early (in situ and occult invasive) breast carcinoma. In: Bland KI, Copeland EM, eds. The Breast: Comprehensive Management of Benign and Malignant Diseases. Philadelphia: WB Saunders, 1991:731–751.
15. Goldhirsch A, Wood WC, Gelber RD, et al. Meeting highlights: Updated international expert consensus on the primary therapy of early breast cancer. J Clin Oncol 2003;21:3357–3365.
16. Cuzick J, Baum M. Tamoxifen and contralateral breast cancer. Lancet 1985;2:282.
17. Baum M, Brinkley DM, Dossett JA, et al. Improved survival among patients treated with adjuvant tamoxifen after mastectomy for early breast cancer. Lancet 1983;2:450.
18. Edinburgh SCTO. Adjuvant tamoxifen in the management of operable breast cancer: The Scottish Trial: Report from the Breast Cancer Trials Committee. Lancet 1987;2:171–175.
19. Fisher B, Costantino JP, Wickerham DL, et al. Tamoxifen for prevention of breast cancer: Report of the National Surgical Adjuvant Breast and Bowel Project P-1 Study. J Natl Cancer Inst 1998;90:1371–1388.
20. Powles TJ, Ashley S, Tidy A, et al. Twenty-year follow-up of the Royal Marsden randomized double-blinded tamoxifen breast cancer prevention trial. J Natl Cancer Inst 2007;99:283–290.
21. Cuzick J, Forbes FJ, Sestak I, et al. Long-term results of tamoxifen prophylaxis for breast cancer -96-month follow-up of the randomized IBIS-1 trial. J Natl Cancer Inst 2007;99:272–282.
22. Cuzick J, Powles T, Veronesi U, et al. Overview of the main outcomes in breast cancer prevention trials. Lancet 2003;361:296–300.
23. Ettinger B, Black DM, Mitlak BH, et al. Reduction of vertebral fracture risk in postmenopausal women with osteoporosis treated with raloxifene: Results from a 3-year randomized clinical trial: Multiple Outcomes of Raloxifene Evaluation (MORE). JAMA 1999;282:637–645.
24. Cummings SR, Eckert S, Krueger KA, et al. The effect of raloxifene on risk of breast cancer in postmenopausal women: Results from the MORE randomized trial. JAMA 1999;281:2189–2197.
25. Gail MH, Brinton LA, Byar DP, et al. Projecting individualized probabilities of developing breast cancer for white females who are being examined annually. J Natl Cancer Inst 1989;81:1879–1886.
26. Vogel VG, Costantino JP, Wickerham DL, et al. The study of tamoxifen and raloxifene (STAR): Report of the National Surgical Adjuvant Breast and Bowel Project P-2 trial. JAMA 2006;295:2727–2741.
27. Goss PE, Strasser-Weippl K. Aromatase inhibitors for chemoprevention. Best Pract Res Clin Endocrinol Metab 2004;18:113–130.
28. Smith RA, Cokkinides V, Eyre HJ. American Cancer Society guidelines for the early detection of cancer, 2006. CA Cancer J Clin 2006;56:11–25.
29. U.S. Preventive Services Task Force. Breast cancer screening. February 2002, *www.ahcpr.gov/clinic/uspstf/uspsbrca.htm.*
30. National Cancer Institute. NCI statement on mammography screening. *http://www.cancer.gov/newscenter/mammstatement31jan02.*
31. Singletary SE, Allred C, Ashley P, et al. Revision of the American Joint Committee on cancer staging system for breast cancer. J Clin Oncol 2002;20:3628–3636.

32. NIH Consensus Development Conference Statement. Adjuvant therapy for breast cancer 2000, November 1–3;17:1–23. *www.nih.gov website.*

33. Ivens D, Hoe AL, Podd TJ, et al. Assessment of morbidity from complete axillary dissection. Br J Cancer 1992;66:136–138.

34. Keramopoulos A, Tsionou C, Minaretzis D, et al. Arm morbidity following treatment of breast cancer with total axillary dissection: A multivariated approach. Oncology 1993;50:445–449.

35. Hsueh EC, Hansen N, Giuliano A. Intraoperative lymphatic mapping and sentinel lymph node dissection in breast cancer. CA Cancer J Clin 2000;50:279–291.

36. Morrow M, Harris JR. Local management of invasive breast cancer. In: Diseases of the Breast, 2nd ed. Lippincott Philadelphia, Williams & Wilkins, 2000:515–560.

37. Persing M, Große R. Current St. Gallen recommendations on primary therapy of early breast cancer. Breast Care 2007;2:137–140.

38. NCCN Practice Guidelines in Oncology – v.1.2009; *www.nccn.org.*

39. Winer EP. Quality-of-life research in patients with breast cancer. Cancer 1994;74:410–415.

40. Levine MN, Gent M, Hirsh J, et al. The thrombogenic effect of anticancer drug therapy in women with stage II breast cancer. N Engl J Med 1988;318:404–407.

41. Smith RE, Bryant J, DeCillis A, et al. Acute myeloid leukemia and myelodysplastic syndrome after doxorubicin-cyclophosphamide adjuvant therapy for operable breast cancer: The National Surgical Adjuvant Breast and Bowel Project experience. J Clin Oncol 2003;21:1195–1204.

42. Henderson IC, Sloss JL, Jaffe N, et al. Serial studies of cardiac function in patients receiving adriamycin. Cancer Treat Rep 1978;62:923–929.

43. Ellence (epirubicin) product information. Pharmacia and Upjohn Co., April 2003.

44. Ravdin PM, Siminoff IA, Harvey JA. Survey of breast cancer patients concerning their knowledge and expectations of adjuvant therapy. J Clin Oncol 1998;16:515–521.

45. Lindley C, Vasa S, Sawyer WT, Winer EP. Quality of life and preferences for treatment following systemic adjuvant therapy for early stage breast cancer. J Clin Oncol 1998;16:380–387.

46. Paik S, Tang G, Shak S, et al. Gene expression and benefit of chemotherapy in women with node-negative, estrogen receptor-positive breast cancer. J Clin Oncol 2006;24:3726–3734.

47. Albain K, Barlow W, Shak S, et al. Prognostic and predictive value of the 21–gene recurrence score assay in postmenopausal, node–positive, ER–positive breast cancer (S8814, INT0100) (abstr 10). Program and abstracts of the 30th Annual San Antonio Breast Cancer Symposium, Dec 13–16, 2007.

48. Marchionni L, Wilson RF, Wolff AC, et al. Systematic review: Gene expression profiling assays in early-stage breast cancer. Ann Intern Med 2008;148:358–369.

49. Hayes DF, Thor AD. c-erbB-2 in breast cancer: Development of a clinically useful marker. Semin Oncol 2002;29:231–245.

50. Pritchard KI, Shepherd LE, O'Malley FP, et al. HER2 and responsiveness of breast cancer to adjuvant chemotherapy. N Engl J Med 2006;354:2177–2179.

51. Paik S, Bryant J, Tan-Chiu E, et al. HER2 and choice of adjuvant chemotherapy for invasive breast cancer. J Natl Cancer Inst 2000;92:1991–1998.

52. Love RR, Mazess RB, Barden HS, et al. Effects of tamoxifen on bone mineral density in postmenopausal women with breast cancer. N Engl J Med 1992;326:852–856.

53. Love RR, Wiebe DA, Newcomb PA, et al. Effects of tamoxifen on cardiovascular risk factors in postmenopausal women. Ann Intern Med 1992;115:860–864.

54. Early Breast Cancer Trialists' Collaborative Group. Tamoxifen for early breast cancer: An overview of the randomized trials. Lancet 1998;351:1451–1467.

55. Albain KS, Green SJ, Ravdin PM, et al. Adjuvant chemohormonal therapy for primary breast cancer should be sequential instead of concurrent: Initial results from intergroup trial 0100 (SWOG-8814) (Meeting abstract). Proc Am Soc Clin Oncol 2002;A143.

56. Fisher B, Dignam J, Bryant J, et al. Five versus more than five years of tamoxifen for lymph node-negative breast cancer: Updated findings from the National Surgical Adjuvant Breast and Bowel Project B-14 randomized trial. J Natl Cancer Inst 2001;93:684–690.

57. Jin Y, Desta Z, Stearns V, et al. CYP2D6 genotype, antidepressant use, and tamoxifen metabolism during adjuvant breast cancer treatment. J Natl Cancer Inst 2005;97:30–39.

58. Schroth W, Antoniadou L, Fritz P, et al. Breast cancer treatment outcome with adjuvant tamoxifen in relation to patient CYP2D6 and CYP2C19 genotypes. J Clin Oncol 2007;25:5187–5193.

59. Goetz MP, Rae JM, Suman VJ, et al. Pharmacogenetics of tamoxifen biotransformation is associated with clinical outcomes of efficacy and hot flashes. J Clin Oncol 2005;23:9312–9318.

60. Goetz MP, Knox SK, Suman VJ, et al. The impact of cytochrome P4502D6 metabolism in women receiving adjuvant tamoxifen. Breast Cancer Res Treat 2007;101:113–121.

61. Gonzalez-Santiago S, Zarate R, Haba-Rodriguez JA, et al. CYP2D6*4 polymorphism as blood predictive biomarker of breast cancer relapse in patients receiving adjuvant tamoxifen (Meeting abstract). J Clin Oncol 2007;A590.

62. Fareston (toremifene) product information. Shire US. May 2003.

63. Hayes DF, Van Zyl JA, Hacking A, et al. Randomized comparison of tamoxifen and two separate doses of toremifene in postmenopausal patients with metastatic breast cancer. J Clin Oncol 1995;13:2556–2566.

64. Early Breast Cancer Trialists' Collaborative Group. Ovarian ablation for early breast cancer: An overview of the randomized trials. Cochrane Database Syst Rev 2000:CD000485.

65. Jonat W, Kaufmann M, Sauerbrei W, et al. Goserelin versus cyclophosphamide, methotrexate and fluorouracil as adjuvant therapy is premenopausal patients with node-positive breast cancer: The Zoladex Early Breast Cancer Research Association Study. J Clin Oncol 2002;20:4628–4635.

66. Jakesz R, Hausmaninger H, Kubista E, et al. Randomized adjuvant trial of tamoxifen and goserelin versus cyclophosphamide, methotrexate, and fluorouracil: Evidence for the superiority of treatment with endocrine blockade in premenopausal patients with hormone-responsive breast cancer—Austrian Breast and Colorectal Cancer Study Group Trial 5. J Clin Oncol 2002;20:4621–4627.

67. Laurentiis MD, Martignetti A, Isernia G, et al. Amenorrhea induced by adjuvant chemotherapy in breast cancer patients strongly correlates with a better survival: A long follow-up study (Meeting abstract). Proc Am Soc Clin Oncol 1998;A519.

68. Winer EP, Hudis C, Burstein HJ, et al. American Society of Clinical Oncology technology assessment on the use of aromatase inhibitors as adjuvant therapy for postmenopausal women with hormone receptor-positive breast cancer: Status report 2004. J Clin Oncol 2005;23:619–629.

69. Giordano SH. Update on locally advanced breast cancer. Oncologist 2003;8:521–530.

70. Assikis VJ, Buzdar AU. Recent advances in aromatase inhibitor therapy for breast cancer. Semin Oncol 2002;29(3 Suppl 11):120–128.

71. Mauras N, O'Brien KO, Klein KO. Estrogen suppression in males: Metabolic effects. J Clin Endocrinol Metab 2000;85:2370–2377.

72. Stenbygaard LE, Herrstedt J, Thomsen JF, et al. Toremifene and tamoxifen in advanced breast cancer—A double-blind cross-over trial. Breast Cancer Res Treat 1993;25:57–63.

73. Osborne CK, Pippen J, Jones SE, et al. Double-blind, randomized trial comparing the efficacy and tolerability of fulvestrant versus anastrozole in postmenopausal women with advanced breast cancer progressing on prior endocrine therapy: Results of a North American Trial. J Clin Oncol 2002;20:3386–3395.

74. Howell A, Robertson JFR, Albano JQ, et al. Fulvestrant, formerly ICI 182,780, is as effective as anastrozole in postmenopausal women with advanced breast cancer progressing after prior endocrine treatment. J Clin Oncol 2002;20:3396–3403.

75. Ingle JN, Krook JE, Green SJ, et al. Randomized trial of bilateral oophorectomy versus tamoxifen in premenopausal women with metastatic breast cancer. J Clin Oncol 1986;4:178–185.

76. Klijn JGM, Blamey RW, Boccardo F, et al. Combined tamoxifen and luteinizing hormone-releasing hormone (LHRH) agonist versus LHRH

agonist alone in premenopausal advanced breast cancer: A meta-analysis of four randomized trials. J Clin Oncol 2001;19:343–353.

77. Michaud LB, Valero V, Hortobagyi G. Risks and benefits of taxanes in breast and ovarian cancer. Drug Saf 2000;23:401–428.

78. Mouridsen H, Harvey V, Semiglazov V, et al. Phase III trial of docetaxel 100 versus 75 versus 60 mg/m^2 as second-line chemotherapy in advanced breast cancer (Meeting abstract). San Antonio Breast Cancer Symposium 2002;A327.

79. Jones S, Erban J, Overmoyer B, et al. Randomized trial comparing docetaxel and paclitaxel in patients with metastatic breast cancer (Meeting abstract). San Antonio Breast Cancer Symposium 2003;A10.

80. Gradishar WJ, Tjulandin S, Davidson N, et al. Phase III trial of nanoparticle albumin-bound paclitaxel compared with polyethylated castor oil-based paclitaxel in women with breast cancer. J Clin Oncol 2005;23:7794–7803.

81. Thomas ES, Gomez HL, Li RK, et al. Ixabepilone plus capecitabine for metastatic breast cancer progressing after anthracycline and taxane treatment. J Clin Oncol 2007;25:5210–5217.

82. Lee FY, Camuso A, Castenada C, et al. Preclinical efficacy evaluation of ixabepilone (BMS-247550) in combination with cetuximab or capecitabine in human colon and lung carcinoma xenografts (Meeting abstract). J Clin Oncol 2006;A12017.

83. Innocenti F, Ratain MJ. Update on pharmacogenetics in cancer chemotherapy. Eur J Cancer 2002;38:639–644.

84. Xeloda (Capecitabine) product information. Roche Pharmaceuticals, April 2003.

85. Esteva FJ, Valero V, Pusztai L, et al. Chemotherapy of metastatic breast cancer: What to expect in 2001 and beyond. Oncologist 2001;6:133–146.

86. Cobleigh MA, Vogel CL, Tripathy D, et al. Multinational study of the efficacy and safety of humanized anti-HER2 monoclonal antibody in women who have HER2-overexpressing metastatic breast cancer that progressed after chemotherapy for metastatic disease. J Clin Oncol 1999;17:2639–2648.

87. Slamon DJ, Leyland-Jones B, Shak S, et al. Use of chemotherapy plus a monoclonal antibody against HER2 for metastatic breast cancer that overexpresses HER2. N Engl J Med 2001;344:783–792.

88. Yeon CH, Pegram MD. Anti-erbB-2 antibody trastuzumab in the treatment of HER2-amplified breast cancer. Invest New Drugs 2005;23:391–409.

89. Vogel CL, Cobleigh MA, Tripathy D, et al. Efficacy and safety of trastuzumab as a single agent in first-line treatment of HER2-overexpressing metastatic breast cancer. J Clin Oncol 2002;20:719–726.

90. Geyer CE, Forster J, Lindquist D, et al. Lapatinib plus capecitabine for HER2-positive advanced breast cancer. N Engl J Med 2006;355:2733–2743.

91. Burris HA III, Hurwitz HI, Dees EC, et al. Phase I study, pharmacokinetics, and clinical activity study of lapatinib (GW572016), a reversible dual inhibitor of epidermal growth factor receptor tyrosine kinases, in heavily pretreated patients with metastatic carcinomas. J Clin Oncol 2005;23:5305–5313.

92. Geyer CE, Martin A, Newstat B, et al. Lapatinib (L) plus capecitabine (C) in HER2+ advanced breast cancer (ABC): Genomic and updated efficacy data (Meeting abstract). Proc Am Soc Clin Oncol 2007;A1035.

93. Campone M, Bourbouloux E, Fumoleau P. Cardiac dysfunction induced by trastuzumab. Bull Cancer 2004;91(Suppl 3):166–173.

94. Grazette LP, Boecker W, Matsui T, et al. Inhibition of erbB2 causes mitochondrial dysfunction in cardiomyocytes: Implications for herceptin-induced cardiomyopathy. J Am Coll Cardiol 2004;44:2231–2238.

95. Hillner BE, Ingle JN, Chlebowski RT, et al. American Society of Clinical Oncology 2003 update on the role of bisphosphonates and bone health issues in women with breast cancer. J Clin Oncol 2003;21:4042–4057.

90 Lung Cancer

Val Adams and Justin Balko

LEARNING OBJECTIVES

● **Upon completion of the chapter, the reader will be able to:**

1. Identify major risk factors for the development of lung cancer.

2. Explain the pathologic progression of lung cancer and its relationship with signs and symptoms of the disease.

3. Make appropriate recommendations for screening or preventative measures in high-risk patients.

4. Understand staging of lung cancer patients and how it influences treatment decisions.

5. List the rationale, advantages, disadvantages, and place in therapy for adjuvant and neoadjuvant chemotherapy.

6. Identify the chemotherapeutic regimens of choice for limited and extensive small cell lung carcinoma, as well as local, locally advanced, and advanced nonsmall cell lung carcinoma.

7. Monitor patients for chemotherapy-associated toxicity, and recommend appropriate management.

8. Distinguish the treatment goals of palliative care versus those of first-line treatment.

KEY CONCEPTS

❶ The most important risk factor for the development of lung cancer is smoking, and the most effective way for high-risk patients to reduce their risk is to stop smoking. Additional recommendations should include an increase in dietary intake of fruits and vegetables.

❷ The signs and symptoms of lung cancer can be classified as pulmonary, extrapulmonary, and paraneoplastic. These classifications relate to disease progression.

❸ The treatment goals in lung cancer are cure (early-stage disease), prolongation of survival, and maintenance or improvement of quality of life through alleviation of symptoms.

❹ The performance status (PS) of the patient represents an important aspect of chemotherapy treatment decisions. Patients with a PS of 0 to 1 may be treated with chemotherapy. Patients with a PS of 2 may be treated with less aggressive regimens that have a decreased risk of major toxicities, whereas patients with a PS 3 and 4 should be treated with supportive care only.

❺ Surgical resection of the tumor is the mainstay of treatment in early-stage nonsmall cell lung cancer and produces the longest survival rates.

❻ Doublet chemotherapy regimens offer superior response rates compared to single-agent regimens and should be used when the patient can tolerate the associated toxicity. Platinum-containing doublets are first-line treatment in most cases.

❼ Knowing when and how to treat adverse events from chemotherapy is an important aspect of patient care. Unmanaged events may cause delays in chemotherapy administration and reduced chemotherapy doses, and may contribute to treatment failure.

❽ While some evidence suggests that the use of a colony-stimulating factor reduces the number of neutropenic fever episodes, hospital stay, and antibiotic administration in certain subsets of lung cancer patients, routine front-line (prophylactic) use of a colony-stimulating factor is not recommended owing to lack of a survival benefit.

INTRODUCTION

Lung cancer has a major health impact both in the United States and worldwide. Prior to 1930, lung cancer was a relatively rare disease, but a sharp incline in industrialization and smoking in the early 1900s has bred an epidemic. Lung cancer has a high mortality rate, and although treatment can cure selected patients, most therapies only prolong survival for months. Recent advances in lung cancer research provide good reason for optimism. However, in spite of the emergence of new therapies, antismoking campaigns still appear to offer the best opportunity to reduce lung cancer incidence and mortality.

EPIDEMIOLOGY AND ETIOLOGY

Incidence and Mortality

Cancer is the second leading cause of death in the United States. Cancers of the lung and bronchus rank first in cancer-related mortality, comprising over 28% of cancer-related deaths.[1] In 2008, over 215,000 new cases of lung cancer were diagnosed. A close correlation exists between incidence and mortality of lung cancer, reflecting the reality that approximately 85% of lung cancer patients ultimately die of the disease.

Gender

Lung cancer incidence and mortality are slightly higher in males, but the rate in females is expected to match that of males in future years owing to changes in smoking patterns.[2] Typically, women with lung cancer are diagnosed at an earlier age, which has raised the question that there may be inherent genetic differences between males and females in susceptibility to lung cancer. Furthermore, there are differences in the prevalence of histological subtypes of tumors. Interestingly, historical studies have shown improved prognosis and survival times for women diagnosed with lung cancer.[3]

Race

While no significant difference is noted in incidence or mortality between black and white females, black males have a markedly higher incidence and mortality rate than white males. Proposed contributions to this gap include differences in smoking habits, such as increased menthol cigarette use.[2] Black Americans also have a significantly lower 5-year survival rate than white Americans regardless of gender. They present with more advanced disease and are less likely to be treated, which suggests that genetic, psychosocial, and socioeconomic components contribute to this disparity. Although it remains a significant health care issue, Asians, Hispanics, and Native Americans have lower rates of lung cancer than both Caucasians and African Americans.[2,4,5]

Clinical Risk Factors

▶ Smoking

❶ *The most important risk factor for the development of lung cancer is smoking.* One of the most predictive factors on lung cancer epidemiology is trends in population cigarette smoking. Because lung cancer is a fatal disease in most cases, both incidence and mortality strongly reflect the smoking trends of the population on a 20- to 30-year lag. In other words, decreases in tobacco use now would be expected to affect lung cancer incidence in 2030. With this knowledge, the current expectation is that lung cancer incidence and mortality will decrease steadily until 2020, reflecting decreases in cigarette smoking between 1970 and 1990. Because smoking has continued at a steady rate since 1990, lung cancer incidence is expected to plateau.[2] Correlation between smoking and lung cancer continues to drive antismoking campaigns and should be considered an investment in the future health care of the nation. Furthermore, smoking cessation plays an important role in reducing lung cancer risk on a patient-to-patient basis, and appropriately guiding such therapy is a crucial part of treating at-risk patients.[6] Total smoke exposure, as well as current use, correlates with the individual's risk of developing malignancy. The risk of lung cancer decreases to near-normal levels 10 to 15 years following successful smoking cessation. Total smoke exposure is reported as pack-years. One pack-year is the equivalent of smoking 1 pack per day for 1 year. A patient who smokes 40 cigarettes per day (2 packs) for 5 years would have a 10 pack-year history (2 packs/day for 5 years).

▶ Other Air-Related Risks

In addition to direct inhalation of cigarette smoke, other environmental factors have been identified as risks for the development of primary lung tumors. Environmental tobacco smoke (ETS) presents a significant occupational hazard for nonsmokers working in environments that have a high-smoking population, such as bars or restaurants. Some states have instituted laws banning public smoking in order to protect individuals working in these locations. Each year approximately 3,000 cases of lung cancer in nonsmokers are due to ETS. Other environmental factors linked to lung cancer include radon, arsenic, nickel, and chloromethyl ethers. Those who live in an urban environment are also at an increased risk for lung cancer owing to exposure to high concentrations of combustion fumes.[4] Asbestos exposure increases the risk of developing a distinct type of lung cancer called mesothelioma, which is rare and beyond the scope of this chapter.

▶ Nutrition

Diet and nutrition have long been suspected to play a role in cancer susceptibility, and many studies have sought to define specific foods or nutrients that influence cancer risk. Because not all heavy smokers develop lung cancer, it is thought that nutritional factors may explain part of this variation. Epidemiologic studies focusing on diet and nutrition in lung cancer have shown reduced rates of lung cancer in individuals who report higher fruit and vegetable consumption. However, studies attempting to identify specific chemical components of fruits and vegetables that are responsible for this effect have not been successful.[7] **❷** *Recommendations to patients who are at risk owing to smoking or other factors or those who are simply interested in reducing their risk of cancer should include an increase in dietary intake of fruits and vegetables.*

Hereditary or Genetic Risk Factors

Although smoking is a key risk factor for lung cancer, the majority of people who smoke never develop lung cancer. Genetic risk factors may predispose certain smokers to lung cancer. After adjustments for age, smoke exposure, occupation, and gender, relatives of a lung cancer patient have approximately a twofold risk of developing lung cancer. The degree of inherited risk inversely correlates with the age of the relative at the time of diagnosis. First-degree relatives of a lung cancer patient diagnosed between the ages of 40 and 59 years have a sixfold relative risk for lung cancer. Familial lung cancer that develops at an early age in nonsmokers fits a Mendelian codominant inheritance model. However, a lung cancer gene has not been identified.

Other genetic links to lung cancer involve metabolic enzymes that process carcinogens. The damaging effects of tobacco smoke are thought be a result of bulky aromatic hydrocarbons that damage DNA. These chemicals are activated by certain phase I metabolic enzymes and are deactivated by phase II conjugating enzymes such as the glutathione-*S*-transferases. People with elevated cytochrome CYP450 2D6, 1A1, or 1A2 have greater risk of DNA damage and subsequent cancer owing to higher formation rates of active carcinogens. Those with deficient phase II metabolism (*GSTM1* or *GSTT1*) similarly may have increased risk owing to lower clearance of carcinogens.[8–10]

Chemoprevention

Chemoprevention refers to the use of prophylactic medications to prevent the development of cancer. Many studies of potential chemopreventatives, including nonsteroidal anti-inflammatory drugs, retinoids, inhaled glucocorticoids, vitamin E, selenium, and green tea extracts, have been conducted, but none has been successful. Large randomized clinical trials have evaluated β-carotene and vitamin E as lung cancer chemopreventative agents in high-risk patients (older smokers). Although vitamin E has no influence on lung cancer, the trials show that older people who smoke have a higher risk of developing and dying of lung cancer if they take a β-carotene supplement. Nonsmokers do not appear to have an altered risk of lung cancer with β-carotene consumption.[11]

Screening and Early Detection

Overall 5-year survival in lung cancer is only 15%, whereas those who are diagnosed at a localized stage exhibit a 5-year survival rate of 50%. Currently, over three-quarters of newly diagnosed lung cancers present with locally advanced or metastatic disease, and therefore, very few patients are able to undergo surgical resection.[1] In an attempt to identify tumors when they are localized and have higher cure rates, many investigators are evaluating different screening modalities. Effective screening methods have the potential to save thousands of lives. To date, no screening study has demonstrated a benefit in overall survival; however, the use of spiral CT scanning has been shown to be sensitive in detecting small nodules. Unfortunately, spiral CT scanning alone is not likely to be of benefit owing to the high rate of false-positive results (i.e., lack of specificity), leading to excessive patient anxiety and workup, which can have a negative effect on morbidity and mortality. Because lung cancer tumors are hypermetabolic, they can typically be visualized with 5-fluorodeoxyglucose (5-FDG) positron-emission tomographic (PET) scanning. The combination of spiral CT scanning and follow-up PET scanning for positive lesions is currently the most promising method. In a recent study, this combination resulted in 90% specificity and 100% sensitivity for detection of cancer when a 3-month follow-up CT was used after a negative PET scan. Furthermore, 92% of nonsmall cell tumors were diagnosed at stage IA or IB.[12] Additional studies evaluating the benefits on mortality of this approach are under way. Spiral CT and PET scanning are currently the most promising screening tools for patients at a high risk for lung cancer. High-risk individuals should be encouraged to enter randomized, controlled trials aimed at demonstrating a survival benefit from screening.

PATHOPHYSIOLOGY

Most lung cancers arise from the epithelium of the airways and are classified as carcinomas. There are four major and several rare histological types of lung cancer. They appear to form through different mutagenic pathways; however, they all appear to undergo transition through a premalignant state. The presence of a transitional state from normal tissue to cancerous tissue is important because the premalignant cells contain damage that is generally thought to be reversible. Researchers are currently trying to develop methods to identify people with premalignant lesions as well as drugs that can reverse the damage.

Continued damage to premalignant cells can lead to cancer. The first appearance of cancer cells that have not yet become invasive is referred to as *carcinoma in situ*. Patients are rarely diagnosed with this early stage of cancer owing to a lack of symptoms and relatively rapid progression from this state to larger invasive tumors. As the tumor grows, cells may become dislodged from the tumor bulk and enter the hematologic or lymphatic circulatory systems where they can travel to either local or distant parts of the body. Hematologic spread usually results in metastatic sites in the bones, liver, and CNS. Lymphatic spread is more orderly in nature, with the hilar and mediastinal lymph nodes in the pleural cavity commonly being involved. Once the tumor has spread to multiple locations, curative treatment is rare because surgical excision and radiotherapy cannot remove all or nearly all the cancer cells.

Histologic Classification

Histologic classification of lung cancer involves determining the cellular origin of the tumor. Knowing the histology of the tumor influences treatment decisions as well as prognosis. In order to carry out a histologic classification, the pathologist must obtain a tissue sample. Methods of tissue sampling are discussed in Table 90–1.

There are four major histologic types of lung cancer that are divided into two classes based on response to treatment and prognosis: small cell lung cancer (SCLC) and nonsmall cell lung cancer (NSCLC). However, it is important to note that certain other rare malignancies as well as mixed-type carcinomas can be seen. The four major types of lung cancer are outlined by class in Table 90–2.[13]

CLINICAL PRESENTATION AND DIAGNOSIS

Clinical symptoms are not commonly seen until lung cancer tumors become large and/or have metastasized. This is a key factor in the poor prognosis associated with lung cancer. Patients who are diagnosed at an earlier clinical stage have improved prognosis compared to those diagnosed at later

Patient Encounter, Part 1

A 53-year-old African American man presents at your clinic complaining of new-onset cough. He has had several upper respiratory infections in the last 2 months, with occasional hemoptysis. He has consistently smoked 1.5 packs per day for the last 20 years. He has worked as a bartender at a local restaurant for most of his life.

What risk factors for lung cancer are present?

Calculate this patient's pack-year history.

Table 90–1

Diagnostic Tools

	Technique	Description
Visualization	CXR	The least expensive visualization method in the diagnosis of lung cancer. Readily accessible and does not require systemic administration of contrast dye. However, it often detects lesions that are not cancerous and is not capable of assessing lymph node status
	CT	More accurate when providing information on size, location, and invasion than CXR. It is recommended as part of the standard workup in most cases
	PET scanning	Uses a substance called 5-FDG to produce a functional image of the lungs. Cells that are actively growing and dividing use greater amounts of glucose and therefore take up more 5-FDG. Focal regions of fluorescence can be visualized in cancerous lesions. PET scanning combined with a CT scan is more accurate than CT scan alone; however, the exact role of PET scanning in staging and monitoring is unclear. The apparent benefit and common role in staging is to evaluate mediastinal disease when it can influence the tumor resectability
Tumor sampling	Fine-needle aspiration	A method of aspirating cells from the tumor via insertion of a small-bore needle into the lesion and aspirating. Commonly used to evaluate lymph nodes or other poorly accessible sites, it has the advantage of being faster and less invasive than other biopsy methods; however, it does not preserve the architecture of the tumor and may return cells that are undergoing cell death, which negates histologic analysis
	Bronchoscopy	A fiber optic camera is inserted through the airways to examine the site of the suspected lesion. Once the lesion is visualized, a tool attached to the camera allows for a tissue biopsy. Newer technologies incorporate fluorescence to differentiate malignant tissue from premalignant lesions
	Core needle biopsy	A method of obtaining tissue and preserving the tumor architecture. A large-bore needle is inserted into a lesion, where it cuts a core of tissue out that then can be evaluated
	Thoracentesis	Involves removal of fluid in the pleural cavity via a needle. The fluid then is assayed for presence cancerous cells. This procedure has low sensitivity and depends on the presence of a pleural effusion
	Sputum cytology	Detects cancerous cells that become dislodged from the airways into the sputum. Sputum cytology is useful because it is not invasive, although it has much lower sensitivity for detecting cancer

CXR, chest x-ray; PET, positron-emission tomography.

From Ref. 13.

Table 90–2

Lung Tumor Histopathology

Tumor Type	Percentage of Tumors	Approximate Cell Doubling Time (Days)	Sensitivity to Chemotherapy and Radiotherapy	Relative Risk of Metastasis
Small cell	15–20	30	High	High
Nonsmall cell				
Adenocarcinoma	30–35	180	Low	Medium
Large cell (giant)	9	100	Low	Low
Squamous (epidermoid)	30–35	180	Low	Low

From Ref. 13.

Clinical Presentation and Diagnosis of Lung Cancer

❷ *Signs and symptoms of lung cancer can be classified into three subdivisions: pulmonary, extrapulmonary, and paraneoplastic syndromes. Distinguishing between these classes of symptoms is important because it can aid in determining the severity of the disease, guide treatment options, and affect prognosis.*

Pulmonary Symptoms

Symptoms owing to the direct effects of the primary tumor are often the first to appear and are the most common. These include:

- Cough
- Chest pain
- SVC obstruction
- Shortness of breath
- Dysphagia
- Hemoptysis
- Pleural effusion

Extrapulmonary Symptoms

Once the tumor invades tissues outside the pleural cavity, it can produce a wide array of symptoms including:

- General bone pain
- Adrenal insufficiency
- Confusion
- Nausea
- Focal neurologic symptoms
- Horner's syndrome
- Personality changes
- Enlarged lymph nodes
- Weight loss
- Seizures
- Fatigue
- Headache
- Vomiting
- Subcutaneous skin nodules

Paraneoplastic Syndromes

Symptoms that are not a result of the direct effects of the tumor are termed paraneoplastic syndromes. They may be caused by substances secreted by the tumor or in response to the tumor and often occur in tissues far from the site of malignancy. Paraneoplastic syndromes are numerous and affect a wide variety of systems, including the endocrine, neurologic, skeletal, renal, metabolic, vascular, and hematologic systems.

Diagnosis

Diagnosis requires visualization of one or more lesions as well as biopsy of the lesion to confirm malignancy. Both visualization and sampling can be performed by invasive or noninvasive methods. These methods are summarized in Table 90–1.

---

stages. Therefore, diagnosing lung cancer earlier through screening and identification of initial signs and symptoms is important. Several screening techniques including CT and PET scanning are being investigated to detect lung cancer at earlier, curable stages in an attempt to reduce mortality. However, screening is not part of the current recommendations. The current approach is based on identifying lung cancer patients on symptomatic presentation or by follow-up of lesions noted from unrelated radiologic scans.

Diagnosis

Diagnosis of lung cancer requires both visualization of the cancerous lesion and tissue sampling for pathologic assessment. Visualization of the suspected tumor provides the clinician with the information necessary to choose the most appropriate sampling technique. While some lung tumors may be apparent using relatively simple techniques such as a chest x-ray (CXR), many can be too small to detect or may be located in an anatomically difficult area to visualize. Therefore, multiple methods of visualization are often used. Once the tumor has been located, sampling provides tissue to confirm malignancy and to determine the histology (e.g., squamous cell, adenocarcinoma, large cell, or small cell). The advantages and disadvantages of various sampling methods must be weighed carefully so that the procedure performed is the least invasive with a high likelihood of providing an accurate diagnosis. Tools used in the diagnosis of lung cancer are outlined in Table 90–1.

Clinical Staging

Once the diagnosis of lung cancer is confirmed through visualization and biopsy, the extent of disease must be determined. NSCLC is staged using the American Joint Committee on Cancer tumor, node, and metastasis (TNM) staging system. SCLC is typically staged using the Veterans Administration Lung Cancer Study Group method. Clinical staging serves two primary purposes: predicting prognosis and guiding therapy.

▶ Nonsmall Cell Lung Cancer

Clinical staging of NSCLC with the TNM system evaluates the size of the tumor (T), extent of nodal involvement (N), and presence of metastatic sites (M). The combination of these three evaluations determines the stage. Clinical stages and associated survival rates are outlined in Table 90–3. Local disease includes tumors that are confined to a single hemithorax and those cancers that have spread to the ipsalateral hilar lymph nodes. Once malignancy invades the mediastinal lymph nodes or contralateral hilar nodes, the disease becomes locally advanced. When signs of cancer are detected outside the pleural cavity, it is classified as advanced

Table 90–3

Clinical Stage and Prognosis

Clinical Stage	TNM staging			Survival Rate (%)	
	Tumor	Node	Metastasis	1 Year	5 Years
Local					
IA	1	0	0	94	67
IB	2	0	0	87	53
IIA	1	1	0	89	40
Locally advanced					
IIB	2	1	0	73	30
	3	0	0		
IIIA	1	2	0	58	15
	2	2	0		
	3	1	0		
	3	2	0		
IIIB	Any	3	0	37	10
Advanced					
IIIB	4	Any	0	37	10
IV	Any	Any	1	18	Less than 5

From Ref. 14.

disease. Local disease is associated with the highest cure and survival rates, whereas those with advanced disease have a 5-year survival rate of less than 10%.

▶ Small Cell Lung Cancer

● The most common system for staging SCLC was developed originally by the Veterans Administration Lung Cancer Study Group. This system categorizes SCLC into two classifications: limited and extensive disease[14]:

- Limited disease: Evidence of the tumor is confined to a single hemithorax and can be encompassed by a single radiation port
- Extensive disease: Any progression beyond limited disease

TREATMENT

Desired Outcome and General Approach to Patient

The treatment of lung cancer depends on tumor histology, stage of disease, and patient characteristics such as age, gender, history, and performance status (PS). All of these aspects must be assessed before appropriate treatment can be recommended. The general approach to treatment of lung cancer is outlined in Figure 90–1. In the development of a patient care plan, keep in mind the ultimate goals of therapy. ❸ *In patients with early-stage disease, a definitive cure is the primary goal of treatment, although this end point is not always met. Additional goals of treating lung cancer patients include prolongation of survival and improvement of quality of life through alleviation of symptoms.* The goals of treatment must be considered when selecting a therapeutic plan. Some treatments may prolong survival by a few months, but at the expense of significant decreases in patient's quality of life.

Patient Encounter, Part 2: Medical History, Physical Examination, and Diagnosis

PMH: Significant for COPD (poorly controlled), GERD (controlled with PPIs), and moderate hypertension

FH: Father died of MI, mother living

Meds: Lisinopril 20 mg daily; Lansoprazole 30 mg daily; Albuterol/ipratropium MDI two puffs twice a day

ROS: (+) light chest pain, shortness of breath, hemoptysis; (–) recent weight loss

PE:

VS: BP 135/69, RR 26, P 80, T 37.2°C (99°F)

CV: RRR

Labs: Slightly elevated ionized calcium and LFTs; all others WNL.

CXR reveals a solitary nodule in right lower lobe.

Fine-needle aspiration confirms adenocarcinoma.

Further evaluation with CT and PET scans reveal a $T_2N_0M_0$ tumor.

What clinical stage is this patient's disease?

What is the estimated survival time for this stage of NSCLC?

Does this patient have any factors that may negatively or positively influence survival?

Treatment decisions must include both the health care team and an informed and well-counseled patient.

▶ Performance Status

The PS of an individual patient predicts response and likelihood of toxicity to chemotherapy as well as overall survival. The PS scaling system used most frequently was developed by the Eastern Cooperative Oncology Group (ECOG) (see Chap. 88). ❹ *Categorizing patients by their ECOG PS allows for an objective measure of capability to tolerate systemic therapies that may severely compromise the patient's health. Patients with a good PS (0–1) are more likely to tolerate intense therapy, whereas patients with a poor PS (3–4) are considered unfit for chemotherapy or surgery. There is some controversy over whether to treat patients with a PS of 2. At this point, treatment is aimed at treating comorbidities to improve the PS or the use of palliative symptomatic therapy.* Patients with less advanced disease may be treated more aggressively in this scenario since the intent of treatment is curative.

Nonpharmacologic Therapy

▶ Surgery

❺ *Of all treatment modalities, surgical resection of the affected lobe or lung leads to the greatest improvement in survival for*

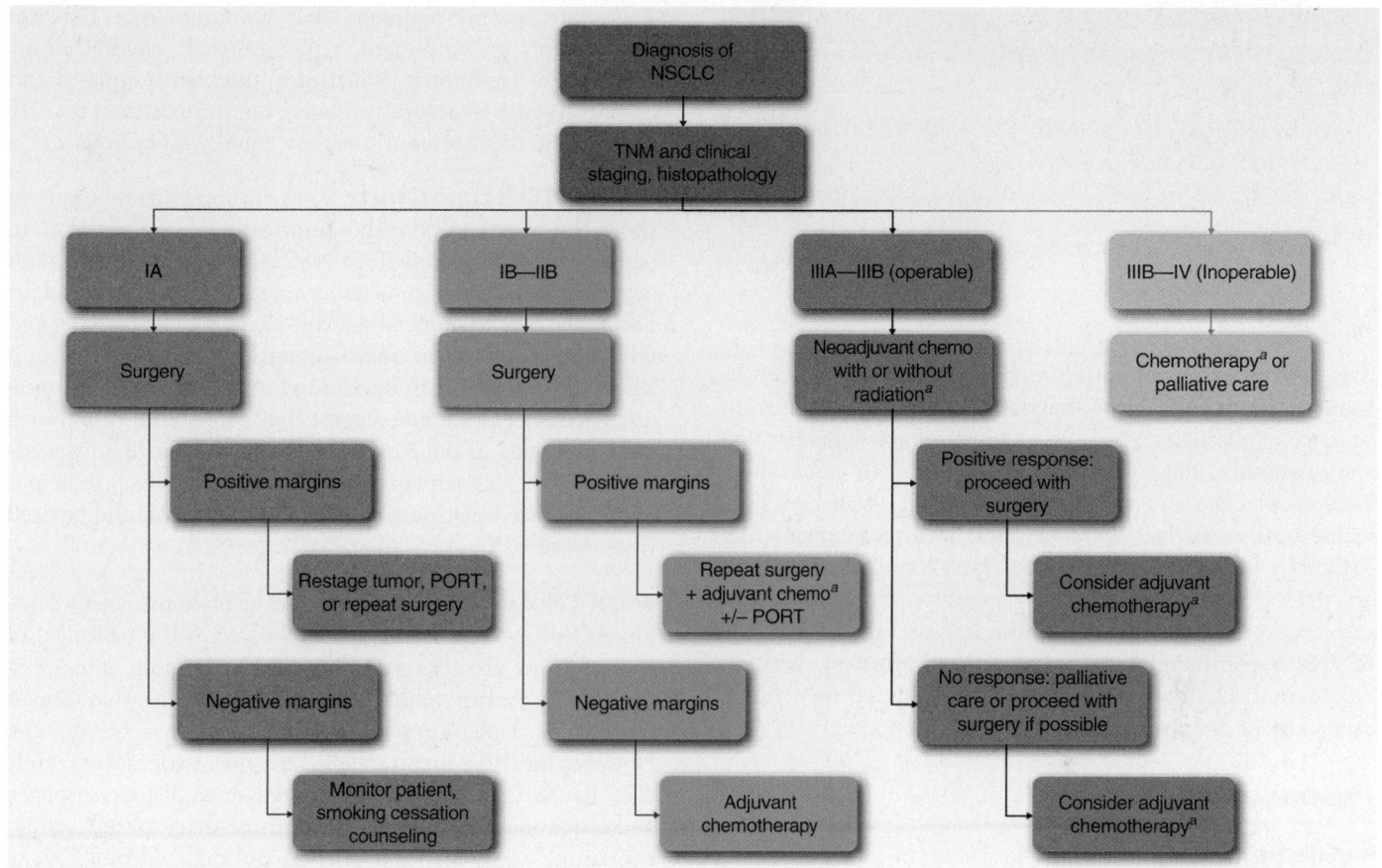

FIGURE 90–1. Clinical pathway for nonsmall cell lung cancer. ªSee text for specific treatment recommendations. (Chemo, chemotherapy; NSCLC, nonsmall cell lung cancer; PORT, postoperative radiotherapy; TNM, tumor node metastasis.)

patients with early-stage and locally advanced NSCLC (clinical stage IA, IB, or IIA). The candidacy of the tumor for resection should only be determined by an experienced thoracic surgeon who routinely works with cancer patients. During surgery, peripheral lymph nodes may be removed if they are thought to be involved, and mediastinal nodes are often dissected for biopsy to determine their involvement. In patients with advanced disease NSCLC, surgery is not curative and as a general approach does not prolong survival. However, surgery for advanced disease is an important palliative treatment that can improve quality of life in some patients. In this respect, surgery is limited to local sites where the tumor is causing significant morbidity (e.g., spinal cord compression). Patients with small cell carcinomas are rarely treated with surgery because the results of a randomized trial published in 1969 showed that surgery did not result in any 5- or 10-year survivors, whereas radiation produced a 4% survival rate at 5 and 10 years.[15] With improved imaging and surgical techniques as well as the use of effective adjuvant therapy, some clinicians believe that surgery does have a role in early-stage SCLC. However, this has yet to be proven in a clinical trial.

▶ Radiotherapy

As mentioned earlier, radiotherapy is the treatment of choice for limited-stage SCLC. Optimal patient outcomes are achieved when radiation is administered concurrently with chemotherapy because of synergy between the two modalities. Limited and extensive stage SCLC patients who respond to therapy should also receive prophylactic cranial irradiation (PCI), which prevents brain metastasis and improves cure rates for limited stage disease. Patients with localized NSCLC are best treated with surgery; however, many of these patients are inoperable because of comorbidities (e.g., lung disease from smoking). In these situations, radiation therapy can be used with curative intent in place of surgery, and the success rate is approximately 50% that of surgery.[16] Similar to SCLC, patients with late-stage NSCLC can receive radiation therapy to palliate symptomatic metastases. Although radiation is less invasive than surgery, it can have marked toxicity on normal tissue and patients may experience esophagitis, pneumonitis, cardiac abnormalities, myelopathies, and skin irritation. These adverse events can be decreased by using stereotactic radiation and/or hyperfractionated administration.[17]

Postoperative radiotherapy (PORT) is thought to eliminate remnants of the resected tumor that might be deposited in nearby tissue. In clinical trials, PORT decreases local recurrence; however, a survival benefit has never been shown. A meta-analysis of investigations evaluating PORT suggested that it may actually be detrimental to patients with stage I or II NSCLC.[18] The meta-analysis evaluated older studies

Patient Encounter, Part 3

The patient's condition has not interfered with his ability to work, and he is able to complete daily activities.

What is this patients ECOG PS score?

Are there any nonpharmacologic interventions you would suggest?

that used outdated radiation techniques, and consequently, some argue that the meta-analysis does not apply to current practice. Nonetheless, no studies to date have demonstrated a survival advantage with the use of PORT. In cases where local recurrence is a significant risk, PORT still may be a viable option. In fact, current guidelines recommend that patients with positive surgical margins (i.e., cancerous cells are detected on the surface of the excised tissue) undergo re-resection or systemic chemotherapy or PORT.[19] Outside of this recommendation, adjuvant radiotherapy without concurrent chemotherapy is not considered beneficial, especially in early-stage disease.

Pharmacologic Therapy

▶ Chemotherapy

Traditional chemotherapeutic agents interfere with processes during cell division or affect DNA replication in nondividing cells, resulting in cell death. Unfortunately, these agents are not specific for cancer cells, and other tissues in the body often are affected. Rapidly cycling cells, both tumor and normal tissue such as bone marrow, epithelial cells of the GI tract, and hair follicles, are most susceptible to chemotherapy toxicity. Because the dose of traditional chemotherapy agents is determined in phase I studies where the maximum tolerated dose is considered the best dose, toxicity is seen with each of these agents. Preventing and managing chemotherapy toxicity are crucial to optimizing patient outcomes (e.g., curing, prolonging life, or palliating symptoms). The decision to start chemotherapy depends greatly on the overall patient picture, with emphasis on PS and comorbid conditions. Knowledge of the major adverse effects of individual regimens is important for anticipation and prophylaxis of such toxicities. Many regimens require appropriate premedication and hydration. Furthermore, decisions to start chemotherapy must include the full consent and understanding of risks by the patient. Counseling on the chemotherapy and risk of toxicity is imperative before dosing. Lung cancer regimens and their associated toxicities are shown in Table 90–4. (See Chap. 88: Cancer Chemotherapy and Treatment for dosing recommendations in renal and hepatic failure.)

❻ *Doublet chemotherapy regimens offer superior response rates compared to single-agent regimens and should be used when the patient can tolerate the increased toxicity. Platinum-containing regimens are the mainstay of multidrug regimens.*

There are several regimens that contain either cisplatin or carboplatin combined with another chemotherapy agent; these are known as platinum doublets. Cisplatin and carboplatin are structurally related, but have distinct toxicity profiles and it is unclear if they are equally efficacious.

Nonsmall Cell Lung Cancer Both carboplatin and cisplatin show the most pronounced improvements in survival in patients with advanced-stage NSCLC when combined with newer agents such as gemcitabine, vinorelbine, docetaxel, or paclitaxel. Due to reduced neurotoxicity, nephrotoxicity, and GI toxicity, many clinicians favor carboplatin over cisplatin.[28] There is also interest in developing nonplatinum-containing doublets. Recent studies suggest that gemcitabine combined with paclitaxel or docetaxel is just as effective in advanced-stage NSCLC as a platinum doublet; however, guidelines maintain that a platinum-containing doublet should be used when feasible.[19]

Small Cell Lung Cancer In SCLC, a platinum agent combined with an older agent (e.g., etoposide) is the treatment of choice. There are also a number of nonplatinum-containing three-drug anthracycline-containing regimens that are as effective as a platinum doublet, in extensive-stage disease. However, the three-drug regimens are more toxic and are rarely used in the United States. In limited-stage disease, cisplatin and etoposide are superior to the three-drug anthracycline-containing regimens, and provide optimal outcomes when combined with concurrent radiation.[29]

A direct comparison of etoposide combined with either cisplatin or carboplatin in SCLC found similar results. This leads some clinicians to consider the agents interchangeable; however, this trial primarily enrolled patients with extensive-stage disease. A direct comparison in patients with limited-stage disease has not been performed, and most clinicians consider cisplatin and etoposide to be the treatment of choice because this combination has been used in nearly all the large comparative trials.

Single-Agent Chemotherapy First-line therapy for advanced-stage NSCLC and SCLC is best done with a two-drug regimen. However, patients who have a recurrence after the initial regimen are best treated with a single-agent chemotherapy. Single-agent therapy is also acceptable for patients with poor health and advanced disease because toxicities tend to be lower with one-drug regimens. Chemotherapeutic agents used in monotherapy in lung cancer include pemetrexed, docetaxel, gemcitabine, paclitaxel, topotecan, and vinorelbine (Table 90–4).

Adjuvant Chemotherapy Surgery has a limited role in the treatment of SCLC making adjuvant chemotherapy primarily applicable to NSCLC. The rationale behind adjuvant chemotherapy is to eradicate micrometastases or other tumor cells that may have been missed during removal of the primary tumor. The recent results of five relatively large prospective trials (n = 344–1,867) suggest that there is benefit from adjuvant chemotherapy. The largest study, the International Adjuvant Lung trial,[30] led

Table 90–4

Chemotherapy Regimens in Lung Cancer and Associated Toxicities

Dose		Neutropenia		
		Cycle Length	Grade III	Grade IV
Nonsmall Cell				
Paclitaxel–carboplatin–bevacizumab	Carboplatin, dose targeted to AUC of 6 IV (day 1), paclitaxel 200 mg/m² IV over 3 hours (day 1), bevacizumab 15 mg/kg IV (day 1)	21		24
Cisplatin–paclitaxel	Paclitaxel 135 mg/m² IV over 24 hours (day 1) and cisplatin 75 mg/m² IV (day 2)	21	18	57
Cisplatin–docetaxel	Cisplatin 75 mg/m² IV (day 1) and docetaxel 75 mg/m² IV (day 1)	21	21	48
Cisplatin–gemcitabine	Cisplatin 100 mg/m² IV (day 1) and gemcitabine 1,000 mg/m² IV (days 1, 8, and 15)	28	24	39
Cisplatin–vinorelbine–cetuximab	Cisplatin 80 mg/m² (day 1) and vinorelbine 25 mg/m² (days 1 and 8) ± cetuximab 400 mg/m² initial dose, then 250 mg/m²/week)	21	14	38
Cisplatin–vinorelbine	Cisplatin 50 mg/m² (days 1 and 8) and vinorelbine 25 mg/m² weekly (days 1, 8, 15, and 22)	28		
Carboplatin–paclitaxel	Carboplatin, dose targeted to AUC of 6 IV (day 1), and paclitaxel 225 mg/m² IV over 3 hours (day 1)	21	20	43
Gemcitabine–paclitaxel	Paclitaxel 200 mg/m² IV (day 1) and gemcitabine 1,000 mg/m² (day 1 and 8)	21	10	5
Gemcitabine–docetaxel	Gemcitabine 1,100 mg/m² IV (days 1 and 8) and docetaxel 100 mg/m² IV (day 8)	21	11	11
Gemcitabine	Gemcitabine 1,125 mg/m² (days 1 and 8)	21		19
Pemetrexed	Pemetrexed 500 mg/m² (day 1), vitamin B₁₂ 1 mg IM 1–2 weeks before treatment initiation and every 9 weeks thereafter, folic acid 1 mg daily beginning 3 weeks before treatment initiation	21		5–6
Paclitaxel	Paclitaxel 200 mg/m² IV over 3 hours (day 1)	21	34	3
Docetaxel	Docetaxel 35 mg/m² IV over 1 hour (days 1, 8, and 15)	28		5
Small Cell				
EP	Etoposide 100 mg/m² IV (days 1–3) and cisplatin 100 mg/m² IV (day 2)	28	85	18
CAV	Cyclophosphamide 800 mg/m² IV (day 1), doxorubicin 50 mg/m² (day 1), and vincristine 1.4 mg/m² (maximum of 2 mg) IV (day 1)	21–28	15	72
EC	Etoposide 100 mg/m² IV (days 1–3) and carboplatin AUC 5–6 IV (day 1)	21	10–20	5–15
IC	Irinotecan 60 mg/m² (days 1, 8, 15) and cisplatin 60 mg/m² (day 1)	28	40	25
Topotecan	Topotecan 1.5 mg/m² IV over 30 minutes (days 1–5)	21	18	70

	Other Significant Toxicities	Nausea/Vomiting Potential
Nonsmall Cell		
Paclitaxel–carboplatin–bevacizumab	Diarrhea, fever, headache, hypertension, hemoptysis, infection, leucopenia, nausea, neuropathy, peripheral neuritis, vomiting, thrombocytopenia, thrombotic events, bleeding, and proteinuria	High (day 1 only)
Cisplatin–paclitaxel	Febrile neutropenia/infection, thrombocytopenia, nausea, vomiting, diarrhea, cardiac toxicity, renal toxicity, neuropathy, weakness, hypersensitivity reactions, and anemia	High (day 2 only)
Cisplatin–docetaxel	Infection, thrombocytopenia, nausea, vomiting, diarrhea, cardiac, renal, neuropathy, weakness, hypersensitivity, and anemia	High (day 1 only)
Cisplatin–gemcitabine	Febrile neutropenia/infection, thrombocytopenia, and nausea, vomiting, diarrhea, cardiac, renal, neuropathy, weakness, and anemia	High (day 1); mild (days 8/15)
Cisplatin–vinorelbine–cetuximab	Data not available, likely to be similar to cisplatin-vinorelbine, with additional rash, infusion reactions, and hypomagnesemia	High (day 1 only)
Cisplatin–vinorelbine	Neutropenia, infection, anorexia, thrombocytopenia, nausea, vomiting, dyspnea, constipation, neuropathy, and anemia	High (day 1 and 8)
Carboplatin–paclitaxel	Infection, thrombocytopenia, nausea, vomiting, diarrhea, cardiac, renal, neuropathy, weakness, hypersensitivity, and anemia	High (day 1 only)
Gemcitabine–paclitaxel	Alopecia, nausea and vomiting, neurotoxicity, and thrombocytopenia	Moderate
Gemcitabine–docetaxel	Nausea and vomiting, diarrhea, thrombocytopenia, asthenia, and neurotoxicity	Moderate
Gemcitabine	Thrombocytopenia	Mild
Pemetrexed	Anemia	Mild
Paclitaxel	Infection, nausea, vomiting, diarrhea, mucositis, arthralgia, asthenia, peripheral neuropathy, alopecia, and cardiovascular	Mild (day 1 only)
Docetaxel	Fatigue, nausea, vomiting, skin toxicity, neuropathy, anemia, hypersensitivity, and alopecia	Mild

(Continued)

Table 90-4		
Chemotherapy Regimens in Lung Cancer and Associated Toxicities (Continued)		
	Other Significant Toxicities	**Nausea/Vomiting Potential**
Small Cell		
EP	Infection, nausea, vomiting, thrombocytopenia, and anemia	High (day 2 only)
CAV	Nausea, vomiting, thrombocytopenia, neuropathy, hepatic, renal, and alopecia	High
EC	Infection, thrombocytopenia, and alopecia	High (day 1 only)
IC	Fever, infection, thrombocytopenia, anemia, diarrhea, nausea and vomiting, and elevated liver enzymes	High (day 1); moderate (days 8/15)
Topotecan	Neutropenic fever, neutropenic sepsis, anemia, thrombocytopenia, nausea, fatigue, vomiting, stomatitis, anorexia, diarrhea, and fever	Mild (days 1–5)

CAV, cyclophosphamide, doxorubicin, and vincristine; EC, etoposide carboplatin; EP, etoposide cisplatin; IC, irinotecan cisplatin.

From Refs. 19–27, 35.

to the conclusion that adjuvant chemotherapy following surgical resection of nonsmall cell tumors results in a 4% improvement in survival. However, the majority of patients in the International Adjuvant Lung (IALT) trial were treated with a cisplatin and etoposide, which has been proven inferior to newer combinations of cisplatin in the advanced disease setting. In support of this criticism, the intergroup JBR-10 study evaluated adjuvant cisplatin–vinorelbine (a current standard regimen for advanced-stage disease) and found a survival advantage of 15%.[20] Consequently, adjuvant therapy has become the standard of care in resectable NSCLC and should be offered to patients after resection, particularly those with stage II–III disease. Although the regimen of choice is unclear, cisplatin–vinorelbine appears to be the regimen with the most evidence.

● **Neoadjuvant Therapy** Neoadjuvant or induction therapy refers to the use of chemotherapy regimens or radiotherapy prior to surgery. Again, because surgery has a limited role in SCLC, this section applies primarily to NSCLC. The rationale behind neoadjuvant therapy is to decrease the size of the tumor so that it can be extracted more easily with clean margins, as well as to eliminate distant micrometastases before invasive local treatment. Furthermore, patients with marginally resectable or nonresectable tumors may respond sufficiently to induction therapy that surgery becomes an option. Neoadjuvant chemotherapy has been shown to yield benefits in NSCLC (i.e., increase in median survival and disease-free survival and decreased risk of metastasis) for both local and locally advanced disease.[31] One concern is that the toxicity of induction regimens may delay surgery, and if the tumor does not respond to the treatment, there is a risk of disease progression. Nonetheless, current data suggest that over 90% of patients who are treated with neoadjuvant therapy maintain their scheduled surgery.[32] This approach is most common in patients with locally advanced tumors (stage III).[33] Current studies are aimed at comparing neoadjuvant with adjuvant therapy in earlier-stage NSCLC patients. The benefit of combining adjuvant therapy with induction therapy and surgery is also being investigated, but is of unknown value at this time.

▶ Monoclonal Antibodies

Bevacizumab and cetuximab are IgG monoclonal antibodies that have activity in NSCLC. Bevacizumab targets vascular endothelial-derived growth factor (VEGF), which facilitates angiogenesis, a process contributing to growth and maintenance of the tumor environment. Bevacizumab has been shown to improve survival of advanced stage nonsquamous cell NSCLC patients in a large phase III trial[34] and has been incorporated into current guidelines.[19] Squamous cell carcinoma of the lung should not be treated with bevacizumab due to the increased risk of bleeding events (an adverse event associated with bevacizumab administration) in this histological subtype.

Cetuximab targets epidermal growth factor receptor (EGFR), a cytokine receptor on tumor cells that is frequently involved with tumor survival and proliferation. This monoclonal antibody has a different and less extensive toxicity profile than traditional chemotherapy agents and appears to be synergistic when combined with chemotherapy. Cetuximab has recently been shown to be beneficial in NSCLC when added to cisplatin and vinorelbine in recurrent or metastatic NSCLC (Stages IIIB–IV).[35]

▶ Tyrosine Kinase Inhibitors

Tyrosine kinase inhibitors (TKIs) work by targeting specific intracellular messenger proteins that transmit growth and survival signals. Two TKIs are currently available for treatment of lung cancer: erlotinib and gefitinib. These agents, like cetuximab, target the EGFR that has been shown to be mutated or overexpressed in some lung tumors. Both gefitinib and erlotinib are structurally related and presumably have the same mechanism of action; however, data show that erlotinib prolongs survival, whereas gefitinib does not in unselected patient populations. Consequently, gefitinib availability is restricted until the FDA determines if there is a predictable way to identify patients who will respond to therapy.

Pharmacogenomics and pharmacogenetics will likely soon play a major role in the selection of NSCLC patients who should receive oral *EGFR* inhibitors such as gefitinib or erlotinib.

Large bodies of preclinical and clinical data demonstrate that certain mutations in the kinase domain of *EGFR* (L858R and del746–750) are associated with significant responses to such agents.[36] The presence of other mutations in *EGFR* (T790M) are associated with resistance to such inhibitors through decreased drug binding to the receptor. *EGFR* mutations are more frequent in females, Asians, patients with adenocarcinoma histology, and nonsmokers. Additionally, the presence of activating mutations in *KRAS*, another oncogene known to play a role in lung cancer, is also associated with clinical resistance to *EGFR* inhibitors. These findings have prompted clinical guidelines to suggest that assessment of the mutation status of *EGFR* and/or *KRAS* may be critical in selecting patients for *EGFR* kinase inhibitor therapy.[19] Patients with mutations in exons 19 or 21 of *EGFR* demonstrate the greatest likelihood of benefit, whereas those with mutations in exon 20 of *EGFR* or those with mutations in exons 1 or 2 of *KRAS* demonstrate the lowest likelihood of benefit. However, use of genotyping *KRAS* and *EGFR* has not yet entered into routine use in lung cancer. In addition to erlotinib and gefitinib, several "multitargeted" TKIs that target the *EGFR* and other cell-signaling cascades are in clinical trials and show promise for the treatment of lung cancer.

Small Cell Lung Cancer

SCLC typically presents as extensive disease (approximately 60–70% of new cases) and progresses very quickly. Small cell carcinomas are very responsive to chemotherapy and radiation, but have a short duration of response. Radiotherapy became the standard in 1969, when a randomized trial showed that it offered the potential for cure, whereas surgery did not.[37] In the vast majority of patients, chemotherapy with or without radiotherapy is the treatment of choice. Even after a complete response to therapy, the cancer usually recurs within 6 to 8 months, and survival time following recurrence is typically short (approximately 4 months). This yields a typical survival rate of 14 to 20 months for limited disease and 8 to 13 months for extensive disease.[21] Figure 90–2 illustrates the general treatment path of SCLC.

▶ *Limited Disease*

● The regimen of choice for limited-disease SCLC is etoposide-cisplatin (EP). In patients who are able to tolerate combined therapy, concomitant chemoradiotherapy offers the greatest survival benefit. Carboplatin may be substituted for cisplatin in patients who cannot tolerate cisplatin toxicity.[38] In European countries, a three-drug combination containing an anthracycline has been the mainstay of therapy; however, mounting clinical evidence shows that these regimens are inferior to EP plus concurrent radiation and have more toxicity. Consequently, the guidelines recommend that the EP regimen be used with concurrent radiotherapy.[21]

Because patients with SCLC commonly have a recurrence in the CNS, trials have been performed to evaluate the benefit of PCI. A pivotal study showed that PCI reduces the incidence of brain metastasis and increases 3-year survival from 15% to 21%.[39] Patients with limited stage SCLC who achieve a complete response with treatment should be offered PCI.

▶ *Extensive Disease*

● Platinum regimens, particularly EP, are the treatment of choice in extensive disease. In one Japanese study, a combination of irinotecan and cisplatin demonstrated an increased median survival time by approximately 3 months

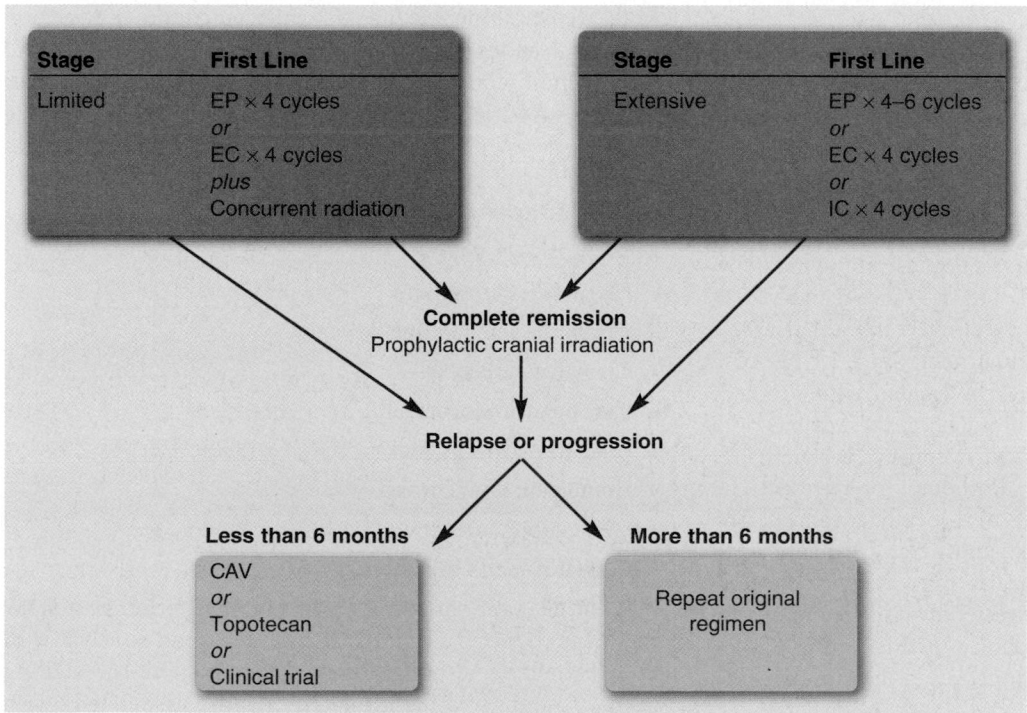

FIGURE 90–2. Small cell lung cancer treatment overview. (CAV, cyclophosphamide, doxorubicin, vincristine; EC, etoposide carboplatin; EP, etoposide cisplatin; IC, irinotecan, cisplatin.) *(From Ref 21.)*

over the EP regimen. This irinotecan–cisplatin regimen also had a lower incidence of severe neutropenic side effects but exhibited higher rates of middle- to high-grade diarrhea.[22] However, this study was repeated in the United States and did not show a similar improvement over the EP regimen.[40] Therefore, EP remains the regimen of choice for treating extensive SCLC in the United States. Due to the high sensitivity of treatment-naive SCLC to chemotherapy, it is imperative that these patients be monitored for signs of tumor lysis syndrome and possibly treated with prophylactic therapy.

Concurrent radiotherapy is not used routinely in extensive disease; however, PCI provides significant benefit in patients responding to chemotherapy. A pivotal study demonstrated that median survival from the time of randomization increased from 5.4 to 6.7 months and 1-year survival rates increased from 13.3% to 27.1% with PCI. An additional benefit was a lower rate of brain metastasis (14.6% versus 40.4%).[41]

▶ Recurrent Disease

The treatment of recurrent SCLC depends on the time to recurrence. If the time to recurrence is less than 6 months, second-line therapy should be considered if the patient has an acceptable PS (see Patient Care and Monitoring). The most widely accepted second-line therapies in SCLC are topotecan alone or CAV [cyclophosphamide, doxorubicin (Adriamycin), and vincristine]. Relapses occurring more than 6 months after treatment warrant a repeat of the initial regimen. Poor PS patients (3–4) are typically treated with palliative care therapies.

Nonsmall Cell Lung Cancer

The first step in treatment of NSCLC involves confirmation of the clinical stage and determination of resectability of the tumor. This decision should always be made by a thoracic surgeon who routinely performs lung cancer surgery. Treatment options depend on the advancement of disease (i.e., local, locally advanced, or metastatic), PS, and eligibility for resection.

▶ Local Disease (Stages 1A, 1B, and IIA)

Local disease encompasses stages IA through IIA and is associated with a favorable prognosis because approximately 40% to 60% of patients are expected to live more than 5 years from diagnosis. Goals of therapy are curative in local disease, and surgery is the mainstay of treatment. Stage IA tumors are rarely seen clinically and may be treated with surgery alone. In this case, neoadjuvant or adjuvant therapy has not been adequately studied to know if it conveys a benefit. If surgical margins are positive, radiotherapy or re-resection is recommended.[19] Stages IB, IIA, and locally advanced IIB NSCLC is treated with adjuvant chemotherapy. Patients who have positive or questionable margins may receive radiation therapy, which typically is administered with the adjuvant chemotherapy. The regimen of choice in this setting is not clear; however, clinical trials demonstrating the most benefit used cisplatin–vinorelbine.[19,42]

▶ Locally Advanced Disease (Stages IIB and IIIA)

Patients with locally advanced disease should also be considered for surgery. Neoadjuvant chemotherapy with concurrent radiotherapy can be used prior to surgery, although this practice varies from institution to institution. Progression of disease during induction therapy may preclude surgery, and the regimen should be altered. If there is a response, surgical resection can be attempted, with or without additional adjuvant chemotherapy. Nonresectable locally advanced disease may be treated with both an active platinum-containing regimen and radiotherapy.

▶ Advanced or Metastatic Disease (Stages IIIB and IV)

Advanced disease is treated with chemotherapy if the patient has an acceptable ECOG PS score (0–1). Platinum-containing doublets have produced the highest overall response rates (25–35%) and survival times (30–40% 1-year survival) in well-performing patients with advanced disease. A number of different platinum doublet treatment regimens have been used in this setting. In some patients with stage IIIB disease, cisplatin and etoposide may be given concurrently with radiotherapy. However, treating unresectable stage III patients with a platinum-containing doublet regimen and omitting the radiation is common. The optimal regimen has yet to be determined. There has been some debate about the equivalence of cisplatin and carboplatin. To address this question, a recent meta-analysis was performed, which indicated that cisplatin was superior to carboplatin when combined with another agent (see below) in advanced-stage NSCLC.[43] As with any meta-analysis, the methodology is subject to limitations leaving clinicians to make their own decision. Additionally, two nonplatinum-containing regimens have been shown to have similar response and survival benefits. Both gemcitabine–paclitaxel and gemcitabine–docetaxel produce response durations and survival times similar to the platinum-containing doublet regimens. These regimens may be substituted when patients are unlikely to tolerate the toxicity of platinum regimens owing to comorbidities or other factors. NSCLC chemotherapy doublets that are considered generally equivalent include:

- Paclitaxel–cisplatin
- Paclitaxel–carboplatin
- Cisplatin–gemcitabine
- Cisplatin–docetaxel
- Carboplatin–docetaxel
- Cisplatin–vinorelbine
- Gemcitabine–paclitaxel
- Gemcitabine–docetaxel
- Cisplatin–pemetrexed

A large randomized trial comparing the first four regimens reported similar response rates and survival with all treatments, although there was less life-threatening toxicity and treatment-related death associated with paclitaxel–carboplatin.[23] Consequently, one may argue that paclitaxel–carboplatin is the treatment of choice. However, the carboplatin–paclitaxel regimen used in the trial infused paclitaxel over 24 hours, which is uncommon in clinical practice. The most common carboplatin–paclitaxel regimen infuses a higher dose of paclitaxel over 3 hours in the clinic rather than admit patients to the hospital for a 24-hour infusion. It is unfair to extrapolate the toxicity advantage from this trial to the commonly used 3-hour paclitaxel infusion, and consequently, there is not a single best regimen.

Taxanes (docetaxel and paclitaxel) are frequently employed in advanced NSCLC. Albumin-bound paclitaxel may be substituted for docetaxel or paclitaxel in patients who have experienced hypersensitivity reactions to taxanes despite antihypersensitivity premedication. The albumin-bound paclitaxel formulation does not include excipients such as Cremophor-EL that are thought to be the primary cause of frequent taxane-related reactions.

● **Targeted Agents** While it is unclear exactly which combination is the best, new research is being aimed at adding targeted agents to platinum regimens. Adding bevacizumab to the carboplatin–paclitaxel (3-hour infusion) regimen increases response rates and prolongs progression-free survival by 1.7 months and overall survival by 2.3 months.[34] Consequently, carboplatin–paclitaxel and bevacizumab are arguably the new standard of care. Based on the inclusion/exclusion criteria for this study, bevacizumab is recommended when the patient meets the following criteria:

- Nonsquamous cell histology (NSCLC only)
- History negative for hemoptysis
- History negative for untreated CNS metastasis
- No concurrent anticoagulation therapy (i.e., enoxaparin, heparin, or warfarin). In clinical trials, low-dose aspirin was permissible.
- Chemotherapy regimen that does not have significant (greater than 10%) risk of thrombocytopenia.

Interestingly, bevacizumab does not show synergy with all regimens; when combined with cisplatin and gemcitabine, no survival advantage is seen. Consequently, it should only be used with carboplatin and paclitaxel.

The anti-EGFR monoclonal antibody cetuximab has been shown to improve survival when combined with cisplatin and vinorelbine. The FLEX trial demonstrated a 1.2-month survival advantage of cetuximab when added to cisplatin and vinorelbine in recurrent or metastatic NSCLC (Stages IIIB–IV).[35] The study population consisted of chemotherapy-naive patients with PS 0 to 2 that demonstrated positive tumor staining for EGFR by immunohistochemistry. It is unclear how this regimen compares to bevacizumab plus carboplatin and paclitaxel. Because bevacizumab was proven effective first and the survival advantage appears superior; cisplatin, vinorelbine, and cetuximab will likely only be used in patients with a contraindication to bevacizumab (squamous cell histology). Adding EGFR TKIs (erlotinib or gefitinib) to chemotherapy provides no benefit.

● **Poorly Performing Patients** Treating patients with a PS of 2 is a subject of debate. While PS 2 patients typically have inferior survival rates and higher toxicity to platinum chemotherapy than higher-performing patients, low-toxicity single-agent regimens may offer a survival advantage in this subset. Use of these regimens also presents a method of providing symptomatic care for advanced-stage patients. Agents such as pemetrexed, gemcitabine, and docetaxel may be used in this scenario. In PS 3 or 4 patients, chemotherapy typically results in high rates of toxicity and fails to convey a survival benefit. Consequently, treatment should be aimed at relief of symptoms instead of a definitive cure.

▶ *Recurrent and Progressive Disease*

● Although patients may experience a response to initial therapy, disease recurs in many cases. If the recurrence is localized, surgery options may be assessed. If the patient's PS remains acceptable (0–1), second-line systemic chemotherapy has been shown to improve survival. Although platinum doublets may be used at this point in care, a single-agent therapy with docetaxel, pemetrexed, or erlotinib is recommended.[44] Recurrences in poorly performing patients (3–4) usually are not treated with chemotherapy and are instead treated with supportive care. Additional recurrences (e.g., third-line therapy) may be treated with erlotinib if not used previously. Otherwise, repeat single-agent therapy or administer best supportive care.

PATIENT CARE AND MONITORING
Management of Toxicity

❼ *Knowing when and how to treat adverse events from chemotherapy is an important aspect of patient care. Unmanaged events may cause delays in chemotherapy administration and reduced chemotherapy doses may contribute to treatment failure.* Given the fatal nature of untreated lung cancer, patients and health care professionals are willing to tolerate high risks of severe and life-threatening side effects, provided that the therapy has been shown to benefit the patient. There are multiple methods of preventing or reducing toxicity from chemotherapeutic agents. These methods usually are agent-specific but commonly include maintenance of adequate hydration, use of appropriate premedications, dose reduction of the causative agent, and use of growth factors to combat toxicities associated with cytopenias.

▶ *Grading Toxicity*

● In order to standardize grading of adverse events, the National Cancer Institute (NCI) has developed the Common Toxicity Criteria (CTC, V3.0) for adverse events (see Chap. 88). In most cases, patients who experience grade 3 or 4 toxicity require a change in therapy with the next cycle of treatment. Common changes include a chemotherapy dose reduction or pharmacologic intervention to prevent or treat the toxicity. The CTC is an invaluable tool to determine what serious toxicity is most likely with a particular regimen, and improves the pharmacist's ability to counsel the patient as well as to determine appropriate toxicity-prevention measures.

▶ Dose Intensity and Growth Factors

● The term dose intensity refers to the percent of drug delivered compared with the planned amount as measured by milligrams per meter squared per week. Maintaining dose intensity (i.e., delivering the planned dose, according to the scheduled time course) has been shown to influence survival in some cancers such as breast cancer; however, the importance of dose intensity in lung cancer is not well established. In order to maintain dose intensity, pharmacologic agents are sometimes used to combat serious toxicities that may prohibit or delay administration of subsequent doses.

With most lung cancer chemotherapy regimens, the most common grade 3 or 4 toxicity is neutropenia. Patients who experience grade 3 or 4 neutropenia are at a high risk of developing a severe or life-threatening bacterial infection. Consequently, patients with neutropenia who develop a fever are empirically given broad-spectrum antibiotics. If a patient experiences neutropenic fever, dose reduction, or intervention with growth factors (e.g., pegfilgrastim, filgrastim, or sargramostim) to maintain dose intensity should occur prior to the next cycle of chemotherapy. In lung cancer patients, no survival benefit has been demonstrated by using a colony-stimulating factor to maintain dose intensity. ❽ *While some evidence suggest that the use of a colony-stimulating factor reduces the number of neutropenic fever episodes, hospital stay, and antibiotic administration in certain subsets of lung cancer patients, routine front-line (prophylactic) use of a colony-stimulating factor is not recommended owing to lack of a survival benefit.*[45,46]

▶ Nausea and Vomiting

● Platinum agents are the most active lung cancer agents and historically have very high rates of nausea and vomiting. This is particularly true of high-dose cisplatin, which is used in many regimens. Understanding how to prevent and treat chemotherapy-induced nausea and vomiting (CINV) in lung cancer patients is crucial because nearly all the regimens are highly emetogenic. Although the pathology of CINV is not fully understood, there are three classifications of CINV based on the time of occurrence in relationship to chemotherapy administration: acute CINV (1–24 hours after the dose), delayed (1–5 days after the dose), and anticipatory (before the dose following one or more previous cycles).

Acute CINV appears to be influenced predominantly by serotonin binding to 5-hydroxytryptamine-3 (5-HT$_3$) receptors on the vagal nerve, where it innervates the GI tract. Delayed CINV has been attributed to a variety of mechanisms but appears to be influenced by substance-P stimulation of neurokinin-1 (NK-1) receptors in the CNS, as well as a corticosteroid-responsive element. Anticipatory CINV is thought to be a learned or conditioned behavior. The major influencing factors appear to be prior acute or delayed CINV and anxiety. Anticipatory CINV may be prevented or treated with benzodiazepines such as lorazepam or alprazolam not because they possess antiemetic properties but rather because they contain amnesic and antianxiety properties.

There are three main drug targets that are antagonized to prevent or treat acute and delayed CINV: 5-HT$_3$ receptors, dopamine type 2 receptors (D$_2$), and NK-1 receptors. 5-HT$_3$-receptor antagonists are the most effective agents for preventing acute CINV. However, they are only recommended for moderate- to high-emetogenic-potential regimens, primarily owing to cost (see Table 90–5 for a comparison of agents). Aprepitant is the only available NK-1-receptor antagonist that is approved to prevent CINV. It has modest but additive activity in acute CINV and appears to be highly active in preventing delayed CINV. It was approved for use in highly emetogenic regimens but also works in patients receiving moderately emetogenic chemotherapy. The use of aprepitant is somewhat limited by the cost. D$_2$ receptor antagonists, which are approved for schizophrenia, also have antiemetic activity in both acute and delayed CINV. As a group, these agents do not appear to be as effective as 5-HT$_3$-receptor antagonist in acute CINV or as effective as aprepitant in delayed CINV. Consequently, their use is frequently limited to patients receiving mild or moderate emetogenic chemotherapy as prevention or as treatment following full-dose 5-HT$_3$-receptor antagonist and/or aprepitant. They are attractive owing to their relatively low cost but cause a significant number of side effects. Interestingly, corticosteroids, most commonly dexamethasone, is an active antiemetic agent that can be used as monotherapy to prevent acute CINV in patients receiving mild-to-moderate emetogenic chemotherapy. They are also synergistic with 5-HT$_3$-receptor antagonists, aprepitant, and D$_2$-receptor antagonists in acute and delayed CINV. Although antiemetic choices typically are guided by chemotherapy, patient-specific risk factors that may play a role include the following high-risk features: very young age, very old age, female gender, emesis associated with pregnancy or motion sickness, and those with low alcohol intake.[47]

▶ Diarrhea

● Chemotherapy-induced diarrhea can be of significant toxicity in cancer patients and should be managed pharmacologically when necessary. The most common offending agent in the treatment of lung cancer is irinotecan. Treatment may include loperamide (4 mg at the onset followed by 2 mg every 2 hours until resolution—may use 4 mg every 4 hours during sleep) or octreotide (starting at 100 mcg subcutaneously every 8 hours and titrated to effect). The goals of therapy are resolution of diarrhea and improvement in quality of life.

Surveillance

Following response to surgery or pharmacologic treatment, the patient should be monitored regularly to detect recurrence. National Comprehensive Cancer Network (NCCN) guidelines suggest a physical examination and CXR every 3 to 4 months for 2 years. If no disease is detected during this time, follow-up frequency can be prolonged

Table 90–5

Pharmacotherapy for CINV

Class	Indication	Drug	Dose	Half-life
NK-1 inhibitors	Acute/delayed NV	Aprepitant	125 mg po on day 1 80 mg po daily on days 2–3	9–13
		Fosaprepitant	115 mg IV on day 1 80 mg po aprepitant daily on days 2–3	9–13
5-HT$_3$ inhibitors	Acute NV	Ondansetron	16–24 mg po or 8–12 mg IV on day 1; 16 mg po daily or 8 mg IV daily on days 2–4	3–6
		Palonosetron	0.25 mg IV on day 1	40
		Granisetron	1–2 mg po or 0.01 mg/kg IV on days 1–4	4–12
		Dolasetron	100 mg po or 100 mg IV daily on days 1–4	8 (active metabolite)
D$_2$ antagonists	Acute/delayed NV, PRN break-through treatment	Haloperidol	1–2 mg po q 4–6 h or 1–3 mg IV q 4–6 h	20
		Olanzapine	Olanzapine 2.5–5 mg po twice a day, as needed	20–50
Corticosteroids	Adjunctive treatment for acute or delayed NV	Dexamethasone	12 mg IV or po on day 18 mg IV or po daily on days 2–4	2–4 biological half-life of 36–54
Benzodiazepines	Anticipatory NV	Lorazepam	0.5–2 mg po once on night before and once on morning of treatment	12–16
	Anticipatory NV	Alprazolam	0.5–2 mg po three times a day starting the night prior to treatment	12–16

CINV, chemotherapy-induced nausea and vomiting; NV, nausea and vomiting.

to every 6 months for 3 years and then annually. Low-dose spiral CT scanning is also recommended annually. Additionally, smoking-cessation counseling with or without pharmacologic treatment should be a priority. While studies have shown that patients who continue to smoke through treatment in NSCLC do not perform more poorly compared to those that quit prior to treatment, those that respond to treatment and continue to smoke probably have increased risk of developing secondary malignancies.[48] In contrast to NSCLC, some data suggest that SCLC patients with limited stage disease have poorer outcomes if they continue to smoke during treatment.[49]

Complications

▶ Cachexia and Anorexia

Cachexia is a severe wasting syndrome that is seen in many cancer patients. Although it is more common in advanced disease, it is often seen in localized disease as well. Cachexia is characterized by a catabolic state that leads to significant loss of body mass, both lean muscle and fat. The causes of cachexia are poorly understood, but it is thought that they involve inflammatory cytokines such as tumor necrosis factor-*a* (originally described as cachexin). Anorexia is the patient's loss of appetite or willingness to eat. The presence of anorexia can aggravate cachexia and contribute to morbidity. When anorexia contributes to cachexia, it is important to assess the patient for the underlying cause of the anorexia.

Causes for anorexia in lung cancer patients can be widespread and include CINV, esophagitis, and mucosal irritation from combined radiotherapy and chemotherapy, GI obstruction owing to tumors, constipation from opioid analgesics, and psychological factors such as anxiety or depression. Many of these issues may be improved with pharmacologic treatment of the underlying cause (i.e., antidepressant therapy for psychological factors) or with palliative treatment of the offending tumor.[50] Additionally, appetite stimulants such as the cannabinoid dronabinol (2.5 mg twice daily with meals, titrated to a maximum of 20 mg/day) and megesterol acetate (400–800 mg/day orally) can aid in increasing caloric intake.

Cachexia is more difficult to treat, although it may resolve following treatment of the underlying malignancy. Nutritional consultation may be of aid, although cachexia is thought to be more attributable to internal pathophysiologic processes than malnutrition.

▶ Paraneoplastic Syndromes

Paraneoplastic syndromes are clinical syndromes caused by nonmetastatic systemic effects of cancer. Tumors make and secrete biologically active products that can stimulate or inhibit hormone production, autoimmunity, immune complex production, or cause immune suppression. Lung cancer, particularly SCLC, is associated with a high rate of paraneoplastic syndromes. Pharmacologic therapy is necessary when the abnormality causes the patient acute physical or psychological stress or adversely affects his or her health. When possible, therapy should be directed at the primary tumor, and a response often leads to resolution of symptoms.

Patient Encounter, Part 4

On the basis of the information provided, develop a care plan for this patient. Include (a) treatment goals, (b) monitoring parameters for anticipated toxicities, and (c) a follow-up plan to determine response to treatment and surveillance.

▶ *Palliative Care*

Ultimately, most lung cancer patients succumb to their disease. Palliative care involves management of symptoms and improvement of quality of life when curative treatment options are no longer available. Often, problematic metastases can be removed by surgery (depending on location) or can be treated with radiotherapy to reduce tumor size. In selecting options at this point in treatment, it is important to keep the goals of therapy in mind, those being maximizing the duration and quality of life. Low-toxicity single-agent chemotherapy, targeted therapy, and best supportive care (including fatigue and pain management) are commonly the mainstays of palliative care.

OUTCOME EVALUATION

Following treatment, evaluate the goals of therapy versus the response that was achieved. Was there response to treatment or progression of disease? If the patient is being treated with supportive care, then alleviation of symptoms and improvement in quality of life should be of primary importance. Be sure to document objective evaluations of the outcome in the care plan.

Abbreviations Introduced in This Chapter

5-FDG	5-Fluorodeoxyglucose
5-HT$_3$	5-Hydroxytryptamine-3
CAV	Cyclophosphamide, doxorubicin, and vincristine
CINV	Chemotherapy-induced nausea and vomiting
CTC	Common toxicity criteria
ECOG	Eastern Cooperative Oncology Group
EGF	Epidermal growth factor
EGFR	Epidermal growth factor receptor
EP	Etoposide, cisplatin
ETS	Environmental tobacco smoke
GM-CSF	Granulocyte-macrophage colony-stimulating factor
G-CSF	Granulocyte colony-stimulating factor
IALT	International Adjuvant Lung trial
NCCN	National Comprehensive Cancer Network
NSCLC	Nonsmall cell lung cancer
PCI	Prophylactic cranial irradiation
PET	Positron-emission tomography

Patient Care and Monitoring

1. Review the patient's medical and social history. Was the patient exposed to clinical risk factors for lung cancer?

2. Verify the histology and clinical stage of disease. Evaluate the patient's PS. Is the patient a surgical candidate? How does this influence your treatment recommendations?

3. Develop a care plan based on treatment goals. If the goal is palliative care, how does treatment-related toxicity influence therapy?

4. If chemotherapy is the treatment of choice, counsel the patient on risks and benefits of undergoing such therapy. Be sure that the patient understands the issues fully before moving forward.

5. Verify dosing of all agents in the chemotherapy regimen. What are the major expected toxicities?

6. Evaluate toxicity as treatment progresses. Is the toxicity severe enough to warrant dose reduction or pharmacologic treatment? Record graded toxicities according to the NCI CTC V3.0 criteria.

7. Evaluate the response to treatment. Did the patient experience a complete response, partial response, stable disease, or disease progression? How does this change future treatment?

8. If the patient is in remission, develop a monitoring plan. What signs or symptoms denote disease progression?

9. Recommend a smoking-cessation program or other risk-reduction plan for the patient.

PORT	Postoperative radiotherapy
PS	Performance status
SCLC	Small cell lung cancer
SVC	Superior vena cava
TKIs	Tyrosine kinase inhibitors
TNM	Tumor, node, and metastasis staging
VEGF	Vascular endothelial growth factor

 Self-assessment questions and answers are available at *http://www.mhpharmacotherapy.com/pp.html*.

REFERENCES

1. Jemal A, Siegel R, Ward E, et al. Cancer statistics, 2008. CA Cancer J Clin 2008;58(2):71–96.

2. Alberg AJ, Brock MV, Samet JM. Epidemiology of lung cancer: Looking to the future. J Clin Oncol 2005;23(14):3175–3185.

3. Fu JB, Kau TY, Severson RK, Kalemkerian GP. Lung cancer in women: Analysis of the national Surveillance, Epidemiology, and End Results database. Chest 2005 Mar;127(3):768–777.

4. Ginsberg MS. Epidemiology of lung cancer. Semin Roentgenol 2005; 40(2):83–89.

5. Tammemagi CM, Neslund-Dudas C, Simoff M, Kvale P. In lung cancer patients, age, race-ethnicity, gender and smoking predict adverse comorbidity, which in turn predicts treatment and survival. J Clin Epidemiol 2004;57(6):597–609.

6. Westmaas JL, Brandon TH. Reducing risk in smokers. Curr Opin Pulm Med 2004;10(4):284–288.

7. Mannisto S, Smith-Warner SA, Spiegelman D, et al. Dietary carotenoids and risk of lung cancer in a pooled analysis of seven cohort studies. Cancer Epidemiol Biomarkers Prev 2004;13(1):40–48.

8. Kufe DW, Holland JF, Frei E, American Cancer Society. Cancer medicine, Vol. 6, 6th ed. Hamilton, Ont.; Lewiston, NY: B.C. Decker, 2003.

9. Landi S, Gemignani F, Monnier S, Canzian F. A database of single-nucleotide polymorphisms and a genotyping microarray for genetic epidemiology of lung cancer. Exp Lung Res 2005;31(2):223–258.

10. Sobti RC, Sharma S, Joshi A, et al. Genetic polymorphism of the CYP1A1, CYP2E1, GSTM1 and GSTT1 genes and lung cancer susceptibility in a North Indian population. Mol Cell Biochem 2004;266(1–2):1–9.

11. Dragnev KH, Stover D, Dmitrovsky E. Lung cancer prevention: The guidelines. Chest 2003;123(1 Suppl):60S–71S.

12. Bastarrika G, Garcia-Velloso MJ, Lozano MD, et al. Early lung cancer detection using spiral computed tomography and positron emission tomography. Am J Respir Crit Care Med 2005;171(12):1378–1383.

13. Ruckdeschel JC, Schwartz AG, Bepler G, et al. Cancer of the Lung: NSCLC and SCLC. In: Abeloff MD, Armitage JO, Niederhuber JE, Kastan MB, McKenna WG, eds. Clinical Oncology, 3rd ed. Orlando: Churchill Livingston, 2004.

14. Micke P, Faldum A, Metz T, et al. Staging small cell lung cancer: Veterans Administration Lung Study Group versus International Association for the Study of Lung Cancer—What limits limited disease? Lung Cancer 2002;37(3):271–276.

15. Fox W, Scadding JG. Medical Research Council comparative trial of surgery and radiotherapy for primary treatment of small-celled or oat-celled carcinoma of bronchus. Ten-year follow-up. Lancet 1973; 2(7820):63–65.

16. Jeremic B, Shibamoto Y, Acimovic L, Milisavljevic S. Hyperfractionated radiotherapy for clinical stage II non-small cell lung cancer. Radiother Oncol 1999;51(2):141–145.

17. Spira A, Ettinger DS. Multidisciplinary management of lung cancer. N Engl J Med 2004, 2004;350(4):379–392.

18. Postoperative radiotherapy for non-small cell lung cancer. Cochrane Database Syst Rev 2005(2):CD002142.

19. NCCN Practice Guidelines in Oncology: Non-small cell lung cancer. National Comprehensive Cancer Network. 2008, *www.nccn.org*.

20. Winton T, Livingston R, Johnson D, et al. Vinorelbine plus cisplatin vs. observation in resected non-small-cell lung cancer. N Engl J Med 2005;352(25):2589–2597.

21. NCCN Practice Guidelines in Oncology: Small Cell Lung Cancer. National Comprehensive Cancer Network. 2008, *www.nccn.org*.

22. Noda K, Nishiwaki Y, Kawahara M, et al. Irinotecan plus cisplatin compared with etoposide plus cisplatin for extensive small-cell lung cancer. N Engl J Med 2002;346(2):85–91.

23. Schiller JH, Harrington D, Belani CP, et al. Comparison of four chemotherapy regimens for advanced non-small-cell lung cancer. N Engl J Med 2002;346(2):92–98.

24. Hanna N, Shepherd FA, Fossella FV, et al. Randomized phase III trial of pemetrexed versus docetaxel in patients with non-small-cell lung cancer previously treated with chemotherapy. J Clin Oncol 2004;22(9):1589–1597.

25. Kosmidis P, Mylonakis N, Nicolaides C, et al. Paclitaxel plus carboplatin versus gemcitabine plus paclitaxel in advanced non-small-cell lung cancer: A phase III randomized trial. J Clin Oncol 2002;20(17): 3578–3585.

26. Scagliotti GV, Kortsik C, Dark GG, et al. Pemetrexed combined with oxaliplatin or carboplatin as first-line treatment in advanced non-small cell lung cancer: A multicenter, randomized, phase II trial. Clin Cancer Res 2005;11(2 Pt 1):690–696.

27. Shepherd FA, Dancey J, Ramlau R, et al. Prospective randomized trial of docetaxel versus best supportive care in patients with non-small-cell lung cancer previously treated with platinum-based chemotherapy. J Clin Oncol 2000;18(10):2095–2103.

28. Milton DT, Miller VA. Advances in cytotoxic chemotherapy for the treatment of metastatic or recurrent non-small cell lung cancer. Semin Oncol 2005;32(3):299–314.

29. Johnson DH. "The guard dies, it does not surrender!" Progress in the management of small-cell lung cancer? J Clin Oncol 2002;20(24): 4618–4620.

30. Arriagada R, Bergman B, Dunant A, et al. Cisplatin-based adjuvant chemotherapy in patients with completely resected non-small-cell lung cancer. N Engl J Med 2004;350(4):351–360.

31. Depierre A, Milleron B, Moro-Sibilot D, et al. Preoperative chemotherapy followed by surgery compared with primary surgery in resectable stage I (except T1N0), II, and IIIa non-small-cell lung cancer. J Clin Oncol 2002;20(1):247–253.

32. Belani CP. Adjuvant and neoadjuvant therapy in non-small cell lung cancer. Semin Oncol 2005;32(2 Suppl 2):S9–S15.

33. De Marinis F, Gebbia V, De Petris L. Neoadjuvant chemotherapy for stage IIIA-N2 non-small cell lung cancer. Ann Oncol 2005;16(Suppl 4): iv116–iv122.

34. Sandler A, Gray R, Perry MC, et al. Paclitaxel-carboplatin alone or with bevacizumab for non-small-cell lung cancer. N Engl J Med 2006;355(24):2542–2550.

35. Pirker R, Pereira JR, Szczesna A, et al. Cetuximab plus chemotherapy in patients with advanced non-small-cell lung cancer (FLEX): An open label randomised phase III trial. Lancet 2009;373:1525–1531.

36. Sequist LV, Joshi VA, Janne PA, et al. Epidermal growth factor receptor mutation testing in the care of lung cancer patients. Clin Cancer Res 2006;12(14 Pt 2):4403s–4408s.

37. Miller AB, Fox W, Tall R. Five-year follow-up of the Medical Research Council comparative trial of surgery and radiotherapy for the primary treatment of small-celled or oat-celled carcinoma of the bronchus. Lancet 1969;2(7619):501–505.

38. Simon GR, Wagner H. Small cell lung cancer. Chest, 2003; 123(90010):259S–271S.

39. Auperin A, Arriagada R, Pignon JP, et al. Prophylactic cranial irradiation for patients with small-cell lung cancer in complete remission. Prophylactic Cranial Irradiation Overview Collaborative Group. N Engl J Med 1999 12;341(7):476–484.

40. Hanna N, Bunn PA, Jr., Langer C, et al. Randomized phase III trial comparing irinotecan/cisplatin with etoposide/cisplatin in patients with previously untreated extensive-stage disease small-cell lung cancer. J Clin Oncol 2006;24(13):2038–2043.

41. Slotman B, Faivre-Finn C, Kramer G, et al. Prophylactic cranial irradiation in extensive small-cell lung cancer. N Engl J Med 2007;357(7): 664–672.

42. Dunant A, Pignon JP, Le Chevalier T. Adjuvant chemotherapy for non-small cell lung cancer: Contribution of the International Adjuvant Lung Trial. Clin Cancer Res 2005;11(13 Pt 2):5017s–5021s.

43. Hotta K, Matsuo K, Ueoka H, et al. Meta-analysis of randomized clinical trials comparing cisplatin to carboplatin in patients with advanced non-small-cell lung cancer. J Clin Oncol 2004;22(19):3852–3859.

44. Pfister DG, Johnson DH, Azzoli CG, et al. American Society of Clinical Oncology Treatment of Unresectable Non-Small-Cell Lung Cancer Guideline: Update 2003. J Clin Oncol 2004;22(2):330–353.

45. Berghmans T, Paesmans M, Lafitte JJ, et al. Role of granulocyte and granulocyte-macrophage colony-stimulating factors in the treatment of small-cell lung cancer: A systematic review of the literature with methodological assessment and meta-analysis. Lung Cancer 2002;37(2):115–123.

46. Kasymjanova G, Kreisman H, Correa JA, et al. Does granulocyte colony-stimulating factor affect survival in patients with advanced non-small cell lung cancer? J Thorac Oncol 2006;1(6): 564–570.

47. Jordan K, Kasper C, Schmoll HJ. Chemotherapy-induced nausea and vomiting: Current and new standards in the antiemetic prophylaxis and treatment. Eur J Cancer 2005;41(2):199–205.

48. Tsao AS, Liu D, Lee JJ, et al. Smoking affects treatment outcome in patients with advanced nonsmall cell lung cancer. Cancer 2006;106(11): 2428–2436.

49. Videtic GM, Stitt LW, Dar AR, et al. Continued cigarette smoking by patients receiving concurrent chemoradiotherapy for limited-stage small-cell lung cancer is associated with decreased survival. J Clin Oncol 2003;21(8):1544–1549.

50. MacDonald N, Easson AM, Mazurak VC, et al. Understanding and managing cancer cachexia. J Am Coll Surg 2003;197(1):143–161.

91 Colorectal Cancer

Patrick J. Medina

LEARNING OBJECTIVES

Upon completion of the chapter, the reader will be able to:

1. Identify the risk factors for colon cancer.

2. Recognize the signs and symptoms of colorectal cancer.

3. Describe the treatment options for colorectal cancer based on patient-specific factors, such as stage of disease, age of patient, genetic mutations, and previous treatment received.

4. Outline the pharmacologic principles for agents used to treat colorectal cancer.

5. Develop a monitoring plan to assess the efficacy and toxicity of agents used in colorectal cancer.

6. Educate patients about the adverse effects of chemotherapy that require specific patient counseling.

7. Outline preventive and screening strategies for individuals at average and high-risk for colorectal cancer.

KEY CONCEPTS

❶ Although there are numerous risk factors for developing colorectal cancer, age is the biggest risk factor for sporadic colorectal cancer.

❷ Diets high in fat and low in fiber are associated with increased colorectal cancer risk, whereas the regular use of aspirin (and nonsteroidal anti-inflammatory drugs [NSAIDs]) and calcium supplementation may decrease the risk of colorectal cancer.

❸ Effective colorectal cancer screening programs incorporate annual fecal occult blood testing in combination with regular examination of the entire colon starting at age 50 for average-risk individuals and should be recommended by all health care providers.

❹ Most patients with colorectal cancer are asymptomatic early but may develop changes in bowel or eating habits, fatigue, abdominal pain, and blood in stool.

❺ The stage of colorectal cancer is determined by the tumor-node-metastasis (TNM) staging system and is the most important prognostic factor for patient survival. Disease stages I to III are curable, whereas patients with stage IV disease are treated with the goal of palliation.

❻ Adjuvant chemotherapy is not needed in patients with stage I colon cancer, may be beneficial in selective high-risk patients with stage II colon cancer, and is standard of care in patients with stage III colon cancer.

❼ 5-Fluorouracil, leucovorin and oxaliplatin chemotherapy (FOLFOX) is the standard regimen used in adjuvant colon cancer. It is usually given for 6 months.

❽ Triple-drug therapy consisting of 5-fluorouracil and leucovorin with oxaliplatin or irinotecan improves survival compared to 5-fluorouracil plus leucovorin alone, and is considered as standard first-line therapy for metastatic disease. The addition of bevacizumab is recommended to be added to 5-fluorouracil-based regimens based on improvements in overall survival.

❾ Treatment of relapsed or refractory metastatic disease uses agents not given in the first-line setting.

❿ Adjuvant therapy consisting of 5-fluorouracil-based chemotherapy in combination with radiation therapy should be offered to patients with stage II or III cancer of the rectum.

INTRODUCTION

Colorectal cancer is one of the three most common cancers diagnosed in the United States and includes cancers of the colon and rectum. In 2008, an estimated 148,810 new cases will be diagnosed and an estimated 49,960 deaths will occur making colorectal cancer the second leading cause of cancer-related deaths in the United States.[1] Prognosis is primarily determined by the stage of disease with the majority of patients with early stage (I or II) disease cured. Treatment options for colorectal cancer include surgery, radiation, chemotherapy, and new targeted molecular therapies.

EPIDEMIOLOGY AND ETIOLOGY

Colorectal cancer occurs at a much higher rate in industrialized parts of the world such as North America and Europe, while the lowest rates are seen in less-developed areas suggesting that environmental and dietary factors influence the development of colorectal cancer.[2] In addition to these environmental factors, colorectal cancers are known to develop more frequently in certain families, and genetic predisposition to this cancer is well known.

The incidence of colorectal cancer is greatest among males, who have an approximately 1.5 times greater risk for developing colorectal cancer than women. Overall, colon and rectal cancers make up approximately 10% of all cancer diagnoses in men and women in the United States.[1] The median age at diagnosis is 72 years with very few cases occurring in individuals less than 45 years of age.[3] ❶ *Age appears to be the biggest risk factor for the development of colorectal cancer with 70% of cases diagnosed in adults older than 65 years of age.*

Though still the third leading cause of cancer death, mortality rates for colorectal cancer have declined over the last 30 years as a result of better and increasingly used screening modalities and more effective treatments.

RISK FACTORS

Besides age, the development of colorectal cancer appears to be caused by variety of dietary or environmental factors, inflammatory bowel disease, and genetic susceptibility to the disease. Table 91–1 lists well-known risk factors for developing colorectal cancer. Epidemiologic studies of worldwide incidence of colorectal cancer suggest that dietary habits strongly influence its development.

❷ *High-fat, low-fiber diets, which usually occur in tandem, have been associated with an increased risk of colorectal cancer.* The association between red meat consumption and colorectal cancer is strongest, possibly a result of the heterocyclic amines formed during cooking or the presence of specific fatty acids in red meat such as arachidonic acid. While data indicate that animal meat and saturated fat intake are associated with an increased risk of colorectal cancer, the exact increase in risk is unknown. The evidence for low-fiber diets as a risk factor is based on the ingestion of large amounts of dietary fiber being associated with a small, inconsistent, reduced colorectal cancer risk. Foods that are high in fiber include vegetables, fruit, grains, and cereals. The protective effects of fiber may be a result of reduced absorption of carcinogens in the bowel, reduced bowel transit time, or a reduction in dietary fat intake associated with high fiber diets.[4,5]

The degree of colorectal cancer risk-reduction associated with increased consumption of vegetables and fruit is variable but generally modest and has ranged from no difference to a 25% decrease in cancer risk in prospective studies.[4–6] A

Table 91–1
Risk Factors for Colorectal Cancer
General Age is the primary risk factor **Dietary** High-fat, low-fiber diets **Lifestyle** Alcohol Smoking Obesity/physical inactivity **Comorbid conditions** Inflammatory bowel disease (ulcerative colitis and Crohn's disease) **Hereditary/genetic** FAP and HNPCC Family history

large pooled analysis of 13 prospective cohort studies found dietary fiber intake to be inversely associated with the risk of colorectal cancer; however, upon multivariate analysis for other dietary risk factors, the benefit was no longer seen.[6] This analysis does not account for the known benefits of a fiber-rich diet for noncancerous conditions like diabetes and coronary artery disease.

❷ *The risk of colorectal cancer appears to be inversely related to calcium and folate intake.* Higher intake of calcium and vitamin D has been associated with a reduced risk of colorectal cancer in epidemiologic studies and polyp recurrence in polyp-prevention trials. However, daily supplementation of calcium (1,000 mg) with vitamin D_3 (400 IU) for 7 years had no effect on the incidence of colorectal cancer among postmenopausal women when compared to a placebo group in the randomized trial involving 18,106 females The benefit of calcium and vitamin D on preventing colon cancer may require longer follow-up.[7]

Calcium's protective effect may be related to a reduction in mucosal cell proliferation rates or through its binding to bile salts in the intestine while dietary folate helps maintain normal bowel mucosa. Based on its role in DNA methylation, folate intake has been associated with modifying the risk of colorectal cancer. Epidemilogic evidence suggests that higher intake of folate will decrease the risk for the development of colorectal cancer. However, studies are inconsistent and whether benefit is limited to certain patient populations requires further study. In addition, the timing of folate intake may be important with early intake preventing colorectal cancer and later intake promoting the progression of disease.[8,9] Additional micronutrient deficiencies have been demonstrated through several studies to increase colorectal cancer risk and include selenium, vitamin C, vitamin D, vitamin E, and β-carotene; however, the benefit of dietary supplementation does not appear to be substantial.[10]

Chronic use of several medications has been shown to influence the risk of developing colorectal cancer. ❷ *Studies have consistently demonstrated that regular (at least two doses per week) nonsteroidal anti-inflammatory drug (NSAID) and aspirin use is associated with a reduced risk of colorectal cancer.*[10–12] Additional studies support these findings that regular aspirin or NSAID use may decrease the risk of colorectal cancer by as much as 50%.[11,12] The potential mechanisms by which these agents exert their protective effects appear to be linked primarily to their inhibition of cyclooxygenase-2 (COX-2), and protective effects may be limited to those precancerous lesions that overexpress COX-2.[13] Colorectal cancers with weak or absent expression of COX-2 may not derive the same benefit from long-term COX-2 inhibition.[13] Exogenous hormone use, particularly postmenopausal hormone replacement therapy, is associated with a significant reduction in colorectal cancer risk in most studies with the greatest benefit in women who are on current hormone replacement therapy.[14] Unfortunately, the known risks of hormone replacement therapy outweigh this benefit and routine use of hormone replacement therapy to prevent colorectal cancer is not recommended.

Personal attributes such as physical inactivity and elevated body mass index (BMI) are associated with up to a twofold increase in the risk of colorectal cancer. Decreased bowel transit time and exercise-induced alterations in body glucose, insulin levels, and perhaps other hormones may reduce tumor cell growth.[10,15] Type 2 diabetes mellitus, independent of body mass size and physical activity level, is also associated with an increased risk of colorectal cancer in women and supports a role for hyperinsulinemia as a possible link between obesity, sedentary lifestyle, diabetes mellitus, and colorectal cancer.[15] Additional lifestyle choices that increase the risk of colorectal cancer include alcohol consumption and smoking that may increase the risk of colorectal cancer by generating carcinogens or their direct toxic effects on bowel tissue.[10]

Inflammatory bowel diseases, such as chronic ulcerative colitis, particularly when it involves the entire large intestine, and to lesser extent Crohn's disease, confer increased risk for colorectal cancer. Overall, persons diagnosed with either disease constitute about 1% to 2% of all new cases of colorectal cancer each year.

Finally, as many as 10% of cases are thought to be hereditary, resulting from genetic mutations. The two most common forms of hereditary colorectal cancer are familial adenomatous polyposis (FAP) and hereditary nonpolyposis colorectal cancer (HNPCC).[4] FAP is a rare autosomal dominant trait that is caused by mutations of the **adenomatous polyposis coli (APC)** gene and accounts for 1% of all colorectal cancers. The disease is manifested by hundreds to thousands of **polyps** arising during adolescence.[16] The risk of developing colorectal cancer for individuals with untreated FAP is virtually 100% and patients will require early screening for the disease, and likely prophylactic total colectomy. HNPCC, also an autosomal dominant syndrome, accounts for up to 5% of colorectal cancer cases.[16] In contrast to FAP, juvenile polyps occur rarely and the average age of colorectal cancer in these patients is closer to that of average risk patients, with most patients diagnosed in their forties. Testing for HNPCC mutations is available but reserved for those individuals who meet strict diagnostic criteria.

Up to 25% of patients who develop colorectal cancer will have a family history of colorectal cancer unrelated to a mutation described above. First-degree relatives of patients diagnosed with colorectal cancer have an increased risk of the disease that is at least two to four times that of persons in the general population without a family history.[17]

Summary of Risk Factors

In summary, the true association between most dietary factors and risk of colorectal cancer is unclear. The protective effects of fiber, calcium, and a diet low in fat are not completely known at this time. NSAID use and hormonal use appear to decrease the risk of colorectal cancer while physical inactivity, alcohol use, and smoking appear to increase the risk of colorectal cancer. Clinical risk factors and genetic mutations are well-known risks for colorectal cancer.

SCREENING

❸ *Health care professionals must be aware of and promote appropriate screening recommendations for colorectal cancer in their patients.* Effective screening programs incorporate fecal occult blood tests (FOBTs) and regular examinations. Appropriate screening of patients at normal and high risk for colorectal cancer leads to the detection of smaller, localized lesions and higher cure rates.[18] Screening techniques include a digital rectal exam, FOBTs, and imaging of the colon. The use of FOBTs annually in combination with digital rectal exams has led to earlier diagnosis of early stages of disease and may reduce colorectal cancer mortality by up to one-third.[18] Two main methods are available to detect occult blood in the feces: guaiac dye and immunochemical methods. The Hemoccult II is the most commonly used FOBT in the United States and is a guaiac-based test. Proper counseling by health care providers is required to receive accurate test results. Table 91–2 lists common reasons for inaccurate results with the guaiac tests and requires appropriate

---

Patient Encounter, Part 1

GW is a 61-year-old man who presents to your clinic with a chief complaint of abdominal discomfort and cramping for the last 3 weeks not relieved with over-the-counter medications. While obtaining your medical history, he states that he also has seen small amounts of blood in his stool on and off for 4 months. He has a medical history positive for hypertension and obesity. He states that he has smoked a pack of cigarettes per day for the last 40 years and drinks 4 to 6 beers every couple of days.

What risk factors does GW have for colon cancer?

Does he have clinical symptoms suggestive of colon cancer?

What additional tests need to be ordered to diagnosis colon cancer?

Table 91–2	
Common Reasons for Inaccurate Results from Guaiac Stool Tests	
False Positives	**False Negatives**
Red meat, blood soup, blood sausage[a]	Vitamin C[a]
Vegetables with peroxidase activity[a]	Dehydrated samples
Iron[a]	
Gastric irritation (NSAIDs)[a]	

[a]Avoid these foods and medications for 3 days prior to test.

Table 91–3	
Colon Cancer Screening Guidelines	
Average risk	Annual DRE after age 50 *and*
	Annual FOBT or FIT after age 50, at the time of DRE. Stool DNA testing may be used as an alternative *and*
	One of the following after age 50:
	Sigmoidoscopy every 5 years
	Colonoscopy every 10 years
	Barium enema every 5 years
	CTC every 5 years
Family history	Screening at ages 35–40
HNPCC	Screening at age 30
FAP	Screening at ages 10–12

FIT, fecal immunochemical tests; FOBT, fecal occult blood tests; CTC, computed tomographic colonography; DRE, digital rectal examination.

counseling on the use of these tests. Fecal immunochemical tests (FIT) (InSure, and others), which use antibodies to detect hemoglobin, are also available for use. One advantage of immunochemical tests is that they do not react with dietary factors or medications. Both FOBTs can be recommended in screening protocols for patients.

In addition, imaging of the colon with a sigmoidoscopy, colonoscopy, or double-contrast barium enema is required every 5 to 10 years in most individuals. Colonoscopy is the preferred procedure as it allows for greater visualization of the entire colon and simultaneous removal of lesions found during screening.[18] A sigmoidoscopy only examines the lower half of the colon, and a double-contrast barium enema requires a supplemental colonoscopy to remove any lesions found during the screening process. Several revisions to the colorectal cancer screening guidelines have been made in an attempt to increase the compliance to screening guidelines. These include the use of computed tomographic colonography (CTC) and stool DNA testing as acceptable screening methods. CTC, also known as "virtual colonoscopy," uses integrated 3D and 2D images to detect and characterize polyps. Although noninvasive compared to colonoscopy, adequate bowel preparation, which is often cited as the reason for noncompliance, is still required. In addition, any lesions found on examination require a follow-up colonoscopy.

Stool DNA testing detects molecular markers associated with advanced colorectal cancer. Because this test is not dependent on the detection of bleeding, which can be sporadic, it requires only a single stool collection. How often and what molecular markers to test for are undergoing further evaluation. ❸ *Table 91–3 is a summary of the current American Cancer Society guidelines for screening and surveillance for early detection of colorectal polyps and cancer.*[18]

COLORECTAL CANCER PREVENTION

Strategies to prevent colorectal cancer can be done with pharmacologic or surgical interventions and involve either preventing the initial development of colorectal cancer (primary prevention) or preventing cancer in patients that demonstrate early signs of colorectal cancer (secondary prevention).

The most widely studied agents for the chemoprevention of colorectal cancer are agents that inhibit COX-2 (aspirin, NSAIDs, and selective COX-2 inhibitors) and calcium

supplementation.[19] COX-2 appears to play a role in polyp formation and COX-2 inhibition suppresses polyp growth. In 1999, the FDA approved the use of celecoxib to reduce the number of colorectal polyps in patients with FAP, as an adjunct to usual care. This may delay the need for surgical intervention in these patients but the results cannot be extrapolated to the general population. The dose of celecoxib for this indication is 400 mg orally twice daily and the risk of cardiovascular damage from COX-2 inhibition needs to be assessed carefully in these patients. The use of aspirin as both a primary and secondary chemoprevention agent has also been studied. In a prospective, randomized trial, low-dose (81 mg/day) aspirin was shown to decrease the incidence of additional polyps by 19% in patients with a previous history of at least one polyp.[20]

Calcium supplementation appears to be associated with a moderate reduction in risk of recurrent colorectal adenomas with prospective studies demonstrating a nonstatistical decrease in adenoma recurrence and its role as a chemoprevention agent remains under investigation.[19]

Additional agents including selenium, folic acid, and HMG-CoA reductase inhibitors (statins) show promise as chemopreventive agents in colorectal cancer and preliminary and confirmatory studies evaluating their effectiveness have been completed or are ongoing.[19]

Surgical resection remains an option to prevent colorectal cancer in individuals at extremely high risk for its development such as patients diagnosed with FAP. Individuals with FAP who are found to have polyps on screening examinations require total abdominal colectomy. In addition, removal of noncancerous polyps detected during screening colonoscopy is considered standard of care to prevent the progression of premalignant polyps to cancer.

PATHOPHYSIOLOGY

Anatomy and Bowel Function

The large intestine consists of the cecum; ascending, transverse, descending, and sigmoid colon; and the rectum

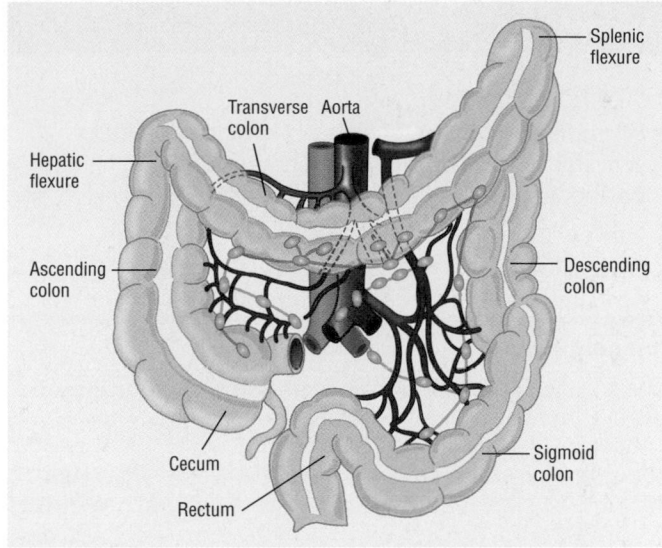

FIGURE 91–1. Colon and rectum anatomy. (From DiPiro JT, Talbert RL, Yee GC, et al., eds. Pharmacotherapy: A Patholphysiologic Approach, 6th ed. New York: McGraw-Hill, 2005; Fig. 127–2.)

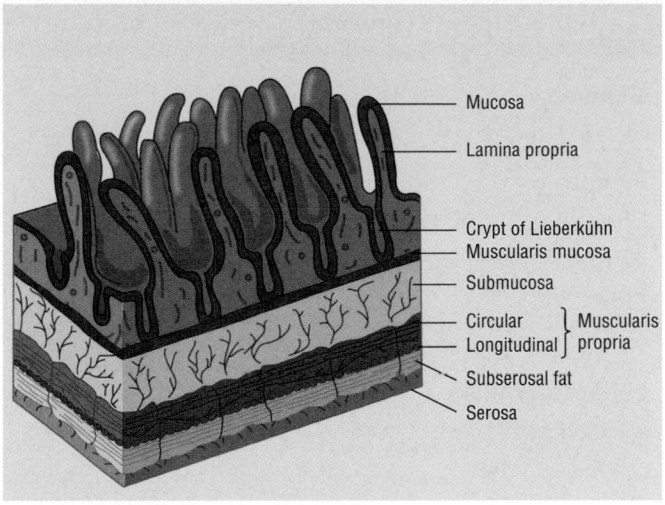

FIGURE 91–2. Cross-section of bowel wall. (From DiPiro JT, Talbert RL, Yee GC, et al., eds. Pharmacotherapy: A Patholphysiologic Approach, 6th ed. New York: McGraw-Hill, 2005; Fig. 127–3.)

(Fig. 91–1). The function of the large intestine is to receive contents from the ileum, absorb water, and package solid waste for excretion. Absorption of materials occurs in segments of the colon proximal to the middle of the transverse colon, with movement and storage of fecal material in the left colon and distal segments of the colon.

Four major tissue layers, from the lumen outward, form the large intestine: the mucosa, submucosa, muscularis externa, and serosa (Fig. 91–2). Complete replacement of surface epithelial cells occurs every 7 to 10 days with the total number of epithelial cells remaining constant in normal colonic tissue. As patients age, abnormal cells accumulate on the surface epithelium and protrude into the stream of fecal matter, their contact with fecal mutagens can lead to further cell mutations and eventual adenoma formation.[16]

Colorectal Tumorigenesis

The development of a colorectal neoplasm is a multistep process of several genetic and phenotypic alterations of normal bowel epithelium leading to unregulated cell growth, proliferation, and tumor development. A genetic model has been proposed for colorectal tumorigenesis that describes a process of transformation from adenoma to carcinoma. This model of tumor development reflects an accumulation of mutations within colonic epithelium that give a selective growth advantage to the cancer cells.[16] Genetic changes include activating mutations of oncogenes, mutations of tumor suppressor genes, and defects in DNA mismatch repair genes.

Additional genes and protein receptors are believed important in colorectal tumorigenesis. COX-2, which is induced in colorectal cancer cells, influences apoptosis and other cellular functions in colon cells, and overexpression of the epidermal growth factor receptor (EGFR), a transmembrane glycoprotein involved in signaling pathways that affect cell growth, differentiation, proliferation, and angiogenesis, occurs in the majority of colon cancers.[11,21] These mechanisms are potentially important because of the availability of pharmacologic agents targeted to inhibit these processes.

Over 90% of colorectal cancers that develop are adenocarcinomas and are assigned a grade of I to III based on how similar they are compared to normal colorectal cells. Grade I tumors most closely resemble normal cellular structure, whereas grade III tumors have frequently lost the characteristics of mature normal cells. Grade III tumors are associated with a worse prognosis than grade I turmors.[22]

CLINICAL PRESENTATION AND DIAGNOSIS

❹ *The signs and symptoms associated with colorectal cancer can be extremely varied, subtle, and nonspecific. Most patients are asymptomatic but may develop changes in bowel or eating habits, fatigue, abdominal pain, and blood in the stool.*

TREATMENT

Desired Outcome

Staging is required to determine the extent of disease and is necessary in developing patient treatment options and determining patient prognosis. The tumor-node-metastasis (TNM) classification system that takes into account T (tumor size and depth of tumor invasion), N (lymph node involvement), M (presence or absence of metastases) is used to stage patients from stage I to stage IV. CT scans and appropriate assessment of lymph node involvment during surgical

Clinical Presentation and Diagnosis of Colorectal Cancer

General

Patients are often asymptomatic in early stages of disease

Symptoms

Changes in bowel habits, abdominal pain, anorexia, nausea and vomiting, weakness (if anemia is severe), and tenesmus

Signs

Blood in stool and weight loss

Laboratory Tests

- Patients may have a low hemoglobin level from blood loss

- Positive FOBT
- Liver function tests (International Normalization Ratio, activated partial thromboplastin time, and bilirubin) may be abnormal if disease has metastasized to the liver.
- Carcinoembryonic antigen (CEA) level may be high. Normal level is less than 2.5 ng/mL (2.5 mcg/L) in nonsmokers and less than 5 ng/mL (5 mcg/L) in smokers

Imaging Tests

Chest x-ray, CT scan, or **position-emission tomography (PET)** scan may be positive if cancer has spread to the lungs, liver, or peritoneal cavity

Patient Encounter, Part 2: Medical History, Physical Examination, and Diagnostic Tests

PMH: Hypertension since age 47, which is not well controlled; obesity; the patient is 65% over his ideal body weight

FH: Mother and father both dead. Father died of a myocardial infarction at age 62; mother died of colon cancer at age 64. Patient states that "many" relatives have cancer in his family

SH: Works as an auto mechanic. Drinks alcohol frequently, and smokes a pack of cigarettes daily. Patient also does no exercise and states that he eats fast food daily. He is married with twin boys aged 29

Meds: Atenolol 50 mg orally once daily

ROS: (+) Abdominal cramping, mild nausea and loss of appetite, blood in stool, and fatigue

PE:

VS: 153/90 mm Hg, P 78, RR 16, T 37.2°C (99°F), ht 183 cm (72 in.), wt 128 kg (282 lb)

Abd: Distended and tender to touch, (+) bowel sounds, and heme (+) stools

Labs: Positive hemoglobin 11.3 g/dL (113 g/L or 7 mmol/L) (decreased from 14.8 g/dL [148 g/L or 9.2 mmol/L] last year)

Imaging and Diagnostic Studies

- Colonoscopy revealed multiple polyps in his transverse colon.
- Biopsy revealed three polyps positive for adenocarcinoma of the colon.
- Staging CT scan revealed metastatic disease in the liver, lung, and bone.
- All other findings negative.

Because GW has stage IV colon cancer, how does this affect your treatment plan compared with stage I–III disease?

What is your treatment goal for him?

What nonpharmacologic and pharmacologic options are available to GW?

resection are essential in determining the stage of disease and subsequent treatment options. At this time, routine MRI and PET scans for initial staging are not recommended. Figure 91–3 depicts how the three categories are used in combination to determine the stage of disease. ❺ *The stage of colorectal cancer upon diagnosis is the most important prognostic factor for survival and disease recurrence. Stages I, II, and III disease are considered potentially curable and are aggressively treated in an attempt to cure these patients. Patients who develop stage IV disease are treated to reduce symptoms, avoid disease-related complications, and prolong survival.*

General Approach to Treatment

● The treatment approaches for colorectal cancer reflect two primary treatment goals: curative therapy for localized disease (stages I to III) and palliative therapy for metastatic cancer (stage IV). Surgical resection of the primary tumor is the most important part of therapy for patients in whom cure is possible.[23] Depending on the stage of disease and whether the tumor originated in the colon or rectum, further **adjuvant** chemotherapy or chemotherapy plus radiation may be needed after surgery to cure these patients. In the metastatic setting, pharmacologic intervention is the main treatment option.

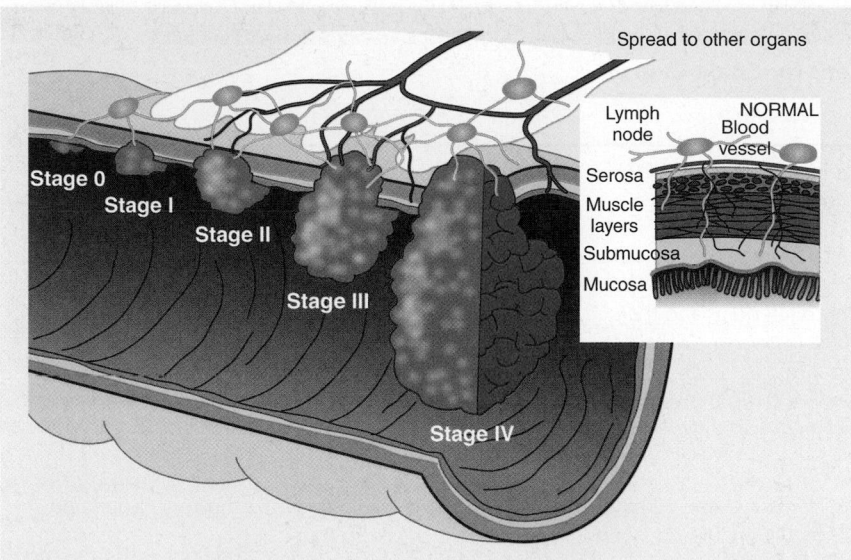

FIGURE 91–3. Stage I: Cancer is confined to the lining of the colon. Stage II: Cancer may penetrate the wall of the colon into the abdominal cavity but does not invade any local lymph nodes. Stage III: Cancer invades one or more lymph nodes but has not spread to distant organs. Stage IV: Cancer has spread to distant locations in the body, which may include the liver, lungs, or other sites. (From *http://www.cancer.gov/cancertopics/pdq/treatment/colon/Patient/page2.*)

Nonpharmacologic Therapy

▶ Operable Disease (Stages I–III)

Surgery Individuals with stage I to III colorectal cancer should undergo a complete surgical resection of the tumor mass with removal of regional lymph nodes as a curative approach for their disease.[23] Surgery for rectal cancer depends on the region of tumor involvement with attempts to retain rectal function as a goal of the surgical procedure. Overall, surgery for colorectal cancer is associated with a low morbidity and mortality rate. Common complications associated with colorectal surgery include infection, anastomotic leakage, obstruction, adhesion formation, and malabsorption syndromes.

Radiation Therapy There is currently no role for adjuvant radiation in colon cancer. However, patients who receive surgery for rectal cancer receive radiation therapy to reduce local tumor recurrence. Adjuvant radiation plus chemotherapy is considered standard treatment for patients with stage II or III rectal cancer after the surgical procedure is complete.[24] Preoperative radiation may be used to reduce the initial size of rectal cancers in order to make the surgical procedure easier.

▶ Metastatic Disease (Stage IV)

Surgery Unlike stages I to III disease, the benefit of surgical resection in most patients with metastatic disease is limited to symptomatic improvement. Select patients who have from one to three small nodules isolated to the liver, lungs, or abdomen may have a prolongation of survival, though cure is rare. Five-year survival for patients who undergo surgical resection of metastases isolated to the liver is approximately double that of patients who are not surgical candidates with approximately 33% of patients alive at 5 years.[25] Alternatives to surgery include destroying the tumor through freezing and thawing (cryoablation), heat (radiofrequency), or alcohol injection though these appear to be less successful than

surgical resection.[23,25] Because the majority of these patients will relapse, many practitioners offer adjuvant chemotherapy to select patients following potentially curative resection, but further studies are needed to determine an optimal treatment regimen.[25] Additionally, **neoadjuvant** approaches to patients with isolated hepatic lesions will be discussed later in the chapter.

Radiation Symptom reduction is the primary goal of radiation for patients with advanced or metastatic colorectal cancer.

Pharmacologic Therapy

Table 91–4 lists common chemotherapy regimens used in colorectal cancer, and the abbreviations used in the literature to describe them.

▶ Operable Disease (Stage I–III)

❻ *Adjuvant chemotherapy is administered after tumor resection to decrease relapse rates and improve survival in patients with colon cancer by eliminating micrometastatic disease that is undetected on imaging studies. Patients diagnosed with stage I colon or rectal cancer are usually cured by surgical resection, and adjuvant chemotherapy is not indicated in these patients.*[23] *The role of adjuvant chemotherapy for stage II colon cancer is controversial but may benefit certain high-risk groups.* Table 91–5 lists adjuvant treatment regimens based on stage and performance status. Adjuvant chemotherapy for patients with stage II disease has not been shown to be superior to surgery alone with the exception of high-risk patients. High-risk patients that may benefit include those with inadequate nodes sampled for staging, bowel perforation upon diagnosis, T4 lesions, and those with unfavorable histology. The use of tumor gene profiling may predict patients with stage II disease that would benefit from adjuvant chemotherapy but requires further validation in prospective trials.[26] Consequently, the American Society of Clinical Oncology

Table 91–4	
Dosing Schedules of Chemotherapy Regimens for Colon Cancer[a]	
Regimen	**Dosing**
5-Fluorouracil	300 mg/m^2/day IV bolus or 250–1,000 mg/m^2/day IV over 24 hours × 5 days
5-Fluorouracil + leucovorin (bolus)	Leucovorin 500 mg/m^2 IV 5-Fluorouracil 500 mg/m^2 IV Every week × 6 weeks, followed by 2-week rest
5-Fluorouracil + leucovorin (continuous infusion)	Leucovorin 200 mg/m^2 IV 5-Fluorouracil 400 mg/m^2 IV bolus and then 600 mg/m^2 of 5-fluorouracil as a 22-hour continuous infusion On days 1 and 2; repeat every 2 weeks
FOLFIRI	Irinotecan 180 mg/m^2 IV day 1 Folinic acid (leucovorin) 400 mg/m^2 IV day 1 5-Fluorouracil 400–500 mg/m^2 IV bolus, after folinic acid; then 2,400–3,000 mg/m^2 of 5-fluorouracil IV over 46 hours Repeat every 14 days
FOLFOX4	Oxaliplatin 85 mg/m^2 IV + leucovorin 200 mg/m^2 IV, followed by 5-fluorouracil 400 mg/m^2 IV bolus and then 5-fluorouracil 600 mg/m^2 IV over 22 hours day 1 Leucovorin 200 mg/m^2, followed by 5-fluorouracil 400 mg/m^2 IV bolus and then 5-fluorouracil 600 mg/m^2 IV over 22 hours day 2 Repeat every 2 weeks
Bevacizumab + 5-fluorouracil regimen	Bevacizumab 5 mg/kg every 2 weeks + a 5-Fluorouracil containing regimen (FOLFOX, FOLFIRI, or 5-fluorouracil + leucovorin) Bevacizumab 7.5 mg/kg every 3 weeks with CAPOX
Cetuximab ± irinotecan	Cetuximab 400 mg/m^2 first infusion, then 250 mg/m^2 weekly ± irinotecan 125 mg/m^2 every week for 4 weeks Repeat irinotecan every 6 weeks (after a 2-week break)
Panitumumab	6 mg/kg every 2 weeks
Capecitabine	1,250 mg/m^2 twice a day orally for 14 days Repeat every 3 weeks
CAPOX	Capecitabine 1,000 mg/m^2 twice a day orally for 14 days Oxaliplatin 130 mg/m^2 IV on day 1 Repeat every 3 weeks
CAPIRI	Capecitabine 1,000 mg/m^2 twice a day for 14 days Irinotecan 100 mg/m^2 IV days 1 and 8 Repeat every 22 days

CAPIRI, capecitabine and irinotecan; CAPOX, capecitabine and oxaliplatin.

[a]Note that many variations exist, and current literature should be checked prior to administering any chemotherapy regimen.

does not recommend the routine use of adjuvant chemotherapy in the general patient population unless part of a clinical trial.[27] Patients with stage II colon cancer should be enrolled into carefully controlled clinical trials to assess the impact of new agents and prognostic models. ❻ *Adjuvant chemotherapy is standard therapy for patients with stage III colon cancer.* The presence of lymph node involvement in the resected specimen places patients with stage III colon cancer at high risk for relapse; the risk of death within 5 years of surgical resection alone is as high as 70%.[23] In this population of patients, adjuvant chemotherapy significantly decreases risk of cancer recurrence and death and is considered standard of care.

❼ *5-Fluorouracil, leucovorin, and oxaliplatin (FOLFOX)-based chemotherapy is the standard regimen used in adjuvant colon cancer. It is usually given for 6 months.* 5-Fluorouracil alone results in a small improvement in survival that can vary based on the method of 5-fluorouracil administration.

Table 91–5	
Treatment Regimens for Adjuvant Colon Cancer	
Stage II[a]	**Stage III**
High Risk • FOLFOX • Capecitabine or 5-fluorouracil plus leucovorin	**Good Performance Status** • FOLFOX • Capecitabine or 5-fluorouracil plus leucovorin
Low Risk[b] • Observation or clinical trial	**Poor Performance Status** • Capecitabine

[a]Individualized assessment of patient risk is necessary to determine if treatment is required. Clinical trials or observation may be an appropriate option.

[b]T3 lesions may be considered high risk by some clinicians.

Studies suggest that continuous IV 5-fluorouracil infusion treatment schedules are more effective as adjuvant therapy.[28]

More often, 5-fluorouracil is administered as part of a combination regimen. The most frequently used combination is that of 5-fluorouracil, oxaliplatin, and leucovorin. The combination of 5-fluorouracil plus leucovorin has undergone extensive study in the adjuvant setting with decreased rates of recurrence and improved survival seen in patients receiving 5-fluorouracil plus leucovorin compared to surgery alone. A pooled analysis demonstrated that 5-year disease-free survival and overall survival were increased by 12% and 7% with adjuvant 5-fluorouracil-based chemotherapy, respectively.[29] 5-Fluorouracil and leucovorin can be administered in a variety of treatment schedules, but none has proven superior with regard to overall patient survival. In the past, the United States has favored bolus regimens based on patient convenience. However, improved availability and comfort in use of portable infusion pumps has led to an increase in use of the continuous IV schedule of 5-fluorouracil commonly advocated in Europe. Patients are treated with 6 months of adjuvant therapy. Longer regimens do not improve patient outcomes. No standard exists for the best schedule of 5-fluorouracil and leucovorin administration, though continuous infusions may be less toxic and have improved response rates (though no survival advantage) when compared to bolus regimens.

Oxaliplatin added to the combination of 5-fluorouracil and leucovorin has further improved response rates in the adjuvant setting. The MOSAIC trial, conducted in over 2,200 patients, demonstrated that the addition of oxaliplatin to 5-fluorouracil and leucovorin decreases disease recurrence and improves disease-free and overall survival in patients with stage III disease.[30] These results led to the approval of the FOLFOX4 regimen, given for 6 months, for the adjuvant treatment of colon cancer. This regimen is considered standard of care for patients with stage III disease unless their performance status is so poor that clinicians do not feel they could tolerate intensive combination therapy. Age alone should not determine whether patients receive combination adjuvant therapy or not as elderly patients have been found to equally benefit from this approach with minimal addition of adverse effects.[31] Every effort should be made to minimize adverse treatment effects and utilize this regimen in patients with stage III colon cancer as this is the only regimen demonstrated to improve overall survival in these patients.[30,31]

Capecitabine is an oral prodrug of 5-fluorouracil that is also effective in the adjuvant setting and is being evaluated as a replacement for 5-fluorouracil for patient convenience and possible economic and safety reasons. Data suggest that capecitabine is at least equivalent to bolus 5-fluorouracil and leucovorin in efficacy and is better tolerated by patients.[32] An increase in hand-foot syndrome and decreased mucositis and neutropenia are seen with capecitabine when compared to bolus 5-fluorouracil. Consequently, most practitioners feel that capecitabine is an acceptable alternative to IV 5-fluorouracil plus leucovorin. However, the role of capecitabine with additional chemotherapy agents such as oxaliplatin or compared to the more common infusional 5-fluorouracil requires further study in the adjuvant setting.

▶ Metastatic Disease (Stage IV)

Traditional chemotherapy and targeted biological therapies are the mainstay of treatment for metastatic colon or rectal cancer and have improved the median survival of these patients to over 20 months.[33] Most often, a combination of chemotherapy agents with biological therapies is administered to these patients. Currently, metastatic colorectal cancer is incurable and treatment goals are to reduce patients' symptoms, improve quality of life, and extend survival. Combination chemotherapy regimens have been demonstrated to result in prolongation of survival with tolerable adverse effects. Similar to the adjuvant setting, 5-fluorouracil plus leucovorin continues to be in most first-line chemotherapy regimens used for metastatic colorectal cancer. A variety of continuous IV infusion 5-fluorouracil and bolus regimens can be used; however, in comparison to IV bolus 5-fluorouracil, response rates with continuous infusion 5-fluorouracil are approximately doubled. In a meta-analysis of six randomized trials evaluating over 1,200 patients with advanced colorectal cancer, continuous infusions of 5-fluorouracil had a significantly higher tumor response rate, a small increase in survival, and lower incidence of myelosuppression, diarrhea, and mucositis when compared to bolus regimens.[33,34]

Additional agents have been added to the 5-fluorouracil and leucovorin regimen with superior response and survival rates compared to the two drugs used alone. The addition of irinotecan to 5-fluorouracil plus leucovorin (IFL) significantly improves response rates and survival, without adversely affecting quality of life. In a landmark trial, this regimen was superior to 5-fluorouracil plus leucovorin with regard to tumor response, survival, and quality of life.[35] As a result, irinotecan received approval from the FDA in 2000 as first-line therapy for metastatic colorectal cancer in combination with 5-fluorouracil and leucovorin. Soon thereafter, oxaliplatin in combination with 5-fluorouracil and leucovorin (FOLFOX4) demonstrated improvement in median survival when compared to the IFL regimen described above. A comparison of oxaliplatin plus 5-fluorouracil and leucovorin (FOLFOX4) to weekly IFL showed superior efficacy with FOLFOX4 compared to IFL with regard to response rates and survival.[36] Several study design questions including the crossover design and differing methods of 5-fluorouracil administration led several practitioners to debate the significance of these results. Patients on the IFL arm received weekly IV bolus 5-fluorouracil, while FOLFOX4 patients received 5-fluorouracil as IV bolus followed by continuous infusion IV, which is thought to increase response rates. A larger European study validated these concerns when it compared a combined bolus and infusional 5-fluorouracil regimen plus irinotecan (FOLFIRI) to the FOLFOX regimen (using a slightly different schedule) with crossover to the opposite arm upon relapse.[37] No difference in patient survival was seen with either regimen and toxicity was as expected. Neuropathy and neutropenia were more common with FOLFOX and diarrhea, nausea, vomiting, dehydration, and febrile neutropenia were more common with FOLFIRI. Based on improved survival data with the FOLFOX and FOLFIRI regimens, irinotecan administered in a bolus fashion, as described in the IFL regimens, is no longer recommended for routine use. When irinotecan-based combination chemotherapy is to be given for the metastatic treatment of colon cancer, it should be as FOLFIRI described in Table 91–4.

Targeted or biologic agents have been approved for use in metastatic colorectal cancer. Bevacizumab, in combination with IV 5-fluorouracil-based chemotherapy, is approved by the FDA for initial treatment of patients with metastatic colorectal cancer. Results from randomized trials show increased benefit compared to chemotherapy alone. One phase III trial of bevacizumab in combination with IFL as first-line therapy in patients with metastatic colorectal cancer has also been completed with a 5-month increase in median survival seen with the addition of bevacizumab with manageable adverse effects.[38] The results of this study show the relevance of **angiogenesis** as an important target for the treatment of metastatic colorectal cancer. Similar to when used without bevacizumab, FOLFIRI is superior to IFL in combination with bevacizumab. Survival was improved by approximately 9 months with FOLFIRI plus bevacizumab compared to IFL plus bevacizumab.[39]

The addition of bevacizumab when added to first-line oxaliplatin-based chemotherapy has also been demonstrated to improve progression-free survival but did not positively impact response rates or overall survival.[40] Based on these results, bevacizumab is recommended as part of all 5-fluorouracil-based chemotherapy regimens used for the first-line treatment of metastatic colorectal cancer unless contraindicated. Bevacizumab should not be used in patients who present with or develop the following conditions until they are stabilized or treated, including patients with GI perforation or fistulas involving a major organ, recent (within 28 days) major surgeries or open wounds, wound dehiscence requiring medical intervention, hypertensive crisis or uncontrolled severe hypertension, hypertensive encephalopathy—serious bleeding, a severe arterial thromboembolic event, moderate or severe proteinuria (2 g or higher of proteinuria/24 hours); nephrotic syndrome, and reversible posterior leukoencephalopathy syndrome.

❽ *In summary, most practitioners select first-line treatment for metastatic colorectal cancer from among these currently approved, triple-drug treatments: oxaliplatin plus 5-fluorouracil plus leucovorin (FOLFOX); irinotecan plus 5-fluorouracil plus leucovorin (FOLFIRI); bevacizumab plus 5-fluorouracil-based chemotherapy (FOLFIRI or FOLFOX).*[41]

The routine replacement of 5-fluorouracil with capecitabine in biologic combination regimens should not be recommended outside of controlled clinical trials. In one phase III trial, capecitabine in combination with irinotecan and bevacizumab was inferior to FOLFIRI plus bevacizumab with no improvement in safety.[39] This inferiority with capecitabine may be specific to its use with irinotecan. When given in combination with oxaliplatin and bevacizumab as the (CAPOX) regimen, improvements in disease control were demonstrated. Based on these results, CAPOX is an acceptable alternative to FOLFOX in most instances; both regimens can be given with or without bevacizumab.[41]

5-Fluorouracil plus leucovorin or capecitabine alone is appropriate first-line treatment only for those individuals for whom three-drug combination regimens are believed too toxic. The site(s) of tumor involvement, history of prior chemotherapy, and patient-specific factors help define the appropriate management strategy. The most important factor in patient survival is not the initial regimen but whether or not patients receive all three active chemotherapy drugs (5-fluorouracil, irinotecan, and oxaliplatin) at some point in their treatment course.[42]

▶ Second-Line Therapy

❾ *Treatment of relapsed or refractory metastatic disease uses agents not given in the first-line setting.* Because most patients will have received a combination of 5-fluorouracil with either irinotecan or oxaliplatin, second-line therapy with the alternate regimen should be considered.[41] If targeted agents such as bevacizumab were not part of the initial regimen, addition to the second-line regimen should be strongly considered.

An additional option includes the use of cetuximab either alone or in combination with irinotecan-based chemotherapy.[41,43] Cetuximab is FDA approved for use in EGFR expressing metastatic colorectal cancer in combination with irinotecan but can be used as a single agent in patients who cannot tolerate irinotecan-based chemotherapy. The results appear to be best when irinotecan is continued due to synergy demonstrated between the two agents.[41,43]

Recent evidence suggests that cetaximab is only effective in *KRAS* wild-type colon tumors. All patients who are candidates for cetuximab should have their tumor tested for *KRAS* mutations, and cetuximab should only be used in those without mutations.

Cetuximab is given as at loading dose of 400 mg/m^2 IV followed by weekly infusions of 250 mg/m^2 IV until disease progression. The incidence of grade 3 or 4 adverse effects was as anticipated based on previous trials; asthenia and rash occurred most commonly with cetuximab alone. The benefit of adding cetuximab to oxaliplatin-based regimens or as part of initial therapy for metastatic colorectal cancer is an area of active investigation. Initial data suggest that cetuximab adds to the response rates in both of these settings and supports its use as initial therapy of metastatic colorectal cancer.[41] However, no direct comparison can be made to bevacizumab-based regimens, and cetuximab should be reserved for relapsed patients or in those for whom bevacizumab is contraindicated.[41] Immunohistochemical (IHC) evidence of EGFR-positive staining in tumors is recommended in the product labeling, though the clinical activity has been seen in EGFR-negative tumors and EGFR status as determined by IHC should not limit its use.[41]

▶ Salvage Therapy

Third-line options for patients with metastatic colorectal cancer are limited. Panitumumab, another EGFR inhibitor, is approved for patients who have progressed after 5-fluorouracil, oxaliplatin, and irinotecan. Compared to best supportive care, it was demonstrated to improved disease progression.[41,44] Like cetuximab, panitumomab should only be used in patients without a *KRAS* mutation. Use in combination with chemotherapy or other biologics is not currently recommended.

Patients who fail standard treatment for metastatic colorectal cancer should be encouraged to participate in a clinical trial evaluating new treatment approaches for this incurable disease. Table 91–6 lists treatment options for first- and second-line treatment of metastatic colorectal cancer. Patients with good performance status are treated more aggressively than those with poor performance status because of their ability to better tolerate chemotherapy.

▶ Metastatic Patients With Isolated Hepatic Metastasis

Patients with metastatic lesions in the liver that remain unresectable have a poor outcome with limited chance for long-term survival. One approach to treating these patients is to resect the lesion and then give adjuvant chemotherapy. Unfortunately, the majority of patients with hepatic lesions are unresectable at diagnosis. For these patients, neoadjuvant chemotherapy should be considered in attempt to convert their tumors unresectable to resectable.[41]

FOLFOX and FOLFIRI have both been demonstrated to allow for an increase in surgical resection and increase the potential for long-term survival.[41] Recent studies have added bevacizumab to combination chemotherapy regimens with success. No more than 8 to 10 weeks of chemotherapy should be given to avoid liver complications associated with it, and health care practitioners should take precautions to ensure that bevacizumab is not given within 6 weeks of surgery in this setting.[41,45]

Hepatic arterial infusion pumps have been used in the setting of isolated liver metastases, but this practice has fallen out of favor given improvements in local therapy such as radiofrequency ablation, cryoablation, and chemoembolization.

SPECIFIC AGENTS USED IN COLORECTAL CANCER

Table 91–7 lists all FDA-approved drugs used in colorectal cancer along with their mechanism of action and common toxicities.

5-Fluorouracil

5-Fluorouracil acts as a "false" pyrimidine inhibiting the formation of the DNA base thymidine.[23,44] The main mechanism by which it accomplishes this is by inhibiting the enzyme thymidylate synthase, the rate-limiting step in thymidine formation. 5-Fluorouracil must first be metabolized to its active metabolite (F-dUMP). Additionally, metabolites of 5-fluorouracil may incorporate into RNA inhibiting its synthesis.

5-Fluorouracil is commonly used in the adjuvant and metastatic treatment of colon and rectal cancers. Various dosing administration techniques and schedules have been developed with 5-fluorouracil including IV bolus every 3 to 4 weeks, IV continuous infusion, weekly IV boluses and IV boluses, followed by continuous infusions of 5-fluorouracil. Clinical studies comparing efficacy of bolus and continuous infusion schedules generally favor continuous infusion of 5-fluorouracil. This is consistent with evidence that suggests that the duration of infusion may be an important determinant of the biologic activity of 5-fluorouracil, particularly because of its short plasma half-life, S-phase specificity, and relatively slow growth of colon tumors.[23,33,44]

Clinical significant differences in toxicity also differ based on the dose, route, and schedule of 5-fluorouracil administration. Leukopenia and mucositis are the primary dose-limiting toxicities of bolus 5-fluorouracil, whereas palmar-plantar erythrodysesthesia ("hand-foot syndrome") and diarrhea occur most frequently with continuous infusions of 5-fluorouracil.[23,33,34] Health care practitioners can offer valuable patient advice to decrease the impact of these

---

Patient Encounter, Part 3: Creating a Care Plan

Based on the information presented, create a care plan for this patient's colon cancer. Your plan should include:

(a) the patient's drug- and nondrug-related needs and problems,

(b) the goals of therapy,

(c) a treatment plan specific to GW that includes strategies to prevent adverse effects of chemotherapy,

(d) a follow-up plan to determine whether the goals have been achieved and the adverse effects of chemotherapy have been minimized, and (e) a plan for treatment options when the initial therapy is no longer achieving the goals of therapy.

Table 91–6

Treatment Options for Metastatic Colon Cancer[a]

First-Line Therapy	Second-Line Therapy
Good Performance Status	**If First-Line Irinotecan**
• FOLFOX with or without bevacizumab	• FOLFOX with or without bevacizumab[b]
• FOLFIRI with or without bevacizumab	• Irinotecan with or without cetuximab
• 5-Fluorouracil + leucovorin with bevacizumab	• Capecitabine or 5-fluorouracil plus leucovorin
Poor Performance Status	**If First-Line Oxaliplatin**
• Capecitabine or 5-fluorouracil plus leucovorin with or without bevacizumab	• FOLFIRI with or without bevacizumab[b]
	• Irinotecan with or without cetuximab

[a]CAPOX may replace FOLFOX in selected patients.

[b]Bevacizumab may be given if not part of the first-line therapy.

Table 91–7

FDA-Approved Drugs Used in Colon Cancer

Generic Name (Trade Name)	Mechanism of Action	Common Toxicities	Dosing Adjustments for Renal or Hepatic Dysfunction or Pharmacogenetic Considerations
5-Fluorouracil	Inhibition of the enzyme thymidylate synthase, the rate-limiting step in thymidine formation	*Dose-limiting:* Myelosuppression and mucositis with bolus administration Diarrhea and hand-foot syndrome with continuous infusion *Additional toxicities:* Skin discoloration, nail changes, photosensitivity, and neurologic toxicity	Do not give if bilirubin greater than 5 mg/dL (86 μmol/L)
Capecitabine (Xeloda)	Orally active prodrug of 5-fluorouracil. Once activated, the mechanism of action is the same	Similar to continuous infusion 5-fluorouracil	CrCl 30–50 mL/min decrease starting dose to 75% of the original dose Do not give if CrCl less than 30 mL/min
Irinotecan (Camptosar)	Topoisomerase inhibitor that forms a complex with the covalently bound DNA topoisomerase enzyme and interferes with the DNA breakage-resealing process	*Dose-limiting:* Early and late diarrhea *Additional toxicities:* Neutropenia, nausea, and vomiting	Decrease dose one level in patients with a homozygous UGT1A1*28 allele. This decreases the hepatic metabolism of irinotecan and increases the toxicity
Oxaliplatin (Eloxatin)	Similar to other platinum analogs (cisplatin) in that it binds to the N-7 position of guanine, which results in cross-linking of DNA and double-stranded DNA breaks	*Dose-limiting:* Acute (within first 2 days) and persistent (greater than 14 days) neuropathies *Additional toxicites:* Anaphylactic-like reactions, dyspnea, nausea, vomiting	No formal dose adjustment though use with caution in patients with mild to moderate renal dysfunction
Bevacizumab (Avastin)	Monoclonal antibody that binds to VEGF and inhibits angiogenesis	*Dose-limiting:* Hypertension, bleeding episodes, thrombotic events *Additional toxicities:* Rare perforation of the bowel, proteinurea	None
Cetuximab (Erbitux)	Binds to the cell surface EGFR, preventing EGF and TGF-*a* binding. This decreased cell proliferation of cancer cells	*Dose-limiting:* Infusion-related reactions, acneiform skin rash *Additional toxicities:* Diarrhea, hypomagnesemia, hypocalcemia, interstitial lung disease	*KRAS* wild-type only
Panitumumab (Vectibix)	Similar to cetuximab	*Dose-limiting:* Acneiform skin rash *Additional toxicities:* Infusion-related reactions, diarrhea, hypomagnesemia, hypocalcemia, interstitial lung disease	*KRAS* wild-type only

adverse effects. Patients can be informed to suck on ice chips prior to and for up to 30 minutes after 5-fluorouracil boluses to decrease the incidence of mucositis. Hand-foot syndrome, characterized by painful swelling and redness of the soles of the feet and palms of the hand, can be minimized with loose fitting clothing and keeping skin moist. Additional toxicities include moderate nausea and vomiting, skin discoloration, nail changes, photosensitivity, and neurologic toxicity.

An additional determinate of 5-fluorouracil toxicity, regardless of the method of administration, is related to its cata-bolism and **pharmacogenomic** factors. Dihydropyrimidine dehydrogenase (DPD) is the main enzyme responsible for the catabolism of 5-fluorouracil to inactive metabolites.[46] A number of polymorphisms in DPD have been identified, in which patients have a complete or near-complete deficiency of this enzyme. This results in unusually severe toxicity, including death, after the administration of 5-fluorouracil. Approximately 3% of patients have a complete lack of DPD activity with other patients demonstrating a partial deficiency in enzyme activity. Although patients may be tested for level of DPD activity, it is not routinely done, but may be considered in patients who develop severe toxicity after 5-fluorouracil administration.

Leucovorin is commonly given with 5-fluorouracil. Leucovorin acts to increase the affinity of 5-fluorouracil to thymidine synthase, thus increasing the pharmacologic activity of 5-fluorouracil.[23] Leucovorin is most effective when administered prior to 5-fluorouracil and can be given by IV bolus or as a continuous infusion. Health care practitioners can also expect an increase in 5-fluorouracil toxicities (leukopenia, mucositis, and diarrhea) when leucovorin is given in combination with 5-fluorouracil.

Capecitabine

Capecitabine (Xeloda) is an oral prodrug of 5-fluorouracil that is designed to be selectively activated by tumor cells. Capecitabine undergoes a three-step conversion to 5-fluorouracil, the last step being phosphorylation by thymidine phosphorylase (TP). TP levels are reported to be higher in tumor cells than normal tissues; therefore, the systemic exposure of active drug is minimized and tumor concentrations of the active drugs are optimized.[32,33] Once the drug is converted to 5-fluorouracil, it has the same mechanism of action. The current FDA-approved indication for capecitabine is for use in metastatic and adjuvant colorectal cancer when monotherapy is desired, though it is actively being investigated as a replacement for 5-fluorouracil in most combinations of colon and rectal cancer regimens. Capecitabine has been demonstrated to be at least equivalent to bolus IV 5-fluorouracil in the metastatic and adjuvant setting with improved patient tolerability.[32,47] Hand-foot syndrome and diarrhea are common with capecitabine as its toxicities (and pharmacologic activity) appear to mimic those of continuous infusions of 5-fluorouracil. Both irinotecan and oxaliplatin have been combined with capecitabine. Capecitabine in combination with oxaliplatin appears to be as safe and effective as IV-based 5-fluorouracil in the treatment of colorectal cancer.[41,44] Combinations with irinotecan have had mixed results and are not routinely recommended.[39,41]

The dose of capecitabine ranges from 1,000 to 1,250 mg/m^2 twice a day when used by itself; lower doses are often used when it is given in combination with irinotecan or oxaliplatin or in patients with renal insufficiency. The dose should be taken on a full stomach with breakfast and dinner. Capecitabine administered with warfarin can result in significant increases in patients' International Normalized Ratio (INR) and requires close monitoring. The convenience of oral administration potentially requiring less clinic visits and an improvement in toxicity makes capecitabine a useful alternative to IV 5-fluorouracil both by itself and incorporated into other regimens used in colorectal cancer.

Irinotecan

Irinotecan (Camptosar) is a topoisomerase-I inhibitor that forms a complex with the covalently bound DNA topoisomerase I enzyme and interferes with the DNA breakage-resealing process.[33,44] Binding permits uncoiling of the double-stranded DNA, but it prevents subsequent resealing of the DNA, resulting in double-stranded DNA breaks. Irinotecan is a prodrug that is converted by carboxlyesterases to its active form SN-38. Irinotecan is indicated for the first-line treatment of metastatic colorectal cancer in combination with 5-fluorouracil and leucovorin or as a single agent in patients who fail first-line therapies. Irinotecan is not recommended as part of the adjuvant treatment of colorectal cancer at this time.

The major toxicity of irinotecan is diarrhea, which can occur both early and late in therapy.[41,44] The early diarrhea is a cholinergic reaction that occurs in the first 24 hours (often during the infusion) in up to 10% of patients and responds to atropine 0.25 to 1 mg IV. The late diarrhea seen in a larger percent of patients occurs 7 to 14 days after the irinotecan infusion. Health care practitioners have to be diligent in counseling patients on this adverse reaction and counseling them on the proper use of antidiarrheals. At the first change in bowel habits, an intensive loperamide regimen should be started by patients (4 mg initially, followed by 2 mg every 2 hours until diarrhea-free for 12 hours). If diarrhea does not stop, or worsens, patients should be instructed to call their health care provider immediately. Late-onset diarrhea may require hospitalization or discontinuation of therapy, and fatalities have been reported. Additional toxicities with irinotecan include leukopenia (including neutropenic fever) and moderate nausea and vomiting. Toxicities of irinotecan appear to be greater when the drug is given weekly when compared to other administration schedules.

Similar to 5-fluorouracil, there is a pharmacogenomic abnormality associated with irinotecan toxicity. UDP-glucuronosyltransferase (UGT1A1) is an enzyme that is responsible for the glucuronidation of SN-38 to inactive metabolites, and reduced or deficient levels of this enzyme correlate with irinotecan-induced diarrhea and neutropenia.[41,44,48] Recently, the FDA approved a blood test that detects variations in this gene. This test may assist health care providers in predicting which patients may develop severe toxicities from "normal" doses of irinotecan and can be ordered prior to patients receiving irinotecan.[41] The package insert recommends dose reductions of one levels in patients who are UGT1A1 homozygous variants. Irinotecan is administered as an IV bolus over 60 to 90 minutes in a variety of dosing schedules.

Oxaliplatin

Oxaliplatin (Eloxatin) is similar to other platinum analogs (cisplatin) in that it binds to the N-7 position of guanine that results in cross-linking of DNA and double-stranded DNA breaks.[23,33,44] Oxaliplatin differs from cisplatin in that the DNA damage induced by oxaliplatin may not be as easily recognized by DNA repair genes, often seen in colorectal cancer. Oxaliplatin, in combination with 5-fluorouracil-based regimens, is indicated for the first- and second-line treatment of metastatic colorectal cancer as well as the adjuvant treatment of colorectal cancer.

The dose-limiting toxicity of oxaliplatin is acute and chronic neuropathy.[49] Acute neuropathies occur within 1 to 2 days of dosing, resolve within 2 weeks, and usually occur peripherally. These acute neuropathies occur in almost all patients to some degree and are exacerbated by exposure to cold temperature or cold objects. Health care providers should instruct patients to avoid cold drinks, use of ice, and to cover skin before exposure to cold or cold objects. In addition, carbamazepine, gabapentin, amifostine, and calcium and magnesium infusions have been used to both prevent and treat oxaliplatin-induced neuropathies, although use of these agents is not widely accepted.[43] Persistent neuropathies generally occur after eight cycles of oxaliplatin and are characterized by defects that can interfere with daily activities (e.g., writing, buttoning, swallowing, and walking). Patients may receive predefined breaks from oxaliplatin to decrease the onset of these toxicities with reinitiation of therapy.[36] This strategy varies among protocols, but involves administering a certain number of predefined oxaliplatin cycles and then stopping. Maintenance therapy with another agent is usually administered and then the oxaliplatin-based regimen is restarted based on the protocol. These neuropathies occur in up to half of patients receiving oxaliplatin but usually resolve with dosage reductions or after oxaliplatin is stopped.[33,49] Oxaliplatin has minimal renal, myelosuppressive effects, and nausea/vomiting when compared to other platinum drugs. Oxaliplatin is given IV in a variety of dosing schedules with a typical dose of 85 mg/m² IV every 2 weeks.

Bevacizumab

Bevacizumab (Avastin) is a recombinant, humanized monoclonal antibody that inhibits vascular endothelial growth factor (VEGF). VEGF is a proangiogenic growth factor found in many cancers including colorectal and is thought to promote blood vessel formation and metastasis of the tumor by binding to VEGF receptors on tumors. Bevacizumab inhibits circulating VEGF, preventing it from binding to receptors and decreasing the formation of new blood vessels.[33] Additionally, bevacizumab may allow for increased concentrations of traditional chemotherapy such as irinotecan to reach the tumor to exert its pharmacologic effect. Bevacizumab is not effective alone and must be used in combination with other agents effective in colorectal cancer. It is indicated for first-line treatment of patients with metastatic colorectal cancer in combination with IV 5-fluorouracil-based regimens. Bevacizumab has also been shown to increase survival in the second-line setting when used in combination with the FOLFOX regimen in patients who have not yet received bevacizumab.[41]

Adverse effects associated with bevacizumab include hypertension which is common but easily managed with oral antihypertensive agents.[38,50] Thrombotic events (including myocardial infarctions, pulmonary embolisms, and deep vein thrombosis) occur more frequently in the elderly patients with cardiovascular risk factors and need to be monitored routinely. Because bevacizumab interferes with normal wound healing, it should not be given shortly before or after surgical procedures.[50] Initiation within 28 days of surgery is not recommended to allow for proper wound healing and decrease the risk of bleeding. The amount of time needed after bevacizumab discontinuation to perform elective surgical procedures is less clear but health care providers should take into consideration bevacizumab's half-life of approximately 20 days when making clinical decisions.[50] Patients should have their urine checked for protein prior to each dose of bevacizumab to check for potential kidney damage. Patients who have developed 2+ protein on the urinalysis require additional testing prior to receiving therapy. These patients will have their 24-hour urine collected and assessed for protein. Therapy is interrupted for 2 g or more of proteinuria/24 hours and resumed when proteinuria was less than 2 g/24 hours. Finally, there is a risk of GI perforation that is rare but potentially fatal. Patients complaining of abdominal pain associated with vomiting or constipation should be counseled to call their physician immediately. Bevacizumab is commonly given at a dose of 5 mg/kg IV every 14 days until disease progression. Once disease progresses and salvage chemotherapy is initiated, the benefit of continuing bevacizumab is unclear.

Cetuximab and Panitumumab

Cetuximab (Erbitux) and panitumumab (Vectibix) are monoclonal antibodies directed against the EGFR. Cetuximab is a chimeric antibody, whereas panitumumab is a fully human monoclonal antibody. The EGFR receptor is overexpressed in colorectal cancers and leads to an increase in tumor proliferation and growth.[23,33,44] Cetuximab received FDA approval for use in EGFR-expressing metastatic colorectal cancer in irinotecan relapsed or refractory patients. Cetuximab should be administered in combination with irinotecan, but can be used as a single agent in patients who cannot tolerate irinotecan-based chemotherapy. Panitumumab is approved as monotherapy agent and should not be used in combination with other agents outside of clinical trials.

Both agents are well tolerated with infusion-related reactions being cetuximab's dose-limiting toxicity and rash most commonly seen with panitumumab. Patients receiving

---

Patient Encounter, Part 4: Screening and Preventing Colon Cancer

GW is concerned about his twin boys developing colon cancer given his disease and his family history of cancer. He asks for advice on preventing colon cancer and ways to detect the disease earlier in his children.

What is the role for chemoprevention for GW's children?

What are the screening recommendations for colon cancer? Do these change for GW's children?

cetuximab require premedication with acetaminophen and diphenhydramine and may require modifications to their adminstration schedule or permanent discontinuation if they develop severe allergic toxicity. A skin rash and diarrhea are also commonly seen with both agents, and health care practitioners should provide counseling to patients about these adverse effects. Treatment options include common medications used to treat acne (doxycycline), topical and systemic steroids, and general skin care. Development of rash may be a surrogate marker of response and clinicians should attempt to minimize the complications of the rash prior to discontinuing therapy.[41] Other toxicities common to both agents include low magnesium, calcium, and potassium levels that require checking levels and replacement therapy as clinically indicated. A rare (less than 1%) interstitial lung disease is seen with all agents that inhibit EGFR and patients should be instructed to report any new onset shortness of breath. Cetuximab has an initial loading dose of 400 mg/m^2 IV infusion. Weekly doses of 250 mg/m^2 are then administered starting the following week. Panitumumab is given 6 mg/kg every 2 weeks.

Recent data have demonstrated specific tumor characteristics that may assist clinicians in predicting who may respond to these agents. Early IHC staining for EGFR status is not useful in predicting response as both EGFR-positive and -negative patients response at the same rate. Fluorescence in situ hybridization (FISH) of EGFR copy number and *KRAS* gene mutation status have recently demonstrated predictive value. Patients with high EGFR gene copy number and wild-type (nonmutated) *KRAS* are more likely to benefit from cetuximab or panitumumab therapy.[41,44] In particular, testing for *KRAS* mutational status is now part of the disease workup to define patients who may derive benefit from cetuximab or panitumumab. Most clinical trials currently underway are now stratifying patients based on *KRAS* status to further assist clinicians in defining appropriate therapy for this subset of patients.

RECTAL CANCER

Although often treated similarly to colon cancer, there are some important differences in the treatment of rectal cancer, especially in the adjuvant setting. Rectal cancer involves those tumors found in distal 15 cm of the large bowel and, as such, is very distinct from colon cancer in that it has a propensity for both local and distant recurrence. The higher incidence of local failure and poorer overall prognosis associated with rectal cancer is due to limitations in surgical techniques. Therefore, multimodality therapies with a combination of chemotherapy, radiation, and surgery are at the forefront in the treatment of rectal cancer with the main goal of survival and quality of life by preserving the function of the anal sphincter. In addition, because treatment with surgery, radiation, or systemic chemotherapy at the time of the recurrence is often suboptimal, adjuvant therapy after tumor resection is an important aspect of treatment of the primary tumor. Similar to adjuvant therapy for colon cancer, 5-fluorouracil provides the basis for chemotherapy regimens for rectal cancer.

⑩ *Adjuvant therapy consisting of 5-fluorouracil-based chemotherapy in combination with radiation therapy should be offered to patients with stage II or III cancer of the rectum.*[51] Radiation therapy decreases the rate of local recurrences whereas the 5-fluorouracil decreases the risk of distant tumor recurrence as well as acting as a radiosensitizer. Toxicities from combined modality therapy include severe hematologic toxicity, enteritis, and diarrhea. Additional trials have sought to determine optimal combinations of concurrent radiation and 5-fluorouracil. Similar to tumors in the colon, continuous infusions of 5-fluorouracil appear to be superior to bolus doses. However, leucovorin does not appear to improve efficacy of adjuvant treatment for rectal cancer. Use of oral alternatives to 5-fluorouracil that are also known to enhance radiation effects, such as capecitabine, are under investigation with preliminary data suggesting the combination of capecitabine and radiation will be safe and effective. In addition, based on the efficacy in colon cancer, FOLFOX regimens have moved into clinical trials in the adjuvant setting.

Another unique aspect of rectal cancer is the use of neoadjuvant therapy. Preoperative radiation (with or without chemotherapy) is given to downstage the tumor prior to surgical resection to improve sphincter preservation.[51] The issue of pre- versus postoperative radiation is a subject of debate and investigation in the United States and will require further data to determine the superiority of a specific neoadjuvant protocol.

Finally, once rectal cancer is metastatic, similar regimens as outlined in the colon cancer section are used for palliation of symptoms.[51]

OUTCOME EVALUATION

The goal of monitoring is to evaluate whether the patient is receiving any benefit from the management of the disease, to detect recurrence, and to minimize the adverse effects of treatment. During treatment for active disease, patients should undergo monitoring for measurable tumor response, progression, or new metastases; these tests may include chest CT scans or x-rays, abdominal or pelvic CT scans or x-rays, depending on the site of disease being evaluated for response, and carcinoembryonic antigen (CEA) measurements every 3 months if the CEA is or was previously elevated.[52] A PET scan can be considered to identify localized sites of metastatic disease in situations where a rising CEA level suggests metastatic disease but CT scans and other imaging studies are negative. Symptoms of recurrence such as pain, changes in bowel habits, rectal bleeding, pelvic masses, anorexia, and weight loss develop in fewer than 50% of patients. Patients who undergo curative surgical resection, with or without adjuvant therapy, require close follow-up because early detection and treatment of recurrence could still result in patient cures. In addition, early treatment for asymptomatic metastatic colorectal cancer appears superior to delayed therapy. Colorectal cancer surveillance guidelines published by the American Society of Clinical Oncology recommend against routinely monitoring liver function tests, CBC,

FOBT, CT scans, annual chest x-rays, or pelvic imaging in asymptomatic patients.[52]

In addition, a complete blood count should be obtained prior to each course of chemotherapy administration to ensure that hematologic values are adequate. In particular, white blood counts and absolute neutrophil counts can be decreased in patients receiving chemotherapy such as irinotecan and 5-fluorouracil. Baseline liver function tests and an assessment of renal function should be evaluated prior to and periodically during therapy. Other selected laboratory tests include checking for the presence of protein in the urine in patients receiving bevacizumab and monitoring of magnesium, calcium, and potassium in patients receiving cetuximab or panitumumab.

Patients should be evaluated during every treatment visit for the presence of anticipated side effects from their treatment, and health care practitioners should anticipate these adverse reactions and aggressively treat and prevent them from occurring. These generally include loose stools or diarrhea from irinotecan, 5-fluorouracil, and capecitabine; hand-foot syndrome from 5-fluorouracil and capecitabine; nausea or vomiting from irinotecan, 5-fluorouracil, and oxaliplatin; mouth sores from 5-fluorouracil; neuropathies from oxaliplatin; bleeding and hypertension from bevacizumab; and skin rash associated cetuximab and panitumumab.

SUMMARY

Recent advances in the treatment of cancer of the colon and rectum now offer the potential to improve patient survival but for many patients, improved disease- and progression-free survival represent equally important therapeutic outcomes. In the absence of the ability of a specific treatment to demonstrate improved survival, important outcome measures should include the effects of the treatment on patient symptoms, daily activities, performance status, and other quality-of-life indicators. Individualized patient care to balance the risks associated with treatment and benefits of a specific treatment regimen is necessary to optimize patient outcomes.

Abbreviations Introduced in This Chapter

APC	Adenomatous polyposis coli
CAPOX	Capecitabine and oxaliplatin
CBC	Complete blood count
CEA	Carcinoembryonic antigen
COX-2	Cyclooxygenase-2
CTC	Computed tomographic colonoscopy
DPD	Dihydropyrimidine dehydrogenase
EGFR	Epidermal growth factor receptor
FAP	Familial adenomatous polyposis
F-dUMP	Fluoro-deoxy-uridine monophosphate
FISH	Fluorescence in situ hybridization
FIT	Fecal immunochemical test
FOBT	Fecal occult blood test

FOLFIRI	Folinic acid, fluorouracil, and infusional irinotecan
FOLFOX	Folinic acid, fluorouracil, and oxaliplatin
HNPCC	Hereditary nonpolyposis colorectal cancer
IFL	Irinotecan, fluorouracil, and leucovorin
IHC	Immunohistochemical
INR	International Normalized Ratio
NSAIDs	Nonsteroidal anti-inflammatory drugs
PET	Positron-emission tomography
TNM	Tumor, node, metastasis
TP	Thymidine phosphorylase
UGT	UDP-glucuronosyltransferase
VEGF	Vascular endothelial growth factor

Patient Care and Monitoring

1. Review any available diagnostic data to determine the status of the colon cancer.

2. Obtain a thorough history of prescription, nonprescription, and natural drug product use.

3. Evaluate patient-specific factors that may dictate treatment regimen. Does the patient have a known pharmacogenomic deficiency? What lifestyle issues are important to the patient?

4. Determine if any dose modifications are required in the chemotherapy regimen prescribed. Does the patient have adequate blood counts to receive chemotherapy?

5. Educate the patient on drug therapy and possible treatment-related adverse effects, and counsel the patient on appropriate recommendations to prevent or minimize these adverse effects. What medications are for the treatment of cancer and what medications are to prevent the adverse effects of chemotherapy?

6. Develop a plan to prevent treatment-related adverse effects. Are the antiemetics appropriate? Does the patient understand the possible adverse effects and when to call the physician versus when patient-directed care is appropriate?

7. Warning signs to report to the physician (depends on regimen used) include fever, diarrhea, mucositis, and hand-foot syndrome.

8. Evaluate the patient for the presence of adverse drug reactions, drug allergies, and drug interactions.

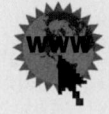

Self-assessment questions and answers are available at *http://www.mhpharmacotherapy. com/pp.html.*

REFERENCES

1. Jemal A, Siegel R, Ward E, et al. Cancer statistics, 2008. CA Cancer J Clin 2008;58:71–96.

2. Pisani P, Bray F, Parkin DM. Estimates of the world-wide prevalence of cancer for 25 sites in the adult population. Int J Cancer 2002;97:72–81.

3. Ries LAG, Eisner MP, Kosary CL, et al., eds. SEER Cancer Statistics Review, 1975–2000, National Cancer Institute. Bethesda, MD, *http://seer.cancer.gov/csr/1975_2000.*

4. Peters U, Sinha R, Chatterjee N, et al. Dietary fibre and colorectal adenoma in a colorectal cancer early detection programme. Lancet 2003;361:1491–1495.

5. Fuchs CS, Giovannucci EL, Colditz GA. Dietary fiber and the risk of colorectal cancer and adenoma in women. N Engl J Med 1999;340:169–176.

6. Park Y, Hunter DJ, Spiegelman D, et al. Dietary fiber intake and risk of colorectal cancer: A pooled analysis of prospective cohort studies. JAMA 2005;294:2849–2857.

7. Wactawski-Wende J, Kotchen JM, Anderson GL. Calcium plus vitamin D supplementation and the risk of colorectal cancer. N Engl J Med 2006;354:684–696.

8. Kim YI. Folate and colorectal cancer: an evidence-based critical review. Mol Nutr Food Res 2007;51:267–292.

9. Cole BF, Baron JA, Sandler RS, et al., for the Polyp Prevention Study Group. Folic acid for the prevention of colorectal adenomas: a randomized clinical trial. JAMA 2007;297:2351–2359.

10. Giovannucci E. Modifiable risk factors for colon cancer. Gastroenterol Clin North Am 2002;31:925–943.

11. Thun MJ, Henley J, Patrono C. Nonsteroidal anti-inflammatory drugs as anticancer agents: Mechanistic, pharmacologic, and clinical issues. J Natl Cancer Inst 2002;94:252–266.

12. Chan AT, Giovannucci EL, Meyerhardt JA, et al. Long-term use of aspirin and nonsteroidal anti-inflammatory drugs and risk of colorectal cancer. JAMA 2005;294:914–923.

13. Chan AT, Ogino S, Fuchs CS. Aspirin and the risk of colorectal cancer in relation to the expression of COX-2. N Engl J Med 2007;356:2131–2142.

14. Nelson HD, Humphrey LL, Nygren P, et al. Postmenopausal hormone replacement therapy: Scientific review. JAMA 2002;288:872–881.

15. Giovannucci E. Metabolic syndrome, hyperinsulinemia, and colon cancer: A review. Am J Clin Nutr 2007;86:s836–s842.

16. Calvert PM, Frucht H. The genetics of colorectal cancer. Ann Intern Med 2003;137:603–612.

17. Fuchs CS, Giovannucci EL, Colditzs GA, et al. A prospective study of family history and the risk of colorectal cancer. N Engl J Med 1994;331:1669–1674.

18. Levin B, Lieberman DA, McFarland B, et al. Screening and surveillance for the early detection of colorectal cancer and adenomatous polyps, 2008: A joint guideline from the American Cancer Society, the US Multi-Society Task Force on Colorectal Cancer, and the American College of Radiology. American Cancer Society guidelines for the early detection of cancer. CA Cancer J Clin 2008;58:130–160.

19. Hawk ET, Levin B. Colorectal cancer prevention. J Clin Oncol 2005;23:378–391.

20. Baron JA, Cole BF, Sandler RS, et al. A randomized trial of aspirin to prevent colorectal adenomas. N Engl J Med 2003;348:891–899.

21. Grunwald V, Hidalgo M. Developing inhibitors of the epidermal growth factor receptor for cancer treatment. J Natl Cancer Inst 2003;95:851–867.

22. Alexander D, Jhala N, Chatla C, et al. High-grade tumor differentiation is an indicator of poor prognosis in African Americans with colonic adenocarcinomas. Cancer 2005;103:2163–2170.

23. Libutti SK, Saltz LB, Tepper JE. Colon cancer. In: DeVita VT, Lawrence TS, Rosenberg SA, eds. Cancer: Principles and Practice of Oncology, 8th ed. Philadelphia: Lippincott Williams & Wilkins, 2008:1235–1285.

24. Libutti SK, Tepper JE, Saltz LB. Rectal cancer. In: DeVita VT, Lawrence TS, Rosenberg SA, eds. Cancer: Principles and Practice of Oncology, 8th ed. Philadelphia: Lippincott Williams & Wilkins, 2008:1285–1301.

25. Simmonds PC, Primrose JN, Colquitt JL, et al. Surgical resection of hepatic metastases from colorectal cancer: A systematic review of published studies. Br J Cancer 2006;94:982–999.

26. Barrier A, Boelle PY, Roser F, et al. Stage II colon cancer prognosis prediction by tumor gene expression profiling. J Clin Oncol 2006;24:4685–4691.

27. Benson AB, Schrag D, Somerfield MR, et al. American Society of Clinical Oncology recommendations of adjuvant chemotherapy for stage II colon cancer. J Clin Oncol 2004; 22:3408–3419.

28. Saini A, Norman AR, Cunningham D, et al. Twelve weeks of protracted venous infusion of fluorouracil (5-FU) is as effective as 6 months of bolus 5-FU and folinic acid as adjuvant treatment in colorectal cancer. Br J Cancer 2003; 88:1859–1865.

29. Gill S, Loprinzi CL, Sargent DJ, et al. Pooled analysis of fluorouracil-based adjuvant therapy for stage II and III colon cancer: Who benefits and by how much? J Clin Oncol 2004;22:1797–1806.

30. de Gramont A, Boni C, Navarro M, et al. Oxaliplatin/5FU/LV in adjuvant colon cancer: Updated efficacy results of the MOSAIC trial, including survival, with a median follow-up of six years. J Clin Oncol 2007; 2007 ASCO Annual Meeting Proceedings Part I;25(18S):Abstract 4007.

31. Wolpin BM, Meyerhardt JA, Mamon HJ, Mayer RJ. Adjuvant treatment for colon cancer. CA Cancer J Clin 2007;57:168–185.

32. Twelves C, Wong A, Nowacki MP, et al. Capecitabine as adjuvant treatment for stage III colon cancer. N Engl J Med 2005;352: 2696–2704.

33. Meyerhardt JA, Mayer RJ. Systemic therapy for colorectal cancer. N Engl J Med 2005;352:476–487.

34. Saltz LB, Cox JV, Blanke C, et al. Efficacy of intravenous continuous infusion of fluorouracil compared with bolus administration in advanced colorectal cancer. Meta-analysis Group in Cancer. J Clin Oncol 1998;16:301–308.

35. Saltz LB, Cox JV, Blanke C, et al. Irinotecan plus fluorouracil and leucovorin for metastatic colorectal cancer. N Engl J Med 2000;343:905–914.

36. Goldberg RM, Sargent DJ, Morton RF, et al. A randomized controlled trial of fluorouracil plus leucovorin, irinotecan, and oxaliplatin combinations in patients with previously untreated metastatic colorectal cancer. J Clin Oncol 2004;22:23–30.

37. Tournigand C, André T, Achille E, et al. FOLFIRI followed by FOLFOX6 or the reverse sequence in advanced colorectal cancer: A randomized GERCOR study. J Clin Oncol 2004;22:229–237.

38. Hurwitz H, Fehrenbacher L, Novotny W, et al. Bevacizumab plus irinotecan, fluorouracil, and leucovorin for metastatic colorectal cancer. N Engl J Med 2004;350:2335–2342.

39. Fuchs CS, Marshall J, Barrueco J. Randomized, controlled trial of irinotecan plus infusional, bolus, or oral fluoropyrimidines in first-line treatment of metastatic colorectal cancer: Updated results from the BICC-C study. J Clin Oncol 2008;26:689–690.

40. Saltz LB, Clarke S, Díaz-Rubio E, et al. Bevacizumab in combination with oxaliplatin-based chemotherapy as first-line therapy in metastatic colorectal cancer: A randomized phase III study. J Clin Oncol 2008;20:2013–2019.

41. NCCN Guidelines—Colon Cancer v.2.2008, *http://www.nccn.org.*

42. Grothey A, Sargent D, Goldberg RM, Schmoll H. Survival of patients with advanced colorectal cancer improves with the availability of fluorouracil-leucovorin, irinotecan, and oxaliplatin in the course of treatment. J Clin Oncol 2004;22:1204–1214.

43. Cunningham D, Humblet Y, Siena S, et al. Cetuximab monotherapy and cetuximab plus irinotecan in irinotecan-refractory metastatic colorectal cancer. N Engl J Med 2004;351:337–345.

44. Wolpin BM, Mayer RJ. Systemic treatment of colorectal. Gastroenterology 2008;134:1296–1310.

45. Kemeny N. Management of liver metastases from colorectal cancer. Oncology (Williston Park) 2006;20:1161–1176.

46. Mercier C, Ciccolini J. Profiling dihydropyrimidine dehydrogenase deficiency in patients with cancer undergoing 5-fluorouracil/capecitabine therapy. Clin Colorectal Cancer 2006;6:288–296.

47. Twelves C. Capecitabine as first-line treatment in colorectal cancer: Pooled data from two large, phase III trials. Eur J Cancer 2002;38(suppl): 15–20.

48. Desai AA, Innocenti F, Ratain MJ. Pharmacogenomics: Road to anti-cancer therapeutics in nirvana? Oncogene 2003;22:6621–6628.

49. Saif MW, Reardon J. Management of oxaliplatin-induced peripheral neuropathy. Ther Clin Risk Manag 2005;1:249–258.

50. Motl S. Bevacizumab in combination chemotherapy for colorectal and other cancers. Am J Health Syst Pharm 2005;62:1021–1032.

51. NCCN Guidelines—Rectal Cancer v.2.2008, *http://www.nccn.org.*

52. Desch CE, Benson AB, Smith TJ, et al. Recommended colorectal cancer surveillance guidelines by the American Society of Clinical Oncology. J Clin Oncol 1999;17:1312–1321.

92

Prostate Cancer

Trevor McKibbin and Jill M. Kolesar

LEARNING OBJECTIVES

● **Upon completion of the chapter, the reader will be able to:**

1. List the risk factors associated with the development of prostate cancer.

2. Compare placebo versus finasteride for the prevention of prostate cancer.

3. Recommend a prostate cancer screening program for a man on the basis of his age and risk factors.

4. Recommend a treatment for initial treatment of prostate cancer on the basis of stage, Gleason score, age, and symptoms.

5. Understand the role of chemotherapy in the treatment of metastatic hormone-refractory prostate cancer.

KEY CONCEPTS

❶ Prostate cancer is the most frequent cancer in U.S. men. African American ancestry, family history, and increased age are the primary risk factors for prostate cancer.

❷ Prostate-specific antigen (PSA) is a useful marker for detecting prostate cancer at early stages, predicting outcome for localized disease, defining disease-free status, and monitoring response to androgen-deprivation therapy or chemotherapy for advanced-stage disease.

❸ The prognosis for prostate cancer patients depends on the histologic grade, the tumor size, and disease stage. More than 85% of patients with stage A_1 disease but less than 1% of those with stage D_2 can be cured.

❹ Androgen ablation with a luteinizing hormone–releasing hormone (LHRH) agonist plus an antiandrogen should be used prior to radiation therapy for patients with locally advanced prostate cancer to improve outcomes over radiation therapy alone.

❺ Androgen ablation therapy, with orchiectomy, an LHRH agonist alone or an LHRH agonist plus an antiandrogen (combined hormonal blockade), can be used to provide palliation for patients with advanced (stage D_2) prostate cancer. The effects of androgen deprivation seem most pronounced in patients with minimal disease at diagnosis.

❻ Antiandrogen withdrawal, for patients having progressive disease while receiving combined hormonal blockade with an LHRH agonist plus an antiandrogen, can provide additional symptomatic relief. Mutations in the androgen receptor have been documented that cause antiandrogen compounds to act like receptor agonists.

❼ Chemotherapy with docetaxel and prednisone improves survival in patients with hormone-refractory prostate cancer.

INTRODUCTION

Prostate cancer is the most commonly diagnosed cancer in U.S. men.[1] For most men, prostate cancer has an indolent course, and treatment options for early disease include expectant management, surgery, or radiation. With expectant management, patients are monitored for disease progression or development of symptoms. Localized prostate cancer can be cured by surgery or radiation therapy; advanced prostate cancer is not yet curable. Treatment for advanced prostate cancer can provide significant disease palliation for many patients for several years after diagnosis. The endocrine dependence of this tumor is well documented, and hormonal manipulation to decrease circulating androgens remains the basis for the initial treatment of advanced disease.

EPIDEMIOLOGY AND ETIOLOGY

❶ *Prostate cancer is the most frequent cancer among U.S. men and represents the second leading cause of cancer-related deaths in all males.*[1] In the United States alone, it is estimated that 192,280 new cases of prostatic carcinoma will be diagnosed and more than 27,360 men will die from this disease in 2009.[1] Although prostate cancer incidence increased during the late 1980s and early 1990s owing to widespread prostate-specific antigen (PSA) screening, deaths from prostate cancer have been declining since 1995.[1]

Table 92–1 summarizes the possible factors associated with prostate cancer.[2,3] The widely accepted risk factors for prostate cancer are age, race ethnicity, and family history of prostate cancer.[2,3] The disease is rare under the age of 40, but the incidence sharply increases with each subsequent decade, most likely because the individual has had a lifetime exposure to testosterone, a known growth signal for the prostate.[3]

Race and Ethnicity

The incidence of clinical prostate cancer varies across geographic regions. Scandinavian countries and the United States report the highest incidence of prostate cancer, while the disease is relatively rare in Japan and other Asian countries.[4] African American men have the highest rate of prostate cancer in the world, and in the United States, prostate cancer mortality in African Americans is more than twice that seen in Caucasian populations.[1] Hormonal, dietary, and genetic differences, as well as differences in access to health care, may contribute to the altered susceptibility to prostate cancer in these populations.[2,3] Testosterone, commonly implicated in the pathogenesis of prostate cancer, is 15% higher in African American men compared with Caucasian males. Activity of 5-α-reductase, the enzyme that converts testosterone to its more active form, dihydrotestosterone (DHT), in the prostate, is decreased in Japanese men compared with African Americans and Caucasian.[2,3] In addition, genetic variations in the androgen receptor exist. Activation of the androgen receptor is inversely correlated with trinucleotide (CAG) repeat length. Shorter CAG repeat sequences have been found in African Americans. Therefore, the combination of increased testosterone and increased androgen receptor activation may account for the increased risk of prostate cancer in African American men.[2,3] The Asian diet generally is considered to be low in fat and high in fiber with a high concentration of phytoestrogens, potentially explaining their decreased risk.[4,5]

Family History

Men with a brother or father with prostate cancer have twice the risk for prostate cancer compared to the rest of the population.[5] There appears to be a familial clustering of a prostate cancer syndrome and genome-wide scans have identified potential prostate cancer susceptibility candidate genes. Male carriers of germline mutations of BRCA1 and BRCA2 are known to have an increased risk for developing prostate cancer.[6] Common exposure to environmental and other risk factors may also contribute to increased risk among patients with first degree relatives with prostate cancer.[5,7]

An alternative explanation for the familial clustering may be polymorphisms in genes important for prostate cancer function and development.[5,7] Candidate polymorphisms include a polymorphism in the androgen receptor, which has two different nucleotide repeat variants, the CAG or the GCC. The CAG repeat varies in repeat number from 11 to 31 repeats in healthy individuals, and the number of repeats is inversely proportional to the activity of the androgen receptor. Some studies have demonstrated that shorter CAG repeats are associated with increased prostate cancer risk. Another candidate polymorphism is SRD5A2, which is the gene that codes for 5-α-reductase, the enzyme that converts testosterone to the more active DHT. A variant in SRD5A2, the Ala49Thr, increases the activity and may increase prostate cancer risk.[5,7]

Diet

A number of epidemiologic studies support an association between high-fat intake and risk of prostate cancer. A strong correlation between national per capita fat consumption and national prostate cancer mortality has been reported, and prospective case-control studies suggest that a high-fat diet doubles the risk of prostate cancer.[5,8] This relationship between high-fat intake and prostate cancer may explain differences in insulin-like growth factor-1 (IGF-1).

Table 92–1	
Risk Factors Associated With Prostate Cancer	
Factor	**Possible Relationship**
Probable Risk Factors	
Age	More than 70% of cases are diagnosed in men above 65 years
Race	African Americans have higher incidence and death rate
Genetic	Familial prostate cancer inherited in an autosomal dominant manner
	Mutations in p53, Rb, E-cahedrin, α-catenin, androgen receptor, KAI1, microsatellite instability, loss of heterozygocity at 1, 2q, 12p, 15q, 16p, and 16q, BRCA1 and BRCA2 mutations
	Candidate prostate cancer gene locus identified on chromosome 1
Possible Risk Factors	
Environmental	Clinical carcinoma incidence varies worldwide Latent carcinoma similar between regions' nationalized males adopt intermediate incidence rates between that of the United States and their native country
Occupational	Increased risk associated with cadmium exposure
Dietary	Increased risk associated with high-meat and high-fat diets
	Decreased intake of 1,25-dihydroxyvitamin D, lycopene, and β-carotene increases risk
Hormonal	Does not occur in eunuchs
	Low incidence in cirrhotic patients
	Up to 80% are hormonally dependent
	African Americans have 15% increased testosterone
	Japanese have decreased 5-α-reductase activities
	Polymorphic expression of the androgen receptor

High-calorie and high-fat diets stimulate production of IGF-1 by the liver. This factor is involved in the regulation of proliferation of cancer cells and may also prevent them from undergoing apoptosis.[5,8] High levels of IGF-1 are associated with an increased risk for prostate cancer.[5]

Other dietary factors implicated in prostate cancer include retinol, carotenoids, lycopene, and vitamin D consumption.[5,7,9] Retinol, or vitamin A, intake, especially in men older than 70, is correlated with an increased risk of prostate cancer, whereas intake of its precursor, β-carotene, has a protective or neutral effect. Lycopene, obtained primarily from tomatoes, decreases the risk of prostate cancer in small cohort studies. Men who developed prostate cancer in one cohort study had lower levels of 1,25(OH)$_2$-vitamin D than matched controls, although a prospective study did not support this. Clearly, dietary risk factors require further evaluation, but because fat and vitamins are modifiable risk factors, dietary intervention may be promising in prostate cancer prevention. Investigations of selenium and vitamin E supplementation are discussed further in the chemoprevention section.

Other Factors

Benign prostatic hyperplasia (BPH) is a common problem among elderly men, affecting more than 40% of men over the age of 70. BPH results in the urinary symptoms of hesitancy and frequency. Since prostate cancer affects a similar age group and often has similar presenting symptoms, the presence of BPH often complicates the diagnosis of prostate cancer, although it does not appear to increase the risk of developing prostate cancer.[2,7]

Smoking has not been associated with an increased risk of prostate cancer, but smokers with prostate cancer have an increased mortality resulting from the disease when compared with nonsmokers with prostate cancer (relative risk 1.5–2).[2,7] In addition, in a prospective cohort analysis, alcohol consumption was not associated with the development of prostate cancer.

Chemoprevention

Currently, the most promising agents for the prevention of prostate cancer are the 5-α-reductase inhibitors, finasteride and dutasteride.[7,10,11] These medications work by inhibiting 5-a-reductase, an enzyme that converts testosterone to its more active form, DHT, which is involved in prostate epithelial proliferation. There are two types of 5-α-reductase, type I and type II; both are implicated in the development of prostate cancer. Finasteride selectively inhibits the 5-α-reductase type-II isoenzyme, whereas dutasteride inhibits both isoenzymes.[11] Both finasteride and dutasteride falsely lower the PSA in patients and this needs to be adjusted for when measuring the PSA in patients on these medications.[7,11]

The Prostate Cancer Prevention Trial (PCPT) compared finasteride 5 mg daily for 7 years to placebo for the prevention of prostate cancer.[7] When compared to placebo, the point prevalence of prostate cancer was reduced for those on finasteride by 24.8% (95% confidence interval [CI]

18.6–30.6%) (hazard ratio 0.75). However, in those that did develop prostate cancer, there was an increase in the number of high-grade (Gleason grade 7–10) tumors detected at biopsy in the finasteride group. Overall, finasteride did reduce the frequency of prostate cancer; however, the prostate cancers that were diagnosed in the finasteride group were more aggressive.

The use of finasteride to prevent prostate cancer is the subject of a recent joint consensus statement. The American Society of Clinical Oncology (ASCO) and the American Urological Association (AUA) used the results from a systematic review of the literature to develop evidence-based recommendations for the use of 5-α-reductase inhibitors for prostate cancer chemoprevention. 5-α-reductase inhibitors decrease the period prevalence of for-cause prostate cancer by approximately 26% (relative risk 0.74; 95% CI, 0.67–0.83). The absolute risk reduction is about 1.4% (4.9% in controls versus 3.5% in the treatment arms), although this may vary with the age of the treated population. On the basis of these outcomes, ASCO and AUA recommend that asymptomatic men with a PSA less than or equal to 3 ng/mL, who are regularly screened with PSA, may benefit from a discussion of both the benefits of 5-α-reductase inhibitors for 7 years for the prevention of prostate cancer and the potential risks (including the possibility of high-grade prostate cancer). Men who are taking 5-α-reductase inhibitors for benign conditions such as lower urinary tract symptoms may benefit from a similar discussion, understanding that the improvement of symptoms should be weighed with the potential risks of high-grade prostate cancer.

Selenium and vitamin E alone or in combination were evaluated in the *Selenium and Vitamin E Cancer Prevention Trial* (SELECT), a clinical trial investigating their effects on the incidence of prostate cancer. The data and safety monitoring committee found that after 5 years selenium and vitamin E taken alone or together did not prevent prostate cancer. On the basis of these data and safety concerns, the trial was halted.[12] Other agents, including vitamin D, lycopene, green tea, nonsteroidal anti-inflammatory agents, isoflavones, and statins, are under investigation for prostate cancer and show promise; however, none are currently recommended for routine use outside of a clinical trial.[13]

Screening

Early detection of potentially curable prostate cancers is the goal of prostate cancer screening. For cancer screening to be beneficial, it must reliably detect cancer at an early stage, when intervention would decrease mortality. Whether prostate cancer screening fits these criteria has generated considerable controversy.[14] Digital rectal examination (DRE) has been recommended since the early 1900s for the detection of prostate cancer. The primary advantage of DRE is its specificity, reported at greater than 85%, for prostate cancer. Other advantages of DRE include low cost, safety, and ease of performance. However, DRE is relatively insensitive and is subject to interobserver variability. DRE as a single screening method has poor compliance and had little effect on preventing metastatic prostate cancer in one large case-control study.[15]

❷ *Prostate-specific antigen is a useful marker for detecting prostate cancer at early stages, predicting outcome for localized disease, defining disease-free status, and monitoring response to androgen-deprivation therapy or chemotherapy for advanced-stage disease.* PSA is used widely for prostate cancer screening in the United States, with simplicity as its major advantage and low specificity as its primary limitation.[16] PSA may be elevated in men with acute urinary retention, acute prostatitis, and prostatic ischemia or infarction, as well as BPH, a nearly universal condition in men at risk for prostate cancer. PSA elevations between 4.1 ng/mL (4.1 mcg/L) and 10 ng/mL (10 mcg/L) cannot distinguish between BPH and prostate cancer, limiting the utility of PSA alone for the early detection of prostate cancer. Additionally, only 38% to 48% of men with clinically significant prostate cancer have a serum PSA outside the reference range.[17]

Neither DRE nor PSA is sensitive or specific enough to be used alone as a screening test. Although the relative predictability of DRE and PSA is similar, the tumors identified by each method are different. Catalona and associates[18] confirmed that the combination of a DRE plus PSA determination is a better method of detecting prostate cancer than DRE alone.

The common approach to prostate cancer screening today involves offering a baseline PSA and DRE at the age of 40 with annual evaluations beginning at the age of 50 to all men of normal risk with a 10-year or greater life expectancy. Men with an increased risk of prostate cancer, including men of African American ancestry and men with a family history of prostate cancer, may begin screening earlier, at age 40 to 45.

Despite this common practice, the benefits of prostate cancer screening are unproven.[19] PSA measurements can identify small, subclinical prostate cancers, where no intervention may be required. Detecting prostate cancer in those not needing therapy not only increases the cost of care through unnecessary screening and workups but also increases the toxicity of therapy, by subjecting some patients to unnecessary therapy.[20,21] Currently, the American College of Physicians recommends that rather than screening all men for prostate cancer as a matter of routine, physicians should describe the potential benefits and known risks of screening, diagnosis, and treatment, listen to the patient's concerns, and then decide on an individual's screening method.

PATHOPHYSIOLOGY

The prostate gland is a solid, rounded, heart-shaped organ positioned between the neck of the bladder and the urogenital diaphragm (Fig. 92–1). The normal prostate is composed of acinar secretory cells arranged in a radial shape and surrounded by a foundation of supporting tissue. The size, shape, or presence of acini is almost always altered in the gland that has been invaded by prostatic carcinoma. Adenocarcinoma, the major pathologic cell type, accounts for more than 95% of prostate cancer cases.[22,23] Much rarer tumor types include small-cell neuroendocrine cancers, sarcomas, and transitional cell carcinomas.

Prostate cancer can be graded systematically according to the histologic appearance of the malignant cell and then grouped into well, moderately, or poorly differentiated grades.[23,24] Gland architecture is examined and then rated on a scale of 1 (well differentiated) to 5 (poorly differentiated). Two different specimens are examined, and the score for each specimen is added. Groupings for total Gleason score are 2 to 4 for well-differentiated, 5 or 6 for moderately differentiated, and 7 to 10 for poorly differentiated tumors. Poorly differentiated tumors grow rapidly (poor prognosis), while well-differentiated tumors grow slowly (better prognosis).

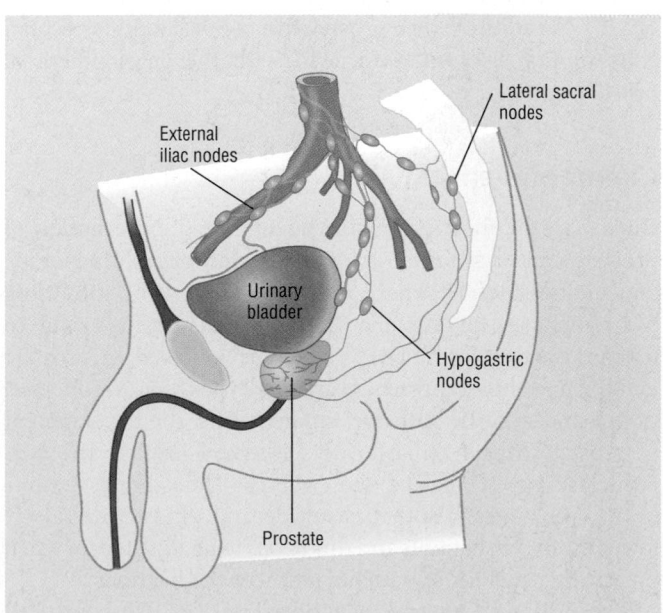

FIGURE 92–1. The prostate gland. (From DiPiro JT, Talbert RL, Yee GC, et al, eds. Pharmacotherapy: A Pathophysiologic Approach, 6th ed. New York: McGraw-Hill, 2005: 1856.)

Patient Encounter 1: Prevention and Screening

OC is a 66-year-old Caucasian male who comes into the pharmacy requesting some "vitamins" for prostate health. He is interested in lycopene, zinc, selenium, and finasteride.

OC does not have a family history of prostate cancer and no symptoms suggestive of BPH. He has never been screened for prostate cancer.

What do you recommend for prostate cancer screening?

What do you recommend for prostate cancer chemoprevention?

Metastatic spread can occur by local extension, lymphatic drainage, or hematogenous dissemination.[24,25] Lymph node metastases are more common in patients with large, undifferentiated tumors that invade the seminal vesicles. The pelvic and abdominal lymph node groups are the most common sites of lymph node involvement (Fig. 92–1). Skeletal metastases from hematogenous spread are the most common sites of distant spread. Typically, the bone lesions are osteoblastic or a combination of osteoblastic and osteolytic. The most common site of bone involvement is the lumbar spine. Other sites of bone involvement include the proximal femurs, pelvis, thoracic spine, ribs, sternum, skull, and humerus. The lung, liver, brain, and adrenal glands are the most common sites of visceral involvement, although these organs usually are not involved initially. About 25% to 35% of patients will have evidence of lymphangitic or nodular pulmonary infiltrates at autopsy. The prostate is rarely a site for metastatic involvement from other solid tumors.

Normal growth and differentiation of the prostate depends on the presence of androgens, specifically DHT.[25,26] The testes and the adrenal glands are the major sources of circulating androgens. Hormonal regulation of androgen synthesis is mediated through a series of biochemical interactions between the hypothalamus, pituitary, adrenal glands, and testes (Fig. 92–2). Luteinizing hormone–releasing hormone (LHRH) released from the hypothalamus stimulates the release of luteinizing hormone (LH) and follicle-stimulating hormone (FSH) from the anterior pituitary gland. LH

complexes with receptors on the Leydig cell testicular membrane and stimulates the production of testosterone and small amounts of estrogen. FSH acts on the Sertoli cells within the testes to promote the maturation of LH receptors and to produce an androgen-binding protein. Circulating testosterone and estradiol influence the synthesis of LHRH, LH, and FSH by a negative feedback loop operating at the hypothalamic and pituitary level.[27] Prolactin, growth hormone, and estradiol appear to be important accessory regulators for prostatic tissue permeability, receptor binding, and testosterone synthesis.

Testosterone, the major androgenic hormone, accounts for 95% of the androgen concentration. The primary source of testosterone is the testes; however, 3% to 5% of the testosterone concentration is derived from direct adrenal cortical secretion of testosterone or C19 steroids such as androstenedione.[24-26]

In early stage prostate cancers, aberrant tumor cell proliferation is promoted by the presence of androgens. For these tumors, blockade of androgens induces tumor regression in most patients. Hormonal manipulations to ablate or reduce circulating androgens can occur through several mechanisms[25,26] (Table 92–2). The organs responsible for androgen production can be removed surgically (orchiectomy, hypophysectomy, or adrenalectomy). Hormonal pathways that modulate prostatic growth can be interrupted at several steps (see Fig. 92–2). Interference with LHRH or LH (by estrogens, LHRH agonists, progesterones, and cyproterone acetate) can reduce testosterone secretion by the testes. Estrogen administration reduces androgens by directly inhibiting LH release, by acting directly on the prostate cell, or by decreasing free androgens by increasing steroid-binding globulin levels.[24-26]

Isolation of the naturally occurring hypothalamic decapeptide hormone LHRH has provided another group of

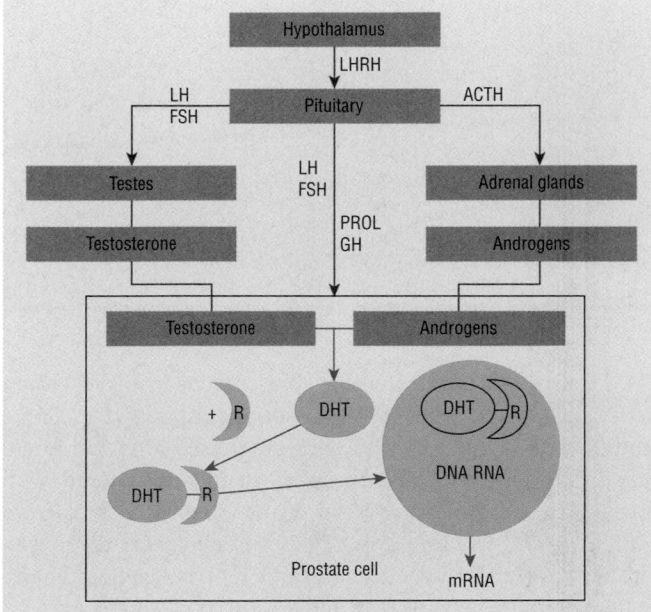

FIGURE 92–2. Hormonal regulation of the prostate gland. ACTH, adrenocorticotropic hormone; DHT, dihydrotestosterone; FSH, follicle-stimulating hormone; GH, growth hormone; LH, luteinizing hormone; LHRH, luteinizing hormone–releasing hormone; PROL, prolactin; R, receptor. (From DiPiro JT, Talbert RL, Yee GC, et al, eds. Pharmacotherapy: A Pathophysiologic Approach, 6th ed. New York: McGraw-Hill, 2005: 1856.)

Table 92–2	
Hormonal Manipulations in Prostate Cancer	
Androgen source ablation	Antiandrogens
Orchiectomy	Flutamide
Adrenalectomy	Bicalutamide
Hypophysectomy	Nilutamide
LHRH or LH inhibition	Cyproterone acetate[b]
Estrogens	Progesterones
LHRH agonists	5-α-reductase inhibition
Progesterones[a]	Finasteride[b]
Cyproterone acetate[b]	Dutasteride[b]
Gonadotropin receptor antagonists	
Abarelix	
Degarelix	
Androgen synthesis inhibition	
Aminoglutethimide	
Ketoconazole	
Progesterones[a]	

LH, luteinizing hormone; LHRH, luteinizing hormone–releasing hormone.

[a]Minor mechanisms of action.

[b]Investigational compounds or use.

effective agents for advanced prostate cancer treatment. The physiologic response to LHRH depends on both the dose and the mode of administration. Intermittent pulsed LHRH administration, which mimics the endogenous release pattern, causes sustained release of both LH and FSH, whereas high dose or continuous IV administration of LHRH inhibits gonadotropin release due to receptor downregulation.[19] Structural modification of the naturally occurring LHRH and innovative delivery have produced a series of LHRH agonists that cause a similar downregulation of pituitary receptors and a decrease in testosterone production.[27]

Androgen synthesis can also be inhibited in the testes or adrenal gland. Aminoglutethimide inhibits the desmolase-enzyme complex in the adrenal gland, thereby preventing the conversion of cholesterol to pregnenolone. Pregnenolone is the precursor substrate for all adrenal-derived steroids, including androgens, glucocorticoids, and mineralocorticoids. Ketoconazole, an imidazole antifungal agent, causes a dose-related reversible reduction in serum cortisol and testosterone concentration by inhibiting both adrenal and testicular steroidogenesis.[28] Megestrol is a synthetic derivative of progesterone that exhibits a secondary mechanism of action by inhibiting the synthesis of androgens. This inhibition appears to occur at the adrenal level, but circulating levels of testosterone also are reduced, suggesting that inhibition at the testicular level also may occur.[28]

Antiandrogens inhibit the formation of the DHT-receptor complex and thereby interfere with androgen-mediated action at the cellular level.[28] Megestrol acetate, a progestational agent, also is available and has antiandrogen actions.[28] Finally, the conversion of testosterone to DHT may be inhibited by 5-α-reductase inhibitors.[7]

In advanced stages of the disease, prostate cancer cells may be able to survive and proliferate without the signals normally provided by circulating androgens.[29] When this occurs, the tumors are no longer sensitive to therapies that are dependent on androgen blockade. These tumors are often referred to as hormone refractory or androgen independent.

CLINICAL PRESENTATION AND DIAGNOSIS

Prior to the implementation of routine screening, prostate cancers were frequently identified on the investigation of symptoms including urinary hesitancy, retention, painful urination, hematuria, and erectile dysfunction. With the introduction of screening techniques, most prostate cancers are now identified prior to the development of symptoms.[30]

The information obtained from the diagnostic tests is used to stage the patient. There are two commonly recognized staging classification systems (Table 92–3). The formal international classification system (tumor, node, metastases; TNM), adopted by the International Union Against Cancer in 1974, was last updated in 2002. The AUA classification is the most commonly used staging system in the United States (Table 92–4). Patients are assigned to stages A through D and corresponding subcategories based on the size of the tumor

---

Clinical Presentation of Prostate Cancer

Localized Disease

Asymptomatic

Locally Invasive Disease

Ureteral dysfunction, frequency, hesitancy, and dribbling

Impotence

Advanced Disease

Back pain

Cord compression

Lower extremity edema

Pathologic fractures

Anemia

Weight loss

Table 92–3

Diagnostic and Staging and Classification Systems Workup for Prostate Cancer

Initial tests	Digital rectal examination (DRE)
	Prostate-specific antigen (PSA)
	Transrectal ultrasound (TRUS) if either DRE is positive or PSA is elevated
	Biopsy
Staging tests	Gleason score on biopsy specimen
	Bone scan
	CBC
	Liver function tests
	Serum phosphatases (acid/alkaline)
	Excretory urogram
	Chest x-ray
Additional staging tests (depends on tumor classification, PSA, and Gleason score)	Skeletal films
	Lymph node evaluation
	Pelvic CT
	^{111}In-labeled capromab pendetide scan
	Bipedal lymphangiogram
	Transrectal MRI

(T), local or regional extension, presence of involved lymph node groups (N), and presence of metastases (M). Some studies classify patients who have progressed after hormonal therapy as stage D_3.[31] On the basis of men diagnosed with prostate cancer at Walter Reed Army Medical Center from 1988 to 1998, including over 2,042 prostate cancer diagnoses, localized prostate cancer (stage T_1 and T_2) was diagnosed more frequently (89% versus 68%), and advanced disease (stages T_3, T_4, and D) was diagnosed less frequently (11% versus 32%) when comparing the incidence rates in 1998 to the 1988 rates[31].

❸ *The prognosis for patients with prostate cancer depends on the histologic grade, tumor size, and local extent of the primary tumor.*[23] The most important prognostic criterion appears to be the histologic grade because the degree of differentiation ultimately determines the stage of disease. Poorly differentiated tumors are highly associated with both regional lymph node involvement and distant metastases.[23]

Table 92–4

Staging and Classification Systems for Prostate Cancer

AUA[a] Stage (A–D)	AJCC-UICC[b] Classification (TNM)
A (occult, nonpalpable)	$T_xN_xM_x$ (cannot be assessed)
	$T_0N_0M_0$ (nonpalpable)
A_1: Focal	T_0: Focal or diffuse
A_2: Diffuse	
B (confined to prostate)	$T_1N_0M_0$, $T_2N_0M_0$
B_1: Single nodule in 1 lobe, less than 1.5 cm	T_1 (Clinically inapparent tumor not palpable or visible by imaging)
	T_{1a}: Tumor incidental histologic finding in 5% or less of tissue resected
	T_{1b}: Tumor incidental histologic finding in 5% or more of tissue resected
	T_{1c}: Tumor identified by needle biopsy (e.g., because of elevated PSA)
B_2: Diffuse involvement of whole gland, greater than 1.5 cm	T_2: (Tumor confined within the prostate[c])
	T_{2a}: Tumor involves half of a lobe or less
	T_{2b}: Tumor involves more than half a lobe, but not both lobes
	T_{2c}: Tumor involves both lobes
C (localized to periprostatic area)	$T_3N_0M_0$, $T_4N_0M_0$
C_1: No seminal vesicle involvement, less than 70 g	T_3: (Tumor extends through the prostatic capsule[d])
	T_{3a}: Unilateral extracapsular extension
	T_{3b}: Bilateral extracapsular extension
	T_{3c}: Tumor invades the seminal vesicle(s)
C_2: Seminal vesicle involvement, greater than 70 g	T_4: Tumor is fixed or invades adjacent structures other than the seminal vesicles
	T_{4a}: Tumor invades any of bladder neck, external sphincter, or rectum
	T_{4b}: Tumor invades levator muscles and/or is fixed to the pelvic wall
D (metastatic disease)	Any T, N_{1-4}, M_0, or N_{0-4}, M_1
D_1: Pelvic lymph nodes or ureteral obstruction	N_1: Metastasis in a single lymph node, 2 cm or less in greatest dimension
D_2: Bone, distant lymph node, organ, or soft tissue metastases	N_2: Metastasis in single lymph node more than 2 cm but not more than 5 cm in greatest dimension; or multiple lymph node metastases, none more than 5 cm in greatest dimension
	N_3: Metastasis in lymph node more than 5 cm in greatest dimension
	M_{1a}: Nonregional lymph node(s)
	M_{1b}: Bone(s)
	M_{1c}: Other site(s)

[a]American Urologic Association.

[b]American Joint Committee on Cancer–International Union Against Cancer.

[c]Tumor found in one or both lobes by needle biopsy, but not palpable or visible by imaging, is classified as T_{1c}.

[d]Invasion into the prostatic apex or into (but not beyond) the prostatic capsule is not classified as T_3 but as T_2.

During 1996 to 2003, 5-year overall survival rates were estimated at 99% for whites and 95% for African Americans.[1] For this same period, the survival rates for localized or regional disease (100%) and distant disease (31%) in white males were about the same as the survival rates for localized or regional disease (100%) and distant disease (26%) in African American males.[1] A 4.1% decline in age-adjusted mortality has been documented for the period 1994 to 2004. 10-year cancer-specific survival is estimated as 95% for stage A_1, 80% for stages A_2 to B_2, 60% for stage C, 40% for stage D_1, and 10% for stage D_2.[32] It is estimated that more than 85% of patients with stage A_1 can be cured, whereas fewer than 1% of patients with stage D_2 will be cured.

TREATMENT

Desired Outcome

The desired outcome in early stage prostate cancer is to minimize morbidity and mortality due to prostate cancer.[33]

The most appropriate therapy of early stage prostate cancer is a matter of debate. Early stage disease may be treated with surgery, radiation, or watchful waiting. While surgery and radiation are curative, they are associated with significant morbidity and mortality. Since the overall goal is to minimize morbidity and mortality associated with the disease, watchful waiting is appropriate in selected individuals. Advanced prostate cancer (stage D) is not currently curable, and treatment should focus on providing symptom relief and maintaining quality of life.[34]

General Approach to Treatment

The initial treatment for prostate cancer depends primarily on the disease stage, Gleason score, presence of symptoms, and life expectancy of the patient.[33] Prostate cancer is usually initially diagnosed by PSA and DRE and confirmed by a biopsy, where the Gleason score is assigned. Asymptomatic patients with a low risk of recurrence, those with a T_1 or T_{2a}, with a Gleason score of 2 through 6, and a PSA of less than 10 ng/mL (10 mcg/L) may be managed by

Table 92–5

Management of Prostate Cancer With Low and Intermediate Recurrence Risk

Recurrence Risk	Expected Survival (years)	Initial Therapy
Low T_1-T_{2a} and Gleason 2–6 and PSA less than 10 ng/mL (10 mcg/L) and less than 5% tumor in specimen	Less than 10	Expectant management or radiation therapy
	Greater than or equal to 10	Expectant management or radical prostatectomy with or without pelvic lymph node dissection or radiation therapy
Intermediate T_{2b}-T_{2c} or Gleason 7 or PSA 10–20 ng/mL (10–20 mcg/L)	Less than 10	Expectant management or radical prostatectomy with or without pelvic lymph node dissection or radiation therapy with or without 4–6 months of androgen deprivation therapy
	Greater than or equal to 10	Radical prostatectomy with or without pelvic lymph node dissection or radiation therapy with or without 4–6 months of androgen deprivation therapy

expectant management, radiation, or radical prostatectomy (Table 92–5). As patients with asymptomatic early stage disease generally have an excellent 10-year survival, immediate morbidities of treatment must be balanced with the lower likelihood of dying from prostate cancer. In general, more aggressive treatments of early stage prostate cancer are reserved for younger men, although patient preference is a major consideration in all treatment decisions. In a patient with a normal life expectancy of less than 10 years, expectant management or radiation therapy may be offered. In those with a normal life expectancy of equal to or greater than 10 years, either expectant management, radiation (external beam or brachytherapy), or radical prostatectomy with a pelvic lymph node dissection may be offered. Radical prostatectomy and radiation therapy generally are considered therapeutically equivalent for localized prostate cancer, although neither has been proven to be better than observation alone.[34,35] Complications from radical prostatectomy include blood loss, stricture formation, incontinence, lymphocele, fistula formation, anesthetic risk, and impotence. Nerve-sparing radical prostatectomy can be performed in many patients; 50% to 80% regain sexual potency within the first year. Acute complications from radiation therapy include cystitis, proctitis, hematuria, urinary retention, penoscrotal edema, and impotence (30% incidence).[23] Chronic complications include proctitis, diarrhea, cystitis, enteritis, impotence, urethral stricture, and incontinence.[23] Since radiation and prostatectomy have significant and immediate mortality when compared with expectant management alone, many patients may elect to postpone therapy until symptoms develop.

Individuals with T_{2b} and T_{2c} disease or a Gleason score of 7 or a PSA ranging from 10 to 20 ng/mL (10–20 mcg/L) are considered at intermediate risk for prostate cancer recurrence.[33] Individuals with less than a 10-year expected survival may be offered expectant management, radiation therapy, or radical prostatectomy with or without a pelvic lymph node dissection, and those with a greater than or equal to 10-year life expectancy may be offered either radical prostatectomy with or without a pelvic lymph node dissection or radiation therapy (see Table 92–5).

The treatment of patients at high risk of recurrence (stages T_3, a Gleason score ranging from 8 to 10, or a PSA value greater

Table 92–6

Management of Prostate Cancer With High and Very High Recurrence Risk

Recurrence Risk	Initial Therapy
High T_{3a}, Gleason 8–10, PSA greater than 20 ng/mL (20 mcg/L)	Androgen ablation (2–3 years) and radiation therapy, or radiation therapy or radical prostatectomy with or without pelvic lymph node dissection
Locally Advanced, Very High T_{3b-T4}	Androgen ablation (2–3 years) or radiation therapy + androgen ablation (2–3 years)
Very High Any T, N_1	Androgen ablation or radiation therapy + androgen ablation
Any T, Any N, M_1	Androgen ablation

Androgen ablation = serum testosterone levels less than 50 ng/mL (1.74 nmol/L).

LHRH agonist (medical castrations or surgical are equivalent).

than 20 ng/mL [20 mcg/L]) should be treated with androgen ablation for 2 to 3 years combined with radiation therapy (Table 92–6). Selected individuals with a low tumor volume may receive a radical prostatectomy with or without a pelvic lymph node dissection.

Patients with T_{3b} and T_4 disease have a very high risk of recurrence and are not candidates for radical prostatectomy because of extensive local spread of the disease.[33]

❹ *Androgen ablation with a luteinizing hormone–releasing hormone (LHRH) agonist plus an antiandrogen should be used prior to radiation therapy for patients with locally advanced prostate cancer to improve outcomes over radiation therapy alone.* Recent evidence suggests that androgen ablation should be instituted at diagnosis rather than waiting for symptomatic disease or progression to occur. In a randomized clinical trial enrolling 500 men with locally advanced prostate cancer, who were randomized to either immediate initiation of androgen ablation with either orchiectomy or androgen

Patient Encounter 2: Initial Presentation and Treatment

FF is a 66-year-old male who presents to the clinic complaining of impotence for the last 1 to 2 months and requesting a prescription for Cialis. Upon questioning, he gives a history of fatigue, gradual weight loss of 10 lb, and difficulty with urination that began about 6 months ago.

Physical exam is positive for a 1-cm nodule in the prostate and his laboratories reveal the following: PSA 12 ng/dL (12 mcg/L); PSA from 1 year ago was 2 ng/dL (2 mcg/L).

A prostate biopsy by transrectal ultrasound (TRUS) reveals adenocarcinoma of the prostate, with a Gleason score of 8. CT scanning and bone scan reveal disease that is metastatic to the bone, and a final stage of T_4 (metastatic) prostate cancer is determined.

What is the pathophysiology underlying his clinical presentation?

Based on his stage, what are treatment options for this patient?

ablation, or deferred hormonal therapy, individuals with immediate therapy had a median actuarial cause-specific survival duration of 7.5 years for immediate treatment and 5.8 years for deferred treatment.[36]

⑤ *Androgen ablation therapy, with either orchiectomy, an LHRH agonist alone or an LHRH agonist plus an antiandrogen (combined androgen blockade), can be used to provide palliation for patients with advanced (stage D_2) prostate cancer.* Estrogens were once widely used; however, the primary estrogen, diethylstilbestrol (DES), was withdrawn from the U.S. market in 1997 due to the increased cardiovascular risk. Secondary hormonal manipulations, cytotoxic chemotherapy, or supportive care is used for the patient who progresses after initial therapy.[37]

Nonpharmacologic Therapy

▶ Expectant Management

Expectant management, also known as observation or watchful waiting, involves monitoring the course of disease and initiating treatment if the cancer progresses or the patient becomes symptomatic. A PSA and DRE are performed every 6 months with a repeat biopsy at any sign of disease progression. The advantages of expectant management are avoiding the adverse effects associated with definitive therapies such as radiation and radical prostatectomy and minimizing the risk of unnecessary therapies. The major disadvantage of expectant management is the risk that the cancer progresses and requires a more intensive therapy.[33]

▶ Orchiectomy

Bilateral orchiectomy, or removal of the testes, rapidly reduces circulating androgens to castrate levels (i.e., serum testosterone levels less than 50 ng/dL [1.74 nmol/L]).[22] However, many patients are not surgical candidates owing to their advanced age, and other patients find this procedure psychologically unacceptable.[22] Orchiectomy is the preferred initial treatment in patients with impending spinal cord compression or ureteral obstruction.

▶ Radiation

The two commonly used methods for radiation therapy are external beam radiotherapy and brachytherapy.[33] In external beam radiotherapy, doses of 70 to 75 Gy are delivered in 35 to 41 fractions in patient with low grade prostate cancer and 75 to 80 Gy for those with intermediate or high-grade prostate cancer. Brachytherapy involves the permanent implantation of radioactive beads of 145 Gy 125-Iodine or 124 Gy of 103-Palladium and is generally reserved for individuals with low-risk cancers.

▶ Radical Prostatectomy

Complications from radical prostatectomy include blood loss, stricture formation, incontinence, lymphocele, fistula formation, anesthetic risk, and impotence. Nerve-sparing radical prostatectomy can be performed in many patients; 50% to 80% regain sexual potency within the first year. Acute complications from radical prostatectomy and radiation therapy include cystitis, proctitis, hematuria, urinary retention, penoscrotal edema, and impotence (30% incidence).[15] Chronic complications include proctitis, diarrhea, cystitis, enteritis, impotence, urethral stricture, and incontinence.[22] Since radiation and prostatectomy have significant and immediate mortality when compared with observation alone, many patients may elect to postpone therapy until symptoms develop.

Pharmacologic Therapy

▶ LHRH Agonists

LHRH agonists are a reversible method of androgen ablation and are as effective as orchiectomy in treating prostate cancer[38] (Table 92–7). Currently available LHRH agonists include leuprolide, leuprolide depot, leuprolide implant, triptorelin depot, triptorelin implant, and goserelin acetate implant. Leuprolide acetate is administered once daily, whereas leuprolide depot and goserelin acetate implant can be administered either once monthly, once every 12 weeks, or once every 16 weeks (leuprolide depot, every 4 months). The leuprolide depot formulation contains leuprolide acetate in coated pellets. The dose is administered intramuscularly, and the coating dissolves at different rates to allow sustained leuprolide levels throughout the dosing interval. Goserelin acetate implant contains goserelin acetate dispersed in a plastic matrix of D,L-lactic and glycolic acid copolymer and is administered subcutaneously. Hydrolysis of the copolymer material provides continuous release of goserelin over the dosing period. A recently approved leuprolide implant is a mini-osmotic pump that delivers 120 mcg of leuprolide daily

Table 92–7 LHRH Agonist		
LHRH Agonist	Usual Dose	Adverse Effects (Similar for All Agents)
Leuprolide depot	7.5 mg every 28 days 22.5 mg every 12 weeks 30 mg every 16 weeks	Gynecomastia Hot flashes Decreased libido, impotence, Fatigue
Goserelin implant	3.6 mg every 28 days 10.8 mg every 12 weeks	Tumor flare in first 2 weeks Osteopenia with long-term use
Triptorelin depot	3.75 mg every 28 days 11.25 mg every 84 days	

for 12 months. After 12 months, the implant is removed and a different implant can be placed. Triptorelin LA is administered as an intramuscular (IM) injection of 11.25 mg every 84 days. Triptorelin depot is administered 3.75 mg once every 28 days.

Several randomized trials have demonstrated that leuprolide, goserelin, and triptorelin are effective agents when used alone in patients with advanced prostate cancer.[26] Response rates around 80% have been reported, with a lower incidence of adverse effects compared with estrogens.[26] There are no direct comparative trials of the currently available LHRH agonists or the dosage formulations, but a recent metaanalysis reported that there is no difference in efficacy or toxicity between leuprolide and goserelin. Triptorelin is a more recent addition but is generally considered equally effective. Therefore, the choice between the three agents is usually made on the basis of cost and patient and physician preference for a dosing schedule.

The most common adverse effects reported with LHRH agonist therapy include a disease flare-up during the first week of therapy, hot flashes, erectile impotence, decreased libido, and injection-site reactions.[26] The disease flare-up is caused by an initial induction of LH and FSH by the LHRH agonist, leading to an initial phase of increased testosterone production, and manifests clinically as either increased bone pain or increased urinary symptoms.[26] This flare reaction usually resolves after 2 weeks and has a similar onset and duration pattern for the depot LHRH products.[39,40] Initiating an antiandrogen prior to the administration of the LHRH agonist and continuing for 2 to 4 weeks is a frequently employed strategy to minimize this initial tumor flare.[27]

LHRH agonist monotherapy can be used as initial therapy, with response rates similar to orchiectomy. There is a lower incidence of cardiovascular-related adverse effects associated with LHRH therapy than with estrogen administration. Patients should be counseled to expect worsening symptoms during the first week of therapy, appropriate pain and symptom management is required during this period and a short course of concomitant antiandrogen therapy may need to be considered prior to initiating the LHRH agonist. Caution

should be exercised if initiating LHRH agonist therapy in patients with widely metastatic disease involving the spinal cord or having the potential for ureteral obstruction because irreversible complications may occur.

Another potentially serious complication of androgen deprivation therapy is a resultant decrease in bone-mineral density, leading to an increased risk for osteoporosis, osteopenia, and an increased risk for skeletal fractures. Most clinicians recommend that men starting long-term androgen deprivation therapy should have a base-line bone-mineral density and be initiated on a calcium and vitamin D supplement.[27]

▶ Gonadotropin-Releasing Hormone (GnRH) Antagonists

An alternative to LHRH agonists is the recently approved GnRH antagonist, degralix. Degralix works by binding reversibly to GnRH receptors on cells in the pituitary gland, reducing the production of testosterone to castrate levels. The major advantage of degralix over LHRH agonists is the speed at which it can achieve the drop in testosterone levels; castrate levels are achieved in 7 days or less with degralix, compared to 28 days with leuprolide, eliminating the tumor flare seen and need for antiandrogens, with LHRH agonists.

In a trial of 610 men with advanced prostate cancer, degralix was shown to be equivalent to leuprolide in lowering testosterone levels for up to 1 year and is approved by the FDA for the treatment of advanced prostate cancer. Degralix is available as a 40 mg/mL and a 20 mg/mL vial for SC injection and the starting dose is 240 mg followed by 80 mg every 28 days. The starting dose should be split into two injections of 120 mg.

The most frequently reported adverse reactions were injection-site reactions, including pain (28%), erythema (17%), swelling (6%), induration (4%), and nodule (3%). Most were transient and mild to moderate, leading to discontinuation in less than 1% of study subjects. Other adverse effects included elevations in lever function tests, which occurred in approximately 10% of study subjects. Like other methods of androgen deprivation therapy, osteoporosis may develop and calcium and vitamin D supplementation should be considered.

Degralix has not been studied in combination with antiandrogens and routine use of the combination cannot be recommended.

Like degralix, abarelix is a GnRH antagonist, with the same advantage of reducing testosterone to castrate levels rapidly and avoiding the tumor flare associated with LHRH agonists. Unfortunately, abarelix is also associated with severe allergic reactions, including syncope and hypotension, which occur in approximately 1% of initial doses and an increased frequency with repeat doses, for an incidence approaching 5% overall. Therefore, abarelix is available only through a restricted distribution program (Plenaxis PLUS Program) and is only indicated for men with advanced prostate cancer who cannot tolerate LHRH agonist therapy and who refuse surgical castration, and have one or more

Table 92-8 Antiandrogens		
Antiandrogen	**Usual Dose**	**Adverse Effects**
Flutamide	750 mg/day	Gynecomastia Hot flushes GI disturbances (diarrhea) Liver function test abnormalities Breast tenderness Methemoglobinemia
Bicalutamide	50 mg/day	Gynecomastia Hot flushes GI disturbances (diarrhea) Liver function test abnormalities Breast tenderness
Nilutamide	300 mg/day for first month then 150 mg/day	Gynecomastia Hot flushes GI disturbances (nausea or constipation) Liver function test abnormalities Breast tenderness Visual disturbances (impaired dark adaptation) Alcohol intolerance Interstitial pneumonitis

of the following: (a) risk of neurologic compromise due to metastases; (b) ureteral or bladder outlet obstruction due to local encroachment or metastatic disease; or (c) severe bone pain from skeletal metastases persisting on narcotic analgesia. The recommended dose of abarelix is 100 mg administered intramuscularly to the buttock on days 1, 15, 29 (week 4), and every 4 weeks thereafter.

Antiandrogens

Three antiandrogens, flutamide, bicalutamide,[39] and nilutamide,[38] are currently available (Table 92-8). Cyproterone is another agent with antiandrogen activity but is not available in the United States. Antiandrogens have been used as monotherapy in previously untreated patients, but a recent metaanalysis determined that monotherapy with antiandrogens is less effective than LHRH agonist therapy.[40] Therefore, for advanced prostate cancer, all currently available antiandrogens are indicated only in combination with androgen-ablation therapy; flutamide and bicalutamide are indicated in combination with an LHRH agonist; and nilutamide is indicated in combination with orchiectomy.[37]

The most common antiandrogen-related adverse effects are listed in Table 92-7. In the only randomized comparison of bicalutamide plus an LHRH agonist versus flutamide plus an LHRH agonist, diarrhea was more common in flutamide-treated patients. Antiandrogens can reduce the symptoms from the flare phenomenon associated with LHRH agonist therapy.[27]

Combined Androgen Blockade

Although up to 80% of patients with advanced prostate cancer will respond to initial hormonal manipulation, almost all patients will progress within 2 to 4 years after initiating therapy.[22] Two mechanisms have been proposed to explain this tumor resistance. The tumor could be heterogeneously composed of cells that are hormone dependent and hormone independent, or the tumor could be stimulated by extratesticular androgens that are converted intracellularly to DHT. The rationale for combination hormonal therapy is to interfere with multiple hormonal pathways to completely eliminate androgen action. In clinical trials, combination hormonal therapy, sometimes also referred to as maximal androgen deprivation or total androgen blockade, or **combined androgen blockade** *(CAB)*, has been used. The combination of LHRH agonists or orchiectomy with antiandrogens is the most extensively studied CAB approach.

Many studies comparing CAB with conventional medical or surgical castration have been performed.[31,41,42] In studies with LHRH agonists, the results have varied, with no consistent benefit demonstrated for CAB. A recently completed National Cancer Institute (NCI) intergroup trial involving 1,387 evaluable stage D$_2$ prostate cancer patients failed to show any significant survival benefits for the combination of orchiectomy plus flutamide over orchiectomy alone.[43] Like other studies of CAB, overall survival was longest in patients with minimal disease. Diarrhea, elevated liver function tests, and anemia were more common in those patients who received flutamide.

A metaanalysis of 27 randomized trials in 8,275 patients (4,803 treated with flutamide, 1,683 treated with nilutamide, and 1,784 treated with cyproterone) comparing CAB with conventional medical or surgical castration showed a small survival benefit at 5 years for those treated with flutamide or nilutamide (27.6%) compared to those with castration alone (24.7%; $P = 0.0005$).[41]

In one of the few combination androgen-deprivation studies comparing two different antiandrogens (bicalutamide versus flutamide), the time to treatment failure (the main study end point), time to progression (as defined by appearance of new or worsening bone or extraskeletal lesions), and time to death were equivalent, suggesting that the two treatments are equally effective.[44]

Although some investigators now consider CAB to be the initial hormonal therapy of choice for newly diagnosed advanced prostate cancer patients, the clinician is left to weigh the costs of combined therapy against potential benefits in light of conflicting results in the randomized trials[37] and the modest benefit seen in the metaanalysis.[41] For those trials that did show an advantage for CAB, whether these effects are specific to the testosterone-deprivation method (orchiectomy vs leuprolide vs goserelin), the antiandrogen, the duration of therapy, or patient selection is not clear. Until further carefully designed studies that use survival, time to progression, quality of life, patient preference, and cost as end points are conducted, it is appropriate to use either LHRH agonist monotherapy or CAB as initial therapy for metastatic prostate cancer. CAB may be most beneficial for improving survival in patients with minimal disease and for preventing tumor flare, particularly in those with advanced metastatic disease. All other patients may be started on LHRH monotherapy, and an antiandrogen may be added after several months if androgen ablation is incomplete.

There is considerable debate concerning when to start hormonal-deprivation therapy in patients with advanced prostate cancer.[26] The original recommendation to start therapy when symptoms appeared was based on the Veterans Administration Cooperative Urologic Research Group (VACURG) trials, in which no overall survival difference was demonstrated in patients who either started DES initially or crossed over to active treatment when symptoms appeared; the excess mortality was attributed to estrogen administration.[44] Because LHRH agonists and antiandrogens are viable therapies with less cardiovascular toxicity, it is not clear whether delaying therapy is justified with these agents. Reanalysis of the original VACURG data[45] and recent combined androgen-deprivation trials demonstrate a survival advantage for young, good-performance status, minimal-disease patients treated initially with hormonal therapy, suggesting that early intervention before symptoms appear may be appropriate.[45] The issue of when best to start hormonal therapy is the subject of several ongoing clinical trials.[45]

Secondary Therapies

Secondary or salvage therapies for patients who progress after their initial therapy depend on what was used for initial management.[33] For patients initially diagnosed with localized prostate cancer, radiotherapy can be used in the case of failed radical prostatectomy. Alternatively, androgen ablation can be used in patients who progress after either radiation therapy or radical prostatectomy.

In patients treated initially with one hormonal modality, secondary hormonal manipulations may be attempted. This may include adding an antiandrogen to a patient who incompletely suppresses testosterone secretion with an LHRH agonist. In patients that have progression while receiving CAB, withdrawing antiandrogens, or using agents that inhibit androgen synthesis may be attempted. Supportive care, chemotherapy, or local radiotherapy can be used in patients who have failed all forms of androgen-ablation manipulations because these patients are considered to have hormone-refractory prostate cancer.

For patients who initially received an LHRH agonist alone, castration testosterone levels should be documented. Patients with inadequate testosterone suppression (greater than 20 ng/dL, 0.7 nmol/L) can be treated by adding an anti-androgen or performing an orchiectomy. If castration testosterone levels have been achieved, the patient is considered to have androgen-independent disease, and palliative androgen-independent salvage therapy can be used.

❻ *Antiandrogen withdrawal, for patients having progressive disease while receiving combined hormonal blockade with an LHRH agonist plus an antiandrogen, can provide additional symptomatic relief. Mutations in the androgen receptor have been documented that cause antiandrogen compounds to act like receptor agonists.*

If the patient initially received CAB with an LHRH agonist with an antiandrogen, then androgen withdrawal is the first salvage manipulation.[33] Objective and subjective responses have been noted following the discontinuation of flutamide, bicalutamide, or nilutamide in patients receiving these agents as part of combined androgen ablation with an LHRH agonist. Mutations in the androgen receptor have been demonstrated that allow antiandrogens such as flutamide, bicalutamide, and nilutamide (or their metabolites) to become agonists and activate the androgen receptor. Patient responses to androgen withdrawal manifest as significant PSA reductions and improved clinical symptoms. Androgen withdrawal responses lasting 3 to 14 months have been noted in up to 35% of patients, and predicting response seems to be most closely related to longer androgen exposure times.[44] Incomplete cross-resistance has been noted in some patients who received bicalutamide after they had progressed while receiving flutamide, suggesting that patients who fail one antiandrogen may still respond to another agent. Adding an agent that blocks adrenal androgen synthesis, such as amino-glutethimide, at the time that androgens are withdrawn may produce a better response than androgen withdrawal alone. Because of the potential for response immediately after antiandrogen withdrawal, a sufficient observation and assessment period (usually 4–6 weeks) is usually required before a patient can be enrolled on a clinical trial evaluating a new agent or therapy for advanced prostate cancer.

Androgen synthesis inhibitors, such as aminoglutethimide 250 mg orally every 6 hours or ketoconazole 400 mg orally three times a day, can provide symptomatic relief for a short time in approximately 50% of patients with progressive disease despite previous androgen-ablation therapy.[37] Adverse effects during aminoglutethimide therapy occur in approximately 50% of patients.[37] CNS effects that include lethargy, ataxia, and dizziness are the major adverse reactions. A generalized morbilliform, pruritic rash has been reported in up to 30% of patients treated. The rash is usually self-limiting and resolves within 5 to 8 days with continued therapy. Adverse effects from ketoconazole include GI intolerance, transient rises in liver and renal function tests, and hypoadrenalism. Additionally, ketoconazole is a strong inhibitor of CYP1A2 and CYP3A4 and is contraindicated in combination with a number of medications that are commonly used in men with prostate cancer, including cisapride, lovastatin, midazolam, and triazolam because ketoconazole inhibits their metabolism and leads to increased toxicity. Arrhythmias often fatal have been reported with the combination of cisapride and ketoconazole. Absorption of ketoconazole requires gastric acidity; therefore, ketoconazole should not be administered with H2-blockers, proton pump inhibitors, or antacids. Additionally, ketoconazole should not be administered with strong CYP3A4 inducers, such as rifampin, as this may reduce the effectiveness of ketoconazole because it is also a substrate for CYP3A4. Ketoconazole is combined with

Table 92–9

First-Line Chemotherapy for Metastatic Hormone-Independent Prostate Cancer

Chemotherapy	Usual Dose	Adverse Effects	Dose Adjustments
Docetaxel	75 mg/m² every 3 weeks	Fluid retention, alopecia, mucositis, myelosuppression, hypersensitivity	*Hepatic* If AST/ALT is greater than 1.5 × the upper limit of normal and alkaline phosphatase is greater than 2.5 upper limit of normal, do not administer *Hematologic* Ensure complete blood count recovered
Estramustine	280 mg three times a day on days 1–5	Edema, gynecosmatia, leucopenia, increased risk of thromboembolic events	*Hematologic* Ensure complete blood count recovered

replacement doses of hydrocortisone to prevent symptomatic hypoadrenalism.[37]

After all hormonal manipulations are exhausted, the patient is considered to have androgen-independent disease, also known as hormone-refractory prostate cancer. At this point, either chemotherapy or palliative supportive therapy is appropriate. Palliation can be achieved by pain management, using radioisotopes such as strontium-89 or samarium-153 lexidronam for bone-related pain, analgesics, corticosteroids, bisphosphonates, or local radiotherapy.[33,45,46]

Skeletal metastases from hematogenous spread are the most common sites of distant spread of prostate cancer. Typically, the bone lesions are osteoblastic or a combination of osteoblastic and osteolytic. Bisphosphonates may prevent skeletal related events and improve bone-mineral density. A randomized, controlled trial of zoledronic acid at a dose of 4 mg every 3 weeks reduced the incidence of skeletal-related events by 25% ($P = 0.021$) compared to placebo.[47] The usual dose of pamidronate is 90 mg every month and the usual dose of zoledronic acid is 4 mg every 3 to 4 weeks. A trial of pamidronate or zoledronic acid can be initiated in prostate cancer patients with bone pain; if no benefit is observed, the drug may be discontinued.[48]

❼ *Chemotherapy with docetaxel and prednisone improves survival in patients with hormone-refractory prostate cancer.*

Docetaxel 75 mg/m² every 3 weeks combined with prednisone 5 mg twice a day improve survival in hormone-refractory metastatic prostate cancer.[49] The most common adverse events reported with this regimen are nausea, alopecia, and bone marrow suppression. In addition, fluid retention and peripheral neuropathy, known effects of docetaxel, are observed. Docetaxel is hepatically eliminated; patients with hepatic impairment may not be eligible for treatment with docetaxel because of an increased risk for toxicity.

The combination of estramustine (280 mg three times a day, days 1–5) and docetaxel 60 mg/m² on day 2 every 3 weeks also improves survival in hormone-refractory metastatic prostate cancer.[50] Estramustine causes a decrease in testosterone and a corresponding increase in estrogen; therefore, the adverse effects of estramustine include an increase in thromboembolic events, gynecomastia, and

Patient Encounter 3: Progressive Disease

AX is a 62-year-old male who was initially diagnosed with metastatic prostate cancer 5 years ago. He was initially started on leuprolide and has progressed through treatment as described in the treatment summary below.

Treatment Summary

Date	PSA	Intervention
9/2/04	25 ng/mL (25 mcg/L)	Started leuprolide 7.5 mg IM q month
12/2/04	2 ng/mL (2 mcg/L)	Continued leuprolide
6/2/06	22 ng/mL (22 mcg/L)	Added bicalutamide 50 mg po daily
9/2/06	5 ng/mL (5 mcg/L)	Continued leuprolide and bicalutamide
10/2/07	32 ng/mL (32 mcg/L)	Continued leuprolide, stopped bicalutamide
1/1/08	7 ng/mL (7 mcg/mL)	Continued leuprolide
1/1/09	67 ng/mL (67 mcg/mL)	

Today he presents to the clinic with bone pain and a serum PSA of 67 ng/mL (67 mcg/L).

Why was bicalutamide discontinued on 10/2/07?

How would you characterize the patient's disease?

What treatment is an option for him?

What long-term complications would you expect from his chronic androgen suppression?

decreased libido (Table 92–9). Estramustine is an oral capsule and should be refrigerated. Calcium inhibits the absorption of estramustine. While both the docetaxel/prednisone and the docetaxel/estramustine regimens are effective in hormone-refractory prostate cancer, most clinicians prefer the docetaxel/prednisone regimen because of the cardiovascular adverse effects associated with estramustine and the improved survival seen with docetaxel/prednisone. In addition, androgen ablation is usually continued when chemotherapy is initiated.[33]

Patient Care and Monitoring

1. Obtain complete past medical history, family history, and social history.

2. Obtain complete list of any concomitant prescription and over-the-counter medications, be sure to include herbal, vitamin, and mineral supplements.

3. Verify completion of prostate-cancer workup and staging.

4. Using information obtained, identify appropriate treatment options.

5. Discuss the benefits and risks of appropriate treatment options with health care team and patient.

6. If drug therapy is selected, review patient medical history for drug–drug, drug–herbal interactions.

7. Initiate therapy, if patient was asymptomatic, monitor PSA and circulating androgens for castration level of testosterone. If patient was symptomatic, monitor symptoms for improvement or worsening.

8. Monitor for any new symptoms and adverse events from therapy.

CAB	Combined androgen blockade
CI	Confidence interval
DES	Diethylstilbestrol
DHT	Dihydrotestosterone
DRE	Digital rectal examination
FSH	Follicle-stimulating hormone
GnRH	Gonadotropin-releasing hormone
IGF-1	Insulin-like growth factor-1
IM	Intramuscular
LH	Luteinizing hormone
LHRH	Luteinizing hormone–releasing hormone
NCI	National Cancer Institute
PCPT	Prostate Cancer Prevention Trial
PSA	Prostate-specific antigen
SELECT	Selenium and Vitamin E Cancer Prevention Trial
TRUS	Transrectal ultrasound
VACURG	Veterans Administration Cooperative Urologic Research Group

 Self-assessment questions and answers are available at *http://www.mhpharmacotherapy.com/pp.html.*

The regimen of mitoxantrone plus prednisone has been shown to be effective in reducing pain from bone metastasis and was a standard therapy prior to the development of docetaxel and prednisone. The effectiveness of mitoxantrone after failure of docetaxel-based therapy has not been scientifically evaluated. Many clinicians will treat patients with radiation therapy for palliation of symptoms after failure of docetaxel-based chemotherapy.[33]

OUTCOME EVALUATION

Monitoring of prostate cancer depends on the stage of the cancer.[33] When definitive, curative therapy is attempted, objective parameters to assess tumor response include assessment of the primary tumor size, evaluation of involved lymph nodes, and the response of tumor markers such as PSA to the treatment. Following definitive therapy, the PSA level is checked every 6 months for the first 5 years, then annually. Local recurrence in the absence of a rising PSA may occur, so the DRE is also performed. In the metastatic setting, clinical benefit responses can be documented by evaluating performance status changes, weight changes, quality of life, and analgesic requirements, in addition to the PSA or DRE at 3-month intervals.

Abbreviations Introduced in This Chapter

ASCO	American Society of Clinical Oncology
AUA	American Urological Association
BPH	Benign prostatic hyperplasia

REFERENCES

1. Jemal A, Siegel R, Ward E, et al. Cancer statistics, 2009. CA Cancer J Clin 2009;59:225–249.
2. Hsieh K, Albertsen PC. Populations at high risk for prostate cancer. Urol Clin North Am 2003;30:669–676.
3. Odedina FT, Ogunbiyi JO, Ukoli FA. Roots of prostate cancer in African-American men. J Natl Med Assoc 2006;98:539–543.
4. Denis L, Morton MS, Griffiths K. Diet and its preventive role in prostatic disease. Eur Urol 1999;35:377–387.
5. Crawford ED. Epidemiology of prostate cancer. Urology 2003;62:3–12.
6. Liede A, Karlan BY, Narod SA. Cancer risks for male carriers of germline mutations in BRCA1 or BRCA2: A review of the literature. J Clin Oncol 2004;22:735–742.
7. Thompson IM, Goodman PJ, Tangen CM, et al. The influence of finasteride on the development of prostate cancer. N Engl J Med 2003;349:215–224.
8. Gurel B, Iwata T, Koh CM, et al. Molecular alterations in prostate cancer as diagnostic, prognostic, and therapeutic targets. Adv Anat Pathol 2008;15:319–331.
9. Marberger M, Adolfsson J, Borkowski A, et al. The clinical implications of the prostate cancer prevention trial. BJU Int 2003;92:667–671.
10. Musquera M, Fleshner NE, Finelli A, et al. The REDUCE trial: Chemoprevention in prostate cancer using a dual 5alpha-reductase inhibitor, dutasteride. Expert Rev Anticancer Ther 2008;8:1073–1079.
11. Kramer BS, Haggerty KL, Justman S, et al. Use of 5-alpha-Reductase Inhibitors for Prostate Cancer Chemoprevention: American Society of Clinical Oncology/American Urological Association 2008 Clinical Practice Guideline Published Ahead of Print on February 24, 2009 as 10.1200/JCO.2008.16.9599.
12. Lippman SM, Klein EA, Goodman PJ, et al. Effect of selenium and vitamin E on risk of prostate cancer and other cancers: the Selenium and Vitamin E Cancer Prevention Trial (SELECT). JAMA 2009;301:39–51.

13. Neill MG, Fleshner NE. An update on chemoprevention strategies in prostate cancer for 2006. Curr Opin Urol 2006;16:132–137.

14. Schmid HP, Prikler L, Semjonow A. Problems with prostate-specific antigen screening: A critical review. Recent Results Cancer Res 2003;163:226–231.

15. Galic J, Karner I, Cenan L, et al. Role of screening in detection of clinically localized prostate cancer. Coll Antropol 2003;27(Suppl 1):49–54.

16. Wilson SS, Crawford ED. Screening for prostate cancer: Current recommendations. Urol Clin North Am 2004;31:219–226.

17. Gohagan JK, Prorok PC, Kramer BS, et al. The prostate, lung, colorectal, and ovarian-cancer screening trial of the National-Cancer-Institute. Cancer 1995;75:1869–1873.

18. Catalona WJ, Smith DS, Ratliff TL, et al. Measurement of prostate-specific antigen in serum as a screening test for prostate cancer. N Engl J Med 1991;324:1156–1161.

19. Screening for prostate cancer: U.S. Preventive Services Task Force recommendation statement. Ann Intern Med 2008;149:185–191.

20. Harris R, Lohr KN. Screening for prostate cancer: An update of the evidence for the U.S. Preventive Services Task Force. Ann Intern Med 2002;137:917–929.

21. Ross KS, Carter HB, Pearson JD, et al. Comparative efficiency of prostate-specific antigen screening strategies for prostate cancer detection. JAMA 2000;284:1399–1405.

22. Khauli RB. Prostate cancer: Diagnostic and therapeutic strategies with emphasis on the role of PSA. J Med Liban 2005;53:95–102.

23. Iczkowski KA. Current prostate biopsy interpretation: Criteria for cancer, atypical small acinar proliferation, high-grade prostatic intraepithelial neoplasia, and use of immunostains. Arch Pathol Lab Med 2006;130:835–843.

24. De Marzo AM, Meeker AK, Zha S, et al. Human prostate cancer precursors and pathobiology. Urology 2003;62:55–62.

25. Culig Z. Role of the androgen receptor axis in prostate cancer. Urology 2003;62:21–26.

26. Marks LS. Luteinizing hormone-releasing hormone agonists in the treatment of men with prostate cancer: Timing, alternatives, and the 1-year implant. Urology 2003;62:36–42.

27. Sharifi N, Gulley JL, Dahut WL. Androgen deprivation therapy for prostate cancer. JAMA 2005;294:238–244.

28. Anderson J. The role of antiandrogen monotherapy in the treatment of prostate cancer. BJU Int 2003;91:455–461.

29. Nieto M, Finn S, Loda M, et al. Prostate cancer: Refocusing on androgen receptor signaling. Int J Biochem Cell Biol 2007;39:1562–1568.

30. Cooperberg MR, Moul JW, Carroll PR. The changing face of prostate cancer. J Clin Oncol 2005;23:8146–8151.

31. Labrie F, Dupont A, Cusan L, et al. Combination therapy with flutamide and medical (LHRH agonist) or surgical castration in advanced prostate cancer: 7-year clinical experience. J Steroid Biochem Mol Biol 1990;37:943–950.

32. Leach FS, Koh MS, Chan YW, et al. Prostate specific antigen as a clinical biomarker for prostate cancer: What's the take home message? Cancer Biol Ther 2005;4:371–375.

33. National Comprehensive Cancer Network. National Comprehensive Cancer Network guidelines for the management of prostate cancer. Prostate Cancer v.1. 2009, *www.nccn.org*.

34. Schroder FH, de Vries SH, Bangma CH. Watchful waiting in prostate cancer: review and policy proposals. BJU Int 2003;92:851–859.

35. Scher HI. Prostate carcinoma: Defining therapeutic objectives and improving overall outcomes. Cancer 2003;97:758–771.

36. The Medical Research Council Prostate Cancer Working Party Investigators Group. Immediate versus deferred treatment for advanced prostatic cancer: Initial results of the Medical Research Council Trial. Br J Urol 1997;79:235–246.

37. Oh WK. Secondary hormonal therapies in the treatment of prostate cancer. Urology 2002;60:87–92.

38. Prostate Cancer Trialists' Collaborative Group. Maximum androgen blockade in advanced prostate cancer: An overview of the randomised trials. Lancet 2000;355:1491–1498.

39. Hedlund PO, Henriksson P. Parenteral estrogen versus total androgen ablation in the treatment of advanced prostate carcinoma: Effects on overall survival and cardiovascular mortality. The Scandinavian Prostatic Cancer Group (SPCG)-5 Trial Study. Urology 2000;55:328–333.

40. Seidenfeld J, Samson DJ, Hasselblad V, et al. Single-therapy androgen suppression in men with advanced prostate cancer: A systematic review and meta-analysis. Ann Intern Med 2000;132:566–577.

41. Moul JW, Fowler JE, Jr. Evolution of therapeutic approaches with luteinizing hormone-releasing hormone agonists in 2003. Urology 2003;62:20–28.

42. Tyrrell CJ, Altwein JE, Klippel F, et al. Comparison of an LH-RH analogue (Goeserelin acetate, "Zoladex") with combined androgen blockade in advanced prostate cancer: Final survival results of an international multicentre randomized-trial. International Prostate Cancer Study Group. Eur Urol 2000;37:205–211.

43. Eisenberger MA, Blumenstein BA, Crawford ED, et al. Bilateral orchiectomy with or without flutamide for metastatic prostate cancer. N Engl J Med 1998;339:1036–1042.

44. Carcinoma of the prostate: Treatment comparisons. J Urol 1967;98:516–522.

45. Crawford ED, Kozlowski JM, Debruyne FM, et al. The use of strontium 89 for palliation of pain from bone metastases associated with hormone-refractory prostate cancer. Urology 1994;44:481–485.

46. Resche I, Chatal JF, Pecking A, et al. A dose-controlled study of 153Sm-ethylenediaminetetramethylenephosphonate (EDTMP) in the treatment of patients with painful bone metastases. Eur J Cancer 1997;33:1583–1591.

47. Saad F, Gleason DM, Murray R, et al. Long-term efficacy of zoledronic acid for the prevention of skeletal complications in patients with metastatic hormone-refractory prostate cancer. J Natl Cancer Inst 2004;96:879–882.

48. Posadas EM, Dahut WL, Gulley J. The emerging role of bisphosphonates in prostate cancer. Am J Ther 2004;11:60–73.

49. Tannock IF, de Wit R, Berry WR, et al. Docetaxel plus prednisone or mitoxantrone plus prednisone for advanced prostate cancer. N Engl J Med 2004;351:1502–1512.

50. Petrylak DP, Tangen CM, Hussain MH, et al. Docetaxel and estramustine compared with mitoxantrone and prednisone for advanced refractory prostate cancer. N Engl J Med 2004;351:1513–1520.

93 Malignant Lymphomas

Christopher Fausel and Patrick J. Kiel

LEARNING OBJECTIVES

● **Upon completion of the chapter, the reader will be able to:**

1. Discuss the underlying pathophysiologic mechanisms of the lymphomas and how they relate to presenting symptoms of the disease.

2. Differentiate the pathologic findings of Hodgkin's lymphoma (HL); follicular indolent non-Hodgkin's lymphoma (NHL); and diffuse aggressive NHL and how this information yields a specific diagnosis.

3. Describe the general staging criteria for the lymphomas and how it relates to prognosis; evaluate the role of the International Prognostic Index (IPI) for providing prognostic information for NHL.

4. Contrast the treatment algorithms for early and advanced-stage disease for HL.

5. Delineate the clinical course of follicular indolent and diffuse aggressive NHL and the implications for disease classification schemes and treatment goals.

6. Outline the general treatment approach to follicular indolent and diffuse aggressive NHL for localized and advanced disease.

7. Interpret the current role for monoclonal antibody therapy in NHL.

8. Assess the role of autologous hematopoietic stem cell transplantation (SCT) for relapsed HL and NHL.

KEY CONCEPTS

❶ B and T cells undergo neoplastic transformation that is governed by specific mutations in their chromosomes that result in populations of malignant lymphoma cells.

❷ Specific pathologic characteristics distinguishing Hodgkin's lymphoma (HL) from non-Hodgkin's lymphoma (NHL) include morphology, cell surface antigens, and chromosomal mutations.

❸ Classic signs and symptoms of the lymphomas include lymphadenopathy and B symptoms (i.e., fever, night sweats, and weight loss).

❹ The diagnosis of malignant lymphomas is established by tumor biopsy sample, analysis of the biopsy tissue, and determination of the extent of the disease in the patient.

❺ The goal of treatment of HL is cure for all stages of disease and first relapse.

❻ Follicular indolent NHL is incurable, so therapy goals focus on inducing and maintaining remission duration while minimizing treatment-related toxicities.

❼ Diffuse, aggressive NHL centers on curative-intent therapy using anthracyline-based combination chemotherapy for initial treatment and high-dose chemotherapy with autologous stem cell transplantation (SCT) for relapsed disease.

❽ The recombinant monoclonal antibody rituximab is an effective treatment option for patients with B-cell origin CD20+ NHL as a single agent and enhances the efficacy of combination chemotherapy regimens.

INTRODUCTION

The malignant lymphomas are a clonal disorder of hematopoiesis with the primary malignant cells consisting of lymphocytes of either B-cell, T-cell, and NK-cell origin. These cells originate from a small population of lymphocytes that have undergone malignant transformation secondary to a series of genetic mutations. Lymphoma cells predominate in the lymph nodes; however, they can infiltrate other tissues, such as the bone marrow, CNS, GI tract, liver, mediastinum, skin, and spleen. A diagrammatic overview of the lymph node regions is depicted in Figure 93–1. Lymphoma is categorized into two general headings: Hodgkin's lymphoma (HL) and non-Hodgkin's lymphoma (NHL), both containing numerous histologic subtypes that are pathologically distinct disease entities. HL is distinguished from NHL by the presence of the pathognomonic Reed-Sternberg (RS) cell. Other lymphomatous disease entities are classified as types of NHL.

The clinical course varies widely among histologies of HL and NHL. More aggressive lymphoma subtypes are highly proliferating tumor cells that require aggressive therapeutic intervention with chemotherapy, radiation therapy, or both. By contrast, certain subtypes of NHL are characterized by a disease course that flares and remits intermittently over a period of several years either with or without treatment.

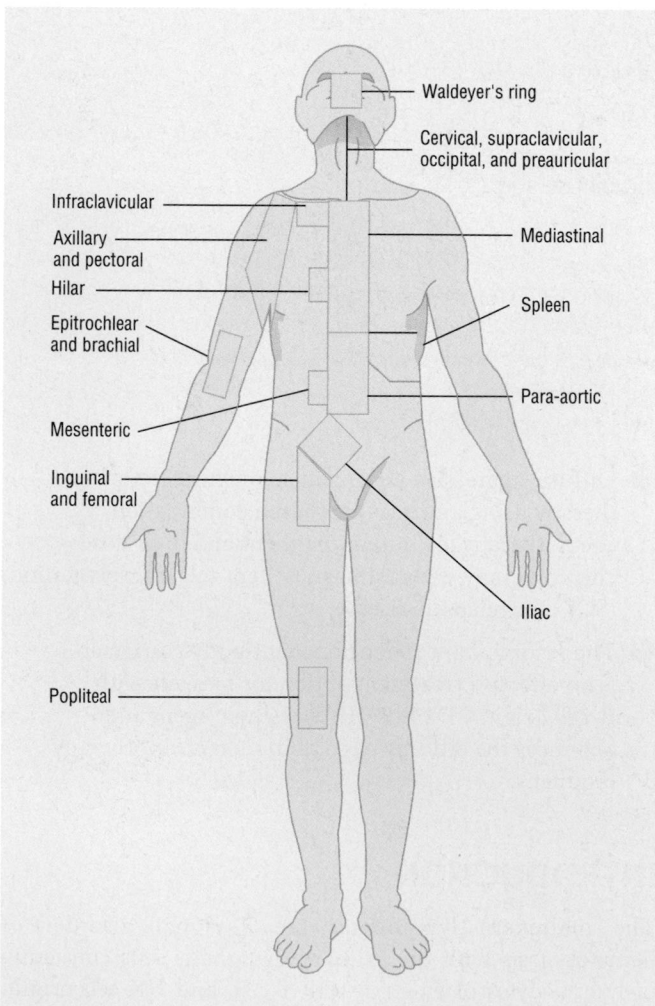

FIGURE 93–1. Representation of the anatomic regions used in the staging of Hodgkin's disease. (From Rosenberg SA. Staging of Hodgkin disease. Radiology 1966;87:146.)

Patient Encounter 1, Part 1

A 33-year-old male professional with no remarkable medical history notes shortness of breath while exercising, which has progressively worsened over the past 3 weeks. Upon review of systems, it is discovered that he has experienced intermittent sensations of shortness of breath over the past 2 months. His only medication is PRN antihistamines and he reports no known drug allergies. A chest x-ray is remarkable for a 10 cm × 12 cm mediastinal mass.

Is this age group at risk for a particular malignant diagnosis that presents as a mediastinal mass?

What is necessary to establish a diagnosis for this patient?

EPIDEMIOLOGY AND ETIOLOGY

Hodgkin's Lymphoma

Approximately 8,510 new cases of HL estimated to be diagnosed in the United States in 2009, with 1,290 deaths attributed to the disease. The age-specific incidence of HL is bimodal, with its greatest peak between ages 16 and 34 and a smaller peak in the fifth decade of life.[1] The precise cause of HL is unknown, but certain associations have been noted to provide insight about possible etiologic factors. Viruses, such as the Epstein-Barr virus (EBV), have been implicated by epidemiologic, serologic, and molecular studies. The EBV genome has been detected in RS cells in up to 50% of cases in developed countries and more in developing nations. To date, no conclusive studies have correlated HL with HIV. Other possible risk factors identified include woodworking and familial factors such as same-sex siblings with HL.[2]

Non-Hodgkin's Lymphoma

There are approximately 65,980 cases of NHL estimated to be diagnosed in the United States in 2009, with the number of deaths approaching 20,000. The incidence of the disease is increasing 4% per year, which has doubled the number of cases in the United States since 1950.[3] This increase is related to the development of aggressive NHL in 20- to 40-year-old men with HIV, although the overall increase is independent of HIV disease, particularly for patients older than 65 years of age. The median age for diagnosis is 50 years, although children and young adults may be affected. The etiology of certain aggressive NHL subtypes is related to specific endemic geographic factors. Follicular or low-grade lymphoma is more common in the United States and Europe and is relatively uncommon in the Caribbean, Far East, Middle East, or Africa. The human T-cell leukemia virus I (HTLV-I) induces T-cell lymphoma/leukemia in both Japan and the Caribbean. Kaposi's sarcoma-associated herpes virus, or human herpes virus 8 (HHV-8), and hepatitis C have been implicated in inducing NHL. Lymphomas of the GI tract are more prevalent in patients with celiac sprue, inflammatory bowel disease, or *Helicobacter pylori* infection. The incidence of Burkitt's NHL is 7 cases per 100,000 population in Africa, compared with 0.1 per 100,000 in the United States. Malaria or EBV is thought to contribute to the chronic B-lymphocyte stimulation that leads to malignant transformation. EBV has been shown to transform lymphocytes in vitro to a monoclonal malignant population, which is believed to drive the development of disease in patients who have received a solid-organ transplant or bone marrow transplant or have other chronic immunosuppressed states. Patients with congenital diseases such as Wiskott-Aldrich syndrome, common-variable hypogammaglobinemia, X-linked lymphoproliferative syndrome, and severe combined immunodeficiency are also at risk.[4] Environmental factors have been identified as contributing to the development of NHL. Certain occupations such as wood and forestry workers, butchers, exterminators, grain millers, machinists, mechanics, painters, printers, and industrial workers have a higher prevalence of disease. Industrial chemicals such as pesticides, herbicides, organic chemicals (e.g., benzene), solvents, and wood preservatives are also associated with NHL.

PATHOPHYSIOLOGY

Pluripotent stem cells in the bone marrow are able to differentiate to both lymphoid and myeloid progenitor cells. Lymphoid progenitor cells undergo gene rearrangement to yield either B-cell or T-cell lineage precursor cells. Normal maturation for naive B cells includes expression of cell surface antibody or the cells typically undergo apoptosis (programmed cell death). These cells are differentiated from other B cells, such as memory cells, by virtue of cell surface antigen (CD5+ or CD5– and CD27–) and bound antibody (IgM+ and IgD+). Once naive B cells recognize antigen with their cell surface antibody, they accumulate in the lymph nodes, spleen, or other lymphoid tissue. The DNA of these B cells is susceptible to three different types of genetic modification: receptor editing, somatic hypermutation, and class switching within the germinal center of the lymph node. Germinal centers are microanatomic structures located within lymph nodes that develop with clonal B-cell expansion secondary to antigen stimulation. Under normal circumstances, these genetic changes allow for adaptation of the immune system to the repeated exposure to environmental antigens.

Hodgkin's Lymphoma

The pathophysiology of HL is defined by the presence of the RS cell in a grouping of lymph nodes. The RS cell is a large cell morphologically with a multinucleated structure with pronounced eosinophilic nucleoli.[5] In the affected lymph nodes, the RS cells are contained in a reactive milieu of T lymphocytes, eosinophils, histiocytes, and plasma cells, which makes them difficult to distinguish from these background cells. The natural course of the disease, if left untreated, is less than a 5% probability of surviving 5 years.

RS cells are genetically derived preapoptotic germinal center B cells. There is evidence to suggest that a protein called c-FLIP that inhibits apoptosis garners protection for RS cells. RS cells express cell-surface antigens CD30 and CD15 while lacking other common B-cell antigens such as CD20. RS cells lack the expression of surface immunoglobulin likely owing to the lack of immunoglobulin transcription factors in normal B cells. The overexpression of a proproliferative and antiapoptotic transcription factor NF-κB is believed to contribute to the expansion and survival of RS cells.[6]

HL is classified into disease subtypes based on the number and morphologic appearance of RS cells and the background cellular milieu. These are listed in the WHO classification of lymphoid neoplastic diseases in Table 93–1.[7] Nodular

Table 93–1
WHO Classification of Lymphoid Neoplasms

B-Cell Neoplasms
Precursor B-cell neoplasm
Precursor B-lymphoblastic leukemia/lymphoma
Mature (peripheral) B-cell neoplasms
B-cell chronic lymphocytic leukemia/small lymphocytic lymphoma
B-cell prolymphocytic leukemia
Lymphoplasmacytic lymphoma
Splenic marginal zone B-cell lymphoma (+/– villous lymphocytes)
Hairy cell leukemia
Plasma cell myeloma/plasmacytoma
Extranodal marginal zone B-cell lymphoma of MALT type
Nodal marginal zone B-cell lymphoma (+/– monocytoid B cells)
Follicular lymphoma
Mantle-cell lymphoma
Diffuse large B-cell lymphoma
Mediastinal large B-cell lymphoma
Primary effusion lymphoma
Burkitt's lymphoma/Burkitt's cell leukemia

T-Cell and NK-Cell Neoplasms
Precursor T-cell neoplasm
Precursor T-lymphoblastic lymphoma/ALL
Mature (peripheral) T-cell neoplasms
T-cell prolymphocytic leukemia
T-cell granular lymphocytic leukemia
Aggressive NK-cell leukemia
Adult T-cell lymphoma/leukemia (HTLV1+)
Extranodal NK/T-cell lymphoma, nasal type
Enteropathy-type T-cell lymphoma
Hepatosplenic gamma-delta T-cell lymphoma
Subcutaneous panniculitis-like T-cell lymphoma
Mycosis fungoides/Sezary syndrome
Anaplastic large-cell lymphoma, T/null cell, primary cutaneous type
Peripheral T-cell lymphoma, not otherwise characterized
Angioimmunoblastic T-cell lymphoma
Anaplastic large-cell lymphoma, T/null cell, primary systemic type

HL
Nodular lymphocyte-predominant HL
Classical HL
Nodular sclerosis HL (grades 1 and 2)
Lymphocyte-rich classical HL
Mixed cellularity HL
Lymphocyte depletion HL

sclerosing HL is the most common form of HL, representing 70% of cases. It is more common in young adults and is marked by the presence of the RS variant cell, the lacunar cell. The second most common form of HL, accounting for approximately 25% of cases, is the mixed-cellularity variant, with others accounting for less than 5% of cases. Factors identified as negative disease prognostic indicators are listed in Table 93–2.[8]

Non-Hodgkin's Lymphoma

The pathophysiology of NHL is governed by numerous environmental and genetic events culminating with a monoclonal population of malignant lymphocytes. B cells represent the cells of origin in excess of 90% of cases of NHL. Figure 93–2 outlines normal B-cell maturation with accompanying cell-surface antigens. **❶** *Evolving data are correlating chromosomal mutations with specific disease subtypes. Cytogenetic abnormalities*

Table 93–2

Negative Prognostic Factors for HL and NHL

International Prognostic Score—Advanced HL
Albumin less than 4 g/dL (40 g/L)
Hemoglobin less than 10.5 g/dL (7.3 μmol/L)
Male sex
Age greater than 45 years
Stage IV disease
WBC greater than or equal to 15,000/mm³ (15 × 10⁹/L)
Lymphocytopenia (count less than 600/mm³ (0.6 × 10⁹/L), or less than 8% (0.08) of white blood cell count or both)

International Prognostic Index—Diffuse, Aggressive NHL
Age greater than 60 years
Stage III/IV disease
Extranodal disease greater than 1 site
ECOG performance status 2 or greater
Serum LDH greater than 1 × normal limit

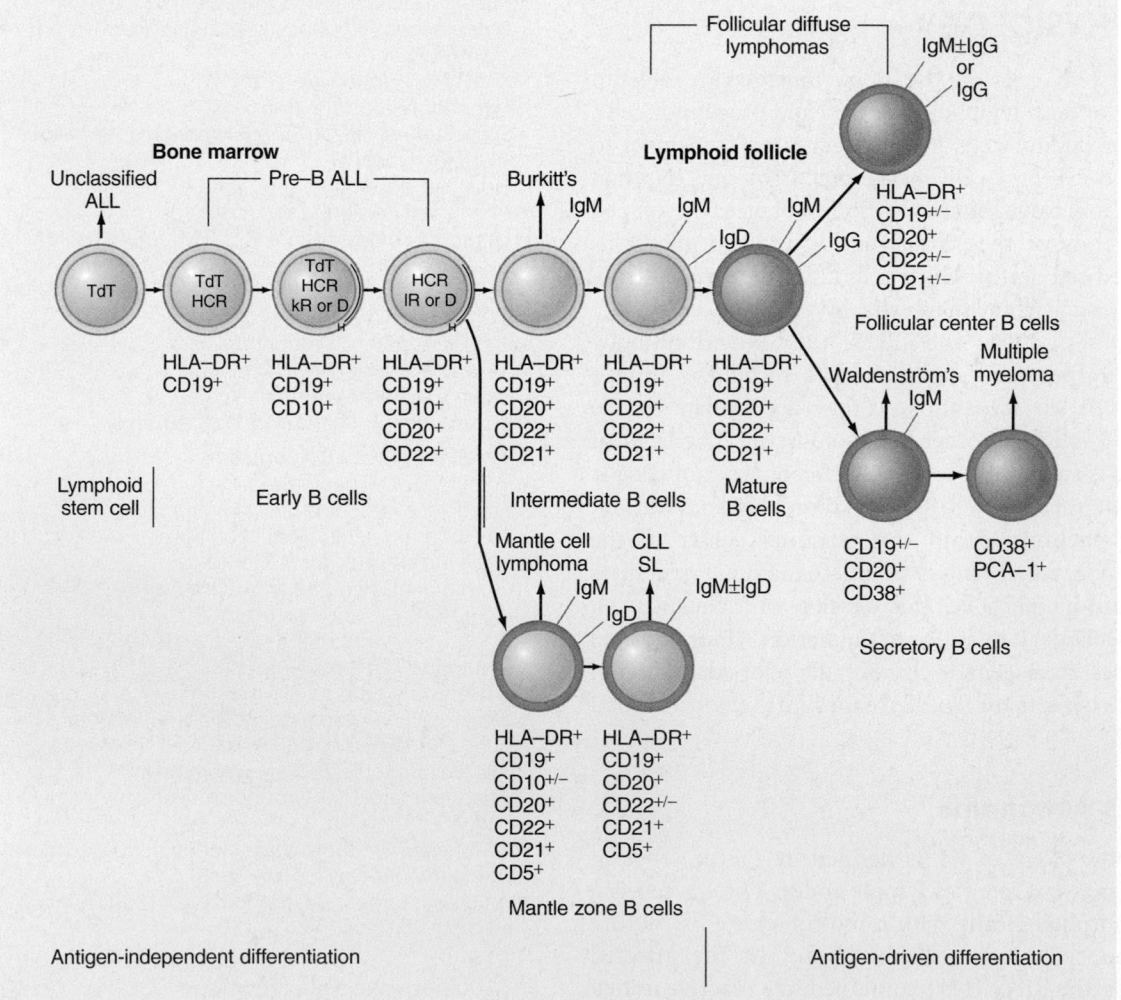

FIGURE 93–2. Pathway of normal B-cell differentiation and relationship to B-cell lymphocytes. (From Armitage JO, Longo DL. Malignancies in lymphoid cells. In: Kasper DL, Braunwald E, Fauci AS, et al., eds. Harrison's Principles of Internal Medicine. 16th ed. New York: McGraw-Hill, 2005:544.)

involving translocations of antigen receptor genes are prevalent in NHL. These include T-cell receptor genes in T-cell lymphomas and immunoglobulin genes in B-cell lymphomas. The principal defect appears to be an error in the assembly of the regulatory gene segment of an antigen receptor gene, resulting in inappropriate binding to an oncogene. This results in dysregulaton of cell growth and proliferation, giving rise to the malignant clone of lymphocytes. Oncogenes that have been identified in different lymphomatous diseases include *c-myc*, a regulator of gene transcription; *bcl-1*, important in the regulation of mitosis; *bcl-2*, a regulator of apoptosis; and *bcl-3*, *NF-κB*, and *bcl-6*, which regulate cell differentiation.[9] Classic translocations for NHL include t(8;14) in Burkitt's lymphoma, t(14;18) in follicular lymphomas, t(11;14) mantle cell lymphoma, and t(11;18)/t(1;14) in mucosa-associated lymphoid tissue (MALT).

❷ *Characterization of the morphology of the lymphocytes, the reactivity of the other cells in the lymph node, and the lymph node architecture is essential in obtaining a diagnosis and predicting disease course.* The nodal presentation of NHL is divided into two main categories: follicular, corresponding with low-grade disease, and diffuse, corresponding with aggressive disease. A follicular disease pattern in the inspected lymph node is indicative of a more indolent or low-grade disease progression that has survival measured in years if left untreated. In contrast, a diffuse pattern of lymph node infiltration is a marker of highly aggressive disease, resulting in death within weeks to months if left untreated. Follicular NHL is the most common indolent subtype, comprising 22% of NHL cases, where diffuse, large B-cell lymphoma is the most common aggressive histology in 31% of cases. The cells of origin for follicular NHL tend to be more mature, nondividing lymphocytes, whereas aggressive NHL is derived from rapidly dividing lymphoid precursors, such as immunoblasts, lymphoblasts, and centroblasts. A unique feature of the biology of NHL is that follicular low-grade histologies can undergo further malignant transformation, and a segment of malignant lymphocytes transforms further into a diffuse, large B-cell lymphoma population. This syndrome, called *Richter's transformation*, may occur in up to 20% of follicular low-grade lymphoma patients and involves multiple genetic events, including abnormalities of chromosomes 11 and 12 and tumor-suppressor genes.[10]

The classification of NHL has undergone several revisions as the histology, molecular biology, and clinical course of the disease have been more precisely defined. Classification schemes such as the *Working Formulation* categorize disease on aggressiveness into three general categories: Low grade—survival estimated in years without treatment; intermediate grade—survival estimated in months without treatment; and high grade—survival measured in days to weeks for untreated disease. This scheme is limited in its clinical applicability because the large number of distinct clinical disease entities is not categorized by this classification. The Working Formulation classification of NHL and diseases unclassifiable by

that system are presented in Table 93–3. The WHO has updated a classification scheme published in 1994 by the International Lymphoma Study Group called the *Revised European American Classification of Lymphoid Neoplasms* (REAL) that broadly categorizes histologic subtypes into B- and T-cell subtypes. This newer classification

Table 93–3	
Working Formulation for NHL	
Classification	**Immunophenotype**
Low Grade	
Small lymphocytic	100% B-cell
Follicular, small cleaved cell	100% B-cell
Follicular, mixed small cleaved cell and large cell	100% B-cell
Intermediate Grade	
Follicular, large cell	100% B-cell
Diffuse, small cleaved cell	75% B-cell, 20% T-cell, 5% null-cell
Diffuse, mixed small and large cell	75% B-cell, 20% T-cell, 5% null-cell
Diffuse, large cell	70% B-cell, 20% T-cell, 10% null-cell
Diffuse, large cell	70% B-cell, 20% T-cell, 10% null-cell
High Grade	
Immunoblastic	50% B-cell, 50% T-cell
Lymphoblastic	5% B-cell, 95% T-cell
Diffuse, small noncleaved cell	100% B-cell

Lymphomas not included in Working Formulation: Mycosis fungoides, mantle-cell lymphoma, monocytoid B-cell lymphoma, mucosa-associated lymphoid tissue (MALT), anaplastic large cell lymphoma, angiocentric lymphoma, angioimmunoblastic lymphadenopathy (AILD), Castleman's disease, adult T-cell leukemia/lymphoma.

Patient Encounter 1, Part 2

PMH: Allergies as a child

FH: Remarkable for colon cancer with maternal grandmother and lung cancer paternal grandfather

SH: Nonsmoker; social drinker

Meds: Loratidine 10 mg orally daily as needed

ROS: As mentioned previously

PE: T 38.0°C (100.4°F)

Labs: WNL, except LDH—2302

CXR: Patient is seen by a hematologist who recommends an open-lung biopsy by a cardiothoracic surgeon. The biopsy is conducted and pathology assessment shows nodular sclerosing Hodgkin's disease. The hematologist then conducts a staging workup with CT scans of the chest, abdomen/pelvis and performs a bone marrow biopsy.

What therapy is appropriate for this patient?

incorporates immunologic, morphologic, genetic, and clinical attributes of various NHL histologies.

Prognostic factors present at diagnosis have been identified for NHL. Age, presence of B symptoms, performance status, number of nodal and extranodal sites, lactate dehydrogenase (LDH) concentration, bulky disease (greater than 10 cm),

advanced stage, and β_2-microglobulin concentration have been correlated with survival. The International Prognostic Index (IPI) is a predictive model for aggressive NHL to be treated with doxorubicin-containing chemotherapy regimens.[11] This index is used as a tool for selecting therapy for patients who may warrant a more intense treatment regimen based on known poor prognostic factors.

TREATMENT OF HL

Desired Outcome

Staging of HL with a standard staging classification is necessary to guide appropriate treatment with chemotherapy, radiotherapy, or both. The number of involved sites, disease involvement on one or both sides of the diaphragm, localized or disseminated extranodal disease, and B-symptoms are factors in assignment of stage. The Cotswald staging system, a revision of the original Ann Arbor classification, is outlined in Table 93–4.[12]

⑤ *The principal goal in treating HL is to cure the patient of the primary malignancy.* HL is a disease sensitive to both radiation and chemotherapy, resulting in an 80% rate of cure with modern therapy. Treatment strategy generally is divided into approaches for early-stage I/II localized disease and stage III/IV advanced disease. Regardless of the stage of the disease, all patients are treated with curative intent. Other goals during treatment include:

- Complete resolution of symptoms of disease
- Minimization of acute treatment-related toxicity

Clinical Presentation and Diagnosis of Malignant Lymphomas

General

Nonspecific; can range from an asymptomatic patient with a less aggressive lymphoma to a patient that is gravely ill with advanced disease

❸ Symptoms

- *Lymphadenopathy, generally in the cervical, axillary, supraclavicular or inguinal lymph nodes*
- *Splenomegaly*
- *Shortness of breath, dry cough, chest pressure (patients with mediastinal mass)*
- *GI complications (nausea, vomiting, early satiety, constipation, and diarrhea)*
- *Back, chest or abdominal pain*

Signs

- *Fever**
- *Night sweats**
- *Weight loss greater than 10% within last 6 months**
- *Pruritis*

Laboratory Tests

- LDH
- Erythroid sedimentation rate (ESR)
- Serum chemistries
- CBC with differential

❹ Other Diagnostic Tests

- *Physical exam with careful attention to lymph node inspection*
- *Imaging—chest x-ray, chest CT, abdominal/pelvic CT; PET scan or gallium scan may be used to confirm presence of active disease after treatment*
- *Bone marrow biopsy*
- *Biopsy of suspected lymph node(s)—either open lymph node biopsy or core biopsy preferred over fine needle aspirate*
- *Hematopathology evaluation of biopsy specimen— morphologic inspection, immunohistochemistry for cell surface antigens to characterize lymphoma cells, cytogenetic analysis.*

---

*Known collectively as B symptoms.

Table 93–4	
Cotswald Staging Classification for Hodgkin's Disease (1989 Revision of Ann Arbor Staging)	
Stage	**Description**
I	Involvement of a single lymph node region of lymphoid structure (e.g., spleen, thymus, Waldeyer's ring)
II	Involvement of two or more lymph node regions on the same side of the diaphragm. The number of anatomic sites is indicated by a subscript
III	Involvement of lymph node regions or structure on both sides of the diaphragm
	III_1: With or without involvement of splenic, hilar, celiac, or portal nodes
	III_2: Involvement of para-aortic, iliac, or mesenteric.
IV	Involvement of extranodal site(s) beyond that designated E
Designations Applicable to All Stages	
A	No symptoms
B	Fever, night sweats, and weight loss
X	Bulky disease: greater than 1/3 the width of the mediastinum or greater than 10 cm maximal dimension of nodal mass
E	Involvement of a single extranodal site, contiguous or proximal to a known nodal site
CS	Clinical stage
PS	Pathologic stage

- Minimization of long-term treatment-related toxicity
- Provision of high-level supportive care to ameliorate the toxicities of chemotherapy and/or radiation therapy to optimize quality of life during treatment
- Selection of palliative therapy for refractory disease.

Nonpharmacologic Therapy

Patients presenting with stage I/II disease generally are curable with subtotal lymphoid irradiation, which involves treatment of the mantle and paraaortic fields. Radiation alone has overall 90% cure rate, with greater than a decade of follow-up. However, up to one-third of patients will relapse at the site of original disease presentation. If a patient relapses, then it likely will occur in the first 3 years after therapy has been completed. Fortunately, most of these patients are still curable with salvage chemotherapy.

Standard doses of radiotherapy for HL generally total 3,600 cGy to each field in daily fractions of 180 cGy over 4 weeks. Clinically involved areas are given boost doses of 550 to 900 cGy in three to five fractions, resulting in a total dose to the involved area of upwards of 4,500 cGy. Radiation may be given as consolidation following completion of a complete course of chemotherapy in patients with advanced HL.[13,14] This treatment typically is reserved for patients who have an unconfirmed response to chemotherapy or who have bulky disease on presentation.

Treatment with these doses of radiotherapy produces significant toxicity. Both acute and late effects of radiotherapy occur. Acute effects of mantle-field irradiation include nausea, vomiting, anorexia, xerostomia, dysgeusia, pharyngitis, dry cough, fatigue, diarrhea, and rash. Prophylaxis with antiemetics such as dexamethasone or prochlorperazine helps to prevent or treat nausea. These effects generally are transient and resolve shortly following completion of treatment. Delayed effects from radiotherapy are more concerning in that they may be permanent and present months to years after therapy is complete. Pneumonitis, pericarditis, hypothyroidism, infertility (with pelvic field irradiation), coronary artery disease, deformities in bone and muscle growth in adolescents and children, herpes-zoster reactivation, Lhermitte's sign, and secondary malignancies are not uncommon. Patients cured with radiotherapy are at increased risk for breast cancer, lung cancer (particularly in smokers), stomach cancer, melanoma, and NHL depending on the involved radiation field.

Pharmacologic Therapy

Chemotherapy compared with radiotherapy for Stage I or II nonbulky HL has produced equivocal results in major clinical trials.[15] A National Cancer Institute (NCI) trial comparing MOPP (mechlorethamine, vincristine, procarbazine, and prednisone) and radiotherapy showed no overall difference in survival. However, an Italian randomized trial comparing radiotherapy and chemotherapy in early-stage HL showed a significant survival advantage for the radiotherapy arm. This difference has been attributed to the higher salvage rate for patients who relapsed in the radiotherapy arm and received subsequent treatment with salvage chemotherapy. A complete listing of chemotherapy regimens used in HL with drugs, dosing, administration, and treatment interval is presented in Table 93–5.

In an attempt to reduce relapse rate and late toxicity, combined-modality therapy using lower doses of radiation and an abbreviated course of chemotherapy has been evaluated.[16] The goal of decreased relapse rate has been achieved, but no overall survival benefit has been documented. A limitation of this approach is exposing patients to the additive toxicities of chemotherapy. Trials that have investigated this approach typically have incorporated between two and four cycles of a standard regimen for HL, such as ABVD (doxorubicin, bleomycin, vinblastine, and dacarbazine) with involved-field radiation. At present, combined-modality therapy is considered to be a standard of care for stage I/II HL.

Table 93–5

Common Treatment Regimens in HL

MOPP—every 28 days
Mechlorethamine 6 m/m² IV × 1, days 1,8
Vincristine 1.4 mg/m² IV × 1, days 1,8
Procarbazine 100 mg orally daily, days 1–14
Prednisone 40 mg orally daily, days 1–14

ABVD—every 28 days
Doxorubicin 25 mg/m² IV × 1, days 1, 15
Bleomycin 10 units IV × 1, days 1, 15
Vinblastine 6 mg/m² × 1, days 1, 15
Dacarbazine 375 mg/m² IV, days 1,15

MOPP/AVD hybrid—every 28 days
Mechlorethamine 6 mg/m² IV × 1 day 1
Vincristine 1.4 mg/m² IV × 1; day 1
Procarbazine 100 mg orally daily, days 1–7
Prednisone 40 mg orally daily, days 1–14
Doxorubicin 35 mg/m² IV × 1 day 8
Bleomycin 10 units IV × 1 day 8
Vinblastine 6 mg IV × 1 day 8

ChlVPP—every 28 days
Chlorambucil 6 mg orally daily, days 1–14
Vinblastine 6 mg/m² IV × 1, days 1–8
Procarbazine 100 mg orally daily, days 1–14
Prednisone 40 mg orally daily, days 1–14

BEACOPP (escalated)—every 21 days
Bleomycin 10 mg/m² IV, day 8
Etoposide 200 mg/m² IV daily × days 1–3
Doxorubicin 35 mg/m², day 1
Cyclophosphamide 1,200 mg/m² IV, day 1
Vincristine 1.4 mg/m² IV, day 8
Procarbazine 100 mg/m² orally daily, days 1–14
Prednisone 40 mg orally daily, days 1–5
Gemcitabine 1,250 mg/m² IV × 1 days 1, 8 every 21 days

BCV (high-dose with autologous SCT)[a]
Carmustine 400 mg/m² IV × 1 day
Etoposide 800 mg/m² IV daily × 3 days
Cyclophosphamide 1,800 mg/m² IV daily × 4 days

BEAM (high-dose with autologous SCT)[a]
Carmustine 300 mg/m² IV × 1day
Etoposide 800 mg/m² IV × 1 day
Cytarabine 1,600 mg/m² IV × 1 day
Melphalan 140 mg/m² IV × 1 day

[a]Used for both HL and NHL.

Advanced Disease

Treatment of advanced-stage (stage III–IV) HL is focused on the use of multiagent chemotherapy for six to eight total cycles. MOPP is of historical significance because it was the first chemotherapy regimen to cure HL when it was introduced in the 1960s. However, the significant toxicity, including sterility and secondary leukemia, prompted investigators to evaluate other regimens. ABVD was compared with MOPP or ABVD alternating with MOPP.[17] This pivotal phase III Cancer and Leukemia Group B (CALGB, an alliance of cancer centers under the supervision of the National Cancer Institute that conducts national clinical trials in cancer) trial comparing these regimens in 361 patients with stage III or IV HL documented a higher complete response (CR) in the ABVD containing arms (82% and 83%) versus MOPP (65%). There was increased hematologic toxicity in the MOPP arm. A recent update of the data show the 8-year freedom from progression of 37% in the MOPP arm and about 50% in the ABVD containing arms. A survival advantage has yet to be demonstrated. ABVD is now considered standard therapy for initial treatment of stage III or IV HL. Further information on ABVD may be found in Table 93–6.

More recently, a German study compared a dose-escalated regimen of BEACOPP (with white blood cell colony stimulating factor support) with standard-dose bleomycin, etoposide, doxorubicin, cyclophosphamide, vincristine, procarbazine, prednisone, gemcitabine (BEACOPP) and COPP alternating with ABVD (C—cyclophosphamide instead of mechlorethamine for MOPP).[18] The escalated BEACOPP was superior to the other arms in freedom from treatment failure at 5 years and was superior to COPP alternating with ABVD in overall survival at 5 years. The escalated BEACOPP regimen had a higher number of cases of secondary leukemia, and the procarbazine increases the risk of infertility. Currently, this regimen has not been adopted widely in the United States, but considerable interest has been generated in evaluating it in patients with advanced-stage HL with a high number of poor prognostic factors.

Relapse in HL has the potential for cure with chemotherapy for both localized and advanced HL. For patients with early-stage HL, the chance of relapse is about 10% to

Patient Encounter 1, Plan 3: Creating a Care Plan

Based on the information presented, create a care plan for this patient including goals of therapy, antineoplastic therapy plan, and necessary supportive care.

30%. Advanced-stage HL patients, who have approximately a one-third chance of relapse within the first 3 years of therapy, still retain a chance for cure. Management of relapsed HL can be broadly subcategorized into three different categories: relapse after treatment for early-stage disease, relapse after treatment with chemotherapy for advanced disease, and relapse in patients with advanced disease who do not achieve a remission. For these patients, the definitive therapy is high-dose chemotherapy with autologous stem cell transplantation (SCT).[19] This treatment offers a cure rate of approximately 40%.

The role of SCT in HL has evolved from data with conventional four-drug regimens demonstrating that patients with lower dose intensity had a higher rate of relapse. Data comparing high-dose chemotherapy with lower doses of the same regimen yielded a significant benefit in the high-dose arm, leading to early closure of the study. High-dose chemotherapy is given to patients who are in first relapse with encouraging results. A series of 58 patients had a progression-free survival of over 60% with a median follow-up of 2.3 years. The safety profile of autologous SCT continues to improve as improvements in supportive care are realized, and current estimates of mortality from autologous SCT for HL approximate 5%. Morbidity commonly associated with the preparative regimens in HL, aside from infectious and bleeding complications, includes the additive pulmonary toxicity of bleomycin coupled with carmustine in inducing potentially fatal pulmonary pneumonitis.

Patients who are not deemed candidates for high dose chemotherapy with autologous SCT may receive multiagent salvage chemotherapy, such as etoposide, methylprednisolone,

---

Table 93–6

Practical Information for ABVD and CHOP

Regimen	Drug Class	Phamacokinetics	Unique Toxicities
ABVD			
Doxorubicin	Anthracycline	Hepatic metabolism	Cardiomyopathy
Bleomycin	Antitumor antibiotic	Renal clearance	Pulmonary fibrosis
Vinblastine	Vinca alkaloid	CYP 3A4/5 metabolism	Neuropathy, constipation
Dacarbazine	Alkylating agent	Hepatic metabolism	Myelosuppression
CHOP			
Cyclophosphamide	Alkylating agent	Prodrug; CYP3A4/5, 2D6	Hemorrhagic cystitis
Doxorubicin	Anthracycline	Hepatic metabolism	Cardiomyopathy
Vincristine	Vinca alkaloid	CYP3A4/5	Neuropathy, constipation
Prednisone	Corticosteroid	100% oral bioavailability	Hyperglycemia, osteopenia

cytarabine, and cisplatin (ESHAP) or dexamethasine, cytarabine, and cisplatin (DHAP). If less aggressive therapy is desired, patients can be offered palliation with single-agent gemcitabine or vinblastine.[20]

TREATMENT OF NHL

Desired Outcome

Treatment of NHL depends primarily on histologic subtype (follicular low grade versus diffuse aggressive) and staging (local stage I/II versus advanced stage III/IV) to guide appropriate treatment strategy with observation, chemotherapy, radiotherapy, or chemotherapy and radiation. As with HL, the number of involved sites, disease involvement on one or both sides of the diaphragm, localized or disseminated extranodal disease, and B-symptoms are factors in staging assignment. The Ann Arbor staging system is outlined in Table 93–7.[21]

Treatment goals for NHL depend on the presence of follicular low-grade versus diffuse aggressive disease. For follicular low-grade NHL, the disease is considered to be incurable with standard therapies There is a small prospect for cure using allogeneic SCT owing to the graft-versus-lymphoma effect of donor T cells. Many patients with follicular low-grade NHL are older than 60 years of age, making allogeneic SCT impractical owing to the high treatment-related mortality for older patients.

❻ *The treatment goals for low-grade NHL include:*

- *Observation of the disease until the patient exhibits obvious progression that limits functional capacity or is life-threatening for low-grade NHL*

- Treatment that induces the disease into remission with resolution of disease symptoms and manageable toxicity

- Judicious selection of treatment options to avoid long-term toxicity because patients may require several different chemotherapy treatment regimens over a period of years for low-grade NHL

- Prevention of infectious complications of treatment

The treatment aim for patients with aggressive histologies is cure of the malignancy. There are some histologic subtypes that exhibit an aggressive clinical course that are not considered to be curable. These patients are still treated with curative-intent chemotherapy or may be considered for a clinical trial.

Nonpharmacologic Therapy

For patients with low-grade follicular NHL, deferring initiation of therapy until progression of disease is standard. The median survival is 6 to 10 years, with some patients waiting several years before the disease becomes symptomatic, making observation a reasonable front-line therapy for most of these patients. Radiation therapy has a limited role in NHL relative to HL. NHL is a systemic disease, and radiation typically has been reserved for consolidation therapy following chemotherapy in patients presenting with a large extranodal mass.

For early-stage diffuse, aggressive NHL, combined-modality therapy was tested versus a longer course of chemotherapy.[22] Overall survival favored the cyclophosphamide doxorubicin vincristine prednisone (CHOP)/radiation arm for 5 years (82% versus 72%). There was a trend toward increased toxicity, particularly hematologic and cardiac toxicity, in the CHOP alone arm. The results of this trial have established combined-modality therapy as first-line treatment for early-stage NHL. Unique presentations of NHL, such as CNS primary disease, may incorporate radiation into treatment algorithms.[23]

Pharmacologic Therapy

▶ Follicular Low-Grade NHL

The management of low-grade lymphomas is an area of controversy. Chemotherapy such as single-agent oral cyclophosphamide or fludarabine is often offered initially. In patients in whom a more rapid response is desired, multiagent chemotherapy such as cyclophosphamide vincristine prednisone (CVP) or cyclophosphamide doxorubicin vincristine prednisone (CHOP) may be used. None of these therapies is associated with an improvement in overall survival, making it impossible to select an unequivocal first-line regimen.[24–26] These regimens are detailed in Table 93–8.

Introduction of the monoclonal antibody rituximab has prompted interest in a novel modality of therapy for this disease. Rituximab is a chimeric murine/human monoclonal antibody that binds specifically to the antigen CD20 expressed on pre-B and mature B lymphocytes.[27] NHL of B-cell origin expresses CD20 in greater than 90% of cases. CD20 is believed to play a role in early differentiation and activation of the cell cycle. After the Fab domain of rituximab binds to CD20, the Fc domain acts to recruit

Stage	Description
Table 93–7	
Ann Arbor Staging of NHL	
Stage	**Description**
I	Involvement of a single lymph node region (I) or a single extralymphatic organ or site (IE)
II	Involvement of two or more lymph node regions on the same side of the diaphragm(II) or localized involvement of an extralymphatic organ or site (IIE)
II	Involvement of two or more lymph node regions on the same side of the diaphragm(II) or localized involvement of an extralymphatic organ or site (IIE)
III	Involvement of lymph node regions on both sides of the diaphragm (III), or localized involvement of an extralymphatic organ or site (IIIE) or spleen (IIIS) or both (IIISE)
IV	Diffuse or disseminated involvement of one or more extranodal organs with or without associated lymph node involvement
Designations Applicable to All Stages	
A	No symptoms
B	Fever, night sweats, and weight loss (greater than 10%)

Table 93–8

Treatment Regimens for Low-Grade, Follicular NHL

Cyclophosphamide (100 mg/m²) orally daily
Fludarabine 25 mg/m² IV daily, days 1–5
Rituximab 375 mg/m² IV day 1 given weekly for 4 or 8 weeks

CVP every 21 days
Cyclophosphamide 800 mg/m² IV, day 1
Vincristine 1.4 mg/m² IV, day 1
Prednisone 100 mg orally daily, days 1–5

rCVP every 21 days
Rituximab 375 mg/m² IV day 1
Cyclophosphamide 800 mg/m² IV, day 1
Vincristine 1.4 mg/m² IV, day 1
Prednisone 100 mg orally daily, day 1–5

CHOP every 21 days
Cyclophosphamide 750 mg/m² IV, day 1
Doxorubicin 50 mg/m² IV, day 1
Vincristine 1.4 mg/m² IV, day 1
Prednisone 100 mg orally daily, day 1–5

rCHOP every 21 days
Rituximab 375 mg/m² IV, day 1
Cyclophosphamide 750 mg/m² IV, day 1
Doxorubicin 50 mg/m² IV, day 1
Vincristine 1.4 mg/m² IV, day 1
Prednisone 100 mg orally daily, day 1–5

complement and other components of the immune system to induce cell-mediated cytotoxicity with subsequent lysis of the bound lymphocytes. Rituximab also may produce apoptosis of the bound lymphocyte with the act of binding to the CD20 receptor. Rituximab has specific affinity for binding to lymphocytes and lymphoid tissue, begins depleting B lymphocytes with the first dose, and results in sustained suppression for 6 to 9 months with as few as three doses. B-cell recovery begins 6 months following administration of the drug. The drug has a half-life of 60 hours with the first dose that increases with subsequent dosing to approximately 150 hours, allowing for weekly dosing. The initial clinical experience with rituximab involved 166 patients with CD20+ low-grade lymphoma treated with four doses of 375 mg/m² of rituximab weekly.[28] The overall response rate was 48%, with 6% representing complete responses and the remainder representing partial responses. The median follow-up of 12 months demonstrated a median time to progression of 13 months by intention-to-treat analysis. Most adverse events were related to intolerance of the first infusion with hypotension, fever, chills, nausea, and bronchospasm. These data established the role of rituximab as a viable treatment option in patients with indolent follicular NHL. Further research has examined rituximab as maintenance therapy administered once every 3 months for up to 2 years following CHOP+/-R in patients with relapsed or resistant disease. Compared to an observational group, rituximab resulted in increased progression-free survival (51 versus 14 months) and 3-year overall survival rates (85% versus 77%).[29]

Novel strategies for treatment of low-grade lymphomas include the combination of monoclonal antibodies directed

against CD20 with a radioactive moiety attached. Two such entities are now approved by the FDA: ibritumomab-yttrium 90 (Zevalin) and tositumomab-iodine[131] (Bexxar). Both agents are active in disease that has become refractory to rituximab. The radiation component necessitates compounding both medications in a nuclear medicine pharmacy. High-dose chemotherapy is being evaluated for low-grade follicular NHL, but its role is currently limited to clinical trials. Bendamustine, a unique alkalyting agent with a novel chemical structure, has been studied in a phase II trial of rituximab-refractory and transformed NHL. Among 74 assessable patients, an overall response rate of 77% was noted with a progression free survival of 7.1 months.[30]

▶ Diffuse, Aggressive NHL

❼ *The mainstay of therapy for diffuse, aggressive NHL has been the administration of anthracycline-based combination chemotherapy, which generally consists of programs of four or more drugs.* Therapy options for intermediate- and high-grade NHL generally are segregated between localized (stage I/II) and disseminated (stage III/IV) disease. Combined-modality therapy with an abbreviated course of CHOP and local radiation is considered a standard of care for stage I/II disease.

The standard therapy for disseminated disease since the 1970s has been CHOP. This regimen conferred a response of 50% to 60%, with a long-term survival of approximately 30%. However, the 1980s were notable for the development of newer combination chemotherapy regimens that incorporated increasing numbers of agents with varying schedules. More complex chemotherapy regimens were shown in phase II trials to have higher response rates than CHOP. The CALGB designed a phase III randomized four-arm trial to assess the impact on survival of three more intensive regimens compared with CHOP.[31] This phase III cooperative group trial randomized 899 patients with intermediate- or high-grade (Working Formulation classification) NHL to CHOP or one of the three more intensive advanced-generation regimens. There were no significant differences in response rate or overall survival, which was consistent among all subgroups. Severe toxicity and death were higher in the advanced-generation treatment programs relative to CHOP. This pivotal trial has cemented CHOP's position as front-line therapy in diffuse NHL.

The next hypothesis tested was whether combining monoclonal antibody therapy with chemotherapy could increase activity against diffuse, aggressive NHL. A French study randomized patients 60 to 80 years of age with newly diagnosed diffuse, large B-cell NHL to either CHOP for eight cycles or CHOP plus rituximab for eight cycles.[32] At relatively early follow-up of 2 years, the combination arm had a superior complete response rate (76% versus 63%) and event-free survival (57% versus 38%), with comparable toxicity in each arm. Similar findings in younger patients have been reported recently, making CHOP plus rituximab first-line therapy for advanced-stage diffuse, aggressive NHL (Table 93–9).

Table 93–9

Treatment Regimens for Diffuse, Aggressive NHL

CHOP every 21 days
Cyclophosphamide 750 mg/m^2 IV, day 1
Doxorubicin 50 mg/m^2 IV, day 1
Vincristine 1.4 mg/m^2 IV, day 1
Prednisone 100 mg orally daily, days 1–5

rCHOP every 21 days
Rituximab 375 mg/m^2 IV day 1
Cyclophosphamide 750 mg/m^2 IV, day 1
Doxorubicin 50 mg/m^2 IV, day 1
Vincristine 1.4 mg/m^2 IV, day 1
Prednisone 100 mg orally daily, days 1–5

m-BACOD every 21 days
Methotrexate 200 mg/m^2 IV, days 8, 15
Bleomycin 4 mg/m^2 IV, day 1
Doxorubicin 45 mg/m^2, day 1
Cyclophosphamide 600 mg/m^2 IV, day 1
Vincristine 1.4 mg/m^2 IV, day 1
Dexamethasone 6 mg orally daily, days 1–5
Leucovorin 10 mg orally q 6 hours, 24 hours following methotrexate ×
   8 doses

ProMACE-CytaBOM every 28 days
Prednisone 60 mg orally daily, days 1–14
Doxorubicin 25 mg/m^2 IV, day 1
Cyclophosphamide 650 mg/m^2 IV, day 1
Etoposide 120 mg/m^2 IV, day 1
Cytarabine 300 mg/m^2 IV, day 8
Bleomycin 5 units IV, day 8
Vincristine1.4 mg/m^2 IV, day 8
Methotrexate120 mg/m^2, day 8
Leucovorin 25 mg/m^2 IV q 6 hours, 24 hours following methotrexate ×
   5 doses

MACOP-B
Methotrexate 400 mg/m^2 IV, day 8
Doxorubicin 50 mg/m^2 IV, days 1, 15
Cyclophosphamide 350 mg/m^2 IV, days 1,15
Vincristine 1.4 mg/m^2 IV, days 8,15
Prednisone 75 mg orally daily, × 12 weeks
Bleomycin 10 units IV, day 28
Leucovorin 15 mg orally q 6 hours, 24 hours following methotrexate × 6 doses

Hyper-CVAD
Cyclophosphamide 300 mg/m^2 IV q 12 hours, days 1–3 (with mesna)
Doxorubicin 50 mg/m^2 IV, day 1
Vincristine 1.4 mg/m^2 IV, days 1,11
Dexamethasone 40 mg orally daily, days 1–4 and 11–14
Methotrexate 15 mg intrathecal, day 2
Cytarabine 30 mg intrathecal, day 2
Hydrocortisone 15 mg intrathecal, day 2

Above drugs given on courses 1,3,5,7
Methotrexate 1,000 mg/m^2 IV over 24 hours, day 1
Cytarabine 3,000 mg/m^2 IV q 12 h, days 2,3
Leucovorin 25 mg IV × 1 then 25 mg orally q 6 hours for 7 doses
Methotrexate 15 mg intrathecal, day 2

Above drugs given on courses 2, 4, 6, 8
Relapsed Disease

ESHAP
Etoposide 40 mg/m^2 IV per day continous infusion, days 1–4
Cisplatin 25 mg/m^2 IV per day continuous infusion, days 1–4
Cytarabine 2,000 mg/m^2 IV × 1, day 5
Methylprednisone 250 mg IV q 12 hours, days 1–4

DHAP
Dexamethasone 40 mg orally or IV daily, days 1–4
Cisplatin 100 mg/m^2 IV continuous infusion, day 1
Cytarabine 2,000 mg/m^2 IV q 12 hours for 2 doses on day 2

ICE
Etoposide 100 mg/m^2 IV daily, days 1–3
Carboplatin AUC 5 (max dose 800 mg) IV, day 2
Ifosfamide 5,000 mg/m^2 IV continuous infusion × 1 on day 2 (with 100%
   replacement with mesna)

▶ *Special Populations*

There are certain histologic subtypes of diffuse, aggressive NHL that respond less well to treatment with conventional regimens such as CHOP. Burkitt's lymphoma, lymphoblastic lymphoma, mantle cell lymphoma, and primary CNS lymphoma are examples of disease that benefit from more intensive therapy. Regimens such as hyper-CVAD, which alternate cycles of hyperfractionated cyclophosphamide, doxorubicin, vincristine, and dexamethasone with high-dose cytarabine and methotrexate, may be substituted for CHOP.

Patients with CNS NHL have disease that is poorly responsive to therapy because of inadequate penetration of standard doses of chemotherapy across the blood–brain barrier. High-dose methotrexate, ranging from 2,500 to 8,000 mg/m^2 is a mainstay of therapy. Treatment may be augmented by direct instillation of intrathecal chemotherapy into the cerebrospinal fluid. Drugs that are commonly instilled intrathecally include methotrexate, cytarabine (conventional formulation and liposomal products) and corticosteroids. Medication errors causing death or permanent disability caused by inadvertent administration of intrathecal vincristine has been extensively reported in the medical literature. The WHO has published specific recommendations aiming to prevent further administration errors associated with vinca alkaloids.[33]

The recent appreciation of the etiology of *H. pylori* in the etiology of peptic ulcer disease and the association between colonization and MALT has spurred the more aggressive treatment of this organism with antibiotics. Generally, 7 to 14 days of combination therapy including; omeprazole, clarithromycin, and amoxicillin or tetracycline, metronidazole, and bismuth subsalicylate have been shown to provide rates of *H. pylori* clearance near 90%.

Mantle cell lymphoma, which comprises 6% of NHL cases, is defined by a chromosomal translocation of t(11;14) (q13;32). This translocation results in the overexpression of cyclin D1 coupled with NF-κB which plays a critical role in intracellular protein regulation and protranscription factors leading to increased cell survival. Bortezomib, a novel proteosome inhibitor disrupts the regulation and degradation of proteins required for cell cycle regulation. Bortezomib was approved by the FDA in 2006 for the treatment of patients with mantle cell lymphoma who have failed initial treatment. A study conducted in 155 patients demonstrated that bortezomib resulted in a overall response rate of 31% with a median duration of survival of 9.3 months.[34]

With over half of patients expected to relapse with disease, salvage therapy plays a major role in the attempt to cure patients with recurrence. Multiple drug programs such as ESHAP and DHAP can induce a complete response, but the long-term cure rates with these regimens are less than 10%. Salvage therapy can induce remissions with subsequent relapses; however, the chance for a CR and the duration of remission is further diminished.

Now high-dose chemotherapy with autologous SCT has been studied as an alternative to standard dose regimens in the setting of first relapse.[35] The best-studied indication for

SCT is for patients with intermediate- or high-grade disease that fails to respond to first-line therapy. A 3- to 5-year survival of upwards of 40% is achieved in patients who have good performance and disease that demonstrates a significant response to one or two cycles of salvage chemotherapy. The procedure-related mortality has ranged from 5% to 10% in published reports. However, as with HL, with more broad application of peripheral blood stem cells and improved supportive care, this figure continues to decline. The role of allogeneic bone marrow transplantation (BMT) in this setting is limited due to donor availability, older age of patients and the high treatment-related morbidity and mortality.

Patients with HIV-related lymphoma represent a therapeutic dilemma in that many have high-grade disease of B-cell origin. A common presentation is that of extranodal disease, frequently in the GI tract, CNS, and bone marrow. Therapy for this population thus far has fared poorly, with a median survival of 6 to 12 months, which decreases to 3 months with CNS involvement.[36] It remains to be seen if improved antiretroviral therapy will have an impact on the incidence and treatment options for these patients. The addition of rituximab to chemotherapy has failed to improve overall survival in this patient population and is associated with increased infectious complications relative to chemotherapy alone.[37]

OUTCOME EVALUATION

Treatment success in lymphoma is measured in successive stages, the first being inducing tumor regression and the degree of that regression: complete response (CR) versus partial response (PR) versus stable disease (SD) versus progressive disease (PD). The RECIST criteria, a uniform criteria assessing tumor response, developed by the National Cancer Institute are the standard methodology that physicians utilize to gauge treatment efficacy. Both HL and NHL may have residual masses following completion of treatment, adding to the difficulty in establishing a definitive remission from treatment. Clinical trials with limited numbers of patients have been published suggesting value of PET scans and/or gallium scans to rule out whether residual tumor masses following treatment contain viable tumor.[38] PET scans hold the promise of a future role because the 2-fluoro-2deoxyglucose contrast material is taken up more avidly by metabolically active tumor cells relative to necrotic tumor cells.

Long-term follow-up monitors patients for continued disease remission or relapse with careful physical examination of the lymph nodes and sites of prior disease involvement and imaging studies. Patients will have routine chest x-rays and CT scans to screen for disease recurrence. Patients require long-term monitoring for toxicities of their primary treatment, either chemotherapy or radiation therapy.

Most patients treated for lymphoma with chemotherapy or radiation notice a regression of palpable lymphadenopathy within days. This is due to the high sensitivity of the rapidly proliferating malignant lymphocytes to chemotherapy and radiotherapy. This necessitates implementation of tumor lysis syndrome precautions with aggressive sodium bicarbonate–containing IV fluid resuscitation and allopurinol for patients with moderate to high tumor burdens. Most chemotherapy treatments for lymphoma have a significant risk of infectious complications. Combination chemotherapy for both HL and NHL is associated with rates of severe leukopenia and/or neutropenia ranging from 20% to 100% of patients. Consideration must be given to supportive care with prophylactic antibiotics and myeloid colony-stimulating factors (CSFs). The American Society of Clinical Oncology has published guidelines stating that CSFs may be used as primary prevention when the incidence of febrile neutropenia with the chemotherapy is approximately 20% and no other equally effective and less myelosuppresive regimen is available or for secondary prevention where the patient already has experienced febrile neutropenia with the previous cycle of chemotherapy.[39] Effective antiemetic support is currently available that can control chemotherapy-induced nausea and vomiting reasonably well for most standard-dose regimens.[40]

For female survivors of HL who are treated with radiation to the thoracic cavity, there is an increase in the incidence of breast cancer, and baseline mammograms are recommended at the conclusion of treatment.[41] For HL patients, exposure to bleomycin can induce pulmonary fibrosis, which often

---

Patient Care and Monitoring

1. Verify chemotherapy regimen dosages with a standardized reference and assess for dose adjustment for renal or hepatic dysfunction.

2. Assess appropriateness of supportive care for each chemotherapy regimens such as antiemetics or CSFs.

3. Prior to initiation of treatment with chemotherapy determine if tumor lysis syndrome precautions need to be implemented.

4. Take a thorough medication history with particular attention to nonprescription or herbal medications.

5. Provide patient education regarding common toxicities associated with chemotherapy such as nausea/vomiting, mucositis, myelosuppression, and alopecia.

6. For doxorubicin-containing regimens, total the cumulative dosage received by the patient to monitor for cardiac toxicity.

7. For bleomycin-containing regimens total the cumulative dosage received by the patient to monitor for pulmonary fibrosis.

8. Educate patients regarding short and long term complications associated with radiation therapy.

9. Monitor patient for signs of response of tumor to chemotherapy.

10. Provide contact numbers for patient in the event of a fever and a response plan if the patient is considered to be at risk for neutropenic fever.

is subclinical. Patients who relapse and require high-dose chemotherapy and are treated with the drug carmustine in the conditioning regimen are at a higher risk of morbidity and mortality from idiopathic pulmonary syndrome/diffuse alveolar hemorrhage during SCT treatment. These patients are also at risk for exacerbation of underlying bleomycin-induced pulmonary damage if they ever require mechanical ventilation with high oxygen requirements. Combination chemotherapy that contains alkylating agents or etoposide carries the risk of a secondary acute myeloid leukemia or myelodysplastic syndrome. The cumulative dose of doxorubicin used for most lymphoma regimens is unlikely to cause cardiac toxicity with the standard six cycles. Neuropathy with vincristine or vinblastine may necessitate its removal from subsequent cycles if severe. Historically, it is more severe with vincristine. Treatment with fludarabine can harbor the risk of opportunistic infections such as *Pneumocystis carinii* pneumonia (PCP) for months following completion of therapy.

A limitation of rituximab treatment is the severe and potentially fatal infusion-related reactions. Deaths have been reported resulting from the profound hypotension and circulatory collapse seen with the drug, particularly on the first dose. The package labeling recommends premedication with acetaminophen and diphenhydramine before each infusion. For the first infusion, the drug should be administered at 50 mg/h. The infusion rate may be increased by 50 mg/h every 30 minutes to a maximum of 400 mg/h if no infusion-related reactions occur. If infusion-related reactions do occur, the manufacturer recommends stopping the infusion or temporarily slowing it until symptoms resolve. The infusion should be reinstituted at a rate that is one-half the previous rate. For subsequent rituxamab infusions, the rate may commence at 100 mg/h and be increased at 100 mg/h increments every 30 minutes for a maximum of 400 mg/h as tolerated. Other associated toxicities of rituxamab include fever, chills, headache, asthenia, nausea, vomiting, angioedema, bronchospasm, and skin reactions. ❽ *Despite these toxicities, rituximab is an effective treatment option for patients with indolent low-grade NHL as a single agent or in combination with standard chemotherapy regimens for more aggressive NHL histologies.* Radiolabeled rituximab causes more myelosuppression than rituximab alone and, similar to combination cytotoxic chemotherapy regimens, has a long-term risk of inducing secondary leukemias.[42]

Abbreviations Introduced in This Chapter

Bcl-1	Important in the regulation of mitosis
Bcl-2	A regulator of apoptosis
Bcl-3	A regulator of nuclear transcription factor
Bcl-6	Regulates cell differentiation
c-myc	Regulator of gene transcription
CALGB	Cancer and leukemia group B
CD	Cluster of differentiation
CHOP	Cyclophosphamide doxorubicin vincristine prednisone
CSFs	Colony-stimulating factors
EBV	Epistein-Barr virus
ESR	Erythroid sedimentation rate
HL	Hodgkin's lymphoma
IPI	International Prognostic Index
LDH	Lactate dehydrogenase
MALT	Mucosa-associated lymphoid tissue
NHL	Non-Hodgkin's lymphoma
RS	Reed-Sternberg
SCT	Stem cell transplant
NF-κB	Nuclear factor-kappa light chain enhancer

 Self-assessment questions and answers are available at *http://www.mhpharmacotherapy.com/pp.html.*

REFERENCES

1. Cartwright RA, Watkins G. Epidemiology of Hodgkin's disease: A review. Hematol Oncol 2004;22:11–26.
2. Yung L, Linch D. Hodgkin's lymphoma. Lancet 2003;361:943–951.
3. Fisher SG, Fisher RI. The epidemiology of non-Hodgkin's lymphoma. Oncogene 2004;23:6524–6534.
4. Evans LS, Hancock BW. Non-Hodgkin lymphoma. Lancet 2003;362:139–146.
5. Kuppers R, Hansmann ML. The Hodgkin and Reed/Sternberg cell. Int J Biochem Cell Biol 2005;37:511–517.
6. Re D, Thomas RK, Behringer K, Diehl V. From Hodgkin's disease to Hodgkin lymphoma: Biologic insights and therapeutic potential. Blood 2005;105:4553–4560.
7. Harris NL, Jaffe ES, Diebold J, et al. World Health Organization classification of neoplastic diseases of the hematopoietic and lymphoid tissue: Report of the Clinical Advisory Committee meeting, Airlie House, Virginia, November 1997. J Clin Oncol 1999;17:3835–3849.
8. Hasenclever D, Diehl V. A prognostic score for advanced Hodgkin's disease. N Engl J Med 1998;339:1506–1514.
9. Kuppers R, Klein U, Hansmann ML, Rajewsky K. Cellular origin of human B-cell lymphomas. N Engl J Med 1999;341:1520–1529.
10. Tsimberidou AM, Keating MJ. Richter syndrome: Biology, incidence and therapeutic strategies. Cancer 2005;103:216–228.
11. The International non-Hodgkin's Lymphoma Prognostic Factors Project. A predictive model for aggressive non-Hodgkin's lymphoma. N Engl J Med 1993;329:987–994.
12. Lister TA, Crowther D, Sutcliffe SB, et al. Report of a committee convened to discuss the evaluation and staging of patients with Hodgkin's disease: Cotswold meeting. J Clin Oncol 1989;7:1630–1636.
13. Alerman BMP, Raemaekers JMM, Tirelli U, et al. Involved-field radiotherapy for advanced Hodgkin's lymphoma. N Engl J Med 2003;348:2396–2406.
14. Horning SJ, Williams J, Bartlett NL, et al. Assessment of the Stanford V regimen and consolidative radiotherapy for bulky and advanced Hodgkin's disease: Eastern Cooperative Oncology Group pilot study 1402. J Clin Oncol 2000;18:972–980.
15. Aisenberg AC. Problems in Hodgkin's disease management. Blood 1999; 93:761–779.
16. Specht L, Gray RG, Clarke MG, Peto R. Influence of more extensive radiotherapy and adjuvant chemotherapy on long-term outcome of early-stage Hodgkin's disease: A meta-analysis of 23 randomized trials involving 3,888 patients. International Hodgkin's Disease Collaborative Group. J Clin Oncol 1998;16:830–843.

17. Canellos GP, Anderson JR, Propert KJ, et al. Chemotherapy of advanced Hodgkin's disease with MOPP, ABVD, or MOPP alternating with ABVD. N Engl J Med 1992;327:1478–1484.

18. Diehl V, Franklin J, Pfreundschuh M, et al. Standard and increased-dose BEACOPP chemotherapy compared with COPP-ABVD for advanced Hodgkin's disease. N Engl J Med 2003;348:2386–2395.

19. Linch DC, Winfield D, Goldstone AH, et al. Dose intensification with autologous bone-marrow transplantation in relapsed and resistant Hodgkin's disease: Results of a BLNI randomised trial. Lancet 1993; 341:1051–1054.

20. Santoro A, Bredenfeld, Devizzi L, et al. Gemcitabine in the treatment of refractory Hodgkin's disease: Results of a multicenter phase II trial. J Clin Oncol 2000;18:2615–2619.

21. Lu P. Staging and classification of lymphoma. Semin Nucl Med 2005;35:160–164.

22. Miller TP, Dahlberg S, Cassady JR, et al. Chemotherapy alone compared with chemotherapy plus radiotherapy for localized intermediate-and high-grade non-Hodgkin's lymphoma. N Engl J Med 1998;339:21–26.

23. DeAngelis LM, Seiferheld W, Schold SC, Fisher B, Schultz CJ. Combination chemotherapy and radiotherapy for primary central nervous system lymphoma: Radiation Therapy Oncology Group Study 93–10. J Clin Oncol 2002;20:4643–4648.

24. Hagenbeek A, Eghbali H, Monfardini S, et al. Phase III intergroup study of fludarabine phosphate compared with cyclophosphamide, vincristine, and prednisone chemotherapy in newly diagnosed patients with stage III and IV low-grade malignant Non-Hodgkin's lymphoma. J Clin Oncol 2006;24:1590–1596.

25. Marcus R, Imrie K, Belch A, et al. CVP chemotherapy plus rituximab compared with CVP as first-line treatment for advanced follicular lymphoma. Blood 2005;105:1417–1423.

26. Peterson BA, Petroni GR, Frizzera G, et al. Prolonged single-agent versus combination chemotherapy in indolent follicular lymphomas: A study of the cancer and leukemia group B. J Clin Oncol 2003;21:5–15.

27. McCune SL, Gockerman JP, Rizzieri DA. Monoclonal antibody therapy in the treatment of non-Hodgkin's lymphoma. JAMA 2001;286:1149–1152.

28. McLaughlin P et al. Rituximab chimeric anti-CD20 monoclonal antibody therapy for relapsed indolent lymphoma: Half of patients respond to a four dose treatment program. J Clin Oncol 1998;16:2825–2833.

29. Van Oers MH, Klasa R, Marcus RE, et al. Rituximab maintenance improves clinical outcomes of relapsed/resistant follicular non-hodgkins lymphoma in patients both with and without rituximab during induction: Results of a prospective randomized phase 3 intergroup trial. Blood 2006;108:3295–3301.

30. Friedberg JW, Cohen P, Chen L, et al. Bendamustine in patients with rituximab-refractory indolent and transformed non-Hodgkin's lymphoma: Results from a phase II multicenter, single agent study. J Clin Orthod 2008;26:201–210.

31. Fisher RI, et al. Comparison of standard regimen (CHOP) with three intensive chemotherapy regimens for advanced non-Hodgkin's lymphoma. N Engl J Med 1993;328:1002–1006.

32. Coiffer B, Lepage E, Briere J, et al. CHOP chemotherapy plus rituximab compared with CHOP alone in elderly patients with diffuse large B-cell lymphoma. N Engl J Med 2002;346: 235–242.

33. *http://www.who.int/patientsafety/highlights/PS_alert_115_vincristine.pdf*

34. Kane RC, Dagher R, Farrell A, et al. Bortezomib for the treatment of mantle cell lymphoma. Clin Cancer Res 2007;13:5291–5294.

35. Stebbing J, Marvin V, Bower M. The evidence-based treatment of AIDS-related non-Hodgkin's lymphoma. Cancer Treat Rev 2004;30:249–253.

36. Thierry P, Guglielmi C, Hagenbeek A, et al. Autologous bone marrow transplant as compared with salvage chemotherapy in relapses of chemotherapy-sensitive non-Hodgkin's lymphoma. N Engl J Med 1995;333:1540–1545.

37. Kaplan LD, Lee JY, Ambinder RF, et al. Rituximab does not improve clinical outcome in a randomized phase III trial of CHOP with or without rituximab in patients with HIV-associated non-Hodgkin's lymphoma: AIDS-Malignancies Consortium Trial 010. Blood 2005;106:1538–1543.

38. Juweid ME, Wiseman GA, Vose JA, et al. Response assessment of aggressive non-Hodgkin's lymphoma by Integrated International Workshop Criteria and fluorine-18-fluorodeoxyglucose positron emission tomography. J Clin Oncol 2005;21:4652–4661.

39. Smith TJ, et al. Update of Recommendations for the Use of White Blood Cell. Growth Factors: An Evidence-Based Clinical Practice Guideline 2006. www.asco.org..

40. Kris MG, Hesketh PJ, Somerfield MR, et al. American Society of Clinical Oncology guideline for antiemetics in oncology: Update 2006. J Clin Oncol 2006;17:2971–2994.

41. Deniz K, O'Mahony S, Ross G, Purushotham A. Breast cancer in women after treatment for Hodgkin's disease. Lancet Oncol 2003;4: 207–214.

42. Armitage JO, Carbone PP, Connors JM, Levine A, Bennett JM, Kroll S. Treatment-related myelodysplasia and acute leukemia in non-Hodgkin's lymphoma patients. J Clin Oncol 2003;21:897–906.

94 Ovarian Cancer

Judith A. Smith

LEARNING OBJECTIVES

● **Upon completion of the chapter, the reader will be able to:**

1. Demonstrate understanding the etiology and risk factors associated with the development of ovarian cancer.

2. Justify the risk and benefits of the surgical and chemoprevention options available for decreasing the potential risk of developing ovarian cancer.

3. Interpret and understand the utility of the screening tests and serological markers for diagnosing ovarian cancer.

4. Distinguish the nonspecific physical signs and symptoms of ovarian cancer.

5. Recommend the appropriate surgical and chemotherapy treatment options for newly diagnosed and relapsed ovarian cancer patients.

6. Compare and contrast chemotherapy options for women with recurrent platinum-resistant ovarian cancer.

7. Compare and contrast the treatment options for management of hot flushes in ovarian cancer patients.

8. Devise a plan for the management of common complications associated with advanced and recurrent ovarian cancer.

KEY CONCEPTS

❶ Ovarian cancer is a sporadic disease, less than 10% of ovarian cancers can be attributed to heredity.

❷ Because CA-125 is a nonspecific marker, there is no standard recommendation for routine screening for prevention of ovarian cancer.

❸ Ovarian cancer is denoted "the silent killer" because of the nonspecific signs and symptoms.

❹ Surgery is the primary treatment intervention for ovarian cancer.

❺ Ovarian cancer is staged surgically using the International Federation of Gynecology and Obstetrics (FIGO) staging algorithm.

❻ After initial surgery, the gold standard of care is six cycles of a taxane/platinum-containing regimen.

❼ Although majority of patients will initially achieve a complete response (CR), more than 50% will recur within the first 2 years.

❽ Because the efficacy of the agents is similar, the selection of agent for treatment of recurrent platinum-resistant ovarian cancer is dependent upon residual toxicities, physician preference, and patient convenience.

❾ Precaution should be used in removal of ascites because of the potential complications associated with rapid fluid shifts.

❿ In ovarian cancer patients, small bowel obstruction (SBO) is a common complication of progressive disease (PD). In general, laxatives should not be used in patients with SBOs.

INTRODUCTION

Ovarian cancer is relatively uncommon but the most fatal gynecologic cancer. The primary reason for the high mortality associated with ovarian cancer is the nonspecific symptoms and difficulty for early detection or screening that result in patients presenting with advanced disease. Majority of ovarian cancers are of epithelial origin. Each time ovulation occurs, the epithelium of the ovary is broken followed by occurrence of cell repair. The *incessant ovulation hypothesis* proposes that the increasing number of times the ovary epithelium undergoes cell repair is associated with the

Patient Encounter 1, Part 1

A 67-year-old female with history of coronary artery disease, diabetes, and GI reflux presents to your clinic complaining of persistent flatulence, bloating, and feels she is "getting fat." After discussing the symptoms with her, you learn that her reflux symptoms are recent onset and her proton pump inhibitor is "working." However, for the past 3 or 4 months, she also has irregular bleeding and occasional "cramping," which has been frustrating for her because she thought that ended years ago when she went through menopause. She reports her menses began when she was 9 and lasted all way until she was 61. She has two sisters in good health and a brother with diabetes. She has been married for 25 years with no children. The physician orders a CA-125 and CT scan that both come back positive and suggestive of ovarian cancer.

What symptoms could be associated with ovarian cancer?

Does she have any known risk factors?

What are your treatment options for this patient after surgery?

increasing risk of mutations and ultimately ovarian cancer. Ovarian cancer is often denoted as the "silent killer" because although the majority of patients will achieve a complete response (CR) to primary surgery and chemotherapy, over 50% will recur in the first year. Ovarian cancers will often cause metastasis via the lymphatic and blood systems to the liver and/or lungs. Common complications of advanced and progressive ovarian cancer include ascites and small bowel obstruction (SBO), which often are associated with the end of life.

EPIDEMIOLOGY AND ETIOLOGY

In 2009, there were an estimated 21,550 new cases of ovarian cancer diagnosed with an associated 14,600 deaths.[1] Ovarian cancer remains the number one gynecologic killer and the fifth leading cause of cancer-related death in women. Despite great efforts and extensive research, there has been little change in the mortality rate associated with ovarian cancer over the past three decades. The high mortality associated with ovarian cancer can be attributed to its insidious onset of nonspecific symptoms resulting in the majority of patients not presenting until the cancer has progressed to stage III–IV disease.

As with many other disease states, a significant risk factor associated with ovarian cancer is aging. A woman's risk increases as her age advances from 40 to 79 years, with the mean age at diagnosis being 63, majority of women being diagnosed between 55 and 64 years.[2]

❶ *Ovarian cancer is a sporadic disease, less than 10% of ovarian cancers can be attributed to heredity.* Majority of the cases of ovarian cancer occur sporadically, thus making it

difficult to screen and prevent. Although hereditary accounts for less than 10% of all ovarian cancer cases, when there is a family history it appears to be an important risk factor in the development of ovarian cancer in some patients.[3] If one family member has a diagnosis of ovarian cancer, the associated risk is about 9%, but this risk increases to greater than 50% if there are two or more first-degree relatives, that is, mother and sister, with a diagnosis of ovarian cancer or multiple cases of ovarian and breast cancer.[3] Both breast cancer activator gene 1 (*BRCA1*) and breast cancer activator gene 2 (*BRCA2*) mutations have been associated with ovarian cancer. However, *BRCA1* is more prevalent, being associated with 90% of hereditary and 10% of sporadic cases of ovarian cancer.[3] Hereditary breast and ovarian cancer (HBOC) syndrome is one of the two different forms of hereditary ovarian cancer and is associated with germ-line mutations in *BRCA1* and *BRCA2*.[3,4] The hereditary nonpolyposis colorectal cancer (HNPCC) or Lynch syndrome is a familial syndrome with germ-line mutations causing defects in enzymes involved in DNA mismatch repair (MMR), which has been associated with up to 12% of hereditary ovarian cancer cases.[4]

Although it is not clearly defined, hormones and reproductive history are associated with the risk of developing ovarian cancer. Nulliparity, infertility, early menarche, or late menopause is associated with an increased risk of ovarian cancer.[5,6]

Ovarian cancer is associated with certain dietary and environmental factors as well. A diet that is high in galactose and animal fat and meat increases the risk of ovarian cancer, whereas a vegetable-rich diet is suggested to decrease the risk.[4,7] Although controversial, exogenous factors such as asbestos and talcum powder use on the perineal area have also been suggested to increase the risk of ovarian cancer.[4,7]

Screening and Prevention

▶ *Screening*

Currently there is no standard effective screening tool that is adequately predictive or sensitive for early detection.

Pelvic examinations are effective for detecting obvious tumors present with a sensitivity of 67% for detecting all tumors; however, minimal or microscopic disease cannot be detected on physical examination.[8] Pelvic examinations are noninvasive and well accepted, but it does not usually detect ovarian cancer until it is in advanced stage. Therefore, routine pelvic examinations will not improve earlier diagnosis or help decrease overall mortality.[8]

Serum cancer antigen-125 (CA-125) is the most extensively evaluated tumor marker for ovarian cancer. Unfortunately, the CA-125 is nonspecific and elevated levels can be associated with a number of other gynecologic and GI related diseases. CA-125 levels in a woman without ovarian cancer are static or tend to decrease over time, while levels associated with malignancy will continue to rise.[9] ❷ *Because CA-125 is a nonspecific marker, there is no standard recommendation for routine screening for prevention of ovarian cancer.*

Patient Encounter 2

A 36-year-old female who has been in good health presents to your clinic complaining of constipation and abdominal pain. She explains to you that she has been feeling stressed lately because her 40-year-old sister is undergoing chemotherapy for breast cancer and they just lost their mother to ovarian cancer a few years ago.

Does she have a hereditary risk factor?

What screening tools could be used to monitor this patient?

Identify the treatment options for prevention of ovarian cancer available to this patient?

Transvaginal ultrasound (TVUS) is a component of current screening practices. Typically, it is used in combination with CA-125 or could be used as a single modality. TVUS releases sonic sound waves that create an image of the ovary to evaluated the size, shape, and detect the presence of cystic or solid masses. Limitations of this technique are lack of specificity and an inability to detect peritoneal cancer or cancer in normal size ovaries.[2,9] Most prevention clinics use this multimodality approach to screen high-risk women and recommend yearly ultrasound in combination with CA-125 blood test every 6 months.

▶ Prevention

Ovulation is considered a hostile event to the ovarian epithelium, making it more susceptible to damage and cancer. Interventions or conditions that limit the number of ovulations in a woman's reproductive history, including multiparity, will have a protective effect.

Chemoprevention Investigational chemoprevention strategies used for ovarian cancer include oral contraceptives (OCs), aspirin and nonsteroidal anti-inflammatory agents, and retinoids, although none of these is currently accepted as standard treatment for the prevention of ovarian cancer. The theory that OCs reduce the number of ovulatory events is a basic explanation of its protective effect. Recent studies have suggested that progestin-induced apoptosis of the ovarian epithelium is responsible for the chemopreventive effect of OCs. The theory is that cells that have genetic damage, but are not yet neoplastic, have an increased chance of undergoing apoptosis.[10] OCs decrease the relative risk to less than 0.4% in women that use OCs for greater than 10 years.[11] However, the maximum protective effect of OC use in women with *BRCA* mutations has been reported to be between 3 and 5 years.[12] However, at the same time, OC use has been associated with an increased risk of breast cancer.[11,12] Thus, women with a family history of breast cancer would not be ideal candidates for this preventative measure.

Nonsteroidal anti-inflammatory agents, aspirin, and acetaminophen have been suggested for use in the prevention of different cancers, especially hereditary nonpolyposis colon cancer.[13] While there have been observational studies linked to a reduction of ovarian carcinoma risk, evidence is still lacking. Potential mechanisms include effects on normal ovulation shed and inhibition of ovulation.[13,14] Other pharmacologic interventions that have been suggested but are still being evaluated include vitamin A, lutein, and other carotenoids.[15–17] The protective effect of these agents is associated with inhibition of cell growth as well as promotion of cellular differentiation.[16]

Prophylactic Surgery Surgical strategies are also used in the prevention of ovarian cancer. The goal is to remove healthy, at-risk organs and ultimately reduce the risk of developing cancer. These surgeries include prophylactic bilateral salpingo-oophorectomy (BSO) or tubal ligation.

Prophylactic oophorectomy should be considered in any woman with a high risk of developing ovarian cancer.[18] The criteria for defining high risk includes any woman with two or more first-degree relatives with epithelial ovarian carcinoma, a family history of multiple occurrences of nonpolyposis colon cancer, endometrial cancer, and ovarian cancer, and a family history of multiple cases of breast and ovarian cancer.[18] Patients undergoing prophylactic oophorectomy need to be made aware that complete protection is not guaranteed.[11,19] Although a 67% reduction in risk has been shown, a potential 2% to 5% risk of peritoneal carcinomatosis remains.[18,20]

Tubal ligation is another procedure that has shown potential for risk reduction. However, it is not recommended as a sole procedure in prophylaxis. Protective effect may be due to the limiting exposure of the ovary to environmental carcinogens. A case-control study conducted by Narod and colleagues found that a history of tubal ligation in BRCA-positive women was associated with a statistically significant 63% reduction in risk.[21]

Genetic Screening Genetic screening is another option available for high-risk patients. Patients can be screened for genes such as *BRCA1*, *BRCA2*, or other genes such as those associated with HNPCC or the HBOC syndrome.[3,21–23] Patient/family counseling and genetic counseling should be available for the patient/family to prepare and deal with the health and psychosocial implications of the genetic test results. Prior to this decision, the potential preventative options should be discussed, such as prophylactic BSO and/or total hysterectomy. Patients specifically positive for *BRCA1* or *BRCA2* may also consider a mastectomy.[24] Cancer risk and patient's health need to be balanced, but typically surgery can be held off until after the childbearing years.[25–27]

PATHOPHYSIOLOGY

The three current theories are the incessant ovulation hypothesis, the pituitary gonadotropin hypothesis, and the chronic inflammatory processes hypothesis.[2] The incessant ovulation hypothesis proposes that the pathogenesis of ovarian cancer is connected to continual ovulation. Ovulation is considered a "hostile" event to the ovary perhaps with not enough time for adequate repair. Each time ovulation occurs, the ovary epithelium is disrupted and cell damage occurs. Thus, repeated ovulations may lead to a greater number of repairs of the ovarian epithelium and increase the possibility of aberrant repairs, mutation, and carcinogenesis.[28-30] The pituitary gonadotropin hypothesis associates the disease with elevations in gonadotropin and estrogen levels.[2] This leads to an increase in the number of follicles and therefore an increased risk of malignant changes. Finally, the chronic inflammatory processes may be involved with various environmental carcinogens to cause cancer.[2,12]

The three major pathologic categories of ovarian tumors include sex-cord stromal, germ cell, and epithelial. About 85% to 90% of ovarian cancers are of epithelial origin. Epithelial ovarian tumors are composed of cells that cover the surface of the ovary such as serous, mucinous, endometrioid, clear cell, and poorly differentiated adenocarcinomas. Germ cell tumors involve the precursors of ova with the most common type being dysgerminoma, which are most commonly diagnosed in women under the age of 40 and generally have a better prognosis.[2] Sex-cord stromal tumors are indolent tumors that produce excess estrogen and androgens but also have a better overall prognosis.[2] Although the histologic type of the tumor is not a significant prognostic factor, it is important to know the histopathologic grade. Undifferentiated tumors are associated with a poorer prognosis than those lesions that are considered to be well or moderately differentiated.

Ovarian cancer is usually confined to the abdominal cavity, but spread can occur to the lung, liver, and less commonly, to bone or brain. Disease is spread by direct extension, peritoneal seeding, lymphatic dissemination, or by blood-born metastasis. Lymphatic seeding is the most common pathway and frequently causes ascites.

Mechanisms of Resistance

The common mechanisms of drug resistance in ovarian cancer include: (a) alteration of drug inactivation by agents such as glutathione S-transferase (GST), (b) enhanced DNA repair, (c) dysregulation of apoptotic pathways through activation of oncogenes or the loss of tumor suppressor gene functions, (d) *p*-glycoprotein (Pgp) multidrug resistance that leads to decreased drug accumulation, and (e) steroid xenobiotic receptor (SXR) that leads to enhanced drug metabolism. At this time, our understanding about the mechanism of drug resistance in ovarian cancer is incomplete and limited mostly to in vitro studies. Ongoing improvements in current technology have allowed development of in vivo studies to

---

Clinical Presentation and Diagnosis of Ovarian Cancer

General

❸ *Ovarian cancer has often been denoted as the "silent killer" because of the nonspecific signs and symptoms.* By the time symptoms become unrelenting and bothersome, patients most likely have advanced stage disease.

Symptoms

Patients may experience episodes or persistent symptoms such as abdominal pain, constipation or diarrhea, flatulence, urinary frequency, or incontinence.

Signs

The degree of abdominal swelling secondary to fluid accumulation may present like "pregnant abdomen" and irregular vaginal bleeding.

Laboratory Test

- *Cancer antigen-125 (CA-125).* The normal level is less than 35 units/mL (35 kilounits/L). Note: this test is associated with a lack of specificity. CA-125 can be elevated in a number of other states such as different phases of the menstrual cycle, endometriosis, and nongynecologic cancers.
- NOTE: It is important to rule out other cancers associated with the abdominal cavity.
- *Carcinoembryonic antigen (CEA).* CEA is marker for colon cancer. Normal value is less than 3 ng/mL (3 mcg/L).

- *CA-19–9* is a marker for many GI tumors such as cholangiocarcinomas.

Chemistries With Liver Function Tests (LFTs)

- LFTs and serum creatinine might be suggestive of extent of disease. Majority of this information is needed to determine if patient is a surgical candidate. Laboratories should be within normal limits.

CBC

- Abnormalities in CBC are not associated with ovarian cancer; however, this information is needed to determine if patient is a surgical candidate. Laboratories should be within normal limits.

Other Diagnostic Tests

To characterize local disease, one or both of the following are completed:

- Transvaginal ultrasound
- Abdominal ultrasound

To evaluate extent of disease, only one of the following is completed:

- CT scan
- MRI
- Positron emission tomography (PET) scan

Chest x-ray is also often done as part of clearance for surgery.

evaluate mechanisms of drug resistance in ovarian cancer. MDR has been one of the major limitations and is one of the ongoing challenges for the successful therapeutic treatment on recurrent and persistent ovarian cancer.

TREATMENT

Desired Outcomes

● Health care providers use a multimodality approach including surgery and chemotherapy in initial treatment of ovarian cancer with a curative intent, or restoring a normal life span. ❼ *Although majority of patients will initially achieve a CR, more than 50% will recur within the first 2 years.*[2,31] CR to treatment is defined as no evidence of disease can be detected by physical examination or diagnostic tests and patient has a normalized CA-125.

The stage of disease at the time of diagnosis is the most important prognostic factor affecting overall survival in ovarian cancer patients.[32] The estimated 5-year survival rate of patients with localized, regional, distant, and unstaged ovarian cancer is 92.7%, 71.1%, 30.6%, and 26%, respectively.[32] The histology of the disease is another predominant prognostic factor influencing treatment outcomes. Clear cell and undifferentiated tumors do not respond as well to chemotherapy.[2] The extent of residual disease and tumor grade are also predictive of response to chemotherapy and overall survival.[2] There are other prognostic factors that may predict how well a patient will respond to adjuvant chemotherapy.

Generally, younger patients with a better performance status tolerate chemotherapy better compared to elderly patients. Caucasian women tend to have a worse prognosis and response to therapy compared to other ethnic backgrounds.[2,4,5]

The treatment goals shift when a patient presents with recurrent ovarian cancer. The desired outcomes focus on relief of symptoms such as pain or discomfort from ascites, slowing disease progression, and prevention of serious complications such as SBO. When a patient relapses, the prognostic factors are similar as post initial surgery except the amount of time that has lapsed since the completion of chemotherapy should be considered to determine if drug resistance is emerging in the tumor. Recurrent platinum-sensitive ovarian cancer patients generally have a better prognosis than platinum-resistant patients.

Nonpharmacologic Therapy

● ❹ *Surgery is the primary treatment intervention for ovarian cancer.*[33-37] A total abdominal hysterectomy with BSO (TAH-BSO) (Fig. 94–1), **omentumectomy**, and lymphonectomy (or lymph node dissection) is the standard initial surgical treatment of ovarian cancer.[33,35] The objective of the surgery is to debulk the patient to less than 1 cm of residual disease remains. Residual disease less than 1 cm correlates with better CR rates to chemotherapy and better overall survival compared to patients with bulky residual disease

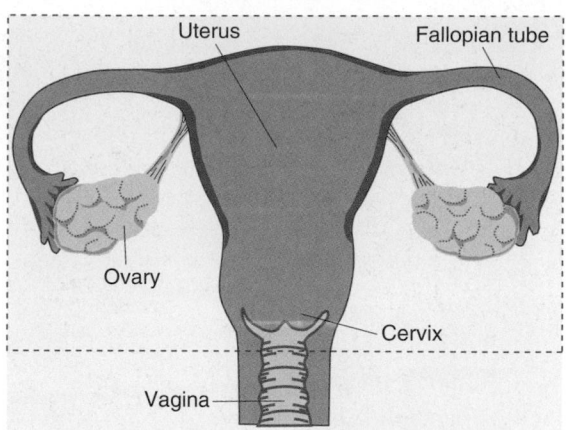

FIGURE 94–1. Diagram of female reproductive tract (uterus, fallopian tubes, ovaries, vagina). Dash-line box outlines what is removed during the total abdominal hysterectomy with bilateral salpingo-oophorectomy (TAH/BSO).

(greater than 1 cm).[36,37] Indeed, the size of residual tumor masses after primary surgery is found to be another important prognostic factor in patients with advanced ovarian cancer.[37]

A thorough exploratory **laparotomy** is essential for the accurate staging of the patient.[33-35] ❺ *Ovarian cancer is staged surgically using the International Federation of Gynecology and Obstetrics (FIGO) staging algorithm* (Fig. 94–2). For certain patients with limited stage disease, surgery may be curative.

Other surgical procedures have been evaluated to improve overall survival. Debulking surgery is intended to relieve symptoms associated with complications such as SBO and help improve the patient's quality of life but does not have a curative intent. Interval debulking that is completed after two to three cycles of chemotherapy has not translated to an improved survival benefit. Often debated, the benefit of the "second-look laparotomy" to evaluate residual disease after completing chemotherapy remains controversial because it has been difficult to establish any impact on patient overall survival. It has questionable benefit because, although approximately 40% of patients with advanced disease will have a negative second look, 50% still relapse.[2] The role of **laparoscopic** surgery is somewhat controversial for initial surgery but is more often considered in debulking of recurrent or advanced disease when the intent is palliative rather than curative.[36]

Pharmacologic Therapy

▶ First-Line Chemotherapy

❻ *After initial surgery, the gold standard of care is six cycles of taxane/platinum-containing regimen for patients with advanced ovarian cancer.*[38-40] Patients with limited disease will have observation alone after surgery (Fig. 94–3). Most often, paclitaxel is the taxane agent used in combination with carboplatin as the preferred platinum agent.[38-40] Depending upon patients' pre-existing comorbidities and how well

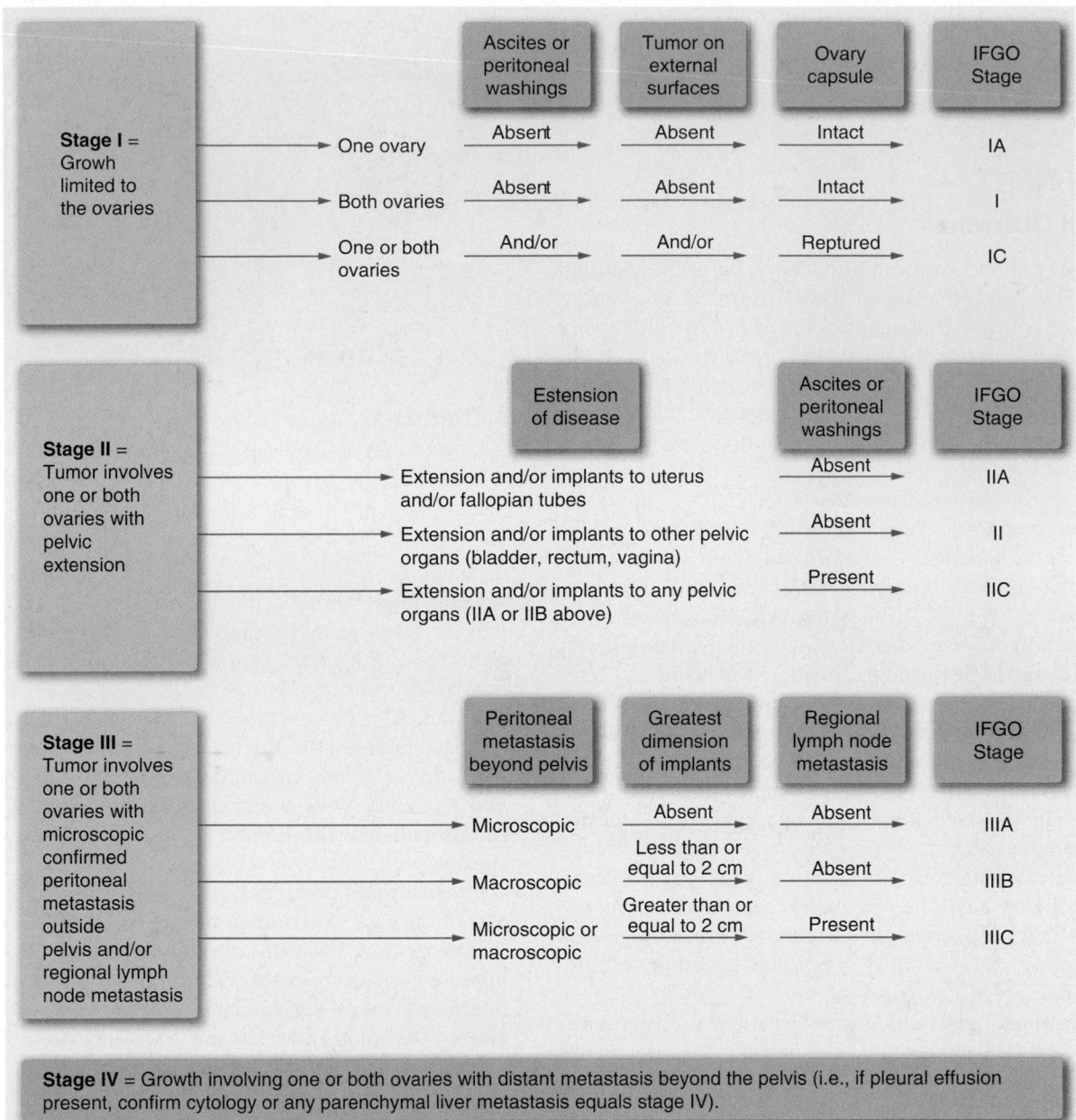

FIGURE 94–2. International Federation of Gynecology and Obstetrics (FIGO) staging algorithm for ovarian cancer.

they tolerate chemotherapy regimens, substitution with docetaxel or cisplatin might be considered. The route of administration should also be discussed. Most often IV administration will be used; however, in some patients **intraperitoneal** (IP) administration may have an advantage to improve overall survival[41] (Table 94–1). Close monitoring of organ function, nausea/vomiting, myelosuppression, and neuropathies is necessary for all taxane/platinum regimens (Table 94–2).

▶ *IP Chemotherapy*

For over three decades, numerous investigators have evaluated the IP route for administration of chemotherapy;

however, it was not until the third report of an improvement in overall survival that brought its use to the forefront in the first-line setting.[42] The principal theory supporting IP administration is to increase drug concentration in the site of disease, specifically the abdominal cavity. Patient characteristics greatly influence response and tolerability of IP chemotherapy. To be selected to receive IP chemotherapy for first-line treatment of ovarian cancer, the patient should have tumor optimally debulked and no bowel resection with primary surgery, normal renal and liver function, younger age, and no significant comorbidities.

If IP therapy is going to be considered, the placement of an IP port should occur at the time of surgery unless otherwise contraindicated. During IP administration,

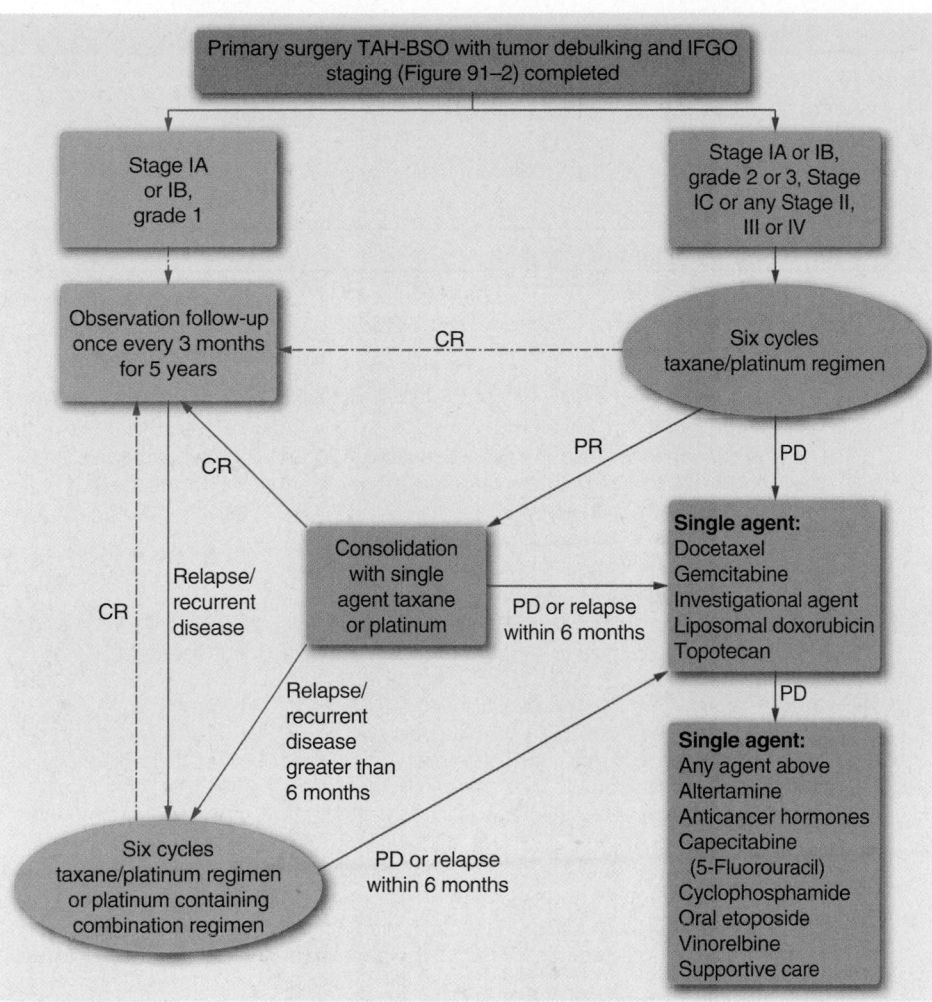

FIGURE 94–3. Summary of chemotherapy treatment algorithm for epithelial ovarian cancer. (CR, complete response; PR, partial response; PD, progressive disease.)

Table 94–1

Summary of First-Line Chemotherapy Regimens for Advanced Ovarian Cancer

Gold standard first-line chemotherapy after initial surgery for treatment of ovarian cancer:
Paclitaxel 175 mg/m² IV infused over 3 hours + carboplatin AUC = IV infused over 1 hour. Regimen is given once every 21 days × 6 cycles

Alternative first-line regimen: Paclitaxel IV with substitution of carboplatin IV with cisplatin IP and addition of paclitaxel IP therapy:
Patient selection is critical: must have optimally debulked disease (less than 1 cm), no significant comorbidities, younger patients tolerate better
Day 1: paclitaxel 135 mg/m² IV infused over 24 hours + day 2: cisplatin 100 mg/m² IP infused over 1 hour + day 8: paclitaxel 60 mg/m² IP infused over 1 hour. Regimen is given once every 21 days × 6 cycles

Alternative first-line regimen: Substitution of cisplatin in place of carboplatin. Consider for patients experiencing difficulty with maintaining platelet counts:
Paclitaxel 135 mg/m² IV infused over 24 hours + day 2: cisplatin 75 mg/m² IV infused over 4 hours. Regimen is given once every 21 days × 6 cycles

Alternative first-line regimen: Substitution of docetaxel in place of paclitaxel. Consider for patients with pre-existing or increased risk of neuropathies:
Docetaxel 75 mg/m² IV infused over 1 hour + carboplatin AUC = 5 IV infused over 1 hour. Regimen is given once every 21 days × 6 cycles

---

chemotherapy is delivered to the peritoneal space in one liter of normal saline (NS) that has been warmed followed by another liter of NS to enhance drug distribution as tolerated.[43,44] In addition, it is recommend to alternate the position of patient every 15 minutes for the first hour after drug IP administration to ensure proper distribution.[43,44] The current standard IP regimen includes the administration of paclitaxel IV on day 1 followed by cisplatin IP on day 2 and then paclitaxel IP on day 8 given on a 21-day cycle for a total of six cycles (Table 94–2). The most common toxicities associated with IP administration include abdominal pain, myelosuppression, neurotoxicity, and catheter-related infections.

▶ Neoadjuvant Chemotherapy

Neoadjuvant chemotherapy is first-line treatment for patients who are poor surgical candidates or patients with bulky or significant tumor burden.[31] For patients who are poor surgical candidates because of significant comorbidities, a combination of taxane with platinum agent is administered every 3 to 4 weeks as tolerated with intent to relieve symptoms and slow progression of disease. In some cases, especially elderly patients, single-agent carboplatin is used

---

Table 94–2

Summary of Chemotherapy Agents Used for First-Line Treatment of Advanced Ovarian Cancer

Mechanism of Action of First-Line Agents

Platinum analogues: Produce intra- and interstrand cross-links and DNA adducts to disrupt DNA replication

Taxanes agents: Stabilize microtubules and prevents depolymerization of tubulin

Agent	Common Adverse Effects	Monitoring/Comments
Paclitaxel	Peripheral neuropathy (DLT), nausea/vomiting, alopecia, hypersensitivity reactions	1. Use caution with any elevation in AST (SGOT) 2. Give proper dosing for liver dysfunction. At least a 50% dose reduction generally recommended 3. Do not give if total bilirubin is greater than 5 mg/dL (86 μmol/L) 4. Premedicate for hypersensitivity reactions: dexamethasone, diphenhydramine, and cimetidine
Docetaxel	Neutropenia (DLT) hyperlacrimation, fluid retention, nail disorders, myelosuppression	1. Use with caution in liver dysfunction. Patients with bilirubin greater than the upper limit of normal (ULN) and/or liver transaminases greater than 1.5 times, the ULN should not receive docetaxel 2. Do not give if biliary tract is obstructed 3. Premedicate for hypersensitivity reactions: dexamethasone
Carboplatin	Myelosuppression (DLT), nephrotoxicity, nausea/vomiting, electrolyte wasting, diarrhea, stomatitis, hypersensitivity reactions	1. Prehydration not required 2. If using BSA dosing, then give proper dosing for renal dysfunction CrCl greater than or equal to 60 mL/min: no dosage adjustment needed. CrCl 41–59 mL/min: give 250 mg/m² CrCl 16–40 mL/min: give 200 mg/m² CrCl less than or equal to 15 mL/min: do not give NOTE: Calvert formula (AUC dosing) is based on renal function, so no additional dose adjustment needed 3. Premedicate for hypersensitivity reactions: dexamethasone, diphenhydramine, and cimetidine 4. Appropriate antiemetic regimen for prevention of acute and delayed nausea
Cisplatin	Neurotoxicity (DLT), nausea/vomiting, ototoxicity, nephrotoxicity, myelosuppression, electrolyte wasting, diarrhea	1. Prehydration and posthydration with electrolyte replacement (i.e., potassium chloride 10 mEq and magnesium sulfate 16 mEq) required 2. Do not use if SrCr greater than 1.5 mg/dL (133 μmol/L) or BUN greater than 25 mg/dL (8.9 mmol/L) 3. Give proper dosing for renal dysfunction CrCl 46–60 mL/min: decrease dose by 50%. CrCl 31–5 mL/min: decrease dose by 75%. CrCl less than or equal to 30 mL/min: do not use 4. Appropriate antiemetic regimen for prevention of acute and delayed nausea

DLT, dose-limiting toxicity.

---

as palliative treatment instead. Chemotherapy alone has not been curative for patients with advanced ovarian cancer.[31]

In patients with bulky disease or significant tumor burden, neoadjuvant chemotherapy can be used to decrease tumor burden to increase the likelihood of optimal tumor debulking during surgery.[31] Typically three cycles of the standard combination taxane/platinum regimen is administered once every 3 weeks. After surgery, patient will receive another three to six cycles depending upon response to chemotherapy.

▶ Consolidation Chemotherapy

Consolidation chemotherapy is the addition of cycles of the taxane/platinum regimen or the addition of single-agent platinum or single taxane after completion of first-line chemotherapy.[45] If the tumor has a partial response (PR) to first-line chemotherapy evident by a significant decline in CA-125 by greater than 50% presurgery level and/or tumor regression/decrease in size, then cancer is still considered taxane/platinum sensitive. Additional cycles of chemotherapy are given until CR is achieved (see Fig. 94–3).

▶ Agents Used in First-Line and Consolidation Chemotherapy of Ovarian Cancer

Taxanes

Paclitaxel. Paclitaxel is a taxane that is naturally derived from the bark of the yew tree. Paclitaxel is cytotoxic to cells by stabilizing microtubules to prevent depolymerization of tubulin causing cell cycle arrest in the M-phase. The two most common regimens used in ovarian cancer is a 3-hour infusion of 175 mg/m² or a 24-hour infusion of 135 mg/m².

Paclitaxel is a water-insoluble drug so alcohol-based diluent, cremophor, is used in the formulation and is associated with increase hypersensitivity reactions. Patients are pretreated with an H_2 blocker, diphenhydramine, and steroids. The dose-limiting toxicity (DLT) of paclitaxel is infusion dependent. For shorter infusion, for example, 3 hours, the DLT is neuropathy and for longer infusions the DLT is myelosuppression. Additional common adverse effects can be found in Table 94–2.

Docetaxel. Docetaxel is another agent in the class of taxanes with a similar mechanism of action as paclitaxel but with differences in affinity for α-tubulin-binding sites, hence more potent.

Because the experience with docetaxel in the treatment of ovarian cancer is limited, it is often considered as a second-line option. However, there are clinical trials ongoing comparing the efficacy and toxicity of docetaxel to paclitaxel in the combination with platinum agents for first-line treatment of ovarian cancer.[46] The dose of docetaxel typically used is 75 mg/m^2 given every 21 days and is reasonably well tolerated. To avoid severe fluid retention or hypersensitivity reactions, patients are premedicated with corticosteroids. The DLT associated with docetaxel primarily is neutropenia. Additional common adverse effects can be found in Table 94–2.

Platinum Analogues

Cisplatin. Cisplatin forms Pt-DNA adducts that intercalate the DNA interrupting DNA synthesis.

The typical dose of cisplatin used for the treatment of ovarian cancer is 75 mg/m^2 when administered via IV route or 100 mg/m^2 if administered via IP route. Because cisplatin is nephrotoxic, regardless of route of administration, prehydration with 1 to 3 L of NS is required, which often requires an inpatient stay. The DLT of cisplatin is neurotoxicity that is nonreversible in many patients. Cisplatin is highly emetogenic but can be minimized with 5HT$_3$-antagonists. Additional common adverse effects can be found in Table 94–2.

Carboplatin. Carboplatin has a similar mechanism of action as cisplatin forming PLT-DNA adducts that intercalate the DNA interrupting DNA synthesis to ultimately cause cell death.

Carboplatin dose is determined using the Calvert formula: *carboplatin dose (mg) = target AUC * (CrCl + 25).* The Calvert formula uses the calculated glomerular filtration rate (GFR) for the estimated creatinine clearance (CrCl) in this equation to individualize the dose and minimize dose-related toxicity. For the first-line treatment of ovarian cancer, the target area under the curve (AUC) is five to seven. Individualized dosing has decreased the incidence and degree of nephrotoxicity associated with carboplatin compared to cisplatin, eliminating the need for intensive prehydration thus allowing for outpatient administration. Myelosuppression, primarily thrombocytopenia, is the DLT of carboplatin. Additional common adverse effects can be found in Table 94–2.

Recurrent Chemotherapy

In the recurrent setting, platinum sensitivity of the tumor is assessed first. If recurrence occurs in less than 6 months or disease progresses while receiving a platinum-based regimen, the cancer is considered to be platinum resistant (see Fig. 94–3). These parameters are also used to determine taxane sensitive or resistant. However, patients resistant to paclitaxel may still respond to docetaxel.[47] If the treatment goal is palliative care, then often single therapy will be used, while curative care typically is an aggressive combination regimen (see Fig. 94–3). Often an investigational study may have more likelihood or

achieving a response as well or better than the current agents used for the treatment of recurrent ovarian cancer.

▶ Platinum Sensitive

In patients who experienced a CR to first-line chemotherapy and have had greater than a 6-month platinum-free interval, retreatment with a platinum containing regimen is appropriate. Current National Comprehensive Cancer Network (NCCN) guidelines recommend the combination of carboplatin with either gemcitabine or paclitaxel for the treatment of platinum-sensitive recurrent ovarian cancer with a curative intent.[41] However, in patients who are unable to tolerate additional combination chemotherapy regimens, carboplatin alone or any one of the second-line agents would be appropriate[48] (see Table 94–2).

▶ Platinum Resistant

Recurrent or persistent ovarian cancer after platinum-based regimens has a discouraging prognosis. Second-line agents have not been successful to date, but any active agent that has not been used during initial treatment is available to use. ❽ *Single-agent chemotherapy is standard practice for recurrent platinum-resistant ovarian cancer.* Active agents include altretamine (formerly hexamethylmelamine), anastrozole, capecitabine (5-fluorouracil), cyclophosphamide, docetaxel, gemcitabine, liposomal doxorubicin, oral etoposide, vinorelbine, topotecan, or investigational agents. There are numerous ongoing investigational studies evaluating the benefit of addition of biologically targeted agents such as bevacizumab to cytotoxic agent regimens to improve outcomes in the recurrent ovarian cancer setting (see Fig. 94–3). ❽ *Since the efficacy of the agents is similar, the selection of agent for treatment of recurrent platinum-resistant ovarian cancer is dependent upon residual toxicities, physician preference, and patient convenience.* Table 94–3 gives a short

---

Patient Encounter 1, Part 2: 1 Year After Initial Diagnosis

This patient was optimally debulked and completed six cycles of paclitaxel/carboplatin after her surgery. Her CA-125 normalized (12 units/mL [12 kilounits/L]) upon completion of her chemotherapy treatment and her CT scan was negative. This patient returns to your clinic for her first 3-month follow-up appointment. Her CA-125 is 45 units/mL (45 kilounits/L) and she reports some mild bloating. CT scan report states mild fluid accumulation in the pelvic cavity.

List the possible chemotherapy treatment options for this patient?

Discuss the side effect profile and administration schedule of each agent and how this information would help in selection of her next chemotherapy regimen?

What is the goal of treatment for this patient?

Table 94–3

Summary of Chemotherapy Agents Used for Second-Line Treatment of Progressive and Recurrent Platinum-Resistant Ovarian Cancer

Agent	Dose	Response Rate (%)	Common Adverse Effects	Monitoring/Comments
Docetaxel	75 mg/m² IV over 1 hour repeat every 21–28 days versus 30–40 mg/m² IV over 1 hour once every week	22 NR	Neutropenia (DLT) hyperlacrimation, fluid retention, nail disorders, myelosuppression	1. Premedicate for hypersensitivity reactions with dexamethasone 2. Use with caution in liver dysfunction. Patients with bilirubin greater than the upper limit of normal (ULN) and/or liver transaminases greater than 1.5 times the ULN should not receive docetaxel 3. Do not give if biliary tract is obstructed
Gemcitabine	800 mg/m² IV infused over 30 minutes once a week on days 1, 8, and 15 followed by 1 week of rest	13.9–27	Myelosuppression (DLT), flu-like symptoms, headache, somnolence, nausea/vomiting, stomatitis, diarrhea, constipation, rash	1. Use with caution in renal or liver dysfunction. No specific guidelines available
Liposomal doxorubicin	40 mg/m² IV infused over 3 hours cycle 1 and 2, then infused over 1 hour thereafter repeat every 28 days	12.3–18	Myelosuppression, stomatitis, mucositis, alopecia, flushing, shortness of breath, hypotension, headaches, cardiotoxicity, hand–foot syndrome	1. Give proper dosing for liver dysfunction. Total bilirubin 1.2–3 mg/dL (21–51 µmol/L): reduce dose by 50%. Total bilirubin greater than or equal to 3 mg/dL (51 µmol/L): reduce dose by 75% 2. Do not give if total bilirubin is greater than 5 mg/dL (86 µmol/L)
Topotecan	1.5 mg/m² IV infused over 30 minutes on days 1, 2, 3, 4, and 5 repeat every 21 days OR 4 mg/m² IV infused over 30 minutes once a week for 3 consecutive weeks followed by 1-week rest	6.5–17 31	Myelosuppression (DLT), nausea/vomiting, diarrhea, stomatitis, abdominal pain, alopecia, SGOT/SGPT elevation	1. Give proper dosing for renal dysfunction CrCl 40–60 mL/min: no dosage adjustment needed. CrCl 20–39 mL/min: reduce dose by 50% 2. Do not give if CrCl less than 20 mL/min
Altretamine (Hexalen™)	260 mg/m² po daily for 14–21 days repeat every 28 days	9.7	Nausea/vomiting, diarrhea, abdominal cramping, myelosuppression	1. Monitor for potential CYP450 drug interactions
Capecitabine	1,800–2,500 mg/m² po as divided dose twice daily for 14 consecutive days followed by 1 week of rest	29	Myelosuppression, hand–foot syndrome, nausea/vomiting, edema, stomatitis, diarrhea, cardiotoxicity, rash	1. Monitor for PPE and recommend regular use of lotions on hands and feet 2. Use with caution in renal dysfunction. CrCl greater than or equal to 51 mL/min: No dose adjustment. CrCl 30–50 mL/min: Reduce dose by 25%. CrCl less than 30 mL/min: Do not give 3. Use with caution in liver dysfunction. No specific guidelines available
Cyclophosphamide	Cyclophosphamide 750 mg/m² IV over 30 minutes	NR	Nausea/vomiting, nephrotoxicity, myelosuppression, cardiotoxicity, alopecia, hemorrhagic cystitis	1. Monitor for potential CYP450 drug interactions 2. Monitor for any signs of blood in urine
Etoposide	50 mg/m²/day po in divided doses given daily for 3 consecutive weeks followed by 1 week of rest	18	Myelosuppression, nausea/vomiting, anorexia, alopecia, headache, fever, hypotension	1. Give proper dosing for liver dysfunction. Total bilirubin 1.5–3 mg/dL (26–51 µmol/L): Decrease dose by 50%. Total bilirubin 3–5 mg/dL (51–86 µmol/L): Decrease dose by 75% 2. Do not give if total bilirubin is greater than 5 mg/dL (86 µmol/L) 3. Give proper dosing for renal dysfunction. CrCl 60–45 mL/min: Reduce dose by 15%. CrCl 44–30 mL/min: Reduce dose by 20%. CrCl less than 30 mL/min: Reduce dose by 25%
Letrozole	2.5 mg once daily	15	Headache, nausea, dyspepsia, skin rash	1. No protective effect on bone, recommend calcium supplementation
Tamoxifen	20 mg po twice a day continuously until PD	10	Thrombocytopenia, anemia, thromboembolism, hot flashes, decreased libido, nausea/vomiting	1. Protective effect on bone and lipids 2. Increased risk for endometrial cancer
Vinorelbine	30 mg/m² IV infused over 15 minutes on days 1 and 8 repeat every 21 days	29	Constipation, neutropenia, anemia, thrombocytopenia, neurotoxicity	1. Consider bowel regimen to prevent constipation

DLT, dose-limiting toxicity; NR, not reported.

summary of the adverse effects and monitoring parameters for chemotherapy agents commonly used for the treatment of recurrent ovarian cancer.

OUTCOME EVALUATION

Overall survival is impacted by success of initial surgery to debulk tumor to less than 1 cm of disease and response to first-line chemotherapy. The CA-125 level should be monitored with each cycle and at least a 50% reduction in CA-125 after four cycles of taxane/platinum chemotherapy is related to an improved prognosis. Patients who achieve CR should have follow examinations once every 3 months, including CA-125, physical examination, and pelvic examination, and appropriate diagnostic scans (i.e., CT scan, MRI, or PET scan) should be evaluated for the detection of disease. Side effects while evaluating patient for resolution of any residual chemotherapy include neuropathies, nephrotoxicity, ototoxicity, myelosuppression, or nausea/vomiting. In younger patients with an active menstrual cycle prior to surgery will encounter "surgical menopause" and often experience intense hot flushes. Since there are concerns about potential of hormones in the pathogenesis of ovarian cancer, the use of hormone replacement therapy is controversial. The use of phytoestrogen supplements, such as black cohosh or soy, is also controversial. An effective alternative has been the use of the class of serotonin reuptake inhibitors such as venlafaxine controlled released once daily.

In the PD or recurrent setting, CA-125 levels should still be monitored with each cycle, but no change in therapy is recommended until after minimum of three cycles of chemotherapy. In addition, appropriate diagnostic scans (i.e., CT scan, MRI, or PET scan) should be evaluated once every three cycles. Patients should also have routine physical examinations with each cycle of chemotherapy to evaluate for any physical toxicity associated with chemotherapy such as neuropathies, fluid retention, palmar-plantar erythrodysesthesia (PPE), myelosuppression, or nausea/vomiting.

Unfortunately, if patients will eventually progress through all chemotherapy options, then supportive care measures should be provided to maintain patient comfort and quality of life. Common complications while developing a plan for treatment of advanced/progressive ovarian cancer include ascites, uncontrollable pain, and SBO. ❾ *Precaution should be used in removal of ascites because of the potential complications associated with rapid fluid shifts.* Liberal use of opioids to control pain is appropriate as ovarian cancer patients cope with PD and approaching end of life. Appropriate bowel regimens with laxatives and stool softeners should be used to prevent constipation. However, when a patient with a well-controlled bowel regimen presents with new onset of constipation, additional workup is required prior to altering bowel regimen. ❿ *In ovarian cancer patients, small bowel obstruction is a common complication of progressive disease. In general, laxatives should not be used in patients with*

Patient Care and Monitoring

1. Assess patient history of nonspecific symptoms to determine if patient should be evaluated by gynecologist.

2. Determine if patient is at high risk for development of ovarian cancer and make appropriate recommendations for screening and prevention.

3. Evaluate patient comorbidities and medications to determine if additional workup is necessary prior to tumor debulking surgery. Do any medications need to be stopped or changed prior to surgery (i.e., aspirin, warfarin, nonsteroidal anti-inflammatory agents)?

4. Develop a plan for preventing and treatment of nausea and vomiting for patient receiving emetogenic chemotherapy.

5. Monitor patient for signs of hypersensitivity reactions to taxane or platinum chemotherapy regimens.

6. Monitor appropriate laboratories to determine

    a. Changes in organ function—adjust chemotherapy doses as indicated

    b. Electrolyte wasting—replace and supplement electrolytes IV or oral as indicated.

7. Provide appropriate patient education on respective chemotherapy agents that will be given for treatment of recurrent ovarian cancer.

    a. What is chemotherapy and how this agent works?

        i. Explain plan for monitoring response to treatment.

    b. What side effects to expect during chemotherapy?

        i. Precautions to take to prevent infection when neutropenic.

        ii. Monitor for signs/symptoms of infection.

    c. When to contact physician/clinic between cycles of chemotherapy?

    d. Drug or food interactions with chemotherapy to avoid.

SBOs. Prior to treating constipation, patients should have a physical examination and abdominal x-ray to rule out SBO. Often, palliative surgery is required to correct SBO and alleviate patient pain. Patients should not eat any solid or liquids until resolution of SBO. If inoperable SBO exists, then parenteral nutrition can be considered but weighed against ultimate treatment objectives. Overall, providing any measures needed to maintain patient comfort is the priority for patients with progressive ovarian cancer.

Abbreviations Introduced in This Chapter

AUC	Area under the curve
BRCA1	Breast cancer activator gene 1

BRCA2	Breast cancer activator gene 2
BSO	Bilateral salpingo-oophorectomy
CA-125	Cancer antigen-125
CA-19	Cancer antigen 19
CEA	Carcinoembryonic antigen
CR	Complete response
CrCl	Creatinine clearance
DLT	Dose-limiting toxicity
FIGO	International Federation of Gynecology and Obstetrics
GFR	Glomerular filtration rate
GST	Glutathione S-transferase
HBOC	Hereditary breast and ovarian cancer
HNPCC	Hereditary nonpolyposis colorectal cancer
IP	Intraperitoneal
LFTs	Liver function tests
MMR	Mismatch repair
MDR	Multidrug resistance
NCCN	National Comprehensive Cancer Network
NS	Normal saline
OC	Oral contraceptive
Pgp	*p*-Glycoprotein
PPE	Palmar-plantar erythrodysesthesia
PD	Progressive disease
PET	Positron emission tomography
PR	Partial response
SBO	Small bowel obstruction
SXR	Steroid xenobiotic receptor
TAH	Total abdominal hysterectomy
TVUS	Transvaginal ultrasound

Self-assessment questions and answers are available at *http://www.mhpharmacotherapy.com/pp.html.*

REFERENCES

1. Jemal A, Siegel R, Ward E, et al. Cancer statistics, 2009. CA Cancer J Clin 2009;59:225–249.
2. Cannistra SA. Cancer of the ovary. N Engl J Med 2004;351:2519–2529.
3. Lux MP, Fashing PA, Beckmann MW. Hereditary breast and ovarian cancer: Review and future perspectives. J Mol Med 2006;84(1):16–28.
4. Runnebaum IB, Stickeler E. Epidemiological and molecular aspects of ovarian cancer risk. J Cancer Res Clin Oncol 2001;127:73–79.
5. Martin VR. Ovarian cancer. Semin Oncol Nurs 2002;18:174–183.
6. Pecorelli S, Odicino F, Maisonneuve P, et al. Carcinoma of the ovary. Annual report on the results of treatment in gynaecological cancer. J Epidemiol Biostat 1998;3:75–102.
7. Edmondson RJ, Monaghan JM. The epidemiology of ovarian cancer. Int J Gynecol Cancer 2001;11:423–429.
8. Cherry C, Vacchiano SA. Ovarian cancer screening and prevention. Semin Oncol Nurs 2002;18(3):167–173.
9. Edwards BK, Brown ML, Wingo PA, et al. Annual report to the nation on the status of cancer 1975–2002, featuring population-based trends in cancer treatment. J Nat Cancer Inst 2005;97(19):1407–1427.
10. Whittemore AS, Balise RR, Pharoah PD, et al. Oral contraceptive use and ovarian cancer risk among carriers of BRCA1 or BRCA2 mutations. Br J Cancer 2004;91(11):1911–1915.
11. Barnes MN, Grizzle WE, Grubbs CJ, et al. Paradigms for primary prevention of ovarian carcinoma. CA Cancer J Clin 2002;52:216–225.
12. McLaughlin JR, Risch HA, Lubinski J, et al. Reproductive risk factors for ovarian cancer in carriers of BRCA1 or BRCA2 mutations: A case control study. Lancet Oncol 2007;8:26–34.
13. Cramer DW, Harlow BL, Titus-Ernstoff L, et al. Over-the-counter analgesics and risk of ovarian cancer. Lancet 1998;351:104–107.
14. Tavani A, Gallus S, La Vecchia C, et al. Aspirin and ovarian cancer: An Italian case-control study. Ann Oncol 2000;11:1171–1173.
15. Prat J, Ribe A, Gallardo A. Hereditary ovarian cancer. Human Pathol 2005;36:861–870.
16. Bertone ER, Hankinson SE, Newcomb PA, et al. A population-based case-control study of carotenoid and vitamin A intake and ovarian cancer. Cancer Causes Control 2001;12:83–90.
17. Harris RE, Beebe-Donk J, Doss H, et al. Aspirin, ibuprofen, and other non-steroidal anti-inflammatory drugs in cancer prevention: A critical review of non-selective COX-2 blockade (review). Oncol Rep 2005;13:559–583.
18. Meeuwissen PAM, Seynaeve C, Brekelmans CTM, et al. Outcome of surveillance and prophylactic salpingo-oophorectomy in asymptomatic women at high risk for ovarian cancer. Gynecol Oncol 2005;97(2):476–482.
19. Cherry C, Vacchiano SA. Ovarian cancer screening and prevention. Semin Oncol Nurs 2002;18(3):167–173.
20. Finch A, Beiner M, Lubinski J, et al. Salpingo-oophorectomy and the risk of ovarian, fallopian tube, and peritoneal cancers in women with a BRCA1 or BRCA2 mutation. JAMA 2006;296:185–192.
21. Narod SA, Sun P, Ghadirian P, et al. Tubal ligation and risk of ovarian cancer in carriers of BRCA1 and BRCA2 mutations: A case control study. Lancet 2001;357:1467–1470.
22. Coukos, G. Gene therapy for ovarian cancer. Oncology 2001;15(9):1197–1208.
23. Tait DL, Obermiller PS, Hatmaker AR, et al. Ovarian cancer BRCA1 gene therapy: Phase I and II trial differences in immune response and vector stability. Clin Cancer Res 1999;5(7):1708–1714.
24. Kuschel B, Lux MP, Goecke TO, et al. Prevention and therapy for BRCA1/2 mutation carriers and women at high risk for breast and ovarian cancer. Eur J Cancer Prev 2000;9:139–150.
25. Pavelka JC, Li AJ, Karlan BY. Hereditary ovarian cancer-assessing risk and prevention strategies. Obstet Gynecol Clin North Am 2007;34(4):651–665.
26. Batista LI, Lu KH, Beahm EK, et al. Coordinated prophylactic surgical management for women with hereditary breast-ovarian cancer syndrome. BMC Cancer 2008;14(8):101–106.
27. Fry A, Busby-Earle C, Rush R, et al. Prophylactic oophorectomy versus screening: Psychosocial outcomes in women at increased risk for ovarian cancer. Psychooncology 2001;10:231–241.
28. Shushan A, Paltiel O, Schenker JG. Induction of ovulation and borderline ovarian cancer: The hormonal connection? Eur J Obstet Gyn 1999;85:71–74.
29. Klip H, Burger CW, Kenemans P, et al. Cancer risk associated with subfertility and ovulation induction: A review. Cancer Causes Control 2000;11:319–344.
30. Whittemore AS, Harris R, Itnyre J. Collaborative Ovarian Cancer Group. Characteristics relating to ovarian cancer risk: Collaborative analysis of 12 US case-control studies. Am J Epidemiol 1992;136:1184–1203.
31. Salzberg M, Thurlimann B, Bonnefois H, et al. Current concepts of treatment strategies in advanced or recurrent ovarian cancer. Oncology 2005;68:293–298.
32. National Cancer Institute. Cancer stat fact sheets. Cancer of the ovary. Available at: *http://seer.cancer.gov/statfacts/html/ovary.html.*
33. Stratton JF, Tidy JA, Paterson MEL. The surgical management of ovarian cancer. Cancer. Treat Rev 2001:27;111–118.
34. Cooper A, DePriest P. Surgical management of women with ovarian cancer. Semin Oncol 2007;34:226–233.
35. Stratton JF, Tidy JA, Paterson MEL. The surgical management of ovarian cancer. Canc Treat Rev 2001:27;111–118.
36. Bristow RE, Tomacruz RS, Armstrong DK, et al. Survival effect of maximal cytoreductive surgery for advanced ovarian carcinoma

during platinum era: A meta analysis. J Clin Oncol 2002;20:1248–1259.

37. Hoffman MS, Griffin D, Tebes S, et al. Sites of bowel resected to achieve optimal ovarian cancer cytoreduction: Implications regarding surgical management. Am J Obstetrics Gynecol 2005;193:582–588.

38. Ozols RF, Bundy BN, Greer BE, et al. Phase III trial of carboplatin and paclitaxel compared with cisplatin and paclitaxel in patients with optimally resected stage III ovarian cancer: A gynecologic oncology group study. J Clin Oncol 2003;21:3194–3200.

39. Neijt JP, Engelholm SA, Tuxen MK, et al. Exploratory phase III study of paclitaxel and cisplatin versus paclitaxel and carboplatin in advanced ovarian cancer. J Clin Oncol 2000;18:3084–3092.

40. National Comprehensive Cancer Network (NCCN) Practice Guidelines in Oncology—Ovarian Cancer—v.1.2008. 3/13/08 *www.nccn.org*

41. Armstrong DK, Bundy B, Wenzel L, et al. Intraperitoneal cisplatin and paclitaxel in ovarian cancer. N Engl J Med 2006;354:34–43.

42. Rao G, Crispens M, Rothenberg ML. Intraperitoneal chemotherapy for ovarian cancer: Overview and perspective. J Clin Oncol 2007;25:2867–2872.

43. National Cancer Institute. NCI Clinical Announcement: Intraperitoneal chemotherapy for ovarian cancer, January 5, 2006. Available at *http://ctep.cancer.gov/highlights/clin_annc_010506.pdf*.

44. Alberts DS, Bookman MA, Chen T, et al. Proceedings of a GOG workshop on intraperitoneal therapy for ovarian cancer. Gynecol Oncol 1006;103:783–792.

45. Gadducci A, Cosio S, Conte PF, et al. Consolidation and maintenance treatments for patients with advanced epithelial ovarian cancer in CR after first-line chemotherapy: A review of the literature. Crit Rev Onc Hematol 2005;55:153–166.

46. Vasey PA, Jayson GC, Gordon A, et al. Phase III randomized trial of docetaxel-carboplatin versus paclitaxel-carboplatin as first-line chemotherapy for ovarian carcinoma. J Natl Cancer Inst 2004;1796(22):1682–1691.

47. Rose PG, GBlessing JA, Ball HG, et al. A phase II study of docetaxel in paclitaxel-resistant ovarian and peritoneal carcinoma: A Gynecologic oncology group study. Gynecol Oncol 2003;88:130–135.

48. Salom E, Almeida Z, Mirashemi R. Management of recurrent ovarian cancer: Evidence-based decisions. Curr Opin Oncol 2002;14:519–527.

95 Acute Leukemia

Nancy Heideman

LEARNING OBJECTIVES

● **Upon completion of the chapter, the reader will be able to:**

1. Describe the pathogenesis of acute leukemia.

2. Compare the classification systems for acute lymphocytic leukemia (ALL) and acute myelogenous leukemia (AML).

3. Identify the risk factors associated with a poor outcome for the acute leukemias.

4. Explain the importance of minimal residual disease (MRD) and its implication on early bone marrow relapse.

5. Explain the role of induction, consolidation, and maintenance phases for acute leukemia.

6. Define the role of CNS preventive therapy for acute leukemia.

7. Recognize the treatment complications associated with therapy for acute leukemias.

8. Describe the late effects associated with the treatment of long-term survivors of acute leukemias.

KEY CONCEPTS

❶ The acute leukemias are hematologic malignancies of bone marrow precursors characterized by excessive production of immature hematopoietic cells. This proliferation of "blast" cells eventually replaces normal bone marrow and leads to the failure of normal hematopoiesis and the appearance of leukemia cells in peripheral blood as well as infiltration of other organs.

❷ Acute leukemias are classified according to their cell of origin. Acute lymphocytic leukemia (ALL) arises from the lymphoid precursors. Acute nonlymphocytic leukemia (ANLL) or acute myelogenous leukemia (AML) arises from the myeloid or megakaryocytic precursors.

❸ The goal is to match treatment to risk and minimize over- or undertreatment. Children with ALL are sorted into prognostic categories based on clinical and biological features that mirror their risk of relapse. Risk assessment is an important factor in the selection of treatment.

❹ Minimal residual disease (MRD) is a quantitative assessment of subclinical remnant of leukemic burden remaining at the end of the initial phase of treatment (induction) when a patient may appear to be in a complete morphologic remission. This measure has become one of the strongest predictors of outcome for patients with acute leukemia. The elimination of MRD is a principal objective of postinduction leukemia therapy.

❺ The initial treatment for acute leukemias is called **induction**. The purpose of induction is to induce a **remission**, a state where there is no identifiable leukemic cells in the bone marrow or peripheral blood with light microscopy. This definition may change as more sensitive techniques come into play.

❻ The current induction therapy for ALL typically consists of vincristine, asparaginase, and a steroid (prednisone or dexamethasone). An anthracycline is added for higher-risk patients.

❼ Leukemic invasion of the CNS is considered to be an almost universal event in patients, even in those whose cerebrospinal fluid (CSF) cytology shows no apparent disease. Thus, all patients with ALL and AML receive intrathecal chemotherapy. Although this is often referred to as "prophylaxis," it more realistically represents treatment.

❽ Marrow relapse is a major complication for 15% to 20% of patients with ALL. Current research suggests that this is the result of residual leukemic cells at diagnosis. Thus the importance of MRD.

⑨ The current induction therapy for AML usually consists of a combination of cytarabine and an anthracycline daunorubicin or idarubicin, with the frequent addition of a steroid and/or an antimetabolite such as 6-thioguanine. The second phase of treatment for AML is called consolidation. The purpose of this phase is to further enhance remission with more cytoreduction.

⑩ Although survival in pediatric cancers has improved dramatically over the last 35 years, 50% to 60% of cancer survivors are estimated to have at least one chronic or late-occurring complication of treatment.

INTRODUCTION

① *The acute leukemias are hematologic malignancies of bone marrow precursors characterized by excessive production of immature hematopoietic cells. This proliferation of "blast" cells eventually replace normal bone marrow and lead to the failure of normal hematopoiesis and the appearance in peripheral blood as well as infiltration of other organs.* These blast cells proliferate in the marrow and inhibit normal cellular elements, resulting in anemia, neutropenia, and thrombocytopenia. Leukemia also may infiltrate other organs, including the liver, spleen, bone, skin, lymph nodes, and CNS. Virtually anywhere there is blood flow, the potential for extramedullary (outside the bone marrow) leukemia exists.

② *Acute leukemias are classified according to their cell of origin. Acute lymphocytic leukemia (ALL) arises from the lymphoid precursors. Acute nonlymphocytic leukemia (ANLL) or acute myelogenous leukemia (AML) arises from the myeloid or megakaryocytic precursors.* As a result of clinical trials defining various prognostic (risk) factors that helped guide treatment modifications, the outcomes of acute leukemias, especially ALL, has improved dramatically over the last 30 years.[1] Risk-based treatment strategies that consider multiple phenotypic and biological risk factors and attempt to match the aggressiveness of therapy with the presumed risk of relapse and death are now the standard of care. Currently, the overall survival (OS) of pediatric patients with ALL is about 80%. For AML, it is significantly less at about 50%. If left untreated, most patients with either of these acute leukemias will die of their disease within 2 to 3 months.

EPIDEMIOLOGY AND ETIOLOGY

Epidemiology

Leukemia is a relatively uncommon disease overall. The current overall age-adjusted annual incidence of acute leukemia in the United States has remained relatively stable at 10 per 100,000. Of the estimated 1.4 million new cancers diagnosed in 2009, only 1% to 2% will be acute leukemia, with 760 cases of ALL and about 12,800 cases of AML.[2,3] Interesting age-related patterns of disease exist in ALL and AML. The average age of diagnosis for AML is about 65 years and is a result of an increasing incidence of AML with age.[4] ALL is a more common process in children than adults and relatively uncommon in adults where its incidence decreases with age.[5,6]

In the pediatric population, leukemia is a common disease, accounting for almost one-third of all childhood malignancies. ALL accounts for 75% to 80% of all cases of childhood leukemia, whereas AML accounts for no more than 20%. Males generally are affected more often than females in all but the infant age group, and its incidence is higher in whites than among other racial groups. The incidence of AML in children is bimodal: It peaks at 2 years of age, decreases steadily thereafter to age 9 years, and then increases again at around age 16.[3]

The 5-year event-free survival (EFS) rate for ALL is nearly 80% in children as compared to only 40% for adults.[1] The success rate for children with ALL is attributed to enrollment in clinical trials, risk-adapted treatment, and integration of presymptomatic CNS prophylaxis.[7] A recent increase in the survival rate for adults has been attributed to the adoption of the principles of treatment that characterize pediatric protocols.[8] For patients with AML, a similar pattern exists. Those younger than 20 years of age have a 5-year survival of 50%.[6] Patients with AML older than age 60 generally have a poorer prognosis with a 5-year survival of less than 20%.[9]

Etiology

The causes of the acute leukemias is unknown; multiple influences related to genetics, socioeconomics, infection, environment, hematopoietic development, and chance all may play a role.[3] Table 95–1 lists the major conditions that have been associated with the acute leukemias. In most cases, however, there is no identifiable cause of the leukemia.

Table 95–1

Clinical Conditions Associated With an Increased Frequency of Acute Leukemias

Drugs	**Chemicals**
Alkylating agents	Benzene
Epidophyllotoxins	**Radiation**
Genetic Conditions	Ionizing radiation
Down's syndrome	
Bloom's syndrome	**Viruses**
Fanconi's anemia	Epstein-Barr virus
Klinefelter's syndrome	Human T-lymphocyte virus
Ataxia telangiectasia	(HTLV-1 and HTLV-2)
Langerhans' cell histiocytosis	
Shwachman's syndrome	**Social Habits**
Severe combined	Cigarette smoking
immunodeficiency syndrome	Maternal marijuana use
Kostmann's syndrome	Maternal ethanol use
Neurofibromatosis type 1	
Familial monosomy 7	
Diamond-Blackfan anemia	

Adapted from Ref. 6.

While leukemia is rarely a hereditary disease some genetic associations are evident. For example, among identical twins, the concordance for ALL in the initially unaffected twin is 20% to 25% within 1 year. While the incidence in fraternal twins is much less, there is still a fourfold increase in the risk of leukemia in the initially unaffected twin as compared with the normal population. One explanation for this association may be a shared placental circulation, which allows for transmission of disease from one twin to the other. Additionally, leukemia is known to be increased in several chromosomally abnormal populations. Patients with Down's syndrome have a 20 times increased risk of developing leukemia compared with the rest of the population. Patients with Klinefelter's syndrome and Bloom's syndrome also have an increased incidence of leukemias.[3]

Exposure to environmental agents such as agricultural chemicals, pesticides, and radiation have also been periodically associated with leukemia, however none of these agents is linked conclusively with the development of leukemia. An increased frequency of ALL is associated with higher socioeconomic status. It is postulated that less social contact in early infancy and thus a late exposure to some common infectious agents may have some impact.[3] In most individual instances, there is no reasonable or obvious explanation for the development of leukemia.

Risk factors for the development of AML include exposure to environmental toxins, Hispanic ethnicity, and genetics.[6] Of greater concern is the increased prevalence of AML as a secondary malignancy, resulting from chemotherapy and radiation treatment for other cancers. Alkylating agents, such as ifosfamide and cyclophosphamide, and topoisomerase inhibitors, such as etoposide, are linked to an increased risk of myelodysplastic syndrome (MDS) and AML.[9]

PATHOPHYSIOLOGY

Hematopoiesis is defined as the development and maturation of blood cells and their precursors. In utero, hematopoiesis may occur in the liver, spleen, and bone marrow; after birth this process occurs exclusively in the bone marrow. All blood cells are generated from a common hematopoietic precursor, or *stem cell*. These stem cells are self-renewing and pluripotent and thus are able to commit to any one of the different lines of maturation that give rise to platelet-producing megakaryocytes, lymphoid, erythroid, and myeloid cells. The myeloid cell line produces monocytes, basophils, neutrophils, and eosinophils, whereas the lymphoid stem cell differentiates to form circulating B and T lymphocytes, NK cells, and dendritic cells. In contrast to the ordered development of normal cells, the development of leukemia seems to represent an arrest in differentiation at an early phase in the continuum of stem cell to mature cell.[1]

Both AML and ALL are presumed to arise from clonal expansion of these "arrested" cells. As these cells expand, they acquire one and often more chromosomal aberrations, including translocations, inversions, deletions, point mutations, and amplifications.[3] The translocation ETS leukemia acutemyeloid leukemia-1 (*TEL–AML1*)

fusion, found in approximately 25% of cases is associated with a favorable prognosis.[7] Another example is the t(9;22) translocation, which underlies the *BCR–ABL* fusion protein. The normal *ABL* gene encodes a growth-promoting protein kinase whose activity is tightly controlled. By contrast, the translocation and fusion of the *BCR* and *ABL* gene sequences produce a kinase that leads to uncontrolled proliferation, survival, and self-renewal of cells. Imatinib is a tyrosine kinase inhibitor that inhibits the activity of *ABL*. It has shown great success given the pathogenic role of *BCR–ABL* tyrosine kinase in chronic myelogenous leukemia (CML), which is characterized by this molecular abnormality. Imatinib also has shown activity in the infrequent, but high-risk patients with ALL in patients who are *BCR–ABL* positive.[3]

AML represents a group of disorders in which both failure to differentiate and overproliferation in the stem cell compartment produce an overabundance of nonfunctional cells termed myeloblasts. While the specific cause for this biological abnormality is unknown, an understanding of the genetic influence of leukemia is leading to a wide variety of targeted therapies.[10]

In AML, there is a substantial difference in clinical and biological features, as well as in response to and tolerance of therapy, by age group. In the elderly, trilineage leukemic involvement is common, indicating that the cell of origin is probably a stem or very early progenitor cell. In the younger population, a more differentiated progenitor becomes malignant, permitting maturation of some granulocytic and erythroid populations. These two forms of AML show different patterns of resistance to chemotherapy, with resistance more frequent in the older adults with AML.[6]

For patients with MDS or AML as a secondary neoplasm, there are often a number of key features characterized by having had prior alkylator-based or etoposide-based chemotherapy. Patients receiving treatment for Hodgkin's disease or solid tumors are often trated with this type of chemotherapy. Many of these patients have an abnormal bone marrow, but have not converted to overt leukemia. Instead, they have a myelodysplastic prodrome, which consists of a marrow that is hypoplastic and in which a monosomy 5 or monosomy 7 is often seen. Secondary AML with the use of epipodophyllotoxin (etoposide) demonstrates mainly M4 or M5 morphology and exhibits translocations within the *MLL* gene with 11q23 chromosomal alterations, which is otherwise an uncommon feature of AML.[9]

Leukemia Classification

For all newly diagnosed patients with leukemia, an aspirate of the liquid marrow and a bone marrow core biopsy are obtained.[5] Morphologic and cytochemical analyses of these samples distinguish three subtypes of ALL (L1, L2, and L3) and eight subtypes of AML (M0–M7) as classified by the French-American-British (FAB) scheme. See Tables 95–2 and 95–3 for the FAB classification of AML and ALL. Another classification system proposed by the World Health Organization (WHO) and the Society of Hematopathology for myeloid neoplasms includes not only morphologic findings,

---

Table 95–2

Morphologic (FAB) Classification of AML

Subtype		Frequency of FAB Subtype[a]		
		Adults (%)	Children Older Than 2 Years (%)	Children Younger Than 2 Years (%)
M0	Acute myeloblastic leukemia, without maturation	5	Low	Low
M1	Acute myeloblastic leukemia with minimal maturation	15	17	25
M2	Acute myeloblastic leukemia with maturation	25		27
M3	Acute promyelocytic leukemia	10		5
M4	Acute myelomonocytic leukemia	25	30	26
M5a	Acute monoblastic leukemia, poorly differentiated	5	52	16
M5b	Acute monoblastic leukemia, well differentiated	5		
M6	Acute erythroleukemia	5		2
M7	Acute megakaryoblastic leukemia	10		5–7

FAB, French-American-British.

[a]Percentages should be compared vertically and not horizontally.

Adapted from Ref. 6.

Table 95–3

Morphologic (FAB) Classification and Immunophenotype of ALL

Subtype	Cell of Origin	Frequency of FAB Subtype[a]	
		Adults (%)	Children (%)
L1	Early pre-B cell Pre-B cell B cell T cell	30	85
L2	Early pre-B cell Pre-B cell B cell T cell	60	14
L3	B cell	10	1

FAB, French-American-British.

[a]Percentages should be compared vertically and not horizontally.

Adapted from Leather HL, Bickert B. Acute Leukemias. In: DiPiro JT, Talbert RL, Yee GC, et al., (eds.) Pharmacotherapy: A Pathophysiologic Approach, 6th ed. New York: McGraw-Hill; 2005: 2485–2511.

Table 95–4

WHO Classification of AML

AML with recurrent genetic abnormalities:
AML with t(8;21)(q22;q22), (*AML1/ETO*)
AML with abnormal bone marrow eosinophils and inv(16)(p13q22) or t(16;16)(p13;q22), (*CBFβ/MYH11*)
Acute promyelocytic leukemia with t(15;17)(q22;q12), (*PML/RARα*) and variants
AML with 11q23 (*MLL*) abnormalities
AML with multilineage dysplasia
Following MDS or MDS/MPD
Without antecedent MDS or MDS/MPD, but with dysplasia in at least 50% of cells in 2 or more myeloid lineages
AML and MDSs, therapy related
Alkylating agent/radiation-related type
Topoisomerase II inhibitor-related type (some may be lymphoid)
Others
AML, not otherwise categorized

Classify as:
AML, minimally differentiated
AML without maturation
AML with maturation
Acute myelomonocytic leukemia
Acute monoblastic/acute monocytic leukemia
Acute erythroid leukemia (erythroid/myeloid and pure erythroleukemia)
Acute megakaryoblastic leukemia
Acute basophilic leukemia
Acute panmyelosis with myelofibrosis
Myeloid sarcoma

AML, acute myeloid leukemia; MDS, myelodysplastic syndrome; MPD, myeloproliferative disorders.

Adapted from Ref. 6.

---

but also genetic, immunophenotypic, biological, and clinical characteristics (Table 95–4). A disadvantage of this system is that it does not account for some of the myeloid disorders in pediatrics.[6]

Classification methods for leukemia have evolved from simple schemes that were largely phenotypic and considered only age, gender, WBC, and blast morphology to now-complex methods that include biological features such as cell-surface receptors, DNA content (ploidy; more or less then normal chromosomal DNA content), and a variety of cytogenetic abnormalities.

Markers on the cell surface or membrane of the lymphoblast can be used to classify ALL. Among the early classification system was the FAB scheme, which was based purely on morphology and apparent degree of cellular differentiation. This system is no longer used, and the current classification of acute leukemias is based on features that can be identified only by immunological and molecular analyses.[3] Markers on the cell surface or membranes of the leukemic cell (lymphoblasts) are now more regularly used to classify ALL and to assign prognosis and, in turn, treatment.

Immunophenotyping by **flow cytometry** has taken on an increasingly important role in the diagnosis of leukemia. Owing to the ease of application, sensitivity, and quantifiable results, flow cytometry is the preferred method for leukemic lineage as well as prognostic assignment.[8] This approach takes advantage of the development of monoclonal antibodies (MABs) to many cell-surface antigens that are differentially expressed during hematopoietic differentiation. The antigens are referred to as antibody *cluster determinants* (CDs) that define cells at various stages of development and can easily separate ALL from AML and T-cell from preB-cell ALL.[5,11] The combined approach of flow cytometric identification and cytogenetic DNA content, much of which is also revealed by flow cytometry and fluorescent in-situ hybridization (**FISH;** microscopic, fluorescence identification of chromosomal features) has facilitated diagnosis and delineation of specific treatments for the major subtypes of the acute leukemias. Common immunophenotypic markers seen in AML and ALL are provided in Table 95–5.

Prognostic Factors

❸ *The goal of treatment is to match treatment to risk and minimize over- or undertreatment. Children with ALL are sorted into prognostic categories based on clinical and biological features that mirror their risk of relapse. Risk assessment is an*

Table 95–5

Common Immunophenotypes in Acute Leukemia

Leukemia	Common Immunophenotypes
AML	CD13, CD15, CD33, CD14, CD64, and C-KIT
B-cell ALL	CD19, CD20, CD10, and CD22
T-cell ALL	CD2, CD3, CD4, CD5, and CD7

ALL, acute lymphoblastic leukemia; AML, acute myeloid leukemia; CD, cluster determinants.

Adapted from Ref. 6.

Clinical Presentation and Diagnosis of ALL[3,6,11]

General

Typically, patients have symptoms for 1 to 3 months before presentation. These include fatigue, fever, and pallor, but patients generally are in no obvious distress.

Symptoms

- The patient may present with weakness, malaise, bleeding, and weight loss.
- Neutropenic patients are often febrile and highly susceptible to infection.
- Anemia usually presents as pallor, tiredness, and general fatigue.
- Patients with thrombocytopenia usually present with bruising, petechiae, and ecchymosis.
- Patients often present with bone pain secondary to expansion of the marrow cavity from leukemic infiltration.
- CNS involvement is common at diagnosis.

Signs

- Temperature may be elevated secondary to an infection associated with a low WBC.
- Petechiae and bleeding are indicative of thrombocytopenia.
- Patients may present with organ involvement, such as peripheral adenopathy, hepatomegaly, and splenomegaly.
- T-lineage ALL may present with a mediastinal mass.

Laboratory Tests

- CBC with differential is performed.
- The anemia is usually normochromic and normocytic. Approximately 50% of children present with platelet counts of less than $50 \times 10^3/mm^3$ ($50 \times 10^9/L$). The WBC may be normal, decreased, or high. About 20% of patients have WBCs over $100 \times 10^3/mm^3$ ($100 \times 10^9/L$), which places them at risk for leukostasis.
- Uric acid is increased in approximately 50% of patients secondary to rapid cellular turnover.
- *Electrolytes:* Potassium and phosphorus often are elevated. Calcium usually is low.
- *Coagulation disorders:* Elevated prothrombin time, partial thromboplastin time, D-dimers; hypofibrinogenemia.

Other Laboratory Tests

Flow cytometric evaluation of bone marrow and peripheral blood is performed to characterize the type of leukemia as well as to detect specific chromosomal rearrangements. The bone marrow at diagnosis usually is hypercellular, with normal hematopoiesis being replaced by leukemic blasts. At diagnosis, a lumbar puncture is performed to determine if CNS leukemia is present.

Patient Encounter, Part 1

RH is a 7-year-old girl who presents to her pediatrician with a 1-week history of runny nose and fever. Her mom has noted a lot of bruising on her lower extremities. Physical examination reveals splenomegaly, multiple petechiae, and pallor. A CBC reveals a normochromic, normocytic anemia with a hemoglobin of 6 g/dL (60 g/L, 3.7 mmol/L; normal 11.7–15.7 g/dL, 117–157 g/L, 7.3–9.7 mmol/L), hematocrit of 18% (0.18; normal 35–47%, or 0.35–0.47), and WBC of 2.6 × 10³/mm³ (2.6 × 10⁹/L). The differential on the WBC reveals 75% (0.75) lymphocytes (normal 20–40%, or 0.2–0.4), 20% (0.2) neutrophils (normal 55–62%, or 0.55–0.62), and 5% (0.05) lymphoblasts (normal 0%). Based on this information, a bone marrow aspirate and biopsy are performed, which reveal 85% (0.85) lymphoblasts and a DNA index of 1.17. A lumbar puncture is also performed, which shows no evidence of leukemia.

What information is suggestive of acute lymphocytic leukemia?

What are the prognostic factors for RH?

What is the goal of induction therapy?

Table 95–6

Prognostic Factors in ALL

| Factor | Risk for Leukemic Relapse | |
	Low	High
Morphology	L1	L2, L3
Immunologic phenotype	Early pre-B cell	Null cell, T cell, pre-B cell, B cell
WBC at diagnosis	Less than 10 × 10³/mm³ (10 × 10⁹/L)	Greater than 50 × 10³/mm³ (50 × 10⁹/L)
Platelets	Greater than 100 × 10³/mm³ (100 × 10⁹/L)	Less than 30 ×10³/mm³ (30 × 10⁹/L)
Patient age	3–7 years	Less than 1 year or greater than 10 years
Cytogenetics	Normal karyotype	t(9;22); t(4;11); −7; +8
Myeloid markers	Absent	Present
CNS leukemia	Absent	Present
Node/liver/spleen enlargement	Absent	Massive
Mediastinal mass	Absent	Present
Time to remission	Less than 4 weeks	Greater than 4 weeks

Adapted from Ref. 6.

important factor in the selection of treatment.[12] Age, WBC, leukemic cell-surface markers, DNA content, and specific cytogenetic abnormalities predict response to therapy and are used to assign risk and associated treatment.[3] On the basis of these prognostic variables, patients are assigned to one of the three risk groups (e.g., standard-, high-, or very high–risk groups) that determine the aggressiveness of treatment.

▶ Prognostic Factors in ALL

In both children and adults with ALL, clinical trials have identified several risk factors that correlate with outcome (Table 95–6). Prognostic features include age, WBC, cytogenetic abnormalities, ploidy (DNA content), leukemic cell immunophenotype, and degree of initial response to therapy (minimal residual disease, MRD).[13] When these factors are combined, they predict groups of patients with varying degrees of risk for treatment failure.

In adults, there is a steady decline in the rate of complete remission (CR) following initial induction therapy with increasing age. When results are corrected for differences in immunophenotype, ALL cells from adults are more resistant to the multiple antileukemic agents than are cells from children in the first decade of life.[8] While induction treatment produces 95% CR in children, it declines to no more than 60% in patients older than 60 years of age. This is due in part to decreased tolerance of assertive induction/consolidation regimens in older patients. Other potentially important factors relate to a higher incidence of poor prognostic factors such as the presence of Philadelphia chromosome (Ph⁺) or t(9;22), in older populations.[5] *BCR–ABL* fusions (Ph⁺) are strongly associated with chemoresistant leukemia in all age groups but are much more prevalent in adults with ALL than in children (30% versus less than 5%).[11]

The association of age and outcome is nowhere more evident than between infants and older patients. Infants (less than 1 year of age) often possess a poor prognostic genotype represented by the presence of the *MLL* gene rearrangement. The *MLL* gene is capable of partnering with many genes, and in virtually every instance the result is a markedly poor prognosis. All cells that have the *MLL* gene rearrangement are highly resistant to the key antileukemic drugs such as glucocorticoids and L-asparaginase. Thus, investigators are now focusing on protocols specifically aimed at infant ALL.[7]

Like age, the WBC at presentation is a reliable indicator of CR rate and outcome. The WBC is indicative of tumor burden, although the underlying biological mechanisms that account for the unfavorable outcomes associated with an elevated WBC are unclear. Patients with WBCs of less than 50 × 10³/mm³ (50 × 10⁹/L) are considered standard risk and have a better outcome than those with a higher WBC at presentation, which is associated with higher risk of treatment failure (Table 95–6).

Specific chromosomal abnormalities in leukemic cells also possess prognostic significance. Blast cells with a translocation of parts of chromosome 12 and 21 (the *TEL–AML1* fusion) or trisomies of 4, 10, and 17 are considered to have favorable genetic features.[3] The presence of specific translocations between chromosome 9 and 22 (Ph⁺) is a high-risk feature, which is present in about 5% of patients with ALL.

The DNA content of blast cells, hyper-, hypo-, or diploid, corresponding to increased-, decreased-, or normal-chromosome numbers, has been considered prognostic. Lower-risk patients with hyperdiploidy (greater than 50 chromosomes per leukemic cell) generally include approximately 25% of children who have B lineage ALL.[7] These children are between the ages of 1 and 9 years, whereas the higher-risk patients with normal diploidy (50 chromosomes) generally are older.

Patients with cell-surface markers indicating that the blasts are early in the B-cell lineage (CD markers) are considered favorable and standard risk, whereas those with mature B-cell and T-cell blasts are considered high risk. T-cell ALL is found in approximately 15% of childhood ALL. Compared to B-lineage ALL, T-cell ALL is relatively resistant to different classes of drugs including methotrexate and cytarabine.

Patients completing induction treatment and in apparent remission still harbor malignant cells in their bone marrow, even though they appear disease-free by peripheral blood and bone marrow morphology. Assuming that most patients present with about a 10^{12} leukemic cell burden at diagnosis, at least 10^{10} or 1% residual disease remains after induction. These residual leukemic cells are below the limits of detection using standard morphologic examination. Measurement of this population of cells has become an increasingly significant prognostic factor and a determinant of the aggressiveness of postinduction therapy. Through flow cytometric analysis

and polymerase chain reaction, it is possible to detect one leukemic cell among 10^4 normal cells, representing a 100-fold greater sensitivity than morphological examination. ❹ *MRD is a quantitative assessment of subclinical remnant of leukemic burden remaining at the end of the initial phase of treatment (induction) when a patient may appear to be in a complete morphologic remission. This measure has become one of the strongest predictors of outcome for patients with acute leukemia. The elimination of MRD is a principal objective of postinduction leukemia therapy.*[14] Several studies in children, in whom ALL is common, have evaluated disease levels at the end of induction and correlated these values with EFS. For example, a patient with detectable MRD less than 0.1% at the end of induction has a EFS greater than 90% at 3 years. Conversely, a patient with high MRD (1%) has a 3-year EFS of only about 25%.[15] Assessment of MRD is also emerging as an important indicator of disease recurrence in the adult population and in patients with AML.

▶ Prognostic Factors in AML

The major prognostic factors in newly diagnosed AML are age, subtype, chromosome status, ethnicity, and body mass

Clinical Presentation and Diagnosis of AML[3,6,11]

General

Patients may have symptoms of AML for 1 to 3 months prior to presentation. These include fatigue, fever, and pallor, but patients generally are in no obvious distress.

Symptoms

- The patient may present with weakness, malaise, bleeding, and weight loss.
- Neutropenic patients are often febrile and highly susceptible to infection.
- Anemia usually presents as pallor, tiredness, and general fatigue.
- Patients with thrombocytopenia usually present with bruising, petechiae, and ecchymosis.
- Chloromas (localized leukemic deposits named after their color) may be seen, especially in the periorbital regions and as skin infiltrates.
- Gum hypertrophy is indicative of AML M4 and AML M5 subtypes.
- Disseminated intravascular coagulation is common in AML M3 and is associated with generalized bleeding or hemorrhage.
- Lymphadenopathy, massive hepatosplenomegaly, and bone pain are not as common in AML as in ALL.

Signs

- Temperature may be elevated secondary to an infection associated with a low WBC.

- Petechiae and bleeding are indicative of thrombocytopenia.

Laboratory Tests

- CBC with differential is performed.
- The anemia is usually normochromic and normocytic.
- Approximately 50% of children present with platelet counts of less than $50 \times 10^3/mm^3$ ($50 \times 10^9/L$).
- The WBC may be normal, decreased, or high. About 20% of patients have WBCs of over $100 \times 10^3/mm^3$ ($100 \times 10^9/L$), which places them at risk for leukostasis.
- Uric acid is increased in approximately 50% of patients secondary to rapid cellular turnover.
- *Electrolytes:* Potassium and phosphorus are often elevated. Calcium is usually low.
- *Coagulation disorders:* Elevated prothrombin time, partial thromboplastin time, D-dimers; hypofibrinogenemia

Other Diagnostic Tests

Flow cytometric evaluation of bone marrow and peripheral blood to characterize the type of leukemia, as well as to detect specific chromosomal rearrangements. The bone marrow at diagnosis usually is hypercellular, with normal hematopoiesis being replaced by leukemic blasts. The presence of greater than 20% blasts in the bone marrow is diagnostic for AML. At diagnosis, a lumbar puncture is performed to determine if CNS leukemia is present.

index. Older adults with AML (greater than 60 years), in comparison with younger patients with the same disease, have a dismal prognosis and represent a distinct population in terms of disease biology, treatment-related complications, and OS. These older patients have a higher incidence of unfavorable chromosomal abnormalities, such as aberrations of chromosomes 5, 7, or 8, and fewer abnormalities that are associated with a more favorable outcome, such as t(8;21) or inv(16) (see Table 95–7).[10]

Even though chromosomal abnormalities correlate with prognosis in adult AML, they appear to have less influence on outcome. Among children, the male gender, platelet count of less than $20 \times 10^3/mm^3$ ($20 \times 10^9/L$), hepatomegaly, more than 15% bone marrow blasts on day 14 of induction, MDS, and FAB subtype M5 all were associated with lower CR rates. The absence of these features and the presence of an abnormal chromosome 16 were associated with more favorable outcomes.[16]

Recent studies suggest that ethnicity may be an important predictor of outcome in children with AML. Investigators found that African Americans treated with chemotherapy had a significantly worse outcome than whites probably suggesting pharmacogenetic differences among the races. Body mass index may also affect the prognosis of children with AML. Underweight patients and overweight patients were less likely to survive than normoweight patients due to a greater risk of treatment-related deaths.[17]

TREATMENT

Desired Outcome

The primary objective in treating patients with acute leukemia is to achieve a continuous complete remission (CCR). Remission is defined as the absence of all clinical evidence of leukemia with the restoration of normal hematopoiesis. For both ALL and AML, remission induction is achieved with the use of highly myelosuppressive chemotherapy that initially induces a state of bone marrow aplasia as the leukemic cells die, followed by a slow return and proliferation of normal cells.[12] Following this period, hematopoiesis is restored. Failure to achieve remission in the first 7 to 14 days of therapy is highly predictive of later disease recurrence.

This again represents the growing importance of MRD in prognosis and treatment.

Nonpharmacologic Therapy

This year, roughly 1.6 million people will be diagnosed with cancer in the United States and Canada. With improvements in detection and treatment, approximately two-thirds of those diagnosed with the disease can expect to be alive in 5 years. With improving longevity, the cumulative adverse effects of both the disease and treatment are becoming an increasingly important issue. "Late-effects" data show that both adult and pediatric cancer survivors are at greater risk for developing second malignancies, cardiovascular disease, diabetes, and osteoporosis than those in the general population. With respect to the growing population of pediatric cancer survivors, data confirm that they are eight times more likely than their siblings to have a severe or life-threatening chronic health condition. For example, the survivors of pediatric ALL have an increased onset of obesity, osteopenia, and associated comorbidities. Thus, it is important to provide supportive care and intervention and counseling related to nutrition, smoking cessation, and exercise as a part of their active treatment. Health care professionals should think beyond the immediate treatment-related issues of their patients and provide appropriate, active assistance to promote healthy lifestyles and encourage patients to take active roles in pursuing general preventive health strategies.[18]

Pharmacologic Therapy: ALL

The treatment for ALL consists of four main elements: Remission induction (the initial tumor reduction leading to morphologic remission), CNS directed treatment and consolidation, delayed intensification, and maintenance phases of treatment all of which are aimed at complete elimination of the residual, but subclinical disease remaining after induction[7] (Table 95–8).

▶ Remission Induction

❺ *The initial treatment for acute leukemias is called induction. The purpose of induction is to induce a remission,*

	Risk Category		
Table 95–7			
Risk Category According to Cytogenetic Abnormalities Present			
Disease	**Good Risk**	**Intermediate Risk**	**High Risk**
AML	t(8;21)(q22;q22); inv(16); t(15;17); t(9;11) trisomy 21	Normal karyotype; trisomy 8; 11q23; del(7q); del(9q); trisomy 22	Complex karyotype; −5; −7; del (5q); inv(3P)
Probability of relapse	Less than or equal to 25%	50%	Greater than 70%
4-Year survival	Greater than or equal to 70%	40–50%	Less than or equal to 20%
ALL	Hyperdiploidy; t(10;14); or 6q		t(9;22); t(8;14); t(4;11); t(1;9)

ALL, acute lymphocytic leukemia; AML, acute myelogenous leukemia.

Adapted from Ref. 6.

a state where there is no identifiable leukemic cells in the bone marrow or peripheral blood with light microscopy. This definition may change as more sensitive techniques come into play.[19] ❻ *The current induction therapy for ALL typically consists of vincristine, asparaginase, and a steroid (prednisone or dexamethasone). An anthracycline is added for higher-risk patients.* Adults, unlike children, are universally considered to be at high risk for relapse, thus their induction regimens include an anthracycline (daunorubicin or doxorubicin) in addition to the standard steroid and vincristine treatment that have been the backbone of treatment for this disease for the last 40 years.[5] Dexamethasone is often replacing prednisone as the steroid of treatment because of its longer half-life and better CNS penetration.[6,20] Even though dexamethasone possesses more favorable pharmacologic characteristics than prednisone, its use may be associated with more aseptic osteonecrosis of the femoral and humoral heads as well as an increase in life-threatening infections and septic deaths.[20]

▶ CNS Prophylaxis

❼ *Leukemic invasion of the CNS is considered to be an almost universal event in patients, even in those whose CSF cytology shows no apparent disease. Thus, all patients with ALL and AML leukemia receive intrathecal (IT) chemotherapy. Although this is often referred to as "prophylaxis," it more realistically represents treatment.*[6] CNS prophylaxis relies on IT chemotherapy (e.g., methotrexate, cytarabine, and corticosteroids), systemic chemotherapy with dexamethasone and high-dose methotrexate, and craniospinal irradiation (XRT) in selected high-risk patients.[11] Cranial radiation was once a common intervention, but it is now reserved for only high-risk patients in whom IT treatment is inadequate. Its use has diminished substantially once the efficacy of IT treatment was evident, and the toxicities associated with radiation, learning disabilities, growth retardation, *and* secondary malignancies, were recognized. IT therapy has replaced cranial XRT as CNS prophylaxis for all except the very high-risk patients.

Inexplicably, the treatment of CNS leukemia has not had the same remarkable impact on the OS of adults as it has for childhood ALL. Although it reduces the incidence of CNS relapse in adults, it has not been associated with a measurable effect on survival.[11]

▶ Consolidation

After completion of induction and restoration of normal hematopoiesis, patients begin consolidation. The goal of consolidation is to administer dose-intensive chemotherapy in an effort to further reduce the burden of residual leukemic cells.[13] It is in this and subsequent treatment phases that the presence of MRD is reduced by increasing the aggressiveness of the drug regimen. Several regimens use agents and schedules designed to minimize the development of drug cross-resistance. Studies have demonstrated that this phase of treatment has proven to be an effective strategy in the prevention of relapse in children with ALL, but its benefits in adults are less clear.

In children, the intensity of the consolidation treatment is now determined not only by the child's risk classification but also by the rate of cytoreduction during induction.[5] Patients who respond slowly to induction therapy (as determined by bone marrow examination early in induction) are at higher risk of relapse and are treated on more aggressive regimens.

▶ Delayed Intensification

The Berlin-Frankfurt-Munster (BFM) Study Group introduced a treatment element called *delayed intensification (or reinduction) therapy.* This therapy consisted of repetition of the initial remission induction therapy administered approximately 3 months after remission. This, like consolidation, has been adopted as a component of treatment by virtually all institutions.[13]

Intensification regimens may vary in their aggressiveness and the drugs they use depending on the patient's risk group and immunophenotype. For example, the use of very-high-dose methotrexate (5 g/m^2) appears to improve outcome in patients with T-cell ALL. The use of intensive asparaginase treatment in T-cell ALL patients also has improved outcomes significantly.[13]

▶ Maintenance

The purpose of maintenance therapy is to further eliminate leukemic cells and produce an enduring CCR. The two most important agents in maintenance chemotherapy are a combination of oral methotrexate and 6-mercaptopurine. Improved outcome has been associated with increasing

---

Patient Encounter, Part 2

RH is admitted to the pediatric oncology service. She is started on allopurinol and IV fluids with sodium bicarbonate to prevent tumor lysis syndrome (TLS). According to her risk status, she will receive a three-drug induction with vincristine, dexamethasone, and pegylated asparaginase. She also will receive intrathecal (IT) chemotherapy for CNS prophylaxis with methotrexate, cytarabine, and hydrocortisone.

What is the role of CNS prophylaxis?

Patient Encounter, Part 3

RH had a bone marrow aspiration performed on days 15 and 29 that showed morphologic remission. The MRD on day 29 was less than 0.1%. RH completed her induction therapy and started intensification therapy.

What is the significance of MRD?

What is the purpose of intensification therapy?

Table 95–8

Representative Chemotherapy Regimens for Adult ALL

Remission Induction		CNS Prophylaxis		Consolidation		Maintenance
Drug and Dose	**Days**	**Prophylaxis**	**Days**	**Drug and Dose**	**Days**	**Drug, Dose, and Timing**
German or Hoelzer Regimen (Adult)[a]						
PRED (oral) 60 mg/m^2	1–28	Cranial irradiation		DEX (oral) 10 mg/m^2	1–28	MP (oral) 60 mg/m^2 daily and
VCR (IV) 1.5 mg/m^{2b}	1, 8, 15, 22	MTX (IT) 10 mg/m^{2c}	31, 38, 45, 52	VCR (IV) 1.5 mg/m^{2b}	1, 8, 15, 22	MTX (oral/IV) 20 mg/m^2 weekly, Weeks 10–18 and 29–130
DNR (IV) 25 mg/m^2	1, 8, 15, 22			DOX (IV) 25 mg/m^2	1, 8, 15, 22	
ASP (IV) 5,000 units/m^2	1–14			CTX (IV) 650 mg/m^{2d}	29	
CTX (IV) 650 mg/m^{2d}	29, 43, 57			Ara-C (IV) 75 mg/m^2	31–34, 38–41	
Ara-C (IV) 75 mg/m^2	31–34, 38–41, 45–48, 52–55			TG (oral) 60 mg/m^2	29–42	
MP (Oral) 60 mg/m^2	29–57					

CALGB 8811 (Adult)[e]

Course I

CTX (IV) 1,200 mg/m^2	1
DNR (IV) 45 mg/m^2	1, 2, 3
VCR (IV) 2 mg	1, 8, 15, 22
PRED (Oral) 60 mg/m^2	1–21
ASP (SC) 6,000 units/m^2	5, 8, 11, 15, 18, 22

Induction chemotherapy for patients greater than or equal to 60 year old, use:

CTX (IV) 800 mg/m^2	1
DNR (IV) 30 mg/m^2	1–3
PRED (Oral) 60 mg/m^2	1–7

Course III

Cranial irradiation	
MTX (IT) 15 mg	1, 8, 15, 22, 29
MP (oral) 60 mg/m^2	1–70
MTX (oral) 20 mg/m^2	36, 43, 50, 57, 64

Course II: Early intensification

MTX (IT) 15 mg	1
CTX (IV) 1,000 mg/m^2	1
MP (Oral) 60 mg/m^2	1–14
Ara-C (SC) 75 mg/m^2	1–4, 8–11
VCR (IV) 2 mg	15, 22
ASP (SC) 6,000 units/m^2	15, 18, 22, 25

Course IV: Late intensification

DOX (IV) 30 mg/m^2	1, 8, 15
VCR (IV) 2 mg	1, 8, 15
DEX (Oral) 10 mg/m^2	1–14
CTX (IV) 1,000 mg/m^2	29
TG (Oral) 60 mg/m^2	29–42
Ara-C (SC) 75 mg/m^2	29–32, 36–39

Course V

VCR (IV) 2 mg day 1 monthly	
PRED (Oral) 60 mg/m^2 days 1–5 monthly	
MTX (Oral) 20 mg/m^2 days 1, 8, 15, 22 monthly	
MP (Oral) 60 mg/m^2 days 1–28 monthly	

ASP, asparaginase; C, cytarabine; CALGB, Cancer and Leukemia Group B; CTX, cyclophosphamide; DEX, dexamethasone; DNR, daunorubicin; DOX, doxorubicin; IT, intrathecal; MP, mercaptopurine; MTX, methotrexate; PRED, prednisone; SC, subcutaneous; TG, thioguanine; VCR, vincristine.

[a]Holzer D, Thiel E, Ludwig WD, et al. Follow-up of the first two successive German multicentre trials for adult ALL (01/81 and 2/84). Leukemia 1993;7(suppl 2):130–134.

[b]Maximum single dose, 2 mg.

[c]Maximum single dose, 15 mg.

[d]Maximum single dose, 1,000 mg.

[e]Larson RA, Dodge RK, Burns CP, et al. A five-drug remission induction regimen with intensive consolidation for adults with acute lymphocytic leukemia. Cancer and leukemia Group B study 8811. Blood 1995;85:2025–2037.

Adapted from Leather HL, Bickert B. Acute leukemias. In: DiPiro JT, Talbert RL, Yee GC, et al., (eds.) Pharmacotherapy: A Pathophysiologic Approach. 6th ed. New York: McGraw-Hill; 2005: 2191–2213.

Patient Encounter, Part 4: Creating a Care Plan

After completion of induction and intensification therapy, RH will begin maintenance therapy for 2.5 years.

Which agents are used in maintenance therapy?

Why is maintenance therapy of such a long duration?

Create a care plan to include: (a) monitoring parameters during maintenance therapy; (b) a list of drug-related problems to access toxicity during maintenance therapy; and (c) goals of maintenance therapy.

6-mercaptopurine dosages to the limits of individual tolerance based on absolute neutrophil count (ANC). The goal is to induce a moderate immunosuppression and leukemic cell kill. 6-Mercaptopurine at usual doses causes significant neutropenia and its use has been associated with increased rates of infection. At lower doses, it is associated with poor leukemic activity and a higher rate of relapse. In both instances, 6-mercaptopurine is associated with the inability to deliver planned appropriate therapy. 6-Mercaptopurine is metabolized by thiopurine methyltransferase (TPMT). TPMT deficiency is inherited as an autosomal recessive trait, with 89% to 94% of whites having high activity, 6% to 11% having intermediate activity, and 0.3% having very low or no activity. This deficiency is explained largely by three polymorphisms in the *TPMT* gene (*2, *3A, and *3C) that also have a profound influence on 6-mercaptopurine tolerance and dose-intensity in children with ALL. While these polymorphisms are rare, they are certainly important, with case reports of toxic deaths attributed to 6-mercaptopurine dating back several decades.

Children who were homozygous for one of the alleles require 6-mercaptopurine dose reductions of 90%, whereas heterozygotes require a dose reduction of approximately 50%. Children with dose reductions had equivalent OS when compared with children receiving full-dose 6-mercaptopurine, suggesting that TPMT polymorphisms are important for drug metabolism and toxicity but play no role in the pathogenesis of ALL. TPMT screening is recommended for children starting therapy with 6-mercaptopurine, with empirical dose reductions for those with genotypes associated with a deficiency. The addition of intermittent "pulses" of vincristine and a steroid (usually dexamethasone) to the antimetabolite backbone improves outcome and is encouraged in most modern continuation regimens.[12]

The optimal duration of maintenance therapy in both children and adults is unknown, but most regimens are given for 2 to 3 years; extension of the regimen beyond 3 years has not shown any additional benefit.

ALL in Infants

Infants account for approximately 5% of all children with ALL, and they experience the worst prognosis of any group

of children with the disease. These patients have several poor prognostic features at diagnosis, including hyperleukocytosis, hepatomegaly, splenomegaly, and CNS leukemia.[6] The bone marrow of infants at day 14 usually shows poor response to therapy. Infants with ALL have increased frequencies of cytogenetic abnormalities; 60% to 70% have a translocation that involves the *MLL* gene located at 11q23. The 11q23 breakpoint abnormality, t(4,11), is the most common structural karyotypic abnormality in infants with ALL. In vitro, blasts from infants with ALL showed greater drug resistance to prednisolone and L-asparaginase than those from older patients, although they are more sensitive to cytarabine.[13] Based on this information, several studies are testing the efficacy of intensified chemotherapy that includes high-dose cytarabine. Another achievement is the prevention of CNS relapse using IT cytarabine in conjunction with high-dose systemic cytarabine. This combination has eliminated the need for cranial XRT in this young population. Even with major advances in cure rates for the general pediatric ALL population, where survival is 80% or more, the long-term EFS of infants is only about 40% (Tables 95–9 and 95–10).

ALL in the Elderly

The proportion of ALL in patients older than age 60 years constitutes between 16% and 31% of all adult leukemias. Treatment of adults largely has followed the conventional chemotherapeutic regimes used in childhood ALL. However, the intensification regimens common in childhood are not suitable for this population because of their associated toxicities in older patients. The adverse prognostic factor, the Ph+, occurs in 15% to 30% of adults and thus is more common in the over 60 age group.[21] Based on the experience achieved in CML, the use of imatinib, a potent inhibitor of the Ph+-associated *BCR–ABL* tyrosine kinase, is becoming a common practice for these older adults. Results show that the combination of imatinib with conventional chemotherapy has improved remission rates compared with the use of conventional chemotherapy alone, although the effect on long-term disease-free survival (DFS) is unclear. With other tyrosine kinase inhibitors, dasatinib and nilotinib, resistance can be overcome, but the remission is not long lasting.[7] Improving the outcomes of these elderly patients with ALL continues to be a challenge.

Relapsed ALL

Relapse is the recurrence of leukemic cells at any site after remission has been achieved. ❽ *Relapse is a major complication for 15% to 20% of patients with ALL. Current research suggests that this is the result of residual leukemic cells at diagnosis. Thus the importance of MRD.*[22] Bone marrow relapse is the principal form of treatment failure in patients with ALL. Extramedullary sites of relapse include the CNS and the testicles.[23] Extramedullary relapse while once common, has decreased to 5% or less because of effective prophylaxis. Site of relapse and the length of the first remission are important predictors of second

Table 95–9

Representative Chemotherapy Regimens for Pediatric ALL

Induction (1 month)

Intrathecal cytarabine on day 0
Prednisone 40 mg/m²/day or dexamethasone 6 mg/m²/day orally for 28 days
Vincristine 1.5 mg/m²/dose (max 2 mg) IV weekly for 4 doses
Pegaspargase 2,500 units/m²/dose IM for 1 dose or asparaginase 6,000 units/m²/dose IM Mon, Wed, and Fri for 6 doses
Intrathecal methotrexate weekly for 2–4 doses

Consolidation (1 month)

Mercaptopurine 50–75 mg/m²/dose orally at bedtime for 28 days
Vincristine 1.5 mg/m²/dose (max 2 mg) IV on day 0
Intrathecal methotrexate weekly for 1–3 doses
Patients with CNS or testicular disease may receive radiation

Interim Maintenance (1 or 2 cycles) (2 months)

Methotrexate 20 mg/m²/dose orally at bedtime weekly
Mercaptopurine 75 mg/m²/dose orally daily on days 0–49
Vincristine 1.5 mg/m²/dose (max 2 mg) IV on days 0 and 28
Dexamethasone 6 mg/m²/day orally on days 0–4 and 28–32

Delayed Intensification (1 or 2 cycles) (2 months)

Dexamethasone 10 mg/m²/day orally on days 0–6 and 14–20
Vincristine 1.5 mg/m²/dose (max 2 mg) IV weekly for 3 doses
Pegaspargase 2,500 units/m²/dose IM for 1 dose
Doxorubicin 25 mg/m²/dose IV on days 0, 7, and 14
Cyclophosphamide 1,000 mg/m²/dose IV on day 28
Thioguanine 60 mg/m²/dose orally at bedtime on days 28–41
Cytarabine 75 mg/m²/dose SC or IV on days 28–31 and 35–38
Intrathecal methotrexate on days 0 and 28

Consolidation Option (2–3-week intervals for 6 courses on weeks 5–24)

Mercaptopurine 50 mg/m²/dose orally at bedtime
Prednisone 40 mg/m²/day for 7 days on weeks 8 and 17
Vincristine 1.5 mg/m²/dose (max 2 mg) IV on the first day of weeks 8, 9, 17, and 18
Methotrexate 200 mg/m²/dose IV + 800 mg/m2/dose over 24 hours on day 1 of weeks 7, 10, 13, 16, 19, and 22
Intrathecal methotrexate on weeks 5, 6, 9, 12, 15, and 18

Late Intensification (weeks 25–52)

Methotrexate 20 mg/m²/dose IM weekly or 25 mg/m²/dose orally every 6 hours for 4 doses every other week
Mercaptopurine 75 mg/m²/dose orally at bedtime
Prednisone 40 mg/m²/day orally for 7 days on weeks 25 and 41
Vincristine 1.4 mg/m²w/dose (max 2 mg) IV on the first day of weeks 25, 26, 41, and 42
Intrathecal methotrexate on day 1 of weeks 25, 33, 41, and 49

Maintenance (12-week cycles)

Methotrexate 20 mg/m²/dose orally at bedtime or IM weekly with dose escalation as tolerated
Mercaptopurine 75 mg/m²/dose orally at bedtime on days 0–83
Vincristine 1.5 mg/m²/dose (max 2 mg) IV on days 0, 28, and 56
Dexamethasone 6 mg/m²/day orally on days 0–4, 28–32, and 56–60
Intrathecal methotrexate on day 0

IM, intramuscular; SC, subcutaneous.

Adapted from Leather HL, Bickert B. Acute Leukemias. In: DiPiro JT, Talbert RL, Yee GC, et al., (eds.) Pharmacotherapy: A Pathophysiologic Approach, 6th ed. New York: McGraw-Hill; 2005: 2458–2511.

remission and OS. Marrow relapses occurring less than 18 to 24 months into first remission are associated with a poor survival, while longer periods of remission, greater than 36 months, have a much higher chance of survival.[22] Treatment strategies for relapsed ALL include chemotherapy or allogeneic hematopoietic stem cell transplant (allo-HSCT). Even though patients undergoing allo-HSCT are less likely to relapse, treatment-related toxicity leads to a higher incidence of morbidity and mortality as compared to chemotherapy alone.[6] Clofarabine, a next-generation deoxyadenosine analog, has shown considerable activity in children and adults with refractory acute leukemias. Of interest, this is the only anticancer drug to receive primary indication for use in pediatrics in the last 10 years.[24]

Treatment: AML

As with ALL, the primary aim in treating patients with AML is to induce remission and thereafter prevent relapse. Treatment of AML is conventionally divided into two phases: induction and consolidation. Despite several strategies to increase the intensity of therapy, the OS rate has reached a plateau at 50% to 60%, suggesting that further intensification of therapy will not improve survival rates greatly.[12] ❾ *The current induction therapy for AML usually consists of a combination of cytarabine and daunorubicin, with the frequent addition of a steroid and/or an antimetabolite such as 6-thioguanine. The second phase of treatment for AML is called* consolidation. *The purpose of this phase is to further enhance remission with more cytoreduction.*

▶ Remission Induction

The goal of induction chemotherapy in AML is essentially identical to that in ALL: "Empty" the bone marrow of all hematopoietic precursors, and allow repopulation with normal cells. The combination of an anthracycline (e.g., daunorubicin, doxorubicin, or idarubicin) and the antimetabolite cytarabine forms the backbone of AML induction therapy. The most common induction regimen (7 + 3) combines daunorubicin for 3 days with cytarabine on days 1 to 7. The remission rate for this combination is approximately 80% in children and younger adults but declines to 40% to 50% in patients older than 60 years of age.[6] Despite studies that have used alternative anthracyclines or substituted high-dose for conventional-dose cytarabine and added etoposide and/or thioguanine, the 7 + 3 regimen remains the standard induction regimen.

▶ Postremission Therapy

Once an initial remission is achieved, further intensive therapy is imperative to prevent relapse. Induction therapy fails to provide adequate cell kill, and leukemia cells survive the initial treatment. Three options available for patients include high-dose chemotherapy, allog-HSCT from

Table 95–10

Chemotherapy for the Acute Leukemias

Agent/Major Uses	Class/Mechanism	Major Side Effects	Drug Interactions
Asparaginase (L-asparaginase; Elspar) Pegaspargase (Oncospar) ALL	Antitumor enzyme, hydrolyzes L-asparagine in bloodstream, depriving tumor cells of the essential amino acid; results in inhibition of protein, DNA, and RNA synthesis and cell proliferation; derived from *Escharichia coli*	Hypersensitivity reactions (fever, hypotension, rash, dyspnea in 25%), much lower risk with polyethylene gycol form; low emetogenic potential; pancreatitis; decreased synthesis of proteins, clotting factors; CNS: lethargy	Increased toxicity has been noted when given concurrently with vincristine and prednisone. Decreased metabolism when used with cyclophosphamide Increased hepatotoxicity when used with mercaptopurine
Cytarabine (Ara-C; cytosine arabinoside; Cytosar-U) ANLL; ALL; Lymphomatous meningitis; NHL; MDS High-dose Ara-C (HiDAC) liposomal cytarabine (DepoCyt) for IT use for lymphomatous meningitis	Antipyrimidine antimetabolite; inhibits DNA polymerase with inhibition of DNA strand elongation and replication; activated in tumor cells in triphosphate form; competes with conversion of cytidine to deoxycytidine nucleotides, further blocking polymerization of DNA; leads to production of short DNS strands; cell-cycle specific (S phase): acts only on proliferating cells	Myelosuppression; alopecia; moderate emetogenic; worse with high dose (greater than 1 g/m^2) or IT administration; diarrhea; mucositis; flu-like syndrome with fever and arthralgias; rash often followed by desquamation on palms and soles HiDAC toxicities; cerebellar direct neurotoxicity:ataxia, slurred speech, nystagmus; conjunctivitis (drug is excreted into tears and blocks corneal DNA synthesis)	Possible increased toxicity when given concurrently with alkylating agents, radiation, purine analogs, and methotrexate
Daunorubicin (daunomycin, Dauno, Cerubidine) *Liposomal daunorubicin (DaunoXome)* ANLL; ALL; KS	Antitumor antibiotic; topoisomerase II inhibitor; DNA intercalator; free-radical formation (thought to be related to cardiac toxicity and tissue injury)	Myelosuppression (dose-related); mucositis (worse with continuous infusion); moderate emetogenic potential; alopecia; vesicant. severe extravasation injury; cardiac toxicities: *acute*—not related to cumulative dose; arrhythmias, pericarditis; chronic—cumulative injury to myocardium (total dose greater than 550 mg/m^2; lower total cumulative doses cause damage to myocardium in children (e.g., 350 mg/m^2)	
Etoposide (VP-16; Vepesid), Etoposide phosphate (Etopophos) Testicular cancer; SCLC; NSCLC; ANLL; KS; HD; NHL; BMT preparative chemotherapy; gastric cancer	Plant alkaloid, epipodophyllotoxin; inhibits DNA binding activity of topoisomerase II, resulting in multiple DNA double-strand breaks	Myelosuppression; moderately emetogenic: may be worse with oral and high-dose regimens; alopecia; mucositis; hypotension: infusion rate-related; etoposide phosphate can be given IV push without hypotension risk; hypersensitivity reactions: especially common in children	Substrate of MDR Cyclosporine may increase levels of etoposide
Gemtuzumab ozogamicin (Mylotarg)	Humanized antiCD33 antibody linked to calicheamicin, a potent toxin; binding to the CD33 receptor results in internalization of the antibody-antigen complex; calicheamicin is then released intracellularly and exerts cytotoxicity by causing DNA double-strand breaks, resulting in cell death	Infusion reactions: fevers, chills, nausea, vomiting, hypotension, dyspnea; myelosuppression may be severe and prolonged; tumor lysis syndrome: WBCs should be reduced to less than 30 × 10^3/mm^3 (30 × 10^9/L) prior to administration if possible, to decrease risk; increased liver function tests and bilirubin, hepatic veno-occlusive disease	
Imatinib mesylate (Gleevec, STI 571) CML (adults and pediatrics); GIST; Ph+ ALL	Tyrosine kinase inhibitor; relatively specific for the tyrosine kinase coded for by the *BCR–abl* translocation in CML patients	Moderate emetogenic potential: take with meals and a full glass of water; edema; periorbital edema is characteristic; pleural effusions, ascites, or pulmonary edema also occur; rash; diarrhea; neutropenia, thrombocytopenia (sometimes difficult to distinguish from CML-induced cytopenias); increased liver function tests	Drug interactions are minimal. Substrate of P450 3A4 Serum concentrations of imatinib may be increased by drugs which inhibit CYP3A4

(Continued)

Table 95–10

Chemotherapy for the Acute Leukemias (*Continued*)

Agent/Major Uses	Class/Mechanism	Major Side Effects	Drug Interactions
6-Mercaptopurine (Purinethol; 6-MP) ALL	Antipurine antimetabolite; purine analog; inhibits DNA, RNA, protein synthesis; metabolized by xanthine oxidase	Myelosuppression: mild, anorexia, low emetogenic potential; dry skin rash, photosensitivity; hepatotoxicity: jaundice and hyperbilirubinemia occur after 1–2 months of therapy and may be dose-limiting	Allopurinol can increase levels of mercaptopurine. Aminosalicylates may inhibit TPMT
Methotrexate (MTX) ALL CNS leukemia (IT) Breast cancer NHL Osteosarcoma Head and neck cancer Bladder cancer Rheumatoid arthritis	Folic acid antagonist; inhibits dihydrofolate reductase (DHFR); blocks reduction of folate to tetrahydrofolate; inhibits de novo purine synthesis; results in arrest of DNA, RNA, and protein synthesis Leucovorin provides reduced folate to bypass the metabolic block	Myelosuppression: can be prevented with leucovorin rescue Mucositis: can be prevented with leucovorin Renal dysfunction: (high-dose regimens) caused by precipitation of drug in renal tubules; hydration (3 L/m²/day) and alkalinization of urine	Salicylates, sulfonamides, probenecid, and high-dose penicillin may decrease clearance of methotrexate
Vincristine (VCR, Oncovin) ALL; HD; NHL; multiple myeloma; breast cancer; SCLC, KS; brain tumors; soft tissue sarcomas; osteosarcomas; neuroblastoma; Wilms' tumor	Antimicrotubule agent/vinca alkaloid; derived from periwinkle plant; disrupts formation of microtubules	Peripheral neuropathy: primary dose-limiting toxicity; motor sensory, autonomic, and cranial nerves may all be affected (paresthesias, ileus, urinary retention, facial palsies); may be irreversible; mild emetogenic; SIADH; vesicant: extravasation injury	Vincristine levels may be increased when given with drugs that inhibit cytochrome P450 3A enzyme (itraconazole)

ALL, acute lymphocytic leukemia; ANLL, acute nonlymphocytic leukemia; BMT, bone marrow transplant; C, cytarabine; CD, cluster determinants; CML, chronic myelogenous leukemia; CYP, cytochrome; DNS, DNS strands; GIST, gastrointestinal stromal tumor; HD, Hodgkin's disease; HiDAC, high-dose Ara-C; IT, intrathecal; KS, Kaposi's sarcoma; MDS, myelodysplastic syndrome; MTX, methotrexate; NHL, non-Hodgkin's lymphoma; NSCLC, non small cell lung cancer; Ph⁺, Philadelphia chromosome; SIADH, syndrome of inappropriate antidiuretic hormone; SCLC, small cell lung cancer; VCR, vincristine; VP, etoposide.

Adapted from McManus Balmer C, Wells Valley A, Iannucci A. Cancer Treatment and Chemotherapy. In: DiPiro JT, Talbert RL, Yee GC, et al., (eds.) Pharmacotherapy: A Pathophysiologic Approach, 6th ed. New York: McGraw-Hill; 2005: 2458–2511.

an human leukocyte antigen matched (HLA-matched) related or unrelated donor, and autologous bone marrow transplantation.[9]

▶ *Postremission Chemotherapy*

In AML, postremission chemotherapy is often referred to as consolidation therapy.[6] Several cycles of intensive postremission chemotherapy combining noncross-resistant agents given every 4 to 6 weeks improves DFS. One of three cytarabine-based regimens has been used in current treatment programs, either alone or in combination with L-asparaginase, mitoxantrone, or etoposide. The following cytarabine dosing schedule is used: 100 mg/m²/day for 5 days by continuous infusion (standard-dose arm), 400 mg/m²/day for 5 days by continuous infusion (intermediate-dose arm), or 3 g/m² twice daily over 3 hours on days 1, 3, and 5 (high-dose arm). The higher-dose regimen for cytarabine can be tolerated only by younger patients (younger than 60 years of age). While the optimal number of courses remains to be determined, at least three are probably required.[11]

Gemtuzumab ozogamicin is an MAB that binds to the CD-33 antigen. Almost all AML cells express this antigen. Phase I and II trials using this agent have shown some success, and current studies using this agent alone or with chemotherapy for the treatment of AML are ongoing.[25]

Allogeneic Hematopoietic Stem Cell Transplantation
Allo-*HSCT* has been used in the treatment of pediatric AML in first complete remission. In most clinical trials, the availability of HLA-matched sibling donors determined whether patients underwent HSCT as postremission treatment. To facilitate this process, it is important to obtain HLA typing on all younger patients with AML and siblings shortly after diagnosis. Patients who do not have an HLA-matched sibling will proceed to postremission therapy with chemotherapy alone.

In HSCT, very high doses of chemotherapy with or without total-body radiation (TBI) are given in an attempt to potentiate leukemia cell kill. Hematopoiesis is restored by the infusion of stem cells harvested from an HLA-compatible donor, thereby rescuing the patient from the consequences of total aplasia.[15] It is the most effective antileukemic therapy currently available.

Transplantations from nonidentical sources have many complications, including graft-versus-host disease (GVHD), delayed or incomplete engraftment, and an increased likelihood of opportunistic infections that increase morbidity and mortality substantially. An immunological effect of the donor marrow on residual host-leukemic cells may translate into antileukemic activity, however, as indicated by the lower relapse rates in patients with GVHD. This graft-versus-leukemia (GVL) effect also accounts for the success of allo-HSCT.

Transplant-related mortality following matched-sibling allo-HSCT is 20% to 30% in most series. Complications from transplantation increase with age; therefore, patients older than 60 years of age are uncommonly considered to receive a myeloablative allo-HSCT. Since the average age of AML patients is 65 years, most patients with this disease are not candidates for this form of therapy. For older patients up to 70 years, a reduced-intensity (mini or nonmyelobative allogeneic) transplant may be an option. These transplants use less intensive preparative regimens and rely on the allogeneic GVL effect to eliminate their disease.[5]

HSCT in first remission is often recommended for patients with a matched-sibling donor because of the lower relapse rate with transplant versus postremission chemotherapy. However, only 30% of patients will have an HLA-matched sibling. Some types of AML patients may be curable with conventional-dose chemotherapy alone. Thus indiscriminate use of allo-HSCT could reduce the rate and quality of survival in these individuals.

Autologous Hematopoietic Stem Cell Transplantation

Since the majority of AML patients lack a HLA-identical donor, investigators began to consider the use of the patient's own bone marrow, obtained while in CR, as a source of hematopoietic regeneration. However, relapse continues to be a problem secondary to the presence of residual disease in the graft. The DFS for patients undergoing autologous bone-marrow transplantation in first remission has been reported at 40% to 60%, with a relapse rate of 30% to 50%. Thus few investigators recommend the use of autologous transplantation, because it failed to improve outcome substantially versus standard postremission chemotherapy.[3,10]

▶ CNS Therapy

The prevalence of CNS disease at diagnosis of AML ranges from 5% to 30% in various treatment series. Features associated with the risk of CNS leukemia include hyperleukocytosis, monocytic, or myelomonocytic leukemia (FAB M4 or M5), and young age. In most cases, IT cytarabine with or without methotrexate and systemic high-dose cytarabine provide adequate CNS prophylaxis.[3] Results from studies have shown that patients with CNS disease at diagnosis can be cured with IT therapy alone without the use of cranial XRT.[11]

AML in Infants

AML in infants younger than 12 months shows clinical and biological characteristics different from AML in older children. The phenotype is more commonly monoblastic or myelomonoblastic (M4, M5), and the patients usually present with hyperleukocytosis. Extramedullary involvement is common, often involving skin and other organs. As in infant ALL, there is a high incidence of translocations involving the *MLL* gene in infant AML. The number of infant AML trials reported is limited, but the EFS is similar to that of older children with AML. This is in marked contrast to the outcomes for infants with ALL, for whom the EFS is much lower than in older children (Tables 92–9 and 92–10).[26]

AML in the Elderly

AML is the most common acute leukemia in the elderly. In comparison with younger patients with the same disease, older adults have a poor prognosis and represent a distinct population with regard to disease biology. Older adults have a lower incidence of favorable chromosomal aberrations and a higher incidence of unfavorable aberrations.[10]

In older adults, AML is either more likely to arise from a proximal bone marrow–stem cell disorder, such as MDS, or present as a secondary leukemia resulting from treatment with prior chemotherapy or radiation for an earlier malignancy. These forms of AML are notoriously less responsive to chemotherapy and thus have a lower CR rate and EFS.[27]

Older adults are not as tolerant of or as responsive to remission induction and consolidation chemotherapy as younger patients. Younger adults treated with a standard-induction regimen of an anthracycline and cytarabine have approximately 70% probability of attaining a CR, whereas patients older than 60 years of age have only a 38% to 62% probability. Further, long-term survival for patients older than 60 years is only 5% to 15% compared with 30% DFS for younger adults.[10]

Relapsed AML

Even though 75% to 85% of patients with AML will achieve a remission, only about 50% will survive. Patients who relapse usually respond less to treatment and have a shorter duration of remission. This is related to drug resistance during induction, certain chromosomal abnormalities, and the length of the first remission. Even though there is no standard therapy for relapse, most studies have shown that the use of high-dose cytarabine containing regimens have considerable activity in obtaining a second remission. Cytarabine has been used in combination with mitoxantrone, etoposide, fludarabine, 2-chlorodeoxyadenosine, and most recently, clofarabine.[28] Once a patient has achieved a second remission with conventional chemotherapy, allo-HSCT is the therapy of choice. For patients without an HLA-matched sibling, a matched unrelated donor (MUD) or cord blood transplant may be a reasonable alternative. The combination of myeloablative high-dose chemotherapy and the GVL effect is thought to offer the best chance of survival in AML.

Complications of Treatment

▶ *Tumor Lysis Syndrome*

Tumor lysis syndrome (TLS) is an oncological emergency that is characterized by metabolic abnormalities resulting from the death of blast cells and the release of large amounts of purines, pyrimidines, and intracellular potassium and phosphorus. Uric acid, the ultimate breakdown product of purines, is poorly soluble in plasma and urine. Deposition of uric acid and calcium phosphate crystals in the renal tubules can lead to acute renal failure. Many patients with acute leukemia, especially those with a high tumor burden, are at risk for TLS during the first few days of chemotherapy. Measures to prevent TLS include aggressive hydration, alkalinization to help solubilize uric acid, allopurinol, and on some occasions, the use of rasburicase. Rasburicase is an enzyme that catalyzes the oxidation of uric acid to allantoin, which are more soluble and excreted more easily than uric acid.[28] Given its high cost, rasburicase generally is restricted to patients with a high WBC (greater than 50 × 10^3/mm^3, 50 × 10^9/L) and uric acid levels greater than 8 g/dL (476 μmol/L).[29]

▶ *Infection*

Infection is a primary cause of death in acute leukemia patients. The majority of chemotherapy used to treat ALL and AML can cause severe myelosuppression, placing the patient at risk for sepsis from otherwise normal bacteria. It is important to recognize that symptoms and signs of infection may be absent in a severely immunosuppressed or neutropenic patient. Fever (greater than 38.3°C [100.9°F]) in a neutropenic patient is a medical emergency. Following chemotherapy, the period of neutropenia usually reaches its nadir approximately 14 days after the beginning of a course of chemotherapy and usually lasts another 7 to 14 days. In a newly diagnosed leukemic, the period of neutropenia may persist until remission is obtained. The most common sites of infection include the GI tract and vascular access devices.[6]

Because the progression of infection in neutropenic patients can be rapid, empirical antibiotic therapy should be administered quickly to such patients once fever is documented. Currently, the most commonly used initial antibiotic agent is cefepime, a fourth-generation cephalosporin that has good antipseudomonal coverage as well as adequate coverage against *viridans* streptococci and pneumococci.[30]

The therapy for AML is extremely myelosuppressive. Children with AML have a 10% to 20% induction mortality rate secondary to infection and bleeding complications. Therefore, patients receiving induction therapy usually are hospitalized for the first 4 to 6 weeks of therapy. The induction therapy for ALL is less myelosuppressive; therefore, these patients recover their counts quicker and usually do not require prolonged hospitalizations.[6]

Trimethoprim-sulfamethoxazole is started in all patients with acute leukemia for the prevention of *Pneumocystis carinii* pneumonia. Patients normally continue this therapy for 6 months after completion of treatment. The use of additional antibiotic prophylaxis is not encouraged in all patients with leukemia because of concerns for antibiotic resistance.

▶ *Secondary Malignancies*

In children, secondary malignancies are a risk of the successful treatment for cancer. The chemotherapy agents used, especially alkylating agents and topoisomerase II inhibitors, predispose the patient to secondary hematopoietic neoplasms. As the aggressiveness of treatment and the number of survivors of ALL increase, the risk of secondary neoplasms also may rise. There are two different types of second malignancies: acute leukemia, which generally is myeloid in origin (or MDS), and solid tumors. The latency period between treatment and the development of a secondary leukemia is often several years, with leukemia being the earlier and solid tumors being the later of such events.

Secondary neoplasms induced by epipodophyllotoxins are characterized by balanced chromosomal translocations and short latency periods (2–4 years). The risk of this leukemia is related to schedule (dose intensity) and the concomitant use of other agents (L-asparaginase, alkylating agents, and possibly antimetabolites). The prognosis for topoisomerase II inhibitor–related secondary leukemia is extremely poor. Only about 10% of these patients survive after chemotherapy, and only 20% survive after HSCT. The incidence of second cancers attributed to alkylators peaks 4 to 6 years after exposure and plateaus after 10 to 15 years. Higher cumulative doses and older age at the time of treatment are risk factors for this type of cancer.[31]

Ionizing radiation therapy is also a cause of secondary malignancies. These secondary tumors generally develop within or adjacent to the previous radiation field. These cancers often have a prolonged latency, typically 15 to 30 years, but shorter latencies (5–14 years) are known. Higher doses of radiation and younger age are associated with an increased risk of secondary malignancy.

Unlike children, adults may have other factors that predispose them to secondary malignancies. Lifestyle choices such as tobacco use, alcohol use, and diet have been implicated in influencing the development of secondary neoplasms in the adult population.

Now that 80% or more of children survive their primary cancers, the incidence of secondary neoplasms may increase. Recognizing this potential, many treatment regimens for children are being modified appropriately to reduce exposure to alkylators, topoisomerase inhibitors, and radiation. Late effects clinics screen for secondary malignancies and other disease and treatment-related disabilities that accompany childhood cancer. Similar screening and educational opportunities are not currently established in adult survivors. The Lance Armstrong Foundation is raising awareness of the concerns of adult and pediatric cancer survivors by providing grants for research and program development in addressing the long-term issues related to disease and treatment.

▶ *Late Effects*

● With increased success in pediatric clinical trials, the OS rate for pediatric cancers has increased significantly over the last 35 years. For certain disease states, the OS rate for specific pediatric malignancies is now up to 80%. ❿ *Although survival in pediatric cancers has improved dramatically over the last 35 years, 50% to 60% of cancer survivors are estimated to have at least one chronic or late-occurring complication of treatment.*[24]

In leukemia, the intensified use of methotrexate and glucocorticoids is responsible for causing an increased frequency of neurotoxicity and, in older children and adults, avascular necrosis of bone. High cumulative doses of anthracyclines can cause cardiomyopathy. Cranial XRT causes neuropsychological deficits and endocrine abnormalities that lead to obesity, short stature, precocious puberty, and osteoporosis.[3] As newer and more intensive treatments enter clinical trials, close observation for long-term side effects will assume even greater importance.[25]

▶ *Supportive Care*

Because of the need for repeated venous access, a central venous catheter or infusion port is placed prior to starting treatment. These devices are useful not only for delivery of chemotherapy but also to support patients during periods of myelosuppression. Infection and bleeding complications are the primary cause of mortality in patients with leukemia.

Platelet transfusions are used to prevent hemorrhage. Patients with uncomplicated thrombocytopenia can be transfused when the platelet count falls below $10 \times 10^3/\text{mm}^3$ $(10 \times 10^9/\text{L})$. Patients who are either highly febrile or actively bleeding may require transfusions at higher levels. Red blood cell transfusions generally are not necessary for a hemoglobin concentration greater than 8 g/dL (80 g/L, 4.96 mmol/L).

There is much controversy regarding the routine use of colony-stimulating factors (e.g., G-CSF and GM-CSF) in neutropenic patients. Even though several clinical trials have shown the time to ANC recovery is decreased with a colony-stimulating factor, none have demonstrated that CSFs statistically influence infection-related mortality. At present, the use of colony-stimulating factors (G-CSF most commonly) generally is limited to those chemotherapy regimens that place the patient at highest risk for prolonged neutropenia.[6]

OUTCOME EVALUATION

Developing strategies for the treatment and monitoring of acute leukemias begins with risk stratification. Understanding the likely risk of relapse determines the aggressiveness and length of therapy. Remission status following the induction phase of treatment should be monitored closely by following bone marrow status and MRD. Failure to obtain morphologic bone marrow remission by day 28 is a bad prognostic sign that dictates further induction treatment. For those with

---

Patient Care and Monitoring

1. Evaluate the patient for response to therapy during induction, consolidation, and maintenance by following hematologic indices closely.

2. Review the treatment plan closely with the patient.

3. Educate the patient on potential adverse reactions and drug interactions.

4. Stress the importance of medication compliance.

5. Provide patient education regarding disease state and drug therapy:

   • Possible complications of leukemia, especially infections.

   • Potential side effects of drug therapy

   • Warning signs to report to the physician (e.g., temperature, bruising, or bleeding)

6. Based on WBCs during ALL maintenance, is the patient receiving the appropriate dose of mercaptopurine?

7. Provide education regarding the long-term sequelae associated with the treatment for the acute leukemias.

---

morphologic remission, quantification of MRD is being used increasingly as a prognostic factor.

It is important to develop a plan to educate patients and families about their drugs and doses. If modifications are necessary secondary to toxicity or inadequate response, establish a plan for treatment change. Remember that individual patients often do not fit the "average" patient profile, and dose modifications are frequently needed. The practitioner should be familiar with dosing ranges, WBC count, and other parameters that indicate "appropriate" treatment response. Based on response to prior phases of treatment, the clinician should recognize potential toxicities in subsequent phases of treatment with the same or different drugs at similar or different doses.

Abbreviations Introduced in This Chapter

ALL	Acute lymphocytic/lymphoblastic leukemia
allo-HSCT	Allogeneic hematopoietic stem cell transplantation
AML	Acute myelogenous leukemia
ANC	Absolute neutrophil count
ANLL	Acute nonlymphocytic leukemia
BFM	Berlin-Frankfurt-Munster
CCR	Continuous complete remission
CD	Cluster determinants
CML	Chronic myelogenous leukemia
CR	Complete remission
CSF	Cerebral spinal fluid
CSF	Colony-stimulating factor

DFS	Disease-free survival
EFS	Event-free survival
FAB	French-American-British
FISH	Fluorescent in-situ hybridization
G-CSF	Granulocyte colony-stimulating factor
GM-CSF	Granulocyte-macrophage colony-stimulating factor
GVHD	Graft-versus-host disease
GVL	Graft-versus-leukemia (effect)
HLA	Human leukocyte antigen
HSCT	Hematopoietic stem cell transplantation
MABs	Monoclonal antibodies
MDS	Myelodysplastic syndrome
MPD	Myeloproliferative disorder
MRD	Minimal residual disease
MUD	Matched unrelated donor
OS	Overall survival
Ph+	Philadelphia chromosome
TBI	Total-body radiation
TLS	Tumor lysis syndrome
WHO	World Health Organization
XRT	Irradiation

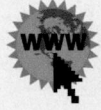 Self-assessment questions and answers are available at *http://www.mhpharmacotherapy.com/pp.html.*

REFERENCES

1. Pui CH, Relling MV, Downing JR. Acute lymphocytic leukemia. N Engl J Med 2004 Apr; 350(15):1535–1548.
2. Jemal A, Murray T, Ward E, et al. Cancer statistics, 2008. CA Cancer J Clin 2008;58:71–96.
3. Campana D, Pui CH. Childhood leukemia. In: Abeloff MD, Armitage JO, Niederhuber JE, et al., eds. Clinical Oncology, 4th ed. Philadelphia, PA: Elsevier, 2008:2139–2169.
4. Schumacher HR, Alvares CJ, Blough RI, Mazzella F. Acute leukemia. Clin Lab Med 2002;22:153–192.
5. Hoelzer D, Gokbudet N. Acute lymphoid leukemia in adults. In: Abeloff MD, Armitage JO, Niederhuber JE, et al., eds. Clinicol Oncology, 4th ed. Philadelphia, PA: Elsevier, 2008:2191–2213.
6. Leather HL, Bickert B. Acute leukemias. In: DiPiro JT, Talbert RL, Yee GC, et al., eds. Pharmacotherapy: A Pathophysiologic Approach, 7th ed. New York City: McGraw-Hill, 2008:2259–2280.
7. Pieters R, Carroll WL. Biology and treatment of acute lymphoblastic leukemia. Pediatr Clin North Am 2008;55(1):1–20.
8. Faderl S, Jeha S, Kantarjian HM. The biology and therapy of adult acute lymphoblastic leukemia. Cancer 2003; 98(7):1337–1354.
9. Lowenberg B, Downing JR, Burnett A. Acute myeloid leukemia. N Engl J Med 1999;341(14):1051–1062.
10. Stone RM, O'Donnell MR, Sekeres MA. Acute myeloid leukemia. Hematology Am Soc Hematol Educ Program 2004;1:98–117.
11. Scheinberg DA, Maslak P, Weiss M. Acute leukemias. In: Devita VT, Hellman S, Rosenberg SA, eds. Cancer: Principles and Practice of Oncology, 6th ed. Philadelphia, PA: Lippincott Williams & Wilkins, 2001:2404–2433.
12. Pui CH, Schrappe M, Ribeiro RC, Niemeyer CM. Childhood and adolescent lymphoid and myeloid leukemia. Hematology Am Soc Hematol Educ Program 2004;1;118–145.
13. Pui CH, Relling MV, Campana D, et al. Childhood acute lymphoblastic leukemia. Rev Clin Exp Hematol 2002;6:161–180.
14. Mandrell BN, Pritchard M. Understanding the clinical implications of minimal residual disease in childhood leukemia. J Pediatr Oncol Nurs 2006;23:38–44.
15. Carroll WL, Bhojwani D, Min DJ, et al. Pediatric acute lymphoblastic leukemia. Hematology Am Soc Hematol Educ Program 2003;1:102–131.
16. Wells RJ, Arther DC, Srivastava A, et al. Prognostic variables in newly diagnosed children and adolescents with acute myeloid leukemia: Children's Cancer Group Study 213. Leukemia 2002; 16:601–607.
17. Rubnitz JE, Gibson B, Smith FO. Acute myeloid leukemia. Pediatr Clin North Am 2008;55:21–51.
18. Demark-Wahnefried W, Jones LW. Promoting a healthy lifestyle among cancer survivors. Hematol Oncol Clin North Am 2008;22:319–342.
19. Pui CH, Campana D, Evans WE. Childhood acute lymphoblastic leukaemia: Current status and future perspectives. Lancet Oncol 2001;2:597–607.
20. Hurwitz CA. Substituting dexamethasone for prednisone complicates remission induction in children with acute lymphocytic leukemia. Cancer 2000;88(8):1964–1969.
21. Robak T. Acute lymphoblastic leukaemia in elderly patients. Drugs Aging 2004; 21:779–791.
22. Bailey LC, Lange BJ, et. al. Bone marrow relapse in pediatric acute lymphocytic leukemia. Lancet Oncol 2008;99:873–883.
23. Pui CH. Acute lymphoblastic leukemia. Pediatr Clin North Am. 1997;44:831–846.
24. Jeha S. Clofarabine for the treatment of acute lymphoblastic leukemia. Expert Rev Anticancer Ther 2007;7:113–118.
25. Gregory J, Arceci R. Acute myeloid leukemia in children: A review of risk factors and recent trials. Cancer Invest 2002;20:1027–1037.
26. Ishii E, Kawasaki H, Isoyama K, Eguchi-Ishimae M, Eguchi M. Recent advances in the treatment of infant acute myeloid leukemia. Leuk Lymphoma 2003;44:741–748.
27. Lancet JE, Willman CL, Bennett JM. Cancer in the elderly. Hematol Oncol Clin North Am 2000;14:251–267.
28. Golub TR, Arceci RJ. Acute myelogenous leukemia. In: Pizzo PA, Poplack DG. eds. Principles and Practice of Pediatric Oncology, 5th ed. Philadelphia PA: Lippincott, Williams& Wilkins; 2006: 591–644.
29. Davidson MB, Thakkar S, Hix JK, et al. Pathophysiology, clinical consequences, and treatment of tumor lysis syndrome. Am J Med 2004;116:546–554.
30. Hughes WT, Armstrong D, Bodey GP, et al. 2002 guidelines for the use of antimicrobial agents in neutropenic patients with cancer. Clin Infect Dis 2002;34:730–751.
31. Hoelzer D, Gokbuget N, Ottmann, et al. Acute lymphoblastic leukemia. Hematology Am Soc Hematol Educ Program 2002:162–192.

96 Chronic Leukemias and Multiple Myeloma

Amy M. Pick

LEARNING OBJECTIVES

● **Upon completion of the chapter the reader will be able to:**

1. Explain the role of the Philadelphia chromosome (Ph) in the pathophysiology of chronic myelogenous leukemia (CML).

2. Describe the natural history of CML.

3. Identify the clinical signs and symptoms associated with CML.

4. Discuss treatment options for CML with special emphasis on tyrosine kinase inhibitors.

5. Describe the clinical course of chronic lymphocytic leukemia (CLL).

6. Describe patients who may be observed without treatment and those who receive aggressive treatment for CLL.

7. Discuss the various treatment options available for CLL.

8. Describe the clinical presentation of multiple myeloma.

9. Discuss treatment options available for multiple myeloma.

KEY CONCEPTS

❶ The Philadelphia chromosome (Ph) is a chromosomal translocation responsible for chronic myelogenous leukemia (CML).

❷ The Ph results in the formation of an abnormal fusion gene, *BCR-ABL*, which encodes an overly active tyrosine kinase.

❸ Allogeneic stem cell transplantation is the only curative treatment option for CML.

❹ Imatinib is a tyrosine kinase inhibitor used as first-line therapy in patients with CML.

❺ Dasatinib and nilotinib are second-generation tyrosine kinase inhibitors used to overcome imatinib resistance or intolerance.

❻ Chronic lymphocytic leukemia (CLL) can have a variable disease course but most patients survive for many years.

❼ Chemotherapy does not improve overall survival in early-stage CLL.

❽ Fludarabine-based chemotherapy is commonly used as first-line therapy for younger patients with CLL.

❾ Autologous transplant either as a single or double transplant offers younger patients with myeloma longer disease-free survival.

❿ Newer therapies for multiple myeloma including thalidomide, lenalidomide, and bortezomib in combination with dexamethasone produce major responses.

INTRODUCTION

Several diseases comprise chronic leukemia. The two most common forms are chronic myelogenous leukemia (CML) and chronic lymphocytic leukemia (CLL). The slower progression of the disease contrasts it from acute leukemia, with the survival of chronic leukemia often lasting several years without treatment. This chapter will cover CML and CLL. There will also be a discussion of multiple myeloma and a brief discussion of Waldenstrom macroglobulinemia.

CHRONIC MYELOGENOUS LEUKEMIA

CML is a hematological cancer that results from an abnormal proliferation of an early myeloid progenitor cell.[1] The clinical course of CML has three phases: chronic phase, accelerated phase, and blast crisis. Chemotherapy can be used to control WBC counts in the chronic phase but as CML slowly progresses the cancer becomes resistant to treatment. Blast crisis resembles acute leukemia and immediate aggressive treatment is required. Table 96–1 describes each of the phases of CML.

Table 96–1		
Clinical Course of CML		
Phase	**Characteristics**	**Median Duration (With Treatment)**
Chronic	Elevated WBC Responsive to treatment	4–6 years[a]
Accelerated	Elevated WBC Unresponsive to treatment Increased symptoms	6–9 months
Blast	Disease transformation to acute leukemia	3–6-month

[a]Prior to imatinib therapy.

EPIDEMIOLOGY AND ETIOLOGY

It was estimated that 5,050 new cases of CML were diagnosed in 2009, accounting for 15% of all adult leukemias.[2] The incidence of CML increases with age, with the median age of diagnosis in the fifth decade of life.[1] In most newly diagnosed cases, the etiology cannot be determined but high doses of ionizing radiation and exposure to solvents such as benzene are recognized risk factors.

PATHOPHYSIOLOGY

Cell of Origin

CML arises from a defect in an early progenitor cell. The pluripotent (noncommitted) stem cell is implicated as the origin of the disease, thus multiple cell lineages of hematopoesis may be affected, including myeloid, erythroid, megakaryocyte, and rarely, lymphoid lineages. These cells remain functional in chronic phase CML, which is why patients in this phase are at low risk for developing infections.

Ph Chromosome

❶ *The Philadelphia chromosome (Ph) results from a translocation between chromosomes 9 and 22, leaving a shortened chromosome 22.* ❷ *The Ph results in the formation of an abnormal fusion gene between the breakpoint cluster region and the abelson proto-oncogene (BCR-ABL), which encodes an overly active tyrosine kinase. The loss of control of tyrosine kinase activity causes abnormal cellular proliferation and inhibition of apoptosis.*[1,3] Molecular tools such as quantitative and qualitative polymerase chain reaction (Q-PCR) and fluorescence in situ hybridization (FISH) are used in the detection and monitoring of CML.[4]

TREATMENT

Desired Outcome

The primary goal in the treatment of CML is to eradicate the Ph positive clones. Elimination of the Ph is termed cytogenetic

Clinical Presentation and Diagnosis of CML

Signs and Symptoms

- 30–50% are asymptomatic at diagnosis.[1,5]
- Symptoms may include fatigue, fever, weight loss, bleeding.
- Organomegaly consisting of splenomegaly and hepatomegaly.

Diagnostic Procedures

- Peripheral blood smear
- Bone marrow biopsy (required for diagnosis)
- Cytogenetic studies
- Molecular testing (Q-PCR and FISH)

Laboratory Findings

- Peripheral blood smear
  - Leukocytosis (most present with WBC greater than 100 × 10⁹/L [100 × 10³/mm³])
  - Thrombocytosis (approximately 50% of patients in chronic phase)[1]
  - Anemia
  - Presence of blasts
- Bone marrow
  - Hypercellularity with presence of blasts
  - Presence of Ph

Poor Prognostic Factors[1]

- Older age
- Splenomegaly
- High percentage blasts in the blood
- High or low platelet count
- Increased eosinophils or basophils

complete remission. If treatment produces Q-PCR negative disease, this is termed molecular complete remission and indicates a several log reduction over cytogenetic complete remission. An early goal of therapy is to achieve hematologic complete remission or to normalize peripheral blood. A cure from CML can only come from complete eradication of the Ph clone.

General Approach to Treatment

There have been significant advances in the treatment of CML since the discovery of the Ph in 1960. The success of therapy is partially dependent on the clinical phase of the disease. Treatment decisions are based on patient's age, phase of CML, comorbidities, and availability of a donor for transplant. Nearly all patients with CML are treated initially with imatinib. Hydroxyurea may be used after diagnosis to rapidly reduce high WBC counts and prevent potentially serious complications (respiratory and neurologic) associated with large numbers of circulating neutrophils. Hydroxyurea, though, does not alter the disease process. Imatinib can also reduce peripheral WBC counts over several weeks, thus many patients are started on imatinib alone. Dasatinib or nilotinib are second-generation tyrosine kinase inhibitors used when patients cannot tolerate or are resistant to imatinib. Prior to the development of the imatinib, interferon-α was once the treatment of choice. With the emergence of more effective therapies in CML, today interferon-α's role is minimal. Interferon-α should be reserved for use in patients who do not respond to tyrosine kinase therapy and do not enroll in a clinical trial. Allogeneic stem cell transplant is the only curative therapy for CML and is used in younger patients with a matched donor. Figure 96–1 illustrates one common method of clinically managing newly diagnosed CML patients.

Nonpharmacologic Therapy

▶ *Hematopoetic Stem Cell Transplantation*

❸ *Allogeneic stem cell transplantation is the only curative treatment option for CML.*[1] It is an option for younger patients (younger than 50 years) in chronic phase CML that have an HLA-matched donor. Cure rates are superior when patients are transplanted in chronic phase within the first year of diagnosis and may be as high as 70%.[5,6] Unfortunately, only 30% to 40% of patients will be candidates for transplantation. There are significant risks associated with allogeneic transplant with a 10% to 20% early mortality, or within 100 days of transplant.[6] Patients may also have

a significant decline in quality of life from chronic graft-versus-host disease and other long-term complications associated with allogeneic stem cell transplantation. For those patients who do not achieve a molecular complete remission or have a relapse after transplant the infusion of donor lymphocytes will usually place the patient back into a durable remission. The National Comprehensive Cancer Network (NCCN) recommends that allogeneic stem cell transplant be reserved for rare cases considering the effectiveness and survival benefit of imatinib and other tyrosine kinase inhibitors.[7]

Pharmacologic Therapy (Table 96–2)

The treatment of CML has experienced a dramatic change since the introduction of first- and second-generation tyrosine kinase inhibitors. These oral agents do not cure CML but are able to produce long-term disease control in the vast majority of patients.

▶ *Imatinib Mesylate (Gleevec)*

❹ *Imatinib mesylate (STI-571; Gleevec) is a tyrosine kinase inhibitor used as first-line therapy in patients with CML.* As a potent first-generation tyrosine kinase inhibitor, imatinib inhibits phosphorylation of various proteins involved in cell proliferation. Imatinib works by binding to the ATP binding pocket of *BCR-ABL.*[8] Data show that the use of imatinib in chronic phase CML results in 89% of patients reaching 5-year survival.[9] The drug induces complete hematologic responses in more than 97% of patients and complete cytogenetic responses in about 87% of patients in chronic phase.[9] As expected in more aggressive disease, lower response rates are reported in accelerated phase and

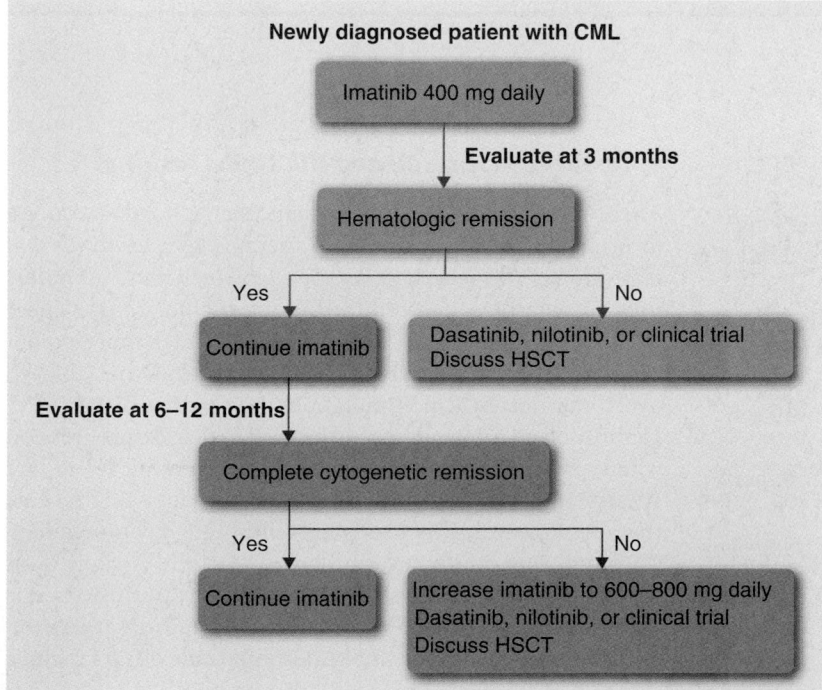

FIGURE 96–1. Algorithm for imatinib therapy in newly diagnosed CML patients. (HSCT, hematopoietic stem cell transplantation.)

Table 96–2

Drugs Used in CML

Drug	Adverse Effects	Comments	Renal Dosing	Hepatic Dosing
Dasatinib (Sprycel)	Thrombocytopenia, neutropenia, headache, rash, edema, pleural effusions	Dose: 100 mg orally once daily for chronic phase CML or 70 mg orally twice daily for accelerated phase/blast crisis Avoid concomitant medications that prolong the QT-interval. Low levels of potassium and magnesium should be corrected prior to initiating therapy Drug interactions: Metabolized by CYP-450 3A4 (e.g., cyclosporine, erythromycin, itraconazole, phenytoin, St. John's wort)	No reductions	No reductions
Imatinib mesylate (Gleevec, STI 571)	Neutropenia, thrombocytopenia, diarrhea, rash, nausea, edema, fatigue, arthralgias, myalgias, headache, increased liver function tests	Dose range: 400–800 mg orally per day depending on phase Take with meals and a full glass of water Drug interactions: Metabolized by CYP-450 3A4 Avoid taking with acetaminophen to reduce hepatic toxicity Diarrhea usually responds to loperamide	CrCl 20–39 mL/min: 50% reduction in dose CrCl less than 20 mL/min: use with caution	Mild-moderate impairment: no adjustment Severe impairment: reduce dose by 25% Discontinue imatinib if liver tranaminases are greater than 5 × upper limit of normal *OR* if serum bilirubin greater than 3 × upper limit of normal
Interferon-α (Intron A, Roferon-A, IFN)	Flu-like symptoms: fever, chills, myalgias, fatigue; depression; insomnia; thrombocytopenia	Premedicate with acetaminophen or an NSAID to lessen flu-like symptoms Dose is given subcutaneously or intramuscularly daily	No reductions	No reductions
Nilotinib (Tasigna)	Thrombocytopenia, neutropenia, elevated bilirubin, elevated serum lipase	Dose: 400 mg orally twice daily Take on an empty stomach Black-box warning for QT-prolongation. Avoid concomitant medications that prolong the QT-interval. Low levels of potassium and magnesium should be corrected prior to initiating therapy Drug interactions: Metabolized by CYP-450 3A4 Pharmacogenomic testing of UGT1A1 polymorphisms can be used to identify patients who may have hyperbilirubinemia	No reductions	Discontinue nilotinib if experiencing Grade 3 or 4 elevations in bilirubin or liver transaminases

blast crisis.[10, 11] Disease progression is typically attributed to imatinib resistance.[12,13]

The dosing of imatinib depends on the phase with 400 mg/ day used in the majority of patients in chronic phase CML. Because lower responses are seen with advanced disease studies are investigating the use of 600 to 800 mg/day of imatinib in accelerated phase and blast crisis. Although these higher doses are used quite often in clinical practice, increased efficacy over standard dose imatinib has not been demonstrated.

Therapy with imatinib is generally well tolerated. Common side effects include myelosuppression (phase and dose-related), rash, nausea, edema, fatigue, arthralgias, myalgias, and headaches. Imatinib is metabolized by CYP-450 3A4 and possible drug interactions include those agents which inhibit or induce 3A4, such as erythromycin, ketoconazole, and phenytoin.[14]

▶ *Dasatinib (Sprycel) and Nilotinib (Tasigna)*

There is a small percentage of patients that will fail to respond to or are intolerant to imatinib therapy. ❺ *Dasatinib and nilotinib are two second-generation tyrosine kinase inhibitors used to overcome imatinib resistance or intolerance.* These inhibitors are anywhere from 10 to 325 times more potent than imatinib in inhibiting *BCR-ABL* and are able to overcome most *BCR-ABL* mutations that lead to resistance.[12,13] Dasatinib and nilotinib should be used in disease progression when patients have failed imatinib therapy. There are studies investigating the role of these agents as first-line therapy, however, this use is currently not recommended.[7] Common side effects are similar to imatinib. A significant and potentially severe side effect of pleural effusions has been reported with the use of imatinib and dasatinib but not with the use of nilotinib. Additional side effects include

QT-prolongation (dasatinib and nilotinib) and increase in indirect bilirubin (nilotinib).[12]

▶ *Interferon-α and Cytarabine*

Prior to the introduction of tyrosine kinase inhibitors, the combination of interferon-α and low-dose cytarabine was the nontransplant treatment of choice for patients in chronic phase CML. The precise mechanism of action of interferon-α remains unknown. The addition of cytarabine to interferon-α improves the response compared to interferon alone. This combination produces cytogenetic response rates of 30%, much lower than imatinib.[15] One of the major drawbacks, in addition to the low response rates, is interferon's toxicity including flu-like symptoms, depression, and thrombocytopenia. Today, interferon-α and cytarabine should only be considered in rare circumstances for those patients who do not respond to any tyrosine kinase inhibitor and are not candidates for stem cell transplantation or a clinical trial.

OUTCOME EVALUATION

Successful treatment for CML depends on the elimination of the Ph. Nearly all newly diagnosed CML patients will initially be placed on imatinib. If patients fail to obtain a cytogenetic response within 12 months, dose escalation of imatinib or a change in therapy to dasatinib or nilotinib is recommended.[7] Patients who do not respond to a tyrosine kinase inhibitor and cannot be transplanted should be encouraged to enroll in a clinical trial. Some patients will not respond to treatment and will progress to blast crisis where they will receive treatment for acute leukemia. Although its use is limited, allogeneic transplant offers the only cure for CML. Allogeneic stem cell transplantation may be discussed with the minority of patients who have a matched donor and are young enough to tolerate transplant.[7]

Patient Encounter, Part 1

A 40-year-old woman well known to you comes into your pharmacy complaining of fatigue. You suggest she see her M.D. to have some blood work done. A CBC shows the following:

Total WBC: 158 × 10⁹/L (158 × 10³/mm³), (20% [0.20] blasts, 70% [0.70] segs, 10% [0.10] lymphs)

HgB/HCT: 9 g/dL (5.6 mmol/L) /32% (0.32)

Platelets: 650 × 10⁹/L (650 × 10³/mm³)

Bone marrow biopsy: Hypercellular, FISH is positive for Ph

What is the treatment of choice for this chronic-phase CML patient?

How would you evaluate response to therapy?

If this patient has suboptimal response to initial therapy what would you recommend?

CHRONIC LYMPHOCYTIC LEUKEMIA

CLL is a cancer that results in the accumulation of functionally incompetent lymphocytes.[15] CLL is considered an indolent, incurable disease where treatment should only be initiated when patients have symptoms. There is a subset of patients who will have aggressive disease and these individuals need to be treated aggressively.

EPIDEMIOLOGY AND ETIOLOGY

CLL is the most common type of leukemia diagnosed in adults. It is estimated that, in 2009, 15,490 new cases were diagnosed in the United States.[2] Median age at diagnosis is the sixth decade with the incidence increasing with age. The etiology of CLL is unknown but hereditary factors may have a role, with family members of CLL patients having a two- to sevenfold increased risk of CLL.[16]

PATHOPHYSIOLOGY

Cell of Origin

CLL is characterized by small, relatively incompetent B-lymphocytes that accumulate in the blood and bone marrow over time. It is the lack of apoptotic mechanisms that leads to the persistence and accumulation of B-lymphocytes. The exact cell of origin is controversial but has been described as an antigen activated B-lymphocyte.[16] Chromosomal abnormalities have been identified in 40% to 50% cases of CLL. Detection of some of these markers may predict clinical course and prognosis and may influence treatment decisions.[16, 17]

Clinical Course

❻ *CLL can have a variable clinical course with survival ranging from months to decades.* Low-risk disease is asymptomatic and median survivals exceed 10 years, intermediate risk is associated with lymphadenopathy and has median survivals of about 7 years, and high-risk patients with anemia have median survivals of only 3 years.[18] The typical low-risk patient is an elderly patient without symptoms who is diagnosed on routine blood draw. The typical high-risk patient is a middle-aged patient in which symptoms have brought them to their physician.

PROGNOSTIC FACTORS

Two staging systems, Rai's and Binet's, have been developed to help practitioners determine the overall prognosis of patients with CLL. They are comparable systems and useful when broadly determining good, intermediate, and poor prognostic disease.[16,17] These systems are less useful in accurately determining prognosis in an individual patient.[19] Increasingly a number of biological markers of the disease such as deletion of chromosome 17p and mutational status of immunoglobulin heavy chain variable region gene (IgVH) are being used to predict likely clinical course.[18]

Clinical Presentation and Diagnosis of CLL

Signs and Symptoms

- 40% are asymptomatic at diagnosis[16]
- Lymphadenopathy
- Organomegaly consisting of splenomegaly and hepatomegaly
- Fatigue, weight loss, night sweats, fevers
- Chronic infections due to immature lymphocytes

Diagnostic Procedures

- Peripheral blood smear
- Bone marrow biopsy (required for diagnosis)
- Cytogenetic studies
- Molecular testing

Laboratory Findings

- Peripheral blood smear
  - Leukocytosis (WBC greater than 100×10^9/L [100×10^3/mm³])
  - Lymphocytosis (absolute lymph count greater than 5×10^9/L [5×10^3/mm³])
  - Anemia
  - Thrombocytopenia
  - Hypogammaglobinemia
- Bone marrow
  - Must have at least 30% lymphocytes

Poor Prognostic Factors

- Lymphocytosis with accompanying:
- Anemia (hemoglobin less than 11 g/dL)
- Thrombocytopenia (platelets less than 100×10^9/L [100×10^3/mm³])
- ZAP-70 and CD38 antigen expression
- Cytogenetics (17p-)

TREATMENT

Desired Outcomes

The primary goals in the treatment of CLL are to provide palliation of symptoms and improve overall survival. Because the current treatments for CLL are not curative, reduction in tumor burden and improvement in disease symptoms are reasonable endpoints particularly in the older patient. A complete response (CR) to therapy can be defined as a resolution of lymphadenopathy and organomegaly, normalization of peripheral blood counts, and elimination of lymphoblasts in the bone marrow.

Nonpharmacologic Therapy

❼ *Chemotherapy does not improve overall survival in early-stage CLL.* In addition, deferring therapy until a patient becomes symptomatic does not alter overall survival.[20,21] For this reason, the notion of "watch and wait" is considered reasonable for older patients with indolent disease. Several factors will influence this approach including the patient's life expectancy, disease characteristics, and the patient's ability to tolerate therapy.[22]

▶ Hematopoietic Stem Cell Transplantation

The use of hematopoietic stem cell transplantation in CLL is limited. Allogeneic transplantation offers longer disease-free remissions than autologous transplantation but neither has demonstrated the ability to cure patients.[16] Several factors must be considered before allogeneic stem cell transplantation. The lack of a donor, older age, and poor performance status makes transplant an uncommon procedure in this population. Allogeneic transplantation may be an option for younger patients who have aggressive disease. NCCN guidelines suggests that patients younger than 70 years of age with the deletion of chromosome 17p or who relapse after initial treatment consider allogeneic stem cell transplantation because these patients have a poor response to conventional therapies.[23] Although its use is currently limited, hematopoietic stem cell transplantation may someday be an important component in achieving a cure for CLL.[16]

Pharmacologic Therapy (Table 96–3)

▶ Single-Agent Chemotherapy

The treatment for CLL has changed with the development of the purine analogue fludarabine (Fludara). Historically, chlorambucil (Leukeran), an alkylating agent, was considered standard treatment for CLL. **❽** *Today, fludarabine-based chemotherapy is used as first-line therapy for younger patients with CLL.* Randomized clinical trials have shown that fludarabine is superior to chlorambucil in achieving higher response rates and producing a longer duration of response (CR 20% versus 4%, respectively).[24] Fludarabine is effective in previously untreated patients as well as patients who have chlorambucil-resistant disease.[25] Although fludarabine is one of the most effective agents in the treatment of CLL, it is rarely used as a sole agent. Instead fludarabine is given in combination with other drugs.[16,23,24]

The most common dose for fludarabine is 20 mg/m² IV daily for 5 consecutive days, whereas chlorambucil can be taken daily as an oral tablet with the dose ranging from 4 to 10 mg/day.[25] Fludarabine is associated with more toxicities than chlorambucil, including myelosuppression and prolonged immunosuppression.[24] Resultant infectious complications may occur during the periods of prolonged immunosuppression. NCCN guidelines recommend that clinicians consider antibacterial and antiviral prophylaxis for *Pneumocystis* and *Varicella* zoster when using fludarabine-based therapy.[23] Today, chlorambucil remains a practical option for the symptomatic elderly patient who requires palliative therapy because of the ease of oral administration and limited side effects profile.

Bendamustine (Treanda) is an alkylating agent approved in 2008 for the treatment of CLL. As first-line therapy for CLL, bendamustine was shown to have superior overall response rates, complete responses and longer progression-free survival than chlorambucil.[23] The efficacy of bendamustine has not been compared to fludarabine-based combination therapy. NCCN guidelines suggest that bendamustine can be given as single-agent therapy or in combination with rituximab.[23] The dosing for bendamustine is 100 mg/m^2 given IV on days 1 and 2 of a 28-day cycle. Table 96–3 lists some of the adverse effects seen with bendamustine.

▶ Monoclonal Antibodies

Rituximab (Rituxan) Rituximab is a naked chimeric monoclonal antibody directed against the CD20 antigen on B-lymphocytes.[25] Similar to other B-cell malignancies, CLL expresses CD20 antigens. Dose escalation studies suggest that higher doses are required than those used in non-Hodgkin's lymphoma.[24,26] The higher doses required in CLL is probably a combined effect of lower CD20 antigen expression and higher concentrations of soluble CD20 antigen than in non-Hodgkin's lymphoma.[16,24] Rituximab is typically given in combination with other therapies since these combinations result in higher complete responses than rituximab alone.[27] The most commonly observed side effects of rituximab include infusion reactions consisting of fever, chills, hypotension, nausea, vomiting, and headache.[16] Premedication with diphenhydramine and acetaminophen is recommended to minimize infusion reactions.

Alemtuzumab (Campath) Alemtuzumab is a humanized monoclonal antibody directed against the CD52 antigen.[27] CD52 antigen is expressed on the majority of B- and T- lymphocytes. Alemtuzumab is FDA-approved for single agent use in the treatment of CLL. Studies have shown alemtuzumab to be effective in fludarabine-resistant disease, in patients with the deletion of 17p and as front-line therapy.[24] Infusion-related reactions can be significant and typically occur with the initial dose and lessen in severity with subsequent doses. To limit acute allergic reactions, subcutaneous administration may be given instead of IV dosing.[16,24] Premedication with oral antihistamines and acetaminophen is recommended. Alemtuzumab also suppresses the T-cells, resulting in prolonged

Table 96–3				
Drugs Used in CLL				
Drug	**Adverse Effects**	**Comments**	**Renal Dosing**	**Hepatic Dosing**
Alemtuzumab (Campath)	Infusion-reactions: fever, chills, nausea, vomiting; hypotension; prolonged immunosuppression (resulting in infectious complications)	Antiviral and PCP prophylaxis should be initiated during treatment. Consider antifungal prophylaxis. Premedicate with acetaminophen, diphenhydramine with or without a steroid to alleviate infusion-related reactions Subcutaneous dosing may lessen acute toxicity	No reductions	No reductions
Bendamustine (Treanda)	Myelosuppression, fever, nausea, vomiting, infusion reactions, tumor lysis syndrome	Consider using allopurinol for tumor lysis syndrome during first few cycles of therapy	CrCl less than 40 mL/min: do not use	Mild impairment: use with caution Moderate-severe impairment: do not use
Chlorambucil (Leukeran)	Myelosuppression; allergic reactions (skin rash); secondary malignancies	Take on an empty stomach since food decreases absorption Dose range: 4–10 mg orally daily	No reductions	No reductions
Fludarabine (Fludara)	Myelosuppression; prolonged immunosuppression resulting in secondary infectious complications; edema; neurotoxicity	Dose: 20 mg/m^2 IV daily for 5 days Often given in combination	CrCl 30–70 mL/min: 20% reduction of dose (IV and oral) CrCl less than 30 mL/min: do not use IV. Reduce dose of oral by 50%	No reductions
Rituximab (Rituxan)	Infusion-reactions: fever, chills, rigors, hypotension	Premedicate with acetaminophen, diphenhydramine with or without a steroid to alleviate infusion related reactions Rate of infusion should be increased gradually to minimize reactions	No reductions	No reductions

immunosuppression. Infectious complications may occur from the reactivation of *Cytomegalovirus* and herpes virus and from infection with *Pneumocystis*. These infections have been shown to occur with both the IV and subcutaneous routes of administrations. Guidelines recommend that patients receive trimethoprim–sulfamethoxazole and famciclovir or valacyclovir to prevent these infections. [16,28]

- **Fludarabine-Based Combination Therapy** Fludarabine-based combination therapy may improve long-term disease free survival. The combination of fludarabine, cyclophosphamide, and rituximab improves CR rates compared to fludarabine alone (70% versus 20%) but at the expense of increased infections. [29,30] The combination of fludarabine and alemtuzumab is also being investigated, with the hopes of improving overall survival. [16] No fludarabine-based regimen has been shown to be superior to another. [24]

OUTCOME EVALUATION

Successful outcomes depend on the appropriate treatment selection for a specific patient. A risk versus benefit analysis should be done in the treatment of older CLL patients. Because CLL is not curable, watch and wait is a reasonable approach for those with indolent disease. Treatment can then begin when the patient becomes symptomatic. Aggressive fludarabine-based therapy is often reserved for younger patients with high-risk CLL, with the goal being prolonged disease-free survival. A desirable response to therapy includes a reduction in lymphocytes, decrease in stage of the disease, and resolution of symptoms.

MULTIPLE MYELOMA

Multiple myeloma is a malignancy of the plasma cell and is characterized by an abnormal production of a monoclonal

Patient Encounter, Part 2

A 72-year-old man presents to his primary care physician for his yearly check-up. He reports feeling fine over the past year. A physical exam appears normal, however, the patient had an abnormal WBC count of 20×10^9/L (20×10^3/mm^3) with 80% (0.80) lymphocytes. The bone marrow exam reports 60% (0.60) lymphocytes and the diagnosis of CLL is made.

What treatment approach do you recommend?

Would your treatment options change if the patient becomes symptomatic? If so, what would be your new options?

Would your treatment options change if the patient were 48 years old? If so, what would be your new options?

protein in the bone marrow. Features of the disease include bone lesions, anemia, and renal insufficiency. [31] Multiple myeloma is an incurable disease; however, advancements in the treatment of myeloma have significantly extended survival.

EPIDEMIOLOGY AND ETIOLOGY

Multiple myeloma is the second most common hematological malignancy. It is estimated that approximately 20,580 new cases of multiple myeloma were reported in 2009, accounting for 1% to 2% of all cancers. [2] The median age at diagnosis is 68 years and less than 2% are diagnosed under the age of 40. [32] The incidence of myeloma is highest in African Americans, lowest in Asians, and occurs more frequently in men than women. [32] The etiology of multiple myeloma is unknown.

PATHOPHYSIOLOGY

The pathogenesis of multiple myeloma is quite complex with multiple step models created to postulate the process. Myeloma must be distinguished from a condition called monoclonal gammopathy of unknown significance (MGUS), which is characterized by a monoclonal immunoglobulin without malignant plasma cells. Yearly, about 1% of patients with MGUS will develop multiple myeloma. The pathophysiology of multiple myeloma involves complex bone-marrow microenvironment and cytokine interactions. Interleukin-6, tumor necrosis factor, vascular endothelial growth factor and stroma-derived factor-1 support the establishment and proliferation of myeloma cells. [32,33] Chromosomal abnormalities and other genetic changes often occur as the disease progresses, which leads to cell cycle dysregulation. [32] It is the understanding of these interactions that has led to the newer agents used in the treatment of multiple myeloma.

PROGNOSTIC FACTORS

Prognostic factors for myeloma include extent of tumor burden and patient performance status. The International Staging System is used to predict outcomes following therapy. Staging is stratified based on the levels of serum β_2-microglobulinemia and serum albumin. High β_2-microglobulinemia and low albumin are poor prognostic factors and are indicative of high tumor load. [34] Cytogenetic abnormalities are not included in the staging system. The older aged patient, renal impairment, and other comorbidities also predict for poorer outcomes. [34] Increasingly, chromosomal changes are being used to predict the high-risk patient with perhaps the most important being deletion of the long arm of chromosome 13. [33]

TREATMENT
Desired Outcomes

The primary goal in the treatment of multiple myeloma is to decrease tumor burden and minimize complications associated with the disease. A watch and wait approach is an

Clinical Presentation and Diagnosis of Multiple Myeloma

Signs and Symptoms

- "CRAB"
  - "C"—hyper**C**alcemia
  - "R"—**R**enal failure
  - "A"—**A**nemia (fatigue)
  - "B"—**B**one pain/lesions (fractures)
- Weight loss
- Recurrent infections

Diagnostic Procedures

- Laboratory
  - CBC, chemistry panel, β_2 microglobulin
  - Peripheral blood smear
  - Serum protein electrophoresis and immunofixation
  - Urine protein electrophoresis and immunofixation
  - Freelite assay
- Radiologic evaluation (MRI, bone densitometry)
- Bone marrow biopsy
  - Cytogenetic studies
  - Molecular testing

Laboratory Findings

- Peripheral blood
  - Monoclonal protein in serum (usually IgG or IgA)

- High β_2 microglobulin
- Low platelets and hemoglobin
- High creatinine, urea, LDH, C-reactive protein, and calcium
- Rouleaux formation
- Urinalysis
  - Bence-Jones Protein
- Bone marrow
  - Plasma cells (greater than or equal to 10%)
  - Abnormal cytogenetics
- Radiologic findings
  - Bone lesions, fractures, osteoporosis

Poor Prognostic Factors

- High serum β_2-microglobulin and low serum albumin
- Elevated C-reactive protein
- Elevated LDH
- IgA isotype
- Low platelet count
- Chromosome 13 deletions and other cytogenetic abnormalities

---

option for asymptomatic patients who have no lytic lesions in the bone. Once symptoms occur, treatment is required. All patients should be evaluated to see it they are eligible candidates for transplant. Autologous stem cell transplantation prolongs overall survival in patients who can tolerate high-dose chemotherapy. Immunomodulators such as thalidomide should be incorporated into initial therapy to reduce tumor burden in patients with symptomatic disease. Almost all patients will become refractory to initial treatment and will require the use of salvage therapies. Table 96–4 lists the treatment options for transplant eligible and ineligible patients.

Nonpharmacologic Therapy

▶ *Autologous Stem Cell Transplantation*

❾ *Autologous stem cell transplantation results in higher response rates and extends overall survival compared to those who receive conventional therapy such as VAD.* Since overall median survival is prolonged from 42 to 54 months, stem cell transplant should be considered in all patients who can tolerate high-dose chemotherapy.[35,36] High-dose melphalan is the most common preparative regimen. Two sequential transplants (tandem transplants) improve overall survival in those patients who do not have a good partial response after one transplant.[32] The use of maintenance therapy after

autologous transplantation with thalidomide or bortezomib is under investigation.[32]

Pharmacologic Therapy (Table 96–5)

▶ *Conventional-Dose Chemotherapy*

Once patients present with symptomatic disease they will be started on therapy. Melphalan and prednisone (MP) was once the most common initial treatment combination for myeloma. Today, MP is often used in combination therapy with immunomodulators as front-line therapy for patients who are not eligible for transplant. Vincristine/doxorubicin/dexamethasone (VAD) is another combination chemotherapy regimen that was often utilized in myeloma. With the advent of thalidomide and other newer agents, the use of VAD has declined. VAD may be used as induction therapy for patients who are transplant eligible because it avoids the alkylating agent melphalan, thus minimizing the risk of secondary malignancies that are associated with chronic alkylating therapy.[32,36]

▶ *Thalidomide (Thalomid)*

Thalidomide as monotherapy or combination therapy is effective in the treatment of multiple myeloma. The precise mechanism of action of thalidomide is unknown, but its

Table 96-4

Possible Combination Therapies for Multiple Myeloma

Frontline Therapy for Transplant-Eligible Candidates (Induction)		Frontline Therapy for Nontransplant-Eligible Candidates	
Drug Regimen	Acronym	Drug Regimen	Acronym
Thalidomide-dexamethasone	Thal-Dex or TD	Melphalan-prednisone	MP
Lenalidomide-dexamethasone	Rev-Dex	Melphalan-prednisone-thalidomide	MPT
Bortezomib-dexamethasone	Vel-Dex	Melphalan-prednisone-lenalidomide	MPR
Bortezomib-thalidomide-dexamethasone	VTD	Melphalan-prednisone-bortezomib	MPV
Bortezomib-lenalidomide-dexamethasone	Vel-Rev-Dex	Thalidomide-dexamethasone	Thal-Dex or TD
Vincristine-doxorubicin-dexamethasone	VAD	Vincristine-doxorubicin-dexamethasone	VAD
Liposomal vincristine-doxorubicin-dexamethasone	DVD	Dexamethasone	Dex

Evaluate patient for adverse effects including peripheral neuropathy and deep vein thrombosis. Prophylactic anticoagulation should be used if on dexamethasone and thalidomide or lenalidomide.

antimyeloma activity may be due to its **antiangiogenic** and anticytokine properties.[33] 🔟 *The combination of thalidomide and dexamethasone has emerged as the one of the most commonly used induction regimens in the treatment of transplant eligible patients with myeloma.* Thalidomide and steroid combinations produce responses in 60% to 80% of previously untreated patients.[37] The addition of thalidomide to MP improves overall response and overall survival in newly diagnosed patients.[38] This combination (MPT) can be used as initial therapy in patients who are not transplant-eligible. Common side effects of thalidomide therapy include somnolence, constipation, peripheral neuropathy, and deep vein thrombosis. Standard dose warfarin or low-molecular-weight heparins are recommended to prevent deep vein thrombosis.[36,39] There are substantial teratogenic effects of thalidomide if used during pregnancy so distribution of the drug is closely monitored through the STEPS program.[33]

▶ *Lenalidomide (Revlimid)*

Lenalidomide is an immunomodulating agent related to thalidomide that is approved for the treatment of relapsed myeloma in combination with dexamethasone. Phase III trials showed that lenalidomide in combination with dexamethasone produced higher response rates and longer

Patient Encounter, Part 3

A 50-year-old male presents with fatigue and back pain. A CBC reveals the following: hemoglobin 8.7 g/dL (5.4 mmol/L), platelets 128×10^9/L (128×10^3/mm), corrected calcium 11.8 mg/dL (2.95 mmol/L), serum creatinine 1.4 mg/dL (124 μmol/L), and serum IgG 3,500 mg/dL (35 g/L) (normal: 620–1,500 mg/dL [6.2–15 g/L]). A subsequent bone marrow biopsy confirms multiple myeloma.

Assuming this patient is a candidate for autologous stem cell transplantation, what would be an appropriate induction regimen?

Assuming this patient is a not a candidate for autologous stem cell transplantation, what would be an appropriate induction regimen?

Discuss whether this patient is a candidate for autologous stem cell transplantation.

time to progression than dexamethasone alone in relapsed and refractory myeloma.[32,40] 🔟 *Lenalidomide–dexamethasone is an alternative to thalidomide–dexamethsone for induction therapy prior to a transplant.* The combination of melphalan, prednisone, and lenalidomide (MPR) is being studied for initial therapy in patients not eligible for transplant. The response rate appears to be quite high at 81% with 24% achieving a complete response.[40] A randomized trial comparing MPR to MPT is currently underway. Lenalidomide has a more favorable safety profile over thalidomide being that it lacks the common side effects of somnolence, constipation, and peripheral neuropathy. Significant adverse effects of lenalidomide include myelosuppression and deep vein thrombosis. Like thalidomide-dexamethasone, DVT prophylaxis is recommended with lenalidomide–dexamethasone combinations.[36,39]

▶ *Bortezomib (Velcade)*

Bortezomib is a **proteosome** inhibitor approved for the treatment of multiple myeloma. Proteosome inhibitors induce myeloma cell death by modulating **NF-kappa-B** products including inflammatory cytokines and adhesion molecules that support myeloma cell growth. Bortezomib also disrupts the myeloma microenvironment by inhibits the binding of myeloma cells to the bone marrow stromal cells.[32] 🔟 *The role of bortezomib in the treatment of myeloma has expanded since the introduction of the agent.* Initially approved in the treatment of relapsed disease, bortezomib produces response rates of 35% in heavily pretreated individuals.[41] Today, bortezomib is frequently given in combination with dexamethasone and thalidomide or lenalidomide as induction therapy prior to a transplant. The response rates have been reported as high as 90% in newly diagnosed myeloma.[32] Bortezomib can also be given in combination with prednisone and melphalan (MPV) in

Table 96–5				
Drugs Used in Multiple Myeloma				
Drug	**Adverse Effects**	**Comments**	**Renal Dosing**	**Hepatic Dosing**
Bortezomib (Velcade)	Constipation; decreased appetite; asthenia; fatigue; fever; thrombocytopenia; dose related, reversible peripheral neuropathy	Dose: 1.3 mg/m² IV bolus twice weekly for 2 weeks; week 3 off; repeat. Consider herpes zoster prophylaxis with daily acyclovir	No reductions	No reductions
Dexamethasone	Hyperglycemia, edema, adrenal cortical insufficiency	Dose given orally once daily	No reductions	No reductions
Doxorubicin (Adriamycin)	Myelosuppression; alopecia; cumulative dose limiting toxicity: myocardium damage	Given in combination with vincristine and dexamethasone (VAD)	No reductions	Bilirubin 1.2–3 mg/dL: 50% reduction in dose. Bilirubin 3.1–5 mg/dL: 75% reduction in dose. Bilirubin greater than 5 mg/dL: use with caution
Lenalidomide (Revlimid)	Possible birth defects (since analogue of thalidomide), neutropenia, thrombocytopenia, deep vein thrombosis, pulmonary embolism, pruritis, fatigue	Dose taken with water once daily. Women of child-bearing age must use two forms of contraception. Pregnancy test must be taken before and during use. Enrollment into monitoring program required	Use with caution	No reductions
Melphalan (Alkeran)	Myelosuppression, secondary malignancies, pulmonary fibrosis, sterility, alopecia	Dose given orally once daily. IV formulation used for stem cell transplantation	No recommendation but may consider an initial dose reduction.	No reductions
Thalidomide (Thalomid)	Severe birth defects, peripheral neuropathy, deep vein thrombosis, somnolence, constipation	Titrate initial doses. Doses are taken nightly. Women of child-bearing age must use two forms of contraception. Pregnancy test must be taken before and during use. Enrollment into monitoring program required	No reductions	No reductions
Vincristine (Oncovin)	Dose limiting toxicity: peripheral neuropathies; paresthesias, constipation, alopecia	Given in combination with doxorubicin and dexamethasone (VAD)	No reductions	Bilirubin greater than 3 mg/dL: 50% reduction in dose

patients who are not transplant eligible. Superior response rates and survival are seen with the combination of MPV compared to MP.[40] Side effects of bortezomib include fatigue, nausea, peripheral neuropathy, and hematologic effects.[42]

▶ Bisphosphonates

Bone disease is a common manifestation of multiple myeloma. Bisphosphonates should be initiated in symptomatic patients with bone lesions to slow osteopenia and reduce the fracture risk associated with the disease. Pamidronate 90 mg and zolendronic acid 4 mg have equivalent efficacy in the management of osteolytic lesions.[43] The use of zolendronic acid decreases pain and bone-related complications and improves quality of life. Osteonecrosis of the jaw is a major concern with bisphosphonate therapy. Risk factors are unclear but osteonecrosis of the jaw is more common in patients receiving IV administration of bisphosphonates and having dental procedures performed. It is recommended that patients have dental restoration work prior to starting bisphosphonate therapy. Several consensus guidelines have been published on the use of bisphosphonates and myeloma. Recommendations on the duration of therapy and which bisphosphonate to use have largely been left up to the practitioner.[44, 45]

OUTCOME EVALUATION

Newly diagnosed, asymptomatic patients with myeloma may be observed without treatment. This asymptomatic period may last for months to a couple years. All patients with multiple myeloma will become symptomatic and once this occurs, treatment is required. All patients should be evaluated for an autologous stem cell transplant. For those patients who are eligible for transplant, induction therapy will often consist of thalidomide or lenalidomide and dexamethasone. For those patients who are not transplant-eligible, therapy may consist of MPT, MPV, or MPR. Nearly all patients will progress at some point and second-line therapy will usually include bortezomib. Monthly bisphosphonates should be given to patients who have bone lesions with the hope of reducing pain and fractures.

Patient Care and Monitoring

CML

1. Patients are placed on imatinib at the time of diagnosis. Patients should be monitored for a dose-dependent myelosuppression, GI intolerance, edema, and rash. Drug interactions with CYP450 3A4 inducers are clinically important and should be monitored.

2. Imatinib resistance should be identified when patients fail to respond to imatinib therapy. A change to dasatinib or nilotinib may be necessary when patients fail to have a complete cytogenetic response at 6 to 12 months.

3. Allogeneic stem cell transplantation may be considered when the patient fails to respond or is intolerant to imatinib. Ideal candidates include younger patients in chronic phase CML that have a HLA-matched related or unrelated donor.

CLL

1. Watch and wait is a reasonable approach if the patient is asymptomatic.

2. Monitor WBC and watch for signs of infection if patients are receiving fludarabine-based chemotherapy.

3. Watch for infusion reactions with rituximab and alemtuzumab. Premedicate with acetaminophen and diphenhydramine to prevent these reactions.

4. Prophylactic trimethoprim-sulfamethoxazole and an antiviral (famciclovir or valacyclovir) are recommended for all patients receiving alemtuzumab. Consider adding an antifungal (fluconazole) if warranted.

Multiple Myeloma

1. During chemotherapy, monitor myeloma monoclonal protein in urine and serum, renal function, hemoglobin, and platelets.

2. Bisphosphonates should be initiated in symptomatic patients. Renal function must be monitored. Patients may need pain medication for bone pain.

3. If a reduction in myeloma protein is not seen with one chemotherapy regimen, another regimen should be used.

WALDENSTROM MACROGLOBULINEMIA

Waldenstrom macroglobulinemia is a rare immunoglobulin disorder that is associated with non-Hodgkin's lymphoma. Approximately 4/1 million individuals are affected with the disease. Waldenstrom macroglobulinemia is characterized by an elevation of serum IgM and the involvement of the lymph nodes, bone marrow and spleen. Patients are typically asymptomatic at the time of diagnosis, with the disease being discovered by routine laboratory examination. Similar to indolent lymphomas, the watch and wait approach is employed for asymptomatic patients. Symptomatic patients experience anemia, fatigue, hepatosplenomegaly, lymphadenopathy, and hyperviscosity syndrome. When these symptoms arise, treatment is necessary with the goal being palliation. Systemic therapy includes alkylating agents, nucleoside analogs, rituximab, thalidomide, or bortezomib.[36] Treatment is often continued until a desired response (reduction in symptoms) is achieved. Plasmapheresis may be required in addition to systemic therapies to alleviate symptoms associated with hyperviscosity syndrome.[46]

Abbreviations Introduced in This Chapter

CD	Cluster of differentiation
CLL	Chronic lymphocytic leukemia
CML	Chronic myelogenous leukemia
CR	Complete response
FISH	Fluorescence in situ hybridization
HLA	Human leukocyte antigen
MGUS	Monoclonal gammopathy of undetermined significance
MP	Melphalan and prednisone
NCCN	National Comprehensive Cancer Network
Ph	Philadelphia chromosome
Q-PCR	Qualitative and quantitative polymerase chain reaction
VAD	Vincristine/doxorubicin/dexamethasone

 Self-assessment questions and answers are available at *http://www.mhpharmacotherapy.com/pp.html.*

REFERENCES

1. Garcia-Manero G, Faderl S, O'Brien S, et al. Chronic myelogenous leukemia: A review and update of therapeutic strategies. Cancer 2003;98:437–457.
2. Jemal A, Siegel R, Ward E, et al. Cancer statistics, 2008. CA Cancer J Clin 2008;58:71–96.
3. Nowell PC. Progress with chronic myelogenous leukemia: A personal perspective over four decades. Annu Rev Med 2002;53:1–13.
4. Kantarjian H, Schiffer C, Jones D, et al. Monitoring the response and course of chronic myeloid leukemia in the modern era of BCR-ABL tyrosine kinase inhibitors: Practical advice on the use and interpretation of monitoring methods. Blood 2007;111:1774–1780.
5. Lowenberg B. Minimal residual disease in chronic myelogenous leukemia. N Engl J Med 2003;96:358–361.
6. Faderl S, Talpaz M, Estrov Z, Kantarjian HM. Chronic myelogenous leukemia: Biology and therapy. Ann Intern Med 1999;131:207–219.
7. National Comprehensive Cancer Network Clinical Practice Guidelines in Oncology. Chronic myelogenous leukemia. Rockland, PA. Version 2009, *www.nccn.org*.
8. Druker BJ, Talpaz M, Resta DJ, et al. Efficacy and safety of a specific inhibitor of the bcr-abl tyrosine kinase in chronic myeloid leukemia. N Engl J Med 2001;344:1031–1037.
9. Druker BJ, Guilhot F, O'Brien S, et al. Five year follow-up of patients receiving imatinib for chronic myelogenous leukemia. N Eng J Med 2006;355:2408–2417.
10. Talpaz M, Silver TR, Druker BJ, et al. Imatinib induces durable hematologic and cytogenetic responses in patients with accelerated phase chronic myeloid leukemia: Results of a phase 2 study. Blood 2002;99:1928–1937.
11. Sawyers CL, Hochhaus A, Feldman E, et al. Imatinib induces hematologic and cytogenetics responses in patients with chronic myeloid leukemia in myeloid blast crisis. Blood 2002;99:3530–3539.
12. Kantarjian HM, Giles F, Quintas-Cardama A, Cortes J. Important therapeutic targets in chronic myelogenous leukemia. Clin Cancer Res 2007;13:1089–1097.
13. Kantarjian HM, Talpaz M, Giles F, O'Brien S, Cortes J. New insights into the pathophysiology of chronic myeloid leukemia and imatinib resistance. Ann Intern Med 2006;145:913–923.
14. Deininger MWN, O'Brien SG, Ford JM, Druker BJ. Practical management of patients with chronic myeloid leukemia receiving imatinib. J Clin Oncol 2003;21:1637–1647.
15. O'Brien SG, Guilhot F, Larson RA, et al. Imatinib compared with interferon and low-dose cytarabine for newly diagnosed chronic-phase chronic myeloid leukemia. N Engl J Med 2003;348:994–1004.
16. Wierda WG, Keating MJ, O'Brien S. Chronic Lymphocytic Leukemias. In: Devita VT, Hellman S, Rosenberg SA, eds. Cancer: Principles and Practice of Oncology, 8th ed. Philadelphia, PA: Lippincott, 2008:2278–2304.
17. Hallek M. Prognostic factors in chronic lymphocytic leukemia. Ann Oncol 2008;19:iv51–iv53.
18. Montserrat E. New prognostic markers in CLL. Hematology Am Soc Hematol Educ Program 2006:279–284.
19. Chiorazzi N, Rai KR, Ferrarini M. Chronic lymphocytic leukemia. N Engl J Med 2005;352:804–815.
20. Dighiero G, Maloum K, Desablens B, et al. Chlorambucil in indolent chronic lymphocytic leukemia. N Engl J Med 1998;338:1506–1514.
21. Chemotherapeutic options in chronic lymphocytic leukemia: A meta-analysis of the randomized trials. CLL Trialists' Collaborative Group. J Natl Cancer Inst 1999;91:861–868.
22. Shanafelt TD, Kay NE. Comprehensive management of the CLL patient: A holistic approach. Hematology Am Soc Hematol Educ Program 2007:324–331.
23. National Comprehensive Cancer Network Clinical Practice Guidelines in Oncology. Non Hodgkin's Lymphoma. Rockland, PA. Version 3. 2008, *www.nccn.org*.
24. Wierda WG. Current and investigational therapies for patients with CLL. Hematology Am Soc Hematol Educ Program 2006:285–294.
25. Ferrajoli A, O'Brien SM. Treatment of chronic lymphocytic leukemia. Sem Oncol 2004;31:60–65.
26. Hillmen P. Advancing therapy for chronic lymphocytic leukemia—The role of rituximab. Sem Oncol 2004;31(Suppl 2):22–26.
27. Byrd JC, Rai K, Peterson BL, et al. Addition of rituximab to fludarabine may prolong progression-free survival and overall survival in patients with previously untreated chronic lymphocytic leukemia: An updated retrospective comparative analysis of CALGB 9712 and CALGB 9011. Blood 2005;105:49–53.
28. Moreton P, Hillmen P. Alemtuzumab therapy in B-cell lymphoproliferative disorders. Sem Oncol 2003;30:493–501.
29. Keating MJ, O'Brien S, Albitar M, et al. Early results of a chemoimmunotherapy regimen of fludarabine, cyclophosphamide, and rituximab as initial therapy for chronic lymphocytic leukemia. J Clin Oncol 2005;23:4079–4088.
30. Wierda W, O'Brien S, Wen S, et al. Chemoimmunotherapy with fludarabine, cyclophosphamide, and rituximab for relapsed and refractory chronic lymphocytic leukemia. J Clin Oncol 2005;23:4070–4078.
31. Sirohi B, Powles R. Multiple myeloma. Lancet 2004;363:875–887.
32. Munshi NC, Anderson KC. Plasma cell neoplasms. In: Devita VT, Hellman S, Rosenberg SA, eds. Cancer: Principles and Practice of Oncology, 8th ed. Philadelphia, PA: Lippincott, 2008:2305–2342.
33. Kyle RA, Rajkumar SV. Multiple myeloma. N Engl J Med 2004;351:1860–1873.
34. Greipp PR, San Miguel J, Durie BGM, et al. International staging system for multiple myeloma. J Clin Oncol 2005;23:3412–3420.
35. Child JA, Morgan GJ, Davies FE, et al. High-dose chemotherapy with hematopoietic stem-cell rescue for multiple myeloma. N Engl J Med 2003;348:1875–1883.
36. National Comprehensive Cancer Network Clinical Practice Guidelines in Oncology. Multiple Myeloma. Rockland, PA. Version 2. 2009, *www.nccn.org*.
37. Weber D, Rankin K, Gavino M, et al. Thalidomide alone or with dexamethasone for previously untreated multiple myeloma. J Clin Oncol 2003;21:16–19.
38. Facon T, Mary JY, Hulin C, et al. Melphalan and prednisone plus thalidomide versus melphalan and prednisone alone or reduced-intensity autologous stem cell transplantation in elderly patients with multiple myeloma (IFM 99–06): A randomized trial. Lancet 2007;370:1209–1218.
39. Palumbo A, Rajkumar SV, Dimopoulous MA, et al. Prevention of thalidomide- and lenalidomide-associated thrombosis in myeloma. Leukemia 2008;22(2):414–423.
40. Kyle RA, Rajkumar SV. Multiple myeloma. Blood 2008:2962–2972.
41. Richardson PG, Barlogie B, Berenson J, et al. A Phase 2 study of bortezomib in relapsed, refractory myeloma. N Engl J Med 2003;348:2609–2617.
42. Blade J, Cibeira MT, Rosinol L. Bortezomib: A valuable new antineoplastic strategy in multiple myeloma. Acta Oncologica 2005;44:440–448.
43. Rosen LS, Gordon D, Kaminski M, et al. Long-term efficacy and safety of zoledronic acid compared with pamidronate disodium in the treatment of skeletal complications in patients with advanced multiple myeloma or breast carcinoma: A randomized, double-blind, multicenter, comparative trial. Cancer 2003;98:1735–1744.
44. Lacy MQ, Dispenzieri A, Gertz MA, et al. Mayo clinic consensus statement for the use of bisphosphonates in multiple myeloma. Mayo Clin Proc 2006;81:1047–1053.
45. Kyle Ra, Yee GC, Somerfield MR, et al. American Society of Clinical Oncology 2007 clinical practice guideline update on the role of bisphosphonates in multiple myeloma. J Clin Oncol 2007;25:2462–2472.
46. Dimopoulos MA, Kyle RA, Anagnostopoulos A, Treon SP. Diagnosis and management of Waldenstrom's macroglobulinemia. J Clin Oncol 2005;23:1564–1577.

97 Skin Cancer

Trinh Pham and Jennifer Nam Choi

LEARNING OBJECTIVES

● **Upon completion of the chapter, the reader will be able to:**

1. Identify the risk factors associated with skin cancer.

2. Describe the common signs and symptoms of skin cancer and identify the features of a mole that are suspicious for melanoma.

3. Identify the key features in the different stages of melanoma and their correlation with prognosis.

4. Explain the goals of therapy for the treatment of nonmelanoma and melanoma skin cancer.

5. Devise a plan of lifestyle modifications for the prevention of skin cancer.

6. Discuss the pros and cons of interferon-α therapy for melanoma, and formulate a monitoring plan for patients receiving interferon-α.

7. Discuss the pros and cons of interleukin-2 (IL-2) therapy for melanoma, and formulate a monitoring plan for patients receiving IL-2.

8. Discuss the different treatment options for melanoma with brain metastasis.

9. Discuss the role of temozolomide in the treatment of stage IV melanoma with or without CNS metastasis.

10. Discuss the different treatment options for nonmelanoma skin cancer.

KEY CONCEPTS

❶ Exposure to ultraviolet radiation from the sun is recognized as one of the primary triggers for skin cancer development.

❷ Staging of malignant melanoma is important to determine prognosis, categorize patients with regard to metastatic potential and survival probability, and aid in clinical decision making.

❸ Determination of lymph node status is important in melanoma staging because it is an independent prognostic factor, and it provides the oncologist with guidance for therapy decisions.

❹ Surgery is the primary treatment modality for nonmelanoma and melanoma skin cancer.

❺ Stages IIB, IIC, and III melanoma are considered to be high risk because of their potential for recurrence and distant metastasis. The primary treatment modality is surgical excision of the tumor and a lymphadenectomy for patients with positive lymph nodes.

❻ Interferon-α2b is approved by the FDA as adjuvant therapy for high-risk melanoma. It is controversial if it should be offered to every patient at high risk for recurrence.

❼ Stage IV melanoma is not curable, and the primary goal of therapy is local control of the disease and relief of identifiable symptoms.

❽ Interleukin-2 (IL-2) therapy is approved by the FDA for the treatment of metastatic melanoma, and it is a reasonable option for patients with this stage of the disease.

❾ Combination chemotherapy or biochemotherapy increases toxicity significantly without offering overall survival benefit; thus, they are not standards of care for stage IV melanoma.

❿ One of the most common sites of metastasis for melanoma is the brain and treatment options for brain metastasis include surgery, radiation, and chemotherapy. The choice of therapy depends on the number of metastatic lesions, accessibility of the lesions for surgery, the presence of neurologic symptoms, and the status of extracranial disease.

Skin cancer is the most prevalent of all malignancies occurring in humans, and in the United States, it accounts for more than 50% of all cancers.[1] The most common cutaneous malignancies are basal cell carcinoma (BCC), squamous cell carcinoma (SCC), and malignant melanoma (MM). BCC and SCC are categorized as nonmelanoma skin cancer. Worldwide, the incidence of nonmelanoma skin cancer (NMSC) and MM is increasing at a rate of 3% to 8% per year in fair-skinned Caucasian populations.[2] The mortality rate for MM is on the rise in North America, Australia, and New Zealand at a pace of 2% to 4% annually.[2] Ultraviolet (UV) radiation exposure is the leading environmental factor causing skin cancer.[3] This is a modifiable risk factor, and prevention of skin cancer development is possible through a sun protection regimen that includes wearing protective clothing, avoidance of prolonged, intense sun exposure and sunburns, and regular application of sunscreen. If skin cancer is detected in its early stage, survival is improved, and the disease is curable. Therefore, campaigns for primary and secondary prevention of skin cancer are important in combating this tumor. NMSC and MM differ with regard to prognosis, metastatic potential, mortality, curability, and treatment options. This chapter will review the pathogenesis and risk factors for the development of skin cancer and provide current data on the recommendations for the prevention and treatment of both NMSC and MM.

MELANOMA

EPIDEMIOLOGY AND ETIOLOGY

MM is ranked as the fifth most common cancer among men and the sixth most common cancer in women.[1] In 2008, it is estimated that 62,480 new cases of invasive melanoma will be diagnosed. MM is a major public health problem of significant worldwide concern because of its dramatic rise in incidence and mortality. In the United States in 1935, the lifetime risk of melanoma was estimated at 1 in 1,500; in 2002, the lifetime risk was 1 in 68 persons.[2] In Australia, the country with the highest incidence of melanoma in the world, the hazard is even higher at an estimated lifetime risk of 1 in 25 persons.[4] The incidence of melanoma is not evenly dispersed among all populations. Race, gender, and age confer different incidence rates.[4] Caucasians have higher risks than Asians, Hispanics, and African Americans.[4] The rate of MM is 10 times higher in whites than in African Americans.[1] MM generally occurs in the young, and is diagnosed primarily in the third or fourth decades of life.[5] Sixty-two percent of cases are diagnosed before patients reach 65 years of age, and the median age of death is 67 years.[6] Overall, in the United States, males have higher incidence rates than females.[5] The incidence rises with age, and older men have the highest melanoma risk in the United States.[5]

RISK FACTORS

The maintenance of cellular homeostasis involves a balance of cell division, differentiation, senescence, and apoptosis.

Patient Encounter 1, Part 1

KM is a 71-year-old man being evaluated in the dermatology clinic for a recent change in a mole on his shoulder. The mole has been on his shoulder for as long as he can remember. A year ago it began to itch, and his wife noted that it seemed to be getting darker in color. On physical examination, it is noted that the primary lesion is a 9-mm nodule, the border is ragged and irregular, and it is brown, black, and white in color. There is no oozing, bleeding, or crusting around the lesion. A couple of years ago, he had a complete excision of an in situ melanoma on his back.

KM has light-brown hair, blue eyes, and fair skin. He has a history of numerous severe blistering sunburns in his childhood. As a teenager and young adult, he spent many hours outdoors as a construction worker and a lifeguard. He lives with his wife in Denver, Colorado, and they enjoy outdoor activities such as hiking, skiing, and canoeing. He does not have a family history of melanoma.

What are KM's risk factors for malignant melanoma (MM)?

What information is suggestive of MM?

What should be done to confirm the diagnosis of MM?

How is the stage of the melanoma determined?

What primary prevention measures are recommended to prevent skin cancer?

Cancer occurs when the growth and function of cells are "out of control" in relation to normal tissue. The combination of genetic alterations and environmental toxins is the most frequent contributor to the process of carcinogenesis. In the development of skin cancer, the risk factors are categorized as environmental (solar UV radiation), genetic (family history), immunosuppression, and previous history of skin cancer.

❶ *Exposure to ultraviolet radiation from the sun is recognized as one of the primary triggers for skin carcinogenesis.* UV radiation (specifically UVB) is absorbed by DNA in the cells in the epidermal layer and may induce DNA lesions by forming dimers between neighboring pyrimidine bases, resulting in the development of cyclobutane pyrimidine dimers (CPDs) and pyrimidine-pyrimidone(6-4) photoproducts.[7] Gene mutations may then transpire, leading to carcinogenesis.[7] Other mechanisms of UV radiation–induced DNA damage include the generation of reactive oxygen species (ROS), e.g., 8-hydroxydeoxyguanosine, (8-OHdG), which can cause oxidative stress to DNA base pairs, and protein–DNA cross-links and single-strand breaks.[7] It is estimated that 60% to 70% of MMs are linked to UV exposure, particularly in the form of severe sunburns and intermittent (recreational or vacation) exposure. The association between sun exposure and melanoma is not clearly defined, though, because cutaneous melanoma can arise frequently in areas of the body not exposed to the sun.[8] Exposure to sources of artificial UV radiation such as tanning beds have also been linked to increased risk of skin cancer.[9]

Genetics play a significant role in the development of MM. Patients with two or more family members with melanoma are significantly more likely to develop melanoma at a younger age and to develop multiple melanomas.[5] The inherited mutation of two highly penetrant melanoma genes has been identified in families with melanoma susceptibility: the *CDKN2A* gene (also known as *INK4/ARF, MTS1,* and *CDK1*) and the *CDK4* gene. Polymorphism of the *MC1R* gene, which is associated with red hair, also increases susceptibility to melanoma.[10] Mutations affecting the serine–threonine kinase *B-RAF* gene have been reported with high rates in individuals with MM.

Another risk factor for the development of melanoma is the dysplastic nevus syndrome (also known as *B-K syndrome, familial atypical mole,* or *Clark's nevus*). This is an autosomal dominant disorder with incomplete penetrance, in which microscopic examination of the nevi shows disordered proliferation of melanocytes with varying degree of atypia without evidence of invasion. An individual typically may have 25 to 75 abnormal nevi present on his or her body. The cumulative lifetime risk for melanoma development in individuals with dysplastic syndrome is almost 100%.

In individuals without a family history of melanoma (sporadic melanoma), the presence of benign melanocytic nevi (benign moles) is consistently identified as the strongest risk factor for the future development of melanoma.[6] The greater the number of benign nevi (greater than 20), the greater the susceptibility to melanoma growth.[11]

Aging is a risk factor for skin carcinogenesis because the passage of time allows more instances for the initiation and promotion of tumor formation through exposure to UV radiation. Furthermore, the capacity to repair DNA decreases with age, and the capability to remove DNA photoproducts such as CPDs and pyrimidine-pyrimodone(6-4) from UV-irradiated skin also diminishes with age, leading to an increased rate of genetic mutations. These characteristics may account for the exponential increase in the incidence of NMSC and MM in the elderly population.

PRIMARY PREVENTION OF SKIN CANCER

Ultraviolet (UV) radiation exposure from the sun is the major cause of NMSC and MM. **Primary prevention** strategies for skin cancer aim at educating people against excessive exposure to the sun and are spearheaded by the American Academy of Dermatology, the American Cancer Society, the Environmental Protection Agency, and the Centers for Disease Control and Prevention. The aims of these programs are to increase public awareness about the harmful effects of sun exposure and the risk of skin cancer, change attitudes about the social norms related to sun protection and tanned skin, and decrease the incidence of skin cancer and deaths related to this malignancy. Recommendations for prevention

of skin cancer are universal and include a variety of simple strategies to minimize exposure to UV rays:[12]

- Avoid direct exposure to the sun between the hours of 10 AM to 4 PM, when UV rays are most intense.
- Wear hats with a broad enough brim to shade the face, ears, and neck.
- Wear protective clothing (especially tightly woven apparel) that covers as much as possible the arms, legs, and torso.
- Cover skin with a sunscreen lotion with a skin protection factor (SPF) of at least 15, protecting against UV radiation (both UVA and UVB).
- Reapply sunscreens every 2 hours (especially if sweating or swimming).
- Avoid sun lamps and tanning beds, which provide an additional source of UV radiation.
- Seek shade when outdoors.

The use of chemical sunscreen is only one of many strategies, and it should not be the sole agent used for cancer prevention. The lay public should be warned not to use sunscreen with a higher SPF with the intent to extend the duration of exposure because it is observed that DNA damage can occur long before sunburn appears, and the long-term effects of increased sun exposure are not known.[13] Sunscreen protective agents have been proven only to reduce the risk of actinic keratosis and SCC. There is no convincing evidence that sunscreen application has protective effect against BCC or MM.[13]

SECONDARY PREVENTION OF SKIN CANCER

Secondary prevention of skin cancer involves early detection of premalignant cancers for early intervention with the hope that it will reduce mortality and increase cure. Skin cancer screening consistently identifies MMs that are, on average, thinner than those found during usual care. Unfortunately, at this time, there is no evidence that skin cancer screening reduces morbidity or mortality.[14] Given this lack of evidence for a beneficial effect of skin cancer screening, recommendations vary with different agencies. The American Cancer Society recommends skin examination as part of cancer-related check-ups every 3 years for people between 20 and 40 years of age and on a yearly basis for those over 40 years of age. The American College of Preventive Medicine recommends total-body skin examination only in high-risk individuals. High-risk individuals are defined as those with a family or personal history of skin cancer, predisposing phenotypic characteristics, increased occupational or recreational exposure to sunlight, or clinical evidence of precursor lesions. The National Institutes of Health Consensus Panel recommends screening for MM as part of routine primary care.[14] Routine self-examination of the skin is a method in which individuals can take responsibility for identifying MM early when it is curable. Pamphlets and online information describing the method of skin self-examination are available from agencies such as the American Cancer Society (*www. cancer.org*), the American Academy of Dermatology (*www. aad.org*), and the Skin Cancer Foundation (*www.skincancer. org*).

PATHOPHYSIOLOGY

Skin Anatomy

The skin contains three layers: the epidermis (top layer), the dermis (middle layer), and the subcutis (innermost layer).[10] The epidermis serves as a barrier to the environment to protect internal organs, and within its layers are squamous cells that produce keratin to provide its protective effect.[10] Melanocytes, cells that synthesize melanin, also reside in the epidermis.[10] Melanin is a brown-black pigment that is distributed to surrounding keratinocytes within the dermis and epidermis via dendritic projections. The dermis gives the skin its strength, resiliency, and resistance to tearing.[10] It is made up of a dense network of collagen and elastic fibers that anchors hair follicles, sweat glands, blood vessels, and nerves. Basal cells separate the epidermis from the dermis, and these cells divide continually to replace the older cells that slough off the skin. The subcutis is composed of collagen and loose adipose connective tissue. It serves to conserve heat and act as a shock absorber to protect the inner organs[10] (Fig. 97–1).

MM involves the abnormal growth and proliferation of melanocytes and begins with the proliferation of a single melanocyte from within the epidermis. After a series of intraepithelial events, the melanocyte migrates to the dermis, possibly deeper into the cutis, and proliferates therein.[15] From within the dermis and subcutis, melanoma may metastasize and spread to distant sites via lymphatic and vascular channels.[15] The overwhelming majority of MMs originate from the skin, although they also may arise less commonly from the retina, meninges, or GI tract.

CLINICAL PRESENTATION, DIAGNOSIS, AND STAGING

There are four major subtypes of MM: superficial spreading, nodular, lentigo maligna melanoma, and acral lentiginous (Table 97–1). They each vary in clinical and growth characteristics.

Data from the Surveillance, Epidemiology, and End Results (SEER) study show that 82% of patients diagnosed with MM present with localized disease, 9% with regional disease, and

---

Table 97–1

Characteristics of Different Types of Skin Cancer

| | Malignant Melanoma | | | | Nonmelanoma Skin Cancer | |
	Superficial Spreading	Nodular	Lentigo Maligna Melanoma	Acral Lentiginous	Basal Cell Carcinoma	Squamous Cell Carcinoma
Frequency	70%	15–30%	4–10%	Less than 10%	60–80%	20%
Location	Trunk in men Legs in women Upper back	Trunk, head, neck	Sun-exposed areas, face	Palms of the hands, soles of feet, nailbeds	Head/neck trunk/ lower limbs	Backs of the hand, bare scalp, lips, ears
Age/gender at presentation	Middle forties Women more than men	Any age (fifth to sixth decades) Men more than women	70s Rare before 50	60s	Incidence increases after age 40	Incidence increases after age 40
Ethnicity	Caucasian	Caucasian	Caucasian	African Americans Asians, Hispanics	Most common in Caucasians, rare in dark-skinned people	Most common in African descendants
Initial growth	Radial	Pure vertical	Radial	Radial	Radial	Radial
Clinical features	Long horizontal growth phase, months to years before invading vertically *Melanoma in situ*—confined to the epidermis	Very aggressive without identifiable horizontal growth phase, deeply invasive at the time of diagnosis, associated with poor prognosis	Lentigo maligna—in situ form of lentigo maligna melanoma; 5–50% transform to malignant melanoma	50% of all melanomas in blacks, Asians, and Hispanics; 10% of melanomas in Caucasians	Four subtypes: 1. Nodular BCC (50–55%), most common subtype 2. Superficial BCC (10%), least aggressive 3. Morpheaform (2–5%), most aggressive 4. Pigmented or metatypical BCC	Usually presents as a painless, erythematous, poorly defined lesion with elevated borders

From Refs. 5, 8, 9, 20, 23.

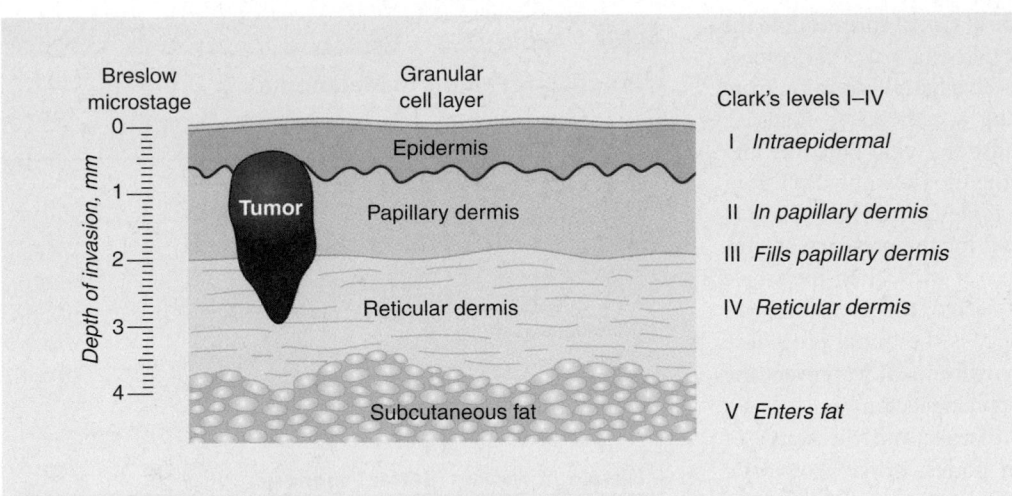

FIGURE 97–1. Skin anatomy: Breslow microstaging and Clark's levels. (From Langley RGB, Barnhill RL, Mihm Jr MC, et al. Neoplasms: Cutaneous melanoma. In: Freedberg IM, Eisen AZ, Wolff K, et al., eds. Fitzpatrick's Dermatology in General Medicine, 6th ed. New York: McGraw-Hill; 2003:938.)

Table 97–2

2002 AJCC Revised Melanoma Staging System

Stage	Histologic Features	Overall Survival 5 Years (%)	10 Years (%)
0	Melanoma in situ (involves only the epidermis layer)	100	100
IA	Less than or 1 mm thickness, no ulceration and Clark's level[a] II or III		
IB	Less than or 1 mm with ulceration or 1 mm with ulceration or Clark's level IV or V or between 1.01 and 2 mm with no ulceration	89–95	79–88
IIA	Between 1.01 and 2 mm with ulceration or between 2.01 and 4 mm with no ulceration	45–79	32–64
IIB	Between 2.01 and 4 mm with ulceration or greater than 4 mm with no ulceration		
IIC	Greater than 4 mm with ulceration		
IIIA	Any tumor thickness with no ulceration with one lymph node involved and micrometastases or any tumor thickness with no ulceration with two to three lymph nodes involved and micrometastases	63–70	57–63
IIIB	Any tumor thickness with ulceration and one to three lymph nodes involved and micrometastases or any tumor thickness without ulceration and one to three lymph nodes involved and macrometastases or any tumor thickness with ulceration with in-transit metastases/satellite lesions without metastatic lymph nodes	46–59	36–48
IIIC	Any tumor thickness with ulceration with one lymph node involved and macrometastases Any tumor thickness with ulceration with two to three lymph nodes involved and macrometastases Any tumor thickness with four or more metastatic lymph nodes or in-transit metastases/ satellite lesions with metastatic lymph nodes	24–29	15–24
IV	M_{1a}: Skin, subcutaneous tissue, or distant lymph nodes with normal lactate dehydrogenase M_{1b}: Lung with normal lactate dehydrogenase M_{1c}: To all other visceral sites (liver) or distant metastasis at any site with elevated serum LDH	7–19	3–16

[a]Clark's level refers to the level of penetration into the dermis (see Fig. 97–1). Breslow classification measures tumor thickness, in millimeters, from the epidermis to the deepest depth of penetration into the dermis (see Fig. 97–1).

From Ref. 20.

4% with distant disease.[4] ❷ *Once skin cancer is diagnosed, it is important to determine the stage of the cancer to find out if the cancer is confined to the original tumor site or has spread to other sites, such as the lymph nodes, liver, brain, lungs, or bone. The purpose of staging cancer is to determine prognosis, categorize patients with regard to metastatic potential and survival probability, and aid in clinical decision making.* As with most solid tumors, the tumor node metastasis (TNM) classification is used to stage MM, and the latest guidelines for staging MM proposed by the American Joint Committee on Cancer were implemented in 2002 (see Table 97–2).

❸ *Determination of lymph node status is important in melanoma staging because it is an independent prognostic factor, and it provides the oncologist with guidance for therapy decisions.*

For patients with melanomas who are at risk of spreading to the lymph nodes, a sentinel lymph node (SLN) biopsy is performed. The SLN, the first lymph node to receive lymph draining from the tumor, is identified by injecting a radioactive material, technetium-99m-labeled radiocolloids, and vital blue dye into the skin next to the tumor and tracing the flow of lymph from the tumor site to the nearest lymph node chain. Once the SLN is located, it is removed and analyzed for the presence of MM cells. If it is positive for the presence of MM, then the whole lymph node basin in that area is dissected; this is also known as lymphadenectomy. An SLN biopsy is the initial procedure to assess the status of lymph node involvement to prevent the morbidity associated with a total lymphadenectomy.

In addition to the stage of the disease and the status of disease involvement in the lymph nodes, other prognostic factors for outcome in MM include patient age and gender, tumor location, and histology of the MM. Specific patient-related and histopathological criteria that have been identified to characterize high-risk patients, in particular among those diagnosed with thin cutaneous melanomas, include male gender, mitogenicity, and evidence of regression.[16] Table 97–3 provides complete information on factors that confer good prognosis for a patient diagnosed with MM.[17]

Skin Examination

The *ABCDE* acronym is a helpful mnemonic for recognizing the signs and symptoms of early MM (Fig. 97–2). It was devised in 1985 by clinicians working in the Melanoma

Table 97–3

Prognostic Factors in Melanoma

Factor (Better Prognosis)

Age (less than 65 years)	5-year survival (%)
Less than 30 years	87
60 years	78
70 years	71
80 years	60
Gender (female)	10-year survival (%)
Female	86
Male	68
Tumor location (extremities)	10-year survival (%)
Extremities	90
Trunk, head, or neck	70

Histologic Factors (Better Prognosis)

Tumor thickness (less than 1 mm)	Clark's level (level I)
Ulceration (none)	Tumor vascularity (absent)
Nodal status (none)	Regression (absent)
Vascular invasion (none)	Mitotic rate (low)
Microsatellites (none)	Tumor infiltrating lymphocytes (present)

From Ref. 17.

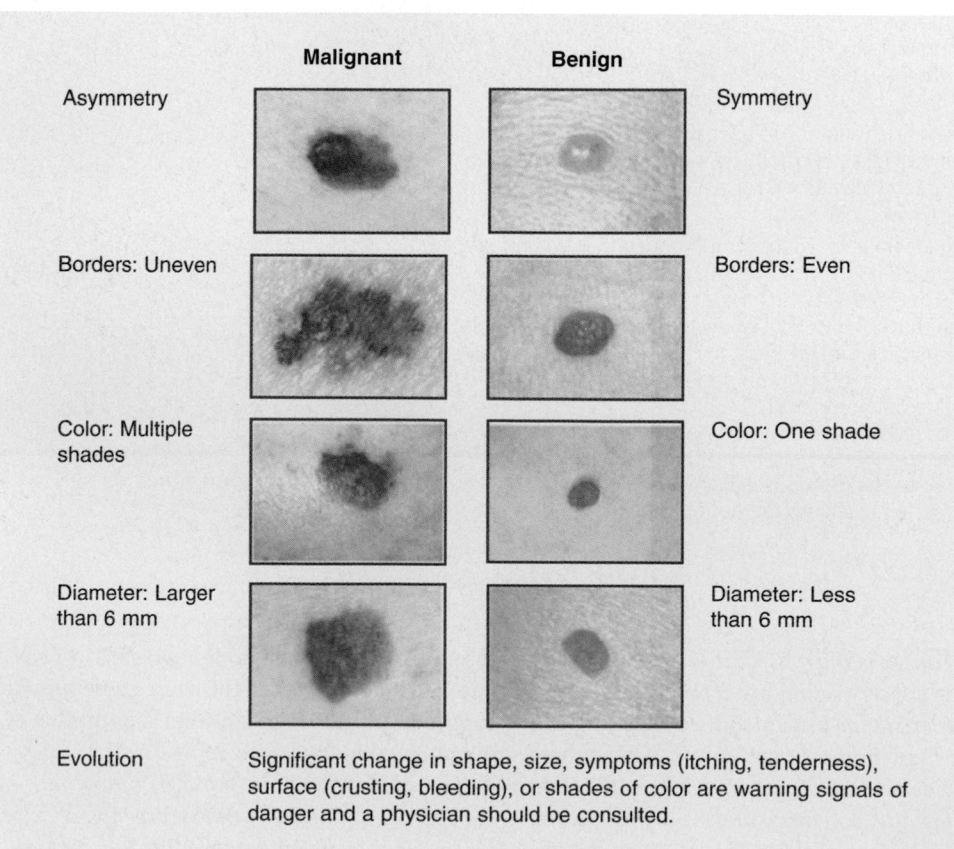

	Malignant	Benign	
Asymmetry			Symmetry
Borders: Uneven			Borders: Even
Color: Multiple shades			Color: One shade
Diameter: Larger than 6 mm			Diameter: Less than 6 mm
Evolution	Significant change in shape, size, symptoms (itching, tenderness), surface (crusting, bleeding), or shades of color are warning signals of danger and a physician should be consulted.		

FIGURE 97–2. ABCDE features of early melanoma. (Images courtesy of the Skin Cancer Foundation, New York, *www.skincancer.org*.)

Clinical Presentation of MM

Patients with skin cancer generally present with a lesion that may be located anywhere on the body. The most common sites are the head, neck, trunk, and extremities. Changes in any characteristics of a lesion are important danger warning signals. Abnormal presentations of a mole/lesion indicate the need for further assessment.

- *Asymmetry*: Half the lesion does not mirror the other half.
- *Border*: Sharp, ragged, uneven, and irregular borders.
- *Color*: Multiple colors of various hues of light brown, dark brown, black, red, blue, or gray.
- *Diameter*: Larger than 6 mm or the size of a pencil head eraser.
- *Evolving*: Significant change in shape, size, symptoms, surface, or shades of color.

Other signs and symptoms to monitor for in a lesion, in addition to ABCDE, include:

- Sudden or continuous enlargement of a lesion or elevation of a lesion
- Changes in the skin surrounding the nevus
- Redness, swelling, itching, tenderness, or pain
- Ulceration: friability of the lesion with bleeding or oozing. This is a danger signal.

Less Common Sites and Manifestations of MM

It is important to examine these sites for "hidden" MM:

- Nailbed
- Mucosal tissue
- Scalp
- Eye

In the nailbed, a black streak or wide variegated brown streak, elevation of nailbed, skin next to nail becomes darker, nail looks deformed or is being destroyed; size of nail streak increases over time.

Diagnostic Tests

- Dermoscopy
- Biopsy

Staging Tests (Depending on Patient's Presentation)

- Baseline chest x-ray
- Lactate dehydrogenase level
- CT of chest, abdomen, pelvis
- Sentinel lymph node (SLN) biopsy: ❸ *The status of the SLN is one of the most powerful independent prognostic factors predicting survival. It also provides the oncologist with guidance for therapy decisions and accurate staging.*
- Positron emission tomography (PET scan)
- Magnetic resonance imaging (MRI)

From Refs. 20, 22.

Clinical Cooperative Group at New York University School of Medicine and is used to educate health care professionals who are not dermatologists in differentiating common moles from cancer.[12] It is also a useful tool to educate the lay public to assess pigmented lesions and screen for suspicious moles to help identify the MM in its early stage when it is curable. Not all MMs, including nodular melanoma, have all four ABCDE characteristics, and it is not meant to provide a comprehensive list of all MM features. The characteristics for each of the letters are described in the "Clinical Presentation" box. It should be noted that evolution of a lesion is one of the most important warning signs of danger in the assessment of moles for MM.

TREATMENT

Diagnostic accuracy and clinical skills are two essential factors in the appropriate management of skin cancer. Early diagnosis of skin cancer is the key to improved prognosis. On presentation to a clinician's office, patients may offer a history of a new growth or an area of irritation. Conversely, the skin cancer may have been present for years undetected by the patient. The definitive diagnosis of any suspected cutaneous malignancy should be confirmed by a biopsy prior to treatment.

The modality of treatment for skin cancer depends on the size, location, and stage of the tumor; the age of the patient; and the type of skin cancer. Treatment options for skin cancer include surgery, radiation, chemotherapy, and immunotherapy. ❹ *Surgery is the primary treatment modality for nonmelanoma and melanoma skin cancer.*

Desired Outcome

The primary goals of therapy for skin cancer are to completely eradicate the tumor and minimize the risk of tumor recurrence and metastasis. Secondary goals of therapy include preserving normal tissue, maintaining function, and providing optimal cosmetic outcomes.[18] Patients with local disease MM (stages I and IIA) are curable with surgical resection of the tumor. Thus the aim is to diagnose patients at the earliest stage in order to increase the probability of cure. Patients with regional disease (stages IIB, IIC, and III) have a high recurrence risk, and the goal of therapy is to prevent relapse of the disease. Disseminated, metastatic MM is not curable, and the goal of therapy is local control of the disease and palliation of symptoms.

Patient Encounter 1, Part 2: Medical History, Physical Examination, and Diagnostic Tests

PMH: Hypertension, currently controlled; gastroesophageal reflux disease

FH: No known family history of cancer; specifically, no NMSC, MM, or hereditary dysplastic nevus syndrome

SH: Patient is retired. His sun-exposure history is as described in Patient Encounter 1, Part 1

Meds: Hydrochlorothiazide 25 mg orally once daily; famotidine 20 mg orally twice daily

ROS: No changes in vision, headaches, SOB, cough, fever, nausea, vomiting, diarrhea

PE:

• **VS:** BP 126/84, P 80, RR 16, T 37°C (98.6°F), ht 68 in. (173 cm), wt 72 kg (158 lb)

• **Skin:** Fair complexion, multiple scattered nevi, 9 mm nodule on shoulder as described

• **HEENT:** PERRLA, EOMI, sclera nonicteric, nose and throat clear without exudates or lesions

• **Neck and lymph nodes:** Supple, no lymphadenopathy

• **Lungs:** CTA bilaterally

• **CV:** RRR without murmurs

• **Abd:** Soft, nontender, nondistended, no hepatosplenomegaly

• **Exts:** No cyanosis, clubbing, edema

• **Neuro:** Alert and oriented × 3. Cranial nerves II–XII are intact, nonfocal.

• **Labs:** Within normal limits

• **CT scan of chest, abdomen, and pelvis:** Negative

• **CXR:** Negative

Treatment: KM underwent surgical resection of the primary tumor, and an SLN biopsy was positive for lymph node involvement. A lymphadenectomy was performed. After extensive discussion with his oncologist, the decision was made to start KM on interferon-α2b.

Given this additional information, what is KM's stage of MM?

What is the goal of therapy for KM?

What are the treatment options for KM after surgery?

What data support the use of high-dose IFN in KM?

Treatment Options for MM (Fig. 97–3)

▶ Stages I and IIA MM

The primary treatment modality for carcinoma in situ (stage I and IIA cutaneous MM) is surgical excision of the tumor.[19] The 5-year survival rates for patients with stages I and II tumors are 78% to 95%.[20] Achieving adequate surgical margins for the primary tumor is important in preventing local recurrence and improving overall survival. The thickness of the tumor dictates the extent of the surgical margin.[21] For tumors that are greater than 1 mm, or if the tumor is less than 1 mm but has ulceration, it is recommended that an SLN biopsy be performed to rule out occult nodal metastasis.[20] There is no recommendation for systemic therapy in patients with stage I or IIA MM.

▶ Stages IIB, IIC, and III MM (High-Risk MM)

❺ *Excision of the tumor with clear margins is the primary treatment modality for stages IIB and IIC. In addition to surgical excision of the primary tumor site, removal of the involved lymph node chain, a lymphadenectomy, is the standard treatment for stage III MM.*[19] *Patients at these stages are considered to be high risk because of their potential for recurrence and distant metastases.* The role of adjunct immunotherapy after surgery to decrease the incidence of recurrence for high-risk melanoma is controversial.

Interferon-α2b for High-Risk MM Interferon-α2b (IFN) has diverse mechanisms of action, including antiviral activity, impact on cellular metabolism and differentiation, and antitumor activity.[22] The antitumor activity is due to a combination of direct antiproliferative effect on tumor cells and indirect immune-mediated effects.[22] IFN is currently approved by the FDA as adjuvant therapy for patients who are free of disease after curative surgical resection but are at high risk of MM recurrence. This includes patients with bulky disease or regional lymph node involvement such as stages IIB, IIC, or III disease.[23] **❻** *It is controversial if IFN should be offered for high risk melanoma, as different doses of IFN have not proved definitively that IFN improves overall patient survival.*

The doses of IFN used in clinical trials can be classified into three groups: high-dose (HDI), intermediate-dose (IDI), and low-dose (LDI) interferon (Table 97–4). Data from many clinical trials assessing LDI in patients with high or intermediate risk of recurrence did not demonstrate an impact on overall survival, and it is unclear if disease-free survival is improved.[24-26] Therefore, at this time, LDI cannot be considered efficacious as adjuvant therapy for high-risk, stage III MM.

HDI has shown activity against MM in the adjuvant setting. In the evaluation of HDI for high-risk MM, data from a pooled analysis of four major clinical trials showed improved relapse-free survival, with an approximate 10% reduction in the risk of recurrence, but no effect on overall survival in patients receiving HDI.[27] A pooled analysis of several high-dose IFN trials and a trial comparing HDI with vaccine (E1694) also confirmed a reduction in the risk of recurrence with HDI without significant improvement in overall survival.[28,29]

HDI has substantial side effects (Table 97–5) and is an expensive therapy.[30] The constellation of side effects associated with the administration of IFN can be divided into acute and chronic manifestations and categorized into four major side-effect groups: constitutional, neuropsychiatric, hematologic,

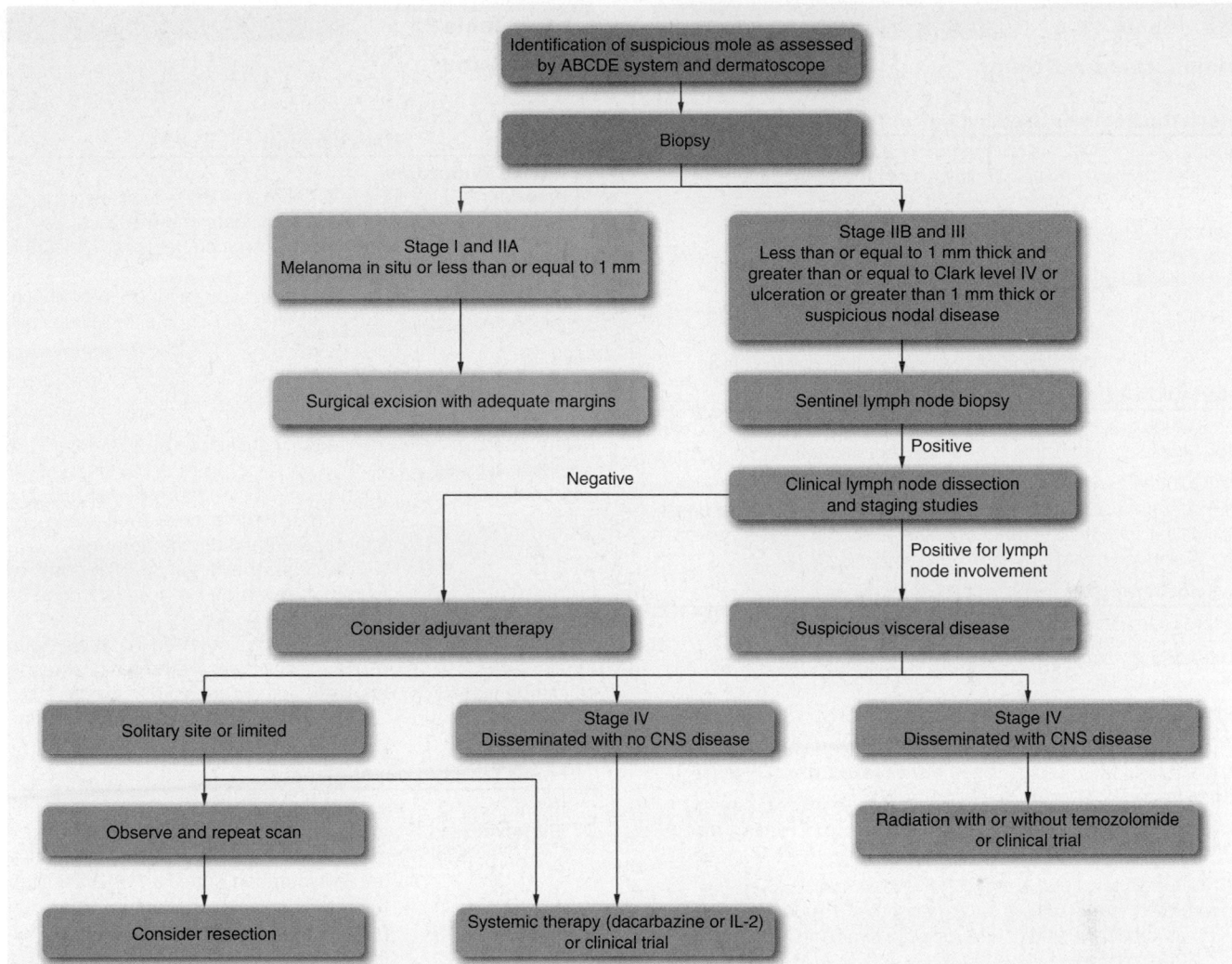

FIGURE 97–3. Algorithm for management of cutaneous melanoma. (From Ref. 39.)

and hepatic.[30] It is very important to educate patients on the side effects to expect and the interventions that are available to minimize the toxicities in order to reassure the patient.

The clinical dilemma in the use of HDI as adjuvant therapy for high-risk MM patients becomes: Is the benefit of preventing recurrence in only a small portion of patients without much improvement in overall survival worth the risk of considerable disabling toxicity? Which MM patient at risk for recurrence should receive HDI as adjuvant therapy? Decision guidelines proposed by Kilbridge and colleagues suggest that the patient should be willing to undergo the side effects of HDI treatment, understanding that it may decrease the chance of MM recurrence in 5 years by 10% or less.[31] Other factors that should be considered in the decision include the patient's comorbidities and/or contraindications to receiving HDI.[31] If the patient is eligible, encouragement to participate in clinical trials designed to address the issues of survival, quality of life, and treatment costs is also reasonable.[31]

▶ Stage IV MM

The prognosis for patients diagnosed with stage IV MM varies with the location of the metastases and the number of metastatic sites. Treatment options for stage IV metastatic MM include surgical excision of the lesion and radiation therapy for palliation of symptoms.

❼ *Surgical excision of the tumor is not curative for metastatic MM, and the primary goal of therapy is local control of the disease and relief of identifiable symptoms.* In highly selected patients, such as those with good performance status, less aggressive tumor biology, prolonged period of disease-free interval from the time of primary tumor treatment, and limited disease that is contained within a single location, complete surgical resection results in a median survival of 2 years and a 5-year survival rate of 10% to 25%.[32] For most other patients with stage IV MM, unfortunately, the survival rate is measured in months rather than years, with overall median survival of 5 to 8 months and a 5-year survival rate of less than 5%.[32]

Table 97–4

Immunotherapy Dosing[a]

Interferon Regimes Used in Clinical Trials

High dose (HDI)	20 million units/m² IV daily × 5 days/week for 4 weeks, followed by 10 million units/m² SC 3 times/week for 48 weeks
Intermediate dose (IDI)	10 million units × 5 days/week for 4 weeks, followed by 10 million units SC 3 times/week for varying durations
Low dose (LDI)	3 million units SC 3 times/week for varying durations 1 million units SC every other day for 1 year

Interleukin 2 Dosing Regimens[a]

IL-2 600,000 or 720,000 IU/kg by 15-minute infusion every 8 hours for 14 consecutive doses over 5 days as tolerated

IL-2 720,000 IU IV over 15 minutes beginning at 6 PM on day 1 and subsequently at 8 AM and 6 PM up to a maximum of 8 total doses on days 1 to 5 (first treatment course) and repeated on days 15 to 19 (second treatment course)

Chemotherapy[a]

Dacarbazine 250 mg/m²/day IV, days 1 to 5, every 21 days

No guidelines exist for dose adjustment in patients with renal or hepatic impairment

Temozolomide 150 to 200 mg/m²/day by mouth × 5 days, every 28 days

Caution should be used in patients with severe renal or hepatic impairment, no specific guidelines exist

Measure absolute neutrophil count (ANC) and platelets on day 22 and 29

If ANC is less than 1,000/L or platelet is less than 50,000/L, postpone therapy until ANC is greater than 1,500/L and platelet is greater than 100,000/L. Reduce dose by 50 mg/m² for subsequent cycle

If ANC is 1,000–1,500/L or platelet is less than 50,000–100,000/L, postpone therapy until ANC is greater than 1,500/L and platelet is greater than 100,000/L; maintain initial dose

If ANC is greater than 1,500/L and platelet is greater than 100,000/L; increase dose to or maintain dose at 200 mg/m²/day for 4 subsequent cycle

SC, subcutaneously

[a]The doses presented here are general. Clinicians should refer to clinical trials to determine the specific dose based on the regimen the patient is receiving.

From Refs. 33, 46, 47, 49, 50.

Table 97–5

IFN Toxicities

Common Acute Toxicity	Management
Flu-Like Symptoms	
Fever, rigors, chills, headaches, myalgia, nausea, emesis	Last 1–12 hours after dose and tolerance develops with continued therapy
	Bedtime administration helps with tolerating side effects
	Premedicate with acetaminophen or NSAID and administer meperidine for severe chills and rigors
	5-HT₃ antagonist, prochlorperazine, metoclopramide, fluids helps with nausea and vomiting
Neutropenia	Weekly CBC; reduce dose by 30–50%
Hepatic enzyme elevation	Liver function tests (LFTs) at baseline, weekly during induction, monthly during first 3 months of maintenance, then every 3 months. Withhold treatment until LFTs normalize; restart at 30–50% dose reduction; reversible on dose reduction or cessation
Cutaneous— alopecia, transient, mild rashlike reaction	Interferon is contraindicated in patients with psoriasis because exacerbation of psoriasis has been noted during IFN therapy

Common Chronic Toxicity	Management
Fatigue, weight loss, anorexia	Reported in 70–100% of patients and increases in intensity as therapy continues
	Increase aerobic activity, light exercise, improve nutrition, increase noncaffeinated fluid intake, stress management technique; pharmacologic intervention—megesterol acetate, methylphenidate, to help with either fatigue or anorexia
Depression, cognitive dysfunction. Rare—mania, mood instability	Psychiatric history prior to therapy and reassess every 4 to 6 weeks; antidepressants—SSRIs, mood stabilizer, bupropion, psychostimulants
Thyroid dysfunction	Initial thyroid function test (TSH), then monthly; if three sequential values are stable or normal, bimonthly or quarterly TSH

From Ref. 40.

• **Interleukin 2 for Stage IV MM** ❽ *Interleukin 2 (IL-2) therapy is approved by the FDA for the treatment of metastatic MM, and it is a reasonable option for patients with this stage of the disease.* IL-2 indirectly causes tumor cell lysis by proliferating and activating cytotoxic T lymphocytes (CTL).[33] The overall objective response rate for patients with metastatic MM receiving high-dose IL-2 is 16%, with a complete response in 6% of patients and a partial response in 10% of patients.[34] The median duration of response is 8.9 months for all responding patients and 5.9 months for patients with a partial response.[35] The median duration of complete response has not been reached but is at least 59 months. Disease progression is not observed in any patient responding for longer than 30 months.[35] Good performance status and no prior systemic therapy are the only prognostic factors that are associated with response, with objective response rate being twice that of patients with poor performance status and who received prior chemotherapy.[34] The site of metastasis did not influence response, and patients had responses in all organ sites, including lung, liver, adrenal, bone, liver, kidney, and spleen.[34] The data are encouraging because for the small number of patients who responded to therapy, the effect is of a long duration, and some patients may be considered to be cured of the disease (Refer to Table 97–4 for an example dosing regimen.)

High-dose IL-2 therapy is associated with severe toxicities.[34,36,37] Table 97–6 lists the most common side effects experienced by patients receiving IL-2 therapy and recommendations for management. Patients receiving IL-2 may be managed on the oncology unit as long as cardiac telemetry is available; however, it is important that all medical staff involved with the care of these patients be well educated on the side effects to monitor for and in the management of critical-care issues such as hypotension.[34]

Chemotherapy for Stage IV MM Dacarbazine, an alkylating agent, is the most active single-agent chemotherapy against MM, achieving response rates of 15% to 25%.[38] It is the only chemotherapy agent approved by the FDA for the treatment of metastatic MM. A recent phase III clinical trial in patients with advanced metastatic MM demonstrated a response rate of 12% and stable disease in 16% of patients treated with dacarbazine alone.[38] The response duration was not long-standing, with a median survival time of 6.4

months.[38] Nausea and vomiting are the most common side effects of dacarbazine. Combining dacarbazine with other chemotherapy agents with activity against MM in single-institution phase 2 trials resulted in response rates of between 30% and 50%.[39] Two phase III clinical trials assessing the CVD (cisplatin, vinblastine, and dacarbazine) regimen and the Dartmouth regimen (carmustine, cisplatin, dacarbazine, and tamoxifen) versus single-agent dacarbazine showed that there was a trend toward improved response rate, but the results were not statistically significant.[40] Furthermore, there was no significant survival advantage over single-agent dacarbazine alone, but toxicity was greater with the combination chemotherapy.[33] Therefore, combination chemotherapy is not a standard of care for stage IV MM.

Biochemotherapy for Stage IV MM Clinical trials combining chemotherapy and immunotherapy are based on the observations of independent clinical activity of each of these treatment modalities in treating metastatic MM. This combination is known as biochemotherapy. Only one phase III clinical trial showed significant improvement in response rate, time to progression, and median survival favoring the

---

Table 97–6

IL-2 Toxicities

Toxicity (% of Patients)	Management
Cardiovascular Hypotension (64%), supraventricular tachycardia (17%)	Discontinue antihypertensive medications. IV fluids to maintain systolic blood pressure greater than 80–90 mm Hg or vasopressor support with an α-agonist such as phenylephrine as indicated. Be judicious in use of IV fluids for hypotension
GI Vomiting and diarrhea (55%), nausea (24%), stomatitis (14%)	5-HT$_3$ antagonist, prochlorperazine for emesis (avoid corticosteroids), H$_2$ blocker for gastritis, antidiarrheal as needed (loperamide, diphenoxylate/atropine, codeine)
Neurologic Confusion (30%), somnolence	Haldol for agitation, lorazepam for anxiety, temazepam or zolpidem for insomnia
Pulmonary Dyspnea (31%), pulmonary edema, and adult respiratory distress syndrome	Advise smokers to quit 2 weeks before therapy; discontinue therapy if requiring greater than 4 LO$_2$ or 40% O$_2$ mask for saturation greater than 95%
Hepatic Elevated bilirubin (51%), transaminase (39%), alkaline phosphatase	Consider discontinuing therapy if severe
Renal Oliguria (49%), elevated serum creatinine (35%), anuria (8%)	Normal saline or dopamine at renal perfusion dose of 2 mcg/kg/min for oliguria; monitor for electrolyte abnormalities and replace as indicated
Hematologic Thrombocytopenia (43%), anemia (29%), leukopenia (21%)	Transfuse with packed red blood cells and platelets as needed
Skin Rash (27%), exfoliative dermatitis (15%), pruritus	Hydroxyzine, diphenhydramine, oatmeal powder baths, Lubriderm lotion
General Fever and or chills (47%), malaise (34%), infection (15%) Hypothyrodism	Acetaminophen and NSAIDs around the clock for fever and chills; add meperidine if chills are severe; clindamycin or cefazolin to prevent infection May occur in one-third of patients; thyroid function tests

From Refs. 46, 47.

biochemotherapy arm versus the combination-chemotherapy arm.[41] A systematic review of the literature to evaluate the use of biochemotherapy for the treatment of metastatic MM was conducted by Hamm and colleagues.[42] The results revealed inconsistent response, time to progression, and survival with consistently high toxicity rates. Therefore, currently, the use of biochemotherapy is not justified outside a clinical trial in patients with stage IV MM.[33,39,43]

In summary, systemic therapy for stage IV MM is controversial. ❾ *Combination chemotherapy and biochemotherapy increase toxicity significantly without offering overall survival benefit; thus they are not the standard of care for stage IV MM. Both high-dose IL-2 and dacarbazine are approved for the treatment of stage IV MM.* High-dose IL-2 may be preferred in patients with a good performance status. Enrollment in a clinical trial and best supportive care are also reasonable alternatives.[44]

▶ MM With Brain Metastases

Radiation for Brain Metastases One of the most common sites of metastasis for MM is the brain, and MM is reported to be the third most common cause of brain metastasis.[45] The incidence of brain metastasis is reported to range from 10% to 40% in clinical studies.[45] ❿ *Treatment options for brain metastases include surgery, radiation (which includes whole-brain radiotherapy and stereotactic surgery [SRS]), or chemotherapy. The choice of therapy depends on the number of metastatic lesions, accessibility of the lesion for surgery, the presence of neurologic symptoms, and the status of extracranial disease.*

Surgery followed by whole-brain radiotherapy (WBRT) is best indicated for patients with an accessible single brain lesion and controlled or limited systemic MM.[45,46] For those patients with multiple metastatic brain lesions and systemic disease, surgery generally is not considered to be appropriate.[44] In some cases, however, it may be necessary to resect the one "dominant" lesion that is causing symptoms such as intracranial hypertension, seizures, hemorrhage, or other severe neurologic side effects.[45,46] WBRT is indicated for patients with multiple (more than three) CNS metastases, surgically inaccessible lesions, and extensive systemic disease.[47] WBRT for metastatic CNS MM does not improve survival or provide a cure; however, it is effective in relieving neurologic symptoms.[47]

Stereotactic radiosurgery (SRS) may be considered over surgery for patients with fewer than three metastatic CNS lesions that are deep, nonsymptomatic, and less than 3 cm in size.[47] SRS delivers high doses of focused ionizing external-beam radiation to a well-defined target area in one session of radiation therapy.[47] This technique maximizes the dose of radiation to the tumor with a rapid dose falloff outside the target area, resulting in sparing of the surrounding nontarget normal tissue.

The median survival for patients with CNS metastasis is 3.5 months with best supportive care and corticosteroids.[48] Patients treated with WBRT and SRS or SRS alone have a median survival of 28 to 40 weeks, and the cause of death for most of these patients is progressive extracranial disease.[45]

Systemic Therapy for Brain Metastases Temozolomide (TMZ) is an oral chemotherapy agent that is structurally and functionally similar to dacarbazine, and it belongs to a new class of alkylating agents known as imidazotetrazines. Temozolomide possesses activity against MM cells and the ability to cross the blood–brain barrier because of its lipophilicity, thus making it an ideal chemotherapy agent to be investigated for the treatment of MM with CNS metastases. It is stable in the acidic pH of the stomach and is absorbed readily in the digestive tract with 100% bioavailability. Once it is in the CNS, temozolomide is hydrolyzed to the active metabolite MTIC (5-[3-dimethyl-1-triazenyl] imidazole-4-carboxamide). MTIC breaks down rapidly to form the reactive methyldiazonium ion, which methylates guanine residues in the DNA molecule causing cytotoxicity. TMZ does not cause cross-linking of DNA strands, making it less toxic to hematopoetic progenitor cells in the bone marrow than the nitrosoureas, platinum compounds, procarbazine, and dacarbazine. A recent phase III clinical trial comparing single-agent TMZ with dacarbazine demonstrated that TMZ is at least as effective as dacarbazine against advanced metastatic MM without CNS involvement.[38] The role of TMZ, either alone or as combination therapy, in the prevention and treatment of MM CNS metastasis is an area of active research.[49–51] In a phase 2 trial involving patients who have not received prior systemic chemotherapy for the treatment of MM brain metastases, single-agent TMZ showed a response rate of 7%, stable disease in 29% of patients, and a median overall survival of 3.5 months.[52] When TMZ was administered in combination with WBRT in patients with CNS metastasis, the response rate was only 10%, with the duration of response ranging from 2 to 7 months.[49] The combination of TMZ and a biochemotherapy regimen that included cisplatin, IL-2, IFN was evaluated in a phase 2 outpatient clinical trial for metastatic MM.[50] The results suggest that the rate of CNS metastasis may be decreased in patients who have either a complete or partial response owing to the addition of a CNS-active agent (TMZ).[50] Thalidomide in combination with TMZ has also been studied, showing a response rate of 12%.[51] In light of these promising data with TMZ, further trials are being conducted to confirm the benefit of TMZ in preventing progression or treating CNS metastases.

OUTCOME EVALUATION

The outcome of patients diagnosed with MM depends on the stage of the disease at diagnosis. The overall 5-year survival rate for patients with localized disease (stages I and IB) is the best at 89% to 95%.[20] For patients with stage IIA to IIIA disease, the 5-year survival rate is greater than 50%, ranging from 63% to 77%.[20] In patients with more advanced regional metastatic disease (stage IIIB to IIIC), the 5-year survival rate ranges from 27% to 53%.[20] Patients with stage IV distant

Patient Encounter 1, Part 3: Create a Care Plan

Create a care plan while KM is receiving INF therapy. Your plan should include: (a) the goal of therapy with INF, and (b) a plan related to dealing with the side effects to expect from this therapy.

What supportive measures should be used to minimize side effects?

What laboratory parameters need to be monitored?

What are the indications to discontinue or hold therapy?

When may the therapy be restarted after the doses were held?

What are the pharmacologic and nonpharmacologic recommendations for managing side effects?

How frequently should KM be monitored while on therapy?

Be able to discuss with the patient the following for INF:

- The differences between acute and chronic side effects
- The side effects that the patient will develop tolerance to
- The best time of the day to administer the drug
- The importance of keeping regular follow-up appointments to monitor for long-term side effects of the therapy and draw blood for routine lab tests
- Reassure the patient that therapy may be stopped at any time if side effects are intolerable
- What is the follow-up plan for KM after he has completed therapy with interferon-*a*2b?

metastatic disease have the worst 5-year survival rate at only 10% to 19%.[20]

After diagnosis and treatment of skin cancer, the next crucial step in management is monitoring for recurrence. Most recurrences materialize in the first 5 years, and the majority appears within the first 2 to 3 years following treatment.[19] The site of recurrence can be at the original site of the disease or in a different, distant anatomic location. Early detection of tumor recurrence is crucial because response rate is decreased significantly with tumor relapse.[18] Recurrences are found equally by physicians and patients, and one study demonstrated that 94% of recurrences were detected by the patient.[53] Thus it is imperative to educate patients on how to perform a total skin self-examination appropriately. Additionally, patients need to understand the importance of scheduling regular follow-up visits with the oncologist or dermatologist after the diagnosis and treatment of skin cancer.

There is no universal guideline for follow-up care for MM. The National Comprehensive Cancer Network recommends annual skin examination for all patients.[44] Educate patients with stage IA disease to have a history and physical examination every 3 to 12 months as clinically indicated and an annual skin examination for life. For stages IB to III disease, schedule a history and physical examination every 3 to 6 months for 3 years, every 4 to 12 months for 2 years, and then annually as indicated. It is optional to obtain a chest x-ray, LDH, CBC, and liver function tests (LFTs) every 3 to 12 months. CT scan can be obtained as indicated clinically.[44]

Patients who received immunotherapy after stage III or IV MM may experience fatigue and other chronic side effects. Develop a plan to order laboratory tests such as LFTs, thyroid-stimulating hormone, and white blood cell count at baseline and on a weekly or monthly basis as indicated. Monitor and evaluate patients for side effects of IL-2 or IFN, and educate patients on what to expect and how the side effects will be managed. Assess the patients' psychological, physical, and social functioning. Counsel patients to contact the hospital's social service department or the American Cancer Society for assistance in dealing with the disease emotionally, and recommend that patients consider attending support group meetings or talking to a counselor if or before they become overwhelmed with the diagnosis.

NONMELANOMA SKIN CANCER

EPIDEMIOLOGY AND ETIOLOGY

NMSC accounts for nearly half of all newly diagnosed cancers in the United States each year, and it is estimated that more than 1 million cases will be diagnosed in 2008. The true prevalence of NMSC may be underestimated because it is treated in outpatient settings, and no formal reporting to cancer registries is required.[54] BCC is the most common form of NMSC in Caucasians and comprises 75% of newly diagnosed NMSC. SCC accounts for 20% of NMSC.[54] NMSCs occur at a lower incidence in darker-skinned people or in descendants of African, Asian, and Mediterranean countries. In African Americans, the most common form of NMSC is SCC.[18] The majority of NMSCs are curable and the mortality rate is low; cure rates approach 98%, and the overall 5-year survival rate is greater than 95%.[18] Metastasis occurs in less than 0.1% of BCCs compared with an average of 3.6% of SCCs. Seventy-five percent of all NMSC deaths are attributed to SCC.[18] NMSC is associated with considerable morbidity owing to functional and cosmetic deformity. In addition, it is an economic burden to the health care system because costs associated with NMSC treatment are estimated at approximately $426 million per year.[55]

RISK FACTORS

It is estimated that 90% of NMSCs are linked to UV exposure and data from epidemiologic studies indicate that greater cumulative lifetime exposure is associated with a higher risk of developing SCC, whereas severe sunburns correlates more with BCC.[6]

Most cases of BCC are sporadic; however, it occurs frequently in the rare individuals with hereditary disorders such as basal cell nevus syndrome (also known as Gorlin's syndrome) and xeroderma pigmentosum (XP). The *patched* gene (*PTCH*), a tumor-suppressor gene, has been shown to be mutated in XP and 50% to 60% of sporadic BCCs.[7] The oncogene *bcl-2*, which suppresses programmed cell death (apoptosis), also has been found to be expressed in high levels in patients with BCC.[56]

There is clear evidence linking defects of the immune system to the development of NMSC. For example, it is observed that patients receiving chronic immunosuppressant therapy for organ transplantation have a 50% risk of developing SCC within 20 years of transplantation, and 30% of these cancers are highly aggressive.[57] Additionally, patients with HIV infection are predisposed to melanoma. Data also support the idea that UV radiation exposure induces immunosuppression and that this is associated with carcinogenesis.[58] Langerhans' cells are responsible for antigen processing and initiation of the immune cascade in the skin, and it has been demonstrated that UVB alters their function.[58] UV radiation also induces suppressor T cells and activates biologic response modifiers by initiating cytokine cascades, ultimately leading to a state of immune tolerance and unsuppressed tumor growth.

PATHOPHYSIOLOGY

NMSCs arise from epidermal keratinocytes and involve primarily squamous cells and basal cells of the epidermis and dermis skin layers. BCCs arise from basal cells or keratinocytes in hair follicles or sebaceous glands.

CLINICAL PRESENTATION, DIAGNOSIS, STAGING

Like MM, BCC is also divided into four main histologic subtypes: nodular, superficial, morpheaform, and pigmented (or metatypical) (Table 97–1). BCC has indolent growth characteristics, with a very low metastatic rate, ranging from 0.0028% to 0.55%.[18] Paradoxically, BCCs can cause extensive local destruction and significant disfigurement.

SCCs are more aggressive than BCCs (Table 97–1). The rate of metastasis for SCC is 2% to 6% and may be as high as 10% to 14% in high-risk sites such as the ear and lip and 30% in the genital area.[18] SCCs are preceded by leukoplakia, actinic keratosis, radiation damage, or sun damage to the skin.[17] Actinic keratosis, a small papule that appears on areas of sun damage on the skin, has a 1 in 400 risk of transforming to SCC.[18]

Lymph Node Consideration in NMSC

In patients with SCC, metastatic spread to the lymph nodes occurs in less than 5%.[59] Patients are still potentially curable with this stage of the disease, but they are at high risk of experiencing regional relapse and distant metastasis to the bones and lungs. A tumor thickness of greater than 4 mm has been suggested as the threshold at which nodal

---

Clinical Presentation of NMSC

Five Warning Signs of BCC

The appearance of some BCCs is similar to plaque, psoriasis, or eczema, and these benign disorders are included in the differential diagnosis.

- An open sore that bleeds, oozes, or crusts and remains open for 3 or more weeks
- A reddish patch or irritated area that may crust, itch, hurt, or persist with no noticeable discomfort
- A shiny bump or nodule that is pearly or translucent and may be pink, red, or white. In dark-haired people, it may be tan, black, or brown and can be confused with a mole
- A pink growth with slightly elevated, rolled border and a crusted indentation in the center
- A scarlike area that is white, yellow, or waxy with poorly defined borders

Warning Signs and Symptoms of SCC[5,26]

- A wartlike growth, a persistent scaly red patch with irregular borders, or an open sore that crusts or bleeds
- An elevated growth with a central depression that bleeds occasionally. This growth type increases in size rapidly
- In situ SCC: red scaling macule or plaque
- Invasive SCC: firm or friable red papule or nodule covered with scale or crust
- Precursor of invasive SCC (actinic keratosis): scaly erythematous macule or papule on areas of chronic sun exposure

From Ref. 22.

---

metastasis should be suspected and an SLN biopsy should be considered.[59]

TREATMENT

In patients diagnosed with BCC and SCC, the primary goal of therapy is to cure the patient and to prevent recurrence. Although NMSC has a low mortality rate, morbidity owing to tissue destruction, functional impairment, and disfigurement is a significant issue. Therefore, secondary goals of therapy for NMSC are preservation of function and restoration of cosmesis.[18]

Nonpharmacologic Therapy

▶ Surgery

Surgery is the primary treatment modality for all patients diagnosed with either BCC or SCC. Full-thickness ablative procedure in the form of surgical excision of the tumor along with a margin of normal tissue surrounding the tumor is the preferred method for high-risk tumors. Obtaining negative surgical margins is critical for cure and decreasing the risk of tumor recurrence. For lesions that are less than 2 cm in diameter, a minimum margin of 4 mm is usually adequate.[21] Depending on the tumor size, degree of differentiation, and invasion of surrounding structures, larger margins of resection may be necessary.

Low-risk tumors can be treated with superficial ablative techniques, including electrodessication and curettage (ED&C) and cryotherapy.[19] ED&C is a simple, cost-effective technique that utilizes repeated cycles of using a curette to cut through malignant tissue, followed by electrodesiccation, which involves the application of high voltage, low current to the skin, causing drying or desiccation of the tissue. ED&C is most appropriate for well-defined superficial lesions that are not located in areas with increased risk for metastasis.

Cryotherapy is a procedure used primarily for smaller, low-risk NMSCs with clearly defined margins. It involves delivering liquid nitrogen at subzero temperatures as a spray or with a supercooled metal probe to destroy the malignant tissue.[18] While cryotherapy is cost-effective and easy to deliver, the recurrence rate is high.[18]

NMSC is considered to be high risk if it has any of the following features: it is recurrent, the location is at a high risk site (e.g., mask areas of the face, lips, ears, hands, and feet), it is larger than 2 cm in diameter or greater than or equal to 4 mm in depth, it is moderately or poorly differentiated, it is fast growing, it has ill-defined borders, there is positive perineural or vascular invasion, the patient is immunosuppressed, or it is the morpheaform or metatypical subtype of BCC.[19] If the tumor is located on the trunk or extremities, less than 2 cm in diameter and less than 4 mm in depth, well differentiated, slow growing, has well-defined borders, and is the nodular or superficial subtype of BCC, then it is considered to be low risk.[19] For high risk NMSC, Mohs' micrographic surgery (MMS) provides the highest cure rate.[18] The goal of this therapy is complete removal of the cancer with preservation of as much surrounding normal tissue as possible. MMS involves careful dissection, staining of frozen sections, and anatomic mapping of the tumor specimen. Sections are assessed immediately under the microscope in the operating theater and the process is repeated until a tumor-free margin is attained.[18]

The 5-year survival rate for surgical excision, electrodesiccation and curettage, and MMS is 90% or better for NMSC.[19]

▶ Radiation

Radiation is not standard therapy for the treatment of skin cancer; however, there are circumstances in which radiation may be preferred. Older patients or patients who are poor candidates for surgery may be offered radiation as an option.[48] Radiation offers good cosmetic results, but it requires multiple visits over the course of several months, making it inconvenient for patients.[19] In the treatment of NMSC, radiation results in poorer cosmetic outcomes than surgery or electrodesiccation and curettage.[7] Disadvantages of radiation include radiation-induced dermatitis, high cost, and the increased risk of secondary malignancy, including SCC and BCC.[7]

▶ Photodynamic Therapy

Photodynamic therapy is a noninvasive treatment option for actinic keratoses and is being investigated in the treatment of superficial BCC and SCC. A photosensitizing agent is administered IV or topically to the target area, followed by exposure to a light source. The energy absorbed by the sensitizer is transferred to molecular oxygen to create an activated form of oxygen called *singlet oxygen*, which reacts with cellular component to cause cell damage and death.[60] One of the most commonly used photosensitizing agents is topical 5-aminolevulinic acid, a solution that is applied for 14 to 18 hours to the lesion and irradiated for 5 to 20 minutes.[61] Response rates for superficial SCC have ranged from 75% to 100%, while those for superficial BCC range from 90% to 100%.[7] Side effects of topical agents are usually limited to local skin reactions, while those of IV agents often include generalized photosensitivity.

Pharmacologic Therapy

Nonsurgical treatment is used frequently for superficial NMSCs. Topical 5-fluorouracil has been used for the treatment of actinic keratoses, superficial BCCs, and SCCs in situ.[62] Fluorouracil interferes with the synthesis of DNA and to a lesser extent RNA by blocking the methylation reaction of deoxyuridylic acid to thymidylic acid, ultimately causing cell death, particularly of more rapidly dividing cells. Topical applications of 5% 5-fluorouracil usually consist of a twice daily dosing for at least 3 to 6 weeks, for up to 12 weeks. Intralesional 5-fluorouracil has also been used successfully in treating SCC using 8 weekly injections.[63] Imiquimod cream is another treatment option for actinic keratoses and low-risk NMSC. It is a Toll-like receptor 7 (TLR7) agonist that promotes Th1-type immunity and induces cytokines, including interferon-α. It is FDA-approved for treatment of actinic keratoses and superficial BCC. Response rates of superficial BCC with application of 5% imiquimod cream five times a week for 6 weeks range from 70% to 88%,[64] with lower cures for nodular BCC.[65] Imiquimod has also been shown to be an effective treatment for SCC in situ; in a placebo-controlled trial, 11 of 15 lesions resolved versus 0 in the placebo-treated group.[66] The most common side effects of both 5-fluorouracil and imiquimod are erythema, itching, pain, and crusting that are mild to moderate. Finally, intralesional injection of interferon-α2b three times weekly for 3 weeks has been used to treat BCC, with cure rates up to 97%.[67]

OUTCOME EVALUATION

BCC and SCC have excellent outcomes, with cure rates approaching 98%.[18] Recurrence of NMSC during a 5-year follow-up is around 30% to 50% and 70% to 80% of recurrence develops within the first 2 years after initial therapy. Therefore, it is crucial to advise patients to schedule routine follow-up visits with their dermatologist and educate them about the value of sun protection and total body skin self-examination. For patients at high risk for recurrence, they should be monitored every 1 to 3 months for the first year, every 2 to 4 months in the second year, every 4 to 6 months for years 3 to 5, then every 6 to 12 months annually for life. The follow-up recommendation for low-risk patients is every 3 to 6 months for 2 years, every 6 to 12 months for year 3, then annually for life.

Patients receiving topical agents such as fluorouracil or imiquimod should be educated to wash the treatment area with mild soap and water before applying the cream, use gloves to apply enough to cover the area with a 1-cm margin and wash their hands thoroughly after each application.

Patient Care and Monitoring

1. Obtain a thorough patient medication history, both prescription and nonprescription, to prevent drug interactions with the current therapy the patient is receiving.

2. Obtain the appropriate baseline laboratory tests, and determine a time interval for reevaluation of specific laboratory tests to determine toxicity.

3. Provide education on the side effects of therapy:
   - What to administer/take to prevent side effects
   - When to administer/take the medication to decrease side effects
   - Nonpharmacologic recommendations to minimize side effects
   - Drugs that may interact with therapy
   - Lab tests that need to be monitored on a regular basis
   - The parameters for discontinuing or holding therapy
   - If therapy is to be reinitiated, the new dose of therapy

4. Assess the patient for adverse drug reactions and drug–drug interactions.

5. Educate the patient on the signs and symptoms of infection.

6. Assess for changes in the patient's quality of life owing to side effects of drug therapy.

7. Educate the patient on measures that should be undertaken to limit sun exposure and prevent skin cancer.

8. Educate the patient on how to do skin self-examination for suspicious moles.

9. Educate the patient on follow-up recommendations after treatment for skin cancer is completed.

They should avoid sun exposure and be counseled to monitor for side effects such as pain, itching, and inflammation. They should consult their dermatologist if the side effects are intolerable.

Abbreviations Introduced in This Chapter

BCC	Basal cell carcinoma
CPDs	Cyclobutane pyrimidine dimers
CTL	Cytotoxic T lymphocyte
ED&C	Electrodessication and curettage
HDI	High-dose interferon-α2b
IDI	Intermediate dose interferon-α2b
IFN	Interferon-α2b
IL-2	Interleukin 2
LDI	Low-dose interferon-α2b
LFTs	Liver function tests
MM	Malignant melanoma
MMS	Mohs' micrographic surgery
MTIC	5-(3-Dimethyl-1-triazenyl) imidazole-4-carboxamide
NMSC	Nonmelanoma skin cancer
ROS	Reactive oxygen species
SCC	Squamous cell carcinoma
SEER	Surveillance, Epidemiology, and End Results
SLN	Sentinel lymph node
SPF	Skin protection factor
SRS	Stereotactic radiosurgery
SSRI	Selective serotonin reuptake inhibitor
TMZ	Temozolamide
UV	Ultraviolet
WBRT	Whole-brain radiation therapy
XP	Xeroderma pigmentosum

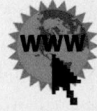 Self-assessment questions and answers are available at *http://www.mhpharmacotherapy.com/pp.html.*

REFERENCES

1. Jemal A, Siegel R, Ward E, et al. Cancer Statistics, 2006. CA Cancer J Clin 2006;56:106–130.
2. Lens MB, Dawes M. Global perspectives of contemporary epidemiological trends of cutaneous malignant melanoma. Br J Dermatol 2004;150:179–185.
3. Armstrong B, Kricker A. The epidemiology of UV induced skin cancer. J Photochem Photobiol B 2001;63:8–18.
4. Beddingfield III FC. The melanoma epidemic: Res Ipsa Loquitur. Oncologist 2003;8:459–465.
5. Desmond RA, Soon S. Epidemiology of malignant melanoma. Surg Clin N Am 2003;83:1–29.
6. Rager EL, Bridgeford EP, Ollila DW. Cutaneous Melanoma: Update on prevention, screening, diagnosis, and treatment. Am Fam Physician 2005;72:269–276.
7. Kuijpers DI, Thissen MR, Neumann MH. Basal cell carcinoma. Treatment options and prognosis, a scientific approach to a common malignancy. Am J Clin Dermatol 2002;3:247–259.

8. Thompson JF, Scolyer RA, Kefford RF. Cutaneous Melanoma. Lancet 2005;365:687–701.

9. Ting W, Schultz K, Cac N, et al. Tanning bed exposure increases the risk of malignant melanoma. Int J Dermatol 2007;46:1253–1257.

10. American Cancer Society, National Comprehensive Cancer Network. Melanoma: Treatment guidelines for patients. Dermatol Nursing 2005;17:119–131.

11. MacKie RM. Risk factors for development of primary cutaneous malignant melanoma. Dermatol Clinic 2002;20:597–600.

12. Poochareon RS, Federman DG, Kirsner RS. Primary prevention efforts for melanoma. J Drugs Dermatol 2004;3:506–519.

13. Gallagher RP. Sunscreens in melanoma and skin cancer prevention. CMAJ 2005;173:244–245.

14. Helfand M, Mahon SM, Eden KB, et al. Screening for Skin Cancer. Am J Prev Med 2001;20:44–58.

15. Friedman R, Heilman ER. The pathology of malignant melanoma. Dermatol Clin 2002;20:659–676.

16. Gimotty PA, Elder DE, Fraker DL, et al. Identification of high-risk patients among those diagnosed with thin cutaneous melanomas. J Clin Oncol 2007;25:1129–1134.

17. Homsi J, Kashani-Sabet M, Messina JL, Daud A. Cutaneous melanoma: Prognostic factors. Cancer Control 2005;12:223–239.

18. Garner KL, Rodney WM. Basal and squamous cell carcinoma. Dermatology 2000;27:447–457.

19. Martinez JC, Otley CC. The management of melanoma and non-melanoma Skin cancer: A review for the primary care physician. Mayo Clinic Proceedings 2001;76:1253–1265.

20. Balch CM, Buzaid AC, Soon SJ, et al. Final Version of the American Joint Committee on Cancer Staging System for Cutaneous Melanoma. J Clin Oncol 2001;19:3635–3648.

21. Nahabedian MY. Melanoma. Clin Plast Surg 2005;32:249–259.

22. Jonasch E, Haluska FG. Interferon in oncological practice: Review of interferon biology, clinical applications, and toxicities. Oncologist 2002;6:34–55.

23. Lawson DH. Choices of adjuvant therapy of melanoma. Cancer Control 2005;12:236–241.

24. Hancock BW, Wheatley K, Harris S, et al. Adjuvant interferon in high risk melanoma: The AIM HIGH study—United Kingdom Coordinating Committee on Cancer Research Randomized Study of Adjuvant Low-Dose Extended-duration interferon alpha 2b in high risk resected malignant melanoma. J Clin Oncol 2004;22:53–61.

25. Kleeberg UR, Suciu S, Brocker EB, et al. Final results of the EORTC 18871/DKG 80-1 randomized phase III trial: rIFN-alpha 2b versus rIFN-gamma versus ISCADOR M versus observation after surgery in melanoma patients with either high-risk primary (thickness > 3 mm) or regional lymph node metastasis. European J of Cancer 2004;40:390–402.

26. Kirkwood JM, Ibrahim GJ, Sondak VK, et al. High and low dose interferon alpha 2b in high risk melanoma: First analysis of intergroup trial E1690/S9111/C9190. J Clin Oncol 2000;18:2444–2458.

27. Kirkwood JM, Manola J, Ibrahim J, et al. A pooled analysis of eastern cooperative oncology group and intergroup trials of adjuvant high-dose interferon for melanoma. Clin Cancer Res 2004;10:1670–1677.

28. Kirkwood JM, Ibrahim JG, Sosman JA, et al. High-dose interferon alpha 2b significantly prolongs relapse free and overall survival compared with the GM2-KLH/QS-21 vaccine in patients with resected stage IIB-III melanoma: Results of Intergroup Trial E1694/S9512/C509801. J Clin Oncol 2001;19:2370–2380.

29. Wheatley K, Ives N, Hancock B, et al. Does adjuvant interferon alpha for high risk melanoma provide a worthwhile benefit? A meta-analysis of the randomized trials. Cancer Treat Rev 2003;29:241–252.

30. Hauschild A, Gogas H, Tarhini A, et al. Practical guidelines for the management of interferon-alpha-2b side effects in patients receiving adjuvant treatment for melanoma. Cancer 2008;112:982–994.

31. Kefford RF. Adjuvant therapy of cutaneous melanoma: The interferon debate. Annals of Oncology 2003;14:358–365.

32. Spanknebel K, Kaufman HL. Surgical treatment of stage IV melanoma. Clinics in Dermatol 2004;22:240–250.

33. O'Day SJ, Kim CJ, Reintgen DS. Cancer Control. Metastatic Melanoma: Chemotherapy to Biochemotherapy 2002;9:31–38.

34. Atkins MB, Lotze MT, Dutcher JP, et al. High dose recombinant Interleukin 2 therapy for patients with metastatic melanoma: Analysis of 270 patients treated between 1985 and 1993. J Clin Oncol 1999;17:2105–2116.

35. Atkins MB, Kunkel L, Sznol M, Rosenberg SA. Cancer J Sci Am. High dose recombinant interleukin 2 therapy in patients with metastatic melanoma: Long-term survival update 2000;6:S11–S14.

36. Buzaid AC, Atkins M. Practical guidelines for the management of biochemotherapy related toxicity in melanoma. Clin Can Res 2001;7:2611–2619.

37. Acquavella N, Kluger H, Rhee J, et al. Toxicity and activity of a twice daily high dose bolus interleukin 2 regimen in patients with metastatic melanoma and metastatic renal cell cancer. J Immunother 2008;31:569–576.

38. Middleton MR, Grob JJ, Aaronson N, et al. Randomized phase III study of temozolomide versus dacarbazine in the treatment of patients with advanced metastatic melanoma. J Clin Oncol 2000;18:158–166.

39. Tsao H, Atkins MB, Sober A. Management of cutaneous melanoma. NEJM 2002;351:998–1012.

40. Kirkwood JM, Bender C, Agarwala S, et al. Mechanisms and management of toxicities associated with high dose interferon alpha 2b therapy. J Clin Oncol 2002;20:3703–3718.

41. Eton O, Legha SS, Bedikian AY, et al. Sequential biochemotherapy versus chemotherapy for metastatic melanoma: Results from a Phase III randomized trial. J Clin Oncol 2002;20:2045–2052.

42. Hamm C, Verma S, Petrella T, et al. Biochemotherapy for the treatment of metastatic malignant melanoma: A systematic review. Cancer Treat Rev 2008;34:145–156.

43. Keilholz U, Punt CJA, Gore M, et al. Dacarbazine, cisplatin, and interferon alpha 2b with or without interleukin 2 in metastatic melanoma: A randomized phase III trial (18951) of the European organization for research and treatment of cancer melanoma group. J Clin Oncol 2005;23:6747–6755.

44. NCCN Melanoma clinical practice guidelines v.1.2006, *www.NCCN.org*.

45. Douglas JG, Margolin K. The treatment of brain metastases from malignant melanoma. Seminars in Oncology 2002;29:518–524.

46. Tarhini AA, Agarwala SS. Management of brain metastasis in patients with melanoma. Curr Opin Oncol 2004;16:161–166.

47. Bafaloukos D, Gogas H. The treatment of brain metastases in melanoma patients. Cancer Treatment Rev 2004;30:515–520.

48. Tsao H, Sober AJ. Melanoma treatment update. Dermatol Clin 2005;23:323–333.

49. Margolin K, Atkins MB, Thompson JA, et al. Temozolomide and whole brain irradiation in melanoma metastatic to the brain: A phase II trial of the cytokine working group. J Cancer Res Clin Oncol 2002;128:214–218.

50. Ready N, Aronson F, Wanebo H, Kennedy T. A low rate of central nervous system progression in a phase II trial of outpatient chemobiologic therapy with cisplatin, temozolomide, interleukin-2, and interferon alpha 2-B for metastatic malignant melanoma. Am J Clin Oncol 2005;28:479–483.

51. Hwu W, Lis E, Menell JH, et al. Temozolomide plus thalidomide in patients with brain metastasis from melanoma. Cancer Control 2005;103:2590–2597.

52. Agarwala SS. Temozolomide for the treatment of brain metastases associated with metastatic melanoma: A phase II study. J Clin Oncol 2004;22:2101–2107.

53. Lang PG. Current concepts in the management of patients with melanoma. Am J Clin Dermatol 2002;3:401–426.

54. Diepgen TL, Mahler V. The epidemiology of skin cancer. Br J Dermatol 2002;146:1–6.

55. Chen JG, Fleischer AB, Smith ED, et al. Cost of non-melanoma skin cancer treatment in the US. Dermatol Surg 2001;27:1035–1038.

56. Abbasi NR, Shaw H, Rigel DS, et al. Early diagnosis of cutaneous melanoma. Revisiting the ABCD Criteria. JAMA 2004;292:2771–2776.

57. Acarturk TO, Edington H. Nonmelanoma skin cancer. Clin Plast Surg 2005;32:237–248.

58. Swanson NA, Lee KK, Gorman A, Lee H. Biopsy techniques. Diagnosis of melanoma. Dermatol Clin 2002;20:677–680.

59. Veness MJ. Treatment recommendations in patients diagnosed with high-risk cutaneous squamous cell carcinoma. Aust Radiol 2005;49:365–376.

60. Danson S, Lorigan P. Improving outcomes in advanced malignant melanoma. Drugs 2005;65:733–743.

61. Brown SB, Brown EA, Walker I. The present and future role of photodynamic therapy in cancer treatment. The Lancet Oncology 2004;5:497–508.

62. Jorizzo J, Carney P, Ko W, et al. Fluorouracil 5% and 0.5% creams for the treatment of actinic keratosis: Equivalent efficacy with a lower concentration and more convenient dosing schedule. Cutis 2004;74:18–23.

63. Morse LG, Kendrick C, Hooper D, et al. Treatment of squamous cell carcinoma with intralesional 5-fluorouracil. Dermatol Surg 2003;29:1150–1153.

64. Burns CA, Brown MD. Imiquimod for the treatment of skin cancer. Dermatol Clin 2005;24:151–164.

65. Peris K, Campione E, Micantonio T, et al. Imiquimod treatment of superficial and nodular basal cell carcinoma: 12-week open-label trial. Dermatol Surg 2005;31:318–323.

66. Patel G, Goodwin R, Chawla BA, et al. Imiquimod 5% cream monotherapy for cutaneous squamous cell carcinoma in situ (Bowen's disease): A randomized, double-blind, placebo-controlled trial. J Am Acad Dermatol 2006;54:1025–1032.

67. Tucker S, Polasek JW, Perri AJ, et al. Long-term follow-up of basal cell carcinomas treated with perilesional interferon α 2b as monotherapy. J Am Acad Dermatol 2006;54:1033–1038.

98 Hematopoietic Stem Cell Transplantation

Amber P. Lawson

LEARNING OBJECTIVES

● **Upon completion of the chapter, the reader will be able to:**

1. Explain the rationale for using hematopoietic stem cell transplant (HSCT) to treat cancer.

2. Compare the different types of HSCTs, specifically (a) the types of donors (i.e., autologous and allogeneic), (b) the source of hematopoietic cells (i.e., umbilical cord, peripheral blood progenitor cells [PBPCs], and bone marrow), and (c) the type of preparative regimen (i.e., myeloablative and nonmyeloablative).

3. List the nonhematologic toxicity to high-dose chemotherapy used in myeloablative preparative regimens, specifically busulfan-induced seizures, hemorrhagic cystitis, GI toxicities, and sinusoidal obstruction syndrome.

4. Develop a plan for monitoring and managing engraftment of hematopoiesis.

5. Explain graft-versus-host disease (GVHD).

6. Recommend a prophylactic and treatment regimen for GVHD.

7. Choose an appropriate regimen to minimize the risk of infectious complications in HSCT patients.

8. Evaluate the long-term health care of HSCT survivors.

KEY CONCEPTS

❶ Hematopoietic stem cell transplantation (HSCT) is a procedure used mainly to treat hematologic malignancies via high-dose chemotherapy and/or a graft-versus-tumor effect.

❷ An autologous HSCT involves the infusion of a patient's own hematopoietic cells and allows for the administration of higher doses of chemotherapy, radiation, or both to treat the malignancy. Infusion of another's hematopoietic cells is an allogeneic HSCT; these cells can be from donors related or unrelated to the recipient.

❸ Umbilical cord blood, peripheral blood progenitor cells (PBPCs), and bone marrow can serve as the source of hematopoietic cells. The optimal cell source differs based on the donor and recipient characteristics.

❹ A myeloablative preparative regimen involves the administration of sublethal doses of chemotherapy to the recipient in order to eradicate residual malignant disease. The recipient will not regain his or her own hematopoiesis and will be at risk for substantial life-threatening nonhematologic toxicity.

❺ A nonmyeloablative preparative regimen is less toxic than a myeloablative regimen in hopes of being able to offer the benefits of an allogeneic HSCT to more patients. A nonmyeloablative HSCT is based on the concept of donor immune response having a graft-versus-tumor effect.

❻ Nonhematologic toxicity differs based upon the preparative regimen administered.

❼ Engraftment is the reestablishment of functional hematopoiesis. It is commonly defined as the point at which a patient can maintain a sustained absolute neutrophil count (ANC) of greater than 500 cells/mm³ (0.5×10^9/L) and a sustained platelet count of greater 20,000/mm³ (20×10^9/L) lasting for three or more consecutive days without transfusions.

❽ Graft-versus-host disease (GVHD) is caused by the activation of donor lymphocytes leading to immune damage to the skin, gut, and liver in the recipient. An immunosuppressive regimen is administered to prevent GVHD in recipients of an allogeneic graft; this regimen is based on the type of preparative regimen and the source of the graft.

❾ Recipients of HSCT are at higher risk of bacterial, viral, and fungal infections and usually receive a prophylactic or preemptive regimen to minimize the morbidity and mortality owing to infectious complications.

⑩ Long-term survivors of HSCT should be monitored closely, particularly for infections and secondary malignant neoplasms.

INTRODUCTION

❶ *Hematopoietic stem cell transplantation (HSCT) is a procedure used mainly to treat hematologic malignancies via high-dose chemotherapy and/or a graft-versus-tumor effect.* An essential component of this procedure is the infusion of hematopoietic cells into the recipient to facilitate an immunologic response against the residual malignancy and/or restore normal hematopoiesis and lymphopoiesis. The first HSCTs were performed using allogeneic bone marrow, which involved administration of high-dose chemotherapy and/or radiation aimed at eradicating residual malignant disease followed by transplantation of bone marrow from one individual to another in order to "rescue" the recipient's immune system from the myelotoxic effects of the treatment. Bone marrow contains pluripotent stem cells and post-thymic lymphocytes, which are responsible for long-term hematopoietic reconstitution, immune recovery, and its associated graft-versus-host disease (GVHD). Subsequently, the dose-intensity concept for cancer treatment was expanded to using myeloablative preparative regimens followed by autologous HSCT.

The type of HSCT performed depends on a number of factors, including type and status of disease, availability of a compatible donor, patient age, performance status, and organ function. In addition to bone marrow, hematopoietic stem cells may be obtained from the peripheral blood progenitor cells (PBPCs) and umbilical cord blood. The essential properties of the hematopoietic cells are their ability to engraft, the speed of engraftment, and the durability of engraftment.

Examples of diseases treated with HSCT are listed in Table 98–1. ❷ *Autologous HSCT, or infusion of a patient's own hematopoietic cells, allows for the administration of higher doses of chemotherapy, radiation, or both to treat the malignancy or autoimmune disorder.* In this setting, the hematopoietic cells "rescue" the recipient from otherwise dose-limiting hematopoietic toxicity. Autologous HSCT is used to treat intermediate- and high-grade non-Hodgkin's lymphoma (NHL), multiple myeloma (MM), autoimmune diseases, and relapsed or refractory Hodgkin's disease.[1] ❷ *Allogeneic HSCT involves the transplantation of hematopoietic cells obtained from a different person's (donor) bone marrow, peripheral blood, or umbilical cord blood to the recipient.* Unless the donor and the recipient are identical twins (referred to as a *syngeneic HSCT*), they are dissimilar genetically. Allogeneic HSCT is used to treat both nonmalignant conditions and hematologic malignancies such as acute and chronic leukemias.[1]

The infusion of hematopoietic cells follows the administration of a combination of chemotherapy and/or radiation, termed the conditioning or preparative regimen. ❹ *A myeloablative preparative regimen involves the administration of sublethal doses of chemotherapy to the recipient in order to eradicate residual malignant disease. The recipient will not regain his*

		Table 98–1
Diseases Commonly Treated With HSCT		
	Autologous Graft	**Allogeneic Graft**
Cancers	Multiple myeloma Non-Hodgkin's lymphoma Hodgkin's disease Neuroblastoma Germ cell tumors	Acute myeloid leukemia Acute lymphoblastic leukemia Chronic myeloid leukemia Myelodysplastic syndrome Myeloproliferative disorders Non-Hodgkin's lymphoma Hodgkin's disease Chronic lymphocytic leukemia Multiple myeloma
Other diseases	Autoimmune diseases Amyloidosis	Aplastic anemia Paroxysmal nocturnal hemoglobinuria Fanconi's anemia Thalassemia major Sickle cell anemia Severe combined immunodeficiency Inborn errors of metabolism

or her own hematopoiesis and will be at risk for substantial life-threatening nonhematologic toxicity. For those undergoing an autologous HSCT, their hematopoietic cells must be harvested and stored before the myeloablative preparative regimen is administered. After the administration of the myeloablative preparative regimen, these hematopoietic cells serve as a rescue intervention to reestablish bone marrow function and avoid long-lasting, life-threatening marrow aplasia. In the setting of an allogeneic HSCT, the preparative regimen is designed to suppress the recipient's immunity, eradicate residual malignancy, or create space in the marrow compartment. Improved survival outcomes have been observed with both autologous and allogeneic HSCT when the hematologic malignancy is in complete remission at the time of HSCT.[2] At most HSCT centers, age younger than 65 years and normal renal, hepatic, pulmonary, and cardiac function are considered eligibility requirements for myeloablative allogeneic HSCT. A myeloablative or nonmyeloablative preparative regimen may be used for allogeneic HSCT; only myeloablative preparative regimens are used for autologous HSCT. Allogeneic HSCT offers the potential for a graft-versus-tumor effect in which immune effector cells from the donor recognize and eliminate residual tumor in the recipient.[1]

The recognition of graft-versus-tumor effect, which likely is caused by cytotoxic T lymphocytes in the donor stem cells, led to investigations with nonmyeloablative transplants, in which less toxic preparative regimens are used in the hope of expanding the availability of HSCT to recipients whose medical condition or age prohibits use of myeloablative regimens.

EPIDEMIOLOGY AND ETIOLOGY

Each year, the number of allogeneic HSCTs is less than the number of autologous HSCTs. Worldwide, approximately

35,000 autologous HSCTs and 20,000 allogeneic HSCTs are performed per year, with 40% of allogeneic HSCTs employing reduced-intensity preparative regimens. In the late 1990s, the number of allogeneic HSCTs reached a plateau, most likely related to the introduction of imatinib (Gleevec) for treatment of newly diagnosed chronic-phase chronic myelogenous leukemia (CML). Furthermore, the limited availability of suitable donors may have contributed to the plateau effect. Recently, however, the number of allogeneic transplants for hematologic malignancies other than CML appears to be increasing.[2]

Autologous PBPC use has increased and essentially has replaced bone marrow as a graft source in many transplant centers. From years 2002 through 2006, over 95% of autologous HSCTs in adults and 80% in children used PBPCs as the source of hematopoietic cells.[2] Patients do not benefit from an immunologic graft-versus-tumor effect while undergoing an autologous transplant; instead, the administration of high-dose chemotherapy followed by an autologous stem cell transplant in chemotherapy-sensitive malignancies relies on the preparative regimen alone to eradicate the malignant disease. Autologous HSCT is used to treat a variety of malignancies; Hodgkin's lymphoma, NHL, and MM are the most common indications for this procedure and represent over one-half of all autologous HSCTs.[2] Autologous HSCT circumvents the need for histocompatible donors, is associated with lower mortality, and is not restricted to younger patients.[3] The use of allogeneic PBPCs is increasing; from years 2002 through 2006, 75% of allogeneic HSCTs performed worldwide used PBPCs as the source of hematopoietic cells rather than bone marrow in adult patients.[3]

PATHOPHYSIOLOGY

For an allogeneic HSCT, the recipient and the donor are dissimilar genetically unless they are identical twins (a transplant between twins is referred to as a *syngeneic HSCT*). The transplanted tissue is immunologically active, and thus there is potential for bidirectional graft rejection. In the first scenario, cytotoxic T cells and natural killer (NK) cells belonging to the host (recipient) recognize minor histocompatibility (MHC) antigens of the graft (donor hematopoietic stem cells) and lead to a rejection response. In the second scenario, immunologically active cells in the graft recognize host MHC antigens and elicit an immune response. The former is referred to as *host-versus-graft disease* and the latter is referred to as GVHD. Host-versus-graft effects are more common in solid-organ transplantation. When host-versus-graft effects occur in allogeneic HSCT, they are referred to as *graft failure* or *rejection,* which results in ineffective hematopoiesis (i.e., adequate ANC and/or platelet counts were not obtained). ❼ *Engraftment is defined as the point at which a patient can maintain a sustained absolute neutrophil count (ANC) of greater than 500 cells/mm³ (0.5 × 10⁹/L) and a sustained platelet count of greater than or equal to 20,000/mm³ (20 × 10⁹/L) lasting greater than or equal to three consecutive days without transfusions.*[4] Therefore, an essential first step for patients eligible for HSCT is finding a human leukocyte antigen (HLA)–compatible graft with an acceptable risk of graft failure and GVHD.

Histocompatibility

Histocompatibility differences between the donor and the recipient necessitate immunosuppression after an allogeneic HSCT because considerable morbidity and mortality are associated with graft failure and GVHD. Rejection is least likely to occur with a syngeneic donor, meaning that the recipient and host are identical (monozygotic) twins. In patients without a syngeneic donor, initial HLA typing is conducted on family members because the likelihood of complete histocompatibility between unrelated individuals is remote. Siblings are the most likely individuals to be histocompatible within a family. The chance for complete histocompatibility occurring in an individual with only one sibling is 25%. Approximately 40% of patients with more than one sibling will have an HLA-identical match. Having a matched-sibling donor is no longer a requirement for allogeneic HSCT because improved immunosuppressive regimens and the National Marrow Donor Program have allowed an increase in the use of unrelated or related matched or mismatched HSCTs. The use of alternative sources of allogeneic hematopoietic cells, such as related donors mismatched at one or more HLA loci or phenotypically (i.e., serologically) matched unrelated donors, has been evaluated.[5] Establishment of the National Marrow Donor Program has helped to increase the pool of potential donors for allogeneic HSCT. Through this program, an HLA-matched unrelated volunteer donor might be identified. Recipients of an unrelated graft are more likely to experience graft failure and acute GVHD relative to recipients of a matched-sibling donor. Determination of histocompatibility between potential donors and the patient is completed before allogeneic HSCT. Initially, HLA typing is performed using blood samples and compatibility for class I MHC antigens (i.e., HLA-A, HLA-B, and HLA-C) is determined through serologic and DNA-based testing methods. In vitro reactivity between donor and recipient also can be assessed in mixed-lymphocyte culture, a test used to measure compatibility of the MHC class II antigens (i.e., HLA-DR, HLA-DP, and HLA-DQ). Currently, most clinical and research laboratories are also performing molecular DNA typing using polymerase chain reaction methodology to determine the HLA allele sequence.[6]

The preparative regimen or GVHD prophylaxis may be altered based on the mismatch between the donor and the recipient. The risk of graft failure decreases with better matches such that those with a class I (i.e., HLA-A, -B, or -C) antigen mismatch have the highest risk of rejection; those with just one class I allele mismatch have a minimal risk. Graft failure does not appear to be associated with mismatch at a single class II antigen or allele.[6] GVHD and survival have been associated with disparity for class I and II antigens and alleles.[7]

Stem Cell Sources

Autologous hematopoietic stem cells are obtained from bone marrow or peripheral blood. The technique for harvesting autologous hematopoietic cells depends on the anatomic source (i.e., bone marrow or peripheral blood). A surgical procedure is necessary for obtaining bone marrow. Multiple aspirations of marrow are obtained from the anterior and posterior iliac crests until a volume with a sufficient number of hematopoietic stem cells is collected (i.e., 600–1,200 mL of bone marrow). The bone marrow then is processed to remove fat or marrow emboli and usually is infused IV into the patient like a blood transfusion.

The shift to the use of PBPCs over bone marrow for autologous HSCT is primarily because of the more rapid engraftment and decreased health care resource use. Because the harvest occurs before administering the preparative regimen, autologous hematopoietic cells must be cryopreserved and stored for future use.

Transplantation with PBPCs essentially has replaced bone marrow transplantation (BMT) as autologous rescue after myeloablative preparative regimens. Autologous PBPCs are obtained by administering a mobilizing agent(s) followed by apheresis, which is an outpatient procedure similar to hemodialysis. Hematopoietic growth factors (HGFs) alone or in combination with myelosuppressive chemotherapy are used for mobilization of autologous PBPCs with similar results. The HGFs granulocyte-macrophage colony-stimulating factor (sargramostim, Leukine) and granulocyte colony-stimulating factor (filgrastim, Neupogen) are used as mobilizing agents. The use of pegylated granulocyte colony-stimulating factor (pegfilgrastim, Neulasta) for mobilization of PBPCs appears more convenient and is promising as a mobilization agent; however, further data are needed regarding graft composition, HSCT outcomes, and donor safety in allogeneic donations before widespread use of this agent can be recommended.

The combination of chemotherapy with an HGF enhances PBPC mobilization relative to HGF alone.[1] In addition to treating the underlying malignancy, this approach lowers the risk of tumor cell contamination and the number of apheresis collections required, but there is a greater risk of neutropenia and thrombocytopenia. The HGF is initiated after completion of chemotherapy and is continued until apheresis is complete. Many centers monitor the number of cells that express the CD34 antigen (i.e., CD34+ cells) to determine when to start apheresis. The CD34 antigen is expressed on almost all unipotent and multipotent colony-forming cells and on precursors of colony-forming cells, but not on mature peripheral blood cells. Apheresis is continued daily until the target number of PBPCs per kilogram of the recipient's weight is obtained. For adult recipients, the number of CD34+ cells correlates with time to engraftment. Lower yield of CD34+ cells is associated with administration of stem cell toxic drugs (e.g., carmustine and melphalan) and intensive prior chemotherapy or radiotherapy.

If patients are unable to obtain an adequate yield of CD34+ cells per kilogram after mobilization attempts fail, then allogeneic transplant may be considered as an alternative. In 2008, plerixafor (Mobozil) was FDA approved for use in combination with granulocyte colony-stimulating factor to mobilize PBPCs for collection and subsequent autologous transplantation in patients with NHL and MM. Plerixafor is an inhibitor of the CXCR4 chemokine receptor which results in more circulating PBPCs in the peripheral blood due to the inability of CXCR4 to assist in anchoring hematopoietic stem cells to the bone marrow matrix. Since administration of plerixafor with granulocyte colony-stimulating factor results in increased yield of CD34+ cells per kilogram compared to granulocyte colony-stimulating factor alone, this combination may serve as an alternative mobilization strategy in patients deemed to be at risk for mobilization failure with conventional methods.

TREATMENT

Desired Outcome

The desired outcome with HSCT is to cure the patient of his or her underlying disease while minimizing the short- and long-term morbidity associated with HSCT.

Nonpharmacologic Therapy

▶ *Harvesting, Preparing, and Transplanting Allogeneic Hematopoietic Cells*

❸ *Bone marrow, PBPCs, and umbilical cord blood can serve as the source of hematopoietic cells. The optimal cell source differs based on the donor and recipient characteristics.*

Bone Marrow Harvesting the bone marrow from an allogeneic donor is conducted via the same process as for an autologous HSCT. The harvest occurs on day 0 of the HSCT such that it is infused into the recipient immediately after processing. The marrow may need additional processing if the donor and recipient are ABO-incompatible, which occurs in up to 30% of HSCTs. Red blood cells (RBCs) may need to be removed before infusion into the recipient to prevent immune-mediated hemolytic anemia and thrombotic microangiopathic syndromes.

Peripheral Blood Progenitor Cells The allogeneic donor first undergoes mobilization therapy with an HGF to increase the number of hematopoietic cells circulating in the peripheral blood. The most commonly used regimen to mobilize allogeneic donors is a 4- to 5-day course of filgrastim, 10 to 16 mcg/kg/day, administered subcutaneously, followed by leukopheresis on the fourth or fifth days when peripheral blood levels of CD34+ cells peak. An adequate number of hematopoietic cells usually are obtained with one to two apheresis collections, with the optimal number of CD34+ collected being a minimum of 5×10^6 cells/kg of recipient body weight. Higher numbers of CD34+ cells are associated with more rapid neutrophil and platelet engraftment; patients who receive less than 2×10^6/kg CD34+ cells experience a higher mortality rate and a decreased overall survival compared to patients who receive at least 2×10^6/kg CD34+ cells.[8] Hematopoietic stem cells obtained from the peripheral blood are processed like bone marrow–derived stem cells and may be infused immediately into the recipient or frozen for future use. In comparison with bone marrow donation, allogeneic PBPC donation leads to quicker hematopoietic recovery. Neutrophil engraftment occurs 2 to 6 days earlier and platelet engraftment occurs approximately 6 days earlier with PBPC grafts compared to bone marrow grafts.[9] The donor may experience musculoskeletal pain, headache, mild increases in hepatic enzyme or lactate dehydrogenase levels related to filgrastim administration. Hypocalcemia may also occur owing to citrate accumulation, which decreases ionized calcium concentrations during apheresis.

Allogeneic PBPC grafts contain approximately 10 times more T and B cells than bone marrow grafts. Historically, there has been significant concern that the greater T- and B-cell content of PBPCs could increase the risk of acute and/or chronic GVHD. In patients with a hematologic malignancy who have an HLA-matched sibling donor, a PBPC graft is optimal relative to bone marrow graft because the PBPC graft is associated with quicker neutrophil and platelet engraftment and potentially improved disease-free survival rates.[10] Grafts from PBPCs are associated with a similar incidence of acute GVHD but an approximately 20% increase in the incidence of extensive-stage and overall chronic GVHD.[10] Similar trends for engraftment and GVHD have been found with unrelated donors.[11]

Umbilical Cord Blood Transplant with umbilical cord blood offers an alternative stem cell source to patients who do not have an acceptable matched related or unrelated donor. When allogeneic hematopoietic cells are obtained from umbilical cord blood, the cord blood is obtained from a consenting donor in the delivery room after birth and delivery of the placenta. The cord blood is processed, a sample is sent for HLA typing, and the cord blood is frozen and stored for future use. Numerous umbilical cord blood registries exist, with the goal of providing alternative sources of allogeneic stem cells. One potential limitation to the use of umbilical cord blood transplants is the inability to employ donor-lymphocyte infusions in the event of relapse. Engraftment is slower in umbilical cord blood transplants, with a potential lower risk of GVHD and similar survival rates relative to BMT.[1,12] In children receiving an umbilical cord blood graft from an unrelated donor, cell dose (e.g., nucleated cells) is related to engraftment, transplant-related morbidity, and survival.[13] Although there were initial concerns regarding whether a umbilical cord blood transplant could provide enough nucleated cells to engraft adequately within an adult, there is growing experience to indicate that a umbilical cord blood transplant is feasible when at least 1×10^7 nucleated cells per kilogram of recipient body weight are administered.[13] The prospective use of dual umbilical cord units and ex vivo expansion of umbilical cord units to obtain adequate engraftment are methods currently under exploration.

T-Cell Depletion Immunocompetent T lymphocytes may be depleted from the donor bone marrow ex vivo before infusion (referred to as *T-cell–depleted hematopoietic cells*) into the recipient as a means of preventing GVHD. Depletion of T lymphocytes in donor hematopoietic cells is completed ex vivo using physical (e.g., density-gradient fractionation)

and/or immunologic (e.g., antithymocyte globulin [ATG] and CAMPATH-1 antibodies) methods. Functional recovery of T cells in the recipient is delayed, and the risk of Epstein-Barr virus–associated lymphoproliferative disorders is higher with the use of T-cell–depleted bone marrow. The use of T-cell–depleted grafts reduces the incidence of GVHD, but graft failure and relapse are more common. The use of donor lymphocyte infusion in patients who relapse after receiving a T-cell–depleted HSCT is being investigated.

Engraftment After chemotherapy and radiation, pancytopenia lasts until the infused stem cells reestablish functional hematopoiesis. The median time to engraftment is a function of several factors, including the source of stem cells such as PBPCs, which can result in earlier engraftment than bone marrow.[9] Myeloablative preparative regimens have significant regimen-related toxicity and morbidity and thus usually are limited to healthy, younger (i.e., usually younger than 50 years) patients. Alternatively, nonmyeloablative transplants are being performed with the hope of curing more patients with cancer by increasing the availability of HSCT with less regimen-related toxicity and by using the graft-versus-tumor effect.[1]

A delicate balance exists between host and donor effector cells in the bone marrow environment. Residual host-versus-graft effects may lead to graft failure, which is also known as graft rejection. *Graft failure* is defined as the lack of functional hematopoiesis after HSCT and can occur early (i.e., lack of initial hematopoietic recovery) or late (i.e., in association with recurrence of the disease or reappearance of host cells after initial donor cell engraftment). Engraftment usually is evident within the first 30 days in patients undergoing an HSCT; however, rejection can occur after initial engraftment. Therapeutic options for the treatment of graft rejection are limited; a second HSCT is the most definitive therapy, although the toxicities are formidable.[14]

▶ *Graft-Versus-Tumor Effect*

A graft-versus-tumor effect occurs owing to the donor lymphocytes, as supported by three observations after myeloablative allogeneic HSCT; namely, (a) lower relapse rates in patients with GVHD relative to those who did not have GVHD; (b) a higher rate of leukemia relapse after T-cell–depleted, autologous, or syngeneic HSCT, and (c) the effectiveness of donor lymphocyte infusions in reinducing a remission in patients who relapsed after allogeneic HSCT. Rapid taper of immunosuppression in patients with residual disease may induce a graft-versus tumor effect. In donor lymphocyte infusion, lymphocytes are collected from the peripheral blood of the donor and administered to the recipient. Eradication of the recurrent malignancy is due to either specific targeting of the tumor antigens or to GVHD, which may affect cancer cells preferentially. Patients with hematologic malignancies (e.g., CML and AML) and certain solid tumors (e.g., renal cell carcinoma) appear to benefit from a graft-versus-tumor effect. These data gave rise to the use of nonmyeloablative preparative regimens.

Pharmacologic Therapy

▶ *Preparative Regimens for HSCT*

Examples of commonly used preparative regimens are included in Table 98–2. ❻ *The nonhematologic toxicity differs based on the preparative regimen administered.*

● **Myeloablative Preparative Regimens** In both autologous and allogeneic HSCT, infusion of stem cells circumvents dose-limiting myelosuppression, maximizing the potential value of the steep dose-response curve to alkylating agents and radiation, suppressing the host immune system, and creating space in the marrow compartment to facilitate engraftment. The preparative regimen is designed to eradicate immunologically active host tissues (lymphoid tissue and macrophages) and to prevent or minimize the development of host-versus-graft reactions. Most allogeneic preparative regimens for the treatment of hematologic malignancies contain either cyclophosphamide, radiation, or both. The combination of cyclophosphamide and total-body irradiation (TBI) was one of the first preparative regimens developed and is still used widely today. This regimen is immunosuppressive and has inherent activity against hematologic malignancies (e.g., leukemias and lymphomas). TBI has the added advantage of being devoid of active metabolites that might interfere with the activity of donor hematopoietic cells. In addition, TBI eradicates residual malignant cells at sanctuary sites such as the CNS. Modifications of the cyclophosphamide-TBI preparative regimen include replacing TBI with other agents (e.g., busulfan) or adding other chemotherapeutic or monoclonal

agents to the existing regimen in hopes of minimizing long-term toxicities. In the case of a mismatched allogeneic HSCT with a substantially increased chance of graft rejection, ATG also may be added to the preparative regimen to further immunosuppress the recipient.

The optimal myeloablative preparative regimen remains elusive. The long-term outcomes of busulfan-cyclophosphamide (BU-CY) and cyclophosphamide-TBI (CY-TBI) in patients with AML and CML, the more common indications for allogeneic HSCT, have been compared in a meta-analysis of four clinical trials.[18] Equivalent rates of long-term complications were present between the two preparative regimens, except that there was a greater risk of cataracts with CY-TBI and alopecia with BU-CY. Overall and disease-free survivals were similar in patients with CML, whereas there was a trend for improved disease-free survival with CY-TBI in AML patients. Thus, the preparative regimen can be tailored to the primary disease and to the degree of HLA compatibility.

Nonmyeloablative Preparative Regimens ❺ *A non-myeloablative preparative regimen is less toxic than a myeloablative regimen in hopes of being able to offer the benefits of an allogeneic HSCT to more patients. A nonmyeloablative HSCT is based on the concept of donor immune response having a graft-versus-tumor effect.*

Because of the severe regimen-related toxicity of a myeloablative preparative regimen, the use of HSCT traditionally was limited to younger patients with minimal comorbidities. Most patients diagnosed with cancer are elderly and thus, myeloablative HSCT could not be offered to

---

Table 98–2

Commonly Used Preparative Regimens for HSCT[a]

Type of HSCT	Preparative Regimen	Dose/Schedule for Adults	Dose/Schedule for Pediatric Patients
Allogeneic[15]	Myeloablative CY-TBI	CY 60 mg/kg/day IV on 2 consecutive days before TBI 1,000–1,575 rads fractionated over 1–7 days	CY 60 mg/kg/day IV on 2 consecutive days before TBI 1,000–1,575 rads fractionated over 1–7 days
Allogeneic, autologous[16]	Myeloablative BU-CY	BU 1 mg/kg per dose po or 0.8 mg/kg per dose IV every 6 hours × 16 doses; CY 60 mg/kg/day IV daily × 2 days following BU	BU 1 mg/kg per dose po or 0.8 mg/kg per dose IV every 6 hours × 16 doses; CY 120–200 mg/kg IV given over 2–4 days following BU
Autologous[17]	Myeloablative BEAM (carmustine/etoposide/-cytarabine/melphalan)	Carmustine 300 mg/m² IV Etoposide 400–800 mg/m² IV given over 4 days Cytarabine 400–1,600 mg/m² IV given over 4 days Melphalan 140 mg/m² IV	Carmustine 300 mg/m² IV Etoposide 400–800 mg/m² IV given over 4 days Cytarabine 400–1,600 mg/m² IV given over 4 days Melphalan 140 mg/m² IV
Allogeneic[3]	Nonmyeloablative BU-FLU	Fludarabine 30 mg/m²/day IV on day –10 to day –5 followed by busulfan 1 mg/kg/dose po every 6 hours × 8 doses on days –6 and –5	Fludarabine 30 mg/m²/day IV on day –10 to day –5 followed by busulfan 1 mg/kg/dose po every 6 hours × 8 doses on days –6 and –5

BU, busulfan; CY, cyclophosphamide; FLU, fludarabine; TBI, total-body irradiation.

[a]Patients undergoing HSCT are required to undergo pretransplant screening to ensure adequate organ function prior to administration of the preparative regimen. Therefore, no standard dosage reductions based on renal or hepatic dysfunction can be recommended for listed preparative regimens. Any dosage reductions based on renal or hepatic dysfunction should be considered on a case-by-case basis per institutional protocols.

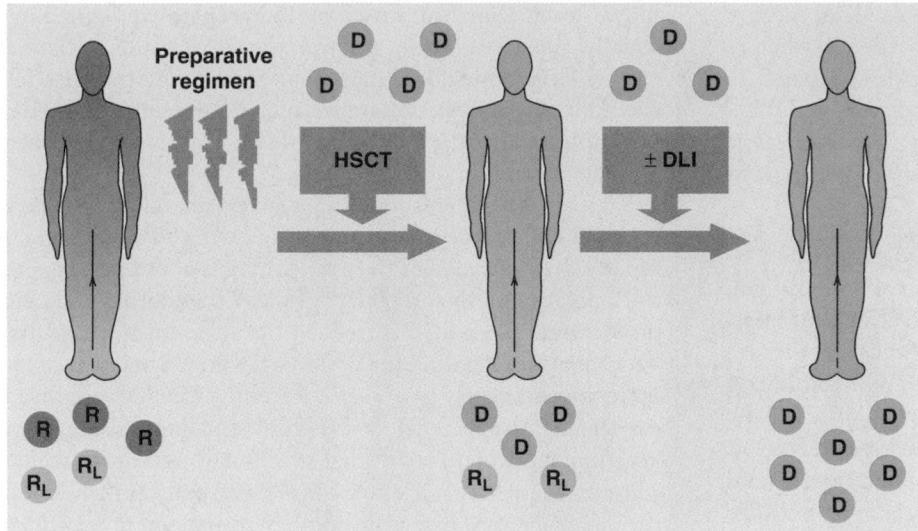

FIGURE 98–1. Schema for nonmyeloablative transplantation. Recipients (R) receive a nonmyeloablative preparative regimen and an allogeneic HSCT. Initially, mixed chimerism is present with the coexistence of donor (D) cells and recipient-derived normal and leukemia/lymphoma (R$_L$) cells. Donor-derived T cells mediate a graft-versus-host hematopoietic effect that eradicates residual recipient-derived normal and malignant hematopoietic cells. Donor-lymphocyte infusions may be administered to enhance graft-versus-tumor effects. (From Ref. 19.)

a substantial portion of cancer patients. The concept of donor immune response having a graft-versus-tumor effect gave rise to the theory that a strongly immunosuppressive, but not myeloablative, preparative regimen (i.e., a nonmyeloablative transplant may result in a state of chimerism in which the recipient and donor are coexisting. The toxicity and efficacy of nonmyeloablative transplants are being evaluated in patients with malignant and nonmalignant conditions who are not eligible for a myeloablative HSCT.

A nonmyeloablative preparative regimen allows for development of mixed chimerism (defined as 5% to 95% peripheral donor T cells) between the host and recipient to allow for a graft-versus-tumor effect as the primary form of therapy (Fig. 98–1). Chimerism is assessed within peripheral blood T cells and granulocytes and bone marrow using conventional (e.g., using sex chromosomes for opposite-sex donors) and molecular (e.g., variable number of tandem repeats) methods for same-sex donors.

The nonmyeloablative preparative regimen does not completely eliminate host normal and malignant cells. Donor cells eradicate residual host hematopoiesis, and the graft-versus-tumor effects generally occur after the development of full donor T-cell chimerism. After engraftment, mixed chimerism should be present and is shown by the presence of both donor- and recipient-derived cells. Autologous recovery should occur promptly if the graft is rejected. The intensity of immunosuppression required for engraftment depends on the immunocompetence of the recipient and the histocompatibility and composition of the HSCT.[19] More intensive conditioning regimens that are required for engraftment in the setting of unrelated-donor- or HLA-mismatched-related HSCT recently have been termed *reduced-intensity myeloablative transplants*. After chimerism develops, donor-lymphocyte infusion can be administered safely in patients without GVHD to eradicate malignant cells.

Nonmyeloablative preparative regimens typically consist of a purine analog (e.g., fludarabine) in combination with an alkylating agent or low-dose TBI. Adverse effects in the early post-transplant period are decreased because of the lower-intensity preparative regimen, thus making HSCT available to patients who in the past were not healthy or young enough to receive a myeloablative preparative regimen. The risk of GVHD remains with nonmyeloablative transplant; the GVHD prophylaxis regimens are reviewed in the GVHD section below. Presently, nonmyeloablative transplant is not indicated as first-line therapy for any malignant or nonmalignant conditions although research is ongoing. Nonmyeloablative transplantation is being evaluated for cancers sensitive to a graft-versus-tumor effect (e.g., CML and AML), in older patients, or for those with comorbidities who would not be able to tolerate a myeloablative HSCT.

Toxicities and Management of Preparative Regimens

Myelosuppression is a frequent dose-limiting toxicity for antineoplastics when administered in the conventional doses used to treat cancer. However, because myelosuppression is circumvented with hematopoietic rescue in the case of patients receiving HSCT, the dose-limiting toxicities of these myeloablative preparative regimens are nonhematologic and vary with the preparative regimen used. Most patients undergoing HSCT experience toxicities commonly associated with chemotherapy (e.g., alopecia, mucositis, nausea and vomiting, and infertility), albeit these toxicities are magnified in the HSCT population.

Busulfan Seizures Seizures have been reported in both adult and pediatric patients receiving high-dose busulfan for HSCT preparative regimens. Anticonvulsants are used to minimize the risk of seizures. Anticonvulsants are begun shortly before busulfan, with the loading dose completed at least 6 hours prior to the first busulfan dose. Oral loading and maintenance regimens generally are sufficient because target phenytoin concentrations of 10 to 20 mcg/mL (40–79 μmol/L) can be achieved by the peak time of seizure risk. If patients are experiencing significant vomiting or have difficulty maintaining therapeutic phenytoin concentrations, IV phenytoin should be substituted. Benzodiazepines such as lorazepam or clonazepam also have been used for seizure prophylaxis during high-dose busulfan therapy before HSCT. Antiseizure medications usually are discontinued 24 to 48 hours after administration of the last dose of busulfan. Seizures still can occur despite the use of prophylactic anticonvulsants and usually do not result in permanent neurologic deficits.

Adaptive Dosing of Busulfan The considerable interpatient variability in the clearance of both oral and IV busulfan, along with the identified concentration-effect relationships, has led to the adaptive dosing of busulfan. Adjusting the oral busulfan dose to achieve a target concentration minimizes the toxicities of the BU-CY regimen, particularly hepatic sinusoidal obstruction syndrome (formerly referred to as *veno-occlusive disease*), while improving engraftment and relapse rates. Complete reviews of these relationships after oral busulfan administration are available elsewhere.[20] An IV busulfan product, Busulfex, was approved by the FDA in February 1999 in combination with cyclophosphamide as a preparative regimen prior to allogeneic HSCT for CML. Recent data with Busulfex in combination with either cyclophosphamide or fludarabine suggest that therapeutic drug monitoring may be needed.[21]

Hemorrhagic Cystitis High-dose cyclophosphamide causes moderate to severe hemorrhagic cystitis; acrolein, a metabolite of cyclophosphamide, is the putative bladder toxin. Preventive measures to lower the risk of hemorrhagic cystitis include vigorous hydration, continuous bladder irrigation, and/or concomitant use of the uroprotectant mesna. The American Society of Clinical Oncology (ASCO) Guidelines for the Use of Chemotherapy and Radiotherapy Protectants recommends the use of mesna plus saline diuresis or forced saline diuresis to lower the incidence of urothelial toxicity with high-dose cyclophosphamide in the setting of HSCT.[22] The optimal mesna dose with high-dose cyclophosphamide in preparation for myeloablative HSCT is unknown.

Chemotherapy-Induced GI Effects Preparative regimens for myeloablative HSCT result in other end-organ toxicities, such as renal failure and idiopathic pneumonia syndrome. In addition, recipients of myeloablative preparative regimens are at risk for severe GI toxicity, specifically chemotherapy-induced nausea and vomiting (CINV), diarrhea, and mucositis. CINV can be due to administration of highly emetogenic chemotherapy over several days, TBI, and also poor control of CINV prior to HSCT. Thus, patients who are undergoing a myeloablative HSCT should receive a prophylactic corticosteroid with a serotonin antagonist, with higher doses of serotonin antagonists potentially being needed in this patient population. In addition, these patients are at high risk for delayed CINV in the immediate post-transplant period and these issues should be addressed accordingly as per published clinical practice guidelines.[23]

Diarrhea is also an adverse effect experienced by a majority of patients undergoing HSCT. Chemotherapy-induced diarrhea occurs due to the effects of the preparative regimen, which results in inflammation and damage to the cells lining the GI tract. Diarrhea caused by the preparative regimen is usually apparent within the first week after the initiation of chemotherapy and/or radiation. Treatment strategies for chemotherapy-induced diarrhea include the administration of antidiarrheals after excluding infectious causes of diarrhea and the prevention of dehydration.

Virtually all patients receiving a myeloablative preparative regimen experience severe mucositis owing to its effects on rapidly dividing cells of the oral epithelium and subsequent inflammation of the oropharyngeal cavity. Routine oral care protocols are indicated to reduce the severity of mucositis, which may onset within the first week of HSCT and persist for up to approximately two weeks. Recently, the FDA approved palifermin (Kepivance), a recombinant human form of keratinocyte growth factor that specifically acts on epithelial cells. In recipients of an autologous HSCT, palifermin lowered the incidence and average duration of severe oral mucositis as well as the incidence and duration of opioid use.[24] Patients still may require parenteral opioid analgesics for pain relief owing to mucositis and total parenteral nutrition may be necessary to prevent the development of nutritional deficiencies.

Sinusoidal Obstruction Syndrome Hepatic sinusoidal obstruction syndrome is a life-threatening complication that may occur secondary to preparative regimens or radiation. The pathogenesis of sinusoidal obstruction syndrome is not understood completely, although several mechanisms have been proposed. The key event appears to be endothelial damage caused by the preparative regimen. The primary site of the toxic injury is the sinusoidal endothelial cells; the endothelial damage initiates the coagulation cascade, induces thrombosis of the hepatic venules, and eventually leads to fibrous obliteration of the affected venules.[25]

The clinical manifestations of sinusoidal obstruction syndrome are hyperbilirubinemia, jaundice, fluid retention, weight gain, and right upper quadrant abdominal pain. To make a clinical diagnosis of sinusoidal obstruction syndrome, these features must occur in the absence of other causes of post-transplant liver failure, including GVHD, viral hepatitis, fungal abscesses, or drug reactions. Most cases of sinusoidal obstruction syndrome occur within three weeks of HSCT and clinical diagnosis can be confirmed histologically via liver biopsy.

Patients with mild sinusoidal obstruction syndrome have an excellent prognosis, whereas those with more severe disease (i.e., bilirubin greater than 20 mg/dL [342 μmol/L] or weight gain greater than 15%) have a high mortality rate. Pretransplant risk factors for sinusoidal obstruction syndrome include a mismatched or unrelated graft, increased age, prior abdominal radiation or stem cell transplant, and increased transaminases prior to HSCT.[25] Interpatient variability in the metabolism and clearance of the chemotherapy (i.e., busulfan and cyclophosphamide) used within the preparative regimen also may be associated with a poor outcome, although the relationships vary within the various preparative regimens.[20] The association of sinusoidal obstruction syndrome with busulfan concentrations is discussed in the section on adaptive dosing of busulfan. Preliminary data suggest that IV busulfan may be associated with a lower risk of sinusoidal obstruction syndrome, although more data are needed.[26] Use of ursodiol, unfractionated heparin, or low molecular weight heparin have been associated with a lower incidence of sinusoidal obstruction syndrome in a limited number of small, randomized studies and may be recommended for sinusoidal obstruction syndrome prophylaxis.[25]

The mainstay of treatment for established sinusoidal obstruction syndrome is supportive care aimed at sodium restriction, increasing intravascular volume, decreasing extracellular fluid accumulation, and minimizing factors that contribute to or exacerbate hepatotoxicity and encephalopathy. Recombinant tissue plasminogen activator administered with or without heparin has been investigated for treatment of sinusoidal obstruction syndrome but life-threatening risk of bleeding precludes any potential benefit.[25] Defibrotide, an oligonucleotide with antithrombotic, anti-ischemic, and anti-inflammatory activity, has shown promising results in the treatment of sinusoidal obstruction syndrome in clinical trials.[25]

Myelosuppression and Hematopoietic Growth Factor Use

Hematopoietic growth factors (HGFs) may be administered in order to mobilize PBPCs prior to an HSCT, to hasten hematopoietic recovery during the period of aplasia after an autologous HSCT, and to stimulate hematopoietic recovery in cases where the patient fails to engraft.[27]

Autologous HSCT is associated with profound aplasia owing to the myeloablative preparative regimen. Aplasia typically lasts 7 to 14 days after an autologous PBPC transplant. During this period of aplasia, patients are at high risk for complications such as bleeding and infection. Filgrastim and sargramostim exert their effects by stimulating the proliferation of committed progenitor cells and accelerating recovery on hematopoiesis. Once engraftment occurs HGFs may be discontinued. The anatomic source of hematopoietic cells predicts the degree of benefit, with the greatest benefit reached when bone marrow is the graft source. With autologous PBPC transplant, the effect of HGF on neutrophil recovery is variable.

The use of HGF after allogeneic HSCT—whether from bone marrow or PBPC grafts—is controversial. The amount of data with sargramostim is limited in this setting; data with filgrastim have shown more rapid neutrophil but slower platelet engraftment in those receiving grafts from bone marrow or PBPCs.[28] The effects of post-HSCT filgrastim use on acute and chronic GVHD have been conflicting, with either no effect or increases in both the incidence of acute and chronic GVHD and treatment-related mortality.[28] Thus, there is little reason to treat allogeneic BMT with filgrastim as prophylaxis after HSCT.

Graft Failure

A delicate balance between host and donor effector cells in the bone marrow is necessary to ensure adequate engraftment because residual host-versus-graft effects may lead to graft rejection. The incidence of graft rejection is higher in patients with aplastic anemia and those undergoing HSCT with histoincompatible marrow or T-cell–depleted marrow.[1] Graft rejection is uncommon in leukemia patients receiving myeloablative preparative regimens with a histocompatible allogeneic donor.

Therapeutic options for the treatment of graft rejection or graft failure are limited. A second HSCT is the most definitive therapy, although the associated complications and toxicities may preclude its use. Graft rejection is best managed with immunosuppressants such as ATG. Primary graft failure occasionally can be treated successfully using HGFs, although patients who received purged autografts are less likely to respond.

Clinical Presentation and Diagnosis of Sinusoidal Obstructive Syndrome

General

- Sinusoidal obstructive syndrome (SOS) usually occurs within the first 3 weeks after HSCT
- Busulfan, cyclophosphamide, pretransplant exposure to gemtuzumab, TBI-containing preparative regimens, and pretransplant abnormalities in liver function tests may increase risk for SOS

Symptoms

- Patients may complain of weight gain and abdominal pain

Signs

- **Fluid retention**: Weight gain due to ascites greater than 2% compared to pretransplant weight
- **Hepatomegaly**: May result in right upper quadrant pain

- **Hepatic**: Jaundice due to hyperbilirubinemia defined as a bilirubin greater than 2 mg/dL (34.2 μmol/L)

Laboratory Tests

- **Hepatic**: Elevation of bilirubin, alkaline phosphatase, and γ-glutamyltransferase (GGT)
- **Hematologic**: CBC with differential may reveal thrombocytopenia, elevated plasminogen activator-1 levels, decreased antithrombin III, protein C, and protein S

Other Diagnostic Tests

- Reversal of blood flow in portal and hepatic veins on Doppler ultrasonography
- Liver biopsy for pathologic review

Patient Encounter 1

LL, a 47-year-old male, was diagnosed with high-risk diffuse large cell B-cell non-Hodgkin's lymphoma (NHL) 12 months ago. LL had a complete response to his initial treatment of six cycles of RCHOP (rituximab, cyclophosphamide, doxorubicin, vincristine, and prednisone). LL is participating in a clinical trial and is randomized to receive a myeloablative autologous HSCT: TBI days –8 to –5, etoposide day –4, rest day –3, cyclophosphamide day –2, rest day –1, with infusion of autologous PBPC on day 0.

What nonhematologic toxicity should be monitored? How long should the patient be monitored for these toxicities?

What pharmacologic management is necessary during administration of the preparative regimen?

It is day +1, and LL has a WBC with differential of 0/mm³, ANCs 0/mm³ (0×10^9/L), platelets 30,000/mm³ (30×10^3/µL), and hemoglobin 9 g/dL (5.6 mmol/L). Renal clearance and liver function are within normal limits. Vital signs are bp 130/80, RR 18, and T 39°C (102.2°F). Medications include meropenem 2 g IV every 8 hours and filgrastim 480 mcg subcutaneously daily.

Develop a monitoring plan for LL's hematologic function.

Identify your treatment goals for LL's hematologic function.

▶ Graft-Versus-Host Disease

8 *GVHD is caused by the activation of donor lymphocytes, leading to immune damage to the skin, gut, and liver in the recipient.* Immune-mediated destruction of tissues, a hallmark of GVHD, disrupts the integrity of protective mucosal barriers and thus provides an environment that favors the establishment of opportunistic infections. **8** *An immunosuppressive regimen is administered to prevent GVHD in recipients of an allogeneic graft; this regimen is based on the type of preparative regimen and the source of the graft.* The combination of GVHD and infectious complications are leading causes of mortality for allogeneic HSCT patients. GVHD is divided into two forms (i.e., acute and chronic) based on clinical manifestations. Traditionally, the boundary between acute and chronic GVHD was set at 100 days after HSCT; however, more recent definitions hinge upon different clinical symptoms rather than the time of onset.[29]

Acute GVHD The degree of histocompatibility between donor and recipient is the most important factor associated with the development of acute GVHD. The pathophysiology for acute GVHD is a multistep phenomenon, including (a) the development of an inflammatory milieu that results from host tissue damage induced by the preparative regimen, (b) both recipient and donor antigen-presenting cells and inflammatory cytokines triggering activation of donor-derived T cells, and (c) the activated donor T cells mediate cytotoxicity through a variety of mechanisms, which leads to tissue damage characteristic of acute GVHD.[30]

Clinically relevant grades II to IV acute GVHD occurs in up to 30% of HLA-matched sibling grafts and 50% to 80% of HLA-mismatched sibling or HLA-identical unrelated donors.[30] Other factors that increase the risk of acute GVHD include increasing recipient or donor age (older than 20 years), female donor to a male recipient, and mismatches in minor histocompatibility antigens in HLA-matched transplants.[30] T-cell depletion or receipt of an umbilical cord blood graft appears to lower the risk of acute GVHD.[1]

Clinical Presentation and Staging of Acute GVHD Acute GVHD must be distinguished accurately from other causes of skin, liver, or GI toxicity in the HSCT patient. Other causes of toxicities affecting the skin, liver, or GI tract may include a drug reaction or an infectious process. A staging system based on clinical criteria is used to grade acute GVHD (Fig. 98–2). The severity of organ involvement is scored on an ordinal scale from 0 (no symptoms) to IV (severe symptoms), and then an overall grade is established based on the number and extent of involved organs.

Immunosuppressive Prophylaxis of Acute GVHD GVHD is a leading cause of morbidity and mortality after allogeneic HSCT and thus, efforts have focused on preventing acute GVHD. The donor graft and preparative regimen influence the prophylactic regimen for acute GVHD, with two approaches having been taken by clinicians over time. One approach involves T-cell depletion, which was discussed more fully in the section on T-cell depletion earlier. The more common method is to use two-drug immunosuppressive therapy that typically consists of a calcineurin inhibitor (i.e., cyclosporine or tacrolimus) with methotrexate after myeloablative HSCT and a calcineurin inhibitor with mycophenolate mofetil after nonmyeloablative HSCT.

After myeloablative conditioning, acute GVHD rates have been similar or lower with triple-drug regimens, but infectious complications are higher and overall survival is similar to that with two-drug regimens.[31] With the two-drug regimen, a short-course of low-dose methotrexate (e.g., on days +1, +3, +6, and day +11) is used and thus, can delay engraftment, increase the incidence and severity of mucositis, and cause LFT elevations. The methotrexate dose is reduced in the setting of renal or liver impairment. The calcineurin inhibitors (i.e., cyclosporine and tacrolimus) should be initiated before donor cell infusion (e.g., day –1) when used for GVHD prophylaxis. This schedule is recommended because of the known mechanism of action of cyclosporine, which entails blocking the proliferation of cytotoxic T cells by inhibiting production of T-helper-cell-derived interleukin 2 (IL-2). Administering cyclosporine before the donor cell infusion allows inhibition of IL-2 secretion to occur before a rejection response has been initiated. Studies comparing cyclosporine and tacrolimus in combination with methotrexate have shown that tacrolimus administration is associated with

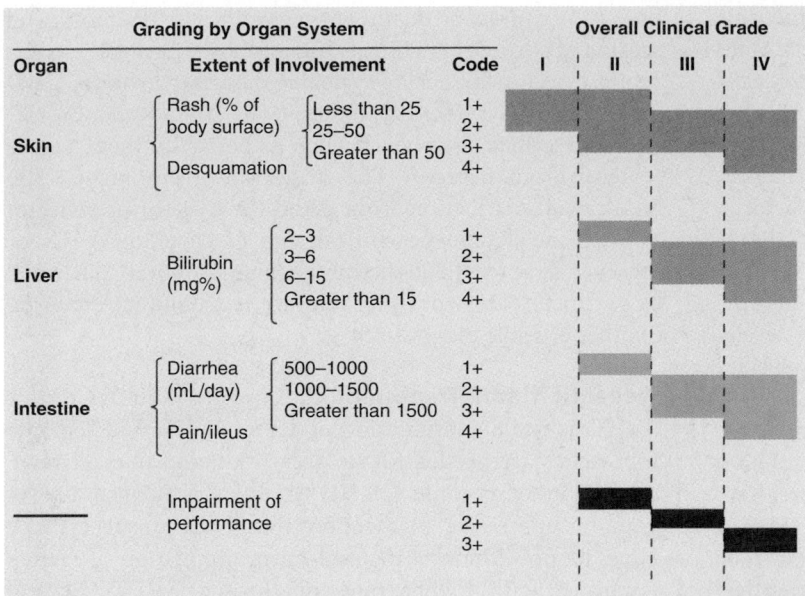

FIGURE 98–2. Clinical grading of acute GVHD. The left panel summarizes the grading of one organ system; the right panel shows the overall clinical grade. With grade I, only the skin can be involved. With more extensive involvement of the skin or involvement of liver and intestinal tract and impairment of the clinical performance status, either alone or in any combination, the severity grade advances from II to IV. (From Perkins JB, Yee GC. Hematopoietic stem cell transplantation. In: DiPiro JT, Talbert RL, Yee GC, et al., eds. Pharmacotherapy: A Pathophysiologic Approach. 6th ed. New York: McGraw-Hill;2005:2552.)

Clinical Presentation and Diagnosis of Acute GVHD

General
- Patients may present with any or all of the following: skin rash, GI complaints, or jaundice
- Signs and symptoms present after engraftment when donor lymphoid elements begin to proliferate

Symptoms
- Patients may complain of nausea, vomiting, bloody diarrhea or itching from skin rash

Signs
- **Skin**: Maculopapular skin rash on the face, truck, extremities, palms, soles, and ears which may progress to generalized total-body erythroderma, bullous formation, and skin desquamation

- **GI**: Ileus, malnutrition, dehydration and electrolyte abnormalities due to nausea, vomiting, and diarrhea
- **Hepatic**: Jaundice due to hyperbilirubinemia

Laboratory Tests
- **Hepatic**: Elevation of bilirubin, alkaline phosphatase, and hepatic transaminases
- **GI**: send stool for bacterial, viral, and parasitic cultures to rule out infectious causes

Other Diagnostic Tests
- Biopsy of affected site for pathologic review

a lower incidence of grade II to IV acute GVHD and a similar incidence of chronic GVHD, but variable effects on overall survival.[32,33] Because of the mucosal toxicity from myeloablative preparative regimens, the calcineurin inhibitors are administered IV until the GI toxicity from a myeloablative preparative regimen has resolved (e.g., for 7–21 days). Most centers use a 1:2 to 1:3 ratio for conversion of IV to oral cyclosporine with the Neoral formulation; the ratio for tacrolimus conversion from IV to oral is often 1:4. Different conversion ratios for IV to oral regimens may be used when patients are receiving concomitant medications that affect cytochrome P-450 3A or p-glycoprotein; these pathways are involved in the metabolism and transport of the calcineurin inhibitors (e.g., voriconazole).

Prophylaxis of acute GVHD for nonmyeloablative preparative regimens is varied, but a calcineurin inhibitor with either methotrexate or mycophenolate mofetil is used.[3] To date, trials evaluating the optimal acute GVHD prophylaxis regimen have not been conducted.

Adaptive Dosing of the Calcineurin Inhibitors Most HSCT centers have their own standardized approach to dose adjust the calcineurin inhibitors cyclosporine and tacrolimus to target concentration ranges. Cyclosporine trough concentrations are associated with the acute GVHD and nephrotoxicity. Cyclosporine trough concentrations usually are maintained between 150 and 400 ng/mL (125–333 nmol/L) in patients undergoing allogeneic HSCT. Tacrolimus trough concentrations are targeted to a range of 10 to 20 ng/mL

(10–20 mcg/L).[34] Dosage adjustments to either calcineurin inhibitor also should be made for elevated serum creatinine (SrCr) regardless of their serum concentrations. Nephrotoxicity can occur despite low or normal concentrations of the calcineurin inhibitor cyclosporine and may be a consequence of other drug- or disease-related factors known to influence the development of nephrotoxicity (e.g., genetic risk factors, concurrent use of other nephrotoxic agents, and sepsis). Careful monitoring for drug interactions via cytochrome P-450 3A4 and p-glycoprotein is also warranted. The calcineurin inhibitor doses are adjusted based on serum drug levels and the calculated creatinine clearance. Common adverse effects to these agents include neurotoxicity, hypertension, hyperkalemia, hypomagnesemia, and/or nephrotoxicity (which may lead to an impaired clearance of methotrexate).

Tapering schedules for the calcineurin inhibitors after myeloablative HSCT vary widely. In patients without GVHD, the calcineurin inhibitor doses usually are stable to day +50 and then are tapered slowly with the intent of discontinuing all immunosuppressive agents by 6 months after HSCT. By this time, immunologic tolerance has developed and patients no longer require immunosuppressive therapy. There is a paucity of information regarding the optimal duration of GVHD prophylaxis after nonmyeloablative HSCT, with data suggesting that a two month duration of cyclosporine with a four month taper lowers the rate of severe acute GVHD.[35]

Treatment of Acute GVHD The most effective way to treat GVHD is to prevent its development. Corticosteroids, usually in combination with a calcineurin inhibitor, are the first-line therapy for treatment of established acute GVHD. Corticosteroids indirectly halt the progression of immune-mediated destruction of host tissues by blocking macrophage-derived IL-1 secretion. IL-1 is a primary stimulus for T-helper-cell-induced secretion of IL-2, which, in turn, is responsible for stimulating proliferation of cytotoxic T lymphocytes. The recommended dosage of methylprednisolone in this setting is 2 mg/kg/day; there is no advantage to higher corticosteroid doses (i.e., 10 mg/kg/day).[30] A partial or complete response is seen in approximately 50% of patients treated with corticosteroids. Once a clinical improvement occurs, there is no consensus on the optimal method for tapering the corticosteroids. Patients with steroid-refractory acute GVHD have a poor prognosis and a number of medications are being studied for salvage therapy.

Chronic GVHD Occurring in 20% to 70% of HSCT recipients surviving over 100 days, chronic GVHD is the most frequent and serious late complication of allogeneic HSCT.[36] Chronic GVHD is the major cause of nonrelapse mortality and morbidity. The clinical course of chronic GVHD is multifaceted, involving almost any organ in the body and its symptoms resemble autoimmune and immunologic disorders (e.g., scleroderma). Chronic GVHD symptoms usually present within 3 years of allogeneic HSCT and often are preceded by acute GVHD.[29] Traditionally, the boundary between acute and chronic GVHD was set at 100 days after HSCT; however, more recent definitions hinge on different clinical symptoms rather than the time of onset.[36] A consensus document regarding the diagnosis and scoring of chronic GVHD has been published recently which proposes a clinical scoring system to describe chronic GVHD as opposed to historical descriptions of chronic GVHD which described the phenomenon as being "limited" versus "extensive" in nature.[29] The diagnosis of chronic GVHD requires (a) distinction from acute GVHD, (b) presence of at least one diagnostic clinical sign of chronic GVHD or presence of at least one distinctive manifestation confirmed by pertinent biopsy or other relevant tests, and (c) exclusion of other possible diagnoses.

Prevention and Treatment of Chronic GVHD Chronic GVHD is not a continuation of acute GVHD and separate approaches are needed for its prevention and management. Prevention of chronic GVHD through prolonged use of immunosuppressive medications has been unsuccessful.[36] Thus, its prevention is focused on minimization of factors associated with higher rates of chronic GVHD. Several recipient, donor, and transplant factors are relevant. Recipient risk factors that are not modifiable include older age, certain diagnoses (e.g., chronic myeloid leukemia), and lack of an HLA-matched donor. Modifiable factors that may lower the risk of chronic GVHD include selection of a younger donor, avoidance of a multiparous female donor, use of umbilical cord blood or bone marrow grafts rather than PBPCs, and limitation of CD34+ and T-cell dose infused.[36] Development of acute GVHD is a major predictor for chronic GVHD, with 70% to 80% of those with grade II to IV acute GVHD developing chronic GVHD.[36]

Relative to no treatment, survival in those with chronic GVHD is improved by extended corticosteroid therapy; however, multiple long-term adverse effects are associated with corticosteroid use. The prednisone dosage is 1 mg/kg/day administered orally in divided doses for 30 days and then slowly converted to an alternate-day therapy by increasing the "on day" and decreasing the "off day" dose until a total of 2 mg/kg/day on alternate days is administered. Once therapy is initiated, one to two months may pass before an improvement in clinical symptoms is noted and therapy usually is continued for 9 to 12 months. Therapy can be tapered slowly after resolution of signs and symptoms of chronic GVHD. If a flare of chronic GVHD occurs during the tapering schedule or after therapy is discontinued, immunosuppressive therapy is restarted. Other potential approaches for patients who are refractory to initial therapy include etanercept (Embrel), infliximab (Remicade), mycophenolate mofetil (Cellcept), rituximab (Rituxan), extended use of calcineurin inhibitors, or extracorporeal photochemotherapy.[36] When immunosuppressive therapy is administered for long periods, the patient must be monitored closely for chronic toxicity. Cushingoid effects, aseptic necrosis of the joints, and diabetes can develop with long-term corticosteroid use. Other severe complications include a high incidence of infection with encapsulated organisms and atypical pathogens such as *Pneumocystis jiroveci*, cytomegalovirus (CMV), and varicella-zoster virus (VZV).

Patient Encounter 2

AS is a 65-year-old female with relapsed acute myeloid leukemia. PMH is significant for type II diabetes and renal hypertension. She is day +1 from a nonmyeloablative HSCT with fludarabine (30 mg/m²/day IV for 3 days) and total-body irradiation (TBI) preparative regimen and a graft from a full HLA-matched sibling.

What preventive measures are needed for the complications of HSCT?

How would you monitor AS for GVHD?

What would you recommend for treatment of GVHD?

▶ Infectious Complications

❾ *Recipients of HSCT are at higher risk of bacterial, viral, and fungal infections and usually receive a prophylactic or preemptive regimen to minimize the morbidity and mortality owing to infectious complications.* After myeloablative and nonmyeloablative HSCT, opportunistic infections are a major source of morbidity and mortality. There are three periods of infectious risks, early (days 0–30), middle (engraftment to day +100), and late (after day +100). From days 0 to 30 after HSCT, particularly for patients undergoing myeloablative HSCT, the primary pathogens are aerobic bacteria, *Candida,* and herpes simplex virus (HSV). Respiratory viruses such as respiratory syncytial virus (RSV), influenza, adenovirus, and parainfluenza virus are recognized increasingly as pathogens causing pneumonia, particularly during community outbreaks of infection with these organisms. To reduce potential exposure of HSCT recipients to such respiratory viruses, visitors and staff members with respiratory signs and symptoms of a viral illness may not be allowed direct contact with patients.

The second period of infectious risk occurs after engraftment to post-transplant day +100. Bacterial infections are still of concern, but pathogens such as CMV, adenovirus, and *Aspergillus* species are common. A common manifestation of infection is interstitial pneumonitis (IP), which can be caused by CMV, adenovirus, *Aspergillus,* and *P. jiroveci.* Suppression of the immune system from acute GVHD and corticosteroids contributes to the risk of such infections during this period. Therefore, patients undergoing nonmyeloablative transplant who are receiving corticosteroids to treat GVHD can be expected to have a similar risk for infection as those undergoing myeloablative HSCT.[37] Invasive fungal infections over the first year after HSCT occur at a similar rate in nonmyeloablative transplant when compared with historical controls receiving a myeloablative preparative regimen.[38]

During the late period (after day +100), the predominant organisms are the encapsulated bacteria (e.g., *Streptococcus pneumoniae, Haemophilus influenzae,* and *Neisseria meningitidis*), fungi, VZV. The encapsulated organisms commonly cause sinopulmonary infections. The risk of infection during this late period is increased in patients with chronic GVHD as a result of prolonged immunosuppression.

Prevention and Treatment of Bacterial and Fungal Infections Due to the need to administer chemotherapy, blood products, antibiotics, and other adjunctive medications, the placement of a semipermanent double- or triple-lumen central venous catheter is necessary prior to HSCT. However, the indwelling IV central catheters put HSCT recipients at increased risk for *Staphylococcus* infections.

Between the time of administration of the preparative regimen and successful engraftment, allogeneic myeloablative HSCT patients undergo a period of pancytopenia that can last from two to six weeks. During this time, multiple transfusions of blood and platelet products are needed to support the patient through the pancytopenic period. Transfusions with multiple blood products place patients at risk for blood product–derived infection (e.g., CMV and hepatitis) and sensitization to foreign leukocyte HLA antigens (i.e., alloimmunization) which can lead to immune-mediated thrombocytopenia. Thus, blood product support in the myeloablative allogeneic HSCT patient must incorporate strategies that reduce the risk of viral infection and alloimmunization by minimizing the number of pretransplant infusions, using of single-donor (rather than pooled-donor) blood products, irradiating blood products in order to inactivate T cells in the product, or filtering blood products with leukocyte-reduction filters. The risk of infection in autologous and allogeneic myeloablative HSCT patients is minimized through a variety of measures. Private reverse isolation rooms equipped with positive-pressure HEPA filters and adherence to strict hand-hygiene techniques reduce the incidence of bacterial and fungal infections.[4] To reduce exposure to exogenous sources of bacteria, immunosuppressed-patient (low-microbial) diets are used and live plants or flowers are not allowed in the patient's room. Chemotherapy-induced mucosal damage serves as a portal of entry for many organisms (e.g., *Streptococcus viridans,* aerobic gram-negative bacteria, and fungi) into the bloodstream. The mouth should be kept clean by using frequent (at least four to six times daily) mouth rinses with sterile water, normal saline, or sodium bicarbonate.[4] Soft toothbrushes may be employed for oral hygiene during periods of neutropenia and thrombocytopenia. The risk of infection is also reduced by aggressive use of antibacterial, antifungal, and antiviral therapy both prophylactically and for the treatment of documented infection. The antibacterial prophylactic regimens vary substantially among HSCT centers. Some HSCT centers use a prophylactic fluoroquinolone (e.g., levofloxacin) on admission for HSCT and then switch to a broad-spectrum IV antibiotic (e.g., meropenem) when the patient experiences his or her first neutropenic fever. Although fluoroquinolones reduce the incidence of gram-negative bacteremia, they have not been shown to affect mortality; the possibility of developing clostridium difficile-associated diarrhea exists with fluoroquinolone use and infectious causes should be ruled out if diarrhea occurs.[4] Concerns with fluoroquinolone use in the prophylactic setting during HSCT include the emergence of resistant organisms and an increased risk for streptococcal infection.[4] Broad-spectrum IV antibiotics should be initiated immediately at the time of the first neutropenic fever under the treatment guidelines endorsed by the Infectious Disease Society of America for management of fever of unknown origin in the neutropenic host.[39]

● **Prevention of HSV and VZV** Patients who are HSV-antibody seropositive before HSCT are at high risk for reactivation of their HSV infection. Acyclovir is highly effective in preventing HSV reactivation, and thus, prophylactic acyclovir is used commonly in HSV-seropositive patients who are undergoing an allogeneic or autologous HSCT.[4] In the setting of HSV prophylaxis, dosing regimens for prophylactic acyclovir vary widely and most centers discontinue acyclovir at the time of hematopoietic recovery.[4] Valacyclovir (Valtrex), a prodrug of acyclovir with improved bioavailability, may allow for adequate serum concentrations to prevent HSV in patients undergoing HSCT as well.

In those with a history of VZV infection, VZV disease occurs in 30% of allogeneic HSCT recipients.[40] The appropriate duration of VZV prophylaxis is controversial. Although VZV infections are reduced by prophylactic acyclovir administered from one to two months until one year after HSCT, the risk of VZV persists in those on continued immunosuppression.[40]

● **Prevention and Preemptive Therapy of CMV Disease** After allogeneic HSCT, CMV disease is common and has high morbidity and mortality rates. Allogeneic patients are at greater risk than autologous recipients primarily because the latter more efficiently reconstitute their immune system after transplantation. However, autologous HSCT recipients who are CMV-seropositive before HSCT are at risk for CMV infection and prophylaxis should be considered in a select minority of patients.[4] Infection due to CMV is usually asymptomatic and develops when CMV replication occurs primarily in body fluids such as the blood (viremia), bronchoalveolar fluid, or urine (viruria). Cytomegalovirus disease is symptomatic and occurs when the virus invades an organ or tissue. Pneumonia and gastritis are the most common types of CMV disease after allogeneic HSCT. The presence of a CMV infection substantially increases the risk for developing invasive CMV disease. Strategies to prevent CMV infection have resulted in dramatic reductions in the incidence of CMV disease.

Primary CMV can be prevented with CMV seromatching, which includes transplanting PBPCs or bone marrow from CMV-seronegative donors and infusing CMV-negative blood products to CMV-negative recipients. Antivirals are essential in those who are CMV-seropositive or have a CMV-seropositive graft, with two available approaches to minimize the morbidity associated with CMV. The first is universal prophylaxis, in which ganciclovir is begun at the time of engraftment and is continued until approximately day +100. The second approach is called preemptive therapy, for which ganciclovir is selectively administered based on detection of CMV reactivation.

Preemptive therapy is the most commonly used strategy for preventing CMV disease after allogeneic HSCT because ganciclovir is used only in patients at highest risk for developing CMV disease. This approach minimizes administration of ganciclovir, thus lowering the risk of ganciclovir-induced neutropenia with its subsequent increased risk of invasive bacterial and fungal infections. With a decreased risk of ganciclovir-induced neutropenia, fewer interruptions of ganciclovir therapy due to myelosuppression may occur with a preemptive approach and the subsequent use of filgrastim to maintain adequate neutrophil counts may be limited. Preemptive therapy hinges on the ability to detect early reactivation of CMV using shell vial cultures, assays of blood for CMV antigens (such as pp65), or viral nucleic acids using polymerase chain reaction (PCR). Antigenemia-based preemptive therapy has similar efficacy in preventing CMV disease as universal ganciclovir prophylaxis and preemptive therapy also has been associated with a significant reduction in CMV mortality. Preemptive strategies typically use an induction course of ganciclovir for 7 to 14 days, followed by a maintenance course until 2 or 3 weeks after the last positive antigenemia result or until day +100 after HSCT.[4] Oral valganciclovir (Valcyte) is an orally bioavailable prodrug of ganciclovir that is converted to ganciclovir in vivo after intestinal absorption and has been used for preemptive therapy. Foscarnet may be given as an alternative to ganciclovir to prevent CMV disease, although its use is complicated by nephrotoxicity and electrolyte wasting.

Fungal Infections

● ***Prevention of Fungal Infections.*** The widespread use of fluconazole prophylaxis since the early 1990s has led to a significant decline in the morbidity and mortality associated with invasive candidiasis in HSCT recipients. However, invasive aspergillosis (IA), zygomycetes, and fluconazole-resistant *Candida* species, such as *C. krusei* and *C. glabrata,* have increased markedly in incidence.[41] Itraconazole, another azole antifungal agent, has better in vitro activity against fluconazole-resistant fungi (e.g., *Aspergillus* and some *Candida* spp.) and is more effective than fluconazole for long-term prophylaxis of invasive fungal infections after allogeneic HSCT; however, itraconazole is used less often due to frequent GI side effects and concern for potential drug interactions.[42] Posaconazole (Noxafil) is a triazole antifungal that has recently been FDA approved for prophylaxis against IA in HSCT patients with GVHD and is now the recommended prophylactic agent for this subset of HSCT patients on immunosuppression.[43] Posaconazole should be given with food for adequate absorption. Micafungin (Mycamine), an agent of the newer class of antifungals known as the echinocandins, has been FDA approved for prophylaxis of *Candida* infections in patients undergoing HSCT.

Risk Factors for Invasive Mold Infections. Invasive mold infections (e.g., Aspergillus spp., Fusarium spp., Zygomycetes, and Scedosporium spp.) are an increasing cause of morbidity and death after allogeneic and autologous HSCT. It has been estimated that up to one-third of febrile neutropenic patients who do not respond to antibiotic therapy after one week are harboring a fungal infection.[39] In HSCT recipients, risk factors for invasive fungal infections include (a) previous history of IA; (b) recipient factors including older age, CMV seropositivity, and type of stem cell transplant; (c) treatment factors (e.g., a fludarabine-based preparative regimen); (d) transplant complications (e.g., prolonged neutropenia, graft failure, and higher-grade GVHD); and (e) host factors (e.g., diabetes, iron overload).[44] Infections with Aspergillus species remain the most common mold infections diagnosed in the HSCT population and optimal treatment must be promptly initiated if indicated.

Treatment of Invasive Aspergillosis. Early diagnosis and initiation of appropriate therapy may reduce the high mortality of IA. Outcomes also depend on recovery of the recipient's immune system and reduction of immunosuppression. Diagnosis is difficult with the use of CT scans and cultures. Research is ongoing to evaluate the benefit of using nonculture-based methods, such as galactomannan and (1,3)-β-D-glucan antigen detection, which are components of the fungal cell wall that can be detected by commercially available assays.

Practice guidelines are available for the treatment of invasive *Aspergillus* infections in immunocompromised patients.[43] Available mold-active agents include triazole antifungals (itraconazole, voriconazole, and posaconazole), echinocandins (caspofungin, micafungin, and anidulafungin), and amphotericin B formulations. Historically, conventional amphotericin B (c-AmB) has been considered the "gold standard" antifungal therapy for any IA infection although the majority of responders eventually died of their infection. Significant toxicity occurs with c-AmB administration, with nephrotoxicity, electrolyte wasting (e.g., potassium and magnesium), and infusion-related reactions being the most troublesome side effects. Lipid analogs of amphotericin B were developed with the specific intent of reducing nephrotoxicity associated with conventional amphotericin B while retaining therapeutic efficacy, albeit at a higher acquisition cost.[45] These products include amphotericin B lipid complex (Abelcet, ABLC), liposomal amphotericin B (Ambisome, L-Amb), and amphotericin B colloidal dispersion (Amphotec, ABCD).

With significant toxicity limiting the overall utility of conventional amphotericin B, voriconazole (Vfend) was compared to c-AmB for treatment of IA. For initial therapy of IA, voriconazole had higher response and survival rates than c-AmB and is now considered the primary option for patients with IA.[46] An advantage of voriconazole is its 96% oral bioavailability, making use of this oral drug an attractive alternative. Common toxicities reported with voriconazole include infusion-related reactions, transient visual disturbances, skin reactions, elevations in hepatic transaminases and alkaline phosphatase, nausea, and headache. In addition, voriconazole increases the serum concentrations of medications cleared by cytochrome P-450 2C9, 2C19, and 3A4 (e.g., cyclophosphamide and calcineurin inhibitors); concomitant use of voriconazole and sirolimus should be carefully monitored. Due to pharmacokinetic and pharmacodynamic relationships, antifungal therapy with triazole antifungals such as voriconazole may be optimized for efficacy and toxicity through the practice of therapeutic monitoring of serum levels of these agents.[43]

In patients who have failed initial therapy (i.e., salvage), lipid formulations of amphotericin products, itraconazole, posaconazole, or an agent from the echinocandin class may be used. The echinocandins have a unique target for their antifungal activity—specifically, β-1,3-glucan synthase, an enzyme that produces an important component of the fungal cell wall. Three agents in the echinocandin class (caspofungin, micafungin, and anidulafungin) are currently FDA approved and are only available as IV formulations. Caspofungin (Cancidas) is the only member of the echinocandin class approved for use in pediatric patients, for patients with persistent neutropenic fever, and for patients with probable or proven IA that is refractory to or intolerant of other approved therapies. The most common adverse effects observed include increased liver aminotransferase enzyme levels, mild to moderate infusion reactions and headache, with a smaller number of patients experiencing dermatologic reactions related to histamine release (e.g., flushing, erythema, and wheals).

The optimal duration of appropriate antifungal therapy for treating IA is individualized to the reconstitution of the patient's immune system and his or her response to antifungal treatment. Most clinicians will continue aggressive antifungal therapy until the infection has stabilized radiographically and may continue with less aggressive "maintenance" therapy (e.g., oral voriconazole) until immunosuppression is lessened or completed. In general, it is not uncommon to require several months of antifungal therapy to treat IA.

P. jiroveci After allogeneic HSCT, prophylaxis for *P. jiroveci* (formerly *P. carinii*) pneumonia (PCP) is used because *Pneumocystis* is a common infection with a high mortality rate if left untreated. The optimal prophylactic regimen in this setting is unclear, with most centers using cotrimoxazole for 6 to 12 months after HSCT.[4] Aerosolized or IV pentamidine and oral dapsone are alternatives for patients who are allergic to sulfa drugs or who do not tolerate cotrimoxazole. Because PCP most often occurs after engraftment, cotrimoxazole usually is begun after neutrophil recovery because of its myelosuppressive effects. Patients receiving prophylactic cotrimoxazole should be monitored closely for rash and unexplained neutropenia or thrombocytopenia. Cotrimoxazole usually is avoided on days of methotrexate administration because the sulfonamides can displace methotrexate from plasma binding sites and decrease renal methotrexate clearance, resulting in higher methotrexate concentrations. Autologous HSCT patients do not receive post-transplant immunosuppression, and thus, their risk of developing PCP is lower.[4] Thus PCP prophylaxis is used often after autologous HSCT in patients with a hematologic malignancy.

▶ Issues of Survivorship after HSCT

The number of long-term HSCT survivors is increasing as 5-year disease-free survival rates improve. Since nonmyeloablative preparative regimens were developed over the past decade, the late effects reported in HSCT survivors

---

Patient Encounter 3

JM is a 44-year-old female who is currently day + 8 following an HSCT from a full HLA-matched sibling for AML in first complete remission. Her preparative regimen consisted of busulfan and cyclophosphamide; tacrolimus and methotrexate are being administered for GVHD prophylaxis. She is currently receiving fluconazole 400 mg daily and acyclovir 400 mg three times daily for infection prophylaxis. She is currently day 4 of cefepime 2 g IV every 8 hours and vancomycin 1,000 mg (15 mg/kg) IV every 12 hours for neutropenic fever; all cultures remain negative. Her ANC today is 20 cells/mm³ (0.02 × 10⁹/L). She remains persistently febrile. Her latest vital signs reveal a temperature of 38.9°C, (102°F), blood pressure 106/70 mm Hg, heart rate 112 bpm, respiration rate of 20 breaths per minute, and an oxygen saturation of 95% on room air. She has no other complaints other than she is experiencing grade II mucositis.

What diagnostic measures are needed to address JM's current signs and symptoms?

Are any changes to JM's anti-infective regimen warranted? What options are available in terms of medication management and what monitoring parameters are necessary with each medication?

---

describe those resulting from myeloablative preparative regimens.[47] HSCT recipients—with either an autologous or an allogeneic graft—have higher mortality than the general population.[48] ❿ *Long-term survivors of HSCT should be monitored closely, particularly for infections and secondary malignant neoplasms.*

HSCT survivors are at higher risk for secondary malignant neoplasms.[47] Long-term impairment of end-organ function, including kidney, liver, and lungs, may be due to the preparative regimen, infectious complications, and/or post-transplant immunosuppression. Many HSCT recipients experience endocrine dysfunction, such as hypothyroidism from TBI, adrenal insufficiency from long-term corticosteroids to treat GVHD, and infertility from radiation and/or high doses of alkylating agents in myeloablative preparative regimens. Osteopenia has been found in over half of HSCT recipients, most likely from gonadal dysfunction and/or corticosteroid administration.

Close monitoring of HSCT recipients for infections is necessary because recovery of immune function is slow, sometimes requiring over two years, even in the absence of immunosuppressants.[47] Fevers should be assessed and treated rapidly to minimize the likelihood of a fatal infection. HSCT recipients—both autologous and allogeneic—lose protective antibodies to vaccine-preventable diseases; the CDC and the European Group for BMT have issued recommendations for reimmunization for HSCT recipients.[49]

HSCT survivors should be monitored routinely for signs of relapse and, if an allogeneic graft was used, chronic GVHD. They should be advised regarding revaccination and obtaining prompt medical care for fevers or signs of infection. Routine evaluations of organ function (i.e., renal, hepatic, thyroid, and ovarian) and osteopenia should occur and the appropriate management strategies initiated if necessary.

OUTCOME EVALUATION

Monitor for symptoms and signs of the disease that is being treated by HSCT in order to assess the effectiveness of the HSCT. For example, the monitoring plan for a patient with CML would be to monitor disease response by PCR of the *BCR-ABL* transcript. The actual clinical outcome monitored, along with the frequency of monitoring, is based on the underlying disease.

Monitor for nonhematologic toxicity of the preparative regimen during its administration. Monitor these symptoms at least daily, with more frequent monitoring if the patient is experiencing these nonhematologic effects. The goal is to prevent or minimize these adverse effects. Specifically,

- *Busulfan*: Seizures, busulfan concentrations if being used with the BU-CY preparative regimen, number of vomiting episodes, and nausea by patient self-report, total bilirubin, and sudden weight changes (sinusoidal obstruction syndrome [SOS])

- *Cyclophosphamide*: ECG during IV administration, RBCs in urine, frequency of urination, pain on urination, urinary output, number of vomiting episodes, and nausea by patient self-report, total bilirubin, and sudden weight changes (sinusoidal obstruction syndrome [SOS])

- *Etoposide*: Blood pressure, respiratory rate, serum pH, serum bicarbonate with arterial blood gases, and evaluation of anion gap if necessary

- *Total-body irradiation*: Number of vomiting episodes, nausea by patient self-report, sudden weight changes (SOS), total bilirubin, and skin assessment for presence of irritation or blister formation

Until the patient has achieved engraftment, monitor the patient for engraftment with at least daily CBCs with differentials; these tests may be needed more often if the patient is critically ill or had a prior low hemoglobin. Patients will require transfusion support with blood products and platelets until engraftment occurs if hemoglobin and/or platelets drop below unsafe levels. Transfusion parameters may differ for individual patients but typically patients will be transfused if the hemoglobin drops below 8 g/dL (4.96 mmol/L); platelets are maintained at least above 10,000/mm³ (10 × 10⁹/L) to prevent spontaneous bleeding.

Until engraftment has occurred, monitor the patient's temperature every 4 to 8 hours for signs of infection. Also guide monitoring signs of focal point of infection based on clinical symptoms. For example, if the patient develops shortness of breath, then imaging of the lungs should occur to assess pulmonary infection. Monitor for the toxicity of prophylaxis and/or treatment of bacterial, fungal, or viral infections.

Patient Care and Monitoring

1. Assess the patient regarding the indication for HSCT, the type of preparative regimen, and the type of donor. Determine the nonhematologic toxicity of the preparative regimen, the expected timing of engraftment after the graft is infused, along with the need for GVHD prophylaxis.

2. Determine the supportive care needs during administration of the preparative regimen, including use of indwelling central venous catheters, blood product support, and pharmacologic management of CINV, mucositis, and pain.

3. After the graft is infused, monitor CBC with differential at least daily to evaluate engraftment. Allogeneic HSCT patients experience an initial period of pancytopenia followed by a more prolonged period of immunosuppression, which substantially increases the risk of bacterial, fungal, viral, and other opportunistic infections.

4. Counsel the patient regarding adherence to prophylactic antibiotic, antifungal, and antiviral regimens. Evaluate the patient for infection and adverse drug reactions to antibiotics, antifungals, and antivirals. Ensure that the patient is appropriately immunized after recovery from HSCT.

5. Counsel the patient regarding adherence to GVHD prophylaxis and treatment. Monitor and manage for adverse drug reactions.

ASCO	American Society of Clinical Oncology
ATG	Antithymocyte globulin
BMT	Bone marrow transplantation
BU-CY	Busulfan-cyclophosphamide
CINV	Chemotherapy-induced nausea and vomiting
CML	Chronic myelogenous leukemia
CMV	Cytomegalovirus
CY-TBI	Cyclophosphamide-TBI
GVHD	Graft-versus-host disease
HGF	Hematopoietic growth factors
HLA	Human leukocyte antigen
HSCT	Hematopoietic stem cell transplant
IA	Invasive aspergillosis
IL-2	Interleukin-2
MHC	Minor histocompatibility
MM	Multiple-myeloma
NHL	Non-Hodgkin's lymphoma
NK	Natural killer
PBPC	Peripheral blood progenitor cells
PCP	Pneumocystis pneumonia
SOS	Sinusoidal obstruction syndrome
SrCr	Serum creatinine
TBI	Total-body irradiation
VZV	Varicella-zoster virus

 Self-assessment questions and answers are available at http://*www.mhpharmacotherapy.com/pp.html.*

Monitor for acute nonhematologic toxicity to the preparative regimen to approximately day +30. Specifically,

- Monitor the inside of the mouth and assess the patient's mouth pain for signs and symptoms of mucositis.

- Monitor weight and skin color daily to observe sudden weight changes suggesting sinusoidal obstruction syndrome. Obtain a total bilirubin determination at least twice weekly or more frequently if sinusoidal obstruction syndrome is suspected based upon weight change.

Monitor for signs of acute GVHD at least daily during engraftment and more often if GVHD is suspected or diagnosed. The patient and his or her caregivers should be educated regarding the signs and symptoms to self-monitor for GVHD. The signs and symptoms for acute GVHD that occur between day +0 and day +100 are rash, nausea, diarrhea, jaundice, elevated liver function tests, and elevated bilirubin.

Abbreviatons Introduced in This Chapter

AML	Acute myeloid leukemia
ANC	Absolute neutrophil count

REFERENCES

1. Copelan EA. Hematopoietic stem-cell transplantation. N Engl J Med 2006;354:1813–1826.
2. Pasquini MC, Wang Z, Schneider L. Current use and outcome of hematopoietic stem cell transplantation: Part I—CIBMTR Summary Slides, 2007. CIBMTR Newsletter [serial online] 2007;13(2):5–9, *http://www.cibmtr.org/PUBLICATIONS/Newsletter/DOCS/2007Dec.pdf.*
3. Baron F, Sandmaier BM. Current status of hematopoietic stem cell transplantation after nonmyeloablative conditioning. Curr Opin Hematol 2005;12:435–443.
4. Centers for Disease Control and Prevention; Infectious Disease Society of America; American Society of Blood and Marrow Transplantation. Guidelines for preventing opportunistic infections among hematopoietic stem cell transplant recipients. MMWR Recomm Rep 2000; 49:1–125, CE1-7.
5. Davies SM, Kollman C, Anasetti C, et al. Engraftment and survival after unrelated-donor bone marrow transplantation: A report from the national marrow donor program. Blood 2000;96:4096–4102.
6. Petersdorf EW, Hansen JA, Martin PJ, et al. Major-histocompatibility-complex class I alleles and antigens in hematopoietic-cell transplantation. N Engl J Med 2001; 345:1794–1800.
7. Morishima Y, Sasazuki T, Inoko H, et al. The clinical significance of human leukocyte antigen (HLA) allele compatibility in patients receiving a marrow transplant from serologically HLA-A, HLA-B, and HLA-DR matched unrelated donors. Blood 2002;99:4200–4206.
8. Kessinger A, Sharp JG. The whys and hows of hematopoietic progenitor and stem cell mobilization. Bone Marrow Transplant 2003;31:319–329.

9. Schmitz N. Peripheral blood hematopoietic cells for allogeneic transplantation. In: Blume KG, Forman SJ, Thomas ED, eds. Hematopoietic Cell Transplantation, 3rd ed. Malden, MA: Blackwell Science, 2004:588–598.

10. Stem Cell Trialists' Collaborative Group. Allogeneic peripheral blood stem-cell compared with bone marrow transplantation in the management of hematologic malignancies: An individual patient data meta-analysis of nine randomized trials. J Clin Oncol 2005;23: 5074–5087.

11. Remberger M, Ringden O, Blau IW, et al. No difference in graft-versus-host disease, relapse, and survival comparing peripheral stem cells to bone marrow using unrelated donors. Blood 2001;98:1739–1745.

12. Barker JN, Davies SM, DeFor T, et al. Survival after transplantation of unrelated donor umbilical cord blood is comparable to that of human leukocyte antigen-matched unrelated donor bone marrow: Results of a matched-pair analysis. Blood 2001;97:2957–2961.

13. Rocha V, Gluckman E. Clinical use of umbilical cord blood hematopoietic stem cells. Biol Blood Marrow Transplant 2006;12:34–41.

14. Wolff SN. Second hematopoietic stem cell transplantation for the treatment of graft failure, graft rejection or relapse after allogeneic transplantation. Bone Marrow Transplant 2002;29:545–552.

15. Clift RA, Buckner CD, Thomas ED, et al. Marrow transplantation for patients in accelerated phase of chronic myeloid leukemia. Blood 1994;84:4368–4373.

16. Woods WG, Neudorf S, Gold S, et al.; Children's cancer group. A comparison of allogeneic bone marrow transplantation, autologous bone marrow transplantation, and aggressive chemotherapy in children with acute myeloid leukemia in remission. Blood 2001;97:56–62.

17. Bierman PJ, Freedman AS. Autologous hematopoietic stem cell transplantation for non-Hodgkin lymphoma. In: Atkinson K, Champlin R, Ritz J, Fibbe WE, Ljungman P, Brenner MK, eds. Clinical Bone Marrow and Blood Stem Cell Transplantation, 3rd ed. New York, NY: Cambridge University Press, 2004:524.

18. Socie G, Clift RA, Blaise D, et al. Busulfan plus cyclophosphamide compared with total-body irradiation plus cyclophosphamide before marrow transplantation for myeloid leukemia: Long-term follow-up of 4 randomized studies. Blood 2001;98:3569–3574.

19. Champlin R, Khouri I, Anderlini P, et al. Nonmyeloablative preparative regimens for allogeneic hematopoietic transplantation. Biology and current indications. Oncology (Williston Park) 2003;17:94–100; discussion:103–107.

20. McCune JS, Gibbs JP, Slattery JT. Plasma concentration monitoring of busulfan: Does it improve clinical outcome? Clin Pharmacokinet 2000;39:155–165.

21. Grochow LB. Parenteral busulfan: Is therapeutic monitoring still warranted? Biol Blood Marrow Transplant 2002;8:465–467.

22. Schuchter LM, Hensley ML, Meropol NJ, et al. 2002 update of recommendations for the use of chemotherapy and radiotherapy protectants: Clinical practice guidelines of the American Society of Clinical Oncology. J Clin Oncol 2002(Jun 15);20(12):2895–2903.

23. Kris MG, Hesketh PJ, Somerfield MR, et al. American Society of Clinical Oncology guideline for antiemetics in oncology: Update 2006. J Clin Oncol 2006(Jun 20);24(18):2932–2947.

24. Radtke ML, Kolesar JM. Palifermin (Kepivance) for the treatment of oral mucositis in patients with hematologic malignancies requiring hematopoietic stem cell support. J Oncol Pharm Pract 2005;11:121–125.

25. Ho VT, Revta C, Richardson PG. Hepatic veno-occlusive disease after hematopoietic stem cell transplantation: Update on defibrotide and other current investigational therapies. Bone Marrow Transplant 2008;41:229–237.

26. Kashyap A, Wingard J, Cagnoni P, et al. Intravenous versus oral busulfan as part of a busulfan/cyclophosphamide preparative regimen for allogeneic hematopoietic stem cell transplantation: Decreased incidence of hepatic venoocclusive disease (HVOD), HVOD-related mortality, and overall 100-day mortality. Biol Blood Marrow Transplant 2002;8:493–500.

27. Smith TJ, Khatcheressian J, Lyman GH, et al. 2006 update of recommendations for the use of white blood cell growth factors: An evidence-based clinical practice guideline. J Clin Oncol 2006(Jul 1);24(19):3187–3205.

28. Ringden O, Labopin M, Gorin NC, et al. Treatment with granulocyte colony-stimulating factor after allogeneic bone marrow transplantation for acute leukemia increases the risk of graft-versus-host disease and death: A study from the Acute Leukemia Working Party of the European Group for Blood and Marrow Transplantation. J Clin Oncol 2004;22:416–423.

29. Filipovich AH, Weisdorf D, Pavletic S, et al. National Institutes of Health consensus development project on criteria for clinical trials in chronic graft-versus-host disease: I. Diagnosis and staging working group report. Biol Blood Marrow Transplant 2005;11:945–956.

30. Couriel D, Caldera H, Champlin R, Komanduri K. Acute graft-versus-host disease: Pathophysiology, clinical manifestations, and management. Cancer 2004;101: 1936–1946.

31. Chao NJ, Schmidt GM, Niland JC, et al. Cyclosporine, methotrexate, and prednisone compared with cyclosporine and prednisone for prophylaxis of acute graft-versus-host disease. N Engl J Med 1993;329:1225–1230.

32. Ratanatharathorn V, Nash RA, Przepiorka D, et al. Phase III study comparing methotrexate and tacrolimus (prograf, FK506) with methotrexate and cyclosporine for graft-versus-host disease prophylaxis after HLA-identical sibling bone marrow transplantation. Blood 1998;92:2303–2314.

33. Nash RA, Antin JH, Karanes C, et al. Phase 3 study comparing methotrexate and tacrolimus with methotrexate and cyclosporine for prophylaxis of acute graft-versus-host disease after marrow transplantation from unrelated donors. Blood 2000;96:2062–2068.

34. Leather HL. Drug interactions in the hematopoietic stem cell transplant (HSCT) recipient: What every transplanter needs to know. Bone Marrow Transplant 2004;33:137–152.

35. Burroughs L, Mielcarek M, Leisenring W, et al. Extending postgrafting cyclosporine decreases the risk of severe graft-versus-host disease after nonmyeloablative hematopoietic cell transplantation. Transplantation 2006;81:818–825.

36. Lee SJ. New approaches for preventing and treating chronic graft-versus-host disease. Blood 2005;105:4200–4206.

37. Junghanss C, Boeckh M, Carter RA, et al. Incidence and outcome of cytomegalovirus infections following nonmyeloablative compared with myeloablative allogeneic stem cell transplantation, a matched control study. Blood 2002;99:1978–1985.

38. Fukuda T, Boeckh M, Carter RA, et al. Risks and outcomes of invasive fungal infections in recipients of allogeneic hematopoietic stem cell transplants after nonmyeloablative conditioning. Blood 2003;102: 827–833.

39. Hughes WT, Armstrong D, Bodey GP, et al. 2002 guidelines for the use of antimicrobial agents in neutropenic patients with cancer. Clin Infect Dis 2002;34: 730–751.

40. Boeckh M, Kim HW, Flowers ME, et al. Long-term acyclovir for prevention of varicella zoster virus disease after allogeneic hematopoietic cell transplantation—A randomized double-blind placebo-controlled study. Blood 2006;107:1800–1805.

41. Richardson M, Lass-Flörl C. Changing epidemiology of systemic fungal infections. Clin Microbiol Infect 2008(May);(Supp l4):5–24.

42. Winston DJ, Maziarz RT, Chandrasekar PH, et al. Intravenous and oral itraconazole versus intravenous and oral fluconazole for long-term antifungal prophylaxis in allogeneic hematopoietic stem-cell transplant recipients. A multicenter, randomized trial. Ann Intern Med 2003;138:705–713.

43. Walsh TJ, Anaissie EJ, Denning DW, et al. Treatment of aspergillosis: Clinical Practice Guidelines of the Infectious Diseases Society of America. Clin Infect Dis 2008;46(3):327–360.

44. Garcia-Vidal C, Upton A, Kirby KA, Marr KA. Epidemiology of invasive mold infections in allogeneic stem cell transplant recipients: Biological risk factors for infection according to time after transplantation. Clin Infect Dis 2008;47:1041–1050.

45. Dupont B. Overview of the lipid formulations of amphotericin B. J Antimicrob Chemother. 2002(Feb); 49(Suppl 1):31–36.

46. Herbrecht R, Denning DW, Patterson TF, et al. Voriconazole versus amphotericin B for primary therapy of invasive aspergillosis. N Engl J Med 2002;347:408–415.

47. Antin JH. Clinical practice. Long-term care after hematopoietic-cell transplantation in adults. N Engl J Med 2002;347:36–42.

48. Bhatia S, Robison LL, Francisco L, et al. Late mortality in survivors of autologous hematopoietic-cell transplantation: Report from the Bone Marrow Transplant Survivor Study. Blood 2005;105:4215–4222.

49. Ljungman P, Engelhard D, de la Camara R, et al. Vaccination of stem cell transplant recipients: Recommendations of the Infectious Diseases Working Party of the EBMT. Bone Marrow Transplant 2005;35:737–746.

99 Supportive Care in Oncology

Sarah L. Scarpace

LEARNING OBJECTIVES

● **Upon completion of the chapter, the reader will be able to:**

1. Describe the impact of various supportive care interventions on the prognosis of patients with cancer.

2. Discuss the scientific basis for providing various supportive care interventions in the oncology patient population.

3. Identify patient-related and disease-related risk factors in defining a population for whom supportive care interventions would be of benefit.

4. Recognize typical presenting signs and symptoms of common complications/emergencies that require supportive care interventions.

5. Outline an appropriate prevention and management strategies for various supportive care interventions.

6. Prepare a monitoring plan to evaluate the efficacy and toxicity of pharmacotherapy interventions for supportive care problems.

KEY CONCEPTS

❶ The optimal method of managing chemotherapy-induced nausea/vomiting (CINV) is to provide adequate pharmacologic prophylaxis given a patient's risk level for emesis.

❷ The fundamental approach to lessen the severity of mucositis begins with basic, good oral hygiene.

❸ A risk assessment should be performed at presentation of febrile neutropenia (FN) to identify low-risk patients for potential outpatient treatment. Patients who do not meet low-risk criteria should be hospitalized for immediate parenteral administration of broad-spectrum antibacterials before culture results are obtained.

❹ The primary goal of treatment of superior vena cava syndrome (SVCS) is to relieve obstruction of the superior vena cava (SVC) by treating the underlying malignancy.

❺ Because patients with spinal metastases are generally incurable, the primary goal of treatment of spinal cord compression is palliation. The most important prognostic factor for patients presenting with spinal cord compression is the underlying neurologic status.

❻ The goals of treatment of brain metastases are to manage symptoms and improve survival by reducing cerebral edema, treat the underlying malignancy both locally and systemically.

❼ The use of effective prevention strategies can decrease the incidence of hemorrhagic cystitis to less than 5% in patients receiving cyclophosphamide or ifosfamide. There are three methods to reduce the risk: administration of mesna, hyperhydration, and bladder irrigation with catheterization.

❽ The primary goal of treatment for hypercalcemia is to control the underlying malignancy. Therapies directed at lowering the calcium level are temporary measures that are useful until anticancer therapy begins to work.

❾ The primary goals of management of tumor lysis syndrome (TLS) are: (a) prevention of renal failure and (b) prevention of electrolyte imbalances. Thus, the best treatment for TLS is prophylaxis to enable delivery of cytotoxic therapy for the underlying malignancy.

❿ Chemotherapy extravasation may be avoided in many cases by the use of successful prevention strategies. The most important preventative measure is proper patient education.

INTRODUCTION

Patients with cancer are at risk for serious adverse events that result from their treatment, the cancer, or both. The management of these complications is generally referred to as supportive care (or symptom management). Treatment-related complications include chemotherapy-induced nausea and vomiting (CINV), febrile neutropenia (FN), extravasation, hemorrhagic cystitis, mucositis, and tumor lysis syndrome (TLS). Tumor or cancer-related complications include superior vena cava (SVC) obstruction, spinal cord compression, and hypercalcemia and brain metastases. In some cases, these events can be life-threatening. SVC obstruction, spinal cord compression, TLS, and hypercalcemia have traditionally been defined as oncologic emergencies. Although some of these conditions are not imminently life-threatening (i.e., chemotherapy extravasation), as a group of treatment- and disease-related complications in the oncology population, they do require rapid assessment and supportive care interventions/treatment. The onset of oncologic emergencies may herald the onset of an undiagnosed malignancy or progression/relapse of a pre-existing malignancy. Optimal management of patients with various oncologic emergencies and complications requiring supportive care interventions can significantly decrease morbidity and mortality in patients with cancer. This chapter provides an overview of these issues. First, an overview of the management of common side effects of treatment will be discussed. Later, a summary of common oncologic emergencies will be presented.

CHEMOTHERAPY-INDUCED TOXICITIES: NAUSEA/VOMITING

Nausea and vomiting are among the most commonly feared toxicities by patients undergoing chemotherapy. One study demonstrated that both nausea and vomiting ranked in the top five bothersome side effects of chemotherapy.[1] ❶ *The optimal method of managing CINV is to provide adequate pharmacologic prophylaxis given a patient's risk level for emesis.* Studies have demonstrated that insufficient control during the first cycle of chemotherapy leads to more difficulty in controlling emesis for subsequent cycles.[2]

EPIDEMIOLOGY AND ETIOLOGY

While it is widely known that chemotherapy causes nausea and vomiting, the rate of emesis varies depending on individual patient risk factors and drug therapy regimen. Therefore, cancer treatments are stratified into varying risk levels: high, moderate, low, and minimal. Agents with a "high" emetic risk cause emesis in greater than 90% of cases if not given any prophylaxis. The rates of emesis for "moderate," "low," and "minimal" are 30% to 90%, 10% to 30%, and less than 10%, respectively. Table 99–1 lists the individual agents and their risk category.[3] With proper prophylaxis using antiemetics, the rate of emesis when receiving a highly emetogenic regimen can decrease to about 30%.[4]

PATHOPHYSIOLOGY

The pathophysiology of nausea and vomiting is described in Chapter 20. Specific to CINV, the key receptors include

Table 99–1	
Emetogenic Potential of Chemotherapy	
Risk	**Agent**
High emetic risk (greater than 90% of patients will vomit without appropriate antiemetics)	Altretamine
	Carmustine greater than 250 mg/m²
	Cisplatin equal to or greater than 50 mg/m²
	Cyclophosphamide greater than 1,500 mg/m²
	Dacarbazine
	Mechlorethamine
	Streptozocin
Moderate emetic risk (30–90%)	Aldesleukin greater than 12–15 million units/m²
	Amifostine greater than 300 mg/m²
	Arsenic trioxide
	Azacitidine
	Bendamustine
	Busulfan grater than 4 mg/m²
	Carboplatin
	Carmustine less than or equal to 250 mg/m²
	Cisplatin less than 50 mg/m²
	Cyclophosphamide less than or equal to 1,500 mg/m²
	Cyclophosphamide (oral)
	Cytarabine greater than 1 g/m²
	Dactinomycin
	Daunorubicin
	Doxorubicin
	Epirubicin
	Etoposide (oral)
	Idarubicin
	Ifosfamide
	Irinotecan
	Imatinib (oral)
	Lomustine
	Melphalan
	Methotrexate greater than 1,000 mg/m²
	Oxaliplatin greater than 75 mg/m²
	Temozolamide (oral)
	Vinorelbine (oral)
Low emetic risk (10–30%)	Amifostine less than 300 mg/m²
	Bexarotene
	Capecitabine
	Docetaxel
	Etoposide
	Fludarabine (oral)
	5-Fluorouracil less than 1,000 mg/m²
	Gemcitabine
	Ixabepilone
	Methotrexate greater than 50 mg/m² and less than 250 mg/m²
	Mitomycin
	Nilotinib
	Paclitaxel
	Pemetrexed
	Topotecan
	Vorinostat
Minimal risk (less than 10%)	Most other agents

serotonin (5-HT₃) receptors (located in the chemoreceptor trigger zone, emetic center of the medulla, and in the GI tract) and neurokinin-1 (NK1) receptors (located in the emetic center of the medulla). Serotonin plays an important role in the genesis of acute vomiting, as some cancer drug therapies can stimulate a release of serotonin from enterochromaffin cells in the GI tract. Serotonin then activates the emetic response by binding to $5HT_3$ receptors in the emetic center. This short-lived release of serotonin likely explains why serotonin antagonists are more beneficial for preventing acute versus delayed vomiting.[5] Other sites that are targeted by antiemetics include dopamine, muscarinic (acetylcholine), histamine, and cannabinoid receptors.

CLINICAL PRESENTATION AND DIAGNOSIS

CINV, though frequently discussed as one syndrome, are two distinct clinical entities. Nauseous patients may present with general GI upset and reflux and may report a sensation or desire to vomit without being able to do so (patients may describe this as having "dry heaves"). Patients with chemotherapy-induced vomiting may experience vomiting with the first 24 hours of chemotherapy administration ("acute" nausea/vomiting) or several days following chemotherapy ("delayed" nausea/vomiting).[3] Patients may additionally experience nausea/vomiting prior to chemotherapy administration ("anticipatory" nausea/vomiting).[3] In all cases, it is important that other causes of nausea and vomiting are ruled out before diagnosing chemotherapy as the source.[6] Other causes of nausea and vomiting may include bowel obstruction, opioids, electrolyte imbalances, brain metastases, and vestibular dysfunction.[6]

Clinical Presentation and Diagnosis of CINV

Acute Nausea/Vomiting
- Occurs within the first 24 hours after chemotherapy administration

Delayed Nausea/Vomiting
- Occurs between 24 hours and 5 days after chemotherapy administration

Anticipatory Nausea/Vomiting
- A learned, conditioned reflex response to a stimulus (sight, sound, smell) often associated with poor emetic control in a previous cycle of chemotherapy

Breakthrough Nausea/Vomiting
- Occurs despite prophylaxis with an appropriate antiemetic regimen

Differential Diagnosis
- Surgery, radiation
- Gastric outlet/bowel obstruction, constipation
- Hypercalcemia, hyperglycemia, hyponatremia, uremia
- Other drugs (opioids)

TREATMENT

Desired Outcomes

The desired outcome is to completely prevent or minimize the severity of nausea, vomiting, and the use of breakthrough antiemetic medications. In clinical trials, a common endpoint is "complete response," defined as having no emesis and no breakthrough medication use within a defined period of time. If patients experience nausea or emesis, the goal is to quickly relieve the episode and prevent future nausea or vomiting, whether in the next few days or for the next cycle of chemotherapy.

General Approach to Treatment

Treatment-related factors and patient-related factors can help define a patient population at risk for developing CINV. Treatment-related factors include those chemotherapy agents with high levels of emetogenecity (see Table 99–1 for a complete listing). CINV is typically a cyclical occurrence. While this section is focused on CINV, it can be helpful for the practitioner to remember that patients undergoing concomitant radiation therapy and chemotherapy are at risk for more severe nausea and vomiting. Radiation (particularly total body irradiation as part of a conditioning regimen for stem cell transplant) can cause a more cumulative (versus cyclical) nausea/vomiting phenomenon.

Specific patient-related factors such as female gender, age (children), history of motion sickness, pregnancy-induced nausea or vomiting, and poor emetic control in previous chemotherapy cycles increase the risk of emesis. Interestingly, patients with a history of alcohol abuse have a reported decreased risk of emesis.[3] It is important to design an antiemetic regimen with consideration of these patient-specific risk factors.

A well-designed regimen includes a prophylactic regimen and a breakthrough antiemetic drug "as needed." Although there are many drugs recommended as "breakthrough" drugs, choose a drug with a different mechanism of action compared to the drugs used for prophylaxis.[6]

▶ Nonpharmacologic Therapy

Nonpharmacologic therapy for nausea and vomiting can be useful adjuncts to drug therapy, particularly in the setting of anticipatory nausea and vomiting. The National Comprehensive Cancer Network (NCCN) recommends behavior therapies such as relaxation, guided imagery, and music therapy as well as acupuncture/acupressure as useful in this setting.[6] Other general measures that can be taken include ensuring adequate sleep before treatment, eating smaller meals, and avoiding greasy foods and foods with strong odors.[7] Nonprescription medications such as antacids, histamine-2-receptor blockers, and proton pump inhibitors can be helpful in reducing gastroesophageal reflux associated with some cancer treatments that may trigger or exacerbate CINV.[8]

Nonprescription antihistamines marketed for nausea associated with motion sickness are not usually helpful in managing CINV.

▶ *Pharmacologic Therapy*

According to the American Society of Clinical Oncology's antiemesis guidelines, there are three drug classes with a "high therapeutic index" to treat CINV: corticosteroids (dexamethasone), serotonin receptor antagonists, and NK1 receptor antagonists (aprepitant).[9] A drug in these three classes will be used either in combination with drugs from the other classes or as a single agent for prophylaxis, depending on the emetic risk level (Table 99–2). Dexamethasone and serotonin antagonists are usually administered 30 minutes before chemotherapy, while aprepitant is administered 60 minutes before chemotherapy. Dexamethasone is the preferred agent to prevent CINV in the delayed setting, and is recommended to be scheduled at a dose of 4 mg orally, twice daily (or 8 mg once daily) for 3 to 4 days following chemotherapy to prevent delayed nausea vomiting. In some cases, the serotonin antagonists may also be continued orally for 3 to 4 days after chemotherapy. For those patients in whom aprepitant is used prechemotherapy (as either 125 mg orally or 115 mg IV as fosaprepitant), the aprepitant is continued as 80 mg orally once daily on days 2 and 3 of the chemotherapy cycle. The other antiemetics are usually prescribed "as needed" for breakthrough nausea or vomiting. The dopamine antagonists prochlorperazine and metoclopramide are usually recommended, as they antagonize a different receptor than the drugs already given for prophylaxis. However, the NCCN guidelines state that other drugs, including serotonin receptor antagonists, cannabinoids, dexamethasone, or olanzapine may be used.[6] For those in any risk group who experience anticipatory nausea and vomiting, the addition of lorazepam for prophylaxis and breakthrough is recommended, for its antiemetic and antianxiety properties. Table 99–3 lists the doses of the antiemetic agents for prophylaxis and breakthrough use.

A prophylactic antiemetic regimen for high emetic risk levels should be with a triple-drug combination using dexamethasone, aprepitant, and 5-HT$_3$ antagonist to prevent both acute and delayed emesis. Dexamethasone should be continued until day 4 and aprepitant is also administered on days 2 and 3.

For moderately emetogenic regimens, acute emesis is still of major concern, but the incidence of delayed emesis is less. Therefore, dexamethasone plus a 5-HT$_3$ antagonist should be given on day 1. On days 2 to 4, choose to continue either the dexamethasone or the 5-HT$_3$ antagonist to prevent delayed emesis. One exception is when palonosetron is given as the 5-HT$_3$ antagonist on day 1. Because its half-life is long, no redosing is necessary on subsequent days. Aprepitant is also FDA-approved for the prevention of CINV in the moderate setting and can be used as described above. For patients with additional risk factors or who had uncontrolled emesis with previous chemotherapy cycles, the same regimen for "high" risk levels may be used.

For low emetic risk regimens, single antiemetic prophylaxis with either dexamethasone or a dopamine antagonist (prochlorperazine, metoclopramide) is recommended. For minimal emetic risk groups, guidelines do not recommend routine prophylaxis with antiemetics; instead, patients should be provided something as needed for nausea and vomiting. Table 99–2 summarizes the NCCN guidelines for antiemetic prophylaxis for the different risk levels.

OUTCOME EVALUATION

It is often difficult to evaluate nausea and vomiting when chemotherapy is given as an outpatient. After drug

Table 99–2

Recommended Therapy by Emetic Risk

Emetic Risk Category (Incidence of Emesis Without Antiemetics)	Antiemetic Regimens and Schedules
High (greater than 90%)	5-HT$_3$ serotonin receptor antagonist: day 1 Dexamethasone: days 1–4 Aprepitant: days 1, 2, 3
Moderate (30–90%)	5-HT$_3$ serotonin receptor antagonist: day 1 Dexamethasone: day 1
Moderate (30–90%) but getting anthracycline, carboplatin, cisplatin, irinotecan cyclophosphamide, methotrxate	5-HT$_3$ serotonin receptor antagonist: day 1 Dexamethasone: day 1, 2, 3 Aprepitant: days 1, 2, 3
Low (10–30%)	Dexamethasone: day 1
Minimal (less than 10%)	As needed

Table 99–3

Antiemetic Dosing

Antiemetic	Single Dose Administered Before Chemotherapy	Daily Schedule
5-HT$_3$ Serotonin Receptor Antagonists		
Dolasetron	Oral: 100 mg IV: 100 mg or 1.8 mg/kg	100 mg po daily
Granisetron	Oral: 2 mg IV: 1 mg or 0.01 mg/kg Topical: 34.3 mg patch (apply 24–48 hours before chemotherapy)	1–2 mg po daily or 1 mg two times a day
Ondansetron	Oral: 16–24 mg IV: 8 mg or 0.15 mg/kg	8 mg po two times a day or 16 mg po daily
Palonosetron	IV: 0.25 mg Oral: 0.5 mg po	
Others		
Aprepitent	Oral: 125 mg	80 mg po days 2, 3
Fosaprepitant	IV: 115 mg	
Dexamethasone	Oral: 12 mg	12 mg po days 2–4

administration, patients return home and may or may not report inadequate control of emesis. Subsequent chemotherapy cycles may also be poorly controlled, especially if patients do not state their experience with the previous cycle. To ameliorate this problem, patients' experiences with CINV should be assessed, particularly after the first and second cycle of chemotherapy. Patients should be asked about their previous emesis control with subsequent cycles of chemotherapy, and a prophylaxis regimen may need to be adjusted. Patients should also be encouraged to self-report poor control of emesis while at home. Side effects of the antiemetic regimen should also be assessed and reported.

Patient Encounter 1: CINV

MJ is a 42-year-old woman diagnosed with stage II hormone-receptor positive, *HER2*-negative breast cancer. She has been treated with lumpectomy and radiation therapy and presents to clinic for cycle 1 day 1 of adjuvant doxorubicin and cyclophosphamide (the "AC" regimen). She appears calm and optimistic about her prognosis with no more than expected mild anxiety about the side effects of chemotherapy. She reports drinking alcohol only on holidays but does report a history of motion sickness. All labs are within normal limits, she has no drug allergies, and is otherwise healthy with no comorbidities.

How would you approach the prevention and monitoring of MJ for CINV?

Patient Care and Monitoring: CINV

Monitoring

- Using a visual analogue or numerical rating scale (0 to 10), have the patient rate the severity of nausea (assess nausea first, then move on to emesis)

- Daily, ask about the number of emesis episodes in the last 24 hours

- Assess scheduled and breakthrough medication adherence

Counsel the patient regarding his or her antiemetics

- Explain which drugs are taken as prophylaxis to prevent nausea and vomiting, and which are taken as needed to treat it

- Have the patient journal when a dose is taken in relation to the chemotherapy. Encourage journaling the severity and frequency of nausea, vomiting, diet and antiemetic adherence

- Discuss expected/common side effects of antiemetic medications

---

MUCOSITIS

Mucositis is the degradation of mucosal lining in the oral cavity and GI tract due to damage from radiation or chemotherapy.[10] Mucositis is a common supportive care issue that deserves attention and is associated with many negative health consequences including pain, inadequate nutritional intake, and risk for infection. Patients with mucositis often require parenteral analgesics, nutrition supplementation, and anti-infectives to treat concomitant bacterial, fungal, or viral infections. Furthermore, mucositis is associated with economic consequences, primarily increased length of hospital stay.[11] An understanding of the current guidelines for prevention and treatment of mucositis can help improve patient outcomes.

EPIDEMIOLOGY AND ETIOLOGY

● The incidence of chemotherapy or radiation-induced mucositis depends mostly on the type and area of radiation, the type of chemotherapy, and the specific cancer. Studies have reported an incidence of about 80% in head and neck cancer patients receiving chemoradiation.[12] The World Health Organization estimates that approximately 75% of patients who are treated with high-dose chemotherapy for stem cell transplantation developed oral mucositis.[10] Specific chemotherapy agents associated with mucositis include taxanes, anthracyclines, platinum analogues, methotrexate, and the fluoropyrimidines.

PATHOPHYSIOLOGY

The classical concept of mucositis pathophysiology asserts that direct cytotoxicity from chemotherapy or radiation to basal epithelial cells results in ulcerative lesions due to a lack of regeneration. These lesions are further complicated by trauma and/or microorganism growth. However, the most recent theory of mucositis pathophysiology is more detailed, and involves a multistage, dynamic process that builds upon the historical model.[13] According to this theory, there are five stages of mucositis: initiation, primary damage response, signal amplification, ulceration, and healing. It is important to note that these stages do not occur sequentially. Rather, they are dynamic and may overlap.

CLINICAL PRESENTATION AND DIAGNOSIS

● Patients with mucositis may present along a continuum of mild, painless, erythematous ulcers to those that are painful and/or bleeding which may interfere with eating and swallowing or which may require treatment with hydration, antibiotics, or even parenteral nutrition in its most severe forms.[13]

TREATMENT

Nonpharmacologic Treatment

The goal of nonpharmacologic measures to prevent mucositis is to reduce the bacterial load of organisms in the mouth

Clinical Presentation and Diagnosis of Mucositis

- Painful, erythematous ulcers develop on lips, cheeks, soft palate, floor of mouth
- Asses mucositis using validated scales, either oral mucositis assessment scale (OMAS), or University of Nebraska oral assessment score (MUCPEAK)
- Symptoms appear within 5 to 7 days after chemotherapy and resolve in 2 to 3 weeks
- Pain may affect ability to swallow and eat
- May have concomitant localized or systemic infection
- Diarrhea can lead to electrolyte imbalances

to prevent infection of the inflamed mucosa. Prevention of mucositis with good basic oral hygiene (brushing with a soft-bristled toothbrush at least twice daily, flossing, bland rinses, and saline substitutes) is key. ❷ *The fundamental approach to lessen the severity of mucositis begins with basic, good oral hygiene.*[10,13,14]

Pharmacologic Treatment

In the setting of radiation therapy, amifostine at doses equal to or greater than 340 mg/m^2 IV prior to each dose of radiation therapy may be considered.[14] Cryotherapy, such as with ice chips, is recommended as a prophylactic measure for patients treated with both standard-dose and high-dose chemotherapy regimens.[14] Antimicrobial lozenges, sucralfate and chlorhexidine rinses, and "magic-mouthwash" compounded rinses are not generally recommended by clinical practice guidelines for mucositis prevention though they are sometimes used in practice.[10,13,14]

Unfortunately, little evidence is available to recommend specific treatments for mucositis. Pain assessment and appropriate management are important.[10,13,14] Pain management may be achieved with oral morphine, topical anesthetic products, and compounded rinses which incorporate lidocaine.[10,13,14] In more severe cases where infection of the oral mucosa is suspected, appropriate antibiotic therapy is necessary to prevent systemic infection.[10,13,14]

Palifermin is FDA-approved for the prevention and treatment of mucositis in patients receiving high-dose chemotherapy for stem cell transplant or leukemia induction. Palifermin is administered as an IV bolus injection at a dosage of 60 mcg/kg/day, for 3 consecutive days before and three consecutive days after myelotoxic therapy for a total of six doses. Administering palifermin within 24 hours of chemotherapy can result in an increased sensitivity of rapidly dividing epithelial cells to the cytotoxic agent. For this reason, palifermin should not be administered for 24 hours before, 24 hours after, or during the infusion of myelotoxic chemotherapy to avoid increasing the severity and the duration of oral mucositis.

OUTCOME EVALUATION

Based on these goals, outcomes measured in clinical trials often assess the incidence, duration, and severity of mucositis with a given intervention intended to prevent or treat mucositis. Agents that are intended to palliate the symptoms of mucositis are usually assessed by measures in pain scales and the ability to eat or drink.

HEMATOLOGIC COMPLICATIONS: FN

INTRODUCTION

FN is a common adverse effect after administration of cytotoxic chemotherapy. The mortality rate in neutropenic patients due to infectious complications currently remains between 5% and 10%; therefore FN is considered a true oncologic emergency. Patients frequently require hospitalization for prompt administration of broad-spectrum antibiotics that are critical to avoid morbidity and mortality.

EPIDEMIOLOGY AND ETIOLOGY

The microorganisms responsible for infections in neutropenic patients have changed significantly in the last 50 years. From the 1960s through the mid-1980s, gram-negative organisms were the most common bacteria isolated. This pattern shifted to the gram-positive organisms in the late 1980s, which remain the most common isolates. Recent data indicate that gram-positive organisms account for 62% to 76% of all bloodstream infections.[15] The causes of this change are attributed to the widespread use of central venous catheters and more aggressive chemotherapy regimens as well as the use of prophylactic antibiotics with relatively poor gram-positive coverage (quinolones). Commonly isolated pathogens are shown in Table 99–4. Although gram-negative infections are less common, they cause the majority of infections in sites other than the blood and are particularly virulent. It should be noted that isolates vary considerably among

Patient Encounter 2, Part 1: FN

FG is a 73-year-old male with extensive stage small cell lung cancer. He has a 100-pack-year history of smoking, hypertension, and has oxygen-dependent chronic obstructive pulmonary disease (COPD). He has poor appetite and has lost 9.1 kg (20 lb) in the last month. He is a 3-year survivor of stage IIIa colorectal cancer (CRC), which was treated with surgery and six cycles of adjuvant combination chemotherapy (5-fluorouracil, leucovorin, and oxaliplatin).

What risk factors for FN does this patient have?

What signs and symptoms of infection would you counsel this patient to watch for following treatment?

institutions thus attention to institutional isolation patterns is prudent.

Fungal infections due to *Candida* species (especially *C albicans*) have emerged as significant pathogens, especially in patients with hematologic malignancies and those undergoing bone marrow transplantation (BMT). In addition, *Aspergillus* species are important pathogens in patients with prolonged and severe neutropenia.

PATHOPHYSIOLOGY

The neutrophils are the primary defense mechanism against bacterial and fungal infection. Most infections in neutropenic patients are a result of organisms contained in endogenous flora, both on the skin and within the GI tract. These organisms are provided access to the blood stream through breakdowns in host defense barriers (mucositis, use of central venous catheters). Mucositis in particular is a significant risk factor for sepsis and is increasingly more common due to the widespread use of aggressive chemotherapy regimens.[18]

Neutropenia is defined as an absolute neutrophil count (ANC) less than $500 \times 10^3/\mu L$ ($500 \times 10^9/L$) cells or an ANC less than $1,000 \times 10^3/\mu L$ ($1,000 \times 10^9/L$) cells with a predicted decrease to less than $500 \times 10^3/\mu L$ ($500 \times 10^9/L$) cells. The ANC is calculated by multiplying the total WBC by the percentage of neutrophils (segmented neutrophils plus "bands"). Fever is defined as a single oral temperature greater than or equal to 38.3°C (101°F) or a temperature greater than or equal to 38.0°C (100.4°F) for at least 1 hour. The combination of these two factors defines FN.[19] The risk of infection during the period of neutropenia depends primarily on two factors:

- The duration of the neutropenia (time period of ANC less than $500 \times 10^3/\mu L$ ($500 \times 10^9/L$) cells)

- The severity of the neutropenia (lowest ANC level reached [nadir])

A multitude of other risk factors for FN have been identified (Table 99–5). Many of these are also risk factors for poor outcome in patients who experience FN. Cancer drug therapy regimens are also categorized as being high risk (greater than 20% incidence of FN reported in clinical trials) or intermediate risk (10–20% risk of FN reported in clinical trials). Similar to the approach to the prevention of CINV, it is important to consider both the regimen and patient-specific risk factors when determining whether a patient should receive prophylactic therapy for FN.

It is clear that patients with FN represent a heterogenous group. Some patients are at lower risk and could potentially be treated as outpatients thereby avoiding the risk and cost of hospitalization. The Multinational Association for Supportive Care in Cancer (MASCC) has validated a risk assessment tool that assigns a risk score to patients presenting with FN (Table 99–6).[21] Patients with a risk-index score greater than or equal to 21 are identified as low-risk and are candidates for outpatient therapy (discussed under Treatment).

Table 99–4	
Commonly Isolated Pathogens in Patients With FN	
Type of Organism	**Comments**
Bacteria	
Gram-positive organisms	Most common isolates in FN
Coagulase-negative staphylococci (i.e., *Staph epidermidis*)	Between 70% and 90% resistance to methicillin; indolent course with low mortality
Staph aureus	Some centers report greater than 50% resistance to methicillin
Enterococcus species	Resistance to vancomycin greater than or equal to 30%
Viridans streptococci	Increasing resistance to penicillin; result of fluoroquinolone prophylaxis; associated with mucositis
Gram-negative organisms	Infections rapidly fatal
	High mortality; increasing resistance to quinolones
Pseudomonas aeruginosa	Increased incidence of β-lactamase producing strains
Escherichia coli	Increased incidence of β-lactamase producing strains
Klebsiella species	
Enterobacter species	
Fungi	Occur primarily after prolonged neutropenia (greater than 1 week)
Yeasts	
Candida albicans	Increasing incidence (approximately 10%); high mortality
Nonalbicans *Candida* (*C. krusei, C. glabrata*)	Resistant to fluconazole; high mortality
Molds	Resistant to fluconazole; high mortality
Aspergillus species	Pulmonary infection common
Fusarium species	Emerging pathogen
Scedosporium species	Emerging pathogen

FN, febrile neutropenia.

From Refs. 16, 17.

Table 99–5	
Risk Factors for FN	
Patient Related	**Therapy Related**
Age 60 years or more	History of prior extensive chemotherapy
Poor performance status	Planned full dose intensity of chemotherapy
Bone marrow involvement by tumor	High-dose chemotherapy (i.e., bone marrow transplant)
Poor nutritional status	
Hematologic malignancy	Greater than 20% incidence of FN reported in clinical trials with treatment regimen
Elevated LDH	
Decreased hemoglobin level	
Baseline or first-cycle low neutrophil counts	10–20% incidence of FN reported in clinical trials with treatment regimen plus presence of patient-specific risk factors
History of previous FN	
Uncontrolled or advanced stage cancer	

FN, febrile neutropenia; LDH, lactate dehydrogenase.

From Ref. 20.

Table 99–6	
MASCC Risk-Index for Identifying Low-Risk Patients With FN	
Characteristic	**Score**
Burden of illness[a]	
No symptoms	5
Mild symptoms	5
Moderate symptoms	3
No hypotension	5
No COPD	4
Solid tumor or hematologic malignancy without fungal infection	4
No dehydration	3
Outpatient onset of fever	3
Age less than 60 years[b]	2

Note: A risk-index score of 21 or higher indicates that the patient is likely to be at low risk for complications and morbidity.

COPD, chronic obstructive pulmonary disease; FN, febrile neutropenia; MASCC, multinational association for supportive care in cancer.

[a]Choose one item only.

[b]Does not apply to patients 16 years of age or below.

From Ref. 21.

CLINICAL PRESENTATION AND DIAGNOSIS

Patients with suppressed immune systems are often unable to mount the same response to infection as normal individuals, thus limiting the expression of typical presenting signs and symptoms.[22] Often fever is the only indicator of infection and diagnosis is made empirically based on the patient's temperature, ANL, and coexisting risk factors for infection such as presence of an indwelling catheter, inpatient status, history of chemotherapy or radiotherapy, peripheral blood stem cell or bone marrow transplant, renal or hepatic compromise, and older age.[22,23]

PREVENTION

Three primary modalities for preventing infection in patients who are expected to become neutropenic have been utilized, the first of which is the least expensive and simplest:

- Vigilant hand hygiene
- Prophylactic antibiotics
- Colony-stimulating factors (CSFs)

The advantages and disadvantages of these strategies will be discussed individually in the following section.

Hand-Hygiene

As previously discussed, most infections in neutropenic patients are a result of endogenous flora; however, prevention of further acquisition of environmental pathogens is also important. Patients who are or will become neutropenic should

---

Clinical Presentation and Diagnosis of FN

General

- Only 50% of patients with FN have a clinically documented infection
- Only 25% of patients with FN have a microbiologically documented infection

Signs and Symptoms

- Fever is typically the only sign of infection, although septic patients may have chills
- Infected catheter sites may be erythematous and tender to the touch

Laboratory Tests

- CBC with differential
- Two blood cultures from *each* access site (peripheral and central), urinalysis, urine culture, chest x-ray, sputum cultures

Other Diagnostic Tests

- Detailed physical exam of oral mucosa, sinuses, skin, catheter access sites, perineal area (no rectal exam due to risk of bacteremia)

---

practice careful hand-washing and avoid contact with people who neglect hand-hygiene. In addition, ingestion of certain fresh fruits and vegetables as well as unprocessed dairy products should be avoided during the neutropenic period.

Prophylactic Antibiotics

Routine antibacterial prophylaxis is controversial and has been attempted primarily with sulfamethoxazole-trimethoprim (SMZ-TMP) and quinolones. SMZ-TMP offers improved prophylaxis for gram-positive organisms compared with quinolones while quinolones are more effective prophylaxis against gram-negative infections. The 2002 Infectious Diseases Society of America (IDSA) guidelines for the use of antimicrobial agents in cancer do not recommend the use of these agents for routine prophylaxis.[19] Reasons for this recommendation include the lack of a clear benefit on mortality rates and concerns regarding increasing antibiotic resistance. One exception is that SMZ-TMP is recommended for prophylaxis of *Pneumocystis jirovesi* (formerly *Pneumocystis carini*) pneumonitis (PCP) in all at-risk patients (i.e., bone marrow transplant recipients, AIDS), regardless of the presence of neutropenia.

Two recent meta-analyses add fuel to the controversy of routine antibiotic prophylaxis.[24,25] Decreases in infection-related mortality and gram-negative bacteremia were demonstrated with the use of quinolones, however overall adverse events were higher and most of the studies were conducted in patients with hematologic malignancies (an inherently high-risk group). Although two additional randomized trials in patients with both solid tumors and hematologic malignancies demonstrated lower rates of FN, infection, and hospitalization with oral prophylactic levofloxacin compared to placebo, the NCCN only recommends prophylactic levofloxacin for patients with expected duration of neutropenia (defined as an ANC less than 1,000/μL) for more than 7 days due to the:

- Unknown long-term consequences on the development of resistant organisms

- Emergence of *Clostridium difficile* and methicillin-resistant *Staphylococcus aureus* (MRSA) from fluoroquinolone overuse

- Ability to treat lower risk patients on an outpatient basis[26–28]

Therefore, the use of prophylactic quinolones in patients who are at high risk for infection (i.e., hematologic malignancies) is reasonable, however, use should not be routine for low-risk patients. If prophylactic quinolone use is adopted, changes in local patterns of resistance should be closely monitored.

Colony-Stimulating Factors

The CSFs stimulate the maturation and differentiation of neutrophil precursors. Three agents are currently approved for use in the United States (Table 99–7). The prophylactic use of these agents decreases days of hospitalization and use of empiric antibiotics by shortening the duration of severe neutropenia (defined as ANC less than $500 \times 10^3/\mu L$ ($500 \times 10^9/L$). There is little to no effect on the depth of neutrophil nadir. A recent meta-analysis found that the use of prophylactic granulocyte CSF (either filgrastim or pegfilgrastim) results in a 46% risk reduction of FN and a 48% risk reduction

in infectious mortality, although absolute differences are small (3.3% versus 1.7%).[29] It is critical to note that patients who receive these agents may still experience FN despite the risk reduction. The primary limitation of the use of these agents is cost. Clinical practice guidelines for the use of CSFs have been developed by the NCCN.[23] These guidelines recommend the use of CSFs beginning with the first cycle (primary prophylaxis) of chemotherapy when the risk of FN is greater than or equal to 20%. This is the point where the use of CSFs is cost effective when balanced against the cost of hospitalization and antimicrobials. Secondary prophylaxis refers to the subsequent prophylactic use of a CSF after a patient has had a prior episode of FN. This strategy should be utilized especially when the chemotherapy is being given in patients with the intention of cure (i.e., Hodgkin's lymphoma, early breast cancer). In this circumstance, administration of full doses of chemotherapy on time without delays has been shown to improve patient outcomes.

Although generally well tolerated, CSFs may cause bone pain in around 25% of patients. This may be managed with acetaminophen or nonsteroidal anti-inflammatory drugs (NSAIDs), although attention to the platelet count is warranted with the use of NSAIDs. Sargramostim in particular may result in low-grade fever and myalgias, perhaps as a result of its wider pattern of effector cell stimulation.

TREATMENT

Desired Outcomes

Because rapid death may occur with certain infections in neutropenic patients, prompt and emergent treatment is indicated. The primary goal is to prevent morbidity and

---

Table 99–7

Overview of CSF

Agent	Effector Cell(s)	Dosage	Common Adverse Effects	Comments[a]
Filgrastim (Neupogen GCSF)	Neutrophil	5 mcg/kg/day SC or IV *OR* round to 300 mcg or 480 mcg vial size	Bone pain (approximately 25%)	Begin 1–3 days after chemotherapy
Pegfilgrastim (Neulasta)	Neutrophil	6 mg SC one time	Bone pain (approximately 25%)	Self-mediated clearance via neutrophils. Once per cycle dosing. Administer 1–3 days after chemotherapy
Sargramostim (Leukine GMCSF)	Neutrophil, eosinophil, macrophage	250 mcg/m²/day SC or IV *OR* round to 250 mcg or 500 mcg vial size	First dose effect (hypotension, flushing). Low-grade fever. Bone pain. Injection-site skin reaction	Indicated for use following induction chemotherapy in older patients with AML. Limited experience and lack of FDA-approval for prevention of FN

AML, acute myeloid leukemia; FN, febrile neutropenia; GCSF, granulocyte-colony stimulating factor; GMCSF, granulocyte-macrophage colony stimulating factor; SC, subcutaneous.

[a]No renal or hepatic dose adjustments are required for any product listed in this table

From Ref. 23.

mortality during the neutropenic period. This is accomplished by effectively treating subclinical or established infections.

General Approach to Treatment

❸ *A risk assessment should be performed at presentation of FN to identify low-risk patients for potential outpatient treatment (Table 99–6). Patients who do not meet low-risk criteria should be hospitalized for parenteral administration of broad-spectrum antibacterials.* The IDSA has published evidence-based guidelines for the management of FN (Fig. 99–1).[19,30] The choice of initial antimicrobial agent(s) depends on the following factors:

- Presence of a central venous catheter
- Drug allergies
- Concurrent renal dysfunction or use of nephrotoxic agents
- Use of prophylactic antibiotics
- Institutional and/or community susceptibility patterns
- Cost

❸ *The administration of empiric therapy should begin immediately after cultures are taken. Therapy should not be withheld until after culture results are obtained.*

As illustrated in Figure 99–1, specific criteria exist for the addition of vancomycin for coverage of resistant gram-positive organisms or agents for coverage of fungal infections. Additional agents are necessary in the setting of continued fever or declining clinical status in neutropenic patients. In general, all empiric therapy is continued until recovery of the ANC to levels above $500 \times 10^3/\mu L$ $(500 \times 10^9/L)$ cells in patients with negative cultures. If a specific etiology is identified, appropriate therapy should be continued until 7 days after neutropenia resolves. Specific regimens with recommended dosages are summarized in Table 99–8.

▶ Nonpharmacologic Therapy

Prevention of infection is key. Hand-washing is critical in the prevention of disease transmission.[26] It is also important to ensure that patients receive annual influenza vaccines and have had a pneumonia vaccine and neutropenic patients should avoid individuals with active respiratory infections.[31] Plants and animal secretions are also sources of infection and should be avoided.[31] Indwelling catheters are often a source of infection; however, the Infectious Disease Society of America acknowledges that catheters do not always need to be removed. Catheters should be removed in the following circumstances: established tunnel infection (subcutaneous tunnel or periport infection, septic emboli, hypotension associated with catheter use, or a nonpatent catheter); recurrent infection; no response to antibiotics within 2 or 3 days.[19] Wound debridement should also be performed upon catheter removal. In the setting of peripheral blood stem cell or bone marrow transplant, the Centers for Disease Control (CDC) recommends the use of high-efficiency particulate air (HEPA) filtration systems in patient rooms and the NCCN suggests that HEPA filters are reasonable to be considered for other patients who experience prolonged neutropenia.[26] HEPA filters are likely to be most useful in preventing mold infections. Though several small studies have attempted to evaluate the effectiveness of isolation of neutropenic patients as a mechanism for infection prevention, no clear data are available to support this practice.[31]

▶ Pharmacologic Therapy

There are two primary choices for the initial management of high-risk FN: monotherapy and dual therapy (Fig. 99–1). Both regimens have been shown to be equivalent in randomized studies and meta-analyses. Monotherapy avoids the nephrotoxicity of the aminoglycosides and is potentially less expensive, but lacks significant gram-positive coverage and may increase selection of resistant organisms. Dual therapy provides synergistic activity, decreased resistance, and dual coverage of *P. aeruginosa*, but requires therapeutic monitoring for aminoglycosides.

Vancomycin adds broad-spectrum gram-positive coverage, however the increasing emergence of vancomycin-resistant organisms (i.e., *Enterococcus* spp) prompts conservative use of this medication. Furthermore, the European Organization for the Research and Treatment of Cancer (EORTC) found that although empiric vancomycin decreased the number of days of fever, it did not improve survival, and also resulted in increased renal and hepatic toxicities.[32] Thus, vancomycin should only be included as part of the initial therapy in the following cases:

- Severe mucositis
- Soft tissue infection
- Quinolone or TMP-SMX prophylaxis
- Hypotension or septic shock
- Colonization with resistant gram-positive organisms (i.e., MRSA)
- Evidence of central venous catheter infection

Vancomycin may be added to the empiric regimen after 3 to 5 days in persistently febrile patients or if cultures reveal gram-positive organisms. Vancomycin should be changed if

---

Patient Encounter 2, Part 2: FN

FG presents to the clinic approximately 8 days after his second cycle of cisplatin-etoposide with a temperature of 38.9°C (102.2°F). He is also hypotensive and coughing up green sputum. His CBC reveals a WBC of 840 $10^3/\mu L$ $(840 \times 10^9/L)$ with 10% (0.10) neutrophils and 15% (0.15) bands. He does not have a central line.

What is FG's ANC?

What treatment goals do you have for FG?

Construct an initial treatment plan for this patient.

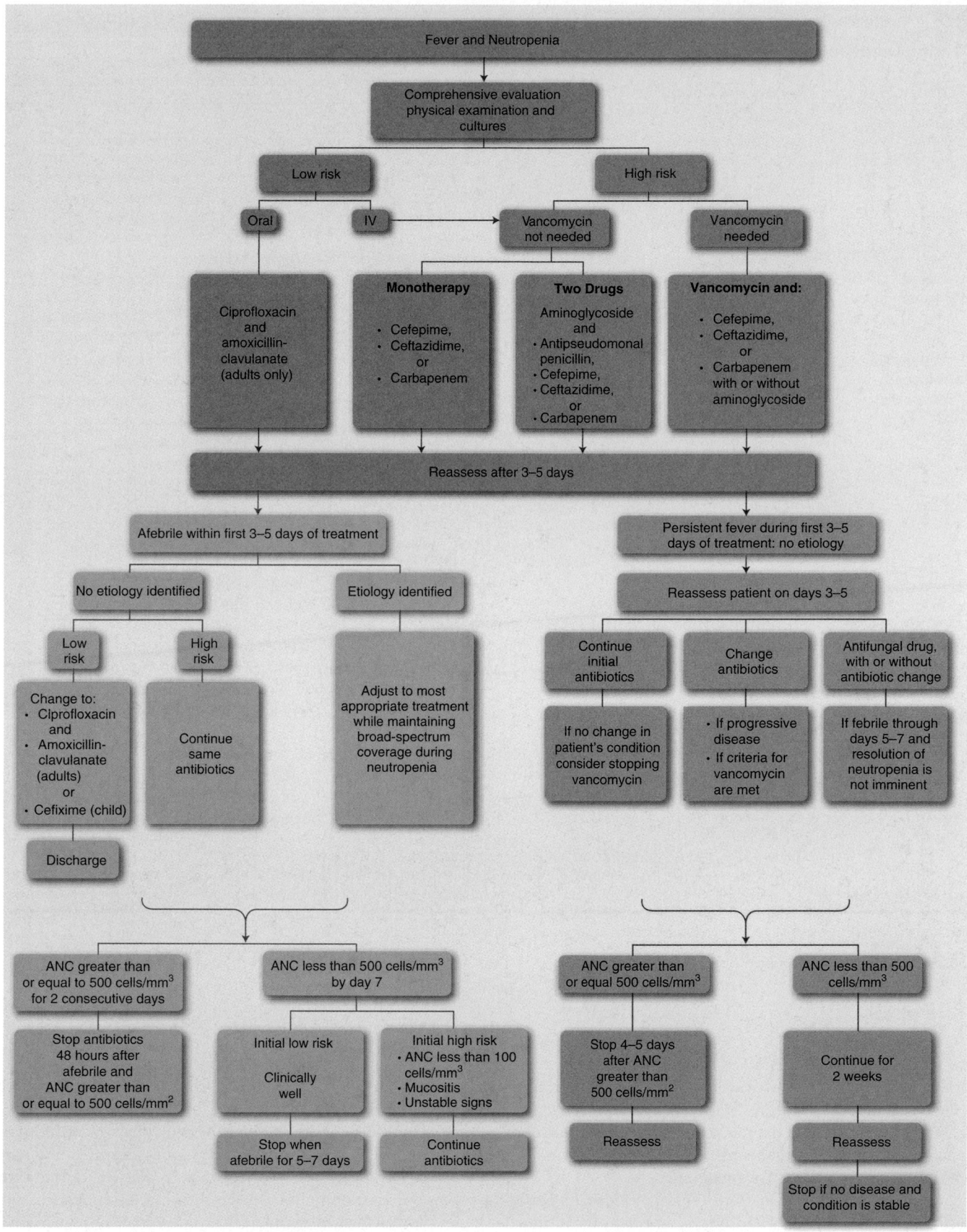

FIGURE 99–1. Management of febrile episodes in neutropenic cancer patients. (From Refs. 5, 12.)

Table 99-8

Dosing Guidelines for Empiric Antimicrobial Agents in FN

Regimen Type	Agents and Dosing[a]	Comments
Antibacterial		
β-lactam monotherapy	Cefepime 2 g IV every 8 hours Ceftazidime 2 g IV every 8 hours Imipenem 500 mg IV every 6 hours Meropenem 1 g IV every 8 hours Piperacillin/tazobactam 4.5 g IV every 8 hours	Although piperacillin/tazobactam is not recommended in the IDSA guidelines, recent data demonstrate equivalence to other monotherapy and dual therapy regimens. All of these agents require renal dose adjustment and none require adjustment in hepatic dysfunction. All except meropenem require adjustment during dialysis
Dual therapy with antipseudomonal β-lactam plus aminoglycoside	Cefepime, ceftazidime, imipenem, meropenem, piperacillin/tazobactam (above dosages), ticarcillin/clavulanic acid 3.1 g IV every 6 hours + gentamicin or tobramycin	Gentamicin or tobramycin 2 mg/kg loading dose followed by doses adjusted by serum concentrations; once daily dosing of aminoglycosides may be utilized. Both gentamicin and tobramycin require renal dose adjustment but are dosed based on serum levels. Neither gentamicin nor tobramycin require hepatic dose adjustment
Empiric regimens containing vancomycin	Cefepime, ceftazidime, imipenem, meropenem (above dosages) + vancomycin 0.5–1 g every 6–12 hours ± aminoglycoside	Vancomycin dosages may be adjusted based on serum levels and are adjusted for renal disease and dialysis. No dose adjustment is recommended for hepatic dysfunction
Dual therapy containing fluoroquinolone	Ciprofloxacin 400 mg IV every 8 hours + piperacillin/tazobactam, ceftazidime (above dosages)	Cannot be used in patients who receive fluoroquinolone prophylaxis. Dose adjusted in renal disease and dialysis but not for hepatic dysfunction
Low-risk oral regimen	Ciprofloxacin 750 mg po every 12 hours + amoxicillin/clavulanate 500–875 mg po every 12 hours	For patients with MASCC score greater than or equal to 21 not receiving fluoroquinolone prophylaxis. Amoxicillin/clavulanate is adjusted in renal disease and dialysis but not hepatic dysfunction
Antifungal		
Amphotericin B deoxycholate	0.5–1 mg/kg IV daily	Premedication with acetaminophen and diphenhydramine; 500 mL normal saline boluses before and after. No dose adjustments are recommended for renal or hepatic dysfunction or during dialysis
Liposomal amphotericin B	3 mg/kg IV daily	Lower incidence of nephrotoxicity and infusion reactions; more expensive. No dose adjustments are recommended for renal or hepatic dysfunction or during dialysis
Caspofungin	70 mg/kg IV loading dose on day 1 followed by 50 mg/kg IV daily	Dosage adjustment in hepatic dysfunction but not for renal disease or dialysis
Voriconazole	6 mg/kg IV loading dose every 12 hours on day 1 followed by 4 mg/kg po/IV every 12 hours	Dosage adjustment in hepatic dysfunction; IV formulation contraindicated if creatinine clearance less than 50 mL/min; multiple drug interactions
Posaconazole	Prophylactic: 200 mg po three times a day with food Salvage: 200 mg po four times a day with food then 400 mg po two times a day once stable	Not FDA-approved for primary or salvage therapy for infasive fungal infections though used clinically; drug of choice per NCCN for prophylaxis in neutropenic patients with AML or MDS. No dose adjustments required for renal or hepatic dysfunction or during dialysis

AML, acute myeloid leukemia; MDS; myelodysplastic syndrome; NCCN, National Comprehensive Cancer Network.

[a]Dosing for adult patients; adjust doses for renal dysfunction.

the gram-positive organism is susceptible to other antibacterials or discontinued in patients with persistent fever after 3 days with negative cultures. Linezolid, quiuprostin/dalfoprostin, tigecycline, and daptomycin may be used in cases of vancomycin-resistant organisms or if vancomycin is not an option due to drug allergy or intolerance.

Empiric antifungal agents are typically added in persistently febrile patients after 5 to 7 days, especially if continued neutropenia is expected. Amphotericin B has historically been the drug of choice due to its broad-spectrum activity against both yeast (*Candida* spp) and mold (*Aspergillus* spp) infections. Because frequent toxicity (nephrotoxicity, infusion

reactions) limits the use of amphotericin B, less toxic alternatives have been studied. Lipid formulations of amphotericin provide decreased toxicity and liposomal amphotericin B (AmBisome) has been shown to be equivalent to conventional amphotericin B as empiric therapy, but is significantly more expensive. The role of voriconazole is unclear at this time; however, caspofungin has been shown to be equivalent with less toxicity when compared to liposomal amphotericin B in a randomized trial and is FDA-approved for this indication.[33] Itraconazole has also been used in some institutions, however, its use is complicated by poor bioavailability of oral preparations and numerous drug interactions. Posaconazole is a newer azole that is preferred by the NCCN for prophylactic use in neutropenic patients with acute myeloid leukemia (AML) or myelodysplastic syndrome (MDS) and for patients with graft versus host disease (GVHD) while receiving intensive immunosuppressive therapy. It is not FDA-approved as primary or salvage therapy for the treatment of invasive fungal infections but it is approved by the European Union for invasive aspergillosis and other fungal infections that are refractory to standard antifungal agents.

As stated earlier, low-risk patients fulfilling the MASCC criteria (Table 99–6) may be treated empirically as an outpatient with a regimen combining amoxicillin/clavulanic acid and ciprofloxacin. Ciprofloxacin and clindamycin are reasonable alternatives for penicillin-allergic patients.

The CSF should not routinely be utilized for treatment of FN in conjunction with antimicrobial therapy.[19] However, the use of CSFs in certain high-risk patients with hypotension, documented fungal infection, pneumonia, or sepsis is reasonable. A recent meta-analysis demonstrated that hospitalization and neutrophil recovery are shortened and infection-related mortality is marginally improved.[34] As with prophylactic use of these agents, cost considerations limit their use to high-risk patients.

Patient Care and Monitoring: FN

1. Counsel patients receiving cytotoxic chemotherapy or alemtuzumab to promptly report fever. Provide patients with a diet to use during the neutropenic period. Counsel patients to avoid close contact with sick friends and relatives and remind the patient and caregivers of the importance of handwashing.

2. If FN occurs, patient history is important:

   a. What chemotherapy did the patient receive and when? Is the ANC on the way down (before nadir) or on the way up (after nadir)? Was the patient receiving prophylactic antibiotics, filgrastim, sargramostim, or pegfilgrastim?

   b. Did the patient have previous episodes of FN? What were the previous culture results to determine colonization status?

3. Assess the patient daily for any new signs or symptoms of infection. Evaluate the patient for adverse drug reactions, drug allergies, and interactions. Have all antibiotics been dose adjusted for renal or hepatic dysfunction?

4. For patients receiving oral antibiotics either prophylactically or as treatment of FN: Counsel patients that initial or persistent fever should be promptly reported and that compliance with the regimen is critical. Patients should also have easy access to medical care and adequate caregiver support. Provide information on drug interactions and adverse effects.

OUTCOME EVALUATION

The success of the treatment of FN depends on the adequate recovery of the ANC and either optimal antimicrobial coverage of identified organisms or empiric coverage of unidentified organisms. Monitor the CBC with differential and Tmax (maximum temperature during previous 24 hours) daily. Assess renal and hepatic function at least twice weekly, especially in patients receiving nephrotoxic agents. Vital signs should be taken every 4 hours. Follow-up on blood and urine culture results daily since many cultures do not become positive for several days. Assess the patient daily for pain that may indicate an infectious source. Conduct daily physical examination of common sites of infection. Repeat cultures and chest X-ray in persistently febrile patients and culture developing sources of infection (i.e., stool cultures for diarrhea).

CARDIOVASCULAR COMPLICATIONS: SUPERIOR VENA CAVA SYNDROME (SVCS)

INTRODUCTION

Superior vena cava syndrome (SVCS) is a relatively rare complication of underlying cancer, although nonmalignant, may also occur in patients with cancer. SVCS is rarely immediately life-threatening except in patients with airway compromise and/or laryngeal or cerebral edema. However, rapid recognition of typical presenting symptoms facilitates referral for tissue diagnosis (if unknown) and treatment.

EPIDEMIOLOGY AND ETIOLOGY

SVCS occurs in around 15,000 patients per year, 90% of which are caused by malignancy. Specific cancers most commonly associated with SVCS are listed in Table 99–9. Lung cancer is the most frequent cause, of which small cell lung cancer (SCLC) is the most frequent subtype associated with SVCS. This is thought to be due its predilection for the central and **perihilar** areas of the lung. Interestingly, right-sided lung cancers are four times more likely than left-sided lesions

Table 99–9	
Tumors Most Commonly Associated With SVCS	
Cause	**Frequency (%)**
Nonsmall cell lung cancer	50
Small cell lung cancer	22
Lymphoma	12
Metastatic cancer (esp. breast)	9
Germ Cell Tumor	3
Thymoma	2
Mesothelioma	1

From Ref. 35.

to cause SVCS. Mediastinal masses from lymphomas are the second most common cause.

The most common nonmalignant etiology of SVCS is catheter-related thrombosis, primarily due to the increasing use of central access devices. Other causes include benign teratoma, tuberculosis, silicosis, and sarcoidosis.

PATHOPHYSIOLOGY

The SVC is the primary drainage vein for blood return from the head, neck, and upper extremities. It is a relatively thin-walled vein that is particularly vulnerable to obstruction from adjacent tumor invasion or thrombosis. The obstruction leads to elevated venous pressure, although collateral veins partially compensate. This is one reason for the relatively slow onset of the classic symptoms of SVCS. In fact, 75% of patients have signs and symptoms for more than 1 week before seeking medical attention.[35]

CLINICAL PRESENTATION AND DIAGNOSIS

Visible swelling of the face, neck, chest, and upper limbs with obvious venous distention are the usual presenting symptoms of SVCS.[35] Patients may also report coughing, hoarseness, sleep disturbances, dyspnea, headache, and confusion.[35] Diagnosis is made with consideration of these symptoms in conjunction with imaging studies which show unusual narrowing of the upper airway.[35]

TREATMENT

Desired Outcomes

❹ *The primary goal of treatment of SVCS is to relieve the obstruction of the SVC by treating the underlying malignancy.* In the case of SVCS caused by thrombosis, the goal is to eliminate the thrombus and prevent further clot formation. Resolution of the obstruction will rapidly relieve symptoms and restore normal SVC function. The final goal of therapy is to avoid potentially fatal complications of SVCS such as cerebral edema from rapid increases in intracranial pressure (ICP) and intracranial thrombosis or bleeding.

General Approach to Treatment

Because the majority of SVCS is not immediately life-threatening, a tissue diagnosis (if malignancy is unknown) to specifically identify the cancer origin is critical since treatment approaches vary considerably according to tumor histology. Thus, therapy can typically be withheld until a definitive tissue diagnosis is established. While biopsy results are pending, supportive measures such as head elevation, diuretics, corticosteroids and supplemental oxygen may be utilized.

▶ *Nonpharmacologic Therapy*

Radiation therapy is the treatment of choice for chemotherapy-resistant tumors such as nonsmall cell lung cancer

---

Clinical Presentation and Diagnosis of SVCS

General
- Presentation depends on the degree of SVCS obstruction
- Almost complete obstruction is necessary to demonstrate classic symptoms

Signs and Symptoms
- Face, neck, and upper extremity edema, dyspnea, cough, dilated upper extremity veins and, orthopnea are most common
- Less common—hoarseness, dysphagia, dizziness, headache, lethargy, chest pain
- Patients with elevated ICP may have mental status changes
- Patients with airway obstruction may have shortness of breath

Diagnostic tests
- Tissue biopsy to determine underlying malignancy (if unknown), chest x-ray, CT scan, bronchoscopy, mediastinoscopy

---

(NSCLC) or in chemotherapy-refractory patients with SVCS. Between 70% and 90% of patients will experience relief of symptoms. Radiation therapy may also be combined with chemotherapy for chemotherapy-sensitive tumors such as SCLC and lymphoma. In the rare emergency situations of airway obstruction or elevated ICP, empiric radiotherapy prior to tissue diagnosis should be used. In most patients, symptoms resolve within 1 to 3 weeks.

Surgical options for the management of SVCS include stent placement and surgical bypass. SVC stenting may provide longer term relief of symptoms than radiotherapy, thus it is often used in the palliative care setting when chemotherapy has failed.[36] One disadvantage of SVC stenting is the need for anticoagulation, especially in patients at high risk for thrombosis. The role of surgical bypass is limited to patients with complete SVC obstruction or patients who are refractory to chemotherapy and radiotherapy, thus it is rarely indicated.

▶ *Pharmacologic Therapy*

Cytotoxic chemotherapy is the treatment of choice for chemotherapy-sensitive tumors such as SCLC and lymphoma. As indicated above, chemotherapy may also be combined with radiotherapy, especially in patients with lymphoma who have bulky mediastinal lymphadenopathy.

Corticosteroids play a key role in the management of SVCS, particularly in cases of lymphoma since these tumors inherently respond to corticosteroid therapy. They are also helpful in the setting of respiratory compromise. Corticosteroids benefit patients who are receiving radiation therapy by reduction of local radiation-induced inflammation and patients with increased ICP. Dexamethasone 4 mg IV or by

Patient Care and Monitoring: SVCS

Surgery provides rapid relief of symptoms within 1 to 7 days of stent placement.[32] Patients who receive chemotherapy and/or radiotherapy will generally experience symptom relief within 1 to 2 weeks. Monitor the patient for relief of symptoms by:

- Daily physical assessment of signs and symptoms
- Daily monitoring of fluid status
- For corticosteroid use: Daily serum glucose, insomnia, fluid retention, GI upset, mental status changes, signs and symptoms of infection.
- Repeat CT scans of the chest after the first cycle of chemotherapy, surgical stenting, or radiotherapy to assess tumor response.

Clinical Presentation and Diagnosis of Spinal Cord Compression

General

- Once neurologic deficits appear, progression to irreversible paralysis may occur within hours to days.
- Around 10% to 38% of patients present with multiple sites of spinal involvement.

Signs and Symptoms

- Back pain is present in more than 90% of patients.
  - Initially localized and increases in intensity over several weeks
  - Aggravated by movement, supine positioning, coughing, sneezing, neck flexion, straight leg raise, Valsalva maneuver, palpation of spine
- Sensory deficit
  - Cervical spine compression—quadriplegia
  - Thoracic spine compression—paraplegia
  - Upper lumbar spine compression—bowel and bladder dysfunction (constipation and urinary retention) and abnormal extensor plantar reflexes
- Weakness

Diagnostic Tests

- MRI with gadolinium enhancement is the gold standard.
- X-rays may be helpful to identify bone abnormalities.

mouth every 6 hours is a frequently used regimen. The dosage should be tapered upon completion of radiation therapy or resolution of symptoms.

The role of diuretics in the management of SVCS is controversial. While patients may derive symptomatic relief from edema, complications such as dehydration and reduced venous blood flow may exacerbate the condition. If diuretics are utilized, furosemide is most frequently used with diligent monitoring of the patient's fluid status and blood pressure.

In the case of thrombosis-related SVCS, anticoagulation is controversial since there is a lack of survival benefit. However, thrombolytics (i.e., alteplase) and anticoagulation with heparin and warfarin may be beneficial in patients with thrombosis due to indwelling catheters if used within 7 days of onset of symptoms, although catheter removal may be required.

OUTCOME EVALUATION

The major measure of outcome of treatment of SVCS is the relief of symptoms, regardless of the therapy utilized.

NEUROLOGIC COMPLICATIONS: SPINAL CORD COMPRESSION

INTRODUCTION

Although not typically life-threatening, spinal cord compression is a true oncologic emergency since delays in treatment by mere hours may lead to permanent neurologic dysfunction. Practitioners must quickly recognize the signs and symptoms of this condition to facilitate rapid management strategies.

EPIDEMIOLOGY AND ETIOLOGY

Around 20,000 cancer patients experience spinal cord compression in the United States every year, most of which involves the thoracic spine (approximately 70%). Cancers that inherently metastasize to the bone (i.e., breast, prostate, and lung) are the most frequent underlying malignancies associated with this complication. Most spinal cord compression occurs in patients with a known malignancy; however 8% to 34% of cases occur as the initial presentation of cancer, especially in patients with non-Hodgkin's lymphoma, multiple myeloma, and lung cancer.[37]

PATHOPHYSIOLOGY

The spinal cord emerges from the brain stem at the base of the skull and terminates at the second lumbar vertebra. The thoracic spine is most vulnerable to cord compression because of natural kyphosis and because the width of the thoracic spinal canal is the smallest among the vertebrae. Most spinal cord compression is due to adjacent vertebral metastases that compress the spinal cord or from pathologic compression fracture of the vertebra. This results in significant edema and inflammation in the affected area.

Patients with spinal cord compression are in acute, severe back and/or neck pain and may present to the emergency department for evaluation. Diagnosis is made based on symptoms and imaging studies that show fractured vertebrae.

TREATMENT

Desired Outcomes

⑤ *Because patients with spinal metastases are generally incurable, the primary goal of treatment of spinal cord compression is palliation. The most important prognostic factor for patients presenting with spinal cord compression is the degree of underlying neurologic dysfunction.* Only around 10% of patients who present with paralysis are able to ambulate following treatment.[37] Therefore, the goals of treatment are recovery of normal neurologic function, local tumor control, pain control, and stabilization of the spine. Therapeutic options depend primarily on the following factors:

- Underlying malignancy
- Prior therapies
- Stability of the spine at presentation
- Overall patient prognosis

▶ *Nonpharmacologic Therapy*

Radiation therapy is generally considered to be the treatment of choice for most patients. Exceptions to this include patients with prior radiation to the treatment site and patients with inherently radio-resistant tumors (i.e., melanoma, renal cell carcinoma). The radiation field should include two vertebral bodies above and below the involved area.

Surgery for spinal cord compression typically involves either laminectomy for posterior lesions or decompression with fixation. Surgery is the treatment of choice for the following patients: (a) patients with unstable spine requiring stabilization; (b) immediately impending sphincter dysfunction requiring rapid spinal decompression; (c) patients who do not respond to or have received their maximum dose of radiotherapy; (d) direct compression of the spinal cord due to spinal bony fragments.[37] Recent evidence suggests that surgery followed by radiation therapy may be superior to radiotherapy alone in terms of increased ambulation time after treatment, maintenance of continence, and rates of nonambulatory patients becoming ambulatory.[38] Surgery is also useful for establishing a tissue diagnosis in cases of unknown malignancy. Overall, the risks and benefits of surgery must be weighed against the expected prognosis of the patient in light of the significant rehabilitation required after surgery.

▶ *Pharmacologic Therapy*

Corticosteroids play a vital role in the management of spinal cord compression. Dexamethasone is most frequently used to reduce edema, inhibit inflammation, and delay onset of neurologic complications. Dexamethasone has been shown to improve ambulation in combination with radiation as compared to radiation alone.[39] Significant controversy exists regarding the optimal dosing of dexamethasone. Oral loading doses of 10 to 100 mg followed by 4 to 24 mg orally four times daily have been used. Higher doses may be used in cases of rapidly progressing symptoms, but adverse

---

Patient Care and Monitoring: Spinal Cord Compression

Monitor patients for:

1. Improved symptoms of sensory loss using physical exam every 4 hours until symptoms improve then daily
2. Improved autonomic system function including urine and bowel control every 4 hours until symptoms improve then daily
3. Improved pain control using detailed pain assessment every 2 to 4 hours during initial titration then daily thereafter
4. For corticosteroid use: Serum glucose, insomnia, fluid retention, GI upset, mental status changes, signs and symptoms of infection daily

effects including GI bleeding and psychosis are more severe. Steroids should be continued during radiation therapy then tapered appropriately.

Pain management is also of critical importance in patients with spinal cord compression. While dexamethasone will provide some benefit, opioid analgesics should also be used and titrated rapidly to achieve adequate pain control.

OUTCOME EVALUATION

Patients who receive definitive treatment with radiation and/or surgery generally derive benefit within days.

COMPLICATIONS OF BRAIN METASTASES

INTRODUCTION

Brain metastases are among the most feared complications of cancer and generally carry a poor prognosis. One serious consequence of brain metastases is elevated ICP, which can rapidly lead to fatal intracranial herniation and death. Rapid identification of the signs and symptoms of brain metastases is critical to improve long-term outcome and avoid mortality. The signs and symptoms of brain metastasis can be confused with common psychological distress or other neurologic problems (such as headaches) that may go unrecognized. It is important that patients who are suspected to have brain metastasis are quickly referred for appropriate management.

EPIDEMIOLOGY AND ETIOLOGY

Brain metastasis is the most common neurologic complication seen in patients with cancer. Approximately 170,000 patients develop brain metastases in the United States each

Table 99–10

Cancers Most Frequently Associated With Brain Metastases

Type of Cancer	Frequency (%)
Lung cancer	18–64
Breast cancer	2–21
Melanoma	4–16
Colorectal cancer	2–11
Hematologic malignancies (i.e., leukemia)	Approximately 10 (primarily due to leptomeningeal spread)

From Ref. 43.

year.[40] Many malignancies are frequently associated with brain metastases (Table 99–10). While melanoma is the tumor type most likely to metastasize to the brain, brain metastases due to lung and breast cancer are seen more often, as they are among the most common cancers. In addition, brain metastases may be diagnosed at the same time as the primary malignancy in around 20% of cases.[41] Around 80% of brain metastases occur in the cerebral hemispheres, 15% in the cerebellum, and 5% in the brain stem.

PATHOPHYSIOLOGY

A delicate balance of normal pressure is maintained in the brain and spinal cord by brain, blood, and cerebrospinal fluid. Since the brain is contained within a confined space (skull), any foreign mass contained within that space causes adverse sequelae. This results in either destruction or displacement of normal brain tissue with associated edema. Most brain metastases occur through hematogenous spread of the primary tumor and around 80% of patients will have multiple sites of metastases within the brain.

CLINICAL PRESENTATION AND DIAGNOSIS

Patients with brain metastases may have no symptoms. Alternatively, they may have severe headaches, vision changes, and personality/mood disturbances depending on the location of the metastasis. Diagnosis is made based on physical signs and symptoms and brain CT or MRI which indicate a mass.

TREATMENT

Desired Outcomes

Therapeutic modalities used for the management of brain metastases may be divided into symptomatic management and definitive management. ❻ *The goals of treatment of brain metastases are to manage symptoms by reducing cerebral edema, treat the underlying malignancy both locally and systemically, and improve survival.*

Clinical Presentation and Diagnosis of Brain Metastasis

General

- Almost all patients with brain metastases are symptomatic.
- New cerebral neurologic symptoms in a cancer patient should initiate evaluation for brain metastases.
- Other causes of brain lesions including hemorrhage, infection, and infarct should be ruled out.

Signs and Symptoms

- Mental status changes (most common)—loss of consciousness, irritability, confusion
- Hemiparesis, aphasia, papilledema, weakness, seizure, nausea, and vomiting
- Headache
  - May be of gradual onset or sudden in the case of hemorrhage

Diagnostic Tests

- MRI with contrast enhancement is the gold standard
- CT scans may be used in patients with pacemakers, but may miss small metastases

General Approach to Treatment

Patients with brain metastases have a poor prognosis. Untreated patients generally have a median survival of 1 month. The choice of treatment depends primarily on the status of the patient's underlying malignancy and the number and sites of brain metastases. The primary definitive treatments for brain metastases are surgery and radiation therapy. Pharmacologic modalities are primarily used to control symptoms, although cytotoxic chemotherapy plays a limited role in the management.

► Nonpharmacologic Therapy

Radiation therapy is the treatment of choice for most patients with brain metastases. Most patients receive whole-brain radiation because the majority of brain metastases are multifocal. Another method known as stereotactic radiosurgery provides intense focal radiation, typically using a linear accelerator or gamma knife, in patients who cannot tolerate surgery or have lesions that are surgically inaccessible (i.e., brain stem). Because brain metastases can occur in up to 50% of patients with small cell lung cancer, prophylactic cranial irradiation is recommended in patients with good performance status who at least partially respond to chemotherapy to both prevent the development of brain metastases and to prolong survival.[42] Although other cancers can metastasize to the brain, the benefits of routine prophylactic cranial irradiation have only been demonstrated in studies conducted in patients with small cell lung cancer.[42]

Surgery plays a key role in the management of patients with brain metastases, particularly in patients whose systemic disease is well-controlled and in patients with solitary lesions. Surgery may also benefit patients with multiple metastatic sites who have a single dominant lesion with current or impending neurologic sequelae.

In cases of elevated ICP due to cerebral herniation, mechanical hyperventilation to decrease the arterial P_{CO_2} down to 25 mm Hg acutely decreases ICP by causing cerebral vasoconstriction. Elevation of the patient bed may also quickly reduce the ICP. It should be noted that these strategies only relieve symptoms and definitive therapy is still required.

▶ Pharmacologic Therapy

Corticosteroids are a mainstay in the management of brain metastases. They reduce edema that typically surrounds sites of metastases thereby reducing ICP. A loading dose of dexamethasone 10 mg IV followed by 4 mg by mouth or IV every 6 hours is typically used. Symptom relief may occur shortly after the loading dose, although the maximum benefit may not be seen for several days (after definitive therapy).

Mannitol is an agent that may be used in patients with impending cerebral herniation. Mannitol is an osmotic diuretic that shifts brain osmolarity from the brain to the blood. Doses of 100 g (1–2 g/kg) as an IV bolus should be used. Repeated doses are typically not recommended since mannitol may diffuse into brain tissue leading to rebound increased ICP.[43]

Twenty percent of patients with brain metastases may present with seizures and require anticonvulsant therapy. Phenytoin is the most frequently used agent with a loading dose of 15 mg/kg followed by 300 mg by mouth daily (titrated to therapeutic levels between 10 and 20 mcg/mL). Diazepam 5 mg IV may be used for rapid control of persistent seizures. Prophylactic anticonvulsants have frequently been utilized; however, a recent metaanalysis did not support their use.[44] Thus, because adverse effects and drug interactions are common, the routine use of prophylactic anticonvulsants is not recommended.

OUTCOME EVALUATION

The success of therapy is based on the ability to decrease symptoms, treat the underlying sites of disease within the brain, and prolong survival.

UROLOGIC COMPLICATIONS: HEMORRHAGIC CYSTITIS

INTRODUCTION

Hemorrhagic cystitis is defined as acute or insidious bleeding from the lining of the bladder. Although therapy with certain medications is the most common cause, it is also the most preventable. Once it occurs, hemorrhagic cystitis causes significant morbidity and mortality rates between 2% and 4%. This section will focus on preventative strategies for chemotherapeutic agents, which rely heavily on pharmacotherapeutic approaches.

EPIDEMIOLOGY AND ETIOLOGY

Numerous etiologies have been linked to hemorrhagic cystitis (Table 99–11).[45] Of these, the oxazaphosphorine alkylating agents (cyclophosphamide and ifosfamide) are most frequently implicated. Incidence rates vary considerably, but generally range between 18% and 40% with ifosfamide and 0.5% to 40% with high-dose cyclophosphamide in the absence of prophylactic measures.[46] Chronic, low-dose oral cyclophosphamide as typically used in autoimmune disorders and chronic lymphocytic leukemia is also infrequently associated with hemorrhagic cystitis.

Patient Care and Monitoring: Brain Metastasis

1. Assess patient symptoms for prompt referral for radiation or surgery.

2. For patients receiving corticosteroids, monitor for adverse effects and drug interactions. Does the patient need GI prophylaxis for long-term treatment? Slowly taper once symptoms improve and/or radiation or surgery is completed.

3. Evaluate the patient for drug interactions, allergies, and adverse effects with phenytoin or corticosteroid therapy.

4. Instruct patients receiving phenytoin about symptoms of elevated serum concentrations (nystagmus, blurred vision, dizziness, drowsiness, lethargy).

5. Provide patient education regarding when to take medications, importance of compliance, and promptly report symptoms of recurrence (mental status changes, seizures).

Table 99–11	
Primary Causes of Hemorrhagic Cystitis	
Pharmacologic	**Nonpharmacologic**
Cyclophosphamide	Pelvic irradiation
Chronic low doses	Viral infection
High-doses used in BMT	Cytomegalovirus
Ifosfamide	Papovavirus
Intravesicular thiotepa	Herpes simplex virus
Chronic oral busulfan	Adenovirus
Anabolic steroids	

BMT, bone marrow transplantation

From Ref. 45.

Twenty percent of patients receiving pelvic irradiation may experience hemorrhagic cystitis, especially with concurrent cyclophosphamide. Viral infections commonly associated with this condition most frequently occur in bone marrow transplant recipients who may also receive cyclophosphamide.

PATHOPHYSIOLOGY

Cyclophosphamide or ifosfamide induced damage to the bladder wall is primarily caused by their shared metabolite known as acrolein. Acrolein causes sloughing and inflammation of the bladder lining, leading to bleeding and hemorrhage. This is most common when urine output is low since higher concentrations of acrolein come into contact with the bladder urothelium for longer periods of time.

CLINICAL PRESENTATION AND DIAGNOSIS

Patients with hemorrhagic cystitis from treatment may present with dysuria, anuria, or hematuria. Diagnosis is made based on symptoms and urinalysis which shows presence of red blood cells in the urine.

PREVENTION

❼ *The use of effective prevention strategies can decrease the incidence of hemorrhagic cystitis to less than 5% in patients receiving cyclophosphamide or ifosfamide. There are three methods to reduce the risk: administration of mesna, hyperhydration, and bladder irrigation with catheterization. Mesna*

is the primary method used with ifosfamide while all three strategies are used with cyclophosphamide.

Mesna is a thiol compound that is rapidly oxidized in the bloodstream after administration to dimesna, which is inactive. However, once filtered through the kidneys, dimesna is reduced back to mesna which binds to acrolein leading to inactivation and excretion. The American Society of Clinical Oncology (ASCO) has published evidence-based guidelines for the dosing and administration of mesna (Table 99–12).[46] The dose of oral mesna must be double the IV dose due to oral bioavailability between 40% and 50%. Because the half-life of mesna (approximately 1.2 hours) is much shorter than that of ifosfamide or cyclophosphamide, prolonged administration of mesna beyond the end of the chemotherapy infusion is critical (Fig. 99–2). Patients should receive at least 2 L of IV fluids beginning 12 to 24 hours before and ending 24 to 48 hours after the last dose of chemotherapy.

Hyperhydration with normal saline at 3 L/m^2/day with IV furosemide to maintain urine output greater than 100 mL/hour has also been used with cyclophosphamide. Continuous bladder irrigation by catheterization uses normal saline at 250 to 1,000 mL/hour to flush acrolein from the bladder. Mesna is equivalent to both strategies in patients receiving high-dose cyclophosphamide and avoids the discomfort and infection risk with catheterization and the intensity of hyperhydration. Thus, mesna is the preventative method of choice.

TREATMENT

Desired Outcomes

If hemorrhagic cystitis occurs, the goals of treatment are to decrease exposure to the offending etiology, establish and maintain urine outflow, avoid obstruction and renal compromise, and maintain blood and plasma volume. Restoration of normal bladder function is the ultimate goal following acute treatment.

General Approach to Treatment

The treatment of hemorrhagic cystitis first involves discontinuation of the offending agent. Agents such as anticoagulants and inhibitors of platelet function should also be discontinued. IV fluids should be aggressively administered to irrigate the bladder. Blood and platelet transfusions may be necessary to maintain normal hematologic values. Pain should be managed with opioid analgesics. Local intravesicular therapies may be necessary if hematuria does not resolve (Fig. 99–3).

▶ *Nonpharmacologic Therapy*

A large-diameter, multihole urethral catheter should be inserted to facilitate saline lavage and evacuation of blood clots. Surgical removal of blood clots under anesthesia may be required if saline lavage is ineffective. Active bleeding

---

Clinical Presentation and Diagnosis of Urologic Complications

General

- Presentation may be mild (microscopic hematuria) or severe (massive hemorrhage) and develops during or shortly after chemotherapy infusion.

Signs and Symptoms

- Suprapubic pain and cramping, urinary urgency and frequency, dysuria and burning, hematuria
- Urinary retention leading to **hydronephrosis** and renal failure may occur if large blood clots obstruct the ureters or bladder outlet

Laboratory Tests

- Urine dipsticks for blood
- Urinalysis reveals more than 3 RBCs per high-power field—microscopic hematuria
- CBC with differential, PT/INR, aPTT, BUN, creatinine

Table 99–12

ASCO Guidelines for the Use of Mesna With Ifosfamide and High-Dose Cyclophosphamide

Chemotherapy Schedule	Dosing Schedule for Mesna	Comments
Low-dose ifosfamide 2 g/m²/day	Oral: 100% of total daily dose of ifosfamide given 20% IV 15 minutes before and 40% po 2 and 6 hours after start of ifosfamide	Available in 400-mg tablets Peak urinary thiol concentrations with oral mesna is at 3 hours If patient vomits within 2 hours of administration, repeat dose orally or IV
Standard-dose ifosfamide 2.5 g/m²/day	Bolus: 60% of total daily dose of ifosfamide given IV in 20% increments 15 minutes before and 4 and 8 hours after start of ifosfamide Infusion: 60% of total daily dose of ifosfamide given 20% IV 15 minutes before and 40% by continuous infusion during and for 12–24 hours after end of ifosfamide	Peak urinary thiol concentrations with IV mesna is at 1 hour Compatible with ifosfamide and cyclophosphamide by Y-site administration or when admixed in the same bag
High-dose ifosfamide Greater than 2.5 g/m²/day	Lack of evidence for dosing, however higher doses for longer duration recommended based on longer half-life of ifosfamide at high doses	
Standard-dose cyclophosphamide	Use of mesna is not routinely necessary	
High-dose cyclophosphamide (bone marrow transplant)	Bolus: 40% of cyclophosphamide dose given IV at hours 0, 3, 6, and 9 after cyclophosphamide Infusion: 100% of cyclophosphamide dose given by continuous infusion until 24 hours after cyclophosphamide	Should be combined with saline diuresis (1.5 L/m²/day of normal saline)

ASCO, American Society of Clinical Oncology.

From Ref. 46.

from isolated areas may be cauterized with an electrode or laser. In severe cases that are unresponsive to local or systemic pharmacologic intervention, urinary diversion with percutaneous **nephrostomy** or surgical removal of the bladder may be required.

▶ *Pharmacologic Therapy*

A number of local or systemic agents are utilized in the treatment of hemorrhagic cystitis.[45] Local (direct instillation into the bladder), one-time administration of hemostatic agents

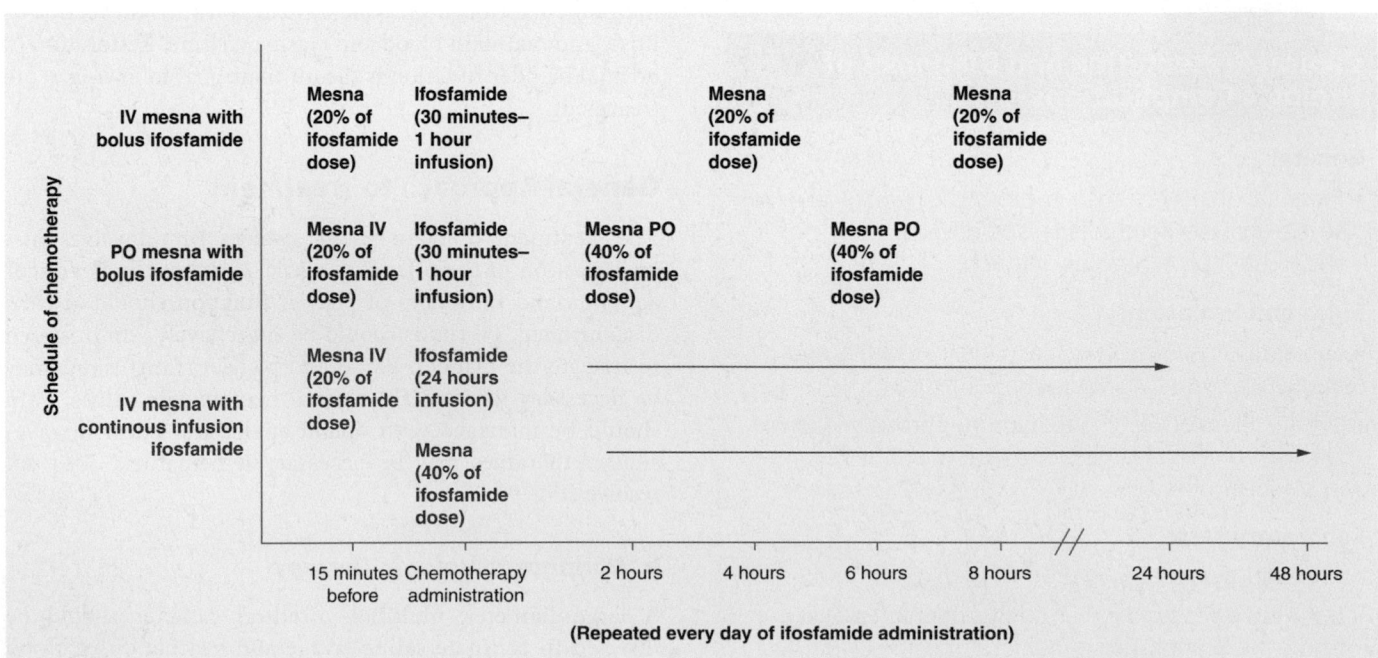

FIGURE 99–2. Examples of mesna administration with ifosfamide.

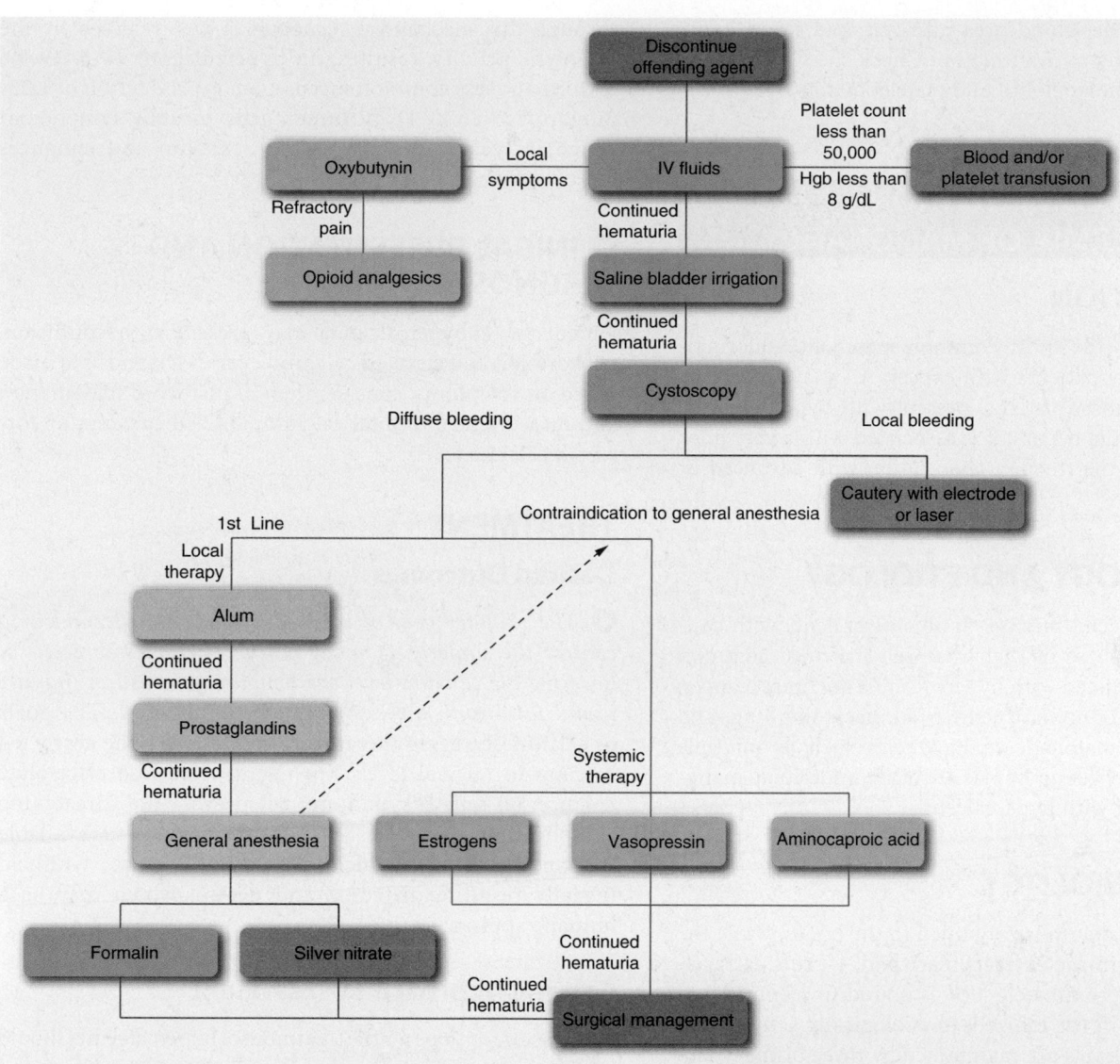

FIGURE 99–3.
Treatment of hemorrhagic cystitis. (From Ref. 27.)

such as alum, prostaglandins, silver nitrate, and formalin may be used; however general anesthesia is required, especially with formalin due to pain. Systemic agents including estrogens, vasopressin, and aminocaproic acid may be used in patients who are refractory to local therapy, although they introduce the risk of systemic side effects. These agents should be continued until bleeding stops.

Antispasmodic agents such as oxybutynin 5 mg by mouth 2 to 3 times daily may be used for bladder spasms. In patients with refractory pain, opioid analgesics should be titrated to adequate pain control.

OUTCOME EVALUATION

The goal of treatment is resolution of bladder symptoms and appropriate pain management.

Monitor the patient for resolution of hematuria after each successive therapeutic intervention. Frequency of monitoring is based on the severity of hemorrhaging. Monitor urinary output and serum chemistries (including sodium,

---

Patient Care and Monitoring: Urologic Complications

1. Assess the patient receiving ifosfamide or cyclophosphamide at least daily for development of hematuria.

2. Ensure administration of adequate hydration and proper doses of mesna.

3. Counsel patient receiving oral mesna on the importance of compliance, when to take doses, and to immediately report any episodes of vomiting for IV readministration.

4. Assess the quantity of urinary bleeding and promptly refer to urologist for local or surgical management.

5. Patients receiving systemic treatment should be monitored every 4 hours for resolution of hematuria. Promptly refer to urologist for refractory hematuria.

6. Evaluate the patient for drug interactions, allergies, and adverse effects with chemotherapy, mesna, or systemic therapies for management.

potassium, chloride, blood urea nitrogen, and serum creatinine) daily for renal dysfunction. Check the CBC at least daily to monitor hemoglobin and platelet count.

METABOLIC COMPLICATIONS: HYPERCALCEMIA OF MALIGNANCY

INTRODUCTION

Hypercalcemia is the most common metabolic abnormality experienced by patients with cancer. A small percentage of as yet undiagnosed patients present with hypercalcemia. Once hypercalcemia occurs, it is associated with a very poor prognosis due to the frequent association with advanced or metastatic disease.[47]

EPIDEMIOLOGY AND ETIOLOGY

Hypercalcemia occurs in 10% to 30% of patients with cancer during the course of their disease. The most common tumor types associated with hypercalcemia are breast cancer, squamous cell carcinomas of the head, neck and lung, and renal cancer. Hematologic malignancies such as multiple myeloma and rarely, lymphomas are other underlying malignances associated with hypercalcemia.

PATHOPHYSIOLOGY

Around 99% of calcium is contained in the bones, while the other 1% resides in the extracellular fluid. Of this extracellular calcium, approximately 40% is bound to albumin and the remainder is in the ionized, physiologically active form. Normal calcium levels are maintained by three primary factors: parathyroid hormone, 1,25-dihydroxyvitamin D, and calcitonin. Parathyroid hormone increases renal tubular calcium resorption and promotes bone resorption. The active form of vitamin D, 1,25-dihydroxyvitamin D, regulates absorption of calcium from the GI tract. Calcitonin serves as an inhibitory factor by suppressing osteoclast activity and stimulating calcium deposition into the bones.

The delicate balance maintained by these factors is altered in patients with cancer by two principal mechanisms: tumor production of humoral factors that alter calcium metabolism (humoral hypercalcemia) and by local osteolytic activity from bone metastases.[48] Humoral hypercalcemia causes around 80% of all hypercalcemia cases and is primarily mediated by systemic secretion of parathyroid hormone-related protein (PTHrP). This protein mimics the action of endogenous parathyroid hormone on bones. Local osteolytic activity causes 20% to 30% of hypercalcemia cases, although local osteolytic activity may also have a humoral component. Local production of various factors directly stimulates osteoclastic bone resorption which releases growth factors and cytokines (i.e., transforming growth factor-β) that are necessary for tumor growth. Thus, these metastatic tumors perpetuate their own growth through this mechanism. Calcium is also released by the osteolytic activity, resulting in hypercalcemia (Fig. 99–4). A third and less common mechanism is production of 1,25-dihydroxyvitamin D by tumor cells (usually lymphoma) which increases GI absorption of calcium and enhances osteoclastic bone resorption.

CLINICAL PRESENTATION AND DIAGNOSIS

Patients with hypercalcemia may present with confusion, dehydration and elevated calcium levels.[47] Diagnosis is made based on symptoms, consideration of history of malignancy, and measurement of total calcium, ionized calcium, or corrected calcium levels.[47]

TREATMENT

Desired Outcomes

❽ *The primary goal of treatment for hypercalcemia is to control the underlying malignancy. Therapies directed at lowering the calcium level are temporary measures that are useful until anticancer therapy begins to work.* The goals of calcium-lowering therapy are to: (a) lower the corrected calcium to normal levels; (b) regain fluid and electrolyte balance; (c) relieve symptoms; (d) prevent life-threatening complications. Patients who are refractory to available therapies may have calcium-lowering therapy withheld (usually resulting in coma and death), which may be a humane approach.[47]

General Approach to Treatment

Therapeutic options for the treatment of hypercalcemia should be directed toward the level of corrected serum calcium and the presence of symptoms (Fig. 99–5). Hypercalcemia may be classified as mild (corrected calcium equal to 10.5–11.9 g/dL [2.6–3 mmol/L]), moderate (12–13.9 g/dL [3–3.5 mmol/L]), and severe (greater than 14 g/dL [3.5 mmol/L]).[47] Adequate treatment of mild or asymptomatic hypercalcemia may be achieved on an outpatient basis with nonpharmacologic measures. Moderate to severe or symptomatic hypercalcemia almost always requires pharmacologic intervention.

▶ *Nonpharmacologic Therapy*

Calciuric therapy in the form of hydration is a key component to the treatment of hypercalcemia, regardless of severity or presence of symptoms.[49] Mild or asymptomatic patients may be encouraged to increase oral fluid intake (3–4 L/day). Patients with moderate to severe or symptomatic hypercalcemia should receive normal saline at 200 to 500 mL/hour according to dehydration and cardiovascular status. Patients should be encouraged to ambulate as much as possible since immobility enhances bone resorption. Although calcium should be discontinued from parenteral feeding solutions, oral calcium supplementation minimally contributes to hypercalcemia, unless it is mediated by vitamin D. In these cases, oral calcium should be

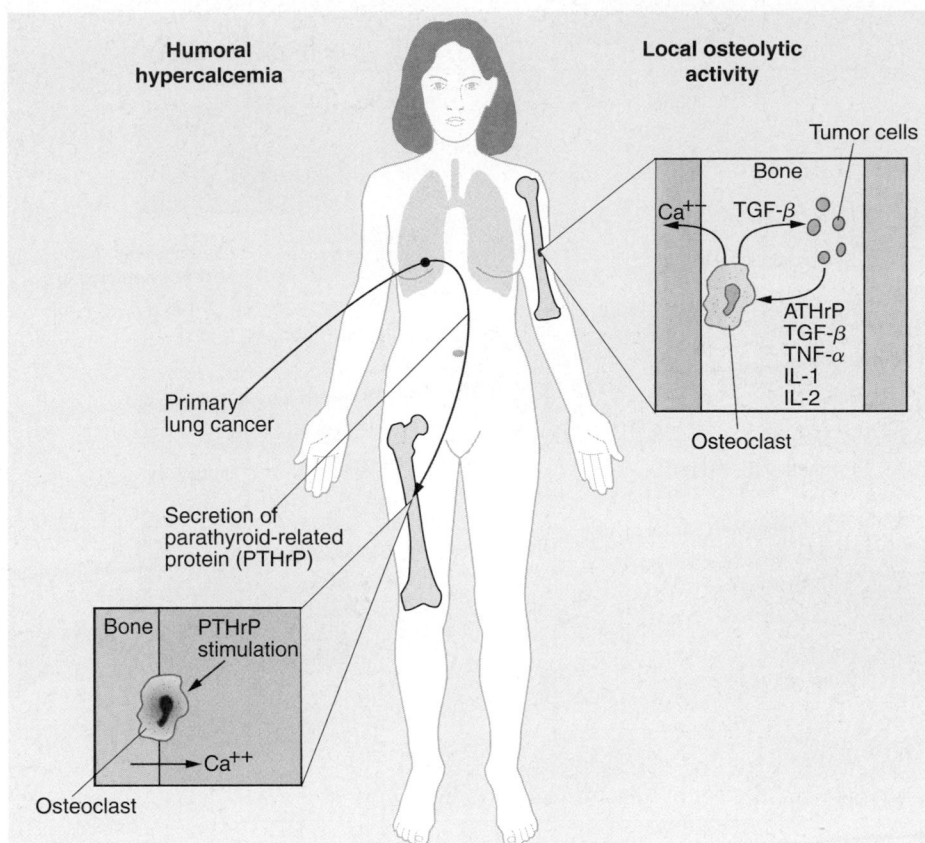

FIGURE 99–4. Pathophysiology of the hypercalcemia of malignancy. (Ca^{2+}, calcium; IL-1, interleukin 1; IL-2, interleukin 2; TGF-β, transforming growth factor β; TNF-α, tumor necrosis factor α; PTHrP, parathyroid hormone-related protein.)

discontinued. Finally, agents that may contribute to hypercalcemia (thiazide diuretics, vitamin D, lithium) or decrease renal function (NSAIDs) should be discontinued. Dialysis may be used in refractory cases or patients who cannot tolerate aggressive saline hydration.

▶ *Pharmacologic Therapy*

Multiple pharmacologic interventions are available for the treatment of hypercalcemia (Table 99–13). Furosemide 20 to 40 mg/day may be added to hydration once rehydration has

---

Clinical Presentation and Diagnosis of Hypercalcemia

General

- Presence of symptoms depends not only on the calcium level but the rapidity of onset
- Normal calcium level is 8.5 to 10.5 g/dL (2.1 to 2.6 mmol/L) (varies by lab)
- Serum calcium level *must* be corrected for albumin level using the following formula:
  - Corrected calcium = (Measured calcium − Measured albumin) + 4

Signs and Symptoms

- Five primary organ systems may be affected:

GI: Anorexia; nausea; vomiting; constipation

Musculoskeletal: weakness; bone pain; fatigue; ataxia

CNS: Confusion; headache; lethargy; seizures; coma

Genitourinary: Polydipsia; polyuria; renal failure

Cardiac: Bradycardia; ECG abnormalities; arrhythmias

Laboratory Tests

- Elevated corrected serum calcium level (greater than or equal to 10.5 g/dL (2.6 mmol/L), serum albumin, low to normal serum phosphate
- Patient may have elevated BUN and serum creatinine
- Elevated alkaline phosphatase may indicate bone destruction
- ECG may indicate prolonged PR interval, shortened QT interval, widened T wave

Other Diagnostic Tests

- Rule out other causes of hypercalcemia including primary hyperparathyroidism, hyperthyroidism, vitamin D intoxication, chronic renal failure

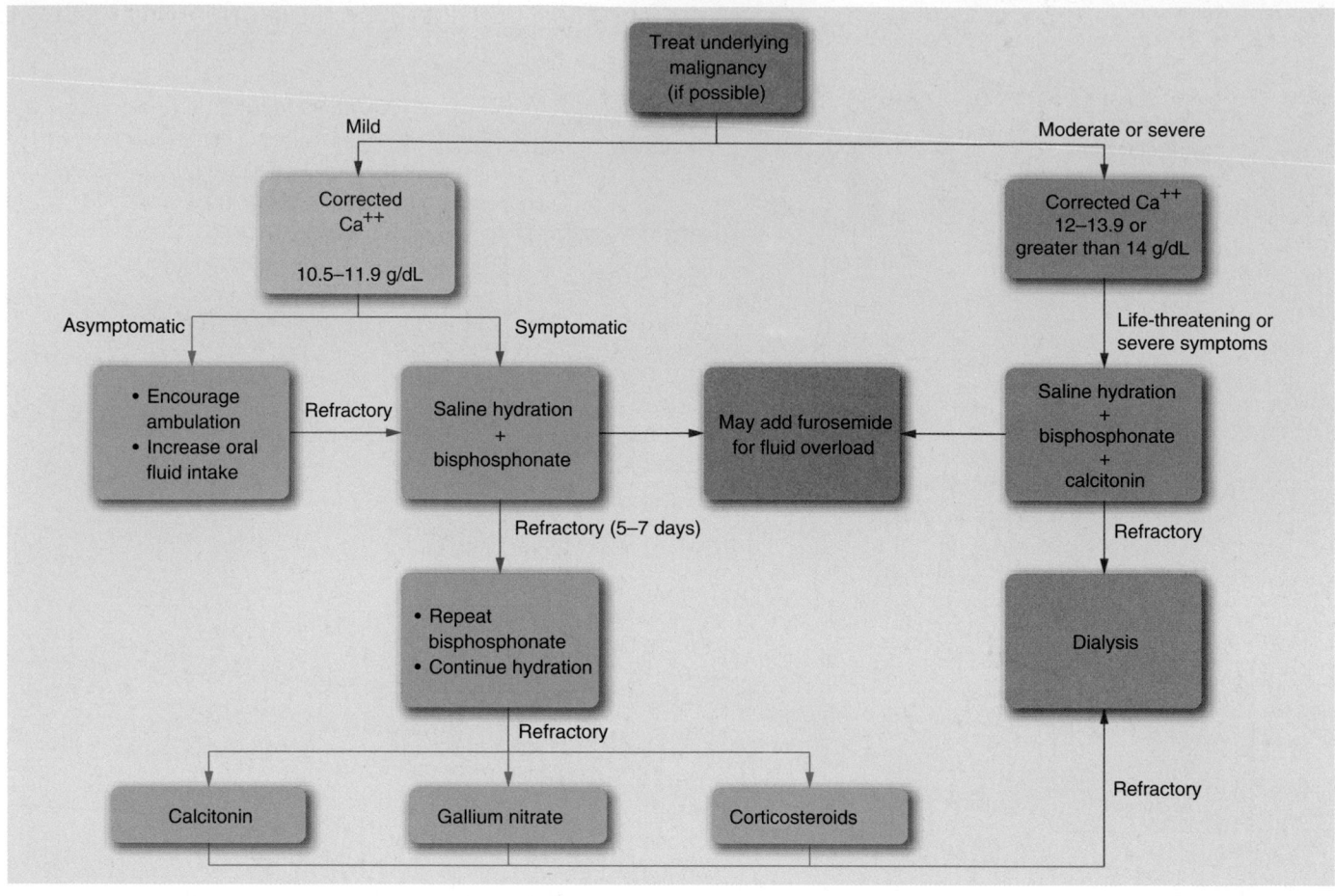

FIGURE 99–5. Treatment algorithm for the hypercalcemia of malignancy.

	Table 99–13

Treatment Options for Hypercalcemia of Malignancy

	Agent	Dosage	Onset	Duration	Reduction in Serum Calcium Concentration	Comments
Calciuric therapy	IV normal saline	200–500 mL/h	24–48 hours	2–3 days	0.5–2 mg/dL	Avoid fluid overload, monitor electrolytes
	Furosemide	20–40 mg IV	4 hours	2–3 days	—	Monitor for hypokalemia, dehydration
Antiresorptive therapy	Pamidronate	60–90 mg IV over 2–24 hours[a]	24–72 hours	3–4 weeks	Greater than 1 mg/dL	Nadir not seen until after 4–7 days; may cause fever, renal dysfunction; pamidronate less expensive
	Zoledronic acid	4 mg IV over 15 minutes	24–48 hours	4+ weeks	Greater than 1 mg/dL	
	Corticosteroids	Prednisone (or equivalent) 50–100 mg daily	5–7 days	3–4 days	0.5–3 mg/dL	Monitor for hyperglycemia, insomnia, immunosuppression
	Calcitonin	4–8 IU/kg SQ or IM every 6–12 hours	2–4 hours	1–3 days	2–3 mg/dL	Salmon-derived formulation preferred; 1 unit test dose recommended; can be given in renal failure; may cause flushing, nausea
	Gallium nitrate	100–200 mg/m² CIV daily for 5 days	24–48 hours	—	—	Do not administer if creatinine greater than 2.5 mg/dL; may cause renal failure

CIV, continuous IV infusion; IM, intramuscularly; SC, subcutaneously.

[a]60 mg of pamidronate may be used in smaller patients or in those patients with mild hypercalcemia or renal dysfunction. May use longer infusion time in patients with renal dysfunction.

From Refs. 47, 49.

been achieved to avoid fluid overload and enhance renal excretion of calcium. Although effective in relieving symptoms, hydration and diuretics are temporary measures that are useful until the onset of antiresorptive therapy, thus hydration and antiresorptive therapy should be initiated simultaneously.

The antiresorptive therapy of choice for hypercalcemia of malignancy is a bisphosphonate. Because of poor oral bioavailability, only IV agents should be used. Pamidronate and zoledronic acid are most commonly utilized and are potent inhibitors of osteoclast activity.[50] The choice of bisphosphonate is a difficult one; zoledronic acid is more efficacious in terms of response rate and longer duration of normocalcemia, but is approximately four times more expensive.[51] Regardless of selection, the bisphosphonates should be administered at diagnosis due to their delayed onset of action.

Calcitonin is the drug of choice in cases of emergent hypercalcemia (patients with life-threatening ECG changes, arrhythmias, or CNS effects) due to its rapid onset of action. Calcitonin inhibits osteoclast activity and decreases renal tubular calcium resorption. Corticosteroids are useful in patients with steroid-responsive malignancies, such as lymphomas or multiple myeloma, and may delay tachyphylaxis to calcitonin. Gallium nitrate was also recently reapproved for treatment, although the 5-day administration regimen and risk of nephrotoxicity limit its use.

OUTCOME EVALUATION

The long-term success of therapy for hypercalcemia is determined primarily by the success of treatment of the underlying malignancy. The goal of treatment is to reduce serum calcium levels to normal range and to relieve patient symptoms if present.

METABOLIC COMPLICATIONS: TLS

INTRODUCTION

Although not as common as hypercalcemia, TLS may cause significant morbidity and mortality if adequate prophylaxis and treatment is not instituted. TLS is the result of rapid destruction of malignant cells with subsequent release of intracellular contents into the circulation.

EPIDEMIOLOGY AND ETIOLOGY

● The overall incidence of TLS is unknown but has been linked to a number of patient-related and tumor related risk factors (Table 99–14).[52] TLS typically occurs in malignancies with high tumor burdens or high proliferative rates. Because of this, children are most frequently affected since they frequently have aggressive malignancies. TLS is typically induced by cancer treatment modalities including chemotherapy, hormonal therapy, radiation, biologic therapy, or corticosteroids, although some patients may present spontaneously before treatment.

PATHOPHYSIOLOGY

Patients with TLS experience a wide range of metabolic abnormalities. The massive cell lysis that occurs leads to the release of intracellular electrolytes resulting in hyperkalemia and hyperphosphatemia. High concentrations of phosphate bind to calcium leading to hypocalcemia and calcium phosphate precipitation in the renal tubule. Purine nucleic acids are also released which are subsequently metabolized to uric acid through multiple enzyme-mediated steps (Fig. 99–6). Uric acid is poorly soluble at urinary acidic pH leading to crystallization in the renal tubule. The precipitation of uric acid and calcium phosphate leads to metabolic acidosis, facilitating further uric acid crystallization. Acute renal failure may be the end result.

CLINICAL PRESENTATION AND DIAGNOSIS

● Patients with TLS are diagnosed based on laboratory monitoring indicating hyperuricemia, hyperkalemia, hyperphosphatemia,

---

Patient Care and Monitoring: Hypercalcemia

1. Determine the disease status of the patient— Is the patient newly diagnosed or has the patient had multiple episodes of hypercalcemia and is becoming refractory to calcium-lowering therapy?

2. Assess the patient's symptoms and serum calcium level to determine appropriate therapy. Is the patient taking any medications that may elevate the calcium level, inhibit its excretion, or affect renal function?

3. Educate the patient regarding the importance of oral hydration and ambulation if an outpatient. Counsel to immediately report any worsening signs or symptoms.

4. Develop a plan to maintain normocalcemia chronically using monthly bisphosphonates.

   • Monitor patients for relief of symptoms and restoration of fluid balance.

   • Monitor the serum calcium level, serum albumin, serum BUN and creatinine, and electrolytes daily during therapy.

   • Assess the fluid balance by daily input/output, weights, and signs of fluid overload.

   • Monitor the ECG in patients with cardiac manifestations until normalized.

   • Repeat doses of bisphosphonate after 5 to 7 days if the patient does not become normocalcemic.

   • Reassess patient status in terms of refractoriness to treatment to determine if treatment should be changed

5. Evaluate the patient for drug interactions, allergies, and adverse effects with calcium-lowering therapy.

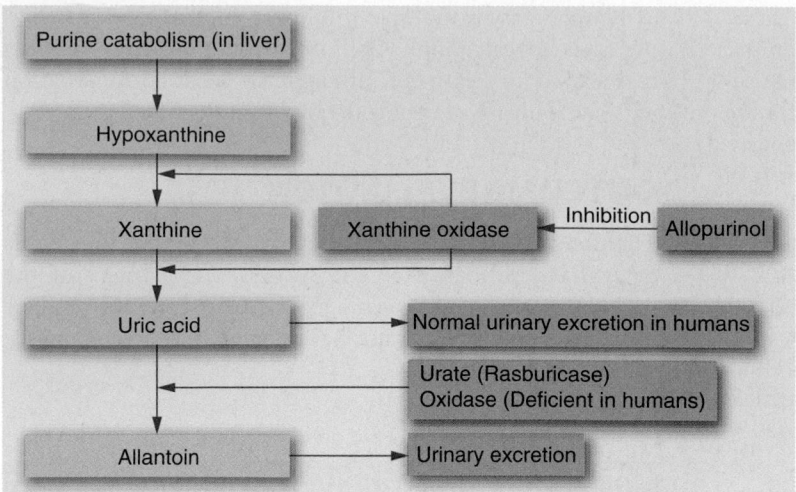

FIGURE 99–6. The role of allopurinol and rasburicase in the enzymatic degradation of purine nucleic acids.

Table 99–14
Risk Factors for TLS

Disease Related

High risk
Acute lymphoblastic leukemia
High-grade non-Hodgkin's lymphoma (i.e., Burkitt's)
Intermediate risk
Chronic lymphocytic leukemia (especially bulky lymphadenopathy)
Acute myeloid leukemia (especially WBC greater than 50,000/mm³)
Multiple myeloma

Low risk
Low- and intermediate-grade non-Hodgkin's lymphoma
Hodgkin's disease
Chronic myeloid leukemia (blast crisis)

Rare
Breast cancer
Small cell lung cancer
Testicular cancer

Patient related
Decreased urinary output, dehydration, or renal failure
Pre-existing hyperuricemia
Acidic urine
WBC greater than 50,000 10³/μL (500 × 10⁹/L)
Lactate dehydrogenase (LDH) levels greater than 1500 IU/L (1500 units/L)
High tumor sensitivity to treatment modalities

From Refs. 52, 54.

hypocalcemia, and renal dysfunction.[53] As a result of these electrolyte abnormalities, patients may present with uremia, visual disturbances, muscle cramping, edema, hypertension, cardiac arrhythmias, seizures, and even sudden death.[53]

TREATMENT

Desired Outcomes

❾ *The primary goals of management of TLS are: (a) prevention of renal failure; (b) prevention of electrolyte imbalances.*

Clinical Presentation and Diagnosis of TLS

General
- Patients present primarily with lab abnormalities
- Normal uric acid is equal to 2 to 8 mg/dL (119–476 μmol/L)
- Most often occurs within 12 to 72 hours of initiation of cytotoxic therapy

Signs and Symptoms
- Most patients are asymptomatic
- Patients may develop edema, fluid overload, and oliguria, which may progress to anuria with acute renal failure
- Some patients with hyperuricemia may have nausea, vomiting, and lethargy
- Hyperkalemia—lethargy, muscle weakness, paresthesia, ECG changes, bradycardia
- Hypocalcemia—muscle cramps, tetany, irritability, paresthesias, arrhythmias

Laboratory Tests (Adults)
- Serum uric acid level greater than 8 mg/dL (476 μmol/L)
- Serum potassium greater than 6 mEq/L (6 mmol/L)
- Serum phosphorus greater than 4.5 mg/dL (1.45 mmol/L)
- Serum calcium less than 7 mg/dL (1.75 mmol/L)
- Elevated BUN and creatinine once renal dysfunction develops

OR

- A change of greater than 25% from baseline in the above lab values[35]

Thus, the best treatment for TLS is prophylaxis to enable delivery of cytotoxic therapy for the underlying malignancy. For patients that present with or develop TLS despite prophylaxis, treatment goals include: (a) decreasing uric acid levels; (b) correcting electrolyte imbalances; (c) preventing compromised renal function. These goals should be achieved in a cost-effective manner.

General Approach to Treatment

Prevention of TLS is generally achieved by increasing the urine output and preventing accumulation of uric acid. Prophylactic strategies should begin immediately upon presentation, preferably 48 hours prior to cytotoxic therapy. Treatment modalities primarily increase uric acid solubility, maintain electrolyte balance, and support renal output.

▶ *Nonpharmacologic Therapy*

Vigorous IV hydration with dextrose 5% in water with ½ normal saline at 3 L/m^2/day to maintain a urine output greater than or equal to 100 mL/m^2/hour is necessary, unless the patient presents with acute renal dysfunction. Alkalinization of the urine to a pH greater than or equal to 7.0 with 50 to 100 mEq/L of sodium bicarbonate has been used to promote uric acid solubility for excretion. This measure is controversial because xanthine and hypoxanthine are less soluble at alkaline pH potentially leading to crystallization, especially during and after allopurinol therapy (Fig. 99–6).[54] Medications that increase serum potassium (angiotensin-converting enzyme [ACE] inhibitors, spironolactone) or block tubular resorption of uric acid (probenecid, thiazides) should be discontinued. Nephrotoxic agents such as amphotericin B or aminoglycosides should also be avoided. Hemodialysis may be required in patients who develop anuria or uncontrolled hyperkalemia, hyperphosphatemia, hypocalcemia, acidosis or volume overload.

▶ *Pharmacologic Therapy*

Pharmacologic prevention strategies for TLS are aimed at low- and high-risk patients (Fig. 99–7). Allopurinol is a xanthine oxidase inhibitor that is used for prevention only because it has no effect on pre-existing elevated uric acid. Rasburicase is a recombinant form of urate oxidase that is useful for both prevention and treatment, but is extremely expensive (Table 99–15). Although the approved dose is 0.2 mg/kg/day for 5 days, recent studies using abbreviated courses (1–3 days) and/or lower doses (0.05–0.1 mg/kg/day) may be equally efficacious with significantly reduced cost.[54] Because uric acid levels generally fall within 4 hours of the first dose, one dose may be administered with frequent, serial monitoring of the uric acid level for repeat dosing if necessary (Fig. 99–7). Of note, rasburicase continues to break down uric acid in blood samples drawn from patients. This can be avoided by immediately placing the sample in an ice bath for processing to avoid falsely lowered uric acid levels.

Electrolyte disturbances that develop in patients with TLS should be aggressively managed to avoid renal failure and cardiac sequelae. One exception pertains to the use of IV calcium for hypocalcemia. Adding calcium may cause further calcium phosphate precipitation in the presence of hyperphosphatemia and should be used cautiously.

OUTCOME EVALUATION

The most successful outcome in TLS is prevention. If the condition is not able to be prevented, the goal of therapy is to avoid renal failure and quickly return electrolytes to normal.

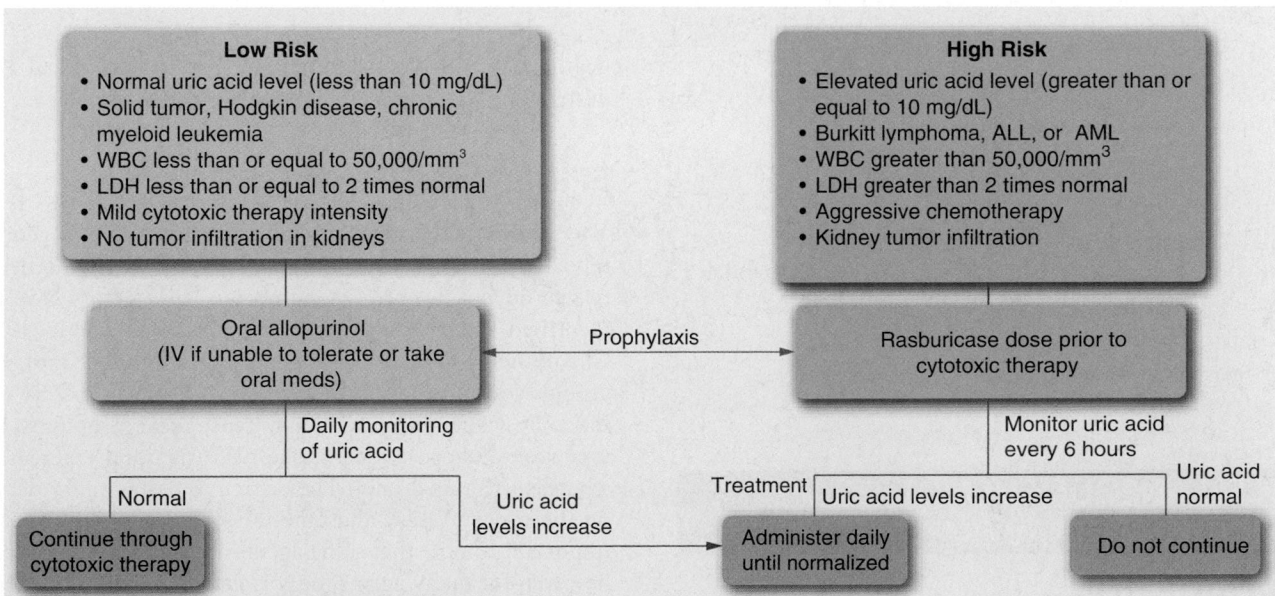

FIGURE 99–7. Prophylaxis and treatment of hyperuricemia associated with TLS. (ALL, acute lymphoblastic leukemia; AML, acute myelogenous leukemia.) (From Refs 35, 36.)

Table 99–15

Comparison of Allopurinol and Rasburicase in TLS

Drug	Dosing	2005 AWP[a]	Comments
Oral allopurinol (Zyloprim)	Adult: 600–800 mg/day in 2–3 divided doses Pediatric: 10 mg/kg/day or 200–300 mg/m²/day	$0.48/day (generic)	Adjust dose for renal impairment Avoid drug interactions (mercaptopurine) Monitor for skin rash
IV allopurinol (Aloprim)	Adult: 200–400 mg/m²/day Pediatric: 200 mg/m²/day	$625–$1,250/day	As above Reserve for patients who cannot tolerate or take oral medications Maximum dose = 600 mg/day
Rasburicase (Elitek)	0.2 mg/kg/day for up to 5 days	$12,000/day	Lower doses and abbreviated schedules may be used to decrease cost (0.05–0.1 mg/kg/day) May rarely cause nausea and vomiting Contraindicated in patients with G6PD deficiency → hemolytic anemia Rare cases of hypersensitivity and antibody formation

AWP, average wholesale price; G6PD, glucose-6-phosphate dehydrogenase

[a]Normalized for 70 kg patient or body surface area = 1.73 m²; all costs are estimated and may vary.

From Ref. 55.

Patient Care and Monitoring: TLS

1. Monitor daily the at-risk patient who presents with normal lab values daily for serum uric acid, electrolytes (Na, K, Ca, Mg, Cl, PO$_4$), BUN, creatinine, and urine output.

2. Monitor for signs of fluid overload during aggressive hydration.

3. Continue hydration and prophylaxis until 2 to 3 days after cytotoxic therapy.

4. In patients undergoing urinary alkalinization with sodium bicarbonate, assess the urine pH every 6 hours and maintain above 7.

5. For patients who present with or develop signs of TLS, monitor these parameters every 6 hours until stable.

6. Order an ECG for patients with hyperkalemia and monitor serially until resolution.

7. Adjust the dose of allopurinol and other renally eliminated medications for patients who develop renal dysfunction.

8. In patients receiving rasburicase, monitor the hemoglobin and hematocrit for signs of hemolysis.

MISCELLANEOUS CHEMOTHERAPY TOXICITIES: EXTRAVASATION

INTRODUCTION

Extravasation is generally defined as leakage of IV fluids into the interstitial tissue.[56] While extravasation does not cause

Table 99–16

Risk Factors for Chemotherapy Extravasation

Presence of multiple venipunctures (common in cancer patients)
Poor needle insertion technique
Poor catheter location (dorsum of the hand, antecubital fossa)
Inability to communicate symptoms (children, sedated patients, language barrier between patient and nurse)
Presence of peripheral neuropathy
Nurse experience and training
Young age or elderly patients (small or fragile veins)
Gross obesity

death, significant morbidity may result from local tissue destruction and immediate management is necessary.

EPIDEMIOLOGY AND ETIOLOGY

The incidence of chemotherapy extravasation is generally reported to be between 0.5% and 6% of all chemotherapy-related adverse events.[57] A number of risk factors have been identified for chemotherapy extravasation (Table 99–16). Chemotherapy agents are generally classified into three groups: vesicants, irritants, and nonvesicants (Table 99–17).[58] Either vesicants or irritants may cause local symptoms, however vesicants cause local tissue necrosis upon extravasation whereas irritants do not. The degree of tissue injury depends on the concentration and amount of fluid extravasated. It is important to note that some agents are well-known vesicants; however, for many agents, only isolated case reports of tissue necrosis exist. Therefore, it is imperative to use caution when administering any chemotherapeutic agent, especially new or investigational agents that have unknown vesicant properties.

Table 99–17

Chemotherapeutic Agents With Vesicant or Irritant Properties

Vesicants	Irritants
Common	Camptothecins
Anthracyclines	Carmustine
Daunorubicin	Cyclophosphamide
Doxorubicin	Dacarbazine
Epirubicin	Epipodophyllotoxins
Idarubicin	Etoposide
Dactinomycin	Fluorouracil
Mechlorethamine	Gemcitabine
Mitomycin C	Ifosfamide
Vinca alkaloids	Irinotecan
Vincristine	Melphalan
Vinblastine	Pentostatin
Vinorelbine	Streptozocin
Rare[a]	Teniposide
Cisplatin	Topotecan
Liposomal doxorubicin	
Mitoxantrone	
Oxaliplatin	
Taxanes	
Docetaxel	
Paclitaxel	

[a]Agents for which there are isolated case reports of local tissue necrosis.

From Ref. 58.

PATHOPHYSIOLOGY

The mechanism of tissue injury is related to the pharmacodynamic characteristics of the extravasated drug. These agents

Clinical Presentation and Diagnosis of Extravasation

General

- Anthracycline, mechlorethamine, and vinca alkaloid extravasations typically cause immediate pain
- Patients may be asymptomatic at the time of extravasation, but return within days to weeks with signs of tissue damage (particularly with mitomycin C)
- Exposure to UV light may worsen some lesions

Signs and Symptoms

- Local pain (burning, tingling, stinging), swelling, erythema, induration
- Lack of blood return
- Ulceration may not develop until after 1 to 2 weeks or longer

Diagnostic Tests

- Usually based on clinical history and presenting symptoms, however tissue biopsy may reveal definitive findings

may be classified into DNA-binding and non–DNA-binding. Examples of DNA-binding agents include the anthracyclines, mechlorethamine, and mitomycin C. These agents first cause cell death through interactions with DNA, and are then released into the surrounding tissue and taken up by adjacent cells. This repeating cycle is perpetuated by the lipophilic nature of these drugs resulting in chronic, slow-healing tissue injury due to long tissue retention. Doxorubicin in particular may remain in tissues for weeks to months.[58]

Non–DNA-binding agents include the vinca alkaloids and etoposide. These agents tend to cause injury in the pattern of a thermal burn and are more easily cleared from interstitial spaces. Thus, they are more readily neutralized and tend to have a better healing prognosis.

CLINICAL PRESENTATION AND DIAGNOSIS

Patients who experience extravasation will report burning pain and discomfort in the limb of the infusion site which can be severe. The area may be erythematous at first. If not quickly treated, the tissue will become necrotic and require amputation. Diagnosis is made based on symptoms.

PREVENTION

🔟 *Chemotherapy extravasation may be avoided in many cases by the use of successful prevention strategies. The most important preventative measure is proper patient education.* Patients must be instructed to promptly report any local symptoms not only during administration, but days to weeks later. Another key factor is the exclusive use of highly trained personnel who are trained to administer chemotherapeutic drugs. The Oncology Nursing Society has developed guidelines for the administration of vesicant drugs as summarized in Table 99–18.[59] Although placement of a central venous catheter is recommended, extravasations may still occur due to dislodged or poorly placed needles or nicked catheters.

TREATMENT

Desired Outcomes

Once extravasation occurs, the primary goals of treatment are to: (a) avoid further tissue damage by using appropriate nonpharmacologic and pharmacologic strategies; (b) promptly refer patients for surgery if required. Optimal pharmacologic and nonpharmacologic treatment of the extravasation will allow the cancer patient to continue with their chemotherapy (Table 99–19).

▶ *Nonpharmacologic Therapy*

If extravasation occurs, the infusion should be stopped immediately with aspiration of fluid from the site, needle, and tubing as much as possible. The affected limb or area should be elevated (if possible). The site should be documented photographically as well as the time, date, site,

Table 99–18

Prevention Strategies for Chemotherapy Extravasation

Central venous catheters should be placed for vesicant administration whenever possible, especially in high-risk patients

Avoid the dorsum of the hand, antecubital fossa, and limbs with significant lymphedema

Use uncovered plastic cannulas or a butterfly needle for peripheral administration

Always test the line with IV fluids before chemotherapy administration and observe site for swelling

Check for blood return prior to and frequently during administration

If venipuncture is repeated, should be proximal to prior needle insertion site

Vesicants given via peripheral vein should be given by IV push rather than by infusion to enable immediate cessation and withdrawal of fluids if extravasation occurs

From Ref. 59.

patient complaints, and estimated volume of extravasated drug.[58] Both hot and cold packs have been used to manage extravasations; however, use of the proper therapy for certain agents is critical. For example, warm compresses have been shown to worsen doxorubicin extravasations; while cold packs may exacerbate vinca alkaloid lesions. Pressure should not be applied to the area as this may facilitate spread. Finally, patients should be referred to a plastic surgeon if pain persists or ulceration develops despite treatment.

▶ *Pharmacologic Therapy*

Therapeutic modalities to treat extravasation events consist of specific antidotes to halt or decrease the severity of local tissue necrosis. It should be noted that only one third of extravasation events will lead to local tissue necrosis and most studies of antidotes are in animal models or isolated case reports. Antidotes either disperse or bind the chemotherapy agent and accelerate the removal of the agent from the tissues. Specific antidotes and their uses are presented in Table 99–19.

Dimethylsulfoxide (DMSO) is the antidote of choice for anthracycline and mitomycin C extravasations. It readily penetrates tissues and increases diffusion in the tissue area. In addition, DMSO is a free-radical scavenger that functions to block this principle mechanism of anthracycline and mitomycin C-mediated tissue injury. DMSO is generally well tolerated but may cause some mild burning and redness. Dexrazoxane is a free-radical scavenger typically used for cardioprotection from anthracyclines. A special formulation of dexrazoxane (Totect) is the only commercially available product that is FDA approved to treat doxorubicin extravasation, though much controversy exists surrounding whether generic dexrazoxane may be equally efficacious than the newer, more expensive alternative.

Hyaluronidase is the antidote of choice for vinca alkaloid and high concentration epipodophyllotoxin extravasations. Hyaluronidase breaks down hyaluronic acid, which functions as "tissue cement." This promotes the absorption of the extravasated drug away from the local site. Hyaluronidase

Table 99–19

Management of Chemotherapy Extravasation

Drug	Application of Heat or Cold	Pharmacologic Antidote	Dose	Comments
Anthracyclines	Cold packs	DMSO 50–99%	Apply 1–2 mL to area of skin twice the size of lesion every 6–8 hours for 7–14 days	Allow to air dry Do not cover
		Alternative: Dexrazoxane	1,000 mg/m² IV within 5 hours of extravasation followed by 1,000 mg/m² on day 2, 500 mg/m² on day 3	Promising new agent; expensive, may not be reimbursed by payors
Mitomycin C	Cold packs	DMSO 50–99%	As above	
Mechlorethamine; concentrated cisplatin	Cold packs	Sodium thiosulfate	Prepare 1/6M solution by adding 4 mL of 10% solution to 6 mL sterile water; inject 2 mL for each mg of mechlorethamine. Follow with 1 mL SC (0.1 mL doses clockwise around area); may repeat every 3–4 hours if needed	Sodium thiosulfate must be diluted prior to administration
Vinca alkaloids	Hot packs	Hyaluronidase	Inject 1–6 mL of 150 units/mL concentration (150–900 units) through IV line or SC if removed; may repeat every 3–4 hours if needed	Dilute with normal saline
Paclitaxel	Cold packs	Hyaluronidase	As above	Hot packs paradoxically shown to worsen lesions in some case reports

DMSO, dimethylsulfoxide; SC, subcutaneously.

From Ref. 58.

Patient Care and Monitoring: Extravasation

1. Upon diagnosis, determine need for administration of chemotherapy with vesicant properties. Refer the patient for surgical placement of a central access device.

2. Insure proper training and certification of all personnel in institution who administer chemotherapeutic agents.

3. Educate the patient regarding signs and symptoms of extravasation and instruct to IMMEDIATELY relate to caregiver.

4. Educate the patient to promptly report increasing pain, spread of the lesion or ulceration.

5. Educate the patient regarding proper application of hot or cold packs as well as topical antidotes. Should the area be allowed to air dry or be covered?

6. Evaluate the patient for allergies and adverse effects of pharmacologic antidotes.

may also be used for paclitaxel extravasations; however, there are conflicting reports regarding its efficacy.[60] Hyaluronidase should not be used with anthracycline extravasations because enhancement of local spread may occur.

The antidote of choice for mechlorethamine extravasations is sodium thiosulfate. This agent binds alkylating agents resulting in neutralization to inactive compounds that are then excreted. Sodium thiosulfate may also be effective for high concentration cisplatin or dacarbazine extravasations.

OUTCOME EVALUATION

The primary outcome is the prevention of extravasation events using proper administration techniques. Instruct patients to promptly report any symptoms of extravasation. If extravasation occurs, select the proper antidote and thermal application for immediate administration. Promptly refer the patient for plastic surgery if pain persists or ulceration develops.

Abbreviations Introduced in This Chapter

ACE inhibitor	Angiotensin converting enzyme inhibitor
ANC	Absolute neutrophil count
AWP	Average wholesale price
BMT	Bone marrow transplantation
BUN	Blood urea nitrogen
CIV	Continuous intravenous infusion
CSF	Colony-stimulating factor
DMSO	Dimethylsulfoxide
G6PD	Glucose-6-phosphate dehydrogenase
G-CSF	Granulocyte-colony stimulating factor
GMCSF	Granulocyte-macrophage colony-stimulating factor
ICP	Intracranial pressure
LDH	Lactate dehydrogenase
NKDA	No known drug Allergies
NSAID	Nonsteroidal anti-inflammatory drug
NSCLC	Nonsmall cell lung cancer
PCP	*Pneumocystis jirovesi* pneumonitis (formerly *Pneumocystis carinii*)
PTHrP	Parathyroid-related protein
SCLC	Small cell lung cancer
SC	Subcutaneous
SVCS	Superior vena cava syndrome

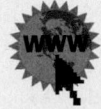 Self-assessment questions and answers are available at *http://www.mhpharmacotherapy.com/pp.html.*

REFERENCES

1. deBoer-Dennert M, deWit R, Schmitz PI, et al. Patient perceptions of the side effects of chemotherapy: The influence of 5HT3 antagonists. Br J Cancer 1997;76:1055–1061.

2. Roscoe JA, Bushnnow P, Morrow GR, et al. Patient experience is a strong predictor of severe nausea after chemotherapy: A University of Rochester Community Clinical Oncology Program study of patients with breast carcinoma. Cancer 2004;101:2701–2708.

3. Hesketh PJ. Chemotherapy-induced nausea and vomiting. N Engl J Med 2008;358:2482–2494.

4. Hesketh PJ, Grunberg SM, Gralla RJ, et al. The neurokinin-1 antagonist aprepitant for the prevention of chemotherapy-induced nausea and vomiting: A multinational, randomized, double-blind, placebo-controlled trial in patients receiving high-dose cisplatin—The Aprepitant Protocol 052 Study Group. J Clin Oncol 2003;21:4112–4119.

5. Geling O, Eichler HG. Should 5-hydroxytryptamine-3-receptor antagonists be administered beyond 24 hours after chemotherapy to prevent delayed emesis? Systematic re-evaluation of clinical evidence and drug cost implications. J Clin Oncol 2005;23:1289–1294.

6. National Comprehensive Cancer Network. Clinical Practice Guidelines in Oncology: Antiemesis. v2.2009, *http://www.nccn.org/professionals/physician_gls/PDF/antiemesis.pdf* .

7. Polovich M, White JM, Kelleher LO, eds. Chemotherapy and Biotherapy Guidelines and Recommendations for Practice, 2nd ed. Pittsburgh, PA: Oncology Nursing Society, 2005.

8. Berardi RR, Kroon LA, McDermott JH, et al. Handbook of Nonprescription Drugs, 15th ed. Washington, DC: American Pharmacists Association, 2006.

9. Kris MG, Hesketh PJ, Somerfield MR, et al. American Society of Clinical Oncology Guidelines for Antiemesis in Oncology: Update 2006. J Clin Oncol 2006;24:2932–2947.

10. Peterson DE, Bensadoun RJ, Roila F. Management of oral and gastrointestinal mucositis: ESMO clinical recommendations. Ann Oncol 2008;19(Suppl 2):ii122–ii125.

11. Nonzel NJ, Dandade NA, Markossia T, et al. Evaluating the supportive care costs of severe radiochemotherapy-induced mucositis and pharyngitis: Results from a Northwestern University costs of cancer program pilot study with head and neck and non-small cell lung cancer patients who received care at a county hospital, a Veterans Administration hospital, and a comprehensive care center. Cancer 2008;113:1446–1452.

12. Troth A, Bellm LA, Epstein JB, et al. Mucositis incidence, severity, and associated outcomes in patients with head and neck cancer receiving radiotherapy with or without chemotherapy: A systematic literature review. Radiother Oncol 2003;66:253–262.

13. Saadeh CE. Chemotherapy- and radiotherapy-induced oral mucositis: Review of preventative strategies and treatment. Pharmacotherapy 2005;25:540–544.

14. Keefe DM, Schubert MM, Elting LS. Updated clinical practice guidelines for the prevention and treatment of mucositis. Cancer 2007;109:820–831.

15. Wisplinghoff H, Seifert H, Wenzel RP, Edmond MB. Current trends in the epidemiology of nosocomial bloodstream infections in patients with hematological malignancies and solid neoplasms in hospitals in the United States. Clin Infect Dis 2003;36:1103–1110.

16. Rolston KVI. Challenges in the treatment of infections caused by gram-positive and gram-negative bacteria in patients with cancer and neutropenia. Clin Infect Dis 2004;40:S246–S252.

17. Picazo JJ. Management of the febrile neutropenic patient: A consensus conference. Clin Infect Dis 2004;39:S1–S6.

18. Elting L, Cooksley C, Chambers M, et al. The burdens of cancer therapy: Clinical and economic outcomes of chemotherapy-induced mucositis. Cancer 2003;98:1531–1539.

19. Hughes WT, Armstrong D, Bodey GP, et al. 2002 Guidelines for the use of antimicrobial agents in neutropenic patients with cancer. Clin Infect Dis 2002;34:730–751.

20. Lyman GH, Lyman CH, Agboola O. Risk models for predicting chemotherapy-induced neutropenia. Oncologist 2005;10:427–437.

21. Klastersky J, Paesmans M, Rubenstein EB, et al. The Multinational Association for Supportive Care in Cancer risk index: A multinational scoring system for identifying low-risk febrile neutropenic patients. J Clin Oncol 2000;18:3038–3051.

22. Greil R, Psenak O, Roila F, et al. Hematopoetic growth factors: ESMO recommendations for the applications. Ann Oncol 2008;2:16–8.

23. National Comprehensive Cancer Network. Clinical Practice Guidelines in Oncology: Myeloid Growth Factors. Version 1.2009, http://www.nccn.org/professionals/physician_gls/PDF/myeloid_growth.pdf.

24. Gafter-Gvili A, Fraser A, Paul M, et al. Meta-analysis: Antibiotic prophylaxis reduces mortality in neutropenic patients. Ann Intern Med 2005;142:979–995.

25. van de Wetering MD, de Witte MA, Kremer LCM, et al. Efficacy of oral prophylactic antibiotics in neutropenic afebrile oncology patients: A systematic review of randomized controlled trials. Eur J Cancer 2005;41:1372–1382.

26. The National Comprehensive Cancer Network (NCCN). Clinical Practice Guidelines in Oncology: Prevention and Treatment of Cancer-Related Infections. V.1.2008, http://www.nccn.org/professionals/physician_gls/PDF/infections.pdf.

27. Bucavene G, Micuzzi A, Menichetti F, et al. Levofloxacin to prevent bacterial infection in patients with cancer and neutropenia. N Engl J Med 2005;353:977–987.

28. Cullen M, Steven N, Billinham L, et al. Antibacterial prophylaxis after chemotherapy for solid tumors and lymphomas. N Engl J Med 2005;353:988–998.

29. Kuderer NM, Crawford J, Dale DC, et al. Meta-analysis of prophylactic granulocyte colony-stimulating factor in cancer patients receiving chemotherapy. J Clin Oncol 2005;23(June 1 Suppl):758s.

30. Fish DN, Goodwin SD. Infections in immunocompromised patients. In: Dipiro JT, Talbert RL, Yee GC, et al., eds. Pharmacotherapy: A Pathophysiologic Approach, 6th ed. New York City: McGraw-Hill, 2005:2191–2215.

31. The Oncology Nursing Society: ONS Putting Evidence into Practice: Prevention of Infection. http://www.ons.org/outcomes/volume1/prevention/pdf/INFECTION-DetailedPEPCard4-06.pdf.

32. National Comprehensive Cancer Network. Clinical Practice Guidelines in Oncology: Small Cell Lung Cancer. V.2.2009, http://www.nccn.org/professionals/physician_gls/PDF/sclc.pdf.

33. Walsh TJ, Teppler H, Donowitz GR, et al. Caspofungin versus liposomal amphotericin B for empirical antifungal therapy in patients with persistent fever and neutropenia. N Engl J Med 2004;351:1391–1402.

34. Clark OAC, Lyman GH, Castro AA, et al. Colony-stimulating factors for chemotherapy-induced febrile neutropenia: A meta-analysis of randomized controlled trials. J Clin Oncol 2005;23:4198–4214.

35. Wilson LD, Detterbeck FC, Yahalom J. Superior vena cava syndrome with malignant causes. N Engl J Med 2007;356(8):1862–1869.

36. Kvale PA, Simoff M, Prakash UB. Lung cancer. Palliative care. Chest 2003;123(Suppl 1):284S–311S.

37. Prasad D, Schiff D. Malignant spinal-cord compression. Lancet Oncol 2005;6:15–24.

38. Patchell RA, Tibbs PA, Regine WF, et al. Direct decompressive surgical resection in the treatment of spinal cord compression caused by metastatic cancer: A randomized trial. Lancet 2005;366:643–648.

39. Loblaw DA, Perry J, Chambers A, et al. Systematic review of the diagnosis and management of malignant extradural spinal cord compression: The Cancer Care Ontario Practice Guidelines Initiative's Neuro-Oncology Disease Site Group. J Clin Oncol 2005;23:2028–2037.

40. Langer CJ, Mehta MP. Current management of brain metastases, with a focus on systemic options. J Clin Oncol 2005;23:6207–6219.

41. Patchell RA. The management of brain metastases. Cancer Treat Rev 2003;29:533–540.

42. Slotman B, Faivre-Finn C, Kramer G, et al. Prophylactic cranial-irradiation in extensive small cell lung cancer. N Engl J Med 2007;357:664–672.

43. Lassman AB, DeAngelis LM. Brain metastases. Neurol Clin North Am 2003;21:1–23.

44. Glantz MJ, Cole BF, Forsyth PA, et al. Practice parameter: Anticonvulsant prophylaxis in patients with newly diagnosed brain tumors. Report of the Quality Standards Subcommittee of the American Academy of Neurology. Neurology 2000;54:1886–1893.

45. West NJ. Prevention and treatment of hemorrhagic cystitis. Pharmacotherapy 1997;17:696–706.

46. Schuchter LM, Hensley ML, Meropol NJ, et al. 2002 Update of recommendations for the use of chemotherapy and radiotherapy protectants: Clinical practice guidelines of the American Society of Clinical Oncology. J Clin Oncol 2002;20:2895–2903.

47. Stewart AF. Hypercalcemia associated with cancer. N Engl J Med 2005;352:373–379.

48. Solimando DA. Overview of hypercalcemia of malignancy. Am J Health Syst Pharm 2001;58(Suppl 3):S4–S7.

49. Davidson TG. Conventional treatment of hypercalcemia of malignancy. Am J Health Syst Pharm 2001;58(Suppl 3):S8–S15.

50. Berenson JR. Treatment of hypercalcemia of malignancy with bisphosphonates. Semin Oncol 2002;29(Suppl 21):12–18.

51. Major P, Lortholary A, Hon J, et al. Zoledronic acid is superior to pamidronate in the treatment of hypercalcemia of malignancy: A pooled analysis of two randomized, controlled clinical trials. J Clin Oncol 2001;19:558–567.

52. Davidson MB, Thakkar S, Hix JK, et al. Pathophysiology, clinical consequences, and treatment of tumor lysis syndrome. Am J Med 2004;116:546–554.

53. Hochberg J, Cairo MS. Tumor lysis syndrome: Current perspective. Haematologica 2008;93:9–13.

54. Cairo MS, Bishop M. Tumor lysis syndrome: New therapeutic strategies and classification. Br J Hematol 2004;127:3–11.

55. Yim BT, Sims-McCallum RP, Chong PH. Rasburicase for the treatment and prevention of hyperuricemia. Ann Pharmacother 2003;37:1047–1054.

56. The National Cancer Institute: Dictionary of Cancer Terms. http://www.cancer.gov/dictionary/

57. Kassner E. Evaluation and treatment of chemotherapy extravasation injuries. J Pediatr Oncol Nurs 2000;17:135–148.

58. Ener RA, Meglathery SB, Styler M. Extravasation of systemic hemato-oncological therapies. Ann Oncol 2004;15:858–862.

59. Oncology Nursing Society. Cancer Chemotherapy and Biotherapy Guidelines and Recommendations for Practice: Module XXII. Pittsburgh, PA: Oncology Nursing Press, 2002.

60. Stanford BL, Hardwicke F. A review of clinical experience with paclitaxel extravasations. Support Care Cancer 2003;11:270–277.

100 Parenteral Nutrition

Michael D. Kraft and Imad F. Btaiche

LEARNING OBJECTIVES

Upon completion of the chapter, the reader will be able to:

1. List the appropriate indications for the use of parenteral nutrition (PN).

2. Describe the components of PN and their role in nutrition support therapy.

3. List the elements of nutrition assessment and factors considered in assessing a patient's nutritional status and nutritional requirements.

4. Explain the pharmaceutical and compounding issues with PN admixtures.

5. Develop a plan to design, initiate, and adjust a PN formulation based on patient-specific factors.

6. Describe the etiology and risk factors for PN macronutrient-associated complications including hyperglycemia, hypoglycemia, hyperlipidemia, and azotemia in patients receiving PN.

7. Describe the etiology and risk factors for the refeeding syndrome.

8. Describe the etiology and risk factors for liver complications and metabolic bone disease in patients receiving PN.

9. Design a plan to monitor and correct fluid, electrolyte, vitamin, and trace element abnormalities in patients receiving PN.

10. Design a plan to assess the efficacy and monitor the safety of PN therapy.

KEY CONCEPTS

❶ Parenteral nutrition (PN), also called total parenteral nutrition (TPN), is the IV administration of fluids, macronutrients, electrolytes, vitamins, and trace elements for the purpose of weight maintenance or gain, to preserve or replete lean body mass and visceral proteins, and to support anabolism and nitrogen balance *when the oral/enteral route is not feasible or adequate.*

❷ Amino acids are provided in PN to preserve or replete lean body mass and visceral proteins, and to promote protein anabolism and wound healing.

❸ Dextrose (D-glucose) is the major immediate energy source in PN and is vital for cellular metabolism, body protein preservation, tissue formation, and cellular growth.

❹ IV lipid emulsions are used as an energy source in PN, and to prevent or treat essential fatty acid deficiency.

❺ PN should not be used to treat acute fluid and electrolyte abnormalities. Rather, PN should be adjusted to meet maintenance requirements and to minimize worsening of underlying fluid and electrolyte disturbances.

❻ Electrolytes, vitamins, and trace elements are essential for numerous biochemical and metabolic functions, and should be added to PN daily unless otherwise not indicated.

❼ PN can be administered via a small peripheral vein (as peripheral PN [PPN]) or via a larger central vein (as central PN).

❽ PN admixtures can be prepared by mixing all components into one bag [3-in-1 admixture or a total nutrient admixture (TNA)] or by mixing and infusing dextrose, amino acids, and all other components together (2-in-1 admixture) and infusing IV lipid emulsion separately.

❾ PN can be associated with significant complications with both short- and long-term therapy.

❿ Patients receiving PN should have specific laboratory values checked to assess electrolyte status, organ function, and nutritional status, and these parameters should be monitored as indicated clinically.

INTRODUCTION

Maintaining adequate nutritional status, especially during periods of illness and metabolic stress, is an important part of patient care. Malnutrition in hospitalized patients is associated with significant complications, including increased infection risk, poor wound healing, prolonged hospital stay, and increased mortality, especially in surgical and critically ill patients.[1] *Nutrition support therapy* refers to the administration of nutrients via the oral, enteral, or parenteral route for therapeutic purposes.[1] ❶ *Parenteral nutrition (PN), also called total parenteral nutrition (TPN), is the IV administration of fluids, macronutrients, electrolytes, vitamins, and trace elements for the purpose of weight maintenance or gain, to preserve or replete lean body mass and visceral proteins, and to support anabolism and nitrogen balance when the oral/enteral route is not feasible or adequate.* PN is a potentially lifesaving therapy in patients with intestinal failure, but also may be associated with significant complications.

DESIRED OUTCOMES AND GOALS

Nutrition support therapy is aimed at meeting patient's nutritional requirements, improving energy and net protein balance, promoting growth or weight maintenance, and improving healing, particularly in malnourished patients. Goals of providing nutrition support therapy include:

- Weight maintenance (potential weight gain in malnourished patients and growing children)
- Preservation (or repletion) of lean body mass and visceral proteins
- Support of anabolism and nitrogen balance
- Correction or avoidance of fluid and electrolyte abnormalities
- Correction or avoidance of vitamin and trace element abnormalities
- Avoidance of further nutritional deficiencies

Indications for PN

PN can be a lifesaving therapy in patients with intestinal failure, but the oral or enteral route is preferred when providing nutrition support therapy ("when the gut works, use it"). Compared with PN, enteral nutrition is associated with lower risk of hyperglycemia and fewer infectious complications (e.g., pneumonia, intra-abdominal abscess, and catheter-related infections).[1,2] However, if used appropriately (i.e., in patients with altered intestinal function or when the intestine cannot be used), PN can be safe, effective, and improves nutrient delivery.[3] Indications for PN are listed in Table 100–1.[1,2] More detailed recommendations on appropriate PN indications in specific disease states, as well as when to initiate PN, can be found in the American Society for Parenteral and Enteral Nutrition (A.S.P.E.N.) Guidelines for the Use of Parenteral and Enteral Nutrition.[1] More recently, A.S.P.E.N. and the Society of Critical Care Medicine (SCCM) published detailed guidelines for nutrition support therapy in critically ill adult patients, including patients undergoing major upper GI surgical procedures.[2]

Table 100–1

Indications for PN[a,b]

- Bowel obstruction
  - Physical/mechanical (e.g., tumor compressing intestinal lumen)
  - Functional (e.g., postoperative ileus)
- Major small bowel resection (e.g., short-bowel syndrome)
  - Adult patients with less than 100 cm small bowel distal to the ligament of Treitz without a colon
  - Adult patients with less than 50 cm of small bowel if the colon is intact
- Diffuse peritonitis
- GI fistulas if enteral nutrition cannot be provided above or below the fistula
- Pancreatitis—if patients have failed enteral nutrition beyond the ligament of Treitz or cannot receive enteral nutrition (e.g., due to intestinal obstruction)
- Severe intractable vomiting
- Severe intractable diarrhea
- Preoperative nutrition support in patients with moderate to severe malnutrition who cannot tolerate enteral nutrition and in whom surgery can be delayed safely for at least 7 days

[a]When anticipated that adequate oral or enteral nutrition will not be possible for approximately 7 days or more, and if anticipated that PN will be used for approximately 7 days or more.

[b]In patients with evidence of malnutrition, nutrition support therapy should be initiated as soon as possible (e.g., within 24–48 hours of hospital admission) after the patient has been resuscitated.

From Refs. 1 and 2.

PN COMPONENTS

PN should provide a *balanced* nutritional intake, including macronutrients, micronutrients, fluid and electrolytes. Macronutrients, including amino acids, dextrose, and IV lipid emulsions, are important sources of structural and energy-yielding substrates. A balanced PN formulation of total daily calories includes 10% to 20% from amino acids, 50% to 60% from dextrose, and 20% to 30% from IV lipid emulsion. Under conditions when patients have higher protein requirements (e.g., severe thermal injury, treatment with continuous renal replacement therapy, hypocaloric feeding—discussed later), amino acids may provide slightly more than 20% of the total daily calories. Electrolytes and micronutrients including vitamins and trace elements are required to support essential biochemical reactions. PN also provides a significant source of fluids. Patients require individual adjustments of PN components based on their nutritional status, nutritional requirements, underlying disease state(s), level of metabolic stress, clinical status, and organ functions.

Amino Acids

Amino acids are the building blocks of body proteins. There is no excess storage form of protein in the body, so amino acids are an essential component of the PN admixture. ❷ *Amino acids are provided to preserve or replete lean body mass and visceral proteins and to promote protein anabolism*

Patient Encounter 1

AA is 45-year-old woman admitted to the hospital with chief complaints of fever, abdominal pain, nausea, and vomiting for 2 days. She also reports decreased appetite and decreased oral intake for the past 3 to 4 days. AA was discharged from the hospital 2 weeks ago after having a small bowel resection for recurrent bowel obstruction.

Medical History

Recurrent intestinal strictures, intestinal obstructions, type II diabetes mellitus

Surgical History

Small bowel resections (less than 100 cm of small intestine remaining, ileocecal valve and colon intact)

Family History and Social History

Noncontributory

Medications Prior to Admission

Glipizide XL 5 mg orally daily

PE:

Height 168 cm (approximately 5 ft, 6 in.), actual body weight 60 kg (132 lb), ideal body weight 60 kg (132 lb), temperature

38.9°C (102°F), heart rate 98 bpm, blood pressure 98/55 mm Hg, respiratory rate 30 breaths/min, alert and oriented × 3, mucous membranes and skin appear cool and dry, tachycardic, tachypneic, lungs clear

Abdomen: slightly tense, diffuse abdominal pain

CT: evidence of interperitoneal free air consistent with perforation.

Diagnoses

Possible intestinal leak/perforation, diffuse peritonitis, sepsis, mild dehydration, and hypovolemic hypotonic hyponatremia

Plan

Admit to the surgical intensive care unit for resuscitation and treatment.

Is PN therapy indicated in this patient?

What other patient data should be collected to help formulate a PN prescription?

---

and wound healing. Amino acids are a source of calories with a caloric value of 4 kcal/g.

Parenteral crystalline amino acid bulk solutions are supplied by various manufacturers in various concentrations (e.g., 3.5%, 5%, 7%, 8.5%, 10%, 15%, and 20%). Different formulations are tailored for specific age groups (e.g., adults and infants) and for some disease states (e.g., kidney and liver disease). Specialized formulations for patients with acute kidney injury contain higher proportions of essential amino acids. Formulations for patients with hepatic encephalopathy contain higher amounts of branched-chain and lower amounts of aromatic amino acids. However, these specialized formulations are not used routinely in clinical practice because their efficacy and role in improving patient outcomes has not been clearly demonstrated. Crystalline amino acid solutions have an acidic pH (pH ≈ 5 to 7) and may contain inherent electrolytes (e.g., sodium, potassium, acetate, and phosphate).

Dextrose

❸ *Dextrose (D-glucose) is the major immediate energy source, and it is vital for cellular metabolism, body protein preservation, and cellular growth.* Several body tissues depend primarily on dextrose for energy, including the central nervous system (CNS), red blood cells, and the renal medulla.

Parenteral dextrose (hydrous dextrose) used in PN compounding typically is provided as a 70% stock solution (70 g/100 mL), although some institutions use a 50% stock

solution. The final dextrose concentration in the central PN solution typically should not exceed 35%. Hydrous dextrose provides 3.4 kcal/g (14.2 kJ/g). A dextrose infusion rate of 2 mg/kg/min in adult patients is sufficient to suppress gluconeogenesis and spare body proteins from being used for energy.[4] Continuous dextrose infusion rate in hospitalized adult patients generally should not exceed 4 to 5 mg/kg/min.[5,6]

IV Lipid Emulsions

❹ *IV lipid emulsions have two main clinical uses: prevent or treat essential fatty acid deficiency and provide an energy source.* IV lipid emulsions currently marketed in the United States consist of long-chain triglycerides. Lipid particles consist of a triglyceride core surrounded by a layer of egg phospholipids (emulsifiers). These particles carry a negative charge on their surface that creates repulsive electrostatic forces between droplets and maintains the stability of the emulsion. Glycerol is added to the emulsion to adjust the tonicity, and water is the solvent. The negative charges on the surface of lipid particles can be disrupted by cations, especially divalent cations such as calcium and magnesium, iron which can exist in divalent or trivalent form,[7] and extreme pH changes, particularly acidic pH. Creaming of the emulsion occurs when lipid particles begin to aggregate and migrate to the surface of the emulsion, but can be reversed with mild agitation. If these particles continue to aggregate, coalescence may occur and destabilize the emulsion. A coalesced emulsion should not be infused into

Table 100–2							
Comparison of IV Lipid Emulsions							
Brand Names	Liposyn II		Liposyn III			Intralipid	
Source	Soybean and safflower oil		Soybean oil			Soybean oil	
Concentration (%)	10	20	10	20	30	20	30
Linoleic acid (%)	65.8	65.8	54.5	54.5	54.5	50	50
Linolenic acid (%)	4.2	4.2	8.3	8.3	8.3	9	9
Phospholipids (egg yolk) (%)	1.2	1.2	1.2	1.2	1.8	1.2	1.2
PL:TG ratio[a]	0.12	0.06	0.12	0.06	0.06	0.06	0.04
Caloric density (kcal/mL)	1.1	2	1.1	2	3	2	3
Approximate osmolarity (mOsm/L)	276	258	284	292	293	350	310
Approximate mean pH (range)	8 (6–9)	8.3 (6–9)	8.3 (6–9)		8.4 (6–9)	8 (6–8.9)	

[a]PL:TG ratio, phospholipid:triglyceride ratio; 1 k cal = 4.18 kilojoules (kj).

a patient because this can result in fat emboli. If coalescence continues, irreversible separation of the emulsion can occur (oiling out or breaking of the emulsion).

IV lipid emulsions differ in their concentration (10%, 20%, and 30%), caloric density, natural source of lipids, and ratio of phospholipids to triglycerides (PL:TG). Table 100–2 shows a comparison of commercially available IV lipid emulsions in the United States. The 10%, 20%, and 30% lipid emulsions provide 1.1 kcal/mL (4.6 kJ/mL), 2 kcal/mL (8.4 kJ/mL), and 3 kcal/mL (12.6 kJ/mL). The 10% and 20% lipid emulsions have a PL:TG ratio of 0.12 and 0.06, respectively; the 30% lipid emulsions have a PL:TG ratio of 0.06 (30% Liposyn III) or 0.04 (30% Intralipid). The lower PL:TG indicates a lower phospholipid content and translates to a better clearance of the 20% and 30% lipid emulsions compared with the 10% lipid emulsion.[8] The 30% lipid emulsion is only approved by the FDA for infusion in a total nutrient admixture (TNA) and should not be infused directly into patients.

Lipid particles are hydrolyzed in the bloodstream by the enzyme lipoprotein lipase to release free fatty acids and glycerol. Free fatty acids are taken up into adipose tissue for storage (triglycerides), oxidized to energy in various tissues (e.g., skeletal muscle), or recycled in the liver to make lipoproteins. The typical daily dose of IV lipid emulsions in adults is 0.5 to 1 g/kg/day. The maximum dose of IV lipid emulsions in adults is 2.5 g/kg/day[6] or 60% of total daily calories, although doses this high are used rarely in practice.

The essential fatty acids in humans are linoleic acid (C18:2 n-6) and α-linolenic acid (C18:3 n-3). Arachidonic acid (C20:4 n-6) is also essential but can be synthesized in vivo from linoleic acid. Adult patients should be provided a minimum of 2% to 4% of total daily calories as linoleic acid and 0.25% to 0.5% of total daily calories as α-linolenic acid to prevent essential fatty acid deficiency.[6] This can be achieved practically by providing a minimum of approximately 500 mL of 20% IV lipid emulsion once weekly (or 250 mL twice weekly, on separate days) for most adult patients. Biochemical evidence of essential fatty acid deficiency (e.g., decreased serum linoleic acid, α-linolenic acid, and arachidonic acid concentrations, elevated mead acid concentrations and elevated triene-to-tetraene ratio) can develop in about 2 to 4 weeks in adult patients receiving lipid-free PN. Clinical manifestations (e.g., dry skin, skin desquamation, hair loss, hepatomegaly, anemia, thrombocytopenia, poor wound healing) generally appear after an additional 1 to 2 weeks, although skin changes may take longer to appear.[9]

Complications and safety concerns related to the administration of IV lipid emulsions include severe hypertriglyceridemia, systemic infection, anaphylactic reactions, and infusion-related reactions. Patients with hypertriglyceridemia, acute kidney injury, chronic kidney disease, and severe metabolic stress may have reduced lipid clearance and are at high risk of developing hypertriglyceridemia. Patients with hepatic dysfunction or pancreatitis (in particular if pancreatitis is caused by hypertriglyceridemia) can also have reduced lipid clearance. IV lipid emulsions should be withheld in adult patients with a serum triglyceride concentration exceeding 400 mg/dL (4.52 mmol/L).

Patients without malnutrition who receive PN may have a higher incidence of infectious complications than patients who do not receive PN.[10] IV lipid emulsions support the growth of common bacterial and fungal pathogens, but bacterial growth is slower in TNAs than in IV lipid emulsions alone.[11,12] This is due to the acidic pH of amino acid solutions and high osmolarity of PN formulations. The Centers for Disease Control and Prevention (CDC) recommends that infusion of IV lipid emulsions separately from PN (i.e., 2-in-1) be completed within 12 hours of initiation (e.g., two lipid containers can be used, with each container infused over 12 hours). If fluid or volume considerations prohibit a reduced infusion time, the lipid infusion can then be completed within 24 hours. Because TNAs support microbial growth at a slower rate than IV lipid emulsions, the CDC recommends that TNA infusion be completed within 24 hours of initiation. Furthermore, a 0.22-micron bacterial retention filter cannot be used on the infusion line because the average size of lipid particles is approximately 0.4 to 0.5 micron. Strict aseptic techniques must be used when handling IV lipid emulsions to minimize the risk of PN contamination and possible infectious complications.

Patients with allergy to eggs or legumes (e.g., soybeans, broad beans, and lentils) may develop allergic reactions with IV lipid emulsions. Rarely, infusion-related adverse effects including fever, chills, headache, palpitations, dyspnea, chest tightness, and nausea also may occur with rapid infusion of IV lipid emulsions. Extending the IV lipid infusion time (e.g., over 12–24 hours) can minimize infusion-related adverse events and improves lipid clearance. Infusion rate of IV lipid emulsions should not exceed 0.12 g/kg/h.[6]

Fluid

❺ *PN should not be used to treat acute fluid abnormalities. Rather, PN should be adjusted to provide maintenance fluid requirements and to minimize worsening of underlying fluid disturbances, taking into account other fluids the patient is receiving.* Daily maintenance fluid requirements for adults can be estimated with the following equation:

Total daily maintenance fluid requirements = 1,500 mL + (20 mL/kg × [wt (kg) − 20])*

For patients with fluid deficits, it is safer, clinically indicated, and more cost-effective to correct fluid abnormalities using standard IV fluids (e.g., sodium chloride 0.9% in water, dextrose 5% in water, dextrose 5% and sodium chloride 0.45% in water, or lactated Ringer's solution). Minimizing fluid volume in PN may be indicated in patients with fluid overload and patients who receive large volumes of fluids from multiple IV medications and fluids (e.g., critically ill, bone marrow transplant), patients with oliguric (urine output less than 400 mL/day) or anuric (urine output less than 50 mL/day) acute kidney injury, and those with congestive heart failure. It is reasonable to provide total daily fluid requirements (both maintenance requirements and GI/other abnormal losses) in the PN admixture in patients who depend on long-term PN. However, caution should be exercised when the PN solution is diluted to an extent that may alter the stability and compatibility of a concentrated solution. Diluting a PN admixture may affect its physical and chemical properties (e.g., the pH, which could affect lipid emulsion stability and calcium–phosphate compatibility); therefore, stability and compatibility data should be confirmed first.

Electrolytes

❻ *Electrolytes are essential for many metabolic and homeostatic functions, including enzymatic and biochemical reactions, maintenance of cell membrane structure and function, neurotransmission, hormone function, muscle contraction, cardiovascular function, bone composition, and fluid homeostasis.* The causes of electrolyte abnormalities in patients receiving PN may be multifactorial, including altered absorption and distribution; excessive or inadequate intake; altered hormonal, neurologic, and homeostatic mechanisms; altered excretion via GI and renal losses; changes in fluid status and fluid shifts; and medications. PN should not be used to treat acute electrolyte abnormalities, but electrolytes in PN should be adjusted to meet maintenance requirements and to minimize worsening of underlying electrolyte disturbances.

Electrolytes that are included routinely in PN admixtures include sodium, potassium, phosphorus (as phosphate), calcium, magnesium, chloride, and acetate. When determi-

---

* For elderly patients (e.g., greater than 60 years old), use 15 mL/kg for every kilogram above 20 kg.

Table 100–3

Approximate Daily Maintenance Electrolyte Requirements for Adults

Electrolyte	Approximate Daily Maintenance Requirements[a]	Electrolyte Salts Used in PN
Sodium	1–2 mEq/kg	Chloride, acetate, phosphate
Potassium	1–2 mEq/kg	Chloride, acetate, phosphate
Phosphorus	20–40 mmol	Sodium phosphate, potassium phosphate
Calcium	10–15 mEq	Gluconate
Magnesium	8–20 mEq	Sulfate
Chloride	b	Sodium, potassium
Acetate	b	Sodium, potassium
Conversions	1 mmol potassium phosphate = 1.47 mEq potassium	
	1 mmol sodium phosphate = 1.33 mEq sodium	

[a]Electrolyte requirements are adjusted based on serum electrolyte concentrations, and vary depending on kidney function, GI losses, nutritional status, specific metabolic and endocrine functions, and medication therapy that affect electrolyte losses or retention.
[b]As needed to maintain acid–base balance; linked to amounts of sodium and potassium provided (as chloride and acetate salts).

From Ref. 6.

ning electrolytes in PN admixtures, the patient's kidney function always must be taken into account. Typical daily electrolyte maintenance requirements for adults with normal kidney function are listed in Table 100–3.

▶ Sodium

Sodium is the most abundant extracellular cation in the body and is the major osmotically active ion in the extracellular fluid. Sodium concentration determines the distribution of water in the extracellular space, and sodium disorders can be caused by many factors. Patients with abnormal GI losses (e.g., gastric, diarrhea, ostomy, and fistula losses) have increased sodium requirements. Patients with fluid overload and hypervolemic hypotonic hyponatremia may require sodium and fluid restriction. Sodium in PN can be provided in the forms of chloride, acetate, and phosphate salts. One millimole (mmol) of sodium phosphate provides 1.33 mEq of elemental sodium. Total sodium concentration in PN should not exceed 154 mEq/L (154 mmol/L, the equivalent of normal saline).

▶ Potassium

Potassium is the second most abundant cation in the body and is found primarily in the intracellular fluid. Potassium has many important physiologic functions, including regulation of cell membrane electrical action potential (especially in the myocardium), muscular function, cellular metabolism, and glycogen and protein synthesis. Potassium in PN can be provided as chloride, acetate, and phosphate salts. One millimole of potassium phosphate provides 1.47 mEq of elemental potassium. Generally, the concentration of potassium in peripheral PN (PPN) admixtures should not exceed 80 mEq/L (80 mmol/L). While it is safer to limit potassium solution concentration to 80 mEq/L (80 mmol/L) for infusion through a central vein, the maximum recommended potassium concentration for infusion via a central vein is 150 mEq/L (150 mmol/L).[13] Patients with abnormal potassium losses (e.g., loop or thiazide diuretic therapy, diarrhea, high gastric fluid output) may have higher potassium requirements, and patients with high gastric fluid output, acute kidney injury or chronic kidney disease may require potassium restriction.

▶ Calcium and Phosphorus

Calcium and phosphorus are essential electrolytes for many physiologic processes and biochemical reactions. Phosphorus is provided as sodium or potassium phosphate in PN. Approximately 10 to 15 mmol of phosphate are needed per 1,000 kilocalories to maintain normal serum phosphorus concentrations (provided the patient is well nourished and has normal kidney function).[14] Patients with decreased kidney function may require phosphorus restriction.

The FDA published a safety alert in 1994 in response to two deaths associated with calcium–phosphate precipitation in PN.[15] Autopsy reports from these patients revealed diffuse microvascular pulmonary emboli containing calcium–phosphate precipitates. Because calcium and phosphate can bind and precipitate in solution, caution must be exercised when mixing these two electrolytes in PN admixtures. Several factors can affect calcium–phosphate solubility, including the following:

- *pH.* Largely affected by the final amino acid concentration, to a lesser extent by the dextrose concentration (unless the final amino acid concentration is very low); the lower the solution pH, the less chance there is for calcium–phosphate precipitation; monobasic phosphates predominate at low pH, leaving fewer free dibasic phosphates for precipitation with divalent calcium; monobasic calcium phosphate is more soluble than dibasic calcium phosphate.
- *Amino acid concentration.* Primary factor that affects pH of the PN admixture; the pH of amino acid stock solutions may vary between commercial products and thus differently affects the final pH of PN admixture; however, in general the higher the final amino acid concentration, the lower the pH of the final admixture (see above), and more phosphates likely bind with amino acids leaving fewer phosphates available to bind with calcium.
- *Calcium salt.* Calcium gluconate is the preferred calcium salt in PN because it is has a low dissociation constant in solution with lesser free calcium available at a given time to bind phosphate (as opposed to calcium chloride, which dissociates rapidly in solution). One gram of calcium gluconate provides 4.5 mEq of elemental calcium.
- *Time.* The longer calcium and phosphate are in solution, the more calcium and phosphate will dissociate over

time and increase the risk for calcium–phosphate precipitation.

- *Temperature.* As temperature increases, more calcium and phosphate dissociate and increase the risk of calcium–phosphate precipitation.
- *Order of mixing.* Calcium and phosphate should be separated when mixing PN admixtures (e.g., add phosphate first, then all other PN components, and then add calcium last); if calcium is added before all other components are in the PN admixture, including lipid emulsion, then the volume in the PN admixture at the time calcium is added must be used to determine the maximum calcium that can be added.

▶ Magnesium

Magnesium is the second most abundant intracellular cation after potassium. Magnesium serves as an essential cofactor for numerous enzymes and in many biochemical reactions, including reactions involving adenosine triphosphate (ATP).[16] Magnesium disorders are multifactorial and can be related to kidney function, disease state(s), and medication therapy. Magnesium in PN typically is provided as magnesium sulfate. One gram of magnesium sulfate provides 8.1 mEq of elemental magnesium.

▶ Chloride and Acetate

Concentration limits for chloride and acetate in PN typically are linked to limitations of sodium and potassium. The usual ratio of chloride:acetate in PN is about 1:1 to 1.5:1. Chloride and acetate primarily play a role in acid–base balance. Chloride is primarily eliminated via the kidneys. Serum chloride concentrations that exceed 130 mEq/L (130 mmol/L) may cause hyperchloremic acidosis. Acetate is converted to bicarbonate at a 1:1 molar ratio. This conversion appears to occur mostly outside the liver. Acetate conversion to bicarbonate is rapid but not immediate, and thus acetate salts should not be used to correct acute severe acidosis. Bicarbonate *never* should be added to or coinfused with PN solutions. This can lead to the release of carbon dioxide and potentially result in the formation of calcium or magnesium carbonate (very insoluble salts).

Vitamins

❻ *The water-soluble and fat-soluble vitamins in the parenteral multivitamin mix are essential cofactors for numerous biochemical reactions and metabolic processes. Parenteral multivitamins are added daily to the PN admixture.* Patients with chronic kidney disease may be at risk for vitamin A accumulation and potential toxicity. Serum vitamin A concentrations should be measured in patients with chronic kidney disease when vitamin A accumulation is a concern. Previously, vitamin K was administered either daily or once weekly because IV multivitamin formulations did not contain vitamin K. However, manufacturers have reformulated their parenteral multivitamin products to provide 150 mcg of vitamin K in accordance with FDA recommendations. There is a parenteral adult multivitamin formulation available without vitamin K (e.g., for patients who require warfarin therapy), but standard compounding of PN formulations should include a parenteral multivitamin that contains vitamin K unless otherwise clinically indicated. Water-soluble vitamins, with the exception of vitamin B12, are generally readily excreted and not stored in the body in significant amounts. Deficiencies of water-soluble vitamins can occur rapidly in the absence of adequate vitamin supplementation in PN. For example, refractory severe lactic acidosis and deaths were reported in patients who were receiving PN without added thiamine. Thiamine is a cofactor of the pyruvate dehydrogenase enzyme that is involved in the aerobic metabolism of pyruvate to acetyl-CoA (via the tricarboxylic acid cycle). Deficiency of thiamine pyrophosphate prevents the formation of acetyl-CoA from pyruvate, which is instead converted to lactate via anaerobic metabolism, resulting in lactic acidosis.

Trace Elements

❻ *Trace elements are essential cofactors for numerous biochemical processes. Trace elements that are added routinely to PN include zinc, selenium, copper, manganese, and chromium.* There are various commercial parenteral trace-element formulations that can be added to PN admixtures (e.g., MTE-5). Zinc is important for wound healing, and patients with high-output fistulas, diarrhea, burns, and large open wounds may require additional zinc supplementation. Patients may lose as much as 12 to 17 mg zinc per liter of GI output (e.g., from diarrhea or enterocutaneous fistula losses); however, 12 mg/day may be adequate to maintain these patients in positive zinc balance.[17] Patients with chronic severe diarrhea, malabsorption, and short-gut syndrome may also have increased selenium losses and may require additional selenium supplementation. Chromium is a cofactor for glucose metabolism, and patients with chromium deficiency may exhibit glucose intolerance; however, chromium deficiency is a rare cause of hyperglycemia. Patients with cholestasis (serum direct bilirubin concentration that exceeds 2 mg/dL [34.2 µmol/L]) should have manganese and possibly copper restricted to avoid their accumulation and possible toxicity, because both elements undergo biliary elimination. Manganese-induced neurotoxicity has been reported in PN patients with cholestasis and those receiving chronic PN. However, copper deficiency resulting in anemia, pancytopenia and death has occurred when copper was omitted from the PN of PN-dependent patients. Because copper deficiency has been reported to occur anywhere between 6 weeks and 12 months following copper elimination from PN,[18] serum copper concentrations need to be regularly monitored (e.g., every 6 weeks at first and 2–3 months thereafter) when copper is omitted from PN admixtures. Trace element status should be monitored at first periodically (e.g., every 2–3 months) in patients at risk for trace element deficiency or accumulation. Once stable, serum trace element concentrations can be monitored less frequently (e.g., every 6–12 months).

PN Additives

▶ *Heparin*

Heparin (0.5–1 unit/mL of final PN volume) may be added to PN admixtures for three reasons:

- To maintain catheter patency, although this effect is debated
- To reduce thrombophlebitis, essentially with PPN infusion
- To enhance lipid particle clearance by acting as a cofactor for the lipoprotein lipase enzyme

The benefits and necessity of adding heparin to PN are unclear, and practices vary between institutions. There are also concerns about the stability and compatibility of IV lipid emulsions with heparin added at concentrations above 1 unit/mL. Heparin should be omitted in patients with active bleeding, thrombocytopenia, heparin-induced thrombocytopenia (HIT), or heparin allergy.

▶ *Regular Insulin*

Regular insulin may be added to PN admixtures for glycemic control. The dose of insulin depends on the severity of hyperglycemia and daily insulin requirements. Generally, once the patient is receiving PN at goal, about 70% of the total insulin administered over the previous 24 hours as sliding scale or continuous infusion can be added to the next PN admixture. The insulin dose should be adjusted based on frequent capillary blood glucose evaluation. Caution should be used when insulin is added to PN to avoid hypoglycemia. Adding insulin to PN rather than administering as a continuous IV infusion does not provide the flexibility of frequent titration of the insulin dose to the desired target blood glucose concentration. As such, severe uncontrolled hyperglycemia is best treated with a continuous insulin infusion.

▶ *Histamine-2-Receptor Antagonists*

IV histamine-2-receptor antagonists such as ranitidine, famotidine, and cimetidine are compatible with PN and can be added to the daily PN when indicated (e.g., prevention of stress-related mucosal damage). This provides a continuous acid suppression and reduces nursing time by avoiding intermittent scheduled infusions.

▶ *Human Albumin*

Human albumin is a colloid used as a plasma volume expander and is *not* a source of nutrition. Albumin should not be added to the PN admixture and should be administered separately from PN because it may increase microbial growth and infectious risk when mixed in the PN admixture. Further, coinfusion of human albumin at the Y-site injection of IV lipid emulsions and TNAs causes disruption and creaming of the IV lipid emulsion.

▶ *Iron Dextran*

Iron-deficiency anemia in chronic PN-dependent patients may be due to underlying clinical conditions and the lack of regular iron supplementation in PN. Parenteral iron therapy becomes necessary in iron-deficient patients who cannot absorb or tolerate oral iron. Parenteral iron should be used with caution owing to its infusion-related adverse effects. A test dose of 25 mg of iron dextran should be administered first, and the patient should be monitored for adverse effects for at least 60 minutes. Iron dextran then may be added to lipid-free PN at a daily dose of 100 mg until the total iron dose is given. Iron dextran is not compatible with IV lipid emulsions and can cause oiling out of the emulsion. Other parenteral iron formulations (e.g., iron sucrose and ferric gluconate) have not been evaluated for compounding in PN and should not be added to PN admixtures.

NUTRITION ASSESSMENT AND NUTRITIONAL REQUIREMENTS

The first step before delivering nutrition support therapy is to perform a nutritional assessment and determine nutrient requirements based on the patient's nutritional status and clinical conditions. Subjective and objective data of dietary intake, functional capacity, anthropometrics, weight changes, GI function, medical history, medication therapy, and laboratory data are collected to determine a patient's nutritional status, identify patients with malnutrition or at risk for malnutrition, and to identify risk factors that may put a patient at risk for nutrition-related problems.[1] A nutrition assessment should include:[1,19]

- Patient history
- Physical assessment including height, weight, ideal body weight (IBW), body mass index (BMI = weight [kg]/height [m²]), and recent weight loss (intentional or unintentional). BMI relates a person's body weight to their height and is a vague indicator of total body fat mass in adults. BMI categories do not account for *frame size*, muscle mass, bone, and water weight. Classifications of weight status in relation to BMI are: underweight less than 18.5 kg/m²; normal 18.5 to 24.9 kg/m²; overweight 25 to 29.9 kg/m²; obese greater than or equal to 30 kg/m²
- Physical examination of the musculoskeletal system (e.g., biceps, triceps, quadriceps, temporalis, deltoid, and interosseus muscles) for loss of muscle mass, and examination of the skin and mucous membranes for abnormalities (e.g., noting dry or flaky skin, bruising, edema, ascites, poorly healing wounds) and loss of subcutaneous fat (e.g., triceps, chest)
- Changes in eating habits and GI function, and associated GI symptoms
- Presence and severity of underlying and concurrent disease(s)
- Serum visceral protein concentrations (e.g., albumin, prealbumin). Hypoalbuminemia at baseline or prior to hospitalization may be indicative of malnutrition, and severe hypoalbuminemia may be associated with poor patient outcome. Serum albumin and prealbumin concentrations are not sensitive and specific markers of nutritional status and protein stores in hospitalized patients under metabolic stress (e.g., postsurgery, organ failure, severe burns, trauma, and sepsis). Albumin and prealbumin are negative acute phase proteins. Their liver synthesis is decreased under stress and they are sensitive to non-nutritional factors including hydration status, and kidney and liver functions. Because prealbumin has a shorter half-life (approximately 2 days) than albumin (approximately 20 days), serum prealbumin concentrations are measured usually once weekly to help evaluate the net anabolism in response to nutrition support therapy.
- Serum concentrations of vitamins, trace elements, and iron as indicated

There are several methods to conducting a nutrition assessment, but one approach that has been validated is the Subjective Global Assessment (SGA).[1] Application of the SGA requires gathering the data listed above and assessing these parameters (i.e., weight change, dietary changes, GI symptoms, functional capacity, and physical examination) and then assigning a subjective rating (A = well nourished; B = moderately malnourished or suspected of being malnourished; C = severely malnourished).[19]

After performing a nutrition assessment, estimate the patient's daily energy and protein requirements (Table 100–4). Indirect calorimetry involves measuring the volumes of oxygen consumption (VO_2) and carbon dioxide production (VCO_2) to determine the resting metabolic rate (RMR) or resting energy expenditure (REE) and respiratory quotient ($RQ = VCO_2/VO_2$). The REE or RMR is the amount of calories required during 24 hours by the body in a nonactive state, and is approximately 10% higher than the basal energy expenditure (BEE, metabolic activity required to maintain life) as it adjusts for the thermic effect of food and awake state. Because critically ill patients may have variable energy expenditure, indirect calorimetry is a valuable tool in assessing energy expenditure in mechanically ventilated patients with multiple and changing clinical conditions. Indirect calorimetry requires expensive equipment and trained personnel to use, and therefore is not feasible in all institutions. Over 200 equations have been developed to determine energy expenditure (EE) for adults. The Harris-Benedict equations, Penn State equations (for nonobese critically ill patients), and the Mifflin St. Jeor equations (for obese noncritically ill patients) are some of the most widely used. Harris-Benedict equations take into account a patient's sex, weight, height, and age to determine the BEE. A "stress" or "injury" factor is then applied to estimate the daily total EE (TEE). Daily energy requirements are about 100% to 130% of the RMR with adequate protein intake. Alternatively, EE can be estimated based on EE per body weight (i.e., kilocalories per kilogram). However, dry weight or admission weight should be used, and this estimation may not be appropriate in patients who are obese or in elderly patients. There is debate over the best method to estimate energy requirements for obese patients. Several equations have been developed to estimate EE in obese

Table 100–4

Estimating Daily Energy and Amino Acid Requirements in Adults

Determining Energy Expenditure

Harris-Benedict equations	Men: BEE = 66.42 + 13.75 (W) + 5 (H) − 6.78 (A)
	Women: BEE = 655.1 + 9.65 (W) + 1.85 (H) − 4.68 (A)
	W = weight in kg, H = height in cm, A = age in years
	Energy expenditure then should be multiplied by a stress factor to estimate the total energy expenditure (TEE):
	Bed rest ≈ 1.2 × BEE
	Ambulatory ≈ 1.3 × BEE
	Anabolic ≈ 1.5 × BEE
	Energy requirements should also be increased ~12% with each degree of fever above 37°C (98.6°F).
Penn State equations (for critically ill nonobese adult patients)	RMR = (0.85 × BEE[a]) + (33 × V_E) + (175 × T_{max}) − 6,433
	RMR = (0.96 × BMR[b]) + (31 × V_E) + (167 × T_{max}) − 6,212
	[a]BEE calculated using Harris-Benedict; [b]BMR calculated using Mifflin-St. Jeor equations; V_E = minute ventilation in liters per minute; Tmax = maximum body temperature in degrees Celsius.
Mifflin-St. Jeor equations (for overweight and obese noncritically ill hospitalized adult patients)	Men BMR = (10 × W) + (6.25 × H) − (5 × A) + 5
	Women BMR = (10 × W) + (6.25 × H) − (5 × A) − 161
	BMR = basal metabolic rate. W = weight (kg); H = height (cm); A = age (years)
Energy expenditure per body weight (i.e., kcal/kg)	Range of ~20–30 kcal/kg/day, possibly up to 35 kcal/kg/day
	Maintenance ~20–25 kcal/kg/day
	Repletion, postoperative wound healing, critical illness, sepsis, severe trauma, severe burns ~25–30 kcal/kg/day, possibly up to 35 kcal/kg/day

Determining Amino Acid Requirements

Patient Clinical Condition	Daily Amino Acid Requirements[a] (g/kg)
Maintenance/nonstressed	0.8–1
Repletion	1.3–1.5
Trauma, burns, sepsis, critical illness	1.5–2
Hepatic failure with encephalopathy	0.8–1
Acute kidney injury, Predialysis	0.8–1
Acute kidney injury receiving intermittent hemodialysis (IHD)	1.2–1.5
Chronic kidney disease receiving continuous ambulatory peritoneal dialysis (CAPD)	1.2–1.5
Acute kidney disease receiving continuous renal replacement therapy (CRRT)	1.5–2.5

[a]Amino acid requirements are based on actual body weight for normal body sized or malnourished adult patients and on ideal body weight (IBW) for obese patients.

From Refs. 1, 6, 18.

patients. Although there is no consensus on the weight used to estimate EE in obese patients, it is reasonable to use an adjusted body weight (AdjBW) in obese patients to avoid overfeeding. Adjusted body weight can be calculated with 25% to 50% of the difference between the actual weight and IBW added to the IBW. Using a 25% difference in calculating the adjusted body weight further avoids overfeeding when estimating energy requirements:

AdjBW = IBW + (0.25 × [actual weight − IBW])

Amino acid requirements are based on the patient's nutritional status, clinical condition(s), and kidney and liver function. There are no evidence-based data on what body weight (actual, ideal, or adjusted) should be used for dosing amino acids in adult patients. It is however suggested to dose amino acids based on actual body weight for normal body sized or malnourished adult patients and based on IBW for obese patients. Amino acids are needed in adequate amounts to facilitate anabolism, restore lean body mass, or promote wound healing while avoiding adverse effects from excessive amino acid loading (e.g., azotemia). Actual body weight is used for amino acid dosing in adult patients with severe malnutrition when their body weight is at or below the IBW.

Hypocaloric nutrition support therapy for obese patients (BMI greater than or equal to 30 kg/m² or actual weight greater than 150% of IBW) is a promising approach. Hypocaloric feeding involves providing high amounts of proteins (approximately 2 g/kg IBW/day) to support anabolism with lower amounts of total calories (average approximately 11–14 kcal/kg [46–59 kJ/kg] actual weight/day, or approximately 22–25 kcal/kg [92–105 kJ/kg] IBW/day) with primary goals to promote net anabolism and avoid hyperglycemia or exacerbation of metabolic stress in critically ill patients.[20] Secondary benefits of hypocaloric feeding could be avoiding fat weight gain or possibly promoting fat weight loss. The role of hypocaloric feeding in patients with acute kidney injury or chronic kidney disease, or in patients with end-stage liver disease and hepatic encephalopathy is unknown. Also, the optimal safe duration of hypocaloric feeding in critically ill obese patients is unknown.

Special Patient Considerations: Ethical and Personal Beliefs

When assessing a patient for PN, attention should be given to patients with special personal dietary choices (e.g., vegetarians, vegans) or religious beliefs (e.g., Jehovah's Witness). These rare situations may present unique challenges for clinicians. Most nutrients used in PN preparations are usually from synthetic sources (e.g., crystalline amino acids) or vegetable sources (e.g., triglycerides used in IV lipid emulsions), with the only exception usually being egg phospholipids used in IV lipid emulsions. Discuss these issues for patients with specific needs who require PN so that a plan can be developed to provide appropriate nutrition support therapy.

PREPARING THE PN PRESCRIPTION: ADMINISTRATION, COMPOUNDING, AND PHARMACEUTICAL ISSUES

After performing a nutrition assessment and estimating nutritional requirements, determine the optimal route to provide nutrition support therapy (e.g., oral, enteral, or parenteral). If PN is deemed necessary, venous access (i.e., peripheral or central; see below) for PN infusion must be obtained. Finally, formulate a PN prescription, and administer PN according to safety guidelines.

Route of PN Administration: Peripheral versus Central Vein Infusion

❼ *PN can be administered via a smaller peripheral vein (e.g., cephalic or basilic vein) or via a larger central vein (e.g., superior vena cava)* (see Fig. 100–1). PPN is infused via a peripheral vein and generally is reserved for short-term administration (up to 7 days) when central venous access is not available. PN formulations are hyperosmolar, and PN infusion via a peripheral vein can cause thrombophlebitis. Factors that increase the risk of phlebitis include high solution osmolarity, extreme pH, rapid infusion rate, vein properties, catheter material, and infusion time via the same vein.[21] The osmolarity of PPN admixtures should be limited to 900 mOsm/L or less to minimize the risk of phlebitis. The approximate osmolarity of a PN admixture can be calculated from the osmolarity of the individual components:

- Amino acids approximately 10 mOsm/g (or 100 mOsm/1% final concentration in PN)
- Dextrose approximately 5 mOsm/g (or 50 mOsm/1% final concentration in PN)

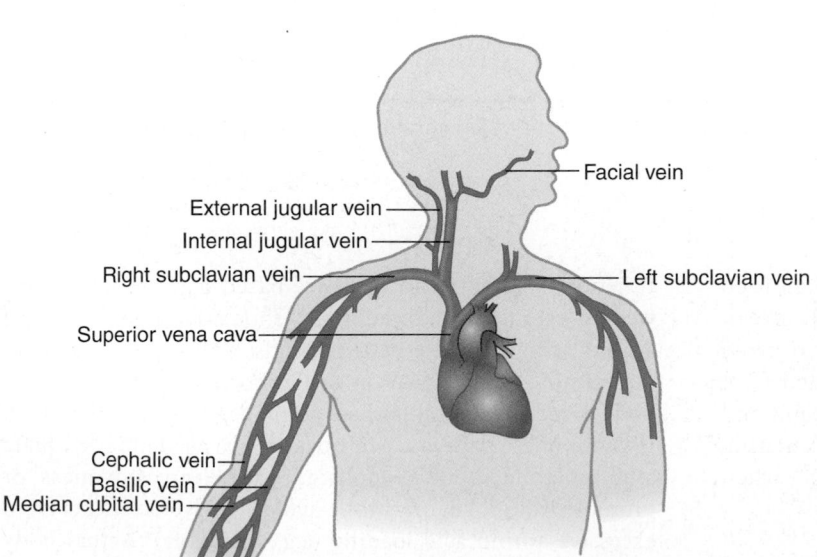

FIGURE 100–1. Selected vascular anatomy. (Reprinted from Krzywda EA, Andris DA, Edmiston CE, Wallace JR. Parenteral Access Devices. In: Gottschlich MM, ed. *The A.S.P.E.N. Nutrition Support Core Curriculum: A Case-Based Approach—The Adult Patient.* Silver Spring, MD: American Society for Parenteral and Enteral Nutrition:2007:300–322 with permission from the American Society for Parenteral and Enteral Nutrition (A.S.P.E.N.). A.S.P.E.N. does not endorse the use of this material in any form other than its entirety.)

- Sodium (chloride, acetate, and phosphate) = 2 mOsm/mEq
- Potassium (chloride, acetate, and phosphate) = 2 mOsm/mEq
- Calcium gluconate = 1.4 mOsm/mEq
- Magnesium sulfate = 1 mOsm/mEq

PPN admixtures should be coinfused with IV lipid emulsion when using the 2-in-1 PN because this may decrease the risk of phlebitis due to the iso-osmolarity and close to neutral pH of IV lipid emulsions (Table 100–2). Infectious and mechanical complications may be lower with PPN compared with central venous PN administration. However, because of the risk of phlebitis and osmolarity limit, PPN admixtures have low macronutrient concentrations and therefore usually require large fluid volumes to meet a patient's nutritional requirements. Given these limitations, every effort should be made to obtain central venous access and initiate central PN when it is unlikely a patient will tolerate enteral or oral nutrition within approximately 7 days.

Central PN refers to the administration of PN via a large central vein, and the catheter tip must be positioned in the vena cava (see Fig. 100–2). Central PN allows the infusion of a highly concentrated, hyperosmolar nutrient admixture. The typical osmolarity of a central PN admixture is about 1,500 to 2,000 mOsm/L. Central veins have much higher blood flow, and the PN admixture is diluted rapidly on infusion, so phlebitis is usually not a concern. Patients who require PN therapy for longer periods of time (greater than 7 days) should receive central PN. One limitation of central PN is the need for placing a central venous catheter and an x-ray to confirm

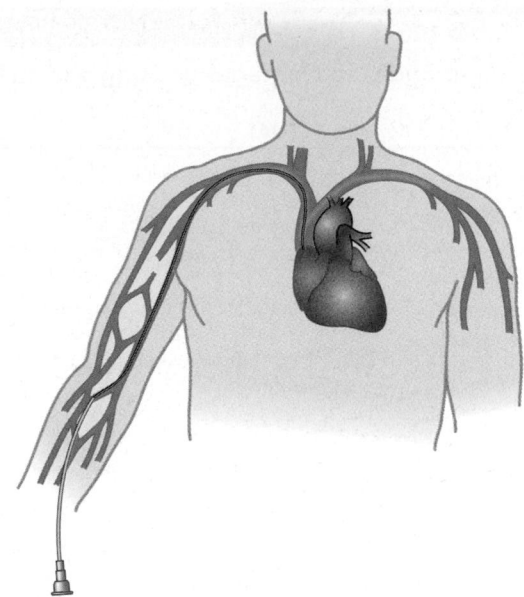

FIGURE 100–3. Peripherally inserted central venous catheter. (Reprinted from Krzywda EA, Andris DA, Edmiston CE, Wallace JR. Parenteral Access Devices. In:Gottschlich MM, ed. *The A.S.P.E.N. Nutrition Support Core Curriculum: A Case-Based Approach—The Adult Patient*. Silver Spring, MD: American Society for Parenteral and Enteral Nutrition:2007:300–322 with permission from the American Society for Parenteral and Enteral Nutrition (A.S.P.E.N.). A.S.P.E.N. does not endorse the use of this material in any form other than its entirety.)

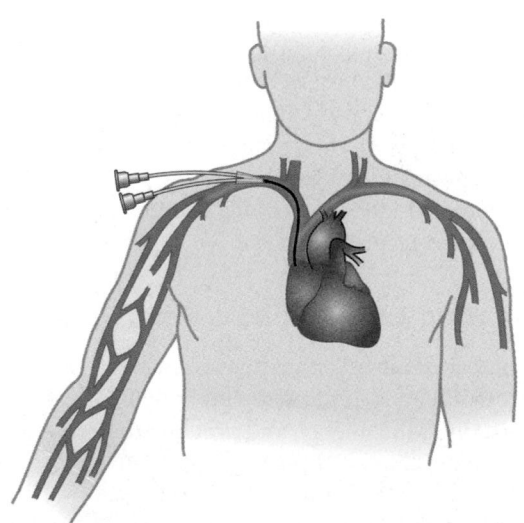

FIGURE 100–2. Percutaneous nontunneled catheter. (Reprinted from Krzywda EA, Andris DA, Edmiston CE, Wallace JR. Parenteral Access Devices. In:Gottschlich MM, ed. *The A.S.P.E.N. Nutrition Support Core Curriculum: A Case-Based Approach—The Adult Patient*. Silver Spring, MD: American Society for Parenteral and Enteral Nutrition:2007:300–322 with permission from the American Society for Parenteral and Enteral Nutrition (A.S.P.E.N.). A.S.P.E.N. does not endorse the use of this material in any form other than its entirety.)

placement of the catheter tip. A commonly used central catheter for PN infusion is a peripherally inserted central venous catheter (PICC) which is inserted into a peripheral vein but the catheter tip is placed in the superior vena cava (see Fig. 100–3). Central venous catheter placement may be associated with complications, including **pneumothorax,** arterial injury, **air embolus**, venous thrombosis, infection, **chylothorax**, and **brachial plexus** injury.[1,21]

Type of PN Formulation: 3-in-1 versus 2-in-1

8 *PN admixtures can be prepared by mixing all components into one bag, or instead, IV lipid emulsion may be infused separately (via a Y-site infusion or through a separate IV catheter or lumen). When all components are mixed together, this is referred to as a 3-in-1 admixture or a TNA.*[22] *When dextrose, amino acids, and all other PN components are mixed together without IV lipid emulsion, this is referred to as a 2-in-1 PN admixture. With a 2-in-1 PN admixture, IV lipid emulsion can be infused separately on a daily or intermittent basis. When lipid emulsion is mixed in the PN, the TNA becomes an emulsion with its physical and chemical characteristics.* There are various advantages and disadvantages to using either 3-in-1 or 2-in-1 PN (Table 100–5).

A primary concern when administering PN is safety. The FDA published a safety alert in 1994 in response to two deaths associated with TNA infusion.[15] Autopsy reports from

Table 100–5

Advantages and Disadvantages of Using 3-in-1 (TNA) or 2-in-1 PN Admixtures

	3-in-1 (TNA)	2-in-1
Advantages	Simplified regimen for patient	Improved stability compared to TNA
	Increased patient compliance at home	Increased number of compatible medications
	Decreased labor (less nursing time)	
	Decreased costs (fewer supplies and equipment needed)	Decreased bacterial growth (in dextrose/ amino acid component) compared to TNA
	Decreased risk of contamination (due to less manipulation, all components aseptically compounded)	
	Inhibited bacterial growth vs. separate IV lipid emulsion	Easier visual inspection
	Minimize infusion-related reactions from IV lipid emulsions and possibly improved lipid clearance (if infused over more than 12 hours)	Can use 0.22-micron bacterial retention filter
	Decreased vein irritation (especially with PPN)	Cost savings if unused (i.e., not spiked or opened) IV lipid emulsion can be reused
Disadvantages	Decreased stability compared to 2-in-1 PN	Increased labor and costs (if IV lipid emulsion infused separately)
	Cannot use 0.22-micron bacterial retention filter, must use 1.2-micron filter	Increased vein irritation, especially if PPN is not coinfused with IV lipid emulsion
	Increased bacterial growth compared to 2-in-1 PN	
	Visual inspection is difficult	
	Limited compatibility with medications	

PPN, peripheral parenteral nutrition; TNA, total nutrient admixture.

these patients revealed diffuse microvascular pulmonary emboli containing calcium–phosphate precipitates. The FDA provided recommendations for safe infusion of PN admixtures containing calcium and phosphate:

- A 0.22-micron air-eliminating in-line filter should be used for infusion of nonlipid-containing PN.

- A 1.2-micron in-line filter should be used for the infusion of 3-in-1 PN (i.e., a TNA) because it can remove large and unstable lipid droplets and also particulate matter.[23]

Another concern is the coinfusion of IV medications with PN admixtures. Many IV medications have limited compatibility with 3-in-1 formulations but may be coinfused with a 2-in-1 formulation.[24,25] Some medications can be coinfused at the Y-site, few medications can be mixed directly into the PN admixture or coinfused with IV lipid emulsion, and some cannot be mixed or coinfused with the PN admixture.[24,25] *Always* consult compatibility data before adding a medication to a PN admixture or coinfusing it with PN. Medications that are compatible should be added to PN only if it is reasonable and safe (i.e., based on toxicity profile, pharmacokinetic/pharmacodynamic considerations).

The United States Pharmacopeia, Chapter 797 (USP 797) is a document that provides guidelines and best practices for pharmaceutical compounding of sterile products.[26] These guidelines address many aspects of compounded sterile preparations (CSPs), including (but not limited to) appropriate training of personnel; appropriate environments for compounding; appropriate storage, handling and labeling of ingredients and final products; and quality assurance. The purpose of USP 797 is to prevent patient harm from CSPs as a result of contamination (including physical, chemical, and bacterial or fungal pathogens), inappropriate ingredients

(variability in strength or quality), or inappropriate preparation, compounding, handling, transportation or storage. CSPs are classified as either low-risk level, medium-risk level, high-risk level, or immediate use. CSPs are also assigned an appropriate beyond-use date (BUD), which is the date or time after which a CSP shall not be stored or transported, and it is determined from the date or time the CSP is compounded. PN admixtures are usually classified as medium-risk products, and they are assigned a BUD of 30 hours at controlled room temperature or 9 days at a cold (refrigerated) temperature. The full details of USP 797 are beyond the scope of this chapter. Pharmacists and other health care professionals involved in the preparation of CSPs should review this document along with institutional policies and procedures regarding CSPs.

Formulating a PN Admixture and Regimen

After completing a full nutrition assessment (e.g., SGA),[1,19] determine if PN is indicated (Table 100–1), estimate the patient's daily fluid, energy, and protein requirements (Table 100–4), and develop a PN prescription.

Initiating PN

Exercise caution when initiating PN to avoid hyperglycemia, and fluid and electrolyte abnormalities. Once the goal daily volume is determined, infuse the PN admixture first over 24 hours. For safety, initiate PN at a lower infusion rate (e.g., approximately 50% of goal for anywhere from approximately 12 to 24 hours) on day 1 with no more than 150 to 200 g of dextrose per day (or a maximum dextrose infusion rate of approximately 2 mg/kg/min). Then increase

Patient Encounter 2

AA was diagnosed with an intestinal leak at the previous surgical site, diffuse peritonitis, sepsis, mild dehydration, and hypovolemic hypotonic hyponatremia.

Laboratory Data

Na = 130 mEq/L (130 mmol/L), K = 3.4 mEq/L (3.4 mmol/L), Cl = 104 mEq/L (104 mmol/L), HCO3 = 21 mEq/L (21 mmol/L), BUN = 14 mg/dL (5 mmol/L), serum creatinine = 0.6 mg/dL (53 μmol/L), blood glucose = 177 mg/dL (9.8 mmol/L), total Ca = 8.3 mg/dL (2.08 mmol/L)], ionized Ca = 2.34 mEq/L (1.17 mmol/L), Mg = 2.1 mg/dL (0.86 mmol/L), phosphorus = 2.1 mg/dL (0.68 mmol/L), TG = 125 mg/dL (1.41 mmol/L), albumin = 3.1 g/dL (31 g/L), WBC count = 14,400/mm³ (14 × 10⁹/L), hemoglobin = 11.2 mg/dL (112 g/L or 6.9 mmol/L), hematocrit = 42% (0.42), and platelets = 164,000/mm³ (164 × 10⁹/L)

AA was taken to the operating room for an exploratory laparotomy, repair of the intestinal leak, and small bowel resection. Postoperatively, a nasogastric (NG) tube was placed and drained 800 to 1,000 mL/day on postoperative days 1 and 2. The surgeons placed a central venous catheter and wanted to start the patient on central PN given her diagnoses of diffuse peritonitis, intestinal leak, evidence of poor intestinal function (given high NG tube output), and history of recurrent bowel obstructions.

Determine appropriate nutritional goals for AA (energy and protein requirements).

What other patient data should be collected to help formulate a PN prescription?

Patient Encounter 3

The surgical team plans to initiate the PN you recommended for AA.

Develop a plan for a complete and balanced PN prescription for AA (including fluid, total calories, dextrose, amino acids, lipid emulsion, electrolytes, vitamins, trace elements, and any additives) and explain the rationale supporting your formulation plan.

How should this PN admixture be initiated and titrated to goal?

PN up to goal over the following approximately 12 to 24 hours, provided that glycemic control is maintained and the patient does not experience any significant fluid or electrolyte abnormalities. Monitor electrolytes daily and correct as needed. Patients with severe malnutrition should be advanced to goal more slowly and cautiously, and they should be monitored for refeeding syndrome (see Complications of PN below).

Cycling PN

PN should be administered over 24 hours in most hospitalized patients to minimize glucose, fluid, and electrolyte abnormalities. However, administering PN via a cyclic infusion over less than 24 hours, or *cycling PN*, may be advantageous in certain patients and situations. Cycling PN typically involves administering the same PN volume to a goal infusion time usually over 12 hours rather than over 24 hours. Taper PN to the goal cycle over 2 to 4 days (e.g., 24 hours, then 18 hours the next day, then 14 hours the next day, and then 12 hours the next day). Titrate the PN infusion rate up over 1 to 2 hours to goal rate to avoid hyperglycemia, and taper down over 1 to 2 hours at the end of the cycle to avoid reactive hypoglycemia. Most home infusion pumps can be programmed to cycle a given PN volume automatically over a given time. However, the pharmacist may have to develop an appropriate PN cycle if the infusion pump cannot be programmed.

Cyclic PN has the following advantages:

- It may help alleviate PN-associated liver cholestasis by avoiding continuous compulsive nutrient overload on the liver.[27]

- It improves the quality of life of patients receiving home PN by allowing the patient time off from PN to engage in normal daily activities. If nocturnal cyclic PN infusion interferes with patient's sleep pattern by causing overdiuresis, the PN cycle can be extended over a longer infusion time or PN can be infused during other times of the day that are most convenient to the patient.

Concerns with cycling PN include hyperglycemia with high infusion rates, reactive hypoglycemia, and fluid and electrolyte abnormalities. Depending on potassium amounts in the daily PN admixture, cyclic PN infusion should also take into consideration the potassium infusion rate that should not exceed 10 mEq/h. Reactive hypoglycemia can be minimized by tapering down PN over 1 to 2 hours before disconnecting. Typically, the nadir will occur around 30 to 60 minutes or even a little over an hour after the PN is stopped. Random capillary blood glucose concentrations should be checked 4 hours into the PN cycle (approximately 2 hours after reaching goal rate), 15 to 60 minutes after PN stops, and intermittently during the PN cycle as needed for glycemic control.

Transition to Oral or Enteral Nutrition

The goal is to transition the patient to enteral or oral nutrition and taper off PN as soon as indicated clinically. When initiating enteral or oral nutrition, monitor the patient for glucose, fluid, and electrolyte abnormalities. When oral nutrition intake is inconsistent, perform calorie counts to determine the adequacy of nutrition via the oral route. When the patient is tolerating more than 50% of total estimated daily calorie and protein requirements via the oral or enteral route, wean PN by about 50%. PN can be stopped once the patient is tolerating at least 75% of total daily calorie and protein requirements via the oral or enteral route, assuming that intestinal absorption is maintained.

A.S.P.E.N SAFE PRACTICES OF PN

Because serious and sometimes fatal adverse events have occurred with inappropriate use of PN, the A.S.P.E.N. has published updated safe practice guidelines for PN.[6] These practice guidelines provide a tool and reference for health professionals for the safe and efficacious use of PN. The guidelines represent the standards of practice as they relate to PN prescribing, compounding, stability, compatibility, labeling, administration, and quality assurance. Although application of these guidelines is voluntary, pharmacists who handle PN should review these guidelines and apply them as they fit in light of the circumstances of their practice sites and individual patient conditions.

COMPLICATIONS OF PN

❾ *PN therapy is associated with significant complications, both with short- and long-term therapy. Many complications are related to overfeeding (Table 100–6). Metabolic complications include hyperglycemia, hypoglycemia, hyperlipidemia, hypercapnia, electrolyte disturbances, refeeding syndrome, and acid–base disturbances. Long-term metabolic complications include liver toxicity, vitamin abnormalities, trace-element abnormalities, and metabolic bone disease. Other complications include infectious and mechanical complications that relate to venous catheters.*

Hyperglycemia

Hyperglycemia is one of the most common complications associated with PN therapy. The rate of dextrose oxidation may be reduced in patients with stress and hypermetabolism, patients with diabetes or acute pancreatitis, and patients receiving certain medications (e.g., corticosteroids, vasopressors, octreotide, and tacrolimus).[28,29] Uncontrolled hyperglycemia can lead to fluid and electrolyte disturbances, hyperglycemic hyperosmolar nonketotic syndrome, hypertriglyceridemia, and increased risk of infection.[30]

Hyperglycemia in critically ill patients may be more a reflection of illness severity than from dextrose infusions, provided that the patient is not being overfed.[31] Critical illness is associated with increased endogenous glucose production (due to increased glycogenolysis and gluconeogenesis) and insulin resistance. Therefore, critically ill patients have lower tolerance for dextrose infusion compared nonstressed patients. In patients with hyperglycemia, it is reasonable to initiate PN with a continuous dextrose infusion rate of approximately 2 mg/kg/min until glycemic control is achieved and then advance to goal.[4] Dextrose infusion rate typically ranges between approximately 3 and 4 mg/kg/min but should not exceed 5 mg/kg/min in the adult stressed patient.[1,5] Adjusted body weight should be used in obese patients rather than actual weight to calculate dextrose infusion rate. A portion of calories can be provided with IV lipid emulsion rather than dextrose to help decrease hyperglycemia, provided that the patient does not have hypertriglyceridemia. Overfeeding (with dextrose and with total calories) always must be avoided.

Hyperglycemia can impair cellular and humoral host defenses and can lead to the development of nosocomial and wound infections.[30] Historically, hyperglycemia has been defined as blood glucose concentrations of more than 200 to 220 mg/dL (11.1–12.21 mmol/L), and concentrations of 150 to 200 mg/dL (8.3–11.1 mmol/L) were considered "acceptable" in critically ill patients. Based on early clinical evidence, tight glucose control (e.g., 80–110 mg/dL or 4.4–6.1 mmol/L) with intensive insulin therapy using continuous insulin infusion in surgical critically ill patients reduced infection rates, patient comorbidities, and mortality.[32] It also appears that the benefits observed are due to glycemic control rather than to the dose of insulin.[33] Achieving a goal serum glucose concentration of 80 to 110 g/dL (4.4–6.1 mmol/L) may be a challenge while avoiding hypoglycemia. A single episode of severe hypoglycemia (blood glucose concentrations less than 40 g/dL or 2.2 mmol/L) could be an independent risk factor for increased patient mortality. Because of the heterogeneity of the critically ill population and the increased hypoglycemia risk with intensive insulin therapy, the exact goal range for optimal glucose control and the effects on hyperglycemia-associated complications in critically ill patients are still debated. However, an upper threshold for serum glucose concentration of 145 mg/dL (8.0 mmol/L) has been suggested as acceptable.[34]

The clinical benefits of tight glucose control (blood glucose concentrations 80–110 mg/dL [4.4–6 mmol/L]) that were derived from the Van den Berghe study were not replicated in the NICE-SUGAR (Normoglycemia in Intensive Care Evaluation—Survival Using Glucose Algorithm Regulation) study.[35] The NICE-SUGAR study was an international, multi-center, prospective, randomized, controlled, unblinded study of 6,104 medical and surgical adult patients admitted to the intensive care units of 42 hospitals. Patients were included in the study if they were expected to be in the intensive care unit for at least 3 days. Patients were randomized to receive intensive insulin therapy to maintain blood glucose concentrations between 81 and 108 mg/dL (4.5–6 mmol/L) or to conventional insulin therapy to keep blood glucose concentrations between 144 and 180 mg/dL (8–10 mmol/L). Blood glucose control was achieved with intravenous insulin infusion. Study results showed a significantly higher 90-day mortality rate (primary outcome) in the intensive glucose

Table 100–6	
Consequences of Overfeeding	
Source of Overfeeding	**Consequences**
Dextrose	Hyperglycemia, hypertriglyceridemia, hepatic steatosis, hypercapnia; hyperglycemia may cause fluid and electrolyte disturbances and increased infection risk
IV lipid emulsions	Hypertriglyceridemia, hyperlipidemia, hepatic steatosis
Amino acids	Azotemia
Total calories	Hepatic steatosis, cholestasis, hypercapnia

control group as compared to the conventional group (27.5% versus 24.9%, respectively; $p = 0.02$). There was no benefit from intensive glucose control on the secondary and tertiary outcomes including length of intensive care unit stay, days on mechanical ventilation, incidence of bloodstream infections, need for renal replacement therapy, and blood transfusions. A significantly higher incidence of severe hypoglycemia (blood glucose concentrations less than or equal to 40 mg/dL [less than or equal to 2.2 mmol/L]) occurred in 6.8% of patients in the intensive glucose control group as compared to 0.5% in the conventional group ($p < 0.001$). Although the NICE-SUGAR study results suggest that optimal blood glucose concentrations in critically ill patients are best maintained between 144 and 180 mg/dL (8–10 mmol/L), it is expected that further data analysis may provide a better explanation of the study findings and their applicability to the diverse critical care patient population.

The use of regular insulin as a continuous infusion rather than adding insulin to PN reduces the risk of prolonged hypoglycemia because the insulin drip can be readily titrated as insulin requirements change. In patients with diabetes, IV insulin doses in the PN admixture to maintain euglycemia range approximately from 0.05 to 0.2 unit of insulin per each gram of dextrose in PN. Starting with a low insulin dose and adjusting the dose daily based on capillary blood glucose evaluation is indicated in order to avoid hypoglycemia. Further and careful reduction to the insulin dose should be made as guided by frequent capillary blood glucose monitoring when metabolic stress decreases, acute pancreatitis resolves, or when corticosteroid doses are tapered off or discontinued.

Hypoglycemia

● Hypoglycemia can occur in patients when PN is interrupted suddenly (reactive hypoglycemia), especially when patients are treated with insulin or as a result of insulin overdosing in PN.[1] It is essential to prevent hypoglycemia and, if it occurs, to identify and treat it promptly. Reactive hypoglycemia typically is rare and usually can be avoided by tapering PN over 1 to 2 hours before discontinuation rather than abruptly stopping the infusion (especially if the patient is receiving insulin in PN or if the patient is not receiving oral or enteral nutrition). Reactive hypoglycemia generally occurs within 15 to 60 minutes after stopping PN (especially in neonatal patients), although it can occur later than this after discontinuing PN.[1] Capillary blood glucose concentrations should be monitored about 15 to 60 minutes after stopping PN infusion in order to detect any potential hypoglycemia. If PN is interrupted abruptly (e.g., due to lost IV access), infusing dextrose 10% in water at the same rate as PN should prevent hypoglycemia. In patients with poor venous access, reduce the PN infusion rate by 50% for 1 hour before discontinuing. Another alternative to prevent reactive hypoglycemia is to provide a glucose source via the oral route (by mouth or sublingually) when feasible. Monitor capillary blood glucose concentrations regularly in patients receiving insulin in PN, and adjust insulin doses accordingly.

Hyperlipidemia

● Patients receiving IV lipid emulsion may be at risk for hyperlipidemia and hypertriglyceridemia. Hyperglycemia can lead to hypertriglyceridemia and is the most common cause of hypertriglyceridemia in patients receiving PN. Hyperlipidemia in patients receiving PN may lead to a reduction in pulmonary gas diffusion and pulmonary vascular resistance (especially in patients with underlying pulmonary and vascular disease).[36] Severe hypertriglyceridemia (especially when serum triglyceride concentrations exceed 1,000 mg/dL or 11.3 mmol/L) can precipitate ● acute pancreatitis.[37] Hypertriglyceridemia may develop as a result of increased fatty acid synthesis due to hyperglycemia or impaired lipid clearance or in patients with history of hyperlipidemia, obesity, diabetes, alcoholism, kidney failure, liver failure, multiorgan failure, sepsis, pancreatitis, or as a result of medications (e.g., propofol, corticosteroids, cyclosporine, and sirolimus).[38] Propofol is formulated in a 10% lipid emulsion (which is not cleared as effectively as the 20% or 30% lipid emulsions) and may lead to hypertriglyceridemia. It also has been proposed that propofol could have direct effects on lipid metabolism, given that hypertriglyceridemia associated with propofol infusion has been observed with lipid doses that are lower than those typically given in PN.[38,39]

A higher PL:TG ratio in the 10% lipid emulsion has been proposed to cause the appearance of the abnormal lipoprotein X particles (rich in phospholipids [approximately 60%] and cholesterol [approximately 25%], small amounts of triglycerides) in the blood.[8,38] Lipoprotein X may compete with lipid particles for metabolism by lipoprotein lipase. Therefore, IV lipid emulsions with a lower PL:TG ratio (i.e., 20% or 30% lipid emulsions) have improved clearance compared with emulsions with a higher PL:TG ratio (i.e., 10% lipid emulsion)[8,38] and should preferentially be used, especially in patients with hypertriglyceridemia. Lipid clearance may be improved by newer formulations of mixed medium- and long-chain triglycerides; however, these products are not yet approved for use in the United States.

● Monitor serum triglyceride concentrations regularly during PN therapy (e.g., at the initiation of PN, then once or twice per week initially, and thereafter depending on clinical condition). If a patient develops hypertriglyceridemia, identify and correct the underlying cause(s) if possible (e.g., treatment of hyperglycemia or reduction of dextrose and/or lipid dose). Prolonging the infusion of IV lipid emulsion (e.g., over 24 hours) may improve clearance; however, this may require hanging two containers daily because each container of lipid emulsion should infuse for only 12 hours based on USP 797 and infection-control policies and practices. If a patient is receiving propofol, take into account the calories administered from the 10% lipid emulsion in propofol (1.1 kcal/mL or 4.6 kJ/mL). For safety reasons, IV lipid emulsion should be withheld in patients receiving ● propofol. It also should be held when the serum is lipemic or when serum triglyceride concentrations are greater than 400 mg/dL (4.5 mmol/L). When this occurs, restart IV lipid emulsions when the serum triglyceride concentration is approximately 200 to 400 mg/dL (2.3–4.5 mmol/L) (or less), and administer IV lipids only two to three times per week to prevent essential fatty acid deficiency.

Hypercapnia

Hypercapnia (abnormally high concentration of carbon dioxide in the blood) can develop as a result of overfeeding with both dextrose and total calories.[1,40] Excess carbon dioxide production and retention can lead to acute respiratory acidosis. The excess carbon dioxide also will stimulate compensatory mechanisms, resulting in an increase in respiratory rate in order to eliminate the excess carbon dioxide via the lungs. This increase in respiratory workload can cause respiratory insufficiency that may require mechanical ventilation. Reducing total calorie and dextrose intake would result in resolution of hypercapnia if due to overfeeding.

Acid–Base Disturbances

Acid–base disturbances associated with PN usually are related to the patient's underlying condition(s). However, acid–base abnormalities may develop as a result of changes in chloride or acetate concentrations in PN admixtures. Because acetate is converted to bicarbonate in the body, excessive acetate salts in PN can lead to metabolic alkalosis; excessive chloride salts in PN can lead to metabolic acidosis. PN should not be used to treat or correct acute underlying disorders. However, adjusting chloride or acetate salts in the PN admixture may help to prevent these acid–base disorders or minimize worsening of any underlying acid–base disorders.

Liver Complications

The incidence of liver complications associated with PN ranges from approximately 7% to 84%, and end-stage liver disease develops in as many as 15% to 40% of adult patients on long-term PN.[38] Patients often develop a mild increase in liver enzymes within 1 to 2 weeks of initiating PN, but this generally resolves when PN is discontinued. Severe liver complications include hepatic steatosis (fat deposition in liver), steatohepatitis (a severe form of liver disease characterized by hepatic inflammation that may progress rapidly to liver fibrosis and cirrhosis), cholestasis, and cholelithiasis.[38]

Hepatic steatosis usually is a result of excessive administration of carbohydrates and/or lipids, but deficiencies of carnitine, choline, and essential fatty acids also may contribute. Hepatic steatosis can be minimized or reversed by avoiding overfeeding, especially from dextrose and lipids.[38] Carnitine is an important amine that transports long-chain triglycerides into the mitochondria for oxidation, but carnitine deficiency in adults is extremely rare and is mostly a problem in premature infants and patients receiving chronic dialysis. Choline is an essential amine required for synthesis of cell membrane components such as phospholipids. Although a true choline deficiency is rare, preliminary studies of choline supplementation to adult patients' PN showed reversal of steatosis.

Cholestasis is a common problem in patients who are dependent on PN. Factors that predispose PN patients to cholestasis include overfeeding, lack of bowel stimulation, bowel rest (decrease in cholecystokinin secretion), long duration of PN, short-bowel syndrome, bacterial overgrowth and translocation, and sepsis.[38] Patients may exhibit increased liver transaminases, increase alkaline phosphatase and gamma-glutamyl transferase concentrations, and mainly increased bilirubin concentrations with jaundice. The most sensitive marker of cholestasis is an increased serum conjugated bilirubin concentration of 2 mg/dL (34.2 μmol/L) or more.[38] Cholestasis generally is reversible if PN is discontinued before permanent liver damage occurs. Serum liver enzyme concentrations may take up to 3 months to return to normal after discontinuing PN. Steps to prevent cholestasis associated with PN include early initiation of enteral or oral feedings, using a balanced PN formulation, avoiding overfeeding, cyclic PN infusion, and treating and avoiding sepsis.[38] Limiting IV lipid emulsion infusion to 1 or 2 times weekly at a dose no less than to prevent essential fatty acid deficiency may also decrease serum bilirubin concentrations and improve cholestasis. Pharmacologic treatments include ursodeoxycholic acid (ursodiol), which may improve bile flow and reduce the signs and symptoms of cholestasis. However, ursodiol is only available in an oral dosage form, and absorption may be limited in patients with intestinal resections. If other measures are not successful, and bacterial overgrowth is thought to be contributing to cholestasis, courses of oral metronidazole, oral gentamicin, or oral neomycin have been used to reduce bacterial overgrowth.

Cholelithiasis can develop as a result of decreased gallbladder contractility, especially in the absence of enteral or oral intake. Lack of intestinal stimulation reduces secretion of cholecystokinin, a peptide hormone secreted in the duodenum that induces gallbladder contractility. The best prevention of cholelithiasis is early initiation of enteral or oral feeding, as stated earlier (to stimulate secretion of cholecystokinin, gallbladder contraction and emptying, and intestinal motility). Pharmacologic treatment with cholecystokinin-octapeptide (sincalide) to stimulate gallbladder contraction and bile flow does not prevent PN-associated cholestasis or improve serum conjugated bilirubin concentrations.

Monitor liver function tests, including serum aspartate aminotransferase (AST), alanine aminotransferase (ALT), alkaline phosphatase, total bilirubin, and conjugated bilirubin, at the initiation of PN and regularly thereafter during PN therapy. The frequency of monitoring liver function tests depends on the presence or absence of liver disease. This varies from one to two times weekly in the acute setting to once weekly to once monthly in the stable home PN patient.

Manganese Toxicity

Manganese is a trace element that serves as a coenzyme in multiple biochemical reactions. Manganese usually is supplied in PN admixtures as part of the trace element package in an adult dose of 0.5 mg/day; however, this may be excessive for longer-term PN patients. Manganese accumulation can occur in patients with cholestasis, and the most common toxicity is neurotoxicity, but liver toxicity also may occur.[38] Neurologic symptoms associated with manganese toxicity include headache, somnolence, weakness, confusion, tremor, muscle rigidity, altered gait, and mask-like face (a Parkinson's-like syndrome).[38] Conversely, some patients with hypermanganesemia may not exhibit symptoms of toxicity. Periodic measurement of blood-manganese concentrations in patients on long-term PN is recommended. Patients with cholestasis receiving PN may require restriction of manganese in PN to prevent its accumulation and possible toxicity.

Metabolic Bone Disease

Metabolic bone disease is a condition of bone demineralization leading to osteomalacia, osteopenia, or osteoporosis in patients receiving long-term PN. Metabolic bone disease, to some degree, may occur in as many as 40% to 100% of patients receiving long-term PN.[38] Often patients are asymptomatic, although symptoms can include bone pain, back pain, and fractures. Patients often will have increased serum alkaline phosphatase concentrations, low to normal parathyroid hormone (PTH) concentrations, normal 25-hydroxy vitamin D, low 1,25 dihydroxyvitamin D concentrations, hypercalcemia or hypocalcemia, and hypercalcuria.[41] Because patients may be asymptomatic, diagnosis can be incidental. Radiologic techniques commonly used in diagnosing bone disease include quantitative computed tomography (CT) and bone mineral density.[41]

Factors that can predispose patients to developing metabolic bone disease include deficiencies of phosphorus, calcium, and vitamin D; vitamin D and/or aluminum toxicity; amino acids and hyperosmolar dextrose infusions; chronic metabolic acidosis; corticosteroid therapy; and lack of mobility.[38,41] Calcium deficiency (due to decreased intake or increased urinary excretion) is one of the major causes of metabolic bone disease in patients receiving PN. Provide adequate calcium and phosphate with PN to improve bone mineralization and help to prevent metabolic bone disease. Administration of amino acids and chronic metabolic acidosis also appear to play an important role. Provide adequate amounts of acetate in PN admixtures to maintain acid–base balance.

Vitamin D toxicity has been suggested as a cause of metabolic bone disease. However, vitamin D deficiency results in bone loss, and data on vitamin D excess and metabolic bone disease remain controversial.

Aluminum toxicity appears to play a role in the development of metabolic bone disease in patients on long-term PN, possibly by impairing calcium bone fixation,[42] inhibiting the conversion of 25-hydroxyvitamin D to the active 1,25-dihydroxyvitamin D, and/or reducing PTH secretion.[38,43] The FDA has been investigating the issue of aluminum contamination in parenteral products and issued a rule specifying acceptable aluminum concentrations in large-volume parenterals in the year 2000.[44] The rule further stated that the package insert ("Precautions") for large-volume parenterals used in making PN should indicate that the product contains no more than 25 mcg/L of aluminum and defined a safe upper limit for parenteral aluminum intake at less than 4 to 5 mcg/kg/day. This has required a great amount of effort by manufacturers to meet these limits and requires pharmacy policies for monitoring aluminum concentrations in PN admixtures. Pharmacies should use products with the lowest labeled aluminum content for the making of PN. Patients who are chronically dependent on PN should have their serum aluminum concentrations routinely monitored or whenever metabolic bone disease is suspected or diagnosed.

Encourage patients on long-term PN to engage in regular low-intensity exercise. Yearly bone density measurements also should be performed on patients on long-term PN and when metabolic bone disease is suspected.

Refeeding Syndrome

Refeeding syndrome describes the metabolic derangements that occur during nutritional repletion of patients who are starved, underweight, or severely malnourished.[45] Hypophosphatemia and associated complications are the classic signs and symptoms, but refeeding syndrome encompasses a constellation of fluid and electrolyte abnormalities affecting multiple organ systems, including neurologic, cardiac, hematological, neuromuscular, and pulmonary function. The most severe cases of refeeding syndrome have resulted in cardiac failure, seizures, coma, and death.[45] The reintroduction of carbohydrates/glucose drives metabolism back to using glucose as the predominant fuel source. This increases insulin secretion, creates a high demand for the production of phosphorylated intermediates of glycolysis (e.g., ATP, and 2,3-diphosphoglycerate [2,3-DPG]), inhibits fat metabolism, and causes an intracellular shift of phosphorus, potassium, and magnesium. These changes, in combination with pre-existing low total body stores of phosphorus, potassium, and magnesium and enhanced cellular uptake of phosphorus during anabolic refeeding, result in hypophosphatemia, hypokalemia, and hypomagnesemia. Vitamin deficiencies (e.g., thiamine) also may exist or be precipitated during refeeding. High carbohydrate intake increases the demand for thiamine, an essential cofactor involved in carbohydrate metabolism. This can precipitate thiamine deficiency with its potential complications, including lactic acidosis and neurologic abnormalities,[45,46] as well as myocardial dysfunction and congestive heart failure. Other metabolic alterations that may occur include expansion of the extracellular water compartment, fluid imbalance, and fluid intolerance.

The primary goal is preventing refeeding syndrome when initiating PN in high-risk patients (e.g., patients with prolonged lack of adequate nutritional intake, significant weight loss, or moderate-severe malnutrition). When initiating nutrition support, the rule of thumb to prevent refeeding syndrome is to "start low and go slow." Initiate PN cautiously (e.g., approximately 25% of estimated nutritional requirements on day 1), and gradually increase to goal over 3 to 5 days. Correct electrolyte abnormalities (e.g., hypophosphatemia, hypokalemia, and hypomagnesemia) before initiating PN, and provide supplemental phosphate, potassium, and magnesium in or outside of PN (if the patient has normal kidney function). Well-nourished patients require 10 to 15 mmol of phosphate per 1,000 kcal to avoid hypophosphatemia,[14] but patients with moderate to severe malnutrition who are at risk for refeeding syndrome will require more aggressive supplementation. Doses of IV phosphate as high as 0.64 to 1 mmol/kg have been used to treat severe hypophosphatemia (provided the patient has normal kidney function).[47,48] Vitamin supplementation also should be provided in addition to the multivitamin provided in PN. Provide supplemental oral or IV thiamine 100 mg/day and folic acid 1 mg/day for about a week. In addition, minimize fluid and sodium intake during the first few days of PN (e.g., total fluid of 1,000 mL/day or less and sodium of 20 mEq/day or less).[49] Assess patients for fluid balance, signs of edema, fluid overload, and weight gain because any gain of more than 1 kg/week likely represents fluid retention.[49] Monitor patients closely for signs and symptoms of refeeding syndrome. Monitor vital signs (i.e., heart rate, blood pressure, and respiratory rate), mental status, and neurologic and neuromuscular function routinely during the first several days of PN until goal is reached. Monitor pulse oximetry and any electrocardiographic changes when indicated clinically.

Infectious Complications

Patients receiving central PN are at increased risk of developing infectious complications caused by bacterial and fungal pathogens.[1,50] Infections may be related to placement of a central venous catheter, contamination of a central venous catheter or IV site (catheter-related infection), and persistent hyperglycemia. Strict aseptic techniques must be used when placing the catheter, along with continuous care of the catheter and infusion site. Catheter-related bloodstream infections are a common complication in long-term PN patients, often requiring hospital admission for parenteral antimicrobial therapy and/or removal of the catheter. Contamination of the PN admixture is possible, although rare if protocols are followed for aseptic preparation of PN admixtures. Lack of use of the intestinal tract also may increase the risk of infection possibly by reducing gut immunity, leading to intestinal bacterial overgrowth and subsequent systemic bacterial translocation.

Mechanical Complications

Mechanical complications of PN are related to venous catheter placement and the system and equipment used to administer PN. A central venous catheter must be placed by a trained professional, and risks associated with placement include pneumothorax, arterial puncture, bleeding, hematoma formation, venous thrombosis, and air embolism.[1,21] Over time, the venous catheter may require replacement. Problems with the equipment include malfunctions of the infusion pump, IV tubing sets, and filters.

MONITORING PN THERAPY

❿ When initiating PN, patients should have important baseline laboratory values checked to assess electrolyte status, organ function, and nutritional status (Table 100–7). Baseline laboratory monitoring should include:

- Basic metabolic panel (i.e., serum sodium, potassium, chloride, bicarbonate, blood urea nitrogen, creatinine, glucose, and calcium), serum phosphorus and magnesium.

- Liver function, including AST, ALT, alkaline phosphatase, lactate dehydrogenase (LDH), total and conjugated bilirubin; a comprehensive metabolic panel can be ordered (i.e., serum sodium, potassium, chloride, bicarbonate, blood urea nitrogen, creatinine, glucose, calcium, AST, ALT, alkaline phosphatase, albumin, and total bilirubin), but phosphorus, magnesium, and fractionated or conjugated bilirubin are not included on this panel and must be ordered separately.

- Serum albumin, prealbumin, and triglycerides.

- Complete blood count (including hemoglobin, hematocrit, red blood cell count, and white blood cell count), and platelets with differential.

❿ *Thereafter, the preceding parameters and other nutritional parameters should be monitored routinely or as indicated* (Table 100–7). Random capillary blood glucose concentrations also should be monitored every 6 to 8 hours when initiating PN, and regular insulin should be administered to control blood glucose concentrations as needed.

Patient Encounter 4

The surgical team plans to initiate PN for AA as you have recommended. Propofol was initiated and the rate titrated for AA adequate sedation. Laboratory data were listed previously.

What other laboratory data or monitoring parameters should be obtained before initiating PN?

How frequently should you monitor each of the various parameters after initiating PN?

What potential complications of PN should you monitor for in AA?

What approaches should be undertaken to prevent and treat hyperglycemia in AA?

How should the PN formulation be adjusted following propofol initiation in AA?

Table 100–7

Suggested Frequency of Monitoring Parameters in Hospitalized Patients Receiving PN

Parameters	Initial	Daily (Unstable)	2–3 × Weekly (Stable)	Weekly	As Indicated
Blood urea nitrogen, creatinine	X	X	X		
Sodium, potassium, chloride, bicarbonate	X	X	X		
Glucose	X	X	X		
Calcium, phosphorus, magnesium	X	X	X		
Albumin, aspartate aminotransferase, alanine aminotransferase, lactate dehydrogenase, alkaline phosphatase, total bilirubin					
Conjugated bilirubin	X			X	
Prealbumin	X			X	
Triglycerides	X			X	X
Red blood cell count, hemoglobin, hematocrit, white blood cell count ± differential, platelets, partial thromboplastin time	X				X
Prothrombin time/International normalized ratio					X
Nitrogen balance					X
Zinc, selenium, chromium, copper, manganese, iron					X
Total iron-binding capacity, ferritin					X
Vitamin concentrations					X
Ammonia					X
Blood cultures					X
Body weight	X	X	X		

SUMMARY AND CONCLUSION

PN is an effective and potentially lifesaving method of administering nutrition support therapy in patients who cannot receive adequate oral or enteral nutrition, but may be associated with several complications. Enteral nutrition is the preferred route of providing nutrition support therapy. Administration of PN is associated with significant adverse effects, and patients must be monitored closely. Patients receiving PN therapy are at risk for metabolic, infectious, and mechanical complications. Optimal design of a PN regimen is essential to minimize the risk of adverse effects and complications, and patients must be monitored closely while receiving PN in order to optimize outcomes.

Abbreviations Introduced in This Chapter

2,3-DPG	2,3-diphosphoglycerate
ALT	Alanine aminotransferase
A.S.P.E.N.	American Society for Parenteral and Enteral Nutrition
AST	Aspartate aminotransferase
ATP	Adenosine triphosphate
BEE	Basal energy expenditure
BMI	Body mass index
BUD	Beyond-use date
C18: 2n-6	Linoleic acid
C18: 3n-3	α-Linolenic acid
C20: 4n-6	Arachidonic acid
CAPD	Continuous ambulatory peritoneal dialysis
CRRT	Continuous renal replacement therapy
CSP	Compounded sterile preparations
HIT	Heparin-induced thrombocytopenia
IBW	Ideal body weight
IHD	Intermittent hemodialysis
LDH	Lactate dehydrogenase
NG	Nasogastric
PICC	Peripherally inserted central venous catheter
PL	Phospholipid(s)
PN	Parenteral nutrition
PPN	Peripheral parenteral nutrition
PTH	Parathyroid hormone
REE	Resting energy expenditure
RMR	Resting metabolic rate
RQ	Respiratory quotient
SGA	Subjective global assessment
TEE	Total energy expenditure
TG	Triglyceride(s)
TNA	Total nutrient admixture
TPN	Total parenteral nutrition
USP 797	United States Pharmacopeia Chapter 797
VO_2	Volume of oxygen consumption
VCO_2	Volume of carbon dioxide production

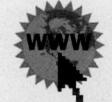 Self-assessment questions and answers are available at *http://www.mhpharmacotherapy.com/pp.html.*

REFERENCES

1. American Society for Parenteral and Enteral Nutrition Board of Directors and the Clinical Guidelines Task Force. Guidelines for the

use of parenteral and enteral nutrition in adult and pediatric patients. JPEN J Parenter Enteral Nutr 2002;26:1SA–138SA.

2. McClave SA, Martindale RG, Vanek VW, et al. Guidelines for the provision and assessment of nutrition support therapy in the adult critically ill patient: Society of Critical Care Medicine (SCCM) and American Society for Parenteral and Enteral Nutrition (A.S.P.E.N.) J PEN J Parenter Enteral Nutr 2009;33:277–316.

3. Woodcock NP, Zeigler D, Palmer MD, et al. Enteral versus parenteral nutrition: A pragmatic study. Nutrition 2001;17:1–12.

4. Wolfe RR, Allsop JR, Burke JF. Glucose metabolism in man: Responses to intravenous glucose infusion. Metabolism 1979;28:210–220.

5. Rosmarin DK, Wardlaw GM, Mirtallo J. Hyperglycemia associated with high, continuous infusion rates of total parenteral nutrition dextrose. Nutr Clin Pract 1996;11:151–156.

6. The American Society for Parenteral and Enteral Nutrition. Task force for the revision of safe practices for parenteral nutrition. Safe practices of parenteral nutrition. JPEN J Parenter Enteral Nutr 2004;28:S39–S70.

7. Driscoll DF, Bhargava HN, Li L, et al. Physicochemical stability of total nutrient admixtures. Am J Health Syst Pharm 1995;52:623–634.

8. Ferezou J, Bach AC. Structure and metabolic fate of triacylglycerol- and phospholipid-rich particles of commercial parenteral fat emulsions. Nutrition 1999;15:44–50.

9. Goodgame JT, Lowry SF, Brennan MF. Essential fatty acid deficiency in total parenteral nutrition: Time course of development and suggestions for therapy. Surgery 1978;84:271–277.

10. The Veteran Affairs Total Parenteral Nutrition Cooperative Study Group. Perioperative total parenteral nutrition in surgical patients. N Engl J Med 1991;325:525–532.

11. Crocker KS, Noga R, Filibeck DJ, et al. Microbial growth comparisons of five commercial parenteral lipid emulsions. JPEN J Parenter Enteral Nutr 1984;8:391–395.

12. D'Angio R, Quercia RA, Treiber NK, et al. The growth of microorganisms in total parenteral nutrition admixtures. JPEN J Parenter Enteral Nutr 1987;11:394–397.

13. Lacy CH, Armstrong LL, Goldman MP, et al., eds. Drug Information Handbook, 14th ed. Hudson, OH: Lexi-Comp, 2006:1292–1294.

14. Sheldon GF, Grzyb S. Phosphate depletion and repletion: Relation to parenteral nutrition and oxygen transport. Ann Surg 1975;182:683–689.

15. Food and Drug Administration. Safety alert: Hazards of precipitation associated with parenteral nutrition. Am J Hosp Pharm 1994;51:1427–1428.

16. Tong GM, Rude RK. Magnesium deficiency in critical illness. J Intensive Care Med 2005;20:3–17.

17. Wolman S, Anderson GH, Marliss EB, Jeejeebhoy YN. Zinc in total parenteral nutrition: Requirements and metabolic effects. Gastroenterology 1979;76:458–467.

18. Spiegel JE, Willenbucher RF. Rapid development of severe copper deficiency in a patient with Crohn's disease receiving parenteral nutrition. JPEN J Parenter Enteral Nutr 1999;23:169–172.

19. Pesce-Hammond K, Wessel J. Nutrition assessment and decision making. In: Merritt R, ed. The A.S.P.E.N. Nutrition Support Practice Manual, 2nd ed. Silver Spring, MD: American Society for Parenteral and Enteral Nutrition, 2005:3–26.

20. Dickerson RN. Specialized nutrition support in the hospitalized obese patient. Nutr Clin Pract 2004;19:245–254.

21. Bodoky A. Parenteral nutrition by peripheral vein, portal vein, or central venous catheter? World J Surg 1986;10:47–52.

22. Driscoll DF. Total nutrient admixtures: Theory and practice. Nutr Clin Pract 1995;10:114–119.

23. Driscoll DF, Bacon MN, Bistrian BR. Effects of in-line filtration on lipid particle size distribution in total nutrient admixtures. JPEN J Parenter Enteral Nutr 1996;20:296–301.

24. Trissel LA, Gilbert DL, Martinez JF, et al. Compatibility of parenteral nutrient solutions with selected drugs during simulated Y-site administration. Am J Health Syst Pharm 1997;54:1295–1300.

25. Trissel LA, Gilbert DL, Martinez JF, et al. Compatibility of medications with 3-in-1 parenteral nutrition admixtures. JPEN J Parenter Enteral Nutr 1999;23:67–74.

26. (797) Pharmaceutical compounding—Sterile preparations. United States Pharmacopeial Convention, Revision Bulletin 2008;1–61.

27. Huang TL, Lue MC, Chen LL. Early use of cyclic TPN prevents further deterioration of liver functions for the TPN patients with impaired liver function. Hepatogastroenterology 2000;47:1347–1350.

28. Watters JM, Norris SB, Kirkpatrick SM. Endogenous glucose production following injury increases with age. J Clin Endocrinol Metab 1997;82:3005–3010.

29. Campbell IT. Limitations of nutrient intake. The effect of stressors: Trauma, sepsis and multiple organ failure. Eur J Clin Nutr 1999;53(Suppl 1):S143–S147.

30. Butler SO, Btaiche IF, Alaniz C. Relationship between hyperglycemia and infection in critically ill patients. Pharmacotherapy 2005;25:963–976.

31. Bjerke HS, Shabot MM. Glucose intolerance in critically ill surgical patients: Relationship to total parenteral nutrition and severity of illness. Am Surg 1992;58:728–731.

32. Van Den Berghe G, Wouters PJ, Weekers F, et al. Intensive insulin therapy in critically ill patients. N Engl J Med 2001;345:1359–1367.

33. Van Den Berghe G, Wouters PJ, Bouillon R, et al. Outcome benefit of intensive insulin therapy in the critically ill: Insulin dose versus glycemic control. Crit Care Med 2003;31:359–366.

34. Finney SJ, Zekveld C, Elia A, et al. Glucose control and mortality in critically ill patients. JAMA 2003;290:2041–2047.

35. The NICE-SUGAR Study Investigators. Intensive versus conventional glucose control in critically ill patients. N Engl J Med 2009;360:1283–1297.

36. Greene HL, Hazlett D, Demaree R. Relationship between Intralipid-induced hyperlipemia and pulmonary function. Am J Clin Nutr 1976;29:127–135.

37. Grundy SM, Billheimer D, Chait A, et al. Summary of the second report of the national cholesterol education program expert panel on detection, evaluation, and treatment of high blood cholesterol in adults. JAMA 1993;269:3015–3023.

38. Btaiche IF, Khalidi N. Metabolic complications of parenteral nutrition in adults, part 1 and part 2. Am J Health Syst Pharm 2004;61:1938–1949, 2050–2059.

39. Devlin JW, Lau AK, Tanios MA. Propofol-associated hypertriglyceridemia and pancreatitis in the intensive care unit: An analysis of frequency and risk factors. Pharmacotherapy 2005;25:1348–1352.

40. Liposky JM, Nelson LD. Ventilatory response to high caloric loads in critically ill patients. Crit Care Med 1994;22:796–802.

41. Buchman AL, Moukarzel A. Metabolic bone disease associated with total parenteral nutrition. Clin Nutr 2000;19:217–231.

42. Vargas JH, Klein GL, Ament ME, et al. Metabolic bone disease of total parenteral nutrition: Course after changing from casein to amino acids in parenteral solutions with reduced aluminum content. Am J Clin Nutr 1988;48:1070–1078.

43. Klein GL. Metabolic bone disease of total parenteral nutrition. Nutrition 1998;14:149–152.

44. Department of Health and Human Services, Food and Drug Administration. Aluminum in large and small volume parenterals used in total parenteral nutrition. Fed Regist 2000(Docket No. 90N-0056);65:4103–4111.

45. Kraft MD, Btaiche IF, Sacks GS. Review of the refeeding syndrome. Nutr Clin Pract 2005;20:625–633.

46. Romanski SA, McMahon M, Molly M. Metabolic acidosis and thiamine deficiency. Mayo Clin Proc 1999;74:259–263.

47. Clark CL, Sacks GS, Dickerson RN, et al. Treatment of hypophosphatemia in patients receiving specialized nutrition support using a graduated dosing scheme: Results from a prospective clinical trial. Crit Care Med 1995;23:1504–1511.

48. Brown KA, Dickerson RN, Morgan LM, et al. A new graduated dosing regimen for phosphorus replacement in patients receiving nutrition support. JPEN J Parenter Enteral Nutr 2006;30:209–214.

49. Apovian CM, McMahon MM, Bistran BR. Guidelines for refeeding the marasmic patient. Crit Care Med 1990;18:1030–1033.

50. Beghetto MG, Victorino J, Teixeira L, de Azevedo MJ. Parenteral nutrition as a risk factor for central venous catheter-related infection. JPEN J Parenter Enteral Nutr 2005;29:367–373.

101 Enteral Nutrition

Sarah J. Miller

LEARNING OBJECTIVES

Upon completion of the chapter, the reader will be able to:

1. Discuss how gut structure and function impact choice of feeding route and outcome of feeding.
2. Evaluate patient-specific parameters to determine whether enteral nutrition (EN) is appropriate.
3. Compare clinical efficacy, complications, and costs of EN versus parenteral nutrition (PN).
4. Choose an appropriate method of EN delivery based on patient-specific parameters.
5. Estimate kilocalorie and protein requirements of an enteral feeding candidate and design an EN regimen to meet these.
6. Choose an appropriate category of EN product given patient-specific parameters.
7. Formulate a monitoring plan for an EN patient.
8. Select appropriate medication administration techniques for an EN patient.

KEY CONCEPTS

❶ EN is the preferred route if the gut can be used safely in a patient who cannot meet nutritional requirements by oral intake.

❷ EN is associated with fewer infectious complications than PN.

❸ For patients intolerant of gastric feedings or in whom the risk of aspiration is high, feedings delivered with the tip of the tube past the pylorus into the duodenum or, preferably, the jejunum are preferred.

❹ Standard EN formulas are polymeric formulas; these are appropriate for most patients.

❺ When choosing an EN formula, the patient's fluid status should dictate the caloric density selected.

❻ Clinical trial data supporting the use of specialty formulas in niche populations typically are unconvincing in terms of patient outcomes.

❼ The role of enteral immunonutrition in clinical practice remains controversial.

❽ GI complications are the most common complications of EN limiting the amount of feeding patients receive.

❾ An important practice to help prevent medication-related occlusion is adequate water flushing of the tube before, between, and after each medication is given through the tube.

❿ Compatibility of medications with an EN formula and, conversely, an EN formula with administered medications is of concern when administering medications through feeding tubes.

Enteral nutrition (EN) is broadly defined as delivery of nutrients via the GI tract. This includes normal oral feeding as well as delivery of nutrients in a liquid form by tube. Sometimes when the term *enteral nutrition* is used, only tube feedings are included; hence the terms *enteral nutrition* and *tube feedings* are often used synonymously. The bulk of this chapter will include information regarding delivery of feedings via tubes. Formulas for EN usually are delivered in the form of commercially prepared liquid preparations, although some products are produced as powders for reconstitution.

It might be expected that EN via tubes would have been used widely before development of parenteral nutrition (PN); however, this was not the case. Modern techniques for enteral access, both placement of the tubes and the materials for making pliable, comfortable tubes, were not developed until the 1960s and 1970s. The National Aeronautics and Space Administration effort in the 1960s led to development of low-residue (monomeric) diets for astronauts. These were adapted for use in sick patients requiring EN. Nonvolitional feedings in patients who cannot meet nutritional requirements by oral intake include EN and PN, which are collectively known as *specialized nutrition support* (SNS).

Several organizations have issued clinical guidelines on the use of EN. These include the American Society for Parenteral and Enteral Nutrition (A.S.P.E.N.), the European Society for Clinical Nutrition and Metabolism (ESPEN), and the Canadian team known as Critical Care Nutrition.[1–4] A.S.P.E.N. has recently teamed with the Society for Critical Care Medicine (SCCM) to release guidelines for SNS in critically ill patients.[5]

GI TRACT STRUCTURE AND FUNCTION
Anatomy and Absorptive Function

With normal volitional feeding, food is ingested via the mouth. Here, the process of breaking down complex foodstuffs into simpler forms that can be absorbed by the small bowel begins. Solid food is chewed in the mouth, and enzymes begin digestion. The trigger for release of many enzymes is presence of food in specific regions of the GI tract. Food is swallowed and passes through the esophagus and the esophageal sphincter to the stomach, where additional digestive enzymes and acids further break it down. The stomach also serves a mixing and grinding function.

The food, now in a liquid form known as *chyme*, passes through the pyloric sphincter into the duodenum, where stomach acid is neutralized. There is wide variation in lengths of the components of the small intestine (i.e., duodenum, jejunum, and ileum) between individuals (Table 101–1). Most absorption of digested carbohydrate and protein occurs within the jejunum. Most fat absorption occurs within the jejunum and ileum. In the small bowel, breakdown of macronutrients (i.e., carbohydrate, protein, and fat) occurs both within the lumen and at the intestinal mucosal membrane surface. The absorptive units on the intestinal mucosal membrane are infoldings known as *villi*. These villi are made up of epithelial cells called *enterocytes*. Projections (striations) from these enterocytes called *microvilli* increase the surface area of the small bowel and make up what is known as the *brush-border membrane*.

Digestive enzymes secreted by the pancreas play a role in food breakdown. The pancreas secretes large amounts of sodium bicarbonate that neutralize stomach acid. These substances flow from the pancreas through the pancreatic duct. The pancreatic duct typically joins the hepatic duct to become the common bile duct that empties through the sphincter of Oddi into the duodenum. Bile secreted by the liver does not contain digestive enzymes, but bile salts help to emulsify fat and facilitate fat absorption. Bile flows through bile ducts into the hepatic duct and common bile duct. Bile is stored in the gallbladder until needed in the gut to aid fat digestion, at which time it empties through the cystic duct to the common bile duct to the duodenum. Pathways through which carbohydrate, protein, and fat are digested and absorbed through the small bowel are illustrated in Fig. 101–1.

After absorption in the small bowel, remaining undigested food passes from the ileum through the ileocecal valve to the colon. A major role of the colon is fluid absorption. Some of the water and sodium absorption achieved by the colon is facilitated by short-chain fatty acids (SFCAs) formed from digestion of certain dietary fibers by colonic bacterial enzymes.

Table 101–1	
Length of the Small Bowel in Adults	
Segment	**Length (ft)**
Total	12–20
Duodenum	1
Jejunum	5–8
Ileum	7–12

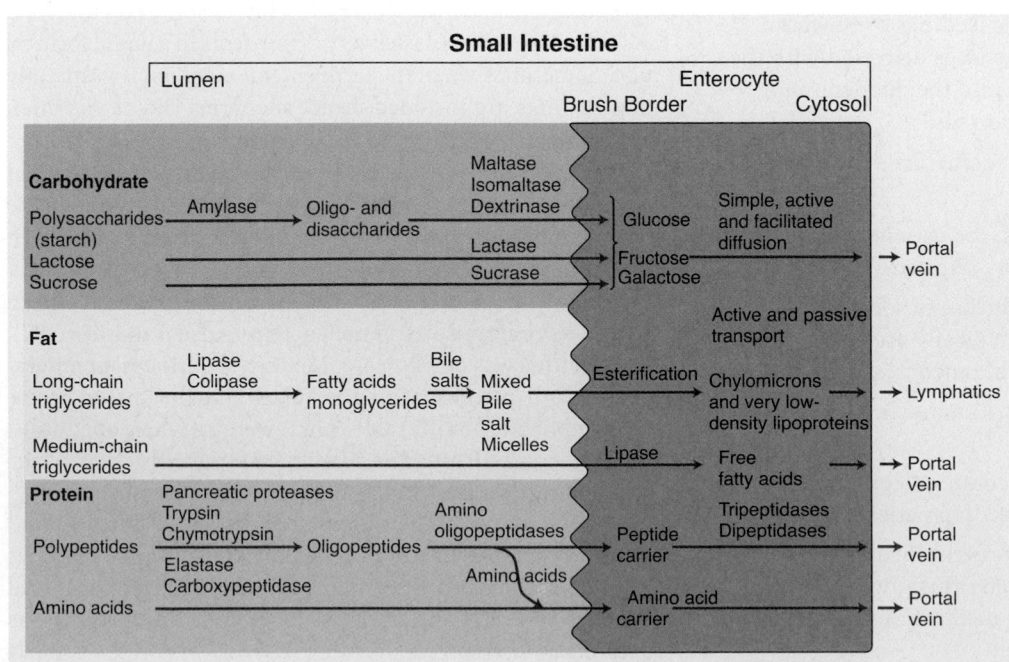

FIGURE 101–1. Schematic of carbohydrate, fat, and protein digestion. (From Kumpf VJ, Chessman KH. Enteral nutrition. In: DiPiro JT, Talbert RL, Yee GC, et al., eds. Pharmacotherapy: A Pathophysiologic Approach, 7th ed. New York: McGraw-Hill, 2008:2400.)

Gut Immune Function

In addition to roles in digestion and absorption, the gut plays significant immune roles. The distal small bowel and colon host many bacteria and their endotoxins, and it is important that these organisms not gain access to the internal systems of the body. This function is known globally as the *gut barrier function* and can be divided into several components.[6] Normal flora of the gut comprise one component. The normal flora, particularly some anaerobes, help to prevent overgrowth of potential pathogens. A second component of the gut barrier involves mechanical factors. These include an epithelial mucus gel layer that prevents adherence of bacteria and peristalsis of the small bowel that prevents stasis of bacteria. Gut-associated lymphoid tissue (GALT), prominent in the small bowel, serves as a local immune system. Secretory immunoglobulin A produced at the mucosal surface prevents bacteria from invading the surface. Bile salts and the reticuloendothelial system of the liver are believed to bind bacterial endotoxin and help clear it from the blood should it be absorbed into the portal circulation.

PATIENT SELECTION

In general, ❶ *if the gut can be used safely in a patient who cannot meet nutritional requirements by oral intake, then EN is the preferred route.* If the gut functions, EN is usually preferred over PN. The timing of SNS (either EN or PN) is controversial, but definitive guidelines for these therapies state that SNS should be started when intake has been inadequate for 7 to 14 days or if inadequate oral intake is anticipated to last at least 7 to 14 days.[1] Prior nutritional status of the patient should be considered. Previously well-nourished patients can better afford not being fed for longer periods of time than those who are previously poorly nourished. Patients in the intensive care unit (ICU) setting probably benefit from early EN started within 24 to 48 hours of admission to the ICU.[3,5] Methods for assessing nutritional status and designing SNS regimens are covered in Chapter 100. In general, non-obese hospitalized patients require 20 to 35 total kcal/kg of body weight/day and 1 to 2 g protein/kg of body weight/day.

Indications

Many potential indications for EN exist (Table 101–2). PN was used extensively previously for many of these conditions. Advances in EN technology now allow many patients with these conditions to receive EN. EN is administered in both institutional and home settings.

Contraindications and Precautions

EN should not be used or should be used with extreme caution in certain conditions (Table 101–3). It is possible to use EN in some patients with these conditions depending on severity of illness, location of abnormality, and experience of practitioners delivering care. Controversy surrounds some of these contraindications and precautions. For example, whereas some clinicians deliberately avoid enteral feedings in

the hemodynamically unstable patient for fear of worsening intestinal ischemia, others believe that early feeding may facilitate intestinal perfusion and is beneficial.[5,7–9] Still others might avoid jejunal feedings in this setting but would proceed with cautious gastric feedings.

Enteral Versus Parenteral Feeding

With the advent of the technique of PN by a large central vein in the late 1960s, this modality of feeding quickly became popular. PN was used originally in patients with

---

Table 101–2

Potential Indications for EN

Neoplastic Disease	**GI Disease**
Chemotherapy	IBD
Radiation therapy	Short bowel syndrome
Upper GI tumors	Esophageal motility disorder
Cancer cachexia	Pancreatitis
Organ Failure	Fistulas
Hepatic	Gastroesophageal reflux disease
Renal	Esophageal atresia
Cardiac cachexia	**Neurologic Impairment**
Pulmonary	Comatose state
Bronchopulmonary dysplasia	Cerebrovascular accident
Congenital heart disease	Demyelinating disease
Hypermetabolic States	Severe depression
Closed head injury	Failure to thrive
Burns	Cerebral palsy
Trauma	**Other Indications**
Postoperative major surgery	AIDS
Sepsis	Anorexia nervosa
	Complications during pregnancy
	Geriatric patients with multiple chronic disease
	Organ transplantation
	Inborn errors of metabolism
	Cystic fibrosis
	Extreme prematurity

From Kumpf VJ, Chessman KH. Enteral nutrition. In DiPiro JT, Talbert RL, Yee GC, et al., eds. Pharmacotherapy: A Pathophysiologic Approach, 7th ed. New York: McGraw-Hill, 2008.

Table 101–3

Contraindications and Precautions for EN

Severe hemorrhagic pancreatitis
Severe necrotizing pancreatitis
Necrotizing enterocolitis
Diffuse peritonitis
Small bowel obstruction
Paralytic ileus
Severe hemodynamic instability
Enterocutaneous fistulae
Severe diarrhea
Severe malabsorption
Severe GI hemorrhage
Intractable vomiting

inflammatory bowel disease (IBD) or congenital bowel abnormalities but was incorporated quickly into care of other types of patients such as the critically ill. The relative ease of PN administration, along with the perception that critically ill patients had prolonged high-energy expenditures, led to complications of overfeeding. In the United States, where no IV fat emulsion was available commercially for several years during the 1970s, the impact of dextrose overfeeding was observed. Complications included hyperglycemia, carbon dioxide overproduction leading to delays in weaning from mechanical ventilation, and liver abnormalities owing to hepatic steatosis.

As complications of PN became evident, the pendulum began to swing toward EN in the late 1980s and early 1990s as clinical studies were published showing better clinical outcomes with EN compared with PN. Some of the potential advantages of EN over PN are included here. First, EN is expected to preserve the gut barrier function better than PN. This, in turn, could prevent translocation of bacteria and endotoxin from the gut lumen into the lymphatic system and systemic circulation, thus preventing infections. Studies from the same era support that ❷ *EN is associated with fewer infectious complications than PN.* EN is cited frequently as having a better overall safety profile than PN. Whereas PN is associated with more severe complications, such as pneumothorax and catheter sepsis, EN is associated with more nuisance complications, such as GI side effects that delay or limit delivery of nutrients. Another major frequently cited advantage of EN over PN is that EN is less expensive. It is true that EN formulas typically are cheaper and less labor intensive to prepare than PN, although some specialty EN formulas approach the cost of PN formulas. However, depending on the method of feeding tube placement, EN costs can mount if the tube must be placed by a radiologist or gastroenterologist rather than a nurse or if the tube must be replaced for some reason.

The arguments in support of EN over PN have been questioned. Part of this questioning relates to the question of whether EN is beneficial compared with PN or whether PN as commonly administered may be detrimental. Overfeeding and hyperglycemia occur easily with PN administration, and the potential harm of hyperglycemia, especially in critical-care populations, has been demonstrated poignantly, although the exact range optimal for glycemic control in the ICU patient remains controversial.[10,11] A high-profile study published in 1991 demonstrated in a mildly malnourished perioperative population that there were more infectious complications in patients randomized to receive PN compared with those randomized to receive no SNS; there was no difference in noninfectious complications between the two groups.[12] Only in severely malnourished perioperative patients were fewer noninfectious complications seen with PN; in these patients, no difference in infectious complications was seen between groups. Whether EN truly prevents infections and improves clinical outcomes or whether PN is detrimental continues to be debated and is probably dependent on the specific patient population. However, at present, EN is preferred by most experts over PN when the gut is functional. In Europe (more so than in North America), PN is used to supplement EN during the first week of intensive care therapy when EN is not yet being tolerated at full rates.[2,13,14] This approach is currently discouraged by the Canadian guidelines and the A.S.P.E.N./SCCM guidelines for SNS in the critically ill patient.[3,4] One meta-analysis did indicate that PN may be superior to delayed EN in critical care.[15] Data are emerging to indicate that caloric and protein deficits early in the critical care stay are associated with increased morbidity and mortality; one method to prevent such deficits would be to augment EN with PN until full EN is tolerated.[13] The Algorithms for Critical-Care Enteral and Parenteral Therapy (ACCEPT) trial showed that use of an evidence-based algorithm for SNS in critical care patients in community and teaching hospitals improved provision of EN and was associated with reduced hospital stay.[16]

ROUTES OF ACCESS[17]

There are several access sites for EN (Fig. 101–2). Nasogastric (NG), orogastric (OG), nasoduodenal (ND), and nasojejunal (NJ) routes generally are for short-term use (less than 1 month), whereas gastrostomy, percutaneous endoscopic gastrostomy (PEG), jejunostomy, and percutaneous endoscopic jejunostomy (PEJ) tubes are preferred for longer-term treatment. The esophagostomy/pharyngostomy is used rarely. Both advantages and disadvantages exist for each EN route (Table 101–4).

Gastric Feeding

Gastric feedings are used commonly. They require an intact gag reflex and normal gastric emptying for safety and success. Certain patients, such as those who have suffered head trauma, may not empty their stomachs efficiently and therefore may not be good candidates for gastric feedings. In these patients, it may be impossible to achieve a gastric tube feeding rate to provide adequate nutrients. In addition, pooling of formula in the stomach could increase risk of aspirating feeding formula into the lungs.

The NG route is used most commonly for short-term (less than 1 month) enteral access. The major advantage of this route is that the tube can be placed quickly and inexpensively by the nurse at the bedside.

Gastrostomy tubes, where an incision is made directly through the abdominal wall, are indicated for patients who can tolerate gastric feedings but in whom long-term (greater than 1 month) feedings are anticipated. The most commonly placed gastrostomy tubes are PEG tubes placed endoscopically. Gastrostomy tubes also can be placed laparoscopically or during an open procedure by a surgeon. Placement of a gastrostomy tube either endoscopically or surgically is more expensive than bedside OG or NG placement but does result in placement of a larger bore tube.

An advantage of feeding into the stomach is that the feedings can be delivered either intermittently or continuously.

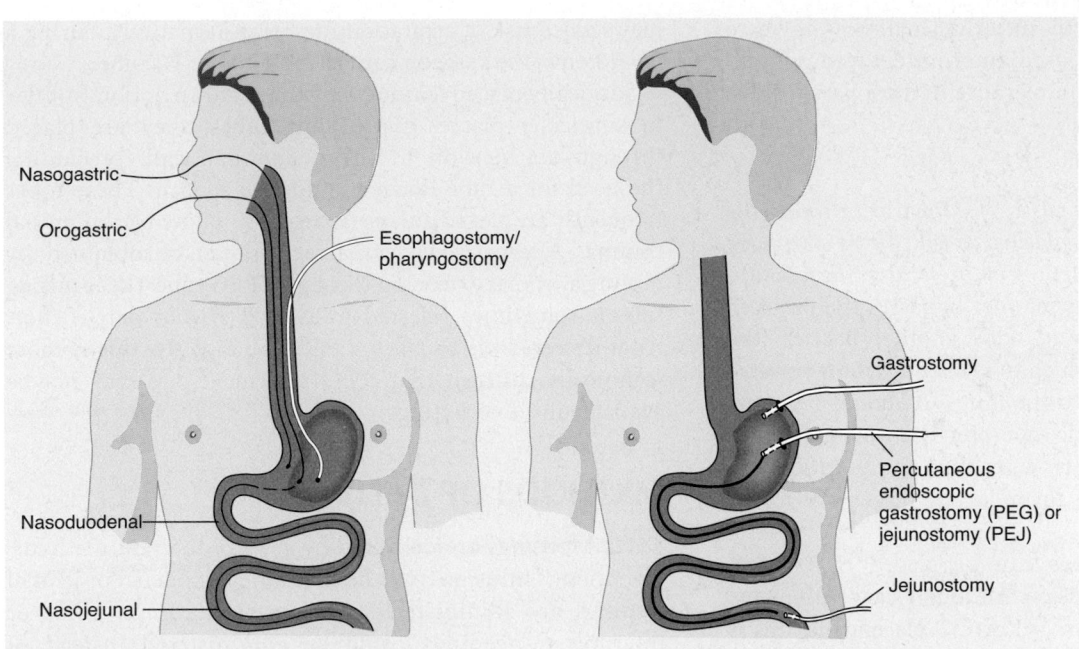

FIGURE 101–2. Access sites for tube feeding. (From Kumpf VJ, Chessman KH. Enteral nutrition. In DiPiro JT, Talbert RL, Yee GC, et al., eds. Pharmacotherapy: A Pathophysiologic Approach, 7th ed, New York: McGraw-Hill, 2008:2403.)

Table 101–4

Options and Considerations in the Selection of Enteral Access

Access	Indications	Tube Placement Options	Advantages	Disadvantages
Nasogastric or orogastric	Short-term Intact gag reflex Normal gastric emptying	Manually at bedside	Ease of placement Allows for all methods of administration Inexpensive Multiple commercially available tubes and sizes	Potential tube displacement Potential increased aspiration risk
Nasoduodenal or nasojejunal	Short-term Impaired gastric motility or emptying High risk of GER or aspiration	Manually at bedside Fluoroscopically Endoscopically	Potential reduced aspiration risk Allows for early postinjury or postoperative feeding Multiple commercially available tubes and sizes	Manual transpyloric passage requires greater skill Potential tube displacement or clogging Bolus or intermittent feeding not tolerated
Gastrostomy	Long-term Normal gastric emptying	Surgically Endoscopically Radiologically Laparoscopically	Allows for all methods of administration Large-bore tubes less likely to clog Multiple commercially available tubes and sizes Low-profile buttons available	Attendant risks associated with each type of procedure Potential increased aspiration risk Requires stoma site care
Jejunostomy	Long-term Impaired gastric motility or gastric emptying High risk of GER or aspiration	Surgically Endoscopically Radiologically Laparoscopically	Allows for early postinjury or postoperative feeding Potential reduced aspiration risk Multiple commercially available tubes and sizes	Attendant risks associated with each type of procedure Bolus or intermittent feeding not tolerated Requires stoma site care

GER, gastroesophageal reflux.

From Kumpf VJ, Chessman KH. Enteral nutrition. In DiPiro JT, Talbert RL, Yee GC, et al., eds. Pharmacotherapy: A Pathophysiologic Approach, 7th ed. New York: McGraw-Hill, 2008.

This is unlike feeding directly into the small bowel, where continuous feedings must be used. Intermittent feedings into the small bowel result in GI intolerance in most patients.

Postpyloric Feedings

❸ *For patients intolerant of gastric feedings or in whom the risk of aspiration is high, feedings delivered with the tip of the tube past the pylorus into the duodenum or, preferably, the jejunum are preferred.* Feeding in this manner bypasses the problem of poor gastric emptying and adds another barrier (the pyloric sphincter) through which tube feedings must traverse before they are aspirated into the lungs. It should be noted that postpyloric feedings do not preclude the possibility of aspiration. Many patients with this complication are not aspirating tube feeding formula but rather their own nasopharyngeal secretions.

ND and NJ feeding tubes can be placed by trained, experienced nurses at the bedside. Although such placements typically take more time than NG or OG placements, this is still a relatively inexpensive method of placement. However, many institutions have not been able to achieve placements consistently at the bedside. In many institutions, ND or NJ placements are done in the radiology suite by a radiologist using fluoroscopy to visualize tube advancement to the appropriate area. This procedure increases the cost of EN therapy. NJ tubes generally are preferred over ND tubes; placement of the tip of the tube distal to the ligament of Treitz (located near the junction of the duodenum and the jejunum)

Patient Encounter, Part 1

A 25-year-old man was involved in a motor-vehicle accident in which he suffered several long bone fractures, a ruptured spleen, and a severe closed-head injury. This 5', 10"- man was well nourished and weighed 75 kg before the accident. During the first surgery to repair his abdominal injuries, the surgeon placed a feeding jejunostomy tube. Following surgery, the patient was taken to the intensive care unit (ICU), where he was mechanically ventilated and had an intracranial pressure monitor. He initially required significant amounts of vasopressor agents to maintain his blood pressure. The decision was made to delay dealing with the long bone fractures until he was more stable.

What would this patient's estimated caloric and protein requirements be?

What is the potential advantage of using EN rather than PN in this patient?

Why is a jejunostomy tube a good access route for feeding this patient?

Would it be prudent to start jejunal feedings immediately after the patient is admitted to the ICU following his abdominal surgery?

---

may reduce risk of aspiration further. Alternatively, during a laparotomy, the surgeon can place an ND or NJ tube.

Surgically placed jejunostomy tubes are an option; similar to surgically placed gastrostomy tubes, they are placed through an incision in the abdominal wall, precluding the need for a tube down the nose or mouth. These tubes frequently are placed during laparotomy following abdominal trauma. Alternatively, jejunal access can be obtained by placing a jejunal extension through a PEG tube; the resulting tube is sometimes referred to as a *PEGJ tube* or *G-J tube*. Another option is to place a PEJ tube directly; this is more technically difficult than PEG placement and may not be available in some settings.

METHODS OF DELIVERY

Enteral feedings are delivered by several different methods. Continuous infusion must be used when duodenal or jejunal feedings are administered. For gastric feedings, bolus or intermittent feedings could be administered instead of continuous feedings. Each method has advantages and disadvantages.

In many hospitals, EN is delivered most commonly as a continuous infusion over 24 hours at a constant rate regulated by an infusion pump. A variation of continuous infusion is cyclic feeding, in which a constant rate is maintained by a pump over a certain number of hours daily. This method of administration is used commonly in long-term care or home settings. Often EN is administered overnight, giving the patient "freedom" from the infusion pump during the day, although this may not be practical for patients with high nutritional needs because it may be difficult to increase the rate of feedings while trying to maintain GI tolerance with limited infusions.

Intermittent feedings are used commonly in long-term care or home settings due to easier administration. Patients frequently are started with continuous feedings, transitioned to intermittent feedings given several times a day over about 30 to 45 minutes for each feeding, and eventually changed to bolus feedings, where feeding is administered several times a day over less than 10 minutes per feeding. An advantage of intermittent feedings is that they may be administered by gravity flow adjusted with a roller clamp, although some institutions may use an infusion pump. Bolus feedings preclude the need for an infusion set or pump and can be administered using a 60-mL syringe, although, again, in some circumstances an infusion set and pump may be used. Intermittent and bolus feedings often are given in amounts of 240 to 480 mL per feeding, corresponding to one to two cans (8 oz each) of formula.

EN FORMULAS

A number of EN formulas are marketed commercially. Hospitals and long-term care facilities usually limit formularies of EN formulas, stocking only a limited number of products. A number of factors should be taken into account when devising a formulary.

Polymeric versus Oligomeric Formulas

A major criterion for categorizing EN products is whether they contain more intact (polymeric) macronutrients or their macronutrient ingredients are present in simpler forms (oligomeric). ❹ *Standard EN formulas are polymeric formulas; these are appropriate for most patients.* Oligomeric formulas should be reserved for patients with GI dysfunction.

Polymeric formulas typically have low osmolality of 300 to 500 mOsm/kg. These formulas usually supply essential vitamins and minerals in amounts similar to the Adequate Intakes or Recommended Dietary Allowances (RDA) for these nutrients when the formula is delivered in amounts adequate to meet macronutrient requirements of most patients. Many polymeric formulas are inexpensive relative to oligomeric formulas. Most polymeric formulas are lactose-free and gluten-free, as are most modern tube feeding products. Products designed to be used as oral supplements generally are polymeric and often have sucrose or other simple sugars added to improve taste.

The oligomeric formulas are also known as *chemically defined formulas*. This class of formulas can be subcategorized based on whether the formula contains all free amino acids (elemental formulas) or peptides (peptide-based) as the protein source. Some formulas contain a combination of free amino acids and small peptides. Actually, dipeptides and tripeptides are absorbed more efficiently than free amino acids. Oligomeric formulas may be better tolerated than polymeric formulas for patients with defects in GI function and may be particularly useful with severe pancreatic dysfunction or significantly decreased GI surface area (e.g., short bowel syndrome).

Oligomeric formulas typically are more expensive than polymeric formulas and have higher osmolality because they contain more osmotically active particles. However, osmolality of these products usually does not exceed 700 mOsm/kg, a value less than that of many oral medications or a regular diet. In the past, there was concern that higher-osmolality EN formulas could cause GI intolerance, particularly diarrhea. This led to dilution of formulas by half or more with water and gradually increasing both the strength and rate of formula administration. This practice is unnecessary and serves only to delay attainment of goal nutritional support. Sometimes enteral feedings are diluted to deliver extra water required by the patient; this practice generally is discouraged because of potential risk of formula contamination. Instead, it is better to give extra water as boluses through the tube. If medications are administered through the feeding tube, generous amounts of water should be used to flush the tube before and after each medication; this practice helps provide extra fluid and prevent problems with occlusion of the tube.

Oligomeric formulas usually are less palatable than polymeric formulas and are not designed for use as oral supplements. Many of the oligomeric formulas provide some fat calories as medium-chain triglycerides (MCTs), a fat source that is more readily absorbed and metabolized than long-chain triglycerides (LCTs) typically found in polymeric formulas. The MCTs do not require bile salts or pancreatic enzymes for absorption. Some of the elemental formulas contain a low proportion of fat (less than 10% of total calories), which makes them useful in certain situations where fat needs to be restricted. The carbohydrate source in oligomeric formulas is also less complex than in polymeric formulas, consisting of oligosaccharides rather than hydrolyzed starch.

Fiber Content

Another distinguishing factor of enteral formulas is whether or not they contain fiber. Both soluble and insoluble fibers may be included in the formula, with insoluble fiber exerting more effect on gut motility by drawing water into the intestine and decreasing transit time, thus preventing constipation. Soluble fiber can help to lower blood cholesterol levels, regulate blood sugar, and prolong gastric emptying. Cellulose gum is an example source of insoluble fiber. Oat fiber and guar gum provide primarily soluble fiber. Soy fiber provides primarily insoluble fiber but also some soluble fiber and is the most commonly used fiber source in tube feeding products. Fiber has been useful for regulating gut motility in some but not all clinical studies; it certainly can be useful in selected patients.[18] Some patients may experience GI discomfort secondary to gas production with introduction of fiber-containing formulas.

Fructooligosaccharides (FOSs) are a form of fiber receiving increasing attention. These pass through the stomach and small bowel undigested and are fermented by colonic bacteria to the SCFAs butyrate, propionate, and acetate. The SCFAs serve as a major fuel source for colonocytes and facilitate water and sodium reabsorption in the colon.[19] The FOSs fit in the category called *prebiotics* that serve as fermentable substrates for the normal flora of the colon. The SCFAs are not added directly to EN products because they would be absorbed completely before reaching the colon; rather FOSs are added, allowing bacterial degradation to form SCFAs.

Caloric Density

Enteral feeding formulas can be categorized based on caloric density. Standard caloric density is 1 to 1.3 kcal/mL. More calorically dense formulas containing 1.5 to 2 kcal/mL are also available and have a higher osmolality. ❺ *When choosing an EN formula, the patient's fluid status should dictate the caloric density selected.* Fluid-overloaded patients may benefit from more calorically dense formulas. It should be recognized that as caloric content of a formula increases, the amount of free water decreases. For example, whereas 1 kcal/mL formulas contain about 850 mL of free water/L, the 2 kcal/mL formulas contain about 710 mL of free water/L.[20]

Protein Content

The protein content is an important factor in choosing an EN formula. The standard protein content in EN formulas is up to about 15% of total calories as protein. High-protein formulas containing up to 25% of total calories as protein are available for highly stressed patients with elevated protein needs. So are low-nitrogen formulas containing less than 10% of total calories as protein for use in patients requiring protein restriction. A wide range of protein is available, from about 35 to 85 g/L.

Fat Content

Both MCTs and LCTs are used in tube feeding products. Corn, soy, and safflower oils have been the mainstay sources of fat, providing mainly ω-6 polyunsaturated fatty acids (PUFAs). Some newer EN products contain higher quantities of ω-3 PUFAs from sources such as fish oil (i.e., docosahexenoic acid [DHA] and eicosapentaenoic acid [EPA]). Other formulas contain higher quantities of monounsaturated fatty acids (MUFAs) from canola oil and high-oleic safflower or sunflower oils. The essential fatty acid (EFA) content (mainly linoleic acid) of EN formulas is important because EFA deficiency can be induced if at least 1% to 4% of total calories are not supplied as EFA. MCT oil does not contain any EFA.

Specialty Formulas

Specialty formulas designed for use in specific clinical situations generally are much more expensive than standard polymeric formulas. ❻ *Clinical trial data supporting use of these specialty formulas in niche populations typically are unconvincing in terms of patient outcomes.*

▶ Stress/Trauma Formulas

Historically, formulas aimed specifically for highly stressed, critically ill patients including those suffering significant

trauma and those undergoing major surgical procedures, were enriched with branched-chain amino acids (BCAAs). The rationale for these products was that skeletal muscle BCAAs are preferentially used for energy in critical illness. Provision of BCAAs was hoped to limit breakdown of muscle in these patients. Clinical data failed to support or refute benefit of these formulas unequivocally in terms of clinical outcomes.[3]

The newer generation of enteral feeding formulas marketed for use in these populations covers a broad spectrum of characteristics (Table 101–5). Whereas some are polymeric, others are oligomeric to address malabsorption that may accompany high stress. Some formulas marketed for use in critical illness are calorically dense (1.5 to 2 kcal/mL) to address fluid restrictions seen in this population, whereas others are less calorically dense. Most products contain generous amounts of protein to address requirements of highly stressed patients (**nonprotein kilocalorie to nitrogen ratios** typically between 75:1 and 125:1). Many products contain ingredients purported to increase immune function; the term *immunonutrition* is sometimes attached to these products.

Immune-enhancing ingredients present in some enteral feeding products include arginine, glutamine, ω-3 fatty acids, nucleic acids, and antioxidants. Few products contain all of these (see Table 101–5). Arginine is an important substrate for nitric oxide (NO) synthesis, and small amounts of NO have beneficial effects on immune function under certain conditions.[21] Arginine has been purported to have positive influence on lymphocyte and macrophage function.

Table 101–5

Selected Enteral Feeding Formulas Marketed for Use in High Stress, Pulmonary Disease, and Trauma

Product Name/Manufacturer	kcal/mL	Protein (g/L)	Enriched Ingredients[a]	Selected Specialized Indications
Polymeric				
Impact/Nestle	1	56	Arginine, nucleotides, ω-3 fatty acids	HS, TR, PD, CI
Impact 1.5/Nestle	1.5	84	Arginine, nucleotides, ω-3 fatty acids	HS, TR, PD, CI
Impact with Fiber/Nestle	1	56	Arginine, nucleotides, ω-3 fatty acids	HS, TR, PD, CI
Nutren Pulmonary/Nestle	1.5	68	55% total kcal as fat	PD, CI
Pulmocare/Abbott	1.5	62.6	55% total kcal as fat	PD
Oxepa/Abbott	1.5	62.7	55% total kcal as fat; ω-3 fatty acids	PD
Isosource 1.5 Cal/Nestle	1.5	68	38% total kcal as fat	PD
Oligomeric				
Impact Glutamine/Nestle	1.3	78	Arginine, nucleotides, ω-3 fatty acids, glutamine	HS, TR, PD, CI
Crucial/Nestle	1.5	94	Arginine, ω-3 fatty acids, MCT	HS, TR
Pivot 1.5 Cal/Abbott	1.5	93.8	Arginine, ω-3 fatty acids	HS, TR
Optimental/Abbott	1	51.3	ω-3 fatty acids	HS, TR
Vivonex Plus/Nestle	1	45	Glutamine	CI
Vivonex RTF/Nestle	1	50	MCT	CI
Vivonex T.E.N./Nestle	1	38		CI
Peptamen 1.5/Nestle	1.5	67.6	MCT	CI
Peptamen AF/Nestle	1.2	75.6	MCT, ω-3 fatty acids	HS, CI, PD
Perative/Abbott	1.3	66.7	Arginine, MCT	HS

CI, critical illness; EPA, eicosapentaenoic acid; GLA, γ-linolenic acid; HS, high stress; MCT, medium-chain triglycerides; PD, pulmonary disease; TR, trauma.

[a]Formula considered enriched if following criteria met: arginine—greater than 10 g/1500 kcal; glutamine—greater than 10 g/1500 kcal; MCT—greater than 30% fat calories; ω-3 fatty acid—ratio of ω-6 to ω-3 less than or equal to 2:1 or greater than 1.5 g/L fish oil.

Glutamine is considered to be conditionally essential in critical illness. This amino acid is a preferred fuel source for enterocytes of the small bowel. Supplementation with glutamine, either parenterally or enterally, may help to maintain the integrity of the gut mucosa. This might prevent translocation of bacteria and endotoxin from the gut lumen into the lymphatic system and systemic circulation, although the importance of translocation in humans remains controversial. The ω-3 fatty acids, primarily from fish oils, are included in many immunonutrition products. The metabolites of ω-6 fatty acids include mediators such as prostaglandins, leukotrienes, and thromboxanes that are primarily proinflammatory and increase coagulation. On the other hand, the mediators produced from ω-3 fatty acids are less proinflammatory and decrease coagulation. Thus ω-3 fatty acids may help preserve the antimicrobial capacity of critically ill patients by downregulating inflammation.[18] Limited data support nucleic acids as immunomodulators. Quantities of antioxidants (particularly vitamin C, vitamin E, and β-carotene) higher than those traditionally found in standard enteral formulas are added to some immunonutrition formulas to protect body systems including the immune system from damage by oxygen-free radicals.[22] Oxygen-free radicals may be produced in high quantities in the setting of injury or infection.

❼ *The role of enteral immunonutrition in clinical practice remains controversial.* A high-profile expert consensus conference held in 2004 concluded that certain populations, particularly malnourished patients undergoing GI surgery and trauma patients, would benefit from this therapy.[23–26] Noteworthy is the fact that this symposium was sponsored by the manufacturer of one of the leading immunonutrition products. Several meta-analyses of the commercial immunonutrition products and/or specific ingredients (e.g., arginine and glutamine) found in these products have been conducted.[3,27,28] In general, these analyses have found no benefit in terms of mortality. However, several have concluded that infection rates, length of stay, and length of time on a ventilator may be decreased with these products. More research will be necessary to further delineate which subpopulations will most likely benefit from these therapies. The best timing (initiation and duration) of delivery also needs to be determined. There is some concern that supplementation with arginine may be detrimental in septic patients.[3]

▶ Pulmonary Formulas

Enteral feeding formulas designed for use in patients with chronic obstructive pulmonary disease or receiving mechanical ventilation contain higher amounts of fat (40% to 55% of total kilocalories) than most formulas. The rationale for high fat content is that burning of fat for energy is associated with less carbon dioxide production compared with burning of carbohydrate. Less carbon dioxide production theoretically would be advantageous in patients with retention of this substance and might facilitate weaning from mechanical ventilation. Since part of the market targeted by the manufacturers of these products comprises mechanically ventilated patients, these products are included in Table 101–5 (e.g., Pulmocare, Nutren Pulmonary, Isosource 1.5 Cal and Oxepa). Carbon dioxide retention owing to carbohydrate administration was a problem previously (particularly with PN) when feeding was overzealous. However, at conservative calorie levels typically administered today, even standard enteral formulas usually can be given without fear of excess carbon dioxide production.

One formula, Oxepa, has been studied specifically in critically ill patients with acute respiratory distress syndrome (ARDS) and acute lung injury.[29,30] This high-fat formula contains high quantities of the ω-3 fatty acids (EPA) and γ-linolenic acid (GLA). γ-Linolenic acid is metabolized to a prostaglandin with vasodilatory properties. EPA is converted to prostaglandins and leukotrienes with primarily an antiinflammatory profile. This formula also contains large quantities of antioxidants. Patients receiving this formula required fewer days of mechanical ventilation than patients receiving a high-fat enteral feeding product as a control.[26,27] Concern that the high-fat product used as a control could actually be detrimental to patients remains. In a preliminary study Oxepa has also demonstrated benefit in patients with severe sepsis.[31]

▶ Diabetic Formulas

Similar to pulmonary formulas, formulas designed for the patient with diabetes or stress-induced hyperglycemia are relatively high in fat and low in carbohydrate (Table 101–6). Macronutrient content of these products does not follow the recommendations of the American Diabetes Association for patients with diabetes (lower carbohydrate content and higher fat content than recommended), which could be an issue if used for more than a couple of weeks. These formulas typically contain fiber (primarily soluble) because it plays some role in glycemic control. They also may contain fructose and MUFAs. Data support improved blood sugar control with use of these formulas in patients with diabetes.[32] The importance of preventing severe hyperglycemia in various clinical settings including intensive care has been

Table 101–6

Selected Enteral Feeding Formulas Marketed for Use in Diabetes and Stress-Induced Hyperglycemia

Product Name/ Manufacturer	kcal/ mL	% kcal as Fat	% kcal as Carbohydrate	Fiber (g/L)
Nutren Glytrol/Nestle Nutrition	1	42	40	15.2
Glucerna 1.0 Cal/ Abbott	1	49	34.3	14.4
Glucerna 1.2 Cal/ Abbott	1.2	45	35	17
Glucerna Select/ Abbott	1	31	49	21.1
Diabetisource AC/ Nestle Nutrition	1.2	44	36	15

recognized. Therefore, whether or not a diabetic EN formula is chosen, avoidance of overfeeding and maintenance of good glycemic control with insulin or other hypoglycemic medications are important in these populations.

▶ Renal Formulas

Each major manufacturer of EN products markets more than one specialty formula for use in renal failure (Table 101–7). These products have high caloric density (2 kcal/mL) in light of the need to decrease fluid in this situation. The products vary in amounts of nutrients of interest in renal failure patients such as protein, potassium, phosphorus, and magnesium. Products low in protein (20 to 35 g/L) may be appropriate in chronic renal failure patients not yet receiving dialysis. On the other hand, removal of protein by dialysis, coupled with the hypercatabolic, hypermetabolic condition seen in many acute renal failure patients, makes use of higher-protein formulas (70 to 85 g/L) appropriate in these situations. Potassium, phosphorus, and magnesium contents of EN formulas designed for use in renal failure tend to be lower than standard formulas because these renally excreted electrolytes accumulate during renal failure.

Historically, elemental formulas designed for renal failure were enriched with essential amino acids (EAAs) and contained lesser amounts of nonessential amino acids (NEAAs) than standard formulas. Theoretically, EAAs could combine with urea nitrogen in the synthesis of NEAAs, leading to a decrease in blood urea nitrogen (BUN). The only situation in which such formulas may be appropriate is in patients with chronic renal failure who are not candidates for dialysis. Even in this setting, use of these products should be limited to no more than 2 or 3 weeks owing to the risk of increased serum ammonia levels.[1] These EAA-enriched formulas have been supplanted largely by polymeric formulas with protein content similar to standard EN formulas. The main difference between these products and standard EN formulas is reduced potassium, phosphorus, and magnesium concentrations.

▶ Hepatic Formulas

Specialized formulas for patients with hepatic insufficiency are limited in number. These are enriched with BCAAs while containing a reduced quantity of aromatic amino acids (AAAs) and methionine compared to standard enteral formulas. These changes address the high levels of AAAs and low levels of BCAAs found in the blood of patients with hepatic insufficiency. Theoretically, these products might help patients with hepatic encephalopathy (HE). One of the mechanisms postulated as a cause of HE is the "false neurotransmitter" hypothesis. According to this hypothesis, high levels of AAAs in the blood allow large quantities of these amino acids to cross the blood–brain barrier and form false neurotransmitters, such as octopamine. Administration of high amounts of BCAAs could competitively inhibit some AAAs from crossing the blood–brain barrier, thus decreasing formation of false neurotransmitters. Hepatic formulas have low AAA content and this distinguishes them from the BCAA-enriched formulas historically used in critical illness and stress. Although some data support the use of these specialty products in treatment of moderate to severe HE, improvement in mortality attributable to them has not been consistent.[1] Therefore, many institutions and clinicians prefer to use less expensive polymeric enteral formulas containing standard protein sources for patients with hepatic insufficiency. The specialty formulas are recommended only for patients with chronic cirrhosis who cannot ingest

---

Table 101–7

Selected Enteral Feeding Products Designed for Use in Renal Failure

Product Name/ Manufacturer	Protein/L	Characteristics
Renalcal/Nestle	34.4	Enriched with EAAs, arginine, histidine; incomplete[a] formula due to negligible electrolytes and lack of fat-soluble vitamins
Nepro with Carb Steady/Abbott	81	Complete formula[b] similar to Novasource Renal
Novasource Renal/ Nestle	74	Complete formula similar to Nepro with Carb Steady
Suplena with Carb Steady/Abbott	44.7	Complete formula with low amounts of protein for patients not yet receiving dialysis

[a]Incomplete formula—contains insufficient amounts of one or more essential nutrients.

[b]Complete formula—contains all nutrients in amounts sufficient to meet needs of most patients in a volume equal to or less than that usually administered.

Patient Encounter, Part 2

By day 2 postoperatively, the patient's intracranial pressures were improving and he had been weaned off the vasopressor agents. He was still being mechanically ventilated and was requiring an insulin drip at 2 units/h to keep his blood sugar below 140 mg/dL. He was started on an immune-enhancing enteral formula containing 1.3 kcal/mL and 80 g protein/L; the beginning rate was 40 mL/h to be advanced as tolerated to goal rate over 24 to 36 hours.

What effect would the enteral feeding be expected to have on the patient's blood sugar?

Is an immune-enhancing formula a good choice for this patient?

Approximately what should be the goal rate for this patient using this enteral formula?

1 g protein/kg/day without becoming encephalopathic.[1] An example of a specialized hepatic formula is Hepatic-Aid II, a product supplied as a powder for reconstitution that requires vitamin, mineral, and electrolyte supplementation. A second product is NutriHep, supplied as a liquid formula containing the recommended amounts of key vitamins, minerals, and electrolytes.

MONITORING AND COMPLICATIONS

Although complications of EN generally are considered less serious than those of PN, some complications nevertheless can be dangerous or can lead to impaired delivery of desired nutrient load. Complications of EN can be divided into four categories: GI, technical, infectious, and metabolic. The first three of these categories, along with common causes, are listed in Table 101–8. Patients on EN must be monitored for prevention of complications (Table 101–9). Note that monitoring of many parameters can become less frequent as the patient's condition stabilizes. Monitoring for efficacy of EN is also important.

GI Complications

❽ *GI complications are the most common complications of EN limiting the amount of feeding that patients receive.* Although diarrhea frequently is blamed on the tube feeding formula or the method of EN administration, other possible causes of diarrhea usually exist (see Table 101–8). Many of these are related to the fact that, particularly in the inpatient setting, patients receiving EN frequently are some of the sickest patients in the hospital. Along these lines, *Clostridium difficile* colitis must be considered as a possible cause of diarrhea, especially in patients who have been receiving antimicrobial therapy or proton pump inhibitors.[33–36] Antibiotic therapy is a major cause of diarrhea in acutely ill patients, including those receiving EN. A medication-related cause of diarrhea largely overlooked until the early 1990s is the sorbitol content of medications.[37] Large quantities of this substance present in many oral liquid medications (often considered the dosage form of choice for administration through a feeding tube) can cause diarrhea. Unfortunately, the sorbitol content of many medications is not listed on their labeling, and some manufacturers state that they frequently reformulate these preparations to contain varying amounts of excipients, such as sorbitol. Determining the cause of the diarrhea is obviously important to know how to address the problem. Whereas *C. difficile* colitis should be treated with metronidazole or vancomycin, sorbitol- or other medication-induced diarrhea can be addressed by removal of the offending agent. Likewise, diarrhea secondary to malabsorption sometimes can be addressed by changing to an oligomeric EN formula. Antiperistaltic agents such as loperamide may be useful in some cases of diarrhea of noninfectious etiology.

On the other hand, constipation may occur in some patients receiving tube feedings, especially the elderly. Increased provision of fluid or fiber may be useful in attaining bowel

Table 101–8	
Complications of Tube Feeding	
Complication	**Causes**
GI	
Diarrhea	Drug related
	Antibiotic-induced bacterial overgrowth
	Hyperosmolar medications administered via feeding tubes
	Antacids containing magnesium
	Malabsorption
	Hypoalbuminemia/gut mucosal atrophy
	Pancreatic insufficiency
	Inadequate GIT surface area
	Rapid GIT transit
	Radiation enteritis
	Tube feeding related
	Rapid formula administration
	Formula hyperosmolality
	Low residue (fiber) content
	Lactose intolerance
	Bacterial contamination
Nausea and vomiting	Gastric dysmotility (surgery, anticholinergic drugs, diabetic gastroparesis)
	Rapid infusion of hyperosmolar formula
Constipation	Dehydration
	Drug induced (anticholinergics)
	Inactivity
	Low residue (fiber) content
	Obstruction/fecal impaction
Abdominal distention/ cramping	Too rapid formula administration
Technical	
Occluded feeding tube lumen	Insoluble complexation of enteral formula and medication(s)
	Inadequate flushing of feeding tube
	Undissolved feeding formula
Tube displacement	Self-extubation
	Vomiting or coughing
	Inadequate fixation (jejunostomy)
Aspiration	Improper patient position
	Gastroparesis/atomy causing regurgitation
	Feeding tube malpositioned
	Compromised lower esophageal sphincter
	Diminished gag reflex
Peristomal excoriation	Improper skin and tube care
	GIT secretions leaking peristomally
Infectious	
Aspiration pneumonia	Same as technical—aspiration comments
	Prolonged use of large-bore polyvinylchloride tube

From Janson DD, Chessman KH. Enteral nutrition. In DiPiro JT, Talbert RL, Yee GC, et al., eds. Pharmacotherapy: A Pathophysiologic Approach, 5th ed. New York: McGraw-Hill, 2005.

Table 101–9

Suggested Monitoring for EN Patients to Prevent the Development of Complications

Parameter	During Initiation of EN Therapy	During Stable EN Therapy
Vital signs	Every 4–6 hours	As needed with suspected change (i.e., fever)
Clinical assessment		
Weight	Daily	Weekly
Length/height (children)	Weekly–monthly	Monthly
Head circumference (less than 3 years of age)	Weekly–monthly	Monthly
Total intake/output	Daily	As needed with suspected changed in intake/output
Tube feeding intake	Daily	Daily
Enterostomy tube site assessment	Daily	Daily
GI tolerance		
Stool frequency/volume	Daily	Daily
Abdomen assessment	Daily	Daily
Nausea or vomiting	Daily	Daily
Gastric residual volumes	Every 4–8 hours (varies)	As needed when delayed gastric emptying suspected
Tube placement	Prior to starting, then ongoing	Ongoing
Laboratory		
Electrolytes, BUN/S_{cr}, glucose	Daily	Every 1–3 months
Calcium, magnesium, phosphorus	3–7 times/week	Every 1–3 months
Liver function tests	Weekly	Every 1–3 months
Trace elements, vitamins	If deficiency/toxicity suspected	If deficiency/toxicity suspected

BUN, blood urea nitrogen; S_{cr}, serum creatinine.

From Knopf VS, Chessman KH. Enteral nutrition. In DiPiro JT, Talbert RL, Yee GC, et al., eds. Pharmacotherapy: A Pathophysiologic Approach, 7th ed. New York: McGraw-Hill, 2008.

regularity. As with diarrhea, constipation may be drug-related, in which case discontinuation or replacement of the offending drug may help alleviate the problem.

Impaired gastric emptying is seen commonly in EN patients receiving gastric feedings and may be associated with nausea and vomiting. Impaired gastric emptying may be related to a disease process (e.g., diabetic gastroparesis or sequelae to head injury) or to drug therapy, most notably narcotics. Gastric residual checks frequently are measured in patients receiving gastric feedings (see Table 101–9). To accomplish such a check, a syringe is attached to the feeding device, and as much liquid as possible is aspirated into the syringe. Much debate is ongoing as to what constitutes a significant gastric aspirate, with numbers between 100 and 500 mL most commonly defended.[4,38–40] Approaches to the patient with delayed gastric emptying might include changing to an enteral formula containing less fat because dietary fat is associated with slower gastric emptying. Metoclopramide often is given to patients receiving gastric feedings to facilitate gastric emptying. Erythromycin is an alternative medication that may be useful in stimulating gastric motility, although it also can be associated with potentially serious drug–drug interactions. Feedings by a PEG tube may be associated with a decreased risk of aspiration compared to NG feedings.[40] Patients with consistently high gastric aspirates are considered to be at higher risk of aspirating feedings into their lungs and should be considered for transition to postpyloric feedings. Postpyloric feedings may help relieve EN-related nausea and vomiting and are preferred for patients without an intact gag reflex. An important practice to help prevent aspiration is elevation of the head of the bed to at least 30 degrees during continuous feedings and during and for 30 to 60 minutes after intermittent and bolus feedings. Adding blue food coloring to tube feeding formulas to help detect aspiration in bronchial or tracheal aspirates has been largely abandoned due to reports of absorption of this supposedly-nonabsorbable substance in patients with sepsis.[41]

Technical Complications

Technical or mechanical complications are encountered frequently in the EN patient. Tube occlusion most commonly is related to formula occlusion or medication administration through the tube. ❾ *An important practice to help prevent medication-related occlusion is adequate water flushing of the tube before, between, and after each medication is given through the tube.* If intermittent feedings are used, water flushing after each feeding is recommended. Tube occlusion can increase cost of EN significantly if the tube has to be removed and replaced. Clearing of the occlusion using water or pancreatic enzymes plus sodium bicarbonate can be attempted, and special devices and kits (e.g., DeClogger) are available for this purpose.[42]

Tube displacement is a potentially significant complication of EN. This may be seen secondary to an agitated patient pulling at the tube, or in some cases the tip of the tube migrates spontaneously. The danger of this complication arises if the tip of the tube is positioned in the tracheobronchial tree and feeding is delivered to this area, potentially leading to pneumonia, pneumothorax, and other problems. Location of the tip of the feeding tube should be confirmed initially by chest radiograph after placement and before use. For ongoing assessment of tube placement, auscultation and measurement of aspirate pH can be used; debate continues as to the best method of monitoring tube placement.

Endoscopic and surgical feeding tubes can be complicated by erosion of the exit site caused by leakage of gastric or intestinal contents onto the skin. This complication must be addressed by good wound care and repair or replacement of the access device. Similarly, NG, ND, and NJ tubes can be complicated by nasopharyngeal irritation or necrosis. This is one reason why such tubes should be considered for short-term use only.

Infectious Complications

Infectious complications of EN include aspiration pneumonia and infections related to delivery of contaminated EN formula. Aspiration is a complication with GI, mechanical, and infectious implications. Although GI infections owing to contamination of enteral formulas have been reported uncommonly, there is ample opportunity for these formulas to be seeded with organisms during the processes of transferring from the can to the delivery bag with ready-to-use formulas and during the process of reconstitution with powdered formulas. The so-called closed systems of delivery, wherein the formulas come from the manufacturer premixed in a delivery bag, should help to decrease the chance of formula contamination.

Metabolic Complications

Metabolic complications of EN most commonly include disorders of fluid and electrolyte homeostasis and hyperglycemia. More severely ill patients require more frequent monitoring (see Table 101–9). Both dehydration and fluid overload can occur with tube feeding. Careful monitoring of fluid inputs and outputs as well as body weight is important. Dehydration may be due either to excessive fluid losses or inadequate fluid intake. The trend in the BUN-to-serum-creatinine ratio can be useful in helping monitor for this complication; a ratio of greater than about 15:1 may be an indicator of dehydration. Attention should be paid to the free-water content of EN formulas; this information usually is included on product labeling. Free-water content of EN formulas varies from about 65% to 85%, with percentage of free water typically dropping as caloric density of the formula rises. If dehydration develops, switching to a less calorically dense formula or using more water flushes may be appropriate. Fluid overload is reflected by increases in weight, lower extremity edema, and pulmonary rales and particularly may be a problem in patients with renal or cardiac insufficiency. Use of an EN formula that is more calorically dense (i.e., contains less free water) may be helpful, and diuretic therapy may be necessary. Fluid imbalances often are associated with abnormalities of sodium homeostasis that should be addressed in concert with fluid imbalance.

Hypokalemia, hypomagnesemia, and hypophosphatemia are some of the most common electrolyte abnormalities in sick, hospitalized patients. These can occur in the context of the so-called refeeding syndrome. This syndrome occurs in chronically malnourished patients when aggressively started on a feeding regime. Although more classically associated with PN, refeeding syndrome can occur with aggressive EN. Careful monitoring of these electrolytes, coupled with a feeding regimen increased gradually to goal rate over a period of several days to a week, should help protect the at-risk patient from this potentially harmful complication. Hypokalemia and hypomagnesemia also may be associated with excessive losses through the GI tract or urine and may be associated with various medication therapies, including diuretics. Repletion of these conditions may be accomplished enterally in the nonsymptomatic patient or parenterally if the patient is symptomatic or the abnormality is severe. Enteral repletion with magnesium and phosphate can be associated with diarrhea. Hyperkalemia, hypermagnesemia, and hyperphosphatemia are encountered less commonly and usually are associated with renal insufficiency and decreased excretion. Hyperkalemia also is associated with several medications, including potassium-sparing diuretics and angiotensin-converting enzyme inhibitors and angiotensin receptor blockers.

Although hyperglycemia is less common with EN than with PN, it can occur. Many severely ill patients (e.g., septic, highly stressed) receiving EN have a metabolic milieu promoting hyperglycemia. In addition, many patients have preexisting or undiagnosed diabetes mellitus. For the ICU patient with hyperglycemia receiving continuous EN, an IV insulin drip may be the most effective way to achieve good glycemic control. Administration of scheduled intermediate or long-acting insulin is preferred over sliding-scale insulin alone in patients requiring insulin after they have been stabilized on their enteral feeding regimen.[43,44] Administration of a higher-fat, lower-carbohydrate EN formula may be useful in selected patients.

Monitoring for Efficacy/Outcome Evaluation

The most useful physical measurement of efficacy of EN in the long-term patient is typically body weight. Depending on the clinical situation, the goal may be weight gain, weight maintenance, or weight loss. Whereas day-to-day fluctuations in weight generally reflect fluid changes, week-to-week variations are more useful in determining if caloric provision is appropriate.

The amount of EN actually administered is often less than the amount ordered owing to interruptions in therapy caused by carrying out of procedures and other daily activities, especially in hospitalized patients. It is imperative to monitor volume of feedings actually received and to make adjustments in rates or amounts of EN as necessary.

Biochemical markers may help the SNS practitioner interpret adequacy of the EN therapy. Albumin frequently is measured as part of standard metabolic lab panels. Its long half-life renders this visceral protein less useful for making decisions regarding adequacy of the nutritional prescription over the short term. Prealbumin, with a much shorter half-life that is expected to increase more rapidly in the setting of sufficient calorie and protein provision, has become the major biochemical monitoring parameter used to determine efficacy of SNS. However, in the acute phase of illness characterized by a proinflammatory state, proteins known as *acute-phase reactants* are preferentially synthesized. One of these acute-phase reactants measured clinically is C-reactive protein (CRP). In some patients with significant illness, prealbumin may not rise, even though the patients are receiving the appropriate EN regimen, until CRP begins to fall. Collection of urine to measure nitrogen balance can help analyze adequacy of caloric and protein provision but must be performed with care to obtain reliable information.

In patients with wounds (e.g., decubitus ulcers), a goal of nutritional therapy is to help facilitate wound healing. Therefore, monitoring the status of the wound becomes part of the ongoing nutritional assessment. In debilitated patients, particularly those on long-term EN, measures of functional status such as grip strength and ability to perform activities of daily living become important parts of the assessment of nutritional adequacy.

MEDICATION ADMINISTRATION IN PATIENTS RECEIVING EN

Medication Administration Through Feeding Tubes

If a patient receiving EN is alert and can swallow oral medications, then, medications should be given by mouth. However, many patients are not able to receive medications by this route, and the feeding tube may be considered as a route of delivery. Although used widely, the effects of medication administration through feeding tubes on the delivery of both the drug and the EN formula nutrients have been inadequately studied, and important questions remain unanswered.[45]

❿ *Compatibility of medication with an EN formula and, conversely, an EN formula with administered medication is of concern when administering medications through feeding tubes.* An important technical complication of EN is tube occlusion, related most commonly to medication administration. Not only must compatibility of the medication and the EN formula be considered, but interactions between these components and the feeding tube itself must be considered. Since either medication or EN formula or some combination thereof can physically stick to the tube itself, strict protocols for flushing the tube before, between, and after administration of medications are important.[5] The best fluid for flushing feeding tubes is warm water. Carbonated beverages and fruit juices are no longer recommended and should be avoided because sugar in these products may stick to the surface of the feeding tube. Between 10 and 30 mL of water should be used as a flush before and after any medication administration through a feeding tube. Medications should be administered one at a time sequentially rather than being mixed together for simultaneous administration down the tube; about 5 mL of water should be used as a flush between each medication. This should help prevent interactions between drugs within the feeding tube itself that could lead to tube occlusion.

Different dosage forms present unique challenges for administration through feeding tubes. Certain solid dosage forms should not be crushed because crushing would significantly alter release characteristics.[46] For example, controlled-release, extended-release, and sustained-release preparations should not be crushed; crushing allows a quicker release of more drug initially than the original dosage form was designed to deliver. Sublingual dosage forms should not be crushed. Enteric-coated dosage forms generally are designed to protect acid-labile medications from stomach acid; when these dosage forms reach the small bowel with its higher pH, the drug then is released into an environment in which it is more stable. Alternatively, enteric-coated dosage forms protect the stomach from medications that could cause irritation. Thus, crushing of the enteric coating for delivery down a gastric feeding tube defeats the purpose of the dosage form and could lead to decreased efficacy or increased adverse events.

Medications available commercially as compressed tablets can be crushed for administration through feeding tubes. After such a tablet is crushed into a fine powder, it should be mixed with 10 to 30 mL of fluid (usually warm water) for administration. A powdered dosage form inside a hard-gelatin capsule similarly can be poured out and mixed with water for administration through feeding tubes. Soft-gelatin capsules can be dissolved in warm water for administration. Some enteric-coated and delayed-release microencapsulated products can be opened, and the individually-coated particles can be administered through the tube without crushing if the tube has a large enough diameter.

If a liquid dosage form of a medication exists, it would seem rational to use this dosage form for administration through a feeding tube. Although this may decrease the potential for tube clogging, it may in some instances decrease tolerability of medication administration. As mentioned above, sorbitol is an excipient found in many liquid medications in amounts sufficient to cause diarrhea. If diarrhea secondary to sorbitol in a liquid medication is suspected, contact with the manufacturer to ascertain sorbitol content may be necessary.

Another potential problem with administration of liquid medications through feeding tubes is high osmolality of some of these products. Dilution of hypertonic medications with 30 to 60 mL of water (depending on osmolality of the medication and dosage volume of the undiluted medication) or administration of smaller dosages more frequently may help prevent diarrhea. Although administration of IV medications through feeding tubes sometimes may be entertained, these dosage forms frequently are hypertonic and contain excipients that can be problematic when given via the GI tract.

It is generally not recommended to mix medications directly into the EN formula because of concerns that physical incompatibilities between the medications and the formula might lead to tube occlusion. There is some evidence that polymeric formulas are more likely to demonstrate physical incompatibility with medications compared with monomeric formulas, although most of the work in this area has used casein or caseinate-based formulas, and other proteins may act differently.[45] Limited data currently available indicate that acidic syrups and elixirs may be most harmful, causing physical incompatibility when admixed with EN formulas. This incompatibility may be due to changes in the protein structure after exposure to acid or alcohol.[45]

It would seem logical that medications considered being absorbed to a greater extent in the fasted state either should be given between feedings on an intermittent feeding schedule or the feedings should be held before and after medication administration. However, results of one provocative study with the antihypertensive medication hydralazine indicated that continuous feeding into the stomach resulted in a situation mimicking fasting in terms of rate of gastric emptying and drug absorption.[45] This issue deserves further study.

The location of the tip of the feeding tube is important when considering medication administration down a feeding tube. This is particularly true if the medication acts locally in the GI tract itself. For example, sucralfate and antacids act locally in the stomach. Therefore, administration of these medications through a duodenal or jejunal tube is not logical. Likewise, for medications such as itraconazole that require acid for best absorption, administration directly into the duodenum or jejunum would be expected to result in suboptimal absorption. Absorption of drugs when administered directly into the small bowel, especially the jejunum, is a topic where more research would be useful.

Problem Medications

▶ *Phenytoin*

Certain medications present specific challenges when administered through feeding tubes. The medication studied most thoroughly is phenytoin. Most studies have shown significant decreases in phenytoin absorption when the medication was administered enterally to patients receiving EN. Several mechanisms have been proposed for this apparent interaction. Many institutions have adopted a policy of holding tube feedings for 1 or 2 hours before and after administration of phenytoin to decrease the interaction, although some EN patients subjected to this routine still will require relatively high dosages of phenytoin to achieve therapeutic serum concentrations. Holding the feeding around medication administration can make meeting nutritional requirements difficult with continuous feedings, especially if the phenytoin is administered several times daily. Diligent monitoring of phenytoin serum concentrations is necessary for the patient on EN receiving this medication. In some cases, use of IV phenytoin or another anticonvulsant medication may be prudent.

▶ *Warfarin*

EN formulas contain vitamin K, which can antagonize the pharmacologic activity of warfarin. Vitamin K content of EN formulas generally has been adjusted down over the past several decades, resulting in products today that contain amounts of vitamin K unlikely to affect anticoagulation by warfarin significantly. However, inadequate warfarin anticoagulation in EN patients receiving formulas containing minimal vitamin K has been reported. There is some thought that a component of certain tube feedings, perhaps protein, may bind warfarin and result in suboptimal activity of the drug. A recent small study indicated a better response in terms of the International Normalized Ratio (INR) when feedings were held for one hour before and after warfarin administration compared to administration of the drug without holding the feedings.[47] When tube feedings are

started, changed, or discontinued, the INR should be monitored closely.

▶ *Fluoroquinolones*

Absorption of antimicrobial agents such as fluoroquinolones and tetracyclines that can be bound by divalent and trivalent cations potentially could be compromised by administration with EN formulas containing these cations. The fluoroquinolones (e.g., levofloxacin and ciprofloxacin) have been best studied in this regard, and results of studies are not consistent.[48,49] Some institutions hold tube feedings for 30 to 60 minutes or more before and after enteral dosages of fluoroquinolones. Because ciprofloxacin absorption has been shown to be decreased with jejunal administration, this drug probably should not be given by jejunal tube.[49]

SUMMARY AND CONCLUSION

EN is an important method of feeding patients who cannot or should not eat enough to meet their nutrient requirements for a prolonged time. When the GI tract can be used safely, EN is preferred over PN. Various types of enteral access devices are available. Whereas tubes inserted through the nose often are adequate for patients expected to receive EN for a short time, more permanent devices (endoscopically or surgically placed) are preferred for longer-term patients. Choice of whether to feed into the stomach or postpylorically is patient-specific. Although numerous EN formulas are available commercially, many products are very similar, making a limited formulary feasible. Data supporting many of the specialized types of EN formulas are limited. Although complications of EN tend to be less serious than those of PN, the adverse effects encountered can be significant, and diligent ongoing monitoring is necessary. Although medications can be administered through feeding tubes, various factors must be taken into account in each individual patient to ensure that this practice is prudent.

Patient Encounter, Part 3

After a week in the ICU, the patient was transferred to a stepdown unit and was switched to a standard polymeric EN formula. He required 3 weeks of inpatient care owing to complications from his injuries, including seizures and a wound infection. He eventually was transferred to a rehabilitation facility still requiring EN.

How should the patient be monitored for adequacy of his EN regimen?

Outline a monitoring plan for tolerance of the EN regimen in the ICU, stepdown unit, and rehabilitation facility.

Discuss work-up of the patient if diarrhea occurs while he is receiving tube feedings.

If the patient requires phenytoin for his seizures, how should this medication be administered?

Patient Care and Monitoring

1. Assess the patient's condition to estimate the amount of time he or she is expected to be unable to eat adequately to meet nutritional requirements. If inadequate intake has occurred or is anticipated for 7 to 14 days, start SNS. The threshold for starting SNS is lower for previously malnourished patients than for previously well-nourished patients. Also, critically ill patients should generally be started on EN within 24 to 48 hours of ICU admission.

2. Assess whether the GI tract is functional. If not, then PN is the first SNS therapy of choice. If the GI tract is functional and no contraindication to EN exists, then EN is the SNS therapy of choice.

3. Does the patient have any condition precluding gastric feeding? If so, then postpyloric feeding should be started.

4. Choose the appropriate type of enteral access device based on the expected duration of SNS.

5. Choose an appropriate feeding formula based on patient-specific factors. This necessitates assessing nutritional requirements. Standard polymeric formulas are appropriate for the majority of patients.

6. Choose the method of feeding administration (e.g., intermittent or continuous) based on the type of feeding access (i.e., gastric versus postpyloric) and other patient factors. For example, in a patient with a gastric access, starting with or later transitioning to intermittent feedings may be preferred if it is anticipated that the patient still receiving these feedings will be discharged to a long-term care facility or to home.

7. Develop a plan to include monitoring at appropriate intervals for metabolic, GI, technical, and infectious complications.

8. Start the tube feeding at full strength and at a low rate, and increase the rate as tolerated to the goal that will meet the patient's nutritional requirements.

9. Develop a monitoring plan for adequacy of the nutritional regimen.

10. If the patient is to be discharged to home on EN, educate the patient or caregiver on
    - Enteral access device care
    - Feeding delivery
    - Troubleshooting
    - Complications to observe for (e.g., fluid overload, dehydration)

Abbreviations Introduced in This Chapter

AAA	Aromatic amino acids
ACCEPT	Algorithms for critical-care enteral and parenteral therapy
ARDS	Acute respiratory distress syndrome
A.S.P.E.N.	American Society for Parenteral and Enteral Nutrition
BCAA	Branched-chain amino acids
BUN	Blood urea nitrogen
CRP	C-reactive protein
DHA	Docosahexenoic acid
EAAs	Essential amino acids
EFAs	Essential fatty acids
EN	Enteral nutrition
EPA	Eicosapentaenoic acid
ESPEN	European Society for Clinical Nutrition and Metabolism
FOSs	Fructooligosaccharides
GALT	Gut-associated lymphoid tissue
GER	Gastroesophageal reflux
GLA	γ-Linolenic acid
HE	Hepatic encephalopathy
IBD	Ideal body weight
ICU	Intensive care unit
INR	International normalized ratio
LCTs	Long-chain triglycerides
MCTs	Medium-chain triglycerides
MUFA	Monosaturated fatty acid
ND	Nasoduodenal
NEAAs	Nonessential amino acids
NG	Nasogastric
NJ	Nasojejunal
NO	Nitric oxide
OG	Orogastric
PEG	Percutaneous endoscopic gastrostomy
PEJ	Percutaneous endoscopic jejunostomy
PN	Parenteral nutrition
PUFAs	Polyunsaturated fatty acids
SCFAs	Short-chain fatty acids
SNS	Specialized nutrition support

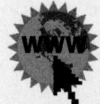 Self-assessment questions and answers are available at *http://www.mhpharmacotherapy.com/pp.html.*

REFERENCES

1. American Society for Parenteral and Enteral Nutrition Board of Directors. Guidelines for the use of parenteral and enteral nutrition in adult and pediatric patients. J Parenter Ent Nutr 2002;26:1SA–138SA.
2. The European Society for Clinical Nutrition and Metabolism. Espen Guidelines on Adult Enteral Nutrition. 2006, *http://www.espen.org/espenguidelines.html.*
3. Critical Care Nutrition. Clinical Practice Guidelines. *http://www.criticalcarenutrition.com/index.php?option=com_content&task=view&id=17&Itemid=40.*
4. Bankhead R, Boullata J, Brantley S, et al. Enteral nutrition practice recommendations. JPEN J Parenter Enter Nutr 2009;33:122–167.
5. McClave SA, Martindale RG, Vanek VW, et al. Guidelines for the provision and assessment of nutrition support therapy in the adult critically ill patient. JPEN J Parenter Ent Nutr 2009;33:277–316.
6. Magnotti LJ, Deitch EA. Mechanisms and significance of gut barrier function and failure. In: Rolandelli RH, Bankhead R, Boullata JI,

Compher CW, eds. Enteral and Tube Feeding, 4th ed. Philadelphia: Elsevier Inc., 2005:23–31.

7. Kudsk KA. Enteral feeding and bowel necrosis: An uncommon but perplexing problem. Nutr Clin Pract 2003;18:277–278.

8. McClave SA, Chang WK. Feeding the hypotensive patient: Does enteral feeding precipitate or protect against ischemic bowel? Nutr Clin Pract 2003;18:279–284.

9. Zaloga GP, Roberts PR, Marik P. Feeding the hemodynamically unstable patient: A critical evaluation of the evidence. Nutr Clin Pract 2003:285–293.

10. van den Berghe G, Wouters P, Weekers F, et al. Intensive insulin therapy in the critically ill patients. N Engl J Med 2001;345:1359–1367.

11. The NICE-SUGAR Study Investigators. Intensive versus conventional glucose control in critically ill patients. N Engl J Med 2009;360;1283–1297.

12. Veterans Affairs Total Parenteral Nutrition Cooperative Study Group. Perioperative total parenteral nutrition in surgical patients. N Engl J Med 1991;325:525–532.

13. Heidegger CP, Romand JA, Treggiari MM, Pichard C. Is it now time to promote mixed enteral and parenteral nutrition for the critically ill patient? Intensive Care Med 2007;33:963–969.

14. Stapleton RD, Jones N, Heyland DK. Feeding critically ill patients: What is the optimal amount of energy? Crit Care Med 2007;35:S535–S540.

15. Simpson F, Doig GS. Parenteral vs. enteral nutrition in the critically ill patient: A meta-analysis of trials using the intention to treat principle. Intensive Care Med 2005;31:12–23.

16. Martin CM, Doig GS, Heyland DK, et al. Multicentre, cluster-randomized clinical trial of algorithms for critical-care enteral and parenteral therapy (ACCEPT). Can Med Assoc J 2004;170:197–204.

17. Byrne KR, Fang JC. Endoscopic placement of enteral feeding catheters. Curr Opin Gastroenterol 2006;22:546–550.

18. Elia M, Engfer MB, Green CJ, Silk DBA. Systematic review and meta-analysis: The clinical and physiological effects of fibre-containing enteral formulae. Aliment Pharmacol Ther 2008;27:120–145.

19. Roy CC, Kien CL, Bouthillier L, Levy E. Short-chain fatty acids: Ready for prime time? Nutr Clin Pract 2006;21:351–366.

20. Charney P, Russell M. Enteral formulations. In: Rolandelli RH, Bankhead R, Boullata JI, Compher CW, eds. Enteral and Tube Feeding, 4th ed. Philadelphia: Elsevier Inc., 2005:216–223.

21. Heyland DK, Dhaliwal R, Suchner U. Immunonutrition. In: Rolandelli RH, Bankhead R, Boullata JI, Compher CW, eds. Enteral and Tube Feeding, 4th ed. Philadelphia: Elsevier Inc., 2005:224–242.

22. Heyland DK, Dhaliwal R, Day AG, et al. Reducing Deaths due to Oxidation Stress (The REDOXS Study): Rationale and study design for a randomized trial of glutamine and antioxidant supplementation in critically-ill patients. Proc Nutr Soc 2006;65:250–263.

23. Zaloga GP. Improving outcomes with specialized nutrition support. J Parenter Ent Nutr 2005;29:S49–S52.

24. Martindale RG, Cresci G. Preventing infectious complications with nutrition intervention. J Parenter Ent Nutr 2005;29:S53–S56.

25. Luiking YC, Poeze M, Ramsay G, Deutz NEP. The role of arginine in infection and sepsis. J Parenter Ent Nutr 2005;29:S70–S74.

26. Cresci G. Targeting the use of specialized nutritional formulas in surgery and critical care. J Parenter Ent Nutr 2005;29:S92–S95.

27. Heyland DK, Novak F, Drover JW, et al. Should immunonutrition become routine in critically ill patients? A systematic review of the evidence. JAMA 2001;286:944–953.

28. Montejo JC, Zarazaga A, Lopez-Martinex J, et al. Immunonutrition in the intensive care unit. A systematic review and consensus statement. Clin Nutr 2003;22:221–233.

29. Gadek JE, Demichele SJ, Darlstad MD, et al. Effect of enteral feeding with eicosapentaenoic acid, gamma-linolenic acid, and antioxidants in patients with acute respiratory distress syndrome. Crit Care Med 1999;27:1409–1420.

30. Singer P, Theilla M, Fisher H, et al. Benefit of an enteral diet enriched with eicosapentaenoic acid and gamma-linolenic acid in ventilated patients with acute lung injury. Crit Care Med 2006;34:1033–1038.

31. Pontes-Arruda A, Aragao AM, Albuquerque JD. Effects of enteral feeding with eicosapentaenoic acid, gamma-linolenic acid, and antioxidants in mechanically ventilated patients with severe sepsis and septic shock. Crit Care Med 2006;34:2325–2333.

32. Elia M, Ceriello A, Laube H, et al. Enteral nutritional support and use of diabetes-specific formulas for patients with diabetes. Diab Care 2005;28:2267–2279.

33. Dial S, Alrasadi K, Manoukian C, et al. Risk of *Clostridium difficile* diarrhea in hospital in-patients prescribed proton pump inhibitors: Cohort and case-control studies. CMAJ 2004;171:33–38.

34. Cunningham R, Dale B, Undy B, Gaunt N. Proton pump inhibitors as a risk factor for *Clostridium difficile* diarrhea. J Hosp Inf 2003;54:243–245.

35. Dial S, Delaney JA, Barkun AN, Suissa S. Use of gastric acid-suppressive agents and the risk of community-acquired *Clostridium difficile*-associated disease. JAMA 2005;294:2989–2995.

36. Jayatilaka S, Shakov R, Eddi R, et al. *Clostridium difficile* infection in an urban medical center: Five-year analysis of infection rates among adult admissions and association with the use of proton pump inhibitors. Ann Clin Lab Sci 2007;37:241–247.

37. Edes TE, Walk BE, Austin JL. Diarrhea in tube-fed patients: Feeding formula not necessarily the cause. Am J Med 1990;88:91–93.

38. McClave SA, Snider HL. Clinical use of gastric residual volumes as a monitor for patients on enteral tube feeding. J Parenter Ent Nutr 2002;26:S43–S50.

39. McClave SA, DeMeo MT, DeLegge MH, et al. North American summit on aspiration in the critically ill patient: Consensus statement. J Parenter Ent Nutr 2002;26:S80–S85.

40. McClave SA, Lukan JK, Stefater JA, et al. Poor validity of residual volumes as a marker for risk of aspiration in critically ill patients. Crit Care Med 2005;33:324–330.

41. Maloney JP, Ryan TA. Detection of aspiration in enterally fed patients: A requiem for bedside monitors of aspiration. J Parenter Ent Nutr 2002;26:S34–S42.

42. Lord LM. Restoring and maintaining patency of enteral feeding tubes. Nutr Clin Pract 2003;18:422–426.

43. Braithwaite SS. Inpatient insulin therapy. Curr Opin Endocrinol Diabetes Obes 2008;15:159–166.

44. Grainger A, Eiden K, Kemper J, Reeds D. A pilot study to evaluate the effectiveness of glargine and multiple injections of lispro in patients with type 2 diabetes receiving tube feedings in a cardiovascular intensive care unit. Nutr Clin Pract 2007;22:545–552.

45. Rollins C, Thomson C, Crane T. Pharmacotherapeutic issues. In: Rolandelli RH, Bankhead R, Boullata JI, Compher CW, eds. Enteral and Tube Feeding, 4th ed. Philadelphia: Elsevier Inc., 2005:291–305.

46. Mitchell JF. Oral Dosage Forms That Should Not Be Crushed. 2008, *www.ismp.org/tools/donotcrush.pdf*.

47. Dickerson RN, Garmon WM, Kuhl DA, et al. Vitamin K-independent warfarin resistance after concurrent administration of warfarin and continuous enteral nutrition. Pharmacotherapy 2008;28:308–313.

48. Rollins CJ. Drug-nutrient interactions. In: Gottschlich MM, ed. The A.S.P.E.N. Nutrition Support Core Curriculum. Silver Spring, MD: A.S.P.E.N., 2007:340–359.

49. Nyffeler MS, Frankel E, Hayes E, Mighdoll S. Drug-nutrient interactions. In: Merritt R, ed. The A.S.P.E.N. Nutrition Support Practice Manual, 2nd ed. Silver Spring, MD: A.S.P.E.N., 2005:118–137.

102 Overweight and Obesity

Maqual R. Graham and Cameron C. Lindsey

LEARNING OBJECTIVES

● **Upon completion of the chapter, the reader will be able to:**

1. Explain the underlying causes of overweight and obesity.

2. Identify parameters utilized to diagnose obesity and other objective information that indicates the severity of disease.

3. Identify desired therapeutic goals for patients who are overweight or obese.

4. Recommend appropriate nonpharmacologic and pharmacologic therapeutic interventions for overweight or obese patients.

5. Implement a monitoring plan that will assess both the efficacy and safety of therapy initiated.

6. Educate patients about the disease state and associated risks, appropriate lifestyle modifications, drug therapy, and surgical options necessary for effective treatment.

KEY CONCEPTS

❶ Body mass index (BMI), waist circumference, comorbidities, and readiness to lose weight are used in the assessment of the overweight or obese patient.

❷ Presence of comorbidities (coronary heart disease [CHD], atherosclerosis, type 2 diabetes mellitus, and sleep apnea) and cardiovascular risk factors (cigarette smoking, hypertension, elevated low-density lipoprotein cholesterol, low high-density lipoprotein cholesterol, impaired fasting glucose, family history of premature CHD, and age) requires identification and aggressive management for overall effective treatment of the overweight or obese patient.

❸ The treatment goals for overweight and obesity are to prevent additional weight gain, reduce and maintain a lower body weight, and control related risks.

❹ Weight loss is indicated for patients with a BMI of 25 to 29.9 kg/m² or an elevated waist circumference with two or more comorbidities or for any patient with a BMI of 30 kg/m² or greater.

❺ Weight maintenance occurs following successful achievement of weight loss.

❻ Treatment of obesity includes lifestyle changes (e.g., dietary modification, enhanced physical activity, and behavioral therapy), pharmacologic treatment, surgical intervention, or a combination of modalities.

❼ Pharmacotherapy, in addition to lifestyle modifications, is reserved for patients with a BMI of 30 kg/m² or greater, or a BMI of 27 kg/m² or greater with other obesity-related risk factors.

❽ Weight likely will be regained if lifestyle changes are not continued indefinitely.

❾ Surgery is warranted when other treatment attempts have failed in severely obese patients (BMI of 40 kg/m² or greater, or 35 kg/m² or greater with other obesity-related risk factors).

Overweight and obesity are terms used to describe weight measurements greater than what is considered healthy for a given height.[1] ❶ *Body mass index (BMI), waist circumference, comorbidities, and readiness to lose weight are used in the assessment of the overweight or obese patient.* The primary modality in defining overweight and obesity is the BMI—a measure of body fat based on height and weight that applies to both adult men and women. The BMI accurately measures body fat when compared with body weight alone.[2] Several surveys were conducted to establish categories of BMI.[3] BMI does not reflect distribution of body fat; therefore, the measurement of **waist circumference** is a more practical method to evaluate abdominal fat before and during weight-loss treatment. Abdominal fat poses a greater health risk over peripheral fat and may be an independent risk predictor when BMI is not elevated significantly.[4,5] Both BMI and waist circumference should be used in the diagnosis and management of weight loss. Evaluation of the patient's risk status involves not only calculation of the BMI and measurement of waist circumference but also determination

Patient Encounter, Part 1

A 35-year-old female presents to your clinic wanting to lose weight. She reports not following any specific diet as they have all failed in the past. She does admit to eating out frequently. This patient does not exercise as her job and her kids are too demanding. Patient does smoke ½ pack of cigarettes per day and consumes low-calorie, caffeinated and alcoholic drinks most days. Her BMI is 32 kg/m² and her waist circumference is 38 in.

What classification of overweight and obesity is appropriate for this patient?

Does she have other risk factors that may contribute to morbidity and/or mortality?

What additional information do you need to know before creating a treatment plan for this patient?

of comorbidities or the presence of cardiovascular disease (CVD) risk factors. ❷ *Presence of comorbidities (coronary heart disease [CHD], atherosclerosis, type 2 diabetes mellitus, and sleep apnea) and cardiovascular risk factors (cigarette smoking, hypertension, elevated low-density lipoprotein cholesterol, low high-density lipoprotein cholesterol, impaired fasting glucose, family history of premature CHD, and age) requires identification and aggressive management for overall effective treatment of the overweight or obese patient.* Obese patients may be at very high risk for mortality if concomitant risk factors exist; therefore, high-risk patients require aggressive modification of risk factors in addition to obesity treatment.[6]

ETIOLOGY AND EPIDEMIOLOGY

Obesity is a multifactorial, complex disease that occurs following an interaction between genotype and the environment. While the etiology is not known completely, it involves overlapping silos of social, behavioral, and cultural influence; pathophysiology; metabolism; and genetic composition.[7] The majority of overweight or obese individuals are adults, but these diseases are also prevalent in children between 2 and 19 years of age. Thirty-two percent of adults 20 years of age and older are considered obese. Almost 5% meet the criteria for extreme obesity. The prevalence of obesity in men and women of various racial or ethnic origins differ. Thirty percent of non-Hispanic white adults are considered obese where approximately 37% of Mexican Americans and 45% of non-Hispanic black Americans are obese.[8]

Among children and adolescents, 17% are considered overweight.[8] Overweight children typically mature to overweight adults, but most obese adults were not overweight as children.[9] Overweight and obesity, when present in young adults, may be a better predictor of prevalence.[9] Additionally, adulthood overweight and obesity contribute to an increased risk of death in the presence of hypertension, hyperlipidemia, diabetes mellitus, coronary artery disease (CAD), stroke, sleep apnea, gallbladder disease, osteoarthritis, and certain cancers.[6] Psychosocial functioning also may be hindered because obese patients may be at risk for discrimination if negatively stereotyped.[6] Pediatric obesity is also associated with significant health-related problems and thus is a risk factor for much of the adult morbidity and mortality discussed previously.[10,11] Cardiovascular (e.g., dyslipidemia and hypertension), endocrine (e.g., hyperinsulinemia, impaired glucose tolerance, type 2 diabetes mellitus, and menstrual irregularities), and mental (e.g., low self-esteem and depression) health problems exist for obese children and adolescents.[12]

PATHOPHYSIOLOGY

While a correlation between body weight in parents and children exists, the specific gene or genes contributing to obesity are unknown.[13] Syndromes where obesity is a major component collectively contribute very little to the incidence of obesity.[14] The key factor in the development of overweight and obesity is the imbalance that occurs between energy intake and energy expenditure. The extent of obesity is determined by the length of time this imbalance has been present. Energy intake is affected by environmental influences, including social, behavioral, and cultural factors, whereas genetic composition and metabolism affect energy expenditure.[15]

Energy Intake

Food intake is regulated by various receptor systems. Direct stimulation of Serotonin 1A subtype (5-HT_{1A}) and noradrenergic α_2-receptors will increase food intake, whereas Serotonin 2C subtype (5-HT_{2C}) and noradrenergic α_1- or β_2-receptor activation decreases food intake. Stimulation of histamine receptor subtypes 1 and 3, and dopamine receptors 1 and 2 result in lower food consumption. Recently, the cannabinoid receptor (CB1), which is a G-protein-coupled receptor in the endocannabinoid system, has been identified and associated with food intake and regulation of energy homeostasis.[16–18] Inhibition of CB1 is shown to decrease the craving for food, resulting in weight loss when coupled with dietary and lifestyle modifications.[19] In addition to receptor-modulated food consumption, higher levels of the protein leptin are associated with decreased food intake.[20] In contrast, elevated levels of neuropeptide Y increase food intake.[20]

It is debatable whether obesity is related to total calorie intake or composition of macronutrients. Of the three macronutrients (i.e., carbohydrate, protein, and fat), fat has received the most attention, given its desirable texture and its ability to augment the flavor of other foods. Food high in fat promotes weight gain, in comparison with the other macronutrients, because fat is more energy-dense. When compared with carbohydrate and protein, more than twice as many calories per gram are contained in fat. In addition, fat is stored more easily by the body compared with protein and carbohydrate.[21]

Energy Expenditure

A person's metabolic rate is the primary determinant of energy expenditure. The metabolic rate is enhanced following food consumption and is directly related to the amount and type.[14] Physical inactivity may predispose an individual to overweight and obesity. In addition, endocrine-related disorders (e.g., hypothyroidism and Cushing syndrome) may lower the metabolic rate, further contributing to the development of overweight and obesity.

CLINICAL PRESENTATION AND DIAGNOSIS

Any interaction between a patient and a healthcare provider presents an opportunity to evaluate the patient's height and weight. From these parameters, the BMI should be determined as well as waist circumference and the presence of comorbidities or associated risks. ❶ *BMI, waist circumference, comorbidities, and readiness to lose weight are used in the assessment of the overweight or obese patient.* The BMI is calculated using the measured weight in kilograms divided by the height in meters squared (kg/m^2) for all adult patients regardless of gender. The BMI distribution changes with age for children just as height and weight. Percentiles specific for age and gender are used to define overweight and obesity as well as healthy and underweight (pediatrics). The BMI is classified according to Table 102–1. Waist circumference should also be determined for adult patients by placing a measuring tape at the top of the right iliac crest and proceed around the abdomen, ensuring that the tape is tight but not constricting the skin. The value is measured following normal expiration.[6] Table 102–2 defines high-risk

waist circumference.[6] Measurement of waist circumference is not recommended for children and adolescents as reference values identifying risk are unavailable.[22] After obtaining patient appropriate parameters, further assess the adult patient for the presence of comorbidities and cardiovascular risk factors. ❷ *Presence of comorbidities (CHD, atherosclerosis, type 2 diabetes mellitus, and sleep apnea) and cardiovascular risk factors (cigarette smoking, hypertension, elevated low-density lipoprotein cholesterol, low high-density lipoprotein cholesterol, impaired fasting glucose, family history of premature CHD, and age) requires identification and aggressive management for overall effective treatment of the overweight or obese patient.* A patient is at very high absolute risk if diagnosed with CHD or other atherosclerotic diseases, type 2 diabetes mellitus, or sleep apnea or if three or more of the risk factors listed in Table 102–3 are present.[6] Aggressive disease management should be initiated and not limited to weight loss. If the patient is a child or adolescent and the BMI is greater than the 85th percentile, determine the patient's risk for future obesity-related problems or presence of obesity-related medical problems such as sleep, respiratory, GI, endocrine, cardiovascular, and psychiatric disorders.[22]

Table 102–2

High-Risk Waist Circumference

Men	Greater than 40 in. (102 cm)
Women	Greater than 35 in. (88 cm)

From U.S. Department of Health and Human Services, NIH-NHLBI. Clinical guidelines on the identification, evaluation, and treatment of overweight and obesity in adults. NIH publication no. 00–4084. Bethesda, MD: National Institutes of Health, 2000.

Table 102–1

BMI Classification

Adult

Underweight	less than 18.5 kg/m^2
Normal weight	18.5–24.9 kg/m^2
Overweight	25–29.9 kg/m^2
Obesity (Class 1)	30–34.9 kg/m^2
Obesity (Class 2)	35–39.9 kg/m^2
Extreme obesity (Class 3)	greater than or equal to 40 kg/m^2

Children (Does Not Pertain to Those Less Than 2 Years of Age[a])

Underweight	less than 5th percentile
Healthy weight	5th–84th percentile
Overweight	85th–94th percentile
Obesity	greater than or equal to the 95th percentile

[a]Weight for height values should be plotted and monitored over time for children less than 2 years of age.

From Refs. 6, 22.

Table 102–3

Risk Factors

- Cigarette smoking
- Hypertension (systolic blood pressure greater than or equal to 140 mm Hg or diastolic blood pressure greater than or equal to 90 mm Hg) or current use of blood pressure lowering medication(s)
- Low-density lipoprotein cholesterol greater than or equal to 160 mg/dL (4.14 mmol/L)
- Low-density lipoprotein cholesterol greater than or equal to 130–159 mg/dL (3.37–4.12 mmol/L) plus two additional risk factors
- High-density lipoprotein cholesterol less than 40 mg/dL (1.03 mmol/L)
- Impaired fasting glucose (fasting blood glucose 100–125 mg/dL [5.6–6.9 mmol/L])
- Family history of premature CHD (first degree male relative less than 55 years of age or first degree female relative less than 65 years of age)
- Males greater than or equal to 45
- Females greater than or equal to 55

From Refs. 6, 23, 24.

Patient Encounter, Part 2: Medical History, Physical Exam, and Diagnostic Tests

PMH: Hypertension for 3 years, currently at goal; depression

FH: Father alive and 58 years of age. Mother also alive with history of obesity and depression.

SH: Registered nurse. Drinks alcohol most days but denies any alcohol-related problems. Smokes ½ pack of cigarettes per day.

Meds: Irbesartan 150 mg once daily; hydrochlorothiazide 25 mg once daily; fluoxetine 20 mg once daily

ROS: (+) Heartburn, regurgitation; (–) chest pain, nausea, vomiting, diarrhea, change in appetite, shortness of breath, or cough.

PE:

VS: BP 120/82 mm Hg, P 82 bpm, RR 16 rpm, T 98.6° F, wt: 240 lb; ht: 64 in

Waist Circumference: 38 in.

CV: RRR; no murmurs, rubs, gallops

Abd: Obese, soft, nontender, nondistended; (+) bowel sounds

Ext: (–) Edema

Labs: All values are within normal limits.

ECG: No evidence of past ischemia.

Given this additional information, what is your assessment of this patient?

Identify your treatment goals for the patient.

What nonpharmacologic and pharmacologic alternatives are available for the patient?

TREATMENT

Desired Outcome

General management of obesity in the adult patient is directed at weight reduction, maintenance of weight loss, and prevention of weight regain. ❸ *The treatment goals for overweight and obesity are to prevent additional weight gain, reduce and maintain a lower body weight, and control related risks.* A 10% weight loss as derived from the patient's current weight is the initial goal of obesity management because favorable outcomes on the negative effects of obesity have been documented.[6,25] Weight loss should occur at a rate of 0.45 to 0.9 kg (1–2 lb) per week, meeting the initial goal within the first 6 months of therapy. ❹ *Weight loss is indicated for patients with a BMI of 25 to 29.9 kg/m² or an elevated waist circumference with two or more comorbidities or for any patient with a BMI of 30 kg/m² or greater.* Weight

then should be maintained (minimal regain of less than 3 kg [6.6 lb] and continued reduction in waist circumference of 1.6 in. [4 cm]). If weight loss has been achieved and/or maintained for 6 months, further therapy promoting weight loss may be inconsidered. Once maximal weight loss has been attained, any therapy used to promote the weight loss must be sustained in order to prevent weight regain.[6] ❺ *Weight maintenance occurs following successful achievement of weight loss.*

It is desirable to achieve a goal of improved long-term physical health for a child or adolescent. A BMI below the 85th percentile is warranted, although difficult to assess in frequent or short time periods. Thus, serial weight measurements may better quantify energy balance. Goals are most likely accomplished through adaptation of lifelong healthy lifestyle habits. In doing so, weight loss or maintenance can be attained for some children. Others may need to incorporate changes that result in a negative energy balance or energy input less than energy output.[22]

General Approach to Treatment

Since the goals for obesity management in the adult population are multifactorial, it should be considered a chronic illness where treatment is maintained for life. Any implemented therapy promoting weight loss should focus on behavior modification directed toward both dietary restriction and increased activity in conjunction with the selective use of pharmacologic or surgical intervention. Before initiating therapy, secondary causes of obesity (e.g., hypothyroidism and Cushing syndrome) must be considered. Current treatment with medications that negatively alter weight should be determined and if present, alternative therapies should be suggested. Table 102–4 provides a list of drugs commonly associated with weight gain. If no secondary cause exists, the presence of other cardiovascular risk factors and comorbidities must be determined to guide clinical decisions. ❷ *Presence of comorbidities (CHD, atherosclerosis, type 2 diabetes mellitus, and sleep apnea) and cardiovascular risk factors (cigarette smoking, hypertension, elevated low-density lipoprotein cholesterol, low high-density lipoprotein cholesterol, impaired fasting glucose, family history of premature CHD, and age) requires identification and aggressive management for overall effective treatment of the overweight or obese patient.* Therapy implemented to minimize associated risk(s) may not enhance weight loss, but weight loss will positively address risk factors. Weight loss should not be initiated in pregnant or lactating patients, decompensated psychiatric patients, or patients in whom reduced caloric intake can exacerbate an acute, serious illness.[6] ❻ *Treatment of obesity includes lifestyle changes (dietary modification, enhanced physical activity, and behavioral therapy), pharmacologic treatment, surgical intervention, or a combination of modalities.*

Four stages have been suggested for the treatment of obesity in children and adolescents. Stage 1 or Prevention Plus is the first step for overweight or obese patients and includes adherence to healthy eating and activity habits.

Table 102–4	
Drugs Contributing to Weight Gain	

Anticonvulsants/mood stabilizers
  Carbamazepine
  Gabapentin
  Valproic acid
  Lithium
Antidepressants
  Monoamine oxidase inhibitors (phenelzine)
  Presynaptic α-2 antagonist (mirtazapine)
  Selective serotonin reuptake inhibitors
  Tricyclics (amitriptyline, imipramine, nortryptyline)
Antidiabetics
  Insulin
  Meglintinides
  Sulfonylureas (glyburide, glipizide)
  Thiazolidinediones
Antipsychotics
  Atypical (clozapine, olanzipine, risperidone, paliperidone, quetiapine)
Others
  Antihistamines
  Corticosteroids
  Hormonal Contraceptives (depo injections)

From Refs. 26–28.

Table 102–5	
Low-Calorie Step I Diet	
Nutrient	**Recommended Intake**
Calories[a]	Approximately 500–1,000 kcal/day reduction from usual intake
Total fat[b]	30% or less of total calories
Saturated fatty acids[c]	8–10% of total calories
Monounsaturated fatty acids	Up to 15% of total calories
Polyunsaturated fatty acids	Up to 10% of total calories
Cholesterol[c]	Less than 300 mg/day
Protein[d]	Approximately 15% of total calories
Carbohydrate[e]	55% or more of total calories
Sodium chloride	No more than 100 mmol/day (approximately 2.4 g of sodium or approximately 6 g of sodium chloride)
Calcium[f]	1,000–1,500 mg/day
Fiber[e]	20–30 g/day

[a]A reduction in calories of 500–1,000 kcal/day will help achieve a weight loss of 1–2 pounds/wk. Alcohol provides unneeded calories and displaces more nutritious foods. Alcohol consumption not only increases the number of calories in a diet but also has been associated with obesity in epidemiologic studies as well as in experimental studies. The impact of alcohol calories on a person's overall caloric intake needs to be assessed and appropriately controlled.

[b]Fat-modified foods may provide a helpful strategy for lowering total fat intake but will only be effective if they are also low in calories and if there is no compensation by calories from other foods.

[c]Patients with high blood cholesterol levels may need to use the Step II diet to achieve further reductions in LDL-cholesterol levels; in the Step II diet, saturated fats are reduced to less than 7% of total calories, and cholesterol levels to less than 200 mg/day. All of the other nutrients are the same as in Step I.

[d]Proteins should be derived from plant sources and lean sources of animal protein.

[e]Complex carbohydrates from different vegetables, fruits, and whole grains are good sources of vitamins, minerals, and fiber. A diet rich in soluble fiber, including oat bran, legumes, barley, and most fruits and vegetables, may be effective in reducing blood cholesterol levels. [5]A diet high in all types of fiber may also aid in weight management by promoting satiety at lower levels of calorie and fat intake. Some authorities recommend 20–30 g of fiber daily, with an upper limit of 35 g.

[f]During weight loss, attention should be given to maintaining an adequate intake of vitamins and minerals. Maintenance of the recommended calcium intake of 1,000–1,500 mg/day is especially important for women who may be at risk of osteoporosis.

From U.S. Department of Health and Human Services, NIH-NHLBI. Clinical guidelines on the identification, evaluation, and treatment of overweight and obesity in adults. NIH publication no. 00–4084. Bethesda, MD: National Institutes of Health, 2000.

Patients should be encourage to eat greater than or equal to five servings of fruits and vegetables daily, limit consumption of sweetened drinks, decrease television or other screen time behaviors, and increase physical activity to greater than or equal to 1 h/day. Stage 2 or Structured Weight Management incorporates Prevention Plus habits while setting specific eating and activity goals. Responsibilities include meal planning, observed physical activity or play daily for 1 hour and, documentation of energy consumption and expenditure. Comprehensive Multidisciplinary Interventions (Stage 3) is directed at increasing the intensity of healthy behaviors. To accomplish goals, the child or adolescent should work closely with the primary care provider, registered dietician, exercise specialist, and behavioral counselor. Stage 4, Tertiary Care Intervention, may be needed for the severely obese adolescents. A very low-calorie diet (LCD), medication or weight control surgery may be warranted.[22]

6 *Treatment of obesity includes lifestyle changes (dietary modification, enhanced physical activity, and behavioral therapy), pharmacologic treatment, surgical intervention, or a combination of modalities.*

Nonpharmacologic Therapy

▶ *Dietary*

A LCD is essential for weight-loss management in overweight and obese patients. The Step-1 Diet (Table 102–5) is a LCD recommended as part of an obesity education initiative from the National Heart, Lung, and Blood Institute.[6] In general, the Step-1 Diet restricts daily calories to a range of 1,000 to 1,200 kcal (4,184–5,021 kJ/day) for women weighing less than 75 kg (165 lb) and 1,400 to 1,600 kcal (5,858–6,694 kJ/day) for all others. However, this daily limit should be considered after assessing a patient's normal daily caloric intake and ensuring that the initial caloric restriction does not exceed 500 to 1,000 kcal (2,092–4,184 kJ/day). For example, a male patient who consumes 3,000 kcal (12.552 kJ/day) should not reduce his daily caloric intake to less than 2,000 kcal (8,368 kJ/day) when initially implementing a dietary program. Further reduction to the target of 1,600 kcal (6,694 kJ/day) can be attempted once the patient has reduced calories successfully as initially recommended for a period agreeable by the provider and the patient.[6] Diets too restrictive in calorie reduction are successful initially but fail long-term because compliance is difficult to sustain.[29] Therefore, this less aggressive approach promotes gradual weight loss and weight maintenance.

Dietary consumption should be balanced in carbohydrates, protein, and fat. Several diet plans exist that promote weight loss through strict limitation or overabundance of only one macronutrient (e.g., low-fat, low-carbohydrate, or high-protein diets); however, overall energy consumption and expenditure will determine the amount of weight alteration. Consultation with a dietician is recommended when implementing a healthy meal plan tailored to the individual's nutritional needs.

▶ Exercise

While diet and exercise contribute to weight loss, combining a LCD with physical activity results in greater weight loss compared with either therapy alone.[25] In addition, physical activity can help to prevent weight regain and reduce related cardiovascular risks.[6] Slow titration of both the amount and intensity of physical activity is recommended for most overweight and obese patients.[6] A program that incorporates daily walking is a viable option for most patients (Table 102–6). Consider 10 min/day 3 days/week with a target of 30 to 45 minutes most days, if not every day.[6,30] This type and amount of activity equate to a 100 to 200 kcal (418–836 kJ/day) caloric expenditure.[6]

▶ Behavioral

Nonadherence with recommended lifestyle changes may result in unsuccessful weight loss for adults.[6,25] Therefore, eliminating these barriers through behavior modification is necessary to gain maximal benefit from both dietary modification and exercise. Components to successful behavioral modification include, but are not limited to, the following steps:[6]

- Determine the patient's readiness to lose weight and willingness to implement a weight-loss plan.
- Build and nurture the patient–provider partnership.
- Restructure cognitive abilities.
- Set achievable goals.
- Contact the patient frequently.
- Instruct the patient on the importance and technique of self-monitoring.

Table 102–6	
Examples of Moderate Physical Activity	
Common Chores[a,b]	**Sporting Activities**[a,b]
Washing and waxing a car for 45–60 minutes	Playing volleyball for 45–60 minutes
Washing windows or floors for 45–60 minutes	Playing touch football for 45 minutes
Gardening for 30–45 minutes	Walking 1¾ miles in 35 minutes (20 min/mile)
Wheeling self in wheelchair for 30–40 minutes	Basketball (shooting baskets) for 30 minutes
Pushing a stroller 1½ miles in 30 minutes	Bicycling 5 miles in 30 minutes
Raking leaves for 30 minutes	Dancing fast (social) for 30 minutes
Walking 2 miles in 30 minutes (15 min/mile)	Water aerobics for 30 minutes
Shoveling snow for 15 minutes	Swimming laps for 20 minutes
	Basketball (playing a game) for 15–20 minutes
	Jumping rope for 15 minutes
Stair walking for 15 minutes	Running 1½ miles in 15 minutes (15 min/mile)

[a]A moderate amount of physical activity is roughly equivalent to physical activity that uses approximately 150 calories of energy/day, or 1,000 calories/week.

[b]Some activities can be performed at various intensities; the suggested durations correspond to expected intensity of effort.

From U.S. Department of Health and Human Services, NIH-NHLBI. Clinical guidelines on the identification, evaluation, and treatment of overweight and obesity in adults. NIH publication no. 00–4084. Bethesda, MD: National Institutes of Health, 2000.

- Control stimuli that negatively affect weight loss or weight maintenance.
- Reward the patient for any amount of weight loss or avoidance of weight regain.

Targeted behaviors should be recommended to pediatric patients and their families as healthy habits help prevent excessive weight gain. These include, but are not limited to:[22]

- Limit the consumption of sugar-sweetened beverages.
- Meet daily fruit and vegetable requirements set forth by the U.S. Department of Agriculture.
- Limit the amount of time watching television to 2 hours or less. Other screen time activities, such as computer play, should also be limited.
- Consume a healthy breakfast daily.
- Limit the number of times the family eats at a restaurant, especially those that serve fast food.
- Parents should eat dinner with their children and limit portion size when preparing and serving a meal.

Pharmacologic Therapy

Pharmacotherapy is not recommended for individuals with a BMI of less than 27 kg/m². If lifestyle changes do not

Table 102–7

Summary of Approved Pharmacologic Weight-Loss Agents

Drug	Class	Daily Dose (mg)	Duration of Therapy
Sibutramine	Noradrenergic/serotonergic agent	5–15	More than 3 months[a]
Orlistat	Lipase inhibitor	360	More than 3 months[b]
Phentermine	Noradrenergic agent	15–37.5	Up to 6 months
Diethylpropion	Noradrenergic agent	75	Up to 12 months

[a]Efficacy and safety have not been determined beyond 2 years of use.

[b]Efficacy and safety have not been determined beyond 4 years of use.

result in weight loss after 6 months, drug therapy, in addition to a healthy lifestyle, is warranted for overweight individuals with other related risks and for obese patients. **❼** *Pharmacotherapy, in addition to lifestyle modification, is reserved for patients with a BMI of 30 kg/m² or greater, or a BMI of 27 kg/m² or greater with other obesity-related risk factors.* Currently available pharmacologic products are classified according to their mechanism of action, which includes the suppression of appetite and the suppression of fat absorption (Table 102–7). Therapy was indicated previously for short-term use; however, as obesity-related risks resurface with weight regain, long-term treatment is recommended to minimize these sequelae. **❽** *Weight likely will be regained if lifestyle changes are not continued indefinitely.* Prolonged use of both fenfluramine and dexfenfluramine monotherapy, and fenfluramine and phentermine in combination (Fen-Phen) resulted in cardiac valvular disease.[31] Therefore, only two drugs are currently approved for long-term use in promoting weight loss and preventing weight regain. Sibutramine (Meridia, Abbott Laboratories) was approved by the FDA in 1997, and orlistat (Xenical, Roche Pharmaceuticals) received FDA approval in 1999. Rimonabant is a new medication entity approved for use in Europe in 2006. In June of 2007, the FDA's Endocrine and Metabolic Drugs Advisory Committee denied approval as there was significant concern for serious psychiatric adverse events, specifically depression, anxiety, psychomotor agitation, and sleep disorders.[32] Approximately 20 days later, Sanofi-Aventis withdrew its application for sale of rimonabant in the United States, but remains committed to working with the FDA to make the drug available.[33]

▶ *Sibutramine*

Sibutramine and its two active metabolites (M_1 and M_2) exert their effect by inhibiting the reuptake of serotonin, norepinephrine, and dopamine.[34] Appetite becomes suppressed because patients feel a sense of satiety.

The effect of prolonged sibutramine use on morbidity and mortality is unknown. Most studies vary in dose and length, from 1 to 30 mg/day and 3 to 12 months of use, respectively.[34] Weight loss appears proportional to the dose of sibutramine used, with greater weight loss observed using higher doses of sibutramine.[34] In one trial, subjects randomized to placebo lost an average of 1.4 kg compared with an average loss of 2.9 and 5 kg using a 5 and 20 mg/day dose of sibutramine,

respectively.[35] Two longer-term studies have documented maximal weight loss following 6 months of sibutramine therapy and sustained weight loss over 12 months of use.[34] Three trials with a study duration of greater than 6 months suggest that subjects losing 4 lb within 4 weeks of sibutramine initiation are more likely to achieve long-term weight loss.[34] Conversely, sibutramine may not be effective for patients who do not achieve a weight loss of 4 lb within the initial 4 weeks.

Safe pediatric use has not been established in patients younger than 16 years of age. The efficacy of sibutramine use in overweight adolescent has been evaluated in several studies, two of which provide data for longer-term use. Patients enrolled in the first randomized trial were titrated to a sibutramine dose of 15 mg/day. Six-month data revealed a weight loss greater than placebo by a mean of 4.6 kg. Subjects taking sibutramine throughout the 12-month study period lost an average of 7 kg. Two subjects in the sibutramine group discontinued therapy after experiencing an adverse effect.[36]

Most recently, a 12-month, randomized double blind trial enrolled and evaluated 498 adolescents aging from 12 to 16 years. Sibutramine was initiated at 10 mg daily and increased to 15 mg if a 10% weight loss was not achieved in 6 months. BMI decreased from baseline significantly in the sibutramine-treated group.[37] Data from this trial was presented by the manufacturer (Abbott Laboratories) in hopes of gaining FDA approval. The FDA determined that the safety of sibutramine could not adequately be addressed resulting in continued investigational use of sibutramine in the adolescent population.[38]

Since an increased waist circumference is associated with increased risk for type 2 diabetes mellitus, hyperlipidemia, hypertension, and CVD, a decrease then should reduce risk. A significant dose-related reduction in waist circumference has been reported in 6- and 12-month sibutramine trials.[34] Blood glucose and lipid parameters are not adversely affected, but a small rise in blood pressure and pulse has been observed in clinical trials. On average, the blood pressure increased by 1 to 3 mm Hg, and the heart rate increased by 4 to 5 bpm. Larger increases have been observed for both blood pressure and heart rate when higher doses of sibutramine were studied. Sibutramine should be used cautiously in patients with hypertension or other disease states resulting in elevated blood pressure and/or pulse. Sibutramine is not recommended for patients with a history of congestive heart failure, CVD, arrhythmias, or stroke. Blood pressure and heart rate should be measured prior to initiating sibutramine and reassessed at regular intervals. A dose reduction or discontinuation of sibutramine should be considered for patients experiencing a sustained elevation in either blood pressure or heart rate. More common adverse reactions include dry mouth, anorexia, insomnia, constipation, and headache.[34]

Although not evaluated systematically, drugs that exhibit their effect on the CNS may interact with sibutramine. Since sibutramine inhibits the reuptake of serotonin, use of this drug in combination with a monoamine oxidase inhibitor (MAOI) can elevate blood levels of serotonin, resulting in a serious, potentially fatal reaction known as the *serotonin syndrome*. This syndrome consists of a collection of symptoms that includes one or more of the following: excitement, hypomania, restlessness, loss of consciousness, confusion, disorientation, anxiety, agitation, motor weakness, myoclonus, tremor, hemiballismus, hyperreflexia, ataxia, dysarthria, incoordination, hyperthermia, shivering, pupillary dilation, diaphoresis, emesis, and tachycardia. 2 weeks should elapse between discontinuation of the MAOI (or sibutramine) and initiation of sibutramine (or MAOI) to avoid this potentially serious interaction. Concomitant administration of other serotonergic drugs (e.g., fluoxetine, fluvoxamine, paroxetine, sertraline, and venlafaxine) or medications for migraine treatment (e.g., sumatriptan) and sibutramine also should be avoided to eliminate the risk of serotonin syndrome.[34] Coadministration of a decongestant and sibutramine may increase blood pressure or heart rate. Cytochrome P450 (CYP450) inhibitors, including ketoconazole, erythromycin, and cimetidine, in combination with sibutramine have resulted in increased blood levels of sibutramine; however, the clinical relevance of this is unknown.[34] Highly protein-bound drugs such as warfarin or phenytoin have the potential to interact with sibutramine because it too is highly protein-bound. No data exist to evaluate the extent of this interaction.[34]

Since no human data exist to determine its safe use in pregnant women, sibutramine is not recommended; therefore, women of childbearing potential should use effective methods of contraception while taking sibutramine. Further, sibutramine is not recommended for lactating mothers because its excretion in breast milk is likewise unknown.[34]

Initiate sibutramine at a dose of 10 mg once daily, preferably in the morning without regard to meals. The dose may be increased after 4 weeks to 15 mg once daily if weight-loss goals are not attained. Doses exceeding 15 mg/day are not recommended. For patients intolerant of the 10 mg/day, a dose of 5 mg once a day may be used.[34]

▶ Orlistat

Orlistat promotes and maintains weight loss by acting locally in the GI tract. Orlistat is a chemically synthesized derivative of lipstatin, a natural product of *Streptomyces toxitricini* that inhibits pancreatic and gastric lipases, as well as triglyceride hydrolysis. As a result, undigested triglycerides are not absorbed, causing a caloric deficit and weight loss.[39]

Several studies have reported significant weight loss for patients receiving orlistat 120 mg three times a day compared with placebo.[40,41] Weight maintenance or prevention of weight regain also has been documented with continued orlistat use.[40,42] After 1 year of treatment, 57% of orlistat-treated patients lost at least 5% of their baseline weight.[39] The long-term weight-loss effect on one obesity-related comorbidity was assessed in a large placebo-controlled study. In 3,000 obese patients, 21% had impaired glucose tolerance at enrollment. After 4 years, weight loss was greater and the incidence of new diabetes was lower in patients receiving orlistat.[43]

One study evaluated the longer-term effect of orlistat in adolescents. In a group of 12- to 16-year-old individuals, orlistat (120 mg three times daily) in combination with diet, exercise, and behavior modification resulted in a significant reduction in BMI and waist circumference when compared to placebo. In addition, orlistat-treated subjects exhibited minimal weight increase after 1 year (0.53 kg) compared with placebo-treated patients (3.14 kg). Common adverse reactions observed were fatty or oily stools, oily spotting, oily evacuation, or abdominal pain and/or flatulence with bowel movements. Soft stools, nausea, increased defecation, and fecal incontinence also were noted.[44]

The safety and efficacy of orlistat have not been determined beyond 4 years of use. Minimal systemic effects exist because orlistat acts locally in the GI tract. Thus, common side effects reported include oily spotting, flatus with discharge, fecal urgency, fatty/oily stools, oily evacuation, increased defecation, and fecal incontinence.[39] Other adverse events include bloating, abdominal pain, dyspepsia, nausea, vomiting, diarrhea, and headache.[45]

Orlistat reduces the absorption of fat-soluble vitamins. Daily intake of a multivitamin containing vitamins A, D, E, and K, as well as β-carotene, is recommended. Patients should take a multivitamin daily and preferably 2 hours prior to or after the dose of orlistat.[39] Since availability of vitamin K may decline in patients receiving orlistat therapy, close monitoring of coagulation status should occur with concomitant administration of warfarin.[39] Administration of orlistat in conjunction with cyclosporine can result in decreased cyclosporine plasma levels. To avoid this interaction, cyclosporine should be taken 2 hours preceding or following the dose of orlistat. Additionally, cyclosporine levels should be monitored more frequently.[36]

Pregnant or lactating women should not take orlistat because no data exist to establish safety. Orlistat is contraindicated in patients with chronic malabsorption syndrome or cholestasis.[39]

Initiate orlistat 120 mg three times a day with a well-balanced but reduced-caloric meal containing no more than 30% of calories from fat. Orlistat may be taken during or up to 1 hour after the meal. If a meal is missed or contains little fat, the dose of orlistat may be omitted. Doses above 360 mg/day provide no greater benefit and thus are not recommended.

▶ Rimonabant

Rimonabant is a selective CB1 receptor antagonist that is currently under investigation in phase III trials. CB1 receptors are found in the brain, adipose tissue, the GI tract, pituitary and adrenal glands, sympathetic ganglia, heart, lungs, liver, and bladder.[15,16] Food cravings are diminished following inhibition of this receptor.[17]

The efficacy of rimonabant was evaluated as part of the Rimonabant in Obesity (RIO) Program. Four studies (RIO-Europe, RIO-Lipids, RIO-North America, and RIO-Diabetes) compared rimonabant 5 mg and 20 mg to placebo in 6,600 patients. Treatment with rimonabant resulted in a 4.7 kg reduction in body weight. All studies observed greater weight loss in the rimonabant treatment groups when compared to placebo.[46] Improvements of waist circumference, HDL cholesterol concentration, triglyceride concentration, and A1C were also demonstrated.[47] Rimonabant's impact on cardiovascular morbidity and mortality is unknown, however, when available, the results of the Comprehensive Rimonabant Evaluation Study of Clinical Endpoints (CRESCENDO) should help fill this information void.

The most frequent side effects reported with rimonabant use include nausea, diarrhea, dizziness, and insomnia.[47] RIO Program patients treated with rimonabant were 1.4 times more likely to experience an adverse effect and 2.5 times more likely to cease study participation secondary to depressive mood disorders. Depression, major depression, depressed mood, and depressed symptoms comprise depressed mood disorders.[46]

Two other drugs with a mechanism of action similar to rimonabant are currently in Phase III trials. Taranabant is a CB1 receptor inverse agonist where CP-945598 is a CB1 receptor antagonist. Expectation for FDA approval is unknown.[48]

▶ *Phentermine*

Phentermine decreases food intake, and hence weight, by increasing norepinephrine and dopamine release in the CNS. This drug is indicated for short-term use—no more than a few weeks—in addition to lifestyle modifications in obese patients with a BMI of 30 kg/m² or greater, or a BMI of 27 kg/m² or greater in the presence of other risk factors.[49]

A recent meta-analysis evaluated patients at doses of 15 mg and 30 mg daily. Patients were analyzed for periods of 2 to 24 weeks. The majority of patients enrolled were female, and more than 80% of the patients evaluated received adjunctive modification in lifestyle. An average weight loss of 3.6 kg (7.9 lb) was demonstrated for patients treated with phentermine compared with placebo. Although modest in amount, this value was statistically significant.[45]

Safety and efficacy have not been determined in pediatric patients less than 16 years of age.[49]

Common adverse reactions seen with phentermine use include heart palpitations, tachycardia, elevated blood pressure, stimulation, restlessness, dizziness, insomnia, euphoria, dysphoria, tremor, headache, dry mouth, constipation, and diarrhea. Phentermine should be avoided in patients with unstable cardiac status, hypertension, hyperthyroidism, agitated states, or glaucoma. In combination with fenfluramine or dexfenfluramine, primary pulmonary hypertension and valvular heart disease have been reported. The risk of developing either serious adverse effect cannot be

ruled out with use of phentermine alone. Since phentermine is related to the amphetamines, the potential for abuse is high; thus, this should be kept in mind when selecting this agent as an aid for weight loss.[49]

Phentermine use should be avoided in patients concomitantly receiving or having received an MAOI within the preceding 14 days. Combination therapy with any stimulant or MAOI has the potential for causing hypertensive crisis. Alcohol is not recommended for patients prescribed phentermine.[49]

Since no studies have been conducted in pregnant women, phentermine should be administered only when clearly indicated. Owing to the potential for severe adverse effects in nursing infants, a decision to stop the drug or discontinue nursing must be made.[49]

Phentermine is available as an immediate-release and a sustained-release product. In conjunction with a healthy lifestyle, 30 to 37.5 mg of phentermine is administered once daily, typically before breakfast or 1 to 2 hours following the morning meal. The dosage should be individualized; some patients may be managed adequately at 15 to 18.75 mg daily, whereas a dose of 18.75 mg twice daily may be used to minimize side effects, excluding insomnia. To lessen the risk of insomnia, dosing phentermine in the evening should be avoided. Timed-release preparations of phentermine are not recommended because phentermine's half-life is approximately 20 hours.[50]

▶ *Diethylpropion*

This sympathomimetic amine exudes similar pharmacologic activity as the amphetamines, resulting in CNS stimulation and appetite suppression. This drug is indicated for short-term use in conjunction with a reduced-calorie diet and exercise in obese patients with a BMI of 30 kg/m² or greater following failed attempts of diet and exercise alone.[51]

One meta-analysis reviewed patients receiving doses of 75 mg daily during periods of 6 to 52 weeks. Similar to study characteristics for phentermine, the majority of patients enrolled were female, and all patients implemented adjunctive lifestyle modifications. The average additional weight loss observed was 3 kg (6.6 lb) compared with diet and exercise alone, resulting in a borderline statistically significant difference.[45]

Safety and effectiveness of diethylpropion have not been established in patients under the age of 16; therefore, its use is not recommended.[51]

Use of diethylpropion for a period longer than 3 months is associated with an increased risk for development of pulmonary hypertension. When used as directed, reported common CNS adverse effects included overstimulation, restlessness, dizziness, insomnia, euphoria, dysphoria, tremor, headache, jitteriness, anxiety, nervousness, depression, drowsiness, malaise, mydriasis, and blurred vision. In addition, diethylpropion can decrease seizure threshold, subsequently increasing a patient's risk for an epileptic event. Other organ systems also can adversely be affected, resulting in tachycardia, elevated blood pressure, palpitations, dry mouth, abdominal discomfort, constipation, diarrhea, nausea, vomiting, impotence or change in libido, gynecomastia, bone marrow suppression, agranulocytosis, and leukopenia. Diethylpropion is contraindicated in patients with pulmonary hypertension, advanced arteriosclerosis, severe hypertension, hyperthyroidism, agitated states, or glaucoma. Since diethylpropion is related to the amphetamines, the potential for abuse is high, and therefore, its use is contraindicated in patients with a history of substance abuse.[51]

As with phentermine, use of diethypropion should be avoided in patients concomitantly receiving or having received an MAOI within the preceding 14 days to prevent hypertensive crisis. Combination with other anorectic agents should be avoided.[51]

No adequate studies have been conducted using diethylpropion in pregnant women; therefore, the drug should be used only if the benefit outweighs potential fetal risk. Use with caution in nursing mothers because the drug is excreted in breast milk.[51]

Diethylpropion is available as both an immediate-release and a controlled-release product. In conjunction with a reduced-calorie diet and/or exercise, dose diethylpropion (immediate-release) 25 mg three times a day before meals or 75 mg (controlled-release) once a day, usually midmorning.[51]

▶ *Other Pharmacologic Therapy*

Other noradrenergic agents—not approved by the FDA and subsequently not recommended for weight loss—include amphetamine salts (e.g., ephedrine and phenylpropanolamine), methamphetamine, and benzophetamine. Although the selective serotonin reuptake inhibitors (e.g., fluoxetine and sertraline) appear to promote weight loss, further study is warranted given the inconsistent results available to date. Dietary supplements containing ephedra or ephedrine alkaloids are banned from sale following the FDA's final ruling.[52] However, ephedrine is available in nonprescription and prescription formulations for the treatment of bronchospasm, nasal congestion, hypotension/shock, and cardiac arrhythmias. Herbal products lack consistency in labeling, vary in effect, and present potentially dangerous health risks. Herbal products are not recommended.

Surgical Intervention

Weight-reduction (bariatric) surgery is an option for patients whose BMIs are 40 kg/m² or greater, or 35 kg/m² or greater in the presence of other comorbid conditions and who have failed more conventional approaches to weight loss.[6,53] ❾ *Surgery is warranted when other treatment attempts have failed in severely obese patients (BMI of 40 kg/m² or greater, or 35 kg/m² or greater with obesity-related risk factors).* There are two basic surgical techniques: (a) gastric bypass—the full partitioning of the proximal gastric segment into a jejunal loop of the intestine—whereby weight loss is induced through both malabsorption of food and limited gastric capacity, and (b) gastroplasty—incomplete partitioning at the proximal gastric segment with the placement of a gastric

outlet stoma of set diameter—which promotes weight loss by limiting gastric capacity.[6,53]

A meta-analysis of surgical options for obesity reported that surgical treatment produces a weight loss of 20 to 30 kg (44–66 lb) that is maintained for 5 to 10 years. Additionally, favorable outcomes for comorbid conditions are observed following surgery. When evaluating the various types of surgery available, pooled data concluded that gastric bypass produces a 10 kg (22 lb) greater weight loss at 12 and 36 months than gastroplasty procedures. Complications are inherent to any surgical procedure. The more common bariatric surgery complications are respiratory problems, wound formation, wound infections, hernia development, deep venous thrombosis, and pulmonary embolism. No differences were observed in mortality rates among various surgical procedures. Postoperative weight loss is much greater when compared with pharmacologic therapies, but no comparative trials exist.[54]

Gastric surgery, either banding or bypass, is an alternative offered to adolescents as it results in substantial weight loss and medical health improvement. Patients with a BMI greater than or equal to 40 kg/m² and an associated medical condition or BMI greater than or equal to 50 kg/m², at or over the age of 13 and 15 years for girls and boys respectively, display emotional and cognitive maturity, and have implemented a behavioral-based weight-loss program are candidates for surgery.[22]

All patients undergoing bariatric surgery should be part of an integrated program of health education, diet, exercise, and behavioral modification before and following surgery.[6] Patients must understand and commit to a substantial change in eating patterns to maintain long-term weight reduction.[22,54]

SPECIAL POPULATION CONSIDERATION
Elderly Patients with Obesity

The majority of obese patients are 40 to 59 years of age.[8] However, the prevalence of obesity in older adults is increasing; therefore, it should not be surprising that more cardiovascular risk factors are present in this group of individuals. Additionally, obesity is a major predictor of functional limitation and mobility problems in older persons. Age alone should not prejudice the clinician from treating geriatric patients, whereas the benefits of cardiovascular health and functionality should be considered. Treatments should be initiated that minimize adverse effects on bone health and nutritional status and should include dietary and activity modifications.[6]

OUTCOME EVALUATION

Successful management of overweight and obesity is determined by the ability the treatment plan has to: (a) prevent weight gain, (b) reduce and maintain a lower body weight, and (c) decrease the risk of obesity-related comorbidities. Since weight is necessary to calculate the BMI, it, as well as waist circumference, should be determined. Obesity management may encompass more than weight loss or maintenance in the presence of other conditions; other pertinent parameters should be assessed at baseline. The presence of hypertension, type 2 diabetes, hyperlipidemia, CAD, sleep apnea, hypothyroidism, osteoarthritis, gallbladder disease, gout, or cancer should be determined. Blood pressure and heart rate should be measured prior to implementation of any therapy. Certain laboratory parameters also should be assessed. A basic metabolic panel, liver function tests, complete blood count, fasting lipid profile, full thyroid function tests, and other laboratory studies as deemed necessary should be obtained. An electrocardiogram should be performed if recent results are unknown.[6]

The patient should be assessed in 2 to 4 weeks following the implementation of therapy to determine effectiveness of and intolerance to treatment. Monthly visits are encouraged during the first 3 months. More frequent follow up may be necessary in the presence of other medical conditions. Less frequent follow up occurs after 6 months of effective weight-loss therapy.[6]

At each follow-up visit, compliance with a healthy lifestyle should be determined, as well as measurement of physical parameters, including weight, blood pressure, and heart rate. Waist circumference should be measured intermittently. A complete assessment also would include identification of adverse drug reactions or drug interactions if weight-loss medications have been initiated.[6]

Once the patient has achieved the recommended weight loss, he or she then enters the weight-maintenance phase, which includes continued contact for education, guidance, and risk-factor assessment. If weight loss is not attained, further assessment is required to determine why the goals of therapy have not been met. The interaction should be directed toward determining the motivation to lose weight, balance between caloric intake and physical activity, adherence to behavioral therapy, and determination of psychological stressors present.[6]

Abbreviations Introduced in This Chapter

5-HT$_{1A}$	Serotonin 1A subtype
5-HT$_{2C}$	Serotonin 2C subtype
BMI	Body mass index
CAD	Coronary artery disease
CB1	Cannabinoid receptor
CHD	Coronary heart disease
CRESCENDO	Comprehensive Rimonabant Evaluation Study of Clinical Endpoints
CVD	Cardiovascular disease
CYP450	Cytochrome P450
GERD	Gastroesophageal reflux disease
LCD	Low-calorie diet
MAOI	Monoamine oxidase inhibitor
NIH-NHLBI	National Institute of Health-National Heart Lung and Blood Institute
RIO	Rimonabant in obesity
RPM	Respirations per minute

Patient Care and Monitoring

1. Determine if history of BMI greater than or equal to 25 kg/m². If unavailable or BMI unknown, obtain weight, height, and waist circumference. Calculate the BMI. Assess the patient's willingness to lose weight.

2. If the BMI is greater than 25 kg/m² or waist circumference greater than 35 in. for females or 40 in. for male patients, determine the presence of risk factors.

3. Prevention of weight gain is recommended in all patients with a BMI greater than or equal to 25 kg/m². Weight loss is indicated for patients with a BMI 25 to 29.9 kg/m², or an elevated waist circumference with two or more risk factors, or for any patient with a BMI greater than or equal to 30 kg/m².

4. Educate the patient regarding a healthy lifestyle, one that includes a balance between caloric intake and energy expenditure as well as suggest methods to modify behavior.

5. If the patient presents with a desire to lose weight, develop treatment goals and weight-loss strategies (nonpharmacologic, drug therapy, or surgical intervention) including control of associated risks.

6. Close monitoring should follow to assess weight, BMI, waist circumference, and presence of complications related to the treatment plan. If weight-loss goals are not attained, determine reasons for failure.

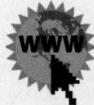
Self-assessment questions and answers are available at *http://www.mhpharmacotherapy.com/pp.html.*

REFERENCES

1. Centers for Disease Control and Prevention. Defining Overweight and Obesity, *http://www.cdc.gov/nccdphp/dnpa/obesity/defining.htm.*
2. Heymsfield SB, Allison DB, Heshka S, Pierson RN Jr. Assessment of human body composition. In: Allison DB, ed. Handbook of Assessment Methods for Eating Behaviors and Weight Related Problems: Measures, Theory, and Research. Thousand Oaks, CA: Sage Publications, 1995: 515–560.
3. McDowell A, Engel A, Massey JT, Maurer K. Plan and operation of the Second National Health and Nutrition Examination Survey, 1976–1980. Vital Health Stat 1981;1: 1–144.
4. Dowling HJ, Pi-Sunyer FX. Race-dependent health risks of upper body obesity. Diabetes 1993;42:537–543.
5. Kissebah AH, Vydelingum N, Murray R, et al. Relation of body fat distribution to metabolic complications of obesity. J Clin Endocrinol Metab 1982;54:254–260.
6. U.S. Department of Health and Human Services, NIH-NHLBI. Clinical guidelines on the identification, evaluation and treatment of overweight and obesity in adults. NIH publication no. 00-4084. Bethesda, MD: National Institutes of Health, 2000.

7. Lew EA, Garfinkel L. Variations in mortality by weight among 750,000 men and women. J Chronic Dis 1979;23:563–576.

8. Ogden CL, Carroll MD, Curtin LR, McDowell MA, Tabak CJ, Flegal KM. Prevalence of overweight and obesity in the United States, 1999–2004. JAMA 2006;295:1549–1555.

9. Power C, Lake JK, Cole TJ. Body mass index and height from childhood to adulthood in the 1958 British born cohort. Am J Clin Nutr 1997;66:1094–1101.

10. Freedman DS, Dietz WH, Srinivasan SR, et al. The relation of overweight to cardiovascular risk factors among children and adolescents: The Bogalusa heart study. Pediatrics 1999;103:1175–1182.

11. Must A, Jacques PF, Dallal GE, et al. Long-term morbidity and mortality of overweight adolescents. A follow-up of the Harvard Growth Study of 1922 to 1935. N Engl J Med 1992;327:1350–1355.

12. American Academy of Pediatrics Committee on Nutrition. Prevention of pediatric overweight and obesity. Pediatrics 2003;112(2):424–430.

13. Comuzzie AG, Allison DB. The search for human obesity genes. Science 1998;280:1374–1377.

14. Flier JS, Foster DW. Eating disorders: Obesity, anorexia nervosa, bulimia, nervosa. In: Wilson JD, Foster DW, Kronenberg HM, Larsen PR, eds. Williams' Textbook of Endocrinology, 9th ed. Philadelphia: WB Saunders, 1998:1061–1097.

15. National Research Council. Committee on Diet and Health. Implications for Reducing Chronic Disease Risk. Washington, DC: National Academy Press, 1989.

16. Di Marzo V, Bifulco M, De Petrocellis L. The endocannabinoid system and its therapeutic exploitation. Nat Rev Drug Discov 2004;3:771–784.

17. Croci T, Manara L, Aureggi G, et al. In vitro functional evidence of neuronal cannabinoid CB1 receptors in human ileum. Br J Pharmacol 1998;125:1393–1395.

18. Bensaid M, Gary-Bobo M, Esclangon A, et al. The cannabinoid CB1 receptor antagonist SR141716 increases Acrp30 mRNA expression in adipose tissue of obese fa/fa rats and in cultured adipocyte cells. Mol Pharmacol 2003;6:908–914.

19. Van Gaal L, Rissanen A, Scheen A, et al. Effects of the cannabinoid-1 receptor blocker rimonabant on weight reduction and cardiovascular risk factors in overweight patients: 1-year experience from the RIO-Europe study. Lancet 2005;365:1389–1397.

20. Woods SC, Seeley RJ, Porte DJ, et al. Signals that regulate food intake and energy homeostasis. Science 1998;280: 1378–1383.

21. Lissner L, Levitsky DA, Strupp BJ, et al. Dietary fat and the regulation of energy intake in human subjects. Am J Clin Nutr 1987;46:886–892.

22. Expert committee recommendations regarding the prevention, assessment, and treatment of child and adolescent overweight and obesity: Summary report. Pediatrics 2007;120:S164–S192.

23. Executive summary of the third report of the National Cholesterol Education Program (NCEP) Expert Panel on Detection, Evaluation and Treatment of High Blood Cholesterol in Adults (Adult Treatment Panel III). JAMA 2001;285:2486–2509.

24. Standards of medical care for patients with diabetes mellitus. Diabetes Care 2008;31(Suppl 1):S13.

25. Orzano AJ, Scott JG. Diagnosis and treatment of obesity in adults: An applied evidence-based review. J Am Board Fam Pract 2004;17(5):359–369.

26. Malone M. Medications associated with weight gain. Ann Pharmacother 2005;39:2046–2055.

27. Janssen, Division of Ortho-McNeil-Janssen Pharmaceuticals, Inc. Invega (Paliperidone) Package Insert. Titusville, NJ: Janssen, Division of Ortho-McNeil-Janssen Pharmaceuticals, Inc., 2007.

28. AstraZeneca Pharmaceuticals LP. Seroquel (Quetiapine) Package Insert. Wilmington, DE: AstraZeneca Pharmaceuticals LP, 2008(July).

29. Wadden TA, Foster DD, Letizia KA. One-year behavioral treatment of obesity: Comparison of moderate and severe caloric restriction and the effects of weight maintenance therapy. J Consult Clin Psychol 1994;62:165–171.

30. Chobanian AV, Bakris GL, Black HR, et al. The seventh report of the joint national committee on prevention, detection, evaluation and treatment of high blood pressure: The JNC 7 report. JAMA 2003;289(19):2560–2572.

31. Connolly HM, Crary JL, McGoon MD, et al. Valvular heart disease associated with fenfluramine-phentermine. N Engl J Med 1997;337:581–588.

32. Medical Week News, Inc. FDA Delay on Diet Pill Acomplia (Rimonabant) Tied to Suicide, Seizures. *http://www.acompliareport.com/News/news-061107.htm.*

33. Medical Week News, Inc. Sanofi Withdraws Bid to Sell Diet Drug Acomplia (Rimonabant) in United States. *http://www.acompliareport.com/News/news-062907.htm.*

34. Abbott Laboratories. Meridia (Sibutramine) Package Insert. North Chicago, IL: Abbott Laboratories, 2007(Oct).

35. Weintraub M, Rubio A, Golik A, et al. Sibutramine in weight control: A dose-ranging, efficacy study. Clin Pharmacol Ther 1991;50(3):330–337.

36. Berkowitz RI, Wadden TA, Tershakovec AM, Cronquist JL. Behavior therapy and sibutramine for the treatment of adolescent obesity: A randomized controlled trial. JAMA 2003;289:1805–1812.

37. Berkowitz RI, Fujioka K, Daniels SR, et al. Effects of sibutramine treatment in obese adolescents: A randomized trial. Ann Internal Med 2006;145:81–90.

38. Beaston P. Clinical review for NDA 20–632,SE5-021. *www.fda.gov/cder/foi/esum/2005/02063s021_sibutramine_hydrochloride_clincal_BPCA.pdf.*

39. Roche Laboratories. Xenical (Orlistat) Package Insert. Nutley, NJ: Roche Laboratories, 2008(July).

40. Sjöström L, Rissanen A, Andersen T, et al. Randomized placebo-controlled trial of orlistat for weight loss and prevention of weight regain in obese patients. Lancet 1998;352:167–173.

41. Davidson MH, Hauptman J, DiGirolamo M, et al. Weight control and risk factor reduction in obese subjects treated for 2 years with orlistat. JAMA 1999;281:235–242.

42. Hill JO, Hauptman J, Anderson JW, et al. Orlistat, a lipase inhibitory, for weight maintenance after conventional dieting: A 1-year study. Am J Clin Nutr 1999;69:1108–1116.

43. Torgerson JS, Hauptman J, Boldrin MN, et al. XENical in the prevention of diabetes in obese subjects (XENDOS) study: A randomized study of orlistat as an adjunct to lifestyle changes for the prevention of type 2 diabetes in obese patients. Diabetes Care 2004;27:155–161.

44. Chapione JP, Hampl S, Jensen C, et al. Effect of orlistat on weight and body composition in obese adolescents: A randomized controlled trial. JAMA 2005;293:2873–2883.

45. Li Z, Maglione M, Tu W, et al. Meta-analysis: Pharmacologic treatment of obesity. Ann Intern Med 2005;142:532–546.

46. Christensen R, Kristensen PK, Bartels EM, Bliddal H, Astrup A. Efficacy and safety of the weight loss drug rimonabant: A meta-analysis of randomized trials. Lancet 2007;370:1706–1711.

47. Padwal RS, Majumdar SR. Drug treatments for Obesity: Orlistat, sibutramine and rimonant. Lancet 2007;369: 71–77.

48. Medical Week News, Inc. What Are Some Options to Acomplia / Zimulti? *http://www.acompliareport.com/Other.htm.*

49. Gate Pharmaceuticals. Adipex-P (Phentermine) Package Insert. Sellersville, PA: Gate Pharmaceuticals, 2005(July).

50. Thompson Healthcare Products. MICROMEDEX Healthcare Series. www.micromedex.com/products/hcs/.

51. Merrell Pharmaceuticals. Tenuate (Diethylpropion) Package Insert. Bridgewater, NJ: Merrell Pharmaceuticals, 2003(Nov).

52. U.S. Food and Drug Administration. Final Rule Declaring Dietary Supplements Containing Ephedrine Alkaloids Adulterated Because They Present an Unreasonable Risk. *http://www.cfsan.fda.gov/~lrd/fr040211.html.*

53. Snow V, Barry P, Fitterman N, et al. Pharmacologic and surgical management of obesity in primary care: A clinical practice guideline from the American College of Physicians. Ann Intern Med 2005;142:525–531.

54. Maggard MA, Shugarman LR, Suttorp M, et al. Meta-analysis: Surgical treatment of obesity. Ann Intern Med 2005;142:547–559.

Appendix A: Conversion Factors and Anthropometrics*

CONVERSION FACTORS

SI Units

SI (*le Systéme International d'Unités*) units are used in *many* countries to express clinical laboratory and serum drug concentration data. Instead of employing units of mass (such as micrograms), the SI system uses moles (mol) to represent the amount of a substance. A molar solution contains 1 mole (the molecular weight of the substance in grams) of the solute in 1 L of solution. The following formula is used to convert units of mass to moles (mcg/mL to µmol/L or, by substitution of terms, mg/mL to mmol/L or ng/mL to nmol/L).

▶ *Micromoles per Liter*

Micromoles per liter (µmol/L) =

$$\frac{\text{drug concentration (mcg/mL)} \times 1,000}{\text{molecular weight of drug (g/mol)}}$$

▶ *Milliequivalents*

An equivalent weight of a substance is that weight which will combine with or replace 1 g of hydrogen; a milliequivalent is 1/1,000 of an equivalent weight.

Milliequivalents per Liter

Milliequivalents per liter (mEq/L) =

$$\frac{\text{weight of salt (g)} \times \text{valence of ion} \times 1,000}{\text{molecular weight of salt}}$$

$$\text{Weight of salt (g)} = \frac{\text{mEq/L} \times \text{molecular weight of salt}}{\text{valence of ion} \times 1,000}$$

Approximate Milliequivalents: Weight Conversions for Selected Ions

Salt	mEq/g Salt	mg Salt/ mEq
Calcium carbonate ($CaCO_3$)	20.0	50.0
Calcium chloride ($CaCl_2 \cdot 2H_2O$)	13.6	73.5
Calcium gluceptate ($Ca[C_7H_{13}O_8]_2$)	4.1	245.2
Calcium gluconate ($Ca[C_6H_{11}O_7]_2 \cdot H_2O$)	4.5	224.1
Calcium lactate ($Ca[C_3H_5O_3]_2 \cdot 5H_2O$)	6.5	154.1
Magnesium gluconate ($Mg[C_6H_{11}O_7]_2 \cdot H_2O$)	4.6	216.3
Magnesium oxide (MgO)	49.6	20.2
Magnesium sulfate ($MgSO_4$)	16.6	60.2
Magnesium sulfate ($MgSO_4 \cdot 7H_2O$)	8.1	123.2
Potassium acetate ($K[C_2H_3O_2]$)	10.2	98.1
Potassium chloride (KCl)	13.4	74.6
Potassium citrate ($K_3[C_6H_5O_7] \cdot H_2O$)	9.2	108.1
Potassium iodide (KI)	6.0	166.0
Sodium acetate ($Na[C_2H_3O_2]$)	12.2	82.0
Sodium acetate ($Na[C_2H_3O_2] \cdot 3H_2O$)	7.3	136.1
Sodium bicarbonate ($NaHCO_3$)	11.9	84.0
Sodium chloride (NaCl)	17.1	58.4
Sodium citrate ($Na_3[C_6H_5O_7] \cdot 2H_2O$)	10.2	98.0
Sodium iodide (NaI)	6.7	149.9
Sodium lactate ($Na[C_3H_5O_3]$)	8.9	112.1
Zinc sulfate ($ZnSO_4 \cdot 7H_2O$)	7.0	143.8

Valences and Atomic Weights of Selected Ions

Substance	Electrolyte	Valence	Molecular Weight
Calcium	Ca^{2+}	2	40.1
Chloride	Cl^-	1	35.5
Magnesium	Mg^{2+}	2	24.3
Phosphate (pH = 7.4)	HPO_4^- (80%) $H_2PO_4^-$ (20%)	1.8	96.0[a]
Potassium	K^+	1	39.1
Sodium	Na^+	1	23.0
Sulfate	SO_4^-	2	96.0[a]

[a]The molecular weight of phosphorus only is 31; that of sulfur only is 32.1.

*This appendix contains information from Appendices 1 and 2 of Anderson PO, Knoben JE, Troutman WG, et al (eds). *Handbook of Clinical Drug Data*, 10th ed. New York: McGraw-Hill, 2002:1053–1058, with permission.

Anion Gap

The anion gap is the concentration of plasma anions not routinely measured by laboratory screening. It is useful in the evaluation of acid–base disorders. The anion gap is greater with increased plasma concentrations of endogenous species (e.g., phosphate, sulfate, lactate, and ketoacids) or exogenous species (e.g., salicylate, penicillin, ethylene glycol, ethanol, and methanol). The formulas for calculating the anion gap are as follows:

$$\text{Anion gap} = (Na^+ + K^+) - (Cl^- + HCO_3^-)$$

or

$$\text{Anion gap} = Na^+ - (Cl^- + HCO_3^-)$$

where the expected normal value for the first equation is 11 to 20 mmol/L and that for the second equation is 7 to 16 mmol/L. Note that there is a variation in the upper and lower limits of the normal range.

Temperature

Fahrenheit to Centigrade: $(°F - 32) \times 5/9 = °C$
Centigrade to Fahrenheit: $(°C \times 9/5) + 32 = °F$
Centigrade to Kelvin: $°C + 273 = °K$

Calories

1 calorie = 1 kilocalorie = 1,000 calories = 4.184 kilojoules (kJ)
1 kilojoule = 0.239 calories = 0.239 kilocalories = 239 calories

Weights and Measures

▶ Metric Weight Equivalents

1 kilogram (kg) = 1,000 grams
1 gram (g) = 1,000 milligrams
1 milligram (mg) = 0.001 gram
1 microgram (mcg, μg) = 0.001 milligram
1 nanogram (ng) = 0.001 microgram
1 picogram (pg) = 0.001 nanogram
1 femtogram (fg) = 0.001 picogram

▶ Metric Volume Equivalents

1 liter (L) = 1,000 milliliters
1 deciliter (dL) = 100 milliliters
1 milliliter (mL) = 0.001 liter
1 microliter (μL) = 0.001 milliliter
1 nanoliter (nL) = 0.001 microliter
1 picoliter (pL) = 0.001 nanoliter
1 femtoliter (fL) = 0.001 picoliter

▶ Apothecary Weight Equivalents

1 scruple (ว) = 20 grains (gr)
60 grains (gr) = 1 dram (ʒ)
8 drams (ʒ) = 1 ounce (fl ʒ)
1 ounce (ʒ) = 480 grains (gr)
12 ounces (ʒ) = 1 pound (lb)

▶ Apothecary Volume Equivalents

60 minims (m) = 1 fluidram (fl ʒ)
8 fluidrams (fl ʒ) = 1 fluid ounce (fl ʒ)

1 fluid ounce (fl ʒ) = 480 minims (m)
16 fluid ounces (fl ʒ) = 1 pint (pt)

▶ Avoirdupois Equivalents

1 ounce (oz) = 437.5 grains
16 ounces (oz) = 1 pound (lb)

▶ Weight/Volume Equivalents

1 mg/dL = 10 mcg/mL
1 mg/dL = 1 mg%
1 ppm = 1 mg/L

▶ Conversion Equivalents

1 gram (g) = 15.43 grains (gr)
1 grain (gr) = 64.8 milligrams (mg)
1 ounce (ʒ) = 31.1 grams (g)
1 ounce (oz) = 28.35 grams (g)
1 pound (lb) = 453.6 grams (g)
1 kilogram (kg) = 2.2 pounds (lb)
1 milliliter (mL) = 16.23 minims (m)
1 minim (m) = 0.06 milliliter (mL)
1 fluid ounce (fl oz) = 29.57 milliliters (mL)
1 pint (pt) = 473.2 milliliters (mL)
1 US gallon = 3.78 liters (L)
1 Can gallon = 4.55 liters (L)
0.1 milligram = 1/600 grain
0.12 milligram = 1/500 grain
0.15 milligram = 1/400 grain
0.2 milligram = 1/300 grain
0.3 milligram = 1/200 grain
0.4 milligram = 1/150 grain
0.5 milligram = 1/120 grain
0.6 milligram = 1/100 grain
0.8 milligram = 1/80 grain
1 milligram = 1/65 grain

▶ Metric Length Conversion Equivalents

2.54 cm = 1 inch
30.48 cm = 1 foot
1 m = 3.28 feet
1.6 km = 1 mile

ANTHROPOMETRICS

Creatinine Clearance Formulas

▶ Formulas for Estimating Creatinine Clearance in Patients With Stable Renal Function

Cockroft-Gault Formula
Adults (age 18 years and older)[1]:

$$\text{CrCl (males)} = \frac{(140 - \text{age}) \times \text{weight}}{Cr_s \times 72}$$

$$\text{CrCl (females) } 0.85 \times \text{above value*}$$

*Some studies suggest that the predictive accuracy of this formula for women is better *without* the correction factor of 0.85.

where CrCl is creatinine clearance (in mL/minute), Cr_s is serum creatinine (in mg/dL [or μmol/L divided by 88.4]), age is in years, and weight is in kilograms.

Children (age 1–18 years)[2]:

$$CrCl = \frac{0.48 \times height \times BSA}{SCr_s \times 1.73}$$

where BSA is body surface area (in m²), CrCl is creatinine clearance (in mL/minute), SCr_s is serum creatinine (in mg/dL [or μmol/L divided by 88.4]), and height is in centimeters.

▶ Formula for Estimating Creatinine Clearance From a Measured Urine Collection

$$CrCl \ (mL/minute) = \frac{U \times V^*}{P \times T}$$

where U is the concentration of creatinine in a urine specimen (in same units as P), V is the volume of urine (in mL), P is the concentration of creatinine in serum at the midpoint of the urine collection period (in same units as U), and T is the time of the urine collection period in minutes (e.g., 6 hours = 360 minutes; 24 hours = 1,440 minutes).

*The product of $U \times V$ equals the production of creatinine during the collection period and, at steady state, should equal 20 to 25 mg/kg/day for ideal body weight (IBW) in males and 15 to 20 mg/kg/day for IBW in females. If it is less than this, inadequate urine collection may have occurred, and CrCl will be underestimated.

▶ MDRD Formula for Estimating Glomerular Filtration Rate (From the Modification of Diet in Renal Disease Study)[3]

Conventional calibration MDRD equation [used only with those creatinine methods that have *not* been recalibrated to be traceable to isotope dilution mass spectrometry (IDMS)]

For creatinine in mg/dL:

$$X = 186 \ creatinine^{-1.154} \times age^{-0.203} \times constant$$

For creatinine in μmol/L:

$$X = 32,788 \times creatinine^{-1.154} \times age^{-0.203} \times constant$$

where X is the glomerular filtration rate (GFR), constant for white males is 1 and for females is 0.742, and constant for African Americans is 1.21. Creatinine levels in μmol/L can be converted to mg/dL by dividing by 88.4.

▶ IDMS-Traceable MDRD Equation (Used Only With Creatinine Methods That Have Been Recalibrated to Be Traceable to IDMS)

For creatinine in mg/dL:

$$X = 175 \times creatinine^{-1.154} \times age^{-0.203} \times constant$$

For creatinine in μmol/L:

$$X = 175 \times (creatinine/88.4)^{-1.154} \times age^{-0.203} \times constant$$

where X is the GFR, constant for white males is 1 and for females is 0.742, and constant for African Americans is 1.21.

Ideal Body Weight

IBW is the weight expected for a nonobese person of a given height. The IBW formulas below and various life insurance tables can be used to estimate IBW. Dosing methods described in the literature may use IBW as a method in dosing obese patients.

Adults (age 18 years and older)[4]:

IBW (males) = 50 + (2.3 × height in inches over 5 ft)
IBW (females) = 45.5 + (2.3 × height in inches over 5 ft)

where IBW is in kilograms.

Children (age 1–18 years)[2]:
Under 5 ft tall:

$$IBW = \frac{height^2 \times 1.65}{1,000}$$

where IBW is in kilograms and height is in centimeters.

Five feet or taller:

IBW (males) = 39 + (2.27 × height in inches over 5 ft)
IBW (females) = 42.2 + (2.27 × height in inches over 5 ft)

where IBW is in kilograms.

REFERENCES

1. Cockcroft DW, Gault MH. Prediction of creatinine clearance from serum creatinine. Nephron 1976;16:31–41.
2. Traub SI, Johnson CE. Comparison of methods of estimating creatinine clearance in children. Am J Hosp Pharm 1980;37:195–201.
3. Levey AS, Bosch JP, Lewis JB, et al. A more accurate method to estimate glomerular filtration rate from serum creatinine: A new prediction equation. Modification of Diet in Renal Disease Study Group. Ann Intern Med 1999;130:461–470.
4. Devine BJ. Gentamicin therapy. Drug Intell Clin Pharm 1974;8:650–655.

Appendix B: Common Laboratory Tests

The following table is an alphabetical listing of some common laboratory tests and their reference ranges for adults as measured in plasma or serum (unless otherwise indicated). Reference values differ among laboratories, so readers should refer to the published reference ranges used in each institution. For some tests, both the Système International Units and Conventional Units are reported.

Lab	Conventional Units	Conversion Factor	Système International Units
Acid phosphatase			
Male	2–12 units/L	16.7	33–200 nkat/L
Female	0.3–9.2 units/L	16.7	5–154 nkat/L
Activated partial thromboplatin time (aPTT)	25–40 seconds		
Adrenocorticotropic hormone (ACTH)	15–80 pg/mL or ng/L	0.2202	3.3–17.6 pmol/L
Alanine aminotransferase (ALT, SGPT)	7–53 IU/L	0.01667	0.12–0.88 μkat/L
Albumin	3.5–5.0 g/dL	10	35–50 g/L
Albumin:creatinine ratio (urine)			
Normal	Less than 30 mg/g creatinine		
Microalbuminuria	30–300 mg/g creatinine		
Proteinuria	Greater than 300 mg/g creatinine		
or	or		
Normal			
Male	Less than 2.0 mg/mmol creatinine		
Female	Less than 2.8 mg/mmol creatinine		
Microalbuminuria			
Male	2.0–20 mg/mmol creatinine		
Female	2.8–28 mg/mmol creatinine		
Proteinuria			
Male	Greater than 20 mg/mmol creatinine		
Female	Greater than 28 mg/mmol creatinine		
Alcohol (ethanol) Blood alcohol level (BAL)	Legal limit: Less than 80 mg/dL (or less than 0.08%)	0.217	Less than 17.4 mmol/L
Aldosterone			
Supine	Less than 16 ng/dL	27.7	Less than 444 pmol/L
Upright	Less than 31 ng/dL	27.7	Less than 860 pmol/L
Alkaline phosphatase			
10–15 years	130–550 IU/L	0.01667	2.17–9.17 μkat/L
16–20 years	70–260 IU/L	0.01667	1.17–4.33 μkat/L
Greater than 20 years	38–126 IU/L	0.01667	0.13–2.10 μkat/L
a-fetoprotein (AFP)	Less than 15 ng/mL	1	Less than 15 mcg/L
a-1-antitrypsin	80–200 mg/dL	0.01	0.8–2.0 g/L

(Continued)

Lab	Conventional Units	Conversion Factor	Système International Units
Amikacin, therapeutic	15–30 mg/L peak	1.71	25.6–51.3 µmol/L peak
	Less than or equal to 8 mg/L trough		Less than or equal to 13.7 µmol/L trough
Amitriptyline	80–200 ng/mL or mcg/L	3.4	272–680 nmol/L
Ammonia (plasma)	15.33–56.20 mcg NH_3/dL	0.5872	9–33 µmol NH_3/L
Amylase	25–115 IU/L	0.01667	0.42–1.92 µkat/L
Androstenedione	50–250 ng/dL	0.0349	1.7–8.7 nmol/L
Angiotensin converting enzyme	15–70 units/L	16.67	250–1167 nkat/L
Anion gap	7–16 mEq/L	1	7–16 mmol/L
Anti-double stranded DNA (anti-ds DNA)	Negative		
Anti-HAV	Negative		
Anti-HBc	Negative		
Anti-HBs	Negative		
Anti-HCV	Negative		
Anti-Sm antibody	Negative		
Antinuclear antibody (ANA)	Negative		
Apolipoprotein A-1			
Male	95–175 mg/dL	0.01	0.95–1.75 g/L
Female	100–200 mg/dL	0.01	1.0–2.0 g/L
Apolipoprotein B			
Male	50–110 mg/dL	0.01	0.5–1.10 g/L
Female	50–105 mg/dL	0.01	0.5–1.05 g/L
Aspartate aminotransferase (AST, SGOT)	11–47 IU/L	0.01667	0.18–0.78 µkat/L
β_2-microglobulin	Less than 0.2 mg/dL	10	2 mg/L
Bicarbonate	22–26 mEq/L	1	22–26 mmol/L
Bilirubin			
Total	0.3–1.1 mg/dL	17.1	5.13–18.80 µmol/L
Direct	0–0.3 mg/dL	17.1	0–5.1 µmol/L
Indirect	0.1–1.0 mg/dL	17.1	1.71–17.1 µmol/L
Bleeding time	3–7 minutes		
Blood gases (arterial)			
pH	7.35–7.45	1	7.35–7.45
PO_2	80–105 mmHg	0.133	10.6–14.0 kPa
PCO_2	35–45 mmHg	0.133	4.7–6.0 kPa
HCO_3	22–26 mEq/L	1	22–26 mmol/L
O_2 saturation	Greater than or equal to 0.95	0.01	0.95
Blood urea nitrogen (BUN)	8–25 mg/dL	0.357	2.9–8.9 mmol/L
B-type natriuretic peptide (BNP)	0–99 pg/mL	1	0–99 ng/L
		Alternate SI: 0.289	0–29 pmol/L
Brain natriuretic peptide—N-terminal Pro (See Pro-BNP)			
BUN-to-creatinine ratio	10:1 to 20:1		
C-peptide	0.51–2.70 ng/mL	331	170–894 pmol/L
		0.331	0.17–0.89 nmol/L
C-reactive protein	Less than 0.8 mg/dL	10	Less than 8 mg/L
CA-125	Less than 35 units/mL	1	Less than 35 kU/L
CA 15–3	Less than 30 units/mL	1	Less than 30 kU/L
CA 19–9	Less than 37 units/mL	1	Less than 37 kU/L
CA 27.29	Less than 38 units/mL	1	Less than 38 kU/L
Calcium			
Total	8.6–10.3 mg/dL	0.25	2.15–2.58 mmol/L
	4.3–5.16 mEq/L	0.50	2.15–2.58 mmol/L
Ionized	4.5–5.1 mg/dL	0.25	1.13–1.28 mmol/L
	2.26–2.56 mEq/L	0.50	1.13–1.28 mmol/L

(Continued)

Lab	Conventional Units	Conversion Factor	Système International Units
Carbamazepine, therapeutic	4–12 mg/L	4.23	17–51 µmol/L
Carboxyhemoglobin (nonsmoker)	Less than 2%	0.01	Less than 0.02
Carcinoembryonic antigen (CEA)		1	
Nonsmokers	Less than 2.5 ng/mL		Less than 2.5 mcg/L
Smokers	Less than 5 ng/mL		Less than 5 mcg/L
CD4 lymphocyte count	31–61% of total lymphocytes		
CD8 lymphocyte count	18–39% of total lymphocytes		
Cerebrospinal fluid (CSF)			
Pressure	75–175 mm H_2O		
Glucose	40–70 mg/dL	0.0555	2.2–3.9 mmol/L
Protein	15–45 mg/dL	0.01	0.15–0.45 g/L
WBC	Less than 10/mm³		
Ceruloplasmin	18–45 mg/dL	10	180–450 mg/L
		0.063	1.1–2.8 µmol/L
Chloride	97–110 mEq/L	1	97–110 mmol/L
Cholesterol			
Desirable	Less than 200 mg/dL	0.0259	Less than 5.18 mmol/L
Borderline high	200–239 mg/dL	0.0259	5.18–6.19 mmol/L
High	Greater than or equal to 240 mg/dL	0.0259	Greater than or equal to 6.2 mmol/L
Chorionic gonadotropin (ß-hCG)	Less than 5 mU/mL	1	Less than 5 units/L
Clozapine	Minimum trough 300–350 ng/mL or mcg/L	3.06	918–1,071 nmol/L
		Alternate SI: 0.003	0.92–1.07 µmol/L
CO_2 content	22–30 mEq/L	1	22–30 mmol/L
Complement component 3 (C3)	70–160 mg/dL	0.01	0.7–1.6 g/L
Complement component 4 (C4)	20–40 mg/dL	0.01	0.2–0.4 g/L
Copper	70–150 mcg/dL	0.157	11–24 µmol/L
Cortisol (fasting, morning)	5–25 mcg/dL	27.6	138–690 nmol/L
Cortisol (free, urinary)	10–100 mcg/d	2.76	28–276 nmol/d
Creatine kinase			
Male	30–200 IU/L	0.01667	0.50–3.33 µkat/L
Female	20–170 IU/L	0.01667	0.33–2.83 µkat/L
MB fraction	0–7 IU/L	0.01667	0.0–0.12 µkat/L
Creatinine clearance (CrCL) (urine)	85–135 mL/minute/1.73 m²	0.00963	0.82–1.3 mL/s/m²
Creatinine			
Male 4–20 years	0.2–1.0 mg/dL	88.4	18–88 µmol/L
Female 4–20 years	0.2–1.0 mg/dL	88.4	18–88 µmol/L
Male (adults)	0.7–1.3 mg/dL	88.4	62–115 µmol/L
Female (adults)	0.6–1.1 mg/dL	88.4	53–97 µmol/L
Cyclosporine			
Renal, cardiac, liver, or pancreatic transplant	100–400 ng/mL or mcg/L	0.832	83–333 nmol/L
Cryptococcal antigen	Negative		
D-dimers	Less than 250 ng/mL	1	Less than 250 mcg/L
Desipramine	75–300 ng/mL or mcg/L	3.75	281–1125 nmol/L
Dexamethasone suppression test (DST) (overnight)	8:00 am cortisol less than 5 mcg/dL	0.0276	Less than 0.14 µmol/L
DHEAS (dehydroepiandrosterone sulfate)			
Male	170–670 mcg/dL	0.0271	4.6–18.2 µmol/L
Female			
Premenopausal	50–540 mcg/dL	0.0271	1.4–14.7 µmol/L
Postmenopausal	30–260 mcg/dL	0.0271	0.8–7.1 µmol/L

(Continued)

Lab	Conventional Units	Conversion Factor	Système International Units
Digoxin, therapeutic	0.5–1.0 ng/mL or mcg/L	1.28	0.6–1.3 nmol/L
Erythrocyte count (blood)			
See under Red Blood Cell count			
Erythrocyte sedimentation rate (ESR)			
Westergren			
Male	0–20 mm/h		
Female	0–30 mm/h		
Wintrobe			
Male	0–9 mm/h		
Female	0–15 mm/h		
Erythropoietin	2–25 mIU/mL	1	2–25 IU/L
Estradiol			
Male	10–36 pg/mL	3.67	37–132 pmol/L
Female	34–170 pg/mL	3.67	125–624 pmol/L
Ethanol, legal intoxication	Greater than or equal to 50–100 mg/dL	0.217	10.9–21.7 mmol/L
	Greater than or equal to 0.05–0.1%	217	
Ethosuccimide, therapeutic	40–100 mg/L or mcg/mL	7.08	283–708 µmol/L
Factor VIII or Factor IX			
Severe hemophilia	Less than 1 IU/dL	0.01	Less than 0.01 units/mL
Moderate hemophilia	1–5 IU/dL	0.01	0.01–0.05 units/mL
Mild hemophilia	Greater than 5 IU/dL	0.01	Greater than 0.05 units/mL
Usual adult levels	60 to 140 IU/dL	0.01	0.60 to 1.40 units/mL
Ferritin			
Male	20–250 ng/mL	1	20–250 mcg/L
Female	10–150 ng/mL	1	10–150 mcg/L
Fibrin degradation products (FDP)	2–10 mg/L		
Fibrinogen	200–400 mg/dL	0.01	2.0–4.0 g/L
Folate (plasma)	3.1–12.4 ng/mL	2.266	7.0–28.1 nmol/L
Folic acid (RBC)	125–600 ng/mL	2.266	283–1,360 nmol/L
Follicle-stimulating hormone (FSH)			
Male	1–7 mIU/mL	1	1–7 IU/L
Female			
Follicular phase	1–9 mIU/mL	1	1–9 IU/L
Midcycle	6–26 mIU/mL	1	6–26 IU/L
Luteal phase	1–9 mIU/mL	1	1–9 IU/L
Postmenopausal	30–118 mIU/mL	1	30–118 IU/L
Free thyroxine index (FT_4I)	6.5–12.5		
Gamma glutamyl transferase (GGT)	0–30 IU/L	0.01667	0–0.5 µkat/L
Gastrin (fasting)	0–130 pg/mL	1	0–130 ng/L
Gentamicin, therapeutic	4–10 mg/L peak	2.09	8.4–21 µmol/L peak
	Less than or equal to 2 mg/L trough		Less than or equal to 4.2 µmol/L trough
Globulin	2.3–3.5 g/dL	10	23–35 g/L
Glucose (fasting, plasma)	65–109 mg/dL	0.0555	3.6–6.00 mmol/L
Glucose, two hour postprandial blood (PPBG)	Less than 140 mg/dL	0.0555	Less than 7.8 mmol/L
Granulocyte count	$1.8–6.6 \times 10^3/mm^3$	10^6	$1.8–6.6 \times 10^9/L$
Growth hormone (fasting)			
Male	Less than 5 ng/mL	1	Less than 5 mcg/L
Female	Less than 10 ng/mL	1	Less than 10 mcg/L

(Continued)

Lab	Conventional Units	Conversion Factor	Système International Units
Haptoglobin	60–270 mg/dL	0.01	0.6–2.7 g/L
HBeAg	Negative		
HbsAg	Negative		
HBV DNA	Negative		
Hematocrit			
Male	40.7–50.3 %	0.01	0.407–0.503
Female	36.1–44.3 %	0.01	0.361–0.443
Hemoglobin (Blood)			
Male	13.8–17.2 g/dL	10	138–172 g/L
		Alternate SI: 0.62	8.56–10.67 mmol/L
Female	12.1–15.1 g/dL	10	121–151 g/L
		Alternate SI: 0.62	7.5–9.36 mmol/L
Hemoglobin A1c	4.0–6.0 %	0.01	0.04–0.06
Heparin			
Via protamine titration method	0.2–0.4 units/mL		
Via antifactor Xa assay	0.3–0.7 units/mL		
High-density lipoprotein (HDL) cholesterol	Greater than 35 mg/dL	0.0259	Greater than 0.91 mmol/L
Homocysteine	3.3–10.4 µmol/L		
Ibuprofen			
Therapeutic	10–50 mcg/mL	4.85	49–243 µmol/L
Toxic	100–700 mcg/mL or more	4.85	485–3,395 µmol/L or more
Imipramine, therapeutic	100–300 ng/mL or mcg/L	3.57	357–1,071 nmol/L
Immunoglobulin A (IgA)	85–385 mg/dL	0.01	0.85–3.85 g/L
Immunoglobulin G (IgG)	565–1,765 mg/dL	0.01	5.65–17.65 g/L
Immunoglobulin M (IgM)	53–375 mg/dL	0.01	0.53–3.75 g/L
Insulin (fasting)	2–20 µU/mL or mU/L	7.175	14.35–143.5 pmol/L
International normalized ratio (INR), therapeutic	2.0–3.0 (2.5–3.5 for some indications)		
Iron			
Male	45–160 mcg/dL	0.179	8.1–28.6 µmol/L
Female	30–160 mcg/dL	0.179	5.4–28.6 µmol/L
Iron binding capacity (Total)	220–420 mcg/dL	0.179	39.4–75.2 µmol/L
Iron saturation	15–50%	0.01	0.15–0.50
Itraconazole			
Trough, therapeutic	0.5–1 mcg/mL	1	0.5–1 mg/L
Lactate (plasma)	0.7–2.1 mEq/L	1	0.7–2.1 mmol/L
	6.3–18.9 mg/dL	0.111	
Lactate dehydrogenase (LDH)	100–250 IU/L	0.01667	1.67–4.17 µkat/L
Lead	Less than 25 mcg/dL	0.0483	Less than 1.21 µmol/L
Leukocyte count	$3.8–9.8 \times 10^3/mm^3$	10^6	$3.8–9.8 \times 10^9/L$
Lidocaine, therapeutic	1.5–6.0 mcg/mL or mg/L	4.27	6.4–25.6 µmol/L
Lipase	Less than 100 IU/L	0.01667	1.7 µkat/L
Lithium, therapeutic	0.5–1.25 mEq/L	1	0.5–1.25 mmol/L
Low-density lipoprotein (LDL) cholesterol			
Target for very high-risk patients	Less than 70 mg/dL	0.0259	Less than 1.81 mmol/L
Target for high-risk patients (optimal)	Less than 100 mg/dL	0.0259	Less than 2.59 mmol/L
Desirable	Less than 130 mg/dL	0.0259	Less than 3.36 mmol/L
Borderline high risk	130–159 mg/dL	0.0259	3.36–4.11 mmol/L
High risk	Greater than or equal to 160 mg/dL	0.0259	Greater than or equal to 4.13 mmol/L

(Continued)

Lab	Conventional Units	Conversion Factor	Système International Units
Luteinizing hormone (LH)			
Male	1–8 mU/mL	1	1–8 units/L
Female			
Follicular phase	1–12 mU/mL	1	1–12 units/L
Midcycle	16–104 mU/mL	1	16–104 units/L
Luteal phase	1–12 mU/mL	1	1–12 units/L
Postmenopausal	16–66 mU/mL	1	16–66 units/L
Lymphocyte count	$1.2–3.3 \times 10^3/mm^3$	10^6	$1.2–3.3 \times 10^9/L$
Magnesium	1.3–2.2 mEq/L	0.5	0.65–1.10 mmol/L
	1.58–2.68 mg/dL	0.411	0.65–1.10 mmol/L
Mean corpuscular volume	80.0–97.6 μm³	1	80.0–97.6 fl
Mononuclear cell count	$0.2–0.7 \times 10^3/mm^3$	10^6	$0.2–0.7 \times 10^9/L$
Nortriptyline, therapeutic	50–150 ng/mL or mcg/L	3.8	190–570 nmol/L
NT-ProBNP (see Pro-BNP)			
Osmolality (serum)	275–300 mOsm/kg	1	275–300 mmol/kg
Osmolality (urine)	250–900 mOsm/kg	1	250–900 mmol/kg
Parathyroid hormone (PTH), Intact	10–60 pg/mL or ng/L	0.107	1.1–6.4 pmol/L
PTH, N-terminal	8–24 pg/mL or ng/L		
PTH, C-terminal	50–330 pg/mL or ng/L		
Phenobarbital, therapeutic	15–40 mcg/mL or mg/L	4.31	65–172 μmol/L
Phenytoin, therapeutic	10–20 mcg/mL or mg/L	3.96	40–79 μmol/L
Phosphate	2.5–4.5 mg/dL	0.323	0.81–1.45 mmol/L
Platelet count	$140–440 \times 10^3/mm^3$	10^6	$140–440 \times 10^9/L$
Potassium (plasma)	3.3–4.9 mEq/L	1	3.3–4.9 mmol/L
Prealbumin (adult)	19.5–35.8 mg/dL	10	195–358 mg/L
Primidone, therapeutic	5–12 mcg/mL or mg/L	4.58	23–55 μmol/L
ProBNP	Less than 125 pg/mL or ng/L	0.118	Less than 14.75 pmol/L
Procainamide, therapeutic	4–10 mcg/mL or mg/L	4.23	17–42 μmol/L
Progesterone		0.0318	
Male	13–97 ng/dL		0.4–3.1 nmol/L
Female			
Follicular phase	15–70 ng/dL		0.5–2.2 nmol/L
Luteal phase	200–2,500 ng/dL		6.4–79.5 nmol/L
Prolactin	Less than 20 ng/mL	1	Less than 20 mcg/L
Prostate-specific antigen (PSA)	Less than 4 ng/mL	1	Less than 4 mcg/L
Protein, total	6.0–8.0 g/dL	10	60–80 g/L
Prothrombin time (PT)	10–12 seconds		
Quinidine, therapeutic	2–5 mcg/mL or mg/L	3.08	6.2–15.4 μmol/L
Radioactive iodine uptake (RAIU)	Less than 6% in 2 hours		
Red blood cell (RBC) count (blood)			
Male	$4–6.2 \times 10^6/mm^3$	10^6	$4–6.2 \times 10^{12}/L$
Female	$4–6.2 \times 10^6/mm^3$	10^6	$4–6.2 \times 10^{12}/L$
Pregnant			
Trimester 1	$4–5 \times 10^6/mm^3$	10^6	$4–5 \times 10^{12}/L$
Trimester 2	$3.2–4.5 \times 10^6/mm^3$	10^6	$3.2–4.5 \times 10^{12}/L$
Trimester 3	$3–4.9 \times 10^6/mm^3$	10^6	$3–4.9 \times 10^{12}/L$
Postpartum	$3.2–5 \times 10^6/mm^3$	10^6	$3.2–5 \times 10^{12}/L$
Red blood cell distribution width (RDW)	11.5–14.5%	0.01	0.115–0.145
Reticulocyte count			
Male	0.5–1.5% of total RBC count	0.01	0.005–0.015
Female	0.5–2.5% of total RBC count	0.01	0.005–0.025

(Continued)

Lab	Conventional Units	Conversion Factor	Système International Units
Retinol-binding protein (RBP)	2.7–7.6 mg/dL	10	27–76 mg/L
Rheumatoid factor (RF) titer	Negative		
Salicylate, therapeutic	150–300 mcg/mL or mg/L	0.00724	1.09–2.17 mmol/L
	15–30 mg/dL	0.0724	
Sirolimus (renal transplant)	4–20 ng/mL	1	4–20 mcg/L
Sodium	135–145 mEq/L	1	135–145 mmol/L
Tacrolimus			
Renal, cardiac, liver, or pancreatic transplant	5–20 ng/mL	1	5–20 mcg/L
Testosterone (total)		0.0347	
Men	300–950 ng/dL		10.4–33.0 nmol/L
Women	20–80 ng/dL		0.7–2.8 nmol/L
Testosterone (free)		0.0347	
Men	9–30 ng/dL		0.31–1.04 nmol/L
Women	0.3–1.9 ng/dL		0.01–0.07 nmol/L
Theophylline			
Therapeutic	5–15 mcg/mL or mg/L	5.55	28–83 μmol/L
Toxic	20 or more mcg/mL or mg/L	5.55	111 or more μmol/L
Thiocyanate	Toxic level unclear. Units are mcg/mL or mg/L	17.2	μmol/L
Thrombin time	20–24 seconds		
Thyroglobulin	Less than 42 ng/mL	1	Less than 42 mcg/L
Thyroglobulin antibodies	Negative		
Thyroxine-binding globulin (TBG)	1.2–2.5 mg/dL	10	12–25 mcg/L
Thyroid-stimulating hormone (TSH)	0.35–6.20 μU/mL	1	0.35–6.20 mU/L
TSH receptor antibodies (TSH Rab)	0–1 units/mL		
Thyroxine (T_4)			
Total	4.5–12.0 mcg/dL	12.87	58–154 nmol/L
Free	0.7–1.9 ng/dL	12.87	9.0–24.5 pmol/L
Thyroxine index, free (FT_4I)	6.5–12.5		
TIBC—see Iron Binding Capacity (total)			
Tobramycin, therapeutic	4–10 mcg/mL or mg/L peak	2.14	8.6–21.4 μmol/L
	Less than or equal to 2 mcg/mL or mg/L trough	2.14	Less than or equal to 4.28 μmol/L
Transferrin	200–430 mg/dL	0.01	2.0–4.3 g/L
Transferrin saturation	30–50%	0.01	0.30–0.50
Triglycerides (fasting)	Less than 160 mg/dL	0.0113	Less than 1.8 mmol/L
Triiodothyronine (T_3)	45–132 ng/dL	0.0154	0.91–2.70 nmol/L
Triiodothyronine (T_3) resin uptake	25–35%		
Uric acid	3–8 mg/dL	59.48	179–476 μmol/L
Urinalysis (urine)			
pH	4.8–8.0		
Specific gravity	1.005–1.030		
Protein	Negative		
Glucose	Negative		
Ketones	Negative		
RBC	1–2 per low-power field		
WBC	3–4 per low-power field		
Valproic acid, therapeutic	50–100 mcg/mL or mg/L	6.93	346–693 μmol/L

(Continued)

Lab	Conventional Units	Conversion Factor	Système International Units
Vancomycin, therapeutic	20–40 mcg/mL or mg/L peak	0.690	14–28 µmol/L peak
	5–20 mcg/mL or mg/L trough	0.690	3–14 µmol/L trough
Trough for CNS infections	15–20 mcg/mL or mg/L trough	0.690	10–14 µmol/L trough
Vitamin A (retinol)	30–95 mcg/dL	0.0349	1.05–3.32 µmol/L
Vitamin B$_{12}$	180–1,000 pg/mL	0.738	133–738 pmol/L
Vitamin D$_3$, 1, 25-dihydroxy	20–76 pg/mL	2.4	48–182 pmol/L
Vitamin D$_3$, 25-hydroxy	10–50 ng/mL	2.496	25–125 nmol/L
Vitamin E (a-tocopherol)	0.5–2.0 mg/dL	23.22	12–46 µmol/L
WBC count	$4–10 \times 10^3/mm^3$	10^6	$4–10 \times 10^9/L$
WBC differential (peripheral blood)			
Polymorphonuclear neutrophils (PMNs)	50–65%		
Bands	0–5%		
Eosinophils	0–3%		
Basophils	1–3%		
Lymphocytes	25–35%		
Monocytes	2–6%		
WBC differential (bone marrow)			
Polymorphonuclear neutrophils (PMNs)	3–11%		
Bands	9–15%		
Metamyelocytes	9–25%		
Myelocytes	8–16%		
Promyelocytes	1–8%		
Myeloblasts	0–5%		
Eosinophils	1–5%		
Basophils	0–1%		
Lymphocytes	11–23%		
Monocytes	0–1%		
Zinc	60–150 mcg/dL	0.153	9.2–23.0 µmol/L

This table is a modification of the Medical Algorithms Project (Chapter 40), unit conversions of the following Excel worksheets: Conversion of Conventional to SI units: Blood Chemistries; Conversion of Conventional to SI units: Urine Chemistries; Conversion of Conventional to SI units: Hematology and Coagulation; and Conversion of Conventional to SI units: Therapeutic Drug Monitoring. Available at http://www.medal.org/visitor/www\Inactive\ch40.aspx; accessed March 30, 2009.

Other references (conventional and SI units from the preceding table were double-checked against the following references and modified as needed):

Système International (SI) Conversion Table. JAMA 2005;294(1):119. Available at http://jama.ama-assn.org/cgi/content/full/294/1/119/DC6; accessed March 31, 2009.

A–Z Health Guide from WebMD. Medical Tests: Brain Natriuretic Peptide (BNP) Test. Available at http://www.webmd.com/heart-disease/brain-natriuretic-peptide-bnp-test?page=2; accessed March 31, 2009.

proBNP ©2005 Roche Diagnostics Roche Diagnostics GmbH, D-68298 Mannheim

Laboratory Test Handbook (DS Jacobs, DK Oxley, WR DeMott, eds.) Lexi-Comp, Inc., Hudson OH.

Reviewed and updated by: Edward W. Randell and Rebecca M.T. Law

Appendix C: Common Medical Abbreviations

These are the abbreviations used commonly in medical practice both in verbal communication and in the medical record.

AA	Aplastic anemia; alcoholics anonymous	ALT	Alanine transaminase (SGPT); alanine aminotransferase
AAA	Abdominal aortic aneurysm	AMA	Against medical advice; American Medical Association; antimitochondrial antibody
AAO	Awake, alert, and oriented		
AAO×3	Awake and orientated to time, place, and person	AMI	Acute myocardial infarction
ABC	Absolute band counts; absolute basophil count; apnea, bradycardia, and cytology; aspiration, biopsy, and cytology; artificial beta cells	AML	Acute myelogenous leukemia
		Amp	Ampule
		ANA	Antinuclear antibody
Abd	Abdomen	ANC	Absolute neutrophil count
ABG	Arterial blood gases	ANLL	Acute nonlymphocytic leukemia
ABO	Blood group system (A, AB, B, and O)	A&O	Alert and oriented
ABP	Arterial blood pressure	AODM	Adult-onset diabetes mellitus
ABW	Actual body weight	AOM	Acute otitis media
ABx	Antibiotics	A&O×3	Awake and oriented to person, place, and time
AC	Before meals (*ante cibos*)	A&O×4	Awake and oriented to person, place, time, and situation
A1C	Hemoglobin A1C		
ACE	Angiotensin-converting enzyme	AP	Anteroposterior
ACE-I	Angiotensin-converting enzyme inhibitor	A&P	Active and present; anterior and posterior; assessment and plans; auscultation and percussion
ACLS	Advanced cardiac life support		
ACS	Acute coronary syndromes	APAP	Acetaminophen (acetyl-*p*-aminophenol)
ACTH	Adrenocorticotropic hormone	aPTT	Activated partial thromboplastin time
AD	Alzheimer's disease; right ear (*auris dextra*)	ARB	Angiotensin receptor blocker
ADA	American Diabetes Association; adenosine deaminase	ARC	AIDS-related complex
		ARD	Acute respiratory disease; adult respiratory disease; antibiotic removal device; aphakic retinal detachment
ADE	Adverse drug effect (or event)		
ADH	Antidiuretic hormone		
ADHD	Attention-deficit hyperactivity disorder	ARDS	Adult respiratory distress syndrome
ADL	Activities of daily living	ARF	Acute renal failure; acute respiratory failure; acute rheumatic fever
ADR	Adverse drug reaction		
AF	Atrial fibrillation	AROM	Active range of motion
AFB	Acid-fast bacillus; aortofemoral bypass; aspirated foreign body	AS	Left ear (*auris sinistra*)
		ASA	Aspirin (acetylsalicylic acid)
AFEB	Afebrile	ASCVD	Arteriosclerotic cardiovascular disease
AI	Aortic insufficiency	ASD	Atrial septal defect
AIDS	Acquired immune deficiency syndrome	ASH	Asymmetric septal hypertrophy
AKA	Above-knee amputation; alcoholic ketoacidosis; all known allergies; also known as	ASHD	Arteriosclerotic heart disease
		AST	Aspartate transaminase (SCOT); aspartate aminotransferase
ALFT	Abnormal liver function test		
ALL	Acute lymphoblastic leukemia; acute lymphocytic leukemia	ATG	Antithymocyte globulin
		ATN	Acute tubular necrosis
ALP	Alkaline phosphatase	AU	Each ear (*auris uterque*)
ALS	Amyotrophic lateral sclerosis		

AV	Arteriovenous; atrioventricular; auditory visual	CMV	Cytomegalovirus
AVR	Aortic valve replacement	CN	Cranial nerve
A&W	Alive and well	CNS	Central nervous system
BBB	Bundle-branch block; blood–brain barrier	C/O	Complains of
BC	Blood culture	CO	Cardiac output; carbon monoxide
BCOP	Board Certified Oncology Pharmacist	COLD	Chronic obstructive lung disease
BCP	Birth control pill	COPD	Chronic obstructive pulmonary disease
BCPP	Board Certified Psychiatric Pharmacist	CP	Chest pain; cerebral palsy
BCPS	Board Certified Pharmacotherapy Specialist	CPAP	Continuous positive airway pressure
BE	Barium enema	CPK	Creatine phosphokinase (BB, MB, and MM are isoenzymes)
bid	Twice daily (*bis in die*)		
BKA	Below-knee amputation	CPP	Cerebral perfusion pressure
BM	Bone marrow; bowel movement; an isoenzyme of creatine phosphokinase	CPR	Cardiopulmonary resuscitation
		CrCl	Creatinine clearance
BMC	Bone marrow cells	CRF	Chronic renal failure; corticotropin-releasing factor
BMD	Bone mineral density		
BMR	Basal metabolic rate	CRH	Corticotropin-releasing hormone
BMT	Bone marrow transplantation	CRI	Chronic renal insufficiency; catheter-related infection
BP	Blood pressure		
BPD	Bronchopulmonary dysplasia	CRNA	Certified Registered Nurse Anesthetist
BPH	Benign prostatic hyperplasia	CRNP	Certified Registered Nurse Practitioner
bpm	Beats per minute	CRTT	Certified Respiratory Therapy Technician
BR	Bed rest	CSF	Cerebrospinal fluid; colony-stimulating factor
BS	Bowel sounds; breath sounds; blood sugar	CT	Computed tomography; chest tube
BSA	Body surface area	cTnI	Cardiac troponin I
BUN	Blood urea nitrogen	CTZ	Chemoreceptor trigger zone
Bx	Biopsy	CV	Cardiovascular
C&S	Culture and sensitivity	CVA	Cerebrovascular accident
CA	Cancer; calcium	CVC	Central venous catheter
CABG	Coronary artery bypass grafting	CVP	Central venous pressure
CAD	Coronary artery disease	Cx	Culture; cervix
CAH	Chronic active hepatitis	CXR	Chest x-ray
CAM	Complementary and alternative medicine	D&C	Dilatation and curettage
CAPD	Continuous ambulatory peritoneal dialysis	D_5W	5% Dextrose in water
CBC	Complete blood count	DBP	Diastolic blood pressure
CBD	Common bile duct	D/C	Discontinue; discharge
CBG	Capillary blood gas; corticosteroid-binding globulin	DCC	Direct-current cardioversion
		DI	Diabetes insipidus
CC	Chief complaint	DIC	Disseminated intravascular coagulation
CCA	Calcium channel antagonist	Diff	Differential
CCB	Calcium channel blocker	DJD	Degenerative joint disease
CCE	Clubbing, cyanosis, edema	DKA	Diabetic ketoacidosis
CCK	Cholecystokinin	dL	Deciliter
CCU	Coronary care unit	DM	Diabetes mellitus
CF	Cystic fibrosis	DNA	Deoxyribonucleic acid
CFS	Chronic fatigue syndrome	DNR	Do not resuscitate
CFU	Colony-forming unit	DO	Doctor of Osteopathy
CHD	Coronary heart disease	DOA	Dead on arrival; date of admission; duration of action
CHF	Congestive heart failure; chronic heart failure		
CHO	Carbohydrate	DOB	Date of birth
CI	Cardiac index	DOE	Dyspnea on exertion
CK	Creatine kinase	DOT	Directly observed therapy
CKD	Chronic kidney disease	DPGN	Diffuse proliferative glomerulonephritis
CLL	Chronic lymphocytic leukemia	DRE	Digital rectal examination
CM	Costal margin	DRG	Diagnosis-related group
CMG	Cystometrogram	DS	Double strength
CML	Chronic myelogenous leukemia	DTP	Diphtheria-tetanus-pertussis

DTR	Deep-tendon reflex	GGTP	γ-Glutamyl transpeptidase
DVT	Deep-vein thrombosis	GI	Gastrointestinal
Dx	Diagnosis	GM-CSF	Granulocyte-macrophage colony-stimulating factor
EBV	Epstein-Barr virus		
EC	Enteric-coated	GN	Glomerulonephritis; graduate nurse
ECG	Electrocardiogram	gr	Grain
ECHO	Echocardiogram	GT	Gastrostomy tube
ECT	Electroconvulsive therapy	gtt	Drops (*guttae*)
ED	Emergency department	GTT	Glucose tolerance test
EEG	Electroencephalogram	GU	Genitourinary
EENT	Eyes, ears, nose, throat	GVHD	Graft-versus-host disease
EF	Ejection fraction	GVL	Graft-versus-leukemia
EGD	Esophagogastroduodenoscopy	Gyn	Gynecology
EIA	Enzyme immunoassay	HAART	Highly-active antiretroviral therapy
EKG	Electrocardiogram	HAMD	Hamilton Rating Scale for Depression
EMG	Electromyogram	H/A	Headache
EMT	Emergency Medical Technician	HAV	Hepatitis A virus
Endo	Endotracheal, endoscopy	Hb, hgb	Hemoglobin
EOMI	Extraocular movements (or muscles) intact	HbA_{1c}	Glycosylated hemoglobin (hemoglobin A_{1c})
EPO	Erythropoietin	HBIG	Hepatitis B immune globulin
EPS	Extrapyramidal symptoms	HBP	High blood pressure
ER	Emergency room	HBsAg	Hepatitis B surface antigen
ERCP	Endoscopic retrograde cholangiopancreatography	HBV	Hepatitis B virus
		HC	Hydrocortisone, home care
ERT	Estrogen-replacement therapy	HCG	Human chorionic gonadotropin
ESLD	End-stage liver disease	HCO_3	Bicarbonate
ESR	Erythrocyte sedimentation rate	Hct	Hematocrit
ESRD	End-stage renal disease	HCTZ	Hydrochlorothiazide
ET	Endotracheal	HCV	Hepatitis C virus
EtOH	Ethanol	HD	Hodgkin's disease; hemodialysis
FB	Finger-breadth; foreign body	HDL	High-density lipoprotein
FBS	Fasting blood sugar	HEENT	Head, eyes, ears, nose, and throat
FDA	Food and Drug Administration	HF	Heart failure
FEF	Forced expiratory flow rate	H flu	*Hemophilus influenzae*
FEV_1	Forced expiratory volume in 1 second	HGH	Human growth hormone
FFP	Fresh-frozen plasma	HH	Hiatal hernia
FH	Family history	H&H	Hemoglobin and hematocrit
FiO_2	Fraction of inspired oxygen	Hib	*Hemophilus influenzae* type b
FOBT	Fecal occult blood test	HIV	Human immunodeficiency virus
FPG	Fasting plasma glucose	HJR	Hepatojugular reflux
FPIA	Fluorescence polarization immunoassay	HLA	Human leukocyte antigen; human lymphocyte antigen
FSH	Follicle-stimulating hormone		
FTA	Fluorescent treponemal antibody	HMG-CoA	Hydroxy-methylglutaryl coenzyme A
F/U	Follow-up	H/O	History of
FUO	Fever of unknown origin	HOB	Head of bed
Fx	Fracture	H&P	History and physical examination
G-CSF	Granulocyte colony-stimulating factor	HPA	Hypothalamic-pituitary axis
G6PD	Glucose-6-phosphate dehydrogenase	HPI	History of present illness
GB	Gall bladder	HR	Heart rate
GBS	Group B *Streptococcus;* Guillain-Barré syndrome	HRSD	Hamilton Rating Scale for Depression
		HRT	Hormone-replacement therapy
GC	Gonococcus	HS	At bedtime (*hora somni*)
GDM	Gestational diabetes mellitus	HSV	Herpes simplex virus
GE	Gastroesophageal; gastroenterology	HTN	Hypertension
GERD	Gastroesophageal reflux disease	Hx	History
GFR	Glomerular filtration rate	IBD	Inflammatory bowel disease
GGT	γ-Glutamyl transferase	IBW	Ideal body weight

ICD	Implantable cardioverter defibrillator		LLQ	Left lower quadrant (abdomen)
ICP	Intracranial pressure		LMD	Local medical doctor
ICS	Intercostal space		LMP	Last menstrual period
ICU	Intensive-care unit		LMWH	Low-molecular-weight heparin
ID	Identification; infectious disease		LOS	Length of stay
I&D	Incision and drainage		LP	Lumbar puncture
IDDM	Insulin-dependent diabetes mellitus		LPN	Licensed Practical Nurse
IFN	Interferon		LPT	Licensed Physical Therapist
Ig	Immunoglobulin		LR	Lactated Ringer's
IgA	Immunoglobulin A		LS	Lumbosacral
IgD	Immunoglobulin D		LUE	Left upper extremity
IHD	Ischemic heart disease		LUL	Left upper lobe
IJ	Internal jugular		LUQ	Left upper quadrant
IM	Intramuscular; infectious mononucleosis		LVH	Left ventricular hypertrophy
INH	Isoniazid		MAP	Mean arterial pressure
INR	International normalized ratio		MAR	Medication administration record
I&O	Intake and output		MB-CK	A creatine kinase isoenzyme
IOP	Intraocular pressure		mcg	Microgram
IP	Intraperitoneal		MCH	Mean corpuscular hemoglobin
IPG	Impedance plethysmography		MCHC	Mean corpuscular hemoglobin concentration
IPN	Interstitial pneumonia		MCV	Mean corpuscular volume
IRB	Institutional Review Board		MD	Medical Doctor
ISA	Intrinsic sympathomimetic activity		MDI	Metered-dose inhaler
ISH	Isolated systolic hypertension		MEFR	Maximum expiratory flow rate
IT	Intrathecal		mEq	Milliequivalent
ITP	Idiopathic thrombocytopenic purpura		mg	Milligram
IU	International units		MHC	Major histocompatibility complex
IUD	Intrauterine device		MI	Myocardial infarction; mitral insufficiency
IV	Intravenous; Roman numeral four; symbol for class 4 controlled substances		MIC	Minimum inhibitory concentration
			mL	Milliliter
IVC	Inferior vena cava; intravenous cholangiogram		MM	Multiple myeloma; an isoenzyme of creatine phosphokinase
IVDA	Intravenous drug abuse			
IVF	Intravenous fluids		MMR	Measles-mumps-rubella; midline malignant reticulosis
IVIG	Intravenous immunoglobulin			
IVP	Intravenous pyelogram; intravenous push		MOM	Milk of magnesia
JODM	Juvenile-onset diabetes mellitus		MPV	Mean platelet volume
JRA	Juvenile rheumatoid arthritis		m/r/g	Murmur/rub/gallop
JVD	Jugular venous distension		MRI	Magnetic resonance imaging
JVP	Jugular venous pressure		MRSA	Methicillin-resistant *Staphylococcus aureus*
K	Potassium		MRSE	Methicillin-resistant *Staphylococcus epidermitis*
kcal	Kilocalorie			
KCL	Potassium chloride		MS	Mental status; mitral stenosis; musculoskeletal; multiple sclerosis; morphine sulfate
KOH	Potassium hydroxide			
KUB	Kidney, ureter, and bladder		MSE	Mental status exam
KVO	Keep vein open		MSW	Master of Social Work
L	Liter		MTD	Maximum tolerated dose
LAD	Left anterior descending; left axis deviation		MIX	Methotrexate
LAO	Left anterior oblique		MVA	Motor vehicle accident
LBBB	Left bundle branch block		MVI	Multivitamin
LBP	Low-back pain		MVR	Mitral valve replacement; mitral valve regurgitation
LDH	Lactate dehydrogenase			
LDL	Low-density lipoprotein		MVS	mitral valve stenosis; motor, vascular, and sensory
LE	Lower extremity			
LES	Lower esophageal sphincter		N&V	Nausea and vomiting
LET	Liver function test		NAD	No acute (or apparent) distress
LHRH	Luteinizing hormone-releasing hormone		N/C	Noncontributory; nasal cannula
LLE	Left lower extremity		NG	Nasogastric
LLL	Left lower lobe		NGT	Nasogastric tube; normal glucose tolerance

NIDDM	Non-insulin-dependent diabetes mellitus	PERRLA	Pupils equal, round, and reactive to light and accommodation
NIH	National Institutes of Health	PERRRLA	Pupils equal, round, regular, and react to light and accommodation
NKA	No known allergies		
NKDA	No known drug allergies	PET	Positron-emission tomography
NHDA	Nonketotic hyperosmolar acidosis	PFT	Pulmonary function test
NL	Normal	pH	Hydrogen ion concentration
NOS	Not otherwise specified	PH	Past history; personal history; pinhole; poor health; pubic hair; public health
NPN	Nonprotein nitrogen		
NPO	Nothing by mouth (*nil per os*)	PHx	Past history
NS	Normal saline solution (0.9% sodium chloride solution); neurosurgery	PharmD	Doctor of Pharmacy
		PID	Pelvic inflammatory disease
NSAID	Nonsteroidal anti-inflammatory drug	PKU	Phenylketonuria
NSR	Normal sinus rhythm	PMH	Past medical history
NSS	Normal saline solution	PMI	Past medical illness; point of maximal impulse
NTG	Nitroglycerin	PMN	Polymorphonuclear leukocyte
NT/ND	Nontender, nondistended	PMS	Premenstrual syndrome
NVD	Nausea/vomiting/diarrhea; neck vein distension; neovascularization of the disk; neurovesicle dysfunction; nonvalvular disease	PND	Paroxysmal nocturnal dyspnea
		po	By mouth (*per os*)
		Po_2	Partial pressure of oxygen
N&V	Nausea and vomiting	POAG	Primary open-angle glaucoma
NYHA	New York Heart Association	POD	Postoperative day
O&P	Ova and parasites	PPBG	Postprandial blood glucose
OA	Osteoarthritis	ppd	Packs per day
OB	Obstetrics	PPN	Peripheral parenteral nutrition
OCD	Obsessive–compulsive disorder	Pr	Per rectum
OD	Right eye (*oculus dexter*)	PRBC	Packed red blood cells
OGT	Oral glucose tolerance test	PRERLA	Pupils round, equal, react to light and accommodation
OPV	Oral poliovirus vaccine		
OR	Operating room	PRN	When necessary, as needed (*pro re nata*)
OR×1	Oriented to time	PSA	Prostate-specific antigen
OR×2	Oriented to time and place	PSH	Past surgical history
OR×3	Oriented to time, place, and person	PST	Paroxysmal supraventricular tachycardia
OS	Left eye (*oculus sinister*)	PSVT	Paroxysmal supraventricular tachycardia
OT	Occupational therapy	PT	Prothrombin time; physical therapy; patient
OTC	Over-the-counter	P&T	Peak and trough
OU	*Oculus uterque* (each eye)	PTA	Prior to admission; percutaneous transluminal angioplasty
P	Pulse; plan; percussion; pressure		
PA	Physician Assistant; posteroanterior; pulmonary artery	PTCA	Percutaneous transluminal coronary angioplasty
P&A	Percussion and auscultation	PTE	Pulmonary thromboembolism
PAC	Premature atrial contraction	PTH	Parathyroid hormone
$Paco_2$	Arterial carbon dioxide tension	PTSD	Posttraumatic stress disorder
Pao_2	Arterial oxygen tension	PTT	Partial thromboplastin time
PAOP	Pulmonary artery occlusion pressure	PUD	Peptic ulcer disease
PC	After meals (*post cibum*)	PVC	Premature ventricular contraction
PCA	Patient-controlled analgesia	PVD	Peripheral vascular disease
PCI	Percutaneous coronary intervention	PVR	Peripheral vascular resistance
PCKD	Polycystic kidney disease	PVT	Paroxysmal ventricular tachycardia
PCN	Penicillin	q	Every (*quaque*)
PCP	*Pneumocystis carinii* pneumonia; phencyclidine	QA	Quality assurance
		qd	Every day (*quaque die*)
PCWP	Pulmonary capillary wedge pressure	QI	Quality improvement
PDE	Paroxysmal dyspnea on exertion	qid	Four times daily (*quater in die*)
PE	Physical examination; pulmonary embolism	QNS	Quantity not sufficient
PEEP	Positive end-expiratory pressure	qod	Every other day
PEER	Peak expiratory flow rate	QOL	Quality of life
PEG	Percutaneous endoscopic gastrostomy; polyethylene glycol	QS	Quantity sufficient
PERL	Pupils equal, react to light		

RA	Rheumatoid arthritis; right atrium	SIDS	Sudden infant death syndrome
RBC	Red blood cell	SJS	Stevens-Johnson syndrome
RCA	Right coronary artery	SL	Sublingual
RCM	Right costal margin	SLE	Systemic lupus erythematosus
RDA	Recommended daily allowance	SMA-6	Sequential multiple analyzer for sodium, potassium, CO_2, chloride, glucose, and BUN
RDS	Respiratory distress syndrome		
RDW	Red cell distribution width	SMA-7	Sodium, potassium, CO_2, chloride, glucose, BUN, and creatinine
REM	Rapid eye movement; recent event memory		
RES	Reticuloendothelial system	SMA-12	Glucose, BUN, uric acid, calcium, phosphorous, total protein, albumin, cholesterol, total bilirubin, alkaline phosphatase, SCOT, and LDH
RF	Rheumatoid factor; renal failure; rheumatic fever		
Rh	Rhesus factor in blood	SMA-23	Includes the entire SMA-12 plus sodium, potassium, CO_2, chloride, direct bilirubin, triglyceride, SGPT, indirect bilirubin, R fraction, and BUN/creatinine ratio
RHD	Rheumatic heart disease		
RLE	Right lower extremity		
RLL	Right lower lobe		
RLQ	Right lower quadrant		
R&M	Routine and microscopic	SMBG	Self-monitoring of blood glucose
RML	Right middle lobe	SNF	Skilled nursing facility
RN	Registered Nurse	SNS	Sympathetic nervous system
RNA	Ribonucleic acid	SOB	Shortness of breath; see order book; side of bed
R/O	Rule out		
ROM	Range of motion	S/P	Status post
ROS	Review of systems	SPF	Sun protection factor
RPh	Registered Pharmacist	SQ	Subcutaneous
RR	Respiratory rate; recovery room	SSKI	Saturated solution of potassium iodide
R&R	Rate and rhythm	SSRI	Selective serotonin reuptake inhibitor
RRR	Regular rate and rhythm	STAT	Immediately, at once
RRT	Registered Respiratory Therapist	STD	Sexually transmitted disease
RSV	Respiratory syncytial virus	SV	Stroke volume
RT	Radiation therapy	SVC	Superior vena cava
RUE	Right upper extremity	SVRI	Systemic vascular resistance index
RUL	Right upper lobe	SVR	Supraventricular rhythm; systemic vascular resistance
RUQ	Right upper quadrant		
RVH	Right ventricular hypertrophy	SVT	Supraventricular tachycardia
S_1	First heart sound	SW	Social worker
S_2	Second heart sound	Sx	Signs
S_3	Third heart sound (ventricular gallop)	T	Temperature
S_4	Fourth heart sound (atrial gallop)	T&A	Tonsillectomy and adenoidectomy
SA	Sinoatrial	TB	Tuberculosis
SAD	Seasonal affective disorder	TBG	Thyroid-binding globulin
SAH	Subarachnoid hemorrhage	TBI	Total-body irradiation; traumatic brain injury
SaO_2	Arterial oxygen percent saturation		
SBE	Subacute bacterial endocarditis	T bili	Total bilirubin
SBFT	Small bowel follow-through	T&C	Type and crossmatch
SBGM	Self blood glucose monitoring	TCA	Tricyclic antidepressant
SBO	Small bowel obstruction	TCN	Tetracycline
SBP	Systolic blood pressure	TFT	Thyroid function test
SC	Subcutaneous; subclavian	TG	Triglyceride
SCr	Serum creatinine	TIA	Transient ischemic attack
SEM	Systolic ejection murmur	TIBC	Total iron-binding capacity
SG	Specific gravity	TID	Three times daily (*ter in die*)
SGOT (AST)	Serum glutamic oxaloacetic transaminase (aspartate transaminase)	TLC	Therapeutic lifestyle changes
		TMJ	Temporomandibular joint
SGPT (ALT)	Serum glutamic pyruvic transaminase (alanine transaminase)	TMP-SMX	Trimethoprim-sulfamethoxazole
		TNTC	Too numerous to count
SH	Social history	TOD	Target-organ damage
SIADH	Syndrome of inappropriate antidiuretic hormone secretion	TPN	Total parenteral nutrition
		TPR	Temperature, pulse, respiration

T PROT	Total protein
TSH	Thyroid-stimulating hormone
TURP	Transurethral resection of the prostate
Tx	Treat, treatment
UA	Urinalysis, uric acid
UC	Ulcerative colitis
UE	Upper extremity
UGI	Upper gastrointestinal
UOQ	Upper outer quadrant
UPT	Urine pregnancy test
URI	Upper respiratory infection
USP	United States Pharmacopeia
UTI	Urinary tract infection
UV	Ultraviolet
VF	Ventricular fibrillation
VLDL	Very low-density lipoprotein
VO	Verbal order

VOD	Veno-occlusive disease
V_A/Q	Ventilation-perfusion
VRE	Vancomycin-resistant *Enterococcus*
VS	Vital signs
VSS	Vital signs stable
VT	Ventricular tachycardia
VTE	Venous thromboembolism
WA	While awake
WBC	White blood cell (count)
W/C	Wheelchair
WDWN	Well-developed, well-nourished
WHO	World Health Organization
WNL	Within normal limits
W/U	Workup
yo	Year-old
yr	Year

Appendix D: Glossary

Ablation: Destruction of part or all of an organ or structure.

Abscess: A purulent (i.e., containing, discharging, or causing the production of pus) collection of fluid separated from surrounding tissue by a wall composed of inflammatory cells and adjacent organs. It usually contains necrotic debris, bacteria, and inflammatory cells.

Acanthosis nigricans: A skin condition characterized by dark, thickened, velvety patches, especially in the folds of skin in the armpits, groin, and back of the neck that is often associated with insulin resistance.

Acaricide: A chemical that kills mites and ticks.

Acetaldehyde: A by-product of alcohol metabolism.

Acetylcholinesterase: An enzyme that breaks down unused acetylcholine in the synaptic cleft. This enzyme is necessary to restore the synaptic cleft so it is ready to transmit the next nerve impulse

Achlorhydria: Low level or absence of gastric acid in the stomach.

Acidemia: An increase in the hydrogen ion concentration in the blood or a fall below normal in pH.

Acidosis: Any pathologic state that leads to acidemia.

Acromegaly: A pathologic condition characterized by excessive production of growth hormone during adulthood after epiphyseal (growth plate) fusions have completed.

Action potential: A rapid change in the polarity of the voltage of a cell membrane from negative to positive and back to negative. A wave of electrical discharge that travels across a cell membrane.

Acute chest syndrome: An acute respiratory complication of sickle cell disease characterized by chest pain, fever, and pulmonary infiltrates.

Acute coronary syndromes: Ischemic chest discomfort at rest most often accompanied by ST-segment elevation, ST-segment depression, or T-wave inversion on the 12-lead electrocardiogram; further, it is caused by plaque rupture and partial or complete occlusion of the coronary artery by thrombus. Acute coronary syndromes include myocardial infarction and unstable angina. Former terms used to describe types of acute coronary syndromes include Q-wave myocardial infarction, non-Q-wave myocardial infarction, and unstable angina.

Acute disorder: An acid–base disturbance that has been present for minutes to hours.

Acute kidney injury: Spectrum of acute changes in kidney function ranging from minor changes to those requiring renal replacement therapy.

Acute otitis media: Inflammation of the middle ear accompanied by fluid in the middle ear space and signs or symptoms of an acute ear infection.

Acute tubular necrosis: Form of acute kidney injury that results from toxic or ischemic injury to the cells in the proximal tubule of the kidney.

Addiction: A primary, chronic, neurobiologic disease, with genetic, psychosocial, and environmental factors influencing its development and manifestations. It is characterized by behaviors that include one or more of the following: impaired control over drug use, compulsive use, continued use despite harm, and craving.

Adenocarcinomas: Malignant tumor originating in glandular tissue.

Adenoma: A nonmalignant tumor of the epithelial tissue that is characterized by glandular structures.

Adenomatous polyposis coli (APC) gene: A tumor suppressor gene (see definition) that is one of the first genes mutated in the development of colon cancer. Patients with familial adenomatous polyposis (FAP) are born with this gene mutated.

Adjuvant chemotherapy: Treatment given after primary surgical treatment and is designed to eliminate any remaining cancer cells that are undetectable with the goal of improving survival.

Adjuvant therapy: Therapy that supplements or follows primary therapy to prevent the risk of recurrence.

Adnexal: Adjacent or appending as the fallopian tubes and ovaries are to the uterus.

Adrenalectomy: Surgical removal of an adrenal gland.

Adrenocorticotropic hormone: A hormone secreted by the anterior pituitary that controls secretion of cortisol from the adrenal glands. Also referred to as corticotropin.

Adverse drug reaction (ADR): Any unexpected, unintended, undesired, or excessive response to a medication that: requires discontinuing the medication; requires changing the medication; requires modifying the dose (except for minor dosage adjustments); necessitates admission to the hospital; prolongs stay in a health care facility; necessitates supportive treatment; significantly complicates diagnosis;

negatively affects prognosis; or results in temporary or permanent harm, disability, or death.

Aeroallergen: An airborne substance that causes an allergic response.

Afterload: The force against which a ventricle contracts that is contributed to by vascular resistance, especially of the arteries, and by physical characteristics (mass and viscosity) of the blood.

Ageism: Discrimination against aged persons.

Air embolus: An obstruction in a small blood vessel caused by air that is introduced into a blood vessel and is carried through the circulation until it lodges in a smaller vessel.

Akathisia: Motor or subjective feelings of restlessness.

Akinesia: Lack of movement.

Alcohol dehydrogenase: An enzyme that degrades ethanol in the gut and liver.

Aldosterone: A hormone produced in and secreted by the zona glomerulosa of the adrenal cortex. Aldosterone acts on the kidneys to reabsorb sodium and excrete potassium. It is also a part of the renin-angiotensin-aldosterone system that regulates blood pressure and blood volume.

Alkalemia: A decrease in the hydrogen ion concentration of the blood or a rise above normal in pH.

Alkalosis: Any pathologic state that leads to alkalemia.

Allodynia: Pain that results from a stimulus that does not normally cause pain.

Allogeneic: In the setting of stem cell transplantation, the scenario in which the donor is a genetically similar but not identical to the recipient.

Allograft: Tissue or organ transplanted from a donor of the same species but different genetic makeup; recipient's immune system must be suppressed to prevent rejection of the graft.

Allograft survival: After the transplant procedure, when the transplanted organ continues to have some degree of function, from excellent to poor.

Allorecognition: Recognition of the foreign antigens present on the transplant organ or the donor's antigen presenting cells.

Alopecia: Hair loss.

Amenorrhea: The absence or discontinuation of regular menstrual periods.

γ-Aminobutyric acid: An inhibitory amino acid found in the central nervous system.

Amotivation: Apathy, loss of effectiveness, and diminished capacity or willingness to carry out complex, long-term plans, endure frustration, concentrate for long periods, follow routines, or successfully master new material.

Amygdala: Part of the limbic system that mediates emotions and helps to coordinate the response to threatening or stressful situations.

Amylase: An enzyme that catalyzes the hydrolysis of starch into simpler compounds.

Amylin: A 37-amino acid polypeptide hormone that is secreted from the β-cells of the pancreas in response to nutrients. Mechanisms of action include slowing gastric emptying, suppressing postmeal glucagon secretion, and suppressing appetite.

Amyloid: Any of a group of chemically diverse proteins which are composed of linear nonbranching aggregated fibrils.

Anaphylactic/anaphylaxis: Immediate, severe, potentially fatal hypersensitivity reaction induced by an antigen.

Anaphylactoid: An anaphylactic-like reaction, similar in signs and symptoms but not mediated by IgE. The drug causing this reaction produces direct release of inflammatory mediators by a pharmacologic effect.

Anastomosis: The connection of two hollow organs to restore continuity after resection or to bypass disease process that is not resectable.

Anemia: A reduction below normal in the concentration of hemoglobin in the body that results in a reduction of the oxygen-carrying capacity of the blood.

Anemia of chronic kidney disease: A decline in red blood cell production caused by a decrease in erythropoietin production by the progenitor cells of the kidney. As kidney function declines in chronic kidney disease, erythropoietin production also declines, resulting in decreased red blood cell production. Other contributing factors include iron deficiency and decreased red blood cell lifespan, caused by uremia.

Anergy: A reduction or lack of an immune response to a specific antigen.

Aneuploidy: Abnormal number of chromosomes.

Angina: Discomfort in the chest or adjacent areas caused by decreased blood and oxygen supply to the myocardium (myocardial ischemia).

Angina pectoris: Severe constricting pain in the chest, often radiating from the precordium to a shoulder (usually left) and down the arm, due to ischemia of the heart muscle usually caused by a coronary disease.

Angioedema: Swelling similar to urticaria (hives), but the swelling occurs beneath the skin instead of on the surface. Angioedema is characterized by deep swelling around the eyes and lips and sometimes of the hands and feet. If it proceeds rapidly, it can lead to airway obstruction and suffocation, and it should therefore be treated as a medical emergency.

Angiogenesis: The formation of new blood vessels.

Anhedonia: Inability to experience pleasure.

Anorexia: An eating disorder generally characterized by distorted body image, fear of weight gain, unwillingness to eat, and restrictive diet; may also refer to loss of appetite and serious weight loss as a result of disease.

Anoxia: A lack of oxygen.

Anterograde amnesia: Memory loss affecting the transfer of new information or events to long-term storage.

Antiangiogenic: Preventing or inhibiting the formation and differentiation of blood vessels.

Anticoagulant: Any substance that inhibits, suppresses, or delays the formation of blood clots. These substances occur naturally and regulate the clotting cascade. Several anticoagulants have been identified in a variety of animal tissues and have been commercially developed for medicinal use.

Antimicrobial prophylaxis: Use of an antimicrobial to prevent an infection.

Antiproteinase: A substance that inhibits the enzymatic activity of a proteinase.

Antrectomy: A surgical excision of the wall of the antrum, the region of the stomach that produces the hormone gastrin.

Anuria: Urine output of less than 50 mL over 24 hours.

Anxiogenic: Something that promotes or causes anxiety.

Aphakia: The absence of a lens in the eye.

Aphasia: Impairment of language affecting the ability to speak and to understand speech.

Aphthous ulcer: A small superficial area of ulceration within the gastrointestinal mucosa, typically found in the oral cavity.

Apoptosis: Programmed cell death as signaled by the nuclei in normally functioning cells when age or state of cell health and condition dictates.

Arcuate scotoma: An arc-shaped area of blindness in the field of vision.

Arthralgia: Pain in joints.

Arthrocentesis: Puncture and aspiration of a joint. Certain drugs can be injected into the joint space for a local effect.

Arthus reaction: Local inflammatory response due to deposition of immune complexes in tissues.

Articular: Related to a joint or joints.

Ascites: Accumulation of fluid within the peritoneal cavity.

Asterixis: A flapping tremor of the arms and hands that is seen in patients with end-stage liver disease.

Astringent: A substance that causes tissues to constrict, resulting in a drying effect of the skin.

Ataxia: Defective muscular coordination, possibly manifested by a staggering gait.

Atelectasis: Decreased or absent air in a partial or entire lung, with resulting loss of lung volume.

Atherosclerosis: Accumulation of lipids, inflammatory cells, and cellular debris in the subendothelial space of the arterial wall.

Atopy: A genetic predisposition to develop type I hypersensitivity reactions against common environmental antigens. Commonly seen in patients with allergic rhinitis, asthma, and atopic dermatitis.

Atresia: Congenital absence of a normal opening or normally patent lumen.

Autograft: A tissue or organ grafted into a new position in or on the body of the same individual.

Autologous: In the setting of stem cell transplantation, the scenario in which the donor and recipient are the same person.

Automaticity: Ability of a cardiac fiber or tissue to spontaneously initiate depolarizations.

Autonomic (nervous system): The parasympathetic and sympathetic nerves that control involuntary actions in the body.

Azoospermic: Having no living spermatozoa in the semen, or failure of spermatogenesis.

Bacteriuria: Presence of bacteria in urine.

Barium enema: A diagnostic test using an x-ray examination to view the lower gastrointestinal tract (colon and rectum) after rectal administration of barium sulfate, a chalky liquid contrast medium.

Basal ganglia: Cluster of nerve cells deep in the brain that coordinate normal movement.

Bence-Jones proteins: Light-chained immunoglobulins found in the urine.

Bilateral: Pertaining to both sides.

Bilateral salpingo-oophorectomy: Surgical excision (removal) of both ovaries.

Bile acids: The organic acids in bile. Bile is the yellowish-brown or green fluid secreted by the liver and discharged into the duodenum where it aids in the emulsification of fats, increases peristalsis, and retards putrefaction; contains sodium glycocholate and sodium taurocholate, cholesterol, biliverdin and bilirubin, mucus, fat, lecithin, and cells and cellular debris.

Biliary sludge: A deposit of tiny stones or crystals made up of cholesterol, calcium bilirubinate, and other calcium salts. The cholesterol and calcium bilirubinate crystals in biliary sludge can lead to gallstone formation.

Bioavailability: The amount of agent that is absorbed orally relative to an equivalent dose administered intravenously.

Biopsy: A procedure that involves obtaining a tissue specimen for microscopic analysis to establish a precise diagnosis.

Blastopore: A fungal spore produced by budding.

Blood dyscrasias: Any abnormality in the blood or bone marrow's cellular components such as low white or red blood cell count or low platelets

Blood urea nitrogen (BUN): A waste product in the blood produced from the breakdown of dietary proteins. The kidneys filter blood to remove urea and maintain homeostasis; a decline in kidney function results in an increase in BUN.

Body mass index (BMI): A calculation utilized to correct weight changes for height and is a direct calculation regardless of gender. It is the result of the weight in kilograms divided by the height in meters squared. If nonmetric measurements are used, it is the result of the weight in pounds multiplied by 703 and then that quantity divided by the product of height in inches squared.

Bone and mineral disorders (BMMD): Altered bone turnover that results from sustained metabolic conditions that occur in chronic kidney disease, including secondary hyperparathyroidism, hyperphosphatemia, hypocalcemia, and vitamin D deficiency. The disease can be characterized by high bone turnover, low bone turnover or adynamic disease, or may be a mixed disorder.

Bone remodeling: The constant process of bone turnover involving bone resorption followed by bone formation.

Bouchard's nodes: Hard, bony enlargement of the proximal interphalangeal (middle) joint of a finger or toe.

Brachial plexus: Collection of nerves that arises from the spine at the base of the neck from nerves that supply parts of the shoulder, arm, forearm, and hand.

Brachytherapy: A procedure in which radioactive material sealed in needles, seeds, wires, or catheters is placed directly into or near a tumor. Also called internal radiation, implant radiation, or interstitial radiation therapy.

Bradykinesia: Slow movement.

Breakpoint: The concentration of the antimicrobial agent that can be achieved in serum after a normal or standard dose of that antimicrobial agent.

Bronchiectasis: Chronic condition of one or more bronchi or bronchioles marked by irreversible dilatation and destruction of the bronchial walls.

Bronchoalveolar lavage: Washing out of the lungs with saline or mucolytic agents for diagnostic or therapeutic purposes.

Bronchoscopy: An examination used for inspection of the interior of the tracheobronchial tree.

Bullectomy: Surgical removal of one or more bullae (air spaces in the lung measuring more than 1 cm in diameter in the distended state).

Bursitis: An inflammation of the bursa, the fluid-filled sac near the joint where tendons and muscles pass over bone.

Cachectic: Physical wasting with loss of weight and muscle mass.

Cachexia: Weight loss, wasting of muscle, loss of appetite, and general debility. Anorexia may or may not be present.

CAM (abbreviation of "complementary and alternative medicines"): Defined as "dietary supplements" by the FDA; are not considered as "drugs" and therefore are not regulated as drugs.

Capillary leak: Loss of intravascular volume into the interstitial space within the body.

Carcinoembryonic antigen (CEA): A protein normally seen during fetal development. When elevated in adults it suggests the presence of colorectal and other cancers. Normal range is less than 2.5 ng/mL (less than 2.5 mcg/L) in nonsmokers but can be elevated in smokers and other nonmalignant conditions such as pancreatitis.

Carcinogenesis: Production or origin of cancer.

Carcinoma: A malignant growth that arises from epithelium, found in skin or the lining of body organs. Carcinomas tend to infiltrate into adjacent tissue and spread to distant organs.

Carcinoma in situ: The cancer is limited to the epithelial cells of origin; it has not yet invaded the basement membrane.

Carcinomatosis: Condition of having widespread dissemination of carcinoma (cancer) in the body.

Cardiac cachexia: Physical wasting with loss of weight and muscle mass caused by cardiac disease. A wasting syndrome that causes weakness and a loss of weight, fat, and muscle.

Cardiac index: Cardiac output normalized for body surface area (cardiac index = cardiac output/body surface area).

Cardiac output: The volume of blood ejected from the left side of the heart per unit of time [cardiac output (L/min) = stroke volume × heart rate].

Cardiac remodeling: Genome expression resulting in molecular, cellular, and interstitial changes and manifested

clinically as changes in size, shape, and function of the heart resulting from cardiac load or injury.

Carotid: The two main arteries in the neck.

Carotid bruit: Abnormal sound heard when auscultating a carotid artery caused by turbulent blood flow usually due to the presence of atherosclerotic plaques.

Carotid intima-media thickness: A measurement of the surface between the intima and media. This is a well-validated measure of the progression of atherosclerosis. Increasing measurements over time correlates with increasing atherosclerosis, whereas a decrease in the measurement is indicative of atherosclerotic regression.

Cataplexy: A sudden loss of muscle control with retention of clear consciousness that follows a strong emotional stimulus (as elation, surprise, or anger) and is a characteristic symptom of narcolepsy.

Causalgia: Persistent burning pain, allodynia, and hyperpathia following a traumatic nerve lesion.

Central pain: Pain that results from a lesion in or dysfunction of the central nervous system.

Cephalalgia: A term for head pain similar to headache.

Cervicitis: Inflammation of the cervix.

Chemoprevention: The use of drugs, vitamins, or other agents to reduce the risk, delay the development, or prevent the recurrence of cancer.

Chemoreceptor trigger zone (CTZ): Located in the area postrema of the fourth ventricle of the brain; it is exposed to cerebrospinal fluid and blood and is easily stimulated by circulating toxins to induce nausea and vomiting.

Chemosis: Edema of the conjunctiva.

Cheyne-Stokes respiration: Pattern of breathing with gradual increase in depth and sometimes in rate to a maximum, followed by a decrease resulting in apnea. The cycles ordinarily are 30 seconds to 2 minutes in duration, with 5 to 30 seconds of apnea.

Chimeric: Composed of parts from different origins.

Chloasma: Melasma characterized by irregularly shaped brown patches on the face and other areas of the skin, often seen during pregnancy or associated with the use of oral contraceptives.

Chlorpromazine equivalents: Dose of a first-generation antipsychotic approximately equivalent to 100 mg of chlorpromazine (relative potency).

Cholecystitis: Inflammation of the gallbladder.

Cholelithiasis: Also known as gallstones. Hard masses formed in the gallbladder or its passages that can block bile blow and cause severe upper right quadrant abdominal pain (sometimes radiating to the right shoulder).

Cholestasis: Reduced or lack of flow of bile, or obstruction of bile flow.

Cholesteatoma: A mass of keratinized epithelial cells and cholesterol resembling a tumor that forms in the middle ear or mastoid region.

Chorea: A type of dyskinesia with rhythmic dance-like movement. The increase in motor activity may be associated with fidgetiness, twitching, or flinging movements.

Chronic disorder: An acid–base disturbance that has been present for hours to days.

Chronic kidney disease (CKD): A progressive, irreversible decline in kidney function that occurs over a period of several months to years.

Chronic stable angina: Manifestation of ischemic heart disease (IHD) that typically results when an atherosclerotic plaque progresses to occlude at least 70% of a major coronary artery. Patients typically present with a sensation of chest pressure or heaviness that is evoked by exertion and relieved with rest or sublingual nitroglycerin.

Chronotropic: Referring to changes in the heart rate.

Chvostek's sign: Noted when a tap on the patient's facial nerve adjacent to the ear produces a brief contraction of the upper lip, nose, or side of the face.

Chylothorax: The presence of lymphatic fluid (chyle) in the pleural cavity.

Circadian: Events that occur over a 24-hour interval.

Circadian rhythm: 24-Hour cycles of behavior and physiology that are generated by endogenous biological clocks (pacemakers).

Circulatory shock: A condition wherein the circulatory system is inadequately supplying oxygen and vital metabolic substrates to cells throughout the body.

Cirrhosis: Hepatic fibrosis and regenerative nodules that have destroyed the architecture of the liver, scarring the liver tissues.

Clinical cure: Resolution of signs and symptoms of a disease.

Clonal expansion: An immunological response in which lymphocytes stimulated by antigen proliferate and amplify the population of relevant cells.

Closed comedo: A plugged follicle of sebum, keratinocytes, and bacteria that remains beneath the surface of the skin. Also referred to as a "whitehead."

Clotting cascade: A series of enzymatic reactions by clotting factors leading to the formation of a blood clot. The clotting cascade is initiated by several thrombogenic substances. Each reaction in the cascade is triggered by the preceding one and the effect is amplified by positive feedback loops.

Clotting factor: Plasma proteins found in the blood that are essential to the formation of blood clots. Clotting factors circulate in inactive forms but are activated by their predecessor in the clotting cascade or a thrombogenic substance. Each clotting factor is designated by a roman numeral, e.g., Factor VII, and by the letter "a" when activated, e.g., Factor VIIa.

Clubbing: A deformity produced by proliferation of the soft tissues at the terminal phalanges of the fingers or toes.

CMV disease: This is the term used when patients who are already infected with cytomegalovirus (CMV) present with the classically associated symptoms that resemble a viral infection and may include fever, malaise, arthralgias, and others.

CMV infection: This is the term used when a patient has anti-CMV antibodies in the blood, when CMV antigens are detected in infected cells, or when the virus is isolated from a culture.

Coalescence: Fusion of smaller lipid emulsion particles forming larger particles, resulting in destabilization of the emulsion.

Cognitive function: Executive function and mental processing such as understanding, perception, reasoning, language, and awareness. Executive function involves a long list of skills, which can be divided into four categories: organization, self-regulation, attention, and problem solving. For example, a patient may have trouble thinking quickly, making decisions, planning, and prioritizing tasks. These functions can be evaluated by various neuropsychological tests.

Coitus: Sexual intercourse.

Collateral damage: The development of resistance occurring in a patient's nontargeted flora that can cause secondary infections.

Colloids: Intravenous fluids composed of water and large-molecular weight molecules used to increase volume in patients with hypovolemic shock via increased intravascular oncotic pressure.

Colon cancer: A disease in which cells in the lining of the colon become malignant (cancer) and proliferate without control. Often referred to as colorectal cancer to include cancer cells found in the rectum.

Colonoscopy: A visual examination of the colon using a lighted, lens-equipped, flexible tube (colonoscope) inserted into the rectum.

Colony forming units: The number of microorganisms that form colonies when cultured and is indicative of the number of viable microorganisms in a sample.

Comedolytic: An agent that is able to break up or destroy a comedo.

Comorbidities: Multiple disease states occurring concurrently in one patient.

Compartment syndrome: The compression of nerves and blood vessels within an enclosed space.

Complex regimen: Taking medications three or more times per day, or 12 or more doses per day.

Complicated disorder: The presence of two or more distinct disorders.

Computed tomography: Radiographic imaging of anatomic information from a cross-sectional plane of the body.

Concreteness: Inability to think in abstract terms. It may be a primary developmental defect or secondary to organic mental disorder or schizophrenia.

Congenital adrenal hyperplasia: A rare inherited condition resulting from a deficiency in cortisol and aldosterone synthesis with resulting excess androgen production. The clinical presentation depends on the variant of the condition but typically manifests as abnormalities in sexual development and/or adrenal insufficiency.

Conidia: Propagating form (spores) of filamentous fungi that are released into soil and air currents. Inhalation of spores is the most common route of infections for endemic fungi and invasive molds.

Conjunctival injection: Erythema of the conjunctiva.

Conjunctivitis: Inflammation of the conjunctiva.

Conjunctivitis medicamentosa: A contact allergy to a topical medication.

Consolidation: A type of high-dose chemotherapy given as the second phase (after induction) of a treatment regimen for leukemia.

Contiguous: Describes two structures that are in close contact, or located next to each other.

Continuous positive airway pressure (CPAP): Therapy delivered using a nasal mask to improve the patency of the upper airway by maintaining sufficient air pressure to alleviate sleep-disordered breathing.

Contralateral: Pertaining to the opposite side of the body.

Convection: The movement of dissolved solutes across a semipermeable membrane by applying a pressure gradient to the fluid transport.

Convulsion: A violent involuntary contraction or series of contractions of voluntary muscles.

Copulation: Sexual union of male and female; coitus; sexual intercourse. Also, conjugation between two cells that do not fuse but separate after mutual fertilization.

Corneal arcus: Accumulation of lipid on the cornea.

Coronary Artery Bypass Graft (CABG) Surgery: Thoracic surgery where parts of a saphenous vein from a leg or internal mammary artery from the arm are placed as conduits to restore blood flow between the aorta and one or more coronary arteries to "bypass" the coronary artery stenosis (occlusion).

Coronary heart disease (CHD): Narrowing of one or more of the major coronary arteries, most commonly by atherosclerotic plaques. Also referred to as coronary artery disease.

Cor pulmonale: Right-sided heart failure, usually due to structural lung disease, e.g., pulmonary fibrosis, emphysema.

Corpus luteum: The small yellow endocrine structure that develops within a ruptured ovarian follicle and secretes progesterone and estrogen.

Corticotropin-releasing hormone: A hormone released by the hypothalamus that stimulates release of adrenocorticotropic hormone by the anterior pituitary gland.

Cortisol: An adrenal gland hormone responsible for maintaining homeostasis of carbohydrate, protein, and fat metabolism.

Cosyntropin: A synthetic version of adrenocorticotropic hormone.

Counterirritant: A substance that elicits a superficial inflammatory response with the objective of reducing inflammation in deeper, adjacent structures.

C-peptide levels: A peptide which is made when proinsulin is split into insulin and C-peptide. They split before proinsulin is released from endocytic vesicles within the pancreas—one C-peptide for each insulin molecule. C-peptide is the abbreviation for "connecting peptide." It is used to determine if a patient has type 1 or type 2 diabetes mellitus.

Creaming: Aggregation of lipid emulsion particles that then migrate to the surface of the emulsion; can be reversed with mild agitation.

Creatine kinase, Creatine kinase myocardial band: Creatine kinase (CK) enzymes are found in many isoforms, with varying concentrations depending on the type of tissue. CK is a general term used to describe the nonspecific total release of all types of CK, including that found in skeletal muscle (MM), brain (BB), and heart (MB). CK MB is released into the blood from necrotic myocytes in response to infarction and is a useful laboratory test for diagnosing myocardial infarction. If the total CK is elevated, then the relative index (RI), or fraction of the total that is composed of CK MB, is calculated as follows: RI equal to (CK MB/CK total) × 100. An RI greater than 2 is typically diagnostic of infarction.

Creatinine: A waste product in the blood produced from the breakdown of protein by-products generated by muscle in the body or ingested in the diet. The kidneys filter blood to remove creatinine and maintain homeostasis. A decline in kidney function results in an increase in creatinine.

Creatinine clearance: Rate at which creatinine is filtered across the glomerulus; estimate of glomerular filtration rate.

Cretinism: Obsolete term for congenital hypothyroidism.

Cross allergenicity: Sensitivity to one drug and then reacting to a different drug with a similar chemical structure.

CRP (C-reactive protein): A globulin produced by the liver that appears in the blood in certain acute inflammatory conditions, such as rheumatic fever and bacterial infections.

Crypt abscess: Neutrophilic infiltration of the intestinal glands (crypts of Lieberkuhn). A characteristic finding in patients with ulcerative colitis.

Crystalloids: Intravenous fluids composed of water and electrolytes, e.g., sodium, chloride, etc., used as intravascular volume expanders for patients with hypovolemic shock.

Culture-negative IE: Implies acute endocardial damage with negative blood cultures. It is common in patients treated with antibiotics before blood cultures are obtained.

Cutis laxis: Hyperflaccidity of the skin with loss of elasticity.

Cyanosis: Bluish discoloration of the skin and mucous membranes due to lack of oxygenation.

Cyclic citrullinated peptide (CCP): A circular peptide (a ring of amino acids) containing the amino acid citrulline. Autoantibodies directed against CCP provide the basis for a test of importance in rheumatoid arthritis.

Cyclooxygenase: An enzyme that catalyzes the conversion of arachidonic acid to prostaglandins and consists of two isoforms, generally referred to as COX-1 and COX-2.

Cystitis: Inflammation of urinary bladder.

Cyst: An abnormal membranous sac within the body that contains liquid or partially solid material.

Cystocele: Hernial protrusion of the bladder, usually through the vaginal wall.

Cytogenetic analysis: Laboratory identification of chromosomes that looks for mutational defects.

Cytokine: Regulatory proteins, such as interleukins and lymphokines, that are released by cells of the immune system and act as intercellular mediators in the generation of an immune response.

Dactylitis ("hand-foot syndrome"): Diffuse swelling of the hands and or feet often associated with pain and tenderness.

Deep vein thrombosis: A disorder of thrombus formation causing obstruction of a deep vein in the leg, pelvis, or abdomen.

Deescalation: Decreasing antimicrobial regimen spectrum of activity to provide coverage against specific antimicrobial-sensitive pathogens recovered from culture.

Delirium: Transient brain syndrome presenting as disordered attention, cognition, psychomotor behavior, and perception.

Dementia: An organic mental disorder characterized by a general loss of intellectual abilities involving impairment of memory, judgment, and abstract thinking as well as changes in personality.

Denervation: Loss of nerve impulse input, e.g., by severing a nerve during surgery or nerve impulse blockade farther up the nerve chain.

Dennie-Morgan line: A line or fold below the lower eyelids associated with atopy.

Dermatophytes: Any microscopic fungus that grows on the skin, scalp, nails, or mucosa but does not invade deeper tissues.

Desensitization: A method to reduce or eliminate an individual's negative reaction to a substance or stimulus.

Desquamation: Peeling or shedding of the epidermis (superficial layer of the skin) in scales or flakes.

Detumescence: The return of the penis to a flaccid state.

Diabetes insipidus: Polyuria due to the failure of renal tubules to reabsorb water in response to antidiuretic hormone.

Diabetic ketoacidosis: A reversible but life-threatening short-term complication primarily seen in patients with type 1 diabetes caused by the relative or absolute lack of insulin that results in marked ketosis and acidosis.

Dialysate: The physiologic solution used during dialysis to remove excess fluids and waste products from the blood.

Dialysis: The process of removing fluid and waste products from the blood across a semipermeable membrane to maintain fluid, electrolyte, and acid–base balance in patients with kidney failure.

Diaphoretic (diaphoresis): Sweating profusely.

Diarrhea: Loose, watery stools occurring more than three times in 1 day.

Diarthrodial joint: A freely moveable joint, e.g., knee, shoulder. Contrast with amphiarthrodial joint (a slightly movable joint, e.g., vertebral joint) and synarthrodial joint (an unmovable joint, e.g., fibrous joint).

Diastolic dysfunction: Abnormal filling of the ventricles during diastole.

Diphasic dyskinesia: Motor fluctuations occur while the plasma levodopa concentrations are rising and when they are falling. In each dosing interval, the patient may experience improvement, dyskinesia, and improvement (IDI) or dyskinesia, improvement, and dyskinesia (DID).

2,3-Diphosphoglycerate: A compound in red blood cells that affects oxygen binding to and release from hemoglobin.

Direct current cardioversion: The process of administering a synchronized electrical shock to the chest, the purpose of which is to simultaneously depolarize all of the myocardial cells, resulting in restoration of normal sinus rhythm.

Disease-free survival: Length of time after treatment during which no disease is found.

Disk diffusion test (D-test): A test performed in the microbiology laboratory to detect antibiotic sensitivity in bacteria.

Disseminated idiopathic skeletal hyperostosis (DISH): Excessive bone formation at skeletal sites subject to stress, generally where tendons and ligaments attach to bone.

DNA mismatch repair genes: Genes that identify and correct errors in DNA base pairs during DNA replication. Mutations in the genes can lead to cancer by allowing abnormal cells to continue to grow.

Dose intensity: Delivery of a predetermined dose per unit of time, i.e., mg/m^2/week.

Downregulation: The process of reducing or suppressing a response to a stimulus.

Drusen: Tiny yellow or white deposits of extracellular material in the eye.

Ductus arteriosus: Shunt connecting the pulmonary artery to the aortic arch that allows most of the blood from the right ventricle to bypass the fetus lungs.

Duodenal: The first of three parts of the small intestine.

Dysarthria: Difficult or defective speech, usually due to impairment of tongue movement or of other muscles essential to speech.

Dysentery: An illness involving severe diarrhea that is often associated with blood in the stool.

Dysesthesia: An unpleasant abnormal sensation.

Dysgeusia: Unpleasant taste in the mouth.

Dyskinesia: Abnormal involuntary movements, which include dystonia, chorea, and akathisia.

Dyslipidemia: Elevation of the total cholesterol, low-density lipoprotein cholesterol or triglyceride concentrations, or a decrease in high-density lipoprotein cholesterol concentration in the blood.

Dysmenorrhea: Crampy pelvic pain occurring with or just prior to menses. "Primary" dysmenorrhea implies pain in the setting of normal pelvic anatomy, while "secondary" dysmenorrhea is secondary to underlying pelvic pathology.

Dyspareunia: Pain during or after sexual intercourse.

Dysphagia: Painful or difficult swallowing, accompanied by a sensation of food being stuck in passage.

Dysphasic: An alteration in normal speech patterns or content.

Dysphonia: Impairment of the voice or difficulty speaking.

Dysphoria: A general mood of depression, dissatisfaction, and unrest.

Dyspnea: Shortness of breath or difficulty breathing.

Dyssynergic defecation: A lack of coordination between the pelvic floor muscles and the anal sphincter.

Dystonia: A type of dyskinesia. Movement is slow and twisting. It may be associated with painful muscle contractions or spasms.

Dysuria: Difficulty or pain related to urination

Ebstein's anomaly: Congenital heart defect in which the opening of the tricuspid valve is displaced toward the apex of the right ventricle of the heart.

Eburnation: A condition in which bone or cartilage becomes hardened and denser.

Ecchymoses: Passage of blood from ruptured blood vessels into subcutaneous tissue causing purple discoloration of the skin.

Ectopic pregnancy: Presence of a fertilized ovum outside of the uterine cavity.

Effector cells: Cells that become active in response to initiation of the immune response.

Ejection fraction: The fraction of the volume present at the end of diastole that is pushed into the aorta during systole.

Electrocardiogram: A noninvasive recording of the electrical activity of the heart.

Electroconvulsive therapy: Administration of electric current to the brain through electrodes placed on the head in order to induce seizure activity in the brain, used in the treatment of certain mental disorders.

Electroencephalogram (EEG): A recording of patterns of electrical impulses in the brain.

Electroencephalography: The recording of brain waves via electrodes placed on the scalp or cortex.

Embolectomy: Surgical removal of a clot or embolism.

Embolism: Sudden blockage of a vessel caused by a blood clot or foreign material which has been brought to the site by the flow of blood.

Embolization: The process by which a blood clot or foreign material dislodges from its site of origin, flows in the blood, and blocks a distant vessel.

Emesis: See vomiting.

End-stage liver disease: Liver failure that is usually accompanied by complications such as ascites or hepatic encephalopathy.

Endarterectomy: Removal of a thrombus from the carotid artery.

Endemic fungi: Fungi that are native or prevalent to a particular area or region.

Endocinch: An endoscopic sewing technique used to improve lower esophageal sphincter tone.

Endometritis: Inflammation of the endometrium.

Endoscopic evaluation: General term used to describe the visual inspection of the inside of hollow organs with an endoscope. Used mainly for diagnostic purposes. Refers to procedures such as gastroscopy, duodenoscopy, colonoscopy, sigmoidoscopy, and others.

Endoscopic retrograde cholangiopancreatography (ERCP): A technique in which an endoscope is passed through the mouth and stomach to the duodenum in order to examine abnormalities of the bile ducts, pancreas, and gallbladder.

Endoscopy: A procedure used to evaluate the interior surfaces of an organ by inserting a small scope into the body through which one can directly examine almost any part of the intestinal tract. Biopsies can be obtained, polyps removed, and clear images obtained.

Endothelial cell: A single layer of cell surrounding the lumen of arteries.

Engraftment: The process by which transplanted stem cells begin to grow and reproduce in the recipient to produce functioning leukocytes, erythrocytes, and platelets.

Enteral nutrition: Delivery of nutrients via the gastrointestinal tract, either by mouth or by feeding tube.

Enterobacteriaceae: A family of enteric gram-negative bacilli, e.g., *Escherichia coli* or *Klebsiella pneumoniae*.

Enterocytes: Cells lining the small intestine.

Enuresis: Incontinence at night.

Enzyme-linked immunoabsorbent assay (ELISA): A solid phase in the form of a microtiter plate or bead to which HIV antigen is attached. The antigen may be either a preparation of lysed whole virus or a combination of recombinant viral antigens.

Epilepsy: A neurologic disorder characterized by recurring motor, sensory, or psychic malfunction with or without loss of consciousness or convulsive seizures.

Epistaxis: Nasal hemorrhage with blood drainage through the nostrils; a nosebleed.

Erectile dysfunction (ED): Condition defined as the inability to achieve or maintain an erection sufficient for sexual intercourse.

Erythema multiforme: A rash characterized by papular (small raised bump) or vesicular lesions (blisters), and reddening or discoloration of the skin often in concentric zones about the lesion.

Erythematous: Flushing of the skin caused by dilation of capillaries. Erythema is often a sign of inflammation and infection.

Erythrocyte sedimentation rate (ESR): A nonspecific inflammatory marker that may be elevated in some infections and inflammatory diseases; specifically, the ESR is obtained from a blood sample by measuring the distance that red blood cells precipitate after 1 hour.

Erythropoiesis stimulating agents (ESAs): Agents developed by recombinant DNA technology that have the same biological activity as endogenous erythropoietin to stimulate erythropoiesis (red blood cell production) in the bone marrow. The currently available agents in the United States are epoetin alfa and darbepoetin alfa.

Erythropoietin: A hormone primarily produced by the progenitor cells of the kidney that stimulates red blood cell (RBC) production in the bone marrow. Lack of this hormone leads to anemia.

Esophageal varices: Dilated blood vessels in the esophagus.

Esophagitis: Inflammation of the esophagus that occurs when the esophagus is repeatedly exposed to refluxed material for prolonged periods of time.

Essential fatty acid deficiency: Deficiency of linoleic acid, linolenic acid, and/or arachidonic acid, characterized by hair loss, thinning of skin, and skin desquamation. Long-chain fatty acids include trienes (containing three double-bonds, e.g., 5,8,11-eicosatrienoic [or Mead] acid, trienoic acids,) and tetraenes (containing four double bonds, e.g., arachidonic acid). Biochemical evidence of essential fatty acid deficiency includes a triene:tetraene greater than 0.2 and low linoleic or arachidonic acid plasma concentrations.

Euthymia: Normal mood.

Euthyroid: State of normal thyroid function or hormone activity.

Event-free survival: This term refers to the length of time after treatment that a person remains free of certain negative events.

Evoked potential testing: A procedure in which sensory nerve pathways are stimulated, and the time lapse to electrical response in the corresponding area of the brain is measured.

Exanthem: Skin eruption.

Exfoliative dermatitis: Severe inflammation of the entire skin surface due to a reaction to certain drugs.

Exophthalmos: Abnormal protrusion of the eyeball, seen in Grave's disease.

Exploratory laparotomy: Surgical incision into the abdominal cavity, performed to examine the abdominal organs and cavity in search of an abnormality and diagnosis.

External beam radiotherapy: Treatment by radiation emitted from a source located at a distance from the body. Also called beam therapy and external beam therapy.

Extra-abdominal: Outside of the abdominal cavity.

Extraction ratio: Fraction of the drug entering the liver in the blood which is irreversibly removed.

Extrapyramidal reaction: A combination of neurologic effects which includes tremor, chorea, athetosis, and dystonia; a common side effect of antipsychotic agents.

Extrapyramidal symptoms: Adverse effects of medications such as antipsychotics. They include dystonia (involuntary muscle contractions), tardive dyskinesia (repetitive, involuntary movements), parkinsonian symptoms (akinesia, rigidity, and tremors), and akathisia (motor or subjective restlessness).

Extravasation: Movement of fluid from inside a blood vessel into the surrounding tissues.

Facultative: Biologically capable but not restricted to a particular function or mode of life, e.g., survival within macrophages.

Facultative anaerobe: An organism that makes ATP by aerobic respiration if oxygen is present, but switches to fermentation under anaerobic conditions.

Felty's syndrome: An extra-articular manifestation of rheumatoid arthritis associated with splenomegaly and neutropenia.

Festination: Walking with short, rapid, shuffling steps.

Fibrin: An insoluble protein that is one of the principal ingredients of a blood clot. Fibrin strands bind to one another to form a fibrin mesh. The fibrin mesh often traps platelets and other blood cells.

Fibrinolysis: A normal ongoing process that dissolves fibrin and results in the removal of small blood clots; hydrolysis of fibrin.

Fibroadenoma: A benign neoplasm which commonly occurs in breast tissue and is derived from glandular epithelium.

Fibrosis: Formation of tissue containing connective tissues formed by fibroblasts as part of tissue repair or as a reactive process.

Fistula: Abnormal connection between two internal organs (e.g., arteriovenous fistula, a connection between an artery and a vein) or between an internal organ and the exterior or skin (e.g., enterocutaneous fistula, a connection between the intestine and the skin); often seen in severe cases of Crohn's disease.

Flight of ideas: A nearly continuous flow of rapid speech and thought that jumps from topic to topic, usually loosely connected.

Floppy iris syndrome: Disorder associated with excessive relaxation of the iris dilator muscle, which results in a flaccid iris.

Flow cytometry: Technology used to study characteristics of individual cells in a suspension.

Fluorescence in situ hybridization (FISH): A laboratory technique used to look at genes or chromosomes in cells and tissues. Pieces of DNA that contain a fluorescent dye are made in the laboratory and added to cells or tissues on a glass slide. When these pieces of DNA bind to specific genes or areas of chromosomes on the slide, they light up when viewed under a microscope with a special light.

Foam cell: Lipid-laden white blood cells.

Forced expiratory volume in 1 second: The volume of air that a patient can forcibly blow out in the first second of forced exhalation after taking a maximal breath.

Forced vital capacity: The maximum volume of air that can be forcibly exhaled after taking a maximal breath.

Fragility fracture: Fracture resulting from a fall from standing height or less amount of trauma.

Frailty: Excess demand imposed upon reduced capacity; a common biological syndrome in the elderly.

Frank-Starling mechanism: One of the mechanisms by which the heart can increase cardiac output.

Freelite assay: A highly sensitive assay that determines the ratio of serum-free light chain kappa to lambda.

Friable: Easily crumbled, pulverized, or reduced to powder.

Friction: Risk factor for pressure ulcers that is created when a patient is dragged across a surface, which can lead to superficial skin damage.

Fronto-temporal: Located to the front or side of the head.

Fructooligosaccharides: Polymers of fructose that reach the colon undigested and are broken down there to short-chain fatty acids by bacterial enzymes.

Functional gastrointestinal disorder: A term used to describe symptoms occurring in the gastrointestinal tract in the absence of a demonstrated pathologic condition. The clinical product of psychosocial factors and altered intestinal physiology involving the brain–gut interrelationship.

Gadolinium: An intravenous contrast agent used with magnetic resonance imaging.

Galactorrhea: Inappropriate breast milk production and secretion.

Gallstone (cholelithiasis): A solid formation in the gallbladder or bile duct (choledocholithiasis if in the bile duct) composed of cholesterol and bile salts.

Gamma knife: A device which uses multiple converging beams of γ-radiation from cobalt-60 to highly focus radiation on small tumors within the brain.

Gastric bypass: A surgical procedure for weight loss that elicits its effectiveness through malabsorption and volume limitation. The procedure involves full partitioning of the proximal gastric segment into a jejunal loop.

Gastritis: Acute or chronic inflammation of the lining of the stomach.

Gastroenteritis: Inflammation of the gastrointestinal tract causing nausea, vomiting, diarrhea, and fever; sometimes referred to as the stomach flu although not related to influenza.

Gastroesophageal reflux disease: Troublesome symptoms and/or complications caused by refluxing the stomach contents into the esophagus. These troublesome symptoms adversely affect the well-being of the patient.

Gastroparesis: A form of autonomic neuropathy involving nerves of the stomach. It may include nausea, vomiting, feeling full, bloating, and lack of appetite. It may cause wide fluctuations in blood sugars due to insulin action and nutrient delivery not occurring at the same time.

Gastroplasty: A surgical procedure for weight loss that elicits its effectiveness through gastric volume limitation. The procedure involves partial partitioning at the proximal gastric segment with the placement of a gastric outlet stoma of fixed diameter.

Gastroschisis: Inherited congenital abdominal wall defect in which the intestines and sometimes other organs develop outside the fetal abdomen through an opening in the abdominal wall.

Gastrostomy: Operative placement of a new opening into the stomach, usually associated with feeding tube placement.

Geniculate nucleus: The portion of the brain that processes visual information from the optic nerve and relays it to the cerebral cortex.

Genotype: The genetic constitution of an individual.

Geriatric syndrome: Age-specific presentations or differential diagnoses, including visual and hearing impairment, malnutrition and weight loss, urinary incontinence, gait impairment and falls, osteoporosis, dementia, delirium, sleep problems, and pressure ulcers. Commonly seen conditions in elder patients.

Gestational diabetes: Diabetes that occurs during pregnancy which may or may not end at delivery.

Gigantism: A condition of abnormal size or overgrowth of the entire body or any of its parts. Characteristic of growth hormone excess that manifests prior to closure of epiphyseal plates.

Glasgow Coma Scale: A scale for evaluating level of consciousness after central nervous system injury (evaluates eye opening and verbal and motor responsiveness).

Glomerular filtration rate (GFR): The volume of plasma that is filtered by the glomerulus per unit time, usually expressed as mL/min or mL/min/1.73 m², which adjusts the value for body surface area. This is the primary index used to describe overall renal function.

Glomerulonephritis: Glomerular lesions that are characterized by inflammation of the capillary loops of the glomerulus. These lesions are generally caused by immunologic, vascular, or other idiopathic diseases.

Glucagon: Hormone involved in carbohydrate metabolism that is produced by the pancreas and released when glucose levels in the blood are low. When blood glucose levels decrease, the liver converts stored glycogen into glucose, which is released into the bloodstream. The action of glucagon is opposite to that of insulin.

Gluconeogenesis: Formation of glucose from precursors other than carbohydrates especially by the liver and kidney using amino acids from proteins, glycerol from fats, or lactate produced by muscle during anaerobic glycolysis.

Glucuronidation: A metabolic pathway in the body that combines a drug (or other compound) that possesses a phenol, alcohol, or carboxyl group with glucuronic acid.

Glutamate: An excitatory amino acid found in the central nervous system.

Glycogenolysis: The process by which glycogen is broken down into glucose in body tissues.

Goiter: An enlargement of the thyroid gland, causing a swelling in the front part of the neck.

Gonioscopy: Examination of the anterior chamber angle. A gonioprism or Goldman lens is used to perform gonioscopic evaluation.

Gout: A group of disorders of purine metabolism, manifested by various combinations of (1) hyperuricemia; (2) recurrent acute inflammatory arthritis induced by crystals of monosodium urate monohydrate; (3) tophaceous deposits of these crystals in and around the joints of the extremities, which may lead to crippling destruction of joints; and (4) uric acid urolithiasis.

Graft-versus-host disease: The phenomenon by which transplanted donor T cells recognize normal host tissues as foreign and attack these tissues, resulting in increased morbidity and mortality in allogeneic transplant patients.

Graft-versus-tumor effect: The phenomenon by which transplanted donor cells recognize host malignant cells as foreign and eradicate the malignant cells through immunologic mechanisms.

Grandiosity: Exaggerated sense of self-importance, ideas, plans, or abilities.

Granulomas: Masses of chronically inflamed tissues with granulations.

Gummatous: A tumor of rubbery consistency that is characteristic of the tertiary stage of syphilis.

Gut-associated lymphoid tissue: Lymphoid tissue, including Peyer's patches, found in the gut that are important for providing localized immunity to pathogens.

Hallucinosis: Auditory hallucinations that occur during a clear sensorium.

Haptenation: The process where a drug, usually of low molecular weight, is bound to a carrier protein or cell and becomes immunogenic.

Health literacy: Degree to which individuals have the capacity to obtain, process, and understand basic health information and services needed to make appropriate health decisions.

Heberden's nodes: Hard, bony enlargement of the distal interphalangeal (terminal) joint of a finger or toe.

Hemarthrosis: Blood in the joint space.

Hematemesis: The vomiting of blood.

Hematochezia: Passage of stool that is bright red or maroon, usually because of bleeding from the lower gastrointestinal tract.

Hematogenous: Spread through the blood.

Hematuria: Presence of blood or red blood cells in urine.

Hemiballismus: A rare movement disorder that can be life threatening. Patients with hemiballismus have a dismal prognosis, with physical exhaustion, injuries, and medical complications often leading to death.

Hemiparesis: Weakness or slight paralysis involving one side of the body.

Hemisensory deficit: Loss of sensation on one side of the body.

Hemithorax: A single side of the trunk between the neck and the abdomen in which the heart and lungs are situated.

Hemolytic uremic syndrome: A disease characterized by microangiopathic hemolytic anemia, acute renal failure, and a low platelet count (thrombocytopenia).

Hemoptysis: The expectoration of blood or blood-tinged sputum from the larynx, trachea, bronchi, or lungs.

Hemorrhagic conversion: Conversion of an ischemic stroke into a hemorrhagic stroke.

Hemostasis: Cessation of bleeding through natural (clot formation or construction of blood vessels), artificial (compression or ligation), or surgical means.

Heparin-induced thrombocytopenia: A clinical syndrome of IgG antibody production against the heparin-platelet factor 4 complex occurring in approximately 1% to 5% of patients exposed to either heparin or low-molecular-weight heparin. Heparin-induced thrombocytopenia results in excess production of thrombin, platelet aggregation, and thrombocytopenia (due to platelet clumping), often leading to venous and arterial thrombosis, amputation of extremities, and death.

Hepatic encephalopathy: Confusion and disorientation that a patient with advanced liver disease experiences due to accumulation of ammonia levels.

Hepatic steatosis: Accumulation of fat in the liver.

Hepatocellular carcinoma (HCC): Cancer of the liver.

Hepatojugular reflex: Distention of the jugular vein induced by pressure over the liver; suggestive of insufficiency of the right heart.

Hepatosplenomegaly: An enlarged liver and spleen secondary to leukemic infiltration.

Hepatotoxicity: Toxicity to the liver causing damage to liver cells.

Herniation: Protrusion of the brain through the cranial wall.

Hesitancy: Difficulty with initiating micturition.

Heterotopic: Placing a transplanted organ into an abnormal anatomic location.

Heterozygous: Having different alleles at a gene locus.

Hirsutism: Excess body hair, especially appearing on the lower abdomen, around the nipples, around the chin and upper lip, between the breasts, and on the lower back.

Histocompatibility: The examination of human leukocyte antigen (HLA) differences between a donor and a recipient in order to determine if the recipient is more likely to accept, rather than reject, a graft from that particular donor.

HIV genotype: A type of resistance testing for HIV in which a patient's blood sample is obtained, the HIV RNA is sequenced, and mutations that may confer resistance to antiretrovirals are reported.

HIV phenotype: A type of resistance testing for HIV in which a patient's blood sample is obtained and the patient's HIV genes that encode for reverse transcriptase and protease are removed and placed in an HIV viral vector. This viral vector is replicated in a cell culture system with varying concentrations of antiretrovirals. A drug concentration-viral inhibition curve is developed and the concentration needed to inhibit 50% of the patient's virus is reported. This is used to predict resistance versus susceptibility.

HIV virtual phenotype: A database of matching HIV genotypes and phenotypes is developed. When an HIV genotype for a patient is obtained, the database is used to predict the patient's phenotype based on their actual genotype using matches that occur in the database.

Homeostenosis: Impaired capability to withstand stressors and decreased ability to maintain physiological and psychosocial homeostasis; a state commonly found in the elderly.

Homonymous: Pertaining to the same side.

Homozygous: Having identical alleles at a gene locus.

Hospice: The provision of palliative care during the last 6 months of life as defined by federal guidelines.

Hot flashes: A feeling of warmth that is commonly accompanied by skin flushing and mild to severe perspiration.

Human leukocyte antigens (HLA): Groups of genes found on the major histocompatibility complex, which contain cell-surface antigen presenting proteins. The body uses HLA to distinguish between self cells and nonself cells.

Humoral: Products secreted into the blood or body fluids.

Hydramnios: Increased amniotic fluid.

Hydronephrosis: Distention of the pelvis and kidney with urine resulting from obstruction of the ureter.

β-Hydroxybutyric acid: A ketone body that is elevated in ketosis, is synthesized in the liver from acetyl-CoA, and can be used as an energy source by the brain when blood glucose is low.

Hyperalgesia: An exaggerated intensity of pain sensation.

Hypercalcemia: Excessive amount of calcium in the blood.

Hypercalciuria: Excessive amount of calcium in the urine.

Hypercapnia: Abnormally high concentration of carbon dioxide in the blood.

Hypercoagulable state: A disorder or state of excessive or frequent thrombus formation; also known as thrombophilia.

Hyperemesis gravidarum: A rare disorder of severe and persistent nausea and vomiting during pregnancy that can result in dehydration, malnutrition, weight loss, and hospitalization.

Hyperglycemic hyperosmolar nonketotic syndrome: Severe increase in serum glucose concentration without the production of ketones, leading to an increase in serum osmolality and symptoms such as increased thirst, increased urination, weakness, fatigue, confusion, and in severe cases, convulsions and/or coma.

Hyperopia: Farsightedness.

Hyperosmolar hyperglycemic state: Blood glucose levels greater than 600 mg/dL without significant ketones where extreme dehydration, insulin deficiency, hyperosmolarity, and electrolyte deficiency are common.

Hyperpathia: A painful syndrome, characterized by increased reaction to a stimulus, especially a repetitive stimulus, as well as an increased threshold.

Hyperpigmentation: A common darkening of the skin that occurs when an excess of melanin forms deposits in the skin.

Hyperplasia: An abnormal or unusual increase in the cells of a body part.

Hyperprolactinemia: A medical condition of elevated serum prolactin characterized by prolactin serum concentrations greater than 20 ng/mL (20 mcg/L) in men or 25 ng/mL (25 mcg/L) in women.

Hypersomnia: Sleeping for unusually prolonged periods of time.

Hyperthermia: An unusually high body temperature.

Hyperthyroidism: State caused by excess production of thyroid hormone.

Hypertrichosis: Excessive growth of hair.

Hypertrophy: An increase in the size of the cells in a tissue or organ.

Hyperuricemia: Elevated serum uric acid concentration, defined as a level greater than 7.0 mg/dL (416 μmol/L); it is a prerequisite for the development of gout and may lead to renal disease.

Hypervigilance: The state of being extremely alert and watchful, possibly to avoid danger or harm.

Hypochlorhydria: Hypoacidity. Decreased hydrochloric acid secretion by the stomach.

Hypocretin: A wake-promoting hypothalamic neuropeptide whose deficiency is involved in the pathophysiology of narcolepsy.

Hypogammaglobinemia: Reduced levels of antibodies.

Hypogonadism: A syndrome associated with testosterone deficiency resulting from either testicular or pituitary/hypothalamic diseases. Presenting symptoms differ according to the timing of disease onset in relation to puberty.

Hypomania: Abnormal mood elevation that does not meet criteria for mania.

Hypopituitarism: A clinical disorder characterized by complete or partial deficiency in pituitary hormone production.

Hypothalamic-pituitary-adrenal axis: A neuroendocrine feedback loop that controls response to stress.

Hypothermia: An unusually low body temperature.

Hypothyroidism: State caused by inadequate production of thyroid hormone.

Hypovolemic shock: Circulatory shock caused by severe loss of blood volume and/or body water.

Hypoxemia: Deficiency of oxygen in the blood.

Hypoxia: Deficiency of oxygen.

Hysterectomy: Excision of the uterus.

Immunocompromised: A condition in which the immune system is not functioning normally. This condition is seen in the very young, the very old, HIV infected individuals, or in transplant patients.

Immunogenicity: The property that gives a substance the ability to provoke an immune response.

Immunoglobulin G index: The ratio of immunoglobulin G to protein in the serum or cerebrospinal fluid.

Immunophenotype: The process of identification and quantitation of cellular antigens through fluorochrome-labeled monoclonal antibodies.

Immunotherapy: Treatment of a disease by stimulating the body's own immune system.

Impedance monitoring: A diagnostic technique used to evaluate esophageal bolus transit. When combined with pH monitoring, impedance monitoring helps identify both acidic and weakly acidic reflux episodes.

Implantable cardioverter-defibrillator: A device implanted into the heart transvenously with a generator implanted subcutaneously in the pectoral area that provides internal electrical cardioversion of ventricular tachycardia or defibrillation of ventricular fibrillation.

Incretin effect: A greater insulin stimulatory effect after an oral glucose load than that caused by an intravenous glucose infusion. The majority of the effect is thought to be due to glucose-dependent insulinotropic peptide (GIP) and glucagon like peptide-1 (GLP-1). Patients with type 2 diabetes have a significant reduction of the incretin effect, implying that these patients either have decreased concentration of the incretin hormones, or a resistance to their effects. GLP-1 concentrations are reduced in patients with type 2 diabetes in response to a meal, while GIP concentrations are either normal or increased, suggesting a resistance to the actions of GIP, thus making GLP-1 a more logical target for therapeutic intervention.

Index patient: The patient originally diagnosed with a disease.

Indirect immunofluorescence assay (IFA): HIV-infected T-lymphocytes are fixed onto a microscope slide, covered with the blood sample to be tested, incubated under heat, and washed. If antibodies to HIV are bound to the fixed viral antigens, they will remain on the slide. FITC-conjugated antihuman globulin is then added, incubated, and washed. If the sample contains antibodies to HIV, the cells will show a bright, fluorescent membrane under the microscope.

Induction: Treatment designed to be used as the first step in eliminating the leukemic burden.

Infarction: The formation of an infarct, an area of tissue death due to a local lack of oxygen.

Infective endocarditis (IE): Historically referred to as bacterial endocarditis, IE is an infection, either acute or subacute, that primarily affects the heart valves, but may extend into other surrounding areas of the heart.

Inotropic: Pertaining to the force of contraction of the heart muscle, or relating to or influencing the force of muscular contractions.

Insulin-like growth factor-I: An anabolic peptide that acts as a direct stimulator of cell proliferation and growth in all body cells.

Insulin resistance: A decreased response to insulin found before or early in the diagnosis of type 2 diabetes mellitus.

International normalized ratio (INR): The ratio of the patient's clotting time to the clinical laboratory's mean reference value; normalized by raising it to the international sensitivity index (ISI) power to account for differences in thromboplastin reagents. Thus, INR = (patient's prothrombin time/laboratory's mean normal prothrombin time)^{ISI}.

Intima: The inner layer of the wall of an artery or vein.

Intra-abdominal: Within the abdominal cavity.

Intra-articular: Administered to or occurring in the space within joints.

Intraperitoneal: Within the peritoneal cavity.

Intrathecal: Within the meninges of the spinal cord.

Intravesicular: Administration directly into the bladder through the urethra.

Intussusception: Infolding, like the closing of a telescope, of a segment of the small intestine into the adjacent but more distal segment of the intestine, reducing blood supply to the affected part of the intestine and eventually causing intestinal obstruction.

Iontophoresis: Introduction of a medication into tissue through use of an electric current.

Ipsilateral: Pertaining to the same side of the body.

Ischemic heart disease (IHD): Imbalance between myocardial oxygen supply and oxygen demand.

Jejunal: A section of the small intestine connecting the duodenum to the ileum.

Jejunostomy: Operative placement of a new opening into the jejunum, usually associated with feeding tube placement.

Kegel exercises: Specific exercises that strengthen the pelvic floor muscles and help to prevent and treat stress incontinence.

Keratinization: The sloughing of epithelial cells in the hair follicle.

Keratinocyte: The epidermal cell that synthesizes keratin; making up 95% of all epidermal cells; commonly called "skin cells."

Keratitis: Infection of the cornea.

Keratoconjunctivitis sicca: Also known as Sjogren's syndrome or dry eye syndrome.

Keratotic: Pertaining to any horny growth such as a wart or callus.

Ketosis: An abnormal increase of ketone bodies present in conditions of reduced or disturbed carbohydrate metabolism.

Kindling: Repeated application of electrical stimulation to specific areas of the brain that leads to an alteration in the seizure threshold and the development of epilepsy. This process is used only in animal experimental models, but a similar phenomenon is thought to occur in humans.

Koebner's phenomenon: The occurrence of psoriatic lesions due to skin trauma.

Korotkoff sounds: The noise heard over an artery by auscultation when pressure over the artery is reduced below the systolic arterial pressure.

Korsakoff's syndrome: May occur as a sequel to chronic alcohol use. Characterized by psychosis, polyneuritis, disorientation, insomnia, delirium, hallucinations. Bilateral foot or wrist drop may also occur, possibly accompanied by pain.

Kyphosis: Abnormal curvature of the spine resulting in protrusion of the upper back; hunchback.

Lacrimation: Tearing and discharge of tears from the eyes.

β-Lactam allergy: Allergy to the β-lactam family, namely penicillins and cephalosporins, but may also include carbapenems.

Lactose intolerance: An inability to digest milk and some dairy products, resulting in abnormal bloating, cramping, and diarrhea; caused by enzymatic lactase deficiency.

Lag-ophthalmos: Poor closure of the upper eyelid.

Lamina cribrosa: A series of perforated sheets of connective tissue that the optic nerve passes through as it exits the eye.

Laminectomy: Excision of the posterior arch of a vertebra to relieve pressure on the spinal cord.

Laparoscopic: Abdominal exploration or surgery employing a type of endoscope called laparoscope.

Laparotomy: Surgical opening of the abdominal cavity.

Latent autoimmune diabetes in adults (LADA): A slow, progressive form of type 1 diabetes mellitus in which a patient does not require insulin for a number of years. In its early stages, LADA typically presents as type 2 diabetes mellitus and is often misdiagnosed as such. However, LADA more closely resembles type 1 diabetes mellitus and shares common physiological characteristics of type 1 diabetes mellitus for metabolic dysfunction, genetics, and autoimmune features. LADA does not affect children and is classified distinctly as being separate from juvenile diabetes.

Lentigines: Plural of lentigo. A small, flat, tan to dark brown or black, macular melanosis on the skin, which looks like a freckle but is histologically distinct. Lentigines do not darken on exposure to sunlight, freckles do.

Leukemoid reaction: An elevated white blood cell count, or leukocytosis, that is a physiologic response to stress or infection (as opposed to a primary blood malignancy, such as leukemia).

Leukocytoclastic: The breaking up of white blood cells.

Leukopenia: A condition where the number of circulating white blood cells are abnormally low due to decreased production of new cells, possibly in conjunction with medication toxicities.

Leukostasis: An abnormal intravascular leukocyte aggregation and clumping seen in leukemia patients. The brain and the lungs are the two most frequent organs involved.

Lewy bodies: Abnormal masses inside some nerve cells. They occur in a variety of locations, and their structure and composition vary depending on location.

Lhermitte's sign: Tingling or shock-like sensation passing down the arms or trunk when the neck is flexed.

Libido: Conscious or unconscious sexual desire.

Ligament of Treitz: Landmark in the proximal portion of the jejunum beyond which it is preferred that postpyloric feedings be delivered for minimization of aspiration.

Linear accelerator: A device that uses microwave technology to accelerate electrons in a highly focused beam to deliver targeted radiation to tumor sites.

Lipase: Any one of a group of lipolytic enzymes that cleave a fatty acid residue from the glycerol residue in a neutral fat or a phospholipid.

Lipophilic: Having an affinity for fatty substances.

Lipoprotein lipase: Enzyme located in the capillary endothelium involved in the breakdown of intravenous lipid emulsion particles.

Liver biopsy: A procedure whereby tissue is removed from the liver and is used to determine the severity of liver damage.

Locus ceruleus: Nucleus of norepinephrine containing neurons located in the brainstem which is responsible for physiologic response to stress and panic.

Luteolysis: Death of the corpus luteum.

Lymphadenectomy: Surgical excision of lymph nodes.

Lymphadenitis: Inflammation of the lymph nodes, which become swollen, painful, and tender.

Lymphangitis: Inflammation of lymphatic channels.

Lymphatic: The network of vessels carrying tissue fluids.

Lymphoproliferative: Of or related to the growth of lymphoid tissue.

Maceration: The softening or breaking down of a solid by leaving it immersed in a liquid.

Macrophages: A large scavenger cell.

Macrovascular complications: Vascular complications that are contributed to by diabetes and include heart attacks, strokes, or peripheral vascular disease.

Macula: The central portion of the retina.

Maculopapular: A rash that contains both macules and papules. A macule is a flat discolored area of the skin, and a papule is a small raised bump. A maculopapular rash is usually a large area that is red and has small confluent bumps.

Magnetic resonance imaging: Method of body imaging that uses a magnetic field and radio waves to create cross-sectional images of one's body, which provides detailed pictures of organs and tissues.

Major malformation: A defect that has either cosmetic or functional significance.

Mastalgia: Tenderness of the breast.

Matrix metalloproteinases: Enzymes responsible for the degradation of connective tissue, normally located in the extracellular space of tissue, that break down proteins (e.g., collagen) and require zinc or calcium atoms as cofactors for enzymatic activity.

Meconium: The first intestinal discharge or "stool" of a newborn infant, usually green in color and consisting of epithelial cells, mucus, and bile.

Media: The middle layer of the wall of an artery or vein.

Mediastinum: The space in the thoracic cavity between the pleural sacs and behind the sternum.

Melanosis: Excessive pigmentation of the skin due to a disturbance in melanin pigmentation; called also melanism.

Melasma: Patchy skin pigmentation, often seen during pregnancy.

Melena: Tarry stools.

Menarche: The onset of cyclic menstrual periods in a woman.

Meningeal: Membranes that surround the brain and spinal cord.

Meninges: Covering of the brain consisting of three layers.

Menopause: Permanent cessation of menstruation.

Menorrhagia: Menstrual blood loss of greater than 80 mL per cycle; a more practical definition is heavy menstrual flow associated with problems of containment of flow, unpredictably heavy flow days, or other associated symptoms.

Mesocortical: A neural pathway that connects the ventral tegmentum to the cortex, particularly the frontal lobes. It is one of the major dopamine pathways in the brain.

Mesocorticolimbic pathway: A neural pathway that loops between the midbrain, the cortex, and limbic areas of the brain. An integral part of the brain reward system.

Mesothelioma: A benign or malignant tumor affecting the lining of the chest or abdomen. Commonly caused by exposure to asbestos fibers.

Metabolic acidosis: A condition in the blood and tissues that is a consequence of an accumulation of lactic acid resulting from tissue hypoxia and anaerobic metabolism.

Metabolic alkalosis: Alkalosis that is caused by an increase in the concentration of alkaline compounds (typically bicarbonate).

Metabolic syndrome: Constellation of cardiovascular risk factors related to hypertension, abdominal obesity, dyslipidemia, and insulin resistance diagnosed by the presence of at least three of the following criteria: increased waist circumference, elevated triglyceride concentrations, decreased high-density lipoprotein (HDL) cholesterol or active treatment to raise HDL cholesterol, elevated blood pressure or active treatment with antihypertensive therapy, or elevated fasting glucose or active treatment for diabetes.

Metastasis: Plural is metastases. Cancer that has spread from the original site of the tumor.

Micelle: A microscopic particle of digested fat and cholesterol.

Microalbuminuria: Loss of small amounts of protein in the urine. An albumin excretion ratio of 30 to 300 mg/24 hour, which is a sign of chronic kidney disease. The normal mean value for urine albumin excretion in adults is 10 mg/day.

Microdialysis: A brain research technique whereby very small probes are inserted into the brain, and the concentration of brain chemicals, such as neurotransmitters, can be measured.

β_2 Microglobulin: A low-molecular-weight protein that may be elevated in multiple myeloma.

Micrognathia: Abnormal smallness of the jaws, especially of the mandible.

Microvascular complications: Vascular complications contributed to by diabetes that include retinopathy, neuropathy, and nephropathy.

Microvascular pulmonary emboli: An obstruction in the small blood vessels in the lung caused by material (e.g., blood clot, fat, air, and foreign body) that is carried through the circulation until it lodges in another small vessel.

Micturition: Voiding, urination.

Migraineur: A person who suffers from migraine headaches.

Migrographia: Small handwriting, often seen in patients with Parkinson's disease.

Minimal residual disease: A quantitative assessment of subclinical remnant of leukemic burden remaining at the end of the initial phase of treatment (induction) when a patient may appear to be in a complete morphologic remission.

Minimum inhibitory concentration: The lowest concentration of an antimicrobial agent that inhibits visible bacterial growth after approximately 24 hours.

Minor malformation: A defect that occurs infrequently (less than 4% of the population) but that has neither cosmetic nor functional significance to the child.

Miosis: Pupillary constriction, "pinpoint" pupils.

Mitogenicity: Producing or stimulating mitosis (a process that takes place in the nucleus of a dividing cell resulting in the formation of two new nuclei, each having the same number of chromosomes as the parent nucleus).

Mixed disorder: The presence of two or more distinct disorders. See also Complicated disorder.

Mixed mood episodes: Symptoms of mania and depression occurring simultaneously or in close juxtaposition.

Mobilization: The release of stem cells into the peripheral blood from the bone marrow compartment for the purpose of collecting these stem cells in anticipation of stem cell transplantation.

Mobitz type I: A type of second-degree AV nodal blockade.

Mobitz type II: A type of second-degree AV nodal blockade.

Moebius (also Möbius) syndrome: An extremely rare congenital neurologic disorder which is characterized by facial paralysis and the inability to move the eyes from side to side.

Monocytes: A variety of white blood cells.

Monoparesis: Slight or incomplete paralysis affecting a single extremity or part of one.

Monosodium urate: A crystallized form of uric acid that can deposit in joints leading to an inflammatory reaction and the symptoms of gout.

Mood lability: Unstable or changeable moods.

Morphology: The science of structure and form of cells without regard to function.

Motor tics: Involuntary brief spasmodic muscular movement or contraction, usually of the face or extremities.

Mu receptors: One of the three major classes of endogenous opioid receptors in the body. Mu receptors appear to be responsible for the majority of both the analgesic and rewarding properties of opioids.

Mucositis: Inflammation of mucous membranes, typically within the oral and esophageal mucosa. Usually associated with certain chemotherapy agents and radiation therapy involving mucosal areas.

Mucous colitis: A condition of the mucous membrane of the colon characterized by pain, constipation or diarrhea (sometimes alternating), and passage of mucus or mucous shreds.

Multiparity: Condition of having given birth to multiple children.

Mydriasis: Pronounced or abnormal dilation of the pupils.

Myelin: A protein and phospholipid sheath that surrounds the axons of certain neurons. Myelinated nerves conduct impulses more rapidly than nonmyelinated nerves.

Myeloablative preparative regimen: Radiation and/or chemotherapy that destroys bone marrow activity in preparation for a stem cell transplant. Patients will not likely recover bone marrow function without an infusion of "rescue" autologous or allogeneic stem cells.

Myelodysplastic syndrome: A disease in which bone marrow does not function properly.

Myeloproliferative disorder: A group of diseases of bone marrow in which excess cells, usually lymphocytes, are produced.

Myelosuppression: Reduction in white blood cells, red blood cells, and platelets.

Myocarditis: Inflammation of the muscular wall of the heart.

Myoclonus: A sudden, involuntary jerking of a muscle or group of muscles.

Myoglobinuria: The presence of myoglobin in urine.

Myonecrosis: Necrotic damage to muscle tissue.

Myopathy: Any disease of the muscle causing weakness, pain, and tenderness.

Myringotomy: A surgical incision in the tympanic membrane to relieve pressure and drain fluid from the middle ear.

Myxedema: Relatively hard edema associated with hypothyroidism.

Nasal scotoma: An area of blindness in the nasal portion of peripheral vision.

Nascent: Immature.

Nasolacrimal occlusion: The closing of the tear duct to decrease systemic absorption of a drug.

Nausea: The subjective feeling of a need to vomit.

Necrotizing enterocolitis: Medical condition primarily seen in premature infants, where portions of the bowel undergo necrosis.

Nelson's syndrome: A condition characterized by the aggressive growth of a pituitary tumor and hyperpigmentation of the skin.

Neoadjuvant therapy: Chemotherapy or radiation therapy given prior to primary surgical treatment. In cancer, it is often used to downstage the tumor to a resectable stage.

Neovascular maculopathy: Proliferation of blood vessels in the macula.

Neovascularization: New blood vessel formation (vascularization) especially in abnormal quantity (some conditions of the retina) or in abnormal tissue (tumor).

Nephrolithiasis: A condition marked by the presence of renal calculi (stones) in the kidney or urinary system.

Nephron: The working unit of the kidney that filters blood to remove fluid, toxins, and drugs. Each kidney contains approximately 1 million nephrons.

Nephrostomy: Insertion of a catheter through the skin into the renal pelvis to bypass ureteral obstruction and facilitate urine drainage.

Neuralgia: Pain which extends along the course of one or more nerves.

Neuritic (senile) plaque: An abnormal cluster of dead and dying nerve cells, other brain cells, and protein. One of the structural abnormalities found in the brains of patients with Alzheimer's disease.

Neuritis: Inflammation of a nerve.

Neurofibrillary tangle: An accumulation of twisted protein fragments inside nerve cells; one of the structural abnormalities found in the brains of patients with Alzheimer's disease.

Neuroimaging: Radiologic studies of the brain, usually referring to computerized tomography (CT) or magnetic resonance imaging (MRI).

Neurologic focality: Symptomatic sensory or motor deficits that point to specific lesions or dysfunction in the brain.

Neuropathic pain: Pain resulting from a lesion or dysfunction of the nervous system.

Neuropathy: An abnormal and usually degenerative state of the nervous system or nerves.

Neurotransmitters: Chemicals in the brain that allow the passage of a message between neurons or nerve cells.

Neutralizing antibodies: Antibodies that develop in response to a therapeutic agent that decrease the efficacy of the agent.

Nf-κB: Nuclear factor kappa B regulates cytokine production.

Nidus: A central point or focus consisting of a fibrin matrix (in the case of infective endocarditis), where bacteria are able to accumulate and multiply, allowing for formation of an infected vegetation.

Nitric oxide: An endogenous vasodilator.

Nociception: The perception of pain.

Nociceptors: Receptors for pain caused by injury from physical stimuli (mechanical, electrical, or thermal) or chemical stimuli (toxins); located in the skin, muscles, or in the walls of the viscera.

Nocturia: Micturition at night. Usually characterized by excessive urination at night.

Nocturnal polysomnography: Visual and electrophysiologic assessment of human sleep minimally composed of electroencephalogram, electrooculogram, and electromyogram that allows determination of sleep stage, breathing events, and muscle movements.

Nodules: When seen in rheumatoid arthritis, nodules are subcutaneous knobs over bony prominences or extensor surfaces.

Nonbacterial thrombotic endocarditis (NBTE): Endocarditis caused by noninfectious vegetations.

Nonmyeloablative preparative regimen: Radiation and/or chemotherapy that does not completely eradicate host bone marrow activity. Host bone marrow activity is suppressed but may recover after approximately 4 weeks even in the absence of "rescue" allogeneic stem cells.

Nonnucleoside reverse transcriptase inhibitor (NNRTI): A noncompetitive inhibitor of the viral reverse transcriptase enzyme by binding to the active site of the enzyme itself, rather than by terminating the enzymatic product. NNRTIs are only active against HIV-1.

Nonpolyposis: Absence of polyps.

Nonprotein kilocalorie-to-nitrogen ratio: Numerical value derived from dividing kilocalories from carbohydrate plus fat by the number of grams of nitrogen in the diet.

Non-REM sleep: A state of usually dreamless sleep that occurs regularly during a normal period of sleep with intervening periods of REM sleep and that consists of four distinct substages and low levels of autonomic physiological activity.

Non-ST-segment elevation: A type of myocardial infarction that is limited to the subendocardial myocardium and is smaller and less extensive than an ST-segment MI. Usually there is no pathologic Q wave on the ECG.

Normal flora: Normal colonizing bacteria of a human host.

Normochromic: Being normal in color; especially referring to red blood cells.

Normocytic: Normal size especially referring to red blood cells.

Nosocomial: An infection acquired within the health care system, e.g., hospital. Generally, symptoms of infection must occur after at least 48 hours of care to be considered nosocomial.

Nuchal rigidity: Neck stiffness.

Nuclear medicine scan: Method of body imaging that uses a radioactive tracer material (e.g., technetium and gallium) to produce body images. For example, bone scans detect uptake and cellular activity in areas of inflammation.

Nucleoside reverse transcriptase inhibitor (NRTI)/nucleotide reverse transcriptase inhibitor (NtRI): A modified version of a naturally occurring nucleoside or nucleotide that prevents HIV replication by interfering with the function of the viral reverse transcriptase enzyme. The nucleoside/nucleotide analog causes early termination of the proviral DNA chain. For activity, an NRTI requires three phosphorylation steps once inside the cell, whereas an NtRI has a phosphate group attached and needs only two phosphorylation steps inside the cell for activity.

Nucleus accumbens: One of three nuclei that comprise the striatum (part of the basal ganglia). It receives dopaminergic input from the ventral tegmental area and is part of the limbic loop that plays a part in the motivational regulation of behavior and emotions.

Nulliparity: Not having given birth to a child.

Nystagmus: Rapid, involuntary movement of the eyes.

Obliterative bronchiolitis: Inflammation of the bronchioles (the small elements of the tracheobronchial tree) characterized by obliteration and/or permanent narrowing of the airways.

Off-label use: Use of a medication outside the scope of its approved, labeled use.

Offloading: Modalities, such as orthotics, that help offweight/load an area of pressure, giving tissues time to heal without repetitive stress, which delays wound healing.

Oiling out: Continued coalescence of lipid emulsion particles, resulting in irreversible separation of the emulsion (or "breaking" of the emulsion).

Olfactory tubercle: Both the olfactory tubercle and the amygdala receive direct input from the olfactory bulb, and together they appear to help regulate the emotional, endocrine, and visceral consequences of odors.

Oligoanovulation: The condition of having few to no ovulatory menstrual cycles.

Oligoclonal bands: Small discrete bands in the γ-globulin region of fluid electrophoresis.

Oligohydramnios: Decreased amniotic fluid.

Oligomenorrhea: Abnormally light or infrequent menstruation.

Oliguria: Reduced urine output. Usually defined as less than 400 mL in 24 hours or less than 0.5 mL/kg/h.

Omentumectomy: Excision of the double fold of peritoneum attached to the stomach and connecting it with abdominal viscera (omentum).

Oncogene: Genes that cause transformation of normal cells into cancer cells by promoting uncontrolled cell growth and multiplication leading to tumor formation.

Oophorectomy: Surgery to remove the ovaries.

Open comedo: A plugged follicle of sebum, keratinocytes, and bacteria that protrudes from the surface of the skin and appears black or brown in color. Also referred to as a "blackhead."

Opsonization: The process by which an antigen is altered so as to become more readily and more efficiently engulfed by phagocytes.

Optic neuritis: Usually monocular central visual acuity loss and ocular/periorbital pain caused by demyelination of the optic nerve.

Orbital/supraorbital: Pertaining to the eye socket and the area directly above it.

Orchiectomy: The surgical removal of the testicles.

Organification: Binding of iodine to tyrosine residues of thyroglobulin.

Orthopnea: Difficulty in breathing that occurs when lying down and is relieved upon changing to an upright position.

Orthostasis: Characterized by a drop in blood pressure when standing up from sitting or lying down, often causing lightheadedness and dizziness.

Orthotopic transplant: Placing a transplanted organ into the normal anatomic location.

Osmolality: A measure of the number of osmotically active particles per unit solution, independent of the weight or nature of the particle.

Osmolar gap: The difference between the measured serum osmolality and the calculated serum osmolality.

Osmophobia: A fear of strong odors and unpleasant smells; also called olfactophobia.

Osteoblasts: Cells involved in bone formation; "builders of bone."

Osteoclasts: Cells involved in bone resorption; "creators of cavities."

Osteomalacia: Softening of the bones.

Osteonecrosis: Death of bone tissue.

Osteopenia: Low bone density, which can lead to osteoporosis.

Osteophytes: Bony outgrowths (bone spurs) into the joint space.

Osteoporosis: Disease of the bones characterized by a loss of bone tissue, resulting in brittle, weak bones that are susceptible to fracture (porous bones).

Ostomy: Surgical operation where part of the abdominal wall is opened and part of the intestine is connected to the opening for intestinal draining, e.g., colostomy, ileostomy.

Otitis media with effusion: Fluid in the middle ear space with no signs or symptoms of an acute infection.

Ovulation: Periodic ripening and rupture of mature follicle and the discharge of ovum from the cortex of the ovary.

Oxygen desaturation: A decrease in the oxygen saturation of the blood. Oxygen saturation is described as the oxygen content of blood divided by oxygen capacity and expressed in volume percent.

Pacemaker: A mass of fibers that possess actual or potential automaticity, which initiates and determines the rate of spontaneous depolarizations.

Palliative care: According to the World Health Organization, the active, total care of patients whose disease is not responsive to curative treatment.

Palmar-plantar erythrodysesthesia (PPE): Syndrome characterized by numbness, tingling or burning sensations with edema, and redness of the hands and feet often resulting in cracked skin and blisters with marked peeling of skin.

Pancolitis: Inflammation that involves the majority of the colon in patients with inflammatory bowel disease.

Pancreatitis: Inflammation of the pancreas.

Panhypopituitarism: A clinical disorder characterized by complete deficiency in pituitary hormone production.

Pannus: Inflamed synovial tissue that invades and destroys articular structures.

Papilledema: Edema of the optic disc typically associated with increased intracranial pressure. Also called a choked disc.

Paracentral scotoma: Blind spots near the center of the visual field.

Parasomnia: Undesirable physical or behavioral phenomena (e.g., sleep walking, bruxism, enuresis, sleep talking, and REM behavior disorder) that occur predominantly during sleep.

Parenchyma: Specific cells or tissues of an organ.

Parenteral nutrition: Delivery of nutrients via the intravenous route.

Paresthesia: An abnormal touch sensation, such as burning or prickling, often in the absence of external stimulus.

Parieto-occipital: Located at the top and back of the head.

Paroxysmal: Intermittent occurrence, initiating suddenly and spontaneously, lasting minutes to hours, and terminating suddenly and spontaneously.

Pars reticulate: Dopaminergic cell bodies located in the substantia nigra that project to the thalamus and cortex. Considered one of the basal ganglia pathways; involved not only with movement but also with emotions, motivations, and cognition that drive movement.

Peak expiratory flow: The maximum flow rate of air leaving the lungs upon forced exhalation.

Pelvic inflammatory disease: Inflammation of the endometrium, uterine tubes, and pelvic peritoneum; often due to a sexually transmitted infection.

Percutaneous coronary intervention (PCI): A minimally invasive procedure whereby access to the coronary arteries is obtained through the femoral artery up the aorta to the coronary os. Contrast media is used to visualize the coronary artery stenosis using a coronary angiogram. A guidewire is used to cross the stenosis and a small balloon is inflated and/or stent is deployed to break up atherosclerotic plaque and restore coronary artery blood flow. The stent is left in place to prevent acute closure and restenosis of the coronary artery. Newer stents are coated with antiproliferative drugs, such as paclitaxel and sirolimus, which further reduce the risk of restenosis of the coronary artery.

Percutaneous endoscopic gastrostomy: Gastric feeding tube placed via endoscopic technique.

Percutaneous endoscopic jejunostomy: Jejunal feeding tube placed via endoscopic technique.

Perihilar: The area surrounding the depression in the medial surface of a lung that forms the opening through which the bronchus, blood vessels, and nerves pass.

Perimenopause: Also known as the climacteric, is the period of time prior to menopause when hormonal and biological changes and physical symptoms begin to occur and usually lasts for 1 year after the last menstrual period. The perimenopausal period may last for an average of 3 to 5 years.

Perimetry: Measurement of the field of vision.

Peripheral artery disease: Atherosclerosis of the peripheral arteries.

Peripheral resistance: The sum of resistance to blood flow offered by systemic blood vessels.

Peritonitis: An acute inflammatory reaction of the peritoneal lining to microorganisms or chemical irritation.

PET scan: A scan that produces images of the body after the injection of a radiolabeled form of glucose. A PET scan is often used to detect cancer or follow response to treatment since tumors use more sugar than normal cells.

Petechiae: Tiny localized hemorrhages from the small blood vessels just beneath the surface of the skin

Phagocytic cell: A cell that absorbs waste material, harmful microorganisms, or other foreign bodies in the bloodstream and tissues.

Phagocytosis: The process of engulfing and ingesting an antigen by phagocytes.

Pharmacodynamics: Describing the actions of a drug on the body or a part of the body, e.g., a receptor or organ.

Pharmacogenomic: The influence of genetic variation on drug response in patients, used to correlate gene expression with a drug's efficacy or toxicity.

Pharmacokinetics: Refers to a mathematical method of describing a patient's drug exposure in vivo in terms of absorption, distribution, metabolism, and elimination.

Pharyngitis: Inflammation and/or infection of the pharynx that causes throat pain.

Phenotype: The visible properties of an organism that are produced by the interaction of the genotype and the environment.

Pheochromocytoma: A tumor arising from chromaffin cells, most commonly found in the adrenal medulla. The tumor causes the adrenal medulla to hypersecrete epinephrine and norepinephrine resulting in hypertension and other signs and symptoms of excessive sympathetic nervous system activity. The tumor is usually benign but may occasionally be cancerous.

Phlebitis: Inflammation of a blood vessel, e.g., vein.

Phonophobia: A fear of sounds, loud noises, and even one's own voice.

Photochemotherapy: The use of phototherapy together with topical or systemic drugs in the treatment of psoriasis.

Photodynamic therapy: Cancer treatment that uses interaction between laser light and a substance that makes the cells more sensitive to light. When light is applied to cells that have been treated with this substance, a chemical reaction occurs and destroys cancer cells.

Photophobia: An abnormal sensitivity to or intolerance of light.

Phototherapy: The use of ultraviolet light applied to the skin, e.g., in treating psoriasis or neonatal hyperbilirubinemia.

Physical dependence: A state of adaptation that is manifested by a drug-class specific withdrawal syndrome that can be produced by abrupt cessation, rapid dose reduction, decreasing blood level of the drug, and/or administration of an antagonist.

Piloerection: Erection of hairs, due to stimulation or contraction of the arrector pili muscles, also described as "gooseflesh."

Pilosebaceous unit: A hair follicle and the surrounding sebaceous glands.

Plasma cell: Antibody producing cells.

Plasmapheresis: The process of separating blood cells from plasma. This process is used to remove the monoclonal antibodies from the blood.

Pleocytosis: A transient increase in the number of leukocytes in a body fluid.

Pleuritis: Inflammation of the lining around the lungs.

Pneumatic otoscopy: A diagnostic technique involving visualization of the tympanic membrane for transparency, position, and color, and its response to positive and negative air pressure to assess mobility.

Pneumothorax: The presence of air in the pleural cavity, often causing part of the lung to collapse.

Polycythemia: An abnormal increase in the number of erythrocytes in the blood.

Polydipsia: Excessive thirst.

Polymorphic metabolism: Genetically determined rates of metabolism (fast versus slow) by selected isozymes of cytochrome P450 drug-metabolizing enzymes.

Polymorphisms: Interindividual variations in the genetic code at the level of one nucleotide.

Polymorphonuclear leukocyte: A subgroup of white blood cells, filled with granules of toxic chemicals that enable them to digest microorganisms by phagocytosis.

Polyphagia: Eating excessively large amounts of food at a meal.

Polypharmacy: Taking multiple medications concurrently.

Polyp: A growth from a mucous membrane commonly found in organs such as the colon, rectum, and the nose. Usually not malignant, these can develop into cancer and require removal once found.

Polyuria: Excessive excretion of urine resulting in profuse micturition.

Portal hypertension: Increased blood pressure within the portal vein that supplies the liver.

Postpyloric feeding: Delivery of nutrients via a tube placed with its tip past the pyloric sphincter separating the stomach from the duodenum.

Prader-Willi syndrome: A genetic disorder characterized by short stature, mental retardation, low muscle tone, abnormally small hands and feet, hypogonadism, and excessive eating leading to extreme obesity.

Prediabetes: An asymptomatic but abnormal state that precedes the development of clinically evident diabetes.

Preload: The stretched condition of the heart muscle at the end of diastole just before contraction. Volume in the left ventricle at the end of diastole estimated by the pulmonary artery occlusion pressure (also known as the pulmonary artery wedge pressure or pulmonary capillary wedge pressure).

Preparative regimen (conditioning regimen): Radiation and/or chemotherapy given to stem cell transplant patients in order to kill malignant cells, create space in the bone marrow compartment, and suppress the immune system of the host in order to prevent graft rejection.

Priapism: A prolonged, painful erection lasting more than 4 hours. Considered a medical emergency.

Primary amenorrhea: Absence of menses by age 16 in the presence of normal secondary sexual development or absence of menses by age 14 in the absence of normal secondary sexual development.

Primary prevention: The removal or reduction of risk factors before the development of disease.

Prinzmetal angina: Vasospasm or contraction of the coronary arteries in the absence of significant atherosclerosis. Also referred to as variant angina.

Probiotics: Dietary supplements containing potentially beneficial bacteria that promote health by stimulating optimal mucosal immune responses.

Proctitis: Inflammation confined to the rectum in patients with inflammatory bowel disease.

Prodrome: Early symptom(s) indicating the onset of an attack or a disease.

Progenitor: A primitive cell.

Prolapse: Protrusion of an organ or part of an organ through an opening, e.g., uterine prolapse occurs when the uterus is displaced downward such that the cervix is within the vaginal opening (first degree), the cervix is outside the opening (second degree), or the entire uterus is outside the opening (third degree).

Proptosis: Forward displacement of the eyeball.

Prostaglandin: Any of a large group of biologically active, carbon-20, unsaturated fatty acids that are produced by the metabolism of arachidonic acid through the cyclooxygenase pathway.

Prostate specific antigen: This secretion of prostatic epithelial cells is used as a tumor marker for prostate cancer. It is not specific for prostate cancer. Thus, serum prostate-specific antigen concentrations may be increased in the face of any inflammatory or infectious disorder of the prostate, benign prostatic hyperplasia, or because of instrumentation of the prostate.

Prostatectomy: Surgical removal of the prostate, which can be performed transurethrally, suprapubically, or retropubically. There are two main types: transurethral prostatectomy (TURP) and radical prostatectomy. TURP removes part of the tissue surrounding the urethra, which may be blocking the flow of urine. Radical prostatectomy removes all of the prostate and the seminal vesicles.

Prostatic hyperplasia: Enlargement of the prostate.

Prosthetic-valve endocarditis (PVE): Endocarditis that occurs in patients with bioprosthetic or synthetic implanted heart valves.

Protease: Any one of various enzymes, including proteinases and peptidases, that catalyze the hydrolytic breakdown of proteins.

Protease inhibitor (PI): A drug that acts by inhibiting the viral protease enzyme, which prevents long strands of protein from being cleaved into the smaller proteins the virus requires for assembly.

Protectant: An agent that forms an occlusive barrier between the skin and surrounding moisture.

Protected specimen brush: Used in bronchoscopy, a brush in the lumen of a tube inside the bronchoscope. The brush is extended into the lung to obtain a sample, then retracted back into the tube for removal from the lung.

Proteinase: Any of numerous enzymes that catalyze the breakdown of proteins. Also called protease.

Proteinuria: The presence of measurable amounts of protein (greater than 150 mg/day) in the urine, which is often indicative of glomerular or tubular damage in the kidney.

Proteoglycan: Any one of a class of glycoproteins of high molecular weight that are found in the extracellular matrix of connective tissue. They are made up mostly of carbohydrate consisting of various polysaccharide side chains linked to a protein and resemble polysaccharides rather than proteins with regard to their properties.

Proteolysis: The hydrolysis of proteins, usually by enzyme action, into simpler substances.

Proteosome: An enzyme complex that degrades intracellular proteins.

Prothrombin: A clotting factor that is converted to thrombin. Also known as Factor II.

Prothrombin time: A measure of coagulation representing the amount of time required to form a blood clot after the addition of thromboplastin to the blood sample. Also known as Quick test.

Prothrombotic state: A state of high coagulation of the blood.

Pruritis: Localized or generalized itching due to irritation of sensory nerve endings.

Pseudoaddiction: A term used to describe patient behaviors (e.g., "drug-seeking," "clock watching," or illicit drug use) that may occur when pain is undertreated. Pseudoaddiction can be distinguished from true addiction in that the behaviors resolve when pain is effectively treated.

Pseudohyphae: Elongated forms created by replicating yeast that form buds but do not detach from one another.

Pseudophakia: Refers to presence of a lens after cataract extraction.

Pseudopolyps: An area of hypertrophied gastrointestinal mucosa that resembles a polyp and contains nonmalignant cells.

Pseudoseizure: Convulsions or seizure-like activity that results from causes other than abnormal electrical activity in the brain.

Psychodynamic: The explanation or interpretation of behavior or mood in terms of mental or emotional forces or processes.

Psychomotor retardation: A slowness of thought and physical movement that is primarily due to the psychological state.

Psychosocial: The interface between psychological and social functioning.

Pulmonary artery catheter: An invasive device used to measure hemodynamic parameters directly, including cardiac output and pulmonary artery occlusion pressure. Calculated parameters include stroke volume and systemic vascular resistance.

Pulmonary artery occlusion pressure: A hemodynamic measurement obtained via a catheter placed into the pulmonary artery used to evaluate patient volume status within the circulation.

Pulmonary embolism: A disorder of thrombus formation causing obstruction of a pulmonary artery or one of its branches and resulting in pulmonary infarction.

Pulsus paradoxus: A large fall in systolic blood pressure and pulse volume during inspiration or an abnormal variation in pulse volume during respiration in which the pulse becomes weaker with inspiration and stronger with expiration.

Purkinje fibers: Specialized myocardial fibers that conduct impulses from the AV node to the ventricles.

Purpura: A small hemorrhage of the skin, mucous membrane, or serosal surface.

Purulent: Containing, consisting of, or being pus.

Pyelonephritis: Inflammation of a kidney.

Pyloroplasty: A surgical procedure for enlarging the opening of the stomach to the duodenum.

Pyuria: Presence of pus in urine when voided.

Quality indicators: A list of indicators used by long-term care facility administrators and government overseers to identify potential problems in patient care.

Quality of Life: Perceived physical and mental health over time.

Radiofrequency catheter ablation: Procedure during which radiofrequency energy is delivered through a catheter positioned at the atrioventricular node for the purpose of destroying one pathway of a reentrant circuit.

Raphe nuclei: Bed of serotonin containing neurons that extend to the hypothalamus, septum, hippocampus, and cingulated gyrus.

Recombinant activated factor VII: A clotting factor manufactured via recombinant technology used off-label (non-FDA approved) to foster clotting in hemorrhagic shock patients with massive hemorrhage refractory to conventional therapies such as fresh frozen plasma.

Rectal prolapse: Sinking of the rectum through the anal sphincter so that it is visible externally.

Recurrence: A relapse that occurs after a clear-cut recovery.

5α-Reductase: Intracellular enzyme in some target cells which activates testosterone to dihydrotestosterone. In these androgen-dependent target cells, dihydrotestosterone is more potent than testosterone.

Reentry: Circular movement of electrical impulses, a mechanism of many arrhythmias.

Refractory periods: The period of time after an impulse is initiated and conducted during which cells cannot be depolarized again.

Regurgitation: A passive process without involvement of the abdominal wall and the diaphragm wherein gastric or esophageal contents move into the mouth.

Relapse: The return of symptoms, satisfying the full syndrome criteria, after a patient has responded, but prior to recovery.

REM sleep: A state of sleep that recurs cyclically several times during a normal period of sleep and that is characterized by increased neuronal activity of the forebrain and midbrain, by depressed muscle tone, and by dreaming, rapid eye movements, and vascular congestion of the sex organs.

Remission: Relief of symptoms and return to full functioning in all areas of life.

Renin-angiotensin-aldosterone system: The hormonal system controlled mainly by the kidneys and adrenal glands that regulates blood pressure, blood volume, and electrolyte balance.

Replication capacity: This term is often used interchangeably with the term "viral fitness" and refers to how quickly HIV reproduces or replicates. The slower HIV replicates, the less likely a patient is to have disease progression. A replication capacity may be reported on a resistance test. It is reported as a percentage of the median replication rate for drug-sensitive (wild-type) HIV strains.

Resorption: The process of bone breakdown by osteoclasts.

Respiratory acidosis: Acidosis that is caused by an accumulation of carbon dioxide.

Respiratory alkalosis: Alkalosis that is caused by a loss of carbon dioxide.

Respiratory disturbance index: A summary measure that quantifies the number of apneas, hypopneas, and respiratory effort-related arousals per hour of sleep.

Response: Refers to a predefined reduction of symptoms from baseline that generally results in significant functional improvement.

Response inhibition: Ability to stay on task.

Restenosis: Renarrowing of the coronary artery after a percutaneous intervention to improve coronary blood flow.

Retching: A process that follows nausea and consists of diaphragm, abdominal wall, and chest wall contractions and spasmodic breathing against a closed glottis.

Reticulocytes: Immature blood cells that mature into erythrocytes.

Reticuloendothelial system: Phagocytic cells excluding granulocytes; widely distributed throughout the body.

Retinopathy: The leading cause of blindness in people aged 20 to 74; occurs when the microvasculature nerve layer that provides blood and nutrients to the retina are damaged.

Retrograde ejaculation: Disorder in which semen flows in a backward fashion up the urethra and into the bladder during climax. The patient will complain of dry sex or no ejaculation during sexual intercourse, which may be worrisome to the patient.

Retroperitoneal fibrosis: An accumulation of fibrotic tissues located behind the organs contained in the abdominal sac.

Reye's syndrome: A sudden, sometimes fatal, syndrome characterized by encephalopathy and liver degeneration, which occurs in children after viral infection and is also associated with aspirin use.

Rhabdomyolysis: A rapid lysis or destruction of skeletal muscles that can be associated with renal failure and death.

Rheumatic fever: An acute inflammatory disease involving the joints, heart, skin, brain, and other tissues caused by an immune response to streptococcal infection in genetically susceptible people, particularly in children.

Rheumatoid factors: Antibodies reactive with the Fc region of IgG.

Rhinorrhea: Nasal secretions; a runny nose.

Rhinosinusitis: Inflammation of the mucous membranes in the nose and sinuses.

Rhonchi: Abnormal, rumbling sounds heard on auscultation of an obstructed airway. They are more prominent during expiration and may clear somewhat on coughing.

Rouleaux formation: The stacking of red blood cells on a peripheral smear when diluted.

Rubefacient: A substance that produces redness of the skin.

Rule of six: A previously used weight-based guideline for calculating intravenous continuous infusions by multiplying body weight (kg) by six and adding this amount of drug to 100 mL of fluid, resulting in a concentration and infusion rate of 1 mcg/kg/min and 1 mL/h.

Salicylism: A toxic syndrome caused by excessive doses of acetylsalicylic acid (aspirin), salicylic acid, or any other salicylate product. Signs and symptoms may include severe headache, nausea, vomiting, tinnitus (ringing in the ears), confusion, increased pulse, and increased respiratory rate.

Scarlatiniform rash: Bright, scarlet-colored skin eruption that occurs in patches over the entire body with eventual peeling as a result of streptococcal infection.

Scleral icterus: Jaundice of the outer layer of the eyeball.

Scleritis: Inflammation of the outer layer of the eyeball.

Scoliosis: A congenital lateral curvature of the spine.

Scotoma: Referring to a partial loss of vision.

Secondary amenorrhea: Absence of menses for three cycles or 6 months in a previously menstruating woman.

Secondary hyperparathyroidism (sHPT): Increased secretion of parathyroid hormone from the parathyroid glands caused by hyperphosphatemia, hypocalcemia, and vitamin D deficiency that result from decreased kidney function. Secondary hyperparathyroidism can lead to bone disease (bone and mineral metabolism disorders).

Secondary prevention: Early detection of the premalignant condition or cancer, leading to earlier intervention.

Secondary transmission: Transferring a disease from the primary source to another person.

Seizure: A sudden attack due to involuntary electrical activity in the brain. It is caused by an uncontrolled burst of electrical activity in the brain that can result in a wide variety of clinical manifestation such as: muscle jerks or twitches, staring, tongue biting, loss of consciousness, and total body shaking.

Semiology: The clinical appearance or symptoms of a seizure.

Sentinel lymph node: The first lymph node to receive lymph draining from a tumor.

Sepsis: A syndrome characterized by a systemic inflammatory response (abnormal increases in body temperature, heart rate, respiratory rate, and/or white blood cell concentration) caused by infection.

Sera: Pertaining to human serum.

Serosa: An enclosing serous membrane of the pericardium, pleura, and peritoneum.

Serum ferritin: Quantifies the iron-binding capacity of transferring.

Serum sickness: A group of symptoms caused by a delayed immune response to certain medications. Arthralgias, fever, malaise, and urticaria may develop usually 7 to 14 days after exposure to the causative antigen.

Shear stress: Risk factor for pressure ulcers that is generated when the head of a patient's bed is elevated and can cause deeper blood vessels to crimp, leading to ischemia.

Sialorrhea: Drooling.

Sick sinus syndrome: Idiopathic sinus node dysfunction leading to symptomatic sinus bradycardia.

Sickle cell anemia: Genetic disorder in which the red blood cells become crescent shaped.

Sickle cell syndrome: Describes a group of autosomal recessive genetic disorders that are characterized by the presence of at least one sickle hemoglobin gene.

Sickle hemoglobin: A defective form of hemoglobin produced as a result of a single substitution of the amino acid valine for glutamic acid at position 6 of the β-polypeptide chain.

Sigmoidoscopy: A visual inspection of the sigmoid colon and rectum with a flexible tube called a sigmoidoscope.

Simple disorder: The presence of a single acid–base disorder, with or without compensation.

Sjogren's syndrome: An autoimmune disorder that causes inflammation of the salivary glands; decreasing the production of saliva, which is a buffer against esophageal erosions.

Sleep apnea: The temporary stopping of breathing during sleep; can be caused by narrowing of the airways resulting from swelling of soft tissue.

Sleep latency: The amount of time it takes to fall asleep.

Sliding scale insulin: An increase or decrease in the number of units of insulin administered to correct a blood glucose level at a particular point in time that does not prevent the problem from occurring and does not take into account differing total daily insulin requirements of patients.

Slit lamp biomicroscope: An instrument that allows for the microscopic examination of the cornea, anterior chamber lens, and posterior chamber.

Somatic hypermutation: The occurrence of multiple point mutations.

Somatotrope: Growth hormone producing cells in the anterior pituitary.

Somnolence: Prolonged drowsiness or sleepiness.

Source control: Removal of the primary cause of an infection such as contaminated prosthetic materials (e.g., catheters), necrotic tissue, or drainage of an abscess. Antimicrobials are unlikely to be effective if the process or source that led to the infection is not controlled.

Spastic colon: A synonym for irritable bowel syndrome.

Spasticity: A motor disorder characterized by an increase in muscle tone with exaggerated tendon jerks, resulting from hyperexcitability of the stretch reflex.

Spectrum of activity: A qualitative term that describes the number of different bacterial species that are susceptible to an antimicrobial regimen. Generally, broad-spectrum activity refers to regimens that possess activity against many bacterial species, whereas narrow-spectrum therapy refers to activity against a few bacterial species.

Sphincter of Oddi: Structure through which the common bile duct empties bile and pancreatic secretions into the duodenum.

Spirometry: Measurement by means of a spirometer of the air entering and leaving the lungs.

Splenomegaly: An enlarged spleen secondary to leukemic infiltration.

Spontaneous bacterial peritonitis: Bacterial infection of the peritoneal fluid without abdominal source.

Sprain: An overstretching of supporting ligaments that results in a partial or complete tear of the ligament.

Status epilepticus: Any seizure lasting more than 30 minutes, with or without a loss of consciousness; or having recurrent seizures without regaining consciousness between seizure episodes.

Steatohepatitis: A severe form of liver disease caused by fat deposition in the liver, characterized by hepatic inflammation that may rapidly progress to liver fibrosis and cirrhosis.

Steatorrhea: Excessive loss of fat in stool.

Steatosis: Excessive fat accumulation.

Stenosis: Blockage of an artery.

Stenting: Placement of a stent to allow blood flow through an artery.

Stereotactic radiosurgery: Radiation technique that uses a large number of narrow, precisely aimed, highly focused beams of ionizing radiation. The beams are aimed from many directions circling the head and meet at a specific point.

Stereotyped behavior: Behavior that is associated with repetitive postures or movements without meaning.

Stevens-Johnson syndrome: A severe expression of erythema multiforme (also known as erythema multiforme major). It typically involves the skin and the mucous membranes with the potential for severe morbidity and even death.

Stimulant: Any amphetamine or amphetamine-like substance (methylphenidate) that causes an increase in dopaminergic and norepinephrine activity in the brain resulting in lessening of hyperactivity, impulsiveness and/or inattentiveness.

Stomatitis: Inflammation of mucous membranes in the mouth.

Strain: Damage to the muscle fibers or muscle sheath without tearing of the ligament.

Stretta procedure: Application of radiofrequency to increase lower esophageal sphincter tone.

Striae: Linear, atrophic, pinkish or purplish, scar-like lesions that later become white (striae albicantes, lineae albicantes), which may occur on the abdomen, breasts, buttocks, and thighs. They are due to weakening of the elastic tissues; commonly called stretch marks.

Stricture: Abnormal narrowing of a tubular structure in the body. An area of narrowing or constriction in the gastrointestinal tract due to buildup of fibrotic tissue, often a result of longstanding inflammation.

Stroke volume: The amount of blood ejected from the heart during systole.

ST-segment elevation: A type of myocardial infarction that typically results in an injury that transects the thickness of the myocardial wall. Following an ST-elevation MI, pathologic Q waves are frequently seen on the ECG, indicating transmural myocardial infarction.

Subchondral: Situated beneath and supporting cartilage.

Substantia nigra: The area in the brainstem with highly pigmented cells that make dopamine.

Surgical margins: An area of tissue surrounding a tumor when it is removed by surgery.

Surgical site infection: Infections occurring at or near the surgical incision within 30 days of the operation; up to 1 year if a prosthesis is implanted.

Suspending agent: An additive used in the compounding of oral liquid medications to suspend drug particles throughout a liquid and enables resuspension of particles by agitation (shaking well).

Synechia: Adhesions or the abnormal attachment of the iris to another structure. Peripheral anterior synechia refers to occurrence of synechia with the trabecular meshwork.

Synovitis: Inflammation of the synovial membrane, often in combination with pain and swelling of the affected joint.

Synovium: Membrane lining the internal surfaces of the joint.

Systolic dysfunction: An abnormal contraction of the ventricles during systole.

Tachycardia: Abnormally fast heart rate.

Tachyphylaxis: Rapid decreasing response to a drug or other physiologically active agent after a few doses.

Tachypnea: Abnormally fast respiratory rate.

Tangentiality: Abandoning one's ideational objective in pursuit of thoughts peripheral to the original goal. Used to describe a thought and speech pattern wherein the individual never gets to the point or answers the question.

Tardive dyskinesia: A chronic disorder of the nervous system characterized by involuntary jerky or writhing movements of the face, tongue, jaws, trunk, and limbs, usually developing as a late side effect of prolonged treatment with antipsychotic drugs.

Telangiectasia: Permanent dilation of preexisting small blood vessels (capillaries, arterioles, and venules), usually in the skin or mucous membranes which presents as a coarse or fine red line.

Tendonitis: Inflammation of the tendon.

Tenesmus: Refers to straining, especially painful, or ineffectual straining with a bowel movement or straining on defecation owing to spasms of an inflamed rectal sphincter as occurs in shigellosis.

Tenosynovitis: Inflammation of the tendon sheath.

Teratogen: An exogenous agent or substance that can modify normal embryonic or fetal development. The manifestation of teratogenicity can include structural anomalies, functional deficit, cancer, growth retardation, and death (spontaneous abortion, stillbirth).

Teratogenic potential: The ability of an agent to cause harm or malformations to a fetus or embryo. Medications are assigned pregnancy categories based on their teratogenic potential.

Teratogenicity: The property of causing malformations in the developing fetus.

Terminal secretions: The noise produced by the oscillatory movements of secretions in the upper airways in association with the inspiratory and expiratory phases of respiration. Also known as "death rattle."

Tetany: Hyperexcitability of nerves and muscles characterized by muscular twitching and cramps, laryngospasm with inspiratory stridor, and hyperreflexia.

Third spacing: Fluid accumulation in the interstitial space disproportionate to the intracellular and extracellular fluid spaces.

Thoracentesis: Removal of fluid that is present in the pleural space. Common procedure to determine cause of the fluid accumulation.

Thrombin: The enzyme formed from prothrombin, which converts fibrinogen to fibrin. It is the principal driving force in the clotting cascade.

Thrombocytopenia: Decrease in platelet concentration in the blood.

Thrombocytosis: Increased number of platelets in the blood.

Thrombogenesis: The process of forming a blood clot.

Thrombolysis: The process of enzymatically dissolving or breaking apart a blood clot.

Thrombolytic: An enzyme that dissolves or breaks apart blood clots.

Thrombophlebitis: Inflammation of a blood vessel (e.g., a vein) associated with the stimulations of clotting and formation of a thrombus (or blood clot).

Thromboplastin: A substance that triggers the coagulation cascade. Tissue factor is a naturally occurring thromboplastin and is used in the prothrombin time test.

Thrombosis: The process of forming a thrombus.

Thrombotic thrombocytopenic purpura: Condition characterized by formation of small clots within the circulation resulting in the consumption of platelets and a low platelet count.

Thrombus: Blood clot attached to the vessel wall and consisting of platelets, fibrin and clotting factors. A thrombus may partially or completely occlude the lumen of a blood vessel compromising blood flow and oxygen delivery to distal tissue.

Thymoma: A tumor derived from the epithelial or lymphoid elements of the thymus.

Thyroglobulin: A thyroid hormone-containing protein, usually stored in the colloid within the thyroid follicles.

Thyroid peroxidase: Enzyme that catalyzes the organification and coupling steps of thyroid hormone synthesis.

Thyroiditis: Inflammation of the thyroid gland.

Thyrotoxicosis: State caused by excess amount of thyroid hormone.

Tocolytic: Medication used to suppress premature labor.

Tolerance: A state of adaptation in which exposure to a drug induces changes that result in a diminution of one or more of the drug's effects over time.

Tonometry: A method by which the cornea is indented or flattened by an instrument. The pressure required to achieve corneal indentation or flattening is a measure of intraocular pressure.

Tophi: Chalky deposits of sodium urate occurring in gout; tophi form most often around joints in cartilage, bone, bursae, and subcutaneous tissue and in the external ear, producing a chronic, foreign-body inflammatory response. If untreated, tophi can lead to joint deformity or destruction.

Topoisomerase: Enzyme that temporarily alters supercoiled DNA by cutting the DNA, causing the DNA to relax the supercoil during DNA replication. Topoisomerase inhibitors prevent the DNA from sealing the cut which causes DNA strand breakage.

Torsade de pointes: Very rapid ventricular tachycardia characterized by a gradually changing QRS complex in the ECG; may change into ventricular fibrillation.

Toxic epidermal necrolysis: A life-threatening skin disorder characterized by blistering and peeling of the top layer of skin.

Toxoid: A modified bacterial exotoxin that has lost toxicity.

Tracheal aspirate: Suctioning of secretions from the trachea.

Transaminases: Hepatocellular enzymes that are released into the bloodstream after hepatic damage.

Transesophageal echocardiogram: Procedure used to generate an image of the heart via sound waves, via a probe introduced into the esophagus (rather than the traditional transthoracic view) in order to obtain a better image of the left atrium.

Transferrin saturation: Indicates the amount of transferrin that is bound with iron.

Transient ischemic attack: Focal neurologic deficit lasting less than 24 hours in which symptoms resolve completely.

Translocation: Movement of bacteria and endotoxin from the intestinal lumen through the gut mucosa and into the lymphatic and systemic circulation.

Transmural: Across the wall of an organ or structure. In Crohn's disease, inflammation may extend through all four layers of the intestinal wall.

Transsphenoidal pituitary microsurgery: Surgery through the nasal cavity to access the pituitary gland through the sphenoid bone.

Transvenous pacing: Insertion of a pacemaker into the heart via venous access for the purpose of pacing.

Traveler's diarrhea: An acute infectious diarrhea that afflicts travelers during or immediately upon return from visits to other countries. The presence of at least three loose stools within 24 hours that are associated with nausea, vomiting, abdominal pain, fecal urgency, or dysentery.

Tremulousness: Exhibiting trembling or shaking.

Trigeminal neuralgia: A disorder of the fifth cranial (trigeminal) nerve characterized by excruciating paroxysms of pain in the face.

Trigeminovascular: The complex of vascular supply to and from the trigeminal nerve. The trigeminal nerve is the fifth cranial nerve responsible for pain perception in the head and face.

Trophic: Stimulatory effect.

Troponins T or I: Proteins found predominately in cardiac and not skeletal muscle which regulates calcium-mediated interaction of actin and myosin. Troponin I and T are released into the blood from the myocytes at the time of myocardial cell necrosis secondary to infarction. These biochemical markers become elevated and are used in the diagnosis of myocardial infarction. Troponin I and T are more sensitive and specific for infarction than creatine kinase, which is found in both skeletal and myocardial cells. The exact value of troponin I or T, which is diagnostic of infarction, differs based upon assay.

Tubal ligation: Surgical process of tying up the fallopian tubes to prevent passage of ova from the ovaries to the uterus.

Tuberoeruptive xanthomas: Small yellow–red raised papules usually presenting on the elbows, knees, back, and buttocks.

Tubulointerstitial: Involving the tubules or interstitial tissue of the kidneys.

Tumor lysis syndrome: A syndrome resulting from cytotoxic therapy, occurring generally in aggressive, rapidly proliferating lymphoproliferative disorders. It is characterized by combinations of hyperuricemia, lactic acidosis, hyperkalemia, hyperphosphatemia, and hypocalcemia.

Tumor suppressor gene: A gene that suppresses growth of cancer cells.

T2-weighted magnetic resonance imaging: A setting of the magnetic resonance imaging machine that shows water as a bright signal.

Tympanocentesis: Puncture of the tympanic membrane with a needle to aspirate middle ear fluid.

Tympanostomy tube: Small plastic or metal tube inserted into the eardrum to keep the middle ear aerated and improve hearing in patients with chronic middle ear effusion.

Uhthoff's phenomenon: Acute worsening of multiple sclerosis symptoms on exposure to heat because high body temperatures may exceed the capacitance of the demyelinated nerve and conduction may fail.

Ulceration: A suppurative or nonhealing lesion on a surface such as skin, cornea, or mucous membrane.

Ultrafiltration: The movement of plasma water across a semipermeable membrane.

Ultrasound: Noninvasive imaging of organ or tissue to detect fluid, masses, or cyst.

Uncomplicated disorder: The presence of a single acid–base disorder, with or without compensation. See also Simple disorder.

Unilateral: Pertaining to one side.

Uremia: A condition that results from accumulation of metabolic waste products and endogenous toxins in the body resulting from impaired kidney function. Symptoms of uremia include nausea, vomiting, weakness, loss of appetite and mental confusion.

Uric acid: A by-product of purine metabolism in mammals, including humans. A high serum uric acid concentration is a major risk factor for gout.

Uricosuric: Pertaining to, characterized by, or promoting renal secretion of uric acid.

Urosepsis: Sepsis resulting from a urinary source.

Urticaria: Itchy, raised, swollen areas on the skin. Also known as hives.

Uveitis: An inflammation of the uvea, including the iris, ciliary body or choroid.

Vagal maneuvers: Stimulate the activity of the parasympathetic nervous system, which inhibits AV nodal conduction. Examples of vagal maneuvers include cough, carotid sinus massage, and Valsalva.

Vagotomy: A surgical procedure that blocks vagal (cholinergic) stimulation to the stomach.

Valsalva maneuver: Vagal maneuver; patient bears down against a closed glottis, as if they were having a bowel movement.

Variceal bleeding: Gastric, esophageal, or rectal bleeding from collateral vessels (varices).

Vasculitis: Inflammation of the walls of blood vessels.

Vasopressors: Medications that cause constriction of blood vessels, increase in vascular resistance, and increase in blood pressure.

Vasospasm: Narrowing (constriction) of a blood vessel causing a reduction in blood flow.

Ventilation/perfusion ratio: A comparison of the proportion of lung tissue being ventilated by inhaled air to the rate of oxygenation of pulmonary blood.

Ventral tegmental area: Part of the basal ganglia, containing dopamine neurons that project to the striatum, specifically the nucleus accumbens. This is part of the reward pathway in the brain.

Ventricular depolarization: Change in the membrane potential of a ventricular myocyte, resulting in loss of polarization. Under normal conditions, depolarization of ventricular myocytes is followed by ventricular contraction.

Vertigo: Sensation of spinning or feeling out of balance.

Vesicants: Chemotherapy drugs that cause significant tissue damage if extravasation occurs.

Virilization: Production or acquisition of virilism or the possession of masculine characteristics.

Volvulus: Twisting of the intestine causing obstruction and possible necrosis.

Vomiting: A reflexive rapid and forceful oral expulsion of upper gastrointestinal contents due to powerful and sustained contractions in the abdominal and thoracic musculature.

Waist circumference: A practical tool to measure the abdominal fat in patients with a BMI of less than 35.

Wernicke's syndrome: A syndrome that can be associated with chronic alcohol use, characterized by loss of memory, disorientation, and confabulation.

Western blot (WB): "Gold standard" for HIV diagnostic testing. Disrupted virus is purified, gel electrophoresed to separate by molecular weight to form bands corresponding to the nine HIV antigens, and blotted onto a membrane support. HIV serum antibodies from the patient are allowed to bind to proteins in the membrane support. If HIV antibodies from the patient are bound, the bands will change color. The test is considered reactive if two of the three major bands (p24, gp41, and/or gp120/160) change color. The test is nonreactive if no viral bands are visible.

Wheeze: A high pitched whistling sound caused by air moving through narrowed airways. Wheezes are usually heard at the end of expiration but may be heard during inspiration and expiration in acute severe asthma.

White coat hypertension: A persistently elevated average office blood pressure of greater than 140/90 mm Hg and an average awake ambulatory reading of less than 135/85 mm Hg.

Wilson's disease: A disorder of copper metabolism, characterized by cirrhosis of the liver and neurologic manifestations.

Xanthoma: Firm, raised nodules composed of lipid-containing histiocytes.

Xerostomia: Dryness of the mouth resulting from diminished or arrested salivary secretion.

ZAP-70 expression: An intracellular tyrosine kinase found in CLL B-cells.

INDEX

Note: Page numbers followed by *f*, *t*, and *a* refer to figures, tables, and algorithms, respectively.

A

Abacavir
  adverse effects of, 1427*t*, 1428*t*, 1437*t*–1440*t*
  dosage of, 1427*t*, 1428*t*
  drug interactions of, 1427*t*, 1428*t*
  in HIV infection, 1425, 1427*t*, 1428*t*, 1433
  mechanism of action of, 1421*f*
Abarelix
  in cancer therapy, 1468
  dosage of, 1545
  mechanism of action of, 1468
  in prostate cancer, 1544
Abatacept
  adverse effects of, 991
  dosage of, 991
  in rheumatoid arthritis, 991
ABCD acronym, for melanoma, 1616–1617, 1616*f*
Abciximab
  in acute coronary syndromes, 141*t*, 141, 145
  adverse effects of, 141, 145
  contraindications to, 141
  dosage of, 141*t*, 141
Ablation, thyroid, 777
Abortion
  DIC with, 1131*t*
  septic, peritonitis in, 1283
Abrasions, 1025
Abscess. *See also specific sites*
  in Crohn's disease, 342
Absidia, 1376*t*
Absolute neutrophil count, 1655
Absorption
  in geriatric patients, 10
  in pediatric patients, 26
ABVD regimen, in Hodgkin's lymphoma, 1557–1558, 1557*t*, 1561*t*
Acamprosate
  adverse effects of, 615
  in alcohol dependence, 615
  dosage of, 615
  mechanism of action of, 615
Acanthosis, in amenorrhea, 858
Acarbose
  adverse effects of, 750–751
  in diabetes mellitus, 748*t*, 750–751
  dosage of, 748*t*
ACAT inhibitors, 247
Accidental ingestion, in pediatric patients, 31
Acebutolol
  in arrhythmias, 162*t*
  dosage of, 122*t*
  in hypertension, 66*a*
  in ischemic heart disease, 122*t*
  in lactation, 829*t*
  mechanism of action of, 162*t*
ACEI. *See* Angiotensin converting enzyme inhibitors
ACE inhibitors. *See* Angiotensin-converting enzyme inhibitors
Acetaldehyde, 391, 624
Acetaminophen, 974
  adverse effects of, 285, 574, 1002, 1024
  in common cold, 1218*t*
  dosage of, 833*t*, 1002, 1002*t*, 1043*t*, 1047
  drug interactions of, 205*t*, 614*t*
  in headache, 588
  in hemophilia, 1126

  hepatotoxicity of, 574, 1002, 1024
  mechanism of action of, 574
  in migraine, 586, 588
  in musculoskeletal disorders, 1024
  nephrotoxicity of, 1002
  in opioid withdrawal, 621*t*
  in osteoarthritis, 1000–1002, 1002*t*
  in otitis media, 1207
  in pain, 572*t*, 574, 833*t*
    in sickle cell anemia/disease, 1043*t*, 1047
  in pregnancy, 833*t*
  premedication for alemtuzumab, 1603–1604, 1603*t*
  premedication for rituximab, 1563, 1603, 1603*t*
  in prevention of ovarian cancer, 1567
  in tension-type headaches, 584
  in thyroid storm, 777
Acetate, for parenteral nutrition, 1685*t*, 1686, 1696
Acetazolamide
  adverse effects of, 1041–1042
  dosage of, 1038*t*
  in glaucoma, 1038*t*, 1042
  hypocalcemia with, 489
  hypophosphatemia with, 491
  mechanism of action of, 1038*t*
  metabolic acidosis with, 501*t*
  metabolic alkalosis with, 502
Acetylcholine, in Alzheimer's disease, 597
Acetylcholinesterase, 597
Acetylcysteine
  in COPD, 297
  in prevention of contrast-induced nephropathy, 441
Achalasia, nausea and vomiting with, 358*t*
Achlorhydria, 10, 1111
Acid–base disorders, 495–505. *See also specific types*
  algorithmic approach in, 498*a*
  case study of, 499, 500
  DIC with, 1131*t*
  etiology of, 501–504
  metabolic, 496
  nomograms for, 498
  with parenteral nutrition, 1696
  pathophysiology of, 497–501
  patient care and monitoring in, 504
  respiratory, 496
  treatment of, 501–504
Acid–base homeostasis, 496
Acidemia, 496
Acidosis, 496
  lactic. *See* Lactic acidosis
  metabolic. *See* Metabolic acidosis
  respiratory. *See* Respiratory acidosis
Acinetobacter, in pneumonia, 1190, 1190*t*, 1194, 1198
Acitretin
  adverse effects of, 1086
  dosage of, 1086
  in psoriasis, 1086
  teratogenicity of, 824*t*, 1086
Acne vulgaris, 1094–1100
  case study of, 1099
  clinical presentation in, 1096
  with corticosteroids, 953*t*
  epidemiology of, 1094

  mild, 1096*t*
  moderate, 1096*t*
  outcome evaluation in, 1100
  pathophysiology of, 1094, 1095*f*
  patient care and monitoring in, 1099
  severe, 1096*t*
  treatment of, 1094–1100
    algorithm for, 1100*a*
    antiandrogens, 1100
    antibacterials, 1097, 1099*t*
    azelaic acid, 1097
    benzoyl peroxide, 1096–1097
    chemical peels, 1099
    corticosteroids, 1099
    estrogens, 1099
    isotretinoin, 1098, 1099*t*
    keratolytics, 1097–1098
    nonpharmacologic, 1095–1096
    oral agents, 1098–1099
    oral contraceptives, 843, 848, 1099
    retinoids, 1097
    topical agents, 1096–1097
AC regimen, in breast cancer, 1483*t*
Acrivastine in allergic rhinitis, 1053
Acrolein, 1667
Acromegaly
  case study of, 809
  clinical presentation in, 805
  diagnosis of, 805
  epidemiology of, 803
  etiology of, 803
  facial features of, 804, 804*f*
  osteoarthritis in, 998*t*
  outcome evaluation in, 808–809, 810*t*
  pathophysiology of, 803–804
  patient care and monitoring in, 810
  treatment of, 804–808, 804*f*
    dopamine agonist, 807*t*, 808
    GH receptor antagonists, 807*t*, 808
    goals of, 804
    radiation therapy, 808
    somatostatin analogs, 805–808, 807*t*
    surgery, 806
ACTH. *See* Adrenocorticotropic hormone
Actinic keratosis, 1613, 1624
Actinobacillus actinomycetemcomitans, in infective endocarditis, 1241
Actinomyces, in bite wound infections, 1232*t*
Action potential, ventricular, 159, 159*f*
Activated partial thromboplastin time, 193, 195*t*, 196–197, 201, 1137
Activated protein C, recombinant human, in sepsis, 1356–1357
Activated protein C resistance, 187, 187*t*
Activities of daily living (ADLs), 16*t*
Acupressure
  in dysmenorrhea, 863
  in nausea and vomiting, 360, 829
Acupressure wrist bands, 360
Acupuncture
  in dysmenorrhea, 863
  in headache, 587
  in nausea and vomiting, 360, 829
  in pain, 579
Acute chest syndrome
  in sickle cell anemia/disease, 1143*t*, 1145, 1148
  treatment of, 1148

Acute coronary syndromes, 110, 126, 131–153. *See
    also* Ischemic heart disease
  biochemical markers in, 134–135
  cardiovascular risk assessment for
    phosphodiesterase inhibitors, 890*t*
  case study of, 136, 138, 148, 149, 151
  clinical presentation in, 135
  complications of myocardial infarction, 134
  cost of, 132
  diagnosis of, 135
  echocardiogram in, 135, 139
  electrocardiogram in, 132–135
  epidemiology of, 132
  etiology of, 132
  evaluation of, 133*a*
  non-ST-segment elevation, 132–135, 138
    TIMI risk score, 138, 139*t*
    treatment of, 139, 142–144
  outcome evaluation in, 151
  pathophysiology of, 112, 132–135, 235
  patient care and monitoring in, 152*t*, 153
  prevention of, 119–121
  reinfarction, 132
  risk stratification in, 135, 139
  secondary prevention of, 149–151
  seeking emergent care in, 126
  spectrum of, 132–133
  with ST-segment elevation, 132–135, 137–138
    treatment of, 137–138, 137*a*
  treatment of, 135–151
    ACE inhibitors, 143*t*, 152*t*
    aldosterone antagonists, 143*t*, 152*t*
    angiotensin receptor blockers, 143*t*, 152*t*
    anticoagulants, 145–146, 147–149
    aspirin, 140*t*, 142, 147, 152*t*
    β-blockers, 142*t*, 146–147, 152*t*
    calcium channel blockers, 142*t*, 147, 152*t*
    clopidogrel, 140*t*, 145, 149–150, 152*t*
    fibrinolytics, 135, 137, 140*t*, 144, 152*t*
    glycoprotein IIb/IIIa receptor blockers, 141*t*,
      14–146, 147, 152*t*
    initial pharmacotherapy, 138*a*, 139–147
    morphine, 143*t*, 152*t*
    nitrates, 142*t*, 146, 149, 152*t*
    percutaneous coronary intervention,
      136–139
    ventricular remodeling in, 134
Acute erythroleukemia, 1582*t*
Acute heart failure. *See* Heart failure, acute
Acute lymphocytic leukemia, 1579–1580
  B cell differentiation and, 1554*f*
  case study of, 1584
  clinical conditions associated with, 1580*t*
  clinical presentation in, 1585
  complications of treatment
    infection, 1594
    late effects, 1595
    secondary malignancy, 1594
    tumor lysis syndrome, 1594, 1674*t*
  cytogenetic abnormalities in, 1584, 1584*t*,
    1586*t*, 1589
  in elderly, 1589
  epidemiology of, 1580
  etiology of, 1580–1581
  FAB classification of, 1581–1583, 1582*t*
  genetic factors in, 1581
  immunophenotype in, 1583, 1584*t*
  in infants, 1589
  outcome evaluation in, 1595
  pathophysiology of, 1581–1586
  patient care and monitoring in, 1595
  in pediatric patients, 1580
  prognostic factors for, 1583–1585, 1584*t*

in remission, 1586
treatment of, 1586–1590
  central nervous system prophylaxis, 1587,
    1588*t*
  chemotherapy, 1586–1590, 1588*t*, 1590*t*,
    1591*t*–1592*t*
  continuation (maintenance), 1588*t*, 1587,
    1589, 1590*t*
  delayed intensification therapy, 1587, 1590*t*
  hematopoietic cell transplant, 1593, 1630, 1630*t*
  imatinib, 1581, 1589
  intensification (consolidation), 1587, 1588*t*,
    1589, 1590*t*
  minimal residual disease, 1586, 1587
  nonpharmacologic therapy, 1586–1587
  radiation therapy, 1587
  relapsed leukemia, 1589–1590, 1593–1594
  remission induction, 1586–1587, 1588*t*, 1589,
    1590*t*
  supportive care, 1595
Acute megakaryoblastic leukemia, 1582*t*
Acute monoblastic leukemia, 1582*t*
Acute myeloblastic leukemia, 1582*t*
Acute myelogenous leukemia, 1579–1580
  clinical conditions associated with, 1580*t*
  clinical presentation in, 1585
  complications of treatment
    infection, 1594
    late effects, 1595
    secondary malignancy, 1594–1595
    tumor lysis syndrome, 1594, 1674*t*
  cytogenetic abnormalities in, 1584, 1586*t*, 1592
  disease-free survival in, 1593
  in elderly, 1593
  epidemiology of, 1580
  etiology of, 1580–1581
  event free survival rate for, 1580
  FAB classification of, 1581–1583, 1582*t*
  genetic factors in, 1581
  immunophenotype in, 1583, 1584*t*
  in infants, 1593
  outcome evaluation in, 1595
  pathophysiology of, 1581–1586
  patient care and monitoring in, 1595
  in pediatric patients, 1580
  prognostic factors in, 1585–1586
  in remission, 1586
  as secondary malignancy, 1581
  treatment of, 1590–1595
    central nervous system prophylaxis, 1593
    chemotherapy, 1590–1592, 1591*t*
    hematopoietic cell transplant, 1593–1594,
      1630, 1630*t*, 1634
    minimal residual disease, 1595
    postremission chemotherapy, 1592
    relapsed leukemia, 1593
    remission induction, 1590–1592
    supportive care, 1595
  WHO classification of, 1582*t*
Acute myelomonocytic leukemia, 1582*t*
Acute nonlymphocytic leukemia. *See* Acute
    myelogenous leukemia
Acute-phase reactants, 1713
Acute promyelocytic leukemia, 1582*t*
Acute respiratory distress syndrome (ARDS)
  DIC with, 1131*t*
  in pancreatitis, 404
  sepsis and, 1350
  treatment of, enteral nutrition, 1708*t*, 1709
Acute tubular necrosis, 433
  treatment of, kidney transplantation, 941
Acyclovir
  adverse effects of, 442, 1178*t*, 1330*t*

dosage of, 831*t*, 1178*t*, 1183, 1329–1330, 1330*t*
  in encephalitis, 1183
  in genital herpes, 831*t*, 834, 1329–1330, 1330*t*
  in lactation, 834
  in meningitis, 1178*t*
  in pregnancy, 831*t*, 834
  in prevention of herpes simplex virus, 1642
  in prevention of varicella-zoster virus, 1642
Adalimumab, 988
  adverse effects of, 987*t*, 1088
  dosage of, 987*t*, 1088
  mechanism of action of, 991, 1088
  monitoring treatment with, 987*t*
  in psoriasis, 1088–1089
  in rheumatoid arthritis, 987*t*, 991
Adapalene
  in acne vulgaris, 1097, 1097*t*
  adverse effects of, 1097*t*
  dosage of, 1097*t*
Addiction. *See* Substance-abuse disorders
Addiction Severity Index, 627
Addison's disease
  anxiety with, 694*t*
  diagnosis of, 788*t*
  hyperkalemia in, 488
  outcome evaluation in, 798
  pathophysiology of, 784
  psychotic symptoms in, 635*t*
  treatment of, 786–791, 788*t*
Adefovir dipivoxil
  adverse effects of, 423, 442
  in chronic hepatitis B, 423
  dosage of, 423
  resistance to, 423
Adenocarcinoma, 1449
  breast cancer, 1478
  colorectal cancer, 1521
  lung cancer, 1502*t*
  prostate cancer, 1538
Adenohypophysis, 802
Adenoidectomy, in otitis media, 1206
Adenoma, villous, 501*t*, 502*t*
Adenomyosis, menstruation-related disorders
    in, 857*t*
Adenosine
  adverse effects of, 169*t*
  arrhythmia with, 163*t*, 166*t*, 177*t*
  dosage of, 175*t*
  drug interactions of, 175*t*
  in heart failure, 95
  mechanism of action of, 175*t*
  in paroxysmal supraventricular tachycardia,
    173–175, 175*t*
Adenovirus
  in diarrhea, 376
  in gastroenteritis, 1277, 1277*t*
  in otitis media, 1204
  in pharyngitis, 1214
  in pneumonia, 1190
ADHD. *See* Attention-deficit hyperactivity
    disorder
Adolescents
  amenorrhea in, 858
  anovulatory bleeding in, 864–866
  blood pressure in, 52*t*
  dysmenorrhea in, 1094
  HIV infection in, 1434
  illicit drug use among, 608, 609*f*
  inflammatory bowel disease in, 352–353
  migraine in, 591
  obesity in, 1720, 1728
  schizophrenia in, 644
Adrenal adenoma, 793

ACTH-secreting, 792, 792t
Adrenal carcinoma, 792, 792t, 793
Adrenalectomy
    adrenal insufficiency in, 786t
    in Cushing's syndrome, 793
    in prostate cancer, 1539t
Adrenal gland
    biochemistry of, 784, 785a
    disorders of, 784–791
    physiology of, 784, 785a
Adrenal hyperplasia
    bilateral nodular, 792t
    congenital, 784, 786t
Adrenal infarction, 786
Adrenal insufficiency, 784–791
    case study of, 790–791
    clinical presentation in
        acute adrenal crisis, 790–791
        chronic disease, 786, 790
    diabetes mellitus and, 787
    diagnosis of
        acute adrenal crisis, 790–791
        chronic disease, 786, 790
    drug-induced, 786t, 786
        prevention of, 798
    epidemiology of, 784–786
    etiology of, 784–786
    in hematopoietic cell transplant recipients,
        1644
    hyperprolactinemia in, 814t
    nausea and vomiting in, 358t
    outcome evaluation in, 786–790
    pathophysiology of, 792
        acute adrenal crisis, 792
        chronic disease, 792
    patient care and monitoring in, 799
    pituitary disorders and, 803
    primary, 784–785, 786t, 788t. See also
        Addison's disease
    secondary, 784–785, 786t, 788t
    in sepsis, 1357
    tertiary, 784–785, 786t
    thyroiditis and, 787
    treatment of, 261, 786–792
        acute adrenal crisis, 790–791
        chronic disease, 786, 789t
        DHEA, 784, 785t
        glucocorticoids, 786–790, 789t
Adrenocorticotropic hormone (ACTH), 784
    in gout, 1015
    in multiple sclerosis, 508
    plasma, in adrenal insufficiency, 788t
    rapid ACTH stimulation test, 788t
Adrenoleukodystrophy, adrenal insufficiency
    in, 786t
Adrenolytic agents, in Cushing's syndrome, 797t
Adrenomyeloneuropathy, adrenal insufficiency
    in, 786t
Adsorbents, in diarrhea, 379
Advair, 296
Advanced glycation end-products, 447
Advanced heart failure, 46
    nonpharmacologic treatment, in palliative
        care, 46
    palliative care considerations, 46
    pharmacotherapy, in palliative care, 46
Adverse drug reaction (ADR), 14–15. See also
        individual entries
    allergic. See Allergic drug reactions
    preventing strategies, 15t
    pseudoallergic. See Pseudoallergic drug
        reactions
Advicor, 247

Advisory Committee on Immunization Practices
    (ACIP), 28
African-Americans. See Ethnicity
African trypanosomiasis, 1303
Afterload, 81
    in heart failure, 81, 81t
    in shock, 252
Age-related changes, in geriatrics, 9
    pharmacodynamic changes, 11–13
    pharmacokinetic changes, 10–11
Agranulocytosis
    with antithyroid drugs, 776–777
    clozapine-induced, 645, 648t, 649
AIDS. See HIV infection
Airflow obstruction, in COPD, 291
Airway clearance therapy, in cystic fibrosis, 307
Airway obstruction
    in asthma, 266–267
    in cystic fibrosis, 307
    respiratory acidosis with, 503t
Airway remodeling, 266–267
AJCC staging, of melanoma, 1615t
Akathisia
    with antipsychotics, 640, 641, 649
    in Parkinson's disease, 563t
Akinesia, in Parkinson's disease, 474
Albendazole
    in cysticercosis, 1297, 1298
    dosage of, 1297, 1298
    in enterobiasis, 1297–1298
    in hookworm disease, 1297
    in strongyloidiasis, 1298
Albumin
    albumin:creatinine ratio in urine, 449, 758
    human, as plasma volume expander, 1687
    in nutritional assessment, 1713
    serum-ascites albumin ratio, 394
Albumin therapy, 483
    adverse effects of, 483
    in hypovolemic shock, 258–259, 258t
Albuterol
    anxiety with, 694t
    arrhythmia with, 166t
    in asthma, 270t, 272, 277t, 283
    in COPD, 294, 295t, 296, 298
    in cystic fibrosis, 307, 308t
    dosage of, 270t, 277t, 295t
    in hyperkalemia, 454
    hypokalemia with, 487
Alcaligenes xylosoxidans, in cystic fibrosis,
        304, 310
Alclometasone dipropionate
    in contact dermatitis, 1103t
    dosage and potency of, 1103t
Alcohol abuse
    anxiety with, 694t
    binge drinking, 408
    case study of, 613
    epidemiology of, 608
    erectile dysfunction with, 885t
    hypocalcemia in, 489
    osteoporosis and, 966t, 967
    pancreatitis and, 405–409
    pathophysiology of, 608–610
    signs and symptoms of intoxication, 611, 612t
    status epilepticus in, 543–544
    treatment of, thiamine, 544
    treatment of dependence
        acamprosate, 625
        disulfiram, 624–625
        naltrexone, 625
    treatment of intoxication, 611–616
    urinary incontinence with, 918t

withdrawal syndrome, 617t, 620t, 621t, 622t,
        616–623, 623t
    alcohol hallucinosis, 619
    alcohol withdrawal seizures, 618
    CIWA-Ar, 616, 617t
    delirium tremens, 616, 618–619
    uncomplicated alcohol withdrawal, 616, 618
Alcohol dehydrogenase, 391
Alcoholic liver disease, 391. See also Cirrhosis
    pathophysiology of, 394
Alcoholism. See Alcohol abuse
Alcohol use
    acute leukemia and, 1580t
    adverse effects of, 84
    arrhythmia and, 166t
    blood glucose level and, 737t
    breast cancer and, 1477
    colorectal cancer and, 1518t, 1519
    drug interactions of, 246, 318, 615t, 660t, 699t
    GERD with, 317t
    in heart failure, 80
    hypertension and, 54t, 58–59
    metabolism of ethanol, 391
    nausea and vomiting with, 296t
    pancreatitis and, 408
    stroke and, 217t
Aldesleukin, 1465
    adverse effects of, 1465
    in cancer therapy, 1465
    mechanism of action of, 1465
    pharmacokinetics of, 1465
Aldosterone, 786. See also Renin-angiotensin-
        aldosterone system
    in acute coronary syndromes, 143t, 152t
    in adrenal insufficiency, 788t
    adverse effects of, 95, 152t
    contraindications to, 143t
    dosage of, 143t
    in heart failure, 83, 92t, 95
    in hypertension, 60t, 65, 66t, 70
    in hypovolemic shock, 254, 254a
    in liver disease, 397
    in prevention of myocardial infarction, 150
Alefacept, 952
    adverse effects of, 1087
    dosage of, 1087
    mechanism of action of, 1087
    in psoriasis, 1087
Alemtuzumab, 947, 953, 1465–1466
    adverse effects of, 1466, 1603–1604, 1603t
    in cancer therapy, 1465–1466
    in chronic lymphocytic leukemia, 1603–1604,
        1603t
    dosage of, 1603t
    mechanism of action of, 1465–1466, 1603
    pharmacokinetics of, 1465–1466
Alendronate
    dosage of, 973t
    GERD with, 317t
    in osteoporosis, 973t, 976, 976
Alfacalcidiol, in hyperphosphatemia, 463
Alfentanil, drug interactions of, 955t
Alfuzosin
    adverse effects of, 902, 903t, 906t
    in benign prostatic hyperplasia, 902
    hepatotoxicity of, 904
    mechanism of action of, 903
    pharmacologic properties of, 903t
    in urinary incontinence, 918
    uroselectivity of, 902, 903t
Alginic acid
    dosage of, 320t
    in GERD, 320t

Aliskiren, 55, 68–69
Alkalemia, 496
Alkalosis, 496
    metabolic. *See* Metabolic alkalosis
    respiratory. *See* Respiratory alkalosis
Alkylating agents, 1454a, 1461–1462
    adverse effects of, 1470, 1580t
    in breast cancer, 1484t
    teratogenic effects of, 824t
Allergen immunotherapy, 1049
Allergic bronchopulmonary aspergillosis, 308
Allergic conjunctivitis, 1068–1070
    etiology of, 1068
    outcome evaluation in, 1070
    pathophysiology of, 1068
    treatment of, 1068, 1069t
        antihistamines, 1068–1069, 1069t
        artificial tears, 1067
        corticosteroids, 1069t, 1070
        decongestants, 1069
        mast cell stabilizers, 1069t, 1069
        NSAID, 1069t, 1069
Allergic drug reactions, 928–936
    anticonvulsants and, 933
    aspirin and, 932–933
    β-lactams and, 931–932, 931t
    cancer chemotherapeutic agents and, 933
    case study of, 931, 934, 935
    cephalosporins and, 929t, 823
    clinical presentation in, 929t, 930
    contrast media and, 930t, 933
    diagnosis of, 930
    Gell and Coombs categories of, 928–929,
        929t
    insulin and, 929t, 933
    multiple antibiotic allergies, 932, 932t
    NSAID and, 932–933
    outcome evaluation in, 936
    pathophysiology of, 928–929
    patient care and monitoring in, 936
    penicillin and, 928–929, 929t, 931t
    sulfonamides and, 929t, 932
    treatment of, desensitization, 930, 933–935
    type I, 928–929, 929t
    type II, 929, 929t
    type III, 929, 929t
    type IV, 929, 929t
Allergic response, 1049
Allergic rhinitis, 1047–1060
    in athletes, 1059
    case study of, 1054–1057
    categories of, 1049t
    clinical presentation in, 1050
    diagnosis of, 1050
    in elderly patients, 1059
    epidemiology of, 1048–1049
    intranasal for, 1051t
    ocular symptoms of, 1059, 1060t
    oral medications for, 1051t
    outcome evaluation in, 1059–1061
    pathophysiology of, 1049
    patient care and monitoring in, 1060
    in pediatric patients, 1057–1059
    perennial, 1048–1049
    in pregnancy, 1059
    risk factors for, 1048
    seasonal, 1048–1049
    treatment of, 1049–1059
        allergen immunotherapy, 1049, 1051
        anticholinergics, 1056–1057
        antihistamines, 1051t, 1052–1054
        antimuscarinic, 1051t, 1056
        combination products, 1054

complementary and alternative medicines,
    1057
    corticosteroids, 1051t, 1051–1053
    cromolyn, 1051t, 1055–1056
    decongestants, 1051t, 1055–1056
    ipratropium, 1051t
    leukotriene receptor antagonists,
        1051t, 1056
    mast cell stabilizer/cromone, 1051t,
        1055–1056
    nonpharmacologic therapy, 1049–1050
    omalizumab, 1057
    pharmacologic therapy, 1050–1051
    prescription vs. OTC/self-treatment, 1049
    routine approach, 1058t
    saline, 1056
    types of, 1048t
Allergy, in pregnancy, 833
Allodynia, 569
Allograft, 940
Allopurinol, 954
    adverse effects of, 1015
    in antihyperuricemic treatment, 1014t, 1015
    cost of, 1677t
    desensitization to, 1015
    dosage of, 1014t, 1015, 1677t
    drug interactions of, 205t, 953, 1015, 1456,
        1592t
    hypersensitivity syndrome with, 1015
    mechanism of action of, 1015, 1674a, 1675
    in tumor lysis syndrome, 1017, 1675, 1677t
Allorecognition, 943
Allyl isothiocyanate, in musculoskeletal
    disorders, 1026t
Almotriptan
    dosage of, 589t
    drug interactions of, 589t
    in migraine, 589t
Aloe vera, adverse effects of, 376t
Alopecia
    chemotherapy-induced, 1485
    methotrexate-induced, 990
Alosetron
    adverse effects of, 384
    dosage of, 384t
    in irritable bowel syndrome, 384, 384t
α-adrenergic agonists
    in glaucoma, 1038t, 1042
    in hypertension, 69, 71t
    in urinary incontinence, 912t, 915
    voiding symptoms with, 900t
α-adrenergic antagonists
    adverse effects of, 901–902, 901t, 906t
    in benign prostatic hyperplasia, 897, 900t,
        901–903
    dosage of, 901, 901t
    drug interactions of, 890, 904
    erectile dysfunction with, 885t
    first-generation, 902
    in hypertension, 65, 71t
    pharmacologic properties of, 903t
    second-generation, 903
    urinary incontinence with, 912t, 915
    uroselectivity of, 902
α-glucosidase inhibitors
    contraindications to, 751
    in diabetes mellitus, 748t, 750–751
    mechanism of action of, 750–751
α₁-acid glycoprotein, 10
α₁-adrenergic receptors, in prostate, 897
α₁-antitrypsin, deficiency of, 290, 297
    liver disease and, 392
    lung transplantation in, 941

treatment of, 296–297
α₂-agonists, central, in hypertension, 62t, 69
5-α-reductase inhibitors, 896, 904, 1536
    adverse effects of, 905, 906t
    in benign prostatic hyperplasia, 896, 901t,
        904–907
    erectile dysfunction with, 885t
    mechanism of action of, 903
    pharmacologic properties of, 905t
    in prevention of prostate cancer, 905, 1537,
        1539t, 1540
Alport's syndrome, kidney transplantation
    in, 941
Alprazolam, 45t
    in anticipatory nausea and vomiting, 1512,
        1513t
    dosage of, 698t
    drug interactions of, 614t, 660t, 699t, 850t, 955t
    in panic disorder, 701
    pharmacokinetics of, 698t
Alprostadil
    adverse effects of, 890–891
    dosage of, 887t
    in erectile dysfunction, 884f, 887t, 890–891,
        891f
    intracavernosal injection of, 890–891, 891f
    mechanism of action of, 890
    transurethral suppository of, 890–891, 891f
Alteplase
    in acute coronary syndromes, 135, 141t, 144
    dosage of, 141t, 222
    in hemodialysis-associated thrombosis, 472
    inclusion and exclusion criteria, 221t
    in stroke, 221–222
    in venous thromboembolism, 195t
Alternative medicine. *See* Complementary and
    alternative medicines
Altretamine, 1463
    adverse effects of, 1463, 1574t
    in cancer therapy, 1463
    dosage of, 1574t
    in ovarian cancer, 1573, 1574t
    pharmacokinetics of, 1463
Alum, in hemorrhagic cystitis, 1669
Aluminum
    drug interactions of, 771t
    in parenteral nutrition products, 1697
    toxicity of, 1697
Aluminum acetate, in contact dermatitis, 1102
Aluminum carbonate
    dosage of, 464t
    in hyperphosphatemia, 464–465, 464t
Aluminum hydroxide
    dosage of, 464t
    in hyperphosphatemia, 464–465, 464t
Aluminum restriction
    in hyperparathyroidism, 462
    in renal osteodystrophy, 462
Alzheimer's Association, 602
Alzheimer's disease, 595–604
    behavioral symptoms in, 598
    case study of, 596, 598
    clinical presentation in, 597
    cognitive impairment in, 599t
    cost of, 596
    depression in, 598
    diagnosis of, 597, 598t
    early onset, 597
    epidemiology of, 596–597, 596f
    etiology of, 596–597
    genetic factors in, 597
    mania with, 676t
    mild, 597

moderate, 597
outcome evaluation in, 602
palliative care treatment for, 39
pathophysiology of, 597
patient care and monitoring in, 604
pharmacoeconomic considerations in, 602
risk factors for, 596
severe, 596
treatment of, 598
  algorithm for, 600a
  antipsychotics, 598
  benzodiazepines, 598
  cholinesterase inhibitors, 598, 600
  donepezil, 600
  galantamine, 599–600, 601t
  memantine, 599, 601t, 602
  NMDA antagonists, 597, 598, 601t
  nonconventional pharmacologic
    treatments, 598
  nonpharmacologic, 598–599
  rivastigmine, 600–602, 601t
  tacrine, 598, 601t
  warning signs of, 596t
Amantidine
  adverse effects of, 560, 563
  dosage of, 516t, 559t, 560
  in fatigue, 516t
  mechanism of action of, 559t
  in Parkinson's disease, 559t, 560, 563
  in pneumonia, 1197
Ambulation, in prevention of venous
    thromboembolism, 192t
Ambulatory blood pressure monitoring, 8
Ambulatory geriatric clinic, 18
Amcinonide
  in contact dermatitis, 1103t
  dosage and potency of, 1103t
Amebiasis, 1294–1297
  clinical presentation in, 377, 1296
  diagnosis of, 1296
  epidemiology of, 1295
  etiology of, 1295
  outcome evaluation in, 1297
  pathophysiology of, 1295
  patient care and monitoring in, 1297
  prevention of, 1297
  treatment of, 1295–1296
Amebicides
  luminally-acting, 1296
  tissue-acting, 1296
Amenorrhea
  in acromegaly, 805
  in adolescents, 858
  in adrenal insufficiency, 787
  clinical presentation in, 858
  definition of, 856
  diagnosis of, 858
  epidemiology of, 856
  etiology of, 856
  outcome evaluation in, 866t, 867
  pathophysiology of, 856–857, 857t
  patient care and monitoring in, 867
  primary, 856, 859t
  with progestin-only pills, 848
  secondary, 856, 858, 859t
  treatment of, 857, 859t
    algorithm for, 860a
American Academy of Clinical Toxicology, 31
American Academy of Pediatrics (AAP), 24, 31,
    828, 829
American College of Cardiology/American Heart
    Association staging of heart failure, 87, 87t
American trypanosomiasis, 1303

clinical presentation in, 1303
diagnosis of, 1303
etiology of, 1303
outcome evaluation in, 1303
patient care and monitoring in, 1303
treatment of, 1303
Amica flower, 206t
Amifostine, in oxaliplatin-induced neuropathy,
    1530
Amikacin
  adverse effects of, 1261t
  clinical parameters for, 1353
  in cystic fibrosis, 309, 310t
  dosage of, 310t, 1199t, 1261t
  drug interactions of, 955t
  in keratitis, 1071t
  in meningitis, 1183
  nephrotoxicity of, 440
  in pneumonia, 1198, 1199t
  in tuberculosis, 1260, 1261t
  in urinary tract infections, 1311t
Amiloride, in hypertension, 65
Amino acids
  branched chain, 1708
  caloric value of, 1683
  crystalline solutions of, 1683
  in enteral feeding formulas, 1710
  essential, 1710
  for parenteral nutrition, 1683, 1686, 1689–1690
Aminocaproic acid
  in hemophilia A, 1124
  in hemorrhagic cystitis, 1669
  in recessively inherited coagulation disorders,
    1124
  in von Willebrand's disease, 1128
Aminoglutethimide
  adverse effects of, 1468, 1546
  in cancer therapy, 1468
  hypothyroidism with, 767
  mechanism of action of, 1468
  in prostate cancer, 1539t, 1540, 1546
Aminoglycosides
  administration of, 1354
  clinical parameters for, 1354
  in cystic fibrosis, 310–311
  extended-interval dosing of, 440, 1354
  hypocalcemia with, 489
  hypomagnesemia with, 492
  in infections in cancer patients, 1660t
  in intra-abdominal infections, 1286,
    1288t, 1289
  in meningitis, 1182–1183
  nephrotoxicity of, 440, 1381
  ototoxicity of, 440
  in peritonitis, 474
  in pneumonia, 1196t, 1198
  respiratory acidosis with, 503t
  in sepsis, 1354, 1353t
  in surgical prophylaxis, 1397
  in urinary tract infections, 1311t, 1314t
5-Aminolevulinic acid
  in actinic keratosis, 1625
  adverse effects of, 1625
Aminosalicylates
  drug interactions of, 953, 1592t
  in inflammatory bowel disease, 346–353, 346t
Aminosalicylic acid
  adverse effects of, 1261t
  dosage of, 1261t
  pancreatitis with, 404t
  in tuberculosis, 1261t, 1262
Amiodarone, 10
  adverse effects of, 169t

arrhythmia with, 162t, 163t, 164t, 175t, 178t
in atrial fibrillation, 166t, 167a, 169t, 170a
dosage of, 169t, 170t, 171t, 178t
drug interactions of, 169t, 170t, 175t, 205t, 244,
    537t, 955t
for facilitation of defibrillation, 178, 179a, 179t
in lactation, 829t
mechanism of action of, 162t, 169t
ocular changes with, 1077t
in paroxysmal supraventricular tachycardia,
    169t
teratogenic effects of, 824t
thyroid disorders with, 767, 767t, 771t, 778–779
in ventricular tachycardia, 176–177, 177t
Amitriptyline
  arrhythmia with, 179t
  dosage of, 384t, 661, 661t
  drug interactions of, 614t
  in insomnia, 714
  in irritable bowel syndrome, 384, 384t
  in pain, 578t
  in prevention of migraine, 590, 590t
Amlodipine
  in acute coronary syndromes, 142t, 149, 152t
  adverse effects of, 61t, 152t
  dosage of, 61t, 124t, 142t
  in heart failure, 96
  in hypertension, 61, 64t, 67
  in ischemic heart disease, 123
  in prevention of migraine, 590t
Ammonia, in hepatic encephalopathy, 391
Ammonia water, in musculoskeletal disorders,
    1026t
Ammonium chloride
  adverse effects of, 503
  metabolic acidosis with, 501t
Amniotic fluid aspiration, 1131t
Amniotic fluid embolism, 253t, 1131t
Amobarbital, drug interactions of, 205t
Amoeba, in intra-abdominal infections, 1286t
Amotivation, in schizophrenia, 635
Amoxapine
  adverse effects of, 554
  dosage of, 661t
Amoxicillin
  adverse effects of, 1208t
  in bacteriuria, 831t, 833
  in Chlamydia, 831t, 1321
  dosage of, 335t, 831t, 832t, 1199t, 1208t, 1212t,
    1215t, 1312t, 1321
  drug interactions of, 850t
  in eradication of Salmonella carriage, 1271
  in Helicobacter pylori eradication, 327, 335t,
    330, 1561
  in infective endocarditis, 1250t
  in otitis media, 1206, 1208t
  in pharyngitis, 1215t
  in pneumonia, 1195, 1197, 1196t, 1199t
  in pregnancy, 831t, 833
  in prevention of endocarditis, 1250t
  in rhinosinusitis, 1211, 1212a, 1212t
  in surgical prophylaxis, 1400t
  in urinary tract infections, 1311t, 1312t, 1313
Amoxicillin-clavulanate
  adverse effects of, 1208t
  in bite wound infections, 1232
  in cellulitis, 1225t
  in COPD, 299t
  in cystic fibrosis, 309, 309t
  dosage of, 309t, 1199t, 1208t, 1212t, 1225t,
    1312t, 1660t
  in infections in cancer patients, 1660t, 1661
  in intra-abdominal infections, 1286

Amoxicillin-clavulanate (*Cont.*)
in otitis media, 1208*t*, 1209
in pharyngitis, 1216
in pneumonia, 1195, 1197, 1196*t*, 1199*t*
in rhinosinusitis, 1211, 1212*a*, 1212*t*, 1213*a*
in urinary tract infections, 1311*t*, 1312*t*, 1313
AMPA receptors, 569
Amphetamines. *See also specific drugs*
abuse of
mania with, 676*t*
pathophysiology of, 609
withdrawal syndrome, 613*t*, 615–616
adverse effects of, 54*t*, 1131*t*
anxiety with, 694*t*
drug interactions of, 614*t*
growth hormone deficiency with, 810
seizures with, 522
for weight loss, 1728
withdrawal syndrome, 619
Amphotericin B
adverse effects of, 1356, 1381, 1385, 1643
in aspergillosis, 1386*t*, 1391, 1643
in blastomycosis, 1379*t*
in coccidioidomycosis, 1379*t*
in cryptococcosis, 1386*t*, 1387
dosage of, 1379*t*, 1381, 1384, 1385, 1386*t*, 1387, 1391, 1643, 1660*t*
drug interactions of, 955
in endemic mycosis, 1380, 1381
in esophageal candidiasis, 1368, 1385
in fungal infections, 957
in fusariosis, 1386*t*
in histoplasmosis, 1379*t*
hypomagnesemia with, 492
in infections in cancer patients, 1660, 1660*t*
in infective endocarditis, 1248
infusion-related reactions to, 1381
in invasive candidiasis, 1384, 1385, 1386*t*, 1387
lipid analogs of, 1643
lipid-based formulations of, 440–441, 1356, 1381
liposomal formulation of, 1643, 1660, 1660*t*
metabolic acidosis with, 501*t*
nephrotoxicity of, 433, 440–441, 1381
in oropharyngeal candidiasis, 1385
in peritonitis, 474
in sepsis, 1356
in zygomycosis, 1386*t*
Ampicillin
adverse effects of, 1175*t*, 1176*t*, 1177*t*
in bacteriuria, 833
dosage of, 831*t*, 832*t*, 1175*t*, 1176*t*, 1177*t*, 1249*t*, 1250*t*, 1342*t*
drug interactions of, 850*t*, 1016
in infective endocarditis, 1247, 1249*t*
in intra-abdominal infections, 1288, 1287*t*
in meningitis, 1171*t*, 1175*t*, 1176*t*, 1177*t*, 1182
in osteomyelitis, 1342*t*
in pregnancy, 831*t*, 833, 836
in prevention of endocarditis, 1250*t*
in *Streptococcus* group B infection, 831*t*, 836
in urinary tract infections, 1311*t*
Ampicillin-sulbactam
in bite wound infections, 1233
in cellulitis, 1225*t*
in COPD, 299*t*
dosage of, 1225*t*, 1333*t*
in infective endocarditis, 1248
in intra-abdominal infections, 1288, 1288*t*
in PID, 1333*t*
in pneumonia, 1195, 1197, 1196*t*
in sepsis, 1353*t*, 1354

in urinary tract infections, 1311*t*
Amprenavir
adverse effects of, 1425, 1430*t*, 1437*t*–1440*t*
dosage of, 1430*t*
drug interactions of, 850*t*, 1430*t*
food interactions of, 1430*t*
in HIV infection, 1430*t*
mechanism of action of, 1421*f*
Amputation, lower extremity, in diabetic foot
infections, 736, 1229
Amsel criteria, for bacterial vaginosis, 1331
Amsler grid, 1074, 1074*f*
Amygdala
in anxiety disorders, 692–693
in reward pathway, 609, 609*f*
Amylase
pancreatic, 404
pancreatic enzyme supplements, 409
serum, 405
Amylin, 738
Amyloid deposition, in cystic fibrosis, 305
Amyloidosis, 1630, 1630*t*
adrenal insufficiency in, 786*t*
arrhythmia with, 163*t*, 164*t*
dry eye in, 1075*t*
heart failure in, 80*t*
Amyloid precursor protein, 597
Amyotrophic lateral sclerosis (ALS), palliative
care treatment for, 39
Anabolic steroids
dyslipidemia with, 236*t*
mania with, 676*t*
Anaerobes
in bite wound infections, 1232*t*
in diabetic foot infections, 1227
in intra-abdominal infections, 1283, 1286*t*
in necrotizing fasciitis, 1226
normal flora, 1157*f*
in osteomyelitis, 1339*t*, 1343*t*
in sepsis, 1348*t*
in surgical site infections, 1397, 1397*t*
Anakinra, 990
adverse effects of, 987*t*
dosage of, 987*t*
mechanism of action of, 991
monitoring treatment with, 987*t*
in rheumatoid arthritis, 987*t*, 991
Analgesics. *See also specific drugs*
constipation with, 372*t*
external, 1024, 1026*t*
in pancreatitis, 406
Anaphylactic shock, 253*t*
Anaphylactoid reaction, allergic drug
reaction, 932
Anaphylaxis, 930
allergic drug reaction, 928–929, 929*t*, 931
DIC with, 1131*t*
reaction to intravenous lipid emulsions, 1684
treatment of, 929*t*
epinephrine, 929*t*
normal saline, 929*t*
Anaplasia, 1449
Anastrozole, 1468
adverse effects of, 1468, 1487*t*, 1489
in breast cancer, 1487, 1487*t*, 1489
in cancer therapy, 1468
dosage of, 1487*t*
mechanism of action of, 1468, 1489
in ovarian cancer, 1573
pharmacokinetics of, 1468
Ancrod, in stroke, 222
Ancylostoma duodenale, 1297
Androgen receptor, in prostate cancer, 1536, 1547

Androgen synthesis inhibitors, in prostate
cancer, 1539*t*, 1540
Androgen therapy
adverse effects of, 86*t*
in breast cancer, 1487*t*, 1491
in cystic fibrosis, 312
teratogenic effects of, 824*t*
voiding symptoms with, 900*t*
Androstenedione, adrenal production of, 786
Anemia, 1109–1118. *See also specific types of
anemia*
in acute myelogenous leukemia, 1585
anxiety with, 694*t*
cancer-related, 1116–1117
treatment of, 1117, 1117*t*
case study of, 1110, 1115, 1116, 1118
chemotherapy-induced, 1110, 1116–1117, 1117*t*
treatment of, 1116, 1117*t*
of chronic disease, 1111, 1114*a*, 1116
treatment of, 1117
in chronic kidney disease, 446–468, 1114*a*, 1117
clinical presentation in, 456
epidemiology of, 455
erythropoiesis-stimulating agents in, 456–457, 458*a*, 459*t*
etiology of, 455
iron therapy in, 456–459, 458*a*
outcome evaluation in, 459
pathophysiology of, 455–456
treatment of, 456–459
clinical presentation in, 1112
in cystic fibrosis, 305
decreased-production, 1111
definition of, 1109
depression with, 655
drug-induced, 425
epidemiology of, 1110
etiology of, 1110
evaluation process, 1114*a*
hypoproliferative, 1111
hypothyroidism and, 1114*a*
laboratory tests in, 1113*t*
macrocytic, 1112
megaloblastic, 1116
microcytic, 1112
normochromic, 1585
normocytic, 1112, 1585
outcome evaluation in, 1117–1118
pathophysiology of, 1110–1111
patient care and monitoring in, 1118
in pregnancy, 827
treatment of, 456, 1111
diet therapy, 1111, 1111*t*
nonpharmacologic, 1112–1113
pharmacologic, 1113–1116
red blood cell transfusion, 1109
Anergy, T-cell, 943
Anesthetics
respiratory acidosis with, 503*t*
in status epilepticus, 548–549
Aneuploidy, 1478
Aneurysm, cerebral, rupture of, 216
Angelica root, 206*t*
Angina-like symptoms, 111, 111*t*
Angina pectoris. *See also* Ischemic heart
disease
anxiety with, 694*t*
cardiovascular risk assessment for
phosphodiesterase inhibitors, 890*t*
chronic stable, 110, 112
clinical presentation in, 114–116
conditions associated with, 111

effort-induced, prevention of, 121
pathophysiology of, 234
Prinzmetal's. *See* variant *below*
treatment of
  calcium channel blockers, 117
  nitrates, 117, 121, 124
  nitroglycerin, 121
  ranolazine, 122
unstable. *See* Unstable angina
variant, 111, 114
  treatment of, 126
Angioedema
  with ACE inhibitors, 68, 92, 150
  allergic drug reaction, 932
Angiogenesis, in cancer, 1448, 1521, 1526
Angiopathy
  in diabetes mellitus, 1227–1228
  DIC with, 1131t
Angiotensin-converting enzyme (ACE)
    inhibitors, 38f. *See also specific drugs*
  in acute coronary syndromes, 143t
  adverse effects of, 62, 91–93, 151, 152t
  blood glucose level and, 737t
  contraindications to, 143t, 152t
  cost of, 151
  dosage of, 91, 143t
  drug interactions of, 679, 953, 1004
  in heart failure, 83, 91–93, 92t
  hyperkalemia with, 450, 485
  in hypertension, 62t, 64–65, 66t, 67–68, 70,
    756, 958
  in ischemic heart disease, 120, 121t
  nephrotoxicity of, 432, 440, 442
  in patients with renal disease, 91
  in pregnancy, 62t
  in prevention of myocardial infarction, 150
  in proteinuria, 450
  teratogenic effects of, 824t, 829t
Angiotensin receptor blockers. *See also specific
    drugs*
  in acute coronary syndromes, 143t, 152t
  adverse effects of, 93, 152t
  contraindications to, 143t
  dosage of, 143t
  drug interactions of, 1004
  in heart failure, 83, 92t, 93
  hyperkalemia with, 450
  in hypertension, 62t, 66t, 68, 70, 758, 958
  in ischemic heart disease, 116, 120, 121t
  mechanism of action of, 93
  nephrotoxicity of, 432, 440, 442
  in pregnancy, 62t
  in prevention of myocardial infarction, 150
  in proteinuria, 451
Angiotensin II, 55, 56a. *See also* Renin-
    angiotensin-aldosterone system
  in chronic kidney disease, 447
  in heart failure, 82
  teratogenic effects of, 824t
Anhedonia, in depression, 655
Anidulafungin, in invasive candidiasis, 1384,
  1385
Animal bite, infected bite wound, 1232–1233
Anion gap, 499
  excess gap, 499
  in metabolic acidosis, 466
Anise, 206t
Ankylosing spondylitis, in inflammatory bowel
    disease, 344
Ann Arbor staging, of non-Hodgkin's lymphoma,
  1559, 1561t
Anorexia nervosa, 1513t
  in lung cancer, 1513

Anovulation, chronic, 856
Anovulatory bleeding
  in adolescents, 866–867
  clinical presentation in, 864
  definition of, 857
  diagnosis of, 864
  epidemiology of, 864
  etiology of, 864
  outcome evaluation in, 866t, 867
  pathophysiology of, 857t, 864–865
  patient care and monitoring in, 867
  treatment of, 865–866
Antacid(s)
  administration through feeding tube, 1715
  aluminum-containing, in lactation, 829t
  constipation with, 372t
  dosage of, 830t
  drug interactions of, 321, 953–955, 1426
  in GERD, 320t, 321, 830t, 833
  in hyperphosphatemia, 492
  in nausea and vomiting, 359
  in pregnancy, 830t, 833
Antacid-alginic acid products, in GERD,
  320t, 321
Antazoline
  adverse effects of, 1068t
  in allergic conjunctivitis, 1068t
  dosage of, 1069t
  mechanism of action of, 1068t
Antenatal steroids, 835
Anterograde amnesia, with benzodiazepines, 698
Anthracyclines, 1459–1461
  in breast cancer, 1484t, 1488, 1491–1492, 1493
  extravasation of, 1677t, 1677, 1678t
  mechanism of action of, 1454a
Anthralin
  adverse effects of, 1084–1085
  in psoriasis, 1084–1085
  short-contact therapy, 1085, 1087
Antiandrogens
  in acne vulgaris, 1100
  in cancer, 1468
  hyperprolactinemia with, 814t
  in prostate cancer, 1539t, 1540, 1542, 1543,
    1545, 1546, 1545t
Antiarrhythmic drugs. *See also specific drugs*
  in pain, 578
  Vaughan Williams classification of, 161–162,
    162t
Antibiotic-associated diarrhea, 1274–1276,
  1711–1712
Antibody, diabetes-related, 737
Anti-CD20 monoclonal antibody, in rheumatoid
    arthritis, 991
Anticholinergics. *See also specific drugs*
  adverse effects of, 276, 296, 558, 559t
  in allergic rhinitis, 1056
  anxiety with, 694t
  in asthma, 269, 270t, 272, 276t
  in benign prostatic hyperplasia, 905
  constipation with, 308t
  in COPD, 294, 295t
  dry eye with, 1075t
  in enuresis, 915
  in extrapyramidal symptoms, 644
  GERD with, 317t
  glaucoma with, 1035
  intranasal, 1056
  in nausea and vomiting, 360, 361t, 366
  ocular changes with, 1077t
  in Parkinson's disease, 557, 558, 559t
  in urinary incontinence, 912t, 914
  voiding symptoms with, 900t, 917t

Anticoagulants. *See also specific drugs*
  in acute coronary syndromes, 140t, 141, 145,
    152t
  bleeding risk with, 204, 205t
  contraindications to, 198t
  in DIC, 1131–1132
  in elderly patients, 13
  in heart failure, 96
  natural, 187
  in peripartum cardiomyopathy, 97
  in prevention of myocardial infarction, 145
  in venous thromboembolism, 194, 194a, 195t,
    196–197, 196t, 197t
Anticoagulation clinic, 204
Anticonvulsants. *See also specific drugs*
  in alcohol withdrawal, 626
  allergic drug reactions, 933
  anxiety with, 694t
  in bipolar disorder, 677t
  drug interactions of, 850t
  nausea and vomiting with, 357, 358t
  osteoporosis with, 967t
  in schizoaffective disorder, 647
  in social anxiety disorder, 704
Antidepressants, 12, 657–665. *See also specific
    drugs*
  adverse effects of, 658, 658t, 659t
  anxiety with, 694t
  augmentation therapy, 662
  in bipolar disorder, 676, 685
  in cataplexy, 716
  combination therapy with, 662
  discontinuation of, 664
  dosage of, 660, 661t
  drug holidays, 658
  drug interactions of, 660, 660t, 683
  dry eye with, 1075t
  duration of therapy with, 664
  efficacy of, 662–663
  erectile dysfunction with, 885t
  in generalized anxiety disorder, 695, 696t
  in insomnia, 714, 716t
  in irritable bowel syndrome, 384, 384t
  in major depressive disorder, 657–665
    algorithm for, 663a
  mechanism of action of, 662, 666t
  in pain, 578
  in panic disorder, 700
  in Parkinson's disease, 560
  partial response to nonresponse to, 662
  in pediatric patients, 665
  pharmacokinetics of, 659, 659t
  in pregnancy/lactation, 665, 829t
  for remission of symptoms, 664
  seizures with, 522
  selection of medication, 662, 663a
  in social anxiety disorder, 703
  suicidality and, 665–666
  time course of response to, 662
  in vasomotor symptoms of menopause, 878, 879t
  withdrawal syndromes, 664
Anti-D immune globulin
  dosage of, 1134, 1134t
  in immune thrombocytopenic purpura, 1134,
    1134t
Antidiuretic hormone, 802. *See also* Vasopressin
  in cirrhosis, 390
  in hypovolemic shock, 254, 254a
Antiepileptic drugs. *See also specific drugs*
  adverse effects of, 528, 531t–535t
    chronic adverse reactions, 535
  autoinduction of metabolism of, 528, 529f
  discontinuation of, 536

Antiepileptic drugs (*Cont.*)
  dosage of, 531*t*–535*t*, 536
  drug interactions of, 537, 537*t*
  drug selection and seizure type, 529, 529*t*
  mechanism of action of, 531*t*–535*t*
  metabolism of, 528–529
  osteoporosis with, 535
  in pain, 578
  in pediatric patients, 537
  pharmacokinetics of, 531*t*–535*t*
  in pregnancy, 537, 537*t*
  in prevention of migraine, 590, 591*t*
  protein binding of, 528
  in status epilepticus, 542–543, 545*t*, 546*t*, 547*t*
  switching drugs, 536
Antiestrogens, in breast cancer, 1485–1486, 1490, 1487*t*
Antifactor Xa assay, 197
Antifolates, 1457
Antigen(s)
  inhaled, 266
  intestinal, in inflammatory bowel disease, 342
Antigen-presenting cells, solid-organ transplantation and, 943
Antihistamines, 12. *See also specific drugs*
  adverse effects of, 1052, 1102
  in allergic conjunctivitis, 1068–1069, 1068*t*
  in allergic rhinitis, 1051*t*, 1052–1054, 1058*t*
  anxiety with, 694*t*
  in common cold, 1218
  in contact dermatitis, 1102
  drug interactions of, 660*t*
  dry eye with, 1075*t*
  first-generation, 1052, 1053, 1057
  in insomnia, 716
  intranasal, 1051*t*, 1052, 1053–1054, 1054*t*
  in lactation, 833
  in nausea and vomiting, 360–361, 361*t*, 366
  nonsedating, 1051
  ocular changes with, 1077*t*
  oral, 1051*t*, 1052, 1053, 1054*t*
  in pregnancy, 833
  in pruritus, 468
  second generation, 1053–1054, 1054*t*, 1057
  voiding symptoms with, 900*t*
Antihyperuricemic treatment, 1014*t*, 1015–1016
  allopurinol, 1014*t*, 1016
  nonpharmacologic, 1015
  outcome evaluation in, 1017
  probenecid, 1014, 1016
Anti-IL-6 receptor monoclonal antibody, in rheumatoid arthritis, 991
Anti-incontinence devices, 914
Antimalarials. *See also specific drugs*
  psoriasis and, 1080
Antimetabolites, 1454–1457
  in breast cancer, 1484*t*
Antimicrobial(s). *See also specific drugs*
  in acne vulgaris, 1097, 1100*t*
  administration through feeding tube, 1715
  adverse effects of, 1156, 1163–1164
  allergies to, 1164
  bacteriocidal, 1163
  bacteriostatic, 1163
  bioavailability of, 1163
  in bite wound infections, 1232–1233
  broad-spectrum, 1156
  in chancroid, 1334, 1334*t*
  in cholera, 1273
  collateral damage in therapy with, 1162
  in common cold, 1217
  compliance with drug regimens, 1165
  concentration-dependent activity of, 1163

concentration-independent activity of, 1163
  in COPD exacerbations, 297–298
  cost of, 1164, 1208*t*
  in cystic fibrosis, 312–313
  deescalation therapy, 1165
  in diabetic foot infections, 1229–1230, 1229*t*
  in diaper dermatitis, 1106
  diarrhea with, 376*t*, 379
  dosage of, 1162
  drug considerations in selecting therapy, 1162–1164, 1162*t*
  drug interactions of, 1163–1164
  effects on nontargeted flora, 1162
  in elderly, 1164
  empirical therapy with, 1162
  failure of, 1165–1167
  fortified, 1071
  in gonorrhea, 1319–1320
  hypocalcemia with, 489
  hypokalemia with, 492
  in impetigo, 1222
  in infected pressure sores, 1231, 1232*t*
  in infections in cancer patients, 1657–1661, 1660*t*
  in infective endocarditis, 1242–1248, 1244*t*
  in intra-abdominal infections, 1285–1289, 1287*t*–1288*t*
  intraperitoneal, 474, 1288
  in keratitis, 1071, 1071*t*
  in lactation, 1164
  in meningitis, 1171*t*, 1175*t*–1178*t*, 1178–1179
  metabolism of, 1163
  modifying therapy based on cultures and clinical response, 1165
  narrow-spectrum, 1156
  nausea and vomiting with, 358*t*
  in necrotizing fasciitis, 1227
  in osteomyelitis, 1341–1344, 1342*t*–1343*t*
  in otitis media, 1205–1207, 1208*t*
  outcome evaluation in, 1165–1167, 1166*a*
  in pancreatitis, 406–407, 407*t*
  patient considerations in selecting therapy, 1162*t*, 1164–1165
  in pediatric patients, 1164
  pharmacodynamic properties of, 1163, 1174–1175, 178
  pharmacokinetic properties of, 1162–1163, 1174–1175, 178
  in pharyngitis, 1215–1216, 1215*t*
  in PID, 1332, 1333*t*
  in pneumonia, 1193–1200
  in pregnancy, 1165
  prophylactic
    in hematopoietic cell transplant recipients, 1641
    in neutropenic cancer patients, 1656
    in surgical patients, 1395–1402
  protein binding of, 1163
  regimen selection, 1155–1168
    algorithm for, 1166*a*
  in rhinosinusitis, 1211–1213, 1212*t*
  in salmonellosis, 1269–1270, 1269*t*
  in sepsis, 1352–1356, 1353*t*
  single vs. combination therapy, 1162
  spectrum of activity of, 1156, 1162
  in syphilis, 1322–1324
  topical, in corneal abrasion, 1063
  in travelers' diarrhea, 1273–1274
  in urinary tract infections, 1310–1313, 1311*t*–1312*t*, 1314*t*
  in variceal bleeding, 388
  in viral conjunctivitis, 1067–1068
Antimicrobial resistance, 1156–1157, 1164, 1165
  in *Helicobacter pylori*, 335

in meningitis, 1178–1179
Antimicrobial susceptibility testing, 1161, 1161*f*
  of *Mycobacterium tuberculosis*, 1255
  proportion method, 1255
Antimicrosomal antibodies, 766
Antimuscarinic, in allergic rhinitis, 1051*t*, 1056
Antioxidants
  in enteral feeding formulas, 1709
  in ischemic heart disease, 125
Antiperistaltic agents, in diarrhea, 379, 379*t*
Antiphospholipid antibodies, 187, 187*t*
Antiplatelet drugs. *See also specific drugs*
  in heart failure, 96
  in ischemic heart disease, 119–120
Antiproteinase, in lung, 290
Antipsychotics, 631–649. *See also specific drugs*
  in adolescents, 644
  adverse effects of, 554, 562, 640, 641–642, 643
    monitoring of, 648*t*, 649
    treatment of, 642
  in Alzheimer's disease, 598
  in bipolar disorder, 675*t*, 678*t*, 685–686
  dosage of, 685
  drug interactions of, 646*t*, 647, 660*t*, 679
  in elderly, 645
  erectile dysfunction with, 885*t*
  first-generation, 636, 640*t*, 640–641
  hyperprolactinemia with, 814*t*
  in lactation, 662, 829*t*
  mechanism of action of, 633–634
  menstruation-related disorders with, 857*t*
  metabolism of, 646*t*
  monitoring therapy with, 678*t*
  pharmacokinetics of, 646–647
  in pregnancy, 646
  second-generation, 632, 636–640, 637*t*, 638*t*, 643*a*
  seizures with, 522
  in stimulant abuse, 613
Anti-reflux surgery, in GERD, 319–322
Antiretrovirals, 828*t*
Antisecretory agents, in diarrhea, 379, 379*t*
Antispasmodics. *See also specific drugs*
  adverse effects of, 384
  in irritable bowel syndrome, 384–385
  in urinary incontinence, 915, 916*t*
Antithrombin, 187
  deficiency of, 196, 196*t*
  in DIC, 1132
Antithrombotic drugs, 186
Antithymocyte globulin equine (eATG), 946
Antithymocyte globulin rabbit
  adverse effects of, 945*t*, 946
  dosage of, 945*t*, 946
  mechanism of action of, 946
  in transplant recipient, 945*t*, 946
Antithyroglobulin antibodies (anti-TGAb), 767
Antithyroid drugs. *See also specific drugs*
  adverse effects of, 776
  agranulocytosis with, 776–777
  in hyperthyroidism, 776–777
Antithyroid peroxidase antibodies (anti-TPOAb), 766, 766*t*
Antitumor antibiotic, 1459
Antrectomy, in peptic ulcer disease, 333
Anuria, definition of, 433
Anxiety, 605
  with corticosteroids, 953*t*
  drug-induced, 694*t*
  meaning of, 40
  medical conditions that cause, 694*t*

nonpharmacologic treatment, in palliative care, 40
palliative care considerations, 40
pharmacotherapy, in palliative care, 40–41
respiratory alkalosis in, 504t
Anxiety disorders, 691–705. *See also* Generalized anxiety disorder
case study of, 694, 695, 703
clinical presentation in, 694
comorbidity, 692
course of illness, 692
diagnosis of, 694
epidemiology of, 692
etiology of, 692
genetic factors in, 692
pathophysiology of, 692–693, 693f
patient care and monitoring in, 705
recurrence of, 692
remission in, 692
Anxiogenic behavior, during withdrawal, 610
Anxiolytics, 45
Aortic aneurysm, DIC with, 1131t
Aortic balloon assist device, 1131t
Aortic dissection, chest pain in, 111
APACHE II score, in acute pancreatitis, 404
APC gene, 1519
Aphakic patient, 1041, 1043
Aphasia, in stroke, 218
Aphthous ulcers, 343
Aplastic anemia, 1114a, 1630, 1630t
Aplastic crisis
in sickle cell anemia/disease, 1149
treatment of, 1149
Apolipoprotein(s), 230, 231f, 231t
Apolipoprotein A-I, 230, 231, 232
Apolipoprotein A-II, 230, 246
Apolipoprotein B, 231f, 232, 233t, 238
Apolipoprotein B-48, 230–231, 231f
Apolipoprotein B-100, 230–231, 232, 233t
familial defective, 231, 231t
Apolipoprotein C, 231
Apolipoprotein C-II, 230–231
Apolipoprotein C-III, 231
Apolipoprotein E, 230–231, 232
Alzheimer's disease and, 597
Apomorphine
adverse effects of, 560–561
dosage of, 559t
mechanism of action of, 559t
in Parkinson's disease, 559t, 560–561
Apoptosis, 514, 1445, 1446, 1553
Appendectomy, antimicrobial prophylaxis in, 1400t, 1402
Appendicitis
intra-abdominal infection and, 1283
nausea and vomiting with, 358t
treatment of, 1288t, 1289
Appetite, 1720
Appetite stimulants, in anorexia, 1513
Apraclonidine
adverse effects of, 1041
dosage of, 1038t
in glaucoma, 1038t, 1041
mechanism of action of, 1038t, 1041
Aprepitant
adverse effects of, 366t
in chemotherapy-induced nausea and vomiting, 1652, 1652t
dosage of, 366t
in nausea and vomiting, 366t, 367
chemotherapy-related, 1512, 1513t
Aprotinin, in pancreatitis, 407
Aqueous humor, in glaucoma, 1033, 1033f

Arachidonic acid pathway, 331, 331a, 1021, 1021f
Arbovirus, in CNS infections, 1183
Arcuate scotoma, 1036
ARDS. *See* Acute respiratory distress syndrome
Arformoterol, in COPD, 295t
Argatroban
for acute coronary syndromes, 146
adverse effects of, 205t
drug interactions of, 205t
in venous thromboembolism, 201–202
Arginine, in enteral feeding formulas, 1708t, 1709
Arginine hydrochloride
adverse effects of, 4503
metabolic acidosis with, 501t
Aripiprazole
adverse effects of, 638t, 639, 685
in Alzheimer's disease, 598
in bipolar disorder, 678t, 684–685
dosage of, 637t, 639, 678t, 685
drug interactions of, 646t
mechanism of action of, 637f, 639
metabolism of, 646t
in schizophrenia, 636, 637f, 637t, 638t, 639
Aromatase inhibitors
in breast cancer, 1487, 1487t
in prevention of breast cancer, 1479
Arrhythmia, 157–181. *See also specific arrhythmias*
anxiety with, 694t
drug-related, 162t
heart failure and, 84t
hyperkalemia and, 163t, 164t
hypertension and, 165, 166t
hypokalemia and, 488
mechanism of
abnormal impulse conduction, 160–161, 161f
abnormal impulse initiation, 160
patient care and monitoring in, 179
shock in, 253t
supraventricular, 162–164
treatment of, 488, 488t
ventricular, 175–179
Arsenic exposure/poisoning, 376t, 1500
arrhythmia with, 179t
Arsenic trioxide, 1464
adverse effects of, 1464
in cancer therapy, 1464
mechanism of action of, 1464
pharmacokinetics of, 1464
Arterial blood gases, 495, 496
in hypovolemic shock, 255
Arteriovenous fistula, vascular access in hemodialysis, 472–473, 473t
Arteriovenous graft, vascular access in hemodialysis, 472–473, 473t
Arteriovenous malformation, 216
Arthralgia
with corticosteroids, 953t
in withdrawal syndromes, 616
Arthritis
in cystic fibrosis, 305
gouty, 1012–1015
hypertrophic. *See* Osteoarthritis
osteoarthritis. *See* Osteoarthritis
psoriatic, 1080, 1087
rheumatoid. *See* Rheumatoid arthritis
Arthritis Foundation, 1000
Arthrocentesis, 1014
Arthus reaction, 1415
allergic drug reaction, 929

Articular disease, in rheumatoid arthritis, 985
Artificial tears
in allergic conjunctivitis, 1076
in dry eye, 1076
Arzoxifene, 976
5-ASA. *See* Mesalamine
Asafoetida, 206t
Ascariasis, 1297
Ascites
case study of, 390
in cirrhosis, 388, 390, 390f, 394, 396
diagnosis of, 394
in end-stage liver disease, 413
low-protein, 399
outcome evaluation in, 400
in ovarian cancer, 1566, 1575
pathophysiology of, 388–389, 388f
peritonitis and, 1282–1283
respiratory acidosis with, 503t
treatment of, 394, 396, 398a
diuretics, 396–397
paracentesis, 396
Ascitic fluid, analysis of, 394
Asherman's syndrome, menstruation-related disorders in, 857t
Asian-Americans. *See* Ethnicity
L-Asparaginase, 1463–1464
in acute lymphocytic leukemia, 1587, 1588t, 1590t, 1591t
in acute myelogenous leukemia, 1592
adverse effects of, 1464, 1591t
allergic drug reactions, 933
in cancer therapy, 1463–1464, 1469
dosage of, 1588t, 1590t, 1594
drug interactions of, 1591t
mechanism of action of, 1454a, 1463, 1591t
pancreatitis with, 404t
pegaspargase, 1464
pharmacokinetics of, 1463
ASPEN safe practice guidelines, for parenteral nutrition, 1690
Asperger's disorder, 635t
Aspergillosis
allergic bronchopulmonary, 308
in cancer patients, 1655, 1655t, 1660
in hematopoietic cell transplant recipients, 1642–1643
invasive, 1376t, 1389–1392
clinical presentation in, 1389–1390
diagnosis of, 1383f
epidemiology of, 1389
laboratory diagnosis of, 1390
pathogenesis of, 1389–1390, 1391f
patient monitoring in, 1392
prophylaxis for, 1391–1392
treatment of, 1386t, 1390
in transplant recipient, 957
treatment of, 1390–1391
Aspergillus
in cystic fibrosis, 304
in infective endocarditis, 1242
in sepsis, 1348
Aspergillus flavus, 1389
Aspergillus fumigatus, 1389
Aspergillus niger, 1389
Aspergillus terreus, 1389, 1390
Aspiration
prevention of, 1712
risk factors for, 1191
with tube feeding, 1711t, 1712, 1713
Aspirin, 10, 30
in acute coronary syndromes, 140t, 142, 147, 152t

Aspirin (*Cont.*)
adverse effects of, 149, 152*t*, 222, 223, 574, 1024
allergic drug reactions, 932–933
in atrial fibrillation, 173*t*
contraindications to, 140*t*
cost of, 149
desensitization to, 930, 933–934, 935*t*
dosage of, 140*t*, 147, 149, 173*f*, 1002*t*
drug interactions of, 205*t*, 1004
GERD with, 317*t*
gout with, 1012
in heart failure, 96
in hemophilia, 1126
in ischemic heart disease, 119–120
low-dose, 96, 147, 149
in musculoskeletal disorders, 1024
in osteoarthritis, 1002*t*
in pain, 574
peptic ulcer disease with, 331
in prevention of colorectal cancer, 1520, 1521–1522
in prevention of myocardial infarction, 149
in prevention of ovarian cancer, 1567
in prevention of stroke, 222
in prevention of venous thromboembolism, 193
in stroke, 173*f*, 222, 225*t*
Aspirin-sensitive asthma, 285
Assisted ventilation. *See also* Pneumonia, ventilator-associated
in ARDS, 1357
in COPD, 300
enteral nutrition in, 1708*t*, 1709
in respiratory acidosis, 503
sedation and neuromuscular blockade in, 1357
Astemizole, arrhythmia with, 180
Asthma, 265–286
acute, 268, 285–286
acute severe, 269
airway inflammation and hyperresponsiveness in, 266
airway obstruction in, 266–267
allergic drug reaction, 932
anxiety with, 694*t*
aspirin-sensitive, 285
atopic, 281
case study of, 268, 281, 283, 285
chronic, 266, 268–269, 272–273, 279–280
clinical presentation in, 267–268
COPD vs., 291–292
cost of, 266
diagnosis of, 267–268
epidemiology of, 266
etiology of, 266
exercise-induced, 267, 278, 280, 283
genetic factors in, 266
GERD and, 323
mortality from, 266, 268
occupational, 266
outcome evaluation in, 285–286
pathophysiology of, 266–267
patient care and monitoring in, 286–287
in pediatric patients, 276
in pregnancy, 283
rhinitis and, 267, 285
severity of, 267–268, 274*t*
sinusitis and, 283
treatment of, 268–285
acute severe asthma, 269, 273, 281–283
α_2-agonists, 266, 267–268, 269, 270*t*, 272–273, 274*t*, 277*t*, 282–283
anticholinergics, 270*t*, 276, 277*t*
chronic asthma, 268–269, 272–273, 279–80

corticosteroids, 267, 269, 271*t*, 273–276, 274*t*, 276*t*
cromolyn, 266, 273, 275*t*, 278, 281, 283
drug delivery devices, 271
emergency department and hospital-based management, 266, 268, 273, 277*t*, 282*t*, 283, 284*t*
Heliox, 283
home management, 271, 282*a*
leukotriene modifiers, 273, 275*t*, 277–278, 285
leukotriene receptor antagonists, 278
magnesium, 492
mild intermittent asthma, 283
nedocromil, 275*t*, 278, 281, 283
omalizumab, 278
oxygen therapy, 269, 283
persistent asthma, 281–282
risk factor avoidance, 269–270
self-management, 271–272
theophylline, 269, 272–273, 275*t*, 278, 281, 283
Astringents, in contact dermatitis, 1102
Astrovirus, in gastroenteritis, 1277, 1277*t*
Ataxia, in alcohol intoxication, 612*t*
Ataxia telangiectasia, acute leukemia and, 1580*t*
Atazanavir
adverse effects of, 1425, 1429*t*, 1437*t*–1440*t*
dosage of, 1429*t*
drug interactions of, 1429*t*
food interactions of, 1429*t*
in HIV infection, 1425, 1429*t*
mechanism of action of, 1421*f*
Atelectasis, in cystic fibrosis, 304
Atenolol
in acute coronary syndromes, 142*t*
adverse effects of, 61*t*, 86*t*
in arrhythmias, 162*t*
dosage of, 61*t*, 122*t*, 142*t*
in hypertension, 61*t*, 65, 66*a*
in ischemic heart disease, 122*t*
in lactation, 829*t*
mechanism of action of, 162*t*
in prevention of migraine, 590*t*
in social anxiety disorder, 618
ATG. *See* Lymphocyte immune globulin, antithymoglobulin equine
Atherosclerosis, 111, 112, 230
coronary artery, 112
pathophysiology of, 232–233, 233*f*
Atherosclerotic plaque
formation of, 110–111, 113*f*, 132, 232
rupture of, 113*f*, 114, 132, 234
stable vs. unstable, 112–113, 234
Athletes allergic rhinitis in, 1059
Atomoxetine
in ADHD, 727*t*, 728*t*, 729, 730*t*
adverse effects of, 728*t*, 729
dosage of, 727*t*, 729
mechanism of action of, 729
Atopic dermatitis, 1070*t*
Atopy, 266
Atorvastatin
adverse effects of, 241*t*
dosage of, 241*t*
drug interactions of, 955*t*
in dyslipidemia, 241*t*, 242*t*
in ischemic heart disease, 120
Atosiban, dosage, 832*t*
Atovaquone
adverse effects of, 956*t*
dosage of, 956*t*
in prevention of *Pneumocystis jiroveci*, 956*t*

Atovaquone-proguanil
dosage of, 1300, 1301*t*
in malaria, 1300
and prevention of, 1301*t*
Atrial fibrillation, 160, 165
clinical presentation in, 166
diagnosis of, 166
drug-related, 166
epidemiology of, 165–166
etiology of, 165–166, 166*t*
heart failure and, 166–167
hemodynamically unstable, 167
lone, 166*t*
outcome evaluation in, 176
paroxysmal, 167, 167*a*, 167–168, 170*a*, 171*t*, 172*a*
pathophysiology of, 166–167
permanent, 167, 167*a*, 170*a*
persistent, 167, 167*a*, 170*a*
stroke and, 167, 172–173, 173*t*
treatment of, 167–172, 168*t*–171*t*
calcium channel blockers, 72
conversion to sinus rhythm, 168–171, 170*t*, 171*a*
direct current cardioversion, 167–168
maintenance of sinus rhythm/reduction in episodes of paroxysmal fibrillation, 171–172, 171*t*, 172*a*
stroke prevention, 172–173, 173*t*
ventricular rate control, 168, 169*t*, 170*a*, 171*a*
Atrial natriuretic peptide therapy, in heart failure, 83, 104
Atrial tachycardia, 160
Atrioventricular dissociation, 164
Atrioventricular nodal block, 164–165
clinical presentation in, 165
complete heart block, 164
diagnosis of, 165
drug-related, 164*t*
epidemiology of, 164
etiology of, 164, 164*t*
first-degree, 164–165
Mobitz type I, 164
Mobitz type II, 164
outcome evaluation in, 165
pathophysiology of, 164
second degree, 164–165
third-degree, 164–155
treatment of, 164–165
Atrioventricular node, 158–160, 158*f*
Atropine
adverse effects of, 169*t*
in atrioventricular nodal block, 165
in diarrhea, 379, 379*t*, 1459, 1529
dosage of, 384*t*
dry eye with, 1075*t*
in irritable bowel syndrome, 384*t*
in pancreatitis, 407
in sinus bradycardia, 164
ATS/ERS guidelines, for COPD, 294
Attachment-effacement lesions, 1272
Attapulgite
in diarrhea, 379, 379*t*
dosage of, 379*t*
Attention-deficit hyperactivity disorder (ADHD), 723–732
in adulthood, 723–724
case study of, 723–724
clinical presentation in, 724–725
combined type, 724, 725*t*
diagnosis of, 724–725, 725*f*
DSM-IV criteria, 724, 725*t*
epidemiology of, 723
etiology of, 723

genetic factors in, 723
hyperactive/impulsive type, 724, 725t
inattentive type, 724, 725t
outcome evaluation in, 731
pathophysiology of, 724
patient care and monitoring in, 728t, 731
in pediatric patients, 723
substance-abuse disorders and, 723
treatment of
    algorithm for, 726a
    atomoxetine, 727t, 728t, 729, 730t
    behavioral therapy, 725
    bupropion, 726t, 728t, 729, 730t
    clonidine, 727t, 728t, 731t, 731–732
    guanfacine, 727t, 728t, 730t, 730–731
    imipramine, 727t, 728t, 729, 730t
    medication adherence, 731
    pharmacoeconomics, 731
    stimulants, 725–726, 726t, 727t, 728t
Aura, 585
AUS classification, of prostate cancer, 1540
Auspitz sign, 1081
Autism, 635t
    thimerosal-containing vaccines and, 1415
Autograft, 940
Autoimmune disease
    DIC with, 1131t
    treatment of, 1630, 1630t
Autoimmune hemolysis, 1114
Automated peritoneal dialysis, 473
Automaticity, of cardiac fibers, 158, 160
Autonomic cephalalgia
    epidemiology of, 584
    pathophysiology of, 584
Autonomic neuropathy, in diabetes mellitus, 757
Avascular necrosis, 998t
Axillary thermometers, 24
Axonal transection, in multiple sclerosis, 508
5-Aza-2′-deoxycytidine, in sickle cell anemia/
    disease, 1146
Azacitidine, 1456
    adverse effects of, 1456
    mechanism of action of, 1456
    in myelodysplastic syndrome, 1456
    pharmacokinetics of, 1456
Azalides, in rhinosinusitis, 1212a, 1213a
Azathioprine, 954, 990
    adverse effects of, 945t, 950
    in cancer therapy, 1452t
    dosage of, 347t, 349t, 945t, 950
    drug interactions of, 953–955, 1016
    in inflammatory bowel disease, 347, 347t, 349t,
        351t, 350–353, 353t
    in immune thrombocytopenic purpura, 1134
    mechanism of action of, 948f, 950
    pancreatitis with, 404t
    in psoriasis, 1087
    in transplant recipient, 945t, 950
Azelaic acid
    in acne vulgaris, 1097
    adverse effects of, 1097
    dosage of, 1097
Azelastine
    adverse effects of, 1068t
    in allergic conjunctivitis, 10680t
    in allergic rhinitis, 1051, 1054, 1054t
    dosage of, 1069t
    mechanism of action of, 1068t
Azithromycin
    adverse effects of, 1208t
    anti-inflammatory action of, 308
    in chancroid, 1334t
    in *Chlamydia*, 831t, 834, 1320, 1321

in cholera, 1273
in conjunctivitis, 1066t, 1067t
in COPD, 299t
in cryptosporidiosis, 1276
in cystic fibrosis, 308
in diarrhea, 380
dosage of, 831t, 1066t, 1067t, 1199t, 1208t,
    1212t, 1215t, 1269t, 1319, 1334t
in gonorrhea, 1319
in infective endocarditis, 1250t
in lactation, 834
in otitis media, 1207, 1208t
in pharyngitis, 1215t
in pneumonia, 1195–1197, 1196t, 1199t
in pregnancy, 831t, 834
in prevention of endocarditis, 1250t
in rhinosinusitis, 1212t
in shigellosis, 1268, 1269t
in travelers' diarrhea, 1274
in typhoid fever, 1270
in urinary tract infections, 1311t
Azithromycin resistance, 1194t
Azoles. *See also specific drugs*
    adverse effects of, 834, 1364, 1381
    drug interactions of, 1364
    in vulvovaginal candidiasis, 1363–1364, 1363t,
        1364t
Azoospermia
    adverse effects of, 1177t
    in cystic fibrosis, 305, 309, 309t
    dosage of, 309t, 1177t
    in meningitis, 1177t, 1183
    in pancreatitis, 407t
    in urinary tract infections, 1311t

B

Bachmann bundle, 158, 158f
Bacille Calmette-Guérin vaccine, 1256
Bacillus cereus, in food poisoning, 1278, 1278t
Bacitracin, in conjunctivitis, 1066, 1066t
Back pain, 568
Backwash ileitis, 342
Baclofen
    dosage of, 516t
    mechanism of action of, 516t
    in musculoskeletal disorders, 1027
    in spasticity, 516t
Bacteremia
    definition of, 1348t
    in infective endocarditis, 1238
    Salmonella, 1270
Bacteria
    intestinal, 1702
    immune response to, 342–343
    translocation in gut, 391
Bacterial mastitis in pregnancy, 837
Bacterial synergism, 1283
Bacterial vaginosis, 1331–1332
    clinical presentation in, 1331
    diagnosis of, 1331
    epidemiology of, 1331
    in lactation, 834
    pathophysiology of, 1331
    patient care and monitoring in, 1332
    in pregnancy, 825, 831t, 833–834
    treatment of, 1331–1332
Bacterial virulence, 1157
Bacteriuria, 1307
    asymptomatic, in pregnancy, 1313
    in pregnancy, 825, 833
    significant, 1307–1308, 1308t
Bacteroides
    in intra-abdominal infections, 1283, 1286t

in necrotizing fasciitis, 1226
normal flora, 1157f
in pneumonia, 1190
in rhinosinusitis, 1209
in surgical site infections, 1397t
Balloon angioplasty, in acute coronary
    syndromes, 137
Balloon tamponade, in variceal bleeding, 395
Balsalazide
    dosage of, 346t
    in inflammatory bowel disease, 346t, 346
Bandemia, 1158
Barbiturate(s), 45t. *See also specific drugs*
    anxiety with, 694t
    GERD with, 259t
    mechanism of action of, 522
    ocular changes with, 1077t
    teratogenic effects of, 829t
Barbiturate coma, in status epilepticus, 548
Bariatric surgery, 1728
Barium enema
    double-contrast, screening for colorectal
        cancer, 1519
    in irritable bowel syndrome, 374
Barrett's esophagus, 315–318, 316f, 319, 321
    stricture of, 316f, 317–318
Barrier contraception, 851
Bartter's syndrome, metabolic alkalosis in, 503t
Basal cell(s), 1614
Basal cell carcinoma, 1611–1626. *See also*
    Nonmelanoma skin cancer
    morpheaform, 1614t, 1624, 1625
    nodular, 1614t, 1624
    pigmented (metatypical), 1614t, 1624, 1625
    superficial, 1614t, 1624
    warning signs of, 1624
Basal cell nevus syndrome, 1624
Basal ganglia, 554
Basiliximab
    adverse effects of, 945t
    dosage of, 945t, 946
    mechanism of action of, 946, 948f
    in transplant recipient, 945t, 946
Bazedoxifene, 976
Bazett's equation, 160
B cells
    activated, 943
    differentiation of, 1554f
    solid-organ transplantation and, 943
Bcl-2 gene, 1624
BCR-ABL fusions, 1581, 1584
BCV regimen, in Hodgkin's lymphoma, 1557t
BEACOPP regimen, in Hodgkin's lymphoma,
    1557t, 1558
BEAM regimen, in Hodgkin's lymphoma, 1557t
Beclomethasone
    in allergic rhinitis, 1051, 1052, 1052t, 1054,
        1059
    in asthma, 276t
    in contact dermatitis, 1103t
    in COPD, 295t
    dosage of, 276t, 295t, 830t, 1103t
Bed alarm, in enuresis, 923, 924t
Bedsore. *See* Pressure sore
Beef tapeworm, 1294, 1298
Beers' criteria, 13
Behavioral therapy
    in ADHD, 725
    in enuresis, 914, 923t
    in obesity, 1724
    in smoking cessation, 622
Bell's palsy, 1075t
    anxiety with, 694t

Bence-Jones protein, 1605
Bendamustine
adverse effects of, 1462
in cancer therapy, 1462
chemically active groups, 1462
in chronic lymphocytic leukemia, 1603, 1603t
dosage of, 1462
Benign childhood epilepsy with centrotemporal
spikes, 525t
Benign neonatal epilepsy, 525t
Benign prostatic hyperplasia, 895–907
case study of, 898, 904–905
clinical presentation in, 897–898
complications of, 897
diagnosis of, 897–898
digital rectal examination in, 897, 900
epidemiology of, 896
etiology of, 896
intravenous pyelogram in, 898
irritative symptoms in, 897
lower urinary tract symptoms in, 896–897
obstructive symptoms in, 897
outcome evaluation in, 906
pathophysiology of, 896–897
patient care and monitoring in, 907
post-void residual urine volume in, 898, 900t
prostate cancer and, 1537
prostate needle biopsy in, 900t
prostate-specific antigen in, 896, 900t
staging severity of, 900t
treatment of, 898–905
algorithm for, 899a
α-adrenergic antagonists, 897, 900t, 901–903
5α-reductase inhibitors, 8963, 901t, 904–907
anticholinergics, 905
combination therapy, 905
finasteride, 1537
nonpharmacologic, 901
surgery, 896, 901
watchful waiting, 899
urinalysis in, 900t
urinary incontinence in, 911
urinary tract infections and, 1313
Benzathine penicillin
dosage of, 1322
informational chart, 1324t
in syphilis, 1322, 1324
Benzathine penicillin G, dosage, 831t
Benzene exposure, 1598
Benznidazole, in American trypanosomiasis, 1303
Benzocaine
in musculoskeletal disorders, 1025
in otitis media, 1207
Benzodiazepine(s), 12. *See also specific drugs*
adverse effects of, 697, 701–702
in alcohol withdrawal, 616, 620
loading technique, 618
in Alzheimer's disease, 598
in amphetamine intoxication, 616
anterograde amnesia with, 698
anxiety with, 694t
in bipolar disorder, 676
comparison chart, 698t
in delirium tremens, 618
discontinuation of, 697
drug interactions of, 318, 614t, 660t, 699t, 850t
in generalized anxiety disorder, 697
hyperprolactinemia with, 814t
in lactation, 829t
mechanism of action of, 522, 698
metabolism of, 698
in nausea and vomiting, 362t, 364
ocular changes with, 1077t

in opioid withdrawal, 621t
in panic disorder, 701
in seizures, 618
in social anxiety disorder, 704
in status epilepticus, 544, 545t, 546t, 547, 547t
teratogenic effects of, 829t
for weight loss, 1728
Benzodiazepine receptor agonists
adverse effects of, 714
discontinuation of, 714
in insomnia, 714, 716t
Benzoyl peroxide
in acne vulgaris, 1096–1097
adverse effects of, 1096
comedolytic effects of, 1096
dosage of, 1096–1097
Benztropine
drug interactions of, 660t
in extrapyramidal symptoms, 647
Bepridil, arrhythmia with, 179t
β₂-agonists
adverse effects of, 272, 294
in anaphylaxis, 931t
in asthma, 266, 267–268, 269, 270t, 272–273,
274t, 277t, 282–283
in COPD, 294, 295t
in cystic fibrosis, 308
drug interactions of, 267
in hyperkalemia, 487
long-acting inhaled, 273, 274t, 294, 295t
short-acting inhaled, 271, 272–273, 294, 295t
β-amyloid protein, 597–598
β-blockers, 38f. *See also specific drugs*
in acute coronary syndromes, 142t, 146–147,
152t
adverse effects of, 65, 84t, 86t, 117, 122, 146,
152t, 1040
in akathisia, 647
with α-receptor-blocking properties, 66
arrhythmia with, 161, 162t, 163t, 165
in asthmatic patient, 267
in atrial fibrillation, 168–169, 169t, 170a
blood glucose level and, 737t
bronchospasms with, 1040
cardioselectivity of, 66–67, 122t
contraindications to, 123, 142t
in diabetic patients, 123
dosage of, 122, 169t, 175t
drug interactions of, 169t, 175t, 245, 267, 1004
dry eye with, 1075t
effect on myocardial oxygen demand and
supply, 122t
erectile dysfunction with, 885t
in glaucoma, 1038t, 1040
in heart failure, 65–67, 89, 92t, 94–95
dyslipidemia with, 236t
in hypertension, 65–67, 69, 70, 72t, 756, 958
in hyperthyroidism, 775–776
intrinsic sympathomimetic activity of, 66, 66a,
121, 122t
in ischemic heart disease, 117, 122–123, 122t
mechanism of action of, 94, 162t, 169t, 175t
membrane stabilizing activity of, 66
in myocardial infarction, 65
ocular changes with, 1077t
in paroxysmal supraventricular tachycardia,
169t
in portal hypertension, 396–397
in pregnancy, 72t
in prevention of migraine, 590, 590t
in prevention of myocardial infarction, 150
psoriasis and, 1080
respiratory acidosis with, 503t

in social anxiety disorder, 704
in thyroid storm, 777
topical, 1040
in ventricular premature depolarizations, 160
in ventricular tachycardia, 176
β-carotene
in macular degeneration, 1073
in prevention of lung cancer, 1501
prostate cancer and, 1537
β-lactam(s)
adverse effects of, 1342t
allergy to, 931–932, 931t, 1397, 1398
drug interactions of, 1342t
in infections in cancer patients, 1660t
β-lactam resistance, 309
in CSF isolates, 1175
β-cells, pancreatic, 737
Betamethasone
in adrenal insufficiency, 789t
antenatal steroids, 832t
dosage of, 832t
Betamethasone benzoate
in contact dermatitis, 1103t
dosage and potency of, 1103t
Betamethasone dipropionate, in psoriasis, 1084
Betamethasone valerate
in contact dermatitis, 1103t
dosage and potency of, 1103t
in psoriasis, 1084
Betaxolol
in arrhythmias, 162t
dosage of, 122t, 1038t
in glaucoma, 1038t, 1040
in hypertension, 66a
in ischemic heart disease, 122t
mechanism of action of, 162t, 1038t
Bethanechol in GERD, 322
Bevacizumab, 1466
adverse effects of, 1466, 1484t, 1507t, 1528t,
1530
in breast cancer, 1484t, 1493
in cancer therapy, 1466
in colorectal cancer, 1524t, 1526, 1527t, 1528t,
1530
dosage of, 1484t, 1507t, 1524t, 1530
in lung cancer, 1507t, 1508, 1511
mechanism of action of, 1466, 1493, 1508,
1528t, 1530
pharmacokinetics of, 1466
Bexarotene
adverse effects of, 1464–1465
in cancer therapy, 1464–1465
pharmacokinetics of, 1464
Bicalutamide, 1468
adverse effects of, 1468, 1545t
in cancer therapy, 1468
dosage of, 1545t
mechanism of action of, 1468
pharmacokinetics of, 1468
in prostate cancer, 1539t, 1545, 1545t
Bicarbonate
in extracellular fluid, 484t
serum, 496–497
in metabolic acidosis, 466
normal range for, 484t
Bicarbonate therapy
in metabolic acidosis, 466
in metabolic alkalosis, 503t
in respiratory acidosis, 503
Bichloroacetic acid
adverse effects of, 1327t, 1328
in genital warts, 1328
Bicitra, in metabolic acidosis, 466

Bifidobacterium, 349
Bigeminy, 176
Biguanides
    adverse effects of, 749*t*
    contraindications to, 750
    in diabetes mellitus, 749*t*, 750
Bile, 1712
Bile acid(s), 230, 231*f*
Bile acid sequestrants, in dyslipidemia, 241*t*, 243*t*,
        244–245, 954
Bile acid transport inhibitors, 247
Bile duct cancer, liver transplantation in, 941
Bile salts, 1702, 1702*f*
Bilevel positive airway pressure, in respiratory
        acidosis, 503
Biliary atresia, liver transplantation in, 941
Biliary disease, in inflammatory bowel disease,
        344
Biliary sludge, octreotide-related, 806
Biliary tract
    anatomy of, 404*f*
    surgery, antimicrobial prophylaxis in, 1400*t*
Bimatoprost
    administration of, 1040
    adverse effects of, 1040–1041
    dosage of, 1038*t*
    in glaucoma, 1038*t*, 918
    mechanism of action of, 1038*t*, 1040
Bioavailability, 1163
Biochemotherapy, in melanoma, 1621–1622
Biofeedback
    in headache prevention, 587
    in pain, 573
Bioidentical hormones, 874–876
Biologic DMARDs, 990–992
Biologic response modifiers
    in pregnancy, 990
    in psoriasis, 1087–1088
    in rheumatoid arthritis, 986*t*, 990–991
    selection of, 990–991
Biologic therapy, in breast cancer, 1485, 1484*t*,
        1493
Bipolar disorder, 669–687
    case study of, 670–671, 674, 686
    clinical presentation in, 670–674
    comorbid psychiatric and medical
        conditions, 674
    diagnosis of, 670–671, 673*t*
    differential diagnosis of, 672
    DSM-IV-TR criteria, 670, 671*t*
    in elderly, 686
    epidemiology of, 670
    etiology of, 670
    genetic factors in, 670
    neurochemical hypothesis of, 670
    outcome evaluation in, 687
    pathophysiology of, 670
    patient care and monitoring in, 687
    patient education in, 687
    in pediatric patients, 685
    in pregnancy, 686
    psychotic symptoms in, 635*t*
    suicidality in, 672, 674
    treatment of, 674–687
        algorithm and guidelines for, 675*t*
        anticonvulsants, 677*t*
        antidepressants, 676, 685
        antipsychotics, 674*t*, 678*t*, 684–685
        carbamazepine, 678*t*, 680*t*–681*t*, 682*t*,
            683–684
        clonazepam, 677*t*, 684
        divalproex sodium, 677*t*, 680*t*–681*t*, 681–683
        gabapentin, 684

        lamotrigine, 677*t*, 680*t*–681*t*, 684
        lithium, 676, 677*t*, 679*t*, 680*t*–681*t*, 686
        lorazepam, 677*t*
        mood-stabilizing drugs, 676
        nonpharmacologic, 674–675
        oxcarbazepine, 678*t*, 680*t*–681*t*, 684
        topiramate, 678*t*, 684
        valproate, 678*t*, 680*t*–681*t*, 681
Bipolar I disorder, 670, 671
Bipolar II disorder, 670, 671
Birth defects, 827
Bisacodyl
    in constipation, 374*t*, 577*t*, 829, 830*t*
    dosage of, 374*t*, 830*t*
    in pregnancy, 829, 830*t*
Bishop score, 825
Bismuth subsalicylate
    in diarrhea, 379, 379*t*
    dosage of, 379*t*
    in *Helicobacter pylori* eradication, 335, 335*t*,
        1561
    in prevention of travelers' diarrhea, 1274
Bisoprolol
    in arrhythmias, 162*t*
    dosage of, 92*t*, 122*t*
    in heart failure, 92*t*, 94
    in hypertension, 66*a*
    in ischemic heart disease, 122*t*
    mechanism of action of, 162*t*
Bisphosphonates, 974. *See also specific drugs*
    administration of, 974
    adverse effects of, 974
    in breast cancer, 1487, 1494
    cost of, 973*t*
    in cystic fibrosis, 312
    in hypercalcemia, 490, 490*t*, 1672*t*, 1673
    hyperphosphatemia with, 492
    injectable, 974
    in multiple myeloma, 1607
    ocular changes with, 1077*t*
    in osteoporosis, 973–974, 973*t*
    in prostate cancer, 1547
Bite wound, infected, 1232–1233
    clinical presentation in, 1232*t*
    complications of, 1232
    epidemiology of, 1232
    etiology of, 1232, 1232*t*
    rabies and tetanus prophylaxis in, 1233
    treatment of, 1232–1233
Bivalirudin
    for acute coronary syndromes, 146
    in venous thromboembolism, 200–201
B-K syndrome, 1613
Black cohosh
    adverse effects of, 879*t*
    dosage of, 879*t*
    hepatotoxicity of, 878
    in vasomotor symptoms of menopause, 878,
        879*t*
Blackhead. *See* Comedo, open
Bladder cancer
    epidemiology of, 1446*f*
    genetic factors in, 1447*t*
Bladder irrigation, in prevention of hemorrhagic
        cystitis, 1667
Bladder outlet obstruction, urinary incontinence
        in, 911–912
Blast cells, leukemic, 1579
Blastomycosis
    clinical presentation in, 1377–1378
    diagnosis of, 1378
    in endemic mycosis, 1380
    epidemiology of, 1376

        geographic localization of, 1377*f*
        pathophysiology of, 1376–1377, 1377*f*
        patient monitoring in, 1381–1382
        prophylaxis for, 1382
        treatment of, 1378–1381, 1379*t*
Blastospores, 1362
Bleeding
    anovulatory. *See* Anovulatory bleeding
    with antiretrovirals, 1438*t*
    with direct thrombin inhibitors, 194
    with factor Xa inhibitors, 194
    with hormone-replacement therapy, 876*t*
    with low-molecular-weight heparin, 193
    with unfractionated heparin, 193–194, 197*t*
    uremic, 467
    variceal. *See* Variceal bleeding
    with warfarin, 201–202
Bleeding time, 1137
Bleomycin, 1463
    adverse effects of, 1463, 1561*t*, 1562, 1563
    in cancer therapy, 1463, 1469
    dosage of, 1557*t*, 1561*t*, 1561*t*
        in renal dysfunction, 1470*t*
    in Hodgkin's lymphoma, 1557, 1557*t*, 1561*t*,
        1562, 1563
    mechanism of action of, 1454*a*, 1463
    in non-Hodgkin's lymphoma, 1561*t*
    pharmacokinetics of, 1463
Bleomycin lung, 1463, 1562
Blepharitis, 1064, 1075*t*
Blink reflex, 1075
Blood
    pH of, 496
    viscosity of, 1141
Blood alcohol levels, 612
Blood-brain barrier, 1171
Blood-CSF barrier, 1171
Blood culture, in sepsis, 1349
Blood dyscrasias, allergic drug reaction, 929
Blood pressure. *See also* Hypertension
    ambulatory, 56
    classification of, 52, 52*t*
    measurement of, 56
    in shock, 251
Blood pressure cuff, 56
Blood products
    contaminated
        hepatitis B, 414
        hepatitis C, 414
        hepatitis D, 414–415
    in hypovolemic shock, 257
    risks from, 259
Blood urea nitrogen
    in chronic kidney disease, 468
    in end-stage renal disease, 468
Blood volume, 253, 253*f*
Bloom's syndrome, acute leukemia and,
        1580*t*, 1581
BODE index, 300, 300*t*
Body fluid compartments, 479–481
    case study of, 481
Body louse, 1304
Body mass index, 119, 736, 1719–1721, 1728
    classification of, 1724*t*
    in psoriasis, 1080
Bogbean, 206*t*
Boil. *See* Furuncle
Bone cement, antibiotic-impregnated, 1398, 1400
Bone disease
    in chronic kidney disease, 449–465
    in cystic fibrosis, 305
    metabolic, 1697
Bone dysplasia, 998*t*

Bone marrow
  as source of hematopoietic stem cells, 1629–1630, 1632–1633
  T-cell depletion, 1633
Bone marrow failure, 1114a
Bone marrow suppression, with antiretrovirals, 1439t
Bone mineral density, 966, 968. *See also* Osteoporosis
  measurement of, 968
Bone pain, 45
Bone remodeling, 967
Bone resorption, 967
Borage seed oil, 206t
Bordetella pertussis, 1406
Boric acid
  dosage of, 1364–1365, 1364t
  in vulvovaginal candidiasis, 1364–1365, 1364t
Bortezomib, 952
  adverse effects of, 1606t, 1607
  mechanism of action of, 1606
  in multiple myeloma, 1606t, 1606–1607
  in non-Hodgkin's lymphoma, 1561
Botanicals
  in irritable bowel syndrome, 318
  in pain, 579
Botulinum toxin
  mechanism of action of, 516t
  in prevention of tension-type headaches, 591
  respiratory acidosis with, 503t
  in spasticity, 516, 516t
Bouchard's nodes, 998
Bowel fistula, metabolic acidosis with, 501t
Bowel obstruction
  case study of, 1683
  parenteral nutrition in, 1682t
Brachial plexus injury, with central venous catheter, 1691
Brachytherapy, in prostate cancer, 1543
Bradykinesia, in Parkinson's disease, 555–556
Bradykinin, 68, 83, 1021
  in heart failure, 45
B-RAF gene, 1613
Brain abscess, 1170, 1183
Brain cancer
  epidemiology of, 1446f
  genetic factors in, 1447t
  mania with, 676t
Brain injury
  adrenal insufficiency in, 786t
  constipation in, 372t
Brain metastasis, 1664–1666
  clinical presentation in, 1665
  diagnosis of, 1665
  epidemiology of, 1664–1665
  etiology of, 1664–1665
  in melanoma, 1622
  outcome evaluation in, 1666
  pathophysiology of, 1665
  patient care and monitoring in, 1666
  treatment of, 1665–1666
Brain stem lesion, 503t
BRCA genes, 1477, 1566, 1567
Breakthrough bleeding, with oral contraceptives, 847, 849
Breast
  disorders of, oral contraceptives and, 846
  fibrocystic disease of, 1476
  infections of, 836
Breast biopsy, in breast cancer, 1479, 1494
Breast cancer, 1475–1495
  adenocarcinoma, 1478

advanced/metastatic disease (stage IV), 1480, 1480t, 1487t, 1488–1494
  alcohol use and, 1477
  case study of, 1477, 1481, 1494
  clinical presentation in, 1478
  contralateral, 1476
  diagnosis of, 1478, 1479
  early detection of, 1478–1479, 1479t
  early disease (stage I, II), 1480–1487, 1480t, 1483t–1484t, 1484t
  endocrine responsiveness of, 1482
  environmental factors in, 1477
  epidemiology of, 1278f, 1476–1477
  etiology of, 1476–1477
  genetic factors in, 1447t, 1476–1477
  HER-2/neu gene expression in, 1478, 1480, 1485, 1489, 1493
  hereditary breast and ovarian cancer, 1566
  hormonal factors in, 1476
  hormone receptor status in, 1480, 1485–1487
  hormone-replacement therapy and, 870–871, 876t, 877, 1476
  hypercalcemia with, 1670–1673
  infiltrating lobular, 1478
  inflammatory, 1488
  invasive, 1478
  lifestyle factors in, 1477
  locally advanced disease (stage III), 1480, 1480t, 1488
  in male, 1476, 1489
  metastasis of, 1478
    to bone, 1663
    to brain, 1665, 1665t
  noninvasive, 1478
  obesity and, 1477
  oral contraceptives and, 846
  outcome evaluation in, 1494
  ovarian cancer and, 1566, 1567
  pathophysiology of, 1477–1478
  patient care and monitoring in, 1494
  pharmacogenomics, 1486t
  prevention of, 1478–1479
  prognosis for, 1480
  risk factors for, 1562
  St. Gallen risk classification and therapy recommendations, 1482, 1482t
  staging of, 1479–1480, 1480t
  superior vena cava syndrome with, 1661t
  treatment of
    biologic therapy, 1484t, 1485, 1493
    bisphosphonates, 1487, 1494
    chemotherapy, 1481–1487, 1483t–1484t
    cytotoxic chemotherapy, 1491–1492
    hormonal therapy, 1482, 1485–1487, 1487t
    mastectomy, 1478
    neoadjuvant chemotherapy, 1482
    radiation therapy, 1481, 1487, 1494
    surgery, 1480, 1481, 1488
  tumor lysis syndrome in, 1674t
Breast Cancer Risk Assessment Tool, 1477
Breast carcinoma in situ, 1478
Breast-feeding. *See* Lactation
Breathing retraining, in panic disorder, 700
Brimonidine
  adverse effects of, 1041
  dosage of, 1038t
  in glaucoma, 1038t, 1041
  mechanism of action of, 1038t, 1041
Brinzolamide
  adverse effects of, 1041
  dosage of, 1038t
  in glaucoma, 1038t, 1041
  mechanism of action of, 1038t

Bromelain, 206t
Bromfenac, ocular, in corneal abrasion, 1064
Bromocriptine
  in acromegaly, 808
  adverse effects of, 816, 818t, 859t
  dosage of, 559t, 560, 816, 818t, 859t
  drug interactions of, 817
  in hyperprolactinemia, 817–818, 818t, 858, 859t
  in lactation, 829t
  mechanism of action of, 559t, 816
  in Parkinson's disease, 559t, 560
Bronchiectasis, 292
  in cystic fibrosis, 304
Bronchiolitis, obliterative, 292
Bronchitis, chronic. *See* Chronic obstructive pulmonary disease
Bronchoalveolar lavage specimen, 1198
Bronchoconstriction, 266–267
Bronchodilators. *See also specific drugs*
  anxiety with, 694t
  in COPD, 294–298, 295t
Bronchopulmonary dysplasia, 1703t
Bronchoscopy
  in lung cancer, 1502t
  in pneumonia, 1192
Bronchospasm
  allergic drug reaction, 933
  with β-blockers, 1040
Brucella, in infective endocarditis, 1242
Brudzinski's sign, 1173
Brush-border membrane, 1702, 1702f
Bruxism, 710, 713
B-symptoms, in lymphoma, 1556
B-type natriuretic peptide, in heart failure, 83, 101
Budesonide
  adverse effects of, 347
  in allergic rhinitis, 1051, 1052, 1052t, 1059
  in asthma, 273, 274t, 275t, 276t, 283
  in COPD, 295t
  dosage of, 274t, 295t, 347t, 351t, 830t
  in inflammatory bowel disease, 347, 347t, 350–352, 351t
  in pregnancy, 830t
  in respiratory disorders, 830t
Bulk agents, in diarrhea, 379, 379t
Bulk-forming laxatives
  in constipation, 373, 374t
  in irritable bowel syndrome, 384
Bullectomy, in COPD, 294
Bullous exanthema, allergic drug reaction, 929t
Bumetanide
  in acute kidney injury, 437–438
  adverse effects of, 437–438
  dosage of, 90t, 91t, 437
  in heart failure, 90, 90t, 91t
  in hypertension, 65
Bundle branches, 158f, 158
Bundle of His, 158f
Bupivacaine
  for epidural analgesia, 576
  in pain, 576
Buprenorphine
  adverse effects of, 621
  dosage of, 621, 615
  drug interactions of, 614t, 1434
  in opioid dependence, 615
  in opioid withdrawal, 619, 621, 621t
Bupropion
  in ADHD, 727t, 728t, 729, 730t
  adverse effects of, 658, 659t, 728t, 730
  anxiety with, 694t
  in bipolar disorder, 685

in depression, 665
dosage of, 622t, 660, 660t, 727t
drug interactions of, 660t
in elderly, 665
mechanism of action of, 657, 657t
pharmacokinetics of, 659t
seizures with, 522, 730
in smoking cessation, 292, –622, 622t
Burkholderia cepacia, in cystic fibrosis, 304, 310
Burkitt's lymphoma, 1353, 1355, 1561
Burn patient
DIC in, 1131t
hyponatremia in, 486
protein requirement in, 1689t
respiratory alkalosis in, 504t
treatment of, enteral nutrition, 1703t
Burow's solution, in contact dermatitis, 1102
Bursitis, 1019
clinical presentation in, 1020
pathophysiology of, 1020
Buspirone
adverse effects of, 698
in alcohol dependence, 615
in Alzheimer's disease, 598
augmentation of antidepressant therapy
with, 662
dosage of, 698
drug interactions of, 699
in generalized anxiety disorder, 694, 697–698
mechanism of action of, 698
Busulfan, 1461
adverse effects of, 1461, 1644
in cancer therapy, 1425t, 1461
dosage of, 1634t
adaptive dosing, 1634–1635
drug interactions of, 1381
hemorrhagic cystitis with, 1666t
mechanism of action of, 1461
pharmacokinetics of, 1461
in preparation for hematopoietic cell
transplant, 1634t, 1634, 1635–1636
seizures with, 1634–1635
sinusoidal obstruction syndrome with, 1636
Butabarbital, drug interactions of, 205t
Butenafine, in tinea infections, 1371
Butoconazole
dosage of, 831t, 1363t
in vulvovaginal candidiasis, 1363t
Butorphanol, 45t, 575
Butyrophenones, in nausea and vomiting, 361t, 363

C
CA19-9, in ovarian cancer, 1568
CA-125 antigen, in ovarian cancer, 1566–1567,
1572, 1575
Cabergoline
in acromegaly, 807t, 808
adverse effects of, 560, 807t, 816, 818t
dosage of, 807t, 816, 818t
drug interactions of, 816
in hyperprolactinemia, 816–817, 818t
mechanism of action of, 817
in Parkinson's disease, 560
Cachexia
in breast cancer, 1491
cardiac, 84–85
enteral nutrition in, 1703t
in lung cancer, 1513
Cadmium poisoning, 376t
Caffeine, 56, 828t
in alcohol intoxication, 613
anxiety with, 694t
intake of, 901

CAF regimen, in breast cancer, 1483t
Calamine lotion
in contact dermatitis, 1102
in lice infestation, 1304
Calcimimetics, in hyperparathyroidism, 463
Calcineurin inhibitors. *See also specific drugs*
adaptive dosing of, 1638
comparative efficacy of, 948
drug interactions of, 955t, 1643
hypertension with, 957–958
in prevention of GVHD, 1638
in transplant recipient, 948–950
Calcipotriol, in psoriasis, 1084–1085, 1087
Calcitonin
adverse effects of, 978
cost of, 973t
dosage of, 491t, 861t, 1673t
in hypercalcemia, 490, 491t, 1673, 1673t
injectable, 975
intranasal, 975
in osteoporosis, 973t, 975
production of, 764
tachyphylaxis to, 1673
Calcitriol, 461
in hyperphosphatemia, 463, 464t
in psoriasis, 1084–1085
Calcium
absorption of, 972
in bone, 489
deficiency of, 1697
dietary, colorectal cancer and, 1518
dosage of, 830t
in extracellular fluid, 480, 484t
food sources of, 969, 969t
in intracellular fluid, 480
for parenteral nutrition, 1685t, 1686, 1697
calcium-phosphate precipitation, 1686,
1691–1692
recommended daily intake of, 969, 969t, 860
requirement for, 969
serum, 484
calculation of, 484
normal range for, 484t
target levels in chronic kidney disease, 461,
462t, 465
Calcium acetate
dosage of, 464t
in hyperphosphatemia, 462, 464t, 492
hypophosphatemia with, 491
in metabolic acidosis, 466
Calcium antagonists, in subarachnoid
hemorrhage, 225
Calcium balance, 490–491
Calcium carbonate
dosage of, 464t
in hyperphosphatemia, 462, 464t, 491
in hypocalcemia, 489
in metabolic acidosis, 466
in osteoporosis, 972, 972t
Calcium channel blockers. *See also specific drugs*
in acute coronary syndromes, 142t, 147, 152t
adverse effects of, 84t, 86t, 152t, 835
in angina pectoris, 117
in arrhythmias, 162t
in atrial fibrillation, 67, 170a
constipation with, 308t
contraindications to, 142t
dosage of, 142t
effect on myocardial oxygen demand and
supply, 124t
GERD with, 317t
heart failure and, 96, 123
in hypertension, 61t, 66t, 67, 70, 756, 951t

in ischemic heart disease, 123–124
mechanism of action of, 123, 162t
negative chronotropic effects of, 123
negative inotropic effects of, 123
in pregnancy, 72t
in prevention of cluster headaches, 591
in prevention of migraine, 590, 591t
in prevention of myocardial infarction, 150
in proteinuria, 451
as tocolytics, 835
urinary incontinence with, 912t
in variant angina, 126
Calcium chloride
in hyperkalemia, 454, 488
in hypocalcemia, 489
Calcium citrate
in hypocalcemia, 489
in osteoporosis, 972, 972t
Calcium gluconate
in hyperkalemia, 454
in hypermagnesemia, 492
in hypocalcemia, 489
in osteoporosis, 972t
Calcium infusion, in oxaliplatin-induced
neuropathy, 1530
Calcium lactate, in osteoporosis, 972t
Calcium phosphate, in osteoporosis, 972t
Calcium-phosphorus product
in chronic kidney disease, 461
target levels in chronic kidney disease, 461,
462t, 465
Calcium supplementation
adverse effects of, 972
in cystic fibrosis, 312
drug interactions of, 771t, 1164
in osteoporosis, 951t, 971–972, 972t
in pregnancy, 830t
in prevention of colorectal cancer, 1520
products available, 972t
Caloric requirement, 1703
Calvert equation, 1462
Camphor
adverse effects of, 1026
in musculoskeletal disorders, 1026t, 1026
in osteoarthritis, 1006
Campylobacter
in diarrhea, 380
in travelers' diarrhea, 1273
Campylobacteriosis, 1271–1272
clinical presentation in, 1271
diagnosis of, 1271
epidemiology of, 1271
monitoring patient with, 1271
pathogenesis of, 1271
treatment of, 1271
Canadian Cardiovascular Society classification, of
ischemic heart disease, 115, 115t
Cancer. *See also specific types and sites*
cardiovascular complications in, 1661–1663
case study of, 1460, 1461, 1472
clinical presentation in, 1450
diagnosis of, 1449, 1450
epidemiology of, 1445–1446, 1446f
etiology of, 1445–1446
febrile neutropenia in, 1654–1661
genetic factors in, 1446, 1446t
hematologic complications in, 1654–1661
hypercalcemia in, 1670–1673
metabolic complications in, 1673–1676
metastasis of, 1445, 1446
neurologic complications in, 1663–1664
oncologic emergencies, 1649–1679
oral chemotherapy with respect to food, 1472t

Cancer (*Cont.*)
  palliative care treatment for, 37
  pathophysiology of, 1449
  patient care and monitoring in, 1472
  RECIST criteria, 1448*t*
  secondary malignancies, 1470, 1594, 1644
  staging of, 1448, 1449*t*, 1450
  treatment of, 1449–1469
    adjuvant therapy, 1449
    chemotherapy, 1451–1454
    hormonal therapies, 1468–1469
    immune therapies, 1465
    monoclonal antibodies, 1465–1467
    neoadjuvant therapy, 1449
    palliative therapy, 1451
    radiation therapy, 1451
    supportive care, 1445–1146
    surgery, 1451
  treatment outcomes in, 1472
  tumor growth, 1448
  urologic complications in, 1666–1670
Cancer pain, 572
Candesartan
  in acute coronary syndromes, 143*t*
  adverse effects of, 62*t*
  dosage of, 62*t*, 92*t*, 121*t*, 143*t*
  in heart failure, 92*t*, 93, 97
  in hypertension, 62*t*
  in ischemic heart disease, 121*t*
  in prevention of myocardial infarction, 150
Candida
  in cystic fibrosis, 304
  in folliculitis, 1223*t*
  in infective endocarditis, 1242
  in sepsis, 1348, 1348*t*, 1355
  species identification, 1384
Candida albicans
  in invasive candidiasis, 1376*t*, 1383, 1384, 1387
  in pancreatitis, 407
  in sepsis, 1348, 1348*t*, 1356
  in surgical site infections, 1397, 1397*t*
  in vulvovaginal candidiasis, 1362
Candida glabrata
  in hematopoietic cell transplant recipients, 1642
  in invasive candidiasis, 1376*t*, 1383, 1384, 1385
  in oropharyngeal/esophageal candidiasis, 1366
  in vulvovaginal candidiasis, 1362, 1364
Candida krusei
  in hematopoietic cell transplant recipients, 1642
  in invasive candidiasis, 1376*t*, 1383, 1384, 1385
  in oropharyngeal/esophageal candidiasis, 1366
  in vulvovaginal candidiasis, 1362
Candida parapsilosis
  in invasive candidiasis, 1376*t*, 1384
  in oropharyngeal/esophageal candidiasis, 1366
  in vulvovaginal candidiasis, 1362
Candida tropicalis
  in invasive candidiasis, 1376*t*, 1384
  in oropharyngeal/esophageal candidiasis, 1366
  in vulvovaginal candidiasis, 1362, 1364
Candidemia, catheter-related, 1383, 1385
Candidiasis
  in cancer patients, 1655, 1655*t*, 1660
  with corticosteroids, 296
  diaper dermatitis, 1106, 1106*f*
  esophageal. *See* Esophageal candidiasis
  in hematopoietic cell transplant recipients, 1642
  invasive, 1376*t*
    clinical presentation in, 1383–1384
    diagnosis of, 1384–1385, 1383*f*
    epidemiology of, 1382–1383

    nosocomial, 1383
    pathogenesis of, 1383–1384
    patient monitoring in, 1387
    prophylaxis for, 1387
    treatment of, 1384–1385
  mucocutaneous, in transplant recipient, 957
  nipple, 826, 833*t*, 837
  oropharyngeal. *See* Oropharyngeal candidiasis
  pregnancy, 837–838
  urinary, 1385
  vulvovaginal. *See* Vulvovaginal candidiasis
Cannabinoid(s)
  adverse effects of, 364
  in chemotherapy-induced nausea and vomiting, 1652
  in nausea and vomiting, 362*t*, 364
Cannabinoid receptor, 1720, 1727
Cannabis, 1580*t*
  abuse of
    epidemiology of, 609
    signs and symptoms of intoxication, 612*t*
  erectile dysfunction with, 885*t*
  withdrawal syndrome, 611, 613*t*
CAPD. *See* Continuous ambulatory peritoneal dialysis
Capecitabine, 1455
  adverse effects of, 1455, 1484*t*, 1528*t*, 1529, 1531, 1574*t*
  in breast cancer, 1452*t*, 1484*t*, 1492, 1493
  in cancer therapy, 1455
  in colorectal cancer, 1524*t*, 1525, 1527*t*, 1528*t*, 1529, 1531
  dosage of, 1470*t*, 1484*t*, 1524*t*, 1529, 1574*t*
  drug interactions of, 1455, 1529
  mechanism of action of, 1454*a*, 1455, 1492, 1528*t*, 1529
  myelosuppression with, 1455
  in ovarian cancer, 1574*t*
Capillary, fluid flow into or out of, 253, 254*a*
Capillary leak, 253
CAPIRI regimen, in colorectal cancer, 1524*t*
Capnocytophaga canimorsus, in bite wound infections, 1232*t*
CAPOX regimen, in colorectal cancer, 1524*t*
Capreomycin
  adverse effects of, 1261*t*
  dosage of, 1261*t*
  in tuberculosis, 1259, 1260, 1261*t*
Capsaicin
  adverse effects of, 1027
  dosage of, 1002*t*
  mechanism of action of, 1021, 1027
  in musculoskeletal disorders, 1026*t*, 1027
  in osteoarthritis, 1002*t*, 1007–1008
  in pain, 578
Capsicum, 206*t*
  in musculoskeletal disorders, 1026*t*, 1027
Capsules, administration through feeding tubes, 1714
Captopril
  in acute coronary syndromes, 143*t*
  adverse effects of, 62*t*
  dosage of, 62*t*, 92*t*, 121*t*, 143*t*
  in heart failure, 92*t*, 93
  in hypertension, 62*t*
  in ischemic heart disease, 120, 121*t*
Caput medusae, 390
Carafate, drug interactions of, 1183*t*
Carbachol
  adverse effects of, 1042
  dosage of, 1038*t*
  in glaucoma, 1038*t*, 1042
  mechanism of action of, 1038*t*

Carbamazepine, 828*t*
  adverse effects of, 530, 531*t*, 683
  in alcohol withdrawal, 616
  allergic drug reactions, 933
  anxiety with, 694*t*
  arrhythmia with, 164*t*
  autoinduction of metabolism of, 529, 530*f*
  in bipolar disorder, 677*t*, 680*t*–681*t*, 678*t*, 683–684
  dosage of, 528, 531*t*, 677*t*, 599
  drug interactions of, 205*t*, 537, 537*t*, 615*t*, 646, 660*t*, 684, 699*t*, 771*t*, 850*t*, 955*t*
  in epilepsy, 528, 529*t*, 531*t*, 535
  erectile dysfunction with, 885*t*
  mechanism of action of, 522, 531*t*, 683
  monitoring therapy with, 678*t*, 683
  in oxaliplatin-induced neuropathy, 1530
  pharmacokinetics of, 531*t*, 680*t*–681*t*
  in pregnancy, 537
  in prevention of migraine, 590
  teratogenic effects of, 824*t*, 829*t*
Carbapenems
  allergic drug reactions, 929*t*
  in intra-abdominal infections, 1286
  in meningitis, 1182
  in sepsis, 1353*t*, 1354, 1355
  in urinary tract infections, 1311*t*
Carbidopa. *See* Levodopa/carbidopa
Carbimazole
  in hyperthyroidism, 776
  mechanism of action of, 776
Carbohydrates
  digestion of, 1702*f*
  metabolism of, growth hormone effects on, 803*t*
Carbonate, dosage, 830*t*
Carbon dioxide
  in blood, 496–497
  total venous, 496
Carbonic anhydrase inhibitors
  in glaucoma, 1038*t*, 1041–1042
  systemic, 1041–1042
  topical, 1042
Carbon monoxide poisoning, 501*t*
Carboplatin, 1462
  adverse effects of, 442, 1462, 1507*t*, 1572*t*
  in breast cancer, 1493
  in cancer therapy, 1462
  dosage of, 1507*t*, 1508*t*, 1561*t*, 1572*t*, 1573*t*
    in renal dysfunction, 1470*t*
  emetogenicity of, 365*t*
  in lung cancer, 1506, 1509–1511, 1507*t*, 1508*t*
  mechanism of action of, 1454*a*, 1462
  in non-Hodgkin's lymphoma, 1561*t*
  in ovarian cancer, 1569–1573, 1572*t*
  pharmacokinetics of, 1462
Carbuncle
  clinical presentation in, 1077*t*
  diagnosis of, 1223*t*
  epidemiology of, 1077*t*
  etiology of, 1077*t*
  treatment of, 1077*t*
Carcinoembryonic antigen
  in colorectal cancer, 1522, 1531
  in ovarian cancer, 1568
Carcinogen(s), 1446, 1501
Carcinogenesis, 1447, 1449, 1568
Carcinoid, 792*t*
Carcinoid syndrome, anxiety with, 694*t*
Carcinoma, 1449
Carcinoma in situ, 1449
  of breast, 1478
  of lung, 1501
Carcinomatosis, peritoneal, 1567

Cardiac arrhythmia. *See* Arrhythmia
Cardiac cachexia, 84–85
Cardiac cycle, 80
Cardiac hypertrophy, in heart failure, 81t, 82
Cardiac index, in heart failure, 91
Cardiac output, 80
  in heart failure, 80–81
  in hypertension, 54
  in shock, 252
Cardiac pacemaker, 158. *See also* Implantable
    cardioverter-defibrillator
  implanted
    in atrioventricular nodal block, 165
    in sinus bradycardia, 163
Cardiac remodeling
  in acute coronary syndromes, 150
  in heart failure, 82, 82t
Cardiac resynchronization therapy, in heart
    failure, 103
Cardiobacterium hominis, in infective
    endocarditis, 1241
Cardiogenic shock, 134, 252, 253t
Cardiomyopathy
  alcoholic, 89
  chemotherapy-related, 1485
  dilated, heart failure and, 80, 80t
  hypertrophic, heart failure and, 80t
  nausea and vomiting with, 296t
  peripartum, 97
  tachycardia-induced, 167
  treatment of, heart transplantation, 940
Cardiopulmonary resuscitation, in ventricular
    fibrillation, 178–179
Cardiorenal model, of heart failure, 83
Cardiothoracic surgery, antimicrobial
    prophylaxis in, 1400–1401, 1400t
Cardiovascular disease
  in cancer patients, 1661–1663
  oral contraceptives and, 846
  rheumatoid arthritis and, 983
  in sickle cell anemia/disease, 1152t
Cardiovascular shock, in pancreatitis, 404
Cardiovascular system, in elderly patients, 12
Cardioverter defibrillator. *See* Implantable
    cardioverter-defibrillator
Caregiver, of person with Alzheimer's disease,
    598, 599, 603
Carisoprodol, in musculoskeletal disorders, 1027
Carmustine, 1461
  adverse effects of, 1461, 1563
  in cancer therapy, 1461
  dosage of, 1557t, 1634t
  emetogenicity of, 365t
  extravasation of, 1677t
  in Hodgkin's lymphoma, 1557t, 1563
  mechanism of action of, 1461
  in melanoma, 1621
  pharmacokinetics of, 1461
  in preparation for hematopoietic cell
    transplant, 1634t
Carnitine deficiency, 1696
Carotid angioplasty, in prevention of stroke, 223
Carotid artery, Doppler studies of, 223
Carotid artery stenosis, 223, 244
Carotid bruit, 115
Carotid endarterectomy
  in prevention of stroke, 223
  in stroke, 220
Carotid sinus hypersensitivity, 162t, 164t
Carotid sinus massage, in paroxysmal
    supraventricular tachycardia, 174
Carteolol
  in arrhythmias, 162t

  dosage of, 1038t
  in glaucoma, 1038t, 1040
  in hypertension, 66a
  mechanism of action of, 162t, 1038t
Carvedilol
  adverse effects of, 61t
  in arrhythmias, 162t
  dosage of, 61t, 92t, 122t
  in heart failure, 92t, 94–95
  in hypertension, 61t, 65, 66a
  in ischemic heart disease, 122t, 123
  mechanism of action of, 162t
Casanthranol-docusate, in constipation, 577t
Cascara sagrada
  in constipation, 374t
  dosage of, 374t
Caspofungin
  adverse effects of, 1643
  in aspergillosis, 1385, 1386t, 1643
  dosage of, 1384, 1221t, 1660t
  in esophageal candidiasis, 1368, 1385
  in fungal infections, 957
  in infections in cancer patients, 1660, 1660t
  in infective endocarditis, 1248
  in invasive candidiasis, 1385, 1386t
  mechanism of action of, 1643
  in oropharyngeal candidiasis, 1385
  in peritonitis, 475
  in sepsis, 1356
Castor oil, in constipation, 374
Cataplexy, 712
  treatment of, 716
Cataract, corticosteroids and, 953t, 1077t
Cat bite, 1232, 1232t
Catecholamines
  in hypovolemic shock, 253
  respiratory alkalosis with, 504t
Catechol-O-methyltransferase, 558f
Catechol-O-methyltransferase inhibitors. *See*
    COMT inhibitors
Catheter-related infection
  in parenteral nutrition, 1698
  in peritoneal dialysis
    outcome evaluation in, 475
    pathophysiology of, 475
    prevention of, 475
    treatment of, 475
  sepsis and, 1353t
Caudate nucleus, 554
Causalgia, 570
Cavitary lesion, in tuberculosis, 1255
CAV regimen, in lung cancer, 1507t
CCR5 receptors, 1420–1421
CD (cluster determinants), 1583
CD4 receptors, 1420
CDK4 gene, 1613
CDKN2A gene, 1613
Cefaclor, in urinary tract infections, 1311t
Cefadroxil
  dosage of, 1073t
  in pharyngitis, 1073t
  in prevention of endocarditis, 1102t
  in urinary tract infections, 1155t
Cefamandole, drug interactions of, 614t
Cefazolin
  in cellulitis, 1225t
  dosage of, 832t, 1225t, 1245t, 1249t, 1287, 1342
  in infective endocarditis, 1245t, 1249t, 1250t
  in intra-abdominal infections, 1287
  in keratitis, 1071t
  in osteomyelitis, 1339t, 1342t
  in peritonitis, 474
  in pregnancy, 832t

  in prevention of endocarditis, 1250t
  in sepsis, 1353t, 1354
  in *Streptococcus* group B, 832t
  in surgical prophylaxis, 1397–1398, 1400, 1400t
Cefdinir
  adverse effects of, 1208t
  in COPD, 299t
  dosage of, 1073t, 1208t, 1212t
  in otitis media, 1208t
  in pharyngitis, 1073t
  in rhinosinusitis, 1212a, 1213t, 1071t
Cefepime
  adverse effects of, 1176t, 1177t
  in COPD, 299t
  dosage of, 1176t, 1177t, 1199t, 1287t, 1289,
    1342, 1660t
  in infections in cancer patients, 1594, 1660t
  in infective endocarditis, 1248
  in intra-abdominal infections, 1287t, 1289
  in meningitis, 1171t, 1176t, 1177t, 1180t, 1182
  in osteomyelitis, 1339t, 1342
  in pancreatitis, 407t
  in peritonitis, 474
  in pneumonia, 1196t, 1197, 1198, 1199t
  in postneurosurgical infections, 1183
  in sepsis, 1353, 1354, 1355
Cefixime
  dosage of, 831t, 1319, 1320
  in gonorrhea, 831t, 834, 1319
  in pregnancy, 831t, 834
  in urinary tract infections, 1311t
Cefoperazone, drug interactions of, 614t
Cefotaxime
  adverse effects of, 1175t, 1176t, 1177t
  in campylobacteriosis, 1272
  dosage of, 1175t, 1176t, 1177t, 1199t
  in infections in sickle cell anemia/disease, 1147
  in intra-abdominal infections, 1287t
  in meningitis, 1171t, 1176t, 1177t
  in osteomyelitis, 1339t, 1342t
  in pneumonia, 1196, 1196t, 1197, 1198, 1199t
  in spontaneous bacterial peritonitis, 397
Cefotetan
  drug interactions of, 614t
  in intra-abdominal infections, 1288, 1288t,
    1289
  in surgical prophylaxis, 1397, 1398, 1399–1400
Cefoxitin
  dosage of, 1232t
  in infected pressure sores, 1232t
  in intra-abdominal infections, 1288, 1288t
  in surgical prophylaxis, 1397, 1397–1400t, 1401
Cefpodoxime
  adverse effects of, 1208t
  in COPD, 299t
  dosage of, 1208t, 1212t
  in otitis media, 1066t
  in pneumonia, 1196, 1196t
  in rhinosinusitis, 1071t, 1212a, 1213t
  in urinary tract infections, 1311t
Cefprozil in COPD, 299t
CEF regimen, in breast cancer, 1484t
Ceftazidime
  adverse effects of, 1040t
  in catheter-related infections, 475
  in cellulitis, 1225t
  in COPD, 299t
  in cystic fibrosis, 309t
  in diabetic foot infections, 1229t
  dosage of, 309t, 1040t, 1079t, 1199t, 1287t,
    1289, 1342t, 1660t
  in infections in cancer patients, 1660t
  in intra-abdominal infections, 1287t, 1289

Ceftazidime (*Cont.*)
  in keratitis, 1071*t*
  in meningitis, 117*t*, 1177*t*, 1183
  in osteomyelitis, 1339*t*, 1342*t*
  in peritonitis, 474
  in pneumonia, 1196*t*, 1197, 1198, 1199*t*
  in postneurosurgical infections, 1183
  prophylactic, in hematopoietic cell transplant
    recipients, 1641
  in sepsis, 1354
Ceftizoxime, in intra-abdominal infections,
    1287*t*, 1288
Ceftriaxone
  adverse effects of, 1175*t*, 1176*t*, 1177*t*
  in cellulitis, 1225*t*
  in chancroid, 1334*t*
  in conjunctivitis, 1067
  in COPD, 299*t*
  in diabetic foot infections, 1083*t*
  dosage of, 831*t*, 1097*t*, 1175*t*, 1176*t*, 1177*t*,
    1199*t*, 1208*t*, 1212*t*, 1225*t*, 1249*t*, 1319,
    1320, 1333*t*, 1334*t*, 1342*t*
  in gonococcal conjunctivitis, 1320
  in gonorrhea, 831*t*, 834, 1319, 1320
  in infections in sickle cell anemia/disease, 1147
  in infective endocarditis, 1243, 1244*t*, 1249*t*,
    1250*t*
  in intra-abdominal infections, 1287*t*
  in keratitis, 1071*t*
  in meningitis, 1040*t*, 1171*t*, 1175*t*, 1176*t*, 1177*t*
  in osteomyelitis, 1339*t*, 1342*t*
  in otitis media, 1027, 1028*t*
  in PID, 1333*t*
  in pneumonia, 1196, 1196*t*, 1197, 1199*t*
  in pregnancy, 831*t*, 834
  in prevention of meningococcal disease, 1181
  in rhinosinusitis, 1212*t*
  in sepsis, 1353*t*
  in spontaneous bacterial peritonitis, 397
  in syphilis, 1320, 1324
Ceftriaxone resistance, 1194*t*
Cefuroxime
  adverse effects of, 1208*t*
  in COPD, 299*t*
  dosage of, 1073*t*, 1199*t*, 1208*t*, 1212*t*
  in intra-abdominal infections, 1287*t*
  in otitis media, 1208*t*
  in pharyngitis, 1215*t*
  in pneumonia, 1195, 1196*t*, 1199*t*
  in rhinosinusitis, 1071*t*, 1212*a*, 1213*t*
  in surgical prophylaxis, 1400, 1400*t*
  in urinary tract infections, 1311*t*
Celecoxib
  adverse effects of, 574, 1004*f*, 1024
  allergic drug reactions, 932
  dosage of, 1002*t*
  in gout, 1014*t*
  in osteoarthritis, 1002*t*, 1004, 1005
  in prevention of colorectal cancer, 1520
  in prevention of NSAID-related ulcers, 337
Celiac disease
  anemia in, 1111
  osteoporosis in, 977
Celiac sprue, 376
  lymphoma and, 1553
Cellulitis
  case study of, 1226
  clinical presentation in, 1222, 1223–1224,
    1224*t*
  complications of, 1224
  diagnosis of, 1223–1224, 1224*t*
  epidemiology of, 1223
  etiology of, 1223

  in immunocompromised patients, 1224
  in intravenous drug users, 1226
  orbital, 1064*t*
  treatment of, 1224–1226
    antibiotics, 1224–1226, 1225*t*
    nonpharmacologic, 1224
Centers for Disease Control and Prevention, 13
Centers for Disease Control and Prevention
    (CDC) Growth Charts, 25*f*
Central α$_2$-agonists, in hypertension, 62*t*, 69
Central nervous system
  disorders of, drug-related, 1441*t*, 1442*t*
  elderly patients, 12
  infections of, 1169–1185. *See also* Meningitis
    risk factors for, 1170
Central nervous system irritability, with opioids,
    577*t*
Central nervous system prophylaxis
  in acute lymphocyte leukemia, 1587
  in acute myelogenous leukemia, 1593
Central pain, 570
Central pontine myelinolysis, 486
Central sensitization, 569
Central venous catheter
  in acute leukemia, 1595
  complications of, 1690, 1691, 1698
  in hematopoietic cell transplant recipients,
    1641
  in hypovolemic shock, 257
  infectious complications of, 1641, 1655, 1698
  for parenteral nutrition, 1690, 1691, 1698
Cephalalgia, 584
Cephalexin
  in cellulitis, 1225*t*
  in cystic fibrosis, 309*t*
  in diabetic foot infections, 1229*t*
  dosage of, 309*t*, 832*t*, 1215*t*, 1225*t*
  in erysipelas, 1225
  in furuncles/carbuncles, 1223*t*
  in infective endocarditis, 1250*t*
  in mastitis, 832*t*
  in pharyngitis, 1215*t*
  in pregnancy, 832*t*
  in prevention of endocarditis, 1250*t*
  in urinary tract infections, 1311*t*, 1313
Cephalosporin(s). *See also specific drugs*
  allergic drug reactions, 929*t*, 931, 1397
  anxiety with, 694*t*
  Clostridium difficile-associated diarrhea and,
    1274
  in cystic fibrosis, 309–310
  dosage of, 1333*t*
  drug interactions of, 205*t*
  in impetigo, 1222
  in intra-abdominal infections, 1286, 1287*t*,
    1288*t*
  in meningitis, 1181–1182
  in peritonitis, 474
  in pharyngitis, 1214
  in PID, 1333*t*
  seizures with, 522
  in sepsis, 1353*t*, 1354
  in shigellosis, 1268, 1270
  in spontaneous bacterial peritonitis, 397
  in typhoid fever, 1274
  in urinary tract infections, 1311*t*
Cephalosporin resistance, 1181
  in CSF isolates, 1181
Cephradine, in urinary tract infections, 1311*t*
Cerebral cortex, 43
Cerebral infarction, 216
  mania with, 676*t*
Cerebral ischemia, 224–225

Cerebral palsy, 1513*t*
Cerebrospinal fluid (CSF), 1170–1171
  in meningitis, 1170–1171, 1171*t*
  in multiple sclerosis, 411*t*
  normal, 1036*t*
Cerebrovascular disease. *See* Stroke
Cerivastatin, in dyslipidemia, 241
Certolizumab, 991
Certolizumab pegol, 988
Cervical cancer
  human papillomavirus and, 1327
  oral contraceptives and, 846
Cervical cap, 851
Cervicitis, 851
Cervix, assessing suitability for labor induction,
    825
Cesarean section, antimicrobial prophylaxis in,
    1400, 1400*t*
Cestodes, 1294, 1297
Cestodiasis, 1298–1299
Cetirizine
  in allergic rhinitis, 1051, 1053, 1054*t*
  dosage of, 830*t*
  in nausea and vomiting, 360
  in pregnancy, 830*t*, 833
  in respiratory disorders, 830*t*
Cetuximab, 1466
  adverse effects of, 1466, 1526, 1528*t*, 1531
  in cancer therapy, 1452*t*, 1466
  in colorectal cancer, 1526, 1527*t*, 1528*t*,
    1530–1531
  dosage of, 1526, 1531
  in lung cancer, 1508, 1511
  mechanism of action of, 1466, 1508,
    1528*t*, 1530
  pharmacokinetics of, 1466
Cevimeline
  dosage of, 1077*t*
  in dry eye, 1076, 1077*t*
CFTR (cystic fibrosis transmembrane regulator),
    304–305, 304*f*
Chagas' disease. *See* American trypanosomiasis
Chamomile, 206*t*
  German, in irritable bowel syndrome, 383
Chancre, syphilitic, 1321
Chancroid, 1333–1334
  clinical presentation in, 1333
  diagnosis of, 1333
  epidemiology of, 1333
  pathophysiology of, 1333
  patient care and monitoring in, 1334
  treatment of, 1333–1334
Charcoal, activated, in pruritus, 468
Cheilitis, angular, 1367
Chelation therapy, in iron overload, 1146
Chemical injury, ocular, 1065*t*, 1075*t*
Chemically defined formula. *See* Oligomeric
    formula
Chemical peels, in acne vulgaris, 1099
Chemoreceptor trigger zone (CTZ), 43, 358
Chemosis, in Graves' disease, 774, 775*f*
Chemotherapy. *See also specific drugs*
  in acute lymphocytic leukemia, 1586–1590,
    1588*t*, 1590*t*, 1591*t*–1592*t*
  in acute myelogenous leukemia, 1590–1593,
    1591*t*
  administration of, 1677
  adverse effects of, grading toxicity, 1511–1512
  in breast cancer, 1481–1487, 1484*t*–1485*t*
  case study of, 1461, 1472
  in chronic lymphocytic leukemia, 1602–1603,
    1603*t*
  in chronic myelogenous leukemia, 1592*t*

in colorectal cancer, 1523–1525, 1524t, 1527t, 1528t
combination, 1452, 1454
Common Terminology Criteria for Adverse Events, 1511
crossover design for, 1525
dose-dense therapy, 1561
dose density of, 1451, 1485
dose intensity of, 1485, 1512, 1655
dosing of, 1451–1452
  cycle, 1451
  in liver disease, 1471t
  in renal disease, 1470t
dry eye with, 1075t
emetogenic potential of, 1650t
extravasation injury with, 1676–1679
in Hodgkin's lymphoma, 1557–1558, 1557t, 1561t
intraperitoneal, 1570
intrathecal, 1561, 1587, 1591t
in lactation, 829t
in lung cancer, 1506–1508, 1507t, 1508t
menstruation-related disorders in, 857t
in multiple myeloma, 1605, 1606t
nausea and vomiting with, 296t, 364–365, 365t
  prevention of, 364
in non-Hodgkin's lymphoma, 1559–1562, 1560t–1561t
in ovarian cancer, 1569–1575, 1571a, 1572t, 1574t
patient care and monitoring in, 1472
payment for, 1451–1452
in prostate cancer, 1547, 1547t
resistance to, 1451
response to
  complete response, 1451, 1514
  cure, 1551
  disease progression, 1451
  overall objective response rate, 1451
  partial response, 1451, 1514
  stable disease, 1451, 1514
safety issues in drug handling, 1470–1472
secondary malignancies and, 1470, 1594
in superior vena cava syndrome, 1662
teratogenicity of, 829t
Chemotherapy-induced nausea and vomiting, 1650–1653
epidemiology of, 1650
etiology of, 1650
pathophysiology of, 1650–1651
clinical presentation in, 1651
diagnosis of, 1651
treatment of
  nonpharmacologic therapy, 1651
  pharmacologic therapy, 1652
outcome evaluation in, 1652–1653
patient care and monitoring in, 1653
Chest pain, 114. See also Angina pectoris
in GERD, 323
nonatherosclerotic conditions that cause, 111t
Chest physiotherapy, in cystic fibrosis, 307
Chest wall disorders
hyperprolactinemia in, 814t
respiratory acidosis with, 503t
Chest x-ray, in lung cancer, 1503, 1502t
Cheyne-Stokes respiration, 86
Chickenpox, 1413
Childhood absence epilepsy, 525t
Childhood epilepsy with occipital paroxysms, 525t
Child-Pugh classification, of cirrhosis, 394, 394t
Chiropractic, 579

Chlamydia, 1320–1321
clinical presentation in, 1321
co-infection with gonorrhea, 1319
diagnosis of, 1320
epidemiology of, 1320
pathophysiology of, 1320
in pregnancy, 825, 831t, 835, 1321
treatment of, 1320–1321
Chlamydia pneumoniae, in pneumonia, 1190, 1190t, 1192, 1194t, 1196t, 1197, 1354
Chlamydia trachomatis
in nongonococcal urethritis, 1320
in PID, 1332
Chloasma, with oral contraceptives, 848
Chloral hydrate, drug interactions of, 205t
Chlorambucil
adverse effects of, 1603t
in chronic lymphocytic leukemia, 1602, 1603t
dosage of, 1602, 1603t
Chloramphenicol
adverse effects of, 1175t, 1176t
in campylobacteriosis, 1272
in cystic fibrosis, 309t, 310
dosage of, 309t, 1175t, 1176t
drug interactions of, 205t
in meningitis, 1175t, 1176t
Chlordiazepoxide
in alcohol withdrawal, 618
dosage of, 618, 698t
drug interactions of, 614t, 699t
pharmacokinetics of, 698t
Chloride
in extracellular fluid, 484t
for parenteral nutrition, 1685t, 1686, 1696
serum, normal range for, 484t
sweat, 305
urinary, 504
Chloromethyl ether, 1500
Chloroquine
in amebiasis, 1295
arrhythmia with, 179t
dosage of, 1301t
in malaria, 1300
ocular changes with, 1077t
in prevention of malaria, 1301t
Chlorpheniramine
in allergic rhinitis, 1051, 1053
dosage of, 830t
in pregnancy, 830
in respiratory disorders, 830t
Chlorpromazine
adverse effects of, 361t, 642t
arrhythmia with, 177t, 179t
in bipolar disorder, 684
dosage of, 361t, 640t
drug interactions of, 647, 955t
in nausea and vomiting, 360, 361t
in schizophrenia, 640t
Chlorpromazine equivalent, 640
Chlorthalidone
adverse effects of, 60t
dosage of, 60t
in heart failure, 89
in hypertension, 60t, 64
ocular changes with, 1077t
ChlVPP regimen, in Hodgkin's lymphoma, 1557t
Cholangiocarcinoma, liver transplantation in, 941
Cholangitis, treatment of, 1288t
Cholecalciferol, 969
Cholecystitis
acute, treatment of, 1288t
with fibrates, 246

nausea and vomiting with, 358t
peritonitis in, 1283
Cholecystokinin, in anxiety disorders, 603
Cholelithiasis. See Gallstones
Cholera, 1272–1273
clinical presentation in, 1273
diagnosis of, 1273
epidemiology of, 1272–1273
monitoring patient with, 1273
pathogenesis of, 1273
treatment of, 1273
Cholera vaccine, 1274
Cholestasis, 1131t
with parenteral nutrition, 1696, 1687
treatment of, 1687
Cholesteatoma, 1205
Cholesterol
in Alzheimer's disease, 597
intestinal absorption of, 231, 231f
metabolism of, 230
reverse cholesterol transport, 232f
serum, 229–247
Cholesterol absorption inhibitors, in dyslipidemia, 243t, 244
Cholesterol ester transfer protein inhibitors, 192
Cholestyramine
adverse effects of, 241t, 244
dosage of, 241t
drug interactions of, 205t, 244, 771t, 955
in dyslipidemia, 241t, 243t, 244
in inflammatory bowel disease, 346
metabolic acidosis with, 501t
in pruritus, 468
removal of leflunomide from body, 990
Choline deficiency, 1696
Cholinergic agents. See also specific drugs
direct-acting, 1042
in glaucoma, 1038, 1042
indirect-acting, 1042
ocular changes with, 1077t
Cholinesterase inhibitors
in Alzheimer's disease, 598
in glaucoma, 1038t
Chondrocalcinosis, 998t
Chondroitin
dosage of, 1002t
in osteoarthritis, 1002t, 1005
in pain, 579
CHOP regimen
in Hodgkin's lymphoma, 1561t
in non-Hodgkin's lymphoma, 1559–1561, 1560t, 1561t
CHOP-14 regimen, in non-Hodgkin's lymphoma, 1561t
CHOP-21 regimen, in non-Hodgkin's lymphoma, 1560t
Chorea, in Parkinson's disease, 556
Chromium, for parenteral nutrition, 1687
Chromosome abnormalities. See Cytogenetic abnormalities
Chronic bronchitis. See Chronic obstructive pulmonary disease
Chronic inflammatory processes hypothesis, of ovarian cancer, 1567–1568
Chronic lymphocytic leukemia, 1601–1604
B cell differentiation and, 1554f
case study of, 1604
clinical course of, 1601
clinical presentation in, 1602
diagnosis of, 1602
epidemiology of, 1601
etiology of, 1601
outcome evaluation in, 1604

Chronic lymphocytic leukemia (*Cont.*)
    pathophysiology of, 1601
    patient care and monitoring in, 1608
    prognostic factors in, 1601
    treatment of, 1601–1603
        chemotherapy, 1602–1603, 1603*t*
        hematopoietic cell transplant, 1602, 1630, 1630*t*
        monoclonal antibodies, 1603, 1603*t*
        tumor lysis syndrome in, 1674*t*
Chronic myelogenous leukemia, 1447*t*, 1597–1601
    case study of, 1601
    clinical course of
        accelerated phase, 1597, 1598*t*
        blast crisis, 1597, 1598*t*
        chronic phase, 1597, 1598*t*
    clinical presentation in, 1598
    diagnosis of, 1598
    epidemiology of, 1598
    etiology of, 1598
    outcome evaluation in, 1601
    pathophysiology of, 1598
    patient care and monitoring in, 1608
    Philadelphia chromosome in, 1598
    treatment of, 1598–1601
        algorithm for, 1599*a*
        chemotherapy, 1591*t*
        cytarabine, 1601
        hematopoietic cell transplant, 1599, 1630, 1630*t*, 1634
        imatinib mesylate, 1581, 1599–1600, 1600*t*
        interferon alfa, 1601, 1600*t*
    treatment outcome in
        cytogenetic complete remission, 1598
        molecular complete remission, 1598
    tumor lysis syndrome in, 1674*t*
Chronic obstructive pulmonary disease (COPD), 289–300
    airflow obstruction in, 291
    anxiety with, 694*t*
    arrhythmia in, 166*t*
    asthma vs., 291–292
    ATS/ERS guidelines for, 294
    case study of, 292, 297
    clinical presentation in, 291
    cost of, 290
    diagnosis of, 291–292
    epidemiology of, 290
    etiology of, 290
    GOLD classification of, 294, 292*t*
    mortality from, 290
    outcome evaluation in, 300–301, 300*t*
    palliative care treatment for, 38
    pathophysiology of, 290–291, 290*a*
    patient care and monitoring in, 301
    respiratory acidosis with, 503*t*
    severity of, 291, 292*t*
    smoking and, 290, 296
    treatment of, 292–300
        N-acetylcysteine, 297
        algorithm for, 293*t*
        α_1-antitrypsin, 296–297
        antibiotics, 298–299
        anticholinergics, 294–296, 295*t*
        assisted ventilation, 300
        α_2-agonists, 294, 295*t*
        bronchodilators, 294–298, 295*t*
        bullectomy, 294
        COPD exacerbations, 297–298, 298*a*
        corticosteroids, 295*t*, 296, 298
        enteral nutrition, 1708*t*, 1709
        glucocorticoids, 295*t*
        leukotriene modifiers, 297

lung transplantation, 941
        nedocromil, 297
        nonpharmacologic, 292–294
        oxygen therapy, 299–294, 298
        pulmonary rehabilitation, 293
        smoking cessation, 292, 293*t*
        stable COPD, 294–297
        theophylline, 295*t*, 296
Chronic stable, 110
Chronotropic response, 82
Chvostek's sign, 489
Chylomicron(s), 230–231, 231*f*, 1702*f*
    physical characteristics of, 231*t*
Chylomicron remnants, 230, 231*f*
Chylothorax, with central venous catheter, 1691
Chyme, 1702
Ciclesonide
    in allergic rhinitis, 1052, 1052*t*
    in COPD, 295*t*
Ciclopirox, in tinea infections, 1371
Ciclopirox lacquer, in onychomycosis, 1371, 1372
Cidofovir
    adverse effects of, 442, 1330*t*
    dosage of, 1330*t*
    in genital herpes, 1330*t*, 1329
    ocular changes with, 1077*t*
Cierny-Mader staging, of osteomyelitis, 1338
Cigarette smoking. *See* Smoking
Cilastatin. *See* Imipenem-cilastatin
Cilostazol
    drug interactions of, 955*t*
    in peripheral vascular disease, 758
Cimetidine
    dosage of, 320*t*, 336*t*
    drug interactions of, 170*t*, 205*t*, 321, 537*t*, 577, 699*t*, 955*t*, 1726
    erectile dysfunction with, 885*t*
    in GERD, 320*t*, 321
    growth hormone deficiency with, 810
    migraines with, 588*t*
    in parenteral nutrition admixture, 1687
    in peptic ulcer disease, 336*t*
Cinacalcet, in hyperparathyroidism, 463
Ciprofloxacin
    administration through feeding tube, 1715
    adverse effects of, 1040*t*
    arrhythmia with, 179*t*
    in chancroid, 1334, 1334*t*
    in cholera, 1273
    in conjunctivitis, 1066, 1067*t*
    in COPD, 299*t*
    in cystic fibrosis, 309*t*
    in diarrhea, 380
    dosage of, 309*t*, 353*t*, 831*t*, 1040*t*, 1067*t*, 1156*t*, 1162, 1182*t*, 1199*t*, 1268*t*, 1269, 1269*t*, 1270, 1273, 1319, 1334, 1334*t*, 1660*t*
    drug interactions of, 205*t*, 537*t*, 561, 646
    in eradication of *Salmonella* carriage, 1273
    in gonorrhea, 831*t*, 1319
    in infections in cancer patients, 1660, 1660*t*
    in infective endocarditis, 1248
    in inflammatory bowel disease, 348, 351, 351*t*
    in intra-abdominal infections, 1286, 1287*t*, 1288*t*
    in meningitis, 1177*t*, 1181, 1183
    in osteomyelitis, 1339*t*, 1342*t*
    in pneumonia, 1196*t*, 1197, 1198, 1199
    in pregnancy, 831*t*
    in prevention of catheter-related infections, 475
    in prevention of meningococcal disease, 1181, 1183
    in prevention of spontaneous bacterial peritonitis, 397

prophylactic, in hematopoietic cell transplant recipients, 1641
    in sepsis, 1353*t*
    in shigellosis, 1268*t*
    in surgical prophylaxis, 1400, 1400*t*
    in travelers' diarrhea, 1274
    in tuberculosis, 1262
    in typhoid fever, 1269, 1270
    in urinary tract infections, 1311*t*, 1312*t*
Circadian rhythm, 710
    of gastric acid secretion, 330
Circadian rhythm disorders, 713, 718
Circulatory shock, 252
Circumstantiality, in schizophrenia, 633
Cirrhosis, 387–397. *See also* Ascites; Hepatic encephalopathy; Spontaneous bacterial peritonitis; Variceal bleeding
    biliary, 236*t*, 392
    case study of, 392–393, 395
    Child-Pugh classification of, 394, 394*t*
    clinical presentation in, 392
    coagulation defects in, 391, 399–400
    diagnosis of, 392–394
    epidemiology of, 387–388
    etiology of, 387–388, 413
    gender and, 388
    genetic factors in, 388, 392
    hyperprolactinemia in, 814*t*
    hyponatremia in, 484
    MELD classification of, 394, 394*t*
    menstruation-related disorders in, 857*t*
    outcome evaluation in, 400
    pathophysiology of, 388–392, 388*f*
    patient care and monitoring in, 400
    peritonitis and, 1283, 1286*t*, 1287*t*
    primary biliary, 392
    steroid hormones in, 389
    treatment of, 394–400
        enteral nutrition, 1710
        lifestyle modifications, 394–395
        liver transplantation, 941
    viral hepatitis and, 415
Cisapride
    adverse effects of, 322
    arrhythmia with, 180
    drug interactions of, 955*t*
    in GERD, 322
Cisplatin, 1462
    adverse effects of, 442, 1462, 1507*t*, 1512, 1572*t*
    arrhythmia with, 162*t*
    in breast cancer, 1493
    in cancer therapy, 1462
    dosage of, 1507*t*, 1508*t*, 1561*t*, 1572*t*, 1573*t*
        in renal dysfunction, 1470*t*
    drug interactions of, 1458
    emetogenicity of, 364*t*, 365
    extravasation of, 1677*t*, 1679
    hypokalemia with, 487
    hypomagnesemia with, 492
    hypophosphatemia with, 491
    in lung cancer, 1506, 1507*t*, 1508–1511, 1508*t*
    mechanism of action of, 1454*a*, 1462
    in melanoma, 1621
    nephrotoxicity of, 1381
    in non-Hodgkin's lymphoma, 1561*t*
    osteoporosis with, 967*t*
    in ovarian cancer, 1570, 1572*t*, 1573*t*
    pharmacokinetics of, 1462
Citalopram
    adverse effects of, 659*t*, 701*t*, 879*t*
    arrhythmia with, 162*t*
    in depression, 598, 665
    dosage of, 661*t*, 696*t*, 701*t*, 879*t*

in generalized anxiety disorder, 696*t*
in panic disorder, 701*t*
pharmacokinetics of, 659, 659*t*
in pregnancy, 665
in social anxiety disorder, 703
in vasomotor symptoms of menopause, 878, 879*t*
Citrate/citric acid
in metabolic acidosis, 463
metabolic alkalosis with, 504
Citrobacter, in infective endocarditis, 1242
Cladribine, 1456
adverse effects of, 1456
in cancer therapy, 1456
dosage in renal dysfunction, 1470*t*
mechanism of action of, 1454*a*, 1456
pharmacokinetics of, 1456
Clarithromycin
adverse effects of, 335, 1208*t*
arrhythmia with, 179*t*
in COPD, 299*t*
in cryptosporidiosis, 1276
dosage of, 335*t*, 1199*t*, 1208*t*, 1212*t*
drug interactions of, 241, 537*t*, 684, 816, 955*t*
in *Helicobacter pylori* eradication, 334, 335*t*,
335, 1561
in infective endocarditis, 1250*t*
in keratitis, 1071*t*
in otitis media, 1208*t*
in pneumonia, 1195, 1196*t*, 1197, 1199*t*
in prevention of endocarditis, 1102*t*
in rhinosinusitis, 1212*t*
Clarithromycin resistance, 335
Clark's nevus, 1613
Class switching, 1553
Clavulanate. *See* Ticarcillin-clavulanate
Clemastine
in allergic rhinitis, 1051
in lactation, 829*t*
Clenched-fist injury, 1232
Clidinium bromide
dosage of, 384*t*
in irritable bowel syndrome, 384*t*
Climacteric. *See* Perimenopause
Clindamycin
in acne vulgaris, 1097–1098, 1098*t*
adverse effects of, 836, 1097–1098, 1098*t*, 1183*t*,
1208*t*
in bacterial vaginosis, 731*t*, 834, 836, 1332
in bite wound infections, 1232
in cellulitis, 1225, 1225*t*
Clostridium difficile-associated diarrhea and, 1274
in cystic fibrosis, 308, 309*t*
in diabetic foot infections, 1229*t*
dosage of, 309*t*, 731*t*, 732*t*, 831*t*, 832*t*, 1098*t*,
1208*t*, 1212*t*, 1215*t*, 1225*t*, 1232*t*, 1300,
1332, 1333*t*, 1342*t*
drug interactions of, 1183*t*
in erysipelas, 1224
in infected pressure sores, 1232*t*
in infections in cancer patients, 1661
in infections in sickle cell anemia/disease, 1147
in infective endocarditis, 1241, 1250*t*
in intra-abdominal infections, 1286, 1287*t*,
1288*t*
in lactation, 834
in malaria, 1300
in necrotizing fasciitis, 1227
in osteomyelitis, 1179*t*, 1342, 1343*t*
in otitis media, 1208*t*
in pharyngitis, 1215*t*, 1216
in PID, 1333*t*
in pneumonia, 1197
in pregnancy, 831*t*, 832*t*

in prevention of endocarditis, 1250*t*
in rhinosinusitis, 1213*t*, 1212*t*
in sepsis, 1354
in *Streptococcus* group B infection, 832*t*
in surgical prophylaxis, 1397, 1400, 1400*t*
Clindamycin-gentamicin
dosage of, 831*t*
in PID, 831*t*
in pregnancy, 831*t*
Clindamycin resistance, 1204, 1224
Clinical breast exam, 1479*t*
Clinical cure, 1367
Clinical Institute Withdrawal Assessment of
Alcohol-Revised, 616, 617*t*
Clinical Opiate Withdrawal Scale (COWS), 619, 620*t*
Clinical Pulmonary Infection Score (CPIS), 1200
Clobazam, in epilepsy, 529*t*
Clobetasol
in contact dermatitis, 1103*t*
dosage and potency of, 1103*t*
in psoriasis, 1084
Clofarabine
adverse effects of, 1456
in cancer therapy, 1456
dosage of, 1456
pharmacokinetics of, 1456
Clofibrate, drug interactions of, 205*t*
Clomiphene
adverse effects of, 859*t*
in anovulatory bleeding, 860
dosage of, 859*t*
in menstruation-related disorders, 859*t*
Clomipramine
adverse effects of, 701*t*
in cataplexy, 716
dosage of, 661*t*, 701*t*
in panic disorder, 701*t*
Clonazepam
adverse effects of, 431*t*, 717*t*
in bipolar disorder, 677*t*, 684
dosage of, 431*t*, 677*t*, 698*t*, 717*t*, 718
drug interactions of, 699*t*, 955*t*
in epilepsy, 429*t*, 431*t*
mechanism of action of, 431*t*
in panic disorder, 702
in parasomnias, 718
in Parkinson's disease, 563
pharmacokinetics of, 431*t*, 698*t*
in restless-legs syndrome, 717, 717*t*
in seizure prophylaxis, 1636
in social anxiety disorder, 704
Clonidine
in ADHD, 728*t*, 729*t*, 730*t*, 731
adverse effects of, 62*t*, 620, 729*t*, 879*t*
arrhythmia with, 162*t*
constipation with, 372*t*
dosage of, 62*t*, 622*t*, 728*t*, 879*t*
drug interactions of, 614*t*, 660*t*
erectile dysfunction with, 885*t*
in hypertension, 62*t*, 69
mechanism of action of, 731
in opioid withdrawal, 621, 622*t*
in pain, 578
in pregnancy, 72*t*
in smoking cessation, 622, 622*t*
in vasomotor symptoms of menopause, 878, 879*t*
Clopidogrel
in acute coronary syndromes, 135, 140*t*, 145,
149–50, 152*t*
adverse effects of, 145, 149, 152*t*, 222
contraindications to, 140*t*
dosage of, 140*t*, 145
drug interactions of, 205*t*

in ischemic heart disease, 119–120
in prevention of myocardial infarction, 150
in prevention of stroke, 224, 225*t*, 226*t*
Clorazepate
dosage of, 698*t*
drug interactions of, 699*t*
pharmacokinetics of, 698*t*
Clostridium
in intra-abdominal infections, 1133*t*
in myonecrosis, 1227
normal flora, 1021*f*
Clostridium botulinum, 28
in food poisoning, 1278, 1278*t*
Clostridium difficile-associated diarrhea, 376,
1274–1276
case study of, 1275
clinical presentation in, 1275
diagnosis of, 1275
epidemiology of, 1274
monitoring patient with, 1275
pathogenesis of, 1274
treatment of, 1274–1275
Clostridium difficile colitis, 1199, 1711
Clostridium difficile infections, in surgical site
infections, 1398
Clostridium perfringens
in food poisoning, 1278, 1278*t*
in myonecrosis, 1227
Clostridium tetani, 1406
Clot formation, in acute coronary syndromes, 133
Clotrimazole
in diaper dermatitis, 1106
dosage of, 831*t*, 832*t*, 833*t*, 1363*t*, 1364*t*
drug interactions of, 955, 955*t*, 1643
in fungal infections, 955*t*
in oropharyngeal candidiasis, 1368, 1385
in pregnancy, 831*t*
in prevention of *Pneumocystis jiroveci*
pneumonia, 1643
in prevention of thrush, 957
in tinea infections, 1371
in vulvovaginal candidiasis, 831*t*, 1363*t*, 1364*t*,
1365
Clotrimazole troche, in oropharyngeal
candidiasis, 1368, 1385
Clotting cascade. *See* Coagulation cascade
Cloves, 206*t*
Clozapine
adverse effects of, 638*t*, 645, 646, 647*t*
blood glucose level and, 737*t*
dosage of, 637*t*, 645
drug interactions of, 614*t*, 646*t*, 647, 660*t*, 684
enuresis with, 920
mechanism of action of, 637*f*
metabolism of, 646*t*
in Parkinson's disease, 563
in schizophrenia, 636–637, 637*f*, 637*t*, 638*t*,
645, 646, 647*t*
Clubbing
in cystic fibrosis, 305
in Graves' disease, 774, 775*f*
in infective endocarditis, 1238
Clue cells, 825
Cluster headache
clinical presentation in, 586, 587
diagnosis of, 587
epidemiology, 584
etiology of, 585–586
outcome evaluation in, 592
pathophysiology of, 585–586
patient care and monitoring in, 592
prevention of, 591
treatment of, 589–590

CMF regimen, in breast cancer, 1485*t*
Coagulase-negative staphylococci
  in infective endocarditis, 1236*t*
Coagulation cascade, 187, 191*f*, 217, 1121, 1122*f*
  extrinsic pathway, 1121, 1222*f*
  intrinsic pathway, 1121, 1222*f*
Coagulation disorders, 1122
  acquired, 1130–1133
  in cirrhosis, 391, 399
  inherited, 1122–1126
  patient care and monitoring in, 1137
  recessively inherited. *See* Recessively inherited
    coagulation disorders
Coagulation factors, 201, 202*f*
  vitamin K-dependent, 201
Coalescence, of intravenous lipid emulsions,
  1683–1684
Coal tar products
  adverse effects of, 1084
  in psoriasis, 1084–1085
Coarctation of aorta, 53
Cocaine
  abuse of, 608
    case study of, 618
    pathophysiology of, 608–609
    signs and symptoms of intoxication, 611*t*
  anxiety with, 694*t*
  arrhythmia with, 162*t*
  drug interactions of, 614*t*, 955*t*
  erectile dysfunction with, 885*t*
  hyperprolactinemia with, 814*t*
  mania with, 676*t*
  seizures with, 522
  stroke and, 217*t*
  withdrawal syndrome, 616, 619–620
Coccidioidomycosis
  clinical presentation in, 1377–1378
  diagnosis of, 1377–1378
  epidemiology of, 1376
  geographic localization of, 1376*f*
  pathophysiology of, 1376–1377, 1377*f*
  patient monitoring in, 1381–1382
  prophylaxis for, 1381
  symptoms and signs, 1378
  treatment of, 1378–1381, 1380*t*
Cockcroft–Gault equation, 11, 362, 434*t*
Cockroach allergens, 269, 1048, 1051*t*
Cocoon immunization, 1406
Codeine
  adverse effects of, 717*t*
  dosage of, 575*t*, 717*t*, 830*t*
  drug interactions of, 660*t*
  mechanism of action of, 576
  metabolism of, 575
  in osteoarthritis, 1006
  in pain, 572*t*, 575*t*, 830*t*
    in sickle cell anemia/disease, 1151
  in pregnancy, 830*t*
  pseudoallergic drug reactions, 933
  in restless-legs syndrome, 717, 717*t*
Cognitive-behavioral therapy
  in depression, 656
  in headache prevention, 587
  in pain, 569, 573
  in panic disorder, 700
  in schizophrenia, 635
  in social anxiety disorder, 703
  in substance dependence, 524
Cognitive function, hormone-replacement
  therapy and, 878
Cognitive impairment
  in Alzheimer's disease, 598, 599–600, 599*t*
  in Parkinson's disease, 558

  in schizophrenia, 631
  urinary incontinence in, 912
Cognitive remediation, in schizophrenia, 635
Cognitive restructuring, in panic disorder, 700
Cognitive therapy, in sleep disorders, 714*t*
Cogwheel rigidity, 555
Coitus, 888
Colchicine
  adverse effects of, 1013
  diarrhea with, 376, 376*t*
  dosage of, 1014*t*
  in gout, 1013, 1014*t*
  intravenous, 1013
  oral, 1013
Colcrys
  dosage of, 1014*t*
  in gout, 1014, 1014*t*
Cold therapy/cold packs
  in chemotherapy extravasations, 1678
  in musculoskeletal disorders, 1002–1003, 1003*t*
  in osteoarthritis, 1000
  in pain, 574
Colectomy, in ulcerative colitis, 350
Colesevelam
  adverse effects of, 241*t*, 244
  dosage of, 241*t*
  drug interactions of, 244
  in dyslipidemia, 241*t*, 243*t*, 244
Colestipol
  adverse effects of, 241*t*, 244
  dosage of, 241*t*
  drug interactions of, 244, 771*t*
  in dyslipidemia, 241*t*, 243*t*, 244
Colistin
  in cystic fibrosis, 308, 309*t*, 310
  dosage of, 309*t*
  in meningitis, 1183
Colitis
  Clostridium difficile, 1199, 1711
  hemorrhagic, 1272
  mucous, 380
Collagen, type I, 969
Collagen vascular disease, 1131*t*
Collateral damage, in antimicrobial therapy, 1162
Colloid(s), 483
  adverse effects of, 259
  colloid vs. crystalloid debate, 259
  in hypovolemic shock, 257–259, 258*t*
  mechanism of action of, 257–259, 258*f*
  in pancreatitis, 405
  in resuscitation of septic patient, 1352
Colloid osmotic pressure, intravascular, 258, 258*f*
Colon
  anatomy of, 1521*f*
  obstruction of, nausea and vomiting with, 358*t*
  polyps of, 1519, 1520
  pseudopolyps of, 342
Colon cancer. *See* Colorectal cancer
Colonization, 1157
Colonoscopy
  in diarrhea, 378
  in inflammatory bowel disease, 344
  in irritable bowel syndrome, 381
  screening for colorectal cancer, 1519–1520
Colony-forming unit, 1237
Colony-stimulating factors
  adverse effects of, 1657, 1657*t*
  cost of, 1657
  in neutropenia, 1595
  prophylactic, in neutropenic cancer patients,
    165, 1657*t*
Colorectal cancer, 1517–1532
  adenocarcinoma, 1521

  alcohol use and, 1518*t*, 1519
  anatomy and bowel function, 1520–1521, 1521*f*
  case study of, 1519, 1522, 1527, 1530
  clinical presentation in, 1522
  diabetes mellitus and, 1519
  diagnosis of, 1522
  diet and, 1518, 1518*t*
  environmental factors in, 1518
  epidemiology of, 1446*f*, 1518
  etiology of, 1518
  genetic factors in, 1447*t*, 1518, 1519
  hereditary nonpolyposis, 1447*t*, 1518*t*, 1519
  inflammatory bowel disease and, 342, 1518*t*,
    1519
  metastasis of, 1525–1527
    to brain, 1665*t*
  nonpolyposis, 1567
  obesity and, 1519
  outcome evaluation in, 1531–1532
  pathophysiology of, 1520–1521
  patient care and monitoring in, 1532
  performance status in, 1527
  prevention of, 1520
    hormone-replacement therapy, 876
  risk factors for, 1518–1519, 1518*t*
  screening for, 1519–1520
  smoking and, 1518*t*, 1519
  staging of, 1450*t*, 1521–1522, 1523*f*
  treatment of, 1521–1531
    adjuvant chemotherapy, 1527
    chemotherapy, 1524*t*, 1525–1526, 1527,
      1527*t*, 1528*t*
    radiation therapy, 1531
    surgery, 1523, 1531
  tumorigenesis in, 1521
Colorectal surgery, antimicrobial prophylaxis in,
  1401–1402
Comedo
  closed, 1094, 1094*f*, 1096
  open, 1094, 1095*f*, 1096
Comedolytic effect, 1096
Commensalism, 1294
Common cold, 1216–1219
  clinical presentation in, 1217
  diagnosis of, 1217
  epidemiology of, 1216–1217
  etiology of, 1216–1217
  outcome evaluation in, 1219
  pathophysiology of, 1217
  patient care and monitoring in, 1219
  in pregnancy, 821, 833
  prevention of, 1219
  treatment of, 1217–1219
    nonpharmacologic therapy, 1217
    pharmacologic therapy, 1217–1219
Common Terminology Criteria for Adverse
  Events, 1511
Complementary and alternative medicines
  (CAMs), 29–30
  in allergic rhinitis, 1057
  in pain management, 579
Complex regional pain syndrome, 570
Compliance, 4
  in ADHD, 731
  with antipsychotic regimens, 634
  with hypertension medications, 68
Compliance-enhancing strategies, 4
Compression, in musculoskeletal disorders,
  1002–1003, 1003*t*
Compression stockings
  graduated, in prevention of venous
    thromboembolism, 191
  in venous thromboembolism, 207

Computed tomography
in Alzheimer's disease, 603
in invasive aspergillosis, 1390
in lung cancer, 1502*t*
in pancreatitis, 405
in pulmonary embolism, 192
in stroke, 225
in venous thromboembolism, 190
Computer physician order entry (CPOE) systems, 29
COMT inhibitors
adverse effects of, 562
in Parkinson's disease, 557, 562, 563*t*
ComVax, 1414
Conception, 822
Concreteness, in schizophrenia, 633
Condom, 852, 1334
efficacy of, 844*t*
Conduction system, cardiac, 158–159, 158*f*
Condyloma acuminata, 1327
Congenital rubella syndrome, 1410–1411
Congestive heart failure. *See* Heart failure *entries*
Conidia, 1376
Conjugated equine estrogens, 874, 875*t*
Conjugated estrogens, 875*t*
Conjugation, 11
Conjunctival injection, in Graves' disease, 774, 775*f*
Conjunctivitis, 1065–1068
allergic. *See* Allergic conjunctivitis
allergic drug reaction, 932
bacterial, 1065
etiology of, 1065, 1065*a*
outcome evaluation in, 1066
treatment of, 1066, 1066*t*
case study of, 1067
diagnosis of, 1065*a*
gonococcal, 1320
viral, 1065*a*, 1066
etiology of, 1066–1067
outcome evaluation in, 1067–1068
prevention of, 1067
treatment of, 1067
Conjunctivitis medicamentosa, 1068
Connective tissue disease, keratitis with, 1070*t*
Consolidation, 1587
Constipation, 371–376
case study of, 376
chronic, 372
clinical presentation in, 372
definition of, 372
diagnosis of, 372–373
drug-related, 372*t*
in elderly, 372
enuresis with, 921*t*
epidemiology of, 372
etiology of, 372, 372*t*
in multiple sclerosis, 516
normal-transit, 372
with opioids, 577*t*, 577
with oral contraceptives, 848
outcome evaluation in, 375–376
palliative care, symptom in, 47
pathophysiology of, 372
patient care and monitoring in, 376
in pregnancy, 372, 375, 825, 829, 830*t*
slow-transit, 372, 375
treatment of, 373–375, 374*t*, 577*t*
bulk-forming laxatives, 373, 374*t*
emollients, 374, 374*t*
laxatives, 373–374, 374*t*
lifestyle modifications, 373
lubiprostone, 374–375
lubricants, 373–374, 374*t*
nonpharmacologic, 373

osmotic laxatives, 373, 374*t*
stimulant laxatives, 374*t*, 374
tegaserod maleate, 374
in tube feeding, 1711–1712, 1711*t*
urinary incontinence in, 912
Consumer Healthcare Products Association, 30
Consumption. *See* Tuberculosis
Contact dermatitis, 1100–1104
agents causing, 1101
allergic, 1100–1101, 1101*f*, 1101*t*
case study of, 1102
clinical presentation in, 1100*a*, 1101*f*, 1102
epidemiology of, 1100–1101
irritant, 1100, 1101*f*, 1101*t*
outcome evaluation of, 1102
pathophysiology of, 1101
patient care and monitoring in, 1105
treatment of, 1101–1102
antihistamines, 1102
astringents, 1102
corticosteroids, 1102, 1103*t*–1104*t*
nonpharmacologic, 1102
Contact lens
bacterial keratitis with, 1070–1071
dry eye and, 1075*t*
Contiguous spread, of pathogens into CNS, 1172
Continuous ambulatory peritoneal dialysis
(CAPD), 473
peritonitis and, 1283, 1288
protein requirement in, 1689*t*
Continuous cycling peritoneal dialysis, 473
Continuous positive airway pressure, in
obstructive sleep apnea, 71–718
Continuous renal replacement therapy
in acute kidney injury, 439
protein requirement in, 1689*t*
Continuous subcutaneous insulin infusion. *See*
Insulin pump
Contraception, 841–853
barrier techniques, 851
case study of, 847, 849, 852
efficacy of contraceptives, 844*t*
emergency, 853
fertility awareness and periodic abstinence, 852
intrauterine devise, 842
nonoral hormonal contraceptives, 850–851
injectable, 850–851
transdermal patch, 850
transvaginal ring, 850
oral. *See* Oral contraceptives
outcome evaluation in, 853
patient care and monitoring in, 853
Contraceptive patch, efficacy of, 844*t*
Contraction alkalosis, 503*t*
Contrast medium
adverse effects of, 190
allergic drug reactions, 930*t*, 933
hypothyroidism with, 767, 767*t*
nephrotoxicity of, 362
Controlled-release preparation, administration
through feeding tubes, 1714
Convection, in hemodialysis, 470
Conventional paclitaxel, in breast cancer, 1491–
1492
Convulsion. *See* Seizure
COPD. *See* Chronic obstructive pulmonary disease
Coping skills, in substance dependence, 524
Copper, for parenteral nutrition, 1687
Copulation, in *Strongyloides stercoralis*, 1298
Core needle biopsy in lung cancer, 1502*t*
Cornea
epithelial abnormalities of, 1070*t*
thickness of, 1032, 1032*t*, 1034

Corneal abrasion, 1063
clinical presentation in, 1064
diagnosis of, 1064
outcome evaluation in, 1063–1064
prevention of, 1063
treatment of, 1063, 1063*t*
antibiotics, 1064
NSAID, 1064
Corneal abscess, 1070
Corneal arcus, 232, 235
Corneal edema, drug-induced, 1077*t*
Corneal perforation, 1070
Corneal ulcer, 1064*t*, 1070
Cornstarch, topical, in diaper dermatitis, 1106
Coronary angiography, in ischemic heart
disease, 116
Coronary artery
anatomy of, 111, 111*f*
vasospasm in, 114
Coronary artery bypass graft surgery
in acute coronary syndromes, 138
in ischemic heart disease, 117, 118
Coronary artery disease. *See* Acute coronary
syndromes; Ischemic heart disease
Coronavirus
in CNS infections, 1183
in pharyngitis, 1214
Cor pulmonale, in COPD, 291
Corpus luteum, 856, 864
Corticosteroids. *See also specific drugs*
in acne vulgaris, 1099
in acute chest syndrome, 1148
administration of, 408
adverse effects of, 273, 296, 308, 347–348, 364,
408, 952, 953*t*, 1051, 1052, 1084, 1102,
1363*t*, 1366, 1694
in allergic rhinitis, 1051*t*, 1051–1054, 1058*t*
antenatal, 830*t*, 835
anxiety with, 694*t*
in asthma, 267, 269, 271*t*, 273–276,
274*t*, 276*t*
in brain metastasis, 1622, 1666
in chemotherapy-induced nausea and
vomiting, 1652
in COPD, 295*t*, 296, 298
in cystic fibrosis, 308
depression with, 655
in diaper dermatitis, 1106
discontinuation (tapering) of, 1015
dosage of, 408, 1673*t*
drug interactions of, 850*t*, 953
in elderly, 352
glaucoma with, 1043
in GVHD, 1640
in headache, 592
in hypercalcemia, 1673, 1673*t*
dyslipidemia with, 236*t*
hypertension with, 957–958
hypocalcemia with, 489
hypokalemia with, 487
hypophosphatemia with, 491
in immune thrombocytopenic purpura, 1132,
1134*t*
in inflammatory bowel disease, 347–352, 347*t*,
349*t*
inhaled, 273, 276*t*, 277*t*, 296
adverse effects of, 273
intraarticular
in gout, 1014, 1014*t*
in osteoarthritis, 1006
intramuscular, in gout, 1014
intranasal, 1052*t*
in allergic rhinitis, 1051*t*, 1051–1052, 1053

Corticosteroids, intranasal (*Cont.*)
  medication administration, 1052, 1053*t*
  in rhinosinusitis, 1211
 mania with, 676*t*
 mechanism of action of, 1640
 in melanoma with brain metastasis, 1622
 metabolic alkalosis with, 503*t*, 504
 in multiple myeloma, 1606*t*
 in multiple sclerosis, 508–510
 in nausea and vomiting, 362*t*, 363, 364, 1512
 in non-Hodgkin's lymphoma, 1561
 ocular changes with, 1077*t*
 parenteral nutrition and, 1694
 in pregnancy, 352
 in prostate cancer, 1547
 in psoriasis, 1084, 1087
 in spinal cord compression, 1664
 in superior vena cava syndrome, 1662
 in thrombotic thrombocytopenic purpura, 1135
 topical
  in allergic conjunctivitis, 1068, 1068*t*
  in contact dermatitis, 1102, 1103*t*–1104*t*
  in dry eye, 1076
  in keratitis, 1071
  potency ratings of, 1103*t*–1104*t*
 in transplant recipient, 952, 953*t*
Corticotropin. *See* Adrenocorticotropic
  hormone
Corticotropin-releasing factor, in substance-
  abuse disorders, 610
Corticotropin-releasing hormone, 786
 in anxiety disorders, 693
 ectopic CRH syndrome, 792*t*
Cortisol
 in anxiety disorders, 693
 drug interactions of, 955*t*
 functions of, 786
 in hypovolemic shock, 254, 254*a*
 late-night salivary, 795*t*
 production of, 786
 24-hour urinary free, 795*t*
 unstimulated serum cortisol measurement,
  788*t*
Cortisol-binding globulin, 786
Cortisone, 786
 in adrenal insufficiency, 789*t*
Corynebacterium diphtheriae, in pharyngitis,
  1214
Costimulation blockers, in rheumatoid
  arthritis, 991
Cosyntropin stimulation test, 788*t*
Cotswald staging system, for Hodgkin's
  lymphoma, 1553*t*, 1556
Cough
 with ACE inhibitors, 68, 92–93, 150
 pregnancy, 833
Counteradaptation, in substance
  dependence, 610
Counterirritants, 569
 in musculoskeletal disorders, 1026, 1026*t*
 in osteoarthritis, 1006
 patient education for, 1025–1026, 1026*t*
 salicylate-containing, 1026
Couplet, 176
COX-1 inhibitors
 allergic drug reactions, 932
 in pain, 574
 peptic ulcer disease with, 330–331
COX-2 inhibitors
 adverse effects of, 84*t*, 86*t*, 126, 1003–1004,
  1003*a*, 1024
 cardiovascular safety of, 336–337, 574,
  1003–1004, 1003*a*

 drug interactions of, 1005
 in gout, 1013
 in ischemic heart disease, 126
 in migraine, 588
 in musculoskeletal disorders, 1024
 nephrotoxicity of, 442
 in osteoarthritis, 1002*t*, 1003–1005
 in pain, 574
 peptic ulcer disease with, 330
 in prevention of colorectal cancer, 1520
 in prevention of NSAID-induced ulcers,
  330–331
 in rheumatoid arthritis, 989
Coxiella burnetii, in infective endocarditis,
  1242
C-peptide, in diabetes mellitus, 736
Crab lice, 1304
Cranial irradiation, prophylactic, in lung cancer,
  1509
Craniospinal irradiation, in acute lymphocytic
  leukemia, 1587, 1595
Craniotomy, 1131*t*
C-reactive protein, 120, 240, 1713
 in infections, 1158
 in osteomyelitis, 1341
 in rheumatoid arthritis, 983
Creaming, of intravenous lipid emulsions, 1683
Creatinine, serum, 68
 in acute kidney injury, 431
 in chronic kidney disease, 448
 in end-stage renal disease, 472
Creatinine clearance
 in geriatric patients, 11
 in pediatric patients, 27
Creatinine clearance
 estimation of, 433–434, 434*t*
 indications for dialysis, 472
Creatinine kinase, CK-MB in acute coronary
  syndromes, 114, 133, 134
Cremophor EL, 1458
Creon products, 311*t*, 409*t*
Cretinism, 669
Crohn's disease. *See also* Inflammatory bowel
  disease
 clinical presentation in, 342
 colorectal cancer and, 1518*t*, 1519
 diagnosis of, 345
 epidemiology of, 342
 etiology of, 342
 mild to moderate, 345, 349–350, 351*t*
 moderate to severe, 345, 351*t*, 351
 outcome evaluation in, 354
 pathophysiology of, 342–343, 343*f*
 patient care and monitoring in, 354
 severe to fulminant, 345, 351–352
 skip lesions in, 342
 treatment of, 350–352, 351*t*
  maintenance of remission, 350
Cromolyn
 adverse effects of, 1068*t*
 in allergic conjunctivitis, 1068*t*
 in allergic rhinitis, 1051*t*, 1055–1056, 1059
 in asthma, 266, 273, 275*t*, 278, 281, 283
 dosage of, 275*t*, 1069*t*
 mechanism of action of, 1055, 1056, 1068*t*
Cromone in allergic rhinitis, 1051*t*, 1055–1056
Cross-allergenicity, allergic drug reactions, 930
Crossover design, of chemotherapy program,
  1525
Crotamiton, in scabies, 1304
Crush injury, 1131*t*, 1233
Cryoprecipitate
 in DIC, 1129

 in recessively inherited coagulation disorders,
  1130*t*
 in uremic bleeding, 468
Cryotherapy
 adverse effects of, 1168*t*
 in genital warts, 1327*t*, 1328
 in nonmelanoma skin cancer, 1625
Crypt abscess, 342
Cryptococcosis, 1386*t*, 1387–1389
 clinical presentation in, 1387–1388
 epidemiology of, 1387
 in invasive candidiasis, 1385
 laboratory diagnosis of, 1388
 pathogenesis of, 1387–1388
 prophylaxis for, 1389
 treatment of, 1389
Cryptococcus, 1387–1389
 in meningitis, 1170
 in sepsis, 1348
Cryptosporidiosis, 1276–1277
 clinical presentation in, 376, 1276
 diagnosis of, 1276
 epidemiology of, 1276
 HIV infection and, 1276
 monitoring patient with, 1276–1277
 pathogenesis of, 1276
 prevention of, 1277
 treatment of, 1276–1277
Crystalline penicillin, in syphilis, 1324
Crystalloids, 481–483
 adverse effects of, 257
 colloid vs. crystalloid debate, 258
 electrolyte and dextrose content of, 482*t*
 in hypovolemic shock, 257–259, 258*t*
 in pancreatitis, 405
 in resuscitation of septic patient, 1352
 tonicity of, 481
Crystalluria, drug-related, 1439*t*
CSF. *See* Cerebrospinal fluid
C-Telopeptides, 969
Culture, bacterial, 1159
Cunninghamella, 1376*t*
 cupping of, 1034
 in glaucoma, 1032, 1034, 1034*f*
 in multiple sclerosis, 508, 510*t*
Cupric oxide, in macular degeneration, 1073
Cushing's disease, 792
 anxiety in, 694*t*
 psychotic symptoms in, 635*t*
Cushing's syndrome, 786*t*, 791
 ACTH-dependent, 792, 793*t*
 ACTH-independent, 792, 793*t*
 case study of, 798
 clinical presentation in, 794
 with corticosteroids, 953*t*
 diagnosis of, 794
 drug-induced, 792, 792*t*, 793
  prevention of, 798*t*
 epidemiology of, 791–792
 etiology of, 791–792, 793*t*
 hypertension and, 53
 mania with, 676*t*
 metabolic alkalosis in, 503*t*
 osteoporosis and, 967*t*
 outcome evaluation in, 798
 pathophysiology of, 792, 792*t*
 patient care and monitoring in, 799
 treatment of, 792, 796*t*–797*t*
  adrenolytic agents, 797*tt*
  neuromodulators of ACTH release, 795
  steroidogenesis inhibitors, 795, 796*t*
  surgery, 793–794
CVD regimen, in melanoma, 1621

CVP regimen, in non-Hodgkin's lymphoma, 1559, 1560t
CXCR4 receptors, 1420
Cyanocobalamin. *See* Vitamin B$_{12}$
Cyanosis
  in asthma, 268
  in COPD, 291
  in cystic fibrosis, 306
Cyclic citrullinated peptide, 983
Cyclizine
  adverse effects of, 361t
  dosage of, 361t
  in nausea and vomiting, 361t
Cyclobenzaprine, in musculoskeletal disorders, 1027
Cyclobutane pyrimidine dimer, 1612, 1613
Cyclooxygenase, 1021f
  COX-1, 1003, 1003a
  COX-2, 1003, 1003a
  in colorectal cancer cells, 1521
Cyclooxygenase-2 (COX-2) inhibitors, in hemophilia, 1126
Cyclooxygenase inhibitors. *See* COX-1 inhibitors; COX-2 inhibitors
Cyclopentolate, in ocular trauma, 1065
Cyclophosphamide, 1461
  in acute lymphocytic leukemia, 1588t, 1590t
  adverse effects of, 86t, 1461, 1484t, 1561t, 1574t, 1581, 1644
  in breast cancer, 1482, 1485, 1484t, 1491
  in cancer therapy, 1461
  in chronic lymphocytic leukemia, 1604
  dosage of, 1484t, 1507t, 1508t, 1557t, 1560t, 1561t, 1574t, 1588t, 1590t, 1634t
  drug interactions of, 955t, 1381, 1591t, 1643
  emetogenicity of, 365t
  extravasation of, 1677t
  hemorrhagic cystitis with, 1636, 1666
  in Hodgkin's lymphoma, 1558, 1557t, 1561t
  in immune thrombocytopenic purpura, 1134
  in lung cancer, 1507t, 1508t, 1510
  mechanism of action of, 1461
  in non-Hodgkin's lymphoma, 1559, 1560t, 1561
  in ovarian cancer, 1573, 1574t
  pharmacokinetics of, 1461
  in preparation for hematopoietic cell transplant, 1634t, 1634, 1636
  urinary incontinence with, 918t
Cycloserine, 954
  adverse effects of, 1261t
  dosage of, 1261t
  in tuberculosis, 1259, 1261t
Cyclosporine
  adverse effects of, 348, 945t, 948, 1087, 1638, 1695
  comparative efficacy of calcineurin inhibitors, 948
  dosage of, 347t, 349t, 351t, 945t, 948, 1086–1087, 1638
    adaptive dosing, 1638
  drug interactions of, 169t, 241, 614t, 953, 1364, 1381, 1591t, 1600t, 1638, 1726
  dyslipidemia with, 236t
  gout with, 1012
  hyperkalemia with, 488
  hypertension with, 958
  hypomagnesemia with, 492
  in immune thrombocytopenic purpura, 1134
  in inflammatory bowel disease, 347–348, 347t, 349t, 352, 353t
  mechanism of action of, 949a, 1638

  nephrotoxicity of, 432, 440–442, 1381
  ophthalmic emulsion, in dry eye, 1076
  in prevention of GVHD, 1638
  in psoriasis, 1086–1087
  in transplant recipient, 945t, 948
Cyclothymic disorder, 671
CYP isozymes, oxidative metabolism by, 954
Cyproterone acetate, in prostate cancer, 1539, 1539t, 1545
Cyst
  Entamoeba histolytica, 1294
  Giardia lamblia, 1294
Cysticercosis, 1298
Cystic fibrosis, 303–314, 1703t
  airway obstruction in, 309
  case study of, 307
  clinical presentation in, 306
  epidemiology of, 304
  etiology of, 304
  hematologic disorders in, 305
  lung disease in, 304, 306
  musculoskeletal disorders in, 305, 312
  osteoporosis and, 967t
  outcome evaluation in, 313
  pancreatitis in, 407
  pathophysiology of, 304–305
  patient care and monitoring in, 313
  reproductive disorders in, 305
  treatment of, 307–312
    airway clearance therapy, 307
    antibiotics, 308–310, 309t
    β2-agonists, 308
    corticosteroids, 308
    diet therapy, 307
    DNase, 308
    insulin, 305
    lung transplantation, 941
    nonpharmacologic, 307
    pancreatic enzyme replacement, 307, 311, 311t
    pharmacokinetic considerations, 310
    vitamin D, 312
Cystic fibrosis-related diabetes, 305
Cystic fibrosis transmembrane regulator (CFTR), 304–305, 304f
Cystitis, 1307, 1309f
  hemorrhagic. *See* Hemorrhagic cystitis
  uncomplicated, 1308
Cystocele, 912
CytaBOM regimen, in non-Hodgkin's lymphoma, 1560, 1561t
Cytarabine, 1455
  in acute lymphocytic leukemia, 1587, 1588t, 1590t, 1591t
  in acute myelogenous leukemia, 1590–1592, 1591t
  adverse effects of, 1455, 1591t
  in cancer therapy, 1455
  in chronic myelogenous leukemia, 1601
  dosage of, 1557t, 1561t, 1588t, 1590t, 1634t
    in renal dysfunction, 1470t
  drug interactions of, 1591t
  emetogenicity of, 365t
  in Hodgkin's lymphoma, 1557t
  mechanism of action of, 1454a, 1455, 1591t
  in non-Hodgkin's lymphoma, 1561t, 1561
  pharmacokinetics of, 1455
  in preparation for hematopoietic cell transplant, 1634t
Cytochrome P450, 27
Cytochrome P450 system, 11
Cytogenetic abnormalities
  in acute lymphocytic leukemia, 1584, 1584t, 1586t, 1589

  in acute myelogenous leukemia, 1586, 1586t, 1592
  in chronic myelogenous leukemia, 1598
  in multiple myeloma, 1602
  in non-Hodgkin's lymphoma, 1554–1555
Cytokines
  in allergic drug reactions, 928
  in CNS infections, 1183
  in DIC, 1350
  in intra-abdominal infections, 1283
  in meningitis, 1172
  in rheumatoid arthritis, 982–983, 982t
  in tuberculosis, 1255
Cytomegalovirus
  adrenal insufficiency in, 786t
  with ATG, 946
  in CNS infections, 1183
  in hematopoietic cell transplant recipients, 1642
  in pneumonia, 1190
  prevention of, 956t, 957
  in transplant recipient, 956t, 957
  treatment of, 957

D

Dabigatran, 201
Dacarbazine, 1461–1462
  adverse effects of, 1462, 1561t, 1621
  in cancer therapy, 1461–1462
  dosage of, 1557t, 1561t, 1620t
  emetogenicity of, 365t
  extravasation of, 1677t, 1679
  in Hodgkin's lymphoma, 1557, 1557t, 1561t
  mechanism of action of, 1454a, 1461
  in melanoma, 1620t, 1621, 1622
  pharmacokinetics of, 1461
Daclizumab
  adverse effects of, 945t, 946
  dosage of, 945t, 946
  mechanism of action of, 946, 948f
  in psoriasis, 1087
  in transplant recipient, 945t, 946
Dactinomycin
  emetogenicity of, 365t
  extravasation of, 1677t
  mechanism of action of, 1454a
Dalfopristin. *See also* Quinupristin-dalfopristin
  dosage of, 1249t
  in infective endocarditis, 1249t
Dalteparin
  in acute coronary syndromes, 146
  dosage of, 192t, 195t, 198
  in venous thromboembolism, 195t, 198
    in prevention of, 192t, 193
Danaparoid, drug interactions of, 205t
Danazol
  drug interactions of, 205t
  teratogenic effects of, 824t
Dane particle, 415
Danshen, 125, 206t
Dantrolene
  dosage of, 517t
  drug interactions of, 955t
  mechanism of action of, 517t
  in spasticity, 517t
Dapsone
  adverse effects of, 956t
  dosage of, 956t
  drug interactions of, 955t
  in prevention of *Pneumocystis jiroveci* pneumonia, 956t, 1643
Daptomycin
  in cellulitis, 1225t

Daptomycin (*Cont.*)
  in diabetic foot infections, 1229*t*
  dosage of, 1225*t*, 1342*t*
  in infective endocarditis, 1241, 1243, 1246, 1249*t*
  in methicillin-resistant *Staphylococcus aureus*, 1355*a*
  in osteomyelitis, 1342*t*, 1344*t*
  in pneumonia, 1197
Darbepoetin
  in anemia
    of chronic disease, 1116
    of chronic kidney disease, 456, 459*t*, 1117
  in cancer/chemotherapy-related anemia, 1114*a*, 1116, 1117*t*
  dosage of, 1117*t*, 1117
Darifenacin
  adverse effects of, 915, 916*t*
  dosage of, 916*t*
  pharmacokinetics of, 916*t*
  in urinary incontinence, 916*t*
Dartmouth regimen, in melanoma, 1621
Dasatinib
  adverse effects of, 1467
  in cancer therapy, 1452*t*, 1467
  in chronic myelogenous leukemia, 1599, 1600–1601, 1600*t*
  pharmacokinetics of, 1467
DASH diet, 58, 59*t*
Daunomycin, adverse effects of, 86*t*
Daunorubicin, 1459–1460
  in acute lymphocytic leukemia, 1587, 1588*t*, 1591*t*
  in acute myelogenous leukemia, 1590, 1591*t*
  adverse effects of, 1459, 1591*t*
  in cancer therapy, 1459
  dosage of, 1588*t*
  in hepatic impairment, 1471*t*
    extravasation of, 1677*t*
  mechanism of action of, 1459, 1591*t*
  pharmacokinetics of, 1459
Daytime sleepiness
  evaluation of, 713
  excessive, 711
    assessment of, 715*a*
    treatment of, 715*a*
DDAVP. *See* Desmopressin
D-dimer test, 189, 190, 192
Death rattle. *See* Terminal secretions
Decitabine
  adverse effects of, 1455
  in cancer therapy, 1455–1456
  in myelodysplastic syndrome, 1455
  pharmacokinetics of, 1455
Decongestant
  adverse effects of, 1055
  anxiety with, 694*t*
  in allergic conjunctivitis, 1039
  in allergic rhinitis, 1051*t*, 1054–1056, 1058*t*
  intranasal, 1055
  oral, 1055
  in rhinosinusitis, 1211
Decubitus ulcer. *See* Pressure sore
Deep brain stimulation, in Parkinson's disease, 557
Deep sleep, 710
Deep vein thrombosis, 185. *See also* Venous thromboembolism
  case study of, 206
  chemotherapy-related, 1485
  clinical presentation in, 188–190
  diagnosis of, 188–190
  outcome evaluation in, 207–209

patient care and monitoring in, 210–211
  poststroke, 220
  prevention of, 190–193, 192*t*
    in septic patients, 1357
    thalidomide-related, 1606
  treatment of, 194–207
    approach to, 207, 208*a*
Deescalation therapy, antimicrobials, 1165
Defecation, dyssynergic, 372, 372*t*
Deferasirox
  dosage of, 1146
  in iron overload, 1146
Deferoxamine
  dosage of, 1146
  in iron overload, 1146
Defibrillation, in ventricular fibrillation, 178, 179*t*
Defibrotide, in sinusoidal obstruction syndrome, 1637
Degenerative joint disease. *See* Osteoarthritis
Degralix
  dosage of, 1544
  in prostate cancer, 1544
Dehydration, 480
  with diarrhea, 377–378
  in gastrointestinal infections, 1267, 1268*t*
  hypernatremia in, 486
  in pediatric patients, 1268*t*
  treatment of, volume of fluid required, 480, 481*t*
  with tube feeding, 1713
  vomiting in, 359
Dehydroemetine, in amebiasis, 1295
Dehydroepiandrosterone, adrenal production of, 784
Dehydroepiandrosterone sulfate, 784
Dehydroepiandrosterone therapy, in adrenal insufficiency, 786, 789*t*
Deiodinase, 764
Delavirdine
  adverse effects of, 1428*t*
  dosage of, 1428*t*
  drug interactions of, 955*t*, 1428*t*
  in HIV infection, 1428*t*
Delayed hypersensitivity reaction, 1101
Delirium, 635*t*
  diagnosis of, 672
  nonpharmacologic treatment, in palliative care, 41
  palliative care considerations, 41
  pharmacotherapy, in palliative care, 41
Delirium tremens, 616, 618–619
  treatment of, 618–619
Delta hepatitis. *See* Hepatitis D
Delta sleep, 710
Delusions, in schizophrenia, 631
Demeclocycline, in SIADH, 486
Dementia
  Alzheimer's disease, 595–605
  anxiety with, 694*t*
  classification of, 596, 596*t*
  diagnosis of, 672
  palliative care treatment for, 39
  in Parkinson's disease, 556, 562
  psychotic symptoms in, 635*t*
Demoxepam, dosage of, 698*t*
Demyelination, in multiple sclerosis, 508, 509*f*
Dendritic cells, 942
Denecarium bromide
  adverse effects of, 1042
  drug interactions of, 1042
  in glaucoma, 1042
Denileukin diftitox, 1465

adverse effects of, 1465
  in cancer therapy, 1465
  mechanism of action of, 1465
  pharmacokinetics of, 1465
  in psoriasis, 1087
Denosumab, 976
Dental procedures
  antimicrobial prophylaxis in, 1400*t*
  endocarditis prophylaxis in, 1239, 1249–1250, 1250*t*
  prophylactic regimens for, 1250*t*
Denture stomatitis, 1366, 1367
Deoxycorticosterone, 784
Deoxypyridinoline, 969
Depo-medroxyprogesterone acetate
  in dysmenorrhea, 859*t*
  in menstruation-related disorders, 859*t*
Depo-Provera, 850–851, 1435
Depo-SubQ Provera, 104, 850–851
Depression. *See also* Bipolar disorder
  in Alzheimer's disease, 603
  anxiety disorders and, 692
  in diabetes mellitus, 747
  drug-induced, 655
  epilepsy and, 536
  erectile dysfunction with, 885*t*
  with hormone-replacement therapy, 876*t*
  in multiple sclerosis, 511–512, 516
  palliative care, symptom in, 47
  in Parkinson's disease, 556, 562
  psoriasis and, 1080
  in stimulant withdrawal, 619
  treatment-resistant, 657
  urinary incontinence in, 912
Depressive disorder, major, 653–667
  case study of, 654, 656, 665
  clinical presentation in, 655
  course of depression, 656, 664, 664*f*
  diagnosis of, 655–656, 655*t*
  differential diagnosis of, 655–656
  in elderly, 665
  epidemiology of, 654
  etiology of, 654–655
  gender and, 654
  genetic factors in, 654
  monoamine hypothesis of, 654
  neurotransmitter receptor hypothesis of, 654
  outcome evaluation in, 666
  partial remission of, 656
  pathophysiology of, 654–65
  patient care and monitoring in, 667
  patient counseling in, 666, 666*t*
  in pediatric patients, 665
  in pregnancy, 665
  psychotic symptoms in, 635*t*
  recurrence of, 654, 664
  relapse of, 654, 664
  treatment of, 656–666
    algorithm for, 663*a*
    antidepressants, 657–666. *See also* Antidepressants
    electroconvulsive therapy, 656
    maintenance treatment, 664
    nonpharmacologic, 656–657
Dermatitis. *See specific types*
Dermatophytes, 1369, 1371
  treatment of, 1223*t*
Dermopathy, in Graves' disease, 774, 775*f*
Desensitization, in allergic drug reactions, 930, 933–935, 1322
Desflurane, in status epilepticus, 549

Desipramine
  in depression, 516, 665
  dosage of, 661, 661*t*
  drug interactions of, 614*t*
  in elderly, 665
  in irritable bowel syndrome, 383
  in pediatric patients, 665
Desirudin in venous thromboembolism,
  200–201
Desloratadine, in allergic rhinitis, 1053, 1054*t*
Desmopressin (DDAVP), 915
  adverse effects of, 467, 923, 1123
  dosage of, 467, 923, 816*t*, 1123, 1127
  in enuresis, 923–924, 816*t*
  in hemophilia A, 1123
  mechanism of action of, 1123
  in uremic bleeding, 467
  in urinary dysfunction, 563
  in von Willebrand's disease, 1127–1128
Desogestrel, 843, 845*t*, 846, 849
Desonide
  in contact dermatitis, 1103*t*
  dosage and potency of, 1103*t*
Desoximetasone
  in contact dermatitis, 1103*t*
  dosage and potency of, 1103*t*
Desquamation, in essential fatty acid deficiency,
  1684
Detrusor muscle
  detrusor hyperactivity with impaired
    contractility, 911, 912
  instability, 897
  overactive, 911
  weakened, 911
Detumescence, 885
Devil's claw, 206*t*
Dexamethasone, 954
  in acute lymphocytic leukemia, 1588*t*, 1589,
    1590*t*
  in adrenal insufficiency, 789*t*
  adverse effects of, 362*t*, 1607*t*
  in allergic reaction to insulin, 933
  in brain metastasis, 1666
  in chemotherapy-related nausea and vomiting,
    1512, 1513*t*, 1652, 1652*t*
  in contact dermatitis, 1103*t*
  dosage of, 362*t*, 832*t*, 952, 1103*t*, 1184, 1588*t*,
    1561*t*, 1590*t*, 1662
  drug interactions of, 955*t*
  in meningitis, 1178, 1183–1184
  in multiple myeloma, 1607*t*
  in nausea and vomiting, 362*t*, 364, 365–366,
    1557
  in non-Hodgkin's lymphoma, 1561, 1561*t*
  osteoporosis with, 977
  premedication
    for docetaxel, 1458
    for paclitaxel, 1458
    for pemetrexed, 1457
  in retinoic acid syndrome, 1464
  in spinal cord compression, 1664
  in superior vena cava syndrome, 1662
  in transplant recipient, 952
Dexamethasone sodium phosphate
  in contact dermatitis, 1103*t*
  dosage and potency of, 1103*t*
Dexamethasone suppression test, low-dose, 794,
  795*t*
Dexfenfluramine, 1725
  hyperprolactinemia with, 814*t*
Dexmethylphenidate
  in ADHD, 727*t*, 730*t*
  dosage of, 727*t*, 730*t*

Dexrazoxane
  dosage of, 1678*t*
  in extravasation injury, 1678*t*
Dextran, 483
  in hypovolemic shock, 258–259, 258*t*
Dextroamphetamine
  in ADHD, 727*t*, 728*t*, 730*t*
  adverse effects of, 728*t*
  dosage of, 727*t*
Dextromethorphan
  in common cold, 1218*t*
  dosage of, 830*t*
  drug interactions of, 660, 660*t*
Dextrose
  caloric value of, 1683
  in hyperkalemia, 454, 489
  in hypoglycemia, 1694
  in intra-abdominal infections, 1285
  for parenteral nutrition, 1683, 1690, 1694
Dextrose therapeutic solutions, 483, 482*t*
DHAP regimen
  in Hodgkin's lymphoma, 1559
  in non-Hodgkin's lymphoma, 1561*t*, 1561
Diabetes insipidus
  enuresis with, 921*t*
  hypernatremia in, 486
  lithium-induced, 679
  urinary incontinence in, 912
Diabetes mellitus, 735–761
  adrenal insufficiency and, 787
  angiopathy in, 1228
  arrhythmia in, 166*t*
  β-blocker use in, 123
  case study of, 744, 758, 759–760
  chronic kidney disease and, 447, 450
  clinical presentation in, 739–741
  colorectal cancer and, 1519
  constipation in, 372*t*
  cystic fibrosis-related, 305, 312
  depression in, 747
  diagnosis of, 739–741, 741*t*
  diarrhea in, 376
  drug-related, 737, 737*t*, 1441*t*
  enteral nutrition in, 1709–1710, 1709*t*
  enuresis with, 921*t*
  epidemiology of, 736–737
    type 1, 736
    type 2, 736–737
  erectile dysfunction and, 885, 885*t*
  etiology of, 736–737
    type 1, 736
    type 2, 736–737
  foot problems in. *See* Diabetic foot
  gestational, 737, 739–740, 740*t*
    diagnosis of, 740*t*
    risk assessment for, 739–740
    treatment of, 744
  glycemic control in, 735, 737*t*, 741
    setting and assessing glycemic targets, 741–743
  glycosuria in, 737
  gout and, 1012
  heart failure and, 88
  honeymoon period in, 736
  in hospitalized patients, 758–759
  hyperglycemia in, 735
  hyperlipidemia and, 236*t*, 737, 743*t*, 750,
    755–756
  hyperosmolar hyperglycemic state in, 757
  hypertension and, 68–70, 737, 743*t*, 756
  hypoglycemia and, 756
  ischemic heart disease and, 111, 111*t*, 112,
    151, 755
  keratitis with, 1070*t*

latent autoimmune diabetes in adults, 736
macrovascular complications of, 741
microalbuminuria in, 758
microvascular complications of, 741
nausea and vomiting in, 358*t*
nephropathy in, 758
neuropathy in, 568, 578, 578*t*, 757–758, 1227
new-onset DM after transplantation, 956*t*, 959
obesity and, 737, 746, 1720–1722
osteoarthritis in, 998*t*
osteomyelitis and, 1338, 1339
osteoporosis and, 966*t*
outcome evaluation in, 759–760
pathophysiology of, 738–739
patient care and monitoring in, 743*t*, 761
peripheral neuropathy in, 568, 578, 578*t*
peripheral vascular disease in, 758
polycystic ovarian syndrome and, 737, 865
polydipsia in, 739
polyphagia in, 739
polyuria in, 739
retinopathy in, 757
screening for, 739, 740*t*
sick days, 759
stroke and, 217*t*
treatment of, 741–759, 959
  α-glucosidase inhibitors, 748*t*, 750–751
  biguanides, 749*t*, 750
  in chronic kidney disease, 450
  dipeptidyl peptidase-4 inhibitors, 751
  exercise program, 746–747
  immunizations, 747
  incretin mimetics, 754–755, 754*t*
  insulin, 450, 743
  insulin secretagogues, 747, 748*t*, 750
  insulin therapy, 751, 753, 752*t*
  kidney transplantation, 941
  medical nutrition therapy, 745–746
  meglitinides, 747
  pancreas transplantation, 941–942
  pramlintide, 754*t*, 755
  psychological assessment and care, 747
  sulfonylureas, 747, 748*t*
  thiazolidinediones, 749*t*, 750
  type 1, 743, 751
  type 2, 743–744, 745*a*, 746*a*, 747–751
  weight management, 746
urinary incontinence in, 912
Diabetic foot, 758
  foot ulcers, 758
  prevention of foot complications, 758
Diabetic foot infection, 1227–1230
  clinical classification of, 1228, 1228*t*, 1229*t*
  clinical presentation in, 1228–1229
  complications of, 1229
  diagnosis of, 1228–1229
  epidemiology of, 1227
  etiology of, 1227
  pathophysiology of, 1227–1228
  prevention of, 1229
  treatment of, 1229–1230
    antibiotics, 1230, 1229*t*
    lower extremity amputation, 1229
    off-loading, 1229
Diabetic ketoacidosis, 424*t*, 739, 756–757, 759
  clinical presentation in, 756
  pathophysiology of, 756
  treatment of, 756–757, 757*t*
Dialysis. *See also* Hemodialysis; Peritoneal dialysis
  in acute renal failure, 439
  adverse effects of, 439
  in end-stage renal disease, 468–475
  indications for, 468–475

Dialysis membrane, 439, 468
Dialyzer, 468
Diamond-Blackfan anemia, 1580t
Diaper dermatitis, 1105–1107
  case study of, 1107
  clinical presentation in, 1105, 1106f
  epidemiology of, 1105
  outcome evaluation in, 1106
  pathophysiology of, 1105
  patient care and monitoring in, 1107
  treatment of, 1105–1106
    algorithm for, 1107a
    antibacterials, 1106
    antifungals, 1106
    corticosteroids, 1106
    nonpharmacologic, 1106
    protectants, 1106
Diaper rash, psoriatic, 1082
Diaphoresis, with corticosteroids, 953t
Diaphragm (contraception), 844t, 851
Diarrhea, 376–380, 1268
  acute, 376–378, 379t
  antibiotic-associated, 1274–1276, 1711–1712
  bacterial gastrointestinal infections,
    1267–1276
  with bisphosphonates, 974
  case study of, 380
  chemotherapy-related, 1512–1513, 1529, 1636
  chronic, 376–378, 379t
  clinical presentation in, 378
  Clostridium difficile-associated. See
    Clostridium difficile-associated diarrhea
  with corticosteroids, 953t
  definition of, 376
  dehydration with, 377, 378
  diagnosis of, 377
  drug-related, 377, 376t, 1459
  epidemiology of, 376–377
  etiology of, 376–377
  inflammatory, 377
  metabolic acidosis with, 424t
  osmotic, 377
  outcome evaluation in, 380
  palliative care, symptom in, 47
  pathophysiology of, 377
  patient care and monitoring in, 380
  in pediatric patient, 377
  persistent, 376
  rotavirus, 1412
  secretory, 377
  shock in, 253t
  sorbitol-related, 1711, 1714
  toxicity criteria, 1453t
  travelers'. See Travelers' diarrhea
  treatment of, 377–380
    adsorbents, 379, 379t
    antibiotics, 380
    antiperistaltic agents, 379, 379t
    antisecretory agents, 379, 379t
    bulk agents, 379, 379t
    diet therapy, 378–379
    fluid and electrolyte therapy, 377
    probiotics, 379–380
  with tube feeding, 1711, 1711t, 1714
Diarthrodial joint, osteoarthritis of, 998, 998f
Diastolic blood pressure, 57
Diastolic dysfunction, 80t, 81, 96–97
  isolated, 81
Diatrizoate, nephrotoxicity of, 411
Diazepam, 10, 45t
  adverse effects of, 545t, 547t
  in alcohol withdrawal, 618
  in delirium tremens, 618

  dosage of, 440t, 544–545, 545t, 546t, 547t, 549t,
    618, 698t
  drug interactions of, 322, 614t, 699t, 955t
  mechanism of action of, 440t
  in panic disorder, 702
  pharmacokinetics of, 698t
  in seizures, 618, 1666
  in spasticity, 440t
  in status epilepticus, 544–545, 545t, 546t,
    547t, 549t
DIC. See Disseminated intravascular coagulation
Dichlorphenamide
  adverse effects of, 1041
  in glaucoma, 1041
Diclofenac
  dosage of, 859t, 1002t
  in dysmenorrhea, 859t
  ocular, in corneal abrasion, 1064
  in osteoarthritis, 1002t, 1004, 1007
Diclofenac gel in musculoskeletal disorders,
    1025
Diclofenac patch in musculoskeletal disorders,
    1025
Diclofenac sodium topical gel in osteoarthritis,
    1007
Dicloxacillin
  in cellulitis, 1225t
  in cystic fibrosis, 309, 309t
  in diabetic foot infections, 1229t
  dosage of, 309t, 832t, 1225t
  drug interactions of, 205t
  in erysipelas, 1224
  in furuncles/carbuncles, 1223t
Dicyclomine
  in irritable bowel syndrome, 383, 384t
  in opioid withdrawal, 621t
Didanosine
  adverse effects of, 1425, 1427t, 1437t–1442t
  dosage of, 1427t
  drug interactions of, 1427t
  food interactions of, 1427t
  in HIV infection, 1425, 1427t, 1433
  mechanism of action of, 1421f
  pancreatitis with, 404t
Diet. See also Nutrition
  colorectal cancer and, 1518, 1343t
  for immunosuppressed patients (low-
    microbial), 1641
  lung cancer and, 1500
  ovarian cancer and, 1566
  peptic ulcer disease and, 329
  prostate cancer and, 1536–1537, 1536t
Dietary fiber, 1518
  in enteral feeding formulas, 1707, 1709
Diethylpropion
  adverse effects of, 1728
  dosage of, 1725t, 1728
  drug interactions of, 1727
  mechanism of action of, 1727
  in obesity, 1725t, 1727–1728
Diethylstilbestrol
  adverse effects of, 1487t
  in breast cancer, 1487t
  dosage of, 1487t
  in prostate cancer, 1543
  teratogenic effects of, 824t
Diet therapy
  in anemia, 1112–1113, 1115t
  in chronic kidney disease, 450
  in cystic fibrosis, 307
  in diabetes mellitus, 745–746
  in diarrhea, 378–379
  in epilepsy, 528

  in heart failure, 88–89, 97
  in HIV infection, 1424–1425
  in hypertension, 58, 59t
  in inflammatory bowel disease, 345
  in irritable bowel syndrome, 383
  in ischemic heart disease, 117
  in nausea and vomiting, 359
  in obesity, 1723–1724, 1723t
  in Parkinson's disease, 557
  in premenstrual syndrome, 863
  in pressure sores, 1231
  in prevention of osteoporosis, 969, 969t
Diffusion
  in hemodialysis, 470
  in peritoneal dialysis, 472
Diflorasone diacetate
  in contact dermatitis, 1103t
  dosage and potency of, 1103t
Diflucortolone valerate
  in contact dermatitis, 1103t
  dosage and potency of, 1103t
Diflunisal, adverse effects of, 574
Digestive enzymes, 1702, 1702f
Digitalis, diarrhea with, 376t
Digital rectal examination
  in benign prostatic hyperplasia, 897, 901t, 907
  in prostate cancer, 1537
  screening for colorectal cancer, 1519, 1520t
Digital thermometer, 24
Digoxin, 38f, 828t
  adverse effects of, 95, 119t
  anxiety with, 694t
  arrhythmia with, 163t, 164, 164t, 177t
  in atrial fibrillation, 168, 169t, 170a
  dosage of, 95–96, 169t, 175t
  drug interactions of, 169t, 170t, 175t, 245, 1164
  in heart failure, 95–96
  mechanism of action of, 95, 169t, 175t
  nausea and vomiting with, 358t
  ocular changes with, 1077t
  in paroxysmal supraventricular tachycardia, 175t
Dihydroergotamine, in migraine, 588
Dihydropyridines, effect on myocardial oxygen
    demand and supply, 122t
Dihydropyrimidine dehydrogenase deficiency,
    1528
Dihydrotestosterone, 896
  in prostate cancer, 1539–1540
Diloxanide furoate
  in amebiasis, 1296
  dosage of, 1296
Diltiazem
  in acute coronary syndromes, 142t, 147, 152t
  adverse effects of, 61t, 119t
  in arrhythmia, 162t, 163t, 164t
  in atrial fibrillation, 168, 169t, 170a
  dosage of, 61t, 124t, 142t, 169t, 175t
  drug interactions of, 169t, 175t, 955t
  effect on myocardial oxygen demand and
    supply, 122t
  in heart failure, 96, 97
  in hypertension, 61t, 67
  in ischemic heart disease, 123
  mania with, 676t
  mechanism of action of, 163t, 169t, 175t
  in paroxysmal supraventricular tachycardia,
    175t
Dilutional acidosis, 424t
Dimenhydrinate
  adverse effects of, 361t
  dosage of, 361t, 830t
  in nausea and vomiting, 361t
Dimethyl sulfoxide. See DMSO

DIOS. *See* Distal intestinal obstruction syndrome
Dipeptidyl peptidase-4 inhibitors, in diabetes
  mellitus, 751
Diphasic dyskinesia, in Parkinson's disease, 556
Diphenhydramine
  adverse effects of, 361t
  in allergic rhinitis, 1053
  in anaphylaxis, 931t
  in contact dermatitis, 1102
  dosage of, 361t, 830t, 931t
  in extrapyramidal symptoms, 647
  in nausea and vomiting, 361t, 577t
  premedication
    for amphotericin B, 1643
    for paclitaxel, 1458
    for rituximab, 1563, 1603, 1603t
  in prevention of contrast media reaction, 933
  in pruritus, 468
Diphenoxylate, dry eye with, 1075t
Diphenoxylate/atropine
  in diarrhea, 379t, 379
  dosage of, 379t
2,3-Diphosphoglycerate, 1697
Diphtheria, 1406
Diphtheria, tetanus, acellular pertussis (Dtap)
  vaccine, 1406, 1407, 1408t, 1414t
Diphtheria toxin, 1406
Diphtheria toxoid, 1406, 1407
Diphtheria toxoid, tetanus toxoid (DT, Td)
  vaccine, 1406, 1408t, 1414t, 1416
Diphtheria toxoid booster, 1233
Diphtheroids
  in intra-abdominal infections, 1283
  normal flora, 1157f
Dipivefrin
  adverse effects of, 1043
  dosage of, 1038t
  in glaucoma, 1038t, 1043
  mechanism of action of, 1038t
Dipyridamole
  adverse effects of, 224
  drug interactions of, 205t
  extended-release, in prevention of stroke, 224,
    226t
Direct current cardioversion (DCC)
  in atrial fibrillation, 167–171
  in paroxysmal supraventricular
    tachycardia, 174
  in ventricular tachycardia, 178a
Directly observed therapy, in tuberculosis, 1258,
  1263
Direct thrombin inhibitors
  adverse effects of, 201
  mechanism of action of, 200, 200f
  oral, 201
  in venous thromboembolism, 200–201
Disability, from rheumatoid arthritis, 993
Disease-modifying antirheumatic drugs
  (DMARD)
  biologic, 990–992
  nonbiologic, 990
  in rheumatoid arthritis, 988, 986t–987t,
    990–992
Disease-modifying therapy, in multiple sclerosis,
  510 517, 513t
Disopyramide
  adverse effects of, 86t
  in arrhythmias, 162t, 177t, 179t
  drug interactions of, 955t
  mechanism of action of, 163t
Disordered thinking, in schizophrenia, 631
Disseminated idiopathic skeletal hyperostosis,
  1086

Disseminated intravascular coagulation (DIC),
    1130–1132
  case study of, 1132
  clinical presentation in, 1131
  diagnosis of, 1131
  epidemiology of, 1130
  etiology of, 1130, 1131t
  outcome evaluation in, 1132
  pathophysiology of, 1130
  in sepsis, 1132
  treatment of, 1130–1132
    anticoagulants, 1130–1132
    cryoprecipitate, 1132
    platelet and fresh-frozen plasma, 1132
Distal intestinal obstruction syndrome (DIOS),
    in cystic fibrosis, 304, 312
Distraction techniques, in pain, 573
Distribution, in geriatric patients, 10–11
Distributive shock, 252
  etiology of, 253t
Disulfiram
  adverse effects of, 625
  in alcohol dependence, 624
  contraindications to, 624
  dosage of, 624
  drug interactions of, 205t, 613, 614t, 699t
  hepatotoxicity of, 625
  mechanism of action of, 624
  in stimulant dependence, 626
Disulfiram-ethanol reaction, 624–625
Diuretic(s), 38f. *See also specific drugs*
  in acute renal failure, 434, 436–437
  adverse effects of, 91, 485
  in ascites, 396
  blood glucose level and, 737t
  in chronic kidney disease, 453
  constipation with, 372t
  drug interactions of, 1004
  dry eye with, 1075t
  in elderly, 64–65
  in heart failure, 89–91, 90t, 97, 100–101, 100t
  in hypertension, 59, 60t, 64–65, 66t, 70,
    756, 958
  metabolic alkalosis with, 502t, 503
  ocular changes with, 1077t
  in pregnancy, 72t
  self-adjusted dosing of, 91
  in superior vena cava syndrome, 1663
  voiding symptoms with, 901t
Diuretic resistance, 91, 100, 437
Divalproex sodium
  adverse effects of, 683
  in bipolar disorder, 677t, 680t–681t, 681, 685
  dosage of, 677t, 681
  drug interactions of, 683
  mechanism of action of, 681
  monitoring therapy with, 681
  pharmacokinetics of, 680t–681t
  in prevention of migraine, 590t, 591
Diverticulitis
  constipation in, 372t
  peritonitis in, 1283
Diverticulosis, diarrhea in, 376
DMARD. *See* Disease-modifying antirheumatic
  drugs
DMSO (dimethyl sulfoxide)
  dosage of, 1678t
  in extravasation injury, 1678, 1678t
DNA repair, 1612, 1613
  in colorectal cancer, 1518
DNase, in cystic fibrosis, 307
Dobutamine
  dosage of, 101t, 102–103, 1356

  in heart failure, 101t, 102–103
  hemodynamic effects of, 101t, 102–103
  in hypovolemic shock, 260
  mechanism of action of, 102
  in sepsis, 1356
Docetaxel, 1458
  adverse effects of, 1458, 1484t, 1491, 1507t,
    1547–1548, 1547t, 1572t, 1574t
  in breast cancer, 1482, 1484, 1483t–1484t,
    1491
  in cancer therapy, 1458
  dosage of, 1483t–1484t, 1491, 1507t, 1547,
    1547t, 1571t, 1572t, 1573, 1574t
    in hepatic impairment, 1471t
  extravasation of, 1677t
  in lung cancer, 1507t, 1510
  mechanism of action of, 1458
  in ovarian cancer, 1570–1573, 1571t, 1572t,
    1574t
  pharmacokinetics of, 1458
  in prostate cancer, 1547–1548, 1547t
Docusate
  in constipation, 374, 374t, 577t
  dosage of, 374t, 830t
Dofetilide
  adverse effects of, 119t
  in arrhythmias, 162t, 179t
  in atrial fibrillation, 170t, 171a, 171t, 172a
  dosage of, 170t
  drug interactions of, 170t
  mechanism of action of, 163t
Dog bite, 1232–1233, 1232t
Dolasetron
  adverse effects of, 362t
  in chemotherapy-related nausea and vomiting,
    1513t, 1652t
  dosage of, 362t
  in nausea and vomiting, 362t, 364
Domino heart transplant, 940
Domperidone
  adverse effects of, 363
  hyperprolactinemia with, 814t
  in nausea and vomiting, 361t, 363
Donepezil
  adverse effects of, 600, 601t
  in Alzheimer's disease, 600, 601t
  arrhythmia with, 163t
  dosage of, 600, 601t
  drug interactions of, 600
Dong quai, 125, 206t, 878, 879t
Donor lymphocyte infusion, 1633, 1635f
Dopa decarboxylase, 558f
Dopamine
  in acute renal failure, 437–439
  in ADHD, 724
  adverse effects of, 439
  in anaphylaxis, 931t
  arrhythmia with, 260t
  in atrioventricular nodal block, 165
  in bipolar disorder, 670
  in depression, 654
  dosage of, 101t, 260t, 931t, 1356
  GERD with, 317t
  in heart failure, 101t, 102–103
  hemodynamic effects of, 101t, 102–103
  in hypovolemic shock, 260, 260t
  low-dose, 437–439
  mechanism of action of, 102
  metabolism of, 557
  in Parkinson's disease, 554–555, 554f
  in sepsis, 1356
  in sinus bradycardia, 164
  in wakefulness, 711

Dopamine agonists. *See also specific drugs*
  in acromegaly, 807t, 808
  in hyperprolactinemia, 816–817, 818t
  mechanism of action of, 560
  metabolism of, 561
  in Parkinson's disease, 557–558, 559t, 560–561
  in pregnancy, 817
  in restless-legs syndrome, 717
Dopamine antagonists
  in chemotherapy-induced nausea and
    vomiting, 1652
  in nausea and vomiting, 361t, 360, 363–364
Dopamine hypothesis, of schizophrenia, 632
Dopamine neural tracts, in reward pathway,
    609, 609f
Dornase alfa, 307
  in cystic fibrosis, 308t
Dorzolamide. *See also* Timolol-dorzolamide
  adverse effects of, 1041
  dosage of, 1038t
  in glaucoma, 1038t, 1041
  mechanism of action of, 1038t
Downregulation, of adrenergic receptors, 83
Down's syndrome, acute leukemia and, 1580t, 1581
Doxapram
  in respiratory acidosis, 503
  respiratory alkalosis with, 427t
Doxazosin
  adverse effects of, 63t, 901, 902, 903t, 906t
  in benign prostatic hyperplasia, 901–904
  dosage of, 63t
  drug interactions of, 904
  in hypertension, 63t, 64, 69
  mechanism of action of, 902
  pharmacologic properties of, 903t
  in urinary incontinence, 918
Doxepin
  arrhythmia with, 179t
  dosage of, 384t, 622t, 661t
  drug interactions of, 614t
  in insomnia, 714
  in irritable bowel syndrome, 383, 384t
  in smoking cessation, 622t
Doxercalciferol, in hyperphosphatemia, 463, 465t
Doxorubicin, 1460
  in acute lymphocytic leukemia, 1587, 1588t,
    1590t
  in acute myelogenous leukemia, 1590
  adverse effects of, 86t, 1460, 1485, 1484t, 1561t,
    1563, 1574t, 1605, 1607t
  in breast cancer, 1482, 1483t–1484t, 1491
  in cancer therapy, 1460
  dosage of, 1483t–1484t, 1485, 1507t–1508t, 1557t,
    1560t, 1561t, 1574t, 1588t, 1590t
  in hepatic impairment, 1471t
  emetogenicity of, 365t
  extravasation of, 1677, 1677t, 1678
  in Hodgkin's lymphoma, 1557, 1557t, 1561t
  liposomal, 1460, 1483t, 1484t, 1574t, 1575
  in lung cancer, 1507t–1508t
  mechanism of action of, 1460
  in multiple myeloma, 1607t
  in non-Hodgkin's lymphoma, 1560t, 1561t, 1561
  in ovarian cancer, 1573, 1574t
  pharmacokinetics of, 1460
Doxycycline
  in acne vulgaris, 1098, 1098t
  adverse effects of, 1098t
  in cellulitis, 1225, 1225t
  in *Chlamydia*, 1320–1321
  in diabetic foot infections, 1229t
  dosage of, 831t, 1098t, 1212t, 1225t, 1300, 1301t,
    1319, 1320, 1322, 1333t

drug interactions of, 205t, 850t
  in gonorrhea, 1319
  in intra-abdominal infections, 1288t
  in malaria, 1300
  in PID, 1333t
  in pneumonia, 1195–1196, 1196t
  in prevention of malaria, 1301t
  in rhinosinusitis, 1212a, 1212t
  in sepsis, 1353t
  in syphilis, 1322
  in urinary tract infections, 1311t
Doxylamine
  dosage, 830t
  in nausea and vomiting, 366
D-penicillamine, 990
Drainage procedures, in intra-abdominal
    infections, 1285
D$_2$ receptor antagonists, in chemotherapy-related
    nausea and vomiting, 1512, 1513t
Drinker Inventory of Consequences, 627
Dronabinol
  adverse effects of, 362t
  in anorexia, 1513
  dosage of, 362t
  in nausea and vomiting, 362t, 364, 365
Droperidol
  adverse effects of, 361t, 363
  arrhythmia with, 179t
  dosage of, 361t
  drug interactions of, 647
  in nausea and vomiting, 361t, 363, 365–366
Droplet nuclei, 1254
Drospirenone, 843, 845t, 849
  in premenstrual dysphoric disorder, 865
Drotrecogin alfa, in sepsis, 1356–1357
Drug abuse. *See* Substance-abuse disorders
Drug Abuse Warning Network, 608
Drug interactions, *See specific drugs*
Drug metabolism
  in geriatric patients, 11
  in pediatric patients, 27
Drug-related problems, in elderly patients, 13
  adverse drug reaction, 14–15
  inappropriate prescribing, 13–14
  nonadherence, 15
  polypharmacy, 13
  undertreatment, 14
Drug-taking behaviors, 4
Drug therapy
  in geriatric patients, 17, 18t
  in pediatric patients, 28
    accidental ingestion, in pediatric
      patients, 31
    administration and drug formulation, routes
      of, 28–29
    CAM and OTC medication use, 29–30
    common errors in, 29
    off-label medication use, 30
    pediatric patients and caregiver education,
      medication administration to, 30–31
Drusen, 1072
  ablation of, 1073
Dry-bed training, in enuresis, 922, 924, 923t
Dry eye, 1074–1077
  case study of, 1076
  clinical presentation in, 1075
  conditions that cause or worsen, 1075t
  diagnosis of, 1075
  drug-induced, 1075t, 1077t
  epidemiology of, 1074
  outcome evaluation in, 1077
  patient care and monitoring in, 1077
  pathophysiology of, 1074–1075

  risk factors for, 1074t
  treatment of, 1075–1076
    artificial tears, 1076
    cholinergic agonists, 1076
    cyclosporine emulsion, 1076
Dry mouth, drug-related, 915
Dry powder inhaler, 271
DSM-IV-TR, criteria for substance dependence,
    610–611
Dual-energy x-ray absorptiometry, 968
Ductus arteriosus, 835
  premature closure of, 592, 1004
Duke criteria, modified, for infective
    endocarditis, 1240t
Duloxetine
  adverse effects of, 917, 918t
  dosage of, 660, 661t, 918t
  drug interactions of, 660, 660t, 917
  mechanism of action of, 657, 657t
  in pain, 578, 578t
  pharmacokinetics of, 659t, 918t
  in urinary incontinence, 917, 918t
Duodenal ulcers, 328, 328t. *See also* Peptic ulcer
    disease
Dust mites, 269, 1048, 1048t
Dutasteride
  in benign prostatic hyperplasia, 896, 906t
  mechanism of action of, 896
  pharmacologic properties of, 906t
  in prevention of prostate cancer, 1537
D$_5$W solution, 482–483, 482t
Dysarthria
  in alcohol intoxication, 612t
  in stroke, 218
Dysentery, 376
  bacillary, 1267
Dysesthesia, in Parkinson's disease, 555
Dysfibrinogenemia, 187t
Dysgeusia, 591
Dyskinesia, in Parkinson's disease, 555, 563t
Dyslipidemia, 111, 111t, 229–248
  case study of, 238, 240, 244
  clinical presentation in, 235
  with corticosteroids, 953t
  diabetes mellitus and, 236t, 737, 743t, 750,
    755–756
  diagnosis of, 235
  drug-related, 236t, 1441t
  erectile dysfunction with, 885t
  familial combined, 231
  genetic disorders, 233t
  hypothyroidism and, 768
  ischemic heart disease and, 111, 111t, 229–248,
    238t
  obesity and, 236t, 1720, 1725
  with oral contraceptives, 848
  outcome evaluation in, 247
  pancreatitis and, 232, 235, 240
  with parenteral nutrition, 1694t, 1695–1696
  pathophysiology of, 230–234
  patient care and monitoring in, 248
  renal disease and, 236t, 446–447, 451–452
  screening for, 235
  secondary conditions that cause, 236t
  stroke and, 217t
  in transplant recipient, 956t, 958–959
  treatment of, 234–247, 958–959
    bile acid sequestrants, 241t, 243t,
      244–245, 959
    cholesterol absorption inhibitors, 241t,
      243t, 244
    in chronic kidney disease, 451–452
    combination products, 24t, 243t, 246–247

ezetimibe, 956t
fibrates, 151, 241t, 243t, 245–246, 959
fish oils, 246
gemfibrozil, 956t
guidelines for, 235–240
investigational agents, 247
lifestyle modifications, 236, 238t, 958
niacin, 151, 241t, 243t, 243t, 245, 959
statins, 151, 26, 240–244, 241t, 243t, 243t,
    246–247, 452, 756, 956t, 959
Dysmenorrhea
in adolescents, 864
clinical presentation in, 862
definition of, 862
diagnosis of, 862
epidemiology of, 862–863
etiology of, 862–863
outcome evaluation in, 866t, 867
pathophysiology of, 863
patient care and monitoring in, 867
treatment of, 845, 859t, 863
    algorithm for, 863a
Dyspareunia, 913t
in genital warts, 1327
in menopause, 872
in vulvovaginal candidiasis, 1362
Dyspepsia
functional, 358t
with NSAID, 574
Dysphagia, 226, 1191
in oropharyngeal candidiasis, 1367
palliative care, symptom in, 47
in Parkinson's disease, 555
Dysphasic speech, with migraine, 586
Dysphonia, with corticosteroids, 273, 296
Dysplasia, 1449
Dysplastic nevus syndrome, familial, 1613
Dyspnea
allergic drug reaction, 933
in asthma, 267
in COPD, 300, 300t
in heart failure, 85
MRC dyspnea scale, 300, 300t
nonpharmacologic treatment, in palliative
    care, 42
palliative care considerations, 41–42
pharmacotherapy, in palliative care, 42–43
Dysregulation hypothesis, of schizophrenia, 632
Dyssynergic defecation, 372, 372t
Dystonia
with antipsychotics, 641
in Parkinson's disease, 556
Dysuria, 913t
in urinary tract infections, 1307

E

Eastern Cooperative Oncology Group Scale, of
    performance status, 1451, 1453
Eating disorders
menstruation-related disorders in, 857t
osteoporosis and, 966t
Ebstein's anomaly, 686
Eburnation, 998
Ecchymosis, with corticosteroids, 953t
Echinacea, 376t
Echinacea purpurea in common cold, 1218
Echinocandins
in esophageal candidiasis, 1368
in invasive aspergillosis, 1391
in invasive candidiasis, 1385
Echocardiogram
in acute coronary syndromes, 135, 139
in infective endocarditis, 1239

transesophageal, 1239
transthoracic, 1239
in stroke, 218
Echothiophate
adverse effects of, 1042
dosage of, 1038t
drug interactions of, 1042
in glaucoma, 1038t, 1042
mechanism of action of, 1038t
Eclampsia, 1131t
treatment of, magnesium sulfate, 492
Ectoparasites, 1303–1304
Ectopic CRH syndrome, 792t
Ectopic pregnancy, 851, 861
Eczema, allergic drug reaction, 929t
Edema
in chronic kidney disease, 453
peripheral, in heart failure, 86
Efalizumab, 953
adverse effects of, 1088
dosage of, 1088
mechanism of action of, 1088
in psoriasis, 1087, 1088
Efavirenz
adverse effects of, 1429t, 1437t–1442t
dosage of, 1429t
drug interactions of, 615t, 1429t
food interactions of, 1429t
in HIV infection, 1425, 1429t, 1434, 1435
teratogenicity of, 1425, 1434
Egg allergy, 1408t, 1684
Eicosanoids, 1021
Eikenella corrodens
in bite wound infections, 1232t
in infective endocarditis, 1241
in pneumonia, 1190
Eisenmenger's syndrome, lung transplantation
    in, 941
Ejaculation disorders
with α-adrenergic antagonists, 903, 905, 903t,
    906t
with 5α-reductase inhibitors, 905, 906t
Ejection fraction, 81
Elderly
acute lymphocytic leukemia in, 1589
acute myelogenous leukemia in, 1593
allergic rhinitis in, 1059
antimicrobials in, 1164
bipolar disorder in, 686
constipation in, 375
depression in, 665
diuretics in, 64–65
drug use by, 4
GERD in, 323
hypertension in, 70, 72
inflammatory bowel disease in, 352
ischemic heart disease in, 126
obesity in, 1728
pain in, 568
    assessment of, 571–572
schizophrenia in, 645
status epilepticus in, 549–550
tuberculosis in, 1256
Electrocardiogram, 159–160
in acute coronary syndromes, 132–134, 136
in ischemic heart disease, 114, 115–116
relationship to ventricular action potential,
    159, 159f
in stroke, 218
Electroconvulsive therapy
adverse effects of, 656
in depression, 656
in schizophrenia, 646

Electrodesiccation and curettage, in
    nonmelanoma skin cancer, 1625
Electroencephalogram
in epilepsy, 523
in status epilepticus, 541, 543
video-EEG, 523
Electrolytes, 479–493. *See also* specific elements
in diabetic ketoacidosis, 756
for parenteral nutrition, 1685, 1685t, 1692
Eletriptan
dosage of, 589t
drug interactions of, 589t, 591
in migraine, 589t
Elimination
in geriatric patients, 11
in pediatric patients, 27–28
Elimination diet, in irritable bowel
    syndrome, 383
Eltrombopag
dosage of, 1135
in immune thrombocytopenic purpura,
    1134–1135
Embolectomy, pulmonary, 206
Embolism, 195
pulmonary. *See* Pulmonary embolism
septic, 1237
Embolization, 193
Embryology, 822–823
phases of embryonic and fetal development,
    822t, 823f
teratogen, 822–823, 824t
Emedastine
adverse effects of, 1069t
in allergic conjunctivitis, 1068t, 1070
dosage of, 1069t
mechanism of action of, 1068t
Emergency contraception, 853
Emesis. *See* Vomiting
Emollients
in constipation, 374, 374t
in contact dermatitis, 1102
in pruritus, 467–468
Emphysema, 289. *See also* Chronic obstructive
    pulmonary disease
Empyema, 1131t
Emtricitabine
adverse effects of, 1425, 1426, 1427t–1428t,
    1437t–1440t
dosage of, 1427t–1428t
drug interactions of, 1427t–1428t
in HIV infection, 1425, 1427t–1428t, 1433,
    1435
mechanism of action of, 1421f
Enalapril
in acute coronary syndromes, 142t
adverse effects of, 62t
dosage of, 62t, 92t, 121t, 142t
drug interactions of, 955t
in heart failure, 93, 92t
in hypertension, 62t
in ischemic heart disease, 121t
Enalaprilat
adverse effects of, 71t
dosage of, 71t
in hypertensive emergency, 71t
Encainide, in ventricular premature
    depolarizations, 176
Encephalitis, 1170
anxiety with, 694t
viral, 1183
    psychotic symptoms in, 635t
Encephalopathy, hepatic. *See* Hepatic
    encephalopathy

Endarterectomy, 220
Endemic fungi, in invasive candidiasis, 1385
Endemic mycosis, 1376–1382, 1376t
    case study of, 1378, 1380
    clinical presentation in, 1377–1378
    diagnosis of, 1377–1378
    epidemiology of, 1376, 1377f
    pathophysiology of, 1376–1377, 1377f
    patient monitoring in, 1381–1382
    prophylaxis for, 1382
    radiographs, 1378
    signs and symptoms, 1378
    treatment of, 1378–1381, 1379t–1380t
Endocarditis
    heart failure and, 84t
    infective. See Infective endocarditis
    nonbacterial thrombotic, 1237, 1237a
Endocrine disease. See also specific diseases
    constipation in, 372t
    nausea and vomiting in, 358t
Endometrial ablation
    in anovulatory bleeding, 865
    in menorrhagia, 861
Endometrial cancer, oral contraceptives
        and, 844
Endometrial polyps, menstruation-related
        disorders in, 857t
Endometritis, 851
    peritonitis in, 1283
Endomyocardial fibrosis, 80t
Endoscopic retrograde cholangiopancreatography,
        pancreatitis and, 404
Endoscopic therapy
    band ligation in variceal bleeding, 395
    in GERD, 321
Endoscopy
    in amebiasis, 1296
    in GERD, 315, 316f, 318
    in peptic ulcer disease, 332
Endothelial cells, in arterial wall, 232
Endothelin, in heart failure, 83, 104
End-stage heart failure, palliative care treatment
        for, 37–38
End-stage liver disease, palliative care treatment
        for, 38–39
End-stage renal disease (ESRD), 445–476. See
        also Kidney disease, chronic
    in diabetes mellitus, 758
    epidemiology of, 446–447
    etiology of, 446–447
    palliative care treatment for, 38
    pathophysiology of, 448
    treatment of
        kidney transplant, 468, 941
        renal replacement therapy, 468–475
Enema, hyperphosphatemia with, 491
Energy expenditure
    basal, 1688, 1689t
    daily, 1688, 1689t
    obesity and, 1721
    per body weight, 1689t
    total daily, 1688, 1689t
Energy intake, obesity and, 1720–1721
Energy requirement, 1703
Enfuvirtide
    adverse effects of, 1431t
    dosage of, 1431t
    drug interactions of, 1431t
    in HIV infection, 1431t
    mechanism of action of, 1421f
Engerix-B, 420, 420t
Engraftment, of hematopoietic stem cells, 1630,
        1631, 1633

Enoxaparin
    in acute coronary syndromes, 140t, 145, 146, 148
    dosage of, 140t, 192t, 195t, 198
    in prevention of venous thromboembolism,
        192t, 193
    in venous thromboembolism, 195t, 198
Entacapone
    dosage of, 559t
    mechanism of action of, 559t
    in Parkinson's disease, 559t, 562
Entamoeba histolytica, 1295–1296. See also
        Amebiasis
Entecavir
    adverse effects of, 423
    in chronic hepatitis B, 423
    dosage of, 423
    resistance to, 423
Enteral feeding formula, 1706–1711
    caloric density of, 1707, 1708t, 1710
    compatibility of medication with, 1714
    contaminated, 1713
    diabetic formula, 1709–1710, 1709t
    dilution of, 1707
    fiber content of, 1707, 1709
    free-water content of, 1713
    hepatic formula, 1710–1711
    immune-enhancing ingredients in, 1708–1709
    lipid content of, 1708
    nonprotein kilocalories to nitrogen ratio, 1708
    oligomeric, 1707, 1708t, 1714
    polymeric, 1707, 1708t, 1714
    products available, 1708t
    protein content of, 1707–1708, 1710
    pulmonary formula, 1708t, 1709
    renal formula, 1710, 1710t
    stress/trauma formula, 1708–1709, 1708t
Enteral nutrition, 1701–1716
    access sites for, 1704–1706, 1705f, 1705t
    bolus feeding, 1706
    case study of, 1706, 1710, 1715
    compared with parenteral nutrition, 1682,
        1703–1704
    complications of, 1711–1713
        gastrointestinal, 1711–17123, 1711t
        infectious, 1711t, 1713
        metabolic, 1713
        refeeding syndrome, 1713
        technical, 1711t, 1712, 1714
        tube displacement, 1711t, 1712
        tube occlusion, 1711t, 1712, 1714
    continuous feeding, 1706
    contraindications and precautions in, 1703, 1703t
    cost of, 1704
    definition of, 1701
    gastric feeding, 1704
    indications for, 1703, 1513t
    in inflammatory bowel disease, 352
    intermittent feeding, 1706
    medication administration through feeding
        tube, 1714–1715
    outcome evaluation in, 1713–1714
    patient care and monitoring in, 1712t,
        1713–1714, 1716
    patient selection for, 1703–1704
    postpyloric feedings, 1706
    safety of, 1704
    in sepsis, 1357
    transition from parenteral nutrition to,
        1693
Enteric-coated dosage form, administration
        through feeding tubes, 1714
Enteric fever, 1269–1270
Enteric nervous system, 381

Enterobacter
    in COPD exacerbations, 298, 299t
    in infections in cancer patients, 1655t
    in infective endocarditis, 1242
    in necrotizing fasciitis, 1226
    in sepsis, 1348t
    in surgical site infections, 1397t
    in urinary tract infections, 1308
Enterobacteriaceae
    in diabetic foot infections, 1227
    in meningitis, 1177t, 1182
    normal flora, 1157f
    in osteomyelitis, 1339t, 1342t
Enterobiasis, 1297–1298
Enterococci
    in diabetic foot infections, 1227
    in infections in cancer patients, 1655t, 1658
    in infective endocarditis, 1236, 1241,
        1247–1248, 1247t, 1250
    in intra-abdominal infections, 1284, 1286t,
        1288, 1356
    normal flora, 1157f
    in osteomyelitis, 1339t, 1342t
    in sepsis, 1348t, 1354
    in surgical site infections, 1397t
    in urinary tract infections, 1308, 1310
    vancomycin-resistant, 1247–1248, 1275, 1658
Enterocolitis, necrotizing, 1131t
Enterocytes, 230, 231f, 1702, 1702f
    duodenal, 230
    jejunal, 230
Enterokinase, 404
Enterovirus
    in CNS infections, 1183
    in pneumonia, 1190
Enuresis, 712, 713, 910, 919–925
    adult, 912, 920
    clinical presentation in, 920
    definition of, 919–920
    diagnosis of, 920
    diurnal, 919
    drug-related, 920
    epidemiology of, 920
    etiology of, 920, 921t
    genetic factors in, 920
    monosymptomatic, 920
    nocturnal, 919
    outcome evaluation in, 924
    pathophysiology of, 920
    patient care and monitoring in, 925
    pediatric, 919–925
    polysymptomatic, 920
    primary, 919–920
    secondary, 920
    treatment of, 921–924
        behavioral treatments, 922–923, 923t
        desmopressin, 923–924, 816t
        ICCS protocol, 922a, 924
        imipramine, 924, 816t
        nonpharmacologic, 922–923, 923t
        oxybutynin, 924, 816t
Environmental factors
    in breast cancer, 1477
    in cancer, 1446
    in colorectal cancer, 1518
    in lung cancer, 1500
    in migraines, 588t
    in non-Hodgkin's lymphoma, 1553
    in psoriasis, 1080
Environmental tobacco smoke, 1500
Environment theory, of multiple sclerosis, 508
Enzyme-linked immunosorbent assay, for HIV,
        1422, 1422t

Eosinophilia, 1159*t*
Ependymoma, 1447*t*
Ephedra, 125–126, 694*t*
  for weight loss, 1728
Ephedrine
  drug interactions of, 660
  in urinary incontinence, 917
  for weight loss, 1728
Epidermophyton, 1369
Epidural analgesia, 576
Epilepsy, 521–539. *See also* Seizure; Status epilepticus
  case study of, 526, 536, 538
  classification and presentation of, 524–526,
    524*a*, 525*t*
  clinical presentation in, 523
  comorbid disease states, 535–536
  definition of, 523
  depression and, 536
  diagnosis of, 523, 526
  electroencephalogram in, 523
  epidemiology of, 521–522
  etiology of, 522
  genetic factors in, 523
  head trauma and, 52
  magnetic resonance imaging in, 523
  outcome evaluation in, 538–539
  pathophysiology of, 524–524
  patient care and monitoring in, 538
  in pediatric patients, 537
  in pregnancy, 537–538, 537*t*
  social impact of, 522
  stroke and, 522
  treatment of, 526–538. *See also* Antiepileptic drugs
    algorithm for, 449*f*
    drug selection and seizure type, 529–531, 531*t*
    ketogenic diet, 528
    nonpharmacologic, 527–528
    stopping antiepileptic drugs, 536
    surgical, 527, 528
    vagal nerve stimulation, 527–528
  in women, 537–538
Epilepsy syndrome, 524, 525, 525*t*
  cryptogenic, 525
  idiopathic, 525
  symptomatic, 525
Epileptogenesis, 523
Epinastine
  adverse effects of, 1069*t*
  in allergic conjunctivitis, 1068*t*
  dosage of, 1069*t*
  mechanism of action of, 1068*t*
Epinephrine, 784
  adverse effects of, 1043
  in anaphylaxis, 931*t*
  arrhythmia with, 260*t*
  in asthma, 277*t*
  in atrioventricular nodal block, 165
  dosage of, 179*t*, 260*t*, 931*t*
  for facilitation of defibrillation, 178, 179*a*, 179*t*
  in glaucoma, 1043
  in hypovolemic shock, 260, 260*t*
  in sepsis, 1356
  in sinus bradycardia, 164
Epipodophyllotoxins
  adverse effects of, 1580*t*
  allergic drug reactions, 933
  extravasation of, 1678
  secondary malignancies and, 1594
Epirubicin, 1460
  adverse effects of, 1460, 1485, 1484*t*
  in breast cancer, 1482, 1483*t*–1484*t*, 1491
  in cancer therapy, 1460
  dosage of, 1483*t*–1484*t*, 1485

emetogenicity of, 365*t*
  extravasation of, 1677*t*
  mechanism of action of, 1460
  pharmacokinetics of, 1460
Episcleritis, in inflammatory bowel disease, 344
Epistaxis
  in allergic rhinitis, 1052
  with corticosteroids, 953*t*
  in hemophilia, 1124
  in von Willebrand's disease, 1128
Eplerenone
  in acute coronary syndromes, 143*t*
  adverse effects of, 60*t*, 150
  cost of, 149
  dosage of, 60*t*, 92*t*, 95, 143*t*
  in heart failure, 92*t*, 95
  in hypertension, 60*t*, 65, 66*t*
  in prevention of myocardial infarction, 150
Epoetin. *See also* Erythropoietin
  in anemia
    of chronic disease, 1116
    of chronic kidney disease, 1117
  in cancer/chemotherapy-related anemia, 1114*a*,
    1116, 1117*t*
  dosage of, 1117*t*
Epoetin alfa in anemia of chronic kidney disease,
  456, 459*t*
Epoetin *β*, in anemia of chronic kidney disease, 456
Epstein-Barr virus
  acute leukemia and, 1580*t*
  in CNS infections, 1183
  dry eye in, 1074*t*
  lymphoma and, 1552–1553
  in pharyngitis, 1214
  posttransplant lymphoproliferative disorder
    and, 960
Eptifibatide
  in acute coronary syndromes, 141*t*, 147
  adverse effects of, 147
  dosage of, 141*t*
Epworth Sleepiness Scale, 713
Erectile dysfunction, 883–893
  with 5*α*-reductase inhibitors, 905, 906*t*
  case study of, 887, 892
  clinical presentation in, 886
  definition of, 883
  in diabetes mellitus, 885, 885*t*
  diagnosis of, 886
  drug-related, 885*t*
  epidemiology of, 884
  etiology of, 884
  in multiple sclerosis, 517
  organic, 881*f*, 885
  outcome evaluation in, 892–893
  pathophysiology of, 884–886, 884*f*
  patient care and monitoring in, 893
  psychogenic, 885
  treatment of, 886–892
    alprostadil, 884*f*, 887*t*, 890–891, 891*f*
    lifestyle modifications, 888
    papaverine, 887*t*, 891
    penile prostheses, 884*f*, 888, 888*f*
    phentolamine, 887*t*, 891
    phosphodiesterase type 5 inhibitors, 884*f*,
      887*t*, 888–890
    psychotherapy, 888
    testosterone therapy, 884*f*, 887*t*, 891–892
    vacuum erection devices, 884*f*, 888, 888*f*
    yohimbine, 887*t*, 891
Ergocalciferol, 973
Ergotamine in prevention of migraine, 590*t*
Ergotamine derivatives
  in cluster headaches, 589

in migraine, 588
  in prevention of migraine, 591, 590*t*
Erlotinib, 1467
  adverse effects of, 1467
  in cancer therapy, 1467, 1452*t*
  drug interactions of, 1467
  in lung cancer, 1511
  mechanism of action of, 1467, 1511
  pharmacokinetics of, 1467
Ertapenem
  in cellulitis, 1225*t*
  dosage of, 1225*t*, 1342*t*
  in intra-abdominal infections, 1287*t*
  in osteomyelitis, 1342*t*
  in pneumonia, 1196,1196*t*, 1198
  in sepsis, 1353*t*, 1354
  in surgical prophylaxis, 1398
  in urinary tract infections, 1311*t*
Erysipelas
  clinical presentation in, 1223–1224, 1224*t*
  diagnosis of, 1223–1224, 1224*t*
  epidemiology of, 1223
  etiology of, 1223
  treatment of, 1224–1226
    antibiotics, 1224–1226, 1225*t*
    nonpharmacologic, 1224
Erythema multiforme, allergic drug reaction, 930
Erythema nodosum, in inflammatory bowel
  disease, 344
Erythematous lesions, 1222
Erythrocytapheresis, in sickle cell anemia/
  disease, 1146
Erythrocyte(s), 1110
  physiology of, 1140–1142, 1140*f*
  viscosity of, 1141
Erythrocyte sedimentation rate
  in infections, 1158
  in osteomyelitis, 1341
Erythromycin
  in acne vulgaris, 1097–1098, 1098*t*
  adverse effects of, 1097–1098, 1098*t*
  arrhythmia with, 179*t*
  in campylobacteriosis, 1271
  in chancroid, 1334*t*
  in *Chlamydia*, 1321
  in conjunctivitis, 1066, 1066*t*
  dosage of, 1066*t*, 1098*t*, 1271, 1321, 1334*t*
  drug interactions of, 205*t*, 241, 458*t*, 647, 684,
    698, 699*t*, 816, 955*t*, 1600, 1600*t*, 1726
  in furuncles/carbuncles, 1223*t*
  in gonorrhea, 1320
  in pneumonia, 1195, 1196*t*
  in preoperative bowel cleansing, 1399
  to stimulate gastric motility, 1712
  in surgical prophylaxis, 1400*t*, 1401
Erythromycin base, dosage, 831*t*, 832*t*
Erythromycin-sulfisoxazole
  adverse effects of, 1208*t*
  dosage of, 1208*t*
  in otitis media, 1208*t*
Erythropoiesis, 1110–1111, 1110*f*
Erythropoiesis-stimulating agents
  administration of, 458
  adverse effects of, 458
  in anemia of chronic kidney disease, 456–459,
    457*a*, 459*t*
  dosage of, 459*t*
Erythropoietin, 445, 1110, 1110*f*, 113*t*. *See also*
  Epoetin
  adverse effects of, 54*t*
  in anemia of chronic kidney disease, 455–459
  decreased production or response, 1111, 1116
  in sickle cell anemia/disease, 1146

Escherichia coli
in COPD exacerbations, 298, 299*t*
in diarrhea, 376, 380
enterohemorrhagic, 1272
clinical presentation in, 1272
diagnosis of, 1272
epidemiology of, 1272
monitoring patient with, 1272
pathogenesis of, 1272
treatment of, 1272
enteropathogenic, 380
enterotoxigenic, 380
in infections in cancer patients, 1655*t*
in infective endocarditis, 1242
in intra-abdominal infections, 1284, 1286*t*
in meningitis, 1171*t*
in necrotizing fasciitis, 1226
O157:H7 serotype, 1272
in osteomyelitis, 1339*t*
in peritonitis, 474
in pneumonia, 1190*t*
in sepsis, 1348*t*, 1354
Shiga toxin-producing, 380
in spontaneous bacterial peritonitis, 391
in surgical site infections, 1397, 1397*t*
in travelers' diarrhea, 1273
in urinary tract infections, 1161, 1308, 1310
Escitalopram
adverse effects of, 696, 701*t*
dosage of, 661*t*, 696*t*, 701*t*
in generalized anxiety disorder, 696, 696*t*
in panic disorder, 701*t*
pharmacokinetics of, 659*t*
in social anxiety disorder, 703
ESHAP regimen
in Hodgkin's lymphoma, 1559
in non-Hodgkin's lymphoma, 1561*t*, 1561
Esmolol
adverse effects of, 71*t*, 119*t*
in arrhythmias, 162*t*
dosage of, 71*t*
in hypertension, 66*a*
in hypertensive emergency, 71*t*
mechanism of action of, 163*t*
in thyroid storm, 777
Esomeprazole
dosage of, 320*t*, 321–322, 336*t*
drug interactions of, 322
in GERD, 320*t*, 321–322
in peptic ulcer disease, 336*t*
Esophageal atresia, 1513*t*
Esophageal cancer, 318
epidemiology of, 1446*f*
Esophageal candidiasis, 1366–1369
clinical presentation in, 1367
epidemiology of, 1366
etiology of, 1366
fluconazole-resistant, 1368
outcome evaluation in, 1369
pathophysiology of, 1366
patient care and monitoring in, 1368
recurrent, 1368–1369
risk factors for, 1366, 1366*t*
treatment of, 1366–1369, 1387
Esophageal clearance, in GERD, 316–317
Esophageal motility disorder, 1513*t*
Esophagitis, 319
with bisphosphonates, 974
erosive, 317–318, 321, 323
toxicity criteria, 1453*t*
Esophagostomy tube, 1705*f*
Essential amino acids, 1710
Essential fatty acid(s), 1708

Essential fatty acid deficiency, 1682, 1695
Estazolam
dosage of, 627*t*
in insomnia, 627*t*
Estradiol, 875*t*
drug interactions of, 955*t*
in menstrual cycle, 856, 856*f*
Estramustine, 1458
adverse effects of, 1458, 1547, 1547*t*
in cancer therapy, 1458
dosage of, 1547, 1547*t*
mechanism of action of, 1458
pharmacokinetics of, 1458
in prostate cancer, 1547–1548, 1547*t*
Estrogen receptor, in breast cancer, 1486
Estrogen therapy. *See also* Hormone-replacement
therapy
in acne vulgaris, 1099
adverse effects of, 86*t*, 467, 874, 876*t*, 918*t*
Alzheimer's disease and, 597, 602
augmentation of antidepressant therapy with,
662
in breast cancer, 1487*t*, 1490
dosage of, 918*t*
drug interactions of, 955*t*
erectile dysfunction with, 885*t*
GERD with, 317*t*
in hemorrhagic cystitis, 1669
hypercalcemia with, 490
hyperlipidemia with, 236*t*
hyperprolactinemia with, 814*t*
in menopause, 874, 875*t*
migraines with, 588*t*
oral, 874, 875*t*
pancreatitis with, 404*t*
pharmacokinetics of, 918*t*
in prostate cancer, 1539, 1546
topical, 875*t*
transdermal preparations, 874, 875*t*
trophic effects on uroepithelium, 910
in uremic bleeding, 467
vaginal, in urinary incontinence, 917, 918*t*
venous thromboembolism with, 187, 187*t*
Estropipate, 875*t*
Estrostep Fe, 849
Eszopiclone
dosage of, 627*t*
in insomnia, 627*t*
pharmacokinetics of, 627*t*
Etanercept, 988
adverse effects of, 986*t*, 991, 1088
dosage of, 986*t*
in GVHD, 1640
mechanism of action of, 991, 1087
monitoring treatment with, 986*t*
in psoriasis, 1087–1088
in rheumatoid arthritis, 986*t*, 991
Ethacrynic acid
in acute renal failure, 437
adverse effects of, 437
dosage of, 100*t*
in heart failure, 100*t*
in hypertension, 65
ototoxicity of, 437
Ethambutol
adverse effects of, 1261*t*
dosage of, 1260*t*, 1261*t*
in tuberculosis, 1258, 1259, 1260, 1260*t*,
1261*t*, 1262
Ethanol. *See* Alcohol *entries*
Ethinyl estradiol, 843, 845*t*, 845, 846,
859*t*, 865
adverse effects of, 1487*t*

in breast cancer, 1487*t*
dosage of, 1487*t*
Ethionamide
adverse effects of, 1261*t*
dosage of, 1261*t*
in tuberculosis, 1261*t*, 1262
Ethnicity
asthma and, 266
cystic fibrosis and, 304
glaucoma and, 1032
heart failure and, 93–94, 97
hepatitis A and, 414
hepatitis C and, 414
HIV infection and, 1420
hypertension and, 52, 70, 72
inflammatory bowel disease and, 342
irritable bowel syndrome and, 381
lung cancer and, 1500
osteoarthritis and, 998
prostate cancer and, 1536, 1536*t*
sickle cell anemia/disease and, 1140
skin cancer and, 1612, 1614*t*
stroke and, 217, 217*t*
tuberculosis and, 1254
Ethosuximide
adverse effects of, 453*t*
anxiety with, 694*t*
dosage of, 453*t*
drug interactions of, 955*t*
in epilepsy, 529–530, 529*t*, 531, 532*t*
mechanism of action of, 453*t*
pharmacokinetics of, 453*t*
Ethylene glycol poisoning, 501, 501*t*, 502
Ethynodiol diacetate, 843, 845*t*
Ethynyl estradiol, 875*t*
Etodolac
dosage of, 1002*t*
in osteoarthritis, 1002*t*
Etomidate
adverse effects of, 796*t*
in Cushing's syndrome, 796*t*
dosage of, 796*t*
mechanism of action of, 796*t*
Etoposide, 1459
in acute myelogenous leukemia, 1591*t*, 1592
adverse effects of, 1459, 1470, 1563, 1574*t*, 1581,
1591*t*, 1644
in cancer therapy, 1459
dosage of, 1507*t*, 1557*t*, 1561*t*, 1574*t*, 1593,
1634*t*
in renal dysfunction, 1470*t*
drug interactions of, 955*t*, 1591*t*
extravasation of, 1677, 1677*t*
in Hodgkin's lymphoma, 1557*t*
in lung cancer, 1506, 1507*t*–1508*t*, 1508
mechanism of action of, 1454*a*, 1459, 1591*t*
in non-Hodgkin's lymphoma, 1561*t*
in ovarian cancer, 1573, 1574*t*
pharmacokinetics of, 1459
in preparation for hematopoietic cell
transplant, 1634*t*
Etravirine
adverse effects of, 1429*t*
dosage of, 1429*t*
drug interactions of, 1429*t*
food interactions of, 1429*t*
in HIV infection, 1429*t*
Etretinate, teratogenic effects of, 824*t*
Euthymia, 656
Euthyroid, 764
Euthyroid sick syndrome, 777
Evening primrose oil, 878, 879*t*
Everolimus, 952

Exanatide
in diabetes mellitus, 754–755, 754*t*
dosage of, 754*t*
Exanthem, allergic drug reaction, 931
Exchange transfusion
in iron overload, 1146
in malaria, 1302
in sickle cell anemia/disease, 1146
Exemestane, 1469
adverse effects of, 1469, 1489, 1487*t*
in breast cancer, 1487, 1489, 1487*t*
in cancer therapy, 1469
dosage of, 1487*t*
mechanism of action of, 1469, 1489
osteoporosis with, 966*t*
pharmacokinetics of, 1469
Exercise electrocardiogram (stress test), in ischemic
heart disease, 114, 116
Exercise-induced asthma, 267, 278, 280, 283
Exercise program
in constipation, 373
in COPD, 293
in diabetes mellitus, 747
in generalized anxiety disorder, 695
in heart failure, 88
in hypertension, 58, 59*t*
in ischemic heart disease, 117–118
in menopause, 872
in musculoskeletal disorders, 1027–1028
in obesity, 1724, 1724*t*
in osteoarthritis, 1000
in Parkinson's disease, 557
in prevention of osteoporosis, 969–970
Exfoliative dermatitis, allergic drug reaction, 933
Exophthalmos, in Graves' disease, 774, 775*f*
Expedited partner treatment, 1318
Extended-release preparation, administration
through feeding tubes, 1714
External analgesics, in musculoskeletal disorders,
1024–1025, 1026*t*
Extracellular fluid, 253, 253*f*, 480
ion concentrations in, 484*t*
volume of, 480
Extracorporeal circulation, 1131*t*
Extraction ratios, 11
Extrapyramidal symptoms, 591
with antipsychotics, 636, 638*t*, 641, 642*t*, 644
with phenothiazines, 360, 363
treatment of, 647
Extrapyramidal system, anatomy of, 554–555, 554*f*
Extravasation injury, 546
chemotherapy drugs, 1469, 1676–1679
clinical presentation in, 1677
diagnosis of, 1677
epidemiology of, 1676
etiology of, 1676
outcome evaluation in, 1679
pathophysiology of, 1677
patient care and monitoring in, 1679
prevention of, 1677, 1678*t*
risk factors for, 1676, 1676*t*
treatment of, 1677–1679
Eye
anatomy of, 1033*f*
drug-induced disorders of, 1077*t*, 1077
dry. See Dry eye
minor ophthalmic disorders, 1063–1077
ocular emergencies. See Ocular emergencies
in sickle cell anemia/disease, 1152*t*
Eyelid edema, drug-induced, 1077*t*
Ezetimibe
adverse effects of, 243*t*
dosage of, 243*t*

in hyperlipidemia, 241*t*, 243*t*, 244, 243*t*,
246–247, 956*t*
mechanism of action of, 244
metabolism of, 244

F
FAB classification
of acute lymphocytic leukemia, 1581–1583, 1582*t*
of acute myelogenous leukemia, 1581–1583,
1582*t*
Fabry's disease, kidney transplantation in, 941
FACES of Pain Rating Scale, 571
FAC regimen, in breast cancer, 1483*t*
Factor II, deficiency of, 1129, 1129*t*, 1130*t*
Factor IX, deficiency of. See Hemophilia B
Factor IX concentrate
in hemophilia B, 991*t*, 1124*t*, 1125
products available, 1124*t*
Factor IX inhibitors, 1125–1126
Factor V, deficiency of, 1129, 1129*t*, 1130*t*
Factor V Leiden, 187, 187*t*
Factor VII, deficiency of, 1129, 1129*t*, 1130*t*
Factor VIIa
in hypovolemic shock, 259
recombinant
in intracerebral hemorrhage, 225
in recessively inherited coagulation
disorders, 1129*t*, 1130*t*
Factor VIII
deficiency of. See Hemophilia A
excess of, 187*t*
Factor VIII concentrate
in hemophilia A, 1124–1125, 1124*t*, 991*t*
porcine factor VIII, 1125–1126
products available, 1124*t*
virus-inactivated, in von Willebrand's disease,
1127–1128
Factor VIII inhibitors, 1125–1126, 1126*a*
Factor X, deficiency of, 1129, 1129*t*, 1130*t*
Factor Xa inhibitors, in venous
thromboembolism, 199–200
Factor XI
deficiency of, 1129, 1129*t*, 1130*t*
excess of, 187*t*
Factor XII, deficiency of, 1129, 1129*t*, 1130*t*
Factor XIII, deficiency of, 1129, 1129*t*, 1130*t*
Fagerström Test for Nicotine Dependence, 622
Failure to thrive, inflammatory bowel disease
and, 352
Falls
drug-related, 970
eye injury in, 1063
prevention of, 970
Famciclovir
adverse effects of, 1330*t*
dosage of, 1330*t*
in genital herpes, 1330*t*
Familial adenomatous polyposis, 1343*t*, 1519, 1520
Famotidine
arrhythmia with, 179*t*
dosage of, 320*t*, 336*t*
in GERD, 320*t*, 321
with pancreatic enzyme supplements, 409
in parenteral nutrition admixture, 1687
in peptic ulcer disease, 336*t*
Fanconi's anemia, 1630*t*
acute leukemia and, 1580*t*
Fasciitis, necrotizing. See Necrotizing fasciitis
Fasting plasma glucose, 740, 741*t*
Fat(s). See Lipid(s)
Fat embolism, 1131*t*
Fatigue
in heart failure, 84, 85

in multiple sclerosis, 515, 516, 516*t*
in Parkinson's disease, 555
treatment of, 440*t*
Fat maldistribution, drug-related, 1442*t*
Fatty acids
in enteral feeding formulas, 1708–1709
essential, 1708
in intravenous lipid emulsions, 1683–1684,
1684*t*
essential fatty acid deficiency, 1683
omega-3 polyunsaturated, 117, 246, 1708–1709
omega-6 polyunsaturated, 1708–1709
short-chain, 1702, 1707
Fatty liver
in alcoholic liver disease, 391–392
in nonalcoholic liver disease, 392
of pregnancy, 1131*t*
Fatty streak, 112, 112*f*, 132, 232
Febuxostat
adverse effects of, 1016
in antihyperuricemic treatment, 1016
dosage of, 1014*t*, 1016
in gout, 1014*t*
Fecal impaction, 376, 921*t*
urinary incontinence in, 912
Fecal occult blood tests, screening for colorectal
cancer, 1519, 1520*t*
FEC regimen, in breast cancer, 1483*t*
Feeding tube, 1701–1716. See also Enteral
nutrition; *specific types of tubes*
flushing of, 1714
medication administered through, 1714–1715
placement of, 1705*t*
Felbamate
adverse effects of, 531, 532*t*, 536, 537*t*
dosage of, 453*t*
drug interactions of, 458*t*, 850*t*
in epilepsy, 453*t*
mechanism of action of, 453*t*
pharmacokinetics of, 453*t*
Felodipine
anxiety with, 694*t*
drug interactions of, 955*t*
in heart failure, 96
in ischemic heart disease, 123
Felty's syndrome, in rheumatoid arthritis, 984
Fenfluramine, 1725
Fenofibrate
adverse effects of, 243*t*
in antihyperuricemic treatment, 1016
dosage of, 243*t*
drug interactions of, 205*t*
in hyperlipidemia, 241*t*, 243*t*, 246
Fenoldopam
in acute renal failure, 439
adverse effects of, 71*t*
dosage of, 71*t*
in hypertensive emergency, 71*t*
Fenoprofen
dosage of, 1014*t*
in gout, 1014*t*
Fentanyl
dosage of, 575*t*
for epidural analgesia, 576
in pain, 575*t*, 576
in sickle cell anemia/disease, 1150
in pancreatitis, 406
in PCA pumps, 576
transdermal, in osteoarthritis, 1006
Fenugreek, 206*t*
Ferric gluconate, 1688
iron content of, 1115*t*
in iron-deficiency anemia, 1115, 1115*t*, 1116

Ferrous fumarate
  iron content of, 1115*t*
  in iron-deficiency anemia, 1115*t*
Ferrous gluconate
  iron content of, 1115*t*
  in iron-deficiency anemia, 1115*t*
Ferrous sulfate
  drug interactions of, 321
  iron content of, 1115*t*
  in iron-deficiency anemia, 1115*t*
Fertile window, 852
Fertility awareness-based methods, 852–853
Fertilization, 843
Festination, in Parkinson's disease, 555
Fetal hemoglobin, 1140, 1141–1142
Fetal hemoglobin inducers, in sickle cell anemia/
    disease, 1143*t*, 1144
Fever
  in infection, 1158
  vaccine-related, 1415
Feverfew, 125, 579
Fexofenadine
  in allergic rhinitis, 1053, 1054, 1054*t*
  in nausea and vomiting, 360
Fiber, dietary, in constipation, 373
Fibrates
  adverse effects of, 246
  drug interactions of, 241, 245–246
  in hyperlipidemia, 151, 241*t*, 243*t*, 245–246, 959
  mechanism of action of, 245–246
Fibrin, 188, 1121, 1122*f*
Fibrinolysis, 188, 1121, 1130
Fibrinolysis inhibitors, in von Willebrand's
    disease, 1128
Fibrinolytic therapy. *See also* Thrombolytic
    therapy; *specific drugs*
  in acute coronary syndromes, 135, 137, 141*t*,
      144, 144*t*, 147, 152*t*
  adverse effects of, 144, 152*t*
  contraindications to, 141*t*, 144*t*
  cost of, 149
Fibroadenoma, of breast, 845
Fibrocystic breast disease, 1476
Fibromyalgia, 568
Fibrothorax, respiratory acidosis with, 426*t*
FIGO staging system, in ovarian cancer, 1569,
    1570*a*
Filgrastim
  adverse effects of, 1657*t*
  dosage of, 1632, 1657*t*
  in mobilization of peripheral blood
      progenitor
  cells, 1632, 1637
  in neutropenia, 1512
  prophylactic, in neutropenic cancer patients,
      1657, 1657*t*
Finasteride
  in benign prostatic hyperplasia, 896, 904, 905*t*,
      1537
  dosage of, 1537
  mechanism of action of, 896
  pharmacologic properties of, 905*t*
  in prevention of prostate cancer, 1537
  in prostate cancer, 1539*t*
Fine-needle aspiration biopsy in lung cancer,
    1502*t*
Fish oils
  in hyperlipidemia, 246
  in pain, 579
Fixed drug eruption, 932
Flank pain, in urinary tract infections, 1307
Flavoxate, in urinary incontinence, 516
Flaxseed, 878

Flecainide
  adverse effects of, 86*t*, 119*t*
  arrhythmia with, 162*t*, 163*t*, 177*t*, 179*t*
  in atrial fibrillation, 170*t*, 171*a*, 171*t*
  dosage of, 170*t*
  drug interactions of, 170*t*
  mechanism of action of, 163*t*
  in ventricular premature depolarizations, 176
Flight of ideas, in cyclothymic disorder, 671
Floppy baby syndrome, 686
Floppy iris syndrome, 904
Flow cytometry, immunophenotyping by, 1583
Fluconazole
  arrhythmia with, 179*t*
  in coccidioidomycosis, 1380*t*
  in cryptococcosis, 1386*t*, 1389
  dosage of, 833*t*, 1363*t*, 1364, 1364*t*, 1367–1368,
      1380*t*, 1384, 1385, 1386*t*, 1387, 1389, 1642
  drug interactions of, 205*t*, 458*t*, 615*t*, 955*t*,
      1380, 1381
  in endemic mycosis, 1381
  in esophageal candidiasis, 1367–1368, 1387
  in fungal infections, 956*t*, 957
  in infective endocarditis, 1248
  in invasive candidiasis, 1384, 1386*t*, 1385,
      1387
  in oropharyngeal candidiasis, 1367–1368, 1385,
      1387
  in pancreatitis, 406
  in peritonitis, 475
  in prevention of cryptococcosis, 1389
  in prevention of endemic mycosis, 1382
  in prevention of fungal infections, 1642
  in prevention of invasive candidiasis, 1387
  in sepsis, 1355
  teratogenic effects of, 824*t*
  in vulvovaginal candidiasis, 1363*t*, 1364, 1365,
      1364*t*
Fluconazole resistance, 1368
Flucytosine
  in cryptococcosis, 1386*t*, 1389
  dosage of, 1386*t*
  in invasive candidiasis, 1386*t*
  in peritonitis, 474
  in vulvovaginal candidiasis, 1365
Fludarabine, 1456
  adverse effects of, 1456, 1602, 1603*t*
  in cancer therapy, 1456
  in chronic lymphocytic leukemia, 1602, 1603*t*
  dosage of, 1560*t*, 1602, 1603*t*, 1634*t*
  mechanism of action of, 1454*a*, 1456
  in non-Hodgkin's lymphoma, 1559, 1560*t*
  pharmacokinetics of, 1456
  in preparation for hematopoietic cell
      transplant, 1634*t*, 1636
Fludrocortisone
  in adrenal insufficiency, 786, 789*t*
  in hyperkalemia, 454
Fluid balance, 479–493, 480*t*
  case study of, 481, 486
  in diarrhea, 377
  enteral nutrition and, 1713
  parenteral nutrition and, 1685
Fluid and electrolyte homeostatic mechanism, in
    elderly patients, 12
Fluid loss
  insensible, 480
  sensible, 480
Fluid management
  in constipation, 373
  in diarrhea, 377, 378
  in hypovolemic shock, 257–259
  indications for, 483

  in intra-abdominal infections, 1285
  monitoring of, 484
  in pancreatitis, 405–406
  in prevention of contrast-induced
      nephropathy, 441
  in sepsis, 1352
  therapeutic fluids, 481–484, 482*t*
Fluid requirement, 481
  calculation of, 481*t*
  in pediatric patients, 25
Fluid restriction
  in chronic kidney disease, 453
  in heart failure, 88–89
Fluid retention, in heart failure, 84
Flukes, 1297
Flumazenil
  in alcohol intoxication, 615
  in hepatic encephalopathy, 399
Flumethasone pivalate
  in contact dermatitis, 1103*t*
  dosage and potency of, 1103*t*
Flunisolide
  in allergic rhinitis, 1052, 1052*t*
  in asthma, 276*t*
  dosage of, 276*t*
Fluocinolone acetonide
  in contact dermatitis, 1103*t*
  dosage and potency of, 1103*t*
Fluocinonide
  in contact dermatitis, 1103*t*
  dosage and potency of, 1103*t*
  in psoriasis, 1084
Fluoroquinolone(s). *See also specific drugs*
  administration through feeding tube, 1715
  adverse effects of, 1342*t*
  in bite wound infections, 1233
  in campylobacteriosis, 1271
  in cellulitis, 1225*t*
  Clostridium difficile-associated diarrhea
      and, 1274
  in corneal abrasion, 1064
  in cystic fibrosis, 309, 310
  in diabetic foot infections, 1229*t*
  drug interactions of, 1114, 1342*t*
  in gonorrhea, 1319
  in infections in cancer patients, 1660*t*
  in intra-abdominal infections, 1286
  in keratitis, 1071, 1071*t*
  in osteomyelitis, 1341
  in peritonitis, 474
  in prevention of infections in neutropenic
      patients, 1657
  prophylactic, in hematopoietic cell transplant
      recipients, 1641
  respiratory, 1095–1097, 1213, 1213*a*
  in sepsis, 1353*t*, 1354
  in shigellosis, 1268
  in surgical prophylaxis, 1397, 1399
  in urinary tract infections, 1310, 1311*t*, 1313
Fluoroquinolone resistance, 1204, 1271
Fluorouracil, 1454–1455
  adverse effects of, 1455, 1484*t*, 1527–1528,
      1528*t*, 1519
  in dihydropyrimidine dehydrogenase
      deficiency, 1527–1529
  in breast cancer, 1482, 1483*t*, 1492
  in cancer therapy, 1452*t*, 1454–1455
  in colorectal cancer, 1524–1525, 1524*t*, 1526,
      1527–1528, 1527*t*, 1528*t*
  dosage of, 1483*t*, 1524*t*, 1527
  drug interactions of, 205*t*
  extravasation of, 1677*t*
  mechanism of action of, 1454, 1454*a*, 1527, 1528*t*

mucositis with, 1455
in ovarian cancer, 1573
pharmacokinetics of, 1455
Fluorouracil/epinephrine/bovine collagen gel, in
genital warts, 1328
Fluoxetine, 828t, 878
adverse effects of, 659t, 701t, 879t
arrhythmia with, 163t
in bipolar disorder, 685
in cataplexy, 716
in depression, 665
dosage of, 660, 661t, 696t, 701t, 879t
drug interactions of, 205t, 646t, 660t, 699t,
955t, 1726
in generalized anxiety disorder, 696t
in irritable bowel syndrome, 383
in panic disorder, 701t
pharmacokinetics of, 659, 659t
in pregnancy, 665
in vasomotor symptoms of menopause, 879t
for weight loss, 1728
Fluoxymesterone, 891
adverse effects of, 1487t
in breast cancer, 1487t
dosage of, 1487t
Fluphenazine
adverse effects of, 642t
dosage of, 640t, 640, 641t
metabolism of, 647
in schizophrenia, 640t, 640, 641t
Flurandrenolide
in contact dermatitis, 1103t
dosage and potency of, 1103t
Flurazepam
dosage of, 627t
drug interactions of, 614t
in insomnia, 627t
pharmacokinetics of, 627t
Flurbiprofen
dosage of, 1014t
in gout, 1014t
Flushing, with niacin, 245
Flutamide, 1468
adverse effects of, 1468, 1545t
in cancer therapy, 1468
dosage of, 1545t
drug interactions of, 955t
mechanism of action of, 1468
pharmacokinetics of, 1468
in prostate cancer, 1539t, 1545, 1546, 1545t
Fluticasone
adverse effects of, 1052
in allergic rhinitis, 1052, 1059
in asthma, 273, 276t
in contact dermatitis, 1103t
in COPD, 295t
dosage of, 276t, 295t, 830t, 1103t
Fluticasone furoate, in allergic rhinitis,
1052, 1052t
Fluticasone propionate, in allergic rhinitis, 1052,
1052t, 1059
Flutter valve device, in cystic fibrosis, 307
Fluvastatin
adverse effects of, 242t
dosage of, 242t
in hyperlipidemia, 241t, 242t
Fluvoxamine
adverse effects of, 701t
dosage of, 661t, 696t, 701t
drug interactions of, 205t, 561, 646t, 660t, 698,
699t, 955t, 1726
in generalized anxiety disorder, 696t
in panic disorder, 701t

pharmacokinetics of, 659t
in social anxiety disorder, 703
Foam cells, 232
FOLFIRI regimen, in colorectal cancer, 1524t,
1525–1526, 1527t
FOLFOX regimen, in colorectal cancer, 1524,
1524t, 1525, 1526, 1527t, 1530
Folic acid
deficiency of, 1111, 1114a, 1118
dietary, colorectal cancer and, 1518
dosage, 830t
food sources of, 1115t
pregnancy, 827
treatment of, 1116
Folic acid supplementation
adverse effects of, 1116
dosage of, 1116
drug interactions of, 245, 1116
in folic acid deficiency, 1116
in ischemic heart disease, 125
with methotrexate therapy, 990
with pemetrexed, 1457
in pregnancy, 538
in prevention of colorectal cancer, 1520
in sickle cell anemia/disease, 1144, 1145
Folinic acid. *See* Leucovorin
Follicle-stimulating hormone
at menopause, 870–871
in menstrual cycle, 843, 856, 856f
Folliculitis
clinical presentation in, 1223t
diagnosis of, 1223t
epidemiology of, 1223t
etiology of, 1223t
treatment of, 1223t
Fondaparinux
for acute coronary syndromes, 146, 149
adverse effects of, 198t, 199–200
dosage of, 192t, 195t, 200
mechanism of action of, 196, 196f, 199–200
in venous thromboembolism, 194a, 195t,
199–200, 207
in prevention of, 192t, 193
Food(s)
calcium-rich, 969, 969t
GERD symptoms caused by, 317t
migraine triggers, 588t
rich in vitamin K, 206t
sources of iron, folic acid, or vitamin B$_{12}$, 1115t
tyramine-containing, 1462
Food intolerance, 376
Food poisoning, 1278, 1278t
clinical presentation in, 1278t
treatment of, 1278t
Foot infection, diabetic. *See* Diabetic foot
infection
Foreign body, in eye, 1064t, 1065
Formalin, in hemorrhagic cystitis, 1669
Formoterol
in asthma, 273
in COPD, 294, 295t
dosage of, 295t
Fosamprenavir
adverse effects of, 1430t
dosage of, 1430t
drug interactions of, 1430t
in HIV infection, 1425, 1430t
mechanism of action of, 1421f
Fosaprepitant, in chemotherapy-induced nausea
and vomiting, 1652t
Foscarnet
adverse effects of, 442, 1178t, 1330t
dosage of, 1178t, 1183, 1330t

in encephalitis, 1183
in genital herpes, 1329, 1330t
hypokalemia with, 487
hypophosphatemia with, 491
in meningitis, 1178t
nephrotoxicity of, 1381
in prevention of cytomegalovirus, 1642
Fosfomycin
dosage of, 1312t
in urinary tract infections, 1311t, 1312t
Fosinopril
dosage of, 92t, 121t
in heart failure, 92t
in ischemic heart disease, 121t
Fosphenytoin
adverse effects of, 545t, 546–547
dosage of, 545t, 546–547, 546t, 549, 549t
in status epilepticus, 545t, 546–547, 546t, 547,
549, 549t
Fractional excretion of sodium, 453
Fracture. *See also* Osteoporosis
fragility, 965–978
hypercalcemia in, 490
Frailty, 9
Framingham point scale, estimating coronary heart
disease risk, 236, 237f
Frank-Starling mechanism, 81
in heart failure, 81, 81t
FRAX, 968
Free thyroxine, 766t
Fremitus, in tuberculosis, 1255
Fresh-frozen plasma, 483
adverse effects of, 1129
in DIC, 1132
dosage of, 1132
in hypovolemic shock, 259
in recessively inherited coagulation disorders,
1129, 1130t
risks of, 483
Friction, pressure sores and, 1231
Frostbite, 1023
Frovatriptan
dosage of, 589t
drug interactions of, 589t
in migraine, 589t
Fructooligosaccharides, 1707
Fulvestrant, 1469
adverse effects of, 1469, 1487t
in breast cancer, 1490, 1487t
in cancer therapy, 1469
dosage of, 1487t
mechanism of action of, 1469
pharmacokinetics of, 1469
Functional bowel disease, 381
Functional pain, 568
Fungal infection
adrenal insufficiency in, 786t
in cancer patients, 1655, 1655t
endemic. *See* Endemic mycosis
of hair, 1369–1373
in hematopoietic cell transplant recipients,
1641–1643
invasive, 1375–1392
of nails, 1369–1373
opportunistic. *See* Opportunistic mycosis
of skin, 1369–1373
superficial, 1361–1373
in transplant recipient, 956t, 957
Fungemia, definition of, 1348t
Furazolidone
dosage of, 335t, 1294
in giardiasis, 1294
in *Helicobacter pylori* eradication, 335t

Furosemide, 10
  in acute renal failure, 437
  adverse effects of, 437
  allergic drug reactions, 932
  in diuretics, 397
  dosage of, 90t, 100t, 437, 414t, 1671, 1672t
  in heart failure, 89–91, 90t, 100t
  in hypercalcemia, 414t, 1671, 1672t
  in hypermagnesemia, 492
  in hypertension, 64–65
  hypophosphatemia with, 491
  ototoxicity of, 437
  pancreatitis with, 404t
  in resuscitation fluid, 483
  in superior vena cava syndrome, 1663
Furuncle
  clinical presentation in, 1223t
  diagnosis of, 1223t
  epidemiology of, 1223t
  etiology of, 1223t
  treatment of, 1223t
Fusariosis, 1348, 1376t, 1386t
  in cancer patients, 1655t
  in hematopoietic cell transplant recipients, 1642
Fusarium oxysporum, 1376t
Fusarium solani, 1376t
Fusion inhibitors, in HIV infection, 1421f, 1423, 1431t
Fusobacterium
  in bite wound infections, 1232t
  in pneumonia, 1190

G

GABA. *See* Gamma-amino butyric acid
Gabapentin
  adverse effects of, 454t, 717t, 879t
  in bipolar disorder, 684
  dosage of, 454t, 704, 717t, 879t
  in epilepsy, 530, 530t, 531, 532t
  mechanism of action of, 454t
  in oxaliplatin-induced neuropathy, 1530
  in pain, 578, 578t
  pharmacokinetics of, 454t
  in prevention of migraine, 590, 590t
  in restless-legs syndrome, 717, 717t
  in social anxiety disorder, 704
  in vasomotor symptoms of menopause, 878, 879, 879t
Gait abnormalities, in Parkinson's disease, 555
Galactomannan test, for aspergillosis, 1390, 1643
Galactorrhea, in acromegaly, 805
Galantamine
  adverse effects of, 601t, 602
  in Alzheimer's disease, 601t, 602
  dosage of, 601t, 602
  mechanism of action of, 602
  pharmacokinetics of, 602
Gallbladder, 1702
Gallbladder disease
  hormone-replacement therapy and, 876t, 877
  obesity and, 1720
  oral contraceptives and, 846
Gallium nitrate
  dosage of, 414t, 1672t
  in hypercalcemia, 490, 490t, 1672t, 1673
Gallstones
  in inflammatory bowel disease, 344
  octreotide-related, 805–806
  pancreatitis and, 404, 407
  with parenteral nutrition, 1694t, 1696
Gamma aminobutyric acid (GABA), 12
  in alcohol abuse, 609
  in anxiety disorders, 693

  in depression, 654
  in seizures, 522, 535t
  in status epilepticus, 542, 547
Gamma knife, 1665
Ganciclovir
  adverse effects of, 442, 956t
  dosage of, 956t, 1642
  in prevention of cytomegalovirus, 956t, 957, 1642
Gardnerella vaginalis, in bacterial vaginosis, 1331
Garlic, 125
  drug interactions of, 206t, 1426
"Gasping syndrome," 27
Gastrectomy, osteoporosis and, 966t
Gastric acid
  basal acid output, 330
  circadian secretion of, 330
  maximal acid output, 320
  in peptic ulcer disease, 329–330
Gastric bypass surgery, 1728
Gastric emptying
  GERD and, 317
  impaired, with tube feeding, 1712
Gastric feeding, 1704
Gastric outlet obstruction, in peptic ulcer disease, 331
Gastric residual checks, 1712
Gastric ulcers, 328, 328t. *See also* Peptic ulcer disease
Gastrinoma, 328
Gastritis
  with corticosteroids, 953t
  Helicobacter pylori and, 328
Gastrocolic reflex, 373
Gastroenteritis, viral, 1277–1278, 1277t
Gastroesophageal reflux disease (GERD), 315–324
  anatomic factors in, 316
  aspiration and, 1191
  asthma and, 267, 323
  atypical, 323
  case study of, 318, 319, 324
  clinical presentation in, 318
  in cystic fibrosis, 305, 311, 312
  diagnosis of, 317–318
  in elderly, 323
  endoscopy in, 315, 316f, 317–318
  epidemiology of, 316
  esophageal clearance in, 316–317
  etiology of, 316
  foods and medications that worsen, 317t
  gastric emptying and, 317
  lower esophageal sphincter pressure in, 316–317
  mucosal resistance in, 317
  nocturnal, 317
  outcome evaluation in, 324
  pathophysiology of, 316–317
  patient care and monitoring in, 324
  in pediatric patient, 323
  refluxate composition in, 317
  treatment of, 318f, 318–324, 320t
    antacid-alginic acid products, 320t, 321
    antacids, 320t, 321
    anti-reflux surgery, 319
    combination therapy, 322
    enteral nutrition, 1513t
    H_2-receptor antagonists, 320t, 321
    lifestyle modifications, 319, 320t
    maintenance therapy, 322–323
    mucosal protectants, 322
    prokinetic agents, 322, 323
    proton pump inhibitors, 320t, 321–322

Gastrointestinal bleeding
  NSAID-related, 329, 574
  in peptic ulcer disease, 331
  warfarin-related, 204
Gastrointestinal bloating, in heart failure, 84
Gastrointestinal disease
  in cystic fibrosis, 304–305, 311–312
  food poisoning, 1278, 1278t
  infections
    bacterial, 1267–1276
    case study of, 1268, 1270, 1271, 1272, 1275, 1277, 1278
    dehydration in, 1267, 1268t
    outcome evaluation in, 1278
    parasitic, 1276–1277
    viral, 1277–1278, 1277t
  nausea and vomiting with, 358t
  osteoporosis and, 977
  treatment of, enteral nutrition, 1513t
Gastrointestinal fistula
  parenteral nutrition in, 1682t
  sodium requirement with, 1685
Gastrointestinal intolerance, of antiretrovirals, 1442t
Gastrointestinal surgery, antimicrobial prophylaxis in, 1400t
Gastrointestinal tract
  absorptive function of, 1702
  anatomy of, 1702, 1702t
  enteral nutrition, 1701–1716
  immune functions of, 1703
  mucosal defense and repair of, 330
  perforation of, 1282, 1287t
Gastroparesis
  in diabetic neuropathy, 757
  nausea and vomiting with, 358t
  with opioids, 577t
  treatment of, 577t
Gastroplasty, 1728
Gastroschisis, 833
Gastrostomy, in cystic fibrosis, 307
Gastrostomy tube, 1704, 1705f, 1705t
  percutaneous endoscopic, 1704, 1705f
Gatifloxacin
  adverse effects of, 1261t
  in conjunctivitis, 1066, 1066t
  dosage of, 1066t, 1261t
  drug interactions of, 647
  in intra-abdominal infections, 1287t
  in keratitis, 1071
  in tuberculosis, 1261t
Gefitinib
  in cancer therapy, 1452t
  in lung cancer, 1508–1509
  mechanism of action of, 1508
Gell and Coombs categories, of allergic drug reactions, 928–929, 929t
Gemcitabine, 1455
  adverse effects of, 1455, 1484t, 1507t, 1574t
  in breast cancer, 1483t, 1491, 1492
  in cancer therapy, 1455
  dosage of, 1483t, 1507t, 1557t, 1574t
    in hepatic impairment, 1471t
  extravasation of, 1677t
  in Hodgkin's lymphoma, 1557t
  in lung cancer, 1507t, 1510, 1511
  mechanism of action of, 1454a, 1455
  in ovarian cancer, 1573, 1574t
  pharmacokinetics of, 1455
Gemfibrozil
  adverse effects of, 243t
  cost of, 149
  dosage of, 243t
  drug interactions of, 205t, 241

erectile dysfunction with, 885*t*
in hyperlipidemia, 151, 241*t*, 243*t*, 246, 956*t*
Gemifloxacin, in COPD, 299*t*
Gemtuzumab ozogamicin, 1466
in acute myelogenous leukemia, 1591*t*, 1592
adverse effects of, 1466, 1591*t*
in cancer therapy, 1466
mechanism of action of, 1466, 1591*t*
pharmacokinetics of, 1466
Gender
cirrhosis and, 388
depression and, 654
schizophrenia and, 632
Generalized anxiety disorder
clinical presentation in, 694
course of illness, 692
diagnosis of, 694
epidemiology of, 692
etiology of, 692
outcome evaluation in, 699
pathophysiology of, 692–693, 693*f*
treatment of, 693–699
antidepressants, 695–697, 696*t*
benzodiazepines, 697
buspirone, 697–698
hydroxyzine, 698
nonpharmacologic, 695
pregabalin, 698
serotonin-norepinephrine reuptake
inhibitors, 696, 696*t*
SSRI, 696–697, 696*t*
tricyclic antidepressants, 696, 696*t*
Genetic factors
in acute leukemia, 1581
in ADHD, 724
in Alzheimer's disease, 596–597
in anxiety disorders, 692
in asthma, 266
in bipolar disorder, 670
in bladder cancer, 1447*t*
in brain cancer, 1447*t*
in breast cancer, 1447*t*, 1476–1477
in cancer, 1446–1448, 1447*t*
in cirrhosis, 388, 392
in colorectal cancer, 1447*t*, 1519, 1521
in depression, 654
in enuresis, 920
in epilepsy, 523
in heart failure, 97
in hemophilia, 1122
in hypertension, 54
in inflammatory bowel disease, 342
in ischemic heart disease, 238*t*
in lung cancer, 1447*t*, 1500–1501
in multiple sclerosis, 407, 408
in non-Hodgkin's lymphoma, 1554–1555
in ovarian cancer, 1447*t*, 1477, 1567
in Parkinson's disease, 554
in prostate cancer, 1536, 1536*t*
in psoriasis, 1080
in rheumatoid arthritis, 982
in schizophrenia, 632
in skin cancer, 1613
in thyroid cancer, 1447*t*
Geniculate nucleus, 1034
Genital herpes, 1328–1331
clinical presentation in, 1329
diagnosis of, 1329
epidemiology of, 1328
first episode of, 1329, 1330*t*
in neonates, 1330–1331
pathophysiology of, 1329
patient care and monitoring in, 1331

in pregnancy, 1329–1330
prevention of transmission of, 1329, 1330*t*
treatment of, 1329–1331, 1330*t*
episodic therapy, 1329
suppressive therapy, 1329
vaccination, 1331
Genital warts, 1327–1328
clinical presentation in, 1327
diagnosis of, 1327
epidemiology of, 1328
pathophysiology of, 1327
patient care and monitoring in, 1328
in pregnancy, 1328
treatment of, 1327–1328, 1327*t*
ablative therapy, 1328
patient-applied, 1328
physician-applied, 1328
Genotype, leukemia cell, 1583
Gentamicin. *See also* Clindamycin/gentamicin
adverse effects of, 1176*t*
in campylobacteriosis, 1272
clinical parameters for, 1353
in conjunctivitis, 1066, 1066*t*
in corneal abrasion, 1064
in cystic fibrosis, 309*t*
dosage of, 309*t*, 1066*t*, 1176*t*, 1180*t*, 1199*t*,
1244*t*, 1246*t*, 1247*t*, 1249*t*, 1289, 1333,
1660*t*
drug interactions of, 954, 1163
in infections in cancer patients, 1660*t*
in infective endocarditis, 1241, 1242, 1243,
1244*t*, 1246*t*, 1247*t*, 1249*t*
in intra-abdominal infections, 1286, 1288*t*,
1289
in keratitis, 1071*t*
in meningitis, 1176*t*, 1180*t*
nephrotoxicity of, 440
in PID, 1333*t*
in pneumonia, 1098, 1199*t*
in prevention of catheter-related infections, 475
in surgical prophylaxis, 1400, 1400*t*, 1402
in urinary tract infections, 1311*t*
Gentian violet 0.5–1% solution, dosage, 833*t*
GERD. *See* Gastroesophageal reflux disease
Geriatric assessment, 15
case study of, 9
documentation, 17
drug therapy monitoring, 17, 18*t*
patient education, 17–18
patient interview, 15–17
Geriatric practice sites
ambulatory geriatric clinic, 18
long-term care, 18–19
Geriatrics, 7
age-related changes, 9
pharmacodynamic changes, 11–13
pharmacokinetic changes, 10–11
drug-related problems, 13
adverse drug reaction, 14–15
inappropriate prescribing, 13–14
nonadherence, 15
polypharmacy, 13
undertreatment, 14
epidemiology of, 7–9
etiology of, 7–9
geriatric assessment, 15
documentation, 17
drug therapy monitoring, 17
patient education, 17–18
patient interview, 15–17
geriatric practice sites
ambulatory geriatric clinic, 18
long-term care, 18–19

health status, 8–9
patient care and monitoring in, 19
sociodemographics, 8
undertreatment, common categories of, 14*t*
"Geriatric syndromes," 17
German regimen, in acute lymphocytic
leukemia, 1588*t*
Germ-cell tumor, 1568, 1630, 1630*t*
superior vena cava syndrome with,
1661*t*
Germ-tube test, 1384
Gestational age (GA), 822
Giardiasis, 376, 1294–1295
case study of, 1294
clinical presentation in, 1295
diagnosis of, 1295
epidemiology of, 1294
etiology of, 1294
outcome evaluation in, 1295
pathophysiology of, 1294
patient care and monitoring in, 1295
in pediatric patients, 1294–1295
treatment of, 1294–1295
Gigantism, 804
Ginger, 206*t*
in pain, 579
Ginkgo biloba, 206*t*
in Alzheimer's disease, 602
Ginseng
adverse effects of, 376*t*
anxiety with, 694*t*
GI tract stimulation, 44
Glasgow coma scale, 1174
Glatiramer acetate
adverse effects of, 513*t*, 514
dosage of, 513*t*
mechanism of action of, 514
in multiple sclerosis, 510*t*, 514, 515*t*
pharmacology of, 514
Glaucoma, 1031–1044
aqueous humor in, 1033–1034, 1033*f*
case study of, 1043
with corticosteroids, 953*t*
drug-induced, 1043
ethnicity and, 1032
intraocular pressure in, 1032, 1034
normal-tension, 1034, 1037
optic nerves in, 1033, 1034, 1034*f*
patient care and monitoring in, 1044
primary, 1031–1032
primary angle-closure, 1032
acute, 1035, 1064*t*
chronic, 1035
epidemiology of, 1032
laser iridotomy in, 1037, 1040
outcome evaluation in, 1044
pathophysiology of, 1035
risk factors for, 1032, 1032*t*
subacute, 1035
treatment of, 1037–1043
primary open-angle, 1032
algorithm for treatment of, 1039*a*
α2-adrenergic agonists in, 1038*t*, 1041
β-blockers in, 1038*t*, 1040
carbon anhydrase inhibitors in, 1038*t*,
1041–1042
cholinergic agents in, 1038*t*, 1042
cholinesterase inhibitors in, 1038*t*
clinical course of, 1036
clinical presentation in, 1036
epidemiology of, 1032
hyperosmotics in, 1042–1043
laser trabeculoplasty in, 1037

Glaucoma, primary open-angle (*Cont.*)
nonselective adrenergic agonists in, 1038*t*, 1043
ocular hypotensive lipids in, 1040–1041
outcome evaluation in, 1043–1044
pathophysiology of, 1033–1036
prostaglandin analogs in, 1040–1041
risk factors for, 1032, 1032*t*
treatment of, 1036–1037, 1038*t*
primary open-angle suspects, 1032, 1037
secondary, 1032
Gleason score, for prostate cancer, 1538, 1541–1542, 1542*t*
Glimepiride
in diabetes mellitus, 749*t*
dosage of, 749*t*
Glioblastoma, 1447*t*
Glipizide
in diabetes mellitus, 749*t*
dosage of, 749*t*
Glitazones. *See* Thiazolidinediones
Glomerular filtration rate (GFR), 27, 1117, 1118
in acute renal failure, 431
calculation of, 433, 446
in chronic kidney disease, 446
in end-stage renal disease, 468
Glomerulonephritis, 433, 435
chronic kidney disease and, 447
Plasmodium malariae, 1300
poststreptococcal, 1215
Glucagon, production of, 736
Glucagon emergency kit, 756
Glucagon-like peptide-1, 751
Glucocorticoids. *See also* Corticosteroids; *specific drugs*
in adrenal insufficiency, 786, 786*t*, 789*t*
adverse effects of, 86*t*, 792*t*, 794, 1595
avoiding hypercortisolism or hypocortisolism, 798*t*
blood glucose level and, 737*t*
in cluster headaches, 590
in COPD, 295*t*
discontinuation of, 795, 798*t*
excess of, 784. *See also* Cushing's syndrome
growth hormone deficiency with, 810
insufficiency of, 784. *See also* Addison's disease
in myxedema coma, 772
osteoporosis with, 966*t*, 967, 976–977, 990
in prevention of lung cancer, 1501
in rheumatoid arthritis, 990–991
Glucometer, 742
Gluconeogenesis, 738
Glucosamine, in pain, 579
Glucosamine sulfate
dosage of, 1002*t*
in osteoarthritis, 1002*t*, 1005
Glucose
blood. *See also* Diabetes mellitus; Glycemic control
categorization of glucose status, 740–741, 741*t*
normal insulin action, 738
self-monitoring of, 742
in CSF, 1172*t*
Glucose intolerance, with oral contraceptives, 846
Glucose metabolism, in elderly patients, 12–13
Glucuronidation, 11, 618
Glutamate
in Alzheimer's disease, 597
in depression, 654
in seizures, 522
in status epilepticus, 542

Glutamine, in enteral feeding formulas, 1708–1709
Glutathione-*S*-transferases, 27
Glyburide
in diabetes mellitus, 748*t*
dosage of, 748*t*
Glycemic control
in critically ill patients, 1694
in diabetes mellitus, 735, 737*t*, 741
in enteral nutrition, 1709–1710, 1713
hemoglobin A$_{1c}$ and, 742
in parenteral nutrition, 1687
in prevention of surgical site infections, 1398
in sepsis, 1357
setting and assessing glycemic targets, 741–743
Glyceriltrinitrate, dosage, 832*t*
Glycerin
adverse effects of, 1042
in glaucoma, 1042
Glycogenolysis, 738
Glycoprotein IIb/IIIa receptor(s), 188
Glycoprotein IIb/IIIa receptor blockers. *See also specific drugs*
in acute coronary syndromes, 141*t*, 145, 147, 152*t*
adverse effects of, 147, 152*t*
contraindications to, 141*t*
cost of, 149
dosage of, 141*t*
Glycosaminoglycan, 1309
Glycosuria, in diabetes mellitus, 737
Goeckerman's regimen, 1084
Goiter, 765
multinodular, 772
toxic multinodular, 774*t*
GOLD classification, of COPD, 289, 292*t*
Gold salts, 990
Gold therapy, ocular changes with, 1077*t*
Golimumab, 988, 991
Gompertzian growth curve, 1448, 1448*f*
Gonadotropin-releasing hormone
at menopause, 870
in menstrual cycle, 843, 856
Gonadotropin-releasing hormone agonists
depression with, 655
Gonadotropin-releasing hormone analogs
hyperprolactinemia with, 814*t*
Gonadotropin-releasing hormone (GnRH) antagonists
in prostate cancer, 1544–1545
Gonioscopy, 1035, 1036
Gonorrhea, 1318–1320
case study of, 1319, 1320
clinical presentation in, 1318
co-infection with chlamydia, 1319
diagnosis of, 1318–1319
disseminated infection, 1320
epidemiology of, 1318
pathophysiology of, 1318
in pediatric patient, 1320
in pregnancy, 1320
treatment of, 1319–1320
Goodpasture's syndrome, kidney transplantation in, 941
Gorlin's syndrome, skin cancer in, 1624
Goserelin, 1468
adverse effects of, 1468, 1487*t*, 1544*t*
in breast cancer, 1487, 1487*t*, 1490
in cancer therapy, 1468
dosage of, 1487*t*, 1544*t*
mechanism of action of, 1468
osteoporosis with, 966*t*
pharmacokinetics of, 1468

in prostate cancer, 1543–1544, 1544*t*
Gout, 1011–1018
antihyperuricemic treatment, 1014*t*, 1015–1017
allopurinol, 1014*t*, 1015
nonpharmacologic, 1015
probenecid, 1014*t*, 1016
case study of, 1014, 1016
clinical presentation in, 1012
diabetes mellitus and, 1012
diagnosis of, 1012
drug-induced, 1012
epidemiology of, 1011
etiology of, 1011
ischemic heart disease and, 1012
outcome evaluation in, 1017
pathophysiology of, 1011–1012, 892*f*
patient care and monitoring in, 1017
primary, 1012
risk factors for, 1012
treatment of, 1013–1015
ACTH, 1015
algorithm for, 1013*a*
colchicine, 1013–1014, 1014*t*
corticosteroids, 1014–1015, 1014*t*
nonpharmacologic, 1013
NSAID, 1013, 1014*t*
tumor lysis syndrome, 1016–1017
Gouty arthritis, acute, 1012
Gram-negative bacteria
in infective endocarditis, 1236*t*, 1241, 1248
in meningitis, 1171*t*, 1182–1183
pathogenic, 1160*a*
in pneumonia, 1194, 1096*t*, 1198
Gram-positive bacteria
in infective endocarditis, 1241
pathogenic, 1160*a*
Gram stain, 1159–1160, 1160*a*
Graft-versus-host disease (GVHD), 1592–1593, 1629, 1631, 1635, 1638–1640
acute, 1638–1640
clinical grading of, 1638, 1639*f*
clinical presentation in, 1638, 1639*f*
diagnosis of, 1638
immunosuppressive prophylaxis in, 1638–1639
monitoring for signs of, 1644
pathophysiology of, 1638
treatment of, 1640
chronic, 1640, 1644
clinical presentation in, 1640
clinical scoring system for, 1640
diagnosis of, 1640
prevention of, 1640
treatment of, 1640
dry eye in, 1075*t*
after hematopoietic cell transplantation, 1599
prevention of, 1638
Graft-versus-leukemia effect, 1592–1593
Graft-versus-tumor effect, 1630, 1633
Grandiosity, in cyclothymic disorder, 671
Granisetron
in chemotherapy-induced nausea and vomiting, 1652*t*
in chemotherapy-related nausea and vomiting, 1513*t*
dosage of, 362*t*
in nausea and vomiting, 362*t*, 364
Granulocyte-monocyte colony-stimulating factor, 1110, 1111*f*
Granuloma
caseating, 1254
in endemic mycosis, 1377
Grapefruit juice, 244, 684, 955*t*

Graves' disease, 766, 772, 774, 774t
    case study of, 775, 776
    clinical presentation in, 774, 775f
    in pregnancy, 777
    treatment of, 776–777
Green tea
    in prevention of lung cancer, 1501
    in prevention of prostate cancer, 1537
"Grey Baby Syndrome," 27
Gripe water, 29
Griseofulvin
    drug interactions of, 205t, 850t
    in onychomycosis, 1372
    in tinea infections, 1371
Group B *Streptococcus* infection in pregnancy, 836
Group therapy, in substance dependence, 624
Growth hormone, 803–813
    deficiency of, 803, 809–813
        in adults, 809–813
        clinical presentation in, 811–812
        diagnosis of, 811–812
        drug-induced, 810
        epidemiology of, 809–810
        etiology of, 809–810
        growth hormone replacement therapy in, 811–813
        IGF-1 therapy in, 813
        outcome evaluation in, 813
        pathophysiology of, 810–811
        patient care and monitoring in, 810, 813–814
        treatment of, 811–813
    effects of, 803, 803t
    excess of. *See* Acromegaly; Gigantism
    secretion of, 803
Growth hormone receptor antagonist, in acromegaly, 807t, 808
Growth hormone-releasing hormone, 803
Growth hormone replacement therapy
    administration of, 811
    adverse effects of, 812
    dosage of, 811
    in growth hormone deficiency, 811–813
Guaiac stool tests, 1519, 1520t
Guaifenesin in common cold, 1218, 1218t
Guanabenz
    adverse effects of, 63t
    dosage of, 63t
    in hypertension, 63t, 69
Guanadrel
    adverse effects of, 63t
    dosage of, 63t
    in hypertension, 63t
Guanethidine, drug interactions of, 660t
Guanfacine
    in ADHD, 727t, 728t, 730t, 730–731
    adverse effects of, 62t, 728t
    dosage of, 62t, 727t
    in hypertension, 62t
    mechanism of action of, 730–731
Guarana, 694t
Guided imagery
    in pain, 573
    in psoriasis, 1083
Guillain-Barré syndrome, 1271, 1408t
    clinical presentation in, 1415
    respiratory acidosis with, 426t
    vaccine-associated, 1415
Gut-associated lymphoid tissue, 1703
Gut barrier function, 1703, 1704
GVHD. *See* Graft-versus-host disease
Gynecologic surgery, antimicrobial prophylaxis in, 1399–1400

Gynecomastia
    with 5α-reductase inhibitors, 905, 906t
    with spironolactone, 95, 150–151

H
HACEK group, in infective endocarditis, 1236t, 1241, 1248
Haemophilus aphrophilus, in infective endocarditis, 1241
Haemophilus ducreyi, 1333–1334. *See also* Chancroid
Haemophilus influenzae, 1407
    in bite wound infections, 1232t
    in conjunctivitis, 1065
    in COPD exacerbations, 298, 299t
    in cystic fibrosis, 304, 309
    in immune thrombocytopenic purpura, 1134
    in infective endocarditis, 1241
    in meningitis, 1170, 1171t, 1176t, 1179, 1181–1182, 1184
    in otitis media, 1204
    in pneumonia, 1190, 1190t, 1193, 1195–1197, 1096t, 1354
    in rhinosinusitis, 1209, 1211
    in sepsis, 1348t
Haemophilus influenzae type b vaccine, 1170, 1181–1182, 1407, 1408t, 1414, 1414t, 1416
Haemophilus paraphrophilus, in infective endocarditis, 1241
Hair, fungal infections of, 1369–1373
Hair follicle, 1094
Halcinonide
    in contact dermatitis, 1103t
    dosage and potency of, 1103t
Half-normal saline, 482
Hallucinations
    in schizophrenia, 631, 644
    in stimulant abuse, 616
Hallucinosis, in alcohol withdrawal, 616, 619
Halobetasol
    in contact dermatitis, 1103t
    dosage and potency of, 1103t
    in psoriasis, 1084
Halofantrine, drug interactions of, 647
Haloperidol
    adverse effects of, 638, 638t, 642t
    in alcohol intoxication, 613
    arrhythmia with, 179t
    in chemotherapy-related nausea and vomiting, 1513t
    in delirium tremens, 619
    dosage of, 619, 640t, 640–641, 641t
    drug interactions of, 646t, 660t
    mechanism of action of, 637f
    metabolism of, 646t, 647
    in nausea and vomiting, 361t
    in schizophrenia, 637f, 640t, 640–641, 641t
Halo sign, 1390
Halzepam, drug interactions of, 614t
Hand-foot syndrome
    fluorouracil-induced, 1527, 1528
Hand washing, prevention of infections in neutropenic patients, 1656
Hapten, 928
Haptenation, 928
Harris-Benedict equations, 1688, 1689t
Hashimoto's thyroiditis, 767t
Hawthorn, 125
HDL. *See* High-density lipoproteins
Headache, 568, 583–593
    case study of, 584, 585, 591
    cluster. *See* Cluster headache
    with hormone-replacement therapy, 876t

migraine. *See* Migraine
    with oral contraceptives, 847–848
    patient care and monitoring in, 592
    in pregnancy, 592, 593
    primary, 583
    red flags necessitating further evaluation, 587, 587t
    secondary, 583
    tension-type. *See* Tension-type headache
    treatment of, 586–591
Headache diary, 587
Head and neck cancer, 1447t
    hypercalcemia with, 1670–1673
Head and neck surgery, antimicrobial prophylaxis in, 1400t
Head louse, 1304
Head trauma
    CNS infections in, 1171t
    DIC with, 1131t
    epilepsy and, 522
    mania with, 676t
    psychotic symptoms in, 635t
    treatment of, enteral nutrition, 1513t
Health Assessment Questionnaire (Stanford), 993
Health care workers, vaccination of, 1416
Health literacy, 4
Health status, of elderly
    health care utilization and cost, 9
    life expectancy, 8–9
Hearing loss, in sickle cell anemia/disease, 1152t
Heart. *See also* Cardiac *entries*
    electrical activity of
        arrhythmias. *See* Arrhythmia
        electrocardiogram, 159–160
        normal conduction, 158–159, 158f
        refractory periods, 160
        ventricular action potential, 159, 159f
    mechanical activity of, 158
Heartburn, 318. *See also* Gastroesophageal reflux disease
    pregnancy, 829, 833
Heart disease
    depression with, 655
    drug-related, 1441t
    ischemic. *See* Ischemic heart disease
    nausea and vomiting with, 358t
    stroke and, 217t
    valvular, 111t, 940
Heart failure, 79–105
    acute
        clinical presentation in, 98–99
        cool, 98
        diagnosis of, 98–99
        dry, 98
        hemodynamic monitoring in, 99, 99t
        laboratory assessment of, 99, 99t
        outcome evaluation in, 104–105
        patient care and monitoring in, 105
        precipitating factors, 98–99
        prognosis for, 80
        treatment of, 99–104
            diuretics, 100t, 100–101
            inotropic agents, 102–103
            investigational, 104
            mechanical, surgical, and device therapies, 103–104
            phosphodiesterase inhibitors, 103
            vasodilators, 100–102, 101t
            warm, 98
            wet, 98
    American College of Cardiology/American Heart Association staging of, 87, 87t

Heart failure (*Cont.*)
　in amyloidosis, 80*t*
　anxiety with, 694*t*
　arrhythmia in, 166*t*, 177*t*
　atrial fibrillation and, 166–167
　calcium channel blockers and, 123–124
　cardiac output in, 80
　cardiomyopathy and
　　dilated, 80, 80*t*
　　hypertrophic, 80*t*
　cardiorenal model of, 83–84
　cardiovascular risk assessment for
　　　phosphodiesterase inhibitors, 889*t*
　case study of, 84, 87–88, 97, 104
　chronic, 83
　　clinical presentation in, 84–88
　　diagnosis of, 84–88
　　outcome evaluation in, 97–98
　　with preserved left ventricular ejection
　　　fraction, 96–97
　　treatment of, 88–97
　　　ACE inhibitors, 91–93, 92*t*
　　　aldosterone antagonists, 92*t*, 95
　　　angiotensin receptor blockers, 92*t*, 93
　　　anticoagulants, 96
　　　antiplatelet drugs, 96
　　　β-blockers, 92*t*, 94–95
　　　calcium channel blockers, 96
　　　control of contributing disorders, 88
　　　digoxin, 95–96
　　　diuretics, 89–91, 90*t*, 97
　　　hydralazine, 93–94, 97
　　　isosorbide dinitrate, 93–94
　　　nonpharmacologic, 88–89
　classification of, 86–88, 87*t*
　compensated, 84
　compensatory mechanisms in, 81–82, 81*t*
　cost of, 80
　decompensated, 84
　diabetes mellitus and, 88
　drugs that precipitate/exacerbate, 86, 86*t*
　epidemiology of, 80
　ethnicity and, 93–94, 97
　etiology of, 80–81, 80*t*
　genetic factors in, 97
　hypertension and, 70, 80–81, 84*t*, 88
　hypokalemia and, 83
　hypomagnesemia and, 83
　hyponatremia in, 485
　ischemic heart disease and, 80, 88
　myocardial infarction and, 80, 80*t*, 91
　nausea and vomiting with, 358*t*
　neurohormonal model of, 82–83
　obesity and, 88
　pathophysiology of, 81–84
　patient history in, 86, 86*t*
　pericardial disease and, 80*t*
　precipitating and exacerbating factors in,
　　84, 84*t*
　in pregnancy, 84*t*, 97
　proinflammatory cytokines in, 84
　renal disease and, 83–84, 84*t*, 432, 442
　respiratory acidosis with, 426*t*
　in sarcoidosis, 80*t*
　treatment of
　　ACE inhibitors, 83
　　angiotensin receptor blockers, 83
　　β-blockers, 65–67, 83
　　heart transplantation, 940
　　vasodilators, 97
Heart rate
　in heart failure, 81
　in shock, 252

Heart transplantation. *See also* Solid-organ
　　transplantation
　acute rejection, signs and symptoms of, 944*t*
　domino heart transplant, 940
　epidemiology and etiology of, 940–942
　in heart failure, 104
　heterotopic, 940
　orthotopic, 940
Heat stroke, 1131*t*
Heat therapy
　in musculoskeletal disorders, 1023
　in osteoarthritis, 1000
　in pain, 573
Heavy-metal compounds, in cancer therapy,
　　1462–1463
Heberden's nodes, 998
Helicobacter pylori
　diagnosis of infection, 331–332
　eradication of, 333, 335*t*, 1561
　etiology of, 1561
　lymphoma and, 1553, 1561
　in peptic ulcer disease, 327–329, 328*t*, 333–335,
　　335*t*, 337
Heliox, in asthma, 283
Hellebore, 125
Helminthic disease, 1297–1299
Hemangioma, giant, DIC with, 1131*t*
Hematocrit, 112, 1113*t*
Hematogenous spread
　of pathogens into CNS, 1171
　of urinary tract infections, 1308
　of viral infections, 1183
Hematologic complications
　in cancer patients, 1654–1661
　with interferon therapy, 424
Hematologic disorders, in cystic fibrosis, 305
Hematoma, prevention in musculoskeletal
　　disorders, 1022
Hematopoiesis, 1581
Hematopoietic cell transplantation, 1629–1645.
　　See also Graft-versus-host disease;
　　Graft-versus-tumor effect
　in acute lymphocytic leukemia, 1593, 1630, 1630*t*
　in acute myelogenous leukemia, 1593, 1630,
　　1630*t*, 1634
　adverse effects of, 1558
　allogeneic, 1592–1593, 1599, 1602, 1630–1632,
　　1630*t*, 1634*t*
　autologous, 1593, 1602, 1630–1632, 1630*t*, 1634*t*
　case study of, 1638, 1641, 1644
　in chronic lymphocytic leukemia, 1602, 1630,
　　1630*t*
　in chronic myelogenous leukemia, 1599, 1630,
　　1630*t*, 1634
　complications of, 1593
　complications of preparative regimens
　　busulfan seizures, 1635–1636
　　gastrointestinal illness, 1636
　　hemorrhagic cystitis, 1636
　　myelosuppression, 1637
　　sinusoidal obstruction syndrome, 1636–1637
　diseases treated with, 1630, 1630*t*
　engraftment of, 1630–1631, 1633
　epidemiology of, 1630–1631
　etiology of, 1630–1631
　graft failure, 1631, 1633, 1637
　harvesting, preparing and allogeneic
　　transplanting cell, 1632–1633
　histocompatibility between donor and
　　recipient in, 1631
　in Hodgkin's lymphoma, 1558, 1630*t*
　infectious complications of, 1641–1643
　　cytomegalovirus, 1642

　　fungal disease, 1641, 1642
　　herpes simplex virus, 1641, 1642
　　Pneumocystis jiroveci pneumonia, 1641–1643
　late effects of, 1643
　in multiple myeloma, 1630, 1630*t*
　myeloablative preparative regimen, 1630, 1634,
　　1634*t*
　in non-Hodgkin's lymphoma, 1559, 1562, 1630,
　　1630*t*
　nonmyeloablative preparative regimen, 1630,
　　1633, 1634–1635, 1635*f*
　outcome evaluation in, 1644–1645
　pathophysiology of, 1631–1632
　patient care and monitoring in, 1645
　reduced-intensity myeloablative transplant,
　　1635
　in sickle cell anemia/disease, 1143*t*, 1147
　stem cell sources, 1631–1632
　survivorship after, 1643–1644
　syngeneic, 1630
　T-cell-depleted grafts, 1633
Hematopoietic growth factors
　after hematopoietic cell transplant, 1637
　in mobilization of peripheral blood progenitor
　　cells, 1632–1633, 1637
Hematopoietic stem cells, 1581
Hematuria, gross, 913*t*
Hemiballismus, in serotonin syndrome, 1726
Hemiparesis, 218
　in meningitis, 1170, 1185
Hemisensory deficit, 218
Hemochromatosis
　adrenal insufficiency in, 786*t*
　dry eye in, 1075*t*
　hereditary, 392
　osteoarthritis in, 998*t*
Hemodialysis, 468–470
　advantages and disadvantages of, 468*t*
　adverse effects of, 236*t*
　complications of
　　hypotension, 470
　　infection, 472, 473*t*
　　muscle cramps, 472
　　thrombosis, 472
　intermittent, in acute renal failure, 439
　mania with, 676*t*
　in metabolic alkalosis, 503
　principles of, 468–470
　in tumor lysis syndrome, 1675
　vascular access in, 470
Hemoglobin, 1109
　normal value of, 111, 1113*t*
　sickle. *See* Sickle cell anemia/disease
Hemoglobin A, 1140, 1141
Hemoglobin A$_{1C}$, evaluation of glycemic control,
　　742
Hemoglobin A2, 1140
Hemoglobin-based oxygen carriers, in
　　hypovolemic shock, 259
Hemoglobin C, 1140
　HbSC genotype, 1140
Hemoglobin F. *See* Fetal hemoglobin
Hemoglobin S. *See also* Sickle cell anemia/disease
　HbS*β*$^+$-thalassemia, 1140
　HbS*β*^{0}-thalassemia, 1140
　HbSC genotype, 1140
Hemolysis, intravascular, 1131*t*
Hemolytic anemia, 1114*a*
　allergic drug reaction, 929*t*
Hemolytic-uremic syndrome
　DIC with, 1131*t*
　in *Escherichia coli* O157:H7 infections, 1272
　in shigellosis, 1268

Hemophilia, 1122–1126
  mild, 1123*t*
  moderate, 1123*t*
  osteoporosis and, 966*t*
  pain associated with, 1126
  severe, 1123*t*
Hemophilia A
  clinical presentation in, 1122
  complications of, 1122
  diagnosis of, 1122
  epidemiology of, 1122
  etiology of, 1122
  with factor VIII inhibitors, 1125–1126,
    1126*a*
  genetic factors in, 1122
  outcome evaluation in, 1126
  pathophysiology of, 1122
  primary prophylaxis in, 1123
  treatment of, 991*t*, 1123–1126, 1124*t*, 1126*a*
    antifibrinolytic therapy, 1124
    desmopressin acetate, 1123
    factor VIII replacement, 1124–1125, 1124*t*,
      991*t*
Hemophilia B
  clinical presentation in, 1122
  complications of, 1122
  diagnosis of, 1122
  epidemiology of, 1122
  etiology of, 1122
  with factor IX inhibitors, 1125–1126
  genetic factors in, 1122
  outcome evaluation in, 1126
  pathophysiology of, 1122
  primary prophylaxis in, 1123
  treatment of, 991*t*, 1123–1126, 1124*t*
    factor IX replacement, 991*t*, 1124*t*, 1125
    prothrombin complex concentrate, 1124*t*,
      1125
Hemoptysis, in pulmonary embolism, 189, 192
Hemorrhagic conversion, in stroke, 220
Hemorrhagic cystitis
  in cancer patients, 1666–1670
  chemotherapy-related, 1636, 1666–1670
  clinical presentation in, 1667
  diagnosis of, 1667
  drug-induced, 1461
  epidemiology of, 1666–1667
  etiology of, 1666–1667, 1666*t*
  outcome evaluation in, 1669
  pathophysiology of, 1667
  patient care and monitoring in, 1669
  prevention of, 1667
  treatment of, 1667–1669
    algorithm for, 1669*a*
Hemorrhagic stroke
  etiology of, 216
  pathophysiology of, 218
  patient care and monitoring in, 226, 226*t*
  risk factors for, 217
  treatment of, 219
Hemorrhagic telangiectasia, 1131*t*
Hemorrhoids
  constipation in, 372*t*
  pregnancy, 829
Hemostasis, 187, 188*a*, 1121, 1122*f*, 1129
Hemostatic therapy, in intracerebral hemorrhage,
  225
Henderson-Hasselbalch equation, 496
Heparin
  adverse effects of, 222
  allergic drug reactions, 929*t*
  in DIC, 1130–1132
  dosage of, 1131–1132

low-molecular-weight
  in acute coronary syndromes, 140*t*, 146,
    147–149, 152*t*
  adverse effects of, 152*t*, 198*t*, 199
  contraindications to, 140*t*
  dosage of, 140*t*, 199
  drug interactions of, 205*t*
  hyperkalemia with, 488
  mechanism of action of, 196*f*
  in patient with renal disease, 199
  in stroke, 222
  in venous thromboembolism, 194*a*, 195*t*,
    198–199, 207, 209*t*
  osteoporosis with, 966*t*
  in parenteral nutrition admixtures, 1687
  plasma concentration of, 196
  in prevention of venous thromboembolism,
    192*t*, 193, 220, 1357
  in stroke, 222
unfractionated
  in acute coronary syndromes, 140*t*, 145,
    147–149, 152*t*
  administration of, 196
  adverse effects of, 145, 152*t*, 197, 197*t*, 198*t*
  in atrial fibrillation, 171
  contraindications to, 140*t*
  dosage of, 140*t*, 192*t*, 196–197, 197*t*
  hyperkalemia with, 488
  monitoring in, 197
  in patient with renal disease, 199
  in venous thromboembolism, 195*t*, 196–197,
    197*t*, 207
Heparin-induced thrombocytopenia, 145, 187*t*,
  198–199, 198*t*
Heparin LMWH, 828*t*
Heparinoids, in stroke, 222
Heparin resistance, 197
Hepatic blood flow, 389
Hepatic encephalopathy
  in cirrhosis, 391, 392, 399
  in end-stage liver disease, 413
  mania with, 676*t*
  pathophysiology of, 391
  treatment of, 399
    antibiotic therapy, 399
    enteral nutrition, 1710
    flumazenil, 399
    lactulose, 399
Hepatitis
  alcoholic, 391–392
  DIC with, 1131*t*
  nausea and vomiting with, 358*t*
  viral. *See* Viral hepatitis
Hepatitis A, 1407, 1409
  diagnosis of, 416, 417*t*
  epidemiology of, 413–414
  ethnicity and, 414
  etiology of, 413–414
  pathophysiology of, 415
  patient care and monitoring in, 426
  prevention of, 418–420
    immune globulin, 418–419
    vaccination, 419–420, 420*t*
  risk factors for acquiring, 414*t*
  transfusion-transmitted, 1146
Hepatitis A vaccine, 395, 419–420, 419*t*, 1407,
  1409, 1408*t*
  adverse effects of, 420
  hepatitis A and B combination vaccine, 421–422
Hepatitis B, 1409, 1446
  chronic, 414, 422–424, 1409
    adefovir dipivoxil in, 423
    entecavir in, 423

    interferon therapy in, 422–423
    lamivudine in, 423
    pegylated interferon in, 422
    tenofovir disoproxil fumarate in, 423
  cirrhosis and, 388
  co-infection with HIV, 1435
  diagnosis of, 416, 417*t*
  epidemiology of, 414
  etiology of, 414
  natural history of, 415
  outcome evaluation in, 426
  pathophysiology of, 415
  patient care and monitoring in, 426
  prevention of, 417, 420–422
    hepatitis B immune globulin, 420
    prevention of perinatal transmission,
      421–422, 421*t*
    vaccination, 420–421
  risk factors for acquiring, 414*t*
  transfusion-transmitted, 1146
  treatment of, 1435
    chronic disease, 422–424
    liver transplantation, 941
Hepatitis B core antigen (HBcAg), 415,
  416, 417*t*
Hepatitis B envelope antigen (HBeAg), 415, 416,
  417*t*, 422, 423
Hepatitis B immune globulin, 420
  adverse effects of, 420
Hepatitis B surface antigen (HBsAg), 415, 416,
  417*t*, 422
Hepatitis B vaccine, 395, 414, 420–422, 420*t*,
  1408*t*, 1409, 1414*t*, 1416
  adverse effects of, 421
  efficacy of, 421
  hepatitis A and B combination vaccine,
    421–422
  prevention of hepatitis D with, 425
Hepatitis C
  chronic, 415
    interferon therapy in, 424–425
    ribavirin in, 424–425
    treatment of, 424–425
  cirrhosis and, 388, 415
  co-infection with HIV, 1435
  diagnosis of, 418, 417*t*
  dry eye in, 1075*t*
  epidemiology of, 414
  ethnicity and, 414
  etiology of, 414
  hepatocellular carcinoma and, 415
  lymphoma and, 1552
  natural history of, 415
  outcome evaluation in, 426–427
  pathophysiology of, 415
  patient care and monitoring in, 426
  prevention of, 424
  risk factors for acquiring, 414*t*
  transfusion-transmitted, 1146
  treatment of
    chronic disease, 424–425
    liver transplantation, 941
Hepatitis D
  diagnosis of, 416, 417*t*
  epidemiology of, 414–415
  etiology of, 414–415
  pathophysiology of, 415–416
  prevention of, 425
  risk factors for acquiring, 414*t*
  treatment of, 425
Hepatitis E
  diagnosis of, 417*t*, 416
  epidemiology of, 415

Hepatitis E (*Cont.*)
etiology of, 415
pathophysiology of, 416
prevention of, 425
risk factors for acquiring, 414*t*
treatment of, 425
Hepatitis E vaccine, 425
Hepatoblastoma, liver transplantation in, 941
Hepatocellular carcinoma, hepatitis C and, 415
Hepatocytes, 387–388, 389*f*
Hepatojugular reflex, 86
Hepatoma, liver transplantation in, 941
Hepatorenal syndrome, 390, 433
Hepatosplenomegaly, in acute myelogenous
leukemia, 1585
Hepatotoxicity, 245
HER-2/neu gene expression, 1478, 1480, 1485,
1489, 1493
Herbal products, 3
anxiety with, 694*t*
in ischemic heart disease, 125–126
in Parkinson's disease, 562
in vasomotor symptoms of menopause, 878
for weight loss, 1728
Herd immunity, 1406
Hereditary breast and ovarian cancer, 1566
Hernia, hiatal, 316
Herniation, brain, 218
Heroin
abuse of
case study of, 627
epidemiology of, 608
withdrawal syndrome, 610
Herpes simplex virus
in encephalitis, 1183
in genital herpes, 1328–1331. *See also* Genital
herpes
in hematopoietic cell transplant recipients,
1641, 1642
in keratitis, 1070*t*
in meningitis, 1178*t*
in pneumonia, 1190
Herpes zoster, 1413
Herpes zoster ophthalmicus, 1070*t*
Hesitancy, in urinary incontinence, 913*t*
Hetastarch, 483
in hypovolemic shock, 258–259, 258*t*
Heterozygote, 304
Hexamethylmelamine. *See* Altretamine
Hextend, in hypovolemic shock, 258*t*
Hiatal hernia, 316
High-density lipoproteins (HDL), 230–231, 232*f*
genetically engineered, 247
low levels of, 246
nascent, 230, 232
physical characteristics of, 231*t*
High-frequency chest compression, in cystic
fibrosis, 307
Hip fracture, 876, 965, 970, 973–974
Hip protectors, 970
Hip replacement, 1340
Hirschsprung's disease, 372*t*
intestine transplantation in, 941
Hirsutism, 864
with corticosteroids, 953*t*
in Cushing's syndrome, 792
with oral contraceptives, 847
Hirudin, 200
Hispanics. *See* Ethnicity
Histamine
in allergic rhinitis, 1049, 1053
in pruritus, 467
in wakefulness, 711

Histamine dihydrochloride
adverse effects of, 1027
in musculoskeletal disorders, 1027
Histocompatibility, in hematopoietic cell
transplant, 1631
Histoplasma capsulatum, 1376–1382, 1376*t*
Histoplasmosis
clinical presentation in, 1377–1378
diagnosis of, 1377–1378
epidemiology of, 1376
geographic localization of, 1377*f*
pathophysiology of, 1376–1377, 1377*f*
patient monitoring in, 1381–1382
prophylaxis for, 1382
treatment of, 1378, 1379*t*, 1381–1382
HIV infection, 1419–1443
acute retroviral syndrome, 1422, 1433
in adolescents, 1433
adrenal insufficiency in, 786*t*
case study of, 1435, 1436
clinical presentation in, 1422–1433
co-infection
with hepatitis B virus, 1435
with hepatitis C virus, 1435
cryptococcosis in, 1387–1389
cryptosporidiosis in, 1276
diagnosis of, 1422–1433, 1422*t*
confirmatory tests, 1422
initial screening tests, 1422*t*
rapid tests, 1422*t*
DIC with, 1131*t*
dry eye in, 1075*t*
epidemiology of, 1420
epilepsy and, 522
ethnicity and, 1420
etiology of, 1420–1421
HIV RNA concentration, 1422–1423, 1422*t*,
1424*t*, 1434
life cycle of virus, 1420–1421, 1421*f*
melanoma and, 1624
monitoring for CD4 counts and HIV RNA,
1422–1423, 1424*t*
neuropathic pain in, 568, 570
non-Hodgkin's lymphoma and, 1552, 1562
opportunistic infections in, 1422
opportunistic mycosis in, 1382
oropharyngeal/esophageal candidiasis in,
1366–1368
outcome evaluation in, 1436
palliative care treatment for, 39
pathogenesis of, 1420–1421
patient care and monitoring in, 1443
in pediatric patients, 1434
in pregnancy, 1434–1435
replication capacity of virus, 1433
risk factors for, 1422
salmonellosis and, 1269–1271
substance-abuse disorders and, 1434
transmission of, 1318, 1420, 1424
parenteral, 1420
perinatal, 1420, 1434
sexual, 1420
treatment of, 1423–1435
antiretroviral-experienced patients, 1426,
1433–1434, 1426*t*
antiretroviral-naïve patients, 1425–1426, 1425*t*
compliance in, 1424, 1426, 1433
diet therapy, 1424–1425
fusion inhibitors, 1421*f*, 1423, 1431*t*
HAART, 1419
nonnucleoside reverse transcriptase
inhibitors, 1421*f*, 1423–1424, 1425–1426,
1426*t*, 1427*t*

nonpharmacologic, 1424–1425
nucleoside/nucleotide reverse transcriptase
inhibitors, 1421*f*, 1423–1424, 1425–1426,
1426*t*, 1427*t*–1428*t*
protease inhibitors, 1421*f*, 1423, 1425–1426,
1426*t*, 1429*t*–1431*t*
resistance testing, 1426, 1426, 1433
tuberculosis and, 1254, 1255, 1258, 1260
vaccination in, 1416
virtual phenotype, 1433
HMG-CoA reductase inhibitors. *See* Statins
Hodgkin's lymphoma, 1551–1563
case study of, 1555, 1558
classical, 1553*t*
clinical presentation in, 1556
diagnosis of, 1556
epidemiology of, 1552
Epstein-Barr virus and, 1552
etiology of, 1552
lymphocyte depletion, 1553*t*
mixed-cellularity, 1553*t*, 1554
nodular lymphocyte-predominant, 1553*t*
nodular sclerosing, 1553–1554, 1553*t*
outcome evaluation in, 1562–1563
pathophysiology of, 1553–1554
patient care and monitoring in, 1562
prognostic factors for, 1554*t*
secondary leukemia after, 1581
staging of, 1552*f*, 1556*t*, 1556
treatment of, 1556–1559
chemotherapy, 1557–1558, 1558*t*, 1561*t*
radiation therapy, 1557, 1562
stem cell transplantation, 1558, 1630*t*
tumor lysis syndrome in, 1674*t*
WHO classification of, 1553, 1553*t*
Homeopathy, 579
Homeostenosis, 7
Homocysteine, 240, 562
elevated serum levels of, 125, 217*t*
Homonymous visual symptoms, with
migraine, 586
Homozygote, 304
Hookworm disease, 1297
Hormonal factors, in breast cancer, 1476
Hormone-replacement therapy, 869–880. *See also*
Estrogen therapy
adverse effects of, 125, 874, 876*t*
in amenorrhea, 858
benefits of, 876–877
breast cancer and, 870, 876*t*, 877, 1476
cognitive function and, 878
contraindications to, 874
gallbladder disease and, 876*t*, 877
ischemic heart disease and, 125, 870, 876*t*
in menopause
continuous estrogen and
progestin, 874
cyclic estrogen and progestin, 874
discontinuation, 878
estrogens, 874, 875*t*
low-dose therapy, 874
outcome evaluation in, 879–880
patient care and monitoring in, 880
osteoporosis and, 876, 876*t*, 956, 975
prevention of osteoporosis, 876
in prevention of colon cancer, 876–877
quality of life and, 877–878
risks of, 877–878
stroke and, 876*t*, 877
venous thromboembolism and, 876*t*, 877
Horner's syndrome, 1503
Horse chestnut, 206*t*
Hospice, 36

Host-graft adaptation, in solid-organ transplantation, 944
Host-versus-graft disease, 1631
Hot antibodies, 1466
Hot flashes, 879t
    in menopause, 871
Hot packs, in chemotherapy extravasations, 1678
H₂-receptor antagonists. *See also specific drugs*
    dosage of, 335t
    in GERD, 320t, 321
    in *Helicobacter pylori* eradication, 333, 335t
    hyperprolactinemia with, 814t
    in pancreatitis, 407, 409
    in parenteral nutrition admixture, 1687
    in peptic ulcer disease, 336t, 337
    premedication for paclitaxel, 1458
    in prevention of NSAID-related ulcers, 336, 989
5-HT₃ antagonists
    in irritable bowel syndrome, 383
    in nausea and vomiting, 365, 1512, 1513t
5-HT₄ antagonists, in irritable bowel syndrome, 383–384
Human bite
    clenched-fist injury, 1232
    infected bite wound, 1232–1233
    occlusal injuries, 1232
Human chorionic gonadotropin, 825
Human herpes virus 6, multiple sclerosis and, 508
Human herpes virus 8, lymphoma and, 1552
Human immunodeficiency virus. *See HIV infection*
Human leukocyte antigens, 942
    in diabetes mellitus, 736
    histocompatibility in hematopoietic cell transplant, 1631
    in rheumatoid arthritis, 982
Human papillomavirus, 1446
    cervical cancer and, 1327
    in genital warts, 1327
Human papillomavirus vaccine, 1408t, 1409–1410
Human T-cell leukemia virus 1, 1552–1553
Human T-lymphocyte virus, acute leukemia and, 1580t
HuMax-CD4, in psoriasis, 1087
Humoral hypercalcemia, 1670
Hungry bone syndrome, 462
Huntington's disease
    mania with, 676t
    psychotic symptoms in, 635t
Hyaline membrane disease, 1131t
Hyalohyphomycetes, 1376t
Hyaluronan, intraarticular, in osteoarthritis, 1005–1006
Hyaluronidase
    dosage of, 1678t
    in extravasation injury, 1678–1679, 1678t
Hydralazine
    administration through feeding tube, 1715
    adverse effects of, 63t, 69, 71t, 94
    diarrhea with, 376t
    dosage of, 63t, 71t
    in heart failure, 93–94, 97
    in hypertension, 63t, 69
    in hypertensive emergency, 71t
    mechanism of action of, 93
Hydramnios, 835
Hydration
    in hypercalcemia, 1670–1671
    in tumor lysis syndrome, 1675
Hydrocephalus, nausea and vomiting with, 358t
Hydrochloric acid therapy
    metabolic acidosis with, 501t
    in metabolic alkalosis, 502

Hydrochlorothiazide
    adverse effects of, 60t
    dosage of, 60t
    drug interactions of, 170t
    in heart failure, 89
    in hypertension, 60t, 64
    hypokalemia with, 487
    hypophosphatemia with, 491
Hydrocodone
    adverse effects of, 717t
    dosage of, 575t, 717t, 1151t
    mechanism of action of, 575
    metabolism of, 576
    in pain, 575t
        in sickle cell anemia/disease, 1151t, 1150
    pseudoallergic drug reactions, 933
    in restless-legs syndrome, 717, 717t
Hydrocortisone
    in adrenal insufficiency, 786, 789t
    in anaphylaxis, 931t
    in contact dermatitis, 1103t
    in diaper dermatitis, 1106
    dosage of, 347t, 349t, 351t, 414t, 931t, 1103t, 1106, 1357, 1561t
    drug interactions of, 850t
    in hypercalcemia, 490, 490t
    in inflammatory bowel disease, 347t, 350, 349t, 351t
    in myxedema coma, 772
    in non-Hodgkin's lymphoma, 1561t
    osteoporosis with, 977
    premedication for amphotericin B, 1643
    in psoriasis, 1084
    in sepsis, 1357
Hydromorphone
    dosage of, 575t
    for epidural analgesia, 576
    mechanism of action of, 575
    in osteoarthritis, 1006
    in pain, 572t, 575t, 576
        in sickle cell anemia/disease, 1151t, 1150
    in PCA pumps, 576
Hydronephrosis, in hemorrhagic cystitis, 1667
Hydroxyapatite, 461
Hydroxychloroquine
    adverse effects of, 986t, 988, 990
    arrhythmia with, 164t
    dosage of, 986t
    monitoring treatment with, 986t
    ocular changes with, 1077t
    in rheumatoid arthritis, 986t, 990
18-Hydroxy-deoxycorticosterone, 784
Hydroxyurea
    adverse effects of, 1087, 1144–1145, 1463
    in cancer therapy, 1463
    dosage of, 1145
    mechanism of action of, 1454a, 1463
    pharmacokinetics of, 1463
    in psoriasis, 1087
    in sickle cell anemia/disease, 1143t, 1144–1145
    teratogenicity of, 1145
Hydroxyzine
    adverse effects of, 361t
    in contact dermatitis, 1102
    dosage of, 361t
    in generalized anxiety disorder, 695, 698
    in nausea and vomiting, 361t, 577t
    in pruritus, 468
Hyoscyamine
    in irritable bowel syndrome, 383, 384t
    in urinary dysfunction, 563
Hyperadrenocorticism
    anxiety with, 694t

    osteoarthritis in, 998t
Hyperaldosteronism
    hypertension and, 54
    metabolic alkalosis in, 426t
Hyperalgesia, 569
Hyperapobetalipoproteinemia, familial, 233t
Hyperbaric oxygen therapy
    in necrotizing fasciitis, 1227
Hyperbilirubinemia, in sepsis, 1349
Hypercalcemia
    with calcium supplementation, 973
    classification of, 1670
    clinical presentation in, 490, 1671
    constipation in, 372t
    definition of, 490
    diagnosis of, 1671
    drug-related, 490, 1084
    epidemiology of, 1670
    etiology of, 490, 1670
    humoral, 1670
    of malignancy, 1670–1673
    nausea and vomiting in, 358t
    outcome evaluation in, 1673
    pathophysiology of, 1670, 1671f
    patient care and monitoring in, 1673
    treatment of, 490, 490t, 1670–1673, 1672t
        algorithm for, 1484f
    with vitamin D supplementation, 972–973
Hypercalciuria
    with calcium supplementation, 973
    with vitamin D supplementation, 973
Hypercapnia
    in COPD, 291
    with parenteral nutrition, 1694, 1694t, 1696
Hypercholesterolemia, 229. *See also Dyslipidemia*
    familial, 231, 233t
    polygenic, 232, 233t
Hypercoagulable state
    venous thromboembolism and, 186, 187t
    in warfarin therapy, 201
Hypercortisolism. *See Cushing's syndrome*
Hyper-CVAD regimen, in non-Hodgkin's lymphoma, 1561t, 1561
Hyperemesis gravidarum, 358, 360, 367, 836
Hyperemia, in esophageal candidiasis, 1367
Hyperglycemia
    with corticosteroids, 953t
    in critically ill patients, 1694
    definition of, 1694
    in diabetes mellitus, 735
    with enteral nutrition, 1713
    hyponatremia and, 485
    with parenteral nutrition, 1694t, 1694, 1704
    pneumonia and, 1191
    stress-induced, 1709, 1713
    with tube feeding, 1713
Hyperglycemic hyperosmolar nonketotic syndrome, 1694
Hyperhydration, in prevention of hemorrhagic cystitis, 1667
Hyperinsulinemia, 738
Hyperkalemia, 487
    with ACE inhibitors, 68, 93
    with aldosterone antagonists, 65, 95
    with angiotensin receptor blockers, 93
    anxiety with, 694t
    arrhythmia with, 163, 163t, 164t
    in chronic kidney disease, 454
    clinical presentation in, 454, 488
    definition of, 488
    etiology of, 488
    outcome evaluation in, 454
    pathophysiology of, 454

Hyperkalemia (*Cont.*)
  with potassium-sparing diuretics, 65
  in transplant recipient, 956*t*
  treatment of, 488
    albuterol, 454
    calcium therapy, 454
    dextrose, 454
    fludrocortisone, 454
    insulin, 454
    loop diuretics, 454
    nonpharmacologic, 454
    sodium polystyrene sulfonate, 454
  in tumor lysis syndrome, 1675
Hyperkeratinization, 1094
Hyperkeratosis, 1081
Hyperlipidemia. *See* Dyslipidemia
Hypermagnesemia
  clinical presentation in, 492
  definition of, 492
  etiology of, 492
  with parenteral nutrition, 1696
  treatment of, 492
Hypernatremia, 486
  case study of, 492
  clinical presentation in, 486
  in diabetes insipidus, 486
  etiology of, 486
  treatment of, 486
Hyperopia, 1032, 1032*t*
Hyperosmolar hyperglycemic state
  in diabetes mellitus, 757
  diagnosis of, 757
  treatment of, 757
Hyperosmotics, in glaucoma, 1042–1043
Hyperparathyroidism
  in chronic kidney disease, 459–465
  clinical presentation in, 462
  epidemiology of, 459–460
  etiology of, 459–460
  hypercalcemia in, 490, 491
  hyperphosphatemia in, 462–464
  hypocalcemia in, 490
  osteoporosis and, 966*t*
  outcome evaluation in, 465
  pathophysiology of, 460–461, 461*a*
  pruritus and, 467
  secondary, 461
  treatment of, 461–465
    calcimimetics, 465
    nonpharmacologic, 462
    phosphate-binding agents, 462–463, 464*t*
    vitamin D, 463, 465, 465*t*
Hyperphosphatemia
  clinical presentation in, 491
  definition of, 491
  drug-related, 491
  etiology of, 491
  in hyperparathyroidism, 462–465
  hypocalcemia and, 489
  outcome evaluation in, 465
  in renal osteodystrophy, 462–465
  treatment of, 462–465, 491
    phosphate-binding agents, 462–463, 464*t*
    phosphorus restriction, 462
    vitamin D, 463, 465, 465*t*
    in tumor lysis syndrome, 1675
Hyperpigmentation
  in acne vulgaris, 1096
  in adrenal insufficiency, 787
Hyperplasia, 1449
  mucus-secreting gland, in COPD, 291
Hyperprolactinemia, 803, 814–819
  case study of, 818

clinical presentation in, 815
diagnosis of, 815
drug-induced, 814*t*, 816
epidemiology of, 814
etiology of, 814, 814*t*
menstruation-related disorders in, 856, 857*t*, 859*t*, 864
outcome evaluation in, 818–819
pathophysiology of, 814–815
patient care and monitoring in, 819
in pregnancy, 816–817
treatment of, 815–817, 818*t*
  algorithm for, 817*a*
  dopamine agonists, 816–817, 818*t*
  radiation therapy, 816
  surgery, 816
Hypersensitivity reactions, 1159*t*
  with antiretrovirals, 1438*t*
  of cancer treatments, 1469–1470
  type III, 1415
Hypertension, 51–73
  alcohol use and, 54*t*, 56–59
  aldosteronism and, 54
  arrhythmias and, 161, 166*t*
  cardiac output in, 54
  case study of, 58, 69, 72
  chronic kidney disease and, 447, 450, 458
  clinical presentation in, 56–57
  with corticosteroids, 953*t*, 957–958
  Cushing's syndrome and, 53
  diabetes mellitus and, 68–70, 737, 743*t*, 756
  drug-induced, 54
  in elderly, 70, 72
  epidemiology of, 52–53
  erectile dysfunction with, 885*t*
  essential, 53
  ethnicity and, 52, 70, 72
  etiology of, 53–54
  genetic factors in, 54
  heart failure and, 70, 80–81, 84*t*, 88
  ischemic heart disease and, 70, 111, 111*t*, 112, 238*t*
  isolated systolic, 70, 72
  microalbuminuria in, 57
  obesity and, 54*t*, 56, 58, 1720, 1721, 1722
  ocular, 1032, 1034
    treatment of, 1037
  oral contraceptives and, 846
  outcome evaluation in, 73–74
  parathyroid disease and, 54
  pathophysiology of, 54–56, 55*a*
  patient care and monitoring in, 73
  in pediatric patient, 52*t*, 70, 72
  peripheral resistance and, 54, 55–56
  pheochromocytoma and, 54
  portal. *See* Portal hypertension
  in pregnancy, 70, 72, 72*t*
  primary, 54
  renal disease and, 53, 57, 70
  renin-angiotensin-aldosterone system in, 55, 56*a*
  renovascular, 54
  resistant, 54, 54*t*, 65, 69
  risk factors for, 56–57
  sleep apnea and, 54, 711
  smoking and, 56
  sodium balance and, 54–55
  stroke and, 70, 217, 217*t*, 220, 220*t*, 223–224, 225*t*
  sympathetic nervous system in, 55
  in thyroid disease, 54
  in transplant recipient, 956*t*, 957–958
  treatment of, 51–52, 57–70
    ACE inhibitors, 62*t*, 66*t*, 67–68, 70, 72, 756, 956*t*, 958

aldosterone antagonists, 60*t*, 64, 65, 66*t*, 70
algorithm for, 53*a*
α₁-blockers, 63*t*, 69
angiotensin receptor blockers, 62*t*, 66*t*, 68, 72, 756, 956*t*, 958
β-blockers, 61*t*, 65–67, 66*t*, 66*a*, 70, 756, 958
calcium channel blockers, 61*t*, 66*t*, 67, 70, 72, 756, 956*t*
central α₂-agonists, 62*t*, 69
in chronic kidney disease, 450
direct vasodilators, 63*t*, 66*t*, 69
diuretics, 57, 60*t*, 64, 65*t*, 70, 756, 958
lifestyle modifications, 58–59, 59*t*, 958
nitrates, 63*t*
target blood pressure, 52, 58
white coat, 57
Hypertensive crisis, 70
  antidepressant-induced, 660
Hypertensive emergency, 70
  treatment of, 71*t*
Hypertensive urgency, 70
Hyperthermia, manifestation of intoxication, 612
Hyperthyroidism, 764, 772–777
  anxiety with, 694*t*
  arrhythmia in, 166*t*
  clinical presentation in, 773, 774
  diagnosis of, 765–766, 766*t*, 767*f*, 773
  dosage, 832*t*
  epidemiology of, 765, 772
  etiology of, 772, 774*t*
  fetal, 777
  heart failure and, 84*t*
  hypercalcemia and, 490
  mania with, 676*t*
  neonatal, 777
  osteoporosis and, 967*t*
  outcome evaluation in, 779
  patient care and monitoring in, 778
  in pediatric patients, 777
  primary, 676*t*
  treatment of, 774–777
    antithyroid drugs, 776–777
    β-blockers, 774
    iodide therapy, 775–776
    radioactive iodine, 777
    reduction of thyroid hormone synthesis, 775–777
    surgery, 777
Hypertonic saline, 482
  in cystic fibrosis, 308*t*
  in hyponatremia, 486
  in hypotension, 471
Hypertonic solution, 481
Hypertrichosis, with ocular hypotensive lipids, 1041
Hypertriglyceridemia. *See also* Dyslipidemia
  etiology of, 1694
  familial, 233*t*
  pancreatitis in, 404
  with parenteral nutrition, 1694–1695
  treatment of, 240
Hypertrophic pulmonary osteoarthropathy, 312
Hyperuricemia, 1011–1018
  drug-induced, 1011
  overproducers, 1011, 1015
  patient care and monitoring in, 1017
  treatment of, 1675*a*
    algorithm for, 1013*a*
    with tumor lysis syndrome, 1675*a*
    underexcretors, 1011, 1015
Hyperventilation, 694*t*
  respiratory alkalosis in, 504, 504*t*
Hypervigilance, in cocaine intoxication, 612*t*

Hyperviscosity syndromes, 433
Hyphema, 1064*t*
Hypnotherapy
  in irritable bowel syndrome, 383
  in nausea and vomiting, 360
Hypnotics, respiratory acidosis with, 426*t*
Hypnozoites, 1299
Hypoadrenalism, hyponatremia in, 486
Hypoalbuminemia, 10, 1688
  hypocalcemia and, 489
  in liver disease, 390
Hypoalphalipoproteinemia, 233*t*
Hypocalcemia
  clinical presentation in, 489
  drug-related, 489
  etiology of, 489
  status epilepticus in, 543
  treatment of, 489
  in tumor lysis syndrome, 1675
Hypochlorhydria, *Helicobacter pylori*-induced, 330
Hypochondriasis, 694*t*
Hypocortisolism. *See* Adrenal insufficiency
Hypocretin, in wakefulness, 711
Hypoglycemia
  anxiety with, 694*t*
  definition of, 756
  diabetes mellitus and, 756
  infant, 744
  with parenteral nutrition, 1695
  reactive, 1695
  seizures with, 522
  status epilepticus in, 543, 544
  in stroke, 220
  symptoms of, 756
  treatment of, 756, 1695
Hypoglycemics, oral
  drug interactions of, 1004
  nausea and vomiting with, 357, 358*t*
Hypogonadism, 803
  osteoporosis and, 967*t*, 967, 976
  testosterone replacement in, 891
Hypokalemia, 487
  arrhythmia with, 163*t*, 164*t*, 177*t*, 488
  clinical presentation in, 487
  definition of, 487
  with diuretics, 91
  drug-related, 487
  etiology of, 487
  heart failure and, 83
  hypomagnesemia and, 487
  metabolic alkalosis with, 426*t*
  respiratory acidosis with, 426*t*
  treatment of, 487, 488*t*
Hypomagnesemia
  arrhythmia in, 177*t*
  clinical presentation in, 491
  definition of, 491
  with diuretics, 91
  drug-related, 492
  etiology of, 492
  heart failure and, 83
  hypocalcemia and, 489
  hypokalemia and, 487
  status epilepticus in, 543
  treatment of, 492
Hypomania, 669
Hyponatremia, 485–486
  anxiety with, 694*t*
  case study of, 486
  causes of, 485
  clinical presentation in, 485
  in cystic fibrosis, 305
  definition of, 485

hyperglycemia and, 485
  hypertonic, 485
  in hypoadrenalism, 486
  hypotonic, 486
  nausea and vomiting in, 358*t*
  seizures with, 522
  in SIADH, 485, 486
  sodium deficit calculation, 486
  status epilepticus in, 542, 543
  treatment of, 485–486
Hypophosphatemia
  clinical presentation in, 414
  definition of, 490
  drug-related, 491
  etiology of, 490–491
  in refeeding syndrome, 1697–1698
  respiratory alkalosis and, 504
  respiratory failure and, 491
  treatment of, 491
Hypophysectomy, in prostate cancer, 1539*t*
Hypophysitis, 814*t*
Hypopituitarism, complication of pituitary
  microsurgery, 804
Hypoprolactinemia, 803
Hypotension
  with ACE inhibitors, 93, 150
  allergic drug reaction, 933
  with α-adrenergic antagonists, 906*t*
  with angiotensin receptor blockers, 93
  arterial, 251
  with hemodialysis, 470–472
  with interleukin-2 therapy, 1441
  with nitrates, 124
  pathophysiology of, 470–471
  treatment of, 471–472
Hypotensive lipids, ocular, in glaucoma, 1040–1041
Hypothalamic-pituitary-adrenal axis, in anxiety
  disorders, 693
Hypothalamic-pituitary-thyroid axis, 764, 765*f*
  during acute illness, 777
Hypothalamic stalk interruption, 814*t*
Hypothalamus, 802
  disorders of
    amenorrhea in, 856
    hypothyroidism in, 767*t*
    menstruation-related disorders in, 857*t*, 856
  hypothalamic-pituitary-target-organ axis, 802,
    802*f*
Hypothermia
  in alcohol intoxication, 612*t*
  arrhythmia with, 163*t*, 164*t*
  DIC with, 1131*t*
Hypothyroidism, 764, 766–772
  anemia and, 1114*a*
  anxiety with, 694*t*
  arrhythmia with, 163, 163*t*, 164*t*
  case study of, 770, 772
  clinical presentation in, 768
  congenital, 765, 767, 772
  constipation in, 372*t*
  depression with, 655
  diagnosis of, 765–766, 766*t*, 767*f*, 768, 773
  dosage of, 832*t*
  drug-related, 767
  epidemiology of, 767
  etiology of, 767, 767*t*
  in hematopoietic cell transplant recipients, 1644
  hyperlipidemia and, 236*t*
  hyperprolactinemia in, 814*t*
  lithium-induced, 679
  menstruation-related disorders in, 856, 857*t*
  patient care and monitoring in, 771*t*, 773
  in pediatric patients, 772

  in pregnancy, 771*t*, 772
  primary, 767*t*
  psychiatric illness in, 768
  respiratory acidosis with, 426*t*
  risk factors for, 767
  screening for, 767
  secondary, 767*t*, 803
  sequelae of, 768
  treatment of, 768–772
    animal-derived thyroid products, 769, 769*t*
    levothyroxine, 769–771, 771*t*
Hypotonic solution, 481
Hypovolemic shock, 251–262
  case study of, 255, 260
  clinical presentation in, 255
  diagnosis of, 255
  epidemiology of, 252–253
  etiology of, 252–253, 252*a*, 253*t*
  in intra-abdominal infections, 1283
  manifestations on major organs, 254, 255*t*
  neurohumoral response in, 253, 254*a*
  outcome evaluation in, 261–262
  pathophysiology of, 253–255, 253*f*, 254*a*
  patient care and monitoring in, 261
  treatment of, 255–261
    algorithm for, 256*a*
    blood products, 259
    colloids, 257–259, 258*t*
    crystalloids, 257, 258*t*
    fluid therapy, 257–259
    supportive care, 260–261
    vasopressors, 260, 260, 260*t*
Hypoxemia
  in asthma, 269, 283
  in COPD, 291
  metabolic acidosis with, 424*t*
  respiratory alkalosis with, 427*t*
Hypoxia
  in cystic fibrosis, 305
  in sepsis, 1349
  in status epilepticus, 542, 543, 544
Hysterectomy
  in anovulatory bleeding,
  antimicrobial prophylaxis in, 1399, 1400*t*
  in menorrhagia, 861
  in prevention of ovarian cancer, 1567
  total abdominal, in ovarian cancer, 1569,
    1569*f*
Hysteria, respiratory alkalosis in, 427*t*

I
Ibandronate
  dosage of, 973*t*
  in osteoporosis, 973, 973*t*, 974
Ibritumomab tiuxetan, 1466
  adverse effects of, 1466
  in cancer therapy, 1466
  mechanism of action of, 1466
  pharmacokinetics of, 1466
Ibuprofen
  anxiety with, 694*t*
  in common cold, 1218*t*
  in cystic fibrosis, 308
  dosage of, 308*t*, 834, 837, 838, 1002*t*, 1014*t*,
    1147
  drug interactions of, 954
  in gout, 1014*t*
  mechanism of action of, 1003
  in migraine, 591
  ocular changes with, 1077*t*
  in opioid withdrawal, 621*t*
  in osteoarthritis, 1002*t*
  in otitis media, 1207

Ibuprofen (*Cont.*)
  in pain, 572t
    in sickle cell anemia/disease, 1151t
  in pregnancy, 834, 1004
Ibutilide
  adverse effects of, 169t
  arrhythmia with, 177t, 179t
  in arrhythmias, 162t
  in atrial fibrillation, 170t, 171a
  dosage of, 170t
  drug interactions of, 170t
  mechanism of action of, 162t
Ice massage, 1023
ICE regimen, in non-Hodgkin's lymphoma, 1561t
Icodextrin, in peritoneal dialysis, 472
Idarubicin
  in acute myelogenous leukemia, 1590
  adverse effects of, 1459
  in cancer therapy, 1459
  dosage in hepatic impairment, 1471t
  emetogenicity of, 365t
  extravasation of, 1676t
  mechanism of action of, 1459
  pharmacokinetics of, 1459
Idiopathic thrombocytopenic purpura,
    menstruation-related disorders in, 857t
IDL. *See* Intermediate-density lipoproteins
Idraparinux, 200
Ifosfamide
  adverse effects of, 1461, 1581
  in cancer therapy, 1461
  dosage of, 1470t, 1561t
  emetogenicity of, 302t
  extravasation of, 1676t
  hemorrhagic cystitis with, 1666–1670
  mechanism of action of, 1461
  in non-Hodgkin's lymphoma, 1561t
  pharmacokinetics of, 1461
Ileitis, backwash, 342
Illicit drugs. *See* Substance-abuse disorders
Imatinib mesylate
  in acute lymphocytic leukemia, 1581, 1589,
    1591t
  adverse effects of, 1591t, 1600, 1600t
  in cancer therapy, 1452t, 1467
  in chronic myelogenous leukemia, 1581, 1599–
    1601, 1600t
  dosage of, 1471t, 1598
  drug interactions of, 1467, 1591t, 1599, 1600t
  mechanism of action of, 1467, 1591t, 1601
  pharmacokinetics of, 1467
Imidazotetrazines, 1622
Imipenem
  in campylobacteriosis, 1272
  dosage of, 1196t, 1660t
  in infections in cancer patients, 1660t
  in infective endocarditis, 1248
  in intra-abdominal infections, 1287t
  in pneumonia, 1196t, 1197, 1198, 1199t
  seizures with, 522
  in sepsis, 1353t
Imipenem-cilastatin
  in cellulitis, 1225t
  in diabetic foot infections, 1229t
  dosage of, 1225t, 1229t, 1288t, 1289, 1342t
  in infective endocarditis, 1248
  in intra-abdominal infections, 1287t, 1288t
  in osteomyelitis, 1339t, 1342t
  in urinary tract infections, 1311t
Imipramine, 10
  in ADHD, 727t, 728t, 729, 730t
  adverse effects of, 701t, 728t, 729, 923
  in cataplexy, 716

dosage of, 661, 661t, 696t, 701t, 727t
  drug interactions of, 614t
  in enuresis, 923, 923t, 924
  in generalized anxiety disorder, 696, 696t
  in panic disorder, 701t
  in urinary dysfunction, 563
Imiquimod
  adverse effects of, 1327t, 1328
  in genital warts, 1328
Immune globulin. *See also specific types*
  adverse effects of, 418
  CMV
    adverse effects of, 956t
    dosage of, 956t
    in prevention of cytomegalovirus, 956t
  dosage of, 419
  hepatitis A, 417–418
    postexposure prophylaxis, 418, 419
    pre-exposure prophylaxis, 418, 419
  vaccine interactions, 418, 419
Immune reconstitution syndrome, 1389
Immune thrombocytopenic purpura
  adult-onset, 1132
  childhood-onset, 1133
  clinical presentation in, 1133
  diagnosis of, 1133
  epidemiology of, 1132–1133
  etiology of, 1132–1133
  outcome evaluation in, 1135
  pathophysiology of, 1133
  treatment of, 1133–1135, 1134t
    anti-D immune globulin, 1134, 1134t
    corticosteroids, 1134, 1134t
    immunosuppressant therapy, 1134
    intravenous immunoglobulin, 1134, 1134t
    splenectomy, 1134
    thrombopoietic growth factors, 1134–1135
Immunization. *See* Vaccination
Immunocompromised patient. *See also* HIV
    infection
  cellulitis in, 1223
  cryptosporidiosis in, 1276
  endemic mycosis in, 1382
  intraabdominal infections in, 1288, 1289
  meningitis in, 1170, 1171t
  opportunistic mycosis in, 1382
  oropharyngeal candidiasis in, 1366–1369
  shigellosis in, 1268
  skin cancer in, 1612–1613
  vaccination of, 1416
Immunogenicity, 1405
Immunoglobulin A, secretory, 1703
Immunomodulators
  in pancreatitis, 407
  in psoriasis, 1084
Immunonutrition, 1708
Immunophenotype
  in acute lymphocytic leukemia, 1581, 1582t
  in acute myelogenous leukemia, 1581, 1582t
  immunophenotyping by flow cytometry, 1581
Immunosuppressive therapy
  cost of, 945t
  drug complications, 955–960
  drug interactions of, 953–955, 955t
  induction therapy, 944–947, 945t, 948f
  in inflammatory bowel disease, 353
  maintenance therapy, 945t, 948–952, 949a
Immunotherapy, allergen, 1050
Impaired fasting glucose, 740
Impaired glucose tolerance, 740
Impetigo
  clinical presentation in, 1222
  diagnosis of, 1222

epidemiology of, 1222
  etiology of, 1222
  treatment of, 1222
Implantable cardioverter-defibrillator
  in heart failure, 103
  after myocardial infarction, 139
  in ventricular tachycardia, 177
Implanted contraceptives, 844t
Impotence, 883
Inactivated influenza vaccine, 1408t
Inamrinone, in heart failure, 103
Inappropriate prescribing, definition of, 13–14
Incessant-ovulation hypothesis, of ovarian
    cancer, 1565, 1567–1568
Incontinence, urinary. *See* Urinary incontinence
Incretin mimetics, in diabetes mellitus, 754–755,
    754t
Indapamide
  adverse effects of, 60t
  arrhythmia with, 179t
  dosage of, 60t
  for hypertension, 60t, 72
  in prevention of stroke, 224, 225t
Index patient, 1318
Indinavir
  adverse effects of, 442, 1426, 1430t,
    1438t–1439t
  dosage of, 1430t
  drug interactions of, 816, 955t, 1430t
  food interactions of, 1430t
  in HIV infection, 1426, 1430t
  mechanism of action of, 1421f
Indirect calorimetry, 1688
Indomethacin
  anxiety with, 694t
  dosage of, 832t, 1002t, 894t
  in gout, 1013, 1014t
  migraines with, 588t
  ocular changes with, 1077t
  in osteoarthritis, 1002t
  peptic ulcer disease with, 331
  in pregnancy, 1004
  as tocolytic, 832t, 832t
Infant. *See also* Pediatric patients
  acute lymphocytic leukemia in, 1589
  acute myelogenous leukemia in, 1593
Infantile spasms, 525, 525t
Infection. *See also specific types and sites*
  in acute leukemia, 1594
  antimicrobial therapy in
    drug considerations, 1162–1164, 1162t
    patient considerations, 1162t, 1164–1165
  case study of, 1158, 1161, 1165, 1167
  clinical presentation in, 1158–1161
  colonization vs., 1157
  diagnosis of, 1158–1161, 1165
    DIC with, 1131t
  endogenous, 1156–1157
  in enteral nutrition patients, 1711t, 1713
  epidemiology of, 1156
  etiology of, 1156
  exogenous, 1157
  fever with, 1158
  imaging studies in, 1158
  laboratory studies in, 1158–1159, 1159t
  microbiologic studies in, 1159–1161, 1160a
  nosocomial, 1156
  outcome evaluation in, 1165–1167, 1166a
  in parenteral nutrition patients, 1698
  pathophysiology of, 1156–1157
  patient care and monitoring in, 1167
  physical examination in, 1158
  secondary, 1167

in sickle cell anemia/disease, 1143*t*, 1149
treatment of
    antimicrobial regimen selection, 1155–1168
      general approach, 1161–1162
      nonantimicrobial, 1161–1162
      source control, 1162, 1165
Infective endocarditis, 1235–1251
  case study of, 1236, 1243, 1248, 1249
  causative organisms, 1239–1242
  clinical presentation in, 1238–1239, 1239*f*
  culture-negative, 1236*t*, 1242, 1248
  diagnosis of, 1239, 1239*f*
  epidemiology of, 1236
  etiology of, 1236
  extracardiac manifestations of, 1238, 1239*f*
  fungal, 1236*t*, 1242, 1248
  HACEK group, 1236*t*
  laboratory studies in, 1238–1239
  modified Duke criteria for, 1240*t*
  outcome evaluation in, 1250
  pathophysiology of, 1297, 1297*f*
  patient care and monitoring in, 1251
  prevention of, 1249–1250, 1250*t*
  sites of infection, 1090, 1090*f*
  treatment of, 1242–1250
    antibiotics, 1242–1248, 1244*t*
    surgery, 1248
Inferior vena cava filter
  in prevention of venous thromboembolism, 193
  in venous thromboembolism, 206–207
Infertility in hematopoietic cell transplant
    recipients, 1644
Inflammation
  in COPD, 289
  in musculoskeletal disorders, 1021
  sepsis and, 1347
Inflammatory bowel disease, 341–355. *See also*
    Crohn's disease; Ulcerative colitis
  anemia in, 1110
  case study of, 345, 348, 350
  clinical presentation in, 343–345
  colorectal cancer and, 1518*t*, 1519
  complications of, 343–344
  depth of disease penetration in, 283*f*
  diagnosis of, 344–345
  diarrhea in, 376
  in elderly, 352
  epidemiology of, 342
  etiology of, 342
  extraintestinal manifestations of, 343–344
  gastrointestinal landmarks and disease
    distribution in, 343*f*
  genetic factors in, 342
  lymphoma and, 1553
  nausea and vomiting with, 358*t*
  osteoporosis in, 977
  outcome evaluation in, 354–355
  pathophysiology of, 342–343
  patient care and monitoring in, 354
  in pediatric patient, 352–353
  peritonitis in, 1283
  in pregnancy, 292
  severity of, 345
  smoking and, 342
  treatment of, 345–354
    aminosalicylates, 346–347, 346*t*
    antibiotics, 348
    biologic agents, 347*t*, 348
    cholestyramine, 346
    corticosteroids, 347, 347*t*, 351*t*, 352
    diet therapy, 343, 345
    enteral nutrition, 1702*t*
    immunosuppressants, 347–348, 347*t*

intestine transplantation, 941
  nicotine, 349
  nonpharmacologic, 345
  surgery, 350
  symptomatic interventions, 346
  venous thromboembolism in, 187
Inflammatory mediators
  in allergic rhinitis, 1049
  in asthma, 266
Inflammatory pain, 568
Infliximab, 988
  adverse effects of, 348, 986*t*, 1088
  dosage of, 347*t*, 349*t*, 351*t*, 986*t*, 1088
  in GVHD, 1640
  in inflammatory bowel disease, 347*t*, 348, 349*t*,
    350, 351, 351*t*
  monitoring treatment with, 986*t*
  in pregnancy, 353
  in psoriasis, 1085, 1088
  in rheumatoid arthritis, 986*t*
Influenza, 1410
Influenza A virus, 1410
  in CNS infections, 1183
  in pneumonia, 1190, 1197
Influenza B virus, 1410
  in CNS infections, 1183
  in pneumonia, 1190, 1197
Influenza vaccine, 271, 293, 395, 1197, 1207,
    1408*t*, 1410
  drug interactions of, 205*t*
  recommendations for, 1197
  in sickle cell anemia/disease, 1143
Influenza virus
  in otitis media, 1204
  in pharyngitis, 1214
  in rhinosinusitis, 1209
Ingram's regimen, 1085
Inhalers, 271
  steps for using, 272*f*
Injection site reactions
  with antiretrovirals, 1442*t*
  with vaccination, 1415
Inodilator, 103
Inotropic agents
  in heart failure, 102–103
  in sepsis, 1356
Inotropic state, of heart, 81
INR. *See* International Normalized Ratio
Insomnia
  clinical presentation in, 712
  with corticosteroids, 953*t*
  diagnosis of, 712
  epidemiology and etiology of, 710
  palliative care, symptom in, 47
  pathophysiology of, 711
  patient care and monitoring in, 719
  primary, 710
  rebound, 714
  secondary, 710
  treatment of, 714–715
    antidepressants, 714–715, 714*t*
    antihistamines, 715
    benzodiazepine receptor agonists, 714, 716*t*
Institute for Safe Medication Practice (ISMP), 29
Instrumental activities of daily living (IADLs), 10*t*
Insulin. *See also* Diabetes mellitus
  action of, 738
  fetal production of, 743
  hexamers, 753
  production of, 738
  secretion of, impaired, 738
Insulin-like growth factors, 803
  in acromegaly, 803

in growth hormone deficiency, 812
  IGF-I, 803
  IGF-II, 803
Insulin pen, 751
Insulin pump, 743, 753–754, 753*f*
Insulin resistance, 112, 238, 305, 736, 738
  in critically ill patients, 1694
  drug-related, 1441*t*
Insulin response
  first-phase, 738
  second-phase, 738
Insulin secretagogues
  adverse effects of, 748*t*
  in diabetes mellitus, 747–750, 748*t*
Insulin syringe, 751
Insulin therapy
  administration of, 751–753, 752*t*
  allergic drug reactions, 929*t*, 933
  combination insulin products, 753, 753*t*
  in cystic fibrosis, 302, 312
  in diabetes mellitus, 743–744, 751–753
  in diabetic ketoacidosis, 756
  in hospitalized patient, 758–759
  in hyperkalemia, 454, 489
  in hyperosmolar hyperglycemic state, 757
  hypokalemia with, 487
  hypomagnesemia with, 492
  insulin aspart, 752*t*, 753
  insulin detemir, 751, 752*t*
  insulin glargine, 751, 752*t*
  insulin glulisine, 751, 752*t*
  insulin lispro, 751, 752*t*
  insulin pump, 743, 753–754, 753*f*
  intermediate-acting insulin, 752*t*, 753
  long-duration insulin, 752*t*, 753
  NPH insulin, 752*t*, 753
  in parenteral nutrition admixtures, 1694,
    1694
  rapid-acting insulin, 752*t*, 753
  regular insulin, 752*t*, 753, 1694, 1694
  short-acting insulin, 753*t*
Insulin tolerance test, 788*t*
Integrase, 1421
Intelence, in HIV infection, 1433
Interferon alfa, 1465
  adverse effects of, 1600*t*, 1601
  in chronic myelogenous leukemia, 1600*t*,
    1601
Interferon alfa-2*a*
  in chronic hepatitis B, 422
  in chronic hepatitis C, 424
Interferon alfa-2b
  adverse effects of, 1618, 1620*t*, 1625
  in chronic hepatitis B, 422
  in chronic hepatitis C, 424
  dosage of, 1618, 1620*t*
    in melanoma, 1618, 1620*t*, 1625*t*
Interferon alfacon-1, in chronic hepatitis C, 424
Interferon gamma, 1465
  in psoriasis, 1081
  in tuberculosis, 1255
Interferon-gamma release assay, 1258
Interferon therapy
  adverse effects of, 422, 424–425, 1465
  blood glucose level and, 737*t*
  in cancer, 1465
  in chronic hepatitis C, 424–425
  depression with, 656
  in hepatitis B, 422
  in hepatitis D, 425
  hypothyroidism with, 767, 767*t*, 779
  intralesional, adverse effects of, 1327*t*
  mechanism of action of, 1465

Interferon therapy (*Cont.*)
peylated interferon
in chronic hepatitis C, 424–425
in hepatitis B, 422
pharmacokinetics of, 1465
Interferon β, 1465
administration of, 512
adverse effects of, 511, 513*t*
dosage of, 513*t*, 514
mechanism of action of, 510
in multiple sclerosis, 510–514, 513*t*, 515*t*
neutralizing antibodies to, 512–513
pharmacology of, 510
Interleukin-1
in meningitis, 1172
in rheumatoid arthritis, 982*t*, 983
Interleukin-1 receptor antagonist, in rheumatoid
arthritis, 982*t*
Interleukin-2. *See also* Aldesleukin
dosage of, 1620*t*
in melanoma, 1620*t*
in psoriasis, 1082
Interleukin-3, 1110, 1110*f*
Interleukin-4, in rheumatoid arthritis, 982*t*, 983
Interleukin-6, 992
in rheumatoid arthritis, 982*t*, 983
Interleukin-10, in rheumatoid arthritis, 982*t*, 983
Interleukin-17, in rheumatoid arthritis, 982*t*, 983
Intermediate-density lipoproteins (IDL), 230, 231
physical characteristics of, 177*t*
Intermittent pneumatic compression, in
prevention of venous thromboembolism,
191–192, 192*t*
International Index model, for non-Hodgkin's
lymphoma, 1556, 1557
International League Against Epilepsy,
classification
of seizures, 524, 525, 525*t*, 529, 530*t*
International Normalized Ratio (INR), 13, 96,
135, 171, 172, 193, 194*a*, 202–205, 223,
278, 400, 1455, 1529, 1715
International Sensitivity Index, 202
Interstitial fluid, 480
volume of, 480
Intestine transplantation. *See also* Solid-organ
transplantation
acute rejection, signs and symptoms of, 944*t*
epidemiology and etiology of, 940–941
Intima, 232
Intoxication. *See* Substance-abuse disorders
Intraabdominal abscess,1281–1291. *See also*
Intraabdominal infection
definition of, 1282
Intraabdominal infection, 1281–1291
case study of, 1282, 1285
clinical presentation in, 1284
diagnosis of, 1284
epidemiology of, 1282–1283
etiology of, 1282–1283
in immunocompromised patients, 1288, 1289
microbiology of, 1283
outcome evaluation in, 1289–1290
pathophysiology of, 1283
patient care and monitoring in, 1290
sepsis and, 1353*t*, 1354–1355
treatment of, 1284–1289
antimicrobials, 1286–1289, 1286*t*,
1287*t*–1288*t*
drainage procedures, 1285
fluid therapy, 1285
Intra-abdominal pressure, 910
Intra-aortic balloon counterpulsation, in heart
failure, 103–104

Intracellular cell adhesion molecules, in
psoriasis, 1081
Intracellular fluid, 253, 253*f*, 257, 480
ion concentrations in, 484*t*
volume of, 480
Intracerebral hemorrhage, 216, 217, 219*a*
treatment of, 221
Intracranial hemorrhage, 222
nausea and vomiting with, 358*t*
warfarin-related, 204
Intracranial hypertension, 1172
nausea and vomiting with, 358*t*
respiratory acidosis with, 426*t*
Intraocular pressure
elevated, 1032, 1033. *See also* Glaucoma
target pressure, 1037
Intrapulmonary percussive ventilation, in cystic
fibrosis, 307
Intrauterine device, 851
contraindications to, 851
efficacy of, 844*t*
for emergency contraception, 853
levonorgestrel-releasing
in dysmenorrhea, 859*t*, 863, 864
in menorrhagia, 859*t*, 861
mechanism of action of, 851
patient monitoring in, 853
side effects of, 851
therapy for menstruation-related disorders, 855
Intravascular fluid, 480
volume of, 252, 253, 480
Intravenous drug user
cellulitis in, 1225
hepatitis C in, 414
hepatitis D in, 415
infective endocarditis in, 1235–1236, 1241,
1242
stroke and, 217*t*
Intravenous immunoglobulin
dosage of, 1134, 1134*t*
in immune thrombocytopenic purpura, 1134,
1134*t*
Intravenous medication, "keep the vein open,"
482–483
Intravenous pyelogram, in benign prostatic
hyperplasia, 898
Intravesicular therapy, in hemorrhagic cystitis,
1667
Intrinsic factor, 1111
Intussusception
in cystic fibrosis, 305
rotavirus vaccine-associated, 1412
Iodide therapy
adverse effects of, 775
dosage of, 775–776
in hyperthyroidism, 775–776
Iodine
deficiency of, 764, 767
excess of, 774*t*
organification of, 764
physiology of, 764
radioactive, 766
adverse effects of, 775
in hyperthyroidism, 775–776
Iodism, 776
Iodoquinol
in amebiasis, 1295–1296
dosage of, 1296
Iohexol, nephrotoxicity of, 441
Ionizing radiation, 1622
Iopamidol, nephrotoxicity of, 441
Iopromide, nephrotoxicity of, 441
Iothalamate, nephrotoxicity of, 441

Ioversol, nephrotoxicity of, 441
iPledge, 1098
Ipratropium
adverse effects of, 276
in allergic rhinitis, 1051*t*, 1056, 1058*t*, 1059
arrhythmia with, 166*t*
in asthma, 270*t*, 276, 277*t*
in common cold, 1218*t*
in COPD, 293*t*, 294–295, 298
dosage of, 295*t*
intranasal, 1056
Ipriflavone, in osteoporosis, 976
Irbesartan
adverse effects of, 62*t*
dosage of, 62*t*
in hypertension, 62*t*
Irinotecan
adverse effects of, 1451, 1459, 1512, 1527*t*, 1529
in UDP-glucuronosyltransferase deficiency,
1529
in cancer therapy, 1452*t*, 1459
in colorectal cancer, 1524*t*, 1525–1526, 1527*t*,
1528*t*, 1529
dosage of, 1507*t*–1508*t*, 1524*t*
in hepatic impairment, 1471*t*
emetogenicity of, 365*t*
extravasation of, 1676*t*
in lung cancer, 1507*t*–1508*t*, 1509
mechanism of action of, 1454*a*, 1459, 1528*t*
pharmacokinetics of, 1459
Iris plateau, 1035
Iritis, in inflammatory bowel disease, 344
Iron
deficiency in restless-legs syndrome, 711, 717
dosage, 830*t*
evaluation of iron status, 1112, 1113*t*
food sources of, 1115*t*
transport and metabolism of, 1111, 1111*f*
Iron-deficiency anemia, 1114*a*
in cancer patients, 1116
in chronic kidney disease, 1117
outcome evaluation in, 1117
in parenteral nutrition patients, 1687–1688
pathophysiology of, 1111
treatment of, 1115–1116, 1115*t*
Iron dextran, 1687–1688
adverse effects of, 459, 1116
in anemia of chronic kidney disease, 459
dosage of, 1115–1116
iron content of, 1115*t*
in iron-deficiency anemia, 1114–1116, 1115*t*
Iron overload, transfusion-related, 1146
Iron sucrose, 1688
in anemia of chronic kidney disease, 459
iron content of, 1115*t*
in iron-deficiency anemia, 1115*t*, 1115
Iron supplementation/therapy
adverse effects of, 459, 1113
in anemia of chronic kidney disease, 456–459,
458*a*, 1117
constipation with, 372*t*
dosage of, 459
drug interactions of, 771*t*, 1113
GERD with, 317*t*
in iron-deficiency anemia, 1113–1116, 1115*t*
parenteral therapy, 1114–1115, 1115*t*, 1688
products available, 1115*t*
Irreversible sickle cells, 1006
Irritable bowel syndrome, 380–385
case study of, 383, 385
constipation in, 372*t*
constipation-predominant, 382
cost of, 381

diagnosis of, 381–382
  Manning criteria, 382
  Rome II criteria, 382
diarrhea-predominant, 382
epidemiology of, 381
ethnicity and, 381
etiology of, 381
outcome evaluation in, 384–385
pain in, 568
pathophysiology of, 381
patient care and monitoring in, 385
treatment of, 383–384
  antidepressants, 383, 384t
  antispasmodics, 383, 384t
  botanicals, 383
  bulk-forming laxatives, 384, 384t
  diet therapy, 383
  5-HT$_3$ antagonists, 384
  5-HT$_4$ antagonists, 384
  nonpharmacologic, 383
  psychological, 383
Irritant, 1676, 1677t
Ischemic heart disease, 109–127. *See also* Acute
    coronary syndromes; Angina pectoris;
    Myocardial infarction
arrhythmia in, 162t, 166t, 177t
Canadian Cardiovascular Society classification
  of, 115, 115t
cardiovascular risk assessment for
  phosphodiesterase inhibitors, 890t
case study of, 115, 116
clinical presentation in, 114–116
COX-2 inhibitors in, 119, 126
diabetes mellitus and, 111t, 114, 149, 150
diagnosis of, 114–116
in elderly, 126
epidemiology of, 110–112
etiology of, 110–112
genetic factors in, 28t
gout and, 1011
heart failure and, 80, 80t
hormone replacement therapy and, 125, 766,
  876t, 877
dyslipidemia and, 111, 111t, 112, 229–249
hypertension and, 65, 11, 11t, 112, 119
laboratory analysis in, 115
myocardial oxygen supply and demand in, 110,
  110f, 121, 122, 122t, 123, 132
obesity and, 111t, 112, 1720–1721
outcome evaluation in, 126–127
pathophysiology of, 112–114, 113f, 230–234,
  230f, 231f, 231t
patient care and monitoring in, 127
risk factors for, 111–112, 111t, 236, 237f, 238t
  emerging risk factors, 240
  life-habit risk factors, 240
smoking and, 111, 111t,
treatment of, 116–126, 117f
  ACE inhibitors, 120–121, 121t
  algorithm for, 118a
  angiotensin receptor blockers, 116–117,
    120, 121t
  antioxidants, 125
  antiplatelet agents, 119–120
  assessing drug effectiveness and safety,
    126–127
  β-blockers, 117, 119, 122–123, 122t, 124, 126
  calcium channel blockers, 123–124
  control of risk factors, 119
  coronary artery bypass surgery, 117, 118–119
  drugs with no benefit or potentially
    harmful, 125
  duration of therapy, 127

folic acid, 125
heart transplantation, 940
herbal products, 125–126
interventional approaches, 118–119
lifestyle modifications, 117–118
nitrates, 121, 122t
nitroglycerin, 121
percutaneous coronary intervention, 117, 118
to prevent acute coronary syndromes and
  death, 119–121
prevention of recurrent ischemic
    symptoms, 124
ranolazine, 125
statins, 120, 126
Ischemic penumbra, 217
Ischemic stroke
etiology of, 216
pathophysiology of, 217–218
patient care and monitoring in, 226, 226t
prevention of, 222–224
risk factors for, 217, 217t
treatment of, 219–222, 219–222, 221t
Isentress, in HIV infection, 1433
Islets of Langerhans, 738
Isoflavones
  in osteoporosis, 976
  in prevention of prostate cancer, 1537
Isoflurane, in status epilepticus, 549
Isolated systolic hypertension, 67, 70–71, 72
Isoniazid
  adverse effects of, 1261t
  anxiety with, 694t
  dosage of, 1259t, 1260t, 1261t
  drug interactions of, 153t, 321, 614t, 955t
  hyperprolactinemia with, 814t
  overdose of, 501t
  in tuberculosis, 1253, 1258–1259, 1259t, 1260t,
    1261t, 1262
Isoproterenol
  anxiety with, 694t
  GERD with, 317t
  growth hormone deficiency with, 810
  in torsades de pointes, 181
Isosorbide
  adverse effects of, 1042
  in glaucoma, 1042
Isosorbide dinitrate
  adverse effects of, 63t, 94
  in angina, 121, 124
  dosage of, 63t, 78t
  in heart failure, 93–94
  in hypertension, 63t
  in ischemic heart disease, 78t
  mechanism of action of, 93
Isosorbide mononitrate
  dosage of, 78t
  in ischemic heart disease, 78t
  in portal hypertension, 396
Isotonic solution, 481
Isotretinoin
  in acne vulgaris, 1098–1099, 1099t
  adverse effects of, 1098, 1098t, 1099t
  dosage of, 1098, 1099t
  dry eye with, 1075t
  hyperlipidemia with, 236t
  in lactation, 824t
  teratogenicity of, 824t, 1098
Isradipine, arrhythmia with, 163t
Itch mite, 1304
Itraconazole
  administration through feeding tube, 1715
  adverse effects of, 86t, 1385–1387, 1642
  in aspergillosis, 1642

in blastomycosis, 1379t
in coccidioidomycosis, 1379t
in cryptococcosis, 1389
dosage of, 1364, 1364t, 1368, 1371, 1372, 1379t,
  1386t
drug interactions of, 205t, 214, 684, 698, 699t,
  955t, 1457, 1592t, 1600t, 1642
in endemic mycosis, 1378, 1381
in esophageal candidiasis, 1368, 1385
formulations of, 1378
in fungal infections, 957
in histoplasmosis, 1379t
in infections in cancer patients, 1660t
in invasive candidiasis, 1384, 1386t
in onychomycosis, 1371
in oropharyngeal candidiasis, 1368, 1385
in prevention of endemic mycosis, 1381
in prevention of fungal infections, 1642
in prevention of invasive candidiasis, 1385
in tinea infections, 1371
in vulvovaginal candidiasis, 1364, 1364t
Ivermectin
  dosage of, 1298
  in lice infestation, 1304
  in scabies, 1304
  in strongyloidiasis, 1298
Ixabepilone
  adverse effects of, 1492, 1459
  in breast cancer, 1491–1492
  in cancer therapy, 1458–1459
  dosage in hepatic impairment, 1471t

J
Janeway lesions, 1237, 1238, 1239f
Jarisch-Herxheimer reaction, 1322
Jejunostomy, in cystic fibrosis, 307
Jejunostomy tube, 1704, 1705f, 1705t, 1706
  percutaneous endoscopic, 1704, 1705f
Jeliffe "bedside" clearance equations, 11
Jelliffe equation, 434t
Jet lag, 718
JNC 7 report, 52, 58
Joint Commission on Accreditation of Healthcare
  Organizations, 29
Jugular venous pressure, assessment of, 85t, 86
Junctional tachycardia, 160
Juvenile absence epilepsy with generalized
  tonic-clonic seizure on awakening, 525t
Juvenile idiopathic arthritis (JIA), diagnostic
  criteria for, 985
Juvenile myoclonic epilepsy, 525, 525t

K
Kanamycin
  adverse effects of, 1261t
  dosage of, 1261t
  in tuberculosis, 1260, 1261t
Kaposi's sarcoma, in transplant recipient, 959
Karnofsky scale, of performance status, 1451,
  1453t
Kegel exercises, 872, 874
Keratinization, 1094
Keratinocytes, 1081
Keratitis, bacterial
  clinical presentation in, 1070
  diagnosis of, 1070
  epidemiology of, 1070
  outcome evaluation in, 1071
  pathophysiology of, 1070
  risk factors for, 1070t
  treatment of, 1070–1071, 1071t
Keratoconjunctivitis sicca, 1075
  in rheumatoid arthritis, 984

Keratolytics
in acne vulgaris, 1097–1098
in psoriasis, 1084
Keratotic manifestations, of genital warts, 1327
Kernig's sign, 1173
Ketamine, in status epilepticus, 549
Ketoacidosis, 501, 501t, 502
diabetic. *See* Diabetic ketoacidosis
Ketoconazole
adverse effects of, 796t, 1364, 1546
in Cushing's syndrome, 795, 796t
dosage of, 796t, 1364t, 1468
drug interactions of, 170t, 537t, 647, 684, 955t, 1467, 1468, 1726
mechanism of action of, 796t
in oropharyngeal candidiasis, 1385
in prostate cancer, 1468, 1539t, 1540, 1546
in tinea infections, 1371
in vulvovaginal candidiasis, 1364t
Ketogenic diet, in epilepsy, 528
Ketoprofen
dosage of, 1014t
drug interactions of, 1457
in gout, 1014t
Ketorolac
adverse effects of, 1068t, 1150
in allergic conjunctivitis, 1068t, 1070
dosage of, 1068t, 1151t
drug interactions of, 954
mechanism of action of, 1068t
ocular, in corneal abrasion, 1064
in pain, in sickle cell anemia/disease, 1149–1150, 1151t
peptic ulcer disease with, 331
Ketosis, in gestational diabetes, 744
Ketotifen
adverse effects of, 1068t
in allergic conjunctivitis, 1068t
dosage of, 1068t
mechanism of action of, 1068t
Kidney. *See also* Renal *entries*
assessment of renal function, 433, 434t
functions of, 445
sodium regulation by, 54–55
Kidney biopsy, in acute renal failure, 435
Kidney cancer
epidemiology of, 1446f
hypercalcemia with, 1670–1673
Kidney disease
acute. *See* Renal failure, acute
chronic, 445–476. *See also* End-stage renal disease; Renal disease; Renal failure, chronic
anemia and, 452, 455–459, 1111, 1114a, 1117
assessment for, 448–449
blood urea nitrogen in, 449
case study of, 452, 456, 460, 469
clinical presentation in, 449
complications of, 449
consequences of, 453–468
creatinine in, 449
definition of, 446
diabetes mellitus and, 447, 450, 758
edema in, 453
epidemiology of, 446–447
etiology of, 446–447
glomerular filtration rate in, 446
glomerulonephritis and, 447
hyperkalemia in, 454
hyperlipidemia and, 446–447, 451–452
hyperparathyroidism in, 459–465
hyperprolactinemia in, 814t
hypertension and, 447, 450, 458

initiation factors in, 447, 447t
metabolic acidosis in, 461, 465
microalbuminuria in, 447, 449
NKF-DOQI classification of, 446, 446t
osteoporosis and, 967t
outcome evaluation in, 452–453
pathophysiology of, 448
patient care and monitoring in, 476
progression factors in, 447, 446t
proteinuria in, 447, 449, 450–451
pruritus in, 467–468
renal osteodystrophy in, 459–465
risk factors for, 446, 446t
smoking and, 447, 452
sodium balance in, 453, 454
susceptibility factors in, 446–447, 446t
treatment of, 449–453
diuretics, 453
kidney transplantation, 941
nutritional management, 450
pharmacologic, 450–451
renal replacement therapy, 468–475
vitamin replacement, 468
uremia in, 455
uremic bleeding in, 467
water balance in, 453
Kidney transplantation. *See also* Solid-organ transplantation
acute rejection, signs and symptoms of, 944t
in end-stage renal disease, 468
epidemiology and etiology of, 941
pancreas-kidney transplantation, 942
Kindling, 523, 616
Kingella kingae, in infective endocarditis, 1241
Klebsiella
in infections in cancer patients, 1655t
in infective endocarditis, 1242
in intra-abdominal infections, 1283, 1286, 1286t
in necrotizing fasciitis, 1226
Klebsiella pneumoniae
in COPD exacerbations, 298, 299t
in meningitis, 1171t
in sepsis, 1348t
in spontaneous bacterial peritonitis, 391
in surgical site infections, 1397t
in urinary tract infections, 1308, 1310
Klinefelter's syndrome, acute leukemia and, 1580t, 1581
Koebner phenomenon, 1080
Korotkoff sounds, 56
Korsakoff's syndrome, 618
Kostmann's syndrome, 1580t
Ku-Zyme products, 409t
Kyphoscoliosis, respiratory acidosis with, 426t
Kyphosis, 966
in cystic fibrosis, 305

L
Labetalol
adverse effects of, 71t
in arrhythmias, 162
dosage of, 71t, 124t
in heart failure, 97
in hypertension, 61t, 67, 70, 71t, 72t
in hypertensive emergency, 71t
in ischemic heart disease, 124t
mechanism of action of, 162t
in pregnancy, 72t
in stroke, 220t
Labor, preterm, 826, 832t, 835–836
Labor induction, 825
Labyrinthitis, nausea and vomiting with, 358t

Lacrimation, in opioid withdrawal, 619
Lactase deficiency, 376
Lactase tablets, 380
Lactated Ringer's solution, 482, 482t
in dehydration, 1268t
in hypovolemic shock, 256a, 257
in intra-abdominal infections, 1285
Lactation, 821–838
AAP table, 829
allergic rhinitis in, 1059
antimicrobials in, 1165
bacterial vaginosis in, 825, 833–834
breast infections in, 837–838
depression in, 665
drug, 829, 829t
effects in breast-fed infants, 828–829
pharmackokinetics, 829
drug use in, 821–838
contraindicated drugs and drugs of concern, 824t
desired outcomes, 823
epidemiology of, 821–822
sources of information for, 826–827, 827t
enhancement of, 836–837
epidemiology, 821–822
etiology, 821–822
milk/plasma ration, 829
pathophysiology, 822–823
respiratory disorders in, 835
risk evaluation, 823–829
Lactic acidosis, 501, 501t, 502
drug-related, 1437t
in hypovolemic shock, 254, 260
with metformin, 750
in sepsis, 1349
treatment of, 260
Lactobacillus, normal flora, 1157f
Lactobacillus acidophilus, 349
Lactose intolerance, 377, 1294
Lactulose
in constipation, 373, 374, 375
dosage of, 830t
in hepatic encephalopathy, 399
Lamina cribrosa, 1034
Laminectomy, in spinal cord compression, 1664
Lamivudine
adverse effects of, 423, 1426, 1427t–1428t, 1437t
in chronic hepatitis B, 423
dosage of, 423, 1427t–1428t
drug interactions of, 1427t–1428t
in HIV infection, 1426, 1427t–1428t, 1434
mechanism of action of, 1421f
resistance to, 423
Lamotrigine, 828t
adverse effects of, 529t, 530, 684
in bipolar disorder, 677t, 680t–682t, 684, 686
dosage of, 677t, 684
drug interactions of, 684
in epilepsy, 529t, 530, 530t, 531, 532t, 537t, 538
mechanism of action of, 522, 684
monitoring therapy with, 682t, 684
pharmacokinetics of, 680t–681t
in pregnancy, 686
in prevention of migraine, 590, 590t
Langerhans cell histiocytosis, acute leukemia and, 1580t
Lanolin, in diaper dermatitis, 1106
Lanreotide
in acromegaly, 807t
adverse effects of, 807t
dosage of, 807t
Lansoprazole
dosage of, 320, 321–322, 323, 335t, 336t

drug interactions of, 321–322
  in GERD, 320, 321–322, 323
  in *Helicobacter pylori* eradication, 335t
  in peptic ulcer disease, 336t
Lanthanum
  adverse effects of, 463
  dosage of, 464t
  in hyperphosphatemia, 463, 464t, 491
Laparoscopic surgery, in ovarian cancer, 1569
Laparotomy, exploratory, 1693
  in ovarian cancer, 1569
Lapatinib
  adverse effects of, 1467
  in breast cancer, 1493
  in cancer therapy, 1452t, 1467
  dosage of, 1467
  pharmacokinetics of, 1467
Large intestine, normal flora of, 1157f
Laryngospasm
  allergic drug reaction, 932
  respiratory acidosis with, 426t
Lasar's paste, 1084
Laser iridotomy, in glaucoma, 1037, 1040
Laser trabeculoplasty, in glaucoma, 1037, 1037t
Lasofoxifene, 976
Latanoprost
  administration of, 1040
  adverse effects of, 1041
  dosage of, 1038t
  in glaucoma, 1038t, 1040–1041
  mechanism of action of, 1038t, 1040
  ocular changes with, 1077t
Latent autoimmune diabetes in adults, 736
Latex allergy, 1100, 1100t
Laxatives. *See also specific types*
  abuse, 372t, 376
  in constipation, 373–374, 374t
  contraindications to, 375
  diarrhea with, 376t
  hyperphosphatemia with, 491
LDL. *See* Low-density lipoprotein(s)
Lead, in calcium products, 972
Lead poisoning, 501t, 1114a
Leflunomide, 953, 988
  adverse effects of, 986t, 988
  dosage of, 986t
  mechanism of action of, 988
  monitoring treatment with, 986t
  in rheumatoid arthritis, 986t, 988
Left ventricular dysfunction, 67, 70, 80–81, 84,
    161. *See also* Heart failure *entries*
Legionella, in infective endocarditis, 1242
Legionella pneumophila
  in pneumonia, 1190, 1190t, 1194, 1196t, 1354
  within pulmonary macrophages, 1163
Legume allergy, 1684
Lenalidomide
  adverse effects of, 1464, 1606t, 1606
  in cancer therapy, 1452t
  dosage in renal dysfunction, 1470t
  in multiple myeloma, 1464, 1606, 1606t
  in myelodysplastic syndrome, 1464
  pharmacokinetics of, 1464
Lennox-Gastaut syndrome, 525t, 525t
Lentigines, PUVA, 1085
Lepirudin
  adverse effects of, 198t
  in venous thromboembolism, 200, 200f, 201
Letrozole
  adverse effects of, 1469, 1487t, 1489, 1574t
  in breast cancer, 1487t, 1489
  in cancer therapy, 1469
  dosage of, 1487t, 1574t

  mechanism of action of, 1469, 1489
  osteoporosis with, 967t
  in ovarian cancer, 1574t
  pharmacokinetics of, 1469
Leucovorin, 1457
  in colorectal cancer, 1524–1526, 1524t, 1527t,
    1529, 1531
  dosage of, 1524t, 1561t
  in non-Hodgkin's lymphoma, 1561t
Leukemia. *See also specific types*
  acute, 1579–1595
    case study of, 1584, 1587, 1589
    phenotypic risk factors for, 1580
  chronic, 1597–1608
  metastasis to brain, 1665t
  with mitoxantrone, 514
  secondary, 1594
Leukemoid reaction, in shigellosis, 1268
Leukocytosis, 1159t
  with corticosteroids, 953t
  in sepsis, 1349
Leukopenia, 1159t
  with ATG, 946
  in sepsis, 1349
Leukostasis, in acute myelogenous leukemia,
    1583
Leukotriene(s), biosynthesis of, 1003a
Leukotriene modifiers
  in asthma, 273, 275t, 273, 275t, 276–278, 283
  in COPD, 297
Leukotriene receptor antagonists
  in allergic rhinitis, 1051t, 1056, 1060t
Leuprolide
  adverse effects of, 1468, 1487t, 1543, 1544t
  in breast cancer, 1487t, 1490
  in cancer therapy, 1468
  dosage of, 1487t, 1544t
  in prevention of priapism, 1149
  mechanism of action of, 1468
  osteoporosis with, 967t
  pharmacokinetics of, 1468
  in prostate cancer, 1543–1544, 1544t
Levalbuterol
  in asthma, 270t, 272–273, 277t
  in COPD, 294, 295t
  dosage of, 295t
Levetiracetam
  adverse effects of, 533t, 536
  dosage of, 533t
  in epilepsy, 529t, 530t, 531, 533t
  mechanism of action of, 533t
  pharmacokinetics of, 533t
Levobunolol
  dosage of, 1038t
  in glaucoma, 1038t, 1040
  mechanism of action of, 1038t
Levocabastine
  adverse effects of, 1068t
  in allergic conjunctivitis, 1068t
  dosage of, 1068t
  mechanism of action of, 1068t
Levocarnitine
  in allergic rhinitis, 1053, 1054t
  supplementation during hemodialysis, 472
Levodopa
  adsorption and metabolism of, 558f
  anxiety with, 694t
  mania with, 676t
  in Parkinson's disease, 556, 557
Levodopa/carbidopa
  adverse effects of, 461, 717t
  controlled-release formulation of, 561
  dosage of, 559t, 717t

  liquid formulation of, 561
  mechanism of action of, 559t
  in Parkinson's disease, 557, 559t, 561
  in restless-legs syndrome, 717, 717t
Levofloxacin
  administration through feeding tube, 1715
  adverse effects of, 1262t
  arrhythmia with, 129t
  in *Chlamydia*, 1321
  in conjunctivitis, 1066, 1066t
  in COPD, 299t
  in cystic fibrosis, 309t
  in diarrhea, 380
  dosage of, 251t, 1066t, 1194t, 1196t, 1199t,
    1212t, 1262t, 1269t, 1311t, 1312t, 1333t,
    1342t
  in gonorrhea, 1319
  in intra-abdominal infections, 1287
  in osteomyelitis, 1339t, 1343t
  in PID, 1333t
  in pneumonia, 1194t, 1195, 1196t, 1197, 1198,
    1199t, 1200
  in rhinosinusitis, 1212t
  in sepsis, 1353t
  in shigellosis, 1269t
  in travelers' diarrhea, 1274
  in tuberculosis, 1262t
  in urinary tract infections, 1311t, 1312t
Levofloxacin resistance, 1194t
Levomethadyl, arrhythmia with, 179t
Levonorgestrel, 843, 845t, 849, 851, 853, 875t
Levorphanol
  dosage of, 575t
  in pain, 575t
Levothyroxine (T4), 828t
  anxiety with, 694t
  dosage of, 769t
  drug interactions of, 771t
  in hypothyroidism, 769–771, 771t
    alterations in LT_4 dose requirement, 771
    bioequivalence and LT_4 product selection,
      769–770
    over- and undertreatment, 771
    patient monitoring, 771–772
  in myxedema coma, 772
  in obesity, 771, 772, 774t
  in thyroid cancer, 765, 777
Lewy bodies, 554
LGB 8811 regimen, in acute lymphocytic
    leukemia, 1405t
Lhermitte's sign, 1557
Libido, 883
  decreased
    with 5α-reductase inhibitors, 905, 905t
    with oral contraceptives, 848
Lice infestation, 1303–1304
Licorice, 54t, 206t
Lidocaine
  adverse effects of, 169t
  in arrhythmias, 162t
  dosage of, 178t, 179t
  drug interactions of, 955t
  for facilitation of defibrillation, 178, 178t,
    179t
  mechanism of action of, 162t
  in musculoskeletal disorders, 1025
  in pain, 578, 578t
  in torsades de pointes, 181
  in ventricular tachycardia, 178t, 178a
Life expectancy, of elderly, 8–9
Lifestyle factors
  in anxiety disorders, 692
  in breast cancer, 1477

Lifestyle modifications
  in allergic rhinitis, 1049–1050
  in cirrhosis, 394
  in constipation, 373
  in erectile dysfunction, 885
  in GERD, 317, 319, 320t
  in hyperlipidemia, 234, 236t, 240, 958
  in hypertension, 58–59, 59t, 957–958
  in ischemic heart disease, 117–118
  in musculoskeletal disorders, 1027–1028
  in osteoarthritis, 1000
  in Parkinson's disease, 557
  in urinary incontinence, 914
Lifting, in enuresis, 923t
Lifting techniques, 1028
Ligament, 1020, 1020f
Ligament of Treitz, 1706
Lightning strike, 1131t
Light therapy, in depression, 657
Linea nigra, 825
Linear accelerator, 1665
Linezolid
  adverse effects of, 1177t
  in cellulitis, 1225t
  in cystic fibrosis, 309, 309t, 310
  in diabetic foot infections, 1229t
  dosage of, 251t, 1177t, 1196t, 1225t, 1229t,
      1249t, 1342t
  drug interactions of, 614t
  in infective endocarditis, 1241, 1249t
  in meningitis, 1177t
  in methicillin-resistant *Staphylococcus aureus*,
      1354
  in osteomyelitis, 1342, 1342t, 1343, 1344t
  in pneumonia, 1196t, 1197
  in postneurosurgical infections, 1183
  in sepsis, 1353t, 1354
Linoleic acid
  in intravenous lipid emulsions, 1684, 1684t
  in pain, 579
α-Linolenic acid, in intravenous lipid emulsions,
    1684, 1684t
Liothyronine
  dosage of, 769t
  in hypothyroidism, 769t
Liotrix
  dosage of, 769t
  in hypothyroidism, 769t
Lipase
  pancreatic, 404
  pancreatic enzyme supplements, 408, 409
  serum, 405
Lipid(s)
  digestion of, 1702f
  in enteral feeding formulas, 1708
  metabolism of, 230–232
    growth hormone effects on, 803t
  serum, 229–248
Lipid emulsion, intravenous, 1683–1685, 1684t,
    1690, 1695
  caloric value of, 1683
  coalescence of, 1683
  complications and safety of, 1684
  creaming of, 1683
  oiling out of, 1683
Lipolysis, 756
Lipophilic drugs, 544–545
Lipoprotein(s). See also specific types
  metabolism of, 230–232, 231f, 232f
  structure of, 230, 230f
Lipoprotein(a), 240
Lipoprotein lipase, 230, 231, 1684
Lipram products, 409t

Liquid dosage forms, administration through
    feeding tubes, 1714
Lisinopril
  in acute coronary syndromes, 142t
  dosage of, 92t, 121t, 142t
  in heart failure, 92t, 93
  in hypertension, 62, 64t
  in ischemic heart disease, 121t
Listeria monocytogenes, in meningitis, 1170,
    1171t, 1176t, 1182
Lithium, 10, 828t
  adverse effects of, 38t, 591, 679, 686
  augmentation of antidepressant therapy with,
      662
  in bipolar disorder, 676–681, 678t, 680t–681t,
      682t, 686
  diabetes insipidus with, 679
  dosage of, 678t, 679
  drug interactions of, 679, 681, 1004
  enuresis with, 920
  erectile dysfunction with, 885t
  hypercalcemia with, 492
  hypermagnesemia with, 492
  hypothyroidism with, 679, 767, 767t, 779
  in lactation, 824t
  mechanism of action of, 679
  metabolic acidosis with, 501t
  monitoring therapy with, 679, 682t
  osteoporosis with, 967t
  pharmacokinetics of, 680t–681t
  in pregnancy, 686
  in prevention of cluster headaches, 591
  psoriasis and, 1080
  in schizoaffective disorder, 646
  seizures with, 522
  teratogenic effects of, 824t
Liver abscess, amebic, 295–297
Liver biopsy, in viral hepatitis, 416
Liver cancer, epidemiology of, 1446f
Liver disease
  alcoholic. See Alcoholic liver disease;
      Cirrhosis
  dosing adjustments for chemotherapy, 1471t
  drug-related, 1437t
  end-stage, 413
    viral hepatitis and, 413, 418
  erectile dysfunction with, 885t
  in inflammatory bowel disease, 344
  obstructive, 236t
  oral contraceptives and, 846
  with parenteral nutrition, 1696
  in sickle cell anemia/disease, 1145t
Liver failure
  DIC with, 1131t
  nausea and vomiting with, 358t
  protein requirement in, 1689t
  respiratory alkalosis in, 504t
  treatment of, enteral nutrition, 1702t, 1710
  tuberculosis and, 1261
Liver transplantation. See also Solid-organ
      transplantation
  acute rejection, signs and symptoms of, 944t
  epidemiology and etiology of, 941
Local anesthetics
  in musculoskeletal disorders, 1025
  in pain, 578
Locus ceruleus, 693
Lodoxamide
  adverse effects of, 1068t
  in allergic conjunctivitis, 1068t
  dosage of, 1068t
  mechanism of action of, 1068t
Loestrin-24 Fe, 848–849

Lomefloxacin
  dosage of, 1312t
  in urinary tract infections, 1312t
Lomustine
  adverse effects of, 1461
  in cancer therapy, 1461
  emetogenicity of, 365t
  mechanism of action of, 1461
  pharmacokinetics of, 1461
Long QT syndrome, 179, 301
Long-term care, of elderly patients, 18–19
Loop diuretics. See also specific drugs
  in acute renal failure, 437
  administration of, 437
  adverse effects of, 60t, 65, 437
  in heart failure, 89–90, 90t, 91, 100
  in hypercalcemia, 492, 414t
  in hyperkalemia, 454
  in hypertension, 64–65
  hypocalcemia with, 489
  hypokalemia with, 487
  hypomagnesemia with, 492
  voiding symptoms with, 900t
Loperamide
  in diarrhea, 379, 379f, 1459, 1512, 1529, 1711
  dosage of, 379t, 384t
  in irritable bowel syndrome, 379, 384, 384t
  in opioid withdrawal, 621t
Lopinavir/ritonavir
  adverse effects of, 1431t, 1438t
  dosage of, 1431t
  drug interactions of, 850t, 1431t, 1434
  food interactions of, 1431t
  in HIV infection, 1426, 1431t, 1434
  mechanism of action of, 1421f
Loratadine
  in allergic rhinitis, 1053, 1054t
  dosage of, 830t, 834
  drug interactions of, 955t
  in lactation, 830t, 834
  in pregnancy, 830t, 834
Lorazepam, 45t
  in acutely psychotic patients, 647
  adverse effects of, 300t, 545t, 547t
  in alcohol withdrawal, 618
  in anticipatory nausea and vomiting, 1512, 1513t
  in bipolar disorder, 677t
  in delirium tremens, 618–619
  dosage of, 300t, 545, 545t, 546t, 547t, 549t,
      618–619, 677t, 698t
  drug interactions of, 699t
  metabolic acidosis with, 501t
  metabolism of, 697
  in nausea and vomiting, 362t, 364, 365
  in opioid withdrawal, 621t
  in panic disorder, 702
  pharmacokinetics of, 698t
  in schizophrenia, 646
  in seizure prophylaxis, 1636
  in seizures, 618
  in status epilepticus, 545, 545t, 546t, 547t,
      549t
Losartan
  adverse effects of, 62t
  in antihyperuricemic treatment, 1016
  dosage of, 62t, 92t
  in heart failure, 92t
  in hypertension, 62t
Loteprednol
  adverse effects of, 1068t
  in allergic conjunctivitis, 1068t
  dosage of, 1068t
  mechanism of action of, 1068t

Lovage root, 154*t*
Lovastatin
  adverse effects of, 242*t*
  dosage of, 242*t*
  drug interactions of, 205*t*, 660*t*, 771*t*, 955*t*
  in hyperlipidemia, 186*t*, 242*t*, 243*t*, 247
  in ischemic heart disease, 120
Low-back pain, 570, 1020, 1028
Low-calorie diet, 1723, 1723*t*
Low-density lipoprotein(s) (LDL), 230–234, 231*t*,
    231*f*, 1702*f*
  physical characteristics of, 177*t*
Low-density lipoprotein cholesterol, 120, 230
  goals for, 120, 151, 236, 755–756
  optimal level for, 230
  oxidation of, 125
Lower esophageal sphincter pressure, in GERD,
    316, 317*t*
Lower respiratory tract, normal flora of, 1157*f*
Lower respiratory tract infection, 1189–1201
Lower urinary tract symptoms, 809
  in benign prostatic hyperplasia, 895–898
Loxapine
  adverse effects of, 642*t*
  dosage of, 640*t*
  in schizophrenia, 640*t*
Lubiprostone
  adverse effects of, 374–375
  in constipation, 374–375
  dosage of, 375
Lubricants
  in constipation, 373–374
  in contact dermatitis, 1102
Lugol's solution, in hyperthyroidism, 776
Lumbar puncture, in CNS infections, 1173
Lumiracoxib, 1004
Lumpectomy, 1478, 1481
Lung cancer, 1499–1514
  anorexia in, 1513
  cachexia in, 1513
  carcinoma, 1501
  case study of, 1502, 1504, 1506, 1514
  clinical presentation in, 1502–1503
  diagnosis of, 1502*t*, 1503
  diet and, 1500
  environmental factors in, 1500
  epidemiology of, 1446*f*, 1500–1501
  ethnicity and, 1500
  etiology of, 1500–1501
  extrapulmonary symptoms in, 1503
  gender and, 1500
  genetic factors in, 1447*t*, 1500–1501
  histologic classification of, 1501–1502, 1502*t*
    Horner's syndrome in, 1503
  hypercalcemia with, 1670–1673
  large cell, 1501, 1502*t*
  metastasis of
    to bone, 1663
    to brain, 1664, 1665*t*
  non-small cell, 1501, 1502*t*, 1503–1504, 1504*t*,
    1506, 1510–1511
    advanced/metastatic disease, 1510
    local disease, 1510
    locally advanced disease, 1510
    recurrent disease, 1510
  outcome evaluation in, 1514
  paraneoplastic syndromes in, 1503, 1513
  pathophysiology of, 1501–1502, 1502*t*
  patient care and monitoring in, 1514
  performance status in, 1504, 1504*t*
  in perihilar area, 1661
  prevention of, 1501
  risk factors for, 1500

small cell, 792*t*, 1501, 1502*t*, 1504, 1504*t*, 1506,
    1509, 1509*a*
    extensive disease, 1509–1510
    limited disease, 1509
    recurrent disease, 1510
  smoking and, 1500
  staging of, 1503–1504, 1504*t*
  superior vena cava syndrome with, 1661,
    1661*f*
  treatment of, 1504–1511
    adjuvant therapy, 1504, 1508
    adverse events from chemotherapy,
      1511–1514
    algorithm for, 1505*a*, 1509*a*
    chemotherapy, 1506, 1507*t*–1508*t*
    combination therapy, 1510–1511
    monoclonal antibodies, 1508
    neoadjuvant therapy, 1508
    palliative therapy, 1510, 1514
    postoperative radiotherapy, 1505–1506
    radiation therapy, 1505–1506
    single-agent chemotherapy, 1506–1508
    surgery, 1504–1505
    tyrosine kinase inhibitors, 1507–1508
    tumor lysis syndrome in, 1674*t*
Lung carcinoma in situ, 1501
Lung disease
  in cystic fibrosis, 303, 304, 306, 308, 309
  in sickle cell anemia/disease, 1145*t*
Lung transplantation. *See also* Solid-organ
    transplantation
  acute rejection, signs and symptoms of, 944*t*
  epidemiology and etiology of, 941
Lupus erythematosus, allergic drug
    reaction, 929*t*
Luteinizing hormone
  at menopause, 870–871
  in menstrual cycle, 843, 856, 856*f*
Luteinizing hormone-releasing hormone, 1546
Luteinizing hormone-releasing hormone
    agonists
  in breast cancer, 1485, 1486*t*
  in cancer, 1468
  in prostate cancer, 1539, 1539*t*, 1543–1544,
    1544*t*
Luteinizing hormone-releasing hormone
    antagonists, in cancer, 1468
Luteolysis, 864
Lycopene in prevention of prostate cancer, 1537
Lymphadenectomy, in melanoma, 1616, 1618
Lymphadenitis, cervical, 1215
Lymphangitis, 1232
Lymph nodes
  anatomic locations of, 1552*f*
  axillary, dissection in breast cancer, 1478
  biopsy in lymphoma, 1555
  sentinel. *See* Sentinel lymph node biopsy
Lymphocyte immune globulin,
    antithymoglobulin equine (ATG)
  adverse effects of, 945*t*, 946, 951*t*
  dosage of, 945*t*, 946
  in transplant recipient, 945*t*, 951*t*
Lymphocytosis, 1159*t*
Lymphoma, 1447*t*, 1551–1563. *See also*
    Hodgkin's lymphoma; Non-Hodgkin's
    lymphoma
  case study of, 1472, 1552, 1555, 1558
  dry eye in, 1075*t*
  superior vena cava syndrome with, 1661*t*
Lymphonectomy, in ovarian cancer, 1569
Lymphopenia, 1159*t*
Lymphoproliferative disease

posttransplant, 960
  rheumatoid arthritis and, 983
Lynch syndrome, 1566

M
Maceration, of skin, 1231
MACOP-B regimen, in non-Hodgkin's
    lymphoma, 1561*t*
Macroglobulinemia, Waldenström's, 1608
Macrolide(s). *See also specific drugs*
  in rhinosinusitis, 1212*a*, 1213*a*
  in sepsis, 1353*t*
Macrolide resistance, 1193–1194, 1204
Macrophages, 942
  in atherosclerosis, 232
Macroprolactinemia, 814*t*
Macula, 1071
Macular degeneration, 1071–1074
  atrophic (dry), 1073
  clinical presentation in, 1072, 1072*f*
  diagnosis of, 1072, 1072*f*, 1074*f*
  epidemiology of, 1071
  etiology of, 1071
  neovascular (wet), 1072–1073
  outcome evaluation in, 1074
  pathophysiology of, 1071–1073
  risk factors for, 1072*t*
  treatment of, 1073–1074
    nonpharmacologic, 1073
    pegaptanib, 1073
Macular edema, 1064*t*
Maculopapular rash, allergic drug reaction,
    929–930, 929*t*
Magnesium
  in extracellular fluid, 484*t*
  in intracellular fluid, 484*t*
  for parenteral nutrition, 1685*t*, 1686
  serum, normal range for, 484*t*
Magnesium balance, 491
Magnesium carbonate
  dosage of, 464*t*
  in hyperphosphatemia, 463, 464*t*
Magnesium citrate
  in constipation, 374*t*
  dosage of, 374*t*
Magnesium hydroxide
  adverse effects of, 361*t*
  in constipation, 374*t*
  dosage of, 320*t*, 374*t*, 464*t*, 830*t*
  in GERD, 320*t*
  in hyperphosphatemia, 463, 464*t*
Magnesium oxide, in hypomagnesemia, 492
Magnesium requirement, 491
Magnesium salicylate, in musculoskeletal
    disorders, 1024
Magnesium sulfate
  in constipation, 374*t*
  contraindications to, 835
  dosage of, 374*t*, 832*t*
  in eclampsia, 492
  in hypomagnesemia, 492
  as tocolytic, 835
Magnesium therapy
  in asthma, 492
  drug interactions of, 1164
  in oxaliplatin-induced neuropathy, 1530
  in torsades de pointes, 180
Magnetic resonance imaging
  in Alzheimer's disease, 598
  in epilepsy, 523, 526
  in multiple sclerosis, 508*t*
  in osteomyelitis, 1341
  in stroke, 218–219

Magnolia, 792t

Ma huang. *See* Ephedra

Maintenance of wakefulness test, 713

Major depressive disorder. *See* Depressive disorder, major

Major histocompatibility complex (MHC)
class I molecules, 942
class II molecules, 942
solid-organ transplantation and, 842

Malabsorption
diarrhea in, 377
in inflammatory bowel disease, 344
osteoporosis and, 967t
in pancreatitis, 408

Malaise, with α-adrenergic antagonists, 903t, 904, 906t

Malaria, 1299–1303
case study of, 1299, 1301–1302
chemoprophylaxis for, 1301t
clinical presentation in, 1300
diagnosis of, 1300
epidemiology of, 1299
etiology of, 1299
outcome evaluation in, 1302
pathophysiology of, 1299–1300
patient care and monitoring in, 1302
sickle cell anemia/disease and, 1140
treatment of, 1300–1302

Malathion, in lice infestation, 1304

Malignant effusion, treatment of, 1463

Mammalian target of rapamycin (mTOR) inhibitors, 1463

Mammogram, screening, 1476–1479, 1477, 1479t

Manganese
for parenteral nutrition, 1687, 1697
toxicity of, 1697

Mania. *See also* Bipolar disorder
secondary causes of, 676t

Manning criteria, diagnosis of irritable bowel syndrome, 382

Mannitol
adverse effects of, 1042
contraindications to, 437
diarrhea with, 376t
in glaucoma, 1042
in hypotension, 471
in intracranial hypertension, 1666

Mantle cell lymphoma, 1561

Mantoux test, 1256, 1257t

MAO inhibitors (monoamine oxidase inhibitors), 701, 701t
nonpharmacologic, 700
reversible inhibitors of monoamine oxidase, 704
serotonin-norepinephrine reuptake inhibitors, 701t, 701

Maprotiline, dosage of, 661t

Maraviroc
adverse effects of, 1432t
dosage of, 1432t
drug interactions of, 1432t
food interactions of, 1432t
in HIV infection, 1432t

Marijuana. *See* Cannabis

MASCC risk index, for patients with febrile neutropenia, 1655, 1656t

Masked facies, in Parkinson's disease, 555

Massage therapy, in pain, 573–574

Mastalgia, with oral contraceptives, 848

Mast cell stabilizer
in allergic conjunctivitis, 1068t, 1069
in allergic rhinitis, 1051t, 1055–1056, 1058t

Mastectomy

bilateral total, in prevention of breast cancer, 1477
in breast cancer, 1478, 1480–1481, 1488
modified radical, 1480
partial (segmental), 1481
simple, 1478
total, 1478

Mastitis, 826

Matrix metalloproteinase, 232, 508, 982, 998

Mattress, pressure-reducing, 1231

m-BACOD regimen, in non-Hodgkin's lymphoma, 1561t

MC1R gene, 1613

McDonald criteria, in multiple sclerosis, 507, 508, 511a

MDRD (Modification of Diet in Renal Disease) equation, 11

Meadowsweet, 206t

Mean arterial blood pressure, 252

Mean cell hemoglobin, 1113t

Mean cell hemoglobin concentration, 1113t, 1140

Mean corpuscular volume, 1112, 1113t, 1145

Measles, 1410

Measles, mumps, rubella (MMR) vaccine, 28, 418, 1408t, 1410–1411, 1414t, 1416

Measles vaccine, 1410, 1498t, 1414t

Mebendazole
in ascariasis, 1297
dosage of, 1297–1298
in enterobiasis, 1298
in hookworm disease, 1297

Mecamylamine, in smoking cessation, 623

Mecasermin, 813

Mechanical ventilation. *See* Assisted ventilation

Mechlorethamine
dosage of, 1557t
emetogenicity of, 365t
extravasation of, 1677t, 1678t, 1679
in Hodgkin's lymphoma, 1377, 1378t

Meclizine
adverse effects of, 361t
dosage of, 361t, 830t
in nausea and vomiting, 361t

Meclobemide
in panic disorder, 701
in social anxiety disorder, 704

Meclofenamate
dosage of, 1014t
in gout, 1014t

Meconium, 304

Meconium aspiration, 1131t

Meconium ileus, 304

Media, 232

Medical nutrition therapy, in diabetes mellitus, 745–746

Medical Research Council Dyspnea Scale, 300, 300t

Medicare, 3, 4

Medicare Hospice Benefit, 37

Medication errors, 4

Medium chain triglyceride supplement, in pancreatitis, 410

Medroxyprogesterone
adverse effects of, 792t, 1487t
in breast cancer, 1487t
dosage of, 1487t
drug interactions of, 170t
in respiratory acidosis, 503

Medroxyprogesterone acetate, 850, 875t
adverse effects of, 859t, 1490
in amenorrhea, 858, 859t
in anovulatory bleeding, 865
in breast cancer, 1490
dosage of, 859t

in dysmenorrhea, 863
in menstruation-related disorders, 859t
osteoporosis with, 967t

Medullary cystic disease, kidney transplantation in, 941

Mefloquine
adverse effects of, 1301
depression with, 656
dosage of, 1301t, 1300
drug interactions of, 647
in malaria, 1300–1301
in prevention of malaria, 1301t

Megacolon, toxic, in inflammatory bowel disease, 344, 346

Megestrol acetate
adrenal insufficiency with, 786t
adverse effects of, 792t, 1487t, 1490
in anorexia, 1513
in breast cancer, 1487t, 1490
in cancer therapy, 1469
dosage of, 1487t
mechanism of action of, 1469
in prostate cancer, 1540

Meglitinides, in diabetes mellitus, 747

Meibomian gland dysfunction, 1075t

Melanin, 1096, 1614

Melanocytes, 1614

Melanoma, 1611–1626
ABCDE acronym, 1616–1617, 1616f
acral lentiginous, 1614t
age and, 1613, 1614t
body sites of, 1614t
brain metastasis, 1664, 1665t
chemotherapy in, 1625
radiation therapy in, 1625
stereotactic radiosurgery in, 1622
surgery in, 1662
case study of, 1611, 1618, 1623
clinical presentation in, 1614–1617, 1614t
diagnosis of, 1614–1617, 1614t
epidemiology of, 1446f, 1623
ethnicity and, 1614t
etiology of, 1623
follow-up care for, 1623
genetic factors in, 1612, 1613
in immunocompromised patients, 1624
lentigo maligna, 1614, 1614t
metastasis of, 1614
nodular, 1614, 1614t, 1617
outcome evaluation in, 1622–1623
pathophysiology of, 1614, 1615f
patient care and monitoring in, 1626
primary prevention of, 1613
prognosis for, 1616t
recurrence of, 1617–1618
risk factors for, 1612–1613, 1614t
secondary prevention of, 1613–1614
sentinel lymph node biopsy in, 1616
staging of, 1614–1617, 1614t
superficial spreading, 1614, 1614t
treatment of, 1617–1622
adjuvant therapy, 1618
algorithm for, 1619a
biochemotherapy, 1621–1622
chemotherapy, 1620t, 1621
full-thickness ablative procedures, 1624–1625
interferon alfa-2b, 1618–1619, 1620t
interleukin-2, 1620–1621, 1621t
Mohs' micrographic surgery, 1625
radiation therapy, 1622
stage IIB, IIC, and III, 1618–1619
stage IV, 1619–1622
surgery, 1624–1625

surgical margins of excision, 1615*t*
Melanoma in situ, 1618, 1619*a*
Melanosis, with PUVA therapy, 1085
Melasma, 848
Melatonin
  in circadian rhythm disorders, 718
  in parasomnias, 718
  in Parkinson's disease, 562
MELD classification, of cirrhosis, 393, 394*t*
Meloxicam, 1002*t*, 1004, 1014*t*
Melphalan
  in breast cancer, 1482, 1491
  dosage of, 1557*t*, 1634*t*
    in renal dysfunction, 1470*t*
  emetogenicity of, 365*t*
  extravasation of, 1677*t*
  in Hodgkin's lymphoma, 1557*t*
  in multiple myeloma, 1607*t*
  in preparation for hematopoietic cell
    transplant, 1634*t*
Memantine
  adverse effects of, 601*t*, 602
  in Alzheimer's disease, 597, 598, 601*t*
  dosage of, 601*t*, 602
Menarche, 864, 1362
  breast cancer and, 1476
  onset of migraine at, 583
Meningioma, 1447*t*
Meningitis, 1169–1185
  bacterial, 1170, 1171*t*, 1172*t*
  case study of, 1171
  clinical presentation in, 1173–1174
  cryptococcal, 1170, 1387–1389
  diagnosis of, 1173–1174
  Enterobacteriaceae, 1177*t*, 1182
  epidemiology of, 1170
  Escherichia coli, 1171*t*
  etiology of, 1170, 1171*t*
  fungal, 1170, 1172*t*
  gram-negative bacilli, 1171*t*, 1182–1183
  group B streptococci, 1170, 1171, 1176*t*, 1182
  Haemophilus influenzae, 1170, 1171*t*, 1176*t*,
    1181–1182, 1407
  herpes simplex virus, 1178*t*
  in immunocompromised patients, 1170, 1171*t*
  Klebsiella pneumoniae, 1171*t*
  Listeria monocytogenes, 1170, 1171*t*, 1176*t*, 1182
  nausea and vomiting with, 356*t*
  Neisseria meningitidis, 1170, 1171*t*, 1175*t*,
    1179–1180, 1411
  neonatal, 1182
  noninfectious causes of, 1170
  outcome evaluation in, 1184–1185
  pathophysiology of, 1170–1173, 1172*a*
  patient care and monitoring in, 1185
  in pediatric patients, 1177*t*–1178*t*
  Pseudomonas aeruginosa, 1171*t*, 1177*t*, 1182
  Staphylococcus aureus, 1171*t*, 1177*t*
  Staphylococcus epidermidis, 1177*t*
  Streptococcus pneumoniae, 1170, 1171*t*, 1176*t*,
    1181, 1184
  treatment of, 1174–1184
    algorithm for, 1179*a*
    dexamethasone, 1179*a*, 1183–1184
    empirical antimicrobial therapy, 1171*t*, 1178,
      1179
    impact of antimicrobial resistance on,
      1178–1179
    pathogen-directed antimicrobial therapy,
      1179–1184
  tuberculous, 1172*t*
  viral, 1172*t*, 1183
Menopause, 870, 1485

breast cancer and, 1476
case study of, 871, 872, 880
clinical presentation in, 871
diagnosis of, 871
dyspareunia in, 872
epidemiology of, 870
etiology of, 870
hormone-replacement therapy in, 869–880
  benefits of, 876–877
  continuous combined estrogen and
    progestin, 874
  cyclic estrogen and progestin, 874
  discontinuation, 878
  estrogens, 874, 875*t*
  low-dose therapy, 874
  outcome evaluation in, 879–880
  patient care and monitoring in, 880
  progestins, 875*t*, 877
  risks of, 877–878
nonhormonal treatment in, 876, 877, 878–879
osteoporosis and, 966, 976
physiology of, 870–871
premature, 1476
stress incontinence in, 872
treatment algorithm for, 873*a*
urinary incontinence and, 911
vasomotor symptoms of, 870–871, 876, 879*t*
vulvovaginal atrophy in, 874
Menorrhagia
  clinical presentation in, 861
  definition of, 861
  diagnosis of, 861
  epidemiology of, 855–856
  etiology of, 855–856
  in hemophilia, 1124
  outcome evaluation in, 866*t*, 867
  pathophysiology of, 857*t*, 861
  patient care and monitoring in, 867
  treatment of, 857–858, 859*t*
    algorithm for, 859*t*
  in von Willebrand's disease, 1128
Menstrual cycle, 842, 842*f*, 856
  hormonal fluctuations in, 856*f*
  regulation with oral contraceptives, 844
Menstruation-related disorders, 855–868. *See
  also specific disorders*
  case study of, 858, 860
Menthol
  adverse effects of, 1026–1027
  in musculoskeletal disorders, 1026–027,
    1026*t*
  in osteoarthritis, 1006
Men who have sex with men, 1318
Meperidine, 45*t*
  abuse of, 616
  adverse effects of, 575
  dosage of, 575*t*
  drug interactions of, 660, 660*t*
  GERD with, 317*t*
  metabolism of, 575
  in pain, 575, 575*t*
  in pancreatitis, 406
  pseudoallergic drug reactions, 933
6-Mercaptopurine, 1456, 950
  adverse effects of, 1456, 1592*t*
  dosage of, 347*t*, 1588*t*, 1590*t*
  drug interactions of, 1016, 1456, 1592*t*, 1592*t*
  in acute lymphocytic leukemia, 1587, 1588*t*,
    1589, 1590*t*, 1592*t*
  in cancer therapy, 1452*t*, 1456
  in thiopurine methyltransferase deficiency,
    1589
  mechanism of action of, 1454*a*, 1456, 1592*t*

pancreatitis with, 404*t*
pharmacokinetics of, 1456
in inflammatory bowel disease, 347, 347*t*,
  349–353, 349*t*
Mercury poisoning, 376*t*
Meropenem
  adverse effects of, 1171*t*, 1175*t*
  in cystic fibrosis, 309*t*, 310
  dosage of, 309*t*, 346, 349, 351, 1171*t*, 1175*t*,
    1176*t*, 1199*t*, 1342*t*, 1660*t*
  in infections in cancer patients, 1660*t*
  in inflammatory bowel disease, 346, 346*t*,
    349–350, 349*t*, 351*t*
  in intra-abdominal infections, 1287*t*, 1288*t*
  in meningitis, 1171*t*, 1175*t*, 1176*t*, 1183
  in osteomyelitis, 1339*t*, 1342*t*
  in pneumonia, 1196*t*, 1197, 1199*t*
  in postneurosurgical infections, 1183
  in sepsis, 1353*t*
  in urinary tract infections, 1311*t*
Merozoites, 1299
Mesalamine, mechanism of action of, 346
Mesial temporal lobe epilepsy, 525
Mesna
  dosage of, 1636, 1667, 1668*t*
  in prevention of hemorrhagic cystitis, 1636,
    1667, 1668*f*, 1668*t*
Mesocortical pathways, 632
Mesocorticolimbic system, in reward pathway,
  609, 609*f*
Mesoridazine
  dosage of, 640*t*
  drug interactions of, 647
  in schizophrenia, 640*t*
Mesothelioma, 1500
Mestranol, 845*t*
Metabolic acidosis, 251, 488, 497*t*, 497–498,
  501–502
  case study of, 499, 500
  in chronic kidney disease, 461
  clinical presentation in, 501
  compensatory changes in, 497*t*
  definition of, 501
  drug-related, 501*t*
  with elevated anion gap, 501, 501*t*
  epidemiology of, 465
  etiology of, 465, 501–502, 501*t*
  mnemonic for differential diagnosis of, 501*t*
  with normal anion gap, 501*t*, 502
  outcome evaluation in, 467
  with parenteral nutrition, 1696
  pathophysiology of, 466
  treatment of, 466–467, 502
Metabolic alkalosis, 497–498, 497*t*, 502, 503
  case study of, 499, 500
  clinical presentation of, 502
  compensatory changes in, 497*t*
  definition of, 502
  drug-related, 502
  etiology of, 502–503, 426*t*
  treatment of, 502–503
Metabolic rate, 1721
Metabolic syndrome, 112, 127, 229, 235, 738–739,
  750
  diagnosis of, 112, 238
  components of, 739*t*
Metal allergy, 1101
Metalloprotease ADAMTS13, 1135
Metastasis, 1448–1449
Metaxalone, in musculoskeletal disorders,
  1027
Metered-dose inhaler, 271, 273, 276, 298
  holding chamber/spacer device with, 271, 273

Metformin
  adverse effects of, 750, 859*t*
  in anovulatory bleeding, 865
  diarrhea with, 376*t*
  in diabetes mellitus, 749*t*, 749*t*, 750
  dosage of, 749*t*, 859*t*
  in menstruation-related disorders, 859*t*
  metabolic acidosis with, 501*t*
Methadone
  adverse effects of, 576
  arrhythmia with, 179*t*
  dosage of, 575*t*
  dose conversions, 498*t*, 578
  drug interactions of, 615*t*, 1434
  metabolism of, 575, 577
  in opioid dependence, 610, 619, 621, 626
  in osteoarthritis, 1006*f*
  in pain, 575*t*, 576
  in sickle cell anemia/disease, 1150
Methamphetamine, for weight loss, 1728
Methanol poisoning, 501–502, 501*t*
Methazolamide
  adverse effects of, 1041–1042
  dosage of, 1038*t*
  in glaucoma, 1038*t*, 1041–1042
  mechanism of action of, 1038*t*
Methimazole
  adverse effects of, 776
  agranulocytosis with, 776
  dosage of, 776
  in hyperthyroidism, 776, 777
  mechanism of action of, 776
  teratogenic effects of, 824*t*
Methocarbamol, in musculoskeletal disorders, 1027
Methotrexate, 1457
  in acute lymphocytic leukemia, 1587, 1588*t*,
    1590*t*, 1591*t*
  in acute myelogenous leukemia, 1593
  adverse effects of, 442, 986*t*, 990, 1086, 1457,
    1483*t*, 1591*t*, 1595
  in breast cancer, 1482, 1484*t*
  in cancer therapy, 1470*t*
  dosage of, 347*t*, 351*t* , 986*t*, 1086, 1457, 1588*t*,
    1590*t*, 1638
    in renal dysfunction, 1483*t*
  drug interactions of, 614*t*, 1457, 1591*t*, 1643
  emetogenicity of, 365*t*
  hepatotoxicity of, 1086
  growth hormone deficiency with, 810
  in inflammatory bowel disease, 347, 347*t*,
    351*t*, 352
  intrathecal, 1457, 1590*t*
  mechanism of action of, 990, 1454*a*, 1457, 1591*t*
  monitoring treatment with, 986*t*
  in non-Hodgkin's lymphoma, 1561
  osteoporosis with, 967*t*
  pharmacokinetics of, 1457
  in prevention of GVHD, 1638
  in psoriasis, 1085, 1086
  in rheumatoid arthritis, 986*t*, 990
  teratogenicity of, 824*t*, 993
Methylcellulose
  in constipation, 373, 374*t*
  in diarrhea, 379
  dosage of, 374*t*, 384*t*
  in irritable bowel syndrome, 379, 384*t*
Methyldopa
  adverse effects of, 62*t*
  allergic drug reactions, 929*t*
  dosage of, 62*t*
  drug interactions of, 660*t*
  erectile dysfunction with, 885*t*
  in hypertension, 62*t*

  pancreatitis with, 404*t*
  in pregnancy, 72*t*
Methyl nicotinate
  adverse effects of, 1027
  in musculoskeletal disorders, 1026*t*, 1027
  in osteoarthritis, 1006
Methylphenidate, 538
  in ADHD, 725, 727*t*, 728*t*, 730*t*
  adverse effects of, 728*t*
  anxiety with, 694*t*
  augmentation of antidepressant therapy
    with, 662
  dosage of, 516*t*, 727*t*
  in fatigue, 516*t*
  growth hormone deficiency with, 810
  in insomnia, 715
  respiratory alkalosis with, 504*t*
Methylprednisolone, 954
  in adrenal insufficiency, 789*t*
  adverse effects of, 362*t*
  anxiety with, 694*t*
  in asthma, 270*t*, 274*t*, 277*t*
  in contact dermatitis, 1104*t*
  drug interactions of, 850*t*
  in endemic mycosis, 1381
  in GVHD, 1640
  in headache, 592
  in immune thrombocytopenic purpura, 1134,
    1134*t*
  in inflammatory bowel disease, 347*t*, 350, 351
  in multiple sclerosis, 508
  in nausea and vomiting, 362*t*, 364, 365, 367
  osteoporosis with, 977
  in transplant recipient, 952
Methylprednisone
  dosage of, 1561*t*
  in non-Hodgkin's lymphoma, 1561*t*
Methyl salicylate
  in musculoskeletal disorders, 1026
Methyl salicylate
  in musculoskeletal disorders, 1026*t*
  in osteoarthritis, 1006
Methyltestosterone, 891
Methylxanthine, 297
  in asthma, 278
  respiratory alkalosis with, 275*t*, 504*t*
Methysergide
  adverse effects of, 591
  in prevention of migraine, 590*t*
Metipranolol
  dosage of, 1038*t*
  in glaucoma, 1038*t*, 1040
  mechanism of action of, 1038*t*
  ocular changes with, 1077*t*
Metoclopramide
  adverse effects of, 322, 362*t*, 363, 554
  arrhythmia with, 179*t*
  in chemotherapy-induced nausea and
    vomiting, 1652
  dosage of, 362*t*, 830*t*
  to facilitate gastric emptying, 1712
  in gastroparesis, 577*t*
  in GERD, 322, 830*t*
  hyperprolactinemia with, 814*t*
  in lactation enhancement, 830*t*, 836
  in nausea and vomiting, 362*t*, 363, 830*t*
  in pregnancy, 830*t*
Metolazone, 60*t*, 89, 91, 101, 438, 469
Metoprolol
  in acute coronary syndromes, 142*t*
  adverse effects of, 61*t*, 86*t*, 169*t*
  in arrhythmias, 162*t*
  dosage of, 61*t*, 92*t*, 122*t*

  in heart failure, 92
  in hypertension, 61*t*, 66*a*
  in ischemic heart disease, 122*t*, 123
  mechanism of action of, 162*t*
  in prevention of migraine, 590*t*
Metronidazole, dosage, 831*t*
Metyrapone
  adverse effects of, 796*t*
  in Cushing's syndrome, 796*t*
  dosage of, 796*t*
  mechanism of action of, 796*t*
  overnight metyrapone test, 788*t*
Mexican-Americans. *See* Ethnicity
Mexiletine
  in arrhythmias, 162*t*
  drug interactions of, 561
  mechanism of action of, 162*t*
Mezlocillin, in intra-abdominal infections, 1288
MHC. *See* Major histocompatibility complex
Micafungin
  in fungal infections, 957
  in invasive candidiasis, 1384, 1385
  in prevention of invasive candidiasis, 1387
Micelle, 230
Michaelis-Menten metabolism, 528
Miconazole
  in breast candidiasis, 832*t*
  in diaper dermatitis, 1106
  dosage of, 831*t*, 832*t*, 833*t*, 1363*t*
  drug interactions of, 205*t*, 955*t*
  in pregnancy, 831*t*
  in vulvovaginal candidiasis, 831*t*, 1363*t*
Microalbuminuria
  in chronic kidney disease, 447, 449
  in diabetes mellitus, 758
  in hypertension, 57
Micrococci, normal flora, 1157*f*
Microdialysis studies, during withdrawal, 610
Micrographia, in Parkinson's disease, 555
Microsomal ethanol oxidizing system, 392
Microsporidium, in diarrhea, 376
Microsporum, 1369
Microthrombi, 1130
Microtophi, 1011
Microvascular pulmonary emboli, 1686, 1692
Microvilli, 1702
Microvillous inclusion disease, intestine
    transplantation in, 941
Micturition, 911
Midazolam
  adverse effects of, 545*t*
  dosage of, 545, 545*t*, 546*t*, 548, 549*t*
  drug interactions of, 1381
Middle cerebral artery embolectomy, in
    stroke, 220
Midodrine
  adverse effects of, 472
  in hepatorenal syndrome, 399
  in hypotension, 471
Mifepristone
  adrenal insufficiency with, 786*t*
  adverse effects of, 797*t*
  in Cushing's syndrome, 797*t*
  dosage of, 797*t*
  mechanism of action of, 797*t*
Mifflin-St. Jeor equation, 1688
Miglitol
  adverse effects of, 750
  in diabetes mellitus, 748*t*, 750
  dosage of, 748*t*
Migraine, 488
  in adolescents, 591
  anxiety with, 694*t*

with aura, 585
without aura, 585
chronic, 585
clinical presentation in, 585–586
diagnosis of, 585
epidemiology of, 584–585
etiology of, 584–585
factors that trigger, 588t
multiple sclerosis and, 507
nausea and vomiting with, 358t
pathophysiology of, 584–585
patient care and monitoring in, 592
in pediatric patients, 591
prevention of, 587–591, 590t
  antiepileptic drugs, 590, 590t
  β-blockers, 590t, 591
  calcium channel blockers, 590, 590t
  ergotamine derivatives, 590t, 591
  in pregnancy, 592
  tricyclic antidepressants, 590, 590t
stroke and, 217t
treatment of, 360, 586–592
  ergotamine derivatives, 588
  NSAID, 587–588
  opioids, 589, 592
  triptans, 586, 587, 588, 589, 589t, 591
Migraineur, 584, 585
Mineral supplementation, in inflammatory bowel
  disease, 345
Mini-cog mental status exam, 16f
Minimum inhibitory concentration, 1161, 1161f,
  1241
Minocycline, 988
in infective endocarditis, 1241
Minoxidil
adverse effects of, 63t, 69
dosage of, 63t
in hypertension, 63t, 69
Miosis
drug-induced, 1077t
in opioid intoxication, 616
Mircette, 849
Mirena, 851
Mirtazapine
adverse effects of, 659, 659t, 714
in depression, 665
dosage of, 661t
drug interactions of, 659, 660, 660t
in elderly, 665
mechanism of action of, 657–658, 657t
pharmacokinetics of, 659t
Miscarriage, 861
Misoprostol, teratogenic effects of, 824t
Mitotane
adverse effects of, 797t
in Cushing's syndrome, 797t
dosage of, 797t
mechanism of action of, 797t
Mitral valve prolapse, 166t, 694t
Mitral valve regurgitation, 253t
Mitral valve stenosis, 80t
Mixed mood episodes, 670, 676
Mobiluncus, in bacterial vaginosis, 1331
Modafinil
augmentation of antidepressant therapy
  with, 662
dosage of, 561
drug interactions of, 850t
in insomnia, 715, 716
in obstructive sleep apnea, 718
in sleep disorders, 715, 716
Modification of Diet in Renal Disease (MDRD), 11
Mohs' micrographic surgery, in skin cancer, 1625

Moisturizers, 872, 1083, 1097
Mold, 1376
Molindone
adverse effects of, 642t
dosage of, 640t
in schizophrenia, 640t
Mometasone
in allergic rhinitis, 1052, 1052t
in asthma, 276t
in contact dermatitis, 1104t
in COPD, 295t
dosage of, 276t, 1052t
Moniliasis. *See* Vulvovaginal candidiasis
Monitoring the Future Survey, 608f
Monoamine hypothesis, of depression, 654
Monoamine oxidase inhibitors. *See* MAO
  inhibitors
Monoclonal antibodies
in cancer therapy, 1465–1467
chimeric, 991, 1088
in chronic lymphocytic leukemia, 1603, 1603t
cold antibodies, 1465
hot antibodies, 1465
in lung cancer, 1508
in non-Hodgkin's lymphoma, 1560
syllable source indicators for, 1294t
Monoclonal gammopathy of unknown
  significance, 1466
Monocytes, in atherosclerosis, 232
Monocytosis, 1159t
Monoparesis, 218
Monosodium urate crystals, 1011, 1012f
Montelukast
adverse effects of, 276
in allergic rhinitis, 308, 1056, 1057, 1059
in asthma, 275t, 278
dosage of, 275t, 308
Mood disorders, 694t
with psychotic features, 634t
Mood lability, in alcohol intoxication, 612
Mood-stabilizing drugs, in bipolar disorder, 676
MOPP regimen, in Hodgkin's lymphoma,
  1557–1558, 1557t
Moraxella catarrhalis
in bite wound infections, 1232t
in conjunctivitis, 1065
in COPD exacerbations, 298, 299t
in otitis media, 1204
in pneumonia, 1190, 1190t, 1354
in rhinosinusitis, 1209, 1211
Moricizine, arrhythmia with, 176
Morphine
in acute coronary syndromes, 143t, 152t
adverse effects of, 152t
contraindications to, 143t
dosage of, 143t, 575t, 576, 1151t
for epidural analgesia, 576
GERD with, 317t
mechanism of action of, 575
metabolism of, 575
in osteoarthritis, 1006
in pain, 572t, 575–576, 575t
  in sickle cell anemia/disease, 1151t
in PCA pumps, 576
pseudoallergic drug reactions, 933
Motion sickness, 358t, 359–360
treatment of, 367
Motivational enhancement therapy, in substance
  dependence, 623
Motor tics, 726
Mouth, normal flora of, 1157f
Moxalactam, drug interactions of, 205t, 614t
MPA-glucuronide (MPAG), 954

μ opioid agonists, 619
μ receptors, 610
Mucociliary clearance, respiratory tract, 1205,
  1210, 1217, 1218
Mucor, 1376t
Mucosal defense, gastrointestinal, 330
Mucosal protectants, in GERD, 332, 336t
Mucositis, 1653–1654
chemotherapy-induced, 1636, 1655
clinical presentation in, 1653
diagnosis of, 1653
epidemiology of, 1653
etiology of, 1653
with fluorouracil, 1455, 1527
pathophysiology of, 1653
treatment of, 1507t, 1525
  nonpharmacologic therapy, 1653–1654
  pharmacologic therapy, 1654
outcome evaluation in, 1654
Mucous colitis, 380
Mucous plugging, in asthma, 267
Mucus, hypersecretion in COPD, 291
Multi-drug resistant pathogens, 1194
risk factors for, 1355a
Multi-organ failure, in pancreatitis, 404
Multiparity, 1567
Multiple myeloma, 1604–1608
case study of, 1606
clinical presentation in, 1604
cytogenetic abnormalities in, 1604
diagnosis of, 1604
epidemiology of, 1604
etiology of, 1604
outcome evaluation in, 1607–1608
pathophysiology of, 1604
patient care and monitoring in, 1608
prognostic factors in, 1604
treatment of, 1604–1607
  bisphosphonates, 1607
  bortezomib, 1606–1607
  chemotherapy, 1605
  corticosteroids, 1605
  lenalidomide, 1606
  thalidomide, 1605–1606
Multiple-organ dysfunction syndrome
definition of, 1348t
in hypovolemic shock, 254
Multiple sclerosis, 507–517
case study of, 512, 516, 517
clinical course of, 508, 512f
clinical presentation in, 510
clinical rating scale for, 512t
depression in, 510
diagnosis of, 510, 511a, 508t
epidemiology of, 507
erectile dysfunction with, 510
etiology of, 507–508
fatigue in, 516
genetic factors in, 507
migraine and, 507
outcome evaluation in, 517
pain in, 516
pathophysiology of, 508, 509f
patient care and monitoring in, 517
primary progressive, 508
progressive relapsing, 508
relapsing remitting, 508, 509
secondary progressive, 508, 510–511
spasticity in, 516
treatment of, 508–517
  acute relapses, 508–510
  disease-modifying therapy, 510–515, 513t, 515t
  glatiramer acetate, 513t, 514, 515t

Multiple sclerosis, treatment of *(Cont.)*
 interferon β, 510–514, 513*t*, 515*t*
 mitoxantrone, 513*t*, 514–515, 515*t*
 outcome evaluation in, 515
 symptomatic therapy, 515–517
 urinary tract symptoms in, 510
Multiple sleep latency tests, 712, 713
Mumps, 1410
Mumps vaccine, 1408*t*, 1410, 1414*t*
Mupirocin
 intranasal, to decrease *Staphylococcus aureus* carriage, 1396
 in prevention of catheter-related infections, 475
 topical, in impetigo, 1222
Murmur, in infective endocarditis, 1238
Muronomab-CD3. *See* OKT-3
Muscle contraction, eccentric, 1020
Muscle cramps
 with hemodialysis, 472
 pathophysiology of, 472
 treatment of, 472
Muscle disorders. *See* Musculoskeletal disorders
Muscle relaxants. *See also specific drugs*
 in musculoskeletal disorders, 1027
 in pain, 578
 in prevention of migraine, 590*t*
 in prevention of tension-type headaches, 591
Muscle weakness, with corticosteroids, 953*t*
Muscular dystrophy, respiratory acidosis with, 503*t*
Musculoskeletal disorders, 1019–1029
 case study of, 1012, 1027–1028
 clinical presentation in, 1022
 diagnosis of, 1022
 epidemiology of, 1019–1020
 inflammation in, 1022
 outcome evaluation in, 1029
 overuse injury, 1022, 1024
 pain in, 1022
 pathophysiology of, 1020–1021, 1020*f*
 patient care and monitoring in, 1028
 treatment of, 1021–1029
  acetaminophen, 1024
  algorithm for, 1023*a*
  aspirin, 1024
  counterirritants, 1025–1027
  exercise program, 1027
  external analgesics, 1024–1025, 1026*t*
  lifestyle and behavioral modifications, 1027–1028
  local anesthetics, 1025
  muscle relaxants, 1027
  NSAID, 1024
  opioids, 124
  RICE therapy, 1022–1024, 1023*t*
  rubefacients, 1025–1026, 1026*t*
Myasthenia gravis, respiratory acidosis with, 503*t*
Mycobacterium tuberculosis. See also Tuberculosis
 antimicrobial susceptibility testing of, 1255
 culture of, 1254
Mycological cure, 1367, 1368
Mycophenolic acid (MPA), 954
 enteric-coated, 950–952
Mycoplasma hominis, in bacterial vaginosis, 1331
Mycoplasma pneumoniae, in pneumonia, 1190, 1190*t*, 1196*t*, 1197
Mycosis, endemic. *See* Endemic mycosis
Mycotic infections
 cultural awareness of treatment for, 1372
Mydriasis, 276, 1069
 with diethylpropion, 1727
 drug-induced, 1077*t*
 in opioid withdrawal, 619
Myelin, 508

Myeloablative preparative regimen, for hematopoietic cell transplantation, 1630, 1634, 1634*t*
Myeloblasts, 1581
Myelodysplastic syndrome
 chemotherapy-related, 1581
 treatment of, 1455, 1464, 1630*t*
Myelosuppression
 with azathioprine, 950
 with capecitabine, 1455
 with methotrexate, 990
Myocardial contractility, in shock, 252
Myocardial infarction, 131–153. *See also* Acute coronary syndromes; Ischemic heart disease
 secondary prevention of, 149–151
  ACE inhibitors, 150
  aldosterone antagonists, 150–151
  angiotensin receptor blockers, 150
  aspirin, 149
  β-blockers, 150
  calcium channel blockers, 150
  clopidogrel, 149–150
  nitrates, 150
  smoking cessation, 151
  statins, 151
 ventricular remodeling in, 85, 134
Myocarditis
 in diphtheria, 1406
 heart failure and, 84*t*
 shock in, 253*t*
Myoclonus, in serotonin syndrome, 1726
Myoglobinuria, 241
Myonecrosis, clostridial, 1226
Myopathy, with statins, 241
Myringotomy, in otitis media, 1207
Myxedema, 768
Myxedema coma, 768, 772

N
Nabilone
 adverse effects of, 362*t*
 dosage of, 362*t*
 in nausea and vomiting, 362*t*, 364
Nab-paclitaxel, in breast cancer, 1491–1492
Nabumetone
 dosage of, 1002*t*
 in osteoarthritis, 1002*t*
Nadolol
 in arrhythmias, 162*t*
 dosage of, 124*t*
 in hypertension, 66*a*
 in hyperthyroidism, 774
 in ischemic heart disease, 124*t*
 mechanism of action of, 162*t*
 in prevention of migraine, 590*t*
Nafarelin, osteoporosis with, 967*t*
Nafcillin
 adverse effects of, 1177*t*
 in cellulitis, 1225*t*
 in cystic fibrosis, 309*t*
 dosage of, 832*t*, 1177*t*, 1180*t*, 1225*t*, 1245*t*, 1246*t*, 1249*t*, 1342*t*
 drug interactions of, 205*t*
 in infective endocarditis, 1241, 1243, 1245*t*, 1246*t*, 1249*t*
 in meningitis, 1177*t*, 1180*t*
 in osteomyelitis, 1339*t*, 1342*t*
 in sepsis, 1353*t*, 1354
 in tinea infections, 1371
Nails
 fungal infections of, 1369–1373
 oil spots, 1081

Nalbuphine, 45*t*
Nalmefene, in opioid dependence, 626
Naloxone
 in opioid dependence, 626
 in opioid withdrawal, 619
 in respiratory acidosis, 503
 reversal of opioid intoxication, 577*t*, 616
Naloxone challenge, 626
Naltrexone
 adverse effects of, 625
 in alcohol dependence, 625
 dosage of, 625
 drug interactions of, 625
 hepatotoxicity of, 625
 mechanism of action of, 625
 in opioid dependence, 626
Naphazoline
 in allergic conjunctivitis, 1068*t*
 in allergic rhinitis, 1051*t*, 1055, 1058*t*
Naproxen
 dosage of, 837, 859*t*, 1002*t*, 1014*t*, 1151*t*
 drug interactions of, 954
 in dysmenorrhea, 859*t*
 in gout, 1014*t*
 ocular changes with, 1077*t*
 in osteoarthritis, 1002*t*
  in sickle cell anemia/disease, 1151*t*
 in pregnancy, 837, 1004
Naratriptan
 dosage of, 589*t*
 drug interactions of, 589*t*
 in migraine, 589*t*
Narcolepsy
 clinical presentation in, 712
 diagnosis of, 712
 epidemiology and etiology of, 710
 pathophysiology of, 711
 patient care and monitoring in, 719
Nasal congestion in pregnancy, 833
Nasal polyps, 266, 285
Nasal scotoma, 1036
Nasoduodenal feeding tube, 1704, 1705*f*, 1705*t*, 1706
Nasogastric feeding tube, 1704, 1705*f*, 1705*t*, 1706
Nasogastric suctioning, metabolic alkalosis with, 502–503, 502*t*
Nasojejunal feeding tube, 1704, 1705*f*, 1705*t*, 1706
Nasolacrimal occlusion, 1077
Nateglinide
 in diabetes mellitus, 748*t*
 dosage of, 748*t*
National Council on Patient Information and Education, 15
National Health Interview Survey (2007), 8
National Marrow Donor Program, 1631
Nausea, 357–358
Nausea and vomiting, 357–368
 anticipatory, 364, 365
 with apomorphine, 560
 case study of, 365, 366, 367
 chemotherapy-related, 296*t*, 364–365, 365*t*, 1485, 1507*t*–1508*t*, 1512, 1513*t*, 1562–1563, 1636
  acute, 1512, 1513*t*
  anticipatory, 1512, 1513*t*
  delayed, 1512, 1513*t*
 complex, 359
 with corticosteroids, 953*t*
 epidemiology of, 357–358
 etiology of, 357–358, 358*t*
 with hormone-replacement therapy, 876*t*

nonpharmacologic treatment, in palliative care, 43
with opioids, 577, 577t
with oral contraceptives, 847
outcome evaluation in, 367–368
palliative care considerations, 43–44, 43f
pharmacotherapy, in palliative care, 43
pathophysiology of, 358–359, 359t
patient care and monitoring in, 305
postoperative, 358, 365–366
in pregnancy, 296t, 358, 366–367, 829
radiation-related, 1557
simple, 359
toxicity criteria, 1453t
treatment of, 359–367, 578t
  antacids, 359
  anticholinergics, 359, 360, 360t, 367
  antihistamines, 359, 360, 361t, 366
  benzodiazepines, 300t, 364
  cannabinoids, 632t, 364
  corticosteroids, 362t, 364
  dopamine antagonists, 360, 363
  5-HT3 receptor antagonists, 359a
  neurokinin-1 receptor antagonists, 359, 363t
  nonpharmacologic, 359–360
  serotonin antagonists, 300t, 363
with tube feeding, 1711, 1711t
Near drowning, 1131t
Nebulizer, 270t, 271, 275t, 277t
Necator americanus, 1297
Necrotizing enterocolitis, 835–836
  intestine transplantation in, 941
Necrotizing fasciitis, 1226–1227
  clinical presentation in, 1226–1227, 1227t
  diagnosis of, 1226–1227
  epidemiology of, 1226
  etiology of, 1226
  treatment of, 1227
Nedocromil
  adverse effects of, 1068t
  in allergic conjunctivitis, 1068tt
  in asthma, 275t, 278, 280, 281
  in COPD, 297
  dosage of, 1068t
  mechanism of action of, 1068t
Nefazadone
  adverse effects of, 659t
  in depression, 665
  dosage of, 661, 661t
  drug interactions of, 244, 660, 661t, 698, 699t,
    955t
  in elderly, 665
  in insomnia, 714
  mechanism of action of, 657, 657t
  pharmacokinetics of, 660, 661t
Neisseria, normal flora, 1157f
Neisseria gonorrhoeae. See also Gonorrhea
  in conjunctivitis, 1065
  in pharyngitis, 1214
  in PID, 1332
Neisseria meningitidis, 1411
  in conjunctivitis, 1065
  in meningitis, 1170, 1171t, 1175t, 1179–1181
Nelarabine
  in cancer therapy, 1456
  drug interactions of, 1456
Nelfinavir
  adverse effects of, 1431t
  dosage of, 1431t
  drug interactions of, 850t, 955t, 1431t, 1434
  food interactions of, 1431t
  in HIV infection, 1426, 1431t, 1434
  mechanism of action of, 1421f
Nelson's syndrome, 793

Nematodes, 1297
Neomycin
  in conjunctivitis, 1066
  drug interactions of, 205t
  in preoperative bowel cleansing, 1399
  in surgical prophylaxis, 1400t, 1401
Neovascularization, in diabetic retinopathy, 757
Nepafenac, ocular, in corneal abrasion, 1064
Nephritis
  interstitial, 433, 435
  radiation, kidney transplantation in, 941
Nephrolithiasis
  drug-related, 1439t
  in inflammatory bowel disease, 344
  kidney transplantation in, 941
  uric acid, 1011, 1015
Nephron, 445
Nephropathy. *See* Kidney disease, chronic
Nephrostomy, in hemorrhagic cystitis, 1668
Nephrotic syndrome, 236t
  hyperlipidemia in, 447
  hyponatremia in, 485
Nervous stomach, 380
Nesiritide
  adverse effects of, 102
  dosage of, 101t, 102
  in heart failure, 99, 101, 101t, 102
  hemodynamic effects of, 101, 101t
Neuralgia, post-herpetic, 568, 570, 578t, 1413
Neural plasticity, 569
Neural tube defects, 537, 686, 827
Neuritis, in diphtheria, 1406
Neuroblastoma, 1447t, 1630, 1630t
Neurochemical hypothesis, of bipolar disorder, 670
Neurocysticercosis, 522, 1298
Neurofibrillary tangles, 597
Neurofibroma, 1447t
Neurofibromatosis, acute leukemia and, 1580t
Neurogenic bladder, 911, 921t
Neurogenic shock, 253t
Neurohormonal model, of heart failure, 82–83
Neurohumoral response, to hypovolemia, 253
Neurohypophysis, 802
Neurokinin-1 (NK1) receptors
  in chemotherapy-induced nausea and
    vomiting, 1651, 1652
Neurokinin-1 receptor antagonists, in nausea and
    vomiting, 359, 363t
Neuroleptic malignant syndrome, 642
Neuroleptics, 12
Neurologic disease/impairment
  in cancer patients, 1663–1664
  constipation in, 372t
  enteral nutrition in, 1703t
  erectile dysfunction with, 885t
  nausea and vomiting with, 358t
  in sepsis, 1349
Neurologic focality, 585
Neuronal adaptation, in substance-abuse
    disorders, 610
Neuronal intestinal dysplasia, intestine
    transplantation in, 941
Neuronal mechanisms, in seizures, 522–523
Neuronal plasticity, 655
Neuropathic pain, 45, 568, 570, 578
  treatment of, 578
Neuropathy
  in diabetes mellitus, 1227
  oxaliplatin-induced, 1530
Neuropeptide Y, in anxiety disorders, 693
Neurosurgical procedures
  antimicrobial prophylaxis in, 1400t
  postoperative infections in, 1170, 1171t, 1183

Neurosyphilis, 676t, 1324, 1325
Neurotransmitter(s). *See also specific compounds*
  in ADHD, 724
  in Parkinson's disease, 554, 554f
  in seizures, 522
  in status epilepticus, 542
Neurotransmitter receptor hypothesis, of
    depression, 654
Neutralizing antibodies, to interferon α, 512–513
Neutropenia
  in cancer patients, 1654–1661
    algorithm for management of, 1659a
    case study of, 1653
    clinical presentation in, 1656
    diagnosis of, 1656
    epidemiology of, 1654
    etiology of, 1654, 1655t
    outcome evaluation in, 1661
    pathophysiology of, 1655
    patient care and monitoring in, 1661
    risk factors for, 1655, 1655t
    treatment of infections, 1451, 1512, 1595,
      1657–1661
  chemotherapy-related, 1451, 1485, 1507t, 1512,
    1513t, 1562, 1594–1595, 1654–1661
  definition of, 1655
  febrile, 1654–1661
  in hematopoietic cell transplant recipients, 1641
  with interferon therapy, 424–425
  prevention of infection in
    colony-stimulating factors, 1657, 1657t
    hand hygiene, 1656–1657
    prophylactic antibiotics, 1654
  toxicity criteria, 1453t
Nevirapine
  adverse effects of, 1429t, 1437t–1438t
  dosage of, 1429t
  drug interactions of, 614t, 955t, 1434
  food interactions of, 1429t
  in HIV infection, 1426, 1429t, 1434
Newborn
  DIC in, 1131t
  genital herpes in, 1330–1331
New York Heart Association Functional
    Classification, of heart failure, 86–87, 87t
Niacin
  adverse effects of, 243t, 245
  dosage of, 243t, 245
  drug interactions of, 240
  formulations of, 245
  gout with, 1012
  hepatotoxicity of, 245
  in high-density lipoprotein, 151, 243t, 245
  mechanism of action of, 245
Nicardipine
  adverse effects of, 71t
  dosage of, 71t, 124t
  drug interactions of, 955t
  in hypertension, 220t
  in hypertensive emergency, 71t
  in ischemic heart disease, 124, 124t
  in stroke, 220t
NICE SUGAR study, 1694
Nickel exposure, 1500
Nicotine, 828t
  in inflammatory bowel disease, 349
  respiratory alkalosis with, 504t
  transdermal, 349
  withdrawal syndrome, 613t, 622, 622t, 623t.
    See also Smoking cessation
Nicotine replacement therapy, 117, 293, 622, 622t
  dosage of, 622t
  products available, 622, 622t

Nicotinic acid, blood glucose level and, 737t
Nifedipine, 828t
    in acute coronary syndromes, 142t
    adverse effects of, 61t
    dosage, 61t, 124t, 142t, 828t, 832t
    drug interactions of, 955t
    in hypertension, 61t
    in ischemic heart disease, 123
    migraines with, 588t
    as tocolytic, 828t, 832t, 835
Nifurtimox, in American trypanosomiasis,
    1303
Night awakening, in enuresis, 923t
Nightly intermittent peritoneal dialysis, 473
Nightmares, 710
Nilotinib
    adverse effects of, 1467
    in cancer therapy, 1467
    in chronic myelogenous leukemia, 1599,
        1600–1601, 1600t
    pharmacokinetics of, 1467
Nilutamide
    adverse effects of, 1468, 1545t
    in cancer therapy, 1468
    dosage of, 1545t
    mechanism of action of, 1468
    pharmacokinetics of, 1468
    in prostate cancer, 1539t, 1545, 1545t, 1546
Nimodipine, in subarachnoid hemorrhage,
    226t
Nipple candidiasis, 826, 826t, 826
Nit(s), 1304
Nitazoxanide
    in cryptosporidiosis, 1276
    dosage of, 1294
    in giardiasis, 1294
Nitrates
    in acute coronary syndromes, 142t, 146, 149,
        150, 152t
    adverse effects of, 121, 146, 152t
    in angina pectoris, 121
    contraindications to, 143t
    dosage of, 142t
    drug interactions of, 121, 126, 142t, 146,
        889–890
    effect on myocardial oxygen demand and
        supply, 122t
    GERD with, 317t
    in hypertension, 63t
    in ischemic heart disease, 121, 122t
    long-acting, 121
    mechanism of action of, 121
    migraines with, 588t
    nitrate-free period, 124
    oral, 124, 124t
    in portal hypertension, 396
    in prevention of myocardial infarction,
        149–151
    short-acting, 121
    tolerance to, 124
    transdermal, 124, 124t
    in variant angina, 126
Nitric oxide, 93, 121, 232
    in ascites, 390
    in cirrhosis, 389, 390
    in erectile function, 885
    in heart failure, 83
Nitric oxide synthase, 805
Nitrofurantoin
    in bacteriuria, 833
    in pregnancy, 833
    in urinary tract infections, 1311t, 1312t, 1313,
        1314t

Nitroglycerin
    in acute coronary syndromes, 139, 142t
    adverse effects of, 71t
    in angina pectoris, 121
    arrhythmia with, 162t
    dosage of, 71t, 101, 101t
    in heart failure, 101, 101t, 102
    hemodynamic effects of, 101, 101t
    in hypertensive emergency, 71t
    intravenous, 142t
    in ischemic heart disease, 121
    patient education about, 121
    spray, 121
    sublingual, 121, 148
    tolerance to, 98, 101
    in variant angina, 126
Nitroprusside
    adverse effects of, 28t, 101
    dosage of, 71t, 101t
    in heart failure, 101–102, 101t
    hemodynamic effects of, 101, 101t
    in hypertension, 220t
    in hypertensive emergency, 71t
    metabolic acidosis with, 501t
    in stroke, 220t
Nizatidine
    dosage of, 320t, 336t
    in GERD, 320t, 321
    in peptic ulcer disease, 336t
NK-1 receptor inhibitors, in chemotherapy-
        related nausea and vomiting, 1512, 1513t
NKF-DOQI classification, of chronic kidney
        disease, 446, 446t
NMDA antagonists
    in Alzheimer's disease, 598, 601t, 602
    in pain, 578
NMDA receptors, 569, 597
    in alcohol abuse, 609
Nociception, in migraine, 584
Nociceptive pain, 568
Nociceptors, 568–569, 1021
Nocturia, 910
    in heart failure, 85, 85t
    in urinary tract infections, 1307
Nocturnal polysomnography, 710, 713
Nocturnal tidal peritoneal dialysis, 473
NOD2 protein, 342
Nodules, subcutaneous, in rheumatoid arthritis,
    984
Nonadherence, in elderly patients, 15
Nonarteritic ischemic optic neuropathy, with
        phosphodiesterase inhibitors, 890
Nonbacterial thrombotic endocarditis, 1237,
    1237a
Nonbiologic DMARDs, 990
Noncompliance. See Compliance
Nongonococcal urethritis, 1320
Non-high-density lipoprotein cholesterol, 229
    goal for, 239
Non-Hodgkin's lymphoma, 1551–1563
    B-cell, 1553t, 1554–1555
    clinical presentation in, 1556
    diagnosis of, 1556
    diffuse, 1555, 1560, 1561t
    environmental factors in, 1553
    epidemiology of, 1552–1553
    etiology of, 1552–1553
    follicular, 1555, 1559–1560, 1560t
    genetic factors in, 1554
    HIV infection and, 1552, 1562
    International Index for, 1556, 1557
    lymphoblastic, 1561
    lymphocyte morphology in, 1555

    mantle cell, 1561
    outcome evaluation in, 1562–1563
    pathophysiology of, 1553–1556
    patient care and monitoring in, 1562
    prognostic factors for, 1556, 1555t
    radiation therapy in, 1559
    Richter's transformation in, 1555
    spinal cord compression with, 1663
    staging of, 1559, 1559t
    T-cell, 1553–1556, 1555t
    treatment of, 1559–1562
        chemotherapy, 1559–1562, 1560t, 1561t
        hematopoietic cell transplant, 1558, 1630,
            1630t
        monoclonal antibodies, 1560
    tumor lysis syndrome in, 1674t
    viral infections and, 1554–1555
    WHO classification of, 1374t, 1555
    Working Formulation classification of,
        1555–1556, 1555t
Nonmelanoma skin cancer
    age and, 1612
        clinical presentation in, 1624
    diagnosis of, 1624
    epidemiology of, 1623
        etiology of, 1623
    genetic factors in, 1613
        lymph node considerations in, 1624
    outcome evaluation in, 1625–1626
    pathophysiology of, 1624
    patient care and monitoring in, 1626
    primary prevention of, 1613
    risk factors for, 1623–1624
    secondary prevention of, 1613–1614
        staging of, 1615t
    treatment of, 1624–1625
        cryotherapy, 1625
        electrodesiccation and curettage, 1625
        full-thickness ablative procedures,
            1624–1625
        imiquimod, 1625
        Mohs' micrographic surgery, 1625
        photodynamic therapy, 1625
        radiation therapy, 1625
        superficial ablative procedures, 1625
        surgery, 1624–1625
    ultraviolet radiation exposure and, 1624
Nonnucleoside reverse transcriptase inhibitors.
        See also specific drugs
    adverse effects of, 1437t–1442t
    drug interactions of, 1434
    in HIV infection, 1421f, 1423, 1426–1433,
        1426t, 1427t–1432t
Nonopioid analgesics, in pain, 573
    combination analgesics, 576
Nonoral hormonal contraceptives, 850–851
    injectable, 850
    transdermal patch, 850
    transvaginal ring, 850
Nonoxynol-9, 852
Nonpharmacologic treatment, in palliative care
    advanced heart failure, 46
    anxiety, 40–41
    delirium, 41
    dyspnea, 42
    nausea and vomiting, 43
    pain, 44
    terminal secretions, 45
Non-REM sleep, 710
Nonspecific (nonselective) adrenergic agonists, in
        glaucoma, 1038t, 1043
Nonsteroidal anti-inflammatory drugs
        (NSAIDs). See also specific drugs

adverse effects of, 12t, 38t, 40t, 574–575, 859t, 985, 1002–1004, 1013
in allergic conjunctivitis, 1068t, 1070t
allergic drug reactions, 932–933
in allergic rhinitis, 1058t
in Alzheimer's disease, 602
anxiety with, 694t
in cystic fibrosis, 312
dosage of, 859t
drug interactions of, 205t, 679, 954
in dysmenorrhea, 859t, 864
gastrointestinal complications of, 1004
GERD with, 317t
in gout, 1013, 1014t
in headache, 592
in hemophilia, 1126
hyperkalemia with, 488
inflammatory bowel disease and, 342
in ischemic heart disease, 126
keratitis with, 1070t
mechanism of action of, 1003, 1024
in menorrhagia, 859t, 861
in migraine, 587–588
in musculoskeletal disorders, 1024
nephrotoxicity of, 432, 440, 442, 574, 1004
nonselective, 574–575
in opioid withdrawal, 621t
in osteoarthritis, 1002–1004, 1002t, 1006
in pain, 572, 574
in sickle cell anemia/disease, 1149
peptic ulcer with, 327, 328t, 329, 329t, 330–331, 333, 574, 985
prevention of, 336
in pregnancy, 824t, 1004
in prevention of colorectal cancer, 1518–1519
in prevention of lung cancer, 1501
in prevention of ovarian cancer, 1567
in prevention of prostate cancer, 1537
psoriasis and, 1080
in rheumatoid arthritis, 988–989
selective, 574–575
in tension-type headaches, 589
teratogenic effects of, 824t
topical, 1007
adverse effects of, 1024
in corneal abrasion, 1064
in musculoskeletal disorders, 1024
patient education for, 1025t
Nonthyroidal illness, 777
Nonvesicant, 1676
Norelgestromin, 850
Norepinephrine, 784
in ADHD, 724
in anxiety disorders, 693
arrhythmia with, 204t
in bipolar disorder, 670
in depression, 654
dosage of, 260t, 1356
in heart failure, 82, 83
in hypovolemic shock, 256a, 260, 260t
in sepsis, 1356
in wakefulness, 710
Norepinephrine neurons, loss, in Parkinson's disease, 554
Norethindrone, 845t, 848
Norethindrone acetate, 843, 849, 875t
Norfloxacin
in conjunctivitis, 1066
dosage of, 1269t, 1312t
drug interactions of, 205t
in shigellosis, 1269t
in urinary tract infections, 1311t, 1312t

Norgestimate, 843, 849, 875t
Norgestrel, 843, 845t, 847
Normal flora, 1156–1157, 1157f, 1703
Normal saline, 481, 483
in anaphylaxis, 931t
in dehydration, 1269t
in diabetic ketoacidosis, 756
dosage of, 414t
in hypercalcemia, 414t, 1670, 1672t
in hypotension, 471
in hypovolemic shock, 256a, 257
in pancreatitis, 405
Normeperidine, 575
Norovirus
in gastroenteritis, 1277, 1277t
in travelers' diarrhea, 1273
Nortriptyline
in depression, 665
dosage of, 622t, 661, 661t
drug interactions of, 614t
in elderly, 665
in prevention of migraine, 590, 590t
in smoking cessation, 622, 622t
Norwalk virus, in diarrhea, 376
Nosocomial infection, 1156
NSAIDs. See Nonsteroidal anti-inflammatory drugs
N-Telopeptides, 969
Nuchal rigidity, in stroke, 217
Nuclear medicine scans, in osteomyelitis, 1341
Nucleoside/nucleotide reverse transcriptase inhibitors. See also specific drugs
adverse effects of, 1437t–1442t
in HIV infection, 1421f, 1423, 1426–1433, 1426t, 1427t–1432t
Nucleus accumbens, in reward pathway, 609, 609f
Nugent criteria, for bacterial vaginosis, 1331
Nulliparity, 870
breast cancer and, 1476
dysmenorrhea and, 862
ovarian cancer and, 1566
Nutrition. See also Diet therapy
enteral. See Enteral nutrition
parenteral. See Parenteral nutrition
preoperative, 1682t
Nutritional requirements, 1688–1690
estimation of, 1688–1690, 1689t
Nutrition assessment, 1688–1690
in tube feeding, 1713–1714
NuvaRing, 850
Nystagmus
drug-induced, 1077t
in status epilepticus, 543
Nystatin
in diaper dermatitis, 1106
dosage of, 831t, 832t, 1363t
in intra-abdominal infections, 1288
in oropharyngeal candidiasis, 1368, 1385
in prevention of thrush, 957
in vulvovaginal candidiasis, 831t, 1363t

O

Oatmeal baths
in contact dermatitis, 1102
in psoriasis, 1083
Obesity, 1719–1729
body mass index in, 1721t
breast cancer and, 1477
case study of, 1720, 1722
clinical presentation in, 1721
colorectal cancer and, 1519
definition of, 736, 1719

diabetes mellitus and, 736, 744, 1720–1721
diagnosis of, 1721, 1721t
in elderly, 1728
epidemiology of, 1721
erectile dysfunction with, 885t
etiology of, 1720
gallbladder disease and, 1720
heart failure and, 88
hyperlipidemia and, 236t, 1720
hypertension and, 54t, 56, 1720
ischemic heart disease and, 111t, 112
osteoarthritis and, 999, 1720
outcome evaluation in, 1728–1729
pathophysiology of, 1720–1721
patient care and monitoring in, 1729
in pediatric patients, 1721, 1728
respiratory acidosis with, 426t
secondary causes of, 1720
sleep apnea and, 712, 718, 1721
stroke and, 217t
treatment of, 1722–1728
behavior modification, 1724
diet therapy, 1723–1724, 1723t
diethylpropion, 1725t, 1727–1728
exercise program, 1724, 1724t
levothyroxine, 771, 772, 774t
orlistat, 1725t, 1726
phentermine, 1725t, 1727
rimonabant, 1726–1727
sibutramine, 1725–1726, 1725t
surgery, 1728
venous thromboembolism and, 187t
Obliterative bronchiolitis, 292
Obsessive-compulsive disorder, 695
Obstetric surgery, antimicrobial prophylaxis in, 1399–1400, 1400t
Obstructive shock, 252, 253t
Obstructive sleep apnea
case study of, 718
clinical presentation in, 712
diagnosis of, 712
enuresis with, 921t
epidemiology and etiology of, 710
hypertension and, 711
obesity and, 712, 718
pathophysiology of, 711–712
patient care and monitoring in, 719
respiratory acidosis with, 426t
treatment of, 717–718
continuous positive airway pressure, 717–718
Occlusal injury, 1232
Occupational asthma, 266
Occupational therapy, in Parkinson's disease, 557
Ochronosis, 998t
Octreotide
in acromegaly, 805–806, 807t
adverse effects of, 379, 590, 805–806, 807t
in cluster headaches, 589–590
in diarrhea, 379, 1512
dosage of, 397, 805, 807t
long-acting formulation of, 805
parenteral nutrition and, 1694
in variceal bleeding, 397
Ocular emergencies
corneal abrasion, 1063–1065
epidemiology of, 1063
etiology of, 1063
loss of vision, 1064t, 1065
splash injuries and chemical exposure, 1064t, 1065
time to follow-up by ophthalmologist, 1064tt
trauma, 1064t, 1065
Office-based opioid treatment, 626

Off-label medication use, 30
Off-loading, in diabetic foot infections, 1229
Ofloxacin
  anxiety with, 694t
  in conjunctivitis, 1066, 1066t
  dosage of, 1066t
  drug interactions of, 205t
Oiling out, of intravenous lipid emulsions, 1683
Oil spots, 1081
OKT-3
  in acute rejection reaction, 946
  adverse effects of, 945t, 946, 951t
  dosage of, 945t, 946
  mechanism of action of, 946
  in transplant recipient, 945t, 946, 951t
Olanzapine
  adverse effects of, 638, 638t, 685
  in Alzheimer's disease, 603
  augmentation of antidepressant therapy with, 662
  in bipolar disorder, 678t, 684–685
  blood glucose level and, 737t
  in chemotherapy-related nausea and vomiting, 1513t, 1652
  dosage of, 603, 637t, 638, 678t
  drug interactions of, 614t, 646t, 647
  mechanism of action of, 637f, 638
  metabolism of, 646t, 647
  in schizophrenia, 635, 637f, 637t, 638, 644t, 646
Olfactory tubercle, in reward pathway, 609, 609f
Oligoanovulation, 865
Oligomenorrhea, in hyperprolactinemia, 815
Oligomeric formula, for enteral feeding, 1707, 1708t, 1711
Oliguria
  definition of, 433
  in hypovolemic shock, 254t, 255
  in sepsis, 1349
Olopatadine
  adverse effects of, 1068t
  in allergic conjunctivitis, 1068t, 1070
  in allergic rhinitis, 1054, 1054t
  dosage of, 1068t
  mechanism of action of, 1068t
Olsalazine
  adverse effects of, 347
  dosage of, 346t
  in inflammatory bowel disease, 346t, 347
Omalizumab
  adverse effects of, 278, 1057
  in allergic rhinitis, 1057
  in asthma, 278, 275t
Omega-3 polyunsaturated fatty acids, 117, 1709
  in dyslipidemia, 246
Omega-6 polyunsaturated fatty acids, 1708
Omentumectomy, in ovarian cancer, 1569
Omeprazole
  dosage of, 320t, 321–322, 323, 335t, 336t, 830t
  drug interactions of, 153t, 321–322, 699t, 955t
  in GERD, 320t, 321–322, 323
  in *Helicobacter pylori* eradication, 335t, 1561
  in peptic ulcer disease, 336t
  in pregnancy, 830t, 833
  in prevention of NSAID-related ulcers, 336
Oncogenes, 1446, 1447t
  in colorectal cancer, 1521
  in non-Hodgkin's lymphoma, 1554–1556
Oncologic emergencies, 1649–1679
Ondansetron
  in alcohol dependence, 626
  in chemotherapy-related nausea and vomiting, 1513t, 1652t
  dosage of, 300t

in nausea and vomiting, 300t, 364, 577t
Onion, drug interactions of, 206t
Onychomycosis, 1369–1373, 1370t
Oophorectomy
  in breast cancer, 1485
  in prevention of breast cancer, 1476
  in prevention of ovarian cancer, 1567
Ophthalmic solution, application of, 1043
Opiates, endogenous, 569
Opioid(s). *See also specific drugs*
  abuse of
    pathophysiology of, 609
    signs and symptoms of intoxication, 612t, 616
    treatment of, 616
    withdrawal syndrome, 611
  addiction to, 576
  administration of, 576
  adverse effects of, 575–576, 575t, 1024, 1150
  allergy to, 576–577
  dependence on, 576
  discontinuation of, 577
  drug interactions of, 577
  in headache, 592
  in hemorrhagic cystitis, 1669
  hyperprolactinemia with, 814t
  mechanism of action of, 575, 610
  in migraine, 587–588
  in musculoskeletal disorders, 1024
  nausea and vomiting with, 357, 358, 358t
  in osteoarthritis, 1006
  in pain, 569, 572, 572t, 575–578
    combination analgesics, 576
    equianalgesic dosing, 577–578, 577t
    opioid rotation, 577
    potency of, 577
    selection of agent, 575–576
    in sickle cell anemia/disease, 1150
  in spinal cord compression, 1664
  in tension-type headaches, 589
  teratogenic effects of, 824t
  tolerance to, 1150
  treatment of dependence on
    opioid agonists, 626
    opioid antagonists, 626
  urinary incontinence with, 912t
  withdrawal syndrome, 619–621, 621t
    COWS, 619, 620t
    ultrarapid opioid detoxification, 622
Opioid agonists, in opioid dependence, 626
Opioid agonists/antagonists, 45t
Opioid analgesics in hemophilia, 1126
Opioid antagonists, in opioid dependence, 626
Opioids, 12
Opportunistic. *See* Opportunistic mycosis
Opportunistic infection
  in hematopoietic cell transplant recipients, 1641–1642s
  in HIV infection, 1422
  in transplant recipient, 955–956, 957t
Opportunistic mycosis, 1376, 1376t, 1382
  case study of, 1382
  risk factors for, 1382
Opsonization, 942
Optic nerve
Oral cavity cancer, 1446f
Oral contraceptives, 843–848
  in acne treatment, 845, 847, 1099
  adverse effects of, 12t, 846–848, 859t, 1099
  in amenorrhea, 858, 859t
  in anovulatory bleeding, 859t, 865
  biphasic preparations, 845t
  blood glucose level and, 737t

breast cancer and, 846
breast disease and, 845
cardiovascular disease and, 846
cervical cancer and, 846
chewable, 849
chloasma with, 848
contraindications to, 846, 847t
depression with, 655
dosage of, 859t
drug interactions of, 684, 699t, 849, 850t, 1434
in dysmenorrhea, 845, 859t, 864
endometrial cancer and, 845
gallbladder disease and, 846
gastrointestinal side effects of, 847
glucose intolerance with, 846
headache with, 847
hyperlipidemia with, 848
hypertension and, 846
liver disease and, 846
mania with, 676t
mastalgia with, 847
mechanism of action of, 843, 844t
melasma with, 848
in menorrhagia, 859t, 861
monophasic preparations, 845t
nausea and vomiting with, 357, 358t
noncontraceptive benefits of, 845–846
ocular changes with, 1077t
ovarian cancer and, 845
ovarian cysts and, 845
in prevention of ovarian cancer, 1567
products available, 844, 845t
progestin-only pills, 850
risks of, 845–846
STDs and, 845–846
triphasic preparations, 845t
unique, 848–849
venous thromboembolism with, 135t, 846
von Willebrand's disease and, 1128
weight gain with, 848
Oral glucose tolerance test, 740–741, 741t, 804
Oral rehydration therapy (ORT), 378, 1269t
  in campylobacteriosis, 1271
  in cholera, 1273
  in salmonellosis, 1269
  in travelers' diarrhea, 1274
  in viral gastroenteritis, 1278
OraSweet®, 28
Orbital cellulitis, 1064t
Orbital pain, in cluster headache, 587
Orchiectomy, in prostate cancer, 1539t, 1542, 1543
Organification, of iodine, 764
Organophosphate poisoning, 426t
Organ transplantation. *See* Solid-organ transplantation
Orlistat
  adverse effects of, 1726
  dosage of, 1725t, 1726
  drug interactions of, 1726
  mechanism of action of, 1726
  in obesity, 1725t, 1726
Ornidazole, in trichomoniasis, 1326
Orogastric feeding tube, 1704, 1705f, 1705t, 1706
Oropharyngeal candidiasis, 1366–1369
  case study of, 1367
  clinical presentation in, 1366, 1367
  epidemiology of, 1366
  etiology of, 1366
  fluconazole-resistant, 1368
  hyperplastic, 1367
  outcome evaluation in, 1369

pathophysiology of, 1366
patient care and monitoring in, 1368
pseudomembranous, 1367
risk factors for, 1366, 1366t
treatment of, 1366–1369, 1385
Ortho-Evra, 850
Orthopedic surgery, antimicrobial prophylaxis
  in, 1400t, 1400
Orthopnea, in heart failure, 85t, 86
Orthostasis, in adrenal insufficiency, 787
Orthostatic hypotension, 970
  in Parkinson's disease, 558
Orthotics, in hemophilia, 1123
Ortho Tri-Cyclen, 848
Oseltamivir, in pneumonia, 1197
Osler nodes, 1237, 1238, 1238f
Osmolality
  plasma, 480
    case study of, 485
  serum, 484
  urine, 453
Osmolar gap, 485
Osmophobia, with migraine, 586
Ospemifene, 976
Osteoarthritis, 997–1008
  case study of, 1000, 1007
  clinical presentation in, 999
  comparison of rheumatoid arthritis and
    osteoarthritis, 984t
  cost of, 997
  diagnosis of, 999
  epidemiology of, 998
  ethnicity and, 998
  joints involved in, 984f
  obesity and, 999, 1720
  outcome evaluation in, 1007
  pathophysiology of, 998–999, 998f
  patient care and monitoring in, 1008
  primary, 998, 998t
  risk factors for, 999
  secondary, 998t, 999
  treatment of, 999–1007
    acetaminophen, 1000–1002, 1002t
    algorithm for, 1001a
    counterirritants, 1006
    COX-2 inhibitors, 1002t, 1004–1005
    exercise program, 1000
    glucosamine and chondroitin, 1002t, 1005
    intraarticular corticosteroids, 1006
    intraarticular hyaluronan, 1005–1006
    lifestyle modifications, 1000
    NSAID, 1002–1004, 1002t, 1006, 1007
    opioids, 1006
    patient education, 1000
    physical therapy, 1000
    rubefacients, 1006
    surgery, 1007
    topical analgesics, 1002t, 1006–1007
Osteoarthrosis. See Osteoarthritis
Osteoblasts, 967, 983
Osteoclasts, 967, 983
Osteodystrophy, renal. See Renal
  osteodystrophy
Osteomalacia, with parenteral nutrition, 1697
Osteomyelitis, 1337–1345
  acute, 1337–1338
  case study of, 1340, 1341, 1344
  chronic, 1338, 1340–1341, 1343
  Cierny-Mader staging system for, 1338
  classification of
    by duration of disease, 1338, 1338a
    by route of infection, 1338, 1338a
  clinical presentation in, 1340–1341

contiguous
  with vascular insufficiency, 1338, 1338a,
    1339t, 1340
  without vascular insufficiency, 1338, 1338a,
    1339t, 1340
  diabetes mellitus and, 1228, 1338
  diagnosis of, 1340–1341
  epidemiology of, 1338–1340
  etiology of, 1338, 1339t
  hematogenous, 1338a, 1339–1341, 1339t
  outcome evaluation in, 1344–1345
  pathophysiology of, 1340, 1340a
  patient care and monitoring in, 1345
  in pediatric patients, 1342t, 1343t
  peripheral vascular disease and, 1338
  in sickle cell anemia/disease, 1147
  treatment of, 1339t, 1341–1344, 1342t–1343t
Osteonecrosis
  with bisphosphonates, 974
  drug-related, 1441t
  of jaw, 1607
  in osteoarthritis, 998
Osteonecrosis of jaw (ONJ), 974
Osteopenia
  in cystic fibrosis, 305
  definition of, 968, 968t
  in hematopoietic cell transplant recipients,
    1644
  in inflammatory bowel disease, 344, 345
  with parenteral nutrition, 1697
  treatment of, 971
Osteophytes, 998
Osteoporosis, 965–978
  with antiepileptic drugs, 533t, 535, 536
  case study of, 967, 971
  clinical presentation in, 967–969
  in cystic fibrosis, 305, 312
  definition of, 968, 968t
  diagnosis of, 967–969
  drug-related, 967t
  epidemiology of, 966–967
  etiology of, 966
  and falls, prevention of, 970
  gastrointestinal disease and, 977–978
  glucocorticoid-induced, 953t, 976–977,
    989–990
  hormone-replacement therapy and, 876
  hypogonadism and, 976
  in inflammatory bowel disease, 344, 345
  medical conditions associated with, 967t
  in men, 976
  menopause and, 967, 976
  outcome evaluation in, 977–978
  with parenteral nutrition, 1697
  pathophysiology of, 967
  patient care and monitoring in, 977
  prevention of
    diet therapy, 969, 969t
    exercise program, 969–970
    hormone-replacement therapy, 876
    primary, 965
  rheumatoid arthritis and, 983
  risk factors for, 966, 966t, 969
  screening for, 968–969
  secondary, 965
  in transplant recipient, 967t
  treatment of, 969–977
    algorithm for, 970a
    bisphosphonates, 973–974, 973t
    calcitonin, 973t, 975
    calcium and vitamin D, 971–973
    combination and sequential therapy, 976
    hormone-replacement therapy, 975

isoflavones, 976
parathyroid hormone, 973t, 975
risk factor modification, 969
SERMs, 973t, 974–975
strontium ranelate, 976
Osteosarcoma, 1447t
  teriparatide-related, 975
Ostomy, sodium requirement with, 1685
OTC medication, 3–4
Otitis media, 1204–1209
  acute, 1204–1205
  case study of, 1204, 1209
  clinical presentation in, 1205
  diagnosis of, 1205
  with effusion, 1204–1205
  epidemiology of, 1204
  etiology of, 1204
  outcome evaluation in, 1208–1209
  pathophysiology of, 1205
  patient care and monitoring in, 1209
  prevention of, 1207–1208
  risk factors for, 1204, 1204t
  treatment of, 1205–1208
    adenoidectomy, 1206
    adjunctive therapy, 1207
    algorithm for, 1206a, 1207a
    antibiotics, 1206–1207, 1208t
    myringotomy, 1207
    nonpharmacologic, 1205–1206
    tympanostomy tube, 1205
    watchful waiting, 1205–1206
Ovarian cancer, 1565–1576
  breast cancer and, 1566–1567
  case study of, 1566, 1567
  chronic inflammatory processes hypothesis of,
    1567–1568
  clinical presentation in, 1568
  diagnosis of, 1568
  diet and, 1566
  drug-resistant, 1568–1569
  epidemiology of, 1446f, 1566–1567
  epithelial tumors, 1568
  etiology of, 1566–1567
  genetic factors in, 1447t, 1476–1477, 1567
  germ-cell tumors, 1568
  hereditary breast and ovarian cancer, 1566
  incessant-ovulation hypothesis of, 1565,
    1567–1568
  metastasis of, 1566
  oral contraceptives and, 845
  outcome evaluation in, 1575
  pathophysiology of, 1567–1568
  patient care and monitoring in, 1575
  pituitary gonadotropin hypothesis of, 1567–1568
  platinum-resistant, 1573, 1575
  prevention of
    chemoprevention, 1567
    genetic screening, 1567
    surgery, 1567
  screening for, 1566–1567
  sex-cord stromal tumors, 1568
  staging of, 1569, 1570a
  treatment of, 1569–1575
    algorithm for, 1571a
    chemotherapy, 1569–1575, 1571a, 1572t,
      1574t
    consolidation chemotherapy, 1573
    IP chemotherapy, 1570–1571
    neoadjuvant chemotherapy, 1571–1572
    palliative surgery, 1573
    recurrent chemotherapy, 1570–1571, 1572t
    surgery, 1569–1570, 1569f
Ovarian cyst, oral contraceptives and, 845

Ovarian failure, amenorrhea in, 856
Ovarian radiation, in breast cancer, 1485
Overfeeding, 1704
Overlearning, in enuresis, 923t, 924
Overnight metyrapone test, 788t
Over-the-counter (OTC), 29–30
Over-the-counter (OTC) medication, 3–4
Overuse musculoskeletal injury, 1020, 1024
Overweight, 736, 1719–1729, 1721t
  definition of, 1719
Ovulation, 856, 1567–1568
Oxacillin
  adverse effects of, 1177t
  dosage of, 832t, 1177t, 1180t, 1245t, 1246t,
    1249t, 1342t
  in infective endocarditis, 1243, 1245t, 1246t,
    1249t
  in meningitis, 1177t, 1180t
  in osteomyelitis, 1342t
Oxaliplatin
  adverse effects of, 1463, 1527t, 1529–1530
  in cancer therapy, 1463
  in colorectal cancer, 1524t, 1525, 1526, 1527t,
    1528t, 1529–1530
  dosage of, 1524t
  emetogenicity of, 365t
  extravasation of, 1677t
  mechanism of action of, 1463, 1524t
  pharmacokinetics of, 1463
Oxazepam
  in alcohol withdrawal, 618
  dosage of, 618, 698t
  metabolism of, 697
  in muscle cramps, 472
  in opioid withdrawal, 621t
  pharmacokinetics of, 698t
Oxcarbazepine
  adverse effects of, 529t, 530, 530t, 684
  in bipolar disorder, 678t, 680t–682t, 684
  dosage of, 454t, 678t
  drug interactions of, 850t
  in epilepsy, 529t, 530, 530t, 531, 533, 535
  mechanism of action of, 533t
  monitoring therapy with, 682t
  pharmacokinetics of, 533t, 680t–681t
Oxidative stress, COPD and, 290
Oxybutynin
  adverse effects of, 915, 916t
  dosage of, 916t, 924
  in enuresis, 915, 916t
  in hemorrhagic cystitis, 1669
  pharmacokinetics of, 916t
  in urinary dysfunction, 563
  in urinary incontinence, 516, 915, 916t
Oxycodone
  adverse effects of, 717t
  dosage of, 577t, 717t
  metabolism of, 577
  in osteoarthritis, 1006
  in pain, 572t, 577t, 577
  in restless-legs syndrome, 717, 717t
Oxygen demand, myocardial, 110, 110f, 121, 122,
  122t, 123, 132
Oxygen supply, myocardial, 110, 110f, 121, 122,
  122t, 123, 132
Oxygen therapy, 1227
  in acute chest syndrome, 1148
  in asthma, 269, 283
  in cluster headaches, 589
  in COPD, 294, 299
  in prevention of surgical site infections, 1398
  in stroke, 220
Oxymetazoline

in allergic rhinitis, 1055
in common cold, 1218t
dosage of, 830t
in pregnancy, 830t1
Oxymorphone
  dosage of, 575t
  in pain, 575t
Oxytocin, 802

P

Paced respiration, 872
Pacemaker, cardiac. *See* Cardiac pacemaker
Pachymetry, 1042
Packed red blood cells, in hypovolemic shock,
  256a, 259
Paclitaxel
  adverse effects of, 1458, 1483t, 1484,
    1491–1493
  albumin-bound, 1458
  in breast cancer, 1482, 1483t, 1484
  in cancer therapy, 1458
  dosage of, 1458, 1483t, 1491, 1507t, 1572t, 1573,
    1574t
    drug interactions of, 955t, 1458
  drug-eluting vascular stents, 118
  extravasation of, 1677, 1677t, 1678t
  in lung cancer, 1507t, 1510–1511
  mechanism of action of, 1458
  in ovarian cancer, 1569, 1571, 1571t, 1572,
    1572t
  pharmacokinetics of, 1458
Paget's disease
  hypercalcemia in, 490
  osteoarthritis in, 998t
Pain
  acute, 569
  central, 569
  chronic, 569–570, 578, 578t
    assessment of, 570–572
    malignant, 570
    nonmalignant, 570
  classification of, 569–570
  clinical presentation in, 569–572
  cost of, 570
  diagnosis of, 569–572
  in elderly, 567
  epidemiology of, 567–568
  etiology of, 567–568
  as fifth vital sign, 570
  functional, 568
  headache. *See* Headache
  inflammatory, 568
  at injection site, 1415
  mechanisms of, 568–569
  modulation of, 569
  in musculoskeletal disorders, 1021
  neuropathic, 568, 570, 578
  nociceptive, 568–569
  nonpharmacologic treatment, in palliative
    care, 44
  palliative care considerations, 44
  pathophysiology of, 568–569, 1021
  pharmacotherapy, in palliative care, 44–45
  perception of, 569
  prevalence of, 567–568
  in sickle cell anemia/disease, 1149–1150,
    1151t
  transmission of, 568–569
  types of, 568
  visceral, 569
Pain assessment, 570–572, 1021
  in children, 571
    in elderly, 571–572

methods of, 571, 571f
mnemonic for, 571
in pediatric patients, 571–572
for specific practice settings, 570
Pain Assessment in Advanced Dementia, 571
Pain management, 567–579
  adjuvant agents for chronic pain, 578, 578t
  algorithm for, 573a
  case study of, 572, 575
  complementary and alternative medicine
    in, 579
  mechanistic approach to, 572
  nonopioid analgesics in, 572t, 574–575
  nonpharmacologic, 573–574
  opioids in, 568, 572t, 575–578
  outcome evaluation in, 579
  patient care and monitoring in, 579
  selection of agent based on severity of pain,
    572–573, 572t
  in sickle cell anemia/disease, 1149–1150, 1150t
  undertreatment of pain, 568
Pain rating scale, 571, 571ff
Palifermin
  in mucositis, 1654
  in prevention of mucositis, 1636
Palliative care, 35
  case study of, 38, 42, 47
  clinical presentation and diagnosis
    Alzheimer and other dementia, 39
    amyotrophic lateral sclerosis (ALS), 39
    cancer, 37
    chronic obstructive pulmonary disease
      (COPD), 38
    end-stage heart failure, 37–38
    end-stage liver disease, 38
    end-stage renal disease (ESRD), 38–39
    HIV/AIDS, 39
    Parkinson's disease, 39
    stroke/cerebral vascular accident (CVA), 39
  definition of, 35–36
  drug use, 38f
  epidemiology, 37
  etiology, 37
  goals of, 36–37
  outcome evaluation, 46
  pathophysiology, 37
  patient care and monitoring, 47
  multi-discipline teamwork, 36f
  treatment, 39–46
    advanced heart failure, 46
    anxiety, 40–41
    delirium, 41
    dyspnea, 41–43
    nausea and vomiting, 43–44
    pain, 44–45
    terminal secretions, 45–46
Palliative care considerations
  advanced heart failure, 46
  anxiety, 40–41
  delirium, 41
  dyspnea, 41–42
  nausea and vomiting, 43
  pain, 44
  terminal secretions, 45
Palmar-plantar erythrodysesthesia. *See* Hand-
  foot syndrome
Palonosetron
  in chemotherapy-induced nausea and
    vomiting, 1652t
  dosage of, 300t
  in nausea and vomiting, 363t, 364, 1513t
Pamidronate
  adverse effects of, 1607

in breast cancer, 1494
in cystic fibrosis, 312
dosage of, 414*t*, 1494, 1547, 1672*t*
in hypercalcemia, 490, 490*t*, 1672, 1672*t*
in multiple myeloma, 1607
in osteoporosis, 973–974
in prostate cancer, 1547
Pancolitis, 342, 343*f*
Pancreas
abscess of, 404
anatomy of, 403*f*
autolysis of, 403, 404
functions of, 403
necrosis of, 404–405, 406, 407*t*
pseudocyst of, 404, 405
Pancrease products, 311*t*, 409, 409*t*
Pancreas transplantation. *See also* Solid-organ
transplantation
acute rejection, signs and symptoms of, 944*t*
epidemiology and etiology of, 941–942
pancreas-kidney transplantation, 942
Pancreatic cancer
epidemiology of, 1446*f*
pancreas transplantation in, 942
Pancreatic enzyme(s), insufficiency in cystic
fibrosis, 304
Pancreatic enzyme replacement
in cystic fibrosis, 304–305, 311, 311*t*
in chronic pancreatitis, 409–410, 409*t*
dosage of, 304–305
enteric-coated products, 409, 410
nonenteric-coated products, 409
Pancreatic juice, 403
Pancreatitis, 403–410
acute, 404–407
APACHE II score in, 405
case study of, 407
clinical presentation of, 404–405
diagnosis of, 405
drug-related, 404*f*
epidemiology of, 405
etiology of, 404
gallstones and, 404
hypocalcemia in, 489
outcome evaluation in, 407
pathophysiology of, 404
treatment of, 405–407
algorithm for, 406*a*
analgesics, 406
antibiotics, 406–407
ineffective therapies, 407
nonpharmacologic, 408
alcohol use and, 405
case study of, 405
chronic, 407–410
alcohol abuse and, 408, 409
case study of, 409
clinical presentation in, 408
diagnosis of, 408
epidemiology of, 407
etiology of, 407
gallstones and, 407
outcome evaluation in, 410
pathophysiology of, 408
treatment of, 408–410
analgesics, 408
nonpharmacologic, 408
pancreatic enzymes, 408, 409–410, 409*t*
drug-related, 1437*t*, 1439*t*
hyperlipidemia and, 232, 235, 239, 240
nausea and vomiting with, 358*t*
parenteral nutrition in, 1682*t*, 1684
peritonitis in, 1283

Pancytopenia, in hematopoietic cell transplant
recipients, 1641
Panhypopituitarism, 803
adrenal insufficiency with, 786*t*
Panic disorder
adverse effects of, 1466
with agoraphobia, 692, 700
without agoraphobia, 692, 700
in cancer therapy, 1452*t*, 1466
clinical presentation in, 694
in colorectal cancer, 1526, 1527, 1528*t*, 1530–1531
course of illness, 692
diagnosis of, 694
epidemiology of, 692
etiology of, 692
outcome evaluation in, 702
pathophysiology of, 692–693, 693*f*
pharmacokinetics of, 1466
respiratory alkalosis in, 427*t*
treatment of, 699–702
algorithm for, 702*a*
antidepressants, 700, 701*t*
benzodiazepines, 704
Pannus, 982
Pantoprazole
adverse effects of, 299*t*
dosage of, 320*t*, 321–322, 335*t*, 336*t*
drug interactions of, 321–322
in GERD, 320*t*, 321–322
in *Helicobacter pylori* eradication, 335*t*
in peptic ulcer disease, 336*t*
Papain, 154*t*
Papaverine
dosage of, 887*t*
in erectile dysfunction, 887*t*, 891
Papilledema, in brain metastasis, 1665
Papules, 1223*t*
Para-aminosalicylic acid, hypothyroidism
with, 767
Paracentesis, in ascites, 396
Paracentral scotoma, 1036
Paragard T 380A, 851
Parainfluenza virus, in pharyngitis, 1214
Paraldehyde poisoning, 501*t*
Paraneoplastic syndrome, in lung cancer, 1503,
1513
Parasitic disease, 1293–1304. *See also specific
diseases*
gastrointestinal parasites, 1276
Parasitism, 1294
Parasomnia
clinical presentation in, 713
diagnosis of, 713
epidemiology and etiology of, 710–711
pathophysiology of, 712
patient care and monitoring in, 719
treatment of, 718
Parathyroid disease
hypertension and, 54
nausea and vomiting in, 358*t*
Parathyroidectomy
in hyperparathyroidism, 462
in renal osteodystrophy, 462
Parathyroid hormone, 459–465
intact, target levels in chronic kidney disease,
461, 462*t*, 465
recombinant human
cost of, 973*t*
in osteoporosis, 973*t*, 975
Parathyroid hormone-related protein, 1670
Parenchyma, lung, 290
Parenteral nutrition, 1681–1699, 1701
administration of, 1690–1694

amino acids for, 1682–1683, 1686, 1689–1690
ASPEN safe practice guidelines for, 1694
case study of, 1683, 1693, 1699
central, 1691, 1698
compared with enteral nutrition, 1682, 1704
complications of, 1694–1698, 1694*t*, 1704
acid–base disturbances, 501*t*, 426*t*, 1696
aluminum toxicity, 1697
bone disease, 967*t*, 1697
calcium-phosphate precipitation, 1686,
1691–1692
hypercapnia, 1696
hyperglycemia, 1694–1695
hyperlipidemia, 1695–1696
hypoglycemia, 1695
infectious, 1684, 1698, 1704
liver disease, 1697
manganese toxicity, 1696
mechanical, 1698
refeeding syndrome, 1697–1698
thrombophlebitis, 1687
compounded sterile preparations, 1692
cycling, 1693
dextrose for, 1683, 1690, 1695
discontinuation of, 1695
drugs added to, 1687, 1693
electrolytes for, 1685–1686, 1685*t*, 1690
ethical and personal beliefs, 1690
as fluid source, 1684–1685
formulations of admixtures, 1692
2-in-1, 1691–1692, 1692*t*
3-in-1, 1691–1692, 1692*t*
indications for, 1682, 1682*t*
initiation of, 1692–1693, 1699
lipid emulsion for, 1683–1684, 1684*t*, 1690,
1695
monitoring in, 1699, 1698*t*
osmolarity of admixtures, 1690
outcomes and goals in, 1682
in pancreatitis, 406
peripheral, 1690–1691
pH of, 1686
safety of, 1690
trace elements for, 1687
transition to oral or enteral nutrition, 1693–
1694
vitamins for, 1686–1687
with fosphenytoin, 547
Paricalcitol, in hyperphosphatemia, 463, 465*t*
Parkinson's disease, 553–565
autonomic problems in, 563
case study of, 554, 556, 564
clinical presentation in, 555–557
constipation in, 372*t*
diagnosis of, 555–557
dry eye in, 1075*t*
epidemiology of, 554
erectile dysfunction in, 885*t*
etiology of, 554
genetic factors in, 554
motor symptoms in, 555
nonmotor symptoms in, 555–556
outcome evaluation in, 564
palliative care treatment for, 39
pathophysiology of, 554–555, 554*f*
patient care and monitoring in, 564
response fluctuations in, 556–557, 563, 563*t*
sleep disorders in, 555, 562–563
treatment of, 557–564, 559*t*
amantadine, 557, 559*t*, 560
anticholinergics, 557, 559*t*, 560
COMT inhibitors, 559*t*, 561–562
diet therapy, 557

Parkinson's disease, treatment of (*Cont.*)
dopamine agonists, 557, 559*t*, 560–561
exercise program, 557
herbs and supplements, 562
levodopa, 561
levodopa/carbidopa, 557, 559*t*, 561
lifestyle modifications, 557
MAO inhibitors, 557, 558, 559*t*, 560
nonmotor symptoms, 562–564
response fluctuations, 563, 563*t*
surgery, 557
Paromomycin
in amebiasis, 1295
dosage of, 1294
in giardiasis, 1294
Paroxetine
adverse effects of, 660*t*, 696, 701*t*, 879*t*
in depression, 665
dosage of, 319*t*, 661*t*, 696*t*, 701*t*, 879*t*
drug interactions of, 646*t*, 661*t*, 699*t*, 1726
in generalized anxiety disorder, 696, 696*t*
in irritable bowel syndrome, 383, 384*t*
in panic disorder, 701*t*
pharmacokinetics of, 660*t*
in pregnancy, 665
in social anxiety disorder, 703
in vasomotor symptoms of menopause, 878, 879*t*
Paroxysmal depolarizing shift, 522–523
Paroxysmal nocturnal dyspnea, in heart
failure, 84
Paroxysmal nocturnal hemoglobinuria, 1131*t*,
1630*t*
Paroxysmal supraventricular tachycardia, 173–175
clinical presentation in, 174
diagnosis of, 174
epidemiology of, 173
etiology of, 173
outcome evaluation in, 175
pathophysiology of, 173–174
treatment of, 174–175
algorithm for, 175*a*
prevention of recurrence, 174
termination of PSVT, 174, 175*t*
Parsley, 206*t*
Pars reticulata, in alcohol abuse, 609
Parvovirus B19, in aplastic crisis, 1149
Passion flower, 206*t*, 878, 879*t*
Pasteurella multocida, in bite wound infections,
1232, 1232*t*
Patient-controlled analgesia (PCA), 575
in pain in sickle cell anemia/disease, 1150,
1151*t*
Patient education, of geriatric patients, 17–18
Patient interview, of geriatric patients, 15–17
Peak expiratory flow, in asthma, 267,
271–272, 277*t*, 282–283, 284*a*
monitoring of, 271
Peak flow meter, 271
Pediarix, 1413
Pediatric patient
acute lymphocytic leukemia in, 1580
acute myelogenous leukemia in, 1580
ADHD in, 723–732
age groups, 24*t*
age terminology, 24*t*
allergic rhinitis in, 1057–1059
antimicrobials in, 1164
asthma in, 276, 276*t*
bipolar disorder in, 685
common pediatric illnesses, 28
constipation in, 372
dehydration in, 1269*t*
depression in, 665

diarrhea in, 376, 377
drug therapy, specific considerations in, 28
accidental ingestion, in pediatric
patients, 31
administration and drug formulation, routes
of, 28–29
CAM and OTC medication use, 29–30
common errors in, 29
off-label medication use, 30
pediatric patients and caregiver education,
medication administration to, 30–31
enterobiasis in, 1297–1298
enuresis in, 919–925
epilepsy in, 537
fluid requirement of, 481*t*
fundamentals of
fluid requirements, 25
growth and development, 24, 25*f*
pediatric patients, classification of, 23–24
vital signs, differences in, 24
GERD in, 323
giardiasis in, 1294
gonorrhea in, 1319
growth hormone deficiency in, 809–811
hepatitis A vaccine in, 420, 419*t*
hepatitis B vaccine in, 420*t*, 421
HIV infection in, 1434–1435
hypertension in, 52*t*, 70, 72
hyperthyroidism in, 777
hypothyroidism in, 771
illnesses, 28
immune thrombocytopenic purpura in, 1133
inflammatory bowel disease in, 352–353
meningitis in, 1175*t*–1178*t*
migraine in, 592
obesity in, 1721, 1728
osteomyelitis in, 1342*t*–1343*t*
otitis media in, 1204
pain assessment in, 571–572
patient care and monitoring of, 32
pharmacokinetic and pharmacodynamic
differences, on drug therapy, 26
absorption, 26
elimination, 27–28
metabolism, 27
volume of distribution, 27
pharyngitis in, 1215*t*
pneumonia in, 1197
rhinosinusitis in, t
screening for high cholesterol, 235
status epilepticus in, 549, 549*t*
tuberculosis in, 1256, 1259, 1261*t*
venous thromboembolism in, 199, 200, 201
weight classification, 2*t*
Pediculosis, 1303
Pediculus humanus capitis, 1304
Pediculus humanus corporis, 1304
PEDIS scale, for diabetic foot infections, 1228,
1228*t*, 1229*t*
Pegaptanib, in macular degeneration, 1073
Pegasparagase, 1464
in acute lymphocytic leukemia, 1590*t*
dosage of, 1590*t*
Pegfilgrastim
adverse effects of, 1657*t*
dosage of, 1657*t*
prophylactic, in neutropenic cancer patients,
1657, 1657*t*
Pegvisomant
in acromegaly, 807*t*, 808
adverse effects of, 807*t*, 808
dosage of, 807*t*, 808
mechanism of action of, 808

Pelvic floor muscle rehabilitation, in urinary
incontinence, 914
Pelvic fracture, erectile dysfunction with, 885*t*
Pelvic inflammatory disease (PID), 1332–1333
clinical presentation in, 1332
diagnosis of, 1332
pathophysiology of, 1332
in pregnancy, 825
treatment of, 1288*t*, 1332, 1333*t*
Pemetrexed, 1457
adverse effects of, 1457, 1507*t*
in cancer therapy, 1457
dosage of, 1507*t*
in lung cancer, 1507*t*, 1510–1511
mechanism of action of, 1457
pharmacokinetics of, 1457
Pemirolast
adverse effects of, 1068*t*
in allergic conjunctivitis, 1068*t*
dosage of, 1068*t*
mechanism of action of, 1068*t*
Pemoline
dosage of, 440*t*
in fatigue, 440*t*
Penbutolol
in arrhythmias, 162*t*
dosage of, 124*t*
in hypertension, 66*a*
in ischemic heart disease, 124*t*
mechanism of action of, 162*t*
Penicillamine, teratogenic effects of, 824*t*
Penicillin, 26
adverse effects of, 1324*t*
allergic drug reactions, 929*t*, 930, 931, 931*t*,
1164, 1398
skin testing, 930, 931*t*
Clostridium difficile-associated diarrhea and,
1274
desensitization to, 1322
drug interactions of, 1592*t*
informational chart, 1324*t*
in intra-abdominal infections, 1286, 1287*t*,
1288, 1288*t*, 1289
mechanism of action of, 1324*t*
pharmacodynamics of, 1324*t*
prophylactic, in sickle cell anemia/disease,
1143–1144, 1143*t*
in sepsis, 1354
in syphilis, 1322–1324
in urinary tract infections, 1311*t*
Penicillin G
adverse effects of, 1175*t*, 1177*t*
dosage of, 831*t*, 832*t*, 1175*t*, 1176*t*, 1177*t*, 1215*t*,
1242–1243, 1244*t*, 1249*t*, 1322–1324, 1342*t*
drug interactions of, 1457
in infective endocarditis, 1246*t*, 1249*t*
in intra-abdominal infections, 1286, 1287*t*,
1288, 1288*t*, 1289*t*
in meningitis, 1175*t*, 1176*t*, 1177*t*, 1180
in necrotizing fasciitis, 1227
in osteomyelitis, 1342*t*
in pharyngitis, 1215*t*
in pneumonia, 1197
in pregnancy, 831*t*, 832*t*, 831*t*, 832*t*, 835, 836
in *Streptococcus* group B infection, 831*t*, 832*t*
in syphilis, 831*t*, 1322–1324
Penicillin resistance, 1193, 1194*t*, 1195, 1197,
1203, 1215
in CSF isolates, 1180
Penicillin V
dosage of, 1144, 1215*t*
in pharyngitis, 1215*t*
Penicillium, 1376*t*

Penile erection, 884f, 885. *See also* Erectile
dysfunction
Penile prostheses, 884f, 888, 888f
Penn State equations, 1688
Pentamidine
adverse effects of, 442, 956t
arrhythmia with, 179t
blood glucose level and, 737t
dosage of, 956t
drug interactions of, 647
pancreatitis with, 404f
in prevention of *Pneumocystis jiroveci*
pneumonia, 956t, 1643
Pentastarch, in hypovolemic shock, 258t, 259
Pentazocine, 45t
mechanism of action of, 575
metabolism of, 575
Pentobarbital
adverse effects of, 545t, 548
dosage of, 545t, 546t, 548, 549t
in status epilepticus, 545t, 546t, 548, 549t
Pentostatin
adverse effects of, 1457
in cancer therapy, 1456–1457
dosage of, 1456–1457
emetogenicity of, 365t
extravasation of, 1677t
mechanism of action of, 1454a
pharmacokinetics of, 1456
Pentoxifylline, in peripheral vascular disease, 758
Peppermint oil, in irritable bowel syndrome, 383
Pepsin, in peptic ulcer disease, 329–330
Pepsinogen, 330
Peptic ulcer disease, 327–338
case study of, 329, 330, 332, 333
clinical presentation in, 331–332
complications of, 331
with corticosteroids, 953t
cost of, 328
diagnosis of, 331–332
dietary factors in, 329
epidemiology of, 328–329
etiology of, 328–329
gastrointestinal bleeding with, 331
Helicobacter pylori and, 328, 328t, 330,
331–332, 337
nausea and vomiting with, 358t
NSAID-related, 327, 328t, 329, 329t, 330–331,
333, 574, 989
outcome evaluation in, 338
pathophysiology of, 329–331
patient care and monitoring in, 337
perforated ulcer, 1287t
prevention of NSAID-related ulcers, 330–331
COX-2 inhibitors, 336–337
misoprostol, 336
proton pump inhibitors, 336
sucralfate, 337
smoking and, 329
stress-related mucosal damage and, 335
treatment of
active duodenal and gastric ulcers, 336
algorithm for, 334a
eradication of *Helicobacter pylori,* 332, 333,
1561
H2-receptor antagonists, 336, 336t
maintenance of ulcer healing, 336t, 337
mucosal protectants, 336t
proton pump inhibitors, 336, 336t
refractory ulcers, 337
surgery, 333
Peptostreptococcus
in necrotizing fasciitis, 1226

normal flora, 1157f
in rhinosinusitis, 1210
Percussion, 307
Percutaneous coronary intervention
in acute coronary syndromes, 136–139
in ischemic heart disease, 117, 118
Percutaneous endoscopic gastrostomy tube, 1704,
1705f
Percutaneous endoscopic jejunostomy tube, 1704,
1705f, 1706
Percutaneous transluminal coronary angioplasty
in ischemic heart disease, 118
Perfluorocarbon emulsions, in hypovolemic
shock, 259
Performance status
of cancer patient, 1451, 1453t, 1655t
in colorectal cancer, 1525
in lung cancer, 1504, 1504t
Pergolide
adverse effects of, 717t
dosage of, 559t, 717t
drug interactions of, 816
mechanism of action of, 559t
in Parkinson's disease, 559t
Pericardial tamponade
heart failure and, 80t
shock in, 253t
Pericarditis
chest pain in, 111t
heart failure and, 34t
Perimenopause, 857t, 870–871
Perimetry, automated static threshold, 1036
Perindopril
adverse effects of, 62t
dosage of, 62t, 92t, 121t
in heart failure, 92t
for hypertension, 62t, 72
in ischemic heart disease, 121t
in prevention of stroke, 224, 225t
Periodic abstinence (sexual behavior), efficacy
of, 844t
Periodic limb movements of sleep
clinical presentation in, 712–713
diagnosis of, 713
pathophysiology of, 711
Peripheral artery disease, 230
Peripheral blood progenitor cells
harvesting of, 1631–1632
preparation and transplantation of, 1632
as source of hematopoietic cells, 1629–1632
Peripheral edema, 85t, 86
Peripheral neuropathy
in diabetes mellitus, 757–758
drug-related, 1442t
Peripheral resistance, in hypertension, 54, 55–56
Peripheral sensitization, 569
Peripheral vascular disease
in diabetes mellitus, 758
DIC with, 1131t
osteomyelitis and, 1338
treatment of, 758
Peritoneal carcinoma, 394
Peritoneal dialysis, 472–475
advantages and disadvantages of, 469t
complications of, 474t
catheter-related infections, 475
peritonitis, 474–475, 474t
peritoneal access in, 473
principles of, 472–473
types of, 473
Peritoneovenous shunt, 1131t
Peritonitis,1281–1291. *See also* Intraabdominal
infection

CAPD and, 1282
cirrhosis and, 1282, 1286t
definition of, 1281
nausea and vomiting with, 358t
outcome evaluation in, 475
pathophysiology of, 474
peritoneal dialysis-related, 473–475, 474t
prevention of, 475
primary, 1282, 1286t, 1287t, 1289
secondary, 1282, 1284, 1286t, 1287t, 1289
spontaneous bacterial. *See* Spontaneous
bacterial peritonitis
tertiary, 1283
treatment of, 474–475
parenteral nutrition, 1682t
tuberculosis, 1283
Peritonsillar abscess, 1214
Periwinkle, 1457
Permethrin
in lice infestation, 1304
in scabies, 1304
Pernicious anemia, 376, 1111, 1114a
Peroxisome proliferator-activated receptors,
246, 750
Perphenazine
adverse effects of, 642t
dosage of, 640t
drug interactions of, 646t
metabolism of, 646t, 647
in schizophrenia, 640t
Perseveration, in schizophrenia, 633
Personality disorders, 672, 694t
Pertussis vaccine, 1406–1407, 1408t
acellular, 1407, 1408t
Pervasive developmental disorder, 634t
Petechiae
with corticosteroids, 953t
in infective endocarditis, 1237, 1238, 1239f
PET scan
in colorectal cancer, 1522
in lung cancer, 1503
Peyronie's disease, 885t
p53 gene, 1447, 1447t
P-glycoprotein, 647, 953
Phaeohyphomycetes, 1376t
Phagocytic cells, 1348
Phagocytosis, antigen for, 942
Pharmacodynamic changes, in geriatrics, 11–13
absorption, 26
anticoagulants, 13
cardiovascular system, 12
central nervous system, 12
elimination, 27–28
fluid and electrolyte homeostatic
mechanism, 12
glucose metabolism, 12–13
metabolism, 27
volume of distribution, 27
Pharmacodynamics, 11–12, 1163
Pharmacogenomic factors, 1528
Pharmacogenomics, 97
Pharmacokinetic changes
in geriatrics therapy
absorption of, 10
distribution of, 10–11
elimination of, 11
metabolism of, 11
in pediatric drug therapy, 26
absorption, 26
elimination, 27–28
metabolism, 27
volume of distribution, 27
Pharmacokinetics, 1162–1163

Pharmacotherapy, in palliative care
advanced heart failure, 46
anxiety, 40
delirium, 41
dyspnea, 42–43
nausea and vomiting, 43–44
pain, 44–45
terminal secretions, 46
Pharyngeal cancer, 1446f
Pharyngitis, 1203, 1214–1216
case study of, 1216
clinical presentation in, 1214
diagnosis of, 1214
epidemiology of, 1214
etiology of, 1214
outcome evaluation in, 1216
pathophysiology of, 1214
patient care and monitoring in, 1216
in pediatric patients, 1215t
treatment of
algorithm for, 1215a
antibiotics, 1215–1216, 1215t
Pharyngostomy tube, 1705f
Phenelzine
adverse effects of, 701t
dosage of, 661t, 701t
drug interactions of, 614t
in panic disorder, 701t
in social anxiety disorder, 703
Pheniramine
adverse effects of, 1068t
in allergic conjunctivitis, 1068t
dosage of, 1068t
mechanism of action of, 1068t
Phenobarbital, 26
adverse effects of, 529t, 531, 545t, 547t
allergic drug reactions, 933
dosage of, 384t, 533t, 545t, 547, 546t, 547t,
549t, 550
drug interactions of, 205t, 537, 537t, 615t, 699t,
771t, 850t, 955t, 1381
in epilepsy, 529t, 533t
hypocalcemia with, 489
hypophosphatemia with, 491
in irritable bowel syndrome, 384t
in lactation, 824t
mechanism of action of, 533t
osteoporosis with, 967t
pharmacokinetics of, 533t
in status epilepticus, 547, 545t, 546t, 547t, 549t,
550
teratogenic effects of, 824t
Phenolphthalein
in constipation, 374t
dosage of, 374t
Phenothiazines. See also specific drugs
adverse effects of, 360, 362
constipation with, 372t
drug interactions of, 660t
erectile dysfunction with, 885t
extrapyramidal symptoms with, 360, 361
hyperprolactinemia with, 814t
in nausea and vomiting, 360, 361
ocular changes with, 1077t
voiding symptoms with, 900t
Phentermine
adverse effects of, 1727
dosage of, 1725t, 1727
drug interactions of, 1727
mechanism of action of, 1727
in obesity, 1725t, 1727
Phentolamine
adverse effects of, 71t

in allergic rhinitis, 1055
in common cold, 1218t
dosage of, 71t, 887t
in erectile dysfunction, 887t, 891
GERD with, 3217t
in hypertensive emergency, 71t
Phenylbutazone, drug interactions of, 205t
Phenylephrine
in allergic rhinitis, 1055
anxiety with, 694t
dosage of, 260t
drug interactions of, 660
in hypovolemic shock, 260t
in sepsis, 1356
voiding symptoms with, 900t
Phenylpropanolamine
arrhythmia with, 164t
drug interactions of, 660
in urinary incontinence, 917
for weight loss, 1728
Phenytoin, 10, 828t
administration through feeding tube, 1715
adverse effects of, 531, 533t, 536, 545t, 546, 547t
allergic drug reactions, 933, 959t
blood glucose level and, 737t
dosage of, 533t, 545t, 546, 546t, 547t, 549, 549t
drug interactions of, 205t, 321, 322, 537, 537t,
577, 614t–615t, 660t, 683, 699t, 771t, 850t,
955t, 1114, 1164, 1364, 1381, 1455, 1458,
1600, 1600t, 1726t
in epilepsy, 529t, 533t
erectile dysfunction with, 885t
hypocalcemia with, 489
hypophosphatemia with, 491
mechanism of action of, 522, 533t
metabolism of, 528
ocular changes with, 1077t
osteoporosis with, 967t
pharmacokinetics of, 533t
in prevention of busulfan seizures, 1635
protein binding of, 528
in seizures, 1666
in status epilepticus, 545t, 546, 546t, 547t, 549,
549t
teratogenic effects of, 824t
in torsades de pointes, 181
Pheochromocytoma, 1447t, 784, 792t
anxiety with, 694t
hypertension and, 54
Philadelphia chromosome, 1584, 1598
Phocomelia, 1464
Phonophobia, with migraine, 587
Phosphate binders
calcium-based, 463
in hyperphosphatemia, 462–463, 462t, 491
Phosphate therapy hypocalcemia with, 489
Phosphodiesterase type 5 inhibitors
cardiovascular risk assessment for, 890t
comparison of inhibitors, 889t
drug interactions of, 121
in erectile dysfunction, 884f, 887t, 888–890
in heart failure, 103
Phospholipids, 230
in intravenous lipid emulsions, 1683, 1684t,
1691
Phosphorus
bone, 490
in extracellular fluid, 480t
in intracellular fluid, 480t, 490
for parenteral nutrition, 1685t, 1686, 1697
calcium-phosphate precipitation, 1686, 1692
serum, 489
normal range for, 480t

target levels in chronic kidney disease, 462,
462t, 466
Phosphorus balance, 490–491
Phosphorus restriction, in hyperphosphatemia, 462
Photochemotherapy in psoriasis, 1082, 1085
Photodynamic therapy
in macular degeneration, 1073
in skin cancer, 1625
Photophobia
in inflammatory bowel disease, 344
in migraine, 587
in stroke, 217
Phototherapy, in psoriasis, 1082, 1085
Physical activity. See Exercise program
Physical therapy
in osteoarthritis, 1000–1002
for pain management, 573
Phytoestrogens, in vasomotor symptoms of
menopause, 878
Phytostanol analogues, 247
PID. See Pelvic inflammatory disease
Pilocarpine
adverse effects of, 1042
dosage of, 1038t, 1077t
in dry eye, 1076, 1077t
in glaucoma, 1038t, 1042
mechanism of action of, 1038t
Pilocarpine iontophoresis, 305
Piloerection, in opioid withdrawal, 619
Pilosebaceous unit, 1094
Pimecrolimus, in psoriasis, 1084
Pimozide
arrhythmia with, 179t
dosage of, 640t
drug interactions of, 647
in schizophrenia, 640t
Pindolol
in arrhythmias, 162t
augmentation of antidepressant therapy
with, 662
dosage of, 122t
in hypertension, 66
in ischemic heart disease, 122t
mechanism of action of, 162t
Pink-eye. See Conjunctivitis, viral
Pinworm infection, 1297
Pioglitazone
adverse effects of, 750, 859t, 860t
in anovulatory bleeding, 865
in diabetes mellitus, 749t, 750
dosage of, 749t, 859t
in menstruation-related disorders, 859t
Piperacillin
in infective endocarditis, 1248
in urinary tract infections, 1311t
Piperacillin-tazobactam
in cellulitis, 1225t
in COPD, 299t
in cystic fibrosis, 309t
in diabetic foot infections, 1229t
dosage of, 309t, 1199t, 1225t, 1229t, 1342–
1343t, 1660t
in infections in cancer patients, 1660t
in intra-abdominal infections, 1287t
in osteomyelitis, 1339t, 1342–1343t, 1342t
in pancreatitis, 407t
in pneumonia, 1196t, 1197, 1199t
in sepsis, 1353t, 1354
in spontaneous bacterial peritonitis, 397
in urinary tract infections, 1311t
Piracetam, in epilepsy, 529t
Pirbuterol
in asthma, 277t

in COPD, 294, 295t
dosage of, 295
Piroxicam
dosage of, 1014t
drug interactions of, 205t
in gout, 1014t
Pituitary adenoma, 792
ACTH-secreting, 793
growth hormone-secreting, 803, 804
macroadenoma, 803, 804, 803
microadenoma, 804
prolactin-secreting (prolactinoma), 814–815,
814t, 857
TSH-secreting, 774t
Pituitary gland
anterior, 802
disorders of, 801–819
hypothyroidism in, 767t
hypothalamic-pituitary-target-organ axis,
802f, 803
physiology of, 801–803
posterior, 802
Pituitary gonadotropin hypothesis, of ovarian
cancer, 1567,1568
Placental abruption, 1131t
Plan B, 853
Plaques, in Alzheimer's disease, 597
Plasma
osmolality of, 482
volume of, 253, 253f
Plasma cells, 1604
Plasma exchange, in thrombotic
thrombocytopenic purpura, 1135
Plasmapheresis, in Waldenström's
macroglobulinemia, 1608
Plasma protein fraction in hypovolemic shock,
258t, 259
Plasmin, 188, 1121
Plasminogen, 1121
Plasminogen activator inhibitor-1, 187t, 188
Plasmodium falciparum, 1299, 1301–1302
Plasmodium malariae, 1299, 1300
Plasmodium ovale, 1299, 1300, 1303
Plasmodium vivax, 1299, 1300
Platelet aggregation, 188, 217
Platelet count, 1135
Platelet disorders, 1132–1137
Platelet transfusion
in DIC, 1132
in hematopoietic cell transplant recipients, 1641
in hypovolemic shock, 259
in immune thrombocytopenic purpura, 1134t
in thrombocytopenia, 1595
Platinum compounds, 1462. See also specific drugs
allergic drug reactions, 933
in ovarian cancer, 1569, 1570, 1572t, 1573
Pleocytosis, 1326
Pleural effusion, respiratory acidosis with, 503t
Pleuritis, in rheumatoid arthritis, 984
Pleurovenous shunt, 1131t
Plication, 321
Pneumatic otoscopy, 1205
Pneumococcal polysaccharide vaccine, 297
Pneumococcal vaccine, 89, 271, 395, 747, 1170,
1201, 1208, 1408t, 1411–1412, 1414, 1416
in sickle cell anemia/disease, 1143, 1143t
7-valent, 1181, 1406, 1408t
23-valent, 1181, 1412
Pneumoconiosis, 426t
Pneumocystis jiroveci pneumonia, 1376t, 1388
in hematopoietic cell transplant recipients, 1643
prevention of, 956, 956t, 1595, 1643
in transplant recipient, 956, 956t

Pneumonia, 1189–1201
anxiety with, 694t
aspiration, 1190t, 1191, 1192–1193, 1197
bacterial, 1190, 1190t
case study of, 1191, 1194, 1195, 1196, 1197
clinical presentation in, 1192–1193
community-acquired, 1190, 1192–1196, 1200
adult inpatient in ICU, 1196–1197, 1196t
adult inpatient not in ICU, 1195–1196, 1196t
adult outpatient with comorbid conditions,
1195, 1196t
adult outpatient previously healthy, 1195,
1196t
pediatric inpatient, 1196t, 1197
pediatric outpatient, 1196t, 1197
sepsis and, 1353t, 1354
diagnosis of, 1192
drug-resistant, 1193–1194
endemic mycosis, 1376
epidemiology of, 1190
etiology of, 1190, 1190t
health care-associated, 1191–1192, 1194,
1197–1200, 1199t
sepsis and, 1353t, 1354
hospital-acquired, 1197–1200, 1199t
sepsis and, 1353t, 1354
in intra-abdominal infections, 1290
outcome evaluation in, 1200
pathophysiology of, 1190–1192
patient care and monitoring in, 1200
pneumococcal, 1411–1412
prevention of, 1200–1201
respiratory acidosis with, 426t
treatment of, 1193–1200
antimicrobials, 1193–1198
duration of therapy, 1199–1200
ventilator-associated, 1197–1200, 1199t
sepsis and, 1353t, 1354
viral, 1190, 1197
Pneumonitis, respiratory acidosis with, 426t
Pneumothorax
with central venous catheter, 1691
chest pain in, 111t
respiratory acidosis in, 426t
respiratory alkalosis in, 504t
Podofilox
adverse effects of, 1327t, 1328
in genital warts, 1328
Podophyllin resin
adverse effects of, 1327t, 1328
in genital warts, 1328
Poison ivy, 1100, 1101t
Poison oak, 1101t
Poison sumac, 1101t
Poliomyelitis, 1412
Poliovirus vaccine, 1408t, 1412
Pollen allergy, 1051t, 1049–1050
Polycarbophil
in constipation, 309t, 829, 830t
in diarrhea, 373, 374t
dosage of, 374t, 379t, 829, 830t
in pregnancy, 829, 830t
Polycitra, in metabolic acidosis, 466
Polycystic kidney disease, kidney transplantation
in, 941
Polycystic ovarian syndrome, 814t
diabetes mellitus and, 737, 865
menstruation-related disorders in, 855, 857t
treatment of, 858, 859t, 865
Polycythemia, in COPD, 291
Polycythemia rubra vera, 1131t
Polycythemia vera, 187, 187t
Polydipsia, in diabetes mellitus, 740

Polyethylene glycol, in distal intestinal
obstruction syndrome, 312
Polyethylene glycol-electrolyte preparations
adverse effects of, 373, 374, 375
in constipation, 373
dosage of, 309t
Polymerase chain reaction, 1173
in acute lymphocytic leukemia, 1585
Polymeric formula, for enteral feeding,
1707, 1708t, 1714
Polymorphisms, genetic, 1536
Polymyositis, respiratory acidosis with, 426t
Polymyxin B
in conjunctivitis, 1066, 1066t
dosage of, 1066t
Polyneuropathy, 568, 569
Polyp. See specific sites
Polyphagia, in diabetes mellitus, 740
Polypharmacy, definition of, 13
Polysaccharide-iron complex
iron content of, 1115t
in iron-deficiency anemia, 1115t
Polysomnography, 712–713
Polyuria
in diabetes mellitus, 740
in heart failure, 85
Poplar, 154t
Pork tapeworm, 1294, 1298
Porphyromonas, in bite wound infections, 1232t
Portal hypertension, 387–400
complications of, 392
diagnosis of, 394
pathophysiology of, 388–392
treatment of, 394–400
β-blockers, 395–396
Portal venous system, 388f
Posaconazole
in aspergillosis, 1386t, 1391, 1642
dosage of, 1386t
in fusariosis, 1386t
in prevention of invasive candidiasis, 1387
in zygomycosis, 1386t
Positive expiratory pressure, oscillating, in cystic
fibrosis, 307
Postconceptional age (PCA), 822
Postgastrectomy state, osteoporosis in, 975
Post-herpetic neuralgia, 568, 570, 578t, 1413
Post-ictal state, 676t
Postoperative nausea and vomiting, 358,
365–366
prevention of, 365
risk factors for, 365
Postoperative radiotherapy in lung cancer,
1505–1506
Postpyloric feeding, 1706, 1712
Post-thrombotic syndrome, 186, 189, 190,
195, 207
Post-transplant lymphoproliferative
disorder, 960
Epstein-Barr virus and, 960
treatment of, 960
Post-traumatic stress disorder, 635t
Postural drainage, 307
Postvagotomy syndrome, 358t
Post-void residual urine volume, in benign
prostatic hyperplasia, 898, 900t
Potassium
in extracellular fluid, 484t
in intracellular fluid, 484, 484t
for parenteral nutrition, 1685–1686, 1685t
serum, 487
normal range for, 484t
in ventricular action potential, 159, 159f

Potassium acetate
  in hypokalemia, 487
  potassium content in, 487t
Potassium balance, 487–489
  impaired, in chronic kidney disease, 454–455
Potassium bicarbonate
  in hypokalemia, 487
  potassium content in, 487t
Potassium chloride
  GERD with, 317t
  in hypokalemia, 487
  in intra-abdominal infections, 1285
  potassium content in, 487t
Potassium citrate, potassium content in, 487t
Potassium gluconate
  in hypokalemia, 487
  potassium content in, 487t
Potassium iodide, in hyperthyroidism, 775
Potassium phosphate, in hypophosphatemia, 488t
Potassium requirement, 487
Potassium restriction, in hyperkalemia, 454
Potassium-sparing diuretics. *See also specific drugs*
  adverse effects of, 65, 454
  hyperkalemia with, 488
  in hypertension, 60t, 65
Potassium therapy
  in hypokalemia, 488, 488t
  oral products, 487t, 488t
Poverty of speech, in schizophrenia, 631
Pramipexole
  adverse effects of, 560, 717t
  augmentation of antidepressant therapy
      with, 662
  dosage of, 559t, 560, 717t
  mechanism of action of, 559t
  in Parkinson's disease, 559t, 560, 563
  in restless-legs syndrome, 717, 717t
Pramlintide
  adverse effects of, 755
  in diabetes mellitus, 754t, 755
  dosage of, 754t
  drug interactions of, 755
Pravastatin
  adverse effects of, 242t
  dosage of, 242t
  in hyperlipidemia, 186t, 187t
  in ischemic heart disease, 120
Prazepam, drug interactions of, 614t
Praziquantel
  dosage of, 1298
  in tapeworm infections, 1298
Prazosin
  adverse effects of, 63t
  dosage of, 63t
  drug interactions of, 660t
  in hypertension, 63t, 69
  in muscle cramps, 472
  in urinary incontinence, 918
Prealbumin, in nutritional assessment, 1713
Prebiotics, 1707
Prediabetes, 736, 740, 746
Prednisolone
  in adrenal insufficiency, 789t
  dosage of, 347t
  in inflammatory bowel disease, 347t
  in viral conjunctivitis, 1067
Prednisone
  in acute lymphocytic leukemia, 1590t, 1591t
  in adrenal insufficiency, 789t
  adverse effects of, 945t, 1561t
  anxiety with, 694t
  in asthma, 270t, 274t, 277
  in breast cancer, 1482

dosage of, 347t, 349t, 351t, 510, 513t, 945t, 952,
    1014, 1014t, 1134, 1134t, 1557t, 1560t,
    1561t, 1590t, 1591t
drug interactions of, 850t, 955t, 1590t
in gout, 1014, 1014t
in Graves' ophthalmopathy, 777
in GVHD, 1640
in headache, 592
in Hodgkin's lymphoma, 1557, 1557t, 1561t
hypokalemia with, 487
in immune thrombocytopenic purpura, 1134,
    1134t
in inflammatory bowel disease, 347t, 349t, 350,
    351, 351t, 354
in multiple myeloma, 1606
in multiple sclerosis, 508
in non-Hodgkin's lymphoma, 1561t,
    osteoporosis with, 977
in prevention of contrast media reaction, 933
in prostate cancer, 1547
in rheumatoid arthritis, 989
in transplant recipient, 945t, 952
Preeclampsia, 592, 1131t
Pregabalin
  adverse effects of, 534t
  dosage of, 534t, 703
  in epilepsy, 530, 534t
  in generalized anxiety disorder, 698
  mechanism of action of, 534t
  in pain, 578t
  pharmacokinetics of, 534t
  in social anxiety disorder, 703
Pregnancy, 821–838. *See also* Contraception
  allergic rhinitis in, 1059
  allergy in, 835
  anemia in, 827
  anomalies, 821–822, 822tcauses, 822
  antimicrobials in, 1165
  asthma in, 283
  bacterial mastitis, 837
  bacterial vaginosis in, 825, 831t, 833–834
  bacteriuria in, 825, 833, 833t
  bipolar disorder in, 686–687
  Candidiasis, 837–838
  case study of, 827, 834, 837
  Chlamydia in, 1320
  clinical presentation in, 825–826
  common cold in, 833
  confirmation of, 825
  constipation in, 372, 374, 829, 830t
  and cough, 833
  dating of, 822, 825
  depression in, 665
  diabetes mellitus in. *See* Diabetes mellitus,
      gestational
  diagnosis, 825
  drug use during, 821–822
    distribution, 828
    drug absorption, 827–828
    metabolism.828
    renal elimination, 828
    sources of information, 826t
  ectopic, 851, 861
  embryology, 822–823, 822t, 823f
  epidemiology, 821–822
  epilepsy in, 537–538, 537t
  etiology, 821–822
  fatty liver of, 1131t
  FDA pregnancy categories, 827t
  folic acid, 827
  genital herpes in, 825, 831t, 834, 1329–1330
  genital warts in, 1328
  gonorrhea in, 1319

Graves' disease in, 777
group B *Streptococcus* infection, 836
headaches in, 592–593
and heartburn, 829, 833
heart failure in, 84t, 97
hemorrhoids in, 829
HIV infection in, 1434–1435
hyperprolactinemia in, 816–817
hypertension in, 60t, 62t, 70, 72, 72t, 826
hypothyroidism in, 771, 772t
inflammatory bowel disease in, 353–354
and nasal congestion, 833
nausea and vomiting in, 358t, 358, 366–367,
    829, 830t
NSAIDs in, 1004
pathophysiology, 822–823
patient care and monitoring, 837
PID in, 825
preterm labor, 835
  antenatal corticosteroids, 835
  antibiotics, 836
  tocolytic therapy, 835–836
respiratory alkalosis in, 504t
respiratory disease in, 835rheumatoid arthritis
    in, 990
rhinitis in, 833
risk evaluation, 823–829
schizophrenia in, 646
sexually transmitted infections
  Chlamydia, 834
  gonorrheal, 834
  herpes simplex, 834–835
  syphilis, 835
  trichomoniasis, 835
status epilepticus in, 550STDs in,
    834–835*Streptococcus* group B in, 825,
    826, 832t, 836, 1182
thyroid disorders, 836
trichomoniasis in, 826, 831t, 835
tuberculosis in, 1256, 1259, 1261t
unintended, 842
urinary tract infections in, 1313
vaccination in, 1416
vulvovaginal candidiasis in, 825, 831t, 834, 1365
Prehypertension, 52, 52t
Preload, 81
  in heart failure, 81, 81t
  in ischemic heart disease, 121
  in shock, 252, 253
Premature atrial contractions, 160
Premature ovarian failure, menstruation-related
    disorders in, 857t, 864
Premature ventricular contractions. *See*
    Ventricular premature depolarizations
Prescription drugs, 3
  cost of, 4
Presenilins, 596
Pressure sore
  epidemiology of, 1230
  infected, 1230
    clinical presentation in, 1230, 1231t
    complications of, 1230
    diagnosis of, 1230
    etiology of, 1230
    treatment of, 1230, 1231t
  prevention of, 1230
  staging of, 1230, 1231t
Preterm labor, 835
  antenatal corticosteroids, 835
  antibiotics, 836
  tocolytic therapy, 835–836
Prevotella
  in bacterial vaginosis, 1331

in bite wound infections, 1231t
in pneumonia, 1190
Priapism, 888
  with alprostadil, 890
  with phosphodiesterase inhibitors, 889
  in sickle cell anemia/disease, 1143t, 1144–1146
  stuttering, 1145
  treatment of, 1145–1146
Primaquine
  dosage of, 1031t
  in prevention of malaria, 1301t
Primary biliary cirrhosis, 392
  liver transplantation in, 942
Primidone
  drug interactions of, 205t, 850t
  in lactation, 824t
PR interval, 159f, 160, 164
Probenecid
  adverse effects of, 1015
  in antihyperuricemic treatment, 1014t, 1015
  dosage of, 1014t
  drug interactions of, 699t, 1457, 1592t
  mechanism of action of, 1015
Probiotics
  in diarrhea, 379–380
  in inflammatory bowel disease, 349
Procainamide
  adverse effects of, 169t
  in arrhythmias, 162t, 177t, 179t
  in atrial fibrillation, 170t, 171a, 171t
  diarrhea with, 377
  dosage of, 170t, 177t
  drug interactions of, 170t
  mechanism of action of, 162t
  in ventricular tachycardia, 177, 177t, 178t
Procaine penicillin G
  dosage of, 1323–1325
  informational chart, 1324t
  in syphilis, 1323–1325
Procalcitonin, in sepsis, 1350
Procarbazine, 1463
  dosage of, 1557t
  in Hodgkin's lymphoma, 1557t
Prochlorperazine
  adverse effects of, 361t
  in chemotherapy-induced nausea and
    vomiting, 1652
  dosage of, 361t
  in nausea and vomiting, 360, 361t, 363, 577t,
    1557
Prochlorpromazine, adverse effects of, 554
Proctitis, in ulcerative colitis, 342, 343f, 349, 349t
Proctosigmoidoscopy, in inflammatory bowel
    disease, 344
Prodrome, 1277
Progenitor cells, 1597
Progesterone
  in amenorrhea, 858, 861
  drug interactions of, 955t
  erectile dysfunction with, 881t
  GERD with, 259t
  in lactation, 823f
  in menorrhagia, 865
  in menstrual cycle, 856, 856f, 864
  micronized, 875t
  respiratory alkalosis with, 504t
Progesterone receptor, in breast cancer, 1486
Progestin(s)
  adverse effects of, 875, 876t
  in breast cancer, 1487t
  hyperlipidemia with, 236t
  hyperprolactinemia with, 814t
  in menopause, 875–876, 875t

oral, 875t
transdermal, 875t
Progestin-only oral contraceptives, 849
Progestogen therapy, in prostate cancer, 1539, 1539t
Progressive systemic sclerosis, respiratory
    acidosis with, 426t
Proguanil. *See* Atovaquone-proguanil
Prohapten, 928
Prokinetic agents, in GERD, 322, 323
Prolactin, 813–819
  in lactation, 823f
  secretion of, 814
  serum, 814
Prolactinoma, 814t, 815, 857t
Prolapse, 913
Pro-MACE regimen, in non-Hodgkin's
    lymphoma, 1559, 1561t
Promethazine
  drug interactions of, 170t
  in migraine, 591
  in nausea and vomiting, 360, 361t, 365
Propafenone
  adverse effects of, 169t
  arrhythmia with, 162t, 164t, 177t, 179t
  in arrhythmias, 162t
  in atrial fibrillation, 170t, 171a, 171t, 170t
  dosage of, 170t
  drug interactions of, 170t, 205t, 660t, 955t
  mechanism of action of, 162t
Propantheline
  dosage of, 384t
  in irritable bowel syndrome, 384t
  in urinary dysfunction, 563
Propionibacteria, in postneurosurgical
    infections, 1146
Propionobacterium acnes, 1094
Propofol
  adverse effects of, 545t, 548
  arrhythmia with, 114t
  dosage of, 545t, 546t, 548, 549t
  hypertriglyceridemia with, 1694
  metabolic acidosis with, 501t
  in status epilepticus, 545t, 546t, 548, 549t
Proportion method, of antimicrobial susceptibility
    testing, 1257
Propoxyphene, 45t
  adverse effects of, 577, 717t
  dosage of, 575t, 717t
  drug interactions of, 205t, 537t
  metabolism of, 577
  in osteoarthritis, 1006
  in pain, 575t, 577
  in restless-legs syndrome, 717, 717t
Propranolol, 10
  in acute coronary syndromes, 142t
  adverse effects of, 61t, 86t, 169t
  in akathisia, 647
  in arrhythmias, 162
  depression with, 656
  dosage of, 61t, 124t, 142t
  drug interactions of, 590, 660t, 699t
  in hypertension, 61t, 66a
  in hyperthyroidism, 775
  in ischemic heart disease, 122, 123t
  mechanism of action of, 162t
  in portal hypertension, 395–396
  in prevention of migraine, 590, 590t
  in social anxiety disorder, 701–702
Proptosis
  in Graves' disease, 774, 775f
  sudden congestive, 1069t
Propylthiouracil
  adverse effects of, 778

agranulocytosis with, 778
dosage of, 778, 832t
in hyperthyroidism, 775–777
mechanism of action of, 775
teratogenic effects of, 824t
in thyroid storm, 777
ProQuad, 1414
Prostaglandin(s), 329, 1021
  biosynthesis of, 1003a
  in hemorrhagic cystitis, 1670
  inhibition of gastric secretion by, 329
  synthesis of, 329, 330f
Prostaglandin analogs, in glaucoma, 1038t, 1040
Prostaglandin E2, 1021
Prostate cancer, 1535–1538
  adenocarcinoma, 1538
  benign prostatic hyperplasia and, 1536
  case study of, 1538, 1543–1544
  classification systems for, 1540t, 1541t
  clinical presentation in, 1540
  diagnosis of, 1540, 1540t
  diet and, 1536t, 1536
  epidemiology of, 1446f, 1536–1538
  ethnicity and, 1536, 1536t
  etiology of, 1536–1538
  genetic factors in, 1536–1537, 1536t
  grading of, 1538
  hormone-refractory, 1548, 1548t
  GnRH antagonists in, 1544–1545
  LHRH agonists in, 1539, 1539t, 1542–1543, 1544t
  metastatic, 1538–1539
    to bone, 1663
  outcome evaluation in, 1548
  pathophysiology of, 1539–1540, 1539f
  patient care and monitoring in, 1548
  prevention of, 1536
    5α-reductase inhibitors, 905
  prognosis for, 1540
  risk factors for, 1546t
  screening for, 1536–1540
  smoking and, 1537
  staging of, 1540, 1541t
  treatment of, 1541–1546, 1542t
    5-α-reductase inhibitors, 1539t, 1540
    androgen synthesis inhibitors, 1539t, 1540
    antiandrogens, 1539t, 1540, 1542–1545,
      1544t
    bisphosphonates, 1545
    chemotherapy, 1545–1546, 1546t
    corticosteroids, 1545
    cyproterone acetate, 1539, 1539t, 1544
    estrogen therapy, 1539, 1545
    expectant management, 1546, 1543
    hormonal manipulations, 1539, 1539t,
      1544–1545
    palliative therapy, 1545
    progestogens, 1539, 1539t
    radiation therapy, 1542–15433, 1545–1546
    second-line therapy, 1545–1546
    surgery, 1539t, 1542–1545
Prostatectomy
  in benign prostatic hyperplasia, 897, 900
  erectile dysfunction with, 881t
Prostate gland, 896–897
  anatomy of, 1538f
  benign hyperplasia. *See* Benign prostatic
    hyperplasia
  hormonal regulation of, 1539, 1539f
  needle biopsy of, 900t
  stromal tissue of, 897
Prostate-specific antigen, 1546
  in benign prostatic hyperplasia, 898, 900t,
    905–906

Prostate-specific antigen (*Cont.*)
elevated, 1538
in prostate cancer, 1537–1538
Prosthetic implants, osteomyelitis and, 1340
Prosthetic valve endocarditis, 1236, 1241–1242, 1245, 1246*t*, 1247*t*
Protamine sulfate, to reverse effects of heparin, 198, 199
Protease, pancreatic enzyme supplements, 409
Protease inhibitors. *See also specific drugs*
adverse effects of, 1437*t*–1440*t*
drug interactions of, 241, 816, 850*t*, 1426
in HIV infection, 1421*f*, 1422, 1426–1434, 1426*t*, 1429*t*–1432*t*
hyperlipidemia with, 181*t*
hyperprolactinemia with, 814*t*
in pancreatitis, 407
Protectants, in diaper dermatitis, 1106
Protected specimen brush, 1198
Protective clothing, 1612
Protein
in CSF, 1172*t*
in enteral feeding formulas, 1708, 1710
in extracellular fluid, 484*t*
in intracellular fluid, 484*t*
metabolism of, growth hormone effects on, 803*t*
requirement for, determination of, 1689, 1689*t*
Proteinase, in lung, 290
Protein C deficiency, 187, 187*t*, 188
Protein:creatinine ratio, urine, 449
Protein-losing enteropathy, intestine transplantation in, 941
Protein restriction, in chronic kidney disease, 450
Protein S deficiency, 187, 187*t*, 188
Proteinuria
in chronic kidney disease, 447, 449, 450–451
definition of, 449
reduction
of ACE inhibitors, 450
angiotensin receptor blockers, 450
calcium channel blockers, 451
in sepsis, 1349
Proteoglycan, 998
Proteolysis, 330, 1021
Proteosome inhibitors, in multiple myeloma, 1606
Proteus
in COPD exacerbations, 299*t*
in infective endocarditis, 1242
in surgical site infections, 1397*t*
in urinary tract infections, 1308, 1310
Prothrombin, 187
deficiency of, 1129–1130, 1129*t*
Prothrombin complex concentrate
in hemophilia B, 1124, 1124*t*
in recessively inherited coagulation disorders, 1129*t*, 1130
in vitamin K-deficiency bleeding, 1137
Prothrombin time, 199, 202, 203*a*, 204, 207, 1136
Prothrombin 20210A mutation, 187*t*, 188
Prothrombotic state, 234*f*, 238
Proton pump inhibitors. *See also specific drugs*
diagnosis of GERD, 318, 321–322
dosage of, 335*t*
drug interactions of, 322
in *Helicobacter pylori* eradication, 336, 336*t*
in pancreatitis, 409
in peptic ulcer disease, 336, 336*t*
in prevention of NSAID-related ulcers, 336, 990, 1004, 1024
in Zollinger-Ellison syndrome, 328
Protooncogenes, 1447

Protriptyline
in cataplexy, 717
dosage of, 661*t*
drug interactions of, 614*t*
Prourokinase, in stroke, 222
Providencia, in infective endocarditis, 1242
Pruritus
in chronic kidney disease, 467–468
in impetigo, 1222
pathophysiology of, 467
treatment of
activated charcoal, 468
antihistamines, 468
cholestyramine, 468
emollients, 467–468
nonpharmacologic, 467
Pseudoaddiction, 576
Pseudoallergic drug reactions
contrast media and, 930
epidemiology of, 928
opioids and, 933
outcome evaluation in, 935
pathophysiology of, 928
patient care and monitoring in, 936
Pseudoallescheria boydii, 1376*t*
Pseudocholelithiasis, 1175*t*
Pseudocyst, of pancreas, 404, 405
Pseudoephedrine
adverse effects of, 917, 918*t*, 1055
in allergic rhinitis, 1055, 1057
anxiety with, 694*t*
in common cold, 1218*t*
dosage of, 830*t*, 918*t*, 1055
drug interactions of, 659
pharmacokinetics of, 918*t*
in pregnancy, 830*t*, 917
in prevention of priapism, 1146
in respiratory disorders, 830*t*, 917
in urinary incontinence, 917, 918*t*
voiding symptoms with, 901*t*
Pseudohyphae, 1363
Pseudomembranous colitis, 1097
Pseudomonas
in cellulitis, 1224, 1225*t*
in folliculitis, 1223*t*
in infective endocarditis, 1242, 1245
in intra-abdominal infections, 1283, 1286*t*
in keratitis, 1070
normal flora, 1157*f*
in peritonitis, 474
in pneumonia, 1195
in sepsis, 1353
Pseudomonas aeruginosa
in catheter-related infections, 474
in COPD exacerbations, 298, 299*t*
in cystic fibrosis, 304, 306*t*, 309, 310
in diabetic foot infections, 1228
in infections in cancer patients, 1655*t*
in meningitis, 1171*t*, 1176*t*, 1146
in osteomyelitis, 1339*t*, 1342*t*
in otitis media, 1204
in pneumonia, 1190, 1197
in postneurosurgical infections, 1146
in sepsis, 1348*t*
in surgical site infections, 1397*t*
in urinary tract infections, 1308
Pseudoparkinsonism, with antipsychotics, 641
Pseudophakic patient, 1040
Pseudopolyp, of colon, 342
Pseudoseizure, 526
Psoriasis, 1079–1090
case study of, 1081, 1085, 1087
clinical presentation in, 1081

depression and, 1080
environmental factors in, 1080
epidemiology of, 1080
erythrodermic, 1081
etiology of, 1080
exacerbation (flare-up) of, 1080
drug-related, 1080
prevention of, 1082
exfoliative, 1087
generalized pustular, 1082
genetic factors in, 1080
guttate, 1081
inverse, 1081
outcome evaluation in, 1089
pathophysiology of, 1081
patient care and monitoring in, 1089
plaque, 1081
pustular, 1081
remission of, 1080
treatment of, 1082–1089
acitretin, 1086
algorithm for, 1083*a*
anthralin, 1084
azathioprine, 1085, 1087
BRM, 1086
coal tar products, 1084
corticosteroids, 1084, 1085
cyclosporine, 1085
efficacy assessment, 1083
hydroxyurea, 1086
immunomodulators, 1084, 1086
keratolytic agents, 1085
methotrexate, 1085
moisturizers, 1083
mycophenolate mofetil, 1086
natural health products, 1089
nonpharmacologic, 1083
oatmeal baths, 1083
photochemotherapy, 1082, 1085
phototherapy, 1083, 1085
rotational therapy, 1084
stress reduction, 1083
sulfasalazine, 1085
systemic therapy, 1086
tazarotene, 1085
topical therapy, 1085
vitamin D analogs, 1085, 1086
Psychiatric disorders
erectile dysfunction with, 881*t*
in hypothyroidism, 786
with interferon therapy, 624
irritable bowel syndrome and, 381
Psychodynamic therapy, in substance dependence, 624
Psychoeducation
in generalized anxiety disorder, 694
in panic disorder, 701
Psychogenic vomiting, 358*t*
Psychomotor retardation, in stimulant withdrawal, 619
Psychosis. *See also* Schizophrenia
in Alzheimer's disease, 603
with corticosteroids, 953*t*
disorders with psychotic symptoms, 635*t*
Psychosocial interventions, in schizophrenia, 635
Psychotherapy
in amenorrhea, 857
in depression, 656
in enuresis, 920
in erectile dysfunction, 888
in generalized anxiety disorder, 694
in irritable bowel syndrome, 383
in nausea and vomiting, 360

in pain, 573
in psoriasis, 1083
Psyllium
in constipation, 373, 374t, 829, 830t
in diarrhea, 379
dosage of, 374t, 384t, 830t
in irritable bowel syndrome, 384, 384t
in pregnancy, 829, 830t
PTH (1–84), 976
Pubic louse, 1304
Pulmonary abscess, 1237
Pulmonary angiogram
in pulmonary embolism, 192
in venous thromboembolism, 189
Pulmonary artery catheter, 255
in heart failure, 99
monitoring in hypovolemic shock, 256a, 257
Pulmonary capillary wedge pressure, in heart
failure, 98, 99
Pulmonary congestion, in heart failure, 85, 86,
93, 100
Pulmonary edema
in heart failure, 85t, 86
respiratory acidosis in, 426t
respiratory alkalosis in, 504t
Pulmonary embolism, 185. See also Venous
thromboembolism
arrhythmia in, 166t
case study of, 207
clinical presentation in, 192
diagnosis of, 192
DIC with, 1131t
heart failure and, 84t
microvascular, 1686, 1692
outcome evaluation in, 207–209
patient care and monitoring in, 210–211
prevention of, 192, 192t
respiratory alkalosis in, 504t
shock in, 253t
treatment of, 194–207
approach to, 207, 208a
Pulmonary fibrosis
lung transplantation in, 942
respiratory acidosis with, 426t
Pulmonary hypertension
in COPD, 291
diethylpropion and, 1727
lung transplantation in, 942
Pulmonary infarction, 1131t
Pulmonary rehabilitation, in COPD, 293
Pulmonary vein, 159, 160
automaticity of, 166
Pulseless ventricular tachycardia, treatment of,
179a
Pulsus paradoxus, in asthma, 268
Punctal occlusion, in dry eye, 1075
Puncture headache, 592
Pupillary block, 1035
Purified protein derivative, 1256, 1256t
Purine(s), in cancer therapy, 1456–1457
Purine antimetabolites, 1456–1457
Purkinje fibers, 158f, 159, 160
Purple glove syndrome, 546
Purple toe syndrome, warfarin-induced, 205
Purulent materials, 1224
Pustular exanthema, allergic drug reaction, 929t
PUVA therapy
adverse effects of, 1085
bath PUVA, 1085
oral, 1085
in psoriasis, 1085
RePUVA, 1085
P wave, 159, 159f, 164, 166

Pyelonephritis, 435, 1308, 1309f
acute, 1310–1313, 1312t
Pyknolepsy, 525t
Pyloric obstruction, 358t
Pyloric sphincter, 1702, 1706
Pyoderma gangrenosum, in inflammatory bowel
disease, 344
Pyrantel pamoate
in ascariasis, 1293
dosage of, 1303
in enterobiasis, 1303
Pyrazinamide
adverse effects of, 1261t
dosage of, 1260t, 1261t
gout with, 1011
in tuberculosis, 1259–1260, 1260t, 1261t, 1261
Pyridinoline, 969
Pyridoxine
dosage, 830t
in nausea and vomiting, 366, 829
in pregnancy, 829
Pyrimidine dimer, 1612
Pyrimidine-pyrimidone(6–4) photoproducts,
1612, 1613
Pyuria, in urinary tract infections, 1309

Q
QRS complex, 159f, 159–160
QT interval, 159–160, 159f
Quadrigeminy, 176
Quality of life, of cancer patient, 1446
Quassia, 206t
Quazepam
dosage of, 716t
in insomnia, 716t
pharmacokinetics of, 716t
Quetiapine
adverse effects of, 638, 638t, 684
in Alzheimer's disease, 603
in bipolar disorder, 677t, 684
dosage of, 637t, 638, 677t
drug interactions of, 646t, 955t
mechanism of action of, 638
metabolism of, 646t, 647
in Parkinson's disease, 562
in schizophrenia, 635, 637t, 638, 644t
Quinacrine
dosage of, 1295
in giardiasis, 1295
Quinapril
dosage of, 92t, 121t
in heart failure, 92t
in ischemic heart disease, 121t
Quinidine
allergic drug reactions, 929t
in arrhythmias, 162t, 179
diarrhea with, 376t
drug interactions of, 169t, 205t, 17, 647, 660t,
955t
GERD with, 259t
in malaria, 1300–1301
mechanism of action, 162t
Quinine
dosage of, 1300–1301
in malaria, 1300–1301
Quinolones
drug interactions of, 321
teratogenic effects of, 743
Quinupristin
in infective endocarditis, 1249t
dosage of, 1249t
Quinupristin-dalfopristin
dosage of, 1231t

in diabetic foot infections, 1229t
in infected pressure sores, 1231t
in infective endocarditis, 1245
Q waves, 132

R
Rabeprazole
dosage of, 320t, 321–322, 336t
drug interactions of, 321, 322
in GERD, 320t, 321–322
in peptic ulcer disease, 336t
Rabies, prophylaxis in bite wounds, 1232
Radiation therapy, 1449
in acromegaly, 808
acute leukemia and, 1580t
in acute lymphocytic leukemia, 1589
adverse effects of, 1505, 1533
in brain metastasis, 1662, 1665
in breast cancer, 1480
in colorectal cancer, 1523, 1531
in Hodgkin's lymphoma, 1533, 1562
in hyperprolactinemia, 816
in lung cancer, 1503, 1506–1508
mediastinal, 1477
in melanoma with brain metastasis, 1662
nausea and vomiting with, 358t
in non-Hodgkin's lymphoma, 1554
pelvic, hemorrhagic cystitis with, 1666, 1666t
in preparation for hematopoietic cell
transplant, 1634t, 1634–1635, 1644
in prostate cancer, 1542–1543, 1545–1546
brachytherapy, 1543
external-beam radiation, 1543
reproductive/fertility effects of, 1269
secondary malignancies from, 1269, 1533,
1594
in skin cancer, 1625–1626
in spinal cord compression, 1663–1664
in superior vena cava syndrome, 1662
Radioactive drugs, in lactation, 824t
Radioactive iodine uptake test, 766
Radiocontrast agents. See Contrast medium
Radiofrequency catheter ablation, in
paroxysmal
supraventricular tachycardia, 174
Radioimmunotherapy, 1465
Radon exposure, 1500
Raloxifene
adverse effects of, 974–975
dosage of, 973t
in osteoporosis, 973t, 975
in prevention of breast cancer, 974–975, 1478,
1479
ral rehydration solution, 378
Raltegravir
adverse effects of, 1432t
dosage of, 1432t
drug interactions of, 1432t
food interactions of, 1432t
in HIV infection, 1432t
Ramelteon
dosage of, 716t
in insomnia, 716t
in Parkinson's disease, 563
pharmacokinetics of, 716t
Ramipril
in acute coronary syndromes, 142t
adverse effects of, 62t
dosage of, 62t, 92t, 142t
in heart failure, 92t
in hypertension, 62t
in ischemic heart disease, 120
Ranibizumab in macular degeneration, 1074

Ranitidine
  in anaphylaxis, 931*t*
  dosage of, 320*t*, 336*t*, 830*t*, 931*t*
  drug interactions of, 170*t*, 699*t*
  in GERD, 320*t*, 321, 323, 829, 830*t*
  in parenteral nutrition admixture, 1688
  in peptic ulcer disease, 336*t*
  in pregnancy, 829, 830*t*
  in prevention of NSAID-related ulcers, 336*t*
Ranitidine bismuth citrate, in *Helicobacter pylori*
    eradication, 335*t*
Ranolazine
  adverse effects of, 125
    contraindications and precautions with, 125*t*
  in angina, 122
  in ischemic heart disease, 236
Raphe nuclei, in anxiety disorders, 693
Rapid ACTH stimulation test, 788*t*
Rasburicase
  cost of, 1676*t*
  dosage of, 1676, 1676*t*
  mechanism of action of, 1674*a*
  in tumor lysis syndrome, 1017, 1594, 1676,
    1676*t*
Raynaud's syndrome, DIC with, 1131*t*
rCHOP regimen, in non-Hodgkin's lymphoma,
    1560*t*, 1561*t*
rCVP regimen, in non-Hodgkin's lymphoma,
    1560*t*
Reactive oxygen species, 1612
Rebound headache, 588
Recessively inherited coagulation disorders
  clinical presentation in, 1130
  diagnosis of, 1130
  epidemiology of, 1129, 1129*t*
  etiology of, 1129, 1129*t*
  pathophysiology of, 1129
  treatment of
    pharmacologic, 1130
    transfusional therapies, 1129*t*, 1130
RECIST (Response Evaluation Criteria in Solid
    Tumors), 1448, 1448*t*, 1562
Recombivax, 420, 420*t*
Rectal cancer, 1531. *See also* Colorectal cancer
  neoadjuvant therapy in, 1531
Rectal prolapse, in cystic fibrosis, 305
Rectum, anatomy of, 1521*f*
Red blood cell distribution width, 1113*t*
Red blood cell indices, 1112, 1113*t*
Red blood cell substitutes, 259
Red blood cell transfusion
  in anemia, 1114–1115
  in hematopoietic cell transplant recipients, 1641
Red clover, 154*t*
Red eye, 1070
Reduced-intensity myeloablative transplant, 1635
Reed-Sternberg cells, 1552–1553
Reentry, 160–161, 161*f*
Refeeding syndrome
  with enteral nutrition, 1713
  with parenteral nutrition, 1697–1698
  prevention of, 1697–1698
Reflex sympathetic dystrophy, 570
Refractory period, cardiac, 160–161, 161*f*
Regurgitation, 358
Relaxation techniques
  in headache prevention, 586
  in irritable bowel syndrome, 383
  in psoriasis, 1082
  in sleep disorders, 714*t*
  in tension-type headaches, 589
REM behavior disorder, 701, 713, 718
Reminfemin, 879*t*

REM sleep, 701
Renal angiogram, in acute renal failure, 435
Renal artery stenosis, 62*t*, 68, 92, 433, 442
Renal cell carcinoma, 1447*t*
  kidney transplantation in, 941
Renal disease. *See also* Kidney disease
  dosing adjustments for chemotherapy, 1507*t*
  drug-related, 1438*t*
  end-stage. *See* End-stage renal disease
  heart failure and, 83, 101*t*
  hyperlipidemia and, 236*t*
  hypertension and, 52, 55, 66, 68
  nausea and vomiting in, 358*t*
Renal failure
  acute, 431–443
    assessment of renal function, 433, 434*t*
    case study of, 436, 440
    clinical presentation in, 435
    diagnosis of, 435
    drug-induced, 432, 440–442
    epidemiology of, 432
    glomerular filtration rate in, 431, 432
    heart failure and, 432, 442
    intrinsic (intrarenal), 433
    nonoliguric, 433
    outcome evaluation in, 442
    pathophysiology of, 432–433
    patient care and monitoring in, 443
    postrenal, 433, 435
    prerenal, 432–433, 435
    prevention of, 440–442
    sepsis and, 1350
    serum creatinine in, 431
    treatment of, 433–439
      algorithm for, 438*a*
      dopamine, 437–439
      fenoldopam, 439
      loop diuretics, 437
      renal replacement therapy, 439
      supportive therapy, 439
    with ACE inhibitors, 68
  chronic. *See also* Kidney disease, chronic
  hyperlipidemia and, 236*t*
  end-stage. *See* End-stage renal disease
  erectile dysfunction with, 881*t*
  hyperkalemia in, 488
  hypocalcemia in, 489
  metabolic acidosis with, 501, 501*t*
  in pancreatitis, 404–405
  protein requirement in, 1689*t*
  with spontaneous bacterial peritonitis, 399
  status epilepticus in, 543
  treatment of
    enteral nutrition, 1703*t*, 1710, 1710*t*
    parenteral nutrition, 1684
  tuberculosis and, 1112–1114
  urinalysis in, 435
  urine output in, 431
Renal osteodystrophy, 459–465
  clinical presentation in, 462
  epidemiology of, 459–460
  etiology of, 459–460
  hyperphosphatemia in, 462–464
  outcome evaluation in, 465
  pathophysiology of, 460–461, 461*a*
  treatment of, 461–465
    calcimimetics, 465
    nonpharmacologic, 462
    phosphate-binding agents, 462–463, 464*t*
    vitamin D, 463, 464, 465*t*
Renal replacement therapy, 468–475
  in acute renal failure, 439
  case study of, 469

  in end-stage renal disease, 468–475
Renal tubular acidosis, 486, 501*t*, 502
Renin-angiotensin-aldosterone system, 784
  in ascites, 390
  in cirrhosis, 390
  in heart failure, 82–83
  in hypertension, 55, 56*a*, 55
  in hypovolemic shock, 253
Renin-angiotensin antagonists, in prevention of
    migraine, 590
Renovascular disease, kidney transplantation
    in, 941
Renovascular hypertension, 54
Repaglinide
  in diabetes mellitus, 747*t*
  dosage of, 747*t*
Repetitive strain injury, 1020, 1027
Repetitive trauma, 1028
Replication capacity, of HIV, 1426
Repositioning, in prevention of pressure sores,
    1231
Reproductive disorders, in cystic fibrosis, 305
Reserpine
  adverse effects of, 63*t*, 69
  dosage of, 63*t*
  erectile dysfunction with, 881*t*
  hyperprolactinemia with, 814*t*
  in hypertension, 63*t*, 69
  migraines with, 588*t*
Resistant hypertension, 54, 54*t*, 65, 69
Resorcinol
  in acne vulgaris, 1097
  adverse effects of, 1097
Respiratory acidosis, 496, 497*t*, 503–504
  case study of, 499, 500
  clinical presentation in, 503
  definition of, 503
  drug-related, 503*t*
  etiology of, 503*t*
  with parenteral nutrition, 1696
  treatment of, 503–504
Respiratory alkalosis, 496, 497*t*, 504
  case study of, 499, 500
  clinical presentation in, 504
  compensatory changes in, 504*t*
  definition of, 504
  drug-related, 504*t*
  etiology of, 504, 504*t*
  hypophosphatemia and, 504
  treatment of, 504
Respiratory depression
  with opioids, 577*t*, 576
  treatment of, 577*t*
Respiratory disease
  aspirin-exacerbated, 930
  DIC with, 1131*t*
  in lactation, 917
  in pregnancy, 830*t*, 917
Respiratory disturbance index, 701
Respiratory failure, hypophosphatemia and,
    491, 492
Respiratory syncytial virus
  in otitis media, 1204
  in rhinosinusitis, 1207
Respiratory tract
  infections of
    lower respiratory tract, 1189–1201
    upper respiratory tract, 1203–1219
  normal flora of, 1157*f*
Respiratory tract procedures, endocarditis
    prophylaxis in, 1249–1250, 1250*t*
Response Evaluation Criteria in Solid Tumors
    (RECIST), 1448, 1448*t*, 1562

Restless-legs syndrome, 562–563
  case study of, 718
  clinical presentation in, 703
  diagnosis of, 703
  epidemiology and etiology of, 701
  pathophysiology of, 701
  patient care and monitoring in, 719
  treatment of, 717, 717t
Restricted affect, in schizophrenia, 631
Resuscitation fluids, 257–258, 258t
  oxygen-carrying, 481
Retained fetus syndrome, 1131t
Retching, 358
Reteplase
  in acute coronary syndromes, 135, 141t, 144
  dosage of, 93t
  in hemodialysis-associated thrombosis, 472
  in venous thromboembolism, 195
Reticular activating system, in anxiety disorders,
      692–693
Reticulocyte(s), 1110
Reticulocyte count, 1113t
Reticulocytosis, 1114a
Reticuloendothelial system, 1703
Retinal detachment, 1069t
Retinoblastoma, 1447t
Retinoic acid syndrome, 1464
Retinoids
  in acne vulgaris, 1097, 1097t
  adverse effects of, 1097, 1097t
  mechanism of action of, 1097
  in prevention of breast cancer, 1478
  in prevention of ovarian cancer, 1567
  systemic, dry eye with, 1074t
Retinopathy
  diabetic, 757
  nonproliferative, 757
  proliferative, 757
Retrograde ejaculation, with α-adrenergic
      antagonists, 901t, 902
Retrograde pyelography, in acute renal failure,
      435
Retroperitoneal fibrosis, with methysergide, 591
Retropharyngeal abscess, 1217
Reverse cholesterol transport, 178a
Reverse isolation rooms, 1641
Reverse transcriptase, 1421
Reversible inhibitors of monoamine oxidase
  in panic disorder, 901
  in social anxiety disorder, 703
Reward pathway, activation by addictive drugs,
      608–610, 609f
Reye's syndrome, 30, 591, 1024
Rhabdomyolysis
  in cocaine intoxication, 612t
  with statins, 241
Rheumatic fever, 1215
Rheumatic heart disease, 166t
Rheumatoid arthritis, 981–994
  anemia in, 1185
  B cells in, 983
  cardiovascular disease and, 983
  case study of, 983, 993
  clinical presentation in, 983
  comorbidities associated with, 983
  comparison of rheumatoid arthritis and
      osteoarthritis, 984f, 984t
  cytokines in, 982–983, 982t
  diagnosis of, 983
  dry eye in, 1074t
  epidemiology of, 982
  etiology of, 982
  genetic factors in, 982

infections and, 982
  joints involved in, 984f
  malignancy and, 983
  osteoporosis and, 983
  outcome evaluation in, 993
  pathophysiology of, 982
  patient care and monitoring in, 994
  in pregnancy, 993
  smoking and, 982
  T cells in, 986
  treatment of, 983–984
    adalimumab, 986t, 988
    anakinra, 986t, 988
    BRM, 986t, 990
    combination therapy, 985
    costimulation blockers, 992–993
    DMARD, 985, 986t, 991
    etanercept, 986t, 991
    glucocorticoids, 990–991
    hydroxychloroquine, 986t, 991
    infliximab, 986t, 991
    investigational agents, 991
    leflunomide, 986t, 991
    methotrexate, 986t, 991
    nonpharmacologic, 983
    NSAID, 985
    rituximab, 986t, 990
    stepdown approach, 985
    sulfasalazine, 986t, 990
Rheumatoid factors, 982
Rhinitis, 1061
  allergic. See Allergic rhinitis
  with α-adrenergic antagonists, 901t, 902, 906t
  in asthma, 267, 285
  in pregnancy, 826, 1057
  vasomotor, 1057
Rhinitis medicamentosa, 1055
Rhinorrhea
  allergic drug reaction, 930
  in cluster headache, 586
  in opioid withdrawal, 619
Rhinosinusitis, 1201, 1207–1209
  bacterial, 1207–1209
  clinical presentation in, 1208
  diagnosis of, 1208
  epidemiology of, 1207–1208
  etiology of, 1207–1208
  outcome evaluation in, 1208–1209
  pathophysiology of, 1208
  patient care and monitoring in, 1209
  in pediatric patients, 1212t
  risk factors for, 1208t
  treatment of, 1208–1209
    adjunctive therapy, 1209
    algorithm for, 1212a, 1213a
    antibiotics, 1208–1209, 1212t
    corticosteroids, 1209
    decongestants, 1209
    nonpharmacologic, 1209
Rhinovirus
  in otitis media, 1204
  in pharyngitis, 1216
  in pneumonia, 1190
  in rhinosinusitis, 1207
Rhizomucor, 1376t
Rhizopus, 1376t
Rhonchi, 291
Rhythm method, 852
Ribavirin
  adverse effects of, 424–425
  in chronic hepatitis C, 424–425
  dosage of, 424–425
Ribonuclease H, 1421

RICE therapy, in musculoskeletal disorders,
      1022–1024, 1023t
Richter's transformation, 1555
Rifabutin
  adverse effects of, 1261t
  dosage of, 335t, 1261t
  drug interactions of, 850t, 955t, 1378
  in Helicobacter pylori eradication, 335, 335t
  ocular changes with, 1077t
  in tuberculosis, 1259, 1261t
Rifampicin, drug interactions of, 1466
Rifampin
  adverse effects of, 1176t, 1261t
  in catheter-related infections, 475
  dosage of, 1176t, 1246t, 1249t, 1260t, 1261t
  drug interactions of, 205t, 537t, 699, 699t, 771t,
      850t, 955t, 1165, 1364, 1378, 1466, 1467
  in infective endocarditis, 1241, 1245, 1246t, 249t
  in meningitis, 1176t
  in osteomyelitis, 1344
  in peritonitis, 474
  in postneurosurgical infections, 1146
  in prevention of Hib meningitis, 1181
  in prevention of meningococcal disease, 1181
  in rhinosinusitis, 1213a
  in tuberculosis, 1258–1260, 1259t, 1260t,
      1261t, 1261
Rifapentine
  adverse effects of, 1261t
  dosage of, 1261t
  in tuberculosis, 1261t
Rifaximin
  dosage of, 1269t
  in prevention of travelers' diarrhea, 1274
  in shigellosis, 1268, 1269t
  in travelers' diarrhea, 1273
Rigidity, in Parkinson's disease, 555
Rimantadine, in pneumonia, 1197
Rimonabant
  adverse effects of, 1726–1727
  dosage of, 1726–1727
  drug interactions of, 1726–1727
  mechanism of action of, 1726–1727
  in obesity, 1726–1727
  in smoking cessation, 622
Ringer's injection, 482t
Risedronate
  dosage of, 973t
  in osteoporosis, 973–974, 973t
Risk-adjusted therapy, 1642
Risperidone
  adverse effects of, 637–638, 638t, 684
  in Alzheimer's disease, 603
  in bipolar disorder, 677t, 684
  dosage of, 603, 637t, 642, 677t
  drug interactions of, 646t, 560t
  enuresis with, 920
  erectile dysfunction with, 881t
  mechanism of action of, 636, 637f
  metabolism of, 646t, 647
  in schizophrenia, 636, 637f, 637t, 642, 644t
Ritanserin
  adverse effects of, 796t
  in Cushing's syndrome, 796t
  dosage of, 796t
  mechanism of action of, 796t
Ritonavir. See also Lopinavir/ritonavir
  adverse effects of, 442, 1426, 1432t, 1439t–1440t
  dosage of, 1432t
  drug interactions of, 816, 850t, 955t, 1426, 1432t
  food interactions of, 1432t
  in HIV infection, 1426, 1432t, 1426
  mechanism of action of, 1421f

Rituximab, 953
  adverse effects of, 986t, 991, 1559, 1563, 1606, 1603t
  in chronic lymphocytic leukemia, 1605–1606, 1606t
  dosage of, 986t, 1559, 1560t, 1561t, 1606, 1606t
  in immune thrombocytopenic purpura, 1134
  mechanism of action of, 991, 1559, 1605
  monitoring treatment with, 986t
  in non-Hodgkin's lymphoma, 1559–1560, 1560t, 1561t, 1563
  in rheumatoid arthritis, 986t, 991
Rivastigmine, 600
  adverse effects of, 598, 601t
  in Alzheimer's disease, 599, 601t
  dosage of, 520, 601t
  mechanism of action of, 520
Rizatriptan
  dosage of, 589t
  drug interactions of, 589t, 590
  in migraine, 589t
Rofecoxib, 1004
  adverse effects of, 126
  in prevention of NSAID-related ulcers, 337
  withdrawal from market, 575
Rome II criteria, diagnosis of irritable bowel syndrome, 382
Romiplostim in immune thrombocytopenic purpura, 1134–1135
  dosage of, 1135
Ropinirole
  adverse effects of, 717t
  dosage of, 559t, 560, 717t
  mechanism of action of, 559t
  in Parkinson's disease, 559t, 560–561
  in restless-legs syndrome, 717t, 717
Rosacea, dry eye in, 1074t
Rosiglitazone
  adverse effects of, 86t, 750
  in anovulatory bleeding, 865
  in diabetes mellitus, 748t, 750
  dosage of, 748t
Rosuvastatin
  adverse effects of, 242t
  dosage of, 242t
  in hyperlipidemia, 242t
Rotavirus
  in CNS infections, 1183
  in diarrhea, 376
  in gastroenteritis, 1278
Rotavirus vaccine, 1279, 1408t, 1412, 1414t
Roth spots, 1238, 1239f
Rotigotine, in Parkinson's disease, 560
Roundworms, 1293
RU 486. See Mifepristone
Rubefacients
  in musculoskeletal disorders, 1026–1027, 1026t
  in osteoarthritis, 1006
Rubella, 1410–1411
Rubella vaccine, 1408t, 1411, 1414t
Rue, 206t
"Rule of six," 29, 240

S

Sacroiliitis, in inflammatory bowel disease, 344
S-adenosylmethionine, in pain, 579
Sage, 878, 879t
St. George's Respiratory Questionnaire, 300
St. John's wort
  adverse effects of, 376t, 652
  anxiety with, 694t
  in depression, 652

drug interactions of, 611t, 850t, 955t, 1426, 1467, 1469, 1600t
Salicylate(s)
  adverse effects of, 86t
  blood glucose level and, 737t
  drug interactions of, 1457, 1592t
  in pain, 574
  respiratory alkalosis with, 504t
Salicylate poisoning, 501t, 502, 1097
Salicylic acid
  in acne vulgaris, 1097
  adverse effects of, 1097
  in psoriasis, 1085
Saline in allergic rhinitis, 1056
Saline flush, of hemodialysis catheter, 472
Saline laxatives, 374
Salivary gland cancer, 1447t
Salmeterol
  in asthma, 273, 274t, 275t
  in COPD, 293t, 294
  dosage of, 295t
Salmonella
  chronic carriers of, 1268–1269
  in diarrhea, 376, 380
  in infective endocarditis, 1242
  nontyphoidal, 1268–1269, 1269t
  in osteomyelitis, 1145
  in travelers' diarrhea, 1273
Salmonella paratyphi, 1269
Salmonella typhi, 1269
Salmonellosis, 1269
  clinical presentation in, 1269
  diagnosis of, 1269
  epidemiology of, 1269
  HIV infection and, 1269
  monitoring patient with, 1268–1269
  pathogenesis of, 1269
  treatment of, 1268–1269, 1269t
Salpingitis, peritonitis in, 1260
Salpingo-oophorectomy
  in ovarian cancer, 1569, 1569f
  in prevention of ovarian cancer, 1567
Salsalate
  dosage of, 1002t
  in osteoarthritis, 1002t
Salt. See Sodium entries
Salt substitutes, 488
Saquinavir
  adverse effects of, 1432t, 1439t–1440t
  dosage of, 1432t
  drug interactions of, 850t, 955t, 1432t
  food interactions of, 1432t
  in HIV infection, 1426, 1432t
  mechanism of action of, 1421f
Sarcoidosis
  adrenal insufficiency in, 786t
  arrhythmia with, 163t, 164t
  dry eye in, 1074t
  heart failure in, 80t
  kidney transplantation in, 941
  psychotic symptoms in, 635t
Sarcoma, 1447t, 1449
Sarcoptes scabiei hominis, 1304
Sargramostim
  adverse effects of, 1469, 1657t
  dosage of, 1657t
  in mobilization of peripheral blood progenitor cells, 1632, 1636
  in neutropenia, 1469, 1509
  prophylactic, in neutropenic cancer patients, 1656, 1657t
Saxagliptin, in diabetes mellitus, 750
Scabies, 1304

Scalp, psoriasis of, 1084
Scars, in acne vulgaris, 1096
Scedosporium, in infections in cancer patients, 1655t
Schilling test, 1114a
Schizoaffective disorder, 634t
  treatment of, 647
Schizophrenia, 631–649
  in adolescents, 642–643
  case study of, 632, 635, 639
  childhood-onset, 643
  clinical presentation in, 633–634
  cognitive impairment in, 631, 632
  course and prognosis in, 633–634
  diagnosis of, 632–633, 634t, 672
  early-onset, 642–643
  in elderly, 643–644
  epidemiology of, 632
  erectile dysfunction with, 881t
  etiology of, 632
  gender and, 632
  genetic factors in, 632
  late-life, 631
  negative symptoms in, 631–630
  outcome evaluation in, 647–648
  pathophysiology of, 632–633
  patient care and monitoring in, 649, 646t
  patient education in, 647
  in pregnancy, 646
  psychiatric emergencies in, 646
  substance-abuse disorders and, 634, 634t, 645
  treatment of, 634
    adjunct pharmacologic treatments, 647
    antipsychotics, 636, 637f, 637t
    aripiprazole, 638–639, 644t
    clozapine, 644t, 644, 647–648, 648t
    decanoates, 640, 641t
    electroconvulsive therapy, 646
    first-generation antipsychotics, 641–642, 641t, 642t
    guidelines and algorithm for, 642, 643a
    olanzapine, 638, 644t, 646
    patient-specific antipsychotic selection, 643, 644t
    psychosocial interventions, 636
    quetiapine, 638, 644t
    risperidone, 636, 642, 644t
    second-generation antipsychotics, 636–637, 637t, 643a
    treatment adherence, 642
    treatment-resistant patients, 645–646
    ziprasidone, 638, 644t, 646
  very early-onset, 642
Schwannoma, 1447t
Schwartz equation, 27
Scleritis, in rheumatoid arthritis, 983
Scleroderma
  arrhythmia with, 163t, 164t
  dry eye in, 1074t
Sclerotherapy, in variceal bleeding, 395
Scoliosis, with growth hormone therapy, 811
Scopolamine
  adverse effects of, 360, 361t
  dosage of, 361t
  in motion sickness, 367
  in nausea and vomiting, 360
Scotoma, in glaucoma, 1036
Seasonale, 849
Seasonique, 849
Sebaceous gland, 1094
Sebum, 1094
Secnidazole, in trichomoniasis, 1326
Secobarbital, drug interactions of, 205t

Secondary malignancy, 1269
Secondary transmission, 1411, 1414
Sedation
    with opioids, 577t, 576
    in respiratory alkalosis, 504
    in sepsis, 1357
Sedative(s), respiratory acidosis with, 426t
Sedative-hypnotic drugs, 45t
    urinary incontinence with, 921t
Seizure. See also Epilepsy; Status epilepticus
    absence, 525, 529–530, 529t
    in alcohol withdrawal, 611, 618
    anxiety with, 694t
    atonic, 525
    with brain metastasis, 1665
    bupropion-related, 729
    busulfan-related, 1635
    classification and presentation of, 524–525,
        524a, 252t
    clozapine-induced, 644
    complex partial, 525
    drug-induced, 522, 658
    etiology of, 522
    metabolic acidosis with, 501t
    myoclonic, 525, 529–530, 529t
    partial, 525, 524a, 529t
    pathophysiology of, 522–524
    primary generalized, 524–525, 524a, 525t,
        525, 529t
    psychotic symptoms with, 635t
    secondarily generalized, 252
    semiology of, 524
    simple partial, 525
    tonic, 529t
    tonic-clonic, 524, 525t, 529t
    treatment of, benzodiazepines, 618
Selective estrogen receptor downregulators, in
    breast cancer, 1486
Selective estrogen receptor modulators (SERMs).
        See also specific drugs
    adverse effects of, 977
    in breast cancer, 1486, 1486
    cost of, 973t
    in osteoporosis, 973t, 974
    venous thromboembolism with, 187, 187t
Selective serotonin reuptake inhibitors (SSRIs).
        See also specific drugs
    adverse effects of, 658, 658t, 859t
    anxiety with, 694t
    "behavioral activation" with, 665
    in depression, 665
    dosage of, 661t, 859t
    drug interactions of, 560, 660, 661t
    in elderly, 665
    erectile dysfunction with, 881t
    in generalized anxiety disorder, 696, 696t
    hyperprolactinemia with, 814t
    in irritable bowel syndrome, 383, 384t
    mechanism of action of, 653, 653t
    in pain, 578
    in panic disorder, 701, 701t
    in pediatric patients, 665
    in premenstrual dysphoric disorder, 859t
    in schizophrenia, 647
    in social anxiety disorder, 703
    in vasomotor symptoms of menopause, 878, 879t
    venlafaxine, 704
Selegiline
    adverse effects of, 560, 563, 665
    in Alzheimer's disease, 603
    in depression, 665
    dosage of, 559t, 665
    drug interactions of, 850t
    in insomnia, 717
    mechanism of action of, 559t
    in Parkinson's disease, 559t, 560
    in sleep disorders, 561
    transdermal patch, 665
Selenium
    for parenteral nutrition, 1686
    in prevention of colorectal cancer, 1520
    in prevention of lung cancer, 1503
    in prevention of prostate cancer, 1537
Selenium sulfide shampoo, in tinea infections, 1371
Self-injection, patient education in, 514t
Self-medication, 4
Selzentry in HIV infection, 1433
Semiology, of seizure, 524
Senescence, cellular, 1446
Senile plaques, 597
Senna, dosage, 830t
Senna
    in constipation, 374, 374t, 577t, 829, 830t
    dosage of, 309t, 830t
    in pregnancy, 829, 830t
Sensitization, in substance dependence, 610
Sentinel lymph node biopsy, 1480
    in melanoma, 1616
    in nonmelanoma skin cancer, 1671
Sepsis, 1347–1355
    in acute pancreatitis, 404
    acute renal failure and, 1350
    ARDS and, 1350
    with bowel obstruction, 1683
    case study of, 1350, 1351, 1352, 1357
    catheter-related infections and, 1353t
    clinical presentation in, 1350
    definitions related to, 1348t
    diagnosis of, 1349
    DIC and, 1350
    epidemiology of, 1348
    etiology of, 1348, 1349t
    fungal, 1348
    hemodynamic compromise in, 1348
    inflammatory mediators in, 1348
    intraabdominal infections and, 1353t, 1354
    laboratory tests in, 1349–1350
    pathophysiology of, 1348
    patient care and monitoring in, 1354
    physical examination in, 1349
    pneumonia and, 1353t, 1355
    prognosis for, 1357–1358
    risk factors for, 1348
    severe, 1348t
    shock in, 253t
    skin and soft tissue infections and, 1353t, 1374
    treatment of, 1350–1357
        adjunctive therapies, 1357
        algorithm for, 1351a
        antifungal therapy, 1355
        anti-infective therapy, 1352–1355, 1353t
        duration of therapy, 1352
        enteral nutrition, 1357, 1703t
        glycemic control, 1357
        hydrocortisone, 1357
        initial resuscitation, 1352
        nonpharmacologic, 1357
        recombinant human activated protein C, 1356
        sedation and neuromuscular blockade, 1356
        vasopressors and inotropic therapy, 1356
    urinary tract infections and, 1353, 1353t
Septic emboli, 1237
Septic shock, 253t, 1347–1358. See also Sepsis
    definition of, 1348t
SERM. See Selective estrogen receptor
        modulators

Serotonin (5-HT3) receptors
    in anxiety disorders, 693
    in bipolar disorder, 670
    in chemotherapy-induced nausea and
        vomiting, 1650–1651, 1652, 1652t
    in schizophrenia, 632
    in sleep, 701
Serotonin antagonists, in nausea and vomiting,
        362t, 363, 364
Serotonin-norepinephrine reuptake inhibitors
    dosage of, 661t
    in generalized anxiety disorder, 696, 696t
    mechanism of action of, 652
    in pain, 578
    in panic disorder, 701t, 702
    in urinary incontinence, 917
    for weight loss, 1737
Serotonin syndrome, 576, 590, 659, 1724
Serratia marcescens
    in infective endocarditis, 1242
    in keratitis, 1070
Sertraline
    adverse effects of, 659t, 696, 701t, 879t
    arrhythmia with, 179t
    in depression, 516
    dosage of, 661t, 696t, 701t, 879t
    drug interactions of, 153t, 660t, 771t, 955t, 1724
    in generalized anxiety disorder, 696, 696t
    in irritable bowel syndrome, 383
    in panic disorder, 701t
    pharmacokinetics of, 659, 659t
    in social anxiety disorder, 703
    in vasomotor symptoms of menopause,
        878, 879t
    for weight loss, 1737
Serum sickness, 928
    allergic drug reaction, 829, 929t, 930
Sevelamer
    adverse effects of, 463
    dosage of, 464t
    in hyperphosphatemia, 463, 464t, 491
Severe combined immunodeficiency, 1630, 1630t
    acute leukemia and, 1580t
Sex-cord stromal tumor, 1568
Sex hormone-binding globulin, 865
Sexual dysfunction, antidepressant-induced, 658,
        659t
Sexually transmitted disease (STD), 843,
        1317–1334. See also specific diseases
    behavioral considerations in, 1318
    expedited partner treatment, 1318
    general approach to, 1318
    index patient, 1318
    oral contraceptives and, 845
    in pregnancy, 816, 831t, 835
        Chlamydia, 834
        gonorrheal, 834
        herpes simplex, 834–835
        syphilis, 835
        trichomoniasis, 835
    prevention of, 1318, 1334
    condom use, 852, 1334
Shear stress, risk for pressure sores, 1231
Shigella
    in diarrhea, 376, 378, 380
    in travelers' diarrhea, 1273
Shigella boydii, 1273
Shigella dysenteriae, 1273
Shigella flexneri, 1273
Shigella sonnei, 1273
Shigellosis, 1267–1269
    clinical presentation in, 1268
    diagnosis of, 1268

Shigellosis (*Cont.*)
  epidemiology of, 1267
  in immunocompromised patients, 1268
  monitoring patient with, 1268–1269
  pathogenesis of, 1267–1268
  treatment of, 1269, 1269*t*
Shingles, 1414
Shock. *See also specific types of shock*
  DIC with, 1131*t*
  metabolic acidosis with, 501*t*
  with myocardial infarction, 134
Short bowel syndrome, 345
  treatment of
    enteral nutrition, 1703*t*
    parenteral nutrition, 1682*t*
Short-gut syndrome, intestine transplantation
  in, 941
Shunt infection, CSF shunts, 1070, 1171*t*, 1146
Shwachman's syndrome, acute leukemia and,
  1580*t*
SIADH (syndrome of inappropriate antidiuretic
  hormone), 485, 486
Sialorrhea, in Parkinson's disease, 556
Sibutramine
  dosage of, 1724, 1725*t*
  drug interactions of, 1724
  mechanism of action of, 1725
  in obesity, 1725, 1725*t*
Sickle cell anemia/disease, 165*t*, 1139–1146
  acute chest syndrome in, 1143, 1143*t*, 1151
  aplastic crisis in, 1149
  case study of, 1145, 1146
  clinical presentation in, 1142–1145, 1143*t*
  complications of
    acute, 1143*t*, 1144*t*, 1155–1146
    chronic, 1144
  diagnosis of, 1144–1145
  epidemiology of, 1139–1140
  ethnicity and, 1143
  etiology of, 1139–1140
  hand-foot syndrome in, 1143
  health maintenance in
    folic acid supplementation, 1148, 1150
    immunizations, 1143*t*, 1144, 1144*t*
    prophylactic penicillin, 1143*t*, 1144
  infections in, 1143*t*, 1144
  inheritance of, 1140, 1140*f*
  malaria and, 1140
  morbidity and mortality in, 1143
  osteomyelitis and, 1340
  outcome evaluation in, 1146
  pathophysiology of, 1140–1142, 1141*f*
    erythrocyte physiology, 1140, 1141*f*
    protective hemoglobin types, 1142
    sickle hemoglobin polymerization, 1142, 1141*f*
    viscosity of erythrocytes and sickle cell
      adhesion, 1142
  patient care and monitoring in, 1152
  priapism in, 1143*t*, 1144–1146
  splenic sequestration crisis in, 1143*t*, 1146
  stroke in, 1147–1148
  treatment of, 1142–1153, 1143*t*
    acute complications, 1143*t*, 1145–1146
    5-aza-2'-deoxycytidine, 1147
    chronic transfusion therapy, 1143*t*, 1147
    fetal hemoglobin inducers, 1143*t*, 1142–1146
    hematopoietic cell transplantation, 1143*t*,
      1145–1146, 1630, 1630*t*
    hydroxyurea, 1143*t*, 1144–1145
    pain management, 1145*t*, 1146–1148
  vasoocclusive crisis in, 1143*t*, 1145*t*, 1146
Sickle cell hemolytic transfusion reaction
  syndrome, 1144

Sickle cell syndrome, 1139
Sickle cell trait, 1139, 1145
Sickle hemoglobin, 1139–1146. *See also* Sickle cell
  anemia/disease
Sick sinus syndrome, 163, 163*t*
Sideroblastic anemia, 1114*a*
Sigmoidoscopy
  in constipation, 381
  in irritable bowel syndrome, 381
  screening for colorectal cancer, 1520, 1520*t*
Sildenafil
  adverse effects of, 888
  comparison of phosphodiesterase inhibitors,
    889*t*
  dosage of, 887*t*
  drug interactions of, 121, 124, 142*t*, 146, 887, 902
  in erectile dysfunction, 563, 887, 887*t*
  mechanism of action of, 888
Silver nitrate, in hemorrhagic cystitis, 1670
Silver sulfadiazine
  dosage of, 1231*t*
  in infected pressure sores, 1231*t*
Simvastatin
  adverse effects of, 242*t*
  dosage of, 242*t*
  drug interactions of, 955*t*, 1467
  in hyperlipidemia, 242*t*, 243*t*, 246, 247
  in ischemic heart disease, 120
Singlet oxygen, 1662
Sinoatrial node, 158
Sinus bradycardia, 162–164
  clinical presentation in, 163
  diagnosis of, 163
  epidemiology of, 162–163
  etiology of, 162–163, 163*t*
  outcome evaluation in, 163
  pathophysiology of, 163
  treatment of, 163
Sinusitis. *See* Rhinosinusitis
Sinusoid(s), hepatic, 388, 389, 389*f*, 389*f*
Sinusoidal obstruction syndrome
  clinical presentation in, 1636–1637
  etiology of, 1636–1637
  treatment of, 1636–1637
Sinus tachycardia, 160
Siplizumab, in psoriasis, 1087
Sirolimus
  adverse effects of, 946*t*, 951*t*, 952, 1694
  dosage of, 946*t*, 952
  drug-eluting vascular stents, 118
  drug interactions of, 953, 955*t*, 1384
  hypertension with, 958
  mechanism of action of, 948*f*, 952
  in transplant recipient, 946*t*, 951*t*, 952
SIRS (Systemic inflammatory response
  syndrome), 1348*t*
Sitagliptin
  adverse effects of, 750
  in diabetes mellitus, 750–751
  dosage of, 750
  mechanism of action of, 750
Sjögren's syndrome, 317
  dry eye in, 1074*t*, 1075
Skeletal disorders. *See also* Musculoskeletal
  disorders
Skin
  anatomy of, 1613, 1615*f*
  disorders of, 1093–1108
  drug-related, 1438*t*
  fungal infections of, 1367–1369
  infections of, 1221–1234
    outcome evaluation of, 1232
    pathophysiology of, 1222

patient care and monitoring in, 1232–1233
  sepsis and, 1353, 1353*t*
  maceration of, 1231
  normal flora of, 1157*f*
  warfarin-induced necrosis of, 205
Skin cancer, 1611–1628
  melanoma. *See* Melanoma
  nonmelanoma. *See* Nonmelanoma skin cancer
  prevention of, 1508, 1611
  sun exposure and, 1508, 1611, 1613–1614, 1624
Skin cancer phenotype, 1614–1615
Skin self-examination, 1413
Skin test
  for penicillin allergy, 931, 931*t*
  for tuberculosis, 1256, 1256*t*
Sleep, types of, 709
Sleep apnea
  in acromegaly, 805
  arrhythmia with, 163*t*, 164*t*
  central, 426*t*
  hypertension and, 54
  obesity and, 1721–1723
  obstructive. *See* Obstructive sleep apnea
  respiratory acidosis with, 426*t*
Sleep diary, 718
Sleep disorders, 709–720
  case study of, 709, 713, 718
  clinical presentation in, 711–712
  diagnosis of, 712
  drug-induced, 718
  epidemiology of, 700–701
  etiology of, 700–701
  outcome evaluation in, 719
  in Parkinson's disease, 556, 561–563
  pathophysiology of, 701
  patient care and monitoring in, 719
  treatment of, 713–719
Sleep hygiene, 714, 714*t*
Sleep latency, 713
Sleep talking, 702, 703
Sleep terrors, 702, 703
Sleep walking, 702, 703
Slipped capital femoral epiphysis, with growth
  hormone therapy, 811
Slitlamp biomicroscopy, 1036
Small bowel, normal flora of, 1157*f*
Small bowel obstruction
  nausea and vomiting with, 358*t*
  in ovarian cancer, 1566, 1575
Smoke inhalation, 426*t*
Smokeless tobacco, in smoking cessation, 622
Smoking
  acute leukemia and, 1580*t*
  assessment of tobacco use, 293*a*
  cancer and, 1508
  chronic kidney disease and, 447, 452
  colorectal cancer and, 1518, 1518*t*
  COPD and, 290, 293
  drug interactions of, 614*t*, 646–647
  environmental tobacco smoke, 1500
  epidemiology of, 608
  erectile dysfunction with, 881*t*
  GERD with, 317*t*
  hypertension and, 56
  inflammatory bowel disease and, 342
  ischemic heart disease and, 111, 111*t*, 28*t*
  lung cancer and, 1500
  macular degeneration and, 1072*t*
  oral contraceptive use and, 845
  pack-years, 1500
  pathophysiology of, 610
  peptic ulcer disease and, 329
  prostate cancer and, 1537

rheumatoid arthritis and, 982
stroke and, 217t
Smoking cessation, 59, 622, 622t, 623t, 1500, 1508
in asthma, 269
in chronic kidney disease, 452
in COPD, 292–293, 293t
in heart failure, 88
in ischemic heart disease, 117
nonpharmacologic treatments for, 622
in peripheral vascular disease, 758
pharmacotherapies for, 119–121, 622, 622t
in prevention of myocardial infarction, 151
signs and symptoms of nicotine withdrawal, 613t
Snake bite, 1131t
Social anxiety disorder
clinical presentation in, 694
course of illness, 691
diagnosis of, 693
epidemiology of, 691
etiology of, 692
outcome evaluation in, 704
pathophysiology of, 692–693, 693f
treatment of, 703–704
algorithm for, 704a
anticonvulsants, 704
antidepressants, 703
benzodiazepines, 704
β-blockers, 704
MAO inhibitors, 704
nonpharmacologic, 704
reversible inhibitors of monoamine
oxidase, 704
Social skills training, in schizophrenia, 636
Sociodemographics, of elderly
economics, 8
education and health literacy, 8
population, 8
Sodium
drugs containing, 86t
in extracellular fluid, 484, 484t
fractional excretion of, 454
for parenteral nutrition, 1685, 1685t
serum, 486
normal range for, 484t
in ventricular action potential, 159, 159f
Sodium balance, 485–487
blood pressure and, 58
case study of, 486, 487, 492
impaired in chronic kidney disease, 454–455
clinical presentation in, 454
Sodium bicarbonate
in diabetic ketoacidosis, 776
dosage of, 466
drug interactions of, 614t
in lactic acidosis, 260
in metabolic acidosis, 466, 502
Sodium chloride, 482t
in hypovolemic shock, 257, 258t
in intra-abdominal infections, 1285
Sodium cromolyn, dosage, 830t
Sodium ferric gluconate, in anemia of chronic
kidney disease, 459
Sodium fluoride, in osteoporosis, 977
Sodium loading, 1381
Sodium oxybate, in cataplexy, 717
Sodium phosphate
in constipation, 374t
dosage of, 374t
in hypophosphatemia, 491, 491t
Sodium polystyrene sulfonate
drug interactions of, 771t
in hyperkalemia, 454, 489
Sodium requirement, 485

Sodium restriction
in cirrhosis, 394
in heart failure, 88, 89, 97
in hypertension, 58, 59t
in ischemic heart disease, 120
Sodium sulfacetamide, in acne vulgaris, 1097
Sodium thiosulfate
dosage of, 1678t
in extravasation injury, 1678, 1678t
Soft tissue infection, 1221–1233
outcome evaluation of, 1232
pathophysiology of, 1222
patient care and monitoring in, 1232–1233
sepsis and, 1353t, 1353
Soft tissue injury, 1019
Solid-organ transplantation, 939–961. See also
    specific organs
acute rejection, 942–943, 944t, 953, 1131t
antigen-presenting cells and, 942
B cells and, 942
case study of, 947, 955, 957, 961
chronic rejection, 944
complications of
diabetes mellitus, 959–960
hyperlipidemia, 958–959
hypertension, 957–958
opportunistic infections, 955–956, 955t
osteoporosis, 953t
posttransplant lymphoproliferative
    disorder, 959
skin cancer, 959
epidemiology of, 942
etiology of, 941
history of, 940, 940t
host-graft adaptation in, 944
humoral rejection, 944
hyperacute rejection, 944
immunosuppressive therapy in
drug complications, 955–960
induction therapy, 946–949, 946t, 949a
maintenance therapy, 946t, 948–953, 949a
treatment of acute rejection, 954
MHC and, 942
outcome evaluation in, 9601–961
pathophysiology of, 942–943
patient care and monitoring in, 961
T cells and, 942
tolerance, 943
vaccination of transplant recipient, 1415
Solifenacin
adverse effects of, 915, 916t
dosage of, 916t
pharmacokinetics of, 916t
in urinary incontinence, 915, 916t
Somatic hypermutation, 1553
Somatomedins. See Insulin-like growth factors
Somatostatin, 803
in pancreatitis, 407
Somatostatin analogs, in acromegaly, 807–808,
    807t
Somatotropes, 803
Somatotropin. See Growth hormone
Somnolence, in delirium tremens, 618
Sorafenib, 1467
adverse effects of, 1467–1468
in cancer therapy, 1467
mechanism of action of, 1467
pharmacokinetics of, 1467–1468
Sorbitol
in constipation, 374t
diarrhea with, 376t, 1710, 1714
dosage of, 374t
Sore throat, 1209. See also Pharyngitis

Sotalol
adverse effects of, 169t
arrhythmia with, 162t, 164t, 177t, 179t
in arrhythmias, 162t
in atrial fibrillation, 171t, 171t
depression with, 656
dosage of, 171t
drug interactions of, 647
mechanism of action of, 162t
Source control
in infectious disease treatment, 1161–1162, 1167
in septic patients, 1356
Soy products
adverse effects of, 879t
dosage of, 879t
drug interactions of, 771t
in vasomotor symptoms of menopause, 878, 879t
Spasm, infantile, 525, 525t
Spasticity
in multiple sclerosis, 516, 517t
treatment of, 516, 517
Specialized nutrition support, 1681, 1703. See also
    Enteral nutrition; Parenteral nutrition
Spectinomycin, dosage, 831t
Spectinomycin
in chancroid, 1334t
dosage of, 831t, 1319, 1334t
in gonorrhea, 831t, 743, 1319
in pregnancy, 831t, 743
Spermicide, 852
Spherule, 1377, 1377f
Sphincter of Oddi, 1702
pain in, 406
Sphygmomanometer, 56
Spider angiomata, 389
Spinal cord compression, in cancer patients,
    1662–1664
case study of, 1664
clinical presentation in, 1663
diagnosis of, 1663
epidemiology of, 1663–1664
etiology of, 1664
outcome evaluation in, 1666
pathophysiology of, 1664
treatment of, 1664–1665
Spinal cord injury
constipation in, 372t
erectile dysfunction with, 881t
pain in, 568
urinary incontinence in, 901
Spiritual counseling, in pain, 573
Spirometry
in acute chest syndrome, 1146
in asthma, 267
in COPD, 292
Spironolactone, 38f
in acute coronary syndromes, 143t
adverse effects of, 61t, 95, 150
in ascites, 397
dosage of, 18t, 92t, 95, 143t
erectile dysfunction with, 881t
in heart failure, 92t, 95
in hypertension, 60t, 65
in prevention of myocardial infarction,
    150–151
Splash injury, ocular, 1069t, 1070
Splenectomy
in immune thrombocytopenic purpura, 1134
in splenic sequestration crisis, 1143t, 1146
in thrombotic thrombocytopenic purpura, 1135
Splenic sequestration crisis
in sickle cell anemia/disease, 1143t, 1146
treatment of, 1143t, 1146

Splenomegaly
    in acute lymphocytic leukemia, 1583
    in cirrhosis, 389
Splinter hemorrhages, in infective endocarditis, 1238, 1239*f*
Sponge, contraceptive, 852
Spontaneous bacterial peritonitis, 391
    in cirrhosis, 391, 397, 398*a*
    pathophysiology of, 391
    renal failure and, 397
    treatment of, 397–399, 398*a*
Sports-related injury, 1020
Spotting, with oral contraceptives, 846–848
Sprain, 1020
    clinical presentation in, 1021
    pathophysiology of, 1020
Sputum culture, in tuberculosis, 1263
Sputum cytology
    in lung cancer, 1504
    in tuberculosis, 1259
Squalene synthase inhibitors, 247
Squamous cell carcinoma, 1611–1626. *See also* Nonmelanoma skin cancer
    warning signs of, 1671
SSKI, in hyperthyroidism, 775
SSRI. *See* Selective serotonin reuptake inhibitors
Staging
    of breast cancer, 1478, 1479*t*
    of cancer, 1448, 1449, 1450*t*
    of colorectal cancer, 1450*t*, 1318, 1521–1522, 1523*f*
    of Hodgkin's lymphoma, 1552*f*, 1556, 1556*t*,
    of lung cancer, 1504, 1504*t*
    of melanoma, 1614–1617, 1616*t*
    of non-Hodgkin's lymphoma, 1559, 1559*t*
    of ovarian cancer, 1570, 1570*a*
    of prostate cancer, 1540, 1541*t*
Staphylococci
    in bite wound infections, 1231*t*
    coagulase-negative, 1171*t*
        in infective endocarditis, 1242
        in surgical site infections, 1397*t*
    coagulase-positive, in infective endocarditis, 1241
    in furuncles, 1223*t*
    in infections in cancer patients, 1655*t*
    in infective endocarditis, 1236, 1236*t*, 1241, 1245, 1245*t*, 1246*t*
    in keratitis, 1070
    normal flora, 1157*f*
    in pneumonia, 1194
    in postneurosurgical infections, 1146
    in sepsis, 1348*t*
Staphylococcus aureus
    in bite wound infections, 1231*t*
    in catheter-related infections, 475
    in cellulitis/erysipelas, 1225, 1225*t*
    in conjunctivitis, 1070
    in cystic fibrosis, 304, 306, 309
    in diabetic foot infections, 1228, 1229*t*
    in diaper dermatitis, 1107
    in folliculitis, 1223*t*
    in food poisoning, 1278, 1278*t*
    in hemodialysis access infections, 472
    in impetigo, 1222
    in infections in cancer patients, 1655*t*
    in infective endocarditis, 1236, 1240–1242, 1245
    in intra-abdominal infections, 1283
    in meningitis, 1171*t*, 1176*t*
    methicillin-resistant, 1176*t*, 1197, 1245, 1339*t*, 1342*t*, 1348*t*, 1355, 1396
        community-acquired, 1224, 1225*t*, 1229*t*
        health care-associated, 1224, 1225*t*, 1229*t*
        normal flora, 1157*f*

    in osteomyelitis, 1146, 1338, 1339*t*, 1341, 1342*t*
    in otitis media, 1204
    in peritonitis, 474
    in pneumonia, 1190, 1196, 1196*t*
    in postneurosurgical infections, 1146
    in rhinosinusitis, 1208
    in sepsis, 1348*t*, 1353, 1355*a*
    in surgical site infections, 1396, 1397*t*
Staphylococcus epidermidis
    in catheter-related infections, 475
    in cellulitis, 1224
    in diabetic foot infections, 1228
    in hemodialysis access infections, 472
    in infective endocarditis, 1242
    in intra-abdominal infections, 1283
    in meningitis, 1176*t*
    normal flora, 1157*f*
    in peritonitis, 474
    in surgical site infections, 1396
Staphylococcus lugdunensis, 1241
Staphylococcus saprophyticus, in urinary tract infections, 1308
Starvation, metabolic acidosis in, 424*t*
Statins. *See also specific drugs*
    adverse effects of, 240–241
    in Alzheimer's disease, 603
    cost of, 149
    drug interactions of, 240, 241, 961, 1378
    in dyslipidemia, 151, 234, 240–244, 241*t*, 242*t*, 243*t*, 246, 247, 452, 776, 961
    in ischemic heart disease, 119, 120, 126
    metabolism of, 244
    in osteoporosis, 977
    pharmacologic properties of, 120
    in prevention of colorectal cancer, 1520
    in prevention of myocardial infarction, 151
    in prevention of prostate cancer, 1537
    in prevention of stroke, 222–223
    vasculoprotective effects of, 116
Status asthmaticus, respiratory acidosis with, 426*t*
Status epilepticus, 541–551
    in alcohol withdrawal, 618
    case study of, 542, 544, 548
    clinical presentation in, 542–543
    cost of, 542
    definition of, 541
    diagnosis of, 542–542
    in elderly, 549–550
    electroencephalography in, 541, 548
    epidemiology of, 542
    etiology of, 542
    generalized convulsive, 541, 547
    nonconvulsive, 541, 547
    outcome evaluation in, 550
    pathophysiology of, 542
    patient care and monitoring in, 550
    in pediatric patients, 549, 549*t*
    phase I, 542
    phase II, 542
    in pregnancy, 550
    refractory, 541
    treatment of, 544–550, 545*t*, 546*t*, 547*t*, 549*t*
        antiepileptic drugs, 545–548, 545*t*, 546*t*, 547*t*
        benzodiazepines, 544–545, 545*t*, 546*t*, 548, 547*t*
        nonpharmacologic, 544
Status migrainosus, 585
Stavudine
    adverse effects of, 1426, 1427*t*, 1437*t*–1440*t*
    dosage of, 1427*t*
    drug interactions of, 1427*t*
    in HIV infection, 1426, 1427*t*, 1426
    mechanism of action of, 1421*f*

STD. *See* Sexually transmitted disease
Steatohepatitis, with parenteral nutrition, 1696, 1704
Steatorrhea, in cystic fibrosis, 304–305
Steatosis, in cystic fibrosis, 305
Stem cell transplantation, hematopoietic. *See* Hematopoietic cell transplantation
Stenotrophomonas maltophilia, in cystic fibrosis, 304, 306, 309, 310
Stent
    intracoronary, in acute coronary syndromes, 136, 137
    vascular
        with carotid angioplasty, 223
        drug-eluting, 118
        in ischemic heart disease, 118
Step 1 Diet, 1723, 1723*t*
Stereotactic radiosurgery, in brain metastasis, 1660, 1662, 1665
Stereotyped behavior, in cocaine intoxication, 612*t*
Steroid hormones, in cirrhosis, 389
Steroidogenesis inhibitors, in Cushing's syndrome, 794, 796*t*
Sterols, plant, 230, 231*f*
Stevens-Johnson syndrome, 684, 829, 930, 1015, 1070*t*, 1437*t*
Stimulant laxatives, in constipation, 374, 374*t*
Stimulants. *See also specific drugs*
    abuse of, 608
        signs and symptoms of intoxication, 612*t*, 612
        treatment of, 615–616
    in ADHD, 725–726, 727*t*, 728*t*, 730*t*
    adverse effects of, 726, 728*t*
    contraindications to, 726
    extended-acting, 726, 727*t*, 730*t*
    intermediate-acting, 726, 727*t*, 730*t*
    rebound effect as drug wears off, 726
    short-acting, 726, 727*t*, 730*t*
    withdrawal syndromes, 619
Stomach, normal flora of, 1157*f*
Stomatitis, methotrexate-induced, 990
Stool softeners, 374, 829
Strain, 1019
    clinical presentation in, 1021
    pathophysiology of, 1020
Streptococci
    β-hemolytic
        in diabetic foot infections, 1228, 1229*t*
        in impetigo, 1222
        in necrotizing fasciitis, 1226
    in bite wound infections, 1231*t*
    in diaper dermatitis, 1107
    group A
        in cellulitis/erysipelas, 1224
        in impetigo, 1222
        in intra-abdominal infections, 1283, 1286*t*
        in lymphangitis, 1222
        in necrotizing fasciitis, 1226
        in pharyngitis, 1217–1218
        in toxic shock-like syndrome, 1227
    group B
        in meningitis, 1070, 1171*t*, 1176*t*, 1146
        in osteomyelitis, 1339*t*, 1342*t*
        in pregnancy, 816, 831*t*, 833*f*, 834*t*, 835
    group C, in pharyngitis, 1217
    group D
        in infective endocarditis, 1241
        in surgical site infections, 1397*t*
    group G, in pharyngitis, 1217
    in infective endocarditis, 1236, 1236*t*, 1241, 1249, 1244*t*

in keratitis, 1070
in pneumonia, 1190
in postneurosurgical infections, 1146
in sepsis, 1348*t*
in surgical site infections, 1396, 1397*t*
viridans
in bite wound infections, 1231*t*
in infections in cancer patients, 1655*t*
in infective endocarditis, 1089, 1241, 1249, 1244*t*, 1249
Streptococcus bovis, 1241
Streptococcus mitis, 1241
Streptococcus mutans, 1241
Streptococcus pneumoniae, 1410. *See also* Pneumococcal vaccine
in conjunctivitis, 1070
in COPD exacerbations, 298, 299*t*
drug-resistant, 1193, 1194*t*
in intra-abdominal infections, 1283, 1286*t*
in meningitis, 1171, 1171*t*, 1175*t*, 1181, 1183
normal flora, 1157*f*
in otitis media, 1204
penicillin-resistant, 1204, 1207, 1209
in pneumonia, 1190, 1190*t*, 1196*t*, 1352
in rhinosinusitis, 1208, 1209
in sepsis, 1348*t*
in spontaneous bacterial peritonitis, 391
Streptococcus pyogenes
in otitis media, 1204
in pharyngitis, 1217
in rhinosinusitis, 1207
in sepsis, 1352
Streptococcus salivarius, 1241
Streptococcus sanguis, 1241
Streptokinase
in acute coronary syndromes, 135, 141*t*, 144
dosage of, 141*t*
in stroke, 221
in venous thromboembolism, 195, 195*t*
Streptomycin
adverse effects of, 1262*t*
dosage of, 1262*t*
in tuberculosis, 1260, 1262*t*
Streptozocin
emetogenicity of, 365*t*
extravasation of, 1678*t*
Stress management
in generalized anxiety disorder, 694
in headache, 586
in psoriasis, 1082
Stress myocardial perfusion imaging, in ischemic heart disease, 114
Stress reflux, 316
Stress-related mucosal damage, 327–328, 328*t*
Stress ulcer, prevention of, 260
in septic patients, 1356
Striae, corticosteroid-induced, 1084
Strictures, in Crohn's disease, 344, 345
Stroke, 215–227
alcohol use and, 217*t*
antiplatelet therapy for, 224
antipsychotic-related, 644
anxiety with, 694*t*
atrial fibrillation and, 165–173, 223
case study of, 218, 223, 224
classification by mechanism, 216–217, 216*t*
clinical presentation in, 218, 221*t*
constipation in, 372*t*
cost of, 216
diabetes mellitus and, 217*t*
diagnosis of, 218
epidemiology of, 215–216
epilepsy and, 522

ethnicity and, 217, 217*t*
etiology of, 216
heart disease and, 217*t*
hemorrhagic. *See* Hemorrhagic stroke
hemorrhagic conversion in, 220
hormone-replacement therapy and, 876*t*, 871
hyperlipidemia and, 165*t*
hypertension and, 65, 70, 217, 217*t*, 220, 222
ipsilateral, 223
ischemic. *See* Ischemic stroke
migraine and, 217*t*
obesity and, 217*t*
outcome evaluation in, 225–226
pain in, 568
pathophysiology of, 217–218
patient care and monitoring in, 226, 226*t*
prevention of, 172–173, 173*t*, 217, 222–224
aspirin, 222, 223–224
blood pressure management, 224, 225*t*
carotid angioplasty, 223
carotid endarterectomy, 223
clopidogrel, 224, 225*t*, 226*t*
extended-release dipyridamole, 224, 225*t*
statins, 222–223
ticlopidine, 223–224
warfarin, 223, 226*t*
recurrent, 223–224
risk factors for, 217, 217*t*
in sickle cell anemia/disease, 1145–1146
smoking and, 217*t*, 223
treatment of, 219–222, 220*t*
algorithm for, 166*f*
ancrod, 222
aspirin, 222, 225*t*
blood pressure management, 220*t*, 221
carotid endarterectomy, 220
heparin, 222, 225
middle cerebral artery embolectomy, 220
nonpharmacologic, 220
rehabilitation guidelines, 225–226
supportive measures, 220, 220*t*
thrombolytic therapy, 220–222
urinary incontinence in, 912
Stroke/cerebral vascular accident (CVA), palliative care treatment for, 39
Stroke-in-evolution, 222
Stroke volume
in atrial fibrillation, 166
in heart failure, 81
in shock, 252
Strongyloidiasis, 1303
Strontium ranelate, in osteoporosis, 977
Struma ovarii, 774*t*
Subarachnoid hemorrhage, 216
treatment of
calcium antagonists, 225, 225*t*
surgery, 223
Subchondral bone, in osteoarthritis, 998
Subdural hematoma, 216
Subjective Global Assessment, 1688
Substance-abuse disorders, 607–618. *See also specific substances*
ADHD and, 726
anxiety with, 694*t*
case study of, 611, 626
clinical presentation in, 611–612, 611*t*
depression with, 656
diagnosis of, 611–612, 612*t*
drug interactions in, 614*t*
emergency department visits for, 608, 608*f*
epidemiology of, 508, 608*f*
HIV infection and, 1426
intoxication, 611, 611*t*

keratitis with, 1070*t*
mania with, 676*t*
outcome evaluation in, 626
pathophysiology of
neuronal adaptation, 610
reward pathway, 608–610, 609*f*
patient care and monitoring in, 627
with physiological dependence, 611
without physiological dependence, 611
schizophrenia and, 635, 635*t*, 644
tolerance, 611
treatment of
intoxication syndromes, 611–616
pharmacologic, 610
psychosocial strategies, 610
withdrawal symptoms, 616–622
Substance dependence, 622–626
diagnosis of, 611
maintenance treatment in, 624
nonpharmacologic therapy, 624
outcome evaluation in, 627
patient care and monitoring in, 628
pharmacologic therapy, 624–627
Substance P, 1021
in anxiety disorders, 693
in wakefulness, 701
Substantia nigra, in Parkinson's disease, 554, 554*f*
Succinylcholine, drug interactions of, 1042
Sucralfate
administration through feeding tube, 1715
dosage of, 277*t*, 830*t*
drug interactions of, 153*t*, 771*t*, 1165
in GERD, 322, 829, 830*t*
hypophosphatemia with, 491
in peptic ulcer disease, 336, 336*t*, 337, 338
in pregnancy, 829, 830*t*
in prevention of NSAID-related ulcers, 337
Sudden cardiac death
prevention of, 177
in ventricular tachycardia, 177
Suicidality
antidepressants and, 665
in bipolar disorder, 671–672, 674
in stimulant withdrawal, 619
Sulbactam. *See* Ampicillin-sulbactam
Sulfa-based drugs, glaucoma with, 1043
Sulfacetamide
in conjunctivitis, 1066, 1066*t*
dosage of, 1066*t*
Sulfamethoxazole. *See* Trimethoprim-sulfamethoxazole
Sulfasalazine, 988, 990
adverse effects of, 346, 986*t*, 990
dosage of, 286*t*, 289*t*, 290*t*, 986*t*, 1085
drug interactions of, 953
in inflammatory bowel disease, 346, 346*t*, 347, 349*t*, 350, 351*t*, 353*t*
mechanism of action of, 346
monitoring treatment with, 986*t*
in pregnancy, 993
in psoriasis, 1085
in rheumatoid arthritis, 986*t*, 990
Sulfate
in extracellular fluid, 484*t*
in intracellular fluid, 484*t*
Sulfinpyrazone
adverse effects of, 442
in antihyperuricemic treatment, 1015
drug interactions of, 205*t*
Sulfonamide(s). *See also specific drugs*
allergic drug reactions, 929*t*, 930
in bacteriuria, 917

Sulfonamide(s) (*Cont.*)
drug interactions of, 1592t
ocular changes with, 1077t
pancreatitis with, 404f
in pregnancy, 917
in urinary tract infections, 1311t
Sulfonamide
resistance, 1204
in urinary tract infections, 1314t
Sulfonylureas, 10
adverse effects of, 747t
allergic drug reactions, 931
in diabetes mellitus, 747–750, 747t
drug interactions of, 321, 750
mechanism of action of, 749
Sulfur preparations
in acne vulgaris, 1097
adverse effects of, 1097
Sulindac
dosage of, 1014t
in gout, 1014t
in osteoarthritis, 1004
pancreatitis with, 404f
in pregnancy, 1004
Sumatriptan
in cluster headaches, 589
dosage of, 589t
drug interactions of, 589t
in migraine, 589t
Sundowning, 41
Sun exposure, skin cancer and, 1508, 1611, 1613–1615, 1624
Sunitinib, 1468
adverse effects of, 1468
in cancer therapy, 1468
drug interactions of, 1468
mechanism of action of, 1468
pharmacokinetics of, 1468
Sunlamp, artificial, 1624
Sunscreen, 1611, 1624
in psoriasis, 1082
Superior mesenteric artery syndrome, 358t
Superior vena cava syndrome, 1661–1662
in cancer patients, 1661–1662
clinical presentation in, 1662
diagnosis of, 1662
epidemiology of, 1661–1662
etiology of, 1661–1662, 1661t
outcome evaluation in, 1662
pathophysiology of, 1662
thrombosis-related, 1662
treatment of, 1662–1662
Supraorbital pain, in cluster headache, 586
Supraventricular arrhythmias, 162–181
Surfactants, in constipation, 374
Surgery
antimicrobial prophylaxis in, 1042, 1395
case study of, 1401
choice of antimicrobials in, 1398
outcome evaluation in, 1402
patient care and monitoring in, 1402
recommendations for specific surgeries, 1401, 1400
route of administration, 1398
scheduling of, 1399
clean operations, 1396, 1397t
clean-contaminated operations, 1396, 1400t
contaminated operations, 1396, 1400t
dirty operations, 1396, 1400t
venous thromboembolism and, 186, 187t, 193
Surgical site infection
case study of, 1401
definition of, 1396

epidemiology of, 1396
etiology of, 1397, 1397t
extra-abdominal operations, 1401
incisional, 1396
intra-abdominal operations, 1395, 1397
organ/space, 1396
prevention of
alternative methods to decrease, 1399
antimicrobials, 1398–1401
reporting of, 1398
risk factors for, 1398, 1397t
treatment of, 1398
Sustained-release preparations, administration through feeding tubes, 1714
Swallowing, esophageal clearance, 316, 317, 318
Sweat, in cystic fibrosis, 305
Sweating, 486
Sweet clover, 154t
Symbiosis, 1294
Sympathetic nervous system
in cirrhosis, 390
in heart failure, 81, 81t, 82
in hypertension, 55
Sympathomimetics. *See also specific drugs*
blood glucose level and, 737t
drug interactions of, 660t
glaucoma with, 1043
ocular changes with, 1077t
seizures with, 522
Syncope, neurocardiac, 163t, 164t
Syndrome of inappropriate antidiuretic hormone (SIADH), 485, 486
Synechia, 1035
Synergism, bacterial, 1283
Synovectomy, arthroscopic, in hemophilia, 1123
Synovitis, in osteoarthritis, 998
Synovium, in rheumatoid arthritis, 982
Syphilis, 1321–1326
cardiovascular, 1322
congenital, 1321–1326
diagnosis of, 1322
epidemiology of, 1321
gummatous, 1322
latent, 1322, 1326
pathophysiology of, 1321
patient care and monitoring in, 1325–1326, 1325a
in pregnancy, 816, 831t, 743
primary, 1321, 1322, 1325–1326
psychotic symptoms in, 635t
secondary, 1322, 1325–1326
tertiary, 1322
treatment of, 1322–1326
algorithm for, 1323a
Systemic corticosteroids, teratogenic effects of, 824t
Systemic inflammatory response syndrome (SIRS), 1348t
Systemic lupus erythematosus
acute renal failure and, 433
anemia in, 1118
anxiety with, 694t
arrhythmia with, 163t, 164t
dry eye in, 1074t
mania with, 676t
venous thromboembolism in, 187
Systemic venous congestion, in heart failure, 86
Systolic blood pressure, 52, 56
Systolic dysfunction, 80t, 81

T

Tablets, administration through feeding tubes, 1714
Tacalcitol, in psoriasis, 1084
Tachyarrhythmia, 160

Tachycardia
in heart failure, 81, 81t, 82
in sepsis, 1349
Tachyphylaxis, to calcitonin, 1673
Tachypnea
in asthma, 268
in sepsis, 1349
TAC regimen, in breast cancer, 1482t
Tacrine, in Alzheimer's disease, 598, 601t
Tacrolimus
adverse effects of, 54t, 946t, 951t
arrhythmia with, 179t
comparative efficacy of calcineurin inhibitors, 949
dosage of, 946t, 949
adaptive dosing, 1683
drug interactions of, 953, 1378
in GVHD, 1640
hyperlipidemia with, 961
hypertension with, 960
in inflammatory bowel disease, 352
mechanism of action of, 948f
nephrotoxicity of, 432, 440, 441–442
osteoporosis with, 953t
parenteral nutrition and, 1694
in prevention of GVHD, 1638
in psoriasis, 1085, 1087
in transplant recipient, 946t, 948–949, 951t
Tadalafil
adverse effects of, 887
comparison of phosphodiesterase inhibitors, 889t
dosage of, 887t
drug interactions of, 121, 124, 142t, 146, 887, 902
in erectile dysfunction, 887t, 888
mechanism of action of, 888
Taenia saginata, 1294
Taenia solium, 1294
Tamm-Horsfall protein, 1309
Tamoxifen, 1469
adverse effects of, 974, 1469, 1486, 1486, 1487t, 1574t
in breast cancer, 1486, 1487t, 1487
in cancer therapy, 1469
dosage of, 1487t, 1574t
drug interactions of, 205t, 955t, 1469
hypercalcemia with, 490
mechanism of action of, 1469
in melanoma, 1662
ocular changes with, 1077t
in ovarian cancer, 1574t
pharmacokinetics of, 1469
in prevention of breast cancer, 1478–1479
Tamsulosin
adverse effects of, 901t, 902
in benign prostatic hyperplasia, 902
dosage of, 901
pharmacologic properties of, 901t
in urinary incontinence, 917
uroselectivity of, 901, 901t, 902
Tangentiality, in schizophrenia, 633
Tanning device, 1613
Tapeworms, 1293–1265
Taranabant in obesity, 1727
Tardive dyskinesia with antipsychotics, 636, 642, 643, 648
Target of rapamycin inhibitors, in transplant recipient, 952
Tarsorrhaphy, lateral, in dry eye, 1075
Taxane
in breast cancer, 1493
Taxanes
allergic drug reactions, 933

in breast cancer, 1484*t*, 1488, 1491
in ovarian cancer, 1389–1392, 1392*t*, 1572–1573
Tazarotene
  in acne vulgaris, 1097, 1097*t*
  adverse effects of, 1084, 1097*t*
  dosage of, 1097*t*
  in psoriasis, 1085
  teratogenicity of, 1085
Tazobactam. *See* Piperacillin-tazobactam
T-cell-depleted hematopoietic cells, 1634
T-cell receptors, 942
T cells
  in allergic drug reactions, 928
  allorecognition, 942
  cytotoxic, 942
  helper, 912
  in psoriasis, 1080
  regulatory, 942
  in rheumatoid arthritis, 982
  solid-organ transplantation and, 942
Tegaserod maleate
  adverse effects of, 374, 384
  in constipation, 374
  diarrhea with, 374
  dosage of, 384*t*
  in irritable bowel syndrome, 384, 384*t*
Telangiectasias, corticosteroid-induced, 1085
Telithromycin
  in COPD, 299*t*
  dosage of, 1212*t*
  in pneumonia, 1196*t*
  in rhinosinusitis, 1212*a*, 1210, 1213*t*
Temazepam
  adverse effects of, 717*t*
  dosage of, 698*t*, 716, 717*t*
  in insomnia, 716*t*
  pharmacokinetics of, 698*t*, 716
  in restless-legs syndrome, 717, 77*t*
Temozolomide, 1462
  adverse effects of, 1462
  in cancer therapy, 1462
  dosage of, 1620*t*
  mechanism of action of, 1462, 1662
  in melanoma, 1620*t*, 1662
  pharmacokinetics of, 1462
Temporal lobectomy, in epilepsy, 527
Temsirolimus
  adverse effects of, 1463
  in cancer therapy, 1463
  pharmacokinetics of, 1463
  in renal cell carcinoma, 1463
Tendinosis, 1020
Tendon, 1020, 1020*f*
Tendonitis, 1019
  clinical presentation in, 1021
  pathophysiology of, 1020
  treatment of, 1025
Tenecteplase
  in acute coronary syndromes, 135, 141*t*, 144
  dosage of, 141*t*
Tenesmus
  in amebiasis, 1296
  in shigellosis, 1268
Teniposide, 1459
  adverse effects of, 1459, 1469
  in cancer therapy, 1459
  extravasation of, 1678*t*
  mechanism of action of, 1460
  pharmacokinetics of, 1460
Tenofovir
  adverse effects of, 442, 1427*t*–1428*t*, 1437*t*–1440*t*
  dosage of, 1427*t*–1428*t*
  drug interactions of, 1427*t*–1428*t*

in HIV infection, 1420, 1426, 1427*t*–1428*t*
  mechanism of action of, 1421*f*
Tenosynovitis, 1020
Tension-type headache
  chronic, 585
  clinical presentation in, 585
  diagnosis of, 585
  epidemiology of, 585
  episodic, 585
  etiology of, 585
  outcome evaluation in, 589
  pathophysiology of, 584
  patient care and monitoring in, 592
  prevention of, 589
  treatment of, 588
Teratogen(s), 550, 592, 820, 823, 824*t*, 993
Teratogenic potential, 366
Terazosin
  adverse effects of, 63*t*, 901, 902, 901*t*, 906*t*
  in benign prostatic hyperplasia, 902
  dosage of, 63*t*
  drug interactions of, 902
  in hypertension, 63*t*, 69
  mechanism of action of, 901
  pharmacologic properties of, 901*t*
  in urinary incontinence, 917
Terbinafine
  adverse effects of, 86*t*
  dosage of, 1372
  in onychomycosis, 1371–1372
  in tinea infections, 1371
Terbutaline
  arrhythmia with, 177*t*
  in asthma, 277*t*
  contraindications to, 834
  in COPD, 294, 395*t*
  dosage of, 295*t*, 831*t*, 832*t*
  in prevention of priapism, 1146
  as tocolytic, 831*t*, 834
Terconazole
  dosage of, 831*t*, 1363*t*, 1364*t*
  in pregnancy, 831*t*
  in vulvovaginal candidiasis, 831*t*, 1363*t*, 1364, 1264*t*
Terfenadine, arrhythmia with, 180
Teriparatide
  adverse effects of, 975, 977
  dosage of, 973*t*, 975
  mechanism of action of, 975
  in osteoporosis, 973*t*, 977
Terminal secretions
  nonpharmacologic treatment, in palliative care, 45
  palliative care considerations, 45
  pharmacotherapy, in palliative care, 46
Testicular cancer, tumor lysis syndrome in, 1674*t*
Testosterone, 897, 1536
  biosynthesis of, 1539
  in erectile function, 885
  metabolism of, 902
  in prostate cancer, 1538, 1544
  teratogenic effects of, 824*t*
Testosterone cypionate, 887*t*
Testosterone enanthate, 887*t*
Testosterone therapy
  adverse effects of, 890
  buccal mucoadhesive system, 890
  dosage of, 887*t*
  drug interactions of, 205*t*, 955*t*
  in erectile dysfunction, 884*f*, 887*t*, 890
  injectable esters, 890
  oral, 890

topical, 890
  voiding symptoms with, 901*t*
Tetanolysin, 1406
Tetanospasmin, 1406
Tetanus, prophylaxis in bite wounds, 1232
Tetanus toxoid, 1405
Tetanus vaccine, 1416
Tetany, in tumor lysis syndrome, 1674
Tetracycline
  in acne vulgaris, 1098, 1098*t*
  administration through feeding tube, 1716
  adverse effects of, 1098, 1098*t*
  in cellulitis, 1224
  dosage of, 335*t*, 831*t*, 1098*t*, 1322
  drug interactions of, 850*t*, 964, 1115
  in gonorrhea, 1320
  in *Helicobacter pylori* eradication, 333, 334, 335*t*, 1562
  pancreatitis with, 404*f*
  in pregnancy, 831*t*
  in syphilis, 831*t*, 1322
  teratogenic effects of, 824*t*, 743
  in urinary tract infections, 1311*t*, 1314
Tetracycline resistance, 1194*t*
Tetracyclines
  in urinary tract infections, 1314*t*
  teratogenic effects of, 824*t*
Tetrahydrozoline in allergic rhinitis, 1055
Texas Implementation of Medication Algorithms, 642
Texas Medication Algorithm Project, 662, 663*a*
T4, dosage, 832*t*
Thalamotomy, in Parkinson's disease, 557
Thalassemia
  α-thalassemia, 1114*a*
  β-thalassemia, 1114*a*
    HbS β⁺-thalassemia, 1140
    HbS β⁰-thalassemia, 1140
  treatment of, 1630, 1630*t*
Thalidomide, 1464
  adverse effects of, 1464, 1607*t*, 1606
  antiandrogenic properties of, 1606
  arrhythmia with, 163*t*
  mechanism of action of, 1464
  in melanoma with brain metastasis, 1662
  in multiple myeloma, 1464, 1606, 1607*t*
  pharmacokinetics of, 1464
  teratogenicity of, 824*t*, 1608
THAM
  in metabolic acidosis, 502
  in respiratory acidosis, 504
Theophylline
  adverse effects of, 278, 296
  anxiety with, 694*t*
  arrhythmia with, 166*t*, 177*t*
  in asthma, 269, 278
  in COPD, 295*t*, 296
  diarrhea with, 376*t*
  dosage of, 295*t*
  drug interactions of, 614*t*, 615*t*, 660*t*, 699*t*, 850*t*, 1015, 1165, 1364
  enuresis with, 920
  GERD with, 317*t*
  migraines with, 588*t*
  nausea and vomiting with, 358*t*
  in respiratory acidosis, 503
  seizures with, 522
Thiamine
  in alcoholism, 544, 616, 618
  deficiency of, 1697
  dosage of, 546*t*
  in parenteral nutrition admixture, 1687
  in status epilepticus, 546*t*

Thiazide diuretics. *See also specific drugs*
  allergic drug reactions, 931
  in chronic kidney disease, 453
  dosage of, 64
  drug interactions of, 245, 679
  erectile dysfunction with, 881*t*
  gout with, 1011
  in heart failure, 89, 91, 101
  hypercalcemia with, 490
  hyperlipidemia with, 236*t*
  in hypertension, 63*t*, 64
  hypokalemia with, 487, 490
  hypomagnesemia with, 492
  in osteoporosis, 977
  pancreatitis with, 404*f*
  voiding symptoms with, 901*t*
Thiazolidinediones
  adverse effects of, 84*t*, 86*t*, 748*t*, 750
  in diabetes mellitus, 748*t*, 750
  mechanism of action of, 750
  in menstruation-related disorders, 859*t*
Thiethylperazine
  adverse effects of, 361*t*
  dosage of, 361*t*
  in nausea and vomiting, 360, 361*t*
Thimerosal, 418, 1415
  in acute lymphocytic leukemia, 1588*t*, 1590*t*
  dosage of, 1588*t*, 1590*t*
Thiopurine methyltransferase deficiency, 1589
Thioridazine
  adverse effects of, 642*t*
  arrhythmia with, 164*t*, 177*t*, 179*t*
  dosage of, 641*t*
  drug interactions of, 646*t*, 647, 660*t*
  metabolism of, 646*t*
  in schizophrenia, 641*t*
Thiotepa, 1462
  adverse effects of, 1462
  in breast cancer, 1491
  in cancer therapy, 1462
  hemorrhagic cystitis with, 1666*t*
  mechanism of action of, 1462
  pharmacokinetics of, 1462
Thiothixene
  adverse effects of, 642*t*
  dosage of, 641*t*
  in schizophrenia, 641*t*
Third spacing, 253, 480, 1260
Thoracentesis, in lung cancer, 1504
Thoracic surgery, arrhythmia in, 166*t*
Thought blocking, in schizophrenia, 633
Thrombectomy, in venous thromboembolism, 206
Thrombin, 187, 196, 1121, 1122*f*
Thrombin inhibitors, direct. *See* Direct thrombin
      inhibitors
Thrombin time, 1136
Thrombocytopenia
  allergic drug reaction, 929*t*
  with ATG, 947
  chemotherapy-related, 1469, 1453*t*, 1594
  contraindication to heparin, 1687
  in hematopoietic cell transplant recipients, 1641
  heparin-induced, 140, 145–146, 187*t*, 196, 198,
      198*t*
  in liver disease, 391
  in sepsis, 1349
  toxicity criteria, 1453*t*
  treatment of, 1469
Thrombocytopenic purpura immune. *See*
      Immune thrombocytopenic purpura
  thrombotic. *See* Thrombotic
      thrombocytopenic purpura
Thrombocytosis, in rheumatoid arthritis, 984

Thromboembolism
  prevention in hypovolemic shock, 260–261
  venous. *See* Venous thromboembolism
Thrombogenesis, 187
Thrombolytic therapy
  adverse effects of, 221
  intra-arterial, 222
  in stroke, 220–222
  streptokinase, 221
  in venous thromboembolism, 195, 195*t*
Thrombophlebitis
  with parenteral nutrition, 1690
  prevention of, 1687
Thromboplastin, 202
Thrombosis, 187, 188*a*
  in hemodialysis, 472
  inhibition by statins, 240
Thrombotic thrombocytopenic purpura
  clinical presentation in, 1135
  clopidogrel-related, 224
  diagnosis of, 1135
  epidemiology of, 1135
  in *Escherichia coli* O157:H7 infections, 1272
  etiology of, 1135
  outcome evaluation in, 1135–1136
  pathophysiology of, 1135
  ticlopidine-related, 223–224
  treatment of, 1135
      corticosteroids, 1135
      plasma exchange, 1135
      splenectomy, 1135
Thrombus, 112, 185, 216, 217, 234
  microthrombi, 1131
Thrush, in transplant recipient, 957
Thymoma, superior vena cava syndrome with,
      1661*t*
Thyroglobulin, 764
Thyroglobulin therapy
  dosage of, 769*t*
  in hypothyroidism, 768, 769*t*
Thyroid (desiccated)
  dosage of, 769*t*
  in hypothyroidism, 768, 769*t*
Thyroid adenoma, 774*t*
Thyroid-binding globulin, 764
Thyroid cancer, 774*t*, 767
  epidemiology of, 1446*f*
  genetic factors in, 1447*t*
  treatment of, 765, 767
Thyroid disorders, 763–779
  diagnosis of, 765–766, 766*t*, 767*f*
      thyroid hormone levels, 766
      thyroid-stimulating hormone levels, 766, 767*f*
  drug-induced, 771*t*, 778–779
  epidemiology of, 765
  hypertension and, 54
  nausea and vomiting in, 296*t*
  patient assessment and monitoring in, 642,
      642*t*, 643*a*
  pregnancy, 836
  spectrum of, 764–765
Thyroidectomy, subtotal, in hyperthyroidism, 777
Thyroid hormone(s)
  biosynthesis of, 765, 767*f*
  physiology of, 765, 767*f*
Thyroid hormone therapy
  anxiety with, 694*t*
  osteoporosis with, 953*t*
Thyroiditis
  adrenal insufficiency and, 778–779
  autoimmune, 767*t*
  silent (painless), 774*t*
  subacute, 774*t*

Thyroid nodule, toxic, 773
Thyroid peroxidase, 764
Thyroid scan, radionuclide, 766
Thyroid-stimulating hormone, 764, 765*f*
  in hyperthyroidism, 767, 767*f*
  in hypothyroidism, 767, 767*f*
  normal range of, 766*t*
Thyroid storm, 777
Thyrotoxicosis, 766, 772–774
  chest pain in, 111*t*
  clinical presentation in, 774
  drug-induced, 776
  etiology of, 773, 774*t*
  gestational, 774*t*
  without hyperthyroidism, 774*t*
  patient care and monitoring in, 773
  psychotic symptoms in, 635*t*
  respiratory alkalosis in, 504*t*
  subclinical, 774
  treatment of, 774–776
Thyrotoxicosis factitia, 774*t*
Thyrotropin-releasing hormone, 764, 765*f*, 813
Thyroxine, 764
  drug interactions of, 245
  in thyroid disorders, 766
Tiagabine
  adverse effects of, 534*t*
  dosage of, 534*t*
  drug interactions of, 537*t*
  in epilepsy, 530, 530*t*, 531, 534*t*, 537*t*
  mechanism of action of, 534*t*
  pharmacokinetics of, 534*t*
Ticarcillin-clavulanate
  in cystic fibrosis, 309*t*, 310
  dosage of, 309*t*, 1199*t*, 1660*t*
  in infections in cancer patients, 1660*t*
  in intra-abdominal infections, 1287*t*
  in pneumonia, 1196, 1199*t*
  in urinary tract infections, 1311*t*
Ticlopidine
  dosage of, 225*t*
  drug interactions of, 205*t*, 537*t*
  in prevention of stroke, 223–224
Tigecycline
  in cellulitis, 1225*t*
  in diabetic foot infections, 1229*t*
  dosage of, 1225*t*
  in methicillin-resistant *Staphylococcus aureus*,
      1354
Tiludronate, in osteoporosis, 973–974
TIMI risk score, for non-ST-segment elevation
      acute coronary syndromes, 136, 1391*t*
Timolol
  in arrhythmias, 162*t*
  dosage of, 124*t*, 1038*t*
  in glaucoma, 1038*t*, 1040
  in hypertension, 66*a*
  in ischemic heart disease, 124*t*
  mechanism of action of, 162, 1038*t*
  in prevention of migraine, 590, 590*t*
Timolol-dorzolamide
  dosage of, 1038*t*
  in glaucoma, 1038*t*, 1040
  mechanism of action of, 1038*t*
Tinea barbae, 1370*t*
Tinea capitis, 1370*t*
Tinea corporis, 1366, 1370*t*
Tinea cruris, 1366, 1370*t*
Tinea infection, 1371
Tinea manuum, 1370*t*
Tinea pedis, 1370*t*
Tinea unguium, 1370*t*
Tinea versicolor, 1370*t*

Tinidazole
adverse effects of, 1326
in amebiasis, 1296
dosage of, 1296, 1326
in giardiasis, 1294
in trichomoniasis, 1326
Tinzaparin
dosage of, 192t, 193, 195t, 199
in prevention of venous thromboembolism,
193, 195t, 198
in venous thromboembolism, 195t, 198, 199
Tioconazole
dosage of, 1363t
in vulvovaginal candidiasis, 1363t
Tiotropium
in asthma, 276
in COPD, 293, 294, 295t, 296
dosage of, 295t
Tipranavir
adverse effects of, 1432t, 1437t–1440
dosage of, 1432t
drug interactions of, 1432t, 1433
food interactions of, 1432t
in HIV infection, 1432t
mechanism of action of, 1421f
Tirofiban
in acute coronary syndromes, 141t, 145, 147
adverse effects of, 147
dosage of, 141t
Tissue factor, 188
Tissue plasminogen activator, 188
in stroke, 226t
in venous thromboembolism, 195
Tizanidine
dosage of, 440t
mechanism of action of, 440t
in spasticity, 440t
TNM staging, 1449, 1450t
of breast cancer, 1478, 1479t
of colorectal cancer, 1450t, 1318
of lung cancer, 1504, 1504t
of melanoma, 1615–1616
of prostate cancer, 1540, 1541t
Tobacco. See Smoking
Tobramycin
clinical parameters for, 1353
in conjunctivitis, 1066, 1066t
in cystic fibrosis, 309, 309t
dosage of, 309t, 1066t, 1199t, 1287t, 1660t
drug interactions of, 955
in infections in cancer patients, 1660t
in infective endocarditis, 1245
inhaled, 309
in intra-abdominal infections, 1287t
in keratitis, 1071t
in meningitis, 1146
nephrotoxicity of, 440
in pneumonia, 1198, 1199t
in urinary tract infections, 1311t
Tocainide
in arrhythmias, 162t
mechanism of action of, 112t
Tocilizumab, 992
Tocolytics, 831t–832t, 834
Today sponge, 852
Toilet mapping, 901
Tolazamide
in diabetes mellitus, 747t
dosage of, 747t
Tolbutamide
in diabetes mellitus, 747t
dosage of, 747t
drug interactions of, 660t

Tolcapone
dosage of, 559t
mechanism of action of, 559t
in Parkinson's disease, 559t, 562
Tolmetin
dosage of, 1014t
in gout, 1014t
Tolterodine
adverse effects of, 915, 916t
in benign prostatic hyperplasia, 905
dosage of, 916t
pharmacokinetics of, 916t
in urinary incontinence, 516, 563, 915, 916t
Tolvaptan, in heart failure, 104
Tonometry, 1036
Topical analgesics, in osteoarthritis, 1002t, 1006
Topiramate
adverse effects of, 529t
in alcohol dependence, 626
in bipolar disorder, 677t, 684
dosage of, 529t, 549, 677t
drug interactions of, 537t, 850t
in epilepsy, 529t, 530t, 531, 534t, 537t
mechanism of action of, 529t
metabolic acidosis with, 501t
pharmacokinetics of, 529t
in prevention of migraine, 590, 590t
in status epilepticus, 549
Topoisomerase inhibitors, 1459
in colorectal cancer, 1529
secondary malignancies and, 1594
Topotecan, 1459
adverse effects of, 1459, 1574t
in cancer therapy, 1459
dosage of, 1507t, 1574t
in renal dysfunction, 1507t
extravasation of, 1678t
in lung cancer, 1507t, 1508, 1509
mechanism of action of, 1459
in ovarian cancer, 1573, 1574t
pharmacokinetics of, 1459
Toremifene, 1469
adverse effects of, 974, 1469, 1487t
in breast cancer, 1486, 1487t
in cancer therapy, 1469
dosage of, 1486, 1487t
mechanism of action of, 1469
pharmacokinetics of, 1469
Torsades de pointes, 179–181
clinical presentation in, 180
diagnosis of, 180
drug-related, 179, 179t
epidemiology of, 179
etiology of, 179
outcome evaluation in, 181
pathophysiology of, 179–180
prevention of, 180
treatment of, 180–181
Torsemide
in acute renal failure, 437
adverse effects of, 437
dosage of, 90t, 100t, 437
in heart failure, 89, 90, 90t, 91, 100, 100t
in hypertension, 65
Tositumomab, 1466
adverse effects of, 1466
in cancer therapy, 1466
mechanism of action of, 1466
Total-body irradiation, in preparation for
hematopoietic cell transplant, 1634–1635, 1644
Total body water, 479–480
estimation of, 484–485
Total iron-binding capacity, 1112, 1113t

Total parenteral nutrition. See Parenteral
nutrition
Toxic epidermal necrolysis
allergic drug reaction, 929, 931
drug-related, 1437t
Toxic megacolon, 1274
Toxic shock-like syndrome, group A streptococci
in, 1227
Toxic shock syndrome, barrier contraception
and, 852
Toxin A, Clostridium difficile, 1274
Toxin B, Clostridium difficile, 1274
Toxoid. See also specific products
definition of, 1415
Trabecular meshwork, 1033, 1035, 1040, 1042
Trace elements, for parenteral nutrition,
1686–1687
Tracheal aspirate, 1198
Tracheostomy, in obstructive sleep apnea, 717–718
Tramadol
adverse effects of, 576, 1006
dosage of, 1002t
drug interactions of, 660, 661t, 1006
mechanism of action of, 575
in osteoarthritis, 1005t, 1006
in pain, 576
seizures with, 522
Trandolapril
in acute coronary syndromes, 142t
adverse effects of, 62t
dosage of, 62t, 92t, 121t, 142t
in heart failure, 92t
in hypertension, 62t
in ischemic heart disease, 121t
Tranexamic acid
in hemophilia A, 1124
in recessively inherited coagulation disorders,
1130
in von Willebrand's disease, 1128, 1129
Transcellular fluid, 480
Transcranial magnetic stimulation, in
depression, 653
Transcutaneous electrical nerve stimulation
in dysmenorrhea, 863
in pain, 568, 574
Transdermal fentanyl in osteoarthritis, 1006
Transesophageal echocardiogram, in atrial
thrombus, 171
Transferrin saturation, 1112, 1113t
Transfusion reaction, DIC with, 1131t
Transfusion therapy
chronic, in sickle cell anemia/disease, 1143t,
1145–1146
risks of, 1145
in splenic sequestration crisis, 1143t, 1146
Transient ischemic attack, 216, 217t
Transjugular intrahepatic portosystemic shunt,
in portal hypertension, 395
Translocation, of bacteria from gut, 1704, 1709
Transplantation. See Solid-organ transplantation
Transsphenoidal adenomectomy, in
hyperprolactinemia, 816
Transsphenoidal pituitary microsurgery
in acromegaly, 804
complications of, 804
in Cushing's disease, 793
Transthyretin, 764
Transurethral incision of the prostate, in benign
prostatic hyperplasia, 898
Transvenous pacing, 164
Tranylcypromine
dosage of, 661t
drug interactions of, 614t

Trastuzumab, 1467
  adverse effects of, 1467, 1484t, 1489
  in breast cancer, 1482, 1484, 1484t, 1489, 1493
  in cancer therapy, 1452t, 1467
  cardiotoxicity of, 1489
  dosage of, 1484t
  mechanism of action of, 1467
  pharmacokinetics of, 1467
  pulmonary reactions with, 1489
Trauma patient, enteral nutrition in, 1708–1709, 1708t
Travelers' diarrhea, 366, 367, 379t, 380, 1273–1274
  clinical presentation in, 1275
  diagnosis of, 1274
  epidemiology of, 1274
  monitoring patient with, 1274
  prevention of, 1274
  treatment of, 1273–1274
Travoprost
  administration of, 1040
  adverse effects of, 1040
  dosage of, 1038t
  in glaucoma, 1038t, 1040
  mechanism of action of, 1038t, 1040
Trazodone
  adverse effects of, 658, 717
  in Alzheimer's disease, 603
  arrhythmia with, 179t
  dosage of, 661t
  drug interactions of, 659t
  in insomnia, 715
  mechanism of action of, 653, 653t
  in prevention of migraine, 590, 590t
Trematodes, 1293
Tremor, in Parkinson's disease, 554, 555
Trendelenburg position, in hypotension, 471
Treponema pallidum, 1321–1326. *See also* Syphilis
Tretinoin, 1464
  in acne vulgaris, 1097, 1097t
  adverse effects of, 1097t, 1464
  in cancer therapy, 1452t, 1464
  dosage of, 1097t
  mechanism of action of, 1464
  pharmacokinetics of, 1464
Triamcinolone
  in adrenal insufficiency, 789t
  adverse effects of, 1059
  in allergic rhinitis, 1052, 1052t, 1059
  in asthma, 276t
  in contact dermatitis, 1104t
  in COPD, 295t
  dosage of, 276t, 295t, 1014t, 1104t
  in gout, 1014t, 1013
  in psoriasis, 1085
Triamterene, in hypertension, 60t, 65
Triazolam
  dosage of, 716t
  drug interactions of, 614t, 955t
  in insomnia, 716t
  pharmacokinetics of, 716t
Trichloroacetic acid
  adverse effects of, 1327t, 1328
  in genital warts, 1328
Trichomoniasis, 1326
  clinical presentation in, 1326
  diagnosis of, 1326
  epidemiology of, 1326
  pathophysiology of, 1326
  in pregnancy, 816, 830t, 834
  treatment of, 1326
Trichophyton, 1369
Trichophyton rubrum, 1369
Trichosporon, 1376t

Tricuspid valve stenosis, 80, 80t
Tricyclic antidepressants. *See also specific drugs*
  adverse effects of, 563, 657, 658t, 701
  anxiety with, 694t
  arrhythmia with, 164t, 177t
  constipation with, 372t
  dosage of, 661t
  drug interactions of, 659, 660t
  in elderly, 665
  in enuresis, 924
  erectile dysfunction with, 881t
  in generalized anxiety disorder, 696t
  hyperprolactinemia with, 814t
  in irritable bowel syndrome, 383, 384t
  mechanism of action of, 653, 653t
  ocular changes with, 1077t
  in pain, 563, 578
  in panic disorder, 701, 701t
  in pregnancy, 665
  in prevention of migraine, 590, 590t
  in prevention of tension-type headaches, 589
  in smoking cessation, 622, 622t
  in urinary incontinence, 516
  voiding symptoms with, 901t, 921t
Trifluoperazine
  adverse effects of, 642t
  dosage of, 641t
  in schizophrenia, 641t
Trifluridine
  adverse effects of, 1330t
  dosage of, 1330t
  in genital herpes, 1329, 1330t
Trigeminal neuralgia, 570, 590
Trigeminovascular system, in migraine, 585
Trigeminy, 176
Triglycerides
  in intravenous lipid emulsions, 1683, 1684t, 1694
  long-chain, 1707–1708
  medium-chain, 1707–1718
  metabolism of, 230
Trihexyphenidyl, in extrapyramidal symptoms, 647
Triiodothyronine, 763, 764
  in thyroid disorders, 767
Trimethobenzamide
  adverse effects of, 362t
  dosage of, 362t
  in nausea and vomiting, 362t, 363, 367
  in opioid withdrawal, 621t
  prior to apomorphine, 561
Trimethoprim
  in conjunctivitis, 1066, 1066t
  dosage of, 1066t, 1312t
  drug interactions of, 170t
  teratogenic effects of, 824t
  in urinary tract infections, 1312t
Trimethoprim-sulfamethoxazole
  adverse effects of, 956t, 1176t, 1208t
  allergic drug reactions, 930
  arrhythmia with, 179t
  in bite wound infections, 1232
  in cellulitis, 1224, 1225t
  in cholera, 1273
  in cystic fibrosis, 309, 310, 311, 309t
  in diabetic foot infections, 1229t
  dosage of, 956t, 1176t, 1208t, 1212t, 1225t, 1312t
  drug interactions of, 205t
  in eradication of *Salmonella* carriage, 1268
  in infective endocarditis, 1241
  in keratitis, 1071t
  in meningitis, 1176t, 1181
  in osteomyelitis, 1341

  in otitis media, 1208t
  in prevention of infections in neutropenic patients, 1656
  in prevention of *Pneumocystis jiroveci* pneumonia, 956t, 957, 1594
  in prevention of spontaneous bacterial peritonitis, 399
  in rhinosinusitis, 1212a, 1212t, 1213a
  in travelers' diarrhea, 1273
  in urinary tract infections, 1311t, 1312, 1312t
Trimethoprim-sulfamethoxazole resistance, 1194t, 1312
Trimipramine
  dosage of, 661t
  drug interactions of, 614t
Tripelennamine, in allergic rhinitis, 1057
Triptans. *See also specific drugs*
  adverse effects of, 588
  in cluster headaches, 589
  drug interactions of, 560
  in migraine, 586, 589t, 590
Triptorelin
  adverse effects of, 1487t, 1544t
  dosage of, 1487t, 1544t
  in breast cancer, 1487, 1487t
  in prostate cancer, 1544t
Trolamine salicylate
  in musculoskeletal disorders, 1026t
  in osteoarthritis, 1006
Troleandomycin, drug interactions of, 955t
Tromethamine. *See* THAM
Trophoblastic tumor, 774t
Trophozoites, 1294, 1295
Tropicamide, in ocular trauma, 1070
Troponins, cardiac, in acute coronary syndromes, 114, 133, 134, 135
Trospium chloride
  adverse effects of, 916t
  dosage of, 916t
  pharmacokinetics of, 916t
  in urinary incontinence, 915, 916t
Trousseau's sign, 489
Trypanosoma cruzi, 1303
Trypanosomiasis, American. *See* American trypanosomiasis
Trypsin, 404
Trypsin inhibitor, 404
T-score, 968, 968t, 970
TSH receptor antibodies, 766t, 767, 783
Tubal ligation
  efficacy of, 844t
  in prevention of ovarian cancer, 1567
Tube feeding, 1701–1716. *See also* Enteral nutrition
Tuberculin reaction, 929t
Tuberculosis, 1253–1263
  active disease, 1261
  adrenal insufficiency in, 786t
  case study of, 1256, 1259, 1261, 1263
  clinical presentation in, 1257–1258
  diagnosis of, 1258–1260, 1258t
  in elderly, 1258
  epidemiology of, 1256
  ethnicity and, 1256
  etiology of, 1256–1257
  extrapulmonary, 1257, 1261
  HIV infection and, 1256–1258, 1261–1262
  latent infection, 1260–1261, 1260t
  liver failure and, 1264
  miliary, 1257
  outcome evaluation in, 1263
  pathophysiology of, 1257
  patient care and monitoring in, 1263
  in pediatric patients, 1258, 1261, 1261t

peritonitis in, 1260–1261
in pregnancy, 1261
primary infection, 1257
progressive primary disease, 1257
reactivation disease, 876, 1257–1258
renal failure and, 1262–1264
risk factors
    for disease, 1256
    for infection, 1256
skin test for, 1258–1259, 1258t
transmission of, 1257
treatment of, 1260–1263
    directly observed therapy, 1260–1261, 1263
    nonpharmacologic, 1260
    pharmacologic, 1260–1263, 1259t, 1260t,
        1261t–1262t
    therapeutic drug monitoring in, 1261, 1163
Tubulin active agents, 1457–1459
Tubulointerstitial nephropathy, 1004
Tumor
    benign, 1449
    growth of, 1442, 1448f
    malignant, 1449
    tissue of origin of, 1449
Tumor embolism, 253t
Tumor lysis syndrome, 1673–1676
    in acute leukemia, 1594
    in antihyperuricemic treatment, 1016–1017
    case study of, 1673–1675
    clinical presentation in, 1675
    diagnosis of, 1675
    epidemiology of, 1674
    etiology of, 1674
    outcome evaluation in, 1677
    pathophysiology of, 1675
    patient care and monitoring in, 1677
    prevention of, 1594, 1675
    risk factors for, 1674t
    treatment of, 1675–1676, 1674a, 1675a, 1676t
Tumor necrosis factor-α
    in cachexia, 1512
    in heart failure, 84
    in meningitis, 1172
    in psoriasis, 1080
    in rheumatoid arthritis, 982, 982t
Tumor necrosis factor-α antagonists, in
        rheumatoid
    arthritis, 990–991
Tumor necrosis factor-α inhibitors, in psoriasis,
    1087
Tumor-suppressor genes, 1446, 1447t, 1520
Turmeric, 206t
Turner's syndrome, menstruation-related disorders
    in, 857t
T wave, 159f, 160
Twelve-step facilitation, in substance
        dependence, 624
Twinrix, 421–422, 1414
Twisthaler, 271
Tympanic temperature readings, 24
Tympanocentesis, 1205, 1207
Tympanostomy tubes, in otitis media, 1205
Typhoid fever, 1268–1269
Typhoid vaccine, 1269
Tyramine, drug interactions of, 659, 660t
Tyrosine kinase inhibitors
    in cancer therapy, 1467
    in lung cancer, 1508–1509

U
UDP-glucuronosyltransferase deficiency, 1529
Uhthoff's phenomenon, 510
Ulcer. See also specific sites and types

aphthous, 343
decubitus. See Pressure sore
foot. See Diabetic foot
peptic. See Peptic ulcer disease
Ulcerations, 327
Ulcerative colitis. See also Inflammatory bowel
        disease
    clinical presentation in, 343–345
    colorectal cancer and, 1518, 1518t
    diagnosis of, 344–345
    epidemiology of, 342
    etiology of, 342
    mild to moderate, 345, 349–350, 352
    moderate, 349, 349t
    outcome evaluation in, 354–355
    pathophysiology of, 342–343, 343f
    patient care and monitoring in, 354
    severe to fulminant, 345, 351–352, 351t
    treatment of, 349–350
        maintenance of remission, 352
Ultrafiltration
    in hemodialysis, 470–471
    in peritoneal dialysis, 472
Ultrase products, 311t, 409t
Ultrasonography
    in acute renal failure, 435
    in breast cancer, 1490
    in cirrhosis, 394
    in pancreatitis, 405
    transvaginal, in ovarian cancer, 1567
    in venous thromboembolism, 190
Ultraviolet light
    skin cancer and, 1613–1614
Umbilical cord blood
    cryopreservation of, 1632
    processing of, 1632
    as source of hematopoietic cells, 1629–1630,
        1632
Undertreatment, in elderly, 14
Underweight, 1721t
Unified Parkinson's Disease Rating Scale, 557
Unilateral pain, with migraine, 585
Universal blood donor, 259
Unstable angina, 110, 113, 119. See also Acute
        coronary syndromes
    clinical presentation in, 113, 114
Unstimulated serum cortisol measurement, 788t
Upper motor neuron spasticity, in multiple
        sclerosis, 516
Upper respiratory tract, normal flora of, 1157f
Upper respiratory tract infection, 1203–1219
Urea breath test, for Helicobacter pylori, 332
Uremia
    bleeding with
        in chronic kidney disease, 467
        pathophysiology of, 467
        treatment of, 467
    in chronic kidney disease, 455
    signs and symptoms of, 435
Ureter, ectopic, 921t
Ureteral diversion, 501t
Urethritis, 1309f
Uric acid, 1011
Uric acid crystals, 1011
Uric acid nephrolithiasis, 1011, 1013
Uricase, polyethylene-bonded, in
        antihyperuricemic treatment, 1015
Uricosurics, 1015
Urinalysis
    in acute renal failure, 435
    in benign prostatic hyperplasia, 900t
Urinary bladder. See also Bladder entries
    neurogenic, 911, 921t

Urinary catheter, indwelling, urinary tract
        infections and, 1314
Urinary incontinence, 909–919
    case study of, 910, 919, 918
    clinical presentation in, 912–913
    diagnosis of, 912–913, 913t
    drug-induced, 912, 921t
    epidemiology of, 912
    etiology of, 912
    functional, 911
    in menopause, 910, 912
    mixed, 912
    in multiple sclerosis, 516
    outcome evaluation in, 918–919
    overflow (urethral overactivity; bladder
        underactivity), 912, 918
    patient care and monitoring in, 919
    stress (urethral underactivity), 910, 910–912,
        917, 918t
    treatment of, 914–918
        α-adrenoceptor agonists, 918
        α-adrenoceptor blockers, 918
        anticholinergics/antispasmodics, 915, 916t
        bethanechol, 917
        duloxetine, 918t, 917
        estrogen therapy, 916, 917, 918t
        nonpharmacologic, 914–915
        surgery, 914–915
    urge (bladder overactivity), 901, 916t
Urinary outflow obstruction, 433
Urinary tract infection, 1158, 1307–1314
    benign prostatic hyperplasia and, 1313
    case study of, 1308, 1311
    in catheterized patients, 1313
    clinical presentation in, 1309
    complicated, 1308, 1312t
    diagnosis of, 1309
    enuresis with, 921t
    epidemiology of, 1307–1308
    etiology of, 1307–1308
    host defense mechanisms against, 1308
    in men, 1313
    outcome evaluation in, 1313
    pathophysiology of, 1308–1309, 1309f
    patient care and monitoring in, 1314, 1314t
    in pregnancy, 1314
    prevention of
        nonpharmacologic therapy, 1310
        pharmacologic therapy, 1310–1313
    routes of infection, 1308, 1309f
    sepsis and, 1353, 1353t
    treatment of, 1312–1313, 1311t, 1312t, 1314t
    uncomplicated, 1310–1312, 1312t
    urinary incontinence in, 901
Urine
    alkalinization in tumor lysis syndrome, 1674
    bacterial growth in, 1309
    output in acute renal failure, 431
Urokinase
    in hemodialysis-associated thrombosis, 472
    in venous thromboembolism, 195, 195t
Urokinase plasminogen activator, 188, 189f
Urolithiasis, drug-related, 1438t
Urologic surgery, antimicrobial prophylaxis in, 1400
Ursodiol
    in prevention of cholestasis, 1696
    in prevention of sinusoidal obstruction
        syndrome, 1637
Urticaria
    allergic drug reaction, 929–933, 929t
    chronic idiopathic, 930
    with opioids, 577t
    treatment of, 577t

Uterine abnormality, menstruation-related disorders in, 857t
Uterine cancer, 1446f
Uterine infection, postoperative, 1283
Uterus
  disorders of, amenorrhea in, 856
  fibroids of, 857t
UVB treatment in psoriasis, 1085
Uveitis
  with β-blockers, 1040
  drug-induced, 1077t
  in inflammatory bowel disease, 344
Uveoscleral outflow, 1033
Uvulopalatopharyngoplasty, in obstructive sleep apnea, 717

V

Vaccination. *See also specific vaccines*
  case study of, 1405, 1410, 1416
  cocoon, 1406
  in COPD, 297
  definition of, 1406
  of health care workers, 1416
  in heart failure patient, 89
  of immunocompromised patients, 1415–1416
  in pregnancy, 1416
  rate in adults and children, 1416
  schedules for, 1414
Vaccine, 1415–1416. *See also specific vaccines*
  administration schedules for, 1414
  attenuated, 1416
  combination, 1414
  cost of, 1416
  safety of, 1414–1415, 1414t
Vaccine Adverse Event Reporting System, 1416
Vacuum erection devices, 884f, 888, 889f
VAD regimen, in multiple myeloma, 1606
Vagal maneuvers, in paroxysmal supraventricular tachycardia, 174
Vaginal discharge, 1331
Vaginal hormonal ring, 848
Vagotomy, in peptic ulcer disease, 333
Vagus nerve stimulation
  in depression, 653
  in epilepsy, 527
Valacyclovir
  adverse effects of, 956t, 1330t
  dosage of, 831t, 956t, 1329, 1330t
  in genital herpes, 1330t
  in prevention of cytomegalovirus, 956t
  in prevention of herpes simplex virus, 1642
  in prevention of transmission of genital herpes, 1329
Valdecoxib, 337
  adverse effects of, 126
  dosage of, 1014t
  in gout, 1014t
  withdrawal from market, 575
Valerian root, 562, 878, 879t
Valganciclovir
  adverse effects of, 956t
  dosage of, 956t
  drug interactions of, 955
  in prevention of cytomegalovirus, 956t, 957
Valproate
  adverse effects of, 528, 529t, 535, 545t, 680, 796t
  in alcohol withdrawal, 611
  augmentation of antidepressant therapy with, 662
  in bipolar disorder, 676t, 678t, 679–680, 682t, 686
  in Cushing's syndrome, 796t
  dosage of, 545t, 546t, 549t, 676t, 679, 796t

drug interactions of, 537, 537t, 680, 699t
  enuresis with, 920
  in epilepsy, 528, 529–530, 529t, 530t, 531, 535, 537, 537t, 538
  mechanism of action of, 456t, 679, 796t
  monitoring therapy with, 679–680, 682t
  pancreatitis with, 404f
  pharmacokinetics of, 678t
  in pregnancy, 537, 686
  in prevention of migraine, 590, 590t
  protein binding of, 528
  in schizophrenia, 647
  in status epilepticus, 547–548, 545t, 546t, 549t
  teratogenic effects of, 824t
Valproic acid, 828t
  teratogenic effects of, 824t
Valsalva maneuver, in paroxysmal supraventricular tachycardia, 174
Valsartan
  in acute coronary syndromes, 143t
  adverse effects of, 62t
  dosage of, 62t, 92t, 121t, 143t
  in heart failure, 92t
  in hypertension, 62t, 67, 69
  in ischemic heart disease, 120, 121t
  in prevention of myocardial infarction, 150
Valvular heart disease, 111t
  heart transplantation in, 942
Vancomycin, 27
  adverse effects of, 1175t, 1176t
  allergic drug reactions, 929t
  in catheter-related infections, 475
  in cellulitis, 1225t
  in *Clostridium difficile*-associated diarrhea, 1274
  in cystic fibrosis, 309t, 310, 310t, 311
  in diabetic foot infections, 1229t
  dosage of, 251t, 831t, 832t, 1175t, 1176t, 1077t, 1199t, 1225t, 1231t, 1244t, 1245t, 1246t, 1247t, 1249t, 1342t
  drug interactions of, 1164
  in infected pressure sores, 1231t
  in infections in cancer patients, 1657, 1660t
  in infective endocarditis, 1241, 1244t, 1245, 1245t, 1246t, 1247t, 1249t
  in intra-abdominal infections, 1287t
  in keratitis, 1071t
  in meningitis, 1171t, 1175t, 1176t, 1077t, 1181
  in methicillin-resistant *Staphylococcus aureus*, 1354
  in osteomyelitis, 1339t, 1342t, 1344t
  in pancreatitis, 407t
  in peritonitis, 474
  in pneumonia, 1197, 1199t
  in postneurosurgical infections, 1146
  in pregnancy, 831t
  in sepsis, 1353, 1353t
  in *Streptococcus* group B infection, 831t
  in surgical prophylaxis, 1399, 1400t, 1041
Vaporization
  adverse effects of, 1327t
  of genital warts, 1327
Vardenafil
  adverse effects of, 887–888
  comparison of phosphodiesterase inhibitors, 889t
  dosage of, 887t
  drug interactions of, 121, 124, 142t, 146, 902
  in erectile dysfunction, 887–888, 887t
  mechanism of action of, 887
Variceal bleeding, 387, 388
  case study of, 400
  in cirrhosis, 391, 392, 393, 394–395

in end-stage liver disease, 413
  outcome evaluation in, 400
  treatment of, 394–395, 397
    algorithm for, 329f
    antibiotics, 399
    octreotide, 399
Varicella vaccine, 418–419, 1408t, 1414, 1414t, 1415–1416
Varicella-zoster virus
  in CNS infections, 1183
  in hematopoietic cell transplant recipients, 1641–1642
  in pneumonia, 1190
Varicose veins, 187t
Vascular disease, in diabetes mellitus, 740
Vascular injury, venous thromboembolism and, 186, 187–188, 187f
Vascular resistance, in shock, 252
Vascular surgery, antimicrobial prophylaxis in, 1400t, 1401
Vasculitis, 433
  allergic drug reaction, 929t
  in rheumatoid arthritis, 982
Vasectomy, 844t
Vasoconstriction, in heart failure, 81t
Vasoconstrictors, in priapism, 1146
Vasodilators. *See also specific drugs*
  adverse effects of, 71t
  dosage of, 71t
  in heart failure, 82, 83, 91, 94, 97, 98, 100–101, 102
  in hypertension, 54t, 63t, 67, 69, 71t
  in hypertensive emergency, 71t
  in priapism, 1146
Vasomotor symptoms, of menopause, 869, 870, 871, 876, 879t
Vaso-occlusive pain crisis
  in sickle cell anemia/disease, 1141, 1143t, 1145t, 1144–1146
  treatment of, 1143t, 1145t, 1144–1146
Vasopressin, 803
  dosage of, 179t
  for facilitation of defibrillation, 178, 179t
  in heart failure, 83, 104
  in hemorrhagic cystitis, 1670
  in sepsis, 1356
Vasopressors. *See also specific drugs*
  adverse effects of, 259
  in barbiturate coma, 548
  in hypovolemic shock, 257, 260, 260t
  parenteral nutrition and, 1694
  in sepsis, 1356
Vasospasm, 111, 114, 123
Vaughan Williams classification of antiarrhythmic drugs, 161, 162t
Vegetations, 1237, 1237a
Venlafaxine
  adverse effects of, 658, 659t, 701t, 879t
  in cataplexy, 717
  in depression, 665
  dosage of, 661t, 696t, 701t, 879t
  drug interactions of, 955t, 1724
  in elderly, 665
  in generalized anxiety disorder, 696, 696t
  mechanism of action of, 653, 653t
  in pain, 578
  in panic disorder, 701t, 702
  pharmacokinetics of, 659, 659t
  in social anxiety disorder, 704
  in vasomotor symptoms of menopause, 878, 879t
Venography, contrast, in venous thromboembolism, 189, 190

Venous catheter
    double-lumen, vascular access in hemodialysis, 470, 472, 473t
    indwelling, 187t
Venous circulation, 186, 186f
Venous stasis, 187, 187t, 193
Venous thromboembolism, 185–211. *See also* Deep vein thrombosis; Pulmonary embolism
    case study of, 194, 206, 207, 209
    clinical presentation in, 188–190
    coagulation cascade, 187, 188, 191f
    cost of, 186
    diagnosis of, 188–190
    epidemiology of, 186–187
    etiology of, 186–187, 187t
    hormone-replacement therapy and, 876t, 871
    hypercoagulable state and, 186–187, 187t
    oral contraceptives and, 845
    outcome evaluation in, 207–209
    pathophysiology of, 187–188
    patient care and monitoring in, 210–211
    in pediatric patient, 199, 200
    pregnancy and, 186, 187, 187t, 194, 196, 198
    prevention of, 186, 190–194, 192t, 222–224
        nonpharmacologic therapy, 191–193, 192t
        pharmacologic therapy, 191–193
    with raloxifene, 974–975
    recurrent, 187, 189, 193, 197
    risk factors for, 187, 187t
    surgery and, 186, 187t, 193
    treatment of, 194–207
        acute phase, 194, 194a
        anticoagulants, 194, 194a, 194, 196, 198, 199–202, 205, 209
        approach to, 207, 208a
        chronic phase, 194, 194a
        compression stockings, 207
        direct thrombin inhibitors, 200–201
        factor Xa inhibitors, 199–200
        subacute phase, 194, 194a
        thrombectomy, 206
        thrombolytics, 194, 195
        vena cava interruption, 206
        warfarin, 201–206, 209t
    vascular injury and, 186, 187–188, 187t, 189f
    venous circulation, 186f
Venous valves, 187
Ventilation-to-perfusion scan
    in COPD, 291
    in pulmonary embolism, 192
    in venous thromboembolism, 190, 191
Ventilatory support. *See* Assisted ventilation
Ventolin, 271
Ventral tegmental area, in reward pathway, 609, 609f
Ventricular action potential, 159, 159f
Ventricular arrhythmia, 175–181
Ventricular assist device, 104
Ventricular depolarization, 158
Ventricular fibrillation, 134, 160, 177–179
    clinical presentation in, 178
    diagnosis of, 178
    epidemiology of, 177–178
    etiology of, 177t, 177–178
    outcome evaluation in, 179
    treatment of, 178–179
        algorithm for, 178a
        defibrillation, 178, 1179t
Ventricular hypertrophy, in heart failure, 80, 81t, 82
Ventricular premature beats. *See* Ventricular premature depolarizations
Ventricular premature depolarizations, 160, 175–176

clinical presentation in, 176
diagnosis of, 176
epidemiology of, 175
etiology of, 175
outcome evaluation in, 176
pathophysiology of, 175
treatment of, 176
Ventricular tachycardia, 160, 176–177
    clinical presentation in, 177
    diagnosis of, 177
    epidemiology of, 176
    etiology of, 176, 177t
    nonsustained, 176
    outcome evaluation in, 177
    pathophysiology of, 176
    sustained, 176
    treatment of, 176–177
        algorithm for, 178t
        prevention of sudden cardiac death, 177
        termination of VT, 176, 177, 178t
Ventriculoperitoneal shunt, 1283
Verapamil, 10
    in acute coronary syndromes, 142t, 147
    adverse effects of, 61t, 86t, 169t
    in arrhythmias, 162t, 164t
    in atrial fibrillation, 166t, 168, 169t
    dosage of, 61t, 142t, 169t, 175t, 124t
    drug interactions of, 169t, 170t, 175t, 244, 590, 660t, 955t
    effect on myocardial oxygen demand and supply, 122t
    in heart failure, 96, 97
    hyperprolactinemia with, 814t
    in hypertension, 61t, 67
    in ischemic heart disease, 123, 124t
    mechanism of action of, 162t, 169t, 175t
    menstruation-related disorders with, 857t
    in paroxysmal supraventricular tachycardia, 175t
    in prevention of cluster headaches, 590
    in prevention of migraine, 590t
Vertebral fracture, 965, 966, 971, 974
Verteporfin, 1073
Vertigo, 360
    with opioids, 577t
    in stroke, 218
    treatment of, 360, 577t
Very low-density lipoproteins (VLDLs), 230–231, 232, 233f
    physical characteristics of, 231t
Vesicant, 1458, 1677, 1678t
    extravasation of, 1469
Vestibular disturbance
    anxiety with, 694t
    nausea and vomiting in, 367
Vestibular nausea and vomiting, 44
Vibrio cholerae, 376, 1272–1273. *See also* Cholera
Vildagliptin, in diabetes mellitus, 750
Villi, intestinal, 1702
Vinblastine, 1458
    adverse effects of, 1458, 1557t, 1563
    in breast cancer, 1491
    in cancer therapy, 1458
    dosage of, 1557t, 1559t
        in hepatic impairment, 1507t
    drug interactions of, 955t
    extravasation of, 1678t
    in Hodgkin's lymphoma, 1533, 1557t, 1559t
    in immune thrombocytopenic purpura, 1134
    in melanoma, 1662
    pharmacokinetics of, 1458
Vinca alkaloids, 1457–1459. *See also specific drugs*
    in breast cancer, 1484t

drug interactions of, 1378
extravasation of, 1678, 1678t, 1678t
Vincristine, 1457
    in acute lymphocytic leukemia, 1588t, 1590t, 1592t
    adverse effects of, 1457, 1559t, 1563, 1592t, 1607t
    in breast cancer, 1482
    in cancer therapy, 1457
    dosage of, 1507t–1508t, 1557t, 1559t, 1560t, 1561t, 1588t, 1590t
        in hepatic impairment, 1507t
    drug interactions of, 1457, 1591t, 1592t
    extravasation of, 1678t
    in Hodgkin's lymphoma, 1533, 1557t, 1559t
    in immune thrombocytopenic purpura, 1134
    in lung cancer, 1507t–1508t, 1509
    mechanism of action of, 1457, 1592t
    in multiple myeloma, 1606, 1607t
    in non-Hodgkin's lymphoma, 1560t, 1561t
    pharmacokinetics of, 1457
Vinorelbine, 1458
    adverse effects of, 1458, 1484t, 1574t
    in breast cancer, 1482, 1482t, 1490
    in cancer therapy, 1458
    dosage of, 1482t, 1574t
        in hepatic impairment, 1507t
    extravasation of, 1678t
    in lung cancer, 1507, 1508–1509, 1511
    in ovarian cancer, 1573, 1574t
    pharmacokinetics of, 1458
Viokase products, 253t, 409t, 409, 410
Viral hepatitis, 387, 388, 413–427. *See also specific types*
    case study of, 418, 425
    cirrhosis and, 414
    clinical presentation of, 416
    diagnosis of, 416, 417t
    end-stage liver disease and, 413, 418
    epidemiology of, 413–415
    etiology of, 413–415
    fulminant, 414
    outcome evaluation in, 425–427
    pathophysiology of, 415–416
    patient care and monitoring in, 426
    prevention of, 417–425
    risk factors for acquiring, 414t
    treatment of, 417–425
Virilization, in Cushing's syndrome, 792
Virtual phenotype, in HIV infection, 1433
Visceral pain, 45, 569
Viscosupplementation, 1005
Vision, acute loss of, 1069t, 1070
Visual analog scale (pain assessment), 571
Vital signs
    differences in, 24
    in hypovolemic shock, 255
Vitamin A
    deficiency of, 1070t
    for parenteral nutrition, 1686
    pruritus and, 467
    teratogenic effects of, 824t
Vitamin A ointments, for diaper dermatitis, 1106
Vitamin A supplementation/therapy, hypercalcemia with, 490
Vitamin B$_3$. *See* Niacin
Vitamin B$_{12}$
    deficiency of, 1110, 1118
        anxiety with, 694t
        treatment of, 1116
    food sources of, 1115t
Vitamin B$_{12}$ supplementation/therapy
    administration route, 1116
    adverse effects of, 1116

Vitamin B$_{12}$ supplementation/therapy (*Cont.*)
dosage of, 1116
with pemetrexed, 1457
in vitamin B$_{12}$ deficiency, 1116
Vitamin C, in ischemic heart disease, 125
Vitamin C supplementation/therapy
for macular degeneration, 1073
for Parkinson's disease, 562
Vitamin D
activation of, 461
deficiency of, 489, 971
dosage, 830t
in prevention of colon cancer, 1518
prostate cancer and, 1538
recommended daily intake of, 969, 969t, 972
requirement for, 977
Vitamin D analogs, for psoriasis, 1084, 1087
Vitamin D ointments, for diaper dermatitis, 1106
Vitamin D supplementation/therapy
adverse effects of, 972, 1697
for cystic fibrosis, 312
hypercalcemia with, 490
for hyperphosphatemia, 463, 465, 465t, 491
for osteoporosis, 970–973, 972t
products available, 972t
Vitamin E
for ischemic heart disease, 125
in prevention of lung cancer, 11503
in prevention of prostate cancer, 1538
Vitamin E supplementation/therapy
for Alzheimer's disease, 603
drug interactions of, 205t, 206t
for macular degeneration, 1073
for muscle cramps, 472
for Parkinson's disease, 562
Vitamin K
in coagulation disorders, 399–400
deficiency of
in fetal, 686
in newborn, 1132
clinical presentation in, 1132
diagnosis of, 1132
epidemiology of, 1131
etiology of, 1131–1132
outcome evaluation in, 1132
pathophysiology of, 1132
prophylactic therapy, 1131
treatment of, 1132
dietary, 202f, 206
in enteral feeding formulas, 1715
for parenteral nutrition, 1686
Vitamin K–deficiency bleeding, 1132
Vitamin K–dependent coagulation factors, 201
Vitamin K supplementation/therapy
adverse effects of, 204–205
drug interactions of, 205t
in vitamin K–deficiency bleeding, 1131
in warfarin overdose, 204–205
Vitamin supplementation/therapy
for chronic kidney disease, 468
drug interactions of, 245
for inflammatory bowel disease, 344, 345
for parenteral nutrition, 1686
for Parkinson's disease, 562
prenatal vitamins, 823
VLDLs. *See* Very low-density lipoproteins
Voiding regimen, scheduled, in urinary
incontinence, 914
Volume of distribution, in pediatric patients, 27
Volume overload, 54t
Volvulus
in cystic fibrosis, 305
intestine transplantation in, 941

Vomiting, 357–358. *See also* Nausea and vomiting
metabolic alkalosis in, 426t
shock in, 253t
Vomiting center, central, 358
von Willebrand's factor, 1126
ultralarge molecules of, 1135
von Willebrand's factor-cleaving protease, 1135
von Willebrand's disease
clinical presentation in, 1126
diagnosis of, 1126
epidemiology of, 1126
etiology of, 1126
menstruation-related disorders in, 857t
outcome evaluation in, 1128
pathophysiology of, 1126
treatment of, 1126–1128
algorithm for, 1128a
antifibrinolytic therapy, 1128
desmopressin, 1127
fibrinolysis inhibitors, 1127
replacement therapy, 1127–1128, 1128t
type 1, 1127t, 1127
type 2, 1127t, 1127
type 3, 1127t, 1127
Voriconazole
adverse effects of, 1384
arrhythmia with, 179t
in aspergillosis, 1386t, 1391, 1384
dosage of, 1384, 1386t, 1660t
drug interactions of, 955t, 1384
in esophageal candidiasis, 1366, 1387
in fusariosis, 1386t, 1392
in infections in cancer patients, 1386, 1660t
in infective endocarditis, 1246
in invasive candidiasis, 1384, 1386t, 1385
in peritonitis, 475
in sepsis, 1356
Vorinostat
adverse effects of, 1465
in cancer therapy, 1465
pharmacokinetics of, 1465
Vulvovaginal atrophy, in menopause, 871
Vulvovaginal candidiasis, 1361–1365
case study of, 1361–1362
clinical presentation in, 1362
complicated, 1362
diagnosis of, 1362
epidemiology of, 1362
etiology of, 1362
nonalbicans, 1362
outcome evaluation in, 1365
pathophysiology of, 1362
patient care and monitoring in, 1365
in pregnancy, 825, 830t, 834, 743, 1365
recurrent, 1362, 1364, 1264t
risk factors for, 1362, 1363t
treatment of
antifungal therapy, 1364, 1363t, 1264t
cultural awareness, 1365
nonpharmacologic, 1363
uncomplicated, 1363, 1364, 1363t
Vytorin, 246

W

Waist circumference, 1719–1721, 1724, 1729
determination of, 1721
high-risk, 1721
Waldenström's macroglobulinemia, 1608
Warfarin, 10
administration through feeding tube, 1715
adverse effects of, 152t, 172, 198t, 201–202
in atrial fibrillation, 171, 172, 173f, 175a
dosage of, 192t, 173f, 202

drug interactions of, 120t, 205–206, 205t, 206t,
245, 246, 278, 321, 322, 383, 574, 614t,
660t, 955t, 1004, 1013, 1015, 1165, 1364,
1378, 1455, 1726
food interactions of, 205, 206t
in heart failure, 96
initiation of therapy with, 202, 203a
laboratory monitoring of therapy with,
202–203
mechanism of action of, 200f, 201
metabolism of, 201, 202f, 205
in pregnancy, 205
in prevention of deep vein thrombosis, 1606
in prevention of myocardial infarction, 149–151
in prevention of stroke, 173f, 223, 225t
in prevention of venous thromboembolism,
193, 198t
teratogenic effects of, 824t
in venous thromboembolism, 194, 194a, 198t,
201–206, 209t
Warts, genital. *See* Genital warts
Water balance, impaired
in chronic kidney disease, 453
clinical presentation in, 453
in heart failure, 83
Water intoxication, 924
Weight gain
drugs contributing to, 1723t
with oral contraceptives, 848
Weight loss, 1721–1737
in hypertension, 58, 59t
in ischemic heart disease, 117
in pancreatitis, chronic, 408
Weight maintenance, 1732
Wernicke's encephalopathy, 613, 618
Western blot, for HIV, 1422, 1422t
West Nile virus, in CNS infections, 1183
West syndrome, 525t
Wheezing, in asthma, 266
Whipple's disease, 376
White blood cell count
in CSF, 1172t
in infections, 1158, 1159t
White blood cell count differential, in infections,
1158, 1159t
White coat hypertension, 57
Whitehead. *See* Comedo, closed
White petrolatum, for diaper dermatitis, 1106
WHO classification, 1556t
of acute myelogenous leukemia, 1582t
of Hodgkin's lymphoma, 1553, 1553t
of lymphoid neoplasms, 1553t
of non-Hodgkin's lymphoma, 1556
WHO oral rehydration solution, 378
Whole blood, in hypovolemic shock, 259
Whole-brain radiotherapy, in melanoma with
brain metastasis, 1622
Whooping cough. *See* Pertussis
Wild yam, 878, 879t
Willow bark, 206t
Wilms' tumor, kidney transplantation in, 941
Wilson's disease, 851
liver disease in, 392
liver transplantation in, 941
osteoarthritis in, 998t
Wind-up phenomenon, 569
Witch hazel in contact dermatitis, 1102
Withdrawal (contraception), 844t
Withdrawal syndromes. *See also specific substances*
diagnosis of, 611
outcome evaluation in, 626
pathophysiology of, 610
patient care and monitoring in, 627

signs and symptoms of, 611, 612*t*
treatment of, 610, 616–623
Wolff-Parkinson-White syndrome, 173
Women who have sex with women, 1318
Working formulation, classification of
non-Hodgkin's lymphoma, 1555–1556, 1555*t*
Wound drainage, 486

X
Xanthoma, 232, 235
tuberoeruptive, 232, 235
Xerostomia, 317, 1366

Y
Yasmin, 848
Yaz, 849
Yeast,1377
facultative, 1377
Yogurt, 379
Yohimbine
dosage of, 887*t*
in erectile dysfunction, 887*t*, 891
mechanism of action of, 891
in sexual dysfunction, 562
Yuzpe regimen, 853

Z
Zafirlukast
adverse effects of, 276
in asthma, 275*t*, 276
dosage of, 275*t*
drug interactions of, 205*t*, 276, 955*t*
Zalcitabine
adverse effects of, 1442*t*
drug interactions of, 1442*t*
in HIV infection, 1442*t*

Zaleplon
adverse effects of, 717*t*
dosage of, 716*t*, 717*t*
in insomnia, 716*t*
pharmacokinetics of, 717*t*
in restless-legs syndrome, 717, 717*t*
Zanamivir, in pneumonia, 1197
ZAP-704 expression, in chronic lymphocytic
leukemia, 1602
Zidovudine
adverse effects of, 1424, 1428*t*,
1437*t*–1438*t*
dosage of, 1428*t*
drug interactions of, 1364, 1428*t*
in HIV infection, 1424, 1428*t*, 1433
mania with, 615*t*
mechanism of action of, 1421*f*
Zileuton
adverse effects of, 276
in asthma, 275*t*, 276
dosage of, 275*t*
Zinc oxide
in diaper dermatitis, 1106
in macular degeneration, 1073
Zinc supplementation
drug interactions of, 1164
for parenteral nutrition, 1687
Ziprasidone
adverse effects of, 638, 639, 638*t*, 684
in bipolar disorder, 679*t*,684
dosage of, 637*t*, 638, 678*t*
drug interactions of, 646*t*, 647
mechanism of action of, 637*f*, 639
metabolism of, 646*t*, 647
in schizophrenia, 636, 637*f*, 637*t*, 639,
644*t*, 646

Zoledronic acid, 974
adverse effects of, 1673
in breast cancer, 1547
dosage of, 490*t*, 1547
in hypercalcemia, 490, 490*t*
in osteoporosis, 973
in prostate cancer, 1547
Zollinger-Ellison syndrome
peptic ulcers in, 323
treatment of, 328
Zolmitriptan
dosage of, 589*t*
drug interactions of, 589*t*
in migraine, 589*t*
Zolpidem
adverse effects of, 717*t*
dosage of, 716*t*, 717*t*
drug interactions of, 955*t*
in insomnia, 716*t*
pharmacokinetics of, 716*t*
in restless-legs syndrome, 717, 717*t*
Zona fasciculata, 784, 785*a*
Zona glomerulosa, 784, 785*a*
Zona reticularis, 784, 785*a*
Zonisamide
adverse effects of, 529*t*
dosage of, 531*t*
drug interactions of, 501*t*
in epilepsy, 529, 529*t*, 531, 535*t*, 537*t*
mechanism of action of, 529*t*
metabolic acidosis with, 501*t*
pharmacokinetics of, 529*t*
Zoster vaccine, 1408*t*, 1413
Z-score, 968
Zygomycosis, 1383*f*, 1386*t*
Zymogens, 404